RHEUMATOLOGY

FIFTH EDITION
RHEUMATOLOGY

Marc C. Hochberg, MD, MPH
Professor of Medicine and Epidemiology and Preventive Medicine;
Head, Division of Rheumatology and Clinical Immunology
University of Maryland School of Medicine
Baltimore, Maryland, USA

Alan J. Silman, MD, MSC, FRCP, FMEDSCI
Medical Director, Arthritis Research UK
Chesterfield, UK;
Professor, Rheumatic Diseases Epidemiology
University of Manchester
Manchester, UK

Josef S. Smolen, MD, FRCP
Professor of Medicine;
Chairman,
Department of Internal Medicine III, Division of Rheumatology,
Medical University of Vienna;
Chairman, Second Department of Medicine
Center for Rheumatic Diseases
Hietzing Hospital
Vienna, Austria

Michael E. Weinblatt, MD
John R. and Eileen K. Riedman Professor of Medicine
Harvard Medical School;
Division of Rheumatology, Immunology and Allergy
Brigham and Women's Hospital
Boston, Massachusetts, USA

Michael H. Weisman, MD
Chief, Division of Rheumatology
Professor of Medicine
Cedars-Sinai Medical Center
David Geffen School of Medicine at UCLA
Los Angeles, California, USA

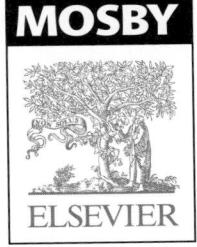

MOSBY

ELSEVIER

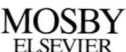

MOSBY
ELSEVIER

1600 John F. Kennedy Blvd.
Ste 1800
Philadelphia, PA 19103-2899

RHEUMATOLOGY   ISBN: 978-0-323-06551-1
Copyright © 2011, 2008, 2007, 2004, 2001, 1996 by Elsevier Ltd.

Library of Congress Cataloging-in-Publication Data

Rheumatology / [edited by] Marc C. Hochberg ... [et al.].—5th ed.
      p. ; cm.
   Includes bibliographical references and index.
   ISBN 978-0-323-06551-1
   1. Rheumatology.   I. Hochberg, Marc C.
   [DNLM: 1. Rheumatic Diseases.   2. Antirheumatic Agents—therapeutic use.   WE 544
R47141 2010]
   RC927.R48215 2010
   616.7'23—dc22

                                                                        2010009823

Volume 1: 9996077691
Volume 2: 9996077756

Acquisitions Editor: Pamela Hetherington
Developmental Editor: Lucia Gunzel
Publishing Services Manager: Linda Van Pelt
Project Manager: Francisco Morales
Design Direction: Louis Forgione

Printed in USA

Last digit is the print number: 9 8 7 6 5 4 3 2 1

ACKNOWLEDGMENTS

We would like to acknowledge the tremendous work of the contributors to *Rheumatology*, without whom this book would not have been possible. In addition, we would like to acknowledge our mentors: Drs. Eva Alberman, Harry Currey (deceased), Lawrence E. Shulman (deceased, OBM), Carl Steffen (deceased), Alfred D. Steinberg, Georg Geyer, Mary Betty Stevens (deceased), and Nathan J. Zvaifler.

We would also like to acknowledge the excellent team at Elsevier led by Kim Murphy and including Pamela Hetherington, Lucia Gunzel, and Frank Morales, as well as our secretaries and administrative assistants (Jacqui Oliver, Aida Medina, Johanna Leibl, and Robin Nichols) for all of their hard work and diligence. Last, but certainly not least, we want to acknowledge our patients, who continue to provide stimulating challenges to us in our clinical practices.

DEDICATION

We would like to dedicate this book to our parents (living or of blessed memory) and our wives, children, and grandchildren:

Susan Hochberg; Francine, Jeffrey, and Eleanor (Nora) Zoe Giuffrida; and Jennifer Hochberg
Ruth Silman; Joanna, Timothy, and Daniel Silman
Alice Smolen; Eva and Daniel Hruschka; Nina, Etienne, and Anna Smolen-Wildson; Daniel Smolen; and Alexander Smolen and Meeri Parikka
Barbara Weinblatt; Hillary and Jason Chapman; and Courtney Weinblatt
Betsy Weisman; Greg, Nicole, Mia, and Joey Weisman; Lisa, Andrew, David, and Thomas Cope; and Annie, Bill, and Caroline Macomber

CONTRIBUTORS

Aryeh M. Abeles, MD
Assistant Clinical Professor of Medicine
Division of Rheumatic Diseases
University of Connecticut School of Medicine
Farmington, Connecticut
USA
Inflammation

Abby G. Abelson, MD
Clinical Assistant Professor of Medicine
Interim Chair
Department of Rheumatic and Immunologic Disease
Vice Chair for Education
Orthopaedic and Rheumatology Institute
Cleveland Clinic
Cleveland, Ohio
USA
Management of osteoporosis

Abhishek Abhishek, MD, MRCP
Academic Rheumatology Unit
School of Clinical Sciences
University of Nottingham Faculty of Medicine and
    Health Sciences
Nottingham
United Kingdom
Calcium pyrophosphate crystal–associated arthropathy

Steven B. Abramson, MD
NYU Langone Medical Center
New York, New York
USA
Inflammation

Michael A. Adams, BSc, PhD
Reader in Spine Biomechanics
Department of Anatomy
University of Bristol Medical School
Bristol
United Kingdom
Biomechanics of the spine

David M. Adlam, MBBS, BDS, FRCS, FDSRCS
Honorary Lecturer in Surgery
University of Cambridge Medical School
Consultant Maxillofacial Surgeon
Addenbrooke's Hospital
Oral and Maxillofacial Surgeon
Spire Cambridge Lea Hospital
Cambridge
United Kingdom
The temporomandibular joint

Thomas Aigner, MD, DSc
Professor of Pathology
Institute of Pathology and Molecular Pathology
Head of Pathology
University of Würzburg/Coburg Medical Center
Coburg
Germany
Pathogenesis and pathology of osteoarthritis

Shizuo Akira, MD, PhD
Professor
Laboratory for Host Defense
World Premier International Immunology Frontier
    Research Center
Osaka University
Osaka
Japan
Principles of innate immunity

Ivona Aksentijevich, MD
Staff Scientist
Laboratory of Clinical Investigation
National Institute of Arthritis and Musculoskeletal and
    Skin Diseases
National Institutes of Health
Bethesda, Maryland
USA
The hereditary recurrent fevers

Daniel Aletaha, MD, MSc
Associate Professor
Department of Medicine
Division of Rheumatology
Medical University of Vienna
Vienna
Austria
*Evaluation and outcomes of patients with rheumatoid
    arthritis*

Antonios O. Aliprantis, MD, PhD
Instructor in Medicine
Harvard Medical School
Associate Physician
Department of Rheumatology, Allergy, and
    Immunology
Brigham and Women's Hospital
Boston, Massachusetts
USA
Relapsing polychondritis

Cornelia F. Allaart, MD, PhD
Associate Professor
Department of Rheumatology
Leiden University Faculty of Medicine
Leiden
The Netherlands
Parenteral gold, antimalarials, and sulfasalazine

Pamela G. Allen, MD
Fellow
Department of Orthopaedics
Union Memorial Hospital
Baltimore, Maryland
USA
The ankle and foot

Roy D. Altman, MD
Professor of Medicine
Department of Medicine
Division of Rheumatology and Immunology
David Geffen School of Medicine at UCLA
Los Angeles, California
USA
*Clinical features of osteoarthritis; Animal models of
    osteoarthritis*

Martin Aringer, MD
Professor of Medicine
Carl Gustav Carus Faculty of Medicine
Dresden University of Technology
Chief
Division of Rheumatology
University Clinical Center Carl Gustav Carus
Dresden
Germany
Signal transduction

Dana P. Ascherman, MD
Professor of Medicine
Department of Medicine
Division of Rheumatology and Clinical Immunology
University of Pittsburgh School of Medicine
Pittsburgh, Pennsylvania
USA
*Clinical features, classification, and epidemiology of
    inflammatory muscle disease*

Shervin Assassi, MD, MCR
Assistant Professor of Internal Medicine–Rheumatology
University of Texas Medical School at Houston
Houston, Texas
USA
Epidemiology and classification of scleroderma

Sergei P. Atamas, MD, PhD
Associate Professor of Medicine and Microbiology and
    Immunology
University of Maryland School of Medicine
Research Health Scientist
Research and Development Service
Baltimore VA Medical Center
Baltimore, Maryland
USA
The principles of adaptive immunity

Alan N. Baer, MD
Associate Professor of Medicine
Johns Hopkins University School of Medicine
Chief of Rheumatology
Good Samaritan Hospital
Baltimore, Maryland
USA
*Metabolic, drug-induced, and other non-inflammatory
    myopathies*

Dominique Baeten, MD, PhD
Professor of Clinical Immunology and Rheumatology
University of Amsterdam Faculty of Medicine
Academic Medical Center
Amsterdam
The Netherlands
*Etiology, pathogenesis, and pathophysiology of
    ankylosing spondylitis*

Nancy Baker, ScD, MPH
Assistant Professor
Department of Occupational Therapy
University of Pittsburgh School of Health and
    Rehabilitation Sciences
Pittsburgh, Pennsylvania
USA
*Principles of rehabilitation: physical and occupational
    therapy*

Alejandro Balsa, MD, PhD
Associate Professor of Rheumatology
School of Medicine
Universidad Autónoma de Madrid
Staff Rheumatologist
Hospital Universitario La Paz
Madrid
Spain
*Septic arthritis, osteomyelitis, and gonococcal and
    syphilitic arthritis*

Les Barnsley, BMed(Hons), GradDipEpi, PhD, FRACP, FAFRM(RACP)
Associate Professor
Department of Medicine
University of Sydney Medical School
Sydney
Head
Department of Rheumatology
Concord Repatriation Hospital
Concord
New South Wales
Australia
Neck pain

Joan M. Bathon, MD
Professor of Medicine
Johns Hopkins University School of Medicine
Baltimore, Maryland
USA
Management of rheumatoid arthritis: synovitis

Michael A. Becker, MD
Professor Emeritus of Medicine
Division of Rheumatology
University of Chicago Pritzker School of Medicine/
   University of Chicago Hospitals
Chicago, Illinois
USA
Etiology and pathogenesis of gout

Professor Jill JF Belch, FRCP, MD
Tayside R&D Director
Head of Institute of Cardiovascular Research, (Vascular
   & Inflammatory Diseases Research Unit)
Ninewells Hospital and Medical School
Dundee
United Kingdom
Raynaud's phenomenon

Nicholas Bellamy, MD, MSc, MBA, DSc
Professor of Rehabilitation Medicine
Director
Centre of National Research on Disability and
   Rehabilitation Medicine (CONROD)
University of Queensland Faculty of Health Sciences
Brisbane, Queensland
Australia
Principles of clinical outcome assessment

Teresita Bellido, PhD
Professor
Department of Anatomy and Cell Biology
Department of Medicine
Indiana University School of Medicine
Indianapolis, Indiana
USA
Bone structure and function

R. Michael Benitez, MD
Associate Professor
Department of Medicine
Division of Cardiology
University of Maryland School of Medicine
Baltimore, Maryland
USA
The heart in rheumatic disease

Michael Benjamin, BSc, PhD
Professor Emeritus of Musculoskeletal Biology and
   Sports Medicine Research
School of Biosciences
Cardiff University
Cardiff
United Kingdom
Enthesopathies

Michael W. Beresford, MBChB, PhD, MRCP(UK), MRCPCH
Senior Lecturer in Paediatric Medicine
Institute of Child Health
University of Liverpool Faculty of Medicine
Honorary Consultant Paediatric Rheumatologist
Clinical Academic Department of Paediatric
   Rheumatology
Alder Hey Children's NHS Foundation Trust
Liverpool
United Kingdom
Connective tissue diseases in children

Brian M. Berman, MD
Professor of Family and Community Medicine
University of Maryland School of Medicine
Medical Director
Center for Integrative Medicine
University of Maryland Medical Center
Baltimore, Maryland
USA
Complementary and alternative medicine

Bonnie Lee Bermas, MD
Assistant Professor of Medicine
Harvard Medical School
Associate Rheumatologist
Brigham and Women's Hospital
Boston, Massachusetts
USA
Drugs and pregnancy

George Bertsias, MD, PhD
Investigator
Rheumatology, Clinical Immunology and Allergy
University of Crete School of Medicine
Crete
Greece
*Systemic lupus erythematosus: treatment—renal
   involvement*

John P. Bilezikian, MD
Professor of Medicine and Pharmacology
Chief
Division of Endocrinology
Department of Medicine
Columbia University College of Physicians and
   Surgeons
New York, New York
USA
*Primary hyperparathyroidism: rheumatologic
   manifestations and bone disease*

Philip E. Blazar, MD
Assistant Professor of Orthopaedic Surgery
Harvard Medical School
Attending Physician
Department of Orthopedic Surgery
Brigham and Women's Hospital
Boston, Massachusetts
USA
The wrist and hand

Jane F. Bleasel, MBBS, PhD, FRACP
Clinical Associate Professor
Department of Rheumatology
University of Sydney Medical School
Head
Department of Rheumatology
Royal Prince Alfred Hospital
Sydney, New South Wales
Australia
Hemophilia and von Willebrand disease

Markus Böhm, MD
Associate Professor
Department of Dermatology
University of Münster Faculty of Health Science
Münster
Germany
Skin in rheumatic disease

Christelle Boileau, PhD
Assistant Professor
Department of Pharmacology
University of Montreal Faculty of Medicine
Postdoctoral Fellow
Osteoarthritis Research Unit
University of Montreal Hospital Research Centre
   (CR-CHUM)
Montreal, Quebec
Canada
Animal models of osteoarthritis

Marcy B. Bolster, MD
Professor of Medicine
Medical University of South Carolina College of
   Medicine
Charleston, South Carolina
USA
Clinical features of systemic sclerosis

Stefano Bombardieri, MD
Professor of Rheumatology and Director of the
   Specialty School of Rheumatology
University of Pisa
Director of Rheumatology Operative Unit and Director
   of the Department of Internal Medicine
Azienda Ospedaliera Universitaria Pisana
Pisa
Italy
Cryoglobulinemia

Sydney Bonnick, MD
Adjunct Professor
Department of Kinesiology and Biological Sciences
University of North Texas
Medical Director
Clinical Research Center of North Texas
Denton, Texas
USA
DXA and measurement of bone

Dimitrios T. Boumpas, MD, FACP
Professor, Internal Medicine
University of Crete School of Medicine
Herakalion
Chief
Internal Medicine and Rheumatology, Clinical
   Immunology, and Allergy
University Hospital of Heraklion
Crete
Greece
*Systemic lupus erythematosus: treatment—renal
   involvement*

Richard D. Brasington, Jr., MD
Professor of Medicine–Rheumatology
Director of Clinical Rheumatology
Washington University School of Medicine
St. Louis, Missouri
USA
Clinical features of rheumatoid arthritis

Ferdinand Breedveld, MD
Professor of Rheumatology
Department of Rheumatology
Leiden University Medical Center
Leiden
The Netherlands
Tyrosine kinase inhibition

Earl W. Brien, MD
Cedars Sinai Medical Center
Los Angeles, California
USA
Bone tumors

Anne C. Brower
Retired
Washington, DC
Seronegative spondyloarthropathies: imaging

Matthew A. Brown, MD, MBBS, FRACP
Professor of Immunogenetics
University of Queensland Faculty of Health Sciences
Brisbane
University of Queensland Diamantina Institute of
    Cancer, Immunology and Metabolic Medicine
Princess Alexandra Hospital
Woolloongabba, Queensland
Australia
Genetics of ankylosing spondylitis

Ian N. Bruce, MD, FRCP
Professor of Rheumatology
School of Translational Medicine
Arthritis Research Council (ARC) Epidemiology Unit
University of Manchester Faculty of Medical and
    Human Sciences
Manchester
United Kingdom
Clinical features of psoriatic arthritis

William D. Bugbee, MD
Associate Professor of Orthopaedic Surgery
University of California, San Diego, School of Medicine
Attending Physician
Division of Orthopaedic Surgery
Scripps Clinic
La Jolla, California
USA
The hip

Marwan A. S. Bukhari, PhD, FRCP
Honorary Senior Lecturer in Clinical Medicine
University of Liverpool Faculty of Medicine
Liverpool
Consultant Rheumatologist
University Hospitals of Morecambe Bay NHS Trust
Lancaster
United Kingdom
Mucopolysaccharidoses

Rubén Burgos-Vargas, MD
Professor of Medicine
Universidad Nacional Autónoma de México
Rheumatologist
Medical Sciences Investigator
Hospital General de México
Mexico City
Mexico
The juvenile-onset spondyloarthropathies

Jane C. Burns, MD
Adjunct Professor
Department of Pediatrics
University of California, San Diego, School of Medicine
La Jolla
Director
Kawasaki Disease Research Center
Rady Children's Hospital San Diego
San Diego, California
USA
Kawasaki disease

David B. Burr, PhD
Professor of Biomedical Engineering
Department of Anatomy and Cell Biology
Indiana University School of Medicine
Indianapolis, Indiana
USA
Bone structure and function

Patricia C. Cagnoli, MD
Clinical Assistant Professor
Department of Internal Medicine
Division of Rheumatology
University of Michigan Medical School/University of
    Michigan Health System
Ann Arbor, Michigan
USA
Treatment of non-renal lupus

Leonard H. Calabrese, DO
Professor of Medicine
Cleveland Clinic Lerner College of Medicine of Case
    Western Reserve University
Vice Chairman
Department of Rheumatic and Immunologic Diseases
R.J. Fasenmyer Chair of Clinical Immunology
Theodore F. Classen DO Chair of Osteopathic Research
    and Education
Cleveland Clinic Foundation
Cleveland, Ohio
USA
Rheumatologic aspects of viral infections

Jeffrey P. Callen, MD
Professor of Medicine–Dermatology
Chief
Division of Dermatology
University of Louisville School of Medicine
Louisville, Kentucky
USA
Cutaneous vasculitis and panniculitis

Juan J. Canoso, MD, FACP, MACR
Adjunct Professor of Medicine
Tufts University School of Medicine
Boston, Massachusetts
USA
Rheumatologist
Department of Medicine
ABC Medical Center
Mexico City
Mexico
Adjunct Professor of Medicine
Department of Medicine
Tufts University School of Medicine
Boston, Massachusetts
USA
*Aspiration and injection of joints and periarticular tissues
    and intralesional therapy*

Sabrina Cavallo, MD
Université de Montréal
Département de Médecine Sociale et Préventive
McGill University Health Center: Montreal Children's
    Hospital
Montreal
Canada
*Rehabilitation and psychosocial issues in juvenile
    idiopathic arthritis*

Tim E. Cawston, BSc, PhD
William Leech Professor of Rheumatology
School of Clinical Medical Sciences
Musculoskeletal Research Group
Institute of Cellular Medicine
Newcastle University
Newcastle upon Tyne
United Kingdom
Tissue destruction and repair

Michael Denis Chard, MD, MB, BS
Consultant Rheumatologist
Worthing Hospital
Worthing
United Kingdom
The elbow

Lan X. Chen, MD, PhD
Clinical Associate Professor of Medicine
University of Pennsylvania
University of Pennsylvania School of Medicine
Attending Physician
Penn Presbyterian Medical Center
Philadelphia, Pennsylvania
USA
Other crystal-related arthropathies

Ernest H. S. Choy, MD, FRCP
Clinical Reader
Academic Department of Rheumatology
King's College London School of Medicine and
    Dentistry
London
United Kingdom
Immunotherapies: T cell and complement

Daniel J. Clauw, MD
Professor
Departments of Anesthesiology and
    Medicine–Rheumatology
University of Michigan Medical School
Ann Arbor, Michigan
USA
Fibromyalgia and related syndromes

Philip J. Clements, MD, MPH
Professor of Medicine
David Geffen School of Medicine at UCLA
Attending Physician
Ronald Reagan UCLA Medical Center
Los Angeles, California
USA
*Immunosuppressives (chlorambucil, cyclosporine,
    cytoxan, azathioprine [Imuran], mofetil, tacrolimus)*

Nona T. Colburn, MD
Guest Researcher
Laboratory of Clinical Investigation
National Institute of Arthritis and Musculoskeletal and
    Skin Diseases
National Institutes of Health
Bethesda, Maryland
USA
The hereditary recurrent fevers

Laura A. Coleman, PhD, RD
Scientist
Epidemiology Research Center
Marshfield Clinic Research Foundation
Marshfield, Wisconsin
USA
Nutrition in rheumatic disease

Philip G. Conaghan, MBBS, PhD, FRACP, FRCP
Professor of Musculoskeletal Medicine
School of Medicine
University of Leeds Faculty of Medicine and Health
Deputy Director
NIHR Musculoskeletal Biomedical Research Unit
Leeds Teaching Hospitals NHS Trust
Leeds
United Kingdom
Imaging of osteoarthritis

Cyrus Cooper, MD, MA, FRCP, FFPH, FMedSci
Professor of Rheumatology
School of Medicine
University of Southampton
Director
MRC Epidemiology Resource Centre
Southampton General Hospital
Southampton
United Kingdom
Epidemiology and classification of metabolic bone disease

Felicia Cosman, MD
Associate Professor of Clinical Medicine
Regional Bone Center
Helen Hayes Hospital
West Haverstraw, NY
USA
Pathogenesis of osteoporosis

Karen H. Costenbader, MD, MPH
Assistant Professor of Medicine
Harvard Medical School
Co-Director
Lupus Center
Brigham and Women's Hospital
Boston, Massachusetts
USA
Epidemiology and classification of systemic lupus erythematosus

Paul Creamer, MD, FRCP
Senior Clinical Lecturer
Department of Rheumatology
University of Bristol Medical School
Consultant Rheumatologist
Southmead Hospital
North Bristol NHS Healthcare Trust
Bristol
United Kingdom
Neuropathic arthropathy

José C. Crispin, MD
Instructor in Medicine
Harvard Medical School
Staff Rheumatologist
Beth Israel Deaconess Medical Center
Boston, Massachusetts
USA
Pathogenesis of lupus

Lindsey A. Criswell, MD, MPH, DSc
Professor of Medicine–Rheumatology and Orofacial Sciences
University of California, San Francisco, School of Medicine
San Francisco, California
USA
The contribution of genetic factors to rheumatoid arthritis

Bruce N. Cronstein, MD
Paul R. Esserman Professor of Medicine
New York University School of Medicine
New York, New York
USA
Pharmacogenomics in rheumatology

Raymond Cross, MD, MS
Associate Professor
Department of Medicine
Division of Gastroenterology and Hepatology
Director
Inflammatory Bowel Disease Program
University of Maryland School of Medicine
Chief
GI Section
VA Maryland Health Care System
Baltimore, Maryland
USA
Gastrointestinal tract and rheumatic disease

Natalie E. Cusano, MD
Postdoctoral Clinical Fellow
Department of Endocrinology
Columbia University Medical Center
New York, New York
USA
Primary hyperparathyroidism: rheumatologic manifestations and bone disease

John J. Cush, MD
Professor of Medicine and Rheumatology
Director of Clinical Rheumatology
Baylor Research Institute
Baylor University Medical Center
Dallas, Texas
USA
Tumor necrosis factor blocking therapies

Maurizio Cutolo, MD
Professor of Rheumatology
Director
Research Laboratory and Academic Unit of Clinical Rheumatology
Department of Internal Medicine
Medical School
University of Genoa Faculty of Medicine
Genoa
Italy
Effects of the neuroendocrine system on development and function of the immune system

Vivette D'Agati, MD
Professor of Pathology
Columbia University College of Physicians and Surgeons
Director
Renal Pathology Division
Columbia University Medical Center
New York, New York
USA
Immunopathology of systemic lupus erythematosus

Hanne Dagfinrud, PhD
Associate Professor
University of Oslo Faculty of Medicine
Senior Researcher
National Resource Center for Rehabilitation in Rheumatology
Diakonhjemmet Hospital
Oslo
Norway
Multidisciplinary approach to rheumatoid arthritis

David I. Daikh, MD, PhD
Associate Professor of Medicine
Department of Medicine
Division of Rheumatology
University of California, San Francisco, School of Medicine
Chief
Rheumatology Section
San Francisco Medical Center
San Francisco, California
USA
Animal models of lupus

Seamus E. Dalton, MBBS, FACRM, FAFRM, FACSP
Consultant in Rehabilitation and Sports Medicine
North Sydney Orthopaedic and Sports Medicine Center
Sydney, New South Wales
Australia
The shoulder

Shouvik Dass, MA, MBBCh, MRCP(UK)
Clinical Research Fellow
Academic Section of Musculoskeletal Disease
Leeds Institute of Molecular Medicine
University of Leeds Faculty of Medicine and Health
Consultant Rheumatologist
Leeds Teaching Hospitals NHS Trust
Leeds
United Kingdom
Rituximab

Jean-Pierre David, PhD
Group Leader
Experimental Bone Pathology
Department of Medicine 3, Rheumatology and Immunology
University of Erlangen-Nuremberg
Erlangen
Germany
Osteoimmunology

Aileen Davis, PhD
Senior Scientist
Division of Health Care and Outcomes Research and Arthritis and Community Research and Evaluation Unit
Toronto Western Research Institute
Toronto, Ontario
Canada
Assessment of the patient with osteoarthritis and measurement of outcomes

Chad L. Deal, MD
Associate Professor of Medicine
Cleveland Clinic Lerner College of Medicine of Case Western Reserve University
Head
Center for Osteoporosis and Metabolic Bone Disease
Cleveland Clinic
Cleveland, Ohio
USA
Management of osteoporosis

Karel De Ceulaer, MD
Department of Medicine
University of the West Indies
Kingston
Jamaica
Joint and bone lesions in hemoglobinopathies

Chris Deighton, MD, FRCP
Special Lecturer
Nottingham University School of Medical and Surgical Sciences
Consultant Rheumatologist
Royal Derby Hospital
Derby
United Kingdom
The contribution of genetic factors to rheumatoid arthritis

Paul F. Dellaripa, MD
Assistant Professor of Medicine
Harvard Medical School
Staff Rheumatologist
Co-Director
Interstitial Lung Disease Center
Brigham and Women's Hospital
Boston, Massachusetts
USA
The lung in rheumatic disease

ix

Alessandra Della Rossa
Clinical Assistant
Azienda Ospedaliera Universitaria Pisana
Pisa
Italy
Cryoglobulinemia

David Dempster, PhD
Professor of Clinical Pathology
Department of Pathology
Columbia University College of Physicians and
    Surgeons
New York
Director
Regional Bone Center
Helen Hayes Hospital
West Haverstraw, New York
USA
Pathogenesis of osteoporosis

Elaine Dennison
MRC Epidemiology Resource Centre
Southampton
United Kingdom
*Epidemiology and classification of metabolic bone
    disease*

Christopher P. Denton, PhD, FRCP
Professor of Experimental Rheumatology
Centre for Rheumatology
Royal Free Campus
University College London
Hampstead
Consultant Rheumatologist
Royal Free Hospital
London
United Kingdom
Pulmonary management of scleroderma

John Denton, MSc
Research Fellow in Osteoarticular Pathology
School of Biomedicine
University of Manchester Faculty of Medical and
    Human Sciences
Honorary Advanced Practitioner in Osteoarticular
    Pathology
Central Manchester University Hospitals NHS
    Foundation Trust
Manchester
United Kingdom
Synovial fluid analysis

Roshan Dhawale, MD, MPH
Fellow
Division of Rheumatology and Clinical Immunology
University of Pittsburgh School of Medicine/University
    of Pittsburgh Medical Center
Pittsburgh, Pennsylvania
USA
T-cell co-stimulation

Michael Doherty, MD, MA, FRCP
Professor of Rheumatology
Academic Rheumatology Unit
School of Clinical Sciences
University of Nottingham Faculty of Medicine and
    Health Sciences
Nottingham
United Kingdom
Calcium pyrophosphate crystal–associated arthropathy

Patricia Dolan, MD, BSc
Reader in Biomechanics
Department of Anatomy
University of Bristol Medical School
Bristol
United Kingdom
Biomechanics of the spine

Rachelle Donn, MBChB, PhD
Reader in Complex Disease Genetics
Arthritis Research Campaign (ARC) Epidemiology Unit
School of Translational Medicine
University of Manchester Faculty of Medical and
    Human Sciences
Manchester
United Kingdom
Etiology and pathogenesis of juvenile idiopathic arthritis

Mary Anne Dooley, MD, MPH
Associate Professor of Medicine
Department of Medicine
Division of Rheumatology and Immunology
Thurston Arthritis Research Center
University of North Carolina at Chapel Hill School of
    Medicine
Chapel Hill, North Carolina
USA
Drug-induced lupus

Maxime Dougados, MD
Medicine Faculty, Paris-Descartes University
Rheumatology B Department
Cochin Hospital
Paris
France
Management of osteoarthritis

Michael F. Drummond, MCom, DPhil
Professor of Health Economics
Centre for Health Economics
University of York
York
United Kingdom
*Principles of health economics and application to
    rheumatic disorders*

George S. M. Dyer, MD
Clinical Instructor in Orthopaedic Surgery
Harvard Medical School
Orthopedic Surgeon
Brigham and Women's Hospital and VA Boston
    Heathcare System
Boston, Massachusetts
USA
The wrist and hand

Brandon E. Earp, MD
Instructor in Orthopedic Surgery
Harvard Medical School
Attending Hand and Upper Extremity Surgeon
Brigham and Women's Hospital
Boston, Massachusetts
USA
The wrist and hand

N. Lawrence Edwards, MD
Professor and Vice Chairman
Department of Medicine
University of Florida College of Medicine
Gainesville, Florida
USA
Clinical gout

Patrick Ellender, MD
Sports medicine: clinical spectrum of injury

Paul Emery, MA, MD, FRCP(UK)
Arthritis Research Campaign (ARC) Professor of
    Rheumatology
Head
Academic Section of Musculoskeletal Disease
Leeds Institute of Molecular Medicine
University of Leeds Faculty of Medicine and Health
Rheumatologist
Leeds Teaching Hospitals NHS Trust
Leeds
United Kingdom
Rituximab

Luis R. Espinoza, MD
Professor and Chief
Section of Rheumatology
Department of Internal Medicine
Louisiana State University School of Medicine
New Orleans, Louisiana
USA
Mycobacterial, brucellar, fungal, and parasitic arthritis

Joshua M. Farber, MD
Cytokines

Anders Fasth, MD, PhD
Professor of Pediatric Immunology
Department of Pediatrics
Institute of Clinical Sciences
Sahlgrenska Academy
University of Gothenburg
Consultant
Division of Immunology
The Queen Silvia Children's Hospital
Gothenborg
Sweden
Consultant
Pediatric Rheumatology and Immunology Service
Hospital Nacional de Niños "Dr. Carlos Sáenz Herrera"
San José
Costa Rica
*Presentations, clinical features, and special problems in
    children*

Debbie Feldman, BScPT, MSc, PhD
Associate Professor
School of Rehabilitation
University of Montreal Faculty of Medicine
Physical Therapist
Montreal Children's Hospital
McGill University Health Center
Epidemiologist
Public Health Department of Montreal
Research Scientist
Center for Interdisciplinary Research in Rehabilitation
    (CRIR)
Montreal, Quebec
Canada
*Rehabilitation and psychosocial issues in juvenile
    idiopathic arthritis*

David T. Felson, MD, MPH
Professor of Medicine and Epidemiology
Chair
Division of Clinical Epidemiology
Boston University School of Medicine
Boston, Massachusetts
USA
Professor of Medicine and Public Health
School of Translational Medicine
Arthritis Research Council (ARC) Epidemiology Unit
University of Manchester Faculty of Medical and
    Human Sciences
Manchester
United Kingdom
*Local and systemic risk factors for incidence and
    progression of osteoarthritis*

G. Kelley Fitzgerald, PT, PhD, FAPTA
Associate Professor
Department of Physical Therapy
University of Pittsburgh School of Health and
    Rehabilitation Sciences
Pittsburgh, Pennsylvania
USA
*Principles of rehabilitation: physical and occupational
    therapy*

Raymond H. Flores, MD
Associate Professor of Medicine
Division of Rheumatology and Clinical Immunology
University of Maryland School of Medicine
Baltimore, Maryland
USA
Entrapment neuropathies and compartment syndromes

David A. Fox, MD
Professor
Department of Internal Medicine
Division of Rheumatology
University of Michigan Medical School
Ann Arbor, Michigan
USA
Emerging therapeutic targets: IL-15, IL-17, IL-18, IL-23

Clair A. Francomano, MD
Associate Professor of Medicine
Johns Hopkins University School of Medicine
Director of Adult Genetics
Harvey Institute for Human Genetics
Greater Baltimore Medical Center
Baltimore, Maryland
USA
Skeletal dysplasias

Anthony J. Freemont, MD, FRCP, FRCPath
Professor of Osteoarticular Pathology
School of Biomedicine
University of Manchester Faculty of Medical and
    Human Sciences
Honorary Consultant in Osteoarticular Pathology
Central Manchester University Hospitals NHS
    Foundation Trust
Manchester
United Kingdom
Synovial fluid analysis

Izzet Fresko, MD
Professor of Medicine
Department of Medicine
Division of Rheumatology
Cerrahpasa Medical Faculty
University of Istanbul
Instanbul
Turkey
Behçet's syndrome

Kevin B. Fricka, MD
Orthopaedic Surgeon
Anderson Orthopaedic Clinic
Clinical Instructor
Adult Reconstruction Fellowship
Anderson Orthopaedic Research Institute
Alexandria, Virginia
USA
The hip

Daniel E. Furst, MD
Professor of Medicine
David Geffen School of Medicine at UCLA
Attending Physician
Ronald Reagan UCLA Medical Center
Los Angeles, California
USA
*Immunosuppressives (chlorambucil, cyclosporine,
    cytoxan, azathioprine [Imuran], mofetil, tacrolimus)*

Cem Gabay, MD
Professor of Rheumatology
University of Geneva School of Medicine
Head
Division of Rheumatology
University Hospitals of Geneva
Geneva
Switzerland
Cytokine neutralizers: IL-1 inhibitors

Sherine E. Gabriel, MD, MSc
Willliam J. and Charles H. Mayo Professor
Professor of Medicine and Epidemiology
Mayo Clinic College of Medicine
Director of Education
Mayo Clinic Center for Translational Science Activities
Mayo Clinic
Rochester, Minnesota
USA
*Principles of health economics and application to
    rheumatic disorders*

Bernat Galarraga, LMC, MRCP(UK), PhD
Hospital Quiron Bizkaia
Erandio
Bizkaia
Spain
Raynaud's phenomenon

Boel Andersson Gäre, MD, PhD
Professor
Department of Quality Improvement and Leadership in
    Health and Welfare
Jönköping Academy for Improvement of Health and
    Welfare
Jönköping University School of Health Sciences
Director
Futurum—The Academy for Healthcare
Jönköping County Council
Jönköping
Sweden
*Presentations, clinical features, and special problems in
    children*

Patrick Garnero, DSc, PhD
Director of Research
Synarc
Lyon
France
Biochemical markers in bone disease

Lianne S. Gensler, MD
University of California, San Francisco (UCSF)
San Francisco, California
USA
Clinical features of ankylosing spondylitis

Danielle M. Gerlag, MD, PhD
Associate Professor
Department of Clinical Immunology and
    Rheumatology
University of Amsterdam Faculty of Medicine
Academic Medical Center
Amsterdam
The Netherlands
Minimally invasive procedures

Piet P. Geusens
Department of Internal Medicine
Subdivision of Rheumatology
Maastricht University Medical Center
Maastricht
The Netherlands
Biomedical Research Institute
University Hasselt
Belgium
Osteoporosis: clinical features of osteoporosis

Jon T. Giles, MD, MPH
Assistant Professor
Department of Medicine
Division of Rheumatology
Johns Hopkins University School of Medicine
Baltimore, Maryland
USA
Management of rheumatoid arthritis: synovitis

Ellen M. Ginzler, MD, MPH
Distinguished Teaching Professor
Department of Medicine
Division of Rheumatology
State University of New York Downstate Medical
    Center College of Medicine
Brooklyn, New York
USA
Clinical features of systemic lupus erythematosus

Alison M. Gizinski, MD
Clinical Lecturer/Research Fellow
Department of Internal Medicine
Division of Rheumatology
University of Michigan Medical School/University of
    Michigan Health System
Ann Arbor, Michigan
USA
Emerging therapeutic targets: IL-15, IL-17, IL-18, IL-23

Garry Gold, MD
Associate Professor of Radiology, Bioengineering, and
    Orthopaedic Surgery
Department of Radiology
Stanford University School of Medicine
Stanford, California
USA
Magnetic resonance imaging

Tania Gonzalez-Rivera, MD
Rheumatology Fellow
University of Michigan Medical School/University of
    Michigan Health System
Ann Arbor, Michigan
USA
Treatment of non-renal lupus

Caroline Gordon, MD, FRCP
Professor of Rheumatology
School of Immunity and Infection
College of Medical and Dental Sciences
University of Birmingham
Birmingham
United Kingdom
*Assessing disease activity and outcome in systemic lupus
    erythematosus*

Rachel Gorodkin, MBChB, PhD
Honorary Lecturer in Rheumatology
School of Translational Medicine
Arthritis Research Campaign (ARC) Epidemiology
    Unit
University of Manchester Faculty of Medical and
    Human Sciences
Consultant Rheumatologist
Kellgren Centre for Rheumatology
Manchester Royal Infirmary
Manchester
United Kingdom
*Complex regional pain syndrome (reflex sympathetic
    dystrophy)*

Jorg J. Goronzy, MD
Professor of Medicine
Stanford University School of Medicine
Stanford, California
USA
Polymyalgia rheumatica and giant cell arteritis

Simon Görtz, MD
Resident Physician
Department of Orthopaedic Surgery
University of California, San Diego Medical Center
San Diego, California
USA
The hip

Elena Gournelos
The Complementary Medicine Program
University of Maryland School of Medicine
Baltimore, Maryland
USA
Complementary and alternative medicine

Rodney Grahame, CBE, MD, FRCP, FACP
Honorary Professor of Rheumatology
Department of Medicine
University College London Medical School
Consultant Rheumatologist
University College Hospital Foundation NHS Trust
Honorary Consultant in Paediatric Rheumatology
Great Ormond Street Hospital for Children
Honorary Consultant in Rheumatology
North West London Hospital NHS Trust
London
United Kingdom
Affiliate Professor of Pathology
University of Washington School of Medicine
Seattle, Washington
USA
Hypermobility syndrome

Andrew J. Grainger, MBBS, MRCP, FRCR
Honorary Senior Lecturer
School of Medicine
University of Leeds Faculty of Medicine and Health
Consultant in Musculoskeletal Radiology
Leeds Teaching Hospitals NHS Trust
Leeds
United Kingdom
Imaging of osteoarthritis

Ellen M. Gravallese, MD
Professor of Medicine and Cell Biology
University of Massachusetts Medical School
Chief
Division of Rheumatology
University of Massachusetts Memorial Medical Center
Worcester, Massachusetts
USA
The rheumatoid joint: synovitis and tissue destruction

Jeffrey D. Greenberg, MD, MPH
Assistant Professor of Medicine–Rheumatology
New York University School of Medicine
Associate Director
Clinical and Translational Sciences
Division of Rheumatology
NYU Hospital for Joint Diseases
New York, New York
USA
Pharmacogenomics in rheumatology

Karlene Hagley, MBBS, MD
Consultant in Internal Medicine
Department of Medicine
University Hospital of the West Indies
Kingston
Jamaica
Joint and bone lesions in hemoglobinopathies

Alan J. Hakim, MBBCh, MA, FRCP
Consultant Physician and Rheumatologist
Director of Strategy and Business Improvement
Whipps Cross Hospital NHS Trust
London
United Kingdom
Hypermobility syndrome

Vedat Hamuryudan, MD
Professor of Medicine
Department of Medicine
Division of Rheumatology
Cerrahpasa Medical Faculty
University of Istanbul
Instanbul
Turkey
Behçet's syndrome

Boulos Haraoui, MD, FRCPC
Associate Professor of Medicine
Department of Medicine
University of Montreal Faculty of Medicine
Montreal, Quebec
Canada
Leflunomide

Adam Harder, MD
Sports medicine: clinical spectrum of injury

John B. Harley, MD, PhD
Professor of Medicine
Chief
Division of Rheumatology, Immunology, and Allergy
Department of Medicine
University of Oklahoma College of Medicine
Chair
Arthritis and Immunology Research Program
Oklahoma Medical Research Foundation
Staff Physician
Oklahoma City VA Medical Center
Oklahoma City, Oklahoma
USA
Genetics of lupus

E. Nigel Harris, MD
Vice Chancellor
The University of the West Ladies
Kingston
Jamaica
Antiphospholipid syndrome: overview of pathogenesis, diagnosis and management

Philip J. Hashkes, MD, MSc
Associate Professor of Medicine and Pediatrics
Cleveland Clinic Lerner School of Medicine of Case Western Reserve University
Cleveland, Ohio
USA
Head
Pediatric Rheumatology Unit
Shaare Zedek Medical Center
Jerusalem
Israel
Management of juvenile idiopathic arthritis

Gillian Hawker, MD, MSc
Professor of Medicine–Rheumatology and Health Policy, Management, and Evaluation
University of Toronto Faculty of Medicine
Physician-in-Chief of Medicine
Women's College Hospital
Toronto, Ontario
Canada
Assessment of the patient with osteoarthritis and measurement of outcomes

Philip N. Hawkins, MBBS, PhD, FRCP, FRCPath, FMedSci
Professor of Medicine
Centre for Amyloidosis and Acute Phase Proteins
University College London Medical School
Head
National Amyloidosis Centre
Royal Free Hospital
London
United Kingdom
Amyloidosis

Turid Heiberg, RN, MNS, PhD
Dean
Lovisenberg Diaconal University College
Research Leader
Oslo University Hospital
Oslo
Norway
Multidisciplinary approach to rheumatoid arthritis

Dick Heinegård, MD, PhD
Professor
Department of Clinical Sciences
Division of Rheumatology–Molecular Skeletal Biology
Lund University Faculty of Medicine
Lund
Sweden
The articular cartilage

Simon M. Helfgott, MD
Associate Professor of Medicine
Harvard Medical School
Director of Education and Fellowship Training
Division of Rheumatology
Brigham and Women's Hospital
Boston, Massachusetts
USA
Rheumatoid manifestations of endocrine and lipid disease

Jenny E. Heller, MPhil
Research Associate
Department of Medicine
Division of Rheumatology, Immunology, and Allergy
Brigham and Women's Hospital/Harvard Medical School
Boston, Massachusetts
USA
Lyme disease

Ariane L. Herrick, MD, FRCP
Senior Lecturer in Rheumatology
School of Translational Medicine
Arthritis Research Campaign (ARC) Epidemiology Unit
University of Manchester Faculty of Medical and Human Sciences
Manchester
Attending
Salford Royal NHS Foundation Trust
Salford
United Kingdom
Complex regional pain syndrome (reflex sympathetic dystrophy)

Laurence D. Higgins, MS, MD
Associate Professor
Harvard Medical School
Chief of Sports Medicine
Harvard Shoulder Service
Boston, Massachusetts
USA
Sports medicine: clinical spectrum of injury

J. S. Hill Gaston, MA, PhD, FRCP, FMedSci
Professor of Rheumatology
Department of Medicine
University of Cambridge School of Clinical Medicine
Honorary Consultant in Rheumatology
Cambridge University Hospitals NHS Foundation Trust
Cambridge
United Kingdom
Cellular immunity in rheumatoid arthritis

Marc C. Hochberg, MD, MPH
Management of osteoarthritis

Markus Hoffmann, PhD
Associate Professor
Researcher
Department of Internal Medicine III
Division of Rheumatology
Medical University of Vienna
Vienna General Hospital
Vienna
Austria
Autoantibodies in rheumatoid arthritis

V. Michael Holers, MD
Professor of Medicine and Immunology
University of Colorado–Denver School of Medicine
Staff Physician
University of Colorado Hospital
Aurora, Colorado
USA
The complement system in systemic lupus erythematosus

Michael F. Holick, PhD, MD
Professor of Medicine, Physiology, and Biophysics
Boston University School of Medicine
Program Director
General Clinical Research Unit
Boston Medical Center
Boston, Massachusetts
USA
Osteomalacia and rickets

Christopher Holroyd, BM, MRCP
Academic Clinical Fellow in Rheumatology
University of Southampton
MRC Epidemiology Resource Centre
Southampton General Hospital
Southampton
United Kingdom
Epidemiology and classification of metabolic bone disease

Osvaldo Hübscher, MD, MACR
Associate Professor of Medicine–Rheumatology
CEMIC Medical School
Buenos Aires
Argentina
Pattern recognition in arthritis

Tom W. J. Huizinga, MD, PhD
Professor and Chairman
Department of Rheumatology
Leiden University Faculty of Medicine
Leiden
The Netherlands
Dapsone, penicillamine, thalidomide, bucillamine, and the tetracyclines

David J. Hunter, MBBS, PhD, FRACP
Assistant Professor of Medicine
University of Sydney Medical School
Sydney, New South Wales
Australia
Chief of Research
New England Baptist Hospital
Boston, Massachusetts
USA
Assessment of imaging outcomes in osteoarthritis

M. Elaine Husni, MD, MPH
Assistant Professor of Medicine
Cleveland Clinic Lerner College of Medicine of Case Western Reserve University
Vice Chair
Arthritis and Musculoskeletal Treatment Center
Department of Rheumatic and Immunologic Diseases
Cleveland Clinic
Cleveland, Ohio
USA
Classification and epidemiology of psoriatic arthritis

Robert D. Inman, MD
Professor of Medicine and Immunology
University of Toronto Faculty of Medicine
Senior Scientist
Toronto Western Research Institute
Toronto, Ontario
Canada
Reactive arthritis: etiology and pathogenesis

Zacharia Isaac, MD
Instructor
Department of Physical Medicine and Rehabilitation
Harvard Medical School
Director
Interventional Physical Medicine and Rehabilitation
Brigham and Women's Hospital and Spaulding Rehabilitation Hospital
Boston, Massachusetts
USA
Lumbar spine disorders

Maura D. Iversen, DPT, ScD, MPH
Professor and Chair
Department of Physical Therapy
Northeastern University
Assistant Professor of Medicine–Rheumatology
Harvard Medical School
Behavioral Scientist
Brigham and Women's Hospital
Boston, Massachusetts
USA
Arthritis patient education and team approaches to management

Douglas A. Jabs, MD, MBA
Professor and Chair
Department of Ophthalmology
Chief Executive Officer and Dean for Clinical Affairs
Mount Sinai Faculty Practice Associates
Mount Sinai School of Medicine
New York, New York
USA
The eye in rheumatic disease

Hayley James, BSc, MSc
Research Fellow
Unit of Behavioural Medicine
University College London
London
United Kingdom
Non-pharmacologic pain management

Rose-Marie Javier, MD
Senior Lecturer
Medical University Louis Pasteur
Senior Attending Physician
Rheumatology Unit
University Hospital Hautpierre
Strasbourg
France
Gaucher's disease

David Jayne, MD, FRCP
Consultant in Nephrology and Vasculitis
Addenbrooke's Hospital
Cambridge
United Kingdom
Churg-Strauss syndrome

Alyssa K. Johnsen, MD, PhD
Instructor/Senior Fellow
Division of Rheumatology, Immunology and Allergy
Brigham and Women's Hospital/Harvard Medical School
Boston, Massachusetts
USA
Methotrexate

Joanne M. Jordan, MD, MPH
Herman and Louise Smith Distinguished Professor of Medicine
Associate Professor of Orthopaedics
Chief
Division of Rheumatology, Allergy, and Immunology
Director
Thurston Arthritis Research Center
University of North Carolina at Chapel Hill School of Medicine
Chapel Hill, North Carolina
USA
Osteoarthritis: epidemiology and classification

Melanie S. Joy, PharmD, PhD, FCCP, FASN
Associate Professor of Medicine and Pharmacy
UNC School of Medicine
Division of Nephrology and Hypertension
Chapel Hill, North Carolina
USA
Drug-induced lupus

Tsuneyasu Kaisho, MD, PhD
Team Leader
Laboratory for Host Defense
RIKEN Research Center for Allergy and Immunology
Kanagawa
Japan
Principles of innate immunity

Cees G. M. Kallenberg, MD, PhD
Head
Department of Rheumatology and Clinical Immunology
University Medical Center Gröningen
Gröningen
The Netherlands
Biology and immunopathogenesis of vasculitis

Yuka Kanno, MD, PhD
Staff Scientist
Laboratory of Clinical Investigation
National Institute of Arthritis and Musculoskeletal and Skin Diseases
National Institutes of Health
Bethesda, Maryland
USA
Principles and techniques in molecular biology

Elizabeth W. Karlson, MD
Associate Professor of Medicine
Harvard Medical School
Associate Physician
Brigham and Women's Hospital
Boston, Massachusetts
USA
Classification and epidemiology of rheumatoid arthritis

Dimitrios G. Kassimos, MD, MSc
Consultant Rheumatologist
Head
Education Department
401 General Military Hospitaa of Athens
Athens
Greece
Neuropathic arthropathy

Daniel L. Kastner, MD, PhD
Clinical Director
Laboratory of Clinical Investigation
National Institute of Arthritis and Musculoskeletal and Skin Diseases
National Institutes of Health
Bethesda, Maryland
USA
Principles and techniques in molecular biology; The hereditary recurrent fevers

Jeffrey N. Katz, MD, MSc
Associate Professor of Medicine and Orthopaedic
    Surgery
Harvard Medical School
Director
Orthopedic and Arthritis Center for Outcomes Research
Brigham and Women's Hospital
Boston, Massachusetts
USA
Lumbar spine disorders

Arthur Kavanaugh, MD
Professor of Medicine
University of California, San Diego
San Diego, California
USA
Tumor necrosis factor blocking therapies

Jonathan Kay, MD
Professor of Medicine
Department of Medicine
Division of Rheumatology
University of Massachusetts Medical School
Director of Clinical Research
Division of Rheumatology
UMass Memorial Medical Center
Worcester, Massachusetts
USA
*Miscellaneous arthropathies including synovial tumors
    and foreign body synovitis and nephrogenic systemic
    fibrosis*

Jennifer A. Kelly, MPH
Statistician and Research Project Director
Arthritis and Immunology Research Program
Oklahoma Medical Research Foundation
Oklahoma City, Oklahoma
USA
Genetics of lupus

Edward Keystone, MD, FRCPC
Professor of Medicine
University of Toronto Faculty of Medicine
Consultant in Rheumatology
Mount Sinai Hospital
Toronto, Ontario
Canada
Leflunomide

Munther A. Khamashta, MD, PhD, FRCP
Reader in Medicine
King's College London School of Medicine
Consultant Physician
Director
Lupus Research Unit
St. Thomas' Hospital
London
United Kingdom
*Antiphospholipid syndrome: overview of pathogenesis,
    diagnosis, and management*

Dinesh Khanna, MD, MSc
Assistant Professor
Department of Medicine
Division of Rheumatology and Immunology
David Geffen School of Medicine at UCLA
Los Angeles, California
USA
Assessing disease activity and outcome in scleroderma

Peter W. Kim, MD, PhD
Clinical Fellow
Laboratory of Clinical Investigation
National Institute of Arthritis and Musculoskeletal and
    Skin Diseases
National Institutes of Health
Bethesda, Maryland
USA
The hereditary recurrent fevers

Ingvild Kjeken, PhD
Senior Researcher
National Resource Center for Rehabilitation in
    Rheumatology
Diakonhjemmet Hospital
Oslo
Norway
Multidisciplinary approach to rheumatoid arthritis

Alisa E. Koch, MD
Staff Physician
VA Ann Arbor Healthcare System
Fredrick G.L. Huetwell and William D. Robinson, MD
    Professor of Rheumatology
Department of Internal Medicine
Division of Rheumatology
University of Michigan Medical School
Ann Arbor, Michigan
USA
Angiogenesis in rheumatoid arthritis

Matthew F. Koff, PhD
Assistant Scientist
Department of Radiology and Imaging–MRI
Hospital for Special Surgery
New York, New York
USA
Biomechanics of peripheral joints

Virginia Byers Kraus, MD, PhD
Associate Professor
Department of Medicine
Division of Rheumatology
Duke University School of Medicine
Durham, North Carolina
USA
*Rare osteoarthritis: ochronosis, Kashin-Beck disease, and
    Mseleni joint disease*

Hillal Maradit Kremers, MD, MSc
Professor of Epidemiology
Mayo Clinic College of Medicine
Mayo Clinic
Rochester, Minnesota
USA
*Principles of health economics and application to
    rheumatic disorders*

Hollis Elaine Krug, MD
Associate Professor of Medicine
Univeristy of Minnesota Medical School
Staff Rheumatologist
Minneapolis VA Medical Center
Minneapolis, Minnesota
USA
*Principles of opioid treatment of chronic musculoskeletal
    pain*

Pradeep Kumar, MD, FRCP
Consultant Rheumatologist
Aberdeen Royal Infirmary
Aberdeen
Scotland
Raynaud's phenomenon

Tore K. Kvien, MD, PhD
Professor of Rheumatology
University of Oslo Faculty of Medicine
Head
Department of Rheumatology
Diakonhjemmet Hospital
Oslo
Norway
Multidisciplinary approach to rheumatoid arthritis

Robert Lafyatis, MD
Professor of Medicine
Boston University School of Medicine
Laboratory Director
Boston University Medical Center
Boston, Massachusetts
USA
Pathogenesis of systemic sclerosis

Talia Landau, BA
Medical Student (Third Year)
University of Maryland School of Medicine
Baltimore, Maryland
USA
Gastrointestinal tract and rheumatic disease

Robert B. M. Landewé, MD
Professor of Rheumatology
Department of Internal Medicine
Division of Rheumatology
Maastricht University Faculty of Medicine
Maastricht
Consultant
Atrium Medical Center
Heerlen
The Netherlands
*Interpreting the medical literature for the rheumatologist:
    study design and levels of evidence*

Carol A. Langford, MD, MHS
Director
Center for Vasculitis Care and Research
Department of Rheumatic and Immunologic Diseases
Cleveland Clinic
Cleveland, Ohio
USA
Takayasu's arteritis

Ronald M. Laxer, MD, FRCPC
Professor of Pediatrics and Medicine
University of Toronto Faculty of Medicine
Staff Rheumatologist
The Hospital for Sick Children
Toronto, Ontario
Canada
Management of juvenile idiopathic arthritis

Thomas J. Learch, MD
Chief of Musculoskeletal Imaging
Department of Imaging
Cedars-Sinai Medical Center
Los Angeles, California
USA
Imaging of rheumatoid arthritis

Marjatta Leirisalo-Repo, MD, PhD
Professor of Rheumatology
University of Helsinki Faculty of Medicine
Chief Physician
Department of Medicine
Division of Rheumatology
Helsinki University Central Hospital
Helsinki
Finland
Reactive arthritis: clinical features and treatment

George T. Lewith, MD, MA, FRCP, MRCGP
Professor of Health Research
School of Medicine
University of Southampton
Honorary Consultant Physician
Southampton Hospitals NHS Trust
Southampton
United Kingdom
Complementary and alternative medicine

Yi Li, MD
Research Assistant
Department of Medicine
University of Florida College of Medicine/Shands at UF
Gainesville, Florida
USA
Autoantibodies in systemic lupus erythematosus

Katherine P. Liao, MD
Research Fellow in Medicine
Harvard Medical School
Fellow in Rheumatology
Brigham and Women's Hospital
Boston, Massachusetts
USA
Classification and epidemiology of rheumatoid arthritis

Geoffrey Littlejohn, MD, MPH
Associate Professor of Rheumatology and Medicine
Monash University Faculty of Medicine, Nursing, and
    Health Sciences
Director
Division of Rheumatology
Monash Medical Centre
Melbourne, Victoria
Australia
Diffuse idiopathic skeletal hyperostosis

Michael D. Lockshin, MD
Professor of Medicine and Obstetrics-Gynecology
Weill Cornell Medical College
Attending Physician
New York-Presbyterian Hospital
Hospital for Special Surgery
New York, New York
USA
*Systemic lupus erythematosus in the pregnant patient
    and neonatal lupus*

Pilar Lorenzo, PhD
Researcher
Department of Clinical Sciences
Lund University Faculty of Medicine
Lund
Sweden
The articular cartilage

Thomas A. Luger, MD
Professor and Chairman
Department of Dermatology
University of Münster Faculty of Health Science
Münster
Germany
Skin in rheumatic disease

Ingrid E. Lundberg, MD, PhD
Professor and Consultant
Rheumatology Unit
Department of Medicine
Karolinska University Hospital
Stockholm
Sweden
*Inflammatory muscle disease—etiology and pathogenesis
    (myositis)*

Harvinder S. Luthra, MD
John Finn Minnesota Arthritis Foundation Professor
Mayo Medical School
Consultant
Division of Rheumatology and Internal Medicine
Mayo Clinic
Rochester, Minnesota
USA
Relapsing polychondritis

Klaus P. Machold, MD
Associate Professor of Medicine
Medical University of Vienna
Deputy Head
Division of Rheumatology
Department of Internal Medicine
Vienna General Hospital
Vienna
Austria
*Evaluation and management of early inflammatory
    polyarthritis*

C. Ronald Mackenzie, MD
Associate Professor of Clinical Medicine
Associate Professor of Public Health
Division of Medical Ethics
Weill Cornell Medical College
Associate Attending Physician
Department of Rheumatology
Hospital for Special Surgery
New York, New York
USA
*Ethics in clinical trials; Perioperative care of the rheumatic
    disease patient*

Maren Lawson Mahowald, MD
Professor
Department of Medicine–Rheumatology
University of Minnesota Medical School
Chief
Rheumatology Section
Department of Internal Medicine
Minneapolis VA Medical Center
Minneapolis, Minnesota
USA
*Principles of opioid treatment of chronic musculoskeletal
    pain*

Alfred D. Mahr, MD
Classification and epidemiology of vasculitis

Joan C. Marini, MD, PhD
Chief
Bone and Extracellular Matrix Branch
National Institute of Child Health and Human
    Development
National Institutes of Health
Bethesda, Maryland
USA
Heritable connective tissue disorders

Eresha Markalanda, MD
Practicing Physician
Colombo
Sri Lanka
*Immunosuppressives (chlorambucil, cyclosporine,
    cytoxan, azathioprine [Imuran], mofetil, tacrolimus)*

Javier Marquez, MD
Professor of Internal Medicine–Rheumatology
Pontifical Bolivarian University School of Health
    Sciences
Staff Physician
Rheumatology Service
Hospital Pablo Tobon Uribe
Medellín
Colombia
Mycobacterial, brucellar, fungal, and parasitic arthritis

Johanne Martel-Pelletier, PhD
Professor of Medicine
Titular Head
Chair in Osteoarthritis
University of Montreal Faculty of Medicine
Co-Director
Osteoarthritis Research Unit
University of Montreal Hospital Research Centre
    (CR-CHUM)
Notre-Dame Hospital
Montreal, Quebec
Canada
Animal models of osteoarthritis

Emilio Martin-Mola, PhD
Associate Professor of Rheumatology
Faculty of Medicine
Universidad Autonoma Madrid
Head
Rheumatology Division
Hospital Universitario La Paz
Madrid
Spain
*Septic arthritis, osteomyelitis, and gonococcal and
    syphilitic arthritis*

Manuel Martinez-Lavin, MD
Professor
Department of Rheumatology
Faculty of Medicine
National Autonomous University of Mexico
Chief
Rheumatology Department
National Institute of Cardiology
Mexico City
Mexico
Digital clubbing and hypertrophic osteoarthropathy

Elena M. Massarotti, MD
Associate Professor of Medicine
Harvard Medical School
Co-Director
Center for Clinical Therapeutics
Division of Rheumatology
Brigham and Women's Hospital
Boston, Massachusetts
USA
Hemochromatosis

Eric L. Matteson, MD, MPH
Professor of Medicine
Mayo Clinic College of Medicine
Chair
Division of Rheumatology
Mayo Clinic
Rochester, Minnesota
USA
*Extra-articular features of rheumatoid arthritis and
    systemic involvement*

Maureen Mayes, MD, MPH
Professor of Medicine
Department of Internal Medicine
Division of Rheumatology
University of Texas Medical School at Houston
Houston, Texas
USA
Epidemiology and classification of scleroderma

Bongani M. Mayosi, PhD, FCP(SA)
Professor of Medicine
Department of Medicine
University of Cape Town
Physician-in-Chief
Groote Schuur Hospital
Cape Town
South Africa
Acute rheumatic fever

Timothy McAlindon, MD, MPH
Professor of Medicine
Tufts University School of Medicine
Chief
Division of Rheumatology
Tufts Medical Center
Boston, Massachusetts
USA
Osteonecrosis

Rex M. McCallum, MD
Professor of Medicine–Rheumatology
Duke University School of Medicine
Attending Rheumatologist
Duke University Hospital
Durham, North Carolina
USA
Cogan syndrome

Geraldine McCarthy, MD, FRCPI
Associate Clinical Professor of Medicine
School of Medicine and Medical Science
University College Dublin
Consultant Rheumatologist
Mater Misericordiae University Hospital
Dublin
Ireland
Basic calcium phosphate crystal deposition disease

W. Joseph McCune, MD
Professor
Department of Internal Medicine
Division of Rheumatology
University of Michigan Medical School/University of
   Michigan Health System
Ann Arbor, Michigan
USA
Treatment of non-renal lupus

Stephany A. McGann, MD
Medical Director
Rheumatology Fellow
University of Maryland School of Medicine
Baltimore, Maryland
USA
Entrapment neuropathies and compartment syndromes

Dennis McGonagle, MD
Professor of Investigative Rheumatology
University of Leeds
Leeds
United Kingdom
*Etiology and pathogenesis of psoriatic arthritis;
   Enthesopathies*

Lachy McLean, PhD, FRCP
Senior Medical Director
Takeda Pharmaceuticals
Lake Forest, Illinois
USA
Etiology and pathogenesis of gout

Philip J. Mease, MD
Clinical Professor of Medicine
University of Washington School of Medicine
Director
Rheumatology Clinical Research
Swedish Medical Center
Chief
Seattle Rheumatology Associates
Seattle, Washington
USA
Management of psoriatic arthritis

Peter A. Merkel, MD, MPH
Associate Professor of Medicine
Boston University School of Medicine
Boston, Massachusetts
USA
Classification and epidemiology of vasculitis

Jamal A. Mikdashi, MD, MPH
Associate Professor of Medicine
University of Maryland School of Medicine
Baltimore, Maryland
USA
Primary angiitis of the central nervous system

Frederick W. Miller, MD, PhD
Chief
Environmental Autoimmunity Group
National Institute of Environmental Health Sciences
National Institutes of Health Clinical Research Facility
Bethesda, Maryland
USA
Management of inflammatory muscle disease

Paul D. Miller, MD, FACP
Distinguished Clinical Professor of Medicine
University of Colorado–Denver School of Medicine
Denver
Medical Director
Colorado Center for Bone Research
Lakewood, Colorado
USA
Renal osteodystrophy

Kirsten Minden, MD
Consultant in Pediatric Rheumatology
Department of Pediatric Pneumology and Immunology
Charité Universitätsmedizin Berlin
Scientist
German Rheumatism Research Center—A Leibnitz
   Institute
Berlin
Germany
*Classification and epidemiology of juvenile idiopathic
   arthritis*

Dimitris I. Mitsias, MD
Research Associate
Department of Pathophysiology
University of Athens School of Medicine
Athens
Greece
Sjögren's syndrome

Girish M. Mody, MD, MBChB, FRCP, FCP
Fellow of the University of Kwa Zulu-Natal
Aaron Beare Family Professor of Rheumatology
Nelson R. Mandela School of Medicine
University of Kwa Zulu-Natal
Durban
South Africa
Acute rheumatic fever

Paul A. Monach, MD, PhD
Rheumatology Fellow
Brigham & Women's Hospital
Boston, MA
USA
The rheumatoid joint: synovitis and tissue destruction

Larry W. Moreland, MD
Margaret Jane Miller Endowed Professor for Arthritis
   Research
University of Pittsburgh School of Medicine
Chief
Division of Rheumatology and Clinical Immunology
Department of Medicine
University of Pittsburgh Medical Center
Pittsburgh, Pennsylvania
USA
T-cell co-stimulation

Haralampos M. Moutsopoulos, MD, FACP, FRCP
Professor and Chairman
Department of Pathophysiology
University of Athens School of Medicine
Athens
Greece
Sjögren's syndrome

Gauthier Namur, MD
Consultant
Department of Nuclear Medicine
University Hospital of Liege
Liege
Belgium
Bone scintigraphy and positron emission tomography

Esperanza Naredo, MD
Professor and Cofounder
Ultrasound School of the Spanish Society of
   Rheumatology
Senior Rheumatologist
Hospital Universario Severo Ochoa
Madrid
Spain
*Aspiration and injection of joints and periarticular tissues
   and intralesional therapy*

David J. Nashel, MD
Professor of Medicine
George Washington & Georgetown
University
VA Medical Center
Washington, DC
USA
Entrapment neuropathies and compartment syndromes

Amanda E. Nelson, MD
Associate Professor of Medicine
University of North Carolina at Chapel Hill School of
   Medicine
Chapel Hill, North Carolina
USA
Osteoarthritis: epidemiology and classification

Stanton P. Newman, DPhil, DipClinPsych, MRCP(Hon)
Professor of Clinical Health and Psychology
Head
Unit of Behavioural Medicine
Division of Research Strategy
University College London Medical School
Honorary Consultant
University College Hospital
London
United Kingdom
Non-pharmacologic pain management

Johannes C. Nossent, MD, PhD
Professor of Medicine
University of Tromsø Faculty of Health Sciences
Institute for Clinical Medicine
Consultant in Rheumatology
University Hospital North Norway
Tromsø
Norway
Adult-onset Still's disease

Ulrich Nöth
Orthopaedic Center for Musculoskeletal Research
Orthopaedic Clinic
König-Ludwig-Haus
Julius-Maximilians-University
Würzburg
Germany
*Principles of tissue engineering and cell- and gene-based
   therapy*

Philip O'Connor, MD, MRCP, FRCR
Consultant in Musculoskeletal Radiology
Leeds Teaching Hospitals NHS Trust
Leeds
United Kingdom
Musculoskeletal ultrasound

Chester V. Oddis, MD
Professor of Medicine
Director
Fellowship Training Program
Department of Medicine
Division of Rheumatology and Clinical Immunology
University of Pittsburgh School of Medicine
Pittsburgh, Pennsylvania
USA
Clinical features, classification, and epidemiology of inflammatory muscle disease

K. Sigvard Olsson, MD, PhD
Associate Professor
Section of Hematology and Coagulation
Sahlgreuslia University Hospital
Gothenburg
Sweden
Hemochromatosis

Michael J. Ombrello, MD
Clinical Fellow
Laboratory of Clinical Investigation
National Institute of Arthritis and Musculoskeletal and Skin Diseases
National Institutes of Health
Bethesda, Maryland
USA
Principles and techniques in molecular biology

Philippe Orcel, MD, PhD
Professor of Rheumatology
Paris-Diderot Faculty of Medicine
University of Paris 7
Head
Rheumatology Department
Medical Coordinator
Musculoskeletal Division
Hospital Lariboisière
Public Assistance Hospitals of Paris
Paris
France
Gaucher's disease

John J. O'Shea, MD
Scientific Director and Chief
Molecular Immunology and Inflammation Branch
National Institute of Arthritis and Musculoskeletal and Skin Diseases
National Institutes of Health
Bethesda, Maryland
USA
Cytokines; Signal transduction

Stephen A. Paget, MD
Profesor of Medicine
Weill Cornell Medical College
Physician-in-Chief Emeritus
Medical Director for Academic, International, and Philanthropic Initiatives
Hospital for Special Surgery
New York, New York
USA
Ethics in clinical trials; Perioperative care of the rheumatic disease patient

Carlo Patrono, MD
Professor and Chair
Department of Pharmacology
Catholic University School of Medicine
Rome, Italy
Nonsteroidal anti-inflammatory drugs

Jean-Pierre Pelletier, MD
Professor of Medicine
Head
Arthritis Centre
University of Montreal Faculty of Medicine
Head
Arthritis Division
University of Montreal Hospital Centre (CHUM)
Notre-Dame Hospital
Director
Osteoarthritis Research Unit
Research Centre
University of Montreal Hospital Research Centre (CR-CHUM)
Montreal, Quebec
Canada
Animal models of osteoarthritis

Silvia Pierangeli, PhD
Professor
Division of Rheumatology, Department of Internal Medicine
University of Texas Medical Branch
Galveston, Texas
USA
Antiphospholipid syndrome: overview of pathogenesis, diagnosis, and management

Heather Pierce, MD
Associate Professor of Pediatrics
University of California, San Diego, School of Medicine
La Jolla
Pediatric Hospitalist
Department of Medicine
Rady Children's Hospital San Diego
San Diego, California
USA
Henoch-Schönlein purpura

Clarissa A. Pilkington, MBBS, BSc, MRCP(Paeds)
Honorary Lecturer
Institute of Child Health
University College London Medical School
Consultant in Paediatric and Adolescent Rheumatology
Great Ormond Street Hospital NHS Trust
London
United Kingdom
Connective tissue diseases in children

Michael H. Pillinger, MD
Associate Professor of Medicine and Pharmacology
Director
Rheumatology Training
Director
Masters of Science in Clinical Investigation Program
New York University School of Medicine
Section Chief
Rheumatology
New York Harbor Health Care System–NY Campus
Department of Veterans Affairs
New York, New York
USA
Inflammation

Carlos Pineda, MD
Subdirector
Biomedical Research
Instituto Nacional de Rehabilitación
Mexico City
Mexico
Digital clubbing and hypertrophic osteoarthropathy

Robert M. Plenge, MD, PhD
Assistant Professor of Medicine
Harvard Medical School
Director
Genetics and Genomics
Division of Rheumatology, Immunology, and Allergy
Brigham and Women's Hospital
Boston, Massachusetts
USA
The contribution of genetic factors to rheumatoid arthritis

Luminita Pricop, MD
Associate Scientist
Hospital for Special Surgery
New York, NY
USA
Immunopathology of systemic lupus erythematosus

Lars Rackwitz
Orthopaedic Center for Musculoskeletal Research
Orthopaedic Clinic
König-Ludwig-Haus
Julius-Maximilians-University
Würzburg
Germany
Principles of tissue engineering and cell- and gene-based therapy

Gautam Ramani, MD
Assistant Professor of Medicine, Cardiology
University of Maryland School of Medicine
Baltimore, Maryland
USA
The heart in rheumatic disease

Angelo Ravelli, MD
Associate Professor of Pediatrics
University of Genoa College of Medicine
Attending
Istituto G. Gaslini
Department of Pediatrics II
Largo G. Gaslini
Genoa
Italy
Evaluation of musculoskeletal complaints in children

Westley H. Reeves, MD
Marcia Whitney Schott Professor of Medicine
Chief
Division of Rheumatology and Clinical Immunology
Department of Medicine
University of Florida College of Medicine
Gainesville, Florida
USA
Autoantibodies in systemic lupus erythematosus

Elaine F. Remmers, PhD
Staff Scientist
Laboratory of Clinical Investigation
National Institute of Arthritis and Musculoskeletal and Skin Diseases
National Institutes of Health
Bethesda, Maryland
USA
Principles and techniques in molecular biology

Heikki Repo, MD
Senior Lecturer in Medicine
Department of Bacteriology and Immunology
University of Helsinki Faculty of Medicine
Attending Physician
Department of Medicine
Helsinki University Central Hospital
Reactive arthritis: clinical features and treatment

Luis Requena, MD
Professor of Dermatology
Universidad Autónoma Medical School
Chairman
Department of Dermatology
Fundación Jiménez Diaz
Madrid
Spain
Cutaneous vasculitis and panniculitis

Clio Ribbens, MD, PhD
Clinic Head
Department of Rheumatology
University Hospital of Liege
Liege
Belgium
Bone scintigraphy and positron emission tomography

Graham Riley, BSc, PhD
Arthritis Research Campaign (ARC) Senior Research
    Fellow
School of Biological Sciences
University of East Anglia
Norwich
United Kingdom
Tendons and ligaments

Christopher Ritchlin, MD, MPH
Professor of Medicine
University of Rochester School of Medicine and
    Dentistry
Attending Physician
University of Rochester Medical Center
Rochester, New York
USA
Etiology and pathogenesis of psoriatic arthritis

Ivan O. Rosas, MD
Assistant Professor of Medicine
Department of Internal Medicine
Division of Pulmonary Medicine
Brigham and Women's Hospital/Harvard Medical
    School
Boston, Massachusetts
USA
The lung in rheumatic disease

Ronenn Roubenoff, MD, MHS
Associate Professor of Medicine
Tufts University School of Medicine
Adjunct Professor of Nutrition
Tufts University School of Nutrition Science and Policy
Boston
Global Head of Translational Medicine
Musculoskeletal Diseases
Novartis Institutes for Biomedical Research
Cambridge, Massachusetts
USA
Nutrition in rheumatic disease

A. D. Rowan, BSc, PhD
Professor of Molecular Rheumatology
School of Clinical Medical Sciences
Musculoskeletal Research Group
Institute of Cellular Medicine
Newcastle University
Newcastle upon Tyne
United Kingdom
Tissue destruction and repair

Martin Rudwaleit, MD
Associate Professor of Medicine
Universitätsmedizin Berlin
Consultant in Rheumatology
University Hospital Charité–Campus Benjamin Franklin
Berlin
Germany
Classification and epidemiology of spondyloarthritis

Kenneth G. Saag, MD, MSc
Jane Knight Lowe Professor of Medicine
University of Alabama at Birmingham School of
    Medicine
Birmingham, Alabama
USA
Systemic corticosteroids in rheumatology

Jane E. Salmon, MD
Associate Clinical Director
Roche
Switzerland
Immunopathology of systemic lupus erythematosus

David C. Salonen, MD, BSc, FRCPC
Associate Professor
Department of Medical Imaging and Orthopedics
University of Toronto Faculty of Medicine
Staff Radiologist
University Health Network, Mount Sinai, and Women's
    College Hospitals
Toronto, Ontario
Canada
Seronegative spondyloarthropathies: imaging

Donald M. Salter, MBChB, MD, FRCPath
Professor of Osteoarticular Pathology
Centre for Inflammation Research
Queen's Medical Research Institute
University of Edinburgh Medical School
Consultant Histopathologist
Royal Infirmary of Edinburgh
Edinburgh
United Kingdom
Connective tissue responses to mechanical stresses

Daniel J. Salzberg, MD, FACP
Assistant Professor of Medicine
University of Maryland School of Medicine
Baltimore, Maryland
USA
The kidney and rheumatic disease

Philip N. Sambrook, MD, FRACP
Professor of Rheumatology
University of Sydney Medical School
Sydney, New South Wales
Australia
Glucocorticoid-induced osteoporosis

Benjamin Sanofsky, MD
Sports medicine: clinical spectrum of injury

Tore Saxne, MD, PhD
Professor
Department of Clinical Sciences
Section of Rheumatology
Lund University Faculty of Medicine
Consultant
Department of Rheumatology
Lund University Hospital
Lund
Sweden
The articular cartilage

Hans-Georg Schaible, MD
Professor of Physiology
Institute of Physiology/Neurophysiology
Friedrich Schiller University of Jena School of Medicine
Director
Department of Neurophysiology
University Hospital
Jena
Germany
Scientific basis of pain

Georg Schett, MD
Professor of Rheumatology and Immunology
Department of Internal Medicine 3
University of Erlangen–Nuremberg Faculty of Medicine
Erlangen
Germany
Osteoimmunology

Nicole Schmitz, PhD
Senior Research Scientist
Department of Pathology
University of Leipzig
Leipzig
Germany
Pathogenesis and pathology of osteoarthritis

Lew C. Schon, MD
Acting Director
Foot and Ankle Fellowship
Department of Orthopaedics
Union Memorial Hospital
Baltimore, Maryland
USA
The ankle and foot

H. Ralph Schumacher, Jr., MD
Professor of Medicine
University of Pennsylvania School of Medicine
Philadelphia, Pennsylvania
USA
*Miscellaneous arthropathies including synovial tumors
    and foreign body synovitis and nephrogenic systemic
    fibrosis; Other crystal-related arthropathies*

David G. I. Scott, MD, FRCP
Professor of Rheumatology
School of Medicine
University of East Anglia
Consultant Rheumatologist
Norfolk and Norwich University Hospital
Norwich
United Kingdom
Polyarteritis nodosa and microscopic polyangiitis

Brooke Seidelmann, BA, MA
Allergy Director
Joan Hisaoka Healing Arts Gallery
Washington, DC
USA
Complementary and alternative medicine

Andrea L. Sestak, MD, PhD
Research Assistant Member
Arthritis and Immunology Research Program
Oklahoma Medical Research Foundation
Oklahoma City, Oklahoma
USA
Genetics of lupus

Margaret Seton, MD
Assistant Professor of Medicine
Harvard Medical School
Director
MGH Rheumatology Fellowship Program
Massachusetts General Hospital
Boston, Massachusetts
USA
Paget's disease of bone

Nancy A. Shadick, MD, MPH
Director of Translational Research Development
Division of Rheumatology, Immunology, and Allergy
Brigham and Women's Hospital
Boston, Massachusetts
USA
Lyme disease

Lauren Shapiro, BA
Research Assistant
Stanford University School of Medicine
Stanford, California
USA
Magnetic resonance imaging

Lewis L. Shi, MD
Orthopedic Surgery Resident
Brigham and Women's Hospital
Boston, Massachusetts
USA
The knee

Prodromos Sidiropoulos, MD
Assistant Professor of Rheumatology
University of Crete School of Medicine
Heraklion
Assistant Professor of Rheumatology
University Hospital of Heraklion
Crete
Greece
*Systemic lupus erythematosus: treatment—renal
    involvement*

Richard M. Siegel, MD, PhD
Senior Investigator
Acting Chief
Autoimmunity Branch
Laboratory of Clinical Investigation
National Institute of Arthritis and Musculoskeletal and
    Skin Diseases
National Institutes of Health
Bethesda, Maryland
USA
Cytokines; Principles and techniques in molecular biology

Joachim Sieper, MD
Professor of Internal Medicine–Rheumatology
Department of Medicine I
Universitätsmedizin Berlin
Head
Division of Rheumatology
University Hospital Charité–Campus Benjamin Franklin
Berlin
Germany
Management of ankylosing spondylitis

Richard M. Silver, MD
Distinguished University Professor
Department of Medicine
Division of Rheumatology and Immunology
Medical University of South Carolina College of
    Medicine
Charleston, South Carolina
USA
Clinical features of systemic sclerosis

Shonni J. Silverberg, MD
Professor of Medicine–Endocrinology and Metabolism
Columbia University College of Physicians and
    Surgeons
Attending
Division of Endocrinology
New York–Presbyterian Hospital
New York, New York
USA
*Primary hyperparathyroidism: rheumatologic
    manifestations and bone disease*

Julia F. Simard, ScD
Department of Medical Epidemiology and Biostatistics
Karolinska Institutet
Clinical Epidemiology Unit
Karolinska University Hospital
Stockholm
Sweden
*Epidemiology and classification of systemic lupus
    erythematosus*

Barry P. Simmons, MD
Associate Professor of Orthopaedic Surgery
Harvard Medical School
Chief
Hand and Upper Extremity Service
Division of Orthopaedic Surgery
Department of Surgery
Brigham and Women's Hospital
Boston, Massachusetts
USA
The wrist and hand

Robert W. Simms, MD
Professor of Medicine
Boston University School of Medicine
Chief
Section of Rheumatology
Boston Medical Center
Boston, Massachusetts
USA
Localized scleroderma and scleroderma-like syndromes

John Sims, PhD
Scientific Executive Director
Amgen
Seattle, Washington
USA
Cytokines

Nora G. Singer, MD
Associate Professor of Pediatrics and Internal Medicine
Case Western Reserve University School of Medicine
Director
Division of Rheumatology
MetroHealth Medical Center
Cleveland, Ohio
USA
Evaluation of musculoskeletal complaints in children

Malcolm D. Smith, MBBS, FRACP, BSc(Hons), PhD
Professor of Internal Medicine–Rheumatology
Flinders University School of Medicine
Regional Head of Rheumatology
Southern Adelaide Health
Adelaide
Consultant in Rheumatology
Repatriation General Hospital
Daw Park, South Australia
Australia
The synovium

Stacy E. Smith, MD
Associate Professor of Radiology
Department of Diagnostic Radiology and Nuclear
    Medicine
University of Maryland School of Medicine
Baltimore, Maryland
USA
Conventional radiography and computed tomography

Josef S. Smolen, MD, FRCP
*Evaluation and outcomes for patients with rheumatoid
    arthritis*

Tim D. Spector, MD, MSc, FRCP
Professor of Genetic Epidemiology
Department of Twin Research and Genetic
    Epidemiology
King's College London School of Medicine
Consultant Rheumatologist
Guy's and St. Thomas' NHS Foundation Trust
London
United Kingdom
Genetics of osteoarthritis

E. William St. Clair, MD
Professor of Medicine and Immunology
Duke University School of Medicine
Durham, North Carolina
USA
Cogan syndrome

Virginia D. Steen, MD
Professor of Medicine
Division of Rheumatology, Allergy and Immunology
Georgetown University School of Medicine
Washington, DC
USA
Management of systemic sclerosis

Günter Steiner, PhD
Professor of Biochemistry
Department of Internal Medicine III
Division of Rheumatology
Medical University of Vienna
Head
Research Laboratory
Group Leader
Vienna General Hospital
Vienna
Austria
Autoantibodies in rheumatoid arthritis

Andre F. Steinert
Orthopaedic Center for Musculoskeletal Research
Orthopaedic Clinic
König-Ludwig-Haus
Julius-Maximilians-University
Würzburg
Germany
*Principles of tissue engineering and cell- and gene-based
    therapy*

John H. Stone, MD, MPH
Associate Professor of Medicine
Department of Medicine
Division of Rheumatology
Harvard Medical School
Clinical Director
Rheumatology Unit
Massachusetts General Hospital
Boston, Massachusetts
USA
Wegener granulomatosis

Millicent A. Stone, MB, MSc, FRCP
Assistant Professor of Medicine
Department of Rheumatology
University of Toronto Faculty of Medicine
Toronto, Ontario, Canada
Clinical Reader
University of Bath School for Health
Bath, United Kingdom
Research Scholar in Rheumatology
Hospital for Special Surgery
New York, New York/Oklahoma City, Oklahoma
USA
Reactive arthritis: etiology and pathogenesis

Rainer H. Straub, MD
Professor of Experimental Medicine
Department of Internal Medicine I
University of Regensburg School of Medicine
Staff Physician
University Hospital Regensburg
Regensburg
Germany
*Effects of the neuroendocrine system on development and
    function of the immune system*

Deborah P. M. Symmons, MD, FFPH, FRCP
Professor of Rheumatology and Musculoskeletal
    Epidemiology
School of Translational Medicine
Arthritis Research Campaign (ARC) Epidemiology Unit
University of Manchester Faculty of Medical and
    Human Sciences
Manchester
United Kingdom
*Epidemiologic concepts and the classification of
    rheumatology*

Zoltán Szekanecz, MD, PhD, DSc
Professor of Rheumatology, Medicine, and
    Immunology
Head
Division of Rheumatology
Third Department of Internal Medicine
University of Debrecen Medical and Health Sciences
    Centre
Debrecen
Hungary
Angiogenesis in rheumatoid arthritis

Ilona S. Szer
Chief of Pediatric Rheumatology at Rady Children's
    Hospital, San Diego
Professor of Clinical Pediatrics
University of California, San Diego, School of Medicine
San Diego, California
USA
Henoch-Schönlein purpura

Paul P. Tak, MD, PhD
Professor of Medicine
Academic Medical Center/University of Amsterdam
Director
Division of Clinical Immunology and Rheumatology
    EULAR & FOCIS Center of Excellence
Amsterdam
Netherlands
Minimally invasive procedures

Antonio Tavoni
Immunology Unit
Department of Internal Medicine
University of Pisa
Pisa
Italy
Cryoglobulinemia

Peter C. Taylor, BMBCh, PhD, FRCP
Professor of Experimental Rheumatology
Head
Clinical Trials
Kennedy Institute of Rheumatology
Imperial College London Faculty of Medicine
Honorary Consultant Physician
Department of Rheumatology and Clinical Trials Unit
Charing Cross Hospital
London
United Kingdom
Tumor necrosis factor blocking therapies

Robert Terkeltaub, MD
Professor of Medicine
University of California, San Diego, School of Medicine
La Jolla
Chief
Rheumatology Section
VA Medical Center San Diego
San Diego, California
USA
The management of gout and hyperuricemia

Mohamed M. Thabet, MD, PhD
Associate Lecturer in Internal Medicine–Rheumatology
Assiut University Medical School
Assiut
Egypt
Clinical Research Fellow
Department of Rheumatology
Leiden University Medical Center
Leiden
The Netherlands
*Dapsone, penicillamine, thalidomide, bucillamine, and
    the tetracyclines*

Jennifer E. Thorne, MD, PhD
Associate Professor of Ophthalmology
Johns Hopkins University School of Medicine
Associate Professor of Epidemiology
Johns Hopkins University Bloomberg School of Public
    Health
Baltimore, Maryland
USA
The eye in rheumatic disease

George C. Tsokos
Division of Rheumatology
Beth Israel Deaconess Medical Center, Harvard Medical
    School
Boston, Massachusetts
USA
Pathogenesis of lupus

Rocky S. Tuan
Department of Orthopaedic Surgery
Center for Cellular and Molecular Engineering
University of Pittsburgh School of Medicine
Pittsburgh, Pennsylvania
USA
*Principles of tissue engineering and cell- and gene-based
    therapy*

Carl Turesson, MD, PhD
Associate Professor
Department of Clinical Sciences
Malmö University Faculty of Medicine
Senior Physician
Department of Rheumatology
Skåne University Hospital
Malmö
Sweden
*Extra-articular features of rheumatoid arthritis and
    systemic involvement*

Athanasios G. Tzioufas, MD
Professor
Department of Pathophysiology
University of Athens School of Medicine
Athens
Greece
Sjögren's syndrome

Patricia A. Uber, BS, PharmD
Assistant Professor
Department of Medicine
Division of Cardiology
University of Maryland School of Medicine
Baltimore, Maryland
USA
The heart in rheumatic disease

Wim B. van den Berg, PhD
Professor of Experimental Rheumatology
Head
Rheumatology Research and Advanced
    Therapeutics
Radboud University Nijmegen Medical Centre Faculty
    of Medical Sciences
Nijmegen
The Netherlands
Animal models of arthritis

Désirée van der Heijde, MD, PhD
Professor of Rheumatology
Leiden University Faculty of Medicine
Leiden
The Netherlands
*Use of imaging as an outcome measure in rheumatoid
    arthritis, psoriatic arthritis, and ankylosing spondylitis
    in clinical trials*

Floris A. van Gaalen, MD, PhD
Fellow in Rheumatology
Leiden University Faculty of Medicine/Leiden
    University Medical Center
Leiden
The Netherlands
Parenteral gold, antimalarials, and sulfasalazine

John Varga, MD
Division of Rheumatology
Northwestern University Feinberg School of Medicine
Chicago, Illinois
USA
Pathogenesis of systemic sclerosis

Dimitrios Vassilopoulos, MD
Assistant Professor of Medicine–Rheumatology
Athens University School of Medicine
Attending
2nd Department of Medicine
Hippokration General Hospital
Athens
Greece
Rheumatologic aspects of viral infections

Archana R. Vasudevan, MD
Clinical Assistant Professor
Department of Medicine
Division of Rheumatology
State University of New York Downstate Medical
    Center College of Medicine
Brooklyn, New York
USA
Clinical features of systemic lupus erythematosus

Patrick J. W. Venables, MD, FRCP
Professor of Viral Immunorheumatology
Kennedy Institute of Rheumatology
Imperial College London School of Medicine
London
United Kingdom
Overlap syndromes

Edward M. Vital, MBChB, MRCP(UK)
Research Fellow in Rheumatology
Academic Section of Musculoskeletal Disease
Leeds Institute of Molecular Medicine
University of Leeds Faculty of Medicine and Health
Leeds
United Kingdom
Rituximab

Richard J. Wakefield, MD, BM, MRCP
Senior Lecturer in Rheumatology
School of Medicine
University of Leeds Faculty of Medicine and Health
Honorary Consultant Rheumatologist
Leeds Teaching Hospitals NHS Trust
Leeds
United Kingdom
Musculoskeletal ultrasound

Jennifer G. Walker, MBBS, FRACP
Senior Lecturer
Flinders University School of Medicine
Adelaide
Senior Consultant in Rheumatology
Repatriation General Hospital and Flinders Medical
    Center
Daw Park, South Australia
Australia
The synovium

Robert J. Ward, MD, CCD
Chief, Musculoskeletal Imaging
Department of Radiology
Tufts Medical Center
Director, Medical Education
Assistant Professor of Radiology and Orthopedics
Tufts University School of Medicine
Boston, Massachusetts
USA
Osteonecrosis

Richard Watts, MA, DM, FRCP
Clinical Senior Lecturer in Health Policy and Practice
School of Medicine
University of East Anglia
Norwich
Consultant Rheumatologist
Ipswich Hospital NHS Trust
Ipswich
United Kingdom
Polyarteritis nodosa and microscopic polyangiitis

Lucy R. Wedderburn, MD, MA, MBBS, PhD, FRCP, MRCPCH
Reader in Paediatric Rheumatology
Institute of Child Health
University College London Medical School
Consultant in Paediatric Rheumatology
Great Ormond Street Hospital NHS Trust
London
United Kingdom
Connective tissue diseases in children

Michael E. Weinblatt, MD
Methotrexate

Matthew R. Weir, MD
Professor of Medicine
University of Maryland School of Medicine
Director
Division of Nephrology
University of Maryland School of Medicine
Baltimore, Maryland
USA
The kidney and rheumatic disease

Claire Y. J. Wenham, BMBS, MRCP
Clinical Research Fellow
NIHR Musculoskeletal Biomedical Research Unit
Leeds Teaching Hospitals NHS Trust
Leeds
United Kingdom
Imaging of osteoarthritis

Sterling G. West, MD
Professor of Medicine
Division of Rheumatology
University of Colorado–Denver School of Medicine
Aurora, Colorado
USA
Sarcoidosis

Cornelia M. Weyand, MD, PhD
Professor of Medicine
Stanford University School of Medicine
Stanford, California
USA
Polymyalgia rheumatica and giant cell arteritis

Kenneth E. White, PhD
Assistant Professor
Department of Medical and Molecular Genetics
Indiana University School of Medicine
Indianapolis, Indiana
USA
Bone structure and function

Frances M. K. Williams, PhD, FRCP(E)
Senior Lecturer
Department of Twin Research and Genetic
  Epidemiology
King's College London School of Medicine
Honorary Consultant Rheumatologist
Guy's and St. Thomas' NHS Foundation Trust
London
United Kingdom
Genetics of osteoarthritis

Kevin L. Winthrop, MD, MPH
Assistant Professor of Infectious Diseases,
  Ophthalmology, and Public Health and Preventive
  Medicine
Department of Medicine
Division of Infectious Diseases
Oregon Health & Science University School of
  Medicine
Portland, Oregon
USA
Infections and biologic therapy in rheumatoid arthritis

Anthony D. Woolf, BSc, MBBS
Professor of Rheumatology
Peninsula Medical School
Universities of Exeter and Plymouth;
Consultant Rheumatologist
Duke of Cornwall Department of Rheumatology
Royal Cornwall Hospital
Truro
UK
History and physical examination

Jane Worthington, PhD
Professor of Chronic Disease–Genetics
School of Translational Medicine
Arthritis Research Campaign (ARC) Epidemiology Unit
Musculoskeletal Research Group
University of Manchester Faculty of Medical and
  Human Sciences
Honorary Research Principal Investigator
Central Manchester and Manchester Children's
  University Hospital
Manchester
United Kingdom
Genetic factors in rheumatic disease

John Wright, MD
Assistant Clinical Professor of Orthopaedic Surgery
Harvard Medical School
Orthopedic Surgeon
Brigham and Women's Hospital
Boston, Massachusetts
USA
The knee

Hasan Yazici, MD
Professor of Medicine
Chief of Medicine and Rheumatology
Department of Medicine
Division of Rheumatology
Cerrahpasa Medical Faculty
University of Istanbul
Istanbul
Turkey
Behçet's syndrome

Yusuf Yazici, MD
Assistant Professor of Medicine–Rheumatology
New York University School of Medicine
Director
Seligman Center for Advanced Therapeutics
Director
Behçet's Syndrome Evaluation, Treatment, and
  Research Center
NYU Hospital for Joint Diseases
New York, New York
USA
Role of laboratory tests in rheumatic disorders

John R. York, MD, FRACP, FRCP(Glasg), GradDipCouns
Clinical Associate Professor
Department of Rheumatology
Institute of Rheumatology and Orthopaedics
Central Clinical School
University of Sydney Medical School
Consultant Emeritus
Department of Rheumatology
Royal Prince Alfred Hospital
Sydney, New South Wales
Australia
Hemophilia and von Willebrand disease

D. A. Young, BSc, PhD
Lecturer
School of Clinical Medical Sciences
Musculoskeletal Research Group
Institute of Cellular Medicine
Newcastle University
Newcastle upon Tyne
United Kingdom
Tissue destruction and repair

Sebahattin Yurdakul, MD
Professor of Medicine
Department of Medicine
Division of Rheumatology
Cerrahpasa Medical Faculty
University of Istanbul
Istanbul
Turkey
Behçet's syndrome

Guangju Zhai, MBBS, MSc, PhD
Genetic Epidemiologist
Department of Twin Research and Genetic
  Epidemiology
King's College London School of Medicine
London
United Kingdom
Genetics of osteoarthritis

Yuqing Zhang, MD
*Local and systemic risk factors for incidence and
  progression of osteoarthritis*

Haoyang Zhuang, PhD
Postdoctoral Fellow
University of Florida College of Medicine/Shands at UF
Gainesville, Florida
USA
Autoantibodies in systemic lupus erythematosus

PREFACE

The fifth edition of *Rheumatology* is:

- The most comprehensive, authoritative rheumatology text, designed to meet the complete needs of all practicing and academic rheumatologists as well as arthritis-related health professionals and scientists interested in disorders of the musculoskeletal system.
- Firmly grounded on modern biomedical science, integrating the relevant basic biology with current clinical practice.
- Easily accessible, user-friendly, and a beautifully illustrated color publication.
- Consistent in style and format, with each chapter written to a strict template and rigorously edited.
- A genuinely international book, with editors, authors, and material drawn from all over the world.
- Fully up-to-date, with carefully selected references to original work and key reviews up to and including articles published in the peer-reviewed literature through 2009.

THE FIFTH EDITION OF RHEUMATOLOGY IS A COMPREHENSIVE AND EXCITING BOOK

The international team of editors representing a broad spectrum of academic and clinical rheumatology and biomedical, clinical, and epidemiological research has again brought together a group of internationally renowned authors to deliver essential information on the scientific basis of rheumatic disease and the definition, epidemiology, pathophysiology, clinical features, and management of all musculoskeletal and rheumatic disorders.

Rheumatology, fifth edition, builds on the success of the fourth edition. As stated by Professor Jan Dequeker in his review: "The fourth edition of *Rheumatology* is the most comprehensive authoritative rheumatology text designed to meet the complete needs of all practicing and academic rheumatologists as well as arthritis-related health care professionals and scientists interested in disorders of the musculoskeletal system. The edition is firmly grounded on modern medical science, integrating the relevant basic biology with current clinical practice, easily accessible, user-friendly and a beautifully illustrated color publication."

For the fifth edition, every chapter has either been carefully revised or, in many cases, completely rewritten. The Editors have pursued a rigorous editorial policy in order to ensure that the content and format of the book remain both consistent and of the highest possible standard so that each chapter contains the latest information in the field. There are 23 new chapters that provide new information on basic biomedical science, including the emerging field of osteoimmunology, clinical therapeutics, including cell- and gene-based therapies, disease and outcome assessment, including new imaging modalities, and patient management and rehabilitation, including new treatments for rheumatoid arthritis. In an effort to streamline the text even further, chapter contributors have provided their "top 50" references in the book only; the remaining references are found online, all with a link to PubMed. We have also continued to improve the index, in order to make it easier for the reader to find the material that she or he wants.

The fifth edition can be found entirely online at www.expertconsult.com. Besides fully searchable text, you will also find a complete library of easily downloadable electronic images, links to PubMed and key society web sites, and continuous content updates from two dedicated web editors.

The production of the fifth edition of *Rheumatology* has been a greatly enjoyable team effort. We would like to thank every one of the authors who have contributed to this or any previous edition of the book, as well as the excellent team at Elsevier. We look forward to bringing you a sixth edition of *Rheumatology* in another 4 years.

The Editors

CONTENTS

1

THE SCIENTIFIC BASIS OF RHEUMATIC DISEASE

Epidemiologic concepts and the classification of musculoskeletal conditions

Deborah P. M. Symmons

- Musculoskeletal epidemiology is concerned with the determinants and distribution of musculoskeletal conditions in different populations.
- Frequency of disease in a population can be expressed in terms of incidence (the number of new cases) and prevalence (the proportion of the population with the disease).
- Most rheumatic diseases are defined using sets of classification criteria.
- Classification criteria are powerful tools for identifying and distinguishing patients with a target disease from those without the condition.
- Rheumatic disease frequency and severity vary with age, gender, ethnic origin, and country.
- Differences in disease or outcome frequency can be explored to yield hypotheses about demographic, genetic, hormonal, environmental, and psychosocial risk factors for development or severity of disease.
- Such hypotheses are best tested in case-control or cohort studies that involve the use of a comparison group.

INTRODUCTION

Epidemiology is the clinical science that studies the distribution and determinants of disease in populations. It involves describing the frequency of diseases and their consequences (including morbidity and mortality) and understanding the risk factors for developing a disease or its complications. There are two basic types of epidemiologic study (Table 1.1).

- *Descriptive* epidemiology describes the number of people who develop the disease in a particular time period or who currently have the disease; what type of people are susceptible (in terms of, e.g., age, gender, or ethnic background); and where and when the disease occurs (geographic variations on a large or small scale, secular trends).[1] Put more succinctly, descriptive studies investigate the distribution of disease in relation to person, place, and time.
- *Analytical* epidemiology tests hypotheses of causation and involves using a comparison group (Fig. 1.1). By comparing the frequency of disease in people who have particular characteristics (such as exposure to certain drugs, pregnancy, or certain genotypes), or exposure characteristics in people with and without a particular disease or outcome, it is possible to identify risk factors for developing disease or attributes that affect outcome or disease severity. In cohort studies subjects are selected on the basis of their exposure status or being disease free and followed to see how many develop the disease. Cohort studies may be prospective, if the outcome has not occurred when the study begins, or retrospective, if the outcome has already happened. In case-control studies groups are selected on the basis of their disease status, those with the disease being the *cases* and those without being the *controls*.

All the subjects are then studied to see how many in each group have been exposed to the risk factor(s) of interest. Each design has its advantages and disadvantages, and the choice is often dictated by the relative prevalence of the disease and the exposure.[2]

This chapter introduces the fundamental concepts of epidemiology and describes how these have been used to study the frequency of musculoskeletal disorders and their burden worldwide. It also discusses how hypotheses concerning risk factors for developing rheumatic diseases or particular outcomes can be generated and tested.

DESCRIPTIVE EPIDEMIOLOGY—HOW MANY PEOPLE HAVE THE DISEASE?

The two most common measures of disease frequency are prevalence and incidence (Table 1.2).[1] Prevalence relates to existing cases of disease. The term *point* prevalence is used to describe the proportion of the population that has the disorder at a particular point in time (sometimes called *prevalence day*). This measure is useful for chronic persistent disorders such as rheumatoid arthritis (RA) and osteoarthritis (OA). For intermittent conditions such as back pain and gout, it is more appropriate to measure *period* prevalence—the proportion of the population that has the disorder at any time during a given time period (usually 1 year). The 1-year period prevalence of back pain includes all those who had back pain at the beginning of the year plus all those who develop back pain during the year regardless of how long any individual episode of back pain lasts. Finally, *cumulative* prevalence is the proportion of the population that has had, or that now has, the disorder up to a specified time point (e.g., by age 60 years) or up to the time of the study.

Prevalence

Prevalence in the population setting is commonly determined by a survey using questionnaires, clinical evaluation, or a combination of both. Such questionnaires may be self-completed or interviewer administered. In the hospital or primary care setting, prevalence is often assessed by identifying diagnosed cases and relating them to the appropriate population base. Although this may be a practical way of measuring prevalence for uncommon conditions,[3] the cases identified in this way are often skewed toward the more severe end of the clinical spectrum because mild cases may not be under current medical review.

Incidence

The term *prevalence* relates to existing disease, whereas the term *incidence* relates to new cases of disease. Investigators of disease etiology will want to know the number of individuals in a defined population who first develop the disorder in a given time period, typically 1 year. This figure is known as the incidence rate or, more accurately, the *first* incidence rate. However, planners and providers of health care services may be more interested in the total number of episodes of a disorder, which is known as the *episode* incidence, than in the number of individuals affected. The episode incidence of back pain would be expected to be higher than the first incidence rate because it includes

TABLE 1.1 QUESTIONS ADDRESSED BY EPIDEMIOLOGIC STUDIES

Question	Methodology
How many?	Descriptive epidemiology
Who?	
Where?	
When?	
Why?	Analytical epidemiology
How does it happen?	

TABLE 1.2 MEASURES OF DISEASE FREQUENCY

Term	Denominator	Numerator
Prevalence (relates to existing disease)	Number of people in the population	Point prevalence (number who have the disorder at a given time point) Period prevalence (number who have the disorder at some time during a given period) Cumulative prevalence (number who have the disorder at some time up to a given time point)
Incidence (relates to disease onset)	Total person-time of observation	First incidence (number who have their first onset of the disorder in a given time period) Episode incidence (number of episodes of the disorder in a given time period) Cumulative incidence (number who have their first onset up to a given time point)

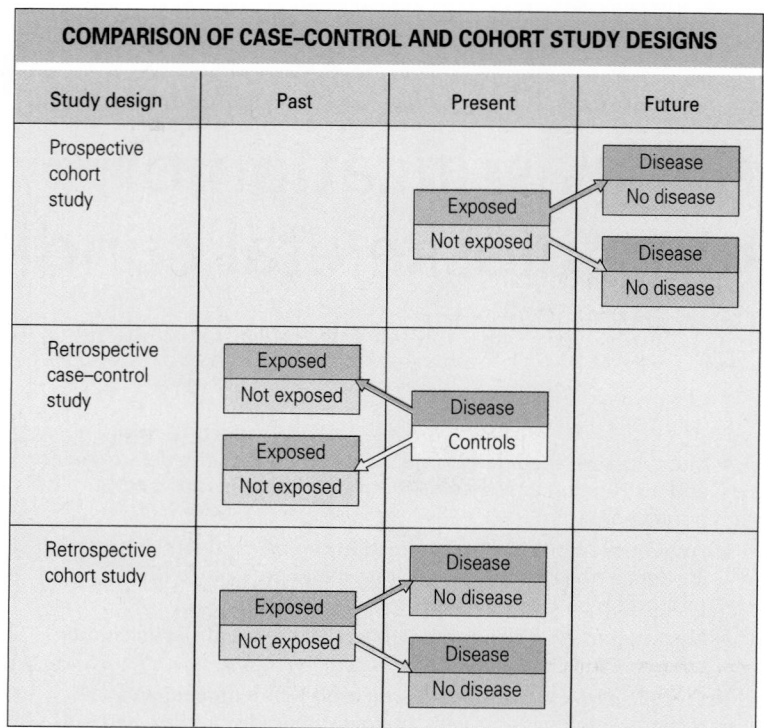

Fig. 1.1 Comparison of case-control and cohort study designs.

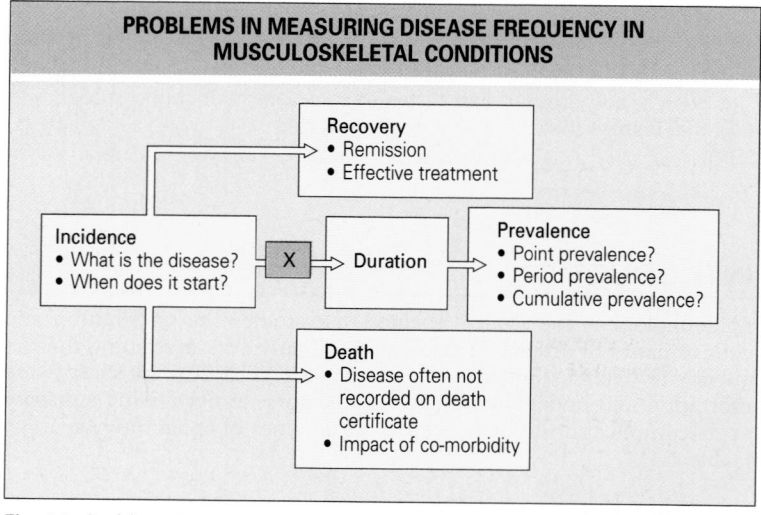

Fig. 1.2 Problems in measuring disease frequency in musculoskeletal conditions.

people who have second or subsequent episodes of back pain and counts more than once those who have repeated episodes during the time frame of interest. Those who are studying outcome may want to consider *cumulative* incidence up to a particular time. This measure can be used, for example, to compare the frequency of certain side effects in patients exposed to antirheumatic drugs.

Incidence is measured either by monitoring for new cases as they are diagnosed or by conducting two cross-sectional surveys some time apart and identifying new cases that have occurred between the two surveys.

Disease incidence and prevalence are related by the formula:

$$\text{Incidence} \times \text{duration} = \text{prevalence}$$

Individuals may leave the prevalent pool of cases through either recovery or death. The mean disease duration is determined by the average length of time to recovery or death. RA has a relatively low incidence but a long duration, so the prevalence is relatively high. The rate of death may be expressed as the mortality rate (the number of deaths from a disease in a given time period divided by the total population) or the case-fatality rate (the number of deaths from a disease in a given time period divided by the number of cases of the disease).

Practical issues in measuring disease frequency

Some of the issues related to measuring disease frequency are highlighted in Figure 1.2 and can be divided into issues related to the numerator and those related to the denominator.

Numerator

1. Case definition
Accurate estimation of incidence and prevalence depends on using a standard nomenclature, a reliable case definition, and complete case ascertainment. The nomenclature in most widespread use is that adopted by the International Classification of Diseases (ICD).[4] The ICD names diseases and groups them in a hierarchy on the basis of the body system. ICD10 is the version in current use.

Most rheumatic diseases do not have a specific diagnostic test, so sets of classification criteria (Table 1.3) have been developed to identify homogeneous patient populations for epidemiologic studies and clinical trials. These sets of classification criteria combine different types of information, including symptoms, signs, laboratory findings, imaging, genetic factors, and etiologic agents (e.g., infectious agents, drugs). Classification criteria have two purposes: first, to separate patients with the target disorder from normal subjects, and second, to distinguish patients with the target disorder from those with other similar disorders (e.g., distinguishing RA from psoriatic arthritis). In the majority of conditions, classification criteria should not be used for the diagnosis of the individual patient.

TABLE 1.3 CLASSIFICATION CRITERIA FOR RHEUMATIC DISEASES

Name of disease	Name of classification criteria	Reference
Ankylosing spondylitis	New York criteria Modified New York Criteria	Bennett et al, 1968[5] Van der Linden et al, 1984[6]
Antiphospholipid syndrome	Sapporo classification Revised Sapporo criteria	Wilson et al, 1999[7] Miyakis et al, 2006[8]
Behçet syndrome	Preliminary classification criteria for Behçet disease	International Study Group, 1992[9]
Benign joint hypermobility syndrome	Revised (Brighton 1998) criteria	Grahame et al, 2000[10]
Churg-Strauss syndrome	ACR 1990 criteria for CSS	Masi et al, 1990[11]
Dermato/polymyositis	Bohan and Peter criteria	Bohan et al, 1975[12] Tanimoto et al, 1995[13]
Fibromyalgia	ACR 1990 classification criteria for fibromyalgia	Wolfe et al, 1990[14]
Giant cell (temporal) arteritis	ACR 1990 criteria for GCA	Hunder et al, 1990[15]
Gout	Preliminary ARA criteria	Wallace et al, 1977[16]
Henoch-Schönlein purpura	ACR 1990 criteria for HSP	Mills et al, 1990[17]
Hypersensitivity vasculitis	ACR 1990 criteria for hypersensitivity vasculitis	Calabrese et al, 1990[18]
Juvenile idiopathic arthritis	ILAR classification criteria for JIA	Petty et al, 1998[19] Petty et al, 2004[20]
Kawasaki syndrome	EULAR/PReS criteria for childhood vasculitides	Ozen et al, 2006[21]
Osteoarthritis hand	ACR classification criteria for hand OA	Altman et al, 1990[22]
Osteoarthritis hip	ACR classification criteria for hip OA	Altman et al, 1991[23]
Osteoarthritis knee	ACR classification criteria for knee OA	Altman et al, 1986[24]
Polyarteritis nodosa	ACR 1990 criteria for PAN	Lightfoot et al, 1990[25]
Polymyalgia rheumatica	Bird/Wood criteria	Bird et al, 1979[26]
Psoriatic arthritis	Moll and Wright CASPAR criteria	Moll and Wright, 1973[27] Taylor et al, 2006[28]
Reiter's syndrome	Preliminary criteria for RS	Willkens et al, 1981[29]
Rheumatic fever	Jones criteria (updated)	American Heart Association, 1992[30]
Rheumatoid arthritis	1987 ACR classification criteria for RA	Arnett et al, 1988[31]
Scleroderma	ARA criteria	*Arthritis Rheum*, 1980[32]
Sjögren's syndrome	Revised European criteria	Vitali et al, 2002[33]
SLE	Revised ACR classification criteria for SLE	Tan et al, 1982[34] Hochberg, 1997[35]
Spondyloarthropathy	ESSG criteria	Dougados et al, 1991[36]
Takayasu arteritis	ACR 1990 criteria for TA	Arend et al, 1990[37]
Vasculitis	ACR 1990 criteria for vasculitis	Hunder et al, 1990[38]
ANCA-associated granulomatous vasculitis	ACR 1990 criteria for WG	Leavitt et al, 1990[39]

TABLE 1.4 SENSITIVITY, SPECIFICITY, POSITIVE AND NEGATIVE PREDICTIVE VALUES OF CRITERIA SETS

		Disease—by "gold" standard	
		Yes	No
	Positive	a (True positive)	b (False positive)
Criterion or criteria set	Negative	c (False negative)	d (True negative)
Sensitivity: the proportion of cases correctly identified		$\dfrac{a}{a+c}$	
Specificity: the proportion of non-cases correctly identified		$\dfrac{d}{b+d}$	
Positive predictive value: the proportion with a positive test who have the disease		$\dfrac{a}{a+b}$	
Negative predictive value: the proportion with a negative test who do not have the disease		$\dfrac{d}{c+d}$	

Historically, most sets of classification criteria in rheumatology were developed by consensus. A panel of experts would compile a list of candidate variables and then assess their ability, either alone or in combination, to distinguish subjects who were judged by their own physician to be cases from those judged to be non-cases (either normal subjects or subjects with similar conditions). The assessment was done by determining the sensitivity and specificity of the criteria (Table 1.4). In more recent times, statistical techniques such as receiver operating characteristic (ROC) curves, discriminant analysis, and logistic regression have been used to eliminate redundant variables and weight the individual characteristics to give maximum sensitivity and specificity. Classification and regression tree (CART) methodology enables the substitution of one variable for another (which helps when some data are missing) and enables attributes to be used more than once in different parts of the tree. In all these methods, the physician's opinion is the gold standard.

These methods assume that physicians (or rheumatologists) share a common construct of the disease in question. If there is no common construct, as perhaps is the issue in psoriatic arthritis, then it may prove impossible to develop criteria by consensus. Similarly, it must be remembered that physicians may share a construct that is wrong. Just because it is possible to develop a set of classification criteria, it does not mean that the disorder so defined, such as fibromyalgia, is a pathologic entity.

There are many problems in interpreting and applying classification criteria. The construction of nearly all the classification criteria sets is such that early or mild cases may not meet the criteria. In addition, some criteria sets require expensive, invasive, or non-standard investigations such as radiography or immunochemical tests, which are not routinely obtained or are not suitable for use in a population setting. This makes it difficult to apply the criteria retrospectively using patients' medical records or to use them unaltered in population surveys.

In inflammatory conditions such as RA or systemic lupus erythematosus (SLE), the criteria were developed using patients with active disease. A population survey of RA prevalence will therefore identify those individuals who currently have active disease plus those people who in the past have had disease that was sufficiently severe to leave stigmata such as joint deformities. People who had mild disease that is now in natural or drug-induced remission will not be detected. Thus the resultant estimate is a cross between point prevalence and cumulative prevalence.

Finally, when conducting population surveys, it is important to recognize that although prevalence does not affect the sensitivity and specificity of classification criteria, it does affect their positive predictive value (see Table 1.4). So in the example given in Table 1.5, the proportion of positives that are false positives is 2% in the clinic setting and 66% in the population setting.

TABLE 1.5 INFLUENCE OF PREVALENCE ON POSITIVE PREDICTIVE VALUE

		Clinic setting			Population setting		
		Prevalence of target disease—50%			Prevalence of target disease—1%		
		Gold standard			Gold standard		
		Yes	No		Yes	No	
Criteria	Positive	490	10	500	98	188	286
	Negative	10	490	500	2	9702	9704
		500	500		100	9900	
		Positive predictive value—98%			Positive predictive value—34%		
		% false positives—2%			% false positives—66%		

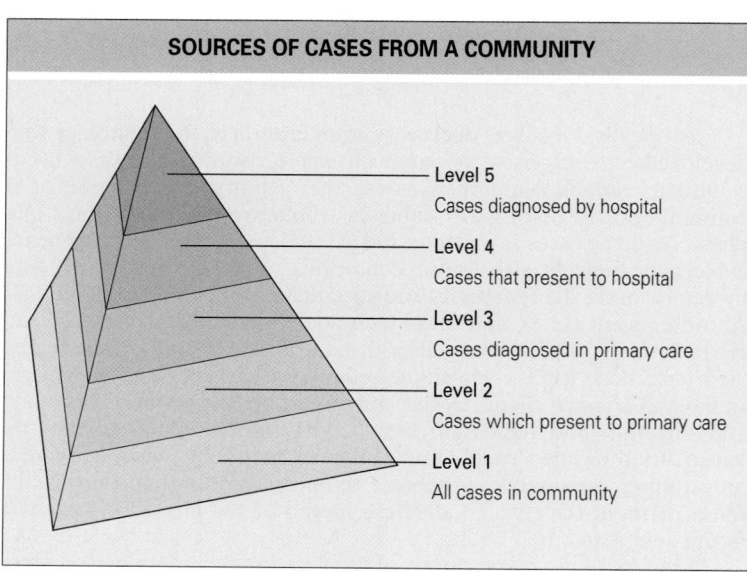

SOURCES OF CASES FROM A COMMUNITY

Level 5
Cases diagnosed by hospital

Level 4
Cases that present to hospital

Level 3
Cases diagnosed in primary care

Level 2
Cases which present to primary care

Level 1
All cases in community

Fig. 1.3 Sources of cases from a community.

2. Determining the *onset date*

Determining the time of disease onset is problematic for some rheumatic diseases. If OA is defined in terms of radiologic change, it is usually impossible to say when this first appeared. The classification criteria for SLE require an individual to satisfy 4 of 11 criteria,[34,35] which may be accumulated over several years. The disease is diagnosed on the day the fourth criterion is met and yet the onset presumably occurred on or before the day that the first feature appeared. It is therefore important to define precisely how the time of onset was determined and to recognize the consequences of this definition when interpreting studies.

3. Completeness of ascertainment

Finally, all cases of the disease within the population should be identified. Disease in the population has a continuum of severity (Fig. 1.3) and ascertainment may not be complete, depending on where it is carried out. Clinic-based studies rely on the patient having sought medical care, being (more or less) correctly diagnosed, and being referred to the appropriate specialist. With severe life-threatening diseases one might reasonably assume that all cases are referred, but this is not the situation with most rheumatic diseases. To overcome this problem, several approaches may be used simultaneously (e.g., ascertaining SLE cases from hospital clinics, self-help groups, and laboratory records of antinuclear antibody results) to try to capture all those with the disorder concerned. Studies that use different case definitions or methods of case ascertainment will not yield comparable results. For example, a study of the prevalence of knee OA that begins by screening

the population by radiography and then evaluates those with abnormal radiographs will not yield the same number of cases as one that screens the population for knee symptoms and then radiographs those who are symptomatic.

Denominator

To calculate rates it is necessary to know the size of the population from which the cases have been identified. This is difficult when cases are identified only from hospital or clinic attenders because many medical facilities do not have defined catchment populations. Many factors determine whether an individual case is referred to a particular center (referral bias). The denominator population should comprise only those individuals at risk of developing the disease. Thus the incidence of juvenile idiopathic arthritis should be expressed per 100,000 children aged 16 and younger, not per 100,000 of the total population.

Sources of data for estimating disease occurrence

Routinely collected data may prove useful in building up a picture of the epidemiology of a musculoskeletal condition. Researchers using routinely collected data need to assess the diagnostic accuracy and level of completeness of these data. Some examples are listed as follows:

1. Death certificates

Mortality records have, with a few exceptions, been of little use in rheumatic disease epidemiology because rheumatologic disorders are an infrequent cause of death and also are often not recorded on the death certificate. Therefore, it is not possible to tell, for example, how many people with RA die each year in a particular country. However, if a cohort of RA patients has already been identified, death certificates will provide valuable information on the number of the cohorts who have died and their attributed causes of death. Because most countries code the cause of death using the ICD, it is possible to make comparisons of the attributed causes of death among RA cohorts in different locations and among RA cohorts and the general populations from which they were drawn.

2. Morbidity registers

Although many countries have cancer registers, the same is not true for the rheumatic diseases. Some Scandinavian countries have registers of people who are disabled or who can claim reimbursable medication and, using a unique personal identity number, investigators are able to link information on these registers with, for example, mortality data. The Mayo Clinic in Rochester, Minnesota, has developed a record linkage system whereby the health care records of all residents in Olmsted County are maintained on a central database. Information from this database, which dates back to 1910, has been used to generate incidence estimates of a number of rheumatic diseases. However, the population of Olmsted County is only about 100,000 and the majority of the population is of Scandinavian descent. The former limits the reliability of estimates for rare diseases and the latter the generalizability of all estimates because the residents of Olmsted County are not representative of the general U.S. population.

3. Health care provider databases

In some countries, health care that is reimbursed by the government or insurance companies is linked to diagnostic codes on large computerized databases. These have provided a rich source of data on the frequency of rare events such as drug toxicity or major complications of orthopedic surgery. They enable the identification of individuals for detailed study. Examples include the data on Medicare patients in the United States or those enrolled in health maintenance organizations such as Kaiser Permanente or Canadians covered by their national health care system. In the United Kingdom, during the 10-yearly census years, a large group of primary care physicians coded the reason for every patient consultation and whether it was the first consultation for the particular diagnosis. These Royal College of General Practitioners (RCGP) morbidity surveys provided unique national primary care–based data on the incidence and prevalence of musculoskeletal diseases. Unfortunately, the last of these surveys was conducted in 1991. U.K. primary care–based data now come from computerized databases such as the General Practice Research Database (GPRD) (www.gprd.com) and The Health Improvement Network (THIN) (www.thin-uk.com) that comprise the pooled anonymized patient data from a large number of GP practices. In all these situations, information about the denominator—the number of people covered by the registers—is known, but standard disease definitions are usually not used.

4. Work absenteeism records

In some countries information on the reason for, and duration of, absence from work for sickness is recorded and can be used to examine the profile of musculoskeletal complaints in the workforce.

5. Population health surveys

In many countries there are regular population surveys (called *health interview surveys* [HIS]) that examine social and demographic trends. These may include health-related information such as number of visits to a physician, self-reported illness, and disability. Examples include the General Household Survey in the United Kingdom. Sometimes an examination phase is included (a health examination survey [HES]). Examples include the National Health and Nutrition Examination Surveys in the United States (www.cdc.gov/nchs/nhanes.htm). There is a move to try to standardize the questions used in HIS across countries to facilitate comparisons.

ANALYTICAL EPIDEMIOLOGY—WHO IS SUSCEPTIBLE TO THE DISEASE?

Differences in disease occurrence arising from descriptive epidemiology provide useful starting points for the investigation of disease causation. Striking differences in age- and sex-specific incidence and prevalence rates are seen in many rheumatic diseases. For example, the annual incidence of RA is twice as high in females as in males[40] and the onset of ankylosing spondylitis is rare after the age of 55 years.[41] Apparent differences in overall or crude (i.e., all ages and sexes combined) incidence and prevalence between populations may simply reflect differences in the proportions of men and women or in the age structures of the populations. It is therefore important, whenever possible, to see epidemiologic data broken down into age- (e.g., 10-year age bands) and sex-specific groups before making inferences. It is then possible to apply the age- and sex-specific incidence rates from one population (the *standard*) to the age/sex distribution of another population (the *index*) in order to calculate an overall rate in the latter, assuming that the age and gender distributions are identical. Frequently, the standard population is based on national data.

Differences in disease frequency or adverse outcomes may also be found among ethnic groups (e.g., SLE is more common in people of African ancestry than in Caucasians)[42]; occupations (e.g., hip OA is more common in farmers)[43]; and social classes (e.g., back pain is more common in lower socioeconomic groups).[44] It can be difficult, however, to determine the relative contributions of race, occupation, and

TABLE 1.6 VARIATIONS IN RHEUMATIC DISEASE FREQUENCY COMPARED WITH EUROPEAN WHITES

	Increased frequency	Decreased frequency
Rheumatoid arthritis	Native American (Pima, Chippewa, Yakima)	Rural African Chinese Indonesian
Juvenile idiopathic arthritis	Canadian Inuit	African-Americans
Ankylosing spondylitis	Haida people	Australian aboriginals
Gout	Polynesians Filipinos	Africans
Systemic lupus erythematosus	African-Americans Afro-Caribbeans Asian Indians Chinese	West Africans
Scleroderma	Southern United States	Australian aboriginals
Polymyalgia rheumatica	Northern European Caucasians	African-Americans
Osteoarthritis of the knee	African-American women	
Osteoarthritis of the hip		Chinese Asian Indians Africans
Osteoporosis	Northern Europeans	Africans

socioeconomic factors to disease etiology because these factors are often interrelated.

WHERE DOES THE DISEASE OCCUR?

Differences in disease rates between countries or regions may be due to genetic, other host-related, and/or environmental factors. Possible environmental factors include macro-environmental variables such as air and water and microenvironmental factors such as diet and socioeconomic factors. Migration studies may suggest whether geographic differences in disease frequency are predominantly due to genetic or environmental factors. If a migrating people have the same frequency of disease in their native and newly adopted countries, this suggests that genetic factors are more important. If the disease frequency changes, especially if it changes within one or two generations, this suggests a change in environment or lifestyle as being important. There are hints of geographic patterns for a number of rheumatic diseases, which are still being unraveled (Table 1.6).

First, RA occurs with similar frequency in most Caucasian populations. However, it has a higher prevalence among some native American peoples such as the Pima and a lower prevalence in West Africa, China, and Indonesia.[45]

Second, most of the geographic variation in the frequency of ankylosing spondylitis can be explained by the varying prevalence of HLA-B27 in different racial groups. By contrast the issue is more complex in explaining the ethnic variation in SLE, although investigation of the frequency and clinical characteristics of SLE in people of African origin can yield important etiologic clues. There is a high frequency of SLE in African-Americans and African Caribbeans but a lower frequency in West Africa.[42] Although this suggests an environmental cause for SLE, it is possible that genetic admixture[46] may play a part in the changing incidence of SLE in this group of people.

WHEN DOES THE DISEASE OCCUR?

Time trends in disease occurrence may also provide important etiologic clues. Clusters of incident cases in a particular season of the year or sporadic time/space clusters suggest that all or most of the cases in the cluster may have been exposed to an etiologic agent from a common source. In rheumatology, Lyme disease provides a good example of a disease identified because of clustering of cases of juvenile and adult inflammatory arthritis in place and time.[47] A rise or fall in disease

TABLE 1.7 ADVANTAGES AND DISADVANTAGES OF VARIOUS EPIDEMIOLOGIC STUDY DESIGNS

Study design	Advantages	Disadvantages
Prospective cohort	Good exposure data Accurate timing of exposure and disease onset Little recall bias	Expensive May be long delay before disease onset Large numbers needed Only suitable for frequent outcomes
Case-control	Relatively inexpensive Quick to perform Useful for rare diseases	Subject to recall bias Cases may not be representative Controls difficult to select and ascertain Exposure data may be unreliable Time of exposure and disease onset may be imprecise
Descriptive prevalence study	Generalizable Quick to perform	Difficult to distinguish cause and effect Biased toward inclusion of chronic cases

TABLE 1.8 ASSESSING CAUSALITY BETWEEN A RISK FACTOR AND A DISEASE OR OUTCOME

An association between an exposure and an outcome may be due to:
- direct causation
- chance
- bias
- confounding

Causality is more likely if:
- exposure precedes the outcome of interest
- association is biologically plausible
- association is strong (high relative risk)
- association is consistent between studies
- association is supported by experimental evidence

incidence year-on-year may suggest a change in the level of exposure to risk factors. Between around 1970 and 1985 there was a marked fall in the incidence of RA in women in the United States and the United Kingdom. This coincided with the increasing use of the oral contraceptive pill and there is evidence to suggest that the two phenomena are linked.[48] Changes in disease prevalence with time are more difficult to interpret because they may be caused by alterations in disease incidence, recovery rates, or survival—or a combination of all three. When considering future health service provision, health care planners must take into account trends in incidence and prevalence, both of which may be affected by increasing life expectancy. For instance, the number of new cases of hip and knee OA in most Western countries is rising steeply. This is due more to the aging population than to any change in age-specific incidence rates of OA.

WHY DOES THE DISEASE OCCUR?

Descriptive epidemiologic studies can generate hypotheses about disease causation but they cannot test those hypotheses. Analytical studies are required to investigate the relationship between exposure to a risk factor (which might be environmental or genetic) and the development of disease. As discussed earlier, such studies may be retrospective or prospective (see Fig. 1.1). In a prospective study the individuals are identified and classified according to their exposure status prior to the development of disease. However, it is sometimes possible to assemble such cohorts retrospectively after the development of disease. For example, it may be possible to identify all men who had an occupational exposure to vinyl chloride over the past 5 years or all children who were immunized with a particular batch of mumps, measles, and rubella vaccine.

A cohort study is more efficient when investigating a rare exposure, whereas a case-control design is more efficient when investigating a rare disease (Table 1.7). The case-control study is best for investigating multiple risk factors simultaneously. Although either incident or prevalent cases can be used for a case-control study, incident cases are usually preferred because it is then clear that any risk factors identified are markers for disease susceptibility rather than chronicity. For example, clinic attenders with RA have a much higher frequency of the *shared epitope* than the general population. Furthermore, combinations of shared epitope alleles (e.g., 0404 homozygosity) are associated with a particularly poor outcome from RA.[49] However, in studies that were confined to incident cases of RA, the association with the shared epitope is only modest.

The most difficult aspect of a case-control study is the selection of appropriate controls. Controls should be individuals who, if they had developed the disease, would have been included among the cases. Thus the cases and controls should be selected from the same catchment population.

The results in longitudinal studies are usually expressed as a relative risk or risk ratio (i.e., the risk [or incidence] of the disease in the exposed cohort [a/a+b] divided by the risk of disease in the unexposed cohort [c/c+d; see Table 1.4]). In a case-control study, however, the relative frequency of risk factors is compared between the cases and controls and so, in this situation, the odds ratio is calculated (i.e., the odds of exposure given disease [a : c] divided by the odds of exposure given no disease [b : d]. The relative risk or odds ratio indicates the strength of the association between the risk factor and the disease. In a case-control study causality cannot be assumed because information about disease state and exposure status is collected cross-sectionally or retrospectively. It is therefore impossible to be certain which came first. In a longitudinal study, the higher the relative risk, the more likely the exposure and the outcome are to be linked in a causal chain. Table 1.8 shows the other factors that should be considered when examining causality.

CLINICAL EPIDEMIOLOGY—WHAT HAPPENS TO PEOPLE WITH THE DISEASE?

The investigation of prognosis is analogous to investigating the development of disease and can be assessed with either cohort or case-control studies. In prognosis studies, all the individuals studied have the disease in question. In longitudinal studies patients are selected on the basis of exposure to a predictor variable (e.g., being HLA-DR4 positive in RA or being overweight in OA) and then followed for the incidence, in those with and without the predictor, of the outcome of interest (e.g., death or the development of disability). Longitudinal observational studies may be subject to right or left censorship.

- Left censorship, a bias in recruitment, occurs when, for example, subjects are recruited as consecutive prevalent cases from a hospital clinic. Patients with mild disease who have been discharged from follow-up and those who have severe disease and have died will be underrepresented in the cohort.
- Right censorship, a bias in follow-up, occurs, for example, in a follow-up study when subjects have been lost to follow-up.

In a case-control study of outcome, patients are selected on the basis of whether or not they have developed a particular complication of their disease (e.g., vasculitis in RA or vertebral fracture in osteoporosis) and then compared with patients without this outcome for predictors such as corticosteroid use.

A summary of some of the etiologic, protective, and prognostic factors for selected rheumatic diseases is shown in Table 1.9. The evidence for some of these factors is more definitive than others, and further study is required.

APPLICATIONS OF EPIDEMIOLOGIC DATA

Determining attributable risk and population attributable risk fraction

The size of the relative risk indicates the strength of association between an exposure and outcome but does not indicate the relative

TABLE 1.9 SOME ETIOLOGIC, PROTECTIVE, AND PROGNOSTIC FACTORS IN RHEUMATIC DISEASE

Condition	Etiologic factors	Protective factors	Risk factors for a poor prognosis
Rheumatoid arthritis	Smoking Breastfeeding Female gender HLA-DR4 PTPN22	Oral contraceptive use High fruit intake	Rheumatoid factor Anti-CCP antibodies HLA-DR4
Ankylosing spondylitis	HLA-B27 Male gender		
Gout	Hyperuricemia Thiazide diuretics Lead exposure		
Systemic lupus erythematosus	Complement deficiency African origin Some drugs (e.g., hydralazine) Female gender		Lower socioeconomic status
Scleroderma	Silica exposure Organic solvents Some drugs (e.g., bleomycin) Female gender		
Osteoarthritis of the knee	Obesity Certain occupations	Smoking	Obesity
Osteoarthritis of the hip	Childhood hip disease (e.g., Perthes) Certain occupations (e.g., farming) Hip dysplasia		
Back pain	Obesity Certain occupations Driving		Previous back pain Psychological factors
Osteoporosis	Early menopause Low body mass index Smoking Corticosteroid use	Obesity African origin Exercise	Falls

importance of the exposure in accounting, for example, for the prevalence of the disease in the population. Patients with Sjögren's syndrome have a relative risk of 44 of developing non-Hodgkin's lymphoma compared with the general population.[50] However, non-Hodgkin's lymphoma is a rare disease in the general population and even when the incidence is increased 44-fold, the actual occurrence is still uncommon. Thus despite this high relative risk, few patients with Sjögren's syndrome develop non-Hodgkin's lymphoma.

From a public health perspective, two other measures are more important: attributable risk and the population attributable risk.

- The attributable risk, which is the difference between the risk of the outcome in the exposed and in the unexposed, gives an estimate of the number of cases among an exposed population that can be attributed to the exposure.

  Example, individuals taking non-selective non-steroidal anti-inflammatory drugs (NSAIDs) have a relative risk of 4 of having a gastrointestinal (GI) bleed or perforation compared with those not taking NSAIDs[51] (i.e., they are four times more likely to have a serious upper GI complication than the general population). However, GI bleeds do occur in those not taking NSAIDs and some of the observed bleeds in NSAID users might have occurred by chance. It is estimated that NSAIDs have an attributable risk of 13/1000 per year for admission to hospital with a GI problem in patients with RA.[52] That is, for every 1000 RA patients who take an NSAID for a year, 13 more will be admitted to the hospital each year for a GI problem than in a comparable group of RA patients not taking NSAIDs.
- The population attributable risk fraction is the proportion of cases of the disease in the population that can be attributed to the risk factor. An example is found in the association between NSAID ingestion and GI bleeding and ulceration. Thus using the earlier example, given data on the population frequency of NSAID use,

it is possible to calculate the proportion of GI problems in a whole population attributable to NSAID use.

Measuring the burden of illness

Information on the age- and sex-specific incidence and prevalence of musculoskeletal conditions can be used to estimate the total number of cases of musculoskeletal illness in a community in which the age and sex structure is known. Measuring the burden of illness within the community also requires information on premature mortality and on the impact of the specific conditions on quality of life.

Planning rheumatology health care services

The ability of a population to benefit from rheumatology health care depends on three things:

1. The incidence and prevalence of musculoskeletal disorders in that community
2. The effectiveness of the regimens available to treat or prevent musculoskeletal disorders
3. The proportion of those affected or potentially affected who might benefit from such interventions

The first step in planning rheumatology services is to compile a profile of the community's musculoskeletal health. Ideally, this would involve conducting a detailed interview with each resident. A reasonable substitute is to perform a survey using a stratified sample of the population. However, even when this is done, it is not possible to cover every aspect of musculoskeletal health in a single survey. Therefore, a picture of the community's burden of illness has to be built up piecemeal using all available sources of data, including published incidence and prevalence data, allowing for modifiers such as socioeconomic group, ethnicity, and cultural factors that may affect the applicability of external data.

KEY REFERENCES

1. Hennekens CH, Buring JE, Mayrent SL. Measures of disease frequency and association. In: Epidemiology in medicine. Boston: Little Brown, 1987: 54-98.
2. Silman AJ, Macfarlane GJ. Epidemiological studies: a practical guide, 2nd ed. Cambridge, Mass: Cambridge University Press; 2002.
3. Safavi KH, Heyse SP, Hochberg MC: Estimating the incidence and prevalence of rare rheumatologic diseases: a review of methodology and available data sources. J Rheumatol 1990;17:990-993.
4. World Health Organization. International statistical classification of diseases and related health problems, 10th revised ed. Geneva: WHO, 1992.
5. Bennett PH, Burch TA. The epidemiological diagnosis of ankylosing spondylitis. In: Bennett PH, Wood PHN, eds. Population studies of the rheumatic diseases. Amsterdam: Excerpta Medica, 1968: 305-313.
6. van der Linden S, Valkenburg HA, Cats A. Evaluation of diagnostic criteria for ankylosing spondylitis. A proposal for modification of the New York criteria. Arthritis Rheum 1984;27:361-368.
7. Wilson WA, Gharavi AE, Koike T, et al: International consensus statement on preliminary classification criteria for definite antiphospholipid syndrome: report of an international workshop. Arthritis Rheum 1999;42:1309-1311.
8. Miyakis S, Lockshin MD, Atsumi T, et al. International consensus statement on an update of the classification criteria for definite antiphospholipid syndrome (APS). J Thromb Haemost 2006;4:295-306.
9. International Study Group for Behcet's Disease, Evaluation of diagnostic ("classification") criteria in Behcet's disease—towards internationally agreed criteria. The International Study Group for Behcet's disease. Br J Rheumatol 1992;31:299-308.
10. Grahame R, Bird HA, Child A. The revised (Brighton 1998) criteria for the diagnosis of benign joint hypermobility syndrome (BJHS). J Rheumatol 2000;27:1777-1779.
11. Masi AT, Hunder GG, Lie JT, et al. The American College of Rheumatology 1990 criteria for the classification of Churg-Strauss syndrome (allergic granulomatosis and angiitis). Arthritis Rheum 1990;33:1094-1100.
12. Bohan A, Peter JB. Polymyositis and dermatomyositis (first of two parts). N Engl J Med 1975;292:344-347.
13. Tanimoto K, Nakano K, Kano S, et al. Classification criteria for polymyositis and dermatomyositis. J Rheumatol 1995;22:668-674.
14. Wolfe F, Smythe HA, Yunus MB, et al. The American College of Rheumatology 1990 Criteria for the Classification of Fibromyalgia. Report of the Multicenter Criteria Committee. Arthritis Rheum 1990;33:160-172.
15. Hunder GG, Bloch DA, Michel BA, et al. The American College of Rheumatology 1990 criteria for the classification of giant cell arteritis. Arthritis Rheum 1990;33:1122-1128.
16. Wallace SL, Robinson H, Masi AT, et al. Preliminary criteria for the classification of the acute arthritis of primary gout. Arthritis Rheum 1977;20:895-900.
17. Mills JA, Michel BA, Bloch DA, et al. The American College of Rheumatology 1990 criteria for the classification of Henoch-Schönlein purpura. Arthritis Rheum 1990;33:1114-1121.
18. Calabrese LH, Michel BA, Bloch DA, et al. The American College of Rheumatology 1990 criteria for the classification of hypersensitivity vasculitis. Arthritis Rheum 1990;33:1108-1113.
19. Petty RE, Southwood TR, Baum J, et al. Revision of the proposed classification criteria for juvenile idiopathic arthritis: Durban, 1997. J Rheumatol 1998;25:1991-1994.
20. Petty RE, Southwood TR, Manners P, et al. International League of Associations for Rheumatology classification of juvenile idiopathic arthritis: second revision, Edmonton, 2001. J Rheumatol 2004;31:390-392.
21. Ozen S, Ruperto N, Dillon MJ, et al. EULAR/PReS endorsed consensus criteria for the classification of childhood vasculitides. Ann Rheum Dis 2006;65:936-941.
22. Altman R, Alarcon G, Appelrouth D, et al. The American College of Rheumatology criteria for the classification and reporting of osteoarthritis of the hand. Arthritis Rheum 1990;33:1601-1610.
23. Altman R, Alarcon G, Appelrouth D, et al. The American College of Rheumatology criteria for the classification and reporting of osteoarthritis of the hip. Arthritis Rheum 1991;34:505-514.
24. Altman R, Asch E, Bloch D, et al. Development of criteria for the classification and reporting of osteoarthritis. Classification of osteoarthritis of the knee. Diagnostic and Therapeutic Criteria Committee of the American Rheumatism Association. Arthritis Rheum 1986;29:1039-1049.
25. Lightfoot RW Jr, Michel BA, Bloch DA, et al. The American College of Rheumatology 1990 criteria for the classification of polyarteritis nodosa. Arthritis Rheum 1990;33:1088-1093.
26. Bird HA, Esselinckx W, Dixon AS, et al. An evaluation of criteria for polymyalgia rheumatica. Ann Rheum Dis 1979;38:434-439.
27. Moll JM, Wright V. Psoriatic arthritis. Semin Arthritis Rheum 1973;3:55-78.
28. Taylor W, Gladman D, Helliwell P, et al. Classification criteria for psoriatic arthritis: development of new criteria from a large international study. Arthritis Rheum 2006;54:2665-2673.
29. Willkens RF, Arnett FC, Bitter T, et al. Reiter's syndrome. Evaluation of preliminary criteria for definite disease. Arthritis Rheum 1981;24:844-849.
30. Special Writing Group of the Committee on Rheumatic Fever, Endocarditis, and Kawasaki Disease of the Council on Cardiovascular Disease in the Young of the American Heart Association. Guidelines for the diagnosis of rheumatic fever. Jones Criteria, 1992 update. JAMA 1992;268:2069-2073.
31. Arnett FC, Edworthy SM, Bloch DA, et al. The American Rheumatism Association 1987 revised criteria for the classification of rheumatoid arthritis. Arthritis Rheum 1988;31:315-324.
32. Subcommittee for scleroderma criteria of the American Rheumatism Association Diagnostic and Therapeutic Criteria Committee. Preliminary criteria for the classification of systemic sclerosis (scleroderma). Arthritis Rheum 1980;23:581-590.
33. Vitali C, Bombardieri S, Jonsson R, et al. Classification criteria for Sjögren's syndrome: a revised version of the European criteria proposed by the American-European Consensus Group. Ann Rheum Dis 2002;61:554-558.
34. Tan EM, Cohen AS, Fries JF, et al. The 1982 revised criteria for the classification of systemic lupus erythematosus. Arthritis Rheum 1982;25:1271-1277.
35. Hochberg MC. Updating the American College of Rheumatology revised criteria for the classification of systemic lupus erythematosus. Arthritis Rheum 1997;40:1725.
36. Dougados M, van der Linden S, Juhlin R, et al. The European Spondylarthropathy Study Group preliminary criteria for the classification of spondylarthropathy. Arthritis Rheum 1991;34:1218-1227.
37. Arend WP, Michel BA, Bloch DA, et al. The American College of Rheumatology 1990 criteria for the classification of Takayasu arteritis. Arthritis Rheum 1990;33:1129-1134.
38. Hunder GG, Arend WP, Bloch DA, et al. The American College of Rheumatology 1990 criteria for the classification of vasculitis. Introduction. Arthritis Rheum 1990;33:1065-1067.
39. Leavitt RY, Fauci AS, Bloch DA, et al. The American College of Rheumatology 1990 criteria for the classification of Wegener's granulomatosis. Arthritis Rheum 1990;33:1101-1107.
40. Gabriel SE, Crowson CS, O'Fallon WM. The epidemiology of rheumatoid arthritis in Rochester, Minnesota, 1955-1985. Arthritis Rheum 1999;42:415-420.
41. Carbone LD, Cooper C, Michet CJ, et al. Ankylosing spondylitis in Rochester, Minnesota, 1935-1989. Is the epidemiology changing? Arthritis Rheum 1992;35:1476-1482.
42. Bae SC, Fraser P, Liang MH. The epidemiology of systemic lupus erythematosus in populations of African ancestry: a critical review of the "prevalence gradient hypothesis." Arthritis Rheum 1998;41:2091-2099.
43. Croft P, Coggon D, Cruddas M, Cooper C. Osteoarthritis of the hip: an occupational disease in farmers. BMJ 1992;304:1269-1272.
44. Mason V. The prevalence of back pain in Great Britain. London: HMSO, 1994.
45. Silman AJ, Hochberg M. Rheumatoid arthritis. In: Epidemiology of the rheumatic diseases. Oxford: Oxford University Press, 2001: 31-71.
46. Rhodes B, Vyse TJ. Systemic lupus erythematosus genetics: what's new? Future Rheumatol 2008;3:103-107.
47. Steere AC, Malawista SE, Snydman DR, et al. Lyme arthritis: an epidemic of oligoarticular arthritis in children and adults in three Connecticut communities. Arthritis Rheum 1977;20:7-17.
48. Spector TD, Hochberg MC. The protective effect of the oral contraceptive pill on rheumatoid arthritis: an overview of the analytic epidemiological studies using meta-analysis. J Clin Epidemiol 1990;43:1221-1230.
49. Symmons D, Harrison B. Early inflammatory polyarthritis: results from the Norfolk Arthritis Register with a review of the literature. I. Risk factors for the development of inflammatory polyarthritis and rheumatoid arthritis. Rheumatology (Oxford) 2000;39:835-843.
50. Kassan SS, Thomas TL, Moutsopoulos HM, et al. Increased risk of lymphoma in sicca syndrome. Ann Intern Med 1978;89:888-892.

REFERENCES

Full references for this chapter can be found on www.expertconsult.com.

Principles of clinical outcome assessment

2

Nicholas Bellamy

- Measurements of pain and other key symptoms, impairment, ability/disability, participation/handicap, patient and physician global assessments, disease activity, and adverse consequences of treatment are all commonly used.

- Outcome measures must be ethical, valid, reliable, and responsive and should be brief, simple, and easy to score, particularly for use in routine clinical care.

- The choice of outcome measures depends on disease state, the response repertoire of the intervention(s) exhibited, and whether for research or routine practice.

- Core sets of outcome measures have been recommended for use in clinical trials for several rheumatic diseases.

INTRODUCTION

Outcome, endpoint, and *health status assessment, measurement,* and *evaluation* are terms that are often used interchangeably.[1] They characterize measurement procedures used to acquire information, which are used to describe, predict, or evaluate. Measurement forms an essential component of health care at all levels, from the treatment of individual patients to policy development. The focus of this chapter is on evaluating clinical health status in individual patients and groups of patients, that is, aspects of the condition that can be appreciated through questioning and clinical examination and that are not dependent on imaging or laboratory determination or ancillary testing. In addition to evaluating individuals and groups of patients, clinical outcome measures find important applications in making formal assessments of the impact of health care decisions on health care costs, quality of care, quality of life, and burden of disease, as measured by morbidity and mortality in the population. Such assessments are an integral part of health care delivery systems.

CLINICAL OUTCOME ASSESSMENT: A CONCEPTUAL FRAMEWORK

The sequence of most chronic diseases is that an etiologic event triggers a pathologic response, resulting in a number of clinical manifestations and outcomes. Clinical outcome measures examine the clinical consequences of a disease, in terms of mortality (survivorship) and morbidity (symptom severity, impact of the condition on various aspects of health-related quality of life [HRQOL], negative consequences of treatment). In painful musculoskeletal conditions the impact on function is particularly important. These concepts were characterized more than 20 years ago by Fries in the paradigm of the "5Ds"—death, disability, discomfort, drug (or other iatrogenic) reactions, and dollar (or economic) costs.[2] The aforementioned outcomes are relevant to all patients, because they are discernible at the individual patient level, represent the key consequences of disease and its treatment, and are the ultimate outcomes of the disease process. The components of health and the consequences of arthritis and musculoskeletal conditions are many and diverse, and it is possible to measure multiple aspects of a patient's condition.[1] Given the diversity of measurement situations, the evaluation procedures selected should be compatible with specific clinical conditions, assessment objectives, and measurement environments.

It is important to appreciate that in the discipline of clinical measurement (syn: clinical metrology) there is variable use of common terminology. Thus, the terms *instrument* and *tool* can refer not only to electromechanical devices but also to questionnaires and other assessment techniques. The questionnaires, in turn, are variably referred to as health status questionnaires (HSQs), health status measures (HSMs), or health status instruments (HSIs). The terms *subjective* (soft) and *objective* (hard) are best avoided, and instead the measurement technique should be referred to according to its measurement characteristics (e.g., type of measure, purpose of measurement, reliability, validity, responsiveness).

Outcome measures may be divided into two broad categories: observer dependent (or assessor-rated) and observer independent (or self-rated). In general, observer-independent clinical measures are based on self-administered questionnaires, whereas observer-dependent clinical measures include interviewer-scored questionnaires, physical examination findings, and tests of performance rated on technical instruments (e.g., grip strength, walk time). Certain techniques, such as face-to-face interview, walk time, grip strength, and articular index, involve an interaction between the assessor and the patient and are not easily classified as either purely subjective or objective.[3]

FUNDAMENTAL PRINCIPLES OF CLINICAL OUTCOME ASSESSMENT

Outcome measurement procedures should fulfill four major criteria[1] that are similar to those proposed by the Outcome Measures in Rheumatology Clinical Trials (OMERACT) group as the OMERACT filter.[4]

Ethics

The measurement process must be ethical.[1] Processes that are potentially hazardous to patients raise ethical issues that must be explained to, and accepted by, patients and study participants. When possible, less invasive procedures should be employed. Furthermore, the importance and necessity of acquiring new information should be weighed against any attendant risks.

Validity

Validity is a measure of the extent to which an instrument specifically measures the phenomenon of interest.[1] In contrast, reliability defines the extent to which the measurement procedure yields the same result on repeated determinations. Validity and reliability are separate clinimetric issues, and it does not follow that because a measure is reliable it is also valid or vice versa (Fig. 2.1). More specifically, validity is concerned with sources of non-random error (i.e., systemic error or bias), whereas reliability is concerned with sources of random error, also known as noise. Systemic error or bias may prevent an instrument from truly measuring what is intended, which results in inaccuracy. A number of different strategies may be employed to determine validity, each conceptually different and relying on different methods of assessment. There are four types of validity: face, content, construct, and criterion.

Face validity

A measure has face validity if experts judge that it measures at least part of the defined phenomenon.[1] In many instances this is self-evident, whereas in others, particularly in questionnaire-based

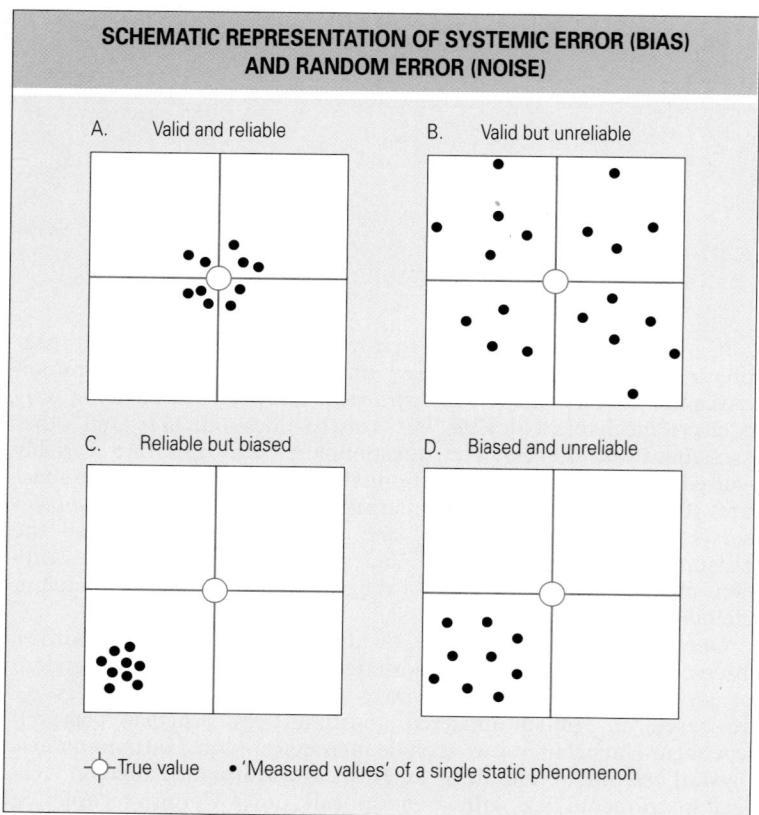

Fig. 2.1 Schematic representation of systemic error (bias) and random error (noise).

measures of functional status, it may not be entirely obvious whether the measurement reflects physical, social, or emotional function.

Content validity

An instrument can have face validity but fail to capture in its entirety the dimension of interest.[1] Content validity, therefore, is a measure of comprehensiveness—the extent to which the measure encompasses all relevant aspects of the defined attribute. Content validity is generally determined by group consensus (e.g., nominal or Delphi techniques). The decision regarding which items should be included in a questionnaire-based instrument and which should be excluded is critical, because it defines the nature of the instrument and its future applicability. Any subsequent addition or deletion results in an instrument that requires further validation.

Given the variability in symptom expression by patients, one of two approaches can be employed to achieve comprehensiveness in questionnaire-based measures. The first is to include a standard battery of measures that probes frequently occurring symptoms that are clinically important to the majority of patients. In the second approach, the measurement process is tailored to the individual by measuring only those items that are important to each person. The issue of importance can be decided by patients, who rate the importance of their symptoms, or by clinical assessors, whose decision is based on their perception of the patient's symptoms.

Construct validity

Construct validity is of two types: convergent and discriminant.[1] Both are tested by demonstrating relationships between measurement scores and a theoretical manifestation (i.e., construct or consequences of an attribute) of the disease. Convergent construct validity testing is assessed by the statistical correlation between scores on a single health component, as measured by two different instruments. If the correlation coefficient is positive and appreciably above zero, the new measure is said to have convergent construct validity.[1] In contrast, discriminant construct validity testing compares correlation coefficients between scores on the same health component, as measured by two different instruments (e.g., separate measures of physical function) and between scores on that health component and each of several other health

components (e.g., measures of social and emotional function). A measure has discriminant construct validity if the proposed measure correlates better with a second measure, accepted as more closely related to the construct, than it does with a third, more distantly related measure.[1]

Criterion validity

Criterion validity is assessed by statistically testing a new measurement technique against an independent criterion or standard (concurrent validity) or against a future standard (predictive validity).[1] Criterion validity is an estimate of the extent to which a measure agrees with a "gold standard" (i.e., an external criterion of the phenomenon being measured). The major problem in criterion validity testing, for questionnaire-based measures, is the general lack of gold standards. Indeed, some purported gold standards may not themselves provide completely accurate estimates of the true value of a phenomenon. In contrast, electromechanical devices such as those evaluating strength, resistance, and range of movement can more often be validated using standard calibration techniques found in the engineering literature.

Reliability

Consistency, reproducibility, repeatability, and agreement are synonyms for reliability.[1] Reliability is the extent to which a measurement procedure yields the same result on repeated determinations (see Fig. 2.1). This determination may be the result of either different measurements performed at the same time (internal consistency) or the same measurements performed at different times (stability). Repeated measurements are rarely exactly the same, because there is usually some random error, noise, or degree of inconsistency. There are various methods of calculating reliability, each method reflecting a different aspect of instrument performance, such that different coefficients are derived using different methods. Defined sources of measurement error include the subject, the assessor, and the measuring instrument. Patient variability often arises from normal variation in symptoms or from fatigue or inattention. When observers are involved in capturing information, both inter-observer and intra-observer reliability are important. Observer variability may be the result of inadequate standardization, the necessity for complex judgments, perceptual elements, or fatigue. When technical instruments are involved in the measurement process, variation in, for example, the cuff configuration of the modified sphygmomanometer or in the mechanical resistance of a dynamometer or dolorimeter may be important sources of error.

Responsiveness (sensitivity to change)

The primary goal of outcome assessment, in evaluative research, is to detect clinically important changes in some aspect of a condition.[1] To detect change, a measurement technique needs to be targeted on aspects of the disease amenable to change, using scaling methods that allow detection of change, and be applied at a point in time when change might have occurred. Validity and reliability are important aspects of all measurement techniques, but the capacity to detect change is the quintessential requirement of a successful outcome measure for evaluating change over time and the patient's response to treatment. An assessment technique may fail to record any clinical improvement for a number of reasons (e.g., patient lacks response potential, lacks compliance with the treatment program, or has received inefficacious treatment; insensitivity of the outcome measure; or occurrence of a type II error due to inadequate sample size).

STATISTICAL ISSUES

It is necessary to have a basic understanding of the statistics used in the development and validation of health status measures. Commonly used statistical tests for reliability, validity, and responsiveness are shown in Table 2.1. Several points are particularly noteworthy:

- Correlation is a measure of the strength of association, not a measure of agreement, such that it is possible to have perfect correlation but zero agreement between two measurements.

TABLE 2.1 STATISTICAL TESTS COMMONLY USED IN OUTCOME MEASURE DEVLOPMENT

- Pearson/Spearman Correlation Coefficients—Estimates of strength of association. Used in evaluating test-retest reliability and construct validity
- Cronbach's alpha—A measure of average inter-item correlation, used to evaluate internal consistency
- Intraclass Correlation Coefficient (ICC)—Used as a measure of reproducibility
- Cohen's kappa—Used to estimate agreement beyond chance in inter-rater and intra-rater agreement studies
- Factor Analysis—Used to examine the structure of the relationship between variables in questionnaires
- Rasch Analysis—Used to test the fit between data and a model, in questionnaire development
- Effect Size (ES)—Used to evaluate responsiveness (Change score/Baseline SD)
- Standardized Response Mean (SRM)—Used to evaluate responsiveness (Change score/Change score SD)
- Relative Efficiency (RE)—Used to evaluate relative responsiveness (Square of the ratio of two t or z statistics)

TABLE 2.2 RELATIVE RESPONSIVENESS OF COMMONLY USED PAIN MEASURES IN OSTEOARTHRITIS (OA) AND RHEUMATOID ARTHRITIS (RA)

Pain measure	Osteoarthritis		Rheumatoid arthritis	
	P	SRM	P	SRM
Visual analog	.0001	.97	.0001	1.08
Continuous chromatic analog	.0001	.94	.0001	1.04
Numerical	.0001	.91	.0001	1.08
Likert	.0001	.84	.0001	.97
Pain Faces Scale (1)	.0001	.78	.0001	.90
MPQ total	.0001	.74	.0001	.68
Pain Faces Scale (2)	.0001	.70	.001	.66

Adapted from Bellamy N, Campbell J, Syrotuik J. Comparative study of self-rating pain scales in rheumatoid arthritis patients. Curr Med Res Opin 1999;15:121-127 and Bellamy N, Campbell J, Syrotuik J. Comparative study of self-rating pain scales in osteoarthritis patients. Curr Med Res Opin 1999;15:113-119.

- Bland and Altman scatter-plots permit the distribution of pairwise data to be appreciated.
- Cohen's kappa statistic, a metric reflecting agreement beyond chance, can be weighted or unweighted and adjustments made for bias and prevalence.
- For continuous data, intraclass correlation coefficients are often used in intra-rater and inter-rater agreement analyses.
- In evaluating construct validity using correlation coefficients, both strength and direction should be considered a priori; otherwise, data interpretation can become complex and biased.
- Factor analysis is a useful procedure for evaluating structure provided that the sample is sufficiently large and is also representative. Repeated factor analyses on the same instrument using different datasets can yield conflicting results.
- Rasch analysis is increasingly being employed to test outcome scales against mathematical models, using a probabilistic form of hierarchical or Guttman scaling. The Rasch model attempts to scale variables along a continuum, but not all Rasch analyses of the same instrument necessarily agree with one another. Although, in general, individuals who can perform tasks of a particular degree of difficulty should be able to perform all tasks of lesser difficulty, this is not always the case.
- Responsiveness may differ between outcome measures used to evaluate different variables or even the same variable and may differ even within an outcome measure when it is presented in different scaling formats (Table 2.2).
- In group-level comparisons random error can, if necessary, be accommodated by increasing the sample size.
- In individual-level comparisons it is necessary to define measurement error such that subsequent measures made on the same individual can be interpreted appropriately based on whether they are entirely within the measurement error or they exceed the measurement error and therefore reflect actual change.

OUTCOME ASSESSMENT TECHNIQUES

There are numerous techniques for assessing the beneficial and adverse outcomes of treatment. A number of health status instruments have been developed to specifically assess certain conditions (Table 2.3), some of which are used routinely in research-based applications. Readers interested in specific measurement issues should consult one or more standard measurement texts.[1,3] In this section a review is presented of the measurement of pain, impairment, ability/disability, participation/handicap, patient and physician global assessments, multidimensional health status instruments (quality of life, utility), and adverse drug reactions. Readers should refer to other sections of this textbook for information on laboratory-based and imaging-based measurement procedures.

Pain

Pain is an entirely subjective phenomenon, the perception of which is modulated by a variety of influences and results in pain behaviors that may be observed.[1] The severity of perceived pain can only be rated by the sufferer. In contrast, pain behavior can be rated by a trained assessor. Complex bidirectional interactions occur between pain and other factors, including personal factors unique to the individual. Pain can be assessed using a variety of techniques (Fig. 2.2), including[1]:

- Likert or adjectival scales
- Visual analog scales
- Ladder scales, numerical rating scales
- Chromatic continuous analog scales
- Pain faces scales
- McGill Pain Questionnaire
- Behavioral observation techniques

Comparative studies of pain rating scales in rheumatoid arthritis (RA) and osteoarthritis (OA) suggest that there is a positive relationship between initial pain rating and subsequent pain relief scores and that all the aforementioned types of scales are responsive.[1] Likert and visual analog scales are the most frequently applied type of scales. Likert scales usually employ an odd (3, 5, 7, or 9) number of descriptors, whereas visual analog scales are most often 100 mm long and horizontal in orientation, with terminal descriptors. The numerical rating scale is often scaled from 0 to 10, displayed in linked boxes, and has terminal descriptors. The focus, phraseology, descriptors, and time frames for recall used in such scales often vary between different questionnaires. In comparative studies in RA and OA, the single-item global numerical rating pain scale appears comparable in responsiveness to the same question presented on a visual analog scale and is slightly more responsive than the corresponding 5-point Likert scale (see Table 2.2).[1]

When applying pain scales, it is important to specify either the global nature of the question or the specific aspect of pain that is being assessed (e.g., while stair climbing, while walking, at rest, during the night, overall) and clearly indicate the time interval over which pain is being evaluated (e.g., 48 hours, 1 week). Several of the standard established segregated multidimensional health status instruments, including the Health Assessment Questionnaire (HAQ),[5] Arthritis Impact Measurement Scales (AIMS and AIMS2),[6,7] Western Ontario and McMaster Osteoarthritis Index (WOMAC),[8] and Australian-Canadian Osteoarthritis Hand Index (AUSCAN),[9] contain distinct pain subscales. These contrast to other instruments that either contain no pain subscale (e.g., FIHOA—Functional Index for Hand Osteoarthritis,[10] Cochin Index[11]) or in which pain is an integral part of an aggregated scoring system combining scores on several different dimensions (e.g., Indices of Clinical Severity [ICS]).[12]

TABLE 2.3 SELECTED HEALTH STATUS MEASURES FOR OUTCOME ASSESSMENT

	Measure	Reference
Rheumatoid arthritis	Disease Activity Score (DAS)	Ann Rheum Dis 1990;49:916-920
	McMaster Toronto Arthritis Patient Preference Disability Questionnaire (MACTAR)	J Rheumatol 1987;14:446-451
	Modified HAQ (MHAQ)	Arthritis Rheum 1983;26:1346-1353
	Rapid Assessment of Disease Activity in Rheumatology (RADAR)	Arthritis Rheum 1992;35:156-162
	Rheumatoid Arthritis Disease Activity Index (RADAI)	Arthritis Rheum 1995;38:795-798
Osteoarthritis	Australian/Canadian Hand Index (AUSCAN)	Osteoarthritis Cartilage 2002;10:863-869
	Cochin Hand Index	Osteoarthritis Cartilage 2001;9:570-579
	Functional Index for Hand Osteoarthritis (FIHOA-Dreiser)	Rev Rheum (Engl Ed) 1995;62(Suppl 1):43S-53S
	Hip Disability and Osteoarthritis Outcome Score (HOOS)	Scand J Rheumatol 2003;32:46-51
	Indices of Clinical Severity (Lequesne)	Semin Arthritis Rheum 1991;20(Suppl 2):48-54
	Knee Injury and Osteoarthritis Outcome Score (KOOS)	Osteoarthritis Cartilage 1999;7:216-221
	Osteoarthritis of Knee and Hip Quality of Life (OAKHQOL)	J Clin Epidemiol 2005;58:47-55
	Western Ontario and McMaster (WOMAC) Osteoarthritis Index	J Rheumatol 1988; 15:1833-1840
Ankylosing spondylitis	Bath Ankylosing Spondylitis Disease Activity Index (BASDAI)	J Rheumatol 1994;21:2286-2291
	Bath Ankylosing Spondylitis Functional Index (BASFI)	J Rheumatol 1994;21:2281-2285
	Dougados Functional Index (DFI)	J Rheumatol 1988;15:302-307
	Dutch AS Index	Br J Rheumatol 1994;33:842-846
	HAQ-S	J Rheumatol 1990;17:946-950
Reactive arthritis related	Disease Activity Index from Reactive Arthritis (DAREA)	Rheumatology 2000;39:148-155
Systemic lupus erythematosus	British Isles Lupus Assessment Group's Index (BILAG)	Q J Med 1998;69:927-937
	Systemic Lupus Activity Measure (SLAM)	Arthritis Rheum 1989;32:1107-1118
	Systemic Lupus Erythematosus Disease Activity Index (SLEDAI)	Arthritis Rheum 1992;35:630-640
Low back pain related	Aberdeen Back Pain Scale	Spine 1994;19:1887-1896
	Oswestry Low Back Disability Questionnaire	Physiotherapy 1980;66:271-273
	Quebec Back Pain Disability Scale	Spine 1995;20:341-352
	Roland and Morris Scale	Spine 1983;8:45-50;141-144
Fibromyalgia related	Fibromyalgia Impact Questionnaire (FIQ)	J Rheumatol 1991;18:728-733
General arthritis measures	Arthritis Impact Measurement Scales (AIMS)	Arthritis Rheum 1980;23:146-152
	Arthritis Impact Measurement Scales (AIMS2)	Arthritis Rheum 1992;35:1-10
	Health Assessment Questionnaire (HAQ)	Arthritis Rheum 1980;23:125-145
Handicap	Disease Repercussion Profile (DRP)	Br J Rheumatol 1996;35:921-932
Fatigue	Functional Assessment of Chronic Illness Therapy Fatigue Scale (FACIT-F)	J Rheumatol 2005;32:811-819
	Multidimensional Assessment of Fatigue (MAF)	Nurs Res 1993;42:93-99
	Piper Fatigue Scale	Oncol Nurs Forum 1990;17:661-662
Coping	Coping with Rheumatic Stressors (CORS)	Br J Rheumatol 1994;33:1067-1073
	Coping Strategies Questionnaire	Pain 1983;17:33-44
	London Coping with RA Questionnaire	Psychol Health 1990;4:187-200
	Self Efficacy Scale	Arthritis Rheum 1989;32:37-44
Helplessness	Arthritis Helplessness Index	J Rheumatol 1988;15:427-432
	Rheumatology Attitudes Index	J Rheumatol 1988;15:418-426
Quality of life	EuroQol	Br J Rheumatol 1994;33:655-662
	Health Utilities Index (HUI)	J Clin Oncol 1992;10:923-928
	Nottingham Health Profile (NHP)	Soc Sci Med 1981;15A:221-229
	Sickness Impact Profile	Med Care 1981;19:787-805
	Short Form 36 (SF-36)	Med Care 1992;30:473-481
	Standard Gamble	Socioecon Planning Sci 1976;10:129-136
	Time Trade-Off	J Health Econ 1986;5:1-30
	WHO Quality of Life Assessment (WHOQOL)	Soc Sci Med 1998;46:1569-1585
	WHO Disability Assessment Schedule II (WHODAS II)	Arthritis Rheum 2008;59:382-390

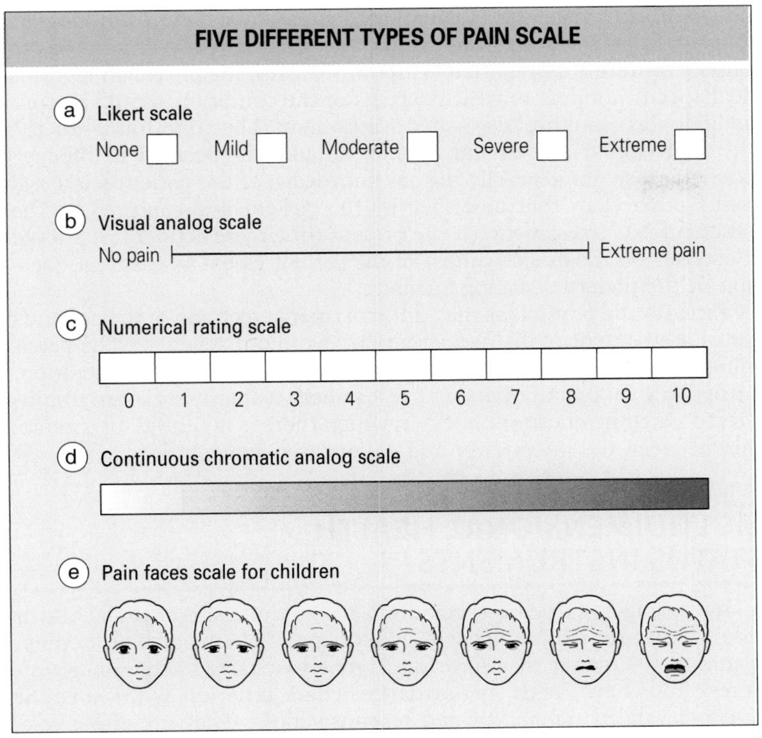

FIVE DIFFERENT TYPES OF PAIN SCALE

(a) Likert scale

None ☐   Mild ☐   Moderate ☐   Severe ☐   Extreme ☐

(b) Visual analog scale

No pain ├──────────────────────────────┤ Extreme pain

(c) Numerical rating scale

| | | | | | | | | | | |
|0|1|2|3|4|5|6|7|8|9|10|

(d) Continuous chromatic analog scale

(e) Pain faces scale for children

Fig. 2.2 Five different types of pain scales.

Impairment, ability/disability, and participation/handicap

The terms *impairment, disability,* and *handicap* may be confused in everyday usage, even though the World Health Organization (WHO) has previously characterized these three different entities.[13] *Impairment* is defined as any loss or abnormality of psychological, physiologic, or anatomic structure or function. It signifies that a pathologic state has reached a stage of detectability. In contrast, *disability* includes any restriction or lack of ability to perform an activity in the manner considered normal. Such disabilities include alteration in behavior, interactive processes such as communication, as well as strictly physical function. A *handicap* is manifest as a disadvantage experienced by an individual as a result of an impairment or disability, such that it limits or prevents the fulfillment of a role considered normal for that individual. In essence, therefore, impairment occurs at an organ level (intellectual, sensory, visceral, musculoskeletal), disability occurs at a personal level (behavior, self-care, locomotion, dexterity), and handicap occurs at a social level (independence, geographic mobility, employability, social integration).[13] The concepts of disability and handicap, in particular, are considered unipolar; and partly for this reason the newer WHO International Classification of Functioning Disability and Health (ICF) is to be preferred, because it considers these same concepts in a bipolar framework of ability and participation.[14] The ICF framework proposed by the WHO is particularly useful in conceptualizing the functional impact of many of the conditions described in other chapters of this text.[1] The ICF framework considers a hierarchy of impairments, activities, and participation, modulated by contextual factors (environmental and personal), and extends the original WHO classification of impairment, disability, and handicap to include positive aspects of health, including physical activity and participation in society.[14]

Impairment

In clinically based musculoskeletal applications in research and practice, measurement is often directed at the assessment of abnormalities in structure (e.g., swelling, tenderness). The most important examination-based measurement procedure is the separate enumeration of swollen and tender joints in patients with inflammatory polyarthritis.[1,3] The usual method employs separate counts of the number of swollen and tender joints, using either the American College of

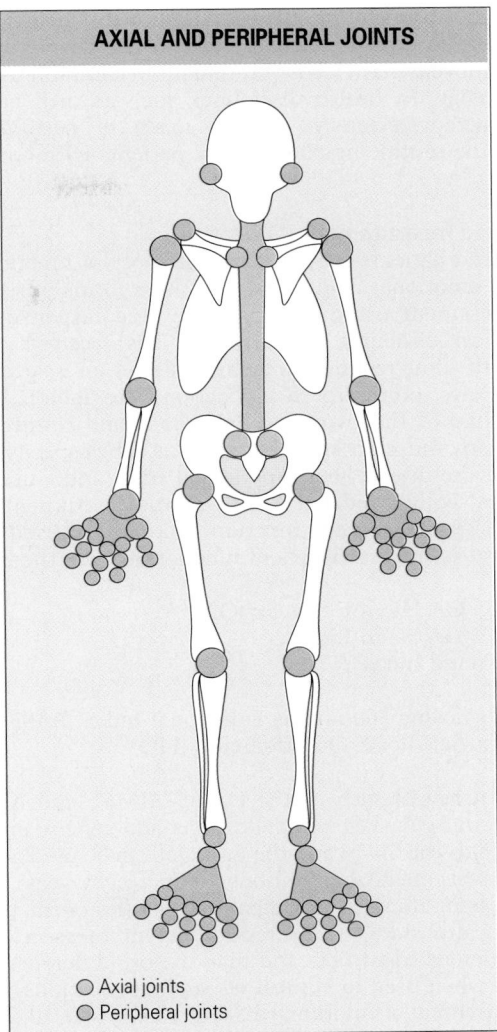

AXIAL AND PERIPHERAL JOINTS

○ Axial joints
○ Peripheral joints

Fig. 2.3 Homunculus for recording joint involvement due to arthritis in routine clinical care.

Rheumatology (ACR) 68 joint count or the European League Against Rheumatism (EULAR) 28 joint count. It is convenient to chart individual joint involvement on a homunculus or mannequin (Fig. 2.3). Other methods have been developed for scoring joint involvement in OA, enthesopathy in ankylosing spondylitis (AS), and tender points in fibromyalgia.[1,3] Methods for assessing other clinical signs, such as heat, erythema, and crepitus, have been less rigorously studied.[1,3] All such procedures are liable to inter-rater and intra-rater error and are best performed by skilled standardized assessors.[3] Nevertheless, various impairment assessments can be conducted at acceptable levels of reliability by trained assessors.[3]

The American Medical Association *Guides to the Evaluation of Permanent Impairment*[15] provide a standardized method to rate impairment at maximum medical improvement (MMI). However, the *Guides* are primarily employed in compensation/litigation applications.

Ability/Disability

Functional measures can be subdivided into those based on observed tests of performance and questionnaires that assess functional capacity.

Performance-based measures

Performance-based measures might at first seem the most direct way to assess the patient's function.[1] However, such measures often involve an interaction between the assessor and subject that may augment or diminish the true performance and raise concern regarding intra-assessor and inter-assessor consistency and the need for assessor standardization. Furthermore, change in performance on the performance test may not correspond to a comparable change in the performance of relevant activities of daily living. The relevance of the change to the patient may therefore require interpretation. Nevertheless, some measures, such as the modified Schober test in AS, grip strength in RA, and range of movement in knee OA, remain in common usage in clinical rheumatology. In health disciplines such as orthopedic surgery and physiotherapy extensive use is made of performance-based measures in the routine management of patients with bone and joint diseases.[1,3]

Capacity-based measurement

Musculoskeletal patients may suffer three types of functional disability: physical, emotional, and social. All three forms are amenable to outcome assessment using valid, reliable, and responsive questionnaires. Physical disability, in particular, has received considerable attention, with some techniques being designed for a specific purpose while others have multipurpose applications (see Table 2.3).[1] Physical disability is one of the two most important and immediate consequences of many musculoskeletal conditions. The capacity to measure this aspect of the disease, both in clinical trials and clinical practice, is paramount. Fully validated health status instruments including separate measures of pain and function are to be preferred over ad hoc scales. Disease-specific measures of function include the following:

- WOMAC OA Hip/Knee Index (OA)[8]
- AUSCAN OA Hand Index[9]
- Cochin Hand Index[11]
- FIHOA[10]
- Bath Ankylosing Spondylitis Functional Index (BASFI)[16]
- Fibromyalgia Impact Questionnaire (FIQ)[17]

In contrast, measures such as the HAQ,[5] AIMS,[6] and AIMS2[7] have multipurpose musculoskeletal applications and generic quality of life measures such as the SF-36 and the EuroQol can be used across a wide variety of diverse medical conditions.[1,18] In recent years, there have been an increasing number of comparative studies of the performance of different health status measures.[1] Different measures are underpinned by different constructs and may impose different sample size requirements when used in clinical research applications.

The measurement of emotional disability in musculoskeletal disease is important, because considerable psychological morbidity has been noted in patients with musculoskeletal disorders. Furthermore, it is not surprising, given the degree of pain, disability, anxiety, depression, and diminished sense of well-being, that many musculoskeletal disorders have social consequences.

Participation/handicap

Measures of handicap reflect the social consequence of disease. Whether an individual is handicapped can be defined either by society or by an individual. The measurement of handicap in the rheumatic diseases has attracted relatively little attention. The Disease Repercussion Profile is a valid and reliable measure of patient-perceived handicap and is a significant contribution to this previously underdeveloped area of musculoskeletal clinical measurement.[1]

Global assessments

Global assessments by patient and physician of the patient's overall condition are commonly used in clinical trials and in clinical practice.[2] It is extremely important to specify in the wording of the global question which aspects of the patient's condition are being considered (e.g., overall health status, symptom severity, disease activity, or an anatomic area). The patient global assessment is particularly important because it can be phrased to assess current status or change in symptom status and be focused on a particular anatomic area, the condition in general, or the patient as a whole. Alternatively, it can be used to assess drug tolerability and/or efficacy or other aspects of the treatment program (palatability, compliance, affordability, convenience). The time frame over which the patient should consider his or her status should be defined (e.g., 48 hours, 1 week). It is debatable whether the physician global assessment of overall health adds much to the measurement process over and above the patient's own global assessment. However, the physician (or other assessor) can consider, in addition, aspects of the condition that are not assessable by the patient (e.g.,

radiographic change and biochemical, hematologic, and immunologic abnormalities) and may have insight into whether the patient tends to amplify or minimize reported symptoms. Again, the physician requires clear specification as to which aspects of the condition should be considered when making his or her assessment. The time frame for the physician global assessment usually should be specified as "today" since the assessor generally has no knowledge of the patient's interval status other than that described by the patient and captured by the patient global assessment. At the present time there is no international consensus on the exact wording of the patient global assessment question or the preferred scaling format.

Patients and physicians may differ in their perception of the patient's global assessment of disease activity or symptom severity.[1] The determinants and consequences of this discrepancy need due consideration, particularly by practitioners and researchers using interviewer-administered outcome questionnaires, in which there is potential for interaction between the interviewer and patient (see Table 2.3).

MULTIDIMENSIONAL HEALTH STATUS INSTRUMENTS

A large number of disease-specific and generic multidimensional health status measures (HSMs) have been developed.[1,3] Many are very sophisticated instruments that have undergone extensive validation procedures and have high performance characteristics with superior levels of validity, reliability, and responsiveness. They are either self-administered or occasionally interviewer administered. It is important for users to contact the originator before initial application for instructions regarding usage (e.g., presentation, scoring, analysis). The latest version of the instrument should be obtained as well as a copy of the user's guide.

Some HSMs have been developed in the form of segregated multidimensional indices, which contain separate, distinct subscales that explore different aspects of the condition, such as HAQ, AIMS, AIMS2, WOMAC, and AUSCAN. They provide subscale scores on each of several separate dimensions. Others are in the form of aggregated multidimensional indices, in which scores from several different dimensions are weighted and aggregated into a single score, such as the Indices of Clinical Severity,[16] Pooled Index,[1] and Disease Activity Score.[1] Health-related quality of life can be assessed either using a multi-item questionnaire, such as Medical Outcomes Study Short-Form (SF)-36 (and its derivatives),[1] Nottingham Health Profile (NHP),[1] EuroQol,[1] or using a utility-based methodology, for example the Health Utilities Index (HUI).[1] A utility is a holistic measure of the quality of life that rates an individual along a continuum from death (0.0) to full health (1.0). Models for predicting utilities from non-utility instrument data are evolutionary. For example, a model has been developed and validated to derive a utility score from WOMAC data that, at the group level, approximates the utility score estimated from the HUI in the same group of patients.[19] This provides opportunity to derive utility scores from previously published studies that contain WOMAC data but that did not include a utility-based measure.

ADVERSE REACTIONS

Adverse reactions caused by treatment can result in symptoms, clinical signs, laboratory abnormalities, or death. Problems often arise in detecting, categorizing, attributing, and grading adverse events. Adverse event rates differ significantly depending on whether the assessment is based on open-ended questioning or structured questionnaires or is determined by a standard protocol. Various systems have been developed for categorizing adverse reactions to treatment. Attribution is the process of ascribing adverse reactions to interventions or other causes. The etiologic relationship is often graded as none, possible, probable, or definite. A number of factors determine the assigned level of the relationship, including prior knowledge of the patient, the pharmacodynamic profile of the intervention, and the duration of treatment. The most difficult attribution decisions are in assigning the grades of "none versus possible" and "probable versus definite" and in grading the intensity of an adverse reaction. Often severity is rated as being mild, moderate, or severe. A mild adverse reaction is one that is easily tolerated by the patient, causes minimal discomfort, and does not interfere with everyday activities. A moderate side effect is an adverse experience that causes sufficient discomfort to interfere with normal everyday activities, whereas a severe reaction is an adverse experience that is incapacitating and prevents normal everyday activities. Finally, it is important to categorize the outcome of an adverse reaction, for example, as resolved, improved, unchanged, worsened, hospitalization required, hospitalization prolonged, or death.

MEASUREMENT IN CLINICAL TRIALS

There are more than 100 different rheumatic disorders, each presenting a different challenge in outcome measurement. Regulatory authorities such as the U.S. Food and Drug Administration (FDA) and the European Medicines Evaluation Agency (EMEA), international non-government organizations, such as the Osteoarthritis Research Society International (OARSI), the Outcome Measures in Rheumatology Clinical Trials (OMERACT) group, the American College of Rheumatology, and the Initiative on Methods, Measurement, and Pain Assessment in Clinical Trials (IMMPACT) group, have pioneered the development of several evidence-based consensus-driven guidance documents. The FDA document on Patient Reported Outcomes is particularly important in understanding the challenges of measuring patient-centered outcomes in regulatory environments.[20] In addition to specifying domains, core set variables (measures), and identifying instruments, some organizations have also initiated investigations leading to the proposal of responder criteria, that is, criteria that could be used to segregate patients according to whether they have experienced a meaningful improvement with treatment.[1] Although improvement with treatment is a very important goal, it is also important to determine the value of the final health state attained. Work in this area is limited. However, proposals are emerging that attempt to identify achievable, acceptable, or desirable health states.

There are a large and continually growing number of outcome measures to evaluate RA, OA, AS, reactive arthritis, systemic lupus erythematosus, low back pain, and fibromyalgia, as well as more generally applicable measures and measures of handicap, coping, helplessness, and quality of life (see Table 2.3). It is beyond the scope of this chapter to describe the development, validation, and scope of application of each of the currently available measures or the exact methods used to develop guidance documents or to develop and propose response and state-attainment criteria. Measurement preferences differ between different disorders, but pain, function, and patient global assessment are often emphasized. Furthermore, several health status questionnaires have been mapped to the ICF framework and, for a limited few, population-based normative values have been elaborated.

Rheumatoid arthritis

In general, RA clinical trials evaluate either fast-acting, symptom-modifying drugs, such as non-steroidal anti-inflammatory drugs (NSAIDs) and analgesics, or slow-acting disease modifying antirheumatic drugs (DMARDs), which include the biologic agents. Measurement tools frequently used in RA studies in rheumatology are shown in Table 2.3. The following recommendation, developed by the OMERACT group,[1] and ratified by the ACR,[21] currently comprise the ACR minimum core set for RA clinical trials (Table 2.4): pain, physical function, number of swollen joints, number of tender joints, patient global assessment, investigator global assessment, erythrocyte sedimentation rate or C-reactive protein, and imaging. Individual response criteria, based on these clinical variables, and referred to as the ACR 20,[22] have been proposed (see Table 2.4) as follows: greater than or equal to 20% improvement in tender and swollen joint counts and greater than or equal to 20% improvement in three of the five remaining ACR core set measures. The above variables should be assessed with validated methods using standardized techniques. Frequently used measurement tools in RA are shown in Table 2.3. The sufficiency of the ACR 20 criteria has been considered,[1] and higher-level response requirements based on the ACR 50 and ACR 70 criteria evaluated.[23] Definitions of remission and minimum disease activity have been

TABLE 2.4 RESPONDER CRITERIA FOR OSTEOARTHRITIS, RHEUMATOID ARTHRITIS, AND ANKYLOSING SPONDYLITIS

Osteoarthritis

High improvement in pain or in function ≥50% and absolute change ≥20 normalized units	or	Improvement in at least two of the three following criteria: Pain ≥20% and absolute change ≥10 normalized units Function ≥20% and absolute change ≥10 normalized units Patient's global assessment ≥20% and absolute change ≥10 normalized units

Rheumatoid arthritis

Required: ≥20% improvement in tender joint count ≥20% improvement in swollen joint count	and	≥20% improvement in three of the following five criteria: Patient pain assessment Patient global assessment Physician global assessment Patient self-assessment disability Acute-phase reactant (ESR or CRP)

Ankylosing spondylitis

Improvement of ≥20% and absolute improvement of ≥1 unit (on a scale of 0-10) in at least three of the following four domains: Patient global assessment Pain Function Inflammation	and	Absence of deterioration in the potential remaining domain, where deterioration is defined as a change for the worse of ≥20% and net worsening of ≥1 unit (on a scale of 0-10)

considered in clinical research and clinical practice applications.[24] The disease activity score using a 28-joint count has been proposed as a remission criterion.[1] ICF core sets have been specified for RA[1] validated from a patient perspective[1] and commonly used instruments mapped to the framework.[1] Normative data for the HAQ have been published[25] and Minimum Clinically Important Improvement (MCII) and Patient Acceptable Symptom State (PASS) estimates explored for RA based on the HAQ.

Osteoarthritis

Clinical trials in OA can be subdivided into those that assess symptom-modifying and those that assess structure-modifying OA drug effects. There is ongoing debate regarding current therapeutic opportunities to prevent, arrest, or repair structural damage in OA. Measurement tools frequently used in OA studies in rheumatology are shown in Table 2.3. Core set measures for OA were proposed by the OMERACT group[26] and ratified,[27] or in the case of hand OA developed,[28] by the OARSI (see Table 2.4). OMERACT and OARSI core set measures for future phase III studies in hip, knee, and hand OA are pain, function, patient global assessment, and, for studies of 1 year or longer, joint imaging using validated methods and standardized techniques. OMERACT and OARSI have jointly proposed responder criteria for hip and knee OA (see Table 2.4), based on combinations of absolute and percentage changes in pain, function, and patient global assessment.[29] The OMERACT-OARSI responder criteria are applicable to both hip and knee OA patients and are not intervention class specific (see Table 2.4). Response criteria developed for OA, and proposed by other groups, include definitions of Minimum Perceptible Clinical Improvement (MPCI),[1] Minimum Clinically Important Difference (MCID),[1] MCII,[1] WOMAC 20-50-70, and AUSCAN 20-50-70.[1] In addition to these definitions based on the degree of change, other definitions have been proposed based on the health state attained, the so-called state-attainment criteria (Table 2.5). Definitions based on PASS[1] and Bellamy Low Intensity Symptom State-Attainment (BLISS) Index[30] are examples of initial attempts to establish working definitions for use in clinical practice and clinical research (see Table 2.5). Observations that

TABLE 2.5 PROPOSED STATE-ATTAINMENT CRITERIA FOR ARTHRITIS AND MUSCULOSKELETAL CONDITIONS

Patient Acceptable Symptom Severity (PASS75) (Preliminary estimates based on REFLECT Study) (All values on 0-100 scales)

Osteoarthritis (hip and knee):
WOMAC Pain = 39.3; WOMAC Stiffness = 44.8; WOMAC Function = 47.7; PGA = 47.1.

Osteoarthritis (hand):
AUSCAN Pain = 41.0; AUSCAN Stiffness =37.8; AUSCAN Function = 44.8; PGA = 41.6.

Rheumatoid arthritis:
Pain = 40.7; HAQ = 39.4; PGA = 41.6.

Ankylosing spondylitis:
Pain = 40.6, PGA = 43.2, BASFI = 40.4, BASDAI = 38.9; PGA = 43.2.

Low back pain:
Pain = 39.4; Roland Morris Disability Questionnaire = 30.7; PGA = 40.3.

Bellamy et al: Low Intensity Symptom State-Attainment (BLISS) Index[30]

Osteoarthritis (knee):
Two components—symptom level based on the WOMAC Osteoarthritis Index (pain, stiffness, function, and total score) and time combined in a state-attainment based analysis.

Magnitude (normalized units [nu] 0-100 scale):
≤25 nu, ≤20 nu, ≤15 nu, ≤10 nu, ≤5 nu

Time:
Time to first BLISS day
BLISS days over 12 months
Patients in BLISS at month 12
Patients in BLISS at any time
BLISS maintained to month 12
Number of BLISS periods over 12 months

---

statistically significant between-group differences are detectable at low or very low symptom intensity levels, so-called BLISS states, are of particular importance in the evaluation of therapeutic interventions,[30] because they provide indicators of achievable health states. Although further research is necessary, observations of BLISS states have been made with the WOMAC and AUSCAN indices and in different classes of interventions and confirm that such states are achievable by some, but not all, patients. ICF core sets for OA have been elaborated and the WOMAC index, ICS, and OAKHQOL mapped to the ICF core set.[1,31] Age- and gender-specific population-based normative data have been elaborated for the WOMAC and AUSCAN index items and MCII and PASS estimates explored for OA based on the WOMAC index for hip and knee OA and the AUSCAN index for hand OA.[1]

Ankylosing spondylitis

Clinical measurement in AS encompasses both the peripheral joints and extra-articular involvement, as well as axial skeletal involvement. Patient-centered measurement tools used in AS are shown in Table 2.3. Through the OMERACT process and the Assessment in Ankylosing Spondylitis (ASAS) Working Group, core set measures have been selected for use in different clinical research settings (see Table 2.4).[1] ASAS has also developed a definition of short-term improvement (ASAS20), based on four domains: physical function, pain, patient global assessment, and inflammation.[1] Based on a scale of 0 to 10, the proposal is as follows: ASAS20 defines improvement as greater than or equal to 20% and greater than or equal to 1 unit (0-10 scale) improvement on at least three of the four domains, with no worsening (defined as ≥20% and ≥1 unit [0-10 scale] deterioration) on the fourth dimension (see Table 2.4).[1] The BASFI, DFI, HAQ-S, and RLDQ instruments have been mapped to the ICF framework,[1] and MCII and PASS estimates have been explored for AS based on the BASFI.

Psoriatic arthritis

Outcome measurement in psoriatic arthritis has received relatively little attention until recently. Through the OMERACT process,

consensus has been reached on a core set of domains for randomized controlled trials and longitudinal observational studies in psoriatic arthritis, namely, peripheral joint activity, skin activity, patient global assessment, pain, physical function, and health-related quality of life.[32] Further research is required in the areas of instrument development and validation, responder and state-attainment criteria, and ICF core sets. Based on qualitative studies, it appears that several aspects of the symptom experience in patients with psoriatic arthritis are not covered by existing measures of functioning.[33]

Systemic lupus erythematosus

Several measures have emerged for conducting outcome measurement in systemic lupus erythematosus[1,34-37] and are shown in Table 2.3. It has been noted that there is moderate agreement between prospective and retrospective evaluations of SLICC/ACR DI scores.[1] Modifications of the SLEDAI, LAI, and SLAM have been proposed for use in systemic lupus erythematosus in pregnancy. These modifications are respectively referred to as SLEPDAI, LAI-P, and m-SLAM.[1]

Core set domains for clinical trials and longitudinal studies have been proposed by the OMERACT group (see Table 2.4) and include (1) disease activity; (2) health-related quality of life; (3) organ damage; and (4) toxicity/adverse events.[1] The ACR has proposed response criteria for systemic lupus erythematosus clinical trials (see Table 2.5).[1] These criteria are based on absolute change, are instrument specific, and have been proposed for the BILAG, SLEDAI, SLAM, ECLAM, SELENA-SLEDAI, and RIFLE instruments. The criteria are in the form of threshold values for improvement and worsening. The Pediatric Rheumatology International Trials Organization and the ACR have proposed provisional response criteria for juvenile systemic lupus erythematosus based on at least 50% improvement in any two of five core set measures, and with no more than one of the remaining measures worsening by more than 30%.[38]

Systemic sclerosis

The current status of outcome measures for clinical trials in systemic sclerosis has been reviewed by the OMERACT group.[1] The HAQ and Scleroderma HAQ (SHAQ) were the only two patient-centered measures considered ready for use in clinical trials.[1] The measurement of disease activity in systemic sclerosis remains challenging. However, the European Scleroderma Study Group have proposed preliminary activity criteria, based on the summation of scores across multiple variables.[1] A Delphi-based consensus estimate has provided initial ranges of estimates for minimal clinically relevant treatment effects in scleroderma for the Modified Rodnan skin score, HAQ-DI, HAQ-Pain, MD global, patient global, and diffusing capacity.[39]

Behçet's disease

To date there has been a paucity of measurement tools to assess disease activity and condition-specific quality of life in Behçet's disease. The development and validation of the Behçet's Disease Activity Index (BDAI)[1] and the Behçet's Disease Quality of Life (BD-QoL) index,[1] represent important contributions to measurement in Behçet's disease.

Sjögren's syndrome

Based on more than a 50% consensus at the Outcome Measures for Sjogren's Syndrome Workshop in 2003, core set measures for Sjögren's syndrome were proposed as follows: sicca symptoms, sicca objective (oral), sicca objective (ocular), HRQOL, laboratory measures, and fatigue.[1] More recently, two new indices for assessing disease in Sjögren's syndrome have been formulated and termed the Sjögren's Syndrome Disease Damage Index (SSDDI) and the Sjögren's Syndrome Disease Activity Index (SSDAI), respectively.[40]

Polymyalgia rheumatica

The European Collaborating Polymyalgia Rheumatica Group developed a specification of core set measures for polymyalgia rheumatica in 2003 that included five measures: pain, physician global assessment, morning stiffness, C-reactive protein, and ability to elevate the upper limbs.[1] From this proposition emerged the proposition for a composite index termed the PMR Activity Score (PMR-AS).[1] A recent evaluation of the PMR-AS suggests it may be useful in monitoring PMR activity in routine practice and in managing corticosteroid tapering.[41]

Inflammatory myopathies

The International Myositis Assessment and Clinical Studies (IMACS) group has proposed three tools for the evaluation of patients with idiopathic inflammatory myopathies.[1] These tools are the Myositis Intention to Treat Index (MITAX), the Myositis Disease Activity Assessment Visual Analogue Scale (MYOACT), and the Myositis Damage Index (MDI). The indices are currently being subjected to validity testing. Preliminary consensus-based estimates of clinically important improvement in adult and juvenile idiopathic inflammatory myopathies have been proposed as follows: muscle strength and physical function, 15%+; physician and patient global assessment, 20%+; and serum levels of muscle associated enzymes, 30%+.[1] The Pediatric Rheumatology International Trials Organization and the ACR have proposed core set measures for juvenile dermatomyositis that include physician global assessment of disease activity, muscle strength, global disease activity measure, parent's global assessment of patient's well-being, functional ability, and health-related quality of life.[42]

Vasculitis

Outcome assessment in the different pathologic entities that collectively form the vasculitides may be difficult with only a single measure. Different conditions may require different indices. Consideration has been given to the development of a Combined Damage Assessment (CDA) Index for vasculitides involving small- and medium-sized vessels.[43] In contrast, other initiatives have resulted in the development of the Birmingham Vasculitis Activity Score/Wegener's Granulomatosis (BVAS/WG) for evaluating patients with Wegener's granulomatosis.[1] The reliability, construct, and discriminant validity of the BVAS/WG have been assessed and the index proposed for use in clinical investigation.[1] It has been suggested that the ability of the BVAS/WG to encompass the spectrum of disease activity might be enhanced by different selection and weighting procedures.[44]

Osteoporosis

Core set measures for bone loss prevention studies (bone mineral density measured at two sites, biochemical markers) and fracture prevention studies (fracture, hip, knee, and spine bone mineral density; biochemical markers; change in height) in osteoporosis have been proposed by the OMERACT group.[1] In addition, ICF core sets have been suggested for osteoporosis[1] and the content of osteoporosis-targeted health status measures compared using the ICF framework.[1]

Low Back Pain

Outcomes in low back pain can be assessed with various instruments (see Table 2.3) as well as with quality of life measures (see Table 2.3). The OMERACT group has proposed preliminary response criteria for chronic low back pain, based on at least 30% improvements in pain and in patient global assessment and no worsening in function.[45] MCII and PASS estimates have been explored for low back pain based on the Roland Morris Disability Questionnaire.

Fibromyalgia

There has been no international agreement on a core set of measures for future phase III trials in fibromyalgia. The most frequently used measures in recent fibromyalgia studies (≤50% of trials) have been tender points, patient global assessment, fatigue, quality of sleep, pain, and stiffness. The Fibromyalgia Impact Questionnaire (FIQ) is probably the most widely used condition-specific measure used in fibromyalgia clinical trials (see Table 2.3).[1]

TABLE 2.6 CHARACTERISTICS OF HEALTH STATUS QUESTIONNAIRES FOR ROUTINE USE IN THE CLINIC

- Health status questionnaires (HSQs) must be short, not use more than minimal staff time, and not disturb the routine of the clinic. They must fit into the routine of the clinic.
- HSQs must help the physician and staff with record keeping, not impede it. They must assist in documentation of clinical care.
- Cost must be minimal.
- The result must be available at the time the patient is seen.
- Comparison with previous data and with other patients must be contemporaneous.
- The results must be intuitive and interpretable.
- The information must be more than just additional data. It must be clinically useful.

With permission from Wolfe F, Pincus T. Data collection in the clinic. Rheum Dis Clin North Am 1995;21:321-358.

OUTCOME MEASUREMENT IN ROUTINE CLINICAL PRACTICE

For many rheumatologists in routine practice the goal will be to efficiently track the progress of individual patients, even if there is no investigational goal. A recent survey of Australian rheumatologists[46] noted that the essential characteristics of, for example, an OA outcome measure for outpatient care were simplicity, rapid completion, easy scoring, reliability, validity, and sensitivity to change.

The major emphasis in clinical metrology has been on the development of instruments for clinical research rather than for routine clinical purposes. The challenge now is to apply these techniques in clinical practice as well as to build on clinical research experience to make available short, simple patient-centered self-completed questionnaires that are easily scored and can be used in office practice (Table 2.6).[47] It will also be important to investigate the extent to which quantitative measurement during routine clinical care results in improved outcomes and is cost effective.[48]

Combinations of disease-specific, generic health-related quality of life and global measures are particularly useful in clinical practice. Six issues of practical importance deserve special consideration:

1. Although measures of discomfort (pain), disability (function), and patient and physician global assessment are common to all rheumatic diseases, conditions with extra-articular consequences may require additional organ-specific assessments (e.g., skin scores in scleroderma).
2. Outcome measurement in children is problematic. It is important to select scales that are valid, reliable, responsive, and comprehensible in this particular group of patients.
3. In addition to defining *a priori* a schedule for assessing the beneficial effects of a treatment program, it is equally important to establish a monitoring schedule for adverse events, particularly for pharmacologic interventions.[1] Such a schedule should be capable of detecting both clinical and non-clinical (laboratory) forms of toxicity in a timely fashion.
4. Methods for handling data are important. For paper-based applications, flow charts are particularly useful in documenting longitudinal change in clinical status, as well as for charting the non-clinical (laboratory) tolerability of antirheumatic drugs. Expanding opportunities for electronic data capture are likely to solve many of the current problems with data capture, storage, and analysis of quantitative data.[49] Electronic data capture has usually employed desktop and laptop computer-based applications. More recently, personal digital assistants and Web-based applications have been used to capture health status information. In recent studies of electronic data capture using mobile (cellular) phones, high levels of correlation between paper and mobile phone-based versions of the WOMAC index and high levels of responsiveness were observed, despite the micro-screen presentation of 11-point Numerical Rating scales.[50]

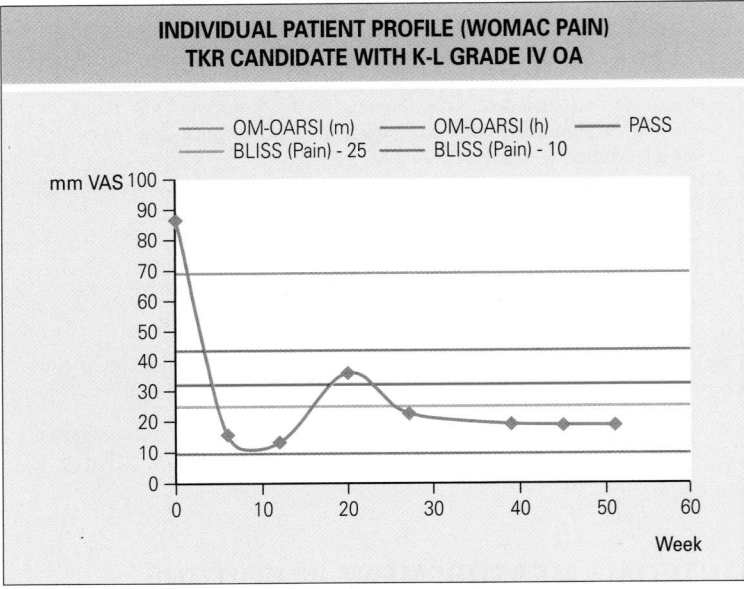

**INDIVIDUAL PATIENT PROFILE (WOMAC PAIN)
TKR CANDIDATE WITH K-L GRADE IV OA**

Fig. 2.4 Response to treatment in osteoarthritis (OA) can be monitored over an extended period, by a combination of responder and state-attainment criteria.

5. The concomitant use of disease-specific, patient and physician global assessments and generic health-related quality of life measures is a particularly powerful combination. In inflammatory polyarthritis these measures can readily be supplemented by an articular index in the form of a simple count of tender and swollen joints.

6. The development of responder criteria, state-attainment criteria, and normative data is an important step in the transfer of measurement procedures used in research environments into routine clinical practice and may permit more effective monitoring of patient progress and response to treatment (Fig. 2.4).

Implementation of what might be termed *quantitative rheumatology* may require the development of new instruments or modifications to existing instruments, measurement processes, and analysis procedures to meet demands in routine clinical practice. However, there is no reason to delay using some of the shorter, user-friendly, patient self-administered questionnaires currently available. The ability to quantitate the clinical condition provides patients, medical practitioners, allied health professionals, third-party payers, and litigators with much important and useful information. Furthermore, proposed definitions of response and state-attainment, the elaboration of population-based normative values, and innovations in electronic data capture all contribute to an expanding capability to capture and interpret health status information in a manner capable of informing shared decision-making and goal setting in clinical practice and the evaluation of new interventions and therapeutic strategies in clinical research.

REFERENCES

1. Bellamy N. Principles of outcome assessment. In: Hochberg M, et al, eds. Rheumatology, 4th ed. London: Mosby, 2008: vol 1, section 1:11-20.
2. Fries JF, Bird HA. The assessment of disability: from first to future principles. Br J Rheumatol 1983;22(Suppl): 48-58.
3. Bellamy N. Musculoskeletal clinical metrology. Dordrecht: Kluwer Academic, 1993:1-367.
4. Boers M, Brooks P, Strand CV, et al. The OMERACT Filter for outcome measures in rheumatology. J Rheumatol 1998;25:198-199.
5. Fries JF, Spitz P, Kraines RG, Holman HR. Measurement of patient outcome in arthritis. Arthritis Rheum 1980;23:137-145.
6. Meenan RF, Gertman PM, Mason JH. Measuring health status in arthritis: the Arthritis Impact Measurement Scales. Arthritis Rheum 1980;23:146-152.
7. Meenan RF, Mason JH, Anderson JJ, et al. AIMS2—the content and properties of a revised and expanded Arthritis Impact Measurement Scales health status questionnaire. Arthritis Rheum 1992;35:1-10.
8. Bellamy N, Buchanan WW, Goldsmith CH, et al. Validation study of WOMAC: a health status instrument for measuring clinically important patient relevant outcomes to antirheumatic drug therapy in patients with osteoarthritis of the hip or knee. J Rheumatol 1988;15:1833-1840.
9. Bellamy N, Campbell J, Haraoui B, et al. Clinimetric properties of the AUSCAN Osteoarthritis Hand Index: an evaluation of reliability, validity and responsiveness. Osteoarthritis Cartilage 2002;10:863-869.
10. Drieser RL, Maheu E, Guillou GB, et al. Validation of an algofunctional index for osteoarthritis of the hand. Rev Rheum 1995;62(6 Suppl):43S-53S.
11. Poiraudeau S, Chevalier X, Conrozier T. Reliability, validity and sensitivity to change of the Cochin Hand Functional Disability Scale in hand osteoarthritis. Osteoarthritis Cartilage 2001;9:570-577.
12. Lequesne MG, Mery C, Samson M, et al. Indexes of severity for osteoarthritis of the hip and knee: validation-value in comparison with other assessment tests. Scand J Rheumatol 1987;65(Suppl):85-89.
13. World Health Organization. Classification of impairments, disabilities and handicaps. Geneva: WHO, 1980.
14. World Health Organization. International classification of functioning, disability and health. Geneva: WHO, 2001.
15. Rondinelli RD, Genovese E, Katz RT, et al, eds. American Medical Association guides to the evaluation of permanent impairment, 6th ed. Chicago: AMA, 2008.

16. Calin A. The individual with ankylosing spondylitis: defining disease status and the impact of illness. Br J Rheumatol 1995;34:663-672.
17. Burckhardt CS, Clark SR, Bennett RM. The fibromyalgia impact questionnaire: development and validation. J Rheumatol 1991;18:728-733.
18. Ware JE Jr, Sherbourne CD. The MOS 36-item Short-Form Health Status survey (SF-36): 1. Conceptual framework and item selection. Med Care 1992;30:473-483.
19. Marshall D, Pericak D, Grootendorst P, et al. Validation of a prediction model to estimate health utilities index Mark 3 utility scores from WOMAC index scores in patients with osteoarthritis of the hip. Value Health 2008;11(3):470-477.
20. Guidance for Industry Patient-Reported Outcome Measures: Use in Medical Product Development to Support Labeling Claims (Draft Guidance). U.S. Food and Drug Administration, February 2006.
21. Felson DT, Anderson JJ, Boers M, et al. The American College of Rheumatology preliminary core set of disease activity markers for rheumatoid arthritis clinical trials. Arthritis Rheum 1993;36:729-740.
22. Felson DT, Anderson JJ, Boers M, et al. American College of Rheumatology preliminary definition of improvement in rheumatoid arthritis. Arthritis Rheum 1995;38:727-735.
23. Felson DT, Anderson JJ, Lange MI, et al. Should improvement in rheumatoid arthritis clinical trials be defined as fifty percent or seventy percent improvement in core set measures, rather than twenty percent? Arthritis Rheum 1998;41:1564-1570.
24. Mierau M, Schoels M, Gonda G, et al. Assessing remission in clinical practice. Rheumatology 2007;46:975-979.
25. Krishnan E, Sokka S, Hakkinen A, et al. Normative values for the Health Assessment Questionnaire Disability Index: benchmarking disability in the general population. Arthritis Rheum 2004;50:953-960.
26. Bellamy N, Kirwan J, Boers M, et al. Recommendations for a core set of outcome measures for future phase III clinical trials in knee, hip and hand osteoarthritis—consensus development at OMERACT III. J Rheumatol 1997;24:799-802.
27. Osteoarthritis Research Society (OARS) Task Force Report. Design and conduct of clinical trials in patients with osteoarthritis: recommendations from a task force of the Osteoarthritis Research Society. Osteoarthritis Cartilage 1996;4:217-243.
28. Maheu E, Altman R, Bloch D, et al. Osteoarthritis Research Society International (OARSI) Task Force

Report. Design and conduct of clinical trials in patients with hand osteoarthritis: recommendations from a task force of the Osteoarthritis Research Society. Osteoarthritis Cartilage 2006;14:303-322.
29. Pham T, van der Heijde D, Altman RD, et al. OMERACT-OARSI Initiative: Osteoarthritis Research Society International set of responder criteria for osteoarthritis clinical trials revisited. Osteoarthritis Cartilage 2004;12:389-399.
30. Bellamy N, Bell MJ, Goldsmith CH, et al. BLISS Index using WOMAC Index detects between-group differences at low intensity symptom states in osteoarthritis. J Clin Epidemiol 2009; 10.1016/j.jclinepi.2009.07.011.
31. Rat AC, Guillemin F, Pouchot J. Mapping the osteoarthritis knee and hip quality of life (OAKHQOL) instrument to the international classification of function, disability and health and comparison to five health status instruments used in osteoarthritis. Rheumatology 2008;47:1719-1725.
32. Gladman DD, Mease PJ, Strand V, et al. Consensus on a core set of domains for psoriatic arthritis. J Rheumatol 2007;34:1167-1170.
33. Stamm TA, Nell V, Mathis M, et al. Concepts important to patients with psoriatic arthritis are not adequately covered by standard measures of functioning. Arthritis Care Res 2007;57:487-494.
34. Yee C, Farewell V, Isenberg DA, et al. British Isles Lupus Assessment Group 2004 index is valid for assessment of disease activity in systemic lupus erythematosus. Arthritis Rheum 2007;56:4113-4119.
35. McElhone K, Abbott J, Shelmerdine J, et al. Development and validation of a disease-specific health-related quality of life measure, the LupusQoL, for adults with systemic lupus erythematosus. Arthritis Rheum 2007;57:972-979.
36. Gutiérrez-Suárez R, Ruperto N, Gastaldi R, et al. A proposal for a pediatric version of the Systemic Lupus International Collaborating Clinics/American College of Rheumatology Damage Index based on the analysis of 1,015 patients with juvenile-onset systemic lupus erythematosus. Arthritis Rheum 2006;54:2989-2996.
37. Meiorin S, Pistoria A, Ravelli A, et al. Validation of the childhood health assessment questionnaire in active juvenile systemic lupus erythematosus. Arthritis Rheum 2008;59:1112-1119.
38. Ruperto N, Ravelli A, Oliveira S, et al. The Pediatric Rheumatology International Trials Organization/American College of Rheumatology provisional criteria for the evaluation of response to therapy in juvenile systemic lupus erythematosus: prospective validation of

the definition of improvement. Arthritis Rheum 2006;55:355-363.

39. Gazi H, Pope JE, Clements P, et al. Outcome measurements in scleroderma: results from a Delphi exercise. J Rheumatol 2007;34:501-509.

40. Vitali C, Palombi G, Baldini, et al. Sjögren's Syndrome Disease Damage Index and Disease Activity Index: scoring systems for the assessment of disease damage and disease activity in Sjögren's syndrome, derived from an analysis of a cohort of Italian patients. Arthritis Rheum 2007;56:2223-2231.

41. Binard A, De Bandt M, Berthelot J, et al. Performance of the Polymyalgia Rheumatica Activity Score for the diagnosing of disease flares. Arthritis Rheum 2008;59: 263-269.

42. Ruperto N, Ravelli A, Pistorio A, et al. The Provisional Paediatric Rheumatology International Trials Organisation/American College of Rheumatology/ European League Against Rheumatism Disease activity core set for the evaluation of response to therapy in juvenile dermatomyositis: a prospective validation study. Arthritis Rheum 2008;59:4-13.

43. Seo P, Luqmani RA, Flossmann O, et al. The future of damage assessment in vasculitis. J Rheumatol 2007;34:1357-1371.

44. Mahr AD, Neogi T, LaValley MP, et al. Assessment of the item selection and weighting in the Birmingham vasculitis activity score for Wegener's granulomatosis. Arthritis Rheum 2008;59:884-891.

45. Simon LS, Evans C, Katz N, et al. Preliminary development of a responder index for chronic low back pain. J Rheumatol 2007;34:1386-1391.

46. Bellamy E, Wilson C, Bellamy N. Osteoarthritis Measurement in Routine Rheumatology Outpatient Practice (OMIRROP) in Australia: a survey of practice style, instrument use, responder criteria and state-attainment criteria. J Rheumatol 2009;36:1049-1055.

47. Pincus T, Sokka T: Quantitative clinical assessment in busy rheumatology settings: the value of short patient questionnaires [editorial]. J Rheumatol 2008;35:1235-1237.

48. Valderas JM, Alonso J, Guyatt GH. Measuring patient-reported outcomes: moving from clinical trials into clinical practice. Med J Aust 2008;189:93-94.

49. Greenwood MC, Hakim AJ, Carson E, et al. Touch-screen computer systems in the rheumatology clinic offer a reliable and user-friendly means of collecting quality-of-life and outcome data from patients with rheumatoid arthritis. Rheumatology 2006;45:66-71.

50. Bellamy N, Wilson C, Hendrikz J, et al. Electronic data capture (EDC) using cellular technology: implications for clinical trials and practice and preliminary experience with the m-WOMAC Index in hip and knee osteoarthritis. Inflammopharmacology 2009;17:93-99.

Principles of health economics and application to rheumatic disorders

3

Hilal Maradit Kremers, Sherine E. Gabriel, and Michael F. Drummond

- Economic evaluation is a systematic appraisal of the costs, the consequences, and the relative cost-effectiveness of alternative courses of action, alternative interventions, or therapies.
- Although economic evaluation is an integral part of the drug development process, postmarketing economic evaluations are critical because they address real-life cost and effectiveness issues.
- The "reference case" is a minimum set of criteria to be included in all economic analyses in order to improve quality, consistency, and comparability of economic evaluations.
- The majority of economic analyses in rheumatic diseases are conducted in osteoarthritis and rheumatoid arthritis and mostly evaluate interventions to reduce gastrointestinal ulcers induced by non-steroidal anti-inflammatory drugs, cost-effectiveness of biologic agents, and the value of arthroplasty. Economic evaluations in osteoporosis focus on the value of hormone replacement therapy for prevention of osteoporotic fractures and cost-effectiveness of screening strategies for different risk populations.
- Economic evaluations in rheumatic diseases are expected to increase in the future.

INTRODUCTION

In the past 2 decades we have witnessed remarkable advances in the field of rheumatology with, for example, the introduction of several biologic treatments for rheumatoid arthritis and other rheumatic diseases. Although many of the biologic agents are quite costly, they may have major long-term benefits, especially slowing disease progression and preventing disability. In our current health care fiscal environment, proof of benefit alone is no longer sufficient. We must also demonstrate that the expected benefits of a new therapeutic agent are worth the costs of that agent. This can only be shown by formal economic evaluation that involves a group of analytical methods that allow us to quantify and compare the benefits, such as prevented disability and improved quality of life, with the costs of medical interventions.

WHAT IS ECONOMIC EVALUATION?

Economic evaluation is about tradeoffs and choices between wants, needs, and the scarcity of resources.[1] It is the systematic appraisal of the costs, the consequences, and the relative cost-effectiveness of alternative courses of action, alternative interventions, or therapies. The methods can be complex, but the general rule is that the difference in costs is compared with the difference in consequences. In health care, costs and consequences of medical interventions can be expressed not only as goods, services, and money but also in clinical or humanistic terms.

Economic evaluation should be viewed as an aid rather than a substitute to medical evaluation and medical decision-making. First, it is heavily dependent on the relevance and validity of the alternatives considered, as well as their costs and consequences. Second, cost-effectiveness is usually not the sole criterion in health care decision-making. For example, equity or fairness in the distribution of health care resources may also be important.

Dimensions of economic evaluation

There are three dimensions of analysis in considering economic evaluation of health care (Fig. 3.1).

The first dimension defines the types of costs and benefits to be evaluated. Costs represent more than just transactions of currency but the sacrifices that result from the consumption of resources that could otherwise be used for alternate purposes. The cost of a resource is valued as the benefits that would be derived from using it in its next best alternative use, which are forgone once the resource has been used. This concept is called *opportunity cost*. In addition, from a societal perspective, not all transactions of money are regarded as costs, especially those that do not involve consumption of resources other than in their administration (e.g., retirement and disability payments, social security payments). These are called transfer payments, and their existence does not change the overall level of resources available to society.

Costs and benefits can be categorized into (1) the direct and (2) the indirect medical costs and benefits, plus (3) direct non-medical costs and benefits, and (4) intangible costs and benefits (Table 3.1). Direct medical costs and benefits are associated with the provision of health care. Typical examples include payments for the drugs, salaries of health care professionals, or the cost of hospital stay. In contrast, indirect medical costs represent the cost of morbidity or mortality associated with the disease. They mostly comprise productivity costs, covering items such as time lost from work, lost wages or death, and premature removal from the workforce. Direct non-medical costs are those incurred due to the disease or the need to seek medical care. Typical examples include cost of transportation to the hospital, home care, or special housing needed due to illness. Intangible costs are those of pain and suffering imposed by the disease and its treatment. These "costs" are difficult to value in monetary terms. Rather, they are reflected in measurements of the impact of interventions on quality of life. However, they influence health care decision-making. Intangible costs and benefits can be included in economic evaluations by using quality-adjusted life years (QALYs) as the effectiveness measure. The latter are calculated by assigning preference weights (or utilities) to various health states relative to perfect health or death.

The second dimension defines the viewpoint, or perspective, of the analysis to determine whose costs and benefits are to be evaluated. Economic analyses can be performed from the perspective of the health care provider, the payer, the employer, the patient, or the society at large. A cost from one point of view may be considered a benefit from another. For example, a hospital's cost of providing a particular service may be less than its charge. If the perspective of the analysis is the hospital, charges would be an overestimation of the actual costs. On the other hand, charges truly reflect the cost of the service if the patient (or the health insurance plan) is paying the full charge. An analysis that takes the society's perspective seeks to determine total costs to all parties. These include opportunity costs (e.g., forgone leisure time of informal careers) that are not easily measured in financial terms, which could have been used for an alternative intervention.

The third dimension defines the methodologic approach. The identification of costs and their measurement in monetary terms are similar across all forms of economic evaluation, but the valuations of consequences arising from alternatives being examined differ considerably. The different analytical approaches are described next.

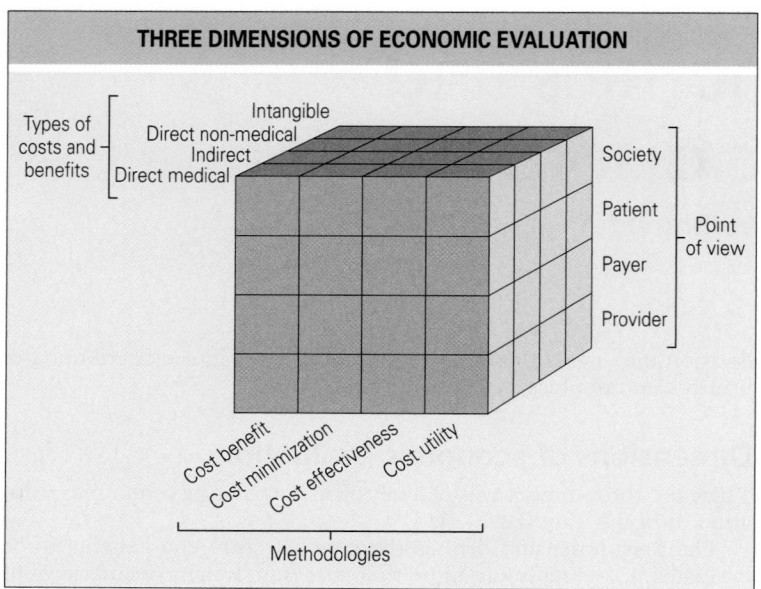

Fig. 3.1 Three dimensions of economic evaluation.

Design features in economic evaluation

An economic evaluation usually starts with identification of alternatives to be compared. For example, in Figure 3.2, the two alternatives considered are treatment strategy A, which may include the new drug(s) or combinations of interest, and treatment strategy B, the current standard of therapy. Treatment strategy B could also be "doing nothing" if no effective therapy currently exists for the disease in question. Once the alternatives are identified, there usually are four key data parameters needed for conducting any economic evaluation: (1) baseline clinical outcome probabilities without the new treatment strategy, (2) the effectiveness of the new treatment strategy in relation to these clinical outcomes, (3) the costs associated with the disease and therapy, and (4) the effect on quality of life in case of a cost-utility analysis.

Depending on the time horizon and the perspective of the analysis, the costs and consequences of the two treatment strategies or interventions are identified, quantified, and valued and the differences in costs are compared with the differences in consequences in an incremental analysis. Finally, various sensitivity analyses are performed to explore the lack of precision of estimates used in analysis. Values of costs and consequences are altered, and the impact of these changes is evaluated.

The time horizon of an analysis is the time over which costs and benefits are considered. It may be short for interventions whose costs and consequences occur immediately, although in most medical situations not all the costs and consequences occur at the same time. For example, preventive programs incur costs now but the benefits may not accrue for several years. Therefore, it is desirable to have a longer time horizon for interventions with long-term consequences and to

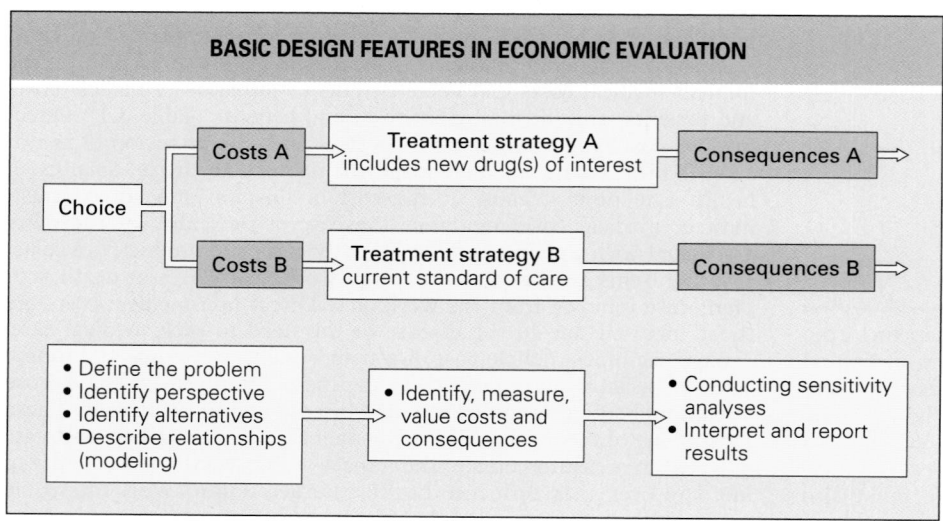

Fig. 3.2 Basic design features in economic evaluation. *(Adapted from Drummond MF, et al. Basic types of economic evaluation. In: Methods for the economic evaluation of health care programmes, 2nd ed. Oxford Medical Publications, Oxford, UK, 1997.)*

TABLE 3.1 TYPES OF COSTS AND BENEFITS CONSIDERED IN ECONOMIC EVALUATIONS

Type of cost or benefit	What is included as costs	What is included as benefits
Direct costs	*Medical:* Costs incurred during provision of medical care. Usually includes inpatient, outpatient, and nursing home care (e.g., physician's fees, salaries of allied health professionals, hospital charges, purchasing of drugs, supplies, equipment, diagnostic tests) *Non-medical:* Costs incurred because of illness or the need to seek medical care (e.g., costs of transportation to the hospital or physician's office, cost of special housing, cost of hotel stays, special clothing or food needed because of illness)	*Medical:* Savings (avoided costs) as a result of therapy (e.g., avoided physician visits and hospitalizations, avoided surgery) *Non-medical:* Costs avoided due to treatment or slowing of progression of illness as a result of therapy (e.g., avoided long-term care)
Indirect costs	Also referred to as *productivity* costs, they represent the costs associated with loss of ability to work or engage in leisure activities due to morbidity (e.g., time lost from work, loss of income, time of family members or volunteers to provide care) and lost economic productivity due to mortality (e.g., death leading to premature withdrawal from the workforce)	Indirect benefits represent reduction of indirect costs (e.g., continued employment, decreased absenteeism, early return to work)
Intangible costs	Costs incurred from changes in quality of life (e.g., pain, suffering, grief) and result from the illness itself or the services used to treat the illness	Improvement in quality of life as a result of the intervention or therapy (e.g., reduced pain, increased mobility)

TABLE 3.2 TYPES OF ECONOMIC ANALYSES

Methodology	Question addressed	Cost measurement unit	Outcome or effectiveness unit
Cost-benefit analysis	The effectiveness of two or more alternatives differs. What is the economic tradeoff between alternatives when all costs and outcomes are measured in monetary terms?	Dollars*	Dollars
Cost-effectiveness analysis	The effectiveness of two or more alternatives differs. What is the comparative cost per unit of outcome for different alternatives?	Dollars	Natural or clinical units (e.g., life-years gained, HAQ score, adverse events averted)
Cost-utility analysis	Same as for cost-effectiveness analysis. The outcome is a preference measure that reflects the value of patients or the society for the outcome.	Dollars	Quality-adjusted life-years or other utilities

*or other currency unit.

INCREMENTAL COST-EFFECTIVENESS RATIO

$$\text{Incremental cost-effectiveness ratio} = \frac{\text{Cost difference}}{\text{Effectiveness difference}} = \frac{\text{Cost of intervention} - \text{cost of alternative}}{\text{Effectiveness of intervention} - \text{effectiveness of alternative}}$$

Fig. 3.3 Incremental cost-effectiveness ratio.

discount future costs and consequences. Discounting adjusts future costs and consequences and allows expression of all in terms of their present value.[2]

Types of economic evaluation

Most authors describe three main economic evaluation methodologies (Table 3.2).[2,3] In addition to these methodologies, cost-minimization analyses can be done when the effectiveness of two or more alternatives or therapies is assumed to be, or shown to be, equal, although in practice such occasions are not very common. There is, however, substantial overlap between these methodologies.

Cost-benefit analysis

All costs and consequences of alternatives are given a financial or monetary value, and the analysis implicitly assumes that each alternative is being compared with a *do-nothing* alternative that entails no costs or benefits. The analysis aims to determine either the ratio of money spent to money saved or the net saving (assuming benefits greater than costs). An intervention is cost beneficial if the monetary value of the benefits outweighs the costs. Cost-benefit analysis can evaluate not only the cost-benefit ratios or net benefits of different alternatives but also the additional or *incremental* cost of an intervention compared with its additional or *incremental* benefit. The main difficulty in cost-benefit analysis is the measurement and valuation of clinical outcomes in monetary units.

Cost-effectiveness analysis

Cost-effectiveness analysis partially deals with the difficulty of assigning a monetary value to health outcomes. Costs are still calculated in monetary units, but effectiveness is determined independently using meaningful clinical terms such as number of lives saved, patients cured, or events prevented. It involves the comparison of alternatives with outcomes of the same type but different in magnitude or achieved to different degrees. It is used to compare variations of a single program, different interventions aimed at the same medical problem, or different programs for different medical problems, but with consequences of the same type. It determines the least cost method of meeting a particular objective.

Like cost-benefit analysis, cost-effectiveness analysis can evaluate not only the cost-effectiveness ratios for individual treatments but also the *incremental* cost-effectiveness of an intervention compared with an alternative (Fig. 3.3). The average cost-effectiveness ratio is calculated by dividing the cost of an intervention by the measure of effectiveness without regard to the alternatives. The incremental cost-effectiveness ratio is an estimate of the cost of per unit of effectiveness of using one alternative in preference to another. For decision-making purposes, the incremental cost-effectiveness ratio is the most relevant because it assesses the extra benefits gained from committing additional resources to a new therapy.

Alternative therapies that cost less and demonstrate equal or better outcomes are said to be *dominant* and should always be preferred. Therapies that are more costly and less effective are said to be *dominated* and should not be preferred. A new therapy that costs more but is also more effective is preferred if both the cost-effectiveness and the incremental cost-effectiveness ratios fall within an "acceptable" range. Acceptable cost-effectiveness thresholds have been proposed,[3] although what is an acceptable cost from one perspective or at one time may be unacceptable from another or at a later time.

Cost-utility analysis

Cost-utility analysis is similar to cost-effectiveness analysis, but the outcome of intervention is measured in terms of both quantity and quality of life. The results are usually expressed as cost per quality-adjusted life-years (QALYs) gained. The QALY is a combined measure of effectiveness that integrates expected increments in quantity of life with the effects on quality of life. It incorporates the preferences of society or patients for certain health states and their willingness to accept a shortening of life to avoid certain diseases or states. It is particularly desirable to use QALYs in rheumatic disorders because most interventions do not necessarily affect mortality but rather the physical, social, and psychological well-being of patients.

Cost-of-illness studies

In addition to these three types of economic evaluation, there are also *cost-of-illness* studies. These estimate the total societal cost of caring for patients with a particular illness compared with people without the illness. No consideration is made of specific interventions. All the direct and indirect costs of an illness are considered and the results provide a baseline against which new interventions can be evaluated.

Conclusion

In summary, economic analysis of a medical intervention or a therapeutic agent compares the monetary costs with the monetary benefits (cost-benefit analysis) or health-related outcomes (cost-effectiveness or cost-utility analyses). The perspective of the analysis determines which costs and benefits are to be taken into account. Direct costs are generated through provision of medical care, whereas indirect (or productivity) costs are considered if the medical intervention has an impact on morbidity and mortality.

Economic evaluation in drug development

The basic approach of economic assessment can be applied to all kinds of medical interventions, but it is particularly relevant to economic evaluation of therapeutic agents. Economic evaluation plays a key role in all phases of drug development—from phase 1 to phase 4 clinical studies. The objective of phase 1 clinical trials is to determine the toxicity profile of drugs in humans. The first phase 1 trials usually consist of administration of single, conservative doses to a small number of healthy volunteers. The effects of increasing the size and number of daily dosages are evaluated to determine the point at which the likely therapeutic dosage has been exceeded. Cost-of-illness studies are carried out during this stage to aid decisions on priority setting and whether to further develop the drug and to gather background data for future economic evaluations.

In phase 2 clinical trials, a drug is administered to limited number of patients with the target disease to explore its potential therapeutic benefit. At this stage, efficacy is still uncertain. Again, cost of illness studies help to determine the potential market for the drug and lay the groundwork for formal economic evaluations. In addition, some of the instruments for gathering economic and quality of life data may be piloted during this phase.

Related applications of phase 1 and phase 2 economic evaluations also include guidance of decisions to focus further development in specific indications or patient groups, strategic positioning in relation to competitors, and determination of optimal sample size and data elements to collect prospectively during the conduct of phase 3 studies.

Phase 3 studies involve large, often multicenter, randomized controlled clinical trials designed to determine efficacy. Such trials typically involve careful patient selection with clearly specified inclusion and exclusion criteria. At this stage of drug development, formal pharmacoeconomic evaluation is indicated to determine the cost-effectiveness of the new drug. Such evaluations are often conducted alongside the randomized controlled clinical trials and used commonly in reimbursement applications.[4-7]

During phase 4 or the postmarketing stage, data are gathered in support of the use of the drug in the community. Postmarketing economic evaluations are critically important, because they allow the study of the costs and consequences of drug therapy outside the strict constraints of controlled clinical trials. In other words, economic evaluations in phase 4 clinical trials address real-world costs, effectiveness, and cost-effectiveness issues, rather than simply the cost-efficacy of a new drug.

Economic data during several phases of drug development are either gathered prospectively as part of the trial protocol or retrospectively after a trial or through modeling using data from various sources.[8-10] However, there remain several methodologic issues that relate to the following:

1. *Atypical nature of trial settings*: Clinical trials are usually performed in specialist centers by highly committed investigators enrolling selected patients who have a higher likelihood of complying with therapy than patients in usual care. Also, patients in the trials are usually selected based on strict inclusion and exclusion criteria that would then limit generalizability of findings (e.g., exclusion of pregnant women, children, the very elderly).

2. *Protocol-driven costs and benefits*: Clinical trial protocols often include close monitoring of enrolled patients through prescheduled extra visits and tests. Protocol-defined testing for efficacy or safety purposes will increase the costs of diagnostic testing in the trial, whereas many of these tests would not be performed in usual care. Protocol-driven tests or procedures may also induce detection of extra cases or adverse events that would otherwise have gone undetected. In addition, detected outcomes may be treated more aggressively than they would be in usual care.

3. *Inappropriate clinical alternatives*: Trials usually compare the new therapy with a placebo or baseline therapy that may not represent the most appropriate alternative in current clinical practice.

4. *Inadequate length of follow-up*: Almost all trials use intermediate or surrogate endpoints such as disease progression or biomedical markers. Ideally, economic analysis should be based on final outcomes such as permanent work disability or mortality.

5. *Inadequate sample size for economic analysis:* Sample size calculations in trials are based on the clinical endpoints that may not be sufficient for highly skewed economic parameters (e.g., length of hospital stay, total cost).

6. *Inappropriate range of endpoints for both costs and consequences*: Ideally, economic analyses require data on resource use and outcomes of direct relevance to patients (e.g., quality of life).

Despite these methodologic problems, clinical trials are still viewed as an appropriate vehicle for economic analysis of drugs. Several methods are currently being investigated to overcome these problems.[6-12] Large and simple outcome trials (pragmatic trials) deal with some of these issues, but they are very expensive to conduct and can only be done in late phase 3 or 4 time frame once the efficacy has been established. With the availability of an extended portfolio of new drugs in treatment of many rheumatic diseases, the focus in recent years has evolved from a simple comparison of single drugs or even drug combinations to comparative effectiveness and cost-effectiveness of alternative treatment strategies over the entire life course of rheumatic diseases. Such an approach considers not only single drugs but also drug combinations and the sequencing and duration of therapy over time. To realize this complex goal, clinical trial–based economic evaluations will be increasingly complemented with utilization and effectiveness data from observational studies and registries.

The reference case

Until the mid 1990s, economic evaluations varied considerably in quality. Regulatory authorities of some countries have established guidelines[10,13-17] to improve comparability. In 1996, the U.S. Public Health Service appointed a panel on Cost-Effectiveness Analysis in Health and Medicine that proposed a "reference case" set of methodologic practices to improve quality and comparability of economic analyses.[18,19] The panel recommended a set of minimum criteria that all analyses should include to allow comparability across studies. Investigators are, however, encouraged to go beyond these minimum criteria in their individual studies.

This reference case analysis, based on a standard set of rules, facilitates comparisons with other similar analyses. It is based on the societal perspective and thus requires that the analysis considers all health consequences and all changes in resource use over a reasonably long time frame. The analysis should compare the new intervention to the existing practice or the best available alternative. It is also recommended that results be presented as incremental, that is, the additional costs incurred, to obtain each additional unit of health (e.g., a QALY).

The panel also outlined all major categories of resource use and health effects to be considered in the numerator and denominator of the cost-effectiveness ratio. The QALY is recommended as a common effect of health measure. Costs and outcomes are recommended to be discounted to present value, and extensive sensitivity analyses are recommended to address uncertainties of estimates and the decision model structure.

APPLICATION TO RHEUMATIC DISEASES

There are many published economic evaluations in rheumatology. However, evaluations, especially those conducted prior to 2000, vary considerably in their methodology and very few comply with the internationally agreed on criteria. This lack of agreement in methods, in turn, limits their validity, usability, and comparability. The methodologic quality and major findings of some of these studies have been reviewed in a number of publications.[20-35]

Source of evaluations

The majority of economic evaluations in rheumatology are conducted in the United States, United Kingdom, and Canada. This is partially due to availability of easily accessible data sources, requirements set by the regulatory bodies, as well as publication of these studies mostly in indexed medical journals in English. It needs to be realized, however, that there are several unpublished* economic evaluations in rheumatic diseases that had been used extensively in decision-making by several parties, including the regulatory authorities.

Therapeutic areas

By far, the most common disease areas for economic evaluations are osteoarthritis and rheumatoid arthritis; and the most common interventions evaluated are prevention of non-steroidal anti-inflammatory drug–induced upper gastrointestinal ulcers and the cost-effectiveness of biologic agents. Osteoporosis is another commonly evaluated disease area. Here, the published economic evaluations mainly focus on the value of various treatment strategies for prevention of osteoporotic fractures and cost-effectiveness of screening strategies in different risk populations. By contrast, there are only a few studies evaluating diagnostic or therapeutic options in common syndromes such as low back pain or the value of preventive or primary care based interventions in the management of rheumatic diseases.

Types of evaluations

Almost all of the economic evaluations in osteoarthritis, rheumatoid arthritis, and osteoporosis are cost-effectiveness or cost-utility analyses with relatively few cost-benefit analyses and thus show the typical spectrum of the economic evaluations in health care. Effectiveness outcomes in cost-effectiveness studies are expressed in clinical terms as the cost of per clinical event avoided or years of life saved (e.g., cost per gastrointestinal ulcer avoided).

Cost-utility analyses report costs per QALYs gained or costs per unit change on certain quality of life scales that combine information on the quantity and quality of life. To calculate QALY, health state utility values are estimated by incorporating preference weights using the commonly used outcome measures in rheumatoid arthritis (Health Assessment Questionnaire [HAQ], Disease Activity Score [DAS], and American College of Rheumatology core response criteria).[36,37] Some cost-utility analyses use directly elicited preferences from patients collected prospectively during the conduct of clinical trials, whereas others use utility weights derived either from the published literature or from expert opinions.

Sources of information

Economic evaluations typically rely on utilization and effectiveness data obtained from a variety of different sources. Earlier economic evaluations in rheumatology tended to rely on the opinion of clinicians in the absence of data, but this has changed dramatically during the past decade. Randomized controlled clinical trials, observational studies, meta-analyses, registries, and administrative databases are currently the most commonly used sources for utilization and effectiveness data. Valuation of resources (or costs) is mainly derived from administrative data sources. True cost data are rarely available and, therefore, the majority of the studies still use market prices such as fee schedules, average payment, charges, and diagnosis-related group reimbursement rates for schemes such as Medicare in the United States to estimate costs.

The analysis perspective is mostly the societal or the third-party payer perspective. The consideration of various relevant cost categories is inconsistent across the majority of the studies. Whereas all studies examined direct medical costs, only a few also examined direct non-medical and/or productivity costs. Differences in cost categories may result in substantial differences in cost-effectiveness estimates.[38] The analysis time frame is typically short in the majority of the evaluations, with only about one fourth of the evaluations considering a lifetime time frame.

Sensitivity analyses

Not all studies include sensitivity analyses or other approaches to allow for uncertainty in estimates. One-way sensitivity analyses are conducted in at least half of the studies, whereas probabilistic sensitivity analyses are rare. Economic evaluations, especially for biologic agents, increasingly rely on modeling techniques to adapt findings to different settings or to extrapolate costs and benefits beyond the time period for which data are available. These models are analytically very complex, with consideration of several treatment regimens, disease stages and health states, treatment periods, compliance and safety outcomes, and sequencing of treatments. Structural features of these models and input parameters can be difficult to tease out and, yet, can significantly impact cost-effectiveness findings.[38]

Evaluation of surgical interventions

Additionally, since the mid 1990s, economic evaluations firmly established the value of total hip and/or knee arthroplasty in patients with arthritis. Cost-effectiveness and cost-utility evaluations in arthroplasty include studies that assess overall cost-effectiveness of primary and revision arthroplasty, comparison of different surgical techniques and prostheses types, antithrombotic and infection prophylaxis, different management and rehabilitation schemes, hospital volume and experience, and interventions to reduce hospital stays and recovery. A 2005 review of cost-utility analyses in arthroplasty[33] highlighted the limitations of cost-utility analyses in orthopedics and concluded that there is limited evidence currently to guide policy in orthopedic practice. One of the main limitations is lack of long-term effectiveness data and, consequently, heavy reliance on assumptions about the effectiveness of alternative strategies. For example, guidelines published by National Institute for Clinical Excellence (NICE) in 2000[39] could not identify the most cost-effective type of prosthesis and concluded that there is "currently more evidence of the long term viability of cemented prostheses, which, in many cases, occupy the lower end of the range of prostheses cost, than there is for uncemented and hybrid prosthesis." It is hoped that the quality, generalizability, and applicability of economic evaluations in arthroplasty will improve with availability of long-term effectiveness data from observational studies and registries.

Conclusion

In conclusion, the science of economic evaluation in rheumatology has developed considerably in recent years but the long-term comparative effectiveness and cost-effectiveness of new therapies, different treatment strategies, and devices are still unclear. In addition, economic evaluations on diagnostic or therapeutic options in common syndromes such as low back pain or the value of primary care based interventions in management of rheumatic diseases are still lacking. There are a number of reasons for this, including the biased selection of comparators, inconsistent use of methodologies across studies, continuing controversy regarding defining meaningful clinical outcomes, lack of identifying optimal sources of effectiveness and utility estimates, lack of long-term comparative effectiveness data, and difficulty in determining the role of mathematical modeling and measuring and incorporating compliance and toxicity. Observational data derived from large cohorts, disease registries, and claims databases are valuable sources of real-world effectiveness data and will be increasingly used in the future for assessing long-term effectiveness of different treatment strategies. Furthermore, emerging methodologic standards for economic evaluations[9,40] would improve the quality of studies, increase comparability across studies, and lead to identification of priorities for methodologic research. Such standards could serve as educational tools and should lead to increased use of such studies in health care decision-making. Indeed, efforts, such as the Economic Evaluation Task Force of the Outcome Measures in Rheumatoid Arthritis Clinical Trials (OMERACT)[41-47] will expedite and enhance both the conduct of the methodologic research itself and, subsequently, the transfer of the results into policy and practice.

---

*Although unpublished in searchable data sources such as PubMed, they may have been published in "grey literature."

THE FUTURE OF ECONOMIC EVALUATION IN THE RHEUMATIC DISEASES

There is no doubt that economic evaluations in health care, including rheumatic diseases, will become increasingly important in the future. There are a number of important reasons for this. First, an increasing number of licensing and reimbursement authorities now require comparative effectiveness and cost-effectiveness data in addition to the usual clinical efficacy data before approval of new drugs.[48] Second, the pharmaceutical industry will use economic arguments more in the future in promotion of their products to the medical professionals and consumers. Third, health care payers will increasingly justify funding (or not funding) certain drugs or interventions in terms of effectiveness and cost-effectiveness. Fourth, the majority of rheumatic diseases are chronic, causing significant disability to patients during their most productive years, and the economic burden to the society is disproportional to their relatively low prevalence. With disability and lost productivity being the major determinants of costs, especially in patients with rheumatoid arthritis, all future therapies will be expected to show economic advantage by delaying onset of disability. Fifth, treatment strategies and the range of available therapeutic options have evolved considerably in recent years. With the expansion of therapeutic possibilities, the choice of rational long-term therapies will increasingly depend on comparative effectiveness, costs weighed against the societal and personal expense of disability, decreased quality of life, and the burden of inpatient and outpatient medical care. In such an environment, it is critically important for clinicians to grasp the basic principles of economic evaluations and actively engage in the debates, the discussions, and the research in an effort to optimize care for patients with rheumatic disease.

REFERENCES

1. Bootman J, Townsend P, McGhan W. Introduction to pharmacoeconomics. In: Principles of pharmacoeconomics, 2nd ed. Harvey Whitney Books, Cincinnati, OH, 1996.
2. Drummond M, O'Brien B, Stoddart G, Torrance G. Basic types of economic evaluation. In: Methods for the economic evaluation of health care programmes, 2nd ed. Oxford Medical Publications, Oxford, UK, 1997.
3. Laupacis A, Sackett DL, Roberts RS. An assessment of clinically useful measures of the consequences of treatment. N Engl J Med 1988;318:1728-1733.
4. Drummond MF, Davies L. Economic analysis alongside clinical trials: revisiting the methodological issues. Int J Technol Assess Health Care 1991;7:561-573.
5. Drummond M, O'Brien B. Economic analysis alongside clinical trials: practical considerations. The Economics Workgroup. J Rheumatol 1995;22:1418-1419.
6. Drummond M. Introducing economic and quality of life measurements into clinical studies. Ann Med 2001;33:344-349.
7. O'Sullivan AK, Thompson D, Drummond MF. Collection of health-economic data alongside clinical trials: is there a future for piggyback evaluations? Value Health 2005;8:67-79.
8. Munin MC, Rudy TE, Glynn NW, et al. Early inpatient rehabilitation after elective hip and knee arthroplasty. JAMA 1998;279:847-852.
9. Weinstein MC, O'Brien B, Hornberger J, et al. Principles of good practice for decision analytic modeling in health-care evaluation: report of the ISPOR Task Force on Good Research Practices—Modeling Studies. Value Health 2003;6:9-17.
10. Ramsey S, Willke R, Briggs A, et al. Good research practices for cost-effectiveness analysis alongside clinical trials: the ISPOR RCT-CEA Task Force report. Value Health 2005;8:521-533.
11. Garrison LP Jr, Neumann PJ, Erickson P, et al. Using real-world data for coverage and payment decisions: the ISPOR Real-World Data Task Force report. Value Health 2007;10:326-335.
12. Manca A, Lambert PC, Sculpher M, Rice N. Cost-effectiveness analysis using data from multinational trials: the use of bivariate hierarchical modeling. Med Decis Making 2007;27:471-490.
13. Guide to the Methods of Technology Appraisal. London: National Institute for Clinical Excellence (NICE), 2004.
14. Canadian Coordinating Office for Health Technology Assessment (CCOHTA). Guidelines for economic evaluation of pharmaceuticals, 2nd ed. Ottawa: CCOHTA, 1997.
15. Drummond M, Dubois D, Garattini L, et al. Current trends in the use of pharmacoeconomics and outcomes research in Europe. Value Health 1999;2:323-332.
16. Hjelmgren J, Berggren F, Andersson F. Health economic guidelines—similarities, differences and some implications [see comment]. Value Health 2001;4:225-250.
17. Murray CJ, Evans DB, Acharya A, Baltussen RM. Development of WHO guidelines on generalized cost-effectiveness analysis. Health Econ 2000;9:235-251.
18. Gold MR, Siegel JE, Russell LB, Weinstein MC. Cost-effectiveness in health and medicine. Vol II. New York: Oxford University Press, 1996.
19. Siegel JE, Torrance GW, Russell LB, et al. Guidelines for pharmacoeconomic studies: recommendations from the panel on cost effectiveness in health and medicine. Panel on Cost Effectiveness in Health and Medicine. Pharmacoeconomics 1997;11:159-168.
20. Ferraz MB, Maetzel A, Bombardier C. A summary of economic evaluations published in the field of rheumatology and related disciplines. Arthritis Rheum 1997;40:1587-1593.
21. Maetzel A, Ferraz MB, Bombardier C. A review of cost-effectiveness analyses in rheumatology and related disciplines. Curr Opin Rheumatol 1998;10:136-140.
22. Rothfuss J, Mau W, Zeidler H, Brenner MH. Socioeconomic evaluation of rheumatoid arthritis and osteoarthritis: a literature review. Semin Arthritis Rheum 1997;26:771-779.
23. Ruchlin HS, Elkin EB, Paget SA. Assessing cost-effectiveness analyses in rheumatoid arthritis and osteoarthritis. Arthritis Care Res 1997;10:413-421.
24. Cranney A, Coyle D, Welch V, et al. A review of economic evaluation in osteoporosis. Arthritis Care Res 1999;12:425-434.
25. Maetzel A. Cost-effectiveness estimates reported for tumor necrosis factor blocking agents in rheumatoid arthritis refractory to methotrexate—a brief summary. J Rheumatol Suppl 2005;72:51-53.
26. Tella MN, Feinglass J, Chang RW. Cost-effectiveness, cost-utility, and cost-benefit studies in rheumatology: a review of the literature, 2001-2002. Curr Opin Rheumatol 2003;15:127-131.
27. Baldwin ML, Cote P, Frank JW, Johnson WG. Cost-effectiveness studies of medical and chiropractic care for occupational low back pain: a critical review of the literature. Spine J 2001;1:138-147.
28. Kobelt G, Andlin-Sobocki P, Maksymowych WP. The cost-effectiveness of infliximab (Remicade) in the treatment of ankylosing spondylitis in Canada. J Rheumatol 2006;33:732-740.
29. Kobelt G, Sobocki P, Sieper J, Braun J. Comparison of the cost-effectiveness of infliximab in the treatment of ankylosing spondylitis in the United Kingdom based on two different clinical trials. Int J Technol Assess Health Care 2007;23:368-375.
30. Fleurence R, Spackman E. Cost-effectiveness of biologic agents for treatment of autoimmune disorders: structured review of the literature. J Rheumatol 2006;33:2124-2131.
31. Chen YF, Jobanputra P, Barton P, et al. A systematic review of the effectiveness of adalimumab, etanercept and infliximab for the treatment of rheumatoid arthritis in adults and an economic evaluation of their cost-effectiveness. Health Technol Assess 2006;10:iii-iv, xi-xiii, 1-229.
32. Doan QV, Chiou CF, Dubois RW. Review of eight pharmacoeconomic studies of the value of biologic DMARDs (adalimumab, etanercept, and infliximab) in the management of rheumatoid arthritis. J Manag Care Pharm 2006;12:555-569.
33. Brauer CA, Rosen AB, Olchanski NV, Neumann PJ. Cost-utility analyses in orthopaedic surgery. J Bone Joint Surg Am 2005;87:1253-1259.
34. Fleurence RL, Iglesias CP, Torgerson DJ. Economic evaluations of interventions for the prevention and treatment of osteoporosis: a structured review of the literature. Osteoporos Int 2006;17:29-40.
35. Zethraeus N, Borgström F, Ström O, et al. Cost-effectiveness of the treatment and prevention of osteoporosis—a review of the literature and a reference model. Osteoporos Int 2007;18:9-23.
36. Bansback N, Ara R, Karnon J, Anis A. Economic evaluations in rheumatoid arthritis: a critical review of measures used to define health states. Pharmacoeconomics 2008;26:395-408.
37. Bansback N, Harrison M, Brazier J, et al. Health state utility values: a description of their development and application for rheumatic diseases. Arthritis Rheum 2008;59:1018-1026.
38. Drummond MF, Barbieri M, Wong JB. Analytic choices in economic models of treatments for rheumatoid arthritis: what makes a difference? Med Decis Making 2005;25:520-533.
39. National Institute for Health and Clinical Excellence. Guidance on the selection of prostheses for primary total hip replacement. National Institute for Clinical Excellence. http://www.nice.org.uk/nicemedia/pdf/Guidance_on_the_selection_of_hip_prostheses.pdf 2000.
40. Philips Z, Bojke L, Sculpher M, et al. Good practice guidelines for decision-analytic modelling in health technology assessment: a review and consolidation of quality assessment. Pharmacoeconomics 2006;24:355-371.
41. Gabriel S, Tugwell P, O'Brien B, et al. Report of the OMERACT task force on economic evaluation. Outcome Measures in Rheumatology. J Rheumatol 1999;26:203-206.
42. Gabriel SE, Drummond MF, Coyle D, et al. OMERACT 5—Economics working group: summary, recommendations, and research agenda. J Rheumatol 2001;28:670-673.
43. Gabriel SE, Tugwell P, Drummond M. Progress towards an OMERACT-ILAR guideline for economic evaluations in rheumatology. Ann Rheum Dis 2002;61:370-373.
44. Drummond M, Maetzel A, Gabriel S, March L. Towards a reference case for use in future economic evaluations of interventions in osteoarthritis. J Rheumatol Suppl 2003;68:26-30.
45. Maetzel A, Tugwell P, Boers M, et al. Economic evaluation of programs or interventions in the management of rheumatoid arthritis: defining a consensus-based reference case. J Rheumatol 2003;30:891-896.
46. Coyle D, Tosteson AN. Towards a reference case for economic evaluation of osteoporosis treatments. J Rheumatol Suppl 2003;68:31-36.
47. Bansback N, Maetzel A, Drummond M, et al. Considerations and preliminary proposals for defining a reference case for economic evaluations in ankylosing spondylitis. J Rheumatol 2007;34:1178-1183.
48. Suarez-Almazor ME, Drummond M. Regulatory issues and economic efficiency. J Rheumatol Suppl 2003;68:5-7.

REFERENCES

Full references for this chapter can be found on www.expertconsult.com.

Biomechanics of the spine

Michael A. Adams and Patricia Dolan

4

- Genes and environment contribute equally to the strength of spinal tissues.
- Moderate mechanical loading strengthens vertebrae and (eventually) intervertebral discs.
- Muscle forces acting on the spine usually exceed gravitational forces, and inertial forces arising during falls are often the greatest of all.
- Intervertebral discs and vertebral bodies resist spinal compression, with the fluid properties of the disc nucleus spreading compressive load evenly on the vertebral bodies in all postures.
- Neural arches protect the intervertebral discs (and spinal cord) from shear, torsion, and bending.
- Intervertebral ligaments limit bending movements but are mostly slack in upright postures so that the spine can move freely within its "neutral zone."
- Compressive overload damages the vertebral body, decompresses the adjacent disc, and can lead to internal disc disruption.
- Combined loading in bending and compression can create radial fissures in the disc anulus and cause disc prolapse, even in macroscopically normal discs.
- Injury to the disc anulus or endplate alters the mechanical environment of disc cells, creating a vicious cycle of matrix weakening, re-injury, and frustrated healing.
- Loss of anulus height can initiate a "degenerative cascade" involving segmental instability, vertebral osteophytosis, and apophyseal joint osteoarthritis.
- In the elderly, vertebral strength depends on physical activity as well as hormonal changes, and fracture patterns depend on disc degeneration.

INTRODUCTION

Relevance of biomechanics

Back pain and spinal deformity are largely attributable to age-related degenerative conditions that are influenced strongly by genetic inheritance. Clinical prognosis depends on psychosocial factors that influence all aspects of human behavior, including the reporting of pain and responses to treatment. The old "injury model" of back pain has been replaced by the *biopsychosocial model*,[1] which recognizes all of the diverse influences in this complex problem. This does not mean, however, that mechanical influences can be disregarded. *Biomechanics* implies an integration between biologic and mechanical influences. As will be discussed later, mechanical loading can make spinal tissues stronger or initiate degenerative changes within them, and genes influence mechanical characteristics as much as biologic ones. There is no reason to doubt that spinal disorders have a real physical basis that needs to be understood if spinal problems are to be avoided or treated successfully. Psychosocial involvement in spinal disorders may represent little more than normal human reactions to unsympathetic or ineffective treatment.

Genes versus environment

Heritability represents that proportion of the variance in "who gets a disease" that can be explained by genetic inheritance, and recent heritability estimates for disc degeneration and vertebral osteoporosis have been reported to be as high as 75%[2] and 83%,[3] respectively. This appears to leave little room for environmental influences such as mechanical loading. However, heritability values depend very much on details of the study. Heritability is high if the population studied is homogeneous for competing environmental influences or if the trait is defined in such a manner that it is biased toward genetic (or other constitutional) factors. For example, heritability of lumbar disc degeneration is 75% if middle-aged women are considered and if degeneration is averaged over all lumbar discs,[2] but heritability falls to 29% in a diverse population of men if the most severe change in a single disc is considered. Similar arguments can be applied to vertebral osteoporosis. A balanced view suggests that genes and environment contribute in approximately equal measure to disc degeneration and spinal osteoporosis; and of the environmental influences, mechanical loading is the best documented and most easily modified. Also, of course, the genetic component includes inherited influences on mechanical factors such as body weight and muscle strength.[3]

Adaptation versus injury

It is simplistic to suppose that mechanical loading is always harmful to the spine, the *injury model*. On the contrary, mechanical loading makes bones stiff and strong according to the principles of adaptive remodeling[4] and there is evidence that articular cartilage[5] and intervertebral discs[6] can also become mechanically conditioned, given enough time. Disc water content *increases* with body mass and muscle strength, suggesting a positive adaptive response to moderate loading.[7] Evidently it is not mechanical loading that should be avoided but mechanical *overload*, which physically disrupts tissues. Epidemiologic studies of the role of occupational loading in spinal pathology and pain usually fail to make this distinction and thus underestimate the influence of mechanical overload on spinal health. Such studies, especially when cross sectional in design, are prone to the "healthy worker effect" (whereby those with back pain move to less arduous occupations leaving only healthy workers behind them[8]), diluting the evidence from cross-sectional surveys that severe loading can injure backs. From a biomechanics standpoint, moderate spinal loading should be encouraged, whereas the risk of severe loading and accidents should be minimized. In the words of Nietzsche: "What does not kill him makes him stronger."

The purpose of the present chapter is not to revive the *injury model*, but to analyze mechanical *influences* in spinal disorders, such as intervertebral disc degeneration, disc prolapse, spinal osteoporosis, and whiplash.

FORCES ACTING ON THE SPINE

Types of loading

The types of loading applied to the spine are illustrated in Figure 4.1. *Compressive* forces are usually defined as those that act down the long axis of the spine, at right angles to the midplane of the intervertebral discs. The curvature of the spine ensures that the direction of the compressive force varies between spinal levels, and this is consistent with the origins of this force, which is primarily tension in the paraspinal muscles. *Shear* acts at right angles to the compressive force and causes vertebrae to slide forward, backward, or sideways relative to adjacent vertebrae. *Bending* moments (measured as a force multiplied by a lever arm, with units in Newton metres [Nm]) cause the spine to bend, usually relative to centers of rotation within each intervertebral disc. *Torsional* moments, or torques, have the same units as bending moment and cause the spine to twist about its long axis (axial rotation).

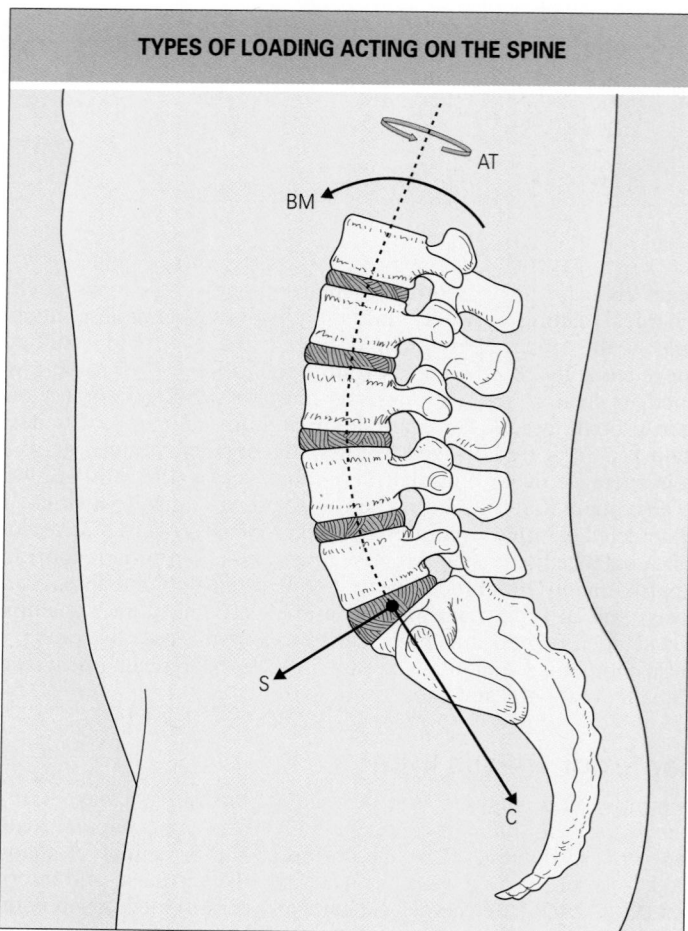

TYPES OF LOADING ACTING ON THE SPINE

Fig. 4.1 The lumbar spine, showing the directions of compressive (C) and shear (S) forces acting on the lumbosacral disc. Spinal compression acts perpendicular to the midplane of the disc, and so its direction varies with spinal level. A bending moment (BM) causes the spine to bend in flexion, extension, or lateral bending. An axial torque (AT) causes axial rotation about the long axis of the spine. (*Reproduced with permission from Adams MA, Bogduk N, Burton K, Dolan P. The biomechanics of back pain, 2nd ed. Edinburgh: Churchill Livingstone, 2006.*)

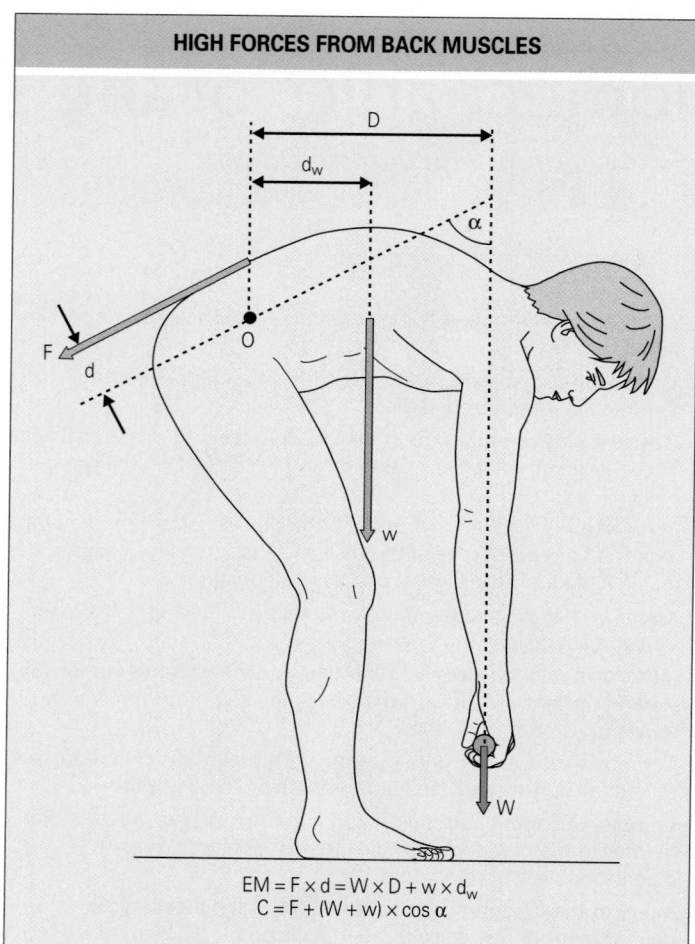

HIGH FORCES FROM BACK MUSCLES

$$EM = F \times d = W \times D + w \times d_w$$
$$C = F + (W + w) \times \cos \alpha$$

Fig. 4.2 During manual handling, a high tensile force (F) must be created by the back muscles to generate an extensor moment (EM) large enough to lift up an external weight (W) and the weight of the upper body (w). Back muscles act on a short internal lever arm (d) compared with the long lever arms (D, d_w) of the objects being lifted. In practice, the muscle force F is often much greater than the weight being lifted, so that the compressive force acting on the spine (C) rises to approximately 500 kg when a weight of 20 kg is lifted. (*Reproduced with permission from Adams MA, Bogduk N, Burton K, Dolan P. The biomechanics of back pain, 2nd ed. Edinburgh: Churchill Livingstone, 2006.*)

Gravitational forces

Gravity exerts a vertical force on each body segment, which is known as its weight. This varies considerably by vertebral level, ranging from approximately 55% of whole-body weight acting at the fifth lumbar vertebral level compared with 7% acting on the first cervical vertebral level. These forces are generally only a small proportion of the total force acting on the spine during vigorous activity.

Inertial or dynamic forces

When a body segment is accelerated or decelerated, the force acting on it is amplified according to Newton's second law of motion:

$$\text{Force} = \text{mass} \times \text{acceleration}$$

Weight can be seen as the special case, when acceleration equals 1 g. Exceptionally high accelerations occur when the human body is ejected from an aircraft, and the compressive force on the lumbar spine can be enough to cause vertebral fracture. More typically, the human body is subjected to high decelerations during falls, especially from a considerable height when the velocity is high just before impact and when the surface is hard so that the velocity is brought to zero in a very short time. Prevention of slips and falls is a prime goal of ergonomics and is probably more important than limiting the maximum weights to be lifted during manual handling.

Muscle forces

Tension in a contracting muscle compresses the bones that lie between the muscle's tendinous insertions. Muscle forces are hidden in the sense that they are internal to the body, but they often reach high levels for the reason illustrated in Figure 4.2. Essentially, muscles act on short internal lever arms and so must exert forces that are several times greater than external loads that often act on much greater lever arms. Often, the external load is dominated by the weight of the upper body, which is why lifting a trivial object (e.g., a pen) from the floor can generate a peak tensile force in the back muscles of over 200 kg![9] This force acts to compress the spine. (Approximately 1 kg = 2.2 lb = 9.81 N.) The highest forces tend to be generated when muscles are accelerating or decelerating body segments, especially during eccentric contractions when the collagenous tissue within muscle is being stretched. This is why forward lunging movements during racquet sports, or during manual handling, so often injure the back. The need to stabilize the body or head in a moving or vibrating environment often requires high levels of co-contraction of the paraspinal and abdominal muscles.

There are a number of practical implications of high muscle forces. In the medicolegal arena, many clinicians underestimate or disregard muscle forces, supposing (quite wrongly) that forces on the spine or neck must be low when external loads are light. A stark warning of the potential danger of muscle contractions comes from the finding that epileptic fits can cause the back muscles to crush vertebrae even when no falls are involved.[10]

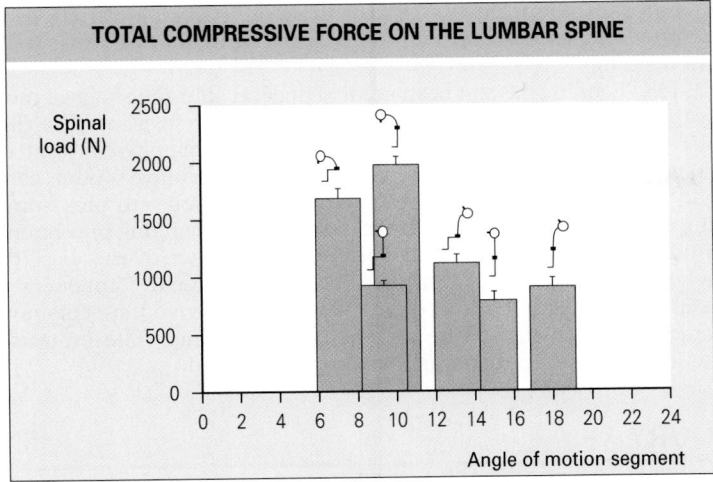

Fig. 4.3 The compressive force acting on the lumbar spine increases to 2000 N (approximately 200 kg) in stooped standing postures. Forces were calculated from pressure in the L4-5 intervertebral disc nucleus, measured in vivo by a miniature pressure transducer. "Angle of motion segment" refers to the relative orientation of the upper and lower endplates of the L4-5 disc. *(Reproduced with permission from Sato K, Kikuchi S, Yonezawa T. In vivo intradiscal pressure measurement in healthy individuals and in patients with ongoing back problems. Spine 1999;24:2468-2474.)*

Intra-abdominal pressure

People struggling to lift a heavy weight usually hold their breath and go red in the face, indicating a common but often unwitting strategy to stabilize the spine and protect it from high forces. Contracting trunk muscles generates a high pressure in the abdominal cavity, which can then transmit a compressive force directly from the thoracic spine and ribs to the pelvis, bypassing the lumbar spine. The mechanism is undoubtedly of benefit but is difficult to quantify because tension in some abdominal muscles acts to compress the spine further. However, raising the intra-abdominal pressure appears to be most beneficial when the spine is flexed, when a thick belt is worn to provide lateral support to the abdomen,[11] and when the pressure is raised primarily by contraction of transversus abdominis (which does not compress the spine).

Overall compressive loading of the spine

The total compressive force acting on the spine of a living volunteer can be measured by inserting a pressure-sensitive needle into an intervertebral disc. Hydrostatic pressure measured in the disc nucleus can then be converted to compressive force by multiplying by disc area, or by calibrating the transducer in cadaveric spines. The average compressive force on the L4-5 disc of healthy subjects (average body weight, 73 kg) ranges from 14 kg when lying prone to over 200 kg in the stooped standing position, as shown in Figure 4.3.[12] Evidently, muscle tension can greatly exceed the weight of the upper body. Relaxed sitting increases spinal compression compared with standing because sitting flexes the lower lumbar spine, generating additional tension in the posterior ligaments, whereas a lordotic standing posture causes some of the compressive force to be resisted by the neural arch.[13]

Diurnal variation

There is an interesting diurnal variation in the forces acting on the spine. In the early morning, discs are swollen with water, so the anulus and intervertebral ligaments resist bending strongly and are most vulnerable to injury. As the day progresses, discs lose 20% of their water and height, so the spine becomes more supple. However, the neural arches then resist more of the compressive force on the spine.[13] These diurnal changes explain why backache often increases after several hours of standing and why recurrent back pain can be reduced by avoiding flexion movements during the early morning.[14]

Measurement of forces

Pressure transducers cannot be used safely when the spine is moved rapidly and forcefully. During manual handling, spine compression can be quantified from the electromyographic (EMG) signal recorded from the skin surface of the back. EMG signals are calibrated against moments and forces generated during isometric exertions and then used to calculate muscle forces acting on the spine during vigorous movements. Peak compressive forces on the lumbar spine vary between 250 and 500 kg when lifting objects weighing up to 30 kg from the floor. Rapid lifts increase peak loading by more than 60% compared with slow lifts,[9] and forces of this magnitude can cause fatigue ("wear and tear") damage to accumulate in some spines.[9] Similar peak forces are reported by mathematical models that calculate spinal loading from optical measurements of the movements and accelerations of various body parts.[15]

Shear forces and torques have not been measured reliably *in vivo*, but mathematical models show that peak anterior shear forces reach 150 to 200 kg in the lower lumbar spine when heavy weights are lifted.[15] Much of this force can be resisted by the back muscles.

Peak bending moments acting on the spine can be estimated by measuring the moment required to bend a cadaveric spine to the same angle as the spine of a living person. The technique has been used to show that bending moments on the lumbar spine rise to 10 to 25 Nm during heavy lifting.[9] Cadaveric spines can be flexed more than this before they are damaged, so, in life, back muscles must normally protect the spine from excessive flexion. Protective muscle reflexes have been demonstrated in animals and humans, but they can be impaired if the spine is flexed repeatedly or for periods of an hour or more.[16] This could be why activities such as gardening and long-distance driving are often associated with back pain.

MECHANICAL FUNCTION

Spinal curvature

Cervical lordosis appears when infants first lift their heads up, and lumbar lordosis develops when walking begins. Thoracic kyphosis appears to be a compensatory mechanism to maintain a level line of sight and to increase volume of the thoracic cavity. Spinal curves probably play a shock-absorbing role during locomotion, because the natural tendency for the curves to flatten and accentuate as the body rises and falls is resisted by the muscles of the trunk. The tendons of these muscles have a great capacity to store strain energy (which is proportional to the tension multiplied by the stretch) so that the tendons of paraspinal muscles are able to act like shock absorbers, minimizing vertical accelerations of the head.[13] A similar mechanism allows the quadriceps tendons to absorb strain energy when the knees are flexed to soften the landing from a jump.

Spinal movements

Intervertebral movements in living people combine angular rotations with small gliding movements (*translation*) in the plane of the disc. Angular rotations involve stretching and compressing the disc anulus in such a manner that the center of rotation (the theoretical pivot point) moves around within the disc nucleus. The oblique surfaces of the apophyseal and uncovertebral joints ensure that certain movements are mechanically coupled: for example, attempted lateral bending normally creates a small axial rotation as well. The cervical spine is the most mobile region, because cervical intervertebral discs are relatively thick compared with the height of adjacent vertebral bodies. Conversely, the thoracic spine is the least mobile because its discs are narrow and because movements are inhibited by ribs and dipping spinous processes. Mobility of the lumbar spine declines by approximately 50% between the ages of 16 and 85 years.[17] This is partly due to disc narrowing, which brings the neural arches of adjacent vertebrae closer together and causes the center of rotation for flexion and extension to migrate posteriorly toward the apophyseal joints.

Intervertebral disc mechanics

The central region of an intervertebral disc, the nucleus pulposus, has such a high water content that it normally behaves like a pressurized fluid, spreading a compressive load evenly on the adjacent vertebral bodies[18] even when the vertebrae are angled in flexion or extension. The layers (lamellae) of the anulus fibrosus act in tension to retain this pressurized nucleus, but the adult human anulus is sufficiently fibrous to resist direct compressive loading as well. The internal mechanical functioning of loaded cadaveric lumbar discs has been investigated by pulling a needle-mounted pressure transducer along their midsagittal diameter: resulting "pressure profiles" are shown in Figure 4.5. The size of the fluid-like region, and the pressure within it, both decrease with age, whereas the direct compressive stress resisted by the anulus increases.[18] Cervical discs are more fibrous than lumbar discs and have a thinner posterior annulus, but they behave in essentially the same way.[19]

Resistance to compression

Compressive loading of the spine is mostly resisted by the discs and vertebral bodies. As the compressive force increases, the disc anulus bulges radially outward and the vertebral endplates bulge vertically into the vertebral bodies.[20] Energy ("shock") absorption by a deformed object is proportional to height change, so the relatively high stiffness of intervertebral discs and vertebral endplates (compared with tendons, for example) ensures that they are not good shock absorbers. A small proportion of the compressive force is resisted by the neural arch, rising to 20% after sustained loading of the disc and when the spine is bent backward slightly to simulate the upright standing posture.

Resistance to shear

Apophyseal joints resist any forward shearing movements of adjacent vertebrae, with the more frontal plane orientation of the lower lumbar joints making them particularly well suited to prevent any forward slip of the overlying vertebra. If the apophyseal joints are removed, or damaged, the intervertebral disc can resist high shearing forces in any direction.

Resistance to torsion

Similarly, the articular surfaces of the apophyseal joints are well orientated to resist axial rotation of the lumbar spine. In the lumbar spine, only 1 to 2 degrees of rotation is permitted before the articular surfaces make firm contact, but considerably more movement is allowed in the thoracic and cervical spine. Stretching of the apophyseal joint capsule and ligaments on the tension side, and deformation of the disc annulus, also contribute substantially to the spine's resistance to torsion. Loss of apophyseal joint articular cartilage after osteoarthritis can allow more free play in these joints and an increased range of axial rotation. The unique shape of the first two cervical vertebrae allows a much greater range of axial rotation.

Resistance to bending

Intervertebral ligaments of the neural arch reorient themselves when the spine is initially flexed. They then resist the movement strongly, with the interspinous and supraspinous ligaments being the first structures damaged in hyperflexion. The strong capsular ligaments of the apophyseal joints resist flexion the most, followed by the disc. The ligamentum flavum has such a high content of elastin that it can be stretched by up to 100% in full flexion, even though it is the only intervertebral ligament to be pre-stressed in the upright "neutral" position. It appears to have a specialist role of protecting the adjacent spinal cord by providing a constant smooth posterior lining to the vertebral canal, a lining that does not overstretch in hyperflexion or become slack (and buckle) in extension. The posterior longitudinal ligament is much weaker than the posterior anulus to which it adheres and so does not protect it from hyperflexion. However, this weak ligament is able to deflect herniated nucleus pulposus tissue away from the spinal cord.[21] A plexus of the mixed (autonomic/sympathetic) sinuvertebral nerve lies in the posterior longitudinal ligament, suggesting that its primary function may be to serve as a "nerve net" that detects abnormalities in the underlying disc.

Backward bending (spinal extension) is resisted by the bony surfaces of the neural arch, with most resistance coming from either the facet

joints or the spinous processes, depending on individual variations in anatomy. The disc and anterior longitudinal ligament also resist backward bending.

Lateral bending has not been studied in detail, but the shape of most discs (wider from side-to-side than front-to-back) suggests that they resist lateral bending strongly, together with the apophyseal joint on the side that is being compressed. In life, lateral bending is often combined with flexion, when individuals bend awkwardly to pick something up that is not directly in front of them. Such bending movements permit extra stretching of one posterolateral corner of the disc (the most usual site of herniation) because the additional component of lateral bending is not resisted by the interspinous and supraspinous ligaments, which lie on the axis of lateral bending. The protective function of these ligaments is therefore diminished.

INJURY

Fracture of the vertebral body

Compressive overload invariably damages the vertebral body before the intervertebral disc, even if the inner anulus of the disc is artificially weakened.[13] In a young or middle-aged person, the vertebral endplate is the most common site of injury, because it is fractured by high pressure in the nucleus of the adjacent intervertebral disc. Cranial endplates are more often injured than caudal because they are thinner and supported by less dense trabecular bone.[22] If nucleus tissue is expressed into the vertebral body (Fig. 4.4b) then it eventually becomes surrounded by a calcified layer known as a Schmorl's node (Fig. 4.4a). These vertical disc herniations are best detected by MRI and are twice as common in patients with back pain.[23] Multiple nodes at adjacent spinal levels are not uncommon in young people[23] and suggest that a single compressive overload event can damage several vertebrae at the same time. Compressive overload injuries to the endplate and underlying trabeculae must be common in life, because damaged trabeculae (some with a healing microcallus) are found in most old cadaveric spines.[24]

Spondylolysis and spondylolisthesis

Spondylolysis represents a fracture of the pars interarticularis and occurs either unilaterally or bilaterally in the lower lumbar spine. It can be reproduced in cadaveric spines by applying a horizontal force of 200 kg to the inferior articular processes so that the neural arch bends backward relative to the rest of the vertebra. In a living person, the injury could be caused by hyperextension of the spine, as in gymnastics. On the other hand, spinal flexion *in vitro* causes the neural arch to be pulled forward and downward by tension in ligaments and muscles. Alternating movements in extension and flexion therefore have the potential to bend the neural arch backward and then forward,[25] creating stress *reversals* in the pars interarticularis that create severe problems for bone metabolism. This probably explains why spondylolysis is particularly associated with sports such as cricket (fast bowling) and gymnastics, which involve extreme flexion *and* extension. Adolescents and young adults are affected the most, because reduced mineralization in their vertebrae allows much greater angular movements at the pars.[25] The L5 disc is affected most because it marks the junction between the mobile spine and relatively immobile sacrum and because it often lies at a steep angle to the horizontal (see Fig. 4.1) so that gravity contributes to the forward shearing force.

Spondylolisthesis is a forward slip of a vertebra. It often follows bilateral spondylolysis in adolescents, but not invariably, suggesting that strong back muscles can keep vertebrae in place.

Apophyseal joint injury

These small joints are most likely to be injured by excessive shear or torsional loading. They are particularly vulnerable to torsion, which concentrates compressive loading on only one of the two joints, so that damage occurs at a torque of 10 to 30 Nm.[13] The inferior and superior margins of the articular surfaces are most frequently affected by cartilage loss and by osteophytes,[26] suggesting that damage also occurs when the spine is heavily loaded in flexion and extension, especially when disc height has been reduced. Hyperextension of the spine can

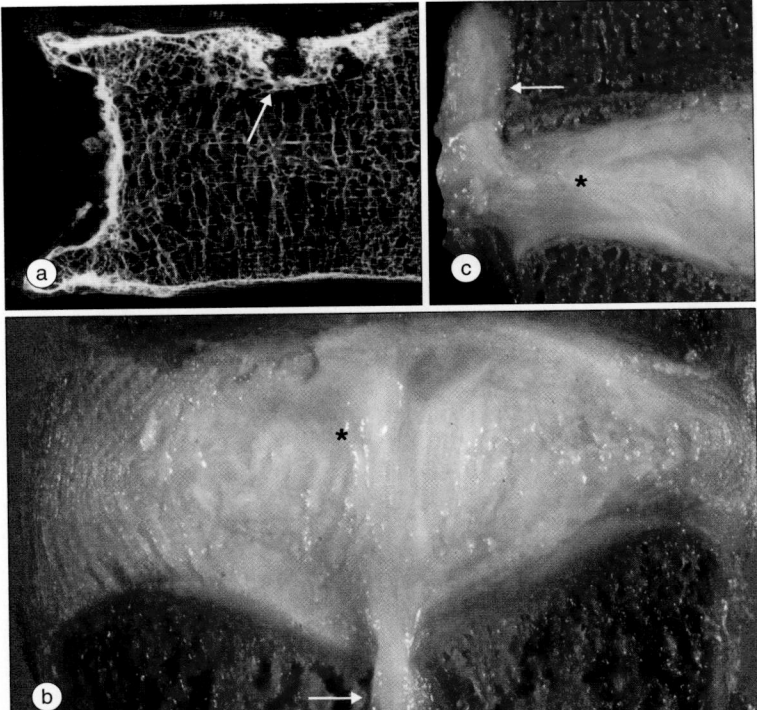

Fig. 4.4 (a) Radiograph of a midsagittal section of a lumbar vertebra (anterior on the left). Note the large Schmorl's node extending from the center of the upper endplate (arrow) and the large osteophytes on the anterior vertebral margins. (b) Midsagittal section through a lumbar disc and vertebrae showing a vertical herniation of nucleus pulposus (arrow) resulting from compressive overload in vitro. In life, calcification around the herniation would create a Schmorl's node. Note the inward collapse of the inner anulus (*). (c) Compressive and bending overload in vitro can cause some nucleus pulposus (arrow) to herniate through a radial fissure in the posterior anulus (*). *(Adapted from Adams MA, Bogduk N, Burton K, Dolan P. The biomechanics of back pain, 2nd ed. Edinburgh: Churchill Livingstone, 2006.)*

cause the inferior articular processes to stretch and probably damage the apophyseal joint capsules.[25]

Disc herniation

Cadaveric experiments have shown that apparently normal discs can be made to prolapse posteriorly by loading them simultaneously in bending and compression.[21] A single application of severe loading can cause an extrusion of nucleus pulposus (see Fig. 4.4c), and discs most readily affected are lower lumbar discs aged 30 to 50 years. In these experiments, either the bending or compression had to exceed normal limits, but not both. More moderate but repetitive loading of discs aged 20 to 40 years creates radial fissures that allow nucleus material to migrate posteriorly but without permitting bulk extrusion of nucleus from the disc space.[13] The underlying mechanism, which is supported by mathematical models,[27] is that spinal bending stretches and thins the opposite wall of the anulus, so that the anulus rather than the vertebral endplate fails when compressive loading increases nucleus pressure. Herniated nucleus material swells by 200% to 300% in just a few hours, before shrinking again over several days as it loses proteoglycans.[13] This transient phenomenon could explain why back pain and sciatica sometimes develop gradually after a back injury. If a radiopaque gel is injected at high pressure into the nucleus of a (bovine) disc, the gel is able to insinuate itself into and between the lamellae of the anulus, eventually reaching the disc periphery.[28] This raises the possibility that compressive loading alone might create a radial fissure in a human disc, but over a time scale of weeks or years rather than hours.

Internal disc disruption

This is more common than disc prolapse and involves internal disruption of the lamellar structure of the anulus. The anulus may develop circumferential or radial fissures (see Fig. 4.4c) or collapse into the nucleus cavity (see Fig. 4.4b). Internal disruption can be caused *in vitro* by traumatic or repetitive loading involving bending and compression.[21] The simplest method is to damage the vertebral body endplate, which is the "weakest link" in the adult spine. Endplate damage allows the pressurized nucleus to expand, reducing pressure within it and allowing inward collapse of the inner anulus (see Fig. 4.4b). The mechanism has been demonstrated in cadavers and animals.[29] Internal disc disruption generates high stress concentrations in the anulus (Fig. 4.5) and sometimes allows nucleus pulposus to reach and sensitize nerves in the peripheral anulus. There is growing evidence that internal disruption plays an important role in discogenic back pain, comparable to the role of disc herniation in sciatica.

Ligament injuries

Excessive flexion tears the interspinous and supraspinous ligaments, followed by the capsular ligaments of the apophyseal joints. Extreme hyperflexion is required to tear the posterior wall of the disc or the ligamentum flavum. The strength of the spine in bending depends on the spinal level. In cadaveric experiments on lumbar spines, approximately 60 Nm is sufficient to reach the elastic limit in flexion and 35 Nm is noted in extension.[13] Equivalent values for the cervical spine are 7 Nm and 8 Nm, respectively.[30] The elastic limit probably marks the end of the physiologic range of motion, at which a clinically relevant injury would be sustained in life. Little is known about injuries to the iliolumbar ligaments or their role in back pain.

Whiplash

The essential feature of whiplash is a painful bending injury to the neck that is caused by a low-velocity insult, such as a car "shunt." Low velocity can be misleading, however, because it does not mean that low forces are involved. Laboratory simulations on cadavers[31] and live volunteers[32] show that a rear impact thrusts the shoulders forward relative to the head, so that the neck is initially distorted into an "S" shape involving hyperextension of lower cervical levels and variable flexion and extension of upper cervical levels (Fig. 4.6). This initial distortion is followed by general hyperextension. Finally, depending on the nature of impact and the presence or absence of a headrest, the neck can be thrown into hyperflexion. The key feature of whiplash is that significant movements occur in less than 50 ms, before the neck muscles can resist them. Consequently the head, which weighs approximately 5 kg, is thrown around relative to the slender neck, rather like a "balloon on a stick." The cervical spine has approximately 45% of the compressive strength of the lumbar spine but only 20% of its strength in bending,[30] suggesting that the neck is particularly vulnerable to bending injury.

The frequent involvement of both flexion and extension ensures that practically any structure in or around the cervical spine can be injured during whiplash.[33] The site of injury would move away from the sagittal midline (perhaps to an apophyseal joint) if the victim was turning his or her head around at the time of impact. Any prior warning (e.g., the sound of braking) would allow the victim to contract the neck muscles in alarm, causing a higher proportion of compression to bending to act on the cervical spine and possibly increasing the risk of injury to muscles and intervertebral discs. As with any other human behavior, the reporting of persisting symptoms after whiplash is subject to a variety of psychosocial influences.

MECHANICAL INFLUENCES IN DISC DEGENERATION AND PROLAPSE

Middle-aged discs are vulnerable to injury

Loss of proteoglycans and water from the aging disc is mostly confined to the nucleus, where it leads to a smaller hydrostatic region (see Fig. 4.5a) that exhibits a lower pressure within it. Consequently,

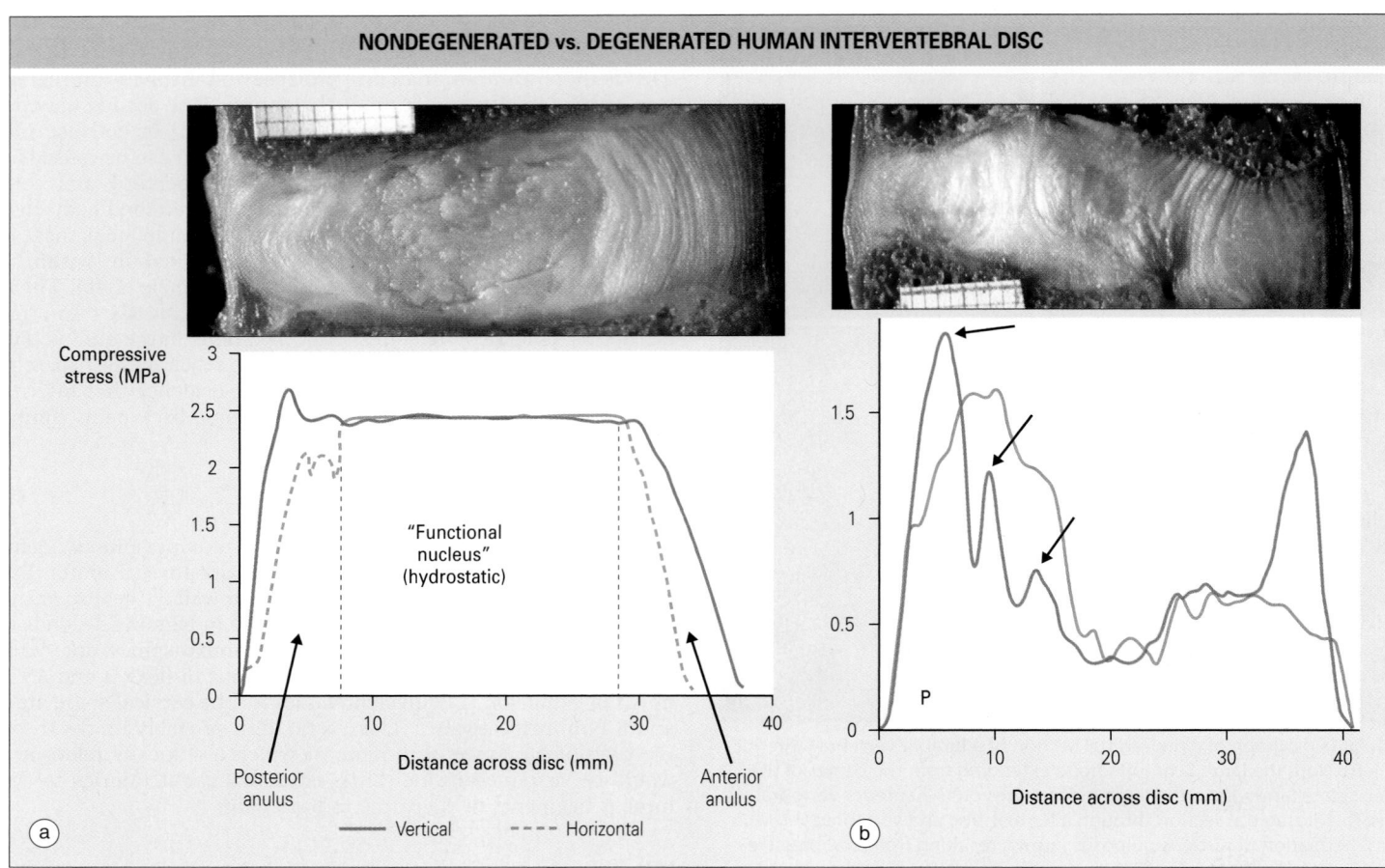

Fig. 4.5 (a) The photograph shows a mature non-degenerated human intervertebral disc cut through in the midsagittal plane. The graph below it shows how the horizontal and vertical components of compressive stress vary within such a disc. There is a central region of hydrostatic pressure (the "functional nucleus") and a small concentration of compressive stress in the posterior anulus. (b) Internal disruption of the anulus lamellae, and the damaged endplate, indicate that this young adult disc is degenerated. Stress distributions in such a disc show a decompressed nucleus and high stress concentrations (arrows) in the anulus. The generally low disc stresses suggest that some compression has been transferred to the neural arch. Approximately 1 MPa = 10 kg/cm². *(Adapted from Adams MA, Bogduk N, Burton K, Dolan P. The biomechanics of back pain, 2nd ed. Edinburgh: Churchill Livingstone, 2006.)*

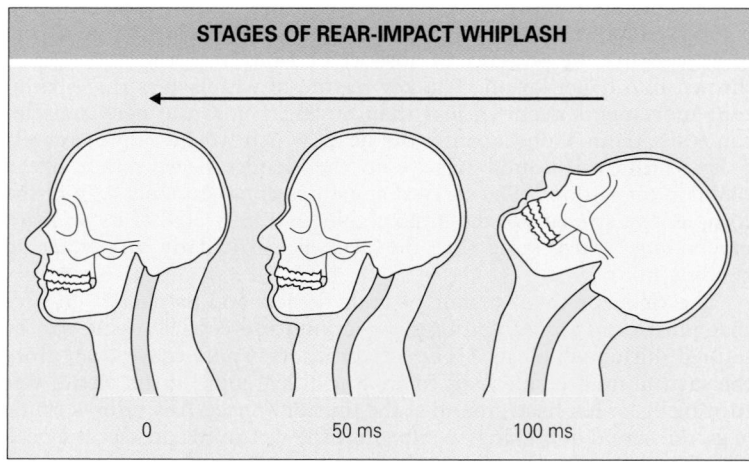

Fig. 4.6 During a rear-impact whiplash injury, the neck adopts an S-shaped deformity after only 50 ms before it can be protected by muscle action. Subsequently, the neck is thrown into hyperextension and possibly also into hyperflexion. *(Reproduced with permission from Adams MA, Bogduk N, Burton K, Dolan P. The biomechanics of back pain, 2nd ed. Edinburgh: Churchill Livingstone, 2006.)*

compressive load-bearing is resisted increasingly by the anulus and high concentrations of compressive stress can develop within it, particularly posterior to the nucleus.[18] Ageing anulus tissue is probably stiffened by increased collagen crosslinking, especially the nonenzymatic glycation reactions that are known to stiffen articular cartilage and render it more vulnerable to injury.[34] The accumulation of small defects in the anulus ensures that its strength does not increase with stiffness; in fact, strength can fall slightly.[6] Vertebral endplates and their supporting trabeculae also weaken with age, in common with most bone structures, and endplates develop an increasing concavity on the disc side. This further reduces nucleus pressure and concentrates stress in the anulus. Hence, increasing stress concentrations, increasing stiffness, and accumulating structural defects make middle-aged discs vulnerable to injury. Injury risk appears to decrease in old age, probably because older people are less active and because sarcopenia reduces the peak forces that can be generated by aging back muscles.[35]

As described earlier, repetitive loading and/or trauma can create radial fissures in the anulus and allow disc herniation. Alternatively, primary endplate damage leads to nucleus decompression and internal collapse of the anulus. Either way, the anulus loses height and the disc bulges radially like a "flat tire."[20] Cadaveric experiments suggest that endplate fracture occurs more readily and has a more immediate effect on stresses within the disc than anulus injury.[36] The distribution of compressive stress (force per unit area) often becomes highly irregular, as shown in Figure 4.5b.

Injury and frustrated healing

Cells within injured discs must respond to their altered mechanical environment. *In vitro*, nucleus and inner anulus cells (which resemble chondrocytes) respond to hydrostatic pressure: they synthesize more matrix in response to moderate and fluctuating pressures and synthesize less matrix when pressures are very high, very low, or static.[37] Outer anulus cells resemble fibroblasts and probably respond to tension rather than to hydrostatic pressure, because they do not normally experience the latter. Applying these principles to human discs *in vivo* suggests that reduced nucleus pressure after injury (see Fig. 4.5b) would inhibit proteoglycan synthesis and lead to steadily lower water content and pressure. This is the reverse of what is required to re-inflate the injured disc. Likewise, high stress concentrations in the injured anulus would inhibit collagen synthesis and repair and also increase the activation of matrix-degrading enzymes.[37] This then provides a mechanism for progressive disc degeneration: injury affects the mechanical environment of disc cells in such a manner that their metabolism becomes aberrant, leading to further weakening of the matrix and re-injury. By responding to their *local* mechanical environment, rather than to the mechanical requirements of the whole disc, cells initiate a degenerative process that resembles frustrated healing rather than a reparative process.[38]

High hydrostatic pressures within a disc would collapse blood vessels, so that discs become avascular at about the time that a child learns to stand upright. However, the loss of pressure in an injured or decompressed disc would allow blood vessels, and therefore nerves, to grow back in again, and this has been reported in severely degenerated discs.[39] Ingrowth is also promoted by proteoglycan loss[40] and by some disc cells.[41] In this way, mechanical factors contribute to discogenic pain as well as to a pathologic process.

Prolapse

As degeneration progresses, radial fissures grow toward the disc periphery, driven by the high gradients in compressive stress (see Fig. 4.5b), whereas increased bulging of a damaged anulus or endplate steadily reduces disc height, by approximately 3% per year.[42] Herniation can occur at any point as a result of injury (see Fig. 4.4c), and the fact that prior degeneration is not a requirement for prolapse is an important medicolegal consideration.

SPINAL DEGENERATIVE CASCADE

Intervertebral discs play such an important role in spine mechanics that disc failure initiates a whole cascade of adverse changes in adjacent structures. This cascade initially leads to adverse mechanical influences but ultimately can lead to a series of pathologic structural changes.

Segmental instability

Loss of nucleus pressure and volume removes tension from the surrounding anulus, and loss of disc height creates slack in intervertebral ligaments. These mechanical changes are sufficient to create "instability" in the motion segment, manifested by a reduced resistance to bending and an increase in horizontal shearing movements.[43] In effect, the segment "wobbles" and has an increased region of free play (or "neutral zone"). The situation is considerably more serious if the endplate becomes damaged, because that causes an immediate and gross decompression of the nucleus[21] as shown in Figure 4.5b. Segmental instability is recognized by many manual therapists, and is associated with back pain. Pain could arise from the stress concentrations in the anulus (and apophyseal joints) that accompany nucleus decompression, rather than from the small movements themselves. Instability should not be confused with hypermobility, which indicates an increased *range* of movement. Hypermobility can be a systemic condition affecting many joints, or it can arise from injury to a restraining ligament.

Vertebral body osteophytes

Spinal instability is generally regarded as a transient phenomenon, because it can be corrected by the growth of osteophytes on the margins of the vertebral bodies (see Fig. 4.4a), adjacent to the "wobbling" disc. Animal experiments have shown that anulus injuries lead to osteophyte growth,[44] presumably because the increased radial bulging and shearing movements of the destabilized anulus pull on the periosteum. The primary mechanical effect of vertebral body osteophytes is to increase the disc's resistance to bending. Osteophytes also increase the disc's resistance to compression by increasing the effective cross-sectional area of the disc, but this is usually a minor effect. Because

osteophytes reduce the abnormal movements that caused them to form in the first place, they can be viewed as adaptive rather than degenerative.

Apophyseal joint osteoarthritis

Height loss by the anulus of a degenerated disc brings adjacent neural arches closer together so that they resist up to 90% of the compressive force acting on the lumbar spine rather than the normal 0% to 20%.[45] Compressive load-bearing creates high concentrations of compressive stress in the inferior margins of the joint, especially in habitual lordotic (upright) postures. In addition, direct bone-on-bone contact between inferior articular processes and the laminae below can lead to gross bone remodeling, including osteophytes. A close relationship has been noted in cadaveric apophyseal joints between high load-bearing and osteoarthritic changes, including cartilage loss, bone eburnation, and sclerosis.[46] Imaging studies *in vivo* have long suggested such a relationship.

Spinal stenosis

The height of the intervertebral foramen is decreased by narrowing of the anulus fibrosus. Its anteroposterior diameter is also decreased as a result of disc radial bulging and by apophyseal joint osteophytosis. These changes can combine to cause a severe reduction in the cross-sectional area of the foramen, trapping the exiting nerve root. The consequences of spinal stenosis are usually most severe at L5-S1, which has a particularly small foramen.

Degenerative scoliosis

The two apophyseal joints at each spinal level often show pronounced asymmetries, a condition known as *tropism*. If the affected joints become heavily load bearing as a result of disc narrowing (see earlier), then their oblique articular surfaces will create an unbalanced torque about the long axis of the spine, leading to axial rotation. Axial rotation is mechanically "coupled" to lateral bending and can be coupled to flexion and extension, so a "triplanar" spinal deformity can develop that involves permanent twisting, lateral bending, and flexion of the thoracolumbar spine. This is a plausible explanation for degenerative scoliosis, but the mechanism is not proved.

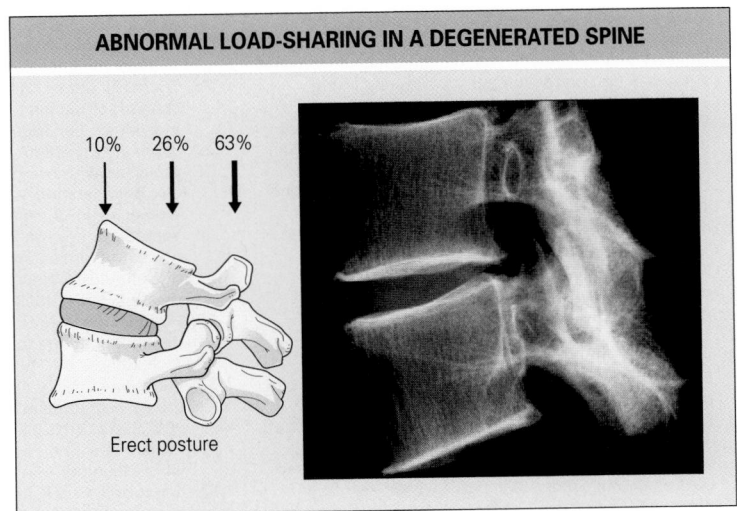

ABNORMAL LOAD-SHARING IN A DEGENERATED SPINE

10% 26% 63%

Erect posture

Fig. 4.7 (Left) The three percentages show how an applied compressive force is distributed between the anterior half of the vertebral body and disc, the posterior half of the vertebral body and disc, and the neural arch. (Average data for cadaveric specimens with severely degenerated discs, tested in the simulated erect standing posture.) (Right) Plain radiograph of such a specimen, showing how image intensity (which reflects bone mineral density) is very low anteriorly and very high in the apophyseal joints. *(Image and data adapted from Adams MA, Pollintine P, Tobias JH, et al. Intervertebral disc degeneration can predispose to anterior vertebral fractures in the thoracolumbar spine. J Bone Miner Res 2006;21:1409-1416.)*

MECHANICAL INFLUENCES IN VERTEBRAL OSTEOPOROSIS

Reduced mechanical loading weakens vertebrae

When a vertebral body is loaded naturally by adjacent intervertebral discs, its compressive strength is closely related to bone mineral density (BMD) and size.[47] Old vertebrae lose BMD and strength, partly as a result of hormonal changes and partly because muscle strength decreases with age (sarcopenia) and so provides a reducing mechanical stimulus to maintain bone mass.[48] Hormone levels and muscle strength are themselves influenced by genetic inheritance, as well as by age and environmental factors. A recent epidemiologic study has shown good correspondence between estimates of habitual mechanical loading and vertebral BMD.[3]

Osteoporotic vertebral deformities

The central region of non-degenerated intervertebral discs presses evenly on adjacent vertebral bodies, even in middle age (see Fig. 4.5a)

and when the spine is flexed or extended. If BMD becomes low, nucleus pressure can drive the central region of the adjacent vertebral endplates outward, creating "biconcave" deformities in the vertebrae. Degenerated discs, on the other hand concentrate compressive stress on the anterior and posterior vertebral body margins (see Fig. 4.5b) in flexion and extension, respectively. If the disc is grossly narrowed, the neural arch resists much of the compressive load on its own, especially in lordotic (upright) postures.[45] These factors combine to stress-shield the anterior vertebral body in upright posture, causing it to lose BMD (Fig. 4.7). Unfortunately, flexion movements disengage the neural arches and transfer high compressive stress onto the weakened anterior vertebral body,[49] creating anterior wedge deformities. The third type of vertebral deformity, "crush fracture," probably results from high compressive impacts when the discs are degenerated. Once one vertebra is damaged, it alters load sharing in the spine in such a manner that it increases the risk of fracture of neighboring vertebrae, in what has been termed a *fracture cascade*.[50]

REFERENCES

1. Waddell G. The back pain revolution, 2nd ed. Edinburgh: Churchill Livingstone, 2002.
2. Sambrook PN, MacGregor AJ, Spector TD. Genetic influences on cervical and lumbar disc degeneration: a magnetic resonance imaging study in twins. Arthritis Rheum 1999;42:366-372.
3. Videman T, Levalahti E, Battie MC, et al. Heritability of BMD of femoral neck and lumbar spine: a multivariate twin study of Finnish men. J Bone Miner Res 2007;22:1455-1462.
4. Frost HM. On our age-related bone loss: insights from a new paradigm. J Bone Miner Res 1997;12:1539-1546.
5. Yao JQ, Seedhom BB. Mechanical conditioning of articular cartilage to prevalent stresses. Br J Rheumatol 1993;32:956-965.
6. Skrzypiec D, Tarala M, Pollintine P, et al. When are intervertebral discs stronger than their adjacent vertebrae? Spine 2007;32:2455-2461.
7. Videman T, Levalahti E, Battie MC. The effects of anthropometrics, lifting strength, and physical activities in disc degeneration. Spine 2007;32:1406-1413.
8. Hartvigsen J, Bakketeig LS, Leboeuf-Yde C, et al. The association between physical workload and low back pain clouded by the "healthy worker" effect: population-based cross-sectional and 5-year prospective questionnaire study. Spine 2001;26:1788-1792; discussion 92-93.
9. Dolan P, Earley M, Adams MA. Bending and compressive stresses acting on the lumbar spine during lifting activities. J Biomech 1994;27:1237-1248.
10. Vascancelos D. Compression fractures of the vertebra during major epileptic seizures. Epilepsia 1973;14:323-328.
11. Cholewicki J, Juluru K, Radebold A, et al. Lumbar spine stability can be augmented with an abdominal belt and/or increased intra-abdominal pressure. Eur Spine J 1999;8:388-395.
12. Sato K, Kikuchi S, Yonezawa T. In vivo intradiscal pressure measurement in healthy individuals and in patients with ongoing back problems. Spine 1999;24:2468-2474.
13. Adams MA, Bogduk N, Burton K, Dolan P. The biomechanics of back pain, 2nd ed. Edinburgh: Churchill Livingstone, 2006.
14. Snook SH, Webster BS, McGorry RW, et al. The reduction of chronic nonspecific low back pain through the control of early morning lumbar flexion: a randomized controlled trial. Spine 1998;23:2601-2607.
15. Bazrgari B, Shirazi-Adl A, Arjmand N. Analysis of squat and stoop dynamic liftings: muscle forces and internal spinal loads. Eur Spine J 2007;16:687-699.
16. Solomonow D, Davidson B, Zhou BH, et al. Neuromuscular neutral zones response to cyclic lumbar flexion. J Biomech 2008;41:2821-2828.
17. Burton AK, Tillotson KM. Reference values for "normal" regional lumbar sagittal mobility. Clin Biomech 1988;3:106-113.

18. Adams MA, McNally DS, Dolan P. "Stress" distributions inside intervertebral discs: the effects of age and degeneration. J Bone Joint Surg Br 1996;78:965-972.
19. Skrzypiec DM, Pollintine P, Przybyla A, et al. The internal mechanical properties of cervical intervertebral discs as revealed by stress profilometry. Eur Spine J 2007;16:1701-1709.
20. Brinckmann P, Grootenboer H. Change of disc height, radial disc bulge, and intradiscal pressure from discectomy: an in vitro investigation on human lumbar discs. Spine 1991;16:641-646.
21. Adams MA, Freeman BJ, Morrison HP, et al. Mechanical initiation of intervertebral disc degeneration. Spine 2000;25:1625-1636.
22. Zhao FD, Pollintine P, Hole BD, et al. Vertebral fractures usually affect the cranial endplate because it is thinner and supported by less-dense trabecular bone. Bone 2009;44:372-379.
23. Hamanishi C, Kawabata T, Yosii T, Tanaka S. Schmorl's nodes on magnetic resonance imaging: their incidence and clinical relevance. Spine 1994;19:450-453.
24. Vernon-Roberts B, Pirie CJ. Healing trabecular microfractures in the bodies of lumbar vertebrae. Ann Rheum Dis 1973;32:406-412.
25. Green TP, Allvey JC, Adams MA. Spondylolysis: bending of the inferior articular processes of lumbar vertebrae during simulated spinal movements. Spine 1994;19:2683-2691.
26. Tischer T, Aktas T, Milz S, Putz RV. Detailed pathological changes of human lumbar facet joints L1-L5 in elderly individuals. Eur Spine J 2006;15:308-315.
27. Schmidt H, Kettler A, Rohlmann A, et al. The risk of disc prolapses with complex loading in different degrees of disc degeneration—a finite element analysis. Clin Biomech 2007;22:988-998.
28. Veres SP, Robertson PA, Broom ND. ISSLS prize winner: microstructure and mechanical disruption of the lumbar disc annulus: II. How the annulus fails under hydrostatic pressure. Spine 2008;33:2711-2720.
29. Holm S, Holm AK, Ekstrom L, et al. Experimental disc degeneration due to endplate injury. J Spinal Disord Tech 2004;17:64-71.
30. Przybyla AS, Skrzypiec D, Pollintine P, et al. Strength of the cervical spine in compression and bending. Spine 2007;32:1612-1620.
31. Panjabi MM, Cholewicki J, Nibu K, et al. Mechanism of whiplash injury. Clin Biomech 1998;13:239-249.
32. Kaneoka K, Ono K, Inami S, Hayashi K. Motion analysis of cervical vertebrae during whiplash loading. Spine 1999;24:763-769; discussion 770.
33. Rauschning W, Jonsson H. Injuries of the cervical spine in automobile accidents: pathoanatomic and clinical aspects. In: Gunzburg R, Szpalski M, eds. Whiplash injuries. Philadelphia: Lippincott-Raven, 1998.
34. DeGroot J, Verzijl N, Wenting-Van Wijk MJ, et al. Accumulation of advanced glycation end products as a

molecular mechanism for aging as a risk factor in osteoarthritis. Arthritis Rheum 2004;50:1207-1215.
35. Sinaki M, Nwaogwugwu NC, Phillips BE, Mokri MP. Effect of gender, age, and anthropometry on axial and appendicular muscle strength. Am J Phys Med Rehabil 2001;80:330-338.
36. Przybyla A, Pollintine P, Bedzinski R, Adams MA. Outer annulus tears have less effect than endplate fracture on stress distributions inside intervertebral discs: relevance to disc degeneration. Clin Biomech 2006;21:1013-1019.
37. Handa T, Ishihara H, Ohshima H, et al. Effects of hydrostatic pressure on matrix synthesis and matrix metalloproteinase production in the human lumbar intervertebral disc. Spine 1997;22:1085-1091.
38. Adams MA, Roughley PJ. What is intervertebral disc degeneration, and what causes it? Spine 2006;31:2151-2161.
39. Freemont AJ, Watkins A, Le Maitre C, et al. Nerve growth factor expression and innervation of the painful intervertebral disc. J Pathol 2002;197:286-292.
40. Johnson WE, Caterson B, Eisenstein SM, et al. Human intervertebral disc aggrecan inhibits nerve growth in vitro. Arthritis Rheum 2002;46:2658-2664.
41. Johnson WE, Sivan S, Wright KT, et al. Human intervertebral disc cells promote nerve growth over substrata of human intervertebral disc aggrecan. Spine 2006;31:1187-1193.
42. Hassett G, Hart DJ, Manek NJ, et al. Risk factors for progression of lumbar spine disc degeneration: the Chingford Study. Arthritis Rheum 2003;48:3112-3117.
43. Zhao F, Pollintine P, Hole BD, et al. Discogenic origins of spinal instability. Spine 2005;30:2621-2630.
44. Lipson SJ, Muir H. Vertebral osteophyte formation in experimental disc degeneration: morphologic and proteoglycan changes over time. Arthritis Rheum 1980;23:319-324.
45. Pollintine P, Przybyla AS, Dolan P, Adams MA. Neural arch load-bearing in old and degenerated spines. J Biomech 2004;37:197-204.
46. Robson-Brown K, Pollintine P, Adams MA. Biomechanical implications of degenerative joint disease in the apophyseal joints of human thoracic and lumbar vertebrae. Am J Phys Anthropol 2008;136:318-326.
47. Brinckmann P, Biggemann M, Hilweg D. Prediction of the compressive strength of human lumbar vertebrae. Spine 1989;14:606-610.
48. Burr DB. Muscle strength, bone mass, and age-related bone loss. J Bone Miner Res 1997;12:1547-1551.
49. Adams MA, Pollintine P, Tobias JH, et al. Intervertebral disc degeneration can predispose to anterior vertebral fractures in the thoracolumbar spine. J Bone Miner Res 2006;21:1409-1416.
50. Briggs AM, Greig AM, Wark JD. The vertebral fracture cascade in osteoporosis: a review of aetiopathogenesis. Osteoporos Int 2007;18:575-584.

Biomechanics of peripheral joints

Matthew F. Koff

5

- A static force analysis of a joint can be performed easily and displays important biomechanical characteristics of the joint.
- Diarthrodial joints in the body act as levers with poor mechanical advantage.
- Joint lubrication is a combination of boundary lubrication, hydrodynamic lubrication, and boundary film lubrication.
- The characteristic stress–strain curve of collagenous tissues, such as tendon and ligament is an initial toe region, followed by a steep linear region prior to eventual failure.
- Many tissues in the body are viscoelastic and exhibit anisotropic behavior.
- The response of a tissue to an applied load or deformation depends on the tissue's structural composition and fluid content.

INTRODUCTION

Biomedical engineering is a large field of study that applies general principles from different engineering backgrounds to the study of the human body. Biomechanics is the application of mechanical engineering principles to living organisms. Biomechanics of organisms can be examined at different levels: cellular level (e.g., response of cells to an externally applied force or deformation), tissue level (e.g., strain of the anterior cruciate ligament during normal gait), and whole-joint level (e.g., joint contact forces during activities of daily living).

Engineering principles may be used to understand the etiology and progression of many rheumatic diseases. A basic understanding of these principles is beneficial for clinicians and medical professionals. This chapter presents a rudimentary background of engineering mechanics pertaining to whole-joint and tissue mechanics in the human body.

BIOMECHANICS OF WHOLE JOINTS

The effects of a rheumatic disease are often seen at the microscopic level, but the symptoms of the disease are commonly found at the whole-joint level. For example, not only does osteoarthritis cause the formation of clefts, fissures, and blisters in articular cartilage, but it also produces symptoms including joint pain, stiffness, and reduced range of motion. Examining the transmission of forces through a diarthrodial joint is one way of determining the changing functional capabilities of the joint during the onset and progression of a rheumatic disease.

Statics and dynamics

Whole-joint force analyses are commonly performed to determine the forces that a diarthrodial joint may experience during activities of daily living. A static analysis of a body or body segment examines the forces and moments (torques) acting on a body at rest. An example of this is the evaluation of forces in the knee during standing, or contact pressures in the thumb when grasping a key. In vector notation, this is written as: $\Sigma \vec{F} = 0$, $\Sigma \vec{M} = 0$ where $\vec{F}$ are the forces acting on the body and $\vec{M}$ are the moments (torques) acting on the body. A dynamic analysis of a body examines the forces and moments acting on a body in motion. A dynamic analysis includes descriptions of the inertial properties of the body being analyzed. In vector notation, this is written as $\Sigma \vec{F} = m\vec{a}$ and $\Sigma M = I\alpha$, where $\vec{a}$ and α are the linear and angular accelerations, respectively, of the body, m is the mass of the body, and I represents the inertial properties (mass distribution) of the body.

An example of a static force analysis is performed for the shoulder joint. Although this analysis is performed in 2-D for ease of analysis, important generalized biomechanical characteristics of whole joints are evident from the results. The goal of this analysis is to calculate the static *in vivo* muscular forces and contact force between the proximal humerus and the glenoid fossa of the shoulder joint. We examine a shoulder at 90 degrees of abduction with a ball held in the hand. An overall picture of our static analysis is shown in Figure 5.1a.

To perform a force analysis (static or dynamic), it is necessary to construct a free-body diagram, which displays all forces and moments acting on a body or body segment of interest. A free-body diagram of a simplified shoulder joint is shown in Fig. 5.1b. For ease of analysis, the radius, ulna, and humerus have been combined into a single bone segment to represent the arm, forearm, and hand. All forces and moments acting on the selected body segment must be included in the free-body diagram. Forces included in the free-body diagram may be separated into four classes:

1. *contact force* from the humerus acting on the glenoid fossa
2. *muscle forces* from muscle groups that flex, extend, and rotate the shoulder joint; only the deltoid muscle is modeled in this analysis
3. *intrinsic weight* of the arm
4. *external forces* such as the weight of the ball in the hand

It is also important to record the lines of action of the forces and moments in the free-body diagram. The point of application, direction (orientation), and magnitude of each force are included in the free-body diagram. The contact force is placed at the proximal end of the humerus; however, its direction (θ_J) and magnitude (F_J) are unknown.

The muscle force of the deltoid muscle is placed at its point of attachment to the humerus at a distance "a" from the glenohumeral joint center. The magnitude of the muscle force (F_M) is unknown. Lines of action of muscle forces (θ_M) are often assumed on the basis of detailed anatomic dissections of joints, which examine points of origin and insertion of muscle groups that cross the joint. The force representing the weight of the arm (W_A) is assumed to be known and is placed at the center of mass of the arm at a distance "b" from the joint center. The force representing the arm weight is directed in the direction of gravity. The same is true for the ball of known weight held in the hand (W_B and distance "c"). The unknown variables in this problem are the magnitude of the contact force (F_J), the direction of the contact force (θ_J), and the magnitude of the muscle force (F_M). These variables are calculated using static force analysis.

A body is considered to be in static equilibrium when all forces and all moments acting on the body sum to zero. The summation of forces and moments may be performed around any point on the free-body diagram. For this 2-D model, the static equilibrium vector equations may be written in terms of their individual x, y, and z components:

$$\sum F_x = 0, \sum F_Y = 0$$

and

$$\sum M_z = 0$$

When the force equilibrium equations are applied to the free-body diagram in Fig. 5.1b, we obtain:

$$\sum F_x = 0 \rightarrow F_J \cdot \cos(\theta_J) = F_M \cdot \cos(\theta_M)$$
$$\sum F_x = 0 \rightarrow F_J \cdot \sin(\theta_J) = F_M \cdot \sin(\theta_M) - W_A - W_B$$

37

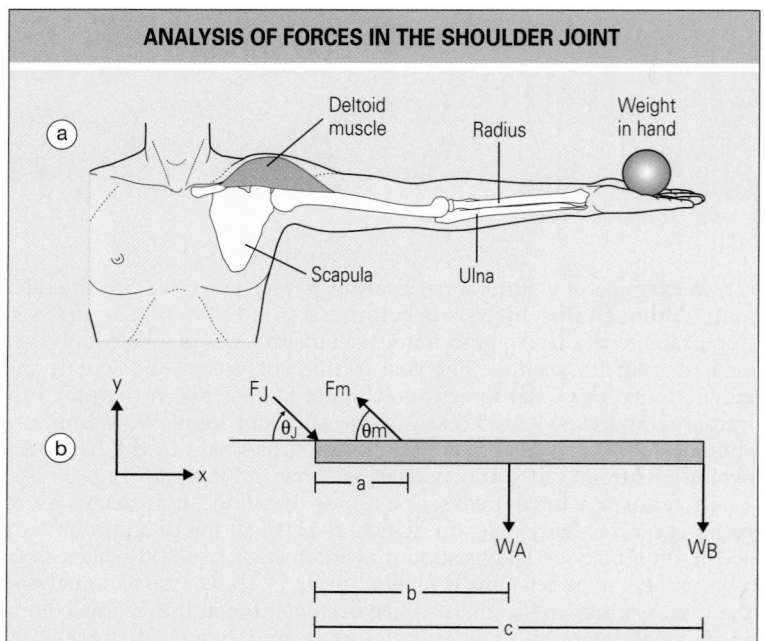

ANALYSIS OF FORCES IN THE SHOULDER JOINT

Fig. 5.1 (a) Person holding a ball in the hand at 90 degrees of shoulder abduction. Relative positions of bones in arm indicated. (b) Free-body diagram of arm in 90 degrees of shoulder abduction (humerus, radius, and ulna grouped together for simplification of analysis). F_J, joint contact force; θ_J, angle of joint contact force; F_M, deltoid muscle force; θ_M, angle of deltoid muscle force; W_A, weight of arm; W_B, weight of ball; a, b, c, distances from the glenohumeral joint center to forces acting on the limb.

In a static analysis, the sum of moments (ΣM_z) may be taken at any coordinate location. In the current analysis, the sum of moments was taken about the point of application of the contact force on the humerus. The sum of moments was taken at this point to preclude the presence of the articulating surface contact force in the moment equation, yielding:

$$\sum M_z = 0 \rightarrow F_M \cdot \sin(\theta_M) a = W_A \cdot b + W_B \cdot c = 0$$

The equations above are then solved using basic algebra and geometric identities to obtain the solutions:

$$F_M = (W_a \cdot b + W_b \cdot c)/(\sin(\theta_M) \cdot a)$$
$$\theta_J = \tan^{-1}((F_M \cdot \sin(\theta_M) - W_A - W_B)/F_M \cdot \cos(\theta_M))$$
$$F_J = \sqrt{(F_M \cdot \cos(\theta_M))^2 + (F_M \cdot \sin(\theta_M) - W_A - W_B)^2}$$

We now substitute values for the known variables: a = 15 cm, b = 30 cm, c = 60 cm, θ_M = 15 degrees, W_A = 40N and W_B = 60N, to solve for the unknown variables F_M, θ_J, and F_J. The calculated values are F_M = 1236.4N, F_J = 1214.3N, and θ_J = 10.4 degrees.

This simple analysis shows a characteristic common to diarthrodial joints throughout the human body: poor mechanical advantage. The poor mechanical advantage of the shoulder is shown when the weight of the ball in the hand is compared with the muscle force required to maintain the ball position. The calculated muscle force is more than 20 times the weight of the ball! Altering two factors of the analysis may increase the mechanical advantage of the system by decreasing the muscle force required to hold the ball. First, an increase of θ_M would increase the component of F_M that resists the downward force of the weight of the arm and the weight of the ball. Another alternative would be to increase the moment arm of F_M, distance "a," but this is often not practical. Second, we can flex the elbow and bring the weight of the arm and the weight of the ball closer to the center of rotation of the shoulder. This would change the resulting value from our moment equation and reduce our effective muscle force and resulting contact force.

A number of limitations to the current static analysis exist due to the number of unknown variables. The number of static equilibrium equations available for use prevented the inclusion of additional muscle or ligamentous forces. That is, for a two-dimensional problem we could only use two force equations ($\Sigma F_x = 0$, $\Sigma F_y = 0$) and one moment equation ($\Sigma M_z = 0$) to solve the unknown variables. Stated differently, only three unknown variables may be determined in a 2-D analysis. If the analysis were performed in 3-D, it would be possible to solve nine unknown variables. Owing to complex human anatomy and numerous muscle forces, we often have a greater number of unknown variables to solve than we have equations to use in the analysis. This results in an indeterminate problem.

Several computational methods have been developed to increase the number of variables that may be solved. One method is the exclusion of selected forces. For example, in the previous analysis, the teres minor muscle, an adducting muscle of the shoulder, was excluded since the shoulder was in pure abduction. It may be reasonable to assume that the force contribution of teres minor to producing shoulder abduction is minimal and may be excluded from the force analysis. A second way to reduce the number of unknown forces is to assume a force relationship between the different muscle units. For example, only the deltoid muscle was included in the above analysis. The supraspinatus is also active during shoulder abduction, but it was excluded to limit the number of unknown variables. We may have assumed a relationship between the deltoid and supraspinatus, such as $F_2 = A \cdot F_1$, where F_2 is the muscle force of the supraspinatus, F_1 is the muscle force of the deltoid, and A is a constant. The relationship between different muscular units not included in the analysis may be formatted in a linear or nonlinear manner.

A third method to decrease the number of unknown variables would be to incorporate direct muscle electromyography (EMG) measurements into the analysis. Some assumptions would be needed to convert EMG measurements to force output but would allow additional unknown variables in the analysis. A fourth method to increase the number of unknown variables is to use numerical optimization. Optimization is performed by minimizing a mathematical function which is defined as the "cost" of performing an activity of daily living. Various cost functions that have been used include minimization of muscular forces; minimization of muscle stress, as calculated by the muscle force divided by physiologic cross-sectional area of the muscle; and minimization of muscle energy. These cost functions have been successful in evaluating muscle forces during various activities of daily living. More advanced methods of optimization have incorporated muscle architecture to accurately predict muscular forces during activities of daily living.

Joint lubrication

The human joints are exposed to a great variation of loading conditions. There can be high-impact, short-duration loads such as in running; moderately low loads with a prolonged loading time such as in standing; and low loads with rapid motion in the swing phase of walking. Over a lifetime there is relatively little wear in the joints, indicating a highly effective lubricating system.

Two types of lubrication exist: boundary lubrication and fluid film lubrication. Boundary lubrication is due to a single layer (monolayer) of lubricant adsorbed on each bearing surface. In the case of a joint, boundary lubrication is achieved by a macromolecular monolayer attached to each articular surface. These layers carry loads and are effective in reducing friction. Fluid film lubrication is due to a thin film of lubricant and produces a greater bearing-surface separation. The pressure developed in the lubricating fluid carries the loads applied to the joint (Fig. 5.2).

In engineering materials such as steel and bronze, the thickness and extent of the fluid film, as well as its load-bearing capacity, are not dependent on the bearing materials. The lubricating characteristics depend on the lubricant properties, such as viscosity, and on the shape of the gap between the two bearing surfaces and the relative velocity of the surfaces. In a human joint, the bearing materials, such as the articular cartilage, are not rigid and are not as stiff as steel and bronze. This results in what is known as *elastohydrodynamic lubrication*. As the joint surfaces move and pressure is developed, the fluid pressure deforms the surfaces (Fig. 5.3). This changes the film geometry by increasing the surface area, reducing escape of the lubricant from

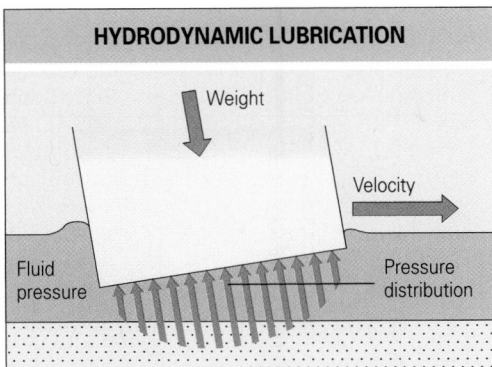

Fig. 5.2 Hydrodynamic lubrication. During motion at sufficiently high velocities, the weight tilts and forms a wedge shape. Because of the viscous properties of the fluid, a pressure will be created within the fluid to support the weight.

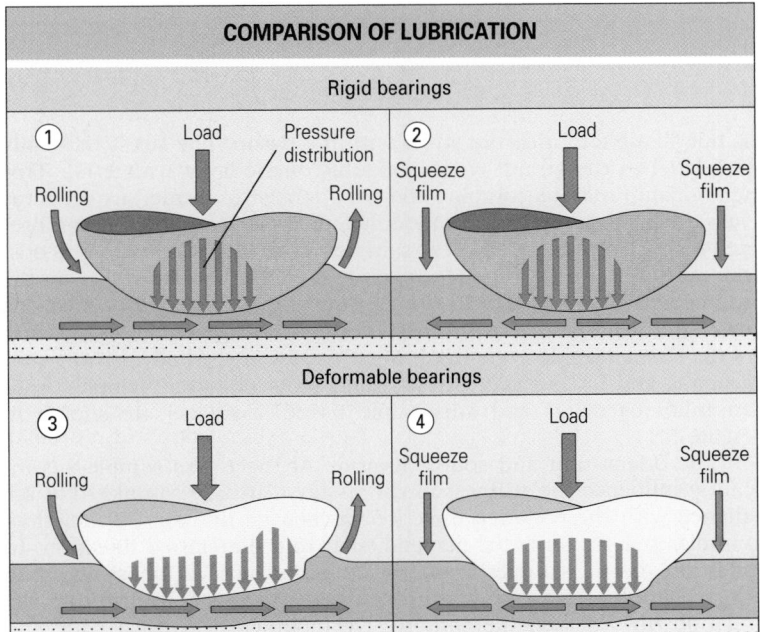

Fig. 5.3 Load carrying by lubricated bearing. A comparison of hydrodynamic lubrication (1) and squeeze film lubrication (2) of rigid surfaces, and elastohydrodynamic lubrication of deformable bearing surfaces under a hydrodynamic (sliding) action (3) and a squeeze film action (4). Surface deformation of elastohydrodynamically lubricated bearings increases the contact area, thus increasing the load-carrying capacity of these bearings.

between the bearing surfaces and generating a longer-lasting film. These factors produce a lower stress within the joint.

In diarthrodial joints, a mixed mode of lubrication occurs, with the joint surface loads being sustained by fluid film pressures in areas of noncontact and by boundary lubrication in areas of contact (Fig. 5.4). In addition, cartilaginous joint surfaces differ from typical engineering bearings in that the cartilage is filled with fluid and is porous and permeable so that the surfaces can exude a lubricating fluid. As the joint moves and the surfaces slide, fluid is exuded in front of and beneath the leading half of the load. Once the peak stresses decrease, fluid is reabsorbed back into the cartilage and it returns to its original dimensions.

The viscosity of a lubricating fluid is important. Synovial fluid undergoes large changes in viscosity, with changes in both temperature and velocity gradient. For very low velocities, a thinner lubricating film is desirable. Being thixotropic, meaning it can become fluid when agitated and then settle when left at rest, synovial fluid can meet these requirements.

If a joint effusion is present, the velocity-dependent properties of the synovial fluid may be lost, resulting in reduced lubrication and subsequent wear of the joint surfaces.

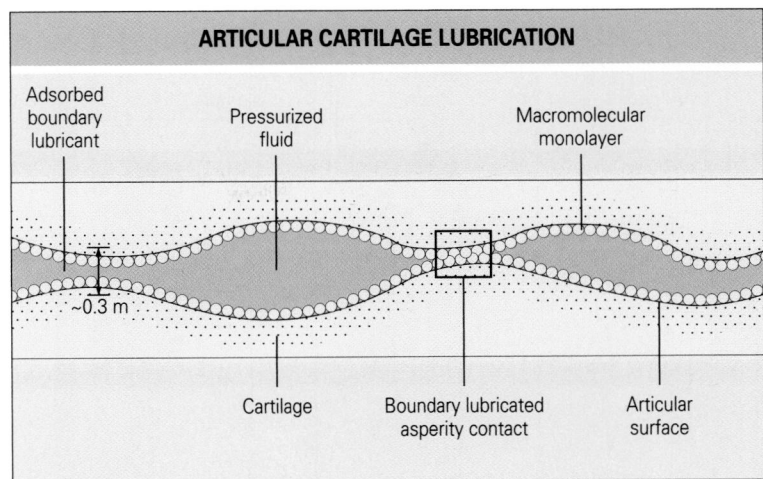

Fig. 5.4 Articular cartilage lubrication. Mixed lubrication operates in articular cartilage: boundary lubrication in which the fluid film is as thick as the roughness of the bearing surfaces, and fluid film lubrication in which surfaces are more widely separated.

BIOMECHANICS OF TISSUES

Understanding how tissues respond to applied loads and deformation often provides insight into the progression of various rheumatic diseases. When a force is applied to a tissue, the tissue will deform in response to the applied load. If a displacement is applied to the tissue, the tissue will produce a resistive force as a reaction to the applied displacement. Different loading modes exist throughout joints and tissues in the body (Fig. 5.5), often in combination. The amount of resulting deformation or reaction force produced by the tissue is directly related to the material composition, size, and shape of the tissue.

Structural properties versus material properties

Tissues can be tested as isolated individual samples (mechanical testing) or in an entire structural complex (structural testing). The structural properties of a tissue incorporate not only the material composition of the tissue but also its geometric configuration and mechanical environment.[1] Output from structural testing is shown as a force-displacement curve. A sample force-displacement curve of a material is shown in Figure 5.6. The units of force are expressed in newtons (N) or pounds force (lbf) and the units of displacement are typically millimeters (mm). Stiffness is a structural property of a body and is calculated as the slope of the elastic region of the force-displacement curve.

On the other hand, material properties of a tissue encompass the inherent material (chemical/physical) composition of the tissue itself (e.g., contribution of collagen fibrils in a tendon).[1] Output from mechanical testing is shown as a stress–strain curve. The units of stress are typically expressed as pascals (Pa, N/m^2), while strain has no assigned units. The mechanical property of modulus is calculated from the stress–strain curve. Stress and strain are considered normalized values of load and displacement, respectively, on the basis of the geometry of the sample being tested (Fig. 5.7). Stress (σ) is calculated as the applied force divided by the initial cross-sectional area of the tissue sample: $\sigma = F/A_o$. Strain (ε) is calculated as change of length of the tissue sample divided by the initial length of the sample: $\varepsilon = \Delta L/L_o$. Stress and strain and force and displacement may be positive or negative values. Additional information about the tissue may be extracted from the stress–strain curve. For example, ductility is a measure of the amount of plastic deformation of a sample when it reaches failure, and resilience is the ability of a material to absorb energy when deformed elastically and to release the energy when unloaded. These mechanical properties are shown in Figure 5.8.

Stress and strain

The stress distribution in a body is a quantitative description of the distribution of external forces acting through the body (Fig. 5.9). In

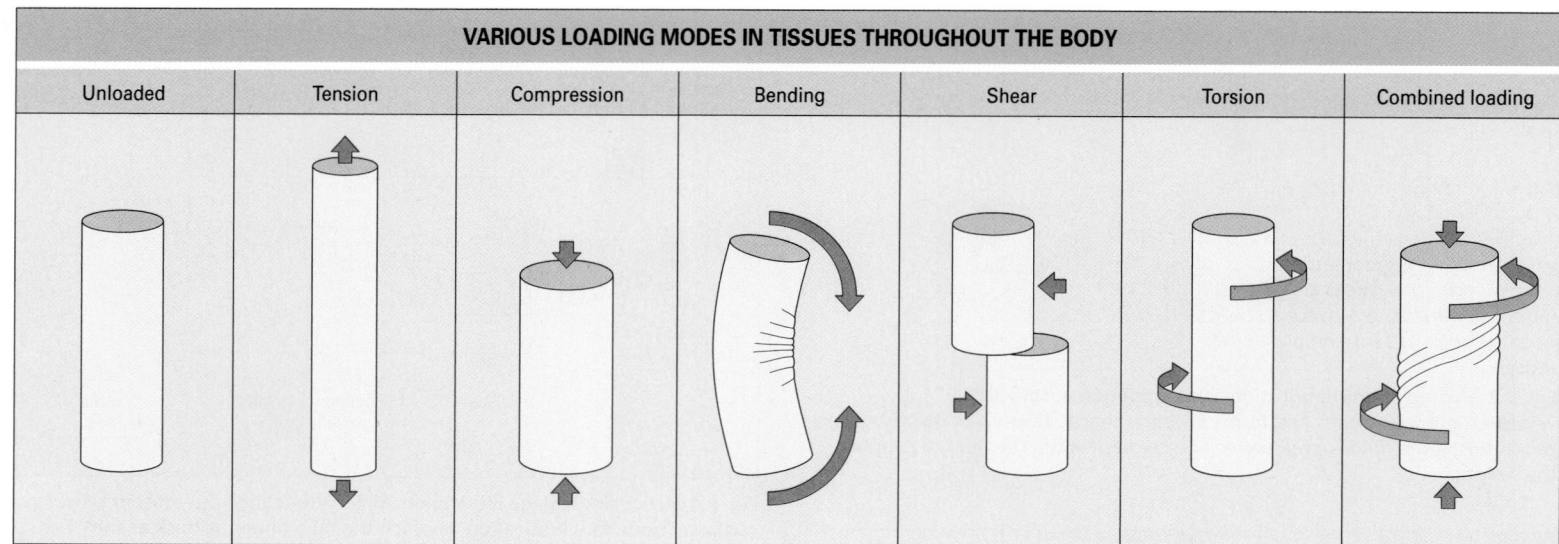

VARIOUS LOADING MODES IN TISSUES THROUGHOUT THE BODY

| Unloaded | Tension | Compression | Bending | Shear | Torsion | Combined loading |

Fig. 5.5 Schematic representation of various loading modes.

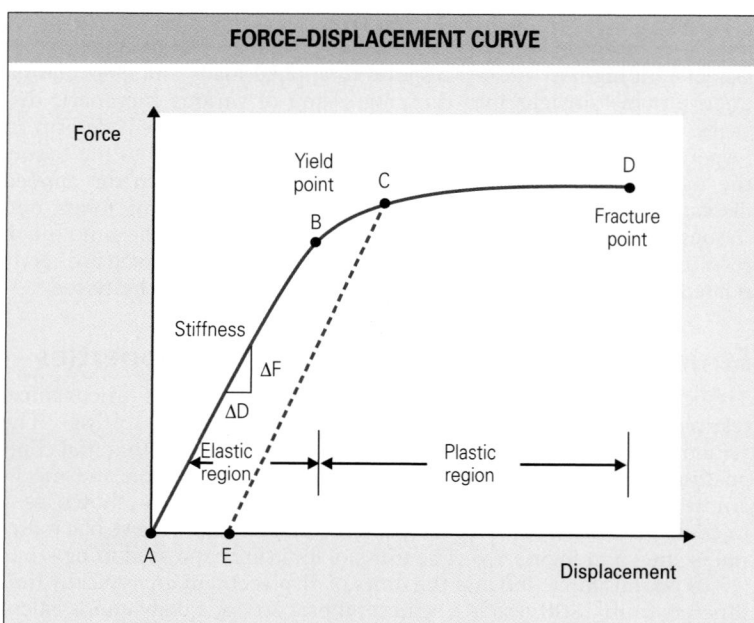

FORCE–DISPLACEMENT CURVE

Fig. 5.6 Force–displacement curve. This is the curve for a structure composed of a pliable material. If a load is applied within the elastic region (A-B) and removed, no permanent deformation occurs. If loading continues past the yield point (B) and into the plastic region (B-D) and is then released, permanent deformation results. The amount of permanent deformation that occurs if the structure is loaded to point C in the plastic region and then unloaded is represented by the distance between A and E. Structural stiffness is calculated as the slope of the linear portion of the elastic region.

is not possible to measure stress within a tissue. The stress in a body is related to the strain by the modulus of the body's material. This relationship may be complex and may consist of numerous modulus values. The exact number of modulus values depends on the homogeneity and isotropy of the test sample.[2] If a tissue is homogeneous, the mechanical properties of the tissue do not differ depending on the source location of the tested tissue sample. If a tissue is isotropic, the mechanical properties of the tissue do not change as the orientation of the tissue sample is changed. Most tissues in the body are inhomogeneous and anisotropic. Stress–strain plots of tissue samples from an inhomogeneous and anisotropic tissue (cartilage) are shown in Figure 5.11.

The orientation and source location of the tissue sample significantly influence the stiffness of the tissue. Cartilage samples that are aligned with the preferred direction of collagen fibrils are stiffer than samples that are oriented perpendicular to the preferred direction. In addition, tissue samples from the articular surface are stiffer than tissue samples from deep within the tissue. As a separate example, the relationship between the compressive modulus of cortical bone and the angle of the tissue sample relative to the long axis of the bone is shown in Figure 5.12. Researchers often assume a tissue to be homogeneous and isotropic. This results in only two variables required to fully describe the force/displacement response of a tissue to mechanical loading. Young's modulus (E_y) and Poisson's ratio (v). In one dimension, Young's modulus is calculated as the slope of the linear portion of the stress–strain curve. Poisson's ratio relates the longitudinal elongation (ε_y) of the material to the lateral contraction (ε_x) of the material (Fig. 5.13). A sample stress–strain curve for a ligament is shown in Figure 5.14. Furthermore, unlike traditional building materials (e.g., steel), soft tissues in the body have an evident viscoelastic component.

Viscoelasticity

For a viscoelastic tissue, the stress–strain response depends not only on the magnitude of the applied stress or strain, but also on the rate of the applied stress or strain. Viscoelastic tissues have three characteristic stress–strain responses: creep, stress–relaxation, and hysteresis. Creep is the deformational response of a tissue sample under a constant load (Fig. 5.15). Stress–relaxation is the stress response of a tissue sample under a constant displacement (Fig. 5.16). Hysteresis is the difference in path between loading and unloading of the tissue sample on a stress–strain diagram (Fig. 5.17). These responses can be shown diagrammatically on a ligament sample. We assume a ligament has been removed from a joint as a bone-ligament-bone (BLB) segment. One end of the BLB has been anchored to the testing system through a load cell to measure applied force, and the other end of the BLB has been attached to the moveable cross-head of the testing system.

three dimensions, six independent stress components are required to describe the state of stress at each point in a body. Three of the stress components are normal stresses (tension–compression), and three stress components are shear stresses.

When an external force acts on the body, the body deforms to resist the applied load. This deformation is called *strain* (Fig. 5.10). In three dimensions, six independent strain components are required to describe the state of strain at each point in a body. Three of the strain components represent longitudinal elongation or compression of the body along the x, y, and z axes of the local coordinate system. The remaining three strain components represent the change of angles between the x-y axes, y-z axes, and z-x axes of the local coordinate system of the body.

We must assume a stress–strain relationship to calculate the stress within a tissue on the basis of experimental strain measurements. It

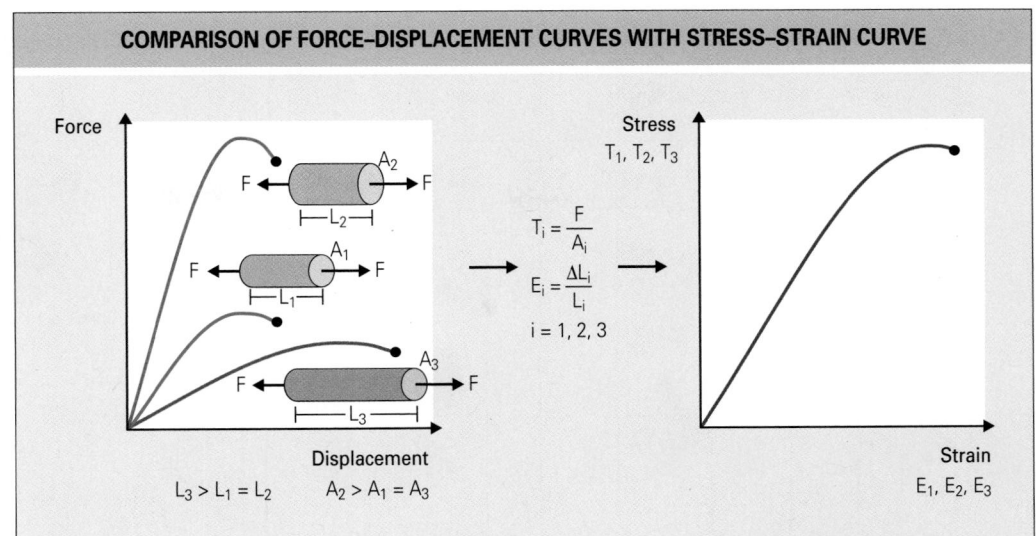

Fig. 5.7 Comparison of force–displacement curves with stress–strain curve. Different continuous structures composed of the same pliable material but with different geometries are tested in a, b, and c. When individual forces are converted to stress and displacements are converted to strains, all loading curves are superimposed onto one another.

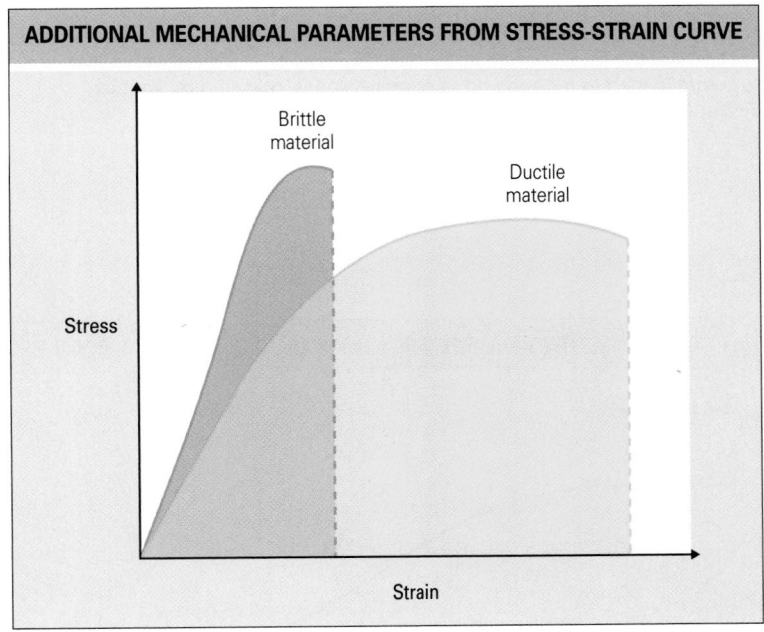

Fig. 5.8 Additional mechanical properties from stress–strain diagram. Ductility is a measure of the amount of plastic deformation at failure and is shown in this figure. Resilience is the ability of a material to absorb energy when deformed elastically and to release the energy when unloaded. Resilience is calculated as the area under the stress–strain curve line. The presence of shear strain in a structure loaded in tension and in compression is indicated by angular deformation.

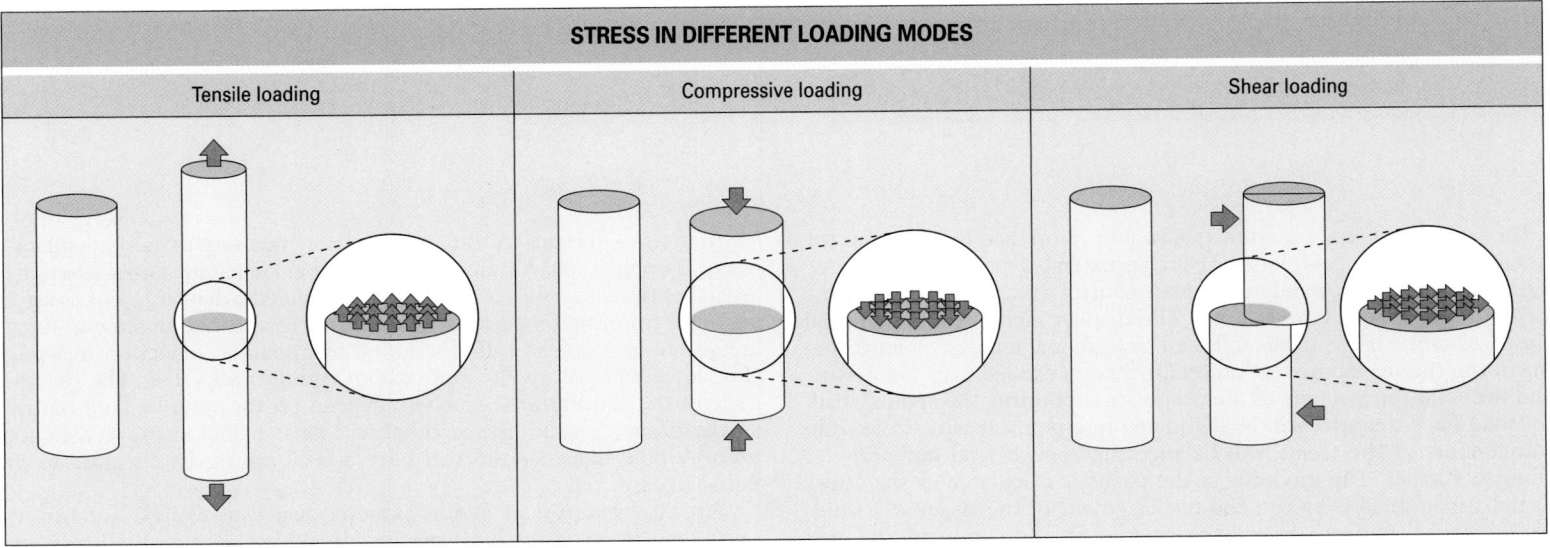

Fig. 5.9 Stress distribution within a material in different loading modes.

STATE OF STRAIN UNDER TENSION AND COMPRESSION LOADING

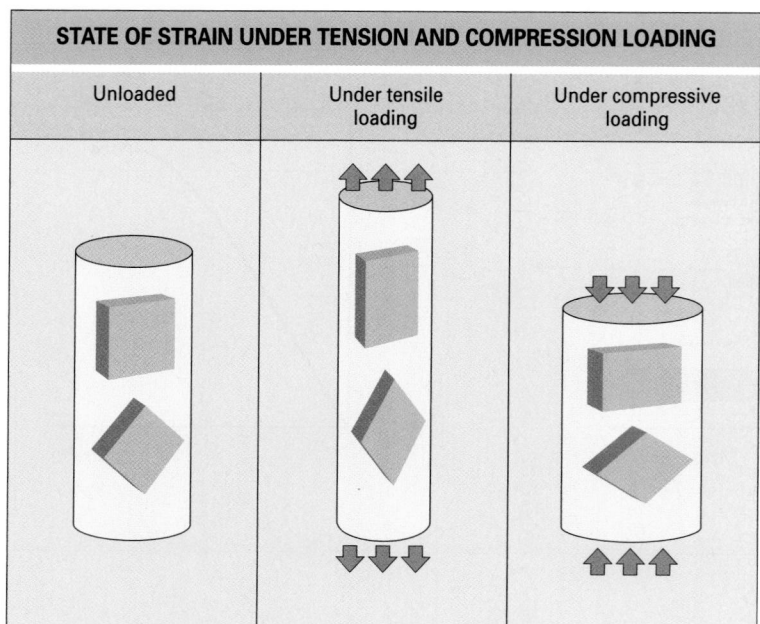

| Unloaded | Under tensile loading | Under compressive loading |

Fig. 5.10 State of strain under tension and compressive loading. Tension and compression strain are indicated by longitudinal elongation or compression of the body of the local coordinate system. The presence of shear strain in a structure loaded in tension and in compression is indicated by angular deformation of the local coordinate system.

ANISOTROPY AND INHOMOGENEITY OF CARTILAGE

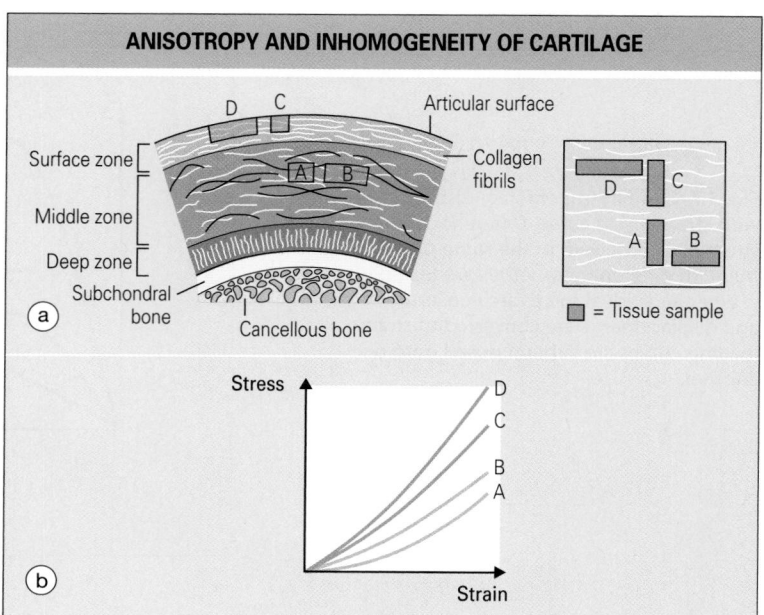

Fig. 5.11 Anisotropy and inhomogeneity of cartilage. (a) Schematic diagram of collagen fiber orientation through the depth of articular cartilage. Superficial fibers are tangent to the articular surface. Fibers in the middle zone have no preferred orientation. Fibers in the deep zone are oriented radially to the subchondral surface. (b) Stress–strain diagram of cartilage testing in tension. Tissue sample A is from the same region as tissue sample B but is oriented 90 degrees to tissue sample B. Tissue sample C is from the same region as tissue sample D but is oriented 90 degrees to tissue sample D. Differences in stress–strain response indicate the anisotropic and inhomogeneous material nature of cartilage.

ORIENTATION-DEPENDENT MODULUS OF CORTICAL BONE IN COMPRESSION

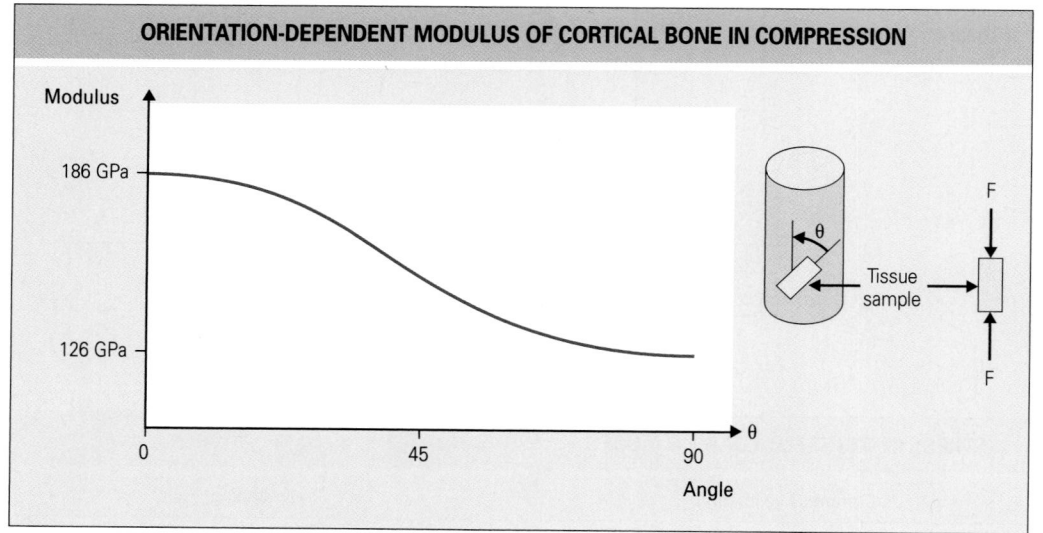

Fig. 5.12 Orientation-dependent modulus of cortical bone in compression. Cortical bone is anisotropic. The apparent compressive modulus of a cortical bone sample depends on the orientation of the sample relative to the longitudinal axis of the whole bone. GPa, gigapascal.

In a creep test, an instantaneous step or ramp load is applied to the tissue sample and held constant for an extended period of time (see Fig. 5.15). This is considered a load control test, and the resulting tissue displacement is measured. The displacement shows an initial elastic response of the tissue followed by a gradual increase of lengthening of the tissue. As the test proceeds, fluid is exuded from the tissue, and the solid components of the tissue are supporting the applied load. A "solid-like" material will be distracted to a point at which the solid components of the tissue will balance the applied load and will not elongate further. The modulus of the tissue is calculated as the stress of the tissue divided by the end displacement of the tissue. A "fluid-like" material will not be able to balance the applied load and will continue to elongate.

In a stress-relaxation test, an instantaneous step or ramp displacement is applied to the tissue sample and held constant for an extended period of time (see Fig. 5.16). This is considered a displacement control test; the resulting tissue force is measured. An initial increase in force measured by the load cell is followed by a gradual reduction in force. The force will eventually approach an equilibrium value. The magnitude of the equilibrium value will depend on the solid or fluid nature of the tissue. A solid-like material will have a final stress that is not zero. A fluid-like material will have a final stress that is close to or equal to zero.

Finally, hysteresis of a soft tissue is displayed while the tissue is cycled to a known force or displacement and back to its initial position (see Fig. 5.17). As shown in the figure, the loading portion of the

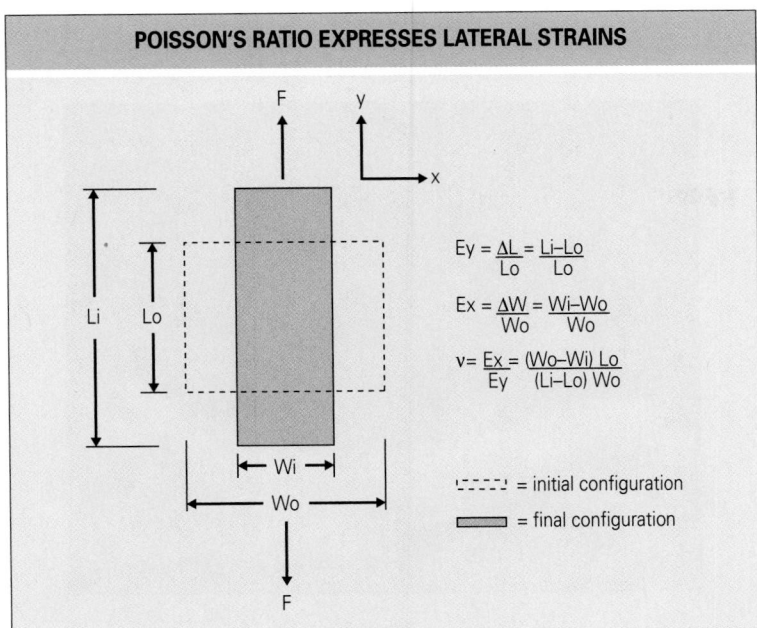

POISSON'S RATIO EXPRESSES LATERAL STRAINS

$$E_y = \frac{\Delta L}{L_o} = \frac{L_i - L_o}{L_o}$$

$$E_x = \frac{\Delta W}{W_o} = \frac{W_i - W_o}{W_o}$$

$$v = \frac{E_x}{E_y} = \frac{(W_o - W_i)}{(L_i - L_o)} \frac{L_o}{W_o}$$

⌐‥‥┐ = initial configuration

▨ = final configuration

Fig. 5.13 Poisson's ratio expresses lateral strains with respect to longitudinal strains. An ideal incompressible material has $v = 0.5$.

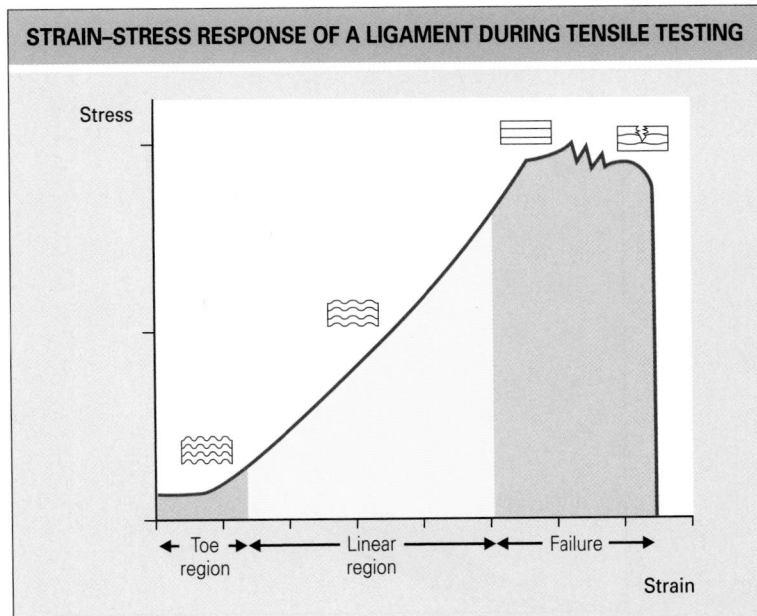

STRAIN–STRESS RESPONSE OF A LIGAMENT DURING TENSILE TESTING

Fig. 5.14 Stress–strain response of a ligament during tensile testing. The stress–strain curve is divided into three regions: toe region, linear region, and failure region. The regions are defined by the uncrimping of collagen bundles in the ligament. In the toe region, the collagen bundles are gradually recruited as force is applied to the ligament. In the linear region, all collagen bundles have been recruited and are resisting the applied load. Additional loading past the linear region will cause the bundles to fail. It is believed that physiological loading of ligaments during activities of daily living is within the toe region and lower limits of the linear region.

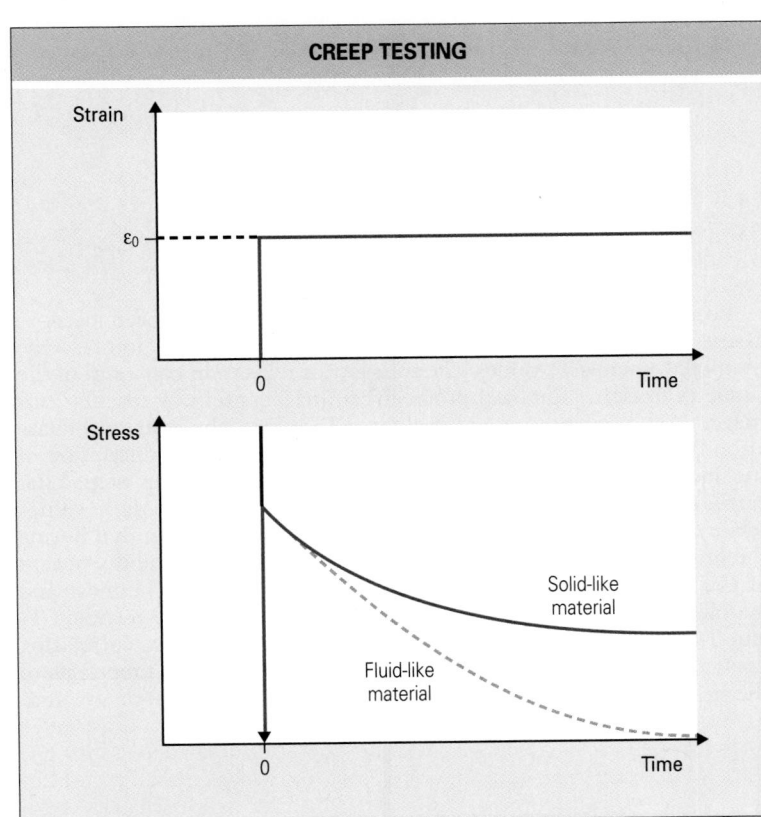

CREEP TESTING

Fig. 5.15 Creep testing. An instantaneous stress (σ_o) is applied to a tissue sample at time t_o and maintained while the resulting tissue strain is recorded. Solid-like materials will exhibit an equilibrium deformation in response to the applied load, whereas fluid-like materials will elongate continuously.

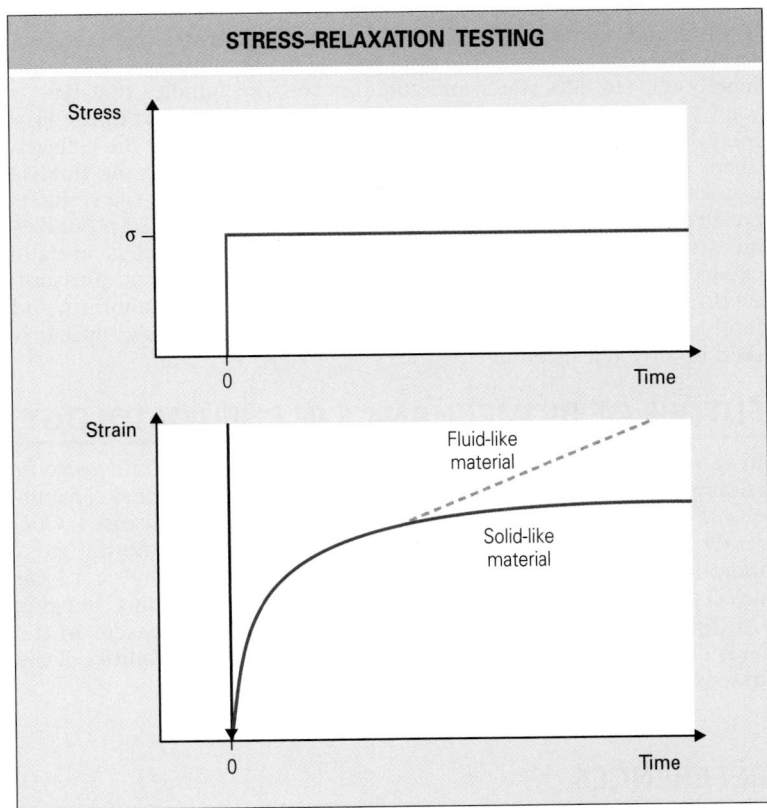

STRESS–RELAXATION TESTING

Fig. 5.16 Stress–relaxation testing. An instantaneous deformation (ε_o) is applied to a tissue sample at time t_o and maintained while the resulting tissue stress is recorded. Tissues in the body have a solid component that will resist the applied deformation after interstitial fluid has been exuded from the tissue.

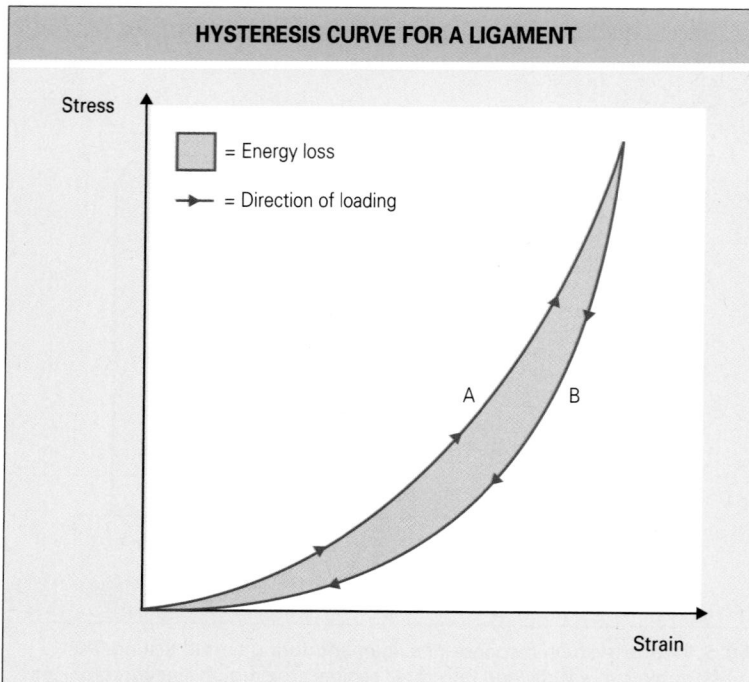

HYSTERESIS CURVE FOR A LIGAMENT

Stress

☐ = Energy loss

➡ = Direction of loading

A   B

Strain

Fig. 5.17 Hysteresis curve for a ligament. The loading portion of the curve (A) is always above the unloading portion of the curve (B). The area between the loading and unloading portions of the curve indicates relaxation of the collagen fibers within the ligament and fluid being exuded from the ligament.

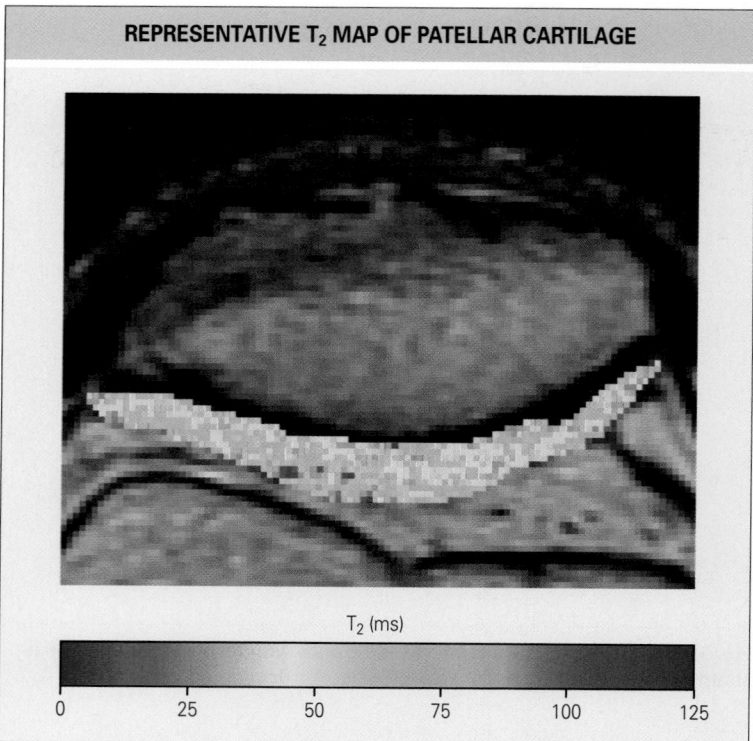

REPRESENTATIVE T₂ MAP OF PATELLAR CARTILAGE

T_2 (ms)

0   25   50   75   100   125

Fig. 5.18 Representative T_2 map of patellar cartilage. Higher values of T_2 indicate fibrillation and degradation of the articular cartilage.

force–displacement curve is always higher than the unloading portion of the curve. The area between the loading and unloading curves represents nonrecoverable energy that is lost during testing.

The viscoelastic responses of the ligament are due to the interaction of fluid and solid components of the ligament: water and collagen, respectively. In a relaxed state prior to loading, the ligament is approximately 60% to 80% water and contains collagen bundles that have a wavy appearance. When a force or displacement is applied to the ligament, the fluid is exuded through pores in the tissue and the collagen fibers begin to straighten. In a creep test, a majority of the fluid is exuded from the tissue and the applied load is balanced by the straightened collagen bundles. In a stress–relaxation test, the collagen bundles are straightened by the imposed displacement and fluid is initially exuded in response to the rapid increase in interstitial fluid pressure. As time passes, the interstitial fluid pressure comes to equilibrium and fluid is no longer exuded. A combination of the fluid–solid effects is seen in a hysteresis loop.

FUTURE OF BIOMECHANICS IN RHEUMATOLOGY

In the future, biomechanics in rheumatology will use noninvasive *in vivo* medical imaging modalities to determine the functional capabilities of tissues during the progression of rheumatologic diseases. Currently, different imaging modalities are used to determine the gross morphologic shape of diarthrodial joints (e.g., radiography) and local defects of soft tissues in the body (e.g., magnetic resonance imaging [MRI]). However, the gross morphologic appearance of tissues in the body does not always directly indicate the functional capabilities of the tissues.

TABLE 5.1 T_2 VALUES OF PATELLAR CARTILAGE AT EACH STAGE OF OSTEOARTHRITIS

Kellgren-Lawrence	T_2 values (ms) radiographic OA stage	n (average ± SD)
0	16	63.02 ± 6.25
1	25	62.15 ± 10.24
2	22	63.72 ± 7.85
3	10	64.18 ± 10.66
4	2	73.97 ± 2.33

Recently, two novel MRI imaging modalities have been used to assess the stage of osteoarthritis (OA) in diarthrodial joints. One method evaluates T_1 values (the spin-lattice relaxation constant) of the tissue to examine the local proteoglycan (PG) content of articular cartilage,[3] and a second method evaluates T_2 values (the spin-spin relaxation constant) of the tissue to examine fibrillation and disruption of the local collagen fibers in cartilage.[4] A sample T_2 map of patellar cartilage is shown in Figure 5.18. Table 5.1 displays how these values relate to radiographic staging of the same joint. It is known that during the progression of OA, the tissue exhibits a loss of PGs and disruption of the superficial collagen fibers. These changes in biochemical and histologic characteristics have been found to change the intrinsic T_1 and T_2 values of cartilage. In addition, current studies are correlating these noninvasive measures of OA with the mechanical properties of the tissue.

REFERENCES

1. Mow VC, Gu WY, Chen FH. Structure and function of articular cartilage. In: Mow VC, Huiskes R, eds. Basic orthopedic biomechanics and mechano-biology, 3rd ed. Philadelphia: Lippincott Williams & Wilkins, 2005: 181-258.

2. Lai WM, Rubin D, Krempl E. Introduction to continuum mechanics, 3rd ed. Oxford: Pergamon Press, 1993.
3. Williams A, Gillis A, McKenzie C, et al. Glycosaminoglycan distribution in cartilage as determined by delayed gadolinium-enhanced MRI of cartilage (dGEMRIC):

potential clinical applications. Am J Roentgenol 2004;182: 167-172.
4. Mosher TJ, Dardzinski BJ. Cartilage MRI T2 relaxation time mapping: overview and applications. Semin Musculoskelet Radiol 2004;8:355-368.

Connective tissue responses to mechanical stresses

6

Donald M. Salter

- Bone, cartilage, tendon, skeletal muscle, and other connective tissues require exposure to physiologic levels of mechanical stresses to remain healthy.
- Moderate exercise improves the strength and function of connective tissues.
- Withdrawal of mechanical stimuli or prolonged exposure to excessive mechanical loads results in tissue degeneration and development of diseases such as osteoarthritis.
- Mechanotransduction is the mechanism by which a mechanical signal is recognized by connective tissue cells and translated into biochemical and molecular responses.
- Connective tissue cells express mechanoreceptors that allow recognition of the physiochemical changes that occur within connective tissue during mechanical loading.
- Activation of mechanoreceptors results in generation of secondary messenger molecules and activation of signaling events that regulate gene expression and control cell function.

Exposure to physiologic mechanical forces is important for the maintenance of most, if not all, connective tissues including bone,[1,2] cartilage,[3] tendon,[4] and skeletal muscle. Movement and mechanical stimulation are essential for normal embryonic development and morphogenesis of the skeleton and joints. Wolff's law states that bone in a healthy person or animal will adapt to the loads it is placed under. When loading increases, the bone remodels to become stronger to resist that sort of loading, whereas if the loading decreases, the bone will atrophy because there is no stimulus for continued remodeling that is required to maintain bone mass. This ability to alter structure in response to mechanical loading is shared with all connective tissues and is referred to as *tissue mechanical adaptation*.

In general, mechanical loading of connective tissues within a physiologic range such as is encountered during normal, everyday activity is sufficient to keep connective tissues healthy. Clinical observations and *in-vivo* studies demonstrate that moderate exercise increases connective tissue performance. Changes in skeletal muscle bulk and strength are obvious but other connective tissues are similarly affected. Differences in bone mass in the dominant and non-dominant arms of tennis players who start training before puberty are a result of the differences in applied mechanical loads.[5] The mechanical strength and collagen content of tendons is increased by physical exercise[6] and exercise promotes proteoglycan synthesis and increases articular cartilage thickness.[7] In contrast, withdrawal of mechanical stimuli results in connective tissue atrophy as can be seen in paraplegics, patients on prolonged bed rest, and in astronauts. The bones in paralyzed and underused limbs are architecturally and mechanically inferior to those subjected to normal mechanical loading. Similarly, immobilization results in a major loss of mechanical properties in tendon[8] and, significantly, both overloading and underloading of articular cartilage are associated with loss of cartilage matrix and development of osteoarthritis.[9]

MECHANOSENSITIVE CONNECTIVE TISSUE CELLS

For tissue adaptation to occur in response to applied mechanical forces, cells within connective tissue need to receive information from their environment and modify that environment appropriately to the mechanical stresses to which it is exposed. This process can be divided into four main phases (Fig. 6.1)[10]: (1) macroscopic forces are translated into local action at the surface of the mechanosensitive cell—mechanocoupling; (2) forces are transduced from the outside of the mechanosensitive cell into biochemical signals within the cell—mechanotransduction; (3) signal transmission from the mechanosensitive cell to effector cells; and (4) extracellular matrix (ECM) modeling/remodeling. Most connective tissue cells have been shown to be mechanosensitive *in vitro*. In cartilage, chondrocytes are the only resident cells and both sense mechanical stimuli and act as effector cells producing both matrix macromolecules and proteases required for tissue turnover and homeostasis. Similarly, the tenocyte appears to have a major role in mechanical tissue adaptation in tendons.[11] In bone the situation is more complex because multiple cell types including progenitor cells, endothelial cells, and bone-forming cells are present. Nevertheless, there is a growing consensus that the osteocyte is likely to be the most important mechanosensitive cell in bone-inducing bone remodeling through paracrine effects on cells of the osteoprogenitor and osteoclast lineage.[1,2]

MECHANOCOUPLING

The mechanical loads applied to connective tissues have been extensively measured *in vivo* and vary in different tissues. In adult bone, peak strain magnitudes of 2000 to 3500 microstrain are encountered during vigorous exercise, whereas in normal activity strains of less than 10 microstrain occur thousands of times a day. Cartilage and tendon are exposed to much greater loads.[12] On normal walking, forces of three to four times body weight are generated in the hip and knee, rising to seven times body weight on rapid walking. During standing or climbing stairs forces up to 20 Mpa are produced in the hip within milliseconds. Tendons, by transmitting forces generated in muscles to bone, are also exposed to large mechanical forces, the Achilles tendon being predicted to encounter forces of 4 to 12 times body weight during walking and running.[13] The cells within connective tissue, however, are not directly exposed to these mechanical forces because they are surrounded by protective extracellular matrix that functions to absorb, transmit, and dissipate these forces. As such, the forces encountered by cells with connective tissues are not entirely clear. Cartilage, for example, consists of type II collagen arranged in a network that imparts tensile strength and proteoglycan that resists compression, allowing it to withstand high compressive and shearing loads.

Dynamic compression of cartilage results in production of a range of physiochemical changes in tissues including hydrostatic pressure gradients, fluid flow, streaming potentials, and alterations in matrix water content, fixed charge density, mobile ion concentrations, and changes in pH and osmotic pressure,[14] as well as chondrocyte deformation. All of these may influence cell behavior. To add further complexity, chondrocytes are enclosed in a specialized pericellular matrix rich in type VI collagen that resists hydrodynamic forces generated upon compression, although differences in the Young's moduli of the pericellular and interterritorial matrix may amplify strain in the vicinity of the chondrocyte by 50%.[15] Loading of bone induces both strain and compression, generating up to 5000 microstrain at the osteocyte cell surface[16] and pressure gradients that stimulate flow of interstitial fluid through the osteocytic lacunar network.[17] Osteocytes may encounter much higher levels of strain as flow of interstitial fluid through the canalicular network is resisted by the non-mineralized pericellular

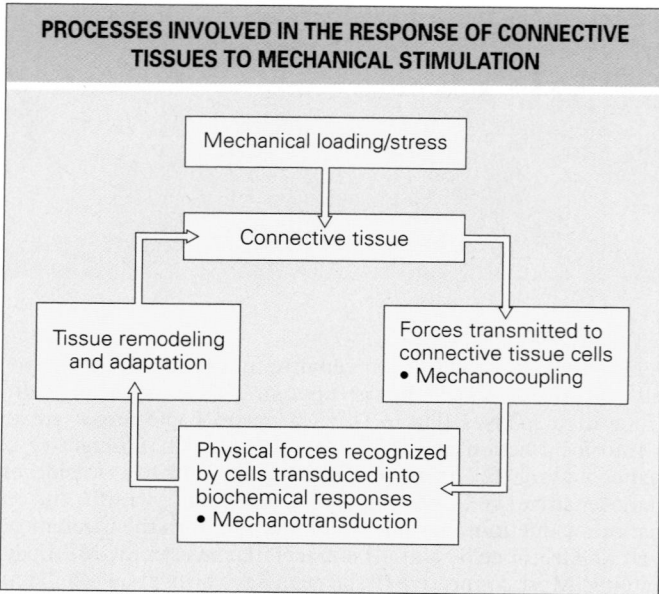

Fig. 6.1 Processes involved in the response of connective tissues to mechanical stimulation.

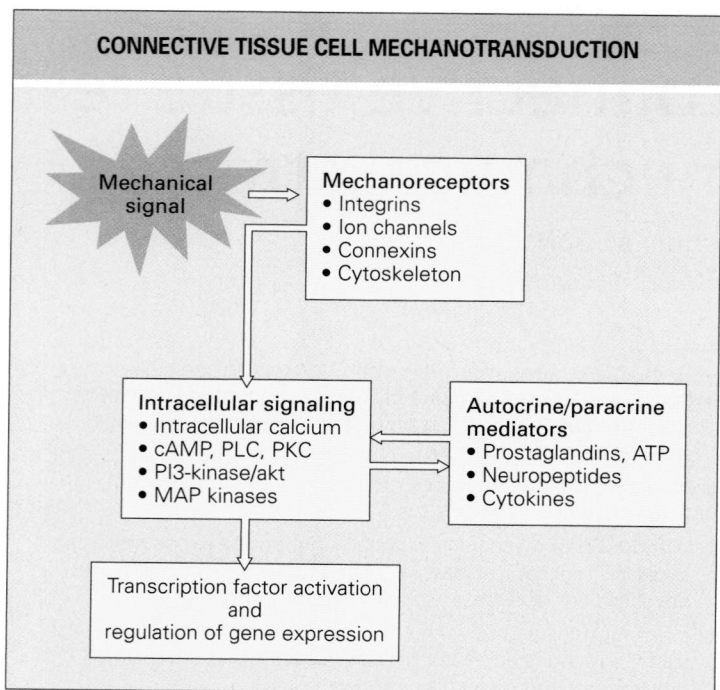

Fig. 6.2 Connective tissue cell mechanotransduction. Mechanical stimuli are recognized by mechanoreceptors that activate a range of intracellular signal pathways, either directly or through autocrine/paracrine signaling, leading to changes in gene expression and tissue remodeling. (*For abbreviations see text.*)

matrix inducing drag forces.[17] Bone cells respond to shear forces and strain *in vitro*, and it is likely that both mechanical stimuli are important *in vivo*. In tendon the complex three-dimensional structure[18] results in a tensile load at the macroscopic level being converted into tensile, shear, and compressive strains encountered by the tenocyte.

MECHANOTRANSDUCTION

Connective tissue cells express mechanoreceptors that allow recognition of the physiochemical changes that occur within connective tissue during mechanical loading. Activation of these receptors results in stimulation of intracellular signaling cascades that regulate gene expression, changes in protein expression, and tissue remodeling (Fig. 6.2). A number of molecules and molecular complexes that recognize physicochemical changes including changes in cell shape, cell membrane deformation, change in local ion concentration, and fluid flow have been identified as candidate mechanoreceptors and include integrins[19,20] mechanosensitive ion channels,[21] and connexins.[22]

INTEGRINS

Integrins are heterodimeric transmembrane glycoproteins comprising α and β subunits. Sixteen α and 8 β subunits may combine to form more than 20 specific integrin receptors. Each α and β subunit consists of an extracellular domain, a single transmembrane region, and a cytoplasmic tail. The extracellular domain provides the ligand-binding site for extracellular matrix protein ligands including fibronectin and collagen. The cytoplasmic tail is coupled to the cytoskeletal network in focal adhesions, specialized large macromolecular assemblies that include actin-associated proteins such as talin, vinculin, paxillin, and zyxin and signaling molecules such as focal adhesion kinase (FAK). This enables the integrin receptor to transduce mechanical signals transmitted through the matrix into biochemical responses within the cell.[23] Integrins have been demonstrated to be involved in cellular responses to stretch, elevated hydrostatic pressure, fluid shear stress, and osmotic forces.[24] Stretch, by increasing tension on integrins, activates these integrins and recruits focal adhesion components. This is followed by activation of a subset of unoccupied integrins inducing their binding to ECM proteins and stimulation of intracellular signaling. Other mechanical forces may act in a similar way, increasing activation of integrins to stimulate cell adhesiveness and signaling.[25] The cytoskeleton also responds mechanically to forces channeled through integrins by rearranging its interlinked actin microfilaments, microtubules, and intermediate filaments.

Chondrocytes and bone cells express a variety of integrin molecules, many of which may function as mechanoreceptors. Roles for α5β1, αVβ5, and αVβ3 have been demonstrated *in vitro* but α5β1 integrin, the classical fibronectin receptor, appears to be the major integrin mechanoreceptor in connective tissues. The anabolic response of human articular chondrocytes to mechanical stimulation is α5β1 dependent and involves phosphorylation of focal adhesion proteins including FAK and paxillin.[26] Integrins may be part of larger mechanoreceptor complexes including accessory molecules such as CD47 that may control integrin activation,[27] and regulate intracellular signaling and gene expression. Conditional knock out of β1 integrin in cortical osteocytes limits the response of bone to disuse, indicating that β1 integrins on osteocytes are active in at least some responses of these cells to mechanical loading.[28]

STRETCH-ACTIVATED ION CHANNELS

Stretch-activated or stretch-sensitive ion channels (SACs) open upon mechanical deformation of the cell membrane.[21] Potassium-selective channels (TREK-1 family of 2P domain channels and ATP-sensitive potassium channels), the Shaker-IR K+ channel, N-type Ca2+ channel, ionotropic *N*-methyl *D*-aspartate (NMDA) receptors (NMDAR), and Ca2+-dependent BK channels have all been shown to act as SACs. SACs are directly activated by mechanical forces applied along the plane of the cell membrane. These forces induce membrane tension and distortion of the cell membrane lipid bilayer, resulting in conformational changes that alter opening or closing rates allowing ion flux.[29] Hydrostatic pressure, in which mechanical forces are applied perpendicular to the cell membrane, appears to be less effective in activating SACs.[21] Opening of calcium-permeable SACs causes an elevation in intracellular calcium levels and stimulation of downstream calcium-dependent intracellular signal cascades. Such changes in intracellular calcium occur rapidly and can be seen in chondrocytes after only one cycle of compression in three-dimensional agarose constructs. SACs sensitive to gadolinium are necessary for load-related increases in prostaglandin and nitric oxide production, cytoskeletal reorganization, and changes in gene expression in response to fluid flow of bone cells and responses of chondrocytes to both strain and compression. Response of connective tissue cells to mechanical stimulation may depend on differential activation of ion channels that are activated as a consequence of changes in membrane potential (voltage-gated) or release of ligands from the cell (ligand gated). L-type calcium channels have roles in bone cell responses to fluid flow rather than strain, whereas K⁺ channels of the TREK family but not gadolinium- or nifedipine-sensitive ion channels are important for stretch-induced elevation of parathyroid hormone (PTH)-related protein gene expression in bone cells. NMDAR are ligand-gated ion channels that are non-selective to *cations* allowing influx of Na⁺ and small amounts of Ca²⁺ ions into the cell and K⁺ efflux when open. Roles for NMDAR in mechanotransduction have been demonstrated in chondrocytes.[30]

CONNEXINS

Connexins, a superfamily of 21 transmembrane proteins, form gap junctions and hemichannels. Connexins assemble in groups of six to form hemichannels, or connexons, that diffuse within the cell membrane to combine with a partner in an adjacent cell to form a gap junction.[22] Gap junctions allow continuity between cells, permitting diffusion of ions, metabolites, and small signaling molecules such as cyclic nucleotides and inositol derivatives. Connexins may also associate directly with intracellular signaling molecules such as c-src and protein kinase C (PKC) and regulate cell function through activation of intracellular signal cascades.

Connexins are widely expressed in connective tissue where networks of cells are seen such as in bone,[31] tendon,[32] and meniscus[33] and probably act to allow propagation of a mechanical stimulus through a tissue. Cx43 is the most abundant connexin family member present in skeletal tissue and believed to be involved in responses to mechanical loading. Conditional deletion of Cx43 reduces mineral apposition rate to mechanical loading, and Cx43 hemichannels are important for fluid shear induced prostaglandin E₂ (PGE₂) and adenosine triphosphate (ATP) release in osteocytic cells.[34] Junctional communication between osteocytes modulates shear stress–induced bone remodeling,[35] and altered expression of connexins by growth factors such as PTH is a route by which signal propagation and effects of mechanical loading can be controlled. Connexins and gap junctions are present at the tip of osteocyte dendritic processes and between these processes and osteoblasts, indicating their potential importance in permitting cell–cell communication among the osteocytic network. Interestingly, connexins are functional in propagating a mechanical signal from osteocytes to osteoblasts but not from osteoblasts to osteocytes.[36]

In view of the limited cell–cell communication evident in mature articular cartilage, the importance of connexins in the mechanical responses of chondrocytes is less clear. Functional unapposed Cx43 hemichannels act as ionic and molecular channels in the absence of a partner cell. As such, they have the potential to provide communication between intracellular and extracellular compartments and by release of small molecules such as glutamate and ATP mediate signal propagation. Cx32 and Cx43 are important in tenocyte mechanotransduction.[37] Cx32 junctions form a communication network arranged along the line of principal loading in the tendon and stimulate collagen production in response to strain. In contrast, the Cx43 network links tenocytes in all directions and is inhibitory for collagen production.

PRIMARY CILIA

Primary cilia are solitary, immotile cilium present in most cells including chondrocytes and bone cells. They are microtubule-based organelles that grow from the centrosome and extend from the cell surface. They contain large concentrations of cell membrane receptors, including integrins, and function as chemosensors and/or mechanosensors.[38,39] The chondrocyte primary cilium projects into the pericellular matrix and, through adhesive receptors, interacts with pericellular matrix components such as fibronectin and collagens. Bending of the cilium upon cartilage compression and deformation of the pericellular matrix is believed to result in the cilium pulling on matrix receptors, and activation of mechanoreceptors. Cx43 hemichannels are also present on chondrocyte primary cilia and by regulating ATP release and activation of the purine receptor P2Y2 may also be involved in mechanotransduction. Similar mechanosensing mechanisms may be present in bone where cilia on osteocytes are deflected during fluid

flow[40] and are required for fluid flow induction of cyclooxygenase-2, osteopontin, and prostaglandin.

MECHANICAL STIMULATION–ACTIVATED INTRACELLULAR SIGNAL CASCADES

Following recognition of a mechanical stimulus by the connective tissue cell mechanoreceptor(s), there is generation of secondary messenger molecules and activation of a cascade of downstream signaling events that regulate gene expression and cell function. A wide range of intracellular signaling molecules have been shown to be activated following mechanical stimulation of connective tissue cells. These include G proteins, protein kinases, and transcription factors that regulate expression of matrix molecules and proteases involved in tissue remodeling. These may be activated directly as a consequence of mechanoreceptor signaling or indirectly following production of autocrine/paracrine acting molecules (see later).

G PROTEIN–COUPLED RECEPTOR SIGNAL TRANSDUCTION PATHWAYS

Heterotrimeric guanine nucleotide binding proteins (G proteins) are associated with a variety of cell surface (G protein–coupled) receptors and, depending on the subclass, activate different intracellular signal cascades. Gs interacts with adenyl cyclase, catalyzing synthesis of cyclic adenosine monophosphate (cAMP) from ATP and activation of the protein kinase A signaling pathway. Gq and Go activate phospholipase C (PLC), leading to production of inositol-triphosphate (IP₃) and diacylglycerol (DAG) from phosphatidylinositol-bisphosphate (PIP₂) with subsequent calcium release from intracellular storage sites and protein kinase C (PKC) activation. There is extensive evidence for the roles for these G protein–associated signaling molecules in mechanotransduction, but limited evidence for G proteins as mechanoreceptors.

cAMP is increased in chondrocytes and bone cells following mechanical stimulation[41,42] and through activation of PKA has roles in regulating at least some of the responses of chondrocytes and bone to mechanical loading. As prostaglandins released by bone cells stimulate the G protein–coupled EP₄ receptor to elevate intracellular cAMP and Cx43 expression, at least some G protein–coupled receptor activity in mechanotransduction is a result of paracrine/autocrine signaling (see later). The PLC/PKC pathway is stimulated as a consequence of mechanical loading of many connective tissue cells. This pathway is required for load-induced aggrecan gene expression in chondrocytes and may be stimulated through integrins.[20]

The phosphoinositide 3-kinase–Akt/Protein kinase B (PKB) pathway

PKB/Akt is a protein family of serine/threonine kinase that has several important effects including inhibition of apoptosis by phosphorylation and inactivation of proapoptotic factors. It is activated by phosphoinositide 3-kinase (PI3K). Mechanical forces activate PI3K via integrin stimulation and through this route can inhibit cell death. Inactivation of the PI3K/PKB pathway may be important in deleterious effects of mechanical overloading of cartilage and bone loss in response to withdrawal of loading.[43]

Mitogen-activated protein kinases

Mitogen-activated protein (MAP) kinases are serine/threonine-specific protein kinases that regulate various cellular activities such as gene expression, mitosis, differentiation, and cell survival/apoptosis. ERK1/2, JNK, and p38 have each been shown to be activated in chondrocytes, bone cells, and fibroblasts[2,44,45] following mechanical stimulation and are of critical importance in regulation of matrix protein and protease gene expression. Upstream pathways involved in MAPK activation by mechanical loading are beginning to be investigated and may depend in part on the nature of the mechanical stimulus and the cell type. ERK1/2 activation in bone cells by mechanical stimulation requires calcium-dependent ATP release, whereas ERK1/2 activation in cartilage appears to be, at least under certain circumstances, dependent on basic fibroblast growth factor-2 (bFGF-2) rather than through integrin mechanoreceptors.[46]

The NF-kappa B pathway

NF-kappa B (NF-κB) is a protein complex that acts as a transcription factor. In bone cells NF-κB is directly stimulated by mechanical stimulation through a pathway involving intracellular calcium release, but not the cytoskeleton.[47] Dynamic biomechanical signals of low-physiologic magnitudes and mechanical stimulation within the physiologic range block NF-κB activity and signaling that promotes chondrocyte responses to proinflammatory cytokines and matrix fragments[48] and regulation of proapoptotic or antiapoptotic pathways. Conversely, high-amplitude dynamic stimulation, a catabolic stimulus, induces rapid nuclear translocation of NF-κB subunits p65 and p50 in a similar manner to interleukin (IL)-1β.

Autocrine/paracrine signaling events in mechanotransduction

In many mechanosensitive connective tissue cells mechanical loading induces secretion of soluble mediators, including prostaglandins, nitric oxide, cytokines, growth factors, and neuropeptides that are involved in downstream tissue modeling and remodeling responses. Production of soluble mediators by connective tissue cells in response to mechanical stimulation, however, may also be intrinsic to mechanotransduction pathways. Rapid production and release of soluble mediators allow autocrine and paracrine activity, permitting crosstalk between different components of a mechanotransduction cascade and regulating the cellular response to the mechanical stimulus.

PROSTAGLANDINS, NITRIC OXIDE, AND ATP

Prostaglandins, predominantly PGE_2, and nitrous oxide (NO) are rapidly produced when bone cells are mechanically stimulated and are required for the anabolic response of bone to mechanical loading *in vivo*. Prostaglandin production is integrin dependent; requires activation of an intracellular signal cascade involving the cytoskeleton, SACs, PKC, and phospholipase A_2 (PLA_2); and may require IL-1β. In bone, PGE_2 may influence bone responses to mechanical loading by regulating gap junction expression[49] and bone mass by effects on RANKL expression and osteoclastogenesis. In contrast to bone, in cartilage PGE_2 is catabolic and physiologic mechanical loading of chondrocytes inhibits production of PGE_2 and NO. Pathologic loading of cartilage such as high-impact loading, however, results in PGE_2 release.[50] ATP is released when bone cells and chondrocytes are mechanically stimulated and may then bind and activate purinergic receptors. Both metabotropic P2Y receptors, which induce intracellular calcium release through activation of G proteins, and ionotropic P2X receptors, which are ligand-gated channels, are involved in mechanical stimulation cascades. $P2X_7$ deficiency results in osteopenia potentially as a result of reduced responsiveness to mechanical loading of the skeleton.

CYTOKINES AND GROWTH FACTORS

IL-4 and IL-1β autocrine/paracrine activity is seen in the integrin-dependent mechanotransduction cascade of chondrocytes (IL-4 and IL-1β) and bone cells (IL-1β) to mechanical stimulation.[51] These molecules are secreted within 20 minutes of the onset of mechanical stimulation, suggesting release from preformed stores. IL-4 release relies on secretion of the neuropeptide substance P, which binds to its NK1 receptor. Both IL-4 and substance P are necessary but not sufficient for the increased expression of aggrecan mRNA and decrease in matrix metalloproteinase-3 mRNA induced by the mechanical stimulus, suggesting crosstalk with other mechanosensitive signaling pathways. IL-1β is involved in the early mechanotransduction pathway of both osteoarthritic chondrocytes and human trabecular bone-derived cells. Mechanical loading may also induce release or activation of sequestered growth factors in extracellular matrix, which will then act on nearby resident connective tissue cells. bFGF-2 is a possible mediator of mechanical signaling in cartilage through such a mechanism.[46]

CONCLUDING REMARKS

Individuals are exposed to a wide range of mechanical stresses during daily activity that are required to maintain connective tissues including bone, cartilage, and tendons in a healthy state. Moderate exercise can improve the strength and function of connective tissues, but withdrawal of mechanical stimuli or prolonged exposure to excessive mechanical loads result in tissue degeneration and development of diseases such as osteoarthritis. The mechanisms by which mechanical stresses regulate connective tissue cell function are beginning to be understood. It is likely that identification of mechanoreceptors and mechanotransduction pathways will increase our knowledge of how adverse mechanical environments have detrimental effects on connective tissue and allow development of novel therapeutic interventions such as mechanomimetics to preserve or reconstitute connective tissue in aging and disease.

REFERENCES

1. Turner CH. Bone strength: current concepts. Ann NY Acad Sci 2006;1068:429-446.
2. Rubin J, Rubin C, Jacobs CR. Molecular pathways mediating mechanical signaling in bone. Gene 2006;367:1-16.
3. Grodzinsky AJ, Levenston ME, Jin M, et al. Cartilage tissue remodeling in response to mechanical forces. Annu Rev Biomed Eng 2000;2:691-713.
4. Wang JH. Mechanobiology of tendon. J Biomech 2006;39:1563-1582.
5. Kannus P, Haapasalo H, Sankelo M, et al. Effect of starting age of physical activity on bone mass in the dominant arm of tennis and squash players. Ann Intern Med 1995;123:27-31.
6. Woo SLY, Ritter MA, Amiel D, et al. The biomechanical and biochemical properties of swine tendons—long term effects of exercise on the digital extensors. Connect Tissue Res 1980;7:177-183.
7. Kiviranta I, Jurvelin J, Tammi J, et al. Weight bearing controls glycosaminoglycan concentration and articular cartilage thickness in the knee joints of young Beagle dogs. Arthritis Rheum 1987;30:801-809.
8. Yamamoto N, Ohno K, Hayashi K, et al. Effects of stress shielding on the mechanical properties of rabbit patellar tendon. J Biomed Eng 1993;115:23-28.
9. Jortikka MO, Inkinen RI, Tammi MI, et al. Proteoglycan alterations in rabbit knee articular cartilage following physical exercise and immobilization. Connect Tissue Res 1983;11:45-55.
10. Duncan RL, Turner CH. Mechanotransduction and the functional response of bone to mechanical strain. Calcif Tissue Int 1995;57:344-358.
11. Screen HRC, Shelton JC, Lee DA, et al. Cyclic tensile strain upregulates collagen synthesis in isolated tendon fascicles. Biochem Biophys Res Commun 2005;336:424-429.
12. Rubin CT, Lanyon LE. Regulation of bone formation by applied dynamic loads. J Bone Joint Surg Am 1984;66:397-402.
13. Giddings VL, Beaupré GS, Whalen RT, et al. Calcaneal loading during walking and running. Med Sci Sports Exerc 2000;32:627-634.
14. Urban JP. The chondrocyte: a cell under pressure. Br J Rheumatol 1994;33:901-908.
15. Nuki G, Salter DM. The impact of mechanical stress on the pathophysiology of osteoarthritis. In: Sharma L, Berenbaum F, eds. Osteoarthritis: a companion to rheumatology. St Louis: Elsevier, 2007: 33-52.
16. Han Y, Cowin SC, Schaffler MB, et al. Mechanotransduction and strain amplification in osteocyte cell processes. Proc Natl Acad Sci USA 2004;101:16689-16694.
17. Burger EH, Klein-Nulend J. Mechanotransduction in bone—role of the lacuno-canalicular network. FASEB J 1999;13:S101-S112.
18. Screen HRC, Lee DA, Bader DL, et al. Development of a technique to determine strains in tendons using the cell nuclei. Biorheology 2003;40:361-368.
19. Ingber D. Integrins as mechanochemical transducers. Curr Opin Cell Biol 1991;3:841-848.
20. Millward-Sadler SJ, Salter DM. Integrin-dependent signal cascades in chondrocyte mechanotransduction. Ann Biomed Eng 2004;32:435-446.
21. Martinac B. Mechanosensitive ion channels: molecules of mechanotransduction. J Cell Sci 2004;17:2449-2460.
22. Müller U. Cadherins and mechanotransduction by hair cells. Curr Opin Cell Biol 2008;20:557-566.
23. Giancotti FG, Ruoslahti E. Integrin signaling. Science 1999;285:1028-1032.
24. Katsumi A, Orr AW, Tzima E, et al. Integrins in mechanotransduction. J Biol Chem 2004;279:12001-12004.
25. Schwartz MA, DeSimone DW. Cell adhesion receptors in mechanotransduction. Curr Opin Cell Biol 2008;20:551-556.
26. Lee HS, Millward-Sadler SJ, Wright MO, et al. Integrin and mechanosensitive ion channel-dependent tyrosine phosphorylation of focal adhesion proteins and beta-catenin in human articular chondrocytes after mechanical stimulation. J Bone Miner Res 2000;15:1501-1509.
27. Orazizadeh M, Lee HS, Groenendijk B, et al. CD47 associates with alpha 5 integrin and regulates responses of human articular chondrocytes to mechanical stimulation in an in vitro model. Arthritis Res Ther 2008;10:R4.

28. Phillips JA, Almeida EA, Hill EL, et al. Role for beta1 integrins in cortical osteocytes during acute musculoskeletal disuse. Matrix Biol 2008;27:609-618.

29. Ingber DE. Cellular mechanotransduction: putting all the pieces together again. FASEB J 2006;20:811-827.

30. Salter DM, Wright MO, Millward-Sadler SJ. NMDA receptor expression and roles in human articular chondrocyte mechanotransduction. Biorheology 2004;41:273-281.

31. Jiang JX, Siller-Jackson AJ, Burra S. Roles of gap junctions and hemichannels in bone cell functions and in signal transmission of mechanical stress. Front Biosci 2007;12:1450-1462.

32. Ralphs JR, Benjamin M, Waggett, et al. Regional differences in cell shape and gap junction expression in rat Achilles tendon: relation to fibrocartilage differentiation. J Anat 1998;193:215-222.

33. Hellio Le Graverand MP, Ou Y, Schield-Yee T, et al. The cells of the rabbit meniscus: their arrangement, interrelationship, morphological variations and cytoarchitecture. J Anat 2001;198:525-535.

34. Roberto Civitelli. Cell-cell communication in the osteoblast/osteocyte lineage. Arch Biochem Biophys 2008;473:188-192.

35. Thi MM, Kojima T, Cowin SC, et al. Fluid shear stress remodels expression and function of junctional proteins in cultured bone cells. Am J Physiol Cell Physiol 2003;284:C389-C403.

36. Yellowley CE, Li Z, Zhou Z, et al. J Bone Miner Res 2000;15:209-217.

37. Waggett AD, Benjamin M, Ralphs JR. Connexin 32 and 43 gap junctions differentially modulate tenocyte response to cyclic mechanical load. Eur J Cell Biol 2006;85:1145-1154.

38. Whitfield JF. The solitary (primary) cilium—a mechanosensory toggle switch in bone and cartilage cells. Cell Signal 2008;20:1019-1024.

39. Poole CA, Jensen CG, Snyder JA, et al. Confocal analysis of primary cilia structure and colocalization with the Golgi apparatus in chondrocytes and aortic smooth muscle cells. Cell Biol Int 1997;21:483-494.

40. Malone AM, Anderson CT, Tummala P, et al. Primary cilia mediate mechanosensing in bone cells by a calcium-independent mechanism. Proc Natl Acad Sci USA 2007;104:13325-13330.

41. Fitzgerald JB, Jin M, Dean D, et al. Mechanical compression of cartilage explants induces multiple time-dependent gene expression patterns and involves intracellular calcium and cyclic AMP. J Biol Chem 2004;279:19502-19511.

42. Carvalho RS, Scott JE, Suga DM, et al. Stimulation of signal transduction pathways in osteoblasts by mechanical strain potentiated by parathyroid hormone. J Bone Miner Res 1994;9:999-1011.

43. Dufour C, Holy X, Marie PJ. Transforming growth factor-beta prevents osteoblast apoptosis induced by skeletal unloading via PI3K/Akt, Bcl-2, and phospho-Bad signaling. Am J Physiol Endocrinol Metab 2008;294:E794-801.

44. Fitzgerald JB, Jin M, Chai DH, et al. Shear- and compression-induced chondrocyte transcription requires MAPK activation in cartilage explants. J Biol Chem 2008;283:6735-6743.

45. Jeon YM, Kook SH, Son YO, et al. Role of MAPK in mechanical force-induced up-regulation of type I collagen and osteopontin in human gingival fibroblasts. Mol Cell Biochem 2009;320:45-52.

46. Vincent T, Saklatvala J. Basic fibroblast growth factor: an extracellular mechanotransducer in articular cartilage? Biochem Soc Trans 2006;34:456-457.

47. Chen NX, Geist DJ, Genetos DC, et al. Fluid shear-induced NFkappaB translocation in osteoblasts is mediated by intracellular calcium release. Bone 2003;33:399-410.

48. Anghelina M, Sjostrom D, Perera P, et al. Regulation of biomechanical signals by NF-kappaB transcription factors in chondrocytes. Biorheology 2008;45:245-256.

49. Cherian PP, Siller-Jackson AJ, Gu S, et al. Mechanical strain opens connexin 43 hemichannels in osteocytes: a novel mechanism for the release of prostaglandin. Mol Biol Cell 2005;16:3100-3106.

50. Jeffrey JE, Aspden RM. Cyclooxygenase inhibition lowers prostaglandin E2 release from articular cartilage and reduces apoptosis but not proteoglycan degradation following an impact load in vitro. Arthritis Res Ther 2007;9:R129.

51. Salter DM, Millward-Sadler SJ, Nuki G, et al. Integrin-interleukin-4 mechanotransduction pathways in human chondrocytes. Clin Orthop Relat Res 2001;391:S49-S60.

The synovium

Malcolm D. Smith and Jennifer G. Walker

- Synovium lines diarthrodial joints, tendon sheaths, and bursae.
- Specialized functions of synovium include non-adherence, control of synovial fluid volume and composition, and chondrocyte nutrition.
- The normal synovium expresses low levels of proinflammatory cytokines and some anti-inflammatory cytokines. In addition, the low levels of RANKL expression with high levels of OPG expression result in a low RANKL-to-OPG ratio suppressing osteoclast formation. This balance is likely to be important in maintaining homeostasis in the normal, non-inflamed synovium.

DEFINITIONS

Synovium is the soft tissue lining the spaces of diarthrodial joints, tendon sheaths, and bursae. The term includes both the continuous surface layer of cells (intima) and the underlying tissue (subintima). The intima is composed of specialized macrophages and fibroblasts, and the subintima contains blood and lymphatic vessels, a cellular content of both resident fibroblasts and infiltrating cells in a collagenous extracellular matrix. Between the intimal surfaces is a small amount of fluid, usually rich in hyaluronan (hyaluronic acid, HA). Together, this structure provides a non-adherent surface between tissue elements. Unlike serosal surfaces, which also have non-adherent properties, synovium is derived from ectoderm and does not contain a basal lamina.

The study of synovial tissue is of major importance in understanding the pathogenesis of a number of inflammatory joint diseases, including rheumatoid arthritis (RA) and the seronegative spondyloarthropathies (SpA). Despite this, our knowledge of the immunohistochemical architecture of the synovial membrane, particularly in normal subjects, is surprisingly limited.

In normal subjects, the synovium comprises an intimal layer, which is 20 to 40 μm thick in cross section, and an areolar subintima, which can be up to 5 mm in thickness. At many sites there is no discrete membrane, especially where subintima consists of fat pad or fibrous tissue.

Synovium is often atypical. Intimal cells may be absent. Superficial bursae contain little or no hyaluronan-rich fluid.[1] Ganglia are sacs containing hyaluronan-rich fluid but do not occur at sites of shearing and do not have a typical intima and so may not be considered to really be synovial tissue. Diseased synovial tissue may lose any recognizable lining structure and only be definable by its relation to a joint. These variations probably reflect interplay of several factors in synovial histogenesis.

EMBRYOLOGY

In the early embryonic limb bud, a central core or blastema that will form the skeleton appears. Within this core, foci of cartilage appear, each destined to become a bone. Blastemal cells around cartilage foci form a perichondrial envelope showing strong expression of CD44. The area where this envelope lies between cartilage elements is known as the interzone, from which synovium forms. The perichondrium forming a sleeve around each cartilage element subsequently invades the cartilage to form bone marrow. Thus synovial and bone marrow stromal cells come from the same embryonic stock.

Shortly before the joint cavity forms, CD55 expression appears on cells along the joint line,[2] followed later by vascular cell adhesion molecule (VCAM)-1 expression. After cavity formation the intimal layer also takes on a higher level of expression of CD44 and β_1 integrins compared with subintima.

The mechanism of cavity formation is not fully understood; a working hypothesis implicates interactions between interzone cells bearing CD44 (a hyaluronan receptor) and hyaluronan itself.[3,4] Shortly before cavity formation, the cells of the potential joint line show high uridine diphosphoglucose dehydrogenase (UDPGD) activity, suggesting increased hyaluronan synthesis. At the time of cavity formation high levels of hyaluronan appear along the joint line. At low concentration extracellular hyaluronan cross-links CD44 molecules on adjacent cells, inducing cell aggregation, but at high levels, hyaluronan saturates CD44 and disaggregation occurs.

Cavity formation might be expected to require lysis of matrix fibers. However, in human joints cavity formation is not associated with high local levels of matrix metalloproteinases at the joint line and matrix fibers appear to run only parallel to the joint line prior to cavity formation. Apoptotic cells are found in the interzone prior to cavity formation but are not localized to the joint line and are unlikely to contribute to cavity formation. It appears, therefore, that development of the joint cavity arises more from differential tissue expansion than through loss of solid elements.

An alternative explanation for the formation of the synovial lining and the synovial-lined joint space has recently been suggested from mouse model work.[5] A study looking at cadherin-11–deficient mice suggests that expression of cadherin-11 on synovial fibroblasts may be critical in the development of the synovial lining by facilitation of cellular organization, compaction, and matrix development to form a recognizable synovial lining. Although these findings have not been replicated in human tissue as yet, it does raise the possibility that cadherin-11 expression by synovial fibroblasts is critical for normal synovial tissue development.

STRUCTURE

The microscopic anatomy of synovial tissue was first fully described by Key,[6] who divided synovium into three main types on the basis of subintimal structure: fibrous, areolar, and adipose (Figs. 7.1 to 7.3). He also noted that subintima may be periosteum, perimysium, or even hyaline or fibrocartilage.

Areolar synovium is the most specialized form (see Fig. 7.1). It is often crimped into folds, which may disappear when stretched. Less often it carries projections or villi. A more or less continuous layer of cells lies two or three deep on the tissue surface.[7,8] Immediately beneath these cells are capillaries. Further into the tissue there is a plexus of small arterioles and venules,[9,10] associated with mast cells. Lymphatic vessels can be found in all types of normal synovial tissue, although they are infrequent in the fibrous type of normal synovium.[11] In normal synovium, most lymphatic vessels are found in the deep subintima and fibrous layers, whereas in synovium from RA patients lymphatic vessels are widespread and numerous. Nerve fibers are present, chiefly in association with blood vessels.[12] Three layers of tissue matrix may be distinguished. The intima is associated with a fine fibrillar matrix with few type I collagen fibers.[13] Beneath this is a layer relatively rich in type I collagen, which forms the physical membrane. Deeper is a loose layer that allows the membrane to move freely. Beyond the loose layer will lie ligament, tendon, or periosteum.

Adipose synovium occurs as fat pads and within villi (see Fig. 7.2). It has a complete intimal cell layer and a superficial net of capillaries. The intima may lie directly on adipocytes but there is usually a band of collagen-rich substratum, whereas the deeper tissue is fat. Villi usually have a central arteriole and venule but can be avascular. The

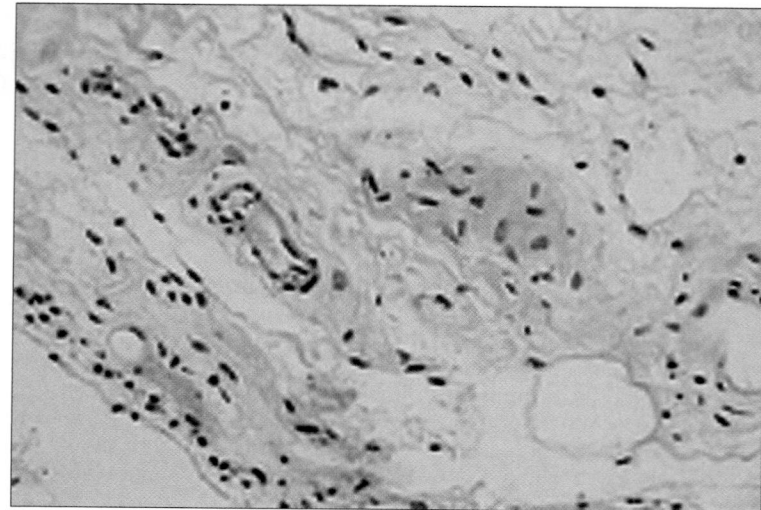

Fig. 7.1 Areolar form of synovium (H&E stain).

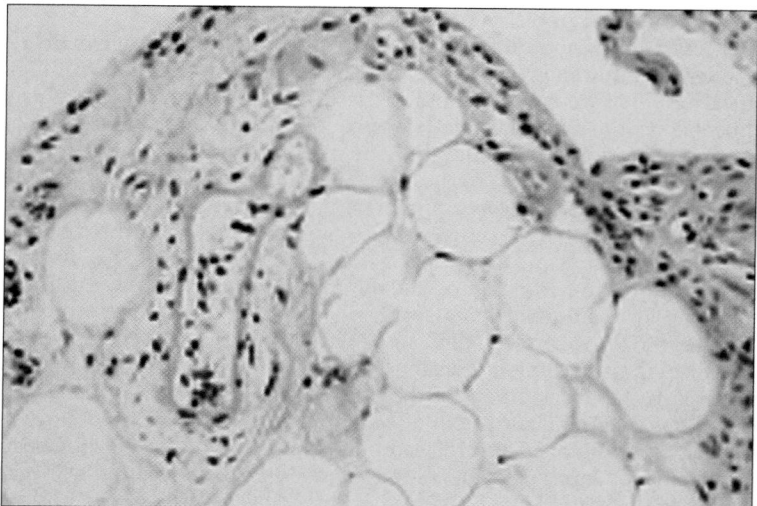

Fig. 7.2 Adipose form of synovium (H&E stain).

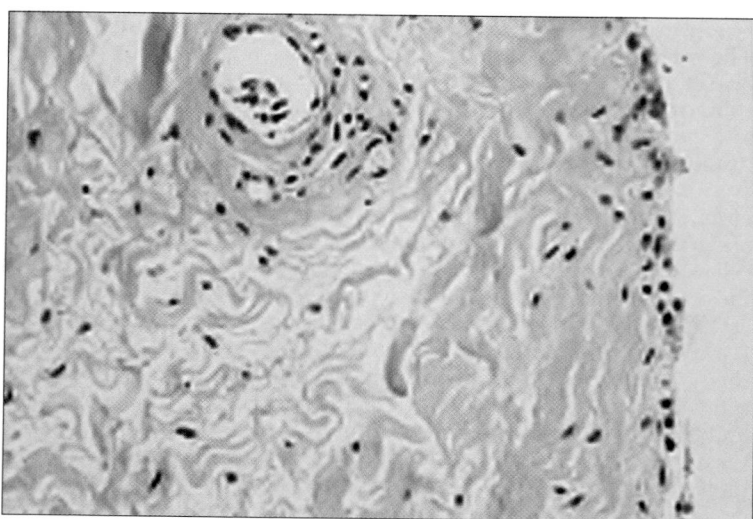

Fig. 7.3 Fibrous form of synovium (H&E stain).

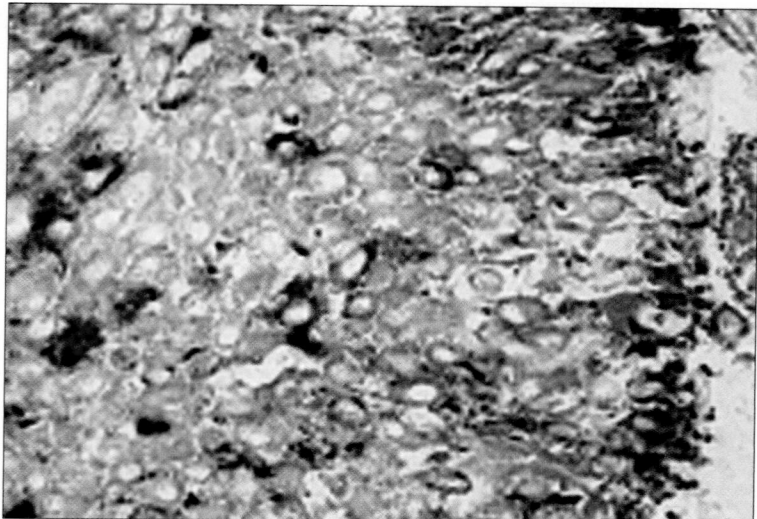

Fig. 7.4 RA synovium (×400 magnification) showing a thickened intimal layer, containing mainly CD68+ macrophages (red) on the surface and weakly CD55+ fibroblastic cells beneath (blue).

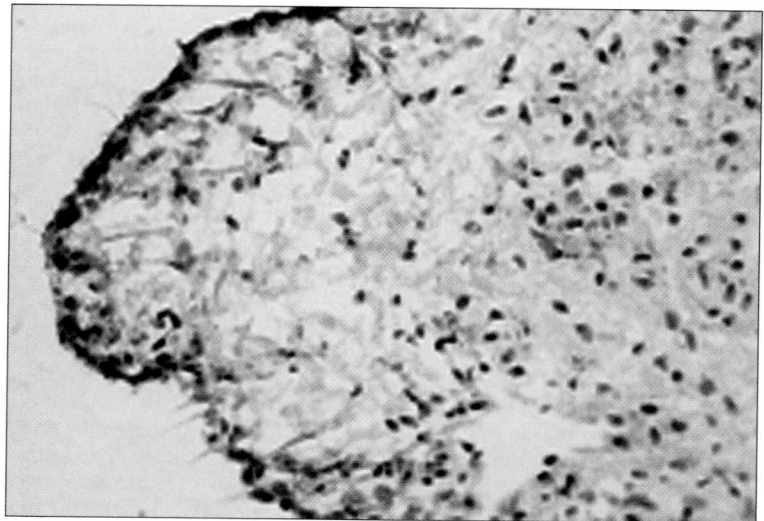

Fig. 7.5 Synovial macrophages. Normal synovium (×200 magnification) stained for CD68+ macrophages (red).

Intimal cells

Two types of intimal cells have been defined by electron microscopy, one consistent with a macrophage (type A) and the other with a fibroblast (type B).[14] It is now generally accepted that intimal macrophages are true macrophages, derived from blood monocytes, whereas the intimal fibroblasts are locally derived.[15]

Immunohistochemical and cytochemical methods have superseded electron microscopy as tools for cell identification.[16] Intimal macrophages can be distinguished by their non-specific esterase (NSE) activity and expression of surface markers such as CD68 and CD163. Intimal fibroblasts show intense activity of the enzyme UDPGD and prominent expression of VCAM-1 and CD55 (complement decay-accelerating factor [DAF]). In most disease states such as rheumatoid arthritis, intimal cells increase in size and number (Fig. 7.4). This is not *hyperplasia* but a complex change in cell populations, in terms of both origin and function, often dominated by macrophage influx.[15]

Synovial macrophages

Macrophages are present in both the intima and subintima. Intimal macrophages carry typical macrophage lineage markers. They show prominent NSE activity and are strongly positive for CD163 and CD68 but less so for CD14 (Fig. 7.5). Macrophages also express the

amount of fat in villi varies and probably decreases with age, with an increase in fibrous tissue.

Fibrous synovium is often difficult to define, consisting of fibrous tissue such as ligament or tendon on which lies an intermittent layer of cells (see Fig. 7.3). Fibrous synovium may be indistinguishable from fibrocartilage, especially in the annular pads found in finger joints.

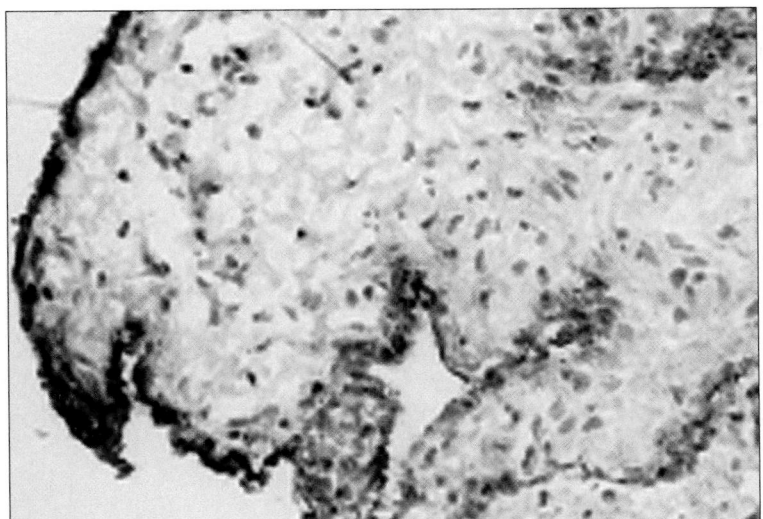

Fig. 7.6 Normal synovium (×200 magnification) stained for CD55+ fibroblasts, which are the predominant cell in the normal synovium intimal layer (contrast with Fig. 7.4).

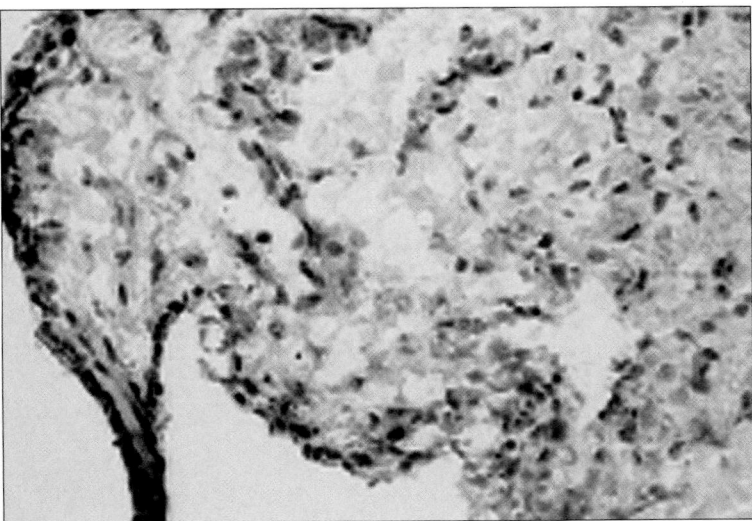

Fig. 7.7 Normal synovium (×200 magnification) stained for VCAM-1.

immunoglobulin receptor FcγRIIIa. Strong FcγRIIIa expression is restricted to a subset of macrophages that correspond closely to sites of macrophage activation in rheumatoid disease: synovial, alveolar, serosal, scleral, salivary gland, lymphoid and bone marrow macrophages, and Kupffer cells.[17] Subintimal macrophages are FcγRIIIa dull or negative.

Macrophages make up a minority of cells in normal intima (Figs. 7.5 and 7.6). In diseased tissue the proportion of macrophages may rise to 80% (see Fig. 7.4). Distribution varies but a common pattern occurs: a superficial layer of macrophages with an intimal phenotype; beneath this a layer of intimal fibroblasts; and further beneath and beyond the limits of the intima, a zone of NSE-weak, strongly CD14+ FcγRI+ macrophages, associated with venules. The deep, strongly CD14+ cells are probably freshly recruited cells and the superficial cells more mature.

In addition to true macrophages, there may be a small number of antigen-presenting interdigitating dendritic cells in normal synovial intima. These are more frequent in diseased tissue but overlap of markers is much greater in disease, making interpretation difficult.[18,19] Cells with features of osteoclasts such as expression of tartrate-resistant acid phosphatase and the vitronectin receptor also often appear in inflamed synovium. However, fully typical osteoclasts with calcitonin receptors may be restricted to pigmented villonodular synovitis and giant cell tumors of tendon sheath.

Synovial fibroblasts

The synovial intima contains cells adapted to the production of hyaluronan. In normal synovium CD68– intimal fibroblasts alone demonstrate high activity of the enzyme UDPGD.[20] UDPGD converts UDP-glucose into UDP-glucuronate, one of the two substrates required by hyaluronan synthase for assembly of the hyaluronan polymer. Unlike many other enzymes, UDPGD activity in intimal fibroblasts is reduced, rather than enhanced, in diseased tissue. Synovial intimal fibroblasts express CD55 (see Fig. 7.6), a feature that can distinguish intimal fibroblasts from intimal macrophages.[21,22]

Cells disaggregated from inflamed synovium and grown in tissue culture display fibroblast characteristics and ramifying processes with production of high levels of metalloproteinases.[23] It is not known whether they derive from intimal or subintimal cells. In tissue sections immunoreactivity for collagenase and gelatinase is patchy and not necessarily confined to the intima.

Synovial intimal fibroblasts also show prominent expression of several adhesion molecules,[7,24] including VCAM-1, intercellular adhesion molecule (ICAM)-1, CD44 and β1 integrins. Expression of VCAM-1 (Fig. 7-7) is particularly unusual, being absent from most other normal fibroblast populations, whereas CD44 and β1 integrins

are present at lower levels. The role of VCAM-1 on intimal fibroblasts is puzzling but it may modulate cell traffic. The ligand for VCAM-1, $\alpha_4\beta_1$ integrin, is present on mononuclear leukocytes but not granulocytes. Intimal fibroblasts may allow transmigration of polymorphs into synovial fluid but not mononuclear cells, potentially trapping inflammatory cell infiltrates within the synovial membrane in disease states such as RA.

The expression of two other surface molecules by synovial fibroblasts is noteworthy. Complement receptor-2 (CR2, CD21) is not expressed by normal intimal fibroblasts but has been induced on synovial fibroblasts in culture, in contrast to other fibroblast populations.[25] DAF, VCAM-1, and CR2 are all involved in B lymphocyte survival, as is a bone marrow stromal cell marker, BST-1, reported to be expressed on fibroblasts in rheumatoid, but not normal, intima.[26] Other molecules associated with bone marrow stromal cells such as the chemokine SDF-1 and bone morphogenetic proteins and their receptors[27-29] are expressed by synovial fibroblasts under various conditions. Moreover, lubricin, otherwise known as *superficial zone protein*, a glycoprotein found in synovium and the superficial zone of articular cartilage,[30] derives from the same gene as megakaryocyte stimulating factor. A defect of this gene leads to joint inflammation, pericarditis, and skeletal dysplasia. As indicated earlier, these patterns of gene expression may reflect a common embryologic origin for synovial and bone marrow stromal cells.

Intimal matrix

Intimal matrix has an amorphous or fine fibrillar ultrastructure. It is poor in type I collagen but contains minor collagens III, IV, V, and VI.[31,32] Intimal matrix also contains laminin, fibronectin, and chondroitin-6-sulfate-rich proteoglycan, which, with collagen IV, are components of basement membrane, although there is no basement membrane beneath the intimal layer. The looser structure of intimal matrix may be explained on the basis of an absence of entactin, which links other components in basement membrane together. Intimal microfibrils are of two types: fibrillin-1 microfibrils form a basketwork around cells, whereas collagen VI microfibrils form a uniform mesh.

Intimal matrix contains large amounts of hyaluronan (Fig. 7.8), which tails off 20 to 50 μm deeper into the tissue. This may indicate diffusion of hyaluronan from the surface toward clearing lymphatics.

Vascular net

A rich microvascular net lies beneath the synovial surface.[9,10] Capillaries occur just below or within the intima (Fig. 7.9). These capillaries are prominent in synovium from children but appear to be lost with increasing age. Some capillaries are fenestrated and fenestrae tend to face the tissue surface[33]; 50 to 100 μm beneath the surface small venules are prominent. About 200 μm beneath the surface, larger

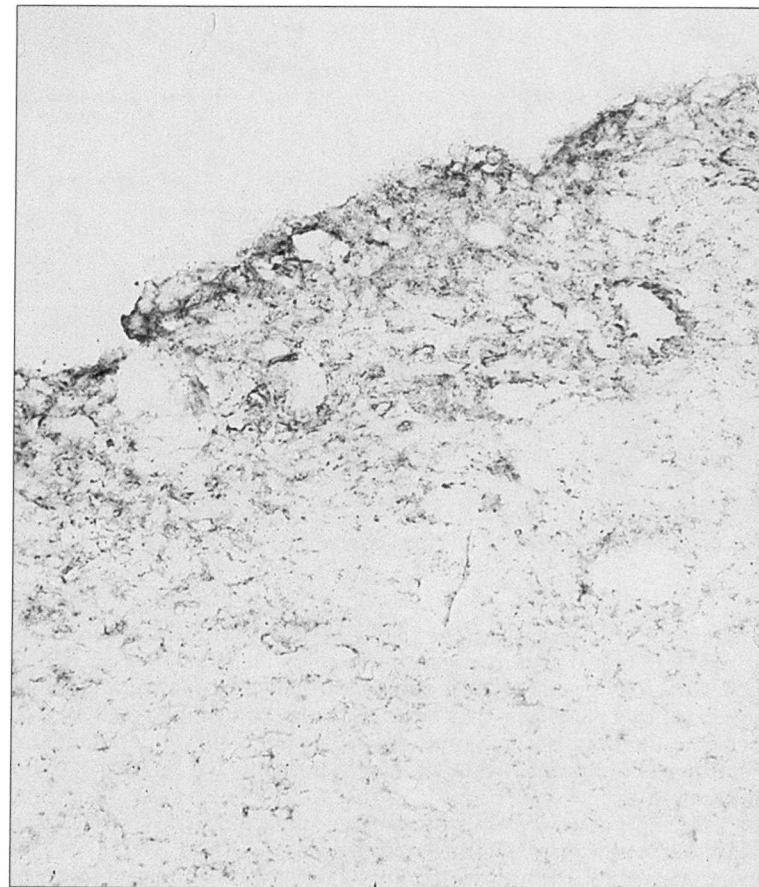

Fig. 7.8 Hyaluronan in normal synovial tissue. Photomicrograph of normal synovial tissue showing hyaluronan stained with a histochemical probe derived from proteoglycan core protein hyaluronan binding region. Staining is most intense surrounding the lining cells and decreases further into the tissue.

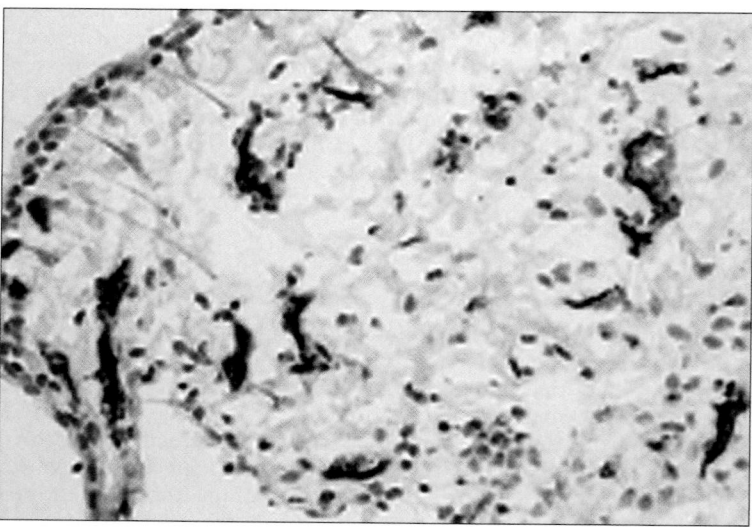

Fig. 7.9 Normal synovium (×magnification) stained with factor VIII to demonstrate the vascular network.

venules, together with arterioles and lymphatics (Fig. 7.10),[11] form an anastomosing quadrilateral array. Vessels with lymphatic staining characteristics are prominent in RA synovium, a disease state in which increased turnover of hyaluronic acid and leukocyte trafficking is seen. It has been proposed that failure of lymphatic drainage of synovial fluid is a cause of villous proliferation in RA synovial tissue. If this is correct, it is likely to be due to overloading of existing lymphatic channels with HA-rich extracellular fluid and leukocytes rather than a lack of lymphatic channels.[11]

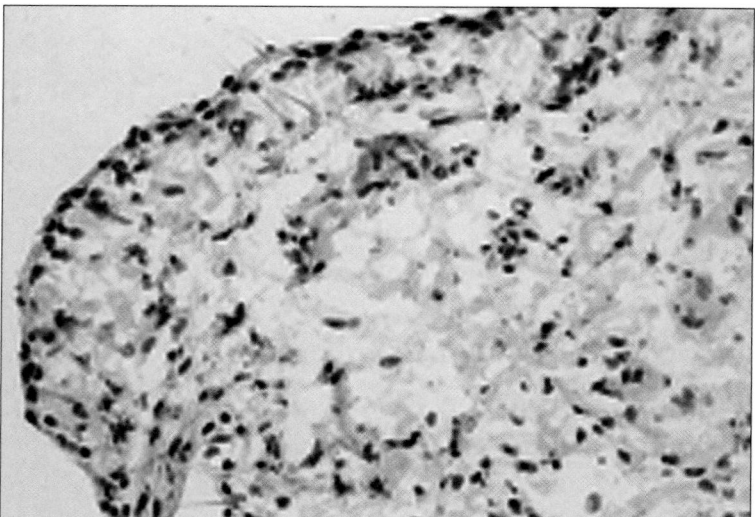

Fig. 7.10 Normal synovium (×magnification) stained with LYV-1 antibody to demonstrate the lymphatic network.

Apart from the fenestration of superficial capillary endothelial cells, there is little evidence of specialization in synovial endothelium. Endothelial cells enlarge in inflamed tissue and microvascular proliferation can occur, but these events are common to inflammation at many sites. Tissue-specific adhesion molecules or *addressins* have been sought, but nothing conclusive has been found. However, there remains the possibility that specialized lymphocyte traffic pathways apply to synovium, possibly based on chemokine-receptor interactions.

CELL ORIGINS AND RECRUITMENT

Evidence to date indicates that both intimal and subintimal macrophages derive from bone marrow via circulating monocytes, many of which probably arrive via subintimal venules and migrate to the intima.

Intimal fibroblasts are thought to arise by division within synovium but the site remains uncertain. Intimal fibroblasts might be a discrete self-replicating population, distinct from subintimal fibroblasts, but several pieces of evidence are against this. Rates of cell division within the intima are very low, even in disease. Following arthroplasty or synovectomy intimal cells reappear and express CD55, UDPGD, and VCAM-1. These may arise from intimal rests but it seems more likely that they are replaced from the subintima. If synovial fibroblasts are disaggregated and cultured in vitro, they lose VCAM-1 and CD55 expression but the majority, apparently including cells of subintimal origin, will readily express these markers following cytokine stimulation. Fibroblasts of dermal or subcutaneous origin express much lower levels of CD55 and VCAM-1 following equivalent stimulation. These findings suggest that synovial fibroblasts, in both the intima and subintima, belong to a specialized population with a propensity to express VCAM-1 and CD55.

Two recent studies[7,8] have demonstrated the range of cells that can be found in the subintimal regions of the normal synovial membrane. CD3+ T cells, including CD4+ and CD8+ cells, can be found within the normal synovial tissue. Some of these cells have memory T-cell phenotype and although they are likely to be simply trafficking through the normal synovium, their role, if any, in the homeostasis of synovial tissue is unknown. It is also possible to detect B cells, plasma cells, and granzyme B-positive cells in normal synovium, although they are present in small numbers.

Although inflammatory cytokine production can be detected in normal synovial tissue, including interleukin (IL)-1, IL-6, and tumor necrosis factor alpha (TNF-α),[7] it is far less than that seen in inflamed synovial tissue such as in RA patients, and the amount of anti-inflammatory cytokine production, at least in the case of IL-1 receptor antagonist (the naturally occurring inhibitor of IL-1), is far greater than the amount of inflammatory cytokine seen (Fig. 7.11). This would achieve the desired result of suppressing an inflammatory process in the normal

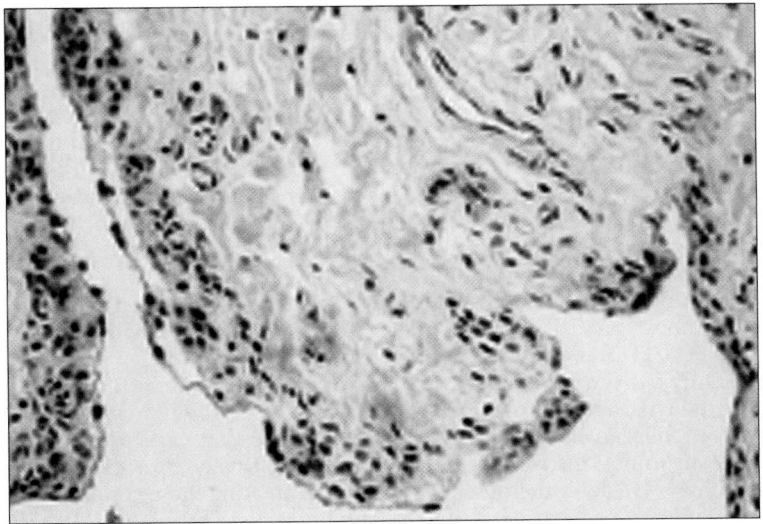

Fig. 7.11 Normal synovium (×200 magnification) stained with an antibody to detect the IL-1 receptor antagonist.

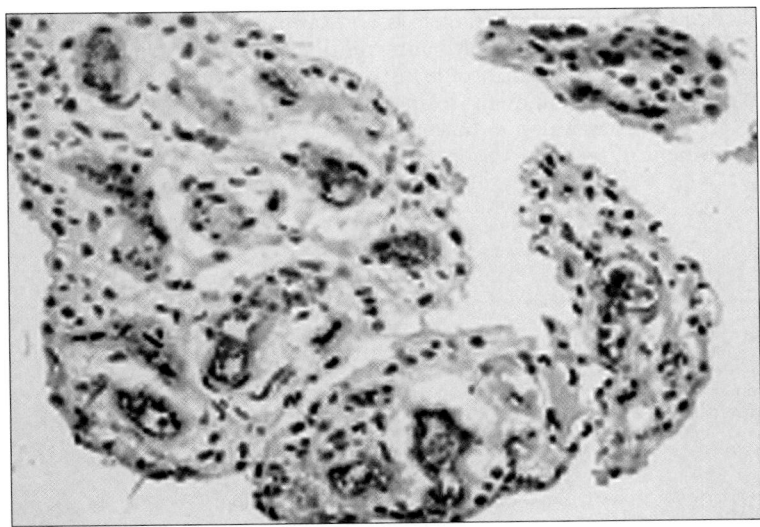

Fig. 7.12 Normal synovium (×200 magnification) stained with an antibody against osteoprotegerin, a naturally occurring inhibitor of osteoclast formation.

synovial tissue. Similarly, the amount of RANKL (an essential factor for the development of osteoclasts) seen in normal synovial tissue is low[7] and far less than that of osteoprotegerin, the naturally occurring inhibitor of RANKL (Fig. 7.12). The net result of this is to suppress the formation of osteoclasts within the normal synovium and preserve homeostasis within the normal joint.

FUNCTION

The functions of synovial tissue are often taken as evident but are remarkably difficult to define.[34] Like other soft connective tissue, synovium provides a deformable packing that allows movement of adjacent, relatively non-deformable tissues. The difference between synovium and other soft connective tissue is that it allows most of the movement to occur between rather than within tissues. Areolar synovium may also have specialized viscoelastic properties for coping with the stretching, rolling, and folding it undergoes during joint movement.

Functions of the tissue relating to the cavity may be considered as:

- maintenance of an intact non-adherent tissue surface
- lubrication of cartilage
- control of synovial fluid volume and composition
- nutrition of chondrocytes within joints

Maintenance of the tissue surface

Synovial surfaces must be non-adherent to allow continued movement. The production of hyaluronan by intimal fibroblasts may be important in inhibiting adhesion. Plasminogen activator and DAF from intimal fibroblasts may also inhibit fibrin formation and scarring. To retain synovial fluid, the intimal matrix must consist of a fibrous mat of a particular porosity that allows free exchange of crystalloids and proteins but inhibits rapid transit of the viscous hyaluronan solution that is an important component of the fluid. These functions presumably reflect the combined activities of the intimal macrophages and fibroblasts. The vasculature is likely to be important in both intimal cell nutrition and recruitment of new cells. New macrophages are derived from blood monocytes that enter the tissue through venules and perivascular fibroblasts may provide the main pool of intimal fibroblast precursors.

Lubrication

The ability of synovial fluid to lubricate cartilage surfaces is dependent on the presence of glycoprotein, especially a glycoprotein known both as *lubricin* and *superficial zone protein* because of its localization to the surface of both synovium and cartilage.[30] Hyaluronan does not appear to contribute to the ability of synovial fluid to lubricate cartilage in *ex vivo* systems, but the glairy quality imparted by hyaluronan may be important in maintaining a film of lubricant on the cartilage surfaces *in vivo*.

Whatever the precise forces acting on fluid volume, the presence of hyaluronan is likely to be the main factor responsible for retaining a constant volume of fluid during exercise.[35] This constant volume is probably important as a cushion for synovial tissue and as a reservoir of lubricant for cartilage. It is likely that the rate of synthesis of hyaluronan and its exportation into the synovial fluid compartment are dependent on the mechanical stimulation of intimal fibroblasts and are influenced by the effectiveness of the synovial fluid cushion. Thus when synovial fluid volume is high, mechanical stresses on intimal fibroblasts are reduced with a resultant reduction in the rate of hyaluronan production and vice versa.

Two distinct mechanisms create joint effusions. When synovium is mechanically irritated by worn bone and cartilage, the composition of the fluid remains reasonably normal. Excessive production of hyaluronan by intimal fibroblasts is stimulated by frictional forces and this excess of hyaluronan retains plasma dialysate in the synovial cavity. In synovitis the effusion is an accumulation of exudate similar to a pleural effusion (i.e., an overspill from the inflammatory edema in synovial tissue created by increased vascular permeability). Recent theories about a possible low-grade inflammatory and immune reaction contributing to the pathogenesis of osteoarthritis would suggest that these two mechanisms of effusion development may not be as distinct as originally thought.[36]

Chondrocyte nutrition

The synovium provides the major route of nutrition for chondrocytes. In normal joints a surprisingly large proportion of hyaline cartilage lies within 50 μm of a synovial surface. In any one position only a small proportion of cartilage is apposed to the other articular surface and synovium packs most of the space between less congruent areas. In immature joints the subchondral plate is incomplete and may contribute to nutrition, but in adult joints this route is unlikely to be significant. Nutrition of areas of cartilage that do not come into close contact with synovium must take an indirect route. This is most relevant to concave articular surfaces. Nutrition may occur by smearing of a thin film of fluid over these surfaces during movement. However, the amount of nutrient carried this way is small. Indirect routes through cartilage matrix and the apposed articular cartilage may be more important.[4]

Despite the fact that the vessels in synovium provide the most direct route for cartilage nutrition, there is no evidence that they are structurally adapted to this function. The fenestrae seen in superficial capillaries are present in tendon sheath synovium at sites where there is no cartilage (or tendon) dependent on their supply of small molecules.

SYNOVIUM AS A TARGET FOR IMMUNOLOGIC DISEASE

Synovial joints are involved in several immunologic or inflammatory disorders, including RA, systemic lupus erythematosus, and the seronegative spondyloarthropathies. Other than relapsing polychondritis, patterns of inflammatory rheumatic disease indicate targeting of synovium or enthesis rather than cartilage. Perhaps the most important reason for studying the biology of synovium is to obtain insight into which immunopathologic processes are likely to be suitable therapeutic targets in inflammatory arthritides.

Autoimmune responses to synovial antigens might theoretically occur but evidence is lacking. Moreover, none of the clinical syndromes indicates targeting of joints alone. Associated targeting of other tissues such as pericardium or uveal tract requires an explanation. Few, if any, synovium-specific antigens are known and when rheumatic disorders are associated with autoantibodies, the antigens involved are ubiquitous. In the seronegative spondyloarthropathies it is doubtful whether there is a true autoimmune response.

Understanding the microarchitecture of the normal synovium, including the wide range of microscopic appearance, cellular infiltrates, production of cytokines, enzymes, and other biologically relevant proteins, will assist in understanding the relevant changes in synovial tissue architecture and immunopathology in disease states. Although the architecture of the normal synovium is not as homogeneous as previously portrayed in rheumatology textbooks, consistencies across the broad spectrum of normal synovial tissues can be contrasted with those seen in the chronically inflamed synovial tissue. The marked increase in synovial lining layer thickness, with a reverse of normal ratio of type A to type B intimal cells, favoring type B cells in normal synovium and type A cells in RA, is an example of this. Numerous other examples can be given, including the changes in subintimal cell content, cytokine, and chemokine production; vascular and lymphatic changes; and production of metalloproteinases and stimulators of osteoclast formation. A recent study on a mouse model of arthritis has also raised the possibility of cadherin-11 expression on synovial fibroblasts as a potential therapeutic target in the treatment of RA,[5] although these results from a murine model may not be directly applicable to human disease.[37] Inhibition of cadherin-11 interactions in this mouse model interfered with both the synovial inflammation and the cartilage invasion by pannus, without any effect on bone erosion, which is predominantly dependent on osteoclast function. The inflammation in this mouse model could be reduced substantially by antibodies to cadherin-11 or a cadherin-Fc fusion protein.

Only two groups of enzymes found in the joint, cysteine cathepsins and matrix metalloproteinases, are capable of degrading native type I and II collagen fibrils. There is some evidence that cathepsin K may play an important role in the pathogenesis of osteoarthritis and RA and may be a potential therapeutic target in treating these conditions.[38] It is important to understand the hierarchy and chronology of these synovial changes in chronic inflammatory arthritides and contrast them with those seen in the normal synovium, to identify suitable therapeutic targets at various stages in the evolution of a chronic inflammatory arthritis. The identification of TNF-α, IL-1β, and IL-6 as two likely therapeutic targets is an example of how such a strategy can lead to useful therapeutic interventions being introduced into the management of several chronic inflammatory arthritides including RA, psoriatic arthritis, and ankylosing spondylitis.

There is still much to be learned about the immunologic microenvironment of articular tissues, particularly the normal synovium.

REFERENCES

1. Canoso JJ, Stack MT, Brandt K. Hyaluronic acid content of deep and superficial subcutaneous bursae of man. Ann Rheum Dis 1983;42:171-175.
2. Edwards JCW, Wilkinson LS. Distribution in human tissues of the synovial lining associated epitope recognised by monoclonal antibody 67. J Anat 1996;188:119-127.
3. Craig FM, Bayliss MT, Bentley G, Archer CW. A role for hyaluronan in joint development. J Anat 1990;171:17-23.
4. Edwards JCW, Wilkinson LS, Jones HM, et al. The formation of human synovial joint cavities: a possible role for hyaluronan and CD44 in altered interzone cohesion. J Anat 1994;185:355-367.
5. Lee DM, Kiener HP, Agarwal SK, et al. Cadherin-11 in synovial lining formation and pathology in arthritis. Science 2007;315(5814):1006-1010.
6. Key JA. The synovial membrane of joints and bursae. In: Special cytology, vol 2. New York: PB Hoeber, 1932: 1055-1076.
7. Smith MD, Barg E, Weedon H, et al. The microarchitecture and protective mechanisms in synovial tissue from clinically and arthroscopically normal knee joints. Ann Rheum Dis 2003;62:303-307.
8. Singh JA, Araysi T, Duray P, Schumacher HR. Immunohistochemistry of normal human knee synovium: a quantitative study. Ann Rheum Dis 2004;63:785-790.
9. Davies DV. The structure and function of the synovial membrane. BMJ 1950;1(4645):92-95.
10. Wilkinson LS, Edwards JCW. Microvascular distribution in normal human synovium. J Anat 1989;167:129-136.
11. Xu H, Edwards J, Banerji S, et al. Distribution of lymphatic vessels in normal and arthritic human synovial tissues. Ann Rheum Dis 2003;62:1227-1229.
12. Mapp PI. Innervation of synovium. Ann Rheum Dis 1995;54:398-403.
13. Ghadially FN. Fine structure of joints. In: Sokoloff L, ed. The joints and synovial fluid. New York: Academic Press, 1978:105-176.
14. Barland P, Novikoff AB, Hamerman D. Electron microscopy of the human synovial membrane. J Cell Biol 1962;14:207-216.

15. Henderson B, Revell P, Edwards JCW. Synovial lining cell hyperplasia in rheumatoid arthritis: dogma and fact. Ann Rheum Dis 1988;47:348-349.
16. Edwards JCW, Wilkinson LS. Immunohistochemistry of synovium. In: Henderson B, Edwards JCW, Pettifer ER, eds. Mechanisms and models in rheumatoid arthritis. New York: Academic Press, 1995:133-150.
17. Bhatia A, Blades S, Cambridge G, Edwards JCW. Differential distribution of FcγRIIIa in normal human tissues and co-localization with DAF and fibrillin-1: implications for immunological microenvironments. Immunology 1998;94:56-63.
18. Poulter LW, Janossy G. The involvement of dendritic cells in chronic inflammatory disease. Scand J Immunol 1985;21:401-407.
19. Wilkinson LS, Worrall JG, Sinclair HS, Edwards JCW. Immunohistochemical reassessment of accessory cell populations in normal and diseased human synovium. Br J Rheumatol 1990;29:259-263.
20. Wilkinson LS, Pitsillides AA, Worrall JG, Edwards JCW. Light microscopic characterisation of the fibroblastic synovial lining cell (synoviocyte). Arthritis Rheum 1992;35:1179-1184.
21. Stevens CR, Mapp PI, Revell PA. A monoclonal antibody (Mab 67) marks type B synoviocytes. Rheumatol Int 1990;10:103-106.
22. Medof ME, Walter EI, Rutgers JL, et al. Identification of the complement decay accelerating factor on epithelium and glandular cells and in body fluids. J Exp Med 1987;165:848-864.
23. Krane SM, Goldring SR, Dayer JM. Interactions among lymphocytes, monocytes and other synovial cells in the rheumatoid synovium. Lymphokines 1982;7:75-87.
24. Edwards JCW. Synovial intimal fibroblasts. Ann Rheum Dis 1995;54:395-397.
25. Leigh RD, Cambridge G, Edwards JCW. Expression of B-cell survival cofactors on synovial fibroblasts. Br J Rheumatol 1996;1(suppl):110.
26. Lee BO, Ishihara K, Denno K, et al. Elevated levels of the soluble form of bone marrow stromal cell antigen 1 in the sera of patients with severe rheumatoid arthritis. Arthritis Rheum 1996;39:629-637.

27. Seki T, Selby J, Haupl T, Winchester R. Use of differential subtraction method to identify genes that characterize the phenotype of cultured rheumatoid arthritis synoviocytes. Arthritis Rheum 1998;41:1356-1364.
28. Fowler MJ Jr, Neff MS, Borghaei RC, et al. Induction of bone morphogenetic protein-2 by interleukin-1 in human fibroblasts. Biochem Biophys Res Commun 1998;248:450-453.
29. Marinova-Mutafchieva L, Taylor P, Funa K, et al. Mesenchymal cells expressing bone morphogenetic protein receptors are present in the rheumatoid arthritis joint. Arthritis Rheum 2000;43:2046-2055.
30. Jay GD, Britt DE, Cha CJ. Lubricin is a product of megakaryocyte stimulating factor gene expression by human synovial fibroblasts. J Rheumatol 2000;27:594-600.
31. Revell PA, Al-Saffar N, Fish S, Osei D. Extracellular matrix of the synovial intimal cell layer. Ann Rheum Dis 1995;54:404-407.
32. Ashhurst DE, Bland YS, Levick JR. An immunohistochemical study of the collagens of rabbit synovial interstitium. J Rheumatol 1991;18:1669-1672.
33. Suter ER, Majno G. Ultrastructure of the joint capsule in the rat: presence of two kinds of capillaries. Nature 1964;202:920-921.
34. Edwards JCW. Functions of synovial lining. In: Henderson B, Edwards JCW, eds. The synovial lining in health and disease. London: Chapman & Hall, 1987: 41-74.
35. Levick JR. Fluid movement across synovium in healthy joints: role of synovial fluid macromolecules. Ann Rheum Dis 1995;54:417-423.
36. Pelletier JP, Martel-Pelletier J, Abramson SB. Osteoarthritis, an inflammatory disease. Potential implication for the selection of new therapeutic targets. Arthritis Rheum 2001;44:1237-1247.
37. Firestein GS. Every joint has a silver lining. Science 2007;315 (5814):952-953.
38. Salminen-Mankonen HJ, Morko J, Vuorio E. Role of cathepsin K in normal joints and in the development of arthritis. Curr Drug Targets 2007;8:315-323.

The articular cartilage

Dick Heinegård, Pilar Lorenzo, and Tore Saxne

8

- The cells in cartilage maintain the extracellular matrix function by a controlled turnover in response to minor damage in fatigue and altered load by removing malfunctioning matrix constituents by breakdown and producing new to achieve repair.
- The cell obtains feedback on the quality of the extracellular matrix via a number of cell surface receptors such as integrins, discoidin receptors, hyaluronan receptors and specific proteoglycans with specificity for different matrix molecules.
- Cartilage extracellular matrix shows different composition close to the cells in the so called territorial matrix compared to the more distant interterritorial matrix.
- Cartilage extracellular matrix contains a specific proteoglycan —aggrecan—providing a very high fixed charge density and therefore an osmotic environment with water retention essential for tissue resilience.
- Fibrillar networks with collagen as the major constituent provide tensile properties essential for load distribution and dissipation. The fibers contain other matrix proteins, e.g. bound at their surface and providing for interactions with other tissue structures including neighboring fibers, thereby enhancing mechanical qualities.
- Cartilage extracellular matrix contains growth factors and proenzymes sequestered by binding to matrix macromolecules and these can be released upon degradation of the carrier molecules.
- As a result of cartilage matrix degradation, fragments formed are released into surrounding fluids and can be used as indicators of the ongoing process, the so called molecular marker technology.

INTRODUCTION

The articular cartilage has key roles in the function of joints. A major function is to take up and distribute load such that a given point of the underlying bone can handle very high strain. Another role of the cartilage is to provide for low friction movement. One key feature of joint diseases is deterioration in joint function. This results from progressive damage of the articular cartilage by degradation of structural components important for the tissue properties. The progressive joint destruction may eventually lead to total loss of the cartilage accompanied by alterations in underlying bone in the common disease of osteoarthritis (Fig. 8.1). Mechanisms triggering this tissue destruction are not known in detail, but it is clear that excessive load may induce a remodeling process that fails to restore normal cartilage. Stimulation of chondrocytes by cytokines like interleukin (IL)-1, IL-6, and tumor necrosis factor (TNF)-α induces the cells to degrade their surrounding matrix and can, over an extended period of time, induce total dissolution of cartilage *in vitro*. The identity of the individual enzyme(s) accomplishing specific fragmentation of a particular matrix protein is (are) not known, although in some cases candidates have been established. There is often a repair response mounted to the ongoing tissue destruction. In the more serious cases this is not sufficient, and results in ensuing tissue failure.

A prerequisite for understanding the mechanisms of tissue destruction and failed repair is to know the functions of the extracellular matrix molecules and how they are assembled into larger networks. It is equally important to understand the mechanisms involved in their degradation. One important and basic clinical observation in joint diseases such as rheumatoid arthritis and osteoarthritis is that upon joint replacement, the inflammation recedes and the symptoms that have been plaguing the patients are ameliorated or disappear in the vast majority of patients. This brings up the question of whether components released from the cartilage actually stimulate the inflammatory reaction.

The main structural entities in cartilage include aggrecan and collagen. The proteoglycan aggrecan has a primary role in taking up load and resisting deformation. The collagen network provides tensile properties, and the type VI collagen network may have a role in protecting the cell and guiding matrix assembly. A set of molecules close to the cells have specific functions in binding to specific cell surface receptors and thereby provide signaling of conditions in the matrix.

This chapter will therefore focus on describing the individual cartilage macromolecules and, when possible, their functional properties and how these have implications for tissue assembly. In some instances candidate enzymes having roles in the degradation of specific macromolecules have been implicated and will be discussed.

OVERALL TISSUE ORGANIZATION

The matrix closer to the cells, the territorial matrix, has a somewhat different composition and structure compared with the matrix at some distance, the interterritorial matrix (Fig. 8.2).[1] Examples of components found in both compartments are collagen type II fibers and aggrecan, whereas collagen type VI is found particularly in the territorial matrix and cartilage oligomeric matrix protein (COMP) as well as cartilage intermediate layer protein (CILP) are primarily found in the interterritorial matrix of normal cartilage. There is also a difference in composition of the cartilage from the superficial to deep layers. The collagen fibers are thinner in the superficial layer and arranged in parallel with the surface of the tissue, while in the deeper layer the fibers are thicker and arranged perpendicularly to the surface, with a transition zone in between (see Figs. 8.1 and 8.3). Certain molecules like CILP are found primarily in the middle portions of the articular cartilage. Although over recent years a number of cartilage components have been described, we still have a very limited understanding of what specific requirements and functions are met by molecules with such a restricted localization in the tissue.

Aggrecan

A major structure of aggrecan, illustrated in Figure 8.4,[1] is approximately 100 chondroitin sulfate glycosaminoglycan chains, each built from a disaccharide unit that is repeated some 50 times. Each disaccharide contains a uronic acid with a negatively charged carboxyl group and an N-acetylgalactosamine with a sulfate either at the 4 or in the 6 position. Each chain will therefore contribute around 100 negatively charged groups. The glycosaminoglycans are linked to a serine residue of the protein core of the proteoglycan via their reducing terminal end. The chains are clustered; this clustering differs between the two regions referred to as CS 1 and CS 2 (see Fig. 8.4). There is an additional glycosaminoglycan, keratan sulfate, with a disaccharide building block of galactose and an N-acetylglucosamine carrying a sulfate in the 6-position. These chains are shorter and particularly enriched closer to the N-terminal end of the protein core, in the so-called keratan sulfate–rich region. There are some 30 such chains in the aggrecan molecule.

The proteoglycan core protein contains globular domains flanking the three domains carrying glycosaminoglycan chains. The one closest to the N-terminal, the hyaluronan-binding domain (G1-globe), contributes specific high-affinity binding of the aggrecan molecule to hyaluronan (see later). After a short interglobular domain there is a second

57

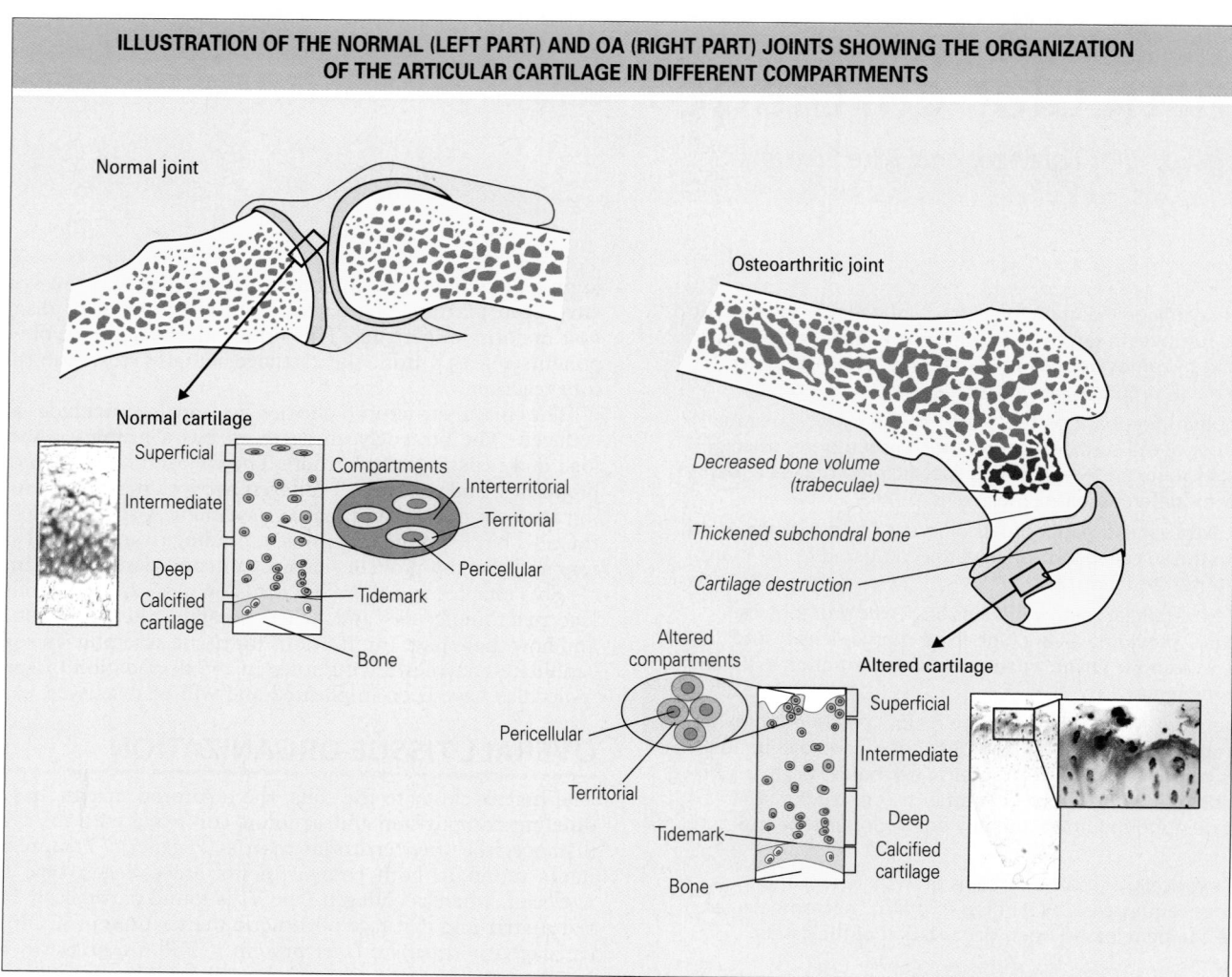

ILLUSTRATION OF THE NORMAL (LEFT PART) AND OA (RIGHT PART) JOINTS SHOWING THE ORGANIZATION OF THE ARTICULAR CARTILAGE IN DIFFERENT COMPARTMENTS

Fig. 8.1 Illustration of a normal joint and an osteoarthritic joint showing the organization of the articular cartilage in different compartments. As an example, one cartilage protein (CILP) shows a distinct change in localization from a distribution in the normal cartilage in intermediate parts of the tissue and rather selectively in the interterritorial matrix to a prominence at the superficial parts and primarily in the pericellular compartment in the diseased cartilage.

globular domain (G2), which shows structural similarities to the G1 globe but does not bind hyaluronan and has no known function. In the very C-terminal end of the aggrecan molecule there is the G3-globe with a lectin homology domain that contributes binding to other proteins (e.g., fibulins and tenascins), which themselves can form molecular complexes involving several such molecules (see Fig. 8.2).

Many aggrecan molecules will bind to a single, very long strand of hyaluronan, thereby forming large aggregates providing an extreme number of charged groups. These are fixed in the glycosaminoglycan chains, which in turn are fixed in aggrecan, in its turn fixed in the aggregate. The interaction of aggrecan via its G1-globe with hyaluronan is stabilized by the link protein having structures similar to the hyaluronan-binding domain of aggrecan. This link protein will bind to this domain of the proteoglycan as well as to hyaluronan.

In normal cartilage turnover, as well as in pathology, the aggrecan molecule is cleaved by enzymes called aggrecanases (i.e., ADAMTS-4 and ADAMTS-5).[2,3] One site of this cleavage is in the interglobular domain between the hyaluronan-binding G1-globe and the G2-globe. This cleavage occurs between the stretches of amino acids EGE and ARG.[4] The new N- and C-terminals formed have been used to develop antibodies recognizing only the fragments produced by the cleavage. These have been used to demonstrate such fragments in body fluids and in tissue extracts.[4,5] The cleavage occurring in the domain carrying the chondroitin sulfate chains will result in shortening of the aggrecan with an ensuing decreased number of fixed charged groups (see Fig. 8.4). With aging there is an accumulation of shorter aggrecan molecules, where the extreme is the hyaluronan-binding domain with no glycosaminoglycan binding structures remaining.[6] Indeed, in an adult,

almost all aggrecan molecules found in the interterritorial matrix at a distance from the cell do not contain the G3, C-terminal globular lectin homology domain (A. Aspberg and D. Heinegård, unpublished observations). On the other hand, the molecules in the territorial matrix close to the cells contain this domain, which is probably a result of the gradual turnover of the aggrecan molecules. At the same time there is substantial accumulation of G1 domain apparently retained bound to hyaluronan.[7] This fragment can be identified in the tissue either via its new C-terminal represented by a—EGE373-COOH sequence formed by the cleavage by aggrecanase or a further matrix metalloproteinase cleavage forming a C-terminal—PEN341-COOH sequence.[8]

Already from the early experiments by Thomas[9] and Hardingham and colleagues,[10] it was clear that the chondrocyte had a remarkable capacity to replace aggrecan molecules removed from the tissue by the use of enzymes cleaving the hyaluronan. It appears that a normal chondrocyte should be able to replace even large amounts of proteoglycans lost unless suppressed by cytokines such as IL-1 and TNF-α.

Collagen fibrillar networks

A major function of the rope-like collagen fiber networks in the cartilage is to provide tensile strength and distribute load essential in preventing local excessive forces on the underlying bone. One type of fiber contains a core of collagen type II with a minor constituent of collagen type XI that is connected via a number of molecules bound at its surface.

The other fibrillar network contains a core of collagen type VI that, by a set of linker molecules, is connected to other molecular assemblies

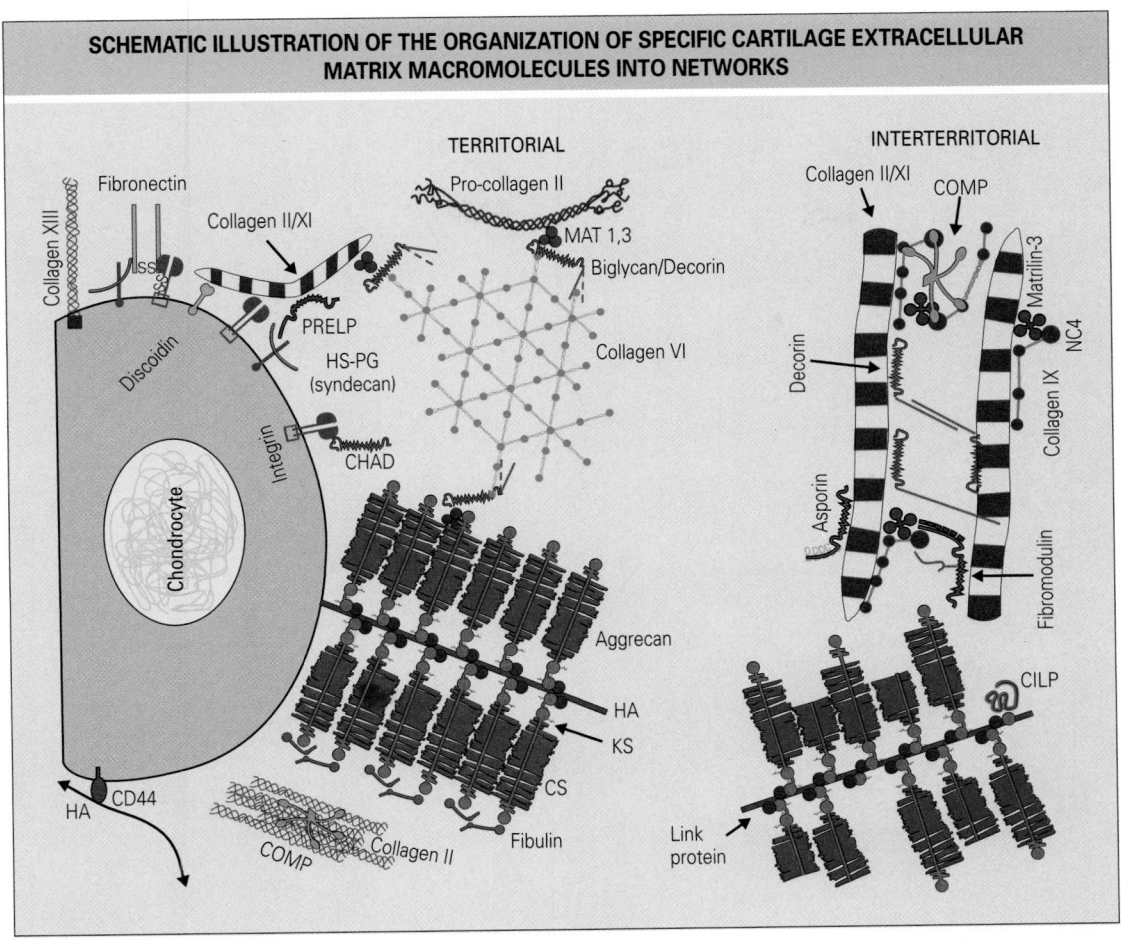

SCHEMATIC ILLUSTRATION OF THE ORGANIZATION OF SPECIFIC CARTILAGE EXTRACELLULAR MATRIX MACROMOLECULES INTO NETWORKS

Fig. 8.2 Schematic illustration of the organization of specific cartilage extracellular matrix macromolecules into networks. Also indicated are the interactions between extracellular matrix proteins and specific receptors at the cell surface. Note the different molecular composition of the territorial matrix closer to the cell compared with the interterritorial matrix at some distance. HS-PG, heparan sulfate proteoglycan; HA, hyaluronan; KS, keratan sulfate; CS, chondroitin sulfate; MAT, matrilin; CHAD, chondroadherin; NC-4, the N-terminal globular domain of collagen 9; CD-44, receptor for hyaluronan.

in the matrix, including the collagen type II fibers and the major proteoglycans. These networks are discussed separately next.

Fibers with collagen type II as the main constituent
Collagen type II and collagen type XI
The major fibrillar network in cartilage contains primarily collagen type II with a minor constituent of collagen type XI.[11] A major feature of both these collagens is that the molecule forming the fibers is made up of three parallel, tightly associated polypeptide chains forming a very stable triple helix, the collagen molecule. This is extremely asymmetric, being 300 nm long and 1.5 nm in diameter. An amino acid quite unique for collagen is hydroxyproline, which is essential for the stability of the molecule due to the hydrogen bonds formed to the hydroxyl group. The collagen type II is produced as a procollagen that does not form fibrils until the propeptides at both ends in the C- and N-termini are cleaved off (see Fig. 8.3). Upon this cleavage the molecules form fibers by interactions with other collagen molecules such that a large part of the surface of the molecule is engaged and the collagen molecules are positioned in relationship to one another to form a so-called quarter stagger arrangement.

The assembly process is regulated by a number of molecules in the matrix, including collagen type XI. It appears that the dimensions of the fiber formed depends on the relative proportion of collagens type II and XI, where the typical ratio is in the order of 50:1. This may depend on the presence of a central core of microfibrils of collagen type II and XI that direct the assembly of the fiber.[12]

The collagen fibers are different in dimensions and in directions between superficial and deep layers of the articular cartilage. Thus, the fibers in the superficial layer of the articular cartilage are thin and run in parallel, while the thicker fibers in the deeper parts of the cartilage

run perpendicular to the surface. In the transition zone layer, fibers run at an angle (see Fig. 8.3).[13] The organization can be seen as Benninghof's arcades on polarized light microscopy.

The collagen fiber formation is influenced by a number of matrix molecules, such as decorin, fibromodulin, and COMP as well as a special variant of an oversulfated CS-chain. In several of these cases, the molecules are also retained bound at the surface of the collagen fiber. This is particularly evident for collagen type IX, which has a part of the molecule extending out from the fiber. These molecules appear to have roles in providing sites for interactions with other matrix molecules including another fiber than the one where the protein is bound (see Fig. 8.2).

An important feature of the collagen fiber network is that the interactions become sealed by covalent crosslink formation once the fibers are assembled outside the cell. This crosslinking depends on oxidation of lysine and hydroxylysine residues by lysyl oxidase, providing an aldehyde function that forms a Schiff base with a neighboring lysine amino group. These are then rearranged to become stable pyridinoline groups that crossbridge between the molecules and within the molecules of a fiber. These crosslinks are important for the mechanical stability of the collagen. Because they are not metabolized on degradation of the collagen, they eventually end up in the urine and can be measured as indicators of collagen breakdown.[14]

Collagen type XI
This fibril forming collagen is an integral component of the fibers forming the main network in cartilage. The collagen consists of a major triple helical portion, similar in size to that of collagens type I and II but contrasting to these collagens in that the N-terminal propeptides are retained with the molecule incorporated into the fiber. There have

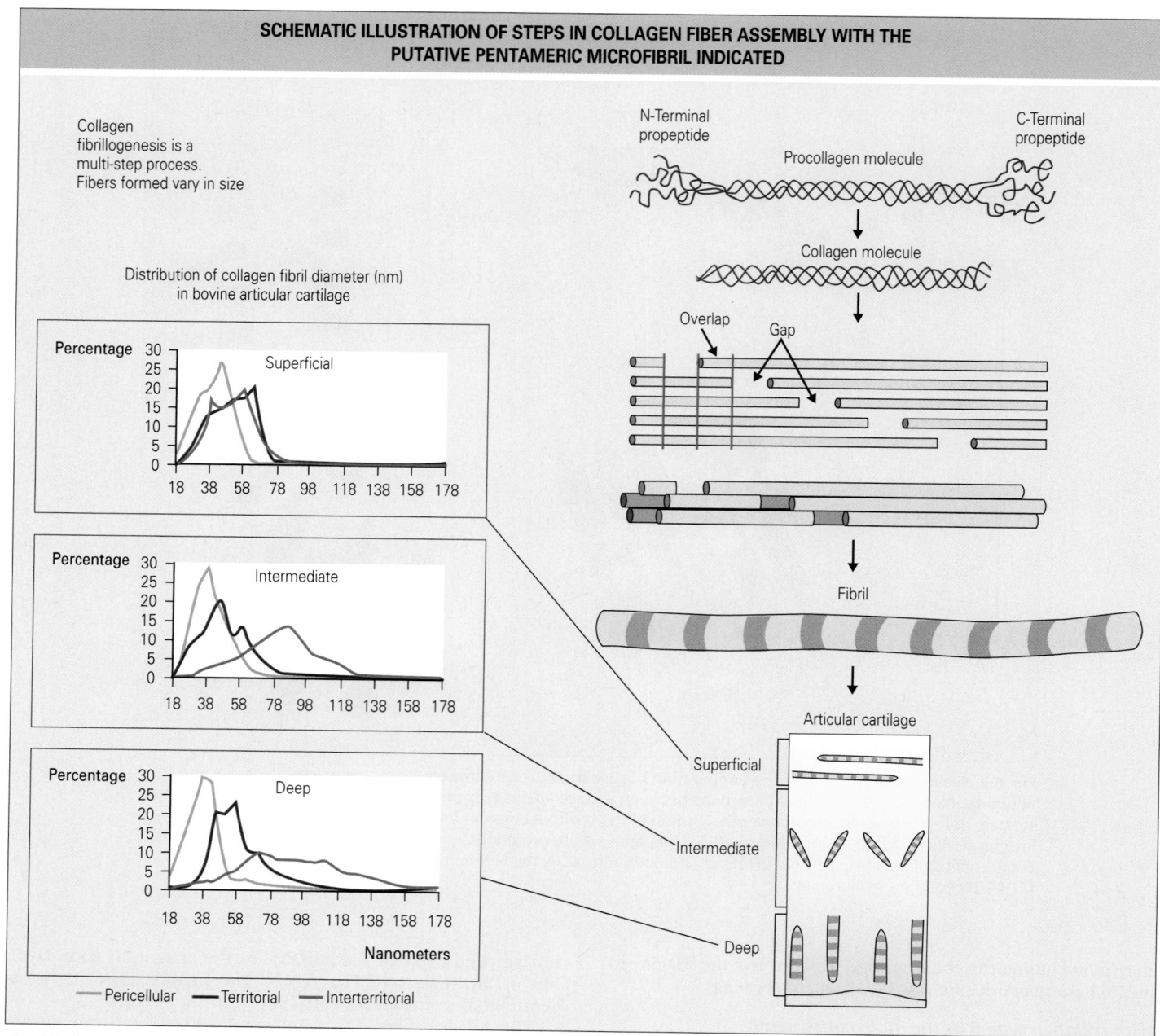

Fig. 8.3 Schematic illustration of steps in collagen fiber assembly with the putative pentameric microfibril indicated. Also shown is the organization of collagen fibers at different distances from the surface of the articular cartilage as well as the differences in fibril diameters between the pericellular, territorial, and interterritorial compartments. (*Data from Hedlund H, Mengarelli-Widholm S, Reinholt FP, Svensson O: Stereologic studies on collagen in bovine articular cartilage. APMIS1993;101(2):133-140.*)

been reports to indicate that the retained N-terminal parts are exposed at the surface of the fibers with collagen type II as the major constituent at the same time as the major triple helical portion occurs more centrally in the fiber.[15] Collagen XI appears to form microfibrils that together with other microfibrils of collagen type II forms the initial assembly regulating the further assembly of the cartilage collagen fiber, at least in skeletal morphogenesis.[12] Interestingly, collagen type XI forms crosslinks to primarily other collagen type XI molecules.[16] There are examples of mutations in collagen type XI chains with ensuing major growth disturbances indicating a role in cartilage growth and stability.[17]

Collagen type IX

This molecule is a member of the FACIT collagens (fibril-associated collagens with interrupted triple helices) and is found in the tissue bound at the surface of the fibrils with collagen type II as the major constituent. Collagen type IX contains three different α-chains with three triple helical domains (col1, col2, and col3), each surrounded by a non-collagenous domain (NC1, NC2, NC3, and NC4). The NC4

domain with its adjacent col3 triple helix protrudes from the fibers and is available for interactions with other molecules in the extracellular matrix (ECM), as is schematically illustrated in Figure 8.2.[18] Examples of such ligands are COMP and the tyrosine sulfate domain of fibromodulin. Collagen type IX often contains a chondroitin sulfate side chain bound at the NC3 domain. Its role in the function of the collagen is not known.

Functionally, collagen type IX has been shown to interact with matrilins, COMP, and, in particular, collagen type II. The collagen is actually covalently crosslinked to collagen type II in the fibers in adult individuals.[19] When collagen type IX is added *in vitro* to fibril-forming systems of collagen type II, assembly and fiber formation is retarded.

Mutations in collagen type IX lead to severe growth disturbances. Some of these are similar to those with a mutated COMP molecule, which is of special interest in view of the high-affinity interaction this protein shows with all four NC domains of collagen type IX. Furthermore, a mouse with a knockout of collagen type IX develops early lesions of articular cartilage similar to those found in osteoarthritis.[20]

THE PROTEOGLYCAN AGGREGATE STRUCTURE AND ORGANIZATION

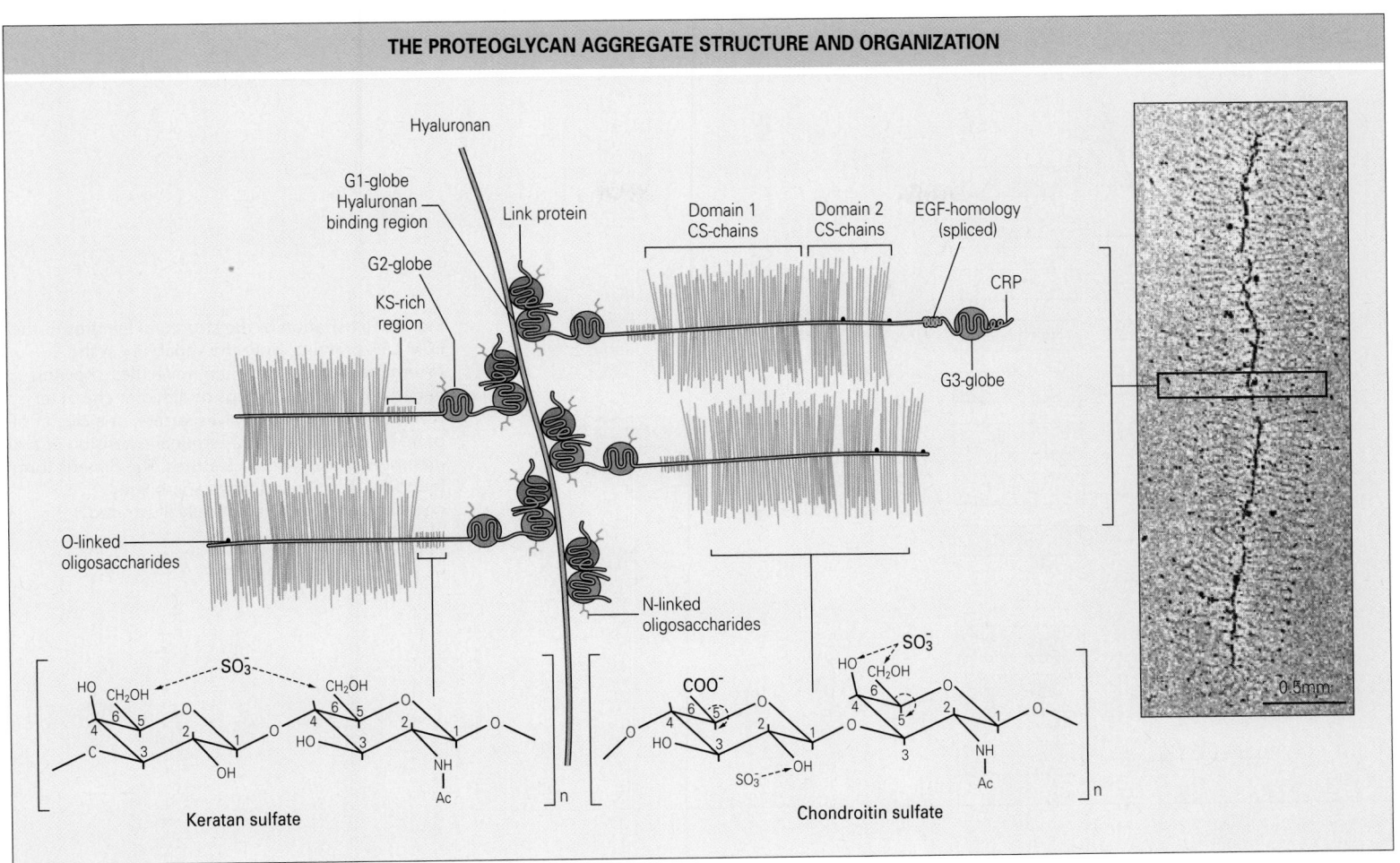

Fig. 8.4 Depiction of the proteoglycan aggregate structure and organization. Also shown is a rotatory shadowing electron microscopic picture of an aggregate isolated from tissue. *(Courtesy of Matthias Mörgelin.)*

Molecules regulating collagen fiber assembly

Collagen fiber dimensions and orientation in the tissue vary between different layers of the articular cartilage. Furthermore, fibers in the territorial matrix close to the cells are thinner and have similar dimensions at different layers of the cartilage. On the other hand, fibers in the interterritorial matrix are thicker and have larger and more variable diameters in the deeper layers. This regulation of fiber diameters is achieved by a number of macromolecules that bind to collagen. The exact role of the individual molecule in achieving the final dimensions and the directions of the fibers is not clear, although there are a number of examples where inactivation of individual genes of involved proteins leads to altered dimensions of collagen fibrils.

The extremely long half-life of collagen type II, in excess of 100 years,[7,21] indicates that there is very little elimination of collagen over the life of an individual, at the same time as fibers defective due to fatigue have to be repaired. It is possible that the very variable dimensions of the fibers in the interterritorial matrix result from adding newly synthesized collagen molecules at the fiber surface, thus gradually increasing the diameter to provide mechanical stability.

A number of molecules bound at the surface of the collagen fibers are likely to prevent further accretion of collagen. It is likely that these molecules will have to be removed before new collagen molecules can be added to a fiber in remodeling or repair.

It appears that while the collagen itself does not turn over, the molecules at the fiber surface are continuously removed and replenished.

Molecules with putative roles in the regulating fibril formation are found among those that can bind collagen *in vitro*.

COMP

COMP is a molecule primarily found in cartilage, where it is quite abundant at a concentration of around 0.1% of the tissue wet weight.

The molecule is made up of five identical subunits, each with a molecular weight of around 87,000 daltons. The five subunits are held together by a coiled domain close to the N-terminal end, and the binding is further stabilized by disulfide bridges. The subunits are made up of several modules that bind calcium. At the C-terminal end, there is a globular domain that is involved in interactions with other proteins in the matrix. The molecule can be viewed as a bouquet of tulips tied together at their stalks (see Fig. 8.2).[22]

COMP, also referred to as thrombospondin-5, is a member of this family of proteins. Cartilage also contains other thrombospondins that share the same properties, where particularly thrombospondin-1 and thrombospondin-4 are abundant. These thrombospondins, however, contain an extension beyond the coiled coil domain in the N-terminal that contains a heparin binding motif adding additional interacting sites. Whereas thrombospondin-4 contains five identical subunits, thrombospondin-1 only contains three.[1]

The 3D structure of the C-terminal domain of thrombospondin-1 has been resolved, demonstrating an organization stabilized by a large number of calcium ions.[23] Because the C-terminal domain of the various thrombospondins shows a great deal of conservation, it is likely that its structure is similar for all five members of the family.

COMP has been shown to bind to collagens type I and II,[1] where an individual C-terminal globular domain provides a high affinity in the nanomolar range. There are four binding sites evenly distributed along the collagen molecule. There is one at each end, and two are located along the filament such that there is a similar distance between the four binding sites. Even though each COMP molecule has five identical binding sites, an individual molecule can only engage one binding site on each collagen molecule and not span over the distance between two such sites. Therefore, each COMP molecule has the potential to bind to five different collagen molecules. The quarter stagger arrangement of the collagen in the fiber and the fact that there

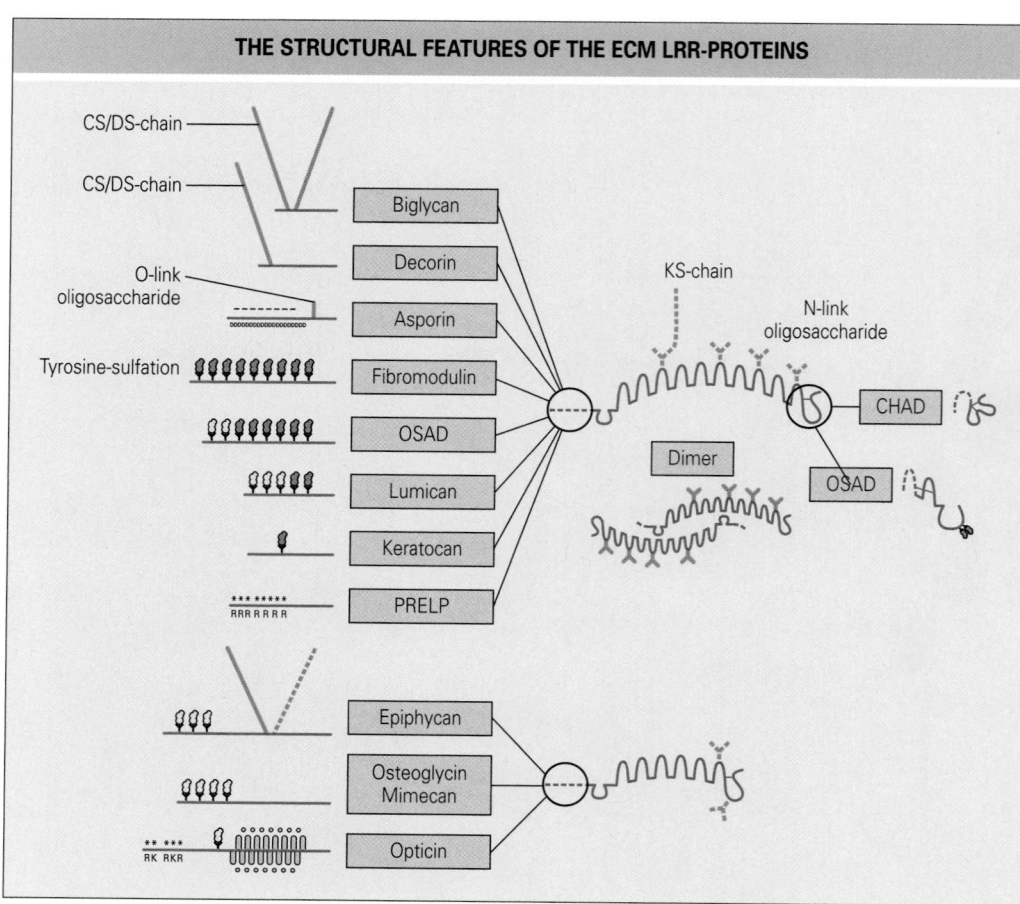

THE STRUCTURAL FEATURES OF THE ECM LRR-PROTEINS

Fig. 8.5 Illustration of the structural features of the ECM LRR-proteins. Note the variability in the N-terminal domain between molecules, showing negatively charged groups of different character (GAG, tyrosine sulfate, polyaspartate, or a cluster of basic amino acids). The C-terminal extension of two members shows distinct features. The dimeric form found for decorin and biglycan on x-ray crystallography is schematically illustrated.

appears to exist a pentameric microfibril unit[24] may relate to the four similarly spaced collagen binding sites in the molecule. COMP will accelerate and provide for a faster collagen fibril formation *in vitro*. It appears that this effect is mediated via the COMP molecule, bringing together several collagen molecules and facilitating their interactions in the forming fiber. The COMP molecule does not remain bound directly to the surface of the forming fiber. The molecule thus appears to function as a catalyst enhancing fibril formation.

In the cartilage of the growing individual and notably in the growth plate, COMP is primarily localized close to the cells in the territorial matrix, where it may have a role in stimulating collagen fibril formation.[25]

COMP has the ability to interact with all four non-collagenous (NC) domains of collagen type IX with similarly high affinity in the nanomolar range. The interaction is mediated via the C-terminal globular domains (see Fig. 8.2).

In the adult individual, COMP is primarily localized in the interterritorial matrix and may be bound to the collagen type IX and/or one of the matrilins that in turn bind to the surface of the collagen fiber (see Fig. 8.2). The role of COMP in adult cartilage appears to be to stabilize the collagen fiber network.

Mutations in the calcium-binding domain of COMP as well as in the C-terminal domain have been shown to lead to severe growth disturbances in the form of pseudoachondroplasia or multiple epiphyseal dysplasia. A feature of these conditions is that material retained in the endoplasmic reticulum of the chondrocytes contains both COMP and collagen type IX.[26]

On the other hand, the COMP null mouse shows no detectable alteration in phenotype.[27] It is possible that other molecules compensate for the lack of COMP function in these mice.

COMP is significantly upregulated in early stages of osteoarthritis,[57] even long before diagnosis, in an apparent repair attempt. At the same time the protein already deposited is cleaved and released from the tissue. Indeed assay for such fragments released to body fluids has been used to measure altered cartilage metabolism as a biomarker for arthritic disease.[28]

Decorin

Decorin was the first molecule within the leucine-rich repeat (LRR) protein family that was cloned and sequenced. This family of molecules in the extracellular matrix contains four subclasses with a total of 12 members, which all appear to share the function of binding to collagen (Fig. 8.5).[1]

One functional domain of these molecules is a central LRR region, where particularly leucine residues are at conserved locations in each repeat of some 25 amino acids, albeit somewhat variably long. Most of these molecules have 10 to 11 such repeats, where the entire domain contains a disulfide loop structure at each end. One subgroup contains molecules with only six repeats.

One variable of almost all the molecules in the family is an N-terminal extension of usually less than 20 amino acids, which may contain a variety of substituents (see Fig. 8.5). Some of the molecules also have a C-terminal extension. There is also variation in the glycosylation of the repeat domain, which usually contains a few N-linked oligosaccharides that may occur with a variably long array of 6-O-sulfated lactosamine repeat disaccharides (see Fig. 8.4) extended to form the glycosaminoglycan keratan sulfate.

The 3D structures of decorin[29] and biglycan[30] have been resolved by x-ray crystallography. These molecules contain one (decorin) or two (biglycan) glycosaminoglycan chains bound at the N-terminal extension. These are chondroitin sulfate or dermatan sulfate depending on the tissue, while very similar between the molecules in a given tissue. In articular cartilage the chain is a lowly epimerized dermatan sulfate where a few of the glucuronic acid residues have been epimerized to iduronic acid, increasing its structural variability. This glycosaminoglycan has capabilities of specific interactions with other molecules in the matrix, including binding other dermatan sulfate chains.[1]

Based on the presented x-ray crystallography data, the LRR family of molecules form a curved structure in which two molecules form a dimer in the crystals that overlap in opposite directions with about 50% of their length such that the N-terminus of one molecule is located in the middle of the curved domain of the other. Support for such a dimeric structure was obtained by other techniques such as gel filtration on line with dynamic light scattering.[29] Electron microscopy indicates that decorin and biglycan as well as chondroadherin may in addition to dimers also exist in a monomeric form at very low concentrations (M. Mörgelin and D. Heinegård, unpublished work).

The presence of the proteoglycan as a monomer or a dimer has specific relevance for interactions and functions. Thus, a monomeric molecule has only one of each interacting site whereas a dimer may exhibit two of each binding site.

Decorin binds tightly to the fibril forming collagens with a K_D in the nanomolar range. Binding is close to the C-terminus of the collagen as shown for collagen type I. Binding occurs via the LRR region and particularly involves repeats 4 and 5.[1] The critical sequence has been identified as SYIRIADTNIT.[31]

Via its binding to collagen, decorin inhibits formation of collagen fibers in vitro in a dose-dependent manner. In accord, mice lacking decorin generated by knockout technology have irregular collagen fibers with increased diameter particularly prominent in skin.[32] They do not show increased early joint pathology, indicating that other molecules may compensate for the lack of decorin in articular cartilage.

Decorin is present bound at collagen fibers in the tissue, where the glycosaminoglycan chains are free to interact with other molecules. Thus, decorin can crossbridge to neighboring collagen fibers as well as to other molecules in the local environment (see Fig. 8.2).

Fibromodulin and lumican

Fibromodulin and lumican belong to the same subclass of the LRR proteins with the gene arrangement distinct from that of decorin. Other members of this subgroup are keratocan, osteoadherin, and PRELP. All these molecules except PRELP contain tyrosine sulfate residues in the N-terminal extension. Notably the number of such sulfate residues is variable both with regard to the relative proportion of candidate tyrosine residues that are sulfated within a given molecule and with regard to the number of such tyrosine residues that may carry a sulfate. One extreme is represented by fibromodulin, which contains up to nine sulfate residues; osteoadherin contains up to eight, lumican up to four, and keratocan only one.[33] PRELP, in contrast, contains a cluster of basic residues contributing heparin-binding activity for this molecule.[34]

The function of this domain with clustered tyrosine sulfate residues is becoming clearer. The domains in fibromodulin and osteoadherin mimic heparin in many interactions and bind growth factors (e.g., fibroblast growth factor [FGF]-2), cytokines (e.g., Oncostatin M and IL-10), matrix metalloproteases [MMPs] (e.g., MMP-13 for fibromodulin), as well as a number of matrix proteins via their heparin-binding domains (e.g., PRELP and chondroadherin).[35] Thus, fibromodulin sitting on a collagen fiber appears to extend its tyrosine sulfate domain, which can bind to molecules with cationic domains. One such charged structure is the NC-4 domain of collagen type IX, which has been shown to interact with the anionic N-terminal extension of fibromodulin,[35] schematically outlined in Figure 8.2.

All of the molecules in this family appear to bind to collagen via their LRR domain, with dissociation constants ranging from 1 to 10 nM.[1] Only in a few cases has it been established where exactly along the collagen the LRR protein binds.

Collagen binding of fibromodulin has been extensively studied. It has been shown that the molecule inhibits fibril formation in vitro. The fibromodulin null mouse shows altered collagen fibril dimensions, particularly apparent in the tail tendon. Unexpectedly, in view of the inhibitory effects observed in vitro, the tendon contained a much larger number of thin fibrils. An explanation appears to be a higher abundance of the related lumican molecule, which could be shown to bind to the same site on the collagen, albeit with somewhat lower affinity. It thus appears that lumican may guide early events in fibril formation. The molecule may then be competed away by fibromodulin to introduce a different function. Because the mRNA levels and therefore synthesis of lumican were lower in the null mouse, it appears that the higher levels of this protein were caused by a retarded elimination apparently caused by the lack of competition by fibromodulin.[1]

These findings illustrate that fibril formation takes place in many steps involving a set of different molecules with different roles.

Fibromodulin is also present at the collagen fiber in the tissue, where it is bound in the gap region.[1] It appears to be bound via

its protein core exposing a keratan sulfate chain as well as the tyrosine sulfate domain, available to interact with PRELP and the NC-4 domain of collagen type IX located on neighboring fibers. Such interactions are important for the stability and properties of the collagen network.

Fibromodulin is a target in joint disease. In a model of articular cartilage destruction using stimulation of cartilage by IL-1 in explant culture, we have been able to show that fibromodulin is degraded after aggrecan and that the molecule is initially cleaved by MMP-13 to release the almost entire N-terminal tyrosine sulfate domain while the remainder of the molecule is initially retained in the tissue, probably bound to the collagen.[36] This loss of the anionic domain is likely to alter the properties and interactions of fibromodulin. At the same time MMP-13 can release the entire NC-4 domain of collagen type IX from cartilage.[37] This results in a loss of function that non-covalently cross-links collagen fibers and stabilizes this network that is essential for the maintenance of structure and function of the cartilage. This may represent a central mechanism in the swelling and surface fibrillation observed in early osteoarthritis.

It is of interest to note that the fragment retained in the tissue is only found in pathology and not in normal tissue, albeit there is continuous turnover of matrix constituents in response to altered load and to remove damaged components. This normal turnover appears to involve different mechanisms of cleavage.

Other LRR proteins

PRELP distinguishes itself by having a basic, heparin binding N-terminal domain.[38] This mediates binding to molecules with heparan sulfate side chains, including perlecan and cell surface syndecan and glypican. At the same time the protein binds via its LRR domain to two sites on fibril-forming collagens type I and II. Thus, the molecule has the potential to bridge from the collagen network back to the cell surface. It thereby has the potential to provide feedback to the cells on the conditions of the matrix. Little is known of alterations of PRELP in joint disease.

Asporin is a close relative of decorin but differs in having a variably long polyaspartate sequence in the N-terminal end. The number of aspartate residues varies between individuals.[39] It has been demonstrated in studies of several cohorts of individuals in Asia that osteoarthritis is overrepresented in individuals having 14 such residues compared with those with 13 residues in the asporin N-terminal structure.[40] In a different study from the United Kingdom no such pronounced relationship could be discerned, indicating that other factors also are involved.[41] One function of the polyaspartate sequence appears to be to bind calcium, where there may be a difference between the 13 and 14 aspartate variants.[42] At the same time asporin binds to collagen to the same sites as decorin,[42] which can provide for its fixation to collagen fibers in the tissue. The molecule may thus have roles in regulating mineralization relevant to the development of osteoarthritis. Asporin, like decorin, biglycan, and fibromodulin, appears to bind transforming growth factor (TGF)-β.

There is a set of LRR-proteins with only six repeats.[1] These include epiphycan, mimecan, and opticin. Also, these molecules appear to have the ability to bind collagen. They all contain N-terminal extensions carrying glycosaminoglycan chains (epiphycan), tyrosine sulfate residues (mimecan), or O-glycosidically linked oligosaccharides (opticin) (see Fig. 8.5). Mimecan has also been named osteoglycin. There is limited knowledge on alterations of these proteins in joint disease. Mimecan and opticin are particularly prominent in connective tissues other than those of the joint.

Heparin/heparan sulfate

A glycosaminoglycan not prominent in cartilage is heparan sulfate, which shows overlapping structural features to heparin. Heparan sulfate is found as side chains of extracellular perlecan (see later), which has a very large protein core with several domains interacting with a number of other proteins in the ECM. The proteoglycan contains an N-terminal domain with some three glycosaminoglycan chains and a C-terminal domain with up to two chains. These may be heparan sulfate or chondroitin sulfate (see later).

Heparan sulfate contains two types of disaccharide repeats of either a glucuronic acid and an N-acetylglucosamine or an iduronic acid and an N-acetylglucosamine. The hexosamine carries an O-sulfate group and some of the residues have an additional N-sulfate instead of the N-acetyl group. Also, the uronic acid may be sulfated, usually in its 2-position. Thus, there is an extensive variability in the building blocks that are then assembled in variably long stretches with different repeat stretches of lowly and highly sulfated residues.

Other heparan sulfate–containing proteoglycans are found at the cell surface of the chondrocyte. These include four different syndecans,[43] which contain a domain intercalated in the cell membrane and some six glypicans that are linked via a glycosylphosphoinositide linkage.[44] The syndecans contain an intracellular signaling domain and, as discussed later, they are involved in signal transduction.

Fibers with collagen type VI as the main constituent

There is a different fibrillar network in cartilage with a more restricted distribution in the tissue. This has collagen type VI as a major constituent and is primarily present in the territorial matrix surrounding the cells (see Fig. 8.1).

Collagen type VI

A distinct network of beaded filaments is represented by collagen type VI. This molecule contains three different α-chains with a central triple helical domain flanked by globular domains. The N-terminal portion, particularly the α_3(VI)-chain, contains nine von Willebrand factor A–like (vWFA) repeats. Also the C-terminal portions of all three chains contain two vWFA repeats, as well as other motifs with less clear functions. The vWFA domain is found in many proteins where it is involved in protein-to-protein interactions.[45]

While still within the cell, two collagen type VI molecules associate in an antiparallel fashion such that the dimer is flanked by the N-terminal domains, with the two C-terminal domains placed to form two interior globular structures along the filament formed by the two triple helices. Two such dimers associate laterally to form a tetramer having globular domains at each end representing a pair of the vWFA-rich globules. Internal in the triple helical central filament are found the two globular structures representing the C-terminals.[45] The tetramer is secreted from the cell, and its N-terminal structures lay the ground for further associations into fibrils involving both end-to-end and side-to-side interactions. This assembly process appears to be governed by other molecules particularly involving the members of the LRR protein family.

Biglycan and decorin

Biglycan and decorin both bind with high affinity to the collagen type VI N-terminal domain independently of their glycosaminoglycan side chains. This binding is a prerequisite for formation of the collagen type VI beaded filament network *in vitro*. The regulation of the collagen type VI assembly also depends on the presence of the chondroitin/dermatan sulfate side chains, where the two present in biglycan provide for a more efficient filament formation than the single chain in decorin. The two closely related proteoglycans appear to bind to the same site, which interestingly does not seem to involve the triple helical domain in this collagen.[46]

Matrilins

Cartilage matrix protein (CMP, matrilin-1) is the first identified of the four matrilins. These proteins[47] contain vWFA domains. Matrilin-1 has two such domains in each of the three identical subunits with a molecular mass of around 50,000 daltons; matrilin-3 with four subunits has only one such domain.

Matrilin-1 and matrilin-3 are quite restricted to cartilage while the others have a more general distribution. Interestingly, matrilin-1 is even further restricted and is not found in articular cartilage and the intervertebral disc, whereas it is particularly prominent in tracheal cartilage. The protein is present in the more immature cartilage of the femoral head during earlier phases of development and can be seen in the early bone anlagen. Its role in cartilage is becoming clearer, and data indicate roles in the collagen network function. Its two vWFA homology domains (only one in matrilin-3) may mediate the ability of the protein to bind to collagen. Matrilin-1 was initially isolated because of its apparent ability to bind to aggrecan.

Matrilin-1 can be isolated from cartilage as a mixed polymer that contains subunits of matrilin-1 as well as matrilin-3. The functional significance of this heterocomplex is not understood.[48]

A module crosslinking to other matrix constituents

Decorin and biglycan appear to have roles also in the completed network. Collagen type VI isolated from a chondrosarcoma cartilage-like tissue contains biglycan or decorin bound at the N-terminal globules. The proteoglycan, in turn, has a bound member of either matrilin-1, matrilin-2, or matrilin-3. This interaction is tight with a dissociation constant in the order of nanomolar. The matrilin, in turn, is binding to a procollagen type II molecule or a completed collagen fiber. Alternatively, the matrilin binds an aggrecan molecule (see Fig. 8.2).[49] Thus, the collagen type VI seems to be a center in a scaffold, which binds to the other major networks in the matrix. The collagen type VI is found only in the territorial matrix closer to the cells and is absent from the interterritorial matrix at some distance from the cell. The information on alterations of collagen type VI in joint disease is limited, but it is important to note that the protein is found particularly enriched in tissues subjected to load.

Molecules interacting at the cell surface and modulating chondrocyte behavior

The chondrocyte has the ability to both degrade the matrix and replenish lost molecules with new constituents in a process of remodeling the tissue in response to material fatigue or to altered load. The cells are guided in this endeavor by receptors at their surface that recognize specific molecules in the matrix (see Fig. 8.2). Binding elicits specific signals, which either will effect cellular spreading and migration by engaging the actin network or lead to alterations in transcription and protein synthesis. Other stimuli that will affect cells include mechanical forces, which provide signals that crosstalk with those from other interactions at the cell surface. Indeed, there are data to indicate that some of the signals elicited by mechanical load involve integrins.[50]

Integrin binding proteins

The integrins contain an α-chain non-covalently bound to a β-chain. The cells in connective tissues either contain a β_1- or β_3-chain in combination with one of many α-chains. The different integrins have different preferred ligand extracellular matrix proteins.[51] As an example of the organization of integrins, members of one such family with four members bind to collagens. They contain a β_1-chain in combination with either an α_1-, α_2-, α_{10}-, or α_{11}-chain. These various integrins show different tissue distribution, such that those with α10 appear unique to cartilage while the others have more ubiquitous distributions. Their binding to collagen may elicit different responses and may either primarily result in an altered production of enzymes degrading the matrix or in production of building blocks like collagen molecules.

There are a number of factors limiting our ability to discern what integrins are present on the chondrocyte in the tissue. One factor is limited accessibility by antibodies used, and another is alterations of integrin presence during the long procedure for cell isolation. Thus, present information on the presence of integrins at the cell surface is variable. It is likely that a number of integrins change their expression on chondrocytes in normal and in pathologic tissue in response to environmental factors.

Many of the molecules binding to integrins are not unique for cartilage. The collagen binding integrins appear not to be specific for a particular fibril-forming molecule. One exception is chondroadherin. This protein appears restricted to cartilage and can bind the $\alpha_2\beta_1$ integrin while not binding to other integrins containing the same β-chain.

Chondroadherin

Chondroadherin is a member of the LRR protein family, forming its own subclass. The protein differs from the other LRR family members in that the C-terminal cysteine loop is double and that the protein has a short C-terminal extension of basic amino acids. The protein has no N-terminal extension. Interestingly, on binding to the cell surface $\alpha_2\beta_1$ integrin the protein elicits signals that do not induce cell spreading, a behavior different from that of most other integrin-binding proteins.[1]

Chondroadherin is present in articular cartilage but particularly enriched during growth in the pre-hypertrophic zone of the growth plate where cell multiplication is slowed, in line with its *in-vitro* effects on cell behavior. Interestingly, the protein appears to be lost early in the process of developing joint damage in osteoarthritis.

Fibronectin

Fibronectin[52] is present in most tissues and can actually form its own fibrils that appear to have roles in guiding matrix assembly and cell migration. The protein contains two identical subunits held together by disulfide bonds close to their C-terminal end.

Fibronectin contains a collagen-binding domain with preference for denatured collagen (gelatin). There are integrin-binding domains, where the RGD (arginine-glycine-aspartic acid) represents the classic motif of integrin binding. This motif in fibronectin preferentially binds the $\alpha_5\beta_1$ integrin, although the $\alpha_v\beta_3$ integrin can also interact. There are also other integrin-binding domains in fibronectin.[53]

Another motif is represented by the two heparin-binding domains of each some 20 kDa on each subunit. These can interact with heparan sulfate proteoglycans at the cell surface, including syndecan, which also represents a signaling molecule.[54]

Although the details are not known, fragments of fibronectin (e.g., those containing either of the heparin-binding domains) when added to cartilage in explant culture as well as injected into the joint will stimulate chondrocytes to produce proteases and cartilage breakdown.[55,56] In contrast, the intact fibronectin molecule will not have these effects on the cells. It is possible that fragmentation of fibronectin is one mechanism for propagating joint destruction in disease. The active fragments have not yet been identified in body fluids.

Fibronectin is upregulated in the articular cartilage already at very early stages of osteoarthritis in many species, including humans.[57] The functional consequences of this upregulation are not known but may represent part of a repair attempt. A result is further availability of fibronectin that may be fragmented to further increase tissue degradation.

Collagen and the discoidin receptors

There is an additional cell receptor for collagen, the discoidin domain receptor 2 (DDR-2). This receptor has been shown to be upregulated in mice developing osteoarthritis. This receptor will bind collagen type II that induces upregulation of MMP-13 production.[58] Exposure of collagen type II may be enhanced by removal of proteins bound at the fibrillar surface, thereby making the molecule available for interactions.

Hyaluronan

Hyaluronan represents an extremely long glycosaminoglycan chain, which is distinct from all the others in that it is not bound to a protein core. It does not contain any sulfate groups. The backbone is made up of one to several thousand repeating disaccharides of glucuronic acid and N-acetylglucosamine. As discussed earlier, this glycosaminoglycan specifically binds to a domain in aggrecan essential for the formation of aggregates.

There is also an interaction with specific cell surface receptors. These are CD-44,[59] which interacts with a minimally long hexasaccharide sequence of the polymer. The interactions with hyaluronan are important for organizing the pericellular environment and provide for signals to the cell. The CD-44 occurs in many different splice forms with different presence on various cells, but a role for such variability in joint disease is unclear. Another receptor for hyaluronan is RHAMM.[60] These are also signaling receptors, but like the CD-44 receptors they are present on a variety of cells.

Ligands for heparan sulfate/syndecans

In addition to heparin-binding domains present in fibronectin, various other matrix proteins contain such domains. Examples are most members of the thrombospondin family, (excluding COMP), many MMPs, CILP, and PRELP.[1] As discussed earlier, isolated heparin-binding domain fragments can induce cartilage breakdown *in vitro* and *in vivo*. The precise role of these interactions or whether they represent a governing factor in tissue breakdown as discussed for fibronectin is not known.

Interestingly, as discussed earlier, the N-terminal tyrosine-sulfate domain of fibromodulin can mimic heparin in many interactions and bind other proteins to crossbridge networks as well as sequester growth factors.

Other molecular functions

In joint disease, inflammation is a frequent component causing pain and limiting function. The inflammation is usually chronic and one issue is whether components from cartilage can propagate the inflammatory activity. It is a long-standing observation that when cartilage is removed in joint arthroplasty the inflammation recedes, indicating that factors released from the tissue have a role in propagating inflammation.

It has been shown that some patients with rheumatoid arthritis have circulating antibodies to collagen type II. Furthermore, an arthritis condition can be elicited by injecting mice and rats with collagen type II (collagen-induced arthritis). The disease can be transferred by antibodies to specific collagen type II epitopes.[61] It is thus possible that antibody binding activates complement and inflammation.

More recent findings indicate that matrix proteins may activate innate immunity. Fibromodulin has been shown to be as active as immune complexes[62] in activating the classical pathway of complement. Although it appears to be as potent as complexes of immunoglobulins, it does not bind to the same site. The protein binds C1q with ensuing deposition and activation of C4 and C3. The fibromodulin binds to the head domains of C1q rather than to the triple helical stalk region.

Interestingly, fibromodulin can also recruit factor H via binding to a different site than that for C1q and thereby inhibit further activation of the complement cascade. Whether different fragments released in disease will have different roles in complement activation remains to be shown.

In other experiments it has been shown that biglycan can inhibit the classical pathway of complement. It appears that other LRR proteins such as biglycan and decorin also can bind factors involved in regulating the complement cascade. One example is a tight interaction to C4BP having roles in regulating complement activity.[63]

Binding and sequestering growth factors in the extracellular matrix

The extracellular matrix of cartilage contains a number of factors that are sequestered there by binding to specific interaction partners. On degradation of the matrix one can envisage that these factors are released and affect cellular activities. In particular, a number of growth factors have been found to have the capacity to bind to matrix proteins.

Transforming growth factor-β

This growth factor has been shown to bind to a number of matrix proteins, where particularly the binding to some members of the LRR protein family has been investigated. All three TGF-β variants bind to bacterially expressed proteins of decorin, biglycan, and fibromodulin as well as to proteins with the full range of post-translational modifications. More recently there are indications that asporin also can bind TGF-β. It has been demonstrated that active TGF-β is released from decorin on treatment with MMP-3. Indeed cartilage contains substantial amounts of TGF-β, which has been extracted and purified from the tissue.

Fibroblast growth factor

There are matrix proteins that contain heparan sulfate side chains, which are likely to bind growth factors within the FGF family. In the case of syndecan at the cell surface, these side chains appear to be involved in presenting the growth factor to its receptor.[64]

Other molecules in the extracellular matrix

Perlecan was found to have a central role in cartilage development when a mouse with the gene inactivated was developed. Most of these mice die during early development from problems with heart and major blood vessels, but those that survive until birth show major growth disturbances, with an extensively altered growth plate, lacking a large proportion of the collagen fibers.[65] Further studies have revealed that chondroitin sulfate side chains specific for perlecan can actually accelerate and catalyze collagen fiber formation.[66]

GP-39 is a protein upregulated in osteoarthritis. It shares homology with a chitinase, but the true activity of the protein is not known.[67] GP-39 is also expressed in a number of other tissues, particularly in disease.

Cartilage matrix also contains a number of proteins that are made elsewhere and are normally primarily found in the circulation. There is a preference for certain proteins, and particularly low-molecular-weight basic proteins (e.g. lysozyme)[68] appear to bind into the matrix. It is not known if these molecules contribute specific functions.

Fragments of matrix proteins released in cartilage breakdown as molecular indicators of disease

In processes resulting in cartilage tissue destruction, extracellular matrix proteins are degraded by proteolytic enzymes. Some of the fragments formed will no longer be retained in the tissue but released to surrounding body fluids. With the use of sensitive immunoassays these fragments can be quantified in synovial fluid or serum. This so-called molecular marker technology (biomarkers) aims at providing new means of assaying ongoing active processes in the articular cartilage. In further developments such techniques may be used in diagnosis, for the estimation of activity of the tissue-destroying process, to document effects of therapeutic intervention, and, most importantly, to discover processes at the early stage before clinical symptoms become apparent. One example is the demonstration that COMP can be used to identify those cases that will lead to the most extensive joint destruction in both osteoarthritis and rheumatoid arthritis.[28,69] Also a number of collagen fragments created by cleavages with collagenases as well as by subsequent gelatinase activity have been used to monitor disease.[70,71] With further developments of the technology we hope to be able to identify indicators specific to a particular pathologic process in a given tissue. Thus, it should be possible to identify activity of a process in the meniscus and activity in the cartilage.

KEY REFERENCES

1. Heinegård D, Aspberg A, Franzén A, Lorenzo P. Non-collagenous glycoproteins in the extracellular matrix, with particular reference to cartilage and bone. In: Royce P, Steinmann B, eds. Connective tissue and its heritable disorders: molecular, genetic, and medical aspects. New York: Wiley-Liss Inc, 2002:271-291.
2. Glasson SS, Askew R, Sheppard B, et al. Deletion of active ADAMTS5 prevents cartilage degradation in a murine model of osteoarthritis. Nature 2005;434:644-648.
3. Stanton H, Rogerson FM, East CJ, et al. ADAMTS5 is the major aggrecanase in mouse cartilage in vivo and in vitro. Nature 2005;434:648-652.
4. Sandy JD. A contentious issue finds some clarity: on the independent and complementary roles of aggrecanase activity and MMP activity in human joint aggrecanolysis. Osteoarthritis Cartilage 2006;14:95-100.
5. Hughes CE, Caterson B, Fosang AJ, et al. Monoclonal antibodies that specifically recognize neoepitope sequences generated by "aggrecanase" and matrix metalloproteinase cleavage of aggrecan: application to catabolism in situ and in vitro. Biochem J 1995;305:799-804.
8. Westling J, Fosang AJ, Last K, et al. ADAMTS4 cleaves at the aggrecanase site (Glu373-Ala374) and secondarily at the matrix metalloproteinase site (Asn341-Phe342) in the aggrecan interglobular domain. J Biol Chem 2002;277:16059-16066.
14. Lohmander LS, Atley LM, Pietka TA, Eyre DR. The release of crosslinked peptides from type II collagen into human synovial fluid is increased soon after joint injury and in osteoarthritis. Arthritis Rheum 2003;48:3130-3139.
16. Eyre DR: Collagens and cartilage matrix homeostasis. Clin Orthop Relat Res 2004;(427 Suppl):S118-S122.
17. Vikkula M, Mariman ECM, Lui VCH, et al. Autosomal dominant and recessive osteochondrodysplasias associated with the COL11A2 locus. Cell 1995;80:431-437.
19. Eyre DR, Pietka T, Weis MA, Wu JJ: Covalent cross-linking of the NC1 domain of collagen type IX to collagen type II in cartilage. J Biol Chem 2004;279:2568-2574.
20. Fässler R, Schnegelsberg PNJ, Dausman J, et al. Mice lacking a1(IX) collagen develop noninflammatory degenerative joint disease. Proc Natl Acad Sci U S A 1994;91:5070-5074.
22. Oldberg Å, Antonsson P, Lindblom K, Heinegård D: COMP (cartilage oligomeric matrix protein) is structurally related to the thrombospondins. J Biol Chem 1992;267:22346-22350.
26. Briggs MD, Chapman KL. Pseudoachondroplasia and multiple epiphyseal dysplasia: mutation review, molecular interactions, and genotype to phenotype correlations. Hum Mutat 2002;19:465-478.
27. Svensson L, Aszodi A, Heinegård D, et al. Cartilage oligomeric matrix protein-deficient mice have normal skeletal development. Mol Cell Biol 2002;22:4366-4371.
28. Saxne T, Månsson B, Heinegård D. Biomarkers for cartilage and bone in rheumatoid arthritis. In: Firestein G, Panayi G, Wollheim F, eds. Rheumatoid arthritis: new frontiers in pathogenesis and treatment. Oxford, Oxford University Press, 2006:301-313.
29. Scott PG, McEwan PA, Dodd CM, et al. Crystal structure of the dimeric protein core of decorin, the archetypal small leucine-rich repeat proteoglycan. Proc Natl Acad Sci U S A 2004;101:15633-15638.
30. Scott PG, Dodd CM, Bergmann EM, et al. Crystal structure of the biglycan dimer and evidence that dimerization is essential for folding and stability of class I small leucine-rich repeat proteoglycans. J Biol Chem 2006;281:13324-13332.
32. Danielson KG, Baribault H, Holmes DF, et al. Targeted disruption of decorin leads to abnormal collagen fibril morphology and skin fragility. J Cell Biol 1997;136:729-743.
35. Tillgren V, Önnerfjord P, Haglund L, Heinegård D. The tyrosine sulfate-rich domains of the LRR proteins fibromodulin and osteoadherin bind motifs of basic clusters in a variety of heparin-binding proteins, including bioactive factors. J Biol Chem 2009;284:28543-28553.
37. Danfelter M, Önnerfjord P, Heinegård D. Fragmentation of proteins in cartilage treated with interleukin-1: specific cleavage of type IX collagen by matrix metalloproteinase 13 releases the NC4 domain. J Biol Chem 2007;282:36933-36941.
38. Bengtsson E, Mörgelin M, Sasaki T, et al. The leucine rich repeat protein PRELP binds perlecan and collagens and may function as a basement membrane anchor. J Biol Chem 2002;277:15061-15068.
39. Lorenzo P, Aspberg A, Önnerfjord P, et al. Identification and characterization of asporin-a—novel member of the leucine rich repeat protein family closely related to decorin and biglycan. J Biol Chem 2001;276:12201-12211.
40. Kizawa H, Kou I, Iida A, et al. An aspartic acid repeat polymorphism in asporin inhibits chondrogenesis and increases susceptibility to osteoarthritis. Nat Genet 2005;37:138-144.
41. Mustafa Z, Dowling B, Chapman K, et al. Investigating the aspartic acid (D) repeat of asporin as a risk factor for osteoarthritis in a UK Caucasian population. Arthritis Rheum 2005;52:3502-3506.
42. Kalamajski S, Aspberg A, Lindblom K, et al. Asporin competes with decorin for collagen binding, binds calcium and promotes osteoblast collagen mineralization. Biochem J 2009;423:53-59.
43. Couchman JR. Syndecans: proteoglycan regulators of cell-surface microdomains? Nat Rev Mol Cell Biol 2003;4:926-937.
47. Segat D, Paulsson M, Smyth N. Matrilins: structure, expression and function. Osteoarthritis Cartilage 2001;9(Suppl A):S29-S35.
49. Wiberg C, Klatt AR, Wagener R, et al. Complexes of matrilin-1 and biglycan or decorin connect collagen VI microfibrils to both collagen II and aggrecan. J Biol Chem 2003;278:37698-37704.
50. Millward-Sadler SJ, Salter DM. Integrin-dependent signal cascades in chondrocyte mechanotransduction. Ann Biomed Eng 2004;32:435-446.
52. Pankov R, Yamada KM. Fibronectin at a glance. J Cell Sci 2002;115:3861-3863.
57. Lorenzo P, Bayliss MT, Heinegård D. Altered patterns and synthesis of extracellular matrix macromolecules in early osteoarthritis. Matrix Biol 2004;23:381-391.
58. Xu L, Peng H, Wu D, et al. Activation of the discoidin domain receptor 2 induces expression of matrix metalloproteinase 13 associated with osteoarthritis in mice. J Biol Chem 2005;280:548-555.
59. Knudson CB, Knudson W, Kresina RL: Hyaluronan and CD44: modulators of chondrocyte metabolism. Clin Orthop Relat Res 2004;(427 Suppl):S152-S162.
60. Nedvetzki S, Gonen E, Assayag N, et al. RHAMM, a receptor for hyaluronan-mediated motility, compensates for CD44 in inflamed CD44-knockout mice: a different interpretation of redundancy. Proc Natl Acad Sci U S A 2004;101:18081-18086.
61. Holmdahl R. Dissection of the genetic complexity of arthritis using animal models. Immunol Lett 2006;103:86-91.
62. Sjöberg A, Önnerfjord P, Mörgelin M, et al. The extracellular matrix and inflammation: fibromodulin activates the classical pathway of complement by directly binding C1q. J Biol Chem 2005;280:32301-32308.
63. Happonen KE, Sjöberg AP, Mörgelin M, et al. Complement inhibitor C4b-binding protein interacts directly with small glycoproteins of the extracellular matrix. J Immunol 2009;182:1518-1525.
64. Allen BL, Filla MS, Rapraeger AC. Role of heparan sulfate as a tissue-specific regulator of FGF-4 and FGF receptor recognition. J Cell Biol 2001;155:845-858.
65. Gustafsson E, Aszodi A, Ortega N, et al. Role of collagen type II and perlecan in skeletal development. Ann N Y Acad Sci 2003;995:140-150.
66. Kvist A, Johnson A, Mörgelin M, et al. Chondroitin sulfate perlecan enhances collagen fibril formation: implications for perlecan chondrodysplasias. J Biol Chem 2006;281:33127-33139.
69. Sharif M, Kirwan JR, Elson CJ, et al. Suggestion of nonlinear or phasic progression of knee osteoarthritis based on measurements of serum cartilage oligomeric matrix protein levels over five years. Arthritis Rheum 2004;50:2479-2488.
70. Garnero P, Charni N, Juillet F, et al. Increased urinary type II collagen helical and C telopeptide levels are independently associated with a rapidly destructive hip osteoarthritis. Ann Rheum Dis 2006;65:1639-1644.
71. Ameye LG, Deberg M, Oliveira M, et al. The chemical biomarkers C2C, Coll2-1, and Coll2-1NO2 provide complementary information on type II collagen catabolism in healthy and osteoarthritic mice. Arthritis Rheum 2007;56:3336-3346.

REFERENCES

Full references for this chapter can be found on www.expertconsult.com.

Bone structure and function

David B. Burr, Teresita Bellido, and Kenneth E. White

9

- Bone is organized differently and for different functions at the organ (whole bone), tissue (material), and molecular (collagen-mineral) levels.
- The non-collagenous proteins function as structural support in the bone matrix and have roles in regulating mineral deposition and crystal growth, as well as cell attachment and growth factor concentration and regulation.
- Bone mineralization is effected through hormonal action (FGF23), as well as through the bioactivity of matrix proteins with emerging roles (DMP1 and MEPE).
- Osteoclasts are the primary bone-resorptive cells and originate from precursors of the hematopoietic lineage upon stimulation with receptor activator of NF-κB ligand (RANKL) and macrophage colony-stimulating factor (MCSF).
- The rate of osteoclast generation determines the extension of the BMU, whereas the life span of osteoclasts determines the depth of resorption.
- Osteoblasts are the cells responsible for bone formation and originate from mesenchymal progenitors that also give rise to chondrocytes, muscle cells, and adipocytes.
- Osteocytes form a network that senses mechanical and hormonal environmental cues and orchestrates the function of osteoblasts and osteoclasts.
- Sclerostin is the first molecular mediator known to mediate the communication between osteocytes and osteoblasts.
- Four dynamic processes control skeletal development and adaptation—growth, modeling, remodeling, and repair—and these are defined by the relationship of bone resorption and bone formation to each other.

Bone is a complex natural composite material that undergoes millions of loading cycles during a lifetime without failure. Its structure is hierarchical, being organized differently at the organ (whole bone), tissue (material), and molecular (collagen-mineral) levels. This sequential hierarchy allows bone to serve a mechanical function. But the organization of its structure at these different levels also allows it to serve physiologically as a blood-forming organ and mineral reservoir and protect vital organs such as the brain and cartilaginous tissues in joints.

The mechanical functions of bone are the most widely recognized and are often described in terms of its strength and stiffness. In reality, bone's design goal is to prevent fracture, which its hierarchical arrangement and composite nature allow it to perform most effectively over a lifetime of use. Although strength and stiffness are important, bone is particularly effective at dissipating energy that could cause a fracture over repeated cycles of loading. Beyond its mechanical function, the marrow cavity and the porous trabecular bone in the ends of long bones and in the vertebrae and iliac crest are regions in which red blood cells are formed and stored. Bone is, in fact, a primary blood-storing organ. Additionally, bone is the body's primary storehouse of calcium and phosphorus; 99% of the body's calcium is stored in bone. These minerals are necessary for the proper function of a variety of systems in the body and are essential for enzyme reactions, blood clotting, the proper function of contractile proteins in muscles, and the transmission of nerve impulses.

ORGANIZATION OF BONE

Macroscopic (organ) level

Bone at the organ level consists of the diaphysis (shaft), metaphysis, and epiphysis (Fig. 9.1). In the long bones of growing children, the growth plate separates the epiphysis from the metaphysis. The primary component of the diaphysis is cortical or compact bone. The Haversian canals in cortical bone create a porosity of about 3% to 5%, although this increases in older age and with osteoporotic changes to the skeleton. Compact bone is also found surrounding the spongy bone of the vertebral body and in the skull. It is strong and provides both support and protection.

Cancellous (trabecular or spongy) bone is found in the metaphyses of the long bones and in the vertebrae, surrounded by cortical bone. During growth, the primary spongiosa are composed mostly of disorganized woven bone, or primary lamellar bone surrounding a core of calcified cartilage. It is separated from the remodeled, more highly oriented secondary spongiosa by an arbitrary boundary. The secondary spongiosa reflects patterns of stress and functions largely to funnel stresses to the stronger and more massive cortical bone. In regions beneath joint surfaces it also attenuates forces generated by mechanical loading and may protect the joint surface from loading-related trauma. The cancellous bone itself is composed of plates and rods of bone, each about 200 μm thick, with a porosity of about 75% to 85%. The marrow in the spaces between the trabecular struts are regions in which red blood cells are formed (i.e., red marrow). In osteoporosis the differentiation of cells in the bone lineage can be partly diverted to adipocytes, and the marrow becomes more fatty (i.e., yellow marrow). Because cancellous bone has a large surface area in contact with vascular marrow, it is ideal for the long-term exchange of calcium ions. In osteopenia, regions of cancellous bone are affected first. This is why the vertebral column, which is mainly composed of cancellous bone, is affected earlier and more severely in osteoporosis than even the femoral neck and hip.

Microscopic (tissue) level

At the microstructural level, bone is organized differently for different functions (Fig. 9.2). In humans bone tissue can be divided into three broad categories partly on the basis of the arrangement of collagen fibers and partly on whether it has replaced preexisting bone: (1) woven bone, (2) primary bone, and (3) secondary bone.

Woven bone is characterized by randomly oriented collagen fibers, which tend to be smaller in diameter than those in more highly organized primary or secondary bone. Woven bone is not lamellar, is porous, and may become highly mineralized because the "loose weave" of the collagen fibers allows deposition of large amounts of mineral. The low density of woven bone, then, is a function of loosely packed collagen fibers and porosity, rather than low mineralization. Woven bone can be deposited *de novo* without any bony or cartilaginous substrate or anlage, but it can also be formed as part of the process of endochondral ossification, either at the growth plate during development or during fracture repair. Woven bone proliferates rapidly because it has a large cell-to-volume ratio, which makes its role in fracture repair ideal. It is often found associated with osteosarcoma, probably because of proliferation, especially of the cellular periosteum. It is also associated with the osteophytosis that occurs in the vertebral column consequent to disk degeneration and composes the bulk of osteophytes found on the margins of joints in osteoarthritis. The function of woven bone is primarily mechanical, rapidly providing both temporary strength and scaffolding on which lamellar bone may be deposited. However, it

67

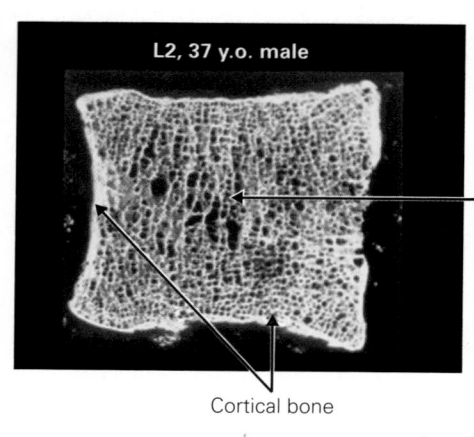

L2, 37 y.o. male

Secondary spongiosa

Cortical bone

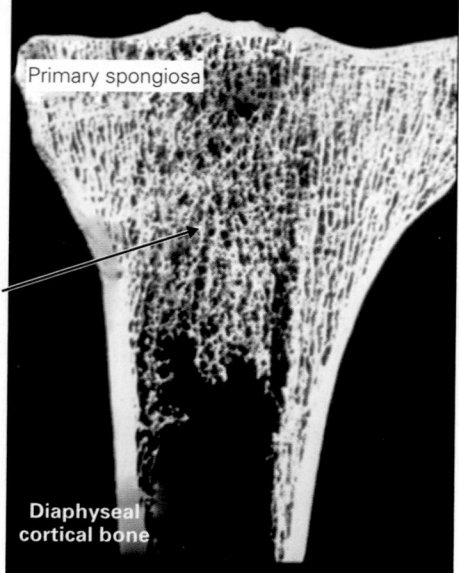

Primary spongiosa

Diaphyseal cortical bone

Fig. 9.1 At the organ level, bone consists of compact (cortical) bone, which forms a shell around the more porous, cancellous (trabecular) bone, or spongiosa. In the cancellous regions of the long bones, such as the proximal tibia shown here, the primary spongiosa is separated from the secondary spongiosa by an arbitrary boundary. Primary spongiosa is composed of primary bone, often laid down during growth on a calcified cartilage core that is subsequently remodeled. Secondary spongiosa is remodeled, reflects patterns of stress, and directs these stresses to the cortical shell.

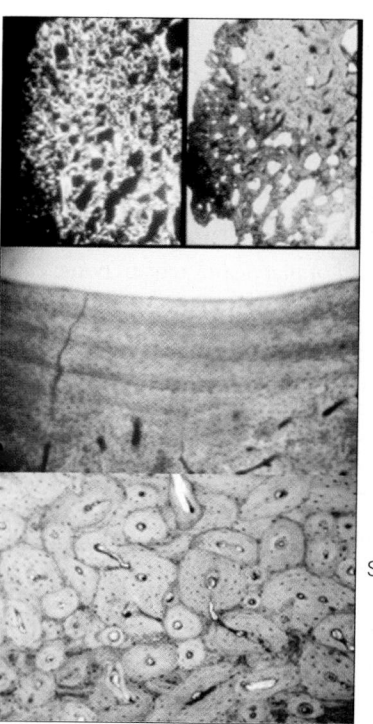

Woven bone

Primary lamellar bone

Secondary osteonal bone

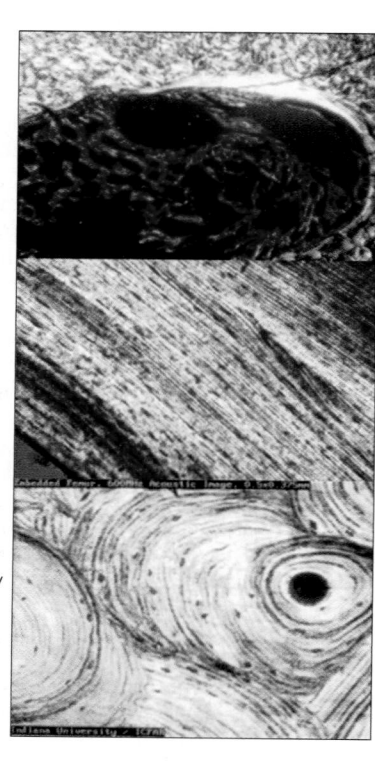

Fig. 9.2 These photomicrographs show the three general microscopic types of bone, defined morphologically. Woven bone is composed of disorganized, randomly oriented collagen fibers. It is found at sites of fracture or inflammation. Lamellar bone can be divided into primary and secondary. Primary bone is deposited in layers by direct apposition on a substrate. It is found circling the endocortical and periosteal circumferences of a long bone and within trabeculae. Secondary bone is formed by replacement of primary bone, through the process of resorption and subsequent new bone formation. Woven bone: polarized light; primary lamellar bone: left—basic fuchsin, right—polarized light; secondary osteonal bone: left—toluidine blue, right—scanning electron microscopic image.

can also be associated with pathologic processes that involve inflammatory cytokines.

Primary bone must be deposited on a preexisting substrate and is organized into lamellar layers. Because of this, trabecular plates, which are mainly composed of primary lamellae, cannot be replaced once they are perforated. This accounts for the loss of trabeculae with age and is part of the reason that it is difficult to reverse osteoporotic changes once trabecular connectivity has been lost. Primary lamellar bone also forms in rings around the endocortical and periosteal surfaces of whole bone (circumferential lamellae). Primary lamellar bone itself is not very vascular and therefore can become dense. However, primary bone often borders highly vascular tissues and therefore the quantity and quality of primary lamellar bone can be affected by hematopoiesis and the body's needs for mineral metabolism. Primary bone can also be arranged in concentric rings around a central canal—much like a secondary Haversian system, except without a definable cement line. Primary osteons tend to be small with few concentric lamellae. In reality, primary osteons are modified vascular channels that have "filled in" by the addition of lamellae to the surface of the vascular space.

Secondary bone is the product of the resorption of preexisting bone and its replacement with new bone. This can occur within dense cortical bone (resulting in a secondary osteon, or Haversian system), or it can begin on the surfaces of trabeculae (resulting in what is sometimes called a *hemiosteon*). The distinction between primary and secondary bone is important because it is likely that control of primary bone apposition is different from that replacing preexisting bone by secondary bone. A secondary Haversian system in cortical bone has a central vascular canal 50 to 90 μm in diameter, known as a *Haversian canal*. The blood vessels in the canal have the characteristics of capillaries and are generally paired within the canal. Venous sinusoids and lymphatic vessels are not found in Haversian canals, although it has been suggested that pre-lymphatic vessels may exist.[1] The vessel walls contain no smooth muscle but are fenestrated capillaries lined by an incomplete layer of endothelial cells, similar to vessels in other blood-forming organs like the spleen and bone marrow.[2] The vessel is accompanied about 60% of the time by two to seven unmyelinated nerve fibers.[3] Because the capillaries have no smooth muscle, these nerves do not serve a vasomotor function. Instead, they are most likely part

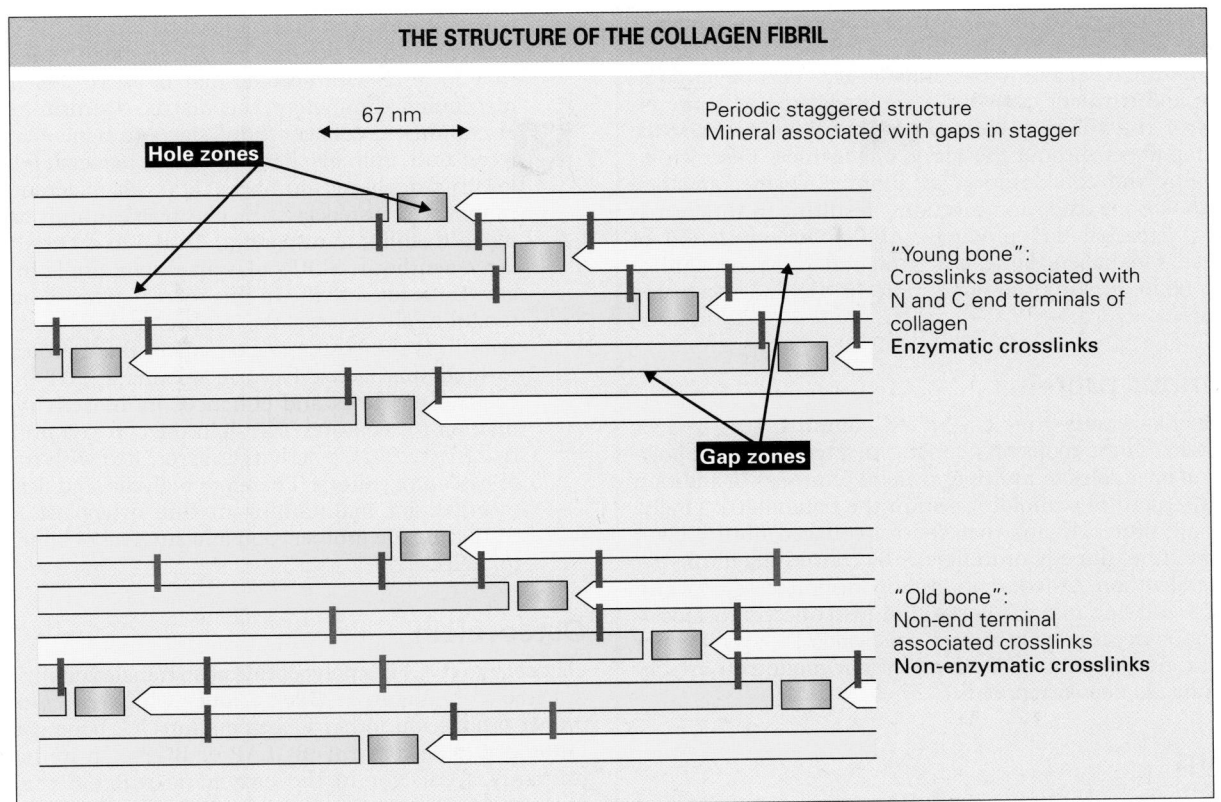

THE STRUCTURE OF THE COLLAGEN FIBRIL

67 nm

Hole zones

Periodic staggered structure
Mineral associated with gaps in stagger

"Young bone":
Crosslinks associated with
N and C end terminals of
collagen
Enzymatic crosslinks

Gap zones

"Old bone":
Non-end terminal
associated crosslinks
Non-enzymatic crosslinks

Fig. 9.3 The structure of the collagen fibril. Molecules are organized in quarter-staggered array, with hole and gap zones between them where mineral can deposit. The hole zones give the collagen fibril its banded appearance when viewed by electron microscopy. Cross-links are formed either through the action of enzymes (divalent and trivalent cross-links) or through non-enzymatic processes, the latter forming advanced glycation end products that can make bone behave in brittle fashion.

of the sympathetic nervous system and may have specialized receptors for stretch or pressure. Nerves in the Haversian canal could act to regulate the exchange of large molecules (e.g., protein polysaccharides or glycoproteins), but they have no direct role in altering blood flow.

The Haversian canal is lined by cells (lining cells, or resting osteoblasts) and is surrounded by a series of concentric lamellae containing bone cells—osteocytes—arranged in a circular fashion. The entire Haversian system is about 200 to 300 μm in diameter. The relationship between the size of the osteon and the size of its canal is a measure of the balance between bone resorption (osteon diameter) and bone formation (canal diameter). The secondary osteon is bounded by a 1- to 5-μm thick cement line, probably composed largely of sulfated glycosaminoglycans and with about 15% less mineral than in surrounding bone.[4] The cement line forms an effective boundary that can arrest cracks in bone and stop them from growing to a critical size.

COMPOSITION OF BONE
Collagen and mineral composite

Bone is composed of organic and mineralized components, mainly consisting of a matrix of cross-linked type I collagen mineralized with nanocrystalline, carbonated apatite. Bone matrix incorporates a small fraction of non-collagenous proteins that serve to control collagen assembly and size, as well as the process of mineralization, and cell attachment. The mineral comprises about 65% to 67% of the bone by weight, the organic component about 22% to 25%, and water the remaining fraction (⊕10%). Within the organic fraction, collagen makes up about 90%, with the remainder accounted for by several minor collagens (types III and V) and a variety of noncollagenous proteins, most of them extracellular, with cell protein accounting for about 15% of the noncollagenous proteins in bone.

Type I collagen in bone is formed by a triple helix composed of two α1 chains and a single α2 chain. At either end of the collagen molecule are an N-telopeptide and a C-telopeptide, which can be cleaved when bone is resorbed, and which are used to measure bone resorption biochemically. These individual triple helical collagen molecules self-associate into a periodic arrangement of parallel molecules spaced in quarter staggered array at distances of 67 nm between their ends to form collagen fibrils (Fig. 9.3). The spaces between the ends of the collagen molecules are known as *hole zones*, and the 35-nm gap zones that run longitudinally parallel between the molecules are known as *pores*. Poorly crystalline hydroxyapatite $(Ca_{10}[PO_4]_6[OH]_2)$ nucleates within these spaces. The initial deposition of mineral—or primary mineralization—occurs rapidly after new bone is deposited, achieving about two thirds of its eventual mineral content within about 3 weeks.[5] As the bone tissue matures, the mineral crystals grow, become more plate-like, and orient themselves parallel to one another and to the collagen fibrils. This process of crystal growth is sometimes called *secondary mineralization* and occurs over the next year or so until full mineralization is achieved. By itself, secondary mineralization can significantly increase the mass and mineral density of the bone. In trabecular bone, the c-axis or long axis of the mineral crystal aligns with the longitudinal axis of the trabeculae, whereas in cortical bone the mineral orients to the long axis of the osteon. Other elements can easily substitute into the hydroxyapatite crystal, changing its character and ability to withstand mechanical loads. As bone matures, carbonate may substitute for the phosphate groups or may be loosely bound to the surface of bone crystals. Ionic substitutions can also occur subsequent to treatment with therapeutic agents for osteoporosis. When sodium fluoride was given to women for osteoporosis, for example, fluoride substituted for the hydroxyl group, and it is now well known that too much fluoride in the crystal will make bone brittle. Likewise, strontium, which is now used in the form of strontium ranelate as a therapeutic agent to treat osteoporosis, can substitute for calcium.

Collagen fibers can become cross-linked through the action of enzymes, resulting in either immature and reducible (divalent) cross-links, or mature and irreducible (trivalent) cross-links such as pyridinoline and deoxypyridinoline, which are formed from divalent forms through the action of lysyl oxidase. Bone retains a large proportion of divalent cross-links throughout life. This is probably the consequence of continuous bone remodeling because divalent cross-links are rapidly converted into mature trivalent cross-links under normal circumstances. Divalent and trivalent cross-links are associated with the N- and C-terminals of the collagen molecule. Cross-links can also be formed between the fibers without the action of enzymes. These cross-links are formed by the condensation of arginine, lysine, and free sugars, or through various oxidation reactions, resulting in the formation of advanced glycation end products (AGEs). Accumulation of AGEs, such as occurs in diabetic bone, is detrimental to the mechanical properties of the bone, making the bone more brittle and increasing the risk of fracture.

Non-collagenous proteins

The skeletal non-collagenous proteins (NCPs) comprise 10% to 15% of total bone protein. These molecules constitute a wide range of polypeptide species and have roles in multiple skeletal processes in addition to functioning as structural scaffolding within the bone matrix. Biglycan and decorin are proteoglycans that control collagen fibril growth and size. Biglycan, either directly or indirectly by controlling fibril size, may inhibit mineralization. Osteocalcin, osteopontin, and osteonectin all play a role in regulating mineral deposition (osteonectin, osteocalcin) and crystal growth (osteopontin and osteocalcin). Several other NCPs such as thrombospondin and fibronectin regulate cell attachment and spreading, as does osteopontin.

Proteoglycans

Proteoglycans (PGs) are a ubiquitous family of molecules composed of a core protein and one or several covalently attached sulfated glycosaminoglycan (GAG) chains. The GAGs are linear polymers of repeated disaccharide units of hexosamine and hexuronic acid, except for keratan sulfate, where hexuronic acid is replaced by galactose. The core proteins attached to the GAGs are a diverse protein group and range in size from 10 to 500 kDa. The wide variety of protein structure may aid in directing the unique functional roles for each PG family.

The bone matrix contains PG families of several primary structures, including the following:

1. *Hyaluronan/CD44-, chondroitin sulfate–containing PGs* are expressed in several regions of bone. Hyaluronan is expressed in focal regions within periosteum and endosteum and surrounding most of the major bone cell types including osteoblasts, osteoprogenitor cells, osteoclasts, and osteocyte lacunae. CD44 is a cell-surface hyaluronan receptor that may play a role in guiding bone development and has been localized to osteoclasts, osteocytes, and bone marrow cells.[6] Versican, a chondroitin sulfate–containing PG, may be enriched during early osteoid formation and may provide a temporary framework in newly formed cartilage matrix during bone development.[7] Results from a mouse model carrying a disrupted versican gene (the "hdf" transgenic mouse) also suggest that mature versican proteoglycan may be essential for precartilage aggregation.[8]
2. *Heparan sulfate PGs* (HSPGs) are produced by osteoblast and osteoclast lineage cells. These molecules play important roles in cell-cell interactions during bone formation by trapping autocrine and paracrine heparin-binding fibroblast growth factor (FGF) family members, as well as acting as co-receptors with the FGF receptors (FGFRs). Also, other secreted molecules bind HSPGs such as transforming growth factor (TGF)-β (betaglycan) and osteoprotegerin (OPG) (syndecans). The bioactivity of these factors is modulated by HSPGs, potentially through focusing concentrations of these potent molecules near differentiating cells.
3. *Small leucine-rich PGs* (SLRPs) are the most abundant of the PGs in bone matrix and include decorin, biglycan, fibromodulin, lumican, and osteoadherin. Their core proteins may form a horseshoe structure to assist interactions with collagen and the mineral components of bone during calcification. These molecules help to provide structural organization of the bone matrix and interact with specific growth factors to increase factor concentration and bioactivity in the matrix (Fig. 9.4). The localization of these proteins in mature bone varies because decorin may localize with specific matrix areas, and biglycan is evenly distributed throughout the matrix. Decorin-null animals have alterations in collagen fibril size and bone shape,[9] whereas biglycan-null animals demonstrated reduced bone mass due to lower osteoblast numbers and also demonstrated reduced numbers of osteoclasts.[10] The biglycan-null animals also have reduced ability to respond to TGF-β in concert with reduced collagen synthesis. SLRPs play an essential role in the regulation of growth factor activity. In this regard, decorin, biglycan, and fibromodulin all possess the ability to bind to TGF-β; however, decorin is the best-characterized of these proteins for the ability to bind this factor. Decorin enhances TGF-β binding with its cognate receptors and enhances its bioactivity, and in concert, may act to sequester TGF-β in the collagen fibrils, thus reducing its activity. TGF-β activity is associated with increased apoptosis of osteoprogenitors. Therefore biglycan and decorin appear to be essential for maintaining mature osteoblast numbers through regulating the proliferation and survival of bone marrow progenitor cells.

Osteocalcin

Osteocalcin (OC) is a polypeptide post-translationally modified to carry di-carboxylic glutamyl (Gla) residue, which relies on vitamin K for proper production (other identifiers for OC: bone gamma-carboxyglutamic acid [Gla] protein [BGLAP or BGP]). In humans, vitamin K is primarily a cofactor in the enzymatic reaction that converts glutamate residues into gamma-carboxyglutamate residues in vitamin K–dependent proteins including osteocalcin, but also in proteins involved in blood clotting such as factor IX. These Gla-containing motifs are thought to enhance calcium binding, which may function to control mineral deposition and bone remodeling. Of note, OC from porcine bone has been crystallized, and this analysis revealed that OC maintains a negatively charged protein surface that has arranged five calcium ions in an orientation spatially complementary to calcium ions in a hydroxyapatite crystal lattice.[11] The interaction of OC with synthetic hydroxyapatite *in vitro* depends on the three residues of gamma-carboxyglutamic acid. A nine-residue domain proximal to the amino-terminus of secreted OC shares high homology with the corresponding regions in known propeptides of the gamma-carboxyglutamic acid–containing blood coagulation factors. This common structural feature may be involved in the post-translational targeting of these proteins for gamma-carboxylation.

Osteocalcin may also act as a hormone to regulate the activity of osteoclasts and their precursors. In support of this, the skeleton of the OC-null animal manifests osteopetrosis when compared with wild type littermates. In humans, osteocalcin is expressed largely by osteoblasts and osteocytes, and the measurement of this protein in serum has been used as a marker for bone turnover. Osteocalcin messenger ribonucleic acid (mRNA) is upregulated by vitamin D through interactions with trans-acting factors in vitamin D response elements (VDREs) in the OC promoter.[12] Due to its cell-specific expression, the OC promoter has proven to be invaluable as an active, functional deoxyribonucleic acid (DNA) to drive foreign cDNAs in osteoblasts in transgenic animals.

Osteopontin

Osteopontin (OPN), also referred to as *secreted phosphoprotein-1* (SPP-1), is a member of the "SIBLING" (Small Integrin Binding Ligand N-linked Glycoprotein) family, which is a group of non-collagenous extracellular matrix proteins involved in bone mineralization. The genes for this family are localized to human chromosome 4q21-25, have similar exon arrangements, and also encode dentin matrix protein-1 (DMP1), dentin sialoprotein (DSP), dentin phosphoprotein (DPP), integrin-binding sialoprotein (IBSP), and matrix extracellular phosphoglycoprotein (MEPE). The SIBLING proteins share common structural features such as multiple phosphorylation sites, a highly acidic nature, the presence of an arginine-glycine-aspartic acid (RGD) cell attachment domain, and proteolytic-resistant acidic serine-aspartate-rich MEPE-associated motif (ASARM motif).

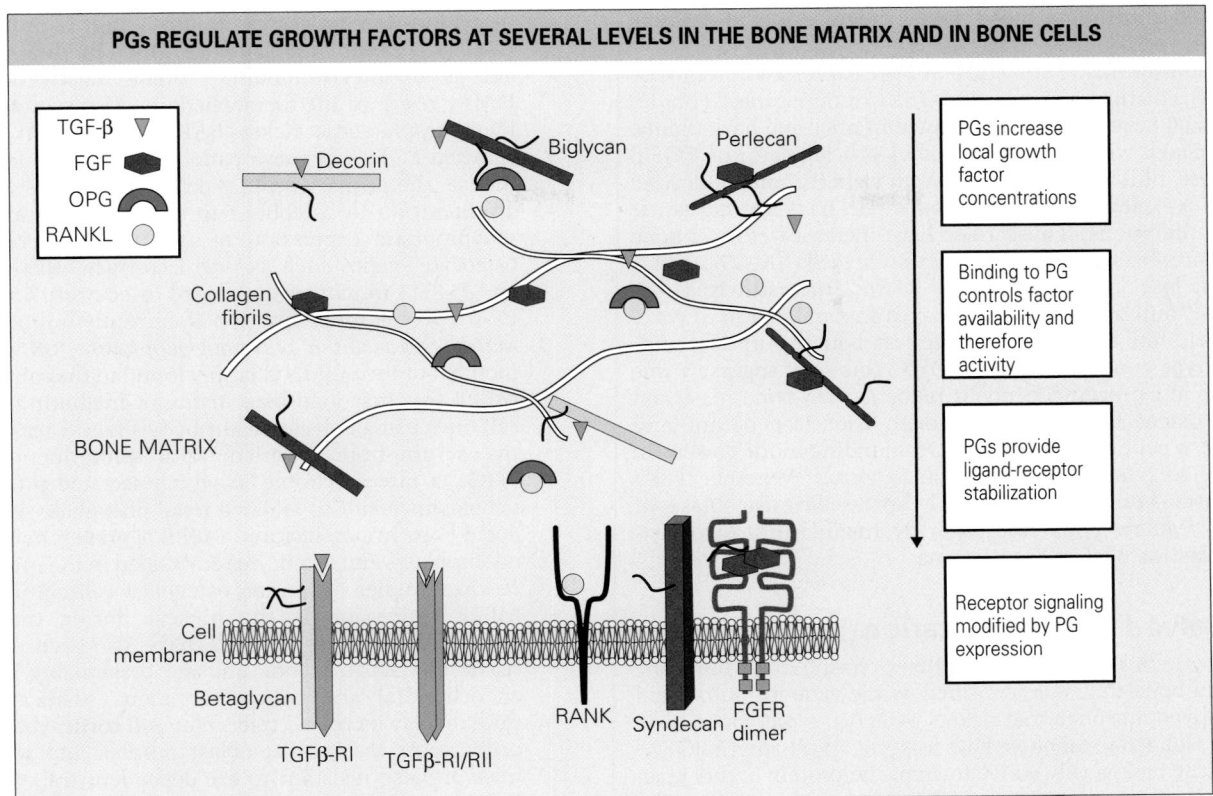

PGs REGULATE GROWTH FACTORS AT SEVERAL LEVELS IN THE BONE MATRIX AND IN BONE CELLS

Fig. 9.4 Proteoglycans (PGs) regulate growth factors at several levels in the bone matrix and in bone cells. These polypeptides trap and locally concentrate endocrine and paracrine growth factors within the matrix. Soluble PGs such as decorin, biglycan, and perlecan also modulate activity through binding, thus controlling the concentrations of bioavailable factor. Membrane-bound PGs such as betaglycan and syndecan modulate ligand-receptor interactions and thus play roles in regulating intracellular signaling. *(Figure adapted from Lamoureux F, Baud'huin M, Duplomb L, et al. Proteoglycans: key partners in bone cell biology. BioEssays 2007;29:758-771.)*

OPN has a high sialic acid content and is produced by osteoblasts under stimulation by calcitriol. The suffix "-pontin" is derived from "pons," the Latin word for bridge, and characterizes the role of osteopontin as a linking protein. In this regard, OPN is expressed within cement lines and may thus act as a promoter of adhesion and allow the arrangement of dissimilar tissues together in biologic composites such as teeth and bone.[13] OPN binds tightly to hydroxyapatite and may be involved in the anchoring of osteoclasts to the mineral of bone matrix. The vitronectin receptor, which has specificity for osteopontin, is focused within the osteoclast plasma membrane in the regions involved in the binding process. OPN-null mice were originally found to have altered wound healing because OPN is also highly expressed in skin. Long bones from OPN-null mice are indistinguishable from those of wild-type littermates by x-ray, but the relative amount of mineral in the more mature areas of the bone (central cortical bone) of the OPN-null mice is significantly increased, as is the mineral maturity (mineral crystal size and perfection) throughout all regions of the bone.[14] *In vitro*, exogenous OPN inhibits pyrophosphate (PP_i)-dependent mineralization of a cultured osteoblast cell line.[15] These findings indicate that OPN is a potent inhibitor of mineral formation, as well as crystal growth and proliferation. OPN is also overexpressed in several cancers and autoimmune disorders and therefore may be a biomarker for these diseases.

Osteonectin

Osteonectin, also referred to as *secreted protein acidic and rich in cysteine*, or SPARC, is a phosphoprotein that is the most abundant non-collagenous polypeptide expressed in bone. The mature protein binds selectively to hydroxyapatite, collagen fibrils, and vitronectin at distinct sites and may allow proper organization of the bone matrix through contacts with the cellular surface. Osteonectin also inhibits cellular proliferation through arrest of cells in the G1 phase of the cell cycle. It may regulate the activity of platelet-derived growth factor

(PDGF), vascular endothelial growth factor (VEGF), and fibroblast growth factor-2 (FGF2). The osteonectin crystal structure has revealed a novel follistatin-like component and an extracellular calcium-binding region. The osteonectin-null mouse develops severe osteopenia, indicating that this gene may have roles in osteoblast proliferation and mineralization.

Alkaline phosphatases

Alkaline phosphatases are widely distributed and are membrane-bound glycoproteins that hydrolyze monophosphate esters.[16] The liver/bone/kidney alkaline phosphatase, referred to as *tissue-non-specific alkaline phosphatase* (encoded by the *ALPL* gene), acts as a lipid-anchored phosphoethanolamine (PEA) and pyridoxal-5-prime-phosphate (PLP) ectophosphatase. Loss of function mutations in the ALPL gene leads to hypophosphatasia, which is characterized by marked defects in bone mineralization and is lethal in the infantile form. The inorganic pyrophosphate (PP_i) produced by cells inhibits mineralization by binding to crystals, and the presence of PP_i may thus prevent the soft tissues from undergoing mineralization. The degradation of PP_i to inorganic phosphate (P_i) by ALPL in bones and teeth may assist crystal growth. Therefore it is thought that loss of function of the ALPL gene in hypophosphatasia results in accumulation of PP_i and reduced skeletal mineralization.

Thrombospondin 1 & 2

The thrombospondins (TSPs) are a family of secreted glycoproteins of high molecular mass. TSP1 and TSP2 share high homology and form 450 kDa homotrimers. Both TSP1 and 2 are expressed by mesenchymal cells and chondrocytes during cartilage formation. As osteoblasts replace the mineralizing cartilage, TSP2 expression decreases in chondrocytes and increases in the matrix within areas undergoing ossification. TSP1 and 2 are strong antiangiogenic factors and therefore may also play a role in controlling blood vessel organization in forming bone.

In the developing animal, TSP1 and TSP2 are expressed in temporal and spatial patterns distinct for each gene. TSP1 (mouse gene: "Thbs1") and TSP2 ("Thbs2") have both been disrupted in mice and have unique phenotypes associated with each gene. Thbs1 is a regulator of TGF-β *in vivo*, and these null animals have lower viability and prolonged wound healing. For skeletal phenotypes, this model has spine curvature and craniofacial alterations. Thbs2 mice have increased cortical bone density, higher numbers of mesenchymal stem cells (MCS), and a resistance to bone loss due to ovariectomy (OVX). Interestingly, osteoblasts from Thbs2-null mice also have delayed mineralization *in vitro*. Because the Thbs2-null mice demonstrate less bone resorption compared with wild-type controls following OVX, this may suggest a role for this molecule in estrogen-dependent reductions in bone mass and in the control of osteoclast function. Although osteoclasts do not bind to TSP1 or TSP2, a peptide encoding a CD36-binding motif present in both TSP1 and TSP2 increases resorption *in vitro*.[17] Whether TSP2 controls osteoclasts is unknown, but TSP2 expressed by osteoblasts or osteoclasts may regulate bone resorption by modulating osteoclast-matrix or osteoclast-osteoblast associations.

Proteins involved in mineralization

1. *Fibroblast growth factor-23 (FGF23)* is a phosphaturic hormone produced in bone that was identified as the gene for autosomal dominant hypophosphatemic rickets (ADHR), a metabolic bone disorder of isolated renal phosphate wasting.[18] Full-length FGF23 (32 kD) is the biologically active form of the protein and is inactivated on cleavage into 20 and 12 kDa protein fragments. The N-terminal region of FGF23 contains the FGF-homology domain, whereas the C-terminus comprises a unique 71-amino acid tail. Intracellular cleavage of FGF23 occurs at a subtilisin-like proprotein convertase (SPC) site ($R_{176}XXR_{179}/S$), which inactivates the protein. The human FGF23 ADHR mutations R176Q, R179Q, and R179W destroy this site and stabilize the full-length active form of the protein. FGF23 acts in the kidney to inhibit phosphate reabsorption through reducing expression of the proximal tubule type I sodium-phosphate co-transporters Npt2a[19] and Npt2c. The subsequent low-serum phosphate results in marked osteomalacia and rickets, fracture, and dental anomalies. Using *in situ* hybridization of adult trabecular bone, FGF23 mRNA was observed in osteocytes and flattened bone-lining cells. In regions of active bone formation, newly formed osteocytes and osteoprogenitor cells also express FGF23.[20] FGF23 is elevated *in vivo* by increased serum phosphate and $1,25(OH)_2$ vitamin D concentrations, and FGF23 then completes the feedback loop by reducing phosphate reabsorption and $1,25(OH)_2$ vitamin D production in the kidney.

   As expected, *Fgf23*-null mice have the reciprocal phenotype to ADHR patients and manifest hyperphosphatemia with elevated $1,25(OH)_2$ vitamin D and often severe ectopic and vascular calcifications due to precipitation of calcium-phosphate crystals. Patients with inactivating mutations in FGF23, or in the FGF23 co-receptor Klotho (KL), have tumoral calcinosis, the human disease correlates to the *Fgf23*-null animal. Whether FGF23 has direct effects on the skeleton is uncertain because KL is predominantly expressed in the kidney and parathyroid glands. However, because FGF23 is produced in bone, FGF23 expression and its actions on serum phosphate concentrations may be coordinated with intraskeletal signals to allow proper bone formation and mineralization.

2. *Dentin matrix protein-1 (DMP1)*, like OPN, is a member of the SIBLING gene family. DMP1 is highly expressed in osteocytes and is composed of 513 residues, but it is secreted in bone and dentin as 37 kD N-terminal (residues 17-253) and 57 kD C-terminal (residues 254-513) fragments from a 94 kD full-length precursor. Recombinant DMP1 binds calcium-phosphate ions and the N-telopeptide region of type 1 collagen with high affinities. Potential roles for DMP1 in bone and teeth may include regulating hydroxyapatite formation and, depending on proteolytic processing and phosphorylation, may regulate local mineralization processes *in vivo*. The C-terminal portion of DMP1 has been implicated in DNA binding, gene regulation, and as an integrin-binding protein. Inactivating mutations in DMP1 result in the metabolic bone disease autosomal recessive hypophosphatemic rickets (ARHR), which is associated with elevated FGF23 in these patients. As shown in the *DMP1*-null mouse, the primary cellular defect due to loss of DMP1 may be an alteration in osteoblast to osteocyte maturation, leading to inappropriate expression of typically "osteoblastic" or "early osteocyte" genes such as type I collagen, alkaline phosphatase, and FGF23 in mature embedded osteocytes. The relationship of DMP1 to cell differentiation is currently unknown.

3. *Matrix extracellular phosphoglycoprotein*, or MEPE, is another member of the SIBLING family found in the mineralizing matrix. MEPE was first identified in tumor medium and osteosarcoma cell lines using polyclonal antibodies raised against the preoperative serum from a patient with tumor-induced osteomalacia (TIO), a rare syndrome in which secreted products of specific neoplasms result in isolated renal phosphate wasting and disordered bone mineralization. MEPE is predominantly expressed in odontoblasts and osteocytes embedded in the mineralized matrix. *In vitro* studies of human osteoblast cell cultures indicate that MEPE expression is the highest during the mineralization phase.[21] High levels of MEPE have also been reported in callus tissue of fractured bone and are presumably involved in both endochondral and intramembranous ossification. *MEPE*-null mice display increased trabecular and cortical bone mass because of increases in both osteoblast number and activity, and these mice are also resistant to age-dependent trabecular bone loss.[22] Taken together, these findings indicate that MEPE likely has a role as an important gene for the negative regulation of skeletal mineralization.

GROWTH FACTORS

Multiple growth factors, either those produced within bone or those that circulate to bone, are critical for skeletal development and function. These factors may be sequestered within bone matrix via the bloodstream or may be produced by the major bone cell types and act as paracrine and autocrine factors.

1. The *insulin-like growth factors* IGF-1 (somatomedin C) and IGF-2 (somatomedin A) are produced primarily in the liver but are also produced in bone. These factors predominantly circulate complexed with binding proteins (IGFBPs) to assist their transport to tissues. IGFBPs can either enhance or inhibit IGF activity. IGF-1 and IGF-2 act through the IGF-1 receptors (IGFR1 and IGFR2) and possess bioactivity that promotes cell proliferation and differentiation.

   The IGF1-null mouse has reduced cortical bone and femur length; however, trabecular density is increased. *In vitro* findings suggest that IGF-1 also increases osteoclastogenesis, and IGF1-null mice have reduced levels of RANKL in osteoblasts isolated from bone marrow. Therefore IGF-1 may regulate osteoclastogenesis through direct and indirect actions. Overexpression of IGF-1 specifically in osteoblasts leads to increased bone mineral density and increased trabecular volume, although osteoblast numbers are not increased.[23] These studies suggest that IGF-1 acts directly on osteoblasts to enhance their function. Specific removal of IGFR1 from osteoblasts results in decreased trabecular number and volume and a dramatic decrease in bone mineralization, further supporting the role of the IGFs on osteoblasts. Less is known regarding the functions of IGF-2 in bone. However, it has been suggested that IGF-2 may be a local regulator of bone cell metabolism.

2. *Bone morphogenetic proteins* (BMPs) are members of the transforming growth factor-β (TGF-β) superfamily. There are now more than 20 BMP-related proteins, which are classified into subgroups on the basis of structure and function. These factors play important roles in skeletal development by directing the fate of mesenchymal cells, through differentiation of these precursor cells into cells of the osteoblastic lineage, and by inhibiting their

differentiation into myoblastic lineage cells. BMPs also increase osteoclastogenesis, which is tightly coordinated with osteoblastogenesis. BMPs activate specific receptors and induce cell signaling by phosphorylating cytoplasmic receptor-regulated Smads, which enter the nucleus to recruit transcription factors and enhance gene expression. The human disorder fibrodysplasia ossificans progressiva (FOP) is a disease of dramatic ectopic bone formation that can be accelerated following blunt trauma. A recurrent mutation in activin receptor IA/activin-like kinase 2 (ACVR1/ALK2), a BMP type I receptor, was reported as the molecular cause of FOP.[24] These findings underscore the potent effects of BMP signaling on bone formation.

3. The *fibroblast growth factor* (FGF) *family* of proteins primarily acts as paracrine and autocrine factors and binds to one or several of four FGF receptors (FGFRs). FGFRs normally exist as an inactivated monomer. With FGF binding in the presence of heparin/heparan sulfate, the FGFRs dimerize, leading to the autophosphorylation of tyrosine residues. The FGF family has potent effects on bone development. This is clearly evident by the fact that activating mutations in FGFR1 and FGFR2 are responsible for disorders of craniosynostosis and limb patterning, and FGFR1 and FGFR3 mutations result in disorders of hypochondroplasia and achondroplasia. The FGFs interact with heparan sulfate PGs (HSPGs) and are sequestered within the mineralizing matrix. In addition, the HSPG syndecan may stabilize FGF-FGFR interactions and promote FGF signaling and bioactivity.

The FGF family members play important roles in bone development and formation. Expression of several FGF ligands including FGF2, FGF5, FGF6, FGF7, and FGF9 has been observed in mesenchyme surrounding initial condensation. In limb buds, FGFR1 and FGFR2 are expressed in condensing mesenchyme. In rat growth plates, mRNAs encoding all four FGFRs and FGF2 can be detected, and FGF2 is also present in osteoblasts. FGF2 treatment of osteoblasts enhances the binding of Runx2 to the Cbfa1 consensus sequence in the osteocalcin promoter and may therefore have a role in differentiation. Transgenic animals have been important for understanding FGF function in bone. Fgf18-null mice show alterations in both endochondral and intramembranous bone. Interestingly, these mice have expanded zones of proliferating and hypertrophic chondrocytes, a similar phenotype to that of Fgfr3-null mice.

4. *Transforming growth factor-β* (TGFβ) controls proliferation, differentiation, and other functions in many cell types. TGF β-1, TGF β-2, and TGF β-3 all function through the type I and type II TGF receptors. The TGFBR1 forms a heterodimer with the TGFBR2 receptor. TGF-β stimulation leads to activation of Smad2 and Smad3, which form complexes with Smad4 that accumulate in the nucleus and regulate the transcription of target genes.

TGF β-1 is the most abundant growth factor in human bone, is localized within the bone matrix, and has functions both during embryonic development and in mature bone. During embryonic development, TGF β-1 plays a role in cell migration, controlling epithelial-mesenchymal interactions, and the formation of cellular condensations, which influence bone shape. This factor also plays a key role in inducing mesenchymal cell differentiation to either chondrocytes or osteoblasts. In adult bone, TGF β-1 controls osteoblast differentiation, which affects matrix formation and mineralization. TGF β-1 inhibits the expression of the differentiation markers Runx2 and osteocalcin in osteoblast cell lines, and its functions interplay with other systems in bone such as the PTH and the Wnt-beta-catenin systems. The relevance of signaling induced by growth factors for osteoblast survival is underscored by decreased bone mass and increased osteoblast apoptosis in mice lacking Smad-3, which mediates TGF β-signaling, and by high bone mass in mice lacking PTEN, the phosphatase that causes osteoblast apoptosis by inactivating the PI3Kinase/IGF survival pathway.

The skeletal disorder Camurati-Engelmann disease (CED) highlights the importance of TGF β1 in skeletal formation. CED is a progressive diaphyseal dysplasia characterized by hyperostosis and sclerosis of the diaphyses of the long bones. The TGF β1 gene was screened and three different heterozygous missense mutations were found in exon 4 in the nine families examined. All of the mutations in the CED patients were located either at (C225) or near (R218), suggesting the importance of this region in activating TGF β-1 in the bone matrix.

5. *Platelet-derived growth factor and vascular-endothelial growth factor* (PDGF and VEGF) are dimers of disulfide-linked polypeptide chains, encoded by nine different genes that direct production of four different PDGF chains (PDGF-A, PDGF-B, PDGF-C, and PDGF-D) and five different VEGF chains (VEGF-A, VEGF-B, VEGF-C, VEGF-D; and placenta growth factor, PIGF). All members of these families carry a growth factor core domain, which is necessary for receptor activation. PDGFs mediate their bioactivity through two receptors, PDGFR-α and PDGFR-β. These receptors both have five extracellular immunoglobulin (Ig) loops for ligand binding and an intracellular tyrosine kinase domain. The VEGFs act through a homologous family of receptors, VEGFRs 1, 2, and 3. PDGFs act primarily as paracrine growth factors.

PDGF is chemotactic and mitogenic for osteoblasts and osteoprogenitor cells, and it upregulates cytokines that are crucial to bone healing. This factor also destabilizes blood vessels during healing to allow sprouting of new vessels. PDGFR-α-null mice develop skeletal abnormalities, including defective vertebral neural arch formation, which results in spina bifida. VEGF is produced by many cell types including fibroblasts, hypertrophic chondrocytes, and osteoblasts. VEGF may act not only in bone angiogenesis and vascular differentiation but also in aspects of development such as chondrocyte and osteoblast differentiation, as well as osteoclast recruitment.

BONE CELLS

Osteoclasts

Osteoclasts are the primary bone-resorptive cells. They are necessary for bone modeling, which leads to changes of the shape of bones, and for bone remodeling, which maintains the integrity of the adult skeleton. Osteoclasts originate from precursors of the monocyte/macrophage family of the hematopoietic lineage that differentiate to multinucleated cells on stimulation with receptor activator of NFκB ligand (RANKL) and macrophage-colony stimulating factor (M-CSF). On completing bone resorption, all osteoclasts undergo programmed cell death or apoptosis and disappear from the bone surface.

Osteoclast function

Osteoclasts have the capacity to adhere firmly to bone by the interaction of osteoclast integrins with bone matrix. Integrins belong to a large family of transmembrane proteins that function as heterodimers of α and β subunits. Several integrins are expressed in osteoclasts and bind to collagen, fibronectin, and other proteins present in the extracellular environment. The expression of integrins αV and β3 is induced by the osteoclastogenic cytokine RANKL during osteoclast differentiation. The αV/β3 dimer recognizes the amino acid sequence Arg-Gly-Asp (RGD) present in osteopontin and bone sialoprotein. Attachment of osteoclasts to the bone surface depends on binding to RGD-containing proteins, as demonstrated by the evidence that competitive RGD ligands block bone resorption.[25] The importance of αV/β3 in bone resorption is underscored by evidence that mice null for integrin β3 develop a progressive increase in bone mass due to osteoclast dysfunction.

The integrin-mediated intimate contact between the osteoclast membrane and the bone matrix creates a space between the osteoclast and the matrix called the "sealing zone." There is also polarization of the osteoclast fibrillar actin into a circular structure called the "actin ring," containing podosomes composed of an actin core surrounded by αV/β3 integrins and associated cytoskeletal and signaling proteins. Thus the area in which the osteoclast apposes the bone is isolated from the general extracellular space and becomes acidified by the activity of a proton pump and a chloride channel.[25] The low pH leads to dissolution of the mineral and exposure of the organic matrix of bone. The matrix, largely consisting of type I collagen, is subsequently degraded by the activity of cathepsin K, an enzyme present in the osteoclast lysosomes, as well as by matrix metalloproteases. These degrading enzymes are transported into acidified vesicles that fuse with the osteoclast plasmalemma forming a villous structure referred to as the *ruffled membrane*. This structure and the actin ring are *sine qua non* features of a resorbing osteoclast, and abnormalities of either structure lead to arrested bone resorption. For example, osteoclasts in β3 null mice exhibit abnormal actin rings and ruffled membranes, fail to spread, and generate fewer and shallower resorptive lacunae on dentin slices than wild-type osteoclasts.

The cytoplasmic domains of integrins serve as platforms for signaling proteins involved in osteoclast function such as the kinase Src, which is crucial for osteoclast attachment and resorption. Src regulates the disassembly of podosomes and the formation of the ruffled membrane, at least in part by its ability to interact with the focal adhesion–related kinase Pyk2 and the proto-oncogene c-Cbl. Rho, Rac, and the guanine nucleotide exchange factor that activates GDPases into GTPases, Vav3, also play a central role in modifying the resorptive capacity of osteoclasts by modulating actin cytoskeleton remodeling.

Products of osteoclast resorption are transported in vesicles through the cytosol to the basolateral surface and are discharged to the extracellular milieu, or directly released to the surrounding fluid after osteoclast retraction from the resorptive pits.

Osteoclast formation and differentiation

Mature, multinucleated osteoclasts are formed by fusion of mononuclear precursors of the monocyte-macrophage lineage. The earliest recognized precursor of the osteoclast is the colony-forming unit, granulocyte-macrophage (CFU-GM), which also gives rise to granulocytes and monocytes. Osteoclast precursors proliferate in response to growth factors such as IL-3 and colony-stimulating factors (CSFs) such as GM-CSF and M-CSF to form postmitotic, committed osteoclast precursors. These committed mononucleated preosteoclasts differentiate and fuse to form multinucleated osteoclasts under the influence of RANKL, a member of the TNF family of ligands. RANKL is produced as a membrane-associated protein or in a soluble form. RANKL is expressed in different cell types including cells of the osteoblastic lineage, as well as T lymphocytes. Expression of RANKL on the surface of osteoblastic cells facilitates osteoclastogenesis via cell-to-cell contact with osteoclast precursors, which express RANK. RANKL expression is upregulated by hormones and cytokines known to induce osteoclast generation. This explains the long-observed property of primary osteoblastic cells or osteoblastic cell lines that, upon treatment with vitamin D, PTH, or interleukin (IL)-11, IL-6, and IL-1, support osteoclast development when co-cultured with osteoclast precursors derived from spleen or bone marrow. RANKL mediates several aspects of osteoclast differentiation, including fusion of mononucleated precursors into multinucleated cells, acquisition of osteoclast specific markers, attachment of osteoclasts to the bone surfaces, stimulation of resorption, and promotion of osteoclast survival. Although M-CSF contributes to RANKL effects, RANKL appears to play a dominant role in bone resorption. Thus whereas M-CSF null mice recover with time from the decreased osteoclast number and activity, RANKL knockout mice do not. Furthermore, RANKL appears to stimulate osteoclast formation and resorption in mice even in the absence of functional M-CSF.[26]

Binding of RANKL (either the membrane-bound or the soluble form) to the trimeric RANK complex expressed in osteoclast precursors leads to activation of several signal transduction pathways involving the recruitment of the adapter protein TRAF6 (TNF receptor associated factor 6) to the intracellular domain of RANK. TRAF6 activates kinase-dependent signaling and transcription factors. Among them, the nuclear factor-κB (NF-KB) has been shown to undergo nuclear translocation leading to upregulation of c-Fos. Fos, in turn, binds to nuclear factor of activated T cells-c1 (NFATc1) and upregulates genes crucial for osteoclast differentiation and function. Although other signaling pathways are activated by RANKL in osteoclasts, the evidence that deletion of NF-KB, c-fos/AP1, and NFATc1 leads to osteoclast dysfunction demonstrates the crucial role of these genes in osteoclasts.[26]

Osteoprotegerin (OPG) is an inhibitor of RANK activation and osteoclastogenesis. Like RANK, OPG is a member of the TNF family of receptors. However, unlike RANK or other members of this family of receptors, OPG is a secreted protein with no transmembrane domain and, therefore, it has no direct signaling capabilities. OPG suppresses osteoclast formation and resorption by binding to its natural ligand RANKL, thereby impeding RANKL interaction with RANK and inhibiting osteoclast differentiation.

Osteoclast differentiation by activating the RANK/RANKL pathway induces the expression of genes required for osteoclast function. Failure of osteoclasts to properly form or function leads to development of osteopetrosis in mice or humans. Mutations in the TCIRG1 gene, which encodes for the a3 subunit of the H+ATPase of the proton pump, accounts for more than 50% of osteopetrosis in humans.

Osteoclast apoptosis

After completing bone resorption, osteoclasts undergo apoptosis and disappear from the bone surface. The types of signals that trigger apoptosis of osteoclasts *in vivo* are not completely understood. High concentrations of extracellular calcium, like the ones present in resorption cavities, induce osteoclast apoptosis *in vitro* and may be the triggering event. Fas ligand stimulates osteoclast apoptosis and Fas-deficient mice exhibit more osteoclasts and decreased bone mass, suggesting that activation of this pathway may also be involved in the control of osteoclast life span *in vivo*.

Alternatively, osteoclast apoptosis might result from loss of survival signals. Indeed, detachment of osteoclasts *in vitro* induces apoptosis, suggesting that changes in integrin expression in osteoclasts on completion of the resorption phase might render osteoclasts more susceptible to apoptosis. However, osteoclast detachment is not sufficient to induce apoptosis, as demonstrated by the induction of detachment and inhibition of resorption induced by calcitonin.

Decreased production of prosurvival cytokines or growth factors in the extracellular milieu surrounding osteoclasts may also lead to osteoclast apoptosis. Potential antiapoptotic factors are M-CSF and RANKL, the same cytokines that induce osteoclast differentiation. TNFα and IL-1 also delay osteoclast apoptosis. All these cytokines activate the extracellular signal-regulated kinases (ERKs), and this activation is crucial for osteoclast survival as demonstrated by using an ERK-specific inhibitor. Another kinase with antiapoptotic effects in several cell types, phosphatidylinositol 3-kinase (PI3K), is also required for survival. PI3K might promote survival by activating the downstream kinase Akt. However, knock-down experiments using short-hairpin RNAs (shRNAs) to reduce Akt expression revealed that Akt is required for osteoclast differentiation but not for survival. Mammalian target of rapamycin (mTOR) is another target of PI3K and is required for the antiapoptotic actions of M-CSF, RANKL, and TNFα in osteoclasts. Because mTOR is also activated by ERKs, it appears to be a point of convergence in the action of prosurvival kinases in osteoclasts.

RANKL, TNFα, and IL-1 also activate NFκB in osteoclasts, and this transcription factor has been shown to inhibit apoptosis in various cell types. In osteoclasts, downregulation of NFκB mRNA inhibits IL-1-dependent survival and blockade of NFκB binding to DNA with specific oligonucleotides induces apoptosis. However, osteoclast precursors lacking NFκB subunits have normal survival rate and inhibition of NFκB activation via a dominant-negative IKK2 did not affect the ability of IL-1 to promote osteoclast survival. Therefore the relevance of NFκB signaling for osteoclast survival is still controversial.

Regulation of osteoclast generation and survival

In the bone remodeling unit (BMU), the rate of osteoclast generation determines the extension of the BMU, whereas the life span of osteoclasts determines the depth of resorption. Whereas both genesis and apoptosis of osteoclasts lead to changes in osteoclast number and bone resorption, alteration of osteoclast life span might represent a more effective mechanism to accomplish rapid changes in bone resorption rate. Several factors regulate osteoclast formation and activity, as well as osteoclast survival.

Sex steroids have profound effects on osteoclasts. Both estrogens and androgens inhibit osteoclast generation by regulating the production of pro-osteoclastogenic cytokines (such as IL-6 and IL-1) by cells of the stromal/osteoblastic lineage. This, together with an inhibitory effect of the hormones on osteoblast generation, leads to attenuation of the rate of bone remodeling. As in the case of sex steroids, glucocorticoids exert opposite effects on the life span of osteoclasts and osteoblasts. In mice receiving excess glucocorticoids, osteoclast progenitors are reduced, but the cancellous osteoclast number does not decrease because glucocorticoids prolong osteoclast life span. This effect may account for the early transient increase in bone resorption in patients with exogenous or endogenous hyperglucocorticoidism. The prosurvival effect of glucocorticoids on osteoclasts is powerful enough to antagonize the proapoptotic effect of bisphosphonates. The antiapoptotic actions of glucocorticoids on osteoclasts are absent in transgenic mice in which the enzyme 11β-HSD2, which inactivates glucocorticoids, is overexpressed, confirming that the steroids act directly on osteoclasts to prolong their life span. In contrast to the rapid prosurvival effect of glucocorticoids on mature osteoclasts, glucocorticoids induce a decrease in osteoclast formation. This effect is likely a consequence of a reduction in the pool of osteoblastic cells that support osteoclastogenesis and leads to the typical low remodeling rate observed in this condition.

Osteoblasts

Osteoblasts are the cells responsible for bone formation. They originate from mesenchymal progenitors, which also give rise to chondrocytes, muscle cells, and adipocytes. Commitment of mesenchymal cells to the osteoblastic lineage depends on the specific activation of transcription factors induced by morphogenetic and developmental proteins that carry out the functions of bone matrix protein secretion and bone mineralization. On completion of bone matrix formation, some mature osteoblasts remain entrapped in bone as osteocytes, some flatten to cover quiescent bone surfaces as bone lining cells, and most die by apoptosis.

Osteoblast function

The main function of osteoblasts is to synthesize bone matrix. Mature osteoblasts actively engaged in this process are recognized by their location on the bone surface and by their morphologic features typical of cells secreting high levels of proteins: cuboidal cells with large nucleus, enlarged Golgi apparatus, and extensive endoplasmic reticulum. Osteoblasts express high levels of alkaline phosphatase and osteocalcin, and the level of expression of these proteins in the circulation reflects the rate of bone formation. Osteoblasts secrete abundant collagen type I and other specialized matrix proteins, which form osteoid. This organic phase of bone serves as a template for the subsequent deposit of mineral in the form of hydroxylapatite.

Interaction of osteoblasts among themselves, with lining cells, and with bone marrow cells are established by adhesion junctions, tight junctions, and gap junctions. Adherens junctions, mainly mediated by cadherins, together with tight junctions serve to join cells and assist their anchorage to the extracellular matrix through the cytoskeleton. Changes in the expression level of the major cadherins expressed in osteoblasts, N-cadherin and cadherin 11, influence osteoblast differentiation and survival. Intercellular communication among osteoblasts and neighboring cells is maintained by cell coupling via gap junctions. Opening of gap junction channels contributes to coupling and the coordination of responses within a cell population. The major gap junction protein expressed in bone cells, and in particular in cells of the osteoblastic lineage, is connexin 43. Its absence or dysfunction leads to impaired osteoblast differentiation, premature apoptosis, and deficient response to hormones and pharmacotherapeutic agents.[27] Furthermore, gap junction communication is fundamental for the maintenance of a continuum from bone, where osteocytes reside, through bone surface cells osteoblasts and osteoclasts, bone marrow cells, and endothelial cells of the blood vessels.[28] This functional syncytium might be responsible for the coordinated response of the bone tissue to changes in physical and chemical stimuli.

Interactions between osteoblasts and the bone matrix via integrins also modulate osteoblast differentiation, function, and survival. In particular, loss of antiapoptotic signals provided by the extracellular matrix causes apoptosis, a phenomenon referred to as anoikis. Thus neutralizing antibodies to the matrix protein fibronectin induce osteoblast apoptosis,[29] and transgenic mice expressing collagenase-resistant collagen type I exhibit increased prevalence of osteoblast and osteocyte apoptosis compared with age-matched wild-type controls.[30] Collectively, this evidence supports the notion that interactions between intact or cryptic sites of matrix proteins with integrins results in "outside-in" signaling that preserves viability.

Osteoblast formation and differentiation

Osteoblast growth and differentiation is governed by an array of transcription factors, resulting in the temporal expression of proteins involved in bone matrix production and matrix mineralization. The entire process can be divided into steps comprising proliferation, extracellular matrix development and maturation, mineralization, and apoptosis. Each stage is characterized by activation of specific transcription factors and genes leading to a succession of osteoblast phenotypic markers. Thus transcription factors of the helix-loop-helix family (Id, Twist, and Dermo) are expressed in proliferating osteoblast progenitors and are responsible for maintaining the osteoprogenitor population by inhibiting the expression of genes that characterize the osteoblast mature phenotype. Transcription factors of the activating protein (AP) family such as c-fos, c-jun, and junD are expressed during proliferation, as well as later in the differentiation pathway, and may activate or repress transcription. Runx2 and osterix are essential for establishing the osteoblast phenotype. Their absence from the mouse genome results in lack of skeletal mineralization and perinatal lethality. Runx2 is expressed earlier than osterix, but both genes regulate the expression of other genes that control bone formation and remodeling including osteocalcin, osteopontin, collagenase 3, osteoprotegerin, and RANKL. Runx2 regulates osteoblast differentiation and function by several signaling pathways, including those activated by Wnts and BMPs, as well as the differentiation and survival of osteoblasts induced by integrins and the PTH receptor.

Osteoblast apoptosis

It is estimated that on completing the process of bone formation, 60% to 70% of osteoblasts die by apoptosis, whereas the remainder become lining cells or osteocytes. Apoptosis appears to begin at the early stages of osteoblast differentiation and continues throughout all stages of osteoblast life. Thus apoptotic mesenchymal progenitors have been found in primary spongiosa of developing long bones of chicks and rabbits and murine calvarial bone, at sites of fracture healing, and in forming bone during distraction osteogenesis.[31] The prevalence of osteoblast apoptosis varies significantly depending on the method used to detect the DNA strand breaks. It has been shown to be as low as 0.5% to 1% in vertebral cancellous bone of adult mice when analyzed with the terminal deoxynucleotidyl transferase enzyme[32] and as high as 10% when using the more sensitive Klenow enzyme.[33]

Apoptosis of cultured osteoblasts has been extensively studied using several methods including increased activity of initiator or effector caspases, presence of cleaved genomic DNA by TUNEL or ISEL, and nuclear fragmentation and chromatin condensation using fluorescent dyes that bind to DNA. Examination of nuclear morphology of cells transfected with fluorescent proteins containing a nuclear localization sequence has proven a particularly useful tool for studying apoptosis in cells co-transfected with genes of interest. Cell detachment from the substrate, changes in the composition of the plasma membrane, and changes revealing cell shrinkage are also features that have been used to detect and quantify apoptotic cells.

Regulation of osteoblast generation and apoptosis

Most major regulators of skeletal homeostasis influence both generation and survival of osteoblasts.

The two major signaling pathways that promote osteoblast differentiation are the ones activated by the bone morphogenetic proteins (BMPs) and Wnts. BMPs play an important role in osteoblast differentiation and also induce apoptosis of mesenchymal osteoblast progenitors in interdigital tissues during the development of hands and feet and of mature osteoblasts. Wnt signaling has a profound effect on bone as shown by the high bone mass phenotype of mice and humans with activating mutations of low-density lipoprotein receptor-related protein 5 (LRP5), which together with Frizzled proteins are receptors for Wnt ligands. Wnts stimulate differentiation of undifferentiated mesenchymal cells toward the osteoblastic lineage and stimulate differentiation of preosteoblasts. Remarkably, Wnt signaling in osteoblasts also affects osteoclasts. Thus canonical Wnt signaling in osteoblastic cells increases expression of the RANKL decoy receptor OPG leading to inhibition of osteoclast development. In addition, Wnt signaling inhibits apoptosis of mature osteoblasts and osteocytes.[34] The increased bone formation exhibited by mice lacking the Wnt antagonist secreted frizzled-related protein-1 (SFRP-1) is associated with decreased osteoblast and osteocyte apoptosis. Likewise, the prevalence of osteoblast and osteocyte apoptosis is decreased in mice expressing the high bone mass activating mutation of LRP5 (G171V). This LRP5 mutant exhibits reduced ability to bind sclerostin—a Wnt antagonist specifically secreted by osteocytes. Consistent with this, sclerostin induces osteoblast apoptosis *in vitro*. Moreover, the ability of PTH and mechanical loading to reduce sclerostin synthesis could contribute to their ability to stimulate osteoblast differentiation and prolong osteoblast life span.[35,36] Activation of Wnt signaling *in vitro* also prevents apoptosis of uncommitted C2C12 osteoblast progenitors and more differentiated MC3T3-E1 and OB-6 osteoblastic cell models. Remarkably, Wnt ligands known to activate the so-called canonical and non-canonical pathways prevent apoptosis of osteoblastic cells by a mechanism that involves the Src/ERK and PI3/AKT prosurvival kinases.

Glucocorticoids (GC) induce rapid bone loss resulting from a transient increase in resorption caused by delayed osteoclast apoptosis. This initial phase is followed by sustained and profound reduction in bone formation and turnover due to decreased osteoblast and osteoclast generation and increased osteoblast apoptosis.

Both chronic excess of parathyroid hormone (PTH), as in hyperparathyroidism, and intermittent elevation of PTH (by daily injections) increase the number of osteoblasts. However, whereas the former condition can lead to bone catabolism, intermittent administration of PTH causes bone anabolism. In both situations, the rate of bone turnover is increased due to simultaneous increase in osteoclast and osteoblast number and a delay in osteoblast apoptosis. However, intermittently administered PTH also causes *de novo* bone formation not coupled to previous resorption. This occurs early, creating the so-called "anabolic window." Additionally, PTH causes an overfilling of erosion pits, creating net bone formation.

The increase in the number of osteoblasts can be achieved by only two mechanisms: an increase in the rate of their production from progenitors or a decrease in the rate of their death by apoptosis, or a combination of the two. Studies in mice indicate that chronic and intermittent PTH increase osteoblast number by different mechanisms. Thus, whereas the increase in osteoblast number and the anabolic effect of intermittent PTH can be accounted for by attenuation of osteoblast apoptosis,[37] chronic elevation of the endogenous hormone resulting from dietary calcium deficiency, or continuous infusion of exogenous PTH, has no effect on osteoblast survival.[37] Therefore, increased osteoblasts with chronic elevation of PTH must result from increased osteoblast generation.

Osteocytes

Osteocytes are former osteoblasts that become entombed during the process of bone deposition and are regularly distributed throughout the mineralized bone matrix. Osteocyte bodies are individually encased in lacunae and exhibit cytoplasmic dendritic processes that run along narrow canaliculi excavated in the mineralized matrix. Osteocytes communicate with each other, with cells on the bone surface, as well as with cells of the bone marrow through gap junctions established between cytoplasmic processes of neighboring cells.

Today, it is accepted that osteocytes are the mechanosensory cells. Osteoblasts and osteoclasts are present on bone only transiently, in low number, and in variable locations. On the other hand, osteocytes are the most abundant resident cells and are present in the entire bone volume. Osteocytes are also the core of a functional syncytium that extends from the mineralized bone matrix to the bone surface and the bone marrow, and all the way to the blood vessels. This strategic location permits the detection of variations in mechanical signals (either through strain or fluid flow), as well as in levels of circulating factors (e.g. Ca^{++}), and allows amplification of the signals leading to adaptive responses.

Osteocyte apoptosis: consequences and regulation

Osteocytes are long-lived cells. However, like osteoblasts and osteoclasts, osteocytes die by apoptosis and decreased osteocyte viability

accompanies the bone fragility syndromes that characterize glucocorticoid excess, estrogen withdrawal, and mechanical disuse.[31] Conversely, preservation of osteocyte viability might explain at least part of the antifracture effects of bisphosphonates, which cannot be completely accounted for by changes in bone mineral density.[33]

Preservation of osteocyte viability by mechanical stimuli

Osteocytes interact with the extracellular matrix in the pericellular space through discrete sites in their membranes, which are enriched in integrins and vinculin, as well as through transverse elements that tether osteocytes to the canalicular wall. Fluid movement in the canaliculi resulting from mechanical loading might induce ECM deformation, shear stress, and/or tension in the tethering elements. The resulting changes in circumferential strain in osteocyte membranes are hypothesized to be converted into intracellular signals by integrin clustering and integrin interaction with cytoskeletal and catalytic proteins at focal adhesions. Physiologic levels of mechanical strain imparted by stretching or pulsatile fluid flow prevent apoptosis of cultured osteocytes. Mechanistic studies indicate that the transduction of mechanical forces into intracellular signals is accomplished by molecular complexes assembled at caveolin-rich domains of the plasma membrane and composed of integrins, cytoskeletal proteins, and kinases including the focal adhesion kinase FAK and Src, resulting in activation of the ERK pathway and osteocyte survival. Intriguingly, a ligand-independent function of the estrogen receptor (ER) is indispensable for mechanically induced ERK activation in both osteoblasts and osteocytes. This observation is consistent with reports that mice lacking the ERα and ERβ exhibit a poor osteogenic response to loading.

In vivo mechanical forces also regulate osteocyte life span. Apoptotic osteocytes are found in unloaded bones or in bones exposed to high levels of mechanical strain. In both cases, increased apoptosis of osteocytes was observed before any evidence of increased osteoclast resorption and accumulated in areas that were subsequently removed by osteoclasts. These findings suggest that dying osteocytes in turn become the beacons for osteoclast recruitment to the vicinity and the resulting increase in bone resorption. In support of this notion, targeted ablation of osteocytes in transgenic mice is sufficient to induce osteoclast recruitment and resorption leading to bone loss.[38] Whether living osteocytes continually produce molecules that restrain osteoclast recruitment or whether in the process of undergoing apoptosis osteocytes produce pro-osteoclastogenic signals remains to be determined. Taken together with the evidence that osteocyte apoptosis is inhibited by estrogens and bisphosphonates,[33,39] these findings raise the possibility that preservation of osteocyte viability contributes to the antiremodeling properties of these agents.

Aging and osteocyte apoptosis

One of the purported functions of the osteocyte network is to detect microdamage and trigger its repair. During aging, there is an accumulation of microdamage and a decline in osteocyte density accompanied by decreased prevalence of osteocyte-occupied lacunae, an index of premature osteocyte death. In view of the evidence discussed earlier on the role of osteocytes in microfracture repair, age-related loss of osteocytes due to apoptosis could be partially responsible for the disparity between bone quantity and quality that occurs with aging. The decline in physical activity with old age could stimulate apoptosis of osteoblasts and osteocytes due to reduced skeletal loading.

Hormonal regulation of osteocyte life span

Estrogen and androgen deficiency lead to increased prevalence of osteocyte apoptosis. Conversely, estrogens and androgens inhibit apoptosis of osteocytes and osteoblasts.[39] This antiapoptotic effect is due to rapid activation of the Src/Shc/ERK signaling pathway through nongenotropic actions of the classical receptors for sex steroids. This effect requires only the ligand-binding domain of the receptor, and unlike the classical genotropic action of the receptor protein, it is eliminated by nuclear targeting.

Increased glucocorticoid activity in bone may also contribute to induction of osteocyte (and osteoblast) apoptosis, as aged mice exhibit higher levels of serum corticosterone, elevated adrenal weight, and increased expression in bone of 11β-hydroxysteroid dehydrogenase type

1 (11β-HSD1), the enzyme that amplifies glucocorticoid action. The apoptotic effect of glucocorticoids is reproduced in cultured osteocytes and osteoblasts in a manner strictly dependent on the glucocorticoid receptor (GR).[31] Induction of osteocyte and osteoblast apoptosis by glucocorticoids can result from the direct action of the steroids because overexpression of the enzyme that inactivates glucocorticoids 11β-HSD2 specifically in these cells abolishes the increase in apoptosis. Strikingly, in osteocytic MLO-Y4 cells the proapoptotic effect of glucocorticoids is preceded by cell detachment due to interference with FAK-mediated survival signaling generated by integrins. In this mechanism, Pyk2 (a member of the FAK family) becomes phosphorylated and subsequently activates proapoptotic JNK signaling. In addition, the proapoptotic actions of glucocorticoids may involve suppression of the synthesis of locally produced antiapoptotic factors including IGF-I and IL-6 type cytokines, as well as MMPs, and stimulation of the proapoptotic Wnt antagonist SFRP-1.

Regulation of bone formation by osteocytes: the sclerostin paradigm

Osteocytes, but no other cells in bone, express sclerostin—the product of the Sost gene. Sclerostin antagonizes several members of the BMP family of proteins and also binds to LRP5/LRP6, preventing canonical Wnt signaling. Loss of Sost in humans causes the high bone mass disorders Van Buchem disease and sclerosteosis. In addition, administration of an antisclerostin antibody increases bone formation and restores the bone lost on ovariectomy in rodents. Conversely, transgenic mice overexpressing Sost exhibit low bone mass.[40] Taken together, these lines of evidence have led to the conclusion that sclerostin derived from osteocytes—the ultimate progeny of the osteoblast differentiation pathway—exerts a negative feedback control at the earliest step of mesenchymal stem cell differentiation toward the osteoblast lineage.

Osteocytes and the skeletal actions of PTH

Recent evidence demonstrates that elevation of PTH dramatically downregulates the expression of the osteocyte-derived Wnt antagonist Sost and its product the protein sclerostin in vivo and in vitro.[35] Together with evidence of the relevance of Wnt signaling for osteoblast function, these findings suggest that the increase in osteoblasts and bone formation induced by chronic elevation of PTH could result from direct actions of the hormone on osteocytes leading to decreased sclerostin and increased Wnt signaling. Consistent with this hypothesis, transgenic mice expressing a constitutively active PTH receptor 1 exclusively in osteocytes (DMP1-caPTHR1 mice)[41] exhibit reduced sclerostin expression, increased Wnt signaling, and a dramatic increase in bone mass. Importantly, the high bone mass of the DMP1-caPTHR1 mice is ameliorated by deletion of the Wnt co-receptor LRP5. DMP1-caPTHR1 mice also exhibit increased remodeling, which has been previously attributed to PTH actions on stromal/osteoblastic cells. Taken together, these findings reveal that osteocytes can mediate two of the recognized skeletal effects of PTH: to increase osteoblast number and bone mass and to increase bone remodeling.

GROWTH, MODELING, REMODELING, AND REPAIR

There are four dynamic processes involved in skeletal development and adaptation, and these are defined in specific ways by the relationship of bone resorption and bone formation to each other (Table 9.1). These general mechanisms include a coordinated system that first involves the activation (A) of cell populations, followed by the resorption (R) of preexisting tissue and/or the formation (F) of new or replacement tissue. Bone growth serves to increase bone mass through bone formation (F). Resorption of tissues is not part of the growth process, and the function of growth is only to increase mass, not to adapt the developing structure to its mechanical needs. Growth can occur on a substrate but may involve ossification directly from fibrous tissue (intramembranous bone formation) or by forming a model with cartilage first, and then replacing the cartilage with bone (endochondral

TABLE 9.1 DYNAMIC PROCESSES OF SKELETAL DEVELOPMENT AND ADAPTATION

Process	Mechanism	Morphology	Function
Growth	F	Woven, lamellar	Increased mass
Modeling	A-F	Primary lamellar	Net increased mass
			or
			Adapt architecture
	A-R	Controls drift and curvature	
Remodeling	A-R-F	Secondary lamellar	Bone maintenance
		(osteons, hemiosteons)	Repair of microdamage
			Prevention of bone loss
Repair	F	Woven	Repair of fractures
		Rapid mechanical adaptation	

A, activation; R, resorption; F, formation.

ossification). Growth involves only the formation of tissues, without regard to shape. Modeling uses the tissue formed during the growth process to further increase bone mass and to shape its geometry to mechanical needs. Modeling occurs through the activation (A) of cells followed by either formation (F) or resorption (R). Formation and resorption are coordinated processes in modeling but do not occur sequentially on the same surface of bone. Remodeling, on the other hand, is defined by the sequential processes on the same bone surface of activation-resorption-formation (A-R-F). The function of remodeling is bone maintenance, not the increase in bone mass. Bone remodeling is also involved in skeletal repair of microdamage. Bone's repair function, which restores its mechanical properties following a complete fracture or trabecular microfracture, usually occurs through the process of endochondral ossification, which forms a cartilage callus that also includes woven bone to bridge the fracture gap. This is eventually replaced through remodeling with replacement by lamellar bone.

Growth, modeling, and remodeling are present concurrently in all growing children. When skeletal maturity is reached, growth naturally stops. Modeling slows down or stops but may still be present at a reduced rate on trabecular surfaces and on the periosteal surface of the bone. However, at maturity, the predominant process is bone remodeling, which serves to maintain the bone that has been formed and repair microscopic damage that may be sustained in bone during normal daily activities. Dysfunction to the remodeling process is associated with the loss of bone found in osteoporosis.

Growth

Growth of bone can occur through two different skeletal processes, one involving formation of bone from fibrous membranes and the other involving the formation of a skeletal anlage, or model. Intramembranous bone formation occurs at centers of ossification via direct mineralization in highly vascular fibrous tissues through the action of mesenchymal cells. The calvarium of the skull is the best example of intramembranous bone formation, with the individual bones of the skull acting as centers that eventually grow together at the sutures. Apposition of bone on the periosteal surface of long bones can also occur through intramembranous ossification and has been demonstrated especially in the region of the femoral neck.[42]

In the long bones, however, development generally occurs by the initial condensation of mesenchyme or hyaline cartilage in the form of the eventual skeletal structure. This cartilage model mineralizes over time and becomes detectable as a primary center of ossification. Some

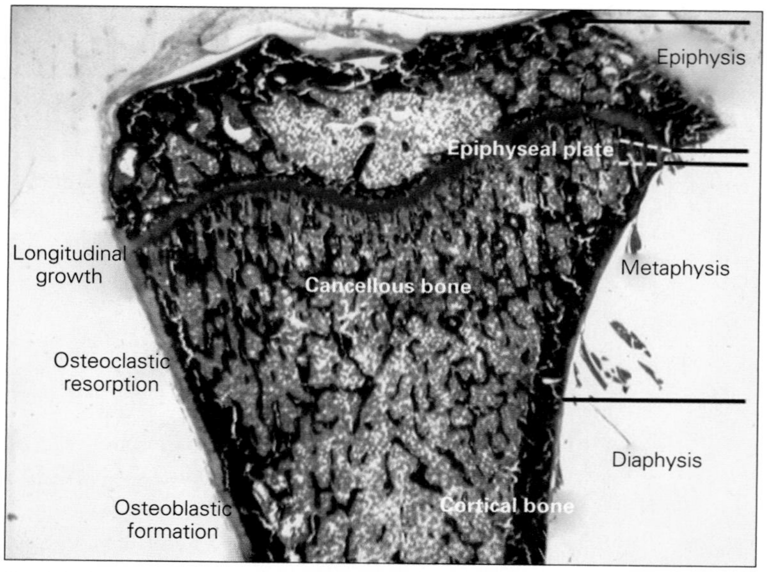

Fig. 9.5 Bone consists of the diaphysis (shaft), metaphysis, and epiphysis. In growing children, the growth (epiphyseal) plate separates the epiphysis from the metaphysis. During growth, the periosteal surface of the metaphysis must be constantly resorbed, while concurrent bone formation occurs on the endocortical surface, to convert the thin-walled but flared metaphysis into the narrower but thicker-walled diaphysis. Stained with McNeal's tetrachrome.

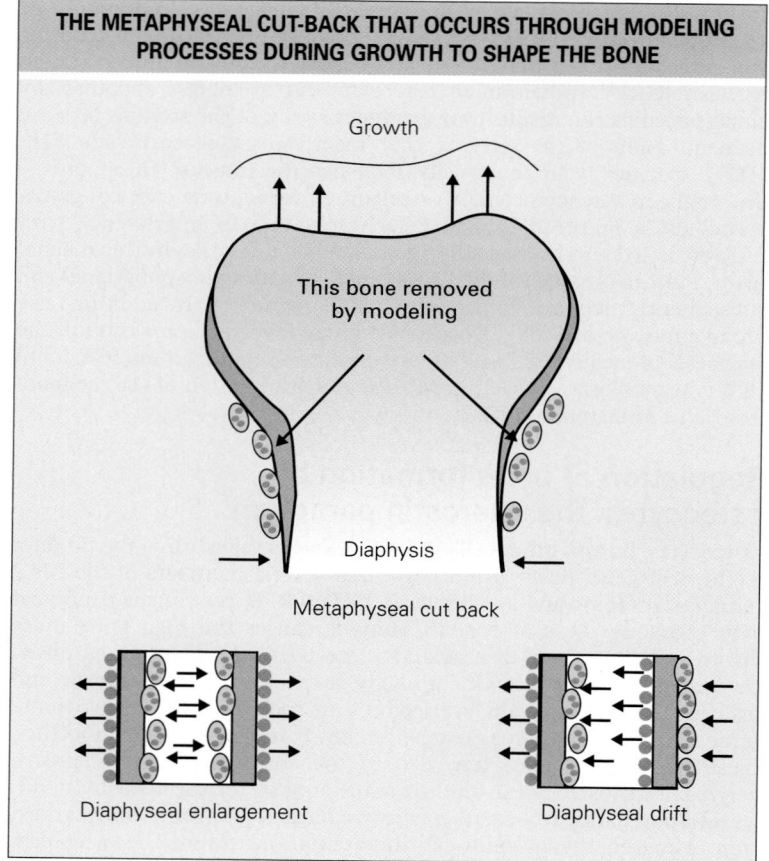

Fig. 9.6 Diagram showing the metaphyseal cutback that occurs through modeling processes during growth to shape the bone. Subsequent enlargement of the diaphysis occurs through direct periosteal apposition, which is often accompanied by resorption on the endocortical surface to enlarge the marrow cavity. Bone can also change its location and curvature through "drift." Arrows indicate direction of drift, with solid cells representing osteoblasts and bone formation, and the open cells representing osteoclasts and bone resorption. *(Reprinted with kind permission of Springer Science+Business Media from Skeletal Tissue Mechanics. RB Martin, DB Burr, NA Sharkey. Skeletal Biology Chapter 2, Figure 19. New York: Springer, 1998:62).*

bones are formed from a single ossification center, although most of the long bones form secondary centers of ossification at the ends (epiphyses), which eventually fuse to the bone that developed from the primary ossification center (diaphysis) (Fig. 9.5). The secondary centers allow growth to occur at a cartilaginous growth plate until skeletal maturity in the late teens or (for the vertebral bodies) in the early part of the third decade. The growth plate slowly converts into primary spongiosa (or trabeculae) that become remodeled into lamellar trabecular plates in the metaphysis of the bone.

Modeling

Long bones must grow both in length and in diameter (Fig. 9.6). At the ends of the long bones—near the epiphyses—growth of bone demands that the wider joint surface continually be reshaped and narrowed as it moves down into the metaphysis and diaphysis. Modeling is a continuous and prolonged process, unlike remodeling, which is episodic, and involves a coordinated process of bone resorption on some surfaces, while other surfaces undergo bone formation. Bone modeling occurs on both periosteal and endocortical envelopes and serves to provide the eventual shape of the bone, as well as to allow for expansion of the marrow cavity and periosteal diameter of the diaphysis. At the metaphysis, this occurs by osteoclastic resorption on the periosteal surfaces. As growth continues, however, bone is added to the periosteal surface by osteoblasts and simultaneously removed from the endocortical surface by osteoclasts. This serves to increase whole bone diameter and expand the marrow cavity, necessary for the formation of blood. It serves a second purpose to increase the mechanical strength of the bone, while at the same time not increasing its mass or weight at the same rate. Bone curvature is also adjusted during growth through a process known as "drift," in which the periosteal surface on one side of the bone is undergoing apposition, while the other is undergoing resorption. Likewise, different portions of the endocortical surface are undergoing formation or resorption in coordination, to maintain cortical thickness of the diaphysis.

Remodeling

The quantum concept of bone remodeling states that bone is replaced in packets through the coupled activity of osteoclasts and osteoblasts. The coupling between osteoclasts and osteoblasts is why it was difficult for so many years to control the processes involved in bone loss. When

bone resorption is suppressed, formation is also suppressed because these activities are linked by intercellular signaling mechanisms that are still little understood. In remodeling, bone resorption and bone formation are coupled, but in fact may not be balanced. Coupling and balance are not the same; balance refers to the relationship between the amount of bone resorbed and the amount formed, whereas coupling only denotes that the processes are linked in some way. Bone resorption and bone formation are in balance in the healthy skeleton, but when these are out of balance the amount of bone that is resorbed can be either more or less than the amount that is subsequently formed. So, bone can be lost or added, even though cells are coupled, in several different ways that alter the balance of resorption and formation. In actuality, one almost never finds a balance in favor of bone formation in a remodeling system, although this has been shown to occur with anabolic treatments for osteoporosis such as the administration of intermittent rhPTH[1-34] (Forteo).[43] More often, the balance is in favor of resorption. This is the case in osteoporosis, in which global resorption is increased, but formation at each of the erosion sites is normal or reduced, leading to a deficit in bone mass.

This coupled system is termed a *bone multicellular unit* (BMU) because different cell populations are involved; bone remodeling is sometimes referred to as BMU-based bone remodeling. A BMU typically consists of about 10 osteoclasts and several hundred osteoblasts. When cut in longitudinal section, the BMU shows the sequential aspects of the A-R-F system, and the various cell populations that are involved (Fig. 9.7). Each of the phases in this sequence is location, magnitude, and rate specific," so alterations in the magnitude or timing of one can produce morphologic features characteristic of specific skeletal abnormalities (Fig. 9.8). Activation is initiated by chemical or mechanical signals (although the latter may be mediated biochemically) but actually involves a series of events that include recruitment of precursor cells, differentiation and proliferation of cells, and eventual migration to the site of activity. In humans, these processes take about 5 to 10 days. Bone resorption by mature osteoclasts takes about 3 weeks at a given site, although osteoclasts moving longitudinally through bone at a rate of about 40 µm/day may live much longer than this. There is a period of reversal, during which there is neither bone resorption nor formation; this may represent a period like the activation period during which osteoblasts are undergoing differentiation and proliferation from their precursors. This is followed by a period of bone formation that lasts about 3 months. As unmineralized bone—or osteoid—is laid down, it subsequently begins to mineralize, quickly at first, and then more slowly over the following years. This sequence of events occurs on all four skeletal envelopes (periosteal, endocortical, trabecular, and intracortical).

Changes in bone mass can occur simply through changes in activation frequency. The greater number of active remodeling sites, the larger the remodeling space (that space actively undergoing remodeling) and the greater the porosity (or the smaller the trabecular bone volume). Changes in activation frequency may lead only to transient changes in bone mass if resorption and formation are in balance, so early losses of bone mass due solely to increased activation frequency may resolve after several months as the new remodeling site leaves the resorption phase and enters the formation phase. Likewise, bone mass may change because some aspect of the recruitment, proliferation, migration, or differentiation of either osteoclasts or osteoblasts is interrupted. These changes may be manifest as alterations of R-F balance but, in fact, may be caused by activation defects during cell maturation.

Repair

Fracture healing involves several stages in the repair (or regeneration) process (Fig. 9.9). The injury is typically followed by the development of a hematoma with associated inflammatory responses. This phase is

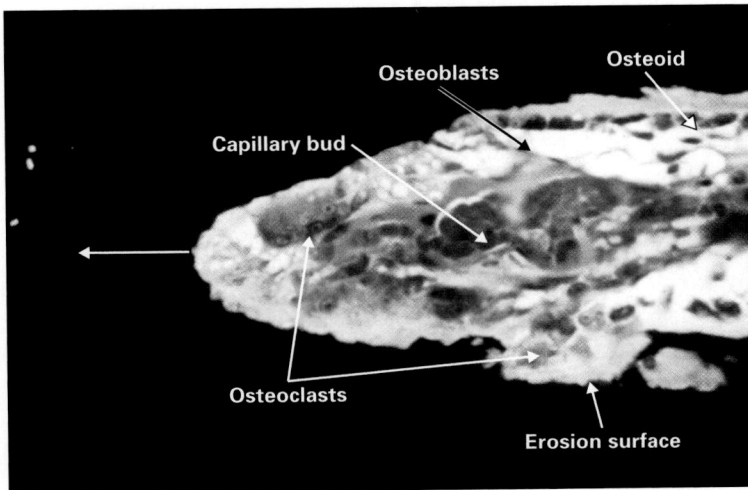

Fig. 9.7 A bone multicellular unit, or BMU. This system shows the sequential aspects of the activation-resorption-formation system and the various cells that are involved. At the head of the resorption front (also called the *cutting cone*), there is a capillary bud that supplies nutrients to the multicellular osteoclasts that are decalcifying and resorbing bone matrix. Behind the resorption front, teams of osteoblasts are lined up along the wall of the BMU, laying down new bone, or osteoid, that will subsequently become mineralized. Some of these osteoblasts will eventually embed themselves and become terminally differentiated osteocytes. Stained with McNeal's tetrachrome.

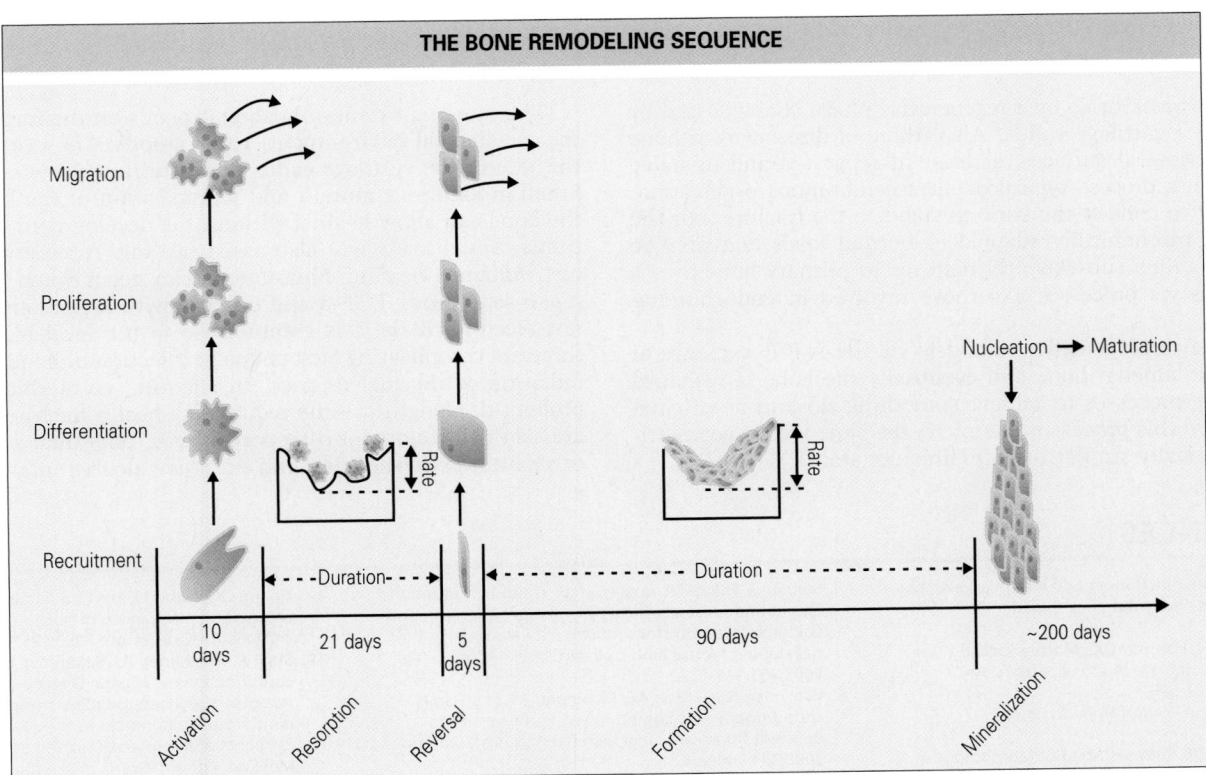

Fig. 9.8 The bone remodeling sequence. The entire sequence, not including mineralization, takes about 4 months in people. Many cellular processes occur during each of the activation-resorption-formation sequence of events. The amount of resorption and formation are determined both by the individual activity of the cells and by the duration of their lifetime. In cross-section, formation requires about four times longer than the resorption of the same amount of bone, and consequently there are many more osteoblasts in bone than osteoclasts. *(Reprinted from "Orthopedic principles of skeletal growth and remodeling." In: Bone biodynamics in orthodontic and orthopedic treatment. Carlson DS, Goldstein SA, eds. Craniofacial growth series. Ann Arbor: Center for Human Growth and Development of the University of Michigan, 1992:15-50.)*

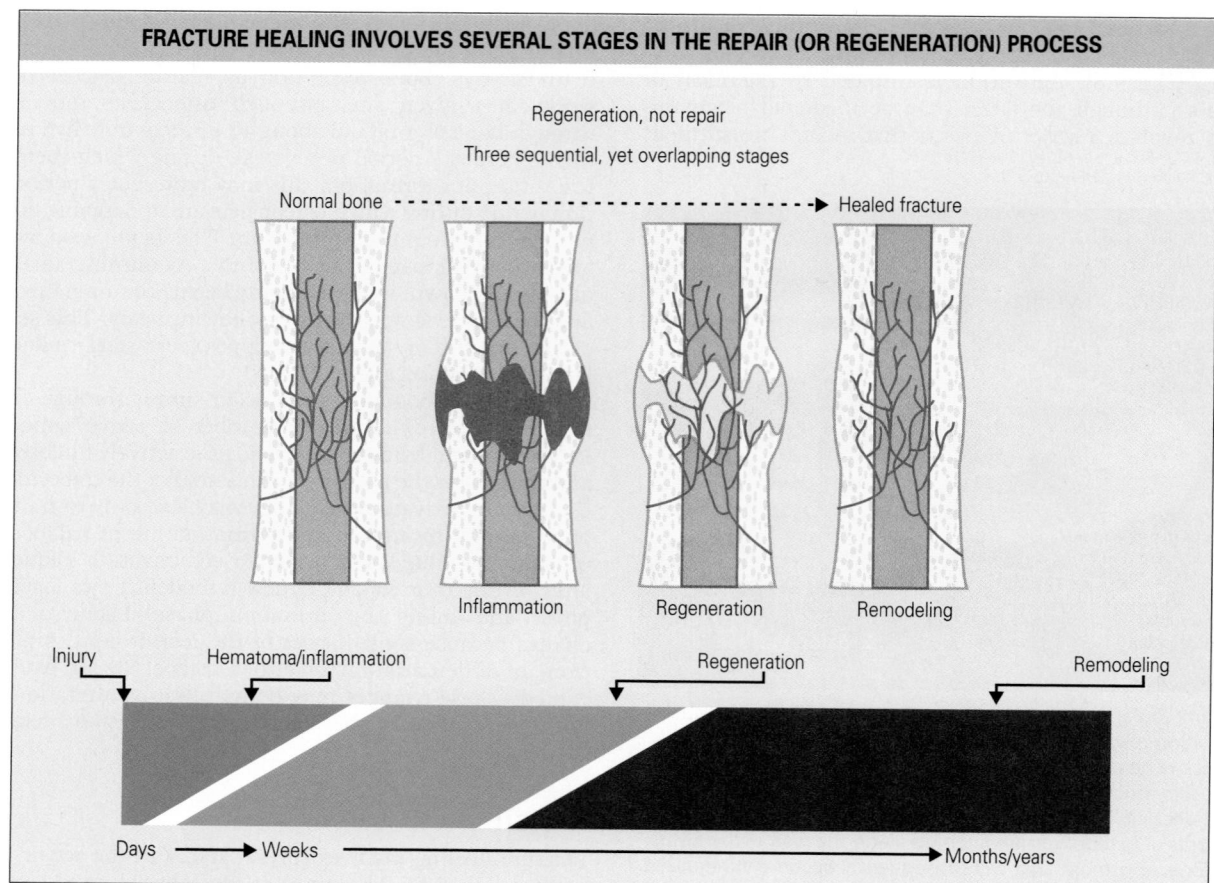

FRACTURE HEALING INVOLVES SEVERAL STAGES IN THE REPAIR (OR REGENERATION) PROCESS

Regeneration, not repair

Three sequential, yet overlapping stages

Normal bone - - - - - - - - - - - - - - - - - - → Healed fracture

Inflammation   Regeneration   Remodeling

Injury   Hematoma/inflammation   Regeneration   Remodeling

Days → Weeks   Months/years

Fig. 9.9 Fracture healing involves several stages in the repair (or regeneration) process. The injury is typically followed by the development of a hematoma with associated inflammatory responses. This phase is followed by the development of a periosteal bridging callus (at least in separated and unstable fractures) that is composed of calcified cartilage. Over time, this cartilage callus remodels to become bone and eventually the bone is reshaped through modeling processes to achieve something close to its original dimensions.

followed within a week or so by a regenerative phase characterized by the formation of a cartilage callus. Also, there is direct woven bone apposition on periosteal surfaces, at least in separated and unstable fractures, through a process typical of intramembranous ossification. This unites the two ends of the bone to stabilize the fracture, but the bone is still not mechanically adapted to normal loads and may be quite weak. The callus subsequently matures to primary bone over a period of months via processes like those involved in endochondral ossification.

Over time, the cartilage callus remodels via the A-R-F sequence of events to become lamellar bone and eventually the bone is reshaped through modeling processes to achieve something close to its original dimensions. When this process is complete, the bone will be geometrically and mechanically similar to its prefracture state.

The rate and extent of healing depends on the fracture and also on the mechanical environment. Large amounts of motion will increase the size of the cartilage callus and interrupt its remodeling to bone. Small amounts of motion and juxtaposition of the fractured ends of the bone can allow healing without the development of much, or any, callus. Small loads will also assist healing. A variety of local factors can influence healing. Non-unions can occur when early signals for repair (e.g., from TGF-β and other growth factors and cytokines) are not received, if there is compromise to the local blood supply, or if there are complicating factors due to infection or bone death caused by radiation or thermal injuries. In addition, co-morbid conditions can prolong the length of time required to heal a fracture. Many of these are also risk factors for osteoporosis (e.g., poor diet, smoking, calcium or vitamin D deficiencies, and excessive alcohol intake).

KEY REFERENCES

1. Casley-Smith JR. The functioning and interrelationships of blood capillaries and lymphatics. Experientia 1976;32:1-12.
2. Bennett HS, Luft JH, Hampton JC. Morphological classifications of vertebrate blood capillaries. Am J Physiol 1959;196:381-390.
3. Cooper RR. Nerves in cortical bone. Science 1968;160:327-328.
4. Schaffler MB, Burr DB, Frederickson RG. Morphology of the osteonal cement line in human bone. Anat Rec 1987;217:223-228.
5. Fuchs RK, Allen MR, Ruppel ME, et al. In situ examination of the time-course for secondary mineralization of Haversian bone using synchrotron Fourier transform infrared microspectroscopy. Matrix Biol 2008;27:34-41.
6. Noonan KJ, Stevens JW, Tammi R, et al. Spatial distribution of CD44 and hyaluronan in the proximal tibia of the growing rat. J Orthop Res 1996;14:573-581.

7. Shibata S, Fukada K, Imai H, et al. In situ hybridization and immunohistochemistry of versican, aggrecan and link protein, and histochemistry of hyaluronan in the developing mouse limb bud cartilage. J Anat 2003;203:425-432.
8. Williams DR Jr, Presar AR, Richmond AT, et al. Limb chondrogenesis is compromised in the versican deficient hdf mouse. Biochem Biophys Res Commun 2005;334:960-966.
9. Corsi A, Xu T, Chen XD, et al. Phenotypic effects of biglycan deficiency are linked to collagen fibril abnormalities, are synergized by decorin deficiency, and mimic Ehlers-Danlos-like changes in bone and other connective tissues. J Bone Miner Res 2002;17:1180-1189.
10. Xu T, Bianco P, Fisher LW, et al. Targeted disruption of the biglycan gene leads to an osteoporosis-like phenotype in mice. Nat Genet 1998;20:78-82.

11. Hoang QQ, Sicheri F, Howard AJ, Yang DS. Bone recognition mechanism of porcine osteocalcin from crystal structure. Nature 2003;425:977-980.
12. Staal A, Van Wijnen AJ, Birkenhager JC, et al. Distinct conformations of vitamin D receptor/retinoid X receptor-alpha heterodimers are specified by dinucleotide differences in the vitamin D-responsive elements of the osteocalcin and osteopontin genes. Mol Endocrinol 1996;10:1444-1456.
13. McKee MD, Nanci A. Osteopontin at mineralized tissue interfaces in bone, teeth, and osseointegrated implants: ultrastructural distribution and implications for mineralized tissue formation, turnover, and repair. Microsc Res Tech 1996;33:141-164.
14. Boskey AL, Spevak L, Paschalis E, et al. Osteopontin deficiency increases mineral content and mineral crystallinity in mouse bone. Calcif Tissue Int 2002;71:145-154.

15. Addison WN, Azari F, Sorensen ES, et al. Pyrophosphate inhibits mineralization of osteoblast cultures by binding to mineral, up-regulating osteopontin, and inhibiting alkaline phosphatase activity. J Biol Chem 2007;282:15872-15883.
16. Weiss MJ, Henthorn PS, Lafferty MA, et al. Isolation and characterization of a cDNA encoding a human liver/bone/kidney-type alkaline phosphatase. Proc Natl Acad Sci U S A 1986;83:7182-7186.
17. Carron JA, Wagstaff SC, Gallagher JA, Bowler WB. A CD36-binding peptide from thrombospondin-1 can stimulate resorption by osteoclasts in vitro1. Biochem Biophys Res Commun 2000;270:1124-1127.
18. White KE, Evans WE, O'Riordan JLH, et al. Autosomal dominant hypophosphataemic rickets is associated with mutations in FGF23. Nat Genet 2000;26:345-348.
19. Shimada T, Mizutani S, Muto T, et al. Cloning and characterization of FGF23 as a causative factor of tumor-induced osteomalacia. Proc Natl Acad Sci U S A 2001;98:6500-6505.
20. Riminucci M, Collins MT, Fedarko NS, et al. FGF-23 in fibrous dysplasia of bone and its relationship to renal phosphate wasting. J Clin Invest 2003;112:683-692.
21. Siggelkow H, Schmidt E, Hennies B, Hufner M. Evidence of downregulation of matrix extracellular phosphoglycoprotein during terminal differentiation in human osteoblasts. Bone 2004;35:570-576.
22. Gowen LC, Petersen DN, Mansolf AL, et al. Targeted disruption of the osteoblast/osteocyte factor 45 gene (OF45) results in increased bone formation and bone mass. J Biol Chem 2003;278:1998-2007.
23. Zhao G, Monier-Faugere MC, Langub MC, et al. Targeted overexpression of insulin-like growth factor I to osteoblasts of transgenic mice: increased trabecular bone volume without increased osteoblast proliferation. Endocrinology 2000;141:2674-2682.
24. Shore EM, Xu M, Feldman GJ, et al. A recurrent mutation in the BMP type I receptor ACVR1 causes inherited and sporadic fibrodysplasia ossificans progressiva. Nat Genet 2006;38:525-527.
25. Teitelbaum SL, Ross FP. Genetic regulation of osteoclast development and function. Nat Rev Genet 2003;4:638-649.
26. Kearns AE, Khosla S, Kostenuik PJ. Receptor activator of nuclear factor kappaB ligand and osteoprotegerin regulation of bone remodeling in health and disease. Endocr Rev 2008;29:155-192.
27. Civitelli R. Cell-cell communication in the osteoblast/osteocyte lineage. Arch Biochem Biophys 2008;473:188-192.
28. Aarden EM, Burger EH, Nijweide PJ. Function of osteocytes in bone. J Cell Biochem 1994;55:287-299.
29. Globus RK, Doty SB, Lull JC, et al. Fibronectin is a survival factor for differentiated osteoblasts. J Cell Sci 1998;111:1385-1393.
30. Zhao W, Byrne MH, Wang Y, Krane SM. Osteocyte and osteoblast apoptosis and excessive bone deposition accompany failure of collagenase cleavage of collagen. J Clin Invest 2000;106:941-949.
31. Jilka RL, Bellido T, Almeida M, et al. Apoptosis in bone cells. In: Bilezikian JP, Raisz LG, Martin TJ. eds. Principles of bone biology. San Diego, San Francisco, New York, London, Sydney, Tokyo: Academic Press, 2008:237-261.
32. Jilka RL, Weinstein RS, Bellido T, et al. Osteoblast programmed cell death (apoptosis): modulation by growth factors and cytokines. J Bone Min Res 1998;13:793-802.
33. Plotkin LI, Weinstein RS, Parfitt AM, et al. Prevention of osteocyte and osteoblast apoptosis by bisphosphonates and calcitonin. J Clin Invest 1999;104:1363-1374.
34. Bodine PV. Wnt signaling control of bone cell apoptosis. Cell Res 2008;18:248-253.
35. Bellido T, Ali AA, Gubrij I, et al. Chronic elevation of PTH in mice reduces expression of sclerostin by osteocytes: a novel mechanism for hormonal control of osteoblastogenesis. Endocrinology 2005;146:4577-4583.
36. Robling AG, Niziolek PJ, Baldridge LA, et al. Mechanical stimulation of bone in vivo reduces osteocyte expression of Sost/sclerostin. J Biol Chem 2008;283:5866-5875.
37. Bellido T, Ali AA, Plotkin LI, et al. Proteasomal degradation of Runx2 shortens parathyroid hormone-induced anti-apoptotic signaling in osteoblasts. A putative explanation for why intermittent administration is needed for bone anabolism. J Biol Chem 2003;278:50259-50272.
38. Tatsumi S, Ishii K, Amizuka N, et al. Targeted ablation of osteocytes induces osteoporosis with defective mechanotransduction. Cell Metab 2007;5:464-475.
39. Kousteni S, Bellido T, Plotkin LI, et al. Nongenotropic, sex-nonspecific signaling through the estrogen or androgen receptors: dissociation from transcriptional activity. Cell 2001;104:719-730.
40. Loots GG, Kneissel M, Keller H, et al. Genomic deletion of a long-range bone enhancer misregulates sclerostin in Van Buchem disease. Genome Res 2005;15:928-935.
41. O'Brien CA, Plotkin LI, Galli C, et al. Control of bone mass and remodeling by PTH receptor signaling in osteocytes. PLoS ONE 2008;3:32942.
42. Allen MR, Burr DB. Human femoral neck has less cellular periosteum, and more mineralized periosteum, than femoral diaphyseal bone. Bone 2005;36:311-316.
43. Dempster DW, Cosman F, Kurland ES, et al. Effects of daily treatment with parathyroid hormone on bone microarchitecture and turnover in patients with osteoporosis: a paired biopsy study. J Bone Miner Res 2001;16:1846-1853.

REFERENCES

Full references for this chapter can be found on www.expertconsult.com.

Tendons and ligaments

Graham Riley

10

- Although tendons and ligaments generally respond similarly to injury, there are anatomic and regional differences in the speed and quality of repair.
- Chronic painful conditions are more common in tendons, but some ligaments may also be affected.
- Most chronic conditions are degenerative, associated with "overuse."
- Although inflammatory cells are usually not present in chronic lesions, various inflammatory mediators are present both in and around the affected tissue.
- Many current therapies for chronic conditions are not supported by good clinical trials.
- Future therapies in development include the use of mesenchymal stem cells to promote better quality repair and regeneration of the extracellular matrix.

INTRODUCTION

Musculoskeletal pain and dysfunction are commonly associated with lesions of soft connective tissues such as ligaments and tendons. These conditions are found in a high proportion of rheumatology patients, affecting not just the middle-aged and elderly but also the young and physically active populations. Current treatments often are not based on a sound scientific knowledge, and the condition frequently responds poorly to treatment, resulting in chronic pain and disability. In this chapter the spectrum of pathology affecting tendons and ligaments is discussed and current and potential novel strategies for treatment are outlined.

GENERAL CONSIDERATIONS

Tendons and ligaments are dense fibrous connective tissues that are important for joint movement and stabilization. They have a similar composition and structure and are composed primarily of a hierarchical arrangement of collagen fiber bundles primarily aligned with the long axis of the tendon. They are metabolically active and capable of responding to extrinsic factors such as mechanical load, exercise, and immobilization. However, there are differences in structure, composition, and function between a tendon and a ligament that make it unwise to extrapolate directly from one tissue to another.[1]

The range of pathology affecting tendons and ligaments is different. Both tissues may be subject to acute injury as a result of trauma, overload, or direct mechanical insult resulting from crushing blows or penetrating objects. The repair response follows the same general pattern, with the important proviso that some ligaments and tendons are apparently able to mount a more effective repair response than others.[2] This has been linked to a number of factors, such as whether tendons are intrasynovial or extrasynovial or whether ligaments are intra- or extra-articular, and the ability to repair may be dependent on the quantity and quality of the vascular network at different sites. Tendons are more prone to chronic, insidious forms of injury than ligaments. These conditions, best described as "tendinopathies," are often associated with repeated strain and repetitive microtrauma ("overuse") rather than a single traumatic episode.[3,4]

ACUTE INJURIES

The cellular events occurring after traumatic injury to a tendon or ligament are similar and common to all soft connective tissues.[1] The response is usually divided into three phases, more for convenience as the phases merge imperceptibly into each other and represent a continuum rather than discrete stages. The first phase, occurring in the first week after disruption of the tendon fibers, is characterized by inflammation. There is edema and infiltration of a variety of cell types attracted to the region by inflammatory mediators. Platelets and mast cells release histamine, a potent agent promoting vasodilation and increasing blood vessel permeability. Serotonin, bradykinin, leukotrienes, and prostaglandins act together to recruit polymorphonuclear leukocytes and lymphocytes from the circulation. Growth factors released by platelets include platelet-derived growth factor (PDGF), transforming growth factor-β (TGF-β), and epidermal growth factor (EGF). Macrophages are present within 24 hours, phagocytosing tissue debris and releasing numerous inflammatory mediators and growth factors, including basic fibroblast growth factor (bFGF), transforming growth factor-α (TGF-α), TGF-β, and PDGF. These growth factors are chemotactic for fibroblasts and other cells and generally act to stimulate matrix synthesis. Angiogenic factors such as bFGF and vascular endothelial growth factor (VEGF) stimulate capillary ingrowth into the fibrous clot. Toward the end of the inflammatory phase, which may last several days, fibroblasts become the predominant cell type. The second phase, generally lasting up to 6 weeks after injury, is characterized by cell proliferation and new matrix synthesis by fibroblasts. This new matrix is different in both quality and quantity from the normal matrix. Described as granulation tissue, it consists of a disorganized matrix with an elevated cell density that fills the tissue defect. The third phase, occurring from 3 to 6 weeks after injury and lasting for at least a year, is a prolonged period of remodeling and maturation in which the matrix components and tissue cellularity revert gradually toward normal. During this stage many cells in the scar are contractile myofibroblasts, which are specialized cells important for the organization of the wound tissue.

LIGAMENT INJURY AND REPAIR

Although ligaments are generally similar to tendons, there are known to be substantial differences in the quality of repair found in ligaments from different anatomic locations.[2] Most ligaments, such as the collateral ligaments of the knee, are extra-articular and in a close relationship with the joint capsule and adjacent vascular structures. This environment is apparently much more conducive to repair than that surrounding the intra-articular cruciate ligaments. Injuries to the cruciate ligaments, for example, provoke a profuse vascular response, but healing by second intention (i.e., the contraction and filling of the defect by the formation of granulation tissue) does not occur. The medial collateral ligament, in contrast, heals spontaneously without the need for surgical repair. A variety of explanations have been proposed, such as the presence of synovial fluid preventing fibrin clot formation and the more dynamic mechanical environment of the cruciate ligament inhibiting repair. There are also thought to be intrinsic differences in cell types from different ligaments, with differences in morphology as well as mitogenic, chemotactic, and synthetic responses. Medial collateral ligament fibroblasts, for example, are more proliferative and produce more type III collagen than cells from the anterior cruciate ligament, and they show a greater response to growth factors such as EGF, TGF-β, and bFGF.[5]

CHRONIC PATHOLOGY

There are a variety of different terminologies for the chronic pathology that is more commonly seen in tendons, although some ligaments (e.g., the patellar) may also be affected. This confusion is partly due to an

83

incomplete understanding of the pathology as well as difficulties of diagnosis, because biopsy specimens are rarely obtained at early stages of the disease. Terms such as *tendinitis* imply that there is inflammation, although there is little evidence of any inflammatory process in histologic studies.[6] Conditions are consequently best considered as either acute or chronic, whether caused by trauma or repeated microtrauma (often attributed to "overuse") or the result of an insidious process of clinically silent (i.e. "pain-free") degeneration. Unless the presence of inflammation or degeneration has been unequivocally demonstrated, most tendon pain and dysfunction is best described as a "tendinopathy."

Sites commonly affected by tendinopathy include the supraspinatus and long head of the biceps in the shoulder, the medial and lateral extensors of the elbow, the patellar ligament, the posterior tibialis, and the Achilles tendon. In most cases, with the notable exception of the Achilles tendon, the site affected is at or near the bone insertion. There are several common features: these sites are more highly stressed, are often exposed to repeated strains, including shear or compressive forces, and are relatively less vascularized than the tendon midsubstance. The insertion also has a different structure and composition compared with the mid-substance; it is fibrocartilaginous, containing matrix components such as type II collagen and aggrecan that are more commonly associated with articular cartilage.[7] The highly specialized structure is thought to help dissipate stress and compressive forces acting on the insertion site.

ETIOLOGY OF TENDINOPATHY

The cause of tendinopathy is still controversial, and many different factors have been implicated. Many lesions are associated with a reduction in vascular perfusion, particularly at specific sites in the supraspinatus and the Achilles. Because most tendon ruptures occur in the fifth decade, age-related changes are also implicated, although ruptures of the Achilles tendon are most common in a younger, physically active population. More tendon ruptures tend to occur in males than females, although it is unlikely that this is directly associated with gender because the age and activity levels of male and female patients are frequently very different.[8] The combination of a more sedentary existence with increased leisure time, recreational sports, and a propensity to obesity may account for the greater incidence of tendinopathy in the developed world. There is a strong association with particular sports and activities that result in high levels of stress being applied to specific sites. Leg-length discrepancies and other anatomic variants, such as the shape and slope of the acromion in the shoulder, are implicated in some individuals. Joint laxity may predispose to some conditions such as rotator cuff lesions. Genetic factors have been recently identified, with an increased risk of tendon injury in individuals with specific variants of genes encoding for the extracellular matrix proteins collagen type V and tenascin C.[9,10]

HISTOPATHOLOGIC FINDINGS

There have been many histopathologic investigations of various kinds of tendinopathy, usually studied in specimens taken from either ruptured tendons or chronic painful tendons. Ruptures are frequently described as "spontaneous," meaning that the rupture occurred without any preceding clinical symptoms, although underlying degeneration of the extracellular matrix is almost always present.[6] Painful tendons frequently do not progress to a frank rupture, and specimens are generally obtained from patients who have failed prolonged conservative treatment before surgery, at which time a specimen was removed for analysis. Painful tendons generally show a much increased cellularity, cell rounding, an increased glycosaminoglycan content ("mucoid degeneration"), decreased matrix organization, and increased blood vessel infiltration (Fig. 10.1). Ruptured tendons show similar degenerative features of the extracellular matrix, although there is generally reduced cellularity and often little evidence of neovascularization. The cell changes in ruptured tendons are consistent with hypoxia, and calcific deposits and lipid droplets are frequently found in the matrix.[6] The calcification, seen in most ruptured tendons, is thought to be a degenerative phenomenon, occurring as a result of precipitation of calcium salts nucleated by cell debris or matrix constituents,[11] although

a cell-mediated process similar to endochondral ossification has been identified in some pathologic tendons.[12] Apoptosis (programmed cell death) is significantly increased in both patellar tendinopathy and in ruptured supraspinatus tendon.[13,14] Most cells in painful tendinopathy specimens are fibroblast-like, albeit generally more rounded or ovoid, and there is an absence of inflammatory cells, at least in the tendon substance. Overall, the histopathologic findings in most tendinopathy are consistent with matrix degeneration, and in painful tendons the cell and vascular response suggests at least some attempt to repair. There is evidence to suggest that the cellular changes, such as the rounder appearance and increased number, occur before any clinical symptoms are apparent.[15]

Extracellular matrix changes in tendinopathy

The extracellular matrix of tendon consists mainly of the structural protein collagen, which comprises around 65% of the dry weight.[1] Around 95% is type I collagen, with lesser amounts of collagen types II, III, IV, V, VI, IX, X, XII, and XIV. In tendinopathy, numerous molecular changes have been identified, consistent with the hypothesis that dynamic changes in the regulation of matrix turnover by the resident tenocytes are responsible for the altered tendon function (Table 10.1). There are changes in the levels of expression of some collagen genes, and increased amounts of collagen type III are found throughout the tendon matrix, not just restricted to the endotenon as in normal tendon.[16-18] Similar changes are found in scar tissue or pathologic fibrosis and have implications for the strength of the tendon, because type III collagen tends to form heterotypic fibrils with type I collagen, which has a smaller average diameter and form a meshwork rather than closely aligned fibril bundles. There are also increases in type V collagen, an increase in denatured collagen, and substantial changes in the crosslinks that stabilize the collagen matrix.[18-20] There is strong evidence for increased turnover of the collagen matrix in tendinopathy, because the collagen carries less of the glycation product pentosidine, which accumulates on long-lived matrix proteins with age.[20] There are differences between tendons, with evidence for higher rates of collagen turnover in supraspinatus tendon compared with the biceps brachii tendon in the forearm, associated with the increased prevalence of tendon injury and pathology in the shoulder, although whether this is cause or effect remains to be established.

Although less abundant than collagen, proteoglycans are important constituents of the tendon matrix, with a range of important functions, including water retention, sequestration of growth factors, and mediating cell-matrix interactions.[1] A diverse family of molecules, they all contain at least one chain of a repeating disaccharide glycosaminoglycan (GAG). Small leucine-rich proteoglycans (SLRPs), such as decorin, fibromodulin, biglycan, and lumican, are present in normal tendon, and they function to modulate fibril growth, fibril diameter, and organization as well as bind growth factors such as TGF-β. The large proteoglycans versican and aggrecan are also present, although aggrecan is more abundant at the insertion or where the tendon is subject to compression.[7] The large proteoglycans carry more GAG chains than the SLRP, aggrecan in particular, and the high negative charge density of the sulfated GAG holds water in the tissue, which is important for viscoelastic properties and resisting shear or compressive load. In tendinopathy, one of the most frequent observations is increased GAG in the matrix, often associated with rounded cells.[21] The identity and processing of the particular proteoglycan associated with the GAG has not been fully characterized at the protein level, although molecular analysis has shown increased expression of genes encoding for aggrecan and biglycan, even in the mid-substance of the Achilles tendon where fibrocartilage is not normally found.[22] These changes are consistent with an adaptive response to shear or compression, suggesting that at least some of the molecular changes are the result of changes in the level and direction of mechanical forces acting on the resident tendon cells (tenocytes). Although most tendinopathies are reported to show similar molecular changes, there may be differences at different sites. For example, levels of gene expression for the large proteoglycan versican were reported to be unchanged in painful Achilles tendons,[23] although increased versican protein has been reported in patellar tendons.[24]

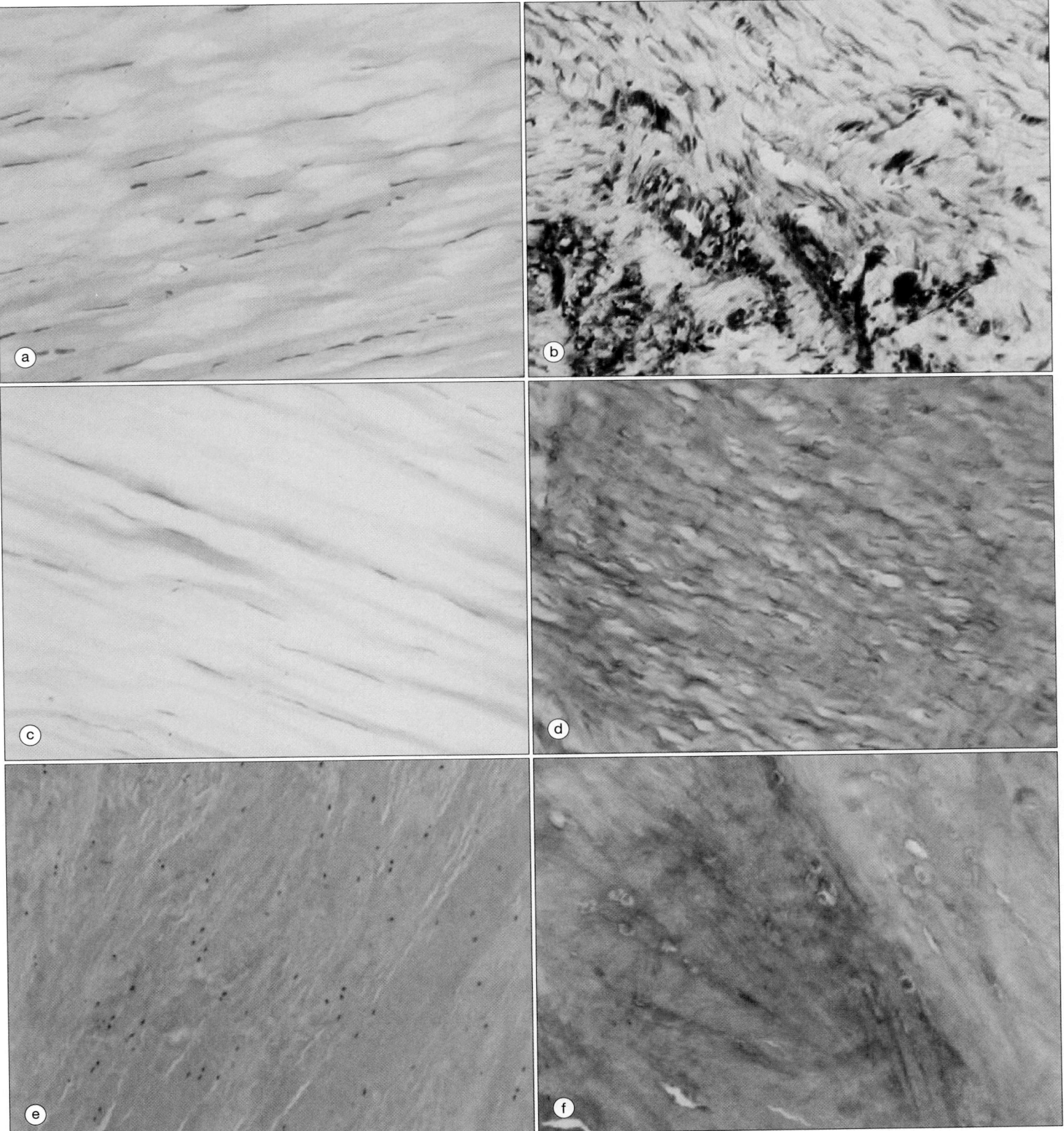

Fig. 10.1 Histologic features of tendinopathy. (a) Normal Achilles tendon, showing dense bundles of highly organized collagen fiber bundles and relatively few tenocytes arranged in columns (H&E). (b) Specimen from patient with painful tendinopathy, showing increased cellularity and vascularity at the site of the lesion (H&E). (c) Normal Achilles tendon, showing low abundance of proteoglycan (toluidine blue). (d) Specimen from patient with Achilles tendinopathy, showing much increased abundance of proteoglycan throughout the tendon matrix (toluidine blue). (e) Degenerate supraspinatus tendon specimen from patient with rotator cuff pathology, showing loss of matrix organization, disruptions in the fibrillar structure, and reduced cellularity (H&E). (f) Specimen of supraspinatus tendon from patient with rotator cuff pathology, showing increased proteoglycan associated with rounded cells in a "fibrocartilaginous" matrix (H&E/Alcian blue).

TABLE 10.1 CHANGES IN EXTRACELLULAR MATRIX IN PAINFUL TENDINOPATHY

Molecule	Potential significance	References
Collagen type I (mRNA) ↑	Attempted repair/adaptation	Ireland et al. Matrix Biol 2001;20:159-169 Corps et al. Rheumatology 2004;43:969-972[23]
Total collagen (protein) →	No significant tendon growth or adaptation	Riley et al. Ann Rheum Dis 1994;53:359-366[17] Samiric et al. Matrix Biol 2009;28:230-236
Collagen type III (mRNA/protein) ↑	Fibrosis/scar formation Smaller diameter fibrils Decreased fibril strength	Riley et al. Ann Rheum Dis 1994;53:359-366[17] Ireland et al. Matrix Biol 2001;20:159-169 Eriksen et al. J Orthop Res 2002;20:1352-1357[16]
Fibronectin (mRNA) ↑	Repair response? Altered cell-matrix interactions	Ireland et al. Matrix Biol 2001;20:159-169 Alfredson et al. J Orthop Res 2003;21:970-975
Tenascin C (mRNA/protein) ↑	Repair response? Altered cell-matrix interactions	Riley et al. Am J Pathol 1996;149:933-943[26] Ireland et al. Matrix Biol 2001;20:159-169
GAG (sugar moiety) ↑	Fibrocartilaginous change Resistance to compression	Riley et al. Ann Rheum Dis 1994;53:367-376 Samiric et al. Matrix Biol 2009;28:230-236
Aggrecan (mRNA/protein) ↑	Fibrocartilaginous change Resistance to compression	Corps et al. Rheumatology 2005;45:291-294[22] Samiric et al. Matrix Biol 2009;28:230-236
Biglycan (mRNA/protein) ↑	Fibrocartilaginous change Resistance to compression	Corps et al. Rheumatology 2005;45:291-294[22] Samiric et al. Matrix Biol 2009;28:230-236
Fibromodulin (protein) ↑	Modulation of collagen fibril formation and fibril diameter	Samiric et al C. Matrix Biol 2009;28:230-236
Versican (mRNA/protein) ↑ →	Increased or no change Significance not known	Ireland et al. Matrix Biol 2001;20:159-169 Corps et al. Rheumatology 2004;43:969-972[23] Samiric et al. Matrix Biol 2009;28:230-236
HP/LP collagen cross links ↑	Fibrosis/scar formation Adaptation to increased load?	Bank et al. Ann Rheum Dis 1999;58:35-41[20]
Pentosidine (AGE) ↓	Replacement of mature collagen and increased matrix remodeling	Bank et al. Ann Rheum Dis 1999;58:35-41[20]

Arrows indicate direction of change (→ indicates no change).
GAG, glycosaminoglycan; HP, hydroxypyridinoline; LP, lysylpyridinoline; AGE, age-related glycation end-product.

Other constituents of the tendon matrix have received relatively little attention in studies of tendinopathy. Fibronectin, a large multi-domain glycoprotein that can form many different interactions with cells and other matrix molecules, is of very low abundance in normal tendon.[25] The large increase reported in ruptured Achilles and supra-spinatus tendons is consistent with a role in the repair response, where fibronectin is involved in cell adhesion and migration at the wound site. Tenascin-C, a multimeric glycoprotein that may function to help organize the matrix, is abundant in normal tendon but is increased in tendinopathy.[26] There are changes in splice variant expression and a strong association of tenascin-C with the rounded cells in the pathologic tendon. In addition, there is evidence for enzyme-mediated degradation of tenascin-C in rotator cuff disease, consistent with the increased matrix remodeling that is associated with the condition.

Matrix turnover and remodeling

Matrix degradation, both in health and disease, is to a large extent mediated by a family of enzymes known as matrix metalloproteinases (MMPs). There are 23 MMPs in humans and a family of four naturally occurring inhibitors known as tissue inhibitors of matrix metalloproteinases (TIMPs). These enzymes have a variety of different substrate specificities, with activity against all the different structural matrix components, although they are also involved in the processing and activation of growth factors and their receptors and implicated in the control of cell activity as well as matrix degradation. In tendinopathy there are changes in the expression and activity of various MMPs and TIMPs that are consistent with increased proteolytic activity and turnover of the matrix (Table 10.2). For example, ruptured rotator cuff tendons showed greatly increased collagenase (MMP-1) activity and reduced gelatinase (MMP-2) and stromelysin (MMP-3) activity compared with normal tendons, and these changes were correlated with levels of collagen turnover in the tissues.[20] A study of gene expression in Achilles tendons showed that painful and ruptured tendons had distinct patterns of expression, consistent with quantitative and qualitative differences in catabolic activity in the different clinical entities.[27] Ruptured tendons showed higher levels of expression of MMP-1, MMP-9, MMP-19, MMP-25, and TIMP-1 and lower levels of MMP-3, MMP-7, TIMP-2, TIMP-3, and TIMP-4. Painful tendons showed reduced expression of MMP-3, MMP-10, TIMP-3, and increased expression of ADAM-12 and MMP-23. Very little is known about the role and function of A disintegrin and metalloproteinase (ADAM)-12 and MMP-23 in tendons, although both have been associated with changes in cell phenotype: ADAM-12 with myogenesis and lipidogenesis and MMP-23 with endochondral ossification.[28,29] In summary, the changes in tendon matrix composition are consistent with changes in cell-mediated matrix remodeling that precede the onset of clinical symptoms, and these changes are mediated at least in part by metalloproteinase enzymes.

Mechanical strain and the regulation of cell activity

The cellular and molecular processes driving the changes in tendon matrix remodeling in tendinopathy are yet to be determined. It is uncertain to what extent the remodeling of the tendon matrix represents a limited repair response to microscopic fiber damage or an adaptive (or potentially maladaptive) response to changes in cell loading. Cyclical tensile loading of tenocytes *in vitro*, simulating overuse, has been shown to elicit the expression of several inflammatory mediators and growth factors as well as metalloproteinase enzymes, and it is suggested that this may trigger neovascularization, inflammation, and increased proteolytic activity in the tendon.[30] However, levels of strain required to elicit this response are high, potentially much higher than the strains experienced by cells *in vivo*. More recently, it has been shown that tenocytes when released from tension will upregulate their expression of the collagenase MMP-13, and that this typically occurs after failure of one or more of the tendon fiber bundles in the stretched tendon.[31] Thus it appears that MMP output is attenuated by normal loading conditions and that damage to tendon fibers releases

TABLE 10.2 CHANGES IN PROTEASES AND THEIR INHIBITORS IN PAINFUL TENDINOPATHY

Molecule	Potential role/ significance	References
MMP-1 ↑	Increased collagen turnover	Riley et al. Matrix Biol 2002;21:185-195 Fu et al. Acta Orthop Scand 2002;73:658-662
MMP-2 ↑	Increased collagen turnover	Ireland et al. Matrix Biol 2001;20:159-169 Alfredson et al. J Orthop Res 2003;21:970-975
MMP-3 ↓	Decreased PG turnover? Reduced activation of MMP?	Ireland et al. Matrix Biol 2001;20:159-169 Jones et al. Arthritis Rheum 2006;54:832-842[27]
MMP-23 (mRNA) ↑	Not known	Jones et al. Arthritis Rheum 2006;54:832-842[27]
ADAM-12 (mRNA) ↑	Not known	Jones et al. Arthritis Rheum 2006;54:832-842[27]
ADAMTS-2 (mRNA) ↑	Pro-collagen peptidase New collagen synthesis	Jones et al. Arthritis Rheum 2006;54:832-842[27]
ADAMTS-3 (mRNA) ↑	Pro-collagen peptidase New collagen synthesis	Jones et al. Arthritis Rheum 2006;54:832-842[27]
ADAMTS-5 ↓	Decreased PG turnover? Cause of increase in PG?	Jones et al. Arthritis Rheum 2006;54:832-842[27]
TIMP-3 ↓	Reduced inhibition of ADAMTS activity	Jones et al. Arthritis Rheum 2006;54:832-842[27]
Caspase-3 ↑	Increased apoptosis	Millar et al. J Bone Joint Surg Br 2009;91:417-424
Caspase-8 ↑	Increased apoptosis	Millar et al. J Bone Joint Surg Br 2009;91:417-424

Arrows indicate direction of change (→ indicates no change).
MMP, matrix metalloproteinase; ADAM, A disintegrin and metalloproteinase; ADAMTS, a disintegrin and metalloproteinase with thrombospondin motifs; TIMP, tissue inhibitor of metalloproteinases; PG, proteoglycan.

TABLE 10.3 CHANGES IN CYTOKINES AND SIGNALING MOLECULES IN PAINFUL TENDINOPATHY

Molecule	Potential role/significance	References
TGF-β ↑	Repair/growth/fibrosis Matrix synthesis	Fenwick et al. J Anat 2001;199:231-240 Fu et al. Clin Orthop Relat Res 2002;73:658-662
VEGF ↑	Associated with angiogenesis and neovascularization	Pufe et al. Scand J Med Sci Sports 2005;15:211-222 Scott et al. Clin Orthop Relat Res 2008;466:1598-1604
IL-1 ↑	Inflammation in surrounding tissues (bursa, synovium)	Gotoh et al. J Orthop Res 2002;20:1365-1371 Ko et al. J Orthop Res 2008;26:1090-1097
IL-6 ↑	Inflammation within tendon	Millar et al. J Bone Joint Surg Br 2009;91:417-424
IL-15 ↑	Inflammation within tendon	Millar et al. J Bone Joint Surg Br 2009;91:417-424
IL-18 ↑	Inflammation within tendon	Millar et al. J Bone Joint Surg Br 2009;91:417-424
COX2 ↑	Production of prostaglandin within and around tendon	Fu et al. Clin Orthop Relat Res 2002;73:658-662
Glutamate ↑	Neurotransmitter—associated with pain and/or apoptosis?	Alfredson et al. J Orthop Res 2001;19:881-886[37] Alfredson et al. Acta Orthop Scand 2000;71:475-479
Substance P ↑	Neurotransmitter—associated with pain perception and edema	Gotoh et al. J Orthop Res 1998;16:618-621[36] Schubert et al. Ann Rheum Dis 2005;64:1083-1086
PGE2 →	Mediator of pain and inflammation	Alfredson et al. J Orthop Res 2001;19:881-886[37] Alfredson et al. Acta Orthop Scand 2000;71:475-479
PDGFR ↑	Mediates cell response to PDGF—cell proliferation	Rolf et al. Rheumatology 2001;40:256-261
NMDAR ↑	Glutamate receptor—affect on tendon cell not known	Alfredson et al. J Orthop Res 2001;19:881-886[37]
TGFβR1 ↓	Mediates cell response to TGF-β—possible reduced response and poor repair?	Fenwick et al. J Anat 2001;199:231-240

Arrows indicate direction of change (→ indicates no change).
TGF-β, transforming growth factor-β; IGF-1, insulin-like growth factor-1; VEGF, vascular endothelial growth factor; IL-1, interleukin-1; COX2, cyclooxygenase-2; PGE2, prostaglandin E2; PDGFR, platelet-derived growth factor receptor; NMDAR, N-methyl-D-aspartate receptor; TGFβR1, transforming growth factor-β type 1 receptor.

the cells from this strain regulation, resulting in increased collagenase expression and the potential for matrix degradation.

Inflammation and inflammatory mediators

Although there is an absence of inflammatory cells, this does not mean that inflammatory mediators are not implicated in tendinopathy, at least at some stage in the disease, and changes in a number of cytokines, growth factors, and signaling molecules have been detected in tendinopathy (Table 10.3). Increased levels of interleukin (IL)-1 have been detected in the tissues surrounding painful tendons, such as the bursa in the shoulder.[32] Prostaglandin E₂ and other inflammatory mediators such as thromboxane, bradykinin, and IL-6 are increased in peritendinous tissue after prolonged periods of intense exercise.[33] There are also increased levels of growth factors such TGF-β and insulin-like growth factor-1 (IGF-1), and these have been shown to have a stimulatory effect on collagen synthesis.[34] However, some or all of these changes may be part of the adaptive response, or involved in tissue repair, and their precise contribution to the pathology is uncertain.

Pain and neuropeptides

Pain in tendinopathy has been associated with the ingrowth of nerve endings and the release of neurotransmitters such as substance P, calcitonin gene–related peptide (CGRP), and glutamate.[35] Levels of substance P were increased in the subacromial bursa fluid of patients with rotator cuff tendinopathy and correlated with the degree of motion pain.[36] Apart from the modulation of pain, substance P and other

neuropeptides regulate the local circulation and may also directly affect tenocyte activity, as well as mediating neurogenic inflammation, potentially accounting for the bilateral occurrence of tendinopathy in many patients. Consequently, antagonists of neuropeptides and neurotransmitters such as glutamate have been proposed for the treatment of tendinopathy.[37] However, nerve ingrowth and increased expression of neuropeptides are part of the normal tendon repair response, and injection of substance P has been used for the treatment of tendon injuries, increasing the organization of collagen fibrils and the strength of the repair.[38]

TREATMENT OF TENDON AND LIGAMENT INJURIES

A great variety of treatments, sometimes quite bizarre, have been used for acute and chronic tendon and ligament injuries, although relatively few have shown clinical benefit in properly controlled clinical trials.[4] Actovegin, a deproteinized extract of calf blood, has been injected around the painful tendons of many top athletes. More evidence exists to support the injection of autologous platelet-rich plasma around tendon injuries, particularly in animal models. Low-energy laser photostimulation stimulates collagen synthesis in healing tendons, possibly mediated by an increase in growth factor activity. Therapeutic ultrasound has been shown to increase the tensile strength and elasticity of healing tendons but only if applied during the early stages of healing. The synthetic polymer glycosaminoglycan polysulfate (GAGPS) was reported to show some benefit in the treatment of chronic tendinopathy, perhaps as a consequence of inhibitory effects on proteolytic activities. Extracorporeal shock wave therapy (ESWT) may have some benefit in the treatment of tendon injury, although the mechanism is not known and there are potential negative effects at high-energy flux density. The injection of a sclerosant, targeting the neovascularization seen in tendinopathy, is advocated by some practitioners,[39] although there is some concern that the vascular response is part of the repair process and may have negative consequences in the long term.

Non-steroidal anti-inflammatory drugs (NSAIDs)

NSAIDs such as ibuprofen are useful for the treatment of pain in ligament and tendon injuries and may be of some benefit in managing pain in chronic tendinopathies. Their pharmacologic target is cyclooxygenase (prostaglandin synthase), a key enzyme in the formation of prostaglandins, which are key mediators of pain and inflammation. Studies of their effects on tendon healing have been inconclusive, with both positive and negative effects reported. The rationale behind NSAID use in chronic tendon pain is uncertain, because inflammation is generally not a feature of these conditions and prostaglandin levels are not increased relative to controls in the fluid surrounding painful tendons. However, because cyclooxygenase 2 (COX-2) was reported to be increased in clinical specimens of patella tendinopathy,[40] and prostaglandin injected around a tendon can induce a form of degenerative tendinopathy,[41] there may be a rational basis for a direct therapeutic effect of NSAIDs, at least in some patients.

Corticosteroids

Corticosteroid injection is a common standby for the treatment of chronic tendon lesions, although once again there is limited evidence to strongly support its use. There are many case reports describing rupture, often bilateral, of Achilles and other tendons after long-term oral corticosteroids and also after local injections. Ruptures are associated with a reduced collagen content and decreased mechanical strength, presumably as a result of the suppression of collagen synthesis and turnover. There are very few controlled studies of the effectiveness of corticosteroid injections, the precise effects on tendon tissue are unknown, and the results of animal studies are often contradictory.

Exercise and mobilization therapies

Controlled motion therapy for acute tendon and ligament injuries is now generally accepted, and also used for the treatment of chronic tendinopathies, particularly in the form of high-loading eccentric exercises.[42] It is well known that prolonged immobilization has deleterious effects on the quality of repair, in addition to other complications such as muscle atrophy, joint stiffness, cartilage deterioration, adhesions, and thrombosis. Tension, applied cyclically or as a constant load, has a positive influence on the intrinsic fibroblast response and the strength of repair. It promotes cell proliferation and migration, facilitating the alignment of fibroblasts and increasing collagen synthesis, presumably mediated by the stimulation of growth factors such as IGF-1, TGF-β, and connective tissue growth factor (CTGF) in and around the tendon.[33] More experimental work with controlled studies is required to define the optimum exercise/loading regimen designed to promote reorganization and remodeling of the damaged tissue so that higher strength and better function can be achieved.

Future therapeutic strategies

The application of exogenous recombinant growth factors to damaged and healing ligaments and tendons has been attempted in a number of animal studies with variable levels of success. Growth factors studied include various bone morphogenetic proteins (BMPs, members of the TGF-β superfamily), PDGF, TGF-β, FGF, and IGF-1.[43-45] However, there are serious questions with the prolonged use of purified growth factors for treatment, including the high cost, problems with delivery systems, and the difficulty maintaining sufficient concentrations of the protein at the site of the lesion. Gene therapy, in which the desired gene for a particular growth factor, for example, is inserted directly into tissue cells, may be an answer to this problem, although issues associated with the transfection of genetic material into human cells remain to be solved.[46] Mesenchymal stem cells, which have the ability to form various types of connective tissue, are currently being evaluated for the treatment of a number of musculoskeletal conditions, including tendinopathy.[47,48] The idea is to replenish the reparative/regenerative capacity of the tendon by injecting stem cell preparations directly into the site of the lesion. Stem cell therapy has been reported to be of some benefit in equine tendinopathy, and future trials in human patients are anticipated. Tissue engineering of new tendon constructs to replace damaged tissue is also a long-term goal being actively pursued, although a number of problems remain to be solved, including the development of scaffolds with the appropriate strength to resist high-tensile loads.[49]

CONCLUSION

Ligaments and tendons are similar but not identical; they respond similarly to acute injury but chronic pain and degeneration are more common in tendons. These tissues are metabolically active and respond to changes in their mechanical and chemical environment, with matrix changes mediated by altered cell synthetic activity and the local production of a variety of matrix-degrading proteases. Injury results in substantial and permanent changes in the quantity and quality of the extracellular matrix. There are regional differences in the response to injury that are related to the tissue cellularity, vascularity, composition, and matrix organization. The repair tissue can be affected and modulated by both physical and chemical factors, although the precise conditions required to optimize repair have not been rigorously defined. In tendons, most pathology is degenerative, resulting either in a "spontaneous" tendon rupture or a chronic painful tendinopathy, sometimes associated with calcification. Degeneration in tendinopathy has been shown to be an active, cell-mediated process involving increased levels of matrix remodeling, with the increased synthesis and degradation of matrix components mediated by a variety of enzymes. The source of pain in chronic tendinopathy is uncertain, because inflammatory mediators may not be present in the tendon, although mediators of pain and inflammation may be increased in the surrounding peritendinous tissues or fluids. Current forms of treatment are based largely on empirical observations, and their effectiveness is in most cases questionable. More clinical and experimental work remains to be done to develop an evidence-based approach to therapy.

REFERENCES

1. Riley GP, Hazleman BL, Speed CA. Tendon and ligament biochemistry and pathology In: Soft tissue rheumatology. Oxford: Oxford University Press, 2004:20-53.
2. Woo SL, Debski RE, Zeminski J, et al. Injury and repair of ligaments and tendons. Annu Rev Biomed Eng 2000;2:83-118.
3. Riley G. The pathogenesis of tendinopathy: a molecular perspective. Rheumatology (Oxford) 2004;43:131-142.
4. Riley G. Tendinopathy—from basic science to treatment. Nat Clin Pract Rheumatol 2008;4:82-89.

5. Schmidt CC, Georgescu HI, Kwoh CK, et al. Effect of growth factors on the proliferation of fibroblasts from the medial collateral and anterior cruciate ligaments. J Orthop Res 1995;13:184-190.
6. Kannus P, Jόzsa L. Histopathological changes preceding spontaneous rupture of a tendon: a controlled study of 891 patients. J Bone Joint Surg Am 1991;73:1507-1525.
7. Benjamin M, Ralphs JR. Fibrocartilage in tendons and ligaments—an adaptation to compressive load. J Anat 1998;193:481-494.

8. Maffulli N, Waterston SW, Squair J, et al. Changing incidence of Achilles tendon rupture in Scotland: a 15-year study. Clin J Sport Med 1999;9:157-160.
9. Mokone GG, Gajjar M, September AV, et al. The guanine-thymine dinucleotide repeat polymorphism within the tenascin-C gene is associated with Achilles tendon injuries. Am J Sports Med 2005;33:1016-1021.
10. Mokone GG, Schwellnus MP, Noakes TD, Collins M. The COL5A1 gene and Achilles tendon pathology. Scand J Med Sci Sports 2006;16:19-26.

11. Riley GP, Harrall RL, Constant CR, et al. Prevalence and possible pathological significance of calcium phosphate salt accumulation in tendon matrix degeneration. Ann Rheum Dis 1996;55:109-115.
12. Fenwick S, Harrall R, Hackney R, et al. Endochondral ossification in Achilles and patella tendinopathy. Rheumatology 2002;41:474-476.
13. Yuan J, Murrell GA, Wei AQ, Wang MX. Apoptosis in rotator cuff tendonopathy. J Orthop Res 2002;20:1372-1379.
14. Lian O, Scott A, Engebretsen L, et al. Excessive apoptosis in patellar tendinopathy in athletes. Am J Sports Med 2007;35:605-611.
15. Cook JL, Feller JA, Bonar SF, Khan KM. Abnormal tenocyte morphology is more prevalent than collagen disruption in asymptomatic athletes' patellar tendons. J Orthop Res 2004;22:334-338.
16. Eriksen HA, Pajala A, Leppilahti J, Risteli J. Increased content of type III collagen at the rupture site of human Achilles tendon. J Orthop Res 2002;20:1352-1357.
17. Riley GP, Harrall RL, Constant CR, et al. Tendon degeneration and chronic shoulder pain: changes in the collagen composition of the human rotator cuff tendons in rotator cuff tendinitis. Ann Rheum Dis 1994;53:359-366.
18. Goncalves-Neto J, Witzel SS, Teodoro WR, et al. Changes in collagen matrix composition in human posterior tibial tendon dysfunction. Joint Bone Spine 2002;69:189-194.
19. de Mos M, van El B, DeGroot J, et al. Achilles tendinosis: changes in biochemical composition and collagen turnover rate. Am J Sports Med 2007;35:1549-1556.
20. Bank RA, TeKoppele JM, Oostingh G, et al. Lysylhydroxylation and non-reducible cross-linking of human supraspinatus tendon collagen: changes with age and in chronic rotator cuff tendinitis. Ann Rheum Dis 1999;58:35-41.
21. Chard MD, Cawston TE, Riley GP, et al. Rotator cuff degeneration and lateral epicondylitis: a comparative histological study. Ann Rheum Dis 1994;35:30-34.
22. Corps AN, Robinson AH, Movin T, et al. Increased expression of aggrecan and biglycan mRNA in Achilles tendinopathy. Rheumatology (Oxford) 2005;45:291-294.
23. Corps AN, Robinson AH, Movin T, et al. Versican splice variant messenger RNA expression in normal human Achilles tendon and tendinopathies. Rheumatology 2004;43:969-972.
24. Scott A, Lian O, Roberts CR, et al. Increased versican content is associated with tendinosis pathology in the patellar tendon of athletes with jumper's knee. Scand J Med Sci Sports 2008;18:427-435.

25. Tillander B, Franzen L, Norlin R. Fibronectin, MMP-1 and histologic changes in rotator cuff disease. J Orthop Res 2002;20:1358-1364.
26. Riley GP, Harrall RL, Cawston TE, et al. Tenascin-C and human tendon degeneration. Am J Pathol 1996;149:933-943.
27. Jones GC, Corps AN, Pennington CJ, et al. Expression profiling of metalloproteinases and tissue inhibitors of metalloproteinases in normal and degenerate human Achilles tendon. Arthritis Rheum 2006;54:832-842.
28. Kawaguchi N, Xu X, Tajima R, et al. ADAM 12 protease induces adipogenesis in transgenic mice. Am J Pathol 2002;160:1895-1903.
29. Clancy BM, Johnson JD, Lambert AJ, et al. A gene expression profile for endochondral bone formation: oligonucleotide microarrays establish novel connections between known genes and BMP-2–induced bone formation in mouse quadriceps. Bone 2003;33:46-63.
30. Archambault J, Tsuzaki M, Herzog W, Banes AJ. Stretch and interleukin-1beta induce matrix metalloproteinases in rabbit tendon cells *in vitro*. J Orthop Res 2002;20:36-39.
31. Arnoczky SP, Tian T, Lavagnino M, Gardner K. *Ex vivo* static tensile loading inhibits MMP-1 expression in rat tail tendon cells through a cytoskeletally based mechanotransduction mechanism. J Orthop Res 2004;22:328-333.
32. Gotoh M, Hamada K, Yamakawa H, et al. Interleukin-1-induced subacromial synovitis and shoulder pain in rotator cuff diseases. Rheumatology 2001;40:995-1001.
33. Kjaer M, Langberg H, Heinemeier K, et al. From mechanical loading to collagen synthesis, structural changes and function in human tendon. Scand J Med Sci Sports 2009;19:500-510.
34. Murphy PG, Loitz BJ, Frank CB, Hart DA. Influence of exogenous growth factors on the synthesis and secretion of collagen types I and III by explants of normal and healing rabbit ligaments. Biochem Cell Biol 1994;72:403-409.
35. Alfredson H, Ohberg L, Forsgren S. Is vasculoneural ingrowth the cause of pain in chronic Achilles tendinosis? An investigation using ultrasonography and colour Doppler, immunohistochemistry, and diagnostic injections. Knee Surg Sports Traumatol Arthrosc 2003;11:334-338.
36. Gotoh M, Hamada K, Yamakawa H, et al. Increased substance P in subacromial bursa and shoulder pain in rotator cuff diseases 10. J Orthop Res 1998;16:618-621.
37. Alfredson H, Forsgren S, Thorsen K, Lorentzon R. *In vivo* microdialysis and immunohistochemical analyses of tendon tissue demonstrated high amounts of free

glutamate and glutamate NMDAR1 receptors, but no signs of inflammation, in jumper's knee. J Orthop Res 2001;19:881-886.
38. Burssens P, Steyaert A, Forsyth R, et al. Exogenously administered substance P and neutral endopeptidase inhibitors stimulate fibroblast proliferation, angiogenesis and collagen organization during Achilles tendon healing. Foot Ankle Int 2005;26:832-839.
39. Alfredson H. Chronic midportion Achilles tendinopathy: an update on research and treatment. Clin Sports Med 2003;22:727-741.
40. Fu SC, Wang W, Pau HM, et al. Increased expression of transforming growth factor-beta1 in patellar tendinosis. Clin Orthop Relat Res 2002;73:174-183.
41. Sullo A, Maffulli N, Capasso G, Testa V. The effects of prolonged peritendinous administration of PGE1 to the rat Achilles tendon: a possible animal model of chronic Achilles tendinopathy. J Orthop Sci 2001;6:349-357.
42. Alfredson H, Pietila T, Jonsson P, Lorentzon R. Heavy-load eccentric calf muscle training for the treatment of chronic Achilles tendinosis. Am J Sports Med 1998;26:360-366.
43. Aspenberg P, Forslund C. Enhanced tendon healing with GDF 5 and 6. Acta Orthop Scand 1999;70:51-54.
44. Duffy FJ Jr, Seiler JG, Gelberman RH, Hergrueter CA. Growth factors and canine flexor tendon healing: initial studies in uninjured and repair models. J Hand Surg [Am] 1995;20:645-649.
45. Molloy T, Wang Y, Murrell G. The roles of growth factors in tendon and ligament healing. Sports Med 2003;33:381-394.
46. Gerich TG, Kang R, Fu FH, et al. Gene transfer to the patellar tendon. Knee Surg Sports Traumatol Arthrosc 1997;5:118-123.
47. Smith RK, Korda M, Blunn GW, Goodship AE. Isolation and implantation of autologous equine mesenchymal stem cells from bone marrow into the superficial digital flexor tendon as a potential novel treatment. Equine Vet J 2003;35:99-102.
48. Awad HA, Butler DL, Boivin GP, et al. Autologous mesenchymal stem cell-mediated repair of tendon. Tissue Eng 1999;5:267-277.
49. Butler DL, Juncosa N, Dressler MR. Functional efficacy of tendon repair processes. Annu Rev Biomed Eng 2004;6:303-329.

REFERENCES

Full references for this chapter can be found on www.expertconsult.com.

Cytokines

John J. O'Shea, John Sims, Richard M. Siegel, and Joshua M. Farber

- Cytokines are critical factors in host defense and immunoregulation.
- Cytokines are key players in autoimmunity and inflammation.
- Cytokines belong to different families and bind structurally distinct receptors.
- Mutation and polymorphisms of cytokines, cytokine receptors, and their signaling pathways are associated with a number of human diseases.
- Targeting cytokines themselves or their signal transduction pathways provides many new opportunities for therapy.

INTRODUCTION

Given the advances in therapy there is no longer a need to convince readers that cytokines play pivotal roles in the pathogenesis of rheumatologic diseases; on the contrary, this area has been one of the most exciting developments in the field, and rheumatologists are well aware of the central role of cytokines. Because of these spectacular developments, the role of the rheumatologist is increasingly that of an "applied immunologist," and other practitioners look to rheumatologists for their expertise in the use of these biologic drugs. However, it is also clear that anti-cytokine therapies are not effective in all patients with a given disease. Furthermore, agents that are efficacious in certain autoimmune disorders are ineffective in others. This suggests different roles of cytokines in various disorders and perhaps subgroups of patients. For all these reasons, it is incumbent on rheumatologists to understand cytokine biology. However, this is a daunting task, given the sheer number of cytokines and the complexity of their actions. In this chapter, our goal is to be reasonably complete but also to provide the reader a conceptual framework for considering the different classes of cytokines. To facilitate the understanding of cytokine action, we provide some details regarding the signal transduction pathways employed by cytokines; however, to try to make the chapter accessible we do not provide an exhaustive discussion of all cytokines and their mechanisms of action.

An additional challenge is that the term *cytokine* does not denote a specific class of structurally or functionally related molecules; on the contrary, many different types of factors produced by immune and non-immune cells can be included in this category of secreted factors. Terms such as *cytokine*, *lymphokine*, *interleukin* (IL), and *interferon* (IFN) have been in use for more than 30 years; however, it is important to recognize the imprecision of the terms and understand that a wide variety of secreted polypeptides can modulate immune and inflammatory responses. Because the problem of intercellular communication is a fundamental problem for homeostasis in all multicellular organisms, the boundary between what we think of as cytokines, growth factors, and hormones is indistinct. For instance, hormones such as growth hormone (GH), prolactin (PRL), erythropoietin (EPO), and leptin are clearly cytokines (see later). Structurally, they are related to interleukins; their receptors are similar and they use the same biochemical pathways to signal. For this reason, it is probably easiest to simply accept that the term *cytokine* is necessarily imprecise and refers to a subset of factors involved in cell-cell communication. Their actions primarily relate to host defense and regulation of immune and inflammatory cells, but evolutionarily these factors are homologous to molecules that influence development and coordinate communication between other tissues and organs.

For this reason, we find it easiest to classify cytokines not by their function but rather by the type of receptor that they bind. This classification is also useful because it reflects the evolutionary relatedness of cytokines, growth factors, and hormones and emphasizes similarities in modes of signal transduction. Thus, we will classify cytokines as following: interleukin (IL)-1, the tumor necrosis factor (TNF), the type I (hematopoietin)/type II (interferon), IL-17, receptor tyrosine kinase, transforming growth factor-β, and chemokine families. In the interest of brevity, cytokines that have important immunologic and inflammatory functions will be stressed; only cursory discussion of other cytokines will be provided.

INTERLEUKIN-1 RECEPTOR FAMILY

Ligand and receptor structure

Cytokines of the IL-1 family are evolutionarily ancient, present in echinoderms, tunicates, and annelids in addition to all species of vertebrates. IL-1 itself is also highly pleiotropic: indeed, the many names this cytokine had before our increasing sophistication led to molecular and nomenclatural consolidation in the 1980s—endogenous pyrogen, osteoclast activating factor, lymphocyte activating factor, leukocyte endogenous mediator, catabolin, and hematopoietin-1—reflect the multiple areas of biology that are profoundly influenced by the actions of IL-1.[1-3]

IL-1 family members form a beta-trefoil structure comprising 12 strands folded into three sheets. These cytokines interact with receptors whose extracellular portions are formed by immunoglobulin domains (typically 3) and whose cytoplasmic domains contain a conserved fold known as the TIR domain. TIR domains are also shared with another important class of molecules in host defense known as Toll-like receptors. Indeed, TIR is an acronym derived from "Toll, IL-1R, plant Resistance genes," all of which contain this ancient fold. The known functional receptor complexes are heterodimeric, such that the cytokine binds its primary receptor subunit (e.g., the IL-1 receptor), which then allows recruitment of a second subunit; in the case of IL-1 itself, the "accessory protein" is required for initiation of signal transduction.

Family members and their action

The IL-1 family consists of 11 members, whereas the IL-1 receptor family has 10 identified members (Figs. 11.1 and 11.2). Most IL-1 family members lack a signal peptide, the exception being IL-1 receptor antagonist (IL-1ra, encoded by *IL1RN*—see later). Most IL-1 family members have prodomains, which, except in the case of IL-1α and IL-33, need to be removed for the cytokine to be biologically active. The prodomains of IL-1β and IL-18 are removed by caspase-1 cleavage within a protein assembly called the inflammasome. Secretion of the active cytokines appears to happen in concert with their cleavage, although the mechanism of how these cytoplasmic molecules are secreted is not well understood. The term *inflammasome* refers to a multiple-protein assembly whose formation results in the activation of caspase-1 and the maturation and secretion of IL-1β and IL-18.[4] There are two key components: caspase-1 itself and a recognition/assembly component that is a so-called NOD-like receptor (NLR). Often another protein called ASC (a simple adapter protein containing both pyrin and CARD domains) is required to facilitate assembly. NLR proteins are intracellular pattern-recognition receptors that contain three domains: a segment with multiple leucine-rich repeats whose role is to recognize the trigger for activation (whether directly or indirectly remains unclear); a portion called a NACHT domain that leads to adenosine

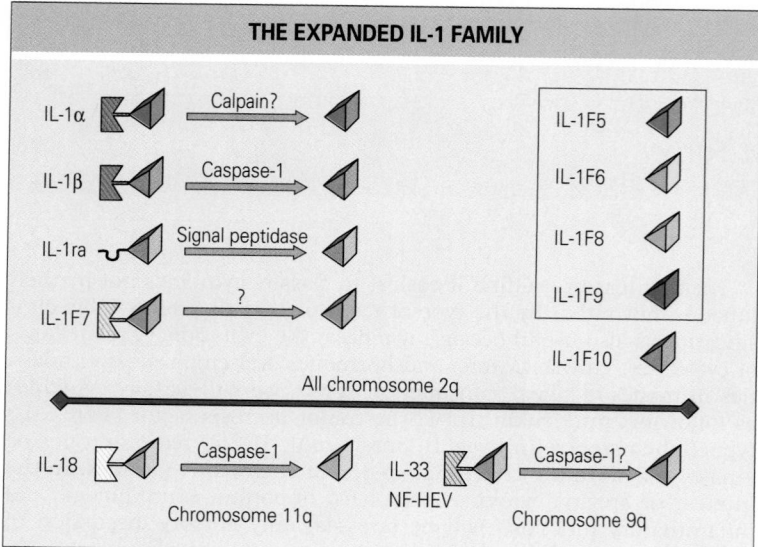

Fig. 11.1 The expanded IL-1 family of cytokines is shown schematically here with the prodomains of each cytokine shown in hatched colors and putative proteases that process the proforms of these cytokines to mature forms indicated as shown. The IL-1 cytokine family has 11 members. IL-1α, IL-1β, IL-18, IL-33, and IL-1F7 have apparent prodomains, although those of IL-1α and IL-33 do not need to be removed for the cytokine to be active. IL-1ra has a signal peptide.

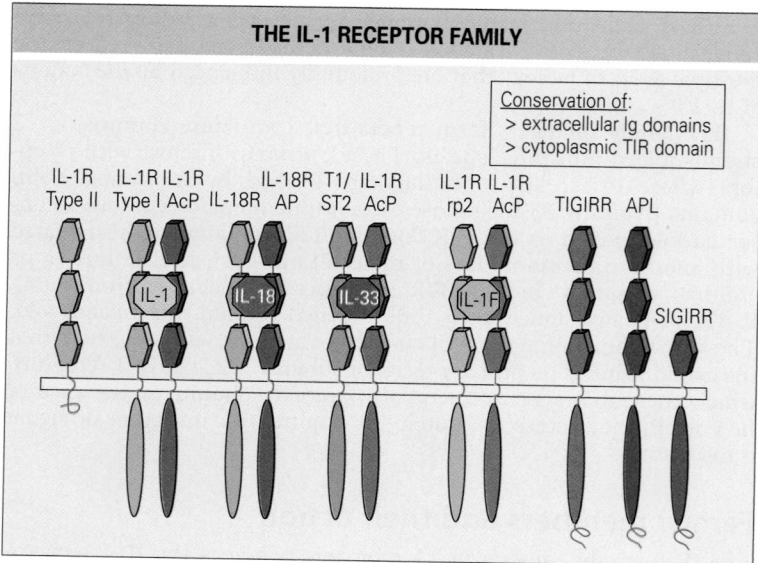

Fig. 11.2 The IL-1 receptor family has 9 members, plus the non-signaling decoy receptor IL-1R type II. All other members have TIR domains cytoplasmically in addition to the extracellular immunoglobulin domains. TIGIRR, APL, and SIGIRR also have an additional 100 to 150 amino acids C-terminal to the TIR domain. IL-1R AcP is shared by the receptors IL-1R type I, IL-1Rrp2, and IL-33R. The receptors that bind members of the IL-1 family are shown schematically here with each subunit of heterodimeric receptors labeled as shown.

triphosphate (ATP)-dependent dimerization of the NLR after trigger recognition; and a protein-protein interaction domain, most commonly either a pyrin or a CARD domain, that recruits caspase-1. The best-studied inflammasome is the so-called NLRP3 inflammasome. Recognition of the trigger by NLRP3 causes its dimerization, recruitment of ASC via interaction of the pyrin domains of NLRP3 and ASC, and subsequent recruitment of caspase-1 via the CARD domains present in both ASC and caspase-1. The dimerization of caspase-1 on inflammasome assembly allows it to autoactivate by cleavage of the proform

to generate active enzyme. The NLRP3 inflammasomes are activated by ATP; components of gram-positive bacterial cell walls, such as muramyl dipeptide; intracytoplasmic DNA, such as occurs during viral infection; molecules resulting from tissue damage, such as hyaluronin fragments; crystals, including those of uric acid (released from necrotic cells), alum (a commonly-used adjuvant); silica and asbestos (environmental contaminants that lead to lung disease); and β-amyloid, a key protein in Alzheimer's disease. Cigarette smoke also leads to activation of caspase-1 in mice, but the mechanism is poorly understood. Mutations in *NLRP3* result in several hereditary periodic fever syndromes, including familial cold autoinflammatory syndrome (FCAS), Muckle-Wells syndrome, and neonatal onset multi-organ inflammatory disease (NOMID; in Europe called chronic infantile, neurologic, cutaneous, articular syndrome [CINCA]). NLRP3 is also called cryopyrin, and these disorders have been collectively referred to as cryopyrinopathies.[5] The consequence of disease-causing mutations is excessive release of IL-1β. Other NLR proteins, including NLRP1, IPAF, and NAIP, assemble into their own inflammasomes, which are triggered by other types of stimuli, such as gram-negative bacteria. Mutations of *NLRP1* are associated with vitiligo. Although IL-1β and IL-18 require cleavage by active caspase-1 to generate their active forms, evidence suggests that the secretion of IL-1α also requires active caspase-1, even though it is not a direct caspase substrate. It is worth noting that although the inflammasome controls production of IL-1 in monocytes and macrophages, IL-1β made by other cells (e.g., neutrophils) is released in its precursor form on cell death and cleaved extracellularly by proteases such as neutrophil protease PR3.

IL-1α and IL-1β

IL-1α and IL-1β are the family members with the most widespread influence. Their biologic activities are identical, although they are made by different cells under different influences. The most abundant sources of IL-1β are monocytes and macrophages. In contrast, IL-1α is made by many types of cells, but keratinocytes and endothelial cells are particularly rich sources. IL-1α often remains associated with the plasma membrane of the cell that produces it, whereas IL-1β is released from cells and diffuses into the surrounding tissue and systemic circulation. The prodomain of IL-1α also has a nuclear localization signal and is thought to influence transcription of certain genes. In general, most of the biology of IL-1 can be rationalized by thinking of it as a coordinator of the early host response to infection or tissue injury. Some of the specific effects of IL-1 on different cell types and organs are discussed next.

IL-1 is strongly induced by pathogens via stimulation of Toll-like receptors on macrophages and other cell types and is strongly induced by tissue damage.[4] IL-1 also induces other inflammatory cytokines, such as TNF and IL-6, which themselves coordinate aspects of the host response, as well as small molecule mediators, including nitric oxide and prostaglandins. IL-1 also induces the synthesis of multiple chemokines (see later), particularly those that attract neutrophils to the site of infection or injury. It also induces adhesion molecules on leukocytes and endothelial cells for the same purpose. Simultaneously, IL-1 promotes release of neutrophils from bone marrow and enhancement of granulopoiesis. In addition, IL-1 enhances adaptive immune responses by increasing the potency with which antigen is presented by monocyte/macrophages and dendritic cells. IL-1 is also a key driver of Th17 cell differentiation (see later) and can also induce Th2 responses. An *IL1B* polymorphism has a large effect on severity of periodontitis. It is noteworthy that most poxviruses have a homolog of the inhibitory IL-1R type II (see later), suggesting that IL-1 plays a role in control of poxvirus infection. Deletion of the IL-1R2 homolog from vaccinia virus leads to greater pathology in mice.

IL-1 is a strong inducer of acute phase proteins, either directly or via induction of IL-6. IL-1 also promotes cartilage destruction by inducing chondrocyte production of aggrecanases and collagenases, and by suppressing the synthesis of new collagen and proteoglycan. It also enhances bone resorption, primarily via induction of RANKL.

IL-1 is a key mediator of injury associated with ischemia and reperfusion, and mouse models demonstrate a significant contribution of IL-1 to atherosclerotic lesion formation.

IL-1 is a potent inducer of fever, through stimulation of central nervous system prostaglandin synthesis. It also causes loss of appetite, enhancement of slow-wave sleep, decrease in energy expenditure, and social withdrawal, a constellation known as "sickness behavior."[6] Inhibition of IL-1 relieves inflammatory and neuropathic pain in rodent models and reverses morphine tolerance. Some of IL-1's effects on pain seem to be mediated via induction of matrix metalloproteinases. Finally, IL-1 also seems to play a role in spatial memory in the hippocampus.

There is evidence linking IL-1 to Alzheimer's disease and stroke. In many animal models, IL-1 inhibition reduces infarct size, probably by preventing recruitment of neutrophils and thus decreasing bystander tissue damage.[7] IL-1 is elevated in Alzheimer's disease brains and induces amyloid precursor protein. In addition, β-amyloid is a trigger for the inflammasome and can induce IL-1. Furthermore, polymorphisms in *IL1A* and *IL1B* alter the risk of developing Alzheimer's disease.

Several hematologic malignancies (multiple myeloma, acute myelocytic leukemia, chronic myelocytic leukemia) constitutively secrete IL-1β, and for early-stage multiple myeloma there is suggestive evidence that IL-1 blockade may reduce the frequency of transition to aggressive disease. Genetic evidence indicates that polymorphisms in *IL1B* and *IL1RN* affect the risk and prognosis of gastric, cervical, pancreatic, and breast cancers. The polymorphisms are thought to increase IL-1β and/or lower IL-1ra levels, contributing to cancer risk by promoting inflammation and cancer progression. These cytokines also induce the secretion of IL-8 and vascular endothelial grown factor (VEGF), which, in turn, promotes angiogenesis.

Negative regulation of IL-1α and IL-1β

The actions of IL-1 are tempered by the actions of a critical natural cytokine antagonist, IL-1 receptor antagonist (IL-1ra) encoded by the *IL1RN* gene. Mutations in *IL1RN* cause a systemic autoinflammatory disease denoted deficiency of IL-1ra (DIRA),[8] and a polymorphism in *IL1RN* is also associated with coronary artery disease and re-stenosis.

A recombinant version of IL-1ra, anakinra, is approved for the treatment of rheumatoid arthritis; however, in most patients the outcome is inferior to treatment with other biologic agents such as TNF inhibitors. By contrast, the systemic-onset form of juvenile idiopathic arthritis (JIA) and its adult counterpart, Still's disease, respond well to IL-1 inhibition. IL-1 inhibition has also been reported to be effective in treatment of cryopyrinopathies, including NOMID, and other autoinflammatory disorders, including Schnitzler's syndrome, Behçet's disease, hyper-IgD syndrome, PAPA (pyogenic arthritis, pyoderma gangrenosum, and acne) syndrome, and TNF receptor–associated periodic syndrome (TRAPS). IL-1 inhibition may also be effective in the treatment of gout.

Early clinical trials suggest that IL-1 inhibition will also be useful in lowering blood glucose and enhancing pancreatic function in type II diabetes.[9] IL-1β is made by the pancreas and at low concentration enhances islet beta cell survival, proliferation, and insulin synthesis. At higher concentrations, which can be induced by elevated glucose levels, IL-1β has cytotoxic effects on islet beta cells. For unknown reasons, in diabetics the pancreatic balance of IL-1β and IL-1ra has shifted in favor of greater agonism. Antagonizing IL-1 is also protective against neointima formation after arterial injury in animal models, and IL-1ra is also being studied in the treatment of stroke.

Rilonacept is a fusion protein containing the extracellular portions of the two IL-1 receptor components IL-1R and AcP, and it has been approved by the U.S. Food and Drug Administration for the treatment of cryopyrinopathies. Other IL-1 antagonists in clinical development include antibodies to IL-1β or to IL-1R.

IL-1 receptor type II is a protein homologous to the IL-1R1, which binds IL-1 but does not signal. The IL-1R2 serves as a decoy receptor to lure IL-1 away from the signaling-competent IL-1R type I. A splice variant of the IL-1 accessory protein, termed *AcPb*, negatively regulates IL-1 responses in the central nervous system. Soluble versions of IL-1R type II and AcP also exist and contribute to negative regulation (in the case of soluble AcP, most likely by competition with full-length AcP for binding to surface IL1/IL-1R complexes). Mice lacking AcPb suffer greater neurodegeneration after a direct inflammatory stimulus to the brain.

Another negative regulator of IL-1 signaling is a cell surface receptor called SIGIRR. SIGIRR-deficient mice have increased susceptibility to infection, asthma, and inflammatory bowel disease and have enhanced signaling by all IL-1 family members that are known agonists (IL-1α and IL-1β, IL-18, IL-33, IL-1F6, F8, and F9). The ST2 receptor may have similar functions.

IL-18

IL-18 is made primarily by dendritic cells and macrophages. Unlike IL-1β, there is a constitutive pool of pro-IL18 in producer cells, so that regulation of secretion is largely determined by inflammasome activation rather than transcription. IL-18 acts to promote Th1 cell activation and enhances the cytotoxic activity of CD8+ T cells and of NK cells by upregulation of FasL.[1] IL-18 is a strong inducer of inflammatory cytokines, especially IFN-γ (its original name was "interferon gamma–inducing factor"). Typically, IL-18 activity is dramatically enhanced by other cytokines, including IL-2, IL-12, IL-15, IL-21, or IL-23. The main reason for the synergy is that IL-18 and the complementing cytokine mutually induce the other's receptors, which normally are expressed at very low levels. In certain circumstances, IL-18 can also lead to induction of Th2 or Th17 cytokines.

IL-18 is elevated in synovium from RA patients and can have a catabolic effect on cartilage. It both induces and is induced by TNF and IL-1. IL-18 is also elevated in inflammatory bowel disease (both Crohn's disease and ulcerative colitis). There is also a connection with vascular disease. After either stroke or myocardial infarction, IL-18 levels are elevated and are correlated with greater extent of atherosclerotic plaque and worse outcome. Individuals carrying an allele in the IL-18 promoter that leads to less IL-18 production have a lower rate of sudden cardiac death. On the other hand, IL-18- or IL-18R-knockout mice, or IL-18bp transgenic animals, all develop a condition similar to human metabolic syndrome (insulin resistance, hyperglycemia, altered lipid metabolism, obesity, and atherosclerosis). Whether this reflects differences between the biology of IL-18 in mice versus humans or is simply a level of complexity greater than we currently understand is not yet clear. The IL-18R is necessary in mice for development of inflammation and emphysema after exposure to cigarette smoke, and levels of IL-18 in the lung are elevated in humans with chronic obstructive pulmonary disease.

The IL-18 receptor (IL-18Rα) and its accessory protein, IL-18Rβ, are both members of the IL-1R family. An entirely separate gene product, IL-18–binding protein (IL-18bp) acts as a decoy receptor that attenuates the actions of IL-18. It circulates with serum levels typically 20 to 30 times greater than IL-18, which is sufficient excess to block any IL-18 activity. Analogous to IL-1R2, poxviruses contain a homolog of the IL-18bp, suggesting a role of IL-18 in controlling viral infection. IL-18bp has been tested in the clinic in psoriasis and rheumatoid arthritis with limited success. Whether this is due to its relatively short half-life or to IL-18 not playing a key role in these diseases is not clear. Antibodies to both IL-18 and IL-18R are in development for several indications by pharmaceutical companies.

Recent evidence suggests the possibility of other ligands in the IL-18 system. IL-18R–deficient mice are reportedly resistant to experimental autoimmune encephalomyelitis (EAE), a model of multiple sclerosis, whereas IL-18 knockout animals are susceptible. On the other hand, IL-18R knockouts have accelerated rejection of transplants and enhanced cytokine production, whereas IL-18 knockouts have the opposite phenotype. Such data suggest the existence of an additional ligand(s) acting through the IL-18R; more work will be required to clarify this picture.

IL-33

IL-33, in contrast to IL-1β and IL-18, is abundant in tissues rather than hematopoietic cells.[1] IL-33 promotes Th2 cell activation and cytokine secretion via a receptor formed by the IL-1R family member IL-33Rα (previously called ST2 or IL-1RL1) and the same AcP used by the IL-1 receptor. In addition, IL-33 promotes survival, maturation, and activation of various cells, including mast cells, eosinophils, basophils, Th2 cells, and NK and NKT cells. Interestingly, the prodomain of IL-33 can bind DNA. Pro-IL33 is localized to the cell nucleus and may serve to affect transcription in endothelial and other cells. It is unclear at present whether processing of full-length IL-33 is required for biologic activity or for release from cells or, indeed, whether it even happens under natural circumstances. If processing does occur, it is unclear what enzyme is responsible, although initial claims that caspase-1 mediates processing seem unlikely. A soluble form of IL-33Rα is generated by alternative splicing and is capable of mediating IL-33 responses. Soluble IL-33Rα levels are elevated in acute asthma attacks compared with stable asthma and are higher in stable asthma than in non-asthmatic individuals. Polymorphisms of IL33RA are associated with asthma incidence and severity and eosinophilia. Soluble IL-33Rα levels are also elevated after myocardial infarction or during destabilized heart failure and are correlated with poor prognosis. Elevated levels of soluble IL-33Rα suggest an attempt by the body, usually unsuccessful, to counteract excessive IL-33 signaling in that disease. In addition to strongly inducing typical Th2 cytokines such as IL-4, IL-5, and IL-13, IL-33 can promote typical Th1 responses such as TNF and IFN-γ production. Accordingly, inhibition of the IL-33/IL-33R pathway is beneficial in mouse models of arthritis.

IL-1F5, IL-1F6, IL-1F8, and IL-1F9

These family members act via a receptor complex formed from the IL-1R homolog IL-1Rrp2 (HUGO nomenclature IL-1RL2) and AcP.[10] They are highly expressed in skin and airway and may be involved in skin diseases such as psoriasis. IL-1F5 serves to antagonize these three ligands in a manner similar to IL-1ra antagonism of IL-1α and IL-1β.

IL-1F7 and IL-1F10

Little is known about these two family members. IL-1F7 has been reported to bind to the IL-18R and IL-18bp. No consequence has been ascribed to IL-18R binding, but the binding of IL-1F7 to IL-18bp reportedly recruits this complex to IL-18Rβ, thereby reducing IL-18 signaling. More generally, IL-1F7 has been suggested to reduce overall levels of inflammatory cytokines produced in response to a variety of stimuli. IL-1F10 has been claimed to bind to IL-1R. The structure of IL-1F10 suggests that it may be an antagonist as well, but there have been no functional studies. IL-1F7 is the only family member that does not have a murine ortholog.

APL and TIGIRR

The remaining members of the IL-1 and IL-1R families are the receptor homologs APL and TIGIRR. Both of these have limited tissue distribution, with TIGIRR found almost exclusively in brain and APL in brain and a small number of other tissues. Nothing is known about the function of TIGIRR or about APL in any organ other than the brain. Most insight into APL has come from the finding that deletions or mutations of this gene cause mental retardation.

Signal transduction

IL-1 signaling is initiated by recruitment of the adapter protein MyD88 to the IL-1R/AcP complex via TIR-TIR domain interactions. MyD88, in turn, recruits the kinase IRAK-4, leading to a chain of protein interactions and complexes that include the molecules IRAK-1 or IRAK-2, Traf6, Tak1, Tab1, and Tab2. This results in activation of the MAP kinases Erk, Jnk, and p38 and the transcription factors NF-κB and AP-1 and related family members. This results in gene induction and mRNA stabilization.[11] PI3 kinase is also activated and contributes via a complementary pathway to the activation of these same MAP kinases and transcription factors. IL-33, IL-1F6, IL-F8, and IL-F9 also activate NF-κB and MAP kinases.

TNF RECEPTOR SUPERFAMILY

Ligand and receptor structure

In the late 1960s, lymphotoxin and TNF were identified as products of lymphocytes and macrophages that mediated lysis of tumor cells. After the cloning of the genes encoding these molecules, it became apparent that they were part of a large gene family.[12] We now know that the TNF family of cytokines and their receptors comprise a structurally related group of molecules that control diverse aspects of cellular function, with a central role in regulation of both adaptive and innate immune responses (Fig. 11.3). The seminal observation that

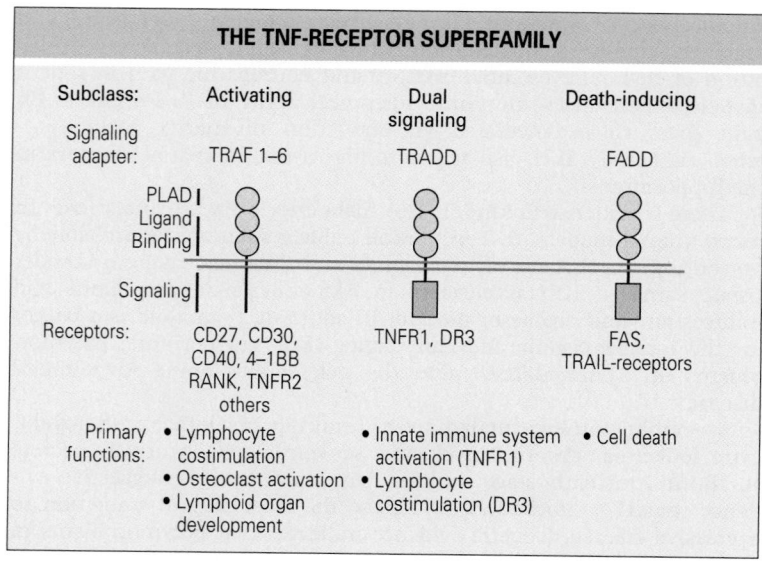

Fig. 11.3 Receptors that bind the tumor necrosis factor (TNF) superfamily cytokines are schematically depicted here, divided into subclasses by the adapter proteins they bind. Key functions for each subclass of receptor are shown at the bottom. Activating receptors induce biologic responses principally through the activation of NF-κB and MAP-kinase signaling pathways initiated by the TRAF (TNF receptor–associated factor) family of adapter proteins. Death-inducing receptors induce cell death principally through activation of caspase-8 through the adapter protein FADD (Fas-associated death domain protein). The dual-signaling class of receptors can activate either cell death or activation through the adapter protein TRADD (TNF receptor–associated death domain protein), which initially interacts with TRAF family proteins and, under certain circumstances, can interact with FADD in a delayed manner to induce cell death.

antibodies to TNF block endotoxic shock in mice paved the way for investigation of TNF blockade in a wide variety of inflammatory conditions, culminating in the widely successful use of TNF-blocking agents in rheumatoid arthritis and other rheumatic diseases. These successes validated TNF family cytokines and receptors as therapeutic targets and led to current studies of blocking the action of other members of the TNF superfamily, which are now coming to fruition with a number of agents in late-stage clinical trials. With such a large number of cytokines and receptors in this family, the translation of knowledge about TNF family cytokines into clinical benefit is only beginning.

Genetically, TNF family members and their receptors are evolutionarily recent, and a case can be made that they co-evolved with the immune system. There are no TNF family members or receptors in single-celled organisms, and in *Drosophila* there is a single TNF ligand, *Eiger*, that binds to a TNFR-like receptor, *Wengen*. In a striking parallel to TNFR1, Wengen can trigger cell death and mediates immunopathology during infection with gram-negative organisms. All TNF-family cytokines are synthesized as type II transmembrane proteins. Despite low primary sequence homology, the structures of all TNF family molecules examined to date share a common "β-jellyroll" structure composed of stacks of beta sheets, with variable loops projecting from the core structure allowing for specificity of interactions between each TNF-family molecule and distinct receptors. The basic structure of TNF-family cytokines whether membrane bound or secreted is a homotrimer stabilized by non-covalent interactions between residues found in the central core of the TNF-homology domain. Lymphotoxin is unique in that it can exist as a heterotrimer composed of one lymphotoxin-α and two lymphotoxin-β subunits. Cleavage by proteases, typically in the metalloprotease family, produces soluble versions of most TNF family cytokines that can circulate systemically, although serum levels of TNF family cytokines are often relatively low and not good biomarkers of their activity.

TNF receptors also share basic structural similarities. The extracellular domains of all TNF-family receptors are composed of variable numbers of cysteine repeat domains (CRD) forming a rod-like structure stabilized by intrachain disulfide bonds. Receptors can have between one and four cysteine-repeat domains, allowing for a large degree of diversity. The relationship between ligands and receptors in the TNF superfamily is not always 1:1. Rather, many TNF family cytokines bind more than one receptor, such as TNF interacting with TNFR1 and TNFR2, and a few receptors, such as TACI, binding more than one ligand (APRIL and BAFF). In all ligand-receptor crystal structures examined to date, the TNF cytokine homotrimer is interdigitated within the receptor chains such that each chain of the ligand makes contact with two chains of the receptor at points within the second and third cysteine-repeat domains of the receptor. This hexameric structure allows for the relatively low affinity of each ligand chain for receptors to be multiplied by the high valency of interactions to result in nanomolar affinities for most TNF-family ligands for their receptors. Interestingly, the N-terminal CRD of receptors containing more than one CRD is not bound by ligand, allowing this domain to participate in homotypic receptor-receptor interactions or interactions between TNF receptors and both pathogen-derived and mammalian molecules outside of the TNF family. These interactions can serve as pathogen entry mediators and also modulate TNFR function.

TNF-family receptor signaling

Unlike many other cytokine receptors, TNF receptors possess no intrinsic kinase activity nor do they stably recruit kinases to their cytoplasmic tails. Instead, TNF receptors signal through the ordered recruitment of a series of signaling complexes that determine the outcome of engagement by their cognate TNF family cytokine ligands.[13] Oligomerization of receptors and downstream signaling proteins is critical for efficient signaling by TNF family receptors, and a number of mechanisms regulate oligomerization of TNF family members.

The majority of TNF family receptors signal through the recruitment of multifunctional adapter proteins termed *TNF receptor–associated factors* (TRAFs). TRAF proteins bind to short consensus sequences in the intracellular tails of the receptors, with the sequence PXQXT (where X is any amino acid) preferentially recruiting TRAFs 1, 2, 3, and 5 and the sequence QXPXEX preferentially recruiting TRAF-6. TRAF proteins are mushroom-shaped homotrimers held together by a coiled-coil "stalk" domain. Each lobe of the TRAF trimer binds one TRAF-interaction motif in the receptor, resulting in a hexameric structure that mirrors the TNF-TNFR complex on the outside of the cell. TRAF6 also interacts with TLRs and IL-1 receptor family members, explaining the more severe phenotype in TRAF6 deficiency. A ring-finger domain in the N-termini of TRAF 2 to 6 allows these proteins to nucleate the assembly of a complex containing the molecules cIAP-1 and cIAP-2, which also contain ring-finger domains.[14] These domains act as E3 ubiquitin ligases to catalyze the addition of K63-linked ubiquitin to many of the components in this signaling complex, including the kinase RIP1 (receptor-interacting protein kinase). RIP1 has multiple functions in TNF-R1 signaling, mediating activation of the NF-κB and p38 MAP kinase signaling pathways, as well as non-apoptotic cell death. Small molecules have been developed that potently alter signal transduction by inactivating some of these molecules. SMAC mimetics, which mimic a short peptide motif in the protein Second Mitochondrial Activator of Caspases (SMAC) that can bind IAP proteins, induce ubiquitin-dependent degradation of IAPs, which potentiates cell death induced by TNF through TNFR1.[15,16] Small molecules termed *necrostatins* bind to RIP1 and inhibit its kinase activity, blocking the ability of RIP1 to induce cell death.[17]

Six TNF-family receptors (Fas, TNFR1, TRAIL receptors 1 and 2, DR6, and EDAR) are termed *death receptors* because of their ability to trigger programmed cell death. The death domain in the cytoplasmic tail of these receptors confers this ability, although the efficiency of cell death induced by these receptors depends on the particular adapter proteins recruited to this domain. The death domain forms a globular structure made up of a knot of six α-helices with multiple protein-protein interaction surfaces. Fas and TRAIL receptors recruit the adapter protein FADD through interactions between death domains present in both proteins. FADD also contains a structurally related domain termed a *death effector domain* that mediates recruitment of

two proteases, caspases 8 and 10, through tandem DEDs at their N-termini. Caspases are cysteinyl proteases defined by their ability to cleave proteins after aspartate residues based on specific tetrapeptide motifs. Caspases can cleave substrates that initiate inflammatory or cell death; and when activated in the signaling complex of TNF receptors, caspases 8 and 10 act as initiator caspases in a cascade of protease activation that amplifies the receptor signal, resulting in efficient death of cells within a few hours after receptor ligation by TNF ligands or agonistic antibodies.[18]

Two TNF-family receptors, TNFR1 and DR3, contain a death domain but combine both apoptotic and non-apoptotic signaling through the recruitment of the adapter protein TRADD. TRADD contains a death domain that mediates recruitment to the death domains of these receptors. However, rather than a death-effector domain, TRADD contains a TRAF-recruitment sequence in its N-terminus, allowing it to recruit TRAF1 and TRAF2, and secondarily cIAP-1, cIAP-2, and RIP, to the primary receptor signaling complex. This signaling complex functions similarly to that recruited by the non–death-domain–containing members of the TNF receptor family. However, after receptor internalization, TRADD dissociates from the receptor and nucleates a second signaling complex containing FADD and caspase-8. Normally, NF-κB upregulates antiapoptotic molecules such as c-FLIP, which blocks caspase-8 activation in "complex-2," but if NF-κB is blocked, caspase-8 becomes activated and initiates apoptosis. It remains to be seen when TNFR1-mediated apoptosis occurs in primary cells, because in those cells TNF-TNFR1 interactions primarily promote production of proinflammatory cytokines and cell death is rarely observed. EDARADD, the adapter protein recruited by the death domain of EDAR, also contains a TRAF recruitment domain and primarily activates NF-κB.

Although these signaling pathways are common to the receptor superfamily, a large number of regulatory mechanisms allow each TNF family ligand to perform distinct functions that can be quite specialized. Expression of TNF family ligands and receptors are under tight control to produce highly dynamic patterns of expression. The subcellular localization and cleavage of TNF family ligands is also regulated, and both TNF family ligands and receptors can be cleaved by proteases to produce soluble forms. Genetically related "decoy receptors" can block signaling through binding to a number of ligands and receptors and may themselves initiate "reverse signaling" on engagement with their receptors. Signaling pathways triggered by other cytokines, environmental factors, or genetic programs allow many TNF family receptors to perform more than one function even in the same cell type, for example, switching from cell death induction to inducing protection from cell death. Not surprisingly, a number of pathogens have evolved proteins that modulate signaling through TNF receptors in a number of interesting ways. Studies with knockout mice and blocking or agonistic agents that affect the function of specific TNF-TNFR interactions as well as genetic diseases stemming from mutations in genes coding for TNF cytokines and their receptors have provided a wealth of knowledge about the functions of TNF family cytokines in the intact immune system.

TNFR family members and their actions

TNF cytokines can be categorized into subgroups according to their function. The lymphotoxin-β receptor (LTβR) and RANK share the property of being important for development of lymphoid structures in the spleen and lymph nodes. Secondary lymphoid structures such as lymph nodes, the white pulp of spleen, and Peyer's patches are induced by the seeding of tissue with specialized bone marrow–derived cells termed *lymphoid-tissue inducer (LTi) cells*. LTα1β2 heterotrimer produced by LTi cells acts through the LTβ receptor on surrounding non-hematopoietic stromal cells to begin this process. In response to lymphotoxin, stromal cells upregulate chemokines and integrins essential for attracting and binding lymphocytes and also secrete RANKL, a TNF family member that, in turn, can act on LTi cells to enhance lymphotoxin expression, perpetuating this cycle. This regulatory circuit for lymphoid tissue was discovered through mouse knockout studies, which showed that mice lacking LTα, LTβ, or LTβ receptors have no lymph nodes, spleen germinal centers, or Peyer's patches. Mice lacking

RANK or RANKL still have lymph nodes but no spleen dendritic cells or Peyer's patches. Lymphotoxin may have distinct functions in the peripheral immune system. LT-LTβ receptor interactions are essential for the ability of dendritic cells to migrate to and proliferate in lymph nodes. Ectopic expression of LTβ promotes "tertiary" lymphoid tissue at sites of inflammation in animal models and a number of disease states.

TNF acting through TNFR1 is a key amplifier of innate inflammatory responses and septic shock. Local injection of TNF produces acute inflammation, and mice deficient in TNF or TNFR1 are defective in innate immune responses to bacteria but resistant to endotoxic shock. Transgenic mice overexpressing TNF develop multiple-organ inflammatory pathology. However, this pathology of TNF in transgenic mice is independent of T and B cells, suggesting that once TNF is produced its actions are primarily on cells of the innate immune system.[19] In rheumatoid arthritis, myeloid cells are the likely source of TNF production, but signals from activated T cells are likely to be important in inducing TNF production within the inflamed joint. Abundant evidence from both mouse and human studies have shown that TNF is a key "master cytokine" in the inflammatory cascade. Patients with RA have elevated levels of TNF-α in their synovial fluid,[20] and TNF levels in synovial fluid correlate with bone erosions. The efficacy of TNF blockade in reducing inflammatory activity and erosions in RA has borne out these correlations.

A third group of TNF family members mediates co-stimulation for lymphocytes and other cells of the immune system. Co-stimulatory signals synergize with TCR and BCR signals on lymphocytes and TLR signals on innate immune cells to enhance the functions of these primary stimuli. Germinal center formation and subsequent B-cell class switching is dependent on interactions between CD40L (CD154) on T cells and CD40 on B cells. CD40L co-stimulation is also important for dendritic cell maturation. CD40L-deficient mice or humans lack germinal centers and have severe defects in B-cell responses (hyper-IgM syndrome). BAFF (also known as BLys) derived from dendritic cells is an additional survival and differentiation factor for germinal center B cells expressing the BAFF receptor. BlyS also binds TACI, which provides additional co-stimulatory signals for B-cell class switching. About 10% of cases of common variable immunodeficiency have been linked to loss of function mutations in TACI. Overexpression of BAFF can induce systemic autoimmunity, and BAFF blockade can inhibit disease in animal autoimmune models. Interestingly, unlike most autoimmune disease models, autoantibody production mediated by BAFF overexpression is independent of T-cell help.[21] Another group of TNF receptors mediates co-stimulation for T cells. This large group of receptors includes DR3, 4-1 BB, HVEM, GITR, TNFR2, CD30, OX40, CD27, and their cognate ligands. Mice deficient for these receptors are defective in specific aspects of T-cell responses, and GITR and TNFR2 may play a role in counteracting suppression mediated by regulatory T cells.[22] Mice lacking DR3, OX40, and CD27 are resistant to a number of T cell–dependent autoimmune disease models, and preclinical and clinical development is underway for blocking agents aimed at these targets.[23,24]

TNF receptors containing death domains that recruit FADD are particularly efficient at triggering programmed cell death. Fas (also known as CD95) triggers programmed cell death in a number of cell types. For T cells, this occurs when activated cells are re-stimulated through the antigen receptor, which triggers both FasL gene synthesis and increased sensitivity to the apoptotic effect of Fas ligation, a process known as re-stimulation–induced cell death (RICD). *In vivo*, this cellular suicide mechanism acts to limit expansion of chronically re-stimulated T cells such as those that recognize ubiquitous self-antigens. This pathway can also be experimentally triggered through repetitive doses of antigen, which has been shown to eliminate autoreactive T cells in mouse models of multiple sclerosis. The importance of Fas/FasL interactions in maintaining immunologic self-tolerance is illustrated by the development of systemic autoimmune disease in Fas-deficient mice and humans harboring dominant-negative mutations in Fas associated with the autoimmune lymphoproliferative syndrome (ALPS). The exquisite sensitivity of chronically activated lymphocytes to Fas-mediated apoptosis may allow strategies to specifically eliminate autoreactive lymphocytes through Fas, although systemic administration of anti-Fas antibodies induces hepatocyte apoptosis and significant liver toxicity in animal models. Receptors for

the TNF-family cytokine TRAIL mediate efficient cell death in tumor cells, but the role of TRAIL in non-transformed cells seems much more restricted. CD8 cells may express TRAIL and undergo TRAIL-mediated autocrine cell death when CD4 T cell help is lacking. However, a non-redundant role for TRAIL in the human immune system has not been clearly identified.

Finally, a group of TNF family receptors mediates development and function of non-immune cells. The TNF-receptor RANK is expressed on osteoclasts and is essential for osteoclast function, as shown by the osteopetrosis seen in RANK or RANKL deficiency, in both mice and humans. In experimental arthritis models, RANKL is expressed by activated CD4 T cells and is important in causing bone erosions. The TNF family receptor EDAR mediates formation of teeth and sweat glands, and ectodermal dysplasias characterized by impaired formation of these structures result from loss of function mutations in EDAR.

TYPE I AND II CYTOKINE RECEPTORS—HEMATOPOIETIN AND INTERFERON RECEPTORS

Cytokines that bind the class of receptors termed the *type I or hematopoietic cytokine receptor superfamily* include hormones such as GH and EPO, colony-stimulating factors (CSF), and many interleukins. Closely related are the interferons, interferon-related cytokines, and IL-10 family cytokines, which bind *type II receptors*. The ligands that bind this receptor superfamily are structurally similar and referred to as the α-helical bundle cytokine family. Structurally, the type I family receptors have a conserved Trp-Ser-X-Trp-Ser motif (where X indicates any amino acid) in their extracellular domains, a single transmembrane domain, and divergent cytoplasmic domains; nonetheless, they utilize the same mode of signal transduction (Fig. 11.4).[25] Some cytokine receptors, such as the EPO and GH receptors, exist as homodimers.

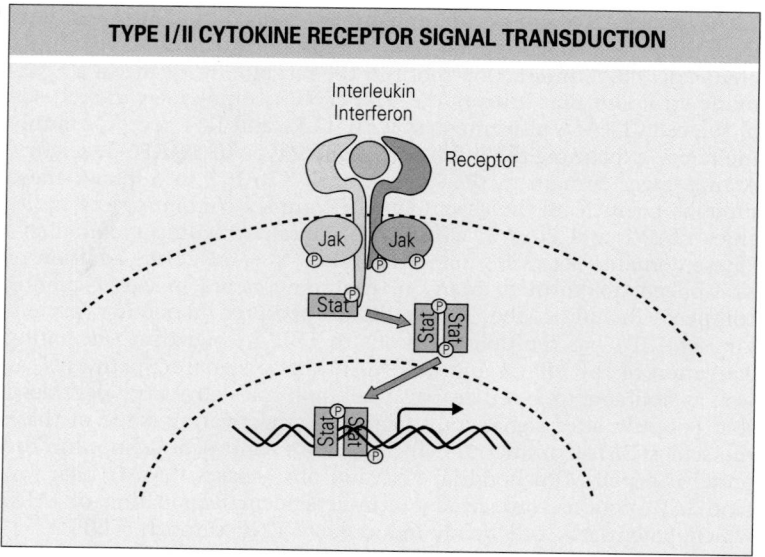

TYPE I/II CYTOKINE RECEPTOR SIGNAL TRANSDUCTION

Fig. 11.4 Cytokine signal transduction. Type I and II cytokine receptors, which bind many cytokines, interleukins, interferons, and colony-stimulating factors, associate with a small family of protein tyrosine kinases known as Janus kinases or Jaks (Jak1, Jak2, Jak3, and Tyk2). Cytokine-binding activates Jaks, which, in turn, phosphorylate cytokine receptors, allowing STAT (signal transducer and activator of transcription) family DNA-binding proteins to dock to cytokine receptors and become phosphorylated. Activated STATs dimerize, translocate to the nucleus, and regulate gene expression. Mutations of *JAK3* underlie autosomal severe combined immunodeficiency. Mutations of *TYK2* are associated with autosomal recessive hyperimmunoglobulin E syndrome (HIES), whereas mutations of *STAT3* result in autosomal dominant HIES or Job's syndrome. Mutations of *STAT1* are associated with atypical mycobacterial infections, and polymorphisms of *STAT4* are linked with susceptibility to systemic lupus erythematosus, rheumatoid arthritis, and Sjögren's syndrome.

However, many cytokines bind receptors that contain two distinct subunits, one of which is often shared by other cytokines. Based on this characteristic, the type I family of receptors can be divided into subfamilies (Tables 11.1 and 11.2).

CYTOKINES THAT USE gp130: IL-6 AS A PROTOTYPE

The shared receptor subunit designated gp130 is a receptor component for a variety of cytokines, including IL-6, IL-11, IL-27, IL-31, leukemia inhibitor factor (LIF), oncostatin M, ciliary neurotrophic factor, and cardiotropin-1. From a rheumatologist's point perspective, IL-6 is the most important cytokine in this subfamily.

The IL-6 receptor (IL-6R) consists of an 80-kDa IL-6–binding protein (α chain) (CD126) and gp130 (CD130). IL-6 is an inducer of febrile and acute phase responses, stimulating production of fibrinogen, serum amyloid A, haptoglobin, C-reactive protein, and complement proteins in the liver. IL-6 decreases synthesis of albumin and transferrin and induces production of hepcidin and thereby contributes to the pathogenesis of anemia of chronic disease. IL-6 is an inducer of IL-17 production and T-helper-17 (Th17) differentiation.[26] IL-6 is a growth and differentiation factor for B cells, inducing immunoglobulin production including IgA. IL-6 also promotes catabolism, induces insulin resistance, and plays a role in osteoporosis by enhancing osteoclast function.

IL-6 is produced by a wide range of cell types, including T cells, macrophages, adipocytes, and muscle cells. It is induced by other

TABLE 11.1 SELECTED HUMAN TNF FAMILY RECEPTORS

Common name(s)	Gene symbol	Chromosomal location	Binds to ligand(s)*	Primary adapter protein	Key functions	Disease and therapeutic associations
Lymph node development						
Lymphotoxin beta receptor (LTβR)	TNFRSF3	12p13	LIGHT (14), LTβ (3)	TRAF	Lymphoid organ formation	Blocking antibodies have been used in clinical trial for RA
Receptor activator of NF-κB (RANK)	TNFRSF11A	18q22.1	RANKL (11)	TRAF	Lymphoid organ formation, dendritic cell co-stimulation, osteoclast maturation and activation	Blocking anti-RANKL (Denosumab) in trial for cancer-associated bone lesions and osteoporosis. Familial osteolytic lesions associated with activating mutations in RANK
Inflammation						
Tumor necrosis factor receptor 1 (TNF-R1), p55, CD120A	TNFRSF1A	12p13.2	TNF-α (2), LTα (1)	TRADD	Mediates TNF-induced inflammation by acting on myeloid cells and non-hematopoietic cells such as hepatocytes (and apoptosis in some cells)	Periodic fever syndrome (TRAPS) associated with heterozygous extracellular mutations. Multiple biologic agents (anti-TNF, TNFR2Fc) effective in RA, spondyloarthropathies, inflammatory bowel disease
Lymphocyte co-stimulation						
Tumor necrosis factor receptor 2 (TNF-R2), p75, CD120b	TNFRSF1B	1p36.3-p36.2	TNF-α (2), LTα (1)	TRADD	CD8 T cell co-stimulation	
OX40, CD134	TNFRSF4	1p36	OX40L (4)	TRAF	T-cell co-stimulation	Anti-OX40L in trials for asthma and other diseases
CD27	TNFRSF7	12p13	CD27L (7)	TRAF	T-cell co-stimulation	Blocking anti-CD70 in development for autoimmune and inflammatory diseases
CD30	TNFRSF8	1p36	CD30L (8)	TRAF	? Inhibition of CD8 T-cell effector function	Agonistic anti-CD30 in trials for cancer immunotherapy
4-1BB, CD137	TNFRSF9	1p36	4-1BBL (9)	TRAF	T-cell co-stimulation	
Herpesvirus entry mediator (HVEM)	TNFRSF14	1p36.3-p36.2	LIGHT (14), herpesviruses	TRAF	T-cell co-stimulation	
Glucocorticoid-induced TNF receptor (GITR)	TNFRSF18	1p36.3	GITRL (18)	TRAF	T-cell co-stimulation, marker for CD4(+)CD25(+) Treg cells, modulates Treg function	
Death receptor 3 (DR3)	TNFRSF25	1p36.2	TL1A (15)	TRADD	T-cell co-stimulation, secondary T cell responses	
CD40	TNFRSF5	20q12-q13.2	CD40L (5)	TRAF	Co-stimulation and differentiation of B cells and APC	Hyper-IgM syndrome associated with CD40L or CD40 mutations. Blocking anti-CD40L used for systemic lupus erythematosus in trials but associated with thrombosis
TACI	TNFRSF13B	17p11.2	APRIL (13), BAFF (13B)	TRAF	May inhibit some of the pro-survival effects of BAFF-R	~10 % of common variable immunodeficiency
BAFF receptor (BAFF-R)	TNFRSF13C	22q13.1-q13.31	BAFF/BlyS (13B)	TRAF		Anti-BAFF in clinical trials for SLE

TABLE 11.1 SELECTED HUMAN TNF FAMILY RECEPTORS—cont'd

Common name(s)	Gene symbol	Chromosomal location	Binds to ligand(s)*	Primary adapter protein	Key functions	Disease and therapeutic associations
Apoptosis						
Fas, CD95	TNFRSF6	10q24.1	FasL (6)	FADD	Apoptosis (chronically stimulated T cells, B cells, dendritic cells, and others)	Autoimmune lymphoproliferative syndrome (ALPS) associated with heterozygous dominant-interfering mutations
Decoy receptor 3	TNFRSF6B	20q13.3	FasL (6), TL1A (15), LIGHT (14)	NA	Soluble decoy receptor for FasL, LIGHT, and TL1A. May have a role in tumor immune evasion	
Death receptor 4 (DR4), TRAIL Receptor 1	TNFRSF10A	8p21	TRAIL (10)	FADD	Mediator of dendritic cell and tumor cell apoptosis	TRAIL and agonistic anti-TRAIL-R antibodies in trials for cancer
Death receptor 5 (DR5)	TNFRFRSF10B	8p22-p21	TRAIL (10)	FADD	Mediator of dendritic cell and tumor cell apoptosis	TRAIL and agonistic anti-TRAIL-R antibodies in trials for cancer
Decoy receptor 1, TRAIL R3	TNFRSF10C	8p22-p21	TRAIL (10)	NA	GPI-linked decoy receptor, interferes with TRAIL function	
Decoy receptor 2, TRAIL-R4	TNFRSF10D	8p21	TRAIL (10)	NA	Transmembrane decoy receptor, interferes with TRAIL function	

*The number in parentheses refers to the gene symbol number for the TNF family cytokine ligand e.g. (6) is for TNFSF6.

TABLE 11.2 CHARACTERISTICS OF MAJOR CYTOKINE FAMILIES

Subfamily	Cytokine	Major sources	Actions
gp130 using cytokines	IL-6	Many cells: T cells, macrophages, adipocytes, and other non-immune cells	Fever, acute phase response, anemia of chronic disease, catabolism, osteoporosis, B-cell growth factor, Th17 differentiation
β_c using cytokines	IL-3	T cells	Growth of hematopoietic precursors, macrophages, mast cells, and megakaryocytes
	IL-5	Th2 cells, mast cells	Eosinophil survival and differentiation
	GM-CSF	T cells, macrophages, mast cells, and endothelial and other cells	Myelomonocytic differentiation
γ_c using cytokines	IL-2	Activated T cells, dendritic cells	Autocrine T cell growth factor, induces IFN-γ, NK cytotoxicity, promotes CD8 memory, induces Foxp3 in Treg cells, B-cell class switching
	IL-4	Th2 cells, NK T cells, dendritic cells, mast cells, and basophils	Th2 differentiation, B-cell class switching, growth factor for mast cells and basophils
	IL-7	Marrow and thymic stromal cells	T-cell development and homeostasis
	IL-9	Th9 cells, mast cells, basophils	Mast cell growth
	IL-15	Mononuclear and other cells	CD8 memory, NK-cell development
	IL-21	Th17 cells, follicular helper T cells	Th17 differentiation, B-cell differentiation and class switching
Homodimeric receptors	Growth hormone	Pituitary gland	Body growth, increased muscle mass and bone density, anabolic effects
	Erythropoietin	Kidney endothelial cells	Erythroid development and survival
Heterodimeric cytokines	IL-12	Dendritic cells	Th1 differentiation, IFN-γ production
	IL-23	Dendritic cells	Th17 cell survival
	IL-27	Dendritic cells	Immunosuppressive, anti-inflammatory
	IL-35	Treg cells	Immunosuppressive
Interferons	Interferon α and β	Plasmacytoid dendritic cells, widely expressed	Anti-viral effects, upregulate MHC Class I, increase NK cytotoxicity
	Interferon γ	Th1 cells, NK cells	Promote Th1 differentiation, increase NK and CD8 cytotoxicity, activate macrophages, B-cell class switching
IL-10 family	IL-10	T cells, other immune cells	Anti-inflammatory

cytokines, including IL-1, TNF, or microbial products. Produced in response to infection, inflammation, and trauma, circulating levels of IL-6 are detectable in serum. Patients with rheumatoid arthritis, cardiac myxoma, Castleman's disease, and other autoimmune diseases have high levels of IL-6 in their sera. Targeting IL-6 using a monoclonal antibody directed against IL-6R (tocilizumab) is efficacious in the treatment of RA, systemic juvenile idiopathic arthritis, and Takayasu's arteritis.[27] LIF is important for blastocyst implantation and the maintenance of stem cell pluripotency in culture. IL-31 is produced by Th2 cells, and overexpression results in atopic dermatitis. IL-27 also signals through gp130 but is a heterodimeric cytokine (see later).

CYTOKINE RECEPTORS UTILIZING THE β$_c$ CHAIN: IL-3, IL-5, AND GM-CSF

The cytokines IL-3, IL-5, and granulocyte-macrophage colony-stimulating factor (GM-CSF) all bind to receptors that share a common β$_c$ receptor subunit (CD131) and also have a ligand-specific α-subunit. IL-3 synergizes with other cytokines to stimulate the growth of immature hematopoietic progenitors. It also promotes survival of macrophages, mast cells, and megakaryocytes. IL-5 promotes the differentiation of eosinophils and thereby contributes to the pathogenesis of allergic disease. GM-CSF promotes myelomonocytic differentiation but also increases microbicidal activity of myeloid cells.

CYTOKINE RECEPTORS UTILIZING THE γ$_c$ CHAIN: IL-2, IL-4, IL-7, IL-9, IL-15, AND IL-21

IL-2, IL-4, IL-7, IL-9, IL-15, and IL-21 all bind to receptors that share the gamma common chain or γ$_c$ (CD132) in association with a ligand-specific subunit. Mutation of the gene encoding γ$_c$ causes X-linked severe combined immunodeficiency (X-SCID), characterized by lack of T cells, NK cells, and poorly functioning B cells.

The IL-2 receptor consists of three subunits: α (CD25), β (CD122), and γ$_c$. T cells, B cells, and other immune cells have inducible expression of the IL-2Rα subunit, which creates a high affinity receptor for IL-2. IL-2 is produced principally by activated T cells and is a prototypical autocrine T-cell growth factor. It augments the cytolytic activity of T and NK cells and induces IFN-γ secretion. IL-2 is also important for CD8+ memory cells. Interestingly, mutation of the genes encoding IL-2 or its receptor results in autoimmune and lymphoproliferative disease.[28] Polymorphisms of IL-2 are associated with type 1 diabetes and other autoimmune diseases. This is thought to be due to impaired expression of the transcription factor Foxp3 and impaired development and function of Treg cells. IL-2 contributes to class switching in B cells and activates macrophages. IL-2 is approved for the treatment of renal cell carcinoma and has been used to boost CD4 T-cell counts in human immunodeficiency virus (HIV) infection, but its clinical utility is limited by toxicities, including hepatic dysfunction and vascular leak syndrome. Anti–IL-2Rα monoclonal antibodies such as daclizumab and basiliximab are approved for use in allograft rejection but are also being studied in the setting of autoimmunity.

The β and γ$_c$ subunits of the IL-2 receptor can bind another cytokine, IL-15. IL-15 is critical for NK cell development and in the generation of memory T cells. IL-15 is produced by hematopoietic and non-hematopoietic cells, and high levels of IL-15 have been associated with several autoimmune diseases while monoclonal anti–IL-15 antibody is being tested in rheumatoid arthritis.

There are two types of IL-4 receptors: one consisting of IL-4Rα and γ$_c$ and a second comprising IL-4Rα and IL-13R. The former is predominantly expressed on hematopoietic cells. IL-4 promotes allergic response and differentiation of naive CD4+ T cells into a subset that produces IL-4 and IL-5. These cells are denoted as T-helper-2 (Th2) cells. IL-4 also promotes B-cell proliferation and class switching, particularly to IgG$_1$ and IgE. With GM-CSF, IL-4 is also a growth factor for mast cells and basophils. IL-4 inhibits macrophages and the production of proinflammatory cytokines. IL-4 is made by the Th2 subset of CD4+ T cells, NK1.1 CD4+ T cells, basophils, and mast cells. The second receptor is more broadly expressed; consequently, IL-13 has actions on many different types of cells and can promote fibrosis.

The IL-7 receptor consists of the IL-7Rα chain (CD127) in association with γ$_c$. It is expressed on both immature and mature thymocytes. Humans with mutations of IL-7Rα have severe combined immunodeficiency characterized by absence of T and B cells (T(−)B+ SCID).[29] IL-7 is also important for memory T cells. IL-7 is produced by a wide variety of cells, including marrow and thymic stromal cells. TSLP is an IL-7–like cytokine expressed by epithelial cells and keratinocytes. Its receptor comprises TSLPR and IL-7Rα, which is expressed primarily on monocytes and dendritic cells, as well as on B cells. TSLP seems to promote Th2 differentiation through its effects on dendritic cells. Polymorphisms of IL7R are associated with multiple sclerosis.

IL-9 synergizes with stem cell factor (SCF) to promote the growth and differentiation of mast cells, and it is a potent regulator of mast cell function. IL-9 also potentiates IgE production induced by IL-4. IL-9 seems to be produced by a subset of T cells, induced by IL-4 and TGF-β1.[30]

IL-21 binds to a receptor composed of the IL-21 α-chain and γ$_c$. IL-21 is produced by Th17 cells and by follicular helper T (Tfh) cells.[31] In T cells, IL-21 promotes Th17 differentiation. It also acts with IL-4 to activate B cells and induce class switching. IL-21 drives the differentiation of B cells into memory cells and terminally differentiated plasma cells.

HOMODIMERIC RECEPTORS

Many of the cytokines that use homodimeric receptors are classic hormones, including the factors GH, PRL, and leptin. EPO is included in this subfamily and is required for erythrocyte growth and development. Similarly, thrombopoietin (TPO) is required for megakaryocytic development. These recombinant cytokines are commonly used drugs.

HETERODIMERIC CYTOKINES

A small number of cytokines are structurally distinct in that they are heterodimers; this family includes IL-12, IL-23, IL-27, and IL-35. These heterodimers consist of one subunit that is homologous to other cytokines and another that is homologous to cytokine receptors. For instance, IL-12 has two subunits, p35 and p40. IL-12 p35 shares homology with cytokines, whereas p40 resembles the IL-6 receptor. Thus, these cytokines can be thought of as a preformed ligand/receptor complex. The receptor for IL-12 consists of two subunits, IL-12Rβ1 and IL-12Rβ2, which are present on T and NK cells. A major action of IL-12 is to promote the differentiation of naive helper T cells to the Th1 subset that makes IFN-γ. Humans with IL-12R mutations have blunted immune responses and are susceptible to infections by intracellular pathogens. In contrast, IL-23 is composed of p19 and IL-12 p40 and its receptor consists of IL-12Rβ1 chain paired with the IL-23R.[32] This receptor is expressed on activated T cells and NK T cells, and IL-23 promotes the production of IL-17. As a result, IL-23 is very important for host defense against extracellular bacteria and the pathogenesis of autoimmune and autoinflammatory disorders.[33] Dendritic cells and macrophages produce IL-12 and IL-23 in response to occupancy of pattern recognition receptors. Polymorphisms of the gene encoding IL-23R are associated with inflammatory bowel disease, spondyloarthropathy, and multiple sclerosis.[34] Ustekinumab targets the shared p40 subunit of IL-12 and IL-23 and has efficacy in inflammatory bowel disease and psoriasis but, interestingly, not multiple sclerosis.[26,35]

IL-27 is composed of two subunits, designated EBI3 and p28. It signals through a receptor comprising gp130 and WSX-1/TCCR (T cell cytokine receptor), which is expressed on naïve CD4+ T cells. IL-27 can promote Th1 differentiation but also has critical Th1 anti-inflammatory properties. An important effect of IL-27 is to induce production of the anti-inflammatory cytokine IL-10.[36] IL-35 is another dimeric cytokine consisting of EBI3 and p19; it is produced by regulatory T cells and appears to be another immunosuppressive cytokine, but the nature of its receptor has not been elucidated.[37]

INTERFERONS

The type I interferons include IFN-α, IFN-ω, and IFN-β; however, there are at least 14 separate IFN-α genes. All these ligands bind to a heterodimeric receptor composed of two subunits—IFNAR1 and IFNAR2—and, therefore, have similar actions. Discovered more than 50 years ago, the major effect of type I interferons is their antiviral action, inhibiting viral replication, protein translation, and cellular proliferation.[38] They also upregulate major histocompatibility complex (MHC) class I expression, downregulate MHC class II expression, and increase the cytolytic activity of NK cells.

Type I interferons are produced ubiquitously, being induced by viral and bacterial infections. A subset of dendritic cells, plasmacytoid dendritic cells, produce especially high levels of IFNs. Type I IFN is used clinically in the treatment of viral hepatitis and leukemia. IFN-β has also been used as an immunosuppressant in the treatment of multiple sclerosis. The IFN signature of gene expression changes is now a well-recognized characteristic of systemic lupus erythematosus, and therapeutic use of type I IFNs has also been associated with the appearance of antinuclear antibodies and the development/exacerbation of autoimmune disease. Blocking type I IFN is currently being tested in systemic lupus erythematosus.

IFN-γ, also known as type II IFN, binds to a dimeric receptor composed of IFNγRα and IFNγRβ subunits. IFN-γ is a major activator of macrophages, enhancing their ability to kill microorganisms. It induces nitric oxide and upregulates MHC class II expression. IFN-γ acts on CD4 T cells to promote Th1 differentiation and inhibit Th2 cell differentiation. It augments NK and CD8 T cell cytolytic activity. In B cells, it promotes switching to IgG$_{2a}$ and IgG$_3$ and inhibits switching to IgG$_1$ and IgE.

IFN-γ is produced primarily by Th1 and NK cells. Humans with mutations of IFNγR subunits are also susceptible to mycobacterial and *Salmonella* infections.[38] Conversely, IFN-γ has been used to treat patients with immunodeficiencies (e.g., chronic granulomatous disease) and disseminated mycobacterial infections. Clinical use of IFN-γ can be associated with production of autoantibodies and a lupus-like syndrome. A monoclonal anti–IFN-γ antibody, fontolizumab, was tested in RA, but the trial was terminated. Other interferon-like cytokines including IL-28A, IL-28B, and IL-29 (also designated IFNλ1, -λ2 and -λ3) have been identified, but their exact functions are less well understood.

The IL-10 receptor consists of two chains, IL-10R1 and IL-10R2. It is a critical immunosuppressive cytokine; mice lacking this cytokine have autoimmunity and inflammatory bowel disease. IL-10 inhibits production of inflammatory cytokines and decreases expression of MHC class II, adhesion molecules, and the co-stimulatory molecules. IL-10 is produced by a wide variety of immune cells and is induced by IL-6, LPS, and TNF. Levels of IL-10 are present in the blood of patients with septic shock and other inflammatory and immune disorders. IL-22 also binds to IL-10R2 but also uses another receptor, termed the IL-22R. It is produced by Th17 cells but is also made by non-conventional NK cells (NKp44/46+). It is important for host defense in the gut but also has critical anti-inflammatory effects. It is also involved in the pathogenesis of psoriasis. Other IL-10–related cytokines include IL-19, IL-20, IL-24, and IL-26 but their biologic actions are less well understood and have considerable sharing of receptors.[39]

Signaling by type I/II cytokine receptors

Type I and II receptors have no intrinsic enzymatic activity but instead are associated Janus kinases (JAKs), which play a pivotal role in signaling via this family of cytokine receptors (see Chapter 13).[25] There are four JAKs—JAK1, JAK2, JAK3, and TYK2—that bind to different cytokine receptor chains. Ligand binding activates the JAKs, and they, in turn, phosphorylate cytokine receptor subunits on tyrosine residues, allowing recruitment of signaling molecules. Deficiency of JAK3 results in autosomal-recessive severe combined immunodeficiency with failure to signal by γ$_c$ cytokines, whereas mutation of *TYK2* is associated with an autosomal recessive form of hyper-IgE syndrome. *JAK2* is important for many cytokines, including EPO, and mutation of *JAK2* underlies most cases of polycythemia vera. Polymorphisms of *TYK2* and *JAK2* are also associated with autoimmune disease. JAK inhibitors represent a new class of immunosuppressant drugs, and clinical trials are currently being done.[40]

An important class of molecules activated by JAKs is the signal transducer and activator of transcription (STAT) family of DNA binding proteins. There are seven mammalian STATs: STAT1, STAT2, STAT3, STAT4, STAT5a, STAT5b, and STAT6. Mutations of STAT1, which is activated by interferons, results in increased susceptibility to *Salmonella* and mycobacterial infections.[38] STAT3 is activated by a variety of cytokines, and mutations of this gene result in an autosomal dominant primary immunodeficiency syndrome referred to as autosomal dominant hyper-IgE (AD-HIES), or Job's syndrome.[41] An important aspect of the susceptibility of these patients to infection is the failure to generate Th17 cells. Conversely, polymorphisms of *STAT3* are associated with IBD. STAT4 is activated by IL-12, and type I has critical functions in Th1 differentiation; polymorphisms of *STAT4* are associated with rheumatoid arthritis, systemic lupus, and Sjogren's syndrome.[42] STAT6 is activated by IL-4 and IL-13 and is important in Th2-mediated responses. STAT5a and STAT5b are homologous and have overlapping functions. STAT5 is important for the expression of Foxp3, and mice lacking these transcription factors have impaired Treg development and autoimmunity. A single patient with *STAT5b* mutations has been identified, and she manifests impaired responses to GH and immune dysregulation.

INTERLEUKIN-17 RECEPTORS

The IL-17 receptor family comprises five receptors (IL-17RA through IL-17RE), which are ubiquitously broadly expressed.[33] IL-17 family ligands include IL-17A-F; IL-17E is also called IL-25.

IL-17 (IL-17A) and IL-17F are produced by a subset of CD4 T cells referred to as Th17 cells but are also produced by γδ T cells, invariant NK cells, and lymphoid tissue inducer cells.[26] These cytokines evoke inflammation by inducing the production of the G-CSF, GM-CSF, and chemokines. As a result, IL-17 is both a major regulator of stress granulopoiesis and recruitment of myeloid cells to sites of inflammation. IL-17A is involved in host defense against gram-negative extracellular bacteria such as *Klebsiella pneumoniae*.[33] Additionally, abundant data point to pathogenic roles of IL-17A in models of immune-mediated disease and in human autoimmune disorders. IL-17E (IL-25) is produced by Th2 cells and mast cells and evokes an inflammatory response characterized by overproduction of Th2 cytokines, mucus production, epithelial cell hyperplasia, and eosinophilia. IL-25 is essential for elimination of helminthic parasites. IL-17B, IL-17C, and IL-17D are less well studied. Studies targeting IL-17 and its receptor are underway in psoriasis, uveitis, Crohn's disease, RA, psoriatic arthritis, and ankylosing spondylitis.

Signaling

IL-17 family receptors have a single transmembrane domain and large cytoplasmic tails, which contain a motif that is similar to the TIR domain of TLRs. This is referred to as an SEFIR domain. The adapter molecule Act-1 also has a SEFIR domain and binds to the IL-17R through a homotypic interaction. Another adapter molecule used by TNF family cytokines, TRAF6, also contributes to IL-17 signaling. Engagement of the IL-17 receptor activates MAP kinases and NF-κB, and IL-17 acts synergistically with TNF.

TRANSFORMING GROWTH FACTOR-β RECEPTOR FAMILY CYTOKINES

The transforming growth factor-β (TGF-β) family comprises more than 40 cytokines, including TGFβ-1, β-2, and β-3, bone morphogenic proteins (BMPs), activins, inhibins, and müllerian-inhibiting substance; only TGFβ-1 is discussed here. The receptor for TGFβ-1 is the dimer of two receptor serine-threonine kinases, TGFβRI and TGFβRII. Functionally, TGFβ inhibits many aspects of lymphocyte function, including T-cell proliferation and cytokine production. TGF-β1 also induces FoxP3 and promotes differentiation of Treg cells. Accordingly, mice lacking this cytokine or its receptor have overwhelming autoimmune disease. The TGF-β family is expressed as biologically inactive disulfide-linked dimers that require processing to be active. The enzyme furin cleaves TGF-β, and deficiency of furin is associated with systemic autoimmunity. Paradoxically, TGF-β1 acting with IL-6 induces the proinflammatory cytokine IL-17.[26] Thus, TGF-β1 has both proinflammatory and anti-inflammatory activities. The TGF-β family also induces fibrosis and may participate in the pathogenesis of diseases such as systemic sclerosis.

Signaling

On ligand binding, the type II receptor phosphorylates the type I receptor, which allows the recruitment of SMAD family transcription factors: SMAD2 and SMAD3. Activated SMADs associate with SMAD4 and the complex translocates to the nucleus to bind promoters of TGFβ-responsive genes. SMADs interact with a variety of other transcription factors, transcriptional co-activators, and transcriptional co-repressors. TGF-β also signals via TAK1 (TGF-β–associated kinase-1), which associates with TAB1 (TAK1-associated binding protein) and activates members of the mitogen-activated protein kinase (MAPK) family of kinases.

RECEPTOR TYROSINE KINASES

Classic growth factors such as the epidermal growth factor and insulin signal through receptors that are themselves tyrosine kinases and thus are called receptor tyrosine kinases (RTKs). Most of the ligands that use these receptors are not classified as cytokines, but some are: CSF-1 (colony stimulating factor-1 or macrophage colony stimulating factor [M-CSF]), stem cell factor (SCF, c-KIT ligand, or steel factor), FMS-like tyrosine kinase 3 ligand (FLT3-L), and platelet-derived growth factor (PDGF). Structurally, SCF and CSF-1 are similar to the four α-helical cytokines, suggesting a common evolutionary ancestor for both groups of cytokines. SCF is widely expressed during embryogenesis, and makes stem cells responsive to other CSFs. It has also important effects for the differentiation of mast cells. FLT3-L acts with SCF to induce proliferation of hematopoietic precursors. It is also important for generation of dendritic cells. Gain-of-function mutations of c-KIT cause systemic mastocytosis and mutations, resulting in a fusion of the *PDGFRA* and *FIP1L1* genes that underlie the hypereosinophilic syndrome. CSF-1 supports the survival and differentiation of monocytic cells. IL-34 is distinct from CSF-1 but binds the same receptor.

CHEMOKINES

As a collection of functionally integrated but anatomically dispersed populations of hematopoietic cells dedicated to defense of the host, the immune system, like any army, depends absolutely on its mobility. Within the immune system, cell migration is necessary during development, homeostasis, and response to pathogen challenge. Several classes of molecules regulate this migration, among them chemoattractants and their receptors. The largest gene family of chemoattractants is that of chemokines (*chemo*tactic cyto*kines*), which contains more than 40 members.[43]

Ligand and receptor structure

Chemokines are small secreted proteins (molecular weights of approximately 10 KDa). Exceptions include CX₃CL1 and CXCL16, which are membrane-anchored through transmembrane domains in addition to having soluble forms generated through proteolytic cleavage. Although chemokines are secreted, they become immobilized by binding to glycosaminoglycans on cell surfaces and extracellular matrix, and it is generally believed that the immobilized chemokines are the active forms, sometimes forming fixed gradients for chemotaxis.

Chemokines can be divided, based on the arrangements of conserved cysteine residues near the N-termini, into CXC, CC, CX₃C, and XC subfamilies, where X is a variable amino acid. The CX₃C and XC subfamilies contain only one and two members, respectively, with all the rest being CXC or CC chemokines. The systematic names for chemokines consist of the subfamily, followed by "L" for ligand, and a number, which generally reflects the order of discovery.

Chemokines signal through seven transmembrane domain G protein–coupled receptors, 19 of which have been identified in humans. The superfamily of G protein–coupled receptors contains almost 1000 members in humans, including the subfamilies of odorant and taste receptors and receptors for light, neurotransmitters, and catecholamines. Because G protein–coupled receptors have been successfully targeted by a large number of small molecule drugs, studies of the chemokine system have always maintained a view to potential therapeutic applications.

An important aspect of receptor-ligand relationships in the chemokine system is promiscuity. One ligand can often bind to more than a single receptor, and receptors generally bind to more than a single ligand. Nonetheless, a given receptor will bind chemokines within a single subfamily only, a feature that underlies the receptor nomenclature: CXCR1-7 and CCR1-10 are receptors for CXC and the CC chemokines, respectively, whereas CX₃CR1 and XCR1 is the receptor for CX₃CL1. In addition to receptor-ligand promiscuity, an additional level of complexity is in the patterns of expression of receptors on leukocytes. Although some receptors are dominant in controlling migration of a given cell type, like CXCR1 and CXCR2 on neutrophils, and CCR3 on eosinophils, all leukocytes express multiple chemokine receptors, so that within a given context, blocking a single receptor may not prevent the cell's recruitment.

As discussed later, clinical trials of antagonists of individual chemokine receptors as anti-inflammatory drugs have not been encouraging, leading to the proposal that "promiscuous" drugs need to be developed that target multiple receptors to overcome the system's redundancy. On the other hand, clinical investigations focused on the chemokine system are still in their early stages, particularly given the complexity of the system and the limited understanding of how the system is functioning in disease. It may, therefore, be premature to abandon the goal of using single-receptor antagonists to treat inflammatory disorders.

Chemokines/chemokine receptors are only one component of the molecular system important for leukocyte trafficking, a critical step of which is movement of cells out of postcapillary venules into tissue. This transendothelial migration has been described using a multiple-step model of selectin-mediated rolling, followed by activation of a chemoattractant G protein–coupled receptor, followed by integrin-mediated firm arrest, followed by diapedesis. Selectins and their ligands are expressed on both leukocytes and endothelial cells. The relevant chemoattractant G protein–coupled receptors and integrins are on leukocytes, with their ligands on endothelial cells—in the case of chemokines, immobilized on the endothelial cell surface. It is generally believed that chemokines also form gradients within tissues which cells move, and there is some direct evidence for such gradients.

Family members and their actions

CXCL12 and CXCR4 and immune cell development

A role for chemokines in leukocyte development has been best shown in studies of CXCL12 and its receptor, CXCR4, which are unusual within the chemokine system in being highly conserved during evolution. Cxcl12–/– mice show defective B lymphopoiesis and bone marrow myelopoiesis. This presumably reflects the role of CXCL12/CXCR4 in homing and retention of hematopoietic stem cells to appropriate niches within the bone marrow. A CXCR4 antagonist, plerixafor (AMD3100/Mozobil), is now being used clinically to enhance stem cell mobilization for subsequent autologous transplantation in individuals with non-Hodgkin's lymphoma or multiple myeloma.

CCR7 and CCR5 and immune anatomy

Roles for chemokines in immune system anatomy and homeostasis are evident in the functions of CCL19 and CCL21 and their receptor CCR7, and CXCL13 and its receptor CXCR5. CCL19 and CCL21 are expressed on high endothelial venules and in the T-cell zones in lymph nodes and other secondary lymphoid organs, and these chemokines are required for the trafficking and positioning of T cells and dendritic cells within secondary lymphoid organs. The counterparts for B cells are CXCL13, which is expressed in B-cell follicles, and CXCR5, which is expressed on B cells and on effector/memory T cells that traffic to B-cell follicles, so-called T$_{FH}$, or follicular helper cells.[44] Because B cells are critical for the formation of lymphoid organs during development, lymph nodes and Peyer's patches in mice lacking CXCR5 are absent or rudimentary.

Sphingosine-1-phosphate

Another key pair of proteins that are not within the chemokine system, but have an important related function in lymphocyte trafficking through lymphoid organs, are sphingosine-1-phosphate and one of its receptors, the G protein–coupled receptor S1P$_1$. Sphingosine-1-phosphate and S1P$_1$ mediate lymphocyte egress from the thymus and lymph nodes. This is of particular interest given the discovery that an immunosuppressive drug, fingolimod (FTY720), acts as a functional antagonist of S1P$_1$ *in vivo*. Fingolimod has shown promise in the treatment of relapsing multiple sclerosis.[45] Although the beneficial effects may be related to fingolimod's activity in blocking the egress of activated cells from lymph nodes, the drug has also been reported to increase numbers of suppressive regulatory T cells and to inhibit Th17 cell differentiation in mouse models.

Other family members

The majority of chemokines and their receptors function in recruiting leukocytes, including myeloid cells, NK cells, and activated/memory lymphocytes into inflamed tissue sites. Most of these chemokines/receptors do not have roles restricted to specific organs or tissues, but there are exceptions. The chemokine best documented as specific for a peripheral tissue is CCL25, the ligand for CCR9A/B, which (in addition to a role on thymocytes) has a role in recruiting lymphocytes specifically to the gut and preferentially to the small intestine. Together with the gut-associated integrin, α4β7, CCR9 is induced on T cells by dendritic cells from Peyer's patches, thereby imprinting activated/memory T cells to home to the bowel.[46] As a result of these and related findings, a CCR9 antagonist is currently being investigated for anti-inflammatory activity as therapy for moderate to severe Crohn's disease (ClinicalTrials.gov identifier NCT00306215).

Major chemokine receptors for recruitment of the principal populations of myeloid "effector" cells are CXCR1 and CXCR2 on neutrophils and CCR2 on monocytes/macrophages. A number of agents have been developed to block CXCR1 or CXCR2 and are being evaluated in clinical trials for diseases with neutrophil-mediated tissue damage, such as chronic obstructive pulmonary disease, ulcerative colitis, and ischemia-reperfusion injury associated with graft dysfunction after transplantation (ClinicalTrials.gov identifiers NCT00748410, NCT00248040). In a novel approach, antibody against CXCL8 (IL-8), a ligand for CXCR1 and CXCR2, has been evaluated as a topical therapy for psoriasis (ABCream), and is being marketed in China for that indication. Based on mouse models, CCR2 and its ligands, particularly CCL2, by recruiting monocytes/macrophages, have been suggested to play important roles in the pathogenesis of disorders such as multiple sclerosis, atherosclerosis, rheumatoid arthritis, systemic sclerosis, and lupus nephritis. Both small molecule antagonists and antibodies to CCR2, as well as agents to block CCL2, have been undergoing clinical evaluation for treating some of these diseases. Although beneficial effects for these drug candidates are not yet clear, many of the clinical investigations of CCR2/CCL2 blockade are in their early stages.

Effector/memory T cells can express at least 15 different types of chemokine receptors to produce complex, combinatorial patterns. Although the factors and mechanisms regulating chemokine receptor expression during T cell activation and differentiation have not been extensively studied, it is clear that some receptors are induced as part of defined pathways for T-cell lineage commitment. Cells of the three principal effector/memory lineages of human CD4+ T cells, Th1, Th2, and Th17, are each wholly contained within the subsets expressing CXCR3 or CCR4 or CCR6, respectively. Not surprisingly then, the *CXCR3*, *CCR4*, and *CCR6* genes are inducible, respectively, by the transcription factors T-bet, GATA-3, and RORγt, which are critical, respectively, for Th1, Th2, and Th17 differentiation. Given the expression of these receptors on subsets of effector/memory Th cells implicated in a broad range of diseases, they might be considered good drug targets. Although antagonists have been developed for CXCR3 and

CCR4, these inhibitors have undergone limited clinical testing with as yet no encouraging results.[47] The recent description of Th17 cells as a separate lineage has engendered tremendous interest owing to the findings that these cells are important mediators of tissue injury in models of autoimmune disease. The recognition of the relationship between Th17 differentiation and CCR6 have led to studies that demonstrate an essential pathogenic role for CCR6 in mouse models of arthritis, multiple sclerosis, and psoriasis. These data are likely to spur the development and testing of CCR6 antagonists in autoimmune disorders.

To date, the most significant clinical outcome from studies of the chemokine system has been unrelated to chemokine physiology but related rather to the use of CCR5 and CXCR4 by HIV-1 as co-receptors, together with CD4, for viral entry. All clinical isolates of HIV-1 use CCR5 and/or CXCR4 as obligate co-receptors. CCR5 is the co-receptor of primary importance, since viruses found in an individual early after infection use CCR5 (and not CXCR4), and individuals who are homozygous for an allele encoding a truncated and inactive CCR5 are highly resistant to HIV-1 infection. The latter observations, together with the apparent absence of deleterious consequences in CCR5-null individuals, has led to the development of CCR5 antagonists that block viral entry in individuals infected with HIV-1. The first of these agents to reach clinical practice has been maraviroc (Pfizer, Inc.), which has been shown effective in reducing viral loads in treatment-experienced individuals with CCR5-using HIV-1. The availability of maraviroc will likely lead to its evaluation as an anti-inflammatory drug. One such trial in rheumatoid arthritis failed to show efficacy (ClinicalTrials.gov identifier NCT00427934). Despite the good general health of CCR5-null individuals, it has recently been reported that CCR5 deficiency is a strong risk factor for symptomatic disease in individuals infected with West Nile virus.[48] These data provide both the first good evidence in humans supporting the presumption that CCR5 and other inflammation-associated chemokine receptors have roles in host defense and a cautionary note on the use of chemokine receptor antagonists.

Signaling

G protein–coupled receptors are defined by the central feature of their signaling pathway, namely, the activation of heterotrimeric G proteins through conformational changes in their cytoplasmic domains that are induced by binding of ligands to their extracellular domains. Heterotrimeric G proteins contain one each of 23 different α-, five β-, and 10 γ-subunits. Receptor-mediated G protein activation leads to replacement of Gα subunit-bound guanosine diphosphate (GDP) with guanosine triphosphate (GTP) and the dissociation of the trimer into Gα-GTP and a βγ dimer. For chemokine receptor–mediated processes (e.g., chemotaxis), the βγ dimer is the critical activator of downstream signaling proteins, such as phosphoinositide-3-kinase, leading ultimately to actin polymerization and formation of lamellipodia at the leading edge and actin-myosin–mediated retraction of the uropod at the trailing edge.[49] The 23 Gα subunits fall within four subfamilies, and heterotrimers are grouped similarly, based on their Gα components, into G$_i$, G$_s$, G$_q$, and G$_{12/13}$ subfamiles. All chemokine receptors signal through G$_i$ proteins, which, by using the specific G$_i$ inhibitor, pertussis toxin, can be shown to be essential for chemotaxis. G$_{12/13}$ proteins have also been implicated in chemotaxis, with activated G$_i$ and G$_{12/13}$ proteins responsible for creating, respectively, the front-specific and back-specific components of migrating cells.

Control of chemokine receptor function also requires limiting the duration of the activating signals, which is achieved through a number of mechanisms. Gα subunits have an intrinsic GTPase activity, and once GTP is hydrolyzed to GDP, the Gα-GDP reassociates with a βγ dimer to form the "resting" heterotrimer. The Gα GTPase activity can be accelerated by GTPase activating proteins (GAPs), including members of the RGS family of proteins.[49] The chemokine receptors themselves are typically desensitized after chemokine binding through the activities of G-protein–coupled receptor kinases (GRKs), which phosphorylate serine/threonine residues in the receptors' C-terminal tails. Receptor phosphorylation leads to recruitment of arrestin proteins, which is typically followed by receptor internalization leading to degradation and/or recycling of receptors to the cell surface. At the same time that they serve to limit receptor-mediated activation of G proteins, arrestins can also activate additional G-protein–independent signaling pathways.[50]

OTHER CYTOKINES

IL-32 is another structurally distinct cytokine that is induced by IL-12 and IL-18. It activates NF-κB and p38, enhances production of other inflammatory cytokines and is found in rheumatoid synovium. The functions of IL-16 and IL-14 are uncertain.

REFERENCES

1. Arend WP, Palmer G, Gabay C. IL-1, IL-18, and IL-33 families of cytokines. Immunol Rev 2008;223:20-38.
2. Dinarello CA. Immunological and inflammatory functions of the interleukin-1 family. Annu Rev Immunol 2009;27:519-550.
3. Sims JE. IL-1 and IL-18 receptors, and their extended family. Curr Opin Immunol 2002;14:117-122.
4. Martinon F, Mayor A, Tschopp J. The inflammasomes: guardians of the body. Annu Rev Immunol 2009;27:229-265.
5. Dinarello CA. Interleukin-1beta and the autoinflammatory diseases. N Engl J Med 2009;360:2467-2470.
6. Dantzer R, O'Connor JC, Freund GG, et al. From inflammation to sickness and depression: when the immune system subjugates the brain. Nat Rev Neurosci 2008;9:46-56.
7. Rothwell N. Interleukin-1 and neuronal injury: mechanisms, modification, and therapeutic potential. Brain Behav Immun 2003;17:152-157.
8. Goldbach-Mansky R, et al. Neonatal-onset multisystem inflammatory disease responsive to interleukin-1beta inhibition. N Engl J Med 2006;355:581-592.
9. Larsen CM, et al. Interleukin-1-receptor antagonist in type 2 diabetes mellitus. N Engl J Med 2007;356:1517-1526.
10. Sims J, Towne J, Blumberg H. 11 IL-1 family members in inflammatory skin disease. Ernst Schering Research Foundation Workshop, 2006:187-191.
11. O'Neill LA. The interleukin-1 receptor/Toll-like receptor superfamily: 10 years of progress. Immunol Rev 2008;226:10-18.
12. Bodmer JL, Schneider P, Tschopp J. The molecular architecture of the TNF superfamily. Trends Biochem Sci 2002;27:19-26.
13. Aggarwal BB. Signalling pathways of the TNF superfamily: a double-edged sword. Nat Rev Immunol 2003;3:745-756.
14. Salvesen GS, Duckett CS. IAP proteins: blocking the road to death's door. Nat Rev Mol Cell Biol 2002;3:401-410
15. Wang L, Du F, Wang X. TNF-alpha induces two distinct caspase-8 activation pathways. Cell 2008;133:693-703.
16. Vince JE, et al. IAP antagonists target cIAP1 to induce TNFalpha-dependent apoptosis. Cell 2007;131:682-693.
17. Degterev A, et al. Identification of RIP1 kinase as a specific cellular target of necrostatins. Nat Chem Biol 2008;4:313-321.
18. Siegel RM. Caspases at the crossroads of immune-cell life and death. Nat Rev Immunol 2006;6:308-317.

19. Kollias G. TNF pathophysiology in murine models of chronic inflammation and autoimmunity. Semin Arthritis Rheum 2005;34:3-6.
20. Chu CQ, Field M, Feldmann M, Maini RN. Localization of tumor necrosis factor alpha in synovial tissues and at the cartilage-pannus junction in patients with rheumatoid arthritis. Arthritis Rheum 1991;34:1125-1132.
21. Mackay F, Schneider P. Cracking the BAFF code. Nat Rev Immunol 2009;9:491-502.
22. Croft M. Co-stimulatory members of the TNFR family: keys to effective T-cell immunity? Nat Rev Immunol 2003;3:609-620.
23. Croft M. The role of TNF superfamily members in T-cell function and diseases. Nat Rev Immunol 2009;9:271-285.
24. Meylan F, et al. The TNF-family receptor DR3 is essential for diverse T cell-mediated inflammatory diseases. Immunity 2008;29:79-89.
25. O'Shea JJ, Murray PJ. Cytokine signaling modules in inflammatory responses. Immunity 2008;28:477-487.
26. Weaver CT, Hatton RD, Mangan PR, Harrington LE. IL-17 family cytokines and the expanding diversity of effector T cell lineages. Annu Rev Immunol 2007;25:821-852.
27. Scheinecker C, Smolen J, Yasothan U, et al. Tocilizumab. Nat Rev Drug Discov 2009;8:273-274.
28. Malek TR, Bayer AL. Tolerance, not immunity, crucially depends on IL-2. Nat Rev Immunol 2004;4:665-674.
29. Buckley RH. Molecular defects in human severe combined immunodeficiency and approaches to immune reconstitution. Annu Rev Immunol 2004;22:625-655.
30. Veldhoen M, et al. Transforming growth factor-beta "reprograms" the differentiation of T helper 2 cells and promotes an interleukin 9-producing subset. Nat Immunol 2008;9:1341-1346.
31. Nurieva RI, et al. Generation of T follicular helper cells is mediated by interleukin-21 but independent of T helper 1, 2, or 17 cell lineages. Immunity 2008;29:138-149.
32. Tato CM, Cua DJ. Reconciling id, ego, and superego within interleukin-23. Immunol Rev 2008;226:103-111.
33. Dubin PJ, Kolls JK. Th17 cytokines and mucosal immunity. Immunol Rev 2008;226:160-171.
34. Burton PR, et al. Association scan of 14,500 nonsynonymous SNPs in four diseases identifies autoimmunity variants. Nat Genet 2007;39:1329-1337.
35. Segal BM, et al. Repeated subcutaneous injections of IL12/23 p40 neutralising antibody, ustekinumab, in

patients with relapsing-remitting multiple sclerosis: a phase II, double-blind, placebo-controlled, randomised, dose-ranging study. Lancet Neurol 2008;7:796-804.
36. Stumhofer JS, Hunter CA. Advances in understanding the anti-inflammatory properties of IL-27. Immunol Lett 2008;117:123-130.
37. Collison LW, Vignali DA. Interleukin-35: odd one out or part of the family? Immunol Rev 2008;226:248-262.
38. Zhang SY, et al. Inborn errors of interferon (IFN)-mediated immunity in humans: insights into the respective roles of IFN-alpha/beta, IFN-gamma, and IFN-lambda in host defense. Immunol Rev 2008;226:29-40.
39. Commins S, Steinke JW, Borish L. The extended IL-10 superfamily: IL-10, IL-19, IL-20, IL-22, IL-24, IL-26, IL-28, and IL-29. J Allergy Clin Immunol 2008;121:1108-1111.
40. Ghoreschi K, Laurence,A, O'Shea JJ. Selectivity and therapeutic inhibition of kinases: to be or not to be? Nat Immunol 2009;10:356-360.
41. Milner JD, et al. Impaired T(H)17 cell differentiation in subjects with autosomal dominant hyper-IgE syndrome. Nature 2008;452:773-776.
42. Remmers EF, et al. STAT4 and the risk of rheumatoid arthritis and systemic lupus erythematosus. N Engl J Med 2007;357:977-986.
43. Murphy PM, et al. International union of pharmacology. XXII. Nomenclature for chemokine receptors. Pharmacol Rev 2000;52:145-176.
44. King C, Tangye SG, Mackay CR. T follicular helper (TFH) cells in normal and dysregulated immune responses. Annu Rev Immunol 2008;26:741-766.
45. Kappos L, et al. Oral fingolimod (FTY720) for relapsing multiple sclerosis. N Engl J Med 2006;355:1124-1140.
46. Mora JR, et al. Selective imprinting of gut-homing T cells by Peyer's patch dendritic cells. Nature 2003;424:88-93.
47. Pease JE, Horuk R. Chemokine receptor antagonists: II. Expert Opin Ther Pat 2009;19:199-221.
48. Lim JK, et al. Genetic deficiency of chemokine receptor CCR5 is a strong risk factor for symptomatic West Nile virus infection: a meta-analysis of 4 cohorts in the US epidemic. J Infect Dis 2008;197:262-265.
49. Kehrl JH. Chemoattractant receptor signaling and the control of lymphocyte migration. Immunol Res 2006;34:211-227.
50. Reiter E, Lefkowitz RJ. GRKs and beta-arrestins: roles in receptor silencing, trafficking and signaling. Trends Endocrinol Metab 2006;17:159-165.

Principles and techniques in molecular biology

12

Elaine F. Remmers, Michael J. Ombrello, Yuka Kanno, Richard M. Siegel, and Daniel L. Kastner

- Restriction enzymes, DNA and RNA polymerases, DNA ligases, reverse transcriptases, phosphatases, kinases, and thermostable DNA polymerases are enzymes used to clone, modify, and amplify DNA in the laboratory.
- Incorporation of exogenous DNA fragments into vectors that can replicate in bacteria, yeast, or insect cells permits large-scale production of the cloned gene or encoded protein.
- Restriction fragment length polymorphisms (RFLPs), minisatellite markers, microsatellite markers, and single nucleotide polymorphisms (SNPs) are common DNA sequence variants that differ among individuals and are therefore useful in genetic analysis of diseases with mendelian and complex inheritance.
- Northern blots and real-time PCR are methods that quantitatively measure the expression of specific genes, whereas microarray expression profiling methods simultaneously evaluate the expression of thousands of genes.
- Electromobility shift assays and chromatin immunoprecipitation assays detect DNA interactions with proteins, such as transcription factors and modified histones that are regulators of gene expression.
- Transfection methods are biochemical, physical, or viral methods for transferring exogenous DNA into cultured cells for expression. In a variant of the experiment, the expression vector directs transcription of short inhibitory RNAs (siRNAs) that block the endogenous gene's expression.
- Transgenic mice are genetically modified animals in which an exogenous DNA construct has been transferred, whereas in knockout mice the endogenous gene has been disrupted, thereby preventing its expression.
- Protein-protein interactions can be analyzed by co-immunoprecipitation and yeast two-hybrid screening. Fluorescence resonance energy transfer (FRET) can be used to evaluate protein-protein interactions in living cells.

INTRODUCTION

In the recent past we have witnessed the publication of the draft sequence of the human genome, affording scientists and physicians extraordinary opportunities to advance our understanding of physiology and pathology.[1] Until just a few years ago these possibilities were more science fiction than science. However, a number of critical technologic breakthroughs have truly revolutionized biomedical research. The opportunities for improving our understanding of rheumatic and autoimmune diseases are now astounding. Moreover, it is likely that recent advances will accelerate the pace at which disease susceptibility genes are identified and their functions analyzed. It is likely that this information will also improve treatment and propel the discovery of new therapeutic modalities.

It is therefore intended in this chapter to review the basic tools that rheumatologists now see being employed when they read the literature.

Given the space constraints, we will not review basic concepts in DNA replication, transcriptional control, or signal transduction. There are several excellent textbooks that cover these topics.[2,3] Rather, we will focus on the methods used to study these processes, but our intent is also not for this to be a laboratory manual or "how to" guide; again there are ample sources that provide detailed protocols of this sort.[4,5] Instead, our goal is to present the principles underlying important techniques with which the average rheumatologist should be familiar to comprehend studies that are pertinent to clinical work. Skimming through the rheumatologic literature one sees references to techniques such as single nucleotide polymorphism (SNP) typing, electrophoretic mobility shift assays (EMSAs), microarrays and gene expression profiling, and tissue-specific knockouts using the cre-lox system. We therefore intend to discuss some of the major techniques and their modifications, to facilitate comprehension of the literature.

THE DRAFT SEQUENCE OF THE HUMAN GENOME AND BIOMEDICAL RESEARCH

The human genome consists of about three billion adenine (A), guanine (G), cytosine (C), and thymine (T) bases (Fig. 12.1) arranged in 23 pairs of chromosomes. A great surprise was that the immense amount of potential genetic information encodes a relatively small number of genes, less than 30,000,[6,7] making humans about twice as complex as model organisms such as yeast and *Drosophila* but less complex than rice. It is important to emphasize, however, that alternative splicing and protein modifications greatly increase the complexity of the polypeptides encoded by the human genome.

The onslaught of information brought about by the Human Genome Project has provided both new opportunities and new challenges to investigators. DNA and protein sequences, sequence variation, expression data, and structural data are among the information being deposited into a growing number of public and private databases. Savvy investigators can mine these databases to obtain useful information with a variety of search and computational tools. Many publicly accessible databases and tools are available at the National Center for Biotechnology website (http://www.ncbi.nlm.nih.gov/). Tools such as BLAST, which facilitates sequence comparisons, can be used, for example, to find additional members of gene families that may have similar functions to one another. Comparisons of homologous genes of several species can identify regions that are conserved among species. These elements may be expressed parts of genes or unexpressed regions that may be conserved because they contain important regulatory elements. Managing and analyzing the data derived from genome-wide approaches to expression profiling and disease-gene linkage and association studies can also require sophisticated computational and organizational approaches. The computational, statistical, and computer programming skills required for development of tools applicable to biologic problems have given rise to the new field of bioinformatics, surely an area that will continue to grow in the near future.[8,9]

The molecular biology revolution, of course, began long before the Human Genome Project. Major steps in the revolution were the development of techniques that permitted the *in-vitro* manipulation of DNA and advances in large-scale DNA sequencing. These advances permitted the identification, sequencing, isolation, and expression of genes, allowing their functions to be rapidly discerned.

BASIC MANIPULATION OF DNA: CLONING VECTORS AND CUTTING AND PASTING DNA USING ENZYMES

Vectors are engineered DNA molecules used to replicate, isolate, and express foreign DNA. There are several general types of vectors commonly used, which were derived from bacteria and bacteriophage.

Plasmids are extrachromosomal, double-stranded circular DNA molecules. Often they are relatively small (3-5 kb), and they have three important features: a drug selection marker, convenient cloning sites, and a replicator that permits autonomous replication in cells (Fig. 12.2). Some plasmids also have mammalian promoters that permit expression of the protein in mammalian cells, whereas others are designed for expression in bacteria, yeast, or insect cells, the last being a very efficient means of generating large quantities of protein for crystallography studies. Sometimes, plasmids are constructed to permit the production of "fusion proteins."

A commonly used vector permits cloning of a given gene in-frame with glutathione S-transferase (GST). Glutathione-coupled agarose beads bind GST with high affinity and allow one to do "pull-down experiments" (see later). Another commonly used technique is to fuse the protein of interest to green fluorescent protein (GFP), a protein made by jellyfish, which can be easily visualized within cells (Fig. 12.3).[10] Remarkably, most fusions to GFP retain the localization properties of the original protein molecule, provided that expression levels are not extremely high. As discussed later, this permits one to visualize trafficking of molecules in cells by live cell imaging. This is aided by the fact that fusion fluorescent proteins are now engineered in a choice of colors, thus permitting simultaneous detection of multiple proteins.

The bacteriophage λ has been a heavily used tool in molecular biology for many years. Its genome is about 50 kb, but the central portion of the viral genome is not essential for lytic growth and can be replaced by 10- to 20-kb inserts; as such, this is a commonly used vector to create libraries of genes. Cosmid vectors are hybrids between lambda and plasmid vectors that can accommodate larger inserts of foreign DNA (35-50 kb). P1 vectors are derived from bacteriophage P1 and are large, circular DNA molecules that can contain 70 to 100 kb of eukaryotic DNA. P1-derived artificial chromosomes (PACs) can

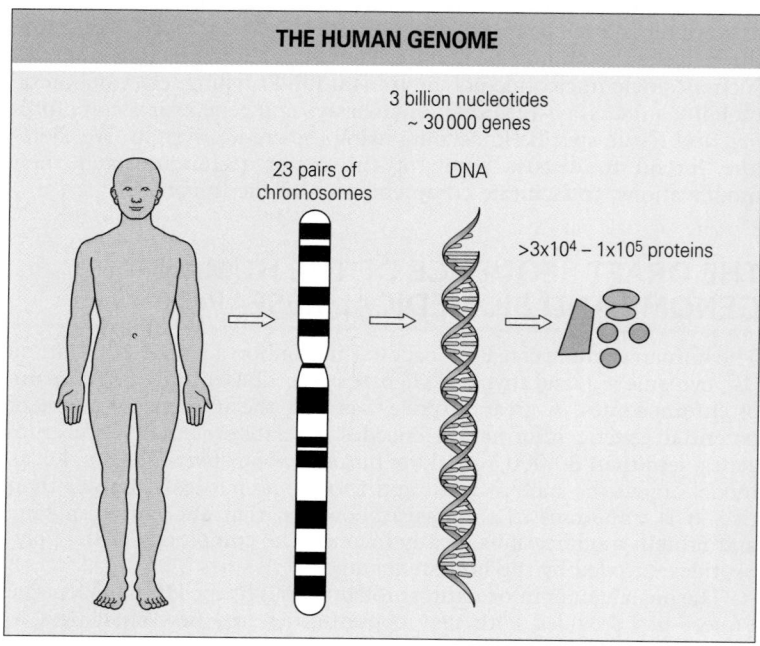

THE HUMAN GENOME

3 billion nucleotides ~ 30 000 genes

23 pairs of chromosomes

DNA

>3x10^4 – 1x10^5 proteins

Fig. 12.1 The human genome. Although less complex than initially thought in terms of the actual number of human genes, regulatory phenomena such as alternative splicing may considerably increase the diversity of proteins produced.

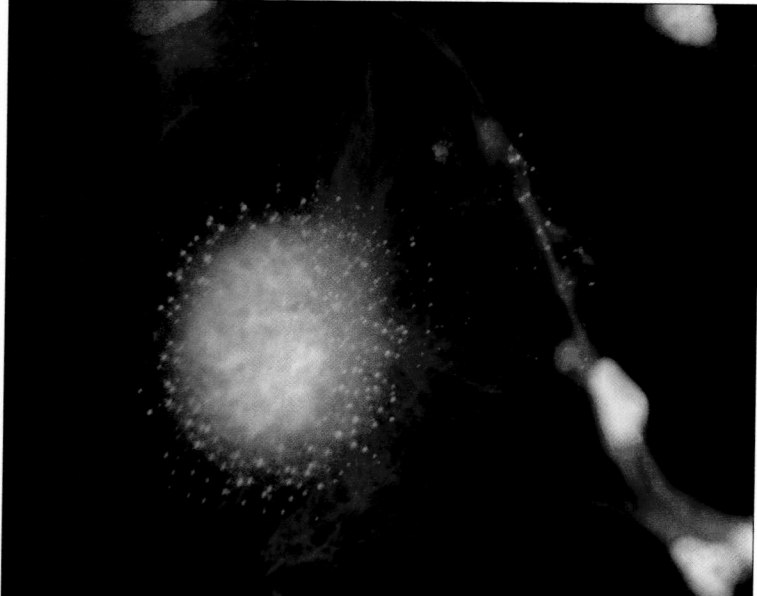

Fig. 12.3 Green fluorescent protein. The ability to visualize the trafficking of cell proteins by tagging them with GFP has revolutionized cell biology and cell signaling. In this case, the Cybr gene is fused to GFP (green). Actin is visualized by binding of rhodamine-labeled phalloidin, and nuclei are stained with DAPI. *(Courtesy of Dr. Massimo Gadina, National Institute of Arthritis, Musculoskeletal and Skin Disease, National Institutes of Health.)*

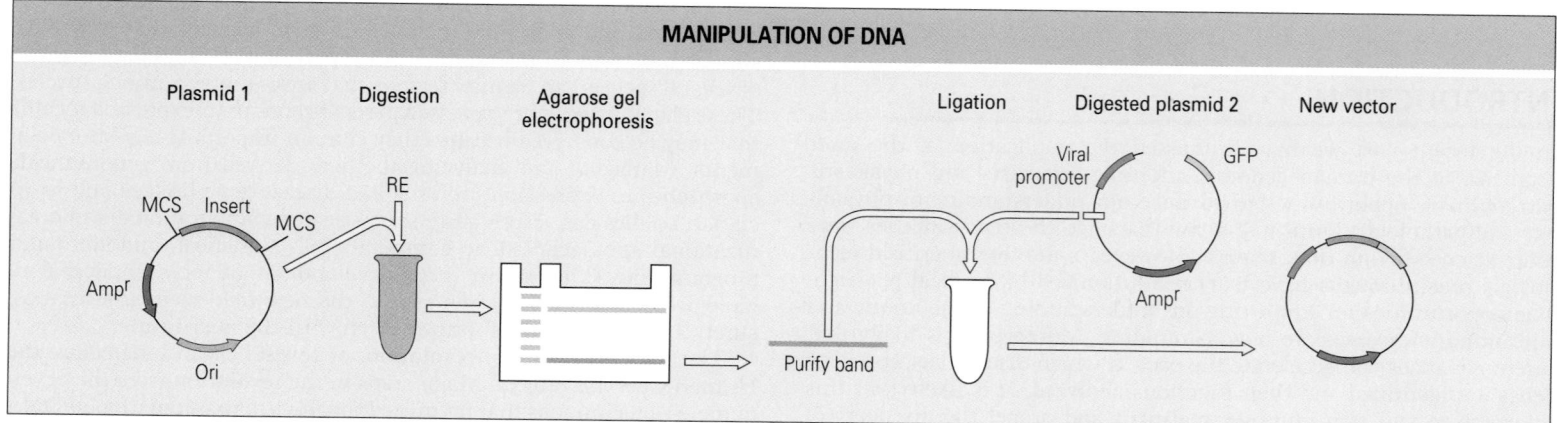

MANIPULATION OF DNA

Plasmid 1 | Digestion | Agarose gel electrophoresis | Ligation | Digested plasmid 2 | New vector

MCS Insert MCS

Amp^r

Ori

RE

Purify band

Viral promoter GFP

Amp^r

Fig. 12.2 Manipulation of DNA. Abundant commercially available enzymes (ligases, polymerases, and restriction enzymes) and vectors make the *in-vitro* manipulation of nucleic acids feasible. Amp^r, ampicillin resistance gene; GFP, green fluorescent protein; MCS, multiple cloning site; Ori, origin of replication; RE, restriction enzyme.

accommodate even larger DNA inserts (up to 150 kb), whereas bacterial artificial chromosomes (BACs) have a still larger insert capacity (up to 200 kb) and have become the preferred vector for sequencing large DNA fragments and are used for multiple purposes, including generating transgenic mice. Although, yeast artificial chromosomes (YACs) can accommodate even larger DNA inserts (about 1 Mb), these vectors are used less frequently because of problems with instability and chimerism. Finally, vectors derived from the M13 filamentous bacteriophage can accommodate small inserts (up to 1 kb) and can be used to produce single-stranded or double-stranded DNA.

Libraries containing many different inserts representing different genes can be made using most of the aforementioned vectors. Libraries are made using genomic or cDNA and in some cases can permit expression of the gene encompassed by the insert.

Many different enzymes are commercially available that permit replication and joining of DNA; such enzymes are termed *DNA polymerases* and *ligases*. Modifying enzymes such as phosphatases and kinases are also important in DNA ligation reactions. Exonucleases and endonucleases cut DNA, whereas restriction enzymes are bacterially derived enzymes that cut DNA at specific sites. These are among the most important tools in molecular biology. Hundreds of restriction enzymes are commercially available, allowing one to cut DNA in a predictable manner.

Using the enzymes just listed, pieces of DNA can be copied and spliced into vectors, allowing large-scale production of the gene or the encoded protein. An example of how these different enzymes can be used to move a piece of DNA from one vector to another is provided in Figure 12.2. RNA can also be synthesized from DNA by DNA-dependent RNA polymerase and the RNA, in turn, can be translated *in vitro* into protein. Conversely, reverse transcriptase, derived from retroviruses, synthesizes DNA from RNA. This enzyme is used to make complementary DNA (cDNA) and to make libraries from mRNA and can be the starting point in the polymerase chain reaction (PCR).

POLYMERASE CHAIN REACTION

The polymerase chain reaction is a rapid procedure for *in-vitro* amplification of DNA; the development of this procedure was another landmark in molecular biology. A large number of applications use PCR, including:

- Cloning of genomic DNA or complementary DNA (cDNA)
- Mutagenesis or modification of DNA
- Assays for the presence of pathogens
- Detection of mutations
- Analysis of allelic sequence variations
- Genetic fingerprinting of forensic samples
- Nucleotide sequencing

A schematic of PCR is shown in Figure 12.4. The reaction includes the following components: a segment of double-stranded DNA to be amplified (template), two single-stranded oligonucleotide primers complementary to the template, and deoxyribonucleoside triphosphates (dNTPs). Another critical component is a heat-stable DNA polymerase such as *Taq* polymerase. Its heat stability is an essential feature because the enzyme must withstand repeated cycles of heating and cooling to denature and replicate the target sequence many times. PCR takes place in a device termed a *thermocycler*, which can rapidly change the reaction temperature.

First, the double-stranded DNA template is heated to generate single-stranded DNA. The primers, added in vast excess compared with the template DNA, anneal or hybridize to opposite strands of single-stranded DNA. The DNA polymerase then synthesizes new strands of DNA complementary to the template. After the first round of synthesis the reaction mix is again heated, with subsequent denaturation of the double-stranded DNA, annealing of primers, and synthesis of DNA. These cycles permit a million-fold amplification of DNA. By designing particular primers, one can mutagenize DNA or add cloning sites.

An important application of PCR is to detect RNA transcripts or to amplify their sequences to permit cloning and/or sequencing. This requires first converting RNA templates to cDNA using reverse transcriptase (RT-PCR).

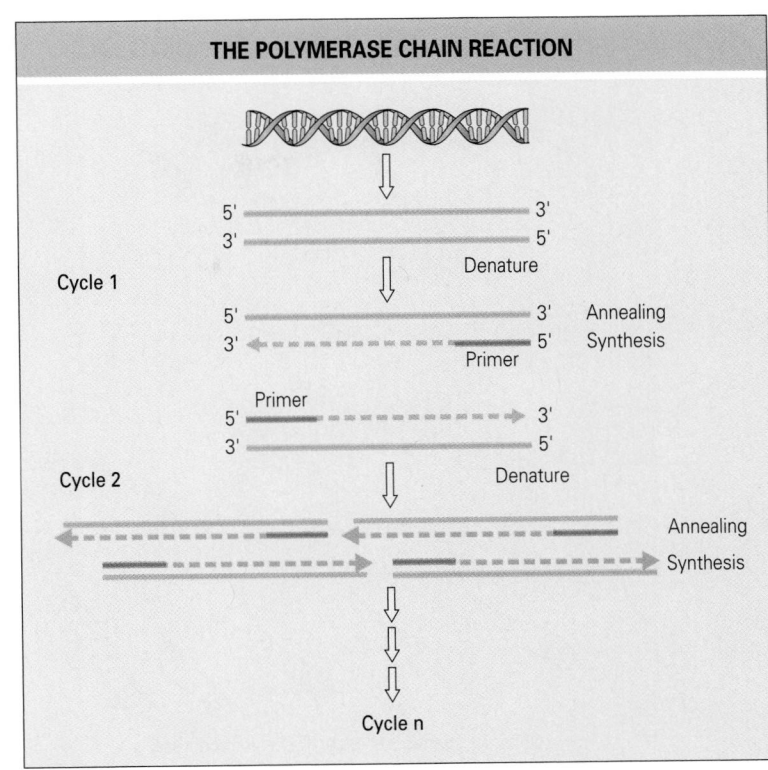

THE POLYMERASE CHAIN REACTION

Fig. 12.4 The polymerase chain reaction. The use of thermostable DNA polymerases and automated thermocyclers permits vast amplification of DNA and RNA templates. Double-stranded DNA (template, light blue) is denatured by heat and, when cooled, primers (dark blue) anneal, allowing synthesis of new cDNA (broken line, lavender). These cycles of denaturing, annealing, and synthesis are repeated with continued amplification of DNA (green). One can start with double-stranded DNA or with mRNA and use reverse transcriptase to generate the first cDNA strand, which is further amplified as above. PCR has many applications, ranging from diagnostics to mutagenesis, and has become an indispensable laboratory tool.

DNA SEQUENCING

Manual techniques to sequence DNA were devised in the 1970s; however, sequencing the human genome was made possible by the development of automated sequencing technology. This technology continues to play an important role in the rheumatology research laboratory and is beginning to be applied as a diagnostic tool. In the research setting, DNA sequencing is being used to refine the human genome sequence and to provide information regarding normal and disease-associated variation in the human genome. Sequencing cDNAs constructed by reverse transcription of mRNA can provide information regarding the structure of gene products. The DNA sequence is also obtained to confirm the structure of cloned DNA and manipulated DNA constructs used for expression, gene transfer, or gene-targeting experiments.

In the clinical setting, several rheumatic diseases are now known to be genetic disorders for which mutations have been identified. These include several members of the periodic fever disease group, as well as some musculoskeletal disorders such as Marfan's syndrome and familial osteochondral dysplasias causing early-onset osteoarthritis. For such disorders, sequencing can be used as a diagnostic tool, for example, to confirm the diagnosis of familial Mediterranean fever, which might be confused with a number of different inflammatory disorders. A definitive diagnosis permits the clinician to apply the most effective therapy as a treatment instead of using response to the therapy as a diagnostic tool.

Sequencing requires isolated DNA fragments specifically amplified by cloning or PCR. Complementary strands are synthesized by complementary base pairing on denatured DNA templates using enzymes (DNA polymerases) that normally perform this job in replicating cells.

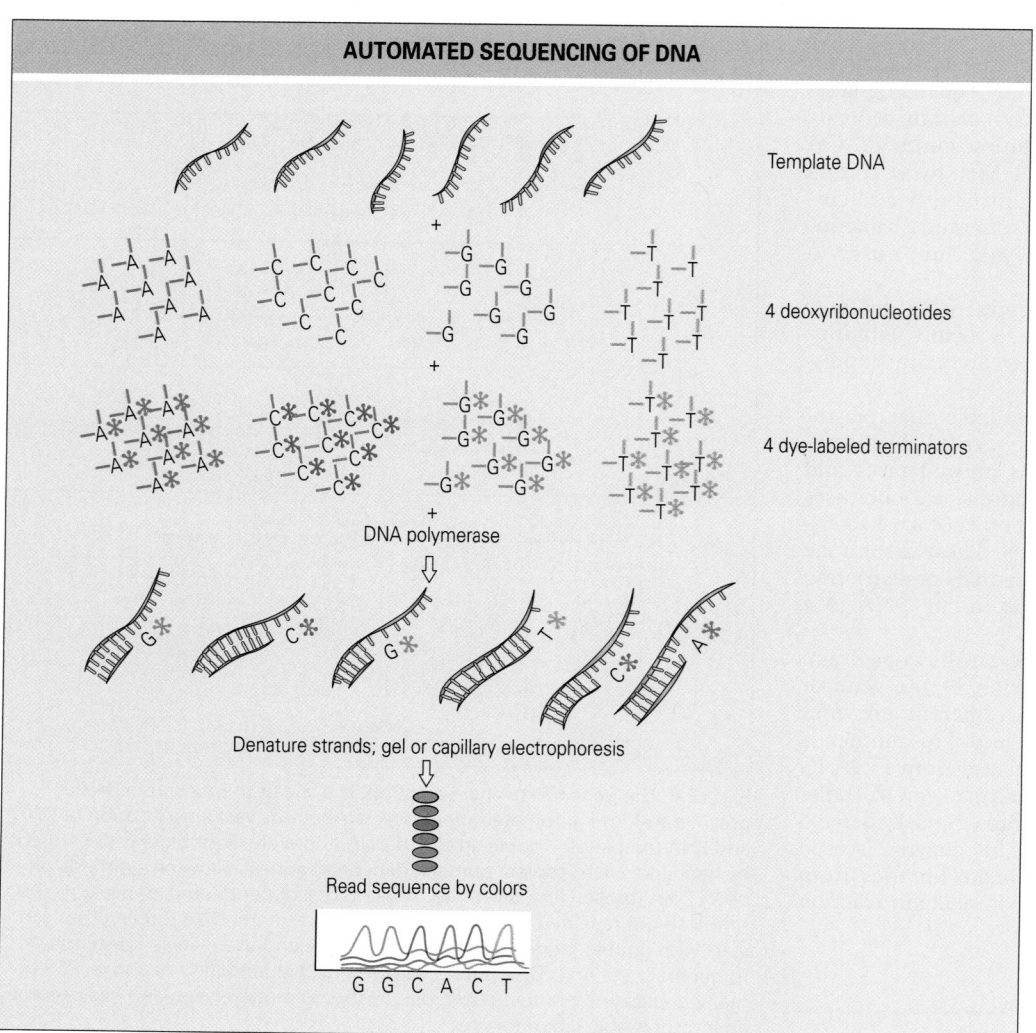

AUTOMATED SEQUENCING OF DNA

Template DNA

4 deoxyribonucleotides

4 dye-labeled terminators

DNA polymerase

Denature strands; gel or capillary electrophoresis

Read sequence by colors

G G C A C T

Fig. 12.5 Automated sequencing of DNA. Sequencing is performed by extending oligonucleotide-primed DNA templates with a thermostable DNA polymerase in the presence of dye-tagged dideoxy terminators that block further extension of the newly synthesized DNA strand and label the strand with one of four different fluorescent dyes identifying the last base incorporated. Automated methods for size fractionating the fragments, detecting the fluors, and reading the DNA sequence have made possible large-scale sequencing required for sequencing the human genome.

There are several variations on the strategy to automatically obtain the sequence of the DNA fragment. In the most common variant, four different fluorescent dye–labeled analogs of the four deoxyribonucleotides are included in the replication mix (Fig. 12.5). When an analog incorporates into a growing complementary DNA strand, the strand is labeled with the associated dye and further extension of the complementary strand is prevented. If, for example, a "red"-labeled deoxyribocytosine analog is used, some fragments will terminate at each location at which a cytosine residue should be incorporated into the growing strand. All these fragments will be labeled with the same "red" fluorescent dye. The four nucleotide analogs are each labeled with a different fluorescent dye, permitting the C, A, T, and G products to be individually identified. The dye-labeled fragments are then separated by size by gel or capillary electrophoresis. The dye associated with each fragment indicates the nucleotide analog incorporated. The sequence can then be automatically read by detecting the succession of dyes detected as the fragments move through the separation medium.

IDENTIFICATION OF DISEASE-ASSOCIATED GENES

An exciting development in rheumatology research is the recently enhanced ability to identify genes associated with rheumatic diseases that has been provided by leveraging information from the human genome project. While these genetic approaches have been most successful for relatively rare genetic diseases that display mendelian inheritance, they are now being successfully applied to identify genes associated with more common rheumatic diseases that fail to demonstrate a simple mendelian mode of inheritance but nevertheless show evidence of a genetic contribution to disease susceptibility.

Positional cloning to identify genes associated with diseases with simple mendelian inheritance

Positional cloning refers to the process of identifying a disease gene by its position in the genome (Fig. 12.6). An example of a successful application of this strategy to a rheumatic disease is the positional cloning of the gene causing familial Mediterranean fever.[11,12] The strength of this technique is that it does not require prior knowledge of the disease mechanism. The first step in positional cloning is to perform linkage analysis. Investigators systematically search the genome for polymorphic genetic markers that co-segregate with disease in families in which the disease occurs (see Fig. 12.6). Polymorphic genetic markers are DNA segments that vary among individuals. There are several kinds. *Restriction fragment length polymorphisms (RFLPs)* are sequence variants that alter a restriction enzyme recognition site and thereby result in different patterns of restriction enzyme digested fragments. *Minisatellite markers* are tandem repeats of 14- to 100-base sequences; the number of tandem repeats varies among individuals. *Microsatellite markers* are tandem repeats of short sequences that are two to four nucleotides in length. The number of these repeats also varies among individuals. *Single nucleotide polymorphisms (SNPs)* are single nucleotides that differ among individuals.[13] SNPs are the most numerous genetic markers available for mapping studies.

If a particular variant of a polymorphic marker tends to occur in family members with the disease, the marker is likely to be linked to the disease locus. Statistical methods are used to evaluate whether a region of the genome is likely to contain a disease gene. Investigators often report LOD scores as evidence supporting linkage of a genetic region to a disease. The LOD score is the logarithm of the ratio of the likelihood of the genotype data assuming linkage versus the likelihood of the data assuming no linkage. For instance, a LOD score of 3 means

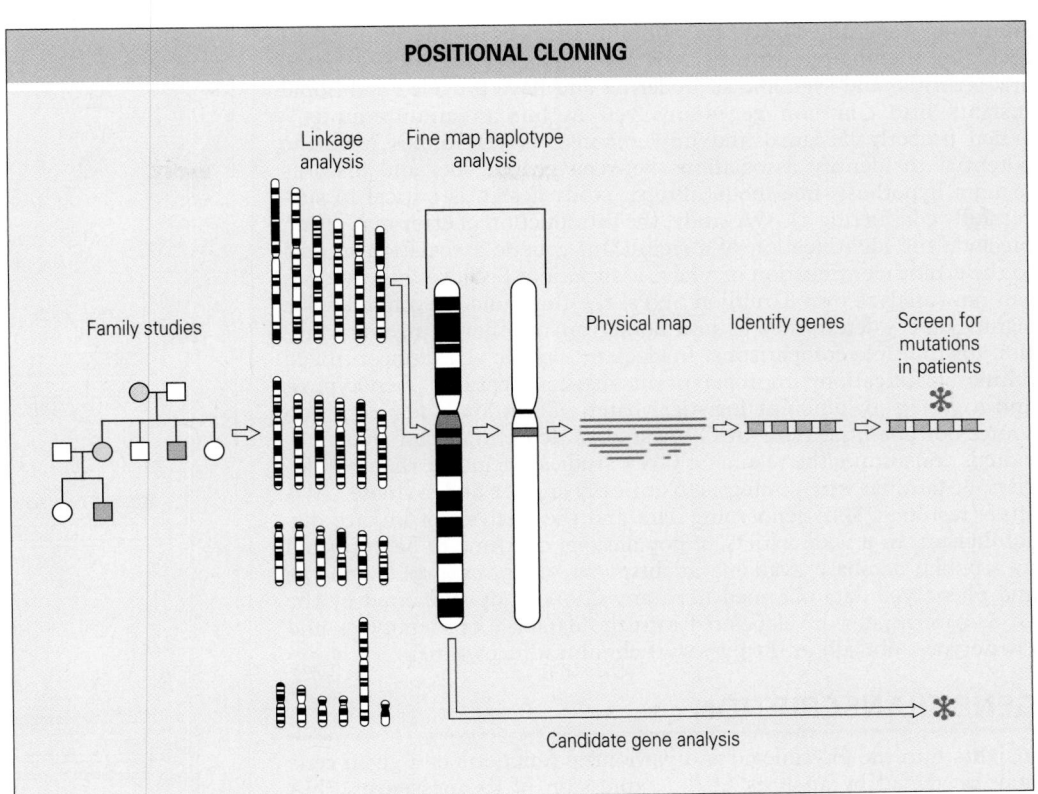

POSITIONAL CLONING

Linkage analysis | Fine map haplotype analysis

Family studies

Physical map | Identify genes | Screen for mutations in patients

Candidate gene analysis

Fig. 12.6 Positional cloning. A disease-associated gene can be identified by its position in the genome. DNAs from multicase families are used for linkage analysis, in which a disease gene location is identified by the locations of genetic markers that co-segregate with the disease. This location can then be refined by fine-mapping and haplotype analysis. The physical map of the refined region is determined and the genes within the interval identified; these steps are being accelerated by the data produced by the human genome project. The genes within the interval are then screened for mutations in patients. Identifying plausible candidate genes within the interval may shorten the process as shown by the long arrow in the figure.

that the likelihood of obtaining the genotype data assuming linkage is 1000 times greater than the likelihood assuming no linkage.

After linkage to a genetic region is established, the location of the disease gene can then be further refined by fine mapping, but the resolution is ultimately limited by the occurrence of recombination events near the locus in families in which the disease occurs. *Linkage disequilibrium* and *ancestral haplotype* analysis can then be used to further narrow the interval in which a specific disease mutation is located. Whereas linkage measures co-segregation of markers and disease in pedigrees, linkage disequilibrium measures marker co-segregation in a population. Because linkage disequilibrium measures the tendency to inherit markers as a group or haplotype after many generations of recombination, the intervals identified by linkage disequilibrium are much smaller than those identified by linkage. When the interval has been sufficiently narrowed, all the genes contained in the interval can be identified. This step has been greatly aided by the products of the Human Genome Project. The genes in the interval can then be screened for mutations in patients. Investigators may select plausible candidate genes for evaluation even before interval narrowing is completed, significantly expediting the disease gene-discovery process (see Fig. 12.6).

Positional cloning to identify genes associated with diseases with complex inheritance

Although positional cloning has successfully identified disease genes for rare mendelian genetic disorders, its application to more common diseases with a complex genetic etiology is less well established. These diseases are thought to result from a variety of genetic and non-genetic factors, and the genetic contribution is predicted to be the result of the sum of multiple genetic variants. These variants may be common in the population and difficult to recognize as disease-causing loci. It is hoped that genetic analysis of large, well-characterized cohorts will permit identification of the most common and most important disease-associated genetic variants.

A number of variations to the positional cloning strategy described earlier are necessary to identify complex disease-associated genes. Use of multiplex/multigeneration families may not be practical because of incomplete disease penetrance, late age at disease onset, and the contribution of non-genetic factors. In the place of multiplex families, affected pairs of siblings can be used for linkage analysis (sib-pair

analysis). Alternatively, collections of trios, an affected child and two parents, can be used in the transmission disequilibrium test (TDT), a statistically robust method that tests for linkage of an allele with disease. In this method, linkage of a disease with genetic markers is evaluated by comparing the frequency at which heterozygous parents transmit the "disease-associated" allele to an affected child with the frequency expected by chance (50%). Another use of trios is to perform an analysis for association by comparing the frequency of marker alleles in affected offspring with the frequency in their parents' untransmitted chromosomes. These family-based tests have the advantage of being insensitive to population stratification problems that can lead to spurious associations in standard case-control association studies. An encouraging result using these techniques identified a disease gene, *NOD2*, associated with a complex disease, Crohn's disease.[14,15]

For late-onset diseases, such as rheumatoid arthritis, it may not be practical to collect a sufficiently large number of well-characterized cases with parents to perform an adequately powered TDT or family-based association analysis, and therefore the standard case-control design may be required. In this instance, the matching of cases to controls is crucial to avoid false-positive results due to different population substructure in the cases compared with the controls. Use of haplotype data as opposed to individual marker genotypes may increase the statistical power to identify associations with disease.

Until recently, adequately powered case-control disease association studies with sufficient markers to evaluate the entire genome for association were considered unwieldy, impractical, and cost prohibitive. In the wake of the *HapMap Project*, which identified and genotyped over 4 million SNPs in four different populations, the *genome-wide association* (GWA) study has emerged as a powerful tool for investigating complex genetic diseases. By employing these widely mapped SNP data, the linkage disequilibrium structure of the human genome can be used to define subsets of SNPs representing virtually all known common variation in the human genome. Rapid technologic advances utilizing the *HapMap* data have quickly emerged and have evolved into cost-effective methodologies for high throughput SNP genotyping. Using hybridization technologies that interrogate genome-wide SNP variation on microarray chips, companies such as Affymetrix (Santa Clara, CA) and Illumina (San Diego, CA) have developed platforms to undertake the whole-genome SNP genotyping necessary for GWA studies. These platforms have now been used to perform GWA studies on a broad range of diseases affecting every medical specialty. GWA studies have identified novel susceptibility genes in rheumatic diseases, including rheumatoid arthritis, systemic lupus erythematosus, psoriatic arthritis, and systemic scleroderma and have provided additional insights into common genes involved in human autoimmunity.[16] When properly designed and implemented, GWA studies have the potential to identify associations between genetic loci and diseases using a hypothesis-free model. Proper study design is critical to successfully conducting a GWA study; the introduction of error may either preclude the identification of a significant genetic association or lead to the errant identification of a false association. Because these studies can now analyze over 1 million SNPs, the threshold for genome-wide significance is determined using a Bonferroni or other stringent correction for multiple comparisons. Inadequate sample sizes, uncontrolled ethnic stratification, improper or inconsistent patient phenotyping, and a variety of different logistical batch effects are a few common sources of potential error in GWA studies. It is important that individuals consuming the results of GWA studies, including rheumatologists, be familiar with strategies to critically analyze and evaluate GWA study results.[17] SNP genotyping data and the analysis of linkage disequilibrium in a wide variety of populations continue to be deposited in a public database available at: http://www.hapmap.org/. Genotype and phenotype data obtained from any GWA study supported by the U. S. government are deposited into the database of Genotypes and Phenotypes (dbGaP) at: http://www.ncbi.nlm.nih.gov/gap.

GENE TRANSCRIPTION

Insights into the physiologic and pathologic functions of a given gene may be gained by analysis of the expression of its messenger RNA (mRNA) in tissue and cells and delineating when, where, and how the gene is regulated. Northern blotting and quantitative real-time PCR are useful to measure the level of gene expression, and *in-situ* hybridization can be used to show the gene expression in tissue.

RNA is often isolated using acid guanidinium-phenol-chloroform–based methods and in some cases is further purified by oligo dT columns, which bind the polyA tail of mRNA. In Northern blotting, RNA is separated by size in an agarose gel, transferred to a membrane, and detected by a labeled probe utilizing RNA-DNA hybridization. The amount of mRNA corresponds to the binding of the radioactive probe, which can be visualized by autoradiography.

In real-time PCR, a quantitative method for measuring mRNA, mRNA is transcribed into complementary DNA by reverse transcriptase (Fig. 12.7). A probe with a fluorescent dye at its 5′ end and a quencher dye at the 3′ end is added to the reaction tube. During the PCR reaction, the reporter dye is separated from the quencher dye; DNA polymerase has 5′ nuclease activity, which degrades the hybridized probe as a new DNA strand is synthesized in its place. When the reporter dye is separated from the associated quencher dye, its fluorescence is detected and accumulates with each successive round of PCR. Generation of the fluorescence is quantitatively dependent on the number of transcript copies in the cDNA sample. A reference probe for a housekeeping gene is also included, allowing this to be a quantitative assay. RNAse protection is another means of measuring mRNA and has the advantage that multiple genes can be analyzed simultaneously. In this method, labeled antisense riboprobes are hybridized to RNA in solution and then digested with RNAse, which digests single-stranded but not double-stranded RNA. The amount of riboprobe protected by the mRNA is therefore a measure of the gene expression.

In-situ hybridization identifies which type of cell in a tissue expresses a particular gene. In this method, one hybridizes a specifically labeled nucleic acid probe to the cellular RNA in individual cells or tissue sections. In principle, this employs the same strategy as Northern blotting (hybridization of RNA with labeled cDNA), but in this case the hybridization is visualized within cells using microscopy. The gene's protein product or other proteins can also be visualized by immunohistochemistry, which may be quite informative in the analysis of clinical samples or in assessing the role of the gene in development.

The steady-state levels of mRNA are influenced by several factors, including the rate of its transcription as well as its stability, transport, and translation. The nuclear run-on assay measures the levels of primary transcript production without influence of other factors, and

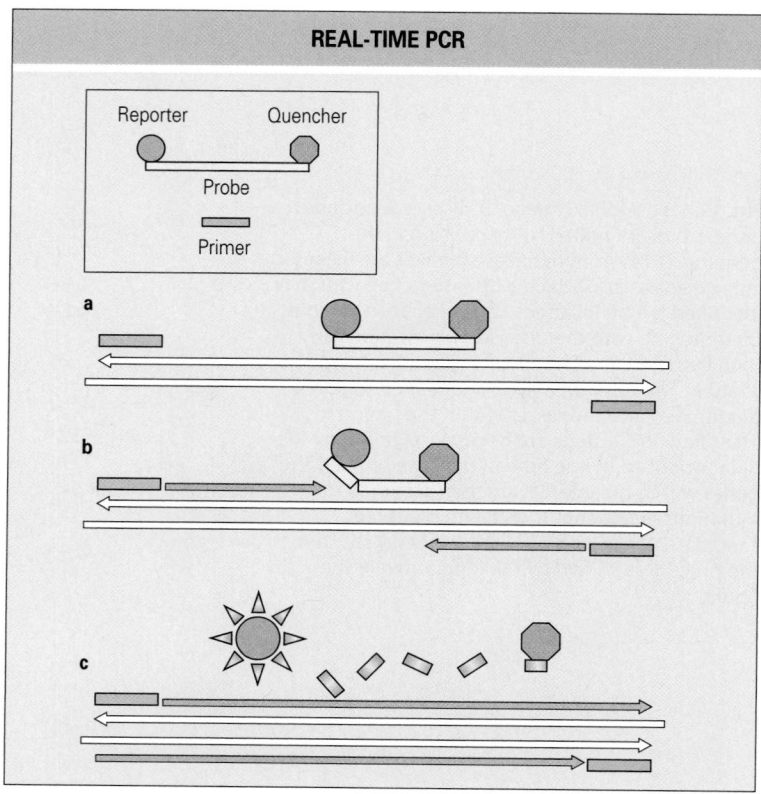

REAL-TIME PCR

Reporter Quencher

Probe

Primer

Fig. 12.7 Quantitative real-time polymerase chain reaction. Oligonucleotide probes coupled to a reporter dye are synthesized along with ordinary primer pairs and used in a PCR reaction. The intact probe does not fluoresce because a quencher is also coupled to the probe. However, the probe is cleaved by DNA polymerase during amplification, separating reporter dye from quencher dye, resulting in increased fluorescence. The amount of PCR products generated can therefore be measured by monitoring the fluorescence intensity with each cycle, because the amount of probe cleaved parallels the amount of PCR products produced. This is a reflection of the initial amount of cDNA generated from mRNA. This test can be further standardized by including probes and primers for "housekeeping genes" and can be made more quantitative by generating a standard curve using known amounts of cDNA encoding the gene of interest.

thus can be used to distinguish if a change in mRNA level is due to induction of transcription *per se* or to other reasons.

EXPRESSION PROFILING AND MICROARRAY TECHNOLOGY

A goal of the human genome sequencing project is to definitively map and identify all the genes encoded within the human genome. Completion of this goal will provide information that will allow us to comprehensively examine gene expression in both health and disease and thereby gain insights into the perturbations of gene expression that may lead to or be a result of different disease pathologies. Studying the function of the aberrantly expressed genes may lead to a better understanding of physiologic and molecular disease mechanisms and, it is hoped, will allow development of new and improved treatments. Although expression of genes can be evaluated by *in-situ* hybridization, RNAse protection assay, Northern blotting, or quantitative real-time PCR (see earlier), the selection of genes for study is limited by the extent of our prior knowledge. New technologies permit expression profiling, that is, analysis of the expression of thousands of genes, including those with unknown function, in a tissue or cell population. Indeed, these newer methods are likely to permit evaluation of expression of not just a few genes but potentially *all* genes.

Several techniques have been developed for expression profiling. In serial analysis of gene expression (SAGE), a small tag (short DNA fragment) is generated from each transcript. The tags are concatenated, and these larger DNA fragments are sequenced to identify the transcripts as well as their frequency in the transcript pool derived from a

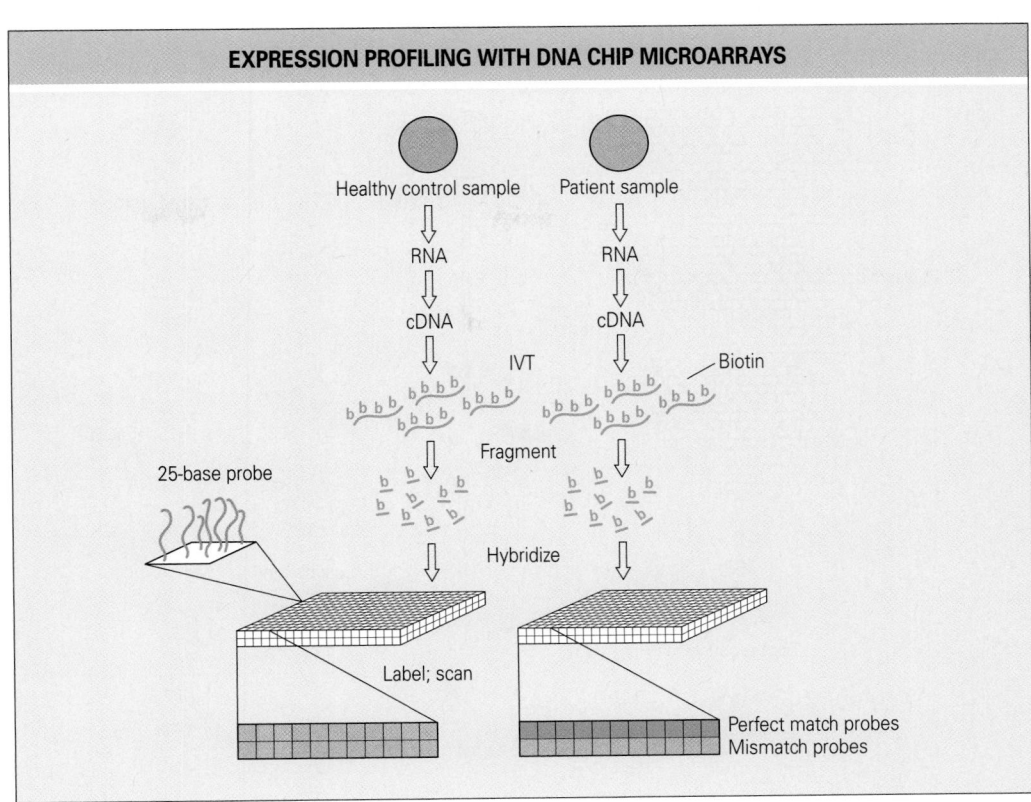

Fig. 12.8 Expression profiling with DNA chip microarrays. Expression of tens of thousands of genes is simultaneously determined using mRNA extracted from samples. The mRNA is reverse transcribed to cDNA, which is *in vitro* transcribed (IVT), producing biotin-labeled cRNA. The cRNA is fragmented and hybridized to oligonucleotide probes that have been synthesized on the surface of a silica chip. The hybridized cRNA is labeled with a streptavidin-conjugated fluor and scanned for detection. Specific hybridization is gauged by comparison of hybridization to pairs of perfect-matched and single-base mismatched oligonucleotides, represented in the figure by the blocks directly above and below one another. Approximately 11 pairs of oligonucleotides on the chip represent each gene. The intensity of the specific hybridization signal is a measure of the gene expression in the sample.

tissue or cell population.[18] Array-based methods of expression profiling use specific nucleic acid probes immobilized in an ordered array on a solid surface. Hybridization techniques in which labeled cDNA or cRNA fragments bind to the immobilized probes are then used to estimate the relative number of copies of each gene transcript in RNA extracted from a tissue or cell sample by the amount of label that binds to the immobilized probe. To achieve probe density sufficient to assay expression of tens of thousands of genes from relatively small tissue or cell samples, microarray technology was developed. There are two commonly used expression profiling microarray techniques; DNA chip microarrays and spotted DNA arrays. In the DNA chip microarray technique the probes are oligonucleotides synthesized on the surface of a DNA chip or attached to the surface of beads that are affixed to the surface of a slide-like BeadChip, and in the second technique they are fragments of cDNA clones or synthetic oligonucleotides that are spotted on the surface of glass microscope slides.[19,20]

DNA chip microarrays

DNA chip microarrays (Fig. 12.8) are manufactured by Affymetrix, Inc. using a proprietary photolithographic process to synthesize 25-base oligonucleotides tethered to the chip surface; each is confined to an 11×11-µm square space. Each gene is represented by 22 squares with oligonucleotide probes covering various parts of the gene. Half the probes are perfect-match, and half are hybridization controls, that is, copies of the perfect match oligonucleotides, each with a single nucleotide mismatch. Probes for up to 47,000 transcripts can be synthesized on a single chip that is less than 1 cm². RNA is extracted from tissue or cells, and cDNA is synthesized. The cDNA is used to produce biotin-labeled complementary RNA (cRNA), which is fragmented and hybridized to the probes on the chip surface. The chips are washed and stained with a streptavidin-conjugated fluorescent dye, which binds to the hybridized biotinylated cRNA. The chips are scanned and the fluorescent signals are processed to determine the expression level of each gene. Normalized expression levels determined from different tissue or cell samples on different chips can then be compared (see Fig. 12.8).

A variant of the DNA chip microarray is the BeadChip microarray (Illumina, Inc.). In this technique beads are coated with oligonucleotides probes (50-mers) attached to an address tag oligonucleotide (30-mers). The beads are randomly affixed to the surface of a slide-like solid support. About 30 of each bead-type (representing a single transcript) are affixed to each BeadChip microarray, and their locations are determined by the address tags. Labeled cRNA is produced and hybridized to the BeadChip. The chips are scanned, and the signal intensity for each probe type is measured.

An advantage of DNA chip or bead microarrays is that, because the microarrays are mass-produced under highly controlled conditions, reproducibility of the expression data obtained from them can be very high. A disadvantage is that production of the microarrays is inflexible (custom arrays are expensive). Furthermore, only genes with sufficient sequence data to generate the probes can be represented on a DNA chip microarray.

Spotted DNA microarrays

A somewhat different technique is used for spotted DNA microarrays (Fig. 12.9). The arrays are produced by robotically spotting cDNA fragments or synthetic oligonucleotides onto glass microscope slides. The cDNA fragments are produced by PCR amplification of collections of cloned cDNA plasmids to obtain the cDNA inserts. Up to 40,000 elements can be printed on a single glass microscope slide. Unlike the DNA chip microarrays, in which transcripts from a single sample are hybridized to the array, cDNA transcripts from two samples the investigator wishes to compare are simultaneously hybridized to the spotted DNA microarray. RNA is extracted from the two samples and converted to cDNA in the presence of either Cy3- or Cy5-labeled nucleotides. The labeled transcripts are then co-hybridized to the DNA probes on the microarray. Hybridization signals from the two dyes are used to determine expression ratios for all the genes on the microarray (see Fig. 12.9).

A variant of the cDNA spotted array technique is to spot long oligonucleotides (60-mers) in the place of the cDNA fragments. This change permits selection of a region or multiple regions of a transcript to be used as probes, thus allowing exclusion of regions that may be involved in non-specific hybridization, as well as allowing separate evaluation of differentially spliced forms of genes.

An advantage of spotted DNA microarrays is that, because the arrays are produced on a small scale, they can be customized, for example to include newly discovered genes. A disadvantage is that the cDNA clone or oligonucleotide libraries must be acquired for production of the arrays. Furthermore, cDNA microarrays are technically difficult to produce and can be subject to reproducibility problems.

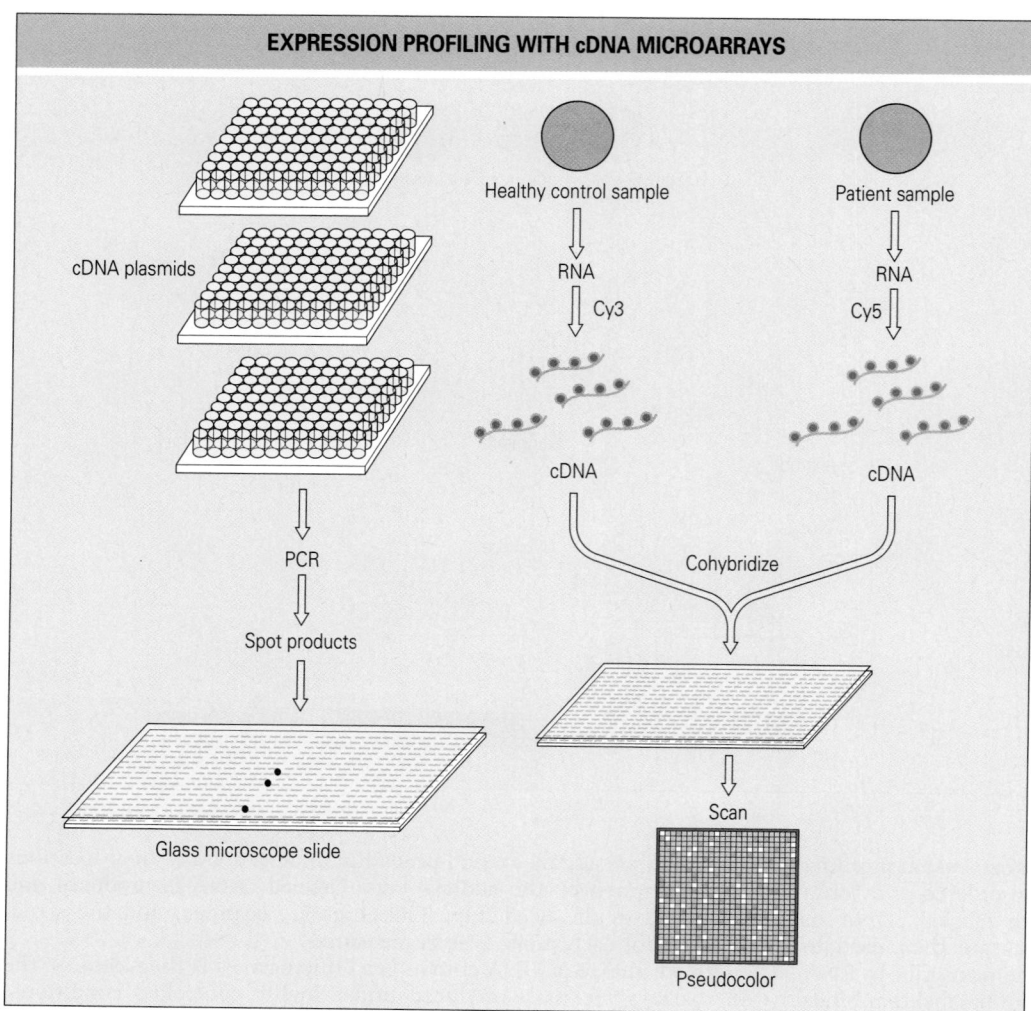

EXPRESSION PROFILING WITH cDNA MICROARRAYS

cDNA plasmids

Healthy control sample

Patient sample

RNA

Cy3

RNA

Cy5

cDNA

cDNA

PCR

Cohybridize

Spot products

Glass microscope slide

Scan

Pseudocolor

Fig. 12.9 Expression profiling with cDNA microarrays. Relative expression of tens of thousands of genes is compared in pairs of samples by extracting RNA from each sample and producing cDNA labeled with one of two different fluorescent dyes (Cy3 or Cy5). The labeled cDNAs are combined and co-hybridized to cDNA library probes (PCR products) that have been spotted onto the surface of glass microscope slides. The relative intensity of the hybridization signal from the two dyes is a measure of relative gene expression in the two samples.

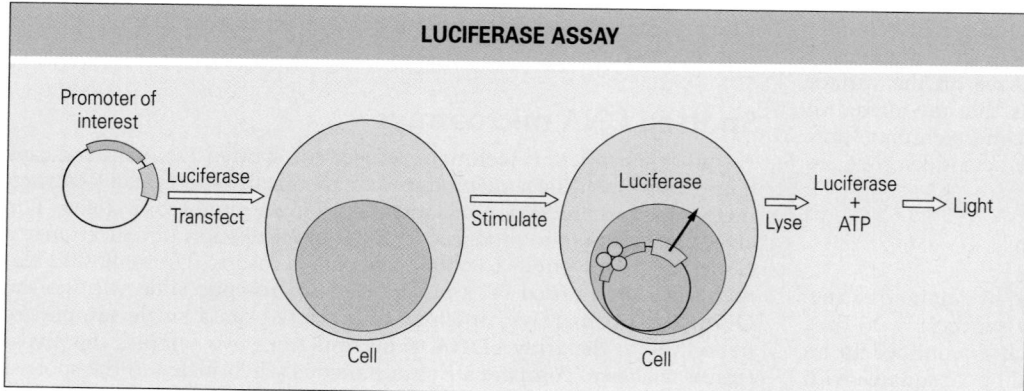

LUCIFERASE ASSAY

Promoter of interest

Luciferase

Transfect

Stimulate

Cell

Luciferase

Lyse

Luciferase + ATP

Light

Cell

Fig. 12.10 Luciferase assay. To determine if a segment of DNA has enhancer/promoter activity, it is cloned upstream of a "reporter gene," which when transcribed will produce the protein encoded by the reporter—in this case the luciferase enzyme. The transcription of this gene and hence the production of the protein is measured by an *in-vitro* assay that produces light, the amount of light produced being proportional to the activation of the promoter.

REGULATION OF GENE EXPRESSION AND PROTEIN-DNA INTERACTIONS

Understanding what controls the expression of a given gene is of considerable interest in the pathogenesis of rheumatic diseases. Typically, the first step in the process involves the identification of the promoter and enhancers of the gene of interest. Generally, this is accomplished by identifying the transcriptional start site and the 5′ untranscribed regulatory portion of the gene. These regions of the gene are then subcloned into reporter systems, which are used as surrogates to measure transcriptional regulation and the interactions of *cis-* and *trans*-acting elements with promoters and enhancers. Typically, regulatory sequences are ligated to reporter genes, such as firefly luciferase, and these plasmids are transfected into cells of interest that are stimulated in various ways. In this manner, the luciferase gene is transcribed

in the place of the native gene, and the level of transcription can be detected by light produced by the translated luciferase protein, which is regulated by stimuli that act on the heterologous promoter (Fig. 12.10). The fine structure of promotor/enhancer regions can be analyzed by introducing a series of mutations and examining the effects on reporter gene expression. The effect of patient-derived mutations/polymorphisms in promoters may also be examined to assess their influence on gene expression.

Identifying transcription factors that bind promotor/enhancer sequences is another important aspect of understanding gene regulation. *Electrophoretic mobility shift assay (EMSA)* is a commonly used technique to detect specific DNA-protein interactions (Fig. 12.11). Nuclear proteins are incubated with radioactively labeled oligonucleotides, electrophoresed on polyacrylamide gels, and visualized by autoradiography. DNA bound to protein "shifts," meaning that it

ELECTROPHORETIC MOBILITY SHIFT ASSAY

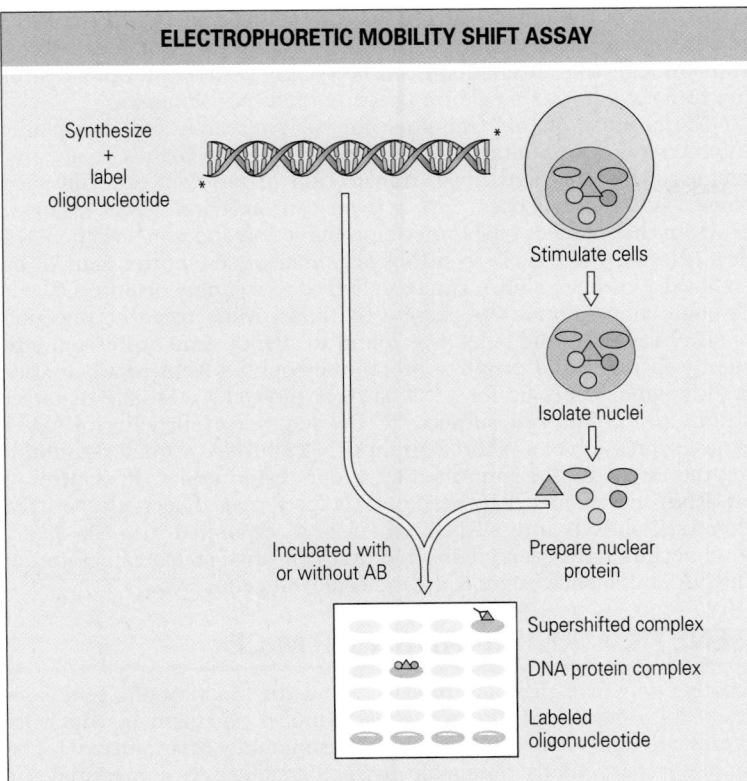

Fig. 12.11 Electrophoretic mobility shift assay. When radiolabeled oligonucleotides are bound by nuclear proteins, their migration in acrylamide gels is retarded or slowed because of their larger molecular weight. This is also referred to as a "shift" in their mobility in the gel. If antibodies against the putative DNA-binding proteins are also included, the complex is said to be "supershifted," and this provides evidence that a particular transcription factor is bound to the oligonucleotide.

migrates more slowly than the unbound radioactive oligonucleotide probe. Bound proteins can be identified by the use of specific antibodies that cause the protein-DNA complex to migrate even more slowly, a so-called super-shift. The *DNAse footprinting assay* is another assay used to look for transcription factors bound to DNA and determine precisely which nucleotides are bound by transcription factors that protect them from degradation by DNAse treatment.

The chromatin immunoprecipitation (ChIP) assay is a technique that detects protein-DNA interaction in cells (Fig. 12.12).[21] In this procedure, nuclear proteins are cross-linked to DNA by formaldehyde. The DNA is sheared and the protein-DNA complexes are immunoprecipitated with antibodies against the proteins that putatively interact with the DNA of interest, thus co-precipitating the DNA bound to these proteins. The cross-links are reversed, and PCR is used to amplify the regions of genes of interest. These products are then run out on agarose gels. Alternatively, real-time PCR can be employed to detect the DNA that was bound by the immunoprecipitated protein. An extension of these principles allows the identification of virtually all the targets of the investigated DNA-binding protein in different cells under different circumstances. This can be accomplished by labeling the immunoprecipitated DNA fragments and hybridizing them to DNA sequences on a microarray slide (ChIP on Chip) or by sequencing all of the immunoprecipitated DNA fragments using efficient "next generation" sequencing technologies. When combined with other "gene expression" data, these experiments provide a powerful genome-wide screening method to identify target genes of transcription factors.

Recent evidence shows that modification of the histone tail (e.g., acetylation, methylation, phosphorylation) is of considerable importance in regulating chromatin structure and the accessibility of genetic loci to transcription factors.[22] Alterations of histone modification are very important in explaining transcriptional on-off states. These changes can be assessed using ChIP with antibodies that detect these modifications. The interaction of other transcription factors with promoters and enhancers can also be determined using ChIP in regions with altered histone modifications. Histone modifications are thought to affect the "accessibility" of genes, and therefore their ability to be

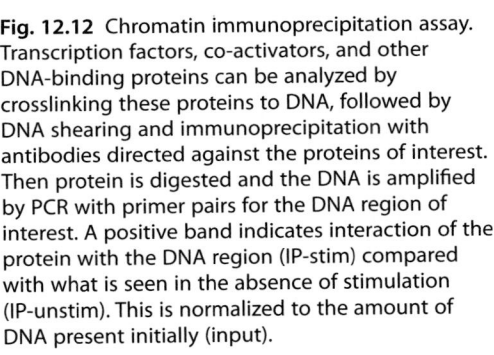

Fig. 12.12 Chromatin immunoprecipitation assay. Transcription factors, co-activators, and other DNA-binding proteins can be analyzed by crosslinking these proteins to DNA, followed by DNA shearing and immunoprecipitation with antibodies directed against the proteins of interest. Then protein is digested and the DNA is amplified by PCR with primer pairs for the DNA region of interest. A positive band indicates interaction of the protein with the DNA region (IP-stim) compared with what is seen in the absence of stimulation (IP-unstim). This is normalized to the amount of DNA present initially (input).

CHROMATIN IMMUNOPRECIPITATION ASSAY

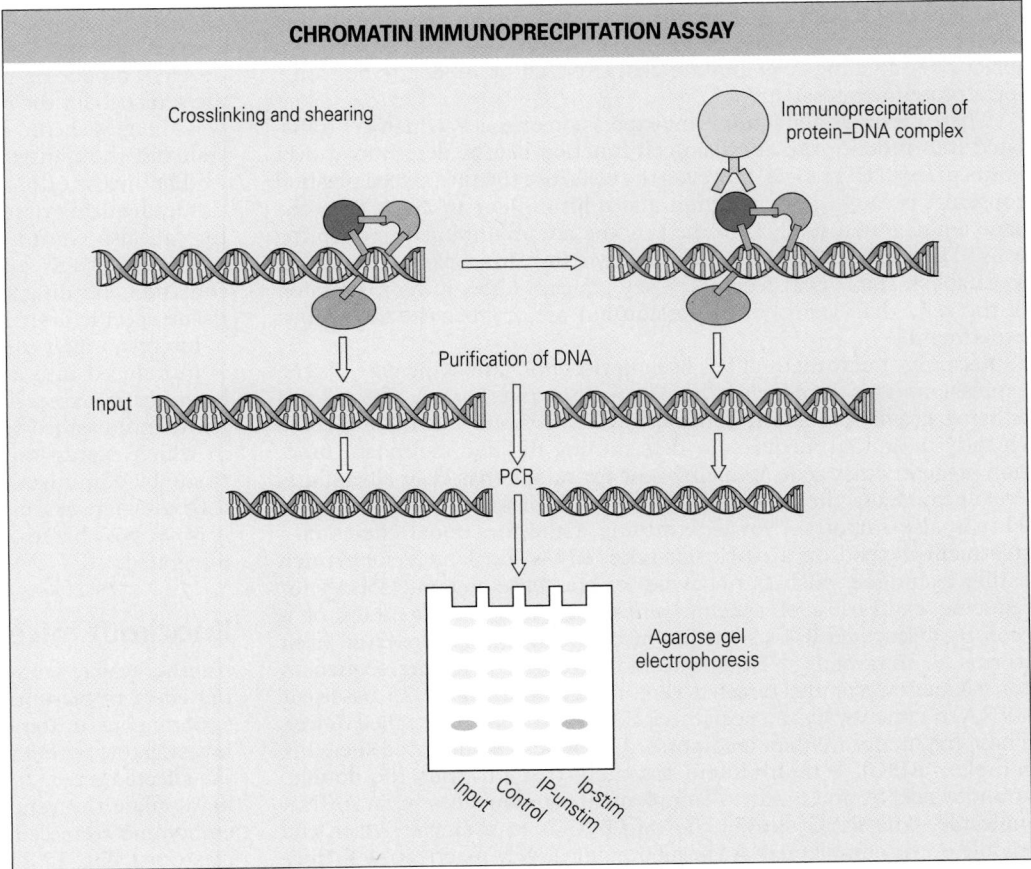

acted on by *cis*-acting transcription factors. Accessibility of genes can also be assessed by their ability to be digested with DNase; *DNAse hypersensitivity* is another means of assessing the transcriptional potential of a locus.

Recent work has illustrated that transcriptional regulation takes place in the context of interactions between disparate genomic loci. *Chromosome conformation capture assay (3C assay)* is designed to detect these interactions of genomic loci *in vivo*.[23] In living cells, two loci that are seemingly far apart on the genome can move into close proximity by "looping out" of the chromosome and sharing DNA binding proteins. A chemical cross-linker is used to stabilize these interactions. Subsequently, the captured DNA is digested and ligated to generate a novel junction between the two interacting DNA loci. PCR is then used to detect these novel ligation products, which are indicative of intrachromosomal interactions between a gene locus and a distant enhancer element and even interactions between two loci on different chromosomes. The 3C assay has the potential to uncover coordinated regulation of genes that are not located close together on the genome yet become physically close together during regulatory remodeling of the chromatin.

ANALYZING GENE FUNCTION

The transfer of genes into mammalian cells has been an essential tool to study gene function. These techniques allow examination of the consequence of expression of a new or altered gene and provide us with a great deal of our knowledge about the action of the encoded protein. cDNAs corresponding to the genes of interest are cloned into expression vectors and are coupled to a strong promoter enabling high expression in cells. For instance, viral promoters are often used to allow high expression in various cell lines. Many different methods are used to transfect these constructs into mammalian cells. These include biochemical methods such as calcium phosphate, DEAE-dextran, and liposome-based methods. Alternatively, for cells that are difficult to transfect by these methods, physical methods such as electroporation and microinjection are used. A third way to transduce genes is by using viral vectors. Developed as tools for gene therapy, these are now widely used for many experiments. The vectors can infect various types of mammalian cells, including cells that are hard to transfect by the other two methods. Adenovirus and retroviruses are representative viruses used for gene transfer. Adenovirus can infect most types of cells and allows transient but high protein expression, whereas retroviruses infect only dividing cells and are characterized by moderate but long-term protein expression.

These methods allow transient expression of genes, which are translated into protein; the effect on cell function can be determined over hours to days. Over time, however, the cells lose the introduced plasmid construct because of degradation and dilution, but in a few cells the gene is integrated stably into the genome and maintained in offspring cells. These rare cells can be selected by using drug selection reagents to establish stable transfectants. They typically show lower expression of the gene than transient expression but are of great use for various experiments.

Recently, a new method has been devised for "knocking down" gene expression. This approach is based on RNA interference (RNAi) and is being heavily employed both with cells in tissue culture and more recently in animal models. For determining the non-redundant function of a particular gene, reducing gene expression has clear advantages over introducing the gene exogenously with plasmid or viral vectors. This is also important for determining if the functional effects of a treatment depend on a particular gene. RNAi has largely supplanted earlier techniques such as ribozymes or antisense oligonucleotides for reducing expression of specific genes. RNAi takes advantage of a recently discovered RNA silencing mechanism that is conserved from worms to mammals.[24] Double-stranded RNA containing sequences complementary to the targeted gene are cut into 21 to 23 base-pair siRNA fragments by a specialized RNAse III enzyme called Dicer. These fragments are then incorporated into the RNA-induced silencing complex (RISC), a multiprotein assembly that unwinds the double-stranded siRNA and binds to complementary sequences in an mRNA molecule. The RISC cleaves the target RNA at a single site in the middle of the complementary sequence, effectively inactivating further translation of the target mRNA. Because a single siRNA in the RISC can inactivate multiple target mRNA's, "knockdown" of gene expression through this mechanism can be potent (>90%) and long-lasting (up to 5 days from a single transfection of siRNA duplexes).

The promise of this technique for basic research and therapeutic intervention is beginning to be realized.[25] In most higher organisms, including humans and mice, transfection of long dsRNA and even some shorter sequences can activate an antiviral gene response program that induces type I interferon induction and non-specific RNA degradation by RNAse L, so siRNA oligonucleotides shorter than 23 bp are used. Synthetic siRNA can be delivered to a variety of cultured cells through conventional transfection methods. More recently, injection of siRNA with a fluid bolus was found to silence gene expression efficiently in mice, and coupling protamine-bound siRNA to a Fab antibody fragment specific for a cell surface molecule was able to target siRNA to specific cell subsets.[26,27] For long-term silencing of target genes, expression of a "short-hairpin" RNA (shRNA) sequence containing the target siRNA connected by a loop region under the control of an RNA polymerase III promoter is preferred. Dicer cleaves the expressed shRNA into siRNA, which is incorporated into the RISC. Viral vectors have been engineered that can drive stable expression of shRNA and silence target RNA molecules in primary cells.[28,29]

GENETIC MANIPULATION OF MICE

Another way investigators can learn about the function of a gene is to study its *in-vivo* function in a genetic model organism in which its expression and structure can be experimentally manipulated. The mouse is particularly amenable to such studies. As a mammal, its genes and gene functions are very similar to those in humans, but it is possible to manipulate its genome by introducing or overexpressing genes in transgenic mice or by using targeted disruption to destroy a gene in knockout mice.[30] Investigators can then study the effects of these genetic alterations in the animals, their tissues, or cells.

Transgenic mice

Transgenic animals are genetically modified animals in which foreign DNA has been experimentally inserted into the transgenic genome. This is accomplished by injecting a DNA construct into the pronucleus of a fertilized oocyte. Blastocysts that develop from these injected oocytes are transferred to pseudopregnant females, in which they develop, producing potentially transgenic pups (Fig. 12.13). The pups are screened for the presence of the transgene and bred. If the transgene was integrated into the genome of its germline, the animal will then transmit the transgene to the next generation.

The investigator can target expression of the transgene to specific tissues by using tissue-specific promoters or enhancers. The investigator can also control expression of a transgene by using an inducible promoter system such as a tetracycline-regulated system, in which a construct encoding a tetracycline-induced factor under the control of a tissue-specific promoter is introduced in one mouse line and the gene of interest, under control of a promoter that is controlled by the factor, is introduced into a second line. The tetracycline-induced factor can be either an expression activator or an expression repressor. The lines are then crossbred to generate animals with both genetic alterations, in which expression of the transgene can be controlled in the target tissue by administering or withdrawing tetracycline. Transgenes typically integrate as a tandemly repeated unit within the recipient genome. It is not possible to control the integration site or the number of copies integrated.

Knockout mice

Another way to study the function of a gene is to determine in animals the effect of disrupting the gene so that its product is not produced. Spontaneous mutations that have this effect on genes have provided investigators with a great deal of information regarding the function of the affected genes. It is now possible for investigators to experimentally manipulate the genomes of mice by disrupting a gene in pluripotent embryonic stem cells and incorporating those cells into a developing blastocyst (Fig. 12.14).

TRANSGENIC MICE

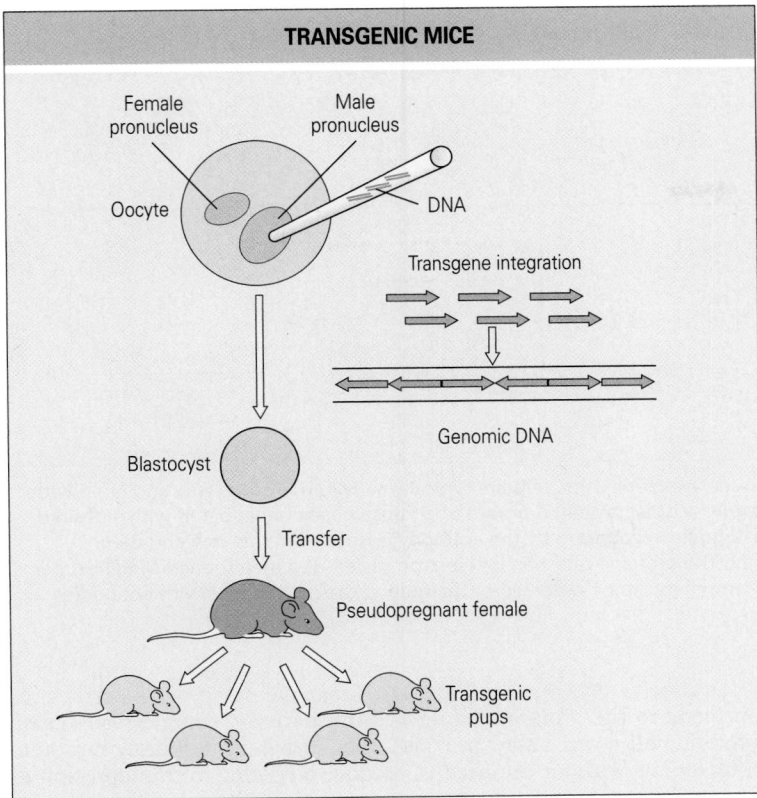

Fig. 12.13 Transgenic mice. Overexpression of DNA constructs in transgenic animals is achieved by injecting a DNA construct (containing the transgene) into the male pronucleus of a fertilized oocyte. The transgene may integrate as a tandem repeat within the recipient genome. Blastocysts are allowed to develop *in vitro* and are then transferred to pseudopregnant female mice. If the transgene has integrated into the genome of the germline, the transgenic offspring (founders) will transmit the transgene to their offspring.

KNOCKOUT MICE

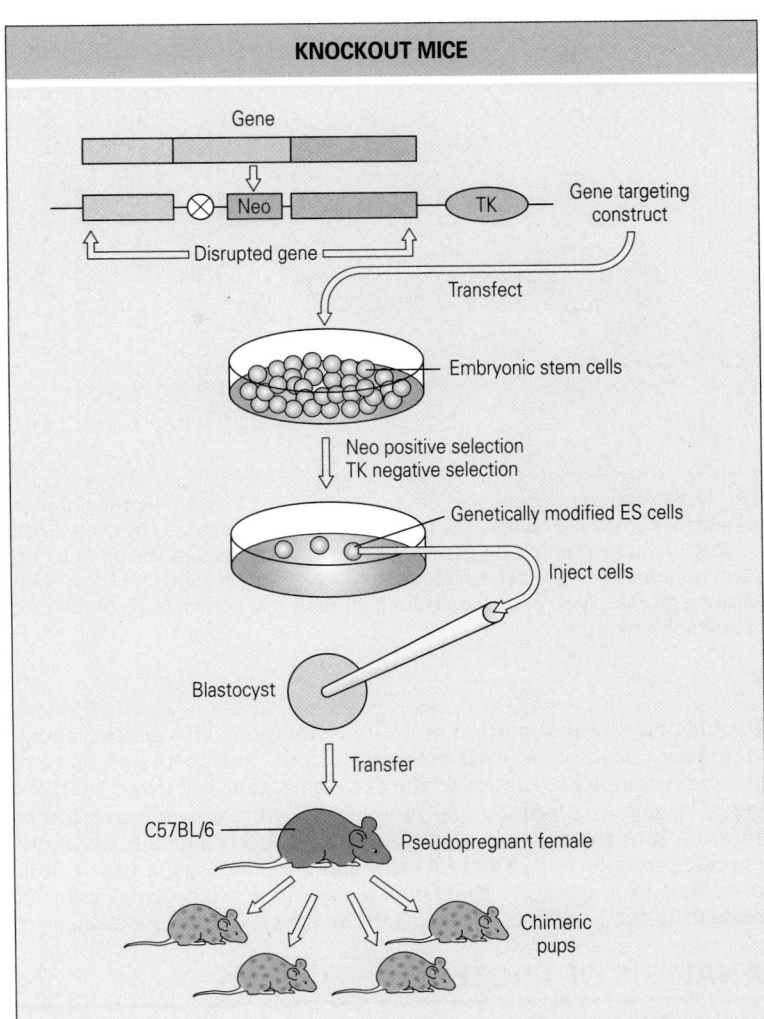

Fig. 12.14 Knockout mice. A gene can be effectively deleted from an animal's genome by disrupting it or deleting an essential domain in embryonic stem cells that can then be transferred to blastocysts, in which they may be incorporated into the germline tissue of the developing embryo. A gene-targeting construct is transfected into embryonic stem cells, and a disruption cassette replaces a part of the cell's gene by the process of homologous recombination. Because this process is inefficient, a positive selection gene (Neo) is incorporated within the disruption cassette and a negative selection gene (TK) is incorporated outside the cassette to eliminate untransfected cells and transfectants with integration of the targeting construct elsewhere in the genome. Rare cells that have undergone homologous recombination are expanded in culture and injected into blastocysts. Chimeric offspring, in which the targeted embryonic stem cells have incorporated, can be recognized by the contribution of agouti (brown) targeted (L129) stem cells to the non-agouti (black) coat of the recipient (B6) blastocyst. If the stem cells have contributed to the offspring germline, the offspring will transmit the disrupted gene to its offspring.

The technique used to disrupt a gene is to transfect the embryonic stem cells *in vitro* with a DNA construct in which a fragment of the gene sequence has been disrupted by incorporating a selectable marker gene, such as the neomycin resistance marker, that can be used for positive selection of cells that have integrated the construct. Disruption of the endogenous gene occurs by the process of homologous recombination, whereby homologous sequences flanking the disruption facilitate the exchange of the disrupted gene fragment with the analogous fragment of the endogenous gene. The construct may include a coding sequence deletion and/or a premature termination and polyadenylation signal, which, when incorporated within the endogenous gene, blocks its expression. The construct also contains, outside of the gene disruption cassette, a second marker, such as the thymidine kinase marker, that can be used for negative selection to eliminate transfectants in which non-homologous recombination occurred.

Cells in which homologous recombination occurred are injected into blastocysts and the blastocysts are transferred to foster mothers. Some of the pups produced may be chimeras, in which the genetically altered embryonic stem cells have expanded and contributed to the developing embryo. By using blastocysts and stem cells from strains with different-colored coats, the chimeric pups can be recognized by the contribution of the stem cells to the coat color.

As with transgenic mice, the chimeric offspring are then bred to determine whether the embryonic stem cells contributed to the development of germ cells and will therefore be transmitted to the next generation. Carriers of the chromosome with the disrupted gene can be interbred to produce knockout or gene-targeted mice, in which both copies of the gene are disrupted.

A variant of the knockout mouse, the knockin mouse, can be used to trace the temporal and spatial expression patterns of a gene and to study regulation of its expression. In this technique the targeting construct includes a reporter gene, such as the β-galactosidase gene, as well as the selectable marker. The targeted animals produce a chimeric protein, in which the reporter gene is fused to a portion of the gene under study. The chimeric gene is expected to be expressed in the same manner as the gene under study. Expression of the chimeric gene can be evaluated by analyzing expression of the reporter gene. This knockin technology can also be used to introduce a disease-associated or other mutation into the gene of interest.

Cre/lox-directed targeted disruption

If disruption of a gene interferes with embryonic development or is lethal, it is difficult to discern its function in knockout mice. Investigators may, however, examine the effect of eliminating the gene's expression from specific tissues or at specific times. These experiments are made possible by the cre/lox recombinase system in which lox sites, recognized by the cre recombinase, are inserted in intron sequences

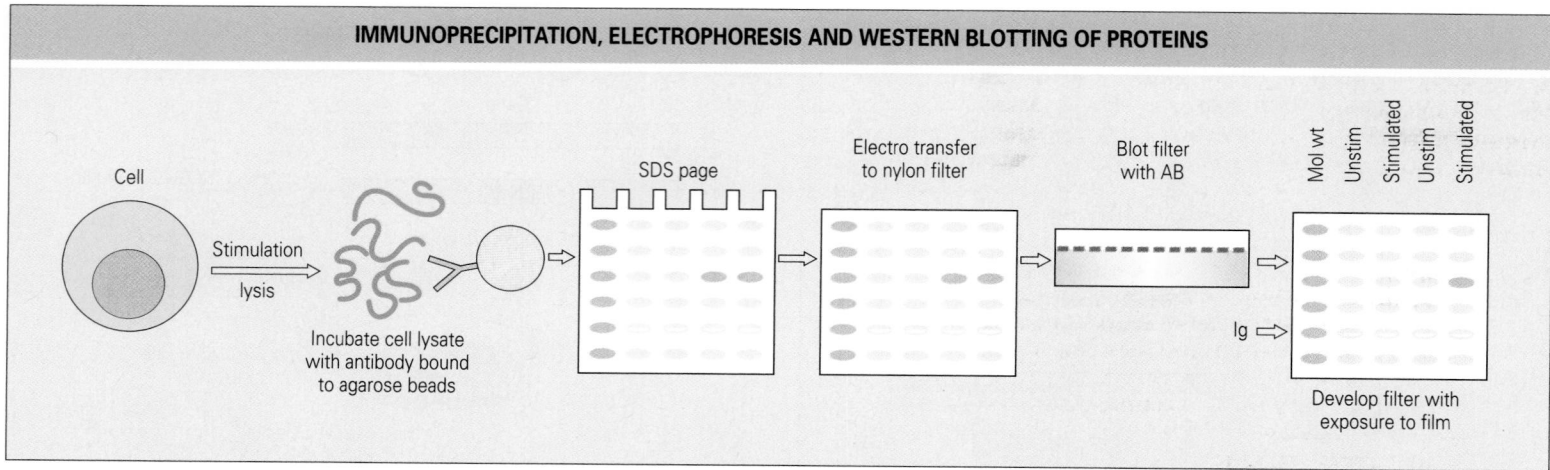

IMMUNOPRECIPITATION, ELECTROPHORESIS AND WESTERN BLOTTING OF PROTEINS

Fig. 12.15 Immunoprecipitation, electrophoresis, and Western blotting of proteins. In these experiments, cells are typically activated in some way and lysed with detergent-containing buffers. The insoluble material is removed by centrifugation. Staphylococcal protein A bound to agarose beads is incubated with a desired antibody, and this complex is then incubated with cell lysates. The protein or protein complex recognized by the antibody is isolated in this way and then electrophoresed on polyacrylamide gels, which separates proteins by molecular weight. The proteins can then be electrotransfered to membranes. Modifications of these proteins (e.g., phosphorylation), proteins that co-associate, or the proteins themselves can be detected by incubating the membranes with antibodies (immunoblotting).

flanking an essential portion of the targeted gene. This genetic alteration does not interfere with the gene's expression. In the presence of the cre recombinase, however, the targeted region is excised from the gene, leaving a non-functional remnant. The cre recombinase can be inserted into the genome as a transgene and an inducible or tissue-specific promoter can direct its expression. In this way, a gene can be disrupted in a specific tissue or at a specific developmental stage by regulating the location and timing of cre expression in the animal.

ANALYSIS OF PROTEINS

The regulation of expression of proteins in cells pertinent to rheumatologic disease is often analyzed. Flow cytometry allows detection of cell surface and intracellular proteins recognized by specific antibodies on a single-cell basis and, with multicolor staining, permits the simultaneous analysis of the expression of several molecules on specific cell populations. Because of the ease of this technique it is commonly employed. To identify the location of a protein of interest within tissues, immunohistochemistry is often used; again, the detection of the protein is dependent on its recognition by specific antibodies. For localization within a cell, electron microscopy or confocal microscopy and immunofluorescence are often employed. Transfection of cells with proteins fused to GFP to detect under video-imaging is a modern technology to track localization and movement of the molecule in a living cell (see Fig. 12.3).

Immunoblotting or Western blotting is still the most widely used technique to identify protein expression, modification, and interactions with other proteins. In brief, proteins are separated by SDS-polyacrylamide gel electrophoresis, transferred to a membrane, and detected by specific antibodies bound to enzymes such as horseradish peroxidase. These antibody-protein complexes are detected by chemilluminescence, autoradiography, or similar methods (Fig. 12.15).

Protein function is regulated by various post-translational modifications and through dynamic protein-protein interactions; indeed a paradigm shift in cell signaling has been the understanding of the importance of these interactions. For instance, tyrosine phosphorylation and serine/threonine phosphorylation are major modifications that regulate protein function and assembly of protein complexes. Increasingly, antibodies against phosphorylated forms of various proteins are being made available for the dissection of signal transduction pathways. These antibodies can be used in immunoblotting (see Fig. 12.15) and even in flow cytometry.

Protein-protein interactions can be analyzed by various techniques. Co-immunoprecipitation of one protein with another is a standard technique, but the interactions can be influenced by the detergents used to lyse the cells. Immunoprecipitation reactions require a specific antibody to the protein of interest. Alternatively, using a GST-fusion protein pull-down assay provides good evidence for protein-protein interactions without the need to produce a specific immunoprecipitating antibody. The GST tagged protein binds with high affinity to glutathione attached to agarose beads. Non-interacting proteins are removed by washing. Proteins that remain bound to the GST-tagged protein can then be assayed by 2D gel electrophoresis or other analytic techniques. A third method for assessing protein-protein interactions is far-Western blotting, in which a labeled, recombinant protein is used to "blot" a membrane in which cell lysates have been separated. If the recombinant protein interacts with a cellular protein, the interaction is visualized as a "band."

Fluorescence resonance energy transfer (FRET) can be used to study protein-protein interactions in living cells as an important complement to strictly biochemical methods. Energy emitted by a fluorophore can be transferred to an acceptor fluorophore causing sensitized emission at a longer wavelength only if the two molecules are in extremely close proximity (<10 nm). Antibodies conjugated to appropriate fluorochromes were originally used to measure protein-protein interactions in this way. More recently, fusion proteins to fluorescent protein pairs with properties suitable for FRET such as cyan fluorescent protein (CFP) and yellow fluorescent protein (YFP) have been used to assess interactions of proteins by microscopy and flow cytometry.[31] In cell-free systems, protein-protein interactions can be quantitatively measured using surface plasmon resonance.[32]

Yeast two-hybrid screening is another method that not only provides a means of detecting interactions between known proteins but also permits the identification of new partners. Most proteins consist of multiple domains with independent functions. Two-hybrid technology takes advantage of these modular functions. Typically, a fusion protein is created in which the DNA binding domain of one protein is linked to a domain from a heterologous protein; this is referred to as the "bait." Either a known protein or a library of cDNAs is fused to a transcriptional activation domain. Interaction of the "bait" and the "prey" allows the activation of transcription of a reporter gene that is bound via the DNA binding domain. Often the reporter gene encodes β-galactosidase, so that protein-protein interaction is visualized by the blue color of the colonies. If the DNA binding domain and activation domain are not in proximity, no activation of the reporter occurs (Fig. 12.16).

PROTEOMICS

Proteomics is a term that connotes some of the same issues as genomics. It is defined as the expressed protein complement of the genome and seeks to gain a global and integrated view of changes in protein

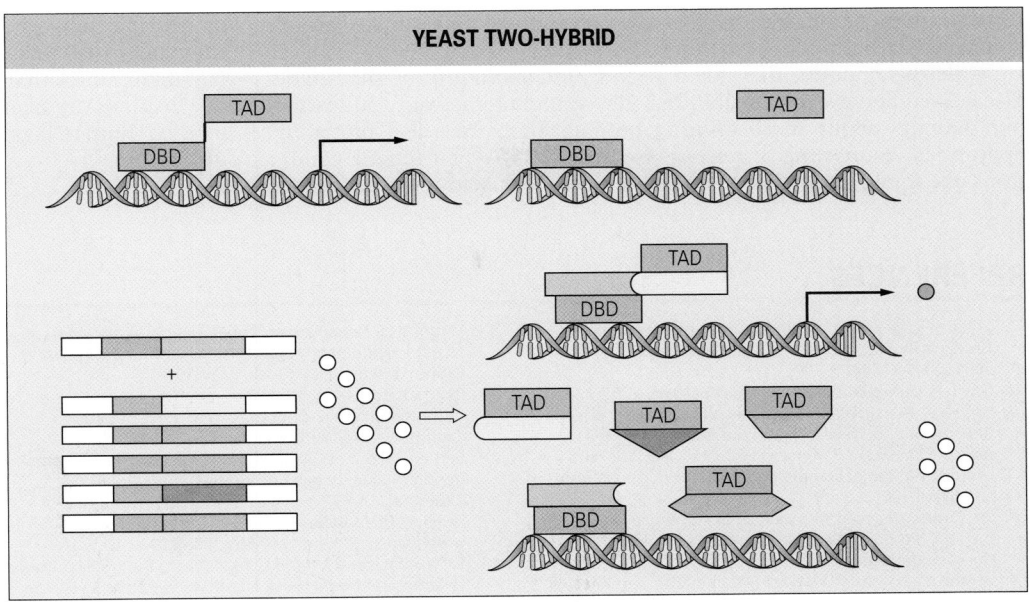

YEAST TWO-HYBRID

Fig. 12.16 Yeast two-hybrid. DNA binding domains (DBD) and transcriptional activation domains (TAD) may be present in a single protein, which regulates gene transcription, whereas transcription does not occur if they are not in proximity. However, these domains may also function as independent modules. When fusion proteins are created that join heterologous polypeptides ("bait" and "prey") to these modules, transcription is driven only when there is physical interaction between these polypeptides. Often the "bait" is used to screen a library of potential "prey"; interacting polypeptides will score as positives in transcription of the reporter gene, in this case β-galactosidase, which will turn colonies blue.

expression in cells or tissues.[33,34] Whereas the human genome comprises about 30,000 genes, alternate splicing and different types of modification probably result in at least 100,000 different proteins. Furthermore, proteomics also includes protein-protein interactions and localization, making this field far more complex than genomics. It is worth emphasizing, in this respect, that proteins and not genes are the regulators of cell function.

2D gel electrophoresis is a multiple-step procedure that can be used to separate hundreds to thousands of proteins with extremely high resolution. It works by separating proteins by their isoelectric points in the first dimension (isoelectric focusing) and then by their molecular weights in the second dimension (polyacrylamide gel electrophoresis). Using sophisticated image analysis methods, the proteins from different samples can be compared to identify differences among the samples. Proteins of interest can then be extracted, identified, and further analyzed.

Sequencing of proteins by Edman degradation has been performed since the 1940s, but automation of this technique and microsequencing of electrophoresed proteins transferred to membranes has greatly improved the ability to identify polypeptides. Mass spectroscopy was devised more than a century ago, but biomolecules are large and polar and are not easily transferred to the gas phase and ionized. However, the development and automation of two methods, electron spray ionization and matrix-assisted laser desorption ionization (MALDI), has facilitated the application of mass spectroscopy to biology. The identification of polypeptides is also greatly enhanced by the availability of amino acid sequence and peptide mass fingerprinting databases; in this respect, advances in genomics facilitate advances in proteomics.

Like genomics, the field of proteomics has been driven by advances in technology. A variety of new techniques involving microarrays of proteins and tissues are permitting large-scale analysis of protein interactions and localization. Spotting cell lysates on microarrays is allowing efficient evaluation of pathways; for example, the kinetics of signal transduction pathways has been probed with phosphorylation-specific antibodies.[35] Of particular interest to rheumatologists, autoantigen microarrays have been used to profile serum autoantibodies in patients with autoimmune diseases.[36]

MOLECULAR BIOLOGY: THE NEW PATHOLOGY FOR THE PRACTICING RHEUMATOLOGIST?

Aside from helping the clinician to understand the research papers that appear in the medical literature, what is the utility of the material presented in this chapter? Or to put it another way, what is the likely impact of the Human Genome Project and the molecular biology revolution on the clinical practice of rheumatology?

At earlier times in the history of medicine, technologic advances have transformed diagnosis and treatment by fostering rational diagnostic schemes based on etiologic or pathogenetic insights. Microscopy and histochemistry led to our basic concepts of pathology at the tissue and cellular level. Later, the emerging field of microbiology permitted a classification of infectious disease based on specific pathogens. More recently, biochemistry has provided the tools to dissect still other classes of illnesses that evaded understanding on the basis of histology or microbiology alone. For instance, our current understanding of amyloidosis is critically dependent on the discovery that amyloid deposits that are indistinguishable under the microscope are actually composed of one of several different possible proteins and that each type of deposit is associated with a different pathogenesis, prognosis, and treatment.

Rheumatology in the 21st century specializes in a number of disorders that have defied understanding by application of current cellular, biochemical, and immunologic techniques. Whereas systemic lupus erythematosus, rheumatoid arthritis, and osteoarthritis are often viewed as single disease entities, there is great clinical heterogeneity among patients, and it is likely that these conditions are actually syndromes that subsume multiple disorders, each with a distinct pathogenesis, prognosis, and treatment.

Although it is unlikely that molecular biology will be the prism that resolves all of the rheumatic syndromes into their etiologic subsets, the genome revolution does provide us with new tools that are already beginning to have an impact. For example, owing largely to the advent of positional cloning, in the past 10 years we have witnessed the discovery of five different genes and over 300 mutations in patients who were previously lumped together under the label of having "hereditary periodic fever." In the field of oncology, lymphomas indistinguishable by light microscopy can now be classified according to gene expression profiles that much more accurately predict prognosis and response to treatment. In many areas of medicine, polymorphisms in drug metabolizing enzymes have been associated with both clinical response and adverse effects of treatment. Proteomics and genomics offer new opportunities to identify biomarkers that provide surrogates of disease activity and response to therapy.

DNA diagnostics, gene expression profiling, and SNP analysis are among the molecular techniques that make up what might be regarded as the "new pathology," and in many cases these approaches promise to redefine the clinical practice of rheumatology. For certain conditions it is already common practice to obtain blood specimens for DNA or RNA extraction for clinically indicated tests. In other conditions, particularly for complex rheumatic diseases such as systemic lupus erythematosus, molecular studies are still at the level of bench research. However, the practitioner can help to catalyze the potential molecular transformation of rheumatology by participating in studies that often require samples from hundreds or even thousands of patients to attain sufficient statistical power.

With the opportunities for a deeper understanding of rheumatic diseases come new responsibilities. These include not only educating our patients about these exciting new advances but also providing appropriate counseling or referrals for counseling when genetic conditions are found. Moreover, as a society we must deal with the issues of possible job or insurance discrimination arising from predictive inferences that may be drawn from genetic test results. As with other paradigm shifts that have overtaken medical science in the past, the implications are likely to be far reaching, both in their impact on many levels of human experience and in the time course over which they will unfold.

REFERENCES

1. Collins FS, McKusick VA. Implications of the Human Genome Project for medical science. JAMA 2001;285:540-544.
2. Lewin B. Genes IX. Boston: Jones & Bartlett, 2007.
3. Lodish H, Matsudaira P, Berk A, et al. Molecular cell biology, 6th ed. New York: WH Freeman, 2007.
4. Ausubel FM, Brent R, Kingston RE, et al., eds. Current protocols in molecular biology. New York: John Wiley and Sons, 2009.
5. Sambrook J, Russell DW. Molecular cloning: a laboratory manual, 3rd ed. Cold Spring Harbor, NY: Cold Spring Harbor Laboratory, 2001.
6. Venter JC, Adams MD, Myers EW, et al. The sequence of the human genome. Science 2001;291:1304-1351.
7. Lander ES, Linton LM, Birren B, et al. Initial sequencing and analysis of the human genome. Nature 2001;409:860-921.
8. Goodman N. Biological data becomes computer literate: new advances in bioinformatics. Curr Opin Biotechnol 2002;13:68-71.
9. Kitano H. Systems biology: a brief overview. Science 2002;295:1662-1664.
10. van Roessel P, Brand AH. Imaging into the future: visualizing gene expression and protein interactions with fluorescent proteins. Nat Cell Biol 2002;4:E15-E20.
11. International FMF Consortium. Ancient missense mutations in a new member of the RoRet gene family are likely to cause familial Mediterranean fever. Cell 1997;90:797-807.
12. French FMF Consortium. A candidate gene for familial Mediterranean fever. Nat Genet 1997;17:25-31.
13. Kwok PY. Methods for genotyping single nucleotide polymorphisms. Annu Rev Genomics Hum Genet 2001;2:235-258.
14. Hugot JP, Chamaillard M, Zouali H, et al. Association of NOD2 leucine-rich repeat variants with susceptibility to Crohn's disease. Nature 2001;411:599-603.
15. Ogura Y, Bonen DK, Inohara N, et al. A frameshift mutation in NOD2 associated with susceptibility to Crohn's disease. Nature 2001;411:603-606.
16. Lettre G, Rioux JD. Autoimmune diseases: insights from genome-wide association studies. Hum Mol Genet 2008;17:R116-R121.
17. Pearson TA, Manolio TA. How to interpret a genome-wide association study. JAMA 2008;299:1335-1344.
18. Saha S, Sparks AB, Rago C, et al. Using the transcriptome to annotate the genome. Nat Biotechnol 2002;20:508-512.
19. Duggan DJ, Bittner M, Chen Y, et al. Expression profiling using cDNA microarrays. Nat Genet 1999;21:10-14.
20. Lipshutz RJ, Fodor SP, Gingeras TR, Lockhart DJ. High density synthetic oligonucleotide arrays. Nat Genet 1999;21:20-24.
21. Orlando V. Mapping chromosomal proteins in vivo by formaldehyde-crosslinked-chromatin immunoprecipitation. Trends Biochem Sci 2000;25:99-104.
22. Jenuwein T, Allis CD. Translating the histone code. Science 2001;293:1074-1080.
23. Osborne CS, Chakalova L, Brown KE, et al. Active genes dynamically colocalize to shared sites of ongoing transcription. Nat Genet 2004;36:1065-1071.
24. Dykxhoorn DM, Novina CD, Sharp PA. Killing the messenger: short RNAs that silence gene expression. Nat Rev Mol Cell Biol 2003;4:457-467.
25. Dykxhoorn DM, Lieberman J. The silent revolution: RNA interference as basic biology, research tool, and therapeutic. Annu Rev Med 2005;56:401-423.
26. Song E, Lee SK, Wang J, et al. RNA interference targeting Fas protects mice from fulminant hepatitis. Nat Med 2003;9:347-351.
27. Song E, Zhu P, Lee SK, et al. Antibody mediated in vivo delivery of small interfering RNAs via cell-surface receptors. Nat Biotechnol 2005;23:709-717.
28. Paddison PJ, Caudy AA, Bernstein E, et al. Short hairpin RNAs (shRNAs) induce sequence-specific silencing in mammalian cells. Genes Dev 2002;16:948-958.
29. Stewart SA, Dykxhoorn DM, Palliser D, et al. Lentivirus-delivered stable gene silencing by RNAi in primary cells. RNA 2003;9:493-501.
30. Mak TW, Penninger JM, Ohashi PS. Knockout mice: a paradigm shift in modern immunology. Nat Rev Immunol 2001;1:11-19.
31. Zacharias DA, Baird GS, Tsien RY. Recent advances in technology for measuring and manipulating cell signals. Curr Opin Neurobiol 2000;10:416-421.
32. McDonnell JM. Surface plasmon resonance: towards an understanding of the mechanisms of biological molecular recognition. Curr Opin Chem Biol 2001;5:572-577.
33. Mann M, Hendrickson RC, Pandey A. Analysis of proteins and proteomes by mass spectrometry. Annu Rev Biochem 2001;70:437-473.
34. Aebersold R, Rist B, Gygi SP. Quantitative proteome analysis: methods and applications. Ann N Y Acad Sci 2000;919:33-47.
35. Chan SM, Ermann J, Su L, et al. Protein microarrays for multiplex analysis of signal transduction pathways. Nat Med 2004;10:1390-1396.
36. Robinson WH, DiGennaro C, Hueber W, et al. Autoantigen microarrays for multiplex characterization of autoantibody responses. Nat Med 2002;8:295-301.

REFERENCES

Full references for this chapter can be found on www.expertconsult.com.

Signal transduction

Martin Aringer and John J. O'Shea

- Introduce principles of relaying messages within cells.
- Provide a systematic overview on signal transduction pathways.
- Define receptors, key enzymes and messengers in signaling.
- Sketch signaling pathways with relevance for rheumatic diseases.
- Relate to novel therapeutics targeting signaling molecules.

INTRODUCTION

A fundamental issue in cell biology is how cells respond to external stimuli and perturbations within the cell. Solutions to this problem underlie the concept of recognition of self/non-self by the vertebrate immune system but also pertain to the notion of immunoregulation and the control of inflammatory responses. Conceptually, one can visualize this problem by considering the nature of the ligands.

Some molecules such as gases or lipid-soluble ligands directly traverse the plasma membrane, exerting their effects in the cytosol and nucleus. For instance, nitric oxide is an important gas that has critical regulatory functions in both non-immune and immune cells. Another subset of these membrane-permeant ligands binds cytosolic or nuclear receptors, which themselves function as transcription factors. Members of the steroid receptor superfamily, such as glucocorticoid receptors, are examples of such factors. In contrast, charged ions are obliged to traverse the plasma membrane via channels.

However, many other ligands require interaction with some kind of membrane receptor. The ligands themselves do not cross the plasma membrane; rather, they initiate a signal transduction cascade. From the point of view of a rheumatologist, most of the relevant ligands fall into this category. For instance, receptors on the cell membrane or inside the cell bind antigen, chemokines, cytokines, products of pathogens (so-called pathogen-associated molecular patterns [PAMPS]), adhesion, and co-stimulatory molecules.

In some cases, signal transduction leads to immediate changes in the cell, such as mobilization of intracellular calcium, actin polymerization, alteration of cell shape and motility, and chemotaxis; caspase activation and initiation of apoptotic pathways; converting enzyme activation and processing of cytokines; and release of preformed mediators (Fig. 13.1). In other cases, signal transduction leads to *de novo* gene expression through the action of latent, cytosolic factors, which bind DNA and regulate transcription (transcription factors).

It is not our goal to comprehensively discuss all aspects of signal transduction, and we will not discuss transcriptional and epigenetic regulation of gene expression[1-4]; interested readers are referred to relevant cell biology and biochemistry texts. Rather, our intent is to discuss this problem from a conceptual point of view, emphasizing what is relevant for rheumatic disorders. By focusing on the different types of receptors and the biochemical pathways they activate, our goal is to try to make a complex topic more accessible. It is hoped that this will serve as a platform for understanding disease pathogenesis and existing and potential therapies.

MEMBRANE PERMEABLE LIGANDS THAT BIND INTRACELLULAR RECEPTORS

As indicated, factors that readily cross the plasma membrane represent the simplest conceptual means of modulating cell function. Nitric oxide, which regulates vascular tone, binds to a soluble, cytosolic receptor that has intrinsic guanylate cyclase activity.[5] This enzyme uses guanosine triphosphate (GTP) to produce cyclic guanosine monophosphate (cGMP), which, in turn, serves as a "second messenger" within the cell. cGMP is known to regulate many cellular proteins, such as protein kinases, ion channels, and phosphodiesterases.

Almost as simple are lipid-soluble ligands that bind to receptors that reside in the cytosol or the nucleus. For instance, the nuclear hormone receptor superfamily includes the receptors for vitamin A, vitamin D, glucocorticoid, estrogen, and thyroid hormone, as well as the peroxisome proliferator-activated receptor.[6,7] These intracellular receptors have ligand-binding, DNA-binding, and transactivation domains and are often associated with co-activators or co-repressors. Arguably, for a rheumatologist, the most important group of ligands in this category are the glucocorticoids. Retinoid receptors are another important group, and Rorα and Rorγt have recently been recognized to be important factors that promote Th17 differentiation.[8,9] Conversely, vitamin A, which binds to other retinoid receptors, inhibits interleukin (IL)-17 and upregulates Foxp3, thereby promoting the function of regulatory T cells.[8,9] Similarly, the immunomodulatory effects of vitamin D are increasingly recognized.[10] Conceivably, drugs that target this family of receptors could emerge as important immunomodulatory agents.

The aryl hydrocarbon receptor (AHR) is a basic, helix-loop-helix transcription factor. Its ligands include aromatic hydrocarbons such as tetrachloro-dibenzo-*p*-dioxen, a product of the defoliant Agent Orange. Additionally, endogenous products of tryptophan generated by ultraviolet light exposure (6-formylindolo [3,2-b] carbazole) also activate AHR. The lipophilic nature of these ligands allows them to permeate the plasma membrane. Prior to ligand binding, AHR is associated with heat-shock protein 90.[11] On activation, AHR dissociates from HSP-90 and binds aryl-hydrocarbon receptor nuclear transporter (ARNT). This complex binds DNA and regulates gene expression. Recently it has been recognized that AHR can regulate IL-17, IL-22, and Foxp3 expression, and thus this receptor provides a means by which environmental toxins and ultraviolet light can have immunoregulatory actions.[12]

RECEPTORS WITH INTRINSIC ENZYMATIC ACTIVITY

Because most ligands are water soluble and cannot simply cross the plasma membrane they must interact with some kind of receptor on the cell surface. From a conceptual framework, the simplest architecture encompasses receptors that have intrinsic enzymatic activity. These enzymes include phosphotransferases (kinases), phosphatases, and guanylate cyclases.

One of the most intensively studied classes of receptor are the receptor tyrosine kinases (RTKs). These receptors have a ligand-binding domain outside the cell with a short transmembrane domain followed by a kinase domain on the intracellular portion of the receptor. Examples of this type of receptors include those for insulin, the epidermal growth factor, and the platelet-derived growth factor. Other ligands that bind to this class of receptor also include stem cell factor and colony-stimulating factor-1. Ligand binding to RTK activates their enzymatic activity, and the receptors themselves become phosphorylated. These receptors are then bound by proteins that have modules that bind phosphotyrosine. This module is called an src homology 2 (SH2) domain. Of the many molecules that have SH2 domains, some have kinase and some have phosphatase activity, but other molecules lack enzyme activity. Instead, they serve as adapter molecules. For instance, the SH2-containing adaptor Grb2 brings the guanine-nucleotide exchange factor Sos into proximity with Ras, which activates downstream kinases including Raf1 and mitogen-activated protein kinase (MAPK).[13] Other adaptors are transmembrane molecules and can

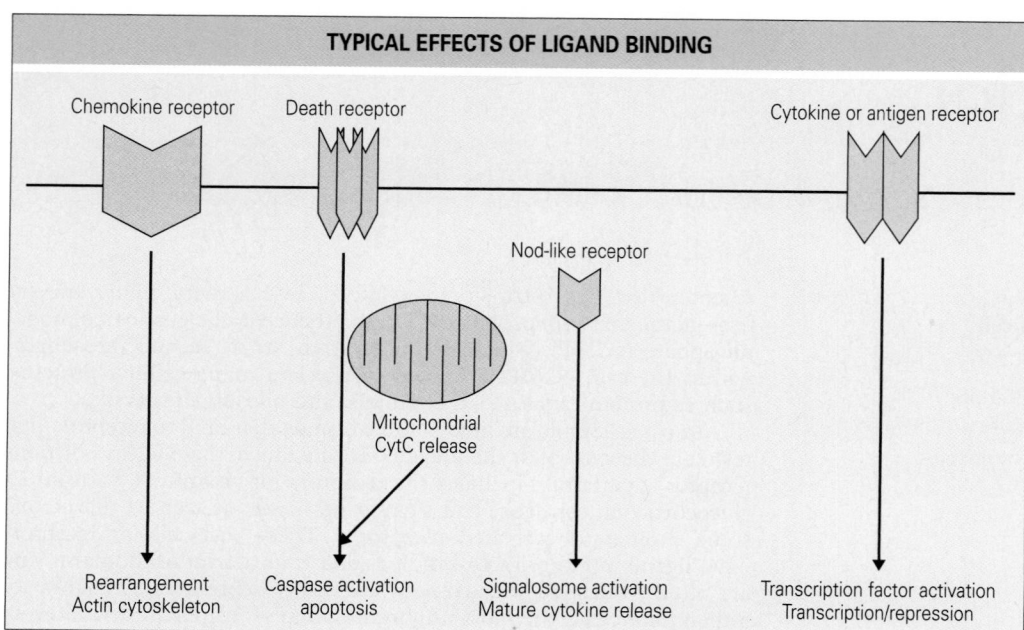

Fig. 13.1 Typical effects of ligand binding to various receptors (in light gray) in the immune system. CytC, cytochrome C.

function as scaffolds to organize several enzymes into larger signaling complexes.[14]

The architecture of the receptor for transforming growth factor (TGF)-β is similar to the RTKs: it, too, contains an extracellular ligand-binding domain, a single transmembrane domain, and an intracellular kinase domain. In this case, however, the enzyme has serine/threonine kinase activity. The TGF-β receptor consists of two subunits, whereby TGF-β type II receptor phosphorylates TGF-β type I receptor upon ligand binding.[15] Whereas the enzymatic activity of the latter does not change, the TGF-β type I receptor is activated by a conformational change following phosphorylation and release of the inhibitory protein FKBP12.[16]

The critical family of substrates for the TGF-β receptors are the Smad family of transcription factors. These are cytosolic DNA-binding proteins that upon phosphorylation translocate to the nucleus and activate gene transcription. The activated TGF-β type I receptor phosphorylates receptor-activated Smads (R-Smads), mostly Smad2 and Smad3, enabling them to complex with the only common Smad (coSmad), Smad4.[17,18] The complex then enters the nucleus and regulates transcription. In addition, the two inhibitory Smads (I-Smads), Smad6 and Smad7, are negatively regulating TGF-β signaling through the inhibition of receptor activity. The many types of bone morphogenic proteins also bind this class of receptor.[19]

Rather than having kinase activity, some receptors have phosphatase activity, meaning they remove phosphate from proteins. A large group of receptors include the receptor protein tyrosine phosphatases. For instance, the CD45 molecule, which is an extremely abundant receptor on the surface of immune cells, is a protein tyrosine phosphatase.[20]

RECEPTORS THAT ASSOCIATE WITH ENZYMES

Some receptors do not have intrinsic enzymatic activity, but they do the next best thing—they associate with enzymes. We will first discuss a large family of receptors that associates with a small family of dedicated kinases.

Type I/II cytokine receptors

More than 30 cytokines, interleukins, colony-stimulating factors, and hormones bind type I/II cytokine receptors (see Chapter 11). These receptors have extracellular ligand-binding domains and a single transmembrane domain. Their intracellular domain lacks motifs indicative of enzymatic activity. Instead, the membrane proximal domain of these receptors serves to bind members of a small family of kinases, the Janus kinases (Jaks) (i.e., Jak1, Jak2, Jak3, and Tyk2).[21]

TABLE 13.1 TRANSCRIPTION FACTORS OF THE SIGNAL TRANSDUCER AND ACTIVATOR OF TRANSCRIPTION FAMILY AND THEIR ROLE IN SIGNALING AND AUTOIMMUNE DISEASE

	Important for signaling of	Associations of mutations/polymorphisms
Stat1	All interferons	Mycobacterial infections[23]
Stat2	Type I interferons	
Stat3	gp130 cytokines	Hyper-IgE syndrome[24]
Stat4	IL-12, IL-23, type I interferons	Systemic lupus erythematosus, rheumatoid arthritis, primary Sjögren's syndrome[25]
Stat5a/Stat5b	Most cytokines, growth factors, hormones	
Stat6	IL-4, IL-13	

IL, interleukin.

On ligand binding, the Jaks become activated and phosphorylate the receptor. This provides docking sites for proteins that have SH2 domains. Some cytokines activate MAPK in a manner similar to RTKs. Additionally, however, phosphorylation of cytokine receptors allows recruitment of members of a family of transcription factors that have SH2 domains known as the signal transducer and activator of transcription (Stat) family. Phosphorylation of Stat factors allows them to reconfigure to a nutcracker-like structure,[22] translocate into the nucleus, and bind cognate sites at various promoter and enhancer regions, regulating gene expression. There are seven members of the Stat family, all with distinct functions (Table 13.1).

It is interesting that one target of Stat family transcription factors is the SOCS (suppressor of cytokine signaling) family of genes. These genes encode small proteins with SH2 domain, which bind to Jaks and cytokine receptors and inhibit signaling; as such, these proteins provide a classic mechanism for feedback inhibition.[26,27]

A classic example of signaling via Jaks and Stats is IL-2 and IL-15 signal transduction (Fig. 13.2). These receptors differ in their ligand-binding α-chains only.[28] They share the same β-chain, which binds Jak1, and the common γ-chain (γc), which binds Jak3 and is also part of the receptors for IL-4, IL-7, IL-9, and IL-21. Jak3 is specific for immune cells, and deficiency in functional Jak3 or γc leads to severe combined immunodeficiency.[29] On IL-2 and IL-15 binding, respectively, their heterotrimeric receptors change their conformation, so that

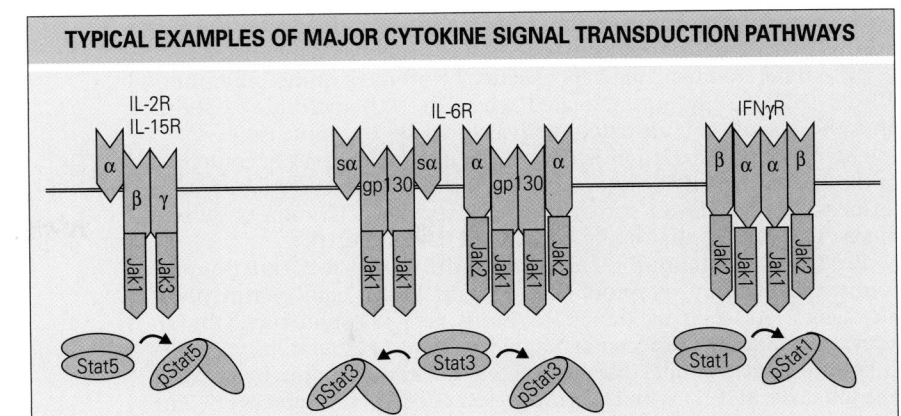

TYPICAL EXAMPLES OF MAJOR CYTOKINE SIGNAL TRANSDUCTION PATHWAYS

Fig. 13.2 Typical examples of major cytokine signal transduction pathways. Receptors are in blue, tyrosine kinases (of the Janus kinase [Jak] family) are depicted as orange arrows, and transcription factors (of the signal transducer and activator of transcription [Stat] family) are shown as blue ovals.

Jak1 and Jak3 phosphorylate each other. They next phosphorylate tyrosine residues on the receptor β-chain, which then bind homodimers or heterodimers of the closely related Stat5a and Stat5b molecules, and finally phosphorylate the Stat dimers. These dimers reconfigure, translocate into the nucleus, and regulate transcription. The IL-2 and IL-15 receptors also bind and activate the phosphatase Shp2[30] and phosphatidyl-inositol-3(OH)-kinase (PI3K).

Other important examples are the receptors for IL-6 and for interferons (IFNs). The IL-6 receptor consists of two molecules of gp130, again shared with other cytokines, and two IL-6 receptor α-chains (membrane bound or soluble) important for ligand binding.[31,32] The gp130 chains bind a Jak1 molecule each; the activation of these Jaks leads to Stat3 phosphorylation and signaling. Stat3 is counter-regulated by SOCS3[33]; deficiency in this counter-regulatory molecule leads to chronic inflammation of the liver. IFN-γ signaling is similar to the signaling of IL-6, but it is Stat1 homodimers that are essential for IFN signaling and SOCS1 molecules that provide counter-regulation; as exemplified for IL-2, other pathways are likewise involved.[34] In addition to SOCS1, which inhibits Jak and Stat1 phosphorylation, PIAS1, a SUMO ligase, binds phospho-Stat1 and inhibits its action.[35] IFN-α receptors also consist of heterodimers of two cognate chains, binding Jak1 and Tyk2. In contrast to IFN-γ, IFN-α induces the phosphorylation of another type of Stat complex, namely, a heterotrimer consisting of Stat1, Stat2, and p48.

Although their receptors are not particularly different from the ones just mentioned, it is worthwhile to briefly mention IL-4/IL-13 and IL-12. Their receptors are peculiar for binding unique Stats, namely, Stat6 and Stat4.[36] Stat6 dimers, which bind to slightly larger-spaced GAS sites, are activated by the prototypical Th2 cytokines IL-4 and IL-13 and essential for Th2 differentiation. Stat4 acts downstream of both IL-12 and IFN-α and is an important prerequisite for Th1 cells.

Multichain immune recognition receptors

Another large group of receptors lacking enzymatic activity that also couple to protein tyrosine kinases are the multi-chain immune recognition receptors (MIRRs).[37] This family encompasses more than 80 receptors, including the T-cell antigen receptor, the B-cell antigen receptor, Fc receptors, killer inhibitor receptors (KIRs), killer-activating receptors (KARs), dectin-1, and co-stimulatory receptors (CD-28, CTLA4). All these receptors have motifs termed immunoreceptor-based tyrosine activation motifs (ITAMs) or immunoreceptor-based inhibitor motifs (ITIMs). Phosphorylated ITAMs generate docking sites for two kinases, Syk and Zap70, which have two SH2 domains in the amino termini.

The T-cell receptor (TCR) is an especially well-studied receptor that serves as a useful model to discuss signaling by an ITAM-containing receptor. Other MIRRs, and the B-cell receptor in particular,[38] work in largely analogous ways. The αβ or γδ TCR recognizes antigen, while, at the same time, the CD4 or CD8 co-receptor binds the major histocompatibility class II or class I molecule, respectively. The TCR neither has kinase function nor is it able to directly bind kinases. Instead, the four CD3 chains and two ζ-chains provide the ITAM motifs required for kinase binding. Each ζ-chain contains three ITAMs, and each CD3

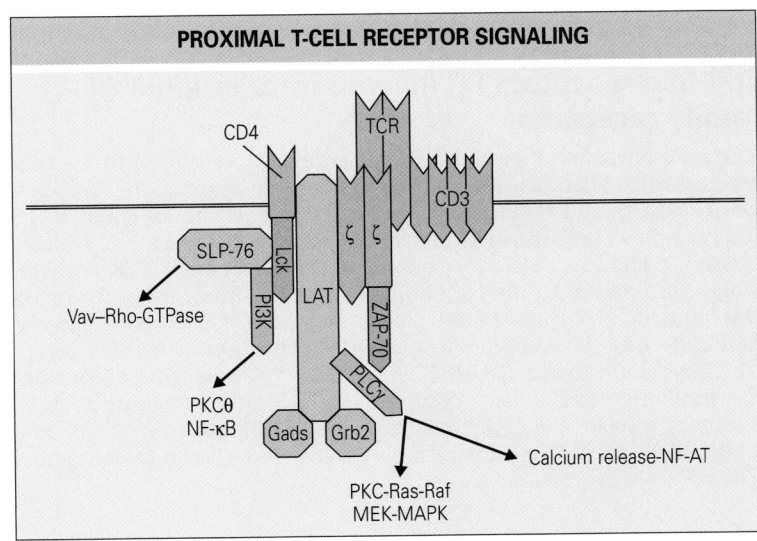

PROXIMAL T-CELL RECEPTOR SIGNALING

Fig. 13.3 Proximal T-cell receptor signaling. Receptor chains are in blue, adapter proteins are depicted as brown octagons (Src family), tyrosine kinases are shown in orange, and phosphatidyl-inositol-3(OH)-kinase and phospholipase Cγ are indicated by green arrows.

chain contains one ITAM. For starting the whole machinery, however, the CD4 (or CD8) co-receptor has to recruit the tyrosine kinase Lck, which phosphorylates the ITAMs, and, consecutively, activates ZAP-70 and Syk, tyrosine kinases likewise essential for TCR signaling[39] (Fig. 13.3).

Lck also directly binds SLP-76 and PI3K, and ZAP-70 similarly has adaptor-like functions. Thus, kinase-dead ZAP-70 is still sufficient for ERK phosphorylation while ZAP-70 kinase activity is necessary for the phosphorylation of the transmembrane adaptor protein LAT, and calcium release via phospholipase-Cγ, which binds LAT and is activated by ZAP-70 and, consecutively, by the Tec family kinase Itk. Like LAT, the cytoplasmic adaptor protein SLP-76 is absolutely required for TCR signaling, whereas Lck and Fyn can replace each other, as can ZAP-70 and Syk. These mechanisms lead into a variety of pathways, including activation of the transcription factor NF-AT, MAPK, and the classic nuclear factor-κB (NF-κB) pathway.

The serine-threonine phosphatase calcineurin is activated by a prolonged increase in cytoplasmic calcium.[40] Calcineurin then dephosphorylates NF-AT, thereby activating this transcription factor and exposing its nuclear import signal. This pathway is of significant importance, best demonstrated by the fact that it is through blocking calcineurin that cyclosporine and tacrolimus exert their well-known immunosuppressive effects.

For the MAPK pathway, the MAPK kinase kinase (MAPKKK or MAP3K) Raf activates the MAPK kinases (MAPKKs) MEK1/2 and the MAPKs ERK1/2, leading to activation (by serine phosphorylation) of the transcription factors Ets, Elk-1, and c-Myc.[41] The scaffolding protein kinase suppressor of Raf (KSR) helps the amplification of this process by assembling the components near the plasma membrane.[14]

NF-κB heterodimers are kept inactive by proteins of the inhibitor of NF-κB (IκB) family and activated when the IκB molecule is serine phosphorylated, ubiquitinated, and digested by the proteasome.[38,42,43] IκB serine phosphorylation is effected by a complex mainly composed of the IκB kinases (IKK) α (or 1) and β (or 2) and their regulatory unit termed IKKγ or NEMO. Proximal events include activation of protein kinase C θ (PKCθ) that binds Lck, MALT-1, and Bcl10.[44]

Receptors containing ITAMs and the associated kinases are counterbalanced by receptors that contain ITIMs and recruit phosphatases.[45] As soon as the ITIM motif gets phosphorylated by an activating kinase, the receptor is able to bind SH2-containing molecules, such as the lipid phosphatase SHIP and the protein tyrosine phosphatase SHP-1, which becomes activated in this process.[46] The importance of this counter-regulation by SHP-1 is illustrated by the fact that deficiency of this phosphatase leads to cellular activation and autoimmunity.[47]

Toll-like receptors (TLRs) and interleukin-1 (IL-1) family receptors

TLRs are one class of pattern recognition receptors (PRRs) that recognize PAMPs such as lipopolysaccharides, glycolipids, or bacterial DNA.[48] TLRs and IL-1 family receptors, such as the IL-1 and IL-18 receptors, also lack intrinsic enzymatic activity; however, these receptors are related in that they both have an intracellular TIR domain. This motif serves to bind a family of adaptors that also encompass this domain, such as Myd88, TRIF, and Mal. TIR-domain adaptor molecules link the receptors to a complex of kinases called IL-1 receptor–associated kinases (IRAKs) 1, 2, and 4.[45] These kinases activate the inhibitor of κB kinase complex (Fig. 13.4).[49] In addition, these receptors activate the ERK, JNK, and p38 MAPK pathways,[41,49,50] and TLRs, like other PRRs, induce type I INFs via INF regulatory factors (IRFs).[51]

Tumor necrosis factor receptor superfamily

TNF and related cytokines bind to a family of more than 20 different receptors. These trimeric receptors also have no enzymatic activity and are also linked to downstream kinases, including those that activate NF-κB. Analogous to the IL-1/TLR family, the TNFR family associates with a family of adaptors referred to as TNFR-associated factors (TRAFs). These proteins have a "TRAF" domain, which is also present in TNFR family receptors, that allows for homotypic interactions. TNFR2, for example, binds TRAF2 and induces the phosphorylation of the MAP3Ks Ask1 and NIK and the MAPKK MKK4, leading to p38 and JNK MAPK as well as to NF-κB activation.[52] TNFR1, in contrast, is an exception in that it has no TRAF domain. Instead, its death domain binds the adaptor protein TRADD, thus coupling to the TRAFs and the serine kinase RIP. This complex leaves the receptor and leads to the activation of the MAP3Ks Tab-associated kinase-1 (Tak1) and MEKK3, as well as of the IKKs, thereby inducing activation of the MAPK Jnk and of NF-κB.[50]

In addition to linking to kinases, some TNFR family members can also recruit a specialized series of proteases. These include TNFR1 (CD120a), Fas (CD95), and the Death receptors DR-3 through DR-6. These receptors associate with an adaptor called Fas-associated protein with death domain (FADD) through a motif termed the *death domain*. FADD also has a "death effector domain" that binds death effector domains of cysteine proteases or caspases, which cleave proteins at asparagine residue.[53] This brings caspase-8, or alternatively caspase-10, into proximity. These caspases cleave each other, which in turn activates effector caspases, namely, caspase-3 or caspase-7. Activation of this pathway culminates in a specialized form of cell death termed *apoptosis*. Alternatively, release of cytochrome C from mitochondria leads to the formation of the Apaf-1 apoptosome, which unleashes caspase-9[54] and likewise leads to caspase-3 activation (Fig. 13.5). Thus, in this case, signal transduction is mediated by the sequential building of complexes through protein interaction domains; this complex of proteins has been referred to as the "apoptosome."

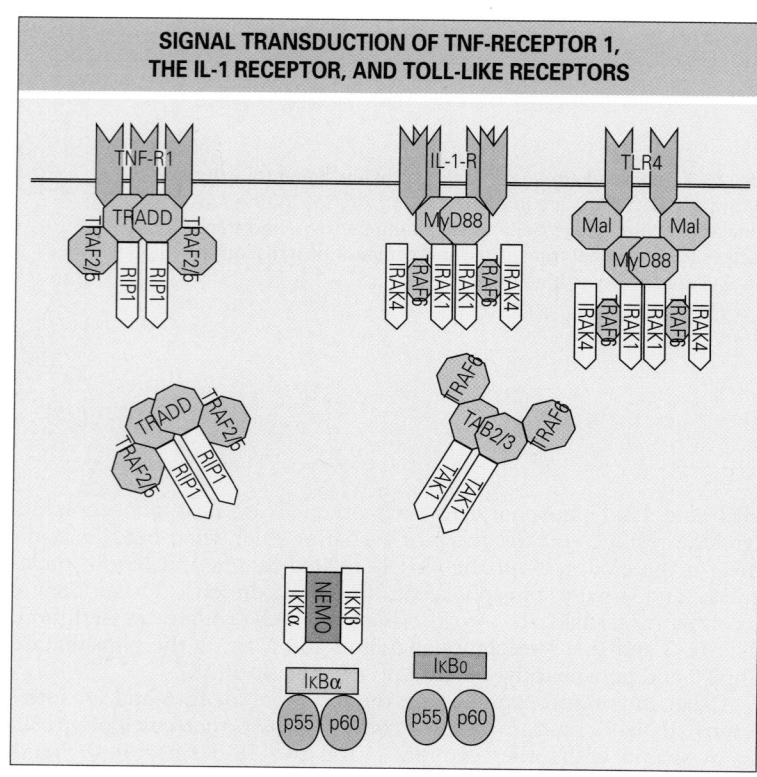

SIGNAL TRANSDUCTION OF TNF-RECEPTOR 1, THE IL-1 RECEPTOR, AND TOLL-LIKE RECEPTORS

Fig. 13.4 Signal transduction of TNF-receptor 1, the IL-1 receptor, and Toll-like receptors. Receptors are in blue, adapter proteins are depicted as brown octagons, serine kinases are indicated by yellow arrows, and transcription factors are shown as blue ovals. The inhibitor of κB protein is shown as a gray bar, which, on phosphorylation, is degraded by the proteasome and releases the transcription factor.

SENSING OF INTRACELLULAR PATHOGENS BY THE INFLAMMASOME

In the past few years, it has become clear that a system analogous to the apoptosis cascade is essential for recognition of products of pathogens and other danger signals. Starting at intracellular receptors that recognize PAMPs, these pathways are relevant for crystal-induced inflammation and, if genetically abnormal, the cause of fever syndromes. These NOD-like receptors (NLRs) activate caspase-1. Caspase-1, also called IL-1 converting enzyme (ICE), cleaves immature IL-1 and IL-18 into their mature forms, which are immediately released.[55,56] NLRs contain a NACHT domain, leucine-rich repeats (LRRs), plus a caspase recruitment domain (CARD) and/or a pyrin domain.[57] Those with a CARD, such as NOD1, NOD2, CIITA, and IPAF, directly bind caspase-1. NALP1 and NALP3 (for NACHT domain, LRR, pyrin domain–containing proteins) use their pyrin domain to bind the adaptor ASC (Fig. 13.6). ASC combines a pyrin domain and a CARD, thus bridging to caspase-1.[58] AIM2, the intracellular sensor for double-stranded DNA, likewise contains a pyrin domain.[59] In contrast, the RIG I–like receptors or helicases (RLRs or RLHs), which are intracellular RNA sensors, use their CARD-like domain for interacting with the adaptor IPS-1, inducing IRFs and the NF-κB pathway similar to the TLRs.[60]

G PROTEIN–COUPLED RECEPTORS

This largest class of receptors, the GPCRs, comprises roughly 350 members divided into 19 groups. GPCRs include receptors that sense light, odor, or taste and receptors for neurotransmitters (serotonin, dopamine, glutamate); epinephrine, norepinephrine, or acetylcholine; hormones; lipids (sphingolipids, leukotrienes, prostanoids); and chemokines.

GPCRs are notable for having seven transmembrane domains. As indicated by their family name, they bind guanine nucleotide binding

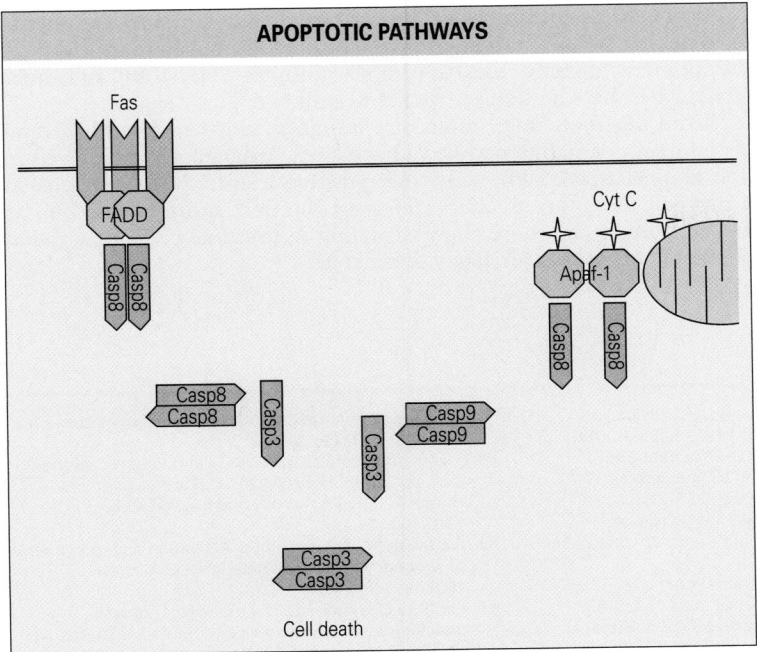

Fig. 13.5 Apoptotic pathways. Death receptors are in blue, adapter proteins are depicted as brown octagons, and caspases appear as red arrows. Yellow asterisks depict cytochrome C (Cyt C) molecules.

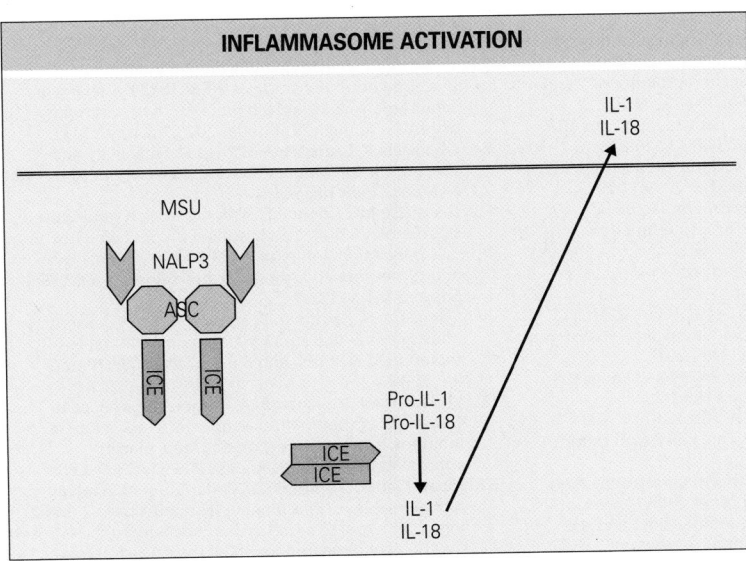

Fig. 13.6 Inflammasome activation. The NOD-like receptor is in blue, the adaptor protein ASC is depicted as a brown octagon, and caspase-1 is shown by a red arrow.

proteins, usually heterotrimers (Gα, β, γ). On activation, the α-subunit exchanges GDP for GTP and dissociates from the β- and γ-subunits, which remain as heterodimers.[13,61] Some family members produce cyclic adenosine monophosphate (cAMP) through the activation of adenylate cyclase, a protein that spans the plasma membrane 12 times. cAMP in turn activates protein kinase A.

Other GPCRs activate phospholipase-Cγ (PLCγ), a major example of another class of enzymes that are involved in the signaling by a variety of receptors, including G-coupled receptors. PLCγ breaks membrane phosphatidyl-inositol-(4,5)-diphosphate down to intracellular diacyl-glycerol (DAG) and inositol-(1, 4, 5)-triphosphate (IP3).

DAG, one of the products, then can activate protein kinase C (PKC) and the Ras-GTPase-MAPK pathway. Ras is a monomeric G protein,

which, when aided by its guanine-nucleotide exchange factor Sos, switches from its (inactive) GDP-bound state to its (active) GTP-bound state,[62] activating the kinase Raf and the Rho family members Rho, Rac, and Cdc42, which are important for cytoskeletal rearrangement.[13]

IP3, the other split product, via a specific receptor linked to calcium pores, provokes the immediate release of calcium (Ca^{2+}) stores from the endoplasmic reticulum into the cytoplasm. This Ca^{2+} stream further activates store-operated calcium channels (SOC) of the plasma membrane, ensuring a prolonged increase in cytoplasmic calcium that activates the serine-threonine phosphatase calcineurin, which dephosphorylates NF-AT.[40]

In addition to inducing calcium mobilization and lipid phosphorylation, these β-γ dimers activate Rho family G proteins, which then directly activate formins, which in turn effect actin filament assembly.[63] Alternatively, promoting factors such as WASP can activate the Arp2/3 complex, which was the first assembly factor to be detected.

Within the immune system, moving immune cells must react rapidly to reach and address their target. Changes within the cytoskeleton, such as induced by chemokine receptors, C5a anaphylotoxin, FMLP receptor, or histamine, are critical and among the most rapid events induced by cell-surface receptors, with changes occurring within seconds to minutes.[64]

For inflammatory disease, one particularly interesting example of a GPCR are the five receptors for sphingosin-1 phosphate (S1P), termed S1P1 to S1P5.[65] These are classic GPCRs, which therefore have a variety of effects, particularly on vascular cells. By mimicking effects of S1P on its receptors, the oral immunomodulatory compound FTY720 downmodulates SP1, significantly reducing inflammatory vessel functions.[66]

For completeness, it should be noted that some GPCRs may also have additional ways to transmit signals. For example, the bradykinin receptor B2 includes an ITIM motif and thereby apparently couples to the phosphatase Shp-2 and to phospholipase-Cγ1 (PLCγ1).[67]

NOVEL THERAPEUTIC APPROACHES IN RHEUMATOLOGY VIA MODIFYING SIGNAL TRANSDUCTION

Through the use of cyclosporine, which targets calcineurin (see earlier), rheumatologists have employed therapeutic interference with cell signaling for some time. In addition to FTY720, the last years have brought a full palette of exciting new agents, which mostly interfere with various enzymes in signaling pathways. Since the successful use of the Abl tyrosine kinase inhibitor imatinib, which also inhibits PDGF-receptor kinase function and may eventually prove useful in connective tissue diseases,[68,69] kinase inhibition has gained momentum. Many such drugs targeting various signaling pathways have recently been tried in patients with rheumatoid arthritis or other rheumatic diseases. At the moment it is not clear which of these drugs will finally make it to routine clinical use; however, animal models and early clinical trials allow for some conclusions.

Among the most promising is blockade of Jaks. As mentioned earlier, Jak3 is essential for IL-2, -4, -7, -9, -15, and -21 signaling. Mutations of Jak3 cause severe combined immunodeficiency (SCID), and Jak3 is limited to immune cells.[21] This was the impetus for developing Jak inhibitors. One such inhibitor, CP-690,550 has efficacy in animal models of allograft transplantation and autoimmunity (rheumatoid arthritis [RA]).[70] The drug has also been studied in humans with RA[71] and psoriasis[72]; preliminary data appear promising in terms of safety and efficacy. Another Jak inhibitor, INCB018424, which preferentially inhibits Jak1 and Jak2, has also been tested in RA and also appears to be reasonably safe and effective.[73] None of these inhibitors is entirely specific for a given Jak. However, selectivity may not always be advantageous for achieving significant therapeutic efficacy while not having major adverse effects.[74] Several MAPK inhibitors are likewise being tested in various diseases, some of them in RA or at least animal models of arthritis or osteoarthritis.[41,75] Among these are inhibitors of MEK1/2 inhibitors (ARRY-438162, PD198306), Jnk (SP600125), and p38 (BIRB 796, FR 167653, RPR200765A, SB 242235,

SB681323, SCIO-496, SD-282, VX-702, VX-745). Most animal data suggested protective effects at least against bone erosion.[41,75] However, elevated liver enzymes and/or disappointing efficacy were seen in some early clinical studies.[76,77]

Another interesting approach is inhibition of the Spleen tyrosine kinase (Syk). Syk is importantly involved in B-cell receptor[78] and Fc-receptor[79] signaling. The relatively selective Syk inhibitor fostamatinib (R788) appeared fairly safe in a first trial and showed efficacy in the 150-mg twice-daily group, with Disease Activity Score remission rates of 47%, compared with 17% on placebo alone.[80]

Although, despite some safety concerns, there are also arguments for blocking NF-κB,[42] there are only limited animal data available at the moment, namely, with the MEK2 inhibitor PHA-408[81] and, indirectly, with the Rho kinase blocker fasudil.[82]

Taken together, small molecules designed to interfere with several of the major signaling pathways have been designed and employed in first clinical trials, some with very positive results. Most likely, such drugs will have considerable impact in the near future. Moreover, as we learn more and more about signaling in immune cells, new therapeutic opportunities are likely to emerge.

KEY REFERENCES

2. van der Maarel SM. Epigenetic mechanisms in health and disease. Ann Rheum Dis 2008;67(Suppl 3):iii97-iii100.

5. Raines KW, Bonini MG, Campbell SL. Nitric oxide cell signaling: S-nitrosation of Ras superfamily GTPases. Cardiovasc Res 2007;75:229-239.

7. Szatmari I, Nagy L. Nuclear receptor signalling in dendritic cells connects lipids, the genome and immune function. EMBO J 2008;27:2353-2362.

9. Mucida D, Park Y, Cheroutre H. From the diet to the nucleus: vitamin A and TGF-beta join efforts at the mucosal interface of the intestine. Semin Immunol 2009;21:14-21.

10. Adorini L, Penna G. Control of autoimmune diseases by the vitamin D endocrine system. Nat Clin Pract Rheumatol 2008;4:404-412.

11. Beischlag TV, Luis MJ, Hollingshead BD, Perdew GH. The aryl hydrocarbon receptor complex and the control of gene expression. Crit Rev Eukaryot Gene Expr 2008;18:207-250.

12. Quintana FJ, Basso AS, Iglesias AH, et al. Control of T(reg) and T(H)17 cell differentiation by the aryl hydrocarbon receptor. Nature 2008;453:65-71.

13. Dustin ML, Chan AC. Signaling takes shape in the immune system. Cell 2000;103:283-294.

14. Shaw AS, Filbert EL. Scaffold proteins and immune-cell signalling. Nat Rev Immunol 2009;9:47-56.

15. Heldin CH, Landstrom M, Moustakas A. Mechanism of TGF-beta signaling to growth arrest, apoptosis, and epithelial-mesenchymal transition. Curr Opin Cell Biol 2009;21:166-176.

17. Hill CS. Nucleocytoplasmic shuttling of Smad proteins. Cell Res 2009;19:36-46.

19. Gazzerro E, Canalis E. Bone morphogenetic proteins and their antagonists. Rev Endocr Metab Disord 2006;7:51-65.

21. Pesu M, Laurence A, Kishore N, et al. Therapeutic targeting of Janus kinases. Immunol Rev 2008;223:132-142.

22. Mertens C, Zhong M, Krishnaraj R, et al. Dephosphorylation of phosphotyrosine on STAT1 dimers requires extensive spatial reorientation of the monomers facilitated by the N-terminal domain. Genes Dev 2006;20:3372-3381.

27. Dimitriou ID, Clemenza L, Scotter AJ, et al. Putting out the fire: coordinated suppression of the innate and adaptive immune systems by SOCS1 and SOCS3 proteins. Immunol Rev 2008;224:265-283.

29. Marodi L, Notarangelo LD. Immunological and genetic bases of new primary immunodeficiencies. Nat Rev Immunol 2007;7:851-861.

30. Gadina M, Sudarshan C, O'Shea JJ. IL-2, but not IL-4 and other cytokines, induces phosphorylation of a 98-kDa protein associated with SHP-2, phosphatidylinositol 3'-kinase, and Grb2. J Immunol 1999;162:2081-2086.

31. Zhang Q, Putheti P, Zhou Q, et al. Structures and biological functions of IL-31 and IL-31 receptors. Cytokine Growth Factor Rev 2008;19:347-356.

35. Liu B, Shuai K. Targeting the PIAS1 SUMO ligase pathway to control inflammation. Trends Pharmacol Sci 2008;29:505-509.

36. O'Shea JJ, Murray PJ. Cytokine signaling modules in inflammatory responses. Immunity 2008;28:477-487.

37. Sigalov AB. Multichain immune recognition receptor signaling: different players, same game? Trends Immunol 2004;25:583-589.

38. Simmonds RE, Foxwell BM. Signalling, inflammation and arthritis: NF-kappaB and its relevance to arthritis and inflammation. Rheumatology (Oxford) 2008;47:584-590.

40. Vig M, Kinet JP. Calcium signaling in immune cells. Nat Immunol 2009;10:21-27.

41. Thalhamer T, McGrath MA, Harnett MM. MAPKs and their relevance to arthritis and inflammation. Rheumatology (Oxford) 2008;47:409-414.

42. Brown KD, Claudio E, Siebenlist U. The roles of the classical and alternative nuclear factor-kappaB pathways: potential implications for autoimmunity and rheumatoid arthritis. Arthritis Res Ther 2008;10:212.

44. Weil R, Israel A. Deciphering the pathway from the TCR to NF-kappaB. Cell Death Differ 2006;13:826-833.

45. Zikherman J, Weiss A. Antigen receptor signaling in the rheumatic diseases. Arthritis Res Ther 2009;11:202.

46. Tabernero L, Aricescu AR, Jones EY, Szedlacsek SE. Protein tyrosine phosphatases: structure-function relationships. FEBS J 2008;275:867-882.

48. Beutler BA. TLRs and innate immunity. Blood 2009;113:1399-1407.

50. Verstrepen L, Bekaert T, Chau TL, et al. TLR-4, IL-1R and TNF-R signaling to NF-kappaB: variations on a common theme. Cell Mol Life Sci 2008;65:2964-2978.

51. Kawai T, Akira S. Toll-like receptor and RIG-I-like receptor signaling. Ann N Y Acad Sci 2008;1143:1-20.

53. Wallach D, Kang TB, Kovalenko A. The extrinsic cell death pathway and the elan mortel. Cell Death Differ 2008;15:1533-1541.

54. Bao Q, Shi Y. Apoptosome: a platform for the activation of initiator caspases. Cell Death Differ 2007;14:56-65.

55. Pope RM, Tschopp J. The role of interleukin-1 and the inflammasome in gout: implications for therapy. Arthritis Rheum 2007;56:3183-3188.

58. Mathews RJ, Sprakes MB, McDermott MF. NOD-like receptors and inflammation. Arthritis Res Ther 2008;10:228.

59. Burckstummer T, Baumann C, Bluml S, et al. An orthogonal proteomic-genomic screen identifies AIM2 as a cytoplasmic DNA sensor for the inflammasome. Nat Immunol 2009;10:266-272.

60. Takeuchi O, Akira S. MDA5/RIG-I and virus recognition. Curr Opin Immunol 2008;20:17-22.

61. Hunter T. Signaling—2000 and beyond. Cell 2000;100:113-127.

62. Frauwirth KA, Thompson CB. Activation and inhibition of lymphocytes by costimulation. J Clin Invest 2002;109:295-299.

63. Chhabra ES, Higgs HN. The many faces of actin: matching assembly factors with cellular structures. Nat Cell Biol 2007;9:1110-1121.

64. Thelen M, Stein JV. How chemokines invite leukocytes to dance. Nat Immunol 2008;9:953-959.

65. van der Giet M, Tolle M, Kleuser B. Relevance and potential of sphingosine-1-phosphate in vascular inflammatory disease. Biol Chem 2008;389:1381-1390.

67. Duchene J, Chauhan SD, Lopez F, et al. Direct protein-protein interaction between PLCgamma1 and the bradykinin B2 receptor—importance of growth conditions. Biochem Biophys Res Commun 2005;326:894-900.

73. Williams W, Scherle P, Shi J, et al. A randomized placebo-controlled study of INCB018424, a selective Janus kinase 1&2 (Jak1&2) inhibitor in rheumatoid arthritis (RA). Arthritis Rheum 2008;58(Suppl):S431.

74. Ghoreschi K, Laurence A, O'Shea JJ. Selectivity and therapeutic inhibition of kinases: to be or not to be? Nat Immunol 2009;10:356-360.

76. Genovese MC, Cohen SB, Wofsy D, et al. A randomized, double-blind, placebo-controlled phase 2 study of an oral p38a MAPK inhibitor, SCIO-496, in patients with active rheumatoid arthritis. Arthritis Rheum 2008;58(9 Suppl):S431-S432.

77. Damjanov N, Kauffman R, Spencer-Green GT. Safety and efficacy of VX-702, a p38 MAP kinase inhibitor, in rheumatoid arthritis. Ann Rheum Dis 2009;67(Suppl II):125-126.

80. Weinblatt ME, Kavanaugh A, Burgos-Vargas R, et al. Treatment of rheumatoid arthritis with a Syk kinase inhibitor: a twelve-week, randomized, placebo-controlled trial. Arthritis Rheum 2008;58:3309-3318.

81. Mbalaviele G, Sommers CD, Bonar SL, et al. A novel, highly selective, tight binding IkappaB kinase-2 (IKK-2) inhibitor: a tool to correlate IKK-2 activity to the fate and functions of the components of the nuclear factor-kappaB pathway in arthritis relevant cells and animal models. J Pharmacol Exp Ther 2009;329:14-25.

REFERENCES

Full references for this chapter can be found on www.expertconsult.com.

Genetic factors in rheumatic disease

14

Jane Worthington

- The majority of rheumatic conditions have a complex etiology in which multiple genetic and environmental effects interact to cause disease.
- Many rheumatic diseases are associated with human leukocyte antigen (HLA) class II or class I locus alleles, suggesting an immune-mediated component to these conditions.
- Some disease-associated genes encode susceptibility, whereas others relate to disease progression, severity, and clinical heterogeneity.
- Genome-wide association studies using hundreds of thousands of single nucleotide polymorphisms genotyped in large samples of cases and controls have successfully identified large numbers of susceptibility loci for the rheumatic diseases.
- Identification of genetic factors for rheumatic disease etiopathogenesis is likely to assist in risk prediction, early diagnosis and intervention, differential diagnosis and resolution of clinical heterogeneity, variation in treatment response, and discovery of novel drug targets.

INTRODUCTION

A genetic basis for the majority of rheumatic conditions is now established, and for a small number of these diseases the genetic contribution is clear and can be attributed to a disease-causing mutation in a single gene. Examples of such monogenic disorders include some cases of multiple epiphyseal dysplasia and periodic fevers. For single-gene disorders the penetrance of the disease-causing allele may not always be complete (i.e., the presence of a mutation may not result in the full disease phenotype), although the conditions are inherited in a strict mendelian fashion in either a dominant or a recessive way.

In contrast, the more common rheumatic diseases are not inherited as a simple mendelian trait but are the cumulative result of multiple genetic and environmental effects. The challenge of identifying risk factors for these complex diseases is significantly greater; however, in the past few years, significant advances in the characterization of variation across the genome and the development of high-throughput, accurate, and affordable technologies for single nucleotide polymorphism (SNP) genotyping have resulted in major advances in the identification genetic loci for complex diseases. The focus of this chapter is to describe the various approaches used to identify susceptibility loci for complex diseases and, in particular, to illustrate how, since the introduction of SNP-based whole-genome association studies in 2007, using rheumatoid arthritis (RA) as an example, knowledge of complex disease risk loci has increased exponentially. The genetics of a number of monogenic disorders and of the complex diseases of ankylosing spondylitis, systemic lupus erythematosus (SLE), and osteoarthritis are described in detail in Chapters 114, 124, and 174, respectively.

COMPLEX RHEUMATIC DISEASES

A large number of rheumatic conditions are now considered to represent complex disease phenotypes, including RA, juvenile idiopathic arthritis, SLE, osteoarthritis, osteoporosis, and ankylosing spondylitis. The evidence for this has largely come from the demonstration of an increased disease risk and clustering in the families of affected cases, in the absence of any clear pattern of mendelian inheritance.

For a number of rheumatic diseases, twin studies have proved to be useful in confirming the existence of a genetic component and also in estimating the relative contributions of both genetic and environmental effects. Monozygotic twins are genetically identical, sharing 100% of their DNA. If a disease is caused solely by genetic factors it would be expected that when one twin develops the condition the co-twin should also be affected. The proportion of monozygotic twins in which both are affected is referred to as the level of disease concordance. Crude monozygotic twin disease concordance figures reflect approximately the relative contribution of genetic factors and environmental/stochastic events. These estimates can be further refined by comparing concordance rates in monozygotic twins with those observed in dizygotic (non-identical) twins, who only have, on average, 50% of their genes in common. Because both monozygotic and dizygotic twins usually share early environmental exposures, monozygotic and dizygotic disease concordance figures can be modeled to more accurately measure disease heritability. Monozygotic and dizygotic twin concordance figures for a number of rheumatic conditions are summarized in Table 14.1.[1-10]

Many twin studies have been based on relatively small datasets and/or have suffered from sampling bias and should be interpreted with caution. For RA, estimates of monozygotic twin disease concordance range from 12% to 34%, but analysis of heritability suggests that up to 60% of disease etiology is likely to be explained by genetic factors.[11]

An alternative strategy for assessing increased familial risk is to compare the levels of disease risk for close blood relatives of probands (affected cases) with that seen in the open population. One measure used is that of the familial disease recurrence risk, and for RA this has been calculated as being approximately 10.[12] Thus, first-degree relatives of RA patients are 10 times more likely to develop the disease than individuals without an RA-affected relative. This approach has been further modified to take account of how rare or common a disease is in the population. The coefficient of familial clustering (λs) was defined by Risch[13] as a measure of how much genetic or shared environment component is involved in the etiology of a disease. This is calculated by dividing the sibling recurrence risk by the population prevalence. Depending on which published figures for RA sibling risk and prevalence are used, the λs for RA has been estimated to be between 2 and 10.[14] The λs values for a range of rheumatologic and autoimmune conditions are summarized in Table 14.2.[14-20]

RATIONALE FOR INVESTIGATING THE GENETIC BASIS OF RHEUMATIC DISEASES

An understanding of the risk factors for disease has the potential to impact on medicine and patient care at a number of points. Knowledge of genetic susceptibility factors could be used to identify individuals in whom modification of lifestyle might be advised to minimize exposure to environmental triggers of disease. Identifying potential cases before the onset of symptoms or at the very earliest stages of the disease process may identify a window of opportunity in which therapeutic interventions might be used to prevent development of the full-blown disease. These possibilities may be futuristic, and more immediately achievable targets include the identification of novel targets for therapies. This has already been illustrated in inflammatory bowel disease (IBD) in which the identification of an association with polymorphisms in genes involved in autophagy highlighted this pathway for the first time in the pathogenesis of this disorder.[21] Sirolimus, which is licensed for use in human organ transplantation, is known to have

TABLE 14.1 TWIN CONCORDANCE RATES

Condition	Monozygotic concordance (%)	Dizygotic concordance (%)	Reference
Rheumatoid arthritis	34	4.9	Harvarld & Hauge 1965[1]
	32	6.0	Lawrence 1970[2]
	12.3	3.5	Aho et al. 1986[3]
	21	0	Bellamy et al. 1992[4]
	15.4	3.6	Silman et al. 1993[5]
Systemic lupus erythematosus	57	0	Block et al. 1975[6]
	24	3	Deapen et al. 1992[7]
	25	0	Grennan et al. 1997[8]
Ankylosing spondylitis	50	15	Jarvinen 1995[9]
	75	13	Brown et al. 1997[10]

TABLE 14.2 SIBLING RECURRENCE RISKS

Condition	λs	Reference
Rheumatoid arthritis	5-10	Ollier & Worthington, 1997[14]
Systemic lupus erythematosus	20	Vyse et al., 1996[15]
Ankylosing spondylitis	46	Brown et al., 1998[16]
Behçet's disease	11.4-52.5	Gul et al., 2001[17]
Juvenile idiopathic arthritis	15	Glass & Giannini, 1999[18]
Systemic sclerosis	11-158	Englert et al., 1999[19]
Paget's disease	14	Ralston, 2002[20]

autophagy-promoting as well as immunosuppressant and antifibrotic activities. In psoriasis and type II diabetes, recently identified genetic associations have been identified in genes encoding proteins that are already the target of successful therapeutics[22]; for example, ustekinemab, a drug that targets *IL12/IL23R*, has been used to treat psoriasis.[23]

RA is an example of a disease showing considerable heterogeneity in terms of clinical presentation and disease course, making it challenging for clinicians to identify those patients who should be targeted for most aggressive therapies and those in whom the condition may relapse with little or no intervention. It seems likely this heterogeneity is genetically determined, and thus the identification of genetic markers to predict outcome would have significant clinical utility. Response to therapies also is likely to be genetically determined, and the identification of markers to predict likely treatment response or identify those at risk of adverse events would have major advantages in improving targeting of expensive therapies. Being able to achieve any or all of the above will have significant impact on the diagnosis and treatment of patients and will lead to a more personalized approach to disease.

APPROACHES FOR IDENTIFYING DISEASE GENES

The search for genetic variants that determine susceptibility to disease has been based on the use of two different scientific strategies: linkage and association studies. Traditional parametric linkage analysis, used with great success to identify loci determining monogenic diseases, relies on the use of multi-case extended pedigrees of the type rarely available for complex rheumatic diseases. In contrast, non-parametric linkage analysis carried out on smaller "affected sibling pair" pedigrees has been widely used to search for complex disease genes. These studies depend on the analysis of hundreds of highly informative genetic markers (usually microsatellites) mapping at regular intervals of the whole genome in large numbers of families. The markers are used to identify regions of the genome shared "identical by descent" by the affected sibling pairs more frequently than expected by chance that are, therefore, likely to contain disease genes. Before the advent of genome-wide association studies (GWAS), linkage studies offered the only method for screening the whole genome in a hypothesis-free approach.[24]

In contrast, association studies are based on the comparison of polymorphic markers in cohorts of cases and controls, with a difference in allele or genotype frequency providing evidence that the polymorphism, or one in linkage disequilibrium with it, is associated with disease. The vast majority of association studies before GWAS were candidate gene investigations based on a limited number of polymorphisms. Sequencing of the human genome and the subsequent exponential increase in the identification and characterization of millions of polymorphic markers were vital to the development of association studies that screened the whole genome. Also critical was the develop-

ment of technologies for rapid and accurate genotyping of single nucleotide polymorphism (SNP) markers in large numbers of samples.

In the past few years, GWAS have largely superceded whole-genome linkage in the study of complex disease genetics; however, a brief description of the linkage approach is presented here because it was used with success to identify a major non-HLA RA susceptibility locus. Candidate gene association studies have also been used with some success, and because many of the methodologic issues relevant to these studies are also considerations for GWAS, these are discussed, followed by an update on current knowledge of RA susceptibility loci revealed by each of the just discussed approaches.

Linkage analysis

The main advantage afforded by linkage studies is that they provide an opportunity to search the whole genome for novel susceptibility loci and require no *a priori* hypothesis for the involvement of a particular gene. Classic parametric linkage analysis that assesses linkage by calculating the logarithm of the odds of linkage (LOD score) has seen relatively limited application to rheumatic diseases because it requires multi-case affected pedigrees, ideally with at least three generations. In addition, parametric linkage analysis requires specification of a model, the mode of transmission (dominant, recessive, additive), and estimates of penetrance and recombination rates between markers and disease loci. Such factors are unknown for complex diseases, and because specification of the wrong model can lead to inaccurate results, this approach should be applied with caution for non-mendelian disorders.

Non-parametric linkage analysis is a model-free approach based on allele-sharing probabilities that allows identification of regions of the genome linked with disease and is much better suited to complex diseases. Evidence of linkage is obtained for genetic markers when analysis of large numbers of affected sibling pairs reveals an increased sharing of alleles inherited "identical by descent" above that expected under random segregation.[25]

Microsatellite-based whole-genome screens analyzing 300 to 1000 markers in affected sibling pair families have been carried out for RA,[26-29] SLE,[30-35] osteoarthritis,[36,37] and ankylosing spondylitis[38]; and in all cases, in addition to strong evidence of linkage to the HLA region on chromosome 6, a number of additional potential disease loci were identified. The regions identified in genome scans may span several centimorgans (1 cM is approximately equal to 1 Mb in physical distance) that may contain hundreds of genes, and it has consistently proved difficult to identify a disease-associated polymorphism under linkage peaks. The early stages of the development of high-throughput SNP genotyping provided an opportunity using a higher density of genetic markers to refine linkage peaks. This was first demonstrated in an SNP-based linkage analysis of RA-affected sibling-pair families.[39] This study was based on only 157 families and was underpowered to detect small effects; however, it demonstrated the utility of SNP-based linkage analysis and resulted in the identification of four novel loci ($P < .05$) and refinement of the major linkage peak over the HLA region from 50 to 31 cM. A second SNP-based linkage screen of RA in a larger number of families identified two peaks on chromosome 11p12 and 2q33.[40] Subsequent dense association mapping of the region on chromosome 2 led to compelling evidence of association to the gene known as signal transducer and activator of transcription 4 (STAT4); interestingly, the same association was also observed in SLE.[41] The effect size observed for the association with RA was small (OR, 1.25) but is now recognized as typical of complex disease loci. The same association to markers in intron 3 of the gene has also been observed in Asian populations, and this together with the role of STAT4 in interleukin (IL)-12 signaling in T cells and natural killer (NK) cells have established it as a key RA susceptibility gene.

Association studies

The direct investigation of associations between gene polymorphisms and disease to study disease susceptibility has been in use for many years. Well before the advent of non-parametric linkage studies, association was the approach by which most of the well-established HLA associations with rheumatic diseases were identified. The principle is simple and is based on the assumption that the marker under investigation is either causally related to disease or strongly correlated with the causal variant (i.e., in linkage disequilibrium). A difference in the allele or genotype frequency between groups of cases and controls provides evidence of disease association of the variant under investigation. Before 2007, disease association studies targeted candidate genes or were the approach used to fine-map linkage peaks. The advent of technologies facilitating accurate, high-throughput genotyping of hundreds of thousands of SNPs has heralded the era of GWAS in which association studies screening the genome in a hypothesis-free manner are carried out using 0.5 to 1 million SNPs and large numbers of cases and controls.

Providing basic epidemiologic principles are followed, both candidate gene and GWAS are robust approaches and the key methods by which new susceptibility loci will be identified and characterized; however, a PubMed search (at www.pubmed.com) for any of the rheumatic diseases will reveal thousands of reports claiming association or lack of association, the large majority of which are almost certain to be false-positive or false-negative results. There are a number of reasons for this observation. The majority of these considerations are relevant to both candidate gene and GWAS.

Selection of cases and controls

Perhaps the most common reason given for false-positive associations is population stratification. This arises when the population studied contains subpopulations that differ both in allele frequency and in the prevalence of the disease under study. Allele frequency differences between ethnic groups are well documented, and most studies will endeavor to take cases and controls from the same ethnic group. The extent to which population stratification, within an ethnic group, might influence the generation of false-positive associations is currently a major topic of debate.[42] A recent study in the United Kingdom suggests that population stratification leads to an 11% inflation of the test statistics, which could be overcome by matching cases and controls within 12 geographically defined regions.[43] This must raise concerns for candidate gene association studies, particularly for those to be carried out in populations considered to be less homogeneous than that of the United Kingdom. Methods to test for and correct for population stratification have been available for some time,[44] and it is envisaged that panels of markers sensitive to population structure, so-called ancestry markers, will be developed and incorporated into future studies to overcome problems arising from population stratification. GWAS have a built-in opportunity to adjust for population-based differences of cases and controls, and the utility of three different approaches for these large datasets—(1) structured association tests; (2) principal components analyses; and (3) multidimensional scaling—has been demonstrated. The availability of such methods brings an additional advantage to GWAS in that it becomes possible to use large common population controls for studies in different diseases and different populations, resulting in significant cost savings.[45] Family-based tests of association such as the transmission disequilibrium test are not subject to such problems and became popular for a while. They are, however, less cost effective and less powerful, and when investigating gene-environment interactions they are probably overmatched for environmental exposures.[46]

A further consideration when sampling subjects for association studies is whether the cases are truly representative of the disease group as a whole. This issue is well illustrated by studies of HLA associations in RA patients. Numerous studies over many years have characterized the HLA-DRB1 associations with RA and have shown quite variable effect sizes.[47] What now emerges is that most of the earlier studies and those showing the highest effect sizes tended to be based on hospital-derived cohorts of patients. Many RA patients are managed by primary care physicians, and only those with more severe disease or complications will be seen in hospital-based specialist centers. It was only by the establishment of prospective primary care–based cohorts with longitudinal follow-up, such as the U.K. Norfolk Arthritis Registry, that it was demonstrated that the HLA shared-epitope alleles are only weakly associated with inflammatory arthritis (OR, 1.8; 95% CI, 1.4-2.4). The risk increases for those cases satisfying American College of Rheumatology criteria (OR, 2.3; 95% CI, 1.7-3.1) but is strongest for hospital-based studies (average fivefold increased risk), suggesting that shared-epitope alleles may be more important in influencing disease progression than susceptibility.[48]

Power/effect sizes

The power of a study to detect a genetic effect size will depend on the sample size of the study and the frequency of the alleles that predispose to disease. Most association studies use similar numbers of cases and controls, although more power is gained by increasing the ratio of controls to cases (a ratio of four times more cases than controls is considered the most efficient). The "common disease/common variant hypothesis" supposes that, because common diseases generally occur after peak reproductive stages of life, the variants responsible are unlikely to have undergone negative selection and will have reached a reasonably high frequency in the population. It is now clear that the effect size for the majority of complex disease loci is very small, with the majority identified so far having odds ratios below 2. These observations serve to confirm that a large proportion of published association studies, particularly from the pre-GWAS era, were underpowered and emphasizes the importance of using adequately powered studies, which for GWAS of most diseases means sample sizes of many thousands.

Selection of genetic markers

Candidate genes for association studies have tended to be selected either on the basis of pathology and biologic processes or because they map to a region of linkage. Potentially any polymorphism (micro- or mini-satellite repeat, insertions or deletions, or SNPs) could be causative. Until recently, the relative paucity of markers characterized for a given gene meant that, other than those prioritized because of known functional effect, available markers were analyzed in the hope that, if not causal, they would be sufficiently correlated with the causal variant for an association to be detected. As a result, many of the negative association studies reported may have failed to detect an effect because no markers in linkage disequilibrium with the causative variant were identified.

SNPs have been the markers most commonly used, largely because they are most easily genotyped. Three major initiatives have focused on the identification and characterization of SNPs, and as a result that it is now possible to select markers in a systematic and efficient manner to ensure coverage of common variation (minor allele frequency > 1%) for a given locus/gene. First, the sequencing of the human genome provided a template against which genetic variation could be studied and mapped; second, the availability of markers was dramatically increased by characterization of millions of polymorphic markers (www.ncbi.nih.gov/SNP), and, third, patterns of linkage disequilibrium between markers (www.hapmap.org) have been defined with data generated from four populations (Yoruba, Nigeria, n = 90; North American whites living in Utah, n = 90; Han Chinese, n = 45; and Japanese, n = 44). More recently the 1000 genomes initiative (www.1000genomes.org), which involves the complete resequencing of the genome in samples from three populations, has begun to reveal further detail of genetic variation between individuals and populations.

The presence and knowledge of linkage disequilibrium between markers means that it is usually unnecessary to type every known variant at a locus of interest, because haplotype tagging methods can be used to select the minimal number of markers to capture all haplotypes of significant frequency within the population. SNP marker sets used for GWAS depend on linkage disequilibrium to achieve coverage of the genome, and although the effectiveness of coverage depends on the population under study it is typically in excess of 75%.

Genotyping of markers/genotyping technology

Another common source of error is poor genotyping quality. The earliest disease association studies were mostly based on restriction fragment length polymorphism (RFLP) assays that depend on a polymorphism introducing or destroying a restriction enzyme cut site. A failure to perform complete enzyme digestion often resulted in inaccurate genotyping, most commonly an increase in heterozygous genotypes. One would expect this to occur with equal frequency in both cases and controls, but this was often not the case and led to false-positive associations. Simple steps such as mixing cases and controls within the same assay and including sequenced controls for each genotype can highlight a problem. Testing for a deviation from Hardy-Weinberg equilibrium can also be used to screen for genotyping error in controls.

There have been major technologic advances for SNP genotyping, with new platforms allowing ever-higher throughput and claiming greater accuracy. Although this is undoubtedly the case, the principles of good experimental design should not be forgotten. A detailed discussion of currently available technologies is beyond the scope of this chapter, but there is clear evidence that insufficient quality control checks can lead to false-positive associations in both candidate gene and GWAS.

Analysis and interpretation of results

As genotyping costs decrease and sample throughput increases, the issue of correction for performing multiple comparisons becomes more pertinent. Applying a significance threshold of $P = .05$ means that 1 in 20 observed associations will have occurred by chance. Performing multiple tests without adjustment of the threshold is certain to generate false-positive findings.[49] Applying a Bonferroni correction is thought to be overly conservative, particularly if SNPs are in linkage disequilibrium with each other. An alternative is to perform permutation testing to empirically test the probability of having observed an association by chance.[50] The issue of multiple testing is key in the interpretation of GWAS based on the comparison of many hundreds of thousands of markers. The setting of significance thresholds for distinction of genuine associations from false-positive results remains a topic of debate, but a generally accepted threshold for the current generation of GWAS (500,000 to 1 million SNPs) is $P < 5 \times 10^{-7}$.

Replication of findings in an independent cohort provides compelling evidence that the original result was real and not a false-positive finding. An interesting phenomenon in this context is the "winner's curse" whereby there is an upward bias in the effect sizes reported in the first published study.[51] This has been shown in a study of 55 meta-analyses, which demonstrated that subsequent studies showed weaker or no association compared with the original studies.[52] Hence follow-up studies should at least be powered to detect effects at the lower limit of the confidence interval around the odds ratio of the first study.

SUCCESSFUL EXAMPLES OF CANDIDATE ASSOCIATION STUDIES

The first genetic associations in rheumatic diseases were identified some 30 years ago and were with alleles of genes located in the HLA region.[53-55] Since then, many other associations between HLA antigens and a wide range of rheumatic diseases have been reported, a considerable number of which have been replicated. A summary of these is reported in Table 14.3. A detailed discussion of how HLA may contribute to the etiology of RA has been given elsewhere (see Chapter 86).

TABLE 14.3 HLA CLASSIC ASSOCIATIONS		
Condition	**HLA association**	**Reference**
Rheumatoid arthritis	DR4, DR1, DR10, DR14 (Native American)	Ollier & Thomson, 1992[47]
Systemic lupus erythematosus	DR3/DQB1*0201; DR2/DQB1*0201	Schur, 1995[93]
Ankylosing spondylitis	B27, B60, DR1	Brewerton et al, 1973[55] Wordsworth, 1998[94]
Juvenile arthritis	A2, DR8, DR11, DR13, DPB1*0201	Donn & Ollier, 1996[95]
Giant cell arteritis	DR4	Dababneh et al, 1998[96]
Polymyalgia rheumatica	DR4, DR13	Dababneh et al, 1998[96]
Reactive arthritis	B27	Aho et al, 1986[3]
Scleroderma	DR11, DR3, DR2 (Japanese)	Tan & Arnett, 2000[97]
Polymyositis/ dermatomyositis	DR3, DQB1*0201, DR13 (black)	Shamim et al, 2000[98]
Primary Sjögren's syndrome	DR3	Kay et al, 1991[99]
Psoriatic arthritis	B27, B38, B17, B13, DR7, CW6	Silman, 2001[100]
Paget's disease	DR2	Singer et al, 1985[101]
Lyme disease	DR7, DR4	Wang and Hilton, 2001[102] Steere et al, 2001[103]
Behçet's disease	B51	Ohno et al, 1982[104]
Erythema nodosum	DR1	Amoli et al, 2001[105]
Kawasaki's disease	B51	Krensky et al, 1983[106]
Takayasu's arteritis	B52 (Japanese)	Kimura et al, 1996[107]
ANCA-associated granulomatous vasculitis	B8	Katz et al, 1979[108]

Protein tyrosine phosphatase N22

PTPN22 is one of a number of protein tyrosine phosphatases involved in regulating the immune response. A functional polymorphism of the PTPN22 gene, 1858C>T, was initially found to be associated with type 1 diabetes.[56] Subsequently, researchers performed a large-scale case-control association study of candidate genes for RA (16,000 SNPs) and found the most significant association was with the same non-synonymous SNP identified in the type 1 diabetes study.[57] The initial association to RA has since been replicated in all the studies that have followed.[58-65] Interestingly, association to the same SNP has been found in juvenile idiopathic arthritis,[58] SLE,[60,66-68] autoimmune thyroid disease,[69-73] and a number of other autoimmune diseases.[74] A number of the studies cited have demonstrated a functional effect of the associated polymorphism in terms of reduced binding of the protein encoded by PTPN22, Lyp, to Csk; and it had been assumed that this might cause a reduced ability to downregulate T-cell activation, resulting in an increased likelihood to develop autoimmunity. However, subsequent investigations of the functional effect of the 1858C>T polymorphism found that the disease-associated allele was, in fact, a more efficient inhibitor of T-cell activation. Based on these observations, it is hypothesized that this may result in less-efficient deletion of autoreactive T cells during thymic development or insufficient activity of T-regulatory cells.[75] Interestingly, the 1858C>T variant is found only extremely rarely in Asian populations and although PTPN22 is clearly established as the major non-HLA RA susceptibility locus for whites there is no evidence that it has a role in RA susceptibility in Asians.

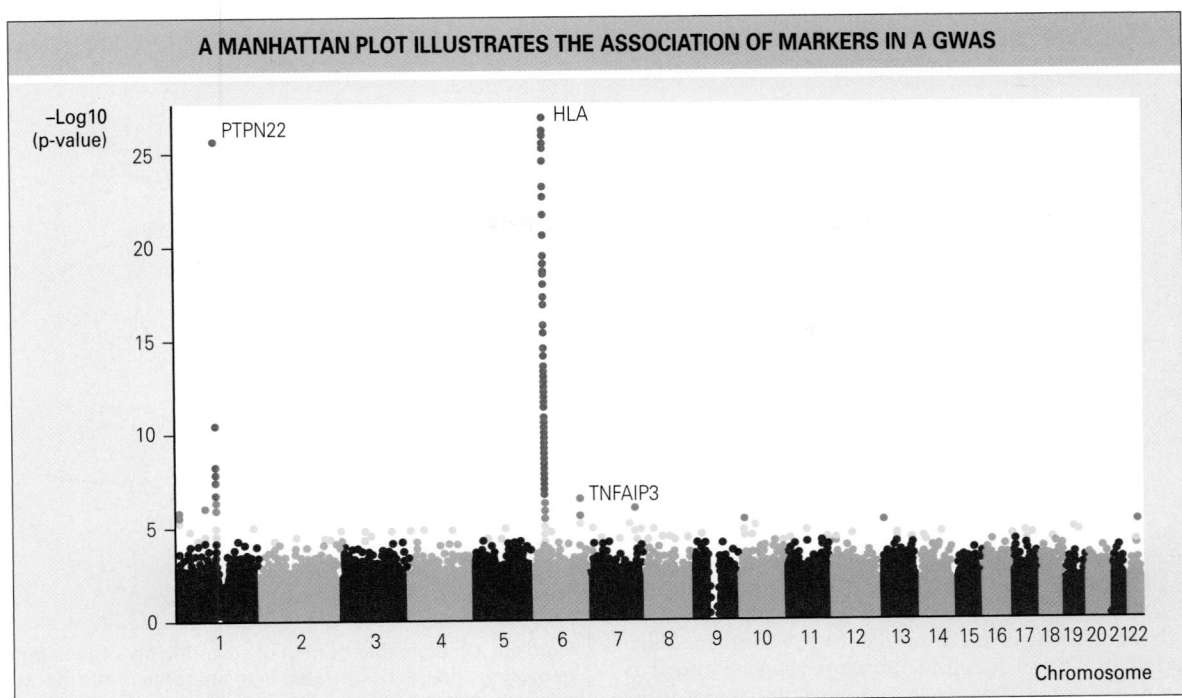

A MANHATTAN PLOT ILLUSTRATES THE ASSOCIATION OF MARKERS IN A GWAS

Fig. 14.1 A Manhattan plot illustrates the association of markers in a genome-wide association study. Each dot represents the *P* value for comparison of genotype frequencies for each marker when comparing cases (n = 2000) and controls (n = 3000). Shades of blue are used to represent alternate chromosomes. Levels of significance of association are indicated. Red spots: $P < 5\times10^{-7}$; green spots: $P < 10^{-5}$-5×10^{-7}; yellow spots: $P < 10^{-4}$.[78]

The *PTPN22* story in many ways exemplifies the modern approach to disease association studies: well-powered experiments, multiple replications in different populations, and experimental data to demonstrate a functional effect of the disease-associated allele. It will not, however, always be so straightforward as in this case where a single amino acid changing polymorphism was successfully targeted. A more likely scenario is extensive linkage disequilibrium–based investigation of multiple markers revealing evidence of association to a number of markers with differences dependent on the population studied.

There are further examples of RA associations that appear to be population specific, a phenomenon that has not been observed in other complex diseases. Replicated evidence for association to SNPs in peptidylarginine deiminase-4 (PADI4)[76] and FCγ-receptor-like (FCRL)3[77] have been identified in Asian but not white populations.

WHOLE-GENOME ASSOCIATION STUDIES OF RHEUMATOLOGIC CONDITIONS

Successful GWAS have now been carried out for all the major rheumatologic conditions, including RA, SLE, and ankylosing spondylitis, and screens are underway for osteoarthritis and psoriatic arthritis, juvenile idiopathic arthritis, and systemic sclerosis. In all cases the studies have both confirmed some of the established associations and identified new susceptibility loci. With the exception of RA, the findings are detailed in later chapters.

Rheumatoid arthritis GWAS

The proof of principle investigation that demonstrated the practicality and utility of GWAS came in 2007 from The Wellcome Trust Case Control Consortium (WTCCC), which undertook a genome-wide analysis of seven common diseases, including RA. Five hundred thousand SNPs were genotyped using the Affymetrix Gene Chip 500k Mapping Array Set in 2000 cases from each of the seven diseases and a set of 3000 common controls, all samples from white U.K. residents.[78] Markers in the *HLA-DRB1* and *PTPN22* gene regions were highly significantly associated with RA ($P < 5\times10^{-7}$). Strong but not incontrovertible evidence of association was detected to over 50 additional loci

($P < 10^{-4}$-5×10^{-7}) (Fig. 14.1). Analysis of markers from these loci in large independent sample sets has since confirmed RA loci at 6q23,[79] 10p15, 12q13, and 22q13,[80] implicating the genes *TNFAIP3, PRKCQ, KIF5A, IL2RB,* and *AFF3*.

The first RA GWAS from the United States used the Affymetrix GeneChip 100-k Mapping Array and in a relatively small study (397 cases and 1,211 controls) also found highly significant association to markers at 6q23.[81] Interestingly, the minor allele of the markers rs10499194 was associated with protection from RA (OR = 0.75), in contrast to rs6920220, the minor allele of which was associated with susceptibility in the U.K. study (OR = 1.2). Further genotyping of SNPs in the region in U.K. samples detected an additional independent association with markers in the *TNFAIP3* gene and illustrated the complexity of the locus and the importance of systematic investigation of loci detected in GWAS.[82] The odds ratio for carriage of risk alleles for both susceptibility markers together with non-carriage of the protective allele was 1.50, confirming 6q23 as the RA locus with the third largest effect, after HLA and *PTPN22*. Further complexity for this locus has been revealed by studies in different populations for both RA and other diseases, including SLE.[83,84]

Data from a second, larger GWAS in a U.S. population was combined with that generated in a GWAS of a Swedish population, and after *HLA-DRB1* and *PTPN22* the most significant association was found to marker rs3761847 (4×10^{-14}) in the *TRAF/C5* gene region.[85] Interestingly, the same region had been targeted for a candidate gene investigation by a Dutch group that found association to rs10818488 (1.4×10^{-8}), providing independent confirmation of this as an RA locus.[86] No markers at this locus were statistically associated with RA in the WTCCC study, although a subsequent replication study in U.K. samples did confirm association to this locus.[87]

The possibility and advantages of meta-analyses of GWAS to increase the power to detect risk alleles with small effect sizes have been clearly demonstrated for RA. Although the U.K., U.S., and Swedish studies all used different genotyping platforms with non-identical sets of SNPs using data from Hapmap and methods for imputing data for SNPs not physically genotyped, together with methods to adjust for population differences a meta-analysis of these datasets revealed further novel RA susceptibility loci at *CD40, CCL21, MMEL, PRKCQ,* and *KIF5A*.[88]

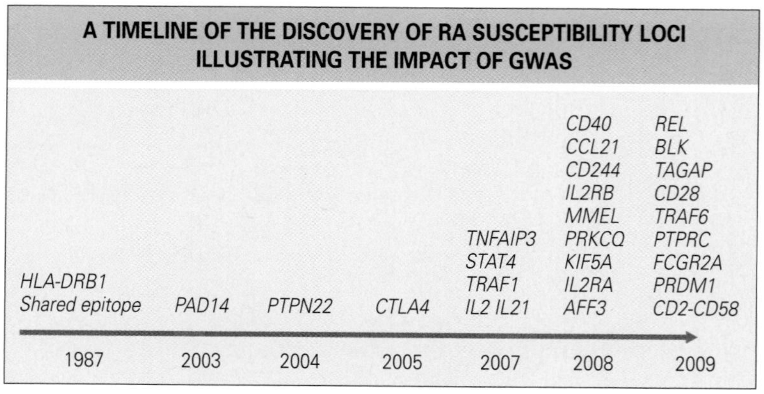

A TIMELINE OF THE DISCOVERY OF RA SUSCEPTIBILITY LOCI ILLUSTRATING THE IMPACT OF GWAS

						CD40 CCL21 CD244 IL2RB MMEL	REL BLK TAGAP CD28 TRAF6
					TNFAIP3 STAT4 TRAF1	PRKCQ KIF5A IL2RA	PTPRC FCGR2A PRDM1
HLA-DRB1 Shared epitope	PAD14	PTPN22	CTLA4	IL2 IL21	AFF3	CD2-CD58
1987	2003	2004	2005	2007	2008	2009

Fig. 14.2 A timeline of the discovery of RA susceptibility loci illustrating the impact of a genome-wide association study.

GWAS can now be carried out as a matter of routine. The challenge remains to distinguish all true-positive associations from among a considerable number of highly significant results arising as false-positives. Increasing sample sizes and meta-analyses offer one solution, but bioinformatics has a great, but as yet largely unexplored, potential to assist with this challenge. Genes for a number of RA-confirmed loci are known to function in T- and B-cell signaling pathways, and it is likely that additional genes on the same or related pathways may harbor risk alleles. A recent paper demonstrated how a computational method (GRAIL) that applies statistical text mining to PubMed abstracts was used to prioritize loci with a functional connection to established RA loci from loci with relatively weak evidence of association in the GWAS data ($P < .001$) for investigation.[89] As a result, further RA loci were identified; *CD2/CD58* (rs11586238), *PRDM1* (rs548234), *CD28* (rs1980422), *PTPRC* (rs10919563), *TAGAP* (rs394581), *RAG1/TRAF6* (rs540386), and *FCGR2A* (rs12746613).

The list of confirmed RA loci continues to grow. Most recently, a further GWAS of Canadian and U.S. samples identified association to c-REL in the nuclear factor-κB (NF-κB) family (Fig. 14.2).[90] As the list grows it is tempting to try to determine what proportion of the genetic component of susceptibility can now be explained; however, until these loci have been fine mapped and all the risk and protective alleles determined, such calculations are likely to be inaccurate. A potentially more useful approach is to consider what insights we can get into the biology of the disease process from the genes revealed so far. The considerable overlap between loci identified for RA and those identified for other autoimmune diseases, including type 1 diabetes, celiac disease, and multiple sclerosis (Fig. 14.3), is quite amazing; and at the moment it appears the vast majority of RA loci are not unique to this disease.[91] Already we can see that multiple genes on key pathways are associated with disease, perhaps best illustrated to date by the identification of four genes (*CD40, TRAF1, TNFAIP3, c-REL*) on the NF-κB signaling pathway and important signaling pathways in T and B cells. The integration of our understanding of genetic variation into our studies of biology will surely enhance our understanding of disease processes.

Although rapid progress has been achieved over the past couple of years advancing our knowledge of RA susceptibility loci from 2 or 3 to over 20, for the most part our understanding of these loci and how associated alleles cause disease is very limited. The next key step will involve in-depth characterization of the genetic architecture at each locus. Subsequently, understanding how associated variants affect function will require an array of approaches but is likely to benefit considerably from the GenCode initiative,[92] a program aimed at annotating all protein coding sequences in the genome.

NEW HORIZONS

Since entering the post-genome era and the new millennium, it is sometimes difficult to comprehend how quickly things are now progressing. Accrual of knowledge about our own DNA code and how this translates into both health and disease susceptibility is almost exponential. Progress has been driven largely by staggering advances in technology and computer-based informatics. Whereas it took a major international consortium 10 years, with teams of scientists and many

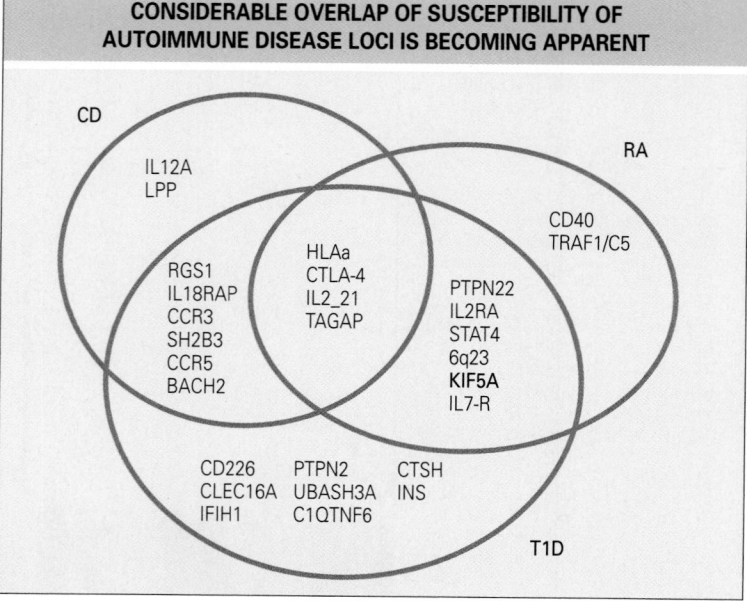

Fig. 14.3 Considerable overlap of susceptibility of autoimmune disease loci is becoming apparent. Illustrated here are some of the loci identified for type 1 diabetes, celiac disease, and rheumatoid arthritis. The specific markers associated with each disease may differ.

DNA-sequencing machines, to complete the sequencing of the human genome, we are now entering an era when re-sequencing the genome of an individual will be possible in a matter of days at affordable prices. The impact that such information could have on medicine in general and rheumatology in particular is hard to imagine.

Furthermore, the post-genome era has led to a greater realization that disease etiology and processes should not just be viewed one-dimensionally from the level of gene sequence but, rather, how these are transcribed differently by differentiated cells and how such transcripts are translated into proteins. The great expansion in complexity that increases from approximately 20,000 genes in the human genome to an estimated 300,000 different proteins, largely through alternative gene splicing and post-translational protein modification, is becoming better appreciated. The way such proteins interact and the metabolic processes and products that result are now providing important insights into unraveling disease processes and pathways. Scientists are now increasingly realizing that a holistic approach has to be taken to fully understand disease etiopathogenesis. The development of genomic technologies such as transcriptomics, proteomics, and metabolomics is being powerfully combined with genomics into an approach called "systems biology." This is increasingly driving translational medicine and is anticipated to have a major impact on rheumatology.

The full translation of the information that resides in our genome and how it relates to complex diseases will only come through understanding how it interacts with environmental factors. These could be gene-nutrient interactions, gene-infection interactions, gene-lifestyle (e.g., alcohol/smoking), or gene-drug interactions (pharmacogenetics). Such studies are difficult, and many can only be appropriately addressed through large longitudinal population-based cohorts. These enable pre-morbid environmental exposure data and biologic samples to be collected. One such study is U.K. Biobank in which environmental and lifestyle data, biological samples, and longitudinal health data are being collected on 5 million volunteers (www.ukbiobank.ac.uk). This may reveal great information for many human diseases, including rheumatologic conditions such as rheumatoid arthritis, osteoarthritis, and osteoporosis.

There is increasing realization that response to drug treatment, in terms of both efficacy and adverse reactions, is largely encoded within our genes; and this is poised to have great impact in the field of rheumatology. Pharmacogenetic studies are already beginning to explain why some patients are multi-drug resistant to some second-line drugs or develop reactions to drugs such as azathioprine. The next 5 years in the genetic study of rheumatic disease will undoubtedly be very interesting.

KEY REFERENCES

5. Silman AJ, MacGregor AJ, Thomson W, et al. Twin concordance rates for rheumatoid arthritis: results from a nationwide study. Br J Rheumatol 1993;32:903-907.

10. Brown MA, Kennedy LG, MacGregor AJ, et al. Susceptibility to ankylosing spondylitis in twins: the role of genes, HLA, and the environment. Arthritis Rheum 1997;40:1823-1828.

13. Risch N. Assessing the role of HLA-linked and unlinked determinants of disease. Am J Hum Genet 1987;40:1-14.

16. Brown MA, Pile KD, Kennedy LG, et al. A genome-wide screen for susceptibility loci in ankylosing spondylitis. Arthritis Rheum 1998;41:588-595.

24. Ollier W, Worthington J. Investigation of the genetic basis of rheumatic diseases. In Hochberg M, Silman AJ, Smolen J, et al, eds. Rheumatology, 4th ed. Philadelphia: Elsevier, 2008:123-131.

26. Cornelis F, Faure S, Martinez M, et al. New susceptibility locus for rheumatoid arthritis suggested by a genome-wide linkage study. Proc Natl Acad Sci U S A 1998;95:10746-10750.

27. Shiozawa S, Hayashi S, Tsukamoto Y, et al: Identification of the gene loci that predispose to rheumatoid arthritis. Int Immunol 1998;10:1891-1895.

28. Jawaheer D, Seldin MF, Amos CI, et al. A genomewide screen in multiplex rheumatoid arthritis families suggests genetic overlap with other autoimmune diseases. Am J Hum Genet 2001;68:927-936.

29. MacKay K, Eyre S, Myerscough A, et al. Whole-genome linkage analysis of rheumatoid arthritis susceptibility loci in 252 affected sibling pairs in the United Kingdom. Arthritis Rheum 2002;46:632-639.

35. Lindqvist AK, Steinsson K, Johanneson B, et al. A susceptibility locus for human systemic lupus erythematosus (hSLE1) on chromosome 2q. J Autoimmun 2000;14:169-178.

37. Greig C, Spreckley K, Aspinwall R, et al. Linkage to nodal osteoarthritis: quantitative and qualitative analyses of data from a whole-genome screen identify trait-dependent susceptibility loci. Ann Rheum Dis 2006;65:1131-1138.

38. Carter KW, Pluzhnikov A, Timms AE, et al. Combined analysis of three whole genome linkage scans for ankylosing spondylitis. Rheumatology (Oxford) 2007;46:763-771.

39. John S, Shephard N, Liu G, et al. Whole-genome scan, in a complex disease, using 11,245 single-nucleotide polymorphisms: comparison with microsatellites. Am J Hum Genet 2004;75:54-64.

40. Amos CI, Chen WV, Lee A, et al. High-density SNP analysis of 642 Caucasian families with rheumatoid arthritis identifies two new linkage regions on 11p12 and 2q33. Genes Immun 2006;7:277-286.

41. Remmers EF, Plenge RM, Lee AT, et al. STAT4 and the risk of rheumatoid arthritis and systemic lupus erythematosus. N Engl J Med 2007;357:977-986.

42. Ardlie KG, Kruglyak L, Seielstad M. Patterns of linkage disequilibrium in the human genome. Nat Rev Genet 2002;3:299-309.

43. Clayton DG, Walker NM, Smyth DJ, et al. Population structure, differential bias and genomic control in a large-scale, case-control association study. Nat Genet 2005;37:1243-1246.

44. Pritchard JK, Rosenberg NA. Use of unlinked genetic markers to detect population stratification in association studies. Am J Hum Genet 1999;65:220-228.

45. Tian C, Gregersen PK, Seldin MF. Accounting for ancestry: population substructure and genome-wide association studies. Hum Mol Genet 2008;17:R143-R150.

46. Spielman R, Ewens W. A sibship test for linkage in the presence of association: the sib transmission/disequilibrium test. Am J Hum Genet 1998;62:450-458.

48. Thomson W, Harrison B, Ollier B, et al. Quantifying the exact role of HLA-DRB1 alleles in susceptibility to inflammatory polyarthritis: results from a large, population-based study. Arthritis Rheum 1999;42:757-762.

49. Colhoun HM, McKeigue PM, Davey SG. Problems of reporting genetic associations with complex outcomes. Lancet 2003;361:865-872.

50. Hirschhorn JN. Genetic approaches to studying common diseases and complex traits. Pediatr Res 2005;57:74R-77R.

51. Lohmueller KE, Pearce CL, Pike M, et al. Meta-analysis of genetic association studies supports a contribution of common variants to susceptibility to common disease. Nat Genet 2003;33:177-182.

52. Ioannidis JP, Trikalinos TA, Ntzani EE, et al. Genetic associations in large versus small studies: an empirical assessment. Lancet 2003;361:567-571.

56. Bottini N, Musumeci L, Alonso A, et al. A functional variant of lymphoid tyrosine phosphatase is associated with type I diabetes. Nat Genet 2004;36:337-338.

57. Begovich AB, Carlton VE, Honigberg LA, et al. A missense single-nucleotide polymorphism in a gene encoding a protein tyrosine phosphatase (PTPN22) is associated with rheumatoid arthritis. Am J Hum Genet 2004;75:330-337.

58. Hinks A, Barton A, John S, et al. Association between the PTPN22 gene and rheumatoid arthritis and juvenile idiopathic arthritis in a UK population: further support that PTPN22 is an autoimmunity gene. Arthritis Rheum 2005;52:1694-1699.

61. Viken MK, Amundsen SS, Kvien TK, et al. Association analysis of the 1858C>T polymorphism in the PTPN22 gene in juvenile idiopathic arthritis and other autoimmune diseases. Genes Immun 2005;6:271-273.

67. Reddy MV, Johansson M, Sturfelt G, et al. The R620W C/T polymorphism of the gene PTPN22 is associated with SLE independently of the association of PDCD1. Genes Immun 2005;6:658-662.

71. Velaga MR, Wilson V, Jennings CE, et al. The codon 620 tryptophan allele of the lymphoid tyrosine phosphatase (LYP) gene is a major determinant of Graves' disease. J Clin Endocrinol Metab 2004;89:5862-5865.

74. Vang T, Miletic AV, Bottini N, et al. Protein tyrosine phosphatase PTPN22 in human autoimmunity. Autoimmunity 2007;40:453-461.

75. Vang T, Congia M, Macis MD, et al. Autoimmune-associated lymphoid tyrosine phosphatase is a gain-of-function variant. Nat Genet 2005;37:1317-1319.

76. Suzuki A, Yamada R, Chang X, et al. Functional haplotypes of PADI4, encoding citrullinating enzyme peptidylarginine deiminase 4, are associated with rheumatoid arthritis. Nat Genet 2003;34:395-402.

77. Kochi Y, Yamada R, Suzuki A, et al. A functional variant in FCRL3, encoding Fc receptor–like 3, is associated with rheumatoid arthritis and several autoimmunities. Nat Genet 2005;37:478-485.

78. Wellcome Trust Case Control Consortium. Genome-wide association study of 14,000 cases of seven common diseases and 3,000 shared controls. Nature 2007;447:661-678.

79. Thomson W, Barton A, Ke X, et al. Rheumatoid arthritis association at 6q23. Nat Genet 2007;39:1431-1433.

80. Barton A, Thomson W, Ke X, et al. Rheumatoid arthritis susceptibility loci at chromosomes 10p15, 12q13 and 22q13. Nat Genet 2008;40:1156-1159.

81. Plenge RM, Cotsapas C, Davies L, et al. Two independent alleles at 6q23 associated with risk of rheumatoid arthritis. Nat Genet 2007;39:1477-1482.

82. Orozco G, Hinks A, Eyre S, et al. Combined effects of three independent SNPs greatly increase the risk estimate for RA at 6q23. Hum Mol Genet 2009;18:2693-2699.

83. Graham RR, Cotsapas C, Davies L, et al. Genetic variants near TNFAIP3 on 6q23 are associated with systemic lupus erythematosus. Nat Genet 2008;40:1059-1061.

84. Musone SL, Taylor KE, Lu TT, et al. Multiple polymorphisms in the TNFAIP3 region are independently associated with systemic lupus erythematosus. Nat Genet 2008.

85. Plenge RM, Seielstad M, Padyukov L et al: TRAF1-C5 as a risk locus for rheumatoid arthritis—a genomewide study. N Engl J Med 2008;40:1062-1064.

86. Kurreeman FA, Padyukov L, Marques RB, et al. A candidate gene approach identifies the TRAF1/C5 region as a risk factor for rheumatoid arthritis. PLoS Med 2007;4:e278.

87. Barton A, Thomson W, Ke X, et al. Re-evaluation of putative rheumatoid arthritis susceptibility genes in the post-genome wide association study era and hypothesis of a key pathway underlying susceptibility. Hum Mol Genet 2008;17:2274-2279.

88. Raychaudhuri S, Remmers EF, Lee AT, et al. Common variants at CD40 and other loci confer risk of rheumatoid arthritis. Nat Genet 2008;40:1216-1223.

89. Raychaudhuri S, Thomson B, Remmers EF, et al: Rheumatoid arthritis risk alleles at CD28, PRDM1, and CD2/CD58. Nat Genet 2009;41:1313-1318.

90. Gregersen PK, Amos CI, Lee AT, et al. REL, encoding a member of the NF-kappaB family of transcription factors, is a newly defined risk locus for rheumatoid arthritis. Nat Genet 2009;41:820-823.

91. Gregersen PK, Olsson LM. Recent advances in the genetics of autoimmune disease. Annu Rev Immunol 2009;27:363-391.

92. Harrow J, Denoeud F, Frankish A, et al. GENCODE: producing a reference annotation for ENCODE. Genome Biol 2006;7(Suppl 1):S4-S9.

REFERENCES

Full references for this chapter can be found on www.expertconsult.com.

The principles of adaptive immunity

15

Sergei P. Atamas

- The adaptive immune system consists of T and B lymphocytes, which produce a large repertoire of T-cell receptors and immunoglobulins using somatic gene recombination.

- In contrast to the innate immune system, the adaptive repertoire of lymphocytes can recognize and eliminate a broad variety of new antigens not previously encountered by the host or the host's species. Clonal selection preserves and expands those lymphocytes whose products prove useful in protecting the host.

- The adaptive immune system has an inherent potential for self-reactivity, or autoimmunity. The potential to induce autoimmunity is usually controlled by a combination of deletional and regulatory mechanisms jointly referred to as immune self-tolerance.

- Immune receptor triggering involves the movement of receptors and co-stimulatory molecules into specialized complexes followed by the assembly of enzymatic cascades within the cells' interior.

- Immune responses can become polarized, depending on the phenotypes of helper T cells, into Th1 (mainly cell-mediated, controlled by interferon-γ), Th2 (mainly humoral, controlled by interleukin-4), Th17 (proinflammatory, controlled by interleukin-17), and Treg (anti-inflammatory and immunosuppressive, controlled by transforming growth factor-β and interleukin-10) types.

- All these processes provide targets for the therapeutic manipulation of autoimmune diseases.

INTRODUCTION

The reason for a rheumatologist to understand the bases of adaptive immunity is that most rheumatic diseases are autoimmune in nature or have an autoimmune component. Although the innate immune mechanisms often deliver the immediate damage in rheumatic diseases, the primary defect leading to autoimmunity—failure to maintain tolerance to the body's own tissues—appears to be in the adaptive immune system. The purpose of the immune system is to provide protection against microscopic invaders and their toxic products. As a result of co-evolution with pathogens, species acquired innate ability to recognize the pathogen-associated molecular patterns (PAMP) and to fight off the microscopic intruders. The innate immunity is not strict in specifically identifying the foreign molecules: anything that resembles commonly occurring infections is considered as a sign of a potential problem. Therefore, general molecular patterns rather than specific molecules are recognized through the innate pattern recognition receptors (PRRs, see Chapter 16). Although the innate immune system is very effective at its job, its limitation is that the spectrum of PRRs is shaped solely by the past history of the host-pathogen interactions. As a result, the innate immunity fails in situations when a new infectious agent that has not been previously encountered in the history of the host species appears. By constantly mutating, pathogens (viruses, bacteria, fungi, and protozoa) generate new molecular patterns that may avoid recognition by the preexisting PRRs. There is a need for a kind of immunity that would be able to adapt to whatever unforeseen pathogens attack the host. The adaptive (to the novelty of the future) immunity developed much later evolutionarily than the innate immunity. As a result of their co-evolution, they are now tightly integrated into a very sophisticated cellular and molecular protective system. The cells of adaptive and innate immunity utilize a complex spectrum of cell-surface molecules and soluble factors to orchestrate a precisely timed and highly effective protection at the microscopic level.

Both innate and adaptive parts of the immune system must first recognize their targets; this process is commonly referred to as "cognitive phase." It is followed by the "effector phase," during which the immune cells respond to the threat. The cognitive phase defines the central difference between the innate and adaptive immunity. In the innate immune system, the PRRs are rather ubiquitously expressed and are ready to immediately bind PAMPs, leading to instant activation of the effector phase. In contrast, the adaptive recognition system is constructed to effectively identify and respond to myriads of unpredictable new foreign molecules (antigens) without confusing them with the body's own molecules. This process is dramatically more complex and less efficient than functioning of the innate immunity, and therefore it is much slower. To save time during the subsequent encounters with the newly "learned" antigens, the adaptive immunity is capable of having specific memory of previous experiences and responds much faster and more effectively the next time a previously encountered antigen threatens the host.

THE ADAPTIVE IMMUNE SYSTEM

The adaptive immune system is composed of B and T lymphocytes, often referred to as *B and T cells.* Numerous subpopulations of lymphocytes exist. When precursors (progenitors) of immune cell undergo maturation and differentiation into numerous subsets of functional cell types, they differentially express various functional molecules—"cluster of differentiation" (CD)—on their cell surface. These molecules are often used as markers of immune cell subtypes. For example, CD19 and CD20 are expressed on B cells, whereas CD3 and CD28 are expressed on T cells.

The B cells mature in the bone marrow and are, in their terminally differentiated state, called *plasma cells*, the sole source of specialized protective molecules synonymically called immunoglobulins (Ig), or antibodies (Ab), or γ-globulins. The secreted antibodies mediate the so-called humoral (or fluid-based) immunity. Their goal is to circulate through the body in fluids, or *humors*, and bind to and neutralize extracellular microbes or any other targets that can be present outside cells. However, some pathogens can evade humoral immunity by hiding in the host's cells as intracellular parasites and thus becoming inaccessible to antibodies. In such cases, cytotoxic T cells (Tc) will recognize and kill the infected host cells, thus preventing further spreading of the infection. Thus, there are the innate immune cells (e.g., macrophages that phagocytize and digest microbes) and adaptive immune cells, such as B cells (antibody producers) and CD8+ cytotoxic T cells (killers of own infected cells), all working together to provide molecular protection to the body. Even at this superficial level of analysis, there appears to be a need to integrate and orchestrate the activities of various cell populations in the humoral and cell-mediated branches of immunity. A major population of T cells acts as such a central regulator of immunity. They are CD4+ helper T cells (Th), the principal regulator of the entire immune response, that produce cytokines regulating activities of other types of immune cells. Unlike B cells that mature in the bone marrow, T cells mature in the thymus.

Despite phenotypic diversity and functional specialization of lymphocytes, each of them is ultimately defined by its antigen receptor, whereas the adaptive immunity as a whole is defined by the vast repertoires of lymphocytes bearing their unique receptors.

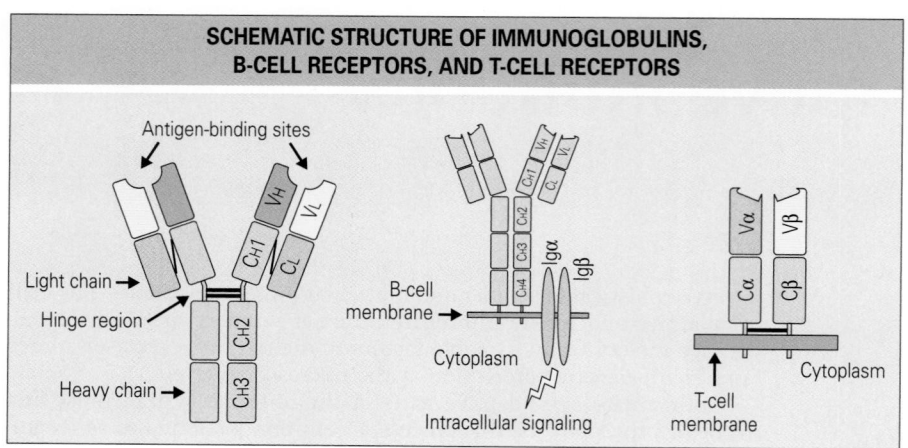

SCHEMATIC STRUCTURE OF IMMUNOGLOBULINS, B-CELL RECEPTORS, AND T-CELL RECEPTORS

Fig. 15.1 A model of IgG is shown on the left, a model of surface IgM B-cell receptor is shown in the middle, and a model of T-cell receptor α/β is shown on the right. Constant (C) and variable (V) domains are indicated, as well as heavy (H) and light (L) chains of immunoglobulins.

Clonal selection and expansion of lymphocytes

The adaptive immune system can respond to previously unencountered antigens. A pre-programmed system such as the innate immune system, by definition, cannot be instructed for dealing with the unknown. The adaptive immune system uses the only successful strategy in the face of the unknown—diversification with subsequent selection of useful elements. The broader a system is diversified, the likelier the possibility that at least one of the diverse elements will, by random chance, be adaptive in a new, changed, environment. Such an adaptive element, no matter how small initially, can be expanded to ensure adaptation of the whole system to the new environment.

Each individual lymphocyte is functionally defined by its antigen-specific receptor, either B-cell receptor (BCR) or T-cell receptor (TCR). On its cell surface, each lymphocyte expresses multiple (tens to hundreds of thousands) copies (molecules) of antigen-binding receptor of only one specificity. Lymphocytes differ from each other: Slight variations in the structure of antigen receptors among individual lymphocytes lead to a tremendous variability of antigen-binding specificities. It has been estimated that about 10^{11} diverse BCRs can be generated in the bone marrow and 10^{18} diverse TCRs can be produced in the thymus, with about 10^7 each BCR and TCR specificities present in a human at any given time. Each of the receptors is stochastically generated and has a binding specificity for a random, unpredictable antigen. As a result of having such a broad repertoire of lymphocytes, chances are that no matter what new antigen is encountered by the organism, at least (or likely more than) one lymphocyte will happen to be responsive to that antigen. In a simplified scenario, binding of an antigen molecule to an antigen receptor stimulates proliferation of the lymphocyte that expresses the receptor. When a lymphocyte proliferates, its offspring inherits the antigen-receptor specificity, thus forming an expanding clone (i.e., multiple copies of a lymphocyte with exactly the same specificity). The proliferating lymphocytes also undergo functional activation and eliminate the antigen in the effector phase of the immune response. Thus antigens select their own killers, lymphocytes that are the "fittest" for dealing with these specific antigens, from a vast variety of the preexisting randomly generated repertoire of lymphocytes. Such clonal selection of lymphocyte repertoires by antigens—a kind of "cellular Darwinism"—is the basis of functioning of the adaptive immune system.

Antigen receptors of lymphocytes

Immunoglobulins can be either membrane bound (acting as the BCRs) or soluble effector molecules (Fig. 15.1). The Y-shaped Ig molecule consists of four chains: two identical heavy chains and two identical light chains (see Fig. 15.1). There are nine heavy chain isotypes (α1, α2, δ, ε, γ1-4, and μ) that determine both immunoglobulin class/subclass (IgA1, IgA2, IgD, IgE, IgG1-4, and IgM, respectively) and the effector mechanisms that a particular antibody can elicit. Two light-chain isotypes (κ and λ) can associate with any heavy chain. The light chains are folded into a variable and a constant domain, whereas the heavy chains are folded into a variable domain in addition to three (α,

γ, and δ) or four (ε and μ) constant region domains. Mature naïve B cells express IgM and IgD with identical variable domains. These cell-surface immunoglobulins are co-expressed with Igα and Igβ chains, forming together a functional BCR capable of antigen recognition and binding (see Fig. 15.1), which lead to initiation of intracellular signaling and subsequent clonal selection of the antigen-specific B cells.

The TCR is a cell-surface heterodimer composed of α and β chains or, in about 5% of T cells, of γ and δ chains. Each of these chains is folded into two domains, one of which is the variable domain that determines antigen specificity, and the other of which is the constant domain that includes hydrophobic sequences that anchor the receptor to the surface of the T cell (see Fig. 15.1). The TCR associates with four other invariant chains at the cell surface: the CD3 proteins γ, δ, ε, and ζ chain. Collectively they are known as the *TCR complex*. Unlike immunoglobulins, the TCRs cannot bind antigens directly. Instead, the TCR chain variable domains bind antigen-MHC complexes, as discussed later.

A functionally important structural similarity between BCRs and TCRs is that they have variable domains that function to bind antigens. Within these variable domains are hypervariable regions, also called *complementarity determining regions* (CDRs), which define complementarity of the antigen receptors to antigens, in terms of geometric shape and spatial distribution of electric charges and/or hydrophobic patches. Variations of amino acid sequences in these hypervariable regions are the basis for the spectrum of antigen-binding specificities within an adaptive immune repertoire.

Generation of diversity of antigen receptors

A newly generated B cell expresses BCRs and a newly generated T cell expresses TCRs of a unique, randomly generated specificity. These immune repertoires develop in a unique process of somatic chromosomal recombination of gene segments in the antigen receptor loci of DNA. This permanent change to DNA, more specifically referred to as *V(D)J recombination*, occurs only in lymphocytes.[1,2] Most genes are composed of protein-coding DNA regions (exons) intermingled with non-coding regions (introns). During transcription, introns and exons are copied into pre-messenger RNA. This process is followed by removal of introns and splicing of exons, to form mature mRNA that can be translated into protein. Splicing of many pre-mRNAs may occur through several alternative pathways, selectively preserving alternative fragments of the coding sequence. Alternative splicing is an important mechanism of generating various protein products from a single gene. However, genetic considerations that go beyond the scope of this chapter prompt that alternative splicing cannot be an effective way of generating the tremendous variety of antigen receptor specificities. Instead, the variable regions of antibodies and TCR chains are encoded in DNA by multiple different variable (V), diversity (D), and joining (J) gene segments. During somatic recombination of DNA, select V, D, and J segments are brought together (Fig. 15.2). Depending on the gene (Ig heavy chain, Ig light chain, TCRα, TCRβ, TCRγ, TCRδ), the number of V segments can vary from dozens to hundreds, D segments from none to a few, and J segments from a few to dozens.[3,4] The random V(D)J recombination leads to combinatorial diversity of antigen receptors. This process is subject to a complex regulation[5,6] by numerous factors including TdT, RAG1, RAG2, Ku70, Ku80, XRCC4, DNA ligase 4, DNA-PKcs, Artemis, and other factors that continue to be vigorously investigated. In addition to combinatorial diversity, even more variability is added by junctional diversity resulting from imprecise joining of the V, D, and J segments (i.e., insertions and deletions that occur during V(D)J gene segment recombination). The mechanisms described earlier take place during lymphocyte maturation. In addition, mature naïve B cells, but not T cells, undergo receptor editing, somatic hypermutagenesis, and isotype switching processes that are briefly discussed in the section devoted to B cells.

B CELLS AND HUMORAL IMMUNITY

B-cell development

Maturation of B cells in the bone marrow (Fig. 15.3) occurs under control of cell-surface molecules and soluble growth factors produced

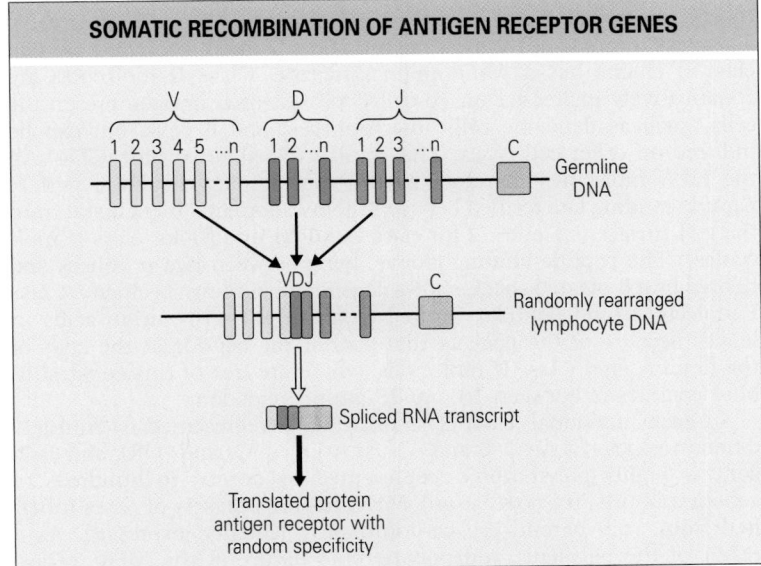

SOMATIC RECOMBINATION OF ANTIGEN RECEPTOR GENES

Fig. 15.2 This diagrammatic representation shows features common to BCR and TCR genes. Gene recombination randomly joins one of each variable (V), diversity (D), joining (J) gene segments together to form a variable domain-encoding V-D-J region. Following transcription of this region, as well as the constant (C) gene segments into pre-mRNA, the final mRNA transcript is formed by RNA splicing.

by bone marrow stromal cells,[7,8] as well as several key transcription factors.[9,10] Pro-B cells begin rearrangement of the Ig heavy-chain (H) genes and express the pro-BCR. DJ rearrangements begin first and V to DJ rearrangements follow. Productively rearranged μ chains are expressed on the cell surface with a surrogate light chain and Igα and Igβ. This pre-BCR induces cell division and the generation of nondividing small pre-B cells. It also suppresses further Ig heavy-chain (H) gene recombination (allelic exclusion) by decreasing RAG expression and appears to make further VH genes less accessible to the recombination machinery. The subsequent rearrangement of the light chain leads to expression of the mature BCR, in which the surrogate light chain in the pre-BCR[11] is replaced by a mature κ or λ chain. Expression of the BCR leads to suppression of further light-chain recombination; however, allelic exclusion at the light chain locus is "leaky" and about 10% of B cells express two separate light chains. At this stage the lymphocyte becomes an immature B cell expressing surface IgM (BCR), and it is at this stage that induction of immune tolerance occurs. Because the mechanism of generating BCR specificity is intrinsically stochastic, the likelihood is high that many (up to 60%[12]) of the newly generated BCRs will, by a random chance, be reactive against own-body molecules. If the BCR on an immature B cell reacts with own-body molecules (self-antigens), then it should be removed, to avoid development of a self-reactive, autoimmune, clone of B cells. Such clonal deletion occurs by apoptosis, but not instantly. First, autoreactive immature B cells become anergic (not able to proliferate in response to stimulation). Then, a unique process called receptor editing occurs, in which Ig rearrangements continue even after assembly of a functional BCR.[12,13] This mechanism, in contrast to anergy or deletion, spares many autoreactive B cells by replacing their receptor with a new one, possibly one that is not self-reactive. However, if the new receptor is also self-reactive, such self-reactive B cell becomes apoptotically deleted. Recent data indicate that censoring of potentially autoreactive B cells may take place even before the BCR is fully matured, at the level of pre-BCR,[14] or in the mature naïve B cell, to maintain peripheral tolerance.[15] The process of receptor editing may be either impaired or accelerated in patients with rheumatic autoimmune diseases. Such impairments contribute to pathogenesis of autoimmune disorders by promoting the uncontrolled emergence and/or persistence of autoreactive B-cell clones.[16,17]

Immature B cells that emigrate from the bone marrow are known as *transitional B cells*. The transitional cell pool is homeostatically controlled to maintain mature B cell numbers. Mature naïve B cells express membrane-bound monomeric IgM (as opposed to soluble IgM pentamer) and IgD with identical variable domains. This is accomplished by alternative RNA splicing. These IgM and IgD co-expressing B cells will survive between 3 and 8 weeks if they successfully enter primary follicles in secondary lymphoid tissues. This is where they will encounter specific antigen. If that happens, the B cell will interact with

Fig. 15.3 Hematopoietic stem cells (HSCs) differentiate into non-self-renewing hematopoietic multipotential progenitors (MPPs), then lymphoid-primed multipotential progenitors (LMPPs), and then into common lymphoid progenitors (CLP). Expression of various markers is shown for each differentiation stage. Immature B cells, which are generated from fraction D cells, exit the bone marrow and reach the spleen, where they mature into peripheral mature B cells and plasma cells. Factors that regulate B cell development at the indicated stages are shown at the bottom. CD20 is a target for therapeutic monoclonal antibodies (rituximab), which deplete B cells in patients with autoimmune, including rheumatic, diseases. This cell-surface molecule is expressed on B cells during the indicated stages of development, as well as on activated and memory B cells, but it is lost during terminal plasma cell differentiation. *(Adapted by permission from Macmillan Publishers Ltd: Nagasawa T. Microenvironmental niches in the bone marrow required for B-cell development. Nat Rev Immunol 2006;6:107–116, copyright 2006.)*

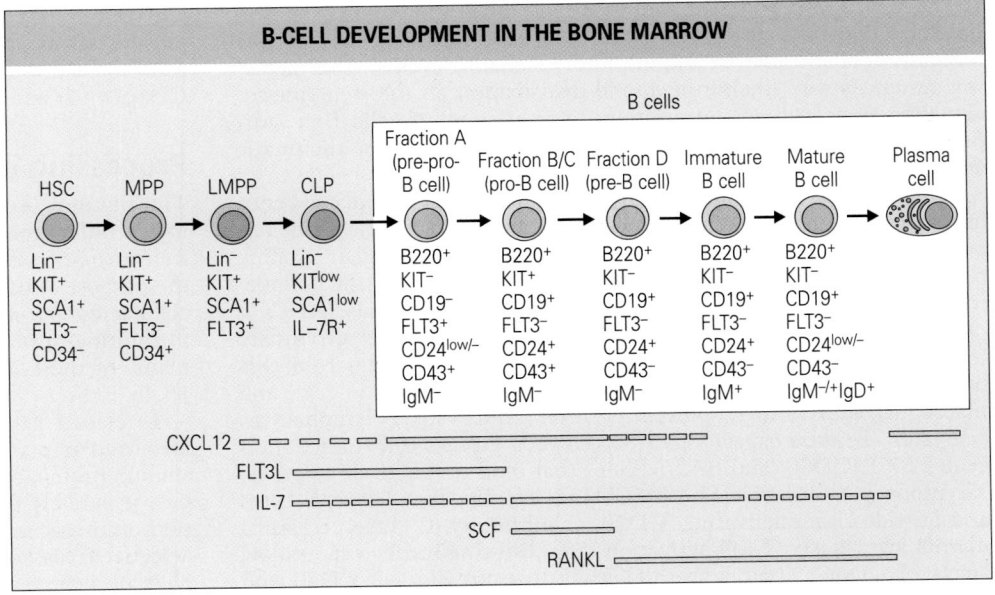

B-CELL DEVELOPMENT IN THE BONE MARROW

Th cells and become activated. Some B cells will proliferate and differentiate directly into Ig-secreting plasma cells, whereas others will enter into nearby primary follicles. These primary follicles become secondary follicles with germinal centers where large proliferating B cells (centroblasts) undergo somatic hypermutation and class switching before becoming non-proliferating centrocytes. Affinity maturation is a phenomenon unique to B cells, in which affinity of antibodies to antigens increases over time. It is mechanistically achieved through somatic hypermutation, where additional sequence variation is introduced into the recombined V(D)J sequence. Activated B cells that have survived the affinity maturation process will home to other secondary lymphoid tissues or bone marrow and differentiate into plasma cells secreting IgG, IgA, or IgE high-affinity antibodies; others will become quiescent, long-lived memory B cells. The Ig class switching, or isotype switching, upon B-cell stimulation involves recombination of so-called switch regions of DNA that are located upstream of each constant heavy-chain gene segment. This process moves the rearranged VDJ segment closer to the intended constant heavy-chain gene segment, by excising the intervening sequence.[18,19] An enzyme activation-induced deaminase (AID) is critical for both somatic hypermutation and isotype switching.[20,21]

The survival of peripheral B cells is critically dependent on B-cell activation factor of the TNF family (BAFF), also called BLyS, and a proliferation-inducing ligand (APRIL). Elevated levels of BAFF and APRIL have been associated with autoimmunity. Inhibitors of BAFF and/or APRIL are promising agents for treating rheumatic diseases.

B-cell activation and functions

Both the BCR and soluble Ig can bind both linear and conformational (three-dimensional) epitopes on a wide variety of molecules, including protein, polysaccharide, and lipid antigens. They recognize such antigens directly, without the need for antigens to be presented to them. Certain antigens (thymus-independent Ag) can activate B cells without the need for helper T cells, but many require T-cell help and are thymus dependent.

Upon BCR ligation with antigen, numerous intracellular signaling molecules become activated, such as kinases of the Src family, Syk, and Btk; also, Ca^{++} mobilization and Ras activation, as well as phosphorylation of Igα and Igβ chains, takes place. Activation of a downstream signaling cascade ensues (see Chapter 13), with final activation of a series of transcription factors, resulting in dramatic changes in the pattern of gene expression, and in overall B-cell activation.[22,23] Engagement of the BCR by an antigen is by itself not sufficient to activate a B cell. Instead, the BCR relies on co-stimulatory receptors to bring about B-cell activation.[24,25] The co-stimulatory receptors CD19 and CD21 form a non-covalent complex that is co-ligated with the BCR to promote B-cell activation. Upon phosphorylation, CD19 recruits PI-3K, Src family kinases, and Vav to facilitate activation of the MAPK pathways and Ca^{++} mobilization. Negatively regulating co-receptors such as CD22, CD72, and FcγIIB1 inhibit B-cell proliferation and Ca^{++} mobilization. Thus the activation state of B cells is determined by the integration of stimulatory and inhibitory signaling events. This signaling system is very finely tuned, and disturbances in the signaling/co-signaling may lead to autoimmune activation of B cells that start producing antibodies against own tissue, particularly in rheumatic diseases.

The principal function of B cells is to differentiate into plasma cells and secrete antibodies. When secreted as soluble molecules, antibodies perform various protective effector functions following their binding to pathogens, such as direct neutralization, activation of the complement system or of antibody-dependent cellular cytotoxicity (ADCC), or opsonization of pathogens for phagocytosis. These are innate immune mechanisms that are discussed in detail in Chapter 16 of this book. In addition, B cells can serve, along with dendritic cells and macrophages, as antigen-presenting cells (APCs) for T lymphocytes (see later). In their capacity as APCs, B cells express cell-surface molecules B7.1 (CD80) and B7.2 (CD86) that bind to CD28 or cytotoxic T-lymphocyte antigen (CTLA)-4 (CD152) expressed on T lymphocytes and provide either activating (CD28) or inhibitory (CTLA-4) co-stimulatory signals (see T-cell activation later). Resting B cells express low levels of CD86. Their activation leads to expression of CD80 and enhanced expression of CD86. Dysregulated expression of these molecules on B cells has been associated with autoimmune and rheumatic diseases.

T CELLS AND CELL-MEDIATED IMMUNITY

Recognition of peptide and lipid antigens by T cells

Unlike immunoglobulins, TCRs cannot bind antigens directly. Instead, antigens for TCRs have to be processed and presented to T cells by a specialized class of molecules called *human leukocyte antigen* (HLA) proteins that are encoded in the major histocompatibility complex (MHC) of genes (Fig. 15.4a). In other words, T cells recognize antigens presented in the context of MHC molecules.[26] The terms HLA and MHC are often used interchangeably to denote the same genomic region and corresponding protein products in humans. There are two classes of these cell-surface heterodimeric glycoproteins: class I (e.g., HLA-A, -B, and -C) and class II (e.g., HLA-DP, -DQ, and -DR). The class I proteins consist of a three-domain α chain non-covalently complexed with β_2-microglobulin. They are expressed on the surface of most nucleated cells and bind the CD8 molecule expressed on T cells. The class II molecules consist of an α and a β chain. Each of these two class II chains has a two-domain structure. Class II molecules are constitutively expressed on so-called professional antigen-presenting cells, such as dendritic cells, macrophages, and B cells, but can be induced on other cell types. They bind a T-cell coreceptor, CD4. All the HLA molecules therefore have a four-domain structure with a peptide-binding site formed between the two domains most distal from the cell surface (α1 and α2 for class I and α1 and β1 for class II molecules). The peptide-binding groove, lying between two α helices and floored by a β-pleated sheet, shows degenerate binding specificity. Class I molecules bind peptides limited to about 8 to 10 amino acids in length because of the pockets that anchor the peptide at the ends of the binding site. Class II molecules, which are free of this constraint, bind peptides of between 13 and 25 amino acids long.

In each individual, each class of MHC is represented by multiple different genes (HLA-A, -B and -C; HLA-DP, -DQ, and -DR), and each gene is highly polymorphic (represented by dozens to hundreds of genetic variants in a population). MHC haplotypes (sets of genes inherited from each parent) are co-dominantly (equally) expressed. As a result of the polygenic and polymorphic nature of the MHC genes, each individual in an outbred population expresses a unique set of MHC proteins. This genetic diversity of the MHC loci defines each individual's unique spectrum of peptides that can be presented to the TCRs.

In contrast to presentation of peptides by MHC molecules, lipid and glycolipid antigens are presented by CD1 molecules. These transmembrane proteins expressed on APCs are homologous to MHC class I molecules and non-covalently paired with β_2-microglobulin.[27] Five CD1 molecules have been identified in humans (CD1a-CD1e). They present self or foreign lipid antigens such as microbial lipids derived from the cell walls of mycobacteria to $\alpha\beta$ and $\gamma\delta$ T cells (CD1a, CD1b, CD1c) or to natural killer T (NKT) cells (CD1d).

Processing of antigens for presentation to T cells

The purpose of the MHC class I pathway is to survey for possible intracellular problems such as viral or bacterial infections or malignant transformation and report such problems to CD8+ T cells. In contrast, the purpose of the MHC class II pathway is to survey the overall extracellular environment and to present it to the central regulating and integrating immune cell type, CD4+ T cells. Respectively, the mechanisms of these antigen processing pathways differ substantially (Fig. 15.4b and c).

In class I pathway, a significant proportion of newly synthesized intracellular proteins is degraded by proteasomes, which are multisubunit protein complexes with a number of different proteolytic activities. It is likely that rapid synthesis of viral proteins in the host cells' ribosomes occurs with numerous errors, leading to accumulation of defective ribosomal products (DRiPs). Such proteins are the major supplier of peptides for the class I pathway.[28] Peptides generated by

ANTIGEN PROCESSING AND PRESENTATION BY MHC MOLECULES

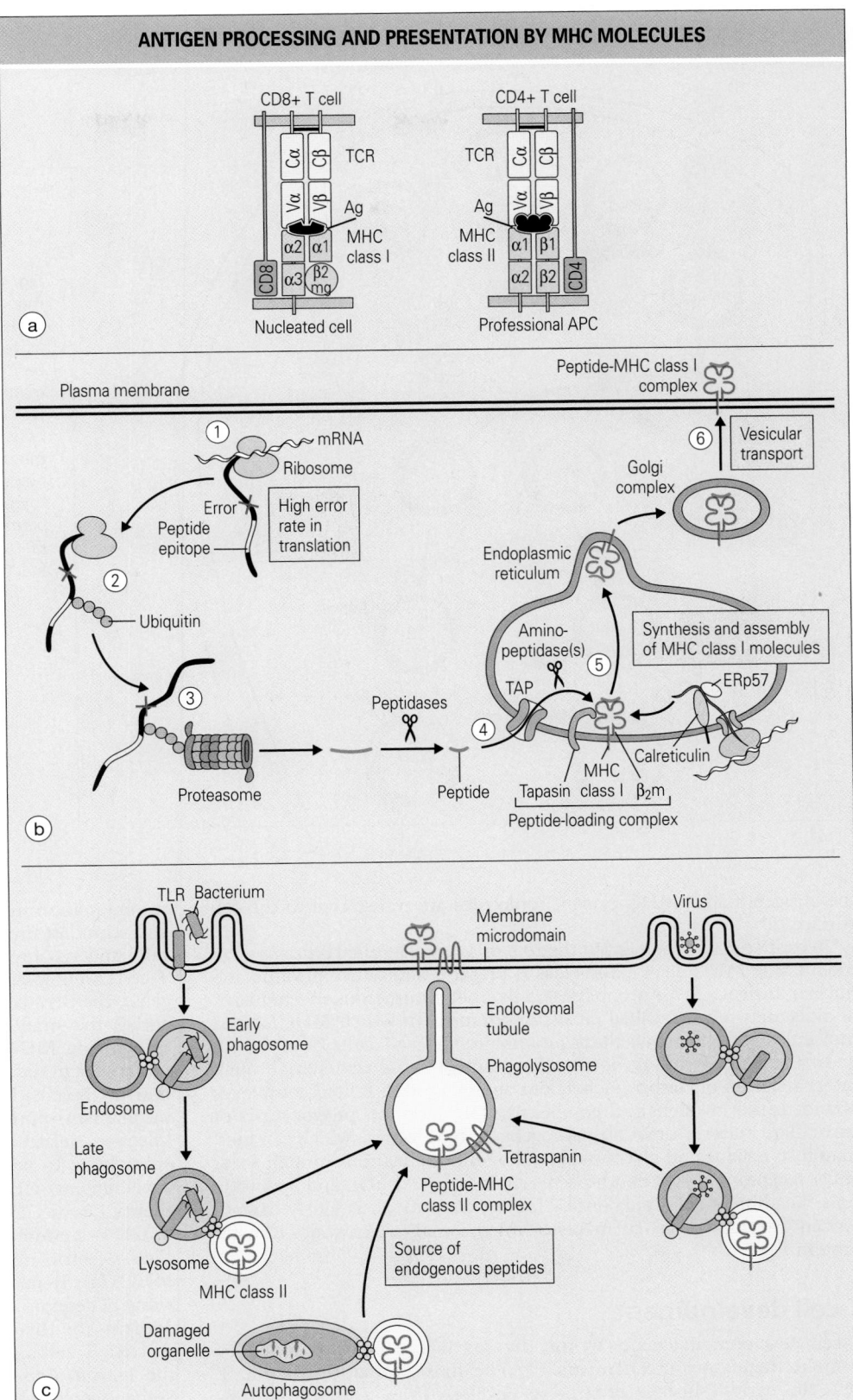

Fig. 15.4 Presentation of antigen peptides by MHC molecules (a), as well as class I (b) and class II (c) antigen processing pathways, are shown. In the class I pathway, proteins with errors are tagged with ubiquitin for degradation and degraded by proteasomes into peptides, which are delivered into endoplasmic reticulum, loaded into nascent MHC class I molecules, and transported via the Golgi complex to the cell surface. In the class II pathway, the internalized pathogens activate toll-like receptors (TLRs) leading to maturation of phagosomes, formation of phagolysosomes, loading of MHC class II molecules with peptide fragments of the bacteria or viruses that are formed by lysosomal proteases, and transport in endolysosomal tubules to the cell surface. Autophagosomes also fuse with lysosomes and serve as an additional source of peptides, including endogenous peptides, for MHC class II presentation. β_2m denotes β_2-microglobulin. (b and c, Adapted by permission from Macmillan Publishers Ltd: Vyas JM, Van der Veen AG, Ploegh HL, et al. The known unknowns of antigen processing and presentation. Nat Rev Immunol 2008;8:607-618, copyright 2008.)

proteasomes are transported by TAP (transporter associated with antigen processing) across the membrane of the endoplasmic reticulum (ER), whereas class I MHC molecules translated by ribosomes at the ER membrane are chaperoned by calnexin until they associate with β_2-microglobulin. Additional chaperones, including calreticulin and tapasin, facilitate peptide loading. The completed MHC-peptide complex is transported through the endoplasmic reticulum and the Golgi apparatus to the cell surface.

Class II MHC molecules present antigens internalized by professional APCs. Protein antigens taken up by phagocytosis, macropinocytosis, endocytosis, and receptor-mediated endocytosis are delivered to an endosomal compartment that contains class II MHC. Peptides are generated from these proteins by proteases that are active in this acidic environment. MHC class II heterodimers, stabilized by their association with the invariant chain (Ii), are targeted to this endocytic compartment through a signal in the cytoplasmic tail of the invariant chain. Once there, the Ii is sequentially digested, leaving only a fragment (class II-associated Ii peptide [CLIP]) in the peptide binding site. HLA-DM and HLA-DO (also encoded in the MHC class II region) then catalyze the exchange of CLIP for antigenic peptides, after which

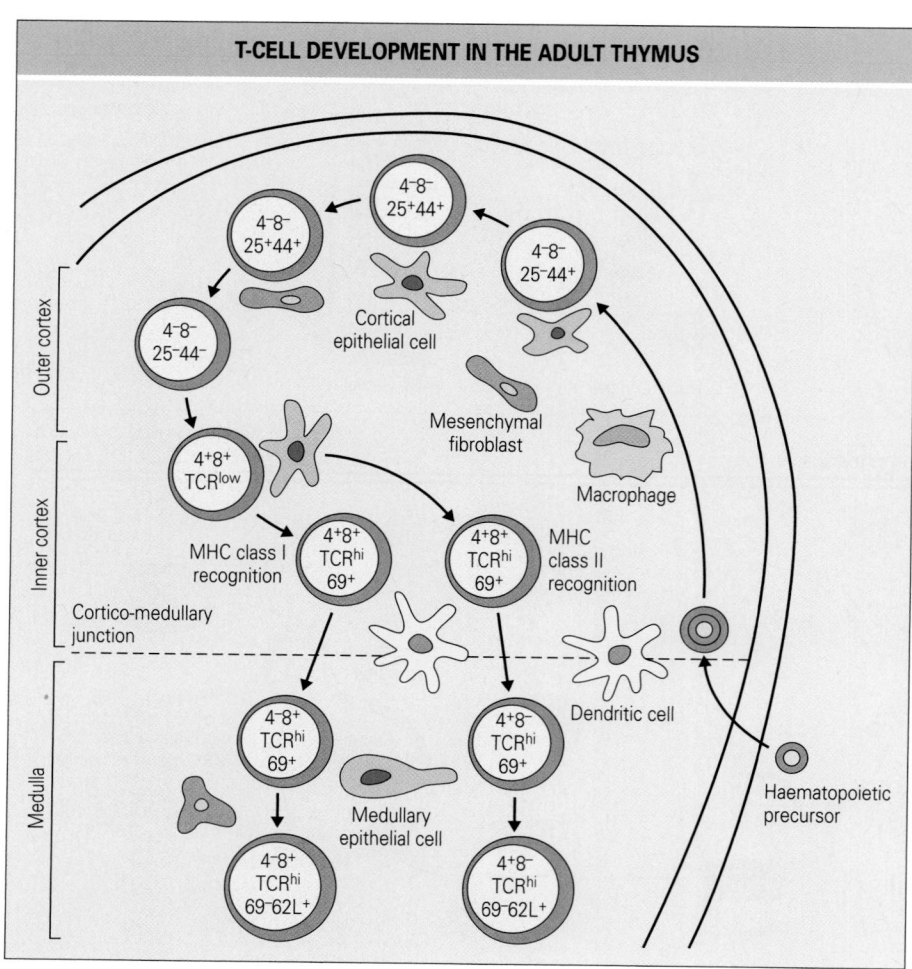

T-CELL DEVELOPMENT IN THE ADULT THYMUS

Fig. 15.5 Thymic lobes are organized into discrete cortical and medullary areas, each of which is characterized by the presence of particular stromal cell types, as well as thymocyte precursors at defined maturational stages. Thymocyte differentiation can be followed phenotypically by the expression of cell-surface markers, including CD4, CD8, CD44, CD25, CD69, and CD62L, as well as the status of the T-cell receptor (TCR). Interactions between thymocytes and thymic stromal cells drive T-cell maturation, resulting in the generation of self-tolerant CD4+ helper and CD8+ cytotoxic T cells, which emigrate from the thymus to establish the peripheral T-cell pool. *(Adapted by permission from Macmillan Publishers Ltd: Anderson G, Jenkinson EJ. Lymphostromal interactions in thymic development and function. Nat Rev Immunol 2001;1:31-40, copyright 2001.)*

the antigen-loaded MHC class II molecules are transferred to the cell surface.

Recent studies emphasized the role of a process called *autophagy* in modulating MHC class I and class II presentation of cytoplasmic and nuclear antigens.[26,29] Autophagy is only one of numerous mechanisms of a peculiar process called *cross-presentation*, in which MHC class I molecules present extracellular proteins to CD8+ T cells.[30,31]

In the CD1 pathway, foreign lipid antigens are uptaken through internalization of clathrin-dependent apolipoprotein E-lipid complexes bound to the low-density lipoprotein (LDL) receptor; phagocytosis of particulate material or whole pathogens; C-type lectins, which can bind mannose residues on glycolipids; and by internalization through scavenger receptors, which can bind modified forms of LDL and apoptotic cells. Loading of self lipids onto CD1 occurs through a poorly characterized mechanism that involves microsomal triglyceride transfer protein.[27]

T-cell development

T-cell development occurs in the thymus (Fig. 15.5), controlled by complex regulatory mechanisms.[32,33] The most immature thymic T cell, the early T-lineage progenitor, develops from a bone marrow–derived hematopoietic cell precursor. These progenitors lack the cell-surface proteins CD4 and CD8 (double-negative cells). They are also negative for the IL-2Rβ chain, CD25, but positive for the adhesion molecule CD44. As the progenitors undergo differentiation, they acquire CD25, lose CD44, and complete somatic rearrangement of the gene loci encoding the TCR β, γ, and δ chains. If both TCR γ and δ chains undergo productive rearrangement, then the T cell expresses this heterodimer and becomes committed to the γδ lineage. If, however, the β chain undergoes production rearrangement first, then the TCR β chain is expressed on the cell surface along with an invariant chain called pre-Tα, forming the pre-TCR complex. Expression of the pre-TCR stimulates proliferation of these T cells, suppresses VDJ

recombination in the second TCR β locus on the allelic chromosome, and stimulates recombination in the TCR α locus. Failure to successfully undergo any of these steps causes apoptotic death of the maturing T cell. After acquiring the CD4 and CD8 co-receptors (double-positive cells), the thymocytes undergo the selection process. Positive selection allows the small percentage of the thymocyte population capable of recognizing MHC-peptide complexes to mature further, leaving the remainder to die by apoptosis. Similar to newly emerging in the bone marrow B cells, many of the TCRs generated through the stochastic mechanisms in the emerging thymic T cells are autoreactive. Negative selection deletes T cells that bind self-peptide-MHC complexes so strongly as to be potentially autoimmune. During the final stage of development, CD4+CD8+ T cells suppress the expression of either their CD4 or CD8 co-receptors to give rise to single positive, CD8+, or CD4+ mature thymocytes, respectively. T cells that express MHC class I–restricted TCRs become CD8+ and lymphocytes that express MHC class II–restricted TCRs become positive for the CD4 co-receptor alone. Therefore along with acting as an environment for T-cell development, the thymus also acts as the principal site of deletion of autoreactive T cell and, as such, shapes the immune repertoire. However, the central thymic elimination of autoreactive T cells is not perfect. Some of such cells leak into the periphery, normally becoming subject to complex regulation by peripheral tolerance mechanisms.

T-cell activation

In order to be successfully activated, T cells require two signals.[34] The first is recognition of antigen by the TCR. On its own, this event can trigger anergy, a non-responsive state in which T cells are resistant to subsequent activation. T-cell activation requires a second signal delivered by co-stimulatory molecules expressed on the surface of T cells. The most potent co-stimulatory signals are delivered when CD28, CD154, or both are ligated on the surface of T cells. Blockade of co-stimulatory signals by monoclonal antibodies or recombinant receptor antagonists confers potent immunosuppression and allows the acceptance of tissue allografts. Simultaneous blockade of both the CD28 and CD154 pathways is significantly more immunosuppressive than blockade of a single co-stimulatory pathway. The ligand for CD154 is CD40, a protein expressed on the surface of activated B cells, dendritic cells, and macrophages. The ligands for CD28 (CD80, CD86) are expressed on the surface of APCs such as dendritic cells, monocytes, and B cells. Their expression is induced when APCs are activated in the course of microbial infection. This property heightens the immune response in the setting of perceived danger (i.e., microbial infection). CD80 and CD86 have overlapping immunostimulatory roles; mice lacking either protein are only partially deficient in generating an immune response to foreign antigen.

Following TCR cross-linking, a series of complex intracellular signaling events takes place (see Chapter 13). The early events following TCR cross-linking include activation of Src-family kinases Fyn and the CD4/CD8-associated Lck, as well as recruitment of a Syk family kinase, ZAP-70. Activated ZAP-70 phosphorylates LAT, allowing for activation of a set of adapter molecules such as PLC-γ1, Grb2, and GADS. Numerous downstream molecules then become activated, leading to cytoskeletal rearrangements; formation of the immune synapse; activation of transcription factors such as ATF-2, NF-AT, NF-κB, and AP-1; changes in gene expression and expression of numerous cell-surface and secreted proteins; and cell cycle entry.

In unstimulated T cells, TCRs and co-receptors are distributed homogeneously over the T-cell surface. At the synapse between T cells and APCs, however, a large number of receptor-ligand pairs, adhesion molecules, and signaling complexes come together in an organized manner to promote cellular activation.[35,36] This immunologic synapse is organized so that the TCR, MHC-peptide complexes, and protein kinase C (PKC)-θ are enriched in a central circle, surrounded by integrins and the adhesion molecule ICAM-1.

The activation signals triggered by TCR ligation are balanced by inhibitory signals that dampen T-cell activation. For example, TCR ligation without CD28 co-stimulation induces induction of an anergic T-cell state rather than stimulation. Moreover, the inhibitory receptor CTLA-4 competes for the same ligands as CD28 (B7 expressed on APCs) and antagonizes TCR signaling via recruitment of PP2A or SHP-2 phosphatase.[37,38] The integration of activation and inhibitory signals determines the state of T-cell activation.

T-cell function

Functionally and phenotypically, T lymphocytes are likely the most diverse known population of cells in the human body. A vast amount of data indicates that disturbances in the specific subsets of T cells are directly involved in pathophysiologic mechanisms of autoimmunity and rheumatic diseases.

Cytotoxic T cells

The main function of CD8+ cytotoxic T cells (Tc) is to induce elimination of "altered-self" cells such as infected or mutated cells. They can also secrete cytokines and participate in regulation (or dysregulation) of immune responses, including in rheumatic diseases. The cytotoxic function is carried out by releasing cytotoxins from lytic granules secreted at the site of target cell contact. These cytotoxins include a family of serine proteases, granzyme A, B, and H, that are capable of inducing caspase-dependent and caspase-independent cell death.[39] The role of another secreted cytotoxin, perforin, is to form pores in the target cell membrane and deliver granzymes into the target cell cytosol.[40] Cytotoxic T cells can also trigger cell death through the Fas-FasL pathway. When stimulated through their TCRs, CD8+ T cells transiently upregulate FasL. Subsequent contact with target cells expressing Fas induces apoptotic cell death.

Helper T cells

There are likely numerous CD4+ helper T-cell (Th) types, but the most characterized, based on the cytokines that they produce, are Th1, Th2, and Th17. Th1 cells secrete interferon (IFN)-γ, interleukin (IL)-2, and tumor necrosis factor (TNF)-α and control protection against infection with intracellular microbes. Maturation of Th1 cells is controlled by IL-12 and transcription factor T-bet.[41] Th2 cells produce IL-4, IL-5,

and IL-13 and promote the humoral immune response necessary to clear parasitic infections, as well as isotype switching to IgG1 and IgE. Maturation of Th1 cells is controlled by IL-4 and transcription factor GATA3.[41] Th1 and Th2 cell responses are functionally opposite. For example, Th2 cytokines promote humoral immunity but suppress Th1 and macrophage function. The cytokine IL-12, which promotes uncommitted helper T cells (Th0) to differentiate into Th1 effector cells, inhibits Th2 commitment. IL-4 acts in the reverse manner. Th17 cells have recently emerged as non-pathogenic regulators of immunity, as well as critical contributors of autoimmunity and inflammation. They produce IL-17A, IL-17F, IL-21, and IL-22 and induce the recruitment of neutrophils and macrophages to tissues.[42,43] Maturation of Th17 is controlled by IL-23; requires IL-1, IL-6, and transforming growth factor (TGF)-β[44]; and is directed by retinoid-related orphan receptor γt (RORγt).[45]

Regulatory T cells

Following activation of the immune response and elimination of pathogen, there is a need to downregulate, or suppress, the activity of lymphocytes. The concept of "suppressor T cells" is old but has undergone a period of neglect, followed by explosive renewed interest during the past decade. The preferred term for these cells now is regulatory T cells (Treg). Tregs comprise a subset of peripheral blood CD4+ T cells that express CD25 (a subunit of the IL-2 receptor) and a transcription factor FOXP3.[46] They suppress the activity of effector T cells (CD4+CD25−) and inhibit autoimmune processes, ensuring immune tolerance to own tissues.[47] The selective removal of CD4+CD25+ T cells from experimental mice results in the development of T cell–mediated autoimmune thyroiditis, gastritis, and diabetes. Tregs regulate effector cells through contact-dependent mechanisms and/or the production of IL-10 and TGF-β.[48] In addition to "natural" thymus-derived Tregs, there are "adaptive" Tregs that can be induced through various modalities in the periphery in vivo, as well as in cell culture, from conventional CD4+ cells. There are numerous subsets of regulatory T cells already described, and more subsets are likely to be found in the future.[49]

AUTOIMMUNITY AND TOLERANCE

The advantage of having adaptive immunity is the ability to fend off new, unpredictable pathogens. The prerequisite for such functioning of the adaptive immune system is formation of stochastic repertoires of B- and T-cell specificities, as discussed earlier. However, because newly generated antigen specificities of lymphocytes are random, the numerous emerging lymphocytes are able to react with the own body's molecules as if they were foreign pathogens. In other words, the first target for the adaptive immune system should be own tissues—the concept of so-called "horror autotoxicus." In most cases, this central problem is successfully avoided through a series of regulatory mechanisms that are collectively called tolerance. If these mechanisms do not function properly, autoimmunity ensues—a process that is so common in rheumatic diseases. Mechanisms that prevent B cell– or T cell–mediated autoimmune damage are complex but can be separated into central and peripheral mechanisms. Central tolerance is achieved by deleting high-avidity autoreactive B cells in the bone marrow and autoreactive T cells in the thymus during their maturation, as discussed earlier. The mechanisms that control central tolerance are being vigorously investigated, with notable achievements in delineating the role of autoimmune regulator (AIRE) in thymic central tolerance.[50]

Peripheral tolerance is even more complex and diverse. Its mechanisms can be grouped into apoptotic deletion of lymphocytes that are repeatedly stimulated by persistent antigens; anergy of lymphocytes (without deletion) through lack of co-stimulation, inhibitory signals (such as CTLA-4), or regulatory action of Tregs; immune indifference, or ignorance, due to low avidity of the antigen receptors, low lymphocyte precursor frequency, or low concentration of the antigen; and homeostatic interactions, including immune deviation (switching of cytokine profiles leading to suppression), interclonal competition of lymphocytes for antigen, and idiotypic network interactions (antibodies developing against other own antibodies). In autoimmune, including rheumatic, diseases, immune tolerance is broken through diverse mechanisms. Such mechanisms may include molecular or cellular defects weakening central and peripheral tolerance; molecular mimicry (confusion of the adaptive immune system regarding non-self versus self-antigens); exposure of normally sequestered antigens from immunologically privileged sites; peculiarities of antigen presentation by particular MHC haplotypes; female sex hormones; and various environmental influences. Once the immune tolerance is broken, autoreactive antibodies, T lymphocytes, and circulating immune complexes deliver damage to the tissues. The damage may be tissue- or organ-specific, or systemic, depending on specifics of a particular disease. In all cases, however, the main cause of autoimmunity is a dysregulation of the adaptive immune system.

CONCLUSION

The adaptive immune system consists of T and B lymphocytes. They produce a large repertoire of immunoglobulins and T-cell receptors using somatic gene recombination. Clonal selection preserves those cells whose products prove useful in fighting off pathogens. Specialized T-helper cells such as Th1, Th2, or Th17 produce characteristic cytokines that polarize immune responses into several distinct types. There is an intrinsic risk of autoimmunity built into the adaptive immune system as a payback for generating virtually unlimited repertoires of immune specificities. The potential of the adaptive immune system to induce autoimmunity is usually controlled by a combination of deletional and regulatory tolerance mechanisms. Regulatory T cells play a central role in maintaining immune tolerance. Failure of tolerance leads to autoimmunity, in which the immune system attacks its own tissues. Autoimmunity commonly occurs in and contributes to mechanisms of rheumatic diseases. By its nature, the adaptive immune system potentially represents the most specific target for therapy in autoimmune diseases. As our understanding of immune function at the cellular and molecular levels increases, we may soon be in a position to modulate the immune response for the benefit of patients with autoimmune rheumatic disease. Although this chapter has outlined basic principles of adaptive immunity in a telegraphic style, leading to inevitable simplifications, the author hopes that there has been enough structure to encourage interest in further independent study of the complexity of immune system processes by practicing rheumatologists.

REFERENCES

1. Bassing CH, Swat W, Alt FW. The mechanism and regulation of chromosomal V(D)J recombination. Cell 2002;109:S45-S55.
2. Jung D, Alt FW. Unraveling V(D)J recombination; insights into gene regulation. Cell 2004;116:299-311.
3. Davis MM, Bjorkman PJ. T-cell antigen receptor genes and T-cell recognition. Nature 1988;334:395-402.
4. Hesslein DG, Schatz DG. Factors and forces controlling V(D)J recombination. Adv Immunol 2001;78:169-232.
5. Jung D, Giallourakis C, Mostoslavsky R, et al. Mechanism and control of V(D)J recombination at the immunoglobulin heavy chain locus. Annu Rev Immunol 2006;24:541-570.
6. Spicuglia S, Franchini DM, Ferrier P. Regulation of V(D)J recombination. Curr Opin Immunol 2006;18:158-163.
7. Nagasawa T. Microenvironmental niches in the bone marrow required for B-cell development. Nat Rev Immunol 2006;6:107-116.
8. LeBien TW, Tedder TF. B lymphocytes: how they develop and function. Blood 2008;112:1570-1580.
9. Nutt SL, Kee BL. The transcriptional regulation of B cell lineage commitment. Immunity 2007;26:715-725.
10. Fuxa M, Skok JA. Transcriptional regulation in early B cell development. Curr Opin Immunol 2007;19:129-136.
11. Mårtensson IL, Keenan RA, Licence S. The pre-B-cell receptor. Curr Opin Immunol 2007;19:137-142.
12. Nemazee D. Receptor editing in lymphocyte development and central tolerance. Nat Rev Immunol 2006;6:728-740.
13. Pelanda R, Torres RM. Receptor editing for better or for worse. Curr Opin Immunol 2006;18:184-190.
14. Keenan RA, De Riva A, Corleis B, et al. Censoring of autoreactive B cell development by the pre-B cell receptor. Science 2008;321:696-699.
15. Rice JS, Newman J, Wang C, et al. Receptor editing in peripheral B cell tolerance. Proc Natl Acad Sci U S A 2005;102:1608-1613.
16. Zouali M. Receptor editing and receptor revision in rheumatic autoimmune diseases. Trends Immunol 2008;29:103-109.
17. Foreman AL, Van de Water J, Gougeon ML, et al. B cells in autoimmune diseases: insights from analyses of immunoglobulin variable (Ig V) gene usage. Autoimmun Rev 2007;6:387-401.
18. Selsing E: Ig class switching: targeting the recombinational mechanism. Curr Opin Immunol 2006;18:249-254.
19. Chaudhuri J, Basu U, Zarrin A, et al. Evolution of the immunoglobulin heavy chain class switch recombination mechanism. Adv Immunol 2007;94:157-214.
20. Peled JU, Kuang FL, Iglesias-Ussel MD, et al. The biochemistry of somatic hypermutation. Annu Rev Immunol 2008;26:481-511.
21. Hackney JA, Misaghi S, Senger K, et al. DNA targets of AID evolutionary link between antibody somatic hypermutation and class switch recombination. Adv Immunol 2009;101:163-189.
22. Engels N, Engelke M, Wienands J. Conformational plasticity and navigation of signaling proteins in antigen-activated B lymphocytes. Adv Immunol 2008;97:251-281.
23. Simeoni L, Kliche S, Lindquist J, et al. Adaptors and linkers in T and B cells. Curr Opin Immunol 2004;16:304-313.
24. Rickert RC. Regulation of B lymphocyte activation by complement C3 and the B cell coreceptor complex. Curr Opin Immunol 2005;17:237-243.
25. Harwood NE, Batista FD. New insights into the early molecular events underlying B cell activation. Immunity 2008;28:609-619.
26. Vyas JM, Van der Veen AG, Ploegh HL. The known unknowns of antigen processing and presentation. Nat Rev Immunol 2008;8:607-618.
27. Barral DC, Brenner MB. CD1 antigen presentation: how it works. Nat Rev Immunol 2007;7:929-941.
28. Yewdell JW, Nicchitta CV. The DRiP hypothesis decennial: support, controversy, refinement and extension. Trends Immunol 2006;27:368-373.
29. Crotzer VL, Blum JS. Autophagy and its role in MHC-mediated antigen presentation. J Immunol 2009;182:3335-3341.
30. Monu N, Trombetta ES. Cross-talk between the endocytic pathway and the endoplasmic reticulum in cross-presentation by MHC class I molecules. Curr Opin Immunol 2007;19:66-72.
31. Ackerman AL, Giodini A, Cresswell P. A role for the endoplasmic reticulum protein retrotranslocation machinery during crosspresentation by dendritic cells. Immunity 2006;25:607-617.
32. Taghon T, Rothenberg EV. Molecular mechanisms that control mouse and human TCR-alphabeta and TCR-gammadelta T cell development. Semin Immunopathol 2008;30:383-398.
33. Abbey JL, O'Neill HC. Expression of T-cell receptor genes during early T-cell development. Immunol Cell Biol 2008;86:166-174.
34. Howard LM, Kohm AP, Castaneda CL, et al. Therapeutic blockade of TCR signal transduction and co-stimulation in autoimmune disease. Curr Drug Targets Inflamm Allergy 2005;4:205-216.
35. Saito T, Yokosuka T. Immunological synapse and microclusters: the site for recognition and activation of T cells. Curr Opin Immunol 2006;18:305-313.
36. González PA, Carreño LJ, Figueroa CA, et al. Modulation of immunological synapse by membrane-bound and soluble ligands. Cytokine Growth Factor Rev 2007;18:19-31.
37. Teft WA, Kirchhof MG, Madrenas J. A molecular perspective of CTLA-4 function. Annu Rev Immunol 2006;24:65-97.
38. Scalapino KJ, Daikh DI. CTLA-4: a key regulatory point in the control of autoimmune disease. Immunol Rev 2008;223:143-155.
39. Chowdhury D, Lieberman J. Death by a thousand cuts: granzyme pathways of programmed cell death. Annu Rev Immunol 2008;26:389-420.
40. Pipkin ME, Lieberman J. Delivering the kiss of death: progress on understanding how perforin works. Curr Opin Immunol 2007;19:301-308.
41. Bowen H, Kelly A, Lee T, et al. Control of cytokine gene transcription in Th1 and Th2 cells. Clin Exp Allergy 2008;38:1422-1431.
42. Fouser LA, Wright JF, Dunussi-Joannopoulos K, et al. Th17 cytokines and their emerging roles in inflammation and autoimmunity. Immunol Rev 2008;226:87-102.
43. Martinez GJ, Nurieva RI, Yang XO, et al. Regulation and function of proinflammatory TH17 cells. Ann N Y Acad Sci 2008;1143:188-211.
44. Lyakh L, Trinchieri G, Provezza L, et al. Regulation of interleukin-12/interleukin-23 production and the T-helper 17 response in humans. Immunol Rev 2008;226:112-131.
45. Miller SA, Weinmann AS. Common themes emerge in the transcriptional control of T helper and developmental cell fate decisions regulated by the T-box, GATA and ROR families. Immunology 2009;126:306-315.
46. Sakaguchi S, Ono M, Setoguchi R, et al. Foxp3+ CD25+ CD4+ natural regulatory T cells in dominant self-tolerance and autoimmune disease. Immunol Rev 2006;212:8-27.
47. Sakaguchi S, Yamaguchi T, Nomura T, et al. Regulatory T cells and immune tolerance. Cell 2008;133:775-787.
48. Romagnani S. Regulation of the T cell response. Clin Exp Allergy 2006;36:1357-1366.
49. Beissert S, Schwarz A, Schwarz T. Regulatory T cells. J Invest Dermatol 2006;126:15-24.
50. Peterson P, Org T, Rebane A. Transcriptional regulation by AIRE: molecular mechanisms of central tolerance. Nat Rev Immunol 2008;8:948-957.

Principles of innate immunity

Tsuneyasu Kaisho and Shizuo Akira

- Innate immunity detects and responds to a variety of microorganism-derived molecular components, which are not expressed in the host.
- Receptor systems for microbial recognition are functionally categorized into three classes: signaling, internalizing, and soluble receptors.
- Signaling receptors, such as Toll-like receptors, trigger signaling pathways for activating immune response genes.
- Internalizing receptors incorporate microorganisms and degrade or process them for presentation to T cells.
- Soluble receptors opsonize microorganisms and make them competent for internalization. They can also activate protease cascades.
- Innate immunity functions as a barrier to microbial invasion and further induces inflammation, triggers adaptive immune responses, and provokes antiviral immunity.
- Innate immune receptors should be considered as therapeutic targets in infection, allergy, and autoimmunity.

INTRODUCTION

Host defense consists of two types of immunity: innate and adaptive (Table 16.1). Adaptive immunity is found only in jawed vertebrates and is mediated by B and T lymphocytes. These cells possess the *RAG* genes that mediate a somatic recombination system, thereby creating a large repertoire of antigen receptors. Antigen receptors with a certain specificity are clonally expressed but, owing to allelic exclusion, each lymphocyte bears only one antigen receptor. Thus, groups of lymphocytes are highly heterogeneous in terms of antigen specificity. During the immune response, receptors with high affinity for an invading antigen are clonally selected and lymphocytes bearing such receptors later stay on as memory cells.

Although highly beneficial for the host, to establish adaptive immunity and to mount an adaptive immune response takes time. Especially early in the course of an infection, an immediate response is required for efficient host defense. This immediate response is mediated by innate immunity. Innate immunity is an evolutionarily ancient system that is found in all multicellular organisms, including plants and insects. In mammals, innate immunity depends on macrophages or dendritic cells, which do not possess rearranged receptors. Insects can develop resistance to infection, indicating that innate immunity is sufficient to effectively eradicate pathogens. In contrast to adaptive immunity, innate immunity is mediated by a group of germline-encoded receptors with a fairly limited repertoire of antigen receptors. In what follows, these receptors are referred to as pattern recognition receptors (PRRs). PRRs can recognize various molecular structures derived from microorganisms.[1] Different from rearranged antigen receptors in the adaptive immune system, any given PRR is expressed on a variety of innate immune cells and each cell possesses a combination of several PRRs. Therefore, innate immune cells are simultaneously or sequentially activated through a variety of PRRs. Here we outline the innate immune system as a sensor system for infection and an activator of host defense.

MICROBIAL RECOGNITION BY INNATE IMMUNITY

Certain groups of microorganisms carry common metabolic pathways, resulting in similar molecular structures. These structures are potential targets for innate immunity and are often referred to as *pathogen-associated molecular patterns* (PAMPs), a term that is somewhat misleading because these structures are expressed both in non-pathogenic as well as pathogenic microorganisms. Importantly, PAMPs are typically not detected in the host and can thus be regarded as nonself. Innate immunity senses the infection by recognizing PAMPs with PRRs.

PAMPs are required for the survival of microorganisms and, therefore, are highly conserved over the course of evolution. Typical examples of PAMPs are constituents of bacterial cell walls. In general, proteins do not function as PAMPs because they are far too diverse for recognition through a limited repertoire of PRRs. For example, in viruses, the structures of many proteins change very rapidly as the virus struggles to escape from immunosurveillance. Thus, for the recognition of viral protein structures, a large repertoire of antigen receptors in the adaptive immune system is inevitable.

PRRs can be functionally divided into three categories: signaling, internalizing, and soluble PRRs (Fig. 16.1).

Signaling PRRs

These PRRs are expressed on the cell surface, in the endosome, or in the cytosol, respectively, where they recognize their various ligands. On recognition, these PRRs can stimulate signaling pathways leading to activation of nuclear factor-kappaB (NF-κB) or mitogen-activated protein kinases (MAPKs). This then leads to expression of a variety of immune response genes, including inflammatory cytokines or co-stimulatory molecules such as CD40 and CD86.

Toll-like receptors

The Toll-like receptor (TLR) family is a typical signaling PRR.[2,3] TLRs are expressed on the plasma membrane or in the endosome and play major roles in activating antigen-presenting cells (APCs). TLRs are type I transmembrane proteins. Their extracellular domain includes a repetitive structure rich in leucine residues, called leucine-rich repeat (LRR), that is involved in the recognition of a variety of TLR ligands. The intracellular region contains a common structure in TLR and interleukin (IL)-1R family members called Toll/IL-1R homologous (TIR) domain that is essential for signal transduction through TLRs.

TLRs can recognize a variety of components derived mainly from bacteria and viruses. TLR ligands can be categorized as lipid, protein, and nucleic acid components (Fig. 16.2). Phylogenetically related TLRs can recognize similar types of ligands. All TLR ligands are potent immune adjuvants that can trigger a vigorous immune response. Therefore, TLRs are also referred to as adjuvant receptors. The most popular and widely investigated TLR ligand is lipopolysaccharide (LPS).[4] LPS is found in outer cell walls of gram-negative bacteria and recognized by TLR4. LPS is first bound to a soluble factor, LPS-binding protein (LBP), in the serum and transferred to target cells such as macrophages. Macrophages express a phosphatidylinositol-anchored cell surface molecule, CD14, which can capture and retain LPS. LPS then activates TLR4. A small secreted molecule, MD-2, is associated with TLR4 and critically involved in forming an LPS-recognizing complex.[5]

Other lipid-containing components from cell walls of a variety of microorganisms are recognized by TLR2 and related TLRs, such as TLR1 or TLR6. Heterodimerization is critical for TLR2-mediated recognition. For example, TLR2 can recognize mycoplasmal macrophage-activating lipopeptide 2 (MALP-2) when associated with TLR6. Meanwhile, a TLR2-TLR1 heterodimer is involved in recognizing bacterial lipopeptides (BLP). MALP-2 and BLP carry a diacylated and triacylated cysteine residue at their amino terminus, respectively, and this subtle difference is discriminated by TLR2-containing heterodimers.

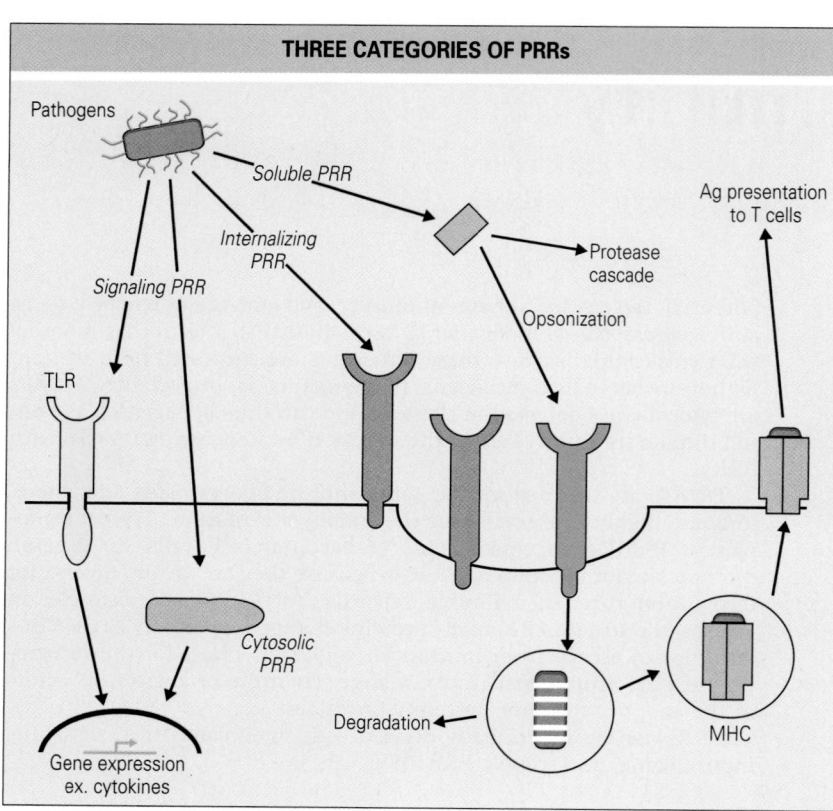

THREE CATEGORIES OF PRRs

Fig. 16.1 Three categories of PRRs. Signaling PRRs trigger signal transduction pathways upon recognition. Internalizing PRRs directly incorporate microbes into the cell. Soluble PRRs attach to the microbes and support the function of internalizing PRRs. Soluble PRRs also activate protease cascades. TLR, Toll-like receptor; Ag, antigen; MHC, major histocompatibility complex.

TABLE 16.1 INNATE AND ADAPTIVE IMMUNITY		
	Innate immunity	**Adaptive immunity**
Evolution	Ancient	Jawed vertebrates or higher
Cells	Macrophages	T and B lymphocytes
	Dendritic cells	
	(Antigen-presenting cells)	
Receptors	Encoded in germline	Rearrangement
	Limited repertoire	Large repertoire
Receptor	Nonclonal	Clonal expression
Memory	No	Yes
Ligands	Molecular structures conserved in a group of microorganisms (LPS, CpG DNA)	Fine structures (peptides)
Responses	Immediate	Slow

LPS, lipopolysaccharide.

TLR5 is involved in recognizing a protein, flagellin, a component of the bacterial flagella that is used for propulsion in a liquid medium. Flagellin can elicit mucosal immune responses by acting on epithelial cells or macrophages. Although flagellin is a protein, its amino acid structure is highly conserved, which suggests it is a target for innate immune recognition.

Nucleic acids are equally important PAMPs recognized by TLRs. Bacterial DNA was long known as a strong immune adjuvant.[6-8] This adjuvant activity depends on an unmethylated CpG motif. The CpG motif is more abundant in bacterial DNA than in mammalian DNA. Furthermore, mammalian CpG DNA is often methylated. Therefore, unmethylated CpG DNA can be regarded as non-self and is recognized by TLR9. Viral DNA is also rich in the CpG motif, and DNA virus infection does indeed trigger TLR9 signaling.

Several small synthetic molecules, including imidazoquinoline derivatives and several anticancer drugs, were long known for their antiviral activity. This activity is dependent on TLR7. Drugs such as imidazoquinoline represent nucleic acid-like structures, suggesting the possibility that TLR7 is involved in the recognition of viral RNA. Indeed, single-stranded RNA (ssRNA) was found to be a ligand for TLR7 and its close relative, TLR8. This interaction is critical for sensing RNA virus infection. RNA virus infection also induces the production of double-stranded RNA (dsRNA) in infected cells, and these dsRNAs can act as immune adjuvants and are recognized by TLR3.

Importantly, TLR2 and TLR4 are mainly expressed on the plasma membrane, whereas nucleic acid-recognizing TLRs are expressed in the endosome. In the endosome, nucleic acids are released from virus or virally infected cells and encounter respective TLRs. Thus, lipid and nucleic acid TLR ligands are recognized in distinct cellular compartments.

Cytosolic signaling PRRs

Signaling PRRs also exist in the cytosol. Retinoic acid–inducible gene I (*RIG-I*)–like receptors (RLRs) are critical cytosolic signaling PRRs for virus-derived nucleic acids and recognize them when virus directly infects the cells. RLRs include *RIG-I* and melanoma-differentiation–associated gene 5 (*MDA5*).[9,10] *RIG-I* and *MDA5* carry tandem caspase recruitment domains (CARDs) and an RNA helicase domain at the amino and carboxy termini, respectively, and the RNA helicase domain is involved in recognizing the ligands. Both *RIG-I* and *MDA5* can recognize virally derived RNA, but they play differential roles in viral infection.[10] *RIG-I* is essential for recognizing various ssRNA viruses, including paramyxoviruses, influenzavirus A, and Japanese encephalitis virus, whereas *MDA5* is critical for sensing other RNA viruses such as picornaviruses. *RIG-I* can recognize 5′-triphosphate ssRNA, which is a typical structure found in viral, non-self RNA. Meanwhile, host-derived self-RNA has a cap structure to mask 5′-triphosphate RNA. Thus, *RIG-I* can distinguish viral RNA from self-RNA.

LGP2 also carries an RNA helicase domain, but not a CARD, and is therefore considered to be a negative regulator for RNA virus–induced responses. However, LGP2 can function as a positive regulator because LGP2-deficient mice have shown impaired responses against certain RNA viruses. Double-stranded DNA (dsDNA), which can function as a potent immune adjuvant, is also recognized by cytosolic sensors such as DNA-dependent activator of interferon regulatory factor (DAI, also

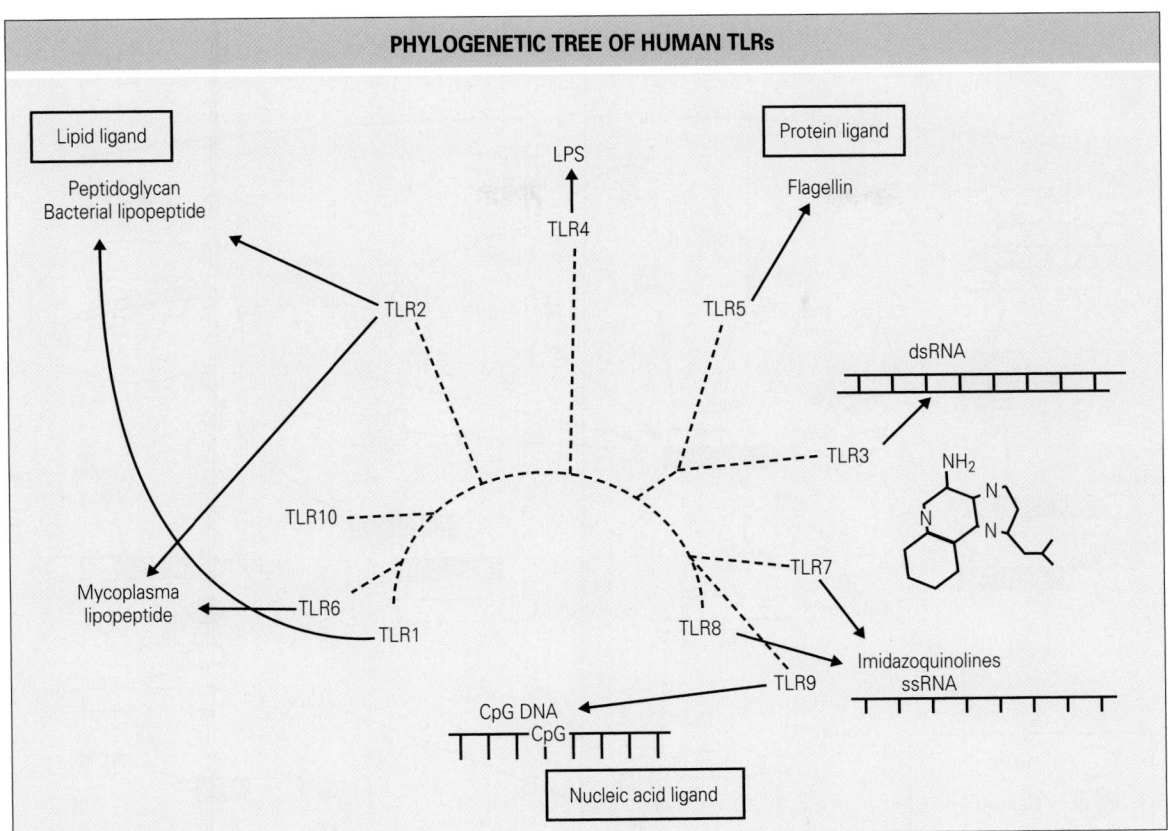

Fig. 16.2 Phylogenetic tree of human Toll-like receptors. Human TLRs are connected with dotted lines based on the phylogenetic analysis of their amino acid structures. Branch length is proportional to evolutionary distances. Arrows indicate representative ligands.

known as Z-DNA–binding protein 1). However, as yet unidentified molecule(s) should also be involved in detecting dsDNA, because DAI-deficient mice can still respond to dsDNA.

Nucleotide-binding oligomerization domain (NOD)-like receptors (NLRs) also belong to cytosolic signaling PRRs (Fig. 16.3).[11] NLRs consist of more than 20 members in humans or mice. They carry a CARD, a pyrin domain, or a baculoviral inhibitor of apoptosis repeat (BIR) domain as a protein interaction domain at the amino terminal, which is followed by a NACHT nucleotide-binding domain (NBD) and an LRR domain. Nod1 and Nod2 are representative NLR members and involved in recognizing bacterial peptidoglycan-derived molecules.[12] Neuronal apoptosis inhibitory protein 5 (NAIP5) and IL-1β-converting enzyme protease-activating factor (IPAF) can sense flagellin derived from intracellular bacteria such as *Salmonella* or *Legionella*. Notably, NACHT, LRR, and pyrin domain–containing protein 3 (NALP3) are required for responses against a variety of immune adjuvants, bacterial products such as RNA or toxin, host-derived nucleic acid metabolites such as adenosine 5′-triphosphate (ATP) or uric acids, environmental substances such as silica crystals or asbestos, and a widely used chemical immune adjuvant, alum. A pyrin domain–carrying protein, absent in melanoma 2 (AIM2), is related to NLRs because it carries a pyrin domain. AIM2 is involved in detecting dsDNA by a hematopoietic interferon-inducible nuclear protein (HIN) domain.

Internalizing PRRs

These PRRs are expressed on the surface of neutrophils, macrophages, or dendritic cells. They bind to and internalize PAMPs or microorganisms, which are subsequently transported to lysosomal compartments (see Fig. 16.1). This process is termed *phagocytosis*, and the group of PRRs involved can thus also be referred to as phagocytic PRRs.[13] After phagocytosis, organism-derived proteins are degraded or processed for presentation to T cells. Internalizing PRRs mainly function to incorporate the organisms or their components, but some internalizing PRRs can also transduce the activation signals.

Lectin

Lectins generically represent carbohydrate-recognizing proteins, and some lectins function as internalizing PRRs. The mannose receptor is a type I transmembrane protein that can bind terminal mannose and fucose residues of glycoproteins or glycolipids, which are found on microbial cell walls. Macrophage scavenger receptor, SR-A, is a type II transmembrane protein. Although originally defined by its ability to bind and mediate endocytosis of oxidized or acetylated low-density lipoprotein (LDL), it can also bind a variety of microorganisms. Macrophage receptor with collagenous structure (MARCO) is structurally and functionally similar to SR-A and can bind to gram-positive and gram-negative bacteria.

Dectin-1 is a C-type lectin and is involved in recognizing β-1,3-linked or β-1,6-linked glucans found in fungal or other microbial cell walls. Dectin-1 carries an immunoreceptor tyrosine-based activation (ITAM) motif in the intracytoplasmic region and also functions as a signaling PRR. Dectin-1 is co-localized with TLR2 in the phagosome and activates macrophages in synergy with TLR2. Macrophage-inducible C-type lectin (Mincle) also carries an ITAM motif and can induce macrophage activation by sensing α-mannose from a pathogenic fungus, *Malassezia*. Notably, Mincle is also involved in detecting damaged cells through the interaction with a nuclear ribonucleoprotein. Another ITAM-motif–carrying C-type lectin, CLEC9A, also known as DNGR-1, is critically involved in sensing necrosis and provoking immune responses through crosspriming (see later).

Soluble PRRs

Soluble PRRs are produced by macrophages or hepatocytes and bind to the cell wall of microorganisms, thus designating them as targets for phagocytosis (see Fig. 16.1). This coating process is termed *opsonization*, and the coating substances are called *opsonins*. The serum levels of certain soluble PRRs, such as C-reactive protein (CRP) or serum amyloid P component (SAP), increase in response to inflammatory cytokines; therefore, these PRRs are also referred to as acute-phase

NLR-MEDIATED RECOGNITION AND SIGNALING

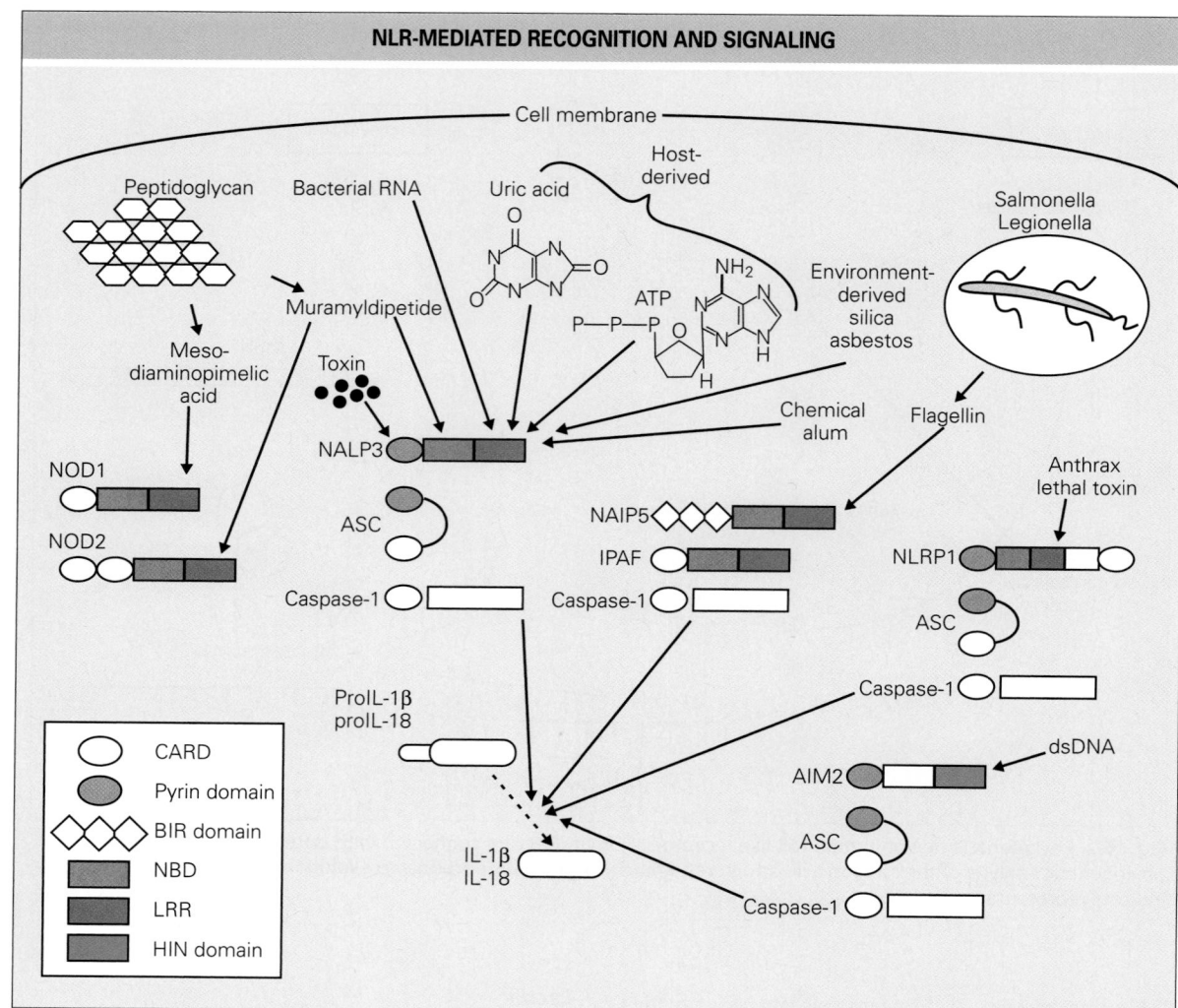

Fig. 16.3 NLR-mediated recognition and signaling. NLRs are cytosolic signaling PRRs and recognize a variety of immune-activating substances. Importantly, NLRs can activate inflammasome and induce production of active IL-1β and IL-18.

proteins.[14] Soluble PRRs are linked to the complement system and can activate protein cascades that are capable of eradicating pathogenic microbes.

Complement system

The complement system consists of more than 35 soluble or membrane proteins (see also Chapter 20).[15] Microbial infection activates three distinct pathways for complement activation (Fig. 16.4). The *classical pathway* is triggered by a complement, C1q, that can detect IgG or IgM antibodies bound to microbes or microbe-related structures. In this situation, antibodies behave as soluble PRRs. CRP and SAA, which belong to a pentraxin family, bind to bacterial phospholipids such as phosphorylcholine and can also activate the classical pathway without antibodies. The *alternative pathway* is triggered by direct recognition of microbial surface structures by C3. This pathway is independent of immunoglobulins and C1q. C3 can recognize almost all kinds of microbes and can be regarded as a soluble PRR. Finally, a collectin family member, mannose-binding lectin (MBL), is involved in the *lectin pathway*.[16] This pathway is triggered by MBL bound to carbohydrates on microbial glycoproteins and glycolipids.

All pathways activate a common pathway that involves cleavage of C3 into C3a and C3b (see Fig. 16.4). C3b attaches to the microbial surface and functions as opsonin. Opsonized microbes are then eliminated by phagocytosis. In addition, C3b also activates a common complement cascade leading to the cleavage of C5 into C5a and C5b. C5b further leads to the formation of the membrane attack complex (MAC). Subsequently, MAC induces direct killing of microbes. The complement system also facilitates host immune reactions. As small molecules, C3a and C5a can act as a chemoattractant for neutrophils and facilitate inflammation.

PHYLOGENETIC COMPARISON OF THE RECOGNITION SYSTEM

TLRs have been named because their molecular structure is similar to that of *Drosophila* Toll.[17,18] Toll is a type I transmembrane protein carrying a LRR repeat and a TIR domain. Toll-deficient flies display increased susceptibility to fungal infection, indicating that Toll is essential for antifungal immunity in insects. Furthermore, both Toll and TLRs can activate signaling pathways leading to the release of antimicrobial substances.

However, the *Drosophila* Toll system is distinct from the mammalian TLR system (Fig. 16.5). Toll does not directly recognize fungi-derived products. The pathogens are recognized by certain, not yet identified, soluble factors. On fungal infection, protease cascades are activated to induce cleavage of a secreted protein, Spaetzle. Processed Spaetzle then binds to Toll. Thus, Toll recognizes a host-derived product.

Toll is also involved in immunity against gram-positive bacteria.[19] A soluble molecule, peptidoglycan recognition protein (PGRP)-SA, recognizes peptidoglycans from bacteria, leading to activation of protease cascades that also cleave Spaetzle. PGRP-SA–deficient flies are susceptible to gram-positive bacteria infection but retain immune responses against fungi, whereas Toll-deficient flies succumb to infection with both organisms, indicating that the discrimination of fungi and bacteria happens upstream of Toll. Thus, flies detect pathogens in the

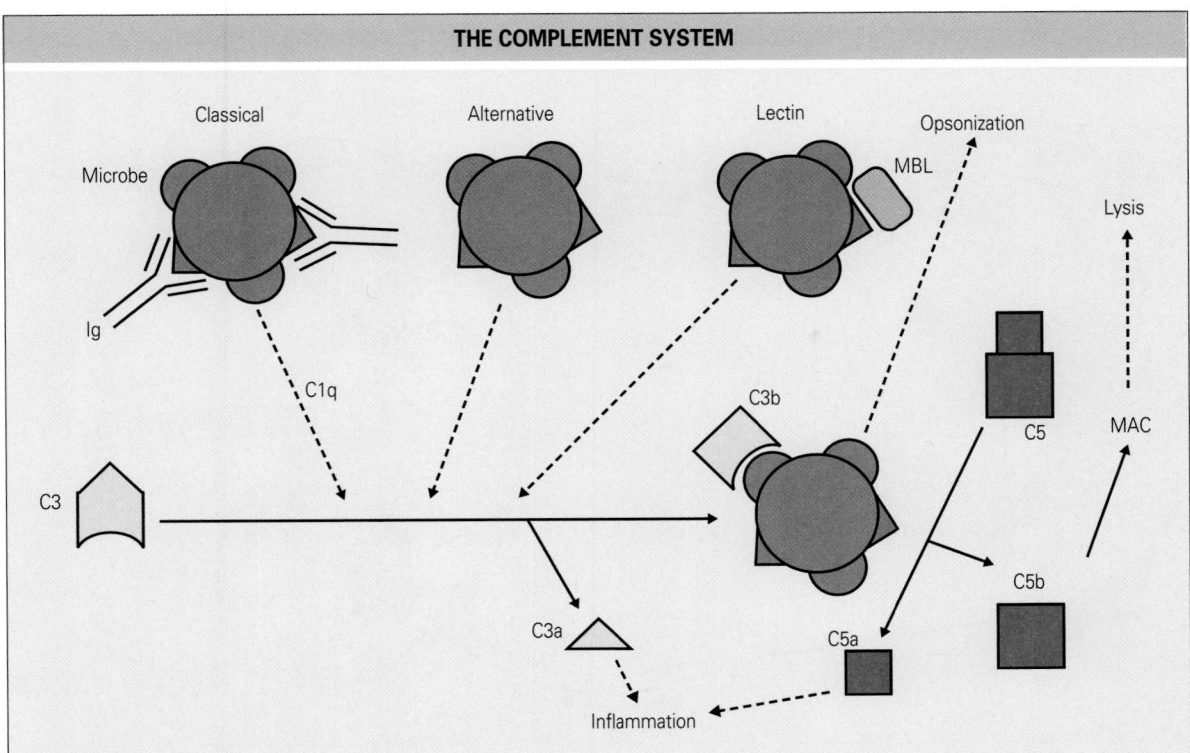

THE COMPLEMENT SYSTEM

Fig. 16.4 The complement system. All pathways lead to the cleavage of C3 and subsequently activation of complement cascades. MBL, mannose-binding lectin; MAC, membrane attack complex.

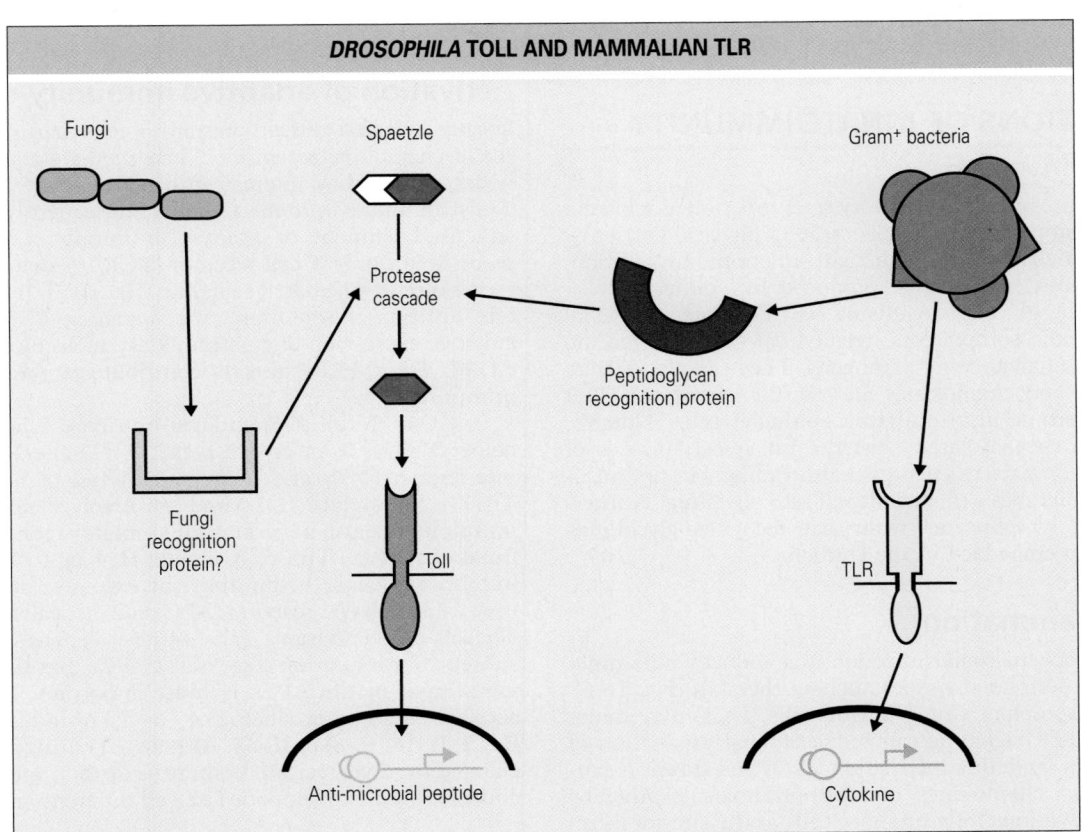

***DROSOPHILA* TOLL AND MAMMALIAN TLR**

Fig. 16.5 *Drosophila* Toll and mammalian TLR. TLRs directly recognize microbial components, while Toll detects a host-derived molecule. In *Drosophila,* microbes are discriminated by soluble factors in the hemolymph, leading to the activation of protease cascades.

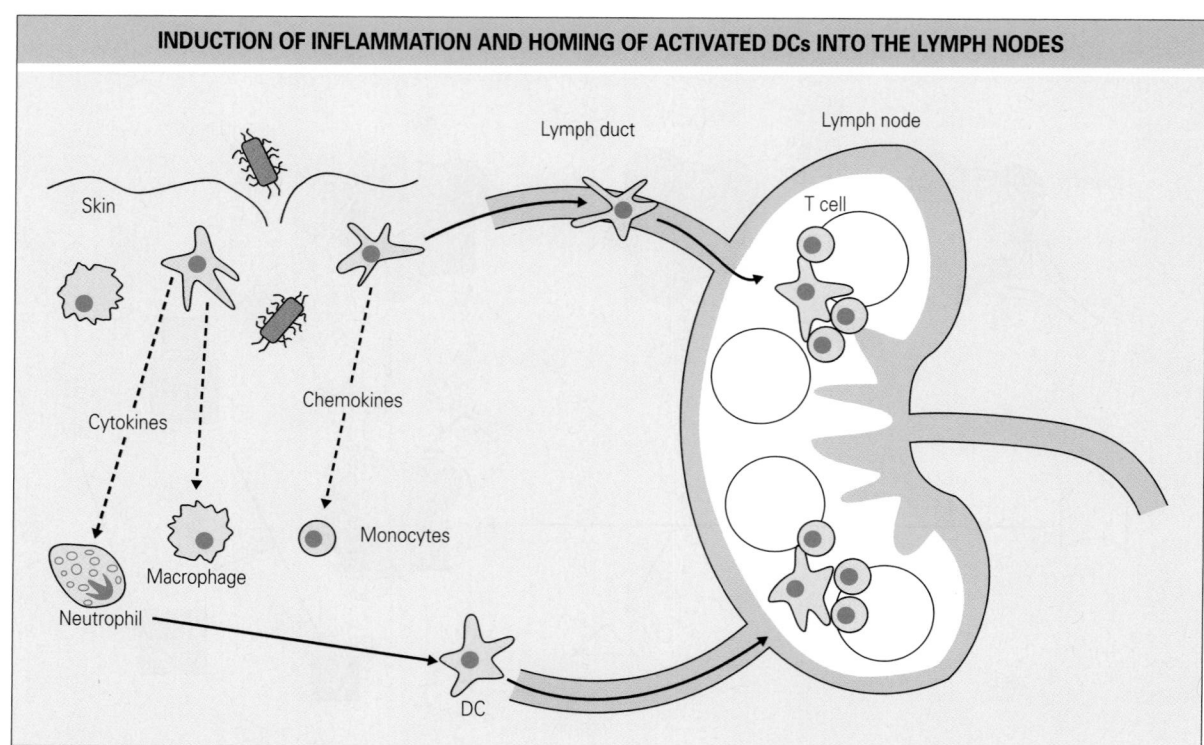

INDUCTION OF INFLAMMATION AND HOMING OF ACTIVATED DCs INTO THE LYMPH NODES

Lymph duct

Lymph node

Skin

T cell

Chemokines

Cytokines

Monocytes

Macrophage

Neutrophil

DC

Fig. 16.6 Induction of inflammation and homing of activated dendritic cells (DCs) into the lymph nodes.

hemolymph, not on the plasma membrane. In mammals, the complement system, rather than the TLR system, is similar to Toll when considering recognition in the fluid and activation of protease cascades.

CRITICAL FUNCTIONS OF INNATE IMMUNITY

Barriers against invasion

Epithelial cells in the intestine or respiratory tract function as a barrier against microbial invasion. Epithelial cells create a physical barrier by connecting with their neighbors through tight junctions. In addition, heavily glycosylated proteins, mucins, produced by epithelial cells, prevent the attachment of microorganisms. Furthermore, epithelial cells can produce peptidic components, termed *defensins*, which are capable of directly killing a variety of pathogens. They can also secrete a variety of cytokines and chemokines and recruit leukocytes. TLR signaling is very important in stimulating epithelial cells. Notably, TLR5 is expressed on the basolateral but not on apical surfaces of epithelia. This expression pattern ensures that invading, but not intraluminal commensal, microbes can stimulate TLR5 signaling. Furthermore, intraepithelial T lymphocytes, which can recognize glycolipids from microbes, are also embedded in the epithelia.

Induction of inflammation

Innate immunity detects microbial infection and induces inflammatory reactions in local peripheral tissues such as the skin (Fig. 16.6). TLRs expressed on macrophages or dendritic cells (DCs) play major roles in this process. TLR signaling can induce robust production of inflammatory cytokines including interleukin (IL)-6 and tumor necrosis factor alpha (TNF-α), chemokines, or adhesion molecules, thereby recruiting or activating various inflammatory cells at the sites of infection. Recruited and activated macrophages or neutrophils then ingest, through internalizing PRRs, and subsequently kill invading pathogens by producing nitric oxide (NO), reactive oxygen species (ROS), or defensins. NLR signaling can induce generation of proinflammatory cytokines such as IL-1β and IL-18 through the activation of inflammasome (see later) and contributes to inflammatory reactions. Inflammation is a critical local response to resolve infection. However,

inflammation is a "double-edged sword," because excessive amounts of cytokines can be lethal for the host, as is the case in endotoxin shock.

Activation of adaptive immunity on infection

Locally activated antigen-presenting cells mature to express a distinct set of chemokine receptors. Then they are transported to the lymph nodes, where they interact with and activate T cells (see Fig. 16.6). Thus, an innate immune response subsequently leads to the activation and establishment of adaptive immunity. Clonal T-cell expansion requires not only T-cell receptor (TCR)-mediated but also co-stimulatory molecule–mediated signaling (Fig. 16.7). Internalizing PRRs facilitate antigen presentation, and signaling PRRs such as TLRs can enhance expression of co-stimulatory molecules, including CD80 and CD86. Thus, PRRs directly contribute to the activation of adaptive immunity.

A CD4+ T cell differentiates into type 1 helper T (Th1), type 17 helper T (Th17), or type 2 helper T (Th2) cells.[20] Th1 cells produce interferon (IFN)-γ and mediate antiviral or antibacterial immunity. Th17 cells produce IL-17 and are involved not only in antibacterial immunity but also in various inflammatory conditions such as autoimmune disorders. Th2 cells secrete IL-4 or IL-13 and are involved in immunity against helminths, but excessive activation of these cells may cause allergic reaction. APCs are critically involved in regulating Th cell differentiation. This activity depends on tissue origin, cell subsets, or maturation stage of the APCs. But the nature of the activating stimuli of the APCs is most important. Most TLR ligands can activate APCs to produce Th1- or Th17-inducing cytokines such as IL-12, IL-18, IL-6, or IL-23. Although Th2-inducing PRRs are not well characterized yet, certain helminths or their products can enhance the ability of APCs to support Th2 cell differentiation.

Antiviral responses

Innate immunity responds to viral infection by producing type I IFNs.[21] Type I IFNs consist of more than 10 IFNs-α and a single IFN-β. IFN-α and IFN-β are produced by different types of cells and regulated by differential combinations of transcription factors and signaling molecules. However, all type I IFNs utilize IFN-α/βR, composed of IFNAR-1

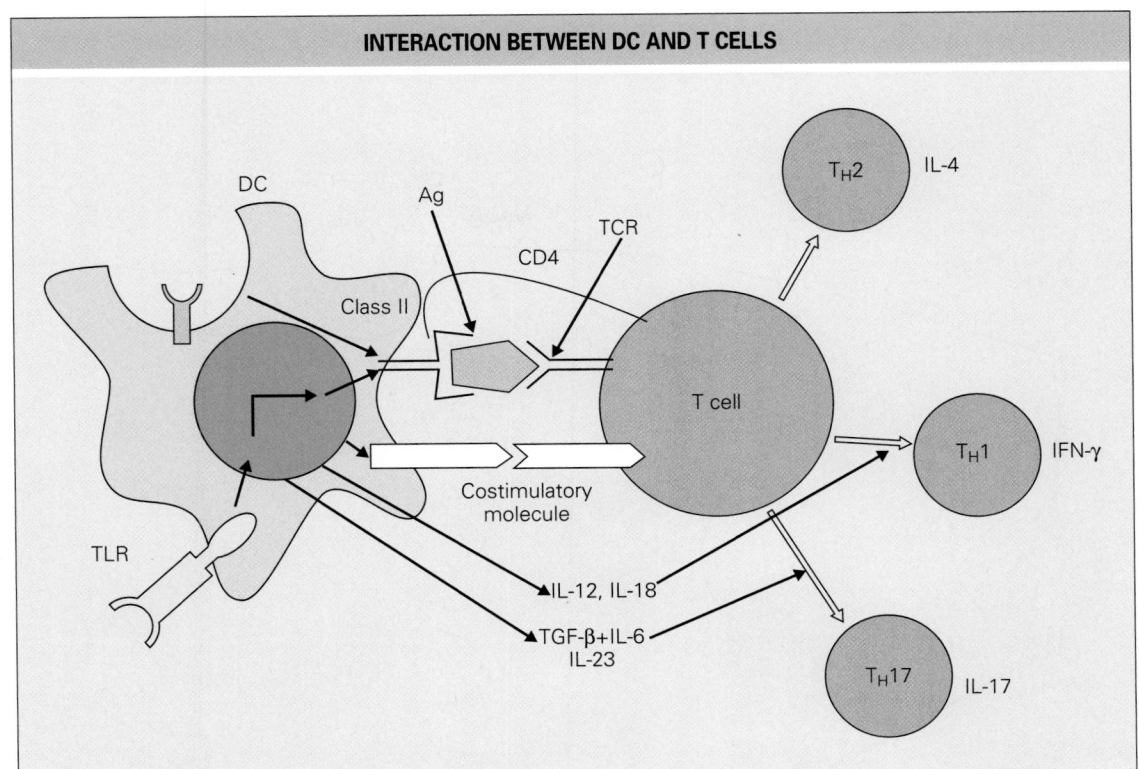

Fig. 16.7 Interaction between dendritic cells (DC) and T cells. Activated dendritic cells induce proliferation of antigen-specific T cells and instruct them in differentiating into Th1, Th2, or Th17 cells depending on the dendritic cell activation stimuli.

and IFNAR2, as a common receptor. The signaling can induce expression of a number of antiviral molecules including 2′-5′-oligoadenylate synthases (OAS) or IFNs themselves. It can also upregulate expression of the major histocompatibility complex (MHC) and induce dendritic cell maturation. These effects contribute to antiviral immune responses.

Type I IFNs are produced in a TLR-dependent and TLR-independent manner. TLR-independent induction depends mainly on cytoplasmic sensors, RLRs. RLRs are potent type I IFN-inducing sensors and are macrophages or conventional dendritic cells, but not plasmacytoid dendritic cells (PDCs) (see later). Among TLRs, TLR7 and TLR9 can induce both IFN-α and IFN-β. The other TLRs, except TLR3 and TLR4, fail to induce type I IFNs. TLR3 and TLR4 can induce only IFN-β but not IFN-α. TLR4-induced IFN-β plays a critical role in shock induction or bacterial infection, but, as a principle, in viral infection TLRs that recognize nucleic acids are more critical than TLR4 in type I IFN production.

PDCs are a distinct DC subset of conventional DC and also known as IFN-α–producing cells.[22] PDCs look like plasma cells and exhibit poor antigen-presenting activity owing to low expression levels of MHC class II and co-stimulatory molecules. PDCs are closely related to a lymphoid lineage, because they express certain lymphocyte-specific genes and carry partially rearranged immunoglobulin genes. PDCs express TLR7 and TLR9 exclusively among TLRs and secrete vigorous amounts of type I IFN, especially IFN-α, in a TLR7/9-dependent manner.

Crosspriming is important in antiviral immunity.[23] Crosspriming is defined as exogenous antigen presentation through MHC class I to induce T-cell activation (Fig. 16.8). Virally infected cells are ingested by antigen-presenting cells. Antigens are processed and transported to MHC class II–containing lysosomes, where antigens associate with MHC class II. The complex becomes competent for presentation to CD4+ T cells. As an alternative to antigen presentation through MHC class II, antigens can be transported from the endosome to the cytosol. It remains unknown if this transport is actively regulated or depends just on a leak from the endosome. In the cytosol, antigens are processed by proteasomes and then incorporated into the endoplasmic reticulum in a transporter associated with antigen processing (TAP)–dependent manner. Then, antigens bind to MHC class I and are presented to

CD8+ T cells. This system ensures that virally infected cells, which do not always possess the ability to present antigen by themselves, can be selected as targets for cytotoxicity. Crosspriming is also believed to be involved in cancer surveillance, because most cancer cells also show poor ability of antigen presentation. Overall, crosspriming plays an important role in host defense. TLR3 is abundantly expressed in a DC subset with high ability to phagocytose dying cells and critically involved in promoting crosspriming.[24]

MOLECULAR MECHANISM OF PRR SIGNALING

TLR signaling requires the intracytoplasmic TIR region.[25] This region associates with cytoplasmic adapters that also possess the TIR region. This association is critically involved in stimulating various pathways leading to activation of NF-κB or interferon regulatory factors (IRFs). There are five TIR domain–containing adapters, and four of them—MyD88, TIR domain-containing adapter protein (TIRAP)/MyD88-adapter-like (MAL), TIR domain-containing adapter protein inducing IFN-β (TRIF), and TRIF-related adapter molecule (TRAM)—are involved in TLR signaling and also shape the pleiotropic function of TLRs (Figs. 16.9 and 16.10). MyD88, characterized first among the TLR adapters, associates with all TLRs except TLR3. MyD88 is essential for TLR-induced cytokine production. TIRAP cooperates with MyD88 downstream of TLR2 and TLR4. MyD88 is critical for all TLR7/9-induced effects, including type I IFN induction (see Fig. 16.10), whereas TRIF, but not MyD88, is essential for TLR3- or TLR4-induced type I IFN production (see Fig. 16.9). TRAM is required for TLR4 to associate with TRIF. TLR3 can directly associate with TRIF and does not require TRAM for its signaling. These adapters differentially stimulate signaling cascades that involve IL-1R–associated kinases (IRAKs) or an adapter molecule, tumor necrosis factor receptor-associated factor 6 (TRAF6), and induce the activation of various transcription factors. Activation and nuclear translocation of NF-κB, IRF-3, and IRF-7 can cause gene expression of proinflammatory cytokines and type I IFNs (see Figs. 16.9 and 16.10).

IκB kinase (IKK) family members play critical roles in linking TLR signaling and activation of transcription factors (see Figs. 16.9 and 16.10). NF-κB activation depends on IKKβ. IRF-3 activation is induced

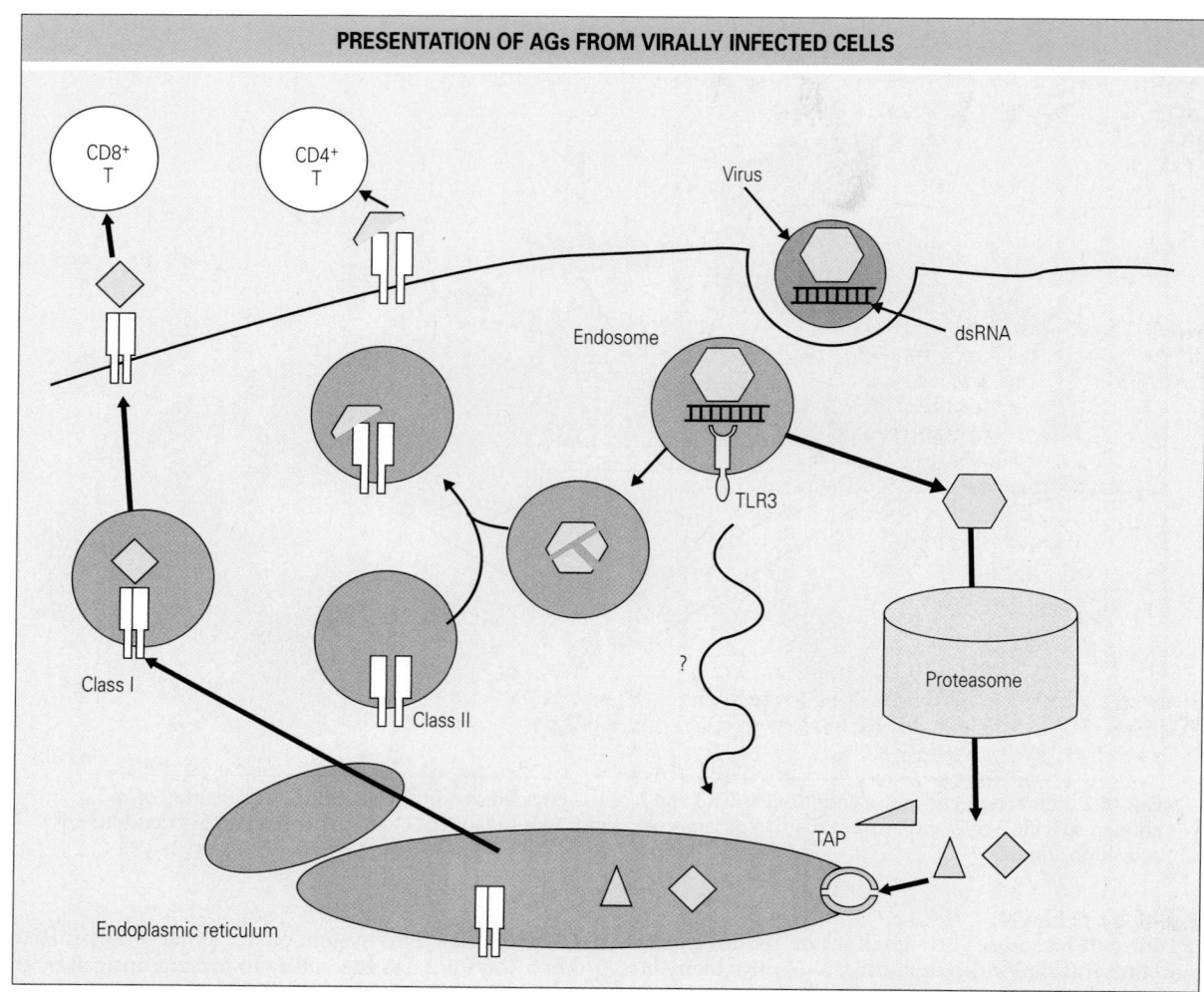

Fig. 16.8 Presentation of antigens from virally infected cells. Infected cells are incorporated into antigen-presenting cells, and antigens are presented through MHC class I or class II. TLR3 can promote crosspriming, which depends on MHC class I, although the mechanism is not clear.

by a heterodimer of IKKε/ι and TBK1. TLR7/9 signaling mechanism in PDC is peculiar in that the MyD88-mediated pathway leads to IRF-7 activation via IKKα and IRAK1.

RLRs do not utilize adapters with the TIR region but require a CARD-like domain carrying adapter, IFN-β promoter stimulator 1 (IPS-1, also known as CARD adapter inducing IFN-β [Cardif], mitochondrial anti-viral signaling [MAVS], or virus-induced signaling adapter [VISA]) (see Fig. 16.10). IPS-1 can induce production of proinflammatory cytokines and type I IFNs through the activation of NF-κB and IRF3/7 via IKKβ and IKKε/ι-TBK1, respectively. The TLR3/4-mediated pathway also converges this cascade by activating IKKβ and IKKε/ι-TBK1 complex via TRIF, but not via IPS-1. DAI signaling can also result in activation of this cascade in a TRIF/IPS-1–independent manner.

Inflammasome is a molecular platform that is activated mainly by NLRs (see Fig. 16.3).[26,27] Inflammasome is activated in several ways, depending on NLRs or NLR-related molecules such as NALP3, NAIP5, NLRP1, or AIM2. Each inflammasome requires apoptosis-associated speck-like protein containing a caspase activation and recruitment domain (ASC) or IPAF as a CARD-containing molecule. ASC and IPAF are critically involved in recruiting caspase-1, which can convert pro-IL-1β and pro-IL-18 to biologic active cytokines, IL-1β and IL-18, respectively.

PRR AND DISEASES

TLR and autoimmunity

Protein or lipid TLR ligands are absent in the host; they are principally non-self components. However, compared with these substances, the structural difference between pathogen and host nucleic acid TLR ligands is not very prominent. For example, unmethylated CpG motifs are still found in mammals although their frequency is very low. Furthermore, ssRNAs irrelevant to viruses also behave as TLR7 agonists. Host cells are phagocytosed after they die, and nucleic acids from ingested cells are then released to endosomes or phagosomes. Thus, hosts potentially expose themselves to the risk of an autoimmune response. However, this risk is contained by several factors. First, these nucleic acids are unstable and easily degraded. Second, TLR7 expression is very low in cells with high phagocytic activity. Third, TLR7/9 expression and released nucleic acids are localized in different cell compartments (Fig. 16.11). Furthermore, the host possesses some DNA sequences that can inhibit TLR9 signaling.[28] In fact, such sequences can be found in the telomere. Thus, several fail-safe mechanisms prevent an autoimmune reaction. Still, it remains unclear how the host tolerates adjuvant effects of self nucleic acids.

The break of this tolerance seems to contribute to the pathogenesis of autoimmune diseases, such as systemic lupus erythematosus (SLE).[22] In SLE, anti–nucleic acid antibodies are produced and immune complexes containing nucleic acids are retained as a stabilized form in the serum, thus creating efficient TLR agonists for PDC stimulation. The immune complexes can activate PDCs to produce IFN-α by co-engaging TLR and FcR. Notably, serum IFN-α levels are often increased in SLE patients and correlate with the severity of the disease. It is also reported that cancer treatment with IFN-α causes SLE-like manifestations. The number of activated PDCs is increased in skin lesions in SLE. It can thus be assumed that prolonged activation of PDCs is involved in elevated production of IFN-α, leading to clinical manifestations. This hypothesis also explains the observed deterioration of SLE after viral infection.

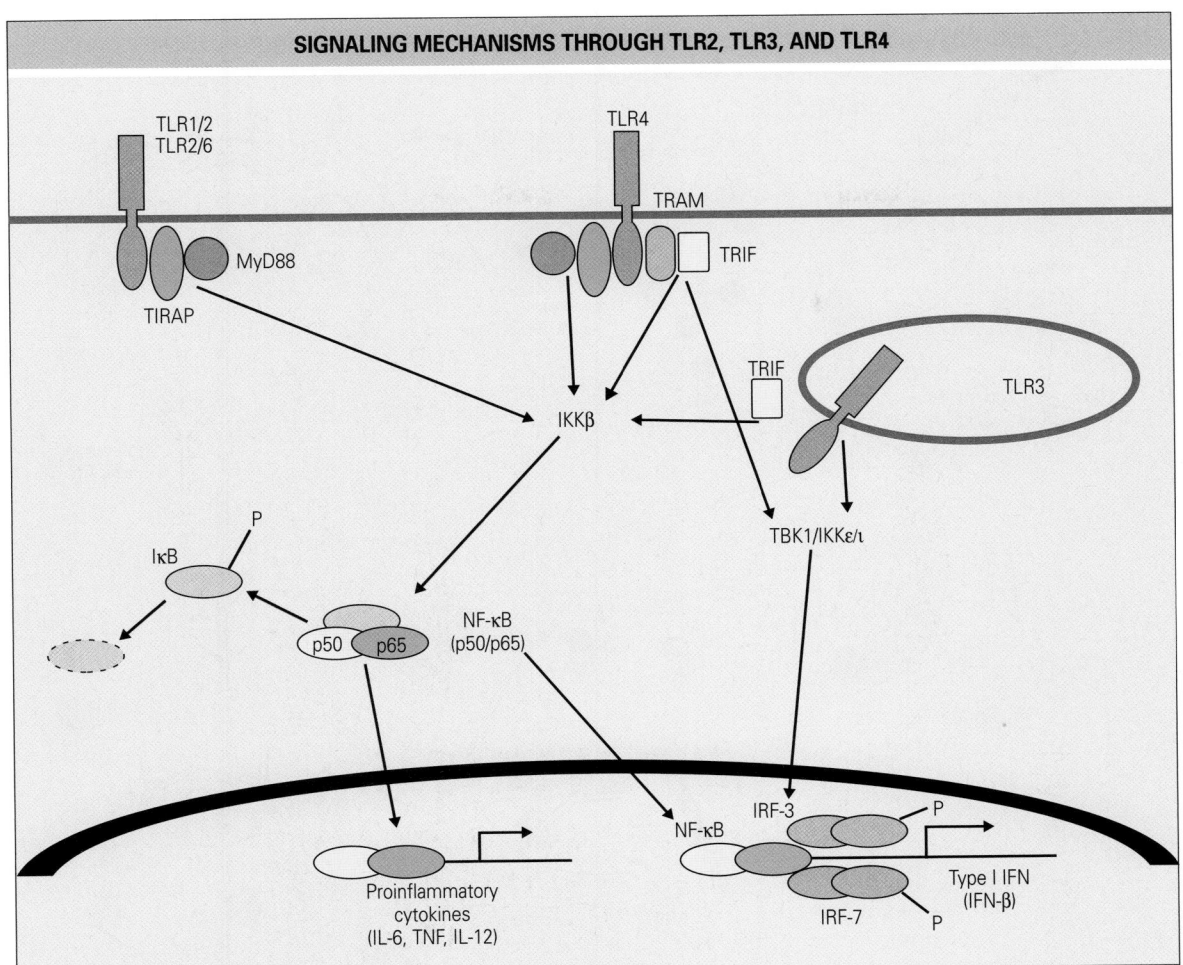

Fig. 16.9 Signaling mechanisms through TLR2, TLR3, and TLR4. These TLRs can induce production of proinflammatory cytokines and IFN-β but not of IFN-α.

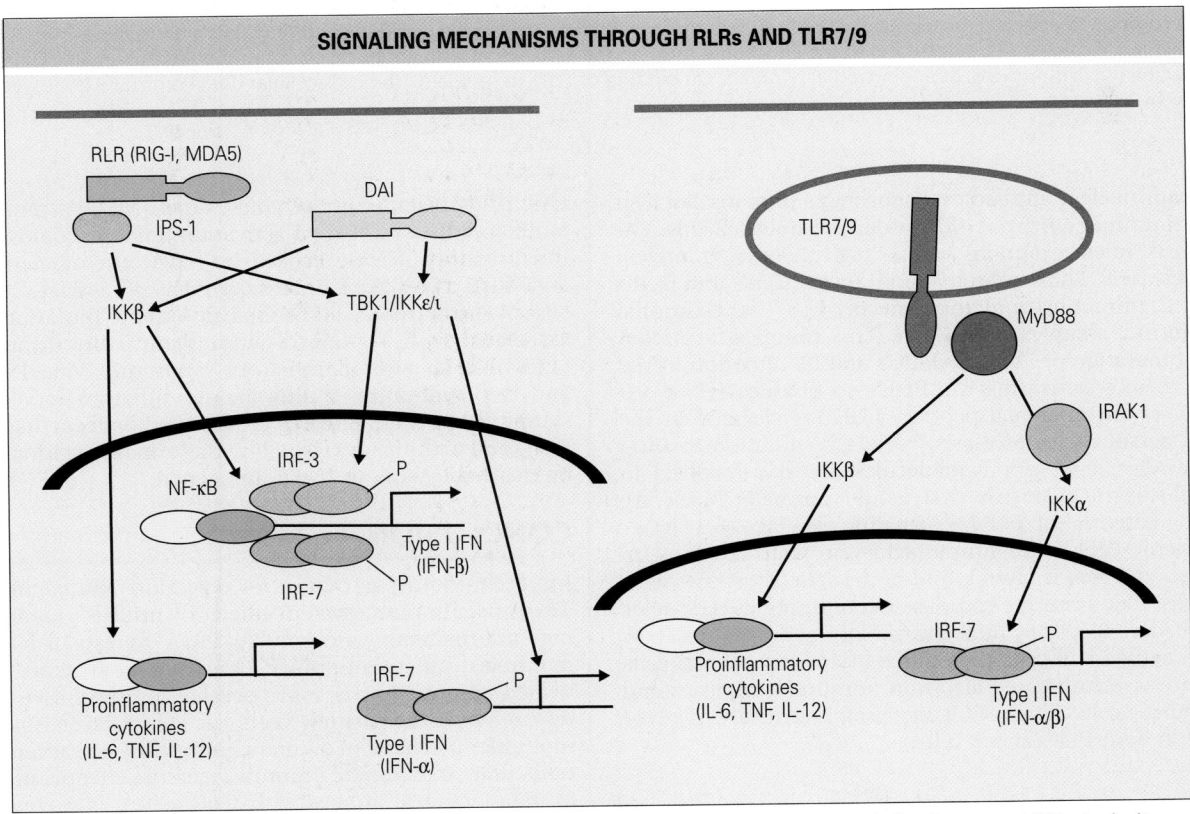

Fig. 16.10 Signaling mechanisms through RLRs and TLR7/9. These PRRs have potent ability to induce type I IFNs, including IFN-α and IFN-β, as well as proinflammatory cytokines. TLR7/9-induced type I IFN induction pathway mainly functions in PDC.

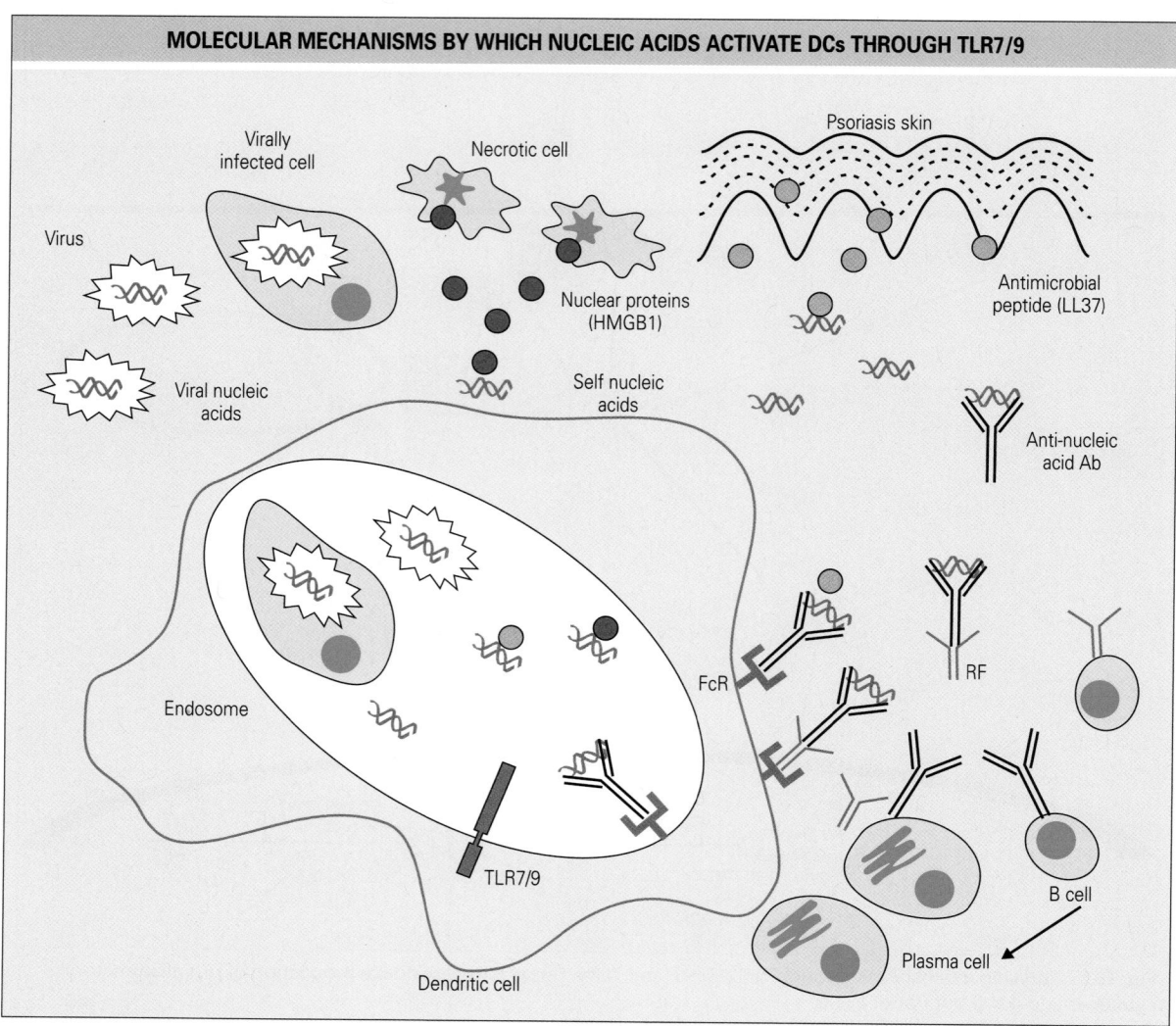

MOLECULAR MECHANISMS BY WHICH NUCLEIC ACIDS ACTIVATE DCs THROUGH TLR7/9

Fig. 16.11 Molecular mechanisms by which nucleic acids activate DCs through TLR7/9. Virus or virally infected cells are incorporated and viral nucleic acids are released in the endosome, where nucleic acid–recognizing TLRs are localized. Self-nucleic acids also gain access to the endosome through the association with antinucleic acid antibodies, rheumatoid factor, nuclear proteins, or antimicrobial peptides. On binding of TLR9 to its ligand, the extracellular domain of TLR9 is cleaved to be activated.

In addition to antinuclear antibodies, endogenous proteins can also manifest the autoimmune potential of host-derived nucleic acids. On massive cell necrosis, nuclear proteins such as high-mobility group box 1 (HMGB1) are released. Those proteins bind nucleic acids and facilitate TLR9-induced immunostimulatory effects. LL37 is a cationic protein and can form a complex with DNA. This complex formation facilitates the incorporation of DNA by PDCs and its retention in the early endosome, thereby activating the PDCs to produce IFN-α via TLR9. Production of antimicrobial peptide, LL37, is elevated in the skin lesions from persons with psoriasis.[29] Thus, in addition to anti–nucleic acid antibodies, endogenous molecules are also involved in bypassing the fail-safe mechanisms that would normally block the immunopathologic potential of TLR7/9 signaling (see Fig. 16.11).

Rheumatoid factor (RF) is an immunoglobulin that can bind to certain types of IgG and that is often found in the sera of patients with an autoimmune disorder. Immune complexes containing nucleic acids can activate RF-positive B cells by dual engagement of a B-cell receptor and TLR9.[30] Such activated B cells then differentiate into plasma cells and produce RF. RF is incorporated also into immune complexes and transferred to dendritic cells. Thus, TLR signaling is critically involved in autoimmunity in both PDC and B cells.

NLR and inflammation

Excessive activation of inflammasome can provoke various inflammatory conditions. Gout is an arthritis accompanied by hyperuricemia.

Uric acid crystals (monosodium urate [MSU]) are precipitated in the joints and lead to NALP3 activation. Pneumoconiosis is a pulmonary inflammatory disease evoked by long-term inhalation of particulate dust such as asbestos or silica, which can activate NALP3 inflammasome. Furthermore, autosomal dominant mutations in NALP3 are associated with a group of autoinflammatory disorders that include familial cold autoinflammatory syndrome, Muckle-Wells syndrome, and neonatal-onset multisystemic inflammatory disease. Clinical symptoms of these diseases are featured by recurring episodes of fever, rash, and arthropathy. Notably, these manifestations are ameliorated by treatment with an IL-1R antagonist.

CONCLUSION

Innate immunity is critical for detecting, and coping with, infection. The innate immune system efficiently utilizes a combination of signaling, internalizing, and soluble PRRs to establish host defense. In mammals, innate immunity represents an ancient, yet highly sophisticated system that is indispensable for the host's survival. Intense research over the past few years has led to the clarification of the basic molecular mechanism of innate immunity, and several clinical applications that target innate immune receptors are now in development. For example, clinical studies with CpG DNA as a powerful adjuvant in allergy or cancer treatments and to boost general immunity are underway. Furthermore, there are indications that various autoimmune manifestations can be improved by manipulating innate immunity.

Further understanding of how innate immune cells function may potentially lead to the development of new treatment strategies in a variety of disease conditions.

ACKNOWLEDGMENTS

We thank all the colleagues in our lab for helpful discussion and Sachiko Haraguchi for secretarial assistance. This work was supported by the Ministry of Education, Culture, Sports, Science, and Technology (MEXT), Japan Society for the Promotion of Science, and the Uehara Memorial Foundation.

REFERENCES

1. Janeway CA Jr. Approaching the asymptote? Evolution and revolution in immunology. Cold Spring Harb Symp Quant Biol 1989;54:1-13.
2. Medzhitov R. Toll-like receptors and innate immunity. Nat Rev Immunol 2001;1:135-145.
3. Takeda K, Kaisho T, Akira S. Toll-like receptors. Annu Rev Immunol 2003;21:335-376.
4. Beutler B. Tlr4: central component of the sole mammalian LPS sensor. Curr Opin Immunol 2000;12:20-26.
5. Miyake K. Endotoxin recognition molecules, Toll-like receptor 4-MD-2. Semin Immunol 2004;16:11-16.
6. Tokunaga T, Yamamoto T, Yamamoto S. How BCG led to the discovery of immunostimulatory DNA. Jpn J Infect Dis 1999;52:1-11.
7. Wagner H. Bacterial CpG DNA activates immune cells to signal infectious danger. Adv Immunol 1999;73:329-368.
8. Krieg AM. The role of CpG motifs in innate immunity. Curr Opin Immunol 2000;12:35-43.
9. Yoneyama M, Kikuchi M, Natsukawa T, et al. The RNA helicase RIG-I has an essential function in double-stranded RNA-induced innate antiviral responses. Nat Immunol 2004;5:730-737.
10. Kato H, Takeuchi O, Sato S, et al. Differential roles of MDA5 and RIG-I helicases in the recognition of RNA viruses. Nature 2006;441:101-105.
11. Ting JP, Lovering RC, Alnemri ES, et al. The NLR gene family: a standard nomenclature. Immunity 2008;28:285-287.
12. Inohara N, Nunez G. NODs: intracellular proteins involved in inflammation and apoptosis. Nat Rev Immunol 2003;3:371-382.
13. Stuart LM, Ezekowitz RA. Phagocytosis elegant complexity. Immunity 2005;22:539-550.
14. Mantovani A, Garlanda C, Bottazzi B. Pentraxin 3, a non-redundant soluble pattern recognition receptor involved in innate immunity. Vaccine 2003;21(Suppl 2):S43-S47.
15. Muller-Eberhard HJ. Molecular organization and function of the complement system. Annu Rev Biochem 1988;57:321-347.
16. Petersen SV, Thiel S, Jensenius JC. The mannan-binding lectin pathway of complement activation: biology and disease association. Mol Immunol 2001;38:133-149.
17. Medzhitov R, Preston-Hurlburt P, Janeway CA Jr. A human homologue of the *Drosophila* Toll protein signals activation of adaptive immunity [see comments]. Nature 1997;388:394-397.
18. Hoffmann JA, Kafatos FC, Janeway CA, Ezekowitz RA. Phylogenetic perspectives in innate immunity. Science 1999;284:1313-1318.
19. Hoffmann JA. The immune response of *Drosophila*. Nature 2003;426:33-38.
20. Bettelli E, Korn T, Oukka M, Kuchroo VK. Induction and effector functions of T(H)17 cells. Nature 2008;453:1051-1057.
21. Taniguchi T, Takaoka A. The interferon-alpha/beta system in antiviral responses: a multimodal machinery of gene regulation by the IRF family of transcription factors. Curr Opin Immunol 2002;14:111-116.
22. Colonna M, Trinchieri G, Liu YJ. Plasmacytoid dendritic cells in immunity. Nat Immunol 2004;5:1219-1226.
23. Heath WR, Carbone FR. Cross-presentation, dendritic cells, tolerance and immunity. Annu Rev Immunol 2001;19:47-64.
24. Schulz O, Diebold SS, Chen M, et al. Toll-like receptor 3 promotes cross-priming to virus-infected cells. Nature 2005;433:887-892.
25. Akira S, Takeda K. Toll-like receptor signalling. Nat Rev Immunol 2004;4:499-511.
26. Petrilli V, Dostert C, Muruve DA, Tschopp J. The inflammasome: a danger sensing complex triggering innate immunity. Curr Opin Immunol 2007;19:615-622.
27. Franchi L, Eigenbrod T, Munoz-Planillo R, Nunez G. The inflammasome: a caspase-1-activation platform that regulates immune responses and disease pathogenesis. Nat Immunol 2009;10:241-247.
28. Lenert P. Inhibitory oligodeoxynucleotides—therapeutic promise for systemic autoimmune diseases? Clin Exp Immunol 2005;140:1-10.
29. Gilliet M, Cao W, Liu YJ. Plasmacytoid dendritic cells: sensing nucleic acids in viral infection and autoimmune diseases. Nat Rev Immunol 2008;8:594-606.
30. Rifkin IR, Leadbetter EA, Busconi L, et al. Toll-like receptors, endogenous ligands, and systemic autoimmune disease. Immunol Rev 2005;204:27-42.

Tissue destruction and repair

Tim E. Cawston, D. A. Young, and A. D. Rowan

17

- Cartilage is made up of collagens, proteoglycans, and glycoproteins. Bone consists of a mineralized collagen matrix. Both tissues can be degraded by active proteinases.

- Different classes of proteinases play a part in connective tissue turnover, but the proteinase that predominates varies with different tissues and resorptive situation.

- Matrix metalloproteinases (MMPs) are potent enzymes that degrade connective tissue and are inhibited by tissue inhibitors of metalloproteinases (TIMPs); the balance between active MMPs and TIMPs determines the extent of degradation. ADAM (a disintegrin and metalloprotease) and ADAMTS (a disintegrin and metalloproteinase with thrombospondin motifs) proteinases are also upregulated in the diseased joint, and cysteine proteinases initiate the breakdown of collagen in bone.

- Various cytokines and growth factors, alone or in combination, inhibit matrix synthesis and stimulate proteinase production and matrix destruction.

- Some growth factors increase the synthesis of matrix and proteinase inhibitors. Growth factor combinations can be used in conjunction with artificial matrices to promote the repair of cartilage defects in large joints.

INTRODUCTION

Cartilage and the underlying subchondral bone are destroyed in severe cases of arthritis, and this limits normal joint function. Cartilage contains different types of collagen, which are composed of rod-shaped molecules that aggregate in staggered arrays to form cross-linked fibers giving connective tissues strength and rigidity.[1] Entrapped within these collagen fibers are the proteoglycans,[2] predominantly aggrecan, which consists of three globular domains interspersed with heavily glycosylated and sulfated polypeptide. In the presence of hyaluronic acid, these form highly charged aggregates, attract water into the tissue, and allow cartilage to resist compression. Chondrocytes in normal adult cartilage maintain a steady state in which the extent of matrix synthesis equals that of degradation. Any change in this steady state will affect the functional integrity of the cartilage. During growth and development, synthesis of matrix components exceeds degradation, whereas in pathology there is an increase in the rate of degradation that is often associated with a reduction in matrix synthesis.

The primary cause of cartilage and bone destruction in the arthritides is elevated levels of active proteinases, secreted from a variety of cells, which degrade collagen and aggrecan. The sources of these proteinases will depend on the type of disease. In osteoarthritis the proteinases produced by chondrocytes play a major role. In contrast, in a highly inflamed rheumatoid joint the chondrocytes, synovial cells, and inflammatory cells all contribute to the proteolytic loss of tissue matrix.

Joint tissues are capable of repair: although aggrecan can be readily resynthesized, the replacement of collagen, after its destruction, is more difficult.[3] A variety of growth factors and cytokines present in the joint are able to upregulate matrix synthesis, and these factors have been studied to determine if cartilage and bone defects can be repaired *in vivo*.

PROTEOLYTIC PATHWAYS OF CONNECTIVE TISSUE BREAKDOWN

Extracellular matrix proteins are broken down by different proteolytic pathways. The five main classes of proteinases[4] are classified according to the chemical group that participates in the hydrolysis of peptide bonds. Cysteine and aspartic proteinases are predominantly active at acidic pH and act intracellularly; threonine proteinases, the proteasome being the most characterized, also act intracellularly at near-neutral pH; and the serine and metalloproteinases, active at neutral pH, mostly act extracellularly. Examples of these enzymes and the matrix proteins they cleave are shown in Figure 17.1. Other enzymes, such as elastase, are released when neutrophils are stimulated. Some enzymes, such as furin, may not participate in the proteolysis of matrix proteins but activate proenzymes that then degrade the matrix. Membrane-bound proteinases are associated with cytokine processing, receptor shedding, and the removal of proteins that are responsible for cell-cell or cell-matrix interactions.

The complete repertoire of human proteases (defined as the degradome)[5] comprises approximately 569 proteinases, and all classes of proteinase have roles in the turnover of connective tissues. One proteinase pathway may act in concert with or precede another, and the pathway that predominates will vary with different resorptive situations. The turnover of the extracellular matrix often involves complex interactions between different cell types. The osteoid layer in bone is removed by osteoblast metalloproteinases before the attachment of osteoclasts, which secrete predominantly cysteine proteinases such as cathepsin K. These degrade bone matrix after the removal of mineral. An intricate series of interactions occur in the rheumatoid joint between T cells, macrophages, synovial fibroblasts, and chondrocytes. In septic arthritis, neutrophils release both serine and metalloproteinases, which exceed the local concentration of inhibitors, resulting in a rapid removal of the cartilage matrix from the joint cavity, in contrast to many other arthropathies. In osteoarthritis (OA), inflammation is typically less marked but nevertheless is thought to contribute to pathology.[6] It is likely, however, that other mechanisms also contribute to joint tissue destruction, especially in OA, including abnormal mechanical loads and mechanotransduction, age-related changes to cartilage matrix such as advanced glycation end products and new gene expression, and factors such as the activation of Toll-like receptors.

EXTRACELLULAR PROTEOLYSIS—NEUTRAL PROTEINASES

Matrix metalloproteinases

The matrix metalloproteinase (MMP) family, when activated and acting collectively, can degrade all the components of the extracellular matrix. MMPs are zinc-dependent endopeptidases, and all contain common domains (Fig. 17.2a).[7] All are produced as latent (inactive) proenzymes, and proteolytic loss of the propeptide leads to activation. The membrane-type MMPs (MT-MMPs) and stromelysin-3 (MMP-11) have a short peptide insert between the propeptide and the N-terminal domain, a sequence recognized by furin, a serine proteinase located in the Golgi apparatus; these MMPs are therefore secreted as active enzymes. Zinc is present at the catalytic center within the N-terminal catalytic domain, which is joined to the C-terminal hemopexin domain by a flexible linking peptide. The hemopexin domain helps to confer substrate specificity, this being especially noteworthy for the collagenases. Two MMPs (collagenase-2/MMP-8 and gelatinase B/MMP-9) are found stored within the specific granules of the neutrophil, whereas

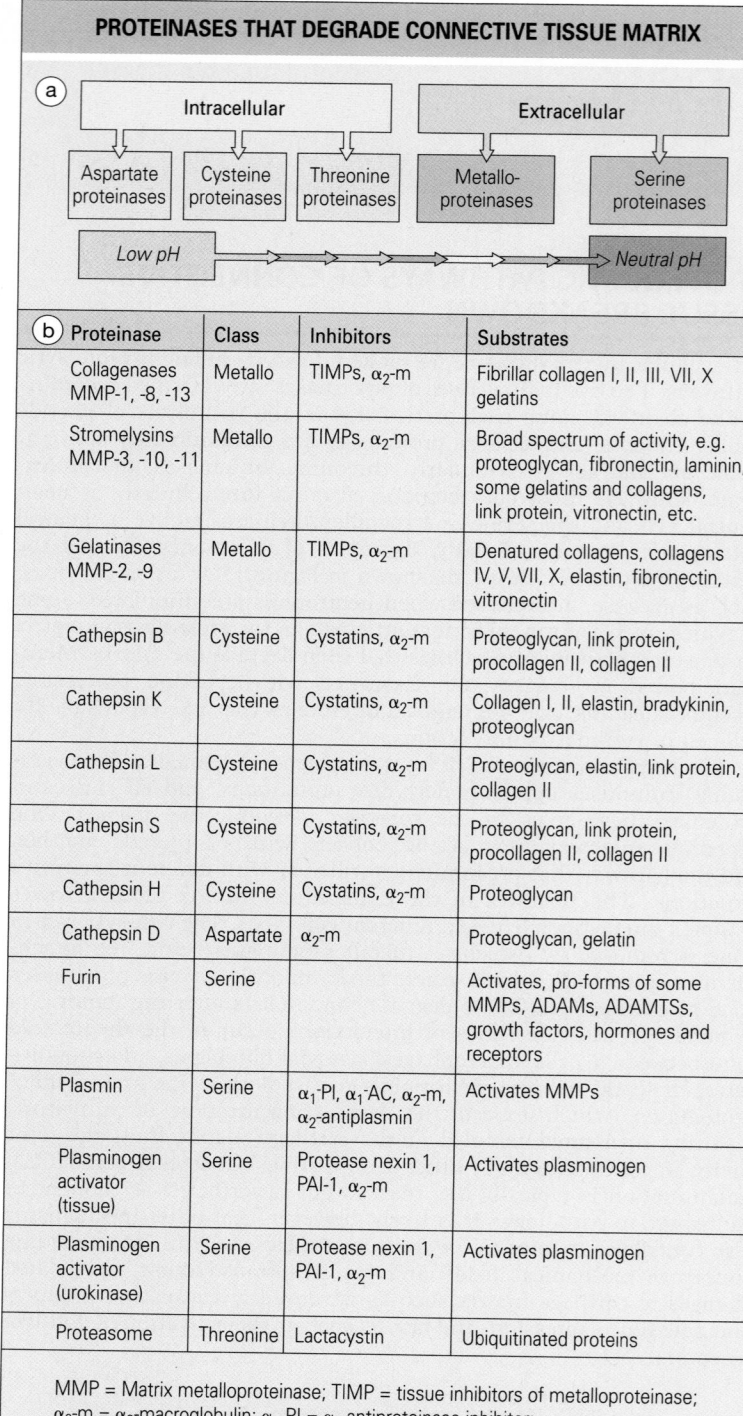

PROTEINASES THAT DEGRADE CONNECTIVE TISSUE MATRIX

(a)

Intracellular			Extracellular	
Aspartate proteinases	Cysteine proteinases	Threonine proteinases	Metallo-proteinases	Serine proteinases

Low pH ⟹⟹⟹⟹⟹ Neutral pH

(b)

Proteinase	Class	Inhibitors	Substrates
Collagenases MMP-1, -8, -13	Metallo	TIMPs, α_2-m	Fibrillar collagen I, II, III, VII, X gelatins
Stromelysins MMP-3, -10, -11	Metallo	TIMPs, α_2-m	Broad spectrum of activity, e.g. proteoglycan, fibronectin, laminin, some gelatins and collagens, link protein, vitronectin, etc.
Gelatinases MMP-2, -9	Metallo	TIMPs, α_2-m	Denatured collagens, collagens IV, V, VII, X, elastin, fibronectin, vitronectin
Cathepsin B	Cysteine	Cystatins, α_2-m	Proteoglycan, link protein, procollagen II, collagen II
Cathepsin K	Cysteine	Cystatins, α_2-m	Collagen I, II, elastin, bradykinin, proteoglycan
Cathepsin L	Cysteine	Cystatins, α_2-m	Proteoglycan, elastin, link protein, collagen II
Cathepsin S	Cysteine	Cystatins, α_2-m	Proteoglycan, link protein, procollagen II, collagen II
Cathepsin H	Cysteine	Cystatins, α_2-m	Proteoglycan
Cathepsin D	Aspartate	α_2-m	Proteoglycan, gelatin
Furin	Serine		Activates, pro-forms of some MMPs, ADAMs, ADAMTSs, growth factors, hormones and receptors
Plasmin	Serine	α_1-PI, α_1-AC, α_2-m, α_2-antiplasmin	Activates MMPs
Plasminogen activator (tissue)	Serine	Protease nexin 1, PAI-1, α_2-m	Activates plasminogen
Plasminogen activator (urokinase)	Serine	Protease nexin 1, PAI-1, α_2-m	Activates plasminogen
Proteasome	Threonine	Lactacystin	Ubiquitinated proteins

MMP = Matrix metalloproteinase; TIMP = tissue inhibitors of metalloproteinase; α_2-m = α_2-macroglobulin; α_1-PI = α_1-antiproteinase inhibitor; α_1-AC = α_1- antichymotrypsin; PAI-1 = plasminogen activator inhibitor-1.

Fig. 17.1 Proteinases that degrade connective tissue matrix. (a) The five main classes of proteinases are named according to the chemical group involved in catalysis. The aspartic and cysteine proteinases act at low pH and are thought to act within the lysosomal system, where they degrade protein intracellularly; these enzymes can also be released into small acidified pockets near the cell membrane to degrade extracellularly. The major threonine proteinase, the proteasome, degrades proteins in the cytoplasm and is an important regulator of many intracellular processes, including proinflammatory signaling pathways. Secreted serine and metalloproteinases act extracellularly at neutral pH. Some enzymes are membrane bound, ensuring that they act locally to the cell. Some serine proteinases also act intracellularly within the Golgi apparatus, activating proenzymes before their secretion. (b) Examples of each enzyme are listed with proteinase class, inhibitors, and major matrix proteins degraded.

most others are produced by different connective tissue cells after stimulation with a variety of mediators.

MMPs are divided into four main groups called the stromelysins, collagenases, gelatinases, and MT-MMPs.[8] The stromelysins have broad substrate specificities (see Fig. 17.1), and the natural substrates of these enzymes are probably proteoglycans, fibronectin, and laminin.[9] Stromelysin-1 (MMP-3) is not normally widely expressed but can be readily induced by growth factors and cytokines such as interleukin (IL)-1 and tumor necrosis factor (TNF)-α. The three stromelysins have a similar substrate specificity, but their expression patterns are often quite distinct.

There are three mammalian collagenases: collagenase-1 (MMP-1), collagenase-2 (MMP-8), and collagenase-3 (MMP-13). The full-length structure of porcine collagenase was solved by x-ray crystallography and is shown in Figure 17.2b.[10] These enzymes, once activated, cleave fibrillar collagens at a single site, producing three-fourths– and one-fourth–sized fragments. The enzymes differ in their specificity for different collagens: collagenase-3 has a much broader substrate specificity than the other collagenases. Both collagenase-1 and collagenase-3 are synthesized by macrophages, fibroblasts, and chondrocytes when these cells are stimulated with inflammatory mediators. Collagenase-2 is predominantly released from neutrophils on stimulation of the cell, but this MMP can also be produced by chondrocytes, and all three collagenases are present in diseased cartilage (Fig. 17.3). Collagenase-3 is often controlled in a different way from collagenase-1; retinoic acid, which downregulates collagenase-1, is known to upregulate collagenase-3 in some cell types.

The two gelatinases cleave denatured collagens, type IV and V collagen, and elastin. Expression of gelatinase A (MMP-2) is the most widespread of all the MMPs; gelatinase B (MMP-9) is expressed in a wide variety of transformed and tumor-derived cells. Both MMP-2 and MT1-MMP (MMP-14) have also been shown to have collagenolytic activity, and the cell-surface location of MT1-MMP ideally situates it for the pericellular proteolysis that is often evident in OA cartilage.

There is an increase in levels of different MMPs in rheumatoid synovial fluid, in conditioned culture media from rheumatoid synovial tissues and cells, in synovial tissue at the cartilage-pannus junction from rheumatoid joints, in osteoarthritic cartilage, and in animal models of arthritis.[11,12] These proteinases are implicated in the pathologic destruction of joint tissue and are involved in the normal turnover of connective tissue matrix that occurs during growth and development. In OA, the rates of both matrix synthesis and breakdown are increased, which leads to the formation of excess matrix in some regions (osteophytes) with focal lesions (loss of matrix) in other areas.

The MMPs, therefore, need careful control[9]; this occurs at a number of critical steps (Fig. 17.4), including synthesis and secretion, activation of the proenzymes, and inhibition of the active enzymes.

Synthesis and secretion

IL-1, TNF-α, and IL-17 stimulate numerous cell types to produce proinflammatory and degradative molecules. The synthesis and secretion of collagenase-1, stromelysin-1, and other MMPs are stimulated by such mediators.[10] Within arthritic joints there are large numbers of different cell types that produce specific cytokines and growth factors that often differ in their action on individual cell types (see Fig. 17.4b). It is also likely that multiple cytokines will be present within such an inflammatory milieu, making it difficult to predict the outcome of blocking the action of an individual cytokine to prevent tissue destruction. TNF-α blockade in some patients with rheumatoid arthritis (RA) successfully reduces inflammation and joint destruction, whereas some studies suggest that blocking other cytokines such as IL-1, IL-6, IL-17, or oncostatin M (OSM) may confer similar benefit, especially in patients unresponsive to a given biologic agent. Cytokines and growth factors mediate their effects on cells by binding to specific cell-surface receptors. A "signal" is transduced to the nucleus via specific intracellular signal transduction pathways that culminate in the activation or repression of target genes. Signaling in inflammation is complex, and multiple signaling cascades are often activated by a given cytokine in different cell types. A further level of complexity is added in that interactions, or "cross talk," between different signaling pathways can occur

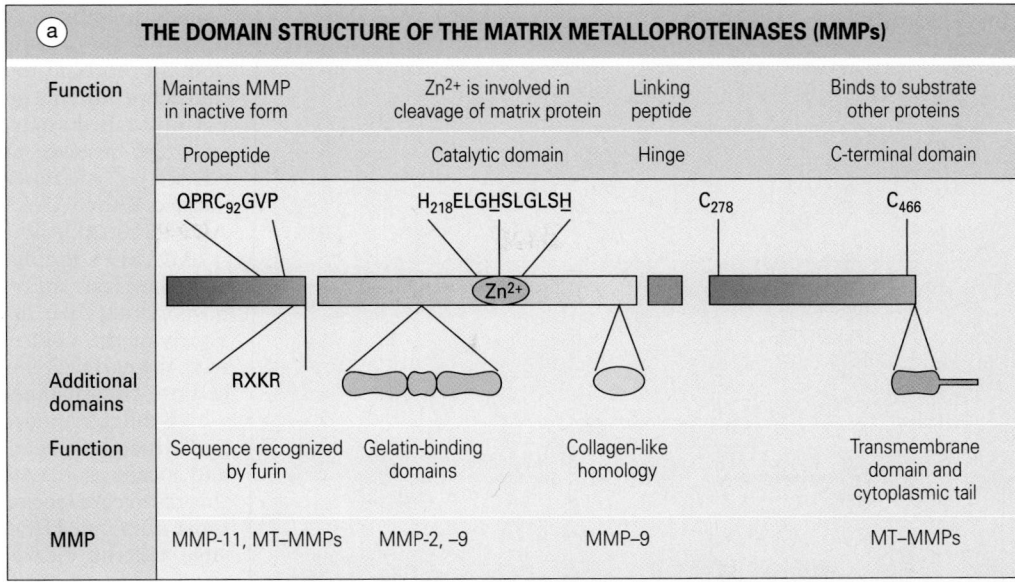

THE DOMAIN STRUCTURE OF THE MATRIX METALLOPROTEINASES (MMPs)

Function	Maintains MMP in inactive form	Zn²⁺ is involved in cleavage of matrix protein	Linking peptide	Binds to substrate other proteins
	Propeptide	Catalytic domain	Hinge	C-terminal domain

$QPRC_{92}GVP$ $H_{218}ELG\underline{H}SLGL\underline{S}H$ C_{278} C_{466}

Zn^{2+}

Additional domains	RXKR			
Function	Sequence recognized by furin	Gelatin-binding domains	Collagen-like homology	Transmembrane domain and cytoplasmic tail
MMP	MMP-11, MT–MMPs	MMP-2, –9	MMP–9	MT–MMPs

Fig. 17.2 The domain structure of the matrix metalloproteinases (MMPs). (a) All MMPs contain a similar domain structure with a zinc-binding domain (yellow), and most contain the C-terminal domain (blue). All are secreted with a propeptide (purple) that maintains the latency of the MMP by a conserved cysteine binding to the active site zinc. Other groups of MMPs build on this core structure. The gelatinases have additional domains inserted (green). The MT-MMPs have a transmembrane domain (pink) that locates the MMP at the cell surface. The MT-MMPs and stromelysin-3 have a sequence of basic amino acids inserted between the pro and catalytic domains that are specifically recognized by furin, a serine proteinase that activates these enzymes intracellularly. Varying the domains ensures that individual MMPs can bind to the matrix components that they cleave. (b) The structure of porcine synovial collagenase-1 is shown. The N-terminal domain (top) contains the active site zinc (purple), a further zinc ion, and three calcium ions (orange). A synthetic inhibitor is shown (yellow) binding to the active site zinc. This is linked by the hinge region to the C-terminal domain (bottom), which is responsible for substrate binding. This is shown as a four-bladed β-propeller with a central calcium ion.

PIG SYNOVIAL COLLAGENASE-1

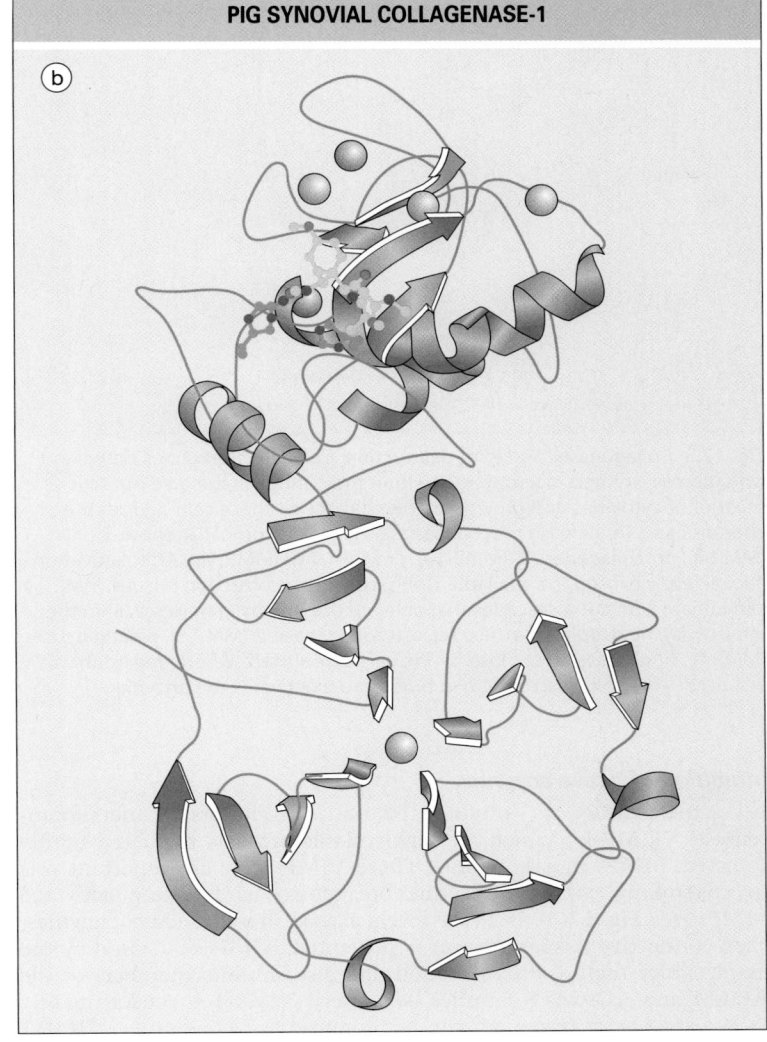

to mediate the gene expression of degradative molecules.[9] Signaling is currently considered an attractive therapeutic target and is therefore the subject of considerable research.[13,14]

Activation of proenzymes

Activation of latent pro-MMPs is an important and understudied control point in connective tissue breakdown. The propeptide is removed proteolytically; this allows the enzyme to hydrolyze peptide bonds, and activation is likely to be achieved in a tightly controlled environment close to the cell surface. Active stromelysin-1 activates procollagenases and other MMPs. Recent data implicate MT1-MMP, which is itself activated by the serine proteinase furin, as an important initiator of MMP activation cascades. Plasmin and possibly other serine proteinases activate some members of the MMP family, and *in vitro* studies have demonstrated that inhibitors of both furin and plasmin can stop cartilage destruction.[15]

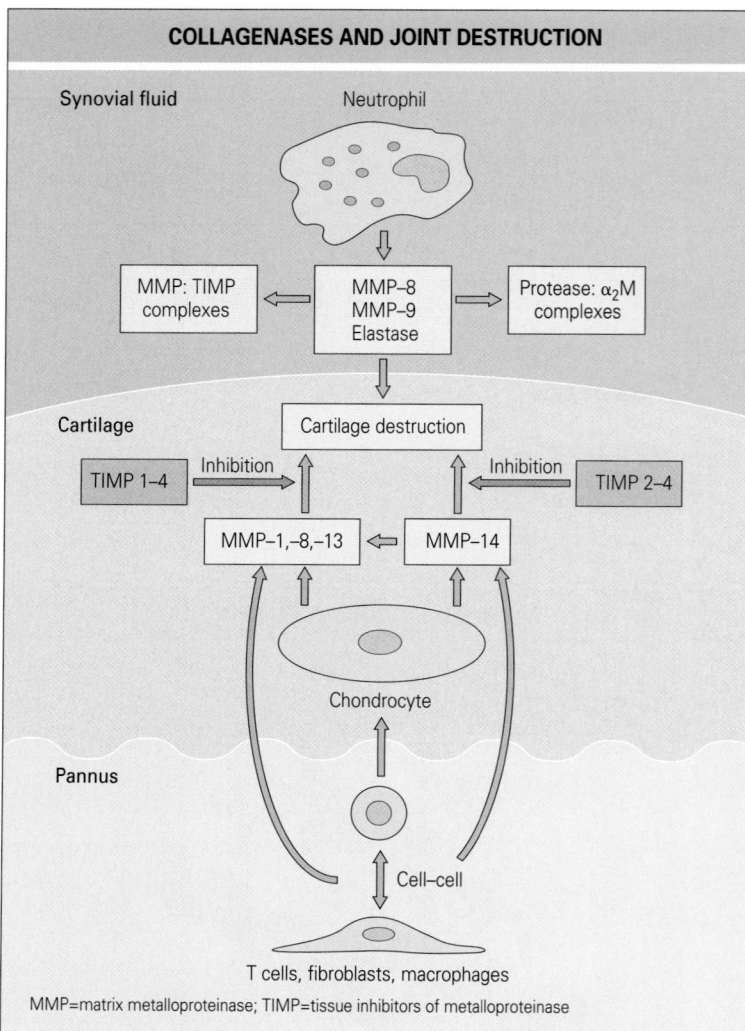

COLLAGENASES AND JOINT DESTRUCTION

Synovial fluid   Neutrophil

MMP: TIMP complexes ← MMP–8 MMP–9 Elastase → Protease: α_2M complexes

Cartilage

Cartilage destruction

TIMP 1–4 — Inhibition → ← Inhibition — TIMP 2–4

MMP–1,–8,–13 ← MMP–14

Chondrocyte

Pannus

Cell–cell

T cells, fibroblasts, macrophages

MMP=matrix metalloproteinase; TIMP=tissue inhibitors of metalloproteinase

Fig. 17.3 Collagenases and joint destruction. Cell-cell interactions between T cells, fibroblasts, and macrophages within the pannus tissue give rise to a mixture of cytokines and growth factors that act on these cells and on the chondrocytes to increase procollagenase-1 (MMP-1), procollagenase-2 (MMP-8), procollagenase-3 (MMP-13), or MT1-MMP (MMP-14). After activation, if local levels exceed the available TIMPs, collagen destruction ensues. MMP-14 can initiate activation cascades that activate the procollagenases. Within the joint cavity, neutrophils can also release collagenase-2 (MMP-8), gelatinase B (MMP-9), or elastase at, or close to, the cartilage surface where degradation will occur unless α_2-macroglobulin binds and inactivates the enzyme.

Inhibition of active enzymes

All active MMPs are inhibited by tissue inhibitors of metalloproteinases (TIMPs),[16] which are highly stable proteins that bind tightly to active MMPs in a 1:1 ratio. These TIMPs play an important role in controlling connective tissue breakdown by blocking activated MMPs (see Fig. 17.3). If TIMP levels exceed those of active enzymes, then connective tissue turnover is prevented. TIMP-3 is bound by the extracellular matrix after secretion and also inhibits members of the ADAM and ADAMTS families (see later). TIMP-4 is predominantly localized in heart tissue but can be produced by joint tissues. TIMP-1 and TIMP-3 are upregulated by growth factors such as transforming growth factor (TGF)-β, insulin-like growth factor (IGF)-1, and OSM; these agents also upregulate matrix synthesis. The mechanisms that control the extracellular activity of the MMPs are illustrated in Figure 17.4.

ADAM and ADAMTS proteinase families

Two additional families of proteinases, both closely related to MMPs, are also implicated in cartilage biology, particularly in relation to proteoglycan turnover. ADAMs (A Disintegrin And Metalloproteinase) are usually membrane-anchored proteinases with diverse functions conferred by the addition of different protein domains. The disintegrin domain can bind to integrins and prevent cell-cell interactions; cysteine-rich, epithelial growth factor (EGF)–like, transmembrane, and cytoplasmic tail domains are also found. Some members are associated with the cleavage and release of cell-surface proteins. For example, ADAM-17 is known for its ability to release TNF-α from the cell surface. Other ADAMs have also been described in cartilage, including ADAM-10, ADAM-12, and ADAM-15.

ADAMTS family members are distinguished from the ADAMs in that they lack these latter three domains but have additional thrombospondin-1–like domains (which can number up to 13), predominantly at the C-terminus, which are thought to mediate interactions with the extracellular matrix.[17] Some ADAMTS proteinases can, under certain circumstances, be produced as alternatively spliced forms, which differ primarily in the number of their thrombospondin repeats and which may give rise to differences in their substrate specificities and localization within the extracellular matrix. Several members of this family are recognized as aggrecanases,[17] and some of these enzymes, most notably ADAMTS4 and ADAMTS5,[18] are thought to be responsible for the cleavage of cartilage proteoglycan (Fig. 17.5). Recent studies suggest that an enzyme is present on the surface of chondrocytes that also cleaves aggrecan and is distinct from ADAMTS4 or ADAMTS5; however, it remains unclear whether it is an ADAMTS family member that is attached tightly via thrombospondin domains or whether a separate enzyme is present. Interestingly, many of the ADAM and ADAMTS family members are inhibited by TIMP-3, which in *in vitro* studies effectively blocks aggrecan release from cartilage.

Serine proteinases

There are almost as many serine proteinases (31%) in the human degradome as there are metalloproteinases (34%),[5] making this proteinase class an increasingly interesting one in terms of joint destruction. Indeed, both direct and indirect roles for serine proteinases have been described, including the regulation of cell signaling and modulating the biologic activity of growth factors; these are events that can significantly alter an inflammatory response.[15] The complement serine proteinase C1s can degrade insulin-like growth factor–binding protein-5 (IGFBP-5) to release active IGF-1, a growth factor integral to controlling cartilage damage. Complement activation components are elevated in the synovial fluid, synovium, and cartilage of arthritis patients, and targeted deletion/inhibition reduces disease severity in murine arthritis models. Therapeutics that target complement components are now being developed for the treatment of RA.[19] As well as a pro-MMP activator, plasmin can active TGF-β, release IGF-1 from IGFBPs, and activate the complement cascade. The serine proteinases neutrophil elastase and cathepsin G are stored in azurophil granules and released after neutrophil exposure to inflammatory stimuli. In mice deficient of both neutrophil elastase and cathepsin G, experimental arthritis is less severe with reduced inflammatory cell infiltration, suggesting that these neutrophil serine proteinases are important in promoting the inflammatory process by establishing chemotactic gradients that recruit immune cells and enhance inflammation. Modulation of the biologic activity of chemokines is another important role,[15] and it is now apparent that serine proteinases are also involved in initiating cell signaling via the proteolytic activation of protease-activated receptors.[20]

INTRACELLULAR PATHWAYS— ACID PROTEINASES

Cathepsin D (an aspartic proteinase) and cathepsin B (cysteine proteinase) are raised in OA cartilage, and raised levels of cathepsins B, H, and L (cysteine proteinases) are reported in antigen-induced rat arthritis models and within the rheumatoid joint.[21] Incubation of resorbing cartilage with specific cathepsin B inhibitors blocked the release of proteoglycan fragments, suggesting the involvement of an intracellular route for cartilage proteoglycan breakdown. Cathepsin K can also cleave collagen, albeit at a different site to the MMPs, and the presence of chondroitin sulfate increases the activity and stability of this enzyme.

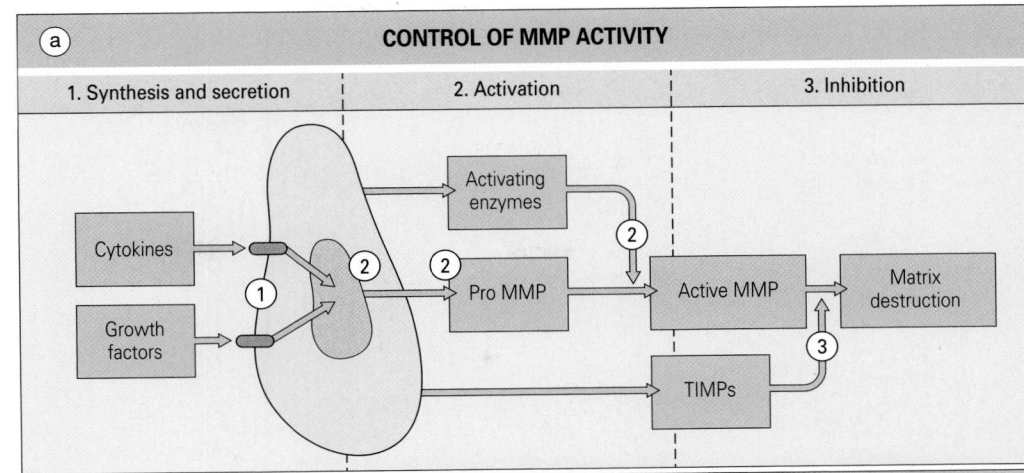

Fig. 17.4 Control of MMP activity. (a) The MMPs are controlled by mechanisms that include upregulation by combinations of cytokines and growth factors, activation of the secreted enzymes, and inhibition by TIMPs. (b) Other factors often alter the cellular response to these stimuli, and different cells can respond to growth factors and cytokines in a number of ways.

A correlation of cathepsin K–generated collagen fragments with increasing age in OA cartilage has been reported.[22] Cathepsin K is now a drug target for the treatment of osteoporosis in which bone resorption is excessive (see later). The relative contribution of intracellular and extracellular pathways to collagen breakdown is controversial. Studies have identified collagen-containing vacuoles within connective tissue fibroblasts.[23] These vacuoles contain either recently synthesized collagen (targeted for intracellular degradation prior to secretion) or collagen phagocytosed from the extracellular space. This occurs when cells form contacts with the collagen fibril and segregate it by cellular processes. Partial digestion of the fibril occurs by membrane-bound MMPs and possibly gelatinases followed by intracellular digestion within the lysosomal system by cathepsin B or L.[24] Tissues with a high matrix turnover (e.g., periodontal ligament) or that have been stimulated to resorb have increased numbers of collagen-containing vacuoles, suggesting that these are linked to resorption. Some workers suggest that the intracellular pathway predominates in normal turnover, whereas the extracellular route is prevalent only under pathologic conditions.[24] A close apposition of intracellular and extracellular pathways will be found in many situations when there is connective tissue turnover (Fig. 17.6).

OSTEOCLASTIC BONE RESORPTION

Bone is also destroyed in RA,[25] and both the MMPs and cysteine proteinases are involved.[26] Osteoblasts respond to parathyroid hormone and other agents that induce bone resorption, such as IL-1 and TNF-α, by increasing the secretion of MMPs to remove the osteoid layer on the bone surface. Osteoclast precursors then adhere to the exposed bone surface, differentiate, and form a low pH microenvironment beneath their lower surface. This removes mineral, and lysosomal proteinases then resorb the exposed matrix (Fig. 17.7). Cathepsins B and L cleave collagen types II, IX, and XI and destroy cross-linked collagen matrix at low pH. Osteoclasts produce cathepsin K, which cleaves type I collagen at the N-terminal end of the triple helix. This enzyme

plays a key role in the degradation of bone collagen, and its expression correlates with bone resorption. It is also produced by synovial fibroblasts and is thought to contribute to synovium-initiated bone destruction in the rheumatoid joint.[27] Bone resorption is impaired in situations in which cathepsin K is deficient, evidence that has made cathepsin K a drug target for the treatment of osteoporosis in which bone resorption is excessive.

There is clear evidence for a central role for receptor activator of the nuclear factor-kappa B ligand (RANKL) in the bone destruction seen in RA. This member of the TNF ligand family of cytokines is abundantly produced by T cells and synovial fibroblasts in RA synovial membrane, and it stimulates the formation of multinucleate osteoclasts. It is upregulated by a variety of cytokines, including IL-1, TNF-α, IL-11, OSM, parathyroid hormone–related peptide (PTHrP), macrophage colony-stimulating factor (M-CSF), and IL-17. It binds to a specific receptor, RANK, on the surface of osteoclast precursors. Increased levels of RANK and RANKL, as well as multinucleate cells, are evident in arthritis models associated with bone erosions. The potent activity of IL-17 in osteoclastogenesis is mediated by the upregulation of RANKL, and its action is antagonized by the decoy receptor osteoprotegerin (OPG). This molecule is effective in blocking bone resorption,[25] and, in rat adjuvant arthritis and the arthritis of TNFtg mice,[28] it protects against the development of bone and cartilage destruction.

MODEL SYSTEMS OF CARTILAGE BREAKDOWN

A large number of animal models are used to study the mechanisms of joint destruction. Initiation of cartilage breakdown can be induced with IL-1, TNF-α, IL-17, retinoic acid, or other proinflammatory cytokine combinations in model systems.[29] Specific proteoglycan fragments are released first from resorbing cartilage (see Fig. 17.5). TIMP-3 blocks this proteoglycan release, supporting a role for ADAMTS enzymes, particularly ADAMTS5, and possibly other chondrocyte membrane metalloproteinases. Cysteine proteinase inhibitors can also block

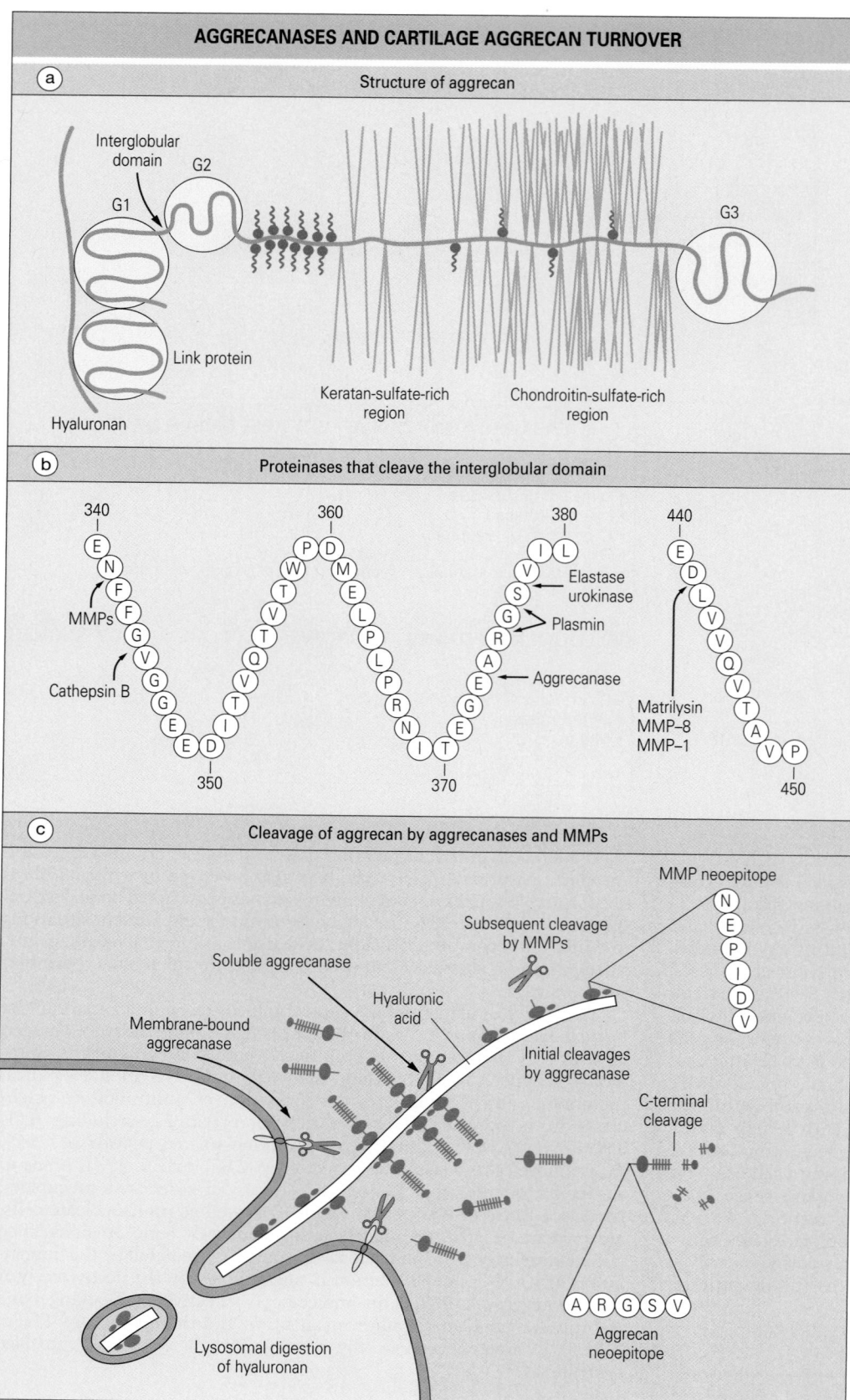

AGGRECANASES AND CARTILAGE AGGRECAN TURNOVER

(a) Structure of aggrecan

(b) Proteinases that cleave the interglobular domain

(c) Cleavage of aggrecan by aggrecanases and MMPs

Fig. 17.5 Aggrecanases and cartilage aggrecan turnover. (a) Structure of aggrecan. The major proteoglycan in human cartilage is aggrecan, a protein with three globular domains: G1 to G3. Between G2 and G3 there is a linear region of polypeptide to which charged sugars are attached that attract water, causing aggrecan to swell. (b) Proteinases that cleave the interglobular domain. Both aggrecanases and MMPs can cleave aggrecan at specific amino acid sequences between the G1 and G2 domains. Cleavage in this region by aggrecanases is thought to be key to the pathologic loss of aggrecan from cartilage. (c) Cleavage of aggrecan by aggrecanases and MMPs. Aggrecanases are metalloproteinases that belong to the ADAMTS family. These are either associated with the chondrocyte membrane or released into the extracellular space where aggrecan is cleaved between the G1 and G2 domains as well as at several sites close to the G3 domain. A specific neoepitope is released and is found in diseased synovial fluids. The G1 domain, which is bound to hyaluronic acid, can be subsequently cleaved by MMPs, leaving a specific MMP neoepitope that can be detected in arthritic cartilage in late-stage disease. TIMP-3 inhibits aggrecan release.

proteoglycan release from cartilage, indicating that they could be involved in upstream activation pathways.[23]

The loss of collagen from cartilage is viewed as the final phase of tissue destruction and is essentially irreversible because attempts at repair do not lead to restoration of normal cartilage. Before the loss of collagen, many of the minor components of the extracellular matrix are first degraded, including molecules that are closely associated with the collagen fibrils such as COMP, decorin, and type IX collagen. It is not known whether this disassembly of the matrix occurs in a defined sequence, but it is evident that a matrix as complex as articular cartilage requires numerous proteolytic activities to effect complete tissue destruction. Although IL-1 and TNF-α are sometimes able to initiate cartilage collagen resorption alone, when these cytokines are combined with OSM a rapid and reproducible release of collagen is found in

THE CONTROL OF COLLAGEN SYNTHESIS AND DEGRADATION

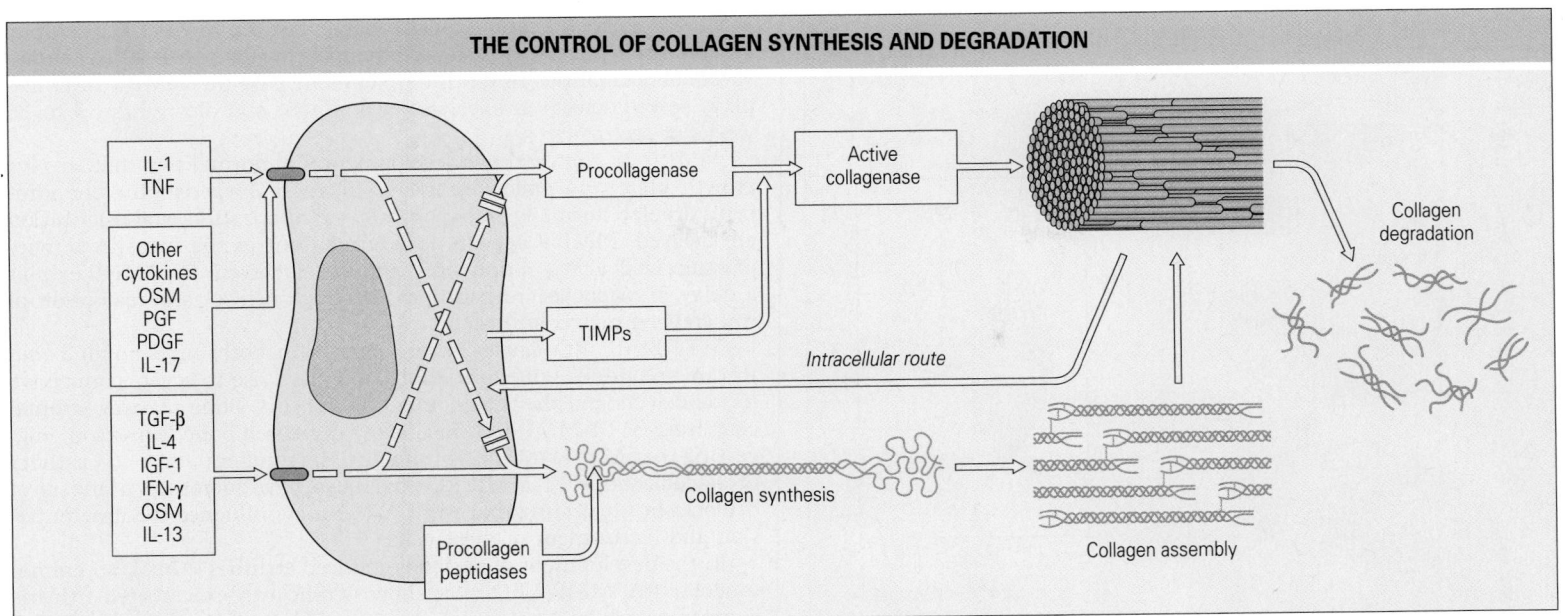

Fig. 17.6 The control of collagen synthesis and degradation. Increased synthesis of collagen or proteinase inhibitors, often linked to reduced production of proteinases, is found after treatment with a variety of growth factors, which include TGF-β, interferon-γ, IGF-1, IL-4, and IL-13. IL-1 and TNF-α increase the production of proteinases and can reduce collagen synthesis. Other agents, such as oncostatin M (OSM), IL-17, basic fibroblast growth factor (bFGF), and platelet-derived growth factor (PDGF), can further influence these processes.

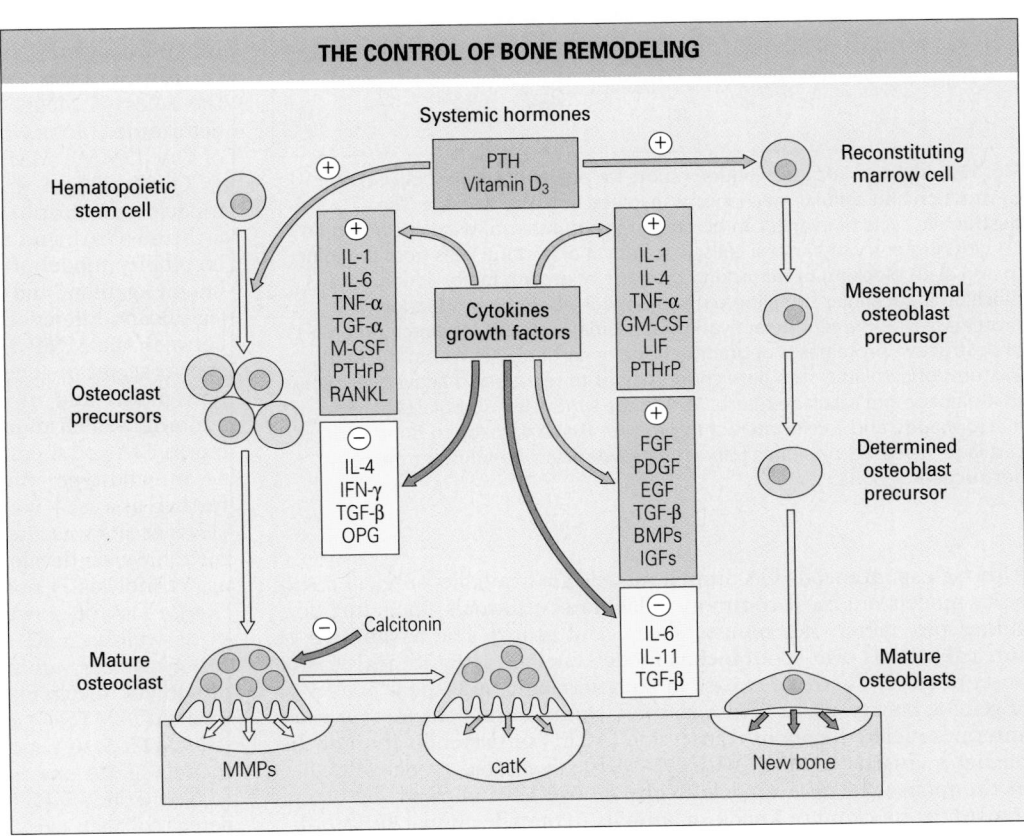

Fig. 17.7 The control of bone remodeling. Hematopoietic stem cells are induced to differentiate into osteoclast precursors by systemic hormones such as parathyroid hormone (PTH) as well as vitamin D₃, and various cytokines and growth factors have stimulatory or inhibitory effects on this differentiation. These precursors mature into osteoclasts that first remove the mineral component of bone via acidification of an extracellular zone on the bone surface and then mediate the breakdown of protein components through the production of MMPs and cathepsin K (catK); calcitonin inhibits osteoclast function. Osteoblasts are derived from reconstituting bone marrow cells that differentiate under certain stimuli into osteoblast precursors that then further differentiate into mature osteoblasts. These cells model and repair bone by producing new mineralized bone matrix. Pathways that promote differentiation are in blue; pathways that inhibit this are in red.

bovine and porcine cartilage. Synthetic MMP inhibitors and TIMP-1 are able to prevent this release,[29] strongly implicating the collagenolytic MMPs in this process; chondrocytes are known to synthesize collagenase-1, -2 and -3.

Murine models of RA include one for collagen-induced arthritis, which has been used for many years. The implantation of RA synovial fibroblasts with normal articular cartilage under the renal capsule of SCID mice leads to maintenance of the aggressive phenotype of the synovial fibroblasts that invade the cartilage, whereas OA synovium

does not.[30] Adenoviral delivery of proinflammatory cytokines intra-articularly can also lead to RA-like tissue destruction with concomitant synovial hyperplasia.[31] These models emphasize the role that synovial fibroblasts play in destroying both bone and cartilage in RA, and methods have also been developed in which synovium and cartilage are co-cultured *in vitro*. The interplay between cartilage, bone, and synovium and the different points at which joint destruction can be blocked are illustrated in Figure 17.8. A role for inflammation and factors such as IL-1 in OA progression is now increasingly recognized.

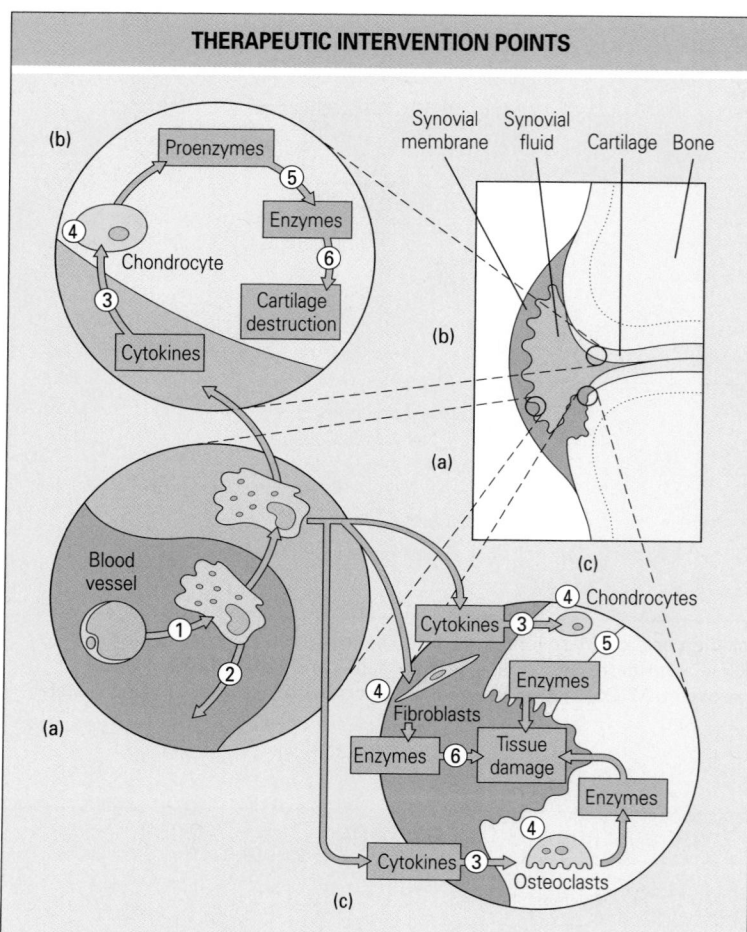

Fig. 17.8 Therapeutic intervention points for preventing connective tissue destruction and cellular mechanisms involved in tissue damage. The destructive cycle of events can be broken in a number of ways, including (a) (1) blocking entry of harmful cells; (2) removal of harmful cells from the joint; (b and c) (3) blocking or mimicking cytokine or growth factor action; (4) blocking intracellular signaling pathways involved in the production of proteinases; (5) preventing activation of proteinases; and (6) direct inhibition of destructive proteinases degrading bone or cartilage. (c) Within the joint, mixtures of cytokines stimulate chondrocytes to release and activate enzymes that damage the cartilage matrix. Within the synovium, fibroblasts, macrophages, and T cells interact to produce tissue damage to bone and cartilage. Released cytokines also activate osteoclasts, leading to the destruction of bone.

Although spontaneous OA animal models are available, surgical instability models are most common in laboratory animals, including dog, guinea pig, rabbit, rat, mouse, sheep, and goat.[32] The advantages of surgical models over spontaneous models include a significantly faster onset of disease with a decrease in both variability and the dependence of genetic background.[33] The two most common models are via either anterior cruciate ligament transection (ACLT) or destabilization of the medial meniscus (DMM), with DMM the suggested model of choice in the mouse.[33] These models in the mouse have allowed the use of transgenic knockout or knock-in animals to provide an insight into the mechanisms that regulate OA pathology.[6,34] Despite these developments, no single model fully replicates human disease, and it is unclear how well any of these resemble the idiopathic OA in the older human population.[6,32]

METALLOPROTEINASE TRANSGENIC MICE IN MODELS OF DISEASE

Targeted gene disruption or knockout (KO) experiments in mice have allowed the investigation of the contribution of individual MMPs to many physiologic and pathologic processes, including arthritis.[35] All

MMP KO mice are embryonically viable, but the MMP-9 KO exhibits an abnormal pattern of skeletal development, the MMP-20 KO shows severe abnormalities in tooth development, and the MMP-14 KO displays severe defects in skeletal development and dies within 3 to 16 weeks of age.

MMP-9 KO mice show developmental abnormalities that involve growth plate and endochondral ossification. Hypertrophic chondrocytes develop normally, but apoptosis, vascularization, and ossification are delayed. MMP-9 appears to be important in the invasive activity of osteoclasts at resorption sites, and mice deficient in MMP-9 exhibit a delay in osteoclast recruitment, although osteoclastic resorption of mineralized matrix still occurs.

MT1-MMP KO causes severe defects in both endochondral and intramembranous bone formations and gives rise to severe connective tissue defects and the development of arthritis. Bone marrow stromal cells from MT1-MMP KO mice show decreased bone formation, suggesting that MT1-MMP may influence the differentiation and activity of osteoblasts. MT1-MMP KO mice also have increased numbers of osteoclasts, suggesting that MT1-MMP may influence the differentiation and recruitment of these cells.

In the development of antibody-induced arthritis (AbIA), an animal model of RA, MMP-2 KO mice show significantly exacerbated arthritis compared with wild-type mice. AbIA could be recovered in the MMP-2 KO mice by injection of wild-type fibroblasts. This suggests a suppressive role for MMP-2 in the progression of AbIA even though MMP-2 is overproduced in the arthritic joint of AbIA in wild-type mice. In contrast to MMP-2 KO mice, MMP-9 KO mice show reduced levels of AbIA, indicating that MMP-9 enhances arthritis in this model. The double KO mice showed no significant difference from the wild-type mice, probably reflecting the effects of both exacerbated arthritis by MMP-2 deficiency and reduced arthritis by MMP-9 deficiency. In AbIA cartilage, erosion was mild even in severely arthritic mice; therefore, the roles of MMP-2 and MMP-9 in cartilage erosion could not be determined. Somewhat counterintuitively, however, in a surgical model of OA (DMM), MMP-9 disruption resulted in more severe OA.

Disruption of the MMP-3 gene has been investigated in several models of arthritis: antigen-induced arthritis (AIA), collagen-induced arthritis (CIA), and the induction of OA by both a collagenase-induced instability model of OA[36] and surgical transection of the medial collateral ligament and partial medial meniscectomy. All studies show no significant differences in either inflammation or proteoglycan depletion between the MMP-3 KO mice and controls. The major MMP cleavage site in aggrecan generates the C-terminal neoepitope VDIPEN. In the AIA model and in collagenase-induced instability models, VDIPEN staining was eliminated or significantly reduced in MMP-3 KO mice, but in CIA and meniscectomized mice, VDIPEN staining was the same as in wild-type mice. MMP-mediated aggrecan cleavage has been further assessed via a knock-in (KI) mouse in which the wild-type cleavage site was altered so as to be impervious to MMP activity. These mice have no developmental problems, implying that MMP-mediated aggrecanolysis is not important in growth plate remodeling. In addition, a lack of growth plate phenotype in KOs for ADAMTS-1, -4 or -5 as well as a KI engineered to resist aggrecanase-mediated aggrecanolysis (the amino-terminal ARGSV neoepitope) supports nonproteolytic mechanisms of aggrecan remodeling in the growth plate.[37] The ADAMTS-4 and ADAMTS-5 KO mice have revealed that ADAMTS-5, at least in mice, plays a major part in tissue turnover in models of OA and inflammatory arthritis.[18,38]

The COL2-3/4C neoepitope (generated by collagenases) was used to detect collagen cleavage, and this was eliminated in the AIA model in MMP-3 KO mice compared with wild-type controls but was unchanged in the meniscectomized model. In the AIA model, MMP-3 appears to have an important role in the mechanisms leading to cleavage of type II collagen. In contrast, the meniscectomized MMP-3 KO mice exhibited accelerated formation of OA lesions compared with that in wild-type mice. These results could suggest that MMP-3 plays an important role in homeostasis in healthy cartilage, balancing anabolism and catabolism of the cartilage matrix, or, alternatively, that the MMP-3 gene is compensated by another similar gene such as MMP-10.

Mice deficient in either TIMP-1 or TIMP-2 exhibit no major phenotype, whereas TIMP-3 KO mice develop a mild but transient OA with increased proteoglycan loss and increased generation of the

VDIPEN neoepitope. As TIMP-3 KO mice age, there is evidence of increased cartilage catabolism; a lack of TIMP-3 will lead to an altered metalloproteinase/TIMP balance, and the higher levels of TNF-α could also be due to a lack of inhibition of the metalloproteinase TNF-α–converting enzyme (TACE).[39]

Studies in KO mice are therefore a powerful approach for defining protein function, and the application of these KO experiments in mouse models of diseases has shown that MMPs serve specific roles in a variety of pathologic processes. These data need to be interpreted carefully because there are significant differences in MMP expression (e.g., MMP-1), gene redundancy, and the distribution of load across joints between mice and humans. However, novel targets for therapeutic intervention can be investigated by using these models.

THERAPEUTIC INHIBITION OF PROTEINASES

The future prospects for the prevention of connective tissue breakdown in the arthritides using synthetic proteinase inhibitors are uncertain. Compounds that inhibit MMPs are the most studied,[9] with the aim of treatment to shift the balance away from matrix degradation to prevent the loss of connective tissue matrix without leading to excess synthesis. Initial problems with the oral availability of MMP inhibitors have been overcome. Despite favorable results in the treatment of some cancers, trials of compounds that inhibit the collagenases in RA patients have not been successful. It may be that the compounds used were unsuitable or that collagenases are not the best target. It is not known if sufficient penetration of cartilage by these compounds was achieved or if their specificity was altered during absorption.

The antibiotic doxycycline and derivatives with no antibiotic activity weakly inhibit MMPs, and these compounds have been licensed for the treatment of periodontal disease. They are also effective in animal models of arthritis and have therefore been proposed as a treatment to prevent cartilage damage. In a randomized placebo-controlled trial of overweight women with unilateral radiographic knee OA, women randomized to doxycycline, 100 mg twice daily, had a 33% reduction in the mean amount of joint space narrowing over 30 months.[40] However, no clinically important differences were noted in symptoms between groups during the study.

It is possible that specific inhibitors of MMPs could be used successfully in the future to halt the progressive and chronic destruction of connective tissue seen in the arthritides. It may be necessary to combine different proteinase inhibitors, either in sequence or with other agents that target different but specific steps in the pathogenesis, before the chronic cycle of joint destruction found in these diseases can be broken (see Fig. 17.8).

Recent interest has begun to focus on compounds that target events before the induction of these destructive genes. Some compounds that block specific signal transduction pathways have been shown to prevent cartilage destruction in vitro. However, more information on the complex interactions that can occur between the different signaling pathways that are activated by the various proinflammatory mediators associated with the arthritides will be required before major advances can be made in this area.[9]

REPAIR OF CONNECTIVE TISSUE MATRIX

Within arthritic tissues there are areas of cartilage in which new matrix synthesis occurs as well as net loss of the extracellular matrix. Growth factors play major roles in regulating normal matrix synthesis and in the processes that protect cartilage in disease. Polypeptide growth factors have direct effects on chondrocytes, and factors such as TGF-β and bone morphogenic proteins (BMPs) are known to be involved in matrix deposition in OA (e.g., osteophyte generation).[41] However, TGF-β is also known to induce MMP-13 expression under some circumstances, and a lack of TGF-β responsiveness with increasing age may also be an important caveat for effective tissue repair in disease. Other factors, such as hormones, corticosteroids, prostaglandins, peptides, or retinoids, may also influence cellular responses to these growth factors.

Cartilage metabolism may be altered by effects on cellular proliferation, migration, or differentiation and the control of individual genes (see Fig. 17.4b). The effect of any particular growth factor will also depend on the differentiation state of the cell. Various types of cells in tissues may respond differently to particular cytokines and growth factors. Other local conditions will affect these responses, such as mechanical loading, oxygen tension, and the presence of other factors (see Fig. 17.4b).

TGF-β and IGF-1 have profound effects on the synthesis of matrix components by chondrocytes.[42] TGF-β can downregulate the production of several matrix-degrading proteinases and upregulate proteinase inhibitors such as TIMP-1 or plasminogen activator inhibitor, suggesting that it may prevent cartilage destruction by both stimulating synthesis and blocking degradative pathways. TGF-β is locally synthesized by chondrocytes, affects protein synthesis, and potentiates the stimulation of DNA synthesis achieved with other growth factors, rather than initiating this itself. IGF-1 mimics many of the actions of TGF-β and has a significant effect on matrix synthesis but does not have the same mitogenic properties or affect protein synthesis to the same extent. Within cartilage, TGF-β and IGF-1 are stored in considerable quantities bound to different matrix components. More recently, connective tissue growth factors and members of the BMP family have been shown to have anabolic effects on cartilage and bone. The source of growth factors will vary. They can be produced by cells outside the cartilage and diffuse in, or they can be produced locally by the chondrocytes. The control mechanisms are complex, and growth factors also exist in a latent form; other proteins, such as IGF-binding proteins, may be present that sequester the factors and prevent them from binding to cellular receptors. The activity of some MMPs can cause the release of growth factors as matrix is degraded. This provides positive feedback mechanisms that redress the balance between degradation and synthesis of matrix components.

Growth factors are recognized as protective to cartilage, stimulating matrix synthesis and blocking the effects of the proinflammatory cytokines. Other factors also protect joint tissues. Interferon-γ inhibits cytokine-stimulated bone resorption and IL-1– or TNF-α–stimulated collagenase production by chondrocytes, as well as reducing IL-1–stimulated prostaglandin release from cartilage. IL-4, IL-13, and IL-10 have all been shown to oppose the effects of these proinflammatory cytokines by blocking MMP secretion or activation and/or increasing inhibitor production and matrix synthesis. Platelet-derived growth factor (PDGF) and basic fibroblast growth factor (bFGF) can also affect cartilage homeostasis by inducing cells to migrate, differentiate, or proliferate. bFGF also stimulates the production of plasminogen activator inhibitors and TIMP-1 in fibroblasts and endothelial cells. All these growth factors are likely to stimulate cartilage repair, and many do not act alone but rather act synergistically to promote new matrix synthesis.

MODELS OF MATRIX REPAIR

Considerable progress has been made in cartilage repair. Defects found in diseased or damaged cartilage can be repaired in model systems after the delivery of agents that will stimulate chondrocytes to synthesize new matrix.[43] Different approaches have been used, including the following:

- The isolation of autologous chondrocytes or stem cells, which are grown and differentiated in culture and then implanted into defects at high density
- Grafting of cartilage into large defects
- Filling of defects with various natural or synthetic polymers
- The addition of growth factors to encourage the migration into the defect and subsequent synthesis of matrix components

Defects in cartilage have been filled with biodegradable matrices that contain low concentrations of a chemotactic or mitogenic factor with a high concentration of TGF-β that is slowly released. Many growth factors have been shown to be effective, including bFGF, PDGF, epidermal growth factor, growth hormone, TGF-β, and IGF-1. A cartilage-like matrix is produced within defects after 6 weeks. Successful induction of cartilage is now achieved in experimental models and could be adapted for clinical use to allow intervention in the disease process. A key issue here is the "quality" of the cartilage matrix generated, and there is an emphasis on ensuring an appropriate ratio of types I and II collagen, where type II should predominate. The potential use of mesenchymal stem cells (non-hematopoietic progenitor cells found in various adult tissues) for tissue engineering to generate replacement tissues to repair joint damage in arthritis is an attractive area of research,[44] but it will still be some time before such stem cell therapies are utilized clinically. However, the successful integration of such matrices with host tissue is often problematic, although advances in regenerative medicine, especially in the area of nanotechnology, have led to novel surface scaffolds for implants that provide specific biofunctionality to better encourage biointegration of implants.[45]

These techniques remain limited because they rely on surgical intervention, which may only be practical in large joints. However, when traumatic injury has resulted in damage to cartilage or when large joints have a discrete and well-defined injury, this procedure may benefit patients by increasing the chances of cartilage repair.

REFERENCES

1. Eyre DR, Weis MA, Wu JJ. Articular cartilage collagen: an irreplaceable framework? Eur Cells Materials 2006;12:57-63.
2. Roughley PJ. The structure and function of cartilage proteoglycans. Eur Cells Materials 2006; 12:92-101.
3. Jubb RW, Fell HB. The breakdown of collagen by chondrocytes. J Pathol 1980;130:159-162.
4. Barrett AJ, Rawlings ND, Woessner JF. Introduction. In: Handbook of proteolytic enzymes. London: Academic Press, 2004:xxxiii-xxxv.
5. Quesada V, Ordóñez GR, Sánchez LM, et al. The Degradome database: mammalian proteases and diseases of proteolysis. Nucleic Acids Res 2009;37(database issue):D239-243.
6. Goldring MB, Otero M, Tsuchimochi K, et al. Defining the roles of inflammatory and anabolic cytokines in cartilage metabolism. Ann Rheum Dis 2008;67(Suppl 3):iii75-iii82.
7. Mott JD, Werb Z. Regulation of matrix biology by matrix metalloproteinases. Curr Opin Cell Biol 2004;16:558-564.
8. Page-McCaw A, Ewald AJ, Werb Z: Matrix metalloproteinases and the regulation of tissue remodelling. Nat Rev Mol Cell Biol 2007;8:221-233.
9. Rowan AD, Litherland GJ, Hui W, Milner JM. Metalloproteinases as potential therapeutic targets in arthritis treatment. Expert Opin Ther Targets 2008;12:1-18.
10. Li J, Brick P, O'Hare MC, et al. Structure of full length porcine synovial collagenase reveals a C-terminal domain containing a calcium-linked four-bladed propeller. Structure 1995;3:541-549.
11. Tetlow LC, Adlam DJ, Woolley DE. Matrix metalloproteinases and proinflammatory cytokine production by chondrocytes of human osteoarthritic cartilage: association with degenerative changes. Arthritis Rheum 2001;44:585-594.
12. Kevorkian L, Young DA, Darrah C, et al. Expression profiling metalloproteinases and their inhibitors in cartilage. Arthritis Rheum 2004;50:4074-4075.
13. Schett G, Zwerina J, Firestein G. The p38 mitogen-activated protein kinase (MAPK) pathway in rheumatoid arthritis. Ann Rheum Dis 2008;67:909-916.
14. Loeser RF, Erickson EA, Long DL. Mitogen-activated protein kinases as therapeutic targets in osteoarthritis. Curr Opin Rheumatol 2008;20:581-586.
15. Milner JM, Patel A, Rowan AD. Emerging roles of serine proteinases in tissue turnover in arthritis. Arthritis Rheum 2008;58:3644-3656.
16. Nagase H, Visse R, Murphy G. Structure and function of matrix metalloproteinases and TIMPs. Cardiovasc Res 2006;69:562-573.
17. Porter S, Clark IM, Kevorkian L, Edwards DR. The ADAMTS metalloproteinases. Biochem J 2005;15:15-27.
18. Stanton H, Rogerson FM, East CJ, et al. ADAMTS5 is the major aggrecanase in mouse cartilage in vivo and in vitro. Nature 2005;434:648-652.
19. Okroj M, Heinegard D, Holmdahl R, Blom AM. Rheumatoid arthritis and the complement system. Ann Med 2007;39:517-530.
20. Mackie EJ, Loh LH, Sivagurunathan S, et al. Protease-activated receptors in the musculoskeletal system. Int J Biochem Cell Biol 2008;40:1169-1184.
21. Vasiljeva O, Reinheckel T, Peters C, et al. Emerging roles of cysteine cathepsins in disease and their potential as drug targets. Curr Pharm Des 2007;13:387-403.
22. Dejica VM, Mort JS, Laverty S, et al. Cleavage of type II collagen by cathepsin K in human osteoarthritic cartilage. Am J Pathol 2008;173:161-169.
23. Sohar N, Hammer H, Sohar I. Lysosomal peptidases and glycosidases in rheumatoid arthritis. Biol Chem 2002;383:865-869.
24. Everts V, Van Der Zee E, Creemers L, Beersten W. Phagocytosis and intracellular digestion of collagen, its role in turnover and remodeling. Histochem J 1996;28:229-245.
25. Walsh NC, Crotti TN, Goldring SR, Gravallese EM. Rheumatic diseases: the effects of inflammation on bone. Immunol Rev 2005;208:228-251.
26. Skoumal M, Haberhauer G, Kolarz G, et al. Serum cathepsin K levels of patients with longstanding rheumatoid arthritis: correlation with radiological destruction. Arthritis Res Ther 2005;7:R65-R70.
27. Morko JP, Soderstrom M, Saamanen AM, et al. Upregulation of cathepsin K expression in articular chondrocytes in a transgenic mouse model for osteoarthritis. Ann Rheum Dis 2004;63:649-655.
28. Schett G, Redlich K, Hayer S, et al. Osteoprotegerin protects against generalized bone loss in tumor necrosis factor-transgenic mice. Arthritis Rheum 2003;48:2042-2051.
29. Koshy PJT, Henderson N, Logan C, et al. Interleukin-17 induces cartilage collagen breakdown: novel synergistic effects in combination with pro-inflammatory cytokines. Ann Rheum Dis 2002;61:704-713.
30. Pierer M, Muller-Ladner U, Pap T, et al. The SCID mouse model: novel therapeutic targets—lessons from gene transfer. Springer Semin Immunopathol 2003;25:65-78.
31. Rowan AD, Hui W, Cawston TE, Richards CD. Adenoviral gene transfer of interleukin-1 in combination with oncostatin M induces significant joint damage in a murine model. Am J Pathol 2003;162:1975-1984.
32. van den Berg WB. Lessons from animal models of osteoarthritis. Curr Rheumatol Rep 2008;10:26-29.
33. Glasson SS, Blanchet TJ, Morris EA. The surgical destabilization of the medial meniscus (DMM) model of osteoarthritis in the 129/SvEv mouse. Osteoarthritis Cartilage 2007;15:1061-1069.
34. Glasson SS. In vivo osteoarthritis target validation utilizing genetically-modified mice. Curr Drug Targets 2007;8:367-376.
35. Milner JM, Cawston TE. Matrix metalloproteinase knockout studies and the potential use of matrix metalloproteinase inhibitors in the rheumatic diseases. Curr Drug Targets Inflamm Allergy 2005;4:636-675.
36. Blom AB, van Lent PL, Libregts S, et al. Crucial role of macrophages in matrix metalloproteinase-mediated cartilage destruction during experimental osteoarthritis: involvement of matrix metalloproteinase 3. Arthritis Rheum 2007;56:147-157.
37. Little CB, Mittaz L, Belluoccio D, et al. ADAMTS-1-knockout mice do not exhibit abnormalities in aggrecan turnover in vitro or in vivo. Arthritis Rheum 2005;52:1461-1472.
38. Glasson SS, Askew R, Sheppard B, et al. Deletion of active ADAMTS5 prevents cartilage degradation in a murine model of osteoarthritis. Nature 2005;434:644-648.
39. Sahebjam S, Khokha R, Mort JS. Increased collagen and aggrecan degradation with age in the joints of Timp3(−/−) mice. Arthritis Rheum 2007;56:905-909.
40. Brandt KD, Mazzuca SA, Katz BP, et al. Effects of doxycycline on progression of osteoarthritis: results of a randomized, placebo-controlled, double-blind trial. Arthritis Rheum 2005;52:1956-1959.
41. Blaney Davidson EN, Vitters EL, van der Kraan PM, van den Berg WB. Expression of transforming growth factor-beta (TGFbeta) and the TGFbeta signalling molecule SMAD-2P in spontaneous and instability-induced osteoarthritis: role in cartilage degradation, chondrogenesis, and osteophyte formation. Ann Rheum Dis 2006;65:1414-1421.
42. Van Der Kraan PM, Buma P, Van Kuppevelt T, Van Den Berg WB. Interaction of chondrocytes, extracellular matrix and growth factors: relevance for articular cartilage tissue engineering. Osteoarthritis Cartilage 2002;10:631-637.
43. Smith GD, Knutsen G, Richardson JB. A clinical review of cartilage repair techniques. J Bone Joint Surg Br 2005;87:445-459.
44. Chen FH, Tuan RS. Mesenchymal stem cells in arthritic diseases. Arthritis Res Ther 2008;10:223.
45. Bonzani IC, George JH, Stevens MM. Novel materials for bone and cartilage regeneration. Curr Opin Chem Biol 2006;10:568-575.

Principles of tissue engineering and cell- and gene-based therapy

18

Ulrich Nöth, Lars Rackwitz, Andre F. Steinert, and Rocky S. Tuan

INTRODUCTION

Tissue engineering and cell-based therapies are rapidly growing disciplines that constitute the principal technologies in the relatively new field of regenerative medicine. These technologies directed toward self-regeneration involve the use of biologically active molecules or biomaterials, application of differentiated or undifferentiated cells, functional tissue engineering, organ transplantation, process technologies, as well as the development of regulatory standards (Fig. 18.1). For the repair of focal articular cartilage defects in the young adult, autologous chondrocyte implantation (ACI) has become an established technique. In contrast, the repair of cartilage lesions arising from rheumatic diseases such as osteoarthritis (OA) or rheumatoid arthritis (RA) represents one of the greatest challenges in orthopedic surgery. The fundamental cause of this challenge is the inflammatory environment that drives the competing anabolic and catabolic processes toward extensive joint and cell-transplant degradation. As a result of intensive research in the past 2 decades, adult mesenchymal stem cells (MSCs) have emerged as a promising candidate cell type for the treatment of rheumatic diseases, owing to their well-characterized ability to differentiate along the chondrogenic pathway and their recently demonstrated anti-inflammatory as well as immune suppressive properties through trophic mediators.

TISSUE ENGINEERING

Tissue engineering is an interdisciplinary research approach that aims for replacement of injured or degenerated human tissues to restore their form, structure, and function, by combining principles and methods of engineering sciences, cell and molecular biology, and clinical medicine.[1,2] From its beginning in the early 1990s, "tissue engineering" has developed into its own scientific and clinical discipline that complements the field of "regenerative medicine," with potential application for almost every tissue of the human body. The central dogma of tissue engineering states that a target-tissue specific template for replacing injured or degenerated tissue relies on three principal components: cells, cell carriers (scaffolds), and external stimuli (e.g., growth factors or mechanobiologic stimuli) (Fig. 18.2).

In the context of tissue engineering, the basic function of the scaffold is to provide a temporary structure for the seeded cells to adhere and subsequently to synthesize new native extracellular matrix (ECM) in a shape and form guided by the scaffold. The main criteria for scaffold design include controlled biodegradability, suitable mechanical strength, and appropriate surface chemistry, as well as the ability to regulate cellular activities, such as proliferation, cell-cell and cell-matrix interactions, and directed differentiation.[3,4] Scaffolds can be manufactured from native or synthetic polymers, with native materials, such as collagen, fibrin, or hyaluronan, exhibiting optimal biocompatibility and biodegradability, whereas synthetic polymers, such as polyglycolic acid (PGA), polylactic acid (PLA), their copolymer poly(lactic-co-glycolic acid) (PLGA), and poly-ε-caprolactone (PCL), have higher primary stability and are more accessible for macro-/microstructure formation. A key requirement for a tissue engineering scaffold is an optimal porosity to facilitate nutrition, proliferation, and migration of cells and to ensure cell colonization of the entire carrier. Although primary, tissue-specific cells (i.e., chondrocytes) are inherently the most suitable cell source for cartilage tissue engineering, they have limitations in practice because of the shortage of supply, loss of phenotype during expansion culture, and potential donor-site morbidity after harvest.[5]

AUTOLOGOUS CHONDROCYTE IMPLANTATION

An established procedure for the treatment of symptomatic chondral or osteochondral defects of the knee joint guided by the principles of tissue engineering is the first generation of autologous chondrocyte implantation (ACI), originally developed by Brittberg and coworkers 2 decades ago.[6] ACI requires two surgical interventions. First, a cartilage biopsy is taken arthroscopically from a small, non–load-bearing area. After enzymatic isolation and chondrocyte expansion in culture *in vitro*, a second surgical procedure is performed involving knee joint exposure via an arthrotomy, débridement of the cartilage defect, and suturing of a periosteal patch/collagen membrane over the defect to obtain a cavity in which the culture-expanded chondrocytes can be injected and secured by sealing with fibrin glue. The long-term results of this technique exhibit predominantly good to very good clinical results in more than 70% of the patients[7] and reveal superior results when compared with a sole débridement or osteochondral cylinder transplantation (OCT).[8]

However, in spite of these encouraging results, ACI exhibits several disadvantages that have to be addressed. The use of periosteum can result in transplant hypertrophy, calcification, and delamination,[9] and the cell suspension has the potential to leak, thus compromising the development of sufficient neo-tissue at the defect site. Given these shortcomings, recent experimental and clinical research has been directed toward the development of matrix-associated procedures of ACI (MACI), whereby biocompatible scaffolds are used as a vehicle for secure delivery of primary chondrocytes to the defect site. Today, clinical experience and promising clinical outcome data using type I collagen membranes or hydrogels, a co-polymer of PGA/PLA, Polyglactin/Vicryl, and polydioxanone, and hyaluronic acid has been reported.[10] For example, the utilization of a type I collagen hydrogel, which minimizes potential chondrocyte dedifferentiation, as seen in monolayer, by providing a 3D environment subsequent to enzymatic cell isolation, results in a homogeneous cell distribution and promotes cartilage-specific cell differentiation and ECM deposition within the scaffold.[11]

In contrast to the surgical treatment of focal articular cartilage lesions, which can result from acute injury or osteochondrosis dissecans, reparative or regenerative approaches for the treatment of OA or RA must take into consideration that cartilage damage arises from an underlying disease process. It is noteworthy that acute cartilage injury and osteochondrosis dissecans often take place in an otherwise healthy joint. The patient may be young and thus a localized treatment may be sufficient to repair the focal defect. On the other hand, in OA and RA, the patient is likely to be older and thus requires the treatment of at least one compartment or the entire articulating surface. Also, inflammatory conditions in the joint are likely to result in degradation of any engineered cartilage. Consequently, unless the underlying disease is treated effectively and technologies are available to restore whole compartments, any cell-based treatment in OA and RA is unlikely to be of long-term benefit.

MESENCHYMAL STEM CELLS

The advantage of adult MSCs, potentially overcoming the shortcomings of chondrocytes, is that they can easily be obtained from a bone marrow aspirate or other mesodermally derived tissues, possess high expansion capacity, and are able to differentiate into a number of mesenchymal lineages.[12] In particular, MSCs have been shown to undergo efficient chondrogenic differentiation *in vitro* and *in vivo*.[4,13]

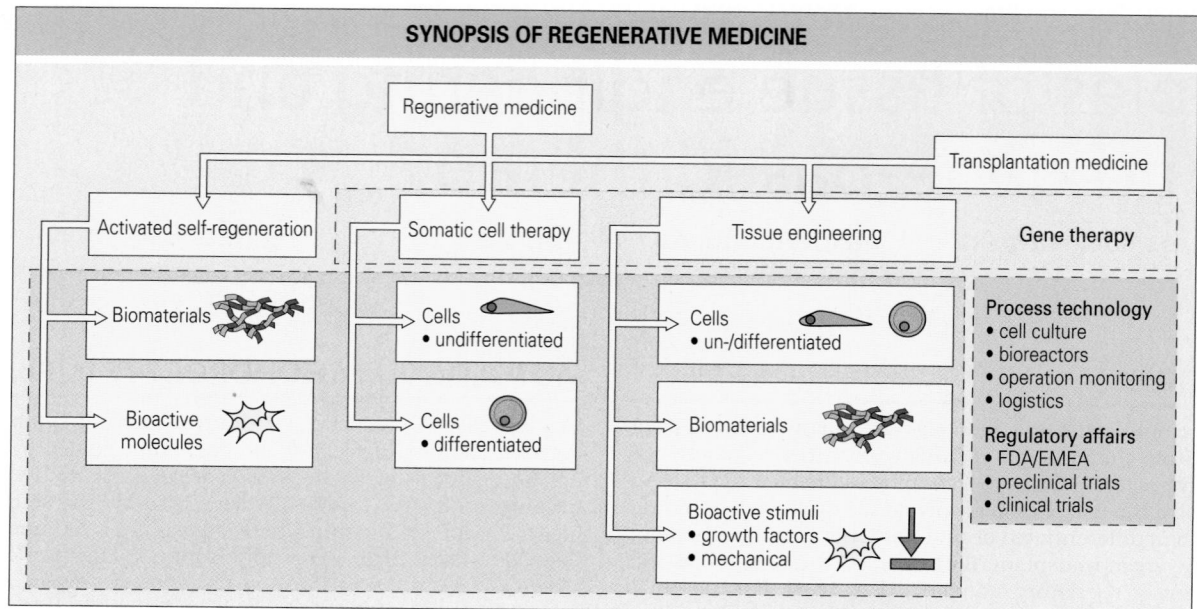

Fig. 18.1 Principal technologies of regenerative medicine aim for the reconstruction of damaged or diseased human tissue and organ function.

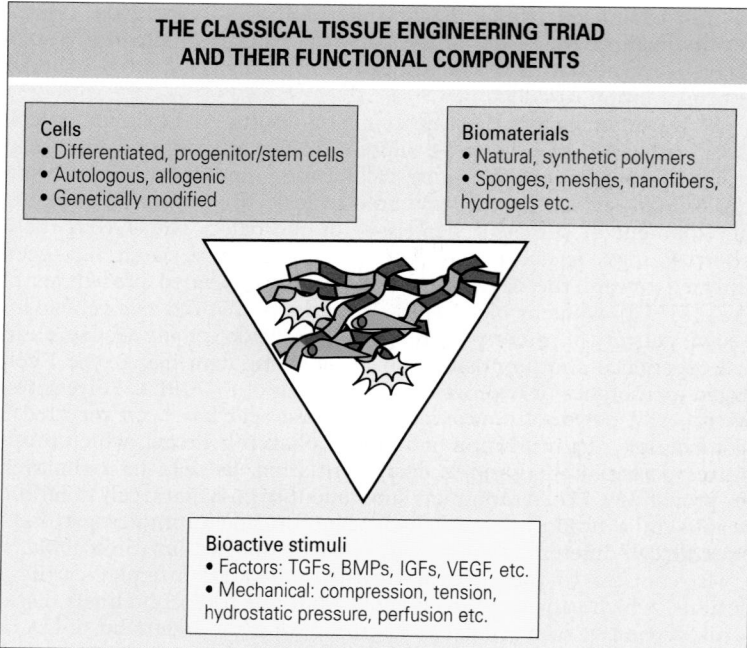

Fig. 18.2 The classical tissue engineering triad and its functional components.

MSCs are commonly isolated from tissue-derived cell mixture by virtue of their avid adherence to cell culture plastic substrate and/or density-gradient fractionation and are therefore intrinsically a heterogeneous cell population. Although no definitive MSC marker(s) has been identified, an immunophenotype positive for STRO-1, CD73, CD146, and CD106 and negative for CD11b, CD45, CD34, CD31, and CD117 has been shown to most reliably characterize the MSC population.[4,13] For the purpose of cartilage regeneration, extensive analyses of microenvironments that promote chondrogenesis in MSCs *in vitro* have been performed. Conditioning the culture medium with growth factors such as fibroblast growth factor-2 (FGF-2) or transforming growth factor-β (TGF-β) during monolayer expansion enhances positive selection for chondroprogenitor cells.[14] The development of effective methods to maintain an articular cartilage phenotype without hypertrophy, ossification, or fibrinogenesis and a delivery system to localize the cells within a lesion without compromising their chondrogenic differentiation or the integrity of the repair tissue are additional requirements for the use of MSCs in articular cartilage regeneration.[15]

Intra-articular injection of mesenchymal stem cells

Intra-articular injection of MSCs into the joint space is, at least conceptually, the simplest approach for their application in rheumatic diseases (Fig. 18.3a). After delivery, MSCs should be distributed throughout the joint space to interact with all available receptive cells and surfaces. Because the synovium lines all the internal surfaces of the joint space, except for cartilage and meniscus, and is highly cellular, it is likely to be a primary tissue for interaction with MSCs.

Only few studies on the direct intra-articular injection of MSCs using animal models of OA have been performed so far. One study describes the delivery of autologous MSCs via a dilute solution of sodium hyaluronan (HA) in knee joints using a goat OA model, induced by a total medial meniscectomy and resection of the anterior cruciate ligament.[16] In cell-treated joints there was evidence of marked regeneration of the medial meniscus and implanted cells were detected in the newly formed tissue. Articular cartilage degeneration, osteophytic remodeling, and subchondral sclerosis also were reduced. There was no evidence of repair of the ligament in any of the joints. Whether the changes observed in the MSC-treated joints result from repair tissue formation by the transplanted cells or the interaction of MSCs with host synovial fibroblasts at the site of injury remains unclear.

In another study, a freshly created partial thickness cartilage defect in the knee joint of the mini pig was treated with a direct intra-articular injection of MSC suspended in sodium hyaluronan.[17] The results demonstrated that the cell-treated group showed improved cartilage healing compared with the control group without cells. The authors postulated that sodium hyaluronan might facilitate the migration and adherence of MSCs or MSC-like cells, probably derived from the synovium, to the defect. This may possibly explain the fact that groups treated with sodium hyaluronan alone demonstrated some form of partial healing at 6 weeks. However, this repair tissue was of inferior quality, possibly due to insufficient MSCs localized to the site of injury, and this was shown to further deteriorate by 12 weeks.

Matrix-guided application of mesenchymal stem cells

A more controlled method of cell application to restore the eroded cartilage surface is via a scaffold (see Fig. 18.3a). Seeding MSCs onto or into a scaffold, such as a biodegradable template, for proliferation and matrix production offers the advantage of providing an accessible, easy-to-manipulate, self-renewing source of otherwise spatially limited progenitor cells.

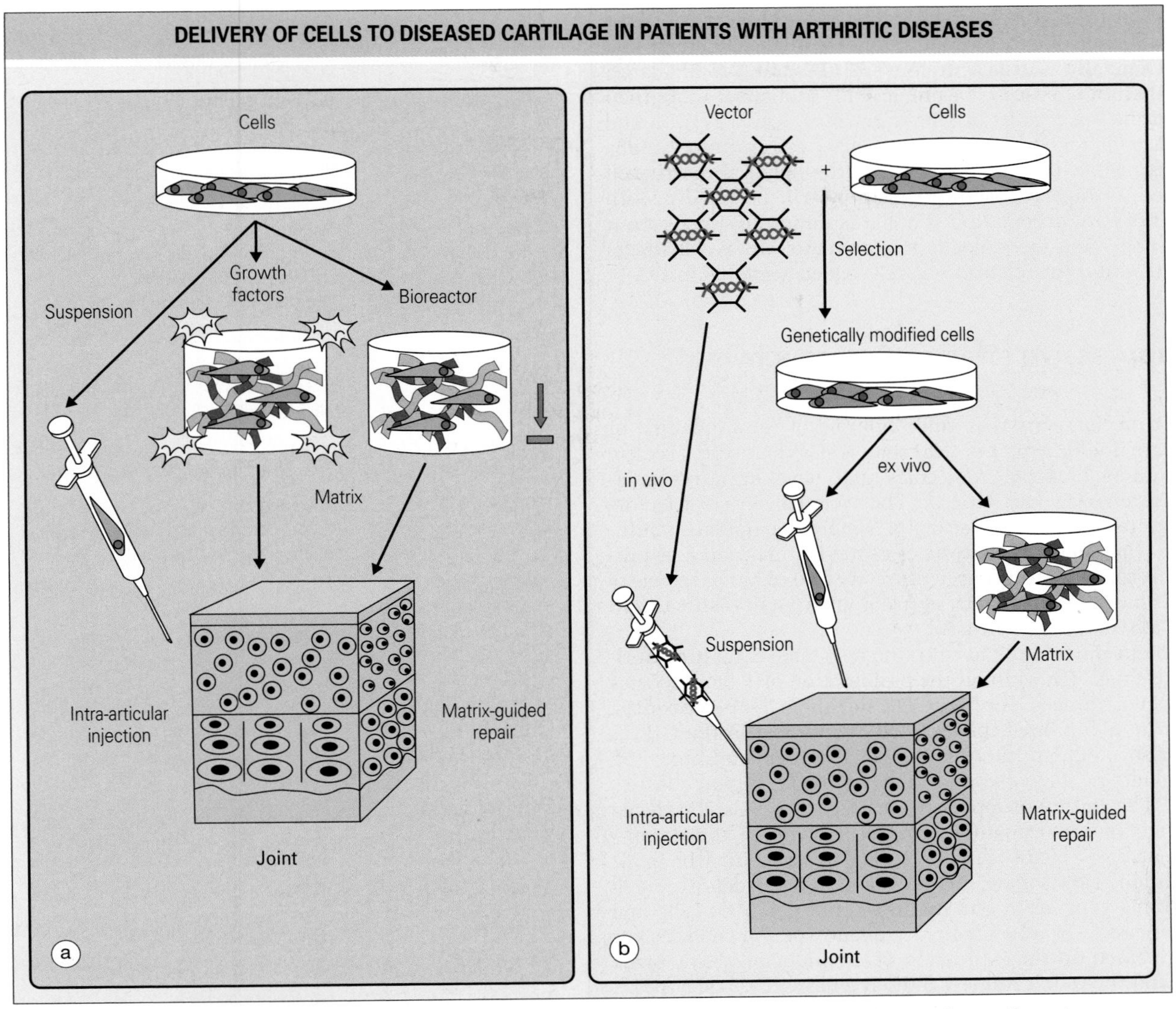

Fig. 18.3 Delivery of cells to diseased cartilage in patients with arthritic diseases. (a) Cell-based therapy for cartilage tissue engineering. Cells in suspension can be injected directly into the joint cavity, where they encounter all intra-articular tissues and might function via trophic mediators and exhibit chondroprotective or regenerative effects. Otherwise, cells (i.e., MSCs/chondrocytes) can be implanted in a matrix-guided manner into the cartilage defect after *ex-vivo* conditioning with biochemical and/or biomechanical stimulation. (b) Gene therapy approach for cartilage tissue engineering. Vectors can be directly injected in an intra-articular mode for *in-vivo* gene delivery, or primary cells are used as vehicles for *ex-vivo* gene delivery. In the latter, successfully transduced cells can be applied to the joint cavity either by intra-articular injection as a suspension or seeded within a matrix that can be implanted into a cartilage defect. Depending on which delivery approach is chosen, ubiquitous or local transgene expression is induced by the *ex-vivo* genetically modified cells or by resident cells that are transduced via intra-articular vector application.

Synthetic scaffolds

Synthetic scaffolds offer the advantage of manipulability in design, such as fiber diameter, pore size, degradation time, and reproducibility in production. Many commonly studied synthetic scaffolds in cartilage repair are fabricated using α-hydroxy polyesters, including PGA, PLA, the copolymer PLGA, and PCL.[18-20] The topography and material properties of these scaffolds play an important role in their ability to support MSC differentiation; for example, nanofibrous scaffold of biodegradable polymers demonstrates enhanced support of MSC proliferative and multilineage differentiative activities.[19,21]

Natural scaffolds

On the other hand, native biomaterials, including collagen type I, hyaluronic acid, chitosan, and alginate[3,22] offer the advantage of presenting a more natural microenvironment. These matrices are biodegradable, can be metabolized by the cells via the action of endogenous collagenases, elicit very limited, if any, inflammatory reaction, and offer a 3D surrounding with material properties similar to those in hyaline cartilage. In particular, collagen gels may be formed to adapt to any desired defect shape. Compared with meshes or fleeces, where cell seeding is often limited to mostly the superficial regions of the scaffold material, seeding in hydrogels permits even distribution of MSCs, thus promoting homogeneous ECM production.[11]

The first clinical results for the transplantation of MSCs seeded with collagen type I hydrogels for the repair of isolated full-thickness cartilage defects were reported by Wakatani and associates.[23] Two patients with a patella defect were treated with collagen gel MSC-constructs, which were covered with a periosteal flap, and fibrocartilaginous defect filling was found after 1 year, as well as a significantly improved patient outcome in the respective follow-ups after 1, 4, and 5 years. In another case report from the same group,[24] a full-thickness cartilage defect in the weight-bearing area of the medial femoral condyle was treated. Histologically, the defect was filled with a hyaline-like type of cartilage tissue, which stained positively with safranin O. One year after surgery, the clinical symptoms had improved significantly.

It is noteworthy that these pilot studies have been performed on isolated or focal articular cartilage defects in an otherwise healthy joint. A very different microenvironment exists as a result of loss of joint homeostasis in OA and thus will influence MSC engraftment and tissue differentiation. The potential role and success of matrix-based cell transplantation in an RA diseased joint is still unclear, as is the impact of the influence of this procedure on disease development and progression.[22] Generally, cartilage lesions in OA and RA are large, unconfined, and often opposed ("kissing lesion") and affect more than one location. In the knee joint, kissing lesions are regularly seen and are frequently accompanied by a varus or valgus deformity or patella maltracking. Because of the direct contact of the opposed matrix-cell transplants, there is high probability that they will be rapidly worn down as a result of joint articulation. Thus it is important to point out that current biologic and technologic developments are as yet inadequate to indicate sufficient retention of cell-loaded scaffolds in OA or RA lesions.

Immune suppressive effects of mesenchymal stem cells

While the exact mechanisms that guide homing of the implanted or mobilized cells are not known, it is clear that MSCs themselves secrete a broad spectrum of bioactive molecules that have immunoregulatory[25,26] and/or regenerative activities.[27] The secreted bioactive factors have been shown to inhibit tissue scarring, suppress apoptosis, stimulate angiogenesis, and enhance mitosis of tissue-intrinsic stem or progenitor cells. This complex, multifaceted activity caused by the secretory activity of MSCs has been referred to as "trophic activity," distinct from the capacity of MSCs to differentiate.[28]

MSCs are potent modulators of immune response, exhibiting antiproliferative capacities. They inhibit the proliferation of T lymphocytes induced by allogens, mitogens, or anti-CD3 and anti-CD28 antibodies. T-cell proliferation is inhibited through cell cycle arrest in the G0/G1 phase.[29] They also modulate the function of the major immune cell populations including CD8+ cytotoxic T lymphocyte, B lymphocytes, and NK cells.[30] The immunosuppressive activity of MSCs is induced by a combination of inflammatory cytokines including interferon-γ (IFN-γ), tumor necrosis factor-α (TNF-α), and interleukin (IL)-1α or IL-1β.[31] In addition, MSCs have significant effects on dendritic cell function by altering generation and maturation of dendritic cells and skewing their function toward a regulatory phenotype.[32] Two other key mechanisms are based on the expression of the inducible nitric oxide (NO) synthase and the indoleamine 2,3-dioxygenase (IDO) enzymes.[33] Another important mediator of immunosuppression secreted by MSCs is HLA-G. HLA-G is a non-classic HLA class I molecule, shown to suppress proliferation of CD4+ T cell, induce apoptosis of CD8+ T cells, and inhibit natural killer (NK) cells.[34] In addition to T cells, B cells also play a major role in the pathogenesis of RA. MSCs can modulate B-cell responses depending on the ratio of both cell types. Indeed, at low ratio, MSCs inhibit the proliferation and activation of B cells, similar to their effect on T cells.[35]

GENE TRANSFER STRATEGIES

Recent advances in cellular, molecular and developmental biology have led to the identification of various gene products that might serve as therapeutic agents for treating rheumatic disorders, some of which are listed in Table 18.1. However, harnessing such factors for clinical use is frequently hindered by their short half-lives, which make them difficult to administer and maintain at functional concentrations for therapeutic effects. Furthermore, certain factors, such as transcription factors, signal transduction molecules, or regulatory RNAs function intracellularly; because cells cannot normally import these molecules, they cannot be readily delivered in soluble form. Gene transfer offers an effective approach to deliver such molecules.

Because exogenous DNA is not spontaneously taken up and expressed by cells in an efficient manner, genes have to be transferred to cells with the aid of vehicles or vectors. These can be assigned to two broad categories: those that are derived from viruses and those that are not. Viral gene delivery is known as transduction, and virus vectors being used in human clinical trials include retrovirus, adenovirus, adeno-associated virus (AAV), and herpes simplex virus. The key features of any viral vector include its host range, ability to infect nondividing cells, ease and cost of production, immunogenicity, whether it integrates into the host genomic DNA, titer, and safety. Overall, it can be stated that no good universal vector exists; instead, the choice

TABLE 18.1 GENE PRODUCTS FOR CARTILAGE RESTORATION AND PROTECTION IN RHEUMATIC DISEASES

Therapeutic target	Gene product (examples)
Chondrogenic induction	Growth factors (e.g., TGF-βs, BMPs, Wnts) Signal transduction molecules (e.g., Smads) Transcription factors (e.g., SOXs, brachyury)
Osteogenic inhibition	Osteogenic inhibitors (e.g., noggin, chordin) Inhibitors of chondrocyte terminal differentiation (e.g., PTHrP, IHH, SHH, DHH) Signal transduction molecules (e.g., Smad 6, 7, mLAP-1)
Apoptosis inhibition	Caspase inhibitors (e.g., Bcl-2, Bcl-XL) FasL blockers (e.g., anti-FasL) NO-induced apoptosis inducers (e.g., Akt, PI-3-kinase) TNF-α, TRAIL-inhibitors (e.g., NF-κB)
Senescence inhibition	Inhibitors of telomere erosion (e.g., hTERT) Free radical antagonists (e.g., NO-antagonists, SOD)
Cartilage matrix synthesis	Growth factors (e.g., TGF-βs, BMPs, IGF-1) ECM component (e.g., collagen type II) Enzymes for GAG synthesis (e.g., GlcAT-1)
Inflammation protection	Cytokine antagonists (e.g., IL-1ra, sIL-1R, sTNFR, anti-TNF-Abs) Proteinase inhibitors (e.g., TIMP1, TIMP2) Anti-inflammatory cytokines (e.g., IL-4, IL-10, IL-11, IL-13) Enzymes inhibiting IL-1 (e.g., GFAT)

TABLE 18.2 VECTOR SYSTEMS FOR GENE DELIVERY APPLICATIONS FOR ARTHRITIC DISEASES

Vector	Comment
Non-viral	Overall weak efficiency, transient, many inflammatory
Adenovirus	High efficiency, transient, inflammatory
Adeno-associated virus	Moderate efficiency, safe, clinical trial for RA
Herpes simplex virus	High efficiency, cytotoxic, transient
Retrovirus	Long-term expression, clinical trial for RA, safety concern
Lentivirus	High efficiency, safety concerns
Spumavirus	Moderate efficiency, no known disease in humans, not yet used in joints

of vector depends on the target application. Non-viral gene transfer is known as transfection and may be as simple as delivery of naked, plasmid DNA or via polymers or delivery by applying biophysical methods, such as electroporation. In general terms, non-viral vectors are less expensive, safer, and simpler than viral vectors but are considerably less efficient. Some of the specific advantages and disadvantages of each available vector system are listed in Table 18.2 and have been reviewed extensively elsewhere.[36] Of note in this context is the occurrence of insertional mutagenesis during human gene therapy trials that has impeded the further use of oncoretroviruses in nonlethal and nonmendelian diseases.[37]

Regardless of the vector, genes may be transferred to their targets by *in-vivo* or *ex-vivo* strategies, the principles of which are illustrated in Figure 18.3. In general, *ex-vivo* approaches are more invasive, expensive, and technically tedious. However, they permit control and expansion of the transduced cells, as well as exhaustive safety testing before reimplantation. *In-vivo* gene transfer entails direct administration of the vector to the body either locally or systemically. It is technically simpler and less expensive but raises safety concerns, because of the direct application of infectious or transfecting agents. The merits of all these strategies in rheumatic diseases depend on a number of variables, including the anatomy and physiology of the target organ(s), the extent of cartilage damage, the pathophysiology of the underlying disease, and the specific features of the gene product, target cell, and vector, among others.

Rheumatoid arthritis

The application of gene transfer to joints was pioneered by Evans and coworkers as a means to treat arthritic disorders.[38,39] For the treatment of RA, biologic therapies that suppress the activities of proinflammatory cytokines such as TNF-α or IL-1β have shown efficacy. However, such therapies are expensive and require repeated administration; only fewer than half of patients achieve a robust therapeutic response, and the issue of side effects remains of concern. Gene therapy offers an alternative approach for the targeted, sustained, and efficient delivery of anti-inflammatory biologic agents.[40] Experimental approaches of this technology have focused on evaluation of methods for gene delivery and identification of appropriate anti-arthritic genes. Although systemic gene delivery was initially considered as an option, most attention has been focused on local, intra-articular administration using ex-vivo and in-vivo modes of gene delivery (see Fig. 18.3). Genes encoding certain anti-inflammatory cytokines such as IL-4, IL-10, and IL-13, antagonists of IL-1 and TNF, or anti-angiogenic proteins have shown efficacy in several animal models of RA (see Table 18.1).[40-46]

Collectively, these studies have established a convincing proof of principle that has led to the development of human gene therapy protocols for RA, seven of which have entered the clinic.[47] The first clinical protocol selected an IL-1 blocker, the IL-1 receptor antagonist (IL-1ra), as the transgene,[39] which was delivered in ex-vivo fashion, using a retrovirus, to the metacarpophalangeal joints of nine individuals with severe RA. This phase I trial was successfully completed without incident, and the procedure was well tolerated by all nine patients included.[38] Although this phase I study was not designed to determine efficacy, intra-articular gene delivery and transgene expression was detected in all joints treated.[38,39] Another phase I protocol almost similar to the just mentioned one that included one patient has been completed in Düsseldorf, Germany,[48] with results very similar to those from the trial in Pittsburgh. A phase I protocol involving the direct, intra-articular injection of a recombinant AAV2 vector into 15 individuals carrying a cDNA encoding a fusion protein comprising two TNF soluble receptors (sTNF-R) combined on an immunoglobulin molecule is now closed and was converted to a first phase II clinical trial using the same vector.[47] This was temporarily halted by the U.S. Food and Drug Administration (FDA) owing to the death of one individual enrolled in the study from a severe histoplasmosis infection.[37] However, the FDA determined that the vector was not to blame and allowed the trial to continue.[47] The only clinical trial of gene therapy in RA using non-viral gene delivery employs the genetic synovectomy approach using DNA encoding the herpes simplex thymidine kinase gene, with one individual treated.[49] This trial is now closed. Two other phase I trials in Korea and the United States involved the use of ex-vivo delivery of TGF-β1 via retrovirus vectors, and 16 individuals have been enrolled without adverse events thus far.[37] It remains to be seen how the clinical results of a genetic synovectomy compare with those of conventional synovectomy.

Osteoarthritis

Because IL-1 is also an important mediator for cartilage breakdown in OA, its inhibitors have been considered likewise useful targets for gene interventions. Several animal studies confirmed the promise of IL-1ra gene delivery in treating OA.[50] Ex-vivo delivery of IL-1ra cDNA via retrovirus vectors and direct delivery of IL-1ra via plasmid DNA to osteoarthritic knee joints of dogs[51] and rabbits,[44] respectively, were shown to slow cartilage loss. Remarkably, in a similar study in horses exploring the effects of adenoviral-mediated gene delivery of IL-1Ra in experimental OA, reduced lameness of the horses receiving gene therapy was observed.[52] Of note is that the localized pathology in OA makes it better suited for local, intra-articular delivery of gene transfer vectors compared with RA, where a systemic condition is typically present. However, in late stages of human OA, it is highly likely that arresting the progress of the disease with an anti-inflammatory and chondroprotective gene, such as IL-1ra, is insufficient. In addition, it may be necessary to repair damaged cartilage, possibly using the gene therapy approaches to restore full joint function, which has been extensively reviewed elsewhere.[5,53]

KEY REFERENCES

1. Langer R, Vacanti JP. Tissue engineering. Science 1993;260:920-926.
2. Vacanti JP, Langer R. Tissue engineering: the design and fabrication of living replacement devices for surgical reconstruction and transplantation. Lancet 1999;354:132-134.
3. Kuo CK, Li WJ, Mauck RL, et al. Cartilage tissue engineering: its potential and uses. Curr Opin Rheum 2006;18:64-73.
4. Chen FH, Rousche KT, Tuan RS. Technology insight: adult stem cells in cartilage regeneration and tissue engineering. Nat Clin Pract Rheumatol 2006;2:373-382.
5. Nöth U, Steinert AF, Tuan RS. Technology insight: adult mesenchymal stem cells for osteoarthritis therapy. Nat Clin Pract Rheumatol 2008;4:371-380.
6. Brittberg M, Lindahl A, Nilsson A, et al. Treatment of deep cartilage defects in the knee with autologous chondrocyte transplantation. N Engl J Med 1994;331:889-895.
7. Peterson L, Minas T, Brittberg M, et al. Treatment of osteochondritis dissecans of the knee with autologous chondrocyte transplantation: results at two to ten years. J Bone Joint Surg Am 2003;85:17-24.
8. Horas U, Pelinkovic D, Herr G, et al. Autologous chondrocyte implantation and osteochondral cylinder transplantation in cartilage repair of the knee joint: a prospective, comparative trial. J Bone Joint Surg Am 2003;85:185-192.
9. Niemeyer P, Pestka JM, Kreuz PC, et al. Characteristic complications after autologous chondrocyte implantation for cartilage defects of the knee joint. Am J Sports Med 2008;36:2091-2099.
10. Iwasa J, Engebretsen L, Shima Y, et al. Clinical application of scaffolds for cartilage tissue engineering. Knee Surg Sports Traumatol Arthrosc 2009;17:561-577.
11. Nöth U, Rackwitz L, Heymer A, et al. Chondrogenic differentiation of human mesenchymal stem cells in collagen type I hydrogels. J Biomed Mater Res A 2007;83:626-635.

12. Pittenger MF, Mackay AM, Beck SC, et al. Multilineage potential of adult human mesenchymal stem cells. Science 1999;284:143-147.
13. Kolf CM, Cho E, Tuan RS. Mesenchymal stromal cells: biology of adult mesenchymal stem cells: regulation of niche, self-renewal and differentiation. Arthritis Res Ther 2007;9:204.
14. Im GI, Jung NH, Tae SK. Chondrogenic differentiation of mesenchymal stem cells isolated from patients in late adulthood: the optimal conditions of growth factors. Tissue Eng 2006;12:527-536.
15. Steinert AF, Ghivizzani SC, Rethwilm A, et al. Major biological obstacles for persistent cell-based regeneration of articular cartilage. Arthritis Res Ther 2007;9:213.
16. Murphy JM, Fink DJ, Hunziker EB, et al. Stem cell therapy in a caprine model of osteoarthritis. Arthritis Rheum 2003;48:3464-3474.
17. Lee KB, Hui JH, Song IC, et al. Injectable mesenchymal stem cell therapy for large cartilage defects—a porcine model. Stem Cells 2007;25:2964-2971.
18. Nöth U, Tuli R, Osyczka AM, et al. In-vitro engineered cartilage constructs produced by press-coating biodegradable polymer with human mesenchymal stem cells. Tissue Eng 2002;8:131-144.
19. Li WJ, Jiang YJ, Tuan RS. Chondrocyte phenotype in engineered fibrous matrix is regulated by fiber size. Tissue Eng 2006;12:1775-1785.
20. Terada S, Yoshimoto H, Fuchs JR, et al. Hydrogel optimization for cultured elastic chondrocytes seeded onto a polyglycolic acid scaffold. J Biomed Mater Res A 2005;75:907-916.
21. Li WJ, Tuli R, Huang X, et al. Multilineage differentiation of human mesenchymal stem cells in a three-dimensional nanofibrous scaffold. Biomaterials 2005;26:5158-5166.
22. Nesic D, Whiteside R, Brittberg M, et al. Cartilage tissue engineering for degenerative joint disease. Adv Drug Deliv Rev 2006;58:300-322.

23. Wakitani S, Mitsuoka T, Nakamura N, et al. Autologous bone marrow stromal cell transplantation for repair of full-thickness articular cartilage defects in human patellae: two case reports. Cell Transplant 2004;13:595-600.
24. Kuroda R, Ishida K, Matsumoto T, et al. Treatment of a full-thickness articular cartilage defect in the femoral condyle of an athlete with autologous bone-marrow stromal cells. Osteoarthritis Cartilage 2007;15:226-231.
25. Chen X, Armstrong MA, Li G. Mesenchymal stem cells in immunoregulation. Immunol Cell Biol 2006;84:413-421.
26. Uccelli A, Pistoia V, Moretta L. Mesenchymal stem cells: a new strategy for immunosuppression? Trends Immunol 2007;28:219-226.
27. Kan I, Melamed E, Offen D. Autotransplantation of bone marrow-derived stem cells as a therapy for neurodegenerative diseases. Handb Exp Pharmacol 2007;(180):219-242.
28. Caplan AI, Dennis JE. Mesenchymal stem cells as trophic mediators. J Cell Biochem 2006;98:1076-1084.
29. Jones S, Horwood N, Cope A, et al. The antiproliferative effect of mesenchymal stem cells is a fundamental property shared by all stromal cells. J Immunol 2007;179:2824-2831.
30. Noël D, Djouad F, Bouffi C, et al. Multipotent mesenchymal stromal cells and immune tolerance. Leuk Lymphoma 2007;48:1283-1289.
31. Ren G, Zhang L, Zhao X, et al. Mesenchymal stem cell-mediated immunosuppression occurs via concerted action of chemokines and nitric oxide. Cell Stem Cell 2008;2:141-150.
32. Djouad F, Charbonnier LM, Bouffi C, et al. Mesenchymal stem cells inhibit the differentiation of dendritic cells through an interleukin-6-dependent mechanism. Stem Cells 2007;25:2025-2032.
33. Alexander AM, Crawford M, Bertera S, et al. Indoleamine 2,3-dioxygenase expression in transplanted NOD Islets prolongs graft survival after adoptive transfer of diabetogenic splenocytes. Diabetes 2002;51:356-365.

34. Selmani Z, Naji A, Zidi I, et al. Human leukocyte antigen-G5 secretion by human mesenchymal stem cells is required to suppress T lymphocyte and natural killer function and to induce CD4+CD25highFOXP3+ regulatory T cells. Stem Cells 2008;26:212-222.

35. Corcione A, Benvenuto F, Ferretti E, et al. Human mesenchymal stem cells modulate B-cell functions. Blood 2006;107:367-372.

36. Thomas CE, Ehrhardt A, Kay MA. Progress and problems with the use of viral vectors for gene therapy. Nat Rev Genet 2003;4:346-358.

37. Evans CH, Ghivizzani SC, Robbins PD. Arthritis gene therapy's first death. Arthritis Res Ther 2008;10:110.

38. Evans CH, Robbins PD, Ghivizzani SC, et al. Gene transfer to human joints: progress toward a gene therapy of arthritis. Proc Natl Acad Sci U S A 2005;102:8698-8703.

39. Evans CH, Robbins PD, Ghivizzani SC, et al. Clinical trial to assess the safety, feasibility, and efficacy of transferring a potentially anti-arthritic cytokine gene to human joints with rheumatoid arthritis. Hum Gene Ther 1996;7:1261-1280.

40. Evans CH, Ghivizzani SC, Robbins PD. Progress and prospects: genetic treatments for disorders of bones and joints. Gene Ther 2009;16:944-952.

41. Ghivizzani SC, Kang R, Georgescu HI, et al. Constitutive intra-articular expression of human IL-1 beta following gene transfer to rabbit synovium produces all major pathologies of human rheumatoid arthritis. J Immunol 1997;159:3604-3612.

42. Ghivizzani SC, Lechman ER, Kang R, et al. Direct adenovirus-mediated gene transfer of interleukin 1 and tumor necrosis factor alpha soluble receptors to rabbit knees with experimental arthritis has local and distal anti-arthritic effects. Proc Natl Acad Sci U S A 1998;95:4613-4618.

43. Ghivizzani SC, Oligino TJ, Glorioso JC, et al. Direct gene delivery strategies for the treatment of rheumatoid arthritis. Drug Discov Today 2001;6:259-267.

44. Fernandes J, Tardif G, Martel-Pelletier J, et al. In vivo transfer of interleukin-1 receptor gene in osteoarthritic rabbit knee joints: prevention of osteoarthritis progression. Am J Physiol 1999;154:1159-1169.

45. Gouze E, Pawliuk R, Pilapil C, et al. In-vivo gene delivery to synovium by lentiviral vectors. Mol Ther 2002;5:397-404.

46. Robbins PD, Evans CH, Chernajovsky Y. Gene therapy for arthritis. Gene Ther 2003;10:902-911.

47. Evans CH, Ghivizzani SC, Robbins PD. Gene therapy of the rheumatic diseases: 1998 to 2008. Arthritis Res Ther 2009;11:209.

48. Wehling P, Reinecke J, Baltzer AA, et al. Clinical responses to gene therapy in joints of two subjects with rheumatoid arthritis. Hum Gene Ther 2008; Nov 5 [Epub ahead of print].

49. Sant SM, Suarez TM, Moalli MR, et al. Molecular lysis of synovial lining cells by in vivo herpes simplex virus–thymidine kinase gene transfer. Hum Gene Ther 1998;9:2735-2743.

50. Evans CH: Gene therapies for osteoarthritis. Curr Rheumatol Rep 2004;6:31-40.

REFERENCES

Full references for this chapter can be found on www.expertconsult.com.

Osteoimmunology

Georg Schett and Jean-Pierre David

19

INTRODUCTION

Two major aspects determine the clinical picture of rheumatic diseases: The first one is that inflammation is a central component of many, especially the most severe, forms of rheumatic diseases. Some rheumatic diseases, such as rheumatoid arthritis (RA), systemic lupus erythematosus, or Sjögren's syndrome, are considered as classic systemic autoimmune diseases based on the observation of autoantibody formation and the accumulation of cells of the adaptive immune system at sites of inflammation. Chronic immune activation is regarded as a central triggering factor for inflammatory rheumatic diseases. The second key aspect is that the consequences of the immune disturbances affect the musculoskeletal tissue, which is the common target of this disease group. Indeed, musculoskeletal tissue experiences progressive local and systemic damages, which are the basis for functional impairment and a high disease burden. Thus, the combination of chronic immune activation and musculoskeletal tissue damage is the hallmark of rheumatic diseases. A detailed understanding of the pathophysiologic processes of rheumatic diseases thus requires understanding the mutual interactions between the immune system and musculoskeletal tissue. These interactions are the basis for osteoimmunology.

CURRENT CONCEPTS OF OSTEOIMMUNOLOGY

Osteoimmunology is the field of research focusing on the crosstalk between the immune and the musculoskeletal system.[1] This field is particularly relevant for the understanding of rheumatic diseases, which are characterized by profound alterations of bone architecture as a consequence of the immune activation. The term *osteoimmunology* is a rather novel one: it was created after landmark observations in the late 1990s that demonstrated T lymphocytes triggering bone loss by inducing the differentiation of bone-resorbing cells, termed *osteoclasts*.[2-4] These concepts put two, at first sight fundamentally different, organ systems—the immune system and the skeleton—in much closer relation to each other as one would ever expect.

Current concepts of osteoimmunology that are of relevance for rheumatology involve (1) the regulation of bone degradation by the immune system, (2) the interaction between inflammation and bone formation, and (3) the role of bone and bone marrow as a niche for immune cells, particularly plasma cells. The first concept, immune-mediated regulation of bone loss, has been studied intensively during recent years and has become a well-developed concept that is instrumental in understanding the different forms of bone loss in the course of rheumatic diseases. In contrast, the second concept, the interactions between inflammation and bone formation, is still much less developed but is important to define the mechanisms of repair of structural damage in the joint and the mechanisms driving the general bone loss as well as to explain the pathophysiology of bony ankylosis. Similarly, the third concept, the bone marrow niche, is still incompletely understood but is particularly relevant to understanding the deregulation of immune cell trafficking during inflammatory diseases (i.e., the triggers for the recruitment of immune cells from the bone marrow into the inflammatory sites) and to explain the formation of a stable microenvironment, which allows longevity and antibody production by long-lived plasma cells.

OSTEOCLASTS AS TRIGGERS OF ARTHRITIC BONE EROSIONS

Erosion of periarticular bone is a central feature of RA and psoriatic arthritis.[5,6] Bone erosion mirrors a destructive process in joints affected by arthritis because it reflects damage triggered by chronic inflammation. Visualization of bone erosions by imaging techniques is important not only for the diagnosis of RA but also for defining the severity of disease and response to antirheumatic therapy.[7] Osteoclasts are bone-specialized macrophages and are the only cell type capable of removing calcium from bone and, consequently, degrading bone matrix. This bone-resorbing function is an essential component of the bone remodeling process that allows not only normal bone development and skeletal growth but also bone maintenance and repair throughout life. Osteoclasts are also required for the bone erosions observed in rheumatic joints. Indeed, osteoclasts are part of the inflamed synovial tissue of human RA and psoriatic arthritis as well as of all major experimental models of arthritis. Gravallese and Goldring first described in great detail the presence and characteristics of osteoclasts in inflamed joints in the late 1990s, showing that mature osteoclasts are localized at the site of bone erosion in RA joints.[8,9] Later, the essential function of osteoclasts in triggering inflammatory bone erosions has been shown by blocking essential molecules for osteoclastogenesis or by using mice deficient in osteoclasts.[10,11] In all these models no bone erosions occurred despite a clear synovial inflammation, when osteoclasts were either effectively blocked or genetically depleted. These findings clearly placed the osteoclasts as the effector cells of bone erosions and structural damage downstream from the inflammation in the affected joints.

MOLECULAR AND CELLULAR MECHANISMS OF INFLAMMATORY BONE EROSION

What are the mechanisms leading to osteoclast formation at a site where they are usually not present, that is, the joints? Two key mechanisms are essential to form osteoclasts in joints: (1) the accumulation of cells, which serve as osteoclast precursors in the joint, and (2) the stimulation of their differentiation into the osteoclast lineage. Osteoclast precursors are mononuclear cells belonging to the monocyte/macrophage lineage.[12] Early monocytic precursor cells have the potential to differentiate into macrophages, dendritic cells, osteoclasts, and other more organ-specific cell lineage types such as Kupffer cells in the liver or microglia in the brain. It is not fully clear whether some monocytes already committed to the osteoclast lineage are entering an inflamed joint or whether monocytes "decide" locally within the inflamed synovium on receiving the appropriate signals to switch toward the osteoclast lineage. Nonetheless, experimental evidence supports that the peripheral monocytic pool changes during inflammation. For instance, the fraction of CD11b-positive cells that serve as osteoclast precursors increases, suggesting that an increased number of cells entering the joint can differentiate into osteoclasts.[13] Moreover, cytokines such as tumor necrosis factor-α (TNF-α) induce the expression on the surface of monocytes of receptors important for osteoclast differentiation. One of them, OSCAR, is an important co-stimulation molecule for osteoclasts.[14] Much less is, in fact, known about surface receptors on monocytes, which can negatively regulate their differentiation to osteoclasts. In fact, one such molecule is CD80/CD86, which effectively blocks osteoclast formation when bound to CTLA4, a negative regulator of T-cell co-stimulation by monocytes.[15,16] This could link regulatory T cells that are highly expressing CTLA4 on their surface to bone homeostasis, because these cells can suppress osteoclast formation independently of the receptor activator of NF-κB ligand (RANKL).

The second mechanism is that monocytic osteoclast precursors that have already entered the inflamed joints find there the ideal environment to further differentiate into osteoclasts because of the presence of the monocyte colony-stimulating factor (M-CSF/CSF-1)

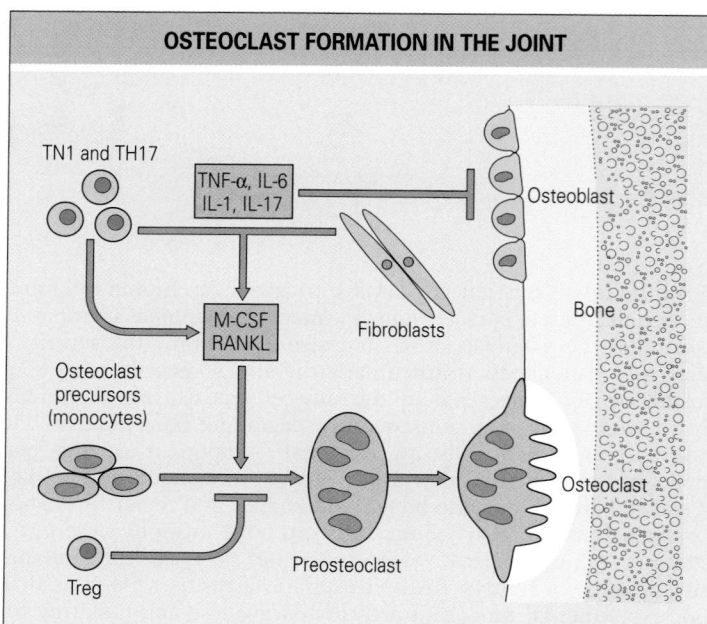

OSTEOCLAST FORMATION IN THE JOINT

Fig. 19.1 Osteoclast formation in the joint. Monocytic cells in the synovium serve as osteoclast precursors. On exposure to M-CSF and RANKL synthesized by T cells and synovial fibroblasts, they fuse to polykaryons, termed *pre-osteoclasts,* which then undergo further differentiation into mature osteoclasts, acquiring specific features such as the ruffled membrane. Inflammatory cytokines such as TNF-α, IL-1, IL-6, and IL-17 increase the expression of RANKL and thus support osteoclastogenesis in the joint while inhibiting systemic bone formation by the osteoblasts. In contrast, Treg blocks osteoclast formation via CTLA4.

and of RANKL, which are both essential stimulating signals for osteoclastogenesis and are also involved in activation of mature osteoclasts (Fig. 19.1). M-CSF, which binds to CSF-1R encoded by the protooncogene *C-FMS* promotes both proliferation and survival of the osteoclast precursors. RANKL binds a surface receptor on the precursor cells named RANK that induces signaling via NF-κB and the AP-1 transcription factor family, both essential for osteoclast differentiation.[2,3] In the joint, this process requires an intensive crosstalk with other cells, particularly with fibroblast-like synoviocytes and activated T cells. Among T cells, both Th1 and Th17 subsets are of importance in this process. Indeed, both cell types inducibly express RANKL.[3,17] This essential osteoclastogenic cytokine is expressed in the synovium of patients with RA, suggesting that it actively contributes to formation of osteoclasts in the synovium.[18,19] A high level of RANKL expression in the synovium is apparently not balanced by expression of regulatory molecules such as osteoprotegerin (OPG), a decoy receptor of RANKL, which blocks osteoclast formation,[20] suggesting this imbalance to be of importance in yielding a negative net effect on local bone mass in the case of arthritis. This concept is supported not only by data obtained in animal models of arthritis showing effective protection from structural damage when blocking RANKL with OPG, despite a clear synovial inflammation, but also by a recent clinical study showing that an antibody against RANKL (denosumab) protects against the progression of bony structural damage in patients with RA.[21]

Apart from RANKL, the osteoclastogenic properties of the inflamed synovial membrane are further enhanced by expression of M-CSF, which is essential for osteoclast formation as well.[22] Moreover, proinflammatory cytokines such as TNF-α and interleukin (IL)-1, IL-6, and IL-17 are all potent inducers of RANKL expression and thus enhance osteoclast differentiation as well. Some of these cytokines additionally exert direct effects on osteoclast precursors; and particularly TNF-α engages TNF-receptor type I on the surface of osteoclast precursors, which increases their differentiation into osteoclasts.[23] This link between proinflammatory cytokines and osteoclast formation is most likely the explanation why cytokine-targeted therapy, particularly blockade of TNF-α, is highly effective to retard the structural damage

in RA. Indeed, TNF-blocking agents virtually arrest radiographic damage in RA and are considered excellent agents for achieving structural protection of joints.[24-29] Although there are yet no data from randomized controlled trials, which define the structure-sparing effect of the IL-6 antagonist tocilizumab in addition to its well-established anti-inflammatory effect,[30,31] one can anticipate such an effect based on the observation that IL-6 drives RANKL expression and thus supports osteoclastogenesis.[32]

PERIARTICULAR AND SYSTEMIC BONE LOSS IN RHEUMATIC DISEASE

Periarticular bone loss has been long known as a radiographic sign of RA and has been explained by paracrine effects of the inflammatory tissue on periarticular bone. Still, periarticular bone loss (also termed *periarticular osteoporosis*) has been poorly defined so far. Apparently, periarticular bone loss is based on a substantial decrease in bone trabeculae along the metaphyses of bones close to inflamed joints, suggesting that the bone marrow cavity along inflamed joints is also part of the disease process of arthritis. This is supported by data from magnetic resonance imaging (MRI) studies in patients with RA, which have unraveled a high frequency of signal alterations in the juxta-articular bone marrow in addition to synovitis outside the cortical bone barrier.[33,34] These lesions are water-rich lesions, which have a low fat content, which suggests that bone marrow fat is locally replaced by a water-rich tissue. Histologic examination of bone marrow lesions has been carried out in joints of patients with advanced-stage RA undergoing joint replacement surgery. They have revealed that the bone marrow lesions visualized in the MRI contain (water-rich) vascularized inflammatory infiltrates, which replace bone marrow fat and harbor aggregates of B cells and T cells. Importantly, very similar, if not identical, MRI changes are found early in the disease process of RA and have shown a link to subsequent bone erosions in the same joints.[35] Bone marrow lesions are often linked to a cortical penetration of inflammatory tissue either by means of bone erosions or by small cortical bone channels, which connect the synovium with the juxta-articular bone marrow. Moreover, bone marrow lesions are associated with an endosteal bone response as they coincide with accumulation of osteoblasts and deposition of bone matrix in the endosteum.[36] These novel data have enhanced our view of arthritis as a disease that is not solely confined to the synovial membrane but also to bone marrow.

It is long known that inflammatory diseases including RA and ankylosing spondylitis (AS) lead to osteoporosis and increased fracture risk. Data obtained during recent years have supported these concepts and have shed a more detailed light on osteoporosis and fracture risk in RA patients. Osteopenia and osteoporosis are frequently observed in patients with RA and even observed in rather high frequency before any disease-modifying antirheumatic drug (DMARD) or glucocorticoid therapy is started. Roughly 25% of patients with RA show an osteopenic bone mineral density at the spine or the hip before onset of therapy in early RA and 10% have osteoporosis, suggesting these symptoms to be an intrinsic component of the diseases.[37] Thus, RA patients are at high risk to develop complications from systemic bone loss because of the increased prevalence of low bone mass at the onset of disease. The reason for this appears to be based on the coincidence of standard risk factors for osteoporosis with the onset of RA such as higher age and female sex. Another explanation is the possibility that low-grade inflammation often long precedes the onset of clinical symptoms of RA. Indeed, even a small elevation of C-reactive protein as a sign of low-grade inflammation in the normal healthy population dramatically increases fracture risk, as independent population-based studies have shown.[38] Fracture risk is indeed higher in RA patients and has been confirmed by a recent meta-analysis of nine prospective population-based cohorts, which showed that fracture risk doubles with the diagnosis of RA independent of whether glucocorticoids are used.[39] Similarly, a large case-control study based on the British General Practice Research Database has shown that RA doubles the risk of hip and vertebral facture, which clearly supports the concept that inflammation is an independent risk factor for osteoporosis.[40]

OSTEOIMMUNOLOGIC ASPECTS OF BONE FORMATION IN RHEUMATIC DISEASE

To gain a balanced view on the interaction between the immune system and bone it is important to better define how immune activation controls bone formation. Given the observation that inflammatory arthritis shows profound changes in joint architecture, covering the whole spectrum from an almost purely erosive disease like RA, to a mixed pattern with erosions and bone formation side by side, to a prominent bone-forming pattern as observed in AS, the regulation of bone formation becomes an interesting aspect of rheumatic diseases. In RA, there is little sign of repair of bone erosions, which is astonishing considering that bone formation is usually coupled to bone resorption and that an increased rate of bone resorption should thus increase bone formation. This, however, is by no means the case in RA, which is virtually a purely erosive disease. Recent data suggest that bone formation is actively suppressed by inflammation. Interestingly, TNF-α is a very potent suppressor of bone formation by enhancing the expression of DKK1, a protein that negatively regulates the Wnt signal transduction pathway.[41] Wnt signals are key triggers for bone formation by enhancing the differentiation of the bone-forming cells, osteoblasts from their mesenchymal cell precursors. Wnt proteins are also involved in the regulation of osteoclastogenesis because they enhance the expression of OPG that blocks osteoclast formation.[42] Thus, influencing the balance of Wnt proteins and their inhibitors is a very potent strategy to disturb bone homeostasis: a low level of Wnt activity yields low bone formation and high bone resorption, whereas a high level of Wnt activity increases bone formation and simultaneously blocks bone resorption. In RA, the former scenarios appear to be relevant because bone resorption is increased and bone formation is decreased. Inhibitors of Wnt, like DKK1, are expressed in the synovial tissue of RA patients, suggesting a suppressive effect on bone formation. This concept is further supported by the paucity of fully differentiated osteoblasts within arthritic bone erosions, which indicates that there is indeed no major bone formation going on in these lesions.

Pure degradation of bone during arthritis is the exception rather than the rule in joint disease. Psoriatic arthritis, AS, but also osteoarthritis and metabolic arthropathies such as hemochromatosis arthropathy are partly or even predominantly characterized by bony spurs along joints and intervertebral spaces. These lesions are based on new bone formation. We have recently perceived that osteophyte formation cannot be easily compared with erosive structural damage observed in RA and those therapies blocking bone erosions such as TNF-α blockade do not influence the formation of osteophytes.[43] Areas that are prone to osteophyte formation are (1) periarticular sites of the periosteum in vicinity of the articular cartilage, (2) edges of vertebral bodies, and (3) the insertion sites of tendons. These sites are particularly rich in fibrocartilage, which is considered a tissue from which osteophyte formation emerges given the interplay of certain triggering factors.[44] Triggers are certainly mechanical factors because osteophytes often emerge at the entheses along the insertion sites of the tendons. Usually, osteophytes are based on endochondral ossification, which first leads to differentiation of hypertrophic chondrocytes from mesenchymal cells and abundant deposition of extracellular matrix, before rebuilding into bone occurs, which requires invasion and resorption of the mineralized cartilage by osteoclasts and then differentiation of osteoblasts that depose the bone. Molecular signals involved in osteophyte formation have recently been defined: transforming growth factor (TGF)-β as well as bone morphogenic proteins (BMPs) along with active BMP signaling through SMAD3 proteins facilitate human osteophyte formation.[45] Moreover, noggin, an inhibitor of BMPs, effectively blocks osteophyte formation, suggesting that this protein family plays a key role in the formation of bony spurs by facilitating osteoblast differentiation.[45] Another essential protein family involved in osteophyte formation is the Wnt protein family. These proteins bind to surface receptors such as LRP5/6 and frizzled proteins on the surface of mesenchymal cells, leading to signaling through β-catenin, which translocates to the nucleus and activated genes involved in bone formation. Nuclear translocation of β-catenin is observed at sites of bony spurs, suggesting its activation by Wnt proteins. There appears to be tight crosstalk between the Wnt proteins and BMP proteins because these two protein families

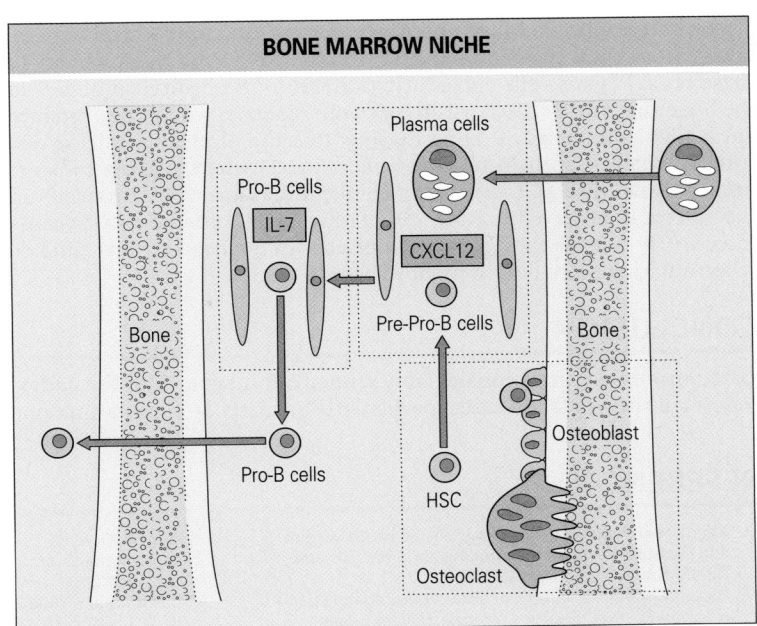

Fig. 19.2 Bone marrow niche. The maintenance and renewal of hematopoietic stem cells (HSCs) depends on a subset of osteoblasts forming the HSCs' niche. HSCs are mobilized by the activity of the osteoclasts and differentiate. Pre-pro-B cells share a common niche with plasma cells based on the expression of CXCL12 by bone marrow stromal cells. On further differentiation into pro-B cells, cells switch to a different niche, which is based on bone marrow stromal cells that express IL-7. Further differentiation of B cells into pre-B cells makes them independent from bone marrow niches before leaving bone marrow to secondary lymphatic organs. Plasma cells reentering the bone marrow share the CXCL12-triggered bone marrow niche with pre-pro-B cells.

act synergistically on bone formation. Moreover, there is crosstalk to the RANKL-OPG system as well, because Wnt proteins induce the expression of OPG, which shuts down bone resorption.[46] It thus appears that the balance between bone-forming factors such as as Wnt and BMP proteins and bone-resorbing factors such as RANKL and TNF is crucial for how a joint remodels during arthritis.

BONE MARROW AS A NICHE FOR B-CELL DIFFERENTIATION AND AUTOANTIBODY FORMATION

The mechanisms that explain the influence of the immune system on bone homeostasis have so far dominated osteoimmunology research; however, there are also other areas in which bone-immune interactions play an important role. Bone is a hematopoietic organ that provides the microenvironment, also called niches, for the maintenance and mobilization of the hematopoietic stem cells (HSCs); it is the site of early B-cell differentiation and of the homing of the long-lived plasma cells. Although the identity of niches and interaction of blood cells is still poorly understood, a subset of the bone-forming cells, or osteoblasts, has been shown to establish the HSC niche and the activity of the bone-resorbing cells or osteoclasts is needed for HSC mobilization. These appear to be important in early B-cell differentiation as well as survival of long-lived B cells and plasma cells.[47] Both the earliest precursors (pre-pro-B cells) and the end-stage B cells (plasma cells) require CXC chemokine ligand (CXCL)-12 to home to the bone marrow (Fig. 19.2). CXCL12-expressing cells are a small population of bone marrow stromal cells, scattered throughout bone marrow, that are distinct from the cells expressing IL-7 adjoining more mature pro-B cells.[48] These cells not only allow homing of memory B cells and plasma cells to the bone marrow but also provide survival signals, which allow longevity of these cells and prevent apoptosis. Thus long-lived memory B cells and plasma cells are dependent not only on affinity maturation but also on an acquired ability to survive. Successful competition for survival niches thus appears to be a key factor explaining the longevity of these cells. Plasma cells apparently traffic into these survival niches in the bone marrow by CXCL12-induced chemotaxis, where they produce antibodies and persist. If bone marrow homing of plasma cells is disturbed, which is seen in murine lupus models where plasma cells are unresponsive to CXCL12, a marked accumulation of plasma cells in the spleen is observed.[47] Also, circulating B cells might only become memory B cells if they find appropriate survival conditions outside re-stimulating secondary lymphoid organs.

CONCLUSION

Osteoimmunology has considerably refined our insights into the pathogenesis of rheumatic diseases, particularly arthritis. It appears that one of the reasons for the preferential targeting of the bone by inflammatory arthritis is the disturbance of the natural interaction of bone and immune systems. This idea gives credence to the old concept of bone remodeling as a controlled inflammatory response despite a clear synovial inflammation.[49] With the help of osteoimmunology, we are now starting to understand the molecular interactions between immune activation and the skeletal system, which links inflammatory diseases with bone loss. Knowledge of these pathways will allow the tailoring of drug therapies to target skeletal damage more specifically and thus more effectively. In addition, further insights in the role bone and bone marrow play in shaping immune responses, particularly in maintaining plasma cells in the bone marrow niche, will open a new perspective in autoimmune diseases.

REFERENCES

1. Takayanagi H. Osteoimmunology: shared mechanisms and crosstalk between the immune and bone systems. Nat Rev Immunol 2007;7:292-304.
2. Lacey DL, Timms E, Tan HL, et al. Osteoprotegerin ligand is a cytokine that regulates osteoclast differentiation and activation. Cell 1998;93:165-176.
3. Kong YY, Yoshida H, Sarosi I, et al. OPGL is a key regulator of osteoclastogenesis, lymphocyte development and lymph-node organogenesis. Nature 1999;397:315-323.
4. Horwood NJ, Kartsogiannis V, Quinn JM, et al. Activated T lymphocytes support osteoclast formation in vitro. Biochem Biophys Res Commun 1999;265:144-150.
5. McInnes I, Schett G. Cytokines in the pathogenesis of rheumatoid arthritis. Nat Immunol 2007;7:429-442.
6. Firestein GS. Evolving concepts of rheumatoid arthritis. Nature 2003;423:356-361.
7. Van der Heijde DM. Joint erosions and patients with early rheumatoid arthritis. Br J Rheumatol 1995;34:74-78.
8. Bromley M, Woolley DE. Chondroclasts and osteoclasts at subchondral sites of erosion in the rheumatoid joint. Arthritis Rheum 1984;27:968-975.
9. Gravallese EM, Harada Y, Wang JT, et al. Identification of cell types responsible for bone resorption in rheumatoid arthritis and juvenile rheumatoid arthritis. Am J Pathol 1998;152:943-951.
10. Pettit AR, Ji H, von Stechow D, et al. TRANCE/RANKL knockout mice are protected from bone erosion in a serum transfer model of arthritis. Am J Pathol 2001;159:1689-1699.
11. Redlich K, Hayer S, Ricci R, et al. Osteoclasts are essential for TNF-alpha–mediated joint destruction. J Clin Invest 2002;110:1419-1427.
12. Teitelbaum SL. Bone resorption by osteoclasts. Science 2000;289:1504-1508.
13. Ritchlin CT, Haas-Smith SA, Li P, et al. Mechanisms of TNF-alpha- and RANKL-mediated osteoclastogenesis and bone resorption in psoriatic arthritis. J Clin Invest 2003;111:821-831.
14. Herman S, Mueller R, Kronke G, et al. OSCAR, a key co-stimulation molecule for osteoclasts, is induced in patients with rheumatoid arthritis. Arthritis Rheum 2008; 58:3041-3050.
15. Zaiss MM, Axmann R, Zwerina J, et al. Treg cells suppress osteoclast formation: a new link between the immune system and bone. Arthritis Rheum 2007;56:4104-4112.
16. Axmann R, Herman S, Zaiss M, et al. CTLA-4 directly inhibits osteoclast formation. Ann Rheum Dis 2008;67:1603-1609.
17. Sato K, Suematsu A, Okamoto K, et al. Th17 functions as an osteoclastogenic helper T cell subset that links T cell activation and bone destruction. J Exp Med 2006;203:2673-2682.
18. Gravallese EM, Manning C, Tsay A, et al. Synovial tissue in rheumatoid arthritis is a source of osteoclast differentiation factor. Arthritis Rheum 2000;43:250-258.
19. Shigeyama Y, Pap T, Kunzler P, et al. Expression of osteoclast differentiation factor in rheumatoid arthritis. Arthritis Rheum 2000;43:2523-2530.
20. Stolina M, Adamu S, Ominsky M, et al. RANKL is a marker and mediator of local and systemic bone loss in two rat models of inflammatory arthritis. J Bone Miner Res 2005;20:1756-1765.

21. Cohen SB, Dore RK, Lane NE, et al. Denosumab treatment effects on structural damage, bone mineral density and bone turnover in rheumatoid arthritis. Arthritis Rheum 2008;58:1299-1309.
22. Seitz M, Loetscher P, Fey MF, Tobler A. Constitutive mRNA and protein production of macrophage colony-stimulating factor but not of other cytokines by synovial fibroblasts from rheumatoid arthritis and osteoarthritis patients. Br J Rheumatol 1994;33:613-619.
23. Lam J, Takeshita S, Barker JE, et al. TNF-alpha induces osteoclastogenesis by direct stimulation of macrophages exposed to permissive levels of RANK ligand. J Clin Invest 2000;106:1481-1488.
24. Klareskog L, van der Heijde D, de Jager JP, et al. Therapeutic effect of the combination of etanercept and methotrexate compared with each treatment alone in patients with rheumatoid arthritis: double-blind randomised controlled trial. Lancet 2004;363:675-681.
25. Smolen JS, Van Der Heijde DM, St. Clair EW, et al. Predictors of joint damage in patients with early rheumatoid arthritis treated with high-dose methotrexate with or without concomitant infliximab: results from the ASPIRE trial. Arthritis Rheum 2006;54:702-710.
26. Keystone EC, Kavanaugh AF, Sharp JT, et al. Radiographic, clinical and functional outcomes of treatment with adalimumab (a human anti–tumor necrosis factor monoclonal antibody) in patients with active rheumatoid arthritis receiving concomitant methotrexate therapy: a randomized placebo-controlled 52-week trial. Arthritis Rheum 2004;50:1400-1411.
27. Lipsky PE, van der Heijde DM, St Clair EW, et al. Infliximab and methotrexate in the treatment of rheumatoid arthritis. Anti-Tumor Necrosis Factor Trial in Rheumatoid Arthritis with Concomitant Therapy Study Group. N Engl J Med 2000;343:1594-1602.
28. Weinblatt ME, Keystone EC, Furst DE, et al. Adalimumab, a fully human anti-tumor necrosis factor alpha monoclonal antibody, for the treatment of rheumatoid arthritis in patients taking concomitant methotrexate: the ARMADA trial. Arthritis Rheum 2003;48:35-45.
29. Maini R, St. Clair EW, Breedveld F, et al. Infliximab (chimeric anti–tumour necrosis factor alpha monoclonal antibody) versus placebo in rheumatoid arthritis patients receiving concomitant methotrexate: a randomised phase III trial. ATTRACT Study Group. Lancet 1999;354:1932-1939.
30. Maini RN, Taylor PC, Szechinski J, et al. CHARISMA Study Group. Double-blind randomized controlled clinical trial of the interleukin-6 receptor antagonist, tocilizumab, in European patients with rheumatoid arthritis who had an incomplete response to methotrexate. Arthritis Rheum 2006;54:2817-2829.
31. Smolen JS, Beaulieu A, Rubbert-Roth A, et al. OPTION Investigators. Effect of interleukin-6 receptor inhibition with tocilizumab in patients with rheumatoid arthritis (OPTION study): a double-blind, placebo-controlled, randomised trial. Lancet 2008;371:987-997.
32. Wong PK, et al. Interleukin-6 modulates production of T lymphocyte–derived cytokines in antigen-induced arthritis and drives inflammation-induced osteoclastogenesis. Arthritis Rheum 2006;54:158-168.

33. McQueen FM, Gao A, Østergaard M, et al. High-grade MRI bone oedema is common within the surgical field in rheumatoid arthritis patients undergoing joint replacement and is associated with osteitis in subchondral bone. Ann Rheum Dis 2007;66:1581-1587.
34. Conaghan P, Bird P, Ejbjerg B, et al. The EULAR-OMERACT rheumatoid arthritis MRI reference image atlas: the metacarpophalangeal joints. Ann Rheum Dis 2005;64:i11-i21.
35. McQueen FM, Benton N, Perry D, et al. Bone edema scored on magnetic resonance imaging scans of the dominant carpus at presentation predicts radiographic joint damage of the hands and feet six years later in patients with rheumatoid arthritis. Arthritis Rheum 2003;48:1814-1827.
36. Jimenez-Boj E, Redlich K, Turk B, et al. Interaction between synovial inflammatory tissue and bone marrow in rheumatoid arthritis. J Immunol 2005;175:2579-2588.
37. Güler-Yüksel M, Bijsterbosch J, Goekoop-Ruiterman YP, et al. Bone mineral density in patients with recently diagnosed, active rheumatoid arthritis. Ann Rheum Dis 2007;66:1508-1512.
38. Schett G, Kiechl S, Weger S, et al. High-sensitivity C-reactive protein and risk of nontraumatic fractures in the Bruneck study. Arch Intern Med 2006;166:2495-2501.
39. Kanis JA, Johnell O, Oden A, et al. FRAX and the assessment of fracture probability in men and women from the UK. Osteoporos Int 2008;19:385-397.
40. van Staa TP, Geusens P, Bijlsma JW, et al. Clinical assessment of the long-term risk of fracture in patients with rheumatoid arthritis. Arthritis Rheum 2006;54:3104-3121.
41. Diarra D, Stolina M, Polzer K, et al. Dickkopf-1 is a master regulator of joint remodeling. Nat Med 2007;13:156-163.
42. Glass DA, Bialek P, Ahn JD, et al. Canonical Wnt signaling in differentiated osteoblasts controls osteoclast differentiation. Dev Cell 2005;8:751-764.
43. Sieper J, Appel H, Braun J, Rudwaleit M. Critical appraisal of assessment of structural damage in ankylosing spondylitis: implications for treatment outcomes. Arthritis Rheum 2008;58:649-656.
44. Benjamin M, McGonagle D. The anatomical basis for disease localization in seronegative spondylarthropathy at entheses and related sites. J Anat 2001;199:503-526.
45. Lories RJ, Derese I, Luyten FP. Modulation of bone morphogenetic protein signaling inhibits the onset and progression of ankylosing enthesitis. J Clin Invest 2005;115:1571-1579.
46. Manz RA, Arce S, Cassese G, et al. Humoral immunity and long-lived plasma cells. Curr Opin Immunol 2002;14:517-521.
47. Tokoyoda K, Egawa T, Sugiyama T, et al. Cellular niches controlling B lymphocyte behavior within bone marrow during development. Immunity 2004;20:707-718.
48. Erickson LD, Lin LL, Duan B, et al. A genetic lesion that arrests plasma cell homing to the bone marrow. Proc Natl Acad Sci U S A 2003;100:12905-12910.
49. David JP. Osteoimmunology: a view from the bone. Adv Immunol 2007;95:149-165.

The complement system in systemic lupus erythematosus

20

V. Michael Holers

- The complement system has multiple functions, both protective and injurious.
- Complement classical pathway deficiencies promote development of systemic lupus erythematosus (SLE).
- SLE is characterized by complement effector function–dependent injury to multiple target organs.

INTRODUCTION

The complement system plays a central role in the pathophysiology of most rheumatic diseases. Because of the potentially dual roles of complement in the pathogenesis of systemic lupus erythematosus (SLE), being both protective and injurious depending on the exact clinical situation, the study of this particular disease has been quite instructive for investigators over the years as the biologic roles of the complement system have been elucidated. Thus, it is appropriate to review the complement system primarily in the context of this disease. However, it is important to point out that many other autoimmune and rheumatic diseases also exhibit evidence of complement-mediated effects, and several are reviewed here as examples.

Complement is a phylogenetically ancient system consisting of soluble activation pathway proteins found in the blood and tissues (Table 20.1), both soluble and membrane-bound receptors (Table 20.2), and regulatory proteins (Table 20.3). The major biologic roles of the complement system include recognition and clearance of foreign pathogens and non-self antigens by promoting humoral and cellular immune responses as well as phagocytosis; clearance of self antigens derived from apoptotic processes in a non-inflammatory manner; immune complex transport; enhancement of tissue regeneration after injury; shaping of the natural antibody repertoire; and the promotion of an autoinflammatory response to injured self tissue.[1-9] The complement system should primarily be considered as a central component of the protective innate immune system but with substantial effects on the evolution and functional capacities of adaptive immunity.[1]

A key concept is that when misdirected, the complement system plays a central role in the tissue damage and pathophysiology of rheumatic diseases, including SLE. In the most common clinical settings in patients with SLE or other inflammatory autoimmune diseases such as rheumatoid arthritis (RA), the powerful effector mechanisms of complement that should be focused on foreign pathogens and antigens appear to be instead re-directed to self and cause tissue damage. However, additional insights into other important roles for this system have been provided by the careful study of complete and partial deficiency states of complement activation and regulatory proteins. For example, complete deficiencies of early complement pathway components are strongly associated with the development of SLE and SLE-like syndromes, likely owing to inefficient clearance of apoptotic self tissues.[5] In addition, the presence of dysfunctional regulatory proteins due to genetic polymorphisms or mutations is associated with systemic vascular injury syndromes such as atypical hemolytic-uremic syndrome,[10,11] hemolytic syndromes such as paroxysmal nocturnal hemoglobinuria,[12] and chronic inflammatory diseases such as macular degeneration.[13]

To help understand these multiple roles of complement, first the complement system is reviewed, focusing on its normal biologic roles in addition to its effector functions and the mechanisms that regulate its activities. Then the specific roles that complement effector functions and deficiencies have been proposed to play in SLE and other rheumatic and autoimmune diseases are discussed.

ACTIVATION PATHWAYS OF COMPLEMENT

Overview

The complement system is activated by any of three pathways: classical, alternative, and lectin (Fig. 20.1). The classical pathway is initiated by IgM- or IgG-containing immune complexes, C-reactive protein (CRP), β-amyloid fibrils, serum amyloid P, or tissue damage products such as mitochondrial membrane proteins that directly bind C1q (Table 20.4). The general order of complement-fixing potential of human antibodies is IgM > IgG3 > IgG1 > IgG2 >> IgG4. IgA can activate the alternative pathway, whereas IgE is not an effective complement activating isotype except under unusual circumstances. Certain autoantibodies designated "C4 nephritic factors" that stabilize C4 convertases (activating enzymes) also promote classical pathway activation.

The alternative pathway does not require a specific initiator but rather undergoes a process of "tickover" that results in activation.[14] Although not required, certain substances such as repeating polysaccharides, endotoxin, IgA-containing immune complexes, C3 nephritic factor (C3Nef) autoantibody, and some immunoglobulin light chains serve to promote alternative pathway activation. This pathway also serves as an "amplification loop" when C3b that is deposited by any pathway serves to bind factor B and initiate further cleavage events through the alternative pathway, with an end result of greatly increased levels of C3 and C5 activation. Notably, the alternative pathway amplification loop, long thought to be a relatively minor contributor to tissue inflammation, has over the past several years been shown to be an essential mechanism for the full elaboration of complement-dependent injury *in vivo*.[15]

The lectin pathway is initiated by mannose-binding lectin (MBL) or by ficolins, which are carbohydrate-binding proteins from a family designated the collectins that are involved in the clearance of foreign organisms such as bacteria and viruses.[16-18] The lectin pathway is initiated when MBL binds to repeating carbohydrate moieties found primarily on the surface of microbial and viral pathogens or by ficolin recognition of specific structural motifs found on pathogens. In addition, the lectin pathway is activated by the protein cytokeratin, which is exposed on ischemic endothelial cells, and by agalactosyl (G0) carbohydrates on IgG in patients with RA.

However the complement system is initiated, convergence on the centrally important C3 protein occurs when multiple-component C3 convertases (activating enzymes) are formed and C3 is cleaved. The presence of a thioester bond in C3 as well as C4 allows the covalent attachment of these two proteins in the C3b and C4b forms through ester or amide linkages to other molecules during the process of activation.[19] This irreversibly "marks" the attached targets as immunologically different and allows the subsequent cleavage of C4b and C3b to forms iC4b/C4d and iC3b/C3dg/C3d and binding of the complex to specific C3/C4 receptors that interact with most of these fragments.[2] The activation of C3 is followed by the formation of a C5 convertase, resulting in C5 cleavage and activation. The pore-like membrane attack complex (MAC) is then assembled by the serial addition of C6 to C9. Importantly, the soluble anaphylatoxins C3a and C5a,[20] which manifest remarkable proinflammatory properties, are also generated during this process.

Sequential events during complement activation

Classical pathway activation steps are shown in Figure 20.2.[21] Regardless of whether antibodies or other molecules bind and activate C1, the same series of events is believed to take place. C1 is a trimolecular complex that consists of three unique protein subunits (C1q, C1r, and C1s) in the stoichiometry of 1C1q:2C1r:2C1s. When C1q binds a target, the first event is autocatalysis and self-activation of C1r, which is then followed by the cleavage of C1s by activated C1r. C1s is then able to cleave nearby C4 into C4a and C4b, the latter which can covalently attach to the target by ester or amide linkages. This property is

TABLE 20.1 COMPLEMENT ACTIVATION PATHWAY PROTEINS

Component	Approximate serum concentration (μg/mL)	Approximate molecular weight
Classical pathway		
C1q	70	410,000
C1r	34	170,000
C1s	31	85,000
C4	600	206,000
C2	25	117,000
Alternative pathway		
Factor D	1	24,000
C3	1,300	195,000
Factor B	200	95,000
Lectin pathway		
MBL	150 (very wide range)	600,000
MASP-1	6.0	83,000
MASP-2	0.5	76,000
MASP-3		95,000
Membrane attack complex		
C5	80	180,000
C6	60	128,000
C7	55	120,000
C8	65	150,000
C9	60	79,000

TABLE 20.2 COMPLEMENT RECEPTORS

Receptors	Approximate molecular weight	Major activities
Complement receptor 1 (CR1, CD35)	190,000-250,000	Immune complex transport (E) Phagocytosis (PMN, Mac) Immune adherence (E) Cofactor and decay acceleration
Complement receptor 2 (CR2, CD21)	145,000	B cell co-activator EBV receptor CD23 receptor
Complement receptor 3 (CD11b/CD18)	170,000 (α chain)*	Leukocyte adherence Phagocytosis of iC3b-bound particles
Complement receptor 4 (CD11c/CD18)	150,000 (α chain)*	Leukocyte adherence
C5a receptor (CD88)	50,000	Cell activation Chemotaxis
C5L2 receptor	50,000	Modulates C5a function
C3a receptor	75,000	Cell activation

E, erythrocyte; PMN, polymorphonuclear neutrophil; Mac, macrophage.
*Common 95,000 β-chain.

TABLE 20.3 COMPLEMENT REGULATORY PROTEINS

Soluble control proteins	Approximate serum concentration (μg/mL)	Approximate molecular weight	Major functions
Positive regulation			
Properdin	25	220,000	Stabilizes alternative pathway
			C3/C5 convertases
Negative regulation			
C1-INH	200	105,000	Inhibits C1r/C1s, MASPs
C4-bp	250	550,000	Decay-acceleration classical pathway, cofactor activity C4b
Factor H	500	150,000	Decay-acceleration alternative pathway, cofactor activity C3b
Factor I	34	90,000	Cleavage of C3b/C4b
Anaphylatoxin inactivator	35	280,000	Generates C3a/C5a desArg (carboxypeptidase H)
S protein (vitronectin)	500	80,000	Blocks MAC formation
SP-40,40 (clusterin)	60	80,000	Blocks MAC formation
Membrane regulatory proteins			
Decay-accelerating factor (CD55)		70,000	Decay-acceleration classical and alternative pathways
Membrane cofactor protein (CD46)		45,000-70,000	Cofactor activity classical and alternative pathways
CD59		20,000	Blocks C8-C9 and C9
CRIT		30,000	Blocks C2

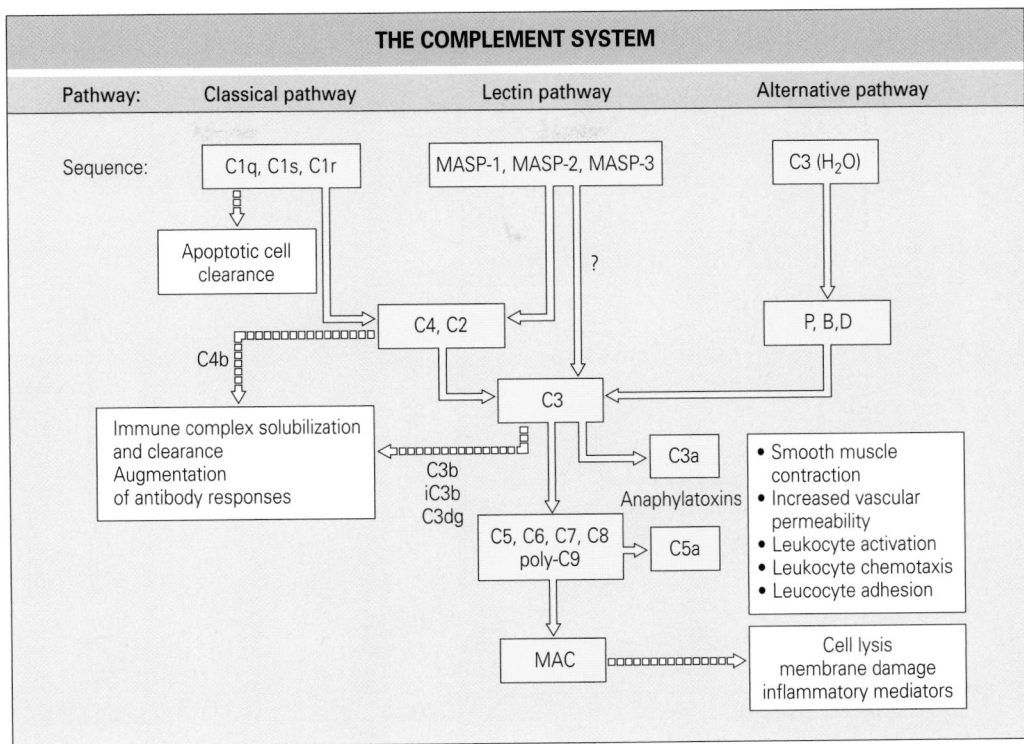

THE COMPLEMENT SYSTEM

Fig. 20.1 Overview of complement initiation and effector pathways. The complement system can be initiated through the classical, lectin, or alternative pathways, resulting in the formation of C3-convertases that cleave and activate this protein. The subsequent activation of C5 and further components of the complement cascade result in formation of the membrane attack complex (MAC). All three initiator pathways can result in C3a and C5a generation. Several examples of effector functions of complement are also shown.

TABLE 20.4 COMPLEMENT PATHWAY ACTIVATORS

Classical pathway	Alternative pathway	Lectin pathway
Immune complexes (IgM, IgG)	"Tickover"	Repeating simple sugars
C-reactive protein (CRP)	Amplification pathway	G0 carbohydrate glycoforms
Apoptotic bodies	Endotoxin	Cytokeratin-1
β-Amyloid fibrils	IgA immune complexes	
Serum amyloid P (SAP)	Polysaccharides	
Mitochondrial products	C3 nephritic factor	
C4 nephritic factor		

due to an internal thioester bond that becomes highly unstable during the cleavage of C4 and allows the covalent attachment to nearby molecules. Because of this dual type of bond formation, the nature of the target surface can modify to some extent the particular site, amount, and type (C4A vs. C4B allotype) of C4b binding and, thus, subsequent complement activation. Approximately 5% of C4 becomes attached to the target, and the rest is inactivated in the surrounding fluid phase by reactivity of the thioester site with H_2O. C1s then cleaves C2 into C2a and C2b, the former of which associates non-covalently with C4b. As part of this C4b2a complex, now designated a C3 convertase, C2a exhibits proteolytic activity for C3, resulting in cleavage into C3a and C3b. C3 also exhibits a thioester bond and can covalently attach to nearby molecules, including C4b. The association of C4b2a with C3b allows the creation of a C4b2a3b C5 convertase, capable of cleaving C5 into C5b and C5a.

In a similar fashion, the lectin pathway is activated by a series of proteolytic cleavage events (see Fig. 20.2).[16-18] In this process, MBL and ficolins are structurally similar to C1q, and the proteases MASP-1 and MASP-2 are similar to C1r and C1s, whereas MASP-3, an alternatively spliced variant of the *MASP-1/3* gene, exhibits different activation requirements. After binding of MBL or ficolins to targets, the MASPs are activated. In this situation, it is not certain yet what are all of the relevant activation steps and protease targets of the MASPs; however,

data exist suggesting that C4 can be cleaved by MASP-2 and C3 can be directly cleaved by MASP-1. Recently, the function of MASP-1 and MASP-3 has been expanded by the suggestion that they are required for the conversion of inactive pro-factor D to active factor D. Regardless of the details, C3 and subsequently C5 are cleaved, both releasing their chemotactic fragments C3a and C5a and resulting in the generation of the MAC.

In contrast to the specific protein/protein or protein/carbohydrate interactions that characterize the initiation mechanisms of the classical and lectin pathways, the alternative pathway can be activated on the surface of any target that manifests neutral or positive charge characteristics and does not contain complement inhibitors. Alternative pathway activation also occurs in the fluid phase in the absence of efficient inhibition. The alternative pathway is capable of this auto-activation because of a process termed *tickover* of C3 (Fig. 20.3). Tickover occurs spontaneously at a rate of about 1% of total C3 per hour, and this process results in the generation of a conformationally altered C3, designated C3(H_2O), that can now bind factor B.

Once factor B associates with C3(H_2O), factor B itself changes conformation and can then be cleaved by the constitutively active serum protease factor D, generating Ba and Bb. Factor D is a member of the serine protease family that, once converted to an active enzyme state by MASP-1 and/or MASP-3, demonstrates an exquisite specificity for conformationally altered factor B and does not efficiently cleave other targets. Once split into two fragments by factor D, Ba diffuses away and Bb remains associated with the complex and can then, through its own serine protease domain, cleave additional C3 molecules, generating a form designated C3b. As part of this cleavage process, C3b can be covalently attached to targets when its thioester bond is broken. Once C3b is generated, it associates with the complex, creating a C3bBbC3b C5 convertase that can now cleave C5 into C5b and C5a. This overall series of successive proteolytic steps is enhanced by the serum protein properdin, which stabilizes protein/protein interactions during the process. The alternative pathway can also be initiated as an "amplification loop" when fixed C3b that is generated by the classical, lectin, or alternative pathways activation binds factor B, again resulting in conformational changes in factor B that allow factor D to cleave it to Ba and Bb similarly to the tickover process.

In addition to the tickover and amplification loop mechanisms, the alternative pathway can be activated when certain antibodies block endogenous regulatory mechanisms or when expression of complement regulatory proteins that control the alternative pathway is

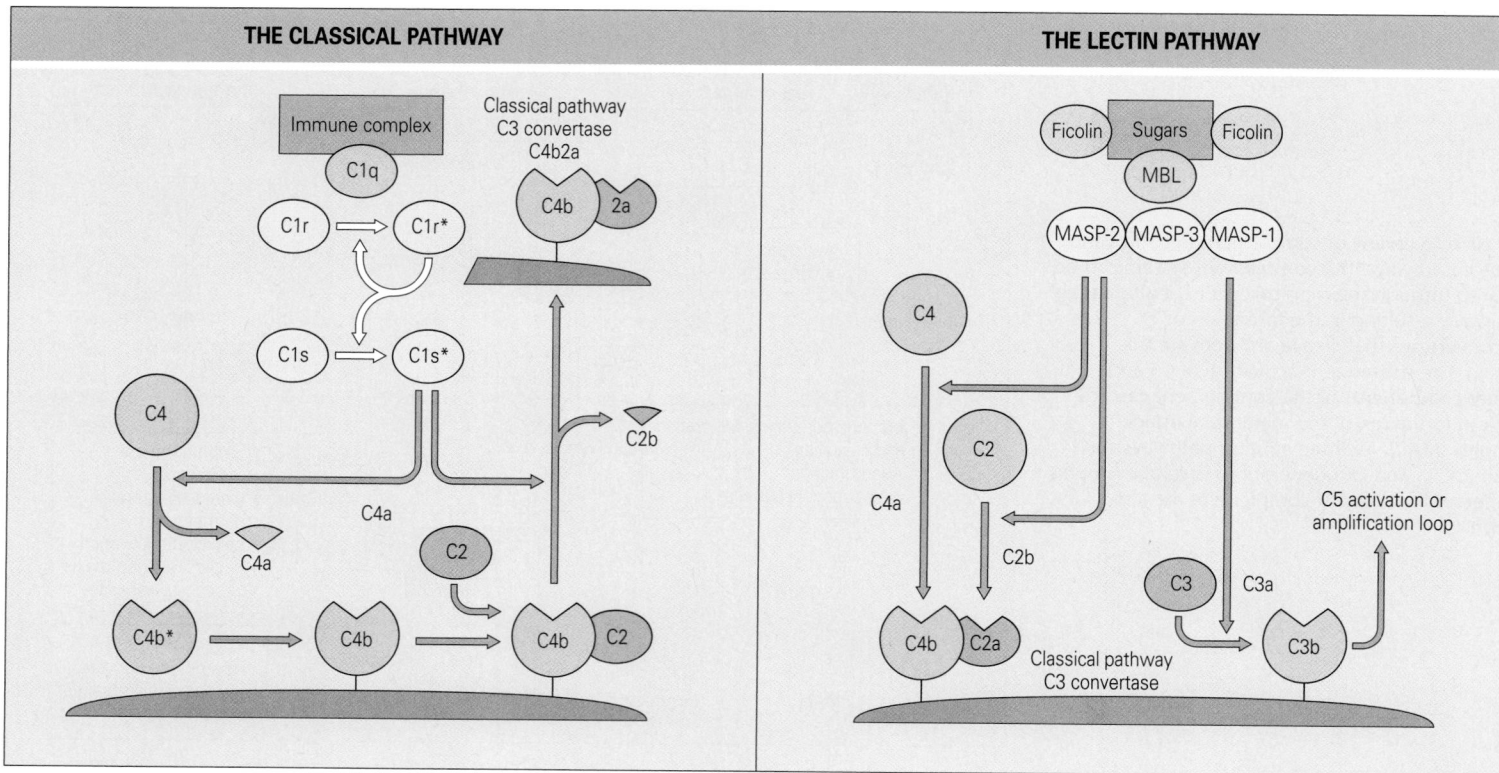

Fig. 20.2 Classical and lectin pathway activation. Sequential activation events that lead to C3 and subsequently C5 activation by the classical and lectin pathways are shown. Exact capabilities of lectin pathway to directly activate C3 as shown are uncertain but possible through MASP-1.

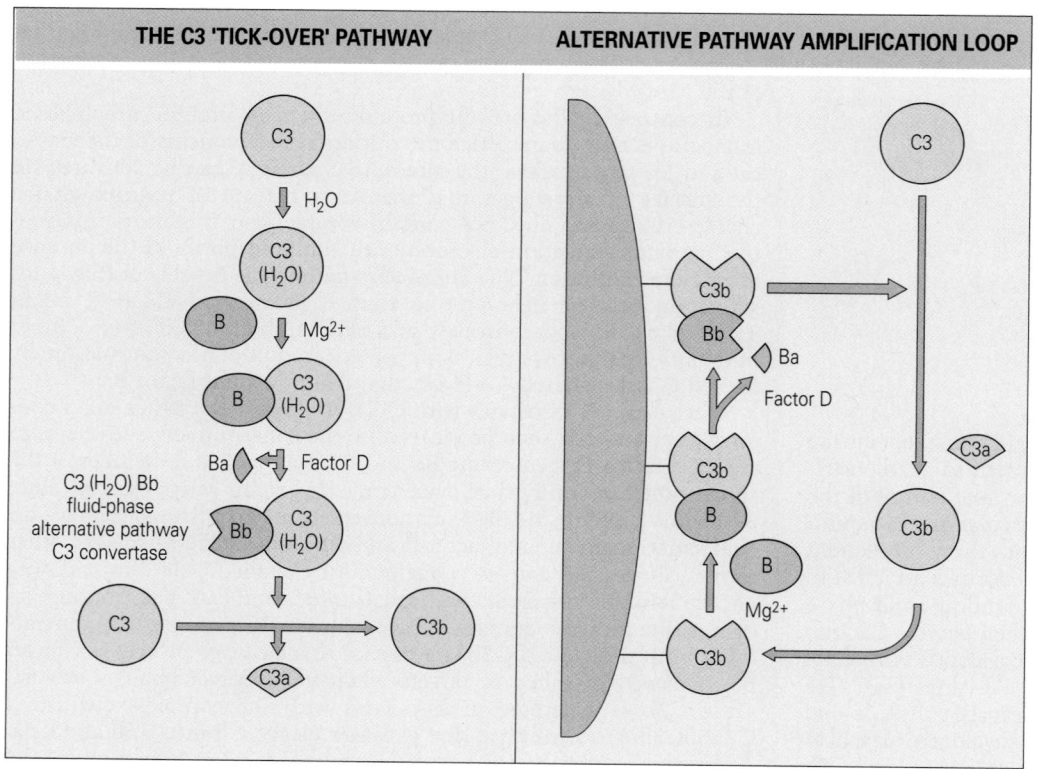

Fig. 20.3 Alternative complement pathway activation events. C3 tickover and amplification loop mechanisms are illustrated. Both depend on the ability of factor B to bind forms of C3, either C3(H₂O) or C3b. The amplification loop can utilize C3b derived from any of the three pathways to increase the downstream generation of effector molecules.

decreased.[22,23] Also, alternative pathway activation is sensitive to changes in pH or ionic strength and conditions such as a low pH can accelerate activation through this pathway. Finally, nucleophilic compounds, such as ammonia, can interact with C3 and promote the development of a C3(H₂O)-like molecule and increase the rate of spontaneous activation of the alternative pathway.

Cleavage of C5 results in the release of C5a, a potent chemotactic and cell-activating molecule, and the noncovalent association of C5b with C3b. This site initiates the assembly of the membrane attack complex (MAC), also designated the terminal complement complex (TCC).[24] The MAC proteins C6-C9 exhibit structural similarities and are built of small subunits of other protein families. In the assembly process, activated C5b is capable of binding C6 and results in a complex that binds C7. The C5b67 complex then associates with the cell membrane. The interaction of C8 with this complex results in the deeper incorporation into the lipid bilayer but incomplete disruption of the cell membrane. To this complex, C9 will bind initially as a monomer and then polymerize. This final process forms the basis for the cell-damaging transmembrane pore.

One interesting difference between the early activation pathway and the later (MAC) components of complement is the absence of proteolytic activity of the later components (after C5). In this regard, C6 through C9 can assemble because each protein can undergo conformational changes that expose new reactive sites. One of the most striking examples is the conformational exposure on C9, a plasma protein, of a hydrophobic lipid interactive face on the α-helices that form the transmembrane pore. In this regard, C9 shares many features with other pore-forming proteins, such as the cytotoxic granule protein perforin.

Local and systemic synthesis of soluble complement components

The liver has traditionally been thought of as being the site of complement component synthesis; however, although this is true of 80% to 90% of the total of most soluble components, many other cell types have been shown to synthesize complement, and there is an emerging understanding that locally produced complement factors are especially important in organ-specific injury. Other cell types that synthesize complement activation and regulatory proteins include monocyte/macrophage, fibroblast, renal mesangial, epithelial, endothelial, and lymphoid, including both T and B cells. Notably, factor D is primarily produced by adipocytes. Both hepatic and tissue specific production is upregulated by the proinflammatory cytokines IL-1, tumor necrosis factor, interleukin (IL)-6, and interferon-γ. Conversely, expression can be decreased by cytokines such as IL-4, platelet-derived growth factor (PDGF) and epidermal growth factor (EGF).

Because of the cytokine-dependent control, complement synthesis typically increases in local sites of inflammation. For example, in the kidney of patients with immune complex glomerulonephritis, C3 synthesis is increased locally whereas C4 is constitutively expressed in tubules in normal persons and patients with disease. Activated macrophages, also driven by the cytokines discussed earlier, increase expression of complement components in tissue sites. Importantly, studies using transplantation of wild type or gene-targeted cells or organs into the converse recipients have demonstrated a key role for local production of complement in immune responses to foreign antigens[25] as well as transplanted organ rejection.[26]

COMPLEMENT RECEPTORS

Receptors for many components of complement have been identified (Fig. 20.4), typically demonstrating high affinity for proteolytic cleavage fragments of specific proteins generated during the activation process (e.g., C3b or C5a) (see Table 20.2). Four distinct receptors, each with preferential binding for different fragments of C3, have been defined.[2,27] CR1 is widely distributed, being found on erythrocytes, polymorphonuclear neutrophils, mononuclear phagocytes, B cells, some T cells, and mesangial phagocytes. CR1 binds C4b and C3b, the initial degradation products of C4 and C3 that are covalently bound to targets, and is also reported to be a receptor for C1q and MBL. CR1 exhibits several important functions. For example, it is clearly important on erythrocytes in binding and processing immune complexes and it acts as a phagocytic receptor on neutrophils and macrophages.

CR2 binds C3dg, a degradation product of iC3b, in addition to iC3b itself, and is expressed on B cells, epithelial cells, follicular dendritic cells, thymocytes, and a subset of peripheral T cells. CR2 is also the receptor for the Epstein-Barr virus (EBV) in addition to the immunoregulatory molecule CD23 that is involved in the production of IgE. CR2 is important in B-cell activation as well as normal trapping of immune complexes in lymphoid tissues.

CR3 and CR4 are members of a group of receptors known as β2-integrins and are composed of two chains: an α-chain of variable size and a common β-chain. Both CR3 and CR4, which bind the C3 degradation product iC3b, are found on fixed tissue macrophages, mononuclear phagocytes, polymorphonuclear neutrophils, and follicular dendritic cells. CR3 and CR4 are probably important in immune complex destruction after erythrocyte CR1-mediated processing of the

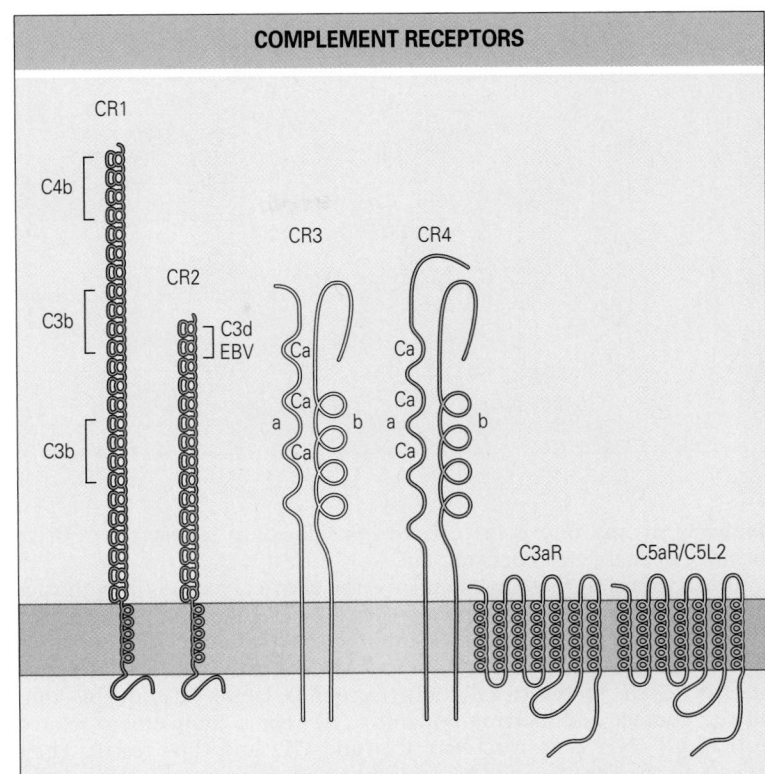

COMPLEMENT RECEPTORS

Fig. 20.4 Complement receptors. CR1 and CR2 are structurally similar molecules composed of the repeating short consensus repeats (SCR). CR3 and CR4 are structurally distinct from CR1 and CR2 and are members of the β2-integrin family of cell surface adhesion molecules. CR3 and CR4, along with LFA-1, share a common β-chain. The C3aR, C5aR, and C5L2 are members of the rhodopsin family, which is characterized by the presence of seven membrane-spanning segments and a functional linkage to G proteins during cell activation processes.

immune complex–bound C3. Deficiency of the family of β2-integrins is associated with loss of adhesive and phagocytic capacity, with severe impairment of host defenses.

Additional types of complement receptors are also important in rheumatic diseases. For example, C5a is a 74-amino acid fragment of C5 that is released during activation and is classified as an anaphylatoxin, and its receptor (C5aR, CD88) is a member of the rhodopsin family.[20] C5a demonstrates potent proinflammatory activities, including leukocyte chemotaxis, aggregation of neutrophils and platelets, release of mast cell mediators, and the generation of leukotrienes, cytokines, and reactive oxygen metabolites. C5L2 is a structurally similar molecule whose biologic role appears to be to modulate C5a functional effects, although it is uncertain as to the exact role that this molecule plays in promoting or limiting complement effects.[28] C3a is a structurally analogous proinflammatory protein derived from C3 that binds the C3a receptor (C3aR) and also plays important roles in diseases such as asthma.[29] Each of these receptors is widely distributed, being expressed on neutrophils, monocytes/macrophages, mast cells, hepatocytes, bronchial and alveolar epithelial cells, vascular endothelium, and astrocytes in addition to other cells.

MECHANISMS OF COMPLEMENT CONTROL

Because of the potent activities manifest by complement, it is a tightly regulated system with inhibitors that act at many steps of the pathway.[30] Figure 20.5 illustrates the specific points at which 11 inhibitors act on the complement pathway. These proteins utilize many molecular mechanisms to block complement activation, including acting as a protease inhibitor, a competitive inhibitor of multiple-component enzymes, and/or cofactor for proteolytic cleavage or as protease itself. Because of the presence of these many inhibitors in sites at which activators can be found or deposited, the state of the complement

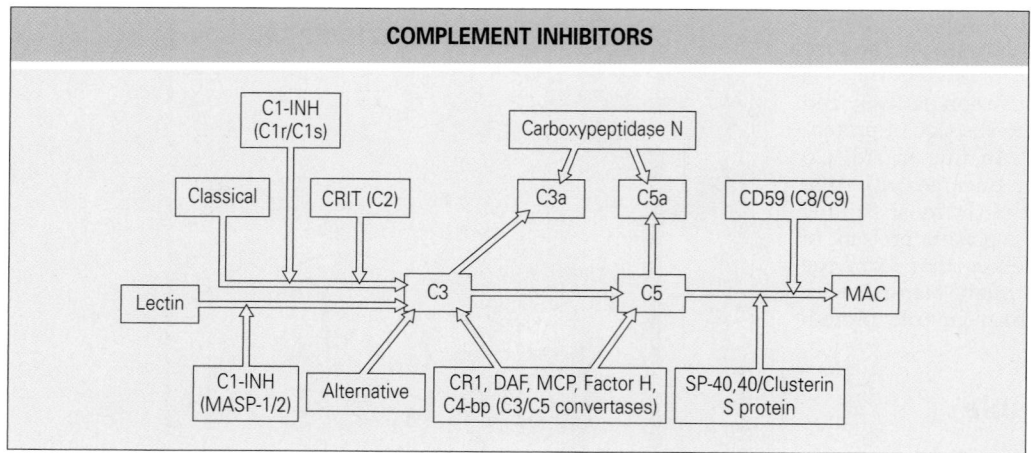

COMPLEMENT INHIBITORS

Fig. 20.5 Naturally occurring inhibitors of the complement pathway. Shown at the sites of action on the complement pathway are the many well-characterized complement inhibitors of this pathway (also included in Table 20.4). Activation pathways are shown in broken lines and sites of regulation in solid lines. Some inhibitors act at multiple points on the pathway, and some activation steps have as many as five proteins that regulate it (e.g., the C3 convertase activation step).

pathway at any one point can be considered to reflect the relative balance of these two opposing forces.

With regard to these mechanisms, the classical and lectin pathways are both blocked at the protease step by C1 inhibitor,[31] which is a member of the serine proteinase inhibitor (serpin) family and serves as an irreversible trap for C1r/C1s and MASP-1/MASP-2. C1-INH also inactivates the proteases kallikrein, factor XIa, factor XIIa, and plasmin of the contact and clotting systems. The major complement-related role of C1-INH is to inactivate C1r and C1s and thus restrict their effects to the specific site of C1 binding and activation.

At the C3/C5 activation steps, several proteins serve to either accelerate the normal decay of C3 and C5 convertases or as cofactors for serum factor I–mediated cleavage. Factor I (C3b inactivator, C3bINA) cleaves C3b and C4b at specific sites and acts on these proteins when they are either free in the fluid phase or target bound. Factor I plays the very important role of cleaving both C3b and C4b in a highly regulated fashion into specific forms of the molecules that can no longer act as part of a C3 or C5 convertase.

In the fluid phase, two major proteins serve to block complement activity at the C3/C5 activation steps. One is factor H, which serves to accelerate the normally slow spontaneous decay of Bb from C3b in the alternative pathway, thus disabling both the C3 and C5 convertases, as well as to exhibit cofactor activity for factor I–mediated cleavage of C3b into the hemolytically inactive form iC3b. Factor H is a 150-kDa serum protein with a structure consisting of 20 repeating units designated short consensus repeats (SCR), or complement control protein repeats (CCP), a structural feature that defines its gene family.[32] Factor H appears to bind to target cells and tissues primarily through initial contact by SCRs 19-20 with tissue that expresses polyanions and fixed C3b/C3d, followed by the elaboration of protective complement alternative pathway C3 convertase inhibitory function on the tissue itself.

Notably, the alternative pathway is also unique in that it is positively affected by a multimeric positive regulatory protein that is designated properdin.[33] Properdin is a polymeric protein that can bind to both C3b and factor B in the C3 convertase and keeps these proteins together and active with regard to additional C3 cleavage. Recent studies have also suggested that properdin can recognize certain target tissues and initiate alternative pathway activation.

With regard to the classical pathway, C4b-binding protein (C4-bp) is a fluid phase protein with parallel activities as factor H but directed toward C4b and the classical pathway rather than C3b and the alternative pathway.[34] C4-bp is also a member of the regulator of complement activation (RCA) protein family that inactivates C4b by serving as an obligate cofactor for factor I–mediated cleavage and also accelerates the spontaneous decay of C2a from C4b. Therefore, C4-bp has both of the functional characteristics of factor H, cofactor activity, and decay acceleration but instead exerts its activities on C4 rather than C3. Of interest, C4-bp can also be utilized by several bacterial species that specifically bind this protein to their surfaces and block complement-mediated killing.

Additional soluble proteins that inhibit the assembly or membrane insertion of the MAC (C5b-9) have also been identified. The two best

characterized are a protein designated SP-40,40 (or clusterin) and S protein (vitronectin). S protein is a multifunctional protein identified by co-purification with C5b-9 from activated human serum. Later studies determined that S protein is identical to vitronectin (serum-spreading factor) and is a widely distributed protein in the intercellular matrix functionally related to fibronectin, laminin, von Willebrand factor, thrombospondin, and collagen. S protein is postulated to act by incorporation into the C5b-7 complex, thus converting the latter to a hydrophilic, non–membrane-binding, and thus inactive, complex. Under these conditions, although C8 and C9 can still bind to the complex, C9 cannot polymerize. SP-40,40 (clusterin) is a disulfide-linked heterodimer that is derived by proteolytic cleavage of a single-chain precursor. It is found free in normal serum and in complement activated serum associated with soluble C5b-9 complexes. SP-40,40 (clusterin) has the same type of complement regulatory activity previously described for S protein.

On the cell membrane, other proteins serve similar functions to block complement activation. These proteins include decay-accelerating factor [DAF] (CD55), membrane cofactor protein [MCP] (CD46), and CD59. DAF is an approximately 70-kDa glycoprotein with a substantial content of O-linked sugars. It acts by binding C3b or C4b on the cell membrane and markedly increasing the spontaneous decay of both the classical pathway C4b2a and alternative pathway C3bBb complexes.[30] DAF is a widely distributed protein that has a glycophosphatidylinositol (GPI) anchor. It has also been shown to have cell-cell adhesion properties by serving as a counter-receptor for CD97. MCP is a widely distributed surface membrane human C3 binding protein that acts as a required cofactor for the cleavage of C3 or C4 into their hemolytically inactive forms, iC3b and iC4b.[30] MCP, therefore, plays a similar biologic role as DAF—protection of cells from inadvertent complement deposition. However, the specific enzymatic activity is different and results in an inactive form of the C3 protein. The expression of MCP is widespread, with the notable exception of erythrocytes; and soluble forms have been found in many biologic tissues.

CD59 is a widely distributed, highly disulfide-linked protein with a GPI anchor and a significant sequence similarity to the Ly-6 mouse antigens.[35] It is found on erythrocytes, monocytes, granulocytes, platelets, endothelial cells, and many cells of the nervous and reproductive tissues. CD59 manifests both complement-related and apparently complement-unrelated activities. With regard to complement regulation, CD59 is able to bind C8 in the C5b-8 complex and to block the effective incorporation of C9. In addition, CD59 is capable of binding C9 already in the MAC and of blocking the subsequent polymerization of C9 and full formation of the transmembrane pore. CD59 is also an adhesion molecule and serves as one counter-receptor for CD2.

Another type of cell membrane protein inhibitor is exemplified by complement C2 receptor inhibitor trispanning (CRIT).[36] This protein binds to C2 and blocks C2 cleavage and thus effectively dampens classical pathway C3 convertase formation. Recent reports suggest that CRIT may also be able to block alternative pathway activation.

Once released, the potent anaphylatoxins C5a and C3a undergo a rapid loss of activity in serum primarily caused by C-terminal cleavage of Arg to make the desArg form.[37] Serum carboxypeptidase-N performs this cleavage, which results in C3a and C5a derivatives with two to three orders of magnitude less cell-stimulating activity.

Each of these inhibitors has an important role in homeostasis of the complement system. This is best demonstrated by the observation that almost every homozygous deficiency, and many heterozygous deficiencies, in humans are accompanied by evidence of uncontrolled complement activation and target organ damage.

BIOLOGIC ROLES OF COMPLEMENT

Complement demonstrates many roles in the immune response. A major role of complement is to identify and mark foreign organisms and antigens as "non-self" using recognition by MBP, C1q, and covalently bound C4b/C3b that is catalyzed by antibody interaction or through lectin and alternative pathway mechanisms. These fragments then play a major role in the clearance of these antigens by binding their cellular receptors. In addition, complement potentiates the B-cell immune response to antigens by providing a co-stimulatory signal for B-cell activation, high-affinity antibody generation, and the establishment of memory. Cleavage fragments like C5a and C3a recruit inflammatory cells such as neutrophils into a tissue site and also provide an activation signal that increases expression of other proinflammatory molecules or the activation of receptors such as CR3 and FcR. C5a also binds receptors on hepatocytes and increases the expression of acute-phase proteins, thus potentiating the effects of proinflammatory cytokines.

Additional effects of complement are found on nucleated cells when they are bound by the MAC. These biologic effects include calcium flux, vesiculation, and the generation of proinflammatory and fibrosis-promoting mediators such as reactive oxygen metabolites, basic fibroblast growth factor (bFGF), and PDGF in addition to cytokines such as IL-1. In the glomerulus, genes such as collagen type IV are activated, and in the central nervous system changes in neuronal cell growth can be detected. Complement also plays a major role in the tissue injury that follows ischemia/reperfusion injury, an area not typically considered to be immune related.[9]

An additional very important process that goes awry in patients with SLE in which complement plays a major role is the proper handling and disposal of immune complexes in the circulation.[38] To prevent disease mediated by immune complex deposition, complement-related protective mechanisms have evolved to effectively eliminate immune complexes from both the circulation and from tissues. The degradation product of the third component of complement, C3b, becomes covalently bound to the immune complex after complement activation and provides the ligand necessary for recognition of the complement-opsonized immune complex by CR1 on erythrocytes. This facilitates binding of immune complexes by erythrocytes and their subsequent transfer to phagocytes in the reticuloendothelial system. Complement activation by immune complexes also leads to their "solubilization," that is, the transformation of larger, preformed complexes into smaller ones and prevention of insoluble complex formation.

More recently, several novel activities have been identified in the complement system that have extended its reach into additional systems. One example has been the finding that, after partial hepatectomy or liver injury, complement activation fragments C3a and C5a demonstrate the capacity to promote regeneration.[7] These data suggest that complement can help not only to initiate inflammation in response to injured tissues but also to promote replacement of that tissue by healthy tissue. Another example of a novel complement effect has been the demonstration that C4-bp protein can activate human B cells by serving as a ligand for the CD40 surface protein.[39] C4-bp also exhibits the ability to bind to apoptotic cell membranes and restrict further complement activation through C4.[40]

Complement receptors demonstrate additional non-complement ligands, perhaps the best demonstrations being EBV binding to CR2 and measles virus binding to MCP. In addition, though, CR2 also interacts with interferon-α and a wide array of complement receptors and regulatory proteins serve as docking mechanisms whereby pathogens bind to and gain entrance to the intracellular compartment through C3-dependent or C3-independent mechanisms in such a manner that they can then infect the cells expressing these complement proteins.[41]

COMPLEMENT AND SYSTEMIC LUPUS ERYTHEMATOSUS

Deficiency of classical pathway activation proteins, a genetic predisposition to the development of SLE

Both inherited and acquired abnormalities in complement classical pathway components have been described in SLE.[5,42] Several different molecular mechanisms can lead to homozygous complement component deficiency, and homozygous deficiencies in the early components of the complement cascade (C1q, C1r/C1s, C4, and C2) are often associated with SLE. Although it is possible to speculate that such a complement deficiency might lead to the decreased generation of pro-inflammatory fragments after antibody-mediated activation and be beneficial, the opposite is clearly true. In particular, patients with complete C1q deficiency demonstrate the most similarity to other patients with SLE in that they often develop severe glomerulonephritis and typical autoantibodies.[5]

Although total homozygous deficiency in any individual component is rare, heterozygous deficiency in C4 is much more common, and patients with SLE show in some studies an increased prevalence of null alleles for C4A. C2-deficient patients have a lupus-like disease with prominent cutaneous manifestations. Homozygous C3 deficiency is extremely rare, with most affected patients suffering from recurrent infections and some having hematuria and/or proteinuria. Interestingly, the presence of a low-producing or dysfunctional MBP allele that cannot efficiently activate complement is also associated with a small increased risk for SLE.[43] In many of these complement deficiencies there is also a predilection for increased rates of infection. Interestingly, individuals with deficiencies of late components (MAC) less frequently have autoimmune features but rather present with recurrent neisserial infections.[44]

These observations that a deficiency in the early components of the classical pathway of complement activation promote the development of SLE have led to two major hypotheses regarding the pathogenic mechanisms. The first is that this leads to a marked decrease in the ability to opsonize, transport, and/or solubilize immune complexes.[45] This dysfunction may predispose to the development of SLE by allowing a cycle to develop in which immune complexes deposit in tissue, inducing inflammation and, over long periods of time, tissue destruction. An alternate hypothesis suggests that autoimmunity is promoted because the inability to clear apoptotic bodies containing nuclear components leads to a break in self-tolerance to these antigens and the development of SLE.[5]

Autoantibodies in patients with SLE have also been found to cause acquired deficiencies, such as C3(Nef), an autoantibody that stabilizes the alternative pathway C3 convertase and results in C3 consumption. In addition, some autoantibodies may be associated with dysfunction of components in the absence of a clearly decreased level. For example, patients with SLE have a strikingly increased incidence of antibodies to the component C1q.[46] These autoantibodies are highly associated with the presence of glomerulonephritis and likely act by potentiating the local effects of C1q fixation to immune complexes.[47] Whether these antibodies promote the further loss of self tolerance by interfering with C1q in a manner that mimics C1q deficiency is also possible.

Lupus nephritis

The complement system is integrally involved in the pathogenesis of tissue injury in SLE, and complement components appear to mediate tissue damage initiated by autoantibodies.[48] Evidence for this includes the presence of complement activation fragments in the glomerulus, tubules, interstitium, and urine in many forms of lupus glomerulonephritis. In the context of the discussion regarding the role of classical pathway deficiencies as a predisposition to SLE, it is important to note that the great majority of patients with SLE have an intact complement system and even those with classical pathway deficiencies have an intact alternative and, likely lectin, pathway. Direct support for a role of complement in lupus nephritis was first provided by the findings that an inhibitory anti-C5 mAb blocks the development of glomerulonephritis in the (NZB × NZW)F₁ model of SLE.[49] Subsequently, a key role for the alternative pathway was suggested by the finding that *fB*–/– and *fD*–/– MRL/*lpr* mice are protected from renal disease.[50]

Although many of the studies have focused on the role of complement in glomerular diseases, substantial evidence exists suggesting additional roles in the pathogenesis of tubulointerstitial inflammation and chronic proteinuric diseases.[51] In particular, emerging evidence strongly suggests that complement activation pathway components that enter the urinary space when the basement membrane is disrupted are capable of being activated on the tubular epithelium that has a relative lack of complement regulatory proteins.

Vasculitis and immune complex abnormalities in SLE

In SLE there are reduced levels of CR1 on erythrocytes.[52] The low levels of CR1 on erythrocytes are thought to be an acquired consequence of disease rather than a cause of disease. That is because normal erythrocytes with high levels of CR1 "acquire" lower levels of CR1 expression with time after transfusion into SLE patients and because CR1 with its bound immune complexes is most probably stripped from erythrocytes as the immune complexes are taken up by phagocytes in the liver. Therefore, the combined presence of genetically determined deficiencies in the complement system, amplified by further acquired deficiencies, leads to a condition of continued complex formation and deposition.

For example, patients with SLE display altered clearance kinetics of tetanus toxoid (TT)/anti-TT, model immune complex that is used to assess complement- and CR1-mediated clearance. This soluble immune complex disappears from the circulation of patients with SLE initially more rapidly than in normal persons, and this difference is thought to reflect rapid deposition in peripheral tissues due to inefficient complement-mediated immune complex removal by the RES. Although abnormal receptor-mediated clearance contributes to immune complex deposition and is correlated with disease activity, many other factors also influence immune complex handling. These factors include the size of the complex, local blood conditions, preexisting tissue inflammation, and the opportunity for charge/charge interactions.

Complement in cutaneous disease of SLE

In general, complement plays an important proinflammatory role in antibody-mediated cutaneous diseases in a similar fashion as other tissue sites.[53] In addition, in patients with SLE the lupus band test commonly demonstrates the deposition of C3 along with immunoglobulin at the dermal/epidermal junction.[54] In lesional skin, complement is often found; in particular, the presence of the MAC may be relatively more specific for SLE.[55]

Atherosclerosis and complement

The complement system is activated during the ischemic and necrotic phases of acute myocardial ischemia, and many studies have supported its role in promoting tissue damage. In addition to being activated during tissue damage caused by infarction, purified recombinant C5a has been found to cause myocardial dysfunction. Therefore, the potential exists for myocardial effects of complement during systemic activation. In addition, complement has also been strongly implicated in the pathophysiology of atherosclerosis, especially in the inflammatory component of the disease.[56] Because of this, it is tempting to speculate that the accelerated atherosclerosis in some patients with SLE may be secondary to or worsened by chronic complement activation.

Pulmonary disease and complement

The lung is particularly sensitive to complement activation occurring either locally or systemically during episodes of sepsis or ischemia/necrosis after vascular occlusion. This is particularly so because neutrophils that have been activated by C5a can agglutinate, adhere to endothelium, and lodge in the capillaries of lung, resulting in at least transient pulmonary dysfunction. Complement deposition is also found in the lungs of patients with SLE who have chronic interstitial lung disease, and an interesting syndrome of transient pulmonary dysfunction associated with increased C3a levels has been described in hospitalized patients with SLE. C3a has many of the same activating effects on neutrophils as C5a.

Role of complement in hemolytic anemia and thrombocytopenia

Complement plays an important role in both intravascular and, along with Fc receptors, extravascular hemolytic anemia in patients with SLE.[57] In addition, complement has important effects on platelet function *in vivo*,[58] especially because complement activation fragments can directly activate platelets. This likely plays a critically important role in clinical situations characterized by microvascular thrombosis and neutrophilic vasculitis. Platelets also express many complement regulatory proteins, including DAF, MCP, CD59, and factor H. There are likely many regulatory proteins because the MAC has dramatic effects on platelet function, such as adhesion, increased Ca^{2+} flux, increased thromboxane synthesis, granule release, and activation of kinases.

Pregnancy, its complications and complement

Analysis of the role of complement in pregnancy and SLE is complicated by a number of issues. First, because the normal fetus is a partial allograft with "foreign" paternal antigens, many immunosuppressive mechanisms are utilized to block the immune response and maintain fetal viability. With regard to complement, the expression of membrane and fluid phase complement inhibitors is increased in the placenta, particularly at sites exposed to the maternal circulation This is presumably a mechanism to block the damaging effects of maternal alloantibodies, which commonly develop during pregnancy.[59] Indeed, even normal pregnancies are associated with the deposition of complement at the maternal/fetal junction. Second, a normal pregnancy is associated with the gradual increase in serum levels of complement components C3, C4, and the levels of total hemolytic complement (THC), all of which are routinely followed in patients with SLE.[60] And third, preeclampsia, which is often a critical differential diagnosis in the acutely ill pregnant patient who may have active SLE with nephritis, is also associated with substantial complement activation.

Because of the varied presentations of patients with SLE and pregnancy, especially in the acute setting that requires one to differentiate a flare presenting with nephritis from preeclampsia alone, substantial efforts have been made to develop better laboratory diagnostic strategies. In particular, the levels of complement split products such as Bb, Ba, and SC5b-9 (soluble MAC) have been examined and found to be elevated in pregnant lupus patients with a flare.[60] Increased levels of Bb and Ba were highly sensitive and predictive of a lupus flare in patients.

In addition to complications with pregnancy due to inflammation, patients with SLE are particularly susceptible to the development of antiphospholipid syndrome (APS), an autoimmune disease characterized by recurrent fetal loss, vascular thrombosis, and thrombocytopenia in the presence of antiphospholipid antibodies. Although the pathogenesis of this syndrome had been attributed to the ability of these antibodies to directly modify clotting-related activities or cell activation, using a murine model of APS in which pregnant mice are injected with human antiphospholipid antibodies containing IgG it was found that inhibition of the complement cascade *in vivo* at the point of complement factor B, C3, or C5 activation, or blockade of C5a, resulted in the absence of fetal loss and growth retardation as well as diminished activation of macrophage tissue factor generation.[61]

Central nervous system disease and complement

Many studies have emphasized the concepts that most if not all complement activation and regulatory proteins are actively synthesized and secreted by central nervous system (CNS) microglial cells and astrocytes.[62] CR1, CR3, and C5aR are also found. Production rates of complement components are increased *in vitro* by proinflammatory cytokines and viral infection. Complement is directly activated by

TABLE 20.5 COMPLEMENT ACTIVATION PROFILES IN INFORMATIVE CLINICAL SITUATIONS

Activated pathway	Profile				Example
	THC	C4	C3	Factor B	
Classical	↓	↓	↓	↓	SLE, serum sickness, RA with vasculitis, essential mixed cryoglobulinemia, systemic vasculitis, hepatitis B antigenemia
Alternative	↓	N	↓	↓	Gram-negative bacteremia, pancreatitis, poststreptococcal glomerulonephritis, factor I or factor H deficiency, C3(Nef)
Classical and alternative	↓	↓	↓	↓	SLE, type I membranoproliferative glomerulonephritis
Fluid-phase classical	↓	↓	N	N	Hereditary angioedema (HAE)
Acute-phase reaction	↑	↑	↑	↑	Acute and chronic infections, inflammatory disorders, pregnancy
Sample mishandling	↓	N	N	N	

Adapted from Whaley K. Measurement of complement activation in clinical practice. Comp Inflamm 1989;6:96-103.

myelin in the absence of antibody. Complement activation products have significant biologic effects, including the opening of transmembrane pores in myelin by the MAC and increasing eicosanoid production by C5a, C3a, and the MAC.

Not surprisingly, therefore, patients with SLE and active CNS disease demonstrate increased levels of complement components in the cerebrospinal fluid in association with other abnormalities such as oligoclonal bands. However, the increase in complement components is not specific for SLE, because C3/C4 levels are increased in other inflammatory disorders such as aseptic meningitis and soluble MAC levels are increased in patients with Guillain-Barré syndrome and multiple sclerosis among others. In addition to not being specific, these complement-related alterations are not sensitive enough to be routinely useful in clinical decisions in patients with SLE. Because of the known damaging effects of complement on neural tissues, however, it is likely that complement plays a role in some forms of lupus CNS disease; and inhibition of complement activation in these patients should have a clinically beneficial effect.

EXAMPLES OF OTHER RHEUMATIC AND INFLAMMATORY DISEASES IN WHICH COMPLEMENT PLAYS A ROLE

Rheumatoid arthritis

The involvement of complement in RA was initially suggested by the observation that the complement activity of joint fluid from patients is significantly lower than in joint fluid from control non-inflammatory subjects and that significant increases in soluble complement activation fragments in joint fluid as well as enhanced local production of complement proteins in synovial tissue are found.[63] As is typical of many diseases, despite evidence of local complement consumption, systemic complement levels are normal or elevated as an apparent acute-phase response.

Evidence of a primary role for complement in inflammatory arthritis came from studies of anti-C5 monoclonal antibody in the collagen-induced arthritis model[64] and both the K/BxN-derived anti–glucose-6-phosphate isomerase (GPI) serum transfer model of RA[65] and the anti–type II collagen antibody–induced arthritis model.[66]

Atypical hemolytic-uremic syndrome

The hemolytic-uremic syndrome (HUS) is a thrombotic microangiopathy usually associated with diarrheal illness caused by Shiga toxin–producing bacteria. However, non–Shiga toxin–associated HUS, or atypical HUS, has been associated with mutations of the fluid phase alternative pathway inhibitor factor H and the membrane-bound inhibitor MCP (CD46) as well as factor I or the presence of autoantibodies to factor H.[67] Alternative pathway activation during the disease has

been detected by decreased levels of C3 and factor B as well as increased levels of C3 activation fragments while C4 levels are unaffected. In addition, C3 but not C4 is also deposited in the glomeruli and arterioles of patients with atypical HUS. The mutations of factor H associated with atypical HUS reduce the ability of the protein to bind polyanion-rich surfaces (e.g., the glomerular basement membrane), perhaps allowing uncontrolled alternative pathway activation after insults from certain infections or drugs.[67]

MEASUREMENT OF COMPLEMENT IN A CLINICAL SETTING

There are many methods to measure complement functional activity and the levels of individual components and activation fragments.[68,69] Most patients are still initially studied using measurements of C3 and C4 levels in addition to the total hemolytic complement (THC) assay. Although a discussion of these is outside the scope of this chapter, there are some points that are important to the management of patients with SLE. First, patients with active disease generally manifest one of two patterns (Table 20.5) reflecting activation of the classical or alternative pathway, or both. Second, decreased levels of these components generally correlate with the clinical disease activity. And third, although many new assays measuring split products are available that are more sensitive and specific in predicting the presence of clinically active disease, no consensus exists yet that it is useful to prospectively follow patients using complement measurements. On the other hand, recent improvements in complement measures such as the finding of decreased CR1 and increased C4d on erythrocytes may provide more sensitive and specific markers than previous assays.[70]

CONCLUSION

Complement as an effector pathway plays a major role in the target organ damage that accompanies SLE. In addition, the classical pathway is necessary to prevent the development of SLE; and, indeed, C1q deficiency represents the most highly penetrant genetic cause of SLE. There remains many questions regarding the complement system. Among these are the relative importance of each activation pathway in individual diseases, the causal relationships between complement activation and tissue damage in many diseases, what is the relative contribution of locally produced versus systemically derived factors in target organ damage, and how this system can both play a role in the initial damage of some organs as well as promote their regeneration. Finally, what is the most appropriate place in the pathway to block complement as a therapeutic strategy in each clinical situation needs to be clarified. Nevertheless, despite these many questions that remain, it is clear that this system plays a key role in SLE and the further study of it in this disease will undoubtedly lead to additional insights.

KEY REFERENCES

1. Fearon DT, Locksley RM. The instructive role of innate immunity in the acquired immune response. Science 1996;272:50-54.

2. Carroll MC. The role of complement and complement receptors in the induction and regulation of immunity. Ann Rev Immunol 1998;16:545-568.

5. Botto M, Walport MJ. C1q, autoimmunity and apoptosis. Immunobiology 2002;205:395-406.

6. Davies KA, Peters AM, Beynon HLC, Walport MJ. Immune complex processing in patients with systemic lupus erythematosus. J Clin Invest 1992;90:2075-2083.

7. Strey CW, Markiewski M, Matellos D, et al. The proinflammatory mediators C3a and C5a are essential for liver regeneration. J Exp Med 2003;198:913-923.

8. Holers VM. Complement receptors and the shaping of the natural antibody repertoire. Springer Semin Immunopathol 2005;26:405-423.

9. Carroll MC, Holers VM. Innate autoimmunity. Adv Immunol 2005;86:137-157.

11. Pickering MC, Cook HT. Translational mini-review series on complement factor H: renal diseases associated with complement factor H: novel insights from humans and animals. Clin Exp Immunol 2008;151:210-230.

12. Rosse WF, Nishimura J. Clinical manifestations of paroxysmal nocturnal hemoglobinuria: present state and future problems. Int J Hematol 2003;77:113-120.

13. Gehrs KM, Anderson DH, Johnson LV, Hageman GS. Age-related macular degeneration—emerging pathogenetic and therapeutic concepts. Ann Med 2006;38:450-471.

14. Muller-Eberhard HJ. Molecular organization and function of the complement system. Ann Rev Biochem 1988;57:321-347.

15. Holers VM. The spectrum of complement alternative pathway-mediated diseases. Immunol Rev 2008;223:316.

16. Runza VL, Schwaeble W, Mannel DN. Ficolins: novel pattern recognition molecules of the innate immune response. Immunobiology 2008;213:297-306.

17. Gadjeva M, Takahashi K, Thiel S. Mannan-binding lectin—a soluble pattern recognition molecule. Mol Immunol 2004;41:113-121.

19. Sahu A, Lambris JD. Structure and biology of complement protein C3, a connecting link between innate and acquired immunity. Immunol Rev 2001;180:35-48.

20. Wetsel RA. Structure, function and cellular expression of complement anaphylatoxin receptors. Curr Opin Immunol 1995;7:48-53.

21. Lachmann PJ, Hughes-Jones NC. Initiation of complement activation. Springer Semin Immunopathol 1984;7:143-162.

22. Xu C, Mao D, Holers VM, et al. A critical role for murine complement regulator crry in fetomaternal tolerance. Science 2000;287:498-501.

23. Linton SM, Morgan BP. Complement activation and inhibition in experimental models of arthritis. Mol Immunol 1999;36:905-914.

24. Shin ML, Rus HG, Nicolescu FI. Membrane attack by complement: assembly and biology of terminal complement complexes. Biomembranes 1996;4:123-149.

25. Gadjeva M, Verschoor A, Brockman MA, et al. Macrophage-derived complement component C4 can restore humoral immunity in C4-deficient mice. J Immunol 2002;169:5489-5495.

26. Pratt JR, Basheer SA, Sacks SH. Local synthesis of complement component C3 regulates acute renal transplant rejection. Nat Med 2002;8:582-587.

27. Holers VM. Complement receptors. Year Immunol 1989;4:231-240.

28. Ward PA. Functions of C5a receptors. J Mol Med 2009;87:378.

30. Liszewski MK, Farries TC, Lublin DM, et al. Control of the complement system. Adv Immunol 1996;61:201-283.

31. Davis AE. C1 inhibitor and hereditary angioedema. Ann Rev Immunol 1988;6:595-628.

32. Hourcade D, Holers VM, Atkinson JP. The regulators of complement activation (RCA) gene cluster. Adv Immunol 1989;45:381-416.

33. Kemper C, Hourcade DE. Properdin: new roles in pattern recognition and target clearance. Mol Immunol 2008;45:4048-4056.

34. Blom AM. Complement inhibitor C4b-binding protein-friend or foe in the innate immune system? Mol Immunol 2004;40:1333-1346.

35. Morgan BP, Berg CW, Harris CL. "Homologous restriction" in complement lysis: roles of membrane complement regulators. Xenotransplantation 2005;12:258-265.

36. Inal JM, Hui KM, Miot S, et al. Complement C2 receptor inhibitor trispanning: a novel human complement inhibitory receptor. J Immunol 2005;174:356-366.

37. Matthews KW, Mueller-Ortiz SL, Wetsel RA. Carboxypeptidase N: a pleiotropic regulator of inflammation. Mol Immunol 2004;40:785-793.

38. Birmingham DJ. Erythrocyte complement receptors. Crit Rev Immunol 1995;15:133-154.

39. Brodeur SR, Angelini F, Bacharier LB, et al. C4b-binding protein (C4BP) activates B cells through the CD40 receptor. Immunity 2003;18:837-848.

40. Trouw LA, Nilsson SC, Goncalves I, Blom AM. C4b-binding protein binds to necrotic cells and DNA, limiting DNA release and inhibiting complement activation. J Exp Med 2005;210:1937-1948.

43. Lee YH, Witte T, Momot T, et al. The mannose-binding lectin gene polymorphisms and systemic lupus erythematosus: two case-control studies and a meta-analysis. Arthritis Rheum 2005;52:3966-3974.

44. Figueroa JE, Densen P. Infectious diseases associated with complement deficiencies. Clin Microbiol Rev 1991;4:359-395.

47. Trouw LA, Groeneveld TWL, Seelen MA, et al. Anti-C1q autoantibodies deposit in glomeruli but are only pathogenic in combination with glomerular C1q-containing immune complexes. J Clin Invest 2004;114:679-688.

48. Quigg RJ. Complement and autoimmune glomerular diseases. Curr Dir Autoimmun 2004;7:165-180.

49. Wang Y, Madri JA, Rollins SA, et al. Amelioration of lupus-like autoimmune disease in NZB/W F1 mice after treatment with a blocking monoclonal antibody specific for complement component C5. Proc Natl Acad Sci U S A 1996;93:8563-8568.

50. Elliott MK, Jarmi T, Ruiz P, et al. Effects of complement factor D deficiency on the renal disease of MRL/lpr mice. Kidney Int 2004;65:129-138.

54. Provost TT, Maddison PJ, Reichlin M. Lupus band test in untreated SLE patients: correlation of immunoglobulin deposition in the skin of the extensor forearm with clinical renal disease and serological abnormalities. J Invest Dermatol 1980;74:407-412.

56. Kao AH, Sabatine JM, Manzi S. Update on vascular disease in systemic lupus erythematosus. Curr Opin Rheumatol 2003;15:519-527.

59. Rooney IA, Oglesby TJ, Atkinson JP. Complement in human reproduction: activation and control. Immunol Res 1993;12:279-294.

60. Abramson SB, Buyon JP. Activation of the complement pathway: comparison of normal pregnancy, preeclampsia, and systemic lupus erythematosus during pregnancy. Am J Reprod Immunol 1992;28:183-187.

61. Girardi G, Yarilin D, Thurman JM, et al. Complement activation induces dysregulation of angiogenic factors and causes fetal rejection and growth restriction. J Exp Med 2006;203:2165-2175.

66. Banda NK, Takahashi K, Wood AK, et al. Pathogenic complement activation in collagen antibody-induced arthritis in mice requires amplification by the alternative pathway. J Immunol 2007;179:4101-4109.

68. Opperman M, Hopken U, Gotze O. Assessment of complement activation in vivo. Immunopharmacology 1992;24:119-134.

69. Whaley K. Measurement of complement activation in clinical practice. Comp Inflamm 1989;6:96-103.

70. Manzi S, Navratil JS, Ruffing MJ, et al. Measurement of erythrocyte C4d and complement receptor 1 in systemic lupus erythematosus. Arthritis Rheum 1994;50:3596-3604.

REFERENCES

Full references for this chapter can be found on www.expertconsult.com.

Inflammation

Aryeh M. Abeles, Michael H. Pillinger, and Steven B. Abramson

21

- Inflammation is the primary process by which the body attacks and destroys microbial invaders, heals wounds, and damages its own tissues.

- The acute, or early, phase of inflammation is characterized by microvascular changes and activation of granulocytic cells (neutrophils, mast cells, eosinophils). Cells from the monocytic lineage predominate in the mature or chronic inflammatory response.

- Activation of platelets and endothelial cells are essential elements of the inflammatory response in tissues.

- Among the most important plasma-derived mediators of inflammation are the products of complement activation, which provoke vasodilation, chemotaxis of granulocytes, and the secretion of mediators from inflammatory cells.

- Multiple inflammatory mediators released from activated cells provoke tissue injury. These include histamine and serotonin, prostaglandins and leukotrienes, superoxide anion, and nitric oxide.

- The inflammatory response involves a complex interaction between the nervous system and inflammatory cells.

INTRODUCTION

Inflammatory processes are necessary for survival and play roles in both maintaining organism homeostasis and warding off infection. Best recognized as a localized response to injury from any number of insults (e.g., microbial pathogens, trauma, neoplasia, toxins), inflammation is also important in tissue remodeling during development, as well as in the clearance of debris during cellular tissue turnover.

For two millennia, inflammation has been clinically recognized by the cardinal signs of calor (heat), rubor (redness), dolor (pain), and tumor (swelling). A fifth sign, functio laesa (loss of function), was proposed by the 19th century German pathologist Virchow and highlights the potential for inflammation to impair an organism functionally. At the cellular level, inflammation involves a series of events, beginning with vasodilation and increased permeability of the microcirculation, that ultimately lead to transmigration of leukocytes, the foot soldiers of inflammation, into the injured tissue.[1] Inflammation at once involves the interplay of multiple cell types, of the innate and adaptive immune responses, of the immunologic and nervous systems, and of the coagulation and fibrinolytic cascades. These responses are regulated, in a complex and integrated manner, by the simultaneous effects of a wide range of molecular mediators. These inflammatory mediators are highly diverse but can be loosely grouped into the following categories: (1) growth factors and cytokines, (2) arachidonic acid derivatives/lipid mediators, (3) the complement system, (4) proteases, (5) neuropeptides, and (6) free radicals/reactive oxygen species.

In health, inflammation is a self-limited response to a specific injury; once the injury is repaired, the inflammatory focus clears and homeostasis is restored. On occasion, however, the inflammatory response is triggered inappropriately, is excessive for the problem at hand, or fails to resolve after the acute trigger is removed. Excessive inflammation may result, for example, in response to a persistent host antigen being mistaken as foreign (as in rheumatic fever or post-streptococcal glomerulonephritis) or from a decreased ability to clear immune system stimulants such as immune complexes (as in systemic lupus erythematosus [SLE]); in these cases, an autoimmune response drives undesirable and potentially destructive inflammation. In other, so-called autoinflammatory syndromes (e.g., familial Mediterranean fever and tumor necrosis factor receptor (TNF)–associated periodic fever syndrome), the inflammatory cells themselves may have defects that lead to undesirable inflammation.[2] In many cases, we still do not fully understand what causes pure inflammatory diseases.

Nonetheless, our understanding of inflammatory processes has increased remarkably over the past several decades; these gains have led to the first targeted therapies for inflammatory diseases, including agents that block the cytokines TNF-α, interleukin (IL)-1β, and IL-6. The more that we learn about the processes of inflammation, the more likely we will be able to develop effective therapies for rheumatic and other inflammatory diseases.

In this chapter we summarize the major cellular participants in inflammation and provide an overview of the mediators that drive inflammatory responses.

THE CELLS OF INFLAMMATION

Acute versus chronic inflammation

Inflammatory responses can be either acute or chronic. The acute, or early, phase of inflammation is characterized by microvascular changes and neutrophilic infiltration, whereas cells from the monocytic lineage predominate in the chronic inflammatory response. These distinctions are somewhat arbitrary, however, with many exceptions. For example, monocytic lineage cells may dominate from the beginning of an inflammatory response (as in tuberculosis), whereas neutrophils may persist in some forms of chronic inflammation (as in polyarteritis nodosa). Resident tissue macrophages from the monocytic line may also provide the early sentinel signals that initiate acute inflammation, as appears to be the case in gout and pseudogout.[3]

Endothelial cell activation

Many of the leukocytes that participate in inflammation circulate within the bloodstream. To localize to extravascular tissue, these cells must exit the vasculature (diapedesis) and migrate to the appropriate extravascular space (chemotaxis). These processes require a complex sequence of events, beginning with the (micro) vascular response to injury. Arterioles vasodilate and endothelial cells contract, exposing the basement membrane; blood flow slows and plasma extravasates.[4] In turn, leukocytes concentrate and gain increased contact with the endothelium.[5]

In response to bacteria or other affront, resident tissue immune cells (macrophages, dendritic cells, and fibroblasts) generate mediators such as IL-1β and TNF-α. These cytokines (Gk. "cell movers") induce local vascular endothelial cells to express surface molecules that contact and bind leukocytes, permitting their egress from the vasculature.[6] Different groups of adhesion molecules sequentially mediate leukocyte rolling, tight adhesion, and passage through the vascular wall, or diapedesis (Fig. 21.1). The first step, leukocyte rolling, occurs via the interactions of the adhesion molecules E-selectin on endothelial cells and L-selectin on leukocytes, with mucin-like sialylated glycoproteins on leukocytes and endothelial cells, respectively.[6] Selectins are expressed constitutively on both leukocytes and endothelium, and their interactions are strong but short-lived, with the result that a percentage of leukocytes are transiently adherent, or marginated, to the endothelium at all times, moving along with a tumbleweed-like progression. At sites of inflammation, after exposure to stimuli such as IL-1β and TNF-α, the expression of E-selectin on endothelial cells increases markedly, leading to an increase in the percentage of leukocytes that marginate

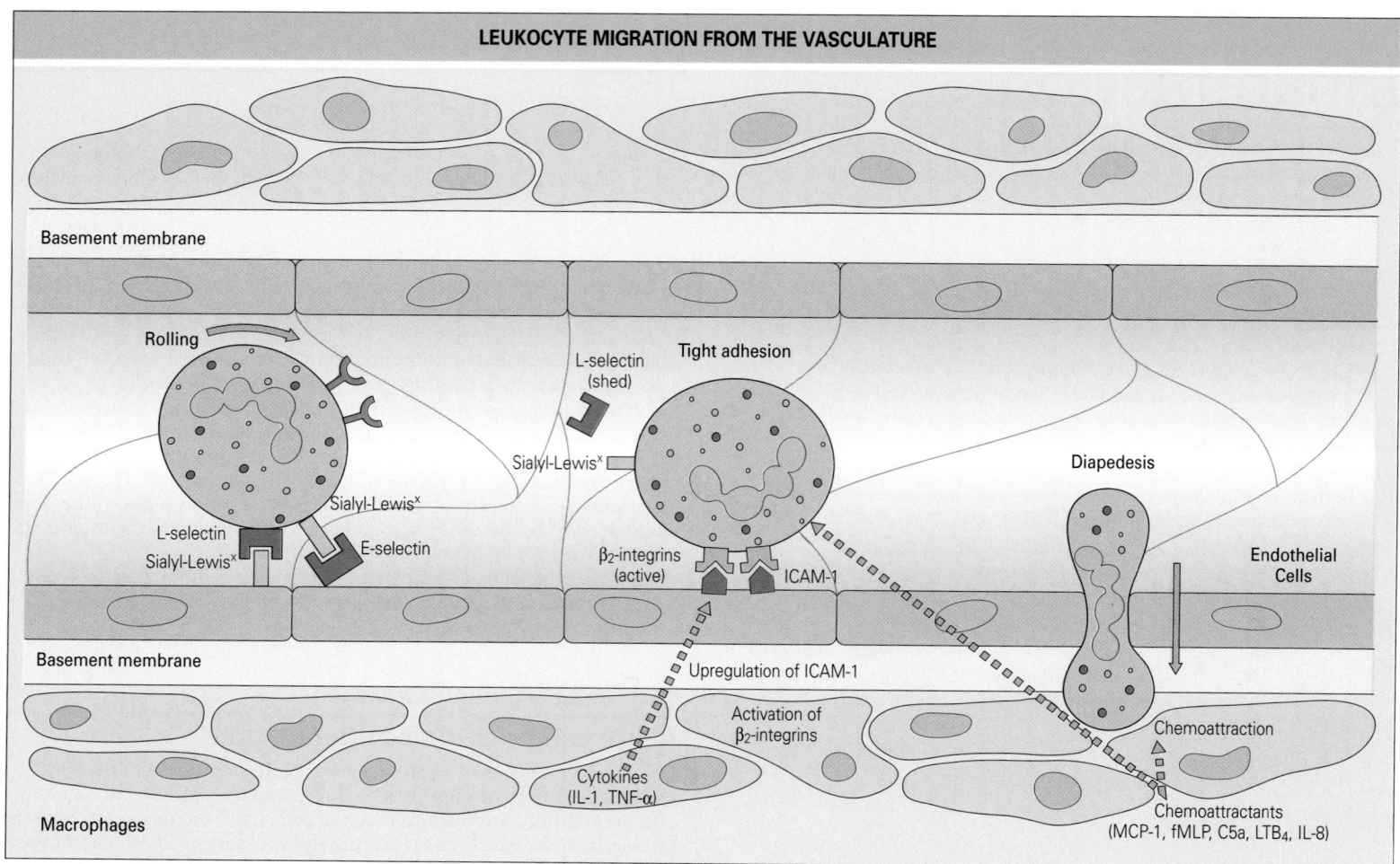

LEUKOCYTE MIGRATION FROM THE VASCULATURE

Basement membrane

Rolling

Tight adhesion

L-selectin
(shed)

Diapedesis

Sialyl-Lewis^x

Sialyl-Lewis^x

L-selectin

Sialyl-Lewis^x E-selectin

β₂-integrins
(active)   ICAM-1

Endothelial
Cells

Basement membrane

Upregulation of ICAM-1

Activation of
β₂-integrins

Chemoattraction

Cytokines
(IL-1, TNF-α)

Macrophages

Chemoattractants
(MCP-1, fMLP, C5a, LTB₄, IL-8)

Fig. 21.1 Leukocyte migration from the vasculature. Leukocytes exit the vasculature through a sequence of interactions with the vascular endothelium. The first step, rolling, guarantees leukocyte-endothelial contact through transient interactions between selectins and sialylated glycoproteins (sialyl-Lewis^x) on cognate cells. Leukocyte tight adhesion results from the interaction of leukocyte adhesion molecules known as integrins with counter-ligands on endothelial cells, such as ICAM-1. In contrast to selectin/glycoprotein interactions, integrin/ICAM interactions are activation and expression dependent. Once tightly adherent to the endothelium, leukocytes transmigrate through the vasculature and into the tissues. Activation of leukocytes, and their transmigration through the endothelium and basement membrane, is mediated by chemoattractants such as MCP-1, C5a, fMLP, LTB₄, and IL-8.

and roll. The next step, leukocyte tight adhesion, results from the interaction of leukocyte adhesion molecules known as integrins (e.g., CD11a/CD18 or LFA-1, CD11b/CD18 or CR3, α4β1, or VLA-4) with counterligands on endothelial cells (e.g., the cellular adhesion molecules [CAMs] ICAM-1 and VCAM-1).[7] This process requires *de novo* expression of CAMs on endothelium and activation of preexisting integrins on leukocytes, both in response to inflammatory mediators. Specific integrin/ligand pairing, in turn, establishes specific cell-cell adhesion events that contribute to the distribution and homing of leukocytes; common integrin/ligand pairs include CD11a/CD18 with ICAM-1 (lymphocytes-endothelium), CD11b/CD18 with ICAM-1 (neutrophils-endothelium), and VLA-4 with VCAM-1 (monocytes-endothelium). Finally, transmigration of leukocytes through the endothelium and basement membrane is driven by chemokines such as monocyte chemoattractant protein (MCP)-1, C5a, and IL-8.[1]

Granulocytes

Neutrophils, eosinophils, and basophils comprise a group of leukocytes known as granulocytes, so named for the presence of highly visible granules—actually highly developed vacuolar structures—in their cytoplasm (Fig. 21.2). Mast cells are similarly equipped with specialized granules, although they are classified separately. The contents of the granules vary with cell type and can be distinguished under routine staining (hematoxylin and eosin) for light microscopy. Granulocytes, also called polymorphonuclear leukocytes because of their multilobed nuclei, form a part of the innate immune system and are crucial to the acute inflammatory response.

Neutrophils

Polymorphonuclear neutrophils (PMNs) are the body's first-line defense against most foreign invaders and constitute the major cell type in most acute inflammatory diseases, as well as in some chronic inflammatory diseases.[5] The importance of neutrophils in bacterial defense is demonstrated by patients who have hereditary defects in neutrophil function and are prone to repeated and often life-threatening infections. Neutrophils are the most prevalent leukocyte in the bloodstream, accounting for more than 50% of all circulating white blood cells; in acute inflammatory conditions such as bacterial infection, the percentage of neutrophils in the bloodstream increases to 80% or more. Unlike most other leukocytes, however, neutrophils are normally not present in significant numbers in extravascular spaces. Neutrophils are also remarkable for their short half-life, which is approximately 7 hours inside the bloodstream and slightly longer in extravascular spaces.

Neutrophil granules contain an impressive arsenal of microbicidal weaponry that is unleashed upon cell activation (Figs. 21.3 and 21.4). As identified by routine staining, neutrophil granules consist of two classes: primary (or azurophilic) granules develop first, followed by secondary (or specific) granules. Azurophilic granules are functionally similar to lysosomes of other cells. Like other lysosomes, azurophilic granules contain a variety of proteases, in this case including elastase, matrix metalloproteinase (MMP)-3, MMP-8, and MMP-9, cathepsins, and lysozyme (Table 21.1).[5] In addition, azurophilic granules contain myeloperoxidase (MPO), a key enzyme for both microbicidal activity and for mediating tissue injury in inflammatory disease. In response to phagocytosis of a bacterium or extracellular material, azurophilic

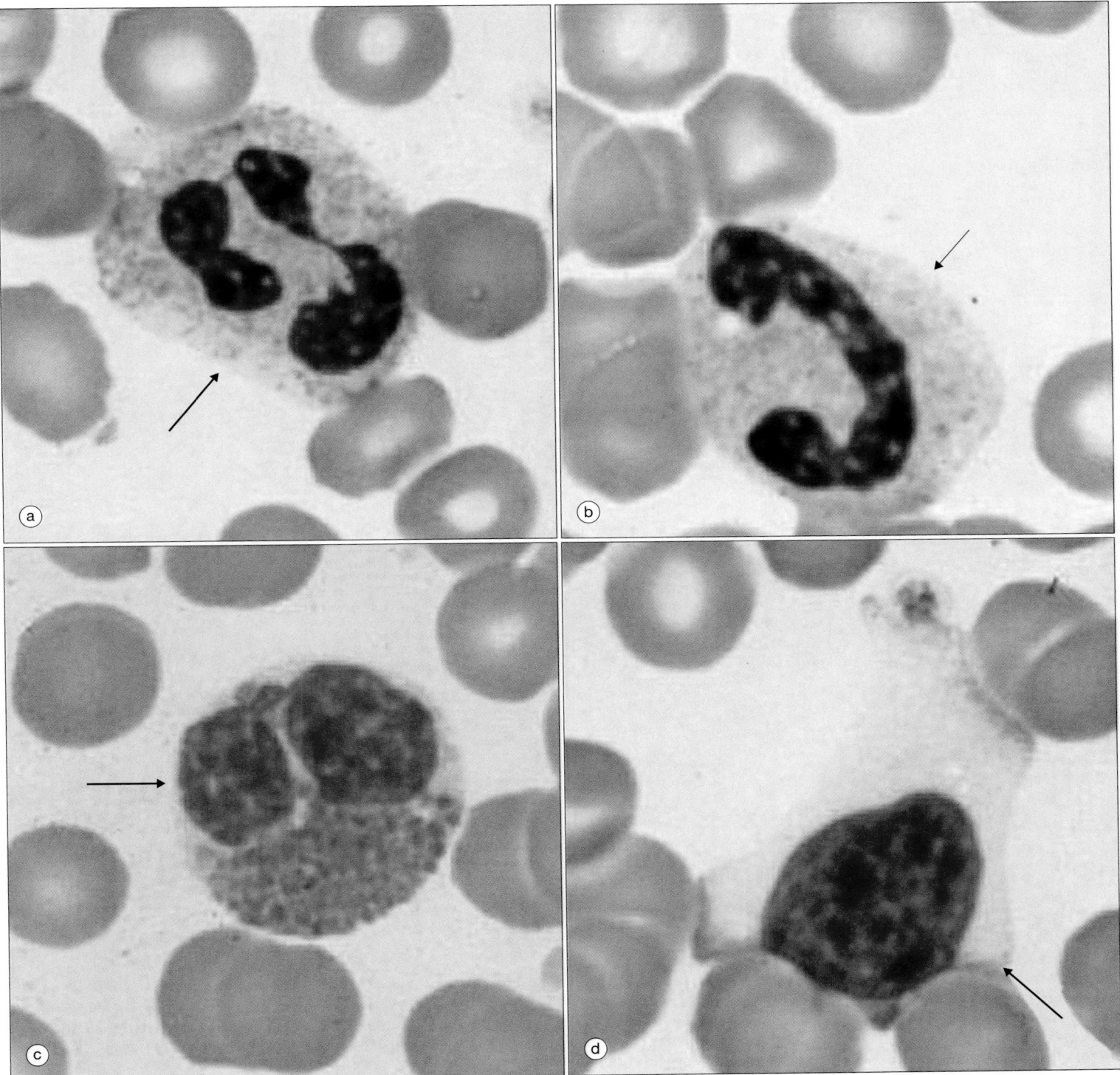

Fig. 21.2 Leukocyte micrographs (light microscopy, H&E staining). (a) A neutrophil, or polymorphonuclear leukocyte. Note that the cytoplasm stains bluish and appears granular secondary to the staining properties of the azurophilic granules. Neutrophils typically have nuclei with three to five lobes; four lobes are seen here. (b) An immature neutrophil, known as a band cell because of the distinctive nuclear shape. Such cells are frequently released prematurely from the bone marrow during acute inflammatory events. (c) An eosinophil, with pink (eosinophilic) granules and a nucleus with two lobes. Eosinophils have multiple lobes, but typically fewer than are seen in neutrophils. (d) A monocyte. Note the lack of obvious cytoplasmic granules, the unilobular nucleus, and the monomorphic nucleus and irregular shape. *(Figure produced with the kind permission of Harold Ballard, MD.)*

granules fuse with the phagosome to direct their contents at the ingested target. In addition, a membrane-bound NADPH oxidase is assembled and activated, resulting in rapid oxygen consumption (the "respiratory burst") and the generation of highly reactive oxygen species (ROS) within the phagolysosome. Simultaneous discharge of MPO from the azurophilic granule into the phagolysosome catalyzes the reaction of ROS and chloride to form hypochlorous acid (HOCl, or chlorine bleach). HOCl and its derivatives are potent oxidizing agents that can, among other things, disrupt bacterial electron-transport

chains and disturb DNA synthesis.[8] Azurophilic granules thus provide potent mechanisms though which microorganisms are destroyed; when inappropriately released into the extracellular environment; however, the content of these granules can cause significant tissue damage.

Whereas specific granules also contain lysozyme, their contents generally differ from primary granules. Specific granule proteases include collagenase (MMP-1) and plasminogen activator; they also contain proteins with poorly defined functions, such as lactoferrin and

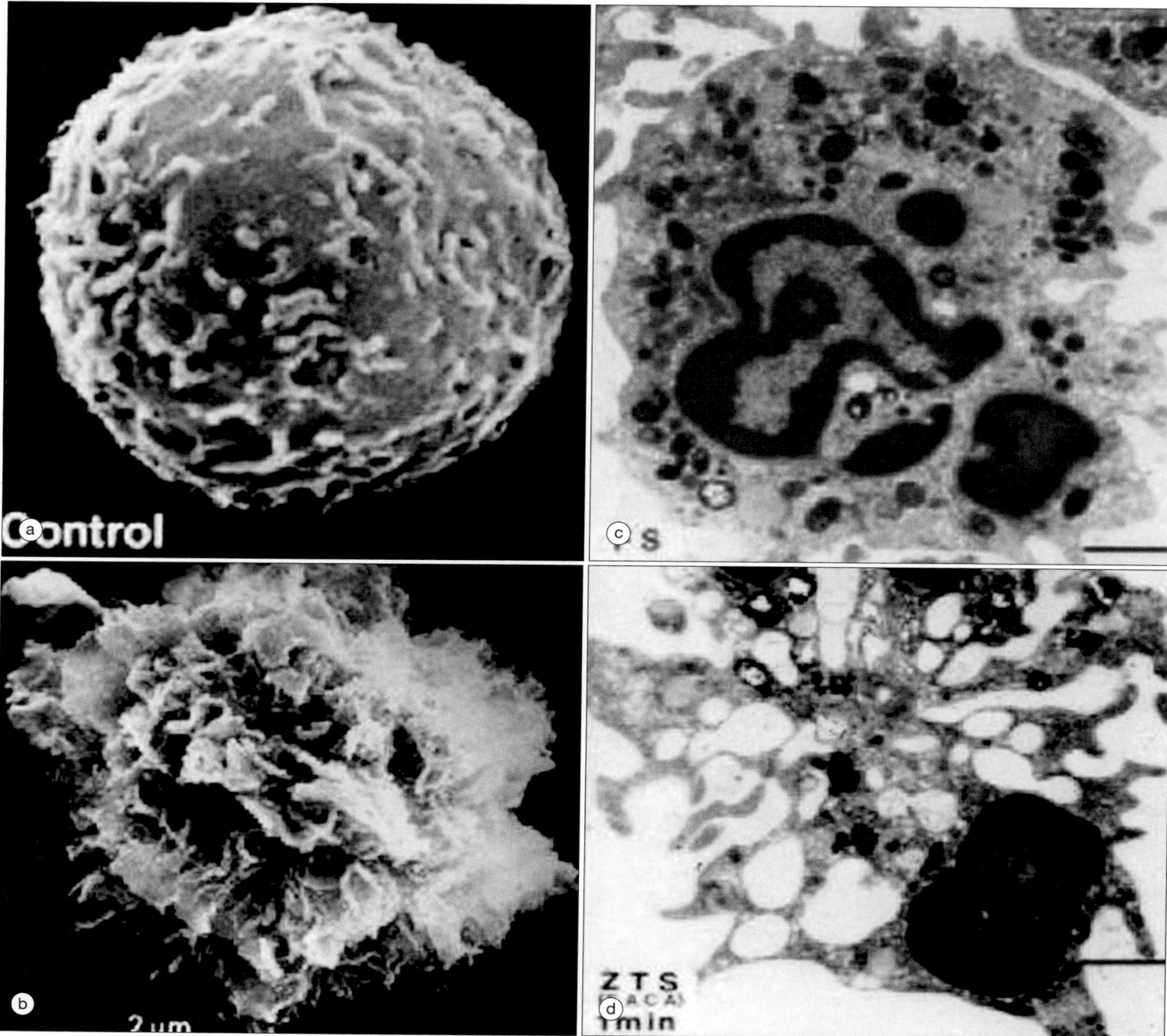

Fig. 21.3 Electron micrographs of neutrophils at rest and after stimulation with fMLP. These electron micrographs highlight the active process of neutrophil disgorgement. When activated, the neutrophil cell surface ruffles as granules and lysosomes merge with the cell surface to release their contents into the extracellular environment. (a and b) Scanning electron micrographs of a resting neutrophil and activated neutrophil, respectively. (c and d) Transmission electron micrographs of the same. Note the numerous empty spaces within the activated neutrophil's cytoplasm; these are indicative of emptied-out granules and resultant expanded surface membrane. *(Figures produced with the kind permission of Gerald Weissmann, MD.)*

β_2-microglobulin.[5] In contrast to azurophilic granules, specific granules possess an extensive array of membrane-associated proteins, including cytochromes, signaling molecules, and receptors; these constitute a reservoir of proteins destined for topologically external surfaces of both phagocytic vacuoles and the plasma membrane.[5]

In addition to primary and secondary granules, more recent studies have identified two other types of neutrophil granules. Gelatinase granules, similar to specific granules in size, are notable for their high concentrations of gelatinase, a latent enzyme with the capacity for tissue destruction. Secretory vesicles are smaller than the other granules and do not appear to contain proteolytic enzymes.[9] In contrast to other granules, which typically fuse with phagolysosomes, secretory granules fuse with the cell membrane and appear to serve as a reservoir of membrane and membrane-associated proteins.

Because neutrophils have such destructive capacity, their localization and activation must be carefully regulated. Chemoattractants for neutrophils include leukotriene B_4 (LTB_4), platelet-activating factor (PAF), IL-8, and the complement split product C5a. At low concentrations, and when distributed in a gradient, these molecules lead neutrophils to migrate toward regions of higher concentrations. At high concentrations, however (i.e., at the bacterial source of the gradient), these same molecules cause neutrophils to cease migration and become activated. Receptors for soluble ligands other than chemoattractants have also been identified on neutrophils, including receptors for growth factors, colony-stimulating factors, and cytokines (see Fig. 21.4); these ligands may modulate neutrophil function. For example, pretreatment of neutrophils with either insulin or granulocyte-macrophage colony-stimulating factor (GM-CSF) results in amplification of subsequent neutrophil responses to chemoattractants.[5]

TABLE 21.1 PRODUCTS OF NEUTROPHILS, MACROPHAGES, AND EOSINOPHILS

Cell	Granule contents	Cytokines produced	Other inflammatory mediators
Neutrophil	**Primary (azurophilic) granules:** Elastase, MMP-3, -8, -9, cathepsins, defensins, bactericidal/permeability increasing protein, proteinase 3, lysozyme, myeloperoxidase **Secondary (specific) granules:** Collagenase, plasminogen activator, lysozyme, lactoferrin, β_2-microglobulin **Gelatinase granules:** Gelatinase	IL-1, IL-6, IL-8, TNF-α, and GM-CSF	Reactive oxygen species (ROS), PAF, PGE_2, LTB_4
Macrophage	Lysozyme (aside from many others mentioned in the text)	IL-1β, TNF-α, IL-6, IL-8, IL-12, MCP-1, MCP-2, RANTES, PDGF, TGF-β, IFN-γ	Complement components, ROS, iNOS, PGE_2, TxA_2, PGI_2, LTB_4, LTC_4, PAF, MMP-1, tissue factor, plasmin inhibitor
Eosinophil	**Specific granules:** Charcot-Leyden crystal protein, major basic protein, eosinophil peroxidase, eosinophil cationic protein, eosinophil-derived neurotoxin, secretory PLA_2 **Small granules:** Arylsulfatase B	IL-4, IL-5, IL-8, IL-10, IL-12, GM-CSF, TNF-α, TGF-β, PDGF, VEGF, MCP-1	LTB_4, LTC_4, PAF, PGE_2, ROS, collagenase

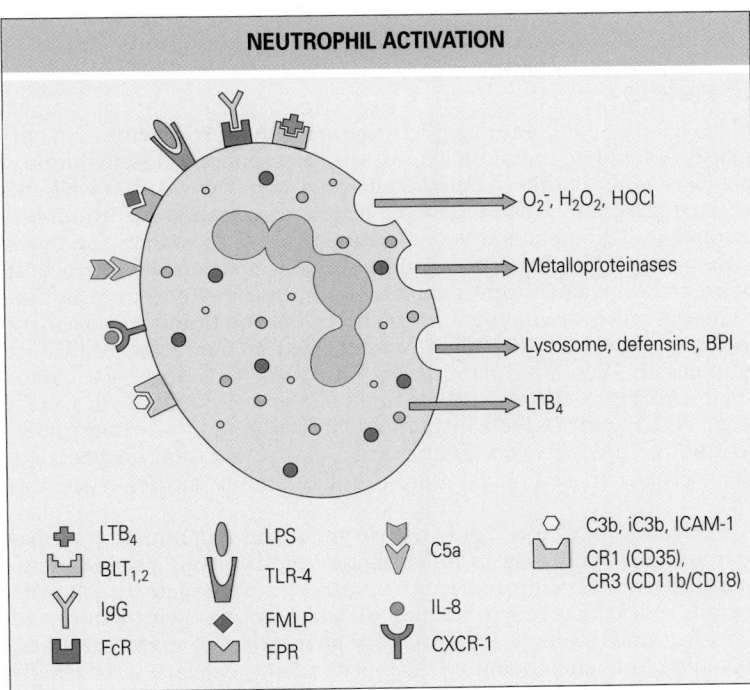

NEUTROPHIL ACTIVATION

O_2^-, H_2O_2, HOCl

Metalloproteinases

Lysosome, defensins, BPI

LTB_4

LTB_4	LPS	C5a	C3b, iC3b, ICAM-1
$BLT_{1,2}$	TLR-4		CR1 (CD35), CR3 (CD11b/CD18)
IgG	FMLP	IL-8	
FcR	FPR	CXCR-1	

Fig. 21.4 Neutrophil activation. Various signals stimulate neutrophil activation via ligation of cell-surface receptors. On activation, neutrophils both degranulate and produce a number of inflammatory mediators. See text for details.

Once localized to its target tissue and activated, the neutrophil is intrinsically inefficient at phagocytosing unmodified targets. Optimal neutrophil phagocytosis depends on opsonization, the modification of a target via its adornment with immunoglobulin, complement components, or both. Neutrophils express complement receptor (CR)1 and CR3 (the integrin CD11b/CD18), which promote phagocytosis by binding complement C3b and iC3b, respectively.[5] In addition, neutrophils express two families of receptors for the Fc portion of complexed or aggregated IgG: low-affinity FcγRIIa and high-affinity FcγRIIIb. During some infections, or after *in-vitro* stimulation with interferon or granulocyte colony-stimulating factor (G-CSF), neutrophils also express the high-affinity receptor FcγRI, which binds monomeric IgG[5] (for an overview of leukocyte receptors, see Table 21.2).

Recently, a completely novel neutrophil function has been identified. In some instances, neutrophils confronted with bacterial invasion may choose to die, and in so doing release neutrophil extracellular nets (NETs) composed of de-condensed chromatin associated with antimicrobial proteins. These NETs have the capacity to trap and kill bacteria, serving both as a physical containment structure to prevent bacterial spread and an antibacterial delivery system. How neutrophils "decide" whether to use their more classical defense systems, or to die and produce NETs, remains an area of intense study.[10]

Eosinophils, basophils, and mast cells

Other granulocytes important in inflammatory responses include eosinophils and basophils. Like neutrophils, these cells also release a variety of lipid and peptide mediators (see Table 21.1). In contrast to neutrophils, these cells are much less common in the bloodstream but are found in greater numbers in extravascular tissue. Eosinophils typically do not phagocytose their targets but are thought to liberate their contents alongside them. Eosinophils are thought to be important in combating parasitic infection and are also involved in the inflammatory response generated by allergic or immediate hypersensitivity reactions; the latter role is shared by mast cells and basophils. Abnormal eosinophil activity is implicated in several inflammatory diseases, including asthma, eosinophilic pneumonia, Churg-Strauss vasculitis, and the idiopathic hypereosinophilic syndrome.[11] Basophils also play roles in allergic reactions.

Mast cells are most commonly localized to perivascular locations within tissues. Their granular contents are similar to those of basophils, and, like basophils, mast cells may play a role in allergic reactions. Recent data from animal models suggest that mast cells may also be important in the pathogenesis of rheumatoid arthritis (RA).

Macrophages

Macrophages play multiple roles in inflammation and immunity, serving both as antigen-presenting cells (APCs) that drive adaptive immune responses and as primary inflammatory cells in chronic diseases such as atherosclerosis and RA. Tissue macrophages derive from circulating monocytes and differentiate and become activated on exiting the vasculature. Although the process of monocyte adhesion to, and diapedesis through, blood vessels is similar in many respects to that of neutrophils, the monocyte responds to a different set of chemotactic factors, including the chemokines RANTES, MCP-1, macrophage inflammatory protein (MIP)-1α and -1β, and the growth factors transforming growth factor (TGF)-β and platelet-derived growth factor (PDGF) (see Table 21.1).[12] Once in tissues, macrophages can live for up to several months.

As actors in the innate immune system, macrophages are stimulated to phagocytose non-encapsulated bacteria via recognition of evolutionarily conserved motifs on bacterial surfaces. To do so, macrophages express surface receptors for pathogen-associated molecular patterns (PAMPS). These include Toll-like receptors, formyl peptide receptors, and scavenger receptors, many of which are also found on neutrophils (see Table 21.2).[13] After phagocytosis, macrophages destroy microbes through mechanisms similar to those that neutrophils employ: lysosomal enzymes, reactive oxygen and nitrogen intermediates, toxic

TABLE 21.2 LEUKOCYTE RECEPTORS, LIGANDS, AND THEIR FUNCTIONS

Receptor type	Examples	Examples of ligands	Functions
FcγR	FcγRI, FcγRIIa, FcγRIIIb	Immunoglobulins	Recognize and bind Fc portions of immunoglobulins
Toll-like receptors	TLR-1 to TLR-11	Pathogen-associated molecular patterns (PAMPS; e.g., LPS)	Recognize pathogens and activate immune responses
Formyl peptide receptors	Formyl peptide receptor I	Bacterial N-formyl-methionyl peptides	Mediate chemotaxis and activation of neutrophils and monocyte-macrophages
Scavenger receptors	Scavenger receptor A	Numerous targets on bacteria, apoptotic cell structures	Stimulate phagocytosis of bacteria and apoptotic cells, adhesion
Mannose receptor	Mannose receptor C type I	Mannose (on pathogens)	Mediates the endocytosis of glycoproteins by phagocytes
Complement receptors	CR1, CR2, CR3, CR4	Complement components	Aid in opsonization and phagocytosis
	C5aR	C5a	Activates inflammatory cells
Integrins	Mac-1 (CD11b/CD18),	ICAM-1	Bind to cell-adhesion molecules and extracellular matrix, resulting in strong adhesion
	LFA-1 (CD11a/CD18)		
Chemokine receptors (CR, CCR, CXCR, CXXXCR classes)	CCR: CCR1 CCR3, CCR5	CC: MCP-1, RANTES, MIP-1a	Recognize chemoattractants, mobilize and activate leukocytes
	CXCR: CXCR1, CXCR2	CXC: IL-8	

radicals, and chloramines. As in the case of neutrophils, macrophage phagocytosis and killing of pathogens is greatly enhanced by pathogen opsonization. Macrophages have surface receptors for multiple opsonins, including the mannose receptor (that directly recognizes glycoproteins on microbial surfaces), CR1, CR3, CR4, FcγRI, FcγRII, and FcγRIII (see Table 21.2).[14,15] Although the majority of macrophage products primarily function to augment inflammation and repel external threats, macrophages, like neutrophils, have the capacity to damage host tissue via release of their digestive and degradative contents.

Macrophages differ from neutrophils in their capacity to serve as "professional" APCs. After phagocytosis, APCs degrade foreign antigens in protease-containing endosomes; vesicles containing major histocompatibility complex (MHC) class II molecules then fuse with the endosomes, allowing membrane-bound MHC class II complexes to become loaded with antigenic peptide fragments; the MHC class II/ peptide complexes are then delivered to the cell surface, where they present antigen to T cells to stimulate the highly specific responses of adaptive immunity.[16]

One of the earliest steps in most inflammatory responses is activation of resident tissue macrophages, whose subsequent production of cytokines alters vasomotor tone and endothelial adhesiveness, as described earlier. Through ligation of various surface receptors, macrophages may be activated by interferon (IFN)-γ, complement components, immune complexes, lipopolysaccharide (LPS), and cytokines such as IL-1β, TNF-α, and IL-6.[13] Once activated, macrophages secrete a dazzling variety of proinflammatory products (see Table 21.1), including proteases (e.g., lysozyme, elastase, and collagenase), inflammatory cytokines (IL-1β, TNF-α, IL-6, IL-12, and others), chemokines (including IL-8, MCP-1, MCP-2, RANTES, and others), and several complement cascade proteins (C1, C2, C3, and C4).[12] Indeed, a vigorous acute-phase response, driven by cytokine production and characterized by high serum levels of acute-phase reactants (as well as a rapid erythrocyte sedimentation rate), is typical of diseases characterized by extensive macrophage involvement. Activated macrophages also produce a number of eicosanoids (e.g., PGE$_2$, thromboxane A$_2$ (TXA$_2$), prostacyclin, LTB$_4$, and PAF) that may contribute to the propagation of inflammation.[17] In addition, activated macrophages produce procoagulant factors such as tissue factor and plasmin inhibitor, linking the inflammatory and clotting responses. Indeed, local intravascular coagulation in response to infection is thought to play a role in limiting the spread of infection; when unchecked, coagulation in the presence of inflammation leads to disseminated intravascular coagulation, a potentially life-threatening condition.

Lymphocytes

For a discussion of lymphocytes, please refer to Chapter 15.

Platelets

Platelets are small, anucleate, circulating cellular fragments that primarily function to maintain hemostasis. In response to vascular injury, platelets adhere to the subendothelial matrix of the vascular wall and become activated, rapidly inducing platelet aggregation and thrombus formation. The rapid and potent nature of these thrombotic events is largely due to platelet degranulation, whereby platelets disgorge a host of preformed factors from α-granules and dense granules into the surrounding microvasculature. In addition to containing procoagulant factors such as von Willebrand factor, fibrinogen, and factor V, platelet granules also contain inflammatory mediators, including chemokines (e.g., RANTES, MCP-3, MIP-1α, and platelet factor 4), growth factors (e.g., PDGF and TGF-β), histamine, and serotonin.[18] Further underscoring the link between inflammation and coagulation, platelets are themselves activated on exposure to inflammatory mediators such as PAF.

Activated platelets not only release preformed inflammatory mediators but also participate in inflammatory processes via plasma membrane activity. Signaling molecules upregulated on the activated platelet include P-selectin, which adheres to and activates neutrophils, and CD40L, which induces inflammatory phenotypes in many cell lines, including the endothelium.[19] On activation, platelets also rapidly produce eicosanoids, such as TXA$_2$ from membrane-derived arachidonic acid, and other lipid membrane-derived inflammatory products, such as PAF. Platelets both participate in cell-cell interactions and release microparticles that contribute to leukocyte-leukocyte and leukocyte–endothelial cell interactions; these interactions play a role in inflammation as well.

Other links between coagulation and inflammation

Inflammation leads to activation of coagulation through additional means. Tissue factor, which stimulates thrombin formation, is overproduced by macrophages in inflammatory conditions such as sepsis and atherosclerosis; blocking tissue factor with a monoclonal antibody abrogates coagulation activity in experimental endotoxemia.[20] Systemic inflammation also inhibits the function of the natural anticoagulant pathways of antithrombin and protein C. Additionally, systemic inflammation inhibits fibrinolysis via generation of plasminogen activator inhibitor type I (PAI-I). Inhibition of fibrinolysis is permissive for microvascular thromboses; PAI-I inhibition prevents both endotoxin-induced microthromboses and experimental coronary thrombosis. Conversely, studies by Salmon and associates have implicated complement activation (see later) as a key player in the evolution of the antiphospholipid syndrome.[21,22] In short, inflammation and coagulation are intricately related processes that exhibit crosstalk at numerous levels, and the role of coagulation needs to be considered when treating systemic inflammatory illnesses.

INFLAMMATORY MEDIATORS

A myriad of soluble mediators coordinate the inflammatory process. These mediators derive from a number of sources, including the inflammatory cells described earlier, plasma proteins, and resident tissue cells such as nerves and endothelium. Some of the more important molecular components are described here.

The complement cascade

Complement was initially discovered by Bordet in 1899 as a heat-labile component of fresh plasma that "complemented" the ability of specific antibodies to lyse red blood cells and bacteria. More than 30 serum proteins and cell surface receptors are now collectively recognized as the complement system. A primary function of the complement system is to coat and opsonize cell membranes and soluble antigens for recognition and digestion by phagocytic cells. Other components, generated during complement activation, independently generate an inflammatory response. These so-called anaphylatoxins (C3a, C5a) can rapidly induce vasodilation, as well as leukocyte activation and chemotaxis (see later). A third function of the system is to act as an independent effector of innate immunity, by directly lysing unencapsulated, gram-negative bacteria.

Three distinct complement cascades—the classical, alternative, and mannose-binding lectin pathways—differ in their mechanisms of target recognition and initial activation but converge at the C5 convertase (Fig. 21.5). Many of the complement plasma proteins are zymogens, which are proteases that become active on undergoing proteolytic cleavage; thus, these proteins generally circulate in a dormant state. Once active, many of these molecules participate in cleavage or activation of subsequent components. Thus, each successive enzymatic step results in rapid and dramatic amplification. In response to this potential for explosive activation, a number of complement regulatory molecules exist to dampen the cascades. Given the importance of complement activation to rheumatic disease, a more detailed understanding of the three complement cascades is important for both researchers and practicing rheumatologists.

Classical pathway

Although it was the first of the three complement pathways to be discovered, the classical pathway was actually the last to evolve and largely depends on a preceding humoral immune response for its activity. Activation of the classical pathway occurs when the C1q component of the multimeric complement 1 complex (C1) binds to the Fc tails of multiple IgG or IgM antibodies complexed to antigen. When at least two of the six globular heads of C1q have bound, the remaining components of the C1 complex (two molecules each of C1r and C1s) undergo a conformational change, unleashing autocatalytic enzyme activity in C1r. Active C1r then cleaves the zymogen C1s to its active form. C1s in turn cleaves soluble C4, then C2, to C4a and C4b and C2a and C2b, respectively.[23] When cleaved, complement components are tagged with the letter "a" for the smaller fragment and the letter "b" for the larger and enzymatically active fragment. Complement molecules in the classical pathway are numbered in the order in which they were discovered, which in most cases corresponds with their place in the complement sequence. The exception is C4, which was discovered after C3 but acts upstream of C2. C4b and C2b combine to form C4b2b (the C3 convertase of the classical pathway), which cleaves C3 to C3a and C3b. C3b combines with C4b2b to form C4b2b3b (C5 convertase), which in turn cleaves C5 to C5b and C5a.[24] Subsequent assembly of the C5b,C6,C7,C8,C9 membrane attack complex (MAC) can form a pore in the cell membrane of some pathogens, and most host cells, leading to their death. C3 performs double duty: while some portion of C3b joins with C4b2b to form the C5 convertase, the majority of C3b serves as opsonin; minutes after activation of the complement cascade, millions of C3b molecules can be covalently attached to a single bacterium's surface, facilitating its phagocytosis by macrophages and neutrophils.

Mannose-binding lectin pathway

The mannose-binding lectin (MBL) pathway evolved before the classical pathway, which appears to have arisen by subsequent duplication and modification of MBL pathway genes. In contrast to the classical pathway, the MBL pathway does not require immunoglobulins but is activated by bacterial surface mannose residues. Because these residues are not accessible on vertebrate cells, the MBL pathway distinguishes "self" from "other" on the basis of a generic pattern, rather than a specific antigen; as such, it represents a bridge between innate and acquired immunity. When a C1q-like component of the MBL complex engages mannose on a pathogen, it activates the mannose-associated serine proteases MASP-1 and MASP-2 (akin to C1r and C1s); thereafter, the MBL complex functions identically to activated C1, cleaving C4 and C2 to form C3 convertase.[25]

Alternative pathway

The alternative pathway is unique in that its activation is not initiated by binding to a pathogen; instead, the alternative pathway is always undergoing activation, via the spontaneous hydrolysis of C3 in plasma. $C3(H_2O)$ binds the alternative pathway component factor B, which is then converted by the associated factor D into Ba and Bb. The $C3(H_2O)$-Bb complex that results is an alternate C3 convertase and converts fluid-phase C3 into C3a and C3b, the latter of which is quickly inactivated by hydrolysis unless it deposits on a cell surface. Once covalently bound to a cell surface (or indeed, any surface), however, C3b binds factor B; factor D cleaves factor B, resulting in the formation of the C3 convertase, C3bBb, which is functionally equivalent to the C3 convertase (C4b2b) of the classic and lectin pathways.[26] Because this primitive pathway fails to distinguish self from other, its specificity resides not in any intrinsic property of foreign particles but in the ability of host cells (but not bacteria) to defend themselves against indiscriminate complement activation (see Complement regulation, later).

C3a and C5a anaphylatoxins

The release of the soluble fragments C3a and C5a, also known as anaphylatoxins, accelerates the inflammatory response in multiple ways: anaphylatoxins engage receptors on mast cells and basophils, triggering release of vasoactive mediators such as histamine and the cysteinyl leukotrienes LTC_4 and LTD_4. C5a and C3a induce vasodilation and increased capillary permeability; upregulate adhesion molecule expression on leukocytes and endothelial cells; and cause smooth muscle contraction. C5a in particular is also a powerful chemoattractant for, and activator of, neutrophils and can stimulate both neutrophil degranulation and the respiratory burst.[27]

Complement regulation

When C3bBb binds to host cells, the host complement-regulatory proteins CR1 and DAF rapidly bind C3b and displace Bb. CR1 and DAF, in combination with the membrane cofactor of proteolysis, also catalyze the cleavage of C3b by the plasma protease factor I to produce inactive C3b. Bacterial surfaces lack these proteins and instead permit binding of properdin, which stabilizes rather than degrades the alternative C3 convertase.

Other proteins have also evolved to inhibit complement activation (Table 21.3). These include fluid-phase proteins, such as C1 inhibitor and the C3 and C5 convertase inhibitors, C4-binding protein and factor H, as well as membrane-bound proteins such as the C3 and C5 convertase inhibitors, and CD59, a glycolipid that prevents insertion of the MAC into plasma membranes.[28]

Complement in disease

Complement deficiencies cause not only susceptibility to bacterial infection but also susceptibility to autoimmune disease. Patients with specific complement deficiencies are especially prone to SLE; approximately 90% of C1q-null, 75% of C4-null, and up to 30% of C2-null individuals develop lupus. Why complement deficiency predisposes to autoimmune disease is not entirely clear but may result from inefficient clearance of apoptotic cells and immune complexes, resulting in either inappropriate exposure to self-antigens or in immune complex deposition.[29] Deficiencies of later complement components may have other effects. For example, deficiencies in C5 result in susceptibility to

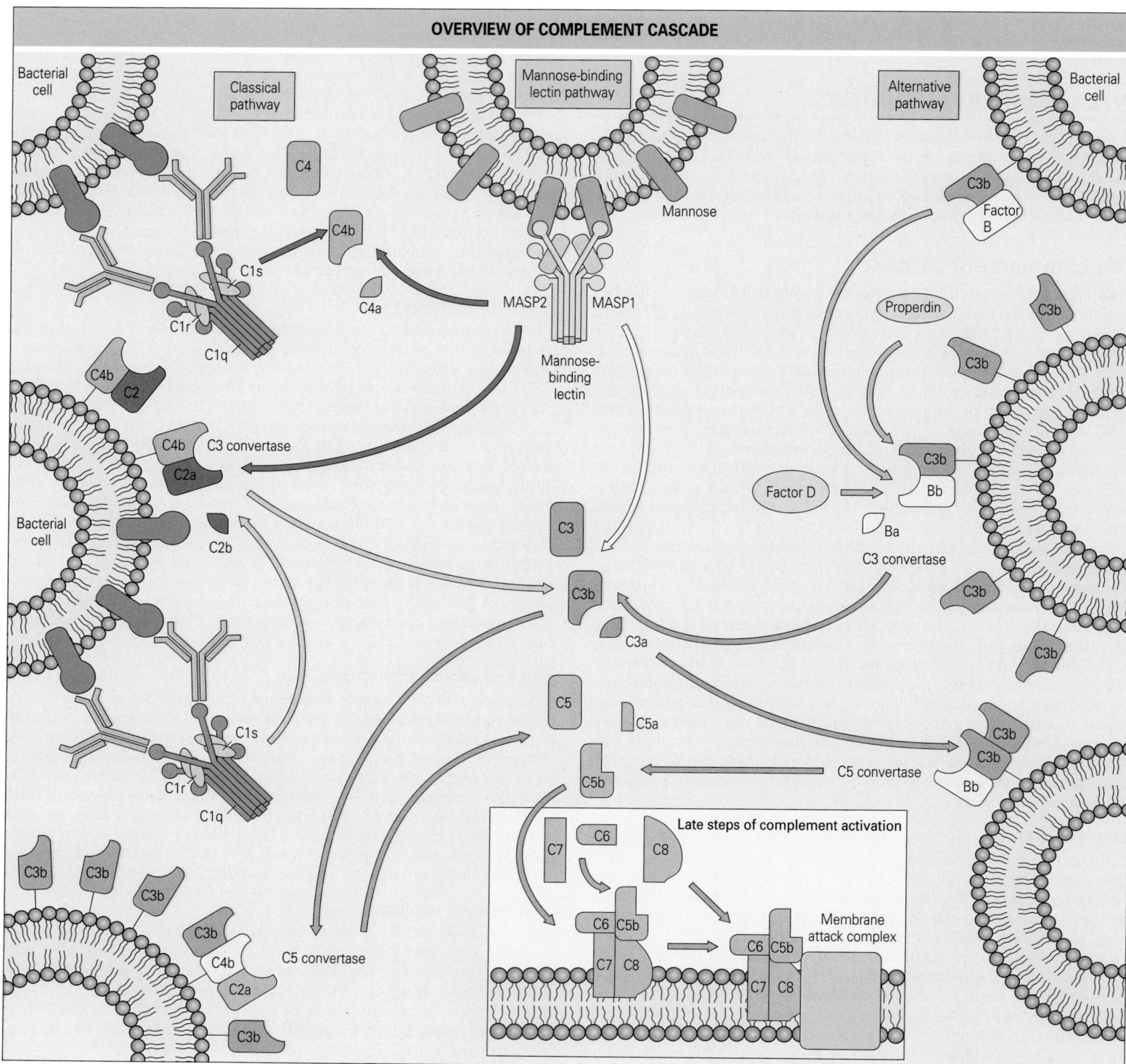

Fig. 21.5 Overview of complement cascade. Three distinct complement cascades—the classic, alternative, and lectin pathways—differ in their mechanisms of target recognition and initial activation but converge at the C3 convertase. Activation of the classic pathway occurs when the C1q component of C1 (which consists of C1q, two molecules of C1r, and two molecules of C1s) binds to multiple Fc portions of IgG or IgM antibodies complexed to antigen. Binding of C1q activates C1r, which in turn cleaves C1s to its active form. C1s then cleaves soluble C4 and C2 to C4a and C4b and C2a and C2b, respectively. C4b and C2b combine to form C4b2b (the C3 convertase of the classic pathway), that cleaves C3 to C3a and C3b. C3b combines with C4b2b to form C4b2b3b (C5 convertase), which then cleaves C5 to C5b and C5a. Subsequent assembly of the C5b, C6, C7, C8, C9 membrane attack complex (MAC) occurs. The mannose-binding lectin pathway is a primitive version of the classic cascade. When the mannose-binding lectin (MBL) component of the MBL complex (analogous in form and function to the C1 complex) binds mannose on a pathogen, it activates the mannose-associated serine proteases MASP-1 and MASP-2 (akin to C1r and C1s); thereafter, the MBL complex functions as does activated C1, cleaving C4 and C2 to form C3 convertase. The alternative pathway is initiated by the spontaneous hydrolysis of fluid-phase C3. C3(H₂O) binds the alternative pathway component factor B, which is then converted by the associated factor D into Ba and Bb. The C3(H₂O)-Bb complex that results is an alternate C3 convertase and converts fluid-phase C3 into C3a and C3b, the latter of which is quickly inactivated by hydrolysis unless it deposits upon a cell surface. If bound to a cell surface, however, C3b can bind factor B; factor D then cleaves factor B, resulting in the formation of the C3 convertase, C3bBb, which is equivalent to the C3 convertase (C4b2b) of the classic and lectin pathways. *(Adapted from Walport MJ. Advances in immunology: complement (first of two parts). N Engl J Med 2001;344:1058-1061.)*

TABLE 21.3 COMPLEMENT REGULATORY PROTEINS

Protein	Complement regulatory function	Comments
C1 inhibitor (C1 INH)*	Membrane-bound serine protease inhibitor that inactivates the C1 complex by binding to C1r and C1s	Deficiency associated with hereditary and acquired angioedema, SLE
C4-bindng protein (C4BP)	Plasma protein that displaces C2b and binds to C4b; cofactor for cleavage of C4b by factor I	
CD35 (complement receptor 1)*	Membrane-bound glycoprotein that displaces Bb and binds C3b, or displaces C2b and binds C4b; promotes C3b and C4b inactivation by factor I	
CD55 (decay-accelerating factor [DAF])*	Membrane-bound protein that regulates the formation of C3 convertase by displacing Bb from C3b and C2b from C4b	Deficiency associated with paroxysmal nocturnal hemoglobinuria
CD59 (protectin)*	Prevents the formation of the membrane attack complex (MAC) on host cells	Deficiency causes paroxysmal nocturnal hemoglobinuria
CD46 (membrane cofactor protein, MCP)*	Membrane-bound protein that binds C3b and C4b and promotes their inactivation by factor I	
Factor H	Plasma protein cofactor for factor I; displaces Bb and binds C3b in plasma and on host cell surfaces	Deficiency leads to recurrent pyogenic infections, hemolytic uremic syndrome
Factor I	Plasma protease that inactivates C3b and C4b; requires CR1, factor H, CD46, or C4BP as cofactor	Deficiency results in recurrent bacterial infections

*Present on host, but not microbial, cell surfaces.

Neisseria infections, testifying to the importance of the MAC in the response to these organisms.

Complement activation almost inevitably results in some degree of tissue destruction; this is seen in rheumatic diseases such as SLE, rheumatoid arthritis, vasculitis, and antiphospholipid antibody syndrome.[30] Complement participates in tissue damage in multiple ways; in reperfusion injury, for instance, excessive MAC deposits in tissues after ischemia. The renascent interest in complement in inflammatory disease has led to the development of pharmacologic complement inhibitors that are currently in trials, including humanized monoclonal C5 antibody and a solubilized CR1 molecule.

A number of inflammatory conditions also result from hereditary or acquired deficiencies of complement regulatory proteins. For example, deficiencies of the C1q inhibitor protein lead to undue complement activity under metabolic stress and the development of intermittent and potentially life-threatening angioedema.

Lipid mediators of inflammation

Given the ubiquity of membrane lipids, it is not surprising that nature has evolved strategies to utilize them for roles in addition to that of membrane structure. Among the most important roles of membrane lipids is their ability to serve as substrates for the generation of hydrophobic proinflammatory and anti-inflammatory mediators.

Arachidonic acid derivatives

Many bioactive lipid mediators are produced through the oxidation of arachidonic acid (AA), including prostaglandins (PGs) and leukotrienes (LTs), as well as the recently recognized anti-inflammatory lipoxins (Fig. 21.6). AA is a polyunsaturated fatty acid normally covalently associated with cell membrane phospholipids; the enzyme phospholipase A_2 (PLA_2) catalyzes its release (phospholipase C2, which liberates diacylglycerol [DAG] from membrane triglycerides, can also indirectly produce AA via the action of lipase on DAG). In any given cell, the products formed from AA will be determined by factors such as cytokine milieu, specific expression of AA-modifying enzymes, and tissue type.

Cyclooxygenase products

Prostaglandins (PGs), so named because they were originally identified in sheep seminal fluid (i.e., from the prostate gland), result from the action of cyclooxygenases (COX-1 or COX-2) on AA. COX enzymes are heterobifunctional: they first incorporate oxygen into C-11 of AA, forming the five-carbon ring common to all prostaglandins, and producing the unstable PGG_2. A second reaction reduces PGG_2 to generate PGH_2 (hence the alternate designation of COXs as PGH synthases).

PGH_2 is converted into stable prostanoids by a variety of specific terminal synthases, which are expressed with some tissue specificity; differentiated cells tend to produce only one PG type in abundance.

COX-1 and COX-2, encoded on separate chromosomes, are structurally and sequentially similar and perform the same enzymatic function but are differentially expressed. COX-1 is generally expressed constitutively and is found abundantly in many tissues and cell types, including renal collecting tubules, gastric epithelial cells, endothelial cells, macrophages, and platelets. COX-1 products typically play roles in organism homeostasis and generally are required for basic physiologic processes (e.g., protection of the gastric mucosa). In contrast, COX-2 is inducible and expressed primarily in cells involved in inflammation (macrophages, fibroblasts, and endothelial cells) in response to stimuli such as IL-1β, TNF-α, PDGF, and EGF.[31] COX-2 products generally contribute to the inflammatory processes that initially drive COX-2 expression. Moreover, COX-2 expression is elevated in many pathologic conditions, including inflammatory arthritis and some neoplasms, such as prostate and colon cancer. On this basis, selective COX-2 inhibitors were developed in the 1990s and were shown to have less gastrointestinal toxicity than non-selective COX inhibitors. However, COX-2 inhibition also appears to convey an increased risk of myocardial infarction, possibly by disturbing the balance between COX-1 and COX-2 products in the vasculature (see Chapter 50 for further discussion of the pharmacology of selective COX-2 inhibitors).

The bioactive prostanoids generated from PGH_2 include PGD_2, PGE_2, PGF_2, PGI_2 (prostacyclin), and TXA_2 (thromboxane), each of which is produced by the action of one or more specific isomerases (terminal synthases). In contrast, PGJ_2 is derived nonenzymatically via dehydration of PGD_2. PGs are short-lived and therefore generally act in an autocrine or paracrine manner. The activities of PG are generally mediated through specific G protein–coupled, seven-transmembrane-domain receptors, which have been classified into five types, according to their responsiveness to selective agonists and antagonists. DP, EP, FP, IP, and TP receptors are preferentially engaged by PGD_2, PGE_2, PGF_2, PGI_2, and TXA_2, respectively.[32]

Prostaglandin E₂

PGE_2 is the most common prostanoid and the one most critical to inflammation. PGE_2 mediates fever, induces smooth muscle contraction, spurs T-cell migration, and, along with PGI_2, produces the vasodilation and vascular hyperpermeability of early inflammation.[33] Production of PGE_2 has been reported in serum and synovial fluids of patients with RA and osteoarthritis and likely contributes to joint damage by promoting osteoclastic bone resorption and inhibition of

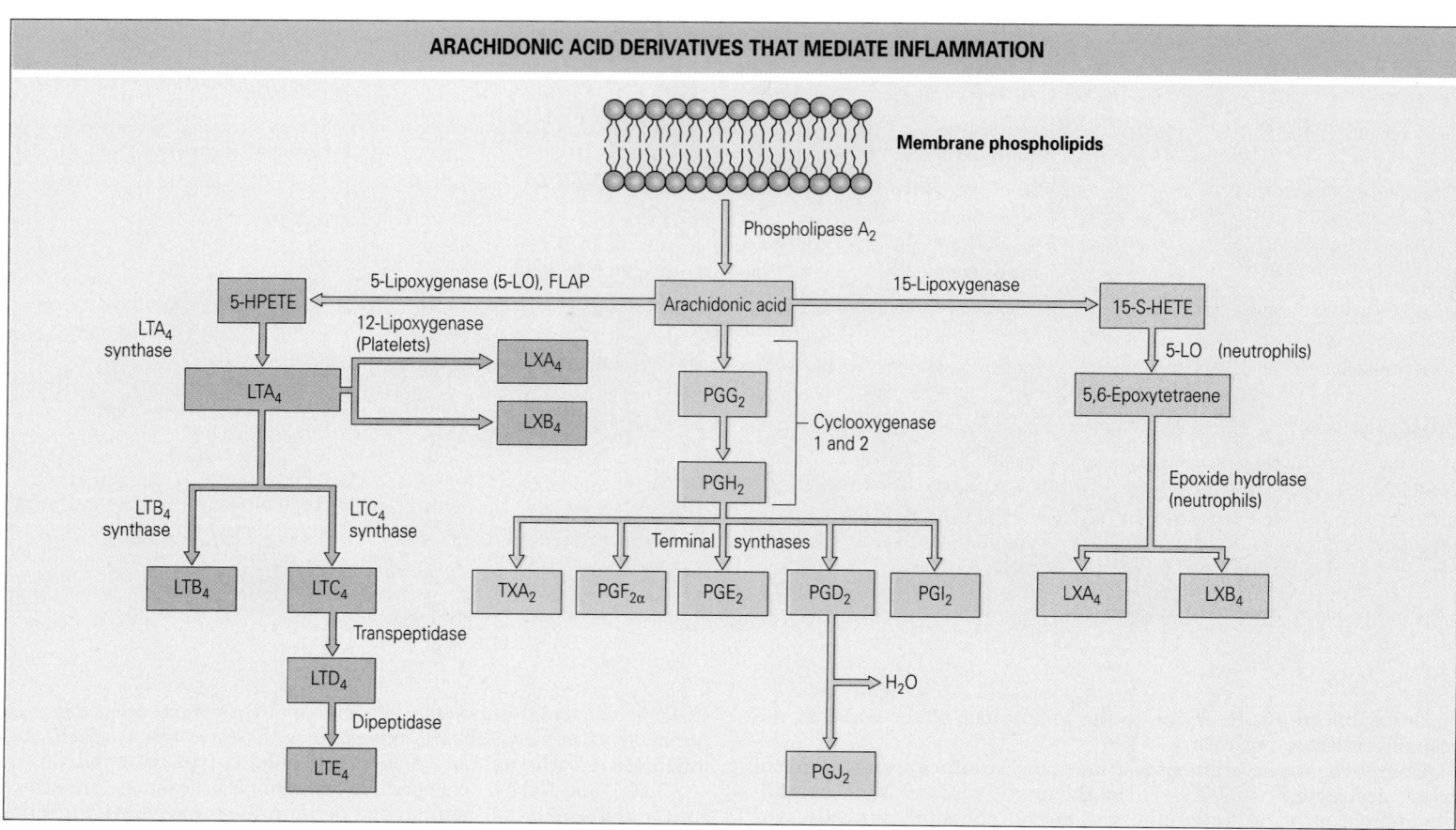

ARACHIDONIC ACID DERIVATIVES THAT MEDIATE INFLAMMATION

Fig. 21.6 Arachidonic acid derivatives that mediate inflammation. Arachidonic acid (AA) is liberated from cell membrane phospholipids via phospholipase A_2 (PLA_2) activity. Three distinct classes of products—prostanoids, leukotrienes, and lipoxins—may be subsequently generated by the action of distinct enzyme systems. *Prostanoid formation*: cyclooxygenase (COX)-1 and -2 convert AA sequentially into PGG_2 and PGH_2. Specific terminal synthases generate all other prostanoid products from PGH_2, with the exception of PGJ_2, which forms from PGD_2 through a dehydration reaction. *Leukotriene formation*: 5-lipoxygenase (5-LO) in concert with 5-lipoxygenase–activating protein (FLAP) act on AA to generate 5-hydroxyeicosapentaenoic acid (5-HPETE), and, subsequently, leukotriene A_4 (LTA_4). LTB_4 is formed from LTA_4 via LTA_4 hydrolase. In contrast, LTC_4 synthase converts LTA_4 into LTC_4. Subsequently, transpeptidase and dipeptidase convert LTC_4 into LTD_4, and LTD_4 into LTE_4, respectively. *Lipoxin formation*: Lipoxins (LX) form through cell-cell interactions during inflammation; two of the several pathways leading to lipoxin formation are shown here. Cells such as airway epithelium produce and release AA-derived 15-S-HETE. 15-S-HETE then diffuses into leukocytes, where it is first converted into 5,6-epoxytetraene by 5-LO, and then into LXA_4 or LXB_4 by the action of epoxide hydrolase. Alternatively, when adherent platelets interact with activated leukocytes in the vascular lumen, LTA_4 released from leukocytes diffuses into platelets, where it is converted to LXA_4 and LXB_4 by 12-LO. In contrast to prostanoids and leukotrienes, lipoxins appear to have largely anti-inflammatory effects. Not shown are the aspirin-triggered lipoxins, which form when acted upon by aspirin-acetylated COX-2.

proteoglycan synthesis. Not all of PGE_2's effects are proinflammatory, however. PGE_2 inhibits T-lymphocyte activation and proliferation, downregulates antibody production, and has variable effects on secretion of MMPs.

PGE_2 is generated from PGH_2 by at least three different isoforms of PGE synthase (PGES), cytoplasmic PGES (cPGES), and microsomal PGES (mPGES-1 and -2). Like COX-1, with which it is functionally coupled, cPGES is constitutively and ubiquitously expressed, whereas mPGES-1 is dramatically upregulated by proinflammatory stimuli and is functionally coupled with COX-2 (mPGES-2, the most recently discovered PGE terminal synthase, has a less clearly defined role and is linked to both COX isoforms).[34] In experimental systems, COX-2 and mPGES increase in tandem and have been found to co-localize to the same subcellular fraction. In human rheumatoid synovial fibroblasts, mPGES-1 expression is induced by both IL-1β and TNF-α and inhibited by dexamethasone.[35,36] mPGES-1-null mice are resistant to both adjuvant arthritis and collagen-induced arthritis.[37] mPGES-1 is therefore an attractive potential therapeutic target.

Other prostaglandins

Whereas PGE_2 is the predominant eicosanoid produced at inflammatory sites, activated cells produce a spectrum of additional prostaglandins with distinctive biologic activities. Prostacyclin (PGI_2) induces vasodilation and inhibits platelet aggregation, qualities that have been exploited in the treatment of pulmonary hypertension. PGD_2 can also produce vasodilation and likely plays a role in allergic inflammation

and asthma; on antigenic stimulation, it is released in large amounts by mast cells. In the CNS, PGD_2 regulates sleep. PGF_2, a powerful uterine constrictor, is not known to participate in inflammatory events.

PGJ_2, the most recently discovered prostanoid, exerts a number of anti-inflammatory effects. Unlike conventional PGs, which signal via G protein–coupled cell surface receptors, PGJ_2 is actively transported into cells, where it acts on the intranuclear peroxisome proliferator activating receptor (PPAR)-γ. Activated PPAR-γ inhibits activation of nuclear factor-κB (NF-κB), an important driver of the transcription of proinflammatory genes. In some cell types, PGJ_2 may also directly inhibit NF-κB. *In vitro*, the addition of PGJ_2 to human macrophages inhibits the production of IL-1β, TNF-α, IL-6, IL-12, and inducible nitric oxide synthase (iNOS). In an animal model of inflammatory arthritis, intraperitoneal administration of PGJ_2 suppressed pannus formation and inflammatory infiltration.[32]

Thromboxane A_2

Thromboxane A_2 (TXA_2) is formed directly from PGH_2 via the terminal enzyme, thromboxane synthase. Unlike prostaglandins, it contains a six-member carbon ring. TXA_2 is a powerful platelet activator, a potent vasoconstrictor, and a smooth muscle contractant. Platelet TXA_2 production is COX-1 dependent and unaffected by COX-2 inhibitors, suggesting that the prothrombotic effects of selective COX-2 inhibitors may be a consequence of TXA_2 production unopposed by PGI_2.[38] Although TXA_2 is conventionally thought of as a product of platelets, thromboxane synthase can be upregulated together with COX-2 in other cell types in response to cytokines, and thromboxane production has been implicated in both asthma and the pathogenesis of murine lupus nephritis.[39-41]

Leukotrienes

Leukotrienes (LTs) are created when 5-lipoxygenase (5-LO), in concert with the AA-binding protein 5-LO–activating protein (FLAP), oxygenates AA at C-5 to generate 5-hydroperoxyeicosatetraenoic acid (5-HPETE), which in turn is converted to LTA_4 (see Fig. 21.6). LTA_4 can then be converted to either LTB_4 or, through an alternative pathway, to LTC_4. LTC_4 is subsequently modified to form LTD_4, itself the precursor for LTE_4. LTC_4, LTD_4, and LTE_4 are also known as cysteinyl LTs (Cys LTs).

LTB_4 is the most important LT in acute inflammatory responses; it both activates leukocytes and prolongs their survival and promotes leukocyte trafficking. LTB_4 is a powerful chemoattractant for neutrophils and macrophages and stimulates leukocyte tight adhesion to vascular endothelium by upregulating leukocyte integrin expression.[42] LTB_4 is found in high levels in the synovial fluid and sera of RA patients, and LTB_4 antagonism inhibits inflammatory arthritis in several animal models. In a phase 2 clinical trial, however, an LTB_4 receptor antagonist was not efficacious for RA.[43]

Cysteinyl (Cys) LTs are produced by eosinophils, basophils, macrophages, and mast cells (and to a lesser extent, T cells and endothelial cells) and have significant biologic effects. They induce vasodilation and increased microvascular permeability; increase bronchoconstriction, wheezing, and mucus secretion; and decrease mucociliary clearance.[44] The leukotriene receptor antagonists montelukast and zafirlukast specifically block Cys LTs from attaching to the CysLT1 receptor and are currently available for treating asthma.

Platelet-activating factor

PAF, like AA, is generated from the plasma membrane. PLA_2, acting on phosphatidylcholine at the cell membrane, releases both AA and the precursor of PAF, lyso-PAF. PAF is synthesized by activated neutrophils, eosinophils, monocytes, platelets, endothelial cells, mast cells, and fibroblasts. It acts in a paracrine and autocrine manner via a G protein–coupled receptor on eosinophils, neutrophils, macrophages, platelets, endothelial cells, and lymphocytes. In addition to activating platelets, PAF is a chemoattractant and cell activator for neutrophils, macrophages, and eosinophils. It also induces bronchoconstriction, increased vascular permeability, and vasodilation.[45] PAF has been implicated in inflammatory arthritis and sepsis, and PAF receptor antagonist (PAF-RA) BN50730 reduces both carrageenan-induced arthritis in rabbits and collagen-induced arthritis in mice.[46,47] In a recent randomized controlled trial, however, BN50730 did not reduce RA disease activity.[48] PAF-RAs also ameliorate animal models of sepsis but have not been successful in phase 3 trials for gram-negative sepsis.

Anti-inflammatory lipids

Accumulating evidence suggests that the resolution of inflammation depends on an organism's ability to produce several novel series of anti-inflammatory mediators. Among this group of mediators are recently discovered AA-derived lipids known as lipoxins (LXs) and aspirin-triggered epi-lipoxins (ATLs). LXs are formed during cell-cell interactions that occur during inflammation (see Fig. 21.6). When adherent platelets interact with activated leukocytes in the vascular lumen, LTA_4 released from the leukocytes diffuses into platelets, where it is converted to LXA_4 and LXB_4 by 12-LO. LXs can also form when cells (e.g., monocytes or airway epithelium) release the 15-LO-dependent AA derivative 15S-HETE, which is then converted to lipoxygenase by neutrophils.[49] This requirement for the presence of two different inflammatory cells for LX formation may be a mechanism for delaying LX production until inflammation has already taken hold, consistent with a role for LX in the resolution phase of inflammation. ATLs, or 15-epi-lipoxins, are similar to other LXs in structure and function and are generated as a consequence of COX-2 modification by aspirin.

LXs and their analogs exert a plethora of anti-inflammatory effects, including inhibition of (1) IL-1β, TNF-α, and IL-8 expression; (2) neutrophil chemotaxis and interaction with endothelial and epithelial cells; (3) monocyte activation; and (4) inflammatory cell proliferation. LXs also promote macrophage clearance of apoptotic leukocytes.[49]

In vivo, lipoxins and their analogs inhibit several animal models of inflammatory disease, including experimental colitis, asthma, and peritonitis.[50] Their actual role in controlling human inflammation is less well established, including the extent to which aspirin's effects are mediated via ATL production.

The resolvins and docosatrienes are recently discovered, non–AA-derived lipid molecules that are potent endogenous anti-inflammatory mediators. Originally isolated in mice during the resolution phase of inflammatory disease models, these lipid products are generated from the essential omega-3 polyunsaturated fatty acids eicosapentaenoic acid (EPA) and docosahexaenoic acid (DHA). Like the lipoxins, they are produced during the later phases of inflammation and hasten its resolution.[51] Resolvin E1, the best-studied molecule of the resolvin series, significantly inhibits leukocyte infiltration in murine models of inflammation and protects against the development of sulfonic acid–induced colitis.[52,53] In a mouse model of ischemic brain injury, docosatrienes inhibited leukocyte infiltration into the brain and were neuroprotective.[54]

Vasoactive amines

Low-molecular-weight amines that are important inflammatory mediators include histamine and serotonin.

Histamine

Histamine is the decarboxylation product of the amino acid histidine and is stored in mast cell and basophil granules. It is released during mast cell activation by various stimuli, most particularly by crosslinking of Fc receptors on the cell surface in response to IgE binding, and promotes immediate hypersensitivity reactions. The biologic effects of histamine are mediated through its interactions with specific receptors. Histamine produces vasodilatation and enhanced permeability of postcapillary venules in addition to bronchoconstriction and the enhanced flow of bronchial mucus.

Serotonin

Serotonin is stored in the dense body granules of platelets. It is a vasoconstrictor but also enhances microvascular permeability. Serotonin also promotes fibrosis by enhancing the synthesis of collagen by fibroblasts and may therefore play a role in the retroperitoneal fibrosis in response to periaortitis. Serotonin also plays an important role as a neurotransmitter.

Proteases

Proteases include cysteine proteases, aspartic proteases, as well as matrix metalloproteinases and related enzymes (ADAMs and ADAMTSs). The proteases are reviewed in detail in Chapter 17.

Reactive oxygen species and nitric oxide

Reactive oxygen species (ROS) and nitric oxide (NO) are small molecules that contain unpaired electrons that are highly reactive with cellular components. It is well established that ROS and reactive nitrogen species function in part as specific intracellular signaling molecules. In inflammatory diseases, however, these unstable intermediates may be overproduced and released by activated immune cells; the subsequent non-specific oxidative reactions that take place between the radicals and biologic targets lead to cell death and tissue damage.

Reactive oxygen species

Inappropriate activation of macrophages and polymorphonuclear neutrophil leukocytes during acute and chronic inflammation can lead to release of ROS into the extracellular milieu, resulting in oxidative stress and damage of extracellular and cellular components, including nucleic acids, lipids, carbohydrates, proteins, and matrix components. ROS are constantly generated in low concentrations in all aerobic cells, which protect themselves from oxidative damage through the presence of antioxidant enzymes, such as catalases, peroxidases, and superoxide dismutases. When ROS are produced at extremely high levels by activated neutrophils and macrophages (via the oxidative burst; see earlier sections on neutrophils and macrophages), however, this machinery is

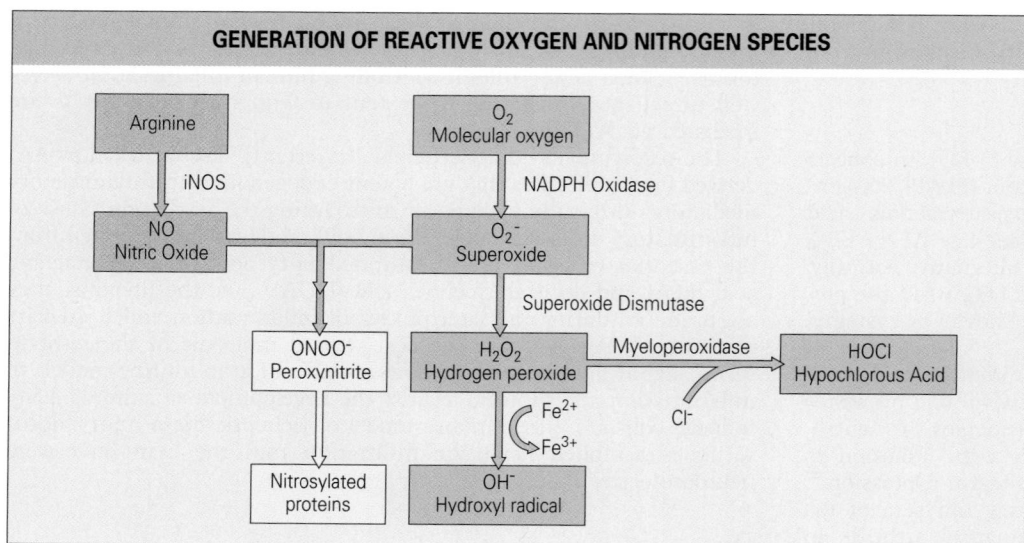

Fig. 21.7 Generation of reactive oxygen and nitrogen species. As shown on the right side of the figure, molecular oxygen is converted to superoxide (O_2^-) by the action of the NADPH oxidase complex. Superoxide dismutase subsequently converts superoxide to hydrogen peroxide (H_2O_2). In the presence of molecular iron, H_2O_2 is spontaneously converted to hydroxyl radical (OH^-), an extremely unstable and reactive oxygen product. Alternatively, reaction of H_2O_2 with molecular chloride is catalyzed by myeloperoxidase in phagolysosomes of macrophages and neutrophils; the product, hypochlorous acid (HOCl), is an extremely potent antibacterial agent. As shown on the left side of the figure, inducible nitric oxide synthase (iNOS) liberates nitric oxide (NO) from the side chain of arginine. Interaction of nitric oxide and superoxide results in the formation of highly reactive peroxynitrites, which can modify, and potentially alter, the function of a wide range of proteins.

overwhelmed and tissue damage can occur. The major ROS formed by cells are, in descending order of stability, superoxide, hydrogen peroxide, and the hydroxyl radical (Fig. 21.7). Of these, by far the least stable species is the hydroxyl radical. It is produced in the presence of iron via the Fenton reaction, has a half-life of less than 10^{-6} second, and is likely responsible for much of the havoc wreaked by oxidative intermediates.[55]

As noted earlier, phagocytes generate ROS in large amounts, in the form of superoxide, from the NADPH oxidase complex. Until recently, it was thought that NADPH oxidases exist only in phagocytic cells (where they are now termed *PHOX*, for phagocytic oxidase), but, in fact, they are ubiquitous; in other cells, NADPH oxidases are termed *NOXs* (for non-phagocytic oxidases), and six variants have been discovered.[56] Over the past decade, studies have shown that ROS produced by NOX influence a number of cellular events, including cell proliferation and apoptosis.[56] They also participate in post-receptor signaling pathways (e.g., PDGF and angiotensin). The proinflammatory transcription factors, activator protein (AP)-1 and NF-κB, were among the first intracellular complexes discovered to be substrates for ROS signaling.[57] These two transcription factors spur the production of literally dozens of proinflammatory mediators, including collagenase, IL-1β, and TNF-α. In line with this discovery, ROS have been demonstrated to cause upregulation of adhesion molecules on endothelium and increase both cytokine and chemokine production by leukocytes.

ROS participate in RA pathology, and their mark is seen in the rheumatoid joint in synovial fluid and tissue, where oxidative products are elevated and antioxidant levels are reduced.[58] Synovial T cells from RA patients show signs of severe oxidative stress, which renders them hyporesponsive. Previously, this oxidative stress had been ascribed solely to exposure from extracellular ROS generated by synovial phagocytes. In actuality, synovial T cells themselves produce intracellular ROS, which may contribute to the overall oxidant stress.[59] Although antioxidants have been shown to ameliorate collagen-induced arthritis in rodents, antioxidant trials for human RA have thus far failed to show benefit.

Nitric oxide

Nitric oxide (NO) is synthesized via the oxidation of arginine by one of three distinct nitric oxide synthase (NOS) isoforms (see Fig. 21.7). The neuronal (nNOS) and the endothelial (eNOS) isoforms are constitutively expressed, with activity regulated by intracellular calcium levels and the calcium-binding protein calmodulin. The third isoform (iNOS) is induced by stimuli that include LPS, IL-1β, TNF-α and IFN-α; its activation leads to a sustained generation of NO.[60] The production of NO plays a vital role in the regulation of physiologic processes, host defense, inflammation, and immunity.[61] Proinflammatory effects include vasodilation, edema, cytotoxicity, and the mediation of cytokine-dependent processes that can lead to tissue destruction. NO-dependent tissue injury has been implicated in a variety of rheumatic diseases, including SLE, RA, and osteoarthritis. Conversely, the production of NO by endothelial cell NOS may serve a protective, or anti-inflammatory, function by preventing the adhesion and release of oxidants by activated neutrophils in the microvasculature.[62]

NO, a gaseous free radical, is labile ($t\frac{1}{2} < 15$ seconds) and in the presence of oxygen is rapidly metabolized to nitrate and nitrite.[63] Given the short half-life of authentic NO gas, the biologic activity of NO in specific tissues will be determined by its reactivity with target molecules. For example, binding of NO to the heme group of soluble guanylate cyclase activates this enzyme, raising intracellular levels of cyclic guanosine monophosphate (cGMP).[64] This action of NO promotes smooth muscle relaxation; it is the mechanism by which NO-donating drugs such as nitroglycerin and drugs that inhibit the degradation of cGMP, such as sildenafil, promote vasodilation. Another important reaction of NO is with free thiols to form *S*-nitrosothiol compounds.[65] *S*-nitrosothiol derivatives, formed both extracellularly and intracellularly, are significantly more stable (e.g., $t\frac{1}{2} > 2$ hours) and retain NO-like vasodilating properties but are less cytotoxic.[65] The reaction of NO with superoxide anion yields peroxynitrite, a highly toxic free radical, which nitrosylates proteins, leading to the accumulation of injurious intracellular oxidants and DNA damage (see Fig. 21.7).[66]

NO and its derivatives play complex roles in immunoregulation. Low levels of NO promote lymphocyte activation and proliferation, whereas high concentrations suppress APC activity and T-cell proliferation.[67,68] There is evidence that NO exerts different effects on discrete subpopulations of T cells, inhibiting secretion of IL-2 by murine Th1 cells while increasing the secretion of IL-4 in Th2 cells. At high concentrations, NO promotes apoptosis in macrophages, CD4+/CD8+ thymocytes, and chondrocytes.[69,70] At lower concentrations (<1 mM), NO inhibits apoptosis of hepatocytes, B lymphocytes, and eosinophils via the inhibition of caspases.[71]

Although excessive NO production is generally associated with tissue injury, it is important to note that NO constitutively produced by endothelium is believed to play a protective role in the microvasculature.[65,72] This protection is afforded by the capacity of NO to inhibit platelet and neutrophil adhesion to endothelial monolayers, as well as to inhibit leukocyte superoxide anion production.[62,72]

Role of nitric oxide in rheumatic diseases

NO has been implicated in the pathogenesis of MRL/lpr model of murine lupus.[73] Splenic and renal tissues from these mice have increased expression of iNOS mRNA and increased amounts of material immunoreactive for iNOS.[73] The administration of NG-monomethyl-L-arginine (L-NMMA), a NOS inhibitor, prevents the development of glomerulonephritis and reduces the intensity of inflammatory arthritis in this model.[73] In human SLE, serum nitrite is elevated during active disease and levels correlate with both SLE Disease Activity Index (SLEDAI) scores and titers of antibodies to double-stranded DNA.[74,75]

The importance of NO is well documented in the development of experimental arthritis. Adjuvant-induced arthritis (AIA) can be

Sham Denervation   Denervation

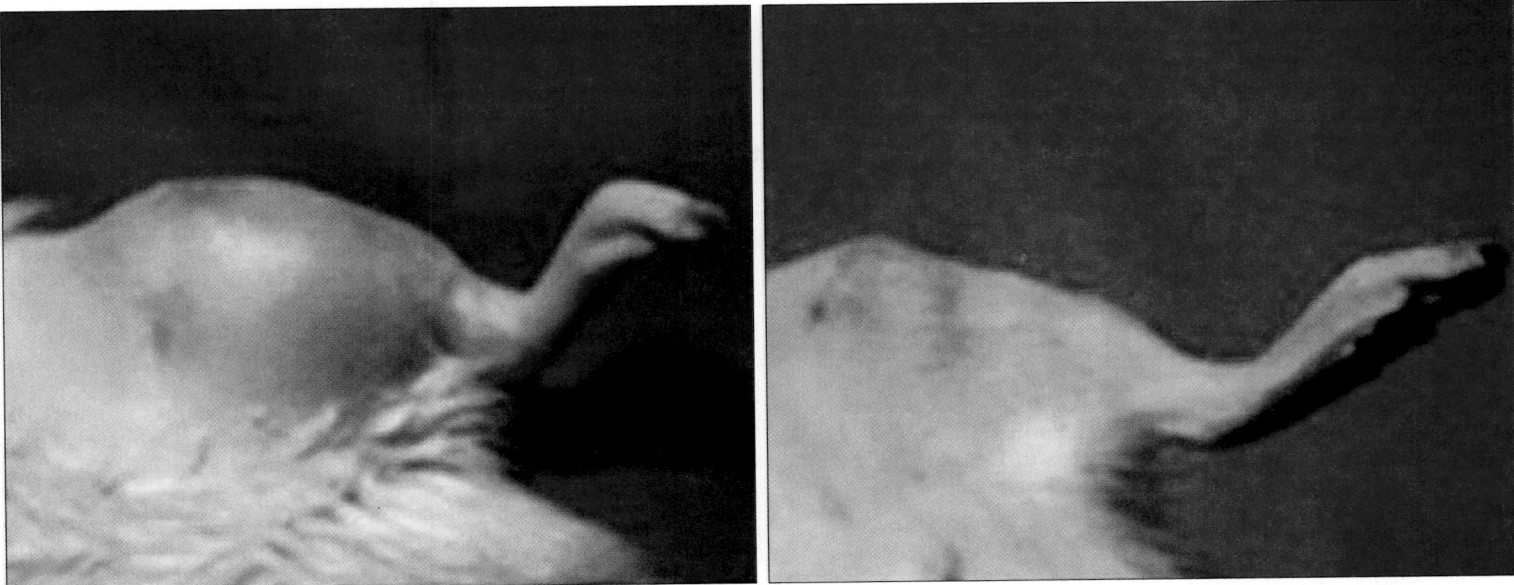

Fig. 21.8 Joint denervation prevents arthritis. Sensory denervation of the rat knee joint prevents development of arthritis. (a) A normal rat knee 24 hours post-carrageenan injection. Note the intense inflammation. (b) A denervated rat knee 24 hours post-carrageenan injection. *(Reproduced with permission from the BMJ Publishing Group.)*

suppressed by the NOS inhibitor L-NMMA.[76] Elevations of NO and amelioration of disease by non-selective NOS inhibitors have also been demonstrated in collagen-induced arthritis and streptococcal cell wall arthritis.[76-78] Inhibition of NO production also attenuates animal models of osteoarthritis.[79,80] In human arthritis, increased concentrations of nitrites have been demonstrated within the joint fluids of patients with osteoarthritis and RA.[81,82] iNOS expression has been demonstrated in both RA and OA synoviocytes and chondrocytes by *in-situ* hybridization and immunohistochemistry.[83] St. Clair and colleagues reported increased expression of blood mononuclear cell iNOS in RA patients.[84] In these studies, the degree of peripheral mononuclear cell nitrite production *ex vivo* correlated with disease activity, leading the authors to suggest that increased iNOS expression and NO generation may be important in the pathogenesis of RA. Subsequently, this group demonstrated that increased PBMC expression of iNOS and iNOS enzyme activity were reduced after treatment with the anti-TNF monoclonal antibody infliximab. Changes in NOS activity after treatment correlated significantly with changes in the number of tender joints.

In osteoarthritis, NO is spontaneously produced by chondrocytes and has been implicated in the progressive cartilage deterioration.[85] Deleterious effects NO exerts on cartilage metabolism include (1) inhibition of collagen and proteoglycan synthesis[86]; (2) activation of metalloproteinases[87]; (3) increased susceptibility to injury by other oxidants (e.g., H_2O_2); and (4) apoptosis.[88,89]

THE NERVOUS SYSTEM IN INFLAMMATION

The immune and nervous systems are in constant communication, and the inflammatory response involves a complex bidirectional interaction between the two. The nervous system registers inflammation in the periphery via sensory nerves and directs the immune system through a variety of messengers, ranging from autonomic neurotransmitters (e.g., acetylcholine) to peripherally synthesized neuropeptides such as substance P (SP); nervous system signals can be either proinflammatory or anti-inflammatory. The CNS also controls inflammatory responses through release of neuroendocrine hormones such as melanocyte-stimulating hormone (MSH) and corticotropin-releasing factor (CRF), which dampen inflammation. Animals that have undergone hypophysectomy or adrenalectomy are sensitized to endotoxemia, and rats deficient in CRF are susceptible to streptococcal antigen-induced arthritis.[90] Conversely, the immune system regulates the CNS through the release of cytokines, growth factors, and other mediators;

cytokine release in the periphery, for instance, can induce the hypothalamic-pituitary-adrenal axis to release glucocorticoids.

Both clinical and experimental evidence support that the peripheral nervous system (PNS) modulates inflammatory arthritis. As early as 1965 it was observed that peripheral nerve transection attenuated distal inflammation in rats with adjuvant arthritis.[91] Carrageenan-induced joint inflammation is also inhibited by joint denervation (Fig. 21.8). Clinically, hemiparetic patients who later develop RA are largely spared from disease on the paralyzed side. That rheumatoid arthritis is characteristically symmetric (indicating cross-spinal reflexes) and predominantly distal (where dense sensory innervation occurs) also suggests CNS involvement.

Joint innervation

Joints are heavily innervated with sensory nerve branches that terminate in the joint capsule, synovium, entheses, subchondral bone, and periosteum (in contrast, cartilage is aneural). Normal synovial tissue is richly innervated with both sensory and sympathetic nerves. Type C sensory nerve fibers containing neuropeptides such as substance P or CGRP are present in the synovial lining and sublining tissue and in the vascularized peripheral parts of the joint menisci, whereas sympathetic fibers are located only around blood vessels.[92] Mast cells and afferent nerve terminals are frequently observed in all parts of the normal synovium; densities of mast cells appear to be greatest at the nerve terminals and perivascularly.

Autonomic influences on inflammation

The autonomic nervous system (ANS) is hard-wired into the immune system; parasympathetic branches from the vagal nerve and sympathetic nerve fibers synapse upon the major organs of immunity, including the spleen, lymph nodes, thymus, bone marrow, and the gut's mucosa-associated lymphoid tissue. Thus, there exists a dense, established network that provides direct lines of communication between the immune and autonomic nervous systems, which permits rapid and robust responses, in response to stimuli, in both directions.

The parasympathetic nervous system: an anti-inflammatory pathway

As noted earlier, activation of leukocytes by foreign or noxious stimuli results in release of mediators. In turn, these mediators activate parasympathetic sensory nerve fibers that ascend in the vagus nerve. By impinging on the nucleus tract solitarius, these afferent signals trigger efferent parasympathetic responses, resulting in the release of acetylcholine, which has potent local anti-inflammatory effects on both macrophages and endothelium.[93]

In vitro, acetylcholine inhibits macrophage production of TNF-α, IL-1β, and IL-18, while permitting the synthesis of the largely anti-inflammatory cytokine IL-10.[90] Acetylcholine also inhibits the release of a recently recognized inflammatory mediator, high-mobility group box-1 (HMGB-1), by macrophages exposed to TNF-α.[94] Acetylcholine anti-inflammatory effects appear to occur via engagement of α-7 nicotinic receptors. Endothelial cells have α-7 nicotinic acetylcholine receptors, and both acetylcholine and the nicotinic acetylcholine receptor agonist CAP55 block TNF-α–stimulated endothelial cell activation (and subsequent leukocyte recruitment).[95] This intimate connection between the nervous and immune systems can therefore profoundly modulate the inflammatory response. The selective cholinergic agonist nicotine improves survival in experimental sepsis[94,96] and has been associated with improvement of ulcerative colitis. Stimulation of the vagal nerve suppresses carrageenan-induced arthritis and endotoxemic shock. These findings may lead to newer and safer cholinergic agonists that may be used to treat inflammatory disease.

Sympathetic nervous system

Sympathetic nerve fibers release norepinephrine, which acts on target cells, including most immune cell types, by engaging α₁-, α₂-, and β-adrenoreceptors. The effects of the sympathetic nervous system on immunity and inflammation are mixed and vary with the cell and clinical context. For instance, norepinephrine effects on macrophages depend on which receptors are being expressed and engaged. Ligation of macrophage β-adrenoreceptors inhibits TNF-α secretion, whereas α₂-receptor engagement induces TNF-α release, and binding of the α₁-receptor stimulates complement production.[97] In addition to inhibiting macrophage function, activated β-adrenergic receptors also inhibit neutrophil and NK cell function. β-Adrenoreceptor ligation can also cause a Th2 shift (alteration of acquired immune response), largely by increasing IL-10 production.[97] Furthermore, norepinephrine is often released en sync with corticotropin release, and glucocorticoids are potentiated in the presence of norepinephrine. On the other hand, stimulation of β-adrenoreceptors also drives IL-8 secretion by monocytes and localized, neurogenic inflammation is promoted by the activation of β-adrenoreceptors.[97] In contrast to the mixed effect of β-adrenoreceptors on macrophages, the function of α-adrenergic receptors on immune cells is largely proinflammatory.

Consistent with these somewhat confusing *in-vitro* observations, animal studies have shown that disrupting sympathetic nervous system signaling can either worsen or improve inflammatory disease, depending on context. Sympathectomy ameliorates early, but exacerbates late, inflammation in collagen-induced arthritis. In contrast, β-adrenergic agonists improve late-stage experimental arthritis. The distinct proinflammatory and anti-inflammatory effects of norepinephrine may, in part, relate to dose, because much higher concentrations of norepinephrine are required to activate the β-adrenergic receptor; a low-density of sympathetic fibers may therefore dictate a primarily α-adrenergic response in the arthritic joint. In this context, it is interesting to note that animals with collagen-induced arthritis demonstrate sympathetic neuron loss in the joint.[98] Similarly, RA patients have a relative paucity of sympathetic nerve fibers in the synovium.[99] Moreover, RA CD8+ T cells have fewer β-adrenoreceptors, suggesting they may be resistant to inhibition by norepinephrine.[100] In contrast, patients with juvenile idiopathic arthritis have immune cells that overexpress α₁-adrenergic receptors. One very small randomized clinical trial in the 1980s used guanethidine to achieve regional sympathetic blockade in a group of 24 RA patients.[101] This study showed that patients receiving active treatment had improved grip strength and decreased pain by the end of the study, which lasted 14 days.

Neuroendocrine mechanisms

The hypothalamus continuously receives data about the body's environment and, in response to stress signals such as IL-1β, releases CRF. CRF activates the pituitary to secrete adrenocorticotropic hormone (ACTH), in turn stimulating the adrenal glands to produce and secrete glucocorticoids, potent endogenous anti-inflammatory immunomodulators. Melanocyte-stimulating hormone (MSH), which derives from the same precursor (POMC) as ACTH, is also secreted by the pituitary gland and can suppress inflammation.[102] Systemic administration of MSH improves inflammatory arthritis, experimental colitis, and experimental allergic encephalomyelitis.[103] Recent studies of crystal-induced arthritis suggests that the anti-inflammatory effects of MSH are mediated through engagement of a specific receptor, MSH-R3, and that not only MSH but also ACTH can engage this receptor, indicating that ACTH has a direct anti-inflammatory effect in addition to its ability to drive cortisol synthesis.[104] Selective MSH-R3 antagonists reduce inflammation in animal models, suggesting a possible future anti-inflammatory strategy.

Peripheral nervous system

Peripheral sensory nerves (Aδ and C fibers) not only transmit pain signaling in response to noxious stimuli such as bradykinin, histamine, and serotonin but also secrete inflammatory mediators from their nerve endings. These mediators, known as neuropeptides, induce a number of critical early inflammatory events, including arteriolar vasodilation, increased microvascular permeability, and leukocyte recruitment (Table 21.4). In recognition of this neuropeptide role, the edema, warmth, and redness seen in early inflammatory lesions are sometimes collectively referred to as neurogenic inflammation. While neuropeptides are neurotransmitters generally thought of as mediating neuron-to-neuron communication, they also can act on (and be produced by) cells outside the nervous system, such as macrophages, dendritic cells, and lymphocytes.

Neuropeptides
Substance P

Substance P, also known as neurokinin, was first discovered and purified in powder form (hence, its full name, substance powder) in 1931. It is widely distributed throughout the peripheral and central nervous systems, where it largely functions as a transmitter of pain signaling. Part of the tachykinin family of peptides, which also includes neuropeptide Y and neurokinins A and B, substance P is formed from an alternate splice of the preprotachykinin I gene.[105] Unmyelinated C-type nerve fibers release substance P in response to noxious stimuli, producing a variety of proinflammatory effects by acting on target cells through binding and activation of the NK-1 receptor (NK-1R). Substance P ligation of NK-1R on postcapillary endothelium increases microvascular permeability and causes edema; it also induces vasodilation in arterioles.[106] Substance P also acts as a chemoattractant and activator for macrophages, lymphocytes, neutrophils, and eosinophils, stimulating the production of cytokines and AA derivatives, and stimulating the oxidative burst in neutrophils and macrophages. Mast cells also possess NK-1R and degranulate in response to substance P, leading to histamine and serotonin release. Lymphocytes proliferate and differentiate when stimulated with substance P, and some leukocytes (e.g., lymphocytes, macrophages, and eosinophils) are themselves capable of substance P expression.[107]

Substantial evidence supports a role for substance P in inflammatory arthritis. In animal models, more severely affected joints have higher levels of substance P than joints with milder disease.[107] Elevated substance P levels are also found in the Achilles tendon enthesis in rats with adjuvant arthritis.[108] Exogenous substance P directly infused into joints exacerbates experimental arthritis, whereas neural depletion of substance P via pretreatment with capsaicin ameliorates joint inflammation.[109-111] Exogenous substance P also mediates vascular changes in non-arthritic joints and stimulates synovial angiogenesis. In a mouse model of adjuvant-induced arthritis, NK-1R knockout mice experienced less joint swelling and plasma extravasation than control littermates.[112]

Increased levels of substance P are found in a number of human inflammatory diseases, including RA, inflammatory bowel disease, and asthma.[106] *In vitro*, RA synovial fibroblasts (RASF) respond to nanomolar concentrations of substance P by releasing PGE₂ and MMP-1 and proliferating.[113] At these same concentrations, substance P also stimulates production of IL-1, TNF-α, and IL-6 in peripheral whole blood from RA patients. Increased levels of both substance P and

TABLE 21.4 INFLAMMATORY EFFECTS OF SELECT NEUROPEPTIDES

Neuropeptide	Where produced (outside the CNS)	Effects on inflammation	Evidence for involvement in arthritis
Substance P (neurokinin)	C-type nerve fibers Lymphocytes Macrophages Eosinophils	Arteriole vasodilation Increased microvascular permeability Chemoattracts and activates macrophages, polymorphonuclear neutrophils, lymphocytes, and eosinophils Mast cell degranulation	Elevated SP in synovial fluid of RA joints RA synovial fibroblasts (RASF) overexpress SP receptor (NK-1R) Stimulates RASF to proliferate and secrete inflammatory products
Calcitonin-gene-related peptide (CGRP)	C-type nerve fibers	Potent arteriole and venous vasodilator	CGRP overexpressed in entheses of animals with adjuvant arthritis Elevated CGRP levels in synovial tissue from OA joints
Neuropeptide Y	Sympathetic nerve fibers	May favor Th2 response: Inhibits IFN-γ and stimulates IL-4 production in lymphocytes	RA synovium has paucity of NPY-containing nerve fibers
Vasoactive intestinal peptide	Peripheral nerves Mast cells Lymphocytes Polymorphonuclear neutrophils Macrophages	Anti-inflammatory peptide Inhibits chemotaxis and activation of macrophages and T cells Stimulates production of IL-4, IL-10, and IL-1ra	Therapeutic in collagen-induced arthritis

NK-1R are found in synovial fluid of the RA joint, and RASF overexpresses NK-1R mRNA. NK-1R antagonists have not yet been studied in the treatment of RA.[106]

Calcitonin gene–related protein

CGRP, an alternative splice product of calcitonin, is a widely distributed neuropeptide that is primarily released from small sensory nerves in the periphery. It acts on the complex of the G protein–coupled calcitonin receptor–like receptor (CL) that must be linked to a receptor activity-modifying protein (RAMP) for functionality. CL is expressed by smooth muscle, endothelial cells, macrophages, and lymphocytes. CGRP is co-localized and co-released with substance P in afferent nerves and is a potent arterial and venous vasodilator, particularly in the microvasculature.[114] In the mouse air-pouch model, a CGRP antagonist inhibits neutrophil accumulation,[115] probably via indirect mechanisms. CGRP is overexpressed at the nerve endings of animals with adjuvant arthritis and in sensory neurons in rats with collagen-induced arthritis.[107,116] Synovial tissue from osteoarthritic joints also contains nerve endings with high concentrations of both substance P and CGRP,[117] consistent with a role in inflammation. However, CGRP may be a mixed proinflammatory/anti-inflammatory agent, because CGRP inhibits T-cell and pre-B-cell differentiation, macrophage antigen presentation, IL-1 production,[114] and RASF activity *in vitro*.[118] At this time, it is unclear what overall role CGRP plays in arthritis.

Neuropeptide Y

Neuropeptide Y is a tachykinin released from sympathetic nerve endings, alone or in combination with catecholamines. Unlike substance P, neuropeptide Y exerts both proinflammatory and anti-inflammatory effects. Neuropeptide Y inhibits IFN-γ and stimulates IL-4 production in rat lymphocytes,[119] suggesting that it may favor Th2 responses, and therefore modify Th1-predominant diseases such as RA and multiple sclerosis. Neuropeptide Y ameliorates disease severity in experimental allergic encephalomyelitis (the animal model for multiple sclerosis) but has not yet been tested in models of inflammatory arthritis.[120] The spinal fluid of patients with multiple sclerosis shows depressed levels of neuropeptide Y, and the synovium of RA patients has a paucity of neuropeptide Y–containing nerve fibers, which may help maintain the Th1 response.

Vasoactive intestinal peptide

Vasoactive intestinal peptide (VIP) is a neuropeptide synthesized and released by immune cells (mast cells, lymphocytes, neutrophils, and monocytes) as well as nerve endings that synapse on central and peripheral lymphoid organs. VIP receptors, of which there are three types, are G protein–coupled receptors found on lymphocytes, monocytes, and macrophages. VIP is a potent anti-inflammatory peptide that inhibits chemotaxis and activation of macrophages and T cells. Consequently, it inhibits production of TNF-α, IFN-γ, IL-6, and IL-12. It also stimulates the production of the anti-inflammatory cytokines IL-10 and IL-Ra.[121] VIP may additionally shift T cells to a Th2 phenotype, as it increases IL-4 production and may promote T regulatory cell production.[121] VIP has been shown to be therapeutic in several inflammatory models, including sulfonic acid–induced colitis, sepsis, and collagen-induced arthritis.[121,122]

KEY REFERENCES

1. Liu Y, Shaw SK, Ma S, et al. Regulation of leukocyte transmigration: cell surface interactions and signaling events. J Immunol 2004;172:7-13.
2. Drappa J, Vaishnaw AK, Sullivan KE, et al. *Fas* gene mutations in the Canale-Smith syndrome, an inherited lymphoproliferative disorder associated with autoimmunity. N Engl J Med 1996;335:1643-1649.
3. Landis RC, Haskard DO. Pathogenesis of crystal-induced inflammation. Curr Rheumatol Rep 2001;3:36-41.
4. Schaible HG, Del Rosso A, Matucci-Cerinic M. Neurogenic aspects of inflammation. Rheum Dis Clin North Am 2005;31:77-101, ix.
5. Burg ND, Pillinger MH. The neutrophil: function and regulation in innate and humoral immunity. Clin Immunol 2001;99:7-17.
6. Gonzalez-Amaro R, Diaz-Gonzalez F, Sanchez-Madrid F. Adhesion molecules in inflammatory diseases. Drugs 1998;56:977-988.
7. Imhof BA, Aurrand-Lions M. Adhesion mechanisms regulating the migration of monocytes. Nat Rev Immunol 2004;4:432-444.

8. Roos D, van Bruggen R, Meischl C. Oxidative killing of microbes by neutrophils. Microbes Infect 2003;5:1307-1315.
9. Bainton DF. Distinct granule populations in human neutrophils and lysosomal organelles identified by nerve-electron microscopy. J Immunol Methods 1999;232:153-168.
10. Papayannopoulos V, Zychlinsky A. NETs: a new strategy for using old weapons. Trends Immunol 2009;30:513-521.
11. Wardlaw AJ, Moqbel R, Kay AB. Eosinophils: biology and role in disease. Adv Immunol 1995;60:151-266.
12. Lefkovits I, Vella AT. Innate immunity. In: Janeway CA, Travers P, Walport M, Shlomchik M, eds. Immunobiology, 5th ed. New York: Garland, 2001:35-91.
13. Ma J, Chen T, Mandelin J, et al. Regulation of macrophage activation. Cell Mol Life Sci 2003;60:2334-2346.
14. Salmon JE, Pricop L. Human receptors for immunoglobulin G: key elements in the pathogenesis of rheumatic disease. Arthritis Rheum 2001;44:739-750.

15. Holers VM. The complement system as a therapeutic target in autoimmunity. Clin Immunol 2003;107:140-151.
16. Geppert TD, Lipsky PE. Antigen presentation at the inflammatory site. Crit Rev Immunol 1989;9:313-362.
17. Bingham CO, Abramson SB. Mediators of inflammation, tissue destruction and repair: cellular constituents. In Klippel J, ed. Primer on the rheumatic diseases, 12th ed. Atlanta: Arthritis Foundation, 2001:51-66.
18. Weyrich AS, Zimmerman GA. Platelets: signaling cells in the immune continuum. Trends Immunol 2004;25:489-495.
19. Wagner DD, Burger PC. Platelets in inflammation and thrombosis. Arterioscler Thromb Vasc Biol 2003;23:2131-2137.
20. Levi M, van der Poll T, Buller HR. Bidirectional relation between inflammation and coagulation. Circulation 2004;109:2698-2704.
21. Peerschke EI, et al. Serum complement activation on heterologous platelets is associated with arterial thrombosis in patients with systemic lupus

erythematosus and antiphospholipid antibodies. Lupus 2009;18:530-538.

22. Salmon JE, Girardi G. Antiphospholipid antibodies and pregnancy loss: a disorder of inflammation. J Reprod Immunol 2008;77:51-56.

23. Arlaud GJ, Gaboriaud C, Thielens NM, et al. Structural biology of the C1 complex of complement unveils the mechanisms of its activation and proteolytic activity. Mol Immunol 2002;39:383-394.

24. Reid KB, Porter RR. The proteolytic activation systems of complement. Annu Rev Biochem 1981;50:433-464.

25. Fujita T, Matsushita M, Endo Y. The lectin-complement pathway: its role in innate immunity and evolution. Immunol Rev 2004;198:185-202.

26. Holers VM, Thurman JM. The alternative pathway of complement in disease: opportunities for therapeutic targeting. Mol Immunol 2004;41:147-152.

27. Guo RF, Ward PA. Role of C5a in inflammatory responses. Annu Rev Immunol 2005;23:821-852.

28. Gasque P. Complement: a unique innate immune sensor for danger signals. Mol Immunol 2004;41:1089-1098.

29. Barilla-LaBarca ML, Atkinson JP. Rheumatic syndromes associated with complement deficiency. Curr Opin Rheumatol 2003;15:55-60.

30. Belmont HM, Abramson SB, Lie JT. Pathology and pathogenesis of vascular injury in systemic lupus erythematosus: interactions of inflammatory cells and activated endothelium. Arthritis Rheum 1996; 39:9-22.

31. Crofford LJ, Lipsky PE, Brooks P, et al. Basic biology and clinical application of specific cyclooxygenase-2 inhibitors. Arthritis Rheum 2000;43:4-13.

32. Scher JU, Pillinger MH. 15d-PGJ2: the anti-inflammatory prostaglandin? Clin Immunol 2005;114:100-109.

33. Tilley SL, Coffman TM, Koller BH. Mixed messages: modulation of inflammation and immune responses by prostaglandins and thromboxanes. J Clin Invest 2001;108:15-23.

34. Fahmi H. mPGES-1 as a novel target for arthritis. Curr Opin Rheumatol 2004;16:623-627.

35. Stichtenoth DO, Thoren S, Bian H, et al. Microsomal prostaglandin E synthase is regulated by proinflammatory cytokines and glucocorticoids in primary rheumatoid synovial cells. J Immunol 2001;167:469-474.

36. Kamei D, Yamakawa K, Takegoshi Y, et al. Reduced pain hypersensitivity and inflammation in mice lacking microsomal prostaglandin E synthase-1. J Biol Chem 2004;279:33684-33695.

37. Trebino CE, Stock JL, Gibbons CP, et al. Impaired inflammatory and pain responses in mice lacking an inducible prostaglandin E synthase. Proc Natl Acad Sci U S A 2003;100:9044-9049.

38. FitzGerald GA, Cheng Y, Austin S. COX-2 inhibitors and the cardiovascular system. Clin Exp Rheumatol 2001;19(6 Suppl 25):S31-S36.

39. Kelley VE, Sneve S, Musinski S. Increased renal thromboxane production in murine lupus nephritis. J Clin Invest 1986;77:252-259.

40. Spurney RF, Fan PY, Ruiz P, et al. Thromboxane receptor blockade reduces renal injury in murine lupus nephritis. Kidney Int 1992;41:973-982.

41. Dogne JM, de Leval X, Benoit P, et al. Therapeutic potential of thromboxane inhibitors in asthma. Expert Opin Invest Drugs 2002;11:275-281.

42. Tager AM, Luster AD. BLT1 and BLT2: the leukotriene B(4) receptors. Prostaglandins Leukot Essent Fatty Acids 2003;69:123-134.

43. Polmar SH, et al. Limited clinical efficacy of a leukotriene B4 receptor antagonist in patients with active rheumatoid arthritis [abstract]. Presented before the annual meeting of the American College of Rheumatology, 2004.

44. Busse W, Kraft M. Cysteinyl leukotrienes in allergic inflammation: strategic target for therapy. Chest 2005;127:1312-1326.

45. Stafforini DM, McIntyre TM, Zimmerman GA, et al. Platelet-activating factor, a pleiotrophic mediator of physiological and pathological processes. Crit Rev Clin Lab Sci 2003;40:643-672.

46. Hilliquin P, Natour J, Aissa J, et al. Treatment of carrageenan-induced arthritis by the platelet activating factor antagonist BN 50730. Ann Rheum Dis 1995;54:140-143.

47. Palacios I, Miguelez R, Sanchez-Pernaute O, et al. A platelet-activating factor receptor antagonist prevents the development of chronic arthritis in mice. J Rheumatol 1999;26:1080-1086.

48. Hilliquin P, Chermat-Izard V, Menkes CJ. A double-blind, placebo-controlled study of a platelet-activating factor antagonist in patients with rheumatoid arthritis. J Rheumatol 1998;25:1502-1507.

49. Serhan CN. A search for endogenous mechanisms of anti-inflammation uncovers novel chemical mediators: missing links to resolution. Histochem Cell Biol 2004;122:305-321.

50. McMahon B, Godson C. Lipoxins: endogenous regulators of inflammation. Am J Physiol Renal Physiol 2004;286:F189-F201.

REFERENCES

Full references for this chapter can be found on www.expertconsult.com.

Scientific basis of pain

Hans-Georg Schaible

22

- Nociception is the encoding and processing of noxious stimuli in the nervous system; the subjective sensation pain is evoked by nociception and influenced by psychological and social factors.

- Clinically relevant pain is classified as nociceptive, when tissue is inflamed or damaged, or as neuropathic, when nerve fibers or nerve cells are affected.

- Peripheral nociceptors are slowly conducting, thinly myelinated or unmyelinated nerve fibers that respond to tissue-damaging mechanical, thermal, and chemical stimuli.

- The central nociceptive system consists of neurons in the spinal cord, the brain stem, the thalamus, and several cortical areas that process noxious stimuli; the conscious pain sensation with its sensory-discriminative and affective components is generated at the thalamocortical level.

- During inflammation, peripheral nociceptors are sensitized to mechanical and/or thermal stimuli by inflammatory mediators (peripheral sensitization).

- Damaged nerve fibers may show action potentials that are evoked at the site of lesion and in the neuronal cell bodies (ectopic discharges).

- Peripheral sensitization and ectopic discharges may induce a state of hyperexcitability in the central nociceptive system (central sensitization) that increases the gain of central nociceptive processing.

- Nerve fibers originating in the brain stem can enhance or inhibit the spinal nociceptive processing (descending facilitation or inhibition).

NOCICEPTION AND PAIN

According to the definition of the International Association for the Study of Pain (IASP), *pain* is an unpleasant sensory and emotional experience that is evoked by actual or potential noxious (i.e., tissue damaging) stimuli or by tissue injury, or is described in such terms. Normally, pain is the subjective result of nociception. *Nociception* is the encoding and processing of noxious stimuli in the nervous system. It can be objectively measured with various techniques (e.g., with electrophysiologic recordings). By contrast, pain as a subjective experience can be only verbally described by humans and it cannot be measured objectively. However, animals (as well as humans) show reflex responses to acute noxious stimuli and these reactions allow an assessment of the relationship between nociception and pain.[1] Under normal conditions the relationship between nociception and pain is relatively precise and predictable; that is, a stimulus that is noxious will usually evoke a subjective pain response. However, under clinically relevant conditions, the relationship between nociception and pain may not be strict, particularly when the pain is chronic (see later).

Neurons in the peripheral and central nociceptive system that encode noxious stimuli form the nociceptive system. A simplified scheme of the nociceptive system is shown in Figure 22.1. The peripheral nociceptive system innervates the skin, deep tissue, and most visceral organs, and the peripheral nociceptive fibers encode noxious stimuli applied to the tissue. The central nociceptive system consists of sensory neurons in the spinal cord, spinal reflex pathways, and ascending tracts that activate the brain stem and supraspinal structures in the thalamus and cortex. Corticothalamic networks produce the conscious pain response.[1,2]

Types of pain

When a noxious stimulus is applied to *normal* tissue, *acute physiologic nociceptive pain* is elicited. This pain protects tissue from being further damaged, because usually withdrawal reflexes are elicited. *Pathophysiologic nociceptive pain* occurs when the tissue is *inflamed* or *injured*. This pain may appear as spontaneous pain (pain in the absence of any intentional stimulation) and/or as hyperalgesia and/or allodynia. *Hyperalgesia* is a higher pain intensity felt with noxious heat stimulation (thermal hyperalgesia) or noxious mechanical stimulation (mechanical hyperalgesia). *Allodynia* is the occurrence of pain that is elicited by stimuli that are normally below the pain threshold. Some authors include the lowering of the threshold in the term *hyperalgesia* in non-neuropathic pain.[2,3]

Whereas nociceptive pain is elicited by noxious stimulation of sensory endings of nociceptors in the tissue, *neuropathic pain* results from injury or disease of neurons in the peripheral or the central nervous system. This pain does not primarily signal tissue damage and is often considered abnormal. It often has a burning or electrical character and can be persistent or occur in short episodes (e.g., trigeminal neuralgia). It may be combined with hyperalgesia and allodynia. In the allodynic state, even touching the skin with a soft brush can cause intense pain. Numerous pathologic processes can cause neuropathic pain (e.g., axotomy, nerve or plexus damage, metabolic diseases such as diabetes mellitus, or herpes zoster). Damage to central pain processing neurons (e.g., in the thalamus) can cause central pain.[2,3]

Chronic pain

Originally pain was called "chronic" when it lasted longer than 6 months.[4] More recently, chronic pain is often defined by its character. Chronic pain may result from a chronic disease and may then actually result from persistent nociceptive processes. However, in many chronic pain states the causal relationship between nociception and pain is not tight and the pain does not strictly reflect tissue damage. Psychological and social factors significantly influence the pain (e.g., in many cases of low back pain).[5] Chronic pain may be accompanied by neuroendocrine dysregulation, fatigue, dysphoria, and impaired physical and even mental performance.[6]

THE PERIPHERAL BASIS OF PAIN

Structure and dual function of nociceptors

Nociceptors are primary afferent neurons with thinly myelinated Aδ or unmyelinated C fiber axons in peripheral nerves. Their cell bodies are located in the dorsal root ganglia. Their peripheral branches form sensory endings in the innervated tissue that are called "free nerve endings" because they are not equipped with corpuscular end organs. Their central branches terminate in the gray matter of the dorsal horn in the spinal cord or in the brain stem, and they activate synaptically secondary dorsal horn neurons (see Fig. 22.1).[7]

Many nociceptors have a dual function. They encode noxious stimuli and transmit this information to the spinal cord (sensory function), and, in addition, they have an efferent function in the innervated tissue. They transport neuropeptides from the cell body to the periphery and release these mediators in the tissue on stimulation. Substance P, calcitonin gene-related peptide (CGRP), and some others are best known. After release, these neuropeptides induce vasodilatation, plasma extravasation, and other effects (e.g., attraction of macrophages or degranulation of mast cells). Such an inflammatory response is called neurogenic inflammation, and it is thought that neurogenic components contribute significantly to many inflammatory diseases.[8]

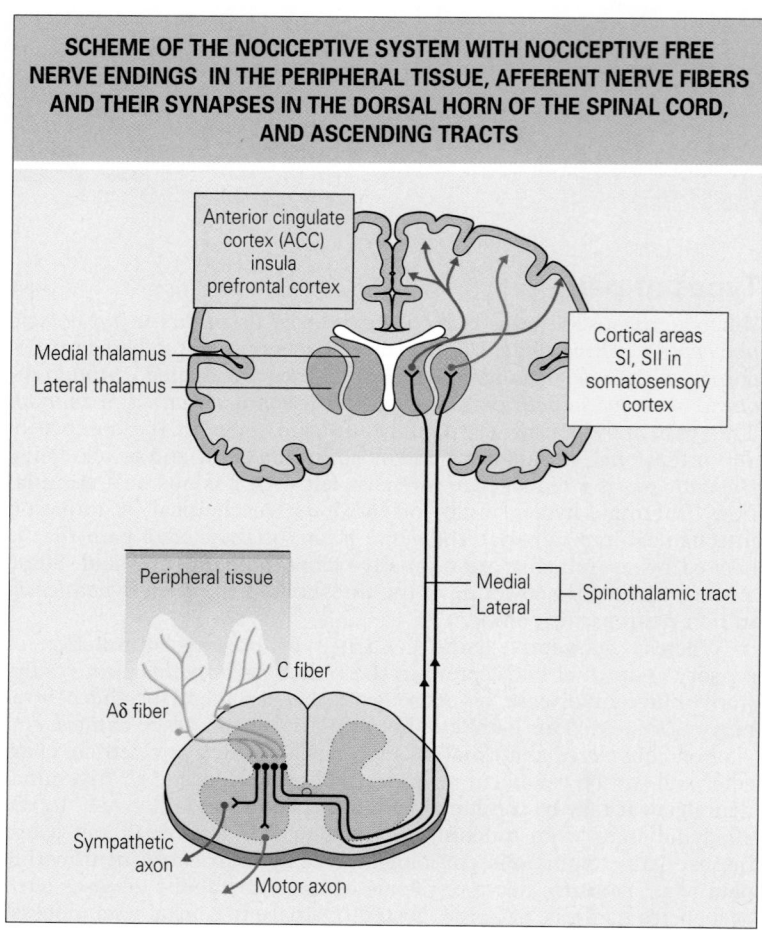

SCHEME OF THE NOCICEPTIVE SYSTEM WITH NOCICEPTIVE FREE NERVE ENDINGS IN THE PERIPHERAL TISSUE, AFFERENT NERVE FIBERS AND THEIR SYNAPSES IN THE DORSAL HORN OF THE SPINAL CORD, AND ASCENDING TRACTS

Fig. 22.1 Scheme of the nociceptive system with nociceptive free nerve endings in the peripheral tissue, afferent nerve fibers, and their synapses in the dorsal horn of the spinal cord. From there the medial and lateral spinothalamic tracts ascend to the medial and lateral thalamus, and interneurons project into motor and sympathetic reflex pathways. Note: other ascending pathways such as the spinoreticular tract and dorsal column pathways are not displayed.

Sensory function of nociceptors

Most nociceptors are *polymodal*, responding to noxious mechanical stimuli (painful pressure, squeezing or cutting the tissue), noxious thermal stimuli (heat or cold), and chemical stimuli. Noxious stimuli evoke a sensor potential in the sensory ending (transduction), and when the amplitude of this depolarization is sufficiently high, action potentials are triggered and conducted by the axon to the dorsal horn of the spinal cord or the brain stem (Fig. 22.2).[7]

In joints, nociceptors innervate mainly the fibrous capsule, ligaments, adipose tissue, and the menisci, and the synovial layer shows some fibers. The cartilage is normally not innervated. A typical joint nociceptor is activated by strong (painful) pressure to the joint (e.g., hitting the joint) and by noxious movements (i.e., by painful rotation against the resistance of the tissue). It is usually not activated by movements and positions in the working range.[9] Nociceptors in the muscle are located near vessels in the muscle belly and in the tendon. A typical muscle nociceptor responds to noxious (painful) compression of the muscle, and it may be activated by muscle contraction under ischemic conditions. Usually it does not respond to innocuous pressure and to contractions of the muscle.[9] When nociceptive fibers in the muscle nerve are stimulated electrically, cramp-like sensations are evoked. Some nociceptive muscle afferents are also activated by noxious thermal stimuli. However, heat responses have been much better studied in cutaneous nociceptors because the skin is more likely exposed to heat than deep tissue. In cutaneous nociceptors, heat responses are encoded in the range of about 42°C to more than 50°C. Cutaneous nociceptors also encode noxious mechanical stimuli.[7] In the viscera, principles of nociception differ to some extent from those in skin and deep somatic tissue. Nociception is less represented by specific nociceptors than in skin and deep somatic tissue.[7]

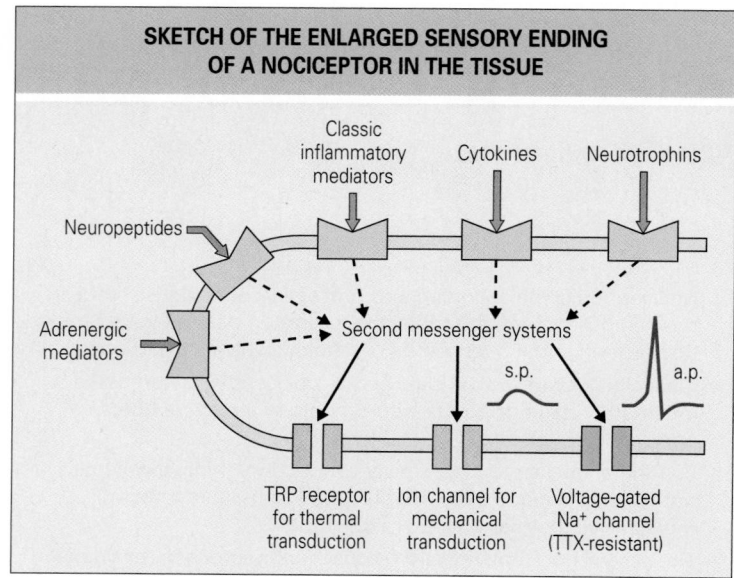

SKETCH OF THE ENLARGED SENSORY ENDING OF A NOCICEPTOR IN THE TISSUE

Fig. 22.2 Sketch of the enlarged sensory ending of a nociceptor in the tissue. It shows ion channels for transduction of thermal and mechanical stimuli and metabotropic receptors for chemical mediators. TRP, transient receptor protein; s.p., sensory potential; a.p., action potential. Classic mediators are bradykinin, prostaglandin E₂, and others.

Notably, not all nociceptors in skin, deep somatic tissue, and viscera are polymodal. An important group of nociceptors is relatively mechanoinsensitive and, in the skin, heat insensitive. Because these nociceptors do not respond to noxious stimuli applied to normal tissue, they were called initially *mechanoinsensitive* or *silent* nociceptors.[3,9] These nociceptors are "recruited" during inflammation (see later).

Sensitization of nociceptors during inflammation

Nociceptors often show a sensitization on repetitive or strong noxious stimulation of the tissue. In the course of inflammation the excitation threshold of polymodal nociceptors drops such that even light, normally innocuous stimuli activate the fibers. In addition, initially mechanoinsensitive (silent) nociceptors are sensitized and become excitable by innocuous and noxious stimuli.[3,9] The sensitization of nociceptors ("peripheral sensitization") causes an enhanced input into the spinal cord and induces a so-called central sensitization (Fig. 22.3). Both peripheral and central sensitization cause a *primary hyperalgesia* and *allodynia* at the site of inflammation, that is, normally non-painful stimuli hurt at this site and noxious stimuli evoke stronger responses than in the non-sensitized state. In addition, central sensitization causes a *secondary hyperalgesia*, that is, enhanced pain sensitivity in healthy tissue surrounding the site of inflammation (see later).

Molecular mechanisms of stimulus transduction and peripheral sensitization

In the past years substantial progress has been made toward the understanding of sensory transduction in nociceptors. Mechanical, thermal, and chemical stimuli activate specific ion channels or receptors in the sensory endings (see Fig. 22-2).

Mechanoreception is thought to result from an opening of cation channels leading to a depolarization of the ending because certain ion channels are sensitive to stretch, membrane deformation, and osmotic swelling. However, it is still unclear which molecules are specifically involved in the transduction of noxious mechanical stimuli.[10,11]

Thermal noxious stimuli are thought to be transduced by transient receptor protein (TRP) molecules. The first receptor that has been cloned is the TRPV1 receptor, previously also called vanilloid receptor (VR)-1. This ion channel is expressed in about 40% of the primary afferent fibers. It is opened by the binding of capsaicin, the compound in pepper that causes burning pain. When this ion channel opens,

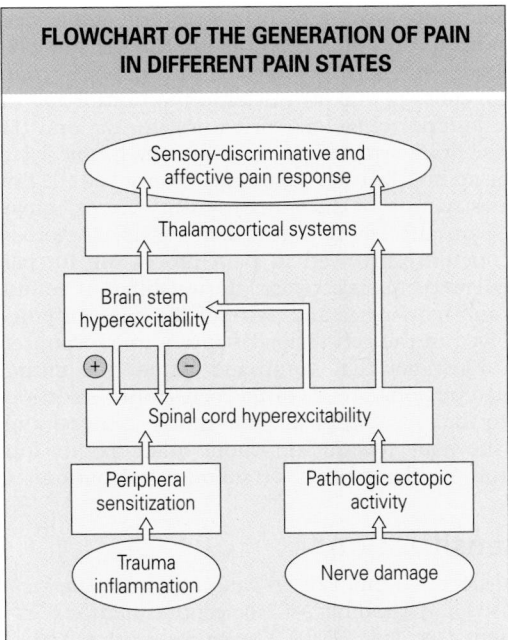

FLOWCHART OF THE GENERATION OF PAIN IN DIFFERENT PAIN STATES

Fig. 22.3 Flowchart of the generation of pain in different pain states. Central sensitization can result both from peripheral sensitization and from pathologic discharges in the afferent nerve fiber. The brain stem provides a feedback to the spinal cord that is either inhibitory or facilitatory.

BOX 22.1 RECEPTORS IN SUBGROUPS OF SENSORY NEURONS

Ionotropic receptors for
■ ATP, H$^+$ (acid-sensitive ion channels [ASICs]), glutamate (AMPA, kainate, NMDA receptors), acetylcholine (nicotinic receptors), serotonin (5-HT$_3$)

Metabotropic receptors for
■ Acetylcholine, epinephrine, serotonin, dopamine, glutamate, γ-aminobenzoic acid, adenosine triphosphate
■ Prostanoids (prostaglandins E$_2$ and I$_2$), bradykinin, histamine, adenosine, endothelin
■ Neuropeptides (e.g., substance P, calcitonin gene-related peptide, somatostatin, opioids)
■ Proteases (protease-activated receptors: PAR1 and PAR2)
■ Neurotrophins (tyrosine kinase receptors)
■ Glial cell line–derived neurotrophic factor (GDNF)
■ Inflammatory cytokines (non–tyrosine kinase receptors)

Data from references 10 and 11.

---

cations, in particular calcium ions, flow into the cell and depolarize it. This ion channel is considered to be one of the transducers of noxious heat because it is also opened by heat at more than 43°C. The sensitivity of TRPV1 receptors is increased (i.e., the threshold is lowered) by numerous inflammatory mediators such as bradykinin and nerve growth factor, suggesting that this molecule is one "final pathway" in heat nociception and thermal hyperalgesia. Indeed, TRPV1 knockout mice do not show thermal hyperalgesia during inflammation.[10,11]

Other members of the TRP family may be transducers of temperature stimuli in nociceptors and thermal receptors. The TRPV2 receptor is thought to be a transducer for extreme heat (threshold > 52°C) that is also present in nociceptors. The TRPA1 receptor is activated by noxious cold. This molecule is often co-expressed with the TRPV1 receptors in nociceptors and may be the basis for cold pain. In contrast, TRPV3 and/or TRPV4 may be transduction molecules for innocuous warmth in warm receptors, and TRPM8 may transduce cold stimuli in innocuous cold receptors.[10]

The *chemosensitivity* of nociceptors allows inflammatory and trophic mediators to act on these neurons. The field of chemosensitivity is extremely complicated owing to the large numbers of receptors that have been identified in primary afferent neurons.[10,11] Receptors that are involved in the activation and sensitization of neurons are either ionotropic (the mediator opens an ion channel) or metabotropic (the mediator activates a second messenger cascade that influences ion channels and other cell functions). Many receptors are coupled to G proteins, which signal via the production of the second messengers cyclic adenosine monophosphate, cyclic guanosine monophosphate, diacylglycerol, and phospholipase C. Other receptor subgroups include receptors bearing intrinsic protein tyrosine kinase domains and receptors that associate with cytosolic tyrosine kinases and protein serine/threonine kinases.[10] Figure 22.2 displays receptors for classes of mediators, and Box 22.1 shows which particular mediator receptors are expressed in subgroups of sensory neurons.[10,11]

Functions of mediators are severalfold. Some of them activate neurons directly (e.g., the application of bradykinin evokes action potentials by itself) and/or they sensitize neurons for mechanical, thermal, and chemical stimuli (e.g., bradykinin and prostaglandins increase the excitability of neurons so that mechanical stimuli evoke more action potentials than under control conditions). For example, prostaglandin E$_2$ activates G protein–coupled receptors that cause an increase of cellular cyclic adenosine monophosphate. This second messenger activates protein kinase A, and this pathway influences ion channels in the membrane, leading to an enhanced excitability of the neuron with lowered threshold and increased action potential frequency elicited during suprathreshold stimulation.[2] More recently, proinflammatory cytokines such as tumor necrosis factor-α and interleukin-6 were shown to exert excitatory and/or sensitizing effects on nerve cells. Other compounds inhibit neurons (e.g., somatostatin, opioids).[2] Possibly the threshold of a neuron results at least partially from the balance between excitatory and inhibitory mediators in the tissue.

Other functions include stimulation of the production of mediators in sensory neurons. For example, nerve growth factor, which is a survival factor during the development of the nervous system, is produced during inflammation of the tissue, and it increases the synthesis of substance P and CGRP in the primary afferents through activation of TrkA receptors. Nerve growth factor may also act on mast cells and thereby activate and sensitize sensory endings by mast cell degranulation.[11] Indeed, many compounds have acute actions on cell excitability as well as more tonic regulatory functions. The expression of mediator substances, ion channels, and receptors is not totally stable but undergoes changes under pathophysiologic conditons.[10] It is conceivable that changes in the expression of ion channels and receptors may contribute to the maintenance of chronic pain.

Although mechanosensitive and thermosensitive ion channels are important in the process of sensory transduction (see earlier), voltage-gated ion channels in the sensory endings are important for the generation and conduction of action potentials in nerve fibers on depolarization. In the focus of interest are voltage-gated Na$^+$ channels (see Fig. 22-2).[12] Although most voltage-gated Na$^+$ channels are blocked by tetrodotoxin (TTX), many small dorsal root ganglion cells (most of which are nociceptors) express TTX-resistant Na$^+$ channels in addition to TTX-sensitive Na$^+$ channels. Both TTX-sensitive and TTX-resistant Na$^+$ channels contribute to the Na$^+$ influx during the action potential. Currently, the TTX-sensitive Na$^+$ channel subtype Na$_v$1.7 and the TTX-resistant Na$^+$ channel subtypes Na$_v$1.8 and Na$_v$1.9 are considered most important for nociception. The TTX-resistant Na$^+$ currents are influenced by some inflammatory mediators. For example, prostaglandin E$_2$ enhances TTX-resistant Na$^+$ currents, and this is thought to contribute to the sensitizing effect of this mediator.

Peripheral mechanisms of neuropathic pain

In some patients pain may also be caused by neuropathic mechanisms (see earlier), for example when an intervertebral disc causes compression of dorsal roots. Although in healthy sensory nerve fibers action potentials are generated in the sensory endings on stimulation of the receptive field, impaired nerve fibers often show pathologic ectopic discharges. These action potentials are generated at the site of nerve injury or in the cell body of impaired fibers in dorsal root ganglia. The discharge patterns vary from rhythmic firing to intermittent bursts.[3] Neuropathic pain may also be generated by intact nerve fibers in the vicinity of injured nerve fibers that are affected by the process of wallerian degeneration.[2,3] Pathologic discharges may also cause a state of central sensitization (see Fig. 22.3).

Different mechanisms are thought to produce ectopic discharges. First, they may be facilitated by changes in the expression of ion channels. After nerve injury, the expression of TTX-sensitive Na$^+$ channels is increased and the expression of TTX-insensitive Na$^+$ channels is decreased. These changes are thought to alter the membrane properties of the neuron such that rapid firing rates (bursting ectopic discharges) are favored.[2] Changes in the expression of K$^+$ channels of the neurons have also been shown.[2] Second, injured axons of primary afferent neurons may be excited by inflammatory mediators (e.g., by bradykinin, nitrous oxide, and cytokines).[11] The source of these inflammatory mediators may be white blood cells and Schwann cells around the damaged nerve fibers. Third, injured nerve fibers may be affected by the sympathetic nervous system. The sympathetic nervous system does not activate primary afferents in normal tissue. Injured nerve fibers, however, may become sensitive to adrenergic mediators because adrenergic receptors are upregulated at the sensory nerve fiber ending. A direct connection between afferent and efferent fibers (so-called ephapses) is considered. Furthermore, sympathetic nerve fibers may sprout in the dorsal root ganglion after nerve injury.[2,3] Currently, the best treatment for peripheral neuropathic pain is the application of drugs that reduce excitability of neurons (e.g., carbamazepine or gabapentin).

THE CENTRAL BASIS OF PAIN

Nociceptive spinal cord neurons

Nociceptors activate synaptically nociceptive dorsal horn neurons (see Fig. 22-1). The latter are either tract neurons that ascend to supraspinal sites or local interneurons that are part of segmental motor or vegetative reflex pathways. As pointed out, a noxious stimulus to normal tissue causes a withdrawal reflex that removes the threatened part of the body from the damaging source. Under inflammatory conditions the inflamed tissue is kept in a position that activates nociceptors as little as possible. Long axons of spinal nociceptive neurons ascend in the spinothalamic and the spinoreticular tract. Interestingly, nociceptive information from the viscera seems to be conducted to supraspinal sites mainly in the dorsal column pathway.[7]

Typically, nociceptive spinal cord neurons receive convergent inputs from numerous primary afferent fibers. Whereas part of the dorsal horn neurons are only activated from the skin, others are only activated from deep tissue (i.e., muscles, tendons, and joints). A large proportion of dorsal horn neurons receives input from both skin and deep tissue, and others are excited by cutaneous, deep tissue, and visceral stimulation. The enormous convergence of afferent fibers onto spinal cord neurons has functional consequences. In many cases the pain is badly localized (in particular in the deep somatic tissue) and may be even projected to the skin. In particular, noxious stimulation of the viscera leads to a projection of pain into skin and deep tissue that are supplied by nociceptors of the same segment.[7,9]

The spinal cord is under the influence of descending tracts that reduce or facilitate the spinal nociceptive processing. Descending influences are formed by pathways that originate from brain stem nuclei (in particular the periaqueductal gray matter and nucleus raphe magnus) and descend in the dorsolateral funiculus of the spinal cord.[1,7]

Generation of the conscious pain response in the thalamocortical system

The conscious pain response is produced by the thalamocortical system (see Fig. 22-1). Electrophysiologic data and brain imaging in humans have provided insights into which parts of the brain are activated on noxious stimulation. As pointed out earlier, pain is an unpleasant sensory and emotional experience and these different components of the pain response are produced by different networks. The analysis of the noxious stimulus for its location, duration, and intensity is the *sensory-discriminative aspect* of pain. This is produced in the *lateral thalamocortical system*, which consists of relay nuclei in the lateral thalamus and the areas SI and SII in the postcentral gyrus. In these regions innocuous and noxious stimuli are discriminated.[13]

The second component of the pain sensation is the *affective aspect;* that is, the noxious stimulus is felt as unpleasant and causes aversive reactions. This component is produced in the *medial thalamocortical system*, which consists of relay nuclei in the central and medial thalamus and the anterior cingulate cortex, the insula, and the prefrontal cortex.[13] These brain structures are part of the limbic system, and the insula may be an interface of the somatosensory and the limbic system. Even when destruction of the somatosensory cortex impairs stimulus localization, pain affect is not altered. It should be noted that limbic regions are not only involved in pain processing. In particular, the anterior cingulate cortex is activated during different emotions, including sadness and happiness, and parts of the anterior cingulate cortex are also involved in the generation of autonomic responses (they have projections to regions that command autonomic output systems). Other cingulate regions are involved in response selection (they have projections to the spinal cord and the motor cortices) and in the orientation of the body toward innocuous and noxious somatosensory stimuli. A role in the process of memory formation/access is also discussed.[14]

Central sensitization

Pathologic nociceptive input often causes *central sensitization*, which is an increase of excitability of nociceptive neurons in the central nervous system (see Fig. 22.3). The process of central sensitization amplifies the synaptic processing of nociceptive inputs and thus facilitates the pain response. Central sensitization has been mainly studied in the spinal cord. The focus here is on *spinal sensitization*, that is, the development and maintenance of hyperexcitability in nociceptive spinal cord neurons. Spinal sensitization leads to increased responses of the neurons to input from the injured or inflamed region as well as to input from regions adjacent to and even remote from the injured/inflamed region, although these areas are in a healthy condition. Often, the total area from which the neuron is activated is enlarged. Another consequence of spinal sensitization is that in the spinal segments with input from the injured regions a higher proportion of neurons respond to stimulation of peripheral tissue.[7,9] Central sensitization is thought to contribute to secondary hyperalgesia, that is, hyperalgesia in healthy tissue surrounding the inflamed area.

In many cases, central sensitization persists as long as the nociceptive input persists and it disappears when the peripheral input is reduced. In other cases, however, central sensitization may outlast the peripheral nociceptive process. Possibly nociceptive inputs have triggered a so-called long-term potentiation, a persistent increase of synaptic efficacy.[15] Such a process could account for pain states that persist even when the peripheral nociceptive process has disappeared.

It is thought that inflammation-evoked sensitization results mainly from an increase of excitatory mechanisms. The intraspinal release of excitatory transmitters and neuropeptides such as substance P and CGRP from sensitized primary afferents is increased (a presynaptic component of spinal sensitization), and excitatory postsynaptic mechanisms are facilitated (see later). In the case of neuropathic pain, it is being discussed whether an important mechanism of spinal sensitization is the loss of segmental inhibition. This is normally provided by γ-aminobutyric acid (GABA)-ergic interneurons.[16,17]

Spinal sensitization is influenced by neuronal systems descending from the brain stem (see Fig. 22.3). Experimental evidence suggests that descending inhibition of neurons with input from inflamed areas is increased, at least in the acute stage of inflammation, keeping spinal sensitization under control. However, secondary hyperalgesia (hyperalgesia outside the inflamed area) may be due to descending facilitation of spinal cord activity. In the case of neuropathic pain, mainly descending facilitation has been observed. Both possibilities are indicated in the flowchart in Figure 22.3. In all, spinal/supraspinal/spinal loops are quite important in the generation of pathologic pain.[18]

Transmitters in the Spinal Cord and Molecular Mechanisms of Spinal Sensitization

Different transmitters and mediators are involved in the induction and maintenance of central sensitization.[19] Glutamate is the main transmitter in nociceptors. It activates ionotropic *N*-methyl-D-aspartate (NMDA) and non-NMDA receptors and metabotropic glutamate receptors in spinal cord neurons.[20] During noxious stimulation both non-NMDA and NMDA receptors are activated. It has been particularly shown that administration of antagonists to the NMDA receptor prevents central sensitization and reduces established hyperexcitability.[9,20] The use of NMDA antagonists in non-operative pain treatment is hampered by side effects such as psychosis because NMDA receptors are expressed throughout the brain.

Neuropeptides and spinal prostaglandins are also involved in the process of central sensitization. Many neurons in the spinal cord express receptors for substance P and CGRP.[7,19] During peripheral inflammation the spinal release of substance P and CGRP from nociceptors is increased and these neuropeptides further the generation of spinal cord hyperexcitability, probably by a facilitation of glutamatergic synaptic transmission.[7,9]

During inflammation in the periphery, prostaglandin E_2 is released in the spinal cord. Topical application of prostaglandin E_2 to the spinal cord causes nociceptive reactions in awake animals.[21] Electrophysiologic recordings showed that topical application of prostaglandin E_2 to the spinal cord causes a central sensitization similar to peripheral inflammation and that application of the prostaglandin synthesis inhibitor indomethacin to the spinal cord before induction of inflammation attenuates the development of spinal hyperexcitability.[22]

Recently it has been revealed that glial cells in the spinal cord contribute significantly to the generation of pain states.[11,23] On stimulation, neuroglia secrete a number of mediators such as nitrous oxide,

neurotrophins, and interleukin-1β.[11] Thus, inflammation or nerve injury in the periphery causes a complex scenario of neuronal events in the spinal cord that ultimately determines central sensitization. Importantly, however, inhibitory transmitters and receptors, such as opioids and opioid receptors, are able to reduce spinal sensitization, by reduction of transmitter release and of the depolarization of postsynaptic neurons.

CONCLUSION

Pain is an important component of suffering from disease, and, therefore, pain treatment is an absolute necessity in clinical medicine. Pain research has revealed multiple mechanisms in the peripheral and central nervous systems that contribute to the generation and maintenance of pain, and there is a continuous challenge to identify new key targets for new therapies.[24] In a wider sense, pain has also been considered an important element of the so-called illness response. It has been suggested that not only are many symptoms of diseases the result of local disease processes but also that the nervous system contributes to the expression of symptoms by responding to challenges such as inflammation, infection, and injury in a coordinated fashion. In fact, there is plenty of evidence for autonomic/endocrine/immune interactions that are related to acute and chronic pain.[25] In this respect, pain therapy may not only just attack a clinical symptom but also modify the further course of disease.

REFERENCES

1. Basbaum AI, Jessell TM. The perception of pain. In: Kandel ER, Schwartz JH, Jessell TM, eds. Principles of neural science, 4th ed. New York: McGraw-Hill, 1999:472-491.
2. Schaible H-G, Richter F. Pathophysiology of pain. Langenbecks Arch Surg 2004;389:237-243.
3. Campbell JN, Meyer RA. Neuropathic pain: from the nociceptor to the patient. In: Merskey H, Loeser JD, Dubner R, eds. The paths of pain 1975-2005. Seattle: IASP Press, 2005:229-242.
4. Russo CM, Brose WG. Chronic pain. Annu Rev Med 1998;49:123-133.
5. Kendall NA. Psychological approaches to the prevention of chronic pain: the low back paradigm. Baillieres Best Pract Res Clin Rheumatol 1999;13:545-554.
6. Chapman CR, Gavrin J. Suffering: the contributions of persistent pain. Lancet 1999;353:2233-2237.
7. Willis WD, Coggeshall RE. Sensory mechanisms of the spinal cord, 3rd ed. New York: Kluwer Academic/Plenum Publishers, 2004.
8. Schaible H-G, Del Rosso A, Matucci-Cerinic M. Neurogenic aspects of inflammation. Rheum Dis Clin North Am 2005;31:77-101.
9. Schaible H-G. Basic mechanisms of deep somatic tissue. In: McMahon SB, Koltzenburg M, eds. Textbook of pain. London: Elsevier, 2006:621-633.

10. Gold MS. Molecular basis of receptors. In: Merskey H, Loeser JD, Dubner R, eds. The paths of pain 1975-2005. Seattle: IASP Press, 2005:49-67.
11. Marchand F, Perretti M, McMahon SB. Role of the immune system in chronic pain. Nature Rev Neurosci 2005;6:521-532.
12. McCleskey EW, Gold MS. Ion channels of nociception. Annu Rev Physiol 1999;61:835-856.
13. Treede RD, Kenshalo DR, Gracely RH, et al. The cortical representation of pain. Pain 1999;79:105-111.
14. Vogt BA. Pain and emotion: interactions in subregions of the cingulate gyrus. Nat Rev Neurosci 2005;6:533-544.
15. Sandkühler J. Learning and memory in pain pathways. Pain 2000;88:113-118.
16. Moore KA, Kohno T, Karchweski LA, et al. Partial peripheral nerve injury promotes a selective loss of GABAergic inhibition in the superficial dorsal horn of the spinal cord. J Neurosci 2002;22:6724-6731.
17. Polgár E, Gray S, Riddell JS, et al. Lack of evidence for significant neuronal loss in laminae I-II of the spinal dorsal horn in the rat in the chronic constriction injury model. Pain 2004;111:144-149.
18. Vanegas H, Schaible H-G. Descending control of persistent pain: inhibitory or facilitatory? Brain Res Rev 2004;46:295-309.

19. Millan MJ. The induction of pain: an integrative review. Progr Neurobiol 1999;57:1-164.
20. Fundytus ME. Glutamate receptors and nociception. CNS Drugs 2001;15:29-58.
21. Vanegas H, Schaible H-G. Prostaglandins and cyclooxygenases in the spinal cord. Progr Neurobiol 2001;64:327-363.
22. Vasquez E, Bär KJ, Ebersberger A, et al. Spinal prostaglandins are involved in the development but not the maintenance of inflammation-induced spinal hyperexcitability. J Neurosci 2001;21:9001-9008.
23. Watkins LR, Maier SF. Glia and pain: past, present, and future. In: Merskey H, Loeser JD, Dubner R, eds. The paths of pain 1975-2005. Seattle: IASP Press, 2005:165-175.
24. Basbaum AI. The future therapy of pain therapy: something old, something new, something borrowed, and something blue. In: Merskey H, Loeser JD, Dubner R, eds. The paths of pain 1975-2005. Seattle: IASP Press, 2005:513-532.
25. Jänig W, Levine JD. Autonomic-endocrine-immune interactions in acute and chronic pain. In: McMahon SB, Koltzenburg M, eds. Textbook of pain. London: Elsevier, 2005:205-218.

Pharmacogenomics in rheumatology

Jeffrey D. Greenberg and Bruce N. Cronstein

23

- Pharmacogenomics is the application of genomics to the optimization of drug design and selection and course of therapy based on individual patients' genetic profiles, whereas pharmacogenetics refers specifically to the elucidation of the roles of individual genetic variations in determining drug response.

- Single nucleotide polymorphisms (SNPs) are single nucleotide variations in the DNA sequence occurring in at least 1% of the population and present in the human genome at a density of one per thousand base-pairs or greater. SNPs may be tested individually for direct association with a phenotype or used as part of a set of markers to identify genomic regions associated with a phenotype and are thus a powerful tool in the field of pharmacogenetics.

- Association studies are population-based studies that test for statistically significant relationships between particular genotypes and phenotypes. Association studies have been widely utilized in efforts to identify putative genetic risk factors for poor or toxic response to commonly administered therapies for rheumatologic diseases.

- The impact of pharmacogenetics on clinical medicine is likely to be substantially enhanced in the near future by the convergence of the availability of larger, better characterized patient populations, continued improvements in the speed and cost-effectiveness of high-throughput genotyping technologies, optimization of marker selection for more complete and efficient coverage of the genome, and an improved understanding of both target disease etiologies and the mechanisms of action of drugs.

PHARMACOGENOMICS

Much attention has recently been given to the role of genetic background in determining patient response to drug therapy. The rapidly growing field of pharmacogenomics focuses on the application of genomics to the optimization of drug design and selection and course of therapy based on individual patients' genetic profiles. Pharmacogenetics, a branch of pharmacogenomics, refers specifically to the elucidation of the roles of individual genetic variations in determining drug response. Although the long-term impact of these fields on clinical medicine is uncertain,[1-4] the principle of particular allelic variants affecting the incidence of poor efficacy and/or adverse response to drug therapy has been established for decades.[5-8] In this chapter we provide a brief introduction to pharmacogenetics with a focus on practical considerations for the researcher in the design and interpretation of pharmacogenetic studies as well as review the current literature on pharmacogenetics research relevant to rheumatology.

In recent years, the availability of detailed sequence data in the wake of the Human Genome Project and the rapid evolution of high-throughput genotyping systems have provided tools that substantially enhance the capabilities of researchers in performing genomics research. Of particular utility toward identifying genetic markers for directing therapy has been a rapidly increasing number of single nucleotide polymorphisms (SNPs) identified throughout the genome at a reported frequency of roughly one per every thousand base-pairs of DNA or higher. Such information is of value for biomedical research on a number of levels. First, the identification of an SNP within a gene of known relevance to a phenotype of interest provides the basis for asking whether an allele of that SNP is associated with the phenotype. This could occur directly, such as through the alteration of a gene's regulatory properties (e.g., promoter region, splice site, mRNA stability) or

by encoding an amino acid change affecting the structure and/or function of the protein. Alternatively, a phenotypic association with an SNP allele could result if the allele is in linkage disequilibrium with (i.e., segregates with) an allele of a second SNP or other genetic variation that confers such an effect. Thus, a single SNP may by itself provide a sufficient basis for uncovering a genotype/phenotype association.

SNPs have also become increasingly useful as genetic markers for use in mapping and genome-wide association studies. In such cases, the SNP is not being utilized on an individual basis but rather as one of a set of SNPs distributed across the genome, such that alleles of particular SNPs within the set that associate with a phenotype of interest serve to identify the region and/or regions of the genome in which the gene or genes responsible for the phenotype lie. Within what gene, if any, an SNP is located is not of direct importance when it is used for this purpose but rather the extent to which the SNP set adequately covers the genome. In general, the smaller the average distance between SNP markers across the set, the greater the likelihood that at least one marker will be in sufficient linkage disequilibrium with each contributing allele for the tract to be mapped. An important caveat to this rule is that varying degrees of linkage disequilibrium exist across the genome, which results in "blocks" of sequence and, with them, SNPs that segregate together. Such strings of contiguous SNP genotypes are referred to as haplotypes, and a large-scale effort has been completed that establishes a human genome "Hapmap" identifying the location and sizes of these blocks of sequence, potentially easing the performance of association studies by reducing the number of markers that need to be genotyped in order to cover the genome.[9-11] Still, SNP density remains a critical factor in determining the success of such mapping projects; and as the density of known SNPs across different populations continues to increase, so does researchers' ability to interrogate the genetic components of pharmacogenetic (and other) phenotypes.

Experimental approaches and considerations regarding study design and data interpretation

Drug response presents unique challenges as a phenotype (see later) and often limits the experimental approaches an investigator may apply to elucidating its genetic basis, but many of the design considerations critical for the success of genetic association studies in general apply to pharmacogenetic studies as well. Briefly, in both cases one must address issues such as the heritability of the phenotype (i.e., fraction of the response phenotype due to genetic rather than non-genetic factors), the size and make-up of the sample population, the choice of markers, the accuracy of genotyping methods used, the accuracy of phenotypic classifications, and the statistical methods applied for data analysis.[12,13] These and other factors impact the statistical power achieved in the analysis,[13] which is central to the success of any genetic association study.

The most common approach to testing for an SNP association with a drug response phenotype is through clinic-based association studies, in which one asks whether the allele frequency of an SNP of interest is significantly different in a group of patients exhibiting a particular response phenotype relative to a control group that does not or, conversely, whether those patients with a particular genotype for an SNP/SNPs have a significantly different incidence of a response phenotype relative to those without it. Such studies are most commonly performed retrospectively, such that chart records of patients given a drug are used to categorize them for a response phenotype, after which allele frequency data for SNPs of interest are determined and appropriate statistical analyses are performed to identify associations. This approach, while pragmatic with regard to time and expense, has a number of weaknesses based in part on the fact that because the objectives of the study were not known at the time of drug treatment, the amount and nature of information available on the patient chart are often lacking.

This issue may be partially resolved through the use of prospective studies, in which a cohort of patients is followed through a course of drug treatment with the particular goal of identifying pharmacogenetic associations, thus allowing for all pertinent information to be appropriately recorded. However, this approach is still vulnerable to flaws that can prevent associations from being identified or, conversely, allow false associations to be observed. For example, in many cases investigators choose to use a "candidate gene" strategy, in which only those genes for which they believe an allelic change would be likely to confer a response phenotype are included in the analysis. Although this approach has yielded useful data, it is inherently limited by the extent to which the complete set of genes involved in conferring the response phenotype is known and all relevant variants have been identified. This issue can be resolved to some degree by taking a whole genome approach, wherein allele frequencies of SNPs distributed throughout the genome are determined with the goal of identifying regions of the genome and, ultimately, particular loci associated with a phenotype in a blinded manner. This option, while clearly favorable with regard to objectivity, may not be available to individual laboratories that lack access to the high-throughput genotyping technology required to perform such a large number of genotype calls. Furthermore, a number of issues regarding the design, execution, and interpretation of such screens remain to be resolved.[14]

The design of association studies may also be flawed by the failure to consider all confounding factors—both genetic and non-genetic—that might influence response and therefore be critical parameters for which the patient populations should be stratified. Examples of such non-genetic factors might include additional drugs being administered, patient age, gender, alcohol/drug consumption, diet, and other such variables. The reliability of such data is often limited by the accuracy of patients' self-assessment, and thus these factors remain a potential source for variation even when appropriately considered.

Irrespective of the degree to which all potential confounding variables are known, the success of the study could still be limited by individual patients' failure to adhere to a prescribed course of treatment. And unlike disease phenotypes, for which specific, objective assessment measures typically exist, drug response phenotypes are often far more qualitative, increasing the potential for inconsistency across clinics and/or individual physicians' standards. This issue is relevant to an additional weakness present in many pharmacogenetic studies, which is that certain drug response phenotypes—particularly adverse events—may occur with extremely low frequency, severely restricting the available sample sizes from individual clinics and thus the statistical power that may be reached. A potential solution may be to utilize data from multiple patient populations in a single analysis,[15] but this option is limited in its utility by the extent to which patient phenotyping standards are consistent across source clinics.

Thus, while the general principle involved in running clinic-based pharmacogenetic association studies is fairly straightforward, numerous potential sources of experimental error necessitate caution in interpreting the results. A substantial number of the associations identified to date have failed to be replicated, and much focus has been placed on addressing this issue.[16-18] For this reason, it is generally accepted that the confirmation of findings in at least one additional study population is necessary to validate the results. Ideally, pharmacogenetic studies are designed as substudies of randomized controlled trials. However, such studies rarely occur in rheumatology trials to date.

PHARMACOGENETICS IN RHEUMATOLOGY

Despite the limitations discussed earlier, pharmacogenetic research has long since begun to impact the field of rheumatology.[19-23] In the following section we review the current literature regarding the pharmacogenetic properties of drugs utilized for rheumatologic disease.

Glucocorticoids

Several studies have been carried out to assess the impact of glucocorticoid receptor (GR) gene variants on glucocorticoid response (Table

TABLE 23.1 REPORTED GENOTYPIC ASSOCIATIONS WITH RESPONSE TO GLUCOCORTICOIDS

Gene	Allele	Phenotype	Reference
Glucocorticoid receptor	22/23 EK	Resistance	Van Rossum[24]
	N363S	Hypersensitivity	Huizenga[27]
	Intron 2 (ex2 + 646bp) – G (*GAT haplotype inclusive of intron 2 SNP allele)	Hypersensitivity	Van Rossum[25]
			Stevens[28]
CRHR1	GAT haplotype	Improved lung function after therapy	Tantisira et al[30]
	rs242941		
	rs1876828		
T-bet transcription factor	rs2240017 G	Increased airway responsiveness after inhaled glucocorticoid therapy	Tantisira et al[31]

23.1). Van Rossum and colleagues have demonstrated that carriers of the glucocorticoid receptor 22/23 EK allele are more resistant to glucocorticoids as measured by dexamethasone suppression tests,[24,25] whereas variant alleles of an intronic polymorphism[26] and N363S[27] were associated with hypersensitivity. In addition, Stevens and associates identified an association between a 3-marker haplotype of hGR, which includes the aforementioned intronic polymorphism, and hypersensitivity to glucocorticoids.[28] Interestingly, an allele of exon 9b has been found to confer increased hGRb mRNA stability *in vitro* and was associated with rheumatoid arthritis,[29] although the effect of this polymorphism on glucocorticoid sensitivity remains uncertain.

Associations of glucocorticoid response with genes other than GR are less well established. Tantisira and coworkers reported that asthma patients who carried SNP alleles of the corticotrophin-releasing hormone receptor 1 (*CRHR1*) gene showed significantly improved lung function after 8 weeks of inhaled glucocorticoid therapy.[30] In a separate study, asthmatic children carrying a variant allele of transcription factor T-bet (T-box expressed in T cells), which has been associated with asthma pathogenesis, were reported to show increased improvement in airway responsiveness after inhaled glucocorticoid therapy relative to non-carriers over a 4-year test period.[31] In addition, two studies have investigated the potential role of polymorphisms in the vitamin D receptor gene (*VDR*), which is involved in intestinal calcium absorption, with glucocorticoid-induced decrease in bone mineral density (BMD) levels.[32,33] In both cases, however, no significant associations were found.

Non-steroidal anti-inflammatory drugs (NSAIDs)

A growing number of studies have examined the pharmacogenetic properties of members of the NSAID family. Genetic factors influencing response to aspirin, in particular, have been investigated by several groups. Perhaps most pertinent to its rheumatologic use is a single report by Halushka and associates identifying an association of cyclooxygenase (COX1) haplotype A842G/C50T with increased inhibition of prostaglandin H$_2$ (PgH$_2$) formation relative to homozygotes for the common allele.[34] The majority of aspirin pharmacogenetic studies, however, have focused on its antiplatelet properties.[34-36] Macchi and coworkers found that the phospholipase A (PLA) allele of platelet glycoprotein IIIa receptor was more common among patients resistant to than those sensitive to the antiplatelet action of aspirin.[37] Conversely, Undas and colleagues reported that the percentage of patients in whom average thrombin levels were decreased after aspirin treatment was higher among those not carrying the PLA2 allele than in those who were,[38] whereas in another study an association was reported of resistance to the reversal of arachidonic acid–induced platelet aggregation by aspirin in carriers of the PLA2 allele relative to those of the PLA1 allele.[39] Interestingly, Michaelson and colleagues found that PLA1/

SINGLE NUCLEOTIDE POLYMORPHISMS IDENTIFIED IN THE HUMAN *MTHFR* GENE

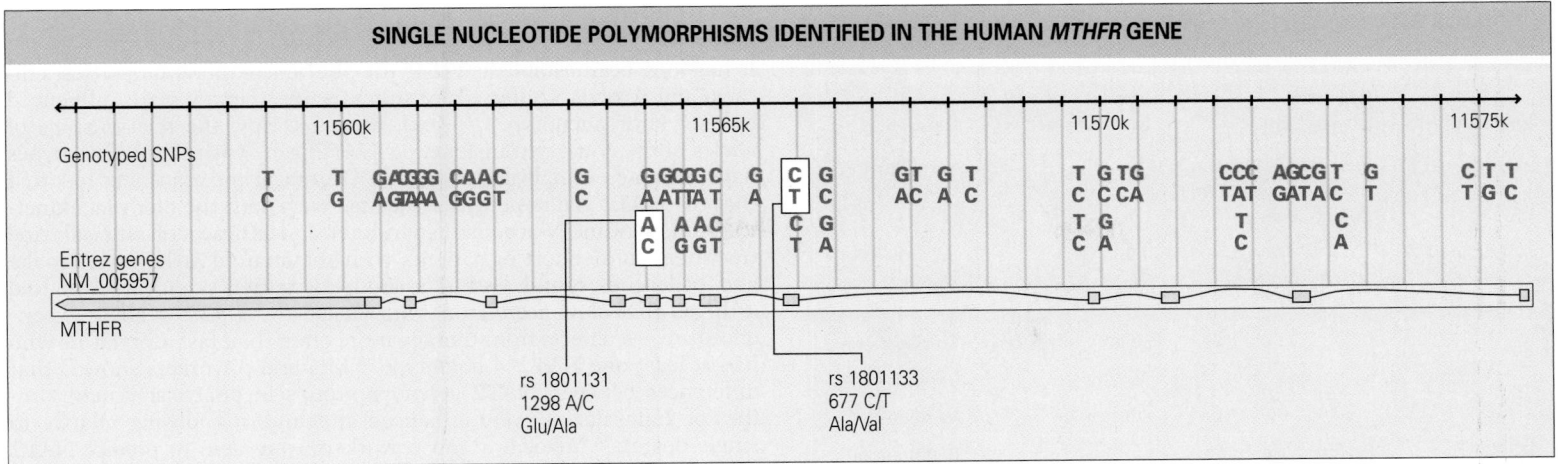

Fig. 23.1 Single nucleotide polymorphisms identified in the human *MTHFR* gene. The locations are indicative of C677T, which encodes an alanine to valine change, resulting in a thermolabile enzyme with reduced activity, and A1298C, which encodes a glutamine to alanine change and reduction in enzyme activity. *(From the International HapMap Consortium. The International HapMap Project. Nature 2003;426:789-796.)*

TABLE 23.2 REPORTED ASSOCIATIONS OF CYP2C8 AND CYP2C9 GENOTYPE WITH RESPONSE TO NSAIDS

Drug	Allele	Phenotype	Reference
Ibuprofen	CYP2C8*3	Low clearance rate	Garcia-Martin et al[41]
	CYP2C9*3		
Flurbiprofen	CYP2C9*3	Low clearance rate	Lee et al[42]
Naproxen	CYP2C9*3, CYP2C9*5	Decreased desmethylnaproxen formation	Tracy et al[44]
Celecoxib	CYP2C9*3	Low clearance rate	Kirchheiner et al[46]
Diclofenac	CYP2C9*3	Diclofenac/4'-OH ratio	Dorado et al[45]

PLA2 platelets showed greater sensitivity to aspirin than those of either homozygous genotype, whereas a similar association was reported by Andrioli and associates.[40] Although these data are together inconsistent and their implications for aspirin's anti-inflammatory efficacy are unclear, attention to future studies may be warranted.

The majority of pharmacogenetic data on other NSAIDs consist of associations of variants of the drug metabolism gene CYP2C8 and CYP2C9 (CYP-cytochrome P) with alterations in the pharmacokinetic profiles of those NSAIDs that are substrates (Table 23.2). Influence of the CYP2C8 and CYP2C9 genotype on the clearance/metabolism of ibuprofen,[41] flurbiprofen,[42] celecoxib,[43] naproxen,[44] and diclofenac[45] have all been reported, although contradictory data for diclofenac[46,47] and celecoxib[46] have arisen as well. Interestingly, Aithal and associates found no association between the CYP2C9 genotype and diclofenac-induced hepatotoxicity[48] but did report an association for this phenotype with alleles of cytokines interleukin-4 and interleukin-10.[49]

Disease-modifying antirheumatic drugs (DMARDs)

Methotrexate

Numerous studies have focused on the pharmacogenetics of low-dose methotrexate (MTX) in rheumatoid arthritis, particularly with regard to common single nucleotide polymorphisms in genes involved with folate metabolism. The data, however, have been somewhat inconsistent.

With regard to MTX-associated toxicity, Van Ede and coworkers reported that the CT and TT genotypes of the methylenetetrahydrofolate reductase (MTHFR) 677 locus were associated with an increased risk of discontinuing MTX treatment due to adverse events, the

majority of which were related to hepatotoxicity.[50] Similarly, Urano and associates found an increased rate of hepatotoxicity in patients carrying the 677T allele.[51] In contrast, Berkun and colleagues reported an association between the MTHFR 1298CC allele and a reduced likelihood of MTX-related side effects, while there was no association between the 677 genotype and toxicity[52] (Fig. 23.1). More recently, Hughes and associates observed an association of the 1298AA genotype with increased risk of toxicity among whites.[53] However, Wessels and colleagues examined the 1298A/C SNP and reported the 1298C allele was associated with toxicity in a cohort of 205 patients with rheumatoid arthritis.[54] Furthermore, Kumagai and colleagues found no association between either the 1298 or the 677 genotype and the likelihood of toxicity.[55] Interestingly, in the latter two studies a substantial portion of patients received folate supplementation and the majority of toxicities reported were non-hepatic, whereas in those patient cohorts for which associations were reported, few if any patients received folate supplementation and the majority of toxicities were hepatic. These observations could be consistent with the findings of Van Ede and associates, who reported that folate supplementation reduces the incidence of hepatic but not non-hepatic MTX-related adverse events[5,56] and may indicate that the pharmacogenetics of MTX-induced hepatic toxicity differ from that of other forms of toxicity. However, further studies will be required to identify and establish the roles of confounding factors influencing the response to MTX.

Associations with MTX efficacy have also been reported. Urano and associates found that among patients with rheumatoid arthritis receiving MTX therapy, those with the MTHFR 1298C allele and those with the 766C-1298C haplotype received lower doses than those without.[51] Kumagai and coworkers reported associations of homozygosity for two alleles of thymidylate synthase (TYMS) with higher MTX dosage and incidence of greater than or equal to 50% improvement in serum C-reactive protein level, respectively.[56] Dervieux and colleagues reported an association of increased "pharmacogenetic index" (a scored value based on genotypes for common alleles of RFC-1 (reduced folate carrier 1), ATIC (AICAR transformylase), and TYMS with the number of tender and swollen joints after MTX treatment in patients. Conversely, Van Ede and coworkers found no association of MTHFR 677 genotype with change in disease activity score (DAS) among MTX-treated patients with rheumatoid arthritis and neither Berkun and coworkers[52] nor Kumagai and colleagues[56] found associations between either MTHFR 677 or 1298 genotype and efficacy. Wessels and associates reported the 1298AA genotype was associated with improved efficacy of methotrexate.[54] Furthermore, a multi-gene pharmacogenetic model was developed by Wessels and coworkers, including genes of MTX metabolism and purine and pyrimidine synthesis.[57]

In the cases of both MTX efficacy and toxicity there has been an apparent lack of consistency in the identification of associations across studies, particularly with regard to *MTHFR* genotype (Table 23-3). To address these inconsistencies that may relate to cohort size and

TABLE 23.3 TESTS FOR ASSOCIATION OF MTHFR SNP ALLELES AND RESPONSE TO MTX

Polymorphism	Reported associations	Lack of associations	Reference
C677T	Increased risk of discontinuing MTX due to adverse events		Van Ede et al[49]
	Increased rate of toxicity		Urano[50]
		Efficacy or toxicity	Kumagai et al[52]
		Toxicity	Berkun et al[51]
		Efficacy	Van Ede[49]
A1298C	Reduced likelihood of MTX-related side effects		Berkun et al[51]
	Lower dose		Urano[50]
		Efficacy or toxicity	Kumagai[52]
		Disease activity	Berkun[51]
	Toxicity		Hughes[53]

MTX, methotrexate.

statistical power, Fisher and Cronstein conducted a meta-analysis of published studies on the *MTHFR* SNPs and risk of toxicity.[58] In the meta-analysis, the C677T SNP was associated with an increased risk of toxicity (odds ratio [OR] 1.71; 95% confidence interval [CI] 1.32-2.21). As discussed earlier, there are a number of factors that may contribute to variability, and in this instance relatively small patient populations and inconsistent phenotyping criteria may be at least partially responsible.

Gold

A number of investigators have reported evidence for HLA genotype influencing propensity toward adverse response to gold therapy. Singal and associates observed an association of HLA-DR3 genotype with gold-induced thrombocytopenia or proteinuria in a population of 520 RA patients,[59] whereas Clarkson and colleagues reported an association of complement C4 null allele but not HLA-DR3 or DR4 with renal or hematologic side effects to gold administration in a cohort of 81 RA patients.[60] Potential genetic risk factors for poor efficacy have not yet been established, but future studies may be aided by continued improvements in the understanding of gold mechanism of action.[61]

Azathioprine

There have been a number of studies on the pharmacogenetic properties of azathioprine, focusing primarily on the role of SNPs in the gene thiopurine methyltransferase (TPMT) in determining susceptibility to toxicity, and the literature in this area has been reviewed elsewhere.[62-65] Among those studies based on data from rheumatologic use, Black and associates reported that 5 of 6 individuals who incurred toxicity out of a cohort of 67 patients receiving azathioprine for rheumatologic disease were heterozygous for mutant TPMT alleles.[65] In another study, among a group of patients with rheumatoid arthritis receiving azathioprine, those experiencing adverse effects showed a significantly decreased level of TPMT activity relative to those who did not and 7 of 8 patients with "intermediate" TPMT activity developed toxicity.[66] In a recent study by Corominas and colleagues in which 40 patients with rheumatoid arthritis were treated with azathioprine, 3 of 6 who developed toxicity were TPMT3A carriers.[67] Similarly, Ishioka and associates reported that in a cohort of 36 patients receiving azathioprine therapy, 3 of 3 carriers for the mutant TPMT*3C allele discontinued treatment owing to leukopenia, relative to 4 of 33 non-carriers.[68] Combined with evidence from the many studies in patients with non-rheumatic diseases, these data strongly support the notion that the TPMT genotype is a useful predictor of azathioprine-associated toxicity.

Sulfasalazine

It has long been established that the pharmacokinetic properties, efficacy, and toxicity conferred by sulfasalazine therapy were influenced by acetylator phenotype,[69-75] and, more recently, the relationships of alleles of the *N*-acetyltransferase 2 (*NAT2*) gene with these phenotypes have been increasingly understood.[76-82] Kumagai and associates reported that the NAT2 genotype was associated with both the pharmacokinetics (sulfapyridine/*N*-acetylsulfapyridine) and efficacy of sulfasalazine treatment in a cohort of patients with rheumatoid arthritis.[77] Tanaka and colleagues found within a group of patients with rheumatoid arthritis that slow acetylators who lacked the NAT2*4 allele experienced adverse effects from therapy more often than fast acetylators who had at least one NAT2*4 haplotype.[80] Kita and coworkers showed that differences between NAT2 genotype groups in pharmacokinetic profiles of sulfasalazine were enhanced after multiple dosing relative to single dosing.[82] Yokogawa and coworkers were able to predict NAT2 genotype among five variants based on observed sulfapyridine metabolism profiles 4 days after onset of sulfasalazine administration.[76] Interestingly, Gunnarsson and associates reported that the NAT2 slow acetylator genotype is associated with propensity for induction of sulfasalazine-induced systemic lupus erythematosus.[83]

Cyclosporine

Bonhomme-Faivre and colleagues reported an association of the multidrug resistance protein 1 (MDR1) transporter C3435T polymorphism with concentration/dose ratio of cyclosporine 3 days after administration in 44 liver transplant patients.[84] In addition, a small study by Min and colleagues showed that mean area under the curve/unit dose (AUC/D) and apparent oral clearance (CL/F) were significantly associated with CYP3A4*1B genotype,[85] whereas in another, similar study, AUC and CL/F after cyclosporine administration were associated with CYP3A5*3C genotype.[86] However, Anglicheau and colleagues found no association of CYP3A5 genotype and cyclosporine pharmacokinetic parameters, although they did find a weak but significant association with the MDR-1 C1236T genotype.[87] The implications of these associations for cyclosporine pharmacokinetics and efficacy in rheumatoid arthritis are worthy of further investigation.

Biologic DMARDs

The vast majority of pharmacogenetic studies of biologic agents have focused on tumor necrosis factor (TNF) antagonists for the treatment of rheumatoid arthritis. Early studies reported associations in relatively small cohorts. Martinez and associates reported associations of the TNF-α a11, b4, and D65273.3 alleles as well as the Bat2_2/D6S273_4 haplotype with response to infliximab after 3 months of therapy in a cohort of 78 RA patients.[88] Mugnier and associates found that among a group of 59 patients with rheumatoid arthritis treated with infliximab, those with the TNF-α −308 G/G genotype showed better response than those with the A/A or A/G genotypes.[89] In a cohort of Crohn's disease patients, homozygosity for a haplotype in the TNF/lymphotoxin A (LTA) region was associated with non-response to infliximab,[90] whereas in a similar study the TNFRI minor allele was associated with lower response to infliximab.[91] In contrast, in a cohort of 226 Crohn's disease patients the TNFα −308 genotype was not associated with response to infliximab[92] and Mascheretti and associates reported that two alleles of TNFRII were associated with lack of response in one (n = 90) but not another (n = 444) cohort of patients with Crohn's disease.[93] In a study based on a population of 123 RA patients, the combination of −308 TNF1/TNF1 and −1087 G/G was associated with response to etanercept, whereas a combination of interleukin-1ra A2 and transforming growth factor-β1 915C alleles was associated with non-response.[94] More recently, larger patient population studies of TNF pharmacogenetics in patients with rheumatoid arthritis have been published. Criswell and colleagues reported that the combination of two HLA-DRB-1 shared-epitope alleles, as well as two extended haplotypes that included the HLA-DRB-1 shared-epitope alleles and six SNPs in the LTA-TNF region were associated with response to etanercept.[95] The significance of any of these findings remains unclear in light of the common clinical observation that individuals who do not respond to one anti-TNF biologic agent may respond to a different one. The largest cohort of TNF antagonist pharmacogenetics was reported by Maxwell and colleagues.[96] They examined 8 SNPs in the region containing the TNF gene among 1050 patients with rheumatoid arthritis, including 455 patients prescribed etanercept and 450 patients prescribed infliximab. An association between the TNF −308 genotype and change in DAS-28 was observed, indirectly validating the TNF −308 finding of other investigators.

Finally, whole genome scans have recently become feasible and have identified a number of novel genes for whom variants are associated with susceptibility to autoimmune diseases. This approach represents an "unbiased" approach that is not subject to publication bias that typically reflects publication of positive findings but not failed studies. A pilot whole genome scan study of TNF antagonist pharmacogenetics was published by Liu and associates on 89 patients and identified by a number of candidate SNPs that require validation in independent cohorts.[97]

CONCLUSION

The work discussed in this chapter provides strong support for the notion that the pharmacogenetic properties of antirheumatic drugs are likely to play an important role in the future of rheumatology. Because the majority of this work consists of studies focusing on single-allele associations, these data may, in fact, represent only the beginning of what such studies will ultimately yield. As is the case in complex disease genetics, it is likely that the genetic components of drug response will in many cases be found to be conferred by multiple genes and, therefore, that response phenotypes will be found to depend on genotypes of multiple alleles rather than just one. Among the challenges for researchers is the difficulty in obtaining patient cohorts of sufficient size that the number of patients in each genotypic category provides adequate statistical power for analysis, as well as the fact that when multiple alleles are conferring a trait, the relative contributions of each are likely to be smaller and therefore more difficult to detect. Resolving these issues will require the implementation of large-scale, prospective association studies; and as the technologies available for cost-effective, high-throughput genotyping, the speed with which new SNPs may be identified, and the knowledge base on how to correctly stratify the study populations for all relevant confounding factors continue to improve, it is likely that the frequency and success of such studies will increase.

Of additional interest in rheumatology is the potential use of pharmacogenetic data as a tool in the elucidation of the etiology of the target disease. As discussed earlier, identifying the appropriate stratification criteria to apply to the study population is a critical factor in an association study's success. Measurement of, and adjustment for, potential confounders is a particular challenge in the case of a disease such as rheumatoid arthritis, in which the etiology is incompletely understood and thus the array of genetic and non-genetic factors likely to influence the course and severity of disease is not entirely defined. In such cases, it is conceivable that response to a drug may be dictated in part by particular disease subphenotypes[98] or clinical presentations indicative of a state or, perhaps, subtype of the target disease in the individual patient. If, as a result, identifying a statistically significant association between a drug response phenotype and a genetic marker depends on the correct subset of patients being included in the study population, then the identification of the required patient stratification criteria combined with the elucidation of contributing alleles and knowledge of the mechanism of action of the drug could together serve to better characterize the target disease and distinguish any existing forms.

The value of pharmacogenetics research to the field of rheumatology, while promising so far, is likely to continue to grow as the tools and knowledge available to investigators continue to evolve. Whereas the genotyping and analysis tools as well as patient cohort data required for large-scale, genome-wide studies capable of teasing out alleles with increasingly small effect sizes continue to improve, so will investigators' understanding of the target diseases as well as the mechanisms of action of drug therapies and their toxicities. The convergence of these data is certain to enhance the power of pharmacogenetics research and thus the promise of rationally individualizing therapy using genetics in the future of clinical medicine.

ACKNOWLEDGMENTS

This work was supported by grants from the National Institutes of Health to Dr. Greenberg (K23 AR054412) and to Dr. Cronstein (GM56268, AR41911, AA13336), King Pharmaceuticals, the General Clinical Research Center (M01RR00096), and the Kaplan Cancer Center of New York University School of Medicine.

KEY REFERENCES

1. Amin AR. Potential impact of pharmacogenomics on the future of drug development and practice of rheumatology: a look from the trenches. Joint Bone Spine 2002;69:1-3.
3. Evans W, Relling M. Moving towards individualized medicine with pharmacogenomics. Nature 2004;429:464-468.
5. Johnson JA. Pharmacogenetics: potential for individualized drug therapy through genetics. Trends Genet 2003;19:660-666.
10. Deloukas P, Bentley D. The HapMap project and its application to genetic studies of drug response. Pharmacogenomics J 2004;4:88-90.
11. International HapMap Consortium. A haplotype map of the human genome. Nature 2004; 437;1299-1320.
12. Newton-Cheh C, Hirschhorn JN. Genetic association studies of complex traits: design and analysis issues. Mutat Res 2005;573:54-69.
14. Hirschhorn JN. Genetic approaches to studying common diseases and complex traits. Pediatr Res 2005;57:74R-77R.
16. Colhoun HM, McKeigue PM, Davey Smith G. Problems of reporting genetic associations with complex outcomes. Lancet 2003;361:865-872.
17. Hirschhorn JN, Altshuler D. Once and again—issues surrounding replication in genetic association studies. J Clin Endocrinol Metab 2002;87:4438-4441.
20. Siva C, Yokoyama WM, McLeod HL. Pharmacogenetics in rheumatology: the prospects and limitations of an emerging field. Rheumatology (Oxford) 2002;41:1273-1279.
23. Hider SL, Buckley C, Silman AJ, et al. Factors influencing response to disease modifying antirheumatic drugs in patients with rheumatoid arthritis. J Rheumatol 2005;32:11-16.

24. Van Rossum EF, Roks PH, de Jong FH, et al. Characterization of a promoter polymorphism in the glucocorticoid receptor gene and its relationship to three other polymorphisms. Clin Endocrinol (Oxford) 2004;61:573-581.
25. Van Rossum EF, Koper JW, Huizenga NA, et al. A polymorphism in the glucocorticoid receptor gene, which decreases sensitivity to glucocorticoids in vivo, is associated with low insulin and cholesterol levels. Diabetes 2002;51:3128-3134.
26. Van Rossum EF, Koper JW, Van Den Beld AW, et al. Identification of the BclI polymorphism in the glucocorticoid receptor gene: association with sensitivity to glucocorticoids in vivo and body mass index. Clin Endocrinol (Oxf) 2003;59: 585-592.
27. Huizenga NA, Koper JW, De Lange P, et al. A polymorphism in the glucocorticoid receptor gene may be associated with an increased sensitivity to glucocorticoids in vivo. J Clin Endocrinol Metab 1998;83:144-151.
28. Stevens A, Ray DW, Zeggini E, et al. Glucocorticoid sensitivity is determined by a specific glucocorticoid receptor haplotype. J Clin Endocrinol Metab 2004;89:892-897.
29. Derijk RH, Schaaf MJ, Turner G, et al. A human glucocorticoid receptor gene variant that increases the stability of the glucocorticoid receptor beta-isoform mRNA is associated with rheumatoid arthritis. J Rheumatol 2001;28:2383-2388.
30. Tantisira KG, Lake S, Silverman ES, et al. Corticosteroid pharmacogenetics: association of sequence variants in CRHR1 with improved lung function in asthmatics treated with inhaled corticosteroids. Hum Mol Genet 2004;13:1353-1359.

40. Andrioli G, Minuz P, Solero P, et al. Defective platelet response to arachidonic acid and thromboxane A(2) in subjects with PI(A2) polymorphism of beta(3) subunit (glycoprotein IIIa). Br J Haematol 2000;110: 911-918.
41. Garcia-Martin E, Martinez C, Tabares B, et al. Interindividual variability in ibuprofen pharmacokinetics is related to interaction of cytochrome P450 2C8 and 2C9 amino acid polymorphisms. Clin Pharmacol Ther 2004;76:119-127.
42. Lee CR, Pieper JA, Frye RF, et al. Differences in flurbiprofen pharmacokinetics between CYP2C9*1/*1, *1/*2 and *1/*3 genotypes. Eur J Clin Pharmacol 2003;58:791-794.
43. Kirchheiner J, Stormer E, Meisel C, et al. Influence of CYP2C9 genetic polymorphisms on pharmacokinetics of celecoxib and its metabolites. Pharmacogenetics 2003;13:473-480.
45. Dorado P, Berecz R, Norberto MJ, et al. CYP2C9 genotypes and diclofenac metabolism in Spanish healthy volunteers. Eur J Clin Pharmacol 2003;59:221-225.
47. Brenner SS, Herrlinger C, Dilger K, et al. Influence of age and cytochrome P450 2C9 genotype on the steady-state disposition of diclofenac and celecoxib. Clin Pharmacokinet 2003;42:283-292.
50. Van Ede AE, Laan RF, Blom HJ, et al. The C677T mutation in the methylenetetrahydrofolate reductase gene: a genetic risk factor for methotrexate-related elevation of liver enzymes in rheumatoid arthritis patients. Arthritis Rheum 2001;44:2525-2530.
51. Urano W, Taniguchi A, Yamanaka H, et al. Polymorphisms in the methylenetetrahydrofolate reductase gene were associated with both the efficacy and the toxicity of methotrexate used for the treatment of rheumatoid

arthritis, as evidenced by single locus and haplotype analyses. Pharmacogenetics 2002;12:183-190.

52. Berkun Y, Levartovsky D, Rubinow A, et al. Methotrexate related adverse effects in patients with rheumatoid arthritis are associated with the A1298C polymorphism of the *MTHFR* gene. Ann Rheum Dis 2004;63:1227-1231.

53. Hughes LB, Beasley TM, Patel H, et al: Racial or ethnic differences in allele frequencies of single-nucleotide polymorphisms in the methylenetetrahydrofolate reductase gene and their influence on response to methotrexate in rheumatoid arthritis. Ann Rheum Dis 2006;65:1213-1218.

54. Wessels JA, de Vries-Bouwstra JK, Heijmans BT, et al. Efficacy and toxicity of methotrexate in early rheumatoid arthritis are associated with single-nucleotide polymorphisms. Arthritis Rheum 2006;54:1087-1095.

56. Van Ede AE, Laan RF, Rood MJ, et al. Effect of folic or folinic acid supplementation on the toxicity and efficacy of methotrexate in rheumatoid arthritis. Arthritis Rheum 2001;44:1515-1524.

57. Wessels JA, van der Kooij SM, le Cessie S, et al. A clinical pharmacogenetic model to predict the efficacy of methotrexate monotherapy in recent-onset rheumatoid arthritis. Arthritis Rheum 2007;56:1765-1775.

58. Fisher MC, Cronstein BN. Meta-analysis of methylenetetrahydrofolate reductase (MTHFR)

polymorphisms affecting methotrexate toxicity. J Rheumatol 2009;36:539-545.

62. McLeod HL, Siva C. The thiopurine S-methyltransferase gene locus: implications for clinical pharmacogenomics. Pharmacogenomics 2002;3:89-98.

65. Black AJ, McLeod HL, Capell HA, et al. Thiopurine methyltransferase genotype predicts therapy-limiting severe toxicity from azathioprine. Ann Intern Med 1998;129:716-718.

66. Stolk JN, Boerbooms AM, de Abreu RA, et al. Reduced thiopurine methyltransferase activity and development of side effects of azathioprine treatment in patients with rheumatoid arthritis. Arthritis Rheum 1998;41:1858-1866.

69. Das KM, Eastwood MA, McManus JP, Sircus W. Adverse reactions during salicylazosulfapyridine therapy and the relation with drug metabolism and acetylator phenotype. N Engl J Med 1973;289:491-495.

78. Wadelius M, Stjernberg E, Wiholm BE, et al. Polymorphisms of NAT2 in relation to sulphasalazine-induced agranulocytosis. Pharmacogenetics 2000;10:35-41.

88. Martinez A, Salido M, Bonilla G, et al. Association of the major histocompatibility complex with response to infliximab therapy in rheumatoid arthritis patients. Arthritis Rheum 2004;50:1077-1082.

89. Mugnier B, Balandraud N, Darque A, et al. Polymorphism at position -308 of the tumor necrosis factor alpha gene influences outcome of infliximab therapy in rheumatoid arthritis. Arthritis Rheum 2003;48:1849-1852.

94. Padyukov L, Lampa J, Heimburger M, et al. Genetic markers for the efficacy of tumour necrosis factor blocking therapy in rheumatoid arthritis. Ann Rheum Dis 2003;62:526-529.

95. Criswell LA, Lum RF, Turner KN, et al. The influence of genetic variation in the HLA-DRB1 and LTA-TNF regions on the response to treatment of early rheumatoid arthritis with methotrexate or etanercept. Arthritis Rheum 2004;50:2750-2756.

96. Maxwell JR, Potter C, Hyrich KL, et al. Association of the tumour necrosis factor-308 variant with differential response to anti-TNF agents in the treatment of rheumatoid arthritis. Hum Mol Genet 2008;17:3532-3538.

97. Liu C, Batliwalla F, Li W, et al. Genome-wide association scan identifies candidate polymorphisms associated with differential response to anti-TNF treatment in rheumatoid arthritis. Mol Med 2008;14:575-581.

REFERENCES

Full references for this chapter can be found on www.expertconsult.com.

Effects of the neuroendocrine system on development and function of the immune system

24

Maurizio Cutolo and Rainer H. Straub

INTRODUCTION

A possible molecular connection between the neuroendocrine system and the immune system was originally predicted on the basis of clinical findings. Independent observations already made in the 19th century by Trousseau, Charcot, and Bannatyne indicating that pregnancy is favorable in rheumatoid arthritis (RA) were summarized in the Nobel Prize lecture of the rheumatologist Philip S. Hench, on December 11, 1950 (http://nobelprize.org/medicine/laureates/1950/hench-lecture.pdf). Dr. Hench wrote[1]:

> ...after 1931, records of these cases [of cases with RA] were more carefully made and assembled...because of my growing belief that this phenomenon of relief [from arthritic disability] was analogous to, if not identical with, that which may occur during jaundice, and that the same agent might be responsible for the relief both during pregnancy and jaundice, although the mechanism...might be different.

For the first time, these observations linked immune/inflammatory diseases to hormones, and this was firmly established by the enormous treatment success obtained through the use of endogenous glucocorticoids at the beginning of the 1950s.[2] In addition, the obvious female-to-male preponderance in prevalence and incidence of autoimmune diseases spoke for the role of sex hormones such as 17β-estradiol, progesterone, and testosterone. This preponderance is particularly evident in the reproductive years, when sex hormones are highest in women and men. Furthermore, the induction of ovulation by gonadotropins, gonadotropin-releasing hormone analogs, or clomiphene can result in flares, embryonic losses, or fetal deaths in patients with systemic lupus erythematosus (SLE) or antiphospholipid antibody syndrome.[3] Again, this indicates that generally an increase of female sex hormones can worsen an autoimmune disease. In sharp contrast seems to be the finding that some women develop an autoimmune disease such as RA after the menopause when serum sex hormone levels dramatically fall. This is not an unsolvable paradox compared with the just-mentioned role of sex hormones, as will be shown, because sex hormones have very different effects on different types of immune cells; in addition, their peripheral metabolism plays an important role.

The clear connection between stressful life events on the one hand and exacerbations of autoimmune diseases on the other demonstrate a role of steroidal hormones or neurotransmitters in these diseases (i.e., cortisol and norepinephrine).[4] Similarly, the phenomenon that in different diseases hemiplegia spares the paretic side from inflammatory signs and symptoms supports an important propagating role of the nervous system.[5] Moreover, the circadian undulation of symptoms in autoimmune diseases links the rhythms of the central nervous and neuroendocrine systems to immunologically mediated phenomena. These clinical findings opened up totally new avenues for understanding the impact of the neuroendocrine system on development and function of the immune system.

THE NEUROENDOCRINE SYSTEM

The neuroendocrine system comprises the central nervous system (CNS), pituitary and pineal hormones, hormones of peripheral glands (mainly adrenal and gonads), the efferent sympathetic and parasympathetic nervous system, and the afferent sensory nervous system. Figure 24.1 is a representation of the different endocrine and neuronal axes. The hypothalamic-pituitary-adrenal (HPA) axis influences many immunologic mechanisms (see later). It comprises the hypothalamic hormone corticotropin-releasing hormone (CRH), the pituitary adrenocorticotropic hormone (ACTH), and adrenal steroids, including the major hormones cortisol, progesterone, dehydroepiandrosterone (DHEA), and androstenedione (ASD), as well as the thyroid axis. Progesterone, DHEA, and ASD are precursor hormones that can be converted to downstream sex hormones. Importantly, sex steroid action can take place in the same cells where conversion takes place (intracrinology).[6] In postmenopausal women, nearly 100% of sex steroids are synthesized in peripheral tissues from precursors of adrenal origin (in older men peripheral conversion depends on age and can be up to 80%). Thus, after the menopause and during aging, the HPA axis can take over various functions of the hypothalamic-pituitary-gonadal (HPG) axis (Fig. 24.2) and influence the immune/inflammatory reactivity. Peripheral conversion of hormones can be influenced by locally produced cytokines, hormones, and neurotransmitters.[7]

In addition to the HPA axis, the HPG axis particularly plays an important role in the reproductive years when gonadal hormones are produced in large amounts from ovaries and testes. The well-known undulation of symptoms of autoimmune diseases during the menstrual cycle demonstrates this important influence. In this situation, gonadally produced estrogens and androgens can bypass the conversion steps via DHEAS, DHEA, and ASD (see Fig. 24.2, yellow box). Beyond steroid hormones, pituitary prolactin and pineal melatonin demonstrate immune-stimulating properties.[8,9] Another important hormonal system is the somatotropic axis with growth hormone–releasing hormone, growth hormone, and peripherally produced insulin-like growth factor-1 (IGF-1), which has proven immunomodulating effects.

The central neuroendocrine system is activated upon peripheral inflammation in which the HPA axis is stimulated (stress response system) and the HPG axis and the somatotropic axis are blocked. The major immune stimulus for the HPA axis is circulating interleukin (IL)-6, interferon-γ, tumor necrosis factor (TNF), and local IL-6 and IL-1β that directly activate sensory afferents. In addition, the neuroendocrine system can be activated by psychological stress (which also includes pain transmitted via sensory afferents). It is important to mention that acute stimulation of neuroendocrine centers can lead to markedly different behavior of these axes when compared with chronic stimulation due to habituation phenomena. Chronic proinflammatory activation can lead to functional and subclinical insufficiency of the HPA axis.

The hypothalamic-pituitary-adrenal axis

Influence of HPA axis hormones on the development of the immune system

There are tight connections between the HPA and somatotropic axes and the thymus.[10] For example, glucocorticoids were long known to inhibit thymocytes, and thymocytes possess all the enzymes to generate glucocorticoids in the thymic microenvironment.[11] ACTH inhibits mitogenesis of immature and mature thymocytes,[12] DHEA suppresses

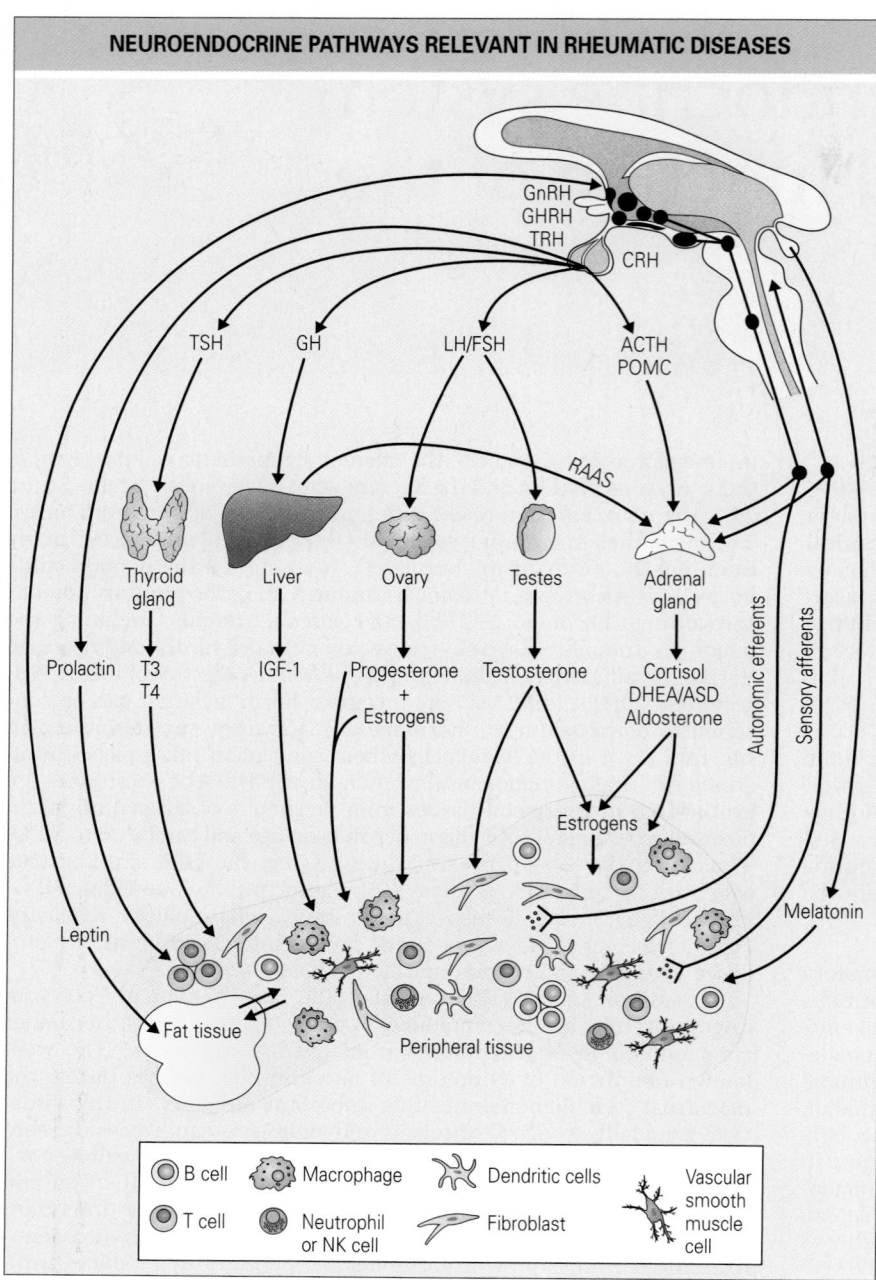

NEUROENDOCRINE PATHWAYS RELEVANT IN RHEUMATIC DISEASES

Fig. 24.1 Neuroendocrine pathways relevant in rheumatic diseases. Neuroendocrine pathways link the central nervous system with the periphery by way of hormones and nerve fibers (neurotransmitters). Some important cells are demonstrated to indicate some targets in inflamed tissue and lymphoid organs. Autonomic efferents comprise sympathetic and parasympathetic nerves with the main sympathetic neurotransmitters norepinephrine (plus neuropeptide Y, adenosine triphosphate, and endogenous opioids) and with the main parasympathetic neurotransmitter acetylcholine. The sensory nervous system bears vesicles with substance P, galanin, and calcitonin gene–related peptide. ACTH, adrenocorticotropic hormone; ASD, androstenedione; CRH, corticotropin-releasing hormone; DHEA, dehydroepiandrosterone; FSH, follicle-stimulating hormone; GH, growth hormone; GHRH, growth hormone–releasing hormone; GnRH, gonadotropin-releasing hormone; IGF-1, insulin-like growth factor-1; LH, luteinizing hormone; POMC, proopiomelanocortin-derived proteins (other than ACTH); RAAS, renin-angiotensin-aldosterone system; T3, triiodothyronine; T4, thyroxine; TRH, thyrotropin-releasing hormone; TSH, thyroid-stimulating hormone (or thyrotropin).

proliferation of thymocytes,[13] and DHEA induces thymocyte apoptosis by upregulation of Fas and Fas-L.[14] Inversely, thymic factors such as thymulin or cytokines influence the hypothalamic-pituitary axis (e.g., GH secretion), which led to the concept of a reciprocal feedback loop between the hypothalamic-pituitary axis and the thymus.[10] In addition, GH and prolactin also were shown to be important connectors of the pituitary gland and the thymus.[10] These interconnections between the hypothalamic-pituitary axis and the thymus most probably play an important role in the aging process when the integration of this network is disrupted and the thymus undergoes involution.[15] Because the thymus is the primary T-lymphopoietic organ during ontogenesis, its age-related involution with morphologic alterations is, in part, responsible for the decline in antigen-specific T-lymphocyte immune functions. Presently, it is unclear whether the neuroendocrine connection between the hypothalamic-pituitary axis and the thymus is altered in human chronic inflammatory autoimmune disease.

Progesterone inhibits differentiation of bone marrow–derived dendritic cells, and it also influences maturation of dendritic cells.[16,17] In addition, progesterone might influence B-lymphocyte development because progesterone receptors have been demonstrated in premature B cells.[18] The inhibiting role of glucocorticoids on B-lymphocyte development has been demonstrated in the mouse.[19] Although most of these

findings play relevant roles in immunophysiology of rodents, their impact has never been demonstrated in humans with or without an autoimmune disease.

The influence of HPA axis hormones on the immune system function: in vivo and in vitro studies

Although CRH, as a major hormone of the hypothalamus, has a strong anti-inflammatory role in the general regulation of the HPA axis, CRH produced locally exerts many proinflammatory effects.[20] Indeed, the use of a CRH receptor type 1 antagonist ameliorated adjuvant arthritis.[21] Typically, stimulation of either CRH receptor type 1 or type 2 triggers activation of adenylyl cyclase and increases cyclic adenosine monophosphate (cAMP) levels mediated by G_s-adenylyl cyclase signaling.[22] However, in certain cells, CRH is unable to activate this anti-inflammatory pathway, and one may observe phosphoinositol hydrolysis, protein kinase C (PKC) activation, stimulation of the p42/p44 and p38 mitogen-activated protein kinases (MAPKs), as well as release of other important proinflammatory signaling molecules, such as Ca^{2+} and nitric oxide synthase.[22] Similarly, local ACTH exerts some stimulatory activities on cytotoxic T cells,[12] and T lymphocytes, B lymphocytes, and macrophages possess melanocortin receptors.[23] ACTH can bind to all melanocortin receptors type 1 to 5, and signaling

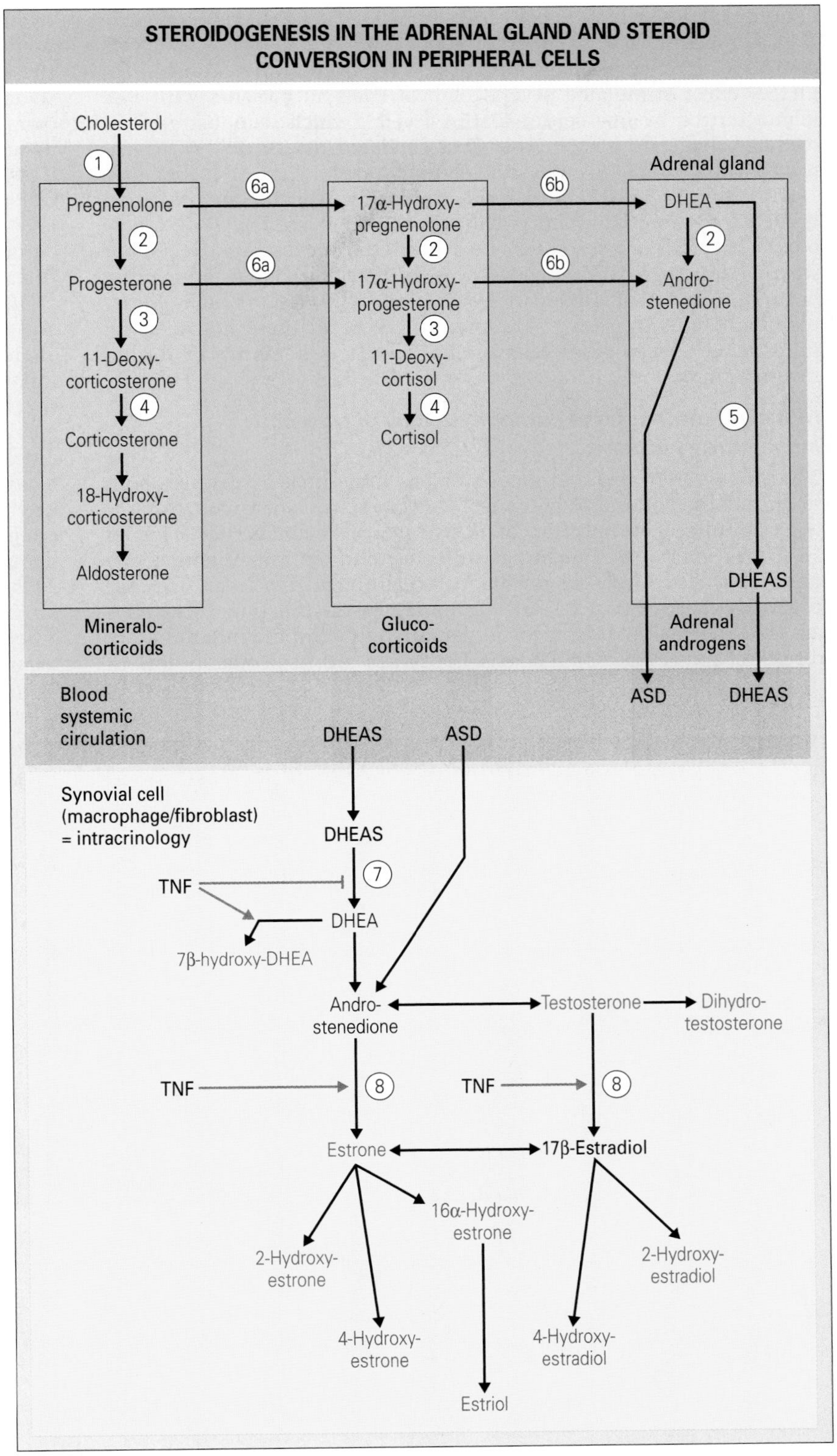

Fig. 24.2 Steroidogenesis in the adrenal gland and steroid conversion in peripheral cells. In the upper part (blue box), steroidogenesis (in adrenal gland) under healthy conditions is demonstrated. In the bottom part (yellow), the conversion of steroid hormones in peripheral cells such as the macrophage or fibroblast is depicted. The violet (and green) color in the yellow boxes indicates a proinflammatory (anti-inflammatory) influence. DHEAS is converted to downstream androgens and estrogens. The proinflammatory TNF interferes with several hormonal conversion steps (a line with a bar at the end indicates inhibition, whereas an arrow indicates stimulation). Numbers: 1 = P450scc, P450 side chain cleavage enzyme; 2 = 3β-HSD, 3β-hydroxysteroid dehydrogenase; 3 = P450c21, 21-hydroxylase; 4 = P450c11, 11α-hydroxylase; 5 = DHEA sulfotransferase; 6a and 6b = P450c17, an enzyme with two activities (17α-hydroxylase and 17/20-lyase); 7 = DHEAS sulfate; 8 = aromatase complex. ASD, androstenedione; DHEA, dehydroepiandrosterone; DHEAS, DHEA sulfate; TNF, tumor necrosis factor.

via type 4 and 5 leads to proinflammatory events via phosphoinositol hydrolysis, PKC activation, and stimulation of the JAK/STAT pathway.[24] This is opposite to the effect of melanocortin receptor type 1, which triggers activation of adenylyl cyclase and increases cAMP levels.[24] Thus, similar to CRH, expression of receptor subtypes and important co-molecules is decisive in modulating the immune response.

In contrast, glucocorticoids possess anti-inflammatory effects *in vitro* on almost all immune cells studied. This is particularly true if concentrations of cortisol or corticosterone are above 10^{-7} mol/L, and if, *in vivo*, this elevation lasts for a longer period of time (days to weeks). In contrast, if, *in vivo*, glucocorticoids rise for only a short period of time (hours), they might exert overall immunostimulatory effects by inducing redistribution and migration of immune cells.[25,26]

Glucocorticoids and progesterone shift the T-cell immune response to a T-helper type 2 (Th2) immune phenotype.[27] This phenomenon is most probably an important factor during pregnancy to save the semiallogenic embryo from the maternal immune system.[28] In addition, this cytokine shift is also an important factor for pregnancy-related amelioration of diseases such as RA and multiple sclerosis (mainly Th1-mediated diseases) but also a stimulating factor in SLE (Th2-mediated disease).

Finally, adrenal androgens were found to have several anti-inflammatory effects by inhibiting cytokines such as IL-2, IL-6, TNF, interferon-γ, and others.[29] These anti-inflammatory effects are attributed to the biologically active DHEA but not its biologically inactive precursor DHEA sulfate (DHEAS). In the circulation, DHEAS is the pool for DHEA, which is converted from DHEAS in peripheral cells. It was thought that biologically active DHEA had opposite effects compared with cortisol by inhibiting Th2 immune reactions. This DHEA effect stimulated several clinical trials in patients with SLE (characterized by low serum DHEA levels), which demonstrated an overall beneficial effect in this Th2-mediated disease.[30,31] A similar positive role of DHEA was not demonstrated in the T-helper type 1/17–driven RA (Th17), which most probably depends on conversion of DHEA to proinflammatory 7β-hydroxy-DHEA (see Fig. 24.2, yellow box).[32] It is still not absolutely clear how DHEA exerts its effects, but we can summarize that a major part is mediated by conversion to other hormones and a smaller part by ligation of DHEA to high-affinity membrane-binding sites.[33] The importance of all these hormones in influencing T regulatory cells or Th17 cells is a matter of further investigations.

HPA axis hormones and pathophysiology of chronic inflammatory diseases

The lack of HPA axis hormones worsens inflammatory diseases both in animal models and in patients.[34,35] Every acute inflammatory event (e.g., simulated by injection of IL-6[36]) increases circulating levels of HPA axis hormones, but in patients with chronic inflammatory diseases, hormone levels are not increased although IL-6 levels are continuously elevated (Fig. 24.3a).[37] Importantly, the function of the HPA axis is abnormal and deficient in patients with chronic inflammatory diseases, and levels of HPA axis hormones are inadequately low in

relation to circulating and stimulating cytokines.[38,39] Habituation phenomena accompanied by cytokine-induced blockade of hormone synthesis lead to their inadequate levels in chronic inflammatory diseases. In addition, concentrations of adrenal androgens are largely decreased owing to reorganization of adrenal steroidogenesis, leading to a preponderance of cortisol relative to other adrenal hormones (stress response). This is most probably due to inhibition of adrenal 17,20-lyase activity of P450c17 (see enzyme 6b in Fig. 24.2). Importantly, the preponderance of cortisol relative to adrenal androgens is a feature of nearly all chronic inflammatory diseases, because the loss of cortisol is life threatening and must be avoided.

In addition to alterations of HPA axis organ function, conversion and degradation of secreted hormones in peripheral tissue is largely altered. For example, glucocorticoids are increasingly degraded in inflamed tissue (i.e., synovial tissue in RA) due to an upregulation of the 11β-hydroxysteroid dehydrogenase type 2 activity and an inadequate reactivation of degraded hormones via 11β-hydroxysteroid dehydrogenase type 1.[40] In cells of inflamed tissue, activation of the biologically inactive DHEAS to the biologically active DHEA is inhibited by TNF[41] (see Fig. 24.2, yellow box), and TNF activates the aromatase complex leading to the formation from androgens of proinflammatory estrogens, such as 16-hydroxylated estrogens (see Fig. 24.2, yellow box).[42] All these peripheral phenomena lead to a more proinflammatory environment in inflamed tissue and might explain otherwise unexpected immune/inflammatory reactions and therapeutic results.

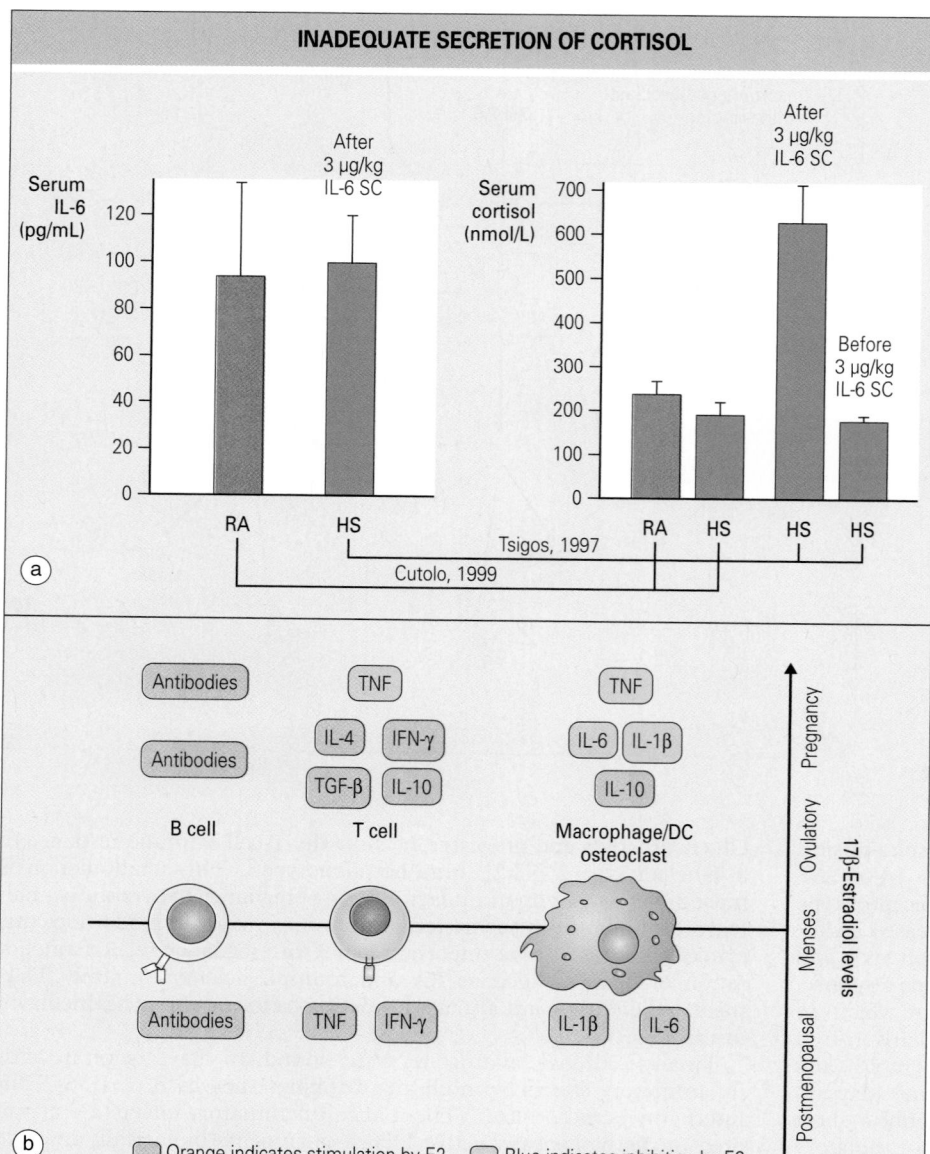

Fig. 24.3 (a) Inadequate secretion of cortisol in relation to inflammation. In the right panel, one can see that subcutaneous (SC) injection of IL-6 leads to a large increase of serum cortisol in healthy individuals (HS).[36] Looking at the left panel, one recognizes that injection of IL-6 leads to very similar serum levels of IL-6 in HS as compared with patients with rheumatoid arthritis (RA).[37] However, serum cortisol levels are not increased in patients with RA as compared with HS, as demonstrated in the right panel.[37] (b) Influence of estrogens on important proinflammatory and anti-inflammatory pathways in different cell types. On the y-axis the concentration of 17β-estradiol is given. Depending on the concentration of 17β-estradiol, factors in orange boxes are stimulated and factors in blue boxes are inhibited by estrogens. DC, dendritic cell; IFN-γ, interferon-γ; IL, interleukin; TGF-β, transforming growth factor-β; TNF, tumor necrosis factor.

The hypothalamic-pituitary-gonadal axis

Influence of HPG axis hormones on the development of the immune system: the animal studies

In animal studies at high concentrations, 17β-estradiol leads to a suppression of B-lymphocyte lineage precursors. In addition, IL-7–responsive B-lineage precursors were greatly expanded in genetically hypogonadal female mice. Estrogen replacement in these mice resulted in a dose-dependent reduction in B-cell precursors.[43] Similarly, pregnancy in mice led to a clear decline in B-cell precursors in the bone marrow, which was blocked by an estrogen receptor antagonist, and an increase was observed in hypogonadal mice. At pregnancy levels, 17β-estradiol induced a downregulation of B lymphopoietic cells in the bone marrow of young ovariectomized mice, which is mediated through both estrogen receptors.[43]

In addition to effects of estrogens on B cells, estrogens have a strong influence on the development and maintenance of thymic function and, thus, on generation of naive CD4+ and CD8+ T cells. Estrogen receptor α–deficient mice have smaller thymuses than their wild-type littermates; and 17β-estradiol–induced thymus atrophy was reduced in these mice.[43] In one study the CD4+/CD8+ phenotype was not changed in estrogen receptor α–deficient mice,[43] but a higher frequency of CD4+CD8+ thymocytes was found in another study.[43] In estrogen receptor–intact animals, 17β-estradiol (pregnancy levels) induced profound thymus involution in normal and adrenalectomized mice.[43] However, 17β-estradiol did not induce lymphocytopenia in the peripheral organs but stimulated extrathymic T-cell numbers in the liver and other organs.[43] Treatment with 17β-estradiol (pregnancy levels) for 4 weeks decreased thymus cellularity and the percentage of CD4+ cells in the spleen, which was not observed in double estrogen receptor–deficient mice.[43] Whether this 17β-estradiol–induced thymic involution is beneficial or harmful in human chronic inflammation remains to be established because autoaggressive but also autotolerant T cells might be eliminated.

Finally, 17β-estradiol has been shown to promote the differentiation of dendritic cells from bone marrow precursors in vitro, and this effect is mediated via estrogen receptor α.[44] Raloxifene and tamoxifen, two selective estrogen receptor modulators, inhibited the differentiation of estrogen-dependent dendritic cells from bone marrow precursors ex vivo in competition experiments with physiologic levels of 17β-estradiol.[45]

In conclusion, these experiments in animals and with cells of rodents demonstrate that 17β-estradiol has inhibitory effects on precursors of B cells and T cells. Similar inhibitory effects were demonstrated for testosterone concerning the thymus.[13] It is presently unclear how these sex hormones influence development of immune cell precursors in patients with autoimmune diseases. This can be an important line of research because sex hormones might bias the immune response toward an autoimmune response already many years before outbreak of the development of the disease.[46]

Androgens and estrogens influence the function of immune system: the human studies

Generally, androgens, in physiologic concentrations, suppress the immune responses.[47] Recent studies have shown that both physiologic (10^{-8} M) and pharmacologic (or high physiologic) (10^{-6} M) concentrations of testosterone inhibit IL-1 secretion by peripheral blood mononuclear cells (PBMC) obtained from RA patients.[48] In addition, physiologic concentrations of testosterone inhibit IL-1 synthesis in primary cultured human synovial macrophages.[49] In other studies, dihydrotestosterone has been found to repress the expression and activity of the human IL-6 gene promoter in human fibroblasts, thus supporting the concept of anti-inflammatory or immunosuppressive effects of androgens. Testosterone treatment does not appear to directly affect isolated B or T cells. However, in a follow-up study of SLE patients, testosterone suppressed both anti–double-stranded DNA IgG and total IgG production of PBMC.[50] Thus, testosterone exerts similar immunosuppressive effects as compared with DHEA mentioned earlier.

Figure 24.3b summarizes the most important effects of high and low concentrations of estrogens on different types of cells involved in chronic inflammation. At pregnancy levels, 17β-estradiol inhibits important proinflammatory pathways such as TNF, IL-1β, IL-6, and MCP-1; inducible nitric oxide synthase expression; production of matrix metalloproteinases (MMPs); and activity of natural killer cells. In contrast, 17β-estradiol at the same concentration stimulates anti-inflammatory pathways such as IL-4, IL-10, TGF-β, tissue inhibitors of MMP (TIMP), and osteoprotegerin. At lower concentrations, 17β-estradiol stimulates TNF, IFN-γ, IL-1β, and activity of natural killer cells. This dichotomy of 17β-estradiol at high versus low concentrations is not observed for B cells, because antibody production is still stimulated throughout the full concentration range (see Fig. 24.3b). Consequences of these 17β-estradiol effects for chronic inflammation are summarized in the next section.

HPG axis hormones and pathophysiology of chronic inflammatory diseases

B cells, T cells, and antigen-presenting cells (macrophages, dendritic cells, and B cells) are needed for the initiation of autoimmune diseases. One might separate two clinically important phases of an autoimmune disease: an asymptomatic phase and a symptomatic phase (after disease development). Disease development means involvement of a target organ/target tissue leading to the classic clinical signs of visible and functionally relevant inflammation.

Recent important work in the field of RA has delineated that autoimmune phenomena are present more than 10 years before disease development.[51,52] In the asymptomatic phase, T cells, B cells, and antigen-presenting cells play an important hidden role because clonal expansion of autoreactive T cells and B cells happens without overt disease symptoms. Because the influence of estrogens on these cell types is different from other cell types, estrogens can have quite opposite roles depending on involved cells. If B cells play a center role by antigen presentation, autoantibody production, and/or bystander cytokine secretion, estrogens will speed up the outbreak of the disease in the early reproductive years. Because men never experience these high estrogen or progesterone levels and counteract these hormones by testosterone, the apparent gender dimorphism of autoimmune disease during the reproductive period of women can be explained. If tissue-destructive T cells and B cells play an equally important role, the onset of disease in a woman will be delayed because 17β-estradiol may inhibit T-cell autoimmunity but always stimulates B-cell autoimmunity. In such a situation, the onset of the disease might be shifted to the late reproductive phase or postmenopausal period. If tissue-destructive T cells play the most important role (no role of B cells), the onset of the disease should be expected in the postmenopausal phase when 17β-estradiol but also progesterone declines. Thus, ovariectomy in animal models and the menopause in women are stimulatory for autoimmune arthritis and other autoimmune diseases of late onset.

The location of tissue inflammation in an autoimmune disease is defined by the major autoantigen (or autoantigens). Once a disease has entered the highly inflammatory symptomatic phase, many other cell types are involved, depending on the major location of the autoimmune disease (e.g., in the brain, in the joint, in the kidney). For example, in the joint, macrophages, fibroblasts, osteoclasts, osteoblasts, adipocytes, endothelial cells, and many more cells are gradually involved in the inflammatory process. Depending on the predominant cell types involved, 17β-estradiol and also progesterone might have quite different effects on these bystander inflammatory activities of participating cells.[43]

All cells (including B cells, T cells, and antigen-presenting cells) might have very different capacities to take up and to metabolize estrogens.[42] Metabolism of estrogens depends on transport into cells, desulfation of sulfated estrogens, sulfatation of non-sulfated estrogens, androgen aromatization, and estrogen conversion to downstream hydroxylated or methylated estrogens (see Fig. 24.2, yellow box). In addition, upregulation or downregulation of estrogen receptors α and β (in cells or on the cell surface) and co-activators and co-repressors might well depend on involved cells and microenvironmental conditions, such as accompanying hypoxia and the surrounding cytokine milieu. In addition, it has nicely been demonstrated in one animal model that 17β-estradiol accelerates immune-complex–mediated glomerulonephritis but ameliorates focal sialadenitis, renal vasculitis, and periarticular inflammation.[53] This indicates that quite different pathologic processes might even be present in the same individual so that estrogens have beneficial effects on one aspect of the disease but a deleterious influence on other mechanisms. This depends most probably on the involved cell types, concentrations, and peripheral metabolism.[7]

Studies in the past decade also demonstrated that the small change of estrogen or progesterone levels during therapy with oral contraceptives or hormone replacement therapy has variable effect to increase the risk or to inhibit an ongoing autoimmune disease (clear effects on overt disease).[43] One understands that estrogens can even stimulate several immune mechanisms at postmenopausal levels owing to their bimodal role (see Fig. 24.3b).

Circadian rhythms and the immune system

The term *circadian rhythm* refers to the 24-hour cycles in the physiologic processes of the living organism. Although circadian rhythms are a fundamental feature of the biology of animals, they were usually not considered as important determinants of disease. In considering symptoms of RA, it is remarkable that the improvement of morning stiffness induced by prednisolone after 6 months is similar in magnitude to the improvement of morning stiffness during a single day (from morning to evening). Under both conditions—the clinical trial and the course of one day—an improvement of 40% to 50% can occur. Imagine,

therefore, a situation in which an investigator in a clinical trial did not pay attention to the time point of examination and recorded improvement that reflected the diurnal variation as much as a sustained treatment effect. Circadian rhythms are a basis for variations of the immune-inflammatory response.

Both IL-6 and TNF display a circadian rhythm (Fig. 24.4a), with maximum levels in the early morning hours.[54] In healthy persons, the peak value of IL-6 is found at about 6 AM; in patients with RA, the peak value of IL-6 appears at 7 AM. In healthy persons IL-6 serum levels are 2 to 4 pg/mL, whereas in RA patients these levels are 20 to 40 pg/mL. Thus, the amplitude of the curve of cytokine production is higher and the curve is broadened in RA as compared with controls.[55] In healthy persons serum levels of IL-6 usually decrease by 9 AM, whereas in RA patients these levels can remain elevated until 11 AM. The increased amplitude and the broadened curve in the morning hours are important for the morning symptoms. In view of these observations the key question is what is driving the circadian oscillation of serum levels of cytokines?

The cycle of the HPA axis has a maximum in the early morning hours at 8 AM and a nadir at midnight (see Fig. 24.4a). Detailed analyses of the circadian curves of cytokines and cortisol have revealed a lag time between the cortisol rise in comparison to the increase of cytokine levels of 60 to 120 minutes.[56] From this study and a recent analysis of

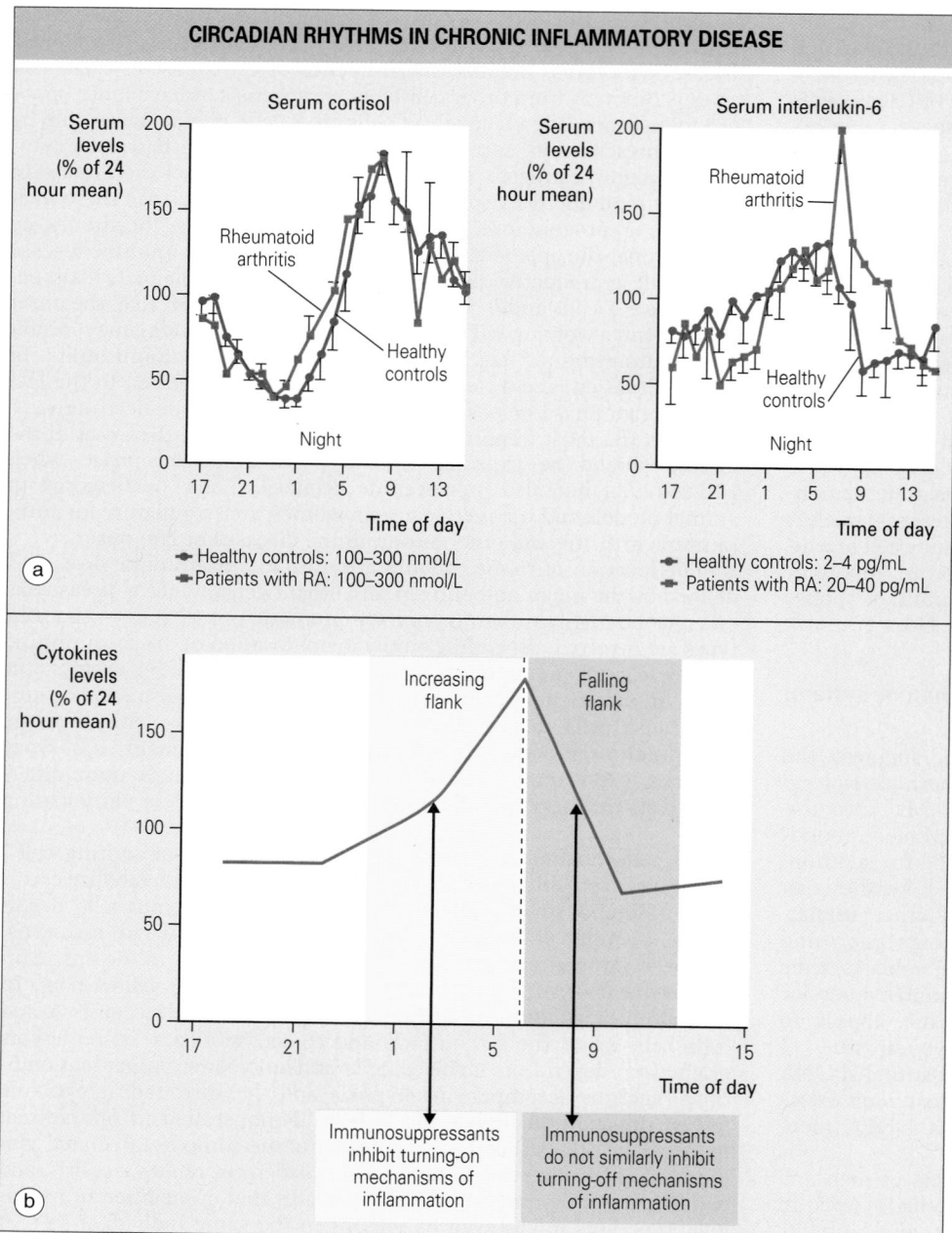

Fig. 24.4 Circadian rhythms in chronic inflammatory disease. (a) Circadian rhythm of cortisol and interleukin-6 (IL-6) in healthy individuals and patients with rheumatoid arthritis (RA). The data are given in percent of the 24-hour mean. The concentration ranges of serum cortisol and serum IL-6 are given in the yellow box below the main graphs. Despite the markedly increased serum levels of IL-6 in patients with RA compared with healthy persons, the circadian rhythm of cortisol is similar in both groups (in amplitude and period). This phenomenon is called "inadequate secretion of cortisol in relation to inflammation." (b) The role of administration of immunosuppressants during the increasing and falling flank of secretion of a proinflammatory mediator such as TNF. This information is derived from a perfusion study of the rat spleen, which demonstrates a very similar time course of TNF increase and decrease.[60] The turning-on phase of a proinflammatory response is more vulnerable to immunosuppressants such as glucocorticoids than the turning-off phase. Administration of immunosuppressants during the turning-on phase has a stronger capacity to inhibit proinflammatory sequelae and related clinical symptoms.[60]

several independent investigations,[54] it appears that morning cytokine levels can drive the increase of cortisol. The cortisol rhythm in healthy subjects does not differ from that of patients with RA when disease activity is relatively low to moderate. This similarity pertains to the period, the amplitude, and the time point of the minimum and peak of the cycle (see Fig. 24.4a).

Although levels of cytokines 10 times higher than normal should drive a stronger cortisol response (see Fig. 24-4a), it is notable that the serum levels of cortisol are similar in healthy controls and patients with RA.[56] This phenomenon was discussed earlier and was called "inadequate secretion of cortisol in relation to inflammation." The reasons for this inadequacy relate in part to an inhibition (or exhaustion) of the HPA axis by chronically elevated cytokines. In other words, secreted cortisol is unable to dampen the proinflammatory response. As such, cytokine levels stay high.

At present, it is thought that the cortisol nadir at midnight and the parallel increase of the proinflammatory hormone melatonin (and possibly prolactin) drive the increase of early nightly morning TNF and IL-6.[55] Subsequently, these two cytokines drive cortisol, and the later cortisol increase finally dampens the cytokine surge, and so forth. Because the circadian rhythm is generated in higher brain centers of the endocrine and nervous systems (in the hypothalamus), the circadian rhythms of cytokines mirror the activity of neuroendocrine centers in the brain. This provides a strong indication that neuroendocrine pathways influence disease-related pathophysiology and might suggest new options for therapeutic intervention.

Interestingly, the circadian activity of the neuroendocrine system seems to serve the different types of immune responses. During the day, the innate immune system is activated as delineated by increased numbers of circulating monocytes and granulocytes. These immune cells play the dominant role of the first-line defense. On take-up of antigens during the day (e.g., bacteria, viruses), macrophages and dendritic cells move to secondary lymphoid organs where the adaptive immune response is initiated and maintained during the night (night immune check-up). Dendritic cells present antigenic material to T and B cells during the night, which start to expand in a clonal manner. Because this is a vastly energy-consuming process, it happens in the night to fully allocate energy to the immune system and not to muscles and viscera.[57]

Finally, circannual variations of the vitamin D endocrine system are now also recognized as an important immune modulatory factor involved in autoimmune rheumatic diseases.[58]

These immunomodulatory and anti-inflammatory activities might be particularly efficient in RA patients and support a therapeutic role of 1,25-dihydroxy vitamin D_3 in such a disease.[58] In addition, vitamin D may play an important role in the maintenance of B-cell homeostasis and the correction of vitamin D deficiency may be useful in the treatment of B cell–mediated autoimmune rheumatic disorders such as SLE.

Translational studies: night-time therapy

One would think that a therapeutic increase of circulating glucocorticoids should alleviate symptoms in patients with RA. Recent data from a double-blind, placebo-controlled randomized study in patients with RA demonstrated a marked effect on morning stiffness and serum IL-6 levels when glucocorticoids were given at 2 AM.[59] The question appears why immunosuppressive treatment with glucocorticoids can inhibit proinflammatory sequelae better when given at an early time point at 2 AM rather than in the morning after awakening.

These observations are very important in understanding anti-inflammatory counter-regulation of immune responses. It has been demonstrated that glucocorticoids induce the transcription of the IκBa gene, which results in an increased rate of IκBa protein synthesis and inhibition of proinflammatory NF-κB effects. Other studies have shown that glucocorticoids can interfere with the transcriptional activation potential of DNA-bound NF-κB complexes, leading to anti-inflammatory effects. These effects appear very early in the turning-on phase of a proinflammatory response (early night). The turning-on phase of a proinflammatory reaction is much more vulnerable to immunosuppressants as compared with the turning-off phase (early morning). Therefore, the regulation of an important proinflammatory factor such as TNF increase must occur very early because otherwise an overwhelming secretion of this harmful cytokine would occur (see Fig. 24-4b).

In view of the circadian rhythms and the impact of the timing of immunosuppressive administration on efficacy, it would be of great interest to explore timed-release forms of cytokine neutralizers (on the basis of small molecules) or hormonal antagonists of melatonin, for example, as therapeutic modalities.[60] Reformulating old drugs in new drug delivery forms could possibly lead to optimized drug release patterns with improved immunosuppressant activities.

CONCLUSION

Clinical observations indicated a strong influence of the neuroendocrine system on the immune function in chronic inflammatory diseases. It is obvious that these neuroendocrine pathways influence the development of the immune system by interfering with the thymus in that almost all hormones of the HPA and HPG axes support the gradual involution of the thymus. Similarly, hormones of these two axes also hinder B-cell lymphopoiesis, which was particularly demonstrated for 17β-estradiol. On the other hand, CRH, ACTH, and 17β-estradiol exert some immunostimulatory effects, whereas glucocorticoids and androgens generally suppress immune responses.

The action of the different hormones is influenced by (1) the immune stimulus (foreign antigens or autoantigens) and subsequent antigen-specific immune responses, (2) the cell types involved during different phases of the disease, (3) the target organ with its specific microenvironment, (4) timing of hormone increase in relation to the disease course (and the reproductive status of a woman), (5) the concentration of hormones, (6) the variability in expression of hormone receptors depending on the microenvironment and the cell type, and (7) intracellular and extracellular peripheral metabolism of hormones leading to important biologically active metabolites with quite different anti-inflammatory and proinflammatory function. Circadian rhythm of disease-related symptoms with a peak in the early morning hours confirms that the neuroendocrine system has a strong influence on these chronic immune/inflammatory diseases. The influence is transferred by the circadian undulation of the activity of hormonal and neuronal neuroendocrine pathways linking the brain to immune cell activation.[61] New therapeutic strategies are based on circadian/circannual rhythms and generally on understanding the complex neuroendocrine/immune system in more detail.[62]

KEY REFERENCES

1. Hench PS. The ameliorating effect of pregnancy on chronic atrophic (infectious, rheumatoid) arthritis, fibrositis, and intermittent hydrarthrosis. Proc Staff Meet Mayo Clin 1938;13:161-167.
2. Hench PS, Slocumb CH, Polley HF, Kendall EC. Effect of cortisone and pituitary adrenocorticotropic hormone (ACTH) on rheumatic diseases. JAMA 1950;144:1327-1335.
4. Cutolo M, Straub RH, Chrousos GP. Stress and autoimmunity. In: Neuroimmunomodulation. Basel: Karger, 2006:13.
5. Miller LE, Wessinghage D, Müller-Ladner U, et al. In vitro superfusion method to study nerve-immune cell interactions in human synovial membrane in long-standing rheumatoid arthritis

and osteoarthritis. Ann N Y Acad Sci 1999;876: 266-275.
6. Labrie F. Intracrinology. Mol Cell Endocrinol 1991;78:C113-C118.
7. Cutolo M, Straub RH, Bijlsma JW. Neuroendocrine-immune interactions in synovitis. Nat Clin Pract Rheumatol 2007;3:627-634.
9. Cutolo M, Maestroni GJ. The melatonin-cytokine connection in rheumatoid arthritis. Ann Rheum Dis 2005;64:1109-1111.
10. Savino W. The neuroendocrine control of the thymus. In: Neuroimmunomodulation. Basel: Karger, 2008:6.
12. Johnson EW, Hughes TK Jr, Smith EM. ACTH enhancement of T-lymphocyte cytotoxic responses. Cell Mol Neurobiol 2005;25:743-757.

14. Liang J, Yao G, Yang L, Hou Y. Dehydroepiandrosterone induces apoptosis of thymocyte through Fas/Fas-L pathway. Int Immunopharmacol 2004;4: 1467-1475.
15. Goya RG, Brown OA, Bolognani F. The thymus-pituitary axis and its changes during aging. Neuroimmunomodulation 1999;6:137-142.
16. Liang J, Sun L, Wang Q, Hou Y. Progesterone regulates mouse dendritic cells differentiation and maturation. Int Immunopharmacol 2006;6:830-838.
17. Butts CL, Shukair SA, Duncan KM, et al. Progesterone inhibits mature rat dendritic cells in a receptor-mediated fashion. Int Immunol 2007;19:287-296.
19. Garvy BA, Fraker PJ. Suppression of the antigenic response of murine bone marrow B cells by

physiological concentrations of glucocorticoids. Immunology 1991;74:519-523.

20. Kalantaridou S, Makrigiannakis A, Zoumakis E, Chrousos GP. Peripheral corticotropin-releasing hormone is produced in the immune and reproductive systems: actions, potential roles and clinical implications. Front Biosci 2007;12:572-580.

22. Grammatopoulos DK, Chrousos GP. Functional characteristics of CRH receptors and potential clinical applications of CRH-receptor antagonists. Trends Endocrinol Metab 2002;13:436-444.

24. Catania A. The melanocortin system in leukocyte biology. J Leukoc Biol 2007;81:383-392.

26. Straub RH, Dhabhar FS, Bijlsma JW, Cutolo M. How psychological stress via hormones and nerve fibers may exacerbate rheumatoid arthritis. Arthritis Rheum 2005;52:16-26.

27. Wilder RL. Hormones, pregnancy, and autoimmune diseases. Ann N Y Acad Sci 1998;840:45-50.

28. Doria A, Iaccarino L, Arienti S, et al. Th2 immune deviation induced by pregnancy: the two faces of autoimmune rheumatic diseases. Reprod Toxicol 2006;22:234-241.

29. Straub RH, Konecna L, Hrach S, et al. Serum dehydroepiandrosterone (DHEA) and DHEA sulfate are negatively correlated with serum interleukin-6 (IL-6), and DHEA inhibits IL-6 secretion from mononuclear cells in man in vitro: possible link between endocrinosenescence and immunosenescence. J Clin Endocrinol Metab 1998;83:2012-2017.

30. van Vollenhoven RF, Engleman EG, McGuire JL. Dehydroepiandrosterone in systemic lupus erythematosus: results of a double-blind, placebo-controlled, randomized clinical trial. Arthritis Rheum 1995;38:1826-1831.

31. Petri MA, Mease PJ, Merrill JT, et al. Effects of prasterone on disease activity and symptoms in women with active systemic lupus erythematosus. Arthritis Rheum 2004;50:2858-2868.

33. Charalampopoulos I, Alexaki VI, Lazaridis I, et al. G protein–associated, specific membrane binding sites mediate the neuroprotective effect of dehydroepiandrosterone. FASEB J 2006;20:577-579.

34. Sternberg EM, Young WS, Bernardini R, et al. A central nervous system defect in biosynthesis of corticotropin-releasing hormone is associated with susceptibility to streptococcal cell wall–induced arthritis in Lewis rats. Proc Natl Acad Sci U S A 1989;86:4771-4775.

36. Tsigos C, Papanicolaou DA, Defensor R, et al. Dose effects of recombinant human interleukin-6 on pituitary hormone secretion and energy expenditure. Neuroendocrinology 1997;66:54-62.

37. Cutolo M, Foppiani L, Prete C, et al. Hypothalamic-pituitary-adrenocortical axis function in premenopausal women with rheumatoid arthritis not treated with glucocorticoids. J Rheumatol 1999;26:282-288.

38. Kanik KS, Chrousos GP, Schumacher HR, et al. Adrenocorticotropin, glucocorticoid, and androgen secretion in patients with new onset synovitis/rheumatoid arthritis: relations with indices of inflammation. J Clin Endocrinol Metab 2000;85:1461-1466.

39. Straub RH, Paimela L, Peltomaa R, et al. Inadequately low serum levels of steroid hormones in relation to IL-6 and TNF in untreated patients with early rheumatoid arthritis and reactive arthritis. Arthritis Rheum 2002;46:654-662.

40. Schmidt M, Weidler C, Naumann H, et al. Reduced capacity for the reactivation of glucocorticoids in rheumatoid arthritis synovial cells: possible role of the sympathetic nervous system? Arthritis Rheum 2005;52:1711-1720.

41. Weidler C, Struharova S, Schmidt M, et al. Tumor necrosis factor inhibits conversion of dehydroepiandrosterone sulfate (DHEAS) to DHEA in rheumatoid arthritis synovial cells: a prerequisite for local androgen deficiency. Arthritis Rheum 2005;52:1721-1729.

42. Cutolo M, Villaggio B, Seriolo B, et al. Synovial fluid estrogens in rheumatoid arthritis. Autoimmun Rev 2004;3:193-198.

43. Straub RH. The complex role of estrogens in inflammation. Endocr Rev 2007;28:521-574.

44. Douin-Echinard V, Laffont S, Seillet C, et al. Estrogen receptor alpha, but not beta, is required for optimal dendritic cell differentiation and [corrected] CD40-induced cytokine production. J Immunol 2008;180:3661-3669.

45. Nalbandian G, Paharkova-Vatchkova V, Mao A, et al. The selective estrogen receptor modulators, tamoxifen and raloxifene, impair dendritic cell differentiation and activation. J Immunol 2005;175:2666-2675.

46. Grimaldi CM, Michael DJ, Diamond B. Cutting edge: expansion and activation of a population of autoreactive marginal zone B cells in a model of estrogen-induced lupus. J Immunol 2001;167:1886-1890.

47. Cutolo M, Sulli A, Villaggio B, et al. Relations between steroid hormones and cytokines in rheumatoid arthritis and systemic lupus erythematosus. Ann Rheum Dis 1998;57:573-577.

49. Cutolo M, Accardo S, Villaggio B, et al. Androgen metabolism and inhibition of interleukin-1 synthesis in

primary cultured human synovial macrophages. Mediators Inflamm 1995;4:138-145.

50. Kanda N, Tsuchida T, Tamaki K. Testosterone suppresses anti-DNA antibody production in peripheral blood mononuclear cells from patients with systemic lupus erythematosus. Arthritis Rheum 1997;40:1703-1711.

52. Nielen MM, van Schaardenburg D, Reesink HW, et al. Specific autoantibodies precede the symptoms of rheumatoid arthritis: a study of serial measurements in blood donors. Arthritis Rheum 2004;50:380-386.

53. Carlsten H, Nilsson N, Jonsson R, et al. Estrogen accelerates immune complex glomerulonephritis but ameliorates T cell–mediated vasculitis and sialadenitis in autoimmune MRL lpr/lpr mice. Cell Immunol 1992;144:190-202.

54. Straub RH, Cutolo M. Circadian rhythms in rheumatoid arthritis: implications for pathophysiology and therapeutic management. Arthritis Rheum 2007;56:399-408.

55. Cutolo M, Straub RH, Buttgereit F. Circadian rhythms of nocturnal hormones in rheumatoid arthritis: translation from bench to bedside. Ann Rheum Dis 2008;67:905-908.

56. Crofford LJ, Kalogeras KT, Mastorakos G, et al. Circadian relationships between interleukin (IL)-6 and hypothalamic-pituitary-adrenal axis hormones: failure of IL-6 to cause sustained hypercortisolism in patients with early untreated rheumatoid arthritis. J Clin Endocrinol Metab 1997;82:1279-1283.

57. Cutolo M, Straub RH. Circadian rhythms in arthritis: hormonal effects on the immune/inflammatory reaction. Autoimmun Rev 2008;7:223-228.

58. Cutolo M. Vitamin D and autoimmune rheumatic diseases. Rheumatology (Oxford) 2009;48:210-212

59. Buttgereit F, Doering G, Schaeffler A, et al. Efficacy of modified-release versus standard prednisone to reduce duration of morning stiffness of the joints in rheumatoid arthritis (CAPRA-1): a double-blind, randomised controlled trial. Lancet 2008;371:205-214.

60. Maestroni GJ, Otsa K, Cutolo M. Melatonin treatment does not improve rheumatoid arthritis. Br J Clin Pharmacol 2008;65:797-798.

61. Kees MG, Pongratz G, Kees F, et al. Via beta-adrenoceptors, stimulation of extrasplenic sympathetic nerve fibers inhibits lipopolysaccharide-induced TNF secretion in perfused rat spleen. J Neuroimmunol 2003;145:77-85.

62. Cutolo M, Straub RH. Insights into endocrine-immunological disturbances in autoimmunity and their impact on treatment. Arthritis Res Ther 2009;11:218.

REFERENCES

Full references for this chapter can be found on www.expertconsult.com.

Interpreting the medical literature for the rheumatologist: study design and levels of evidence

25

Robert B. M. Landewé

INTRODUCTION

In medicine there is a strong belief that randomized controlled trials (RCTs) are superior to observational studies. Randomization does provide indisputable strengths, but data show that RCTs and observational studies often arrive at the same conclusion. Furthermore, there are theoretical and practical problems that preclude the acceptance of RCTs as the only source of useful information: (1) RCTs often address research questions that do not serve the main interest of clinicians; (2) many research questions cannot be solved by RCTs; and (3) an RCT has methodologic requirements that should be met to favor its benefits optimally. Large observational studies are often considered second rate; however, observational cohort studies are sometimes the only source of data available and can often supply useful information to complement RCTs.

Although fundamental theory underlying the RCT—and the primary analysis of a RCT—is relatively simple, practical trial conduct faces a lot of potential pitfalls that may eventually result in the violation of prognostic similarity and introduce bias. Examples are inadvertent unblinding of a study drug (e.g., if the study treatment is very effective while the placebo is not), unbalanced non-random discontinuation (e.g., if the study drug is responsible for adverse drug reactions that cause selective dropout), or simply poor trial conduct or overt misconduct (e.g., if patients do not show up for visits, assessors do not measure outcomes with scrutiny, or, at worst, non-existing or virtual patients with faked response patterns are reported). It is the investigators' responsibility to optimize trial conduct and data collection, to perform a correct analysis of the data, and to transparently describe the process and results of the trial in the medical literature: this is "good clinical practice." The consumers of these reports, peer-reviewers, scientists, rheumatologists, workers in pharmaceutical industry, regulatory authorities, and others have their own responsibility. They have the obligation to interpret the data carefully, weighing their integrity and importance, unprejudiced with respect to the investigators' interpretations, and to translate trial information into useful, clinically applicable information. This process has gained attention as "critical appraisal," and the literature provides superb guidance as to how to critically appraise the report of an RCT.[1,2] Medical journals have agreed on guidelines with respect to trial report (e.g., CONSORT guidelines[3]), thus tremendously improving critical appraisal. Good clinical practice and critical appraisal are applicable to observational research without prejudice, although the focus may be slightly different. Recently, for example, the checklist for STrengthening in Reporting of OBservational Studies in Epidemiology (STROBE) was published in an attempt to improve the quality of reports in this field.[4,5]

In this chapter the focus primarily is on those methodologic elements that in my opinion are most important in critically appraising the results of clinical trials and observational studies with respect to application in clinical practice. Because some of these elements specifically pertain to RCTs, others primarily refer to observational studies, whereas there is also a generic category pertaining to both types of research, there will be three categories of critical appraisal: one primarily referring to RCTs, one referring to observational studies, and one referring to both.

LEVELS OF EVIDENCE

During the past decade the accessibility of medical literature has tremendously improved. It is safe to say that the majority of practicing rheumatologists nowadays can almost immediately get access to (abstracts of) almost every medical study that has been reported in the literature. In addition, meta-analysis and systematic literature review, in which the available literature is weighed and judged in a systematic manner and data are pooled, have become an art of science. In an attempt to bring some order to the quality of epidemiologic research, and consequently to prioritize types of research with respect to methodologic rigor, several scales have been developed. One of the more comprehensive scales (with most differentiation) is the Oxford Center for Evidence-Based Medicine Scale, which applies levels of evidence to five different study scenarios (therapy, prognosis, diagnosis, differential diagnosis, and economic analysis).[6] In general, such scales rate systematic reviews and appropriately conducted meta-analyses higher than individual RCTs, followed by observational studies, followed by case series, with expert opinion at the lowest level. Although level of evidence scales can be very helpful in prioritizing (the quality of) studies, a note of caution is given. Often, a study is inappropriately rated. An unplanned subgroup observation in the context of an RCT, for example, should not be rated level 1, because the result is not obtained in an unbiased manner (see later), whereas a methodologically weak RCT also does not deserve a rate of 1. Sometimes, "low-grade evidence" is the only kind of evidence that can be obtained, for example, if the disease under study is very rare or if an RCT is considered unethical. Those who have been involved in the development of guidelines realize that a lot of what physicians do on an everyday basis is based on "expert opinion" and not substantiated by any study at all.

Instead of relying entirely on levels of evidence, readers of the medical literature should rather rate the studies themselves and try to get some insight in what the aim of the study is, how the study has been performed, and what should be the impact of the results with regard to their own patients.

RCTs OR OBSERVATIONAL STUDIES?

A typical RCT investigates whether a new drug, strategy, or intervention is efficacious and safe in comparison with an equivalent treatment or placebo. The trial involves patient selection and randomization before the treatment begins and, thereafter, a predetermined follow-up time to establish whether the primary endpoint (the measure of the treatment effect) has been met. The most characteristic feature, and the major advantage of the RCT, is randomization. Technically, this process divides patients according to all known and unknown prognostically important factors across treatment groups and thereby creates a situation of similarity with respect to likely prognosis, at baseline. Or, in other words, treatment groups are similar for everything except allocated treatment. Prognostic similarity at baseline is important for attributing an observed effect to a particular treatment rather than to an imbalance in an unrelated, but prognostically important, factor.

RCTs also have important drawbacks. These trials might lack external validity, or generalizability. Inclusion criteria and exclusion criteria ensure that the trial population is a particular selection of the entire population with a certain disease. An RCT includes patients that are "prone to change," that might have a high level of adherence to the protocol so as to ensure retention, or that have a low probability of adverse reactions from co-morbidity and/or co-medication. Consequently, such a trial population comprises highly motivated, often educated individuals who have a high level of disease activity but who are otherwise healthy. This scenario usually does not appropriately reflect the normal clinical situation.

Another disadvantage of RCTs is their often relatively short follow-up time. There are several trivial explanations, but probably the most important argument is that true prognostic similarity only exists at baseline and gets increasingly lost over time. Take, for example, co-medication or other coincident interventions. A short follow-up period is methodologically advantageous (see internal validity, later) but may in rheumatology reflect only a small period of the entire duration that a patient is under observation for a chronic disease in real practice. As a consequence, RCTs often use surrogate endpoints rather than endpoints that truly reflect the clinical outcome of the disease. An appropriate example in this respect is the use of bone mineral density as a surrogate outcome measure for fractures in osteoporosis trials. It largely depends on the study question whether an RCT will provide the most appropriate answer. RCTs do provide a reliable impression of short-term efficacy and safety of drugs in a selection of patients. They do not, however, provide information about an individual patient's prognosis, long-term results on relevant outcomes, and data about rare events. It is here that observational studies, with many patients and long follow-up, might prove their value.

CRITICAL APPRAISAL I: ISSUES PERTAINING TO RCTs

Internal validity and external validity

A trial is a rather artificial construct that usually serves one main purpose: to investigate whether a particular treatment is efficacious. In general, elements of trial design, such as the selection of patients, the sample size, the choice of the comparative intervention, and the duration of the trial, are chosen in such a manner that the trial can optimally demonstrate a treatment effect, that is, a difference in efficacy between the new treatment and the control intervention. The methodologic rigor of a trial, which is dependent on these elements of trial design, is referred to as *internal validity*.

Understandably, trials often do not resemble clinical practice. Rheumatoid arthritis (RA) trials, for example, often include patients with a high level of disease activity, which may form only a minority in clinical practice. The extent to which clinical trial results can be extrapolated to the common clinical practice is referred to as *external validity*. External validity is much more diffuse than internal validity. It depends on how the consumer of the data interprets the results, how these results are presented, how convincingly the investigators have argued their message, and how credible they are in the eyes of the beholder. It depends on whether the reader thinks the data of the trial are applicable to an individual patient in the reader's own practice. Undoubtedly, external validity will be judged as unsatisfactory if internal validity falls short. The opposite is not necessarily true. A trial with high internal validity can easily have insufficient external validity. An increasingly common example in RA is the RCT with 1000 patients with high disease activity that tests a new treatment against the "currently best available disease modifying treatment for RA" and finds a small, statistically significant difference in favor of the new treatment that is not very clinically relevant. Such a new treatment will probably be approved by drug registration authorities if it is considered safe, because it has proven superiority in a well-conducted trial with high internal validity. Needless to say, this effective treatment with doubtful advantage over existing treatments should not be broadly applied in common clinical practice without further consideration (external validation). Readers of trial reports should weigh the balance between internal and external validity, which of both prevails, where one falls short in favor of the other, and which elements are important in translating the trial result into clinical practice.

Efficacy versus effectiveness

It is obligatory to be informed about the underlying aim of the trial, which is not necessarily the same as the primary study objective. Drug registration trials under the auspices of the pharmaceutical industry serve a different purpose than investigator-initiated trials with treatment strategies. The former are often referred to as explanatory or efficacy trials and are characterized by a high level of internal validity, whereas the latter—pragmatic trials or effectiveness trials—more closely resemble clinical practice, often find their basis in questions emerging from clinical practice, and, as a consequence, have a higher level of external validity.[7]

The results of explanatory trials are often very robust and confirm the efficacy of the tested drug beyond statistical doubt but may fall short in terms of clinical significance. Examples are numerous and include any trial that presents results of a "new drug" tested against placebo or an active comparator.

Effectiveness trials often have a more understandable trial result that is more easily applicable in individual patients, but results may be biased, for example, by imperfections in blinding and changes in kind and intensity of treatment during the trial. An interesting type of trial that belongs to this group is the *benchmark trial* in RA. The essential characteristic of the benchmark trial is that treatment (kind and/or intensity) is not kept constant during the course of the trial but is dependent on the clinical response of the individual patient (whether the benchmark is met or not). Such a trial mimics everyday clinical practice very well but is in conflict with fundamental theory underlying RCTs, namely, that patient groups in a trial are prognostically similar during the trial. The methodologic robustness of the trial is to some extent jeopardized by increased clinical face validity. Readers should have knowledge of these elements because they are relevant for the interpretation of the results and the decision about their usefulness for application in individual patients.

Superiority trials and non-inferiority trials

Textbooks in clinical trial design teach that the underlying null hypothesis should be carefully formulated during the design phase of the trial. The formulation of the null hypothesis, which is in theory the hypothesis that is challenged by experimentation (the trial), tells immediately whether the basic design of the RCT aims at proving superior efficacy of a new treatment (the superiority design) or at proving that a new drug treatment is as effective as a comparator drug, for ethical reasons often the current standard of therapy (the non-inferiority design). The RCTs we have seen during the past decade in rheumatology most often had a superiority design, with the null hypothesis that the new treatment was as efficacious as placebo or a comparator treatment. The design of the trial and the sample size are dependent on a *minimally important difference,* which is determined upfront by the investigators and serves as the basis for sample size calculations. In rheumatology, many consecutive RCTs have resulted in a number of treatments that have proven efficacy against placebo or against the standard of care therapy.

An affluence of effective treatments such as in RA has its other side of the coin. First, there is increasing sympathy for the ethical argument that progress in the treatment of rheumatic diseases should have its consequences for the standard of care in this disease. The immediate implication with regard to trial design is that conventional RCTs with placebo as therapy in the control group will be considered unethical. The more effective the therapy in the control group is, the more difficult it is to surpass the effect in the control group with a new treatment: the classic superiority trial will be increasingly unfeasible.

Second, although we have that affluence of effective drugs such as in RA, there is a knowledge gap with respect to drug efficacy in mutual comparison. Using previous argumentation, these pregnant clinical questions cannot be solved with classic trial designs. Therefore we will probably see an increasing number of non-inferiority trials in rheumatology in the near future.[8] Such trials have as a null hypothesis that the new drug is inferior to the effective treatment in the control arm and embark on the determination of an appropriate *non-inferiority margin*. More than the choice of a minimally important difference in superiority trials, the choice of a non-inferiority margin in a non-inferiority trial is a highly subjective decision that includes elements of efficacy, safety, and costs and can make or break the interpretability of such a trial. It is crucial that readers know about elements of the null hypothesis, such as choices and considerations relating to the design type of the trial (superiority vs. non-inferiority) and relating to levels of minimally important difference and non-inferiority margin.

Statistical power

Every RCT should technically be able to reject the null hypothesis if the alternative hypothesis reflects the truth: it should have sufficient statistical power. One could justifiably argue that trials with insufficient power should not have been executed. It is unethical to expose patients to potentially harmful drugs if the trial is not able to demonstrate superiority or non-inferiority of that drug, it fills medical literature with data that are inconclusive, with the risk of misinterpretation and inappropriate application for patient care, and it is extremely cost ineffective to execute trials that do not meet their goals. So, it seems obvious that the reader of a trial report ascertains that statistical power was appropriate. Many do not realize that statistical power is more than sample size alone. Although the latter is of most importance, statistical power is, among other factors, dependent on the outcome measure (the responsiveness and discriminatory capacity) and the expected effect size (the anticipated difference between the new treatment and the control treatment). The wording justifying the sample size of the trial gives to some extent resolution about the power considerations. In sample size calculations, patient numbers are calculated for a given primary outcome measure with an assumption for its *variability*, for given values of *beta* (1-statistical power) and for a predefined *effect size*. Sometimes, the anticipated effect size is based on realistic assumptions stemming from previous studies, but all too often an effect is chosen that has no scientific precedent ("20% between-group difference"). Some investigators want 80% statistical power, others choose 90% power as preference, and all too often the reader is left with the impression that convenience outweighs theoretical arguments about power: "the calculation should fit." Rather than only describing the sample size calculation *per se* (which is often done inappropriately), the trial report should include argumentation for the chosen assumptions, such as the level of the minimal clinically important difference, the non-inferiority margin, the level of beta, the historic precedents, and so on, and the reader should try to interpret this cautiously.

Intention-to-treat analysis

Every investigator, every trial designer, and every clinician knows about the dogmatic character of the intention-to-treat (ITT) principle underlying the main analysis of a clinical trial. Although occasionally a paper mentions a surrogate of ITT (e.g., "modified ITT analysis"), the definition of ITT is crystal clear. It means that every patient in the trial is considered to belong to the group that he or she was originally allocated to by randomization, regardless of what has happened with this patient during the trial. The justification for this somewhat dogmatic principle is that the ITT analysis is the most conservative analysis because it preserves at least the prognostic similarity that was created at baseline by randomization. All other types of analyses, including "modified ITT," are second rate because they allow retrograde patient selection at baseline. The typical *completers analysis*, for example, only includes those patients who have done well on the allocated study treatment and ignores the patients who have discontinued, and may differ from the completing patients in terms of prognosis (prognostic dissimilarity). In fact, the completers of an RCT form a selected group of patients and should be considered as an observational cohort rather than a trial group (see later).

ITT is not a certificate for an appropriate trial analysis. The trial report should spell out how patients who do not provide actually measured trial data are handled (see Missing data, later). It should mention how data generated by patients who discontinued trial medication but showed up at visits are handled. And last, but not least, there is no generic means of data manipulation in this regard. For example, considering every dropout as not having changed (improved) in a clinical trial with RA patients and the ACR20 as the primary outcome measure is probably conservative, because a proportion of these patients will

CHAPTER 25 ● Interpreting the medical literature for the rheumatologist: study design and levels of evidence

TABLE 25.1 EXAMPLE OF INTENTION-TO-TREAT ANALYSIS

	Treatment A (N = 100)	Treatment B (N = 100)
Number of patients who discontinued the trial	15	15
Number of patients who completed the trial	85	85
With clinical response	25	20
Number of patients taking rescue medication	10	30
With clinical response	2	20
Response percentages based on:		
ITT analysis	25% (25/100)	20% (20/100)
Completers analysis	29% (25/85)	24% (20/85)
Per protocol analysis	31% (23/75)	9% (5/55)

have had a clinical response. However, considering these dropouts as not having changed in a clinical trial with radiographic progression as the outcome measure is all but conservative, because it looks as if the dropouts do not have progression, and a trial arm with a high proportion of premature discontinuations may be spuriously benefited.

In summary, ITT together with appropriate handling of data, including appropriate imputation, works conservatively in that it tends to reduce a treatment contrast.

Conservatism, however, is not necessarily a guarantee for a more truthful trial result. In the non-inferiority trial, ITT may spuriously lead to a conclusion of non-inferiority, whereas in truth unbalanced withdrawal, poor trial conduct, or unintended co-interventions may be responsible for the absence of a difference between treatment groups. An example may clarify this (Table 25.1). Suppose that two analgesic drugs (A and B) are compared with respect to their ability to relieve pain in an RCT and that drug A is in truth more effective than drug B (which of course you do not know in reality). The primary outcome measure is the number of patients with 40% decrease in pain on a visual analog scale. Suppose also that patients take additional acetaminophen if they experience too much pain ("rescue analgesia"). Expectedly, the proportion of patients taking additional medication is lower in group A (the better treatment) as compared with group B (10 patients vs. 30 patients). Also expectedly, only 2 of these 10 patients in group A needing additional drug experienced a response (the severe cases), whereas 20 of the 30 patients needing additional drug (the milder cases) in group B experienced a response (attributable to co-medication). Table 25.1 shows how different types of analysis (ITT vs. per-protocol) work with regard to response percentages and treatment effect. Keep in mind that in reality drug A is more efficacious than drug B. The unbalanced use of co-medication resulted in (only) 5% more responses in group A versus group B if analyzed by ITT. This is a small difference, probably not compatible with a conclusion of superiority of drug A in a trial with a superiority design but easily compatible with a conclusion of non-inferiority of drug B in a trial with a non-inferiority design. The picture changes, however, if you repeat the analysis on a per-protocol basis. Now, the treatment effect is almost 20% more responders in group A versus group B, probably compatible with the superiority of drug A in a trial with a superiority design and incompatible with the non-inferiority of drug B in a trial with a non-inferiority design: ITT analysis is conservative with respect to concluding superiority of a drug in a superiority design (even if in reality superiority exists). Per-protocol analysis is conservative with respect to concluding non-inferiority in a non-inferiority design.

The analysis of non-inferiority trials is not yet a closed book, but experts are in favor of simultaneously presenting ITT and per-protocol analyses, so that the reader can judge for himself or herself. It is always wise to be careful with interpretation if both analyses differ importantly (such as in this example).

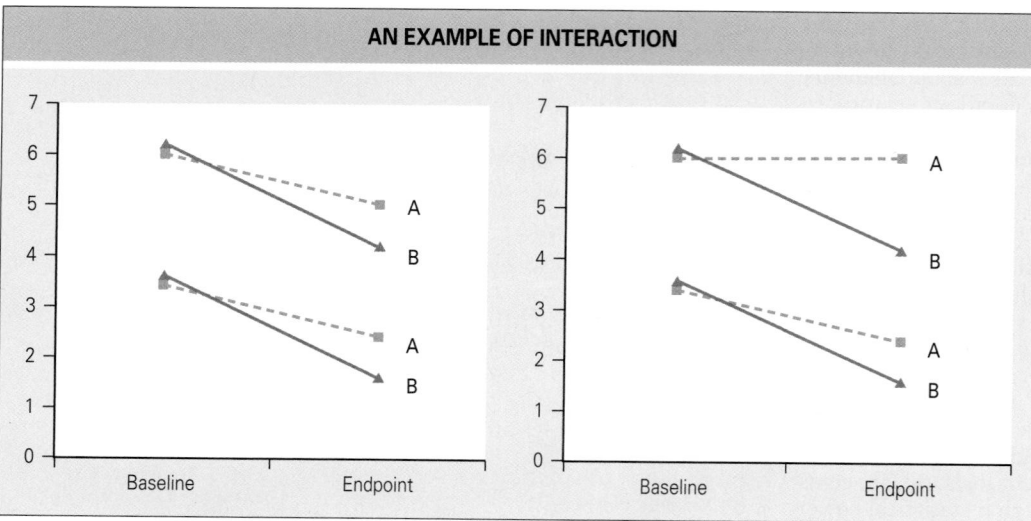

Fig. 25.1 An example of interaction. Results of a subgroup analysis of an imaginary clinical trial comparing two treatments (dashed line with squares: treatment A, solid line with triangles: treatment B) in a subgroup with high baseline disease activity and a subgroup with low baseline disease activity. See text for clarification.

Subgroup analyses

The issue of subgroup analysis in clinical trials is controversial. The proponents of subgroup analysis point to its hypothesis-generating potential. The opponents argue that subgroup analysis is irresponsible data-mining by looking for statistically significant differences by splitting up the trial population into smaller subgroups. Both parties are right to some extent. Subgroup analysis can sometimes help to disentangle incomprehensible trial results and can raise attention to new, previously unacknowledged phenomena. But inappropriate subgroup analysis can also provide spurious results, either by coincidence (multiple testing effects) or by unintended patient selection mechanisms. An example of the latter is as follows: the investigators of an RCT compare radiographic progression in a subgroup of patients with an early clinical response and a subgroup of patients without an early response and find that progression is significantly lower in the first subgroup. This result, however, may easily be confounded by less severe disease at baseline in the favorable subgroup.

It is relevant to some extent to divide subgroup analysis into pre-planned and *post-hoc* subgroup analysis. The former refers to the design phase of the trial and includes analyses in subgroups that are of potential relevance, such as the treatment effect tested in men and women separately or in rheumatoid factor positive and negative patients. Importantly, and in contrast to *post-hoc* subgroup analysis, the decision to perform and report such an analysis cannot be driven by knowing the data. In practice, however, it is often difficult to find out whether a preplanned subgroup analysis is truly preplanned or not. Methodologically, preplanned subgroup analysis is only superior to *post-hoc* analysis if subgroups of interest were created by *stratified randomization*, which means randomization within the subgroups. It is hoped that stratified randomization creates prognostic similarity within the strata (a trial within a trial), and—if performed appropriately—provides sufficient statistical power to detect a meaningful difference within the subgroup.

Usually, subgroup analysis is not performed in subgroups created by stratified randomization. If subgroup analysis is performed, and the question of interest is whether a particular treatment performs differently in subgroup X as compared with subgroup Y, it is important to realize that the analytical translation of this question refers to testing statistical interaction.

Figure 25.1 shows an example of such an interaction. In the first panel, treatment A is less effective than treatment B, both in the subgroup of patients with high disease activity and in the subgroup of patients with low disease activity. The treatment effect is similar in both subgroups: no interaction.

In the second panel, however, the treatment effect is dependent on the subgroup of disease activity. Although treatment A seems effective in patients with low disease activity, though less effective than

treatment B, it seems completely ineffective in patients with high disease activity, whereas treatment B is still effective in this subgroup: interaction. Very often, the absence of efficacy in the subgroup of patients with high disease activity is found and reported while the other subgroup is ignored, so that it is not clear whether a presumed effect is truly attributable to a specific subgroup. This type of subgroup analysis only makes sense if the interaction is demonstrated and confirmed statistically. The issue of how to statistically test interaction is beyond the scope of this chapter.

In summary, subgroup analysis can be informative but there are certain rules of play, among which the most important probably is to interpret subgroup analyses cautiously and with reservation.

CRITICAL APPRAISAL II: ISSUES PERTAINING TO OBSERVATIONAL STUDIES

Types of cohorts

Usually, observational research involves the prospective follow-up of a group of individuals (cohort) with regard to a particular outcome. That outcome can be an event (e.g., death, clinical remission) but can also be a disease activity state over time (e.g., time-averaged disease activity state, mean swollen joint count). The types of cohorts that can be encountered in literature can grossly be divided into two: healthy cohorts and clinical cohorts. It is relevant for the reader of an article to realize what type of cohort is studied.

Healthy cohorts

Healthy cohorts are large cohorts of individuals that are healthy with respect to the outcome of interest (although possibly not in other aspects). Often study subjects belong to some group of easily traceable individuals (e.g., nurses or physicians). The outcome of interest is usually simple and unequivocal (e.g,. mortality), cohorts are large, and follow-up is typically long. The research question of interest might refer to an intervention but also to a potential risk factor or an exposure. Famous examples of healthy cohort studies are the Baltimore Longitudinal Study of Aging, the Framingham study, the Johns Hopkins Precursors Study, and the Nurses Health Cohort. Very often, and understandably, these large cohorts are used to address multiple different study questions and are, sometimes, therefore, referred to as "multipurpose cohorts."

Clinical cohorts

Clinical cohorts include patients with one or more features in common who are followed for a definite or indefinite time with respect to one or more primary outcomes. There are several types of clinical cohorts. Inception cohorts include and follow all patients in whom a particular disease is diagnosed (disease duration at baseline = 0). Prevalence cohorts include and follow patients with a particular disease at a certain point in time (disease duration at baseline > 0). Patient registries include and follow patients with a particular disease and a particular feature (e.g., patients with RA who start a particular treatment). The distinction between cohorts and registries is subtle and often, but not always, relates to the time of follow-up. A cohort has usually a previously defined (limited) follow-up (although often this follow-up duration is adjusted over time); a registry has, in principle, an undefined (unlimited) follow-up duration.

A special form of observational prevalence cohort that is frequently seen in rheumatology is the follow-up cohort of an RCT, the purpose of which is often to investigate whether a particular effect seen in an RCT can be maintained over a longer period of time. Occasionally, trial arms of the original RCT are preserved during the follow-up period, but often they are not. Importantly, results from follow-up studies of RCTs should not be interpreted as if they have the same scientific rigor as the RCT itself. The prognostic similarity created by randomization only exists at baseline but is increasingly lost over time, particularly when trial blinding is unveiled and patients are asked to continue in a follow-up study. The type of longitudinal bias that might arise is discussed in the next section. One specific limitation of such cohorts with regard to generalizability is that the patients in the cohort stem from a clinical trial and reflect a population with relatively severe disease, high disease activity at baseline, and so on. One should keep in mind that the relatively mild cases are by definition not included in the cohort, which has implications for the interpretability of prognostic variables derived from such cohorts.

Selection bias

Looking at the characteristics of observational studies as outlined earlier, it is obvious that they are a better reflection of common clinical practice than RCTs are, perhaps with the exception of follow-up studies of RCTs. That is also their major advantage. But cohorts and registries are not unselected populations. A number of selection mechanisms might influence the interpretation of results, and three well-known examples will be discussed.

Left-censorship bias

Left-censorship bias can occur if patients with particular characteristics are inadvertently excluded from the observational cohort because they are simply not available. Suppose you want to investigate the relationship between cyclooxygenase-2 (COX-2) inhibitors and cardiovascular morbidity in a database of 10,000 patients, including all prevalent patients with osteoarthritis. The study does not include patients who were at such a high risk of cardiovascular death that the outcome (death) has already occurred before entry into the study. As a consequence, the observed mortality rate in this cohort might be an underestimate of the truth, especially if COX-2 inhibitors are particularly dangerous in high-risk patients.

In general, left-censorship bias occurs at the formation of the cohort, or before the cohort is formed, it refers to selection based on differences in disease severity, and it is important only if severity is related to the outcome of interest. By definition, its influence is difficult to quantify and it is impossible to adjust for left-censorship bias in the analysis.

Right-censorship bias

Right-censorship bias is also known as "selective dropout" or "attrition." Suppose, in an RCT using a COX-2 inhibitor that patients at higher risk of adverse gastrointestinal events had a higher dropout rate than those at low risk. This would lead to a spuriously low rate of adverse gastrointestinal events in those patients who remain in any open follow-up. A kind of right-censorship bias that most readers will be familiar with is bias by trial completion, or "completers" bias, which is often seen in follow-up studies of RCTs. Only those patients who perceive that their treatment is effective, and/or tolerate it best, remain in the study, which provides favorable study results for that drug.

Right-censorship bias occurs after the composition of the cohort, during follow-up, refers to selection based on differences in disease severity or disease activity, and is important if severity or activity is associated with outcome. Right-censorship bias can be quantified and adjusted for in the analysis to some extent.

Confounding by indication

Confounding by indication refers to the question of which patient begins treatment with which drug. Suppose, in a clinical practice setting, that patients at high risk of gastrointestinal events are initially given COX-2 inhibitors, whereas those at lower risk are given conventional non-steroidal anti-inflammatory drugs (NSAIDs). A higher event rate is found in patients with COX-2 inhibitors as compared with patients treated with NSAIDs; however, the rate in these high-risk patients might still be lower than it would have been if they had been treated using conventional NSAIDs.

Confounding by indication can occur before, but also after, the composition of the cohort; it refers to situations in which the severity of the disease determines the choice of treatment, and it is important if treatment and disease severity are both related to outcome. There are techniques that quantify the severity of disease so that it is possible to adjust for confounding by indication.

CRITICAL APPRAISAL III: ISSUES PERTAINING TO RCTs AND OBSERVATIONAL STUDIES

Generalizability

As argued earlier, the type of patients included in a study is of pivotal importance with respect to the interpretation of the trial results. In efficacy trials, statistical power—the probability that the trial confirms the superiority of a new treatment if this superiority truly exists—is of eminent importance. Discriminatory ability and sensitivity to change of outcome measures are determinants of statistical power. The outcome measures propagated for clinical trials in RA, such as American College of Rheumatology (ACR)[9] and European League Against Rheumatism (EULAR)[10] response criteria, perform best—and have been validated—in patient groups with high levels of disease activity, which is why most efficacy trials include these patients. In the spectrum of patients with RA, however, these patients do not constitute a majority, which may have implications for the interpretation of trial results. It is possible, if not likely, that many RA patients with less active disease do not necessarily need the "new treatment" that tested most effectively in the efficacy trial but can do very well with the comparator drug.

Another discrepancy between observational studies (clinical practice) and RCT is the paucity of clinically relevant co-morbid conditions in RCTs as compared with clinical practice, because patients with relevant co-morbidities are usually excluded. Similar reasoning can be followed regarding compliance or, in general, any reason that increases the probability of premature discontinuation and/or non-response.

It is very important when appraising a report of a clinical trial to realize that the patients in the trial do not necessarily resemble the individual patient in clinical practice and that such discrepancies may have consequences for the translation of trial results. Study reports should include all necessary information about disease activity, severity, and prognosis (which they often do) but also information about relevant co-morbidity and co-medication (which they often exclude) to allow the reader an appropriate interpretation of generalizability.

Missing data

Ideally, RCTs and observational studies should provide complete data. Practically, studies without missing data do not exist. Patients miss planned visits for whatever reason and do that more frequently than any investigator would consider acceptable. Or patients withdraw consent, lose motivation, and drop out. Or patients report adverse events to the investigator, who decides to discontinue the patient from the study. Or the investigator and the patient are disappointed with regard to a drug effect and decide to stop. Or a patient moves and gets lost to follow-up. All these examples create missing data. Although the examples given here will be very familiar to every reader (and will be considered inherent to clinical practice), methodology, statistical analysis, and interpretation of study results do not very well comply with the problem of missing data. It is crucial to realize the issue of missing data before the study starts and to consider scenarios of how to handle missing data. There is not one acceptable generic solution, but by far the worst solution is to entirely withdraw the patient from the analysis. Usually, discontinuation is a non-random process, which means that the reason why patients withdraw is somehow associated with disease severity and therefore with the probability of achieving an outcome or a treatment response (confounding). Ignoring these patients means that, in a trial, treatment groups cannot be considered prognostically similar anymore, which is probably the most important violation of trial methodology you can commit, and, in observational studies, that your results may be biased by selection.

Data imputation is the only alternative. Imputation means that an imaginary value is attributed to missing assessments, so that the patient with missing data remains in the analysis, but the question obviously is what to impute. *Non-responder imputation* is a popular and conservative means of data imputation in clinical trials with a response measure (e.g., ACR20) as primary outcome variable. It simply attributes non-response to every patient that discontinues from the trial, irrespective of the reason for discontinuation. *Last-observation-carried forward (LOCF)* and *baseline-observation-carried forward (BOCF)* are popular means of imputing continuous data, in which the last value or the baseline value that was actually measured, respectively, are imputed as a substitute for subsequent missing assessments. *Worst-case scenarios* impute the worst group value or the value representing the 95th percentile. Imputation of group means or group medians is also used. *Linear interpolation* can be useful if in-between data points are missed, and *linear extrapolation* is used if the expected time course follows an approximately linear trend. Finally, sophisticated computer algorithms (e.g., Bayesian, Markov chain, Monte Carlo multiple imputation procedure) exist that use multiple imputation techniques. A discussion of such techniques is beyond the scope of this chapter.

As argued, there is not a single acceptable means of imputation. Non-responder imputation usually works well if a predefined response is the outcome of interest, and LOCF seems a reasonably conservative approach for imputation of missing continuous data in a setting in which treatment should improve a preexistent state (e.g., disease activity, physical function). Linear extrapolation is frequently used to impute missing radiographic data, because the natural course of radiographic damage is compatible with worsening, and LOCF would result in a spurious inhibition of progression. In theory, trial results (i.e., the treatment contrast) should not be dependent on what means of data imputation for missing data is used. The only transparent way of confirming the robustness of the study result is to perform and show sensitivity analyses for missing data. This means that you perform different means of imputation and check the consequences with regard to the outcome of interest.

Data interpretation

Probably the most important means of communicating study results is by graphs. A well-designed graph provides far more information than a table with comprehensive descriptive data, such as means, standard deviations, and so on. An appropriate graphic representation of treatment results can give you a good idea about the relative efficacy of a new treatment in comparison with a control drug at first glance. Every reader of RA clinical trial articles will be familiar with the informative bar graph representation of ACR20/50/70 responses per group. More cumbersome is the graphic representation of radiographic progression. The most frequently used Sharp–van der Heijde progression score usually has a *skewed* distribution, meaning that the data are not normally distributed. Very often, a dataset of radiographic progression scores includes a high number of zero scores and a relatively low number of positive scores, with a minority of extreme progression scores at the right side of the spectrum. This feature means that the usual parametric descriptive statistics such as means and standard deviations do not appropriately reflect what has actually happened in the group. Medians and percentiles (25%, 75%) do a better job in that respect, but median progression in modern clinical trials in RA is often zero in the intervention as well as the control group, whereas progression is statistically significantly different. Recently, probability plots have been proposed to fill in this gap of communication.[11] A probability plot shows every individual change score per trial arm that is ordered from the lowest through the highest observed value and is plotted against its cumulative probability. By superposing the plots of the trial arms in one graph, it is clear at first glance how the groups have performed with respect to radiographic progression.

Tabulation of data is important for several reasons: (1) to underscore the author's conclusions and make them transparent to critical appraisal; (2) to make additional inferences for data interpretation (examples are calculations for *number-needed-to-treat* (NNT) and *effect sizes* for researchers interested in the performance of outcome measures), and (3) as a source for the meta-analyst. It is critical that the authors of a trial report realize that their data may be used for several scientific purposes, and they should provide sufficient information. It is difficult to give exact guidelines, because prerequisites are different for different outcome measures, but a few examples may help. When the ACR response is used as an outcome measure, it is crucial to report not only proportions but also crude numbers (nominator as well as denominator). When continuous outcome measures (e.g., swollen joint count, disease activity state) are reported, data about status as well as change should be provided as means and appropriate standard deviations (rather than standard errors of the mean), as well as the actual number of patients who were used in the analysis. When distributions of continuous outcome measures are overtly skewed (e.g., radiographic progression scores), the investigators should not only present means and standard deviations but also medians and key percentiles (e.g., 25th, 75th). With regard to reporting on radiographic progression, there is consensus that—in the interest of the meta-analyst—also logarithmically transformed progression scores are reported in the tables.[12]

The statistical test

The main goal of the statistical analysis in the report of a trial or an observational study is to challenge the null hypothesis or, in other words, to find probabilistic support for a difference observed between treatments (trial) or for a (predictive) association (observational study). A second aim of statistical testing is to find out about the robustness of a demonstrated effect.

In flagrant contrast to what is often done, in reality the statistical analysis should only take a modest place in the report of a study. However, many authors cannot resist the attractiveness of "$P < .0001$" and build their article around the statistical test result rather than the opposite. Unfortunately, many of these authors are unable to reproduce the correct interpretation of $P < .0001$ and counter critical questions about the relevance of the effect with "It is highly statistically significant, though, isn't it?" .implying that the effect is clinically important.

The P value is a probability, namely, the probability that, assuming that the null hypothesis is correct, this null hypothesis is nevertheless rejected. This sentence is only comprehensible if one realizes that the clinical trial one is looking at is only one (random) example of many, let us say 1000 imaginary similar trials. Who accepts this will also accept that all 1000 imaginary trials will have 1000 different results. The majority only slightly differ, but a few will have more deviant results, simply by coincidence, and a very few will even have extremely deviant results in either direction, whereas in truth the difference should be zero! In theory, such differences could be of such a magnitude that they lead to rejecting the null hypothesis. We talk about erroneous rejection of the null hypothesis, or type I error. The P value is the probability of type I error. $P < .0001$ means that there is very, very small chance of type I error. You could say that the result is very robust, and such a P value adds to the credibility of the trial (internal validity). It does not say that the difference that was found is a relevant difference or that an effect is meaningful. Current efficacy trials are often so powerful in statistically underscoring small differences that very good P values can be obtained with treatment effects that are negligible when considered in the context of patient care. So, statistically significant does not imply clinically relevant. The opposite is also true: not statistically significant does not mean not relevant or in other words: "The absence of evidence is not the same as the evidence of absence (of a meaningful effect)," a statement referring to type II error (see later).

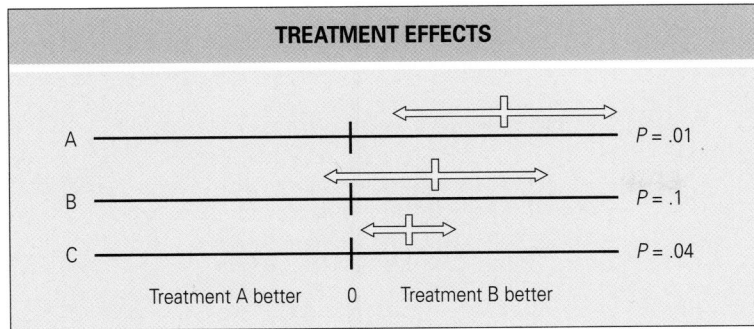

Fig. 25.2 Treatment effects and 95% confidence intervals of three potential scenarios (A, B, and C) for an imaginary clinical trial comparing treatment A and treatment B. See text for clarification.

95% confidence intervals around the mean improvements in disease activity state. Note that the 95% CIs of scenarios A and C lie entirely right from zero. Both treatment effects are statistically significant ($P < .05$): The null hypothesis of "no difference" is rejected. Note that the 95% CI in scenario B crosses zero. The treatment effect is not statistically significant ($P > .05$); the null hypothesis is not rejected. Note also that notwithstanding a *smaller* treatment effect in scenario C as compared with B, the treatment effect in C is statistically significant, as represented by a narrower 95% CI. We say that the trial result is more *precise*. It is the combination of statistical information and information about the preciseness of the treatment effect that make 95% CIs such attractive tools in clinical trials. To improve information exchange and interpretation of trial results, it is almost mandatory to present 95% CIs around the mean treatment effects and not only P values. As with many generic rules, occasionally, the balance dips to the other side: it is not particularly useful and often confusing to present 95% CIs of variables not related to treatment effects (or related to hypothesis testing). An example is the presentation of 95% CIs around the mean disease activity score 28 (DAS28) at baseline.

CONCLUSION

In this chapter, a wide array of points to consider in the critical appraisal of RCTs and observational studies have been addressed. Emphasis is placed on issues referring to external validity or generalizability, because that is what most rheumatologists need to know. As mentioned in the introduction, the choice of the addressed issues is subjective and is by no means intended to cover everything that is important in appraising study data.

It is hoped that the points that are raised will increase the awareness of the importance of the interplay between the clinical investigator responsible for the study report and the consumer of the data, often the clinician, who has to decide about the application of study results in the area of clinical medicine, that which affects the individual patient. Only an appropriate communication in this area will ultimately improve patient care.

The second aim of statistical analysis is to find out about how robust the trial results are. Actually you are interested in the implications with respect to the size of the treatment effect. Usually, a 95% confidence interval (CI) is used to describe the bandwidth for the estimate of the treatment effect. Elaborating on the discussion about P value, the 95% CI is best understandable by imagining that a particular trial is done 1000 times. In 95% of the times the trial result (the estimate of the treatment effect) will lie between the limits of the 95% CI, but in 5% of the times the treatment effect will take a more extreme value. The relation between P value and 95% CI is further clarified in Figure 25.2. Suppose a clinical trial in RA patients with two treatment arms (A vs. B) and (improvement in) disease activity state as the outcome measure. Three possible treatment effects are plotted in a diagram that a reader of meta-analysis may be familiar with. The zero treatment effect reflects the level of equivalence. All three scenarios represent a trial result in which treatment B is better than treatment A (more improvement in disease activity state with B as compared with A). The P values are presented per scenario. The arrows represent the

REFERENCES

1. Guyatt GH, Sackett DL, Cook DJ. Users' guides to the medical literature: II. How to use an article about therapy or prevention: A. Are the results of the study valid? Evidence-Based Medicine Working Group. JAMA 1993;270:2598-2601.
2. Guyatt GH, Sackett DL, Cook DJ. Users' guides to the medical literature: II. How to use an article about therapy or prevention: B. What were the results and will they help me in caring for my patients? Evidence-Based Medicine Working Group. JAMA 1994;271:59-63.
3. Begg C, Cho M, Eastwood S, et al. Improving the quality of reporting of randomized controlled trials—the CONSORT statement. JAMA 1996;276:637-639.
4. von Elm E, Altman DG, Egger M, et al. The Strengthening the Reporting of Observational Studies in Epidemiology (STROBE) statement: guidelines for reporting observational studies. Ann Intern Med 2007;147:573-577.
5. Vandenbroucke JP, von Elm E, Altman DG, et al. Strengthening the Reporting of Observational Studies in Epidemiology (STROBE): explanation and elaboration. Ann Intern Med 2007;147:W163-W194.
6. Oxford Centre for Evidence-Based Medicine. Levels of evidence. 1995. Available at http://www.cebm.net/index.aspx?o=1025.
7. McMahon AD. Study control, violators, inclusion criteria and defining explanatory and pragmatic trials. Stat Med 2002;21:1365-1376.
8. D'Agostino RB Sr, Massaro JM, Sullivan LM. Non-inferiority trials: design concepts and issues—the encounters of academic consultants in statistics. Stat Med 2003;22:169-186.
9. Felson DT, Anderson JJ, Boers M, et al. American College of Rheumatology. Preliminary definition of improvement in rheumatoid arthritis. Arthritis Rheum 1995;38:727-735.
10. van Riel PL, van Gestel AM, van de Putte LB. Development and validation of response criteria in rheumatoid arthritis: steps towards an international consensus on prognostic markers. Br J Rheumatol 1996;35(Suppl 2):4-7.
11. Landewe R, van der Heijde D. Radiographic progression depicted by probability plots: presenting data with optimal use of individual values. Arthritis Rheum 2004;50:699-706.
12. van der Heijde D, Simon L, Smolen J, et al. How to report radiographic data in randomized clinical trials in rheumatoid arthritis: guidelines from a roundtable discussion. Arthritis Rheum 2002;47:215-218.

Ethics in clinical trials*

C. Ronald MacKenzie and Stephen A. Paget

26

The objective of clinical research is the acquisition of generalizable knowledge in order to increase understanding of human biology or to improve health. Although the participation of human subjects is required to achieve these ends, the attainment of the goals of clinical research does not ensure benefits to those who participate. Indeed, it is self-evident that the research subject may be placed at some risk for the good of others, a reality at the core of the ethical dilemmas in human subject research. It is therefore incumbent on those who formulate, conduct, and report such research that their work adhere to the highest of ethical standards. This chapter reviews the ethical dilemmas arising in the research setting and presents principles that should guide this activity.

GENERAL ETHICAL PRINCIPLES

Extensive literature and experience serve to inform the philosophical and practical paradigms that guide current human subject research.[1-7] Theorists interested in this area have looked to the field of moral philosophy and ethical theory to derive principles that provide a foundation for ethical judgments concerning research involving human subjects.[8] Rooted in the Nazi experimentation revealed in Nuremberg, these efforts have been bolstered by a number of seminal documents beginning with the *Nuremberg Code (1949)*,[9] the *Declaration of Helsinki (2000)*,[10] the *Belmont Report (1979)*,[11] the *International Ethical Guidelines for Biomedical Research Involving Human Subjects*,[12] and most recently *Guidelines for Good Clinical Practice for Trials on Pharmaceutical Products* of the World Health Organization.[13] Malfeasance and ethical lapses typified by the Tuskegee study have also provided a potent stimulus for change.[1,2,14] Thus ethically designed and conducted research now rests on principles articulated in these foundational documents. The *Belmont Report*, a particularly influential statement in the current era, added the notions of respect for persons, beneficence, and justice to the enduring principle of informed consent established in Nuremberg more than 30 years before. Indeed, these core ethical tenants provide the foundational elements guiding the current regulation of human subject research, whether that be of the Department of Health and Human Services, the Food and Drug Administration, or locally at the level of the Institutional Review Board.

WHAT IS ETHICAL RESEARCH?

The multifaceted nature and broad scope of ethical controversy concerning the conduct of human subject research cannot simply be articulated by an examination of these principles. For instance, the reconsideration of the ban on the use of women[15] and children,[16] the unresolved debate about the appropriate role of placebos,[17-20] and the problems arising from the globalization of clinical research[21-25] cite just a few of the current ethical challenges that impel discourse beyond an analysis of general principles.

A systematic framework for understanding the ethics of human subject research has been developed by Emanuel and colleagues.[26] Derived from an examination of the relevant literature and incorporating the concepts espoused in the aforementioned declarations and codes, seven requirements are presented to ensure that research subjects are treated with respect and are not exploited in doing so. Table 26-1 summarizes the seven requirements, their rationale, and the ethical value justifying their inclusion. The ethical considerations inherent in these requirements could be framed in the form of questions[6,26]:

1. Does the anticipated societal and scientific value of the research justify the resources required to conduct the research?
2. Does the research employ valid scientific methodology and is it practically feasible?
3. Is the selection of subjects fair and equitable?
4. What potential harms and risks are imposed on the research subjects? Are the risks minimized? Are the potential societal benefits in proportion to the risks imposed on the participants?
5. Has the study undergone independent review?
6. Is informed consent sought from the research subjects?
7. Are there safeguards to ensure the respect for research subjects during their participation in the research?

These requirements and the questions derived from them are premised on ethical values that include those of the *Belmont Report* but also other defining statements concerning research ethics. Introduced are such considerations as exploitation, public accountability, and conflict of interest.

In the setting of drug trials, the traditional stages (phase 1 to 4) of scientific development present phase-specific ethical challenges.[3,5] Although all of the aforementioned ethical constructs apply at each level of drug development, there is some fluidity concerning which constructs are dominant as a drug (device) works it way through the approval cycle. Phase 1 trials represent the phase of drug or device development in which therapeutic intervention is first being introduced for testing in human subjects. Such trials are characterized by a small number of subjects who are often, but not always, healthy volunteers. As such, safety and toxicity in contrast to efficacy are the primary objectives. Given these characteristics, the ethical concepts of informed consent, risk-benefit, and scientific validity are particularly relevant. Because they receive no benefit and may experience significant adverse consequences, subjects participating in phase 1 clinical trials are dedicating themselves to the "greater good."

Phase 2 clinical trials differ from phase 1 studies in that they include more subjects who suffer from the disease for which the treatment is intended and may include efficacy as an active endpoint. The ethical considerations are similar to those of the phase 1 investigation. Phase 3 trials involve not only larger numbers of patients but also an ever-widening range of participants, bringing the ethical construct of fair subject selection to the forefront. Clinical trials at this stage of development focus on efficacy and safety. With both phase 3 and 4 clinical investigations, the latter conducted after the drug has been approved, respect for enrolled subjects becomes a primary consideration raising concerns such as voluntary withdrawal from participation, privacy protection, and informing subjects of new risks and benefits, as well as the results of the research. Further, an ethical concern of particular relevance to the phase 4 clinical trial is the postmarketing investigation conducted by the pharmaceutical industry. Although a subject of some criticism, these are considered justified because they may provide important data on serious but low-prevalence adverse advents associated with the approved therapy.

RANDOMIZED CLINICAL TRIALS

Randomized clinical trials (RCTs) remain the "gold standard" methodology for the demonstration of efficacy and safety in the development of new therapies. This format is defined by a number of design characteristics including randomization, blinding, and the comparison of two (or more) interventions, used in order to demonstrate therapeutic

---

*Adapted from MacKenzie CR, Paget SA: Ethics in clinical trials. In: Hochberg M, Silman AJ, Smolen JS, et al, eds. Rheumatoid arthritis. Mosby/Elsevier, Philadelphia, PA, 2009, 413-418.

TABLE 26.1 ETHICAL REQUIREMENTS FOR ETHICAL RESEARCH

Requirement	Ethical values
1. Social or scientific value	Scarce resources, non-exploitation
2. Scientific validity	Scarce resources, non-exploitation
3. Fair subject selection	Justice
4. Favorable risk-benefit ratio	Non-maleficence, beneficence, and non-exploitation
5. Independent review	Public accountability, minimizing influence of potential conflicts of interest
6. Informed consent	Respect for autonomy
7. Respect for potential and enrolled subjects	Respect for autonomy and welfare

equivalence or superiority of one treatment over another. Despite the advantages, this research design presents a unique spectrum of ethical challenges to the investigator.[3,26] These include such considerations as the treatment versus research dichotomy,[27-31] equipoise (no convincing evidence that one intervention is superior to another),[6,29] choice of control (the use of placebo is one aspect of this issue),[3,5,17-20] randomization (which does not allow for autonomous preferences in treatment),[3] blinding,[3] and the sharing of preliminary information. Each ethical challenge disserves more discussion.

Levine defines *practice* as activities "designed solely to enhance the well-being of an individual patient," whereas the intent of *research* is to contribute to a base of knowledge that can be generalized to all those who suffer from the disease under investigation.[31] In the setting of clinical research, this distinction can be easily blurred, especially when existing treatments for the disease under study are unsatisfactory or when the proposed treatment under study is highly innovative. Because practice and research commonly coexist—most often with new cancer therapies but also in the care and treatment of patients with rheumatoid arthritis with biologic agents—it is virtually instinctive that physicians might wish to employ such therapy despite the lack of formal validation. In so doing, the line that demarcates research from treatment may be breached.

Of all the principles that unite codes of medical ethics, the physician's duty to the individual patient remains a central doctrine. Dating back to Hippocrates, this notion is deeply embedded in how medicine expresses its professionalism. The physician's duty is communicated primarily through the clinical transaction, a patient-centered exercise that relies on physician-based characteristics that could be considered virtuous.[32-35] Against this backdrop, there is the contrasting duty of the researcher—the promotion of human welfare through the rigorous application of the scientific methods in the conduct of research. Tension between these roles and conflicting points of view is especially evident when one considers the RCT. An important and problematic feature of this trial design arises from the process of randomization itself, a practice in which treatment is apportioned by chance rather than the physician recommendation of clinical practice. Although there are scientific, ethical, and practical advantages to the random assignment of treatment, it can be argued that a patient's needs and values become subverted and sacrificed for the greater good of others. An approach to resolving this dilemma is the concept of *clinical equipoise*, first articulated by Freedman.[32] The construct of equipoise requires a researcher to have no justifiable reason for preferring one treatment arm of the study over another. Clinical equipoise expands this concept, examining it from a broader perspective, taking the focus off the researcher and placing it on the greater community of physicians. Instead of the requirement that the treatments being compared exist in exact balance (circumstances in which the researcher would have no preference), clinical equipoise is based on an honest disagreement among knowledgeable professionals; as long as a genuine dispute exists concerning the superiority of one treatment over another, an RCT can be considered permissible.

Another problematic aspect of clinical trials concerns control treatments, particularly the use of placebos. In the setting of new therapies, or where current treatment is ineffective or unsatisfactory for a condition, the use of placebos does not raise ethical concern. However, their use becomes increasingly more problematic when new therapies are being compared with established treatment, circumstances in which currently accepted therapy could be employed as the comparator. The authors of the *Declaration of Helsinki* may have recognized this issue when they stated that the "benefits, risk, burdens, and effectiveness of a new method should be tested against those of the best current ... methods."[10] The U.S. Food and Drug Administration (FDA), however, has generally been supportive of the use of placebos as studies designed in this fashion produce more "purified" knowledge.[17] Thus the role of placebos in clinical research continues to provoke active ethical debate.[17-20] An approach toward a reconciliation of these conflicting positions has been to suggest that the burden of proof lies with those who propose depriving patients of standard care.[17] In addition, a "middle ground" has been advocated by Emanuel and Miller.[20] In their analysis these polarized views—the *placebo orthodoxy*, which promotes the use of placebos on the basis of methodologic considerations, is contrasted to the *active-control orthodoxy*, in which placebos are viewed as sacrificing the rights and welfare of patients in the name of scientific rigor—can be reconciled if specific ethical and methodologic criteria are met. Thus in situations in which life-saving therapy is available, placebo-controlled studies are *prima facie* unethical. In contrast, for conditions that are not thought to be serious, and the risk associated with the use of placebos seems minimal, a placebo comparator can be ethically employed. Placebo use becomes most problematic in those conditions in which effective treatments do exist, and some potential for harm may arise as a consequence of using a placebo. In these circumstances, compelling methodologic advantages must exist in order to justify the use of a placebo control. This would include the study of conditions in which there is a high placebo response rate; a waxing and waning course or frequent spontaneous remissions; those for which existing therapies are only partly effective or have very serious side effects; or the low frequency of the condition means that an equivalency trial would have to be so large as to compromise enrollment and completion of the trial.[20] Many of these disease characteristics are germane to chronic rheumatic diseases, including rheumatoid arthritis.

Other methodologic features of the RCT raise ethical concerns. For instance, there is the defining element of the RCT, the randomization. Randomization is usually performed in a blinded manner, either single (subject does not know what treatment/intervention he or she is receiving), or double-blind (neither subjects nor investigators know which treatment/intervention is being employed). Random assignment and blinding are employed to minimize bias and to enhance the internal validity of the study. Although compatible with the goals of the RCT (to enhance unbiased knowledge), such procedures are not necessarily compatible with the patient's best interests and desires, nor do they respect the subject's autonomy.[5] Two ethical concerns arise from this procedure: (1) preferences and information concerning what intervention the subject is receiving are necessary for autonomous decision-making and (2) information pertaining to which intervention the subject is receiving may be important in the assessment of adverse events or medical emergency. Informed consent addresses concern number one, while providing the appropriate safeguards concerning adverse events requires specification in the research protocol of the conditions, thresholds, and consequences of breaking the code (unblinding the study). A related problem with ethical implications is the sharing of preliminary information. As evidence accumulates in a clinical trial, the understanding of the risks and benefits of the study therapy may change, potentially altering equipoise. Study monitors and independent data safety monitoring boards (DSMBs) are therefore employed to make decisions regarding the early termination of a clinical investigation, thus taking the decision out of the hands of the investigator. Arising in the context of international research, a more recent problem with important ethical dimensions concerns the investigator's (and sponsor's) obligation to study subjects to ensure ongoing access to the investigational therapy upon completion of the clinical trial.[5,33]

Another recent phenomenon of relevance to clinical trials is the advent of the role of contract research organizations (CROs) in drug development.[36,37] CROs are commercial organizations that, as independent contractors, offer clients (usually drug companies) a wide range of pharmaceutical research services. These may include some or all of the following: protocol design, clinical trial (phases 1 through 6) management, centralized laboratory services for processing of clinical trial samples, data analysis, and assistance with the approval status of a drug through the FDA. In effect they offer an important "outsourcing" function to the pharmaceutical industry, which provides for cost savings while bypassing the academic medical center, the traditional (and possibly safer) site for the conduct of clinical trials. CRO-industry revenues have grown dramatically since their inception in the early 1990s.[36,37] However, along with their development, ethical questions have also arisen. Problems such as the preferential enrollment of the economically disadvantaged (through pretrial monetary inducements), "backloading" payment approaches in which the largest payments are made to study subjects at the end of the trial (inhibiting patients who may wish to terminate their participation), disquiet pertaining to the comprehension of non–primary-English-speaking subjects (raising concerns regarding informed consent), inadequate monitoring of adverse events, and concerns about the depth, diversity, and medical knowledge of the workforce that make up the CRO have all been mentioned. Further, whether this model, premised mainly on the desire to reduce costs, compromises ethical oversight remains open to question. Lastly, uncertainty exists with respect to the role and scope of the regulatory mechanisms that oversee the activity of the CROs—that is, do CROs answer to the federal agencies responsible for monitoring clinical trials (a mandated requirement for academic medical centers) or to the drug company for whom they are clients? Little data exist on the degree to which clinical trials in the rheumatic diseases may have been affected by the phenomenon of the CRO. However, reliance on this model remains strong and this practice is likely to grow.

CONFLICT OF INTEREST

The term *conflict of interest* encompasses a spectrum of behaviors and actions involving personal gain, usually but not limited to financial benefit.[38-40] Arising over the past 2 decades from the complex relationships that have developed among industry,[40,41] investigators,[40,41] and the academic institutions where they are employed,[42] such conflicts raise a variety of ethical challenges. The fact that financial and other inducements might influence, and at times overpower, professional judgment comes as no surprise given the pressures accompanying modern life, yet the circumstances and determinants of such behavior are not fully understood. Barnes and Florencio[42] cite a number of considerations including conflict of interest increasing with the value of the secondary interest, as professional judgment becomes more specialized and less amenable to supervision, as the decision-making process becomes less transparent, and when there is a long-standing relationship between the participants. It is well documented that financial and other incentives influence physicians in the clinical environment.[43-45] Although their influence in other arenas of academic medicine may be less appreciated, such influences are pervasive and affect virtually every corner of the academic medical enterprise: physician-industry interactions, investigator-industry relationships, and the academic center itself. Journal publication and continuing medical education are likewise not immune.[46,47]

Efforts to control or manage these conflicts have taken center stage at academic institutions. Initially, simple disclosure was considered sufficient. Whether the context was clinical research, a lecture, or grand rounds, physicians were expected to disclose outside financial interests. More recently, however, institutions have established committees to develop policy, review reported conflicts, and on occasion require the divestment of equities, the termination of consulting relationships, and the imposition of methods of monitoring. Medical journals have also followed suit requiring disclosure and implementing other methods such as the rejection of medical reviews by those believed to have conflicts.[39] Despite these safeguards, breaches are often seen supporting the need to be ever vigilant.

OBSERVATIONS FROM CLINICAL TRIALS

Due to their systemic nature, treatment paradigms for many of the connective tissue diseases require aggressive and increasingly sophisticated therapy that targets the inflammatory response and may produce significant perturbations in the immunologic status of the patient. In the case of rheumatoid arthritis, treatment paradigms have employed multiple disease-modifying drugs (DMARDs), administered early in the onset of disease. Further therapy of such important rheumatic diseases as systemic lupus erythematosus, myositis, and the vasculitides employ an array of other medications that also suppress the patient's immune system. Cyclophosphamide, mycophenolate mofetil, and corticosteroids are just a few of the well-known examples of such therapies. Newer approaches to the suppression of the inflammatory response have focused on a variety of potential molecular targets including cytokines, B and T cells, osteoclasts, and additional immunologic factors, all of which have dual importance in the perpetuation of the disease state and maintaining health.[48] Thus the modulation of immune responses with such biopharmaceuticals as the monoclonal antibodies (mAbs) has become an important therapeutic strategy in the autoimmune diseases. Because many of these new therapies have potentially significant toxicities, patient safety and the ethical considerations arising in the context of clinical trial participation will remain at the forefront of the effort to find more effective treatment for this disease. In order to discuss some of the important ethical considerations arising in this research setting, two recent clinical trials involving agents relevant to rheumatologic practice are illustrative. The clinical details of these cases are summarized in Boxes 26.1 and 26.2.

BOX 26.1 CLINICAL CASE

The patient was a 36-year-old Caucasian female enrolled in an open-label phase 1/2 clinical trial (safety/efficacy study) of a genetically engineered adenovirus encoded with a TNF receptor construct under development by a biotech company as an intra-articular injection for RA. The patient had developed RA 15 years before her enrollment, had previously been treated with etanercept (2002-2004), and at the time of her recruitment to the study had been managed with adalimumab, methotrexate, and prednisone. She previously had surgery on her toe but not her knee, although she had been treated with multiple (10) knee injections of corticosteroids. Randomized to the highest-dose group, she received her first dosage of the study drug on Feb. 26, 2007 without incident. Her second intra-articular injection was administered on July 2, 2007 and on the same evening the patient developed fever and diarrhea. Due to the persistence of the fever, Levaquin was prescribed (July 5, 2007), but within 48 hours she remained febrile (104° F) and was experiencing nausea and vomiting. By July 9, 2007 her knee had become tender, she was tachycardic, and she had a white blood cell count of 29,000/mm³ (predominantly lymphocytes) and exhibited mild liver function abnormalities. Her fever persisted despite aggressive antibiotic therapy, and subsequently (July 16, 2007) her liver function was further deteriorating. She remained febrile and the Hgb was noted to be dropping to a low of 4.6. Hypotension and respiratory distress ensued and she was transferred to another center.

By July 19, additional laboratory and radiologic testing revealed a coagulopathy, retroperitoneal hemorrhage, and further deterioration in the liver function. At this time the question of liver transplantation was raised but dismissed. Serologies for HSV-1 were negative, as were nasopharyngeal cultures. On July 19 a liver biopsy was performed and revealed small areas of acute necrosis and inflammatory lesions, and it was positive for *Histoplasma*. Her deterioration continued and she expired on July 24, 2007. An autopsy revealed disseminated *Histoplasma capsulatum* involving all organs without granuloma (a feature typical for histoplasmosis in the immunocompromised), a large retroperitoneal hematoma, and a minimal swelling of the knees.

BOX 26.2 CLINICAL CASE

Six healthy young male volunteers were enrolled in a phase 1 study of the safety of TGN1412, a superagonist anti-CD28 monoclonal antibody that directly stimulates T cells. Within 90 minutes of receiving a single intravenous dose of the drug, all six volunteers developed a severe systemic inflammatory response secondary to the rapid induction of proinflammatory cytokines. Patients reported headache and myalgia and developed nausea, diarrhea, vasodilatation, and hypotension. Over the ensuing 24 hours, all patients became critically ill with diffuse pulmonary infiltrates, renal failure, and disseminated intravascular coagulation. All patients were admitted to the intensive care unit, where they received aggressive supportive therapy including dialysis, high-dose intravenous corticosteroids, and an anti-interleukin-2 receptor antagonist antibody. Prolonged shock and respiratory distress syndrome developed in two patients, who required intensive support for 8 and 16 days. All patients ultimately survived.

As a consequence of these experiences, both protocols have undergone intense scrutiny from the lay press[49,50] and the scientific community,[51,52] an assessment that has included an examination by the National Institutes of Health (NIH) Recombinant DNA Advisory Committee and the European Medicine Agency (EMEA).[53] Numerous questions have arisen: Was the science underlying the proposed therapy flawed? What factors or conditions associated with the clinical trial contributed to this outcome? Was the patient adequately informed about the risks of participation? Was the patient sufficiently protected against these risks?

An ethical analysis of these events begins with the informed consent. Under the current guidelines for research participation in the United States, all research subjects must be informed of the risks and benefits of their participation in a research study, a requirement fulfilled by the process of informed consent.[54] It is this process that demonstrates respect for the research subject as a person and recognition of his or her autonomy. Three primary elements support this requirement: information, comprehension, and voluntariness. Once these elements are achieved, the subject's authorization is sought.[11,54] Information provided to the research subject should be adequate to explain the rationale for and the procedures involved in the study and should meet a *reasonable volunteer* standard. In order to do so, the investigator may need to consider factors such as the subject's age, educational level, and other barriers to communication such as language. Informed consent continues throughout the subject's participation in the research.

Indications have suggested that there may have been problems with respect to the informed consent process in the case described in Box 26.1. For instance, it has been reported that the subject participated in the clinical trial because of a perceived benefit, primarily the alleviation of knee pain.[49,50] This problem, often referred to as the *therapeutic misconception*, is not uncommon.[28,29] It refers to a mistaken belief held by the research subject that participation will directly benefit him or her and certainly produce no harm. Thus it is possible that this patient believed she was receiving state-of-the-art, even novel therapy, to which others would not have access. Such beliefs are strong inducements to participation and must be adequately tempered by the primary investigator through a thoughtful, considered process of informed consent. Statements such as "you cannot expect to benefit directly from your participation in this study," so often found in consent forms, cannot be regarded as sufficient to mitigate the problem of therapeutic misconception.

Another important consideration relates to the prestudy risk assessment of the developers of the drug and the primary investigators. Although this subject's death is not believed to have been a direct consequence of the adenovirus vector employed to deliver the anti-TNF medication, the patient's immunosuppression, a consequence of the totality of her therapy, as well as the risk of infection with histoplasmosis in a patient living in an endemic region for this condition, may not have been sufficiently appreciated by the investigators.[55,56]

Concerns pertaining to the ethical oversight of this investigation are compounded by the circumstances of its approval. Ethical review was conducted by an independent Institutional Review Board (IRB), one not affiliated with an academic medical center. Two issues are raised in this context. First is the quality of scientific review given the complexities of therapy in this disease setting. Was there sufficient rheumatologic, immunologic, and infectious disease expertise on the IRB to adequately assess the potential for adverse outcomes with this new therapy? The second concern pertains to the for-profit nature of this IRB. Could the IRB process have been influenced by circumstances in which the investigators were being paid directly by the company seeking approval for the drug?

In this study a third issue relating to coercion has also been raised. The research subject was approached directly by her rheumatologist concerning her willingness to participate in this investigation. In the trial presented, the study sponsor had agreed in principle to the use of a neutral party in the recruitment of patients, although this procedure was not employed.[57] This practice has the potential for placing undue influence on the patient to agree to enroll in the study. In order to reduce this form of influence, the NIH recommends that physicians should not recruit their own patients into clinical trials they are conducting. In circumstances where this cannot be avoided, it has been suggested that an impartial third party explain the study and obtain informed consent.[58] This practice is particularly relevant to studies involving novel therapies that are deemed risky, in circumstances when the individual's condition is not life-threatening, and is especially of interest in studies in which the investigator has a financial interest (as was the case in the rheumatoid arthritis [RA] trial discussed in Box 26.1).

A final concern has to do with the assumption of risk. As in the case of the earlier and now well-documented study involving gene therapy with fatal consequences,[59,60] the RA study subject had a mild, or at least well-controlled, disease with standard therapy. Thus the degree of assumed risk may have been out of proportion to the potential benefit, provoking concern in general as to which subsets of diseases should even be considered for innovative therapies that employ emerging technologies.[57]

Turning to the second example (Box 26.2), the investigation was a phase 1 study of the safety of a novel immunomodulatory therapy using healthy volunteers. In this research setting (phase 1 trial), the ethical accountability of the investigator to the (healthy) study participant is especially high, a responsibility magnified by the difficulty in quantifying risks. Indeed, one of the major impediments to drug development in this arena (mAbs) is the risk of adverse immune-mediated reactions in humans that include immunosuppression, autoimmunity, and, in the case presented, cytokine storm, a topic extensively reviewed recently.[53] Dosing for such "first-in-human" clinical trials is based on preclinical safety studies, primarily in nonhuman primates combined with *ex vivo* studies. Dose selection nonetheless remains challenging because of differences between the primate and human systems, species selection, scientific considerations pertaining to the receptor model employed, calculations based on what is known as the *minimal anticipated biological effect level* (MABEL), and a number of additional considerations relevant to mAbs and their pharmacology and immunology.[53] The TGN1412 experience, coupled with a growing science pertaining to safer dosage predictions in mAbs therapy, should have addressed this important safety consideration. Although these problems will require scientifically based solutions, the problems imposed by this currently inexact science compound the ethical challenges.

An important practical matter arising in this study was the decision to administer the drug to all six participants virtually simultaneously. Clearly, had the administration of the drug been performed in a sequential fashion, thus allowing for observation of each patient individually, fewer of the six study participants would have been subjected to the life-threatening adverse effects of the study drug. This methodologic caution has obvious ethical implications concerning the safety of the study participants and appears to have been recognized in the recently published EMEA guidelines concerning first-in-human clinical trials.[61]

KEY REFERENCES

3. Emanuel EJ, Crouch RA, Arras JD, et al. Ethical and regulatory aspects of clinical research: readings and commentary. Johns Hopkins Univ Press, 2003.

5. Grady C. Ethical principles in clinical research. In Gallin JI, Ognibene FP, eds. Principles and practice of clinical research, 2nd ed. London: Elsevier Acad Press, 2007.

6. Derenzo E, Moss J. Writing clinical research protocols: ethical considerations. London: Elsevier Acad Press, 2006.

9. The Nuremberg Code, 1949. Available at www.hhs.gov/ohrp/references/nurcode.htm.

10. Office of Human Subjects Research: NIH Regulations and Ethical Guidelines: World Medical Association Declaration of Helsinki: Revised 09/10/2004. Available at http://ohsr.od.nih.gov/guidelines/helsinki.html.

11. National Commission for the Protection of Human Subjects of Biomedical and Behavioral Research. The Belmont report: ethical principles and guidelines for the protection of human subjects of research. Washington, DC: US Government Printing Office, 1979.

12. International Ethical Guidelines for Biomedical Research Involving Human Subjects. Geneva: Council for International Organizations of Medical Sciences/SHO, 2002. Available at www.cioms.ch.

13. International Conference on Harmonisation of Technical Requirements for Registration of Pharmaceuticals for Human Use, ICH Harmonised Tripartite Guideline—Guideline for Good Clinical Practice (ICH-GCP Guideline), Geneva, 1996. Available at www.vadscorner.com/internet29.html.

14. Brandt AM. Racism and research: the case of the Tuskegee Syphilis Study. Hastings Center Report 1978;6:21-29.

15. U.S. Department of Health and Human Services, National Institutes of Health. Recruitment and retention of women in clinical studies. A report of the workshop sponsored by the Office of Research on Women's Health, NIH Publication No. 95-3756. Bethesda, Md: U.S. Department of Health and Human Services, National Institutes of Health, 1995.

16. NIH Policy and Guidelines on the Inclusion of Children as Participants in Research Involving Human Subjects, Notice 98-024. March 6, 1998. Available at http://grants.nih.gov/grants/guide/notice-files/not98-024.html.

18. Temple R, Ellenberg SS. Placebo-controlled trials and active-control trials in the evaluation of new treatments, part I: ethical and scientific issues. Ann Intern Med 2000;133:455-463.

20. Emanuel EJ, Miller FG. The ethics of placebo-controlled trials: a middle ground. N Engl J Med 2001;345:915-919.

21. Glickman SW, McHutchison JG, Peterson ED, et al. Ethical and scientific implications of the globalization of clinical research. N Engl J Med 2009;360:816-823.

22. Koski G, Nightingale SL. Research involving human subjects in developing countries. N Engl J Med 2001;345:136-138.

23. Shapiro HT, Meslin EM. Ethical issues in the design and conduct of clinical trials in developing countries. N Engl J Med 2003;345:139-142.

26. Emanuel EJ, Wendler D, Grady C. What makes clinical research ethical? JAMA 2000;283:2701-2711.

27. Hellman S, Hellman DS. Of mice but not men: problems of the randomized clinical trial. N Engl J Med 1991;324:1585-1589.

28. Appelbaum PS, Roth LH, Lidz CW, et al. False hopes and best data: consent to research and the therapeutic misconception. Hastings Cent Rep 1987;17:20-24.

30. Freedman B, Fuks A, Weijer C. Demarcating research and treatment: a systemic approach for the analysis of the ethics of clinical research. Clin Res 1992;40:653-660.

31. Levine RJ. The distinction between research and treatment. In: Ethics and regulation of clinical research, 2nd ed. Baltimore: Urban and Schwarzenberg, 1986.

32. Freedman B. Equipoise and the ethics of clinical research. N Engl J Med 1987;317:141-145.

33. Barondess JA. Medicine and professionalism. Arch Int Med 2003;163:145-149.

34. Pellegrino ED. Professionalism, profession and the virtues of the good physician. Mt Sinai J Med 2002;69:378-384.

35. MacKenzie CR. Professionalism and medicine. HSS J 2007;3:222-227.

36. Grady C. The challenge of assuring continued post-trial access to beneficial treatment. Yale J Health Policy Law Ethics 2005;5(1):425-435.

37. Shuchman M. Commercializing clinical trials—risks and benefits of the CRO boom. N Engl J Med 2007;537:1365-1368.

39. MacKenzie CR, Cronstein BN. Conflict of interest. HSS J 2006;2:198-201.

40. Korn D. Conflicts of interest in biomedical research. JAMA 2000;284:2234-2237.

41. Bekelman JE, Li Y, Gross CP. Scope and impact of financial conflicts of interest in biomedical research. JAMA 2003;289:453-465.

42. Barnes M, Florencio P. Financial conflicts of interest in human subjects research: the problem of institutional conflicts. J Law Med Ethics 2002;30:1-13.

43. Hillman AL, Pauly MV, Kerslein B. How do financial incentives affect physician's clinical decisions and the financial performance of health maintenance organizations. N Engl J Med 1989;321:86-89.

44. Hillman AL, Joseph CA, Mabry MR, et al. Frequency and costs of diagnostic imaging in office practice: comparison of self-referring and radiologist referring physicians. N Engl J Med 1990;323:1604-1608.

45. Chren MM, Landefeld CS. Physicians' behavior and their interactions with drug companies: a controlled study of physicians who request additions to a hospital formulary. JAMA 1994;271:684-689.

46. International Committee of Medical Journal Editors. Uniform requirements for manuscripts submitted to biomedical journals. Nov 2001: Available at www.lcmje.org.

47. The Editors. Financial associations of authors. N Engl J Med 2002;346:1901-1902.

48. Savage C, St. Clair W. New therapeutics in rheumatoid arthritis. In Paget SA, Crow MK, eds. Disease modification in rheumatic diseases. Rheum Dis Clin N Am 2006;32:57-74.

49. Weiss R. Death points to risks in research. Washington Post, 8/6/07, pg A01.

50. Weiss R. Fungus infected woman who died after gene therapy. Washington Post, 8/17/07, pg A10.

51. Frank KM, Holgarth K, Miller J, et al. Investigation of the cause of death in a gene-therapy trial. N Engl J Med 2009;361:161-169.

52. Suntharalingam G, Perry MR, Ward S, et al. Cytokine storm in a phase 1 trial of anti-CD28 monoclonal antibody TGN1412. N Engl J Med 2006;355:1018-1028.

53. Muller PY, Brennan FR. Safety assessment and dose selection for first-in-human clinical trials with immunomodulatory monoclonal antibodies. Clin Pharm Ther 2009;85:247-258.

54. U.S. Department of Health and Human Services, National Institutes of Health, and Office for Human Research Protections, The Common Rule, Title 45 (Public Welfare), Code of Federal Regulations, Part 46 (Protection of Human Subjects). Washington, DC: DHHS, revised Nov 13, 2001; effective Dec 13, 2001.

55. Lee JH, Slifman NR, Gersho SK, et al. Life-threatening histoplasmosis complicating immunotherapy with tumor necrosis factor alpha antagonists infliximab and etanercept. Arth Rheum 2002;46:2565-2570.

56. Wook KL, Hage CA, Know KS, et al. Histoplasmosis after treatment with anti-tumor necrosis factor-alpha therapy. Am J Resp Crit Care Med 2003;167:1279-1282.

57. Hughes V. Therapy on trial. Nature Med 2007;13(9):1008-1009.

58. Editorial. Uninformed consent? Nature Med 2007;13:999.

59. Baron J. Against bioethics. Cambridge, Mass: MIT Press, 2006.

60. Stolberg SG. "The biotech death of Jesse Gelsinger." NY Time Magazine, November 28, 1999.

61. Milton MN, Horvath CJ. The EMEA guidelines on first-in-human clinical trials and its impact on pharmaceutical development. Toxicol Pathol 2009;37:363-371.

REFERENCES

Full references for this chapter can be found on www.expertconsult.com.

2

CLINICAL BASIS OF RHEUMATIC DISEASE

History and physical examination

Anthony D. Woolf

27

- History taking is the most important skill in rheumatology.
- The physical examination is pivotal in confirming the cause and effect of musculoskeletal problems.
- Assessment of the musculoskeletal system should form part of any general medical examination.
- The consultation involves a patient-centered phase for his or her story, a physician-centered phase to clarify the story by interrogation and examination, and an interactive phase during which the patient and physician discuss their concerns, findings, conclusions, and plans.
- The consultation must meet the expectations of the patient.
- Musculoskeletal conditions cause a broad range of problems, which need to be assessed by a multidisciplinary team to develop an appropriate plan of management.

INTRODUCTION

Musculoskeletal complaints are among the most common symptoms, and their cause and effect need to be established. The physician to whom the patient presents needs to characterize the problem and its impact, establish the cause, develop a management plan, assess response to treatment, and be able to recognize the lack of expected response. If the physician is not able to identify the cause, he or she must at least be able to describe the abnormality and recognize whether it is important and whether it requires a more skilled assessment. Musculoskeletal conditions are also frequent co-morbidities that need to be identified and treated. Many common musculoskeletal problems are effectively managed by a primary care physician but other less common or more serious problems will require specialist management, often within the context of a multidisciplinary team. Different competencies are needed for these different levels of care. All physicians should be able to recognize an abnormality of the musculoskeletal system and whether it is important by being able to perform a screening assessment in combination with basic knowledge of musculoskeletal conditions. More expert management will require a greater competency in clinical assessment and more detailed knowledge of the possible causes; such an assessment will be made by a specialist physician (rheumatologist).

In this chapter we provide information on a basic screening assessment of the musculoskeletal system that is appropriate as part of a general examination to identify if there is any abnormality. A more detailed evaluation of a person presenting with a musculoskeletal problem is also presented.

SCREENING ASSESSMENT

Musculoskeletal conditions should always be sought as part of any general history and examination by a routine screen. Once an abnormality has been identified, a more detailed assessment is necessary. This screen takes only a few minutes. It has been validated in a general medical setting and within undergraduate training.[1]

Screening history

The common symptoms of any musculoskeletal condition are pain, stiffness, and limitation of function. Joint disease is often associated with swelling. Sensitive functional tests are (1) ability to dress without difficulty, including socks and shoes, which is a complex activity that utilizes both upper and lower limbs and (2) ability to ascend and descend stairs without difficulty, which is sensitive to detecting abnormality in the lower limbs. The following screening questions will establish quickly the presence or absence of major musculoskeletal problems.

- Do you suffer from any pain or stiffness in your arms or legs, neck, or back?
- Do you have any swelling of your joints?
- Do you have any difficulty with washing and dressing?
- Do you have any difficulty with going up or down stairs or steps?

Musculoskeletal conditions are often associated with systemic features, and general inquiry should be made about the person's health.

Screening examination

Any significant abnormalities in the spine, arms, or legs should be identified by inspection at rest and during certain movements, with brief palpation and stress tests of selected joints. Normality is looked for in appearance, posture, and resting position of the joints and in smooth movement through the expected normal range. When any joint is affected by a musculoskeletal condition, there is usually one movement that is nearly always affected and it is these movements that are assessed in this screen. For such a screen to be part of the routine examination of all patients, it has to be quick, simple, and easy to annotate. This screen was developed to meet these criteria.[1] The gait, arms, legs, and spine (G, A, L, S) should be assessed.

- *Gait.* Observe the patient walking forward for a few feet, turning, and walking back again. Abnormalities of the different phases should be recognized: heel-strike, stance phase, toe-off, and swing phase (Fig. 27.1). Look for abnormalities of movement of the arms, pelvis, hips, knees, ankles, and feet during these phases.
- *Inspection of standing patient.* View the patient from the back, side, and front, looking for any abnormalities, in particular of posture and symmetry. Examine for tenderness by applying pressure in the midpoint of each supraspinatus muscle and rolling an overlying skinfold.
- *Spine.* Ask the patient to flex the neck laterally to each side. Place several fingers on the lumbar spinous processes and ask the patient to bend forward and attempt to touch the toes while standing with the legs fully extended, observing and feeling for normal movement.
- *Arms.* Ask the patient to place both hands behind the head with elbows right back. This is a sensitive test of many components of the shoulder apparatus. Straighten the arms down the side of the body and then inspect with the patient's elbows bent to 90 degrees with palms down and fingers straight. Turn hands over and make a tight fist with each hand. Place, in turn, the tip of each finger on to the tip of the thumb. Squeeze the metacarpals from the second to the fifth.
- *Legs.* With the patient reclining on an examination table, flex each hip and knee in turn while holding and feeling the knee. Then passively rotate the hip internally. With the patient's leg extended and resting on the couch, examine for tenderness or swelling of the knee by pressing down on the patella while cupping it proximally. Squeeze all the metatarsals and finally inspect the soles of the feet for callosities.

Any abnormalities identified should be documented to be more fully assessed.

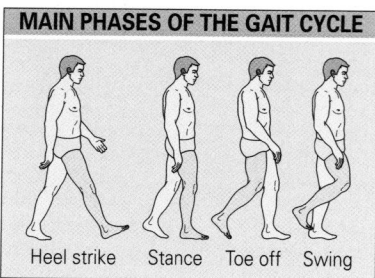

MAIN PHASES OF THE GAIT CYCLE

Heel strike Stance Toe off Swing

Fig. 27.1 Main phases of the gait cycle. The phases relate to the shaded leg.

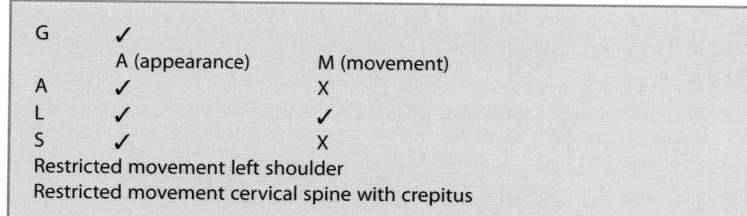

G	✓	
	A (appearance)	M (movement)
A	✓	X
L	✓	✓
S	✓	X

Restricted movement left shoulder
Restricted movement cervical spine with crepitus

ASSESSING A MUSCULOSKELETAL PROBLEM

General principles

The aim of the consultation is to fully characterize the problem the person is complaining of and to make a clinical diagnosis (or at least offer a differential diagnosis) if possible. This requires not just good clinical skills but also knowledge of functional anatomy, the features of common musculoskeletal conditions, their differential diagnosis, risk factors and complications, and their likely prognosis. Musculoskeletal conditions are common and can coexist. It should not be assumed that each symptom relates to a single diagnosis.

The impact of the musculoskeletal problem must be identified in terms of symptoms such as pain, physical disability, depression, and fatigue, as well as the effect on activities of daily living and how it impacts on the person's ability to participate in what he or she wants and needs to do. In addition, interpersonal relationships with family, caregivers, and friends may be affected and there is often fear of the future.

The patient's concerns must also be identified if the consultation is to fulfill the expectations of the patient as well as those of the physician (Table 27.1). It is important to show empathy and gain the confidence of the person to establish a relationship of trust and understanding. If the condition is chronic there is a dependency on the physician for ongoing health issues and future quality of life.

The consultation to assess a musculoskeletal problem

The process of the consultation can be divided into several phases: listening and observing, inquiring, performing an examination, ordering investigations, and making a conclusion. History taking is by far the most important part of the evaluative process, complemented by the examination to confirm the nature of the musculoskeletal problem. One should listen throughout the consultation to understand the patient's concerns and expectations. Observe the patient's overall appearance, movements, and manner. In the majority of cases it is necessary to make a full assessment of the whole person, particularly because an apparently simple local problem may be the manifestation of a more generalized condition or the symptoms may be referred from a distant site. Investigations when dealing with a musculoskeletal problem are usually necessary only to confirm clinical suspicions regarding diagnosis and to help gauge disease activity, prognosis, and choice of treatment. They should follow logically from the findings of the consultation and be performed only if the results will influence decision-making. Further consultations will be more focused on monitoring response to treatment, with appropriate adjustment. There are many standardized assessments for musculoskeletal conditions to measure impact[2] and monitor response to treatment,[3] which are considered within the relevant disease area elsewhere in this book.

TABLE 27.1 WHAT IS THE EXPECTATION OF THE CONSULTATION?	
Patient expectation	**Clinician expectation**
■ What is wrong?	■ Is there an abnormality?
■ What will happen? *Will I get better? Will I become worse and unable to do what I want and need to do?*	■ What is the abnormality?
	■ What is the cause?
	■ What effect is it having?
■ What can you do about it? *Can it be cured or just relieved?*	■ Are there any predisposing or risk factors?
■ What can I do about it? *Will a diet or complementary therapies help? Should I exercise?*	■ Are there any complications?
	■ What treatment is indicated?
	■ What has been the response to previous treatment?
■ Am I getting better?	■ Is there a response to current treatment?
■ Am I receiving the best treatment, because I am not improving?	■ What is the prognosis?

BOX 27.1 CHARACTERIZATION OF A MUSCULOSKELETAL PROBLEM
■ What are the symptoms?
■ Site and distribution of symptoms
■ Chronology
■ Associated symptoms
■ Preceding illnesses or injuries and other relevant clues
■ Response to health interventions
■ What is its impact on activities, participation and quality of life?

Any consultation should close with a full discussion of the findings and conclusions so that the person understands the cause, the treatment, and its likely benefits and risks; what he or she can do; and the likely outcome. This needs to include the patient's needs and expectations. Because many musculoskeletal conditions are chronic or recurrent, the patient will need more a detailed explanation to enable active participation in the care. Other health care professionals, written material, the Internet, and patient support groups can give further support.

History

First one should clarify what has brought the patient to the consultation and what his or her expectations are. The nature of the condition and its impact is discerned. Other potentially relevant factors are explored, such as medical history, risk factors related to lifestyle or occupation, and factors that may influence impact such as the patient's expectations and socioeconomic environment (Box 27.1).

What are the symptoms?

Symptoms specifically related to musculoskeletal conditions are most often pain and stiffness, frequently accompanied by loss of function and mobility, which can limit activities and restrict participation, but there may be non-specific symptoms as well. Red flags for potentially serious conditions must be recognized (Box 27.2).

Analysis of these symptoms helps the physician to differentiate a musculoskeletal complaint into:

- Inflammatory musculoskeletal disease
- Mechanical joint problem
- Periarticular/soft tissue problem
- Bone disorder
- Non-rheumatic disease causing musculoskeletal symptoms
- A disorder of unknown cause

Pain

Pain should be characterized to identify its cause and effect. Nociceptive pain results from a stimulus or lesion in peripheral tissues that causes a painful impulse to be transmitted by an intact nervous system, whereas neuropathic pain arises as a direct consequence of a lesion or disease affecting the nervous system. These need distinguishing; different causes of nociceptive pain have their own characteristics. Pain may also be referred from another site.

TABLE 27.3 PATTERNS OF PAIN

Type	Pain pattern	Cause
Bone pain	Pain at rest and at night	Tumor, Paget's, fracture
Mechanical joint pain	Pain related to joint use only	Unstable joint
Osteoarthritic joint pain	Pain on joint use, stiffness after inactivity, pain at end of day after use	Osteoarthritis
Inflammatory joint pain	Pain and stiffness in the joints in the morning, at rest, and with use	Inflammatory Infective
Neuropathic	Diffuse pain and paresthesia in dermatome, worsened by specific activity	Root or peripheral nerve compression
Referred	Pain unaffected by local movement	

diffuse and described as superficial burning, stinging, or prickling pain; as deep aching pain; or as paroxysmal, electric shock-like pains. It is often evoked by a specific activity such as skin stimulation, pressure over affected nerves, and changes in temperature or emotion and associated with paresthesia in the dermatome. It may include allodynia (pain due to a stimulus that does not normally provoke pain), hyperalgesia (an increased response to a stimulus that is normally less painful), and hyperesthesia (an increased response to a stimulus that is normally less painful). Bone pain is typically present at rest and at night. These types of pain give clues but are not diagnostic.

The evolution of pain should be established in conjunction with the development of any other symptoms—how the patient has arrived at the present situation.

What is the site and distribution?

Ask the patient to demonstrate where the pain is felt and where it is most severe. Is the pain generalized or localized? How easily can it be localized? Articular and periarticular pain often radiates widely and presents far from its origin. Such referred pain is felt in the dermatome relating to the myotomal or sclerotomal origin of the affected structure (Table 27.2). Pain from bone and periosteum radiates little and is localized more reliably. Widespread pain can be due to fibromyalgia or polymyalgia rheumatica, whereas pain in several joints suggests an arthropathy. Myeloma or metastatic malignancy must be considered with multiple sites of pain that are not just related to joints. Examination of the patient is necessary to clarify the anatomic site of origin of pain.

What are its characteristics and pattern?

The features of the pain, the time and mode of onset, and the diurnal pattern provide diagnostic clues. Severity is subjective and is not diagnostic alone, although its perceived severity indicates the likely impact that it is having. Certain musculoskeletal conditions are characterized by specific patterns of pain (Table 27.3). For example, gout usually begins in the middle of the night with a pricking sensation in the great toe, which quickly builds up into an intolerable persistent burning pain, whereas osteoarthritis is characterized by use-related pain and inactivity stiffness of the affected joints. Mechanical pain is generally related to use. Inflammatory joint pain is present at rest and with use and is usually worse at either end of the day. Neuropathic pain is

What precipitates, worsens, or improves pain?

Periarticular problems are often induced by a specific type of repetitive activity. Spinal stenosis can be suspected from the history of activity-related buttock and leg pain that improves rapidly with rest only to recur after further activity, and walking downhill (which extends the spine) causes more pain than walking uphill or cycling. The response to exercise in contrast to rest is a typical feature of sacroiliitis or spondylitis. Rest usually improves pain due to osteoarthritis but has little effect on inflammatory pain. The response to anti-inflammatory analgesics compared with simple analgesics can help distinguish an inflammatory cause of symptoms, such as ankylosing spondylitis, from mechanical back pain; the response of polymyalgia rheumatica to glucocorticosteroids is also characteristic.

What is its effect on the person?

Pain is a subjective sensation that cannot be felt by others. It can be measured using a visual analog scale, but the degree to which it disrupts the person's life in terms of activities and participation gives a more meaningful indication of severity. Pain often disturbs sleep, which magnifies its impact.

Stiffness

People often describe a generalized "stiffness" after prolonged rest or the day after an unusual level of exercise, which is more common as people age. More specifically, people often describe stiffness related to symptomatic joints. An inflammatory joint disorder is generally associated with severe and prolonged morning and evening joint stiffness, whereas osteoarthritis is associated with short-lived but severe stiffness after inactivity. Morning stiffness of the girdle muscles is characteristic of polymyalgia rheumatica, which can be so severe that it is virtually impossible to roll out of bed, although a few hours after getting up the patient may be virtually asymptomatic. The duration of morning stiffness can indicate the activity of rheumatoid arthritis or polymyalgia rheumatica.

Stiffness of movement of the fingers can relate to tenosynovitis (sometimes with triggering), joint disease, or tightening of the soft tissues, such as in systemic sclerosis or with Dupuytren's contracture.

TABLE 27.2 COMMON PATTERNS OF REFERRED PAIN

Source of pain	Pattern of referral
Cervical spine	Occiput, shoulders
Shoulder	Lateral aspect of arm
Lateral epicondyle	Mid forearm
Carpal tunnel	Radial fingers, occasionally forearm or arm
Lumbar spine	Sacroiliac joints, buttocks, posterior thigh, lower leg, foot
Hip joint	Groin, medial thigh, medial knee, greater trochanter, buttock above gluteal fold
Trochanteric bursa	Lateral thigh, buttock

"Stiffness" can also be used to describe a reduced or limited range of movement or by the patient to describe the difficulty in movement associated with muscle disease such as inflammatory myositis, Parkinson's disease, and motor neuron disease. A careful examination is necessary to be certain as to the correct attribution of this symptom.

"Locking" describes the sudden inability to perform a particular movement and suggests a specific mechanical event in which some internal derangement actually causes the joint to lock in one position until a trick movement or help is used to free it up. This is a classic symptom of a loose body or torn meniscus of the knee joint, but it also occurs in the finger with triggering due to stenosing tenosynovitis.

Swelling and deformity

Swelling may be of the soft tissues, the joint, or bone. Did it follow an injury? Did it appear rapidly or slowly? Is it painful? Does it come and go, or is it gradually enlarging? Any swelling needs careful examination to establish its nature and cause. Joint swelling is a sign of disease, and examination is necessary to confirm whether it is related to the joint or a periarticular structure and to establish if it is due to an effusion, synovial proliferation, or bony growth. Imaging may be required. Recognition of any deformity requires familiarity with the musculoskeletal system to separate normal variation from abnormal findings.

Weakness and instability

Weakness can be an important clue to a muscle disorder such as inflammatory myositis or a neuropathy. The pattern of muscle weakness, whether generalized or in a central or peripheral distribution, should be established. Regional weakness is more likely to have a specific cause. However, "weakness" may be used by a patient to describe different things, such as general fatigue, difficulty with movement because of joint disease or pain, the feeling of insecurity that is associated with many forms of joint disease, or the regional weakness of a joint or limb caused by the local muscle wasting that can accompany joint damage. A sensation of "giving way" and general instability of the lower limbs can result from weak quadriceps muscles. A joint may be unstable and suddenly give way because of muscle weakness, or this may relate to the ligaments being ruptured or lax in hypermobility. Examination is needed to characterize what is being described.

Loss of movement or function

Musculoskeletal conditions often cause difficulty in performing various activities, and this may be the presenting complaint. It is uncommon for these limitations to arise in the absence of a complaint of pain and/or stiffness, but the painless loss of movement suggests a tendon rupture or a neurologic cause. Inquiry should establish if any particular movements and functions are restricted and whether this relates to pain and stiffness or if it is a primary problem.

Fatigue and malaise

Fatigue is a manifestation of most generalized rheumatic disorders, including rheumatoid arthritis, systemic lupus erythematosus (SLE), and, most notably, fibromyalgia. Fatigue is sometimes functional and related to depression. Fatigue may also be the consequence of poor sleep, often related to pain. It may be severely disabling and is very distressing to the person. The fatigue of rheumatoid arthritis or SLE is a good indicator of the systemic disease activity. The time at which fatigue becomes a problem is sometimes used, along with the duration of morning stiffness, as one of the indicators of disease activity.

People with inflammatory arthritis are often able to function well for several hours but then suffer overwhelming fatigue. The fatigue of fibromyalgia is usually associated with lack of concentration and poor-quality sleep. Polymyalgia rheumatica is often associated with a feeling of sudden aging, with rapid rejuvenation with a moderate dose of corticosteroids.

Emotional lability

Fear and anxiety are common accompaniments of a musculoskeletal problem, influenced by factors such as the knowledge of possible diagnosis, expectations of prognosis, future aspirations, and fear of losing independence. Emotional lability, depression, and other psychiatric disturbances can also be the direct result of a rheumatic disease, such as SLE. Sleep disturbance secondary to pain can also affect mood.

What is the pattern and chronology of symptoms?

The distribution and chronologic pattern of each symptom need to be established. How did the patient arrive at the present situation? When and how did it start—was the onset sudden or gradual, spontaneous, or after some specific event such as trauma or an infection? What was the subsequent course with respect to time and pattern of distribution of symptoms? If articular, is it peripheral small joints, large joints, or axial? Has it followed an additive, intermittent, or flitting course? Is it symmetric or asymmetric? What associated symptoms or signs have developed, and when? Do the symptoms fit some recognized pattern? It is important, however, to avoid forcing the symptoms into a pattern—musculoskeletal conditions are common, and different conditions can co-exist.

The pattern is important in identifying the possible cause. For example, a traumatic condition obviously relates to a specific event whereas a degenerative pathology usually presents in a slow, insidious fashion. Crystal-related inflammation is particularly rapid in onset and severe but self-limiting, whereas untreated sepsis causes a steadily worsening situation over a few days. Many of the idiopathic inflammatory or immune-mediated rheumatic diseases have a variable course with spontaneous remissions and exacerbations, whereas others, such as reactive arthritis, follow a more predictable course with the sequential development of mucocutaneous and joint inflammation over a period of a few weeks after the initiating event, which gradually subsides over a period of months. Other specific patterns include that of palindromic rheumatism, which, as the word implies, involves episodes of arthritis affecting one or two joints that come and go spontaneously over a few days.

Associated symptoms, preceding factors, and other clues

Musculoskeletal conditions often have systemic features, and systemic disorders often have musculoskeletal symptoms. It is therefore important to ask about the patient's general health and inquire of the presence of systemic symptoms, such as fever, night sweats, or weight loss and other "red flags" (see Box 27.2), which may indicate the presence of a serious systemic disorder such as a malignancy, infection, or active inflammatory disease (Table 27.4). Questions should be directed by knowledge of conditions under consideration. For example, one should inquire about a recent diarrheal illness, urethritis, or psoriasis and mucocutaneous problems in the seronegative spondyloarthritides; dry eyes and mouth in sicca syndrome; and a variety of systemic features in the connective tissue disorders, including rashes, mouth ulcers, Raynaud's phenomenon, neuropsychiatric disturbances, and many others. Was there any preceding trauma or repetitive or unusual use? The previous medical history may include past events that give clues to the present problem, such as a previous attack of unexplained epilepsy in someone with SLE, fetal loss or thrombosis in antiphospholipid syndrome, or a story of a swollen ankle in childhood in a young man with back pain who has now developed ankylosing spondylitis. In other cases, relevant previous medical events may relate to the associations between disorders, such as bronchiectasis preceding rheumatoid arthritis or hypermobility in childhood and past joint trauma as risk factors for osteoarthritis.

The family history can help toward the differential diagnosis in some situations, although almost everyone has a relative with arthritis and familial associations are seldom predictive. A family history also gives personal experience of the potential impact of a rheumatic condition and affects the person's anxieties about his or her own diagnosis and prognosis. Useful clues include a recent flu-like illness in the family or other close contacts, which raises the possibility of a viral arthritis; nodal arthritis affecting the mother when deciding if small joint polyarthralgia of the hands is early rheumatoid arthritis or nodal osteoarthritis; a family history of ankylosing spondylitis, iritis, or psoriasis in a young man presenting with back pain; or a family history of gout.

There are recognized risk factors for the development and outcome of musculoskeletal conditions. These include obesity, lack of physical activity, poor diet, smoking, and excess alcohol intake, as well as activities that expose people to sprains and strains, such as sports or occupation. There are recognized "yellow flags" for chronicity of back pain, such as job dissatisfaction, unavailability of light work, depression, and

TABLE 27.4 ASSOCIATED SYMPTOMS, SIGNS, AND CONDITIONS

	Symptom	Possible diagnosis
Neurologic	Headaches	SLE, temporal arteritis
	Numbness or paresthesia	Neuropathy—compression
	Weakness	Myositis, neuropathy
	Stroke	Antiphospholipid syndrome
	Epilepsy	SLE
Mouth	Dry mouth	Sjögren's syndrome
	Mouth ulcers	Reactive arthritis, Behçet's disease, inflammatory bowel disease
Eyes	Dry eyes	Sjögren's syndrome
	Red eyes	Spondyloarthropathy
	Visual loss	Temporal arteritis
Skin	Rashes	
	Psoriasis	Psoriatic arthritis
	Livedo reticularis	SLE
	Erythema nodosum	Acute sarcoid or erythema nodosum arthropathy
	Telangiectasia	Systemic sclerosis
	Other	Viral
	Photosensitivity	Connective tissue disease
	Ulcers	Behçet's disease, vasculitis
	Raynaud's phenomenon	Connective tissue disease
	Nodules	Osteoarthritis, rheumatoid arthritis, gout, hyperlipidemia, SLE, rheumatic fever, polyarteritis nodosa, multicentric histiocytosis
	Alopecia	SLE
Respiratory	Pleuritis	Connective tissue disease
	Breathlessness	Pulmonary involvement with inflammatory disease, e.g., systemic sclerosis, rheumatoid arthritis
Gastrointestinal	Indigestion, history of peptic ulcer	Nonsteroidal gastritis or ulceration
	Diarrheal illness	Reactive arthritis, inflammatory bowel disease
Genitourinary	Renal stones	Gout
	Dysuria	Reactive arthritis, Behçet's disease, acute gonococcal arthritis
	Genital ulcers	Reactive arthritis, Behçet's disease, acute gonococcal arthritis
	Vaginal discharge	Reactive arthritis, Behçet's disease, acute gonococcal arthritis
Trauma	Fracture	
	Ligament rupture	
Non-specific symptoms	Malaise	Inflammatory disease, malignancy
	Fever	SLE, septic arthritis
	Weight loss	Inflammatory disease, malignancy
	Fatigue	Inflammatory disease
	Anorexia	Inflammatory disease, malignancy
	Aging	Polymyalgia rheumatica
Hematologic	Thrombosis/thromboembolism	Antiphospholipid syndrome
	Anemia	Inflammatory disease
Obstetric history	Fetal loss—early and late	Antiphospholipid syndrome
	Intrauterine growth retardation	Antiphospholipid syndrome
	Pre-eclampsia	Antiphospholipid syndrome

SLE, systemic lupus erythematosus.

low educational level. All this information may need to be considered when fully evaluating someone's musculoskeletal condition.

Previous health interventions and symptom response
Previous and present management should be reviewed. What has the patient been told: what knowledge and understanding does he or she have? What interventions have been tried—prescription and over-the-counter pharmacologic treatments, physiotherapy, supplements, or complementary therapies? What was the response to them? Did the patient benefit or sustain any adverse effects? What is the patient's attitude to and likely compliance with any treatment?

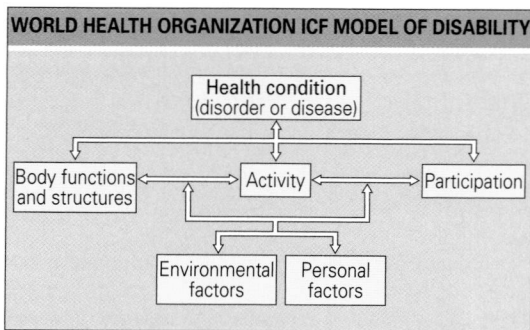

Fig. 27.2 WHO ICF model of disability. *(Adapted from World Health Organization. International classification of functioning and health. Geneva: WHO, 2001.)*

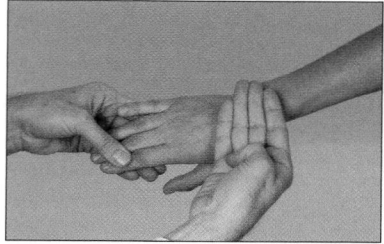

Fig. 27.3 Testing for warmth, using the back of the hand.

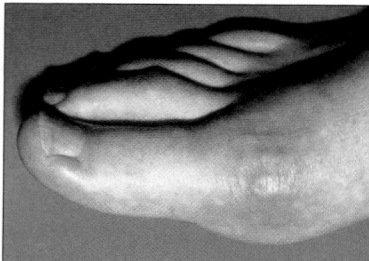

Fig. 27.4 Redness as seen in gout. This is a valuable indicator of the intensity of underlying joint inflammation.

The response to treatment can be of great relevance to understanding the nature of the problem, such as the response to anti-inflammatory therapy of many inflammatory disorders such as ankylosing spondylitis or the rapid and almost miraculous response to corticosteroids that is typical of polymyalgia rheumatica. Drugs themselves may also be the cause of the problem, as in drug-induced lupus and thiazide diuretics in gout.

What is its impact?

The impact of the musculoskeletal condition must be assessed in relation to the patient's needs and aspirations. The framework of the World Health Organization (WHO) International Classification of Functioning, Disability, and Health (ICF)[4] (Fig. 27.2) provides a useful way to look at the effect of any health condition on the functioning of an individual in terms of loss of function, limitation of activities, and restriction of participation within the personal and environmental context of the person's life.

Explore what the patient needs to do and would like to do in everyday activities, in relation to personal care, the home environment, the work whether paid or unpaid, and personal, social, and leisure activities. What is difficult, requires assistance, or has become impossible to do? Many people work around these challenges and still achieve a modified goal, but it is not meeting their needs or aspirations. Musculoskeletal problems often affect mobility and dexterity. Pain disturbs sleep. Talk a patient through a typical day and also remember to ask about any problems in participating in work or leisure activities as well as personal activities such as toileting or sexual activity. Find out the patient's frustrations and concerns.

Learn if and how the patient has gotten around limitations. Establish the amount of physical and emotional support the patient has from family, friends, other caregivers, or social services. Does this meet the patient's needs? How has the condition affected the patient's economic situation?

The effect on health-related quality of life can be formally assessed using various validated generic and disease-specific questionnaires such as the Health Assessment Questionnaire (HAQ).[2]

Social history and occupation

Knowing the patient's social history is important in assessing the condition and its impact and in planning management. The personal and environmental context plays an important role in the impact. Occupation is also important, because it may have a causal role or an effect on the symptoms or, alternatively, the symptoms may have an effect on occupation. Understanding the person's occupation can also give a clearer idea of his or her needs.

Examination

A careful examination is necessary to confirm clinical suspicions gained from the history. It also complements a screening assessment, characterizing any abnormality of the musculoskeletal system that has been identified. Examination of the musculoskeletal system is principally an exercise in applied anatomy. Is the pain originating from the bone, muscle, joint, or periarticular structures? Is the joint pain inflammatory or mechanical in origin? Is the origin of pain local with

tenderness or pain on movement or is it referred? How painful is it to touch or move, and is this consistent with the history? The examination may focus around the symptomatic structures, but it is usually most informative to do this as part of a general examination of the musculoskeletal system and of the whole patient.

Aims of examination

The aim of the examination of the musculoskeletal system is to answer four questions.

1. Is it normal?
2. What is the abnormality?
3. What is the pattern of distribution?
4. What other features of clinical importance are there? These, in combination with the history, should establish the differential diagnosis.

Is it normal?

The expected appearance and ranges of movement of the musculoskeletal system need to be recognized. Abnormalities observed may be abnormal resting position, swelling, deformity, muscle wasting, or abnormal movement. There may be warmth, crepitus, or tenderness on palpation, instability, or weakness.

What is the abnormality?

The nature of the abnormality needs to be established. What structure is involved? What are the characteristics of the abnormality? Is there evidence of inflammation, damage, deformity, and/or biomechanical abnormalities? These are not mutually exclusive; a combination of them may be found.

Inflammation

An inflamed joint is characterized by pain, tenderness, warmth, redness, and swelling. Pain is often apparent by observing movement, and tenderness is elicited by gentle palpation. Warmth is mainly detectable in medium-sized and large joints, for example, the knee, ankle, and wrist joints (Fig. 27.3). Redness is uncommon but is seen in gout, especially around the big toe (Fig. 27.4), and in sepsis. Swelling of an inflamed joint is characterized by its articular origin, is fluctuant because of synovial proliferation or effusion, and is tender, whereas there may be bony swelling along the joint line in osteoarthritis. There are a number of specific techniques for detection of synovitis and effusion at different joints (Fig. 27.5). One must identify the inflamed structure. Inflammation of periarticular structures such as a bursa or enthesis must be carefully distinguished from inflammation of the joint. Inflammation of muscle is characterized by tenderness.

TABLE 27.5 CHARACTERISTIC PATTERNS OF INVOLVEMENT OF THE MUSCULOSKELETAL SYSTEM

Diagnosis	Symmetry	No. of joints involved*	Large or small	Distribution	Upper or lower limbs
Rheumatoid arthritis	Symmetric	Polyarthritis	Large/small	Peripheral	Upper/lower
Ankylosing spondylitis	Asymmetric	Oligoarthritis	Large	Central and peripheral	Lower
Psoriatic arthritis	Asymmetric	Oligo/polyarthritis	Large/small	Peripheral	Upper/lower
Reactive arthritis	Asymmetric	Oligo/polyarthritis	Large/dactylitis	Peripheral	Lower
Gout	Asymmetric	Mono/oligoarthritis	Large/small	Peripheral	Lower/upper

Oligoarthritis ≤ 5 joints affected; polyarthritis > 5 joints affected.

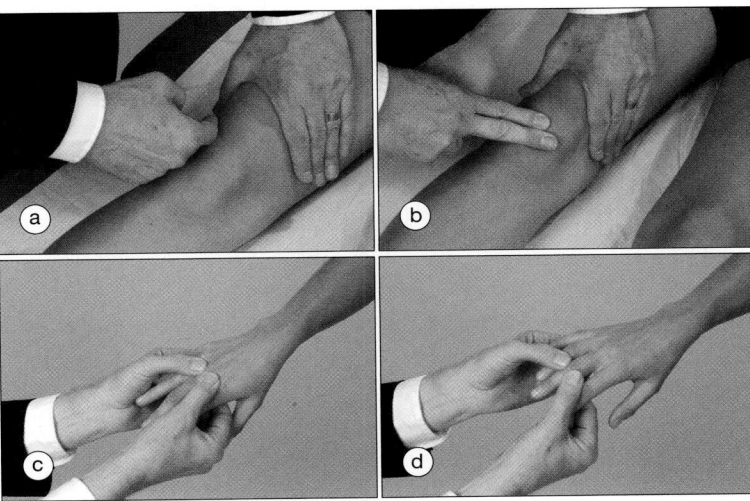

Fig. 27.5 Testing for swelling. (a) The bulge sign in the knee. The back of the hand gently pushes the fluid from one side of the knee to the other, filling out the "dimples" on either side of the patella. This is most helpful in detecting small knee effusions. (b) The patellar tap. One hand is used to cup the patella and compress the suprapatellar pouch, and the fingers of the other hand press down on the patella to feel for cross-fluctuation. (c and d) Swelling/fluctuation of the small joints of the hand. Detect cross-fluctuation at the joint line with the index fingers and thumbs, with the examiner's fingers squeezing and feeling each side of the joint (as illustrated) or one index finger/thumb squeezing and feeling from side to side and the other from the palmar to the dorsal aspect ("interlocking C").

Damage
Joint damage is recognized by the presence of deformity, crepitus, movement in an abnormal plane, and loss of joint range of movement not due to pain and in the absence of features of current inflammation. Crepitus is an audible and palpable sensation resulting from the movement of one roughened surface on another. In osteoarthritis, the crepitus has a fine quality. This should be distinguished from the coarser, clicking sensation encountered in normal joints.

Deformity
Joint deformity usually refers to malalignment or subluxation of two articulating bones in relation to one another and is identified by abnormal posture, often more apparent on weight-bearing or with certain movements, such as developmental scoliosis of the spine. There may be movement in an abnormal plane of a severely damaged joint from rheumatoid arthritis or osteoarthritis. For example, the elbow is a simple hinge joint; hence its normal range is flexion/extension only and any other movement, such as elbow abduction, is abnormal and likely to indicate gross joint disruption. There may be bone deformity in Paget's disease.

Biomechanical abnormalities
For every joint there is a normal posture and a spectrum of normal range of joint motion, which varies with age, gender, genetics, and ethnic origin. Outside this range, there may be hypermobility or hypomobility. Biomechanical abnormalities can result in symptoms, such

TABLE 27.6 CLINICAL SIGNS OF MUSCULOSKELETAL CONDITIONS

- Attitude
- Deformity
- Swelling
- Skin changes
- Muscle wasting
- Tenderness
- Movement restricted
- Crepitus
- Warmth
- Muscle weakness
- Instability
- Function limited

as scoliosis and back pain; joint hypermobility syndrome is associated with joint pain; and foot pain is often caused by abnormal biomechanics. The joint range is reduced by joint inflammation (the bulk of inflamed synovium and the effusion) or by irreversible damage to the joint structures (articular cartilage and subchondral bone). Movement is first lost from the extremes of the range. Complete loss of movement is described as ankylosis.

What is the pattern of distribution?
The distribution of involvement of the musculoskeletal structures is important in the diagnosis of musculoskeletal conditions, because certain patterns are characteristic (Table 27.5 and Chapter 28). Several different problems may affect an individual; the apparent pattern may be a false clue to the diagnosis. Examination is needed to confirm the pattern of distribution and to establish whether the various problems relate to a single diagnosis or to several coincident problems, such as the co-existence of nodal osteoarthritis and rheumatoid arthritis.

What other features of diagnostic importance are there?
There may be systemic features (see Table 27.4) of diagnostic importance or of value in assessing severity. Many of them are easily visible skin signs such as psoriasis, nail fold capillary abnormalities, or telangiectasia, whereas others, such as a pulmonary fibrosis or neuropathy will need to be identified by careful general examination.

Method of examination
One should look at the whole person, including posture and movement. Then each region is examined, comparing one side with the other. It is usually necessary to examine the full musculoskeletal system to correctly assess the problem, but most emphasis is placed on the likely origins of the symptoms, remembering that pain is frequently referred and that any examination must consider all possible causes. Explain to the patient what you are about to do and ask him or her to tell you if he or she thinks any part of the examination is likely to be painful.

The key elements of the examination to identify the clinical signs of musculoskeletal conditions (Table 27.6) are to look, feel, move, and stress (Table 27.7). These are usually performed in an integrated way. Special tests may be necessary to identify specific problems.

TABLE 27.7 SYSTEM FOR EXAMINATION OF THE MUSCULOSKELETAL SYSTEM

Look	At rest for: Swelling Deformity Wasting Attitude Skin During movement
Feel for:	Tenderness Swelling Movement—crepitus Temperature
Move	Active Passive Resistance Listen
Stress	Stability
Tests	

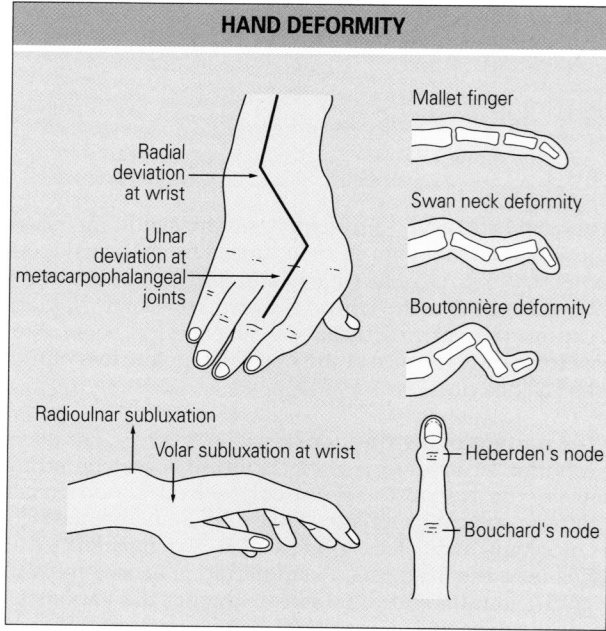

HAND DEFORMITY

Radial deviation at wrist

Ulnar deviation at metacarpophalangeal joints

Radioulnar subluxation

Volar subluxation at wrist

Mallet finger

Swan neck deformity

Boutonnière deformity

Heberden's node

Bouchard's node

Fig. 27.6 Common deformities of the hand.

TABLE 27.8 ASSOCIATED SKIN LESIONS

Region	Type of skin lesions	Associated conditions
Torso/limbs	Livedo reticularis	SLE, antiphospholipid syndrome, vasculitis
	Erythema ab igne	Sign of external heat applied to relieve pain
	Erythema migrans	Lyme arthritis
	Palpable purpura	Leukocytoclastic vasculitis
	Psoriasis	Psoriatic arthritis
	Erythema nodosum	Acute sarcoid
	Nodules	Heberden's, rheumatoid arthritis, gout, hyperlipidemia, SLE, rheumatic fever, polyarteritis nodosa, multicentric histiocytosis, sarcoidosis
	Ulcers	Vasculitis, Behçet's disease, Crohn's disease?
	Calcinosis cutis	Limited cutaneous systemic sclerosis
Face and mouth	Butterfly rash	SLE
	Psoriasis	Psoriatic arthritis
	Heliotrope discoloration	Dermatomyositis
	Oral ulcers	SLE, reactive arthritis, Behçet's disease
	Telangiectasia	Limited cutaneous systemic sclerosis
Nails	Clubbing	Hypertrophic pulmonary osteoarthropathy
	Pitting	Psoriatic arthritis
	Onycholysis	Psoriatic arthritis
	Splinter hemorrhages	Small vessel vasculitis, endocarditis
Hands	Raynaud's phenomenon	SLE, scleroderma, mixed connective tissue disease
	Nail fold capillary abnormalities	Scleroderma, dermatomyositis
	Palmar erythema	Active rheumatoid arthritis, SLE
	Gottron's papules	Dermatomyositis
	Telangiectasia	Limited cutaneous systemic sclerosis
	Sclerodactyly	Limited cutaneous systemic sclerosis
	Vasculitic lesions	Rheumatoid arthritis, connective tissue diseases
Feet	Keratoderma blennorrhagica	Reactive arthritis

SLE, systemic lupus erythematosus.

Look

Attitude and spontaneous movement

Observe the person when sitting and undertaking various functional movements during the consultation for any abnormalities associated with musculoskeletal conditions. An inflamed joint is most comfortable when the periarticular structures are at greatest laxity and the intracapsular pressure is least. Pain is most severe when intracapsular pressure is greatest. An indication of the severity of pain is given by the protection with which the person treats the affected region. Is ease of movement in keeping with the severity of pain described?

Swelling and deformities

Look for swelling, but palpation is necessary to characterize whether it is due to synovial thickening, joint effusion, or bony enlargement or a combination of these features. Look for any deformities of the joints, bones, or spine. There are a number of terms in common use to describe deformities.

- *Kyphosis:* a forward curvature of the thoracic spine
- *Scoliosis:* a lateral curvature of the spine

- *Dislocation:* articulating surfaces are displaced so that they are no longer in contact with one another
- *Subluxation:* partial dislocation
- *Fixed flexion:* loss of extension, so that the joint is permanently flexed
- *Valgus:* a lower limb deformity whereby the distal part is directed away from the midline (e.g., hallux valgus)
- *Varus:* a lower limb deformity whereby the distal part is directed toward the midline (e.g., genu varum).

Examination is necessary to determine if these deformities are correctable. Commonly encountered specific deformities of the hand are shown in Figure 27.6.

Skin

Look at the skin, both overlying the affected region and generally. Redness overlying the joint indicates marked inflammation, such as with infection or crystal arthropathy. Other skin changes include

TABLE 27.9 POSSIBLE CAUSES OF TENDERNESS

Site	Possible cause
Muscular: localized	Myofascial lesion
Muscular: generalized	Fibromyalgia Myositis
Joint line: generalized	Arthropathy or capsular disease
Joint line: localized	Abnormality of intracapsular structure, e.g., medial knee joint line tenderness with a meniscal tear
Periarticular	Bursitis, enthesiopathy, sarcoid
Bone	Bone pathology: osteoporotic fracture or invasive lesion
Vertebral	Bone pathology: osteoporotic fracture or invasive lesion

psoriasis, ulceration, livedo reticularis, and nodules such as tophi, erythema nodosum, and rheumatoid nodules (Table 27.8). Look carefully at the hands and nails because many abnormalities can be seen, such as Raynaud's phenomenon, nail fold capillary changes, telangiectasia, sclerodactyly, clubbing, pitting, or onycholysis.

Wasting
Look for loss of muscle bulk. Arthropathy can cause widespread wasting around the joint. More localized wasting suggests a tendon, muscle, or peripheral nerve lesion. Swelling of a joint can give a false impression of loss of muscle.

Feel
Warmth
First feel gently for warmth, which is best elicited by using the back of the fingers and comparing the finding to a normal structure (see Fig. 27.3). Warmth is a cardinal sign of inflammation but may be detected only over large joints.

Tenderness
The presence and localization of tenderness are important in identifying the cause of the problem (Table 27.9). Examine carefully to establish if it is the joint line or periarticular. Is it muscular, either generalized, such as in myositis, or localized, such as the characteristic tender spots of fibromyalgia? Is it the temporal artery or temporomandibular joint? Is there no tenderness despite pain? Feel for tenderness by gradually increasing pressure while watching the person for any reaction and releasing as soon as the presence of tenderness is established. Only use pressure until blanching of the nail of the examining fingers. Percuss the vertebrae to detect localized tenderness.

Swelling
Characterize any swelling to determine its precise location and anatomic associations, if it is tender, and whether it is fluid, soft tissue, or bone. Different types of swelling have typical characteristics. Swelling of a joint is confined by the capsule and is most apparent at any weaknesses in this; for example, an effusion of the knee may be associated with a popliteal cyst. Fluid and soft tissue are ballotable; this is the principle of the patellar tap and the interlocking-C examination of the interphalangeal joints (see Fig. 27.5).

Movement
Feeling the joint and periarticular structures while moving gives further information about pain and tenderness, as well as detecting crepitus from the joint or tendon sheaths.

Move
There are three methods of assessing joint movement—active, passive, and against resistance.

- To examine joints, a combination of active and passive is recommended.

- To detect lesions in tendons or at tendino-osseous junctions, the against-resistance method is principally of use.
- To measure muscle power, the against-resistance method is the principal technique.

First establish the active range, and, if reduced, then see if it is greater with passive movement, but be cautious because this may be painful. Familiarity with the normal ranges and planes of movement of the joints is needed. If the problem is unilateral, compare the affected with the unaffected side. Formal measurement of range of motion is of limited value. Involvement of the joint, in particular synovitis, usually restricts all movements. Restriction of movement in one plane is characteristic of periarticular lesions, tenosynovitis, or internal derangement of the joint. Pain in all directions of movement is associated with synovitis. Pain in just one plane of movement indicates a localized articular or periarticular problem. Pain throughout the range of movement is more characteristic of mechanical problems such as osteoarthritis.

Resisted active movement is valuable in identifying problems that relate to the muscle tendon or enthesis. This should be performed with the joint in a neutral position. The reproduction of pain indicates that it is originating from the muscle, tendon, or tendon insertion relating to that movement. Passively stretching the tendon or ligament may also reproduce the pain.

Listening during joint movement may detect fine crepitus due to cartilage damage, cracking associated with hypermobility, or clonking due to a loose body or irregular surfaces such as severe damage. Audible tendon friction rubs may be heard in patients with systemic sclerosis.

Stress
Joint stability should be assessed by stressing a joint. This can be abnormal because of generalized hypermobility, ligament rupture subsequent to trauma or inflammation, capsular inflammation, or loss of articular cartilage and bony changes due to osteoarthritis or rheumatoid arthritis.

Special tests
There are various special tests for specific diagnoses that are not within the scope of this overview but are considered elsewhere (see Chapters 68 through 80 as appropriate).

General examination
A full general examination forms an important part of the assessment of a person with a musculoskeletal problem. More frequent problems relate to the skin and nails, neurologic system, and eyes (see Tables 27.4 and 27.8).

Regional examination of the musculoskeletal system
A systematic approach to examination should be taken, but be sure to address any questions raised by the history or screening examination. The sequence can vary, but in general it is easiest to look at the patient as a whole and during walking and standing to observe gait and posture. Then work from the head downward, first with the patient standing to examine the upper limbs, spine, and pelvis and then supine to complete the examination of the pelvis and spine and to examine the lower limbs, comparing one side with the other for each limb (Boxes 27.3 through 27.6, Figs. 27.7 through 27.77).

BOX 27.3 REGIONAL EXAMINATION OF THE MUSCULOSKELETAL SYSTEM

Gait
- Observe the patient walking forward for a few feet, turning, and walking back again.

Posture
- Observe the patient from the back, side, and front, looking for any abnormalities, in particular of posture and symmetry.

BOX 27.4 REGIONAL EXAMINATION OF THE MUSCULOSKELETAL SYSTEM

Head, spine, and pelvis

Cervical spine

Look	Look for hyperextension due to a thoracic kyphosis or loss of normal lordosis.
Feel	Percuss the vertebrae for tenderness.
	Palpate the paraspinal muscles for spasm or tenderness.
Move	Actively turn head to right, left, flexion, extension, rotation to left and right, and lateral flexion to left and right with examiner gently guiding the head to ensure maximum range is reached.
Tests	Problems related to the cervical spine are often associated with neurologic symptoms and signs that should be elicited.

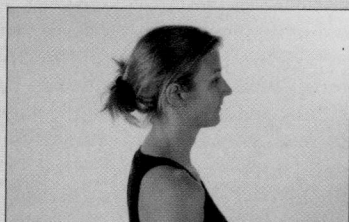 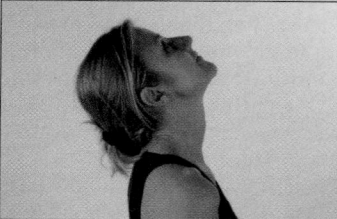

Fig. 27.7 Posture and alignment of the head and neck. **Fig. 27.8** Extension.

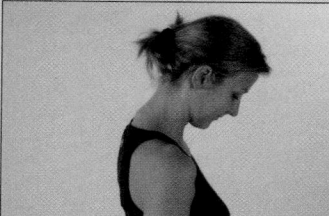 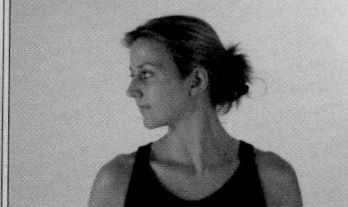

Fig. 27.9 Flexion. **Fig. 27.10** Right rotation.

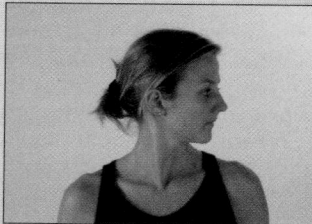 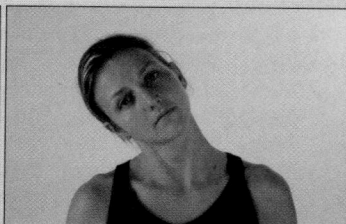

Fig. 27.11 Left rotation. **Fig. 27.12** Right lateral flexion.

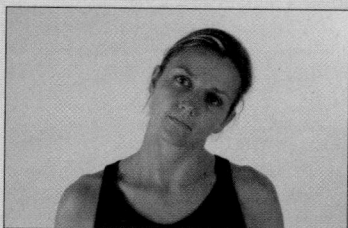

Fig. 27.13 Left lateral flexion.

Temporomandibular joints

Feel	Palpate over the joint line for tenderness, crepitus or clicking. The joint can be palpated anterior to the tragus or from within the external auditory meatus. Feel for crepitus or clicking on movement.
Move	Open mouth wide. Deviate lower jaw side to side.

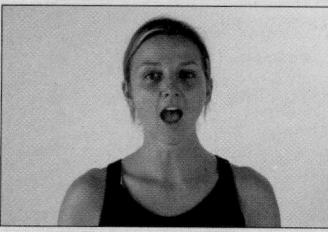 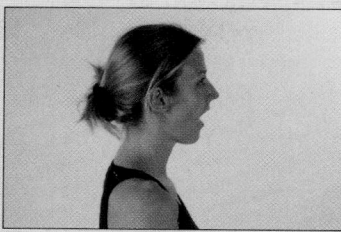

Fig. 27.14 Mouth opening. **Fig. 27.15** Mouth opening.

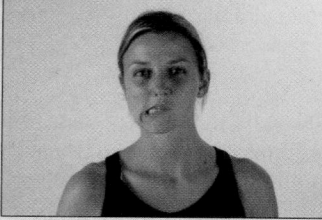 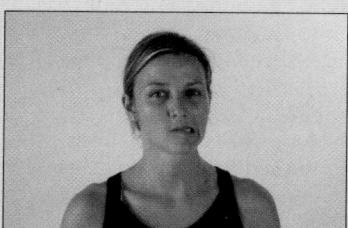

Fig. 27.16 Side-to-side movement of jaw. **Fig. 27.17** Side-to-side movement of jaw.

Dorsal spine

Look	Look for any kyphosis or scoliosis. Look for any asymmetry of scapulae.
Feel	Percuss the vertebrae for tenderness.
	Palpate the paraspinal muscles for spasm or tenderness.
Move	Fix the pelvis by sitting and rotate the upper body to right and left with examiner gently guiding the shoulders to ensure maximum range is reached.

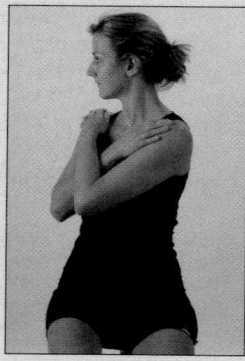 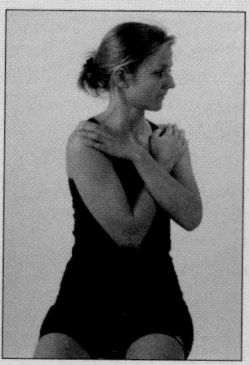

Fig. 27.18 Right rotation. **Fig. 27.19** Left rotation.

Lumbar spine

Look	Look for a normal lordosis or any scoliosis. Look for any asymmetry of pelvic brim or the crease of the buttocks.
Feel	Percuss the vertebrae for tenderness.
	Palpate the paraspinal muscles for spasm or tenderness.
Move	While standing in an erect posture, bend forward as if trying to touch the toes, bend backward to arch the back, and bend from side to side. The person may be able to place the hands flat on the ground if hypermobile.

BOX 27.4 REGIONAL EXAMINATION OF THE MUSCULOSKELETAL SYSTEM—cont'd

Flexion can be more formally assessed by the Schober test with measurement of the extension of a line drawn when upright between 10 cm above and 5 cm below the level of the posterior iliac spines identified by the dimples of Venus.

Stress Tests for tension of the lumbar roots should be performed when patient is lying down.

Femoral nerve stretch test: With the person lying prone, hold the ankle and passively flex the knee as far as it will go. The test is positive if pain is felt in the isolateral anterior thigh.

Sciatic nerve stretch test: With the person lying supine, gently raise the straight leg to the maximum angle achievable without significant pain and then dorsiflex the ankle. An increase in pain indicates sciatic nerve root tension.

Tests The lumbar spine houses the lumbar spinal nerve roots and neurologic symptoms and signs should be elicited.

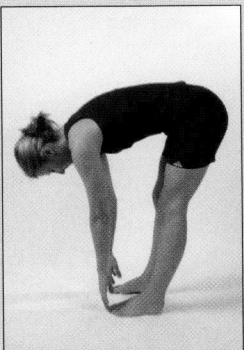

Fig. 27.20 Lumbar flexion.

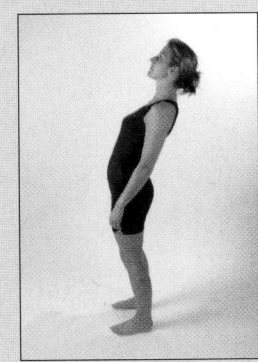

Fig. 27.21 Lumbar extension.

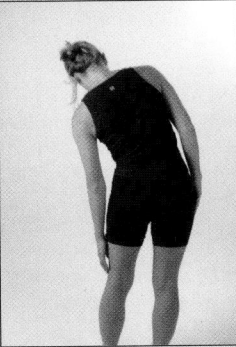

Fig. 27.22 Left lateral flexion.

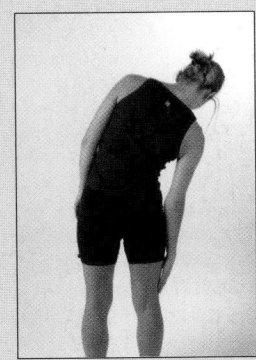

Fig. 27.23 Right lateral flexion.

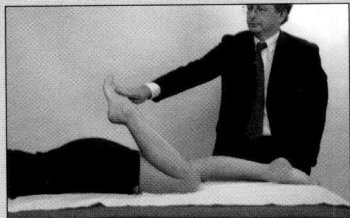

Fig. 27.24 Test for cruralgia.

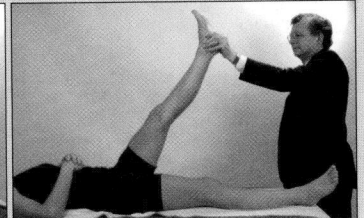

Fig. 27.25 Test for sciatica.

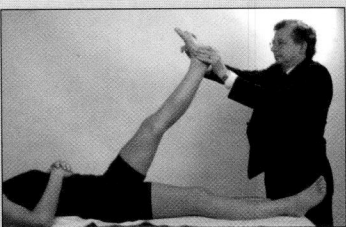

Fig. 27.26 Test for sciatica.

Pelvis and sacroiliac joints

Look Look for asymmetry of the pelvic brim and of the lower part of buttock.

Feel Palpate for tenderness in the buttocks.
Palpate the sacroiliac joints for tenderness.

Stress Stress the sacroiliac joints for tenderness. There are various methods to compress or distract the joint to elicit tenderness such as pushing on both iliac wings when the person is lying supine.

BOX 27.5 REGIONAL EXAMINATION OF THE MUSCULOSKELETAL SYSTEM

Upper extremity

Shoulder

Look Look for any asymmetry of scapulae, posture, or muscle wasting.

Feel Palpate over the midpoint of each trapezius and the supraspinatus to identify tender spots.
Palpate over the acromioclavicular joint line, glenohumeral joint line, and bicipital groove.

Move Actively elevate arms into air.
Actively place hands behind head.
Actively place hands behind back.
Steady scapula and with the elbow at 90 degrees rotate internally and externally; then passively abduct, flex, and internally and externally rotate the shoulder.

Tests There are several methods to establish if there is impingement.

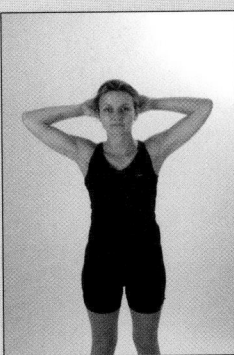

Fig. 27.27 Abduction and external rotation.

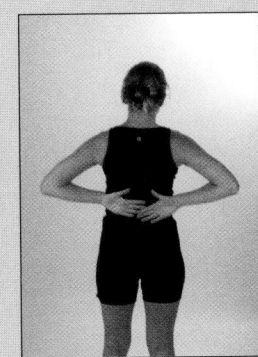

Fig. 27.28 Adduction, extension and internal rotation.

Continued

BOX 27.5 REGIONAL EXAMINATION OF THE MUSCULOSKELETAL SYSTEM—cont'd

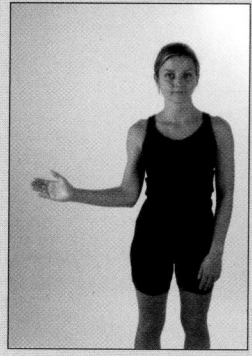

Fig. 27.29 External rotation.

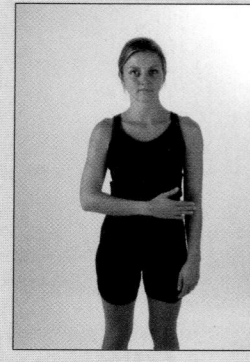

Fig. 27.30 Internal rotation.

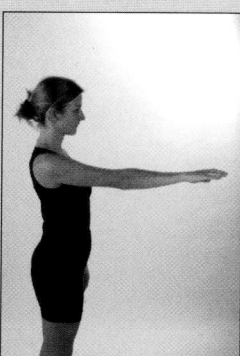

Fig. 27.31 Flexion.

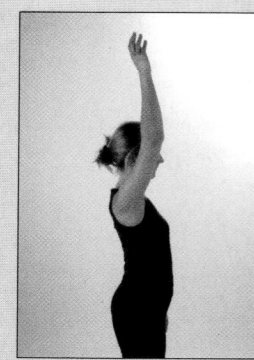

Fig. 27.32 Elevation.

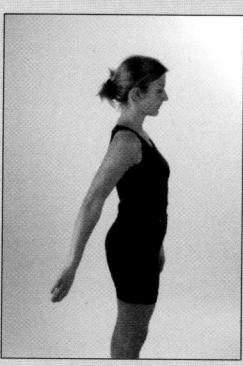

Fig. 27.33 Extension.

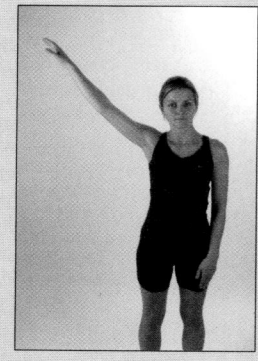

Fig. 27.34 Abduction.

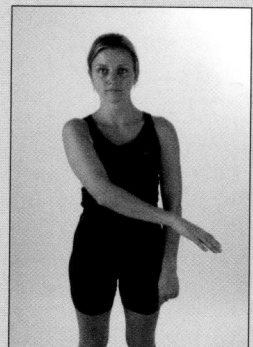

Fig. 27.35 Adduction.

Elbow

Look   Look for any swelling or deformity. Joint swelling is first apparent in the para-olecranon groove. The olecranon is a common site for bursitis and rheumatoid nodules.

Feel   Palpate over the para-olecranon groove for synovial swelling or tenderness. Palpate over the medial and lateral epicondyles for tenderness.

Assess the laxity of the skin if considering hypermobility.

Move   Passively extend and flex the elbow and look for hyperextension.

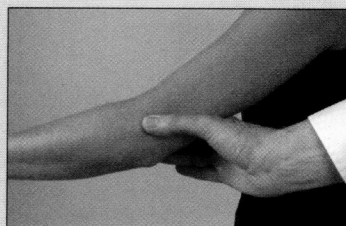

Fig. 27.36 Palpate over the medial and lateral epicondyles for tenderness.

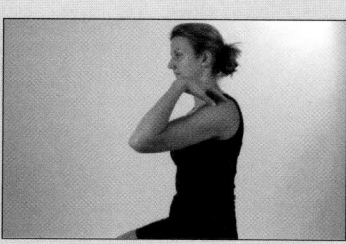

Fig. 27.37 Elbow flexion.

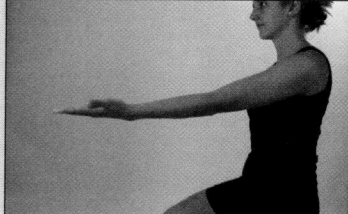

Fig. 27.38 Elbow extension.

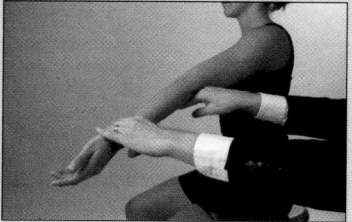

Fig. 27.39 Assess for elbow hyperextensibility.

Wrist

Look   Look for any swelling or deformity.

Swelling over the dorsum is of the joint or extensor tendon sheath. With active extension of the fingers, swelling of the extensor tendon sheath moves—the tuck sign.

Look for squaring of the palm base because of swelling of the carpometacarpal joint seen in osteoarthritis. Typical deformities in established rheumatoid arthritis are volar subluxation and radial deviation at the wrist with dorsal subluxation of the ulnar styloid.

Feel   Palpate over the joint line for tenderness or synovial swelling.

Move   Passively flex and extend the wrist.

Assess for hypermobility by passively moving the thumb toward the volar aspect of the forearm with the wrist in full flexion.

Use resisted flexion, extension, or pronation if assessing epicondylitis at the elbow.

Stress   Assess stability of the inferior radioulnar joint by demonstrating movement with pressing down on the radial head—the piano key sign.

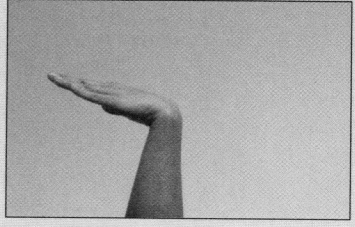

Fig. 27.40 Wrist flexion.

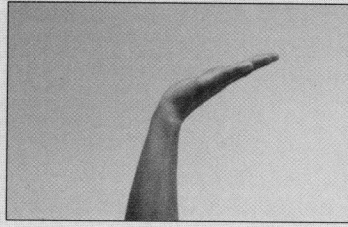

Fig. 27.41 Wrist extension.

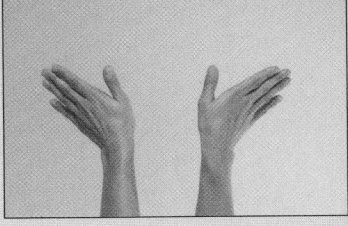

Fig. 27.42 Wrist ulnar movement.

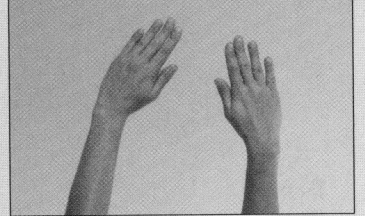

Fig. 27.43 Wrist radial movement.

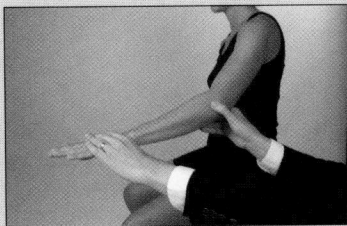

Fig. 27.44 Resisted active wrist extension to test for lateral epicondylitis.

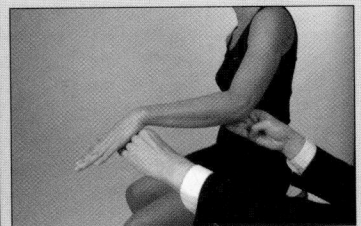

Fig. 27.45 Resisted active wrist flexion to test for medial epicondylitis.

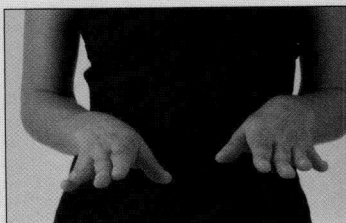

Fig. 27.46 Assess supination.

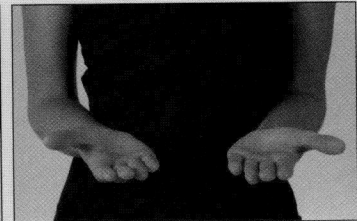

Fig. 27.47 Assess pronation.

Hand

Look Look for any swelling or deformity. Is the swelling specific to joints or tendons or is it diffuse?

Look for any associated clues. Much can be learned from the hand. Look for wasting of the small muscles; inspect the skin, nails, and nail beds.

Typical deformities in established rheumatoid arthritis are ulnar deviation of the fingers at the metacarpophalangeal joints, hyperextension at the proximal interphalangeal joint with flexion at the distal interphalangeal (swan-neck deformity) joint or flexion at the proximal interphalangeal joint with hyperextension at the distal interphalangeal joint (boutonniere deformity). A Z-deformity of the thumb can be seen in systemic lupus erythematosus.

Feel Palpate over each joint line for tenderness or bony or synovial swelling. Squeezing across all the knuckles together can be used as a composite assessment for tenderness of the metacarpophalangeal joints.

Palpate the tendon sheaths during movement to detect crepitus or tendon nodules. Feel the quality of the skin for induration, thickening, or laxity.

Move Actively make a tight fist with palmar aspect uppermost to see if all fingers fully flex and estimate strength of grip by observing the blanching of the palmar surface of the hand on release of the fist.

Actively make a firm pinch grip between the thumb and the fingers individually.

Passively extend the fifth finger to assess for hypermobility.

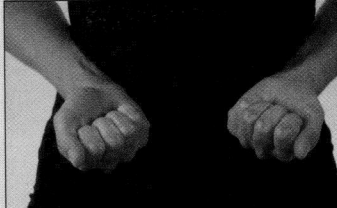

Fig. 27.48 Actively make a fist.

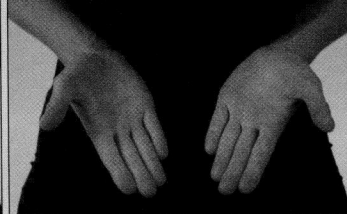

Fig. 27.49 Release grip and observe palm for blanching.

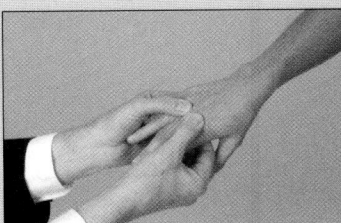

Fig. 27.50 Palpate the metacarpophalangeal joints.

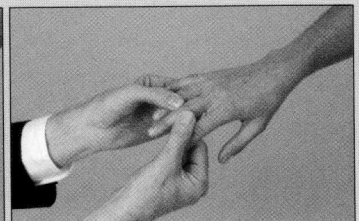

Fig. 27.51 Palpate the proximal interphalangeal joints.

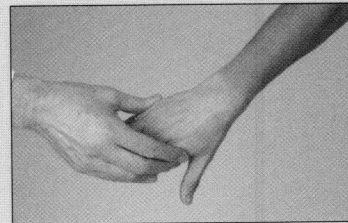

Fig. 27.52 Squeeze across the metacarpophalangeal joints.

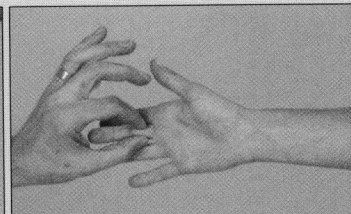

Fig. 27.53 Palpate the tendon sheaths.

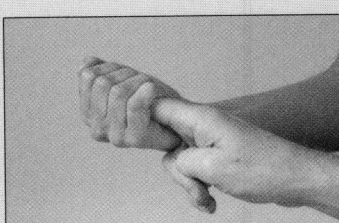

Fig. 27.54 Assess grip strength.

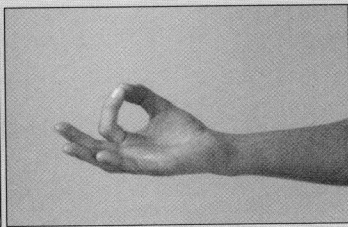

Fig. 27.55 Assess pinch grip.

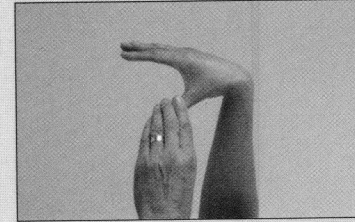

Fig. 27.56 Assess for hypermobility of the thumb and wrist.

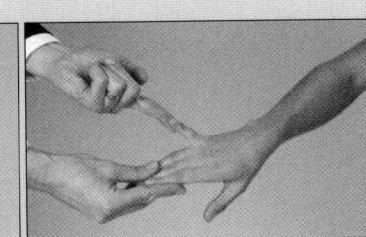

Fig. 27.57 Assess hyperextensibility of fifth finger.

BOX 27.6 REGIONAL EXAMINATION OF THE MUSCULOSKELETAL SYSTEM

Lower extremity

Observing the gait is an important part of assessing the lower limbs. Examination should be done with the person lying on a bench. Measure leg length if a pelvic tilt when standing suggests shortening or if there is a discrepancy in position of medial malleoli with straightened pelvis. Pain in the hindquarter is often called "hip pain" but can have many origins that need elucidating by examination.

Hip

Look Observation of the person walking will have given some information about the hips. There may be wasting of the buttock or thigh muscles from disuse.

Feel Palpation should be used to clarify the origin of any symptoms. The "hip" is used to describe symptoms anywhere in the hindquarter. Tenderness is usually related to tendinitis or bursitis.

Move With the person supine, actively and then passively flex the hip as far as possible with the knee in flexion looking for contralateral movement.

With the hip passively flexed to 90 degrees, rotate it internally and externally by holding the foot, supporting the thigh, and moving the lower leg inward and outward, careful to not inflict pain. Internal rotation is often affected first in disorders of the hip joint.

With the person lying supine with the leg fully extended, hold the contralateral anterior superior iliac spine to prevent movement of the pelvis and passively abduct and adduct the leg.

With the person lying prone or on the side, passively extend the straightened leg.

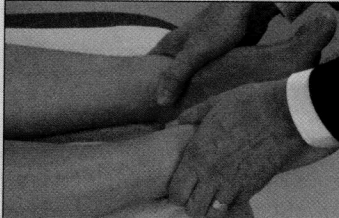

Fig. 27.58 Assess leg length by relative position of medial malleoli with straightened pelvis.

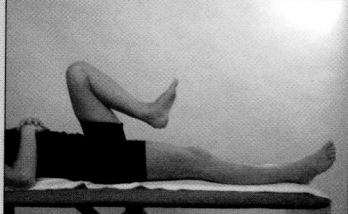

Fig. 27.59 Hip flexion—active.

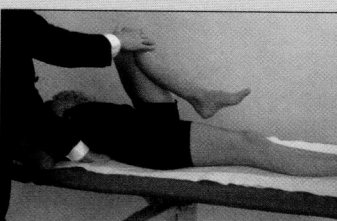

Fig. 27.60 Hip flexion—passive, looking for contralateral movement.

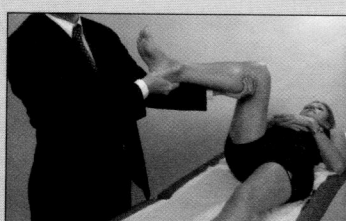

Fig. 27.61 Internal rotation.

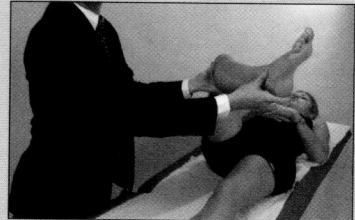

Fig. 27.62 External rotation.

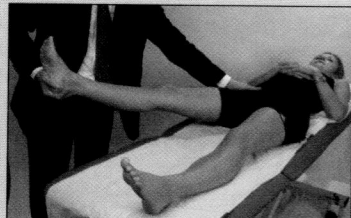

Fig. 27.63 Abduction.

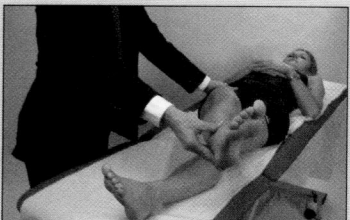

Fig. 27.64 Adduction.

Knee

Look Observation of the person walking will have given some information about the knees. There may be wasting of the thigh muscles from disuse. There may be instability. Look for any swelling and its exact site because it may relate to the joint or periarticular structures. Look for any deformity. Typical deformities are fixed flexion, valgus, or varus.

Feel Palpate for tenderness or swelling and establish the affected structures. Palpate the joint line for tenderness. Assess for articular swelling and effusion by the bulge sign or patella tap (see Fig. 27.5). Palpate for a popliteal cyst.

Move With the person supine, passively flex the knee as far as possible with the hip in flexion. If the hip is also abnormal, hang the leg over the side of the bench to examine flexion of the knee without hip flexion.

With the person lying supine, fully extend the leg in an attempt to touch the back of the knee onto the bench. Assess passively if the knee will hyperextend.

Stress Anterior and posterior stability should be tested to assess the cruciate ligaments.

Medial and lateral stability should be tested to assess the collateral ligaments and for loss of joint space.

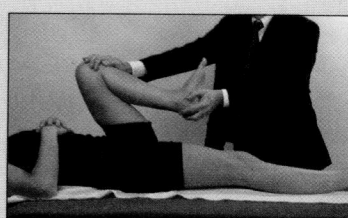

Fig. 27.65 Knee flexion.

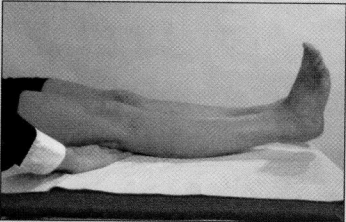

Fig. 27.66 Knee extension.

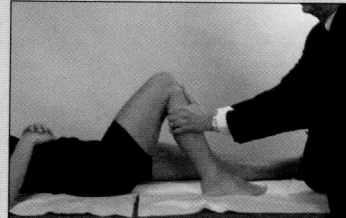

Fig. 27.67 Stress the cruciate ligaments.

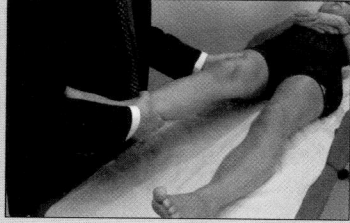

Fig. 27.68 Stress the collateral ligaments.

Foot and ankle

Look Observe the feet when standing and during walking. Look for a normal longitudinal arch and during the gait cycle look for normal heel strike and take off from the forefoot. Look for any callosities beneath the metatarsal heads and for any swelling and redness of the toes.

Swelling of the metatarsophalangeal joints can separate the toes and daylight becomes visible between them. Look for any deformities.

BOX 27.6 REGIONAL EXAMINATION OF THE MUSCULOSKELETAL SYSTEM—cont'd

	Deformities include pes planus (flattening of the longitudinal arch), pronation of the foot, valgus deformity of the hindfoot (eversion of the subtalar joint, pes cavus (high longitudinal arch), talipes equinovarus, hallux valgus, subluxation of the metatarsophalangeal joints, and "claw," "hammer," and "mallet" deformities of the toes.
Feel	Symptoms may relate to the joint; the periarticular bone; the tendons, their sheaths and insertions; or bursae. Palpate for tenderness or swelling and establish the affected structures. Squeeze across the metatarsus, and if there is tenderness, examine the metatarsophalangeal joints individually.
Move	Actively flex and extend the ankle. Actively invert and supinate and then evert and pronate the foot. Passively deviate the heel medially (inversion) and laterally (eversion) by grasping the heel between the examiner's thumb and index finger of one hand and moving it while anchoring the lower leg with the other hand. Passively rotate the forefoot on the hindfoot by grasping the forefoot between the examiner's thumb and fingers while anchoring the heel with the other hand to assess the midtarsal joint. See if the patient is able to stand on the toes, which requires an intact posterior tibialis tendon.

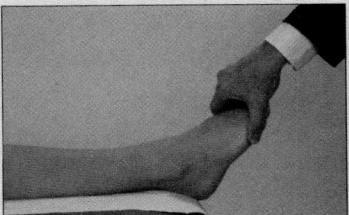 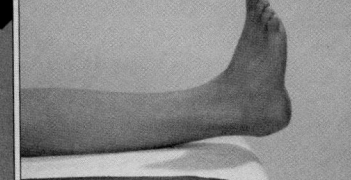

Fig. 27.69 Metatarsal squeeze. **Fig. 27.70** Ankle flexion.

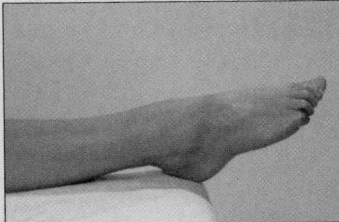 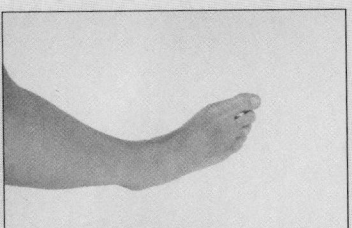

Fig. 27.71 Ankle extension. **Fig. 27.72** Inversion and supination.

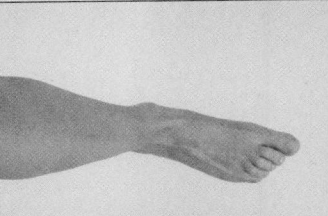 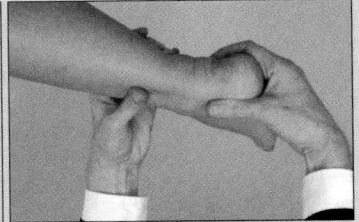

Fig. 27.73 Eversion and pronation. **Fig. 27.74** Subtalar inversion.

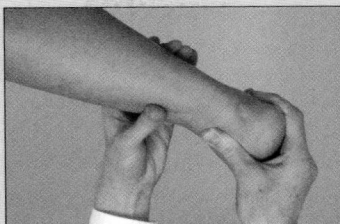 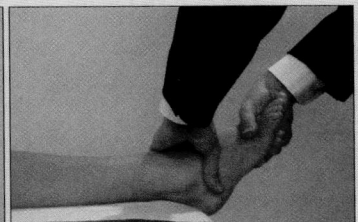

Fig. 27.75 Subtalar eversion. **Fig. 27.76** Midtarsal rotation.

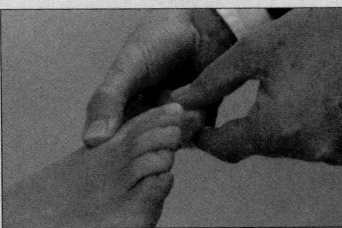

Fig. 27.77 Assessing the first metatarsophalangeal joint.

Gait

The gait demonstrates the integrated function of the lower limbs and will reveal abnormalities of the musculoskeletal system (see Fig. 27.1). Further assessment of the lower limbs will be necessary to identify the specific cause of any abnormality of gait.

Certain abnormal patterns of gait are well recognized. Pain in one limb causes the avoidance of weight bearing by that limb and shortening of that phase of the gait cycle. The cycle is asymmetric, with shorter steps on the painful limb, and is described as an antalgic gait. Weakness of the hip adductors results in dipping of the pelvis to the other side when weight bearing on the affected limb. During the gait cycle the person leans the upper body over the weak hip to compensate for this to keep his or her balance. This Trendelenburg gait is apparent as side-to-side movement of the shoulders when walking. Such movement of the shoulders is also seen if there is an inequality of leg length, leading to tilting of the pelvis during the gait cycle. An alternative gait with leg-length inequality is to flex the knee of the longer leg to clear the ground during the swing phase, with consequent dipping of the person up and down. A dropfoot results in a high-stepping gait to avoid tripping on the toes during the swing phase.

Posture

The normal symmetry of the body helps identify abnormalities of posture. Observe the whole person standing undressed in underwear and look for equality of height of landmarks—the shoulder tips, the scapulae, the pelvic brim, the crease of the buttocks. Inspect the spine carefully for its normal curves and identify any scoliosis. Look at the feet during normal posture.

Documentation

The history and examination need to be documented. The history should form a clear story that another clinician can read, assess, and interpret. The examination is documented most easily on a homunculus. A standardized approach is recommended to denote deformities, restricted movement, joint swelling, and joint tenderness (Fig. 27.78).

There are various disease-specific standardized assessments that can be used to evaluate conditions such as rheumatoid arthritis, ankylosing spondylitis, or SLE. These are considered elsewhere in this text.

CONCLUDING THE CONSULTATION

Interpretation

The aim of the consultation is to identify the cause of the person's problems, assess impact and response to any treatment, plan

ANNOTATING THE EXAMINATION FINDINGS

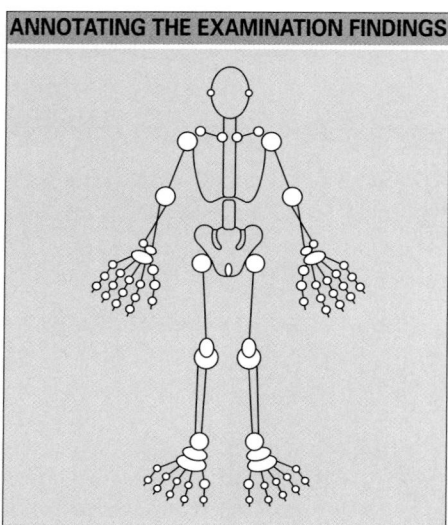

Fig. 27.78 Annotating the examination findings. A homunculus can be used to annotate the abnormal findings made during examination.

management, and fully discuss this and the expected outcome with the patient.

Making a diagnosis requires the integration of the history and findings on examination with knowledge of the possible causes and results of appropriate investigations. Pattern recognition plays a key role (see Chapter 28). Knowing what is likely at different stages of life in different individuals and looking for clues throughout the consultation is important. Because musculoskeletal conditions are common, it must be remembered that multiple pathologic processes are possible.

Communicating the findings

The most important part of the consultation, especially for the patient, is the communication of the findings and conclusions. Ensure that the person feels that all his or her problems have been listened to, questions answered, and expectations met as far as is possible. It is sometimes difficult to explain all of a person's symptoms with precise tissue-based causes, and this can cause concern and loss of confidence in the physician. Concepts of mechanical back pain and fibromyalgia can be difficult for the person to grasp. This part of the consultation needs the most time but is usually the most hurried part. A specialist nurse can supplement the information that the person wants, and there is a lot of material available about musculoskeletal conditions from support organizations, such as the Arthritis Foundation or Arthritis Care and through the Internet.

REFERENCES

1. Doherty M, Dacre J, Dieppe P, Snaith M. The "GALS" locomotor screen. Ann Rheum Dis 1992;51:1165-1169.
2. Fries JF, Spitz PW, Kraines RG, Holman HR. Measurement of patient outcome in arthritis. Arthritis Rheum 1980;23:137-145.

3. Van Der Heijde DMFM, Van't Hof MA, Van Riel PLCM, Van De Putte LBA. Development of a disease activity score based on judgement in clinical practice by rheumatologists. J Rheumatol 1993;20:579-581.

4. World Health Organization. International classification of functioning and health. Geneva: WHO, 2001.

FURTHER READING

Doherty M, Hazleman BL, Hutton CW, et al. Rheumatology examination and injection techniques, 2nd ed. London: WB Saunders, 1999.

McRae R. Clinical orthopaedic examination, 4th ed. Edinburgh: Churchill Livingstone, 1997.

Pattern recognition in arthritis

Osvaldo Hübscher

28

- Pattern recognition is the key to diagnosis of the rheumatic disorders: the central questions that need to be asked are:
  - Is there a musculoskeletal problem or a disease of another system?
  - Is the condition articular or periarticular?
  - Is the condition mechanical (arthrosis) or inflammatory?
  - Does it affect appendicular or axial structures or both?
- These questions can be answered from a synthesis of data from the history and physical examination, in particular:
  - *From the history:* the mode of onset, the sequence of development of different features, and the duration and pattern of the symptoms
  - *From the physical examination:* the number, distribution, and pattern of the affected joints or periarticular structures and the nature of any systemic involvement

INTRODUCTION

The history and physical examination are the two most important components of the diagnostic process for patients complaining of musculoskeletal pain, stiffness, or other symptoms.[1] Clinical judgment in interpreting the findings elicited from the history and physical examination should allow the physician to answer several key questions:

- Do the symptoms originate in the musculoskeletal system or do they reflect diseases primarily affecting other systems (e.g., neurologic disorders, vascular disease, Pancoast's syndrome)?
- Is it an articular or non-articular process? A substantial number of patients will have localized mechanical problems or non-specific soft tissue conditions. Muscular syndromes or pain originating in periarticular foci can often mimic an articular origin (sometimes affecting more than one site). Examples are unilateral or bilateral anserine bursitis, resembling an intra-articular knee joint disorder, and extensor tendinitis of the thumb (de Quervain's tenosynovitis), mimicking wrist involvement. Primary bone conditions (e.g., Paget's disease, osteoid osteoma, osteomalacia) as well as infiltrative (e.g., lymphomas) and lytic (e.g., metastatic disease, osteitis fibrosa cystica) lesions may also provoke pain referred to a joint. Osteonecrosis or infection and stress fractures may also generate confusion.
- Does the patient have arthralgias or arthritis? Arthralgia refers to pain localized to a joint, whereas arthritis refers to the objective evidence of an inflammatory change of the joint. Arthritis is a much more specific sign of an articular disorder.
- Is there evidence of other organ involvement (e.g., systemic connective tissue disorders), or does it appear to be a disorder restricted to the musculoskeletal system (e.g., osteoarthritis)?
- Is the articular problem inflammatory, mechanical, degenerative, or something else?
- Does the disease affect axial or appendicular structures or both?

Once the physician has established that the disorder originates in the joints, several other aspects of the history and physical examination should be considered to delineate a diagnostic pattern of arthropathy (Table 28.1). The attributes of joint involvement that are considered in this section focus on those dominating the clinical picture during the early phases of rheumatologic disorders, when treatment could be of greater benefit. Moreover, the diagnostic value of pattern recognition will be considered without taking into account other characteristics of the patient (e.g., gender, age, family history) or the presence or absence of extra-articular features of disease normally contributing to diagnostic certainty.

MODE OF ONSET AND DURATION OF SYMPTOMS

Some arthropathies typically present as an acute onset of pain with the peak intensity reached within hours or a few days, whereas in others maximum severity is reached gradually (over several weeks or months). Variations may occur, and the same disorder may have a sudden onset in some patients and be gradual in others. Rheumatoid arthritis (RA), for instance, may present as an acute polyarthritis (especially in the elderly) and psoriatic arthritis as an acute monoarthritis resembling gout, whereas in most cases both disorders begin insidiously. Examples of disorders with an acute onset also include bacterial arthritis, rheumatic fever, reactive arthritis, sarcoidosis, palindromic rheumatism, and crystal-induced arthritis (the best example being nocturnal attacks of gout). An arthritogenic virus (e.g., rubella virus and hepatitis B virus) may also cause acute synovitis. An insidious pattern is common in early-onset pauciarticular juvenile idiopathic arthritis (EOPA-JIA), as well as in the polyarticular-onset type and in osteoarthritis (OA), hypertrophic osteoarthropathy, mycobacterial and fungal arthritis, and most cases of neuropathic arthropathy (Charcot's joints).

Arthritic disorders lasting less than 4 to 6 weeks are considered to be self-limiting in practical terms, whereas those lasting longer are considered to be chronic. In self-limiting arthritic disorders the duration of symptoms and signs may be a valuable discriminating feature. Early episodes of monoarticular gout tend to subside spontaneously after 7 to 10 days and resolution is complete; acute or subacute attacks of pseudogout (calcium pyrophosphate dihydrate crystal deposition disease [CPPD]) may last from 2 to 3 days to 3 to 4 weeks; most articular or periarticular episodes of palindromic rheumatism disappear within hours to several days with no articular sequelae. Parvovirus-associated arthritis is usually of acute onset and self-limited, resolving in 1 to 3 weeks. A steady inflammation in an individual joint for more than a few days or a week in children is highly unlikely to be due to rheumatic fever.

THE NUMBER OF AFFECTED JOINTS

The clinical pattern may be monoarticular, oligoarticular, or polyarticular, reflecting involvement restricted to a single, a few, and several joints, respectively.

Although almost any individual arthropathy may begin as monoarthritis, the initial pattern of some disorders is characteristically monoarticular regardless of the subsequent course. In particular, patients with an acute painful synovitis of a single joint and varying degrees of overlying redness represent a challenging subset in clinical rheumatology.[2,3] Although redness may occur in any acute monoarthritis regardless of the cause, its presence usually evokes a restricted list of possible diagnoses (Table 28.2). The most common are crystal-induced synovitis (including acute calcific periarthritis),[4] bacterial infectious arthritis (Fig. 28.1), traumatic conditions, psoriatic arthritis, and palindromic rheumatism (in which the joint may reach a dark, bluish redness).

Owing to the frequency of the underlying disease, it should be remembered that the uncommon occurrence of a red-hot joint in the context of RA may be due to superimposed infectious synovitis and not to the disease process itself.[5] Nonetheless, a syndrome of acute

TABLE 28.1 MAJOR DIAGNOSTIC FEATURES OF JOINT DISORDERS

Mode of onset	Acute
	Insidious
Duration of symptoms	Self-limiting
	Chronic
Number of affected joints	Monoarthritis
	Oligoarthritis (two to four joints)
	Polyarthritis
Distribution of joint involvement	Symmetric
	Asymmetric
Localization of affected joints	Axial
	Appendicular
	Both
Sequence of involvement	Additive
	Migratory
	Intermittent
Local pattern of involvement (in individual joints)	

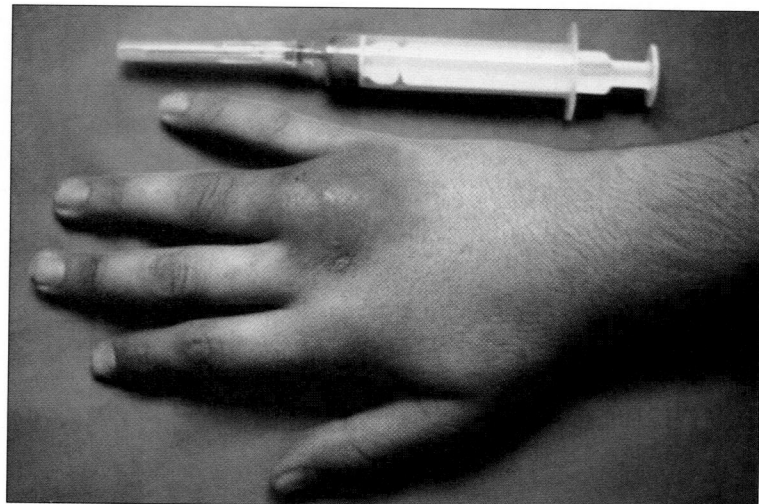

Fig. 28.1 The red-hot joint. Septic arthritis of the ring finger metacarpophalangeal joint showing swelling and intense redness of the skin.

TABLE 28.2 THE RED-HOT JOINT

Type	Subtypes/examples (if applicable)
Infectious	Bacterial
	Neisserial (may be preceded by transient polyarticular disease)
	Mycobacterial
	Virus
	Lyme disease
Crystal induced	Gout
	CPPD (pseudogout type)
	Hydroxyapatite (acute calcific periarthritis)
Traumatic/fracture	
Palindromic rheumatism	
Psoriatic arthritis	
Reactive arthritis	
Bacterial endocarditis	
Sarcoidosis	

TABLE 28.3 SELECTED CAUSES OF CHRONIC MONOARTHRITIS

Type	Subtypes/examples (if applicable)
Infectious arthritis	Mycobacterial, fungal, bacterial, viral, Lyme disease
Inflammatory arthritis	Crystal induced
	Monoarticular RA
	EOPA-JIA
	Seronegative spondyloarthropathies (ankylosing spondylitis, reactive arthritis, colitic arthritis, undifferentiated spondyloarthropathy)
	Psoriatic arthropathy
	Foreign body synovitis (e.g., plant thorn synovitis)
	Sarcoidosis
Non-inflammatory arthritis	Osteoarthritis
	Internal derangement
	Osteonecrosis
	Synovial osteochondromatosis
	Reflex sympathetic dystrophy
	Hemarthrosis (e.g., coagulopathy, anticoagulants)
	Neuropathic (Charcot's joint)
	Stress fracture
	Transient regional osteoporosis
	Juvenile osteochondroses
Tumors	Pigmented villonodular synovitis
	Lipoma arborescens
	Synovial metastasis from solid tumors
	Synovial sarcoma
Undiagnosed	

sterile arthritis mimicking articular infection may occur in RA patients and respond to anti-inflammatory therapy.[6] Although systemic lupus erythematosus (SLE) may cause a number of articular problems, the occurrence of monoarthritis suggests infection or osteonecrosis.

Chronic monoarthritis is often the presenting manifestation of a variety of joint disorders (Table 28.3); histologic elucidation may be necessary to make the correct diagnosis. In a substantial number of patients the cause remains undetermined.[7]

Involvement of two to four separate joints is referred to as oligoarthritis. In general, rheumatologic disorders manifesting as monoarthritis may also be oligoarticular. Despite this overlap, there are examples in which involvement of two or three joints (rather than one) may significantly narrow the diagnostic spectrum. As an example, lower limb oligoarthritis (especially of the knees and ankles) in an asymmetric fashion is reminiscent of the HLA-B27–associated seronegative spondyloarthropathies.[8] An asymmetric oligoarthritis affecting scattered distal interphalangeal (DIP), proximal interphalangeal (PIP), and metacarpophalangeal (MCP) joints of the hands characterizes a common subgroup of patients with psoriatic arthritis.

The third articular pattern is the one in which polyarticular involvement dominates the clinical picture. A wide variety of inflammatory and non-inflammatory disorders, both common and uncommon, may present as polyarthritis (Table 28.4).[9]

TABLE 28.4 DISTRIBUTION OF SELECTED OLIGOARTHRITIS AND POLYARTHRITIS	
Symmetric	**Asymmetric**
Inflammatory	
RA; JIA (systemic and polyarticular types)	Ankylosing spondylitis
	Reactive arthritis
Adult-onset Still's disease	Psoriatic arthritis (oligoarticular type)
Systemic lupus erythematosus	Enteropathic arthritis
Mixed connective tissue disease	Undifferentiated spondyloarthropathy
Polymyalgia rheumatica	JIA (pauciarticular types)
Rheumatic fever (adult onset)	Palindromic rheumatism
Jaccoud's arthritis	
Degenerative/crystal induced	
Osteoarthritis (primary generalized, erosive and nodal types)	Gout (especially oligoarthritis)
	CPPD (pseudogout type)
CPPD (pseudo-RA type)	
"Milwaukee shoulder"	
Hemochromatosis arthropathy	
Infectious	
Viral arthritis	Bacterial arthritis
	Bacterial endocarditis
	Lyme disease (late phase)
Miscellaneous	
Hypertrophic osteoarthropathy	Cancer-associated arthritis
Amyloid arthropathy	Pancreatic disease–associated arthritis
Myxedematous arthropathy	
Sarcoid arthritis (acute type)	
Cancer-associated arthritis	

Most asymmetric arthritides may be, or are characteristically, initially monoarticular

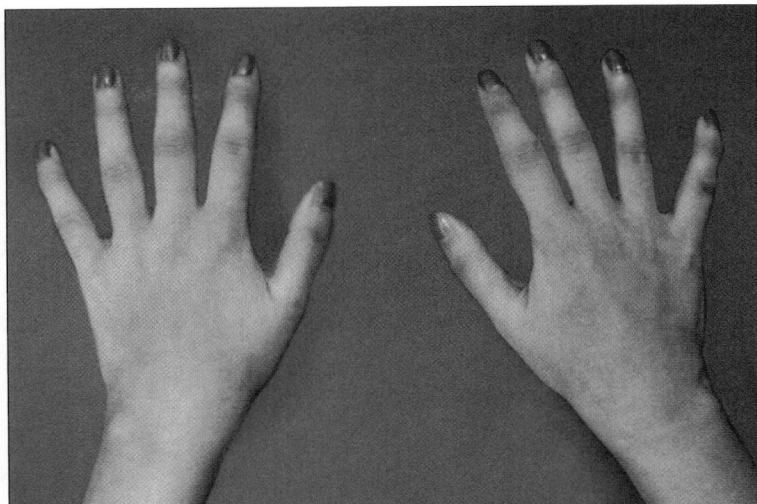

Fig. 28.2 Symmetric interphalangeal synovitis in a woman with seropositive RA.

TABLE 28.5 CHRONIC ARTHROPATHIES WITH PERIPHERAL AND AXIAL INVOLVEMENT	
Type	**Subtypes/examples (if applicable)**
Inflammatory	
Spondyloarthropathies	Ankylosing spondylitis
	Reactive arthritis
	Psoriatic arthropathy (a subset of patients)
	Enteropathic arthritis
	Undifferentiated
Juvenile idiopathic arthritis	Systemic and polyarticular onset
Adult-onset Still's disease	
SAPHO syndrome	
Non-inflammatory	
Osteoarthritis	
Diffuse idiopathic skeletal hyperostosis	
Acromegaly	
Ochronosis	
Spondyloepiphyseal dysplasia	

IS IT A SYMMETRIC OR AN ASYMMETRIC ARTHRITIS?

This distinction is very helpful in the differential diagnosis of oligoarticular and polyarticular conditions, with RA being the classic example of symmetric arthritis (Fig. 28.2), meaning simultaneous inflammatory signs in pairs of peripheral joints (e.g., both knees, both wrists). Symmetry is not necessarily strict in the hands; the same MCP or PIP joint may not be equally affected in both extremities of RA patients. Erosive inflammatory OA, pachydermodactyly, parvovirus arthritis, and many cases of SLE may resemble RA, whereas reactive arthritis, psoriatic arthritis, and polyarticular gout usually present as asymmetric involvement of appendicular joints. Both symmetric and asymmetric seronegative oligoarthritis/polyarthritis have been seldom described in association with neoplasia.[10]

This feature of the articular pattern has obvious limitations; every patient with a symmetric disorder may have an initial asymmetric phase. Table 28.4 lists a number of conditions classified according to the most characteristic pattern.

LOCALIZATION OF AFFECTED JOINTS

Axial involvement

Axial structures include, apart from the spine, centrally located joints such as the sacroiliac, sternoclavicular, and manubriosternal joints and the rest of the chest wall and sometimes shoulders and hips.

In the presence of peripheral arthritis, one of the most helpful clues in the differential diagnosis is to determine the presence of concomitant axial involvement. Whereas some rheumatologic conditions rarely affect the axial segments (e.g., gout, SLE, systemic vasculitis), a combined pattern is often seen in others (Table 28.5). Osteoarthritis of the facet joints of the spine often coexists with appendicular involvement. Diffuse idiopathic skeletal hyperostosis (DISH) affects mainly dorsal and lumbar spinal segments and may be accompanied by OA in atypical upper limb joints (elbow, shoulder, MCP).[11] Patients with ankylosing spondylitis, psoriatic arthritis, reactive arthritis (after both enteric and sexually transmitted infection), and arthritis accompanying inflammatory bowel disease may also exhibit varying degrees of combined axial and peripheral involvement. Polyarticular and systemic-onset juvenile idiopathic arthritis (JIA) as well as adult-onset Still's disease commonly affect the apophyseal joints of the cervical spine in addition to peripheral joints. The SAPHO syndrome (synovitis, acne, pustulosis, hyperostosis, and osteitis) is a further example among the much less frequent arthritides.[12] Acute involvement of a sternoclavicular joint (one of the less frequently involved joints) suggests septic arthritis in intravenous drug users.

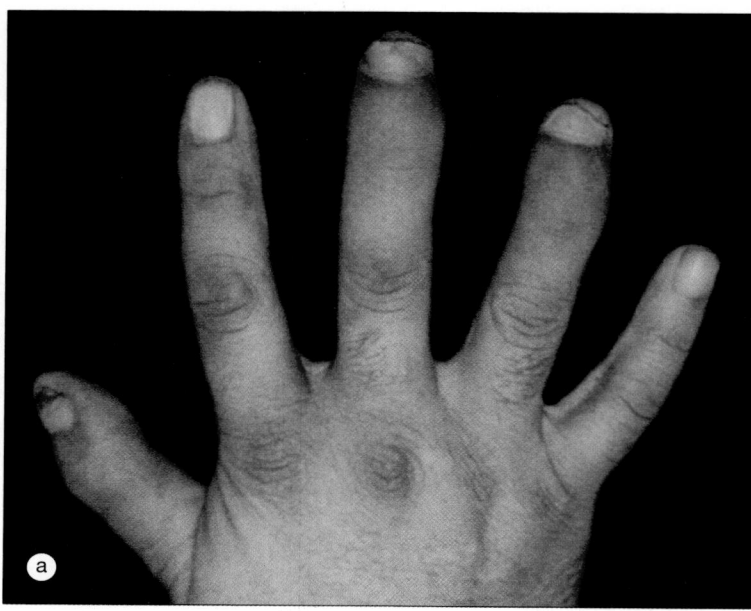
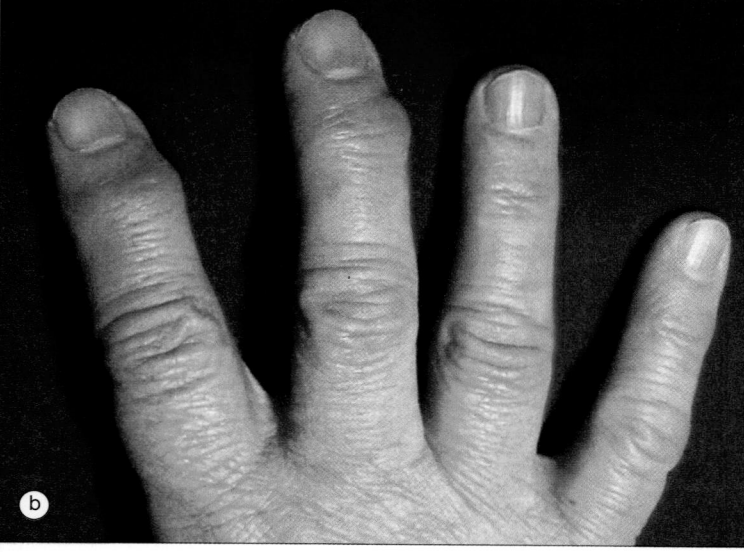

Fig. 28.3 Rheumatic disorders affecting the DIP joints. (a) Psoriatic arthropathy of two DIP joints and the interphalangeal joint of the thumb, together with nail dystrophy. (b) Osteoarthritis is the most common disorder affecting this segment (Heberden's nodes).

Involvement of the cervical spine structures is frequent in RA patients, whereas the dorsal and lumbar segments are spared. Persistent pain in these areas should lead to other diagnoses (e.g., osteoporotic insufficiency fractures of the spine, sacrum, or iliac bones).[13]

Peripheral involvement

Although a large number of related and unrelated rheumatologic diseases may eventually affect any individual joint, tendon sheath, or bursa, the general pattern of joint involvement may be of predominance in the lower or upper limbs. Moreover, some specific joints are closely associated with an individual disease or group of diseases. Understandably, these topographic characteristics refer to the early phases when diagnostic clues are much needed. Most arthritides may later expand to other articular segments, rendering the clinical scenario less clear.

Common examples in clinical rheumatology include the following.

Upper limbs

- Bilateral and symmetric involvement of small and large joints is typical of RA. The MCP and PIP joints of the fingers and wrists are commonly affected. Distal joints are less frequently involved. Patients with SLE or other systemic rheumatologic diseases may occasionally present with a "rheumatoid" pattern of disease. The small joints of the upper extremities are by far the most commonly affected in parvovirus-associated arthritis.
- Exclusive inflammatory DIP joint involvement of the fingers is a relatively infrequent, although important, clue to the diagnosis of a subset of patients with psoriatic arthritis. Nodal OA (Heberden's nodes) is the most frequently encountered disorder affecting this segment (Fig. 28-3).
- Bilateral bony enlargement of the second and third MCP joints with restricted motion is characteristic of hemochromatosis arthropathy.[14]
- Severe proximal pain (neck and shoulders) with minimal objective findings in an appropriate setting is highly indicative of polymyalgia rheumatica, although the onset of RA in the elderly may be difficult to differentiate from this entity.[15]
- Bilateral shoulder disease with striking joint enlargement (shoulder pad sign) is very typical of amyloid arthropathy.[16]

Lower limbs

- Podagra: the metatarsophalangeal joint of the big toe is typically affected in acute gouty attacks (Fig. 28.4). Less frequently, CPPD

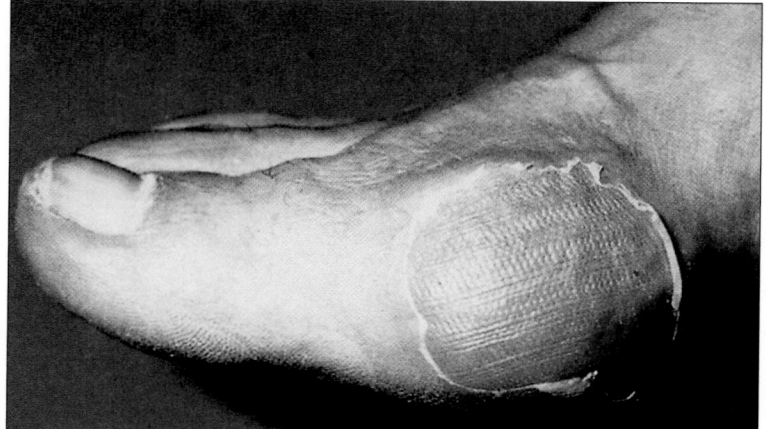

Fig. 28.4 Acute gout. The first MTP joint is involved at some time in approximately 75% of patients. Desquamation of the skin often occurs.

and other crystalline disorders[17] as well as OA, psoriatic arthritis, and a wide variety of conditions, may mimic the podagra of gout.[18] The occurrence of "pseudopodagra" is one of the best examples of how the specific site of the index joint, although helpful, can only suggest the diagnosis.
- Pain and swelling of knees and ankles (often asymmetric) may be seen in the seronegative spondyloarthropathies, including reactive arthritis after infection with *Chlamydia* and enteric organisms.[19] In both of the latter conditions, involvement of the toes is also frequent and the clinical appearance of dactylitis ("sausage" toe) is most typical.
- Juxta-articular pain and tenderness (symptoms of inflammatory enthesopathies) may dominate the clinical picture in some patients with seronegative spondyloarthropathies. An enthesopathy is a pathologic process at the sites of tendinous, ligamentous, or articular capsule attachment to bone and can be inflammatory, degenerative, crystalline, or metabolic.[20] Achilles tendon and plantar fascia insertions into the calcaneum (heel pain) are principally involved. The costosternal areas, iliac crests, ischial tuberosities, greater trochanters, and manubriosternal joint may also be affected. The finding of an enthesopathic digit or dactylitis strongly suggests psoriatic arthritis or reactive arthritis (Fig. 28.5).
- Intermittent synovitis of the knee is a relevant feature of late Lyme disease and seldom becomes chronic. The knee and/or

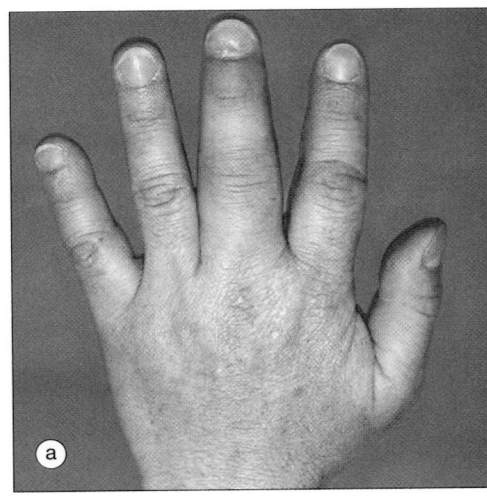
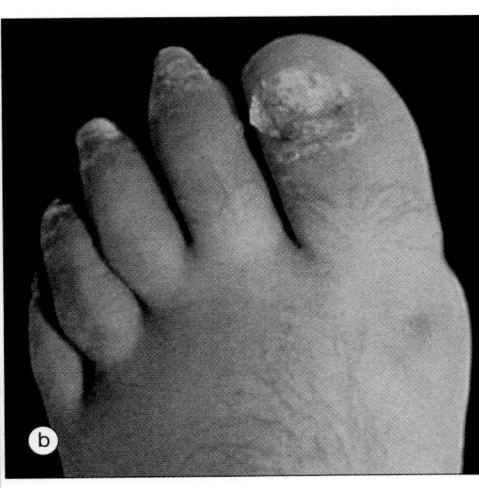

Fig. 28.5 Sausage fingers and toes. (a) Psoriatic arthropathy/dactylitis at the third finger. (b) Reactive arthritis/dactylitis more evident at the second and third toes. Note nail dystrophy.

ankle are also the most commonly involved joints in early EOPA-JIA.

SEQUENCE OF JOINT INVOLVEMENT

Clinical involvement of joints may follow three major patterns: additive, migratory, and intermittent. An additive pattern refers to the involvement of more joints while the previous joints remain symptomatic. Polyarticular OA, reactive arthritis, and RA are typical examples of this progressive sequence.

A migratory pattern means that the process ceases or abates in one joint while simultaneously, or immediately after, starting in a previously normal joint. Whipple's disease and neisserial arthritis may present as a migratory arthritis and tenosynovitis, whereas the fleeting arthritis of rheumatic fever in children is a classic example.

In the intermittent rheumatologic disorders there is complete remission of symptoms and signs until the next recurrence in the same or other joints. No evidence of active disease or residual signs can be detected during intervals. Crystal-induced arthritis, familial Mediterranean fever, Muckle-Wells syndrome, the arthritis seen in Whipple's disease, and palindromic rheumatism usually follow this pattern for years with asymptomatic periods that vary in length. Patients with SLE often show complete resolution of synovitis (commonly polyarthritis) and follow a discontinuous pattern of arthropathy. Adult-onset Still's disease may also run a polycyclic clinical course.[21]

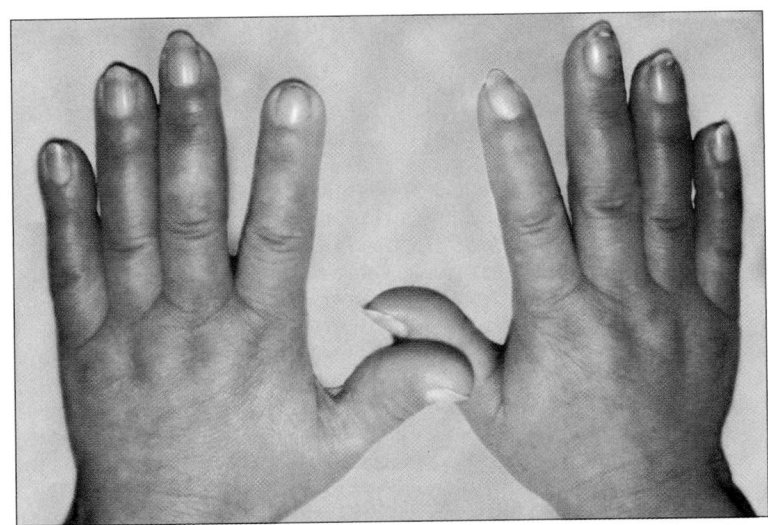

Fig. 28.6 Reflex sympathetic dystrophy syndrome. There is diffuse edematous swelling of the entire right hand.

LOCAL PATTERN OF JOINT DISEASE

Some local signs may be of great diagnostic help. In the same manner as the presence of redness often suggests a particular group of diagnoses (see earlier), the occurrence of skin desquamation when inflammation declines is suggestive of acute gouty monoarthritis. Additional findings that may be of diagnostic value include the following:

- Enlargement of a given individual joint may be symmetric or asymmetric. This physical sign is more obvious in the finger joints. Fusiform swelling of PIP joints in RA is the best example of symmetric involvement, as opposed to Heberden's nodes, erosive OA, chronic sarcoidosis, and tophaceous gout, which often produce asymmetric enlargement of the affected joint.
- The local signs of inflammation may extend beyond the anatomic limits of the joint. This feature may be a major diagnostic contribution, as illustrated by the presence of dactylitis, a characteristic sign of an enthesopathic process (see earlier). A diffusely painful swollen hand or foot may indicate reflex sympathetic dystrophy syndrome in that extremity (Fig. 28.6). Bilateral symmetric puffy swelling of hands and fingers (and sometimes the feet) may be seen in the early phases of systemic sclerosis and mixed connective tissue disease (Fig. 28.7). In a totally different clinical context, diffuse swelling of both hands with pitting is a

Fig. 28.7 Swollen hands in mixed connective tissue disease. The presence of symmetric puffy hands is a common early finding. Similar changes are often seen in the early stages of scleroderma.

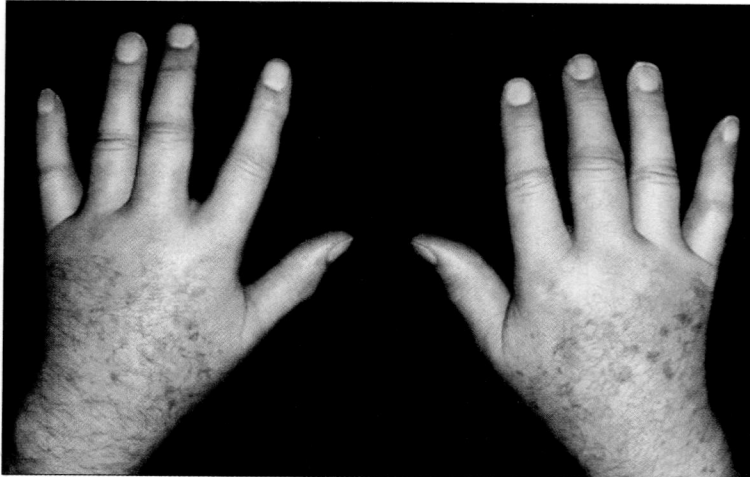

Fig. 28.8 Remitting seronegative symmetric synovitis with pitting edema. Note massive acute painful edema of both hands in an 80-year-old man.

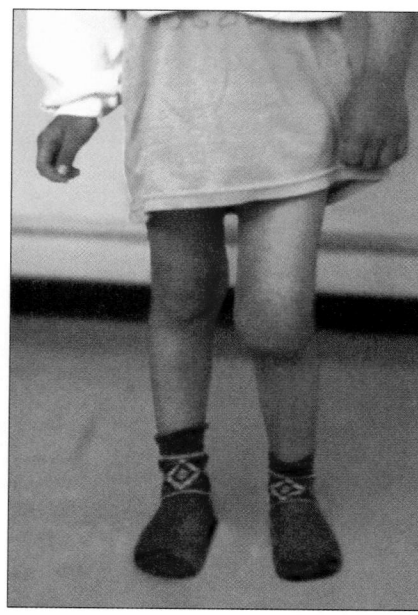

Fig. 28.10 EOPA-JIA in a young girl with monoarthritis. This patient had associated asymptomatic iridocyclitis. In some cases a synovial biopsy is mandatory to exclude other disorders.

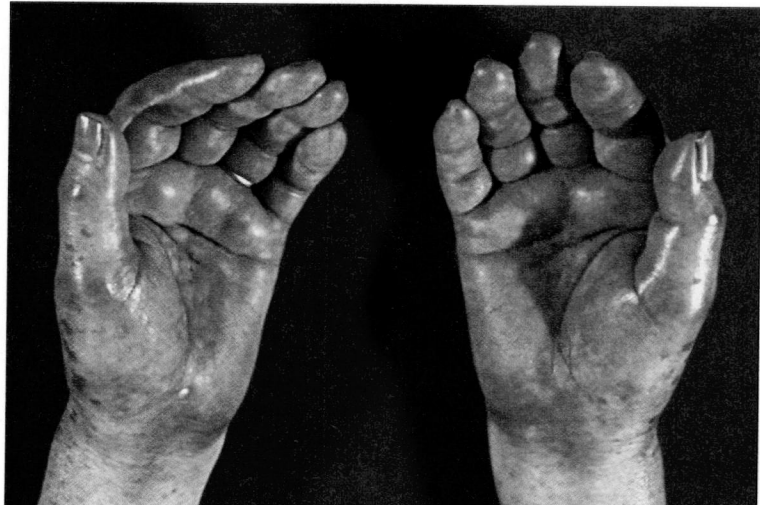

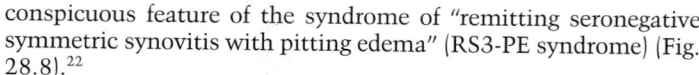

Fig. 28.9 Flexion contractures of all fingers in carcinoma-associated fasciitis. A 50-year-old woman developed painful swelling and contractures of both hands secondary to marked hardening and thickening of the palmar fascia. Palmar erythema is also present. Investigations revealed ovarian carcinoma, the most commonly associated neoplasm in these patients.

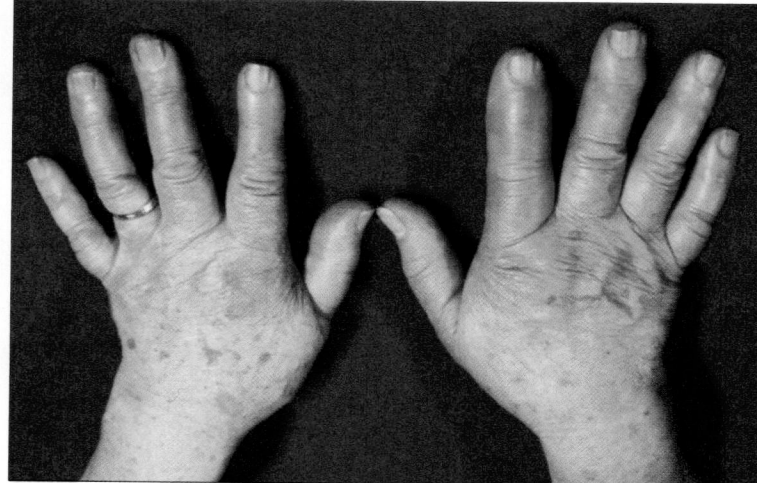

Fig. 28.11 Gouty attack superimposed on a Heberden node. The clinical combination may be found in elderly patients treated with diuretics, as seen in the distal interphalangeal joint of the right index finger in this 78-year-old woman. Note mild desquamation of the overlying skin.

conspicuous feature of the syndrome of "remitting seronegative symmetric synovitis with pitting edema" (RS3-PE syndrome) (Fig. 28.8).[22]

- Symmetric enlargement of hands and feet associated with variable degrees of pain is seen from time to time by rheumatologists.[23] Digital clubbing and local signs of inflammation may or may not be prominent. Hypertrophic osteoarthropathy, pachydermoperiostosis, acromegaly, and the rare thyroid acropachy should be considered when encountering these cases.
- Flexion contractures of the fingers (plus other segments in some cases) due to structural changes in soft tissues lead to a number of clinical diagnoses apart from systemic sclerosis and eosinophilic cutaneous fibroses. β_2-Microglobulin amyloidosis, nephrogenic systemic fibrosis (both entities in patients in hemodialysis), diabetic cheiroarthropathy, and the syndrome of cancer-associated palmar fasciitis are among the diagnostic options (Fig. 28.9).[24] The syndrome of camptodactyly, arthropathy, coxa vara, and pericarditis also includes this type of deformity.

THE CLINICAL VALUE OF PATTERNS OF ARTHROPATHY

Evidence of some distinct articular patterns focuses the spectrum of diagnostic options and reduces unnecessary diagnostic testing.[25] These patterns are not diagnostic *per se,* and they must always be viewed only as a rough guide for various reasons.

First, unrelated arthropathies may share one or more clinical patterns. As an example, EOPA-JIA, tuberculous arthritis, and foreign body arthritis (e.g., plant thorn synovitis)[26] may all present as a chronic monoarthritis of the knee (Fig. 28.10). Both gout and pseudogout can mimic septic arthritis in the setting of febrile acute monoarthritis or polyarthritis.[27]

Second, some major arthritides have more than one mode of onset. It should be remembered, for example, that chronic or intermittent monoarthritis and oligoarthritis (with no involvement of the small joints of the hands) may occasionally dominate the early course of RA before a symmetric polyarthritis evolves. The same presentation may also precede the appearance of typical inflammatory low back pain in patients with ankylosing spondylitis. Moreover, CPPD has many clinical patterns, with pseudogout and pseudo-osteoarthritis being the most frequent.[28]

Third, the articular pattern may change with time in the course of a single disorder. In these cases the correct diagnosis is facilitated when the patient is seen during the "typical" phase of the disease and may be hampered during the "atypical" phases. Early gout, for instance, is an acute, intermittent, monoarticular arthropathy. As the disease progresses, however, the patient may present with a chronic additive, relatively symmetric, polyarticular disease leading to confusion with RA on physical examination.[29] Finally, a single clinical pattern of joint disease may correspond to more than one diagnosis. Chronic gout superimposed on Heberden's nodes[30] and the coexistence of crystals and infection in cases of subacute monoarthritis[31] are examples of this clinical situation (Fig. 28.11).

The combination of features just analyzed can often contribute to the accurate diagnosis of an arthropathy. A deeper knowledge of each of the individual disorders is necessary to enhance the specificity of the diagnostic process. However, this may require the addition of laboratory studies, joint fluid examination, imaging techniques, and other tests to refine the analysis. The more varied the articular patterns possible in a given arthropathy, the more necessary complementary studies become. Systemic vasculitis, SLE, bacterial endocarditis, human immunodeficiency virus infection, solid tumors and leukemia, Behçet's syndrome, sarcoidosis, relapsing polychondritis, and pancreatic-associated arthritis are examples of disorders in which several patterns of arthropathy have been described and which may require a panoply of investigations in addition to the physical findings. However, a careful history and physical examination remains the cornerstone of a diagnostic evaluation for all patients who present with rheumatologic complaints.

REFERENCES

1. American College of Rheumatology Ad Hoc Committee on Clinical Guidelines. Guidelines for the initial evaluation of the adult patient with acute musculoskeletal symptoms. Arthritis Rheum 1996;39:1-8.
2. Rogachefsky RA, Carneiro R, Altman RD, et al. Gout presenting as infectious arthritis. J Bone Joint Surg Am 1994;76:269-273.
3. Baker DG, Schumacher HR. Acute monoarthritis. N Engl J Med 1993;329:1013-1020.
4. Claudepierre C, Rahmouni A, Bergamasco P, et al. Misleading clinical aspects of hydroxyapatite deposits: a series of 15 patients. J Rheumatol 1997;24:531-535.
5. Goldenberg D. Infectious arthritis complicating RA and other chronic rheumatic disorders. Arthritis Rheum 1989;32:496-502.
6. Singleton JD, West S, Nordstrom D. "Pseudoseptic" arthritis complicating RA. J Rheumatol 1991;18:1319-1322.
7. Inaoui R, Bertin P, Preux P, et al. Outcome of patients with undifferentiated chronic monoarthritis: a retrospective study of 46 patients. Joint Bone Spine 2004;71:209-213.
8. Dougados R, Van Der Linden S, Juhlin R, et al. The European Spondyloarthropathy study group preliminary criteria for the classification of spondyloarthropathy. Arthritis Rheum 1991;34:1218-1227.
9. Pinals RS. Polyarthritis and fever. N Engl J Med 1994;330:769-774.
10. Morel J, Deschamps V, Toussirot E, et al. Characteristics and survival of 26 patients with paraneoplastic arthritis. Ann Rheum Dis 2008;67:244-247.
11. Mader R. DISH: time for a change. J Rheumatol 2008;35:377-378.
12. Kahn MF. Why the "SAPHO" syndrome? J Rheumatol 1995;22:2017-2019.
13. Kay L, Holland T, Platt P. Stress fractures in rheumatoid arthritis: a case series and case-control study. Ann Rheum Dis 2004;63:1690-1692.
14. Valenti A, Fracanzani A, Rossi V, et al. The hand arthropathy of hereditary hemochromatosis is strongly associated with iron overload. J Rheumatol 2008;35:153-158.
15. Bahlas S, Ramus-Remus C, Davis P. Clinical outcome of 149 patients with PMR and GCA. J Rheumatol 1998;25:99-104.
16. Prokaeva T, Spencer B, Kaut M, et al. Soft tissue, joint and bone manifestations of AL amyloidosis. Arthritis Rheum 2007;56:3858-3868.
17. Fam A, Stein J. Hydroxyapatite pseudopodagra in young women. J Rheumatol 1992;19:662-664.
18. Bomalaski JS, Schumacher HR. Podagra is more than gout. Bull Rheum Dis 1984;34:77-84.
19. Hamdulay S, Glynne S, Keat A. When is reactive arthritis? Postgrad Med J 2006;82:446-453.
20. Eshed I, Bollow M, McGonagle D, et al. MRI of enthesitis of the appendicular skeleton in spondyloarthritis. Ann Rheum Dis 2007;66:1553-1559.
21. Cush J, Medsger T, Christy W, et al. Adult-onset Still's disease. Arthritis Rheum 1987;30:186-194.
22. Dudley J, Gerster D, So A. Polyarthritis and pitting edema. Ann Rheum Dis 1999;58:142-147.
23. Kirsner R, Goodless D, Kerdel F, et al. Enlargement of the hands and feet in a chronic smoker. Arthritis Rheum 1993;36:569-571.
24. Kay J. Nephrogenic systemic fibrosis. Ann Rheum Dis 2008;67(Suppl iii):66-69.
25. Suarez-Almazor M, Homik J. Reducing serologic testing for rheumatic diseases: feasible goal or utopian dream? J Rheumatol 1999;26:2505-2508.
26. Reginato A, Ferreiro JL, Riester O'Connor C, et al. Clinical and pathologic studies of 26 patients with penetrating foreign body injury to the joints, bursae and tendon sheaths. Arthritis Rheum 1990;33:1753-1762.
27. Ho G, DeNuccio M. Gout and pseudogout in hospitalized patients. Arch Intern Med 1993;153:2787-2790.
28. Doherty M, Dieppe P. Clinical aspects of calcium pyrophosphate crystal deposition. Rheum Dis Clin North Am 1988;14:395-414.
29. Schapira D, Stahl S, Izhak O, et al. Chronic tophaceous gouty arthritis mimicking rheumatoid arthritis. Semin Arthritis Rheum 1999;29:56-63.
30. Fam A, Stein J, Rubenstein J. Gouty arthritis in nodal osteoarthritis. J Rheumatol 1996;23:684-689.
31. Zyskowski L, Silverfield J, O'Duffy JD. Pseudogout masking other arthritides. J Rheumatol 1983;10:449-453.

Role of laboratory tests in rheumatic disorders

29

Yusuf Yazici

- Laboratory tests in rheumatic diseases are used for diagnosis, prognosis, and monitoring of treatment efficacy and safety.
- Even though many tests are commonly ordered by rheumatologists, the diagnosis of most rheumatic conditions is mainly clinical, and the same is true for disease monitoring.
- Virtually all the tests discussed in this chapter will have abnormal results in a certain percentage of the healthy population and among people with diseases other than those for which the test has been ordered.
- A positive test alone is rarely sufficient to make a diagnosis.

INTRODUCTION

In this chapter the focus is on commonly used laboratory tests that are relevant to major disorders seen by rheumatologists rather than an "all inclusive" list of possible tests.

Every test has to be evaluated in the setting it was ordered, keeping in mind the bayesian principles, where the pretest odds of the diagnosis in question are an important factor in determining the importance of the results of the test. Furthermore, as will be discussed below, most of the laboratory tests ordered by rheumatologists are for monitoring adverse events related to medication use. This use of laboratory tests is standard in many clinical guidelines; however, hard evidence behind this from longitudinally followed cohorts is often lacking.

Because laboratory tests are commonly part of the classification/ diagnostic criteria, it is important to understand some key conceptual issues before using results of these tests in making diagnostic and treatment decisions.

Sensitivity is the percentage of *true positives* correctly identified. For example, if 80% of patients with rheumatoid arthritis (RA) have a positive test for rheumatoid factor (RF), the sensitivity of RF for RA is 80%.

Specificity, on the other hand, is the percentage of *true negatives* correctly identified. For example, if 80% of patients without RA do not have RF, then the specificity of RF for RA is 80%.

The *likelihood ratio* (LR) incorporates both the sensitivity and specificity of the test and provides a direct estimate of how much a test result will change the odds of having a disease. The likelihood ratio for a positive result (LR+) provides the odds of the disease increase when a test is positive. The likelihood ratio for a negative result (LR–) provides the odds of the disease decrease when a test is negative. The pretest odds is the likelihood that the patient would have a specific disease before testing and is usually related to the prevalence of the disease. The likelihood ratio can be combined with information about the prevalence of the disease, characteristics of the patient pool, and information about this particular patient to determine the post-test odds of disease.

The more frequent a condition, or a laboratory test, is positive in the healthy population, the more likely there will be a diagnosis. The Bayes theorem is simply a mathematical way of expressing this. Clinicians only seldom appreciate the importance of disease frequency (the pretest probability in bayesian terms) in making a diagnosis.[1] Knowing the prevalence of a certain blood test positivity in the healthy population is required to be able to correctly interpret the results of any rheumatologic screening tests (Table 29.1).

The concepts of false-negative and false-positive are the converse, respectively, of sensitivity and specificity but are useful in clinical decision-making. For example, inflammatory rheumatologic diseases, for which patients are often "screened" with laboratory tests, are seen in about 1% of the population, perhaps 2% if gout is included.[2] However, even a 1% false-positive rate of serologic tests for systemic lupus erythematosus (SLE) or Lyme disease, for example, will result in many people being "labeled" as having SLE or Lyme disease without any clinical evidence of disease. False-positive results of antinuclear antibodies (ANA) testing constitute one frequent reason for rheumatology consultations. The prevalence of SLE in the general population is around 1 in 2000, whereas 1 in 20 have a positive ANA. Thus, given the frequency of non-specific musculoskeletal symptoms in the general population only a minority (1 in 15) of such patients, even if they are ANA positive, will have SLE (Table 29.2).[3] The problem of false-positive interpretations of laboratory data in rheumatic diseases extends beyond serologic tests. For example, gout is often misdiagnosed on the basis of an elevated serum uric acid level rather than on the finding of urate crystals in synovial fluid. Most people with an elevated uric acid level do not have gout and do not need to be treated for hyperuricemia.

False-negative problems are more unusual but may have serious consequences. Patients with RA who have a negative RF test and/or normal erythrocyte sedimentation rate (ESR) may suffer joint destruction while treatment is deferred on the basis of "normal" laboratory values. As will be discussed, up to 40% of RA patients may have a normal ESR at presentation. Similarly, patients with vasculitis and other life-threatening rheumatic diseases may develop irreversible end-organ renal failure or stroke, or even die, while undergoing extensive laboratory evaluation.

Finally there is always the risk of measurement error in any test, and this applies to all laboratory tests in rheumatic diseases. Whenever clinical signs and symptoms do not match the laboratory test results, before accepting the latter as providing "the truth," the tests should be considered possibly in error and should be repeated.

LABORATORY TESTS IN RHEUMATIC DISEASES

Hematology and acute-phase response

The most common use of blood cell counts is for monitoring side effects of the various immunosuppressive medications used for the treatment of rheumatic conditions. American College of Rheumatology (ACR) guidelines have been developed for monitoring hematologic side effects of various drugs; however, there is no consensus, and some guidelines (e.g., those for methotrexate) have been expanded to include medications during the administration of which the guidelines for adverse effect monitoring may be unduly strict.[4]

White blood cells

Increased concentrations of neutrophils are typically seen in bacterial infections (e.g., infectious arthritis, septicemia, pneumonia) but also in active phases of RA and Still's disease. It is also quite rare for a patient to have an active primary systemic vasculitis and not to have neutrophilia. By contrast, neutropenia is a characteristic of Felty's syndrome but the presence of neutropenia should always raise suspicion of a drug-related bone marrow suppression and/or drug-induced removal of neutrophils by the spleen. Lymphocytosis is present during several viral infections, whereas lymphopenia is commonly seen in active phases of SLE and Sjögren's syndrome.

TABLE 29.1 LABORATORY TESTS USED IN INFLAMMATORY RHEUMATIC DISEASES: LIKELIHOOD OF DISEASE IN A PATIENTS WITH A POSITIVE TEST

Blood test	Suspected disease	Patients with positive test	Prevalence of positive test in normal persons	Disease prevalence	Likelihood of disease if test is positive	Likelihood of disease if test positive and joint pain present
Rheumatoid factor	RA	80/100	2/100	1/100	1/2	1/1.5
ANA	SLE	99/100	1/100	1/2000	1/20	1/5
HLA-B27	Ankylosing spondylitis	90/100	6/100	1/300	1/18	1/4.8 (1/3 for back pain)
Elevated uric acid	Gout	80/100	5/100	1/200	1/10	1.3

Adapted from Pincus T. A pragmatic approach to cost-effective use of laboratory tests and imaging procedures in patients with musculoskeletal symptoms. Prim Care 1993;20:795-814.

TABLE 29.2 DIAGNOSIS OF RHEUMATIC DISEASES

Diagnosis	History & physical examination	Blood tests	Radiographs	Synovial fluid
RA	Symmetric polyarthritis Morning stiffness	RF$^+$ in ~80% Elevated ESR in 50-60%	Demineralization Erosions Joint space narrowing	Inflammation WBC > 10,000/mm^3
SLE	Multisystem disease	ANA$^+$ in >99% DNA antibodies in 60-75%	Generally nondestructive	Mild inflammation
Ankylosing spondylitis	Back pain Axial involvement	HLA-B27 in ~90%	Sacroiliitis Vertebral squaring	Inflammation WBC 5,000-20,000/mm^3
Gout	Recurrent attacks	Uric acid elevated in 75-90%	Erosions, cysts	Negatively birefringent crystals
OA	Pain ± swelling ± limited motion	Nonspecific abnormalities	Joint space narrowing Osteophytes	Non-inflammatory WBC <10,000/mm^3
Scleroderma	Skin tightness on dorsum of hand Facial skin tightening	ANA$^+$ in > 90% with Hep-2 cells	±Pulmonary fibrosis ±Esophageal dysmotility ±Calcinosis	Non specific
Polymyositis	Muscle weakness ± pain	CPK elevated in 80% ANA$^+$ in 33%	Not helpful	Non specific

Adapted from Pincus T. Laboratory tests in rheumatic disease. In Klippel JH, Dieppe PA, eds. Rheumatology, 2nd ed. London: Mosby International, 1997:10.1-10.8.

Eosinophilia, commonly seen in some infectious diseases, can be useful for the diagnosis of Churg-Strauss syndrome and help distinguish it from other eosinophilic disorders (e.g., parasitic infections, drug reactions, acute and chronic eosinophilic pneumonia, allergic bronchopulmonary aspergillosis, idiopathic hypereosinophilic syndrome). Peripheral blood eosinophilia also can be a marker of disease activity.

Platelets

Thrombocytosis can accompany active phases of RA, Still's disease, and infections. Thrombocytopenia may be a feature of SLE or represent a hematologic disease, but again this result should raise suspicion of a drug-induced reaction. In patients with thrombocytopenia, the peripheral smear may suggest the cause. If the smear shows abnormalities other than thrombocytopenia, such as nucleated red blood cells or abnormal or immature white blood cells, bone marrow aspiration is indicated. Bone marrow aspiration reveals the number and appearance of megakaryocytes and is the definitive test for many disorders causing marrow failure. However, normal number and appearance of megakaryocytes does not always indicate normal platelet production. For example, in patients with immune thrombocytopenic purpura, platelet production is frequently decreased, or not appropriately increased, despite the normal appearance of megakaryocytes. If the bone marrow is normal but the spleen is enlarged, increased splenic sequestration is the likely cause of thrombocytopenia; if the bone marrow is normal and the spleen is not enlarged, excess platelet destruction is the likely cause. Some patients may have platelet dysfunction; a drug cause is suspected if symptoms began only after patients started taking a potentially causative drug. Some medications such as NSAIDs can interfere with platelet function and lead to bleeding complications.

A hereditary cause is suspected if there is a lifelong history of easy bruising and bleeding after tooth extractions or surgery. In the case of a suspected hereditary cause, von Willebrand's antigen and factor activity studies are obtained.

Hemoglobin

Anemia in the rheumatic diseases most commonly reflects decreased production of red blood cells in the bone marrow due to continued inflammation, characteristically seen as decreased iron deposits in the bone marrow. Anemia of chronic disease commonly is manifested by normocytic normochromic indices; however, microcytic hypochromic indices also can be associated with anemia of chronic disease. Hypochromic microcytic anemia is commonly seen with iron deficiency and other causes such as thalassemia and lead poisoning. Macrocytic anemia, commonly caused by vitamin B_{12} deficiency, folate deficiency, liver disease, and hypothyroidism, is not common in rheumatologic conditions. However, hemolytic anemia is common, especially in SLE and other immune-complex mediated conditions. NSAIDs can lead to chronic and acute blood loss due to their effects on the gastrointestinal mucosa and be a common reason for anemia. Concurrent use with corticosteroids increases the risk of this type of blood loss.

Acute-phase reactants

The acute-phase response occurs in a wide variety of inflammatory conditions, including various infections, trauma, malignancies, inflammatory rheumatic disorders, and certain immune reactions to drugs.[5]

The acute-phase proteins are mainly produced by hepatocytes on stimulation by cytokines (e.g., interleukin-6 [IL-6], IL-1, and tumor necrosis factor [TNF]). The most important acute-phase proteins that increase during inflammation (positive reactants) are C-reactive protein (CRP), fibrinogen, α_1-antitrypsin, haptoglobin, ceruloplasmin, serum amyloid protein A, and several complement components, especially complement C3. The increased plasma level of fibrinogen gives rise to an increased erythrocyte sedimentation rate (ESR) by causing aggregation of red blood cells. In patients with polycythemia, too many red blood cells lower the ESR. An extreme elevation of the white blood cell count as observed in chronic lymphocytic leukemia has also been reported to lower the ESR. Hypofibrinogenemia, hypergammaglobulinemia associated with dysproteinemia, and hyperviscosity may each cause a marked decrease in the ESR. Currently, the most widely used laboratory monitors of inflammation are ESR and CRP. Serial measurements of these may be valuable for monitoring the level of inflammation in patients with disorders such as RA and giant cell arteritis/polymyalgia rheumatica. In each of these conditions some patients can show signs of clinical disease activity but have normal CRP and ESR values or show no signs and symptoms of clinical activity and yet have elevated values. In such instances the clinical picture should be the determining factor in decision-making regarding treatment. It is essential to note that ESR is an indirect measure of acute phase protein concentrations. Although CRP concentrations may increase and decrease very rapidly, ESR values change slowly on control of inflammation. Also, ESR values increase with age in the normal population whereas CRP concentrations tend not to. Finally both have been reported to be higher among obese patients.

Although the presence and pattern of an acute-phase response has been proposed as being of diagnostic value, some reports suggest no differences in ESR or CRP levels between patients with RA, SLE, and osteoarthritis.[6] Both elevated ESR and CRP were seen in similar percentages of patients with each diagnosis, as were combinations of normal ESR with elevated CRP, elevated CRP with normal ESR, or normal levels of both ESR and CRP. In addition, up to 40% of RA patients at presentation may have normal ESR and/or CRP levels yet need treatment as much as those who present with elevated values.[7] Again the most important variables in determining course of action are the clinical signs and symptoms.

ESR and CRP may prove useful in individual patients when it has been demonstrated that their inflammation markers increase with active disease and then return to normal after treatment. This would make it more like to follow a similar trend the next time disease activity is increased.

SEROLOGY

Autoantibodies

Autoantibodies are frequently used in the diagnosis of rheumatic conditions and sometimes for monitoring of disease activity (Table 29.3). Some of these are more specific for one disease whereas others can be found in several diseases. Both of these categories of autoantibodies may be valuable tools for clinical workup. Research into autoantibodies has yielded considerable information about the pathogenesis of various rheumatic conditions, but serologic testing for autoantibodies in clinical practice remains generally more an adjunct to diagnosis and management rather than a precise clinical guide.

Rheumatoid factor

Rheumatoid factor (RF) is the traditional name for autoantibodies directed to the Fcγ chains of IgG molecules. In clinical practice,

TABLE 29.3 COMMON AUTOANTIBODIES AND ASSOCIATED RHEUMATIC DISEASES	
Disease	Associated autoantibodies
Rheumatoid arthritis	RF, ACPA
Systemic lupus erythematosus	ANA, dsDNA, anti-Ro, anti-La
Sjögren's syndrome	Anti-Ro, anti-La
Antiphospholipid syndrome	Anti-cardiolipin, lupus anticoagulant
ANCA-associated granulomatous vasculitis	c-ANCA
Microscopic polyangiitis	p-ANCA

laboratories tend to test only for IgM RF but RF can belong to all major immunoglobulin classes (IgG, IgA, IgM) and in some cases IgD and IgE as well. All these classes of RF are produced locally in the rheumatoid synovial membrane, at which site IgG RF predominates. In peripheral circulation, however, the main immunoglobulin classes of RF that can be easily detected are IgA and IgM RFs.

Today enzyme-linked immunosorbent assay (ELISA) or nephelometric assays have become the most common methods for quantifying RF. IgM RF is produced in many chronic inflammatory conditions (long-standing infections, e.g., bacterial endocarditis, hepatitis B and C, tuberculosis and chronic bronchitis, but also in fibrosing alveolitis, silicosis, primary biliary cirrhosis, and chronic autoimmune hepatitis) and thus is not specific for a particular rheumatic disease such as RA. It can also be seen in 5% to 6% among the elderly in the normal population. Considering RA is seen in 0.5% to 1% of the population, there are at least as many individuals who have RF who do not have RA as have the disease.

The main indications for RF tests in diagnostics are suspicion of RA and Sjögren's syndrome but they commonly appear also in mixed connective tissue disease (MCTD), SLE, cryoglobulinemia, and the polyarticular-onset form of juvenile inflammatory arthritis (JIA). It is thus apparent that the specificity of RF for RA is poor in differentiating some other rheumatologic conditions from RA. However, with higher titer of RF the specificity increases and it becomes a more useful laboratory tool. Higher titers are also associated with more aggressive and erosive disease. Yet up to 20% to 30% of RA patients may be negative for RF and yet have the full clinical picture with the potential poor prognosis when not treated. RF may appear up to several years before the onset of clinical RA. It is rare for RF titers to change with treatment, except possibly with anti–B-cell therapies such as rituximab, and it is usually used as a single time test, at diagnosis to determine prognosis and to help with diagnosis in early and borderline disease.

Antibodies to citrullinated proteins

In 1964, antibodies directed to keratohyaline granules of human buccal mucosa cells were described as a specific marker for RA. They were termed *anti-perinuclear factor* (APF). Several years later antibodies reacting with upper mucosal cells of the esophagus, so-called anti-keratin antibodies (AKA), were found at a similar prevalence and these were found to be as specific for RA as were APF. In the late 1990s anti-Sa antibodies were described in Canada and anti-citrullinated peptide antibodies (ACPAs) in Holland and France. All these antibodies (APF, AKA, anti-Sa, ACPA) have now been shown to target citrullinated parts of proteins such as trichohyalin and filaggrin in buccal mucosa, keratin in esophagus, vimentin in macrophages, and fibrin in the RA joint.

Citrullination is the result of deimination of arginine residues in these proteins by activation of Ca^{2+}-dependent peptidyl-arginine-deiminase enzymes during inflammation-induced apoptosis (programmed cell death) of cells. Leakage of these active enzymes into cells or onto synovial structures causes citrullination of proteins in many types of synovial inflammation. However, only RA patients react to such modified proteins by producing significant amounts of ACPAs. This is likely to depend on the specific presentation of citrullinated peptides to T cells by shared epitope motifs on HLA-DR molecules.

ACPAs can be detected by ELISA and immunoblotting methods using citrullinated proteins or peptides. Because autoantibodies recognize their cognate antigens by their three-dimensional (conformational) structure, the use of a cyclic citrullinated peptide (called CCP-2) has become the most widely used surrogate antigen for detection of anti-citrulline antibodies, thus designated ACPAs. The sensitivity of the ACPA test is around 50% at the onset of RA and can rise up to 85% later in the course of the disease. Several studies have shown the presence of ACPAs up to a decade before the onset of clinical disease.[8] When found in patients with early undifferentiated arthritis, a positive ACPA test predicts later development of classic erosive RA. It is especially prevalent in RF-positive patients but can be found in around 25% of RF-negative RA patients as well.

The ACPA test is helpful in discriminating between RA and SLE with erosive arthritis and also between RA-associated and hepatitis C–associated polyarthritis. Yet in the setting of a positive RF, a positive

TABLE 29.4 RF AND ACPA TABLE OF SENSITIVITY COMPARISONS

	RA (n = 102)	Non-RA (n = 98)	Sensitivity (%)	Specificity (%)	PPV (%)	LR+
RF > 20 U/mL	56	11	55	89	84	5.0
RF ≥ 50 U/mL	46	4	45	96	92	11.3
ACPA (+)	42	2	41	98	96	20.5
RF < 50 U/mL + ACPA (+)	14	2	25	98	88	12.5

PPV, positive predictive value; LR, likelihood ratio.
Adapted from Nell VP, Machold KP, Stamm TA, et al. Autoantibody profiling as early diagnostic and prognostic tool for rheumatoid arthritis. Ann Rheum Dis 2005;64:1731-1736.

TABLE 29.5 FREQUENCY OF ANTINUCLEAR ANTIBODIES IN AUTOIMMUNE AND NON-RHEUMATIC DISEASES

	Sensitivity (%)
Autoimmune disease	
Systemic lupus erythematosus	95-100
Scleroderma	60-80
Mixed connective tissue disease	100
Polymyositis/dermatomyositis	60
Rheumatoid arthritis	50
Rheumatoid vasculitis	30-50
Sjögren's syndrome	40-70
Drug-induced lupus	90
Discoid lupus	15
Pauciarticular juvenile chronic arthritis	70
Non-rheumatic diseases	
Hashimoto's thyroiditis	45
Graves' disease	50
Autoimmune hepatitis	50
Primary pulmonary hypertension	40

TABLE 29.6 ANTINUCLEAR ANTIBODY DISEASE ASSOCIATIONS

	DsDNA	Sm	RNP	Ro	La
Systemic lupus erythematosus					
Sensitivity	70%	25-30	45	40	15
Specificity	95%	Mod	99	87-94	
RA					
Sensitivity	1%	1%	47	Low	Low
Specificity					
Scleroderma					
Sensitivity	<1%	<1%	20		
Specificity					
Polymyositis/dermatomyositis					
Sensitivity	<1%	<1%		Low	
Specificity					
Sjögren's syndrome					
Sensitivity	1-5%	1-5%	5-60	8-70	14-60
Specificity				87	94

ACPA test adds little,[9] especially once a decision to treat has been made, which should be the course of action in any patient suspected of having RA (Table 29.4). Some data suggest, in very early disease, that ACPA-positive patients may respond better to methotrexate and this might also prevent some of these patients from developing the full spectrum of RA, compared with patients who are ACPA negative and were treated with methotrexate. This has been shown in a small cohort and needs further confirmation.[10] A recent association between ACPA positivity, HLA-DR alleles, and smoking has been suggested[11]; however, this has not been confirmed by others.[12]

Antinuclear antibodies

ANAs are seen in many rheumatologic conditions as well as in many healthy people (Table 29.5). They are usually detected by immunofluorescent (IF) techniques (FANA), utilizing monolayers of HEp-2 cells. Specific ANAs are detected by solid-phase immunoassays, such as ELISA. FANA is reported as titers (i.e., 1:40, 1:80). This has been found to be useful in symptomatic patients as a screening tool. In the absence of clinical findings there is no need to test for any of the ANAs.

ANAs can be found in SLE, Sjögren's syndrome, MCTD, scleroderma, undifferentiated connective tissue disease, and similar diseases. However, finding antibodies by itself does not signify disease, because many healthy people (especially family members of patients with connective tissue diseases, elderly, women, patients using drugs such as sulfasalazine, isoniazid, etc.) have positive antibodies and never develop SLE or other connective tissue diseases (Table 29.6).

High titer increases the likelihood that the presence of antibodies is related to a disease. In such cases further workup with testing for anti-dsDNA, anti-Ro (SS-A), anti-La (SS-B), and anti-ribonucleoprotein (RNP) may be indicated. In patients in whom a diagnosis cannot be made based on clinical symptoms, watchful waiting is recommended.

ANAs also produce a wide range of staining patterns; however, these have found to have low specificity and sensitivity for different autoimmune conditions (Figs. 29.1 to 29.3). Antibodies to specific nuclear antigens are usually more useful.

DNA antibodies

These can be against single- or double-stranded DNA; and of the two, double-stranded DNA (dsDNA) antibody has more applications in rheumatic conditions. ssDNA is seen in many conditions and does not correlate with disease activity.

Anti-dsDNA is very specific (95%) but not as sensitive (70%) for SLE, making it useful in the diagnosis of SLE when positive. It also might have a pathogenic role in SLE nephritis and is commonly associated with disease activity in lupus nephritis. The usual picture in active SLE nephritis is increased anti-dsDNA along with decreased C3 and C4, all tending to normalize with control of active kidney disease.

Anti-Sm and anti-RNP antibodies

These antibodies are most commonly detected using solid-phase immunoassays. Anti-Sm antibodies are found almost exclusively in SLE patients, in 10% to 40% of patients, so the majority of SLE patients do not have them. When the test is negative it is not helpful in ruling out SLE, but their presence is very strong evidence of possible SLE.

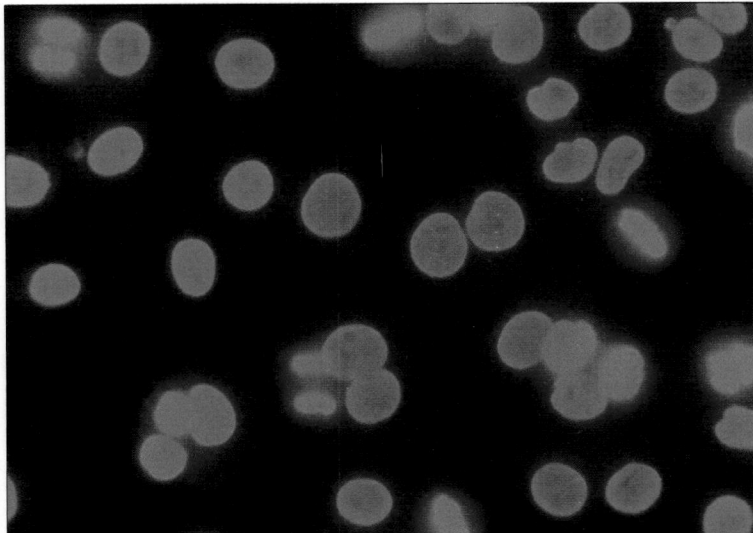

Fig. 29.1 ANA homogeneous staining.

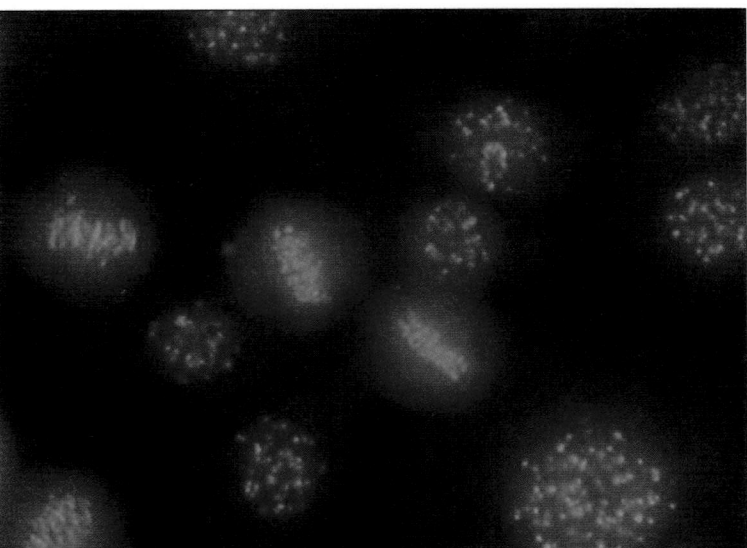

Fig. 29.3 ANA centromere staining.

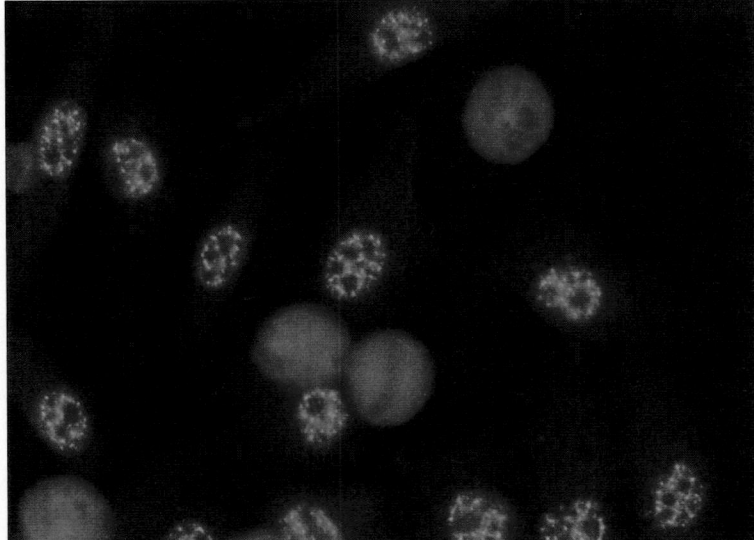

Fig. 29.2 ANA speckled staining.

Anti-RNP antibodies are found in 40% to 60% of SLE patients but are not specific to SLE: however, they can be useful in diagnosing mixed connective tissue disease (MCTD).

Anti-Ro (SS-A) and anti-La (SS-B) antibodies

Anti-Ro and anti-La antibodies are frequently seen in SLE and Sjögren's syndrome patients. They have been particularly associated with sub-acute cutaneous lupus and photosensitivity. Anti-Ro and anti-La antibodies have also been associated with neonatal lupus and congenital heart block. Yet they can be seen in mothers with no evidence of connective tissue disease and there are infants who develop congenital heart block with no detectable antibodies. They do have a role in screening patients planning to get pregnant for possible closer follow-up during pregnancy, but the diagnosis of congenital heart block is still established by electrocardiogram, ultrasonography, and physical examination.

Anti-centromere and anti–Scl-70 antibodies

Anti-centromere antibodies are virtually exclusively noted in patients with limited cutaneous scleroderma, the CREST variant. As such they are also associated with pulmonary hypertension. Anti–Scl-70 is found in about 20% of systemic sclerosis patients and may increase the risk for pulmonary fibrosis in these patients.

Diagnostic utility of antinuclear antibodies

Some ANAs are included as criteria for diagnosis of disease (e.g., SLE, MCTD, and Sjögren's syndrome). A prominently expressed ANA, as indicated by strong fluorescent staining or a high titer, can antedate the establishment of a clinical diagnosis by many years[13] and may serve as a tool for selecting an appropriate diagnostic workup and planning a follow-up strategy. Yet, as with RF, ANA can be positive in around 10% of the healthy population, and, given the prevalence of SLE in the population, a person with a positive ANA test is many more times likely not to have SLE or a connective tissue disease. As is discussed elsewhere in this text, the diagnosis of SLE, for example, can be made on clinical grounds alone. Most SLE patients have a high positive ANA result, but most positive ANA test results are not indicative of SLE.

Antiphospholipid antibodies

Antiphospholipid antibodies (APAs) bind to certain serum proteins complexed to phospholipid molecules.[14] The assays most widely used to show APAs are the anticardiolipin assay (ELISA format) and the lupus anticoagulant functional test (LAC, also called lupus inhibitor). Presence of functionally procoagulant APAs can be screened for by finding an abnormally prolonged activated partial thromboplastin time.

APAs were originally detected by false-positive tests for syphilis using the Wassermann reaction. Subsequently, positive reactivity in the anticardiolipin ELISA assay and in the lupus anticoagulant test was shown to depend on binding of autoantibodies to a serum cofactor, which in the case of the anticardiolipin ELISA is β_2-glycoprotein I and in the lupus anticoagulant assay may be either β_2-glycoprotein I or prothrombin.

Lupus anticoagulant (LAC) is an inappropriate name for the procoagulant autoantibodies because they appear not only in SLE but also in other autoimmune diseases and in the so-called primary antiphospholipid syndrome. These are patients experiencing venous or arterial thrombotic events, recurrent fetal loss, and thrombocytopenia in the absence of clinical features of another chronic inflammatory rheumatic disorder. The name is misleading because LACs are not anticoagulants but procoagulants. They block the assembly of the prothrombinase complex, giving rise to prolonged coagulation assays *in vitro* (e.g., prolonged activated partial thromboplastin time, dilute Russell viper venom time, or kaolin clotting time). This abnormality cannot be corrected by mixing the patient plasma 1:1 with normal plasma, while this procedure corrects clotting properties in patients with coagulation factor deficiencies.

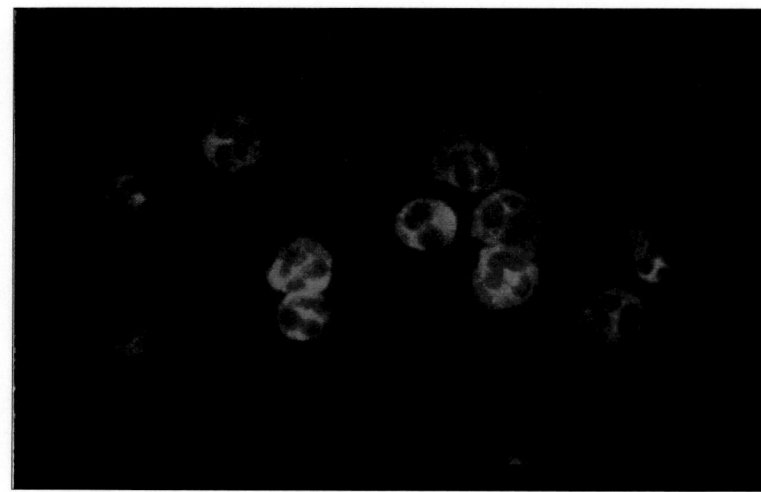

Fig. 29.4 c-ANCA staining.

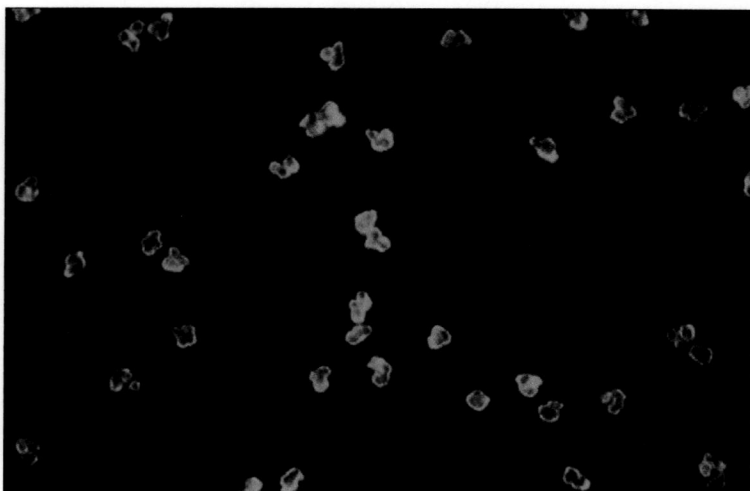

Fig. 29.5 p-ANCA staining.

Anticardiolipin (aCL) antibodies are detected by ELISA using cardiolipin-coated microtiter plates that are then flooded by dilute bovine serum to secure binding of bovine proteins to the phospholipid. The most important phospholipid binding protein attaching to the cardiolipin is β_2-glycoprotein I, which acts as a cofactor in the test. Autoantibodies to β_2-glycoprotein I and to the cardiolipin/β_2-glycoprotein I complex give rise to positive results of importance for diagnosing a procoagulant state, whereas antibodies directed to the cardiolipin itself show no such relationship. Antibodies to the naked cardiolipin appear transiently in several infections and permanently in syphilis. The antibodies may belong to all three major immunoglobulin classes, but IgG aCL antibodies are those most closely related to procoagulant activity and thus presence of LAC activity. To be able to discriminate between diagnostically important aCL antibodies, it is now common to search for specific anti–β_2-glycoprotein I antibodies using ELISA plates coated with purified β_2-glycoprotein I protein. Presence of anti–β_2-glycoprotein I antibodies correlates better with a positive LAC test and with manifestations of antiphospholipid syndrome.

Antinuclear cytoplasmic antibodies

ANCAs represent a subgroup of neutrophil-specific autoantibodies. It is commonly directed to the azurophil granule proteins myeloperoxidase (MPO) and proteinase 3 (PR3). ANCAs are characteristic of patients suffering from necrotizing vasculitides such as Wegener's granulomatosis (WG), microscopic polyangiitis, and Churg-Strauss syndrome. ANCAs directed to PR3 usually give rise to a coarse granular fluorescence pattern on neutrophils and monocytes using ethanol-fixed leukocytes, therefore called cytoplasmic ANCA (c-ANCA) (Fig. 29.4). MPO-ANCA mostly give rise to a perinuclear ANCA (p-ANCA) staining pattern on neutrophils and monocytes (Fig. 29.5).

The usefulness of ANCAs in monitoring disease activity in WG has been controversial.[15,16] They are useful in diagnosing ANCA-associated vasculitides but may not be that helpful in individual patients in predicting remission or relapse and are not currently recommended to be used for these reasons.

Complement

The most frequent clinical parameters used for judging complement activation are the protein levels of C3 and C4, although these values are of limited use because they represent increased production during inflammation (acting as positive acute-phase reactants) but sometimes also consumption by immune complexes. Total hemolytic complement (CH50) is a functional assay used to measure the intactness and consumption of the entire classic pathway. Decreased complement levels are useful in the setting of SLE nephritis where low levels are associated with persistent nephritis and normalization is associated with better outcomes. Hypocomplementemia is also a feature of preeclampsia/eclampsia, which is an important point to remember when

taking care of pregnant patients with SLE with and without antiphospholipid syndrome.

Inherited complement deficiencies are very rare. Interestingly, some complement-deficient patients show signs of lupus-like illness.

To show normal values of the CH_{50} assay all components from C1 to C9 need to be present and be functionally intact. The CH_{50} assay is a good screening tool for detecting deficiencies in the classic pathway. To give optimal information, specimen collection needs to be done appropriately, owing to the lability of several complement components. Assays should thus be done as soon as possible on the day of serum or plasma collection or samples should be immediately frozen at −70°C until the test can be done.

BIOCHEMISTRY

Liver function tests

Liver function tests are ordered frequently to monitor side effects of medication. Aspartate aminotransferase (AST), formerly called serum glutamic oxaloacetic transaminase (SGOT), and alanine aminotransferase (ALT), formerly known as serum glutamic pyruvic transaminase (SGPT), are included in guidelines developed initially for monitoring methotrexate-related adverse events but have been used for monitoring any and all immunosuppressive medications.[17] Albumin levels can also be measured when chronic liver disease or damage to the liver from medications is suspected. There is evidence to suggest that liver function test abnormalities seen with methotrexate in RA may not be as high as previously suggested, with very few patients discontinuing methotrexate treatment owing to liver function test abnormalities over 10 to 15 years of use.[18,19]

Alkaline phosphatase

Alkaline phosphatase is made mostly in the liver and in bone, with some made in the intestines and kidneys. It also is made by the placenta of a pregnant woman. Conditions that lead to rapid bone growth (during puberty), bone disease (osteomalacia or Paget's disease), hyperparathyroidism, or damaged liver cells can lead to increases in alkaline phosphatase levels. Values of 1.5 to 3.0 times the upper limit of normal (ULN) are consistent with hepatocellular (viral infection, drug toxicity, alcohol) etiology, whereas values greater than 3.0 times the ULN are usually associated with biliary involvement. Bone involvement can be found at any value.

Uric acid

Uric acid measurement is commonly included in the workup of patients with arthritis and may be elevated in 90% of patients with gout. Yet healthy people can have elevated levels also, and the definite diagnosis

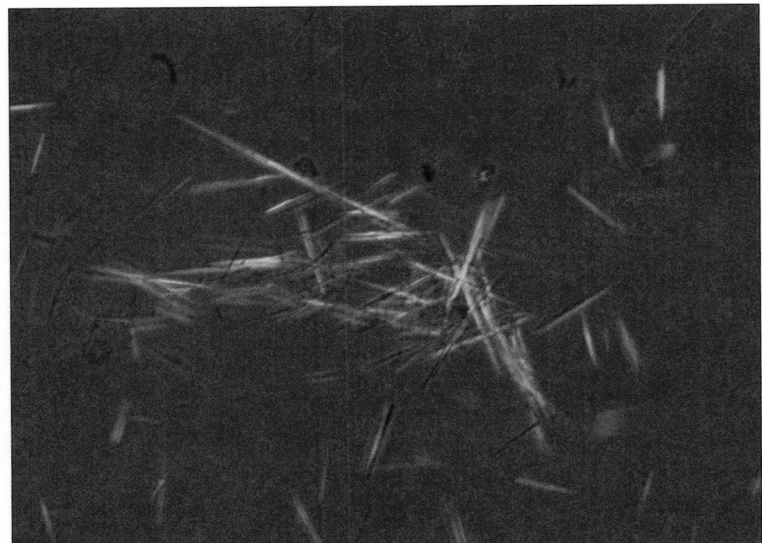

Fig. 29.6 Uric acid crystals in synovial fluid.

of gout depends on demonstration of uric acid crystals in synovial fluid (Fig. 29.6). Uric acid is useful in monitoring allopurinol response; and once the levels have come down to normal, further increase in allopurinol dose may not be necessary to control disease activity.

Calcium and vitamin D

Calcium and vitamin D levels are part of the workup of osteoporosis and high or low bone turnover states and may be considered in patients at risk for these conditions and for monitoring treatment. Calcium absorption, use, and excretion are regulated and stabilized by a feedback loop involving parathyroid hormone vitamin D. Conditions and diseases that disrupt calcium regulation can cause inappropriate acute or chronic elevations or decreases in calcium and lead to symptoms of hypercalcemia or hypocalcemia. Renal insufficiency or failure, symptoms of hypercalcemia (e.g., fatigue, weakness, loss of appetite, nausea, vomiting, constipation, abdominal pain, urinary frequency, and increased thirst) or hypocalcemia (e.g., muscle cramps, or tingling in fingers), gastrointestinal disease leading to poor absorption, thyroid disease, malignancies, and poor nutrition may be reasons for monitoring calcium levels. Monitoring may also be needed during vitamin D supplementation.

In the past 25 years, more than 50 metabolites of vitamin D have been described. To date, only a few of these have been quantified in blood, but this has widened our understanding of the pathologic role that altered vitamin D metabolism plays in the development of diseases of calcium homeostasis. Currently, awareness is growing of the prevalence of vitamin D insufficiency in the general population in association with an increased risk of several diseases. However, for many researchers, it is not clear which vitamin D metabolites should be quantified and what the information gained from such an analysis tells us. Two metabolites, namely, 25-hydroxyvitamin D [25(OH)D] and 1,25-dihydroxyvitamin D [1,25(OH)2D], have received the greatest attention. Of these, the need for measuring serum 1,25(OH)2D is limited, and this metabolite should therefore not be considered as part of the standard vitamin D testing regimen. On the other hand, serum 25(OH)D provides the single best assessment of vitamin D status, and thus should be the only vitamin D assay typically performed.[20]

CONCLUSION

Laboratory tests are useful tools to help monitor adverse events related to medications and diagnosis of some rheumatic conditions. They are secondary to clinical signs and symptoms and should not replace or detract from a good history and physical examination. Most rheumatic conditions can be diagnosed clinically and do not require a laboratory test. As always, any test that will not change the diagnosis, prognosis, or treatment of a rheumatic condition probably should not be done.

KEY REFERENCES

1. Reid MC, Lane DA, Feinstein AR. Academic calculations versus clinical judgments: practicing physicians' use of quantitative measures of test accuracy. Am J Med 1998;104:374-380.
2. Pincus T. A pragmatic approach to cost-effective use of laboratory tests and imaging procedures in patients with musculoskeletal symptoms. Prim Care 1993;20:795-814.
3. Pincus T. Laboratory tests in rheumatic disease. In Klippel JH, Dieppe PA, eds. Rheumatology, 2nd ed. London: Mosby International, 1997:10.1-10.8.
4. Yazici Y, Erkan D, Paget SA. Monitoring by rheumatologists for methotrexate-, etanercept-, infliximab-, and anakinra-associated adverse events. Arthritis Rheum 2003;48:2769-2772.
5. Gabay C, Kushner I. Acute phase proteins and other systemic responses to inflammation. N Engl J Med 1999;340:448-454.
6. Keenan RT, Swearingen CJ, Yazici Y. Erythrocyte sedimentation rate and C-reactive protein levels are poorly correlated with clinical measures of disease activity in rheumatoid arthritis, systemic lupus erythematosus and osteoarthritis patients. Clin Exp Rheumatol 2008;26:814-819.
7. Wolfe F, Michaud K. The clinical and research significance of the erythrocyte sedimentation rate. J Rheumatol 1994;21:1227-1237.
8. Rantapää-Dahlqvist S, de Jong BA, Berglin E, et al. Antibodies to cyclic citrullinated peptide and IgA rheumatoid factor predict the development of rheumatoid arthritis. Arthritis Rheum 2003;48;2741-2749.
9. Nishimura K, Sugiyama D, Kogata Y, et al. Meta-analysis: diagnostic accuracy of anti-cyclic citrullinated peptide antibody and rheumatoid factor for rheumatoid arthritis. Ann Intern Med 2007;146:797-808.
10. van Dongen H, van Aken J, Lard LR, et al. Efficacy of methotrexate treatment in patients with probable rheumatoid arthritis: a double-blind, randomized, placebo-controlled trial. Arthritis Rheum 2007;56:1424-1432.
11. Klareskog L, Stolt P, Lundberg K, et al. A new model for an etiology of rheumatoid arthritis: smoking may trigger HLA-DR (shared epitope)-restricted immune reactions to autoantigens modified by citrullination. Arthritis Rheum 2006;54:38-46.
12. Lee HS, Irigoyen P, Kern M, et al. Interaction between smoking, the shared epitope, and anti-cyclic citrullinated peptide: a mixed picture in three large North American rheumatoid arthritis cohorts. Arthritis Rheum 2007;56:1745-1753.
13. Arbuckle MR, McClain MT, Scofield RH, et al. Development of autoantibodies before the onset of systemic lupus erythematosus. N Engl J Med 2003;349:1526-1533.
14. Roubey RAS. Autoantibodies to phospholipid-binding plasma proteins: a new view of lupus anticoagulants and other antiphospholipid autoantibodies. Blood 1994;84:2854-2867.
15. Stegeman CA. Predictive value of antineutrophil cytoplasmic antibodies in small-vessel vasculitis: is the glass half full or half empty? J Rheumatol 2005;32:2075.
16. Finkielman JD, Merkel PA, Schroeder D, et al. Antiproteinase 3 antineutrophil cytoplasmic antibodies and disease activity in Wegener granulomatosis. Ann Intern Med 2007;147:611-619.
17. Yazici Y, Erkan D, Paget SA. Monitoring for methotrexate hepatic toxicity in rheumatoid arthritis patients: is it time to update the guidelines? J Rheumatol 2002;29:1586-1589.
18. Yazici Y, Sokka T, Kautiainen H, et al. Long-term safety of methotrexate in routine clinical care: discontinuation is unusual and rarely due to laboratory abnormalities. Ann Rheum Dis 2005;64:207-211.
19. Yazici Y, Erkan D, Harrison MJ, et al. Methotrexate use in rheumatoid arthritis is associated with few clinically significant liver function test abnormalities. Clin Exp Rheumatol 2005;23:517-520.
20. Zerwekh JE. Blood biomarkers of vitamin D status. Am J Clin Nutr 2008;87:1087S-1091S.

REFERENCES

Full references for this chapter can be found on www.expertconsult.com.

Synovial fluid analysis

Anthony J. Freemont and John Denton

■ Normal synovial fluid (SF) is a hypocellular, avascular connective tissue.

■ In disease, the SF increases in volume and can be aspirated.

■ Changes in SF composition reflect the pathogenesis of the arthropathy.

■ SF microscopy is a simple, inexpensive, and accurate test that yields information of diagnostic and prognostic significance.

■ Biomarkers of disease processes are becoming increasingly studied in SF and may bring about a revolution in understanding and recognizing joint disease.

INTRODUCTION

Normal synovial fluid

Synovial fluid (SF) is a transudate of plasma supplemented with high-molecular-weight, saccharide-rich molecules, notably hyaluronans, produced by fibroblast-derived type B synoviocytes. The fluid is kept free of debris by macrophage-derived type A synoviocytes, which also synthesize bioactive molecules such as cytokines. Formation of SF is balanced by its removal via synovial lymphatics.

An incomplete cell layer with no underlying basement membrane covers the surface of synovium. This distinguishes it from the lining of most body cavities, where epithelium or mesothelium, supported by an intact basement membrane, regulates fluid flux between the lumen and the underlying tissue. Because cartilage also lacks a regulatory cell covering, there is a relatively homogeneous chemical environment within the joint. Because of this unusual arrangement, it is perhaps better, in terms of pathologic mechanisms, to think of SF as a tissue rather than a true body fluid. In the normal joint, the SF contains few cells (<200/mm³), mainly chondrocytes and synoviocytes, together with migratory defense cells (usually lymphocytes). The nature and regulation of the chemical composition of SF are poorly understood and complex.

Synovial fluid in diseased joints

Variation in the volume and composition of SF reflects pathologic processes within the joint. Because of the anatomic relationships of the tissues in the joint, events such as inflammation and enzyme-mediated degradation within the synovium and cartilage are reflected in changes in the cellular and chemical composition of SF. Both the cell and chemical changes have been studied to obtain a better understanding of disease processes and to identify aspects of diagnostic and prognostic utility.[1]

Synovial fluid microscopy

Synovial fluid microscopy has been carried out as a diagnostic test for many years.[2] Histologic and cytologic analysis of human tissues and body fluids is usually the exclusive realm of the pathologist. This is not the case with SF microanalysis, because it is possible to perform the test without recourse to complex technology; and, indeed, some of the most expert exponents of SF analysis are also highly respected clinicians.[3-5]

Detailed microscopic analysis of SF can yield significant information about the nature of joint diseases and their prognosis.[1] By comparison with other investigations (e.g., MRI, C-reactive protein, autoantibodies), SF microscopy is very simple and inexpensive and gives useful and important clinical data across the whole spectrum of inflammatory and non-inflammatory joint diseases.

SF microscopy gives diagnostic information with different levels of precision, varying from a single precise diagnosis at one end of the spectrum to simply distinguishing between inflammatory and non-inflammatory arthropathies at the other. This should not be seen as detracting from the value of the test because the clinical question may be answered by knowing if the cause of joint swelling is inflammatory or not (e.g., Does my rheumatoid arthritis [RA] patient with long-standing disease who now presents with a red, hot joint have a rheumatoid flare or osteoarthritis [OA]?). In expert hands, SF microscopy viewed "blind" (i.e., without any knowledge of any patient data) will give a precise diagnosis (e.g., a specific crystal arthritis, RA, OA, torn meniscus, septic arthritis) in about 40% of cases. In a further 20% it allows relevant and clinically significant differential diagnoses to be made (e.g., 45% of cases of seronegative spondyloarthropathies have a specific SF cytology that enables them to be distinguished with certainty from other forms of inflammatory arthropathy, including rheumatoid disease, even at initial presentation[6]; and in all but 2% to 3% of the remainder SF microscopy can distinguish inflammatory from non-inflammatory arthropathies). If these limitations of SF microscopy are properly considered and applied, the false-positive rate is very low (typically < 5%) and the false-negative rate almost zero.

At the same time it has to be acknowledged that access to laboratories specializing in SF analysis is, at best, patchy and many rheumatologists and pathologists have to undertake SF analysis without expert support. Therefore, the information in the next section of this chapter, which is based on the authors' experiences of training young clinicians, technical staff, and nurses, will assist those clinicians who find themselves needing to set up and use a small laboratory for analyzing SF specimens using microscopy to obtain reliable diagnoses.

THE BASIC APPROACH TO SYNOVIAL FLUID MICROSCOPY

There are four elements to SF analysis, each requiring different types and complexity of equipment. The following approach will yield the maximal information for relatively little outlay and minimal time input on behalf of the staff undertaking the work. The equipment required is relatively simple: a microscope with polarizers and an interference plate, a hemocytometer chamber, and a cytocentrifuge.

It is important to recognize that SF should be examined unfixed, and as such it should be treated with the same level of care as all other fresh body fluids. For health and safety reasons the samples should be handled in a biological safety cabinet and, because fresh samples deteriorate rapidly even if kept refrigerated, examined within 24 hours of aspiration. Because SF from inflamed joints has a tendency to clot, it should also be anticoagulated. The best anticoagulant is lithium heparin.

The four elements of SF analysis are (1) visual inspection, (2) nucleated cell count, (3) "wet preparation," and (4) cytocentrifuge preparation.

Visual inspection

Synovial fluid should be examined for color and clarity.

Color

Normally, SF is pale yellow. In hemarthroses it will be red or orange, and in inflammatory arthropathies it is cream or white. In septic arthritis it may be colored by bacterial chromogens.

Clarity

Normal SF is clear but with increasing numbers of particles (e.g., crystals) and/or cells it becomes cloudy.

Nucleated cell count

For simplicity and speed the nucleated cell count is best performed manually using a hemocytometer chamber, although it is possible to use automated counters[7] and even "dip sticks."[8] For convenience, the nucleated cell count of SF is expressed as cells/mm³ (directly equivalent to cells/μL). Normal SF contains fewer than 200 cells/mm³. In inflammatory joint disease the cell count is greater than 1000 cells/mm³, and in non-inflammatory arthropathies it is lower. Cell counts in excess of 50,000 cells/mm³ are virtually restricted to four conditions: acute rheumatoid "flares" (including breakdown of disease control by anti–tumor necrosis factor), and septic, acute crystal, and reactive arthritis.

"Wet preparation"

Synovial fluid aspirates often contain visible particles. These are usually fibrin clots of fragments of cartilage. In making the "wet preparation," the specimen should be agitated and a small aliquot containing as many particles as possible placed on a microscope slide. It can then be gently squeezed flat beneath a coverslip and viewed unstained with a conventional microscope. For optimal results the condenser diaphragm is closed to produce diffused light in which the unstained cells and particles are clearly seen. This preparation is examined for one cell type, the ragocyte, several different classes of crystals, and other non-cellular particulate material.

Classes of crystalline material

Several classes of crystalline material are found in the joints,[1] and their detection is not as straightforward as is sometimes believed (Fig. 30.1).[9] Monosodium urate monohydrate ("urate") crystals are needle shaped, 5 to 30 μm long, and highly birefringent. They can be distinguished from other crystals by their properties in polarized light with an interference plate in the system. (For ease, it is useful to have to hand a microscope preparation made by smearing the contents of a superficial tophus onto a slide, because this known sample of urate crystals can then be used to standardize the optics of the microscope). When viewed between crossed polarizers with an interposed interference plate, the background of the microscope image is pink and the urate crystals appear either yellow or blue, depending on the direction of their long axes. Other crystals, notably calcium pyrophosphate ("pyrophosphate") crystals, are also yellow and blue, but the yellow crystals are orientated with their axes in the same direction as the blue-appearing urate crystals and vice versa. Urate crystals, especially when intraleukocytic, are diagnostic of gout.

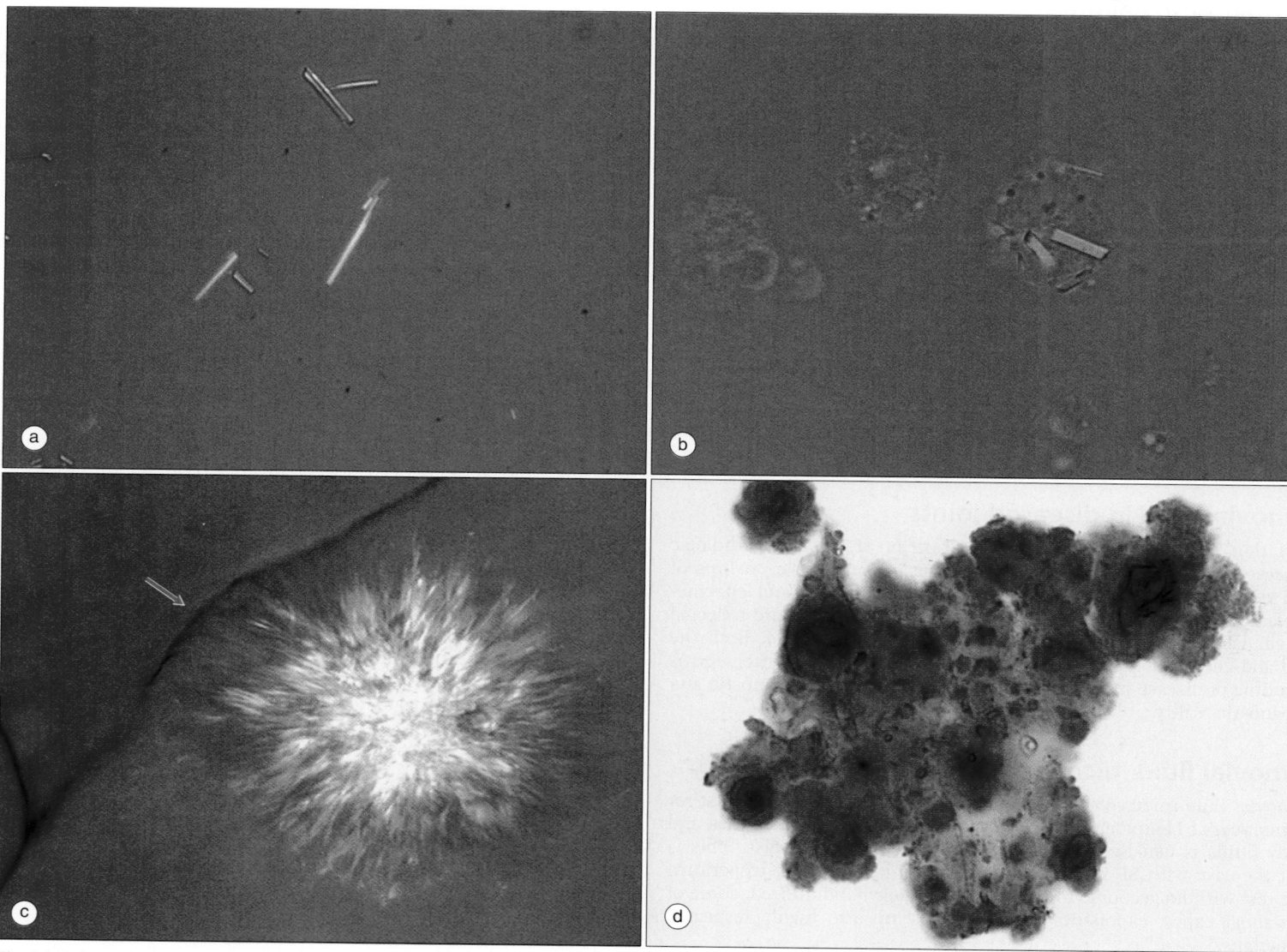

Fig. 30.1 A montage of common crystals. (a) "Urate" crystals viewed in polarized light with an interposed quarter-wave plate. (b) Pyrophosphate crystals viewed in the same system. Note that the crystals appear duller and that the apparent color of the crystal is the opposite of the urate crystals when related to the long axis of the crystal. (c) A lipid droplet (edge arrowed) containing a "beach ball" of needle-like crystals. (d) Hydroxyapatite crystals stained with alizarin red.

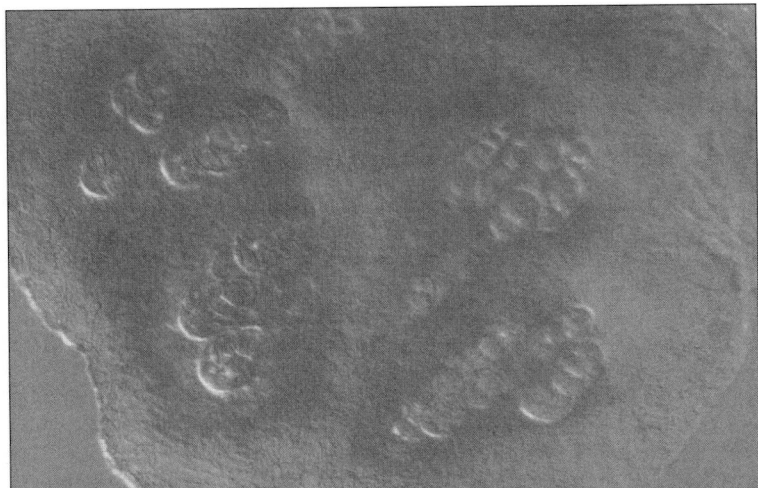

Fig. 30.2 Cartilage seen in a wet preparation shows chondrocyte clusters typical of osteoarthritis.

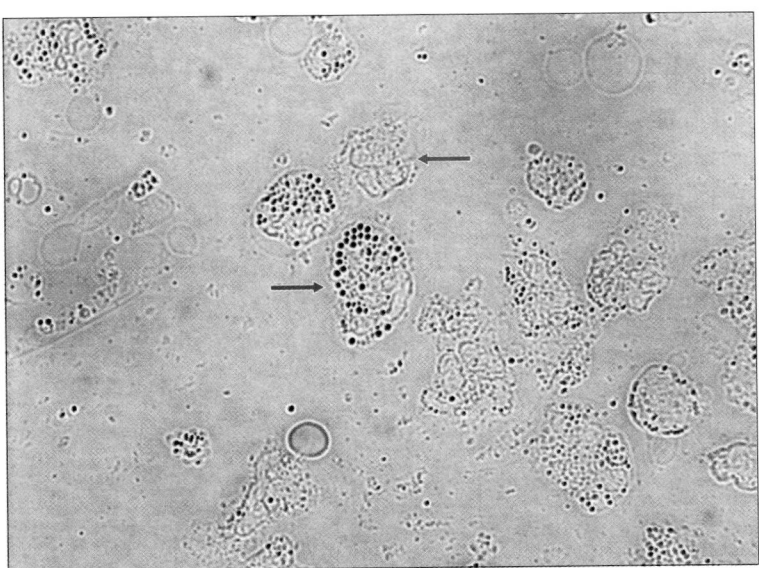

Fig. 30.3 Ragocyte (blue arrow) from a patient with rheumatoid arthritis, showing the typical granules. An adjacent cell does not contain ragocyte granules (green arrow). This photograph was taken using a conventional microscope with the condenser iris almost fully closed (pseudophase). The preparation is unstained.

Pyrophosphate crystals accumulate within joints with advancing age. In acute pseudogout, the crystals are associated with a high nucleated cell count. The presence of calcium pyrophosphate crystals in association with otherwise typical features of OA characterizes hypertrophic OA.[10]

Hydroxyapatite within SF indicates damage to calcified cartilage or underlying subarticular bone. Loss of cartilage sufficient to expose these structures is seen most commonly in OA[11] and RA. The crystals are too small and amorphous to be seen with the light microscope, but staining with alizarin red produces a birefringent red product that is easily visualized. A specific arthropathy, "Milwaukee shoulder" (and its equivalent in other joints), is associated with larger apatite microspheroids.[12]

Lipids enter SF from the blood in inflammatory joint disease and hemarthroses, and by damage to synovial fat in trauma. They are usually present either as droplets with a Maltese cross pattern (liquid spherical crystals) or as needle-shaped crystals within a droplet of neutral fat. After intra-articular injection of depot corticosteroids, lipid crystalloids remain within the joint for up to 10 weeks and may mislead the unwary if their true nature is not recognized.

Other crystals are found within SF but are too numerous and rare to describe here. For a further description see the work by Freemont and Denton.[1]

Non-crystalline particles

Synovial joints are lined by cartilage and synovium and may be crossed by ligaments and bands of fibrocartilage. In disease, small fragments of these structures may appear within the SF. Most common are fragments of articular cartilage or, particularly in the knee, internal ligament and meniscal fibrocartilage.[1]

Articular cartilage has a silken sheen in polarized light. In OA, the most common disorder in which cartilage is found free in the joint, fragments typically show the crimping of fibrillation in polarized light. The typical clusters of chondrocytes can be seen in diffused transmitted light (Fig. 30.2).

With the advent of prosthetic surgery, and particularly as the number of aging prostheses increases, wear of implanted material leads to the presence of foreign material within the joint. Many modern plastics used in prostheses (e.g., high-density polyethylene), methylmethacrylate cement, and composites such as Dacron and carbon fiber mimic crystals if they fragment and can cause diagnostic problems. Metal debris from metal-based prostheses, particularly aluminium/titanium/vanadium alloys and chrome steel, appear as tiny black particles. Although difficult to recognize, these may be important harbingers of imminent prosthetic failure.

Occasionally, peculiar extraneous material such as plant fibers or other foreign bodies introduced accidentally are found within SF and need to be distinguished from diagnostically important particles.

Ragocytes

Ragocytes are cells of various lineages characterized by the presence of large cytoplasmic, refractile granules (Fig. 30.3). Ragocytes were first described in RA (hence the name),[13] in which they have been shown to contain immune complexes. They are not restricted to RA, being a feature of all inflammatory arthropathies, so their diagnostic value is somewhat limited. However, with the exception of RA, septic arthritis, gout, and pseudogout, ragocytes rarely account for more than 50% of all nucleated cells. If a crystal arthropathy is excluded, ragocyte counts above 70% are very strongly suggestive of RA[14] and, if above 95%, of septic arthritis (necessitating very careful examination for organisms by microscopy and culture).

Cytocentrifuge preparation

Synovial fluid cytoanalysis can be adequately conducted only on monolayers made using a cytocentrifuge. Optimal preparations are made by diluting the fluid to 400 cells/mm³ with isotonic saline and staining with Jenner-Giemsa stain. The one exception is when septic arthritis is suspected, when the greatest likelihood of identifying organisms is afforded by diluting the fluid to 1200 cells/mm³ and staining with Gram stain.

Many different cell types are found within SF, reflecting the differing pathogenetic mechanisms of the various joint diseases. Although epitope-defined subclasses of inflammatory cells are being characterized by immunocytochemistry and found to have disease-specific distributions,[15] this has yet to be fully exploited diagnostically. This is, in part due to problems in performing immunocytochemistry on cytocentrifuge preparations. Therefore, cell recognition in SF preparations is based largely on morphologic criteria.

Generally, in inflammatory arthropathies, polymorphs dominate the cytologic picture. Septic arthritis is the only disorder in which both ragocytes and neutrophils account for more than 90% of nucleated cells.

In non-inflammatory arthropathies, lymphocytes, macrophages, and synoviocytes are the most commonly encountered cells.

In a patient with RA, an SF in which over 80% of the nucleated cells are small lymphocytes, is indicative of less destructive and more slowly progressive disease. If lymphocytes account for more than 70% of nucleated cells and LE cells are present in the fluid, a diagnosis of systemic lupus erythematosus has to be seriously considered.

Macrophages are the predominant cell (>80% of nucleated cells) in viral arthritis, "Milwaukee shoulder," and prosthetic-debris–induced

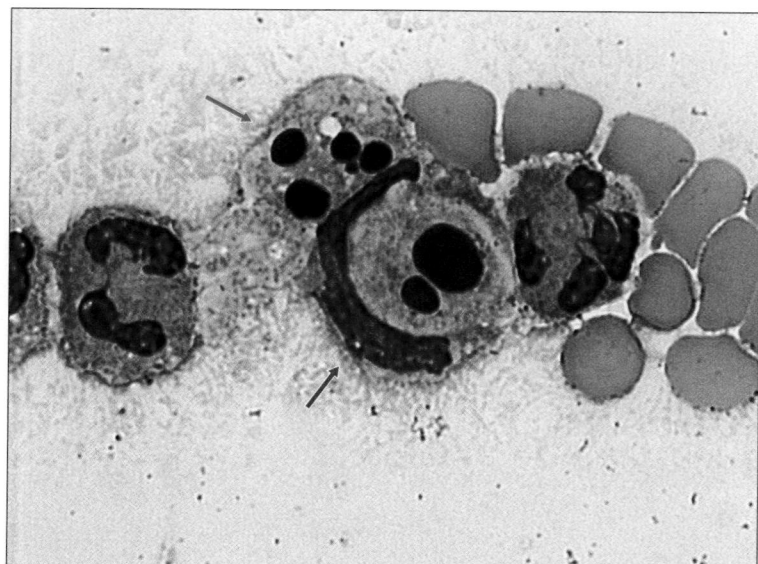

Fig. 30.4 Cytophagocytic mononuclear cell (blue arrow) in which an apoptotic polymorph has been phagocytosed by a macrophage. An apoptotic polymorph is adjacent to it (green arrow).

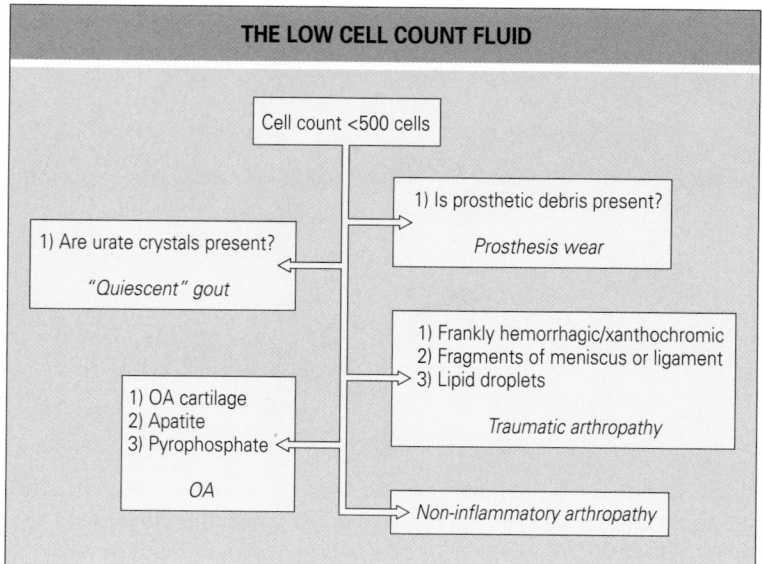

Fig. 30.5 The low cell count fluid.

arthropathy. The presence of macrophages that have phagocytosed apoptotic polymorphs (cytophagocytic mononuclear cells) (Fig. 30.4) is diagnostic of the seronegative spondyloarthropathies.[16]

In RA, extensive apoptosis occurs in the absence of the formation of cytophagocytic mononuclear cells, a feature of such universal occurrence that it can be used diagnostically.

Mast cells, although found in most arthropathies, are seen most commonly in the seronegative spondyloarthropathies and in traumatic arthritis.[16]

THE PLACE OF SYNOVIAL FLUID MICROSCOPY IN DIAGNOSIS

Synovial biopsy is the investigation of choice in diseases with specific synovial appearances,[17] such as granulomatous inflammation or pigmented villonodular synovitis. However, even experienced histopathologists can find difficulty sometimes in distinguishing inflammatory from non-inflammatory arthropathies, and there are very few features in a synovial biopsy that will allow a specific diagnosis to be made from within one of these two groups.[18]

On this background SF microscopy is of greatest value for:

- Differentiating between inflammatory and non-inflammatory arthropathies
- Identifying specific inflammatory and non-inflammatory arthropathies even before the full clinical syndrome develops
- The diagnosis of unexplained monoarthritis and oligoarthritis
- The rapid diagnosis of joint disease, in particular in suspected cases of septic arthritis in which prognosis is inversely related to the delay in diagnosis

Figures 30.5 to 30.7 present simple algorithms showing how the information obtained using the examinations outlined previously can be used to derive diagnoses.

THE DIAGNOSIS OF INTRA-ARTICULAR INFECTION

Infection in joints is a common cause of joint effusion, a major clinical concern, and very difficult to diagnose. As such it warrants specific discussion.

Bacterial arthritis

Of all forms of infective arthritis, bacterial infective arthritis is the most common diagnostic problem. SF microscopy has an important

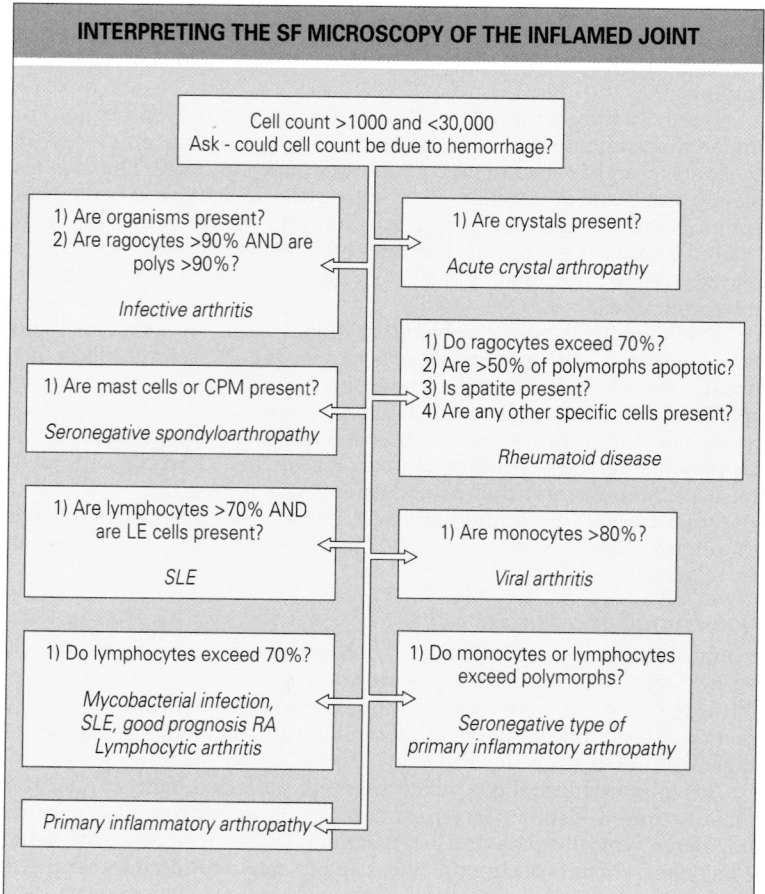

Fig. 30.6 Interpreting the SF microscopy of the inflamed joint.

role to play, because of the speed of turnaround of the test, which in specialist laboratories such as ours is typically less than 2 hours from receipt, and its ability to screen out disorders that mimic bacterial infection. Not all bacterial infections lead to septic arthritis, which is defined as the formation of pus within the joint. In septic arthritis careful microscopic examination of SF allows microorganisms to be identified in approximately 85% of instances of septic arthritis using the Gram stain (most infective arthritis is caused by gram-positive cocci[19]). The greatest problems in diagnosing septic arthritis are caused

THE SYNOVIAL FLUID WITH A VERY HIGH CELL COUNT

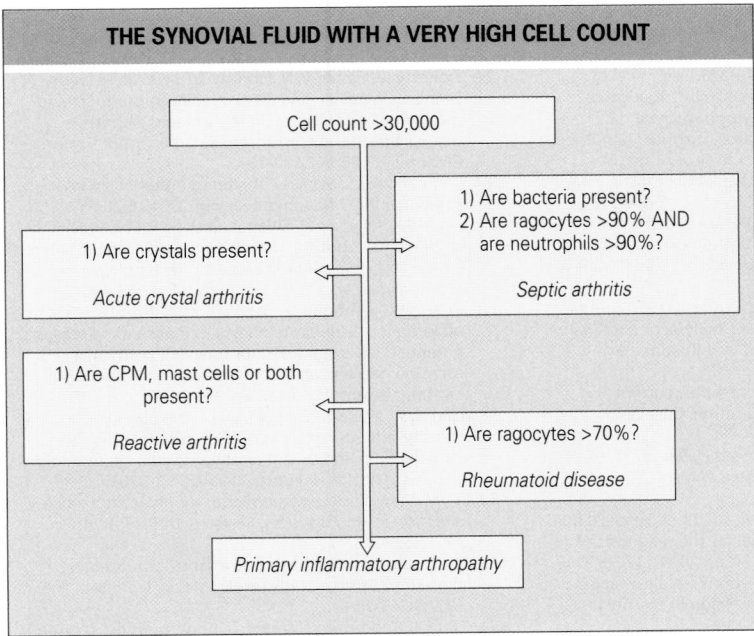

Fig. 30.7 Synovial fluid with a very high cell count.

TABLE 30.1 WELL-INVESTIGATED GROUPS OF SYNOVIAL FLUID BIOMARKERS

Biomarker	Reference
Type II collagen related epitopes	24
Matrix metalloproteinases (and TIMPS)	25
Calprotectin (leukocyte protein)	25
Cytokines	26
Complement	27
Aggrecan and aggrecan fragments	28, 29, 30
Keratan sulfate	28
Hyaluronan	28
Cartilage oligomeric matrix protein	30

by the relative paucity of organisms in most cases, recognition of gram-negative organisms, and identifying gram-positive cocci rendered gram-negative by incomplete antibiotic therapy. In these settings nothing can compensate for patience and experience. Microbiologic culture is also important,[20] but there is little benefit in sending all SF specimens for culture; and in this respect SF microscopy can be used as a rapid test to identify organisms and also to exclude other causes of an acutely severely inflamed single joint, such as a crystal arthropathy or reactive arthritis. Even in the absence of identifiable organisms, SF microscopy can be very useful in identifying those patients with a high probability of having infection, using criteria such as the proportion of ragocytes, the cell count, and the proportion of polymorphs.[21] Thus, we carefully assess all cases in which the ragocyte count is greater than 90%, total nucleated cell count is greater than 20,000 cells/mm³, or polymorphs make up more than 90% of nucleated cells using Gram-stained cyto-centrifuge preparations and recommend that samples are sent for culture.

The reliance on quantitative cytology to make diagnoses of bacterial infective arthritis in the absence of identification of organisms has been taken further in joints with prostheses after researchers at the Mayo Clinic showed that a nucleated cell count of more than 1700/mm³ had a sensitivity of 94% and a specificity of 88% for diagnosing prosthetic joint infection in the knee and a differential count showed more than 65% neutrophils had a sensitivity of 97% and a specificity of 98%.[22]

Other increasingly common bacterial joint pathogens (e.g., *Neisseria*, *Salmonella*, *Mycobacterium* [including atypical forms]) are not typically associated with septic arthritis, and they can be identified in the SF by both culture and direct microscopic examination of appropriately stained cytologic preparations.

Non-bacterial infections

Fungal infections are diagnosed by the same approaches suggested earlier for bacteria. In contrast, viral infections are more difficult to diagnose, although an interest in the arthritides associated with HIV infection has shown the diagnostic importance of some features such as coexistence of a septic arthritis and a seronegative spondyloarthropathy in the same joint that are seen in no other disorder.

Future techniques

New techniques such as proteomics or polymerase chain reaction employing organism-specific primers or amplifying widely expressed bacterial nucleic acid sequences (e.g., 16S ribosomal component) may expand the diagnostic armamentarium in the future.[23]

CHEMICAL CHANGES IN THE SYNOVIAL FLUID IN DISEASE

Biochemical changes in the SF in disease may reflect abnormalities in the blood or result from the production of an excess of normal, or the presence of abnormal, products in the synovium, cartilage, or the fluid itself. In general, products of normal or abnormal joint metabolism will be in dynamic equilibrium with the serum and dependent on a complex set of variables, such as the hydrostatic and osmotic gradients across the joint, so that isolated single estimations of a product are not easy to interpret. This is compounded by a lack of availability of normal SF for comparison with disease samples.

Thirty years ago when biochemical analysis of SF was first studied in earnest, small molecules (e.g., glucose), ions, and pH were the focus of research but, for the reasons given previously, never gained favor diagnostically.

Since then there have been phases of interest in measuring drug levels and antibodies, which again proved of limited value diagnostically. However, recently there has been a burgeoning interest in the discovery and analysis of novel biomarkers (molecules indicative of specific pathologic processes) that may help to pinpoint specific disease processes within a joint. To date, the range of biomarkers that have been investigated is based on studies of specific molecules predicted to be important from the current understanding of molecular drivers of disease processes. Some of the most investigated groups of biomarkers are listed in Table 30.1[24-30] The references in the table will guide the reader to more information. However, many of these findings lack consistency and/or specificity, particularly as markers of the presence or activity of disease in individuals or specific joints.

There can be little doubt that the advent of widely available proteomics[31-33] (or metabolomics[34]) coupled with robust bioinformatics will see a huge increase in the number of biomarkers and peptide/protein "fingerprinting" of disease processes. There is already some evidence of the success of this type of approach when applied to SF, but the opportunities that these technologies open up could herald a revolution in identification of disease processes and subtypes, a reclassification of joint disease, and advances in diagnosis and prognostication.

REFERENCES

1. Freemont AJ, Denton J. Atlas of synovial fluid cytopathology, vol 18, current histopathology. Dordrecht: Kluwer, 1991.
2. Pascual E, Doherty M. Aspiration of normal or asymptomatic pathological joints for diagnosis and research: indications, technique and success rate. Ann Rheum Dis 2009;68:3-7.
3. Swan A, Amer H, Dieppe P. The value of synovial fluid assays in the diagnosis of joint disease: a literature survey. Ann Rheum Dis 2002;61:493-498.
4. Nalbant S, Martinez JAM, Kitumnuaypong T, et al. Synovial fluid features and their relations to osteoarthritis severity: new findings from sequential studies. Osteo Cart 2003;11:50-54.

5. McCarty DJ, Halverson PB, Carrera GF, et al. Milwaukee shoulder: association of microspheroids containing hydroxyapatite crystals, active collagenase, and neutral protease with rotator cuff defects: II. Synovial fluid studies. Arthritis Rheum 1981;24:474-483.

6. Freemont AJ, Denton J. The cytology of synovial fluid. In: Gray W, McKee GT, eds. Diagnostic cytopathology, 2nd ed. Edinburgh: Elsevier Science, 2003;929-939.

7. de Jonge R, Brouwer R, Smit M, et al. Automated counting of white blood cells in synovial fluid. Rheumatology 2004;43:170-173.

8. Revaud P, Hudry C, Giraudeau B, et al. Rapid diagnosis of inflammatory synovial fluid with reagent strips. Rheumatology 2002;41:815-818.

9. Lumbreras B, Pascual E, Frasquet J, et al. Analysis of the crystals in synovial fluid: training of the analysts results in high consistency. Ann Rheum Dis 2005;64:612-615.

10. Yavorsky A, Hernandez-Santana A, McCarthy G, McMahon G. Detection of calcium phosphate crystals in the joint fluid of patients with osteoarthritis—analytical approaches and challenges. Analyst 2008;133:302-318.

11. Freemont AJ, Hoyland JA. Morphology, mechanisms and pathology of musculoskeletal ageing. J Pathol 2007;211:252-259.

12. Rood MJ, van Laar JM, de Schepper AM, Huizinga TW. The Milwaukee shoulder/knee syndrome. J Clin Rheumatol 2008;14:249-250.

13. van de Stadt RJ, van de Voorde-Vissers E, Feltkamp-Vroom TM. Metabolic and secretory properties of peripheral and synovial granulocytes in rheumatoid arthritis. Arthritis Rheum 1980;23:17-23.

14. Davis MJ, Denton J, Freemont AJ, et al. Comparison of serial synovial fluid cytology in rheumatoid arthritis: delineation of subgroups with prognostic implications. Ann Rheum Dis 1988;47:559-562.

15. Bakakos P, Pickard C, Wong WM, et al. Simultaneous analysis of T cell clonality and cytokine production in rheumatoid arthritis using three-colour flow cytometry. Clin Exp Immunol 2002;129:370-378.

16. Freemont AJ, Denton J. The disease distribution of synovial fluid mast cells and cytophagocytic mononuclear cells in inflammatory arthritis. Ann Rheum Dis 1985;44:312-315.

17. Bresnihan B. Are synovial biopsies of diagnostic value? Arthritis Res Ther 2003;5:271-278.

18. Johnson JS, Freemont AJ. A 10 year retrospective comparison of the diagnostic usefulness of synovial fluid and synovial biopsy examination. J Clin Pathol 2001;54:605-607.

19. Ryan MJ, Kavanagh R, Wall PG, et al. Bacterial joint infections in England and Wales: analysis of bacterial isolates over a four year period. Br J Rheumatol 1997;36:370-373.

20. Mathews CJ, Coakley G. Septic arthritis: current diagnostic and therapeutic algorithm. Curr Opin Rheumatol 2008;20:457-462.

21. Margaretten ME, Kohlwes J, Moore D, Bent S. Does this adult patient have septic arthritis? JAMA 2007;297:1478-1488.

22. Trampuz A, Hanssen AD, Osmon DR, et al. Synovial fluid leukocyte count and differential for the diagnosis of prosthetic knee infection. Am J Med 2004;117:556-562.

23. Boyce JD, Cullen PA, Adler B. Genomic-scale analysis of bacterial gene and protein expression in the host. Emerg Infect Dis 2004;10:1357-1362.

24. Birmingham JD, Vilim V, Kraus VB. Collagen biomarkers for arthritis applications. Biomarker Insights 2006;1:61-76.

25. Landewé R. Predictive markers in rapidly progressing rheumatoid arthritis. J Rheumatol Suppl 2007;80:8-15.

26. Punzi L, Calo L, Plebani M. Clinical significance of cytokine determination in synovial fluid. Crit Rev Clin Lab Sci 2002;39:63-88.

27. Doherty M, Richards N, Hornby J, Powell R. Relation between synovial fluid C3 degradation products and local joint inflammation in rheumatoid arthritis, osteoarthritis and crystal associated arthropathy. Ann Rheum Dis 1988;47:190-197.

28. Lohmander LS. Markers of altered metabolism in osteoarthritis. J Rheumatol Suppl 2004;70:28-35.

29. Poole AR, Ionescu M, Swan A, Dieppe P. Changes in cartilage metabolism in arthritis are reflected by altered serum and synovial fluid levels of the cartilage proteoglycan aggrecan. J Clin Invest 1994;94:25-33.

30. Morozzi G, Fabbroni M, Bellisai F, et al. Cartilage oligomeric matrix protein level in rheumatic diseases: potential use as a marker for measuring articular cartilage damage and/or the therapeutic efficacy of treatments. Ann N Y Acad Sci 2007;1108:398-407.

31. Liao H, Wu J, Kuhn E, et al. Use of mass spectrometry to identify protein biomarkers of disease severity in the synovial fluid and serum of patients with rheumatoid arthritis. Arthritis Rheum 2004;50:3792-3803.

32. Ali M, Manolios N. Proteomics in rheumatology: a new direction for old diseases. Semin Arthritis Rheum 2005;35:67-76.

33. De Ceuninck F. The birth and infancy of proteomic analysis in osteoarthritis research. Curr Opin Mol Ther 2007;9:263-269.

34. Ellis DI, Goodacre R. Metabolic fingerprinting in disease diagnosis: biomedical applications of infrared and Raman spectroscopy. Analyst 2006;131:875-885.

Minimally invasive procedures

Danielle M. Gerlag and Paul P. Tak

31

- Various small invasive procedures, ranging from arthrocentesis to synovial biopsy, can be used in daily rheumatology practice to determine the diagnosis or to monitor the response to treatment.
- Analysis of joint fluid can distinguish between an inflammatory and non-inflammatory cause of arthritis and is especially helpful in the case of monoarthritis, when septic arthritis or crystal-induced arthritis is suspected.
- In the diagnostic workup of patients with rheumatologic disease, especially when systemic disease is suspected, histologic samples can be of great additional value.
- Abdominal fat pad fine-needle aspiration is a relatively non-invasive, simple, and safe technique with an excellent specificity and positive predictive value in establishing amyloidosis.
- When inflammatory myositis syndromes, such as polymyositis (PM), dermatomyositis (DM), and inclusion body myositis (IBM), need to be distinguished from other myopathic syndromes, a histologic sample of the involved muscle(s) often leads to the definite diagnosis.
- Minor salivary gland biopsy of sublabial glands is a simple technique that can be performed in an outpatient setting when histologic confirmation of suspected Sjögren's syndrome, sarcoidosis, and other infiltrative processes is necessary.
- Synovial tissue biopsy samples can be taken safely on an outpatient basis using blind needle or arthroscopic techniques. Analysis of synovial tissue can be used for diagnostic reasons in selected cases, to study the pathogenetic processes in various types of arthritis, and to evaluate the response to (experimental) treatment in a research setting.

INTRODUCTION

Several small invasive procedures can be used in daily rheumatology practice to determine the diagnosis or monitor the response to treatment. These techniques include arthrocentesis and biopsies of skin, muscle and fascia, salivary gland, abdominal fat pad, and synovium. In this chapter we review and describe the processes to be followed for each of these techniques and discuss the indications and potential complications of the procedures.

ARTHROCENTESIS

Since its introduction in 1951 by Hollander, the aspiration of fluid from a joint cavity is performed on a routine basis by rheumatologists for both diagnostic and treatment reasons. Analysis of joint fluid can distinguish between an inflammatory and non-inflammatory cause of arthritis and is especially helpful in the case of monoarthritis, when septic arthritis or crystal-induced arthritis is suspected. In addition, arthrocentesis can be used therapeutically when fluid accumulation in a joint causes painful distention of the joint capsule. Intra-articular therapy with corticosteroids or other preparations can be of adjunctive value in the treatment of several types of arthritis.

Usually, physical landmarks and a thumbnail, ballpoint pen, or marker can be used to carefully determine and indicate the site of puncture. In some cases, such as the hip and sacroiliac joint, or when the synovial fluid is loculated, imaging techniques are necessary to ensure the right position of the needle in the joint cavity. Although the risk of contaminating the joint through the arthrocentesis itself is extremely low, aseptic measures to prevent this complication are necessary. After determining the aspiration or injection site, the skin over this area should be disinfected. This can be done using iodine solution or an alcohol-based disinfectant. It is important to allow the disinfectant fluid to dry. The use of gloves is generally advisable to protect oneself from possibly infected body fluids, but routine use of sterile gloves is unnecessary. However, when it is necessary to palpate the joint after disinfecting the area, the clinician should also disinfect his or her hands or use sterile gloves. When a relatively small joint is to be punctured, use of a local anesthetic—such as a 1% or 2% lidocaine solution without epinephrine—to anesthetize the skin, subcutaneous tissue, and joint capsule can minimize discomfort during the procedure. When rapid insertion of the needle into a joint is possible, the use of a local anesthetic is not necessary or can be mixed with the corticosteroid or other agent to be injected. The use of local anesthetics can also yield diagnostic information about the exact localization and nature of the pain. A 21-gauge needle can be used for most aspirations, and a 19-gauge needle can be chosen when large and viscous effusions are aspirated. Smaller (23-gauge) needles can be used for small joints, such as metacarpophalangeal or interphalangeal joints. If the needle is inserted into the joint correctly but no fluid can be aspirated, this could be the result of clogging of the needle because of fibrin or so-called "rice bodies." Irrigation of the joint with isotonic saline or some lidocaine can sometimes result in fluid that contains enough crystals or bacteria to establish the diagnosis. If a therapeutic agent is to be injected after the aspiration has been completed, the syringe can be removed and replaced by the syringe with the medication. After ensuring that the needle is still in the joint cavity, the medication can be injected.

Complications of arthrocentesis are extremely rare and include idiopathic infection and bleeding.

BIOPSIES

In the diagnostic workup of patients with rheumatologic disease, histologic samples can be of great additional value. Especially when systemic disease is suspected, combining the clinical symptoms with the characteristic features of the affected tissue gathered with minimally invasive techniques can lead to the correct diagnosis.

Skin and subcutaneous tissue

Technique

Although many skin lesions may suggest a direct diagnosis combining the clinical information with the aspect and specific location of the lesion, histologic evaluation of skin abnormalities can help to differentiate between different syndromes. Skin biopsies are best taken from a recently developed lesion and should contain normal-appearing skin alongside the edge of the lesion.[1] Using a disposable punch biopsy tool of 3 to 6 mm in diameter, diagnosis of dermal and subdermal abnormalities can be determined. After anesthetizing the skin around the biopsy site with 1% to 2% lidocaine, a small cylinder of tissue is removed with a twisting movement of the punch. After achieving hemostasis, the wound can be closed primarily or left to heal by secondary intention. Both procedures will lead to small scar formation. Complications of the procedure are rare and include bleeding, especially when anticoagulants or non-steroidal anti-inflammatory drugs are used, and infection.

If vasculitis or panniculitis is suspected, excision biopsies using scalpel and forceps are more reliable in revealing the diagnosis because a larger amount of tissue that contains panniculus can be examined, leading to a greater chance of finding abnormalities.[1] A larger amount of tissue also allows for additional studies, using, for

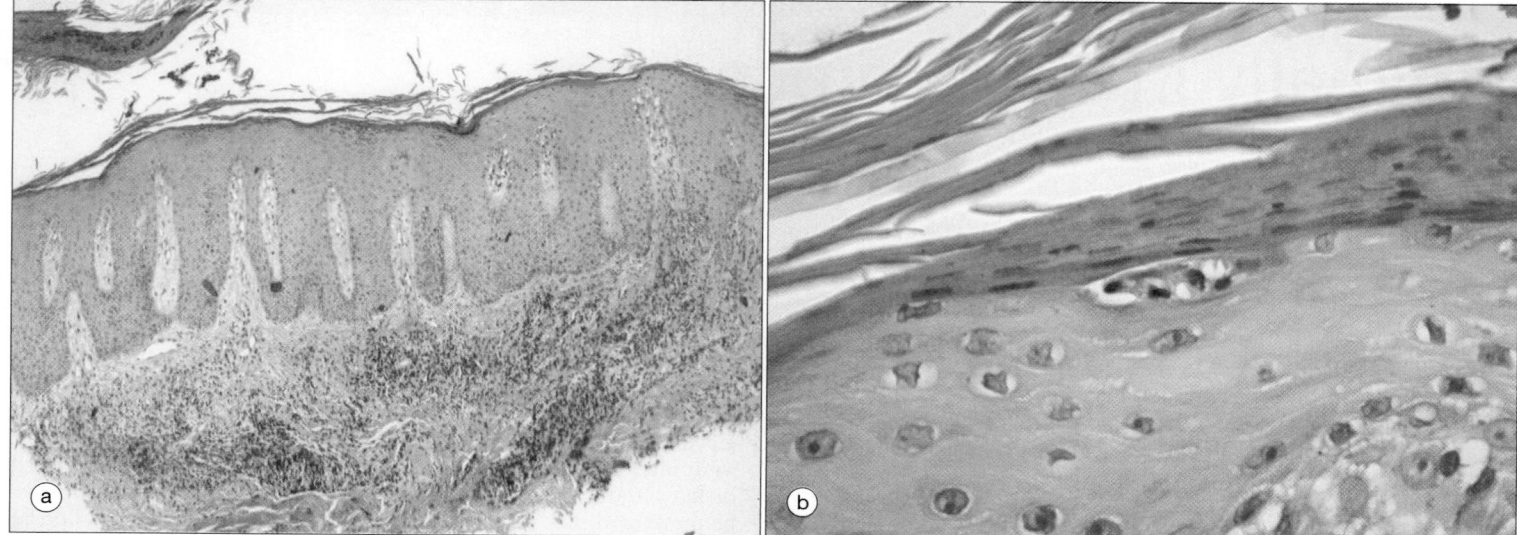

Fig. 31.1 (a) Psoriasis. The epidermis shows regular elongation of the epidermal rete ridges. The cornified layer shows confluent parakeratosis. There is a superficial perivascular lymphocytic infiltrate. (b) Psoriasis detail. Exocytosis of neutrophils.

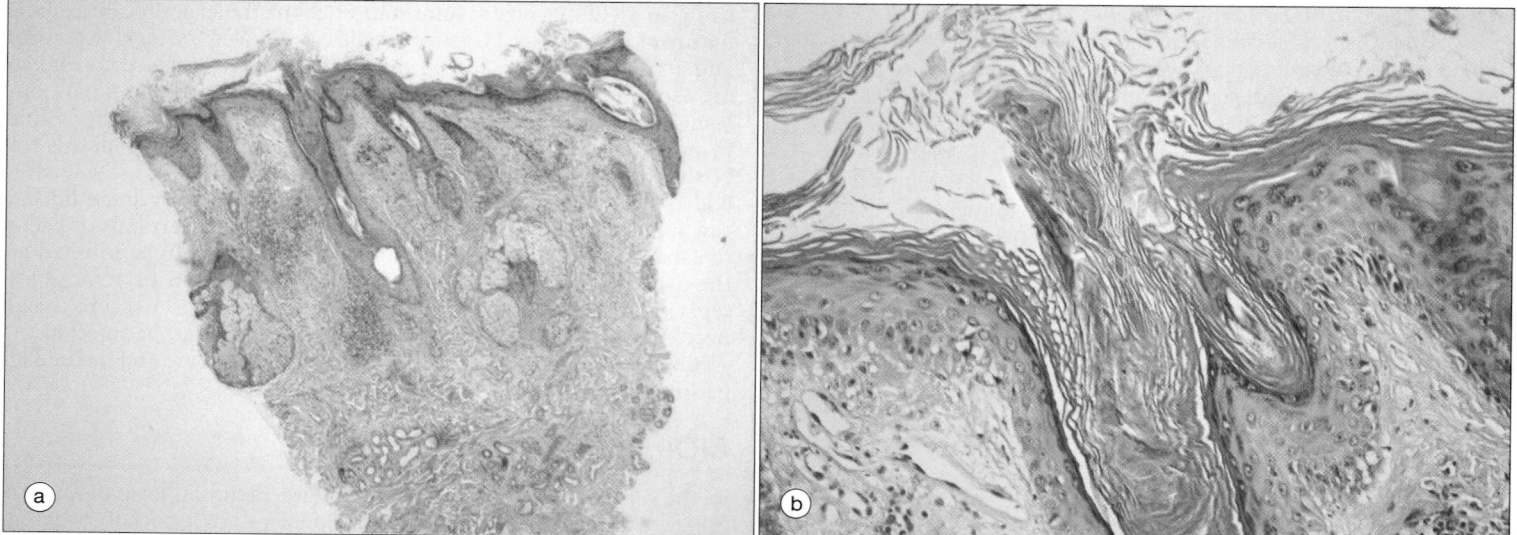

Fig. 31.2 (a) Chronic discoid lupus erythematosus (CDLE). The epidermis shows hyperkeratosis, follicular plugging, atrophy, and basal layer vacuolization. A dense perivascular lymphoid infiltrate is present. (b) CDLE detail.

instance, immunohistochemistry, immunofluorescence, and electron microscopy. For cosmetic reasons, the line of incision should follow the natural lines of the skin.

Skin biopsy in specific rheumatologic disorders

In *psoriasis*, the epidermis is characterized by thickening of the viable cell layers (acanthosis), marked hyperkeratosis (thickening of the corni-fied layer), loss of the granular layer, and parakeratosis (nuclei in the stratum corneum). In addition, the contorted dermal blood vessels are increased in number and size, reaching up to the epidermis. Further-more, leukocyte infiltration is found in the dermis and epidermis, where some leukocytes form Munro microabscesses underneath the stratum corneum (Fig. 31.1a and b). Immunostaining with anti-CD3 antibodies (a T-lymphocyte marker) has shown that these infiltrates comprise many T cells.[2]

In lupus erythematosus (LE), lesions can be diverse and a biopsy can help to distinguish between different lesions. Discoid skin lesions show characteristic features: follicular *p*lugs, *a*trophy, *s*cale, *t*elangiec-tases, and *e*rythema (*"paste"* features) (Fig. 31.2a and b).

Direct immunofluorescence (DIF) techniques can be helpful in various subsets of LE and vasculitis because the site, morphology, and frequency of deposition vary among these subsets.[3,4] DIF requires fresh

tissue, which potentially can be substituted by the application of paraf-fin tissue-based immunohistochemistry. This latter technique can be used as an adjunct in the assessment of select inflammatory skin dis-eases, including vasculopathic conditions and collagen vascular disease.[5]

In discoid lupus, the immune deposits of mainly IgG and IgM are found in various patterns along the dermoepidermal junction in about 60% to 94% of the biopsies of lesional skin.[6] Prior treatment, sun exposure, and duration of the lesion may influence the frequency of positive immunofluorescence. Therefore, the most appropriate biopsy site is an older, untreated lesion that has not been exposed to the sun.

Skin lesions in systemic lupus erythematosus (SLE) may show immune deposits in various sites. SLE may show the so-called lupus band: Granular deposits of immunoglobulins and complement proteins are found at the dermal-epidermal junction.[7] Other deposition sites include superficial dermal blood vessel walls, cytoid bodies in the papil-lary dermis, and nuclei of the epidermal keratinocytes.[8]

In *scleroderma*, mononuclear infiltrates, mainly consisting of T cells located around the blood vessels, and increased collagen, synthe-sized by activated fibroblasts leading to tissue fibrosis, can be seen in early lesions.[9] These findings can be found in localized processes, such as morphea.

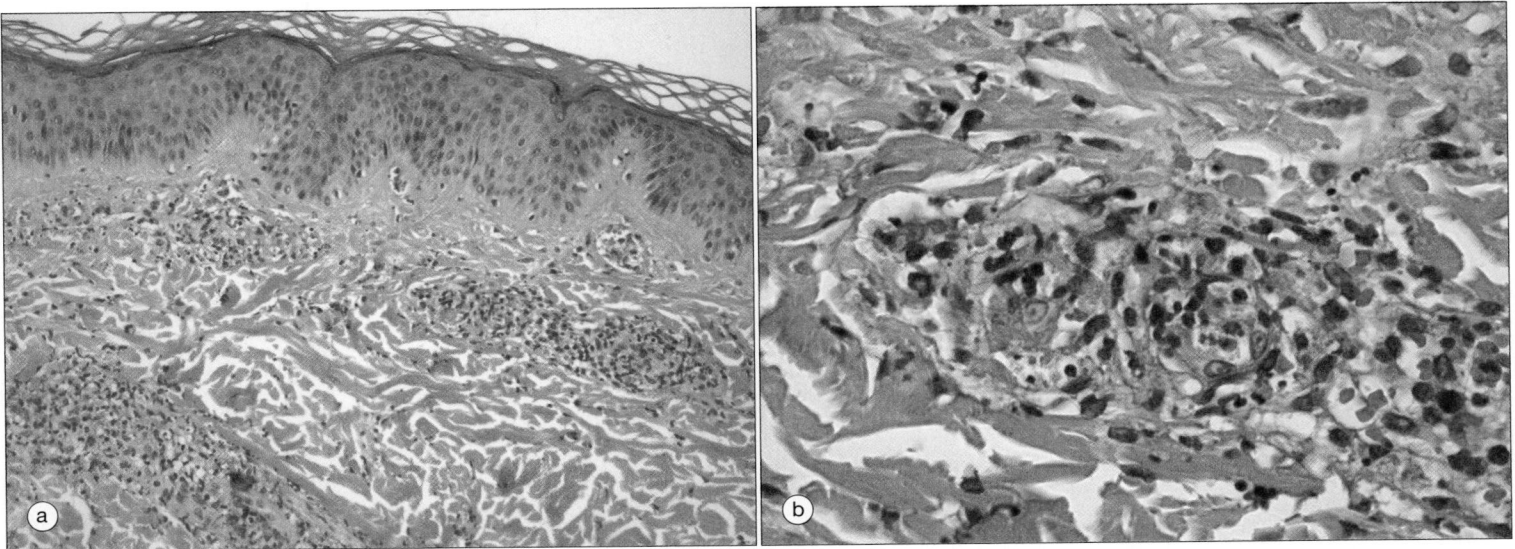

Fig. 31.3 (a and b) Leukocytoclastic vasculitis. Vascular damage with perivascular neutrophilic infiltrate, nuclear debris, and extravasation of erythrocytes is seen.

Various types of *vasculitis* (leukocytoclastic, eosinophilic, Henoch-Schönlein, polyarteritis nodosa) can be distinguished by histologic analysis of the skin or the subcutaneous lesion in which representative vessels are caught. The tissue sample should be of adequate size. When taken from an active lesion, the chance of a false-negative result will be less than when taken from normal skin (Fig. 31.3a and b). Additional immunofluorescent techniques will classically show immunoglobulin (Ig) A depositions in *Henoch-Schönlein purpura* (Fig. 31.4), but this can also be seen in other IgA-associated forms of vasculitis such as lymphocytic vasculopathy.[10]

Rheumatoid nodules show palisading fibroblasts surrounding a central area of necrosis. These fibroblasts are in turn surrounded by chronic inflammatory cells, mainly lymphocytes. Various proinflammatory cytokines, components of the complement system, and rheumatoid factor can be found in these granulomas.[11,12]

Abdominal fat pad fine-needle aspiration

Abdominal fat pad fine-needle aspiration is a relatively non-invasive, simple, and safe technique in establishing amyloidosis.[13,14] This technique, described by Westermark and Stenkvist, has an excellent specificity and positive predictive value. Using an 18- to 23-gauge needle,

aspiration is performed two to five times on different locations from the xiphoid process to the symphysis. The aspirated material is gently distributed on a glass slide and allowed to dry.[15] When stained with Congo red, a specific apple-green birefringence caused by binding to the amyloid can be seen under polarized light. The amyloid deposits are distributed mainly perivascularly, ranging from massive to subtle (Fig. 31.5). Fluorescent microscopy can improve the detection of amyloid in fat pad smears.[16] Sensitivity and specificity of the fine-needle aspiration technique range from 55% to 75% and up to 92% to 100%, respectively.[14,17] No complications of this technique have been reported.

Variants of this technique include Tru-Cut needle biopsy or excision biopsy. Other possible biopsy sites to confirm amyloidosis are the rectal mucosa, labial salivary gland, and compromised organs (kidney, liver, and endomyocardium). The latter sites should be reserved for patients in whom the aforementioned techniques failed to establish the diagnosis.

Biopsy of the temporal artery

The gold standard for diagnosis of giant cell arteritis is a biopsy of the temporal artery. This should be performed as soon as the diagnosis is

Fig. 31.4 IgA deposition in Henoch-Schönlein disease. Immunofluorescence examination reveals IgA deposits in small vessels.

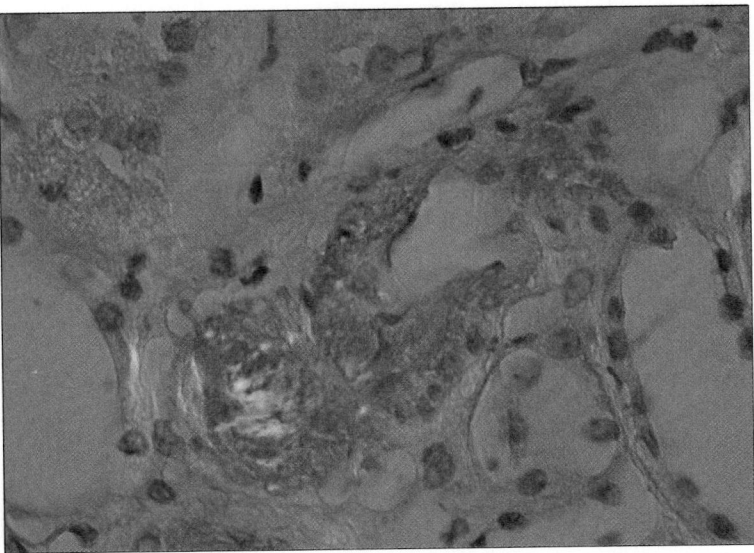

Fig. 31.5 Amyloidosis. Congo red stain observed under polarized light shows greenish birefringence of Congo red–stained amyloid fibrils.

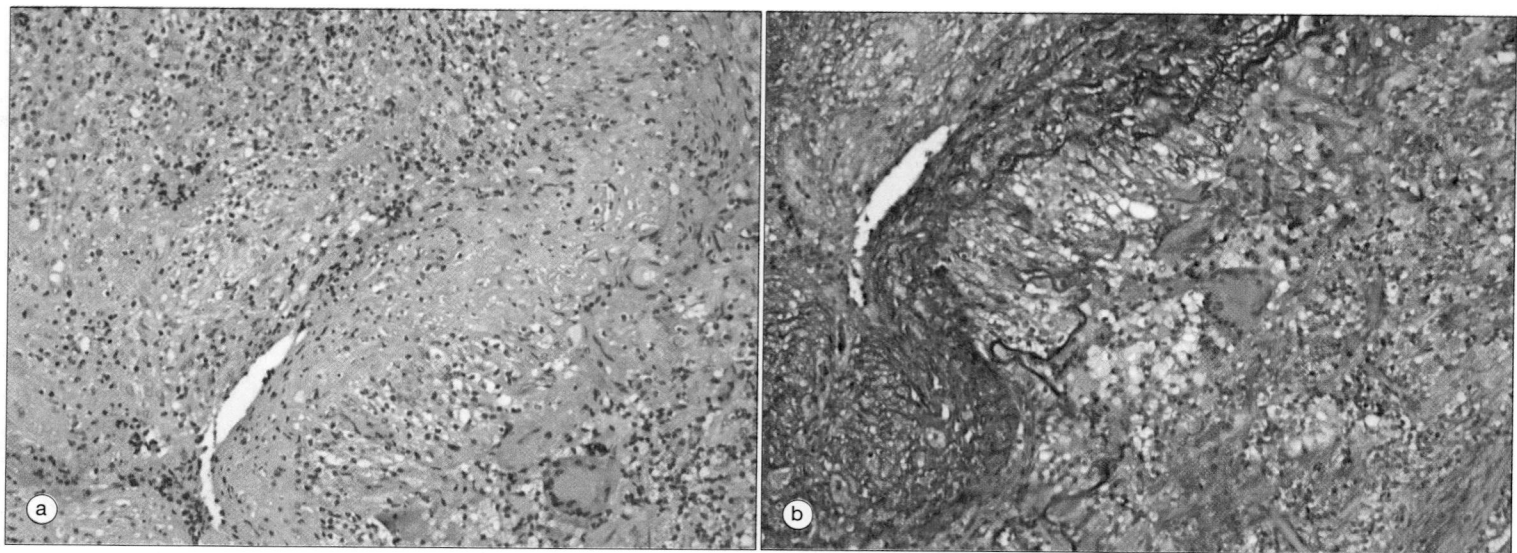

Fig. 31.6 (a) Arteritis temporalis. Low magnification shows partial destruction of the wall by an inflammatory infiltrate containing multinucleated giant cells leading to fragmentation of the internal elastic lamina and extreme narrowing of the lumen (H&E staining). (b) Arteritis temporalis (detail, EvG staining).

suspected, but without delaying treatment. After shaving the patient's hair over the appointed biopsy area and applying standard aseptic measures and local anesthetics, an incision is made directly over the artery in a cautious way. Skin hooks are used to spread the edges of the incision and the subcutaneous fat, if present. When the fascia of the temporal area is encountered, this is gently opened with the tips of the scissors and carefully widened to find the artery. This is dissected free and isolated over a length of 3 to 5 cm. After cutting or tying off small branches and main proximal and distal parts with sutures, the artery can be transected. The ligated ends can be electrocoagulated. The wound is closed with cutaneous sutures after hemostasis is obtained. A bandage can be applied after the procedure. Complications of temporal artery biopsy are rare.

The suggested sample size is 2.5 to 5 cm because the inflammation is discontinuous, causing skip lesions (reported in about 10% of cases).[18] Biopsy of the contralateral side is suggested if the first biopsy is negative. The sensitivity of a positive biopsy was reported to be not significantly decreased after 2 weeks of steroid therapy,[19] and several case reports suggested the persistence of histologic abnormalities even after months of treatment.[20]

A meta-analysis of the sensitivity and specificity of clinical signs and symptoms showed various clinical features, such as jaw claudication, diplopia, and erythrocyte sedimentation rate (ESR), predicting high or low probability of a positive temporal artery biopsy.[21] Several other variables influence the reported incidence of 3% to 10% false-negative results: the length and number of biopsies taken, the presence of skip lesions, pathologic sectioning techniques, and the duration of treatment before biopsy.[22] Using a Bayesian analysis, the sensitivity of a single temporal artery biopsy was calculated to be 89.1% (95% confidence interval, 81.8% to 91.7%).[23] The use of imaging techniques, such as B-flow ultrasound, may perhaps be of help in defining the artery segment to be biopsied to decrease sampling error.[24]

Mononuclear infiltrates penetrating all layers of the arterial wall, causing panarteritis, with activated T cells and macrophages arranged in granulomas can be seen.[25] In 50% of cases multinucleated giant cells are found grouped along the fragmented internal elastic lumina (Fig. 31.6a and b). Temporal artery biopsy is a safe procedure with a low complication rate. Complications include postoperative hematoma, wound infection or dehiscence, and facial nerve damage.[26]

Muscle/fascia

When inflammatory myositis syndromes, such as polymyositis (PM), dermatomyositis (DM), and inclusion body myositis (IBM), need to be distinguished from other myopathic syndromes, a histologic sample of the involved muscle(s) often leads to the definite diagnosis. Furthermore, atypical inflammatory myopathies such as pyomyositis, parasitic

diseases, and granulomatous myositis in sarcoidosis can be identified.[27]

Site selection is crucial when taking a muscle biopsy. A muscle biopsy should be taken from an involved muscle identified by physical examination, but not a fully atrophic or severely weakened one. Also, care should be taken not to obtain samples from a muscle that was injected or has recently been evaluated by electromyography (EMG) because of the chance of focal traumatic myositis. Taking a muscle sample from the side contralateral to the one found to be abnormal on EMG may increase the yield of finding diagnostic abnormalities. The quadriceps or deltoid muscles are involved in most myopathies and are the easiest to access.

Furthermore, the use of magnetic resonance imaging (MRI) in identifying affected areas that show an increased T2 signal may also help to reduce sampling error. The value of fat-suppressive (STIR) image signal intensity was studied in 40 patients with idiopathic inflammatory myopathies and correlated significantly with clinical activity and the presence of inflammation on muscle biopsy.[28] In this study, signal intensity scores were found to be more sensitive in detecting clinical disease activity than the presence of pathologic changes on muscle biopsy (89% vs. 66%).

Open biopsy has several advantages because a larger tissue sample can be obtained under direct vision. This reduces the chance of sampling error and allows for multiple diagnostic tests.[29] In spite of these advantages, 25% to 30% of patients with myositis still have negative biopsy results.[30] For suspected inherited metabolic myopathies, when multiple quantitative assays need to be performed, open biopsy is recommended.[31]

After local anesthestic has been administered, a longitudinal incision is made and the subcutaneous tissue is dissected. Under direct vision, a muscle sample of approximately 2 × 1 × 1 cm is taken, stabilized in a clamp, and kept moist until it is processed. Although the procedure is well tolerated and safe, there are some limitations: It requires the assistance of a surgeon and local or regional anesthetics; it can only be done on superficial muscles; it is not suitable for serial biopsy assessment; and it leads to scar formation. Alternatively, various percutaneous needle muscle biopsy techniques that have been developed are more cost effective, are more convenient for daily practice, and yield adequate tissue samples for histology, histochemistry, and electron microscopy.[29] Some procedures require a skin incision, such as when a disposable Tru-Cut biopsy needle, the suction-assisted reusable device with a side-cutting window and inner cutting cylinder (University College Hospital instrument) (Fig. 31.7), or a sharp-jawed surgical instrument (called a conchotome) is used.[32]

Using the suction-assisted and spring-loaded needles (Bard Biopty-Cut instrument), originally described by Coté,[33] more samples can be taken from the same or more than one muscle, which may improve

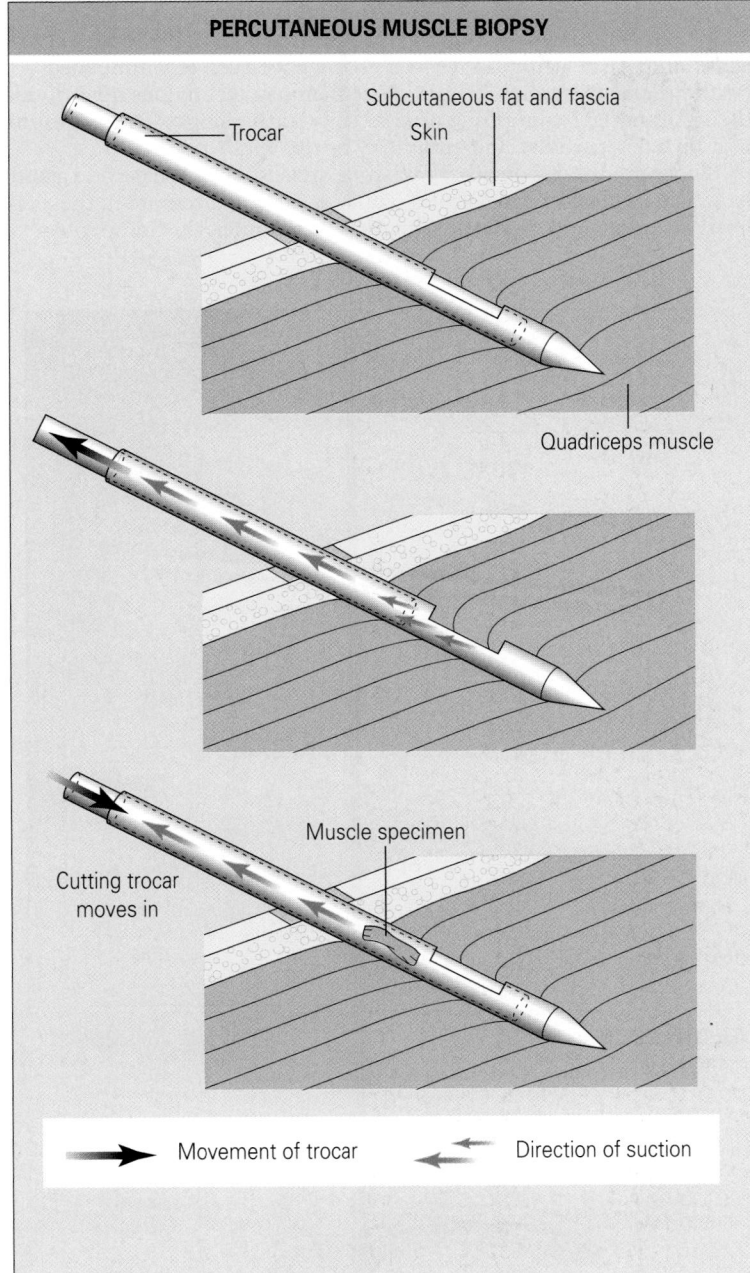

PERCUTANEOUS MUSCLE BIOPSY

Trocar — Skin — Subcutaneous fat and fascia

Quadriceps muscle

Cutting trocar moves in

Muscle specimen

→ Movement of trocar   ← Direction of suction

Fig. 31.7 Percutaneous muscle biopsy using suction-assisted instrument.

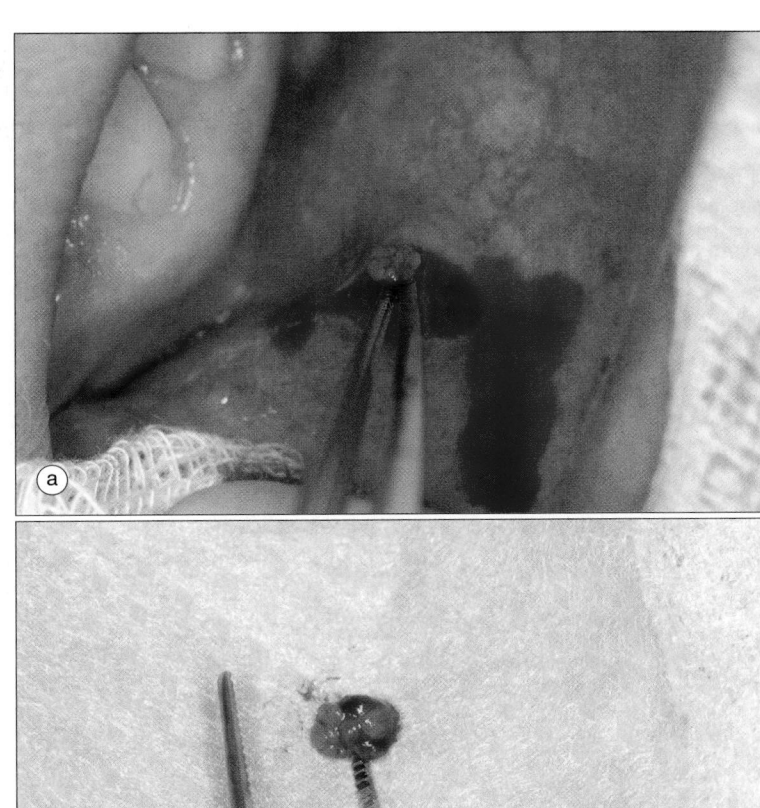

Fig. 31.8 (a) Lip biopsy: incision of the lower lip. (b) Biopsy specimen.

sensitivity.[30,31,33,34] Additional advantages include the ability to perform this method at the patient's bedside, the fact that no skin incision is required, and the possibility of taking serial biopsies to evaluate treatment. Complications from this technique, such as small hematomas, are rare.

Although some controversy exists about the diagnostic value of specific histopathologic features found in muscle biopsies from inflammatory syndromes,[35-37] the combination of clinical information and histologic aspects may result in different therapeutic options and prediction of prognosis.

In inflammatory myopathies, myofiber degeneration, regeneration, and an inflammatory infiltrate consisting of mononuclear cells are usually found. In PM, invasion of cytotoxic T cells into non-necrotic myofibers can be seen. Typical histologic changes in DM consist of perimysial perivascular inflammation with B and T cells, capillary involvement, and atrophy of the fibers due to ischemia. In IBM, chronic myopathic features, endomysial lymphocytic inflammation, and rimmed vacuoles are present. Filamentous inclusions may be seen in ultrastructural studies. Immunohistochemistry can be of help in determining the diagnosis. With the increasing availability of various

antibodies to proteins, both paraffin-embedded and (sequential) cryosections can be used for immunohistochemical analysis of the inflammatory infiltrates.[38] In most metabolic myopathies, immunohistochemistry is not advantageous.

Salivary gland

The main indication for salivary gland biopsy is histologic confirmation of suspected Sjögren's syndrome, sarcoidosis, and other infiltrative processes, such as amyloidosis and hemochromatosis. Various techniques have been described, each with its advantages and disadvantages.

Minor salivary gland biopsy of sublabial glands is one of the most widely used procedures. It is a simple technique that can be performed in an outpatient setting. The patient is seated or lying with the upper half of the body upright. The lower lip is everted, and the mucosa is inspected. The biopsy site should contain normal-appearing mucosa and enlarged labial glands (1- to 2-mm firm nodules), as determined by palpation. The area is infiltrated with local anesthetics (e.g., lidocaine 2%, with or without epinephrine/adrenaline) and a small superficial incision of 0.1 to 1 cm is made (Fig. 31.8a and b). The salivary glands (preferably 5 to 10) are bluntly dissected by grasping the glands carefully at the base with a forceps and applying gentle upward traction.[39] Light pressure can help to bulge the gland from the incision wound.[40] Care should be taken not to damage the sensory nerves, which can be easily distinguished during the procedure. The incision can be closed with dissolvable sutures, but several physicians leave the incision open, allowing it to heal spontaneously. Possible complications include bleeding due to an incision that is too deep; damaging the sensory nerve, leading to permanent hypoesthesia of the lower lip; and burning of the mouth after the procedure owing to drinking hot beverages while still anesthetized.

The glands are fixed in formalin, embedded in paraffin, and stained with hematoxylin and eosin (H&E). For evaluation of the diagnosis of Sjögren's syndrome, the inflammatory infiltrate is scored and graded according to the method of Greenspan and Daniels,[41] which is based on the number of inflammatory cells (foci) within the biopsy section. These foci are usually found perivascularly or periductally, adjacent to the acini of the glands. Classically, a single tissue section is taken to evaluate the infiltrate, but despite standardization of the methodology of sampling, processing, and examining the biopsies, reproducibility of

the histologic scores remains low. To increase the diagnostic accuracy of this test, multilevel sectioning (three different levels, at least 200 μm apart) and use of a cumulative focus score have been recommended.[42,43] Furthermore, the use of immunohistochemical techniques quantifying the IgA- and IgG-containing plasma cells in the biopsy sample results in a higher sensitivity and specificity of the test.[44]

Biopsy procedures on other salivary glands, such as the parotid gland, have also been described. Parotid biopsy is safe and accurate in the diagnosis of adult and pediatric Sjögren's syndrome.[45,46] Comparison of

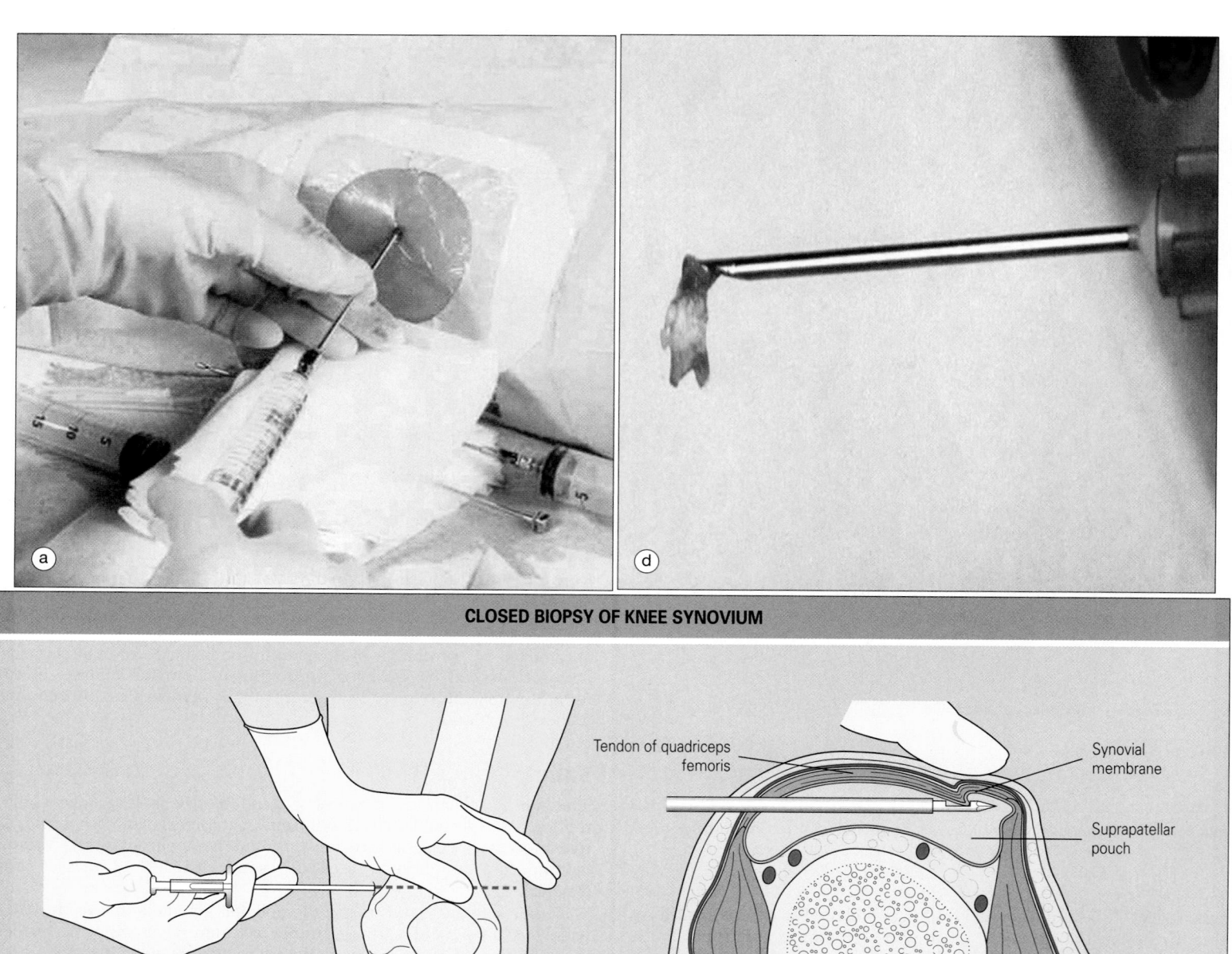

Fig. 31.9 (a) Parker-Pearson needle. (b) Procedure of blind needle biopsy of the knee. (c) Schematic drawing of blind needle biopsy procedure of the knee. (d) Synovial tissue specimen.

parotid and minor salivary gland biopsy shows little added value of the former, especially if other diagnoses such as lymphoma or sarcoidosis are suspected.[47,48]

Synovium

Because the synovial tissue is easily accessible, biopsy samples can be taken safely using blind needle or arthroscopic techniques. Subsequent analysis of synovial tissue can be used for diagnostic reasons in selected cases[49-52] to study the pathogenetic processes in various types of arthritis and evaluate the response to (experimental) treatment in a research setting.[53,54]

Blind or *closed needle biopsy* has been successfully performed with the Parker-Pearson needle, which is a simplified 14-gauge biopsy needle that does not require a skin incision (Fig. 31.9a).[55] This technique is safe, tolerated well, technically easy, and inexpensive. After employing standard aseptic technique and anesthetizing skin, subcutaneous tissue, and joint capsule with 1% or 2% lidocaine (see also earlier discussion on arthrocentesis), the trocar is inserted into the joint and the biopsy needle is introduced into the trocar (Fig. 31.9b and c). Applying suction to a Luer-Lok syringe attached to the biopsy needle helps in obtaining the specimen (Fig. 31.9d). When the angle of the needle is altered, multiple biopsies can be obtained. Taking six or more biopsy samples from multiple locations reduces the chance of sampling error and leads to a variability of less than 10%.[56] In the case of minimal or no clinical evidence of inflammation or effusion, the use of 10 to 20 mL of isotonic saline to fill the joint cavity before introducing the trocar may be helpful. Most investigators use this technique to biopsy the knee joint, but biopsy of other joints such as the ankle, wrist, elbow, and shoulder has also been described. Smaller joints can be approached with a modified short needle.[57] In most cases this technique yields adequate tissue samples, with signs of inflammation generally similar to samples taken under direct vision using an arthroscopic technique.[58] It can fail, however, when joints are not swollen. In a series of more than 800 samples, no complications (such as infection or hemarthrosis) were seen.[51] Several modifications to this technique have been described, such as use of the Tru-Cut needle for a variety of soft tissue biopsies. This is an inexpensive, disposable item that can retrieve synovial tissue through an action similar to that described earlier.

Arthroscopic biopsy

Because there are limitations to the use of blind needle biopsies (e.g., restriction to larger joints, potential sampling error due to the blind character of the procedure, and the difficulty of obtaining adequate tissue when the joint is not clinically inflamed), it may be advantageous to obtain synovial tissue using a small-bore arthroscope (Fig. 31.10).

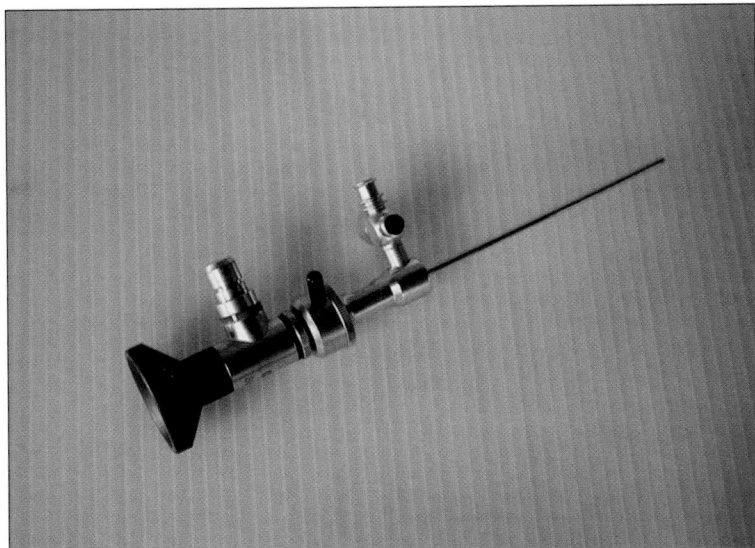

Fig. 31.10 Needle arthroscope.

Knee arthroscopy can be performed when a small-bore arthroscope or needle arthroscope, ranging from 4.5 to 2.7 mm, is introduced into an infrapatellar skin portal, which is created after disinfecting and anesthetizing the skin, subcutis, and knee joint (Fig. 31.11a). For the grasping forceps, a suprapatellar second skin portal is installed. This technique allows macroscopic examination of the synovial tissue and biopsy of different sites in the joint under direct vision. It can also be applied when biopsy samples of an ankle joint are taken, using a medial

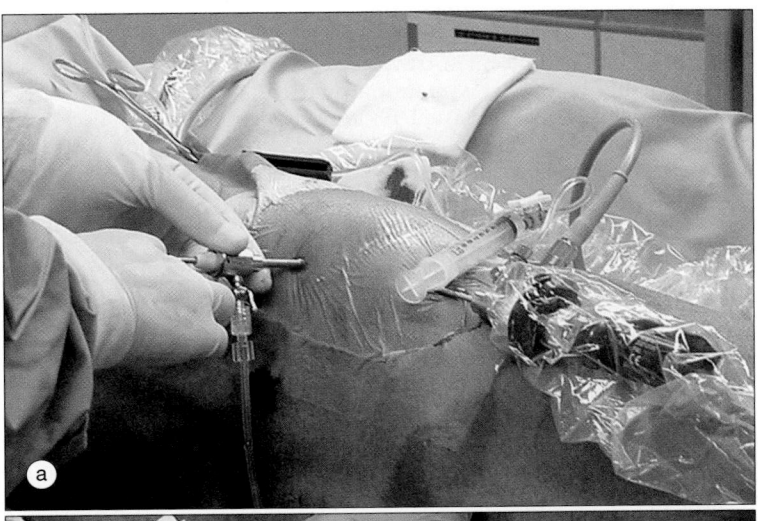

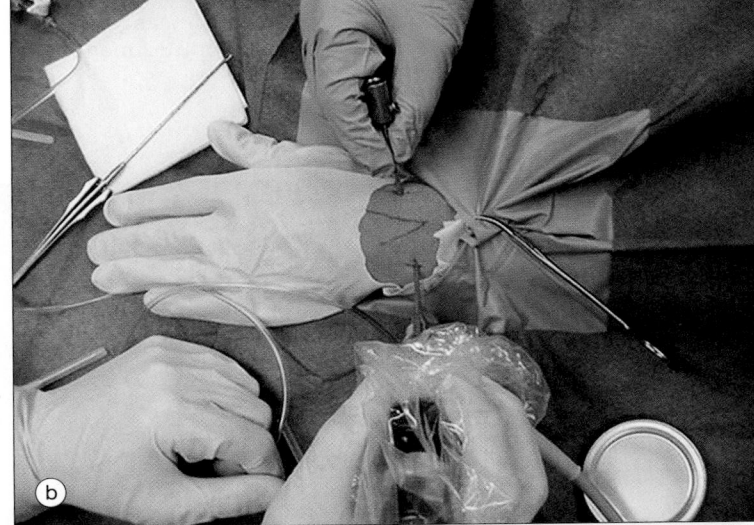

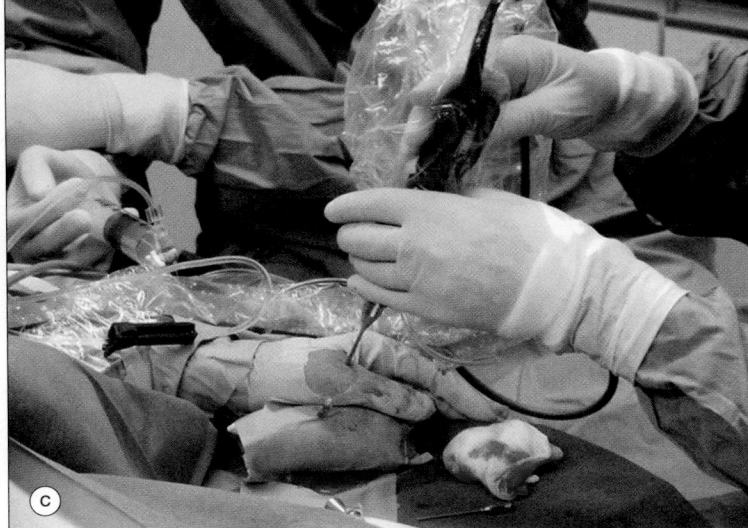

Fig. 31.11 (a) Needle arthroscopy of the knee. (b) Needle arthroscopy of the wrist. (c) Needle arthroscopy of the MCP1 joint.

and lateral malleolar portal. A small-bore arthroscope of 1.9 mm can be used for a smaller joint, such as the metacarpophalangeal joint or the wrist through radial and ulnar skin portals (Fig. 31.11c and 31.11b). Inflammatory markers are generally comparable between biopsy samples taken from a knee and a smaller joint such as the wrist.[59]

This technique, performed in an outpatient setting under local or regional anesthesia, is done by an increasing number of rheumatologists and is well tolerated by patients. Minimal pain and discomfort during the procedure and minor complications such as vasovagal reactions and temporary swelling of the joint are reported by 35% to 36% and 5% to 10% of the patients, respectively.[60] The total complication rate mentioned in a recent survey was 15.1/1000 arthroscopies, which is comparable to the rates mentioned in the orthopedic literature.[61] These complications consisted of joint infection (0.1%), deep vein thrombosis (0.2%), and hemarthrosis (0.9%). A correlation of wound infection and total complication rate with the amount of irrigation fluid was found, possibly a reflection of the duration of the procedure.

ARTHROSCOPIC JOINT LAVAGE

Joint lavage can be considered for different conditions, such as persistent arthritis after needle aspiration, osteoarthritis, and septic arthritis. The therapeutic effect of joint lavage is attributed to the removal of proinflammatory cells and their destructive enzymes, as well as cartilage degradation products. Although various uncontrolled, retrospective studies have reported a beneficial therapeutic effect of joint lavage for osteoarthritis of the knee joint, a randomized, placebo-controlled trial did not show superiority of this procedure compared with placebo.[62] Moreover, joint lavage alone or combined with infiltration of corticosteroids is similarly effective for the symptomatic management of osteoarthritis of the knee; the effects persisted for 3 to 12 months.[63,64]

For inflammatory arthritis, such as rheumatoid arthritis, the efficacy of joint lavage is still somewhat controversial. Retrospective analysis of the therapeutic effect of needle aspiration and joint lavage in 50 patients revealed that arthroscopic lavage had a superior effect.[65] This seems to be dependent on the volume of physiologic fluid used during the procedure, with 5 to 10 liters giving the best results.[66,67] Furthermore, the effects of joint lavage are more beneficial in patients with milder disease.

ULTRASOUND-GUIDED SYNOVIAL BIOPSY

Another method increasingly used to obtain synovial biopsies is the recently developed office-based, mini-invasive, ultrasound-guided technique.[68] This technique uses ultrasound guidance as an aid to acquire synovial tissue percutaneously by means of a portal and a rigid forceps technique.[69] This approach combines the advantages of being minimally invasive and being able to sample inflamed synovial tissue under indirect visual inspection. When a multifrequency linear transducer is applied, effusion and synovitis can be identified. The sensitivity of this technique can be enhanced by applying power Doppler techniques.[70] Under standard sterile conditions and after infiltrating the skin and subcutaneous tissue with local anaesthetics, a 14-gauge needle can be inserted into the designated area under ultrasound guidance. After creating a portal by means of a flexible wire followed by a percutaneous sheath, synovial samples can be acquired using a rigid forceps (Fig. 31.12).[68,69]

ACKNOWLEDGEMENT

The authors would like to acknowledge Dr. L. Schot and Prof. Dr. S. Florquh for the illustrations of the lip biopsy and histology of the skin.

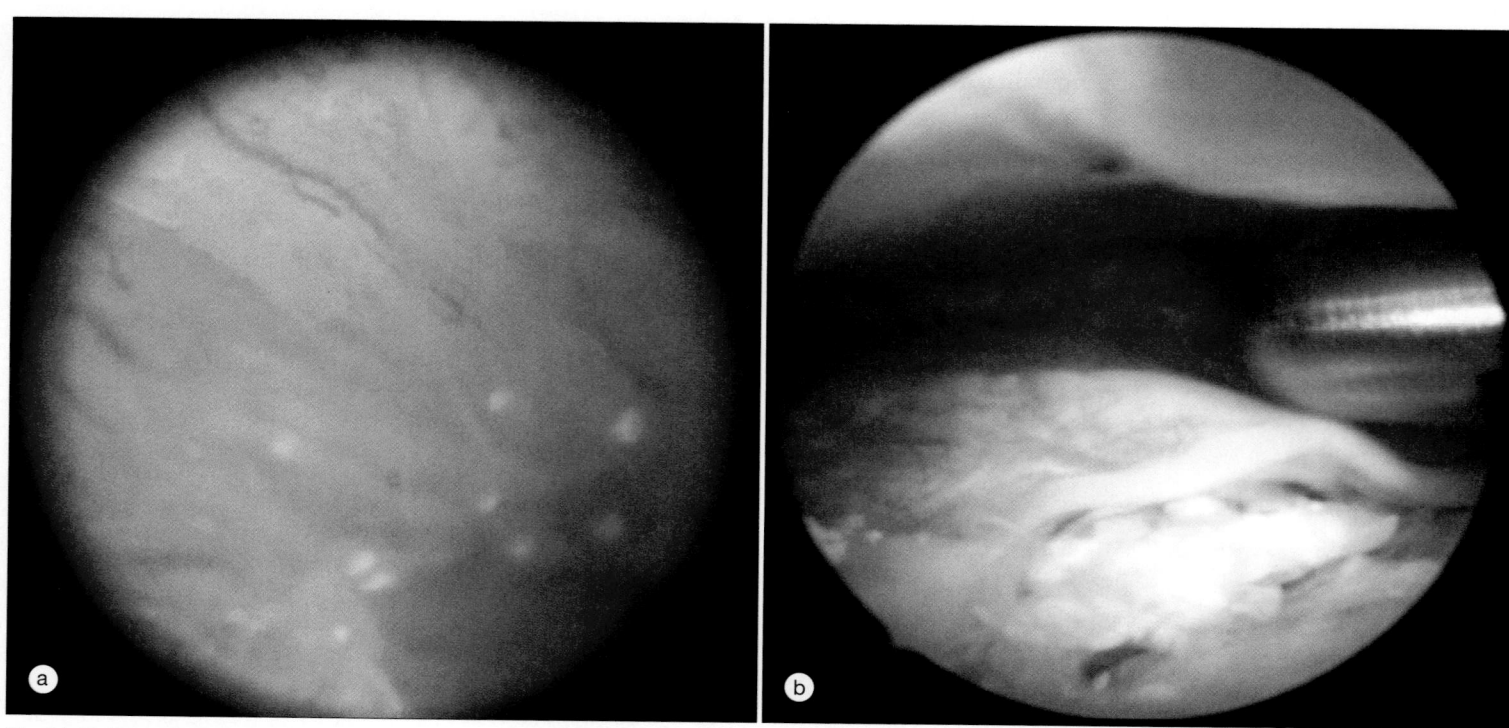

Fig. 31.12 Examples of intra-articular pathology seen at needle arthroscopy. (a) Deposits of monosodium urate crystals (tophi) on the inflamed synovium in a patient with gout. (b) Deposits of calcium pyrophosphate dehydrate crystals on inflamed synovium in a patient with chondrocalcinosis.

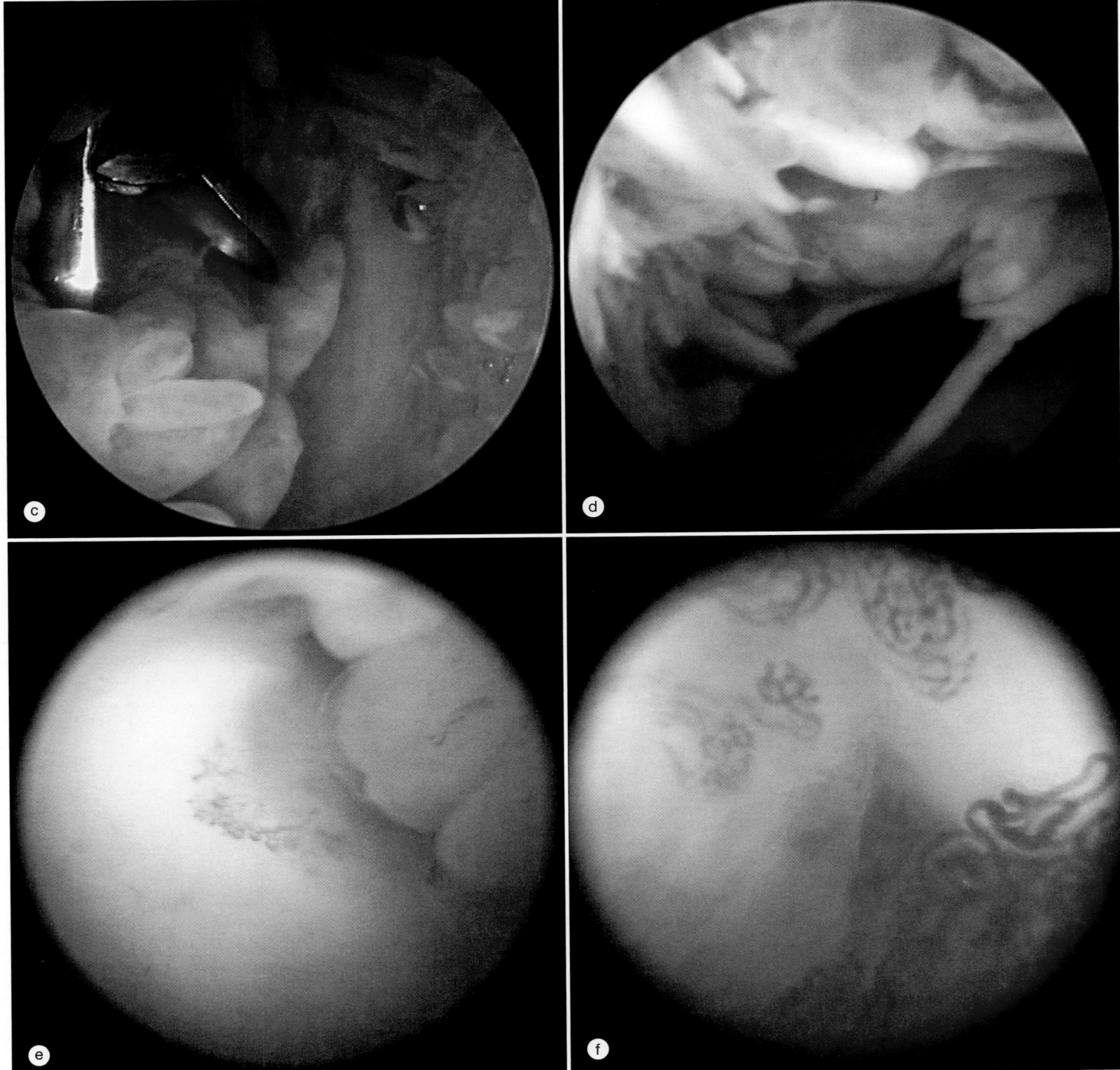

Fig. 31.12, cont'd (c) Villous synovitis in a patient with rheumatoid arthritis plus forceps. (d) Villous synovitis with vascular and avascular villi in a patient with rheumatoid arthritis. (e) Overgrowth of cartilage by synovial tissue at the cartilage-pannus junction in a patient with rheumatoid arthritis/invading synovium at the cartilage-pannus junction. (f) Villous synovitis with tortuous vascular pattern.

Continued

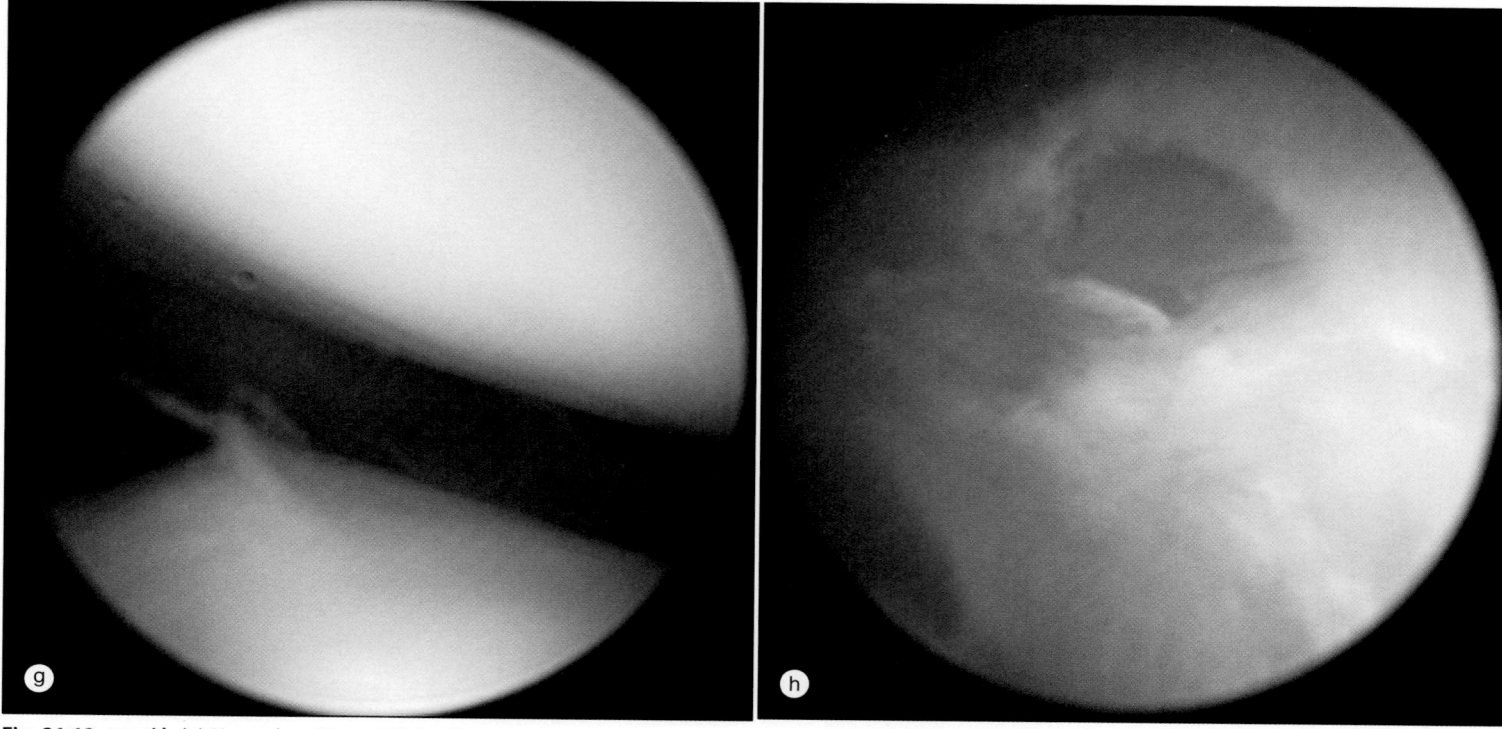

Fig. 31.12, cont'd (g) Normal cartilage. (h) Cartilage erosion in a patient with osteoarthritis without synovitis.

KEY REFERENCES

1. Peters MS, Winkelmann RK. The biopsy. Dermatol Clin 1984;2:209-217.
2. Schon MP, Boehncke WH. Psoriasis. N Engl J Med 2005;352:1899-1912.
4. Dahl MV. Immunoglobulin deposition in skin of patients with lupus erythematosus: clinical correlates and indications for direct immunofluorescence. Adv Dermatol 1986;1:247-266.
5. Magro CM, Dyrsen ME. The use of C3d and C4d immunohistochemistry on formalin-fixed tissue as a diagnostic adjunct in the assessment of inflammatory skin disease. J Am Acad Dermatol 2008;59:822-833.
6. Dahl MV. Usefulness of direct immunofluorescence in patients with lupus erythematosus. Arch Dermatol 1983;119:1010-1017.
7. Burnham TK, Fine G. The immunofluorescent "band" test for lupus erythematosus. Br J Dermatol 1971;84:176-177.
8. Sontheimer RD, Provost TT. Lupus erythematosus. In: Jordon RE, ed. Immunologic diseases of the skin. Norwalk, Conn: Appleton & Lange, 1991: 355-378.
9. Anonymous: Systemic sclerosis: current pathogenetic concepts and future prospects for targeted therapy. Lancet 1996;347:1453-1458.
10. Crowson AN, Magro CM, Usmani A, McNutt NS. Immunoglobulin A–associated lymphocytic vasculopathy: a clinicopathologic study of eight patients. J Cutan Pathol 2002;29:596-601.
11. Hessian PA, Highton J, Kean A, et al. Cytokine profile of the rheumatoid nodule suggests that it is a Th1 granuloma. Arthritis Rheum 2003;48:334-338.
13. Stenkvist B, Westermark P, Wibell L. Simple method of diagnostic screening for amyloidosis. Ann Rheum Dis 1974;33:75-76.
14. Ansari-Lari MA, Ali SZ. Fine-needle aspiration of abdominal fat pad for amyloid detection: a clinically useful test? Diagn Cytopathol 2004;30:178-181.
16. Giorgadze TA, Shiina N, Baloch ZW, et al. Improved detection of amyloid in fat pad aspiration: an evaluation of Congo red stain by fluorescent microscopy. Diagn Cytopathol 2004;31:300-306.
18. Poller DN, van Wyk Q, Jeffrey MJ. The importance of skip lesions in temporal arteritis. J Clin Pathol 2000;53:137-139.
19. Achkar AA, Lie JT, Hunder GG, et al. How does previous corticosteroid treatment affect the biopsy findings in giant cell (temporal) arteritis? Ann Intern Med 1994;120:987-992.
21. Smetana GW, Shmerling RH. Does this patient have temporal arteritis? JAMA 2002;287:92-101.

22. Weyand CM, Bartley GB. Giant cell arteritis: new concepts in pathogenesis and implications for management. Am J Ophthalmol 1997;123:392-395.
23. Niederkohr RD, Levin LA. A Bayesian analysis of the true sensitivity of a temporal artery biopsy. Invest Ophthalmol Vis Sci 2007;48:675-680.
24. Volpe A, Caramaschi P, Marchetta A, et al. B-flow ultrasound in a case of giant cell arteritis. Clin Rheumatol 2007;26:1955-1957.
25. Weyand CM, Goronzy JJ. Medium- and large-vessel vasculitis. N Engl J Med 2003;349:160-169.
26. Bhatti MT, Goldstein MH. Facial nerve injury following superficial temporal artery biopsy. Dermatol Surg 2001;27:15-17.
27. Lacomis D. The utility of muscle biopsy. Curr Neurol Neurosci Rep 2004;4:81-86.
28. Fraser DD, Frank JA, Dalakas M, et al. Magnetic resonance imaging in the idiopathic inflammatory myopathies. J Rheumatol 1991;18:1693-1700.
32. Dorph C, Nennesmo I, Lundberg IE. Percutaneous conchotome muscle biopsy. A useful diagnostic and assessment tool. J Rheumatol 2001;28:1591-1599.
33. Coté AM, Jimenez L, Adelman LS, Munsat TL. Needle muscle biopsy with the automatic Biopty instrument. Neurology 1992;42:2212-2213.
35. Miller FW, Rider LG, Plotz PH, et al. Diagnostic criteria for polymyositis and dermatomyositis. Lancet 2003;362:1762-1763.
36. Dalakas MC, Hohlfeld R. Polymyositis and dermatomyositis. Lancet 2003;362:971-982.
37. Hengstman GJ, van Engelen BG. Polymyositis, invasion of non-necrotic muscle fibres, and the art of repetition. BMJ 2004;329:1464-1467.
39. Friedman JA, Miller EB, Huszar M. A simple technique for minor salivary gland biopsy appropriate for use by rheumatologists in an outpatient setting. Clin Rheumatol 2002;21:349-350.
40. Laiho K, Sorsa S. A technique for minor salivary gland biopsy used in the diagnosis of Sjögren's syndrome. Clin Rheumatol 2003;22:164.
41. Greenspan JS, Daniels TE, Talal N, Sylvester RA. The histopathology of Sjögren's syndrome in labial salivary gland biopsies. Oral Surg Oral Med Oral Pathol 1974;37:217-229.
42. Al Hashimi I, Wright JM, Cooley CA, Nunn ME. Reproducibility of biopsy grade in Sjögren's syndrome. J Oral Pathol Med 2001;30:408-412.
43. Morbini P, Manzo A, Caporali R, et al. Multilevel examination of minor salivary gland biopsy for Sjögren's syndrome significantly improves diagnostic

performance of AECG classification criteria. Arthritis Res Ther 2005;7:R343-R348.
44. de Wilde PC, Kater L, Baak JP, et al. A new and highly sensitive immunohistologic diagnostic criterion for Sjögren's syndrome. Arthritis Rheum 1989;32:1214-1220.
45. Biasi D, Mocella S, Caramaschi P, et al. Utility and safety of parotid gland biopsy in Sjögren's syndrome. Acta Otolaryngol 1996;116:896-899.
47. Wise CM, Agudelo CA, Semble EL, et al. Comparison of parotid and minor salivary gland biopsy specimens in the diagnosis of Sjögren's syndrome. Arthritis Rheum 1988;31:662-666.
49. Kroot EJ, Weel AE, Hazes JM, et al. Diagnostic value of blind synovial biopsy in clinical practice. Rheumatology (Oxford) 2006;45:192-195.
51. Gerlag D, Tak PP. Synovial biopsy. Best Pract Res Clin Rheumatol 2005;19:387-400.
54. Gerlag DM, Tak PP. Novel approaches for the treatment of rheumatoid arthritis: lessons from the evaluation of synovial biomarkers in clinical trials. Best Pract Res Clin Rheumatol 2008;22:311-323.
55. Parker HR, Pearson CM. A simplified synovial biopsy needle. Arthritis Rheum 1963;6:172-176.
56. Dolhain RJ, Ter Haar NT, De Kuiper R, et al. Distribution of T cells and signs of T-cell activation in the rheumatoid joint: implications for semiquantitative comparative histology. Br J Rheumatol 1998;37:324-330.
58. Youssef PP, Kraan M, Breedveld F, et al. Quantitative microscopic analysis of inflammation in rheumatoid arthritis synovial membrane samples selected at arthroscopy compared with samples obtained blindly by needle biopsy. Arthritis Rheum 1998;41:663-669.
59. Kraan MC, Reece RJ, Smeets TJ, et al. Comparison of synovial tissues from the knee joints and the small joints of rheumatoid arthritis patients: implications for pathogenesis and evaluation of treatment. Arthritis Rheum 2002;46:2034-2038.
61. Kane D, Veale DJ, Fitzgerald O, Reece R. Survey of arthroscopy performed by rheumatologists. Rheumatology (Oxford) 2002;41:210-215.
62. Moseley JB, O'Malley K, Petersen NJ, et al. A controlled trial of arthroscopic surgery for osteoarthritis of the knee. N Engl J Med 2002;347:81-88.
64. Smith MD, Wetherall M, Darby T, et al. A randomized placebo-controlled trial of arthroscopic lavage versus lavage plus intra-articular corticosteroids in the management of symptomatic osteoarthritis of the knee. Rheumatology (Oxford) 2003;42:1477-1485.
65. Van Oosterhout M, Sont JK, Van Laar JM. Superior effect of arthroscopic lavage compared with needle aspiration

in the treatment of inflammatory arthritis of the knee. Rheumatology (Oxford) 2003;42:102-107.

67. Tanaka N, Sakahashi H, Hirose K, et al. Volume of a wash and the other conditions for maximum therapeutic effect of arthroscopic lavage in rheumatoid knees. Clin Rheumatol 2006;25:65-69.

68. Scire CA, Epis O, Codullo V, et al. Immunohistological assessment of the synovial tissue in small joints in rheumatoid arthritis: validation of a minimally invasive ultrasound-guided synovial biopsy procedure. Arthritis Res Ther 2007;9:R101.

70. Taylor PC. The value of sensitive imaging modalities in rheumatoid arthritis. Arthritis Res Ther 2003;5: 210-213.

REFERENCES

Full references for this chapter can be found on www.expertconsult.com.

Skin in rheumatic disease

Markus Böhm and Thomas A. Luger

32

- The skin is frequently involved in a variety of rheumatic diseases.
- Skin manifestations can be hallmark features in rheumatic diseases, especially in lupus erythematosus, dermatomyositis, and systemic sclerosis.
- Skin changes occurring in rheumatic diseases are said to be specific when characterized by a distinct clinical and dermatohistopathologic picture.
- Non-specific skin manifestations include a diversity of cutaneous changes that also occur in non-related disorders.
- Skin involvement may indicate a different course and prognosis of a rheumatic disease.

INTRODUCTION

Skin changes occur in a variety of systemic rheumatic diseases and are of particular relevance for the dermatologist, as well as the rheumatologist, for several reasons. First, the skin can be the initial site of manifestation in rheumatic disease, thus providing the clinician with important clues to diagnosis and differential diagnosis. Second, in a number of rheumatic diseases skin involvement may serve as an indicator for systemic disease activity. Third, skin manifestation in rheumatic diseases can be associated with a high degree of morbidity and severe impact on quality of life. Finally, awareness and elucidation of the underlying nature of skin manifestations will shed light on the pathogenesis of many rheumatic disorders.

The skin changes as seen in systemic rheumatic diseases are said to be specific when they display highly characteristic and sometimes even pathognomonic features along with a typical histopathology encountered only in a distinct rheumatic disease. On the other hand, cutaneous manifestations can be non-specific and occur in a diversity of rheumatic and non-rheumatic systemic diseases. It is also well established that some skin diseases have an increased incidence in patients with selected systemic rheumatic diseases. These dermatoses are best referred to as *associated skin diseases*. In most cases, however, only a combination of specific and non-specific skin changes, occasionally in the presence of an associated skin disorder, will help to establish the final diagnosis of a rheumatic disease. We have therefore designated these skin changes as "key dermatologic signs" at the beginning of each section.

In this chapter we highlight the skin manifestations of the major systemic connective tissue disorders: systemic lupus erythematosus, dermatomyositis, systemic sclerosis, and Sjögren syndrome (SjS), followed by a heterogeneous group of other systemic rheumatic diseases (rheumatoid arthritis, systemic onset juvenile rheumatoid arthritis, and relapsing polychondritis). It is beyond the scope of this chapter to describe all rheumatic diseases with skin manifestations. Emphasis is on the key dermatologic signs of the previously mentioned diseases rather than on rare variants. To assist understanding, the most common dermatologic terms are explained in Box 32.1. Because of space limitations, it is impossible to discuss in depth the pathogenesis of the presented rheumatic diseases or to describe the clinical pictures of the differential diagnoses. It is therefore apparent that the experienced dermatologist can not only make a meaningful contribution to the correct diagnosis of systemic rheumatic diseases but also deliver the newest and most effective therapy for the treatment of patients with cutaneous involvement of these diseases.

MAJOR SYSTEMIC CONNECTIVE TISSUE DISORDERS

Systemic lupus erythematosus

Key dermatologic signs: photosensitivity; malar dermatitis; discoid rash; other forms of specific cutaneous lupus erythematosus, localized or generalized, involving the epidermis, dermis, or subcutaneous fat of the skin; oral ulcerations.

Dermatologic changes involving the skin, mucous membranes, and hair are a common manifestation of systemic lupus erythematosus (SLE). Experts estimate that 85% of patients with SLE develop such changes during the course of their disease. The classification of the cutaneous LE (CLE) lesions, however, is complex because similar types of skin involvement can occur both in SLE and in patients with non-systemic forms of LE. A widely accepted classification divides LE-specific skin disease into three major clinical subtypes according to their disease activity: acute CLE (ACLE), subacute CLE (SCLE), and chronic cutaneous LE (CCLE) (Box 32.2).[1] These subtypes are further specified according to the extent of their skin involvement (local versus generalized) and the localization of the inflammatory infiltrate in the skin (e.g., LE panniculitis indicating LE-specific infiltration of the adipose tissue). It is important to note that in patients with SLE (as in patients with CLE only), different forms of LE-specific skin lesions can be present simultaneously (e.g., a butterfly rash as a manifestation of localized ACLE plus chilblain LE as a variant of CCLE).

The hallmark skin lesion of ACLE in patients with SLE is malar dermatitis, which is a reddish maculopapular eruption in a characteristic butterfly distribution of the face (Fig. 32.1). In most cases patients recall induction or exacerbation of the rash by exposure to ultraviolet light (UV), indicating photosensitivity as an important diagnostic clue and pathogenetic component. Lesions tend to be transient, lasting from several hours to weeks, and heal without scarring. Occasionally, poikiloderma can result from dyspigmentation. When generalized, ACLE can involve the trunk with accentuation of the UV-exposed areas (Fig. 32.2) but may be localized elsewhere, including the hands, where knuckles are typically spared (Fig. 32.3). A recently recognized life-threatening variant is toxic-epidermal necrolysis (TEN)-like ACLE. This may be regarded as a fulminant form of generalized ACLE in which a massive epidermal injury occurs, possibly due to severe alterations of the dermoepidermal junction and subsequent apoptosis. Another variant is Rowell syndrome, which was originally described as an erythema multiforme–like eruption in patients with disseminated lupus erythematosus (DLE) and positive anti-Ro/La antibodies. However, subsequent reports and our own observations suggest that similar skin lesions can also develop in patients with SLE and SCLE, as well as in the presence or absence of anti-Ro/La antibodies. Oral lesions are a common mucocutaneous manifestation in patients with SLE and are part of the American College of Rheumatology (ACR) criteria. Typically they consist of painful aphthoid lesions and ulcerations, especially on the lips and buccal and palatal mucosa (Fig. 32.4), but may be localized elsewhere in the oral cavity. Some palatal lesions may be asymptomatic.

Patients with clinical features of SCLE usually have circulating anti-Ro and anti-La antibodies and the HLA-B8 and -DR3 haplotype. Two variants have been identified: an annular variant consisting of slightly raised erythemas with central clearing, and a papulosquamous variant consisting of psoriasis-like or eczematous-like lesions, both typically located on UV-exposed skin, including the lateral aspects of the face, the "V" of the neck (often with sparing of the area under the chin), the upper ventral and dorsal part of the trunk (Fig. 32.5), and the dorsolateral aspects of the forearms. SCLE lesions never lead

BOX 32.1 FREQUENTLY USED DERMATOLOGIC TERMS

Macule—a flat localized discoloration of the skin. When the discoloration is red, it is called *erythema*.

Papule/nodule/plaque—a raised, localized, solid skin lesion. When the raised lesion has spread horizontally, it is referred to as a *plaque*.

Vesicle/bulla—a localized, raised lesion of the skin filled with exudate, either serous or hemorrhagic fluid. When more than 0.5 cm in diameter, the vesicle is called a *bulla*.

Pustule—a vesicle filled with pus.

Urtica/wheal—a transient raised skin lesion due to dermal edema. The center of the lesion is pale and the borders are erythematous.

Erosion—a superficial tangential defect of the epidermis.

Ulcer—a substantial defect of the epidermis and deeper layers of the skin (dermis, subcutaneous), inevitably leading to scar formation.

Purpura/petechia—localized intradermal hemorrhage. When less than 3 mm in diameter, it is called *petechia*.

Poikiloderma—a combination of hyperpigmentation, hypopigmentation, telangiectasia, and skin atrophy.

Sclerosis—induration of the skin.

Squama—localized area of abnormal shedding of the corneal layer of the epidermis.

Köbner/pathergy phenomenon—induction of skin lesions by a non-specific trauma such as scratching or venipuncture.

BOX 32.2 CLASSIFICATION OF LUPUS ERYTHEMATOSUS–SPECIFIC SKIN LESIONS

A. Acute cutaneous lupus erythematosus (ACLE)
   1. Localized ACLE
   2. Generalized ACLE
   3. Toxic epidermal necrolysis-like ACLE
B. Subacute cutaneous lupus erythematosus (SCLE)
   1. Annular
   2. Papulosquamous
C. Chronic cutaneous lupus erythematosus (CCLE)
   1. Discoid lupus erythematosus (DLE)
      a. localized
      b. generalized
   2. Hypertrophic/verrucous lupus erythematosus
   3. Lupus erythematosus tumidus
   4. Lupus panniculitis/profundus
   5. Chilblain lupus erythematosus
   6. DLE–lichen planus overlap

Modified from Sontheimer RD. Skin manifestations of systemic autoimmune connective tissue disease: diagnostics and therapeutics. Best Pract Res Clin Rheumatol 2004;18:429-462.

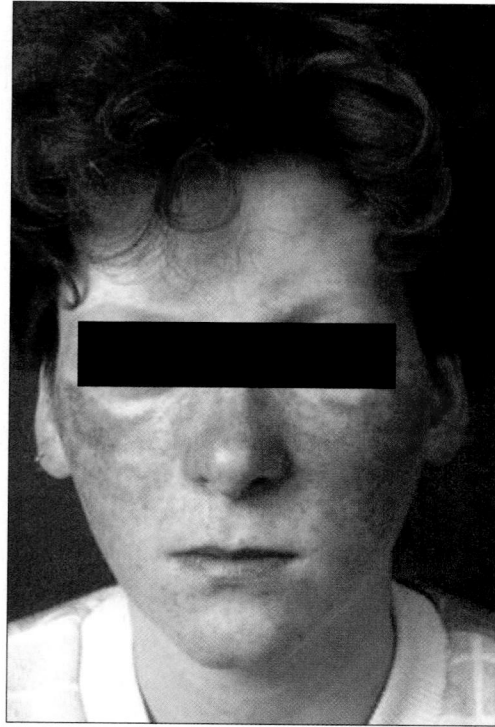

Fig. 32.1 Malar (butterfly) rash in young woman with systemic lupus erythematosus.

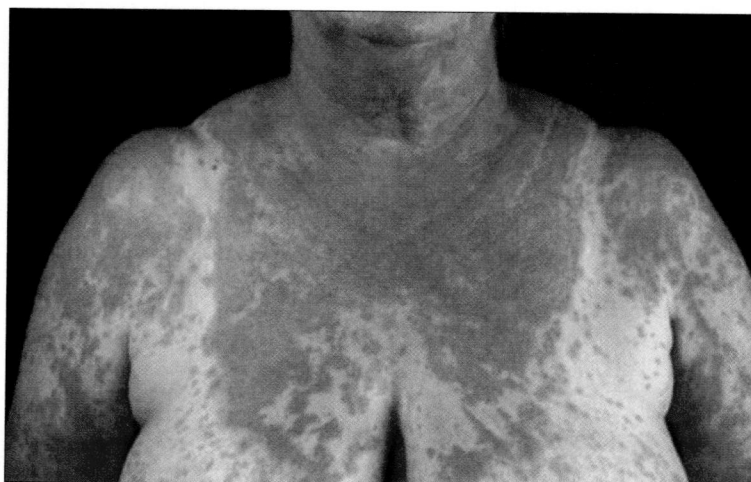

Fig. 32.2 Generalized acute cutaneous lupus erythematosus. Note accentuation of the lesions in the ultraviolet light-exposed area.

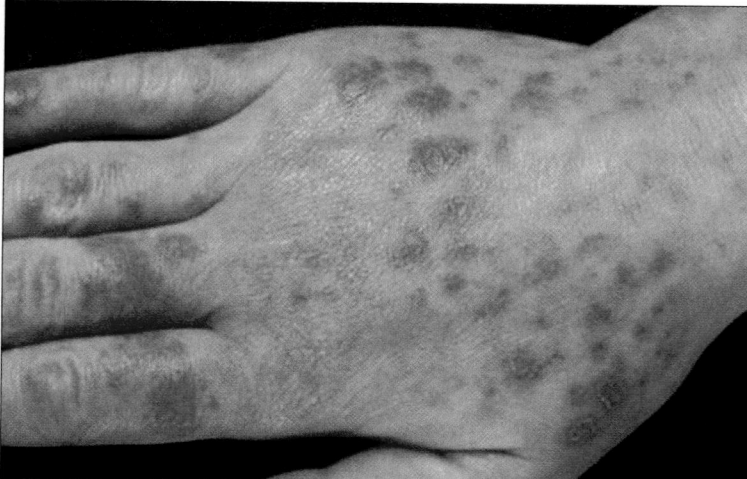

Fig. 32.3 Generalized acute cutaneous lupus erythematosus. Note typical distribution with sparing of the knuckles.

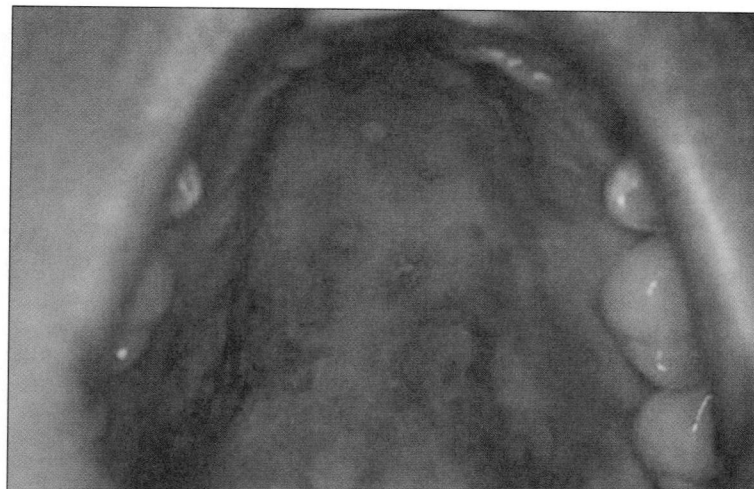

Fig. 32.4 Oral aphthoid lesions and ulcerations of the palatal mucosa in a patient with systemic lupus erythematosus.

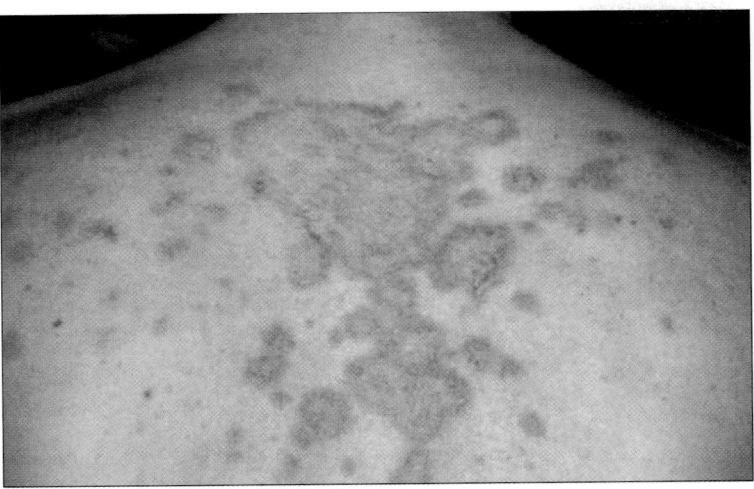

Fig. 32.5 Subacute lupus erythematosus (annular subtype). Note characteristic distribution in the ultraviolet light-exposed area.

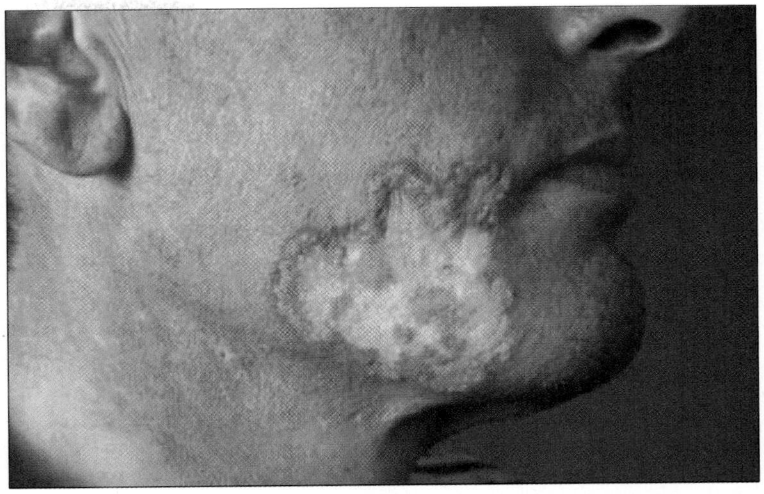

Fig. 32.6 Classic discoid lupus erythematosus of the face. Note central scarring and erythematous hyperkeratotic borders.

to scarring but hypopigmentation or depigmentation is common, resulting in vitiligo-like leukoderma. A substantial proportion of patients with SCLE exhibit mild systemic symptoms, especially arthralgias and musculoskeletal complaints. Data from several studies further indicate that the percentage of patients with SCLE fulfilling four or more ACR criteria for SLE ranges from 30% to 62%.

The prototypical skin lesion of the classic form of CCLE, also known as discoid CLE, is an erythematous discoid plaque that becomes hyperkeratotic and eventually leads to atrophy and scarring (Fig. 32.6). Dyspigmentation, including hypopigmentation and hyperpigmentation, is common. Discoid lesions have a predilection for the face, ears, and neck but may be widespread, without a clear-cut relation to UV exposure. Disfigurement can be a serious problem, especially in patients with facial involvement. Mucosal membranes including the lips, mucosal surfaces of the mouth, nasal membranes, conjunctivae, and genital mucosa may also be involved with characteristic discoid lesions resembling leukoplakia. Although DLE is primarily considered a form of cutaneous LE without systemic involvement, patients with SLE may have classic DLE lesions. Long-term follow-up of patients with DLE is also necessary because 5% to 10% will develop SLE in the course of their disease, on the basis of retrospective analysis from a number of studies.

As outlined in Box 32.2, several other subtypes of CCLE can occur in patients with SLE and non-systemic LE. In hypertrophic/verrucous CCLE, epidermal hyperkeratosis is prominent, resulting in lesions with a thick scaling. LE tumidus describes the presence of photosensitive erythematous, sometimes urticarial plaques and nodules without epidermal hyperkeratosis or follicular plugging. Lesions are usually located on the face, upper trunk, and extremities. The majority of patients with LE tumidus do not have antinuclear antibodies, and diagnosis relies mainly on the clinical and histomorphologic picture. Only rarely will patients with LE tumidus develop SLE.[2] LE panniculitis is an intense inflammation of the adipose tissue of the skin resulting in indurated plaques and lipotrophy. Lesions are commonly seen on the face, proximal parts of the extremities, upper trunk, and buttocks and can be disfiguring. When the overlying dermis and epidermis are involved in LE panniculitis, this is called *LE profundus*. As shown by a retrospective study of 40 patients with this CCLE variant, few patients (10%) fulfill the ACR criteria for SLE.[3] An often unrecognized variant of CCLE is chilblain LE, which denotes pernio-like skin lesions (i.e., red to violaceous plaques located on the distal parts of the extremities—fingertips, toes, and occasionally other parts of the body), which are typically induced and aggravated by cold exposure (Fig. 32.7). These patients should be carefully monitored because up to 24% of them will develop SLE.[4]

The exact pathogenesis of the various LE-specific skin manifestations is complex and incompletely understood. Several lines of evidence suggest that autoantibodies detected in patients with LE play an important role in the development of the LE-specific skin lesions.

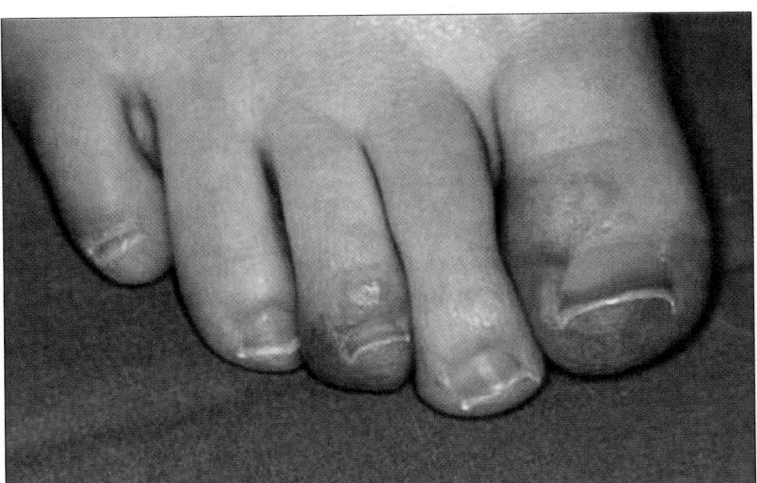

Fig. 32.7 Chilblain lupus erythematosus of the toes.

Accordingly, it is well known that pregnant women with circulating anti-Ro antibodies may deliver babies with SCLE-like lesions (neonatal LE) that are indistinguishable from the skin lesions seen in adults.[5] Data from *in vitro* studies further demonstrate that UVB irradiation of human keratinocytes is capable of translocating autoantigens such as Ro to the plasma membrane and to apoptotic blebs, possibly promoting an immune response and the occurrence of cutaneous LE lesions by sun exposure.[6] Another pathogenetic factor closely related to the occurrence of LE skin lesions is complement C1q. Complete deficiency of C1q is a major risk factor for the development of SLE, and most individuals with homozygous congenital deficiency of C1q develop early-onset SLE with cutaneous LE lesions.[7] Accordingly, deficiency of C1q may result in altered clearance of autoantigens and immune complexes associated with UVB-exposed or cytokine-stimulated epidermal keratinocytes. There is also recent evidence for a role of tumor necrosis factor-α (TNF-α) in the pathogenesis of LE. Accordingly, the use of anti–TNF-α strategies for the treatment of rheumatoid arthritis in several instances has led to the occurrence of autoantibodies, lupus-like syndrome, and in rare cases even to the development of LE or dermatomyositis.[8,9]

Histopathologic examination is a cornerstone in the correct diagnosis of the skin lesions encountered in patients with LE. However, it should be noted that proper classification of the CLE lesions relies substantially on the overall clinical picture and laboratory analysis because, especially in acute forms of cutaneous involvement, LE-specific histologic changes can be subtle. ACLE lesions show vacuolar degeneration of the dermoepidermal junction, dead keratinocytes

("Civatte bodies") and a sparse lymphohistiocytic infiltrate of the upper dermis. Dermal blood vessels are dilated with extravasation of erythrocytes. In SCLE, these findings are often associated with epidermal atrophy. The lymphohistiocytic infiltrate is located in the upper dermis with an interface and perivascular pattern. In classic DLE lesions, there is additional epidermal hyperkeratosis and thickening of the dermoepidermal and follicular basement membranes. The lymphohistiocytic infiltrate is often prominent, involving hair follicles, which may also show hyperkeratotic plugging. Mucin may be deposited in the dermis. Deeper forms of CCLE are characterized by a lymphohistiocytic infiltrate situated in the lower dermis, often with mucin deposits (LE tumidus), whereas in lupus panniculitis, the infiltrate is located primarily in the subcutaneous fat tissue.

The differential diagnosis of ACLE lesions includes erythema solare (sunburn), photoallergic and phototoxic drug eruptions, dermatomyositis, atopic eczema, seborrheic dermatitis, contact eczema, and rosacea. SCLE lesions have to be distinguished from photoallergic and phototoxic drug eruptions, as well as other forms of annular erythemas (erythema annulare centrifugum, erythema gyratum repens, granuloma annulare, eczema, psoriasis, and tinea).

In addition to the previously described LE-specific skin lesions, there is a plethora of non-specific skin signs and associated skin diseases that can be present in patients with SLE. These skin signs include harmless vascular changes such as nailfold abnormalities (large and tortuous capillaries together with areas of avascularity) but also more serious complications such as vasculitis (leukocytoclastic vasculitis, urticarial vasculitis, nodular vasculitis) and other forms of vasculopathy (atrophie blanche, livedo reticularis, Degos disease-like lesions, ulcerations, and thromboses), the latter developing especially in patients with antiphospholipid syndrome. Non-scarring alopecia ("lupus hair") may be seen in patients with SLE, whereas scarring alopecia typically occurs in patients with DLE involving the scalp. Raynaud phenomenon, calcinosis cutis, scleroderma-like changes, and rheumatoid nodules may indicate the presence of an overlap syndrome.

Dermatomyositis

Key dermatologic signs: heliotrope rash, Gottron papules, Gottron sign, poikiloderma atrophicans vasculare, periungual telangiectasia, dystrophic cuticles, calcinosis cutis.

Involvement of the skin is essential to the diagnosis of dermatomyositis (DM) because characteristic cutaneous lesions belong to the diagnostic criteria of DM, according to Bohan and Peter.[10] Importantly, skin manifestations precede the clinical symptoms of muscle weakness, electromyopathic abnormalities, or increased levels of creatine phosphokinase in 30% of patients with DM, and in 10% to 20% of all patients with DM, specific skin changes may occur for longer than 6 months without systemic involvement. This group of patients has been referred to as *DM sine myositis* (or *amyopathic DM*). Although a variety of skin manifestations occur in DM, none of the skin signs allow discrimination between idiopathic DM and the paraneoplastic form.

One highly specific skin sign that can be regarded as the cutaneous hallmark feature of DM is the heliotrope rash (Fig. 32.8). This is an often pruritic, sometimes burning, violaceous, confluent erythema resembling the color of the heliotrope, a red/purple-colored flower tracking the course of the sun. The heliotrope rash of DM has a characteristic distribution, involving especially the periorbital area. Other sites of predilection are the malar area of the face, the posterior neck and shoulders (referred to as the "shawl sign"), and the scalp. DM often also affects the extensor surfaces of the extremities, knuckles and dorsal aspects of the interphalangeal joints, and periungual area of the fingers in a symmetric fashion (Fig. 32.9). The characteristic violaceous color and the periorbital distribution of the heliotrope rash distinguish DM from the butterfly rash (malar rash) in patients with ACLE. It is also important to recognize that the skin lesions of DM when affecting the fingers tend to be located over the joints and not on the interphalangeal areas, as in patients with generalized ACLE (compare Figs. 32.3 and 32.9).

Depending on the intensity of inflammation, the violaceous macules of DM may evolve into plaques, often covered with a fine silvery scale, especially on the knees and elbows. When such lesions occur over the

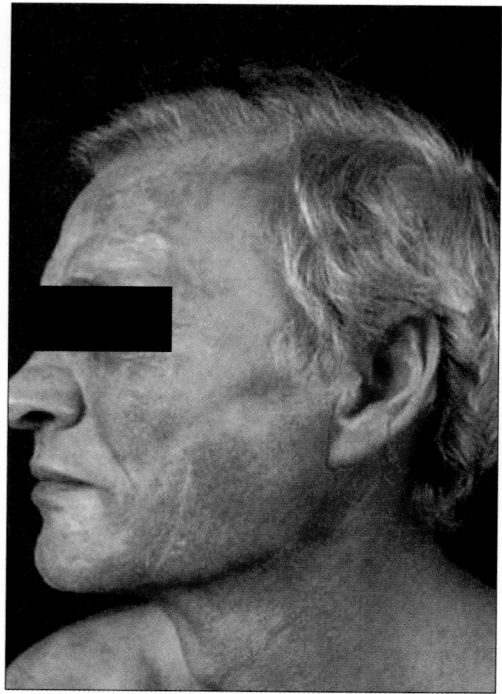

Fig. 32.8 Heliotrope rash of the face in a man with dermatomyositis.

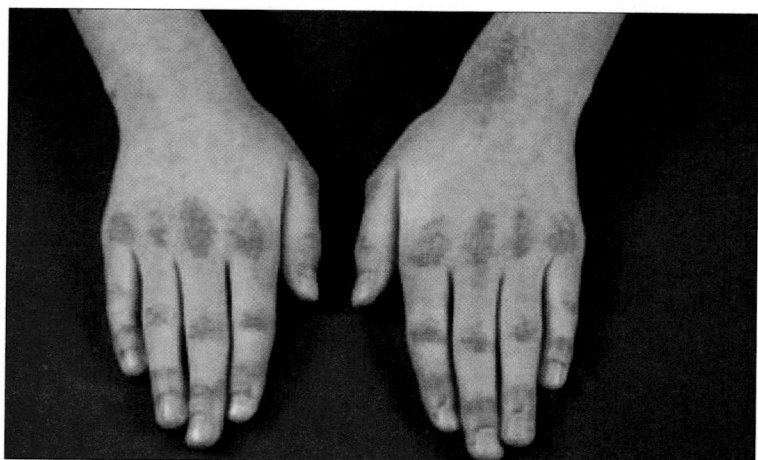

Fig. 32.9 Gottron papules of dermatomyositis on the fingers. Note accentuation over the knuckles.

knuckles, in interphalangeal joints, and in the periungual area, they are known as *Gottron papules* (see Fig. 32.9). Violaceous macules developing over the knuckles and the elbows and/or knees have been referred to as the *Gottron sign* (Fig. 32.10). Intensely inflamed skin lesions of DM may develop into erosions, subepidermal blisters, and ulcers (Fig. 32.11), the latter having to be distinguished from hemorrhagic necrotizing vasculitis, a non-specific sign of DM. Furthermore, the term *poikiloderma atrophicans vasculare* has been coined to describe patients with DM and a combination of violaceous erythema, hyperpigmentation, hypopigmentation, telangiectasia, and atrophy.

In addition to these specific skin signs, many patients with DM show prominent nailfold telangiectasias (Fig. 32.12) and dystrophic ("ragged") cuticles. Moreover, gingival telangiectases have recently been identified as a sign of juvenile DM. Other less frequently encountered cutaneous manifestations of DM include panniculitis leading to lipotrophy, papular and pustular lesions, and centripetal flagellate erythema. The term *mechanic's hand* (Fig. 32.13) has been applied to the occurrence of chronic eczematous skin lesions located on the fingers of patients with myositis.[11] A high proportion of patients with mechanic's hands turned out to have the so-called *antisynthetase syndrome*

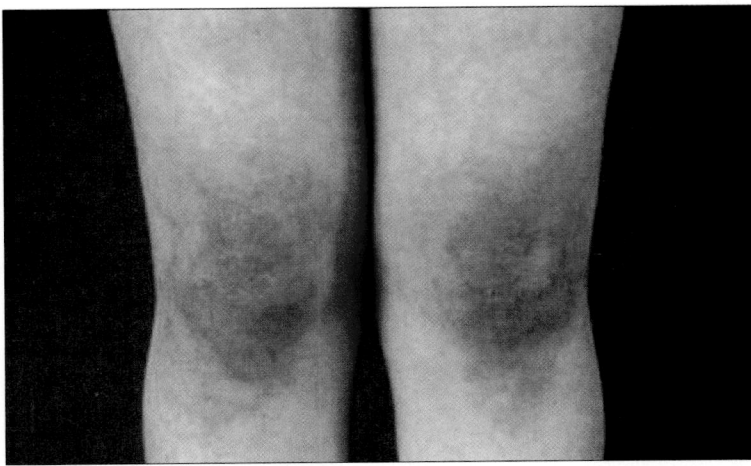

Fig. 32.10 Violaceous plaques on the knees in a patient with dermatomyositis. (Gottron sign).

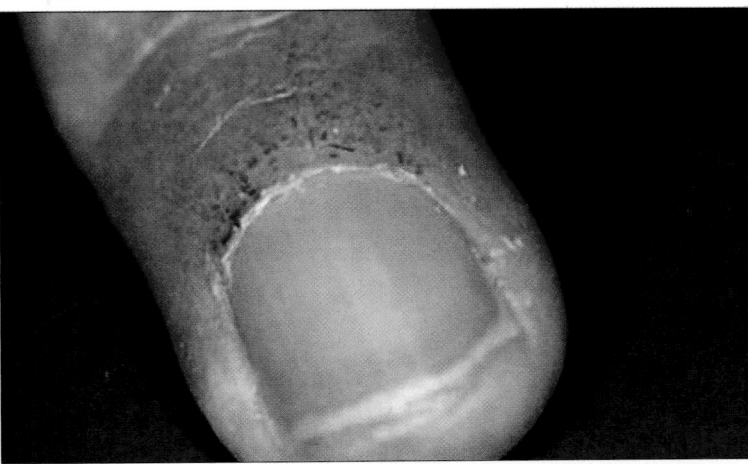

Fig. 32.12 Enlarged nailfold capillaries in a patient with dermatomyositis.

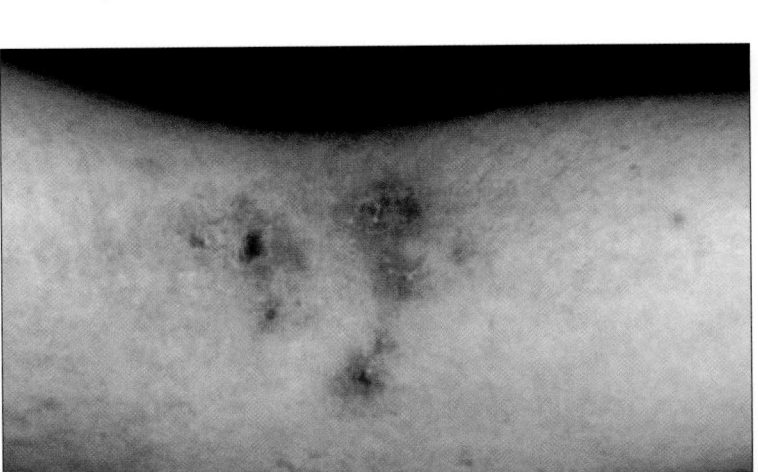

Fig. 32.11 Skin ulcerations in a young female with paraneoplastic dermatomyositis.

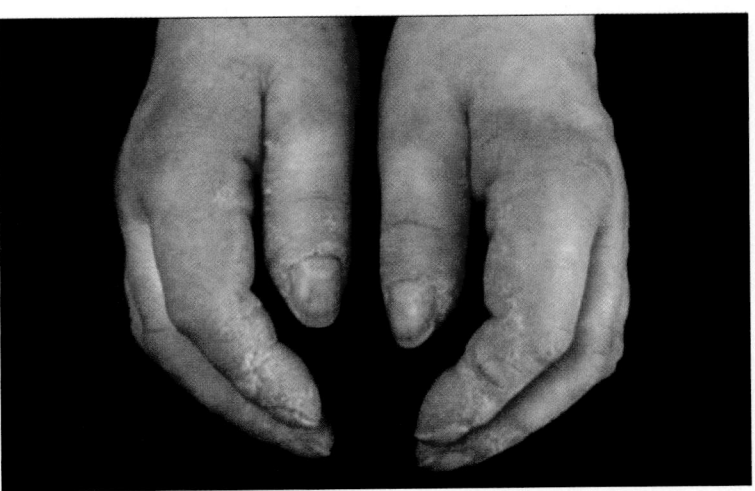

Fig. 32.13 Mechanic's hands in a woman with dermatomyositis-scleroderma overlap syndrome.

(an overlap syndrome consisting of antisynthetase antibodies, erosive polyarthritis, interstitial lung disease, fever, Raynaud phenomenon, and inflammatory myositis). Another subset has anti-PM-SCL antibodies, indicating a polymyositis-scleroderma overlap syndrome. However, recent observations have questioned the specific association of the previously mentioned antibodies with mechanic's hands, suggesting that these skin manifestations may also occur in related systemic connective tissue disorders.

Calcinosis cutis can be an extremely painful and devastating skin manifestation of DM. It occurs most often at sites of friction and trauma such as on the elbows, trochanters, knees, and fingers and presents as hard, irregular nodules that eventually drain chalky material to the skin surface. It is more prevalent in juvenile DM than in the adult form. Of note, calcinosis is also a key feature of the *C*alcinosis, *R*aynaud phenomenon, *E*sophageal hypomotility, *S*clerodactyly, *T*elangiectasia (CREST) syndrome and can be a manifestation of overlap syndromes.

The pathogenesis of DM is poorly understood. The intense B-cell infiltrate together with CD4⁺ T cells in the muscle perivascular areas strongly suggests an abnormal immune response. Antinuclear antibodies are frequently found in DM, and approximately 20% of the patients have anti–Mi-2 antibodies. In addition, the occurrence of several antisynthetase autoantibodies has been described. These are highly specific for DM and polymyositis but do not occur in other connective tissue diseases. However, the precise role of these antibodies in eliciting the characteristic skin manifestations of DM is unknown.

Histopathologic examination of a heliotrope erythema typically reveals an interface dermatitis with a sparse lymphocytic infiltrate,

epidermal atrophy, vacuolar alteration of the basal keratinocytes, basement membrane degeneration, and interstitial mucin deposition. More inflamed lesions (i.e., Gottron papules) also show lichenoid infiltrate and acanthosis of the epidermis. Immunohistologic studies have demonstrated that the infiltrate in skin and muscle lesions of patients with DM consists mainly of CD8⁺ lymphocytes, supporting the concept of a lymphocyte-mediated disease in the pathogenesis of DM.

The differential diagnosis of DM includes SLE, psoriasis, atopic dermatitis, photoallergic and phototoxic drug eruption, contact dermatitis, cutaneous T cell lymphoma, systemic sclerosis, and trichinosis.

Systemic sclerosis

Key dermatologic signs: Raynaud phenomenon, symmetric cutaneous sclerosis, finger swelling, sclerodactyly, digital pits and ulcers, dilated/atrophic nailfold capillaries, calcinosis cutis, hyperpigmentation.

The term *sclerosis* describes hardening or induration due to excessive deposition of interstitial collagen leading to tissue fibrosis. By definition, systemic sclerosis (SSC) is a multisystem disorder involving the skin and internal organs. However, it should be noted that sclerosis of the skin ("scleroderma") is a common reaction pattern of several fibrotic skin disorders, some of which are benign and only localized to the skin, whereas others are systemic conditions. Thus, in the context of the clinical pattern, internal organ abnormalities, and laboratory tests, the diagnosis of systemic sclerosis should always exclude these differential diagnoses (see later).

There is striking heterogeneity within the clinical spectrum of cutaneous thickening in patients with SSC, and subtypes with distinct

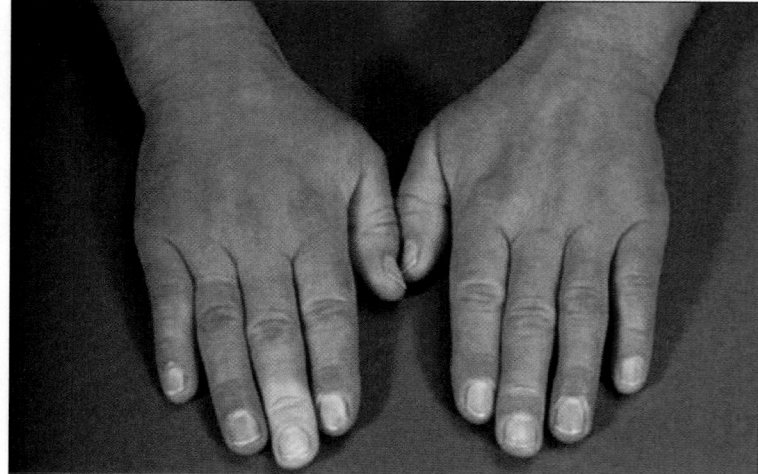

Fig. 32.14 Raynaud's phenomenon.

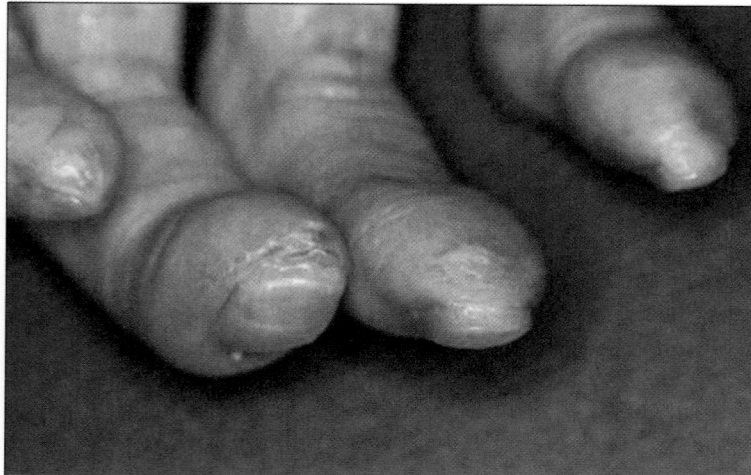

Fig. 32.16 Digital pits of the fingertips.

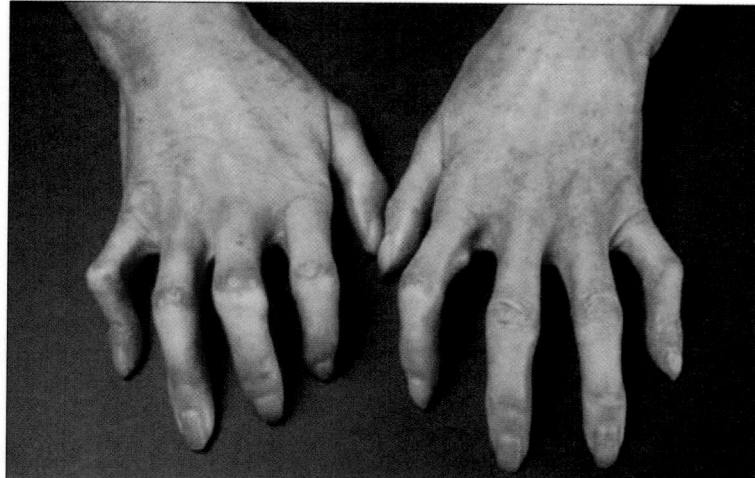

Fig. 32.15 Sclerodactyly in a patient with systemic sclerosis.

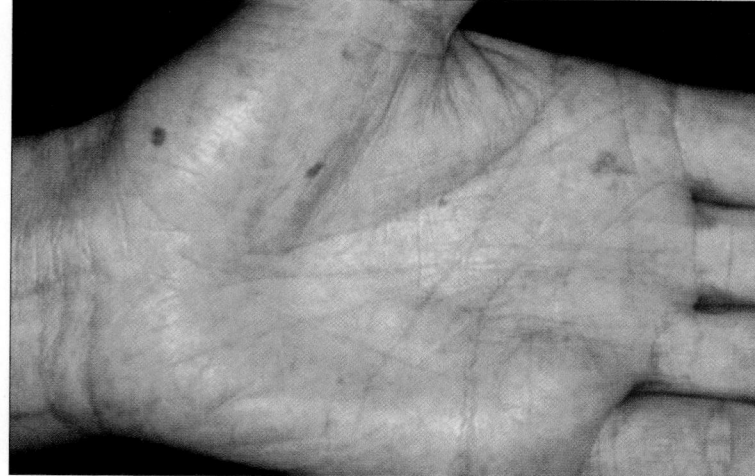

Fig. 32.17 Telangiectatic mats in a patient with systemic sclerosis.

clinical and prognostic features have been delineated. In patients with diffuse SSC, skin thickening involves the trunk and proximal portions of the extremities, whereas in patients with limited SSC, the skin induration is confined to the face and distal portions of the extremities. However, in many cases overlaps do exist between these two widely accepted clinical forms of SSC. A distinct form of limited SSC with induration of the fingers ("sclerodactyly") is the CREST syndrome. These patients typically have detectable anticentromere antibodies and show a generally favorable prognosis compared with patients with diffuse SSC. Finally, an unusual variant called *scleroderma sine scleroderma*, in which affected patients have evidence of SSC due to SSC-related antibodies and internal organ involvement but no skin involvement, has been described. The prognosis of these patients is similar to those with limited SSC.

Often years before the onset of skin induration, patients with SSC experience Raynaud phenomenon (Fig. 32.14). Although a non-specific sign that is present in other connective tissue diseases and closely related overlap syndromes, Raynaud phenomenon is present in 90% to 99% of patients with diffuse or limited SSC. When cutaneous involvement proceeds, there is often an edematous phase of the affected sites, especially on the fingers ("puffy fingers"). Similar changes may also be seen on the forearms, legs, feet, face, and trunk. This is followed by gradual thickening of the skin, in which the initial inflammation is replaced by interstitial fibrosis due to abnormal collagen metabolism (indurative phase), leading to sclerodactyly and dermatopathic contractures (Fig. 32.15). Impaired acral blood flow in sclerodactyly may lead to digital pits and ulcers (Fig. 32.16). A recent study further revealed that patients with SSC and digital ulcers developed internal organ involvement 2 to 3 years earlier than those without digital ulcers.[12]

Among the other common cutaneous key signs of SSC are telangiectasias, which also form a diagnostic cornerstone in patients with CREST syndrome. The telangiectasias seen in patients with SSC are often located on the face, including the lips, but may also be detected on the neck, volar aspects of the fingers, and palms and tend to be matted (Fig. 32.17). Dilated nailfold capillaries, often alternating with areas of capillary loss, can be easily detected using a dermatoscope. Calcinosis is another key feature of the CREST syndrome and tends to be located on the extremities, especially at the fingertips and over joints (Fig. 32.18).

A relatively unappreciated skin sign of SSC is skin hyperpigmentation. This mostly occurs as a diffuse brownish discoloration resembling a suntan and is usually accentuated in areas of friction and pressure (Fig. 32.19). Variants of skin discoloration in patients with diffuse SSC do occur and include "salt and pepper," which describes a combination of hyperpigmentation and hypopigmentation often found on the upper trunk (see Fig. 32.19).

The pathogenesis of SSC is incompletely understood. Many investigators believe that endothelial cell damage is crucial in initiating an inflammatory response, which subsequently leads to the fibrotic stage of the disease.[13] Repetitive vascular injury (as clinically exemplified by Raynaud phenomenon in patients with SSC) may lead to tissue hypoxia, which triggers the induction of several proinflammatory cytokines, including transforming growth factor-β_1 (TGF-β_1).[14] TGF-β_1 plays a central role in collagen metabolism because it is a key profibrotic cytokine that upregulates collagen synthesis in dermal fibroblasts at the transcriptional and non-transcriptional levels and also leads to induction of other mediators of fibrosis, especially connective tissue growth factor.[15] Recent *ex vivo* studies on dermal fibroblasts established from

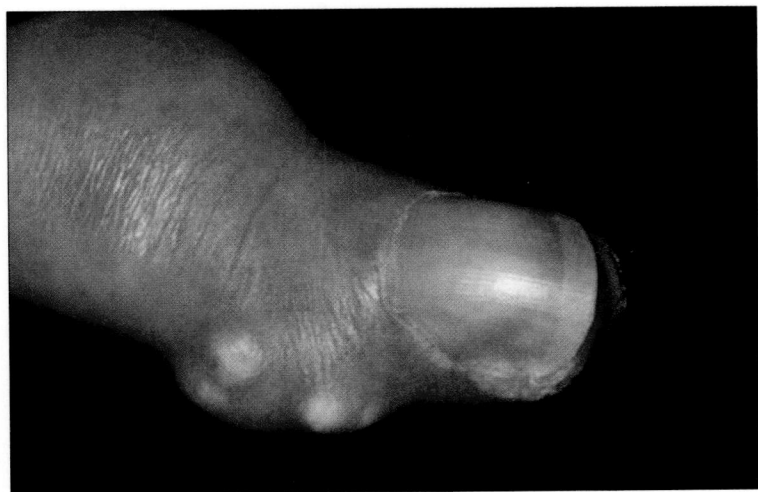

Fig. 32.18 Calcinosis cutis.

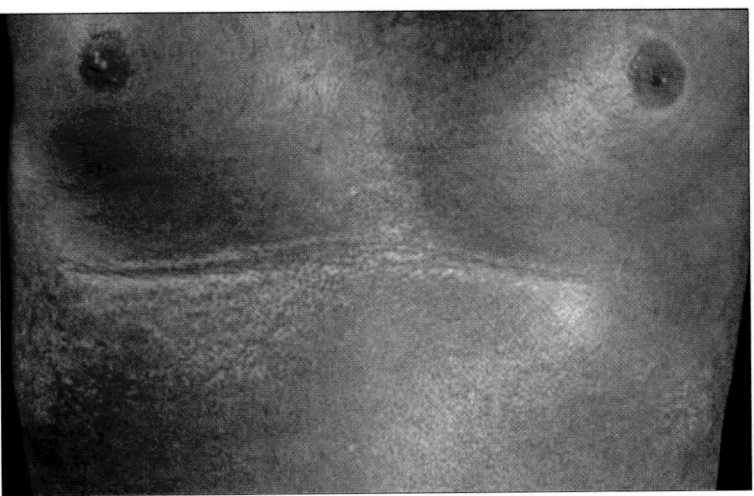

Fig. 32.19 Diffuse hyperpigmentation of the skin in a patient with systemic sclerosis. Note also depigmentation in the submammary region.

patients with SSC, as well as *in situ* studies on lesional skin of SSC patients, have indicated alterations in regular TGF-β_1 function and/or TGF-β_1–induced signaling of the so-called *smad signal molecules*.[16,17] Other cytokines such as endothelin-1 and hepatocyte growth factors appear to be involved in the development of diffuse hyperpigmentation as well as vascular alterations in patients with SSC. Recent observations have also drawn attention to the role of several autoantibodies in the pathogenesis of SSC. For example, it was recently shown that antifibroblast antibodies, which are detectable in 46% of affected patients, are internalized into dermal fibroblasts and induce a proadhesive and proinflammatory cellular phenotype.[18,19] Moreover, the presence of autoantibodies against platelet-derived growth factor receptor was detected in SSC patients. They induced tyrosine phosphorylation, reactive oxidative stress, and collagen type I gene expression.[20] Other scientists, however, could not find such antibodies in patients with SSC.[21] Histopathologic examination of sclerotic skin from patients with SSC demonstrates excessive collagen deposits within the dermis and subcutaneous tissue, often entrapping the adnexal structures, as the predominant finding. In earlier inflammatory phases (edematous phase), a dense lymphocytic infiltrate may be seen at the interface of the deep dermis and adipose tissue.

The differential diagnosis of SSC includes scleromyxedema; eosinophilic fasciitis (Shulman syndrome); scleredema adultorum and diabeticorum; diabetic thick skin; sclerosing chronic graft-versus-host disease; sclerosing forms of porphyria; *P*olyneuropathy, *O*rganomegaly, *E*ndocrinopathy, *M* component, and *S*kin changes (POEMS) syndrome; nephrogenic fibrosing dermopathy; eosinophilia myalgia syndrome; toxic oil syndrome; carcinoid syndrome; pansclerotic localized scleroderma (morphea); exposure to bleomycin; aromatic chlorinated hydrocarbons or vinyl chloride; phenylketonuria; various progeria syndromes; and reflex sympathetic dystrophy.

Sjögren syndrome (Mikulicz disease, sicca syndrome)

Key dermatologic signs: xerostomia, xerosis cutis, angular stomatitis (perlèche), various forms of cutaneous vasculitis, annular erythema.

Mucocutaneous symptoms are usually the first clinical presentation of Sjögren syndrome (SjS), a systemic autoimmune disorder primarily affecting the secretory glands. Although a non-specific sign, dryness (xerosis) of the mucous membranes in context with the other diagnostic criteria is a key component for establishing the diagnosis of this multisystem disease. Xerosis can involve not only the mouth (xerostomia) and the eyes, leading to keratoconjunctivitis sicca, but also the vagina. Regarding the mouth, patients typically complain of dryness, soreness, and burning sensations. Vaginal xerosis can likewise result in dryness, burning, and dyspareunia, but patients frequently do not report these unless asked about them specifically. Owing to diminished salivary production, angular stomatitis (perlèche) of the mouth with *Candida* infection is common. Although dental and gingival problems

are said to be more frequent in patients with SjS, a recent study did not indicate an increased risk for caries and gingivitis, probably because of increased awareness and dental care of the affected patients.[22]

The pathogenesis of the mucocutaneous changes in patients with SjS is incompletely understood. It is well known that patients have positive anti-SSA (Ro) (30% to 95%) and anti-SSB (La) (15% to 60%) antibodies, but their precise role in the pathogenesis of the disease remains unknown. A genetic disposition is suggested by the increased prevalence of HLA-B8, -DR3, -DQ2, and -DRw52a haplotypes, some of which also occur in other systemic connective tissue disorders.[23] As demonstrated by the histopathologic picture of specimens from minor salivary glands, the interaction between lymphocytes and salivary gland epithelia appears to be central in the pathogenesis of SjS. Recent studies focused on the underlying mechanism of "epithelitis," which could be due to aberrant expression of molecules crucial for lymphocyte recruitment and activation, thereby leading to increased apoptosis of salivary gland epithelia in patients with SjS.[24] For example, increased levels of several co-stimulatory molecules including CD40, CD40 ligand (CD154), and B7 have also been noted in salivary gland biopsies of affected patients. The infiltrating lymphocytes showed elevated levels of the apoptotic regulators bcl-2 and bcl-x, which may favor increased survival of the cells and eventually development of marginal B cell lymphoma in the salivary glands.[25] As in other connective tissue diseases, there is accumulating evidence that various neuroendocrine alterations (e.g., a blunted hypothalamic-pituitary-adrenal (HPA) axis, lack of estrogens, or an enrichment of the exocrine glands with distinct neuromediators) exist in patients with SjS.[26]

In addition to the aforementioned key signs in the mucous membranes, several *bona fide* skin manifestations are frequently observed in patients with SjS. All of them are again non-specific. Xerosis cutis is found in 50% of patients, but the underlying pathomechanism remains obscure. It may lead to generalized pruritus. In the authors' experience, various forms of non-cutaneous vasculitis, most likely due to an immune complex mechanism, are frequently encountered in patients with SjS. They include palpable and non-palpable purpura on the legs and buttocks (Fig. 32.20). This form of cutaneous vasculitis is characteristically induced or aggravated by physical exertion. Other forms of cutaneous vasculitis include lymphocytic vasculitis and urticarial vasculitis (either hypocomplementemic or, less commonly, normocomplementemic). By definition, urticarial lesions of urticarial vasculitis last longer than 48 hours (in contrast to common urticaria) and often have a purpuric component. Patients frequently complain of burning and painful sensations. Lesions often heal with hyperpigmentation. Histologically, the lesions of lymphocytic vasculitis display a mononuclear cell infiltration with disruption of the architecture of the small blood vessels, whereas those of leukocytoclastic vasculitis, including urticarial lesions, show the expected well-described changes.

An unusual skin manifestation of SjS was originally described in Japanese children and has been coined annular erythema of SjS. It

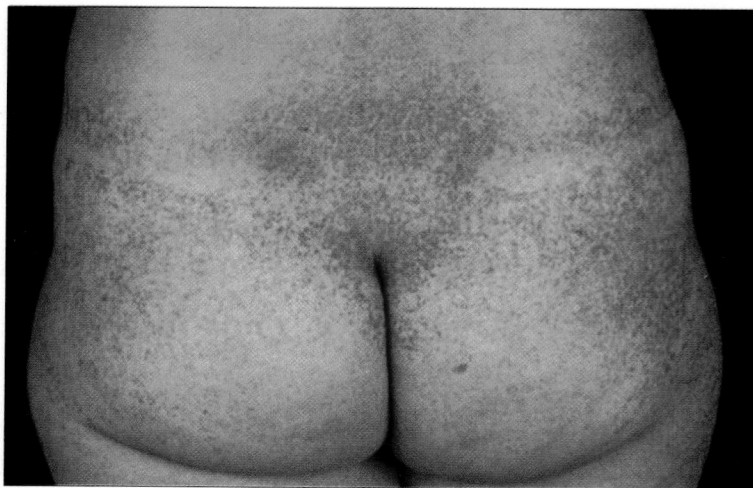

Fig. 32.20 Palpable and non-palpable purpura in patient with Sjögren's syndrome.

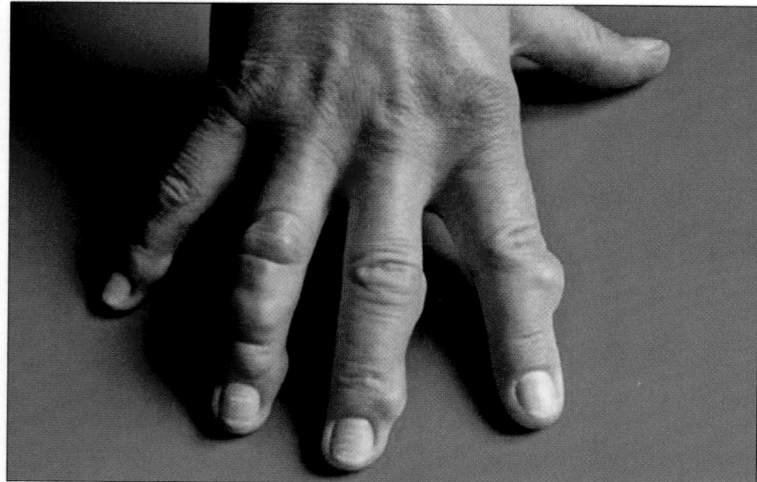

Fig. 32.21 Classic rheumatoid nodules in a patient with rheumatoid arthritis.

appears to be highly associated with the presence of anti-Ro antibodies. Clinically and histologically, these lesions may be indistinguishable from annular SCLE. Recent observations indicate that identical lesions can also occur in white individuals.

Regarding other cutaneous manifestations, it is important to note that SjS can be not only primary but also secondary and therefore associated with a number of other diseases including LE, DM, SSC, rheumatoid arthritis, primary biliary cirrhosis, fibromyalgia, and others. The specific skin signs of these associated disorders must therefore be distinguished from the *bona fide* skin manifestations of SjS.

OTHER SYSTEMIC RHEUMATIC DISEASES

Rheumatoid arthritis

Key dermatologic signs: rheumatoid nodules, accelerated rheumatoid nodulosis, rheumatoid neutrophilic dermatosis, rheumatoid vasculitis, pyoderma gangrenosum, and granulomatous dermatitis.

The characteristic clinical features of rheumatoid arthritis (RA) are frequently associated with skin manifestations, which may not only serve as helpful diagnostic clues but also indicate the severity of the disease. Rheumatoid nodules, accelerated rheumatoid nodulosis, rheumatoid neutrophilic dermatosis, and rheumatoid vasculitis are regarded as RA-specific skin manifestations.

Classic rheumatoid nodules are present in about 25% of patients with RA and are more frequent in the white male population.[27] Most patients with rheumatoid nodules are rheumatoid factor (RF) positive. In seronegative RA, nodular lesions mostly turned out to be granuloma annulare or other palisading granulomas. Genetic predisposition seems to play a role because patients with the HLA-DR4 haplotype and those with heterozygosity for HLA-DRB1 alleles are at high risk for nodular disease, as well as severe RA prognosis.[28] Rheumatoid nodules measuring from a few millimeters up to several centimeters generally develop as subcutaneous, firm, and painless lesions. Usually they occur on periarticular locations over extensor surfaces (Fig. 32.21), but they may appear in any location including lung, heart, and muscle.

The pathogenesis of rheumatoid nodules is not well defined. They may be caused by minor trauma of small vessels that results in immune complex aggregation and focal vasculitis. Furthermore, proinflammatory cytokines such as interleukin (IL)-1 have been implicated in nodule development. Recent evidence indicates that a given cytokine environment triggers the formation of nodules consisting of Th1 granulomas.[29] Complications that sometimes may occur include infection, ulceration, gangrene, bursitis, and synovial rupture.

The differential diagnosis of rheumatoid nodules includes chronic gouty tophi, rheumatic fever nodules, subcutaneous nodules found in SLE, nodular or keloidal scleroderma, and nodules seen in necrobiosis lipoidica and granuloma annulare. In addition, tumoral calcinosis, fibromas, xanthomas, subcutaneous sarcoidosis, metastatic tumors,

> **BOX 32.3 SKIN MANIFESTATIONS OF RHEUMATOID VASCULITIS**
>
> Petechiae or purpura
> Digital infarcts
> Nailfold telangiectasias and infarctions
> Gangrene
> Non-specific maculopapular or nodular erythema
> Hemorrhagic blisters
> Livedo reticularis
> Erythema elevatum et diutinum
> Atrophie blanche
> Allergic venulitis
> Necrotizing granulomatous vasculitis
> Urticaria vasculitis

amyloidosis, ganglion cysts, foreign body granulomas, basal cell carcinomas, epidermoid cysts, and synovial cysts should be considered.

The characteristic symptomatic complex of arthritis, leukopenia, and splenomegaly, which develops in 1% of RA patients, is known as Felty syndrome. Rheumatoid nodules (76%), hyperpigmentation, and therapy-resistant leg ulcers (22%) may also occur.[30] However, cutaneous hyperpigmentation and leg ulceration may be multifactorial and often related to underlying chronic venous insufficiency. Importantly, Felty syndrome is associated with an increased risk of cutaneous and systemic infections that may be difficult to treat and be the cause of sepsis. Differential diagnosis includes SLE, drug-induced leukopenia, viral infection, amyloidosis, leukemia, lymphoma, subacute bacterial endocarditis, aplastic anemia, splenic abscess, hemolytic anemia, tuberculosis, and SjS. In addition, cutaneous ulcerations and hyperpigmentation may also be caused by systemic treatment with methotrexate.

Accelerated rheumatoid nodulosis was initially reported in patients receiving methotrexate (MTX) therapy for RA or juvenile rheumatoid arthritis.[31] It is characterized by the development of painful nodules mainly on the hands of RA patients being treated with MTX; it has not been found to be associated with other immunosuppressive drugs such as azathioprine. RA patients treated with hydroxychloroquine, D-penicillamine, colchicine, and sulfasalazine were found to be protected against the development of MTX-induced accelerated rheumatoid nodulosis. Interestingly, the occurrence of similar nodules has been observed during MTX therapy of a patient with psoriatic arthritis. Recently, accelerated rheumatoid nodulosis also has been described in patients receiving etanercept.[32]

Rheumatoid vasculitis is a late complication of rheumatoid arthritis that may involve the skin as well as other organs and may affect vessels of any size. Accordingly, rheumatoid vasculitis can result in a variety of cutaneous skin signs (Box 32.3). It occurs in seropositive and mainly male RA patients with long-standing disease.[33] Small vessel disease

BOX 32.4 NON-SPECIFIC SKIN MANIFESTATIONS AND ASSOCIATED SKIN DISORDERS IN RHEUMATOID ARTHRITIS

Pyoderma gangrenosum
Rheumatoid neutrophilic dermatosis
Palisaded neutrophilic and granulomatous dermatitis
Interstitial granulomatous dermatitis
Atrophic and fragile skin
Pale and transparent skin
Palmar erythema
Livide (Raynaud-like) fingertips
Onychorrhexis and clubbing of the nails
Onycholysis
Periungual erythema
Yellow nail syndrome
Splinter hemorrhages and nailfold thromboses
Pressure ulcers
Hyperpigmentation
Transient macular erythema
Erythromelalgia
Non-inflammatory purpura
Erythema multiforme
Urticaria
Erythema nodosum
Vitiligo
Alopecia areata
Non-melanoma skin cancer
Intralymphatic histiocytosis of the skin

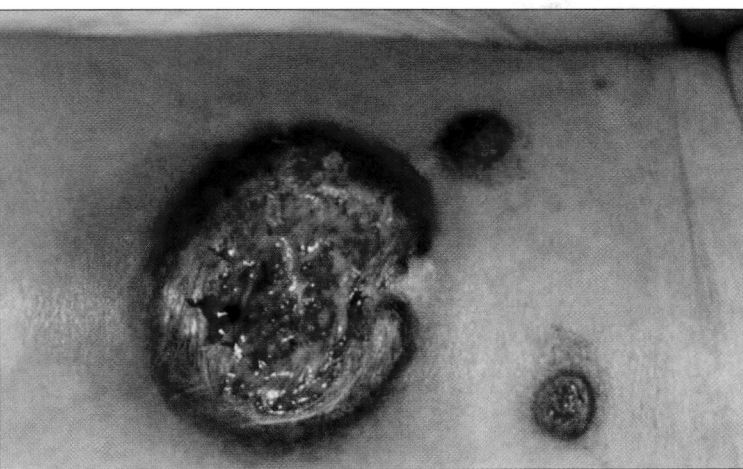

Fig. 32.22 Pyoderma gangrenosum. Note undermined hemorrhagic borders.

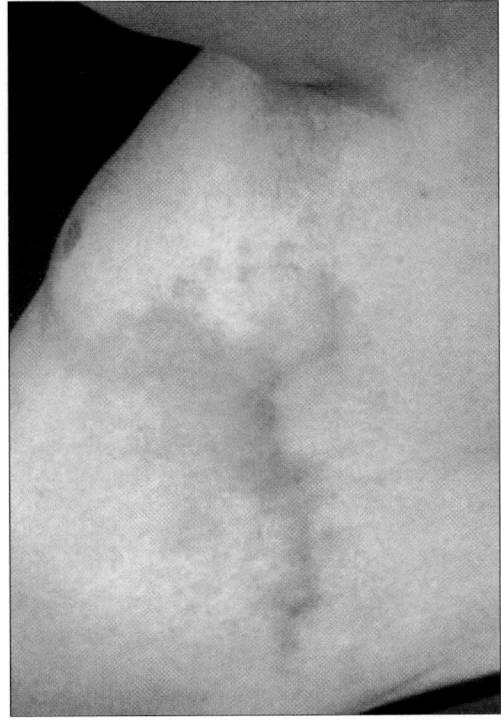

Fig. 32.23 Rope sign in a patient with interstitial granulomatous dermatitis.

clinically represents palpable and non-palpable purpura, localized petechiae, splinter hemorrhages, nailfold infarctions (Bywaters lesions), and peripheral neuropathy. In medium-sized vessel disease, cutaneous findings include nodules, ulcerations, livedo reticularis, and digital infarcts. The pathogenesis of rheumatoid vasculitis may be attributed to IgG-RF complex-mediated vasculitis.[34] Recently, it has been suggested that Th1 lymphocytes and TNF-α also play a role.[35] The course of rheumatoid vasculitis is associated with high morbidity and mortality and therefore requires early and intensive immunosuppressive therapy. The biopsy of cutaneous lesions, preferentially nodules, and immunohistochemical examination are often helpful in establishing the diagnosis. Because the incidence of peripheral neuropathy is frequently observed in cases where vasculitis cannot be identified, nerve conduction studies and sural nerve or muscle biopsies can be performed. Differential diagnosis of rheumatoid vasculitis includes polyarteritis nodosa, pyoderma gangrenosum, SLE, ANCA-associated granulomatous vasculitis, and erythema elevatum et diutinum.

In addition to the previously mentioned specific skin manifestations of RA, large numbers of non-specific skin signs and associated dermatoses have been described (Box 32.4). Pyoderma gangrenosum (PG) is frequently associated with both seronegative and seropositive RA. Clinically it begins as a tender erythematous or violaceous papule, which rapidly expands into a purulent necrotic ulcer with ragged edematous edges (Fig. 32.22). Usually PG occurs as a single painful lesion on the lower extremities. Köbner and pathergy phenomena are characteristic. The presence of chronic relapsing lesions in unusual sites such as the face, upper extremities, or abdomen may indicate another underlying disease such as inflammatory bowel disease or hematologic disorders. The idea that PG is a true skin manifestation of RA has been challenged because it also occurs in other systemic disorders, has no relation in its clinical manifestation with the course of RA, and involves no histology specific for RA.[36] Histologic examination of early lesions demonstrates a neutrophilic infiltrate and small abscesses.

Differential diagnosis for PG includes venous or arterial ulcers, vasculitis, drug reactions, antiphospholipid syndrome, halogenodermas, factitial diseases, deep fungal infections, mycobacterial infections, gummatous syphilis, viral infections, amebiasis, arthropod bites, and tumors.

Rheumatoid neutrophilic dermatosis is a rare cutaneous sign in patients with severe and seropositive RA.[37] Clinically it presents as asymptomatic erythematous urticarial papules and plaques, which may persist and sometimes ulcerate. They are usually distributed on the forearms and hands. Rheumatoid neutrophilic dermatosis resembles Sweet syndrome.

Palisaded neutrophilic and granulomatous dermatitis, originally described by Winkelmann, represents a condition of unknown cause with a variety of clinical pictures in the context of systemic rheumatic diseases. Skin manifestations usually appear symmetrically on the extensor surfaces of the elbows and fingers and present as skin-colored, erythematous, or violaceous papules, nodules, and plaques, sometimes with central umbilication and crusts or perforation.[38]

Another clinical presentation often observed on the trunk of patients with RA consists of erythematous to violaceous indurated linear cords ("rope sign") (Fig. 32.23). This condition is also known as *interstitial granulomatous dermatitis with arthritis.*[39] Lesions may perforate with extrusion of the necrobiotic collagen. The pathologic features consist of palisading histiocytes around basophilic collagen in the dermis and superficial subcutis. Sometimes orderly palisading may not be detected. The dermal interstitial and perivascular mixed infiltrate (in which neutrophils predominate), leukocytoclasis, histiocytes, lymphocytes, and sometimes eosinophils are present. This condition may be associated not only with RA but also with other autoimmune disorders or neoplastic diseases.

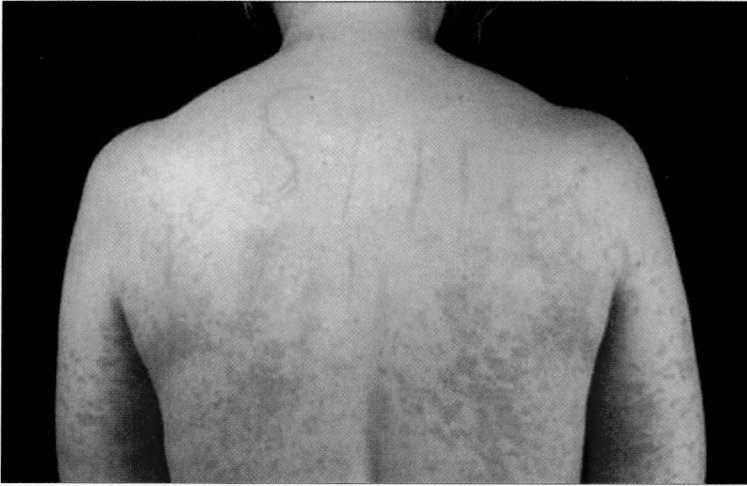

Fig. 32.24 Exanthema of a child with Still's disease.

The differential diagnosis of granulomatous dermatitis of RA includes mainly granuloma annulare, necrobiosis lipoidica, granulomatous slack skin, and interstitial granulomatous drug reactions.

Systemic onset juvenile rheumatoid arthritis (juvenile rheumatoid arthritis, juvenile chronic arthritis, Still disease)

Key dermatologic signs: macular or maculopapular exanthema, rheumatoid nodule-like lesions.

The diagnosis of systemic onset juvenile rheumatoid arthritis (SOJRA) can be challenging. Because skin manifestations can precede arthralgias by years, their early recognition can be crucial in establishing the diagnosis. SOJRA has two clinical presentations: an acute febrile systemic variant and an oligoarticular variant with low-grade persistent fevers. In the acute-onset variant, in which high episodic fevers above 38.9° C are characteristic, 90% of patients develop a non-pruritic transient exanthema that recurs with fevers.[40] It consists of discrete macular or maculopapular lesions, often located on the trunk (Fig. 32.24). The color of the lesions is pink to red, and Köbnerization is common. The histopathologic findings of the rash are non-specific and consist of a discrete perivascular mixed infiltrate with edema of the upper dermis. Another skin sign in patients with SOJRA is rheumatoid nodule-like lesions with a predilection for the extensor surfaces of the extremities.[41] The lesions can be both clinically and histologically indistinguishable from those of patients with RA.

The pathogenesis of SOJRA is fragmentary. It was shown that blood mononuclear cells from patients with SOJRA constitutively and after stimulation with various antigens *in vitro* induce a higher secretion of IL-4 and IL-10 with a characteristic deficiency of IL-2 and interferon-γ, suggesting a Th1/Th2 imbalance.[42] Elevated levels of IL-6 and TNF-α and the beneficial effects of the novel anti–TNF-α and anti–IL-6 receptor therapies on SOJRA disease activity indicate that both cytokines are important players in the pathogenesis of the disease.[43,44] In addition, various circulating autoantibodies have been detected in patients with SOJRA, but it is unclear whether these observations are of pathogenetic relevance or represent an epiphenomenon.

The differential diagnosis of the typical exanthema of SOJRA in combination with fever and arthralgias includes rheumatic fever, familial Mediterranean fever, hyper-IgD syndrome, tumor necrosis factor receptor–associated periodic syndrome (TRAPS), familial Hibernian fever, autosomal dominant periodic fever with amyloidosis, and benign autosomal dominant familial periodic fever.

Relapsing polychondritis (atrophic polychondritis, systemic chondromalacia, polychondropathia)

Key dermatologic signs: erythema, swelling, and pain of the cartilaginous portion of the ear with sparing of the earlobe; auricular and nasal deformity.

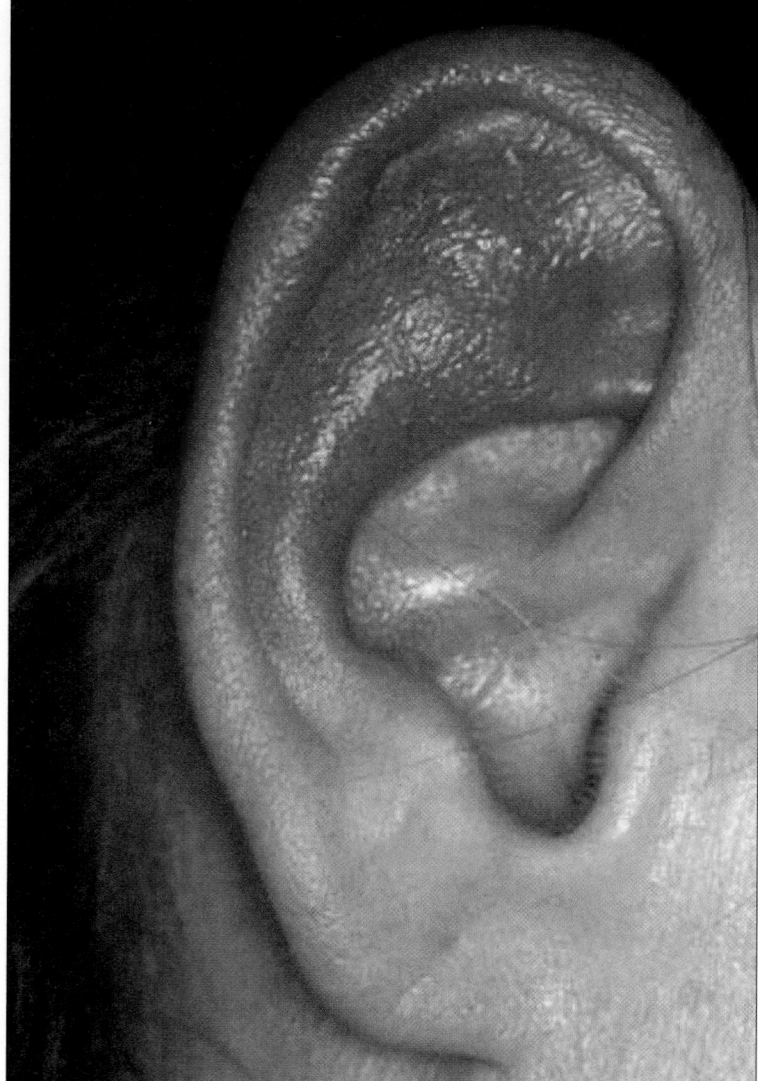

Fig. 32.25 Inflamed helix and anthelix in a patient with relapsing polychondritis. Note sparing of the earlobe.

Relapsing polychondritis (RP) is a chronic inflammatory multisystem disorder that can lead to significant morbidity owing to destruction of the cartilaginous tissue in many organs. In a significant number of RP cases, cutaneous involvement is the first clinical presentation.

The hallmark cutaneous features of RP are erythema, swelling, and pain of the cartilaginous part of the ear that typically spares the earlobe (Fig. 32.25). The vast majority of patients with RP suffer from auricular involvement during the course of their disease. Persistent inflammation will lead to destruction of the auricular cartilage, resulting in so-called "cauliflower ears." Involvement of the nasal cartilage occurs in 70% of affected patients, eventually leading to a saddle nose deformity.[45] Glomerulonephritis may accompany RP.

An autoimmune process is implicated in the pathogenesis of RP in light of the presence of circulating autoantibodies recognizing native type II collagen.[46] The association with the HLA-DR4[47] haplotype also suggests an immunologic mechanism responsible for the destruction of cartilaginous tissue. Histopathologic examination of inflamed cartilage shows basophilic staining, loss of the normal lacunar structures, and a neutrophilic infiltrate. At later stages lymphocytes and plasma cells are more prominent and the cartilage is replaced by granulation tissue and fibrosis.

Several non-specific skin signs have been reported to occur in 36% of affected RP patients.[48] However, a significant proportion may be related to associated diseases (myelodysplastic syndrome, Behçet disease, and other systemic disorders) and/or adverse effects of concomitant systemic treatment. These skin manifestations include various forms of vasculitis, including palpable purpura; livedo reticularis and erythema elevatum et diutinum; non-inflammatory vasculopathies such as livedo reticularis; panniculitis; and aphthosis (oral or complex).

The differential diagnosis of RP includes primarily traumatic and infectious forms of chondritis and ANCA-associated granulomatous vasculitis, which may also lead to cartilage destruction, especially of the nose. The combination of features of RP and Behçet disease has led to the designation *Mouth And Genital ulceration with Inflamed Cartilage* (MAGIC) *syndrome.*[49]

REFERENCES

1. Sontheimer RD. Skin manifestations of systemic autoimmune connective tissue disease: diagnostics and therapeutics. Best Pract Res Clin Rheumatol 2004;18:429-462.
2. Kuhn A, Richter-Hintz D, Oslislo C, et al. Lupus erythematosus tumidus—a neglected subset of cutaneous lupus erythematosus: report of 40 cases. Arch Dermatol 2000;136:1033-1041.
3. Martens PB, Moder KG, Ahmed I. Lupus panniculitis: clinical perspectives from a case series. J Rheumatol 1999;26:68-72.
4. Viguier M, Pinquier L, Cavelier-Balloy B, et al. Clinical and histopathologic features and immunologic variables in patients with severe chilblains. A study of the relationship to lupus erythematosus. Medicine 2001;80:180-188.
5. Lee LA. Neonatal lupus erythematosus. J Invest Dermatol 1993;100:9S-13S.
6. Casciola-Rosen L, Rosen A. Ultraviolet light-induced keratinocyte apoptosis: a potential mechanism for the induction of skin lesions and autoantibody production in LE. Lupus 1997;6:175-180.
7. Walport MJ, Davies KA, Botto M. C1q and systemic lupus erythematosus. Immunobiology 1998;199:265-285.
8. Eriksson C, Engstrand S, Sundqvist KG, Rantapa-Dahlqvist S. Autoantibody formation in patients with rheumatoid arthritis treated with anti-TNF alpha. Ann Rheum Dis 2005;64:403-407.
9. Flendrie M, Vissers WH, Creemers MC, et al. Dermatological conditions during TNF-α-blocking therapy in patients with rheumatoid arthritis: a prospective study. Arthritis Res Ther 2005;7:R666-R676.
10. Bohan A, Peter JB. Polymyositis and dermatomyositis (first of two parts). N Engl J Med 1975;292:344-347.
11. Stahl NI, Klippel JH, Decker JL. A cutaneous lesion associated with myositis. Ann Intern Med 1979;91:577-579.
12. Sunderkötter C, Herrgott I, Brückner C, et al. Comparison of patients with and without digital ulcers in systemic sclerosis: detection of possible risk factors. Br J Dermatol 2009;160:835-843.
13. Kahaleh MB. Vascular involvement in systemic sclerosis (SSc). Clin Exp Rheumatol 2004;22:S19-S23.
14. Falanga V, Zhou L, Yufit T. Low oxygen tension stimulates collagen synthesis and COL1A1 transcription through the action of TGF-beta1. J Cell Physiol 2002;191:42-50.
15. Denton CP, Abraham DJ. Transforming growth factor-beta and connective tissue growth factor: key cytokines in scleroderma pathogenesis. Curr Opin Rheumatol 2001;13:505-511.
16. Dong C, Zhu S, Wang T, et al. Deficient Smad7 expression: a putative molecular defect in scleroderma. Proc Natl Acad Sci USA 2002;99:3908-3913.
17. Mori Y, Chen SJ, Varga J. Expression and regulation of intracellular SMAD signaling in scleroderma skin fibroblasts. Arthritis Rheum 2003;48:1964-1978.
18. Ronda N, Gatti R, Giacosa R, et al. Antifibroblast antibodies from systemic sclerosis patients are internalized by fibroblasts via a caveolin-linked pathway. Arthritis Rheum 2002;46:1595-1601.
19. Chizzolini C, Raschi E, Rezzonico R, et al. Autoantibodies to fibroblasts induce a proadhesive and proinflammatory fibroblast phenotype in patients with systemic sclerosis. Arthritis Rheum 2002;46:1602-1613.
20. Baroni SS, Santillo M, Bevilacqua F, et al. Stimulatory autoantibodies to the PDGF receptor in systemic sclerosis. N Engl J Med 2006;354:2667-2676.
21. Classen JF, Henrohn D, Rorsman F, et al. Lack of evidence of stimulatory autoantibodies to platelet-derived growth factor receptor in patients with systemic sclerosis. Arthritis Rheum 2009;60:1137-1144.
22. Boutsi EA, Paikos S, Dafni UG, et al. Dental and periodontal status of Sjögren's syndrome. J Clin Periodontol 2000;27:231-235.
23. Provost TT, Watson R. Cutaneous manifestations of Sjögren's syndrome. Rheum Dis Clin 1992;18:609-616.
24. Kapsogeorgou E, Manoussakis MN. The central role of epithelial cells in Sjögren's syndrome or autoimmune epithelitis. Autoimmun Rev 2004;3(suppl 1):S61-S63.
25. Nakamura H, Kawakami A, Tominaga M, et al. Expression of CD-40/CD-40 ligand and Bcl-2 family proteins in labial salivary glands of patients with Sjögren's syndrome. Lab Invest 1999;79:261-269.
26. Tzioufas AG, Tsonis J, Moutsopoulos HM. Neuroendocrine dysfunction in Sjögren's syndrome. Neuroimmunomodulation 2008;15:37-45.
27. Ziff M. The rheumatoid nodule. Arthritis Rheum 1990;33:761-767.
28. Ahmed SS, Arnett FC, Smith CA, et al. The HLA-DRB1*0401 allele and the development of methotrexate-induced accelerated rheumatoid nodulosis: a follow-up study of 79 Caucasian patients with rheumatoid arthritis. Medicine 2001;80:271-278.
29. Hessian PA, Highton J, Kean A, et al. Cytokine profile of the rheumatoid nodule suggests that it is a Th1 granuloma. Arthritis Rheum 2003;48:334-338.
30. Sienknecht CW, Urowitz MB, Pruzanski W, Stein H. Felty's syndrome. Clinical and serological analysis of 34 cases. Ann Rheum Dis 1977;36:500-507.
31. Kremer JM, Lee JK. The safety and efficacy of the use of methotrexate in long-term therapy for rheumatoid arthritis. Arthritis Rheum 1986;29:822-831.
32. Cunnane G, Warnock M, Fye KH, Daikh DI. Accelerated nodulosis and vasculitis following etanercept therapy for rheumatoid arthritis. Arthritis Rheum 2002;47:445-449.
33. Voskuyl AE, Zwinderman AH, Westedt ML, et al. Factors associated with the development of vasculitis in rheumatoid arthritis: results of a case-control study. Ann Rheum Dis 1996;55:190-192.
34. Elson CJ, Scott DG, Blake DR, et al. Complement-activating rheumatoid-factor-containing complexes in patients with rheumatoid vasculitis. Ann Rheum Dis 1983;42:147-150.
35. Flipo RM, Cardon T, Copin MC, et al. ICAM-1, E-selectin, and TNF alpha expression in labial salivary glands of patients with rheumatoid vasculitis. Ann Rheum Dis 1997;56:41-44.
36. Von Den Driesch P. Pyoderma gangrenosum: a report of 44 cases with follow-up. Br J Dermatol 1997;137:1000-1005.
37. Ichikawa MM, Murata Y, Higaki Y, et al. Rheumatoid neutrophilic dermatitis. Eur J Dermatol 1998;8:347-349.
38. Sangueza OP, Caudell MD, Mengesha YM, et al. Palisaded neutrophilic granulomatous dermatitis in rheumatoid arthritis. J Am Acad Dermatol 2002;47:251-257.
39. Long D, Thiboutot DM, Majeski JT, et al. Interstitial granulomatous dermatitis with arthritis. J Am Acad Dermatol 1996;34:957-961.
40. Calabro JJ, Marchesano JM. Rash associated with juvenile rheumatoid arthritis. J Pediatr 1968;72:611-619.
41. Lubbe J, Hofer M, Chavaz P, et al. Adult-onset Still's disease with persistent plaques. Br J Dermatol 1999;141:710-713.
42. Raziuddin S, Bahabri S, Al-Dalaan A, et al. A mixed Th1/Th2 cell cytokine response predominates in systemic onset juvenile rheumatoid arthritis: immunoregulatory IL-10 function. Clin Immunol Immunopathol 1998;86:192-198.
43. Moore TL. Immunopathogenesis of juvenile rheumatoid arthritis. Curr Opin Rheumatol 1999;11:377-383.
44. Mihara M, Nishimoto N, Ohsugi Y. The therapy of autoimmune diseases by anti-interleukin-6 receptor antibody. Expert Opin Biol Ther 2005;5:683-690.
45. McAdam LP, O'Hanlan MA, Bluestone R, Pearson CM. Relapsing polychondritis: prospective study of 23 patients and review of the literature. Medicine 1976;55:193-215.
46. Foidart JM, Abe S, Martin GR, et al. Antibodies to type II collagen in relapsing polychondritis. N Engl J Med 1978;299:1203-1207.
47. Zeuner M, Straub RH, Rauh G, et al. Relapsing polychondritis: clinical and immunogenetic analysis of 62 patients. J Rheumatol 1997;24:96-101.
48. Frances C, El Rassi R, Laporte JL, et al. Dermatological manifestations of relapsing polychondritis. A study of 200 cases at a single center. Medicine 2001;80:173-179.
49. Firestein GS, Gruber HE, Weisman MH, et al. Mouth and genital ulcers with inflamed cartilage: MAGIC syndrome. Five patients with features of relapsing polychondritis and Behçet's disease. Am J Med 1985;79:65-72.

The eye in rheumatic disease

Jennifer E. Thorne and Douglas A. Jabs

33

- Ocular inflammation is common in rheumatic disease and often varies with the rheumatic disease in question.
- The most common ocular manifestations of rheumatic disease are uveitis, scleritis, and keratoconjunctivitis sicca.
- In select rheumatic diseases (i.e., Wegener's granulomatosis or Beçhet's disease), the eye disease may be severe enough to dictate therapy for the systemic disease.

INTRODUCTION

The rheumatic diseases are a heterogeneous collection of immune-mediated, multisystem disorders. Ocular involvement is common and often varies with the rheumatic disease in question.[1] The major manifestations of ocular involvement in rheumatic disease include uveitis, scleritis, retinal vascular disease, neuro-ophthalmic lesions, orbital disease, keratitis, and Sjögren syndrome.[1] This chapter deals with each of these disease entities separately. The eyes can also be affected by several drugs used in the therapy of inflammatory rheumatic diseases, such as corticosteroids or antimalarial agents; these abnormalities are discussed in the appropriate chapters.

UVEITIS

Uveitis denotes inflammation inside the eye, which can be classified by the anatomic site where the inflammation primarily occurs.[2] Uveitis detected primarily in the anterior chamber is termed *anterior uveitis* (Fig. 33.1). Inflammation primarily involving the vitreous is termed *intermediate uveitis*, and uveitis located in the retina or choroid is *posterior uveitis*. Uveitis that involves all three compartments but does not have a primary focus of inflammation is termed *panuveitis*.[2] The onset of uveitis may be sudden or insidious, and the duration of the attack may be limited (≤3 months' duration) or persistent (>3 months' duration). The course of uveitis is described as acute, recurrent, or chronic. Acute uveitis has a sudden onset with a limited duration, as in acute anterior uveitis seen with the seronegative spondyloarthropathies. Recurrent uveitis describes a course of multiple attacks of sudden onset and limited duration alternating with periods of remission, when the uveitis is inactive and the patient is not on therapy for the disease. Chronic uveitis typically has an insidious onset and a persistent duration, such as chronic anterior uveitis associated with juvenile rheumatoid arthritis (JRA), also termed *juvenile idiopathic arthritis* (JIA).[1,2]

Acute anterior uveitis (AAU) is also known as *iritis* or *iridocyclitis*. Typically, the patient presents with a red, painful, and photophobic eye. Slit-lamp examination reveals cells in the anterior chamber. These cells may deposit on the posterior corneal endothelium, called *keratic precipitates*. The cellular inflammation in the anterior chamber may be so severe as to produce a hypopyon or a layering of inflammatory cells within the anterior chamber. Protein exudation into the anterior chamber, known as *flare*, also may be seen and may be so marked that a fibrin clot forms in the anterior chamber. A complication of anterior uveitis is the formation of adhesions between the posterior iris and the lens surface (posterior synechiae). Posterior synechiae frequently persist after the inflammation has settled (Fig. 33.2). Acute anterior uveitis also may lead to the development of peripheral anterior synechiae, scar tissue that forms between the peripheral iris and the posterior cornea.

Anterior synechiae may be so extensive as to block the drainage angle of the eye, causing an increase in intraocular pressure and secondary glaucoma. Typically AAU affects one eye at a time, although rarely both eyes may be affected simultaneously. Although only one eye is affected at a time, both eyes may suffer attacks, in which case the uveitis is termed *recurrent, unilateral alternating AAU*.[1,2]

Acute anterior uveitis is most commonly associated with the seronegative spondyloarthropathies.[1,3] The annual incidence of AAU is 8.2 new cases per 100,000 population.[4] Approximately one half of these patients will possess the HLA-B27 gene, and 60% will have a diagnosis of seronegative spondyloarthropathy.[3] The seronegative spondyloarthropathies include ankylosing spondylitis (AS), reactive arthritis (including Reiter syndrome), arthritis with inflammatory bowel disease (IBD), and psoriatic arthritis.[1,3,5] Acute anterior uveitis occurs in 25% to 40% of patients with AS.[6-8] Conversely, studies of patients with AAU have reported that AS is present in 18% to 34%.[1,9] Acute anterior uveitis is said to occur in 5% to 20% of patients with Reiter syndrome at the initial attack and in up to 50% of Reiter patients with long-term follow-up.[6,8,10] Of patients with arthritis related to IBD, those patients with ankylosing spondylitis associated with IBD appear to be at greatest risk for developing AAU. Spondylitis occurs in 20% of patients with Crohn disease and in 10% to 15% of patients with ulcerative colitis.[11,12] Approximately 50% to 70% of patients with spondylitis and IBD are HLA-B27 positive.[12] Of the HLA-B27–positive patients with IBD, 50% will develop AAU.[5,11,12] Recent investigations indicate that a genetic marker, on another chromosome, may be responsible for the AAU that occurs in ankylosing spondylitis.[13] Among patients with psoriatic arthritis, AAU occurs in approximately 7% to 10%.[8,14,15] Although unilateral, alternating AAU is the most typical type of uveitis associated with the seronegative spondyloarthropathies; chronic and bilateral uveitis also occurs occasionally and may be seen more frequently in women with IBD or with psoriatic arthritis.[8,16,17]

Chronic anterior uveitis (CAU) is less frequent than AAU and may be seen with several disorders, most often with sarcoidosis. The rheumatic disease most commonly associated with CAU is JRA, also known as *juvenile idiopathic arthritis*.[18] Approximately 12% to 17% of children with JRA have uveitis.[19,20] A population-based study performed in Finland reported the mean annual incidence and prevalence rates for JRA-associated uveitis as 0.2 and 2.4 cases per 100,000 population, respectively.[21] Although recurrent AAU is seen with HLA-B27–associated subgroups of JRA, CAU is more commonly associated with JRA and is seen with antinuclear antibody (ANA)–positive oligoarticular disease, in which frequencies have been reported to range from 20% to 56%.[22-27] Although CAU typically has been reported in patients with antinuclear antibody (ANA)–positive oligoarticular disease, one study suggested a similar frequency among those with ANA-positive polyarticular disease, suggesting that the presence of ANA and not the type of arthritis was the marker for CAU.[27] Although traditionally it has been said that cases of JRA-related CAU occur more frequently in girls, one retrospective study of 90 children with JRA found no gender difference in the risk of developing CAU.[19] The CAU tends to be insidious and minimally symptomatic (the "white eye" uveitis; Fig. 33.3); therefore it is recommended that patients with ANA-positive oligoarticular JRA be evaluated every 3 months in an effort to detect the uveitis early.[28] Two thirds of patients have bilateral disease, and in patients with unilateral disease, the majority will develop uveitis in the fellow eye within 1 year of presentation.[1] The chronic uveitis typically requires chronic therapy. Although initial therapy typically is with topical corticosteroids, some children will require systemic treatment such as methotrexate to control the disease.[29,30]

Sight-threatening ocular complications may develop in patients with CAU, with band keratopathy and cataracts each occurring in up

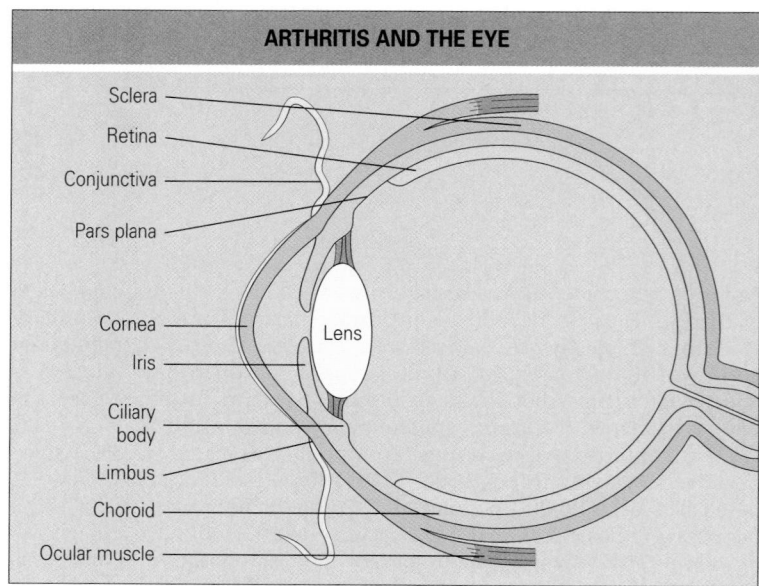

Fig. 33.1 Arthritis and the eye. The structural elements of the eye that may be primarily involved in rheumatic disease processes are shown.

Sclera
Retina
Conjunctiva
Pars plana
Cornea
Lens
Iris
Ciliary body
Limbus
Choroid
Ocular muscle

ARTHRITIS AND THE EYE

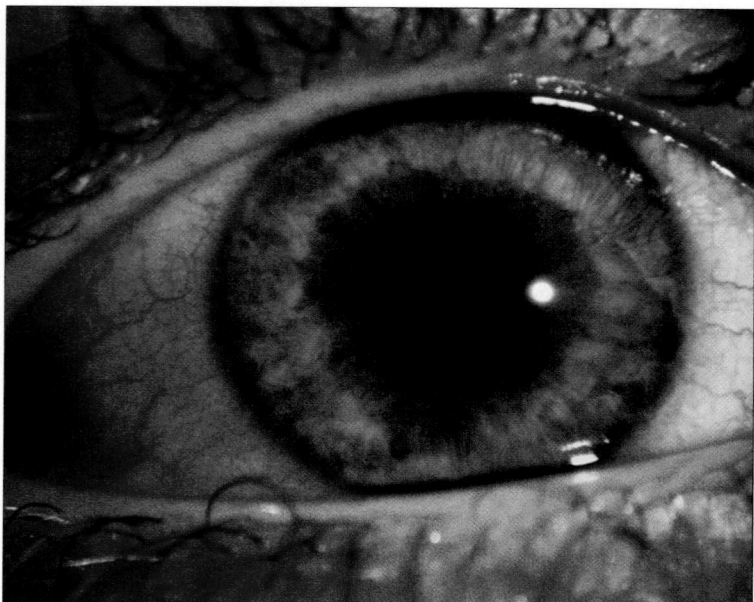

Fig. 33.3 Chronic uveitis in oligoarticular juvenile rheumatoid arthritis: "white eye" uveitis.

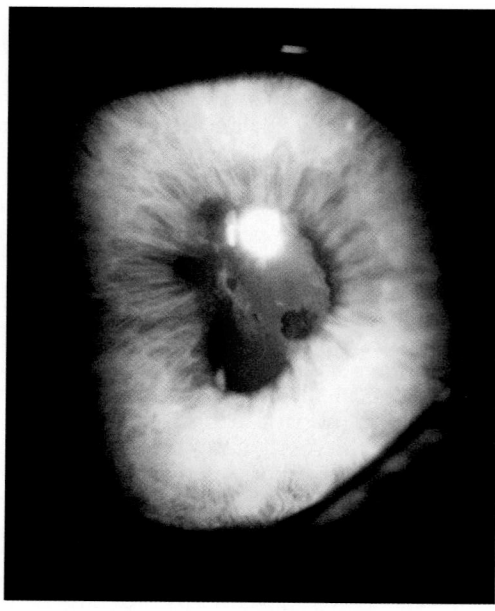

Fig. 33.2 Wide-beam slit-lamp view of "old" posterior synechiae (adhesions between iris and lens) causing pupil distortion.

to one third of patients.[1,19,26,29-31] Secondary glaucoma occurs in 10% to 20% of patients with JRA-associated uveitis and is a poor prognostic finding.[23,24,26,31-33] Posterior synechiae are common.[29,30,34] Other complications include macular edema in 8% to 10% of cases and phthisis in 4% to 10%. Although blindness developed in 40% of patients reported in early series, more recent series have reported a better prognosis, with blindness occurring in about 10%.[19,20,23,26,29-31,33-35] The improved prognosis appears to be due to earlier detection, better treatment, and better surgical management of the complications.[34,36-38] Nevertheless, about 25% of patients with JRA-associated CAU will suffer some degree of visual impairment.

Uveitis is a primary manifestation of Behçet disease.[39] The uveitis in Behçet disease may be anterior (56% to 79% of cases depending on series), intermediate (18% to 66% of cases), posterior (3% to 29% of cases), or panuveitis with retinal vasculitis (29% to 41% of cases).[1,39] The presence of retinal vasculitis confers a poor prognosis for vision and is described further later (see "Retinal Vascular Disease"). Anterior uveitis with or without hypopyon is the most common ocular finding in Behçet disease. Although studies from the 1960s and early 1970s

reported hypopyon uveitis in up to 88% of patients, more recent studies have shown a decreased frequency of hypopyon to as low as 9%.[1,39,40] This reported decrease probably represents earlier diagnosis and more aggressive therapy. Uveitis associated with Behçet disease is typically bilateral. In one series, 81% of patients had bilateral uveitis after 1 year, and 93% of patients had bilateral disease by 2 years.[39-41]

Bilateral CAU also may occur in essential mixed cryoglobulinemia,[42] hypocomplementemic urticarial vasculitis syndrome (HUVS),[43] and familial juvenile systemic granulomatosis (FJSG).[44-46] Essential mixed cryoglobulinemia, or type II cryoglobulinemia, is a small vessel vasculitis, which may result in palpable purpura, arthralgias or arthritis, lymphadenopathy, hepatosplenomegaly, peripheral neuropathy, and hypocomplementemia.[47] Renal disease also may be seen in up to 60% of patients with essential mixed cryoglobulinemia.[47] Most cases of essential mixed cryoglobulinemia are associated with hepatitis C virus (HCV) infection, with an estimated 85% to 95% of patients having circulating antibodies to HCV.[48,49] Diagnosis is made by the presence of a cutaneous small vessel vasculitis confirmed by biopsy and the presence of serum cryoglobulins in a patient with typical clinical features.

An uncommon systemic small-vessel vasculitis, HUVS is characterized by recurrent urticarial lesions associated with a cutaneous vasculitis, constitutional symptoms, arthralgias or arthritis, angioedema, and glomerulonephritis.[50] The joint and kidney disease may be indistinguishable from that found in systemic lupus erythematosus (SLE), and, in fact, low titers of antinuclear antibody (ANA) are often found in patients with HUVS.[50] Diagnosis of HUVS is suggested in a patient with recurrent urticaria accompanied by a leukocytoclastic vasculitis, constitutional symptoms, arthralgias, and hypocomplementemia. A continuous granular deposition of immunoreactants along the basement membrane zone seen on skin biopsy using direct immunofluorescence technique helps to confirm the diagnosis.[51] Ocular findings in HUVS have been reported and include conjunctivitis, episcleritis, anterior uveitis, and diffuse anterior scleritis.[50-52]

Familial juvenile systemic granulomatosis (MIM 186580), also known as *Jabs syndrome* or *Blau syndrome*, is an uncommon autosomal dominant genetic disease characterized by granulomatous polysynovitis, skin rash, vascular disease, and uveitis.[44-46] The syndrome is caused by mutations in the NOD2 (CARD15) gene, which is involved in apoptosis. The uveitis associated with FJSG may be a bilateral CAU[44,45] or a chronic panuveitis with multifocal choroiditis.[46] Patients with FJSG and CAU often are misdiagnosed as having JRA or pediatric sarcoidosis. Patients may require aggressive medical therapy to control the uveitis, including immunosuppressive drugs.[46] Ocular complications such as cataract and macular edema are common.[46]

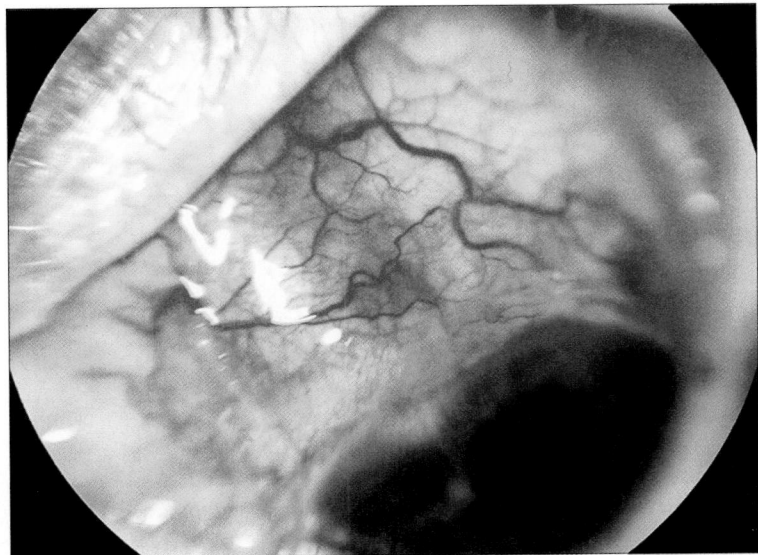

Fig. 33.4 Diffuse and nodular scleritis involving predominantly the upper temporal quadrant of the globe.

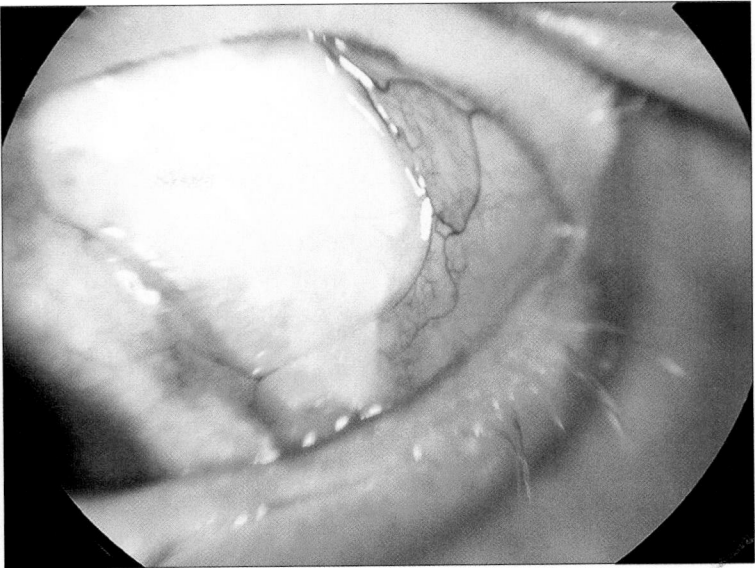

Fig. 33.5 Necrotizing scleritis in severe rheumatoid arthritis.

Management

Anterior uveitis usually responds to topically applied corticosteroids, which reduce the inflammatory response, and mydriatics, which prevent the sequelae of the disease such as posterior synechiae. For the initial flare of uveitis, corticosteroid drops may be required on an hourly basis while awake. Topical corticosteroids have good penetration into the anterior chamber and are therefore useful in treating anterior uveitis. However, because they have limited penetration to the back of the eye, topical corticosteroids are inadequate for intermediate or posterior uveitis. Periocular corticosteroid injections may provide high concentrations of corticosteroids to the eye and are useful in treating intermediate uveitis and cystoid macular edema, a common vision-threatening complication from uveitis. For patients who do not tolerate periocular corticosteroid injections, or if more sustained control of the uveitis is needed, oral corticosteroid therapy is used. Severe acute episodic uveitis occasionally may need treatment with a short course of oral prednisone in addition to intensive topical corticosteroids, as in the case of severe AAU. In patients with chronic posterior uveitis, panuveitis, or anterior uveitis unresponsive to topical corticosteroids, high-dose prednisone (e.g., 1 mg/kg/day) is administered until the inflammation is suppressed, followed by tapering to a lower dose. In many cases, long-term (low-dose) prednisone is needed to suppress the inflammation. If systemic corticosteroids are insufficient to control more severe forms of uveitis, immunosuppressive drug therapy may be required.[1,39,53]

SCLERAL DISEASE

Scleral disease may be classified as episcleritis or scleritis. Episcleritis presents with discomfort rather than pain, more superficial ocular inflammation, and less frequent ocular complications, and typically has a less frequent association with systemic disease.[54] The clinical presentation depends on whether only the episclera is involved or whether there is deeper tissue involvement. Episcleritis may be nodular or simple and is usually a self-limiting condition, which often resolves without treatment. Resolution of the inflammation may be expedited by the use of topical corticosteroids. In severe or recurrent cases, nonsteroidal anti-inflammatory agents (NSAIDs) have also been used. Slit-lamp examination is required to differentiate this condition from other causes of "red eye," such as conjunctivitis and iritis.[39,54-56]

Scleritis often is characterized by pain, presents with deeper inflammation and edema in the sclera, often has ocular complications, and is associated with an infectious or systemic disease in approximately 50% of cases.[54-56] Unlike episcleritis, which is typically self-limiting and spontaneously remitting, scleritis typically requires therapy. Scleritis may be classified as diffuse anterior, nodular anterior (Fig. 33.4), posterior, or necrotizing (Fig. 33.5). Scleromalacia perforans is a

separate category, in which there is an insidious but destructive scleral process, and is seen in patients with long-standing rheumatoid arthritis (RA). Any of the previously mentioned types of scleritis may be seen in association with RA, although diffuse anterior scleritis is most common.[54]

Approximately 10% of patients with scleritis will have an associated infection, such as syphilis, Lyme disease, or herpes zoster ophthalmicus.[55] Patients with scleritis appear to have a higher frequency of rheumatic disease.[57] Forty percent of patients with scleritis will have a rheumatic disease, the most frequent of which is RA.[55] Scleritis affects an estimated 1% to 6% of patients with RA and 14% of patients with rheumatoid vasculitis.[55,58-60] Although estimates of the frequency of scleritis in patients with RA have been as high as 6%, large series have shown that approximately 1% of patients with RA have scleritis.[54,60] Patients with RA and scleritis tend to have a longer and more severe disease and a higher prevalence of extra-articular disease.[56,58-60] One study of patients with necrotizing scleritis or necrotizing keratitis and RA suggested an increased mortality among these patients.[58]

The second most frequent systemic disorder associated with scleritis is the systemic vasculitides (most commonly antinuclear cytoplasmic antibody (ANCA)-associated granulomatous vasculitis); other associated diseases include SLE, IBD, and relapsing polychondritis.[54-56] Any type of vasculitis may be present with scleritis, but one half of vasculitis-associated scleritis is due to ANCA-associated granulomatous vasculitis.[55] Furthermore, in one half of patients with vasculitis and scleritis, the scleritis will be the presenting feature of the disease.[55] Scleritis is common in ANCA-associated granulomatous vasculitis, occurring in 16% to 38% of patients, and is either the first or second most frequent ocular feature, depending on the series.[39,61-64] The scleritis can be of any type, particularly diffuse anterior or necrotizing scleritis. Marginal corneal ulcers often are seen in association with the scleritis (necrotizing sclerokeratitis) and occasionally without scleritis (see "Corneal Disease").[58,63] Posterior scleritis also has been reported.[1]

All types of scleritis have been associated with IBD, including necrotizing scleritis and posterior scleritis.[65-68] The scleral inflammation may parallel the activity of the underlying bowel disease.[66,68] Scleral involvement is the most common ocular manifestation of relapsing polychondritis and occurs in approximately 35% to 41% of patients.[69-71] Most often, diffuse anterior scleritis is the type present, but recurrent episcleritis, necrotizing scleritis, or posterior scleritis also can be seen. An association between scleritis and ankylosing spondylitis and other seronegative spondyloarthropathies has been reported.[55]

Management

Treatment for episcleritis can be observation only or a short course of topical corticosteroids because the disease usually is self-limiting.

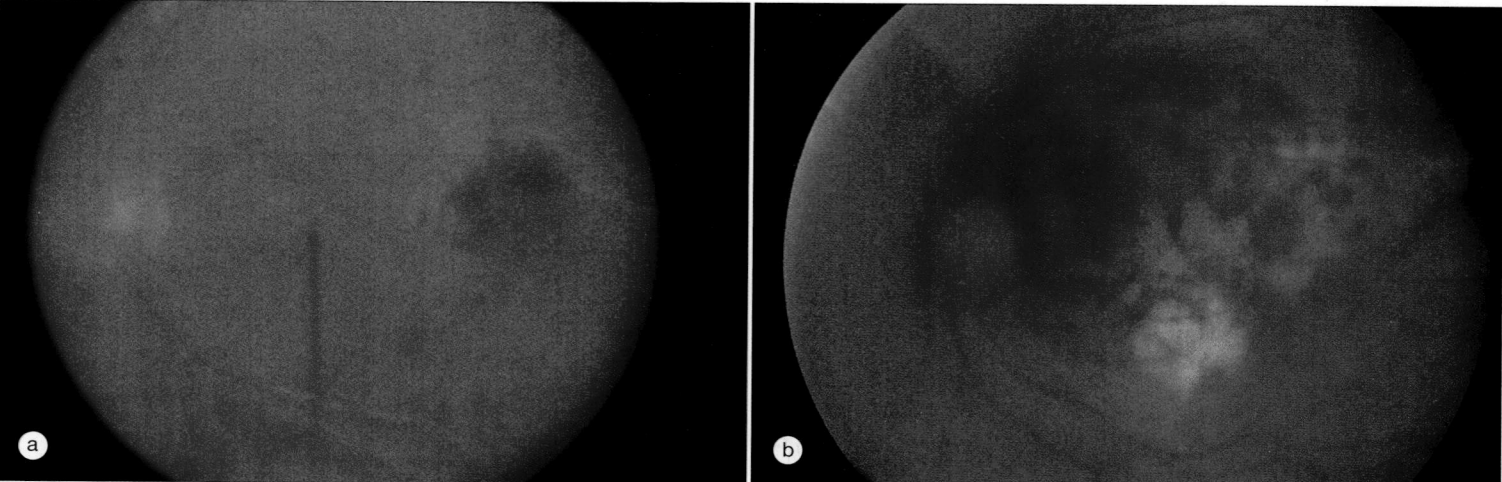

Fig. 33.6 Fundus photographs from a patient with Behçet disease demonstrating retinal vasculitis. Panel (a) shows early macular lesion, and (b) shows progressive disease 1 month later. *(From Thorne JE, Jabs DA. Rheumatic diseases. In: Ryan SJ, ed. The retina, 4th ed. London: Elsevier, 2006:1383-1408.)*

Scleritis typically requires systemic therapy and may require treatment directed at controlling the underlying systemic disease, as in vasculitis.[54-56,58,64] NSAIDs, particularly flurbiprofen and indomethacin, are effective in the initial management of anterior scleritis in approximately one third of patients.[54] If NSAID therapy fails to control the anterior scleritis or if there is posterior or necrotizing scleritis, oral prednisone therapy starting at 1 mg/kg/day (60 to 80 mg daily) is needed.[53,54,72] For cases in which oral prednisone does not control the scleritis, or when it cannot be tapered to an acceptably low daily dose, a steroid-sparing immunosuppressive agent may be required.[53,54] Approximately one third of patients with scleritis require immunosuppressive drug therapy; historically, cyclophosphamide has been the drug used most often.[54,60,72] However, antimetabolites such as mycophenolate mofetil (Cellcept) also may be effective.[73] Necrotizing scleritis and scleritis with an underlying systemic vasculitis nearly always require immunosuppressive drug therapy.[54-56,58,63]

RETINAL VASCULAR DISEASE

Ophthalmologists often use the term "retinal vasculitis" to encompass most retinal vascular inflammatory diseases whether or not there is true vasculitis present. For the purposes of this chapter, retinal vasculitis is defined as inflammation of the retinal vessels accompanied by intraocular inflammation and retinal vessel occlusion. Although most ophthalmologists do not distinguish among the different types of retinal vascular disease, we distinguish retinal vasculitis from the occlusive vasculopathies such as the antiphospholipid antibody syndrome associated with SLE (where there is no intraocular inflammation).

Retinal vasculitis may involve retinal arteries, capillaries, or veins, and it may cause significant visual loss.[74,75] Retinal vasculitis can be seen in the systemic vasculitides, but it is an uncommon complication except for Behçet disease. In Behçet disease, inflammation may involve both veins and arteries with arterial occlusion and retinal necrosis (Fig. 33.6). Occasionally, secondary neovascularization and retinal detachment develop.[40,41,75,76] The end-stage of the disease is a blind, painful eye with secondary glaucoma, rubeosis, and retinal detachment. The natural history of ocular Behçet disease without treatment is poor. The majority of patients will lose all or part of their vision within 5 years, with 74% of eyes in one series having vision worse than 20/200.[76] For eyes that deteriorated to no light perception, vision declined to this level over a period of 3.6 years.[40,76]

Corticosteroid therapy appears to delay the progression of the disease but does not alter the ultimate outcome, and therefore immunosuppressive drug therapy is used in the treatment of retinal vasculitis complicating Behçet disease.[39,53] Initially, chlorambucil was used, typically at a dose of 0.1 to 0.2 mg/kg/day.[53,77-84] Uncontrolled case series of chlorambucil therapy for Behçet disease have shown long-term, drug-free remissions after 2 years of treatment.[53,77,78] Fewer published

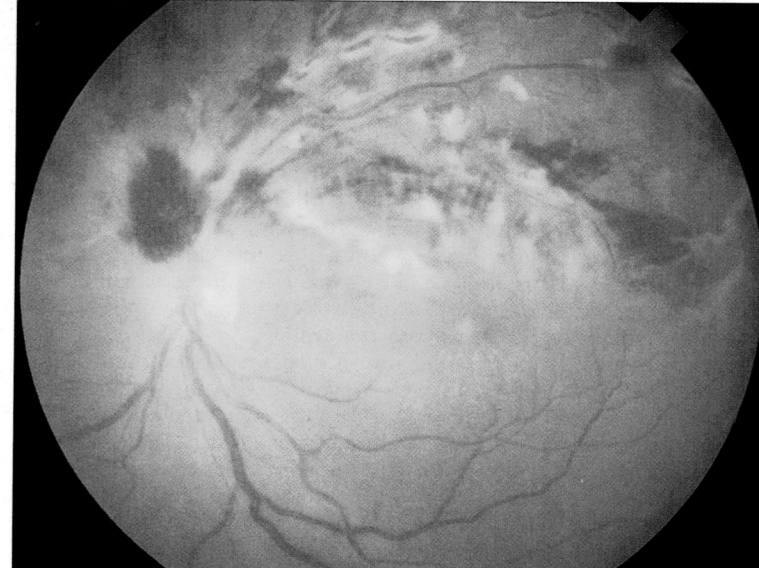

Fig. 33.7 Acute, severe, retinal vaso-occlusive disease affecting the upper temporal retinal vessels. A large number of hemorrhages and white choroidal and retinal infiltrates are present.

data are available on cyclophosphamide in the treatment of ocular Behçet disease, but some clinicians have found it as effective as chlorambucil and easier to use.[53] Cyclosporine and azathioprine have also been reported to be effective in the treatment of ocular Behçet disease, and their efficacy has been shown in randomized clinical trials.[53,82-85] However, nearly 25% of patients treated with azathioprine either had no benefit in terms of the frequency and severity of ocular attacks or required additional therapy, and only 50% of patients treated with cyclosporine had a good response.[53,82,84,85] Uncontrolled case series of patients with ocular Behçet disease treated with infliximab (Remicade) have suggested that it may be effective, although the required dose appears to be 5 mg/kg/month or higher.[86]

Microvascular vaso-occlusive disease also can affect the retinal vasculature. In SLE the retinal capillaries are involved, primarily resulting in cotton-wool spots or microinfarcts of the nerve fiber layer of the retina.[87] The prevalence of retinopathy varies widely depending on the patient population studied, from 3% of ambulatory outpatients to 28% of hospitalized patients with SLE having retinal vascular findings.[88-90] These findings occur in the absence of intraocular inflammation. More extensive retinal and vaso-occlusive disease can occur with active SLE or as a result of the antiphospholipid antibody syndrome (Fig. 33.7).[91-96]

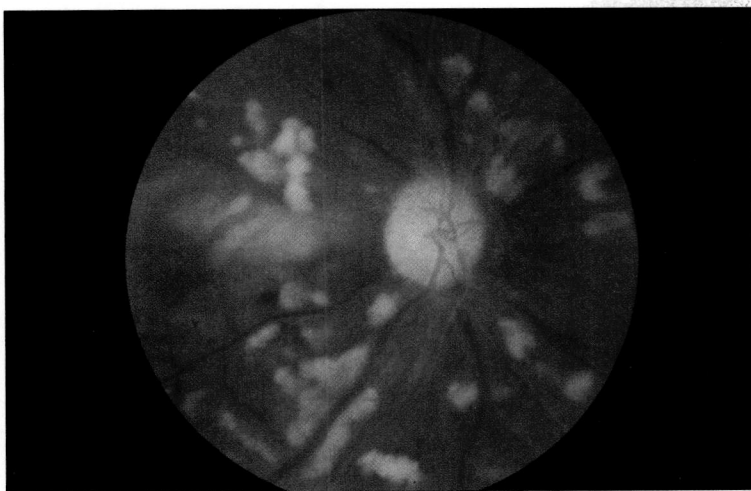

Fig. 33.8 Fundus photograph demonstrating diffuse vaso-occlusive disease in a patient with systemic lupus erythematosus. *(From Jabs DA, Fine SL, Hochberg MC, et al. Severe retinal vaso-occlusive disease in systemic lupus erythematosus. Arch Ophthalmol 1986;104:558-563.)*

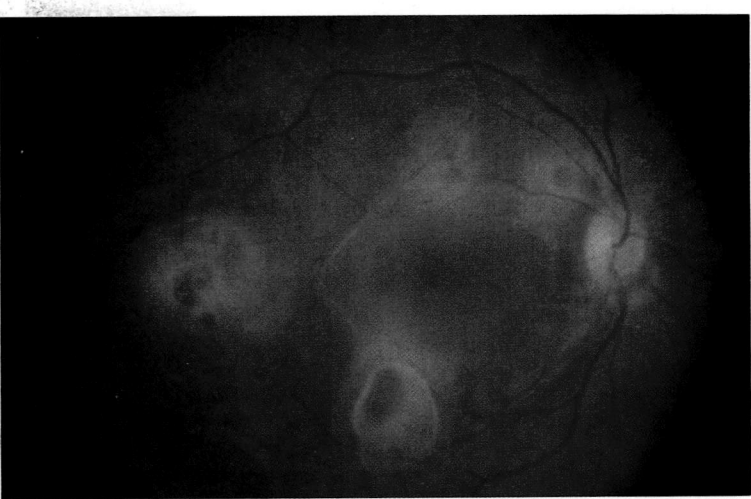

Fig. 33.9 Fundus photograph of a patient with choroidopathy and systemic lupus erythematosus. *(From Jabs DA, Hanneken AM, Schachat AP, Fine SL. Choroidopathy in systemic lupus erythematosus. Arch Ophthalmol 1988;106:230-234.)*

This more severe retinal vaso-occlusive disease occurs in less than 1% of patients with SLE, appears to be associated with central nervous system lupus,[94] and includes central retinal artery occlusion, central retinal vein occlusion, branch artery occlusion, and a diffuse retinal vaso-occlusive disease (Fig. 33.8).[97] With severe retinal vascular disease, the prognosis for vision is poor, and retinal neovascularization commonly develops. Even less common than retinopathy is lupus choroidopathy (Fig. 33.9).[91,96,98,99] The clinical changes seen in patients with lupus choroidopathy involve serous elevations of the retina, most often of the neurosensory retina; serous elevations of the retinal pigment epithelium and combined elevations may also be seen. These clinical findings are associated with a systemic vascular disease, either hypertension from lupus nephritis or systemic vasculitis.[99] Treatment of the underlying disease with systemic corticosteroids, immunosuppressive agents if needed, and control of the hypertension can lead to resolution of the serous retinal detachments.[99]

Central retinal artery occlusions can be seen in patients with giant cell arteritis (GCA), although ischemic optic neuropathy is a more classic finding (see later).[39,73,75,100]

Arteriovenous anastomoses result from shunting of blood from artery to vein without an intervening capillary bed. These are seen commonly in the midperiphery of the retina in patients with Takayasu arteritis.[1,37,101-103] The arteriovenous anastomoses can shunt blood away from the peripheral retina, which occasionally leads to areas of retinal non-perfusion with subsequent neovascularization of the retina and vitreous hemorrhage.[1,101-103]

OPTIC NERVE DISEASE

Optic nerve disease associated with rheumatic diseases includes ischemic optic neuropathy and optic neuritis.[39] The characteristic features of ischemic optic neuropathy are painless sudden loss of vision, decreased color vision, and an altitudinal visual field defect. A relative afferent pupillary defect is present in the affected eye. The optic nerve head may be swollen (as found in anterior ischemic optic neuropathy) or may appear normal initially (as in retrobulbar optic neuropathy). The visual acuity and visual field loss usually are permanent, and the optic nerve head becomes atrophic and pale (e.g., optic nerve pallor) over time. In some cases of ischemic optic neuropathy, however, partial recovery of visual acuity was seen after large doses of pulse intravenous corticosteroids (e.g., 1 g per day of methylprednisolone for 3 days).[104,105] Although ischemic optic neuropathy may occur with any type of vasculitis, as well as in SLE,[106] it is seen most commonly in GCA.[107]

Optic neuritis is characterized by acute or subacute visual loss associated with retrobulbar pain, especially with pain on movement of the affected eye. Examination of the eye reveals decreased vision, a relative afferent pupillary defect, decreased color vision, and visual field loss.

The optic nerve head may be swollen or appear normal initially, depending on whether the optic neuritis is anterior or retrobulbar. Visual symptoms result from optic nerve demyelination. Unlike ischemic optic neuropathy, up to 95% of patients with optic neuritis have a visual acuity of 20/40 or better 1 year after the event.[39] Optic neuritis most typically is associated with multiple sclerosis and responds to pulse intravenous corticosteroids with more rapid improvement of vision. Optic neuritis may also occur in SLE; such patients typically have a steroid-responsive, but also steroid-dependent, process.[1,108]

ORBITAL DISEASE

Orbital disease in rheumatic disease may include primary inflammation of the orbital tissue (e.g., orbital pseudotumor or orbital inflammatory syndrome), inflammation of the extraocular muscles (e.g., orbital myositis), or contiguous spread of inflammation from the sinuses, which most typically occurs in ANCA-associated granulomatous vasculitis.[109-111] The most common presenting sign of orbital disease is proptosis or an anterior displacement of the eye caused by a space-occupying lesion or inflammatory process. Associated symptoms and signs include pain, blurred vision, diplopia (double vision) as a result of restriction of eye movements, eyelid swelling, and displacement of the globe.[110] In ANCA-associated granulomatous vasculitis, orbital involvement is common, ranging from 15% to 50% of patients, and in some series is the most common form of ophthalmic involvement.[109,111,112] Orbital disease may be an extension of the granulomatous inflammation from the sinus into the orbit. This inflammation can lead to a compartment syndrome within the orbit, proptosis, orbital apex syndrome, compressive optic neuropathy and subsequent irreversible vision loss. Orbital pseudotumor, separate from the sinus inflammation, also may be seen.[110,112]

Systemic corticosteroids or immunosuppressive drug therapy aimed at controlling the underlying disease can decrease proptosis, improve mobility, and reduce associated symptoms, as well as improve visual acuity. Rarely, orbital decompression may be necessary if the inflammatory process has caused proptosis severe enough to compromise the optic nerve (orbital apex syndrome).

CORNEAL DISEASE

Corneal manifestations of rheumatologic disease include forms of keratitis (inflammation in the cornea) and dry eye disease or keratoconjunctivitis sicca (described in a separate section later). Keratitis is classified as interstitial keratitis (IK) or peripheral ulcerative keratitis (PUK). The diagnosis of IK includes diffuse stromal keratitis, sclerosing keratitis, and deep keratitis. PUK also is known as *marginal keratitis, marginal corneal ulceration,* or *limbal guttering.* Limbal vasculitis may

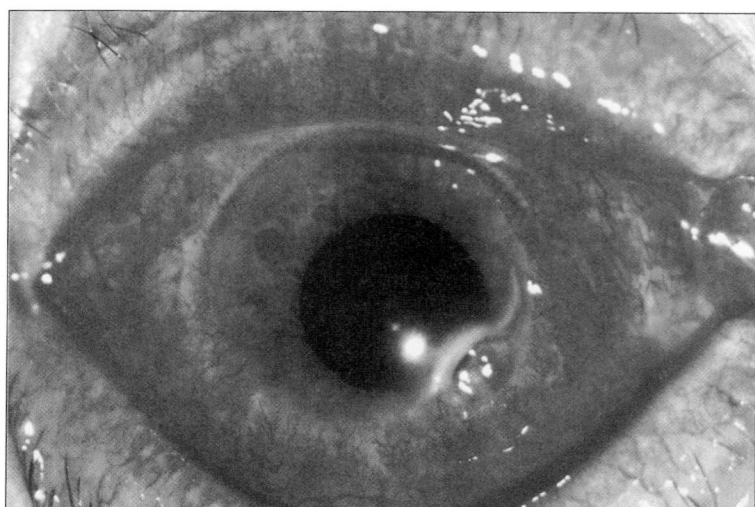

Fig. 33.10 Active corneal ulceration with corneal infiltrates at the "leading edge" of an ulcer and associated conjunctival injection.

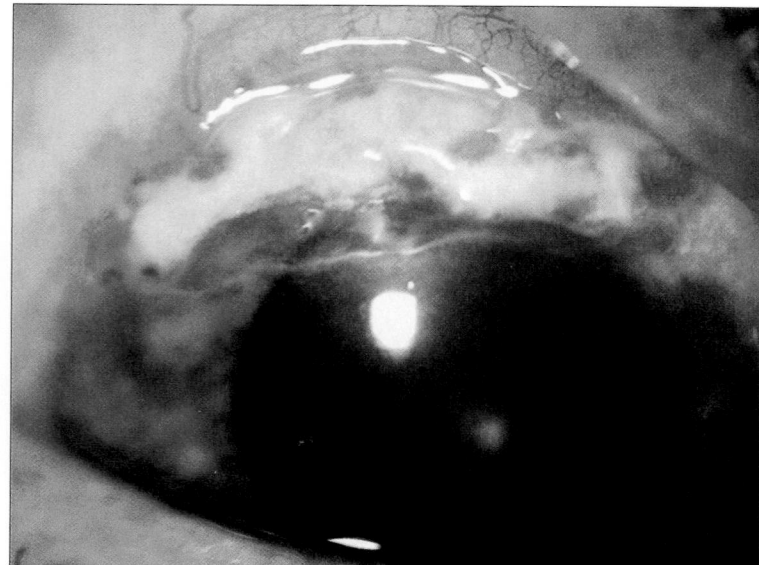

Fig. 33.11 Marginal ulceration of cornea.

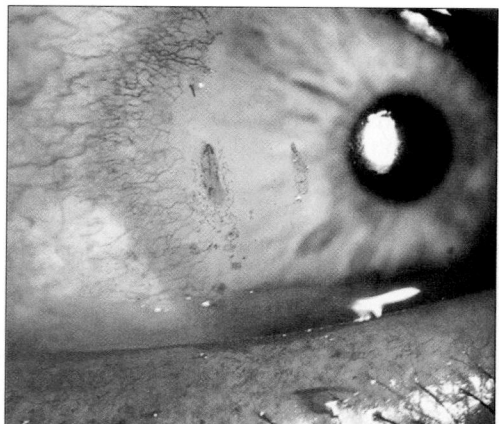

Fig. 33.12 Keratoconjunctivitis sicca.

also be seen as a rare manifestation and is not discussed further here. Keratitis may occur on its own or in association with scleritis, in which case it is termed *sclerokeratitis*. Although PUK and sclerokeratitis often are associated with rheumatic disease, infectious causes such as herpes simplex and syphilis also need to be considered.

Interstitial keratitis is characterized by a non-suppurative inflammation, usually with vascularization of the corneal stroma. It is usually caused by an immunologic response to an infectious agent (e.g., syphilis) but occasionally occurs in systemic disease, with the most common etiology being Cogan syndrome.[113] It also may occur as a common corneal complication of scleritis.[54,55,71] Pericorneal or limbal inflammation is accompanied by peripheral corneal vessels, which advance across the central cornea preceded by superficial stromal opacities. In nodular scleritis the corneal involvement may be restricted to one segment, but in diffuse scleritis the entire cornea may be involved, producing a dense corneal leukoma. The symptoms of IK include pain, tearing, photophobia, and conjunctival injection. The IK associated with Cogan syndrome typically responds to topical corticosteroid therapy.

Clinically, PUK typically presents with pain, although not always. Peripheral corneal infiltrates may develop. There is epithelial breakdown of the cornea followed by corneal ulceration and stromal thinning, which may progress circumferentially and then centrally (Fig. 33.10).[114-116] If left untreated, the lesion progresses and leads to corneal perforation and loss of vision. A bacterial corneal infection must be excluded first, particularly in patients with compromised corneal epithelia (e.g., keratoconjunctivitis sicca secondary to Sjögren syndrome). PUK typically occurs in RA and often involves the lower half of the cornea in a furrowing of the corneal periphery (Fig. 33.11). The development of PUK in patients with RA has been linked to immunologically mediated small-vessel vasculitis of the pericorneal vessels and is associated with advanced RA, elevated rheumatoid factor titers, and an increased risk of mortality.[58] PUK also has been reported to occur in other connective tissue disorders such as ANCA-associated granulomatous vasculitis, relapsing polychondritis, SLE, and progressive systemic sclerosis.[39]

Treatment of PUK is aimed at the underlying disease. Local therapy such as the use of cyanoacrylate adhesive glue and corneal or scleral patch grafts often is needed to prevent perforation and to maintain the tectonic support of the globe.[115,117-119] However, these measures eventually will fail if the underlying inflammation is not controlled. Very small central corneal perforations (<1.5 mm in diameter) may be sealed with a tissue adhesive such as cyanoacrylate glue. Larger perforations usually require emergency keratoplasty if any useful vision is to be salvaged. Topical corticosteroids usually are ineffective in the treatment of PUK and may accelerate corneal thinning and increase the risk of corneal perforation.[115,116]

KERATOCONJUNCTIVITIS SICCA

A common ocular complication of rheumatologic disease is keratoconjunctivitis sicca (KCS), or dry eye syndrome. Symptoms of KCS include dryness, ocular irritation, foreign body sensation, photophobia, and rarely pain. Sometimes patients complain of excessive tearing, which may merely describe a sensation or may be real due to tear spillover. Clinically the eyes may appear minimally affected with loss of surface luster, mild conjunctival redness, and perhaps some accumulation of mucus at the medial canthus (Fig. 33.12). Conjunctival and corneal punctate erosions occur secondary to the failure of aqueous tear secretion and chronic damage to the oil-secreting glands of the palpebral conjunctiva, which induces more rapid evaporation of tears from the ocular surface. In severe cases discrete corneal filaments may develop (filamentary keratitis), which represent tags of exfoliated epithelium still attached at one end and intermixed with surface mucin. Patients with KCS are more vulnerable to bouts of recurrent infectious conjunctivitis, perhaps as a result of reduced antibacterial tear lysozyme and lactoferrin. Thus, patients are more likely to develop corneal ulcer and perforation.

The diagnosis of KCS is made by an abnormal Schirmer test demonstrating decreased tear production (typically < 5 mm of wetting at 5 minutes in an anesthetized eye) and by demonstrating damage to the ocular surface using rose Bengal staining. The presence of KCS in association with evidence of salivary gland dysfunction, such as a positive minor salivary gland biopsy or abnormal salivary flow study, as well as the presence of a defined connective tissue disease such as rheumatoid arthritis, SLE, or scleroderma, constitutes Sjögren syndrome (Chapter 134).[120] Secondary Sjögren syndrome is diagnosed when a defined connective tissue disease is present, and primary Sjögren syndrome when no definable connective tissue disease is present. Sjögren syndrome affects approximately 11% to 13% of patients with RA and approximately 20% of patients with SLE.[1] The cause of the dry eyes and dry mouth in patients with Sjögren syndrome is a chronic lymphocytic and mononuclear inflammatory infiltrate of the lacrimal and salivary glands resulting in glandular destruction and dysfunction.[120-122] Immunohistologic studies have suggested that most cells in this infiltrate are $CD4^+$ T cells, with lesser numbers of $CD8^+$ T cells and B cells.[121,122]

The treatment of KCS includes tear replacement therapy with artificial tears, punctal occlusion, effective treatment of secondary lid disease such as blepharitis, and the use of topical cyclosporine eye drops. Topical cyclosporine appears to benefit patients with severe dry eye due to Sjögren syndrome by improving tear film break-up times and decreasing rose Bengal staining of the corneal surface.[123,124] It has been suggested that the mode of action for topical cyclosporine may be decreased inflammation of the lacrimal gland leading to improved lacrimal gland function and an increase in tear production.[123]

KEY REFERENCES

1. Thorne JE, Jabs DA. Rheumatic diseases. In: Ryan SJ, ed. The retina, 4th ed. London: Elsevier, 2006:1383-1408.
2. The Standardization of Uveitis Nomenclature (SUN) Working Group. Standardization of uveitis nomenclature for reporting clinical data. Results of the first international workshop. Am J Ophthalmol 2005;140:509-516.
3. Rosenbaum JT. Acute anterior uveitis and spondyloarthropathies. Rheum Dis Clin North Am 1992;18:143-151.
4. Smit RLMJ, Baarsma GS. Epidemiology of uveitis. Curr Opin Ophthalmol 1995;6:57-61.
6. Khan MA. Update on spondyloarthropathies. Ann Intern Med 2002;136:896-907.
8. Tay-Kearney ML, Schwam BL, Lowder C, et al. Clinical features and associated systemic diseases of HLA-B27 uveitis. Am J Ophthalmol 1996;121:47-56.
11. Bernstein CN, Blanchard JF, Rawsthorne P, et al. The prevalence of extraintestinal diseases in inflammatory bowel disease: a population-based study. Am J Gastroenterol 2001;96:1116-1122.
17. Banares A, Hernandez-Garcia C, Fernandez-Gutierrez B, et al. Eye involvement in the spondyloarthropathies. Rheum Dis Clin North Am 1998;24:771-784.
21. Paivonsalo-Hietanen T, Tuominen J, Vaahtoranta-Lehtonen H, et al. Incidence and prevalence of different uveitis entities in Finland. Acta Ophthalmol Scand 1997;75:76-81.
27. Ravelli A, Felici E, Magni-Manzoni S, et al. Patients with antinuclear antibody-positive juvenile idiopathic arthritis constitute a homogeneous subgroup irrespective of the course of joint disease. Arthritis Rheum 2005;52:826-832.
28. Cassidy J, Kivlin J, Lindsley C, Nocton J. Ophthalmologic examinations in children with juvenile rheumatoid arthritis. Pediatrics 2006;117:1843-1845.
29. Woreta F, Thorne JE, Jabs DA, et al. Risk factors for ocular complications and poor visual acuity at presentation among patients with uveitis associated with juvenile idiopathic arthritis (JIA). Am J Ophthalmol 2007;143:647-655.
30. Thorne JE, Woreta F, Kedhar SR, et al. Juvenile idiopathic arthritis (JIA)-associated uveitis: incidence of ocular complications and visual acuity loss. Am J Ophthalmol 2007;143:840-846.
34. Edelsten C, Lee V, Bentley CR, et al. An evaluation of baseline risk factors predicting severity in juvenile idiopathic arthritis associated uveitis and other chronic anterior uveitis in early childhood. Br J Ophthalmol 2002;86:51-56.
35. Heiligenhaus A, Niewerth M, Mingels A, et al. Epidemiology of uveitis in juvenile idiopathic arthritis from a national paediatric rheumatologic and ophthalmologic database. Klin Monatsbl Augenheilkd 2005;222:993-1001.

39. Thorne JE, Jabs DA. Ocular manifestations of vasculitis. Rheum Dis Clin North Am 2001;27:761-779.
40. Mamo JG, Bagghdassarian A. Behçet's disease: a report of 28 cases. Arch Ophthalmol 1964;71:4-14.
44. Jabs DA, Houk JL, Bias WB, Arnett FC. Familial granulomatous synovitis, uveitis, and cranial neuropathies. Am J Ophthalmol 1985;78:801-806.
45. Blau EB. Familial granulomatous arthritis, iritis, and rash. J Pediatr 1985;107:689-693.
46. Latkany PA, Jabs DA, Smith JR, et al. Multifocal choroiditis in patients with familial juvenile systemic granulomatosis. Am J Ophthalmol 2002;134:897-904.
53. Jabs DA, Rosenbaum JT, Foster CS, et al. Guidelines for the use of immunosuppressive drugs in patients with ocular inflammatory disorders: recommendations of an expert panel. Am J Ophthalmol 2000;130:492-513.
54. Jabs DA, Mudun A, Dunn JP, et al. Episcleritis and scleritis: clinical features and treatment results. Am J Ophthalmol 2000;130:469-476.
55. Akpek EK, Thorne JE, Qazi FA, et al. Evaluation of patients with scleritis for systemic disease. Ophthalmology 2004;111:501-506.
58. Foster CS, Forstot SL, Wilson LA. Mortality rate in rheumatoid arthritis patients developing necrotizing scleritis or peripheral ulcerative keratitis. Ophthalmology 1984;91:1253-1263.
62. Fauci AS, Haynes BF, Katz P, et al. ANCA-associated granulomatous vasculitis: prospective clinical and therapeutic experience with 85 patients for 21 years. Ann Intern Med 1983;98:76-85.
63. Sainz de la Maza M, Foster CS, Jabbur NS. Scleritis associated with systemic vasculitic diseases. Ophthalmology 1995;102:687-692.
66. Hopkins DJ, Horan E, Burton IL, et al. Ocular disorders in a series of 332 patients with Crohn's disease. Br J Ophthalmol 1974;58:732-737.
69. Hoang-Xuan T, Foster CS, Rice BA. Scleritis in relapsing polychondritis: response to therapy. Ophthalmology 1990;97:892-897.
73. Thorne JE, Jabs DA, Qazi FA, et al. Mycophenolate mofetil therapy for inflammatory eye disease. Ophthalmology 2005;112:1472-1477.
74. Stanford MR, Verity DH. Diagnostic and therapeutic approach to patients with retinal vasculitis. Int Ophthalmol Clin 2000;40:69-83.
76. Mamo JG. The rate of visual loss in Behçet's disease. Arch Ophthalmol 1970;84:451-452.
78. Tessler HH, Jennings T. High-dose short-term chlorambucil for intractable sympathetic ophthalmia and Behçet's disease. Br J Ophthalmol 1990;74:353-357.
80. Mamo JG. Treatment of Behçet's disease with chlorambucil. Arch Ophthalmol 1976;94:580-583.
82. Nussenblatt RB, Palestine AG, Chan CC, et al. Effectiveness of cyclosporin therapy for Behçet's disease. Arthritis Rheum 1985;28:671-679.

83. Masuda K, Nakajima A, Urayama A, et al. Double-masked trial of cyclosporine versus colchicine and long-term open study of cyclosporine in Behçet's disease. Lancet 1989;1:1093-1096.
84. Whitcup SM, Salvo EC, Nussenblatt RB. Combined cyclosporine and corticosteroid therapy for sight-threatening uveitis in Behçet's disease. Am J Ophthalmol 1994;118:39-45.
85. Yazici J, Pazarli H, Barnes CG, et al. A controlled trial of azathioprine in Behçet's syndrome. N Engl J Med 1990;322:281-285.
86. Braun J, Baraliakos X, Listing J, Sieper J. Decreased incidence of anterior uveitis in patients with ankylosing spondylitis treated with the anti-tumor necrosis factor agents infliximab and etanercept. Arthritis Rheum 2005;52:2447-2451.
87. Nguyen QD, Foster CS. Systemic lupus erythematosus and the eye. Int Ophthalmol Clin 1998;38:33-60.
92. Klinkhoff AV, Beattie CW, Chalmers A. Retinopathy in systemic lupus erythematosus: relationship to disease activity. Arthritis Rheum 1986;29:1152-1156.
97. Jabs DA, Fine SL, Hochberg MC, et al. Severe retinal vasoocclusive disease in systemic lupus erythematosus. Arch Ophthalmol 1986;104:558-563.
99. Jabs DA, Hanneken AM, Schachat AP, et al. Choroidopathy in systemic lupus erythematosus. Arch Ophthalmol 1988;106:230-234.
100. Abu El-Asrar AM, Tabbara KF. Retinal vasculitis. Curr Opin Ophthalmol 1997;8:68-79.
102. Chun YS, Park SJ, Park IK, et al. The clinical and ocular manifestations of Takayasu arteritis. Retina 2001;21:132-140.
104. Borruat FX. Neuro-ophthalmologic manifestations of rheumatologic and associated disorders. Curr Opin Ophthalmol 1996;7:10-18.
107. Hayreh SS, Podhajsky PA, Zimmerman B. Ocular manifestations of giant cell arteritis. Am J Ophthalmol 1998;125:509-520.
112. Bullen CL, Liesegang TJ, McDonald TJ, et al. Ocular complications of ANCA-associated granulomatous vasculitis. Ophthalmology 1983;90:279-290.
115. Shiuey Y, Foster CS. Peripheral ulcerative keratitis and collagen vascular disease. Int Ophthalmol Clin 1998;38:21-32.
116. Tauber J, Sainz de la Maza M, Hoang-Zuan T, et al. An analysis of therapeutic decision-making regarding immunosuppressive chemotherapy for peripheral ulcerative keratitis. Cornea 1990;9:66-73.
120. Fox RI, Törnwall J, Michelson P. Current issues in the diagnosis and treatment of Sjögren's syndrome. Curr Opin Rheumatol 1999;11:364-371.

REFERENCES

Full references for this chapter can be found on www.expertconsult.com.

The heart in rheumatic disease

34

R. Michael Benitez, Gautam Ramani, and Patricia A. Uber

- There are several causes of chest pain in patients with systemic rheumatic disease; several are benign but others may indicate significant cardiovascular disease.
- Cardiovascular involvement has been most commonly associated with rheumatoid arthritis and systemic lupus erythematosus (SLE), though it has been described in a wide variety of systemic rheumatic diseases.
- There is an increased incidence of coronary artery disease in patients with systemic lupus erythematosus and rheumatoid arthritis, independent of traditional atherosclerotic risk factors.
- Anticardiolipin antibody syndromes can present difficult diagnostic and therapeutic challenges and may occur independently of SLE or other systemic rheumatic diseases.
- Heart and great vessel disease may present in an indolent fashion and must be suspected in patients with unexplained cardiovascular symptoms and rheumatoid arthritis, giant cell arteritis, or sarcoidosis.

THE HEART IN RHEUMATIC DISEASE

The heart is frequently involved in the most common rheumatic illnesses, as a result of direct inflammatory disease, secondary proatherosclerotic effects of inflammation, or medications directed at treatment of the systemic disease. The resulting cardiac complications range in spectrum from subclinical involvement to overt myocardial infarction or stroke and contribute significantly to morbidity and mortality in patients with rheumatic disease. Recognition of cardiac involvement in rheumatic disease is crucial to therapeutic decision-making in obtaining the best outcomes in these patients.

GENERAL APPROACH TO THE PATIENT

History and physical

Chest discomfort, dyspnea, dizziness, palpitations, and edema are the most common presenting symptoms referable to cardiovascular disease. A directed history with regard to these cardinal symptoms may provide important clues to etiology. Chest pain related to ischemic coronary artery disease is most classically a vague, visceral discomfort, located retrosternally, beginning slowly during exertion and increasing in crescendo fashion. Relief is obtained with rest or nitroglycerin. The overall duration of the discomfort is generally longer than 5 minutes and less than 30. Myocardial infarction should be considered when typical ischemic discomfort is present for longer than 30 minutes. The discomfort of myocardial ischemia must be distinguished from pericardial or pleuritic pain or esophageal spasm. Pericardial pain is generally described as sharp, tends to be worse when supine, and may be lessened by sitting upright and leaning forward. The discomfort may be present at rest and may endure for hours or days. Auscultation may disclose the characteristic leathery friction rub, present in systole and diastole, although this finding can be highly positional and evanescent. Sharp localized discomfort present during deep inspiration or cough is more typical of pleural involvement. Physical examination may disclose moderate or large effusions characterized by dullness to percussion associated with diminished breath sounds. Small effusions may avoid physical detection. Pericardial and pleuritic pain does not respond to nitroglycerin and relief is more likely with anti-inflammatory medica-

tions. Esophageal spasm may produce retrosternal visceral discomfort that can be difficult to differentiate from myocardial ischemia and which may be relieved with nitroglycerin. Important historical clues suggestive of esophageal spasm include an association with eating or drinking (especially hot or cold beverages) rather than with physical exertion. Typical anginal discomfort may also occur, especially with exertion, in patients with severe pulmonary hypertension.

Dyspnea may result from widely varied pathophysiologic processes, including myocardial dysfunction, valvular heart disease, pericardial disease, pulmonary parenchymal disease, venous thromboembolism, and pleural effusion. Cardiac causes of dyspnea are more likely in the patient who describes orthopnea, the sensation of breathlessness while supine.

Palpitations, the subjective awareness of one's heart beat, are common and range in significance from a manifestation of occasional benign ectopy to the sentinels of significant underlying structural heart disease. When palpitations are associated with dizziness, syncope, dyspnea, or chest pain, further directed cardiac evaluation is appropriate. Single, rare palpitations without associated symptoms are more likely to be benign in origin.

A directed cardiovascular examination should include palpation of all peripheral pulses. Blood pressure should be recorded in both arms and in the legs if there is asymmetry or discordance of the pulses. A regularly irregular pulse may reflect atrioventricular block, whereas an irregularly irregular pulse usually reflects atrial fibrillation, which often accompanies significant valvular heart disease, myocardial disease, or pericardial disease. Auscultation of the carotid and subclavian arteries, as well as the abdominal aorta, should be performed with special attention to the presence of bruits. Asymmetric blood pressures or pulses or vascular bruits over large vessels are important potential signs of a large-vessel vasculitis such as Takayasu. The sternum and the point of maximal impulse should be palpated with the palm to assess for a right ventricular heave associated with pulmonary hypertension or evidence of left ventricular enlargement. The degree of jugular venous distention and the jugular waveform should be inspected in each patient. Elevation of the jugular venous waveform confirms high right heart pressure; this may result from left ventricular dysfunction of any cause or may reflect pulmonary hypertension or significant pericardial disease. Further cardiac auscultation may provide important clues such as a third heart sound in patients with myocardial dysfunction. The presence of any diastolic murmur is pathologic and may reflect aortic regurgitation due to aortitis or pulmonic insufficiency due to severe pulmonary hypertension. Any systolic murmur of grade III intensity or greater deserves further investigation to exclude significant mitral regurgitation, tricuspid regurgitation (due to pulmonary hypertension), or aortic stenosis. The presence of an enlarged liver with systolic expansion is characteristic of pulmonary hypertension, either primary or secondary. The presence of ascites on physical examination should alert the clinician to the possibility of constrictive pericarditis, especially in the patient with longstanding rheumatoid arthritis. The lower extremities should be inspected for edema, which may accompany left ventricular dysfunction, pulmonary hypertension, or pericardial disease. Lower extremity edema without concomitant jugular venous distention or a cardiac gallop on examination is more likely to be related to venous or lymphatic disease or hypoalbuminemia. Unilateral lower extremity edema suggests the possibilities of deep venous thrombosis or rupture of a popliteal cyst.

Laboratory testing

The electrocardiogram (ECG) is an inexpensive and widely available tool that can provide insight regarding cardiac involvement in patients with rheumatic disease. One should be obtained as part of the evaluation of any patient with chest pain, dyspnea, palpitations, or findings on examination that suggest cardiac disease such as pulmonary rales, jugular venous distention, a significant murmur, a gallop, or peripheral edema. The ECG can provide information regarding prior infarction, repolarization abnormalities that may indicate ischemia or pericarditis, and important information about atrioventricular conduction and arrhythmias.

Palpitations are best evaluated using either an ambulatory (Holter) monitor or longer-term event monitor. Holter monitors, which are typically worn for 24 to 48 hours, are useful for documenting the mechanism of palpitations when they occur on a nearly daily basis. When palpitations occur less frequently or in an unpredictable fashion, event monitors may be used for up to 30 days, thereby increasing the chance of accurate determination of cardiac rhythm during symptoms. An implantable loop recorder may be inserted subcutaneously, if needed, in order to determine cardiac rhythm during infrequent but clinically worrisome events that have not been electrocardiographically documented by Holter or event recorder. Loop recorders may remain in place for up to a year and are "interrogated" with a transcutaneous wand for data retrieval.

When cardiac disease is suspected, posteroanterior and lateral chest radiograms can yield important information regarding cardiac chamber size. Left atrial dilatation, left ventricular hypertrophy, left ventricular dilatation, and right heart enlargement can all be deduced on the basis of the cardiac silhouette. Additionally, a "water-flask" silhouette may suggest pericardial effusion, and pericardial calcification may disclose constrictive disease. Inspection of the pulmonary arteries may suggest the presence of pulmonary hypertension, and pleural effusions may be documented, especially on the lateral film.

Transthoracic echocardiography yields robust information regarding ventricular cavity size, mass, systolic function, and diastolic filling. Additionally, valvular structure and function can be assessed, along with quantitative analysis of stenotic and regurgitant lesions. Pulmonary artery systolic pressure can be accurately assessed from Doppler measurements of a tricuspid regurgitant jet. Echocardiography is useful in the evaluation of pericardial effusions and can yield important information regarding its hemodynamic significance when present. Directed Doppler echocardiographic techniques including tissue Doppler can also be useful in evaluating patients for suspected pericardial constriction and differentiating this from restrictive cardiomyopathy. Current guidelines from the American College of Cardiology Foundation and the American Society of Echo state that a transthoracic echocardiographic evaluation is appropriate in patients with:

- Dyspnea, dizziness, syncope, or cerebrovascular events
- Significant atrial or ventricular dysrhythmias (not single PACs/PVCs)
- Known or suspected pulmonary hypertension
- Any diastolic, late-systolic, or holosystolic murmur
- Suspected pericardial disease, including constriction or pericardial tamponade
- Heart failure or suspected infiltrative cardiomyopathy (such as amyloid)

Transesophageal echocardiograms often provide increased clarity and definition of cardiac structures and the aorta and have shown increased sensitivity for the detection of infective and non-infective endocarditis and cardiac thrombus. They may also be useful for more accurate quantification of regurgitant valvular lesions, especially with respect to mitral regurgitation. However, transesophageal echocardiography is not routinely warranted as an initial form of testing, with a few exceptions:

- Evaluation of suspected acute aortic pathology, including aortic dissection, penetrating atheroma, or intramural hematoma
- To diagnose and manage endocarditis in a patient with a moderate or high pretest probability
- Evaluation of a patient with atrial fibrillation/flutter to assist clinical decision-making with regard to anticoagulation and cardioversion

Computed tomography (CT) can be useful for imaging the pericardium in cases of suspected constriction, both to document pericardial

thickening and calcification. Multidetector CT can also be useful for the detection and quantitative measurement of coronary calcium, which has been employed for coronary risk assessment. With the use of intravenous contrast, CT coronary angiography can provide a non-invasive means of visualized coronary stenosis. There is continued debate with regards to the appropriate use of these tools, and future study should help us to better understand who should undergo these types of tests versus stress testing or conventional angiography.

Cardiac catheterization should be reserved for patients with unstable coronary syndromes or in whom there is a non-invasive test indicating a high probability of significant coronary disease. Right and left heart catheterization can also be useful, in tandem with echocardiography, in establishing a diagnosis of pericardial constriction and in differentiating this from restrictive cardiomyopathy.

CARDIAC ILLNESS AND MEDICATIONS USED FOR RHEUMATIC DISEASE

Several pharmacologic therapies used in rheumatologic disease have been reported to adversely influence cardiovascular outcomes either in the setting of experimental clinical trials or during postmarketing surveillance. Several mechanisms could be operative in determining this adverse influence, including a direct mechanistic effect of the drugs used or an important interaction with concomitant medications. In patients with preexisting cardiovascular risk markers, subclinical disease, or overt disease, the adverse consequences of these agents may be further compounded.

Cyclooxygenase-2 (COX-2) inhibitors were initially considered better tolerated than more traditional nonsteroidal anti-inflammatory agents (NSAIDs), but evidence of accelerated risk of major cardiovascular events, including acute myocardial infarction and sudden death, surfaced postmarketing. The Vioxx GI Outcomes Research (VIGOR) study investigated rofecoxib versus naproxen on gastrointestinal tolerability in patients with rheumatoid arthritis.[1] This trial was halted early due to a higher rate of cardiovascular adverse events seen with rofecoxib. An increased risk for cardiovascular death, myocardial infarction, or stroke of nearly twofold was seen with rofecoxib compared with placebo in the colonic polyp prevention Adenomatous Polyp Prevention on Vioxx (APPROVe) trial, leading to the removal of this agent from the market.[2] Celecoxib, a coxib with relatively low COX-2 selectivity, was also used in colon polyp prevention trials that revealed a significantly higher risk of cardiovascular death, myocardial infarction, stroke, or heart failure combined endpoint, depending on the dosing strategy assigned. When celecoxib was prescribed at a dose of 400 mg once a day, the level of cardiovascular risk was less pronounced, suggesting a dose-response relationship.[3] An imbalance between thromboxane and prostacyclin leading to a prothrombotic state has been proposed as the mechanism for the increase in cardiovascular risk. The data with NSAIDs are not entirely sanguine. NSAIDs have been associated with myocardial infarction in large retrospective studies or case-controlled studies and may be attributable to a variable degree of platelet COX-1 inhibition allowing for reversible platelet inhibition during the dosing interval.[4] Both NSAIDs and coxibs are associated with new-onset hypertension, as well as attenuated control of blood pressure management. This interaction is worsened by the presence of renal disease and the use of antihypertensives such as angiotensin-converting enzyme (ACE) inhibitors, which act on the renin-angiotensin-aldosterone cascade.[5] Administration of coxibs or NSAIDs to heart failure patients has been linked with clinical deterioration and increased risk of heart failure–related hospitalization.

The introduction of anti–tumor necrosis factor (TNF)-α agents has culminated in clinical improvement in many rheumatologic illnesses. Although proinflammatory cytokines such as TNF-α and interleukin (IL)-6 are recognized as important components in the development and progression of atherosclerosis and heart failure, these agents have not shown clinical benefits with regard to cardiovascular disease. The use of TNF-α antagonist in patients with heart failure has not led to improved clinical status and, in one study, was linked to a dose-related increase in death and hospitalization for heart failure.[6] Reports of new-onset heart failure linked to TNF-α antagonist agents prescribed to patients for rheumatoid arthritis in the Food and Drug Administration

MedWatch program have emerged.[7] In more than half of the observed cases, congestive heart failure (CHF) has developed without associated hypertension, diabetes, or myocardial infarction and may not be age related. The use of TNF-α antagonists in patients with existent heart failure is discouraged and clinical monitoring for signs or symptoms of new heart failure is prudent.

RHEUMATOID ARTHRITIS

Rheumatoid arthritis (RA) is the most common chronic inflammatory polyarthritis and is estimated to affect approximately 1% of the adult population. Survival among patients with rheumatoid arthritis is significantly worse than in the general population, and this disparity has remained constant in recent decades. This excess mortality is primarily due to ischemic cardiovascular disease[8] and is not attributable solely to traditional risk factors.[9] Chronic systemic inflammatory responses in rheumatoid arthritis are similar to those occurring in atherosclerotic plaque, suggesting that such systemic inflammation contributes to accelerated cardiac risk. T-cell activation occurs in both processes, including an expanded population of $CD4^+CD28^-$ T cells,[9] which can directly injure endothelium.[10] Repair of injured endothelium, in part, is accomplished by circulating endothelial progenitor cells (EPC)—however, such repair may be impaired in rheumatoid arthritis due to reduced numbers of circulating EPCs.[11] Macrophage activation is also characteristic of both rheumatoid arthritis and atherosclerotic plaque, with elaboration of the proinflammatory cytokines TNF-α and IL-6. Endothelial dysfunction is apparent early in the natural history of rheumatoid arthritis,[12] and the use of antagonists to proinflammatory cytokines has been associated with improvement in vascular function in patients with RA.[13] RA is also associated with increased expression of adhesion molecules such as VCAM-1 and ICAM-1, which are important in endothelial adhesion of monocytes, the precursors of tissue macrophages, which form an integral part of the atherosclerotic plaque.

Although patients with RA are at increased risk of atherosclerotic coronary events, they may not behave in similar fashion to matched cohorts without RA with respect to clinical manifestations. Specifically, patients with RA are less likely to present with typical angina and are more likely to suffer silent infarction or sudden cardiac death as the initial presentation of ischemic heart disease. It is not clear whether ischemic disease is perceived differently in patients with RA, if pain is masked by the chronic use of other analgesics, or if physician response to complaints of discomfort from patients with RA is responsible for this apparent discrepancy.

It is critical for health care providers to recognize the increased ischemic cardiovascular risk inherent in patients with RA. Efforts to minimize the risk of ischemic events should include the use of HMG-CoA reductase inhibitors (statins) whenever levels of low-density lipoprotein (LDL) are elevated despite reasonable dietary measures. Because statins have anti-inflammatory effects, as well as lipid-lowering effects, it seems reasonable to conclude that high-dose statin use in patients with RA may lead to long-term reduction in cardiac risk. To date, no study to specifically address the optimal LDL level or dose of statin in patients with RA has been completed to address this issue. The best data to date regarding statin use in RA come from the Trial of Atorvastatin in Rheumatoid Arthritis (TARA), in which patients were randomized in double-blind fashion to receive either atorvastatin 40 mg daily, or placebo, for 6 months.[14] The TARA trial was not designed to test the hypothesis that atorvastatin would reduce major cardiovascular events, but it did yield important data regarding safety and rheumatologic disease activity. Interestingly, despite relatively high-dose statin use, no elevation of transaminases was noted, even in patients concomitantly using methotrexate. Additionally, no patients demonstrated new elevation of creatine kinase while on statin therapy. C-reactive protein (CRP) levels fell by an average 50% in the statin treatment group in comparison with placebo, and erythrocyte sedimentation rates (ESRs) and levels of IL-6 were significantly reduced. Additionally, subjects receiving atorvastatin showed significant improvement in a disease activity score (DAS28) compared with placebo. The combination of ezetimibe/simvastatin has recently shown similar improvement in disease activity score and markers of inflammation with one other added benefit: measured improvement in aortic stiffness and endothelial function.[15] Whether long-term statin therapy should be routinely used as an adjunct anti-inflammatory and whether such use will lead to reduction in cardiovascular mortality is yet to be determined.

In addition to consideration of statin use, current clinical guidelines have suggested limitation of glucocorticoid use to the minimal effective dose, following two case-control studies that have suggested it may increase cardiovascular risks in patients with RA.[16,17] These same guidelines have suggested that routine use of aspirin is not indicated in patients with RA for primary prevention. In patients for whom secondary prevention with aspirin is indicated, it should be recognized that concomitant use of NSAIDs may decrease the antiplatelet effects of aspirin. Interestingly, methotrexate may have cardioprotective effects as compared with other forms of therapy for RA. A retrospective cohort study of veterans with either RA or psoriasis suggested that low to moderate doses of methotrexate bore lower itinerant cardiovascular risk than other disease-modifying antirheumatic drugs,[18] and similar findings were noted in a prospective observational study.[19]

Recent data yield hope that progress is being made with regard to cardiovascular risk in patients with RA.[20] Death rates and time trends in mortality caused by acute myocardial infarction with respect to successive incidence in a large cohort of patients followed for 17 years were examined. During the period of observation, the use of methotrexate increased substantially while glucocorticoid use remained stable. The risk of acute infarction declined in successive incidence years, with the risk for incident years after 1990 being equal to the general population. A similar but smaller analysis suggests that glucocorticoid use results in higher cardiovascular event rates only in patients who are rheumatoid factor positive—raising the possibility that within this specific cohort, glucocorticoid-sparing regimens may be preferable in reducing ischemic risk.[21] The use of statins and aspirin within this cohort have not been examined.

Pericarditis is reportedly common in RA, with estimates (derived from either autopsy or echocardiogram) of involvement of up to 50% of patients. However, these estimates were all derived in the late 1960s and early 1970s, when disease-modifying regimens including methotrexate and anti-TNF-α were not available. Despite this high frequency of disease, few patients present with acute symptoms typical of pericarditis and a more indolent effusive inflammation is more common. Given that acute symptomatic pericarditis is less common, there are no comparative treatment trials and the mainstay of therapy for acute disease without hemodynamic compromise remains glucocorticoid and/or NSAID therapy. Colchicine is safe and effective in the treatment of recurrent idiopathic pericarditis. Although it has not been studied extensively in RA, case reports have promoted its benefit for relief of recurrent pericarditis/tamponade and the safety profile of the drug makes it attractive. Pericardiocentesis is not routinely indicated without evidence of hemodynamic compromise, unless clinical suspicion of an infectious pathogen is high, and should generally be reserved as part of the acute treatment of tamponade. The characteristics of pericardial fluid in RA may be quite variable; leukocyte counts vary considerably, although almost always with neutrophil predominance. The glucose level may be low (as in pleural effusions) but is not invariably so. The presence of rheumatoid factor in the fluid does not confirm the process as being related to RA. Neither does a high level of cytokines such as IL-6, which may be found in a rheumatic process. Chronic, indolent, or recurrent pericarditis may progress to mixed effusive-constrictive or frankly constrictive pericardial disease and must be differentiated from amyloid-related restrictive cardiomyopathy. Echocardiographically derived tissue Doppler velocities, as well as invasive hemodynamic studies, may be useful in conjunction with imaging of the pericardium by CT or magnetic resonance imaging (MRI) to help establish the correct diagnosis. Systemic corticosteroids and, more recently, the use of an antagonist to TNF-α[22] have met with modest success in the treatment of hemodynamically significant effusive-constrictive disease, and in patients without severe compromise such treatment may be warranted before committing them to surgical pericardiectomy. Patients with pure constriction, particularly those with calcific constriction, are likely to obtain relief only through pericardiectomy.

Clinical congestive heart failure is twice as common in patients with RA compared with matched populations without the disease.[23] However, definition of this increased incidence of clinical CHF has been established using Framingham Heart Study criteria, which do not effectively discriminate between systolic and diastolic dysfunction. Some echocardiographic studies have demonstrated that RA is associated with increased left ventricular mass but not with reduced ejection fraction, whereas others have suggested that definite systolic dysfunction (left ventricular ejection fraction < 40%) is much more likely in patients with RA than the general population. Regardless of systolic function, mortality among RA patients with a clinical diagnosis of CHF is significantly higher than in a matched general population, with cumulative 1-year mortality for RA in excess of 30%.[24] The mechanism involved in the cardiomyopathy of RA is not well understood, appears to be independent of coronary artery disease, and may be directly related to the systemic inflammatory state. Observation of patients free of heart failure at the index of RA diagnosis has demonstrated a significant elevation of ESR during the 6-month interval preceding a clinical diagnosis of CHF.[25]

Secondary (AA) amyloidosis deserves separate consideration as a form of cardiomyopathy. Cardiac amyloidosis has long been considered a rare extra-articular manifestation of RA. However, a recent re-evaluation of autopsy specimens from RA patients demonstrated a remarkably high incidence of 30%, with cardiac amyloid being as frequent as renal.[26] Within this series, an antemortem diagnosis of amyloidosis was made in only 37% of patients with histologically proven disease. In part, this demonstrates a difference between pathologically present versus clinically relevant amyloid. Whether earlier detection and treatment would alter cardiac outcomes is unclear, although some studies of RA patients with novel AA amyloid polymorphisms suggest that this holds true[27] and that aggressive therapy with cyclophosphamide and prednisolone or etanercept may improve outcomes.[28] Cardiac amyloidosis appears to be more frequent in male patients with long-lasting RA of increased disease activity and may contribute to atrioventricular conduction block, as well as CHF.

VASCULITIS

Takayasu arteritis

Takayasu arteritis (TA) principally affects the aorta and its major branches in young, predominantly Oriental women. Once thought to be related to infectious etiologies, including tuberculosis, studies among identical twins have suggested a genetic predisposition, and there appears to be a significant association of TA with the antigens Bw52 and DR12,[29] as well as particular HLA haplotypes.[30] The disease is uncommon, the onset is insidious, and a high degree of suspicion should be maintained in young women with hypertension, asymmetric upper arm blood pressures, and vascular bruits. Diagnosis is established in young patients (<40 years) by the combined presence of subclavian stenosis and constitutional signs and symptoms. Although subclavian stenosis is the most common arterial manifestation, TA may also involve the ostia of the coronary arteries or the proximal portions of the renal arteries, resulting in cardiac ischemia and renovascular hypertension, respectively. The descending thoracic aorta may be narrowed in a "rat-tail" fashion and, uncommonly, ascending aortic aneurysms may form, resulting in aortic valvular incompetence caused by annuloaortic dilatation. The latter appears to be more common among Japanese patients and is an important risk factor for mortality within that population.[31] Pathologically, inflammation begins within the vasa vasorum, followed by T-cell infiltration of the media and/or adventitia. Subsequent inflammatory changes closely resemble a typical atherosclerotic cascade, and a "burnt-out" inflammatory lesion may be indistinguishable from usual atherosclerosis.

Medical treatment with corticosteroids remains the mainstay of therapy during the acute inflammatory period of the disease, but long-term use of steroids may adversely affect atherosclerotic transformation. Tapering of steroids every 2 weeks to the minimal dose effective in suppressing inflammation as evidenced by serum markers such as ESR or CRP has been recommended. Non-steroidal immunosuppressive agents have been recommended as adjuncts for patients resistant to steroid withdrawal or cessation.[32] Aspirin use during the acute inflammatory phase has been recommended to prevent thrombosis superimposed on the arteritis. During the chronic occlusive stage of TA, percutaneous techniques have become the treatment of choice for

dilatation and/or stenting of coronary ostial lesions, renovascular lesions, and subclavian lesions.[33] Although restenosis is always a concern, the high degree of initial procedural success, coupled with low procedural morbidity, have made these interventions attractive in comparison with surgery. Surgical repair has long been the mainstay of treatment for aortic complications such as "pseudo-coarctation" and aneurysm and remains the only current choice for repair of annuloaortic ectasia with valvular incompetence. Recently, percutaneous balloon dilatation has been reported,[34] with mixed initial success, for treatment of aortic pseudo-coarctation and percutaneous stent-grafts have been deployed for descending aortic aneurysm.[35] Although these techniques hold promise, long-term outcome data, as compared with surgery, have not yet accrued.

Kawasaki disease

Kawasaki disease (KD) is an acute febrile illness that affects predominantly boys, aged 6 months to 4 years, with involvement of the skin, mucosa, lymph nodes, and coronary arteries. Although the precise etiology of KD is not known, most data suggest genetic predisposition coupled with a suspected infectious trigger. In response to this unknown stimulus, mononuclear cells and platelets interact with vascular endothelial cells. Expression of adhesion molecules and chemo-attractants promote further inflammatory cell interaction with the endothelium, increased vascular permeability, and infiltration into the media.[36] Increased expression of cytokines and production of matrix metalloproteinases and elastase contribute to destruction of the arterial wall and coronary aneurysm formation.[37,38]

The diagnosis of KD, or the "mucocutaneous lymph node syndrome," should be considered in the setting of fever, conjunctivitis, cervical lymphadenopathy, erythema, edema or desquamation of the palms and soles, and mucosal changes such as a "strawberry tongue" or fissured lips. Standard therapy for the acute phase of the illness is a single infusion of high-dose γ-globulin.[39] Corticosteroids do not appear to improve coronary outcomes or influence the duration of clinical illness. Coronary artery aneurysms form in approximately 5% of treated children and 20% to 30% of untreated children. Coronary artery aneurysms can often be identified in pediatric patients through echocardiography, and those with a diameter of greater than 6 mm are more likely to be associated with clinically significant sequelae. Coronary artery lesions may evolve in a number of different manners during the late phase of KD (>2 years from index), including regression, localized stenosis, occlusion of the aneurysm, extension, and, rarely, rupture.[40] Catheter-based intervention has been recommended as first-line treatment for late ischemic disease and high-grade proximal stenosis of the left anterior descending coronary artery, regardless of demonstrable ischemia.[41] Aspirin, clopidogrel, dipyridamole, and warfarin have all been used in patients with coronary aneurysms as a means to prevent thrombotic occlusion, although there is no compelling comparative literature. Aspirin has been the most commonly used agent, although there is an increased risk of Reye syndrome, given the population and duration of therapy. Covered stents have also been employed for prevention of thrombotic coronary artery occlusion associated with large aneurysms, though experience is limited.[42]

Vasculitis of small and medium-sized vessels

Although there is debate regarding the nosology of vasculitis of small and medium-sized vessels, there can be significant cardiac involvement in patients with polyarteritis nodosa (as distinguished from microscopic polyangiitis) and the Churg-Strauss syndrome. The medium-sized vasculitis classically defined as polyarteritis nodosa is associated with clinical symptoms related to myocardial dysfunction, pericarditis, or coronary arteritis in 10% to 30% of patients. Of these, clinical congestive heart failure is the most common and may be due to coronary arteritis, compounded with hypertension and renal insufficiency. In autopsy studies, coronary arteritis has been reported to occur in up to 50% of patients. However, angina pectoris and clinically apparent myocardial infarctions are uncommon.

The Churg-Strauss syndrome is characterized by eosinophilic granulomatous infiltrates and a small vessel vasculitis of unknown cause.

Cardiac involvement was noted in 60% of patients in the original series described by Churg and Strauss, and mortality is due to cardiovascular causes in a high percentage of patients. Cardiomyopathy may result from either small vessel vasculitis or eosinophilic granulomatous myocarditis and may be dilated or restrictive.[43] As with other hypereosinophilic cardiomyopathies, large ventricular thrombi may develop in association with the myocarditis.

Treatment of both Churg-Strauss and polyarteritis nodosa is similar, with pulsed high-dose intravenous steroids. In patients who are critically ill, a second immunosuppressive agent should be added. Warfarin should be initiated in patients with ventricular thrombus formation.

SYSTEMIC LUPUS ERYTHEMATOSUS

Systemic lupus erythematosus (SLE) can affect all cardiac structures in the inflammatory process, including pericardium, myocardium, valvular structures, the conduction system, and the coronary arteries. Pericardial involvement is by far the most common clinically. Clinical pericarditis, manifest by chest pain, fever, and signs such as muffled heart sounds, pericardial friction rub, or electrocardiographic changes, is most common either during the index presentation of SLE, or during a clinical "flare" of disease activity. Subclinical involvement is much more common, as noted from echocardiographic and autopsy studies. The pericardial fluid associated with SLE is not diagnostically unique in any fashion, and pericardiocentesis will not establish the diagnosis, though it may exclude other important causes. Pericardiocentesis is not routinely warranted and should be reserved for cases in which there is a high suspicion of a malignant or infectious etiology, or for relief of hemodynamic compromise. Associated pleural effusions are common, and diagnostic needle drainage of such may prove safer. Pericardial effusions caused by SLE rarely progress to tamponade or constriction, though both can occur, particularly if there is associated renal failure. Treatment with NSAIDs or corticosteroids is usually effective in mild cases, whereas high-dose pulsed steroids may be necessary in more severe cases such as those associated with tamponade. Chronic recurrent pericarditis may require the addition of non-steroidal immunomodulating drugs such as methotrexate, azathioprine, or mycophenolate mofetil.[44,45]

Myocardial involvement in SLE may be manifest by overt dysfunction, with a cardiac gallop, fever, dyspnea, and jugular distention, or it may be disclosed in asymptomatic patients by echocardiography. Patients with SLE are at increased risk for development of ischemic heart disease, and this must be excluded as a potential cause of myocardial dysfunction. Regional electrical abnormalities, by ECG, or regional contractile abnormalities, by echo, are more likely in the setting of coronary artery disease. Uncommonly, patients may present with acute myocarditis, manifested by symptomatic heart failure, elevation of cardiac biomarkers (such as cardiac troponin and B-natriuretic peptide), and imaging evidence of ventricular dysfunction. SLE patients with circulating anti-Ro (SSA) or anticardiolipin antibodies and those with prior skeletal myositis may be at increased risk for myocarditis (experts disagree).[45-48] Although endomyocardial biopsy in such cases may demonstrate mononuclear cell infiltrates, fibrosis, and myocyte necrosis, these changes are not diagnostic of SLE myocarditis. Immune complex and complement deposition in perivascular tissue can be demonstrated in SLE,[49] and these changes may be more characteristic of lupus than of other etiologies. Myocarditis as the only manifestation of SLE would be quite rare; in such patients thorough investigation for another etiologic explanation is warranted. In patients with known or suspected SLE and new myocardial dysfunction, myocarditis should be suspected, and, in the absence of an alternative explanation, treatment with pulsed intravenous steroids should be considered. Azathioprine, cyclophosphamide, and intravenous IgG may be useful adjuncts in severe cases[50] and unremitting cases may respond to plasmapheresis or immunoadsorption of autoantibodies.[51] There are little data regarding long-term outcomes of patients successfully treated for lupus myocarditis.

Arrhythmias may complicate severe myocarditis in patients with SLE, as in myocarditis of any cause, and atrial dysrhythmias may complicate severe cases of valvulopathy with significant mitral regurgitation. Isolated involvement of the conduction system is extraordinarily rare in adults as a consequence of SLE, whereas the neonatal lupus syndrome, though something of a misnomer, deserves attention with regard to congenital complete heart block. There is a small but well-established risk of congenital complete heart block developing during the second trimester in fetuses of women who express autoantibodies specifically directed at ribonucleoproteins 48-kDa SSB/La, 52-kDa SSA/Ro, or 60 kDa-SSA/Ro.[52] These women may have SLE or Sjögren syndrome, or they may be asymptomatic, and despite similar serum concentration of autoantibody, they do not suffer conduction abnormalities themselves. The fetal heart seems to be uniquely vulnerable in this regard, though given the low overall incidence of occurrence even in mothers with such autoantibodies, there is likely an element of fetal genetic predisposition as well. The cascade of events leading to complete heart block appears to involve fetal cardiocyte apoptosis, translocation of Ro and La antigens, binding of maternal autoantibodies, and subsequent fibrosis related to scavenging macrophages. Fetal mortality has been estimated at 15% to 30%, and two thirds of live births will require permanent pacing.[53] The recurrence of congenital complete heart block in future pregnancies of women at risk is low, and this has confounded efforts to evaluate the efficacy of immunosuppressive therapy. Although fetal echocardiography conceivably can demonstrate mechanical delay in atrioventricular transport (the equivalent of a first-degree atrioventricular block on ECG), there has been no study to date demonstrating that recognition of an early stage of heart block leads to an effective treatment algorithm.

More than 80 years ago, Emanuel Libman and Benjamin Sacks described the now eponymous verrucous lesions commonly found along the valvular closure line in patients with SLE. Libman-Sacks vegetations (LS) are non-bacterial thrombotic valvular lesions that affect up to 10% of patients with SLE, most frequently involving the mitral valve. The pathogenesis is related to subendothelial immune-complex and complement deposition, increased endothelial cell expression of integrins, localized neovascularization, thrombosis, and fibrosis.[54] Their incidence is related to the duration of lupus, disease activity, and the presence of anticardiolipin or antiphospholipid antibodies,[55] in part due to upregulation and expression of adhesion molecules, as well as decreased production of proteins C and S. Although the mitral valve is most frequently involved, any of the cardiac valves may be targeted and lesions may also be found on endocardial surfaces and chordae tendineae. Although uncommon, significant mitral insufficiency and aortic stenosis have been reported as complications. More common complications include thrombotic events and bacterial superinfection. Over the course of their illness, patients with SLE have a greater than 15% risk of stroke or transient ischemic attack. Valvular thickening or vegetation is two to four times more commonly found by transthoracic echo in SLE patients with cerebrovascular events when compared with SLE controls. The risk of cerebrovascular embolization in LS may be further increased by the presence of antiphospholipid antibodies.[56] The role of antiplatelet or antithrombotic therapy for primary prevention of embolic events in patients in whom LS is identified has not been defined. During active valvulitis, immunosuppressive therapy directed at the systemic illness is recommended, although data supporting outcome differences with such a strategy are limited. In patients who have incurred stroke or transient ischemia, anticoagulation with warfarin to a relatively high international normalized ratio (3-4) has been recommended. Valve repair and replacement with a biologic prosthesis have been disappointing, and when valve surgery is indicated a mechanical prosthesis should be strongly considered.

In addition to the risk of valvulitis, patients with the antiphospholipid antibody syndrome are at risk of venous and arterial thrombotic events, related to antibody-induced endothelial dysfunction, increased platelet aggregation, activation of both intrinsic and extrinsic coagulation pathways, and decreased fibrinolysis. Venous thromboembolic disease is by far the most common complication, but other thrombotic complications may include spontaneous atrial echo "contrast" (considered to be a precursor to thrombosis), adherent or free-floating intracardiac thrombus, or microvascular or epicardial coronary thrombosis. A recent prospective randomized placebo-controlled trial demonstrated that asymptomatic patients with persistent antiphospholipid antibodies do not benefit from low-dose aspirin as a means of primary prevention of thrombotic complications.[57] Treatment of significant valvular or intracardiac thrombotic complications remains high-dose anticoagulation with heparin followed by chronic warfarin.[58] In patients who require cardiovascular surgery, there is a high risk of thrombotic perioperative events despite aggressive antiplatelet and antithrombotic therapy.[59]

Patients with SLE are at increased risk of atherosclerotic coronary and cerebrovascular disease. Although SLE patients have a high prevalence of hypertension, hyperlipidemia, and smoking, the atherosclerotic risks remain significantly elevated in statistical analysis after controlling for these traditional risk factors. A prospective, cross-sectional study using electron beam tomography has demonstrated a threefold increased frequency of coronary calcifications and more severe coronary calcification in patients with SLE as compared with matched controls.[60] A similarly designed study demonstrated a twofold higher ultrasound prevalence of carotid plaque.[61] In large population studies, women with SLE have a fourfold to eightfold increased risk of myocardial infarction compared with matched controls.[62] Patients with SLE should have aggressive management of traditional risk factors, including the use of a statin if dyslipidemia is present during a period of stable disease.

POLYMYOSITIS AND DERMATOMYOSITIS

Cardiac complications of polymyositis/dermatomyositis (PM) include myocardial involvement and conduction system abnormalities. When subclinical involvement is evaluated, including non-invasive studies and autopsy series, the incidence of cardiac complications related to PM has been estimated to be as high as 75%. The true incidence of clinically overt involvement with PM is uncertain, but cardiac death has been documented to occur in 10% to 20% of patients. Congestive heart failure occurs in 3% to 45% of patients with PM, and disorders of cardiac conduction occur in approximately one third of patients.[63-65] As with many rheumatologic illnesses, the incidence of fatal myocardial infarction appears to be substantially elevated within this group of patients.

Cardiac involvement in PM appears to be pathologically similar to the inflammation of skeletal muscle characteristic of the disease, with mononuclear infiltrates localized to the endomysium and perivascular areas, cellular dropout, and fibrosis. Lymphocytic infiltration and fibrosis of the conduction tissues can also be demonstrated pathologically. Coronary vasculitis with intimal proliferation and medial sclerosis, as well as small vessel disease with luminal encroachment due to smooth muscle proliferation, have been documented.

Congestive heart failure is the most common clinical cardiac complication of PM, which may result from either systolic or diastolic dysfunction. Diastolic dysfunction may be severe and restrictive left ventricular physiology can result. Echocardiography can help define systolic and diastolic function and can demonstrate if systolic dysfunction is global or segmental. When segmental systolic dysfunction is present, atherosclerotic coronary artery disease should be included in the differential diagnosis. The onset of heart failure has most commonly been linked to active skeletal muscle involvement, but it may occur any time, including periods of stable disease activity or clinical remission.

Conduction block, when present, usually involves either prolongation of the PR interval, right bundle branch block, left anterior fascicular block, or combinations of these three. Permanent pacemakers are rarely necessary, but PM patients with unexplained syncope and ECG evidence of conduction disease should undergo further cardiac electrophysiologic evaluation. Vasospastic angina and pericarditis have been reported to rarely complicate polymyositis/dermatomyositis.

Corticosteroids have been used most commonly for treatment of clinically significant cardiac complications of PM, but with mixed results. Despite corticosteroid therapy, studies have demonstrated progression of conduction disturbances and autopsy data have suggested that myocarditis may occur independent of steroid use. Regardless, in patients with new signs and symptoms of active myocarditis, corticosteroids should be considered. In patients with systolic dysfunction, the use of ACE inhibitors or angiotensin receptor blocking agents should also be considered because they have demonstrated mortality benefit in general populations with systolic heart failure. Trials specific to heart failure in patients with PM have not been undertaken.

SARCOIDOSIS

Sarcoidosis is a systemic, infiltrative disease characterized histologically by the presence of non-caseating granulomas. The disease is characterized by a female preponderance and is most common in the Scandinavian countries, with an incidence there approaching 60/100,000.[66] The etiology of sarcoidosis and the risk factors for its development are poorly understood. Various environmental and infection triggers, genetics, and cytokine responses appear to be involved in the disease pathophysiology.[67] Histologically, CD4+ T cells interact with antigen-presenting cells (APCs) to initiate the formation of granulomas, the pathologic hallmark of sarcoid.[68] Multiple organs may be involved, including the lung, skin, eyes, and heart. Cardiac sarcoidosis (CS) is the most common myocardial infiltrative disease encountered in clinical practice.[69]

The overall incidence of CS is difficult to estimate. The diagnostic gold standard, endomyocardial biopsy, is not routinely performed in clinical practice. More commonly, a variety of non-invasive imaging studies are employed, with varying diagnostic accuracies. A widely cited postmortem study of 84 consecutive patients with sarcoidosis identified myocardial granulomas in 23 subjects (27%) but only 15 (17%) had an antecedent history of heart failure, arrhythmias, or electrocardiographic abnormalities to suggest cardiovascular involvement.[70] Although the true prevalence of CS in patients with sarcoid remains uncertain, it is clear that cardiac symptoms underestimate the total disease burden. Although mortality from sarcoidosis is primarily driven by pulmonary disease progression, cardiovascular complications, including heart failure and arrhythmias, are important clinical entities to identify because they may present suddenly and catastrophically in previously healthy individuals.[71]

The clinical presentation of CS is variable and unpredictable. Constitutional symptoms, including weight loss, malaise, and myalgias, are nonspecific and frequently present. Additional symptoms, including palpitations, dyspnea, or dizziness, may be related to the extent and location of myocardial involvement. Patients may present with CHF resulting from granulomatous involvement of the myocardium or from progression of valvular heart disease.[72] Valvular disease may reflect direct granulomatous involvement or may follow alterations in left ventricular geometry.

Pulmonary hypertension is increasingly recognized as a complication of sarcoidosis. Similar to CS, the reported prevalence is highly variable depending on clinical definitions and methods of diagnostic testing.[73,74] The pathophysiology is complex and may involve granulomatous involvement of the pulmonary vasculature, occlusion of pulmonary veins, or reaction to progressive fibrosis and interstitial lung disease. This complex etiology makes classification of sarcoid-related pulmonary hypertension challenging, and ongoing debate exists regarding nosology and treatment. A subset of patients with pulmonary hypertension in the absence of interstitial lung disease may respond favorably to pulmonary arterial vasodilator therapy, but data are lacking in the other groups. Untreated, pulmonary hypertension creates right ventricular pressure overload, resulting in dilatation, dysfunction, and eventual cor pulmonale.

All patients with a diagnosis of sarcoidosis should be screened for cardiac disease with a careful history and physical examination, as well as diagnostic testing including a transthoracic echocardiogram (TTE) and an ECG. Abnormalities in these screening tests may prompt additional diagnostic testing. Although neither sensitive nor specific, the ECG is a readily available, noninvasive, and inexpensive test that should be performed in all patients with sarcoidosis. Electrical abnormalities are common in CS and can affect all areas of the conduction system, including the bundle branches, atrioventricular node, or sinus node. Atrial arrhythmias may result from granulomatous involvement, atrial dilation, or valvular heart disease. Granulomatous involvement and fibrosis of myocardial tissue create the substrate for ventricular arrhythmias, including ventricular tachycardia and fibrillation, which may result in sudden cardiac death. Ambulatory ECG monitoring in patients with suspicious symptoms and normal electrocardiograms may help identify high-risk arrhythmias including non-sustained ventricular tachycardia and high-degree atrioventricular block.

The echocardiogram is an essential component in the diagnostic evaluation of CS, providing a non-invasive means of evaluation of the pericardium, left ventricular function, right heart function, and pulmonary artery pressures. Ventricular aneurysms may occur and are differentiated from those related to ischemic disease by their non-coronary artery distribution. Pericardial effusions are not uncommon, and cases of pericardial constriction and tamponade have been reported.[75]

The presence of non-caseating granuloma in an endomyocardial biopsy (EMB) sample supports a diagnosis of CS. However, this procedure is no longer routinely performed in clinical practice. When performed, an EMB is obtained from the right side of the heart, typically directed toward the interventricular septum. However, CS typically infiltrates the basal septum and free wall of the left ventricle, and sampling error reduces the negative predictive value of normal tissue obtained by this technique. Furthermore, EMB in a dilated heart carries an increased risk of perforation and tamponade. EMB should still be considered in patients with unexplained cardiomyopathy who fail to respond to a reasonable course of medical therapy and in whom CS is suspected because a positive biopsy would prompt specific therapy with corticosteroids.[76]

Characteristic myocardial perfusion abnormalities, using either technetium 99m (^{99m}Tc) or thallium 201 (^{201}Tl), have been described in CS, both with intermediate sensitivity and specificity. Abnormal perfusion may reflect granuloma formation or fibrosis when present in a distribution that does not reflect coronary anatomy. Interestingly, perfusion defects related to CS may improve following vasodilator testing ("reverse redistribution"), further delineating this from coronary artery disease.[77] Positron emission tomography (PET) imaging with ^{18}F-fluorodeoxyglucose (^{18}F-FDG) has superior sensitivity and specificity when compared with SPECT and provides both structural and metabolic information.[78] Typically, increased metabolic activity is noted in relation to granuloma coupled with impaired perfusion in fibrotic regions. Importantly, fibrotic myocardium may not improve with therapy. Cardiac MRI has diagnostic properties comparable with PET but has the advantage of superior tissue characterization without the use of ionizing radiation. Gadolinium enhancement can identify areas of inflammation, myocardial nodules, aneurysms, and fibrosis.[79]

In patients with preserved systolic function, 5-year survival ranges between 60% and 90%. Predictors of increased risk include advanced New York Heart Association (NYHA) functional class, reduced left ventricular ejection fraction (LVEF), and sustained ventricular tachycardia (VT).[80] In patients with non-sustained VT or atrioventricular block on ambulatory ECG monitoring, or unexplained syncope, an invasive electrophysiology study may identify the need for pacemaker or defibrillator implantation. Recently published guidelines suggest that an implantable defibrillator should be considered in CS patients with either an unexplained ECG abnormality or abnormal ventricular wall thickness or function.[81]

The cornerstone of treatment for CS is corticosteroid therapy, which suppresses inflammation and granuloma formulation.[82] Small studies and case reports suggest both clinical and structural improvement following treatment with steroids. In a small group of patients with atrioventricular block, corticosteroid therapy resulted in preservation of LVEF and increased freedom from VT.[83] Dosing, treatment duration, and criteria for therapy initiation remain unclear. In patients with LV dysfunction, standard heart failure therapy consisting of ACE inhibition, beta blockade, and diuretics as needed should be continued.

Orthotopic heart transplantation is an option for patients with advanced cardiomyopathy. Careful attention to the extent of pulmonary involvement and pulmonary hypertension is necessary in determining transplant suitability. Sarcoidosis may recur in the allograft and is typically responsive to corticosteroids. Patients who undergo transplantation for cardiac sarcoidosis share outcomes comparable with the transplant population at large.[84]

PROGRESSIVE SYSTEMIC SCLEROSIS

"Scleroderma" suggests hardening and thickening of the skin. When these findings occur with visceral organ involvement, the terms "diffuse cutaneous systemic sclerosis"(dcSSc) and "limited cutaneous systemic sclerosis" (lcSSc) are used. LcSSC is associated more frequently with distal cutaneous involvement and with the CREST syndrome, which has several vascular manifestations including pulmonary arterial

hypertension and Raynaud phenomenon. Cardiovascular involvement confers a poor prognosis in patients with SSc, with a 5-year mortality rate approaching 75%.[85] The etiology of cardiovascular involvement is multifactorial, resulting from inflammation, microvascular dysfunction, and fibrosis related to collagen overproduction by altered fibroblasts. Cardiovascular involvement is seen in both sclerosis subtypes, with a greater incidence of cardiovascular symptoms in dcSSc.

SSc can affect the pericardium, myocardium, and conduction system but is not associated with premature development of coronary artery disease. A spectrum of pericardial diseases has been described, including acute and chronic pericarditis, tamponade, and pericardial constriction. Necropsy studies estimate the prevalence of pericardial involvement in SSc to be approximately 78%.[86] However, only a small fraction of patients are symptomatic. Pericardial effusions are often exudative, without the complement activation seen in RA or SLE. The presence of a pericardial effusion has been correlated with the development of renal failure. However, pericardial histopathology in such cases is not characteristic of uremia, suggesting primary SSc involvement.

Postmortem studies have identified myocardial fibrosis in 80% of patients with SSc.[87] MRI with gadolinium enhancement is highly sensitive for detecting myocardial fibrosis and identifies cardiovascular involvement in 66% of patients, with similar incidence in both dcSSc and lcSSc.[88] Myocardial SPECT is less sensitive for detecting fibrosis, but exercise-induced perfusion defects identified by ^{201}Tl SPECT are predictive of symptomatic cardiovascular disease and death.[89] The etiology of myocardial fibrosis is unclear; it is hypothesized that coronary vasospasm ("myocardial Raynaud phenomenon") may precipitate contraction band necrosis and fibrosis.[90] The clinical significance of such fibrosis remains undefined. Systolic dysfunction is rare, occurring in less than 2% of patients, but echocardiography has demonstrated more common occurrence of myocardial hypertrophy and diastolic dysfunction.[91] The biomarker N-terminal brain natriuretic peptide (NT-pro BNP) appears to be sensitive in identifying patients with cardiovascular involvement, including systolic dysfunction, right ventricular dysfunction, and pulmonary hypertension.[92]

Pulmonary hypertension or interstitial lung disease may occur and accounts for most mortality in patients with SSc.[93] The incidence of pulmonary arterial hypertension (PAH) in SSc ranges between 10% and 20%. Annual screening for pulmonary hypertension is recommended with both pulmonary function testing and echocardiography because pulmonary artery pressures tend to rise over time.[94] Abnormal carbon monoxide diffusion capacity (DLCO) often predicts the development of pulmonary hypertension.[92] Echocardiography provides a noninvasive assessment of right ventricular size, function, and systolic pressure. The arterial pathology in SSc-associated PAH is similar to that seen in idiopathic PAH (IPAH), and vasodilator therapy appears to be effective. However, even with vasodilator therapy, outcomes in patients with SSc are worse than IPAH, and this subset constitutes a high-risk group.[95] The prognosis is especially poor in patients with pulmonary hypertension and concomitant interstitial lung disease, with a fivefold increase in mortality.[96] Although right ventricular (RV) dysfunction is common in SSc, the severity of dysfunction does not fully correlate with pulmonary artery pressures, suggesting that disturbances of myocardial circulation and RV fibrosis may be contributory.[97] Advanced cases of pulmonary hypertension may require lung transplantation.

Multiple electrocardiographic abnormalities have been described in SSc and occur in similar frequency between lcSSc and dcSSc. A large series of 436 patients with SSc identified ECG abnormalities in 25% of patients, the most common of which were left anterior fascicular block, PR interval prolongation, and intraventricular conduction defects.[98] Myocardial fibrosis affects multiple areas of the conduction system, and cases of high-degree heart block have been reported.[99] Patients with involvement of both skeletal and cardiac muscle appear to be at increased risk of fatal complications from arrhythmias and may constitute a higher-risk group.[100] Treatment guidelines for pacemaker implantation are identical to those for the general population.

No specific recommendations exist for the management of scleroderma heart disease. ACE inhibitors lower blood pressure and have beneficial effects on the renal system, particularly in scleroderma renal crisis, and may yield secondary cardiovascular benefits. Calcium channel blockers appear to have beneficial effects on myocardial perfusion and might limit progression of overall disease status.[101]

SPONDYLOARTHROPATHIES

The spondyloarthropathies are a heterogeneous group of inflammatory disorders of unclear etiology and include ankylosing spondylitis, reactive arthritis, and arthritis associated with psoriasis or inflammatory bowel disease. Observational data suggest that 2% to 10% of patients with spondyloarthropathies will develop cardiovascular disease. Despite a shared immunologic mechanism, the spectrum of cardiovascular disease differs significantly between the disorders.[102]

Ankylosing spondylitis is associated with a sclerosing inflammatory process and deposition of scar tissue typically affecting the mitral and aortic valves.[103,104] Echocardiography identifies valvular thickening and regurgitation in 40% and 50% of patients, respectively.[103] Aortic root involvement is frequently encountered, with dilation in up to 80% of patients[103] and the occasional development of sinus of Valsalva aneurysms.[105] Although dilation may be asymptomatic, careful monitoring of aortic diameter and valvular regurgitation is necessary. Clinical predictors of cardiovascular involvement include age older than 45 years and disease duration in excess of 15 years.[103] Importantly, the rate of cardiovascular disease progression is often unpredictable and unrelated to the severity of extracardiac disease.[103]

Minor cardiac arrhythmias, including premature ventricular contractions, are common in patients with spondyloarthropathies, although their clinical significance is unclear.[106] Conduction abnormalities, including varying degrees of atrioventricular block, and bundle branch block are well described and are related to fibrosis with extension into the conduction system. Coronary artery disease and systolic dysfunction are not frequently encountered, although diastolic dysfunction has been described in asymptomatic patients, even in the absence of valvular heart disease.[107]

Extracutaneous involvement in psoriasis is common. Coronary artery disease is the most common cause of death within this population[108] and may be correlated with the severity of cutaneous disease.[109] Obesity and hypertension occur with twice the frequency of the general population.[110,111] Atherogenic dyslipidemia, including high LDL and low high-density lipoprotein cholesterol, is frequently encountered, along with insulin resistance and the metabolic syndrome.[112] These traditional cardiovascular risk factors, coupled with the highly inflammatory nature of psoriasis, contribute to the risk of accelerated atherosclerosis. Patients with moderate or advanced psoriasis may benefit from cardiovascular screening and aggressive risk factor modification.[108]

Reactive arthritis, formerly termed *Reiter syndrome*, refers to an arthritis that develops following an infection. Aortitis and valvular heart disease have been described, though much less commonly than in other connective tissue diseases.[113] A small echocardiographic study detected no significant structural heart disease in a group of 18 patients with reactive arthritis.[114] Conduction abnormalities, including atrioventricular block, have been described.

KEY REFERENCES

1. Bombardier C, Laine L, Reicin A, Shapiro D, et al. Comparison of upper gastrointestinal toxicity of rofecoxib and naproxen in patients with rheumatoid arthritis. VIGOR Study Group. N Engl J Med 2000;343:1520-1528, 2 p following 1528.
2. Bresalier RS, Sandler RS, Quan H, et al. Cardiovascular events associated with rofecoxib in a colorectal adenoma chemoprevention trial. N Engl J Med 2005;352:1092-1102.
3. Solomon SD, McMurray JJ, Pfeffer MA, et al. Cardiovascular risk associated with celecoxib in a clinical trial for colorectal adenoma prevention. N Engl J Med 2005;352:1071-1080.
3a. Solomon SD, Pfeffer MA, McMurray JJ, et al. Effect of celecoxib on cardiovascular events and blood pressure in two trials for the prevention of colorectal adenomas. Circulation 2006;114:1028-1035.
4. Reicin AS, Shapiro D, Sperling RS, et al. Comparison of cardiovascular thrombotic events in patients with osteoarthritis treated with rofecoxib versus nonselective nonsteroidal anti-inflammatory drugs (ibuprofen, diclofenac, and nabumetone). Am J Cardiol 2002;89:204-209.
4a. Johnsen SP, Larsson H, Tarone RE, et al. Risk of hospitalization for myocardial infarction among users of rofecoxib, celecoxib, and other NSAIDs: a population-based case-control study. Arch Intern Med 2005;165:978-984.
5. Sowers JR, White WB, Pitt B, et al. The effects of cyclooxygenase-2 inhibitors and nonsteroidal anti-inflammatory therapy on 24-hour blood pressure in patients with hypertension, osteoarthritis, and type 2 diabetes mellitus. Arch Intern Med 2005;165:161-168.
6. Mann DL. Inflammatory mediators and the failing heart: past, present, and the foreseeable future. Circ Res 2002;91:988-998.
7. Kwon HJ, Coté TR, Cuffe MS, et al. Case reports of heart failure after therapy with a tumor necrosis factor antagonist. Ann Intern Med 2003;138:807-811.
8. Gabriel SE. Cardiovascular morbidity and mortality in rheumatoid arthritis. Am J Med 2008;121:S9-S14.
9. del Rincon ID, Williams K, Stern MP. High incidence of cardiovascular events in a rheumatoid arthritis cohort not explained by traditional cardiac risk factors. Arthritis Rheum 2001;44:2732-2745.
10. Martens PG, Goronzy JJ, Schaid D, Weyand CM. Expansion of unusual CD4+ T cells in severe rheumatoid arthritis. Arthritis Rheum 1997;40:1106-1114.
11. Grisar J, Aletaha D, Steiner CW, et al. Depletion of endothelial progenitor cells in the peripheral blood of patients with rheumatoid arthritis. Circulation 2005;111:204-211.
12. Bergholm R, Leirisalo-Repo M, Vehkavaara S, et al. Impaired responsiveness to NO in newly diagnosed patients with rheumatoid arthritis. Arterioscler Thromb Vasc Biol 2002;22:1637-1641.
13. Hurlimann D, Forster A, Noll G, et al. Anti-tumor necrosis factor-α treatment improves endothelial function in patients with rheumatoid arthritis. Circulation 2002;106:2184-2187.
14. McCarey D, McInnes I, Madhok R, et al. Trial of atorvastatin in rheumatoid arthritis (TARA): double-blind, randomised, placebo-controlled trial. Lancet 2004;363:2015-2021.
15. Maki-Petaja KM, Booth AD, Hall FC, et al. Ezetimibe and simvastatin reduce inflammation, disease activity, and aortic stiffness and improve endothelial function in rheumatoid arthritis. J Am Coll Cardiol 2007;50:852-858.
16. Wei L, MacDonald TM, Walker BR. Taking glucocorticoids by prescription is associated with subsequent cardiovascular disease. Ann Intern Med 2004;141:764-770.
17. Souverein PC, Berard A, Van Staa TP, et al. Use of oral glucocorticoids and risk of cardiovascular and cerebrovascular disease in a population based case-control study. Heart 2004;90:859-865.
18. Prodanowich S, Ma F, Taylor JR, et al. Methotrexate reduces incidence of vascular diseases in veterans with psoriasis or rheumatoid arthritis. J Am Acad Dermatol 2005;52:262-267.
19. Choi HK, Hernan MA, Seeger JD, et al. Methotrexate and mortality in patients with rheumatoid arthritis: a prospective study. Lancet 2002;359:1173-1177.
20. Krishnan E, Lingala VB, Singh G. Declines in mortality from acute myocardial infarction in successive incidence and birth cohorts of patients with rheumatoid arthritis. Circulation 2004;110:1774-1779.
21. Davis JM, Kremers HM, Crowson DS, et al. Glucocorticoids and cardiovascular events in rheumatoid arthritis: a population based cohort study. Arthritis Rheum 2007;56:820-830.
22. Aslangul E, Perrot S, Durand E, et al. Successful etanercept treatment of constrictive pericarditis complicating rheumatoid arthritis. Rheumatology 2005;44:1581-1583.
23. Nicola PJ, Maradit-Kremers H, Roger V, et al. The risk of congestive heart failure in rheumatoid arthritis. A population based study over 46 years. Arthritis Rheum 2005;52:412-420.
24. Davis JM, Roger V, Crowson CS, et al. The presentation and outcome of heart failure in patients with rheumatoid arthritis differs from that in the general population. Arthritis Rheum 2008;58:2603-2611.
25. Maradit-Kremers H, Nicola PJ, Crowson CS, et al. Raised erythrocyte sedimentation rate signals heart failure in patients with rheumatoid arthritis. Ann Rheum Dis 2007;66:76-80.
26. Koivuniemi R, Paimela L, Soumalainen R, et al. Amyloidosis is frequently undetected in patients with rheumatoid arthritis. Amyloid 2008;15:262-268.
27. Tanaka R, Migita K, Honda S, et al. Clinical outcome and survival of secondary (AA) amyloidosis. Clin Exp Rheumatol 2003;21:343-346.
28. Nakamura T. Clinical strategies for amyloid A amyloidosis secondary to rheumatoid arthritis. Mod Rheumatol 2008;18:109-118.
29. Kerr GS, Hallahan CW, Giordano J, et al. Takayasu arteritis. Ann Intern Med 1994;120:919-929.
30. Numano F. Takayasu arteritis, Buerger disease and inflammatory abdominal aortic aneurysms: is there a common pathway in their pathogenesis? Int J Cardiol 1998;66(suppl 1):S5-S10.
31. Morooka S, Takeda T, Saito Y, et al. Dilatation of the aortic valve portion in aortitis syndrome: angiographic evaluation of 70 patients. Jpn Heart J 1981;22:517-526.
32. Ito I. Medical treatment of Takayasu arteritis. Heart Vessels 1992;7(suppl):133-137.
33. Ogino H, Matsuda H, Minatoya K, et al. Overview of late outcome of medical and surgical treatment for Takayasu arteritis. Circulation 2008;118:2738-2747.
34. Tyagi S, Kaul UA, Nair M, et al. Balloon angioplasty of the aorta in Takayasu's arteritis: initial and long-term results. Am Heart J 1992;124:876-882.
35. Baril DT, Carroccio A, Palchik E, et al. Endovascular treatment of complicated aortic aneurysms in patients with underlying arteriopathies. Ann Vasc Surg 2006;20:464-471.
36. Burns JC. Kawasaki syndrome. Lancet 2004;364:533-544.
37. Senzaki H, Masutani S, Kobayashi J, et al. Circulating matrix metalloproteinases and their inhibitors in patients with Kawasaki disease. Circulation 2001;104:860-863.
38. Gavin PJ, Crawford SE, Shulman ST, et al. Systemic arterial expression of matrix metalloproteinases 2 and 9 in acute Kawasaki disease. Arterioscler Thromb Vasc Biol 2003;23:576-581.
39. Newburger JW, Takahashi M, Beiser AS, et al. The treatment of Kawasaki syndrome with intravenous gamma globulin. N Engl J Med 1986;315:341-347.
40. Senzaki H. Long-term outcome of Kawasaki disease. Circulation 2008;118:2763-2772.

41. Newberger JW, Takahashi M, Gerber MA, et al. Committee on Rheumatic Fever, Endocarditis and Kawasaki Disease; Council on Cardiovascular Disease in the Young; American Heart Association; American Academy of Pediatrics. Diagnosis, treatment and long-term management of Kawasaki disease: a statement for health professionals from the Committee on Rheumatic Fever, Endocarditis and Kawasaki Disease, Council on Cardiovascular Disease in the Young, American Heart Association. Circulation 2004;110:2747-2771.

42. Waki K, Baba K. Transcatheter polytetrafluoroethylene-covered stent implantation in a giant coronary artery aneurysm of a child with Kawasaki disease: a potential novel treatment. Catheter Cardiovasc Interv 2006;68:74-77.

43. Terasaki F, Hayashi T, Hirota Y, et al. Evolution to dilated cardiomyopathy from acute eosinophilic pancarditis in Churg-Strauss syndrome. Heart Vessels 1997;12:43-48.

44. Doria A, Iaccarino L, Sarzi-Puttini P, et al. Cardiac involvement in systemic lupus erythematosus. Lupus 2005;14:683-686.

45. Tincani A, Rebaioli CB, Taglietti M, Shoenfeld Y. Heart involvement in systemic lupus erythematosus, anti-phospholipid syndrome and neonatal lupus. Rheumatology 2006;45:iv8-iv13.

46. Nihoyannopoulos P, Gomez PM, Joshi J, et al. Cardiac abnormalities in systemic lupus erythematosus. Association with raised anti-cardiolipin antibodies. Circulation 1990;82:369-375.

47. Logar D, Kveder T, Rozman B, Dobovisek J. Possible association between anti-Rho antibodies and myocarditis or cardiac conduction defects in adults with systemic lupus erythematosus. Ann Rheum Dis 1990;49:627-629.

48. Borenstein DF, Fye WB, Arnett FC, Stevens MB. The myocarditis of systemic lupus erythematosus: association with myositis. Ann Intern Med 1978;89:619-624.

49. Bidani AK, Roberts JL, Schwartz MM, et al. Immunopathology of cardiac lesions in fatal systemic lupus erythematosus. Am J Med 1980;69:849-858.

50. Shere Y, Levy Y, Shoenfeld Y. Marked improvement of severe cardiac dysfunction after one course of intravenous immunoglobulin in a patient with systemic lupus erythematosus. Clin Rheumatol 1999;18: 238-240.

REFERENCES

Full references for this chapter can be found on www.expertconsult.com.

The lung in rheumatic disease

Paul F. Dellaripa and Ivan O. Rosas

35

- All components of the respiratory system can be involved in the lung manifestations of rheumatologic disease.
- Lung disease may precede overt musculoskeletal features by several years.
- The pathologic pattern is variable: Different patterns may coexist.
- Pneumonitis due to drugs or opportunistic infection due to immunosuppression can complicate diagnosis of lung manifestations of rheumatologic disease.
- Each rheumatologic disease has lung patterns of abnormality that are more "typical" for that disease.
- High-resolution computed tomography with or without bronchoalveolar lavage can be helpful in differentiation of lung manifestations: Surgical biopsy may be required where there is residual doubt.
- Treatment approaches depend on the dominant pattern of disease.
- Outcome tends to be better than in the idiopathic interstitial pneumonias that share common pathologic patterns.
- Rarely, more explosive diffuse lung disease mimicking acute respiratory distress syndrome can occur: The outcome of this manifestation is often poor.

INTRODUCTION

Pulmonary manifestations of rheumatic diseases are among the most significant challenges for the practicing rheumatologist. Specifically, interstitial lung disease (ILD) is one of the most worrisome and challenging complications due to the progressive nature of the disease and variable response to therapy and prognosis. Importantly, recent evidence suggests that early disease detection may affect response to treatment, especially in cases where inflammatory lung disease is present. Rheumatologists will encounter these patients most frequently; hence it is incumbent on them to maintain vigilance for the diverse clinical presentations and gamut of lung complications associated with the rheumatic diseases. This chapter highlights major areas of lung involvement in specific rheumatic diseases including airway, pleural, vascular and ILD, the latter of which is the main focus of this chapter given its importance in rheumatologic practice.

Interstitial lung disease or parenchymal lung disease

ILD represents a significant challenge in the management of patients with rheumatic diseases. Prognosis is variable and strongly depends on the histopathologic pattern noted, some studies suggest that ILD associated with rheumatic diseases has a better prognosis than idiopathic pulmonary fibrosis (IPF), whereas other studies suggest that prognosis is similar.[1-3] In order of frequency, ILD in rheumatic disease occurs most commonly in scleroderma (SSc), followed by polymyositis/dermatomyositis (PM/DM), rheumatoid arthritis (RA), and less frequently in Sjögren syndrome (SS) and systemic lupus erythematosus (SLE). ILD may precede the development of a specific rheumatic syndrome or present as part of a poorly defined or undifferentiated rheumatic syndrome that the rheumatologist may be asked to evaluate in the setting of active ILD.

Pathologic features in interstitial lung disease

An understanding of the histopathologic classification in ILD is important because different histologic subtypes portend a different prognosis. The two most common types of ILD associated with rheumatic diseases are non-specific interstitial pneumonia (NSIP) and usual interstitial pneumonia (UIP), followed by lymphocytic interstitial pneumonia (LIP), cryptogenic organizing pneumonia (COP), and less frequently diffuse alveolar damage (DAD).

UIP is associated with a patchy heterogeneous process with fibrotic areas interposed with normal or near normal lung. The distribution is predominately subpleural and associated with honeycombing on chest computed tomography (CT) (Figs. 35-1 and 35-3). Pathology specimens are notable for characteristic fibroblastic foci (Fig. 35-2). Although UIP is the classic pathologic lesion observed in IPF patients, it can also be seen in RA, SSc, and other rheumatic syndromes; the presence of UIP in RA portends a worse prognosis than other histopathologic patterns.[3] NSIP is characterized by a more uniform, homogeneous pattern, with variable degrees of inflammation (cellular NSIP) or fibrosis (fibrotic NSIP) and a noted paucity of fibroblastic foci on pathology (Fig. 35-4). Typically, ground-glass opacities are noted and are often associated with a reticular pattern and traction bronchiectasis but a lack of honeycombing on chest CT scan (Fig. 35-5). NSIP is the histopathologic lung pattern seen more frequently in patients affected with rheumatic diseases and appears to have a better overall prognosis than UIP.[4] COP or cryptogenic organizing pneumonia, formerly known as *bronchiolitis obliterans organizing pneumonia* (BOOP), is an inflammatory disease that predominately involves the distal airways (acini and respiratory bronchioles) and is characterized by its responsiveness to steroids. Histologically it is characterized by alveolar and duct granulation tissue. It can be seen in association with many rheumatic diseases including SLE, RA, and PM/DM. It has also been associated with the use of numerous medications including gold and sulfasalazine.[5]

LIP is characterized by extensive lymphocytic infiltration associated with peribronchial lymphoid follicles; it is most often seen in SS and RA and may be a feature of ILD in undifferentiated forms of autoimmune disease as well.

DAD is notable for the development of hyaline membranes. It can develop in a variety of rheumatic syndromes including SLE and DM/PM. DAD can occur *de novo* or in patients with preexisting lung disease; the presence of DAD is usually associated with severe respiratory failure and overall poor prognosis.

It is important to note that it is more difficult to predict progression in ILD associated with rheumatic syndromes compared with the more predictable steady decline associated with idiopathic pulmonary fibrosis.

EVALUATION OF PATIENTS WITH LUNG INVOLVEMENT IN THE RHEUMATIC DISEASES

Radiographic studies

Chest roentgenography is not particularly sensitive in detecting mild forms of ILD; however, it may be useful to exclude other conditions such as congestive heart failure, pleural disease, and pneumonia. Chest CT scan with high-resolution images (HRCT) is the test of choice in detecting ILD, and findings on CT may predate the onset of clinical symptoms.[6,7] The most common finding in ILD is the presence of ground-glass opacities, which are characteristic of inflammatory disease and most often associated with NSIP. Another important finding is the presence of honeycombing (cystic spaces within clearly definable walls),

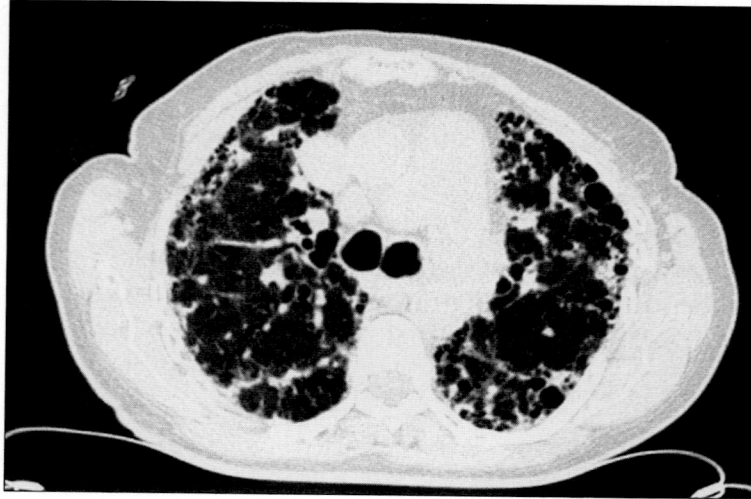

Fig. 35.1 Computed tomography showing the pattern associated with usual interstitial pneumonia. Note the peripheral coarse honeycomb pattern that is the hallmark of usual interstitial pneumonia.

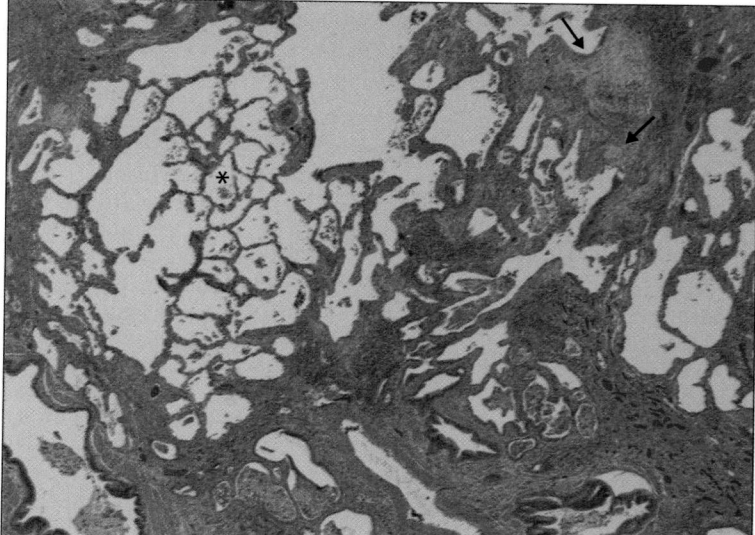

Fig. 35.2 40× view shows characteristic features of usual interstitial pneumonia (UIP) with the presence of normal lung (indicated by asterisk) next to fibrotic lung, illustrating the temporal heterogeneity of UIP. Fibroblastic foci, commonly seen in UIP, are noted by the arrows.

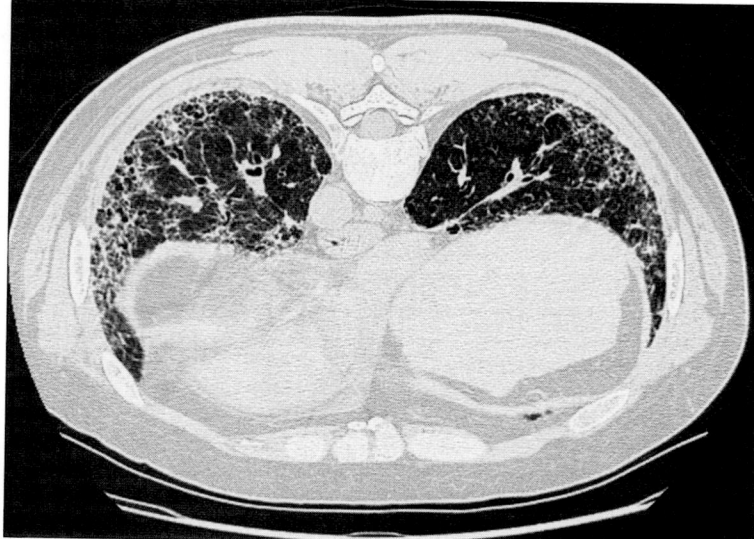

Fig. 35.3 High-resolution computed tomography scan of the chest shows fibrotic changes in a subpleural distribution with honeycombing consistent with usual interstitial pneumonia.

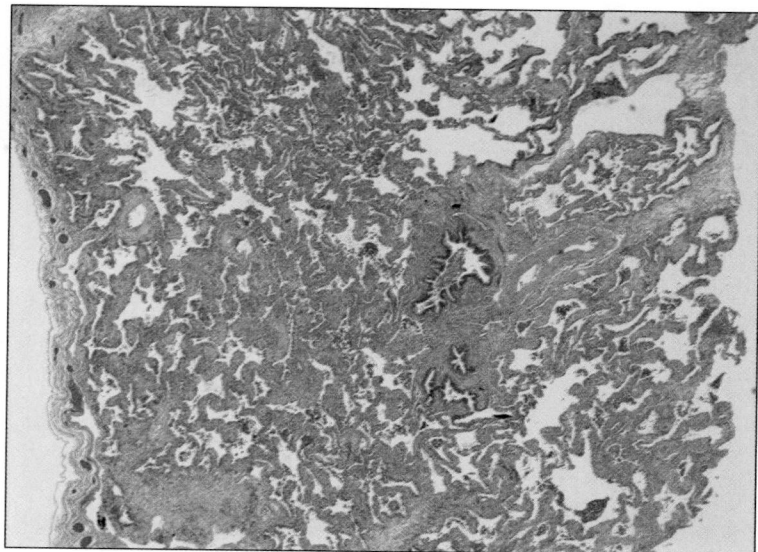

Fig. 35.4 40× power view shows homogeneous inflammation and fibrosis of the interstitium of the lung, characteristic of non-specific interstitial pneumonia or NSIP. *(Courtesy Lynette Sholl, M.D., Brigham and Women's Hospital.)*

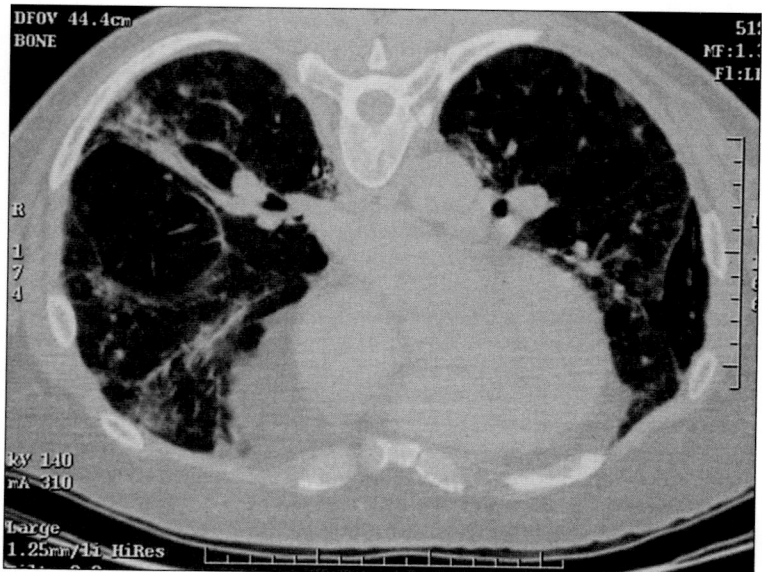

Fig. 35.5 High-resolution computed tomography scan of the chest shows bilateral ground-glass opacities without honeycombing in a patient with dermatomyositis, consistent with non-specific interstitial pneumonia.

which is pathognomonic for UIP and is found typically in a subpleural distribution. There is reasonable correlation of the radiographic appearance on chest CT with histopathologic changes in UIP and NSIP.[8] When performing a chest CT scan, it is important to perform images in the prone position to negate the potential effects of gravity, which can give the false impression of ILD changes at the bases. Emerging technologies using CT-PET and MRI are being investigated. They may help to better define and distinguish areas of inflammation and fibrosis when compared with standard chest CT scans.

Pulmonary function testing

ILD is characterized by the presence of restriction on spirometry and plethysmography (reduced forced vital capacity [FVC], increased ratio of forced expiratory volume in 1 second [FEV_1] to FVC, a low total lung capacity, and low carbon monoxide diffusion capacity [D_LCO]).[9] The 6-minute walk test is a useful and simple test that can detect early interstitial or pulmonary vascular disease when oxygen saturation drops below 95%; however, the use of the 6-minute walk test in clinical practice for this purpose has yet to be validated.[10]

Bronchoalveolar lavage

The main role of bronchoscopy, bronchoalveolar lavage (BAL), and transbronchial biopsy in interstitial lung disease is mainly to determine if there is concomitant infection. In rare instances an alternative diagnosis is established. It can explain part or all of the underlying lung dysfunction. Assessment of cell differentials and specific cell type predominance, such as a predominance of neutrophils, does not serve as an independent predictor of disease progression or response to treatment as noted in the Scleroderma Lung Study.[11,12]

Lung biopsy

In many cases, where the disease pattern on HRCT clearly favors one diagnosis and the clinical features are straightforward, lung biopsy may not be necessary or advised. However, when the clinical presentation is atypical or poorly differentiated or where other diagnoses such as COP or infection are being entertained, a lung biopsy may offer important information that can influence treatment decisions.

Systemic sclerosis

Pulmonary disease is the leading cause of mortality and morbidity in SSc. Although ILD is the most common pulmonary manifestation, other complications such as aspiration pneumonia and pulmonary hypertension can occur separately or concomitantly with ILD.

ILD is the most common pulmonary complication in SSc. The prevalence of disease varies from 25% to 90% depending on the subtype and definition of scleroderma, although clinically significant ILD in scleroderma occurs in about 40% to 50% of patients with diffuse disease and in about 30% of patients with limited disease.[13,14] Most of the morbidity and progression of ILD in diffuse SSc occurs in the first 4 to 5 years, and severe ILD can occur in patients with limited disease and also in patients without cutaneous involvement of scleroderma, known as *sine scleroderma*.[15,16] The predominant pathologic pattern seen is fibrotic NSIP followed by UIP, and rarely COP and DAD may be seen.[3,17] The pathogenesis of the development of fibrosis is not well understood, but both transforming growth factor beta (TGF-β) and platelet-derived growth factor amplification likely play an important role in disease progression.[18-20]

At this time there are no clearly identified treatments that are beneficial in ILD associated with scleroderma. After multiple small trials and a retrospective analysis suggested a potential benefit of cyclophosphamide in ILD and scleroderma, two prospective clinical trials using cyclophosphamide have failed to show clinically significant benefit in terms of survival or clinically significant improvement in pulmonary function based on HRCT or pulmonary function tests (PFTs). In the Scleroderma Lung Study oral cyclophosphamide was used for a duration of 1 year, and a small improvement in FVC was noted after 1 year, although this benefit was not maintained by the end of year 2.[21,22] In another prospective trial, a trend toward improvement in FVC was noted in a study using intravenous cyclophosphamide 600 mg/m^2 monthly for 6 months with prednisone 20 mg on alternate days followed by azathioprine for an additional 6 months.[23] In a systematic review of multiple studies using cyclophosphamide in SSc ILD measuring mean changes in FVC and D_LCO as an outcome, no significant improvement was noted in pulmonary function or quality of life.[24,25] On balance, despite numerous efforts to assess the potential benefit of cyclophosphamide in ILD in scleroderma, it appears that the potential benefits are modest and those benefits must be weighed against significant toxicity associated with treatment. Novel approaches for the treatment of ILD associated with scleroderma include tyrosine kinase inhibition, pirfenidone, mycophenolate mofetil, and endothelin antagonists.[26,27]

Aspiration related to esophageal dysmotility is commonly seen in SSc and may play a role in either the pathogenesis or exacerbation of ILD in SSc. In one study, SSc patients with ILD had higher levels of esophageal acid exposure and reflux episodes compared with those with normal HRCT.[28] Although no prospective trials have measured progression of lung function in response to control of reflux, it may be beneficial to minimize the risk of reflux by using high-dose proton pump inhibitors or consider antireflux surgery in patients with evident ILD.

Pulmonary hypertension occurs most frequently in patients with limited SSc, especially of long-standing disease duration, affecting about 10% of patients with limited SSc.[29] In some patients, severe pulmonary hypertension and ILD can occur concomitantly, representing among the most challenging prognostic and therapeutic scenarios. Early recognition is important given the now numerous therapeutic options available to treat pulmonary hypertension, which may enhance survival and quality of life including phosphodiesterase inhibitors, endothelin antagonists, and prostacyclin inhibition either alone or in combination.[30]

In summary, the initial pulmonary assessment of all patients with scleroderma involves baseline pulmonary function testing, HRCT, and echocardiography. Assessment using an algorithm combining findings on PFTs and HRCT can aid in prognostication and decisions regarding treatment.[31] If significant ILD is present with predominantly inflammatory disease that appears to be progressive, then a trial of cytotoxic or other immune-modulating therapy either with or without steroids may be considered, though data supporting their benefit is limited on the basis of clinical trials in scleroderma. An approach that affects both ongoing inflammation and fibrosis together may ultimately offer a more effective therapeutic option. Finally, there are several ongoing trials assessing the use of stem cell transplant in patients with aggressive disease and patients with rapidly progressive disease may be considered for lung transplant in selected centers.[32]

Rheumatoid arthritis

Pulmonary disease is relatively common in RA. Although morbidity is more readily apparent in the articular system, increased mortality, observed in the first decade, can mostly be attributed to extra-articular organ involvement, in particular of the cardiopulmonary system.[3,33,34] Extra-articular manifestations occur in 40.6% of patients affected with RA, and in this subset 12.8% are considered severe and potentially disabling. A history of ever-smoking is a strong predictor of extra-articular organ involvement and may help explain why the cardiopulmonary system may be responsible for the decreased survival observed in a subset of RA patients.[35]

The lung parenchyma, vasculature, airways, and pleura can be involved in RA; however, the most significant pulmonary complication is rheumatoid arthritis–associated interstitial lung disease (RA-ILD).[36] The histopathologic patterns associated with RA-ILD are diverse, but the two most common patterns are UIP and NSIP. Most interstitial pneumonias associated with collagen vascular disease have a slower rate of progression and better prognosis than patients with idiopathic interstitial pneumonias (i.e., IPF) independent of histopathology classification[3,37,38]; however, RA-ILD associated with UIP has a worse prognosis than that observed with NSIP. Interestingly, UIP histology in lung biopsies of patients with RA-ILD may be more frequent in smokers than non-smokers, further supporting the notion that cigarette smoke exposure is an environmental risk factor for the development of articular and extra-articular disease and may negatively affect outcomes in RA patients.[39,40] There is disparate evidence regarding the significance of anti-CCP antibodies and citrullination in ILD associated with RA.[41,42]

Clinical evidence suggests that the onset of RA-ILD occurs in a bimodal distribution with a majority of patients developing ILD a decade after the onset of articular manifestations and a minority of subjects who develop clinically apparent disease shortly after the development of articular disease.[43] Remarkably, NSIP is the predominant histology found in lung biopsies of the former phenotype while UIP is frequently observed in the latter, which may suggest that early development of RA-ILD is an indicator of poor prognosis. In a small subset of patients lung involvement is the first disease manifestation of RA. These patients will usually present with a syndrome consistent with idiopathic interstitial pneumonia and NSIP on lung biopsy, with subsequent development of articular symptoms and seropositivity. In general this atypical presentation has a similar clinical course, response to treatment, and prognosis of other RA-ILD patients.[44,45] These diverse clinical phenotypes suggest that genetic and environmental (i.e., smoking) determinants are potential disease modifiers that influence outcomes; future clinical studies that focus on molecular phenotyping (genetics, gene expression, and proteomics) of patients affected with RA-ILD could help us better understand the clinical heterogeneity observed in RA-ILD.

Preclinical ILD is relatively common in RA, and studies in which open lung biopsies or chest CT scans were performed demonstrate lung involvement in greater than 40% of the study population.[46-48] In one study, 33% of RA patients without dyspnea or cough had interstitial lung disease identified by chest CT scans; preclinical ILD like RA-ILD was associated with a history of ever-smoking. Importantly, disease progression was observed in 57% of those patients after mean length of follow-up of 1.5 years,[43] suggesting that clinically significant pulmonary fibrosis is likely to develop in a subset of patients affected with preclinical RA-ILD. These findings are consistent with a prospective study of 29 patients with RA, which showed that 34% of patients followed for 24 months had progressive interstitial lung disease[49]; further studies are required to determine the natural history of preclinical interstitial lung disease and what patients will go on to develop clinically significant pulmonary fibrosis.

Bronchiectasis or bronchiolectasis is observed in up to 30% of patients with RA studied with chest CT scans, though sputum production and disease progression is less severe than that observed in idiopathic bronchiectasis.[50-52] Similarly, obliterative bronchiolitis (OB) is more common in RA when compared with other rheumatologic diseases. Although the prevalence of OB is low, the prognosis is poor due to the lack of effective treatments. A genetic predisposition appears likely, and an association between obliterative bronchiolitis and the use of penicillamine has been postulated.

Pulmonary nodules are usually an incidental chest CT finding or, less frequently, in an open lung biopsy.[50,53] Nodule cavitation may result in hemoptysis or pneumothorax, through the rupture of subpleural nodules. Caplan syndrome consists of nodules associated with coal miners' pneumoconiosis. Pleural disease is common in RA, and pleuritic pain occurs at some time in at least 20% of patients. Pleural disease is found in 50% of autopsies. However, clinical evidence of pleural disease is found in less than 5% of patients, usually in males, and is often asymptomatic.

Dermatomyositis/Polymyositis

The idiopathic inflammatory myopathies are a group of disorders predominantly characterized by immune-mediated destruction and dysfunction of muscle[54]; however, the disease frequently involves the skin, joints, and cardiopulmonary system.[55] The most common variant of connective tissue disease–associated ILD is the anti-synthetase syndrome in which antibodies directed against Jo-1 (histidyl-tRNA synthetase) and other amino-acyl tRNA synthetases such as PL-12 are associated with a clinical syndrome characterized by myositis, fever, Raynaud phenomenon, "mechanic's hands," arthritis, and interstitial lung disease.[56,57] As observed in other connective tissue diseases, lung involvement precedes other systemic disease in approximately 16% of patients.[58]

Although estimates of the overall incidence of ILD associated with inflammatory myopathy range from 5% to 45%,[59] lung involvement is clearly more prevalent among patients possessing anti-synthetase antibodies. In the anti-synthetase syndrome most reports consist of small case series in which the prevalence of ILD is as high as 80% to 95% depending on the clinical, functional, and radiographic criteria used to define ILD.[60] Pathologic case series have shown that ILD associated with the anti-synthetase syndrome encompasses a variety of histopathologic subtypes, including NSIP, COP, UIP, and DAD.[61-63] As expected, response to therapy and overall prognosis largely reflects the underlying lung histology. The predominance of NSIP in the majority of myositis-associated ILD case series may explain increased survival rates when compared with more common idiopathic interstitial pneumonias like IPF.[56,64]

Despite these data, recent evidence suggests that there is a subset of anti-Jo-1 antibody–positive individuals who present with a rapidly progressive form of ILD that is reminiscent of the acute disease exacerbations observed in IPF patients.[65] In a study of 90 patients treated in a tertiary referral center, 86% met criteria for ILD. Chest CT scans revealed patterns predominantly suggestive of UIP or NSIP; however, a review of histopathologic abnormalities in a subset of 22 individuals who underwent open lung biopsy demonstrated a preponderance of UIP and DAD. Furthermore, these subjects had worse survival than that previously reported in myositis-associated ILD. In light of the accelerated disease progression associated with a high incidence of DAD on biopsy, these findings suggest that a subset of anti-synthetase syndrome patients may develop acute clinical exacerbations, as has been previously reported in IPF patients.[66,67] Similarly, COP, which is common in DM/PM, tends to have a worse outcome when associated with clinical or CT features suggestive of fibrosing alveolitis.[39] These patients are likely to fail anti-inflammatory and immunosuppressive therapy due to rapidly progressive disease and therefore if otherwise eligible should be referred early for a lung transplant evaluation.

Systemic lupus erythematosus

Pleuritic and chest wall symptoms are common in SLE and usually not of serious consequence, but more serious lung problems such as pneumonitis, pulmonary hemorrhage, and pulmonary hypertension may occur and can present significant clinical challenges. As such, they are the focus of this discussion.

Chest wall, costochondral pain, and pleurisy are common in SLE, are often part of the initial presenting symptoms, and clinically may be difficult to distinguish between musculoskeletal or pleuritic pain. Pleurisy occurs in up to 50% of patients with SLE but only a small percentage will actually develop effusions, which are typically exudative with modestly low glucose concentration and complement levels.[68] The testing of antinuclear antibodies in pleural fluid is generally not indicated and usually reflects what is detected in the serum. Treatment is only for symptomatic patients and includes non-steroidal anti-inflammatory drugs (NSAIDs) in mild cases and corticosteroids in more severe cases.

Acute pneumonitis is a rare, poorly understood but feared complication of SLE. It is characterized by fever, cough, dyspnea, and progressive hypoxemia. Sometimes, hemoptysis may be noted and chest roentenograms show diffuse infiltrates and pleural effusions. Chest CT scan may show ground-glass opacities and consolidation. Biopsy of specimens may show DAD with or without alveolar hemorrhage and capillaritis. The mortality associated with this syndrome is high, reported as 50% in one study of 12 patients.[69] Such patients who present with this syndrome should be treated aggressively with high-dose steroids and consideration for additional immunosuppressive agents such as cyclophosphamide, though no controlled trials exist to guide therapy. A more chronic interstitial lung disease may rarely develop in SLE, which may or may not occur following an acute pulmonary process, and as in scleroderma, lung biopsy specimens may show UIP, NSIP, and rarely LIP. Treatment considerations are similar as noted earlier with ILD related to scleroderma.

Diffuse alveolar hemorrhage can occur in SLE in up to 4% of patients.[70] It typically occurs in a patient with known SLE who presents with dyspnea, cough, and often hemoptysis, though some patients will present with anemia and bilateral infiltrates without hemoptysis. In patients with known SLE, one must consider underlying infection, pulmonary embolism, and capillaritis. Biopsy may reveal bland hemorrhage, immune complex deposition, or capillaritis. Distinguishing this syndrome from acute pneumonitis can be difficult and is a source of considerable controversy. Mortality can be high and treatment involves the use of steroids, cyclophosphamide, and in some cases plasmapheresis.[71,72]

Acute reversible hypoxemia can occur in patients with SLE who present with unexplained hypoxemia and normal chest roentenograms. It is postulated that elevated levels of C3a and upregulation of adhesion molecules result in pulmonary leukoaggregation and a leuko-occlusive vasculopathy. Treatment with corticosteroids and aspirin can be effective.[73,74] Shrinking lung syndrome has been noted in SLE and is characterized by dyspnea, pleuritic pain, and progressive decrease in lung volume. The pathology of this disorder is the subject of controversy, thought by some to be due to a myositis or myopathy of the diaphragm, whereas others have thought it is due to a primary loss of lung compliance. The syndrome should be thought of in those patients with SLE with dyspnea, clear chest roentgenograms, and elevated diaphragms. PFTs may show an abnormal diffusion capacity that corrects for alveolar volume, and esophageal manometry may be useful to identify an abnormality in lung compliance. Corticosteroids, theophylline, and other immunosuppressive therapy may be beneficial, though generally the disorder is self-limiting.[75]

Pulmonary hypertension occurs in a small but significant portion of patients with SLE. Mild to moderate disease may occur in up to 40% of patients. Pulmonary function testing may show restriction, reduced D_LCO, desaturation with exercise, and evidence of right ventricular hypertrophy by echocardiography, though right heart catheterization is required to confirm the diagnosis.[76] In addition, recurrent thromboemboli can result in pulmonary hypertension, especially in those with the antiphospholipid antibody (APLA) syndrome. In those patients with APLA and pulmonary hypertension, assessment with ventilation-perfusion scanning or CT with pulmonary artery protocol should be performed. Treatment in pulmonary hypertension is similar to that described for scleroderma.[77,78] In some cases pulmonary hypertension in SLE may be due to pulmonary vasculitis as opposed to a plexogenic vasculopathy, and cyclophosphamide and rituxan may be useful therapeutic interventions.[79,80]

Sjögren syndrome

SS may have a variety of pulmonary manifestations, including bronchial and airway narrowing, interstitial lung disease, and lymphoproliferative disease including in rare cases lymphoma.

Patients with SS frequently complain of a dry cough, with evidence of hyperactive airways secondary to inflammatory infiltration of bronchial submucosa.[81] Interstitial lung disease includes NSIP, UIP, COP, and LIP with NSIP noted most frequently.[82] LIP, though rare in general, can be seen in SS in addition to other rheumatic diseases and findings on CT include ground-glass opacities, centrilobular nodules, subpleural nodules, and patchy areas of consolidation. On histopathology, T and B lymphocytic infiltrates are notable and rarely can progress to end-stage interstitial fibrosis. In certain cases, the distribution of lymphocytic infiltration is more localized to the bronchial tree, known as *follicular bronchiolitis.*

Nodular lymphoid hyperplasia (pseudolymphoma) may also occur in SS and is characterized by pulmonary nodules or infiltrates containing reactive lymphoid cells. The presence of such lesions on CT may be difficult to distinguish from B-cell lymphoma of the extranodal marginal zone B-cell type (MZCL) of MALT type or more aggressive forms of non-Hodgkin lymphoma and thus biopsy may be required.[83] Treatment options for ILD associated with SS include corticosteroids and additional agents such as cyclophosphamide, azathioprine, mycophenolate mofetil, and emerging agents using B-cell deletion.

Drug-induced lung injury

A host of medications used in rheumatologic practice have been implicated in lung injury, most notably methotrexate (MTX). MTX lung toxicity usually presents within the first 1 to 2 years of initiation of the drug, and clinical presentations can range from a cough to fulminant presentations with fever, progressive dyspnea, and life-threatening respiratory failure. X-ray and CT findings may show diffuse or focal infiltrates and pathologic findings include prominent lymphocytic infiltration, acute interstitial pneumonia, and sometimes COP. Although a chronic fibrotic lung reaction to MTX has been implicated, there is no clear evidence to support this concept and many cases labeled as chronic MTX fibrotic disease probably represent progression of underlying ILD in patients with RA. Risk factors for MTX lung disease include older age, diabetes hypoalbuminemia, and perhaps previous lung disease, though it is unclear if preexisting lung disease is a risk factor for the development of MTX-induced lung toxicity.[84] In patients with minimal underlying lung disease it is reasonable to consider using MTX, though with careful observation and monitoring.

Leflunomide may have an incidence of pneumonitis in up to 1% of patients and this occurrence may be more common in patients previously treated with methotrexate.[85,86] Other agents used in rheumatologic practice that may result in pulmonary toxicity include azathioprine, sulfasalazine, minocycline, NSAIDs, D-penicillamine, gold, and cyclophosphamide. In all cases of suspected drug-induced lung toxicity, treatment involves cessation of therapy in mild cases, consideration of underlying infection using bronchoscopy, BAL if needed, and use of corticosteroids in more severe cases.

The use of tumor necrosis factor (TNF) modulating agents in patients with RA associated with ILD is a matter of significant controversy. A number of case reports have noted progression of underlying ILD in patients given TNF inhibitors (mostly infliximab), and there have also been reports that ILD has either remained stable or actually improved on TNF inhibitors.[87,88] RA patients may also have a higher risk of bronchiectasis and in more severe cases are at higher risk for infectious complication. Therefore in the RA patient with significant ILD or bronchiectasis complication, caution should be exercised in the use of TNF inhibitors.

The lung and vasculitic syndromes

Diffuse alveolar hemorrhage (DAH) as a result of capillaritis is an important feature of various vasculitic syndromes including antineutrophil cytoplasmic antibody (ANCA)–associated granulomatous vasculitis, microscopic polyangiitis, Goodpasture syndrome, SLE, and rarely in RA, cryoglobulinemia, and the antiphospholipid antibody syndrome.[89] Capillaritis may manifest clinically with hemoptysis, though there may be no clinical evidence of bleeding even on bronchoscopy. Capillaritis should be suspected in patients with respiratory symptoms, falling hematocrit, and radiographic abnormalities including diffuse lung infiltrates, ground-glass opacities, and elevated diffusion capacity as the main clues to active bleeding in the lung. In cases of ANCA-associated vasculitis and anti-GBM disease, these findings are often accompanied by active glomerulonephritis, the so-called *pulmonary renal syndrome.* Lung biopsy may be helpful to distinguish pauci-immune disease associated with ANCA versus immune complex– and complement-mediated diseases seen in SLE or anti-GBM disease seen in Goodpasture syndrome, though tissue is often more accessible from the kidney or other sources with less morbidity. Fibrosis and airflow obstruction as a result of chronic inflammation have been noted in ANCA-associated lung disease.[90,91] Treatment involves high-dose corticosteroids, cyclophosphamide, rituxan, or other immunomodulating agent and consideration in severe cases for plasmapheresis, especially in Goodpasture syndrome, though its utility in ANCA-associated pulmonary hemorrhage syndromes is uncertain.

TREATMENT OF INTERSTITIAL LUNG DISEASE ASSOCIATED WITH THE RHEUMATIC DISEASES

Outside of scleroderma, there are no prospective, randomized trials for the treatment of ILD in the rheumatic diseases. Therapeutic choices in ILD and the rheumatic disease have therefore been extrapolated from the scleroderma experience, which may not be appropriate given the varied histopathologic patterns and natural history seen in the lung of the different rheumatic diseases. In patients with active clinical symptoms and evidence of ground-glass opacities on CT scan and/or cellular NSIP on lung biopsy, a trial of anti-inflammatory therapy with high-dose steroids and a second agent such as cyclophosphamide, mycophenolate mofetil, azathioprine, or a calcineurin inhibitor such as tacrolimus or cyclosporine are reasonable options. In patients with predominantly fibrotic ILD, no clear therapeutic regimen can be recommended, though agents such as N-acetyl cysteine, mycophenolate mofetil, pirfenidone, or other emerging agents that have antifibrotic effects may prove beneficial. New and emerging T and B cell–based therapies (e.g., used in RA) may have a beneficial effect on coexisting lung disease.[92-95] In all such patients who are treated, prophylaxis for *Pneumocystis jiroveci* pneumonia should be considered and immunization against influenza and pneumococcal pneumonia is strongly recommended.

In summary, great challenges still exist in our understanding of the natural history and treatment of ILD and other pulmonary manifestations in the rheumatic diseases. A close interaction between rheumatologist and pulmonologist can be particularly helpful in those patients with pulmonary disease who have either overt or subtle findings that may suggest a rheumatic syndrome. Expertise in capillary microscopy, eliciting subtle clues on clinical examination and interpretation of sophisticated immunologic testing are of great importance in establishing the appropriate diagnosis and tailoring treatment. Working in close collaboration with pulmonologists, radiologists, and pathologists, rheumatologists have much to offer to this most challenging group of patients.

KEY REFERENCES

1. Wells A, Cullinan P, Hansell D, et al. Fibrosing alveolitis associated with systemic sclerosis has a better prognosis than lone cryptogenic fibrosing alveolitis. Am J Respir Crit Care Med 1994;149:1583-1590.
3. Park JH, Kim DS, Park I-N, et al. Prognosis of fibrotic interstitial pneumonia: idiopathic versus collagen vascular disease-related subtypes. Am J Respir Crit Care Med 2007;175:705-711.
4. Kinder BW, Collard HR, Koth L, et al. Idiopathic nonspecific interstitial pneumonia: lung manifestation of undifferentiated connective tissue disease? Am J Respir Crit Care Med 2007;176:691-697.
5. Wells A, Dubois RM. Bronchiolitis in association with connective tissue disorders. Clin Chest Med 1993;14:655-666.
8. Flaherty KR, Thwaite EL, Kazerooni EA, et al. Radiological versus histological diagnosis in UIP and NSIP: survival implications. Thorax 2003;58:143-148.
9. Alhamad EH, Lynch JP, Martinez FJ. Pulmonary function tests in interstitial lung disease. 2001;22:715-750.
10. Garin MC, Highland KB, Silver RM, Strange C. Limitations to the 6 minute walk test in interstitial lung disease and pulmonary hypertension in scleroderma. J Rheumatol 2009;36:330-336.
15. Fischer A, Swigris JJ, Groshong SD, et al. Clinically significant interstitial lung disease in limited scleroderma. Chest 2008;134:601-605.
16. Fischer A, Meehan RT, Feghali-Bostwick CA, et al. Unique characteristics of systemic sclerosis sine scleroderma-associated interstitial lung disease. Chest 2006;130:976-981.
21. Tashkin DP, Elashoff R, Clements PJ, et al. Cyclophosphamide versus placebo in scleroderma lung disease. N Engl J Med 2006;354:2655-2666.
22. Tashkin DP, Elashoff R, Clements PJ, et al. Effects of 1-year treatment with cyclophosphamide on outcomes at 2 years in scleroderma lung disease. Am J Respir Crit Care Med 2007;176:1026-1034.
23. Hoyles RK, Ellis RW, Wellsbury J, et al. A multicenter, prospective, randomized, double-blind, placebo-controlled trial of corticosteroids and intravenous cyclophosphamide followed by oral azathioprine for the treatment of pulmonary fibrosis in scleroderma. Arthritis Rheum 2006;54:3962-3970.
24. Nannini C, West C, Erwin P, et al. Effects of cyclophosphamide on pulmonary function in patients with scleroderma and interstitial lung disease: a systematic review and meta-analysis of randomized controlled trials and observational prospective cohort studies. Arthritis Res Ther 2008;10:R124.
27. Gerbino AJ, Goss CH, Molitor JA. Effect of mycophenolate mofetil on pulmonary function in scleroderma-associated interstitial lung disease. Chest 2008;133:455-460.
28. Savarino E, Bazzica M, Zentilin P, et al. Gastroesophageal reflux and pulmonary fibrosis in scleroderma: a study using pH-impedance monitoring. Am J Respir Crit Care Med 2009;179:408-413.
30. Denton CP, Pope JE, Peter H-H, et al. Long-term effects of bosentan on quality of life, survival, safety and tolerability in pulmonary arterial hypertension related to connective tissue diseases. Ann Rheum Dis 2008;67:1222-1228.
33. Gabriel SE, Crowson CS, Kremers HM, et al. Survival in rheumatoid arthritis: a population-based analysis of trends over 40 years. Arthritis Rheum 2003;48:54-58.
36. Brown KK, Rheumatoid lung disease. Proc Am Thorac Soc 2007;4:443-448.
38. Kocheril SV, Appleton BE, Somers EC, et al. Comparison of disease progression and mortality of connective tissue disease-related interstitial lung disease and idiopathic interstitial pneumonia. Arthritis Care Res 2005;53:549-557.
39. Shirley AA, Ernesto S-S, Michael HW. Cigarette smoking and rheumatoid arthritis. Semin Arthritis Rheum 2001;31:146-159.
40. Klareskog L, Stolt P, Lundberg K, et al. for the Epidemiological Investigation of Rheumatoid Arthritis Study Group. A new model for an etiology of rheumatoid arthritis: Smoking may trigger HLA-DR (shared epitope)–restricted immune reactions to autoantigens modified by citrullination. Arthritis Rheum 2006;54:38-46.
41. Inui N, Enomoto N, Sudat T, et al. Anti-cyclic citrullinated peptide antibodies in lung diseases associated with rheumatoid arthritis. Clin Biochem 2008; 41(13):1074-1077.
42. Alexiou I, Germenis A, Koutroumpas A, et al. Anti CCP citrullinated peptide-2 (CCP2) autoantibodies and extra-articular manifestations in Greek patients with RA. Clin Rheumatol 2008;27(4):511-513.
43. Gochuico BR, Avila NA, Chow CK, et al. Progressive preclinical interstitial lung disease in rheumatoid arthritis. Arch Intern Med 2008;168:159-166.
45. Park IN, Jegal Y, Kim DS, et al. Clinical course and lung function change of idiopathic nonspecific interstitial pneumonia. Eur Respir J 2009;33:68-76.
48. Gabbay E, Tarala R, Will R, et al. Interstitial lung disease in recent onset rheumatoid arthritis. Am J Respir Crit Care Med 1997;156:528-535.
49. Dawson JK, Fewins HE, Desmond J, et al. Predictors of progression of HRCT diagnosed fibrosing alveolitis in patients with rheumatoid arthritis. Ann Rheum Dis 2002;61:517-521.
51. Vergnenegre A, Pugnere N, Antonini M, et al. Airway obstruction and rheumatoid arthritis. Eur Respir J 1997;10:1072-1078.
54. Arahata K, Engel A. Quantitation of subsets according to diagnosis and sites of accumulation and demonstration and counts of muscle fibers invaded by T cells. Ann Neurol 1984;16:193-208.
55. Oddis C. Idiopathic inflammatory myopathy. In: Wortmann RL, ed. Diseases of Skeletal Muscle, 1st edition. Philadelphia: Lippincott, Williams & Wilkins, 2000:45-86.
57. Kalluri M, Sahn SA, Oddis CV, et al. Clinical profile of anti-PL-12 autoantibody. Chest March 2009 (epub).
58. Cottin V, Thivolet-Bejui F, Reynaud-Gaubert M, et al. Interstitial lung disease in amyopathic dermatomyositis, dermatomyositis and polymyositis. Eur Respir J 2003;22:245-250.
59. Marie I, Hachulla P, Chérin S, et al. Interstitial lung disease in polymyositis and dermatomyositis. Arthritis Care Res 2002;47:614-622.
61. Tansey D, Wells AU, Colby TV, et al. Variations in histological patterns of interstitial pneumonia between connective tissue disorders and their relationship to prognosis. Histopathology 2004;44:585-596.
64. Fathi M, Vikgren J, Boijsen M, et al. Interstitial lung disease in polymyositis and dermatomyositis: longitudinal evaluation by pulmonary function and radiology. Arthritis Care Res 2008;59:677-685.
65. Richards TJ, Eggebeen A, Gibson K, et al. Characterization and peripheral blood biomarker assessment of Jo-1 antibody-positive interstitial lung disease. Arthritis Rheum 2009;60(7):2183-2192.
71. Santos-Ocampo AS, Mandell BF, Fessler BJ. Alveolar hemorrhage in systemic lupus erythematosus. Chest 2000;118:1083-1090.
75. Warrington KJ, Moder KG, Brutinel WM. The shrinking lungs syndrome in systemic lupus erythematosus. Mayo Clin Proc 2000;75:467-472.
82. Parambil JG, Myers JL, Lindell RM, et al. Interstitial lung disease in primary Sjögren's syndrome. Chest 2006;130:1489-1495.
83. Papiris SA, Kalomenidis I, Malagari K, et al. Extranodal marginal zone B-cell lymphoma of the lung in Sjögren's syndrome patients: reappraisal of clinical, radiological, and pathology findings. Respir Med 2007;101:84-92.
84. Alarcon GS, Kremer JM, Macaluso M, et al. Risk factors for methotrexate-induced lung injury in patients with rheumatoid arthritis: a multicenter, case-control study. Ann Intern Med 1997;127:356-364.
85. Kamata Y, Nara H, Kamimura T, et al. Rheumatoid arthritis complicated with acute interstitial pneumonia induced by leflunomide as an adverse reaction. Intern Med 2004;43:1201-1204.
87. Ostor AJ, Chivers ER, Somerville MF, et al. Pulmonary complications of infliximab therapy in paitents with rheumatoid arthritis. J Rheumatol 2006;33:622-628.
89. Specks U. Diffuse alveolar hemorrhage syndromes. Curr Opin Rheumatol 2001;13:12-17.
90. Seo P, Yuan IM, Holbrook JT, et al. for the WGET Research Group. Damage caused by Wegener's granulomatosis and its treatment: prospective data from the Wegener's Granulomatosis Etanercept Trial (WGET). Arthritis Rheum 2005;52:2168-2178.
92. Nannini C, Ryu JH, Matteson EL. Lung disease in rheumatoid arthritis. Curr Opin Rheumatol 2008;20:340-346.
93. Saketkoo L, Espinoza L. Experience of mycophenolate mofetil in 10 patients with autoimmune-related interstitial lung disease demonstrates promising effects. Am J Med Sci 2009 (Mar 18 Epub).
94. Swigris JJ, Olson AL, Fischer A, et al. Mycophenolate mofetil is safe, well tolerated, and preserves lung function in patients with connective tissue disease–related interstitial lung disease. Chest 2006;130:30-36.

REFERENCES

Full references for this chapter can be found on www.expertconsult.com.

Gastrointestinal tract and rheumatic disease

36

Talia Landau and Raymond Cross

- Abdominal symptoms in a patient with arthritis may reflect several different etiologies.
- Inflammatory bowel diseases, particularly Crohn disease and ulcerative colitis, are often complicated by the development of peripheral or axial arthritis.
- Most systemic rheumatic diseases can be associated with intermittent inflammation involving the gastrointestinal tract.
- A number of antirheumatic drugs can produce gastrointestinal symptoms; gastropathy induced by non-steroidal anti-inflammatory drugs is by far the most common such adverse event.
- Tumor necrosis factor-α blockade produces a rapid significant clinical effect both on the intestinal symptoms of Crohn disease (CD) and on the manifestations of peripheral and axial arthritis of inflammatory bowel disease–associated spondyloarthropathy.

INTRODUCTION

Gastrointestinal illnesses have long been recognized to be associated with extraintestinal manifestations of disease. It is not known why extraintestinal complications of disease occur; however, because many of these complications occur in patients with active gastrointestinal inflammation, it has been postulated that increased intestinal permeability resulting from the underlying inflammatory process allows luminal antigens to be presented to the systemic immune system. Alternatively, because many inflammatory gastrointestinal illnesses cause a systemic inflammatory response, it is possible that the joint and other sites are "innocent" bystanders in the inflammatory process. Recent evidence has linked adhesion molecules, vascular adhesion protein-1, and T cells bearing B7 integrin to joint synovial fluid,[1] providing a direct link between intestinal and joint inflammation. Gastrointestinal diseases that have been linked to inflammatory arthritis include but are not limited to inflammatory bowel disease, composed of ulcerative colitis and Crohn disease, celiac disease, bacterial enteritis, Whipple's disease, vasculitides, Behçet's syndrome, and microscopic colitis. This chapter briefly reviews the gastrointestinal diseases associated with inflammatory arthritis and describes the joint findings associated with each disease.

INFLAMMATORY BOWEL DISEASE: CROHN DISEASE AND ULCERATIVE COLITIS

Inflammatory bowel diseases (IBD), composed of ulcerative colitis and Crohn disease, are chronic inflammatory conditions of the intestines typically affecting young adults. The etiology of IBD is unknown. However, a combination of a genetic predisposition, dysregulated immune system, and environmental antigens are thought to play a role in development of IBD. Crohn disease (CD) and ulcerative colitis (UC) are usually easily distinguished from each other by clinical symptoms, endoscopic findings, and histologic findings. However, in approximately 15% of cases, differentiation between CD and UC is difficult. These patients are classified as having IBD type undetermined or indeterminate colitis. The extraintestinal manifestations, treatment options, and prognoses differ by disease.

Ulcerative colitis usually presents with bloody diarrhea. UC is seen more often in never smokers and former smokers, as opposed to active smokers. The onset of bloody diarrhea after a patient has quit smoking is consistent with the diagnosis of UC until proven otherwise. The extent of colonic involvement determines the UC patient phenotype. UC phenotype is typically broken down into three groups: inflammation limited to the rectum (ulcerative proctitis), inflammation limited to the left colon (left-sided colitis), and inflammation proximal to the splenic flexure (extensive or pancolitis). The amount of colonic involvement is important because patients with pancolitis are more likely to be treated with steroids, become hospitalized for UC, undergo colectomy, and develop colorectal cancer.[2,3] Patients with UC have disease limited to the colon only; endoscopic examination reveals inflammation beginning at the anal verge and extending proximally in a continuous fashion. The inflammatory process in UC tends to be more superficial compared with Crohn disease. Decreased anatomic markings, friability, and erosions are endoscopic hallmarks of the disease (Fig. 36.1). Patients with severe disease can have large or confluent ulcerations, making differentiation from CD difficult. Small bowel involvement does not occur except in patients with pancolitis who have "backwash ileitis" (inflammation in the distal 5 cm of terminal ileum). Skip lesions should not be seen; however, once patients undergo medical therapy, especially with oral or topical agents, the inflammation can appear patchy. Biopsies typically reveal both acute and chronic inflammation; active colitis is defined by the presence of neutrophils in the crypts (cryptitis and crypt abscess), whereas chronicity is established by expansion of the basal surface with plasma cells and lymphocytes, with distortion of the architecture (Fig. 36.2).

Crohn disease can affect any location in the gastrointestinal tract from the mouth to the anus. The terminal ileum is the most commonly affected site. CD is distinguished from UC by the presence of small bowel involvement, development of strictures and/or fistulas, endoscopic appearance, and histopathologic findings (Table 36.1). Symptoms of CD are heterogeneous and depend on the patient's phenotype.[4] Patients with *inflammatory* CD usually present with nonbloody diarrhea and crampy lower abdominal pain. Systemic symptoms may or may not be present. Patients with *obstructing* CD usually present with intermittent abdominal pain, bloating, borborygmi, and obstipation. The symptoms are usually exacerbated by eating. Nausea and emesis can be seen as the strictures become more severe. The diarrhea associated with obstructive CD usually occurs after an episode of pain and is associated with relief of symptoms (postobstructive diarrhea). Patients with *penetrating* CD present with fistulas from a segment of bowel to adjacent organs or to another loop of intestine. Sinus tracts or severe transmural inflammation can result in intra-abdominal abscess formation. Twenty to forty percent of patients develop perianal fistulas with or without abscess.[5] This complication results in perianal pain and drainage from the fistula sites. Fistulas associated with abscess are often associated with severe pain and systemic symptoms. The endoscopic appearance in patients with CD is usually easily distinguishable from UC. Small bowel imaging can demonstrate ulcerations, stricture, or fistula in the small bowel. Rectal involvement is less common and patients typically have "skip lesions" with areas of normal intervening mucosa. The ulcerations seen in CD are typically large, deep, and can be serpiginous. The earliest lesions in CD are aphthous ulcers similar to those seen in the oral mucosa (Fig. 36.3). On histopathology, an acute and chronic inflammatory process is seen as in patients with UC; however, surgical specimens can reveal transmural inflammation and transmural lymphoid aggregates. Mucosal biopsies reveal pathognomonic noncaseating granulomas in 30% to 50% of patients (Fig. 36.4).[6]

TABLE 36.1 CROHN DISEASE AND ULCERATIVE COLITIS

	Symptoms	Gastrointestinal involvement	Endoscopic findings	Pathology
Crohn disease	Abdominal pain, non-bloody diarrhea, perianal and internal fistulas, active smokers	Can involve intestine from mouth to anus	Skip lesions, serpiginous or deep ulcerations, strictures, fistulas, small bowel involvement	Transmural inflammation, non-caseating granulomas, skip lesions
Ulcerative colitis	Bloody diarrhea, tenesmus, never or former smokers	Colon only	Superficial erosions or smaller ulcerations, continuous involvement from rectum to proximal colon	Continuous histologic inflammation from rectum to proximal colon

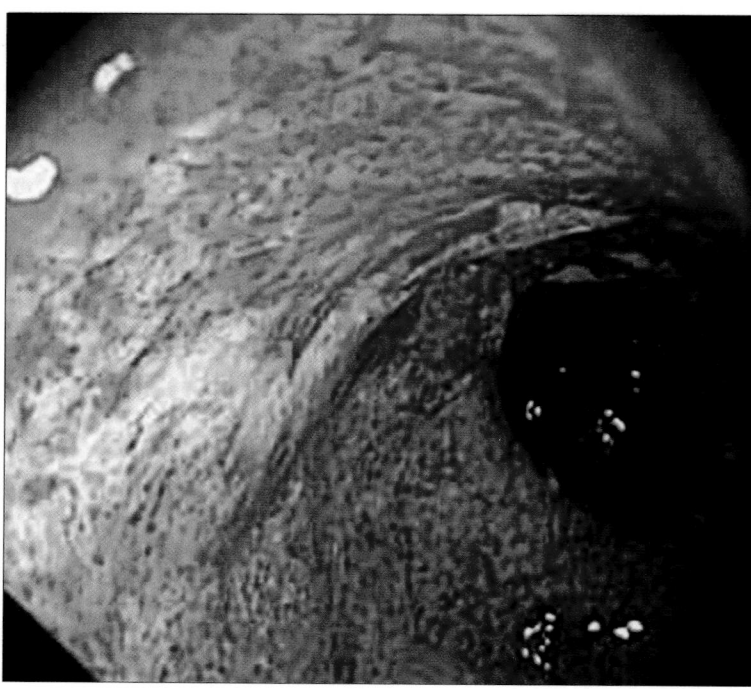

Fig. 36.1 Endoscopic findings in a patient with ulcerative colitis. The entire visualized mucosa is affected in a continuous fashion with loss of the normal vascular markings and light reflex. The mucosa is erythematous, friable, and ulcerated.

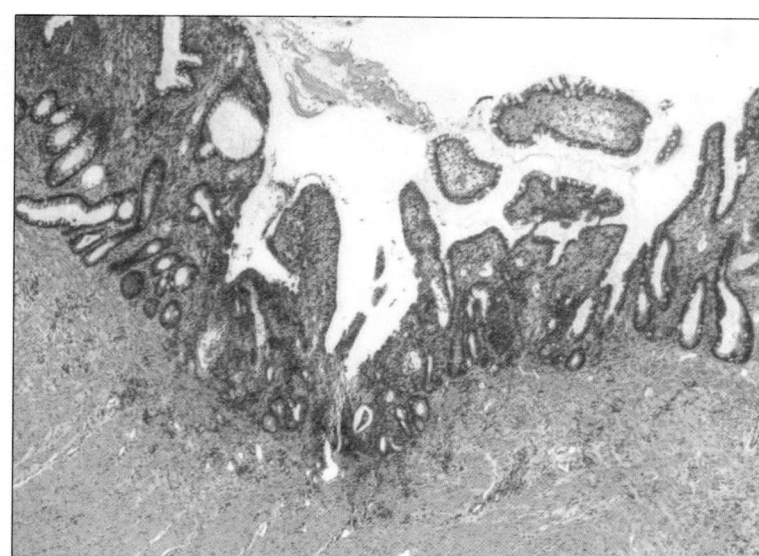

Fig. 36.2 Section of colon showing classic features of active chronic disease including marked architectural distortion (crypt branching, crypt atrophy, crypt dropout), as well as expansion of lamina propria by lymphoplasmacytic infiltrate and focal crypt abscesses (original magnification: 40×). *(Photo courtesy Harris Yfantis, M.D.)*

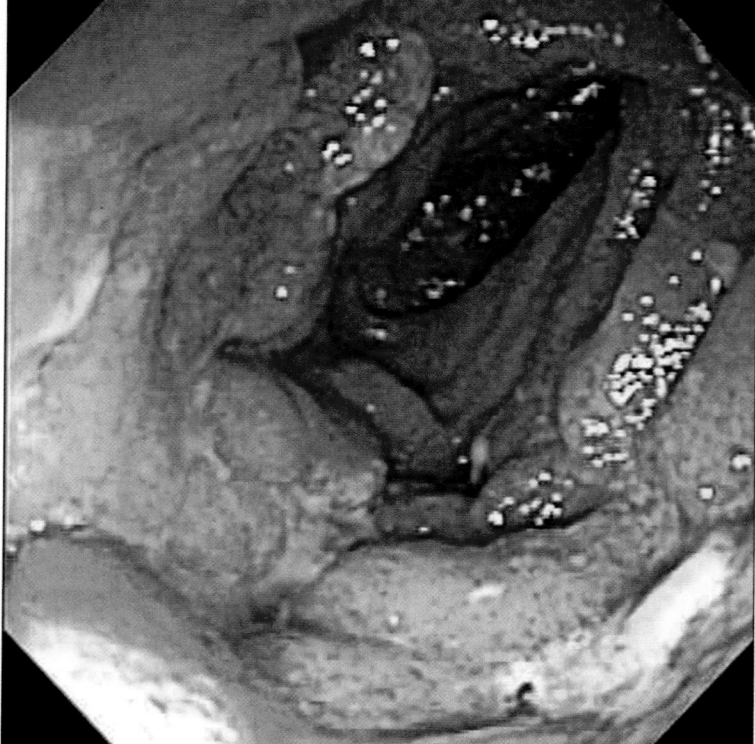

Fig. 36.3 Endoscopic findings from the ileum in a patient with Crohn disease. Deep linear and serpiginous ulcers with intervening edematous mucosa are present ("cobblestoning").

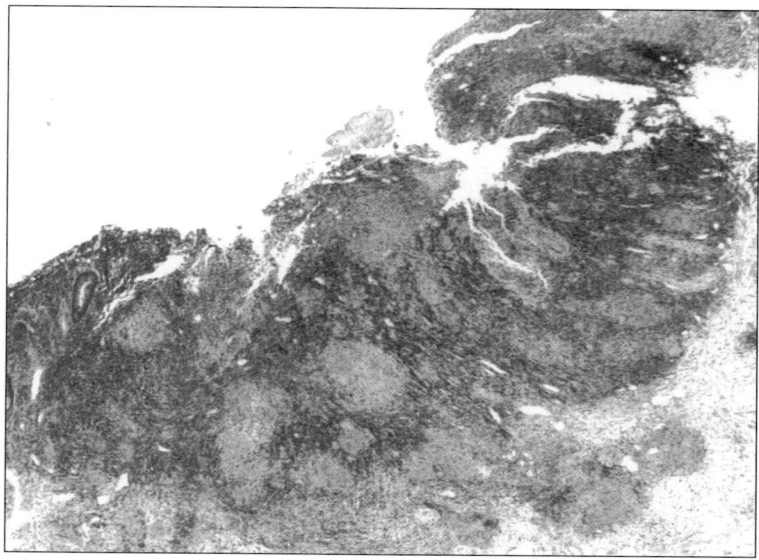

Fig. 36.4 Section of colon showing multiple epithelioid granulomas with surrounding chronic inflammation (original magnification: 40×). *(Photo courtesy Harris Yfantis, M.D.)*

TABLE 36.2 EXTRAINTESTINAL MANIFESTATIONS OF DISEASE IN PATIENTS WITH INFLAMMATORY BOWEL DISEASE

EIM	Description	Epidemiology	Presentation	Treatment
Erythema nodosum	Painful, tender, raised, red nodules, often found on the anterior lower legs	1%-9% UC 6%-15% CD 5:1 female-to-male	90% are associated with active bowel disease	Resolve with treatment of active bowel disease
Pyoderma gangrenosum	Ulcers on lower limbs, trunk, and adjacent to surgical stomas	0.5%-2% IBD	Not associated with active bowel disease	Immunosuppressive therapy; occasionally have spontaneous resolution
Aphthous ulcers	Oral ulcerations in buccal mucosa	20%-30% CD	Associated with active bowel disease Associated with ocular and articular symptoms	Resolve with treatment of active bowel disease[12]
Uveitis	Eye pain, redness, loss of visual acuity, floaters	3:1 female-to-male[13]	Anterior uveitis: 30% associated with erythema nodosum Posterior uveitis: 90% associated with arthritis; particularly ankylosing spondylitis[13]	Topical corticosteroids; systemic immune suppressants for severe cases
Episcleritis	Eye redness, irritation, and watering	3:1 female-to-male 5%-8% IBD	Associated with active bowel disease	Resolve with treatment of active bowel disease or topical corticosteroid therapy
Primary sclerosing cholangitis	Recurrent biliary sepsis, abdominal pain, pruritus, complications of portal hypertension and end-stage liver disease	Male preponderance 7% UC[11]	Not associated with active bowel symptoms; associated with colorectal cancer	Supportive therapy, manage complications of disease

CD, Crohn disease; IBD, inflammatory bowel disease; UC, ulcerative colitis.

EXTRAINTESTINAL MANIFESTATIONS OF INTESTINAL BOWEL DISEASE

In addition to the effects that IBD has on the gastrointestinal tract, extraintestinal manifestations (EIMs) associated with CD and UC are common, occurring in 20% to 30% of patients.[7] Although joint manifestations are the most common EIMs, the oral cavity, eyes, skin, bone, kidneys, and biliary tract can also be involved. The incidence of EIMs differs between CD and UC, and the presentation of extraintestinal symptoms varies with regard to onset, site, and activity of the bowel disease. With regard to extent of the disease, widespread bowel involvement is associated with greater odds of developing EIMs than more limited bowel disease. For example, patients with extensive UC experience EIMs, 22% of the time, whereas patients with left-sided colitis and proctitis have EIMs 12% and 5% of the time, respectively.[9] Likewise, patients with ileocolonic CD have EIMs 37% of the time compared with 25% of the time in patients with isolated ileal disease.[10] Some EIMs, such as large joint monoarticular arthritis tend to occur when the bowel disease is active, whereas other EIMs, such as small joint symmetric arthritis occur prior to diagnosis of IBD or when the disease is quiescent. There are some trends in gender differences and age of presentation seen with certain EIMs. For example, women are more likely to have erythema nodosum and ocular manifestations whereas men are more likely to have primary sclerosing cholangitis and ankylosing spondylitis.[11] A description of the most common EIMs in patients with IBD is provided in Table 36.2.[11,12,13] We discuss the joint manifestations in detail and have divided these disorders into peripheral and axial arthritis.

PERIPHERAL ARTHRITIS ASSOCIATED WITH INFLAMMATORY BOWEL DISEASE

Peripheral arthritis, both polyarticular and pauciarticular, is estimated to occur in 10% to 20% of patients with IBD, with a higher prevalence of peripheral arthritis in CD compared with UC.[14,15] Recent studies have suggested several etiologies of IBD-associated peripheral arthritis. HLA-DR103 and HLA-B*27 have been associated with pauciarticular arthritis, and HLA-B44 has been associated with polyarticular arthritis.[8] Further, increased gut permeability to bacterial antigens may result in the induction of articular symptoms, primarily pauciarticular

arthritis. IBD-related peripheral arthritis is diagnosed clinically because radiology is often normal and shows no signs of joint erosion or deformity. Pauciarticular arthritis in IBD is more common than polyarticular arthritis. Men and women are affected equally. Pauciarticular arthritis tends to be acute and self-limited, commonly affecting large joints such as the knees, wrists, and ankles. Its presentation coincides with active disease and often emerges on relapses of IBD. The duration of arthritis can last for up to 10 weeks, with a mean of 5 weeks; however, 10% to 20% of patients with pauciarticular arthritis will develop persistent joint symptoms.[15] Pauciarticular arthritis is associated with an increased risk of other EIMs such as erythema nodosum and uveitis (see Table 36.1).

Polyarticular arthritis commonly affects the small joints in the hand, particularly the metacarpophalangeal (MCP) joints.[13] Its presentation is independent from the activity of the disease.[16] In fact, polyarticular arthritis can occur before the diagnosis of IBD. The presentation can be insidious with symptoms lasting for years, with a mean of 3 years. Polyarticular arthritis is associated with uveitis (see Table 36.1).

AXIAL ARTHRITIS ASSOCIATED WITH INFLAMMATORY BOWEL DISEASE

The axial arthritides are composed of sacroiliitis and ankylosing spondylitis. Sacroiliitis occurs in 4% to 32% of patients with IBD, although it is often asymptomatic and detected radiographically.[17] The varying incidences can be explained by whether the diagnosis is made on the basis of clinical symptoms, by plain radiograph, or by cross-sectional imaging with computed tomography (CT) scan (Fig. 36.5). Patients typically present with stiffness and/or pain in the buttocks that is worse in the morning or after rest. The symptoms typically improve with exercise. Initial plain radiographs will show unilateral or bilateral iliac erosion, followed by fusion of the sacroiliac joint from chronic inflammation. Sacroiliitis occurs more commonly in patients with CD than in patients with UC.[18] Patients with CD-related sacroiliitis are more likely to develop peripheral arthritis.[19]

IBD-associated ankylosing spondylitis (AS) manifests identically to idiopathic ankylosing spondylitis and is estimated to occur in 4% to 10% of IBD patients,[20,21] although it has been theorized that this number would be larger if all patients suffering from ankylosing

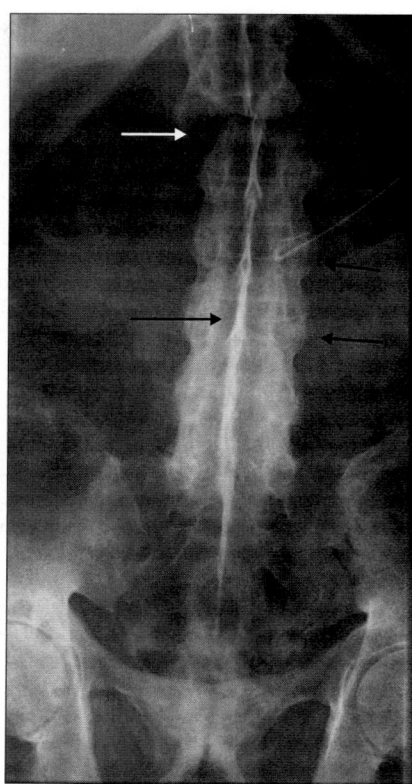

Fig. 36.5 Frontal radiograph of the lumbar spine shows fine bridging bone (syndesmophytes) across the intervertebral disc space (short black arrows), as well as ossification of the posterior interspinous ligaments (long black arrow). This results in a bamboo spine that predisposes to spinal fractures (*white arrow*). The sacroiliac joints are fused. *(Photo courtesy Jade Wong, M.D.)*

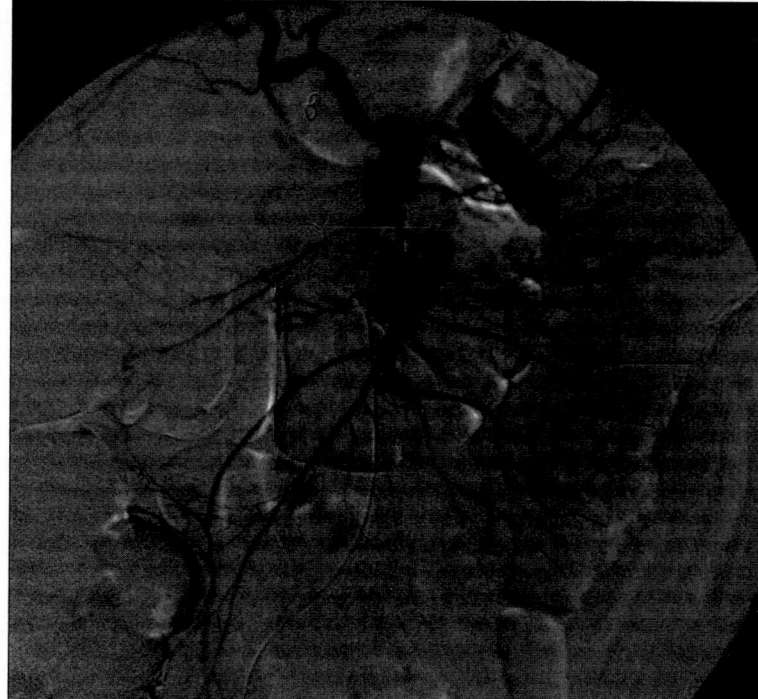

Fig. 36.6 Frontal view obtained during mesenteric arteriography in a patient with polyarteritis nodosa who presented with a gastrointestinal bleed from a gastroduodenal artery aneurysm that was embolized. There are microaneurysms in the branches of the superior mesenteric artery (large arrows) and areas of saccular vessel dilatation (small arrows). *(Photo courtesy Jade Wong, M.D.)*

spondylitis were assessed for IBD.[22] Males and females are equally affected. IBD-related ankylosing spondylitis has a strong genetic susceptibility, with a strong correlation to the HLA-B*27 antigen. Symptoms of AS may include thoracic or lumbar pain, alternating buttock pain or chest pain, and morning stiffness of the spine and thorax. The spinal vertebrae of the lumbar, thoracic, and cervical regions may fuse, forming a "bamboo spine" that limits mobility, causes changes in posture, and a loss of flexibility.[23,24] The spine can easily fracture in response to minor trauma (Fig. 36.6). Radiographically, formation of characteristic syndesmophytes between the vertebral bodies will be seen, as the annulus fibrosus gradually ossifies.[21] Axial arthritic symptoms manifest several years before active IBD is detected, and they are considered independent in their disease course from the underlying bowel disease.[14,25]

Arthralgias without frank arthritis occur in 14% of CD patients compared with 5% of UC patients.[15] Arthralgias can affect any joint. Their presentation coincides with active disease and emerges on relapses of IBD. The only exception is in the case of arthralgias associated with steroid withdrawal (pseudorheumatism or steroid withdrawal syndrome). In this clinical situation, joint pain coincides with steroid withdrawal requiring escalation of the corticosteroids.

We have described extraintestinal joint manifestations in relation to inflammatory bowel disease; now the discussion focuses on non-IBD enteropathies and their associated EIM, including articular symptoms.

BACTERIAL ENTERITIS

Bacterial enteritis refers to infection and inflammation of the intestines, caused by infection with a variety of bacterial pathogens including *Campylobacter jejuni*, *Clostridium difficile*, *Yersinia enterocolitica*, *Yersinia pseudotuberculosis*, *Shigella*, and *Salmonella*. A list of all organisms associated with reactive arthritis is shown in Table 36.3. Symptoms related to bacterial enteritides usually present acutely and include nonbloody or bloody diarrhea, abdominal cramping, and systemic symptoms. Patient history is important in the determination of

TABLE 36.3 ORGANISMS ASSOCIATED WITH REACTIVE ARTHRITIS	
Campylobacter jejuni	*Clostridium difficile*
Yersinia enterocolitica	*Chlamydia trachomatis*
Yersinia pseudotuberculosis	*Salmonella typhimurium*
Shigella flexneri	*Salmonella enteritidis*
Shigella dysenteriae	

the causative bacteria. Benefits of empiric antibiotic treatment are questionable in healthy adults; further antibacterial treatment can precipitate hemolytic uremic syndrome in patients with enterohemorrhagic *Escherichia coli*.

Approximately a quarter to a third of patients with bacterial enteritis will develop reactive arthritis,[26] usually within a few days to a few weeks following infection.[27] In the majority of patients, the arthritis involves multiple joints, is migratory, and involves large joints. The arthritis tends to be asymmetric and usually affects the lower extremities more than the upper extremities. In addition, patients can develop an enthesitis or sacroiliitis. The arthritis is usually self-limiting, lasting a week to several months[28]; however, a chronic, relapsing arthritis occurs in a minority of patients.[29] The presence of HLA-B27 is associated with an increased likelihood of developing reactive arthritis, an increase in its severity, and likelihood of chronicity.[26] Treatment of the underlying bacterial enteritis with antibiotic therapy has not proven to hasten resolution of the joint symptoms.[30]

CELIAC DISEASE

Celiac disease is a chronic inflammatory condition of the proximal small intestine resulting from exposure to gluten in a genetically predisposed host. Celiac disease occurs primarily in Caucasians of Northern European descent, with a prevalence in North America of 1 in every 133 people affected, with a higher prevalence among first degree

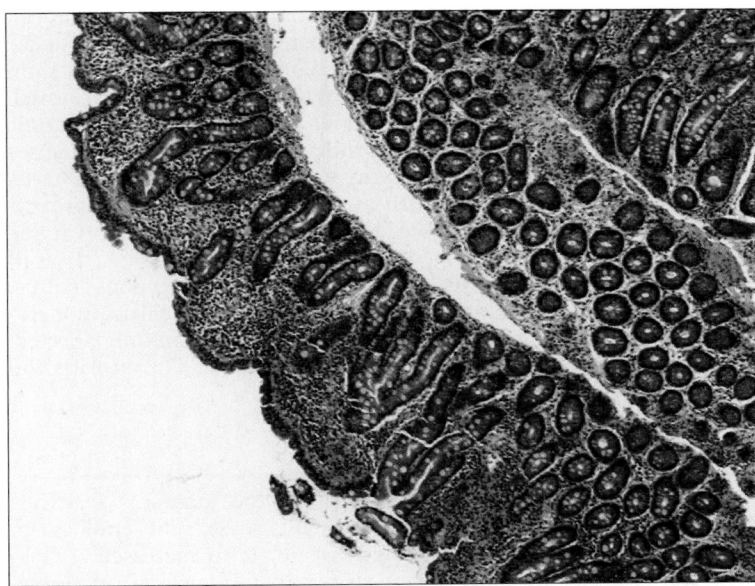

Fig. 36.7 Duodenal mucosa with marked villous blunting and crypt elongation. There is intraepithelial lymphocytosis, and the lamina propria is expanded by increased numbers of lymphocytes and plasma cells (original magnification: 4×). *(Photo courtesy William Twaddell, M.D.)*

relatives of people with Celiac disease.[31] However, the prevalence may even be underestimated because a significant proportion of patients are either undiagnosed or asymptomatic. The disease is associated with HLA class II alleles DQA1*0501 and DQB1*0201.[32] Ingestion of gluten leads to an inappropriate T cell–mediated inflammatory response, causing damage to the small intestine and eventual destruction of the intestinal villi. Destruction of the villi results in a malabsorption syndrome. Symptoms of celiac disease include chronic nonbloody diarrhea, weight loss, abdominal bloating and distention, and overall failure to thrive.[33] In adults, the presentation can be more protean. The most common clinical presentation in adults is iron deficiency anemia.[34] Celiac disease is diagnosed by biopsy of the small intestine, which reveals increased lymphocytes, crypt hyperplasia, and varying degrees of villous atrophy (Fig. 36.7). The treatment for celiac disease is a gluten-free diet, which almost always leads to resolution of symptoms. Celiac disease is associated with a variety of extraintestinal manifestations, including aphthous ulcers, dermatitis herpetiformis, and development of reactive arthritides.[35]

Celiac disease–associated arthritis can be peripheral, axial, or both[36] and commonly affects the lumbar spine, hips, and knees.[37] The joint symptoms often precede the diagnosis of celiac disease. Treatment with a gluten-free diet not only improves the intestinal symptoms and anemia but has been shown to decrease the duration of joint symptoms resulting in resolution of the arthritis within 6 months.[34]

WHIPPLE'S DISEASE

Whipple disease is a rare, chronic systemic infection caused by the actinomycete *Tropheryma whippelii*. Approximately 12 new cases are diagnosed annually around the world,[38] occurring predominantly in Caucasian males between 40 and 60 years of age.[39] *T. whippelii* is thought to cause chronic infection by evading the immune system; there may be a correlation between Whipple disease and the host's defective ability to clear the bacteria.[39] Patients with Whipple disease typically present with diarrhea secondary to fat malabsorption (steatorrhea), weight loss, fever of unknown origin, and arthritis. Neurologic symptoms are present in a minority of cases. Whipple disease is diagnosed by biopsy of the small intestine revealing lymphatic dilation, with periodic acid–Schiff (PAS)-positive macrophages and gram-positive, acid-fast–negative bacilli in the lamina propria. Whipple disease is successfully treated with long-term use of antibiotics such as trimethoprim-sulfamethoxazole.

Arthritis is estimated to occur in 65% to 90% of cases of Whipple disease, with approximately 25% of patients presenting with axial

involvement, either sacroiliitis or spondylitis.[40] Large joints are more commonly affected over small joints. The arthritis is migratory and the same joint is not always affected. Joint destruction does not occur. Joint involvement tends to occur several years before development of other clinical signs of the disease, and the duration of involvement is transient—spanning from hours to days. Treatment of Whipple disease with antibiotics will also result in resolution of joint symptoms.

POLYARTERITIS NODOSA

Polyarteritis nodosa (PAN) is a necrotizing vasculitis that affects small and, predominantly, medium-sized arteries. The typical age at presentation ranges from 40 to 60 years. There is no known etiology for this vasculitis, although numerous infectious agents have been implicated in the pathogenesis; for example, PAN develops within the first 6 months of an HBV infection as a result of immune-complex formation.[41] PAN causes transmural inflammation of blood vessels, leading to fibrinoid necrosis and formation of cutaneous nodules along superficial arteries. PAN can manifest systemically, with multi-organ involvement, including the gastrointestinal tract, kidneys, joints, brain, and heart. Patients often present with systemic constitutional symptoms such as fever, fatigue, weight loss, arthralgias, and myalgias. Gastrointestinal symptoms usually affect the small intestine, manifesting in approximately 50% of patients with PAN.[42] The symptoms are highly variable from postprandial periumbilical pain to nausea and vomiting secondary to bowel infarction and perforation. PAN is treated with systemic steroids and immunosuppressive drugs.

Joint disease can also result from PAN, with more extensive joint involvement the longer PAN is present. It is estimated that 50% of patients with PAN present with arthralgias/arthritis, with large joints preferentially affected.[43] Males tend to present with articular symptoms almost twice as frequently as women. The systemic manifestations of polyarteritis nodosa, including joint symptoms, often resolve with treatment of PAN.

HENOCH-SCHÖNLEIN PURPURA

Henoch-Schönlein purpura (HSP) is an immunoglobulin A–mediated small vessel necrotizing vasculitis that is also characterized by fibrinoid destruction of blood vessels. HSP is the most common vasculitis of childhood, seen predominantly in children from the age of 3 to 10 years following a streptococcal upper respiratory tract infection. However, the disease may occasionally manifest in adults. Males are twice as likely to be affected as females. Like polyarteritis nodosa, the etiology of this vasculitis has yet to be discovered. HSP will often present with a tetrad of symptoms, including palpable purpura around the buttocks and lower extremities, arthritis or arthralgias, abdominal pain, and renal disease, most commonly hematuria with or without proteinuria. Any of the four major symptom complexes can be the initial presenting symptom. Additionally, the classic tetrad of symptoms is not seen in each case. Diagnosis is usually based on clinical symptoms, but if there is any doubt, a skin biopsy can be used to confirm the diagnosis. Because HSP is self-limiting in 50% of patients, some argue that supportive care is the only indicated therapy, whereas others contend that medical treatment with corticosteroids and immunosuppressants improves renal outcomes in patients with HSP.[46,47]

Joint symptoms are the second most common manifestation of HSP, occurring in approximately 70% of patients,[48] with a higher frequency in adult-onset HSP.[49] In 25% of patients, the arthritis precedes the purpura by approximately 1 week.[50] The symptoms are transient and non-deforming and vary from mild arthralgias to debilitating arthritis; however, inflammatory arthritis is more commonly seen than arthralgias alone. Larger joints are more commonly affected such as the ankles, knees, and wrists. Retrospective studies have shown that HSP-associated arthritis is effectively relieved with corticosteroids.[47]

BEHÇET'S SYNDROME

Behçet syndrome is a rare, chronic, multisystem vasculitis involving both the arterial and venous circulations, with a particular predilection for blood vessels in the oral and genital mucosa. Behçet syndrome is most frequently seen in the Middle East, Far East, and Mediterranean, in patients 25 to 35 years of age. There is no known cause for this syndrome, but hypotheses range from autoimmune etiologies, immune circulating complexes, and chemical agents.[51] Behçet syndrome is characterized by recurring and remitting symptoms that include aphthous ulcers, genital ulcers, and uveitis, as well as associated skin, joint, gastrointestinal, and neurologic manifestations. Surgical resection of an aneurysm resulting from Behçet-mediated destruction is indicated in 10% of patients. Currently, there is not a specific diagnostic test for Behçet syndrome; diagnosis is based on clinical findings and recurrence of the disease over time. Treatments are customized to each patient's clinical symptoms and may include glucocorticoids, colchicine, 5-aminosalicylates, thalidomide, azathioprine, and infliximab.[51]

Joint manifestations occur in approximately 57% to 75% of Behçet syndrome patients and are the presenting symptoms in 11% to 18% of cases.[53,54] Large joints such as the knees and ankles are most commonly affected. Polyarthritis, involving large and small joints, occurs in 17% of the cases, while mono- or oligoarthritis occur in 11% and 16% of the cases, respectively. The arthritis is self-limiting after a few weeks and does not cause permanent damage.

MICROSCOPIC COLITIS

Microscopic colitis, comprising collagenous colitis (CC) and lymphocytic colitis (LC), is characterized by chronic, watery diarrhea. CC primarily affects middle-aged women at around 65 years of age; women are almost five times more likely to be affected than men.[55] Similarly, LC affects middle-aged women, but the female-to-male ratio is less, 2 to 3 : 1. The cause of microscopic colitis is unknown and is thought to be multifactorial, occurring in individuals who are susceptible to certain noxious luminal agents that result in microscopic mucosal inflammation. Clinically, CC and LC are indistinguishable from each other, causing chronic, non-bloody, watery diarrhea that may be associated with diffuse abdominal pain and significant weight loss. Approximately 40% of the patients with microscopic colitis have another associated autoimmune condition, most commonly thyroid disorders, celiac disease, diabetes mellitus, or rheumatoid arthritis.[56] Microscopic colitis is differentiated on the basis of colonic mucosal biopsies from the colon and rectum; the endoscopies in both CC and LC are normal. CC manifests as excess subepithelial collagen deposition, with chronic mononuclear inflammation in the lamina propria, whereas LC causes increased intraepithelial lymphocytes with a normal collagen layer. Microscopic colitis is treated with antidiarrheals, bismuth subsalicylate, 5-aminosalicylates, budesonide, or corticosteroids with varying successes.

Articular symptoms will rarely accompany collagenous colitis, occurring in up to 7% of patients.[57] The arthritis is transient, nonerosive, and oligoarticular. Peripheral joints are most commonly affected, including the MCP, interphalangeal, and wrist joints. The arthritis will resolve with treatment of the collagenous colitis.[58]

CONCLUSION

Extraintestinal involvement, particularly of the joints, is relatively common in patients with gastrointestinal disease. The etiology for joint involvement is not known but may relate to increased antigen presentation to the immune system secondary to increased gut permeability or action of systemic cytokines on the joint. The list of gastrointestinal illnesses that affect the joints is extensive. The presentation of arthritis is highly variable and may affect the peripheral versus axial joints and one, few, or many joints. It may or may not correspond to the underlying gastrointestinal symptoms. Most of the arthritides do not result in progressive joint destruction; improvement in the joint symptoms often coincides with treatment of the underlying disorder. The prognosis for many of these forms of arthritis is excellent. Internists, gastroenterologists, and rheumatologists need to be aware of the relationship between joint symptoms and gastrointestinal disease to improve accuracy of diagnosis and improve clinical outcomes.

KEY REFERENCES

1. Elewaut D, De Keyser F, Van Den Bosch F, et al. Enrichment of T cells carrying beta7 integrins in inflamed synovial tissue from patients with early spondyloarthropathy, compared to rheumatoid arthritis. J Rheumatol 1998;25:1932-1937.
2. Skrede B, Raknerud N, Aadland E. Ulcerative colitis. Complications and sequelae in relation to the extent of the disease. A 10-year material. Tidsskr Nor Laegeforen 1997;117:3205-3207.
3. De Dombal FT, Watts J M, Watkinson G, Goligher JC. Local complications of ulcerative colitis: stricture, pseudopolyposis, and carcinoma of colon and rectum. Br Med J 1966;1:1442-1447.
4. Silverberg MS, Satsangi J, Ahmad T, et al. Toward an integrated clinical, molecular and serological classification of inflammatory bowel disease: Report of a Working Party of the 2005 Montreal World Congress of Gastroenterology. Can J Gastroenterol 2005;19(suppl A):5-36.
5. Steinberg DM, Cooke WT, Alexander-Williams J. Abscess and fistulae in Crohn's disease. Gut 1973;14:865-869.
5a. Farmer RG, Hawk WA, Turnbull RB Jr. Clinical patterns in Crohn's disease: a statistical study of 615 cases. Gastroenterology 1975;68:627-635. Rankin GB, Watts HD, Melnyk CS, Kelley ML Jr. National Cooperative Crohn's Disease Study: extraintestinal manifestations and perianal complications. Gastroenterology 1979;77:914-920.
6. Yao K, Yao T, Iwashita A, Matsui T, Kamachi S. Microaggregate of immunostained macrophages in noninflamed gastroduodenal mucosa: a new useful histological marker for differentiating Crohn's colitis from ulcerative colitis. The American Journal of Gastroenterology 1000;95(8):1967-1973.
7. Rankin GB, Watts HD, Melnyk CS, et al. The National Cooperative Crohn's Disease Study: Extraintestinal manifestations and perianal complications. Gastroenterology 1979;77:914-920.
7a. Monsen U, Sorstad J, Hellers G, Johansson C. Extracolonic diagnosis in ulcerative colitis: An epidemiological study. Am J Gastroenterol 1990;85:711-716.

8. Orchard TR, Thiyagaraja S, Welsh KI, Wordsworth BP, Hill Gaston JS, Jewell DP. Clinical phenotype is related to HLA genotype in the peripheral arthropathies of inflammatory bowel disease. Gastroenterology 2000;118:274-278.
9. Wright V, Watkinson G. The arthritis of ulcerative colitis. Medicine 1959;38:243-259.
10. Greenstein AJ, Janowitz HD, Sachar DB. The extraintestinal complications of Crohn's disease and ulcerative colitis: a study of 700 patients. Medicine 1976;55:401-412.
11. Olsson R, Danielsson A, Jarnerot G, Lindstrom E, Loof L, Rolny P, et al. Prevalence of primary sclerosing cholangitis in patients with ulcerative colitis. Gastroenterology 1991;100:1319-1323.
12. Kaufman I, Caspi D, Yeshurun D, Dotan I, Yaron M, Elkayam O. The effect of infliximab on extraintestinal manifestations of Crohn's disease. Rheumatol Int 2005 Aug;25(6):406-410.
13. Lyons JL, Rosenbaum JT. Uveitis associated with inflammatory bowel disease compared with uveitis associated with spondyloarthropathy. Arch Ophthalmol 1997;115:61-64.
14. Gravallese EM, Kantrowitz FG. Arthritic manifestations of inflammatory bowel disease. Am J Gastroenterol 1988;83:703-709.
15. Orchard TR, Wordsworth BP, Jewell DP. Peripheral arthropathies in inflammatory bowel disease: their articular distribution and natural history. Gut 1998;42:387-391.
16. Paredes JM, Barrachina MM, Román J, Moreno-Osset E. Joint disease in inflammatory bowel disease. Gastroenterol Hepatol 2005;28:240-249.
17. McEniff N, Eustace S, McCarthy C, et al. Asymptomatic sacroiliitis in inflammatory bowel disease. Assessment by computed tomography. Clin Imag 1995;19:258-262.
18. Agnew, JE, Pocock DG, Jewell DP. Sacroiliac joint uptake ratios in inflammatory bowel disease: relationship to back pain and to activity of bowel disease. Br J Radiol 1982;55:821.
19. Peeters H, Vander Cruyssen B, et al. Clinical and genetic factors associated with sacroiliitis in Crohn's disease. J Gastroenterol Hepatol 2008;23:132-137.

20. Dekker-Saeys BJ, Meuwissen SG, Van Den Berg-Loonen EM, et al. Ankylosing spondylitis and inflammatory bowel disease. II. Prevalence of peripheral arthritis, sacroiliitis, and ankylosing spondylitis in patients suffering from inflammatory bowel disease. Ann Rheum Dis 1978;37: 33-35.
21. Bernstein CN, Blanchard JF, Rawsthorne P, Yu N. The prevalence of extraintestinal diseases in inflammatory bowel disease: a population-based study. Am J Gastroenterol 96(4):1116-1122.
22. Jayson MI, Salmon PR, Harrison WJ. Inflammatory bowel disease in ankylosing spondylitis. Gut 1970;11:506-511.
23. Gorman J. Spondyloarthropathies. In: Imboden JB, Hellmann DB, Stone JH. Current rheumatology diagnosis and treatment. New York: McGraw-Hill Professional, 2004:157-169.
24. Ward M. Prospects for disease modification in ankylosing spondylitis: do nonsteroidal anti-inflammatory drugs do more than treat symptoms? Arthritis Rheum 2005;52:1634-1636.
25. Dekker-Saeys BJ, Meuwissen SG, Van Den Berg-Loonen EM, et al. Ankylosing spondylitis and inflammatory bowel disease. III. Clinical characteristics and results of histocompatibility typing (HLA B27) in 50 patients with both ankylosing spondylitis and inflammatory bowel disease. Ann Rheum Dis 1978;37:36-41.
26. Gumpel JM, Martin C, Sanderson PJ. Reactive arthritis associated with campylobacter enteritis. Ann Rheum Dis 1981;40:64-65.
27. Müller KD. Value of microbiologic studies for diagnosis of post-enteritis reactive arthritis Z Rheumatol 1990;49:364-368.
28. Schaad UB. Reactive arthritis associated with Campylobacter enteritis. Pediatr Infect Dis 1982;1:328-332.
29. Bremell T, Bjelle A, Svedhem A. Rheumatic symptoms following an outbreak of campylobacter enteritis: a five year follow up. Ann Rheum Dis 1991;50:934-938.
30. Locht H, Kihlstrom E, Lindstrom FD. Reactive arthritis after Salmonella among medical doctors—study of an outbreak. J Rheumatol 1993;20:845-848.

31. Fasano A, Berti I, Gerarduzzi T, et al. Prevalence of celiac disease in the United States among both at risk and not at risk groups. Arch Int Med 2003;163:286-292.

32. Sollid LM, Markussen G, Ek J, et al. Evidence for a primary association of celiac disease to a particular HLA-DQ alpha/beta heterodimer. J Exp Med 1989;169:345-350.

33. Fasano A. Systemic autoimmune disorders in celiac disease. Curr Opin Gastroenterol 2006;22:674-679.

34. Corazza GR, Valentini RA, Andreani ML, et al. Subclinical celiac disease is a frequent cause of iron-deficiency anemia. Scand J Gastroenterol 1995 Feb;30(2):153-156.

35. Parke AL, Fagan EA, Chadwick VS, Hughes GR. Coeliac disease and rheumatoid arthritis. Ann Rheum Dis 1984;43:378-380.

36. Lubrano E, Ciacci C, Ames PR, et al. The arthritis of coeliac disease: prevalence and pattern in 200 adult patients. Br J Rheumatol 1996;35:1314-1318.

37. Bourne JT, Kumar P, Huskisson EC, et al. Arthritis and coeliac disease. Ann Rheum Dis 1985;44:592-598.

38. Dutly F, Altwegg M. Whipple's Disease and "Tropheryma whippelii". Clin Microbiol Rev 2001;14:561-583.

39. Fantry GT, Fantry LE, James SP. Chronic infections of the small intestine. In: Yamada T, Alpers DH, Loren L, Kaplowitz N, eds. Textbook of gastroenterology, 4th ed. Philadelphia: Lippincott Williams & Wilkins, 2003:1561-1580.

40. Lange U, Teichmann J. Whipple arthritis: diagnosis by molecular analysis of synovial fluid—current status of diagnosis and therapy. Rheumatology (Oxford) 2003;42:473-480.

41. Stone J. Polyarteritis nodosa. JAMA 2002;288:1632-1639.

42. Pagnoux C, Mahr A, Cohen P, Guillevin L. Presentation and outcome of gastrointestinal involvement in systemic necrotizing vasculitides: analysis of 62 patients with polyarteritis nodosa, microscopic polyangiitis, Wegener granulomatosis, Churg-Strauss syndrome, or rheumatoid arthritis-associated vasculitis. Medicine 2005(2):115-128.

43. Stone J. Polyarteritis nodosa. JAMA 2002;288:1632-1639.

46. Foster BJ, Bernard C, Drummond KN, Sharma AK. Effective therapy for severe Henoch-Schönlein purpura nephritis with prednisone and azathioprine: a clinical and histopathologic study. J Pediatr 2000;136:370-375.

47. Flynn JT, Smoyer WE, Bunchman TE, et al. Treatment of Henoch-Schönlein purpura glomerulonephritis in children with high-dose corticosteroids plus oral cyclophosphamide. Am J Nephrol 2001;21:128-133.

48. Jennette JC, Falk RJ. Small-vessel vasculitis. N Engl J Med 1997;337(21):1512-1523.

49. Blanco R, Martínez-Taboada VM, Rodríguez-Valverde V, et al. Henoch-Schönlein purpura in adulthood and childhood: two different expressions of the same syndrome. Arthritis Rheum 1997;40:859-864.

50. Saulsbury FT. Henoch-Schönlein purpura. Curr Opin Rheumatol 2001;13:35-40.

REFERENCES

Full references for this chapter can be found on www.expertconsult.com.

The kidney and rheumatic disease

Daniel J. Salzberg and Matthew R. Weir

37

- Rheumatic diseases often involve the kidneys.
- Kidney disease is frequently asymptomatic; thus routine testing is imperative.
- Many drugs used in rheumatology are potentially nephrotoxic.
- Patients with kidney disease experience distinctive joint and soft tissue complications.

SIGNS AND SYMPTOMS OF KIDNEY DISEASE

The kidneys are involved in many homeostatic functions, including the maintenance of acid-base balance, electrolyte concentrations, and osmolarity; excretion of toxins and metabolic wastes; and the elaboration of certain hormones, including erythropoietin, 1,25-dihydroxycalciferol, and renin. As one would expect, diseases of the nephron manifest through dysregulation of these systems. Unlike rheumatologic diseases, the signs and symptoms of kidney disease tend not to present as obvious physical findings until late in the course of disease but are usually discovered through laboratory assessment. Table 37.1 is a list of the renal syndromes that occur in persons with rheumatic diseases.

The functional unit of the kidney is the nephron, which consists of a glomerulus followed by a long network of tubules. The glomerulus has a somewhat unusual anatomy in that its capillary bed is sandwiched between two arteries. This explains why glomerulonephritis is a frequent manifestation of systemic vasculitides such as systemic lupus erythematosus (SLE), Henoch-Schönlein purpura, Churg-Strauss syndrome, microscopic polyangiitis, ANCA-associated granulomatous vasculitis, and cryoglobulinemic vasculitis.

Signs and symptoms of proteinuria

Proteinuria usually reflects an increase in the permeability of the glomerular barrier to normally non-filtered molecules, such as albumin. When proteinuria is severe, it usually manifests as diffuse peripheral edema. However, if the proteinuria is of a lesser degree it may not manifest with any symptoms or signs and is often only detected on urinalysis.

Massive proteinuria is typical in the nephrotic syndrome. This syndrome is characterized by (1) nephrotic-range proteinuria, defined as greater than or equal to 3.5 g/day/1.73 m², (2) hypoalbuminemia, (3) hypercholesterolemia, (4) edema, and (5) lipiduria. Nephrotic-range proteinuria is almost always due to a glomerular pathologic process, because tubulointerstitial kidney disease will result in a more modest degree of protein spillage.

With the nephrotic syndrome the edema tends to be generalized, unlike the edema seen with congestive heart failure, which is dependent, or cirrhosis, which is primarily restricted to the abdomen. Despite massive proteinuria, some patients do not develop edema. Pleural effusions, when present, tend to be painless, unlike serositis.

Nephrotic syndrome is associated with a hypercoagulable state,[1] which may manifest clinically as stroke, deep venous thrombosis, or renal vein thrombosis.[2] In patients with nephrotic syndrome, one must maintain a high index of suspicion for renal vein thrombosis, because it infrequently presents as the classic triad of flank pain, overt hematuria, and worsening kidney function. Patients with SLE with nephrotic syndrome who have had previous episodes of thrombophlebitis are particularly at risk for renal vein thrombosis.[3]

The predominant cause of nephrotic syndrome in children is minimal change disease. In adults, the most frequent causes include diabetic nephropathy, focal segmental glomerulosclerosis (FSGS), and immunoglobulin A (IgA) nephropathy.[4] It is also common in patients with lupus nephritis and amyloidosis.[5,6]

Signs and symptoms of hematuria

Hematuria is usually asymptomatic and not visible to the naked eye (i.e., microscopic). Therefore, it often goes unnoticed until urinalysis is performed. Macroscopic or "gross" hematuria is suspected when the urine is red, brown, or tea colored. As with microscopic hematuria, macroscopic hematuria tends to be asymptomatic and rarely presents as obstructive symptoms. Both are seen in rheumatologic disorders as a feature of a renal vasculitis or acute glomerulonephritis. More frequently, hematuria is due to nephrolithiasis, urinary tract infection (UTI), trauma, polycystic kidney disease, genitourinary cancer, or benign prostatic hypertrophy (Table 37.2). Because the most common presentation of transitional cell cancer is hematuria, its presence in an adult obligates the assessment for an underlying carcinoma.

Signs and symptoms of renal hypertension

Hypertension is a common consequence of kidney disease, including the glomerular damage seen with autoimmune disorders. Renovascular disease accounts for 10% to 45% of acute, severe, or refractory hypertension,[7] although less than 1% of mild hypertension.[8] Severe hypertension may present clinically as visual disturbances, headaches, or angina pectoris. Both left ventricular hypertrophy and microalbuminuria are clinically silent and therefore require appropriate diagnostic testing. Aggressive control of blood pressure is of paramount importance in all individuals with hypertension, but particularly so in those with underlying kidney disease. Treatment with an effective antihypertensive regimen that includes either an angiotensin-converting enzyme (ACE) inhibitor or an angiotensin receptor blocker may prevent the progression of kidney failure.[9]

Signs and symptoms of renal failure

Renal failure is arbitrarily divided into acute, subacute, and chronic, based on the time course. Acute renal failure (ARF) suggests an elevation in serum creatinine concentration that develops over days to weeks, whereas chronic kidney disease (CKD) extends over months to years. With CKD, the symptoms of uremia tend to occur insidiously. These symptoms include easy fatigability, daytime somnolence, night-time sleep disturbances, nausea, anorexia, diffuse pruritus, easy bruising, mucosal bleeding, and dysgeusia. Because these symptoms tend to be nonspecific, they are frequently attributed to other disorders, such as depression or hypothyroidism. They may not be attributed to kidney failure until some estimate of kidney function is obtained (see later). Fluid retention and a reduction in urine volume are not frequent features of CKD until an advanced stage of CKD is reached. In contrast, ARF is frequently associated with oliguria, which is defined as less than 500 mL of urine per day. This is the volume of maximally concentrated urine required to completely excrete the normal dietary acid load. As with CKD, the symptoms of ARF tend to be relatively nonspecific and depend on the underlying disease process. The constellation of worsening or new-onset hypertension and hematuria in the setting of ARF suggests an acute glomerulonephritis and/or vasculitis. Other potential symptoms include fever, arthralgias, or hemoptysis.

TABLE 37.1 RENAL SYNDROMES IN PATIENTS WITH RHEUMATIC DISEASES*

Renal syndrome	Clinical features	Laboratory features	Course
Asymptomatic urinary abnormalities or "subacute"	None	Proteinuria and/or microscopic hematuria	Persistent; may evolve to nephrotic
Nephrotic syndrome	Edema ± ascites, effusions	Proteinuria > 3.5 g/day, low serum albumin and elevated cholesterol levels	Persistent, or remitting and relapsing
Acute nephritic syndrome	Reduced urine output, ± discolored urine, ± fluid retention	Elevated plasma creatinine value, microscopic hematuria, red cell casts	Post-streptococcal form resolves; acute episodes in lupus may recur
Rapidly progressive glomerulonephritis	Progressive oliguria, discolored urine, systemic symptoms	Rapidly rising plasma creatinine level, falling GFR, hematuria, red cell casts	Progresses to renal failure in weeks or months
Persistent "subacute" glomerulonephritis (mixed nephrotic/nephritic)	± Edema, ± discolored urine, ± hypertension	Proteinuria, ± low serum albumin, microscopic hematuria	Persistent; may progress to renal failure (in years)
Renal vasculitis	± Discolored urine, ± visible hematuria, ± hypertension	Elevated plasma creatinine value, proteinuria, hematuria, ± red cell casts	Variable with treatment; may mimic RPGN
Tubulointerstitial nephritis	± Discolored urine	Elevated plasma creatinine value, sterile pyuria (white blood cells), microscopic hematuria	Acute (resolves in months) or chronic (persistent)
Chronic renal failure (mild to moderate)	Few or none, ± hypertension	Elevated plasma creatinine value, reduced GFR, ± urinary abnormalities	Persistent; renal failure usually worsens
Chronic renal failure (severe)	Subclinical to severe uremic symptoms, ± hypertension	Plasma creatinine > 6 mg/dL, GFR < 10 mL/min, ± urinary abnormalities	Imminent need for dialysis or renal transplant

GFR, glomerular filtration rate (measured by creatinine clearance or other methods); RPGN, rapidly progressive glomerulonephritis.
*Some of the principal syndromes of renal involvement are shown. For each syndrome, typical clinical signs and symptoms are listed, together with the distinguishing findings on routine laboratory screening. Some degree of proteinuria is present in the vast majority of cases in all these syndromes and is mentioned in the table only where it is a constant and defining feature of the syndrome. The typical course of evolution of each syndrome over time is also shown because it helps characterize the syndromes and is integral to the definition of some of them (e.g., RPGN). This information cannot be used as a basis for prognosis in individual cases, which varies widely. The laboratory features listed here are only those obtainable from tests used routinely for renal surveillance (blood chemistry, urinalysis, and urine microscopy), plus the results of 24-hour urine chemistry (timed protein quantitation and creatinine clearance to estimate GFR). The latter should be obtained at initial evaluation of patients at risk of renal involvement, whenever new elevations of proteinuria or plasma creatinine are detected, or periodically in nephrotic and renal failure patients. Laboratory studies beyond those listed are appropriate for full diagnosis in all cases and may include additional chemical and serologic tests, imaging studies, and histologic evaluation of renal biopsy material.

Recognition of kidney involvement

As kidney disease tends to be asymptomatic, one is particularly dependent on laboratory tests in detecting kidney involvement in systemic disease. By integration of laboratory and clinical findings, one can classify the kidney involvement into one of the renal syndromes listed in Table 37.1. Each of these syndromes has many different causes. Diagnosis and full evaluation of the underlying disease process often requires further investigation, which may include assessment of serologic findings and complement studies, renal imaging, and histologic assessment of the kidney via biopsy.

TESTING FOR KIDNEY DISEASE

Proteinuria

Normal proteinuria

Ordinarily, a normal healthy adult excretes 84 ± 24 mg of protein per day,[10] which represents less than 0.002% of the total protein filtered. This remarkable conservation results from the charge and size barrier of the glomerular filtering apparatus.[11] The proteins that are normally able to cross this barrier are the low-molecular-weight (LMW) proteins, defined as less than 40,000 daltons, which are reabsorbed by the proximal renal tubules.[12] Therefore, the small amount of protein that appears in normal urine consists of albumin, immunoglobulins, products of hormone metabolism, and Tamm-Horsfall proteins.[13]

Glomerular proteinuria

Glomerular proteinuria results from loss of the charge and size selectivity of the glomerular filter. The abnormal glomerular barrier results in an increased filtered load of albumin and high-molecular-weight proteins. As more proteins enter the filtrate, the capacity for tubular protein reabsorption is exceeded, resulting in significant proteinuria. Glomerular proteinuria can certainly exceed 10 g/day, although in adults just 3.5 g/day can be enough to deplete the serum albumin to the point where its oncotic force is no longer sufficient to prevent peripheral edema. Whether or not edema is present depends on other factors, such as nutritional status. For example, young women with

lupus nephritis may have nephrotic-range proteinuria but with adequate protein intake and hepatic synthetic function they are able to maintain their serum albumin levels and thus avoid edema.

With glomerular proteinuria there is also excessive filtration of lipids, which overwhelms tubular reabsorption. The damaging effect of increased lipid uptake into proximal tubular cells is responsible for some of the tubulointerstitial pathology seen in the nephrotic syndrome.[14] Lipid-lowering agents may improve renal and cardiovascular prognosis in these patients.[15]

The degree of proteinuria, together with the degree of tubulointerstitial damage, is the most powerful predictor of the progression of CKD, regardless of the underlying disease process. Therefore, every effort must be made to minimize or extinguish proteinuria.[16] ACE inhibitors and/or angiotensin receptor blockers should be considered first-line agents in the treatment of all cases of proteinuria.[17]

Tubular proteinuria

Tubular proteinuria occurs in the setting in which glomerular protein sieving is normal but there is impaired tubular reabsorption of normally filtered LMW proteins. As opposed to glomerular diseases, the range of proteinuria is much less, usually in the range of 1 to 2 g/day. Tubular proteinuria can be associated with tubulointerstitial disease, resulting from uric acid nephropathy, Sjögren's syndrome, essential hypertension, and drugs, such as aminoglycoside antibiotics.

Measurement of proteinuria

In clinical practice, urinary protein is most often detected on urinalysis, which employs a colorimetric method.[18] Urine dipsticks have a pad impregnated with tetrabromophenol blue that, when bound to proteins, changes color from yellow to green to green-blue. The intensity of the color change correlates with the degree of proteinuria, which is reported as 0 to 4+. This is a semiquantitative result, because the measurement is dependent on how concentrated the urine specimen is. For example, dilute urine with 3+ protein is likely to have more absolute protein, compared with concentrated urine with the same 3+ protein. To address this issue, newer dipsticks have an additional pad that detects urinary creatinine, which helps control for the degree of

TABLE 37.2 CAUSES OF HEMATURIA

- Glomerulonephritis and other glomerular diseases
- IgA nephropathy
- Membranoproliferative (= mesangiocapillary) glomerulonephritis
- Mesangial proliferative glomerulonephritis
- Lupus glomerulonephritis
- Glomerulonephritis with other rheumatic diseases:
  - Rheumatoid arthritis
  - Polymyositis/dermatomyositis, etc.
- Crescentic glomerulonephritis
- Glomerulonephritis with renal vasculitis:
  - ANCA-associated granulomatous vasculitis
  - Microscopic polyangiitis, etc.
- Alport's syndrome
- Thin basement membrane nephropathy
- Fabry's disease
- Renal vascular diseases
- Renal vasculitis (polyarteritis nodosa, etc.)
- Renal thromboembolism or infarction
- Hypertension
- Familial telangiectasia
- Arteriovenous malformations
- Renal vein thrombosis
- Renal vein occlusion
- Interstitial and medullary diseases
- Tubulointerstitial nephritis
- Polycystic kidney diseases
- Papillary necrosis from:
  - Analgesic nephropathy
  - Sickle cell disease
  - Diabetes mellitus
- Medullary sponge kidney
- Disorders of coagulation
- Anticoagulants
- Bleeding disorders (hemophilia, etc.)
- Renal and urinary tract tumors
- Wilms' tumor
- Renal cell carcinoma
- Transitional cell carcinoma
- Prostatic carcinoma
- Urethral carcinoma
- Infections
- Acute pyelonephritis
- Acute cystitis
- Prostatitis
- Urethritis
- Renal tuberculosis
- Schistosomiasis
- Bacterial endocarditis
- Stones and crystals
- Stones anywhere in the urinary tracts
- Urate crystalluria
- Calcium oxalate crystalluria
- Hypercalciuria
- Miscellaneous
- Trauma
- Release of obstruction
- Loin pain hematuria syndrome
- Endometriosis
- Chemical cystitis (e.g., with cyclophosphamide)
- Meatal ulcers
- Urethral caruncle
- Foreign body
- Factitious (added blood)

is more sensitive to albumin proteins than other types of proteins, such as Bence Jones proteins. Therefore, false-negative results may occur despite the presence of significant proteinuria, for example, in multiple myeloma or Waldenström's macroglobulinemia, in which the majority of protein being spilled is not albumin but a monoclonal protein (M protein).

Another method used to detect urinary proteins is the turbidimetric method. Use of a weak acid, such as sulfosalicylic acid (SSA), when mixed with urine, will denature proteins, resulting in a turbid solution. Like the dipstick test, this method is semiquantitative. Unlike the dipstick test, the SSA method is equally sensitive to non-albumin and albumin proteins.[13]

After protein spillage has been detected, the absolute amount of protein excreted should be measured, because this will help distinguish between glomerular and tubulointerstitial disease. Quantification is accomplished either by a timed (usually 24-hour) urine collection or by analysis of a spot urine sample. The 24-hour urine has been the gold standard method for quantification but is being replaced by the protein-to-creatinine ratio on a "spot" urine sample. The spot protein-to-creatinine method is less cumbersome for the patient and is less prone to collection errors. A protein-to-creatinine ratio of 0.2 correlates with a protein excretion rate of approximately 200 mg/day, a ratio of 2 with 2000 mg/day, and a ratio of 3.5 with 3500 mg/day (i.e., nephrotic-range proteinuria).[21]

The detection of microalbuminuria has become extremely important with the appreciation of its clinical correlation with cardiovascular and kidney disease. It is defined as an elevated urine albumin excretion rate (UAER), as measured by a specific assay that uses antibodies targeted against albumin. The normal range of UAER is less than 20 mg/min on an overnight timed urine collection or 30 mg/day on a 24-hour collection. The abnormal microalbuminuria range is 20 to 200 mg/min (30-300 mg/day). Values above 300 mg/day suggest "overt" proteinuria. First studied in diabetic patients, microalbuminuria has now been found to be a harbinger of renal involvement in many other diseases (see later). Microalbuminuria is present in the majority of patients with SLE, even in those with apparently normal urine and kidney function[22]; biopsy may reveal histologic changes, and some of these patients subsequently develop overt nephritis.

Urine protein electrophoresis and immunofixation

The primary use of the UPEP is to assess for the presence of monoclonal gammopathies, as seen with clonal proliferation of plasma cells. If an M protein is identified on UPEP, then immunofixation should be used for further identification of the abnormal protein.

Hematuria

Hematuria, unlike proteinuria, may arise from anywhere in the urinary tract[23] (see Table 37.2). For example, even strenuous exercise can lead to the appearance of blood in the urine.[24] The first step in assessing hematuria is to confirm its presence, that is, to rule out transient hematuria from physiologic stressors such as a UTI or exercise. Common causes of hematuria in children include acute infection and glomerular diseases. In adults, cystitis, urethritis, and prostatitis account for approximately 25% of hematuria, with nephrolithiasis accounting for another 20%. Hematuria in adults, unlike children, must be regarded as a sign of a tumor of the genitourinary tract until proven otherwise. Therefore, positive identification of the source of hematuria is important.[25] However, in young adults with hematuria unaccompanied by proteinuria, who are otherwise well, the likelihood of finding a significant lesion is very small.[26]

Hematuria can be divided into upper tract bleeding (i.e., glomerular or tubulointerstitial) and lower tract bleeding (i.e., extrarenal). Diagnostic clues such as red blood cell (RBC) casts, significant proteinuria, or abnormal kidney function suggest upper tract bleeding.[27] In patients with rheumatic diseases, microscopic hematuria will often be accompanied by proteinuria, suggesting upper tract bleeding. Patients who are taking anticoagulants may also present with hematuria. In these cases, cystoscopic imaging of the genitourinary tract is necessary to assess for culprit lesions.[28]

concentration. Additionally, it allows for the determination of the protein-to-creatinine ratio, which correlates extremely well with timed urine quantification of proteinuria (see later).[19]

Urine dipsticks can detect albumin at a minimum concentration of 15 to 30 mg/dL.[20] It is important to note, however, that this method

Testing for blood in the urine

In clinical practice, microscopic hematuria, like protein, is detected by a colorimetric method. The dipstick has a pad impregnated with two reagents, diisopropyl-benzene dihydro-peroxide and tetramethylbenzidine. Detection of blood is based on the Fenton reaction. The iron moiety of hemoglobin, which has peroxidase-like activity, reacts with diisopropyl-benzene, generating hydroxyl radicals. These oxidize tetramethylbenzidine, the colorimetric indicator. The intensity of the color change correlates with the degree of oxidation, ranging from orange (negative) to green to blue. The sensitivity of this test for hemoglobin is as low as 0.015 to 0.062 mg/dL but may be reduced in the setting of high specific gravity. Because the Fenton reaction is equally sensitive to unbound hemoglobin and myoglobin, when compared with intact RBC, both hemolysis and rhabdomyolysis will result in a positive urine dipstick for blood. Urine microscopy helps to distinguish among these possibilities.

Urine microscopy

Urine microscopy is best done on fresh urine, because casts and cellular components tend to degenerate after 1 hour. A urine sample is centrifuged at 2000 rpm for 5 minutes; the supernatant is discarded and, after re-suspending the sediment with a fixed volume, is decanted onto a glass slide. After application of a coverslip, the wet-mount unstained sediment is examined at 100 and 400 μm. Use of a phase-contrast and polarizing microscope may improve determination of RBC morphology.

Red blood cells

Red cell morphology offers a clue as to the site of origin of the hematuria.[29] Hematuria will typically have less than 1% dysmorphic erythrocytes.[30] However, hematuria of glomerular origin usually contains a high proportion of abnormally shaped RBCs with vesicle-shaped protrusions (acanthocytes) and considerable anisocytosis.[31] Acanthocytes are best appreciated by use of phase-contrast microscopy (Fig. 37.1).

Other urine microscopy findings

Pyuria, that is, the presence of white blood cells (WBC), suggests an infection within the genitourinary tract and mandates a urine culture. Sterile pyuria has classically suggested renal tuberculosis but also can be seen with tubulointerstitial nephritis, for example, from allergic interstitial drug reactions, Sjögren's syndrome, and lupus interstitial nephritis. Hansel's stain of the urine is the recommended test to detect eosinophils in the urine. However, as an indicator of acute interstitial nephritis, eosinophiluria has limited sensitivity.[32]

Urinary casts are formed in the renal tubules from aggregation of proteins, primarily Tamm-Horsfall proteins. Not all casts are pathologic; for example, hyaline casts can be seen in normal urinary sediment. When intact cells or cellular debris become trapped within the protein matrix, various "cylindricals" result: "muddy brown" granular casts with or without renal tubule epithelial casts are associated with acute tubular necrosis; WBC casts are classically associated with pyelonephritis or interstitial nephritis; and RBC casts are pathognomonic of intraparenchymal bleeding, such as from glomerulonephritis or

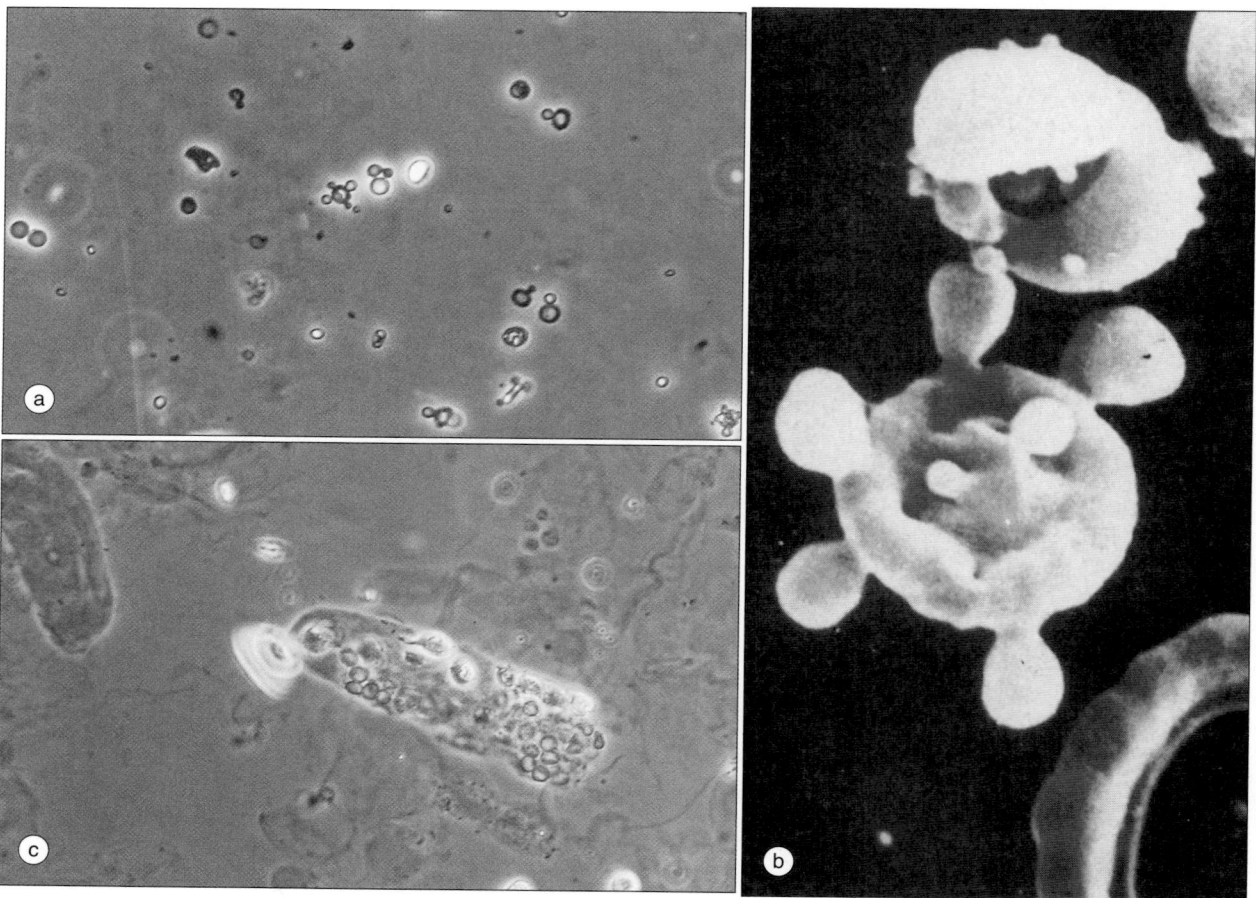

Fig. 37.1 Microscopy of urine. (a) Acanthocytes are seen through the microscope, which indicate a renal (probably glomerular) origin for the hematuria (phase contrast, original magnification ×640). (b) Acanthocytes seen by scanning electron microscope: details of the "knobs" and protrusions can be seen. (c) A tubular cast containing red cells, which usually indicates a glomerular origin for concomitant hematuria[27] and, in general, an active proliferative/infiltrative glomerular disease (phase contrast, original magnification ×400). *(a and c, courtesy of Dr. G.B. Fogazzi; b, reproduced with permission of Blackwell Science from Fassett RG, Owen JE, Fairley J, et al. Urinary red-cell morphology during exercise. BMJ 1982;285:1455-1457.)*

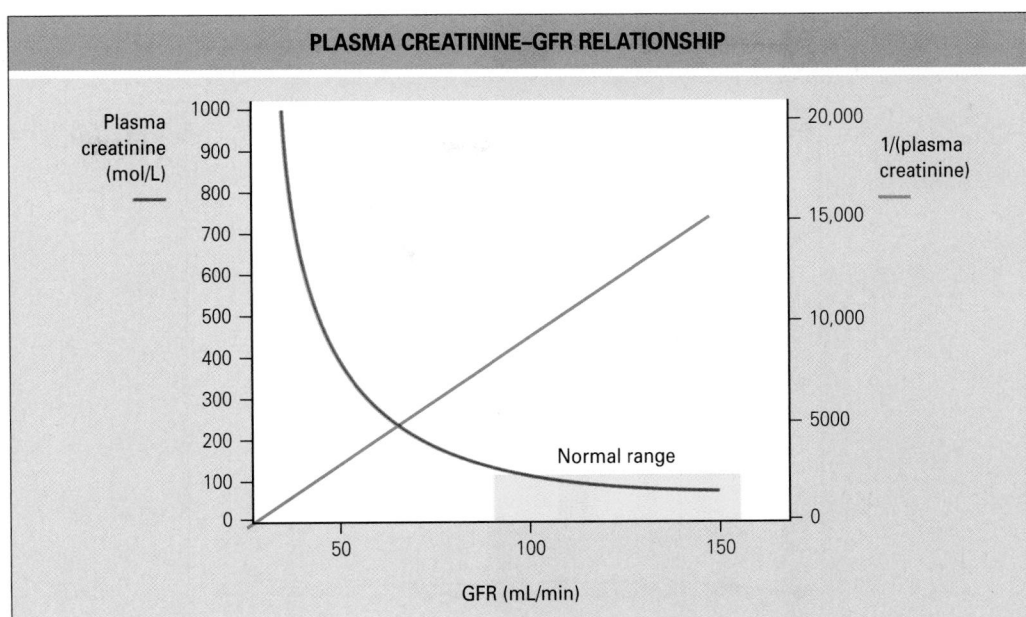

PLASMA CREATININE–GFR RELATIONSHIP

Fig. 37.2 The relationship of plasma creatinine to glomerular filtration rate (GFR). As GFR decreases, plasma creatinine rises, but in a hyperbolic fashion, so that plasma creatinine levels only become abnormal (normal range shaded) after a considerable loss of renal function. One way of compensating for this hidden information is to use the reciprocal of the plasma creatinine, which is approximately linear.

vasculitis. Broad and waxy casts, which are both acellular, strongly suggest CKD.

With nephrotic-range proteinuria, one may see lipid droplets.[33] If seen within renal tubule epithelial cells, they are called oval fat bodies. These fat bodies, when viewed under polarized light, have a characteristic "Maltese cross" appearance.

Kidney function testing

Kidney function is a term usually applied to the principal function of the kidneys, the elimination of nitrogenous wastes by the glomerulus, that is, the glomerular filtration rate (GFR). The GFR is generally considered to be the best index of overall kidney function, because impairment in GFR correlates with severity of structural abnormalities observed on histologic examination of kidney tissue. The normal GFR is 100 to 140 mL/min in men and 85 to 115 mL/min in women. The GFR is not an all-inclusive index of function because many kidney diseases exist that do not alter GFR. Other tests that assess renal tubular function are infrequently assessed,[23] but a few that are relevant to the rheumatic diseases are discussed here.

Plasma creatinine measurement

The plasma creatinine concentration (P_{CR}) is a simple and useful correlate of GFR. Creatinine is derived from both the non-enzymatic degradation of creatine in skeletal muscle and from dietary protein intake. It is released into the circulation at a relatively constant rate. Because creatinine is primarily cleared by glomerular filtration, its clearance will be equal to $P_{CR} \times$ GFR. In steady state, creatinine production must equal elimination. Therefore, $P_{CR} \times$ GFR is equal to a constant. Hence, P_{CR} is inversely proportional to GFR. Plasma creatinine is an inexpensive and widely used test of kidney function; when it is repeated serially in an individual it may give significant insight into changes in kidney function.

Normal ranges of creatinine are between 0.6 and 1.0 mg/dL (53-88 mmol/L) and 0.8 to 1.3 mg/dL (70-114 mmol/L) for women and men, respectively.[34] Recent data on normal non-hypertensive, non-diabetic adults show a mean plasma creatinine of 0.93 mg/dL and 1.13 mg/dL in women and men, respectively.[35]

Despite its appeal, there are significant problems with using P_{CR} as a sole marker of GFR. Specifically, in the lower range, small increases in P_{CR} reflect major reductions in GFR (Fig. 37.2). Thus, in some cases, up to one half of renal function can be lost before the P_{CR} exceeds the upper limits of normal. Also, when GFR changes abruptly, output no longer equals input and it may take several days before the system achieves a new steady state. Because 10% to 20% of creatinine is excreted by tubular secretion, there are cases in which elevations of P_{CR}

are unrelated to changes in GFR. Drugs that block tubular secretion, such as trimethoprim and cimetidine, are associated with such elevations in P_{CR} despite not affecting glomerular function.[36] Other drugs such as cefoxitin and flucytosine may cause false elevations in measured creatinine by interfering with the laboratory chemical assays for creatinine. Finally, in some disease states, there is hyperexcretion of creatinine by the proximal tubule, as is the case with sickle cell disease.

Another concern about the use of P_{CR} as the sole marker of kidney function is that, although GFR decreases markedly with age, the plasma creatinine barely rises (Fig. 37.3). This is due to a decrease in creatinine production as muscle mass decreases with age.[37] Thus the average P_{CR} at 100 years of age is close to that at age 25, despite a reduction in GFR by greater than two thirds (see Fig. 37.3). This problem holds for other states in which muscle mass is lost, such as with anorexia nervosa, amputations, and chronic illnesses. Therefore, the National Kidney Foundation Kidney Disease Outcome Quality Initiative (K/DOQI) recommends that P_{CR} alone should not be used to assess GFR.[38]

Equations of GFR

Cockcroft-Gault formula

Formulas that take into account the P_{CR} and other variables, such as age, gender, and body size are better predictors of GFR. The best-validated and most reproducible formula for GFR is that of Cockcroft and Gault.[39] The Cockcroft-Gault formula takes into account plasma creatinine, age, weight, and gender:

$$GFR\ (mL/min) = \frac{[(140 - \text{Age in years}) \times (\text{Weight in kg}) \times (0.85\ \text{if female})]}{[72 \times P_{CR}]\,(\text{in mg/dL})}$$

or

$$GFR\ (mL/min) = \frac{[1.2 \times (140 - \text{Age in years}) \times (\text{Weight in kg}) \times (0.85\ \text{if female})]}{P_{CR}\,(\text{in mmol/L})}$$

MDRD equation

Using data from the Modification of Diet in Renal Disease (MDRD) study, a formula to predict GFR was developed using a multiple regression model. Like the Cockcroft-Gault formula, the MDRD equation takes into account variables other than P_{CR} but does not require weight[40]:

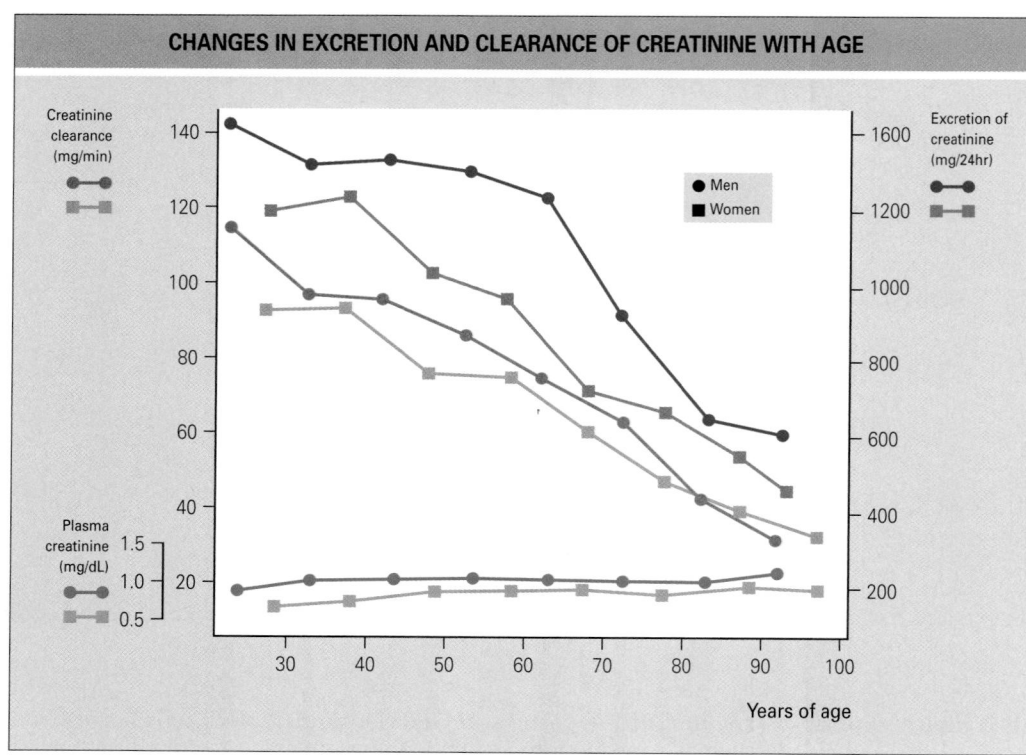

CHANGES IN EXCRETION AND CLEARANCE OF CREATININE WITH AGE

Fig. 37.3 The "hidden" reduction in renal function with age. Although the normal creatinine clearance decreases dramatically with age to a mean of only 40 mL/min in the very elderly, the plasma creatinine value remains constant up to 100 years of age because of a concomitant reduction in excretion (and, by inference, production) of creatinine due to reduction in muscle mass. *(Data from Kampmann J, Siersbaek-Nielsen K, Kristensen M, Hansen JM. Rapid evaluation of creatinine clearance. Acta Med Scand 1974;196:517-520.)*

$$\text{GFR}\,(\text{mL/min/1.73 m}^2) = 186 \times (P_{CR})^{-1.154} \times (\text{Age})^{-0.203} \times (0.742 \text{ if female}) \times (1.210 \text{ if African-American})$$

Because the MDRD equation is most accurate in the setting of some degree of renal insufficiency, the National Kidney Disease Education Program recommends only reporting numerical values when the calculation results in a predicted GFR of less than 60. If using the MDRD equation, for values above 60 mL/min/1.73 m², one should report the result as merely, "above 60 mL/min/1.73 m²." A study comparing the Cockcroft-Gault formula and the MDRD equation to radionuclide-labeled chromium ethylenediaminetetraacetic acid (^{51}Cr-EDTA) determination of GFR in 2095 non-black individuals demonstrated good global agreement. It appeared that the Cockcroft-Gault formula overestimated GFR by 1.94 mL/min/1.73 m², whereas the MDRD equation underestimated it by 0.99 mL/min/1.73 m².[41] Given these results, it seems reasonable to preferentially use the MDRD equation.

Stages of chronic kidney disease

Given the improved determination of GFR by use of formulas like the MDRD equation, the National Kidney Foundation has established stages of CKD, listed in Table 37.3.[42]

Creatinine clearance

The creatinine clearance (C_{CR}) has been the gold standard for estimating GFR[34] but has largely been replaced by formulas that estimate GFR because they avoid collection errors and are less cumbersome for the patient. Additionally, the validity of the C_{CR} appears to be questionable in patients with lupus nephritis (see earlier).[43]

The C_{CR} measurement depends on an accurately timed urine collection and a P_{CR} that is representative of the average creatinine over the collection period. The method assumes that creatinine is freely filtered by the glomerulus (true) and is neither secreted (false, tubular secretion) nor reabsorbed (true) from the ultrafiltrate. If this were the case, then the amount of creatinine in the glomerular filtrate ($P_{CR} \times$ GFR) would equal the amount in the final urine ($U_{CR} \times V$, where U_{CR} is the urine creatinine concentration and V is the urine flow rate).

Thus:

$$P_{CR} \times \text{GFR} = U_{CR} \times V$$

TABLE 37.3 CHRONIC KIDNEY DISEASE: A CLINICAL ACTION PLAN

Stage	Description	GFR (mL/min/1.73 m²)	Action*
	At increased risk	≥90 (with CKD risk factors)	Screening CKD risk reduction
1	Kidney damage with normal or ↑ GFR	≥90	Diagnosis and treatment, treatment of co-morbid conditions, slowing progression, CVD risk reduction
2	Kidney damage with mild or ↓ GFR	60-89	Estimating progression
3	Moderate ↓ GFR	30-59	Evaluation and treating complications
4	Severe ↓ GFR	15-29	Preparation for kidney replacement therapy
5	Kidney failure	<15 (or dialysis)	Replacement (if uremia present)

GFR, glomerular filtration rate; CKD, chronic kidney disease; CVD, cardiovascular disease
Stages 1 through 5 identify patients who have chronic kidney disease; the first row designates individuals who are at increased risk for developing chronic kidney disease. Chronic kidney disease is defined as either kidney damage or GFR < 60 mL/min/1.73 m² for ≥ 3 months. Kidney damage is defined as pathologic abnormalities or markers of damage, including abnormalities of blood or urine tests or imaging studies.
*Includes actions from preceding stages.

Rearranging the formula for GFR:

$$\text{GFR (in mL/min)} = U_{CR}/(P_{CR} \times V)(\text{in mL/min})$$

or

$$\text{GFR (in mL/min)} = U_{CR}/(P_{CR} \times V)(\text{in mL/24 hr/1440})$$

Fortuitously, the error introduced by tubular secretion of creatinine is largely offset by the overestimate of P_{CR} caused by other chromogens in the blood. However, as GFR declines, tubular secretion of creatinine increases, resulting in overestimates of GFR. Normal values of C_{CR} are 95 ± 20 mL/min in women and 120 ± 25 mL/min in men.

Like the 24-hour urine protein test, the measurement of C_{CR} is subject to technical errors in collection. The creatinine index is an "internal control" that helps identify incomplete urine collections. Men tend to excrete 20 to 25 mg of creatinine per kilogram of body weight per day, regardless of kidney function. Women tend to excrete slightly less creatinine, between 15 and 20 mg/kg/day, owing to a lower percentage of muscle mass per body weight. Therefore, if the creatinine index is below these ranges, one should suspect an incomplete collection and discount the results of the C_{CR}.

Isotope measurement of GFR

The GFR can be measured by injection of iohexol, ^{51}Cr-EDTA,[44] or ^{131}I-iothalamate.[45] Inulin clearance, the gold standard for measuring GFR, is an impractical method for clinical medicine.

Tests for renal tubular dysfunction

The renal tubular disorders most likely to be encountered in rheumatic disease patients are renal tubular acidosis (RTA) and either hypokalemia or hyperkalemia. These are seen in several autoimmune diseases, including the interstitial nephritis of SLE and Sjögren's syndrome. About 10% of patients with SLE develop these problems, although subclinical defects in the handling of potassium, sodium, or hydrogen ions can be demonstrated in up to 60% of cases.[46] RTA manifests as a hyperchloremic, non-gap acidosis with a low plasma bicarbonate concentration. With a distal, type 1 RTA there is reduced ammonium ion secretion into the urine. This is determined by measurement of the urine net charge (also called urinary anion gap):

$$(U_{Na} + U_K) - U_{Cl}$$

In the setting of a metabolic acidosis and an appropriate renal response, the urine net charge should be negative (usually ranging between -20 to -50 mEq/L), which represents increased excretion of ammonium (NH_4^+). However, in type 1 RTA the urine net charge is positive, suggesting an inability to effectively secrete ammonium or hydrogen ions. The RTA seen in lupus is usually due to proton secretion defects in distal tubules.[46]

Persistent hyperkalemia is invariably associated with renal tubular dysfunction, resulting in impaired urinary potassium excretion. This occurs with advanced kidney failure, with any cause of hypoaldosteronism, or with marked volume depletion. Assessment of renal potassium handling will help determine the cause of the hyperkalemia. Measurement of the urinary sodium and chloride concentrations will give some insight as to the effective intravascular volume. Calculation of the transtubular potassium gradient (TTKG)[47] allows for a semiquantitative assessment of the activity of the secretory process of potassium. The TTKG is calculated as follows:

$$TTKG = (Urine_K / Plasma_K)/(Urine_{Osmolality} / Plasma_{Osmolality})$$

In the setting of hyperkalemia, a TTKG below 7 confirms a renal cause.[48]

Hypocomplementemia and kidney disease

The identification of hypocomplementemia is sometimes used to help narrow the differential of kidney diseases. The list of glomerulonephritis associated with hypocomplementemia includes lupus nephritis, membranoproliferative glomerulonephritis, mixed cryoglobulinemia, postinfectious glomerulonephritis, membranous nephropathy due to hepatitis B infection, and serum sickness.[49] Complement levels tend to be normal in Goodpasture's syndrome, ANCA-associated granulomatous vasculitis, microscopic polyangiitis, and Henoch-Schönlein purpura.[49]

Renal imaging

Kidney ultrasonography

Ultrasonography is the most commonly used technique to image the kidneys because it is non-invasive and does not depend on kidney function. It allows determination of kidney size, degree of echogenicity, anatomic abnormalities, and obstruction. Normal kidneys are between 11 and 12 cm in length. The findings of bilateral small kidneys, defined as less than 8.5 cm, and increased echogenicity, suggest significant chronicity of the kidney disease. Increased echogenicity with normal or large kidneys suggest a more acute process. Large kidneys are seen in diseases that lead to deposition of material in the kidney, such as multiple myeloma, HIV infection, or amyloid. Ultrasonography may also delineate nephrolithiasis or nephrocalcinosis, although the gold standard remains helical computed tomography (CT).[50] Papillary necrosis, as seen in association with non-steroidal anti-inflammatory drugs (NSAIDs), may also be picked up on ultrasonography, although intravenous pyelogram is the gold standard. Additionally, signs of obstructive uropathy, such as pelvocaliectasis and hydronephrosis, are easily seen on an ultrasound examination.

Assessment of renal vasculature

To assess for renal vasculitis, the best imaging studies include angiogram, magnetic resonance angiography (MRA), and CT. The advantage of MRA is that it avoids the radiocontrast load and therefore the risk of contrast-associated nephropathy. For the assessment of the renal vasculature in patients with rheumatic diseases, duplex Doppler ultrasonography is better at detecting stenoses of the major branches of the renal arteries[51] than at demonstrating vasculitis or aneurysms. Renal vein thrombosis may be diagnosed by Doppler ultrasonography, but the sensitivity and specificity are suboptimal; spiral CT and MRA are better but the gold standard remains selective venography.

Kidney biopsy

Indications

The percutaneous kidney biopsy is an essential tool for determining the diagnosis, prognosis, and treatment options for patients with kidney disease.[52] The introduction of spring-loaded biopsy systems and the use of real-time ultrasound guidance have made obtaining kidney tissue increasingly safe and effective.[53] However, indications for performing a percutaneous biopsy still vary among nephrologists.[54] One of the strongest indications to perform a kidney biopsy is in the setting of rapidly progressive glomerulonephritis (RPGN). The syndrome is defined clinically as a rapid decline in kidney function associated with an active urinary sediment, typically with RBC casts. Delays in diagnosis and subsequent initiation of treatment of RPGN may result in irreversible loss of kidney function. Common rheumatologic causes of RPGN include lupus, antineutrophil cytoplasmic antibody (ANCA)-related vasculitis (including ANCA-associated granulomatous vasculitis), and Henoch-Schönlein purpura. Other indications for obtaining a biopsy in patients with rheumatic disease include unexplained renal failure, acute nephritic syndrome, persistent proteinuria, persistent hematuria, and nephrotic syndrome. Nephrologists also use kidney biopsy to help diagnose unspecified systemic diseases, as typified by *seronegative lupus*.[55] This term is used to describe patients with an active sediment and renal histology typical of lupus but at the time of presentation no other clinical or serologic evidence of SLE. Patients with lupus may need more than one kidney biopsy in the course of their illness. Of note, the World Health Organization's classification of lupus nephritis has recently been modified (see SLE section, later).

Contraindications and precautions

A percutaneous kidney biopsy is generally contraindicated with an uncorrectable bleeding disorder, severe hypertension, horseshoe-shaped kidney, severe obesity, hydronephrosis, or bilaterally small, echogenic kidneys.[51] Previously, a single kidney was regarded as an absolute contraindication to percutaneous biopsy, but with improvements in technique it is now considered to confer only a relative contraindication.[56]

Because each kidney receives approximately one fifth of the cardiac output, it is not surprising that bleeding is the major risk of a kidney biopsy. Additionally, azotemia is associated with a functional defect in platelet adhesiveness. Therefore, every effort should be made to minimize the risk of hemorrhage. Drugs that affect hemostasis should be stopped before planned kidney biopsy: 10 days for aspirin, 5 days for warfarin, and at least 5 half-lives or 7 days for NSAIDs to allow normal platelet function. The platelet count, prothrombin time (PT), and activated partial thromboplastin time (aPTT) must be checked and, if abnormal, corrected before biopsy. Although historically a bleeding time has been used to assess the risk of bleeding, it is not a reliable screening test and should not be used for this purpose.[57] Another factor that can contribute to lack of obtaining hemostasis is uncontrolled hypertension. Therefore, antihypertensive medications should not be withheld on the morning of biopsy and supplemental therapy may be needed.

Procedure

The preferred method of obtaining kidney tissue for histologic evaluation is by use of an ultrasound-guided percutaneous biopsy system. Laparoscopic, CT-guided, open surgical, or transvenous transjugular biopsies are alternative methods occasionally employed in class 3 obesity, with uncorrectable bleeding diatheses, or when a subject has a solitary kidney.

Two or three cores of kidney tissue, measuring approximately 15 mm in length and 15 or 18 gauge in diameter, are obtained and sent for light microscopy (LM), immunofluorescence (IF) microscopy, and electron microscopy (EM). Light microscopy is done using various stains, which routinely include hematoxylin and eosin (H&E), periodic acid–Schiff (PAS), and trichrome Masson. Additional "special stains" include the Jones silver stain, used to evaluate for tram tracking, and the Congo red stain, used to detect amyloid. Immunohistochemical techniques are used to demonstrate the presence of immunoglobulins, complement fractions, and allied proteins, mainly in the glomerulus but also within the tubules and renal vasculature.

Patterns seen on immunofluorescence microscopy

There are three patterns of IF staining: linear, granular, and pauci-immune. The primary cause of a linear pattern is when there are antibodies directed against the glomerular basement membrane (GBM), as is the case with anti-GBM disease. When associated with pulmonary hemorrhage, this constellation of findings is known as Goodpasture's syndrome. On IF, there is linear deposition of IgG all along the basement membrane. In contrast to a linear deposition, diseases where there is immune complex formation and deposition will have a granular, "lumpy-bumpy" appearance. This occurs with SLE and postinfectious glomerulonephritis. The term *pauci-immune* implies that there are no or minimal immunoglobulins present and is seen with ANCA-associated granulomatous vasculitis, microscopic polyangiitis, and other ANCA-related vasculitides.[58]

Transmission EM allows significant enhanced resolution compared with LM and can delineate the precise location and size of electron dense deposits. Deposits can be divided into (1) subepithelial, in which accumulation of material occurs on the external aspect of the glomerular basement membrane, between the basement membrane and the visceral epithelial cell, (2) subendothelial, in which accumulation occurs between the basement membrane and the fenestrated endothelial cell, and (3) transmembranous or intramembranous, in which the deposits are within the glomerular basement membrane. Electron microscopy can also reveal other ultrastructural features of diagnostic importance, such as tubuloreticular structures, so-called virus-like particles, in the glomerular endothelial cells in SLE nephritis.[59]

Interpretation

The renal cortical parenchyma contains three different domains: the glomeruli, the tubules and interstitium, and the vasculature. Small and medium-sized vessel vasculitis can be distinguished from changes due to atherosclerosis, hypertension, diabetes mellitus, or systemic sclerosis. Tubulointerstitial changes can range from acute inflammation with edema to chronic fibrosis with scarring or may include granuloma formation, as seen with renal sarcoidosis.

Terminology

When describing glomerular changes, it is important to understand a somewhat confusing nomenclature. Specific terms have been assigned to describe the pattern of involvement in one glomerulus (segmental or global), and other terms have been assigned to describe the proportion of glomeruli involved with a pathologic process (focal or diffuse). The term *focal* is applied when less than 50% of all glomeruli are

TABLE 37.4 NEPHROPATHOLOGY MORPHOLOGIC TERMINOLOGY

		All glomeruli	
		Focal (<50%)	Diffuse (≥50%)
One glomerulus	Segmental (<50%)	Focal-segmental	Diffuse-segmental
	Global (≥50%)	Focal-global	Diffuse-global

involved, and the term *diffuse* is used when more than 50% of all glomeruli are involved. The term *segmental* is applied to a lesion that involves a portion of one particular glomerulus, and the term *global* is applied to a lesion that involves the whole glomerulus. For example, if a total of 20 glomeruli are examined under LM, and only 5 of them have pathologic changes, this would be referred to as a focal lesion. If these 5 glomeruli have only partial involvement, then the process is further defined as segmental (Table 37.4).

Glomerular pathology is divided into primary or idiopathic lesions and secondary lesions. There are five histologic patterns of primary glomerular lesions:

1. Minimal change disease: as its name implies, minimal change disease has minimal to no pathologic changes on LM or IF. On EM, there is diffuse effacement of the visceral epithelial cell (podocyte) foot processes. Minimal change disease presents as nephrotic syndrome with massive edema and is the most common cause of nephrotic syndrome in young children. In rheumatology practice, it may be seen as a complication of NSAID use (see later).

2. Focal segmental glomerulosclerosis (FSGS): as its name implies, FSGS initially affects only a portion of each glomerulus and tends to involve some but not all the glomeruli. On LM, there are lesions in some glomeruli (focal) with areas of glomerulosclerosis in only parts of the glomerular tufts (segmental). On IF, there may be deposition of IgM and C3 in the areas of sclerosis. EM demonstrates diffuse fusion or effacement of podocyte foot processes. FSGS can present as either a nephritic or nephrotic syndrome or as progressive decline in GFR. Secondary causes of FSGS include HIV infection, reflux nephropathy, and obesity.

3. Membranous glomerulonephritis: On LM, the characteristic finding of membranous glomerulonephritis is thickening of the capillary walls due to subepithelial deposits (seen as spikes on Jones silver stain). On IF, one can see granular deposits of IgG and C3 along the glomerular capillary walls. On EM, there are electron-dense deposits along the capillary wall with associated foot-process effacement. Membranous glomerulonephritis tends to present as massive proteinuria (nephrotic syndrome) and edema and not with nephritic syndrome. Secondary causes of membranous glomerulonephritis include SLE (class V nephritis), mixed connective tissue disease, gold therapy, solid tumors, and hepatitis B infection.

4. Mesangial proliferative glomerulonephritis: On LM, there is no or little involvement of the capillary lumina but the mesangium is expanded with increased cellularity and matrix. The findings on EM mirror that seen on LM, with electron-dense deposits within the mesangium. Immunofluorescence may demonstrate mesangial deposition of IgA, IgM, or IgG, with or without C3. When the predominant finding on IF is IgA deposits, the lesion is referred to as IgA nephropathy or Berger's disease. The clinical presentation of a mesangial proliferative glomerulonephritis is variable, because it spans the spectrum from isolated hematuria through RPGN and from no proteinuria through nephrotic syndrome. Important secondary causes include lupus nephritis, Henoch-Schönlein purpura (systemic Berger's disease), rheumatoid arthritis, and ankylosing spondylitis.

5. Membranoproliferative glomerulonephritis (MPGN): This lesion has also been called mesangiocapillary glomerulonephritis and is divided into type 1, type 2 (dense deposit disease), and type 3

based on microscopy findings. They can all present as an RPGN, as macroscopic hematuria, less commonly as nephrotic syndrome, or as isolated proteinuria and/or microscopic hematuria. Typical LM findings include capillary wall thickening due to the presence of deposits, which frequently take the form of a duplicated or split basement membrane (double contours or "tram tracking"). On IF, deposits located along the capillary wall and mesangium vary in amount, distribution, and appearance. They may be granular, short linear, or a combination of the two and typically include C3 and may include IgG, IgA or IgM. On EM, there are often electron-dense deposits within the mesangium and subendothelium. In some cases, there are also subepithelial deposits. Secondary causes of MPGN include lupus (class III and IV), and a rare form associated with hypocomplementemic partial lipodystrophy.[60]

Another significant abnormal finding is the presence of cells, fibrin, and/or collagen in the urinary space of the glomeruli. When this process involves more than 50% of the circumference of the glomerular tuft, it is termed a *crescent* (fibrous, fibrocellular, or cellular crescent, depending on the predominant finding). The presence of crescents is a marker of severe kidney injury and usually is the pathologic equivalent of the clinical syndrome of RPGN. Crescentic glomerulonephritis may be associated with other forms of primary glomerulonephritis, such as MPGN or IgA nephropathy, or secondary glomerulonephritis, such as SLE and ANCA-associated granulomatous vasculitis.

RHEUMATOLOGIC DISEASES AFFECTING THE KIDNEYS

Details of the pathogenesis, pathology, clinical features, diagnosis, and management of the renal manifestations of rheumatic diseases are given in specific chapters throughout this book. This section lists the principal renal entities for the purpose of correlating and summarizing their key features (Table 37.5).

Systemic lupus erythematosus

Renal involvement is common in SLE, with approximately one third of patients initially presenting to a nephrologist rather than a rheumatologist.[61] The incidence of lupus nephritis likely exceeds 90%, because some kidney involvement may be silent.[62,63] Subgroups of patients with SLE at increased risk for development of nephritis include men younger than 33 years of age at the time of diagnosis of SLE and non-European Americans.[64] The presence of anticardiolipin antibody activity correlates with a worse kidney prognosis.[65]

The principal different renal lesions are summarized in Table 37.5. Of note, the World Health Organization's classification of lupus nephritis has recently been modified[66] (Table 37.6). The primary advantage of the revised classification system is that it provides a clearer description of the lupus nephritis classes.

Treatment and prognosis are different for each type of nephritis.[5,67] Additionally, transitions between the different classes of glomerulonephritis occur frequently but do not occur in a stepwise fashion. Most renal abnormalities emerge soon after diagnosis.[15] As an example, in one study of 1000 patients seen in rheumatologic practice, kidney involvement was initially present in 16% and increased to 50% during follow-up.[68] However, if a subject does not have overt nephropathy, urinalysis and determination of GFR (see earlier) should be performed routinely. Acute nephritis exacerbations require immediate evaluation and usually require a kidney biopsy. Unfortunately, renal vasculitis and thrombotic microangiopathy are rarely demonstrable on biopsy.[69] Renal vein thrombosis in patients with lupus nephritis may similarly be clinically inapparent.[3]

About 10% of patients with lupus nephritis develop an overt distal RTA and hyperkalemia, although subclinical defects are present in a large number of individuals.[46] The hyperkalemia may be exacerbated by use of potassium-sparing diuretics or agents that interfere with the renin-angiotensin system blockade, such as ACE inhibitors and angiotensin receptor blockers. Strategies to decrease hyperkalemia include limiting dietary potassium intake; use of fludrocortisone; and use of loop diuretics.[70]

Mixed connective tissue disease

Although originally described as a syndrome without renal involvement,[71] mixed connective tissue disease (MCTD) is now recognized as having kidney involvement in 25% to 50% of cases.[72] The most common lesion is membranous glomerulonephritis,[72] presenting similarly to that seen in SLE. Individuals with more systemic manifestations from MCTD appear to be at higher risk for kidney involvement than those without. Patients with MCTD may also develop hypertensive crises similar to those seen with "scleroderma kidney."[73]

Rheumatoid arthritis

The existence of a glomerulopathy associated with untreated rheumatoid arthritis is now generally accepted,[74] in addition to renal disease secondary to medications used to treat the underlying disorder. The most common kidney lesion is mesangial proliferative glomerulonephritis, but other renal lesions include membranous glomerulonephritis, focal proliferative glomerulonephritis, and secondary amyloidosis.[74] Rheumatoid arthritis may also present as an RPGN with either crescentic[75] or necrotizing glomerulonephritis,[76] or as a pauci-immune glomerulonephritis.[77] Nephrotic syndrome in patients with rheumatoid arthritis most often reflects either membranous glomerulonephritis from gold or penicillamine toxicity[78] or more often the development of systemic amyloidosis with glomerular involvement[74] (see later).

Sjögren's syndrome

Sjögren's syndrome typically does not result in glomerular pathology but more frequently produces an interstitial nephritis and defects in tubular function. The findings of an interstitial nephritis in association with eye findings should raise the specter of tubulointerstitial nephritis associated with uveitis syndrome. This tubular pathology associated with Sjögren's syndrome can manifest clinically as a reduction in GFR, a distal RTA, or hypokalemia or as mild nephrogenic diabetes insipidus.[79] MPGN and membranous glomerulonephritis have been diagnosed in patients with Sjögren's syndrome.[80]

Relapsing polychondritis

Kidney disease is a variable feature of relapsing polychondritis and may present as proteinuria, hematuria, or a decline in kidney function. Lesions associated with relapsing polychondritis may be associated with coexisting disease such as SLE. Renal pathology has included mesangial proliferative glomerulonephritis, crescentic necrotizing glomerulonephritis, and tubulointerstitial nephritis.[81] Treatments of both the primary condition and the renal disease are controversial, and the role of immunosuppressive therapy is unclear.

Behçet's disease

Kidney involvement in Behçet's disease appears to be less frequent than with other types of vasculitis. However, there is an association with focal or diffuse proliferative and membranous glomerulonephritis.[82] Amyloidosis is a more common renal complication of Behçet's disease and may present as the nephrotic syndrome. Intrarenal microaneurysms have also been described in association with Behçet's disease. In a retrospective review of urinalyses in patients with Behçet's disease, urinary abnormalities (proteinuria and/or hematuria) were present in about 10% of patients but less than 1% developed serious kidney lesions.[83]

Classic polyarteritis nodosa

The kidneys are the most commonly involved organs with polyarteritis nodosa, leading to hypertension and a variable decline in GFR. There may be patchy cortical infarctions, and renal artery aneurysms may rupture. Glomerulonephritis is not a feature of polyarteritis nodosa, because it tends not to be a small vessel disease.

ANCA-associated vasculitides

ANCA-associated granulomatous vasculitis, microscopic polyangiitis, and idiopathic pauci-immune glomerulonephritis likely represent the

TABLE 37.5 PRINCIPAL TYPES OF RENAL PATHOLOGY IN THE RHEUMATIC DISEASES

	Glomerular diseases	Renal vascular diseases	Tubulointerstitial diseases
Systemic lupus erythematosus	Mesangial glomerulonephritis (WHO class II) Focal proliferative glomerulonephritis (WHO class III) Diffuse proliferative glomerulonephritis (WHO class IV), incl. membranoproliferative glomerulonephritis (= mesangiocapillary glomerulonephritis), and crescentic and necrotizing glomerulonephritis (WHO class V)	Vasculitis of the kidney Thrombotic microangiopathy (with thrombotic thrombocytopenic purpura or anticardiolipin syndrome) "Lupus vasculopathy" (see text) Renal vein thrombosis	Lupus tubulointerstitial nephritis Drug-induced (NSAIDs, cyclosporine, etc.) Membranous glomerulonephritis
Mixed connective tissue disease	Membranous glomerulonephritis Mesangial glomerulonephritis	"Scleroderma kidney" (see later)	
Rheumatoid arthritis	Focal proliferative glomerulonephritis Crescentic necrotizing glomerulonephritis (with vasculitis) Membranous glomerulonephritis (gold, penicillamine) Renal amyloidosis (see later)	Vasculitis (rheumatoid) of the kidney Other drug-induced (NSAIDs, methotrexate, cyclosporin, etc.)	Analgesic nephropathy (NSAIDs)
Sjögren's syndrome	Membranoproliferative glomerulonephritis (= mesangiocapillary glomerulonephritis) (with cryoglobulinemia)		Lymphocytic tubulointerstitial nephritis (with hypokalemic renal tubular acidosis)
Relapsing polychondritis	Mild mesangial glomerulonephritis; focal sclerosing glomerulonephritis		Tubulointerstitial nephritis
Behçet's disease	Crescentic glomerulonephritis, or milder proliferative glomerulonephritis Renal amyloidosis (see later)	Renal artery aneurysms and intrarenal microaneurysms	
Polyarteritis nodosa (classic)	Ischemic sclerosis of glomeruli	Arteritis and aneurysms of medium-sized vessels	
Microscopic polyarteritis (polyangiitis)	Focal necrotizing and crescentic glomerulonephritis (pauci-immune)	Vasculitis of small vessels (arterioles, capillaries, and venules)	
ANCA-associated granulomatous vasculitis	Focal necrotizing and crescentic glomerulonephritis (pauci-immune)	Vasculitis of small vessels (arterioles, capillaries, and venules)	Granulomas, lymphocytic infiltrates (periglomerular)
Churg-Strauss syndrome	Focal glomerulonephritis Focal necrotizing and crescentic glomerulonephritis	Vasculitis	Granulomas, eosinophil infiltrates
Essential mixed cryoglobulinemia	Cryoglobulinemic glomerulonephritis Membranoproliferative glomerulonephritis	Small vessel vasculitis	Tubulointerstitial nephritis (= mesangiocapillary glomerulonephritis)
Henoch-Schönlein purpura	Diffuse proliferative glomerulonephritis with mesangial IgA deposits		
Ankylosing spondylitis	Focal proliferative glomerulonephritis with mesangial IgA deposits (= mesangial IgA nephropathy) Renal amyloidosis (see later)		
Reactive arthritis	Focal proliferative glomerulonephritis with mesangial IgA deposits (= mesangial IgA nephropathy)		
Progressive systemic sclerosis ("scleroderma")	Ischemic glomeruli	Concentric layered thickening of arterial walls, with narrowed lumens	
Amyloidosis	Mesangial expansion due to accumulation of amyloid fibrils		Peritubular amyloid deposits
Gout (chronic urate nephropathy)			Chronic interstitial inflammation and fibrosis

spectrum of disease presentation of the ANCA-associated vasculitides. Classic ANCA-associated granulomatous vasculitis involves the upper and lower respiratory tracts and the kidney.[84] When the vasculitis has a more limited systemic involvement but still affects the kidney, it is termed *microscopic polyangiitis*. When only the kidneys are affected by the vasculitis, the condition is termed an *idiopathic pauci-immune glomerulonephritis*. The view that these three entities represent a spectrum of presentations of a unified disease is supported by several facts:

1. A positive test for ANCA is typically present in all three conditions.
2. The glomerular pathology is indistinguishable.
3. Patients diagnosed with idiopathic pauci-immune glomerulonephritis or microscopic polyangiitis may later develop typical pulmonary lesions consistent with ANCA-associated granulomatous vasculitis.
4. Patients with "limited" ANCA-associated granulomatous vasculitis, in which clinical findings are isolated to the pulmonary

TABLE 37.6 WORLD HEALTH ORGANIZATION CLASSIFICATION OF LUPUS NEPHRITIS

Class	Description
Class I	Mesangial immune deposits without mesangial hypercellularity
Class II	Mesangial immune deposits with mesangial hypercellularity
Class III Subdivisions for active and sclerotic lesions	Focal glomerulonephritis (involving < 50% of total number of glomeruli)
Class IV	Diffuse glomerulonephritis (involving ≥50% of total number of glomeruli)
Class IV-S Subdivisions for active and sclerotic lesions	Segmental involvement
Class IV-G Subdivisions for active and sclerotic lesions	Global involvement
Class V	Membranous
Class VI	Advanced sclerosing lesions

Data from Weening JJ, D'Agati VD, Schwartz MM, et al. The classification of glomerulonephritis in systemic lupus erythematosus revisited. Kidney Int 2004;65:521-530.

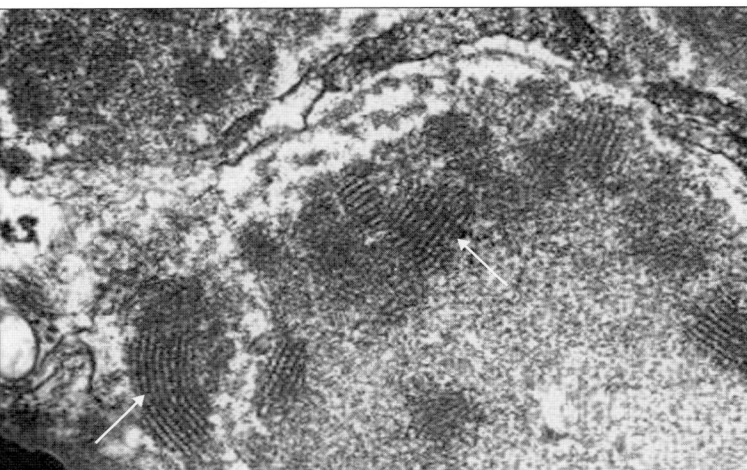

Fig. 37.4 Electron micrograph of subject with cryoglobulinemia demonstrating electron dense deposits of tubular fibrils in a "fingerprint" appearance (arrows).

system, may later develop systemic manifestations, including kidney involvement.

The renal lesion with these conditions typically presents as an RPGN. Renal vessels other than glomerular capillaries can also be involved by the necrotizing vasculitis.

Allergic granulomatosis and angiitis, better known as Churg-Strauss syndrome, is typified by allergic rhinitis, asthma, eosinophilia, and a small vessel vasculitis. As in ANCA-associated granulomatous vasculitis and microscopic polyangiitis, patients tend to be ANCA positive. Although the most common organ involved is the lung, kidney involvement occurs more frequently than previously thought, with a prevalence as high as 84%.[85] Unlike ANCA-associated granulomatous vasculitis, renal failure is rare. The predominant glomerular pathology is FSGN and may be associated with necrotizing features and crescents.[85] Granulomas and eosinophilic infiltrates in the kidney are infrequent.

Essential mixed cryoglobulinemia

Essential mixed cryoglobulinemia (formerly known as Meltzer's syndrome) is often an epiphenomena of a chronic viral infection, such as with hepatitis C or HIV infection.[86,87] Cryoglobulins are immunoglobulins that precipitate in the cold and lead to deposition of antigen-antibody complexes in small and medium-sized arteries. This leads to hypocomplementemia, palpable purpura, arthralgias, hepatosplenomegaly, and peripheral neuropathy. Kidney involvement occurs in upward of 60% of cases of mixed cryoglobulinemia.[88] Histologic examination of the kidney reveals an MPGN with some unique features.[89] On LM, one may see intraluminal thrombi, which are composed of cryoglobulins. Also, on LM, there tends to be diffuse IgM deposits in the glomerular capillary loops. On EM, the majority of deposits are found in the subendothelial zone. These deposits bulge into the capillary lumen and likely lead to the formation of the characteristic thrombi seen on LM. The majority of cryoglobulin deposits have a characteristic substructure, containing curved annular-tubular structures that measure approximately 30 nm in diameter and appear like a "fingerprint" (Fig. 37.4).

Kidney involvement can manifest as asymptomatic hematuria and proteinuria but can progress to nephrotic-range proteinuria or deterioration of kidney function.

Henoch-Schönlein purpura

Henoch-Schönlein purpura is a small vessel vasculitis characterized by tissue deposition of IgA-containing immune complexes.[90] It more frequently affects children than adults and has a classic tetrad of rash (palpable petechiae or purpura), arthralgias, abdominal pain, and kidney disease. The clinical severity of kidney disease varies from mild proteinuria and hematuria to the development of nephrotic syndrome or RPGN. The most common glomerular lesion seen with Henoch-Schönlein purpura is mesangial proliferative glomerulonephritis, with the characteristic finding of moderate to intense diffuse deposits of IgA in the mesangium. Less commonly, it can present as a crescentic glomerulonephritis. Henoch-Schönlein purpura nephritis is an important cause of end-stage kidney (renal) disease (ESRD) in children.[91] In a retrospective, single-center study examining kidney sequelae in adult patients with Henoch-Schönlein purpura and biopsy-proved cutaneous vasculitis, patients with hematuria at disease onset or renal involvement during the course of the disease more commonly developed renal sequelae.[92]

The "seronegative spondyloarthropathies" (ankylosing spondylitis, reactive arthritis)

The spondyloarthropathies, ankylosing spondylitis and reactive arthritis, are infrequently associated with IgA nephropathy.[93] Clinically, this can manifest as microscopic hematuria with or without progressive decline in GFR. Ankylosing spondylitis may also be complicated by the development of secondary amyloidosis.[94] These patients tend to present with nephrotic syndrome, which can progress to ESRD.

Progressive systemic sclerosis (scleroderma)

Scleroderma causes progressive mucoid thickening of the walls and narrowing of the vascular lumen of arteries, which results in severe hypertension and ischemic kidney disease. Diminished kidney blood flow is an early manifestation of scleroderma and appears before the development of hypertension, urinary abnormalities, or renal failure. "Scleroderma renal crisis" is characterized by acute renal failure associated with marked hypertension in the setting of relatively bland urinary sediment. There appears to be a significant association between antecedent high-dose corticosteroid therapy and the development of scleroderma renal crisis.[95] Kidney biopsy demonstrates arterial changes that resemble thrombotic microangiopathy with edematous arteriolar intimal thickening and fibrinoid necrosis. Another classic finding seen on histology is the "onionskin" concentric hypertrophy seen in the interlobular arteries. Because the hypertension is primarily due to ischemic activation of the renin-angiotensin system, ACE inhibitors are the mainstays of treatment.[96] Ten to 15 percent of patients with scleroderma will develop the renal crisis, but a much larger percentage will have some kidney involvement.[97]

Nephrogenic systemic fibrosis

Nephrogenic systemic fibrosis is a relatively newly described disorder that can mimic systemic sclerosis or scleromyxedema.[98] It is only seen in individuals with significant kidney failure and is characterized by thickening and hardening of the skin and marked expansion and fibrosis of the dermis. Originally called nephrogenic fibrosing dermopathy, the name was changed because pathologic findings are not limited to the skin.[99] Although the cause of nephrogenic systemic fibrosis remains unclear, there appears to be a high association with the use of gadolinium, which is used in magnetic resonance imaging (MRI) and MR angiography. It is hypothesized that individuals with marked azotemia cannot eliminate the free gadolinium, which is highly toxic, resulting in tissue damage.[100] Clinically, nephrogenic systemic fibrosis is characterized by skin involvement with or without systemic involvement. The skin manifestations tend to be symmetric, initially affecting bilateral extremities (ankles, lower legs, feet, and hands) with fibrotic indurated plaques or nodules.[99,101] There may be sclerodactyly.[102] However, livedo reticularis is not a feature, unlike in autoimmune sclerosing conditions. The systemic involvement of nephrogenic systemic fibrosis includes muscle induration and joint contractures[103] and fibrosis of lungs,[102] myocardium, pericardium, pleura, and dura mater. Patients with systemic manifestations may have elevated erythrocyte sedimentation rate and C-reactive protein values.[104] Diagnosis of nephrogenic systemic fibrosis is established by histopathologic examination of a punch or incisional biopsy of affected skin, in the correct clinical setting. There are no specific laboratory tests for this disorder. The differential diagnosis includes systemic sclerosis, calciphylaxis, scleromyxedema, and eosinophilic fasciitis. Unfortunately, the course of nephrogenic systemic fibrosis appears to be progressive and unremitting,[104] except in individuals who have recovered kidney function. There is no proven therapy, and current strategies are directed at prevention. Given the link between this disorder and gadolinium, the U.S. Food and Drug Administration (FDA) has made the following recommendations in patients with CKD stage 5[105]: (1) Gadolinium-containing contrast agents should be used only if clearly necessary; (2) gadolinium should be avoided in patients with a diagnosis or clinical suspicion of nephrogenic systemic fibrosis; and (3) prompt initiation of hemodialysis after gadolinium exposure hastens its elimination and may be prudent. The FDA defines individuals at risk as those with acute or chronic kidney disease (estimated GFR < 30 mL/min) or patients with acute kidney injury of any severity due to the hepatorenal syndrome.[105] The risk of nephrogenic systemic fibrosis after gadolinium administration in patients with earlier stages of CKD (i.e., stages 2 and 3) has not been defined.

Amyloidosis

Secondary amyloidosis, due to deposition of amyloid A (AA), tends to occur in concert with inflammatory rheumatologic conditions,[6,95] including rheumatoid arthritis, juvenile idiopathic arthritis, ankylosing spondylitis, psoriatic arthritis, and familial Mediterranean fever. However, it is almost unknown in SLE, in which only a handful of cases have been reported. This probably arises from the fact that in lupus there is no increase in serum AA proteins during inflammatory episodes, which are increased in the other conditions just listed.[106] In familial Mediterranean fever there is evidence that colchicine therapy may prevent the appearance of proteinuria and renal damage.[107]

Clinically, renal amyloidosis presents as nephrotic syndrome and progressive renal failure. On imaging, the kidneys tend to be larger than expected owing to amyloid deposition (see section on kidney imaging). On LM, there is deposition of amyloid fibrils within the mesangial regions, which demonstrate dichroic birefringence under polarized light in tissue stained with Congo red. Amyloid can also infiltrate the tubulointerstitial compartment, leading to renal tubular defects. On EM, amyloid deposits are non-branching, randomly oriented, twisted fibrils that measure 8 to 12 nm in diameter.

Gout

In the majority of cases, monosodium urate crystal deposition disease, better known as gout, results from diminished kidney tubular secretion of uric acid. In addition to intrinsic abnormalities, a number of pharmacologic agents can alter tubular function, resulting in hyperuricemia, such as cyclosporine, diuretics, and low-dose salicylates. Chronic hyperuricemia may involve the kidney in two distinct forms: chronic urate nephropathy and uric acid nephrolithiasis.

Prior to effective anti-hyperuricemic treatment, the prevalence of uric acid nephrolithiasis in patients with gout was about 20%.[108] The stones tend to be radiologically nonopaque and may be passed as gravel or stone. Clinically, gout presents as classic renal colic with paroxysms of waxing and waning severe pain in the flank or groin, typically with hematuria.

Chronic urate nephropathy is secondary to urate deposition in the renal interstitium, which results in a chronic inflammatory reaction and varying degrees of fibrosis (tubulointerstitial disease). Clinically, this can manifest as mild proteinuria, concentrating deficits, and potentially CKD.[109]

As opposed to chronic urate nephropathy, which occurs in patients with gout, acute uric acid nephropathy tends to occur in patients with bulky cancers who undergo tumor lysis syndrome. It is characterized by oliguric ARF due to precipitation of uric acid crystals within the tubules.[110] Classic measures used to prevent tumor lysis syndrome have included the use of allopurinol, alkalinization of the urine, and aggressive volume expansion. Newer medications, such as uricase (Rasburicase), catalyzes uric acid into allantoin,[111] which is more readily excreted by the kidney and thereby may decrease the incidence of tumor lysis syndrome.

The presence of gout in concert with CKD warrants consideration of these potential underlying disorders:

- Familial juvenile hyperuricemia
- Chronic lead intoxication
- Deficiency of hypoxanthine-guanine phosphoribosyltransferase (HPRT)

Familial juvenile hyperuricemia is an autosomal dominant disorder localized to chromosome 16[112] and is characterized by severe underexcretion of filtered urate and renal failure. The renal failure is from tubulointerstitial disease, but this does not appear to be due to urate deposition. Early treatment with allopurinol may improve the kidney prognosis.[113]

Chronic lead intoxication leads to tubulointerstitial damage with resulting impairment of tubular function. This can present clinically as saturnine gout due to decreased urate secretion,[114] renal glucosuria, or aminoaciduria. Continued lead exposure produces progressive tubular atrophy and fibrosis, hypertension, and decline in kidney function. Therefore, occult chronic lead exposure should be suspected when the constellation of hypertension, gout, and CKD is uncovered.

HPRT deficiency is an X-linked disorder. Deficiencies of HPRT lead to an inability to recycle hypoxanthine and guanine and result in overproduction of uric acid. Clinically, its most severe form is known as Lesch-Nyhan syndrome, which is characterized by mental retardation, choreoathetosis, and self-mutilating behavior with signs of gouty arthritis and uric acid stone disease. Less severe forms of HPRT deficiency may present as early-onset gout and sometimes have a positive family history.

Renal lesions with other rheumatic diseases

Individuals who contract acute rheumatic fever rarely develop poststreptococcal glomerulonephritis (PSGN), because the nephritogenic and rheumatogenic strains of β-hemolytic streptococci are different. However, cases of mesangial proliferative glomerulonephritis have been described.[115]

Patients with polymyositis and dermatomyositis sometimes get a persistent mesangial proliferative glomerulonephritis, manifested clinically as non–nephrotic-range proteinuria associated with microscopic hematuria.

A variety of renal abnormalities have been described in patients with psoriatic arthritis that include secondary amyloid and membranous glomerulonephritis.[116]

The common renal manifestations of sarcoidosis include hypercalcemia-associated nephrolithiasis and interstitial nephritis with granuloma formation.[117,118] Infrequently, sarcoidosis can present as an obstructive uropathy secondary to retroperitoneal lymph node involvement.[119] The tubulointerstitial nephritis and uveitis syndrome is relatively uncommon and presents as eye pain associated with renal failure in young women.[120] The differential diagnosis for interstitial nephritis associated with ocular findings should also include a number of rheumatologic disorders: sarcoidosis, ANCA-associated granulomatous vasculitis, SLE, Sjögren's syndrome, and Behçet's disease.

RENAL COMPLICATIONS OF DRUGS USED IN RHEUMATOLOGY

Rheumatologists are well aware of the potential nephrotoxicity of the medications they prescribe. In addition, many over-the-counter (OTC) non-prescription drugs have significant potential for adversely affecting kidney function. It is estimated that on any given day, one in five adults uses an analgesic medication.[121] The use of such drugs is even more prevalent among patients with rheumatologic disorders, and many use them without informing their doctor. Therefore, periodic assessment of kidney function is warranted.

Acetaminophen (paracetamol)

Acetaminophen (paracetamol) is believed to have no significant nephrotoxicity, unlike its parent compound, phenacetin.[122] Phenacetin was removed from the market because of its link to analgesic nephropathy. Acetaminophen overdoses that are associated with acute hepatic failure are often accompanied by ARF.[123] Additionally, occasional cases of ARF are described without obvious hepatic failure[124] or with dosages of acetaminophen that do not appear to be excessive.

Non-steroidal anti-inflammatory drugs

NSAIDs are frequently taken as OTC pain relievers in addition to being prescribed, typically at higher doses than OTC doses. Traditional NSAIDs inhibit both isoforms of the cyclooxygenase (COX) enzyme (COX-1 and COX-2), thereby impairing the production of prostaglandins (PGE_2), prostacyclin (PGI_2), and thromboxanes. The cyclooxygenase inhibitors were developed specifically in an attempt to decrease the gastrointestinal side effects of NSAIDs. By focusing on inhibition of COX-2 to maintain anti-inflammatory efficiency but avoiding inhibition of COX-1, there was also the consideration that these drugs might be more sparing of the kidneys. However, clinical models have demonstrated that COX-2 is likely the key sodium-regulating enzyme within the salt handling parts of the kidney.[125] Consequently, inhibition of COX-2 tends to produce a consistent reduction in the natriuretic effects of endogenous prostaglandins. A meta-analysis examining 19 randomized trials using COX-2 inhibitors demonstrated that they increased systolic blood pressure when compared with placebo (3.85 vs. 1.06 mm Hg, respectively) and traditional NSAIDs (2.83 vs. 1.34 mm Hg, respectively).[126] Additionally, cyclooxygenase inhibitors induce reversible reductions in GFR similar to that seen with traditional NSAIDs.[127-130] As with nonselective NSAIDs, these effects are rarely of clinical significance unless they occur in a patient with compromised kidney function. Rare anatomic inflammatory responses have also been reported with cyclooxygenase inhibitors, which can lead to a significant worsening of kidney function. Based on these data, one can assume that all NSAIDs, whether traditional or COX-2 specific, have a dose-dependent effect on blood pressure, which is likely to be more relevant during the circumstances of a high salt intake. Both cyclooxygenase isoforms are present in the kidney.

Functional effects
Reduction in GFR
The most common renal side effect of NSAIDs is a functional reduction in GFR. In the setting of volume depletion, the renin-angiotensin-aldosterone and sympathetic nervous systems are activated, resulting in neurohumorally mediated systemic vasoconstriction. Prostaglandin E_2 modifies this vasoconstriction in the kidneys and thereby preserves renal perfusion.[131] NSAIDs inhibit the protective prostaglandin-mediated renal vasodilatory effect,[131] compromising GFR. Clinically, this manifests as a clinical spectrum of mild azotemia

to frank oliguric ARF.[132] Typically, the azotemia is reversible once the NSAID is discontinued. Unfortunately, the functional azotemia may progress to acute tubular necrosis, which may take weeks to resolve, or, on rare occasions, can result in permanent kidney failure.[133] The risk of ARF due to NSAIDs is dose dependent and is most often manifest within the first few weeks.[134]

The major risk for developing functional azotemia with NSAID use is preexisting kidney disease or when used in combination with other nephrotoxic agents. Additionally, NSAIDs are relatively contraindicated in settings of preexisting renal hypoperfusion that occur with effective intravascular volume depletion, either absolute or relative, such as nephrotic syndrome, congestive heart failure, cirrhosis, and protein-wasting enteropathies. Finally, because of progressive CKD with aging, one should use NSAIDs judiciously in the elderly. Renal function should be monitored closely in high-risk patients treated with NSAIDs.

Hyperkalemia
Under normal conditions, PGI_2 stimulates renin-angiotensin-aldosterone secretion. Inhibition of PGI_2 may result in severe hyperkalemia, especially in patients with underlying CKD.

Peripheral edema
Inhibition of PGE_2 results in increased sodium reabsorption, which manifests as edema.[135] Edema typically occurs within the first week of therapy and is associated with a 1- to 2-kg weight gain.[136]

Interstitial nephritis and nephrotic syndrome
Less frequent than their functional effects, NSAIDs can produce overt histologic lesions of the kidneys, specifically allergic interstitial nephritis, minimal change disease,[137] and probably membranous nephropathy.[138]

Allergic interstitial nephritis
Allergic interstitial nephritis occurs as an idiosyncratic reaction to NSAIDs and was commonly associated with fenoprofen use. Clinically, patients present with ARF associated with mild proteinuria, usually less than 1 g/day.[139] Rash, eosinophilia, and other systemic features are usually absent.[133]

Nephrotic syndrome
NSAID-induced minimal change disease typically presents as anasarca and nephrotic-range proteinuria associated with a tubulointerstitial nephritis.[140] Membranous nephritis also presents as massive proteinuria.[138] A kidney biopsy is needed to distinguish between these two histologic lesions because both present as nephrotic syndrome.

Analgesic nephropathy and papillary necrosis
Analgesic nephropathy is characterized by renal papillary necrosis and chronic interstitial nephritis caused by prolonged and excessive consumption of combination analgesics,[141] typically containing phenacetin. Analgesic nephropathy is characterized by patchy interstitial ischemia and fibrosis in the renal medulla.

Chronic use of NSAIDs is generally safe.[133] However, daily NSAID use for more than one year may be associated with an increased risk of CKD, perhaps due to papillary necrosis.[142]

In settings of ARF, NSAID therapy should be discontinued immediately. Hemodynamically mediated alterations typically improve relatively quickly, but NSAID-related glomerulopathy and CKD may persist after discontinuation of the offending agent.

Calcineurin inhibitors: cyclosporine and tacrolimus
Acute renal failure
Cyclosporine, which is approved as a treatment for rheumatoid arthritis, is associated with both acute and chronic renal toxicity.[143] The other major calcineurin inhibitor, tacrolimus (FK506), has the same nephrotoxicity potential as cyclosporine.[144] Both agents cause a dose-dependent renal afferent artery vasoconstriction with subsequent acute decreases in GFR.[145,146]

Hypertension

In addition to hemodynamically mediated ARF, both calcineurin inhibitors can induce hypertension through a variety of mechanisms: acting as powerful vasoconstrictors of preglomerular vasculature, inducing sodium retention and volume expansion,[147] activating the sympathetic nervous system,[148] stimulating vasoconstrictor prostaglandin production,[149] upregulating intrarenal renin biosynthesis,[150] stimulating endothelin,[151] activating cytosol calcium after binding calmodulin,[152] and enhancing vascular responsiveness to vasopressin and angiotensin.[153,154]

Chronic kidney disease

The long-term nephrotoxicity of calcineurin inhibitors appears to be both time and dose dependent, results from interstitial fibrosis, and tends to be irreversible. Although studied primarily in transplant recipients, this chronic nephrotoxicity is also well documented in non-transplant cases, including patients with rheumatoid arthritis.[144]

Hemolytic-uremic syndrome

Although an infrequent complication, both calcineurin inhibitors have been implicated as causing hemolytic-uremic syndrome or a microangiopathic syndrome.

Hyperuricemia

Cyclosporine causes hyperuricemia and may lead to gout in both individuals with and without an organ transplant.[155,156] Afferent artery constriction from cyclosporine results in increased proximal tubular uric acid absorption and hyperuremia.[157] Calcium channel blockers such as amlodipine significantly reduce the hyperuricemia associated with cyclosporine usage.[157] Additionally, use of traditional drugs such as uricosuric agents or allopurinol may be beneficial.

RHEUMATOLOGIC COMPLICATIONS OF KIDNEY DISEASE

As a rule, most disorders of the soft tissues, joints, and bones that are referable to kidney disease occur in the setting of a diminished GFR, that is, with chronic kidney disease or in the post–kidney transplant setting. The cause of most can be traced to the biochemical imbalances classically associated with kidney failure. These include disturbances in calcium and phosphorus homeostasis due to alterations in the vitamin D and parathyroid hormone (PTH) axes and the retention of uremic toxins, such as β_2-microglobulin. An exception to this rule is the syndrome of hereditary hypophosphatemic rickets, in which GFR is normal but there is excessive renal tubular wasting of phosphorus.

Rheumatologic complications in patients with ESRD are very common, with more than 70% of patients having joint pain.[158] Additionally, there is a temporal relationship between the length of kidney disease and the prevalence of rheumatologic conditions.

Etiologic factors specific to kidney failure

β_2-microglobulin amyloidosis

β_2-microglobulin is an 11.8-kDa protein that is a component of the major histocompatibility complex (MHC) type 1 antigen. It is normally filtered by the glomerulus and reabsorbed and catabolized by renal tubular cells. In ESRD, production exceeds excretion, which can result in a 60-fold increase in plasma β_2-microglobulin concentration. The β_2-microglobulin protein then appears to be modified by 3-deoxyglucose to form a glycosylated protein, which resists further catabolism and is found in amyloid deposits.[159]

β_2-microglobulin has a high affinity for collagen, which may explain its predilection for deposition in bones, joints, and synovium.[160] An autopsy study demonstrated a direct correlation of amyloid deposition with the number of years on dialysis (21%, 33%, 50%, 90%, and 100% with dialysis durations of less than 2, 2 to 4, 4 to 7, 7 to 13, and more than 13 years, respectively).[161]

Clearance of plasma β_2-microglobulin in patients on hemodialysis has increased with the use of dialysis membranes that have increased hydraulic conductivity (i.e., more porous than older, cellulosic membranes). Additionally, these membranes tend to be more biocompatible and may lead to less stimulation of β_2-microglobulin production.

As a result, patients dialyzed with high-flux membranes develop evidence of amyloid much less frequently than those using low-flux membranes.[162,163]

Calcium, phosphorus, and parathyroid hormone derangements

As GFR declines, the filtered load of phosphate decreases, leading to a positive phosphate balance. This can be seen in as early as stage 2 CKD (see Table 37.3). Phosphate retention increases as GFR declines. Prolonged hyperphosphatemia can lead to soft tissue and vascular calcifications, related to an increase in the calcium-phosphate product.[164,165] An elevated calcium-phosphorus product is associated with increased morbidity and mortality.[166]

In addition to hyperphosphatemia, patients with CKD often suffer from hypocalcemia. The etiology of the hypocalcemia is multifactorial and is related to decreased production of 1,25-dihydroxyvitamin D as well as to diffuse deposition of calcium (see later) due to increased calcium-phosphate product. The combination of hypocalcemia, reduced 1,25-dihydroxyvitamin D synthesis, and hyperphosphatemia results in parathyroid gland proliferation with subsequent secondary hyperparathyroidism.[167,168]

Strategies aimed at reducing hyperphosphatemia may ameliorate the development of secondary hyperparathyroidism. To this effect, current K/DOQI guidelines recommend with stages 3 and 4 CKD that the serum phosphorus concentration should be maintained between 2.7 and 4.6 mg/dL, primarily through dietary phosphorus restriction between 800 to 1000 mg/day.[38] However, dietary phosphorus restrictions are often not sufficient and oral phosphate binders are needed. In the past, aluminum-based phosphate binders were commonly used, but this led to significant toxicity, including aluminum bone disease. Now, the most commonly used phosphate binders are calcium-based phosphate binders (calcium acetate and calcium carbonate) and phosphate-binding resin (sevelamer).

Oxalate deposition

Urinary excretion of oxalate is markedly impaired once the GFR is reduced below 20 mL/min (stage 4 CKD).[169] Secondary oxalosis, due to CKD, shares many features with primary genetic from of hyperoxaluria, with increased vascular and osteoarticular calcification due to deposition of the poorly soluble calcium-oxalate complex. Avoiding carrots, spinach, cocoa, peanut butter, nuts, chocolate, megadose vitamin C, and tea will reduce dietary oxalate.[170] Use of oral phosphate binders also will bind to oxalate and decrease its serum level.

Clinical features of β_2-microglobulin amyloid

Carpal tunnel syndrome in dialyzed patients

A frequent feature of β_2-microglobulin deposition in patients with CKD and ESRD is carpal tunnel syndrome.[163] After 9 years on hemodialysis, more than 30% of patients appear to be affected.[171] The symptoms are indistinguishable from carpal tunnel symptoms from other causes, and the intensity tends to be quite severe. Only transient relief is gained from local injections or by use of splints; surgical decompression appears to be the only effective treatment. Transient carpal tunnel syndrome sometimes occurs after creation of an upper extremity arteriovenous anastomosis dialysis access, owing to altered venous and lymphatic return.

Spondyloarthropathy due to β_2-microglobulin amyloid

A destructive cervical spondyloarthropathy develops in patients with ESRD. The findings correlate strongly with the presence of β_2-microglobulin deposits,[172] which can be demonstrated in the intervertebral discs and paravertebral ligaments and sometimes within the vertebral bodies and around the odontoid process. Ten to 20 percent of dialysis patients have β_2-microglobulin deposits in the cervical spine; thoracic and lumbar spinal involvement is also described.[172] Neck pain is the first feature, but radiculopathy is also seen. MRI demonstrates narrowed disc spaces and other typical findings that differentiate β_2-microglobulin amyloid deposits from osteomyelitis.

Bone cysts and fractures due to β_2-microglobulin amyloid

Bone lesions that arise from β_2-microglobulin deposition are typically cystic and occur at the ends of long bones, to include the humerus, femur, tibia, and carpals. The cysts contain amyloid and tend to enlarge with time, predisposing to pathologic fractures. They may be confused with "brown tumors" of secondary hyperparathyroidism.

Other joint and soft tissue manifestations of β₂-microglobulin amyloid

Shoulder pain afflicts a significant percentage of patients on long-term maintenance hemodialysis. Periarticular deposits of β₂-microglobulin may lead to adhesions to the joint capsule, with joint tenderness and loss of mobility. Similarly, adhesions due to β₂-microglobulin deposition in the flexor tendons of the hand can cause contractures and thickening. Joint effusions are common with periarticular deposition of β₂-microglobulin, especially in the shoulders and knees. On aspiration, these effusive arthropathies tend to be non-inflammatory. Under polarizing microscopy, fibrils of β₂-microglobulin may be seen in the joint fluid. Examination of the joint aspirate may therefore help distinguish shoulder pain due to β₂-microglobulin from calcium hydroxyapatite crystal arthropathy (see later).

Crystal arthropathies

Gout

With CKD, gout is paradoxically uncommon, in part because the fractional excretion of urate rises steadily as GFR falls.[173] Nevertheless, hyperuricemia is the rule in advanced CKD, suggesting that the uremic milieu suppresses the acute inflammatory response to urate crystals.[174] The acute gout attack in patients with CKD should be treated with either intra-articular or systemic corticosteroids, depending on the number of joints involved. Colchicine is relatively contraindicated in patients with the later stages of CKD. Additionally, the use of NSAIDs may precipitate either hemodynamically mediated or tubulointerstitial ARF and should therefore be avoided in patients with CKD.

The long-term management of chronic gout with allopurinol requires dose adjustment for the diminished GFR in patients with CKD.[175] Allopurinol hypersensitivity syndrome also appears to be more likely in patients with CKD.[176] The uricosuric agents sulfinpyrazone and probenecid are ineffective when the GFR is less than 30 mL/min, but benzbromarone may still be effective.[177]

Calcium pyrophosphate dihydrate (CPPD) deposition disease

In patients with CKD, calcium pyrophosphate dihydrate (CPPD) deposition disease is more common than gout. Chondrocalcinosis, defined as articular cartilage calcification, is often present and may be associated with the second hyperparathyroidism of renal failure. Pseudogout, characterized by self-limited acute arthritis attacks, primarily involves the knee joint and other joints of the extremities.[178] As with gout, treatment of the acute arthritis is best accomplished with intra-articular injections; NSAIDs are relatively contraindicated. Management of chronic pseudogout is not well established but should include strategies to improve associated secondary hyperparathyroidism (see later).

Hydroxyapatite arthropathy

Acute episodes of joint pain, particularly in the shoulders, can punctuate the more chronic course of periarthropathy due to calcium hydroxyapatite deposits. Seen in patients with ESRD, this strongly correlates with prolonged hyperphosphatemia and an elevated calcium-phosphorus product. Crystals are usually absent on synovial fluid examination. Periarticular deposits may become large complex masses, called tumoral calcinosis.

The aims of therapy are threefold: (1) reduction of acute inflammation with intra-articular injections and cautious use of anti-inflammatory drugs, (2) joint rest, and (3) reduction in calcium-phosphorus product by increasing phosphate binders and stopping vitamin D analog administration.

Oxalate arthropathy

Arthritis associated with articular and periarticular deposits of calcium oxalate occurs secondary to CKD.[179,180] Oxalate crystals are deposited in renal parenchyma, skin, bone, and blood vessels and in and around joints. There they cause chondrocalcinosis, synovial calcification, and chronic or acute arthropathy.

Clinical features of renal bone disease

Renal osteodystrophy

Renal osteodystrophy is a term used to describe the skeletal complications of ESRD due to a complex amalgam of various pathologic processes. The four principal types are osteitis fibrosa (formally known as osteitis fibrosa cystica), osteomalacia, adynamic bone disease, and mixed disease. Mixed osteodystrophy is an amalgam of osteitis fibrosa and osteomalacia (see later).

The classic histologic form of renal osteodystrophy is osteitis fibrosa, a lesion directly attributable to the secondary hyperparathyroidism seen with CKD. The hallmark lesion is peritrabecular fibrosis in the setting of accelerated bone resorption and formation. Clinically, this can present as bone tenderness and proximal muscle weakness.[177] Radiographic findings include subperiosteal bone resorption, best observed in the middle phalanges, and osteosclerosis.

Osteomalacia, as opposed to osteitis fibrosa, is characterized by a reduced rate of bone turnover associated with increased osteoid volume and defective mineralization. Because osteomalacia is associated with aluminum intoxication, it incidence is decreasing.[180] Clinically, osteomalacia tends to present as more severe bony pain than that with osteitis fibrosa and is also associated with pathologic fractures.[181] In addition to bone symptoms, aluminum toxicity may manifest as microcytic anemia resistant to iron therapy[182] and as acute or chronic (encephalopathy) neurotoxicity.[183] Osteomalacia tends to have minimal radiographic findings but may be associated with pseudofractures, which are radiolucent bands that run perpendicular to the long axis of bones.[181]

Adynamic bone disease, also known as aplastic bone disease, is now the most common type of renal osteodystrophy.[184] The pathogenesis of this condition is poorly understood, but a key factor appears to be excessive suppression of PTH. Bone turnover is markedly decreased, but unlike osteomalacia there is no increase in osteoid formation. Clinically, adynamic bone disease may be asymptomatic[185] or manifest as hypercalcemia or increased risk for hip fractures.[186,187]

Management is based on the type of renal osteodystrophy. Although tests of PTH and serum aluminum levels may be suggestive of the underlying pathologic process, the diagnostic gold standard is dual-labeled bone biopsy. General management should include normalization of serum phosphorus levels; correction of acidemia; avoidance of prolonged use of aluminum-containing phosphate binders, including sucralfate; and control of hyperparathyroidism with judicious use of vitamin D analogs. Despite effective therapy, intractable hyperparathyroidism may require parathyroidectomy.

"Brown tumors"

Severe hyperparathyroidism may lead to the development of osteoclastomas, also known as "brown tumors." They typically occur at the medial end of the clavicle but can occur anywhere in the calvaria, long bones, sternum, or spine.[188]

Calcification of soft tissues and vessels

Soft tissue calcification

Ectopic deposition of calcium, also known as metastatic calcification, is common in patients with CKD and ESRD. The crucial factors include secondary hyperparathyroidism and a high calcium-phosphate product. Calcification may occur in a variety of soft tissues, to include skin, where it manifests as diffuse pruritus; around joints; within the lungs, where calcium is found in the alveolar capillary basement membrane; and in the heart. Of major concern is when calcifications occur within blood vessels. In patients with CKD, the presence and extent of arterial calcifications are independently predictive of subsequent cardiovascular disease (CVD).[189] Coronary artery calcification is much more common in patients on hemodialysis when compared with age- and gender-matched controls,[190] with CVD accounting for approximately half of the deaths.[191]

Calciphylaxis

Calciphylaxis is a poorly understood syndrome characterized by ischemic necrosis of skin and muscle associated with extensive vascular calcifications.[192] Its presentation may be similar to that seen with warfarin-induced skin necrosis.[193] It is associated with hyperparathyroidism and CKD, either dialysis or non-dialysis dependent. The incidence appears to be increasing[194] associated with the increased use of vitamin D analogs. The diagnosis of calciphylaxis is one of exclusion and is suggested by the characteristic ischemic skin lesions in association with biopsy demonstrating arterial calcification and occlusion without vasculitic changes. The ischemia may first manifest as livedo reticularis in the legs or arm. Often there are nodular areas of painful subcutaneous fat necrosis. Extension of this process leads to necrosis of large areas of skin and subcutaneous tissue. Lesions may be prominent on the abdominal wall, thighs, and buttocks.[195] The primary cause of mortality from calciphylaxis syndrome is from severe secondary infections. Treatment is directed toward both the ischemic wounds as well as the underlying cause. Wound care should include appropriate débridement, antibiotic therapy, and pain management. In addition, therapy should be directed at correction of calcium and phosphorus concentrations and discontinuation of vitamin D analogs. The role for urgent parathyroidectomy is poorly defined.[196]

Other arthropathies in dialysis patients

Typical erosive osteoarthritis, mainly of the interphalangeal joints, is common in individuals on dialysis. The clinical and radiologic presentations are indistinguishable from those of individuals without CKD. As in the general population, there is a female predominance and an increased incidence with age. However, erosive osteoarthritis appears to be more common in patients with ESRD.[197] This increased incidence may be related to a higher incidence of hyperparathyroidism and/or iron overload.[198]

Because uremia leads to a bleeding diathesis, patients may bleed into a large joint, resulting in hemarthrosis. An additional risk of bleeding is incurred from the use of anticoagulation during hemodialysis. In some patients, bleeding appears to be associated with β_2-microglobulin deposition of periarticular structures. The incidence of osteonecrosis appears to be increased in patients with ESRD[199] as well as after kidney transplant.[200]

Tendonitis is common in patients on hemodialysis; hyperparathyroidism appears to be the predisposing factor. Tendon rupture is common, principally of the quadriceps tendon but also of the patellar, Achilles, triceps, or finger extensor tendons.[201]

The differential diagnosis of generalized muscle weakness in a patient on dialysis is extensive and includes life-threatening processes such as severe hyperkalemia, severe hypophosphatemia, and bacteremia. More chronic or progressive weakness, if not neuropathic in origin, suggests a possible myopathy[202] that may be due to vitamin D deficiency, possible aluminum toxicity (see earlier), progressive malnourishment, or hyperparathyroidism.

Lupus tends to become more quiescent with the development of ESRD, although symptoms may continue.[203] Additionally, patients with rheumatoid arthritis may continue to have arthritis while on hemodialysis. Individuals on dialysis who have previously received extended courses of corticosteroids for lupus or similar rheumatic conditions are at particular risk for hip osteonecrosis.

Arthropathies in renal transplant patients

Gout

Gout is just one of several arthropathies that are prevalent in kidney transplant recipients.[204] The incidence of gout is increased in individuals who have received a kidney transplant treated with cyclosporine.[205] It appears that use of cyclosporine results in renal vasoconstriction and subsequent decreased capacity to excrete uric acid.[206] The addition of diuretic therapy can lead to intravascular volume contraction and further increases in serum uric acid concentrations. Although tacrolimus has similar immunosuppressive effects as cyclosporine, the incidence of gout appears to be less in patients treated with tacrolimus.

Osteopenia after transplantation

Before kidney transplantation, patients with CKD often have low bone mineral density owing to renal osteodystrophy. After renal transplantation there is a rapid decline in bone mineral density.[207] This rapid decline is due primarily to the use of glucocorticoids[205] and persistent hyperparathyroidism. Clinically, there is an increased incidence of fractures within the first 6 months after transplantation.[208] There is some evidence that bone loss may be prevented by the use of corticosteroid-free or ultra-low-dose corticosteroid regimens.[209] Additionally, use of calcium, vitamin D, and bisphosphonates should be considered in all recipients of kidney transplants.

KEY REFERENCES

1. Crew RJ, Radhakrishnan J, Appel G. Complications of the nephrotic syndrome and their treatment. Clin Nephrol 2004;62:245-259.
4. Haas M, Meehan SM, Karrison TG, Spargo BH. Changing etiologies of unexplained adult nephrotic syndrome: a comparison of renal biopsy findings from 1976-1979 and 1995-1997. Am J Kidney Dis 1997;30:621-631.
8. Safian RD, Textor SC. Renal-artery stenosis. N Engl J Med 2001;344:431-442.
16. D'Amico G, Bazzi C. Pathophysiology of proteinuria. Kidney Int 2003;63:809-825.
31. Kohler H, Wandel E, Brunck B. Acanthocyturia—a characteristic marker for glomerular bleeding. Kidney Int 1991;40:115-120.
42. Levey AS, Coresh J, Balk E, National Kidney Foundation, et al. National Kidney Foundation practice guidelines for chronic kidney disease: evaluation, classification, and stratification. Ann Intern Med 2003;139:137-147.
49. Hebert LA, Cosio FG, Neff JC. Diagnostic significance of hypocomplementemia. Kidney Int 1991;39:811-821.
58. Jennette JC, Falk RJ. The pathology of vasculitis involving the kidney. Am J Kidney Dis 1994;24:130-141.
66. Weening JJ, D'Agati VD, Schwartz MM, et al. The classification of glomerulonephritis in systemic lupus erythematosus revisited. Kidney Int 2004;65:521-530.
67. Najafi CC, Korbet SM, Lewis EJ, et al. Significance of histologic patterns of glomerular injury upon long-term prognosis in severe lupus glomerulonephritis. Kidney Int 2001;59:2156-2163.
68. Cervera R, Khamashta MA, Font J, et al. Systemic lupus erythematosus: clinical and immunologic patterns of disease expression in a cohort of 1,000 patients. The European Working Party on Systemic Lupus Erythematosus. Medicine (Baltimore) 1993;72:113-124.
69. Descombes E, Droz D, Drouet L, et al. Renal vascular lesions in lupus nephritis. Medicine (Baltimore) 1997;76:355-368.

74. Helin HJ, Korpela MM, Mustonen JT, Pasternack AI. Renal biopsy findings and clinicopathologic correlations in rheumatoid arthritis. Arthritis Rheum 1995;38:242-247.
77. Qarni MU, Kohan DE. Pauci-immune necrotizing glomerulonephritis complicating rheumatoid arthritis. Clin Nephrol 2000;54:54-58.
79. Bossini N, Savoldi S, Franceschini F, et al. Clinical and morphological features of kidney involvement in primary Sjögren's syndrome. Nephrol Dial Transplant 2001;16:2328-2336.
82. Akpolat T, Akkoyunlu M, Akpolat I, et al. Renal Behçet's disease: a cumulative analysis. Semin Arthritis Rheum 2002;31:317-337.
84. Hoffman GS, Kerr GS, Leavitt RY, et al. Wegener granulomatosis: an analysis of 158 patients. Ann Intern Med 1992;116:488-498.
93. Garcia-Porrua C, Gonzalez-Louzao C, Llorca J, Gonzalez-Gay MA. Predictive factors for renal sequelae in adults with Henoch-Schönlein purpura. J Rheumatol 2001;28:1019-1024.
94. Lance NJ, Curran JJ. Amyloidosis in a case of ankylosing spondylitis with a review of the literature. J Rheumatol 1991;18:100-103.
95. Steen VD, Medsger TA Jr. Case-control study of corticosteroids and other drugs that either precipitate or protect from the development of scleroderma renal crisis. Arthritis Rheum 1998;41:1613-1619.
97. Traub YM, Shapiro AP, Rodnan GP, et al. Hypertension and renal failure (scleroderma renal crisis) in progressive systemic sclerosis: review of a 25-year experience with 68 cases. Medicine (Baltimore) 1983;62:335-352.
100. Deo A, Fogel M, Cowper SE. Nephrogenic systemic fibrosis: A population study examining the relationship of disease development to gadolinium exposure. Clin J Am Soc Nephrol 2007; 2:264.

104. Mendoza FA, Artlett CM, Sandorfi N, et al. Description of 12 cases of nephrogenic fibrosing dermopathy and review of the literature. Semin Arthritis Rheum 2006;35:238.
109. Johnson RJ, Kivlighn SD, Kim YG, et al. Reappraisal of the pathogenesis and consequences of hyperuricemia in hypertension, cardiovascular disease, and renal disease. Am J Kidney Dis 1999;33:225-234.
110. Arrambide K, Toto RD. Tumor lysis syndrome. Semin Nephrol 1993;13:273-280.
116. Alenius GM, Stegmayr BG, Dahlqvist SR. Renal abnormalities in a population of patients with psoriatic arthritis. Scand J Rheumatol 2001;30:271-274.
118. Muther RS, McCarron DA, Bennett WM. Renal manifestations of sarcoidosis. Arch Intern Med 1981;141:643-645.
122. Henrich WL, Agodoa LE, Barrett B, et al. Analgesics and the kidney: summary and recommendations to the Scientific Advisory Board of the National Kidney Foundation from an Ad Hoc Committee of the National Kidney Foundation. Am J Kidney Dis 1996;27:162-165.
123. Blakely P, McDonald BR. Acute renal failure due to acetaminophen ingestion: a case report and review of the literature. J Am Soc Nephrol 1995;6:48-53.
125. Catella-Lawson F, Reilly MP, Kapoor SC, et al. Cyclooxygenase inhibitors and the antiplatelet effects of aspirin. N Engl J Med 2001;345:1809-1817.
133. Bennett WM, Henrich WL, Stoff JS. The renal effects of nonsteroidal anti-inflammatory drugs: summary and recommendations. Am J Kidney Dis 1996;28: S56-S62.
136. Harris RC Jr. Cyclooxygenase-2 inhibition and renal physiology. Am J Cardiol 2002;89:10D-17D.
138. Radford MG Jr, Holley KE, Grande JP, et al. Reversible membranous nephropathy associated with the use of nonsteroidal anti-inflammatory drugs. JAMA 1996;276:466-469.

139. Neilson EG. Pathogenesis and therapy of interstitial nephritis. Kidney Int 1989;35:1257-1270.

143. de Mattos AM, Olyaei AJ, Bennett WM. Nephrotoxicity of immunosuppressive drugs: long-term consequences and challenges for the future. Am J Kidney Dis 2000;35:333-346.

151. Kon V, Sugiura M, Inagami T, et al. Role of endothelin in cyclosporine-induced glomerular dysfunction. Kidney Int 1990;37:1487-1491.

152. Kopp JB, Klotman PE. Cellular and molecular mechanisms of cyclosporin nephrotoxicity. J Am Soc Nephrol 1990;1:162-179.

156. Clive DM. Renal transplant-associated hyperuricemia and gout. J Am Soc Nephrol 2000;11:974-979.

159. Miyata T, Inagi R, Iida Y, et al. Involvement of beta 2-microglobulin modified with advanced glycation end products in the pathogenesis of hemodialysis-associated amyloidosis: induction of human monocyte chemotaxis and macrophage secretion of tumor necrosis factor-alpha and interleukin-1. J Clin Invest 1994;93:521-528.

162. Jadoul M, Garbar C, Noel H, et al. Histological prevalence of beta 2-microglobulin amyloidosis in hemodialysis: a prospective post-mortem study. Kidney Int 1997;51:1928-1932.

165. Mazhar AR, Johnson RJ, Gillen D, et al. Risk factors and mortality associated with calciphylaxis in end-stage renal disease. Kidney Int 2001;60:324-332.

177. Perez-Ruiz F, Calabozo M, Fernandez-Lopez MJ, et al. Treatment of chronic gout in patients with renal function impairment. J Clin Rheumatol 1999;5:49-55.

184. K/DOQI clinical practice guidelines for bone metabolism and disease in chronic kidney disease. Am J Kidney Dis 2003;42:S1-S201.

187. Sherrard DJ, Hercz G, Pei Y, et al. The spectrum of bone disease in end-stage renal failure—an evolving disorder. Kidney Int 1993;43:436-442.

194. Fine A, Zacharias J. Calciphylaxis is usually non-ulcerating: risk factors, outcome and therapy. Kidney Int 2002;61:2210-2217.

196. Roe SM, Graham LD, Brock WB, Barker DE. Calciphylaxis: early recognition and management. Am Surg 1994;60:81-86.

198. Duncan IJ, Hurst NP, Disney A, et al. Is chronic renal failure a risk factor for the development of erosive osteoarthritis? Ann Rheum Dis 1989;48:183-187.

REFERENCES

Full references for this chapter can be found on www.expertconsult.com.

3

EVALUATION: IMAGING TECHNIQUES

Conventional radiography and computed tomography

38

Stacy E. Smith

- Conventional radiography has a major role in, and remains the mainstay of, initial evaluation and follow-up of rheumatologic disease.

- Although the majority of joints may be adequately assessed using orthogonal radiographic plain film views, specialized views may be required for some joints (e.g., Norgaard views for the hand and a modified AP Ferguson view for the sacrum).

- Multidetector CT (MDCT) provides excellent contrast and delineation of cortical and trabecular bone and is established as a superb diagnostic tool for visualization of subtle cortical or intraosseous lesions not visible on standard radiography due to projectional superimposition.

- CT-guided facet, joint, or bursal injections or aspirations are often utilized in the diagnosis and treatment of rheumatologic disease.

- CT angiography is useful for diagnosis and evaluation of the large vessel vasculitides, particularly giant cell arteritis and Takayasu arteritis, with some studies stating utility in monitoring treatment response.

CONVENTIONAL RADIOGRAPHY

Conventional radiography is the most common and least expensive modality for imaging and evaluating patients with rheumatologic disorders. In particular, it is the mainstay of initial evaluation of the hands, wrists, feet, and sacroiliac (SI) joints.

Uses

The radiographic assessment of bones and joints includes evaluation of all the following criteria: presence/absence of bone loss or bone production, joint space narrowing (an indirect sign of articular cartilage thinning) or widening, presence/absence of calcification—chondrocalcinosis, ankylosis, subluxation, dislocation, changes in bone mineral density, and, finally, gross soft tissue abnormalities (Fig. 38.1). Interpretation of the radiographs requires a sound knowledge of radiographic anatomy, the patient's clinical presentation, symptoms, and laboratory information, as well as disease pathology to provide the most correct diagnosis and/or differential diagnosis. The comparison of bilateral joints can further enhance the detection of subtle abnormalities, allowing for assessment of bilateral involvement and symmetry (Fig. 38.2). Serial radiographs can be utilized for staging, monitoring, and assessing treatment efficacy. Validated scoring methods of radiologic damage in joints have been developed by several authors and used extensively in clinical trials, particularly with respect to osteoarthritis and rheumatoid arthritis (see Chapter 43).[1,2]

Limitations of conventional radiography do exist, however, including a wide variation in image quality, an inability to evaluate the very early stages of inflammatory disease in bone and soft tissue (i.e., synovitis), and the projectional superimposition of structures due to the two-dimensional (2D) representation of three-dimensional (3D) structures in a single plane. Wide variations in image quality (differences in film projection and penetration) make it vital to have proper film exposure and accurate positioning of serial radiographs to obtain accurate results and to provide a true comparison with prior studies.

The inability to evaluate the very early stages of inflammatory disease (early erosions, articular cartilage abnormalities, and synovitis) is due to the insensitivity of radiographs to both the trabecular bone loss and the intramedullary component of early bone erosions as well as its lack of soft tissue detail. Magnetic resonance imaging (MRI) and ultrasonography have both been reported to be more sensitive than conventional radiography with respect to these early changes, particularly articular cartilage abnormalities and early erosions.[3] Radiographs have been found to be more suitable for detecting cortical bone loss, which is a later phenomenon. As a result, radiographs have proven useful as the mainstay for confirming established disease and for following the known disease process, with MRI being more sensitive in predicting non-progressors of disease in clinical trials and in detecting those predisposed to disease (early soft tissue changes).[4]

Projection views

The projectional nature of radiography can lead to superimposition of overlapping structures. In rheumatoid arthritis this can obscure *en face* erosions. It is for this reason that articular disorders and disorders affecting the axial skeleton should be evaluated in at least two orthogonal planes (sometimes three, depending on the specific joint or anatomy) to increase the diagnostic sensitivity and fully evaluate the extent of the disease process. The majority of patients therefore are imaged with two orthogonal views: a routine anteroposterior (AP) or posteroanterior (PA) view and an accompanying 90-degree lateral view (Fig. 38.3). Specialized views and techniques have also been developed that have been invaluable in allowing assessment of specific disease processes for certain joints. Such specialized views include the Norgaard view for the hand and wrist (see Fig. 38.3) and the modified AP Ferguson view for the SI joints (Fig. 38.4). Suggested routine radiographic techniques as well as some of the more specialized techniques and projections are listed in Box 38.1.[5]

Hand and wrist

Although the PA view of the hand and wrist is the best conventional view for assessment of malalignment, joint space narrowing, soft tissue abnormalities, and mineralization, it is limited with regard to the assessment of erosive changes. The Norgaard view (sometimes referred to as the "ball catcher's" view) (see Fig. 38.3) is an AP oblique view of the hand and wrist that profiles both the radial aspect of the base of the proximal phalanges in the hand and the triquetral pisiform joint, two areas where the earliest erosive changes of any inflammatory arthropathy occur. Because the fingers are not rigidly positioned by the radiographer in this view, the reducible subluxations of inflammatory arthropathies and systemic lupus arthropathy may also be easily seen.

Sacroiliac joints

The modified AP Ferguson view (see Fig. 38.4) allows the best visualization of the anteroinferior most portion of the SI joints. This is important histologically because the lower half to two thirds of the SI joint is a true synovial joint and is the area most frequently affected by rheumatologic disorders. To obtain the Ferguson view, the patient is placed supine with knees and hips flexed. The x-ray tube is centered at L5/S1 and angled 25 to 30 degrees toward the head to best profile the SI joint. It is essentially a centrally coned-down modification of a pelvic outlet view directed perpendicular to the sacral inclination to allow *en face* visualization of the entire sacrum.

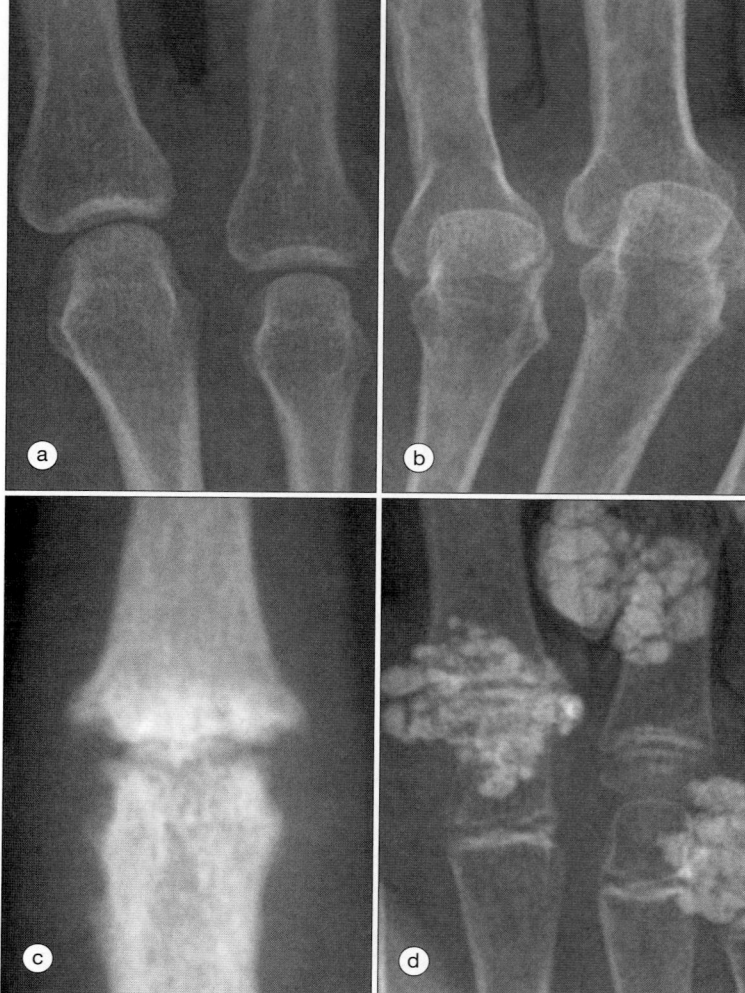

Fig. 38.1 Radiographic assessment criteria. (a) AP view of the metacarpophalangeal (MCP) joints in a disease/trauma-free patient depicts normal joint spaces, soft tissues, and cortical/intramedullary integrity. (b) AP view of the MCP joints with narrowing and subluxation of the joints, periarticular osteopenia, and subtle marginal cortical erosions in a patient with rheumatoid arthritis. Lupus can present as similar subluxation but without cortical erosion. (c) AP view of an MCP joint with soft tissue swelling, cortical erosions, and destruction of both sides of the joint in a patient with chronic joint infection. (d) AP view of the MCP joints with osteopenia and multiple soft tissue calcifications about the joints in a pediatric patient with rheumatoid factor–positive mixed connective tissue disease.

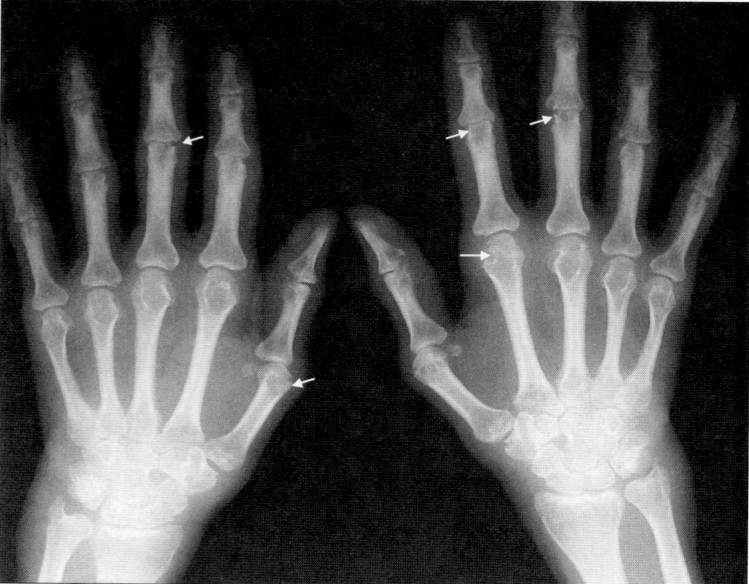

Fig. 38.2 Rheumatoid arthritis. Bilateral PA hand radiographs demonstrate multiple erosions involving predominantly the proximal interphalangeal and metacarpophalangeal joints. Assessment of bilateral involvement and symmetry is helpful in narrowing the differential diagnosis.

BOX 38.1 STANDARD AND SPECIALIZED RADIOGRAPHIC PROJECTIONS
Adequate radiographic evaluation requires at least two orthogonal projections.

Standard radiographs
Finger:
■ PA projection
■ Lateral projection
Hand:
■ PA projection
■ Oblique projection (45-degree semi-pronated or semi-supinated)
■ Lateral projection
  Magnification views are more sensitive for evaluating erosive disease, if available.
Wrist:
■ PA projection (arm abducted 90 degrees from trunk and forearm flexed at 90 degrees to the arm)
■ Oblique projections
■ AP oblique view (Norgaard or "ball catcher's" view)
■ Lateral projection

Foot:
■ AP, oblique, and lateral views
Shoulder:
■ AP views (in true external and internal rotation)
Knee:
■ AP (standing semiflexed position to allow accurate evaluation of cartilage loss)
■ Flexed lateral (non-standing to allow patellofemoral evaluation) ± sunrise or Merchant patellar view and ± tunnel views
Hip:
■ AP (best for femoral neck evaluation)
■ Frog-leg lateral projection (best for femoral head evaluation and investigation of avascular necrosis)
SI joints:
■ Modified AP Ferguson view
Spine:
■ AP and lateral views
Survey radiographs*
Hands:
■ PA projection
■ Semi-pronated oblique view
Wrists:
■ PA projection
■ Lateral projection
■ Obliques (semi-pronated and semi-supinated)
Shoulders:
■ AP 40-degree posterior oblique view
Feet:
■ Medial oblique view
Ankles:
■ Lateral view to include heel
Knees:
■ AP projection
■ Lateral projection
Pelvis:
■ AP projection
Cervical spine:
■ Lateral with neck flexion

---

*The survey requires modification depending on specific diagnosis and clinical questions (i.e., suspected ankylosing spondylitis) or emphasis on axial skeleton including SI joints (i.e., suspected CPPD), symphysis pubis, PA wrist, and AP knees.

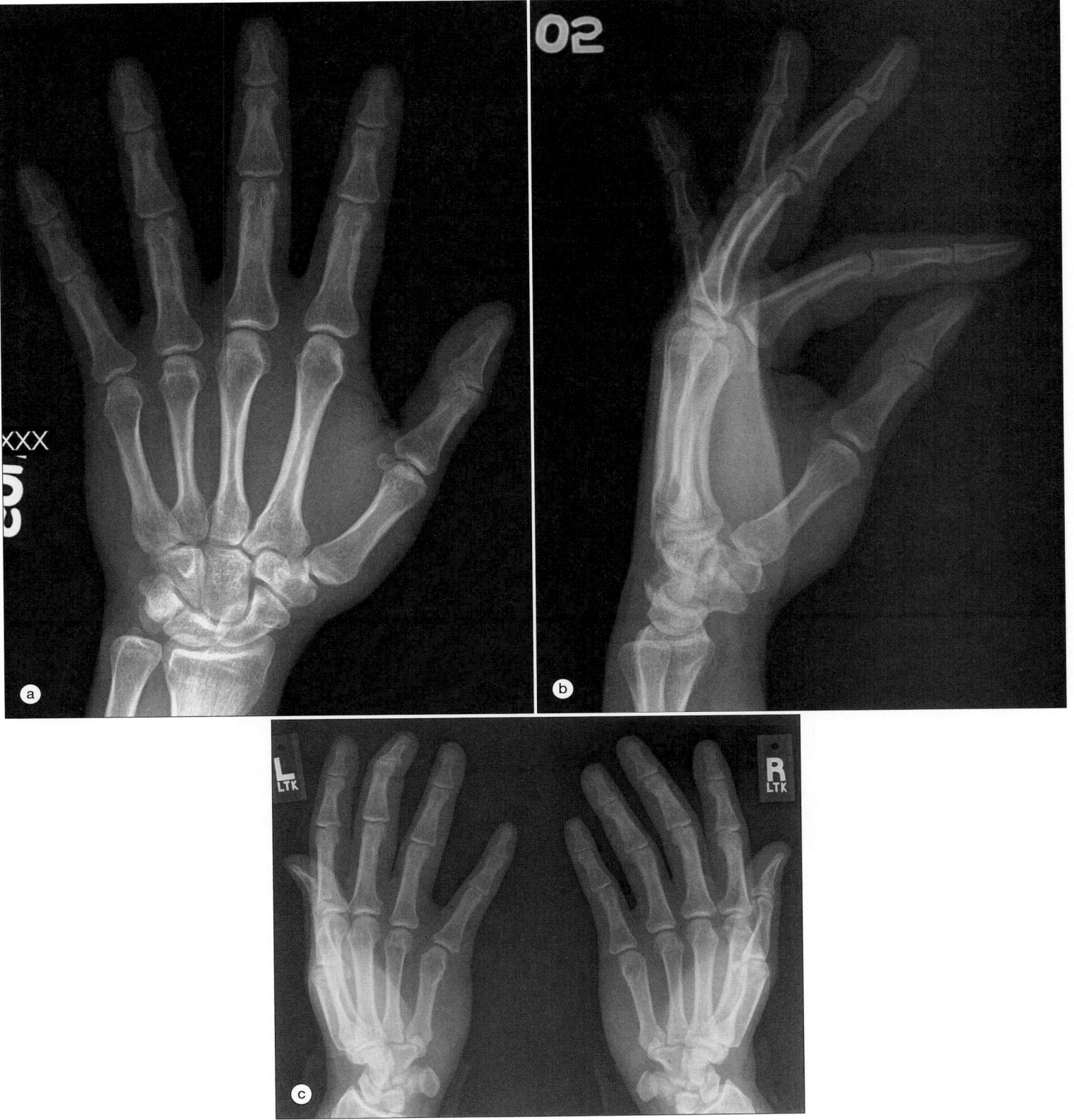

Fig. 38.3 Standard orthogonal views and specialized radiographic views. AP (a) and lateral (b) views of a normal hand depict 3D anatomic structures in 2D projection correcting for possible overlap of structures if imaged in only one plane. (c) Norgaard view (ball catcher's view) of bilateral normal hands and wrists allows better visualization of the pisotriquetral joint, first and second carpometacarpal joints, and lateral cortical margins of the second to fifth proximal phalangeal bases. Early erosive changes are best seen at these locations.

Knees

Another modification of radiographic technique involves the imaging assessment of the knees. AP or PA semiflexed views of the knees are best performed in the standing (weight-bearing position) rather than supine position so as to best assess for cartilage loss. Medial and lateral femoral tibial joints may appear symmetric and normal in a supinely positioned patient, whereas with the standing images true early joint space loss can be assessed. Joint space width of less than 4 mm has been reported to be consistent with cartilage loss.

Choice of joints

In patients with suspected polyarticular disorders, some authors suggest that survey radiographs of the hand and forefoot will typically

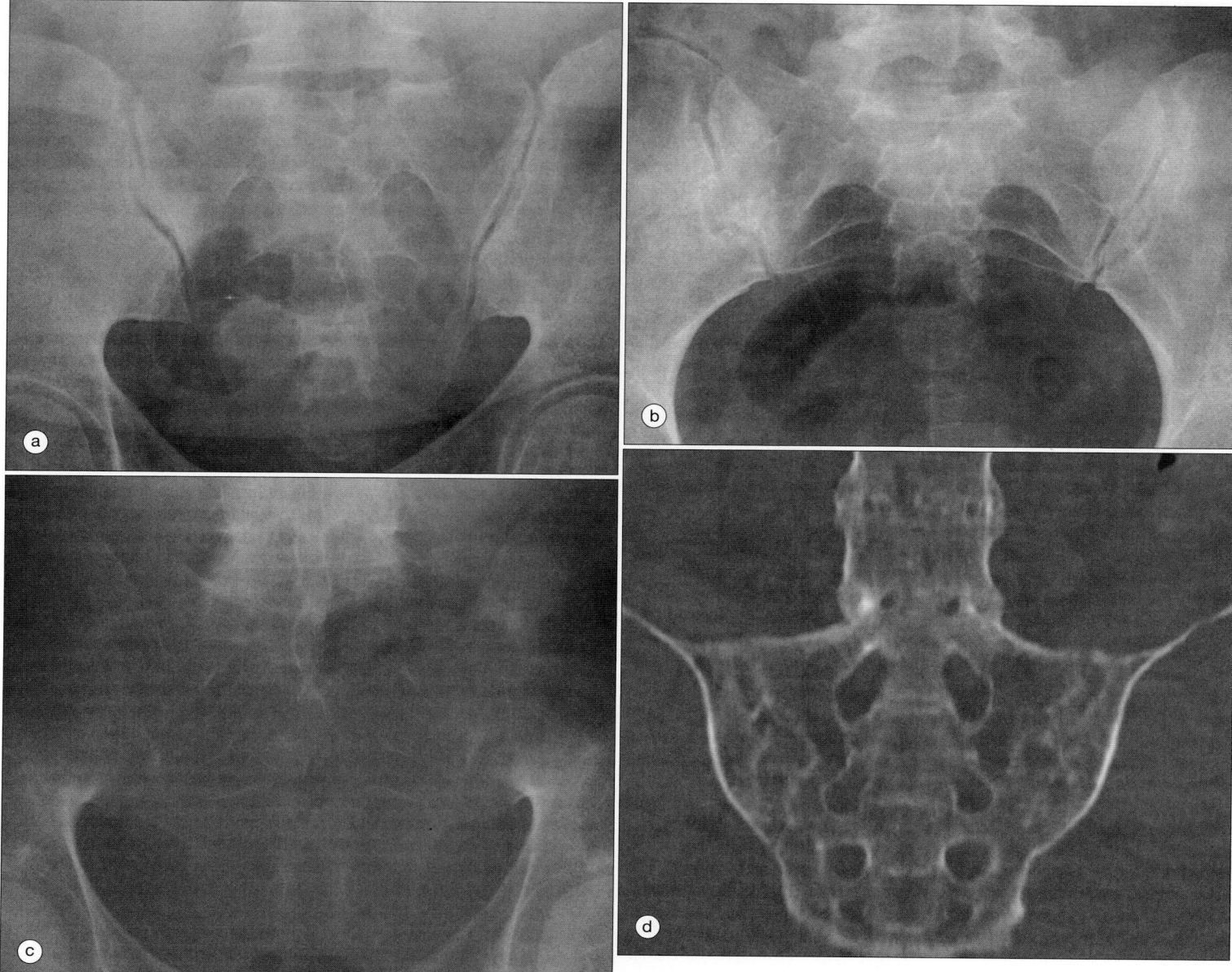

Fig. 38.4 Ferguson view of the sacrum and SI joint evaluation. (a) Better visualization of the anteroinferior SI joints is noted on the specialized Ferguson view in comparison to (b) the standard AP view of the sacrum in a normal patient. (c) Ferguson view in patient with ankylosing spondylitis shows apparent complete fusion of bilateral SI joints. (d) Coronal multiplanar reconstructed CT image of the SI joints in the same patient better depicts near-complete fusion of the SI joints.

provide the highest yield with the least amount of radiation exposure. Survey radiographs may be obtained for initial evaluation and at various intervals during subsequent examinations. Anatomic regions included in the survey depend on the specific disorder suspected clinically, its distribution, and laboratory findings and as a result must reveal enough information to delineate the type and extent of the disorder without representing an overuse of the patient's, technician's, and physician's time or of radiation and expense. Sartorius and Resnick suggest a minimum detailed high-yield radiographic survey for such investigations (see Box 38.1).[6] Modifications to the survey are expected depending on the clinical and laboratory scenario, and follow-up radiographs are not as extensive as the initial survey because they are tailored to the regions of specific interest.

Techniques and physics

X-rays are produced when highly energetic electrons interact with matter and convert their kinetic energy into electromagnetic radiation. The combination of an x-ray tube, x-ray tube housing (for shielding), x-ray field, and a generator (the energy source that supplies the voltage to accelerate the electrons and also controls voltage, current, and exposure time contributing to x-ray output) creates an x-ray beam of well-defined intensity for penetrability and spatial distribution (Fig. 38.5). Projection imaging (acquisition of a 2D image of the patient's 3D anatomy, i.e., radiography) compresses anatomic structures, concentrating the entire thickness of the patient into one single image known as the radiograph. Modern radiography systems still predominantly use the film-screen combinations, which consist of a cassette, one or two intensifying screens (decreases the radiation dose to the patient but can cause loss of spatial resolution), and a sheet of film (single or double photosensitive emulsion) (Fig. 38.6). Double-screen, double-emulsion film-screen systems are most commonly used for routine clinical radiography, whereas high-efficiency single-screen, single-emulsion film-screen combinations or single-emulsion film without screens is preferred for high-quality, high-resolution radiography, particularly in assessing therapeutic response to treatment of disease (see Fig. 38.6).

Magnification radiography

The quality of the radiographic image is important for accurate and detailed assessment of subtle skeletal abnormalities. High-resolution

X-RAY TUBE

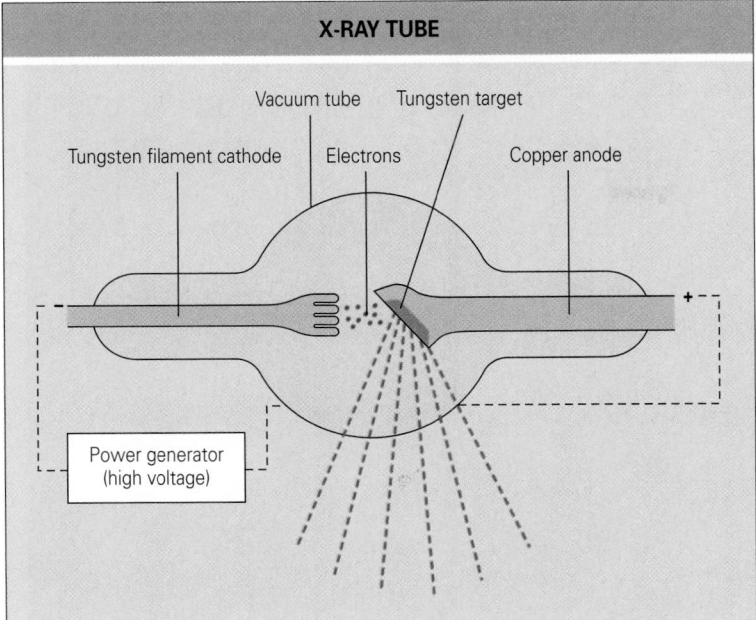

Fig. 38.5 X-ray tube. The tube consists of a cathode tube filament producing electrons, a tungsten target in a copper anode, and a vacuum tube.

INFLUENCE OF SCREEN THICKNESS

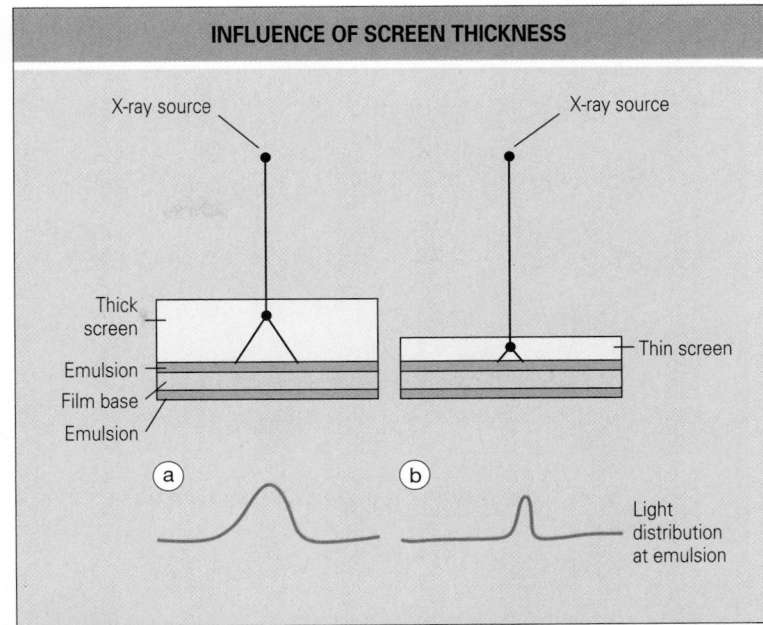

FILM–SCREEN COMBINATION

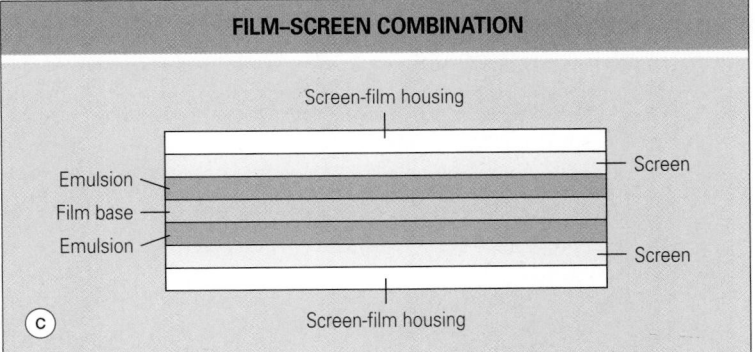

Fig. 38.6 Influence of screen thickness and film-screen combinations. The thicker screen (a) absorbs more incident x-rays. However, the resultant light spreads out over a wider area than with a thinner screen (b), resulting in a loss of spatial resolution. (c) Dual-emulsion and dual-screen system seen in cross section.

magnification radiography and fine detail radiographs have been developed to maximize diagnostic information. These are particularly useful in the hands, fingers, and feet. Magnification radiography is a highly specialized, not commonly available, radiographic technique that results in higher resolution (sharpness), better contrast, and lower quantum noise than conventional radiographs.[7] Image magnification up to 10 times that seen on conventional radiographs can be obtained. It is more sensitive than conventional radiographs in detecting erosions, patterns of bone resorption, early bone proliferation, chondrocalcinosis (i.e., crystal deposition disease [CPPD]), and the presence of soft tissue swelling and is useful when conventional radiographs are negative or equivocal. Fine detail radiography is more sensitive for the subtle early subperiosteal resorption, cortical striation, or tunneling seen in hyperparathyroidism.[6] It may also be helpful in monitoring the course of this disease and its response to therapy.

Two forms of magnification radiography have been used:

1. *Optical magnification of fine grain films.* The exposure, obtained with conventional radiographic equipment and fine grain industrial films, is viewed with optical enlargement. Although increased radiation dose is noted with this technique, it has been utilized in both metabolic and arthritic disorder investigations by Genant[8] and others, with good reproducibility.
2. *Direct radiographic magnification for skeletal radiography.* A small focal spot (100-150 μm) is utilized in this technique, which has received less attention than optical magnification, with only few reports in the literature.[9,10] Because of its fourfold increase in skin dose (exposure per surface area), the utilization of rare earth screen-film system and single-emulsion, single-screen systems as well as a decreased field of view can significantly counteract and reduce the total-body irradiation of this technique.

Digital radiography

Digital radiography has been growing in popularity over the past 10 years, particularly with the current trend for many departments to become "filmless." This technique is more expensive because it requires high luminance and high-resolution monitors to view the digital image, has large datasets that require large amounts of space on digital storage media, and depends on a high network bandwidth for picture archiving and communication systems (PACS).

The four main systems currently available for acquisition of digital radiographs are

1. Computed radiography (CR), which uses photostimulable phosphor detector (PSP) systems in which images are stored and viewed on PACS yet can be printed directly via a laser printer
2. Charged coupled devices (CCDs) utilized in fluoroscopy
3. Direct detection flat panel systems
4. Indirect detection flat panel systems

Direct detection systems utilize a photoconductor material (usually selenium) applied on top of a thin film transistor (TFT) array, whereas the indirect systems utilize an x-ray intensifying screen that converts x-rays to light, which is then detected by the flat panel detector. The principal advantage of direct over indirect detection flat panel systems is a decrease in blurring, with direct detection systems having a higher spatial resolution than either CR or indirect systems, a reduced radiation dose than conventional plain film radiography, and improved tolerance for overexposure or underexposure (too bright or too dark) of images because of a wider dynamic range (Fig. 38.7). Anatomic detail, contrast, and spatial resolution of these digital techniques have been found to be sufficient for the evaluation of arthritis.[11]

Computerized x-ray image analysis methods (computer-aided analysis)

Computer-aided analysis or computer-aided detection (CAD) of radiographic data was developed to fulfill the need for quantitative surrogate outcome measures in clinical research. Large numbers of radiographic images could be digitally imaged and stored for evaluation and training by the computer software system. These methods were initially utilized in mammographic and chest imaging over the past 2 decades. The

Text continued on p. 358

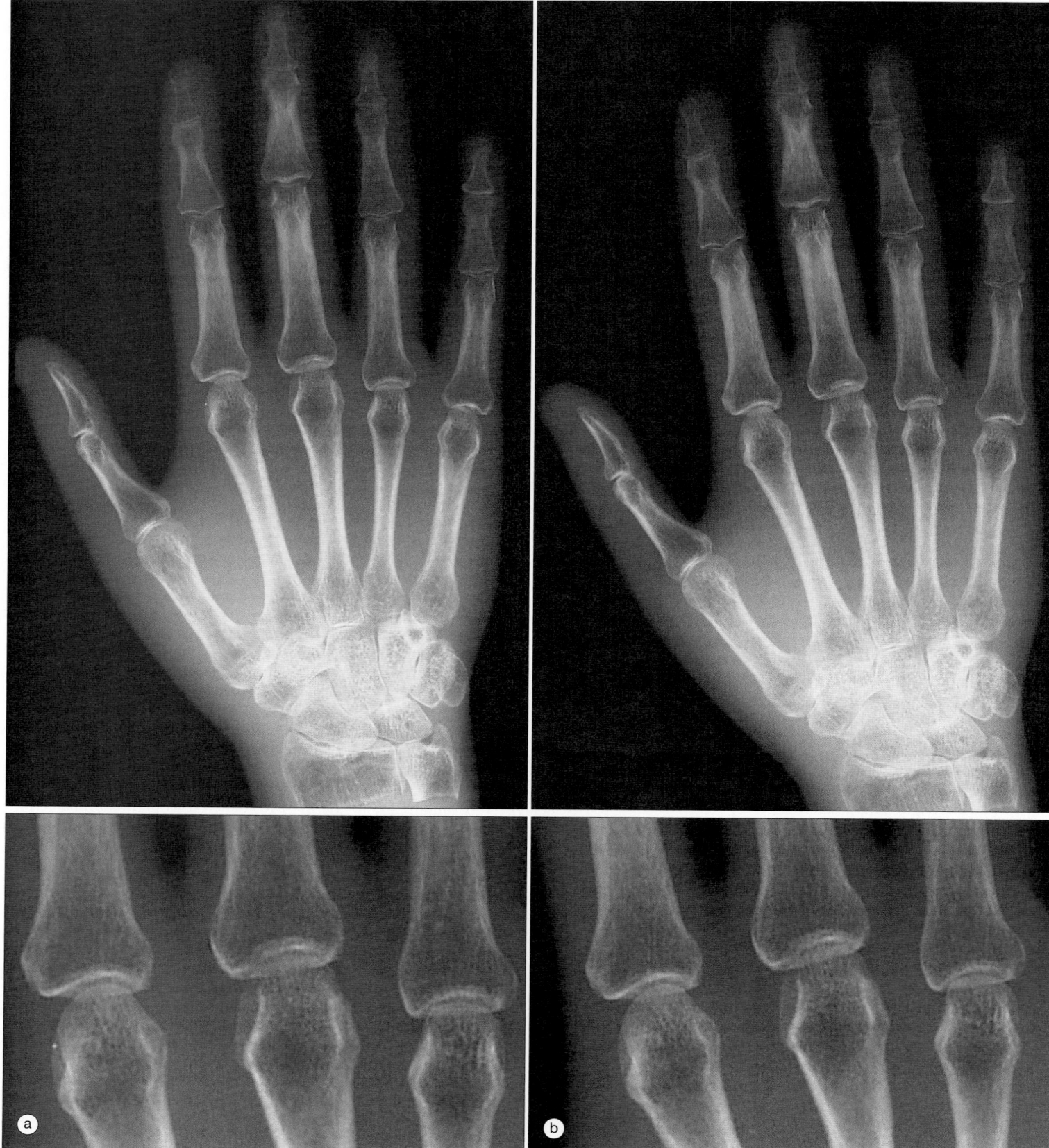

Fig. 38.7 Comparison of 100-speed conventional film-screen combination (a-d) and direct detection flat panel system using selenium detectors (e-h). The voltage is 50 kV in every case. The exposure has been progressively cut from 4.0 mAs (a, e) through 2.8 mAs (b, f) and 2.0 mAs (c, g) to 0.56 mAs (d). Note that the conventional film-screen combination provides no diagnostic information on bone and articular structures with 50 kV, 0.56 mAs exposure. However, the direct detection flat panel system (h) provides images of diagnostic quality because of its greater dynamic range.

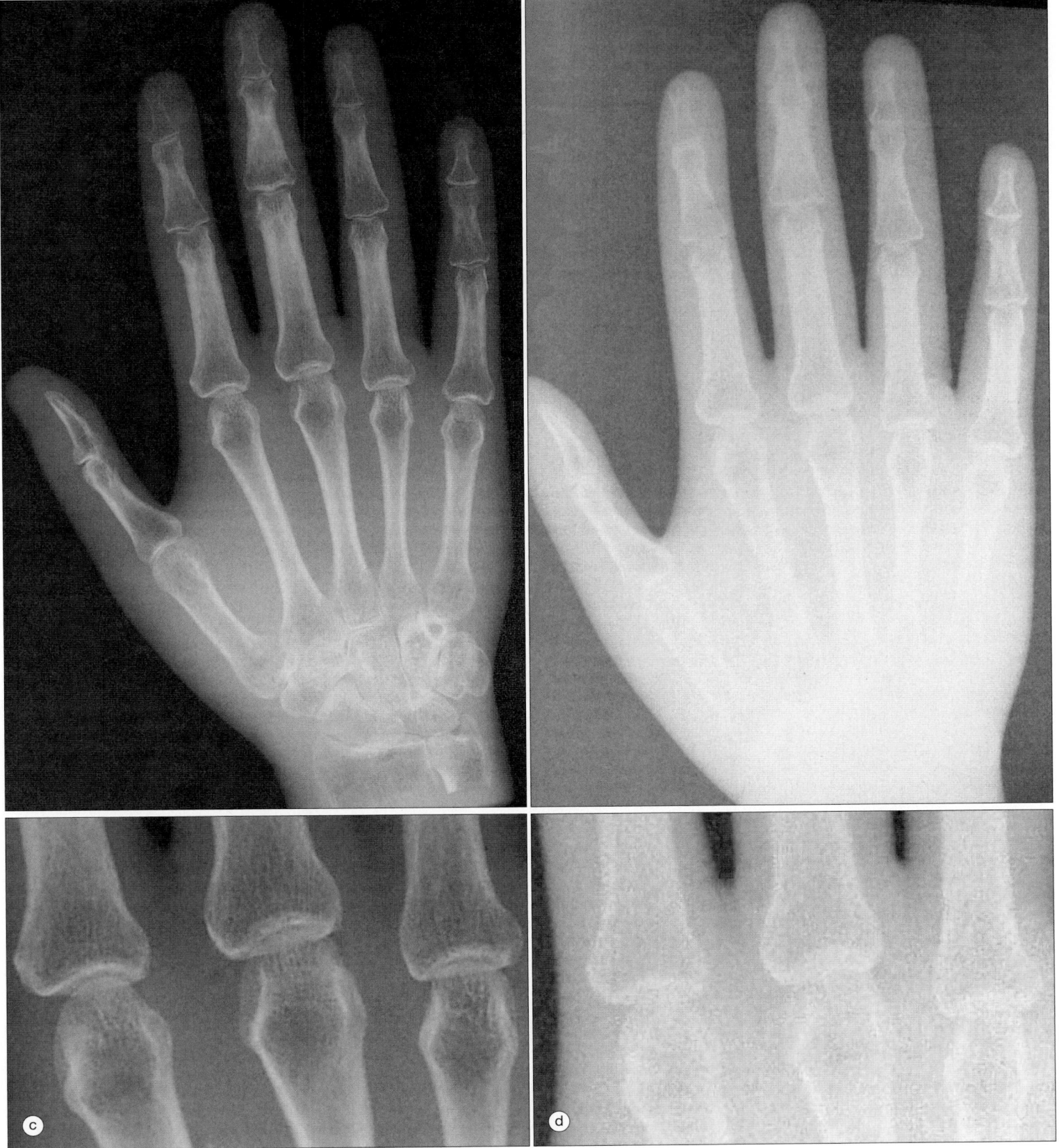

Fig. 38.7, cont'd

Continued

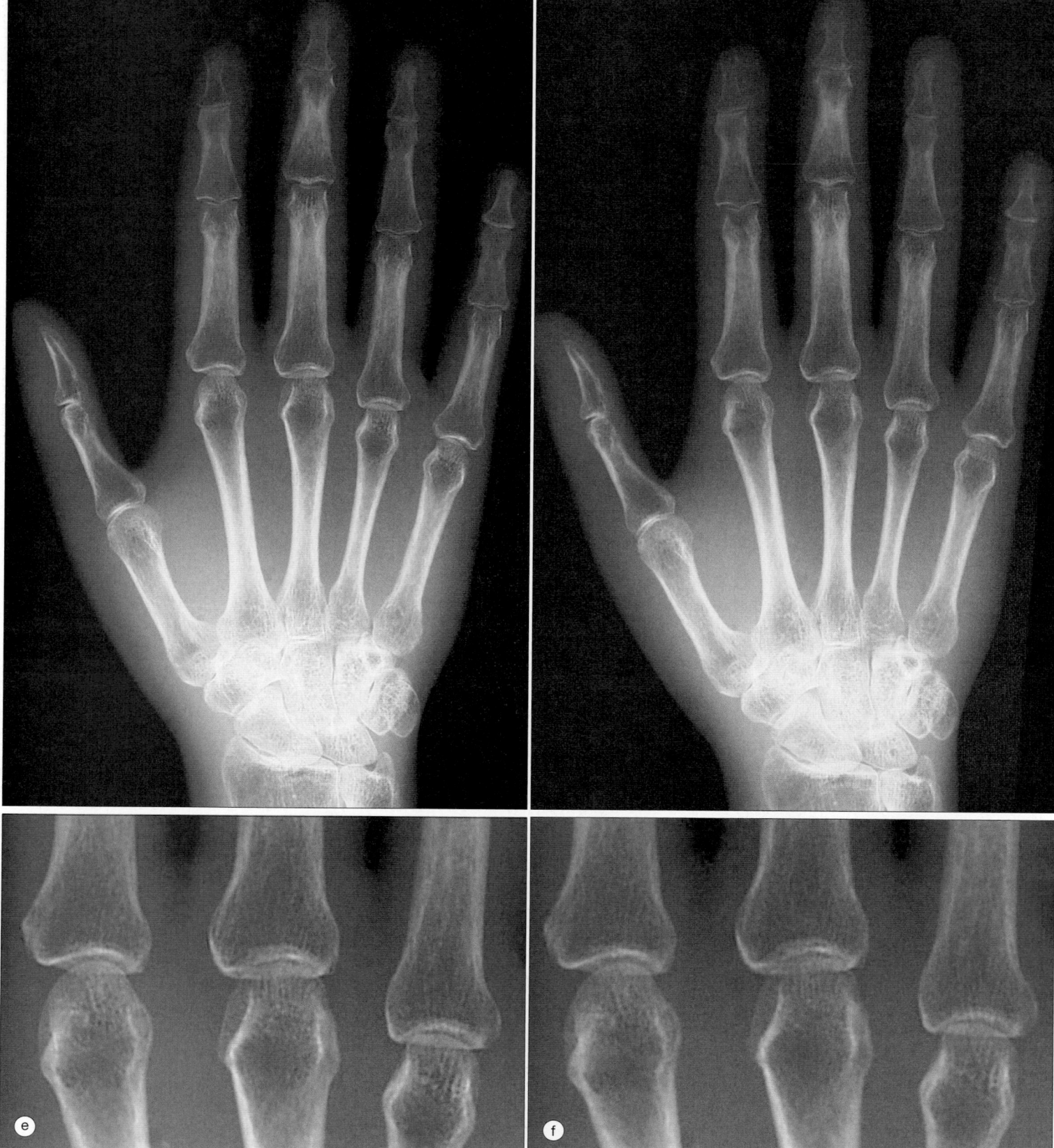

Fig. 38.7, cont'd Comparison of 100-speed conventional film-screen combination (a-d) and direct detection flat panel system using selenium detectors (e-h). The voltage is 50 kV in every case. The exposure has been progressively cut from 4.0 mAs (a, e) through 2.8 mAs (b, f) and 2.0 mAs (c, g) to 0.56 mAs (d). Note that the conventional film-screen combination provides no diagnostic information on bone and articular structures with 50 kV, 0.56 mAs exposure. However, the direct detection flat panel system (h) provides images of diagnostic quality because of its greater dynamic range.

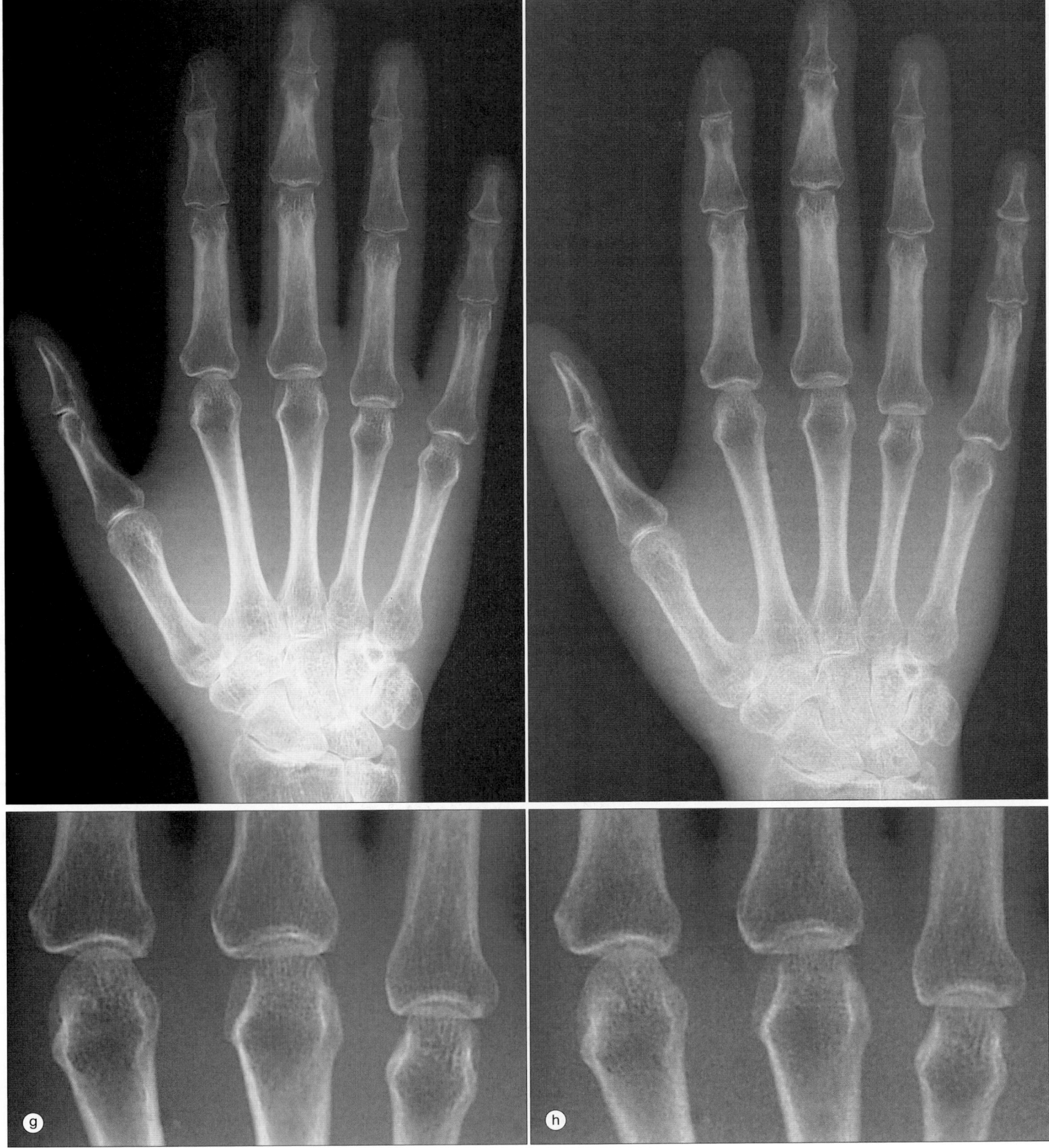

Fig. 38.7, cont'd

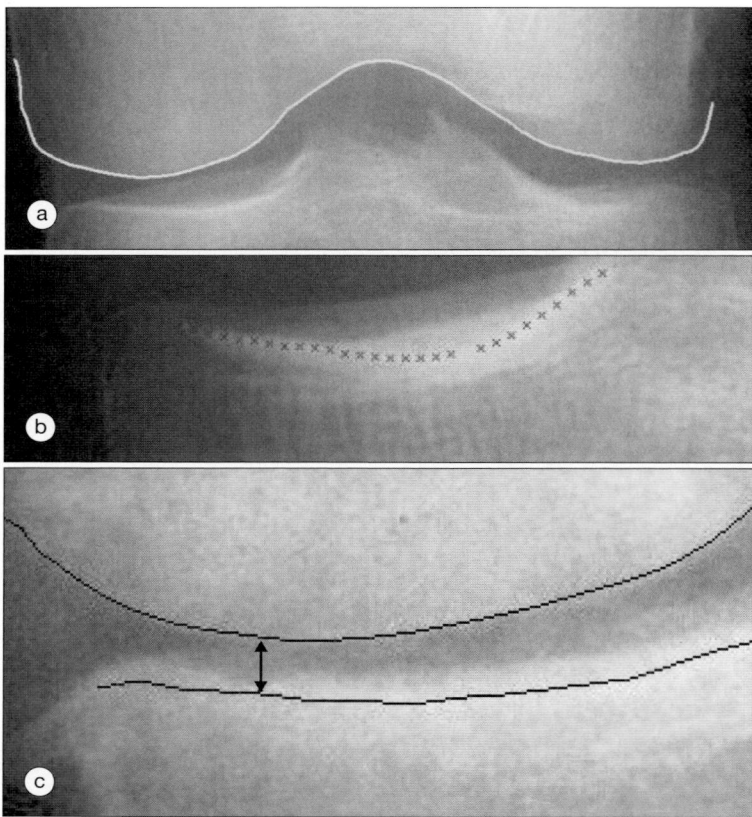

Fig. 38.8 Computerized x-ray image analysis for joint space narrowing. (a) Computer-delineated femoral condyle shown as the white line overlaid on the knee radiograph. (b) The computer-determined joints along the bright band corresponding to the base of the tibial plateau. (c) Computerized determination of minimum joint space width. The points on the tibial plateau have been connected. The shortest distance between the femoral condyle and the tibial plateau is automatically detected.

computer algorithm was developed to be able to find nodules and lesions and classify them as benign or malignant. Their utility in arthritis research is increasing.[12] Most of the work in developing computerized digital radiograph–based techniques in rheumatology has been focused on the evaluation of osteoarthritis of the knee, with more recent studies involving the hip and hand, with the latter focusing on analyses of the metacarpophalangeal and proximal interphalangeal joints in rheumatoid arthritis (RA).[13,14]

The general goal of such systems is to quantify arthritis progression by measuring the radiographic minimum joint space width by way of a computer software algorithm that can delineate the opposing margins of a joint on a digital radiographic image (Fig. 38.8). Although computerized techniques are objective and fast, they are prone to the occasional error, and, as a result, a quality assurance step is necessary that allows for correction. Overall, however, these systems are reproducible, providing a more objective measurement with improved inter- and intra-reader reproducibility and are more efficient and cost effective than manual scoring systems.[12]

Interventional techniques

There is an increasing use of interventional conventional radiography in rheumatology, of which fluoroscopically guided injection of joints for diagnosis or for therapeutic intervention is the most important. Although advanced imaging (MRI or CT) is more commonly used for assessment of synovial thickening, ligament degeneration/tear, or osteochondral bodies, fluoroscopically guided arthrography can be used in those patients who are claustrophobic or who are not candidates for MRI. Indeed, this latter technique can be useful, for example, in demonstrating some reliable indicators of synovial inflammation, such as corrugated irregularity of injected intra-articular contrast material within the wrist or glenohumeral joint, enlargement of the joint, as well as opacification of lymphatic vessels.[15] Degeneration of the triangular fibrocartilage complex (TFCC) with eventual tear can be

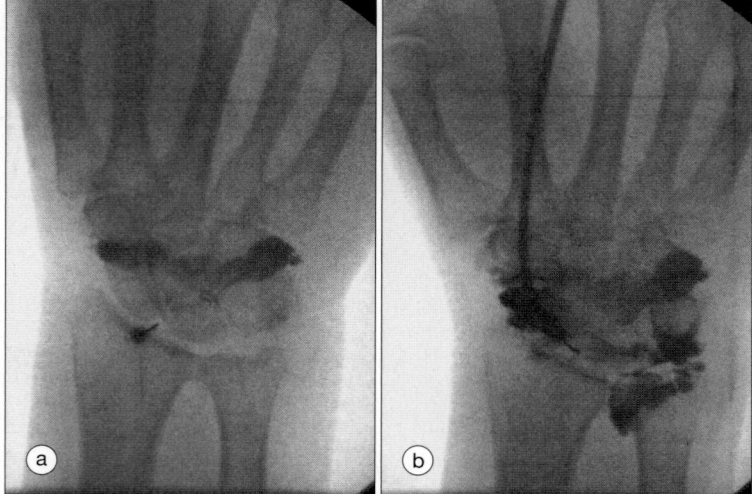

Fig. 38.9 Fluoroscopy. (a) AP view of a wrist arthrogram performed under fluoroscopy demonstrates prior injection of the midcarpal joint without abnormal extravasation with needle now repositioned within the radioscaphoid joint. (b) Contrast medium injection within the proximal radiocarpal joint shows abnormal flow of the agent into the distal radioulnar joint consistent with triangular fibrocartilage tear.

documented under fluoroscopy after injection of the radiocarpal joint as visualized leakage of contrast agent into the distal radial ulnar joint (Fig. 38.9). Osteochondral bodies can be seen as filling defects within the joints on arthrography of the shoulder, helping in diagnosis of osteochondromatosis.

Therapeutic injections include corticosteroid or analgesic injections of the joints, most commonly the shoulder, SI joints, or hips. Other substances that have been injected under fluoroscopy include cartilage "stimulating" or "replacement" substances for patients with little or no cartilage remaining in the knees or hips. Injection of the joint of interest under fluoroscopic guidance may be utilized before MRI or CT for cartilage, joint space, ligament, and soft tissue integrity assessment in arthritic patients.

COMPUTED TOMOGRAPHY

The first head CT scanner was invented by Godfrey Hounsfield (United Kingdom) and Allan Cormack (United States) and introduced in 1972. CT was the first advanced imaging modality to be utilized in the imaging of arthritis long before the advent of MRI. CT has evolved tremendously from its initial first-generation scanner. The former incorporated a rotate/translate system and a pencil x-ray beam that essentially allowed for the acquisition of 360 radiographs acquired at 1-degree intervals around a patient or extremity. Second, third, and fourth-generation developments led to the advent of helical or spiral scanners in 1992. These were followed by the multidetector array CT (MDCT) scanners of today.

All modern CT scanners incorporate a fan beam geometry in which the x-rays at a given projection angle diverge, having the appearance of a fan. In third- and fourth-generation scanners, a single axial image included a large number of transmission measurements (acquisitions), each taken at a specific axial portion of the body while the gantry stopped, then the CT scanner table would advance in a craniocaudal direction and the same process would repeat. This was followed by tomographic reconstruction (filtered backprojection most commonly) to create the final CT image.

Helical or spiral CT scanners incorporate a slip ring technology whereby the gantry continuously rotates, with the x-ray source moving in a helical rather than a circular motion around the patient, acquiring data while the table is moving. This creates shorter scan times.

MDCT

MDCT, also referred to as multislice, multidetector row, or multisection CT, is the latest, most widely used version that is now a true 3D

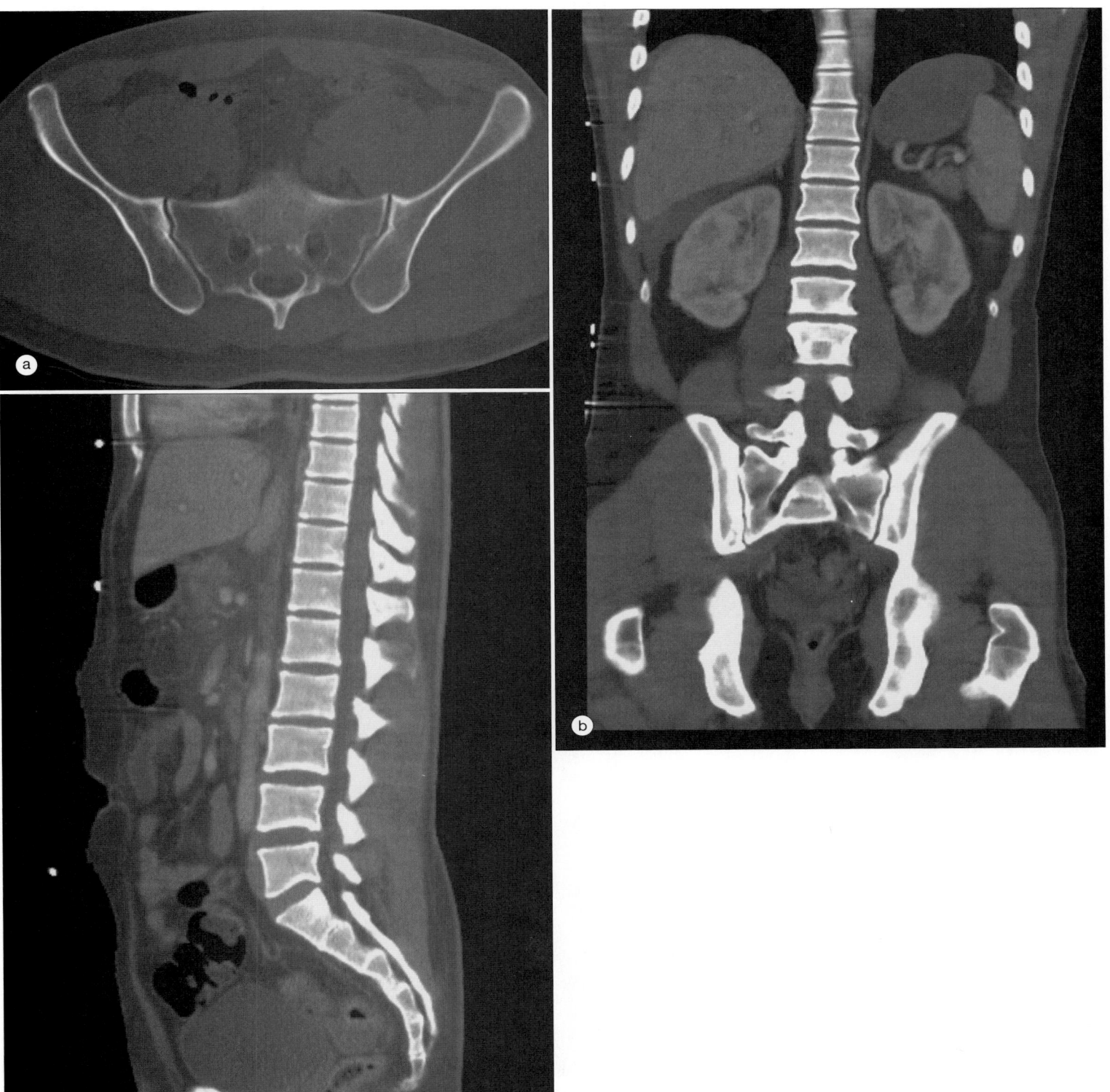

Fig. 38.10 MDCT: 2D and 3D applications. (a) Axial MDCT image of the pelvis, just one of many thin slices in the original study database in this patient. Coronal (b) and sagittal (c) multiplanar reconstruction (MPR) CT images of the spine and pelvis created from the original scanned data.

Continued

imaging modality. Gains over transaxial cross-sectional technique include reduced scan time, section collimation, and increased scan length with high spatial resolution. Multislice CT allows extended anatomic coverage with thinner slices (0.5-mm slice width). This makes it possible to acquire isovolumetric data (arbitrary imaging planes). Thus, techniques such as multiplanar reconstructions (MPR)

and 3D rendering (volume rendering [VR], shaded surface display [SSD], and maximum intensity projections [MIPs]) become an integral part of the examination (Fig. 38.10).[16] In practical terms, the multidetector scanners obviate the need for scanning patients in multiple positions to achieve true 2D sagittal, coronal, axial, or oblique images. Multiplanar reformatted images can be reconstructed in any plane from

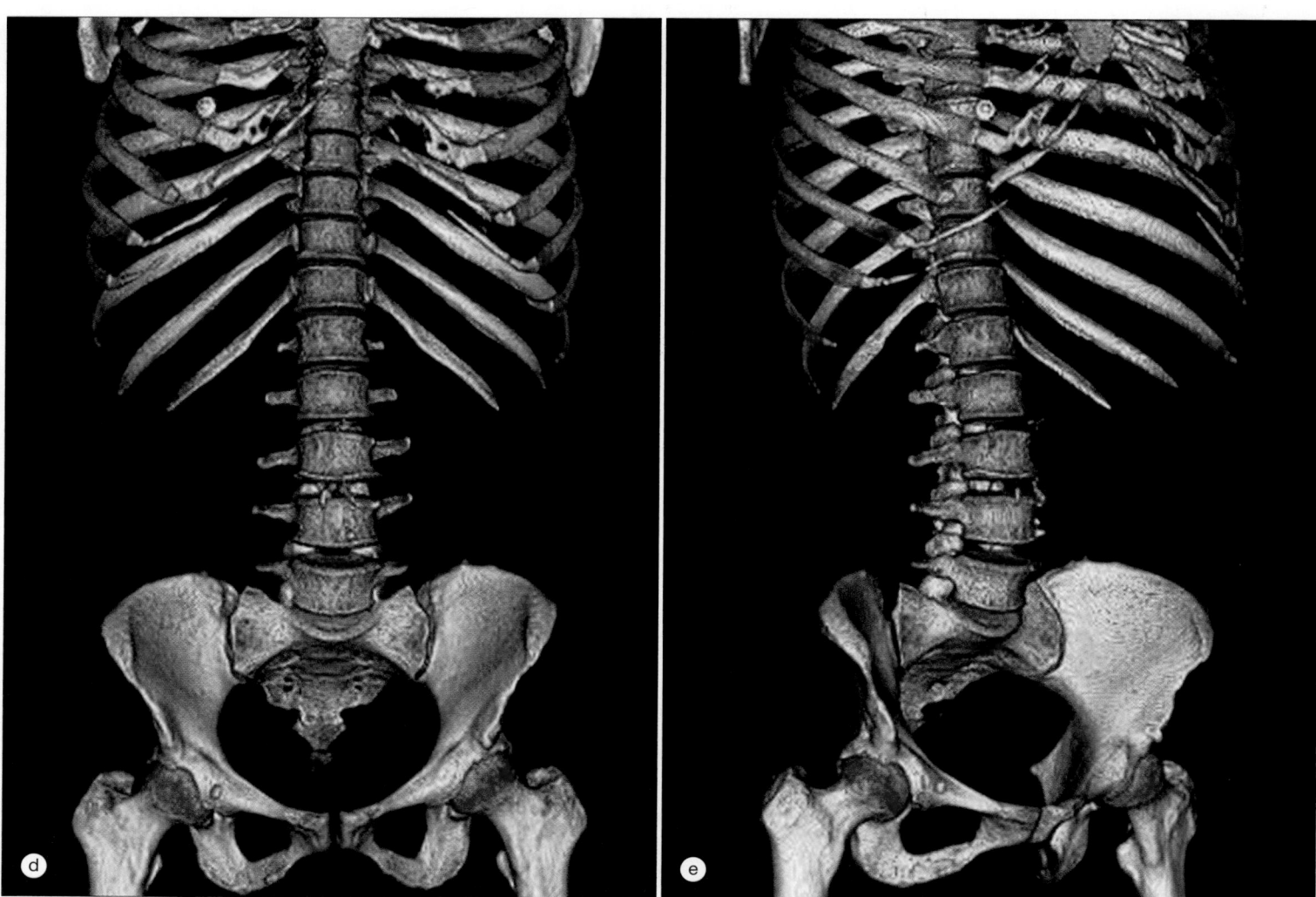

Fig. 38.10, cont'd MDCT: 2D and 3D applications. (d-f) 3D MDCT rendering of the spine and pelvis in the same patient utilizing volume rendering (VR) technique in AP, right anterior oblique, and left anterior oblique projections. Volume-rendered 3D CT image of the pelvis (coronal) (g) and spine (sagittal) (h) using bone windows.

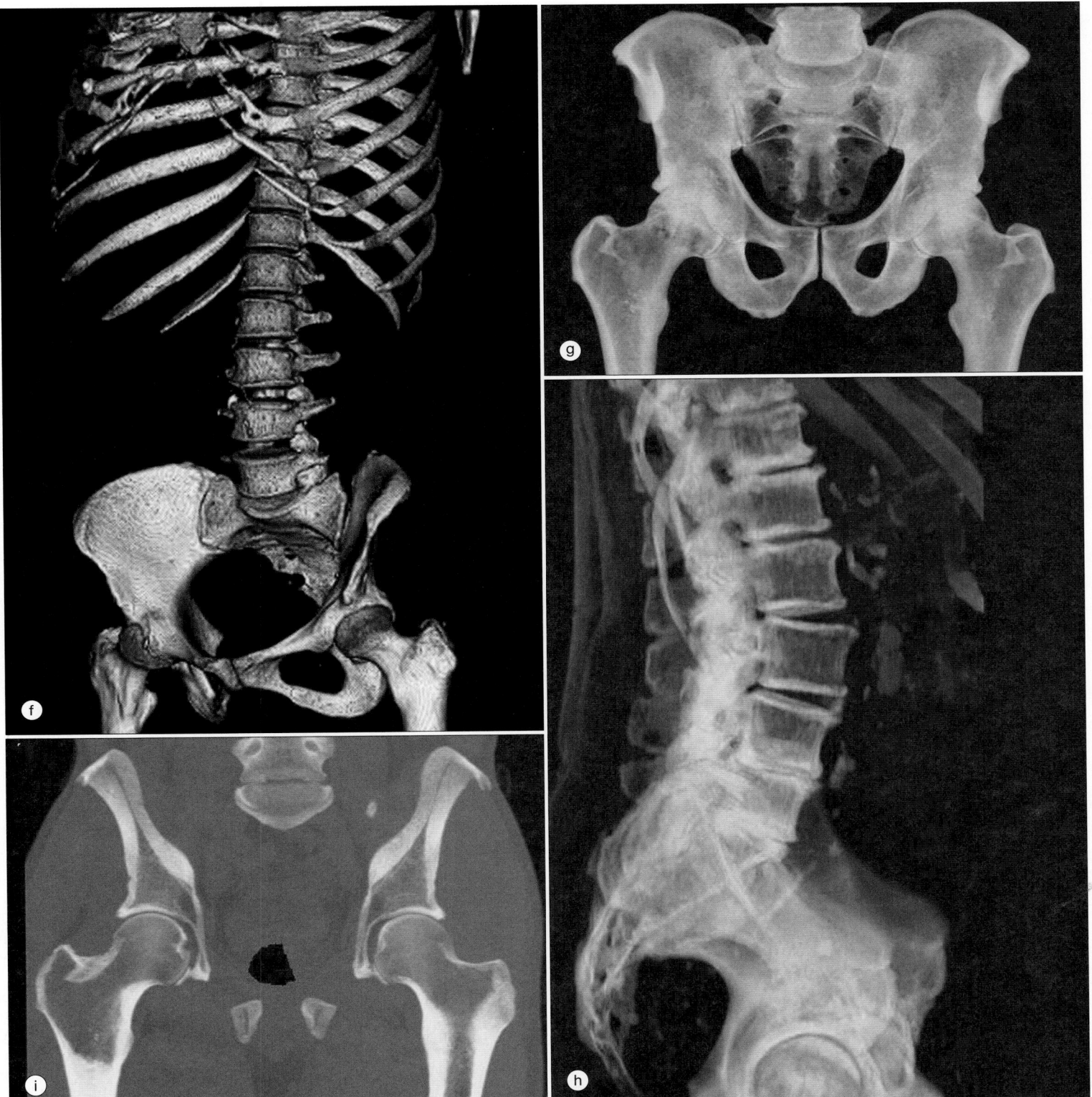

Fig. 38.10, cont'd

Continued

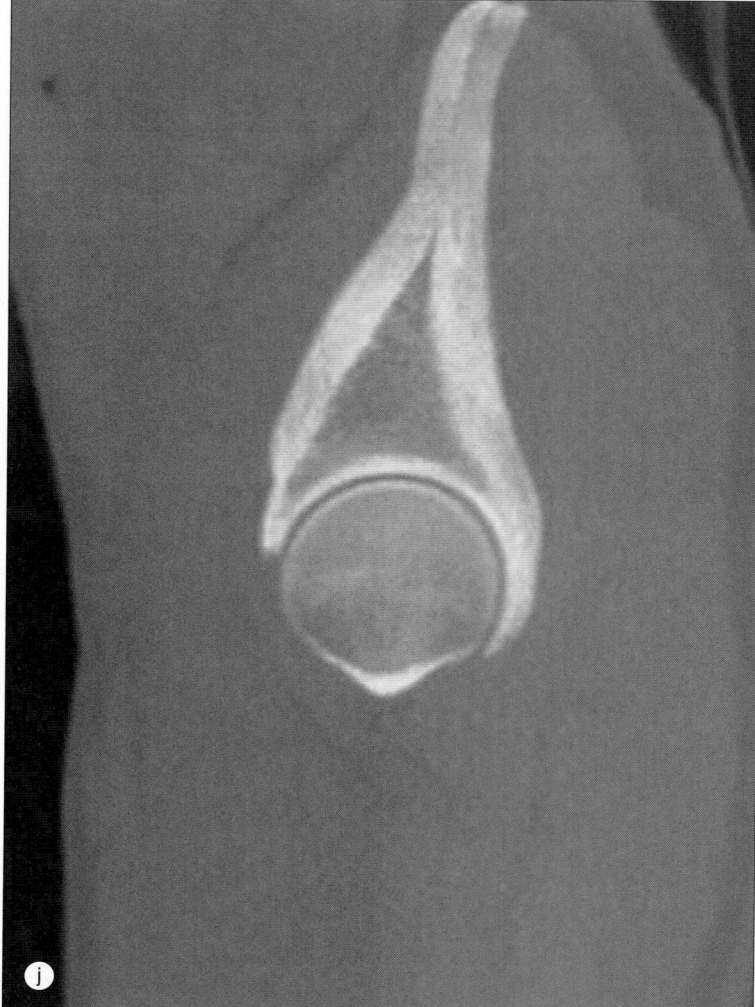

Fig. 38.10, cont'd (i, j) Maximum intensity projection images of the pelvis and hips in coronal and sagittal projections respectively, clearly delineating the joint space and cortical integrity of the hips.

the original dataset acquired during the initial scan. This provides not only sagittal and coronal images but also oblique coronal or even 3D images for further evaluation of the study to provide a diagnosis.

Beginning with 4-, 6-, 8-, and 10-detector array scanners, 16-, 40-, and now 64-detector array scanners are becoming the mainstay of radiology departments. Higher detector arrays result in less possibility of movement artifact, which is not only of benefit in children, ill patients, and claustrophobics but also especially important in imaging of small joints so as not to lose data or critical information during the study.

One of the problems with MDCT is that image noise is increased with sectional collimation reduction (thin slices), requiring either an increase in the radiation dose or thickening of image sections to decrease the noise. This feature is diminishing with higher detector array scanners. Also, thinner slice widths are more commonly utilized in the extremities, which do not contain radiosensitive tissue, making radiation dose less of an issue in these cases.[15]

Applications in rheumatology

Bone

MDCT provides excellent contrast and delineation of cortical and trabecular bone evaluation and is established as a superb diagnostic tool for the visualization of subtle cortical or intraosseous lesions not visible on radiographs due to projectional superimposition (see Fig. 38.10). Whereas MRI and ultrasonography in experienced hands have been found to be superior to CT with regard to erosion detection, one

study found the scoring of erosions in the rheumatoid hand was higher on MDCT than MRI at the metacarpal bases owing to its ability to clearly delineate cortical bony margins and areas of sclerosis.[17] MDCT provides validation of the bone damage or destruction suspected on MRI or ultrasonography and may be useful in treatment follow-up because sclerosis may be indicative of reparative changes.[18]

CT is less expensive than MRI and it has a shorter scanning time, which may benefit some patients, although the radiation dose is higher for CT than MRI. Because of its ability to assess both cortical and trabecular bone, CT can be used to assess for osteopenia or osteoporosis. This can be subjectively assessed on a CT study performed for other purposes. Quantitative CT (QCT) of the spine is one such objective method for volumetric evaluation of bone mineral density, but it is generally reserved for research purposes. Bone mineral density evaluation and its methods are discussed in detail elsewhere (see Chapter 42).

Peripheral and axial joints

Joints that are difficult to visualize with usual imaging techniques (apophyseal, costovertebral, sternoclavicular, and temporomandibular joints) may be better evaluated with MDCT and the use of reformatted images, MIPs, or MPR images for visualization and evaluation of ligaments and bone, spinal cord compression, erosions of the odontoid process, subluxation, and presence of calcification (Fig. 38.11). The 3D analysis of standard joints such as the glenohumeral or hip joint with suspected osteoarthritis, RA, CPPD, or ischemic necrosis can be useful in assessment of subtle bone or joint changes as well as in detecting

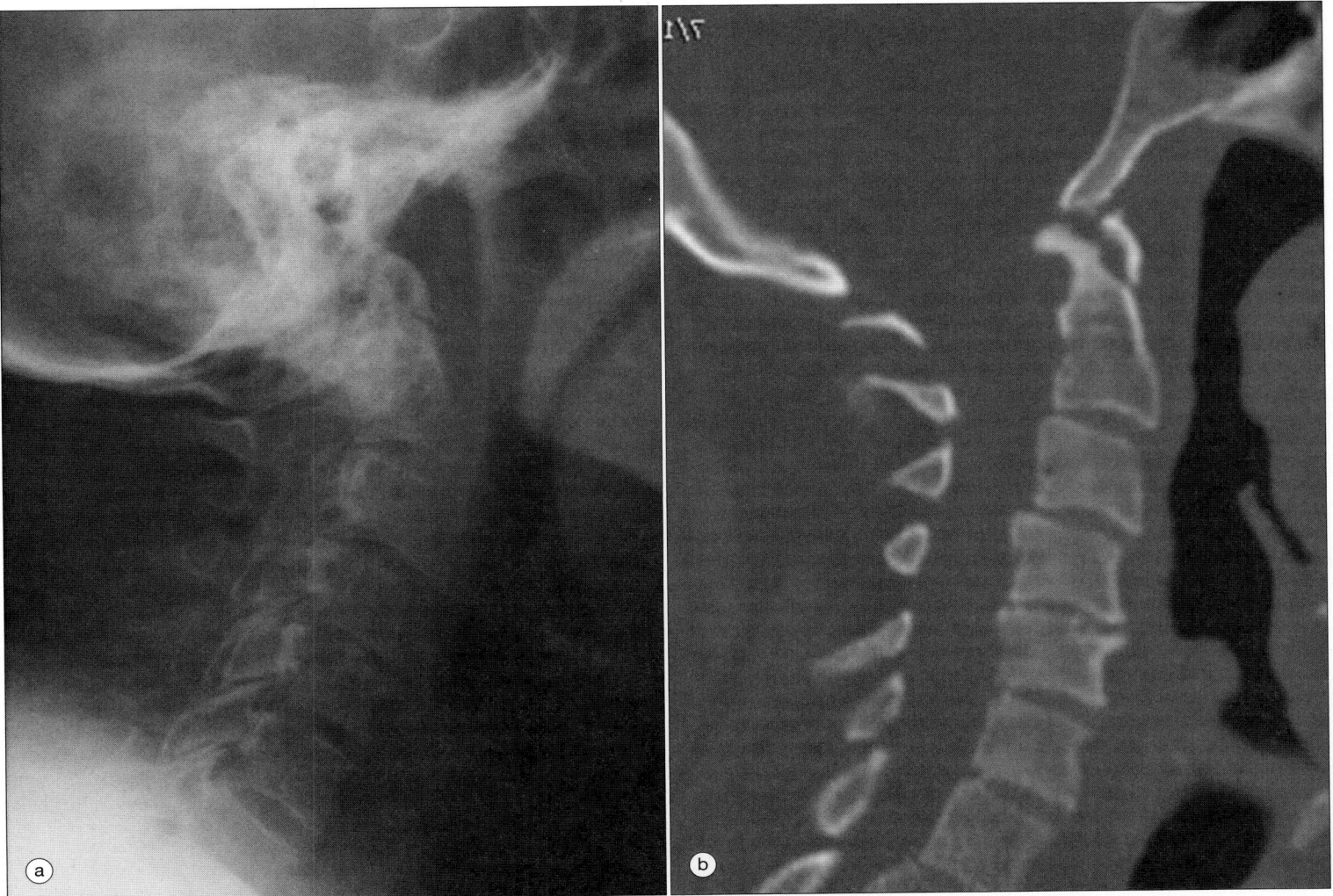

Fig. 38.11 Rheumatoid arthritis of the odontoid. (a) Lateral radiograph of the cervical spine depicts narrowing of the preodontoid space, osteopenia, and midcervical disc space narrowing. MDCT sagittal (b, c) and axial soft tissue and bone window (d, e) CT images of the odontoid better demonstrate the soft tissue pannus about the odontoid with external erosions of the odontoid. Erosions are also noted within the right facet joint on the axial bone window image.

Continued

any periarticular soft tissue masses or synovial cysts. The use of MDCT after intra-articular injection of a contrast agent has proved to be useful in these latter situations because even articular cartilage abnormalities can be visualized secondary to increased spatial resolution and increased delineation of bone versus cartilage (Fig. 38.12).[19]

The CT findings of sacroiliitis are similar to those seen on conventional radiographs, including erosions, sclerosis, and eventual ankylosis if the disease progresses. Several studies indicate that CT is more sensitive than radiographs in identifying sacroiliitis, leading to an earlier diagnosis of sacroiliitis and earlier implementation of treatment.[20] CT is also useful in septic arthritis because irregular bone destruction and intra-articular or periarticular fluid are well seen, particularly after intravenous administration of a contrast agent in which the infected fluid collection demonstrates a characteristic peripheral rim enhancement pattern.[19]

CT-guided facet, joint, or bursal injections are often utilized in the diagnosis and treatment of rheumatologic disease. CT fluoroscopy combines the careful delineation of anatomy with the real-time cineradiography of fluoroscopy, allowing finer visualization of placement and orientation of the procedural needle for appropriate injection or aspiration as required.

Soft tissues and vessels

Whereas CT is usually used for the evaluation of bone, the soft tissue system can also be evaluated, although typically MRI may be a more appropriate modality for these tissues. One of the more common soft tissue indications for CT in rheumatology is the evaluation of the large vessel vasculitides using CT angiography.[21] These disorders, particularly giant cell arteritis or Takayasu arteritis, can be visualized, detected, analyzed, and, according to some studies, even monitored, using CT angiography, because it can evaluate both the vessel wall and the lumen and may show vessel wall alterations even when the lumen appears unaffected on standard angiography.[22] CT has a role in diagnosing both early and advanced Takayasu arteritis. In early Takayasu arteritis, CT may show arterial wall thickening with mural enhancement and low-attenuation ring on delayed images, whereas in advanced Takayasu arteritis, CT shows the typical late-stage complications, including vessel stenosis, occlusion, and aneurysm.[23] Aortic wall enhancement was shown to resolve after immunosuppressive therapy in 7 of 13 Takayasu patients in one study.[24] CT angiography, however, cannot visualize relatively small vessels and therefore is limited to deep large vessel evaluation.[25]

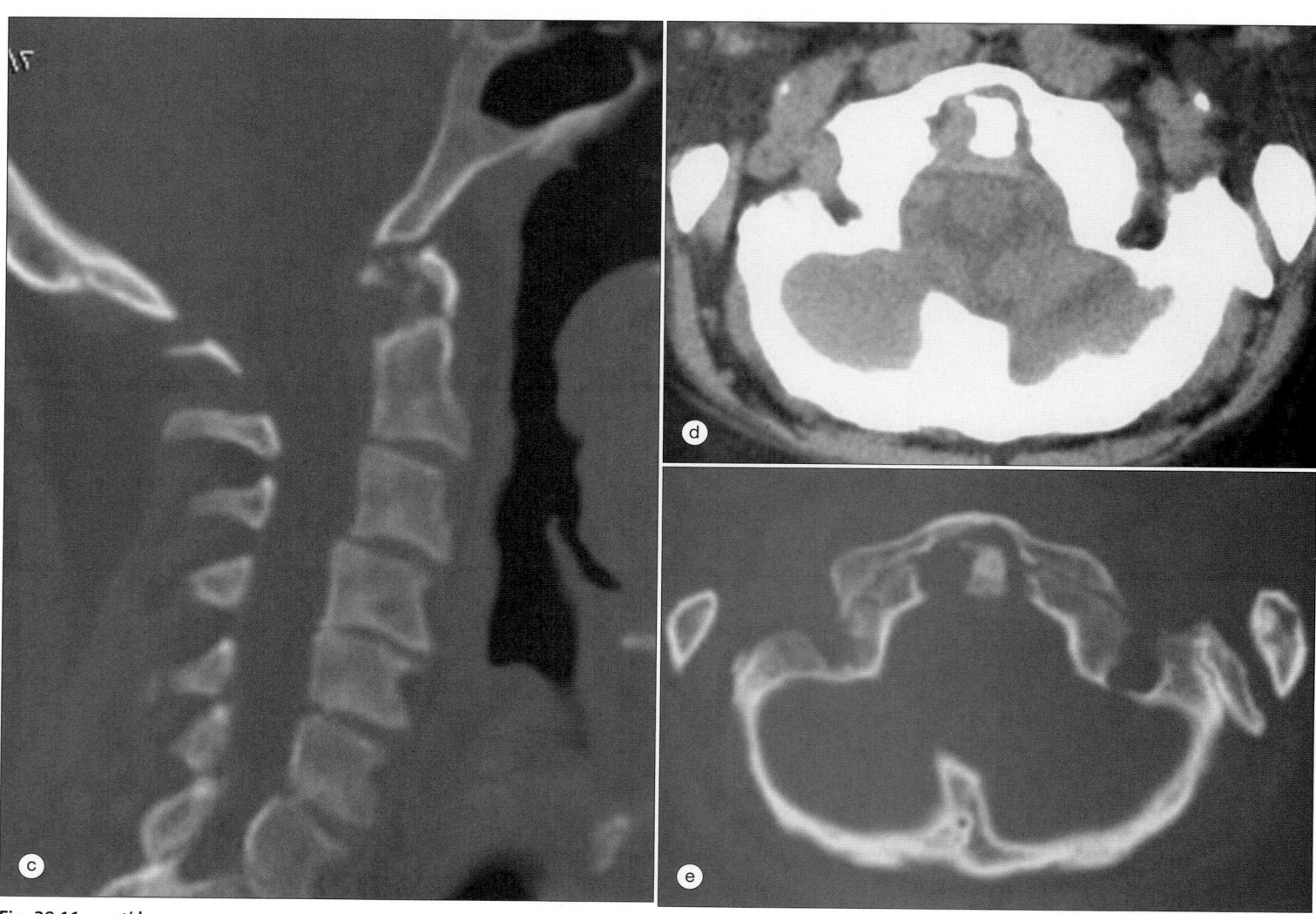

Fig. 38.11, cont'd

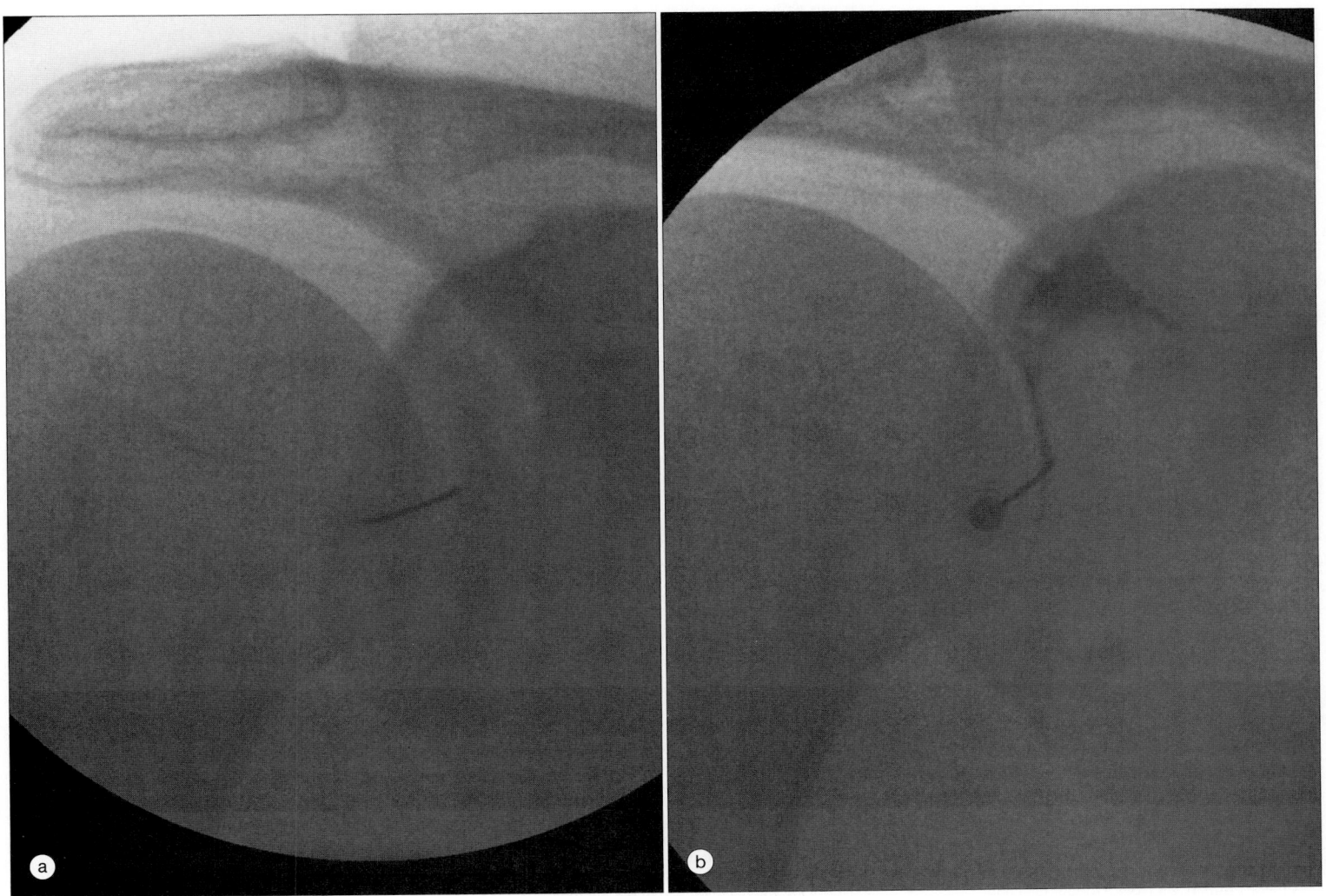

Fig. 38.12 CT arthrography of the shoulder. (a) AP fluoroscopic image of the right shoulder showing needle placement in the mid-distal third of the glenohumeral joint. (b) Subsequent injection of contrast material into the glenohumeral joint is seen flowing along the curvilinear contour.

Continued

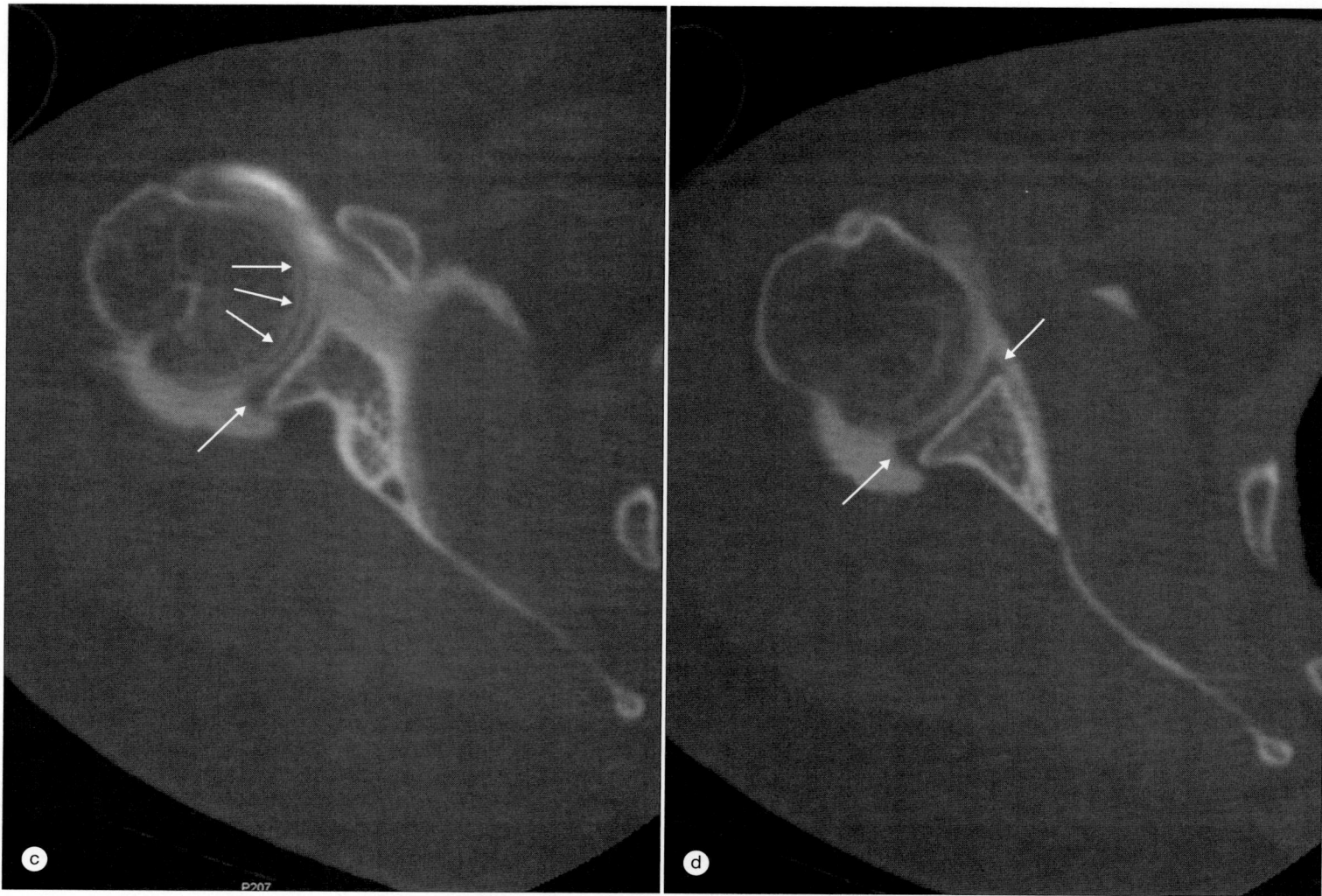

Fig. 38.12, cont'd (c) Axial MDCT scan acquired through the right shoulder joint after intra-articular injection of dilute radiographic contrast agent demonstrates the articular cartilage of the humeral head as a low-density structure (arrowheads) clearly outlined by the high-contrast material. The posterior labrum is well visualized (arrow). (d) A more distal slice demonstrates the anterior and posterior portion of the glenoid labrum (arrows).

REFERENCES

1. Sharp JT. Measurement of structural abnormalities in arthritis using radiographic images. Radiol Clin North Am 2004;42:109-119.
2. Lane NE, Nevitt MC, Genant HK, Hochberg MC. Reliability of new indices of radiographic osteoarthritis of the hand and hip and lumbar disc degeneration. J Rheumatol 1993;20:1911-1918.
3. Hoving JL, Buchbinder R, Hall S, et al. A comparison of magnetic resonance imaging, sonography and radiography of the hand in patients with early rheumatoid arthritis. J Rheumatol 2004;31:663-675.
4. Ostergaard, M, Ejbjerg B, Szkudlarek M. Imaging in early rheumatoid arthritis: roles of magnetic resonance imaging, ultrasonography, conventional radiography and computed tomography. Best Pract Res Clin Rheumatol 2005;19:91-115.
5. Brower AC, Flemming DJ. Arthritis in black and white, 2nd ed. Philadelphia: WB Saunders, 1997.
6. Sartorius DJ, Resnick D. Plain film radiography: routine and specialized techniques and projections. In: Diagnosis of bone and joint disorders, 3rd ed. Philadelphia: WB Saunders, 1995:(1):3-40.
7. Weiss A. A technique for demonstrating fine detail in bones of the hands. Clin Radiol 1972;23:185.
8. Genant HK. Methods of assessing radiographic change in rheumatoid arthritis. Am J Med 1983;75:35-47.
9. Sundaram MB, Brodeur AE, Burdge RE, et al. The clinical value of direct magnification radiography in orthopedics. Skel Radiol 1978;3:85.
10. Genant HK, Doi K, Mall JC, et al. Direct radiographic magnification for skeletal radiology: an assessment of image quality and clinical application. Radiology 1977;123:47.
11. Van Der Jagt EJ, Hofman S, Kraft BM, Van Leewen MA. Can we see enough? A comparative study of film-screen vs digital radiographs in small lesions in rheumatoid arthritis. Eur Radiol 2000;10:304-307.
12. Gupta KB, Duryea J, Weissman BN. Radiographic evaluation of osteoarthritis. Radiol Clin North Am 2004;42:11-41.
13. Conrozier T, Vignon E. Quantitative radiography in osteoarthritis: computerized measurement of radiographic knee and hip joint space. Baillière's Clin Rheumatol 1996;10:429-433.
14. Duryea J, Jiang Y, Zakharevich M, Genant HK. Neural network based algorithm to quantify joint space width in joints of the hand for arthritis assessment. Med Phys 2000;27:1185-1194.
15. Arndt RD, Horns JW, Gold RH. Clinical arthrography. Baltimore: Williams & Wilkins, 1981.
16. Buckwalter KA, Rydberg J, Kopecky KK, et al. Musculoskeletal imaging with multislice CT. AJR Am J Roentgenol 2001;176:979-986.
17. Perry D, Stewart N, Benton N, et al. Detection of erosions in the rheumatoid hand: a comparative study of multidetector computerized tomography versus magnetic resonance scanning. J Rheumatol 2005;32:256-267.
18. Guermazi A, Taouli B, Lynch JA, Peterfy CG. Imaging of bone erosion in rheumatoid arthritis. Imag Arthritis 2004;8:269-285.
19. Farber J. CT arthrography and postoperative musculoskeletal imaging with multichannel computed tomography. Semin Musculoskel Radiol 2004;8:157-166.
20. Bennett DL, Ohashi K, El'Khoury GY. Spondyloarthropathies: ankylosing spondylitis and psoriatic arthritis. Radiol Clin North Am 2004;42:121-134.
21. Pipitone N, Versari A, Salvarani C. Rheumatology 2008;47:403-408.
22. Gotway MB, Araoz PA, Macedo TA, et al. Imaging findings in Takayasu's arteritis. AJR Am J Roentgenol 2005;184:1945-1950.
23. Chung JW, Kim HC, Choi YH, et al. Patterns of aortic involvement in Takayasu arteritis and its clinical implications: evaluation with spiral computed tomography angiography. J Vasc Surg 2007;45:906-914.
24. Paul JF, Fiessinger JN, Sapoval M, et al. Follow-up electron beam CT for the management of early phase Takayasu arteritis. J Comput Assist Tomogr 2001;25:924-931.
25. Schmidt WA, Both M, Reinhold-Keller E. Imaging in vasculitis. Rheumatol Z 2006;65:652-661.

Magnetic resonance imaging

Lauren Shapiro and Garry Gold

39

- Magnetic resonance imaging (MRI), with its versatility and high sensitivity, allows for a comprehensive assessment of the anatomy and pathology of the musculoskeletal system.
- Three dimensional (3D) imaging sequences have been developed and can be used to obtain isotropic resolution allowing for imaging reformation in oblique planes.
- Measurement of cartilage thickness and mapping using 3D imaging and subsequent segmentation can be used to track the progress of osteoarthritis.
- T2 relaxation time measurements can be useful in characterizing the state of fibrocartilage tissues such as the menisci and ligaments by detecting changes in the cartilage matrix.
- Tirho imaging is another physiologic MR imaging technique that can help visualize some of the earliest biomarkers of osteoarthritis through changes in macromolecular content such as proteoglycan depletion.
- Sodium imaging, another physiologic MR imaging technique, is sensitive to fairly small changes in proteoglycan depletion and provides a strong method with which to study, diagnose, and treat early stage osteoarthritis.

INTRODUCTION

Magnetic resonance imaging (MRI) is an extremely versatile and highly sensitive imaging modality that is used to evaluate soft tissue and bone in pathology of the musculoskeletal system.[1] The wide range of contrast mechanisms available for MRI and the continuing development of new software and hardware have resulted in improvements in resolution and sensitivity. Unlike radiography and computed tomography (CT), MRI does not use ionizing radiation and, therefore, involves no significant patient risk when used within the U.S. Food and Drug Administration guidelines. The drawbacks to MRI include high costs of equipment and scanning, long imaging times, and potential for motion and other artifacts that may decrease image quality. Despite these limitations, the overall soft tissue contrast and flexibility have helped to establish MRI as the modality of choice for assessment of the musculoskeletal system.

OVERVIEW OF BASIC PRINCIPLES

The fundamental basis of MRI and the property that makes it possible is known as the MR phenomenon. Atoms that possess a net nuclear spin as a result of having an odd number of protons and/or neutrons exhibit this property. Although a number of different nuclei exhibit the nuclear magnetic resonance phenomena and are candidates for MRI, because of its natural abundance, almost all clinical MRI is done with protium (^{1}H).

MRI requires the application of a strong external magnetic field (B_0) within which protons behave like bar magnets with magnetic moments or "spins." The magnetic moment of a single proton is not detectable, but the additive effects of many protons are able to be measured (Fig. 39.1). In the absence of the external magnetic field, proton magnetic moments are oriented randomly and present a net zero moment when summed together. With an applied B_0 field, however, the spins align either parallel (with the magnetic field) or anti-parallel (against the magnetic field). Because a slightly greater number of protons align with the field than against the field, a small net magnetization results in the direction of B_0.

The spins aligned with the external B_0 field precess at a known angular frequency *w*, given by the Larmor equation where $w = \gamma \cdot B_0$. An external radiofrequency (RF) field is applied at the resonant frequency that causes the spins to tip into the transverse plane perpendicular to the main B_0 field. After the spins have been tipped, they begin to relax back toward the z-axis aligned with the B_0 field. This relaxation results in the emission of the MRI signal and is characterized by two exponential decay constants, T1 and T2. These relaxation rates depend on the tissue properties of the sample, and it is these differences in intrinsic T1 and T2 relaxation times that are often exploited to generate MRI contrast. Free induction decay, the process of the relaxation of the spins in the transverse plane, is illustrated in Fig. 39.2.

T2 relaxation

The process of free induction decay is characterized by the exponential time constant T2. The B_1 RF pulse tips the longitudinally oriented spins into the transverse plane. The angle of the tip away from the z-axis is known as the *flip angle*. When tipped into the transverse plane, the spins are coherent and aligned in one direction. Over a period of time, the spins lose phase coherence in the transverse plane and the net magnetization in the x-y plane becomes zero. This is referred to as *spin-spin relaxation*, and the exponential time constant that governs this loss of phase coherence is the T2 relaxation time. The elapsed time between the peak signal and 37% of the peak signal is the T2 decay constant (Fig. 39.3). From a practical perspective, different tissues in the musculoskeletal system have different T2 relaxation times, which greatly impacts their appearance on MR images. T2* relaxation is another important component that contributes to the generation of image contrast. It is defined as the observed time constant for the free induction decay as a result of the loss of phase coherence. T2* decay, which is present on gradient-echo MR images, is shorter than T2 decay.

T1 relaxation

Loss of transverse magnetization or T2 decay occurs relatively quickly, whereas the recovery of the longitudinal magnetization to equilibrium takes longer. This occurs along the z-axis and is referred to as T1 relaxation. As this occurs, individual spins must release their energy to the local tissue by way of a process that is called *spin-lattice relaxation*. The T1 relaxation time constant is the time needed to recover 63% of the longitudinal magnetization after a 90-degree B_1 pulse tips the spins into the x-y plane. Just as different tissues have different T2 relaxation times, they have different T1 relaxation times that impact their appearance on MR images. Measured T2 and T1 relaxation times for common tissues in the musculoskeletal system are available.[2]

MRI contrast

In most MRI experiments, image contrast is determined by a combination of intrinsic proton density of the tissues and the T1, T2, and T2* relaxation times. The operator of the scanner can influence the appearance of the images by changing the timing of the signal acquisition after excitation (known as *echo time* [TE]) or the time between the excitations (known as *repetition time* [TR]). Images are typically acquired using different parameters that take advantage of the different relaxation types. For example, images with a relatively short TE and TR emphasize differences in T1 relaxation times and are therefore referred to as T1-weighted images. Along the same lines, images with a long TR and long TE emphasize differences in T2 relaxation times

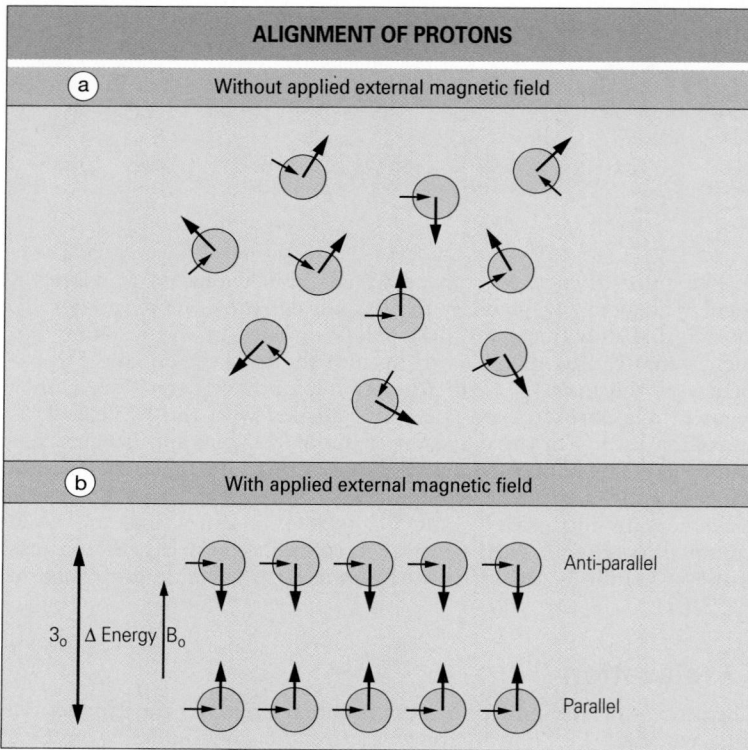

Fig. 39.1 Diagram of the alignment of protons (a) without the applied B_0 field, and (b) after the applied B_0 field. Slightly more protons align parallel with the B_0 field than anti-parallel, resulting in a net magnetization.

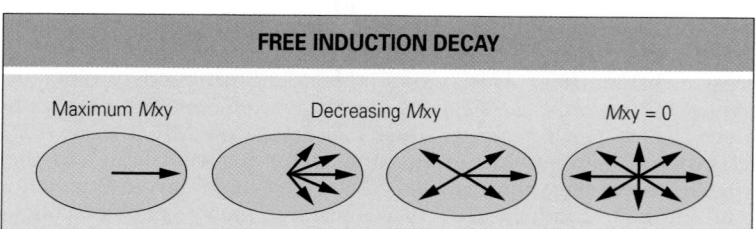

Fig. 39.2 Diagram of free induction decay in MRI. Immediately after excitation, the magnetization in the xy plane (Mxy) is a coherent vector, resulting in the maximum magnetization. As the decay proceeds, the spins lose coherence and eventually are ordered in random directions, giving a net Mxy of zero.

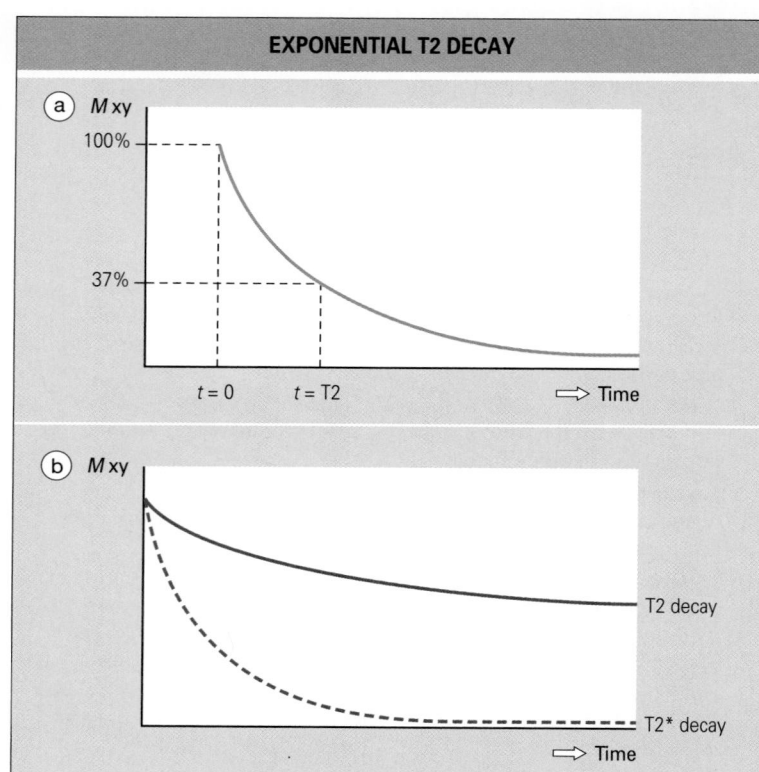

Fig. 39.3 Diagram of exponential spin-spin (T2) decay. (a) After one exponential time constant T2, the magnetization in the xy plane (M xy) has decayed to 37%. (b) Gradient-echo methods demonstrate T2* decay, which is faster than T2 decay. Spin-echo methods in MRI refocus the T2* decay, resulting in T2 decay.

used method is to divide the standard deviation of background noise from a certain region of interest into the mean signal from another region of interest from the same image. SNR is dependent on numerous different variables, including but not limited to field of view, type of coil used, slice thickness, and magnetic field.

CONVENTIONAL MRI METHODS

MRI has emerged as the leading modality for imaging soft tissue structures around joints.[3,4] One of the major advantages of MRI is the ability, as stated earlier, to manipulate contrast to highlight different tissue types. The common contrast mechanisms used in MRI include two-dimensional (2D) multi-slice T1-weighted, proton-density–weighted, and T2-weighted imaging, all of which can be derived with or without fat suppression. Developments in imaging hardware and software have increased considerably in recent years, including improved gradients and RF coils, fast or turbo spin-echo imaging, and techniques such as water-only excitation, thus providing significant advancements in the field of MRI.

Although the tissue relaxation times and imaging parameters are the major determinants of contrast between different types of soft tissue within the joint, lipid suppression increases contrast between non-lipid and lipid-containing tissues and affects how the MR scanner sets the overall dynamic range of the image. The most common type of lipid suppression is fat saturation, in which fat spins are excited and then dephased before imaging. Another type of lipid suppression that can selectively excite water-only spins is known as spectral-spatial excitation.[5] Finally, in areas of magnetic field inhomogeneity, a technique called *inversion recovery* provides a way to suppress lipids that comes at the expense of signal-to-noise and contrast-to-noise ratios.

The type of contrast used in musculoskeletal imaging is critical for the visibility of a pathologic process and the SNR of the tissues. Although T2-weighted imaging creates contrast between short T2 tissues and synovial fluid, it does so at the expense of the MRI signal. The high signal from fluid is useful to highlight defects such as fissuring or tears, but variation in internal short T2 signal is poorly depicted.

and are therefore termed T2-weighted images. Images with a long TR and short TE are proton-density weighted because contrast in these images is generated as a result of differences in tissue proton density rather than differences in T1 or T2.

IMAGE QUALITY

An essential aspect of MRI deals with the ability to evaluate and compare images obtained from different techniques. A variety of strategies are available with which to assess image quality; however, the three most valuable means for comparison include contrast sensitivity, spatial resolution, and signal-to-noise ratio (SNR). Contrast sensitivity is one of the primary reasons as to why MRI is so useful. As a result of MRI's versatility, contrast sensitivity can be altered to the parameters necessary for viewing the desired anatomy or pathologic process by changing the T1, T2, flow velocity properties, and spin densities. Spatial resolution is known as the ability of an imaging system to distinguish between two objects as they decrease in size and move closer together. Spatial resolution is dependent on matrix size, field of view, and slice thickness. SNR is used to measure the amount of the desired signal to the amount of background noise (or "random" signal). There are several technologically advanced and more robust, precise methods of calculating SNR, but the general idea and most commonly

Also, T2-weighted scans are often 2D, leaving small gaps between slices that may contain small areas of tissue damage.

Another technique, called three-dimensional spoiled gradient-recalled-echo imaging with fat suppression (3D-SPGR), destroys or spoils the transverse magnetization between successive TRs. This method produces high cartilage signal but low signal from adjacent joint fluid. Currently, this technique is the standard for quantitative morphologic imaging of cartilage.[6] This technique is useful for cartilage volume and thickness measurements but does not adequately highlight surface defects with fluid and does not allow thorough evaluation of other joint structures such as ligaments or menisci.

MRI of joints requires close attention to imaging spatial resolution. For example, to see early morphologic degenerative changes in cartilage, imaging with resolution on the order of 0.2 to 0.4 mm is required.[7] The ultimate resolution achievable is governed by the SNR possible within a given imaging time and system. Use of high field strength and dedicated phased-array or surface coils usually results in the best possible resolution *in vivo*. Eventually, a high-resolution imaging technique that provides morphologic and physiologic information together would be ideal in the evaluation of joints. Given current techniques, it is likely that a combination of a high-resolution morphologic imaging sequence with a sequence for evaluation of tissue physiology will be the most useful.

2D fast spin-echo imaging

Currently, imaging of the musculoskeletal system with MRI is often limited to 2D multi-slice acquisitions acquired in multiple planes. This is commonly done with turbo or fast spin-echo (FSE) methods. These methods provide excellent SNR and contrast between tissues of interest, but the voxels produced are anisotropic and have slice gaps, resulting in the inability to reformat the images into multiple, oblique planes. For example, a typical sagittal image may have 0.3 to 0.6 mm in-plane resolution but a slice thickness of 2 to 5 mm. FSE techniques show excellent results in detection of cartilage lesions (Fig. 39.4).[8] These methods provide excellent depiction of structures in the imaging plane, but evaluation of oblique or small structures across multiple slices can be challenging. For these reasons, 3D acquisitions with thin slices are more appealing.

2D FSE methods are the primary clinical sequences used for internal derangements of joints. These methods are used for detection of bone marrow edema,[9] effusions, synovium,[3] and ligament and meniscal tears.[4] Several scoring systems for osteoarthritis have been developed based on this acquisition method, including the Whole-organ Osteoarthritis Scoring (WORMS), Boston-Leeds Osteoarthritis Knee Scoring (BLOKS), and Knee Osteoarthritis Scoring System (KOSS).[10,11]

3D gradient-echo techniques

3D MRI sequences are extremely valuable because they produce images with isotropic voxels that do not contain slice gaps. Because of these characteristics the images can be reformatted into various, oblique planes, thereby improving the visualization of the anatomy while shortening the examination time. Traditional 3D gradient-recalled-echo (3D-GRE) methods have the potential to acquire data with isotropic voxel sizes but suffer from a lack of contrast, especially when compared with 2D spin-echo approaches. High accuracy for cartilage lesions has been shown with 3D-SPGR imaging[1,12,13]; however, there are two main disadvantages to this approach: (1) lack of reliable contrast between tissue and fluid that outlines defects and (2) long imaging times that may require up to 8 minutes. Because of the lack of reliable fluid sensitivity, 3D-GRE methods are less useful for diagnosis of ligament or meniscal tears than spin-echo techniques. Despite the previously mentioned limitations, 3D-SPGR is considered the standard for morphologic imaging of cartilage.[6]

The SPGR and GRE techniques can be combined with water-fat separation methods such as iterative decomposition of water and fat with echo asymmetry and least squares estimation (IDEAL) to produce excellent-quality water and fat images with high resolution (up to 0.3 × 0.3 × 1.0 mm). The SPGR method suppresses signal from joint fluid, whereas the GRE method accentuates it (Fig. 39.5). Compared with balanced steady-state free precession (see later), these methods are less SNR efficient but also less sensitive to magnetic field inhomogeneity. Therefore, an ideal 3D cartilage imaging sequence that provides an optimal combination of resolution, SNR efficiency, and minimal artifacts has yet to be established. As such, a number of newer techniques have been established to improve cartilage imaging.

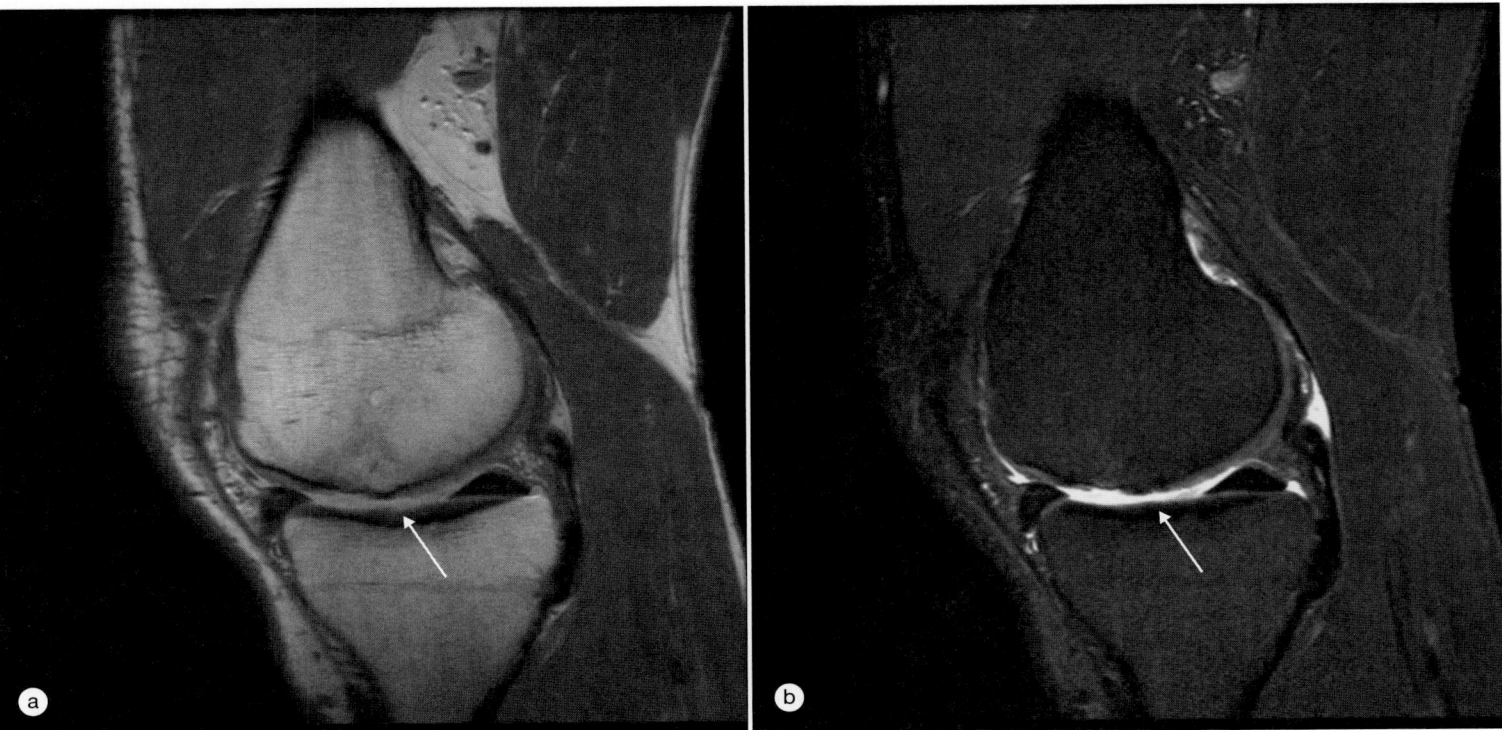

Fig. 39.4 Two-dimensional fast spin-echo MR images from a patient with cartilage damage. (a) Sagittal proton-density image showing medial compartment cartilage loss (arrow). (b) Sagittal T2-weighted image with fat suppression showing the same medial compartment damage (arrow).

Continued

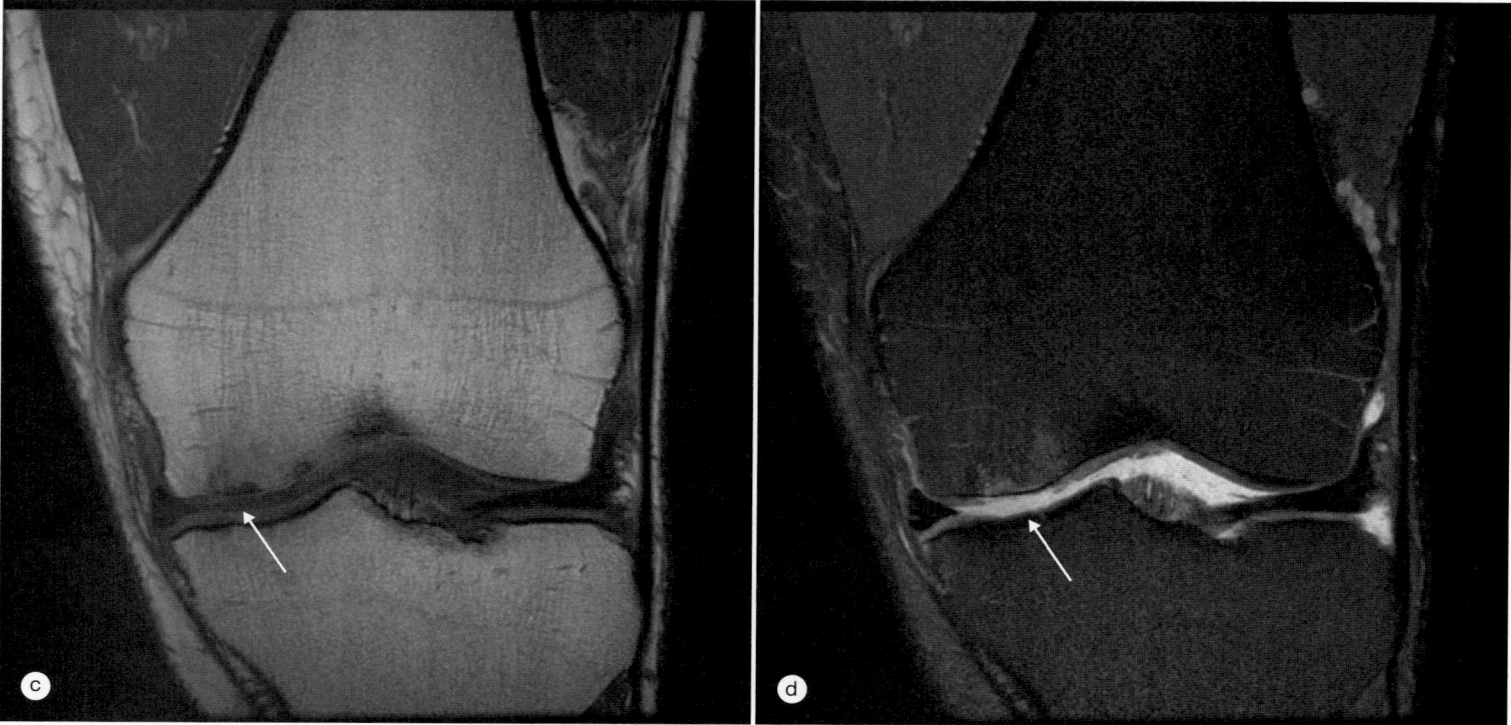

Fig. 39.4, cont'd (c) Coronal T1-weighted image showing medial compartment damage (arrow). Fluid is dark on this image. (d) Coronal T2-weighted image with fat suppression showing medial compartment damage (arrow).

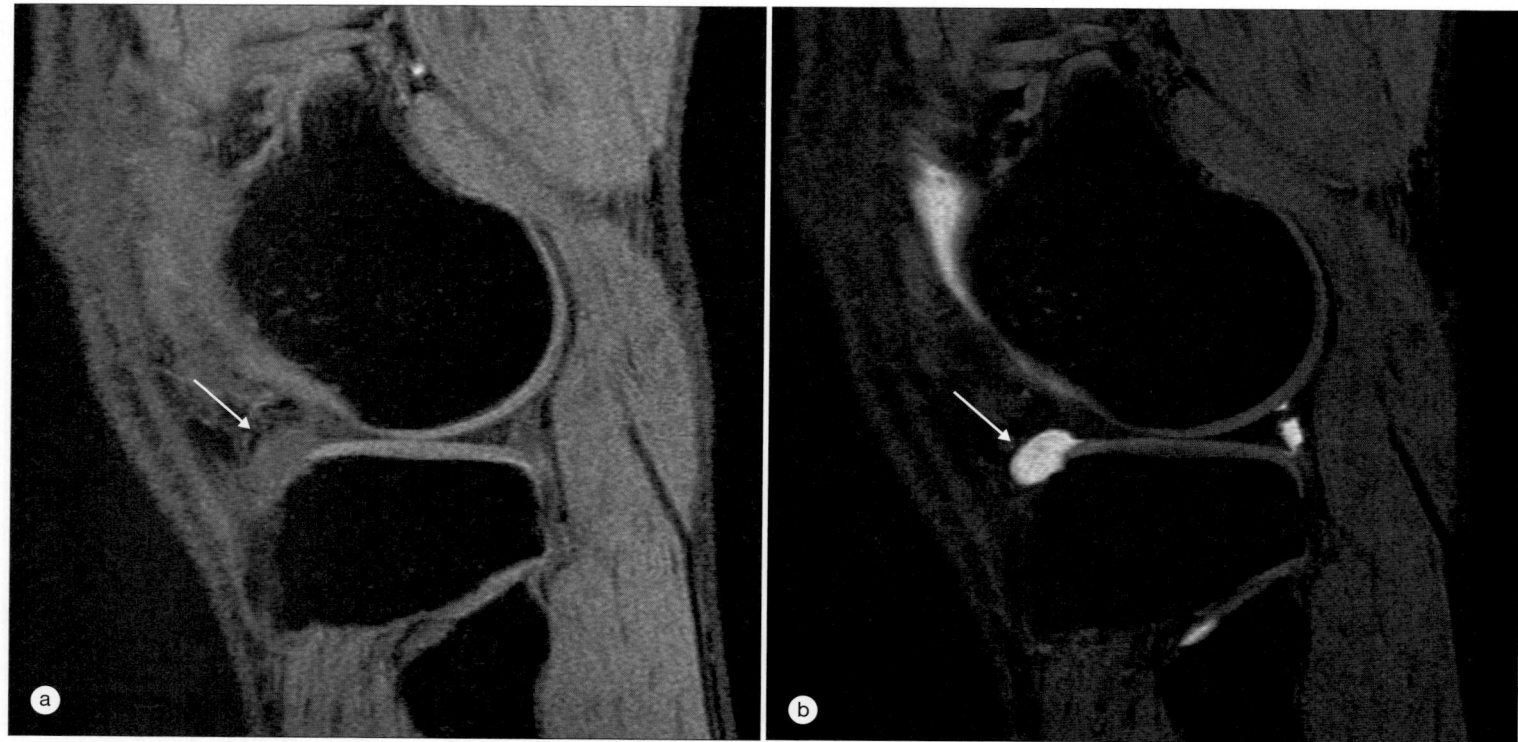

Fig. 39.5 Three-dimensional gradient-echo images of a healthy volunteer. (a) Sagittal spoiled gradient-recalled-echo (SPGR) showing bright cartilage but intermediate to dark fluid (arrow). (b) Sagittal gradient-recalled-echo (GRE) showing bright cartilage and brighter fluid (arrow).

ADVANCED MRI TECHNIQUES

Dual-echo steady-state imaging

Dual-echo steady-state (DESS) imaging has proven useful for evaluation of cartilage morphology, for both volumetric and degradation assessment, due to its ability to maximize contrast between cartilage and synovial fluid.[13a,b,c] This technique acquires two or more gradient echoes separated by a refocusing pulse and then combines both echoes into the image. This results in an image with higher T2* weighting, which has bright signal from both cartilage and synovial fluid. This is currently the imaging method of choice for cartilage evaluation in the Osteoarthritis Initiative.[12]

Driven equilibrium Fourier transform imaging

Driven equilibrium Fourier transform (DEFT) imaging has been used in the past as a method of signal enhancement in spectroscopy.[1] The sequence uses a 90-degree pulse to return magnetization to the z-axis, increasing signal from tissues with long T1 relaxation times such as synovial fluid. Unlike conventional T1- or T2-weighted MRI, the contrast in DEFT is dependent on the ratio of the T1/T2 of a given tissue. For musculoskeletal imaging, DEFT produces contrast by enhancing the signal from synovial fluid, rather than attenuating the signal from cartilage as in T2-weighted sequences. This results in bright synovial fluid at short TR. At short TR, DEFT shows much greater cartilage-to-fluid contrast than SPGR, proton-density FSE, or T2-weighted FSE.[14] DEFT imaging has been combined with a 3D echoplanar readout to make it an efficient 3D cartilage imaging technique. Unlike T2-weighted FSE, cartilage signal is preserved owing to the short TE. A high-resolution 3D dataset of the entire knee using 512 × 192 matrix, 14 cm field-of-view, and 3-mm slices can be acquired in about 6 minutes. Initial studies of cartilage morphology have been done using DEFT imaging,[13] but this technique has not been conclusively proven to be superior to 2D approaches. A sequence similar to DEFT that has been used in musculoskeletal imaging is FSE with driven equilibrium pulses, referred to as a DRIVE sequence.[1,14]

Balanced steady-state free precession imaging

Balanced steady-state free precession (bSSFP) MRI is an efficient, high signal method for obtaining 3D MR images.[1] Depending on the manufacturer of the MRI scanner, this method is also called True-FISP (Siemens), FIESTA (General Electric), or balanced FFE imaging (Phillips).[15] With recent advances in MR gradient hardware, it is now possible to use bSSFP without suffering from the banding or off-resonance artifacts that were previously a problem with this method. However, banding artifacts due to off-resonance are still an issue as TR increases, or at 3.0 T. Hence, TR is usually kept below 10 ms with these techniques, which limits overall image resolution. Multiple acquisition bSSFP can be used to achieve higher resolution at the cost of additional scan time.[1]

Many methods have been proposed to provide fat suppression with bSSFP imaging. If the TR is sufficiently short and the magnetic field is homogeneous, conventional fat suppression or water excitation pulses can be used.[16] Linear combinations of bSSFP[17] and fluctuating equilibrium MRI (FEMR)[18] use the frequency difference between fat and water and do multiple acquisitions to separate fat and water. Intermittent fat suppression uses transient fat saturation pulses to suppress lipid signal.[19] IDEAL uses multiple acquisitions to separate fat and water but does not depend on the fat-water frequency difference to constrain the TR.[20] Rapid separation of water and fat can be achieved with phase detection.[21]

Several studies have demonstrated the utility of bSSFP imaging for articular cartilage and other musculoskeletal tissues.[22] Because of the bright synovial fluid and 3D nature of the acquisition, bSSFP is also useful for internal derangements, including ligaments and menisci, making it more generally useful than SPGR. A variant of bSSFP imaging known as vastly interpolated projection reconstruction imaging (VIPR) has been shown to be useful in imaging the cartilage, ligaments, and menisci in a rapid manner with isotropic resolution (Fig. 39.6).[23]

3D fast spin-echo imaging

2D FSE is a powerful clinical tool but, as stated previously, this method suffers from anisotropic voxels, slice gaps, and partial volume effects. 3D acquisitions with FSE were applied in brain imaging several years ago.[24] 3D FSE, with flip angle modulation to reduce blurring and parallel imaging to reduce imaging time, has made isotropic imaging with spin-echo contrast a clinical reality.[24,25] Preliminary studies demonstrating the effectiveness of using 3D FSE with isotropic resolution in the knee[24] and ankle[26] have been published. Images from this method show isotropic resolution with the ability to obtain high-quality multiplanar reformatted images (Fig. 39.7). A recent study involving more than 100 patients with arthroscopic correlation revealed that 3D FSE was equal to a combination of multiple planes of 2D FSE in the diagnosis of ligament, menisci, and cartilage defects.

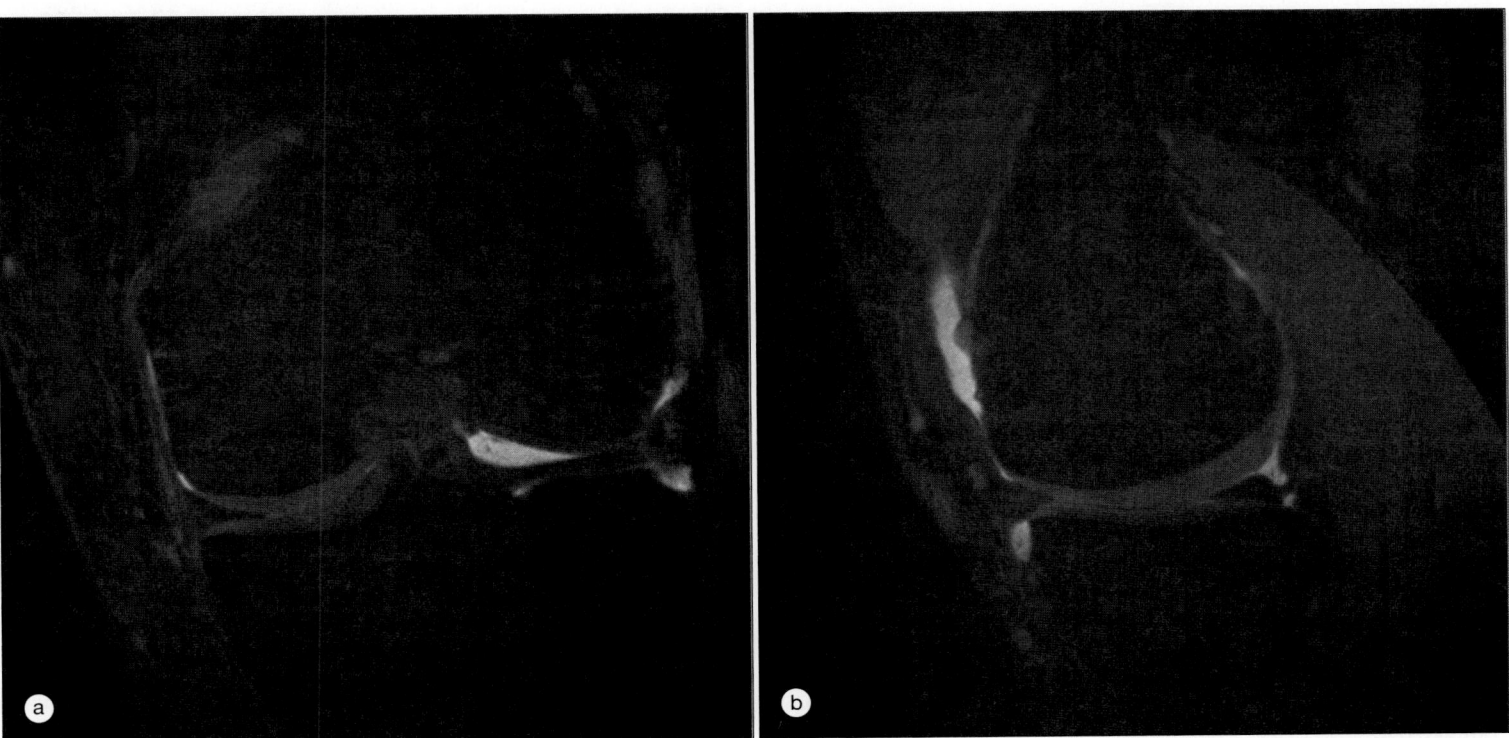

Fig. 39.6 Vastly interpolated projection reconstruction (VIPR) balanced steady-state free precession (bSSFP) images of the knee at 3.0 T in a healthy volunteer. This technique produces isotropic 0.4-mm resolution across the knee, allowing reformatted images in any imaging plane. Scan time was only 5 minutes. (a) Coronal image, 2-mm section thickness. (b) Sagittal reformatted image, 2-mm section thickness.

Continued

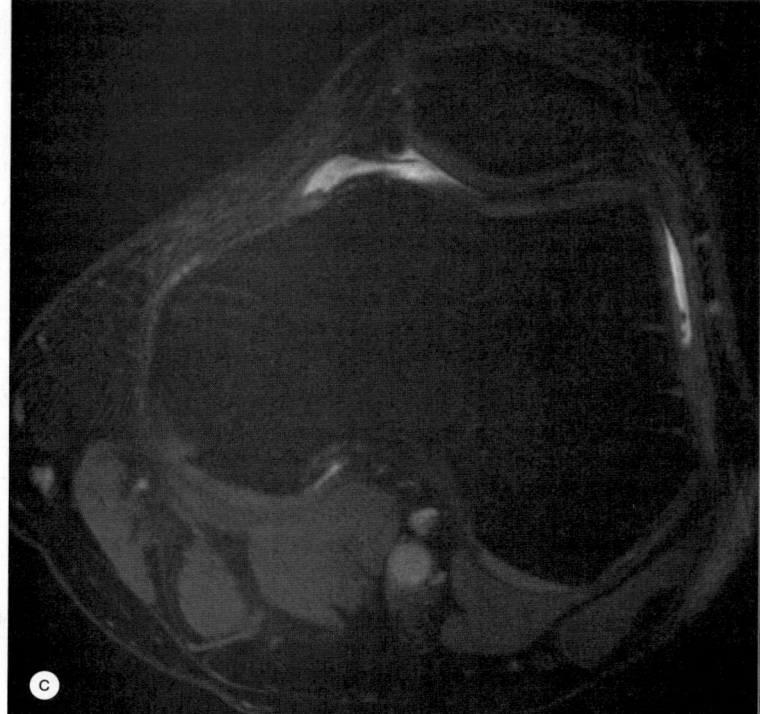

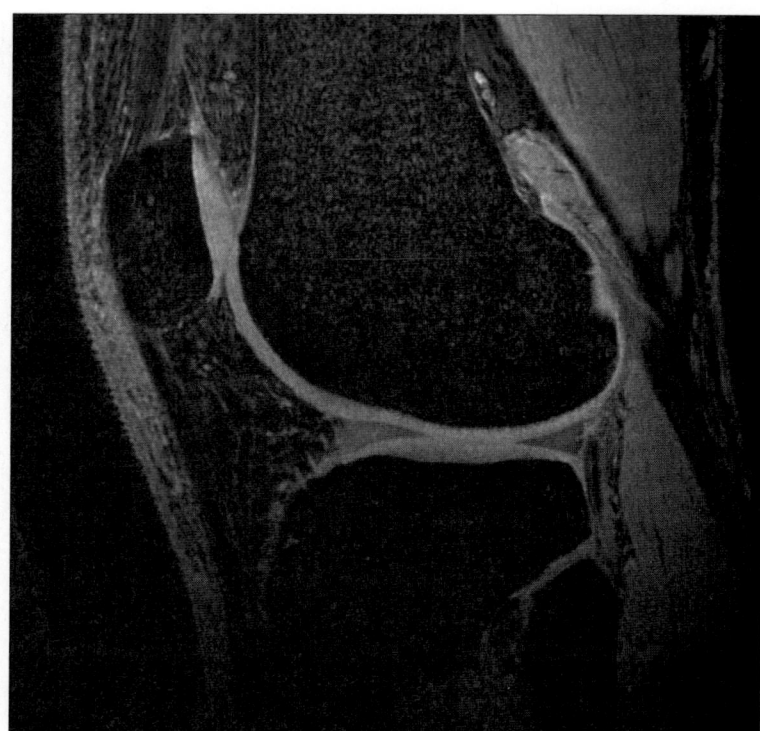

Fig. 39.6, cont'd (c) Axial reformatted image, 2-mm section thickness. *(Courtesy of W. Block, University of Wisconsin, Madison.)*

Fig. 39.8 Sagittal image of a healthy volunteer at 7.0 T using a 3D spoiled gradient-echo (SPGR) method. Resolution was 0.3 × 0.3 × 1.0 mm. *(Courtesy of R. Regatte, New York University.)*

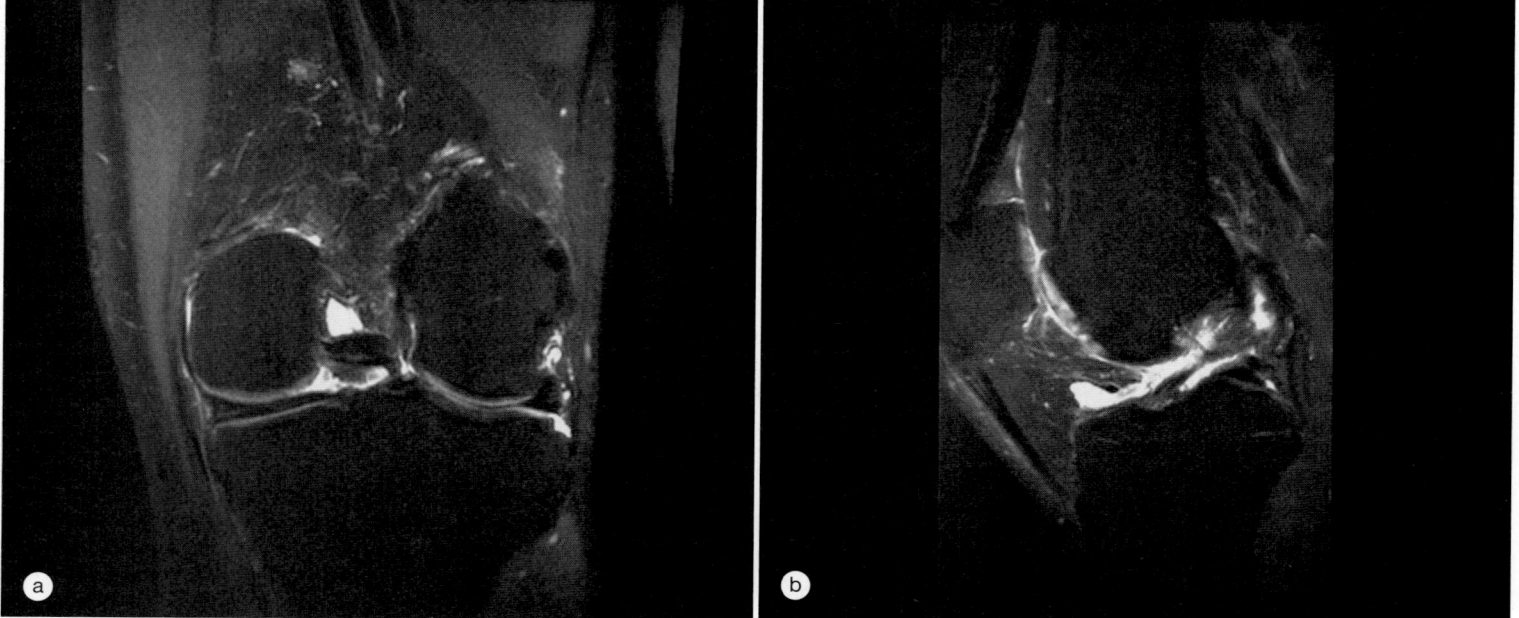

Fig. 39.7 Three-dimensional fast spin-echo imaging using flip-angle modulation and parallel imaging. This acquisition was done at 3.0 T with an imaging time of 5 minutes and an isotropic 0.6-mm resolution. (a) Coronal image, 2-mm section thickness. (b) Sagittal reformatted image, 2-mm section thickness.

High-field MRI

Several centers currently have 7.0-T human MRI systems available for research purposes. Although these systems suffer from problems of RF penetration and high power deposition, they have a considerable SNR advantage over lower field systems.[27] These systems are able to get to a higher resolution in a shorter period of time and may be useful for showing tissue ultrastructure. Fig. 39.8 shows a representative dataset at 7.0 T from a healthy volunteer using a SPGR acquisition. This example shows it is possible to acquire high-resolution (0.3 × 0.4

× 1.5 mm) morphologic data in as little as 3 minutes with excellent SNR.

Cartilage thickness and volume mapping

Measurement of cartilage thickness and volume can be useful in tracking the progress of osteoarthritis. Multicenter studies such as the Osteoarthritis Initiative use high-resolution 3D imaging of cartilage followed by manual or semi-automated segmentation of the images, demonstrating that changes in cartilage thickness in high-risk populations can be visualized in as little as 1 year.[28] Fig. 39.9 shows a 3D reconstruction of knee cartilage from MRI data.

MR Imaging to demonstrate physiologic activity

Contrast-enhanced imaging

Intravenous contrast agents in MRI often contain gadolinium coupled to a large molecule to prevent toxicity. These agents reduce the T1 relaxation time of tissue that is vascular, and areas of enhancement show up as bright on T1-weighted images. These images are often acquired with fat suppression to improve the dynamic range and conspicuity of the enhancing tissues. This technique is especially useful in the area of inflammatory arthritis because synovium and pannus are quite vascular and show considerable contrast enhancement (Fig.

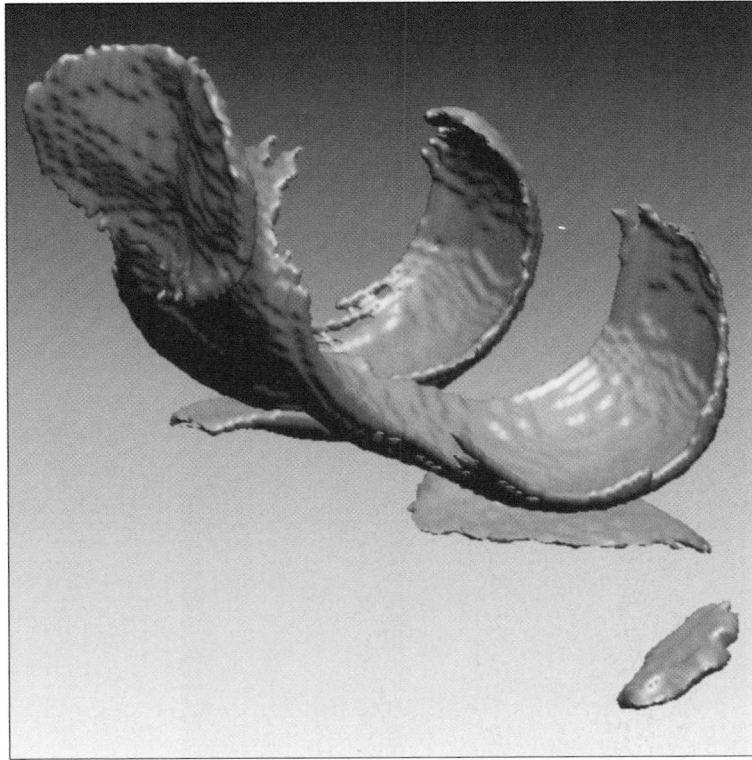

Fig. 39.9 Three-dimensional volume rendering of cartilage from segmented high-resolution MRI. Segmentation allows quantitative measurements of thickness and volume.

39.10). This method can be used to track synovitis in osteoarthritis as well as the activity of drugs for inflammatory arthropathies.[29]

T2 relaxation time mapping

The T2 relaxation time is a function of both the water content and collagen ultrastructure of the tissue. Measurement of the spatial distribution of the T2 relaxation time may reveal areas of increased or decreased water content, correlating with tissue damage. To measure the T2 relaxation time with a high degree of accuracy, attention must be taken with the MR technique. Typically, a multi-echo spin-echo technique is used and signal levels are fitted to one or more decaying exponentials, depending on whether it is believed that there is more than one distribution of T2 within the sample.[30] However, for TEs used in conventional MRI, a single exponential fit is adequate. An image of the T2 relaxation time is then generated with either a color or a gray-scale map representing the relaxation time, as shown in Fig. 39.11.

Several investigators have measured the spatial distribution of T2 relaxation times within articular cartilage. Aging appears to be associated with an increase in T2 relaxation times in the transitional zone.[31] Relaxation time measurements have also been shown to be anisotropic with respect to orientation in the main magnetic field.[32] Focal increases in T2 relaxation times within cartilage have been associated with matrix damage, particularly loss of collagen integrity. Studies on T2 relaxation times documenting the effects of age,[31] gender,[33] and activity[34] have also been published. T2 relaxation time measurements may also be useful in characterizing the state of fibrocartilage tissues such as the menisci and ligaments.[35]

T1rho mapping

A promising technique for evaluating cartilage and other tissues is T1rho imaging, which involves the relaxation of spins under the influence of an RF field.[36] This technique may be sensitive to early proteoglycan depletion.[36,37] In typical T1rho imaging, magnetization is tipped into the transverse plane and "spin locked" by a constant RF field. Recent advances in T1rho imaging have led to rapid cartesian acquisition strategies for 3.0 T.[38,39] An example of a T1rho map from the tibia of a healthy volunteer is shown in Fig. 39.11. This method has also been shown to be useful in detection of early meniscal pathology.[40]

Delayed contrast-enhanced imaging

One of the most common MRI contrast agents, Magnevist or Gd-DTPA2− (Berlex, Richmond, CA), has a negative charge. After intravenous injection of Gd-DTPA2−, it penetrates into cartilage and concentrates where the cartilage glycosaminoglycan (GAG) content is relatively low. Subsequent T1 imaging (which is reflective of Gd-DTPA2− concentration) therefore yields an image depicting GAG distribution. This technique is referred to as delayed gadolinium enhanced MRI of cartilage (dGEMRIC), with the "delay" referring to

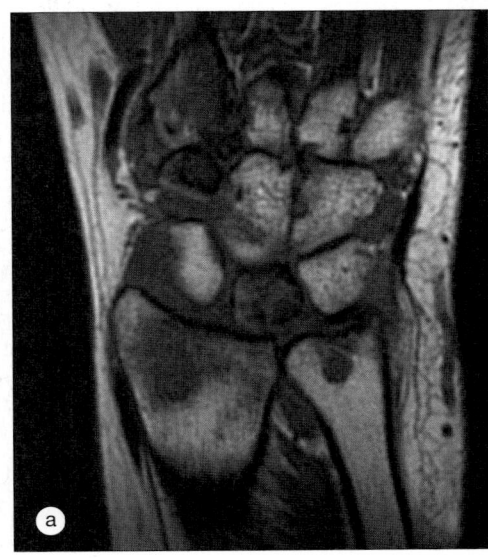
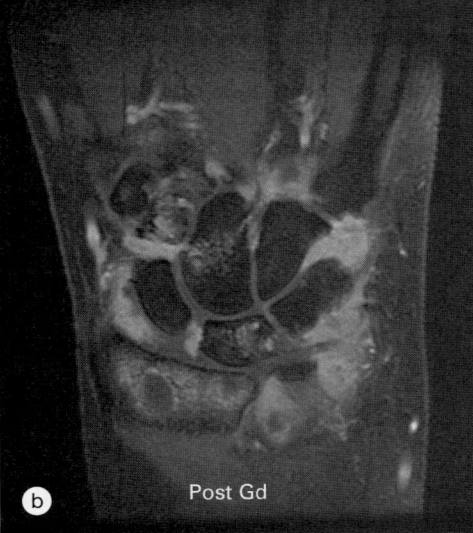

Fig. 39.10 Coronal MR images from a patient with rheumatoid arthritis. (a) T1-weighted image shows bone erosions as areas of signal loss in the marrow fat. (b) Contrast-enhanced image of the wrist shows brightly enhancing synovium and pannus.

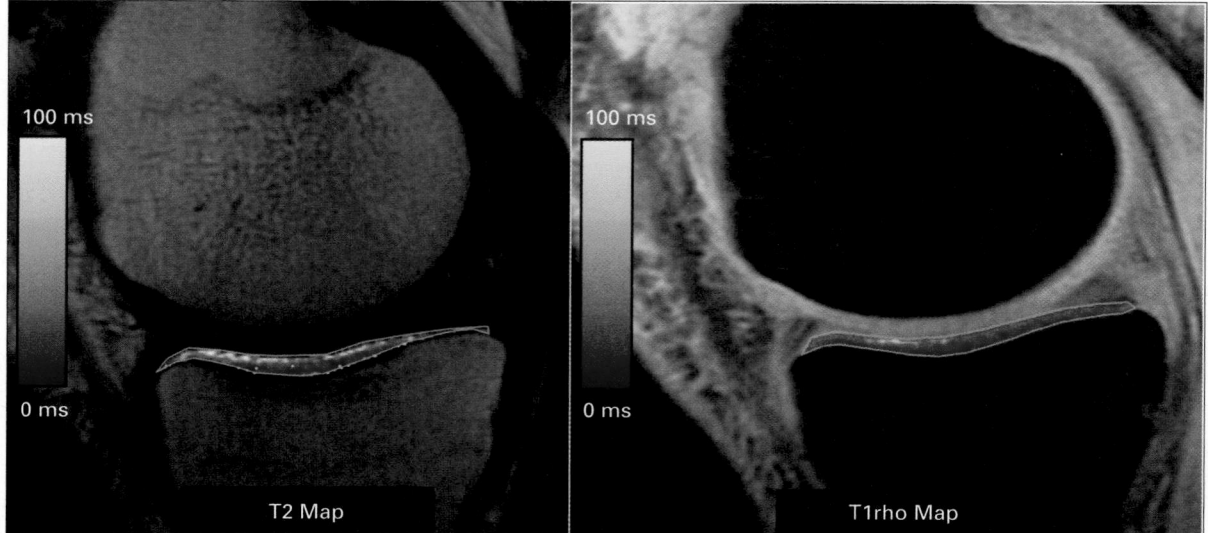

Fig. 39.11 Measurements of tissue physiology with MRI. T2 map (left) and T1rho map (right) of the tibia cartilage in a healthy volunteer. The color scale shows relative relaxation time values between 0 and 100 ms. Changes in T2 relaxation time are correlated with collagen matrix status; changes in T1rho are correlated with proteoglycan content.

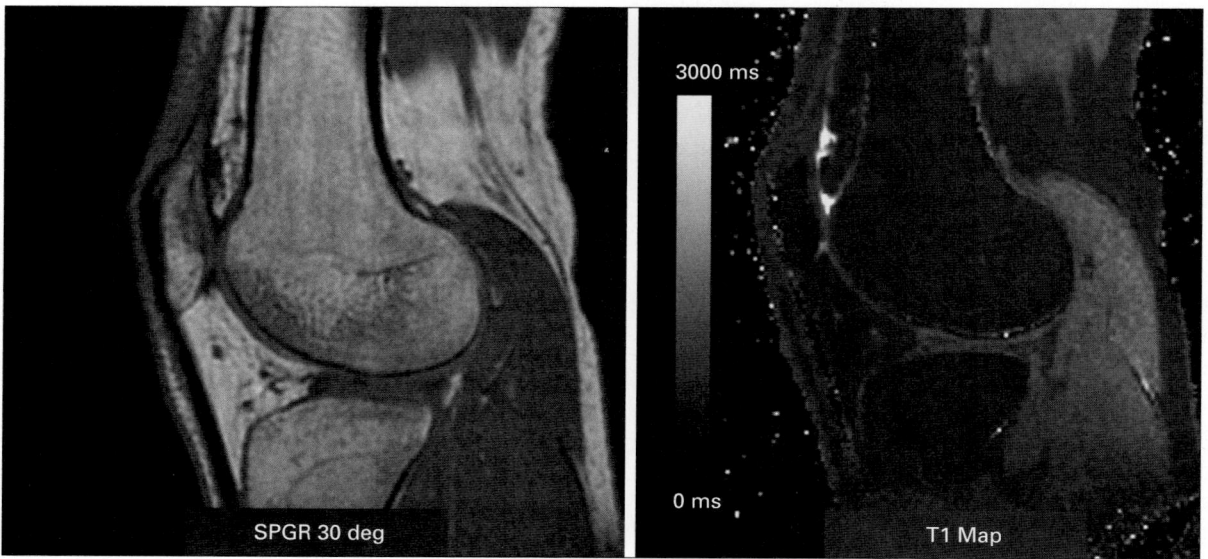

Fig. 39.12 Delayed gadolinium-enhanced MRI of cartilage (dGEMRIC) in a healthy volunteer. The left image is a spoiled gradient-echo image used to map the T1 relaxation times. The right image is a T1 relaxation time map with a gray scale from 0 to 3000 ms.

the time needed for the Gd-DTPA2− to penetrate the cartilage tissue.[41] A T1 map of the cartilage allows assessment of GAG content, with lower values corresponding to areas of GAG depletion.

A number of clinical cross-sectional studies on specified populations have provided interesting observations. For example, a recent study reported that individuals who exercise on a regular basis have higher dGEMRIC indices (denoting higher GAG) than individuals who are sedentary. In a relatively large study of patients with hip dysplasia, measures of the severity of dysplasia (the radiographically determined lateral center edge angle) and of pain both correlated with the dGEMRIC index but not with the standard radiologic parameter of joint space narrowing. In another study, lesions in patients with osteoarthritis were more apparent with the dGEMRIC technique relative to standard MRI scans.[42] A recent study relevant to osteoarthritis showed that dGEMRIC correlated with Kellgren/Lawrence radiographic grading of osteoarthritis.[43] Combining dGEMRIC methods with T2 mapping requires careful attention to technique.[43] It is important to note that, as a free ion, Gd-DTPA2− can be toxic; however, FDA approved Gd-DTPA2− contrast agents are chelated, which greatly reduces their toxicity. Those patients with renal insufficiency or dysfunction should avoid imaging with this contrast agent.[43a]

Physiologic methods such as dGEMRIC and T2 mapping can be time consuming and difficult to perform on a routine basis. dGEMRIC is often performed using a variable flip angle 3D-SPGR approach, as shown in Fig. 39.12.[43,44] SSFP methods also show promise in improving the speed and SNR of T1 and T2 relaxation time measurements.[45]

Sodium MRI

Because sodium-23 ([23]Na) consists of an odd number of protons and/or neutrons it possesses a net nuclear spin and, like ^{1}H, can exhibit the MR phenomenon. [23]Na MRI has been shown to be useful in musculoskeletal imaging owing to the natural abundance of sodium in articular cartilage. As a result of the opposing charges associated with sodium and GAG, [23]Na MRI can be used to estimate the GAG content in cartilage. Despite being both accurate and non-invasive, [23]Na MRI requires high-field MRI systems (3.0 or 7.0 T). The concentration of [23]Na in normal human cartilage is about 320 µM, with T2 relaxation times between 2 and 10 ms.[46] The combination of lower resonant frequency, lower concentration, and shorter T2 relaxation times than ^{1}H make *in vivo* imaging of [23]Na challenging. A limitation of [23]Na MRI is that it requires the use of special transmit and receive coils, along

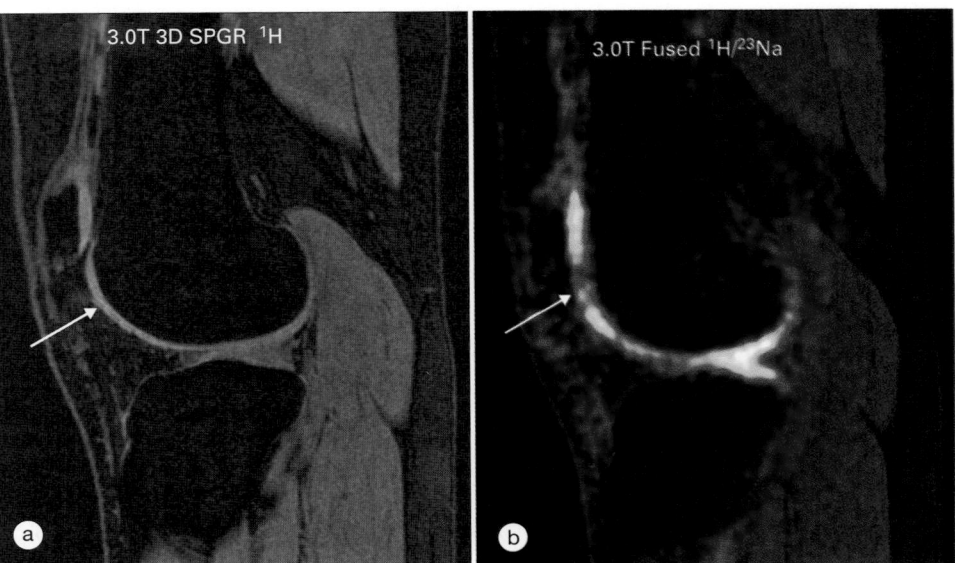

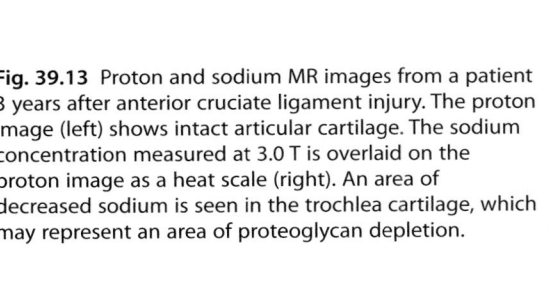

Fig. 39.13 Proton and sodium MR images from a patient 3 years after anterior cruciate ligament injury. The proton image (left) shows intact articular cartilage. The sodium concentration measured at 3.0 T is overlaid on the proton image as a heat scale (right). An area of decreased sodium is seen in the trochlea cartilage, which may represent an area of proteoglycan depletion.

with the fact that relatively long imaging times are needed to achieve adequate SNR.

^{23}Na MRI has recently shown some promising results in the imaging of articular cartilage as a result of its ability to depict regions of proteoglycan depletion.[46] The ^{23}Na atoms are associated with the high fixed-charge density present in proteoglycan sulfate and carboxylate groups. Some spatial variation in ^{23}Na concentration is present within normal cartilage.[46] Because of the short T2 relaxation times of sodium, imaging is often done with a non-cartesian trajectory.[47] Fig. 39.13 shows proton and sodium images from the knee of a patient with a prior ligament injury. These were acquired at 3.0 T with a 3D cones technique.[48] High sodium concentration is seen throughout most of the cartilage, but an area of lower sodium signal is seen in the trochlea. In cartilage samples, sodium imaging has also been shown to be sensitive to small changes in proteoglycan concentration.[49] This method shows promise to be sensitive to early decreases in proteoglycan concentration in osteoarthritis and can be even more sensitive to early changes through the use of triple-quantum-filtered imaging.[50]

CONCLUSION

MRI provides a powerful tool for the imaging and understanding of musculoskeletal tissue. Improvements have been made in morphologic imaging of joints, in terms of contrast, resolution, and acquisition time. This allows for the development of detailed tissue maps and the ability to quantify both thickness and volume. Much progress has been made in the imaging of joint physiology. Important areas include the detection of changes in proteoglycan content and collagen ultrastructure in cartilage and other tissues.

The choice of a particular MRI protocol for imaging joints depends greatly on patient factors. For many patients with internal derangement, imaging with standard FSE and/or 3D-SPGR sequences may suffice. For patients being considered for surgical or pharmacologic therapy, however, a more detailed evaluation may be required. For example, fast morphologic imaging along with evaluation of cartilage physiology may allow for non-invasive evaluation of cartilage implants at different points in time.

Current musculoskeletal MRI protocols include multiple planes of 2D-FSE and 3D-GRE images. The new morphologic methods presented here such as VIPR, 3D-FSE, and bSSFP achieve isotropic resolution for an entire joint in a single acquisition. The isotropic data can then be reformatted into standard or oblique planes as needed, using slice averaging to improve SNR. Combining these methods with fat/water separation methods such as IDEAL provides water, fat, and combined images, which has a variety of different advantages. Overall, it has become apparent that isotropic imaging using reformatted images has the ability to significantly decrease imaging time while still providing several advantages.

Additional studies are required to validate these isotropic methods for their sensitivity to common joint disorders such as meniscal tears. Isotropic acquisitions could improve patient throughput or allow detailed studies of tissue physiology when used in combination with methods such as T2 mapping, T1rho mapping, or sodium MRI. The integration of fast, high-resolution morphologic imaging methods with newer physiologic techniques has the potential to expand the sensitivity of MRI to early cartilage degeneration. Ideally, the combination of these techniques will lead to an MRI examination for cartilage that is brief and well tolerated but contains important morphologic and physiologic data.

REFERENCES

1. Gold GE, Hargreaves BA, Reeder SB, et al. Balanced SSFP imaging of the musculoskeletal system. J Magn Reson Imaging 2007;25:270-278.
2. Gold GE, Han E, Stainsby J, et al. Musculoskeletal MRI at 3.0 T: relaxation times and image contrast. AJR Am J Roentgenol 2004;183:343-351.
3. Frick MA, Wenger DE, Adkins M. MR imaging of synovial disorders of the knee: an update. Radiol Clin North Am 2007;45:1017-1031, vii.
4. Fox MG. MR imaging of the meniscus: review, current trends, and clinical implications. Radiol Clin North Am 2007;45:1033-1053, vii.
5. Meyer CH, Pauly JM, Macovski A, Nishimura DG. Simultaneous spatial and spectral selective excitation. Magn Reson Med 1990;15:287-304.
6. McCauley TR, Disler DG. Magnetic resonance imaging of articular cartilage of the knee. J Am Acad Orthop Surg 2001;9:2-8.

7. Rubenstein JD, Li JG, Majumdar S, Henkelman RM. Image resolution and signal-to-noise ratio requirements for MR imaging of degenerative cartilage. AJR Am J Roentgenol 1997;169:1089-1096.
8. Bredella MA, Tirman PF, Peterfy CG, et al. Accuracy of T2-weighted fast spin-echo MR imaging with fat saturation in detecting cartilage defects in the knee: comparison with arthroscopy in 130 patients. AJR Am J Roentgenol 1999;172:1073-1080.
9. Garnero P, Peterfy C, Zaim S, Schoenharting M. Bone marrow abnormalities on magnetic resonance imaging are associated with type II collagen degradation in knee osteoarthritis: a three-month longitudinal study. Arthritis Rheum 2005;52:2822-2829.
10. Hunter DJ, Lo GH, Gale D, et al. The reliability of a new scoring system for knee osteoarthritis MRI and the validity of bone marrow lesion assessment: BLOKS

(Boston Leeds Osteoarthritis Knee Score). Ann Rheum Dis 2008;67:206-211.
11. Kornaat PR, Ceulemans RY, Kroon HM, et al. MRI assessment of knee osteoarthritis: Knee Osteoarthritis Scoring System (KOSS)—inter-observer and intra-observer reproducibility of a compartment-based scoring system. Skeletal Radiol 2005;34:95-102.
12. Peterfy CG, Schneider E, Nevitt M. The osteoarthritis initiative: report on the design rationale for the magnetic resonance imaging protocol for the knee. Osteoarthritis Cartilage 2008;16:1433-1441.
13. Hargreaves BA, Gold GE, Lang PK, et al. MR imaging of articular cartilage using driven equilibrium. Magn Reson Med 1999;42:695-703.
13a. Eckstein F, Hudelmaier M, Wirth W, et al. Double echo steady state (DESS) magnetic resonance imaging of knee articular cartilage at 3 tesla—a pilot study for the Osteoarthritis Initiative. Ann Rheum Dis 2006;65:433-441.

13b. Hardy PA, Recht MP, Piraino, Thomasson D. Optimization of a dual echo in the steady state (DESS) free-precession sequence for imaging cartilage. J Magn Reson Imaging 1996;6:329-335.

13c. Ruehm S, Zanetti M, Romero J, Hodler J. MRI of patellar articular cartilage: evaluation of an optimized gradient echo sequence (3D-DESS). J Magn Reson Imaging 1998;8:1246-1251.

14. Woertler K, Rummeny EJ, Settles M. A fast high-resolution multislice T1-weighted turbo spin-echo (TSE) sequence with a DRIVen equilibrium (DRIVE) pulse for native arthrograpic contrast. AJR Am J Roentgenol 2005;185:1468-1470.

15. Duerk JL, Lewin JS, Wendt M, Petersilge C. Remember true FISP? A high SNR, near 1-second imaging method for T2-like contrast in interventional MRI at .2 T. J Magn Reson Imaging 1998;8:203-208.

16. Kornaat PR, Doornbos J, van der Molen AJ, et al. Magnetic resonance imaging of knee cartilage using a water selective balanced steady-state free precession sequence. J Magn Reson Imaging 2004;20:850-856.

17. Vasanawala SS, Pauly JM, Nishimura DG. Linear combination steady-state free precession MRI. Magn Reson Med 2000;43:82-90.

18. Gold GE, Hargreaves B, Vasanawala SS, et al. MR imaging of articular cartilage of the knee using fluctuating equilibrium MR (FEMR)—initial experience in healthy volunteers. Radiology 2006;238:712-718.

19. Scheffler K, Heid O, Hennig J. Magnetization preparation during the steady state: fat-saturated 3D TrueFISP. Magn Reson Med 2001;45:1075-1080.

20. Reeder SB, Pelc NJ, Alley MT, Gold GE. Rapid MR imaging of articular cartilage with steady-state free precession and multipoint fat-water separation. AJR Am J Roentgenol 2003;180:357-362.

21. Vasanawala SS, Hargreaves BA, Pauly JM, et al. Rapid musculoskeletal MRI with phase-sensitive steady-state free precession: comparison with routine knee MRI. AJR Am J Roentgenol 2005;184:1450-1455.

22. Gold GE, Reeder SB, Yu H, et al. Articular cartilage of the knee: rapid three-dimensional MR imaging at 3.0 T with IDEAL balanced steady-state free precession—initial experience. Radiology 2006;240:546-551.

23. Kijowski R, Blankenbaker DG, Klaers JL, et al. Vastly undersampled isotropic projection steady-state free precession imaging of the knee: diagnostic performance compared with conventional MR. Radiology 2009;251:185-194.

24. Gold GE, Busse RF, Beehler C, et al. Isotropic MRI of the knee with 3D fast spin-echo extended echo-train acquisition (XETA): initial experience. AJR Am J Roentgenol 2007;188:1287-1293.

25. Busse RF, Brau AC, Vu A, et al. Effects of refocusing flip angle modulation and view ordering in 3D fast spin echo. Magn Reson Med 2008;60:640-649.

26. Stevens KJ, Busse RF, Han E, et al. Ankle: isotropic MR imaging with 3D-FSE-cube—initial experience in healthy volunteers. Radiology 2008;249:1026-1033.

27. Stahl R, Krug R, Kelley DA, et al. Assessment of cartilage-dedicated sequences at ultra-high-field MRI: comparison of imaging performance and diagnostic confidence between 3.0 and 7.0 T with respect to osteoarthritis-induced changes at the knee joint. Skeletal Radiol 2009;38:771-783.

28. Wirth W, Hellio Le Graverand MP, et al. Regional analysis of femorotibial cartilage loss in a subsample from the Osteoarthritis Initiative progression subcohort. Osteoarthritis Cartilage 2009;17:291-297.

29. Cohen SB, Dore RK, Lane NE, et al. Denosumab treatment effects on structural damage, bone mineral density, and bone turnover in rheumatoid arthritis: a twelve-month, multicenter, randomized, double-blind, placebo-controlled, phase II clinical trial. Arthritis Rheum 2008;58:1299-1309.

30. Smith HE, Mosher TJ, Dardzinski BJ, et al. Spatial variation in cartilage T2 of the knee. J Magn Reson Imaging 2001;14:50-55.

31. Mosher TJ, Dardzinski BJ, Smith MB. Human articular cartilage: influence of aging and early symptomatic degeneration on the spatial variation of T2—preliminary findings at 3 T. Radiology 2000;214:259-266.

32. Xia Y. Magic-angle effect in magnetic resonance imaging of articular cartilage: a review. Invest Radiol 2000;35:602-621.

33. Mosher TJ, Collins CM, Smith HE, et al. Effect of gender on in vivo cartilage magnetic resonance imaging T2 mapping. J Magn Reson Imaging 2004;19:323-328.

34. Mosher TJ, Smith HE, Collins C, et al. Change in knee cartilage T2 at MR imaging after running: a feasibility study. Radiology 2005;234:245-249.

35. Robson MD, Gatehouse PD, Bydder M, Bydder GM. Magnetic resonance: an introduction to ultrashort TE (UTE) imaging. J Comput Assist Tomogr 2003;27:825-846.

36. Duvvuri U, Charagundla SR, Kudchodkar SB, et al. Human knee: in vivo T1(rho)-weighted MR imaging at 1.5 T—preliminary experience. Radiology 2001;220:822-826.

37. Wheaton AJ, Dodge GR, Borthakur A, et al. Detection of changes in articular cartilage proteoglycan by T(1rho) magnetic resonance imaging. J Orthop Res 2005;23:102-108.

38. Zuo J, Li X, Banerjee S, et al. Parallel imaging of knee cartilage at 3 Tesla. J Magn Reson Imaging 2007;26:1001-1009.

39. Witschey WR, Borthakur A, Elliott MA, et al. T1rho-prepared balanced gradient echo for rapid 3D T1rho MRI. J Magn Reson Imaging 2008;28:744-754.

40. Rauscher I, Stahl R, Cheng J, et al. Meniscal measurements of T1rho and T2 at MR imaging in healthy subjects and patients with osteoarthritis. Radiology 2008;249:591-600.

41. Burstein D, Bashir A, Gray ML. MRI techniques in early stages of cartilage disease. Invest Radiol 2000;35:622-638.

42. Stevens K, Hishioka H, Steines D, et al. Contrast enhanced MRI measurement of GAG concentrations in articular cartilage of knees with early osteoarthritis. In Proceedings of the Radiology Society of North America, 2001:275.

43. Williams A, Sharma L, McKenzie CA, et al. Delayed gadolinium-enhanced magnetic resonance imaging of cartilage in knee osteoarthritis: findings at different radiographic stages of disease and relationship to malalignment. Arthritis Rheum 2005;52:3528-3535.

43a. Bartolini ME, Pekar J, Chettle DR, et al. An investigation of the toxicity of gadolinium based MRI constrast agents using neutron activation analysis. J Magn Reson Imaging 2003;21:541-544.

44. Deoni SC, Rutt BK, Peters TM. Rapid combined T1 and T2 mapping using gradient recalled acquisition in the steady state. Magn Reson Med 2003;49:515-526.

45. Deoni SC, Ward HA, Peters TM, Rutt BK. Rapid T2 estimation with phase-cycled variable nutation steady-state free precession. Magn Reson Med 2004;52:435-439.

46. Shapiro EM, Borthakur A, Gougoutas A, Reddy R. 23Na MRI accurately measures fixed charge density in articular cartilage. Magn Reson Med 2002;47:284-291.

47. Boada FE, Shen GX, Chang SY, Thulborn KR. Spectrally weighted twisted projection imaging: reducing T2 signal attenuation effects in fast three-dimensional sodium imaging. Magn Reson Med 1997;38:1022-1028.

48. Gurney PT, Hargreaves BA, Nishimura DG. Design and analysis of a practical 3D cones trajectory. Magn Reson Med 2006;55:575-582.

49. Borthakur A, Shapiro EM, Beers J, et al. Sensitivity of MRI to proteoglycan depletion in cartilage: comparison of sodium and proton MRI. Osteoarthritis Cartilage 2000;8:288-293.

50. Borthakur A, Hancu I, Boada FE, et al. In vivo triple quantum filtered twisted projection sodium MRI of human articular cartilage. J Magn Reson 1999;141:286-290.

Musculoskeletal ultrasound

Richard J. Wakefield and Philip O'Connor

40

- Ultrasound is increasingly used in rheumatology.
- It is available in the clinic, allowing rapid decision making.
- It has the ability to scan multiple joints in short periods of time.
- It can visualize many different tissues (e.g., synovium, tendons, bone, and blood vessels).
- It allows morphologic and functional tissue assessments.

Musculoskeletal ultrasound (MUS) is now a routine technique for investigating patients with rheumatic diseases and has become a compulsory part of rheumatology training in some European countries. It has a wide spectrum of potential uses from disease diagnosis and monitoring to guiding interventional procedures. Recent developments in technology, including use of Doppler, continue to redefine its role.

Ultrasound is ideal for a clinical setting in that it can be directly performed by the rheumatologist as an extension to standard clinical assessment.[1] In addition, it can simultaneously image soft tissues and bone; produce multiplanar, "real-time" dynamic images; and, because it lacks ionizing radiation, it allows repeated examinations to be performed safely at multiple anatomic sites. Compared with magnetic resonance imaging (MRI), it is inexpensive, better tolerated by patients, and more readily available.

This chapter discusses the development of MUS and the fundamentals of the technology and describes the current and potential clinical uses of the technique.

ULTRASOUND MILESTONES

One of the earliest observations pertaining to ultrasound is attributed to an Italian priest and biologist named Lazzaro Spallanzani (1729-1799). He found that bats were able to avoid thin wires stretched across a dark room. Subsequent experiments including blinding the bats and putting wax in their ears made him conclude that bats "see with their ears." He did not, however, consider that the bats were using sound to achieve this.

Doppler is a technique for making non-invasive measurements of blood flow, the principles of which were first noted by Austrian physicist Christian Doppler in 1842. He described the effect of motion on a wave (sound or light) when he observed a change in the frequency of a wave as a result of movement of either its source or receiver. The rise in pitch of an emergency vehicle as it approaches is a familiar example.

The first major technologic breakthrough leading to the development of modern ultrasound probes was in 1880, five years before the discovery of x-rays. This was when the Curie brothers discovered the phenomenon of piezoelectricity[2]—the property exhibited by certain materials of generating electrical potentials when mechanically stressed. Conversely, they generate mechanical strains when electrically stressed. One of the first practical uses of ultrasound occurred in the unsuccessful attempt to locate the Titanic, which sank in 1912. In 1916 Langevin developed a method of underwater communication, which later led to the discovery of SONAR—**so**und **na**vigation and **r**anging. The development of sophisticated sonar equipment during World War II helped spur the growth and development of medical ultrasound.[3,4]

Unlike x-rays, which were in clinical use soon after its discovery, ultrasound has been relatively slow to develop in medicine. The first practical imaging unit was developed in Austria in 1957 by Dussik. He attempted to locate brain tumors and the cerebral ventricles, but the method proved impractical because of attenuation of sound by the skull. In 1958 Dussik demonstrated for the first time that ultrasound could be used to differentiate between different articular tissues.[5]

The first clinically relevant ultrasound study pertaining to musculoskeletal disease was published by McDonald and Leopold in 1972.[6] They described the use of a 2.25 MHz contact B-mode (gray-scale) scanner in three patients to successfully differentiate between a ruptured Baker cyst and thrombophlebitis as potential causes of a painful swollen calf. In 1978 Cooperberg and colleagues[7] published the first major paper on rheumatoid arthritis (RA), which described the potential use of ultrasound for the evaluation of knee synovitis.

Despite a steady increase in the number of publications since that time, the widespread use of ultrasound did not significantly escalate until the late 1980s.[8-10] These developments arose from the production of more powerful computers, a change from analog to digital processing systems and the availability of higher frequency (7.5 to 20 MHz) and smaller transducers that were better adapted for superficial structures like tendons and the small joints.

BASIC PRINCIPLES OF ULTRASOUND

What is ultrasound?

Ultrasound waves are a type of "supersonic" or high-frequency sound wave, which is inaudible to the human ear. By definition, they travel at greater than 20,000 cycles/second (20,000 Hz or 20 kHz), although diagnostic equipment uses a much higher frequency range. For comparison, the note of the lowest pitch on a piano has a frequency of about 30 Hz while the highest is 4000 Hz. In musculoskeletal imaging, higher frequencies are preferred and range from 5 to 18 MHz (5 to 18 million Hz).

Properties of an ultrasound wave

Sound is a longitudinal, mechanical wave that abides by the same physical properties as any other wave, particularly in that it requires a medium or material to travel through. An exception to this is the electromagnetic waves, which can travel through a vacuum. An ultrasound wave may be likened to an impulse traveling along a spring (Fig. 40.1). As one coil moves forward, it collides with the next and the next and so on until the end of the spring is reached. The movement of the wave along the spring is not linear. At any time point, some of the coils are close together (compression) while others are farther apart (rarefaction). The closer the coils are together, the more efficiently and more rapidly the sound waves travel through the spring. Therefore denser materials such as solids, in which the molecules are closer together, transmit sound more efficiently than liquids or gases.

The wavelength is the length of a cycle in space. In diagnostic imaging, this corresponds to 0.1 to 1.0 mm in tissue. The frequency of the wave is the number of complete cycles the wave goes through in 1 second.[11] This is measured in hertz (Hz). However, the amount of energy a wave has depends on its amplitude and not the frequency.

Ultrasound waves travel through different media at different speeds; for example, sound travels through bone and water faster than it does through air. The relative "propagation" speeds of sound through different tissues are listed in Table 40.1. They remain constant whatever the amplitude of the sound wave.

The average propagation speed in soft tissues (excluding lung and bone) is taken as 1540 m/sec. The speed of sound through any material depends on the density and compressibility of the material. The denser and more compressible the material, the slower the wave will travel through it. Each tissue therefore has its own acoustic properties, known

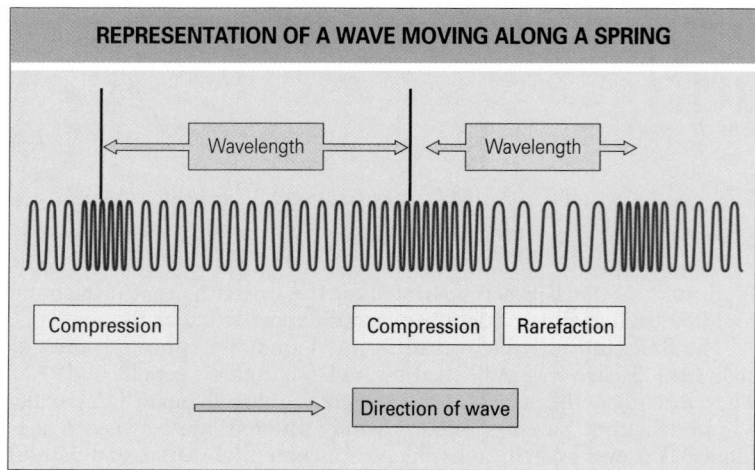

Fig. 40.1 Representation of a wave moving along a spring. Sound is a longitudinal, mechanical wave that is propagated through tissue by a series of compressions and rarefactions, like movement through a spring. One wavelength is the distance between two adjacent compressions or rarefactions. Frequency (expressed in hertz or Hz) is the number of wavelengths that pass through a given point in tissue in 1 second.

TABLE 40.1 PROPAGATION SPEEDS OF SOUND THROUGH DIFFERENT BIOLOGIC MATERIALS	
Biologic material	Speed (m/s)
Air	330
Fat	1450
Water	1480
Soft tissue	1540
Blood	1570
Muscle	1585
Bone	4080

Adapted from Bushong SC, Archer BR. Diagnostic ultrasound: physics, biology and instrumentation. St Louis: Mosby Year Book, 1991:1-4.

as *acoustic impedance* (Z) where Z = density × speed of sound (Table 40.2).

Sound is reflected back to the transducer at interfaces between tissues of different acoustic impedances, as demonstrated in Fig. 40.2. The time delay between the initiation of the pulse and return of the echo is proportional to the distance the beam has traveled. The distance can be calculated from the velocity of sound in tissues. Reflection of sound is greatest when there is a large difference between the acoustic impedances of two structures (e.g., air and skin). This is the reason why acoustic gel is applied to the skin to minimize this difference.

As the sound wave passes through the tissues, it gradually diminishes in intensity, a process known as *attenuation*. The major loss of energy results from absorption (and subsequent conversion to heat) and to a lesser extent reflection, refraction, diffraction, and scattering. Adjustments to the controls are sometimes made, therefore, to increase the reception power of the transducer for those signals that return later from the deeper tissues. Knowledge of such properties helps to explain and overcome some of the artifacts encountered and therefore prevent misinterpretation of the images.

Gray-scale and Doppler ultrasound imaging

Most ultrasound images are presented in "black and white" or "gray-scale" where the brightness of the white dot corresponds to the intensity of reflected wave. This is known as B-mode or brightness-modulated ultrasound. Doppler imaging, which is being used increasingly in rheumatology, is superimposed on the B-mode image.

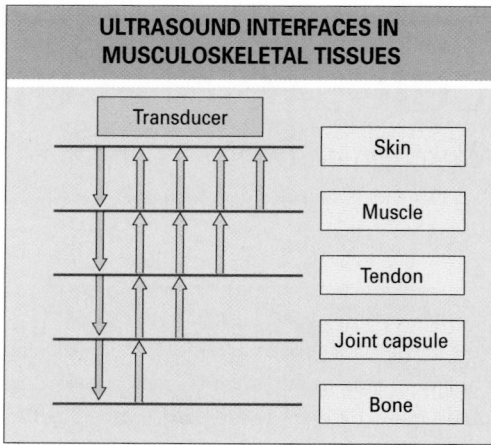

Fig. 40.2 Ultrasound interfaces in musculoskeletal tissues. This diagram demonstrates the different acoustic interfaces a sound wave encounters when passing through musculoskeletal tissues. Reflections occur where two adjacent tissues have different acoustic impedances.

TABLE 40.2 ACOUSTIC IMPEDANCE VALUES (Z) FOR DIFFERENT BIOLOGIC MATERIALS	
Material	Z (kg/m²/sec or Rayls)
Air	0.0004
Fat	1.38
Soft tissue (average)	1.63
Blood	1.61
Bone	7.80

Adapted from Bushong SC. Diagnostic ultrasound. New York: McGraw-Hill, 1999:18.

There are two main types of Doppler ultrasound: color flow Doppler (CFD) and power Doppler (PDS). Both produce a similar color spectral map superimposed onto the gray-scale image (the colors being related to the difference in frequency between the transmitted sound wave and that reflected from the moving interface [the Doppler frequency shift]), but they actually encode different information. CFD represents an estimate of the mean Doppler frequency shift and relates to velocity and direction of red blood cells, whereas PDS denotes the amplitude of the Doppler signal, which is determined by the volume of blood present. In this way CFD is better suited for evaluating high-velocity flow in large vessels (e.g., carotids), whereas PDS is better suited for assessing low-velocity flow in small vessels (e.g., synovium).

A number of particular advantages for using PDS in musculoskeletal assessment exist. It provides increased sensitivity to low-volume, low-velocity blood flow at the microvascular level, so it is particularly useful for measuring and detecting changes in joints and soft tissue as a consequence of inflammation. PDS also increases the specificity of an ultrasound assessment as it aids differentiation among tissue debris, blood clot, fibrin, and a complex effusion, which can mimic features of synovial proliferation. In addition, when compared with CFD, the PDS signal is independent of the transducer angle, there is no aliasing (an image artifact reflecting inadequate signal sampling), and background noise is reduced. PDS also provides superior depiction of the continuity and boundaries of blood flow and improved definition of vessel characteristics such as tortuosity that are suboptimally imaged with conventional CFD.

Artifacts

Artifacts are echoes that do not correspond to a real target in either distance or direction. Several different types of artifact (both gray-scale and color) need to be considered when interpreting images (Table 40.3).

TABLE 40.3 COMMON TYPES OF ARTIFACT SEEN IN MUS IMAGING

Anisotropy	Occurs when transducer or object is not perpendicular
Refractile shadowing	Occurs when ultrasound beam hits structure of different acoustic impedance at oblique angle
Acoustic enhancement	Occurs when there is overcompensation of returning signal in cases of "enhanced through transmission" (e.g., fluid collection)
Acoustic shadowing	Occurs distal to highly reflective surface
Reverberation	Occurs when ultrasound beam hits two highly reflective surfaces
Beam width artifact	Occurs when object is narrower than ultrasound beam

Artifacts of gray-scale imaging

1. Anisotropy

This is the most common artifact observed in musculoskeletal scanning. It occurs when the region of interest is not perpendicular to the transducer, due to either the angle of transducer or the angle of object. It is corrected by adjusting the angle of either the transducer in relation to the object or the object in relation to the transducer. It is most commonly associated with bone and tendon imaging (Fig. 40.3) and can erroneously indicate bone erosion or tendon pathology. Therefore particular care needs to be taken when scanning these tissues. This is one reason why scanning in multiple planes (e.g., longitudinal and transverse planes) is essential.

2. Refractile shadowing

This is reflection away from the transducer when the ultrasound beam hits a structure with different acoustic impedance, at an oblique angle. This most commonly occurs when scanning tendons, when the edge of the tendon and tendon sheath may look erroneously hypoechoic.

3. Acoustic enhancement

The intensity of the echoes returning to the transducer normally decreases exponentially with increasing depth in the tissues being examined. This discrepancy is usually automatically corrected because otherwise there is a rapid decline in image integrity. In the case of tissues with enhanced through transmission of sound waves (e.g., where there is a fluid collection), there is overcompensation with distal enhancement.

4. Acoustic shadowing

This occurs distal to a highly reflective surface where there is a failure of echo return. This often occurs with areas of calcification in soft tissues (Fig. 40.4).

5. Reverberation

This occurs when an ultrasound beam encounters two highly reflective interfaces. Most of the sound waves are reflected back from the first surface to the transducer, but some pass through and are reflected from the second. These waves may pass back to the transducer but may also be reflected back by the first surface and so on. Because there is a time delay for these reflections to reach the probe, they successively appear deeper. Each line on the screen also appears less bright. The classic reverberation artifact is known as the "comet tail." It is due to repeated reflections between the anterior and posterior portions of an object that is strongly reflective such as glass or metal (as with a needle). The thickness of bands equals thickness of object.

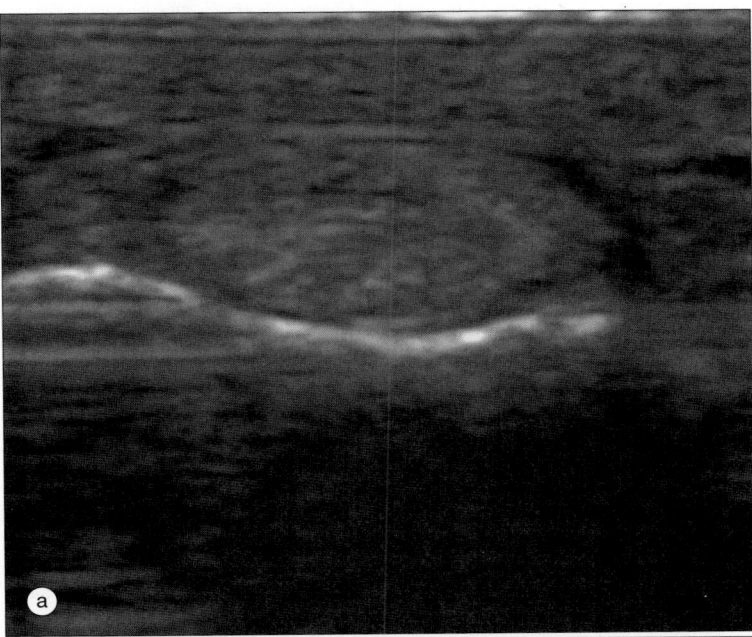

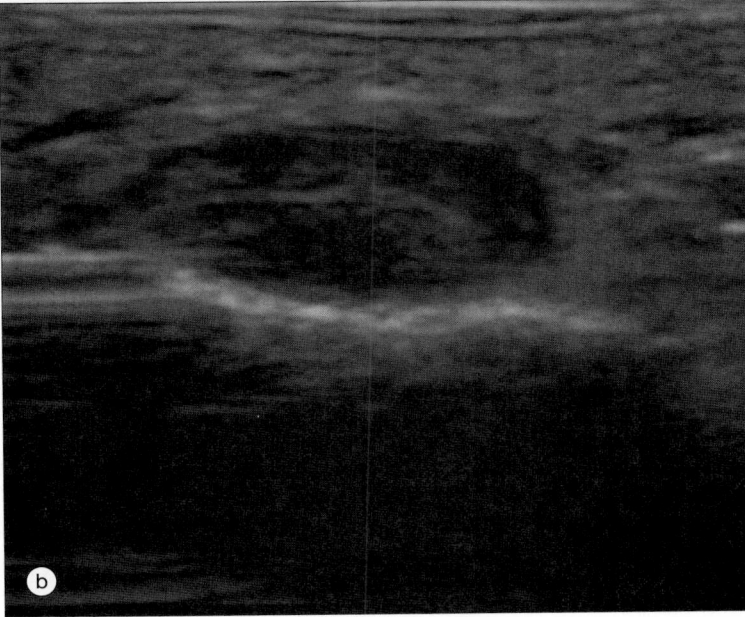

Fig. 40.3 Demonstration of anisotropy. Flexor tendon of finger appears white when the ultrasound beam is perpendicular (a) and dark when the transducer is moved 30 degrees (b).

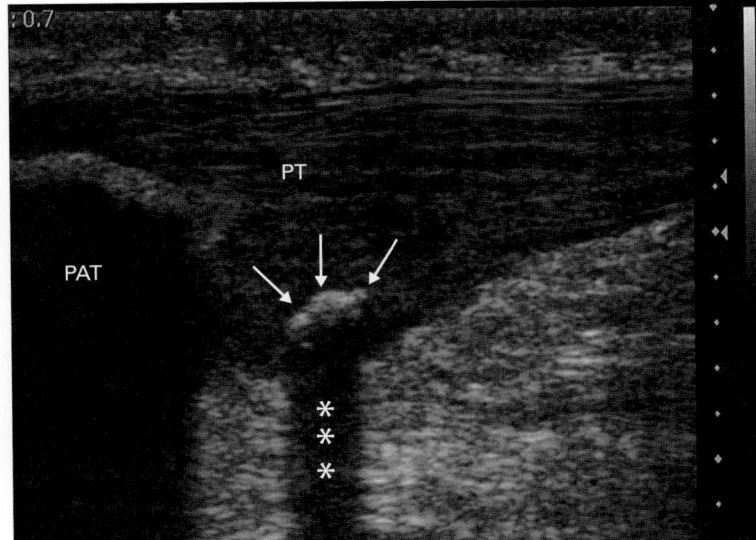

Fig. 40.4 Acoustic shadowing. This is a longitudinal image through the proximal patella tendon (PT) in a patient with jumper's knee. There is involvement of the deep portion of the tendon; a focal area of dense calcification (arrows) within casts a distal acoustic shadow (asterisks).

6. Beam width artifact

This occurs when the object is narrower than the ultrasound beam. Echoes from surrounding tissues can fill in missing gaps (e.g., distal acoustic shadows in the case of small calcifications). In computed tomgraphy (CT) or MRI, this is known as *volume averaging*.

Artifacts of Doppler imaging

Several important artifacts are seen when applying Doppler to studies. Care must be taken when interpreting images; this requires a good understanding of how the machine works and meticulous technique. Common artifacts are mentioned as follows, but the reader is directed to a recent review by Torp-Pedersen and Terslev[12] for details.

1. Random noise

This occurs when the color gain is set too high. Random color signals occur on the screen but do not reappear in the same location as true flow does. The random noise is used to set the Doppler gain. A correct setting is at or just below the level that generates a little random noise.

2. Motion

Doppler depends on the movement of the target tissue (i.e., normally blood cells). It follows therefore that if the patient or transducer moves, then there will be a corresponding Doppler signal. Motion artifacts are minimized when the patient is comfortably positioned with the area under investigation resting. It is also mandatory that the examiner's scanning arm is resting comfortably.

3. Mirror

Any highly reflective smooth surface may act as an acoustic mirror. In rheumatology, the mirror is usually the bone surface. Doppler flow is just as prone to mirroring as the gray-scale image. The mirror artifact is easily seen as such when the true image, as well as the mirror and mirror image, are all in the image.

4. Aliasing

This arises when the Doppler shift is higher than half of the pulse repetition frequency (PRF). It only occurs with CFD and not power Doppler ultrasound (PDUS) and is much more important when scanning larger vessels. Aliased signals are displayed with the wrong directions (red instead of blue and vice versa) and with incorrect relative velocity (the hue of the color). If present, this would lead to decreased sensitivity to slow flow.

5. Blooming

The blooming artifact describes the phenomenon in which the color in a vessel expands beyond the vessel wall edge, making the vessels look larger than they really are. It is gain dependent, and lowering the Doppler gain will decrease the blooming artifact. However, by lowering the gain, the weakest Doppler signals will be lost and important flow information may be lost. It is recommended that the Doppler gain be set by looking at random noise and not by looking at blooming artifacts.

ULTRASOUND TECHNOLOGY

An ultrasound machine consists of a computer processing unit and a transducer (Fig. 40.5). The computer generates the electrical impulses, which are sent to the transducer, and converts the returning impulses into images, as discussed earlier.

Arguably the most important part of the machine is the transducer or scan head, which is the transmitter-receiver section.[13] The nature of the transducer materials and their internal arrangement influence the sensitivity and physical properties of the ultrasound system. The transducer is composed of multiple elements arranged one after another in a row. The most common of these piezoelectric materials used is the ceramic lead zirconate titanate (PZT). Work is currently under way to develop lead-free crystals, which may be potentially less harmful to the environment. Linear (flat) or convex (curved) arrangements of these elements create different fields of view. In general, flat or linear transducers are preferred because they maximize the collection of signals reflected back from the tissue. High-frequency transducers increase the near-field resolution but at the cost of tissue penetration. Most machines in use today have broadband transducers, which means that

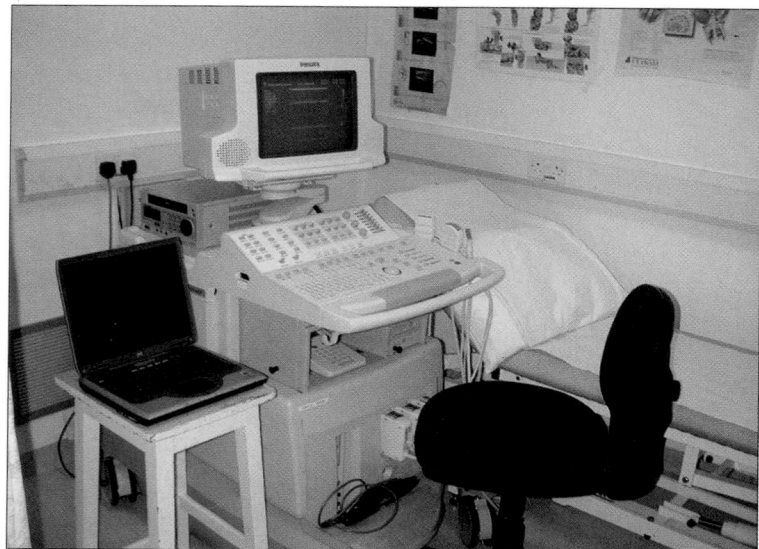

Fig. 40.5 Ultrasound equipment. Ultrasound equipment consists of a computer processing unit and monitor. This is a more expensive, relatively large machine, although machines are becoming increasingly smaller and even laptop sized. Ultrasound rooms should be spacious and preferably air conditioned (to prevent overheating of equipment). Adjustable couches and chairs allow for more comfortable examinations.

one transducer covers a range of frequencies with the chosen frequency being selected automatically by the machine.

Choosing an ultrasound machine

There are many factors to consider when choosing a machine including cost, Doppler sensitivity, and portability. The cost of a good ultrasound machine has decreased considerably in recent years, although the cost does broadly represent the quality. Portable machines may be acquired for as little as $16,000, although those with high specifications may be as high as $165,000. Factors that increase the cost of the machine include additional software packages such as extended field of view or three-dimensional capabilities. For most routine clinical work these are not essential. Operating costs are generally low, but hidden costs include annual service agreements (typically 10% of the cost of the machine), which are important because they include updated software, replacement of worn or broken parts, and general technical support. Doppler capability is now considered an essential aspect of ultrasound imaging, so even though a good gray-scale image remains important, a sensitive Doppler is also crucial. Finally, unlike MRI, ultrasound can be performed anywhere and does not require a special environment, other than a darkened, preferably air-conditioned room. Therefore portable machines are becoming increasingly attractive because they have the versatility to be moved from one clinical area to another and can be locked away for safety. In general, portable machines have suffered from a reduction in image quality when compared with the stand-alone machines, but this difference is now much less when compared with the past.

MUS is widely used in rheumatology imaging in Europe and Australasia. Utilization of ultrasound in the United States and Canada is limited, with MRI being the predominant modality employed. The technology underpinning MUS continues to develop with improvements in the spatial and temporal resolution of ultrasound images. In addition, the clinician's acceptance of ultrasound images has benefited tools allowing extended field of view or panoramic imaging (Fig. 40.6). However, the user must have a full understanding of its advantages and limitations to make appropriate use of it and other modalities.

ADVANTAGES OF ULTRASOUND

Clinical correlation

Ultrasound allows close clinical correlation between patient's symptoms and ultrasound findings. In general, it is best at investigating focal

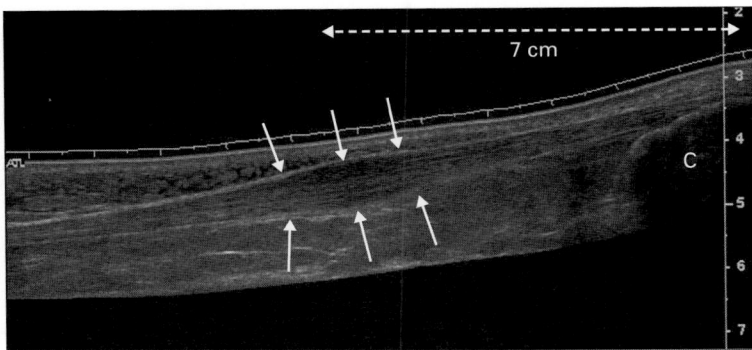

Fig. 40.6 Panoramic longitudinal view through the Achilles tendon. The arrows indicate a fusiform swelling which is 7 cm proximal to the insertion into the calcaneum (C). This is classic for a degenerated tendon. The panoramic view allows a large portion of the tendon to be visualized simultaneously.

symptoms; if the patient can point with one finger at the site of symptoms, ultrasound is more likely to be of value. However, if the patient rubs a large area such as over a knee, then ultrasound is likely to be less specific.

Spatial resolution and tissue visualization

The spatial resolution of ultrasound varies directly with probe frequency—the higher the frequency, the greater the spatial resolution. Most musculoskeletal structures requiring imaging in rheumatology are fairly superficial and thus can be imaged with high-frequency, high-resolution probes. In comparison with conventional magnetic resonance sequences, the typical in-plane resolution is much greater with high-frequency ultrasound imaging.

As a result of its high spatial resolution, the degree of anatomic detail demonstrated by ultrasound is a strength. For example, visualization of most peripheral nerves and tendons is also good. By contrast, the internal architecture of the tendon, particularly early tendonopathic change, is difficult to appreciate with MRI. Ultrasound is particularly good at demonstrating calcification in tissues, which is of value in diagnosing the nature of small bone fragments in sports injury and in the early diagnosis of myositis ossificans and calcific tendonitis.

Edema in muscle tears on MRI can obscure the degree of architectural disruption, making accurate grading difficult. Ultrasound's insensitivity to muscle edema can be an advantage in staging grade 2 and 3 tears but clearly means that it misses less important grade 1 tears.

Dynamic examination

The dynamic nature of ultrasound means tissues can be assessed moving in real time. Movement-related symptoms, especially those related to tendon disease, are best assessed with ultrasound. Tissues can be stressed, allowing assessment of the true extent of muscle damage in either the acute or healing phase. In tendon injury, movement allows improved differentiation between partial and complete tears. It shows the degree of tendon separation in differing positions, which can be of value in deciding between conservative and surgical management of Achilles tears.

Ability to scan multiple joints

A significant advantage of ultrasound relates to its ability to image many joints in a short period of time. This is particularly relevant for the investigation of patients with polyarticular inflammatory joint diseases like rheumatoid arthritis (RA). It may take an experienced operator 30 minutes to scan most joints for synovitis including hands and feet, whereas it may take 30 minutes to scan one joint group (e.g., wrist and metacarpophalangeal joint of one hand only with MRI).

Intervention

Ultrasound allows exceptionally accurate needle-tip placement to a site determined either clinically (clinician request to inject a particular site)

or from imaging findings (MRI or ultrasound demonstration of inflammatory change). Injections can either be diagnostic or therapeutic.

LIMITATIONS OF ULTRASOUND

Acoustic access

Ultrasound needs an acoustic window for the sound waves to reach the region of interest. It is therefore unable to fully see inside some joints and as a result may not be able to appreciate the full extent of an abnormality or may miss some structures altogether. Structures that ultrasound finds difficult to see include the full surface of the menisci or cruciate ligaments in the knee. This can have important implications, especially for sport and related injuries in which problems are frequently complex. Here ultrasound may find an abnormality but may miss the underlying cause. For example, it might demonstrate a lateral ligament injury in the ankle but would miss the more important intra-articular osteochondral injury. This needs to be constantly borne in mind; hence ultrasound is frequently used in combination with MRI. Ultrasound is also unable to visualize bone below the cortical surface, so radiography/CT and MRI are the preferred choices.

Inflammation

Ultrasound can demonstrate soft tissue inflammatory change but is accepted as being less sensitive than MRI. This can be an advantage in muscles where the degree of edema interferes with staging the degree of architectural disruption present in tissues but is a limitation in subtle early muscle disease and other soft tissue inflammation such as synovitis and enthesitis. Power Doppler allows visualization of revascularization and is likely to be as sensitive as MRI in demonstrating new vessels; however, the vessels take time to develop and are more often seen in chronic conditions. MRI is more sensitive to increases in the extracellular fluid volume in tissues, as well as being able to demonstrate neovascularity, which probably accounts for its superior sensitivity.

Reliability

Ultrasound has often been perceived as an operator-dependent tool. This is true because much of the information depends on how the operator acquired and subsequently interpreted the image. These issues, in the context of inflammatory arthritis, have recently been addressed by the Outcome Measures in Rheumatoid Arthritis Clinical Trials (OMERACT) Ultrasound Task Force.[14] Exercises conducted by the group have demonstrated that by standardizing definitions and scoring systems, reliability can dramatically improve.[15] Currently an OMERACT Atlas is in preparation for the scoring of synovitis in RA.

Clinician acceptance

The images from ultrasound are less readily interpreted after the imaging event. Clinicians find it easier to look at tomographic magnetic resonance and CT images with an ensuing instinctive preference for MRI. It is hard to persuade clinicians of the value of ultrasound, but this can be overcome by scanning with the clinician in the examination room to improve understanding of the modality.

CLINICAL APPLICATIONS OF ULTRASOUND IN RHEUMATOLOGY

In the early years, ultrasound was used to investigate mainly orthopedic-related disorders such as rotator cuff tears and tendon ruptures. This still remains an important use, but with the development of smaller, higher-frequency transducers and acknowledgment of the importance of inflammatory arthritis, recent attention has been directed toward the investigation of inflammatory rheumatic diseases and their sequelae, including the detection of synovitis, bone erosions, tenosynovitis, enthesitis, and cartilage pathology. In addition, ultrasound has been used to detect a number of other inflammatory

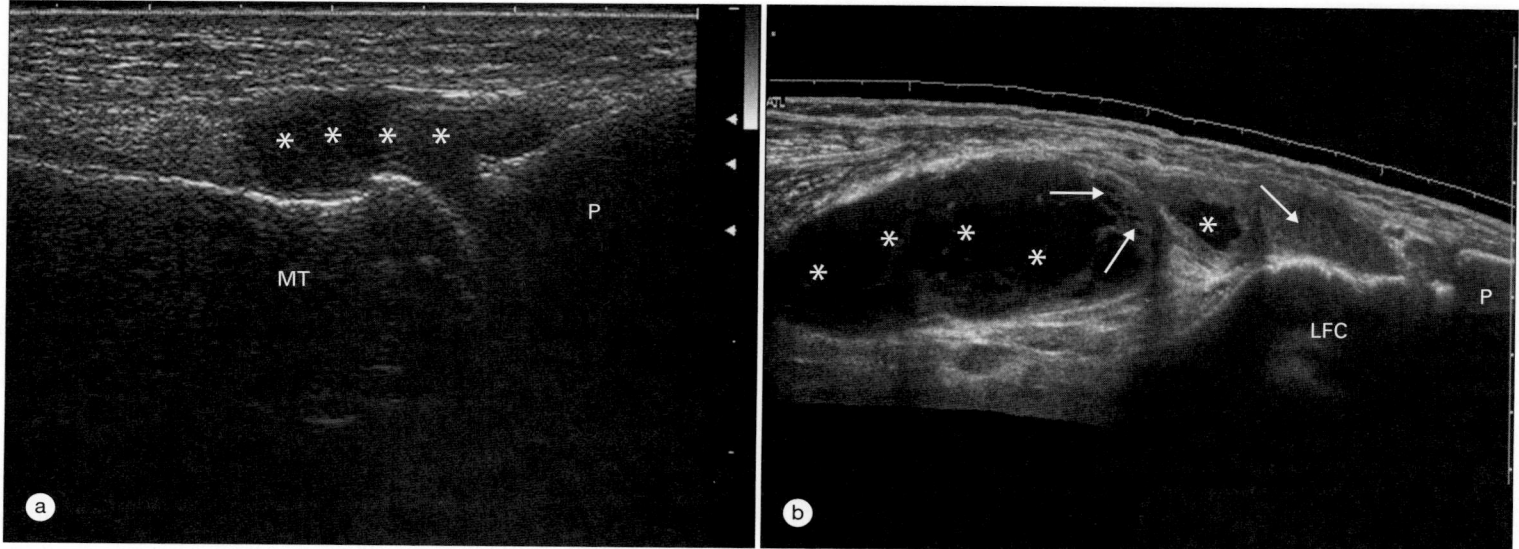

Fig. 40.7 Ultrasound-detected synovitis. (a) This is a longitudinal image through a metatarsophalangeal joint of a patient with rheumatoid arthritis. The asterisks mark a mixed hypoechogenic area representing the distended joint space. The area was partially compressible and displaceable consistent with synovial hypertrophy. (b) This is a longitudinal section through the lateral recess of the suprapatellar pouch of a patient with rheumatoid arthritis. There is a combination of synovitis (arrows) and fluid (asterisks). LFC, lateral femoral condyle; P, patella.

pathologies involving blood vessels, peripheral nerves, muscle, skin, and other organs such as the salivary and parotid glands.

Joint-related structures

Synovial fluid and hypertrophy

The ability to detect fluid or synovial tissue within a joint is an essential requirement of the clinician. Clinical examination may be inaccurate, particularly when there are low levels of disease activity or examination is hampered by the deep location of the joint or surrounding adipose tissue or fluid. Several reports demonstrating the superiority of ultrasound over clinical examination for both fluid and synovial hypertrophy in both small and large joints have been published.[16-18] Until recently there has been no clear consensus on ultrasound definitions of synovitis, synovial effusion, or hypertrophy.[19]

These proposed definitions of synovitis are purely qualitative, and as yet there is no published agreement on quantitative definitions: however, the OMERACT/European League Against Rheumatism (EULAR) Ultrasound Task Force will soon submit a proposal for this. One difficulty has been the limited data on normal individuals,[20] and it is unclear how to define the upper end of normal. It is also likely that as technology continues to improve, these definitions may need to be modified with image resolution improvement. Synovitis defined by ultrasound tends to refer to synovial proliferation and/or effusion—usually they coexist (Fig. 40.7).

Doppler ultrasound, by its ability to detect blood flow, offers interesting pathophysiologic insights into the joint. Several studies have now shown good correlation between Doppler flow with histologic[21-23] and dynamic gadolinium-enhanced MRI[24,25] appearance, as well as with serologic markers. It is well recognized, however, that not all symptomatic, swollen joints with marked gray-scale ultrasound changes exhibit Doppler signal and also that there may be significant variations between machines. Color Doppler and power Doppler have both been used to detect blood flow. Power Doppler has traditionally been more popular because it is more sensitive at lower flow levels (Fig. 40.8). Recently, however, particularly with more expensive machines, there is less of a difference in sensitivity between modalities.

Recent reports have shown that both gray-scale and power Doppler ultrasound of synovial tissue are sensitive to change following both corticosteroids[26] and anti–tumor necrosis factor (anti-TNF) agents,[27,28] suggesting that they may be used for disease monitoring in patients with RA. Limited data exist, however, comparing their use to MRI, although some reports suggest that power Doppler may be more sensitive. The predictive capacity of ultrasound has been suggested by Taylor and colleagues,[29] who demonstrated that a change in gray-scale and

PDS signal correlated with radiologic damage at 54 weeks. In addition to clinical trials, the ability of ultrasound to detect subclinical disease has been shown to be potentially helpful in reclassifying oligoarthritis into polyarticular disease, suggesting that these may need more aggressive therapy.[30] More recently, Naredo and colleagues[31] reported that a time-integrated assessment of PDUS parameters demonstrated a highly significant correlation with radiographic progression ($r = 0.59$ to 0.66, $P < 0.001$) when compared with clinical and laboratory parameters ($r < 0.5$). Two interesting papers by Brown and colleagues[32,33] have shown that subclinical synovitis is common in RA patients in clinical remission and that this synovitis (especially that with power Doppler) is more likely to erode joints. This raises important implications as to what should be used as our treatment endpoints.

Bone erosion

The first major report describing the ability of ultrasound to detect bone erosions in RA was by de Flaviis and colleagues.[34] In this study, 20 patients with early RA underwent ultrasound using a 5- to 7.5-MHz linear or curvilinear transducer and radiography of the wrist and hands. The authors reported radiographic bone erosions being visible in 11 patients, with 6 of these also having ultrasound erosions. The next reports, also of the hand and wrist, occurred some time later. Grassi and colleagues[35] and Lund and colleagues[36] described the ultrasound findings of 20 and 29 patients, respectively, with long-standing RA. The former study highlighted the ability of ultrasound to detect bone erosions and noted that 18 of 20 patients with radiographic erosions also had erosions on ultrasound.

Alasaarela and colleagues[37] published one of the first studies comparing ultrasound with imaging modalities other than radiography alone. They compared ultrasound with conventional radiography, CT, and MRI for the detection of humeral head erosions in patients with long-standing RA. They found MRI, CT, and ultrasound were all more sensitive than conventional radiography, with MRI and ultrasound superior to CT in detecting small erosions. Backhaus and colleagues[38] compared conventional radiography, scintigraphy, ultrasound, and contrast-enhanced MRI for the detection of bone erosions in 60 patients with inflammatory arthritis including 36 with RA. However, this study did not show an overall superiority of ultrasound in those patients already found to have radiographic erosions. There was a small advantage in those patients with no radiographic erosions.

Since then, several other papers have confirmed the greater sensitivity of ultrasound over radiography in both hands and feet.[39-41] Wakefield and colleagues,[42] in a study of 100 RA patients, found that 80% of the ultrasound lesions not seen on radiographs could be identified as bony abnormalities such as cysts, but because of their *en-face* position they

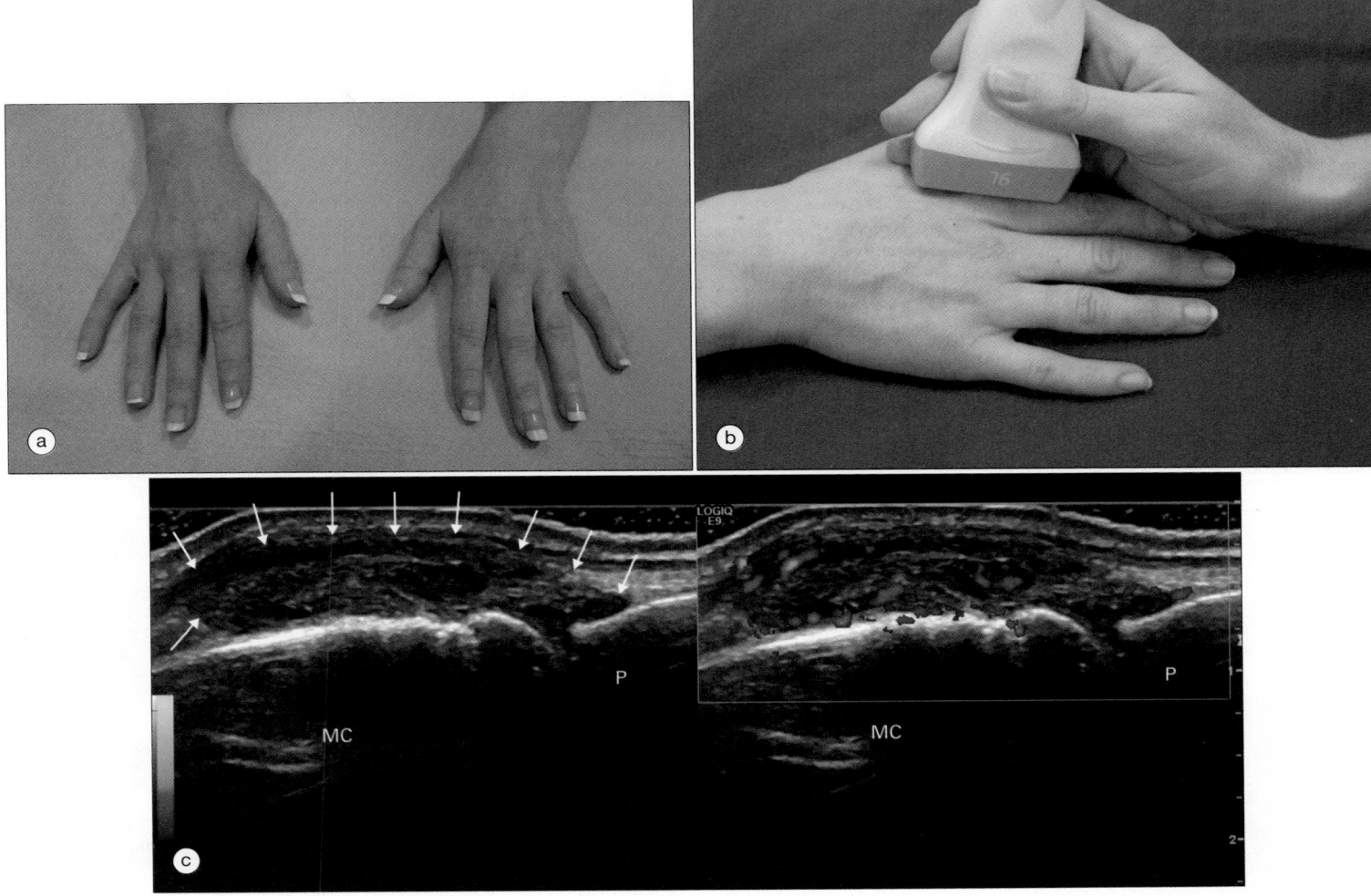

Fig. 40.8 (a) Patient with puffy fingers and arthralgia. (b) Technique of performing an ultrasound examination on an MCPJ. The dorsal, longitudinal plane is shown. (c) Marked grayscale synovitis is demonstrated (white arrows), in longitudinal view. There is also marked Doppler signals within the synovium.

could not be labeled as erosions because no cortical breaks were demonstrated. Recently, a working group of OMERACT has defined an ultrasound bone erosion as an intra-articular discontinuity of the bone surface that is visible in two perpendicular planes (Fig. 40.9).[19] Ultrasound and MRI lesions were comparable where ultrasound had a good access to the tissue under investigation.

One problem of ultrasound is that the transducer may not be able to be adequately angulated in order to visualize the whole bone and may miss erosions as a consequence. This is probably why a study by Hoving and colleagues[43] failed to show a benefit of ultrasound over radiography in the wrist—the ultrasound beam was unable to get between the small carpal bones. In the author's unit, as a consequence, ultrasound has not replaced x-ray but is performed in those in whom the radiographs are normal.

There are limited reports following bone erosions prospectively,[44] which may reflect the difficulty of scoring. Two scoring methods have been proposed. The first is to count individual erosions, while the second is to report global scores of the percentage of bone surface area affected with erosions. Both methods have limitations for use in clinical practice and research. This is especially true of studies including more damaged joints; here it might be considered less sensitive at detecting change. Backhaus and colleagues and later, Scheel,[44] using a subset of the same cohort, showed an increase in the number of joints (wrist, metacarpophalangeal, and proximal interphalangeal joints) with erosions after 2 and 7 years, respectively. Lopez-Ben and colleagues recently found a doubling of erosions after a mean of 6 months when the second and fifth metacarpophalangeal and fifth metatarsophalangeal joints were assessed.[40] Hoving and colleagues, however, showed ultrasound to be inferior to radiographs at detecting changes in the number of bone erosions after 6 months[43] despite it being a relatively

early RA group. The reason behind this could be the inclusion of carpometacarpal and carpal joints in the protocol because they are less accessible to ultrasound. Recently Reynolds and colleagues[29] found no correlation between ultrasound-detected joint synovitis with the progression of the number of ultrasound-detected bone erosions.

Tendon disease

A limited number of studies have highlighted the value of ultrasound for the detection of tendon disease in RA[45-47] and, indeed, some have described it as the gold standard imaging method for assessing tendon involvement in rheumatic diseases.[47] The most common earliest finding appears to be tenosynovitis, while later the tendon becomes thicker and loses its normal fibrillar characteristics. Increased Doppler signal may be seen in the tendon sheath. Small hypoechogenic foci representing tears can sometimes be seen and may be exaggerated by a dynamic examination. In early RA, one of the commonest tendons to be involved is the flexor carpi ulnaris tendon of the wrist. An early paper by de Flaviis demonstrated flexor or extensor tenosynovitis in 18 of 20 (90%) patients with early RA.[34] Grassi and colleagues noted 9 of 20 (45%) patients to have flexor tenosynovitis of the fingers and noted two complete extensor tendon ruptures in two patients with long-standing disease.[45] By contrast, more recent comparisons of ultrasound with gadolinium-enhanced MRI in the hand have shown the former to be less sensitive. In a study of patients with inflammatory arthritis,[32] MRI was found to detect tendon sheath widening in 34% of flexor tendons and 10% of extensor tendons compared with 21% and 5%, respectively, using ultrasound. In a study of 50 early, untreated RA patients, Wakefield and colleagues[48] made similar observations. They also observed that the flexor tendons of the second and third fingers were the most commonly affected. Currently,

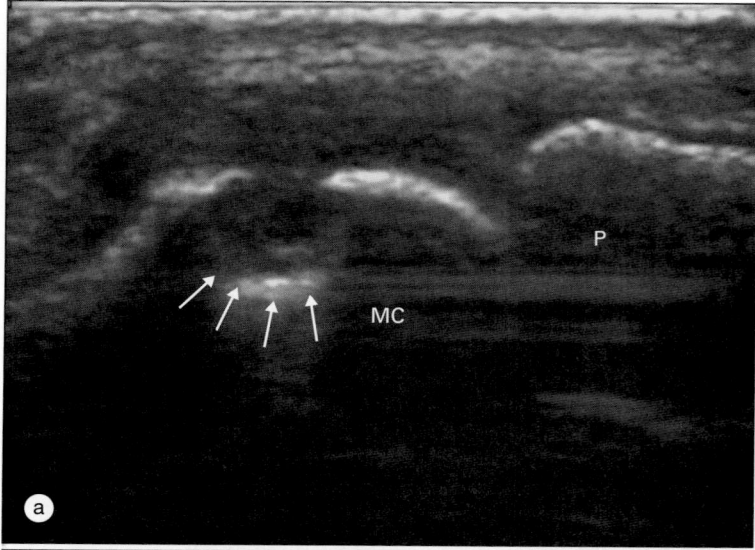

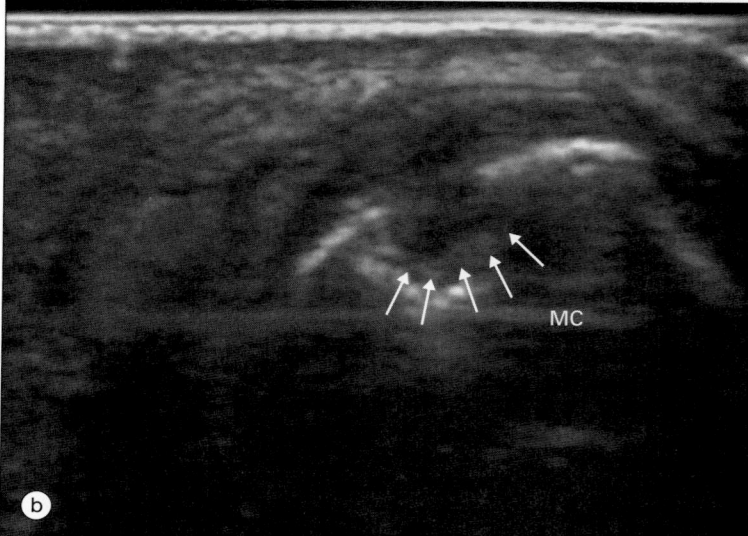

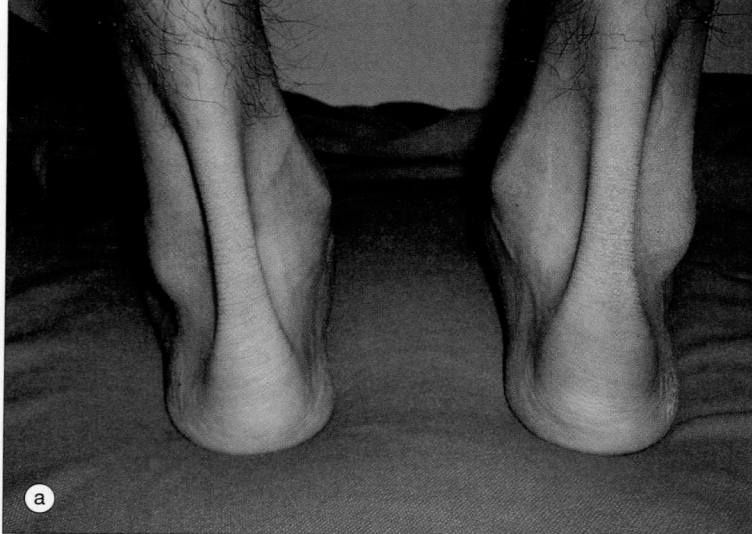

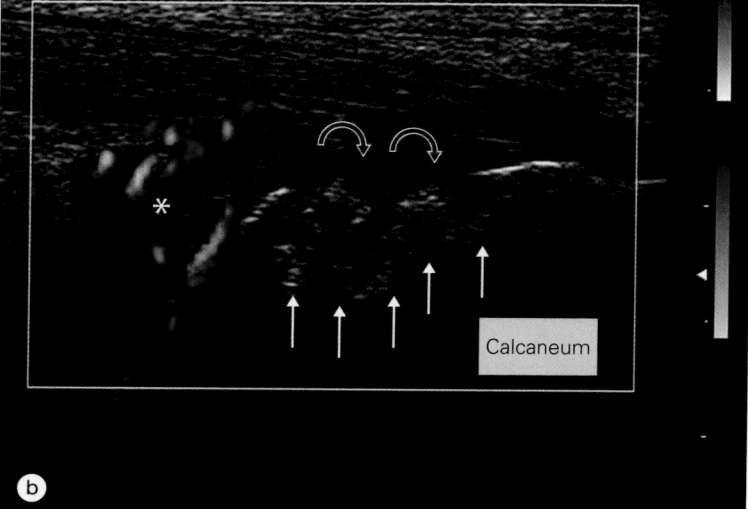

Fig. 40.9 Ultrasound-detected erosion. (a) Longitudinal section through the lateral aspect of the fifth metatarsophalangeal joint of a patient with rheumatoid arthritis demonstrating a large bone erosion (white arrows). MC, metacarpal; P, phalangeal. (b) Transverse section through the same joint demonstrating the same erosion (white arrows). MC, metacarpal.

Fig. 40.10 Achilles enthesitis. (a) Acutely painful posterior heel on right in a young man with a 6-week history of diarrhea and weight loss secondary to underlying Crohn disease. (b) Longitudinal ultrasound section through the Achilles tendon. There is bony irregularity (straight arrows) of the calcaneum, hypoechogenicity, and loss of fibrillar pattern of the tendon at the bony insertion (curved arrows) and increased power Doppler signal seen in the region of the retrocalcaneal bursa (asterisk).

no validated scoring system exists for scoring tenosynovitis with ultrasound.

Enthesitis

Enthesitis is the hallmark of the spondyloarthropathies (SpA) but may also be secondary to mechanical stress. The current diagnosis of SpA is based in part on the clinical ability to detect enthesitis by palpation. Several studies have recently demonstrated the greater sensitivity of ultrasound over clinical examination.[49,50]

The preliminary OMERACT ultrasound definition of enthesopathy is an abnormally hypoechoic and/or thickened tendon or ligament at its bony attachment seen in two perpendicular planes that may exhibit Doppler signal and/or bony changes including enthesophytes, erosions, or irregularity (Fig. 40.10).[19] This definition of enthesitis is based on gray-scale images, which include soft tissue and bone findings. Soft tissue abnormalities, often considered a sign of disease activity, include tendon/ligament thickening, loss of fibrillar pattern, hypoechogenicity, loss of edge definition, intrasubstance calcifications, and associated bursitis. It is not yet proven how well fibrocartilage is visualized on ultrasound. Bone findings that represent structural damage include erosions and enthesophytes.

As with synovitis, Doppler ultrasound is being increasingly used and some reports suggest that if abnormalities are detected at the bony insertion, then this adds greater specificity to the diagnosis of SpA.[50]

Enthesitis on power Doppler has also been shown to improve 3 months after infliximab.[51] Cortical bone erosion and bone spurs may also be clearly seen on ultrasound (often when the radiograph is normal), the positions of which probably relate to the underlying biomechanics of the joint. McGonagle and colleagues[52] recently demonstrated that bone erosions occur proximally on the calcaneum, whereas enthesophytes are more distal. Bone spurs are not specific to the SpAs, and small bone erosions may be seen in normal, especially athletic, individuals.

Sacroiliitis

Preliminary data suggest that ultrasound may be useful in the diagnosis of sacroiliitis.[53,54] The relative deep nature and angulation of the joint means that clear visualization with ultrasound is not always possible and Doppler may be difficult to elicit. Recently studies have suggested relatively good accuracy can be achieved using bubble contrast agents.[55] Ultrasound may also be used to direct needles into the joint space to deliver local therapies, biopsy tissue, or aspirate fluid collections.[56] In the author's opinion, MRI is the preferred method for diagnosing sacroiliitis because it is not only tomographic but able to identify pathology below the surface of the bone (i.e., bone marrow edema, which may predate the synovitis). Ultrasound, however, may have a place in institutions where there is poor access to MRI.

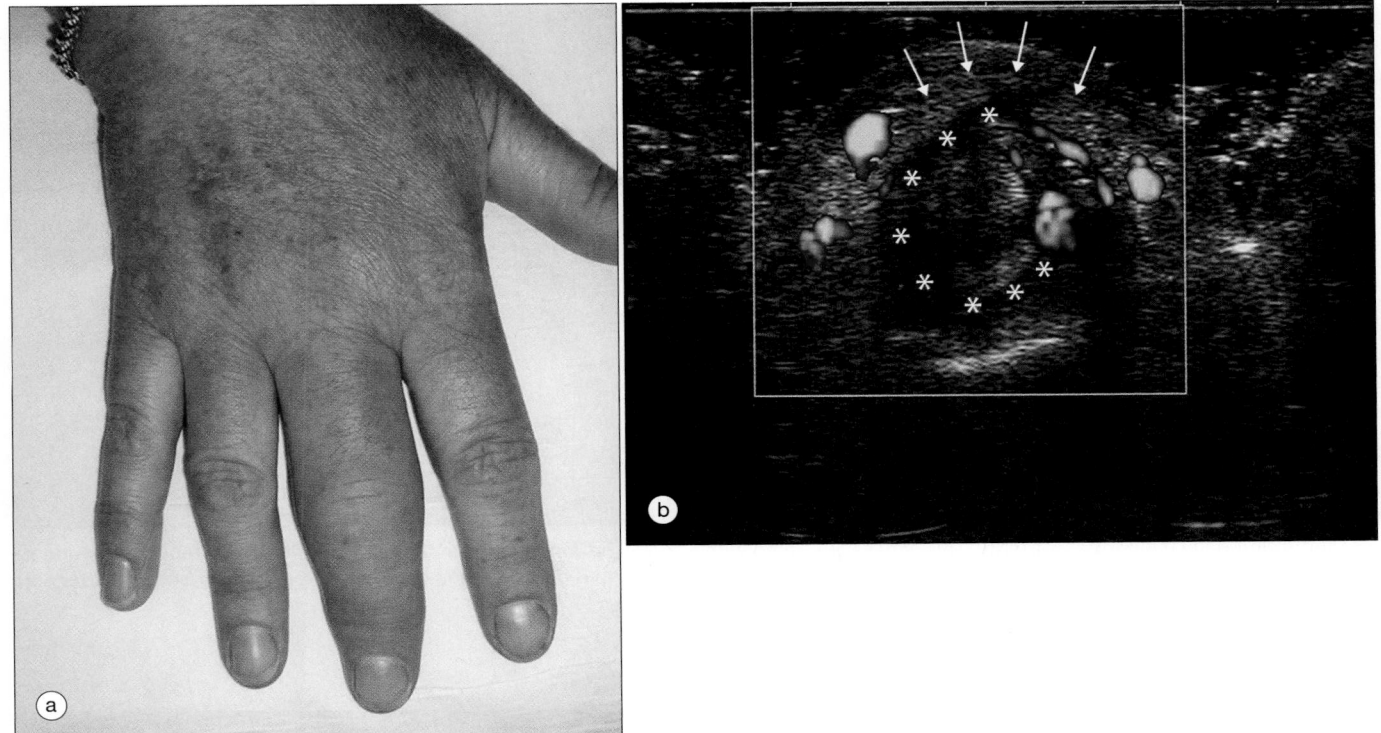

Fig. 40.11 Ultrasound findings in dactylitis. (a) Dactylitis of the third finger of a patient with psoriatic arthritis. (b) Corresponding transverse ultrasound image through the volar aspect of the finger. It demonstrates hypoechogenic thickening of the flexor tendon sheath (asterisks), with increased Doppler signal. In addition there is thickening of the surrounding soft tissue (arrows) with increased vascularity. (a, Courtesy Dr. Sandy Fraser, University of Leeds.)

Dactylitis and bursitis

Dactylitis of the fingers and toes is a common feature of the spondyloarthropathies. The most usual findings on ultrasound are flexor tenosynovitis and subcutaneous edema[57] with synovitis occurring in some but not all joints (Fig. 40.11).[58,59] Bursitis is also a common finding in SpA, particularly in the retrocalcaneal bursa. The lining is synovial based (except the posterior portion), so the ultrasound appearance is of fluid and/or synovial hypertrophy. Doppler signal may also be elicited. Elsewhere, bursae are commonly seen in the shoulder, over the olecranon and patella, and in the feet. It should be noted that normal bursae often contain a small amount of fluid, which can be visualized on ultrasound.[60] Some bursae are adventitial rather than synovial based and occur at sites of mechanical pressure such as in the submetatarsal region of the feet.

Cartilage

Ultrasound has been used to visualize both hyaline (articular) and fibrocartilage. Hyaline cartilage appears anechoic or hypoechoic relative to surrounding subdermal fat. Fibrocartilage such as the menisci of the knee or labrum of the shoulder is more hyperechoic than hyaline cartilage. Ultrasound of cartilage is able to show thinning, osteochondral defects, and, in the case of fibrocartilage, cysts and tears. However, ultrasound is limited by its need for an acoustic window. Therefore full visualization of articular cartilage is not possible; here MRI or arthroscopy is the investigation of choice.

One promising role of ultrasound is in the detection of crystal deposits, especially those not seen by radiography.[61] The pattern of crystal deposition within the cartilage may be helpful. Very high-frequency transducers suggest that in gout, the hyperechoic crystal may lie on the superficial or articular surface of the cartilage and in chondrocalcinosis, the crystals lie within the deeper layers of the cartilage. This may be either diffuse or focal.[62] Recently, diagnostic criteria for CPPD have been proposed using ultrasound.[63]

Non–joint-related structures

Vasculitis

Ultrasound is able to visualize the relatively superficial temporal, carotid, axillary, brachial, and femoral arteries very well (compared with CT and MRI), but the subclavian, iliofemoral, superior and inferior mesenteric, and celiac arteries less well, partly due to the overlying air-filled structures (lungs and bowel). Ultrasound can show morphologic changes of the vessel wall (thickening or increased brightness) and plaques, as well as decreases in flow and vessel elasticity. The role of ultrasound has been explored in a number of vasculitides,[64] most notably temporal arteritis. Here the presence of the "macaroni" halo phenomenon is said to be helpful in the diagnosis, and a recently published meta-analysis suggested a sensitivity of 69% and specificity of 82% for ultrasound when compared with biopsy (Fig. 40.12).[65] The technique of ultrasound requires standardization and as yet, although being helpful, should probably not replace biopsy.

Parotid and salivary glands

Several reports have demonstrated specific parenchymal and duct changes on gray-scale in patients with Sjögren disease.[66-69] There have also been reports of a possible role of Doppler.[70,71]

The technique may have the future potential to be incorporated into diagnostic criteria. Ultrasound has occasionally been useful in identifying parotid abscesses, usually in the severely immunocompromised patients with RA.

Peripheral nerve pathology

The use of ultrasound for detecting peripheral nerve pathology was first proposed by Fornage in 1988.[72] Its routine use is not widespread, but it is an area that is steadily expanding as image resolution improves. High-quality machines can detect almost any mid-size or larger nerves as long as they are accessible to the transducer. Ultrasound can follow the course of the nerve, often through a tortuous route. The most commonly studied nerve is the median nerve in the investigation of carpal tunnel syndrome. Various criteria have been proposed (e.g., bowing of the flexor retinaculum, proximal swelling of the nerve as it enters the carpal tunnel, distal flattening). The cross-sectional area of the nerve appears to be the most consistent association, and a cross-sectional area of 1 cm² has a specificity of 82%, with this figure rising with increased area over this.[73] Our preference is to use a cutoff of about 1.5 cm². Occasionally ultrasound can detect causes of nerve compression such as synovitis, tenosynovitis, ganglia, tumor, or osteophyte.

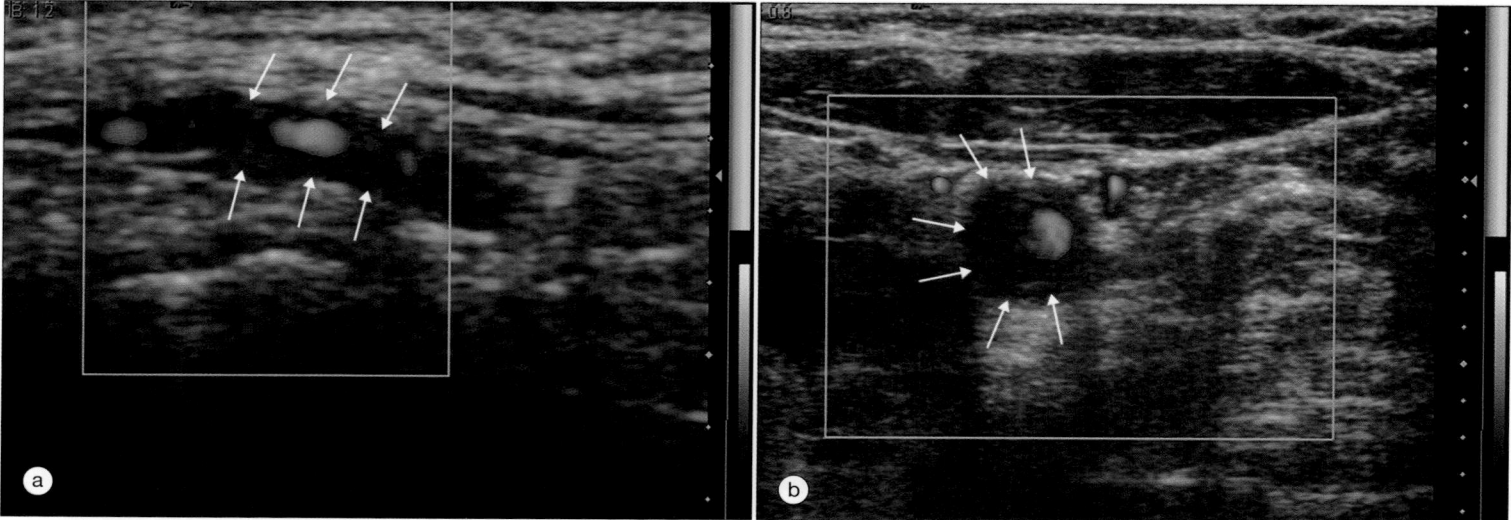

Fig. 40.12 Ultrasound-detected temporal arteritis. This patient presented with a headache consistent with temporal arteritis. These longitudinal and transverse images demonstrate a thickened temporal artery with reduced blood flow. The "halo" sign is demonstrated on transverse section. A temporal artery biopsy confirmed the diagnosis.

Soft tissue disorders of the shoulder and other areas

The most frequent rheumatologic use of ultrasound is in the differential diagnosis of painful shoulder and other soft tissue disorders. This aspect is discussed in detail later.

Rotator cuff disease

Traditionally, the most common indication for shoulder ultrasonography is to evaluate the rotator cuff. In the hands of a good operator, sensitivities and specificities may be as high as 90% to 95%,[74] although they are better for full-thickness than partial-thickness tears (Fig. 40.13).[75] Several studies have shown a good correlation between both MRI[76] and arthroscopy,[75] and in many centers ultrasound has replaced these as a first-line diagnostic tool. However, ultrasound has limitations when viewing the shoulder, including an inability to visualize the labrum-ligamentous complex to diagnose internal derangement.[77]

Calcific tendonitis

Ultrasound can be helpful for identifying and localizing calcific deposits in the rotator cuff. These deposits actually consist of calcium apatite crystals and vary somewhat in ultrasound appearance. Often an abnormality is seen on the radiograph, but ultrasound is used for more accurate localization. The most common site is the supraspinatus tendon followed by the subscapularis tendon, though deposits can be localized in the bursa. Calcifications are usually well defined and cast a clear distal shadow. Early, less-established lesions may cast only a faint shadow or sometimes none at all. The source of pain in these patients is multifactorial involving local inflammation from the crystals, secondary impingement, or frozen shoulder. Ultrasound gives information as to whether the lesion is acute or chronic, is causing thickening of the tendon or is associated with bursa which may result in secondary impingement. This is valuable information when constructing patient treatment plans.

Subacromial-subdeltoid bursitis

The SA-SD bursa covers a large area of the shoulder. The normal bursal membrane is not visualized; the bursal complex appears as a hypoechoic line surrounded by a superficial and deep layer of peribursal fat. Typical fluid collections appear in the most dependent areas of the bursa and more commonly along the edge of the greater tuberosity, producing a typical teardrop appearance. Bursitis may be present as a result of mechanical or inflammatory conditions. Recently, reports have highlighted the high prevalence of bursitis in polymyalgia rheumatica.[78]

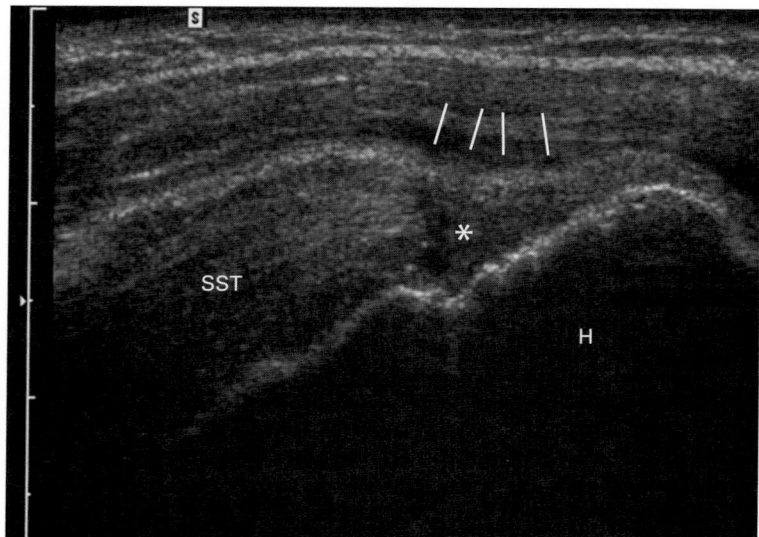

Fig. 40.13 Longitudinal section through the supraspinatus tendon (SST) of a patient with shoulder pain. There is loss of normal convexity of the superficial portion of the tendon (arrows) and an underlying hypoechogenic region (asterisk) consistent with a full-thickness tear extending down to the humerus (H).

Bicipital tendon pathology

The distal long head of biceps is easily visualized by ultrasound until it passes through the rotator cuff to become intra-articular within the glenohumeral joint; the tendon passes between the subscapularis and supraspinatus tendons through what is termed the *rotator cuff interval*. Ultrasound may be used to determine if the tendon is intact, subluxes with movement, or is surrounded by fluid/synovial hypertrophy. Fluid around the tendon may be present and is indicative of either local irritation of the tendon sheath or glenohumeral effusion. Full-thickness rotator cuff tears allow communication of fluid between the joint and subacromial bursa; when there is fluid in both the tendon sheath and bursa, full-thickness cuff tears are present in 95% of cases.[77] A presumptive clinical diagnosis of bicipital tendonitis often has normal ultrasound findings, suggesting that the former is subject to error.

Other soft tissue syndromes

Trochanteric bursitis is better described as a pain syndrome because there are many potential underlying causes. Ultrasound rarely demonstrates a true fluid-distended bursa. Occasionally bone irregularity or soft tissue calcifications are observed around the greater trochanter, but these are often seen in normal controls. The main role of ultrasound in trochanteric bursitis is to exclude other causes of pain and to guide diagnostic and therapeutic trochanteric injections. Ultrasound can sometimes demonstrate a friction bursa as the iliotibial band courses over the greater trochanter. Gluteal muscle tears that have been identified on MRI as common[79] in this syndrome may occasionally be visualized on ultrasound. Ultrasound has also been used to identify pes anserine bursitis, although one study showed that scans are often normal in symptomatic patients.[80] Lateral[81] and medial epicondylitis[82] of the elbow may both be visualized by ultrasound. Findings include tendon thickening, intratendinous calcifications, enthesophytes or erosions, and focal intrasubstance areas of hypoechogenicity. Increased Doppler activity may increase the diagnostic specificity of lateral epicondylitis, may serve as a predictive marker, or may be used as a marker of therapy response.[83]

Interventional procedures

Ultrasound can be used to accurately aspirate fluid collections and introduce needles for diagnostic or therapeutic injections or biopsy.[84] Diagnostic injections are those performed into or around a structure where local anesthetic is instilled to determine whether the patient's symptoms arise from that area. Two published studies showed extremely poor accuracy of joint injections without imaging guidance, reporting an accuracy of 42% to 51% for large joint injection[85] and only 29% for subacromial bursal injections.[86] Ultrasound allows the operator to dynamically image the needle placement (direct approach), although it may be used to simply mark the point of injection and provide an estimation of required angle of needle insertion and distance to target (indirect approach).

Insertion technique

The needle placement technique is similar in all applications regardless of the type of needle being positioned or whether the intention is to aspirate, inject, or biopsy. Aseptic techniques must be adhered to at all times, especially when injecting synovial joints or tendon sheaths; this may or may not require the use of a sterile transducer cover. Needle visualization in musculoskeletal ultrasound is generally good due to the reflective nature of the needle surface and the generally superficial position of the target. Needle placements into deeper structures such as the greater trochanteric bursa or the hip joints are more difficult, but even in these cases the use of probe guides is rarely necessary.

Joint aspiration

Ultrasound-guided joint aspirations are frequently performed to confirm or exclude the presence of infection or crystal disease (Fig. 40.14). The majority of joints can be aspirated under direct visualization of the needle. The hip is the most common joint requiring ultrasound-guided aspiration for the suspicion of infection in adults. On occasion this can be difficult in the adult because lower-frequency (3- to 5-MHz) transducers are required to achieve the beam penetration necessary to visualize the hip. This transducer inherently has a lower spatial resolution that, combined with an oblique needle approach, makes visualization of the needle more difficult. From a diagnostic viewpoint this also makes differentiation between complex fluid and synovial or capsular thickening problematic, with aspiration often the only diagnostic option.

An 18- or 20-gauge needle should be inserted under ultrasound guidance. If no effusion can be aspirated, then there are two possible maneuvers. First, a small amount of sterile saline (2-3 mL) may be injected into the joint with reaspiration of the fluid for microbacteriologic assessment. If there is difficulty with reaspirating this fluid from the joint, then asking the patient to take the weight of the leg on the affected side increases the intra-articular pressure in the joint, allowing easier reaspiration. This maneuver can also be of value during the initial aspiration because effusions often pool posteriorly, with the increased intra-articular pressure redistributing any joint fluid present. Samples can then be sent for routine microbacteriologic analysis either in dry sample pots or in blood culture medium.

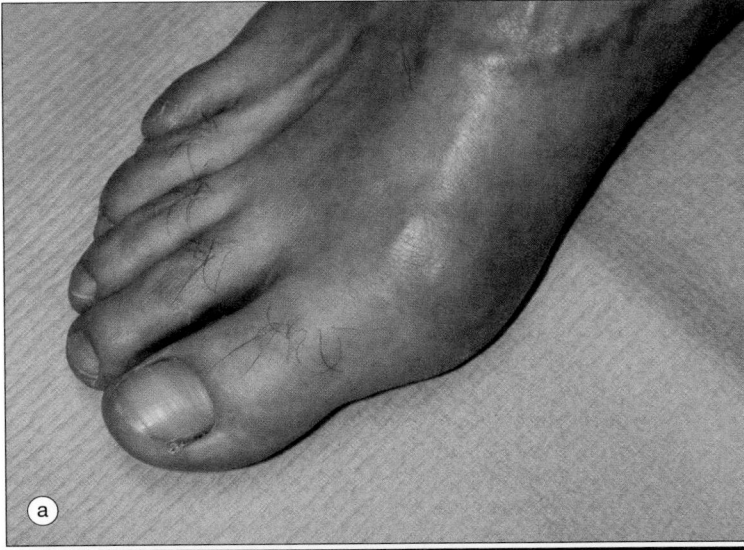

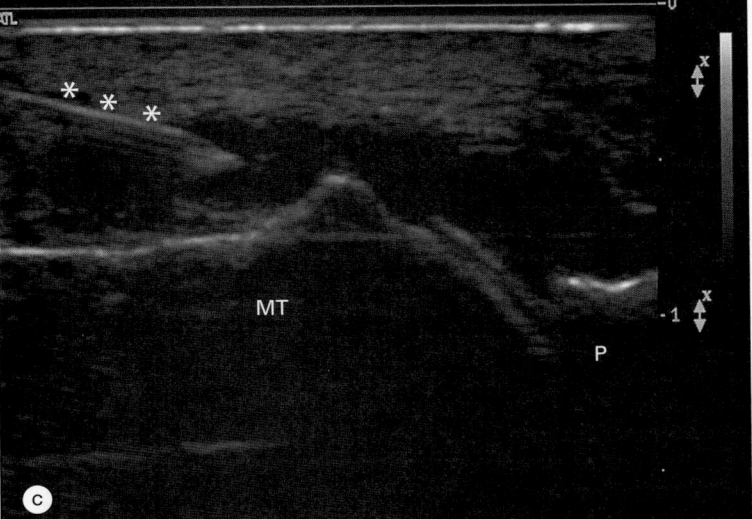

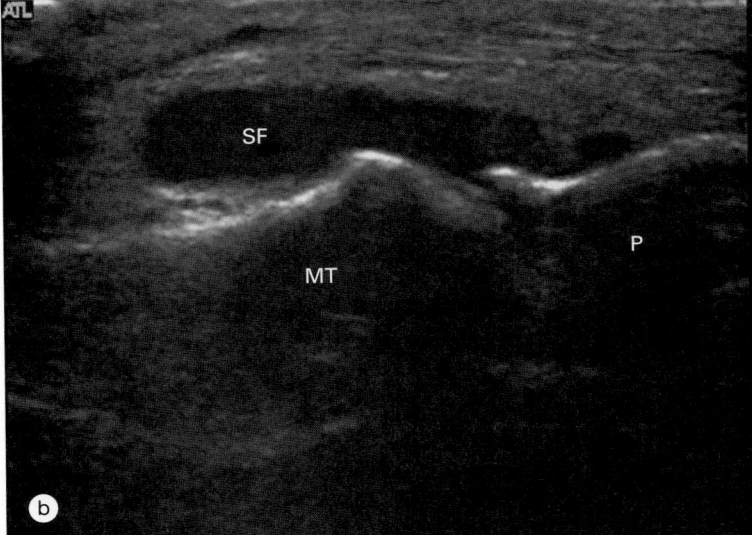

Fig. 40.14 Inflammation of first metatarsophalangeal joint, presumed to be gout. (a) This patient had acute swelling of the big toe with pain, erythema, and swelling. The diagnosis of gout was suspected but the serum urate was within normal limits. (b, c) This longitudinal image through the toe demonstrated a hypoechogenic collection in the joint that was compressible and displaceable and consistent with an effusion. A needle was subsequently introduced into the joint under ultrasound guidance and withdrew a small amount of fluid. Analysis confirmed the presence of urate crystals. MT, metatarsal head; P, phalanx; asterisk denotes needle.

Joint injections

In addition to introducing a needle to aspirate fluid, ultrasound can guide therapies. Diagnostic injections are those that target a particular site with long-acting local anesthetic such as bupivacaine hydrochloride (Marcaine). Combined with either re-examination or a symptom log postinjection, these can give valuable information as to the source of pain. Therapeutic injections contain both steroid and local anesthetic. Intuitively, a more accurate needle placement should increase the success of these injections but there still remains a paucity of studies demonstrating this potential benefit, particularly over a sustained period. The most common injection given is into the subacromial-subdeltoid space, but ultrasound may be used to inject any joint. In particular, it has been used to inject the plantar fascia,[87] glenohumeral joint,[88] wrist,[89] and sacroiliac joints.[90] Ultrasound may also be chosen to guide therapies that may be irritant if introduced outside the joint (e.g., hyaluronic acid).[91]

Needle biopsy

As with aspiration and injections, ultrasound can visualize needle placement in real time. It is increasingly being considered as an alternative to arthroscopy as a source of synovial biopsy.[92] In rheumatology, it has also been used to biopsy bone erosions[93] and early entheseal lesions[94] and to guide nerve biopsies.[95]

Training and education

The wider availability of high-quality, affordable ultrasound machines and the potential to have an immediate positive impact in patient management[96] has meant that rheumatologists are now performing or wanting to perform ultrasound examinations as part of their routine clinical practice. This has created controversy and some unease between rheumatologists and radiologists.[97] However, as time has passed, it is the author's view that this tension has begun to subside as each party has started to understand that its scanning practices are different and largely not conflicting. Many radiologists do not want (or have the resources) to scan multiple joints, while rheumatologists are largely conservative and tend to not scan beyond their level, and refer on where appropriate. This has probably also led to more efficient service in radiology because the rheumatologists only tend to refer on the most important cases. At a European level, the European Society of Skeletal Radiologists (ESSR) is now forging strong links with EULAR, which is likely to lead to collaborations in teaching and research.

The importance of MUS training for rheumatologists was recently recognized at a European level by EULAR, and training guidelines were established for running EULAR courses.[31] Similar guidelines will soon emerge from the Pan-American Congress of Rheumatology (PANLAR) and the Asian Pacific League of Associations for Rheumatology (APLAR). Short MUS courses are now available in most countries, but some countries are currently not in a position to run intermediate or advanced courses, which is why international courses like the EULAR courses remain valuable. New methods of delivering teaching or assessing uploaded images have begun to appear through some e-learning programs. One of the main barriers to learning is a current lack of qualified people to supervise and mentor others. This should change over time as the technique becomes more established; however, there also needs to be a cultural change in institutions where trainers are given time and resources to be allowed to train others. Currently, competency is assessed by ongoing observation by a mentor with a logbook/portfolio review of cases. There is currently no internationally recognized competency examination in rheumatology.

KEY REFERENCES

11. Kremkau FW. Doppler ultrasound: principles and instruments. Philadelphia: WB Saunders, 1990:13.

13. Rizzatto G. Ultrasound transducers. Eur J Radiol 1998,27:S188-S195.

16. Karim Z, Wakefield RJ, Quinn M, et al. Validation and reproducibility of ultrasonography in the detection of synovitis in the knee: a comparison with arthroscopy and clinical examination. Arthritis Rheum 2004;50:387-394.

17. Koski JM, Isomaki H. Ultrasonography may reveal synovitis in a clinically silent hip joint. Clin Rheumatol 1990;9:539-541.

18. Weidekamm C, Koller M, Weber M, Kainberger F. Diagnostic value of high-resolution B-mode and Doppler sonography for imaging of hand and finger joints in rheumatoid arthritis. Arthritis Rheum 2003;48:325-333.

19. Wakefield RJ, Balint P, Szkudlarek M, et al. Musculoskeletal ultrasound including definitions for ultrasonographic pathology. J Rheumatol 2005;32:2485-2487.

20. Schmidt WA, Schmidt H, Schicke B, Gromnica-Ihle E. Standard reference values for musculoskeletal ultrasonography. Ann Rheum Dis 2004;63:988-994.

21. Schmidt WA, Volker L, Zacher J, et al. Colour Doppler ultrasonography to detect pannus in knee joint synovitis. Clin Exp Rheumatol 2000;18:439-444.

22. Walther M, Harms H, Krenn V, et al. Correlation of power Doppler sonography with vascularity of the synovial tissue of the knee joint in patients with osteoarthritis and rheumatoid arthritis. Arthritis Rheum 2001;44:331-338.

23. Koski JM, Saarakkala S, Helle M, et al. Power Doppler ultrasonography and synovitis. Correlating ultrasound imaging with histopathological findings and evaluating the performance of ultrasound equipments. Ann Rheum Dis 2006;65:1590-1595.

24. Szkudlarek M, Narvestad E, Klarlund M, et al. Ultrasonography of the metatarsophalangeal joints in rheumatoid arthritis: comparison with magnetic resonance imaging, conventional radiography, and clinical examination. Arthritis Rheum 2004;50:2103-2112.

25. Terslev L, Torp-Pedersen S, Savnik A, et al. Doppler ultrasound and magnetic resonance imaging of synovial inflammation of the hand in rheumatoid arthritis: a comparative study. Arthritis Rheum 2003;48:2434-2441.

26. Terslev L, Torp-Pedersen S, Qvistgaard E, et al. Estimation of inflammation by Doppler ultrasound: quantitative changes after intra-articular treatment in rheumatoid arthritis. Ann Rheum Dis 2003;62:1049-1053.

27. Ribbens C, Andre B, Marcelis S, et al. Rheumatoid hand joint synovitis: gray scale and power Doppler US quantifications following anti-tumour necrosis factor-alpha treatment: pilot study. Radiology 2003;229:563-569.

28. Hau M, Kneitz C, Tony H-P, et al. High resolution ultrasound detects a decrease in pannus vascularisation of small finger joints in patients with rheumatoid arthritis receiving treatment either soluble tumour necrosis factor a receptor (etanercept). Ann Rheum Dis 2002;61:55-58.

29. Taylor PC, Steuer A, Gruber D, et al. Comparison of ultrasonographic assessment of synovitis and joint vascularity with radiographic evaluation in a randomized, placebo-controlled study of infliximab therapy in early rheumatoid arthritis. Arthritis Rheum 2004;50:1107-1116.

30. Wakefield RJ, Green MJ, Marzo-Ortega H, et al. Should oligoarthritis be reclassified? Ultrasound reveals a high prevalence of subclinical disease. Ann Rheum Dis 2004;63:382-385.

31. De Flaviis L, Scaglione P, Nessi R, et al. Ultrasonography of the hand in rheumatoid arthritis. Acta Radiol 1988;29:457-460.

35. Grassi W, Titarelli E, Pirani O, et al. Ultrasound examination of the metacarpophalangeal joints in rheumatoid arthritis. Scand J Rheumatol 1993;22:243-247.

36. Lund PJ, Heikal A, Maricic MJ, et al. Ultrasonographic imaging of the hand and wrist in rheumatoid arthritis. Skeletal Radiol 1995;24:591-596.

37. Alasaarela E, Suramo I, Tervonen O, et al. Evaluation of humeral head erosions in rheumatoid arthritis: a comparison of ultrasonography, magnetic resonance imaging, computed tomography and plain radiography. Br J Rheumatol 1998;37:1152-1156.

38. Backhaus M, Kamradt T, Sandrock D, et al. Arthritis of the finger joints. A comprehensive approach comparing conventional radiography, scintigraphy, ultrasound, and contrast-enhanced magnetic resonance imaging. Arthritis Rheum 1999;42:1232-1245.

39. Alarcon GS, Lopez-Ben R, Moreland LW. High resolution ultrasound for the study of target joints in rheumatoid arthritis. Arthritis Rheum 2002;46:1969-1981.

40. Lopez-Ben R, Bernreuter WK, Moreland, L, Alarcon GS. Ultrasound detection of bone erosions in rheumatoid arthritis: a comparison to routine radiographs of the hands and feet. Skeletal Radiol 2004;33:80-84.

41. Magnani M, Salizzoni E, Mule R, et al. Ultrasonography detection of early bone erosions in the metacarpophalangeal joints of patients with rheumatoid arthritis. Clin Exp Rheum 2004;22:743-748.

42. Wakefield RJ, Gibbon WW, Conaghan PG, et al. The value of sonography in the detection of bone erosions in patients with rheumatoid arthritis—a comparison with conventional radiography. Arthritis Rheum 2000;43:2762-2770.

43. Hoving JL, Buchbinder R, Hall S, et al. A comparison of magnetic resonance imaging, sonography, and radiography of the hand in patients with early rheumatoid arthritis. J Rheumatol 2004;31:663-675.

44. Scheel AK, Hermann KG, Ohrndorf S, et al. Prospective 7 year follow up imaging study comparing radiography, ultrasonography, and magnetic resonance imaging in rheumatoid arthritis finger joints. Ann Rheum Dis 2006;65:595-600.

45. Grassi W, Tittarelli E, Blastetti P, et al. Finger tendon involvement in rheumatoid arthritis. Evaluation with high frequency sonography. Arthritis Rheum 1995;38:786-794.

46. Swen WA, Jacobs JWG, Hubach PCG, et al. Comparison of sonography and magnetic resonance imaging for the diagnosis of partial tears of finger extensor tendons in rheumatoid arthritis. Rheumatology 2000;39:55-62.

47. Grassi W, Filippucci E, Farina A, Cervini C. Sonographic imaging of tendons. Arthritis Rheum 2000;43:969-976.

49. Balint PV, Kane D, Wilson H, et al. Ultrasonography of entheseal insertions in the lower limb in spondyloarthropathy. Ann Rheum Dis 2002;61:905-910.

50. D'Agostino MA, Said-Nahal R, Hacquard-Bouder C, et al. Assessment of peripheral enthesitis in the spondyloarthropathies by ultrasonography combined with power Doppler: a cross-sectional study. Arthritis Rheum 2003;48:523-533.

51. D'Agostino MA, Breban M, Said-Nahal R, Dougados M. Refractory inflammatory heel pain in spondylarthropathy: a significant response to infliximab documented by ultrasound. Arthritis Rheum 2002;46:840-841.

53. Arslan H, Sakarya ME, Adak B, et al. Duplex and color Doppler sonographic findings in active sacroiliitis. AJR 1999;173:677-680.

54. Klauser A, Halpern EJ, Frauscher F, et al. Inflammatory low back pain: high negative predictive value of contrast-enhanced color Doppler ultrasound in the

detection of inflamed sacroiliac joints. Arthritis Rheum 2005;53:440-444.

57. Olivieri I, Barozzi L, Favaro L, et al. Dactylitis in patients with seronegative spondylarthropathy. Assessment by ultrasonography and magnetic resonance imaging. Arthritis Rheum 1996;39:1524-1528.

58. Kane D, Greaney T, Bresnihan B, et al. Ultrasonography in the diagnosis and management of psoriatic dactylitis. J Rheumatol 1999;26:1746-1751.

59. Wakefield RJ, Emery P, Veale DJ. Ultrasonography and psoriatic arthritis. J Rheumatol 2000;27: 1564-1565.

60. Nazarian L, Rawool N, Martin C, et al. Synovial fluid in the hindfoot and ankle: detection of amount and distribution with ultrasound. Radiology 1995;197:275-278.

61. Monteforte P, Brignone A, Rovetta G. Tissue changes detectable by sonography before radiological evidence of elbow chondrocalcinosis. Int J Tissue React 2000;22:23-25.

62. Sofka CM, Adler RS, Cordasco FA. Ultrasound diagnosis of chondrocalcinosis in the knee. Skeletal Radiol 2002;31:43-45.

63. Frediani B, Filippou G, Falsetti P, et al. Diagnosis of calcium pyrophosphate dihydrate crystal deposition disease: ultrasonographic criteria proposed. Ann Rheum Dis 2005;64:638-640.

64. Schmidt WA. Use of imaging studies in the diagnosis of vasculitis. Curr Rheumatol Rep 2004;6:203-211.

65. Karassa FB, Matsagas MI, Schmidt WA, Ioannidis JP. Meta-analysis: test performance of ultrasonography for giant-cell arteritis. Ann Intern Med 2005;142:359-369.

66. De Vita S, Lorenzon G, Rossi G, et al. Salivary gland echography in primary and secondary Sjogren's syndrome. Clin Exp Rheumatol 1992;10:351-356.

67. Makula E, Pokorny G, Rajtar M, et al. Parotid gland ultrasonography as a diagnostic tool in primary Sjogren's syndrome. Br J Rheumatol 1996;35:972-977.

68. Yonetsu K, Takagi Y, Sumi M, et al. Sonography as a replacement for sialography for the diagnosis of salivary glands affected by Sjogren's syndrome. Ann Rheum Dis 2002;61:276-277.

69. Mandel L, Orchowski YS. Using ultrasonography to diagnose Sjogren's syndrome. J Am Dent Assoc 1998;129:1129-1133.

72. Fornage BD. Peripheral nerves of the extremities: imaging with US. Radiology 1988;167:179-182.

REFERENCES

Full references for this chapter can be found on www.expertconsult.com.

Bone scintigraphy and positron emission tomography

41

Clio Ribbens and Gauthier Namur

- Bone scintigraphy with technetium-labeled diphosphonates is a nuclear medicine technique widely used for the investigation of bone and joint diseases. It is highly sensitive for depicting foci of increased bone turnover and increased blood flow, but uptake is non-specific and the combination with other imaging modalities is necessary for differential diagnosis.

- Positron emission tomography (PET) is a technique using molecules labeled with isotopes that emit positrons from their nucleus, the most widely used being 2-deoxy-2-[^{18}F]fluoro-D-deoxyglucose (^{18}F-FDG). ^{18}F-FDG accumulates in foci of increased glucose consumption, such as inflammatory lesions, allowing for a direct identification of increased metabolic activity.

- Recent PET devices are combined with computed tomography (PET/CT), allowing for a precise localization and even frequently a morphologic description of the lesions with increased metabolic activity.

- The clinical applications of ^{18}F-FDG-PET include the detection of inflammation in various rheumatic diseases such as vasculitis, arthritis, lupus, or sarcoidosis, as well as the workup of fever of unknown origin.

INTRODUCTION

Imaging in rheumatology has greatly evolved these past 2 decades, resulting in major advances in the clinical management of patients. Concurrently to the improvement of radiographic techniques with ultrasonography, computed tomography (CT), and magnetic resonance imaging (MRI) being added to conventional radiography, nuclear medicine techniques have made progress not only in the research area but also in the clinical world. They play a role for both diagnosis and follow-up of inflammatory diseases.[1,2] The most common nuclear medicine technique used in rheumatology is bone scintigraphy, but more recent methods such as positron emission tomography (PET) have emerged, providing information regarding the metabolic status of tissues in addition to the morphologic information provided by the other imaging modalities.

BONE SCINTIGRAPHY

Principles

The high affinity of diphosphonates for bone led to their use as an imaging modality with technetium-99m (^{99m}Tc) labeling for bone scintigraphy in the early 1970s. The energy of the photon emitted by the ^{99m}Tc nuclide (140 keV) is well adapted to the physical properties of the current gamma cameras. On decay, radionuclides emit a gamma ray at their characteristic energies in different directions. Some of these rays interact with the gamma camera, whereas others may scatter, lose direction, or never interact with the camera.[3] Gamma cameras acquire data in a single plane. The resultant images are therefore a two-dimensional representation of a three-dimensional subject, referred to as planar imaging. ^{99m}Tc-methylene diphosphonate (MDP) and ^{99m}Tc-hydroxymethylene diphosphonate (HMDP) are the most commonly used radionuclides for bone scintigraphy. Diphosphonates are either taken up by bone or rapidly cleared through the kidneys. Approximately 50% of the dose is distributed in the skeleton within 3 hours after intravenous injection, the remainder being excreted in the urine.[4] In a normally hydrated subject, less than 5% of the dose remains in the blood 3 hours after injection.[4]

Single-photon emission computed tomography

The disadvantage of planar images obtained with scintigraphy can be overcome by single-photon emission computed tomography (SPECT), which acquires volumetric data by rotating the gamma camera around the patient or by using multidetector systems. It offers images in three planes and has better spatial resolution. The main current clinical applications focus on evaluation of the skull and spine. The advent of gamma cameras with tomographic capabilities combined with a CT scanner (SPECT-CT) in 1998 introduced the concept of blended imaging devices, providing complementary information, that is, a fusion image with functional (SPECT) anatomic (CT) correlation. This technique will probably improve the clinical usefulness of bone scintigraphy, but rigorous extensive data are still lacking.

Uses

Because the uptake of ^{99m}Tc-diphosphonates in bone is dependent on the osteoblastic activity as well as on the regional blood flow, bone scintigraphy is highly sensitive for many disorders causing increased bone turnover (Table 41.1; Fig. 41.1). It lacks, however, specificity and distinguishing for example metastatic disease from osteoarthritis requires the use of other imaging modalities.

It is particularly useful where the arthritis is difficult to detect clinically, such as sacroiliitis. Sacroiliitis may be detected on the basis of an increased uptake of ^{99m}Tc-diphosphonates in the sacroiliac joints. A high uptake in the these joints is, however, also found in normal individuals,[5] and the ratio of the peak sacroiliac joint to the peak sacrum count is usually used, although normal values of this ratio can vary significantly depending on age and gender. Even so, the specificity is low and other imaging modalities such as MRI are of better value for diagnosis of sacroiliitis in spondyloarthropathies.[6] Increased uptake of ^{99m}Tc-diphosphonates in arthritis, whether septic or not, is linked to increased blood flow, expanded blood pool volume, and vascular permeability; and the hyperemia involves not only the synovial membrane but also the juxta-articular bones.[7] This technique can therefore not discriminate accurately between actively inflamed joints and chronically damaged joints[8] and does not allow correct evaluation of inflammatory arthritis.

Use of other tracers

Given the limitation of ^{99m}Tc, other radiotracers have been investigated for the evaluation of arthritis: gallium (^{67}Ga) citrate, indium-111 chloride (^{111}InCl$_3$), ^{99m}Tc-hexamethylpropylene amine oxime (HMPAO)-labeled leukocytes, ^{99m}Tc-liposomes, ^{99m}Tc-polyclonal human immunoglobulin G (IgG) monoclonal antibodies to granulocytes, and ^{99m}Tc-labeled anti-CD4 monoclonal antibodies.[7] Indium and gallium possess a high affinity for iron-binding proteins and probably bind to transferrin receptors abundant in the inflamed synovium, explaining their affinity for the inflammatory site compartment.[9] A combination

TABLE 41.1 DISORDERS EXHIBITING INCREASED UPTAKE ON BONE SCINTIGRAPHY

- Bone tumors: primary (benign/malignant), secondary
- Bone or joint infection
- Traumatic bone or joint injuries
- Metabolic bone diseases (e.g., Paget's disease, hyperparathyroidism, osteomalacia)
- Arthritis: inflammatory or degenerative
- Avascular necrosis
- Orthopedic joint prosthesis
- Reflex sympathetic dystrophy

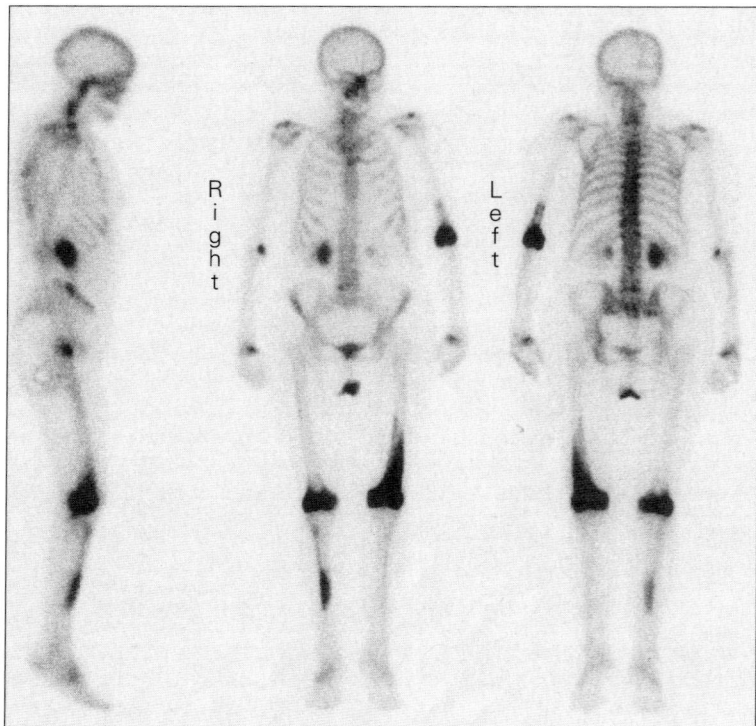

Fig. 41.1 Right lateral, anterior, and posterior whole-body bone scintiscans in a patient with Paget's disease show involvement of the distal parts of both femurs, distal part of the left humerus, and right tibial diaphysis.

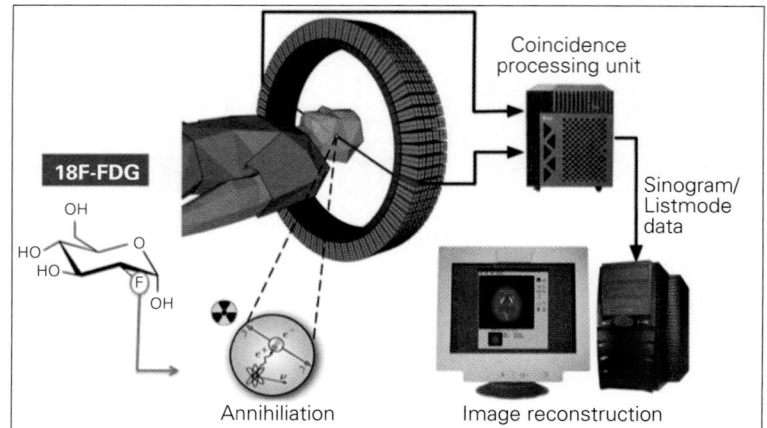

Fig. 41.2 Principles of PET. 2-Deoxy-2-[^{18}F]fluoro-D-deoxyglucose (^{18}F-FDG) is a labeled glucose analog in which the hydrogen in the 2-position is replaced by the ^{18}F radioisotope, a positron emitter. A positron is the antiparticle of an electron, with opposite charge. ^{18}F-FDG accumulates in cells proportionally to their glucose consumption. ^{18}F-FDG decays by emitting a positron from its nucleus. After traveling a short distance into the patient's body, this positron encounters an electron, resulting in an annihilation process. This process involves the emission of two photons of 511 keV in diametrically opposite directions. These photons are registered by the PET "camera" as soon as they arrive at the detector ring. After the registration, the data are forwarded to a processing unit that decides if two registered events are selected as a so-called coincidence event. All coincidences are forwarded to the image processing unit where the final image data are produced via mathematical image reconstruction procedures.

of gallium scintigraphy and ^{99m}Tc-diphosphonate scintigraphy could be helpful because an association of a positive gallium scan with a negative ^{99m}Tc-MDP scan has been suggested to be characteristic of (although not 100% specific for) infection of an orthopedic prosthesis, whereas a negative gallium scan associated with a positive ^{99m}Tc-MDP scan can be seen in synovial giant cell foreign-body reaction in total-knee arthroplasties.[10] However, gallium scans necessitate a 24-hour delay before imaging, entailing two patient visits; imply a relatively high radiation exposure; and exhibit a limited image quality. Scintigraphy with labeled leukocytes has raised concerns due to hazards associated with blood withdrawal, labeling and reinjecting cells under non-physiologic conditions, and performing delayed imaging up to 24 hours after the administration of the cells. Bone scintigraphy with ^{99m}Tc-labeled diphosphonates therefore remains the standard nuclear medicine approach for assessing joint involvement in a whole-body approach.

POSITRON EMISSION TOMOGRAPHY

Background

In contrast to scintigraphy or SPECT in which molecules are "tagged" with radioisotopes emitting gamma rays, PET utilizes molecules labeled with isotopes that emit positrons from their nucleus. These

relatively short-lived positron-emitting isotopes are created in a cyclotron, a device used to accelerate charged particles, and include ^{15}O (half-life of 2 minutes), ^{13}N (10 minutes), ^{11}C (20 minutes), and ^{18}F (110 minutes). The most commonly used radiolabeled molecule, referred to as a probe or tracer, is 2-deoxy-2-[^{18}F]fluoro-D-deoxyglucose (FDG) in which one of the hydrogens has been replaced by the ^{18}F radioisotope. ^{18}F-FDG is an analog of glucose and after intravenous injection it is taken up by cells according to their level of glucose metabolism. ^{18}F-FDG is transported through the cell membrane via glucose transporters into the cytosol and is phosphorylated by the enzyme hexokinase into ^{18}F-FDG-6-phosphate. In contrast to glucose, ^{18}F-FDG-6-phosphate cannot proceed further in the glycolytic pathway and ^{18}F-FDG-6-phospate is not further dephosphorylated and accumulates in the cell, proportionally to the cell glucose consumption. ^{18}F decays by emitting a positron from its nucleus. This positron eventually collides with a nearby electron, resulting in an annihilation event where two 511-keV photons in the form of gamma rays are emitted approximately 180 degrees apart.[3] These photons are detected by the PET "camera," a ring array of detectors (composed of scintillation crystals and photomultiplier tubes) around the patient. Detection of a single annihilation event results in the activation of detectors opposing one another, which is recorded as a "coincident event." Mathematical analysis of the coincident events yields the location of cell populations or tissues that have accumulated ^{18}F-FDG (Fig. 41.2). The spatial resolution of the most recent clinical PET scanners is 4 to 6 mm.

Uses

The development of PET was closely linked to that of ^{18}F-FDG in the 1970s. First used in cardiology and neurology, the clinical application of PET was extended to oncology in view of the increased glucose metabolism in tumoral cells. The use of ^{18}F-FDG-PET for evaluating infection and inflammation arose from false-positive findings encountered in patients undergoing evaluation for malignancy as well as from the demonstration of an increased glucose metabolism in many inflammatory cell types and of the ^{18}F-FDG uptake by inflammatory tissues. Animal studies showed that ^{18}F-FDG uptake by tumors is due not only to the tumor cells themselves but also to the inflammatory cells (macrophages, neutrophils, fibroblasts, endothelial cells) appearing in association with growth or necrosis of the tumor.[11,12] This glucose utilization by inflammatory cells is made possible by their increased expression of glucose transporters when they are activated.[13,14] ^{18}F-FDG-PET is therefore a fully tomographic technique, offering 3D visualization of the glucose metabolism. Compared with scintigraphy, it offers several advantages for the assessment of patients with inflammation. First, the ^{18}F-FDG uptake is directly related to the activity of metabolically active inflammatory cells whereas bone scintigraphy detects the indirect hyperemia. Second, the spatial resolution and count rates of ^{18}F-FDG-PET are much improved when compared with planar scintigraphy.[15] Finally, the uptake phase of ^{18}F-FDG is shorter than with ^{99m}Tc-MDP, allowing a whole-body examination to be completed within 90 minutes while more than 4 hours (uptake + acquisition) is needed for a bone scintiscan. Furthermore, ^{18}F-FDG has a 110-minute half-life, permitting its use in centers distant from a cyclotron, and delivers a dose to the patient that is acceptable when compared with ^{99m}Tc-MDP.

PET/CT

The advent of the combination of PET with CT in 2000 has allowed for a precise anatomic location (revealed by CT) of the increased metabolic activity (provided by PET). The optimal methodology for performing and interpreting the PET/CT studies remains to be defined. To fully contribute to the diagnostic information, the CT scan should be acquired with the appropriate parameters in terms of beam collimation (which is related to the slice thickness) and dose, possibly with intravenous contrast agents. Whether such a full diagnostic CT is really needed in addition to the low-dose CT remains an unanswered question and probably depends on the exam justification. Still, there are no procedure guidelines for PET imaging of inflammation, in contrast to established procedure guidelines for tumor imaging with ^{18}F-FDG-PET specifying duration of fasting, activity of ^{18}F-FDG to be injected, and delay for image acquisition.[16,17]

Finally, PET/MRI may become the blended modality choice of the future,[18] allowing for an even more precise soft-tissue anatomic location of the increased metabolic activity with lower radiation than PET/CT, which could be of particular relevance in pediatric patients. The development of targeted MRI contrast agents based on certain tissue metabolic properties leading to enhanced tissue contrast could further improve our knowledge of functional tissue properties and anatomic consequences of pathologic processes and hence of the etiology and outcome of diseases.[18]

Applications of ^{18}F-FDG-PET in inflammatory diseases

PET can be used in the detection of inflammation in various rheumatic disorders, with articular or extra-articular involvement, such as vasculitis, lupus, sarcoidosis, myositis, or arthritis, and can also be of help for the workup of fever of unknown origin.[1,2]

Large-vessel vasculitis

The diagnosis of the large-vessel vasculitides, giant cell arteritis and Takayasu's arteritis, relies on a spectrum of clinical, biologic, angiographic, and histopathologic features. It can be troublesome in some patients, and American College of Rheumatology criteria combining these various features have therefore been established. However, they do not bear a specificity or sensitivity of 100% and were originally designed for classification purposes and not for the diagnosis of individual patients. Histopathologic features cannot be obtained for Takayasu's disease and can be missed in giant cell arteritis in which biopsies should be performed bilaterally and in an extended manner. Imaging modalities are available but can have limitations. Doppler ultrasonography can be useful if vasculitis is suggested and is particularly helpful in the evaluation of temporal artery inflammation but is of limited use at the large thoracic vessels. Angiography and gadolinium-enhanced MRI can show luminal narrowing and mural thickening of the aorta and its branches in Takayasu's disease, but these abnormalities can also be found in early arteriosclerosis or connective tissue diseases, whereas false-negative angiograms can be found in early vasculitis. Because glucose metabolism is increased in active vasculitis,

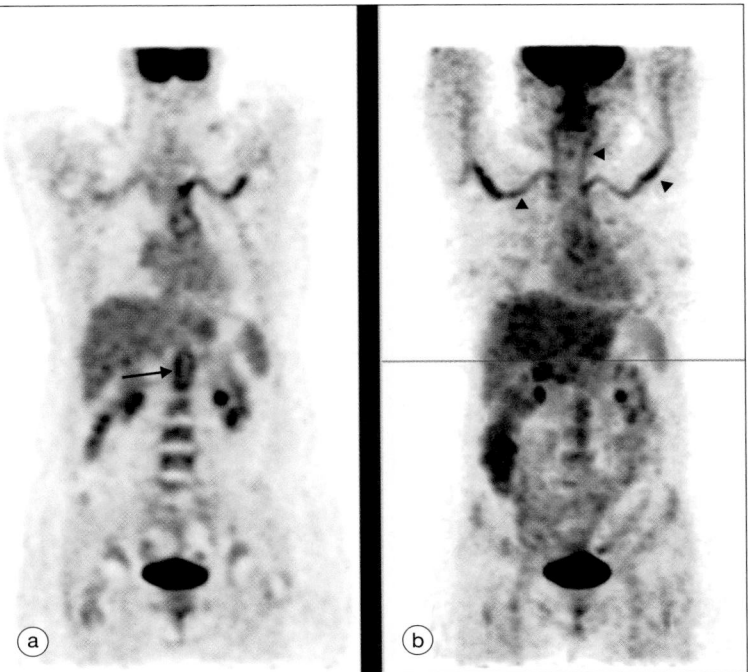

Fig. 41.3 ^{18}F-FDG-PET images of a patient with giant cell arteritis. (a) The arrow in the coronal image points to an intense hypermetabolism of the abdominal aortic wall. (b) The arrowheads in the maximal intensity projection image indicate hypermetabolism of subclavian, axillary, and carotid arteries.

^{18}F-FDG-PET has been used in recent years in the evaluation of giant cell arteritis and Takayasu's arteritis[19-21] and could become a first-line investigation technique for shorter and more successful diagnostic workup in the near future.[21] ^{18}F-FDG vascular uptake is not specific for vasculitis because it can also be found in atherosclerotic plaques. The two conditions can however be differentiated by taking into account the vascular distribution of the ^{18}F-FDG uptake pattern and the intensity of ^{18}F-FDG accumulation. A grading system has been developed by Meller and associates[22] and is based on the comparison of ^{18}F-FDG uptake by vessels and by the liver: grade I, vascular uptake present but lower than liver uptake; grade II, similar to liver uptake; and grade III, uptake higher than liver uptake. In this manner, grade I thoracic aorta uptake can be attributed to atherosclerosis and grade II or III uptake in thoracic aorta or in any other segments to active large vessel inflammation. Asymptomatic extracranial vessels can be affected in giant cell arteritis (Fig. 41.3).[20,23] The common uptake pattern in great vessels in this disease is linear and continuous and predominantly of grade II, with thoracic vessels being the most frequently affected, followed by abdominal vessels. ^{18}F-FDG-PET has been shown to identify significantly more affected regions than MRI. The whole-body evaluation procedure of ^{18}F-FDG-PET could therefore be of use for vascular screening and for identification of aortic uptake in these patients known to develop more frequently aortic aneurysms. ^{18}F-FDG-PET can evaluate the response to treatment (Fig. 41.4). However, it has not been shown to be useful for the prediction of relapses of giant cell arteritis.[20] Furthermore, pathophysiologic insights could be investigated because subclinical vasculitis has been highlighted by ^{18}F-FDG-PET in patients with polymyalgia rheumatica (Fig. 41.5), closely related to giant cell arteritis.

In Takayasu's arteritis, the uptake pattern of ^{18}F-FDG is linear and continuous in the early phase (Fig. 41.6) but can become patchy in the late phase. In this disease, the metabolic imaging with PET has been shown to be able to identify more vascular injured foci than does the morphologic imaging with MRI. The latter, however, may give information about changes in the wall structure or luminal blood flow. The hybrid PET/CT or PET/MRI could therefore be of particular interest in large-vessel vasculitis. The combination of PET and CT has already shown to be of value in Takayasu's disease.[24] The CT can increase the

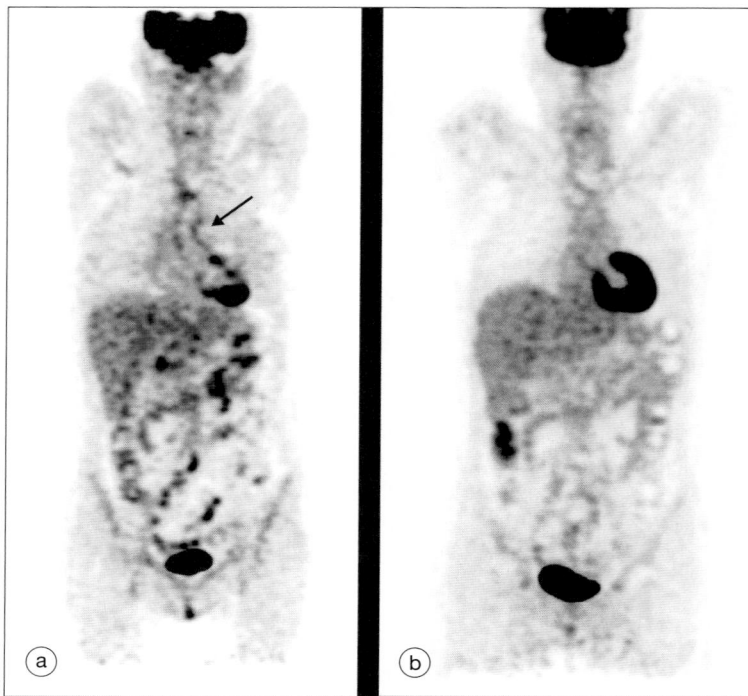

Fig. 41.4 Coronal ¹⁸F-FDG-PET images of a patient with vasculitis before (a) and after (b) treatment with corticosteroids. Note the disappearance of the aortic wall hypermetabolism on the post-therapeutic scan.

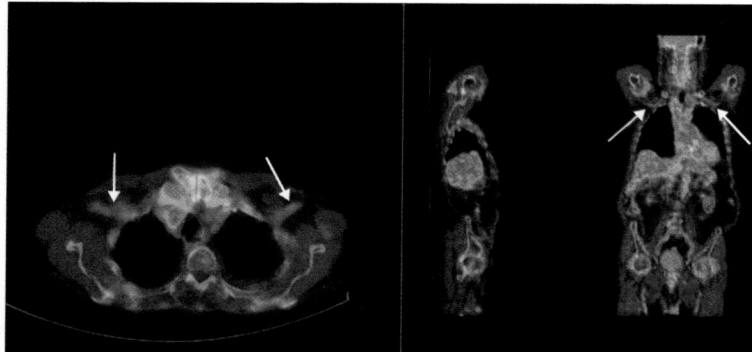

Fig. 41.5 ¹⁸F-FDG-PET/CT fusion images of a patient referred for fever of unknown origin. Bilateral shoulder and hip hypermetabolism is highlighted, consistent with a diagnosis of polymyalgia rheumatica. Note the hypermetabolism of the subclavian arteries (arrows).

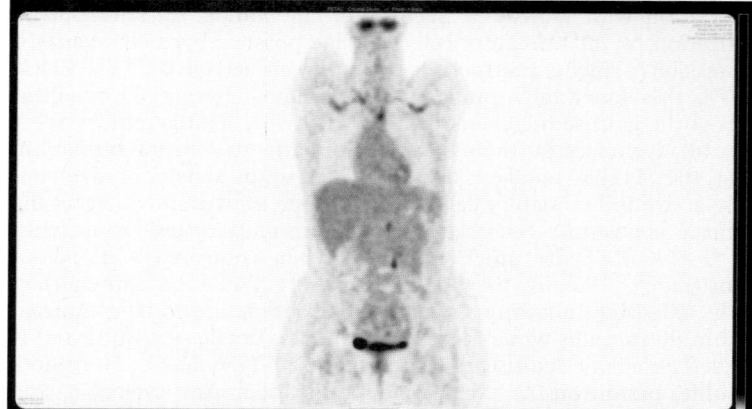

Fig. 41.6 ¹⁸F-FDG-PET coronal image showing an intense hypermetabolism of the aortic arch and both subclavian arteries in a patient with Takayasu's arteritis.

sensitivity of the PET modality in diseased vessels with weak ¹⁸F-FDG uptake and can also help to localize accurately a mediastinal ¹⁸F-FDG uptake coming from pulmonary arteries. On the other hand, FDG accumulation can be found in arteries without vascular wall thickening on CT (i.e., areas of inflammation that have not yet progressed to vascular thickening).[24] In summary, ¹⁸F-FDG-PET is highly effective in evaluating in a single procedure the activity and extent of large-vessel vasculitis and may become a first-line imaging modality technique in patients suspected to present with such vasculitis.

Systemic lupus erythematosus

¹⁸F-FDG-PET is used in systemic lupus erythematosus (SLE) mainly to demonstrate central nervous system (CNS) involvement. Although MRI is the current gold standard for evaluating neuropsychiatric SLE, there are still problems with regard to sensitivity and specificity.[25] The most common white matter hyperintensities can also be associated with hypertension and increase with age in the general population. Periventricular lesions associated with the antiphospholipid syndrome can be impossible to differentiate from multiple sclerosis. Other

neuroimaging techniques such as magnetic resonance spectroscopy, magnetization transfer imaging, SPECT, or PET have therefore been evaluated.[25] PET can detect subtle brain changes in lupus patients. In a study of 22 lupus patients with severe or mild CNS symptoms, brain hypometabolism was detected by PET in all patients, most often affecting the parieto-occipital regions, whereas only half of the patients displayed abnormal MRI images.[26] The change of brain metabolism on follow-up PET scans correlated with the clinical outcome of cerebral symptoms.[26]

Lymph node involvement can also be detected by PET in SLE,[27] as it can in amyloidosis secondary to SLE or to Sjögren's syndrome[28] or in rheumatoid arthritis[29]; and differential diagnosis with lymphoma needs to be made. PET can also assess the distribution of activated lymphocytes and thus provide insight in pathophysiologic immune mechanisms of disease. Increased ¹⁸F-FDG uptake has been found in lymph nodes in both active and inactive SLE patients, suggesting an enhanced metabolic and probably immunologic activity in lymphoid organs in SLE, even when clinically quiescent.[30] Furthermore, an increased ¹⁸F-FDG uptake was observed in the thymus of some SLE patients, even adults, but only in active SLE, suggesting a role of thymus in SLE disease activity.[30]

Sarcoidosis

The classical workup of patients with suspected sarcoidosis includes chest CT, which can demonstrate bilateral hilar and mediastinal lymphadenopathy with or without lung parenchymal infiltrates or interstitial disease. However, the precise distribution of sarcoid disease cannot be obtained by a single CT examination. ⁶⁷Ga scintigraphy has been widely used for the diagnosis of sarcoidosis, with the typical "lambda sign" attributable to mediastinal and hilar lymphadenopathy, as well as for the management of the disease with detection of clinically silent sites and monitoring of therapeutic response.[2] PET can also provide a whole-body evaluation and detect unsuspected sites of involvement. It can detect sarcoid lesions undetected by ⁶⁷Ga scintigraphy,[31] in particular in the abdomen. Both thoracic and extrathoracic sarcoid granulomas are detected with great sensitivity by PET/CT, except for skin lesions, which can be identified visually.[32] Response to treatment can also be evaluated with PET.[2,32] ¹⁸F-FDG-PET/CT is therefore a valuable tool for the management of sarcoidosis, allowing for a complete morphofunctional cartography of active inflammatory sites and for the follow-up of treatment efficacy, especially in atypical, complex, and multisystemic forms of the disease (Fig. 41.7).[32]

Arthritis

The main application of ¹⁸F-FDG-PET in arthritis concerns rheumatoid arthritis (RA). The first reports on the imaging of ¹⁸F-FDG uptake in RA patients concerned incidental findings in rheumatoid patients undergoing PET for cancer screening or follow-up, with uptake in joints alone[33] or also in lung by rheumatoid nodules.[34] The first specific studies on rheumatoid joints go back to 1995 by Palmer and

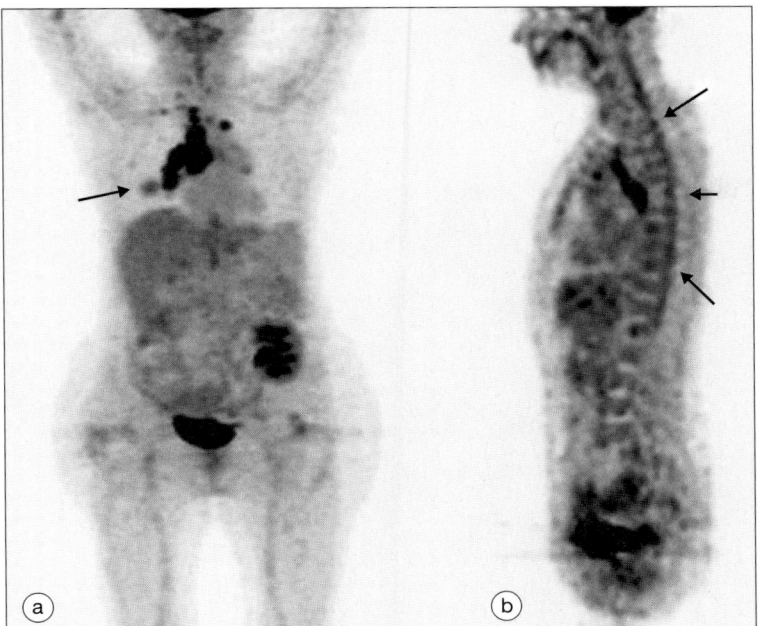

Fig. 41.7 ^{18}F-FDG-PET of a patient referred for fever of unknown origin, associated with dyspnea and headache. (a) The coronal slice shows multiple intense hypermetabolic mediastinal and right hilar lymphadenopathies, as well as a right pulmonary lesion (arrow). Transbronchial biopsies highlighted non-necrotizing granulomas. (b) The sagittal slice shows an unusual increased spinal cord uptake (arrows). The cerebrospinal fluid analysis highlighted a lymphocytic meningitis. The final diagnosis was pulmonary-mediastinal and neuro-sarcoidosis.

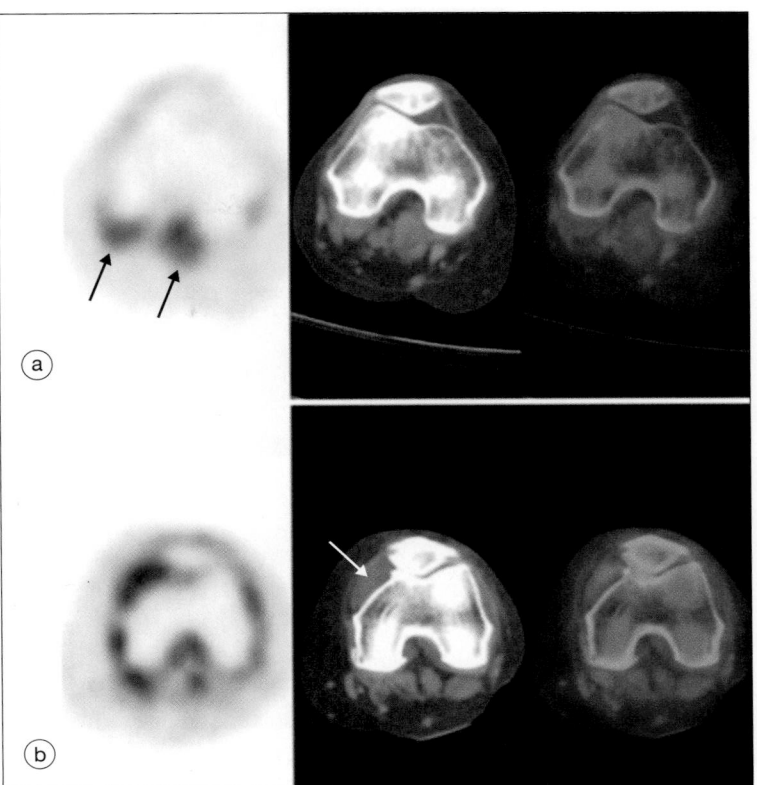

Fig. 41.8 (a) ^{18}F-FDG-PET, CT, and fused PET/CT transverse sections of a normal knee. The CT helps to identify foci of relative hyperactivity seen on PET images posterior to the internal condyle and intercondylar notch (black arrows) as physiologic muscle uptake. (b) ^{18}F-FDG-PET, CT, and fused PET/CT transverse sections of a RA patient. The PET (left) and fusion (right) images show a vast hypermetabolic "ring-like" lesion surrounding the condyles, consistent with a synovitis. Note the thickening of the synovium recognizable on the CT image (white arrow).

associates,[35] who showed that PET could be used to quantify joint inflammation, with ^{18}F-FDG uptake in rheumatoid wrists being correlated to gadolinium uptake evaluated by MRI. Similarly, rheumatoid knees with FDG uptake (Fig. 41.8) (i.e., PET-positive RA knees) exhibit higher ultrasound-measured synovial thickness and higher gadolinium-enhancement MRI parameters than PET-negative knees.[36] Significant correlations are found between the standardized uptake values (SUVs), which are correlated to ^{18}F-FDG tissue concentrations, and MRI parameters, synovial thickness measured by ultrasonography, and serum levels of C-reactive protein and matrix metalloproteinase-3, a synovial-derived parameter reflecting joint inflammation.[36] These data clearly relate to animal studies showing that joint ^{18}F-FDG accumulation increases with the progression of arthritis and is correlated with the pannus rather than with the inflammatory cells around the joint, the main cell type responsible for FDG uptake being fibroblasts, and a dramatic increase in FDG uptake being induced by proinflammatory cytokines in fibroblasts and macrophages.[37] The main interest of ^{18}F-FDG-PET in RA resides, however, in the fact that it allows a whole-body evaluation of inflammation. Beckers and associates[38] studied RA synovitis in 21 patients with active RA, evaluating knees as well as ankles and metatarsophalangeal joints or wrists, and metacarpophalangeal and proximal interphalangeal joints. A "metabolic" rheumatoid disease activity was evaluated by the cumulative SUV (i.e., the sum of SUVs in PET-positive joints). This cumulative SUV was significantly correlated to clinical parameters (numbers of swollen and tender joints), biologic parameters (erythrocyte sedimentation rate and C-reactive protein levels), composite indices of disease activity (the 28-point Disease Activity Score [DAS$_{28}$] and Simplified Disease Activity Index [SDAI]), and ultrasound parameters (cumulative synovial thickness, number of Doppler-positive joints). Goerres and associates[39] also used ^{18}F-FDG-PET for global evaluation of RA, attempting to develop a simple score without using SUVs, by adding the scores graded from 0 to 4 for each of the 28 joints included in the DAS$_{28}$. The precise method for the global evaluation of RA disease activity has not yet been standardized. The use of devices combining PET and CT will further

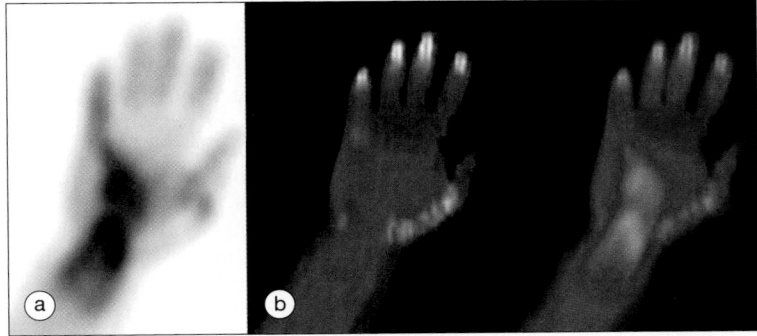

Fig. 41.9 (a) ^{18}F-FDG-PET/CT coronal slice of the distal part of the right upper extremity in a RA patient. (b) The PET (left) and fusion (right) images are strongly suggestive of inflammation of the ulnar bursa, in continuity with the flexor sheath of the fifth digit.

increase the localization of metabolic activity and will be of great interest in small joints such as hands, allowing one to determine whether foci of increased activity are due to synovitis, inflammation of tendon sheaths (Fig. 41.9), or increased muscular intake (Fig. 41.10b). Another potential future point of interest for ^{18}F-FDG-PET could be an eventual prognostic value of SUV. In oncology, pretherapeutic SUV values have been shown to predict response to treatment and overall survival.[40,41] The advent of effective but expensive biologic therapies in rheumatology has prompted the interest in methodologies able to detect change to treatment with great sensitivity. The usefulness of PET in the assessment of the therapeutic response has been shown with low-dose

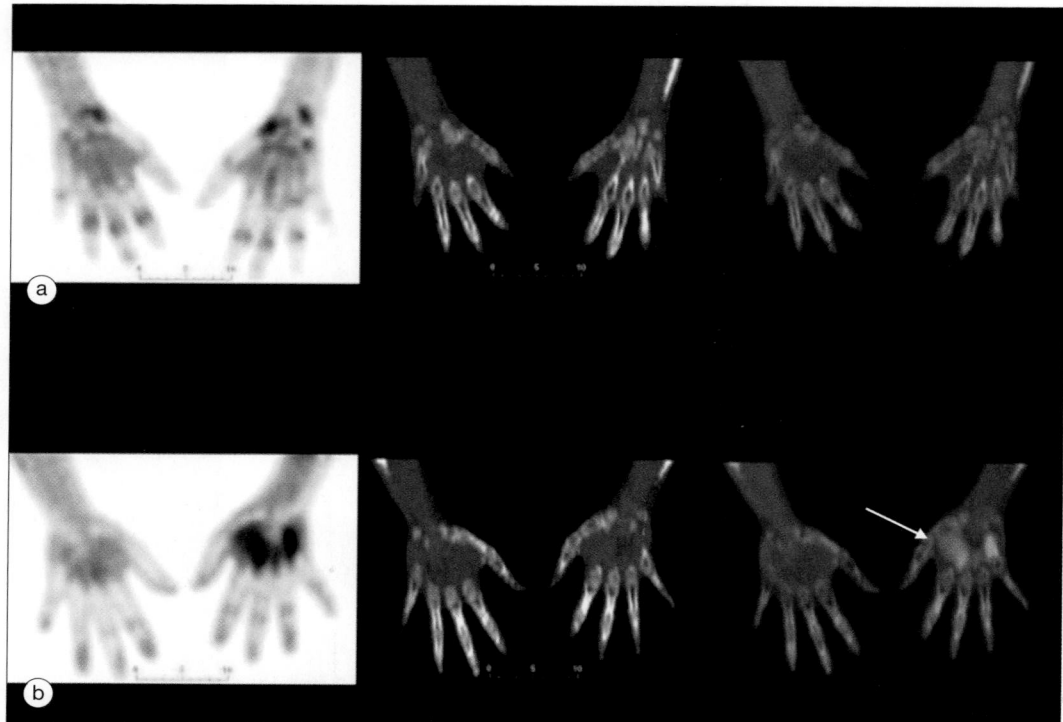

Fig. 41.10 ^{18}F-FDG-PET, CT, and fused PET/CT coronal slices of the distal upper extremities in a RA patient. (a) Inflammatory involvement of several proximal interphalangeal joints of both hands and multiple joints of both wrists. (b) Response to rituximab treatment. After 16 weeks, there is a complete metabolic response in the wrists and a partial response in the interphalangeal joints. Zones of relative hyperactivity in the left hand (arrow) correspond to physiologic muscle uptake.

prednisone and methotrexate,[42] intra-articular injections,[43] and, recently, anti–tumor necrosis factor (TNF). In RA patients treated with anti-TNF, changes in ^{18}F-FDG uptake in knees were significantly correlated with changes in MRI parameters as well as with biologic parameters (C-reactive protein and matrix metalloproteinase-3 levels) after 4 weeks of treatment.[36] Global ^{18}F-FDG-PET joint score was decreased after three infusions of infliximab in clinical responders but not in clinical non-responders.[39] Figure 41.10 illustrates the response to rituximab. Whether PET will be able to identify patients at need for biologic therapies or to detect an early response to these treatments remains to be shown.

^{18}F-FDG-PET can visualize joint inflammation in other inflammatory arthritides such as psoriatic arthritis[44] and ankylosing spondylitis.[45] ^{18}F-FDG accumulation can also be found in various joints due to a local inflammatory reaction, even in degenerative disorders. Wandler and coworkers evaluated shoulder uptake in 24 patients undergoing oncologic assessment.[46] Three recognizable patterns of FDG uptake were identified in 12 of the 14 patients with clinical findings consistent with a shoulder pathology: (1) a circumferential/diffuse uptake in 10 patients (7 of whom had a clinical diagnosis of osteoarthritis and one bursitis) (Fig. 41.11); (2) asymmetric localized uptake at the greater tuberosity in 4 patients (2 had known rotator cuff injuries and one frozen shoulder); and (3) a pattern of focal glenoid uptake in 4 patients (2 with frozen shoulder, one with osteoarthritis). Three patients had more than one pattern. The circumferential/diffuse uptake in 7 of the 8 patients with clinical osteoarthritis of the shoulder was hypothesized to be related to a chronic, non-specific synovitis. The maximum SUV was significantly correlated to age, but there was no significant difference in maximum SUVs between patients with or without clinical symptoms.[46] ^{18}F-FDG uptake in osteoarthritic joints has also been found in hands[47] and knees,[48] localizing in the latter in the intercondylar notch along the posterior cruciate ligament, around osteophytes, or in the subchondral bone.[48] The cost/benefit ratio of PET for these diseases remains to be proven.

Fever of unknown origin

Many non-infectious inflammatory disorders taken care of by rheumatologists, such as arthritis or vasculitis (giant cell arteritis, ANCA-associated granulomatous vasculitis, polyarteritis nodosa), can give rise to fever of unknown origin (see Figs. 41-5 and 41-7). Although ^{18}F-FDG-PET alone is sometimes unable to reliably distinguish between aseptic inflammatory disease and infectious disease or malignancy, it can localize active lesions and in conjunction with other imaging modalities identify the tissue or organ to be sampled to establish a diagnosis.[2]

PRACTICAL ISSUES

As a rule, when ionizing radiations are being used in human studies, dosimetry has to be carefully taken into account. The effective dose resulting from a bone scan with ^{99m}Tc-labeled diphosphonates is 0.0057 mSv/MBq. The administered dose is typically 740 MBq, which gives an effective dose of approximately 4 mSv.[49] PET studies are within the same range (i.e., 5 mSv for 250 MBq of ^{18}F-FDG). The radiation associated with the CT part of the PET/CT study highly depends on the acquisition protocol. Low-dose studies such as those performed in our institution and shown in Figures 41.5 and 41.8 to 41.11 result in an additional dose of 4.5 mSv.[50] Overall, the radiation burden may be considered as minimal and the theoretical risks are largely counterbalanced by the clinical benefits.

The cost of nuclear medicine techniques is linked to the high cost of the sophisticated machines themselves as well as to that of the isotopes used. The technetium-labeled isotopes used for scintigraphy are inexpensive, but their production is subject to recurrent shortage. The isotopes used for PET are generated by a cyclotron, which needs to be within a few hours reach of the user for practical purposes. Their cost can be highly variable but tend to decrease thanks to greater availability.

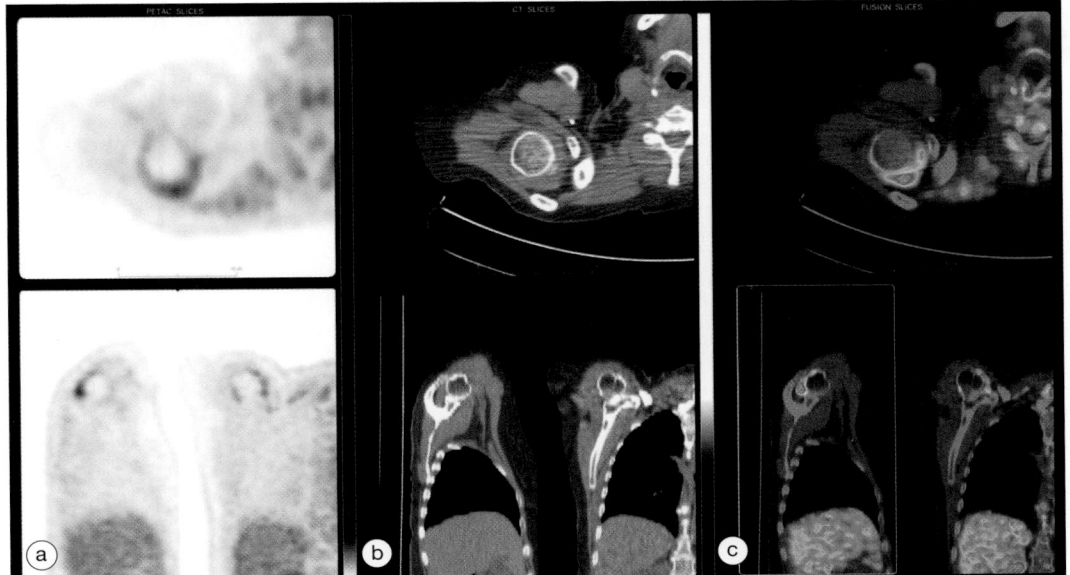

Fig. 41.11 ^{18}F-FDG-PET (a), CT (b) and fused PET/CT (c) of a patient referred for oncologic reasons. Uptake in the right shoulder is incidentally highlighted.

REFERENCES

1. Zhuang H, Alavi A. 18-Fluorodeoxyglucose positron emission tomographic imaging in the detection and monitoring of infection and inflammation. Semin Nucl Med 2002;32:47-59.
2. Basu S, Zhuang H, Torigian DA, et al. Functional imaging of inflammatory diseases using nuclear medicine techniques. Semin Nucl Med 2009;39:124-145.
3. Biswal S. Molecular imaging of musculoskeletal diseases. Semin Musculoskelet Radiol 2003;7:317-350.
4. O'Connor MK, Brown ML, Hung JC, et al. The art of bone scintigraphy: technical aspects. J Nucl Med 1991;32:2332-2341.
5. Spencer DG, Adams FG, Horton PW, et al. Scintiscanning in ankylosing spondylitis: a clinical, radiological and quantitative radioisotopic study. J Rheumatol 1979;6:426-431.
6. Song IH, Carrasco-Fernandez J, Rudwaleit M, et al. The diagnostic value of scintigraphy in assessing sacroiliitis in ankylosing spondylitis: a systematic literature research. Ann Rheum Dis 2008;67:1535-1540.
7. Rosenthall L. Nuclear medicine techniques in arthritis. Rheum Dis Clin North Am 1991;17:585-597.
8. Helfgott S, Rosenthall L, Esdaile J, et al. Generalized skeletal response to [99m]technetium methylene diphosphonate in rheumatoid arthritis. J Rheumatol 1982;9:939-941.
9. Sewell KL, Ruthazer R, Parker JA. The correlation of indium-111 joint scans with clinical synovitis in rheumatoid arthritis. J Rheumatol 1993;20:2015-2019.
10. Rosenthall L, Lisbona R, Hernandez M, et al. ^{99m}Tc-PP and ^{67}Ga imaging following insertion of orthopedic devices. Radiology 1979;133:717-721.
11. Kubota R, Yamada S, Kubota K, et al. Intratumoral distribution of fluorine-18-fluorodeoxyglucose *in vivo*: high accumulation in macrophages and granulation tissues studied by autoradiography. J Nucl Med 1992;33:1972-1980.
12. Yamada S, Kubota K, Kubota R, et al. High accumulation of fluorine-18-fluorodeoxyglucose in turpentine-induced inflammatory tissue. J Nucl Med 1995;36:1301-1306.
13. Gamelli RL, Liu H, He LK, et al. Augmentations of glucose uptake and glucose transporter-1 in macrophages following thermal injury and sepsis in mice. J Leuk Biol 1996;59:639-647.
14. Mochizuki T, Tsukamoto E, Kuge Y, et al. FDG uptake and glucose transporter subtype expressions in experimental tumor and inflammation models. J Nucl Med 2001;42:1551-1555.
15. Hustinx R, Malaise MG. PET imaging of arthritis. PET Clin North Am 2006;1:131-139.
16. Schelbert HR, Hoh CK, Royal HD, et al. Procedure guideline for tumor imaging using fluorine-18-FDG.

Society of Nuclear Medicine. J Nucl Med 1998;39:1302-1305.
17. Bombardieri E, Aktolun C, Baum RP, et al. FDG-PET: procedure guidelines for tumour imaging. Eur J Nucl Med Mol Imaging 2003;30:BP115-124.
18. Bolus NE, George R, Washington J, et al. PET/MRI: the blended-modality choice of the future? J Nucl Med Technol 2009;37:63-71.
19. Webb M, Chambers A, Al-Nahhas A, et al. The role of ^{18}F-FDG PET in characterising disease activity in Takayasu arteritis. Eur J Nucl Med Mol Imaging 2004;31:627-634.
20. Blockmans D, de Ceuninck L, Vanderschueren S, et al. Repetitive ^{18}F-fluorodeoxyglucose positron emission tomography in giant cell arteritis: a prospective study of 35 patients. Arthritis Rheum 2006;55:131-137.
21. Walter MA. [^{18}F]fluorodeoxyglucose PET in large vessel vasculitis. Radiol Clin North Am 2007;45:735-744.
22. Meller J, Strutz F, Siefker U, et al. Early diagnosis and follow-up of aortitis with [(^{18}F]FDG PET and MRI. Eur J Nucl Med Mol Imaging 2003;30:730-736.
23. Belhocine T, Kaye O, Delanaye P, et al. Horton's disease and extra-temporal vessel locations: role of [18]FDG PET scan: report of 3 cases and review of the literature [in French]. Rev Med Interne 2002;23:584-591.
24. Kobayashi Y, Ishii K, Oda K, et al. Aortic wall inflammation due to Takayasu arteritis imaged with ^{18}F-FDG PET coregistered with enhanced CT. J Nucl Med 2005;46:917-922.
25. Peterson PL, Axford JS, Isenberg D. Imaging in CNS lupus. Best Pract Res Clin Rheumatol 2005;19:727-739.
26. Weiner SM, Otte A, Schumacher M, et al. Diagnosis and monitoring of central nervous system involvement in systemic lupus erythematosus: value of F-18 fluorodeoxyglucose PET. Ann Rheum Dis 2000;59:377-385.
27. Fey GL, Jolles PR, Buckley LM, et al. 2-deoxy-2-[^{18}F]-fluoro-D-glucose positron emission tomography uptake in systemic lupus erythematosus–associated adenopathy. Mol Imaging Biol 2004;6:7-11.
28. Serizawa I, Inubushi M, Kanegae K, et al. Lymphadenopathy due to amyloidosis secondary to Sjögren syndrome and systemic lupus erythematosus detected by F-18 FDG PET. Clin Nucl Med 2007;32:881-882.
29. Seldin DW, Habib I, Soudry G. Axillary lymph node visualization on F-18 FDG PET body scans in patients with rheumatoid arthritis. Clin Nucl Med 2007;32:524-526.
30. Nowak M, Carrasquillo JA, Yarboro CH, et al. A pilot study of the use of 2-[^{18}F]-fluoro-2-deoxy-D-glucose-positron emission tomography to assess the distribution of activated lymphocytes in patients with systemic

lupus erythematosus. Arthritis Rheum 2004;50:1233-1238.
31. Xiu Y, Yu JQ, Cheng E, et al. Sarcoidosis demonstrated by FDG PET imaging with negative findings on gallium scintigraphy. Clin Nucl Med 2005;30:193-195.
32. Braun JJ, Kessler R, Constantinesco A, et al. ^{18}F-FDG PET/CT in sarcoidosis management: review and report of 20 cases. Eur J Nucl Med Mol Imaging 2008;35:1537-1543.
33. Yasuda S, Shohtsu A, Ide M, et al. F-18 FDG accumulation in inflamed joints. Clin Nucl Med 1996;21:740.
34. Bakheet SMB, Powe J. Fluorine-18-fluorodeoxyglucose uptake in rheumatoid arthritis–associated lung disease in a patient with thyroid cancer. J Nucl Med 1998;39:234-236.
35. Palmer WE, Rosenthal DI, Schoenberg OI, et al. Quantification of inflammation in the wrist with gadolinium-enhanced MR imaging and PET with 2-[F-18]-fluoro-2-deoxy-D-glucose. Radiology 1995;196;647-655.
36. Beckers C, Jeukens X, Ribbens C, et al. ^{18}F-FDG PET imaging of rheumatoid knee synovitis correlates with dynamic magnetic resonance and sonographic assessments as well as with the serum level of metalloproteinase-3. Eur J Nucl Med Mol Imaging 2006;33:275-280.
37. Matsui T, Nakata N, Nagai S, et al. Inflammatory cytokines and hypoxia contribute to ^{18}F-FDG uptake by cells involved in pannus formation in rheumatoid arthritis. J Nucl Med 2009;50:920-926.
38. Beckers C, Ribbens C, André B, et al. Assessment of disease activity in rheumatoid arthritis with ^{18}F-FDG PET. J Nucl Med 2004;45:956-964.
39. Goerres GW, Forster A, Uebelhart D, et al. F-18 FDG whole-body PET for the assessment of disease activity in patients with rheumatoid arthritis. Clin Nucl Med 2006;31:386-390.
40. Downey RJ, Akhurst T, Gonen M, et al. Preoperative F-18 fluorodeoxyglucose-positron emission tomography maximal standardized uptake value predicts survival after lung cancer resection. J Clin Oncol 2004;22:3255-3260.
41. Pandit N, Gonen M, Krug L, et al. Prognostic value of [^{18}F]FDG-PET imaging in small cell lung cancer. Eur J Nucl Med Mol Imaging 2003;30:78-84.
42. Polisson RP, Schoenberg OI, Fischman A, et al. Use of magnetic resonance imaging and positron emission tomography in the assessment of synovial volume and glucose metabolism in patients with rheumatoid arthritis. Arthritis Rheum 1995;38:819-825.
43. Danfors T, Bergström M, Feltelius N, et al. Positron emission tomography with ^{11}C-D-deprenyl in patients with rheumatoid arthritis. Scand J Rheumatol 1997;26:43-48.

44. Yun M, Kim W, Adam L, et al. F-18 FDG uptake in a patient with psoriatic arthritis: imaging correlation with patient symptoms. Clin Nucl Med 2001;26: 692-693.

45. Wendling D, Blagosklonov O, Streit G, et al. FDG-PET/CT scan of inflammatory spondylodiscitis lesions in ankylosing spondylitis, and short term evolution during anti-tumor necrosis factor treatment. Ann Rheum Dis 2005;64:1663-1665.

46. Wandler E, Kramer EL, Sherman O, et al. Diffuse FDG shoulder uptake on PET is associated with clinical findings of osteoarthritis. Am J Roentgenol AJR 2005;185:797-803.

47. Elzinga EH, van der Laken CJ, Comans EFI, et al. 2-deoxy-2-[F-18]fluoro-D-glucose joint uptake on positron emission tomography images: rheumatoid arthritis versus osteoarthritis. Mol Imaging Biol 2007;9:357-360.

48. Nakamura H, Masuko K, Yudoh K, et al. Positron emission tomography with ^{18}F-FDG in osteoarthritic knee. Osteoarthritis Cartilage 2007;15:673-681.

49. ICRP Report 80. Ann ICRP 1999;28:75.

50. Brix G, Lechel U, Glatting G, et al. Radiation exposure of patients undergoing whole-body dual-modality ^{18}F-FDG PET/CT examinations. J Nucl Med 2005;46:608-613.

DXA and measurement of bone

42

Sydney Bonnick

- Clinical guidelines are based on dual-energy x-ray absorptiometry (DXA) measurements of the posterior-anterior lumbar spine and proximal femur, reducing other skeletal sites and techniques to a lesser role.
- The World Health Organization (WHO) criteria remain the standard for diagnosing osteoporosis on the basis of bone mineral density (BMD).
- The WHO 10-year absolute fracture risk prediction algorithm, FRAX, has refined fracture risk prediction.
- Understanding precision and the least significant change is critical to the interpretation of serial bone density measurements.
- New imaging applications for lateral spine DXA have extended the utility of DXA beyond the measurement of BMD.

Dual-energy x-ray absorptiometry (DXA) was approved by the Food and Drug Administration (FDA) for clinical use in 1988. Because of its versatility and relative ease of use, DXA has become the dominant technology used to quantify bone density in clinical practice. Other technologies such as radiographic absorptiometry, radiogrammetry, quantitative ultrasound (QUS), quantitative computed tomography (QCT), and finite element analysis, each of which is used to evaluate slightly different attributes or parameters of bone, have seen their utility diminish in the face of societal guidelines reliant on measures derived with DXA. Additionally, although virtually any skeletal site can be assessed with DXA, such guidelines tend to focus on DXA measures of the posterior-anterior (PA) lumbar spine and proximal femur, diminishing the utility of non-PA lumbar spine and proximal femur sites.

HISTORY OF BONE DENSITOMETRY

Bone densitometry can be traced to the field of dentistry in the late 1890s,[1] but the modern era began with the publication by Cameron and Sorenson[2] in 1963 describing the methodology for single photon absorptiometric (SPA) measurements of bone mass in vivo. Bone mineral content (BMC) was based on the difference in the beam intensity of a monochromatic or single-energy beam before and after passage through a skeletal region of interest. The magnitude of the attenuation of the photon energy was compared with attenuation standards derived from dried, defatted, ashed human bone of known weight in order to calculate the BMC in the path of the beam. This technique required uniform soft tissue thickness surrounding the skeletal region of interest. To achieve this, it was necessary to surround the region to be studied with water or another soft tissue–equivalent material. Although effective, this limited the application of SPA to the distal appendicular skeleton.

Dual photon absorptiometry (DPA), DXA's immediate predecessor, overcame SPA's restriction to the distal appendicular skeleton by using an isotope or isotopes that generated photon energy at two distinct energy peaks, one of which was preferentially absorbed by bone. In this manner, any contribution to beam attenuation by soft tissue in the region of interest could be mathematically subtracted.[3] This subsequently made it possible to quantify the BMC in skeletal regions surrounded by large or irregular soft tissue masses such as the lumbar spine and proximal femur.

DXA uses the same principles as DPA, except that the photon energy is generated with an x-ray tube rather than a radioactive isotope or isotopes. The advantages of DXA compared with DPA were imme-

diately obvious. The need for periodic replacement of the costly DPA isotope because of source decay was eliminated. The greater photon flux produced by the x-ray tube and smaller focal spot resulted in better beam collimation. This produced less overlap among scan lines, better image resolution, shorter scan times, and superior precision.

In order to produce the two beam energies necessary for separating bone from soft tissue, DXA manufacturers have used rare earth filters or a pulsed power source. Technologic advances since the clinical introduction of DXA in 1988 have resulted in even faster scan times and dramatic improvements in image resolution. Scan times have progressively shortened, such that typical scan times for a PA lumbar spine study or proximal femur study are less than 60 seconds. Initially viewed as a quantitative technique only, the current imaging capabilities of modern DXA devices have resulted in FDA approval for structural diagnosis in the spine and detection of abdominal aortic calcification. The bone mineral density (BMD) can be quantified in virtually every region of the skeleton, as well as the skeleton as a whole. Body composition analysis can also be accomplished with DXA and is considered by some to have replaced the previous gold standard of underwater weighing for this purpose. The primary applications of DXA, however, remain the diagnosis of osteoporosis and the prediction of fracture risk.

DIAGNOSIS OF OSTEOPOROSIS

World Health Organization criteria

Conceptual definitions of osteoporosis have been present in the medical literature for decades. Such definitions largely reflected the recognition that both a decrease in mass and architectural deterioration combined to cause skeletal fragility, the outcome of which was fracture. The practical result of such definitions, however, was that osteoporosis was not diagnosed until the patient had clinical proof of skeletal fragility, which was a low trauma fracture. In the late 1980s and early 1990s, a bone density that was two or more standard deviations (SDs) below the young-adult mean bone density had become the *de facto* working definition of osteoporosis. However, in 1994, the World Health Organization (WHO)[4] issued guidelines for the diagnosis of osteoporosis, also based on the number of SDs below the young-adult mean bone density. These guidelines are shown in Table 42.1. The arbitrary threshold of 2.5 SDs or more below the young-adult mean was selected because it created a prevalence of osteoporosis that was similar to previously observed lifetime risks for fracture. A normal bone density was a bone density that was not more than 1 SD below the young adult mean. The WHO also created a diagnostic category between these two cutoffs of normal and osteoporosis, which they termed *osteopenia*. Finally, a fourth category termed *severe* or *established osteoporosis* was created to include those individuals who satisfied the above bone density criterion for osteoporosis and had also suffered a fracture. In creating these four categories with finite cut points, the WHO maintained the recognized gradient of risk for fracture with declining bone density and the additional effect of prevalent fracture on fracture risk. Bone densitometry T scores of less than or equal to −1, greater than −1 to less than −2.5, and greater than or equal to −2.5 reflect the WHO diagnostic categories of normal, osteopenia, and osteoporosis, respectively.

Limitations of WHO criteria

Although the WHO criteria were to be used to determine the prevalence of osteoporosis in populations, they could also be applied to individuals. In 1994 the WHO cautioned that variations in the skeletal

TABLE 42.1 1994 WHO CRITERIA FOR THE DIAGNOSIS OF OSTEOPOROSIS BASED ON THE MEASUREMENT OF BONE DENSITY AND T SCORE EQUIVALENT CUT POINTS

Diagnostic category	Standard deviations below the young-adult mean	T score
Normal	≤1 SD	Equal to or better than −1
Osteopenia (low bone mass)	Between 1 and 2.5 SD	Between −1 and −2.5
Osteoporosis	≥2.5 SD	Equal to or poorer than −2.5
Severe (established) osteoporosis	≥2.5 SD + a fragility fracture	Equal to or poorer than −2.5 + a fragility fracture

site measured, the technique used, and the reference database employed would all influence individual diagnosis. This was because the WHO criteria were derived from SPA, DPA, and DXA bone density studies of the spine, proximal femur, and radius in Caucasian women. There was also substantial variation in diagnostic category when the WHO criteria were applied to data from the same skeletal site such as the proximal femur but from different DXA manufacturers. However, the substitution of the now-accepted Caucasian standard proximal femur reference database, the National Health and Nutrition Examination Study (NHANES) III database, largely eliminated the differences in diagnostic category assignment.[5] Differences in diagnostic category assignments based on measurements of PA lumbar spine BMD among manufacturers are minimal compared with pre-NHANES III assessments of BMD at the proximal femur.

Controversy on the applicability of the WHO criteria to men and non-Caucasian women remains, given that the original thresholds were chosen on the basis of reconciling fracture risk and prevalence established in Caucasian women. Similarly, the application of WHO criteria to bone density studies of the spine, proximal femur, and radius with other techniques or made at other skeletal sites with any technique remains controversial. In such cases, a given T score may only reflect the variability of bone density in the population rather than some level of fracture risk. In 1999 Faulkner and colleagues[5] compared the T-score regression on age for women for heel QUS, QCT of the spine and DXA of the proximal femur, PA and lateral lumbar spine and forearm on the basis of the reference database provided by the manufacturer of the specific device. The expected T score for an average 60-year-old woman ranged from −0.7 at the heel by QUS to −2.5 by QCT at the spine. This same dilemma has been demonstrated in men.[6]

These findings have led various organizations to recommend restricting the use of the WHO criteria to specific skeletal sites measured with DXA. The International Society for Clinical Densitometry (ISCD)[7] recommended that the WHO criteria be applied only to measurements at the PA lumbar spine, total hip, or femoral neck, using the lowest of the three. The WHO[8] itself suggested that the criteria be applied only to measurements made at the proximal femur, emphasizing the femoral neck region of interest, whereas the International Osteoporosis Foundation (IOF)[9] has stated a preference for the total hip region of interest.

Several authors have attempted to define T-score cut points on the basis of non-spine, non–proximal femur measurements of bone density that would identify individuals with osteopenia or osteoporosis of the PA lumbar spine and/or proximal femur.[10] The data that emerged confirmed that the use of the WHO criteria at sites other than the spine or proximal femur and with techniques other than DXA can be inappropriate and misleading. This does not reflect a lack of accuracy or precision of such measurements but reflects the effects of attempting to apply criteria developed by wholly different means. As a consequence, such alternative techniques have seen their clinical utility diminish.

ISCD currently recommends the use of the WHO criteria in men older than age 50 with a gender-specific reference database. However,

the IOF recommends the use of a Caucasian female reference database in conjunction with the WHO criteria for the diagnosis of osteoporosis in men.[9] This recommendation stems largely from the recognition that the difference in fracture rates between women and men is primarily due to non–bone density factors, not from differences in bone density. At a given level of bone density, the risk for fracture imparted by that level of bone density appears to be the same in both women and men. Therefore, if the purpose of diagnosing osteoporosis based on some level of bone density is to imply a certain level of fracture risk imparted by that bone density, the use of the Caucasian female reference database in men would be appropriate.[11] This concept is gaining acceptance, although it is not the current standard in the United States.

PREDICTION OF FRACTURE RISK

The prediction of fracture risk with DXA bone density measurements is a separate entity from the diagnosis of osteoporosis. The range of bone densities is too wide within the WHO diagnostic categories to use a category to accurately characterize fracture risk for an individual.

The ability to predict fracture risk with a single bone density measurement was considered controversial until 1993 when two sentinel studies clearly demonstrated a statistically significant increase in fracture risk per SD decline in BMD, for different types of fracture and measurement sites.[12,13] The statistical measure called *relative risk* (RR) was appropriately used in these studies, but the ability to apply such relative risk data to individuals in clinical practice is severely limited. The actual RR per SD decline from any given study is really only applicable to that study population. Without knowing the baseline risk to which they are being compared, interpretation of an individual's RR based on his or her reported T or Z score is impossible.

FRAX: WHO 10-year absolute fracture risk prediction algorithm

Sufficient data now exist to assess absolute risk precluding the need to use RR for decision making. There is still controversy on the time frame (e.g., 1, 5, or 10 years) predicted and whether that risk should be a global fracture risk or a site-specific (e.g., hip) fracture risk. However, in 2008 the WHO introduced FRAX, which is a 10-year absolute fracture risk prediction algorithm for the prediction of any major osteoporotic fracture (including hip, wrist, clinical spine, and humerus) and for hip fracture.[14]

FRAX is unique in that it not only provides a fracture risk prediction in the form of absolute risk but also combines validated clinical risk factors with BMD to better predict an individual's fracture risk. The risk factors were chosen on the basis of reviews of the medical literature to establish the magnitude of the relationship between the risk factor and fracture risk.[15-21] Ultimately, the data used to create FRAX came from 9 different study cohorts around the world and were validated in 11 other cohorts in similar geographic locations.[22] To be included as a risk factor in the FRAX algorithm, a therapeutic intervention must be able to reduce its impact or it must not adversely affect the fracture risk reduction efficacy of such interventions. The specific risk factors that were ultimately chosen came to be known as the WHO 8: age, body mass index (BMI), prior fracture, parental hip fracture, current smoking, glucocorticoid use, rheumatoid arthritis, and excessive alcohol consumption.

Although FRAX may be incorporated into bone density software in the future, at present it is an Internet-based application, available at http://www.shef.ac.uk/FRAX/. FRAX algorithms are available for different countries and, in some cases, for different ethnicities within a country. The FRAX data entry algorithm page from the Web site for U.S. Caucasians is shown in Fig. 42.1. After entering either the patient's age or date of birth and gender, height and weight must be entered in the appropriate units. Weight and height conversion utilities are available if the original measurement units were not kilograms and centimeters. The presence or absence of seven of the eight clinical risk factors is then indicated by clicking on the yes or no radio button. The algorithm is designed to provide an absolute fracture risk assessment in the absence of a measurement of BMD; however, the risk

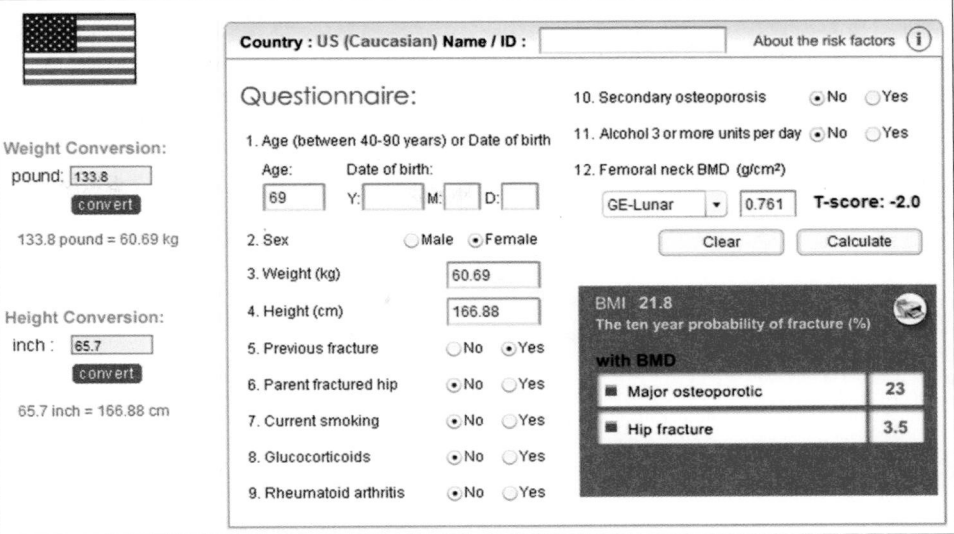

Fig. 42.1 FRAX, a 10-year absolute fracture risk prediction algorithm developed by the World Health Organization, incorporating clinical risk factors for fracture and femoral neck BMD. Reproduced with the kind permission of the World Health Organization Collaborating Centre for Metabolic Bone Diseases, University of Sheffield, United Kingdom. These data are for the patient whose bone density studies are seen in Fig. 42.6a and b.

assessment is improved by inputting the femoral neck BMD. After clicking on "calculate," the 10-year absolute fracture risks are presented for hip fracture and for any major osteoporotic fracture.

FRAX will accept a value for ages 50 to 90. The BMI is automatically calculated from the data entered for height and weight. The risk factors have been reduced to dichotomous variables, requiring a "yes" or "no" response. The risk factor of "prior fracture" refers to a low trauma fracture occurring as an adult. The subjectivity of this assessment is unavoidable. Captured in this assessment are prior morphometric spine, clinical spine, non-spine, and hip fractures. The number, location, and type of the preexisting fracture(s) are not captured. If multiple fractures have occurred, the algorithm may underestimate the 10-year fracture probability. When the risk factors are reduced to dichotomous variables, the inability to convey the effects of a "dose-response" are inevitable. This limitation also applies to the risks of smoking, use of glucocorticoids, and alcohol consumption. Rheumatoid arthritis is considered separately from other causes of secondary osteoporosis because rheumatoid arthritis imparts a fracture risk that is independent of the BMD.[17] Other secondary causes of osteoporosis only contribute to the calculation of fracture risk if no BMD data are entered.

There are several caveats to the current clinical implementation of FRAX. The T score that is actually used to calculate the 10-year fracture risks is derived from the 1998 NHANES III proximal femur database for Caucasian women. This created an obvious dilemma in using data generated from bone density studies performed in men in which T scores are based on a male reference database, and it also posed a dilemma for data from bone density studies performed in Caucasian women in the United States. This is because bone densitometers in the United States use the 1997 and not the 1998 NHANES III proximal femur reference database. To address this issue, the FRAX patch, initially developed by the Oregon Osteoporosis Center, converts the measured BMD at the femoral neck, regardless of the type of DXA device used to measure it or the gender or ethnicity of the patient in whom it was measured, into a 1998 NHANES III Caucasian female T score. Therefore, in using FRAX, the manufacturer of the DXA device must be selected from the drop-down box and the femoral neck BMD must be entered. The recalculated T score, based on the 1998 NHANES III Caucasian female database, then appears to the right of the BMD.

The FRAX algorithm is not intended for use in patients who are already receiving therapy. In such cases, fracture risk would almost certainly be overestimated. FRAX should never substitute for clinical judgment in assessing fracture risk. It also in no way indicates the necessity for treatment. Separate guidelines[23] that incorporate FRAX have been developed to help clinicians identify individuals who would benefit from pharmacologic interventions to reduce fracture risk.

MONITORING CHANGES IN BONE DENSITY

Changes in bone density can be quantified with any of the currently available techniques. However, measured changes cannot be properly interpreted and, therefore, any clinical significance attached, without applying the concepts of precision and the least significant change (LSC). Changes also need to be measured at a clinically relevant skeletal site, with relevance determined by the condition, disease, or drug that may cause the change in bone density.

Precision is an attribute of every quantitative serial measurement and is not unique to densitometry. In densitometry, precision refers to the ability to reproduce a quantitative measurement when the measurements have been performed under identical conditions in the setting of no real biologic change. In 1994 the International Organization of Standardization (ISO)[24] defined two subcategories of precision: repeatability and reproducibility.

- Repeatability refers to the closeness of agreement between test results when the tests were performed by the same technologist, on the same equipment, at the same location within a short period of time on the same subjects.
- Reproducibility refers to the closeness of agreement between test results when the tests were performed on the same subject using the same method but by different technologists, using different equipment at different locations.

As commonly used in densitometry, precision is synonymous with the ISO subcategory of repeatability.

Even if an individual underwent several bone density studies within minutes of each other and each test was performed in an identical fashion by the same technologist, the results of each test would not be the same. There is intrinsic variability in the measurement, although the variability is expected to be small, but this small, intrinsic variability must be quantified before concluding that a real biologic change has occurred. This can be done by performing a short-term precision study.

To perform a short-term precision study, individuals undergo repeated bone density testing within a short period of time. The number of individuals and the number of bone density studies per individual are ultimately based on narrowing the resulting confidence interval for the calculated precision value as much as is reasonably possible. In general and for practical purposes, the number of individuals and number of studies per individual are chosen to achieve 30 degrees of freedom (d.f.). Although one individual undergoing 31 studies would fulfill this criterion, such an approach is not appropriate because of the radiation associated with the larger number of studies, as well as the likelihood of learned positioning by the individual. An intermediate number of individuals is often chosen, such as 15 individuals studied three times each or 10 individuals studied four times

TABLE 42.2 NUMBER OF PATIENTS AND STUDIES PER PATIENT TO ACHIEVE 30 D.F. FOR A SHORT-TERM PRECISION STUDY*

No. patients	No. studies per patient
1	31
5	7
10	4
15	3
30	2

*Note that in the precision study in the case presentation in the text, the combination of 10 patients and 4 studies per patient was used.
D.F., degrees of freedom.
Reproduced from Bonnick SL. Bone densitometry in clinical practice, 2nd ed. Totowa NJ: Humana Press, 2004, with permission of the publisher.

each. Various combinations of numbers of patients and number of studies per patient to achieve 30 d.f. are shown in Table 42.2.[25] A short-term precision study with 30 d.f. results in upper and lower error limits for the 95% confidence interval of the calculated precision of 1.34 and 0.80, respectively.[26] An additional 20 d.f. would be required to reduce the upper error limit to 1.24, whereas a total of 200 d.f. would be required for an upper error limit of 1.11. The studies are completed on each individual on the same day or within a few weeks, such that the time period is too short to expect a real biologic change in bone density. The individuals participating in the precision study should also be representative of the patient population in whom the resulting precision value will be applied.

Using data generated during the short-term precision study, the root-mean-square (RMS) precision, rather than the arithmetic mean precision, is calculated because the latter results in an underestimation of the true Gaussian error. To illustrate the calculation of the RMS precision, assume that 15 individuals have been studied three times each. First, the SD for each set of three measurements is found. Then the RMS-SD or precision is calculated, using the following equation:

$$SD_{RMS} = \sqrt{\frac{\sum_{i=1}^{m}(SD^2)}{m}} \qquad (1)$$

in which m is the number of patients in the precision study, or in this case, 15. The RMS-SD has the units of the measurement, which for DXA is g/cm². The precision value can now be used to calculate the LSC, defined as the value that must be equaled or exceeded before a real biologic change can be said to have occurred.

The magnitude of the LSC is determined not only by the precision but by the level of statistical confidence that is required and the number of measurements made at baseline and at follow-up. The formula for calculating the LSC is shown in equation 2:

$$LSC = Z'(\text{Pr})\sqrt{\frac{1}{n_1} + \frac{1}{n_2}} \qquad (2)$$

in which Z' (pronounced "z-prime") is chosen from a z-distribution table found in many statistical texts on the basis of the desired level of statistical confidence, Pr is the precision expressed as the RMS-SD, n_1 is the number of measurements performed at baseline, and n_2 is the number of measurements performed at follow-up. ISCD[27] recommends that the LSC be calculated at 95% confidence, using a two-sided approach. The Z' value for such a calculation is 1.96. Because common clinical practice is to perform one measurement at baseline and one again at follow-up, the value under the square root sign becomes 2. The formula for calculation of the LSC at 95% confidence with one measurement at baseline and one at follow-up then becomes:

$$LSC = 1.96(\text{Pr})1.414 = 2.77(\text{Pr}) \qquad (3)$$

The LSC will also have the same units as the units for precision.

The interpretation of the LSC is straightforward. If the LSC has been equaled or exceeded, then a statistically significant change in the BMD is said to have occurred, at whatever level of statistical confidence the LSC was calculated. When the LSC is calculated using a two-sided approach, as recommended by ISCD, then an increase or a decrease in BMD that equals or exceeds the LSC would be considered a significant increase or decrease. It is possible to calculate an LSC using a one-sided approach and at levels of statistical confidence other than 95%, but this is not current clinical practice. If the LSC is not known, serial measurements of bone density cannot be interpreted because it is simply not possible to know if the variability in the measurement has been sufficiently exceeded to determine if a real change has occurred in the patient.

The inherent precision of DXA is superb. Few, if any, quantitative tests are used in clinical medicine with superior precision. Nevertheless, the precision at every skeletal region of interest that might be used to monitor bone density must be established at every densitometry facility. The same study population can be used for every skeletal site, but precision must not be assumed to be the same at every skeletal site. Precision tends to be the best at the total hip and proximal forearm sites. The lumbar spine, trochanteric region, and femoral neck follow, generally in that order.

The better the precision, the smaller will be the LSC. In general, that means less time is required between measurements to detect a statistically significant change in bone density. However, the anticipated rate of change in the bone density at a particular site, whether it is due to a disease process or therapeutic intervention, profoundly affects the time required to see a significant change. For example, even though precision is superb at the proximal forearm, the rate of change at that site from commonly used bone active agents is much too slow for that site to have any clinical utility in monitoring the effects of those agents on bone. In contrast, although the precision of the lumbar spine or trochanteric region is generally not as good as at the proximal forearm, the rate of change at those highly trabecular sites is greater, resulting in a much shorter and clinically reasonable interval needed to detect a statistically significant change in bone density.

In 2000 a concept called *regression to the mean* was suggested as invalidating serial measurements of bone density.[28] Unfortunately, there was a failure to appreciate that regression to the mean was a group statistical phenomenon only, which could be created by an errant analysis design. It is not a biologic phenomenon, however, and has no application whatsoever to the monitoring of bone density in individuals in clinical practice.

FAN-ARRAY SPINE IMAGING WITH DXA

Although bone densitometry began as a quantitative measurement technique, improvements in image resolution with fan-array DXA have resulted in clinically useful imaging applications. With fan-array DXA spine imaging, the spine can be imaged from T4 to L5 in seconds to minutes, depending on the scan mode, but always at a fraction of the radiation exposure of conventional spine radiographs. Fan-array DXA imaging also largely avoids the problem created by parallax in plain radiography of the spine. Because the movement of the scan arm allows the DXA beam to be passed parallel to the vertebral endplates through-out the entire length of the spine, the vertebral dimensions are not distorted by the angle of the beam. If the patient has severe scoliosis, however, some parallax effect may be unavoidable. Lateral spine imaging with DXA is used for two relatively new applications: ver-tebral fracture assessment (VFA) and abdominal aortic calcification assessment.

Vertebral fracture assessment

When the spine is imaged with DXA from T4 to L5, T4 to T6 may be poorly visualized, but this is not a major problem because the majority of osteoporotic fractures occur below these levels. Of considerable importance is the finding that a significant percentage of women with non-osteoporotic bone densities may have vertebral fractures. In a study from Schousboe and colleagues[29] using WHO criteria, in which 342 women age 60 and older underwent lateral spine imaging with

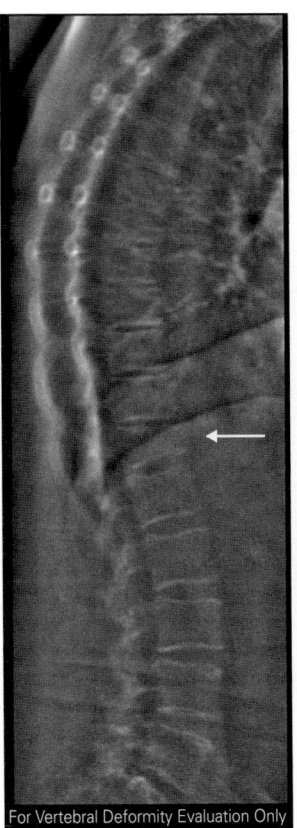

For Vertebral Deformity Evaluation Only

Fig. 42.2 Lateral spine dual-energy x-ray absorptiometry (DXA) imaging for vertebral fracture assessment. This study was performed on a Hologic Dephi DXA device in a matter of seconds. An SQ2 wedge deformity is seen at T12. *(Case courtesy Hologic, Inc., Bedford, Mass.)*

DXA, 27% with osteopenia and 42% with osteoporosis had vertebral deformities consistent with a diagnosis of fracture. Other studies have documented that the majority of morphometric vertebral fractures are undiagnosed. This seems to be true even in patients who have had radiographs in which the spine was visualized.[30,31] An assessment for previously undiagnosed vertebral fracture is imperative for accurate diagnosis, fracture risk prediction, and therapeutic assessment. VFA imaging with DXA is a convenient modality with which to accomplish this.

In 2007 ISCD published extensive guidelines on patient selection for VFA.[32] The guidelines assume that plain films of the spine have not previously been done and that knowledge of a vertebral fracture would change patient management. These guidelines are summarized in Box 42.1. Of note is the recommendation for VFA in patients on chronic glucocorticoid therapy. The "Genant" visual semiquantitative (SQ) method was the preferred method for the assessment of vertebral fracture. In the Genant SQ method the vertebrae are characterized as normal or deformed on the basis of their appearance rather than their measured dimensions.[33] There are three deformation grades: SQ grade 1 (mild), SQ grade 2 (moderate), and SQ grade 3 (severe). Deformed vertebrae are also described on the basis of the shape of the deformation as wedged (anterior fracture), biconcave (middle fracture), or crushed (posterior fracture). Although physical measurements are not made with this technique, a grade 1 deformity roughly corresponds to a 20% to 25% reduction in the anterior, middle, or posterior height of the vertebra and a 10% to 20% reduction in vertebral area. A grade 2 deformity is the result of a 25% to 40% reduction in any of the three heights and a reduction in vertebral area of 20% to 40%. A grade 3 deformity occurs when there is a 40% reduction in any of the three heights and a 40% reduction in vertebral area. The Genant SQ method has been used traditionally with plain radiography. Some DXA VFA software now provides an automated SQ assessment of deformed vertebrae. In Fig. 42.2 a previously undiagnosed SQ2 wedge deformity is seen at T12. This patient's bone densities at the PA lumbar spine and proximal femur were osteopenic on the basis of WHO criteria. However, the finding of a vertebral fracture indicated a much higher risk for future fracture than indicated by the BMD and the finding of a vertebral fracture met NOF criteria[23] for pharmacologic intervention. The VFA study in Fig. 42.3 is from a 66-year-old man. No vertebral deformities are seen in this study. Because of the superb image resolution, small anterior osteophytes are seen at T8. The Genant SQ assessment is illustrated on the lower right of the image.

Abdominal aortic calcification assessment

An extension of the imaging capabilities of the lateral spine with fan-array DXA is the ability to visualize calcification in the abdominal aorta. Although several studies have suggested a relationship between aortic calcification and low bone density, a more important prognostic attribute of aortic calcification is its relationship to the risk of myocardial infarction (MI) and stroke. A significant increase in the hazard ratio for MI and in the RR for stroke with increasing aortic calcification was found in the Rotterdam study, a prospective population-based cohort study of almost 8000 men and women age 55 and older.[34,35] The risk for congestive heart failure or coronary heart disease was also shown to be significantly related to the degree of aortic calcification in the Framingham Heart Study.[36,37] Using the 24-point grading system for abdominal aortic calcification (AAC) seen on radiographs developed by Kauppila and colleagues,[38] an AAC-24 score greater than or equal to 5 was associated with a significant increase in the risk for congestive heart failure or coronary artery disease.[37,38]

Although the AAC-24 point scoring system can be used with DXA VFA images (Figs. 42.4 and 42.5), Schousboe and colleagues[39] proposed an eight-point grading system to improve the ease of use. In this approach, a point score is awarded on the basis of the number of vertebrae from L1 to L4 spanned by the total length of aortic calcification in the anterior and posterior aortic walls separately. A possible score for each wall can range from 0 to 4, such that a maximum worst-case total score is 8. The AAC-8 scoring system is shown in Table 42.3.

The potential identification of aortic calcification is not a major factor in deciding to perform lateral spine imaging with DXA. No medical organization currently recommends the performance of DXA lateral spine imaging for the sole purpose of aortic calcification assessment. Nevertheless, the opportunity to assess this important risk factor for heart disease and stroke presents itself every time VFA is performed. It is an opportunity that should not be missed. In 2006 Hologic, Inc. received 510(k) clearance from the FDA for aortic

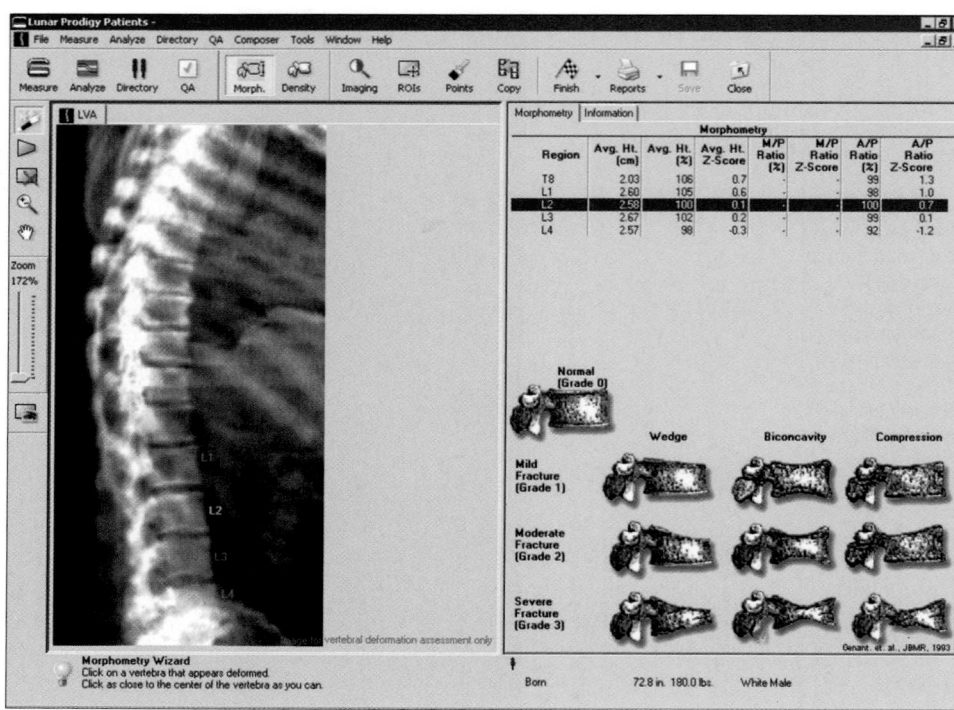

Fig. 42.3 Lateral spine dual-energy x-ray absorptiometry (DXA) imaging for vertebral fracture assessment in a 66-year-old man. This study was performed on a GE Lunar Prodigy DXA device. No deformities are seen. The AAC-8 score is 0. Small osteophytes are visible anteriorly at the T8-T9 level. The Genant semiquantitative grading system is seen in the lower right portion of the image.

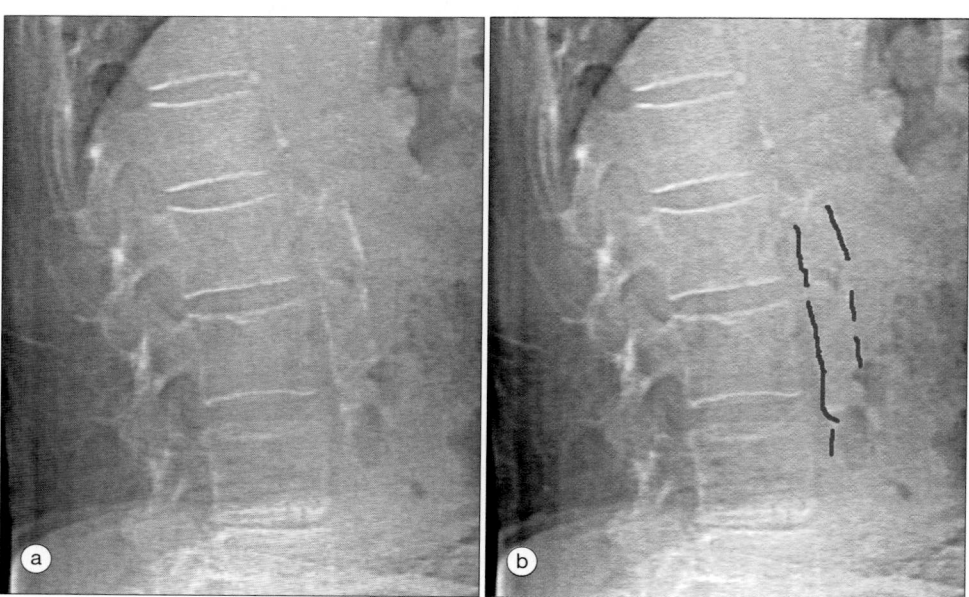

Fig. 42.4 (a) Lateral spine dual-energy x-ray absorptiometry image performed for vertebral fracture assessment in which abdominal aortic calcification is seen. In (b), the aortic calcification has been highlighted. The AAC-8 score was 3. *(Case provided courtesy Hologic, Inc., Bedford, Mass.)*

TABLE 42.3 AAC-8 SCORING SYSTEM*	
Abdominal aortic calcification length relative to lumbar vertebral height	**Score**
None	0
1 vertebra	1
>1 but ≤2 vertebrae	2
>2 but ≤3 vertebrae	3
>3 vertebrae	4

*A point score is awarded for the anterior abdominal aortic wall and the posterior abdominal aortic wall on the basis of the number of vertebrae spanned by the length of the aortic calcification. The worst possible score for both walls combined is 8.

calcification assessment on lateral spine imaging for its fan-array DXA devices.

APPLICATION OF BONE DENSITOMETRY IN CLINICAL PRACTICE

Influence of manufacturer

Although the appearance of screen images and computer printouts from the various manufacturers of DXA equipment may differ, the information that is provided is actually quite similar. Layouts from any one manufacturer may change with updates to the software, but the content generally does not.

Figs. 42.6, 42.7, and 42.8 are screen images of PA lumbar spine and proximal femur bone density studies from GE Lunar, Norland, and Hologic DXA devices. The three studies are not of the same patient.

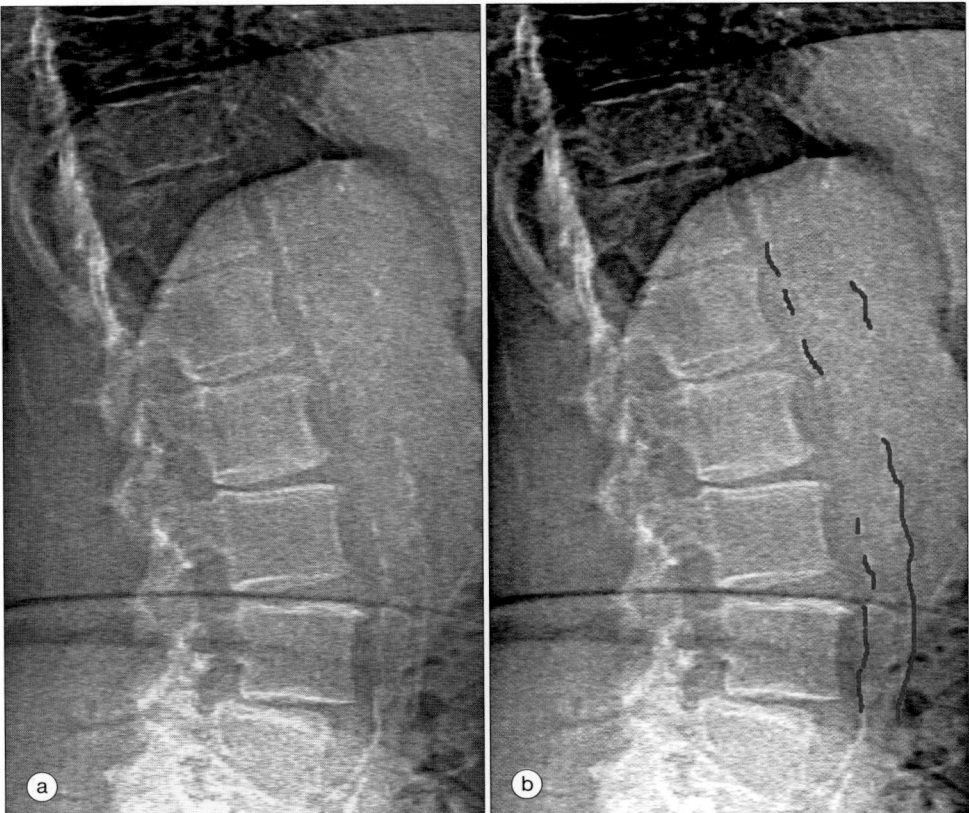

Fig. 42.5 (a) Lateral spine dual-energy x-ray absorptiometry image performed for vertebral fracture assessment in which abdominal aortic calcification is seen. In (b), the aortic calcification has been highlighted. The AAC-8 score was 6. *(Case provided courtesy Hologic, Inc., Bedford, Mass.)*

Nevertheless, a careful review of the images will reveal that, although the initial appearance is quite different among the three devices, the nature of the information provided is the same.

Fig. 42.6a and b are based on a PA lumbar spine and left proximal femur study performed on a GE Lunar DXA device. On the left, the image of the studied region can be seen. On the lower right are the bone density results and standard score comparisons for various regions of interest. On the upper right is the age-regression graph. Above the graph is the notation that indicates from which region of interest the data that have been plotted on the graph came. The graph, although colorful, does not actually provide any additional information beyond the numbers seen on the lower right. On the bottom portion of the screen, relevant biographic data are seen. The patient's name would also normally be seen here.

On the Norland PA lumbar spine and left proximal femur DXA studies seen in Fig. 42.7a and b, the layout is similar but not identical. An obvious difference is that the image of the spine and proximal femur are in color, although this image can be changed to a gray-scale image if the user desires. The age-regression graph is seen in the upper right of the image and the numeric data are seen across the bottom of the image.

Fig. 42.8a and b are PA lumbar spine and left proximal femur studies obtained on a Hologic DXA device. The age-regression graph is not seen on this particular screen image, but it is provided on the computer printout. Patient biographic data are clearly seen on the upper right and once again, the numeric data are seen on the lower right.

On the GE Lunar spine study in Fig. 42.6a, a BMD value is given for each of the four lumbar vertebrae and for every possible combination of contiguous lumbar vertebrae. This is not the case on the Norland DXA spine study seen in Fig. 42.7a. Note that on the Hologic PA spine study in Fig. 42.8a, the L1-L4 BMD is referred to as the "Total," rather than L1-L4 as it is on the GE Lunar and Norland studies. In the proximal femur studies shown here, all of the manufacturers provide results for the total hip, femoral neck, and trochanteric regions of interest. On the GE Lunar and Norland proximal femur studies, values are provided for Ward's area. This is not seen on the Hologic study. This difference is of little consequence because Ward's area, although of historical interest, has little, if any, clinical utility.

The age-regression graphs seen on these images are simply plots of the BMD from the selected region of interest versus the patient's age. The center regression line indicates the expected BMD for age. This center regression line has an upper and lower boundary that, in the case of the GE Lunar graph, is ±1 SD and, in the case of the Norland graph, is ±2 SD. The physician can therefore immediately tell visually how the patient compares with age- and gender-matched peers. This can also be ascertained from the numeric data. In the case of the Norland graph, the background color scheme of green, yellow, and red also corresponds to the WHO T-score diagnostic category cut points. Fracture risk characterizations are made within these different-colored zones. Note, however, that these colored zones span the entire age range shown on the graph and thus they must be interpreted with extreme caution.

All of the manufacturers provide standard score comparisons for the BMDs from the various regions of interest. Percentile comparisons are provided as well. The standard score comparisons indicate the number of SDs above or below the average value that the patient's value lies. The T score is a comparison with the average for a young adult and the Z score is a comparison with the average for the patient's age-matched peers. The T score is, of course, used with the WHO diagnostic criteria. A Z score poorer than −2 strongly suggests the need to evaluate a patient for secondary causes of bone loss. However, a Z score of −2 or better does not negate this possibility such that an evaluation for secondary causes of bone loss should always be considered in an individual with low bone density. Thus the Z score also has limited clinical utility in an adult.

The image of the skeleton should be reviewed on the computer or computer printout to ascertain proper patient positioning, labeling of the regions of interest, and identification of any potential artifacts or structural changes that would affect the accuracy of the bone density measurement. It may be necessary to review the image on the computer itself rather than the printout because the resolution of the image will be superior. Bone density images are not FDA approved for structural diagnosis, but the near-radiographic quality of these images makes such a structural review possible. Once the image has been reviewed and the physician is satisfied with the technical quality of the study, only then should the all-important numeric data be addressed.

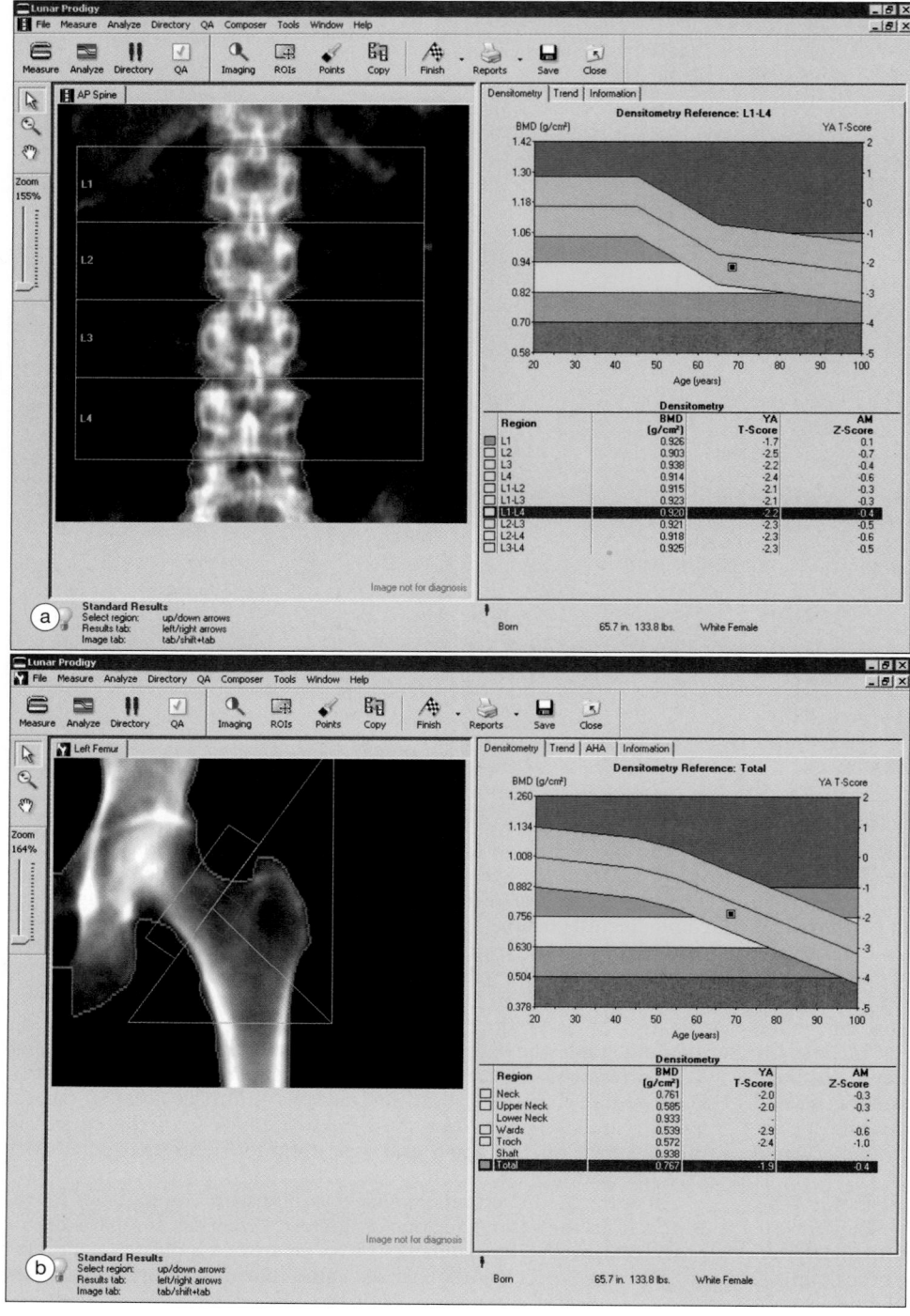

Fig. 42.6 (a) Postero-anterior lumbar spine study performed on a GE Lunar Prodigy DXA device in a 69-year-old woman. The bone mineral density (BMD) and standard scores are given for each vertebra, as well as every possible combination of contiguous vertebrae. The L1-L4 BMD is plotted on the age-regression graph. (b) A left proximal femur study performed on a GE Lunar Prodigy on the same patient.

On the PA lumbar spine study, the L2-L4 or L1-L4 BMD value is preferred to BMD values from a single vertebra or from only two contiguous vertebrae for reasons of accuracy and precision. All three major manufacturers of DXA equipment provide the L1-L4 BMD, although as noted earlier, in the case of Hologic, this is called the "total." At the proximal femur, Ward's area is the least accurate of all the proximal femur measures because of its small size. Because of the localization routines used in these devices, Ward's area should be expected to have the lowest BMD. Ward's area is also placed slightly differently from manufacturer to manufacturer. This is true for the femoral neck as well. The most similar region of interest among the manufacturers in the proximal femur is the total femur region of interest. Even so, the actual measured BMDs at a given skeletal site should never be directly compared among the manufacturers because of the differences in machine calibration. At the proximal femur, a rough comparison of total hip T scores can be attempted only if the T scores are derived from the NHANES III database.

CASE STUDY

The following case study illustrates the application and interpretation of DXA studies of the PA lumbar spine and proximal femur in a 69-year-old woman. This patient was referred for her initial evaluation at the age of 69 after a wrist fracture, which she suffered in a fall on a wet surface. Her baseline studies are the GE Lunar studies previously seen in Fig. 42.6a and b. A review of the spine image indicated good positioning and no degenerative changes, artifacts, or vertebral deformities that would affect the accuracy of the study. The vertebral labeling also appeared to be correct. A review of the left proximal femur study also indicated good positioning and no artifacts that would affect the accuracy of the study. The L1-L4 BMD was 0.920 g/cm^2 with a T score of −2.2 and a Z score of −0.4. At the total hip, the BMD was 0.767 g/cm^2 with a T score of −1.9 and a Z score of −0.4. At the femoral neck, the BMD was 0.761 g/cm^2 with a T score of −2.0 and a Z score of −0.3. In this case, the lowest T score is −2.2 at L1-L4.

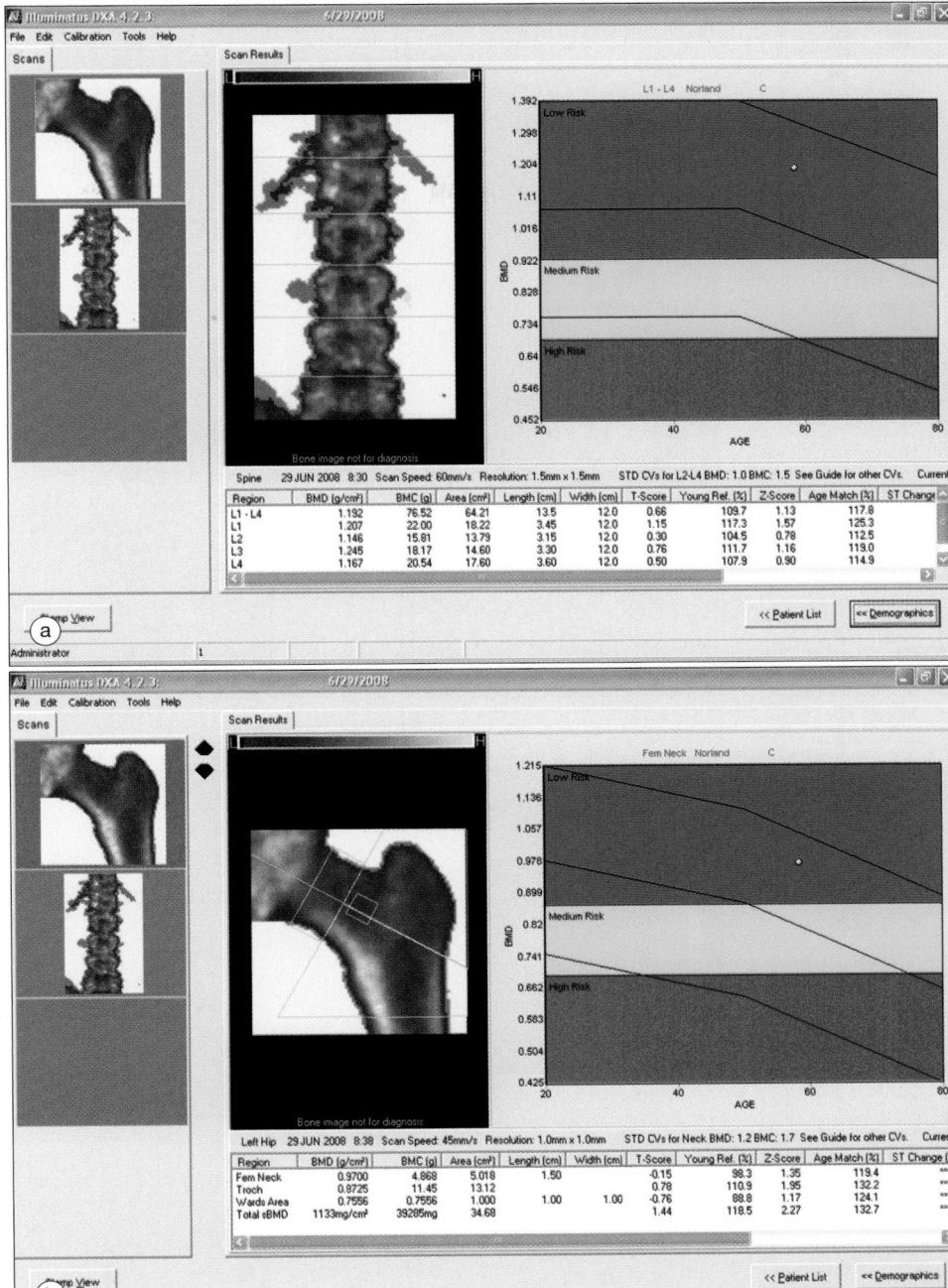

Fig. 42.7 (a) Postero-anterior lumbar spine study performed on a Norland DXA device. (b) A left proximal femur study on the same patient. Note the density-modulated color images of the skeleton. The chosen region of interest is plotted on the age-regression graph. The boundaries of the graph are twice as wide as seen on the GE Lunar studies. *(Case provided courtesy Cooper-Surgical Norland, Trumbull, Conn.)*

Applying the WHO criteria for diagnosis and ISCD guidelines for diagnostic site selection, this patient has osteopenia based on the L1-L4 T score. Her FRAX 10-year absolute fracture risk for hip fracture was 3.5% and for any major osteoporotic fracture, 23%, as shown in Fig. 42.1.

This patient meets the guideline from the U.S. National Osteoporosis Foundation (NOF) for treatment of postmenopausal women based on the combination of osteopenia and a FRAX 10-year absolute hip fracture risk of greater than or equal to 3% or a 10-year major osteoporotic fracture risk of greater than or equal to 20%.[23] Treatment was subsequently begun in this patient with an antiresorptive agent.

To assess therapeutic efficacy, the patient underwent bone density testing after 2 years of therapy. Her follow-up bone density studies are shown in Fig. 42.9a and b. The L1-L4 BMD is now 0.971 g/cm^2, the total hip BMD is 0.796 g/cm^2, and the femoral neck BMD is 0.797 g/cm^2. The BMDs in the three regions appear to have increased. Before the physician can conclude that this has indeed happened, several things must be considered.

First, what machine was used for the baseline and follow-up studies? If machines from different manufacturers were used, the BMDs cannot be compared. If different machines from the same manufacturer were used, a comparison can be made but the LSC cannot be calculated directly and must be assumed to be greater than it otherwise would be. Ideally, exactly the same machine was used. Second, was there adequate quality control of the machine or machines during the time period in question? Has there been adequate quality control monitoring (at least as often as recommended by the manufacturer with results tracking to detect drifts and shifts in machine values)? Third, were there any software changes in the interim that could potentially affect the values? Finally, were comparable regions of interest identified on the two sets of scans? The images from both sets of studies should be compared to determine similar region of interest identification and labeling. Once all of these preliminary issues have been resolved, the final issue to undertake is to determine if the measured change equals or exceeds the LSC, which requires that the precision of testing at a given skeletal site is known.

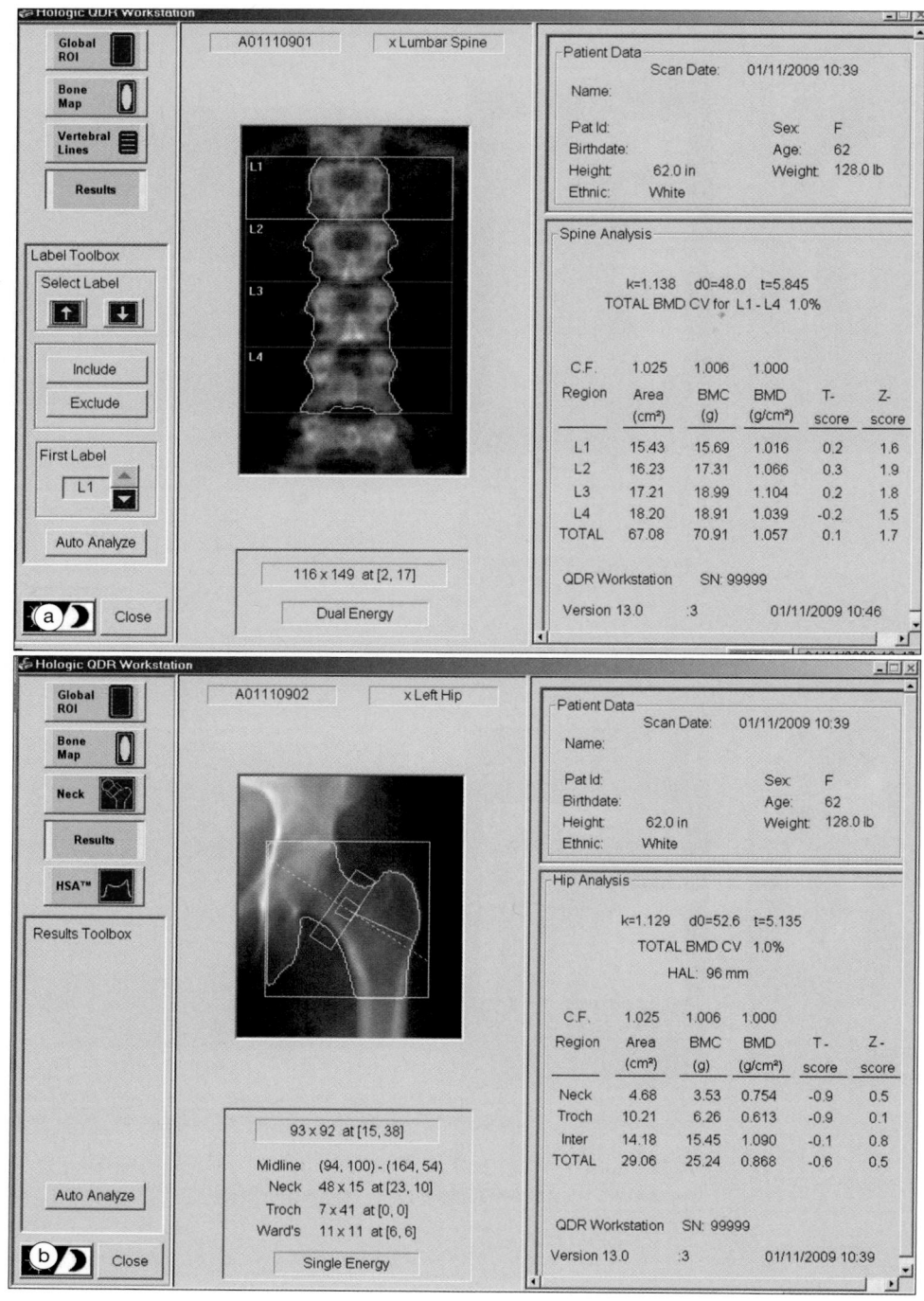

Fig. 42.8 (a) Postero-anterior lumbar spine study performed on a Hologic DXA device. Note that the L1-L4 BMD is called the *total BMD*. BMD values and standard scores are provided for each vertebra as well. (b) A left proximal femur study on the same patient. *(Case provided courtesy Hologic, Inc., Bedford, Mass.)*

In this particular case, a short-term precision study had previously been performed at the bone densitometry facility. The study was performed in 10 postmenopausal women from 50 to 70 years of age. Each of the women underwent four DXA studies of the PA lumbar spine and left proximal femur. The precision at L1-L4, the total hip, and femoral neck was calculated as the RMS-SD in g/cm². The resulting precision values were 0.012 g/cm² at L1-L4, 0.006 g/cm² at the total hip, and 0.011 g/cm² at the femoral neck. On the basis of equation 3, the resulting LSCs were 0.033 g/cm² at L1-L4, 0.017 g/cm² at the total hip, and 0.031 g/cm² at the femoral neck. The observed changes at L1-L4, total hip, and femoral neck all exceed the LSC for that region of interest. Thus there was a statistically significant increase in BMD at all three regions of interest and, on the basis of the intermediate endpoint of BMD, the antiresorptive therapy was deemed efficacious. No change in BMD would also suggest therapeutic efficacy. If, however, a decline in BMD had been observed that equaled or exceeded the LSC, the physician would have concluded that a statistically significant loss in BMD had occurred, a circumstance which should prompt a re-evaluation of the patient.

LIMITATIONS OF DXA BONE DENSITY TESTING

The limitations of DXA bone density testing do not generally detract from the extraordinary clinical utility of the technology. DXA is a two-dimensional measurement. As a consequence, measurements of bone density are mixed measurements of trabecular and cortical bone, unlike three-dimensional QCT, in which the trabecular and cortical densities can be separated. DXA is an x-ray based technology and therefore exposure to ionizing radiation is unavoidable. However, radiation exposure is extremely low and, from a practical clinical perspective, virtually negligible. The accuracy and precision of bone density measurements can unquestionably be affected by degenerative skeletal changes, which are common in the spine after age 60. Less reliance must be placed on PA lumbar spine BMD in men and women of this age, and greater reliance placed on proximal femoral measurements. Surgical hardware or prior fracture will also render a measurement invalid.

Perhaps the greatest limitation of DXA, which also applies to measurements of bone density by any technique, is that the measurement of bone density, although predictive of fracture risk, does not capture

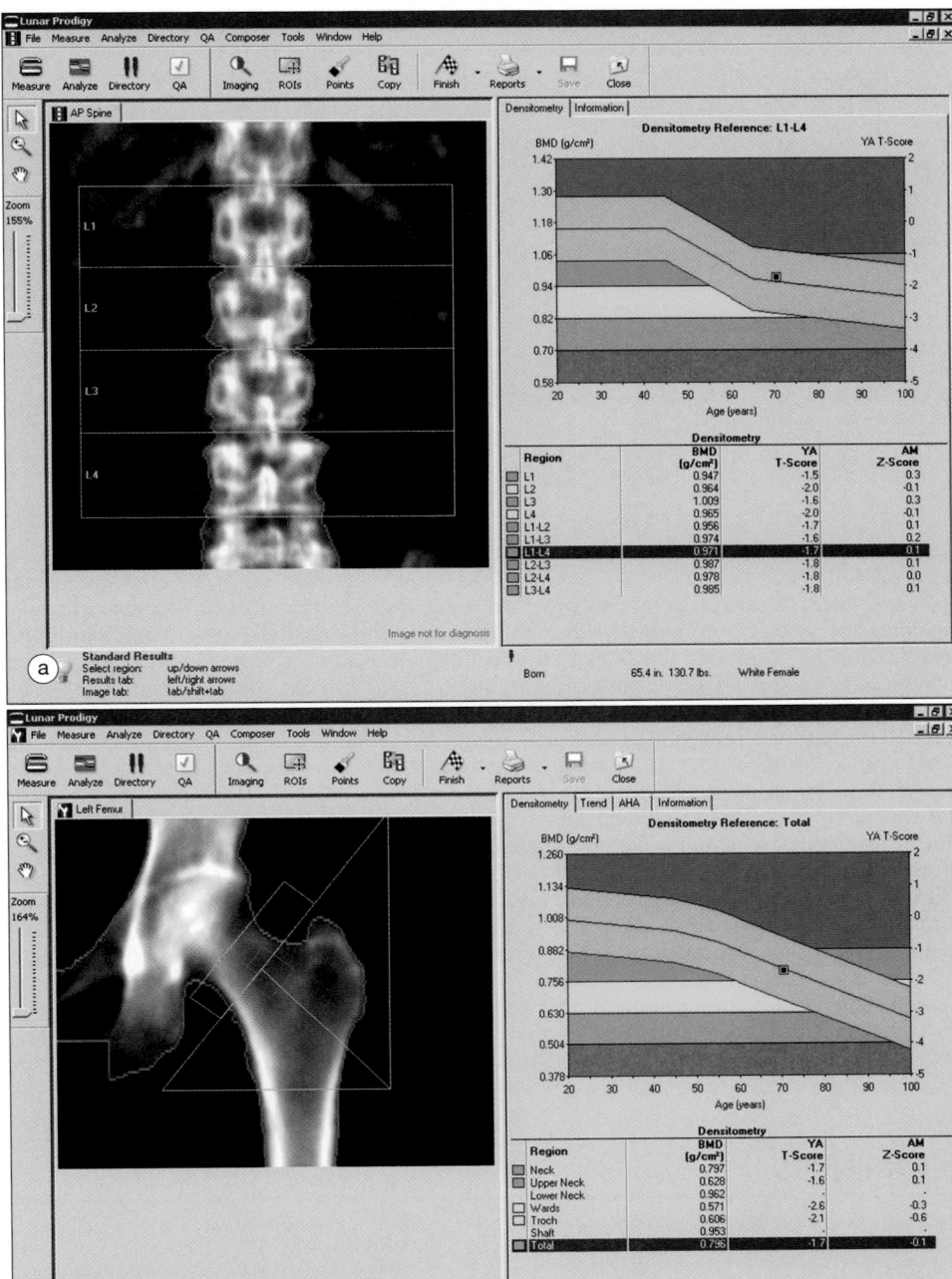

Fig. 42.9 (a) Postero-anterior lumbar spine study performed on a GE Lunar Prodigy on the same patient seen in Fig. 42.6a. (b) A left proximal femur study performed on a GE Lunar Prodigy on the same patient seen in Fig. 42.6b. These studies were performed 2 years later than the studies seen in Fig. 42.6.

every determinant of fracture risk and conversely does not capture every aspect of the therapeutic efficacy of bone active agents in reducing that risk.[13,14] Absolute fracture risk prediction algorithms like FRAX go beyond the recognized limitations of the measurement of BMD to refine fracture risk prediction. Because no agent reduces risk to 0, the presence or absence of a fracture on therapy cannot be used as a measure of efficacy. BMD is considered an intermediate or surrogate endpoint in assessing therapeutic efficacy of a bone active agent in reducing fracture risk. There is a statistically significant relationship between increases in BMD on therapy versus placebo and decreases in fracture risk.[40-42] It is only the magnitude of this relationship that remains controversial.[43]

INDICATIONS FOR BONE DENSITY TESTING

Several organizations have published guidelines or positions on patient selection for bone density testing. There are more similarities among the guidelines from various organizations than there are differences, with some of the differences resulting from an organization's focus on a particular patient population. In general, most guidelines reflect the positions taken by the NOF, which issued its first guidelines for physicians on the use of bone densitometry in 1988 with the most recent guidelines issued in 2010.[23] Guidelines have been produced by other organizations such as ISCD, the American Association of Clinical Endocrinologists (AACE), the North American Menopause Society (NAMS), and the American College of Rheumatology (ACR).[44-47] Guidelines from AACE[45] and NAMS[46] are provided in the context of the prevention and treatment of postmenopausal osteoporosis and are therefore understandably focused on postmenopausal women only, whereas guidelines from the NOF,[23] ISCD,[44] and ACR[47] address bone density testing in general in both men and women. In all of the guidelines, however, bone density testing is recommended in women age 65 and older, regardless of other risk factors. In guidelines from the NOF, ACR, and ISCD bone density testing is recommended

TABLE 42.4 COMPARISON OF CURRENT GUIDELINES FROM MAJOR MEDICAL ORGANIZATIONS FOR USE OF BONE DENSITY TESTING IN CLINICAL PRACTICE

	Women ≥age 65	Postmenopausal women ≤age 64 and at least 1 risk factor	Postmenopausal women with fractures	Men ≥ age 70	Technique for diagnosis	Site for diagnosis
NOF 2010	√	√	√	√	DXA	PA lumbar spine, total hip or femoral neck
AACE 2003	√	√	√*	—	DXA/QCT	Spine, proximal femur
NAMS 2010	√	√	√	—	DXA	PA lumbar spine, total hip or femoral neck, whichever is lowest
ISCD 2007	√	√	√	√	DXA	PA lumbar spine, total hip or femoral neck, whichever is lowest

*Consideration was limited to low-trauma fractures.
AACE, American Association of Clinical Endocrinologists; ISCD, International Society for Clinical Densitometry; NAMS, North American Menopause Society; NOF, National Osteoporosis Foundation;
— indicates no comment.

in men age 70 and older. A comparison of the guidelines is shown in Table 42.4.

Various organizations have also provided guidelines regarding the frequency of testing when monitoring changes in bone density. No organization recommends the use of an appendicular skeletal site for this purpose. Instead, bone density measurements at the lumbar spine or proximal femur are preferred. As noted earlier, this recommendation is based on both the precision of testing at a site, as well as the anticipated rate of change in the BMD at that site from either a therapeutic intervention or disease process. In most cases, the bone density is followed to determine therapeutic efficacy with the notable exception of monitoring changes in bone density to detect glucocorticoid-induced bone loss.

In 2001 the Ad Hoc Committee on Glucocorticoid-Induced Osteoporosis of the ACR recommended that patients initiating glucocorticoid therapy with a planned duration of longer than 6 months undergo baseline bone density testing followed by serial measurements at 6-month intervals.[48] If the patient was receiving therapy to prevent glucocorticoid-induced bone loss, annual follow-up measurements were recommended. ISCD,[44] although noting that 1 year after initiation or change in therapy was an appropriate monitoring interval, also stated that in conditions associated with rapid bone loss such as glucocorticoid therapy, more frequent testing was appropriate. Both AACE and NAMS, focusing on postmenopausal osteoporosis, provided different recommendations on the basis of treatment or bone density status of the woman. NAMS recommended a monitoring interval of 3 to 5 years in untreated women and a monitoring interval of 2 years in women receiving treatment.[46] AACE recommended a 3- to 5-year monitoring interval in women with a normal BMD (based on WHO criteria).[45] For women in an osteoporosis prevention program, however, AACE recommended a follow-up measurement every 1 to 2 years until stability was demonstrated, followed by a 2- to 3-year monitoring interval. In women being treated for osteoporosis, yearly measurements were recommended for a minimum of 2 years and until stability was demonstrated. Thereafter, a monitoring interval of 2 years was recommended. The guiding principle behind all of these recommendations is reflected in the ISCD guidelines[44] in which it is noted that "follow-up BMD testing should be done when the expected change in BMD equals or exceeds the LSC."

REFERENCES

1. Dennis J. A new system of measurement in x-ray work. Dental Cosmos 1989;39:445-454.
2. Cameron JR, Sorenson G. Measurements of bone mineral in vivo: an improved method. Science 1963;142:230-232.
3. Nord RH. Technical considerations in DPA. In Genant HK, ed. Osteoporosis update. San Francisco: University of California Printing Services, 1987:203-212.
4. World Health Organization. Assessment of fracture risk and its application to screening for postmenopausal osteoporosis. WHO Technical Report Series [843]. Geneva: WHO, 1994:1-129.
5. Faulkner KG, von Stetten E, Miller P. Discordance in patient classification using T-scores. J Clin Densitom 1999;2:343-350.
6. Faulkner KG, Orwoll E. Implications in the use of T-scores for the diagnosis of osteoporosis in men. J Clin Densitom 2002;5:87-93.
7. Hans D, Downs RW, Duboeuf F, et al. Skeletal sites for osteoporosis diagnosis: the 2005 ISCD official positions. J Clin Densitom 2006;9:15-21.
8. World Health Organization. Prevention and management of osteoporosis. WHO Technical Report Series [921]. Geneva: WHO, 2003:1-192.
9. Kanis JA, Glüer C-C. An update on the diagnosis and assessment of osteoporosis with densitometry. Committee of Scientific Advisors, International Osteoporosis Foundation. Osteoporos Int 2000;11:192-202.
10. Bonnick SL. Diagnosing osteoporosis. In: Bonnick SL. Bone densitometry in clinical practice, 2nd ed. Totowa, NJ: Humana Press, 2004:217-232.
11. De Laet CEDH, Van Der Klift M, Hofman A, Pols HAP. Osteoporosis in men and women: a story about bone mineral density thresholds and hip fracture risk. J Bone Miner Res 2002;17:2231-2236.
12. Melton LJ, Atkinson EJ, O'Fallon WM, et al. Long-term fracture prediction by bone mineral assessed at different skeletal sites. J Bone Miner Res 1993;8:1227-1233.
13. Cummings SR, Black DM, Nevitt MC, et al. Bone density at various sites for prediction of hip fracture. Lancet 1993;341:72-75.
14. Kanis JA, Johnell O, Oden A, et al. FRAX and the assessment of fracture probability in men and women from the UK. Osteoporos Int 2008;19:385-397.
15. Kanis JA, Johansson H, Oden A, et al. A family history of fracture and fracture risk: a meta-analysis. Bone 2004;35:1029-1037.
16. Kanis JA, Johnell O, De Laet C, et al. A meta-analysis of previous fracture and subsequent fracture risk. Bone 2004;35:375-382.
17. Kanis JA, Johansson H, Oden A, et al. A meta-analysis of prior corticosteroid use and fracture risk. J Bone Miner Res 2004;19:893-899.
18. Kanis JA, Johansson H, Oden A, et al. A meta-analysis of milk intake and fracture risk: low utility for case finding. Osteoporos Int 2005;16:799-804.
19. Kanis JA, Johansson H, Johnell O, et al. Alcohol intake as a risk factor for fracture. Osteoporos Int 2005;16:737-742.
20. Kanis JA, Johnell O, Oden A, et al. Smoking and fracture risk: a meta-analysis. Osteoporos Int 2005;16:155-162.
21. De Laet C, Kanis JA, Oden A, et al. Body mass index as a predictor of fracture risk: a meta-analysis. Osteoporos Int 2005;16:1330-1338.
22. Kanis JA, Oden A, Johnell O, et al. The use of clinical risk factors enhances the performance of BMD in the prediction of hip and osteoporotic fractures in men and women. Osteoporos Int 2007;18:1033-1046.
23. National Osteoporosis Foundation. Clinician's guide to prevention and treatment of osteoporosis. Washington, DC: National Osteoporosis Foundation, 2010.
24. International Organization of Standardization: Accuracy (trueness and precision) of measurement methods and results—part 1: general principles and definition. ISO 5725-1, 1st ed. Switzerland: International Organization of Standardization, 1994:1-17.
25. Bonnick SL. Monitoring changes in bone density. In: Bonnick SL. Bone densitometry in clinical practice, 2nd ed. Totowa, NJ: Humana Press, 2004:267-285.
26. Glüer C-C, Blake GM, Lu Y, et al. Accurate assessment of precision errors: how to measure the reproducibility of bone densitometry techniques. Osteoporos Int 1995;5:262-270.
27. Lenchik L, Kiebzak GM, Blunt BA. What is the role of serial bone mineral density measurements in patient management? J Clin Densitom 2002;5:S29-S38.
28. Cummings SR, Palermo L, Browner W, et al. Monitoring osteoporosis therapy with bone densitometry. Misleading changes and regression to the mean. JAMA 2000;283:1318-1321.
29. Schousboe JT, DeBold CR, Bowles C, et al. Prevalence of vertebral compression fracture deformity by x-ray absorptiometry of lateral thoracic and lumbar spines in a population referred for bone densitometry. J Clin Densitom 2002;5:239-246.
30. Majumdar SR, Kim N, Colman I, et al. Incidental vertebral fractures discovered with chest radiography in the emergency department. Arch Intern Med 2005;165:905-909.

31. Morris CA, Carrino JA, Lang P, Solomon DH. Incidental vertebral fractures on chest radiographs. Recognition, documentation, and treatment. J Gen Intern Med 2006;21:352-356.

32. Schousboe JT, Vokes T, Broy SB, et al. Vertebral fracture assessment: the 2007 ISCD official positions. J Clin Densitom 2008;11:92-108.

33. Genant HK, Wu CY, Van Kuijk C, Nevitt MC: Vertebral fracture assessment using a semiquantitative technique. J Bone Miner Res 1993;8:1137-1148.

34. van der Meer IM, Bots ML, Hofman A, et al. Predictive value of noninvasive measures of atherosclerosis for incident myocardial infarction: the Rotterdam Study. Circulation 2004;109:1089-1094.

35. Hollander M, Hak AE, Koudstaal PJ, et al. Comparison between measures of atherosclerosis and risk of stroke: the Rotterdam Study. Stroke 2003;34:2367-2372.

36. Walsh CR, Cupples LA, Levy D, et al. Abdominal aortic calcific deposits are associated with increased risk for congestive heart failure: the Framingham Heart Study. Am Heart J 2002;144:733-739.

37. Wilson PW, Kauppila LI, O'Donnell CJ, et al. Abdominal aortic calcific deposits are an important predictor of vascular morbidity and mortality. Circulation 2001;103:1529-1534.

38. Kauppila LI, Polak JF, Cupples LA, et al. New indices to classify location, severity and progression of calcific lesions in the abdominal aorta: a 25-year follow-up study. Atherosclerosis 1997;132:245-250.

39. Schousboe JT, Wilson KE, Kiel DP. Detection of abdominal aortic calcification with lateral spine imaging using DXA. J Clin Densitom 2006;9:302-308.

40. Wasnich RD, Miller PD. Antifracture efficacy of antiresorptive agents are related to changes in bone density. J Clin Endocrinol Metab 2000;85:231-236.

41. Cummings SR, Karpf DB, Harris F, et al. Improvement in spine bone density and reduction in risk of vertebral fractures during treatment with antiresorptive drugs. Am J Med 2002;112:281-289.

42. Hochberg MC, Greenspan S, Wasnich RD, et al. Changes in bone density and turnover explain the reductions in incidence of nonvertebral fractures that occur during treatment with antiresorptive agents. J Clin Endocrinol Metab 2002;87:1586-1592.

43. Miller PD, Hochberg MC, Wehren LE, et al. How useful are measures of BMD and bone turnover? Curr Med Res Opin 2005;21:545-553.

44. Baim S, Leonard BM, Bianchi ML, et al. Official positions of the International Society for Clinical Densitometry and Executive Summary of the 2007 ISCD pediatric position development conference. J Clin Densitom 2008;11:6-21.

45. Hodgson SF, Watts NB, Bilezikian JP, et al. American Association of Clinical Endocrinologists medical guidelines for clinical practice for the prevention and treatment of postmenopausal osteoporosis: 2001 edition, with selected updates for 2003. Endocr Pract 2003;9:544-564.

46. Management of osteoporosis in postmenopausal women: 2010 position statement of The North American Menopause Society. Menopause 2010;17:25-54.

47. American College of Rheumatology. Bone density measurement. Available at: http://www.rheumatology.org/publications/position/BoneDensityMeasurement.asp. Accessed January 7, 2009.

48. American College of Physicians Ad Hoc Committee on Glucocorticoid-Induced Osteoporosis. Recommendations for the prevention and treatment of glucocorticoid-induced osteoporosis. Arthritis Rheum 2001;44:1496-1503.

Use of imaging as an outcome measure in rheumatoid arthritis, psoriatic arthritis, and ankylosing spondylitis in clinical trials

43

Désirée Van Der Heijde

INTRODUCTION

Imaging is an important way to assess efficacy of treatment in clinical trials. Depending on the imaging technique it can be used to assess inflammation and/or structural damage. The focus of this chapter will be predominantly on structural damage. It is especially this aspect that makes imaging an important outcome measure in clinical trials. To prove that a drug has disease modification capabilities there needs to be a reduction in signs and symptoms (of inflammation), preservation of physical function, and inhibition of structural damage progression. There are some general concepts about using imaging as an outcome measure that will be discussed first. Because assessment of structural damage on radiographs is well established in rheumatoid arthritis, this will be frequently used to illustrate the concepts. This will then be followed by a discussion of specific issues by disease for rheumatoid arthritis (RA), psoriatic arthritis (PsA), and ankylosing spondylitis (AS) and by imaging method (conventional radiography, magnetic resonance imaging, and ultrasonography).

GENERAL ASPECTS FOR CLINICAL TRIALS

With respect to clinical trials there are general aspects that apply to all imaging methods and scoring in general as well as handling of the data. These are summarized as points to consider and include:

- Different phases of drug development
- Different phases of disease
- Readers
- Statistical aspects of reader agreement
- Grouping of films—read sessions
- Blinding time sequence
- Statistical handling of missing data
- Statistical analyses
- Minimum duration of trial
- Placebo versus active comparator
- Presentation of data
- Repair

Different phases of drug development

The choice of the imaging method depends on what feature will be assessed (inflammation vs. damage), duration of the follow-up, and experience with various imaging techniques in the centers including patients. In early phases of development the most important question is the proof of concept. This might apply to imaging of inflammation and structural damage. For the first, only MRI and ultrasonography are applicable; for damage, radiographs also can do the job. MRI is more widely standardized and applied than ultrasonography in clinical drug development. Damage information on bone (edema and erosions) in RA can be obtained from MRI, whereas radiographs provide insight on the effect on bone (erosions) and indirectly on cartilage (joint space narrowing [JSN]). In later phases of drug development, the data will be used for filing to the drug agencies. At the moment radiographs are used for this purpose. Acceptance of MRI needs to be discussed upfront.

Different phases of disease

In principle, the same imaging techniques can be used in early and advanced disease. Progression of structural damage on radiographs is most prominent in patients who have structural damage already. On theoretical grounds, it might be especially useful to apply MRI in the early phases of the disease before structural damage can be visualized on radiographs.

Readers

Because precision of reading is important it is advised to have two readers score all images independently. The average data of the two readers will be used for the primary analysis. Ideally, these are the same two readers scoring all images, but if this is not possible three or four readers can score the images so that there is a set of two scores for each film. Preferably, the readers score a similar number of images and all possible reader combinations are made. Which reader should read which image should already be decided before the start of the reading. Increasing the number of readers to three or more for all images would improve the precision further but at the cost of feasibility (including time and costs). For pivotal clinical trials the optimum number of readers is two; however, for observational studies or early-phase development scores one reader could be sufficient. It is also important to use experienced, well-trained readers because the consequent reduction in random error increases the power of a study in comparison to the use of untrained readers.

Statistical aspects of reader agreement

An important aspect is the assessment of the agreement of the readers. Traditionally this is done by a correlation coefficient. The intraclass correlation coefficient (ICC) is the preferred measure and can be defined as the proportion of all the variance explained by differences between subjects, that is, suggesting a small contribution from observer variation. The Pearson and Spearman correlation coefficients should be avoided because these latter two give only a measure of association, not agreement. Nevertheless, the ICC also clearly has limitations because it is largely influenced by the dataset: a dataset with great variation in the data gives higher ICCs when compared with a dataset with minor variation, although this is not a reflection of better agreement between the readers. This is especially an issue when comparing the agreement of progression scores, which are typically small. Consequently, the presented ICC might suggest poor agreement while this is actually caused by the lack of variation in the data. Additional analyses to check agreement between readers is the use of Bland and Altman plots (where the difference between the two readers is plotted against their mean), which assess real agreement in the units of the measurement scale.[1] An example is presented in Figure 43.1. Calculating the 95% limits of agreement provides a value that is also referred to as the smallest detectable difference (SDD). This is the value that can be used as a cutoff to determine if a change beyond measurement error is present. The SDD reflects the situation to test if a change in patient A is different from a change in patient B. Mostly, we are interested in

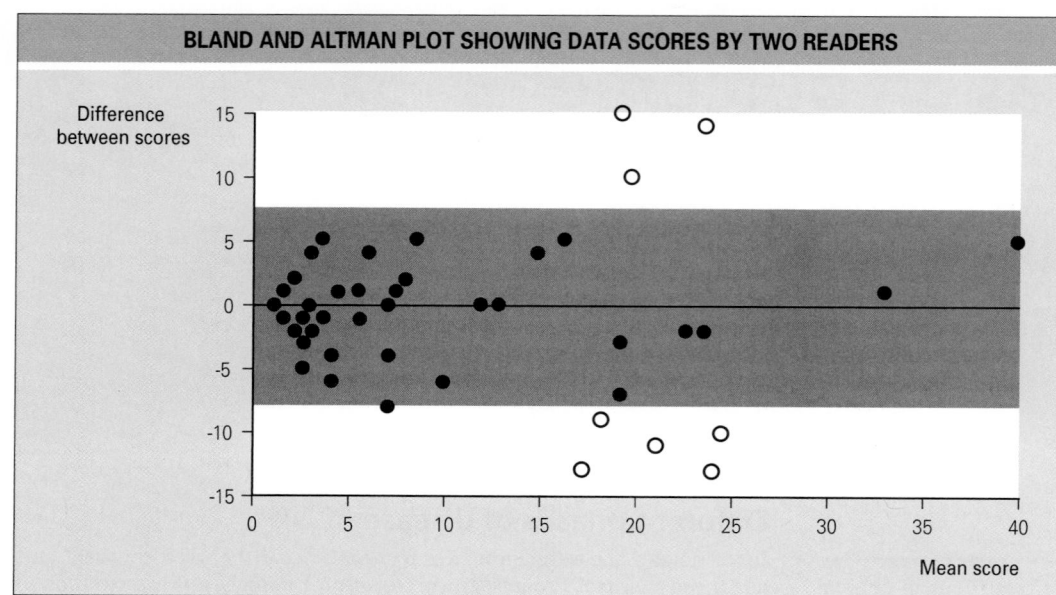

BLAND AND ALTMAN PLOT SHOWING DATA SCORES BY TWO READERS

Fig. 43.1 Bland and Altman plot showing data scores by two readers. This can be applied to status scores and to change scores. On the x-axis the mean score of the two readers is depicted and plotted against the difference between the scores of reader 1 and reader 2 on the y-axis. If there is no variation, all data will be on the line $x = 0$ (this indicates that the difference between the readers is 0 for all values). If the mean difference is not equal to 0, one of the readers is scoring systematically higher than the other reader. It is important to check if the variation between the readers is equal over the entire range of the scores. The limits of agreement do include 95% of the data, and this is a value for the random variation (the gray zone in the figure). This forms the basis for the calculation of the SDD and SDC.

the question if a change in patient A is a real change, in other words if there is a change beyond measurement error in this particular patient. For this purpose the smallest detectable change (SDC) should be used.[2] This can be derived from the SDD by dividing by $\sqrt{2}$. The disadvantage of both the SDD and SDC is that these are frequently relatively high numbers and they underestimate real progression, because progression detected by clinicians judged as clinically relevant (e.g., sufficient to change treatment) is usually below the SDD/SDC. So the best value of the SDD and SDC is the information to judge the level of agreement of reader pairs, but if used as a cutoff to determine progression it most likely underestimates the number of patients with progression.

Grouping of films—read sessions

Typically, all the images from different time points that will be analyzed together are scored in the same read session and are offered simultaneously to the reader. For example, a one-year trial with images at weeks 0, 24, and 52 are offered at the same time to the reader. Although most scoring methods provide absolute scores, the option to compare images of various time points is an important aspect of scoring; also by doing so differences in imaging technique (e.g., over/underexposure; rotation) can be taken into account. Moreover, the change scores are the most important for the analysis of the treatment effect. A consequence of this is that if for the trial in the example the week 104 film comes available, this requires a rescoring of the earlier time points. A rule is that all the data that will be used in one analysis/comparison need to be included in the same read. It is of major importance to define upfront which time periods need to be compared to select the correct images for follow-up read sessions. Especially in the current trial environment with minor progression in many patients, the optimal read circumstances are of major importance.

Blinding time sequence

The advantage of images is that they can easily be blinded for patient identity and treatment group and rescored at later points in time (e.g., when new images become available). An important aspect is the blinding of the time sequence. The sets of images per patient can be offered to the reader with information on which image belongs to baseline and to which follow-up dates. However, in most trials the dates of the images are also blinded. Scoring with chronologic order can be feasible, for example, in observational cohorts in which new annual follow-up images become available. If scoring in blinded time order, each new radiograph would mean a new scoring of all the images. In the case of scoring with known time sequence, scoring of the new images is performed with the baseline and two previous images presented at the same time with the scores of the previous scoring session provided.

In clinical trials, scoring with blinded time sequence is preferred because this avoids bias, although it may lead to errors such as nonexisting repair of erosions. Moreover, most statistical tests require that scoring errors are equally likely to occur in both directions (over and underscoring), which is with blinded reading the case. This is also a prerequisite for the proposed assessment of possible repair in a trial arm. Finally, both the regulatory agency in the United States and in Europe requires blinding order of the images.

Presentation of data

For each trial, information on mean and median (with appropriate assessment of variation) should be presented, because both give additive information. Moreover, the graphic representation of all individual patient data in a so-called cumulative probability (or frequency) plot shows you all information in a comprehensive way.[3] In a probability plot, the scores per group (usually the change scores over a defined period) are ordered from the lowest to the highest scores (Fig. 43.2). This provides an opportunity to appreciate the full range, the median, and the corresponding value for every percentile you might be interested in. The plot can also be used to determine the percentage of patients showing progression above a certain limit. Preferred cutoffs can be applied. This methodology is much more powerful than simply representing patients above 0.5 (if the average of two readers is being used) or 0 (if one reader is used) or above the SDC. Moreover, the coherence of the data can be appreciated, and it illustrates the prevalence and influence of outliers well.

Statistical handling of missing data

Missing data is a significant issue in clinical trials, especially with long-term follow-up. This pertains to clinical as well as imaging data. However, how to deal with missing imaging data is fundamentally more challenging. Theoretically, clinical data on follow-up have three options: no change, improvement, or worsening. Structural damage, however, is largely irreversible; consequently there are in fact only two options: no change or worsening. Moreover, in most trials there is a preferential dropout in the comparator arm of the trial (either placebo or the frequently less effective standard treatment). In case of inefficacy, this is usually based on clinical data: a high level of disease activity. By applying the Last Observation Carried Forward (LOCF) technique this high level of disease activity is captured in the analysis of the clinical efficacy data. Also the imputation of a non-responder status in the clinical analysis provides the correct information that this patient did not respond well to treatment. However, applying the LOCF to imaging data underestimates the real progression because it might be expected that it is more likely that these patients show worsening as

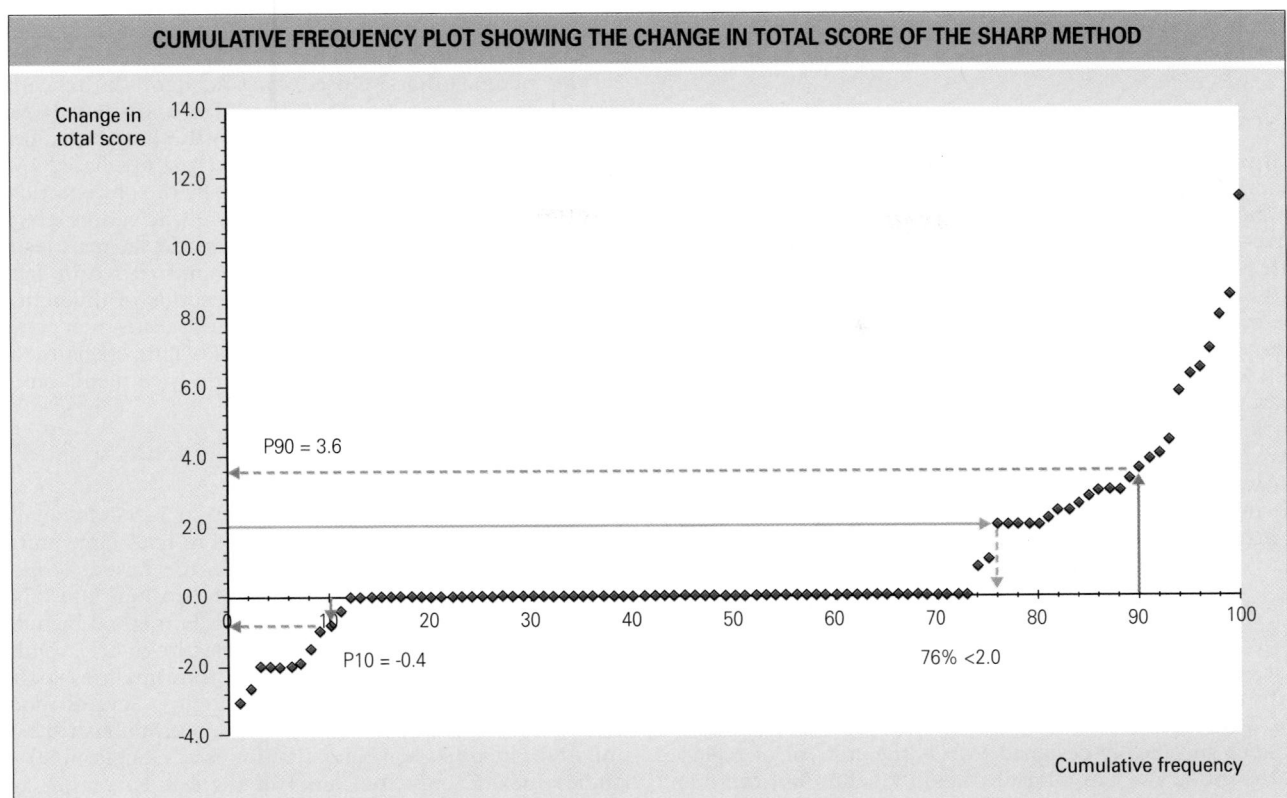

CUMULATIVE FREQUENCY PLOT SHOWING THE CHANGE IN TOTAL SCORE OF THE SHARP METHOD

Fig. 43.2 Cumulative frequency plot showing the change in total score of the Sharp method on the y-axis and the scores of all individual patients depicted as diamonds. These are ordered from the lowest to the highest score and are presented on the x-axis as cumulative frequency. If you want to read the 10th percentile, you draw a line starting at 10% cumulative frequency and connect at the crossing with the figure with the y-axis. The corresponding score on the y-axis (−0.4) can be read. Similarly, the 90th percentile corresponds to a change in score of 3.6, and the median is a change of 0. You can also start with a certain change in score (e.g., +2.0) and read the corresponding percentage on the x-axis: 76% of the patients show a change in score of 2.0 or less. The magenta lines indicate scores belonging to percentiles; the orange line indicates the percentage of patients belonging to a certain score.

compared with no change. Responder data for imaging are not frequently used, certainly not as a primary endpoint, because this greatly decreases the power of a trial. The most widely used "best approach" is the linear extrapolation of the progression. To be able to apply this technique at least one follow-up film needs to be available. Although progression in individual patients is not always linear, it is on a group level and suffices for the analyses of structural damage data. With the use of early escape trial designs, the control group has frequently only a short follow-up before they are switched to open label of the treatment under investigation. With the primary endpoint for imaging at 24 or 52 weeks, and an early escape between 12 and 16 weeks, linear extrapolation is an important aspect in the analyses of the data. In trials with treatment that suppress structural progression effectively, the progression in the control arms determines the power of the study. This progression can only be picked up in the first 12 to 16 weeks until early escape for those patients who opt for early escape, which might be a very high number as shown in recent trials. It has been convincingly shown that radiographs are sufficiently sensitive to pick up changes over 12 to 16 weeks. It should be stressed that it is crucial to obtain follow-up radiographs in all patients regardless of premature discontinuation and to limit data imputation as much as possible.

Missing data on individual joints have to be handled within the same joint group. For example, if data on metacarpophalangeal (MCP) joints are missing, these data will be substituted by data from the remaining MCP joints. The imputation is based on progression scores. Most frequently, missing of up to 20% to 30% of the joints of a particular joint group is accepted before the entire time point is set as missing.

Statistical analyses

For the primary analysis, the average of two readers is used. The scores of the single readers can be applied as sensitivity analyses. Because

radiographic progression is typically not normally distributed, nonparametric testing should be applied. The primary endpoint is the change in progression (extrapolated if necessary) based on the average score of two readers. This can be done by an analysis of covariance (ANCOVA) using the ranks of change with factors at baseline that are expected to influence the structural progression. Baseline structural damage score is such a factor. Mixed effect modeling is another way of analyzing the data because it allows longitudinal interpretations (development in time) of the data because it uses all time points instead of only one predefined endpoint. Under certain conditions, mixed effect models provide more statistical power. Both ANCOVA and mixed effect models can be fit to raw scores as well as after logarithmic transformation.

To confirm the robustness of the data, an LOCF analysis can be confirmed, although it should be realized that statistical significance might be lost.

Minimum duration of trial

For RA, the minimum follow-up for an agent to be able to demonstrate an effect on structural damage is set at 1 year by the U.S. Food and Drug Administration (FDA) and 2 years by the European Medicines Evaluation Agency (EMEA). However, it has been demonstrated that the effects can already be demonstrated after 6 months and even after 3 to 4 months. At the moment structural damage, as assessed on radiographs, is considered the gold standard. The challenge with the early escape design is the length of duration of the control arm. It is being accepted more and more that if the difference obtained during the period with a control arm is sustained over the follow-up period, this is sufficient to fulfill the required longer follow-up period. In practice this means that a significant difference at week 24 (with or without extrapolated data) with a maintenance of the difference between the originally randomized trial arms over the next half year is sufficient for the FDA and over the next 18 months for the EMEA. However, this needs to be discussed with the agencies for each trial specifically.

Placebo versus active comparator

True placebo arms with a sufficient long follow-up to assess structural damage are no longer accepted for ethical reasons. The closest to this assessment is the partial responder trial design in which patients who have still active disease are randomized to continue with the same treatment with placebo added or with the treatment under investigation added. Also in this situation, only short periods of follow-up are accepted to be ethical and patients have a possibility to opt for early escape at a fixed time of follow-up, usually between 12 and 16 weeks. Until now this was sufficient to pick up change in the control arm. There is, however, a trend that patients with less active and less severe disease are included in trials. Consequently, the progression in the control arm is smaller, which results in larger trials to maintain the same power. Alternative trial designs that are expected to come in practice in the near future are non-inferiority design trials. Here it is critical to set a realistic non-inferiority boundary to decide when the new treatment is non-inferior to the known, effective treatment.

Repair

Although most emphasis is on detection of progression of structural damage, over the past decades it became apparent that repair of damage is also possible. This could be observed in individual joints and patients but also in studies specifically designed to test the concept of repair, as well as on the group level in clinical trials. By definition, there is proof of repair on a group level if the mean change over time including the 95% confidence interval is below zero, indicating that there is a statistically significant improvement for the group. Determining definite repair in an individual joint or patient is more difficult. Based on data obtained in a trial, there is circumstantial evidence that repair is a real phenomenon because it is almost exclusively observed in joints without swelling, can be reproduced in independent read sessions, and is predominantly prevalent in patients treated with tumor necrosis factor blockers.

RHEUMATOID ARTHRITIS

Conventional radiography

Films of hands and feet

Structural damage, especially erosions, is frequently present in the joints of both hands and feet. Moreover, these are the sites that structural damage can easily be detected because of the size of the joints. Very importantly, these are the sites that show the first erosions, and this is even more frequent in the feet than in the hands. The wrist is the predilection joint for early JSN. Therefore, it is recommended to always take films of hands and feet. By doing so a large number of joints are available for evaluation. It is not necessary to take films of the large joints routinely for the assessment of the course of disease because it has been proven that damage in the joints of the small joints is representative of the damage in the large joints. Important in this respect is that patients with normal radiographs of hands and feet do not have structural damage in any of the large joints.[4]

For scoring it is sufficient to take films of the hands in the postero-anterior view and the feet in the anteroposterior view. It is of utmost importance to standardize the positioning and technical aspects to ensure comparable images at follow-up. Additional views for the hands such as the Nørgaard or Brewerton (ballcatcher's) views are not recommended because it is hard to standardize and get comparable images over time.

Scoring methods

Information from radiographs only can be used as an outcome in clinical trials if this is quantified. Several scoring methods that will be discussed later in this chapter are available for this purpose. The selection of the most appropriate scoring method is largely dependent on the setting in which it will be applied. For example, in clinical practice

and large cohort studies, feasibility is of major importance, while in clinical trials sensitivity to change is driving the selection of a method.

The methods that are used most frequently in recent research and clinical practice are described here. For a historical overview of all published scoring methods we refer to the literature.[5] Below, first the methods applying a global score and mainly based on the Larsen method are presented. This is followed by the presentation of the more detailed scoring methods. An overview of the various characteristics of the scoring methods, such as the joints and the features included, the range per joint, and the total score is summarized in Table 43.1.[6,7]

Because erosions and JSN are reflections of different disease processes, it is advantageous to score these features independently, which is done in the detailed scoring methods. This opens the possibility to assess a differential effect of specific treatment on bone versus cartilage.

Global assessment per joint

Larsen score

The Larsen score applies a grade from 0 to 5 to individual joints.[8] This is the only method that can be applied to both large and small joints, and a reference atlas with the grades for the various joints is available. The scoring is a combination of mainly erosions and JSN resulting in a global grade. The original Larsen scoring method includes soft tissue swelling and juxta-articular osteoporosis in grade 1. Only from grade 2 onward are there definite structural abnormalities such as erosions. Grade 5 represents mutilating abnormality. Several modifications of the scoring system by the authors have been published, with the most important modification being that for use in longitudinal studies. Most studies include only the joints of the hands, wrists, and feet. The information in Table 43.1 is based on the original method applied to hands, wrists, and feet. Originally, the wrist is evaluated as a single joint. In total, 32 joints are scored, and this leads to a scoring range for hands and feet from 0 to 160. The modification published by Larsen and associates in 1995 has modified both the sites to be evaluated as well as the grading. Most striking is the deletion of soft tissue swelling and osteoporosis for grade 1.[9] Now erosions less than 1 mm and slight JSN are graded as 1. The number of areas in both hands and feet has been changed. The interphalangeal (IP) and MCP joints of the thumb are no longer included, nor are the IP and MTP joints of the big toe. In this modification the wrist is scored in quadrants. Therefore, the number of joints assessed remains 32.

Scott modification of Larsen's method

The modification by Scott and coworkers is frequently used when the "Larsen" method is applied.[10] These researchers redefined the grading and applied it to the same 32 joints as in the original Larsen method. Moreover, the wrist is scored as a single joint but is weighted by a factor of 5 to obtain the total score. This brings the range for hands and feet from 0 to 200.

Ratingen score

In this modification of the Larsen score, the grading is entirely based on the surface area of the joints destructed by erosions.[11] This is graded from 0 to 5 (grade 1, < 20%; grade 2, 21%-40%; up to grade 5, > 80% destroyed). In total, 38 joints of the hands are scored, resulting in a range of 0 to 190.

Detailed scoring methods

Sharp's method

This is the first published method describing a detailed scoring system for erosions and JSN separately for joints in the hands and wrists. The Sharp method that is used at present is in fact the modification described in 1985.[12] This reduced the number of joints scored from originally 27 for both erosions and JSN to 17 areas for erosions and 18 for JSN per hand.

Moreover, the method was developed and validated for scoring the joints of the hands, but nowadays the same methodology is also applied to the joints of the feet. Erosions are scored from 0 to 5 per joint and are counted when discrete, and surface erosions are scored according to the surface area involved. JSN is scored on a 0-4 scale, representing focal narrowing (score 1), joint space loss of less than 50% (score 2), joint space loss of more than 50% (score 3), and complete

TABLE 43.1 COMPARISON OF RADIOGRAPHIC SCORING METHODS FOR RHEUMATOID ARTHRITIS

	Larsen method	Scott modification of Larsen method	Ratingen method	Sharp method	Genant modification of Sharp method	van der Heijde modification of Sharp method	Simple Erosion Narrowing Score (SENS)
Films							
Hands	X	X	X	X	X	X	X
Feet	X	X	–	–	X	X	X
Large joints	X*	–	–	–	–	–	–
Joints included							
PIP/IP	X	X	X	X	X	X	X
MCP	X	X	X	X	X	X	X
Wrist	X	X	X	X	X	X	X
MTP	X	X	–	–	X	X	X
IP1	X	X	–	–	X	X	X
Features scored							
Erosions	–	–	X	X	X	X	X
JSN	–	–	–	X	X	X	X
Malalignment	–	–	–	–	–	X	X
Global	X	X	–	–	–	–	–
No. of joints per hand/foot scored for							
Erosions	–	–	19	17	14	22	22
JSN	–	–	–	18	13	21	21
Malalignment	–	–	–	–	–	†	†
Global	16	16	–	–	–	–	–
Range per joint							
Erosions	–	–	0-5	0-5	0-3.5‡	0-5/0-10§	0-1
JSN	–	–	–	0-4	0-4‡	0-4	0-1
Malalignment	–	–	–	–	–	†	†
Global	0-5	0-5	–	–	–	–	–
Total	0-160	0-200	0-190	0-314	0-292	0-448	0-86

JSN, joint space narrowing.
*Large joints are assessed separately; remaining information in this table based on hands and feet.
†Combined with the JSN score
‡Scored per 0.5.
§Erosions for hands 0-5, for feet 0-10.
Reproduced with permission from van der Heijde D. Quantification of radiological damage in inflammatory arthritis: rheumatoid arthritis, psoriatic arthritis and ankylosing spondylitis. Best Pract Res Clin Rheumatol 2004;18:847-860.

joint space loss or ankylosis (score 4). Subluxation or luxation is not included in the score. The erosion score and the JSN score can be used separately but is usually summed to get the total score (range for hands: 0 to 314).

Genant's modification of Sharp's method

A modification of the Sharp method is described by Genant, which extended the scale for progression from a 6-point scale to an 8-point scale with 0.5 increments from 0 to 3+ for erosions and from a 5-point scale to a 9-point scale with 0.5 increments from 0 to 4 for JSN.[13] This score is applied in 14 joints of each hand and wrist for erosions and in 13 joints for JSN. This results in a total score range from 0 to 202 for the hands. Frequently, this is normalized to a 200-point scale. If the feet are scored, this is applied to the 5 metatarsophalangeal (MTP) joints and the IP joint of the first toe. The maximum of the score of hands and feet is 292, frequently normalized to 290.

van der Heijde's modification of Sharp's method

The main modification by van der Heijde was the addition of 6 joints per foot (5 MTP joints and the IP joint of the first toe) to the scoring system. Moreover, 2 sites for erosions and 2 sites for JSN were deleted from the scoring areas as compared with Sharp's method as described

in 1985, leaving 16 sites for erosions and 15 for JSN per hand.[14] The scoring of erosions in the hands remained the same, with a range of 0 to 5 per joint. However, for the scoring of erosions in the feet the scoring range was expanded to 10 per joint, with a maximum of 5 for the metatarsal and phalangeal sites of the joint. Another major difference is that subluxation and luxation (malalignment) are integrated in the grading of JSN. JSN is scored on a 0 to 4 scale, with the same grading as described for the Sharp method, but in this modification a score of 3 can also be applied in case of subluxation of a joint, with a score of 4 in case of complete luxation. These features are mostly scored in MCPs and MTPs. The scoring range for the total score is 0 to 448. An example of scoring the MCP joints is presented in Figure 43.3.

Figure 43.4 shows a comparison of the sites in the hands included in Sharp's method, van der Heijde's modification of Sharp's method, and Genant's modification of Sharp's method. The major differences are in the sites in the wrist, both for erosions and for JSN. Table 43.2 shows the weighting of the erosions and JSN scores in the three scoring methods. The Genant scores apply a normalization, and thereafter the weight for erosions and JSN are equal. The van der Heijde modification has the largest weight on erosions, whereas for the Sharp method this is in between.

Simple Erosion Narrowing Score (SENS)

This method is based on the joints included in the van der Heijde modification of Sharp's method for hands and feet. Instead of scoring the joints for erosions and JSN, this is a simple counting of the number of eroded joints and the number of narrowed joints.[15] A score of 1 is applied if a site is eroded and also per narrowed site. In total, 15 joints per hand are scored for erosions and 16 for JSN and 6 joints per foot for both erosions and JSN, leading to a scoring range from 0 to 86.

MRI and ultrasonography

Conventional radiography, although the most widely used imaging method to assess structural damage in RA, has limitations. It does not visualize the earliest stages of bone erosion. In contrast, MRI and ultrasonography allow direct visualization of early destructive joint changes in RA. For ultrasonography there are no widely accepted scoring methods available for use in clinical trials, although validation of several methods is underway. For MRI, the RAMRIS (RA MRI scoring system) is the validated scoring method of choice. It is a semi-quantitative assessment of synovitis, bone erosions, and bone edema in hands and wrists.[16] A minimum set of MRI sequences (Table 43.3) as well as consensus MRI definition of important joint pathologic processes (Table 43.4) were also suggested. There is an atlas available with reference images for scoring. The main features of the RAMRIS are presented in Table 43.5.

MRI sum-scores

Sum-scores of synovitis, erosion, and edema, respectively, can be calculated by summation of individual joint scores, as a total sum or separately in the evaluated wrist and second to fifth MCP joints. For synovitis, the possible range of sum scores of unilateral second to fifth MCP joints, wrist joint, and both are 0-12, 0-9, and 0-21, respectively. Corresponding values for bone erosion are 0-80, 0-150, and 0-230, whereas for bone edema they are 0-24, 0-45, and 0-69.

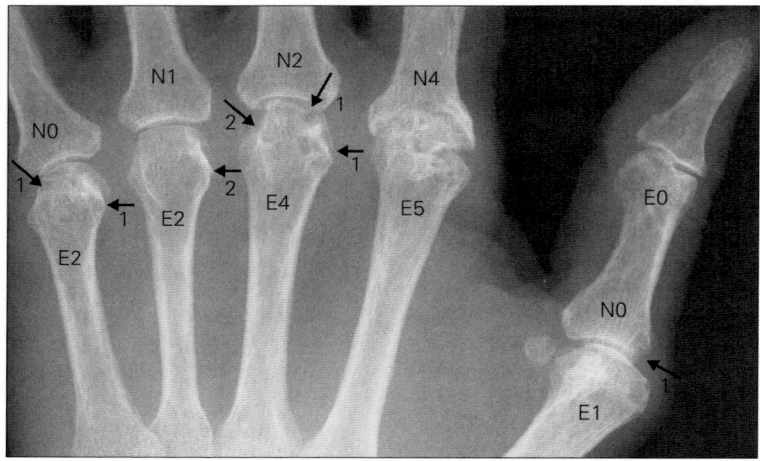

Fig. 43.3 Scores according the van der Heijde's modification of Sharp's method of the metacarpophalangeal and interproximal phalangeal joints of the left hand. The arrows indicate the location of an erosion; the number indicates the score of the erosion. The sum of the erosions per joint is depicted as "E." The score for the joint space narrowing per joint is presented as "N." The interproximal joint is not scored for joint space narrowing.

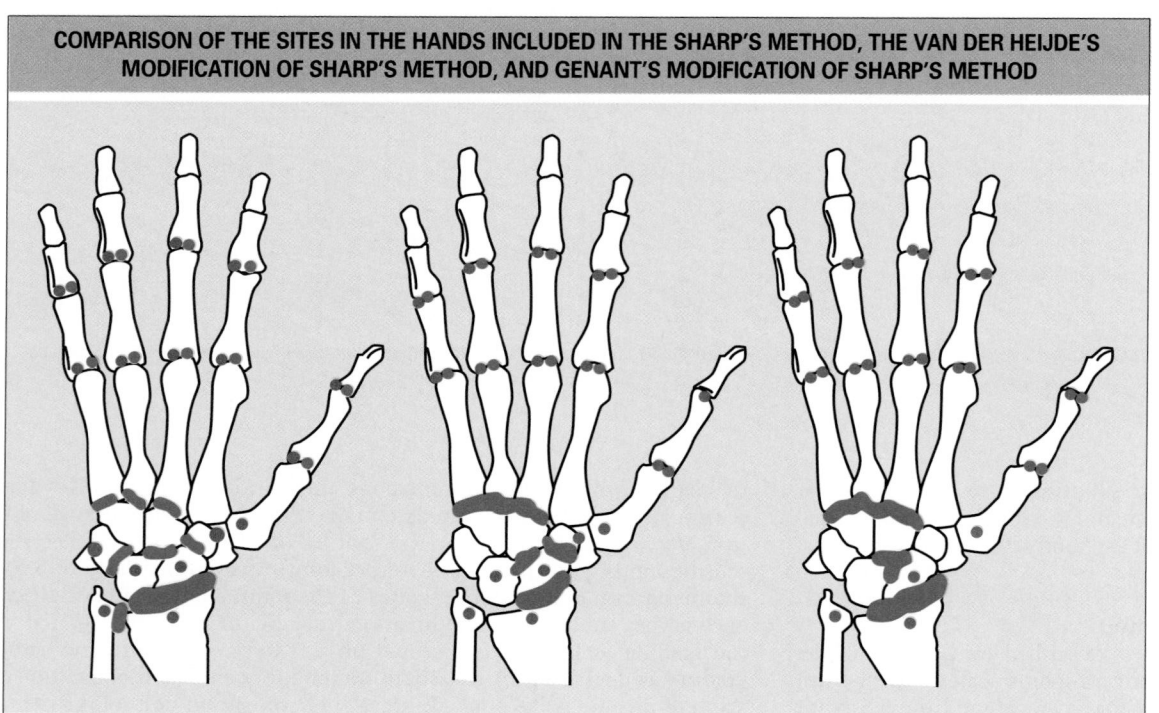

COMPARISON OF THE SITES IN THE HANDS INCLUDED IN THE SHARP'S METHOD, THE VAN DER HEIJDE'S MODIFICATION OF SHARP'S METHOD, AND GENANT'S MODIFICATION OF SHARP'S METHOD

Fig. 43.4 Comparison of the sites in the hands included in the Sharp's method, van der Heijde's modification of Sharp's method, and Genant's modification of Sharp's method.

TABLE 43.2 COMPARISON OF THE WEIGHT OF EROSIONS AND JOINT SPACE NARROWING (JSN) IN THE SHARP, VAN DER HEIJDE'S MODIFICATION OF SHARP'S METHOD, AND GENANT'S MODIFICATION OF SHARP'S METHOD

	Hands erosions	Hands JSN	Hands total score	Hands and feet erosions	Hands and feet JSN	Hands and feet total score
Sharp's method	170	144	314	230	192	422
van der Heijde's modification	160	120	280	280	168	448
Genant's modification	98→100*	104→100	200	140→145	152→145	290

*The scores indicated by → are normalized into the indicated number.

TABLE 43.3 MINIMUM SET OF BASIC MRI SEQUENCES

- Imaging in two planes* with T1-weighted images before and after intravenous administration of gadolinium[†]
- A T2-weighted fat-saturated sequence or, if this is not available, a short tau inversion recovery (STIR) sequence.

*Imaging in two planes can be acquired by obtaining a 2D sequence in two planes or a 3D sequence with isometrical voxels in one plane allowing reconstruction in other planes.
[†]Intravenous injection of gadolinium is probably not essential if destructive changes alone (bone erosions) are considered important.
Reproduced with permission from Østergaard M, Peterfy C, Conaghan P, et al. OMERACT Rheumatoid Arthritis Magnetic Resonance Imaging Studies: Core set of MRI acquisitions, joint pathology definitions, and the OMERACT RA-MRI scoring system. J Rheumatol 2003:6:1385-1386.

TABLE 43.4 DEFINITIONS OF IMPORTANT RHEUMATOID ARTHRITIS JOINT PATHOLOGIC PROCESSES ON MRI

Synovitis: An area in the synovial compartment that shows above-normal post-gadolinium enhancement of a thickness greater than the width of the normal synovium.
- Enhancement (signal intensity increase) is judged by comparison of T1-weighted images obtained before and after intravenous administration of gadolinium.

MRI bone erosion: A sharply marginated bone lesion, with correct juxta-articular localization and typical signal characteristics, which is visible in two planes with a cortical break seen in at least one plane.
- On T1-weighted images there is loss of normal low signal intensity of cortical bone and loss of normal high signal intensity of trabecular bone. Quick post-gadolinium enhancement suggests the presence of active, hypervascularized pannus tissue in the erosion.
- Other focal bone lesions, including metastases, must obviously be considered but are generally distinguishable with associated imaging and clinical findings.

MRI bone edema: A lesion within the trabecular bone, with ill-defined margins and signal characteristics consistent with increased water content.
- This may occur alone or surrounding an erosion or other bone abnormalities.
- There is high signal intensity on T2-weighted fat-saturated and STIR images and low signal intensity on T1-weighted images.

Reproduced with permission from Østergaard M, Peterfy C, Conaghan P, et al. OMERACT Rheumatoid Arthritis Magnetic Resonance Imaging Studies: Core set of MRI acquisitions, joint pathology definitions, and the OMERACT RA-MRI scoring system. J Rheumatol 2003:6:1385-1386.

TABLE 43.5 RAMRIS SCORING SYSTEM

- *Bone erosions:* Each bone (wrists: carpal bones, distal radius, distal ulna, metacarpal bases; MCP joints: metacarpal heads, phalangeal bases) is scored separately. The scale is 0-10, based on the proportion of eroded bone compared with the "assessed bone volume," judged on all available images: 0 = no erosion; 1 = 1-10% of bone eroded, 2 = 11-20% etc. For long bones, the "assessed bone volume" is from the articular surface (or its best estimated position if absent) to a depth of 1 cm, whereas in carpal bones it is the whole bone.
- *Bone edema:* Each bone is scored separately (as for erosions). The scale is 0-3 based on the proportion of bone with edema, as follows: 0 = no edema; 1 = 1-33% of bone edematous; 2 = 34-66%; 3 = 67-100%.
- *Synovitis:* Synovitis is assessed in three wrist regions: (1) the distal radioulnar joint; (2) the radiocarpal joint; (3) the intercarpal and carpometacarpal phalangeal joints) and in each MCP joint. The first carpometacarpal phalangeal joint and the first MCP joint are not scored. The scale is 0-3. Score 0 is normal, whereas 1-3 (mild, moderate, severe) is by thirds of the presumed maximum volume of enhancing tissue in the synovial compartment.

Reproduced with permission from Østergaard M, Peterfy C, Conaghan P, et al. OMERACT Rheumatoid Arthritis Magnetic Resonance Imaging Studies: Core set of MRI acquisitions, joint pathology definitions, and the OMERACT RA-MRI scoring system. J Rheumatol 2003:6:1385-1386.

ratio of nearly 2 : 1. Erosive changes and bone proliferation in the feet usually involve the IP and MTP joints: the IP joint of the first toe is most often affected. Radiographs of the hand are most important in the follow-up of patients, but the addition of films of the feet makes the picture more complete.

Scoring methods
Development and validation of scoring methods for PsA are less well worked out than for RA. All the presently used methods find their basis in scoring methods for RA. There are two global scoring methods and two detailed scoring methods, which are summarized in Table 43.6, and will be described below.

Global assessment per joint
Modified Steinbrocker score
This method has been developed at the PsA clinic at the University of Toronto.[17,18] Each joint is scored on a 0 to 4 scale: 0 = normal, 1 = juxta-articular osteopenia or soft tissue swelling, 2 = erosion, 3 = erosion and JSN, and 4 = total joint destruction, either lysis or ankylosis. This score is applied in 14 joints in each hand and 6 joints in each foot. The range of the score is from 0 to 160.

Psoriatic Arthritis Ratingen Score (PARS)
This method includes 40 joints of the hands and feet.[18,19] All joints are scored separately for destruction and proliferation. The destruction score is based on the amount of joint surface destruction on a 0–5 scale: 0 = normal, 1 = one or more definite erosions with an interruption of the cortical plate of more than 1 mm but destruction of less than 10% of the total joint surface, 2 = destruction of 11% to 25%, 3 = destruction of 26% to 50%, 4 = destruction of 51% to 75%, and 5 = destruction of more than 75% of joint surface. The proliferation score considers any kind of bony proliferation typical for PsA on a 0-4 scale: 0 = normal, 1 = bony proliferation measured from the original bone surface of 1 to 2 mm or, if the margins of the proliferation cannot be distinguished from the original bone surface, clearly identifiable bone growth not exceeding 25% of the original diameter of the bone, 2 = bony proliferation of 2 to 3 mm or bone growth between 25-50%, 3 = bony proliferation more than 3 mm or bone growth more than 50%, and 4 = bony ankylosis. The destruction score with a range from 0 to 200 and the proliferation score with a range from 0 to 160 are summed to give the total score (range: 0–360).

Detailed scoring methods
PsA scoring method based on Sharp scoring method for RA
The erosion scale used in RA has a range of 5 per joint. Scores are applied as 0 = no erosion, 1 = one discrete erosion or involvement of

PSORIATIC ARTHRITIS
Conventional radiography
Typical lesions and site of lesions
Although there are similarities with RA there are also major differences in the type and site of lesions as well as the joints involved. Whereas RA is characterized by mainly osteodestructive lesions, in PsA there are both osteodestructive and osteoproliferative manifestations that may even co-exist not only in the same patient but even in the same joint. Characteristic radiographic features of PsA include joint erosions, JSN, and bony proliferation, including periarticular and shaft periostitis, osteolysis, ankylosis, spur formation, and spondylitis. Abnormalities are seen in the phalangeal tufts and at the sites of attachments of tendons and ligaments of the bone. Although erosive changes in early PsA are marginal as in RA, they become irregular and ill defined with disease progression because of periosteal bone formation adjacent to the erosions. In severe cases, erosive changes may progress to development of "pencil-in-cup" deformity or gross osteolysis. These features are typical of arthritis mutilans.

Joint involvement in PsA is often asymmetric and may be oligoarticular. Asymmetric erosions may be visible radiographically in the carpus and in the MCP and proximal (PIP) and distal IP (DIP) joints of the hands, but the DIP joints are often the first to be affected. The hands tend to be involved much more frequently than the feet, with a

TABLE 43.6 COMPARISON OF RADIOGRAPHIC SCORING METHODS FOR PSORIATIC ARTHRITIS

	Modified Steinbrocker's method	Ratingen's method	Sharp's method	van der Heijde's modification of Sharp method
Films				
Hands	X	X	X	X
Feet	–	X	X	X
Large joints	–	–	–	–
Joints included				
DIP	X	X	X	X
PIP/IP	X	X	X	X
MCP	X	X	X	X
Wrist	X	X	X	X
MTP	–	X	X	X
IP1	–	X	X	X
Features scored				
Erosions	–	X	X	X
JSN	–	–	X	X
Malalignment	–	–	–	X
Proliferation	–	X	–	–
Global	X	–	–	–
No. of joints per hand/foot scored for				
Erosions	–	40	27	26
JSN	–	–	25	26
Malaignment	–	–	–	*
Proliferation	20	40	–	–
Global	–	–	–	–
Range				
Per joint for erosions	–	0-5	0-5	0-5/0-10[†]
Per joint JSN	–	–	0-4	0-4
Per joint malalignment	–	–	–	*
Per joint proliferation	–	0-4	–	–
Per joint global	0-4	–	–	–
Total	0-160	0-360	0-470	0-528

JSN, joint space narrowing.
*Combined with the JSN score.
[†]Erosions for hands 0-5, for feet 0-10.
Reproduced with permission from van der Heijde D. Quantification of radiological damage in inflammatory arthritis: rheumatoid arthritis, psoriatic arthritis and ankylosing spondylitis. Best Pract Res Clin Rheumatol 2004;18:847-860.

less than 21% of the joint area by erosion, 2 = two discrete erosions or involvement of 21% to 40% of the joint, 3 = three discrete erosions or involvement of 41% to 60% of the joint, 4 = four discrete erosions or involvement of 61% to 80% of the joint, and 5 = extensive destruction involving more than 80%.[18,20] The erosion scale was expanded with the scores of 6 and 7 to accommodate more extensive bone destruction seen in many cases of PsA, such as gross osteolysis or a "pencil-in-cup" lesion. However, the scores of 6 and 7 are not added to get the total erosion score but these features are kept separately. The erosion score is applied in 21 joints in each hand and in 6 joints in each foot, resulting in a range of 0 to 210 for hands and 60 for feet. The scoring of JSN is on a scale of 0 to 4 as is used for RA. The JSN scores are 0 = normal joint, 1 = asymmetric and or minimal narrowing, 2 = definite narrowing with loss of up to 50% of the normal space, 3 = definite narrowing with loss of 51% to 99% of the normal space, and 4 = absence of a joint space, presumptive evidence of ankylosis. A score of 5 is added in case of widening, which is automatically scored when gross osteolysis is present. Again the score for widening is not included in the total narrowing score but analyzed as a separate feature. The JSN score is applied to 20 joints in each hand and 5 joints in each foot, leading to a range of 160 for hands and 40 for feet.

Sharp-van der Heijde modified scoring method for PsA

A similar scoring system as used in RA is applied to PsA.[18] The same joints are scored for erosions and JSN, with the addition of the eight DIPs for erosions and the eight DIPs and two IPs of the thumb for JSN. Again, the maximum score for erosions is 5 in the joints of the hands and 10 in the joints of the feet. Scores for erosions are applied as follows: 0 = no erosions, 1 = discrete erosion, 2 = large erosion not passing the middle line, and 3 = large erosion passing the middle line; a combination of the above scores may lead to the maximum of 5 per entire joint in the hands and 5 at each site of the joint (for the entire joint a maximum of 10) in the feet. The so-called JSN score is based on the following features: 0 = normal, 1 = asymmetric or minimal narrowing up to a maximum of 25%, 2 = definite narrowing with loss of up to 50% of the normal space, 3 = definite narrowing with loss of 50 to 99% of the normal space or subluxation, and 4 = absence of a joint space, presumptive evidence of ankylosis or complete luxation. Gross osteolysis and "pencil-in-cup" lesions are scored separately. In the final summary score, joints with one of these abnormalities get the maximum score assigned for both erosions and for JSN. The total range for erosions is 200 for the hands and 120 for the feet; the total range for JSN is 160 for the hands and 48 for the feet. Total erosion score is 360, total JSN score is 168, and total score is 528.

MRI and ultrasonography

Both MRI and ultrasonography have not been widely applied in PsA, although similar advantages as described for RA and AS can be expected. No generally accepted or validated methods for assessment of PsA activity or damage exist. Recently an OMERACT PsA scoring system (PsAMRIS) has been developed for use in PsA hands, including discussions on appropriate MRI sequences and consensus definitions of important pathologic processes. The scoring system needs further testing and validation in longitudinal studies.

ANKYLOSING SPONDYLITIS

Conventional radiography

Scoring methods

Three methods have specifically been designed for the assessment of structural damage in AS. An overview of the various characteristics of the scoring methods is summarized in Table 43.7. All methods are suitable to assess damage in the spine. In addition, scoring methods for the sacroiliac joints exist, as well as one specific method for assessment of the hips in AS.

Global assessment of the spine

Bath Ankylosing Spondylitis Radiological Index (BASRI)

The BASRI-spine has three components: the lumbar, the cervical spine, and the sacroiliac joints.[21] To assess the lumbar spine, a lateral and anteroposterior view are used. The score for the lumbar spine, from the lower border of T12 to the upper border of S1, is a composite score of both views, taking all the affected levels into account in the score. The cervical spine was defined as extending from the lower border of C1 to the upper border of C7. A global score ranging from 0 to 4 (normal, suspicious, mild, moderate, and severe) is applied to both the lumbar and cervical component. The grades are summarized in Table 43.8. Squaring, sclerosis, erosions, syndesmophytes, and fusion are the features that are included. Syndesmophytes and fusion are the most important parts driving the scoring method. The sacroiliac joints are scored according to the four grades of the modified New York criteria. The BASRI-spine is the sum of the mean score of the right and left sacroiliac joint (in one decimal) plus the score of the lumbar spine plus the score of the cervical spine. The range for the BASRI-spine is 2 to 12 (because patients with AS have sacroiliitis by definition, the minimum is 2). A similar grading system has been developed for the hips: BASRI-hip. The sum of the BASRI-spine and BASRI-hip is called the BASRI-total, with a range from 2 to 16.

Detailed assessment of the spine

Stoke Ankylosing Spondylitis Spine Score (SASSS)

The SASSS is a detailed scoring system for the anterior and posterior site of the lumbar spine and includes the lower border of the 12th thoracic vertebra, all five lumbar vertebrae, and the upper border of the sacrum on a lateral view.[22] All four corners of each vertebra are examined and scored 1 if one or more of the following features is present: erosion, sclerosis, or squaring; scored 2 for a syndesmophyte; and scored 3 for total bony bridging, giving a maximum possible score of 72.

Modified Stoke Ankylosing Spondylitis Spine Score

This method is a modification of the SASSS, and scores the anterior site of the lumbar and cervical spine at a lateral view.[23] The anterior site of the same vertebrae of the lumbar spine as described for the SASSS is scored, and the anterior site of the cervical spine from the lower border of the second cervical vertebra up to the upper border of the first thoracic vertebra is scored. The scoring of features is identical to that for the SASSS. The range is also 0 to 72. The modified SASSS

TABLE 43.7 COMPARISON OF RADIOGRAPHIC SCORING METHODS FOR ANKYLOSING SPONDYLITIS

	BASRI	SASSS	Modified SASSS
Films			
Anteroposterior pelvis	X	–	–
Lateral cervical spine	X	–	X
Lateral lumbar spine	X	X	X
Anteroposterior lumbar spine	X	–	–
Joints/vertebrae included			
Sacroiliac	X	–	–
Hip	X	–	–
Cervical spine	X	–	X
Lumbar spine	X	X	X
Features scored			
Erosions	–	X*	X*
Squaring	–	X*	X*
Sclerosis	–	X*	X*
Syndesmophyte	–	X	X
Global	X	–	–
No. of sites per film scored for:			
Erosions	–	6*†	12*‡
Squaring	–	6*	12*
Sclerosis	–	6*	12*
Syndesmophyte	–	6	12
Global	3-4§	–	–
Range			
Per vertebra for erosions	–	0-1	0-1
Per vertebra squaring	–	0-1	0-1
Per vertebra for sclerosis	–	0-1	0-1
Per vertebra syndesmophyte	–	2-3	2-3
Per joint/vertebra global	0-4	–	–
Total	2-12/16‖	0-72	0-72

BASRI, Bath Ankylosing Spondylitis Radiological Index; SASSS, Stoke Ankylosing Spondylitis Spine Score.
*The maximum score per corner is 1, either erosion or sclerosis or squaring can be scored.
†Four corners of six vertebrae are scored.
‡The two anterior corners of 12 vertebrae are scored.
§Without the hips three sites (cervical, lumbar spine, and sacroiliac joints) are scored; including the hips, four sites are scored.
‖Without the hips the range is up to 12; including the hips the range is up to 16.
Reproduced with permission from van der Heijde D. Quantification of radiological damage in inflammatory arthritis: rheumatoid arthritis, psoriatic arthritis and ankylosing spondylitis. Best Pract Res Clin Rheumatol 2004;18:847-860.

TABLE 43.8 BASRI GRADING FOR THE SPINE OF ANKYLOSING SPONDYLITIS PATIENTS*

Score	Grade	Description
0	Normal	No change
1	Suspicious	No definitive change
2	Mild	Any number of erosions, squaring, or sclerosis with or without syndesmophytes ≤ 2 vertebrae
3	Moderate	Syndesmophytes on ≥ 3 vertebrae, with or without fusion involving 2 vertebrae
4	Severe	Fusing involving ≥ 3 vertebrae

*The scores are applied to the lateral cervical spine and to the lateral and anteroposterior lumbar spine combined. The scores for the sacroiliac joints are added to obtain the BASRI-total (range 2-12).

has been selected as the preferred method to assess structural damage in the spine by ASAS and OMERACT based on favorable reproducibility and sensitivity to change in comparison to the BASRI and SASSS.[24,25] An example of scoring the cervical spine is presented in Figure 43.5.

MRI and ultrasonography

MRI is a very important imaging modality in AS, through its ability to visualize inflammatory changes in bone and soft tissues. It is the most sensitive imaging modality for imaging spine and sacroiliac joint changes. AS may also involve peripheral arthritis and enthesitis, which can also be visualized by MRI. Typical AS lesions of the spine, which can be visualized by MRI, are spondylitis, spondylodiscitis, and

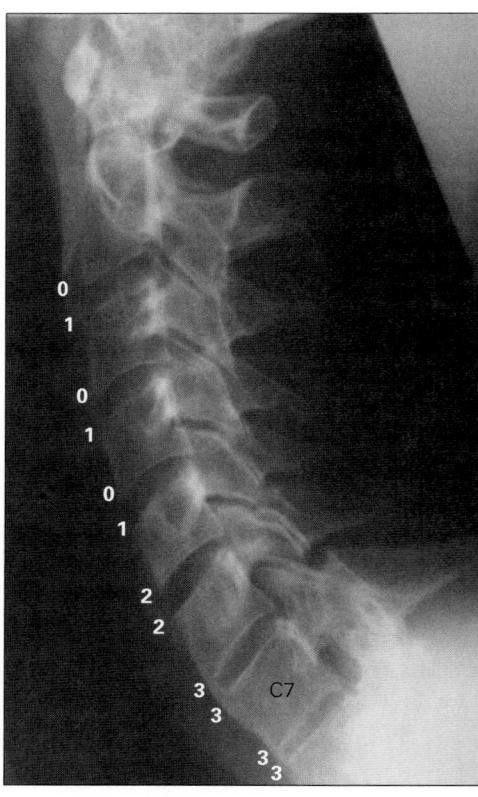

Fig. 43.5 Scores according to the modified Stoke Ankylosing Spondylitis Spine Score of the cervical spine. The numbers are related to each corner at the anterior site of each vertebral body starting at the lower border of cervical 2 to the upper border of thoracic 1. The vertebral body of cervical 7 is indicated by C7.

arthritis of the apophyseal joints, the costovertebral and costotransverse joints. Findings indicating active disease in the sacroiliac joints (sacroiliitis) include juxta-articular bone marrow edema, capsulitis, enhancement of the joint space after contrast medium administration, whereas visible chronic changes include bone erosions, sclerosis, periarticular fatty tissue accumulation, transarticular bone bridges, and ankylosis. Enthesitis is also common and may affect the interspinal and supraspinal ligaments of the vertebral spine and the interosseous ligaments in the retroarticular space of the sacroiliac joints.

The majority of MRI studies of the sacroiliac joint have used only one imaging plane (semi-coronal, i.e., parallel with the axis of the sacral bone). To be maximally sensitive for changes in the ligamentous portion of the sacroiliac joints, imaging in two perpendicular planes is required. This is particularly important when MRI is used for diagnostic purposes while probably less so when used as an outcome measure in trials. Similarly, the majority of MRI studies of the AS spine involves only sagittal images, which are not optimal for visualizing changes in the apophyseal and costovertebral joints. The importance of such changes remains to be determined.

There is general agreement that adequate MRI of the spine in AS, as of the sacroiliac joint, must at least include a T1-weighted sequence without fat saturation and a short tau inversion recovery (STIR) sequence in one plane. To which extent further sequences, including postcontrast sequences and/or more planes, are needed is debated and depends on the goal of the examination.

Ultrasonography is not used as an outcome in clinical trials in AS.

Scoring methods

Several scoring systems for assessment of disease activity in the sacroiliac joints and in the spine have been proposed. These have been tested against each other by the OMERACT-ASAS MRI in AS group. These will be described next, followed by a description of the few available systems for assessment of chronic damage.

Activity—spine

Three different scoring systems have been developed and validated: The Ankylosing Spondylitis spine Magnetic Resonance Imaging–activity (ASspiMRI-a) score, grading activity from 0 to 6 per vertebral unit in 23 units[26]; the Berlin modification of the ASspiMRI-a score, grading activity 0 to 3 per vertebral unit in the same 23 units[27]; and the Spondyloarthritis Research Consortium of Canada (SPARCC) scoring system, scoring only the 6 vertebral units considered by the reader as the most abnormal, with additional points for "depth" and high "intensity" of the lesion (Table 43.9).[28] In an OMERACT-ASAS multi-reader exercise, the feasibility, reliability, sensitivity to change, and discriminatory capacity of all three scoring systems in patients with AS were demonstrated. The SPARCC method had the highest sensitivity to change, as judged by Guyatt's effect size, and the highest reliability as judged by the inter-reader intraclass correlation coefficient (ICC), but not if judged by the smallest detectable change.[29] All of the

	Activity			Damage
	SPARCC[28]	ASspiMRI-a[26]	Berlin[27]	ASspiMRI-c[35]
Images	Sag STIR	Sag post-Gd T1W FS + sag STIR	Sag post-Gd T1W FS + sag STIR	Sag T1W
Area	6 most affected DVUs	All 23 DVUs	All 23 DVUs	All 23 DVUs
Features	Bone marrow edema	Bone marrow edema/enhancement and bone erosion	Bone marrow edema/enhancement	Sclerosis, squaring, syndesmophytes, and bridging/fusion
Grades	0-1 per DVU quadrant + 1 for depth ≥ 1 cm and 1 for high intensity of lesion	0-6 per DVU	0-3 per DVU	0-6 per DVU
Total score range	0-108	0-138	0-69	0-138

TABLE 43.9 MRI SCORING METHODS FOR ASSESSMENT OF THE SPINE IN ANKYLOSING SPONDYLITIS

SPARCC, Spondyloarthritis Research Consortium of Canada; ASspiMRI-a, Ankylosing Spondylitis spine Magnetic Resonance Imaging–activity; ASspiMRI-c, Ankylosing Spondylitis spine Magnetic Resonance Imaging–chronicity. DVU, discovertebral unit defined as the region between two virtual lines through the middle of each vertebra and includes the intervertebral disc and the adjacent vertebral end plates; FS, fat saturated; Gd, intravenous injection of gadolinium-containing contrast agent; sag, sagittal; STIR, short tau inversion recovery; T1W, T1 weighted.

TABLE 43.10 MRI SCORING METHODS FOR ASSESSMENT OF THE SACROILIAC JOINTS IN ANKYLOSING SPONDYLITIS

	Activity			Damage	
	SPARCC[31]	*Puhakka–activity*[33]	*Hermann–activity*[32]	*Puhakka–damage*[33]	*Hermann–damage*[32]
Images	Semicoronal STIR	Pre- and post Gd semicoronal and semiaxial T1W FS; semicoronal STIR	Semicoronal pre- and post-Gd T1W FS, and STIR	Pre-Gd semicoronal and semiaxial T1W and T1W FS	Semicoronal pre- and post-Gd T1W and T1W FS
Area	SI joints, 6 consecutive semicoronal slices	SI joints, in 2 planes	SI joints, in semicoronal plane	SI joints, in 2 planes	SI joints, in semicoronal plane
Features	Bone marrow edema	Bone marrow edema, bone marrow enhancement, joint space enhancement	Bone marrow edema, bone marrow enhancement	Erosion, sclerosis, joint space width	Erosion, sclerosis, joint space width, bone bridging/ankylosis
Grades	In each slice: 0-1 per quadrant + 1 for depth ≥ 1 cm and 1 for high intensity	Marrow edema 0-3 per quadrant; marrow enhancement: 0-3 per quadrant; joint space enhancement: 0-3 per joint	Global: 0-3 per quadrant	Erosion: 0-3 per quadrant, sclerosis: 0-3 per quadrant; joint space: 0-3 per joint	Global: 0-4 per joint
Total score range	0-108	0-60	0-24	0-60	0-8

SPARCC, Spondyloarthritis Research Consortium of Canada; FS, fat saturated; Gd, intravenous injection of gadolinium-containing contrast agent; sag, sagittal; SI, sacroiliac; STIR, short tau inversion recovery; T1W, T1 weighted.

methods perform well, and none of them was selected as a preferred method.[30]

Activity—sacroiliac joints

Three main scoring approaches have been proposed, based on either global scores per quadrant or individual scores in consecutive semi-coronal images through the joint (Table 43.10). The presence and extent of bone marrow edema in the cartilaginous portion of the joint is the primary MRI feature that is scored, although one method also scores inflammation in the joint space and the ligamentous portion of the joint.[31-33] In an OMERACT-ASAS multi-reader exercise, agreement between readers and sensitivity to change were compared and found somewhat better for the most detailed scoring method (the SPARCC-method).[34]

Damage—spine and sacroiliac joints

The only method proposed for scoring the AS spine is the Ankylosing Spondylitis spine Magnetic Resonance Imaging–chronicity (ASspiMRI-c) score, grading chronic changes (sclerosis, squaring, syndesmophytes, and fusion) from 0 to 6 per vertebral unit in 23 units (see Table 43.9).[35]

Two scoring methods to assess chronic changes in the sacroiliac joints are described but not widely used. The first scores bone erosions and sclerosis at four osseous positions per joint (the iliac and sacral sides of the cartilaginous and ligamentous portions of the joints, respectively), as well as joint space width.[31,32] The second method scores each sacroiliac joint from 0 to 4 based on a global assessment of erosion, sclerosis, joint space width, and bone bridging/ankylosis (see Table 43.10). The validation of the methods for damage assessment is limited, and their value is not yet clarified.

REFERENCES

1. Bland JM, Altman DG. Statistical methods for assessing agreement between two methods of clinical measurement. Lancet 1986;8476:307-310.
2. Bruynesteyn K, Boers M, Kostense P, et al. Deciding on progression of joint damage in paired films of individual patients: smallest detectable difference or change. Ann Rheum Dis 2005;64:179-182.
3. Landewé R, van der Heijde D. Radiographic progression depicted by probability plots: presenting data with optimal use of individual values. Arthritis Rheum 2004;50:699-706.
4. Drossaers-Bakker KW, Kroon HM, Zwinderman AH, et al. Radiographic damage of large joints in long-term rheumatoid arthritis and its relation to function. Rheumatology 2000;39:998-1003.
5. van der Heijde D. Plain x-rays in rheumatoid arthritis: overview of scoring methods, their reliability and applicability. Bailliere Clin Rheum 1996;10: 435-453.
6. van der Heijde D. Quantification of radiological damage in inflammatory arthritis: rheumatoid arthritis, psoriatic arthritis and ankylosing spondylitis. Best Pract Res Clin Rheumatol 2004;18:847-860.
7. van der Heijde D, Østergaard M. In Bijlsma JWJ, Burmester GR, daSilva JA, Faarvang KL, Hachulla E, Mariette X, eds. EULAR Compendium on Rheumatic Diseases. BMJ Publishing Group and European League Against Rheumatism, 2009:182-201.
8. Larsen A, Dale K, Eek M. Radiographic evaluation of rheumatoid arthritis and related conditions by standard reference films. Acta Radiol Diagn Stockh 1977;18:481-491.
9. Larsen A: How to apply Larsen score in evaluating radiographs of rheumatoid arthritis in long-term studies. J Rheumatol 1995;22:1974-1975.
10. Scott DL, Coulton BL, Popert AJ. Long-term progression of joint damage in rheumatoid arthritis. Ann Rheum Dis 1986;45:373-378.
11. Rau R, Wassenberg S, Herborn G, et al. A new method of scoring radiographic change in rheumatoid arthritis. J Rheumatol 1998;25:2094-2107.
12. Sharp JT, Bluhm GB, Brook A, et al. Reproducibility of multiple-observer scoring of radiologic abnormalities in the hands and wrists of patients with rheumatoid arthritis. Arthritis Rheum 1985;28:16-24.
13. Genant HK, Peterfy CG, Westhovens R, et al. Abatacept inhibits progression of structural damage in rheumatoid arthritis: results from the long-term extension of the AIM trial. Ann Rheum Dis 2008;67:1084-1089.
14. van der Heijde D. How to read radiographs according to the Sharp/van der Heijde method. J Rheumatol 1999;26:743-745.
15. van der Heijde D, Dankert T, Nieman F, et al. Reliability and sensitivity to change of a simplification of the Sharp/van der Heijde radiological assessment in rheumatoid arthritis. Rheumatology 1999;38:941-947.
16. Østergaard M, Peterfy C, Conaghan P, et al: OMERACT Rheumatoid Arthritis Magnetic Resonance Imaging Studies. Core set of MRI acquisitions, joint pathology definitions, and the OMERACT RA-MRI scoring system. J Rheumatol 2003;6:1385-1386.
17. Rahman P, Gladman DD, Cook RJ, et al. Radiological assessment in psoriatic arthritis. Br J Rheumatol 1998;37:760-765.
18. van der Heijde D, Sharp J, Wassenberg S, Gladman D. Psoriatic arthritis imaging: a review of scoring methods. Ann Rheum Dis 2005;64(Suppl 2):ii61-ii64.
19. Wassenberg S, Fischer-Kahle V, Herborn G, et al. A method to score radiographic change in psoriatic arthritis. Z Rheumatol 2001;60:156-166.
20. Ory PA, Gladman DD, Mease PJ. Psoriatic arthritis and imaging. Ann Rheum Dis 2005;64(Suppl 2):ii55-ii57.
21. Calin A, Mackay K, Santos H, et al. A new dimension to outcome: application of the Bath Ankylosing Spondylitis Radiology Index. J Rheumatol 1999;26:988-992.
22. Taylor HG, Beswick EJ, Dawes PT. Sulphasalazine in ankylosing spondylitis: a radiological, clinical and laboratory assessment. Clin Rheumatol 1991;10:43-48.
23. Creemers MC, Franssen MJ, van't Hof MA, et al. Assessment of outcome in ankylosing spondylitis: an extended radiographic scoring system. Ann Rheum Dis 2005;64:127-129.
24. Wanders AJ, Landewé RB, Spoorenberg A, et al. What is the most appropriate radiologic scoring method for ankylosing spondylitis? A comparison of the available methods based on the Outcome Measures in Rheumatology Clinical Trials filter. Arthritis Rheum 2004;50:2622-2632.
25. van der Heijde D, Landewé R, and the ASAS working group. Selection of a method for scoring radiographs for AS clinical trials by ASAS and OMERACT. J Rheumatol 2005;32:2048-2049.
26. Braun J, Baraliakos X, Golder W, et al. Magnetic resonance imaging examinations of the spine in patients with ankylosing spondylitis, before and after successful therapy with infliximab: evaluation of a new scoring system. Arthritis Rheum 2003;48:1126-1136.
27. Rudwaleit M, Schwarzlose S, Listing J, et al. Is there a place for magnetic resonance imaging (MRI) in predicting a major clinical response (BASDAI 50%) to TNF alpha blockers in ankylosing spondylitis? Arthritis Rheum 2003;50:S211-S212.
28. Maksymowych WP, Inman RD, Salonen D, et al. Spondyloarthritis Research Consortium of Canada

magnetic resonance imaging index for assessment of spinal inflammation in ankylosing spondylitis. Arthritis Rheum 2005;53:502-509.

29. Lukas C, Braun J, van der Heijde D, et al. Scoring inflammatory activity of the spine by magnetic resonance imaging in ankylosing spondylitis: a multireader experiment. J Rheumatol 2007;34:862-870.

30. van der Heijde D, Landewé R, Hermann KG, et al. Is there a preferred method for scoring activity of the spine by magnetic resonance imaging in ankylosing spondylitis? J Rheumatol 2007;34:871-873.

31. Maksymowych WP, Inman RD, Salonen D, et al. Spondyloarthritis research Consortium of Canada magnetic resonance imaging index for assessment of sacroiliac joint inflammation in ankylosing spondylitis. Arthritis Rheum 2005;53:703-709.

32. Hermann KG, Braun J, Fischer T, et al. Magnetic resonance tomography of sacroiliitis: anatomy, histological pathology, MR-morphology, and grading. Radiologe 2004;44:217-228.

33. Puhakka KB, Jurik AG, Egund N, et al. Imaging of sacroiliitis in early seronegative spondylarthropathy: Assessment of abnormalities by MR in comparison with radiography and CT. Acta Radiol 2003;44:218-229.

34. Landewé R, Hermann K-G, van der Heijde D, et al. Scoring sacro-iliac joints by magnetic resonance imaging, a multiple-reader reliability experiment. J Rheumatol 2005;32:2050-2055.

35. Braun J, Baraliakos X, Golder W, et al. Analysing chronic spinal changes in ankylosing spondylitis: a systematic comparison of conventional x rays with magnetic resonance imaging using established and new scoring systems. Ann Rheum Dis 2004;63:1046-1055.

REFERENCES

Full references for this chapter can be found on www.expertconsult.com.

PRINCIPLES OF MANAGEMENT

4

Arthritis patient education and team approaches to management

44

Maura D. Iversen

DEFINITION OF PATIENT EDUCATION AND MODES OF DELIVERY

Patient education is an integral component of disease management, especially in individuals who suffer from chronic illness. In the broadest sense, patient education is a purposeful learning experience that may include any combination of teaching, counseling, and behavioral techniques in order to influence patients' knowledge and health behaviors.[1] Patient education often includes the provision of information, instruction in self-management skills, behavioral motivation strategies, and techniques to enhance or develop social support for health behaviors. Patient education activities are essential for collaborative patient care. Patients have a right to receive information about their medical conditions and the spectrum of treatment options available to them[2] and to actively engage in decision-making about their care.[3] Patients who understand their condition and are knowledgeable about how and when to use their medications are more adherent to treatments and in the short term demonstrate improved health outcomes.[4]

Effective patient education programs are based on psychobehavioral theories and incorporate techniques designed to actively engage patients in their care and to enhance their problem-solving skills.[5] Patient education can be provided by one or more individuals involved in the patient's care and may occur in many settings, beginning with the clinical encounter and expanding to public-based mediums such as television and print campaigns, Internet, and personal electronic devices. The focus of this chapter is on the role of patient education in various settings, the evidence for the effectiveness of patient education, and the use of team approaches to management.

Patient education during the clinical visit

Patient education begins the instant the provider and patient engage in dialogue. The tone, words, and pattern of talk influence the manner in which information is conveyed and received.[6] In general, the provider and patient enter the visit anticipating a successful encounter. The goals of the encounter are to establish a rapport, to formulate and receive a diagnosis/prognosis, to understand the impact of the condition on the patient's life, to discuss and understand treatment options and preferences for treatments, and to develop a plan of care that is acceptable to both the provider and patient. One technique used to enhance adherence to the plan of care is to engage in a discussion regarding the resources available to the patient (e.g., community exercise, self-management programs) and to identify barriers to adherence to develop contingency plans to address these barriers.[7]

Good communication between patients and providers has many benefits. Good communication leads to a more accurate diagnosis and prognosis,[8] improves adherence to treatments,[9] increases satisfaction with care,[10,11] and improves health outcomes.[8,10] Although physicians are not always comfortable providing counseling, research demonstrates that good communication skills can be learned.[12] Simple strategies such as sharing your assessment of the patient's understanding of the information provided, exploring patients' expectations of care, actively listening to patients' concerns, and clarifying patient preferences are essential for successful communication and patient education.[12-15] These conversations can help illuminate patients' decision-making processes and facilitate greater understanding of factors impacting adherence and treatment choices.

Research on provider-patient communication in arthritis

Research on provider-patient communication has focused on the attributes of the participants as well as the processes and outcomes of discussions. Patient concerns extend beyond managing symptoms and medications to social, emotional, and psychological effects of their disease, yet physicians are frequently unaware of the psychosocial and work issues impacting arthritis patients and may fail to address these issues during the visit.[16] Failure to elicit these issues increases the likelihood the patient will raise concerns late in the visit.[8,16]

Patient expectations of how and what should be discussed during the clinical encounter along with their expectations of treatments influence health outcomes, adherence to therapies, and satisfaction with the clinic visit.[14,17,18] Unfortunately, provider and patient expectations of the medical visit differ. Rao and associates[14] surveyed rheumatology patients, noting 58 patients (33%) reported unmet expectations. Nearly half reported unmet expectations with regard to general information and 31% for new medications. Patient expectations of the efficacy of treatments also influence outcomes. In one study, patients' preoperative expectations of function and pain relief for spinal surgery influenced their pain and function up to 6 months after surgery.[18] A review of patient-physician communication studies, including studies in rheumatic disease, supports these findings.[17]

Clinical discussions inform patients of the purposes of treatments as well as how and when to take medications or engage in exercise. Unfortunately, patients often misunderstand the purpose of treatments. A study of first visits to an arthritis clinic found that 15% of patients failed to understand the purpose of their prescriptions. These patients were less likely to adhere to prescriptions after 4 months than patients who understood the purpose of the medication.[19] Patients may not understand or may forget how to take medication properly. Information regarding the purpose of medications, how to take medications properly, and whether a latency period exists before the drugs take effect is necessary to understanding and adhering to therapy. Unfortunately, most patients forget about 50% of the medical instructions in a very short time.[20] To enhance understanding of medical advice and adherence, information should be provided using simple, non-threatening language and clear written instructions.

Patients and providers disagree with respect to the value of nutritional supplements, need for referrals, and use of drugs and surgical therapy.[21] Studies of patient preferences for medications have helped elucidate issues related to patient adherence to drug therapies.[15] Perceptions about the need for medications and fear of overuse of medications influences adherence more than medical demographic factors (e.g., age, disease activity).[15] Patients' beliefs also impact how they interpret information, their perceptions of how they are treated during visits, their recall of information, and what they do with clinical advice.[6] Data also indicate providers' beliefs, and attitudes toward treatments also influence the content of discussions and likelihood of receiving a prescription.[22]

Patients' desire for participation in decision-making is not routinely recognized and may vary based on the circumstances.[12,23] Communicating information about risks in understandable terms (e.g., frequencies vs. probabilities),[24] clarifying patients' beliefs and attitudes toward treatments and preferences for participation in decision-making, and allowing patients to actively negotiate treatment alternatives impacts satisfaction and outcomes of care.[8,16] Even patients who would rather be passive during clinical discussions are

IMPROVING COMMUNICATIONS IN PATIENT EDUCATION PRACTICE

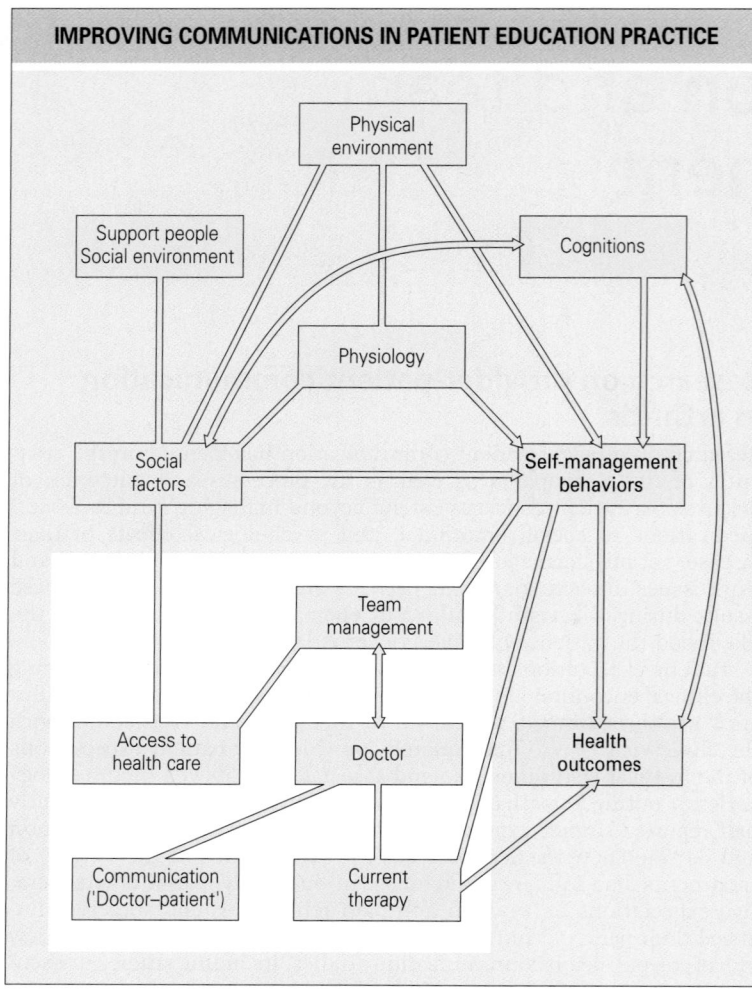

Fig. 44.1 Arthritis patient education: a social learning framework.

TABLE 44.1 SETTINGS FOR ARTHRITIS PATIENT EDUCATION

Setting	Type of patient education
Medical care	Patient education delivered by physicians as part of the medical consultation
Inpatient surgical education	Preoperative or perioperative education for patients with arthritis undergoing joint surgery (may be individual or small group)
Ancillary to medical care	Patient education delivered by a team approach, involving allied health professionals, often including physical therapists, occupational therapists, and nurses; this occurs in practice settings, outpatient clinics, and hospital settings.
Structured small group education	Patient education delivered by trained patient educators as well as other clinician and health professionals, usually through multiple-session, multidisciplinary education; this can occur in the outpatient or community setting.
Other forms of individual education	Broader program reaching a wider target audience, comprising other forms of arthritis education, such as books, pamphlets and other resources, written self-instructional material, audiovisual material, computer-assisted learning, and Internet resources
Community resources	Dissemination, public education, and mass media campaigns and activities and support-group development; activities carried out by national arthritis foundations and societies

more satisfied with their providers when they participate more fully in negotiations about disease management.[23] In a recent cross-sectional study of 420 arthritis patients who were taking disease modifying antirheumatic drugs (DMARDs) or a biologic agent, Lim and colleagues[5] reported that only 64% of patients were satisfied with their level of participation in the decision-making process, although a substantial number (25%) said that information from different sources was conflicting.

DESIGNING PATIENT EDUCATION PROGRAMS

Patient education is well grounded in behavior change theory, derived from a range of disciplines, including psychology and the principles of adult learning. Theory-based approaches, including cognitive behavioral and self-management programs, hold the most promise for successful arthritis education.[20,25] Social learning theory[26] provides a framework for arthritis education (Fig. 44.1). This theory posits that health-enhancing behaviors result from the interplay between physiologic, social, and physical factors as well as an individual's cognitions about his or her disease.[26] This approach integrates program components often applied in isolation, such as cognitive behavior change strategies and a self-management framework.[25] A key cognitive dimension is self-efficacy, an individual's situation-specific confidence in performing a task. Perceptions of the possible consequences of carrying out the behavior are also key to adoption of health behaviors.[26] Increases in self-efficacy frequently lead to increases in appropriate health behaviors and health outcomes.[27] A range of factors across environments (see shaded area of Fig. 44-1) may contribute to the adoption of effective self-management behaviors that may lead to improved health outcomes.

Conducting a needs assessment is the first step in developing arthritis patient education.[25] A needs assessment is the process of defining the knowledge, skills, resources, motivation, and barriers to effective management that influence patients' response to their condition. The needs assessment in turn is influenced by the demographic and environmental factors of the participants.[4,28] Patients with a chronic condition such as arthritis seek attributions for their disease and develop construct models of illness to explain symptoms.[7] They describe and conceptualize their disease and symptoms in terms of their lives, their understanding of how their bodies work, social networks, and the mass media.

Patient education and self-management programs seek to engage participants as active learners. Skills are taught through practice, modeling, group problem-solving, and interactive discussions with other patients. Peer leaders may be selected to role model behaviors. Small group programs usually consist of 6 to 10 members to allow enough time for individual needs, as well as group processes. Groups comprising patients with similar conditions and needs allow discussion and cross-fertilization of ideas and skills to occur.[7]

The program length, learning objectives and goals, selection of leaders, and use of reinforcement sessions need to be considered. Short-term programs can increase knowledge and skills. Longer programs, although better able to transfer knowledge and skills, may discourage attendance.[7] Outcomes of patient education programs tend to be short lived and may require periodic reinforcements to maintain skills and behaviors. A mix of caregiver-based individual counseling and small group education will generally be optimal.[7]

CONTENT OF ARTHRITIS EDUCATION PROGRAMS

There are three major components of patient education programs: knowledge transfer, behavioral change/skill development, and psychosocial counseling (Table 44.1). Helping patients understand their diagnosis and prognosis and to critically appraise new information and seek resources is a goal of patient education. However, patient education alone does not result in cognitive or behavioral changes.[23] Therefore, most programs emphasize the development of self-management skills to promote and adapt behaviors based on patient symptoms and disease activity. Self-management skills include the use of splints and adaptation of exercise in the presence of hot swollen joints in persons with arthritis. These skills are learned through observation, performance and practice of the behaviors, and consequences of the behavior,[25,26] for example when patients who exercise regularly report improved function and decreased pain and stiffness.

Psychosocial counseling seeks to help patients to cope with their arthritis and to feel more confident about their ability to maintain an active social and functional lifestyle. The recruitment and training of lay leaders with arthritis to conduct patient education programs has shown positive short-term psychological effects for participants and leaders.[29] Although efforts to enhance social support do not consistently improve outcomes, family members and significant others may have a role in facilitating understanding and recall of information as well as emotional support and reinforcement of behaviors.[7]

Special considerations: health literacy

Written materials are frequently used to educate patients about their disease. Unfortunately, low literacy is common in the United States. The 2003 National Adult Literacy Survey (NALS) indicates that roughly 75 million adults demonstrated basic or below-basic skills in health literacy.[30] Health literacy encompasses a person's ability to read, comprehend, and use information to receive adequate care. Functional literacy, a component of health literacy, refers to the ability to find information or numbers in a lengthy text, integrate multiple pieces of information, or find two or more numbers in a chart and perform a calculation.[23,31] In a study of literacy among patients with rheumatoid arthritis it was found that 1 in 6 patients were illiterate and struggled to understand patient education materials and prescription labels. These patients had significantly more hospital visits.[32] A second study designed to assess reading levels of 80 patients with rheumatoid arthritis[33] reported that 10% of the patients had difficulties reading patient materials and 31% scored at or below the 9th grade reading level. These results are consistent with research indicating poor health, poor understanding of treatment, greater use of health services, and low adherence to treatment regimens among patients with limited literacy.[34]

Most patient education materials are written at the level of the 11th grade or higher,[34] whereas the average reading level of the general public is below the 8th grade. The following strategies are recommended to enhance patient education and improve adherence to treatments[7]:

- Speak using simple language, avoid medical jargon, and repeat instructions.
- Provide easy-to-read materials in plain English (5th to 8th grade reading level) with illustrations.[30]
- Include significant others or family members in discussion (with consent of the patient).
- Motivate and enhance patient self-efficacy through discussing the pros and cons of treatment from the patient's perspective.
- Demonstrate problem-solving strategies to address potential barriers to adherence and help develop contingency plans for dealing with treatment failure.

Cultural considerations

Social, cultural, and environmental factors as well as past health care experiences influence the manner in which care is provided and perceived.[7] A study of arthritis beliefs and self-care among an urban American Indian population[35] revealed that verbal communication about pain was subtle and under-reported. These findings suggest providers need to be cognizant about information sharing regarding pain and disability in this population. Zhang and associates[36] examined illness management strategies among Chinese immigrants living with arthritis and found management strategies fluctuate between Western and traditional Chinese medicine. Western medicine was believed to be less effective than traditional medicine for chronic conditions such as arthritis. Data indicate patient education programs may be more effective when cultural factors are included in the design to address specific populations[37] and when materials are assessed for readability.[34] Designing culturally relevant educational materials is especially important in groups with low literacy, because interpretation of illustrations and behavioral modeling may be particularly sensitive to cultural context among persons who cannot read accompanying text that could clarify the meaning of illustrations.[7] For tips on designing easy-to-read materials, see Table 44.2.

TABLE 44.2 CONTENT AREAS OF STRUCTURED ARTHRITIS PATIENT EDUCATION

Content area	Examples of specific content
Knowledge	Anatomy, disease process, inflammation Symptoms and signs for improvement or deterioration in disease; understanding of disease monitoring Pharmacologic therapy: use, effects, side effects; alternative therapy Understanding of benefits of surgical intervention Use of heat and cold, joint protection, podiatry Understanding of nutrition, diet and hazardous diets; weight control Understanding of where to find community resources, helping agencies, potential assistance from government agencies
Skills and behaviors	Role of exercise, rest, joint protection skills, TENS, acupuncture Specific goal setting; daily routines established Making domestic tasks easier; domestic environmental modifications Self-monitoring or adherence; when to take additional medication Pain management; use of hot/cold; relaxation, other pain management behaviors Work and occupational simplification (where possible)
Problem solving (linked to self-management skills)	Psychosocial and communication dimension Communicating with health care providers; learning assertiveness and when to ask questions Reducing anxiety, increasing confidence (efficacy) for specific tasks, reducing feelings of helplessness and fear Learning to cope with chronic illness and depression Eliciting support from spouse/family members; learning to cope with disease management in the domestic context

Use of Internet for patient education

Delivering of patient education and self-management advice through the Internet has received less formal evaluation. Generational acceptance of technology and multimedia approaches to patient education exist and can be explored to better understand cost effective and efficacious delivery modes. In a recent study[38] assessing the acceptability of an Internet-based self-management program for adolescents with juvenile idiopathic arthritis, 36 children of various ages, disease severity, and subtypes were recruited from four pediatric centers and participated in structured focus groups. These adolescents reported that a Web-based intervention was a promising avenue to improve accessibility and availability of self-management techniques, such as gaining control over their disease, developing social supports, and learning to communicate with their providers. However, in a study of 71 older adults with arthritis, Tak and Hong[39] reported 39% of older adults used the Internet to obtain arthritis information and only 28% had a home computer.

An important consideration when referring patients to Internet sites for information is the quality of the material provided. Ansani and colleagues[40] evaluated the quality of arthritis information on the Internet using a standardized rubric. They reported that the quality of information varied widely and that the best sources of information were located on Websites with URLs having suffixes of .gov and .edu. Kim and associates[41] examined the impact of Web-based arthritis information on arthritis patients' knowledge and medical practice. First, they reviewed and scored Websites based on authorship, type of publication, contents, and financial interests. Next, 257 Korean arthritis patients and rheumatologists were surveyed about the use of the information from these sites. Twenty-eight percent of patients surveyed reported they searched for arthritis information on the Internet. Significant correlates of Web-based information use were younger age, being employed, and having a higher income and higher education. Ratings of the accuracy of Web-based arthritis information did not differ between physicians and patients. However, only 16.1% of physicians believed their patients understood the content, and physicians' attitudes toward Web-based information were also less positive than those of patients.

Evidence for effectiveness of arthritis education programs

Patient education programs range from the provision of information to the use of cognitive behavioral strategies, exercise, and psychosocial support. The variability in content, target populations and disease conditions, duration, and frequency complicate systemic evaluation of programs. Systematic reviews include a mix of study designs, definitions of patient education, and health outcomes or included heterogeneous patient populations with respect to disease.[7] Patients with osteoarthritis or rheumatoid arthritis are most often included in patient education trials. Comparisons of patient education programs by diagnosis indicate differences in the outcomes that are not consistent across studies.[7,28] Notably, patient education programs with behaviorally based interventions appear to be more effective than instructional programs alone.[4]

In a systematic review[4] of randomized controlled trials of arthritis patient education in which patient education was defined as an intervention that includes formal structured instruction on arthritis and ways to manage the disease, such as psychobehavioral strategies, exercise, biofeedback, or psychosocial support, 31 randomized controlled trials were included. The results indicated modest improvements in functional disability, joint counts, global assessment, psychological status, and depression in the short term (up to 2 months) but no difference at follow-up (3 to 14 months). Improvements in functional disability translated into a 10% improvement on the Health Assessment Questionnaire. This review is unique because separate analyses were performed based on the type of intervention. Data indicated behavioral interventions showed the greatest improvements compared with no intervention. The overall quality rating of the trials was not very high, leaving the findings open to the potential for selection bias.[4] These results are similar to the systematic review of self-management in chronic illness by Warsi and colleagues,[27] who evaluated the outcomes of 71 trials and found small to moderate effects. Mulligan and coworkers[42] believed the randomized controlled trial may not be the best design for examining self-management programs. Few studies have examined the impact of patient education programs on health care use and cost-effective arthritis education.[43]

The research indicates that structured patient education programs based on commonly accepted principles of education and psychology and applied consistently by trained personnel produce small improvements in knowledge, behavior, physiologic measures, and health outcomes beyond the effects of medications and incidental education to which patients have already been exposed.[4,7,42] Effects tend to be strongest when programs include behavioral strategies. Well-designed patient education programs can be effective and should be an integral part of arthritis management. A randomized controlled study examining the outcomes of a small group arthritis patient self-management versus tailored-print education found slightly better results for the tailored-print program in the first year and attenuated over time.[44] This study suggests the benefit of well-designed, tailored education print materials in increasing patient education and allows for greater dissemination of information.

Limitations of research and conclusions

Most evaluations of patient education programs include programs with mixed interventions (information only, information plus behavioral strategies), consist of patients with differing diagnoses, and are often based on small samples.[19] There is no core set of outcomes for patient education trials, and as such variability exists in the outcomes assessed. These outcomes also may not measure changes occurring with the intervention. Literacy assessments of patient education materials are not consistently performed or are infrequently considered in program implementation. These concerns warrant further investigation in subsequent evaluation designs but do not negate the role and importance of arthritis education.[7] Further research is needed to assess the impact and cost-effectiveness of arthritis patient education on specific populations, for patients with specific arthritis diagnoses, and that includes a comprehensive set of outcomes to capture factors addressed in behavioral interventions.

MULTIDISCIPLINARY TEAM APPROACHES TO MANAGEMENT AND ROLES OF PROVIDERS

Arthritis team care improves health care delivery and outcomes.[45] The multidisciplinary team care concept began more than 50 years ago when new pharmacologic approaches were not yet introduced. The philosophy behind team care is to rely on the knowledge and expertise of each health professional to maximally address the patient's needs. Scandinavian countries such as Sweden and Finland were the first to initiate the team care approach. Multidisciplinary team care may be provided during hospital admission by the inpatient team or on an outpatient basis in regular or day care facilities.[10]

The notion of team care varies across the globe. *Team care* is defined here as care involving the patient, a health care provider plus at least one other health care provider or family member and that incorporates a team approach to information sharing, decision-making, and goal setting. The composition of the team may include a primary care physician, rheumatologist, nurse practitioner, physical therapist, occupational therapist, social worker, psychologist, podiatrist, vocational rehabilitator, patient's family, and the patient. Although team composition varies, the central member of the team is the patient and/or patient's family. For the team to be effective, team members need to understand and respect each other's role (Table 44.3) and be cognizant

---

TABLE 44.3 STRATEGIES TO DESIGN EFFECTIVE PATIENT EDUCATION MATERIALS NEEDS ASSESSMENT

Consider interviewing patients
- How do you describe your illness?
- What do you wish you had known?
- What strategies are most useful in helping you learn?
- What skills do you use to manage your disease?
- What is the best format for delivery (brochure, Internet)?

Elicit information to create messages that are culturally relevant

Do not mix formats in the layout

Write for your reader
- Use plain language/simple short sentences.
- Use simplest tense.
- Use "must" to convey requirements.
- Avoid abbreviations.
- Avoid calling the same thing by different names (e.g., medicine, drug, therapy)
- Do use contractions (e.g., don't vs. do not).

Focus on key information

Use a question and answer format
- Helps readers to scan the document and find the information they want
- May see a question that they didn't consider but needed to know the answer

Use "you" and other pronouns
- Personalizes message

Use the active voice

Use the appropriate tone
- Don't talk down to your audience.
- Write in positive not negative terms.
- Avoid ALL CAPS—appears as if you are yelling at the person (especially true for Web formats)

Provide information about when medication/therapy will take effect

Keep subjects and objects close to their verbs

Place conditional words after the main thought
- "Take 3 aspirin if you have pain more than 5 hours and are not taking another NSAID" and NOT "if you have pain more than 5 hours and are not taking another NSAID, take 3 aspirin."

Complex information may be better presented in tables

Adapted from Rudd RE. How to create and assess print materials. Harvard School of Public Health: Health Literacy Website. 2002. Available at: http://www.hsph.harvard.edu/healthliteracy/materials.html. Accessed May 20, 2005.

of the information they have imparted to prevent communication breakdown, prevent overlap and omission of services, and maximize patient care. In theory, team care allows different professionals to motivate and reinforce learning, providing care across a range of patient care settings. Team functioning is important and is becoming a stronger emphasis in health professional education and training.[46]

Although team care is prevalent in Europe, this is not the case in North America, partly owing to budgetary constraints, shortage of health care professionals, and reimbursement issues. Consequently, innovative team care models, such as the clinical nurse-specialist model[47] and the primary therapist model,[48] have emerged. In the primary therapist model and the nurse-specialist model extensions of clinical practice are promoted.[46,47] These models have been developed directly in response to limited access to rheumatology providers. Study results suggest that patients referred to receive treatment from a primary therapist might receive better outcomes than those who were referred to receive traditional therapy.[48] Studies of the use of health care professionals in extended clinical roles are promising and warrant further investigation.

Telemedicine is an emerging model of care to service rural and remote communities. Findings from the literature review suggest that rheumatology telemedicine is a viable model to promote access to care for all persons with arthritis. More research into the benefits, costs, and delivery of these programs is warranted.

PUBLIC HEALTH APPROACHES TO ARTHRITIS PATIENT EDUCATION

The increasing recognition of the role of health education and health promotion as primary prevention is evident by the growing emphasis on public health approaches to arthritis management from the Centers for Disease Control and Prevention and the National Arthritis Foundation. Public health approaches provide population-based programs, enabling access to all individuals to reduce social inequalities and promote health. These approaches include health care professional and physician training (Table 44.4), community education programs, environmental modifications, health policies, and the use of mass media to provide low-intensity but widely disseminated messages about arthritis.[7]

The Americans with Disabilities Act (ADA) is designed to reduce disability and discrimination, allowing individuals to remain active contributors to society. The policies arising from the ADA call for environmental modifications such as ergonomic assessments and the use of functional aids or assistive devices and handicap-accessible sidewalks and buses to maximize functional independence. However, in a study of individuals with arthritis, only 7% to 10% of patients used the ADA even though 47% experienced an ADA-resolvable barrier to community activity and 63% needed a job accommodation or had experienced health discrimination.[49]

A main objective of a public health approach to arthritis is to reach all population segments, including socially disadvantaged groups, those who speak minority languages, and those who cannot access specialist medical care. To provide education to patients with all types of arthritis, we need to develop programs and materials for the less common but serious varieties of rheumatic disease. Health care providers and patients must advocate for policies and programs that reach the majority of individuals with arthritis in a cost-efficient and cost-effective manner. In the United States, the nation's health objectives, as stated in *Healthy People 2010*[50] now includes a section devoted to arthritis and the Centers for Disease Control and Prevention have a dedicated

TABLE 44.4 INTERDISCIPLINARY ROLES: TEAM APPROACHES TO ARTHRITIS EDUCATION

Professional	Role in patient education (examples)
Nurse/pharmacist	Has primary care role in explaining and demonstrating medication use, action, interactions, side effects and medication administration devices
Rheumatologist and/or family physician	Explains the disease, its physiology, natural history, and range of therapies available; the need for disease monitoring; the place of intra-articular injection, surgery, etc. In some countries this is the role of community general practitioners, especially for uncomplicated and prevalent conditions (e.g., osteoarthritis, osteoporosis) and providing adjunctive care for complicated or multisystem disease
Physical therapist	Uses static and dynamic exercises, mobility, prevention of contracture or weakness, acupuncture, TENS, modification of physical activity during active phases of disease; pain management strategies
Nutritionist	Explains role of diet; "alternative" diets and their potential risks; weight control strategies
Occupational therapist	Provides training in relearning routine activities of daily living, recreation, and leisure pursuits; use of technical devices; joint support and when to rest and partially to immobilize joints
Social workers	Helps with "patients' rights" to treatment, arranging time off work, support from caregivers in the family and community and government, and sometimes provision of individual or family counseling
Counselor or psychologist	Provides anxiety and/or depression counseling and aids in dealing with denial or with disease crises, coping with sexuality, and pain management

arthritis initiative.[7] The Arthritis Prevention, Control, and Cure Act is legislation currently being reintroduced in the U.S. Senate to provide public access to arthritis patient education.

THE FUTURE OF ARTHRITIS PATIENT EDUCATION

In the coming years we will experience an expansion in the application and dissemination of technology-based arthritis patient education. New devices are currently being implemented to dispense patient education and provide educational reinforcement opportunities by relaying information through personal digital assistants, home cable boxes, or cell phones. These systems convey an auditory signal or text signal to engage the patient and seek to empower patients to take a more active role in their care. Newer technologies are also expanding to allow providers to remotely monitor patients while improving communication and maintaining a high level of personalized care.

We will continue to expand our development, adaptation, and evaluation of patient education programs for specific populations such as minorities, those with limited literacy,[34] and individuals with rare forms of arthritis. With increasing health care constraints and workforce issues in rheumatology, we will need to explore innovative models of patient care delivery and patient education and assess their cost-effectiveness and health benefits. As we expand patient education and its delivery mechanisms we will continue to define outcomes that reflect the learning process and can capture the psychosocial dimensions and skill developments anticipated with education.

REFERENCES

1. Bartlett EE. Forum: patient education: Eight principles from patient education research. Prev Med 1985;14:667-669.
2. Albrecht TL, Franks M, Ruckdeschel JC. Communication and informed consent. Curr Opin Oncol 2005;17:336-339.
3. Bauman AE, Fardy HJ, Harris PG. Getting it right: why bother with patient-centred care? Med J Aust 2003;179:253-256.
4. Reisma RP, Kirwan JR, Taal E, Rasker JJ. Patient education for adults with rheumatoid arthritis. Cochrane Database Syst Rev 2007;1:0075320.
5. Lim AY, Ellis C, Brooksby A, Gaffney K. Patient satisfaction with rheumatology practitioner clinics: can we achieve concordance by meeting patients' information needs and encouraging participatory decision making? Ann Acad Med 2007;36:110-114.
6. Iversen MD, Eaton HM, Daltroy LH. How rheumatologists and patients with rheumatoid arthritis discuss exercise and the influence of discussions on exercise prescriptions. Arthritis Care Res 2004;51:63-72.
7. Daltroy LH, Barclay GR. Health promotion and patient education for people with arthritis. In: Hochberg MC, Silman AJ, Smolen JS, et al, eds. Rheumatology, 3rd ed. St. Louis: Mosby, 2003:361-368.

8. Du Pre A. Communicating about health: current issues and perspectives. Mountain View, CA: Mayfield, 2000.
9. Heidenreich PA. Patient adherence: the next frontier in quality improvement. Am J Med 2004;117:130-132.
10. Harrington J, Noble LM, Newman SP. Improving patients' communication with doctors: a systematic review of intervention studies. Patient Educ Couns 2004;53:7-16.
11. Bidaut-Russell M, Gabriel SE, Scott CG, et al. Determinants of patient satisfaction in chronic illness. Arthritis Care Res 2002;47:494-500.
12. Maguire P, Pitceathly C. Key communication skills and how to acquire them. BMJ 2002;325:697-700.
13. Neame R, Hammond A, Deighton C. Need for information and for involvement in decision making among patients with rheumatoid arthritis: a questionnaire survey. Arthritis Care Res 2005;53:249-255.
14. Rao JK, Winberger M, Anderson LA, Kroenke K. Predicting reports of unmet expectations among rheumatology patients. Arthritis Care Res 2004;51:215-221.
15. Fraenkel L, Bogardus ST, Concato J, et al. Patient preferences for treatment of rheumatoid arthritis. Ann Rheum Dis 2004;63;1372-1378.
16. Marvel MK, Epstein RM, Flowers K, Beckman HB. Soliciting the patient's agenda: have we improved? JAMA 1999;281:283-287.
17. Suarez-Almazor ME. Patient-physician communication. Curr Opin Rheumatol 2004;16:91-95.
18. Iversen MD, Daltroy LH, Fossel AH, Katz JN. The prognostic importance of patient pre-operative expectations of surgery for lumbar spinal stenosis. Patient Educ Couns 1998;34:169-178.
19. Daltroy LH. Doctor-patient communication in rheumatological disorders. Baillière's Clin Rheumatol 1993;7:221-239.
20. Ley P. Psychological studies of doctor-patient communication. In: Rachman S, ed. Contributions to medical psychology. Oxford: Pergamon Press, 1977:9-42.
21. Lambert BL, Butin DN, Moran D, et al. Arthritis care: comparison of physicians' and patients' view. Semin Arthritis Rheum 2000;30:100-110.
22. Iversen MD, Fossel AH, Daltroy LH. Rheumatologist-patient communication about exercise and physical therapy in rheumatoid arthritis. Arthritis Care Res 1999;12:180-192.
23. Vahabi M. The impact of health communication on health-related decision making. Health Commun 2007;107:27-41.

24. Trevena LJ, Davey HM, Baratt A, et al. A systematic review on communicating with patients about evidence. J Eval Clin Pract 2006;12:13-23.
25. Lorig K. Patient education: a practical approach, 3rd ed. Thousand Oaks, CA: Sage, 2000.
26. Bandura A. Social foundations of thought and action: a social cognitive theory. Englewood Cliffs, NJ: Prentice-Hall, 1986:142-181.
27. Warsi A, Wang PS, LaValley MP, et al. Self-management education programs in chronic disease. JAMA 2004;164:1641-1649.
28. Superio-Cabuslay E, Ward M, Lorig K. Patient education interventions in osteoarthritis and rheumatoid arthritis: a meta-analytic comparison with non-steroidal anti-inflammatory drug treatment. Arthritis Care Res 1996;9:292-301.
29. Hainsworth J, Barlow J. Volunteers' experiences of becoming arthritis self-management lay leaders: "It's almost as if I've stopped aging and started to get younger!" Arthritis Care Res 2001;45:378-383.
30. Kutner M, Greenberg E, Jin Y, Paulsen C. The health literacy of America's adults: results from the 2003 National Assessment of Adult Literacy. U.S. Department of Education. Washington, DC: National Center for Education Statistics, 2006.
31. Parker RM, Baker DW, Williams MV, Nurss JR. The test of functional health literacy in adults: a new instrument for measuring patients' literacy skills. J Gen Intern Med 1995;10:537-541.
32. Gordon MM, Hampson R, Capell HA, et al. Illiteracy in rheumatoid arthritis patients as determined by the Rapid Estimate of Adult Literacy in Medicine (REALM) score. Rheumatology 2002;41:750-754.
33. Buchbinder R, Hall S, Youd JM. Functional literacy of patients with rheumatoid arthritis attending a community-based rheumatology practice. J Rheumatol 2006;33:879-886.
34. Rudd R, Rosenfeld L, Gall V. Health literacy and arthritis research and practice. Curr Opin Rheumatol 2007;19:97-100.
35. Kramer BJ, Harker JO, Wong AL. Arthritis beliefs and self-care in an urban American Indian population. Arthritis Care Res 2002;47:588-594.
36. Zhang J, Verhoef MJ. Illness management strategies among Chinese immigrants living with arthritis. Social Sci Med 2002;55:1795-1802.
37. Wong AL, Harker JO, Lau VP, et al. Spanish arthritis empowerment program: a dissemination and effectiveness study. Arthritis Care Res 2004;51:332-336.

38. Stinson JN, Toomey PC, Stevens BJ, et al. Asking the experts: exploring the self-management needs of adolescents with arthritis. Arthritis Rheum 2008;59:65-72.
39. Tak SH, Hong SH. Use of the Internet for health information by older adults with arthritis. Orthop Nurs 2005;24:134-138.
40. Ansani NT, Vogt M, Henderson BA, et al. Quality of arthritis information on the Internet. Am J Health Syst Pharmacy 2005;62:1184-1189.
41. Kim HA, Bae YD, Seo YI. Arthritis information on the Web and its influence on patients and physicians: a Korean study. Clin Exp Rheumatol 2004;22:49-54.
42. Mulligan K, Newman SP, Taal E, et al. The design and evaluation of psychoeducational/self-management interventions. J Rheumatol 2005;32:2470-2474.
43. Lorig KR, Mazonson PD, Holman HR. Evidence suggesting that health education for self-management in patients with chronic arthritis has sustained health benefits while reducing health care costs. Arthritis Rheum 1993;36:439-446.
44. Lorig KR, Ritter PL, Laurent DD, Fries JF. Long-term randomized controlled trials of tailored-print and small-group arthritis self-management interventions. Med Care 2004;42:346-354.
45. MacKay C, Veinot P, Badley EM. Characteristics of evolving models of care for arthritis: a key informant study. BMC Health Serv Res 2008;8:147.
46. Iversen MD, Petersson IF. Design issues and priorities in team and non-pharmacologic arthritis care research. J Rheumatol 2006;33:1904-1907.
47. Tijhuis GJ, Zwinderman AH, Hazes JMW, et al. A randomized comparison of care provided by a clinical nurse specialist, inpatient team care and day patient team care in rheumatoid arthritis. Arthritis Rheum 2002;47:525-531.
48. Li LC, Iversen MD. Outcomes of patients with rheumatoid arthritis receiving rehabilitation. Curr Opin Rheum 17:172-176.
49. Allaire SH, Evans SR, LaValley MP, Merrigan DM. Use of the Americans with Disabilities Act by persons with rheumatic diseases and factors associated with use. Arthritis Rheum 2001;45:174-182.
50. U.S. Department of Health and Human Services. Healthy people 2010. Washington, DC: U.S. Government Printing Office, 2000.

Nutrition in rheumatic disease

Ronenn Roubenoff and Laura A. Coleman

45

- Systemic inflammatory diseases cause major disruptions in nutritional status, at both the macronutrient (protein, fat, carbohydrate) and micronutrient (vitamins, minerals, trace elements) levels.
- Rheumatoid cachexia is a very common complication of rheumatoid arthritis, although it is seldom recognized or treated. A combination of diet and resistance exercise is effective at reversing the muscle wasting of rheumatoid cachexia.
- Dietary requirements for vitamin B_6, protein, calcium, and vitamin D are increased with systemic rheumatic diseases and with corticosteroid therapy.
- Dietary components may provide anti-inflammatory and antioxidant benefits as adjuvants to pharmacotherapy of rheumatic diseases, although most claims of benefit remain to be proven.
- Obesity is both a cause and a complication of osteoarthritis and, to a lesser extent, gout. Weight reduction can help both diseases, and strengthening exercise can ameliorate joint pain in osteoarthritis.

RELEVANCE OF NUTRITION TO RHEUMATIC DISEASES

In any chronic disease, the interplay between the disease and the host is the major determinant of disease impact. Although clinicians usually focus on the severity of the pathologic insult, wise physicians have long been aware that the physiologic and psychological makeup of the patient has a large effect on both survival and quality of life. Rheumatoid arthritis (RA), by virtue of its systemic, body-wide inflammation, has been the paradigm for understanding how chronic inflammation alters host metabolism and physiology. Host resistance to illness is probably controlled by both genetic and environmental factors: as one of the key environmental exposures, nutritional status is thus an important determinant of how well the patient can withstand the ravages of RA and other chronic rheumatic diseases. Conversely, overnutrition and obesity are the major causes of osteoarthritis (OA) of the knees and hips. Moreover, some nutrients offer the promise of directly affecting the disease process by offering variable amounts of anti-inflammatory activity. Although not working on the same magnitude as anti-inflammatory drugs, dietary anti-inflammatory and antioxidant nutrients are of great interest for patients trying to gain control over their disease. Because these nutrients may support or counteract the effectiveness of medications, a solid understanding of drug-nutrient interactions can be important to both practice and research in the rheumatic diseases.

Undernutrition and rheumatic diseases

Weight loss and muscle wasting are common features of untreated RA, originally described by James Paget in the 19th century as rheumatoid cachexia.[1] Occasionally, a patient with RA will present with weight loss and adenopathy and be diagnosed initially with lymphoma; only after lymph node biopsy fails to identify a malignancy does a rheumatic disease enter the differential diagnosis. Vasculitis, especially medium-vessel vasculitides such as polyarteritis nodosa and ANCA-associated granulomatous vasculitis, is often associated with weight loss. Similarly, both adult and juvenile forms of Still's disease often present as weight loss. Systemic lupus erythematosus (SLE), scleroderma, and reactive arthritis are less commonly associated with weight loss.

Evidence from cancer, heart failure, and HIV infection strongly points to weight loss as an independent predictor of poor outcome.[2]

There is evidence that RA causes significant muscle loss, reduced physical activity, and a trend toward increased fat mass.[3] Loss of lean mass and higher fat mass are each associated with greater disability,[4] and low body mass index (BMI) in patients with RA is associated with threefold higher mortality.[5] Rheumatoid cachexia is found in 25% to 50% of patients with RA; in our experience, all patients with RA develop some degree of muscle loss, although it may only be detectable by specialized methods (see later).[6]

In addition to a disruption in macronutrient status (i.e., protein, carbohydrate, and fat stores), chronic inflammation often leads to abnormal micronutrient status as well. Both RA and SLE are associated with abnormalities of vitamin B_6 status, homocysteine metabolism, and, to a lesser extent, folate metabolism.[7-9] In addition, chronic inflammation leads to increased production of free radical species and oxidative stress, with attendant decreases in antioxidant vitamins such as vitamins C and E.[10-12]

Overnutrition in rheumatic diseases

In contrast to the situation with most of the chronic systemic inflammatory diseases, the major nutritional problem in osteoarthritis and gout is weight gain and obesity. In gout, even a moderate degree of weight gain is a substantial risk factor for development of gouty arthritis.[13] With osteoarthritis, the load factor at the knee (three to six times body weight) and the hip (two to three times body weight) makes weight gain a disproportionate burden on these joints, increasing the stress on the cartilage and promoting degenerative changes.[14] From a public health perspective, the obesity epidemic in both developed and developing countries suggests that OA will follow diabetes and heart disease as a consequence of weight gain (Fig. 45.1).

The interplay of diet and exercise

It is important to think of nutritional status as the present result of a lifelong series of balances, reflecting intake and output of protein, energy, and micronutrients on a daily, weekly, monthly, and long-term basis. These balances are controlled by environmental, genetic, and hormonal influences (Fig. 45.2). Dietary intake reflects the input side of these balances, but physical activity, environmental stress such as heat or cold, and inflammation-driven changes in the internal hormonal milieu account for much of the output side. Thus, any consideration of a patient's nutritional and physiologic status should include an evaluation of his or her level of habitual physical activity, aerobic power, and muscle strength.

BASICS OF NUTRITIONAL ASSESSMENT FOR PATIENTS WITH RHEUMATIC DISEASES

The basic principles of nutritional assessment can be applied to patients with rheumatic diseases, although with some caveats (described later). A complete discussion of nutritional assessment techniques is beyond the scope of this chapter, and more information on the topic can be found elsewhere.[15] Briefly, standard methods for performing a nutritional evaluation include anthropometric, biochemical, clinical, and dietary assessments (summarized in Table 45.1).

Anthropometric and body composition techniques

Anthropometric measurements may be used to assess either growth, primarily in the case of children and adolescents, or body composition. The cellular components of standard man are illustrated in Figure 45.3a. Body cell mass, consisting primarily of muscle, and to a lesser

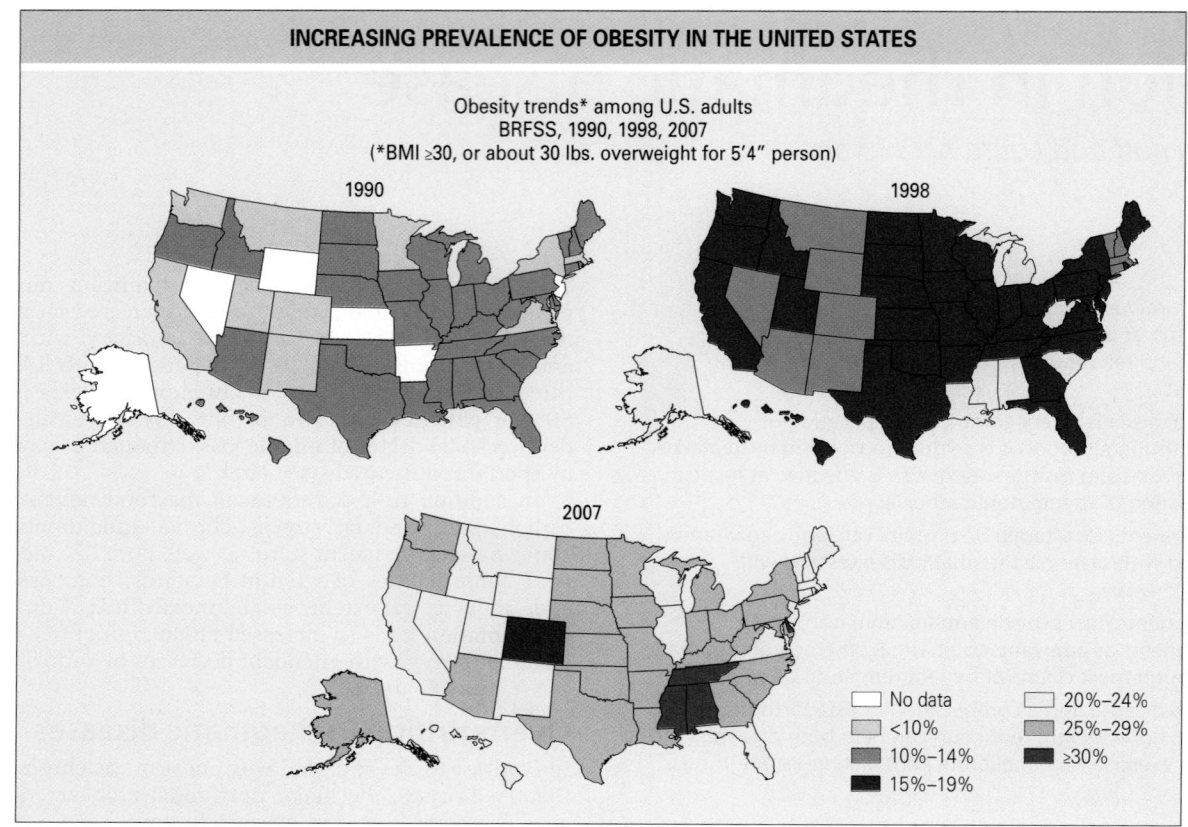

Fig. 45.1 Increasing prevalence of obesity in the United States. *(From BRFSS, Behavioral Risk Factor Surveillance System. Available at http://www.cdc.gov/brfss/)*

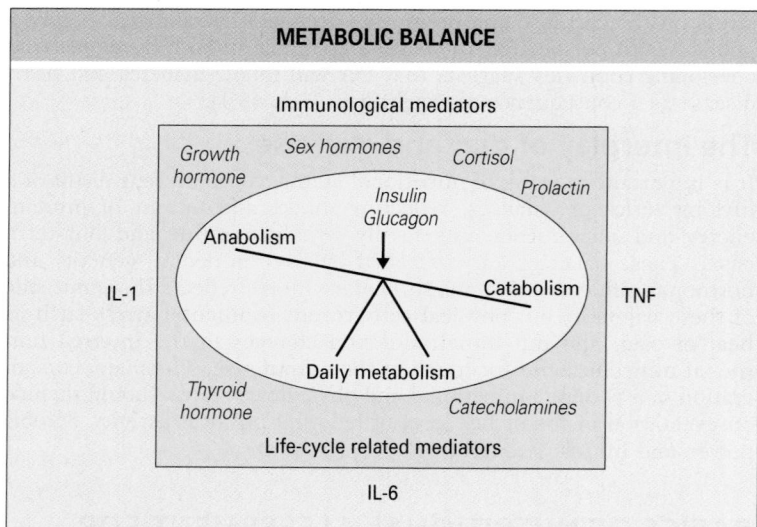

Fig. 45.2 The metabolic balance of the body is determined by a variety of regulators operating on vastly different time scales: daily, yearly, and over decades. TNF, tumor necrosis factor; IL, interleukin.

TABLE 45.1 NUTRITIONAL ASSESSMENT SUMMARY

Parameter	Examples
Anthropometric	Height, weight (current, usual, ideal), knee height, body mass index, waist/hip ratio, arm circumference, triceps skinfold
Biochemical	Serum albumin, hemoglobin, hematocrit, transferrin, plasma pyridoxal-5´-phosphate, folic acid, and 25 OH-vitamin D
Clinical	Co-morbidities, medications, mobility, disease severity, ability to perform activities of daily living by Health Assessment Questionnaire
Dietary	Total energy and protein intake, micronutrient intake by 24-hr recall or food records, dietary supplement use

extent visceral mass and immune cell mass, comprises the largest cellular component of the human body. Body cell mass is also the site of 95% of all metabolic activity. Fat mass and extracellular water make up the next largest compartments, with the remaining mass coming from bone and connective tissue (cartilage, fibrous tissues, and skeletal tissues). These structural proteins are not readily exchangeable with other pools of protein in the body, so changes that may occur in body cell mass during disease, for example, cannot be counteracted by mobilization of extracellular connective tissue.

Intracellular proteins turn over constantly in the body, such that the rates of protein synthesis and protein breakdown determine whether net anabolism or catabolism will occur. Even a small decrease in synthesis or a small increase in degradation, if sustained over the long

term, can result in a marked loss of mass to the organism as a whole. This is important because in all clinical situations in which it has been investigated (e.g., starvation, critical illness, cancer, HIV infection), a loss of greater than 40% of baseline body cell mass is associated with death.[2] Furthermore, even a more modest loss of body cell mass, although not fatal, is known to compromise muscle strength, balance, function, mobility, and immune function, with the net result being a loss of independence, increased risk of clinical depression, and reduced quality of life for the patient.

Anthropometric assessment of body composition essentially involves measuring one of two major compartments in the body: body fat or fat-free mass. There are a variety of specific indices available for assessment, and selection of a particular method depends on the purpose of the assessment (e.g., nutritional screening, surveillance, or evaluation of an intervention). Regardless of the particular method chosen, it is important to remember that any method using prediction equations or a reference population is not necessarily going to be readily applicable to patients with rheumatic disease, because these standards were developed on healthy, lean subjects, and both sensitivity and specificity may be reduced when these methods are applied to other populations.

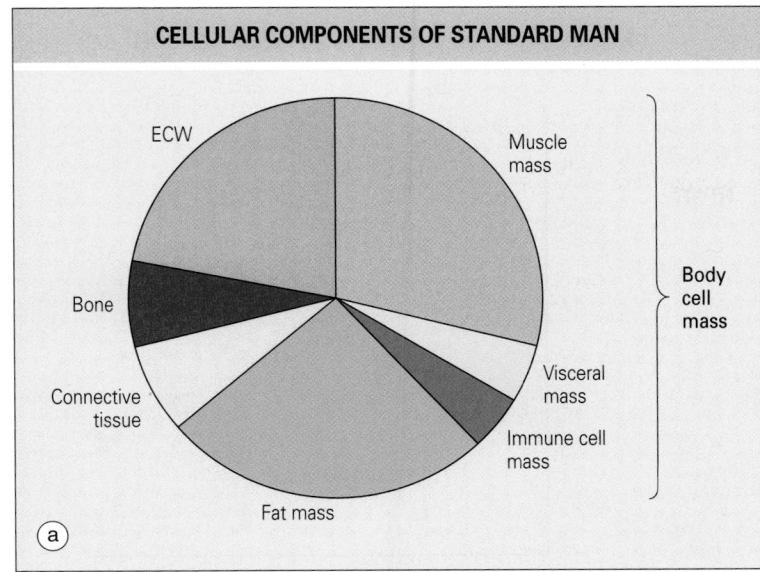

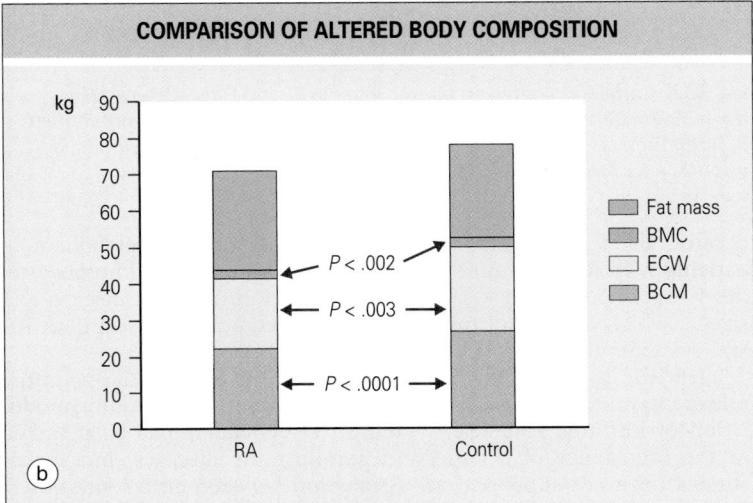

Fig. 45.3 (a) Cellular components of standard man. (b) Altered body composition in patients with rheumatoid arthritis (RA) compared with age, sex, weight, and race-matched healthy controls. BMC, bone mineral content; ECW, extracellular water; BCM, body cell mass. *(a, Adapted from Protection ICoR. Report of the Task Group on Reference Man, No. 23. Oxford, UK: Pergamon Press, 1975; b, based on data from Roubenoff R, et al. Rheumatoid cachexia: depletion of lean body mass in rheumatoid arthritis; possible association with tumor necrosis factor. J Rheumatol 1992;19:1505-1510.)*

Simple and low-cost methods for performing anthropometric assessment of body composition include the use of skinfold measurements (to estimate total body fat from subcutaneous fat), height, weight, waist-hip circumference ratio (for subcutaneous and intra-abdominal adipose tissue), and arm circumference (to estimate total body muscle and fat-free mass). In general, a combination of several skinfold measurements provides a more valid assessment of body fat than a single skinfold measurement, but none of these measures is sensitive enough to detect small changes in body fat or fat-free mass after short-term nutritional support or deprivation.[15] Other, more accurate methods for measuring body composition are available primarily for research purposes; these include total-body potassium using potassium-40, total-body water using isotope dilution, underwater weighing, and dual-energy x-ray absorptiometry, for example. Even with these methods, however, basic assumptions about the model may be invalid in patients with chronic disease and precision and accuracy may be reduced.

Biochemical assessment

Patients with RA often have lower concentrations of serum albumin and other markers of visceral protein status as a result of systemic inflammation. In addition, anemia of chronic disease is often associated with disordered iron metabolism, leading to low hemoglobin and hematocrit values. Vitamin B_6 status (determined by plasma pyridoxal-5′-phosphate) has also been shown to be abnormal in patients with RA and is associated with tumor necrosis factor-α (TNF-α) production by peripheral blood mononuclear cells.[16]

Clinical assessment

Clinical assessment consists of a medical history and physical examination of the patient. Disability can be measured using the disability scales of the Health Assessment Questionnaire (HAQ).[17] Self-reported pain scores can be determined using the HAQ visual analog pain scale. Balance and gait can be evaluated using the Tinetti Balance and Gait Evaluation,[18] and habitual gait speed can be assessed during a 4-meter walk. If a patient is limited by his or her disease in terms of activities of daily living, then physical activity will be reduced and overall nutritional status may be compromised.

Dietary assessment

Dietary assessment of patients' nutritional status is important, particularly if patients are following an alternative diet (see later for dietary therapies). A variety of methods are available, and the choice of which method to use depends on the goal of determining the intake. Repeated 24-hour recalls or replicated weighed or estimated food records can be used to determine actual or usual nutrient intakes of an individual.[15] A thorough dietary assessment also includes an evaluation of factors that may affect dietary intake, such as appetite, taste/smell changes, food allergies or intolerances, dental problems, dysphagia, or odynophagia.

RHEUMATOID CACHEXIA

Rheumatoid cachexia, meaning "bad condition" (literally translated from Greek), was not recognized as a common problem among patients with RA until relatively recently. It refers to the loss of body cell mass, predominantly skeletal muscle, that occurs in RA (see Fig. 45.3b). Loss of body weight does not always occur; in fact, loss of body cell mass is often accompanied by increased fat mass and stable body weight. In patients with RA, these changes predispose to a condition termed *rheumatoid cachectic obesity*, which, although seemingly contradictory, appears to be a common metabolic consequence of RA, affecting up to two thirds of all patients.[6,19,20] The average loss of body cell mass among patients with RA is between 13% and 15%,[19,20] which is approximately one third of the maximum survivable loss of body cell mass. Thus, rheumatoid cachexia should be viewed as an important contributor to increased morbidity and premature mortality in RA. Of note, features that often accompany loss of body cell mass in other disease states are noticeably absent in rheumatoid cachexia; these features may include renal or hepatic impairment, malabsorption, or high corticosteroid use.

A number of factors are likely involved in the pathogenesis of rheumatoid cachexia, including sarcoactive ("muscle active") cytokines, energy expenditure, protein metabolism, physical activity levels, and hormones.

Cytokines

The inflammatory cytokines TNF-α and interleukin (IL)-1β are centrally involved in the pathogenesis of RA, but in addition these cytokines exert a powerful influence on whole-body protein and energy metabolism. Other sarcoactive cytokines include IL-6, interferon (IFN)-α, tumor growth factor-β_1, and MyoD. We have shown that subjects with RA have higher rates of whole-body protein breakdown compared with young and elderly healthy subjects and, furthermore, that protein breakdown rates are directly associated with TNF-α production by peripheral blood mononuclear cells.[21] More recent research has suggested that skeletal muscle protein loss is dependent on the signaling activities of both TNF-α and IFN-α and that nuclear factor-kappa B (NF-κB) activity is needed for these cytokines to induce muscle damage.[22]

Energy expenditure

Total daily energy expenditure is determined by the following equation:

$$TEE = REE + EEPA + TEF,$$

where TEE is total energy expenditure, REE is resting energy expenditure, EEPA is energy expenditure of physical activity, and TEF is the thermic effect of food. In patients with RA, REE is elevated[19,20] but EEPA is reduced, such that TEE is also lower compared with healthy control subjects.[23] The implication of this is that patients need to be cautioned to maintain a diet that is adequate, but not excessive, in terms of protein and calories in an attempt to maintain muscle but prevent fat gain.

Protein metabolism

Adults with RA have increased whole-body protein breakdown rates (measured by ^{13}C-leucine infusion), which are directly associated with TNF-α production by peripheral blood mononuclear cells.[21] This finding is consistent with the reduced body cell mass that is found in subjects with RA.

Physical activity

Patients with RA often have reduced physical activity as a result of joint pain and stiffness, metabolic changes leading to loss of muscle mass and strength, and simple disuse, perhaps related to general cautiousness with regard to physical activity.

Hormones

Although the role of the growth hormone (GH)/insulin-like growth factor-1 (IGF-1) axis in altering muscle mass and strength during healthy aging is not fully understood, GH is known to decline with aging and has been suggested to play a role in the pathogenesis of sarcopenia (age-related muscle loss).[24] However, persistent GH deficiency does not appear to be the cause of rheumatoid cachexia.[24] Like GH, insulin is a potent anabolic hormone, and insulin resistance has been shown to occur in inflammatory arthritis.[25,26] It is possible that the metabolic milieu created by a state of insulin resistance may permit cytokine-driven muscle loss, although this remains speculative.[27] Of note, although the etiology of insulin resistance in RA is unclear, TNF-α has been shown to interfere with insulin receptor signaling and may be a contributing factor.[28] However, although anti-TNF therapy improves insulin resistance in RA it does not seem to reverse rheumatoid cachexia.[29,30]

MICRONUTRIENT ABNORMALITIES IN THE RHEUMATIC DISEASES

Our understanding of the impact of chronic inflammation on vitamin, mineral, and trace element nutrition is largely based on studies of RA and, to a lesser extent, SLE. There has been little systematic study of the nutritional status of most of the other rheumatic diseases. However, to the extent that systemic inflammation is common to a large group of rheumatic disorders, it is likely that the lessons of RA can be applied with reasonable success.

Vitamins

Inflammation increases metabolic rate, and thus the consumption of vitamin B_6 and vitamin C.[7,12] In addition, the excess production of free radicals in RA coincides with declines in antioxidant vitamins C and E.[11] It is tempting to conclude that these vitamins are consumed in an attempt to prevent oxidative damage to tissues, but this is unproven.

Vitamin B_6 appears to have the greatest sensitivity to inflammation, because it is markedly reduced in both animal models of arthritis and in humans with RA; the reduction correlates with disease severity and levels of acute-phase reactants (Fig. 45.4), and treatment with oral vitamin B_6 can reverse this drop, although it does not influence RA disease activity. Decreased vitamin B_6 appears to represent a true nutritional deficiency and not simply another acute-phase marker,

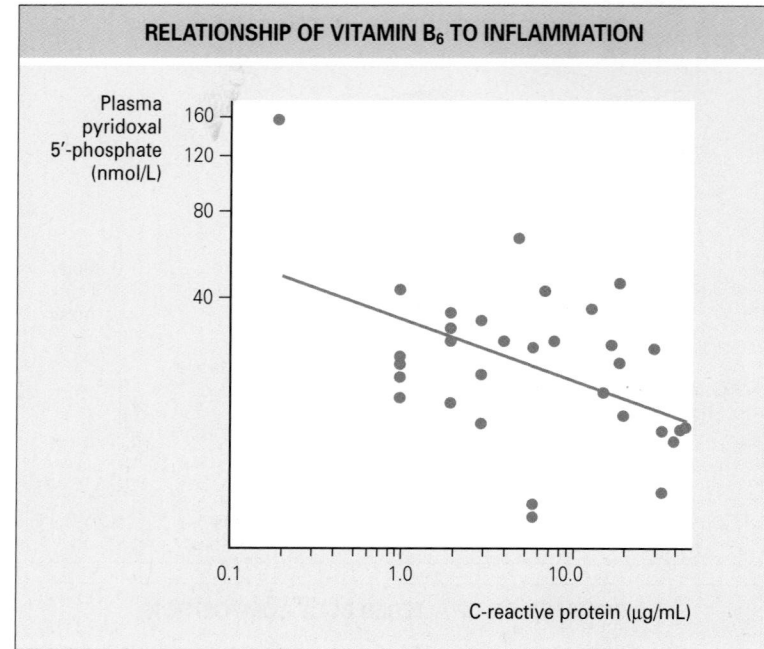

Fig. 45.4 Correlation between plasma vitamin B_6 and C-reactive protein ($r = -.39$, $P = .02$). *(From Chiang E-PI, Bagley P, Selhub J, et al. Abnormal vitamin B_6 status is associated with severity of symptoms in patients with rheumatoid arthritis. Am J Med 2003;114:283-287, with permission.)*

because there is evidence of deranged homocysteine metabolism in patients with low vitamin B_6 indices.[9] An elevated level of homocysteine is an important risk factor for atherosclerotic heart disease and stroke, which can be an important cause of complications in both RA and systemic lupus, as well as in the general population.[8]

Over the past decade, evidence has accumulated for the potential role of vitamin D in a variety of non-classic functions, including modulation of immune response.[31] Vitamin D deficiency has been linked to the occurrence of a variety of autoimmune diseases, but recent studies have not supported an association between either vitamin D intake[32] or vitamin D concentrations[33] and risk of RA or RA-related autoimmunity.

Vitamin E is the major fat-soluble antioxidant vitamin and acts with its water-soluble counterparts, vitamin C, and beta-carotene, to protect against free radical–mediated damage to cell membranes, DNA, and proteins. Although some observational studies have suggested that vitamin E may reduce the risk of developing RA due to its antioxidant properties, a recent, large, randomized controlled trial of women consuming 600 IU of vitamin E every other day found no association between vitamin E and risk of developing RA.[34]

There are also important drug/nutrient interactions that affect vitamin status in patients with rheumatic diseases. For example, corticosteroids antagonize vitamin D effects in the gut and kidney, exacerbating their direct calcium-wasting effects and promoting osteoporosis.[35] Methotrexate and sulfasalazine antagonize folic acid function in cells.[9] Oral contraceptives can interfere with vitamin B_6 and folic acid absorption. Coumadin, of course, works by antagonizing vitamin K and is used in patients with antiphospholipid syndrome and SLE. Grapefruit juice can increase the absorption of many drugs, including nifedipine, sirolimus, tacrolimus, and cyclosporine, leading to unexpected toxicity if taken intermittently.[36]

Minerals

Not surprisingly, calcium is the most important dietary mineral for patients with inflammatory diseases. The combination of systemic inflammation, with activation of cytokines such as TNF-α, IL-1β, and receptor activator of NF-κB ligand (RANKL), reduced physical activity due to joint pain, and corticosteroid therapy conspires to cause negative calcium balance and osteoporosis, especially in postmenopausal women. Women taking corticosteroids should take at least 1200 mg/day of calcium using diet and supplements, and 1500 mg may be preferable.

Iron is also a concern in rheumatic diseases, especially in RA. Iron deficiency is the most common micronutrient deficiency in women, occurring in up to 11% of menstruating women.[37] Chronic inflammation interferes with normal iron handling by bone marrow erythroblasts, leading to anemia of chronic disease. However, because RA and other inflammatory arthritides often occur in premenopausal women, iron deficiency may also be present. Distinguishing the two is very difficult unless a bone marrow biopsy is performed; more recently, the transferrin receptor has been used to help distinguish the two, although this test has a specificity of about 90% and it may not be universally available.[38]

Trace Elements

Trace and ultra-trace elements are present in the normal human diet in milligram and microgram concentrations, respectively.[39] The major trace elements affected by inflammation are zinc, copper, and selenium. These are all acute-phase reactants, and it is difficult to establish whether true deficiency of any of them occurs commonly in rheumatic diseases. All three can be toxic if taken in large doses, and excessive administration of supplements containing them should be discouraged. Copper and zinc behave reciprocally, so that excessive intake of one can lead to deficiency of the other. Selenium, an important part of the body's antioxidant defenses, is next to arsenic on the periodic table of elements and is dangerous in high doses.[40]

OBESITY AND RHEUMATIC DISEASE

Obesity is the major risk factor for OA of the knees and hips,[41] and there is evidence that this association is stronger with body fat than with total weight.[42] Weight loss seems to improve OA symptoms in patients with mild to moderate OA at least.[42-44] On the other hand, several studies have demonstrated that exercise training can improve the symptoms of knee OA, and there is a beneficial interaction with weight loss in this regard.[14,43] Although hip OA has not been as rigorously examined, it is likely that it also benefits from weight reduction.

Weight gain during young adulthood is also a risk factor for gout,[13] primarily in men. It is not known whether weight loss can reduce serum uric acid levels substantially, but some patients may benefit from this advice for a variety of reasons related to the gouty diathesis, such as hyperlipidemia, insulin resistance, and hypertension that often occurs with gout.

NUTRITION IN THE ROUTINE CARE OF THE RHEUMATIC DISEASE PATIENT

Although a comprehensive nutrition screening and evaluation is beyond the requirements of routine rheumatology care, a focused and systematic approach to nutritional assessment can be of great benefit to both patient and doctor in understanding the physiologic status of the patient and treating it properly. This should be neither time consuming nor avoided: if a major nutritional deficiency is found, referral to a registered dietitian is appropriate and should be done in a positive and professional manner. Patients care deeply about their diet and nutritional health, and physicians who dismiss or avoid this topic may jeopardize needlessly the doctor-patient relationship.

Simple habits that offer big returns

The first and most important point is to weigh the patient at every visit and record the weight; recording height once a year is also an excellent idea. This facilitates identification of nutritional risk: loss of more than 10% of body weight in a year or 5% in 6 months without intentional dieting is a red flag indicating a catabolic disease. This may be a rheumatic disease, a complication such as infection, or an unrelated malignancy. With the height, calculating the BMI in kilograms of weight/height per meters squared is simple and patients can be identified as underweight (BMI < 18.5 kg/m^2), overweight (BMI > 25 kg/m^2), or obese (BMI > 30 kg/m^2). Amazingly, such simple analyses are often forgotten in the haste to focus on the joints.

Another simple test is the serum albumin concentration. Although not directly a marker of malnutrition, because it is heavily influenced by cytokine levels, the serum albumin concentration is an excellent marker of overall physiologic status. A serum albumin level less than 3.0 mg/dL (30 g/L) is never normal and suggests ongoing stress with redirection of visceral protein synthesis toward immunoglobulins and away from homeostatic protein repletion.

Evaluation of micronutrient status can be done easily by selectively measuring two or three water-soluble vitamins (red blood cell folic acid, plasma vitamin B_6 [as pyridoxal phosphate], and plasma vitamin B_{12}) and one fat-soluble vitamin (25-hydroxyvitamin D_3), all of which are clinically available assays. These only need to be checked once every few years if patients are clinically stable. Patients at risk of osteoporosis—postmenopausal women, patients on long-term glucocorticoid therapy, smokers, and women with BMI less than 21 kg/m^2—should have their bone density measured by dual x-ray absorptiometry.

It is also important to ascertain what dietary supplements patients are taking and whether they are restricting their diet in any meaningful way. This information is rarely volunteered but is easy to elicit. On the other hand, failure to recognize that a patient is taking St. John's wort or other "nutritional" supplements may lead to untoward drug interactions that are otherwise very puzzling.

When to refer a patient for nutritional consultation

The most common reason for referring a patient to a nutritional professional—dietitian or physician—is for prescribing weight loss. This is certainly appropriate for patients with knee or hip OA and a BMI greater than 30 kg/m^2. Patients with OA and a BMI greater than 40 kg/m^2 (or >35 kg/m^2 with complications such as diabetes or metabolic syndrome) are candidates for bariatric surgery if they cannot lose weight by dieting alone. No clinical trials have compared the efficacy of weight reduction surgery with joint replacement surgery for patients with moderate to severe OA, but it is a reasonable hypothesis that weight loss may improve OA symptoms in some patients. New medications for weight loss are in development and are likely to become part of routine clinical care in the next decade. Medications should be used as part of a comprehensive treatment program that includes behavioral therapy, diet, and exercise.

Conversely, unintentional weight loss or persistent low weight (BMI < 18.5 kg/m^2) should also promote a referral. Nutritional evaluation in this setting can help by documenting whether typical daily dietary energy intake explains the weight loss. If not, then malabsorption or catabolic illness should be considered. A dietitian can estimate average dietary caloric and nutrient intakes, compare these to expected expenditures, and prescribe a diet appropriate to the patient's goals. The rheumatologist can facilitate this through encouragement and demonstrating that this is an important facet of the patient's management.

NUTRITIONAL TREATMENT IN THE RHEUMATIC DISEASES

Rheumatoid cachexia

Although the specific mechanism(s) by which rheumatoid cachexia develops have not been fully described, what is clear is that the functional consequences of this condition are to increase morbidity and mortality in patients with RA. Accordingly, efforts to slow and/or reverse the loss of body cell mass that occurs in RA must be made if functional status is going to be improved. There are essentially three possible interventions: exercise, diet, and pharmacology.

Exercise

Strength training should be considered an important aspect of the nonpharmacologic treatment of RA and should be routinely prescribed. Studies have found that high-intensity strength training is feasible and safe in patients with well-controlled disease and that there can be significant improvements in strength, pain, and fatigue without exacerbation of disease activity or joint symptoms.[45]

Diet

Dietary intake appears to be adequate in terms of energy and protein intake among most patients with RA[3,21]; this, in combination with a reduced TEE, provides evidence that clinicians should not routinely recommend increased dietary energy intake to patients with RA.

Further studies are needed to determine optimal protein intakes for overcoming the catabolic process in RA, particularly when patients participate in an ongoing exercise program. As a general rule, we recommend 1.2 to 1.5 g/kg protein per day, which is 50% to 85% above the Dietary Reference Intake and comparable to the U.S. average intake of 1.2 g/kg/day. There is no evidence that higher protein intakes are useful, and they may cause harm by increasing the metabolic load on the kidneys and liver.

Micronutrient deficiencies

Most vitamin deficiencies in patients with arthritis and connective tissue diseases are adequately treated with daily multivitamin preparations that provide the Recommended Dietary Allowance (RDA) of vitamins and minerals. There is no convincing evidence that larger doses than the RDA are required for patients with rheumatic diseases as long as they eat a healthy and varied diet with adequate fresh fruits, vegetables, and appropriate amounts of high-quality protein. In other words, the U.S. Government's diet pyramid (http://www.mypyramid.gov/) is a reasonable starting point for keeping patients nutritionally healthy.

Treating nutritional deficiencies in patients with inflammatory disease

There are legitimate debates about the value of additional nutrients that could help support the host faced with chronic inflammation in the setting of RA and other inflammatory diseases. Most rheumatologists treat patients taking methotrexate with daily folic acid or weekly folinic acid to minimize the side effects of the drug. Fortification of the U.S. food supply with folate in the mid 1990s substantially improved the population's folate status and coincided with an increase in methotrexate dosing in our clinic.[46] At the same time, we have shown that supplementing the diet with 50 mg/day of vitamin B_6 normalizes low vitamin B_6 levels in patients with RA.[47] However, there is no anti-inflammatory or clinical benefit of this supplementation.

Patients with diseases that increase sedentary behavior should be counseled to avoid high saturated fats and excessive cholesterol in their diets. In addition, they should meet the age-specific recommendations for calcium and iron intake. Patients taking prednisone should take at least 1200 mg/day of calcium as supplements or food, and 1500 mg would be better for young women. Adequate dietary phosphate, such as that found in milk products, enhances the bioavailability of dietary calcium. Excess phosphates, such as those in carbonated sodas, do not have this benefit. Adequate vitamin D is also essential, and it is likely that 800 IU/day is more appropriate than 400 IU/day.[48] Physicians must do their part by measuring bone density at 2-year intervals in patients taking corticosteroids who are at risk of osteoporosis and prescribing antiresorptive agents as necessary. Prevention of fractures in these patients is a crucial way to preserve their quality of life.

Obesity should be treated as a separate health issue in patients with arthritis and treated aggressively. Arthritis reduces the interest in exercise and teaches people to stay sedentary, thus facilitating further weight gain and more joint pain. Patients with RA who achieve good disease control are subject to weight gain and the combination of low lean body mass and rising fat mass—"sarcopenic obesity"—which gives them the worst of both worlds in terms of risk factors for frailty and loss of independence.[49] Diet and exercise programs have been developed and tested that are safe for home use in patients with arthritis, including our own.[50] The cost is minimal and we have found the results quite satisfactory.

NUTRITION AS AN ANTI-INFLAMMATORY TREATMENT

The field of nutritional treatment of rheumatic diseases is one that is of intense interest to patients and often of profound ignorance among physicians. The published literature in this area is contradictory, often confused by poor methodology and sometimes difficult to find. One important resource is the Arthritis Foundation[51]; another is the National Institutes of Health's Office of Dietary Supplements (http://dietary-supplements.info.nih.gov). Most dietary supplements for treating arthritis must be considered unproven remedies; this is charitable—many are quack nostrums designed to separate patients from their money. A few have been investigated rigorously, and we will describe these. A discussion of glucosamine and chondroitin sulfate, which are dietary components used as pharmaceutical treatment of OA, is found in Chapter 47.

Diet therapy of inflammatory arthritis

Dietary modifications that have been proposed as therapy for patients with RA include fasting, vegetarianism, and various forms of nutrient supplementation.[52] A recent systematic review on this topic concluded that the benefits of various diets, including vegetarian, vegan, Mediterranean, elemental, or elimination diets, remain unclear and that some dietary manipulations may even be harmful.[44]

Although there are no specific diet therapies that have been shown to successfully treat RA, a considerable amount of research has investigated the possible therapeutic benefits in terms of symptomatic relief. Some patients may benefit from supplementation of specific nutrients, particularly if dietary intake is not varied enough to provide adequate amounts of micronutrients.

Antioxidant nutrients

Most studies involving vitamin or mineral supplementation in inflammatory arthritis have focused on the antioxidant nutrients, including vitamin C, vitamin E, beta carotene, and selenium. Vitamin D has also generated considerable interest recently. In general, randomized controlled trials have been of relatively short duration and have led to conflicting results, so there continues to be a lack of concrete evidence to support nutrient supplementation at a particular dose.[53] Furthermore, providing individual nutrients in the form of supplements does not necessarily offer the same overall health benefit as when nutrients are consumed from whole foods. It is possible that the combination of nutrients that are present in whole foods, or even some unidentified components of a food, are responsible for any observed beneficial effects. Patients with RA should be encouraged to increase their intake of foods high in antioxidant nutrients, such as vitamin E–rich edible vegetable oils (sunflower, safflower, canola, olive) and unprocessed cereal grain, and of fresh fruits and vegetables rich in vitamin C and beta carotene. Foods high in *trans* fats, high fructose corn syrup, or other calorie-dense ingredients, should be limited.

Dietary fatty acids

Omega-3 fatty acids, derived primarily from marine sources (fish and shellfish) may affect the immunologic and inflammatory responses of RA as a result of altered cellular eicosanoid production. Specifically, the fatty acids eicosapentaenoic acid (EPA) and docosahexaenoic acid (DHA) act as competitive substrates with arachidonic acid (AA), thereby inhibiting the oxidation of AA by cyclooxygenase and lipoxygenase enzymes. Arachidonic acid is the predominant fatty acid found in the typical Western diet, and the net result of a substrate shift from AA to EPA (or DHA) is a change in the regulation of various homeostatic functions mediated by the eicosanoids, including inflammation and cytokine synthesis. Randomized clinical trials of fish oil in RA have shown that EPA supplementation at doses ranging from 3 to 6 g/day may lead to improvement in the number of tender joints and morning stiffness.[54] Additional benefit may be achieved by combining a diet low in AA with fish oil supplements.[44,55] Symptomatic relief may be delayed by several months after starting fish oil supplementation, and relief may occur in a dose-related manner; non-steroidal anti-inflammatory drug sparing has also been reported with the use of fish oil supplements.[56]

CONCLUSION

Nutrition is a crucial determinant of the health of all people; ignoring it in chronic disease removes an important tool from the rheumatologist's "belt." With a few minor efforts, nutritional evaluation and therapy can be part of routine rheumatologic care, with important benefits to patient and caregiver. The impetus for paying attention to nutrition comes from our patients; as clinicians, we can empower patients with correct information and scientifically based treatments that can have far-ranging physiologic benefits.

KEY REFERENCES

1. Paget J. Nervous mimicry of organic diseases. Lancet 1873;2:727-729.
3. Walsmith J, Abad L, Kehayias J, Roubenoff R. Tumor necrosis factor-alpha production is associated with less body cell mass in women with rheumatoid arthritis. J Rheumatol 2004;31:23-29.
4. Giles J, Bartlett S, Anderson R, et al. Association of body composition with disability in rheumatoid arthritis: impact of appendicular fat and lean tissue mass. Arthritis Care Res 2008;59:1407-1415.
5. Kremers H, Nicola P, Crowson C, et al. Prognostic importance of low body mass index in relation to cardiovascular mortality in rheumatoid arthritis. Arthritis Rheum 2004;50:3450-3457.
6. Engvall I-L, Elkan A-C, Tengstrand B, et al. Cachexia in rheumatoid arthritis is associated with inflammatory activity, physical disability, and low bioavailable insulin-like growth factor. Scand J Rheumatol 2008;37:321-328.
7. Chiang E-PI, Bagley P, Selhub J, et al. Abnormal vitamin B_6 status is associated with severity of symptoms in patients with rheumatoid arthritis. Am J Med 2003;114:283-287.
8. Petri M, Roubenoff R, Nadeau M, et al. Homocysteine: an independent risk factor for stroke in systemic lupus erythematosus. Lancet 1996;348:1120-1124.
9. Roubenoff R, Dellaripa P, Nadeau M, et al. Abnormal homocysteine metabolism in rheumatoid arthritis. Arthritis Rheum 1997;40:718-722.
10. Blake D, Merry P, Unsworth J, et al. Hypoxic-reperfusion injury in the inflamed human joint. Lancet 1989;1:289-293.
11. Comstock GW, Burke AE, Hoffman SC, et al. Serum concentrations of alpha tocopherol, beta carotene, and retinol preceding the diagnosis of rheumatoid arthritis and systemic lupus erythematosus. Ann Rheum Dis 1997;56:323-325.
12. Burnham R, Russell A. Nutritional status in patients with rheumatoid arthritis. Ann Rheum Dis 1986;44:788-789.
13. Roubenoff R, Klag M, Mead L, et al. Incidence and risk factors for gout in white men. JAMA 1991;266:3004-3007.
14. Baker K, Nelson M, Felson D, et al. The efficacy of home-based progressive strength training in older adults with knee osteoarthritis: a randomized controlled trial. J Rheumatol 2001;28:1655-1665.
15. Gibson RS. Principles of nutritional assessment. New York: Oxford University Press, 1990.
16. Roubenoff R, Roubenoff R, Selhub J, et al. Abnormal vitamin B_6 status in rheumatoid arthritis: association with tumor necrosis factor-α production and markers of inflammation. Arthritis Rheum 1995;38:105-109.
18. Tinetti M. Performance-oriented assessment of mobility problems in elderly patients. J Am Geriatr Soc 1986;34:119-126.
19. Roubenoff R, Roubenoff R, Cannon J, et al. Rheumatoid cachexia: cytokine-driven hypermetabolism

accompanying reduced body cell mass in chronic inflammation. J Clin Invest 1994;93:2379-2386.
20. Roubenoff R, Roubenoff R, Ward L, et al. Rheumatoid cachexia: depletion of lean body mass in rheumatoid arthritis: possible association with tumor necrosis factor. J Rheumatol 1992;19:1505-1510.
21. Rall L, Rosen C, Dolnikowski G, et al. Protein metabolism in rheumatoid arthritis and aging: effects of muscle strength training and tumor necrosis factor-alpha. Arthritis Rheum 1996;39:1115-1124.
22. Guttridge D, Mayo M, Madrid L, et al. NF-kappaB–induced loss of MyoD messenger RNA: possible role in muscle decay and cachexia. Science 2000;289:2363-2366.
23. Roubenoff R, Walsmith J, Lundgren N, et al. Low physical activity reduces total energy expenditure in women with rheumatoid arthritis: implications for dietary intake recommendations. Am J Clin Nutr 2002;76:774-779.
24. Rall L, Roubenoff R, Veldhuis J, et al. Cachexia of rheumatoid arthritis is not explained by decreased growth hormone. Arthritis Rheum 2002;46:2574-2577.
25. Dessein P, Joffe B. Insulin resistance and impaired beta cell function in rheumatoid arthritis. Arthritis Rheum 2006;54:2765-2775.
26. Chung C, Oeser A, Solus J, et al. Inflammation-associated insulin resistance. Arthritis Rheum 2008;58:2105-2112.
28. DeAlvaro C, Teruel T, Hernandez R, Lorenzo M. Tumor necrosis factor alpha produces insulin resistance in skeletal muscle by activation of inhibitor kappa B kinase in a p38 MAPK-dependent manner. J Biol Chem 2004;279:17070-17078.
29. Straub R, Harle P, Sarzi-Puttini P, Cutolo M. Tumor necrosis factor–neutralizing therapies improve altered hormone axes. Arthritis Rheum 2006;54:2039-2046.
30. Metsios G, Stavropoulos-Kalinoglou A, Douglas K, et al. Blockade of tumor necrosis factor-alpha in rheumatoid arthritis: effects on components of rheumatoid cachexia. Rheumatology 2007;46:1824-1827.
31. Bikle D. Nonclassic actions of vitamin D. J Clin Endocrinol Metab 2009;94:26-34.
32. Costenbader K, Feskanich D, Holmes M, et al. Vitamin D intake and risks of systemic lupus erythematosus and rheumatoid arthritis in women. Ann Rheum Dis 2008;68:446-447.
34. Karlson E, Shadick N, Cook N, et al. Vitamin E in the primary prevention of rheumatoid arthritis: the Women's Health Study. Arthritis Rheum 2008;59:589-595.
35. Hahn T, Halstead L, Teitelbaum S, Hahn B. Altered mineral metabolism in glucocorticoid-induced osteopenia: effect of 25-hydroxyvitamin D administration. J Clin Invest 1979;64:655-666.
36. Hollander A, van Rooij J, Lentjes G, et al. The effect of grapefruit juice on cyclosporine and prednisone metabolism in transplant patients. Clin Pharmacol Ther 1995;57:318-324.

39. Nielsen F. Ultratrace elements in nutrition: current knowledge and speculation. J Trace Elements Exp Med 1998;11:251-274.
41. Felson D, Zhang Y, Hannan M, et al. Risk factors for incident radiographic knee osteoarthritis in the elderly. Arthritis Rheum 1997;40:728-733.
42. Toda Y, Toda T, Takemura S, et al. Change in body fat, but not body weight or metabolic correlates of obesity, is related to symptomatic relief of obese patients with knee osteoarthritis after a weight control program. J Rheumatol 1998;25:2181-2186.
43. Messier S, Loeser R, Miller G, et al. Exercise and dietary weight loss in overweight and obese older adults with knee osteoarthritis. Arthritis Rheum 2004;50:1501-1510.
44. Hagen K, Byfuglien M, Falzon L, et al. Dietary interventions for rheumatoid arthritis. Cochrane Database Syst Rev 2009;1:CD006400.
45. Rall L, Meydani S, Kehayias J, et al. The effect of progressive resistance training in rheumatoid arthritis: increased strength without changes in energy balance or body composition. Arthritis Rheum 1996;39:415-426.
46. Arabelovic S, Sam G, Dallal G, et al. Folic acid fortification of the food supply may interfere with the effectiveness of methotrexate for the treatment of rheumatoid arthritis. J Am Coll Nutr 2007;26:453-455.
47. Chiang E-P, Bagley P, Selhub J, et al. Efficacy of pyridoxine supplementation on biochemical and functional status of vitamin B_6 in patients with rheumatoid arthritis. Arthritis Res Ther 2005;7:R1404-R1411.
48. Bischoff-Ferrari H, Willett W, Wong J, et al. Fracture prevention with vitamin D supplementation: a meta-analysis of controlled trials. JAMA 2005;293:2257-2264.
49. Roubenoff R. Sarcopenic obesity: does muscle loss cause fat gain? Ann N Y Acad Sci 2000;904:553-557.
50. Nelson M, Baker K, Roubenoff R, Lindner L. Strong women and men beat arthritis. New York: Putnam, 2002.
51. Horstman J. The Arthritis Foundation's guide to alternative therapies. Atlanta: Arthritis Foundation, 1999.
52. Rall L, Roubenoff R, eds. Dietary aspects of the aetiology and nutritional management of inflammatory degenerative arthritis. London: Academic Press, 1999.
53. Rennie K. Nutritional management of rheumatoid arthritis: a review of the evidence. J Hum Nutr Dietetics 2003;16:97-109.
54. Cleland L, James M, Proudman S. The role of fish oils in the treatment of rheumatoid arthritis. Drugs 2003;63:845-853.
55. Adam O, Beringer C, Kless T, et al. Anti-inflammatory effects of a low arachidonic acid diet and fish oil in patients with rheumatoid arthritis. Rheum Int 2003;23:27-36.
56. Proudman S, Cleland L, James M. Dietary omega-3 fats for treatment of inflammatory joint disease: efficacy and utility. Rheum Dis Clin North Am 2008;34:469-479.

REFERENCES

Full references for this chapter can be found on www.expertconsult.com.

Principles of rehabilitation: physical and occupational therapy

G. Kelley Fitzgerald and Nancy Baker

46

- Rehabilitation is the process of enabling persons with impairments, activity limitations, or disabilities which cause suboptimal participation in various life situations (self-care, work, recreation and leisure, or community life) to regain or obtain the capacities necessary to participate at an optimal level. Rehabilitation, therefore, requires determining the optimal level of function, identifying the barriers that prevent the individual from obtaining that level of function, and providing interventions which facilitate the attainment of that optimal level.

- Rehabilitation interventions can be classified as either remedial or adaptive processes.
    - Remedial rehabilitation works to *restore* or *establish* capacity or ability. It focuses on improving impairments in muscular strength and endurance, joint motion, cardiorespiratory fitness, balance and coordination, cognitive function (depression, anxiety, fear, self-efficacy), and may also refer to retraining in lost skill sets, such as self-care, dexterity, and/or work skills.
    - Adaptive rehabilitation works to *compensate* for lost or absent capacity or ability. It focuses on providing alternative or supplementary methods to perform a task or activity to optimize the performance. Adaptive rehabilitation includes use of equipment that substitutes for lost capacities, teaching new methods of performing tasks which incorporate existing capacities, altering the environment to facilitate performance, and/or changing the requirements of the task.

- Most rehabilitation therapists use a combination of remedial and adaptive rehabilitation methods to obtain optimal function.

- Because rehabilitation is a multi-factorial process it will often require a multi-disciplinary team approach to optimize the restoration of function for people with rheumatologic disorders.

DEFINITION OF REHABILITATION

The United Nations defines rehabilitation as "a goal-orientated, time-limited process aimed at enabling an impaired person to reach an optimum mental, physical, and/or social level."[1] Rehabilitation is the process of enabling persons with impairments, activity limitations, or disabilities that cause suboptimal participation in various life situations (self-care, work, recreation and leisure, or community life) to regain or obtain the capacities necessary to participate at an optimal level. Rehabilitation, therefore, requires determining the optimal level of function, identifying the barriers that prevent the individual from obtaining that level of function, and providing interventions that facilitate the attainment of that optimal level.

PATIENT-CENTERED APPROACH TO REHABILITATION

Rehabilitation therapists should use a patient-centered approach to determine the optimal level of function in a patient with arthritis because each person's optimal level of function depends on what that person *needs* to be able to do as well as what the person *wants* to be able to do. Thus, a 75-year-old woman with moderate to severe knee osteoarthritis who lives in the community may have different "needs to be able to do" than a comparable woman living in a nursing home, although their "wants to be able to do" may be very similar. The optimal level of function for these two women may be very different: one may have to complete physically demanding tasks related to home care such as vacuuming or making beds, meal preparation, and drive or use public transportation to interact within the community, whereas the other may need to have the physical capacity to perform basic self-care tasks. To determine the optimal level of function, the rehabilitation therapist must work with the patient to identify the types of activities that the patient needs or wants to perform as well as the environmental or social context in which the activities will be enacted.

Once the patient's optimal level of function has been targeted, the next step is to identify barriers that prevent the patient from achieving this optimal level. Both the rehabilitation therapist and patient work together using a thorough examination process to identify these barriers. Patient-reported measures of pain and function as well as performance-based measures of function should be used to identify the types of functional tasks that are problematic and to quantify the severity of these problems. Physical examination procedures are used to identify the presence of physical impairments (e.g., muscle weakness, loss of joint motion and joint stiffness, joint instability, balance and coordination deficits) that may be associated with the functional problems. An assessment of the patient's living or work environments may be undertaken to identify environmental or social support factors that could be either potential barriers or potential assets in obtaining optimal function. Assessment of biobehavioral characteristics (e.g., anxiety, fear, depression, self-efficacy) may be helpful to determine if any of these factors are influencing physical activity or responsiveness to rehabilitation interventions.

After specific barriers have been identified through the examination process, the rehabilitation therapist and patient design and implement a rehabilitation intervention program that addresses the specific barriers to optimal function. Rehabilitation interventions can be classified as either remedial or adaptive processes. *Remedial* rehabilitation works to *restore* or *establish* capacity or ability. It focuses on improving impairments in muscular strength and endurance, joint motion, cardiorespiratory fitness, balance and coordination, and cognitive function (depression, anxiety, fear, self-efficacy) and may also refer to retraining in lost skill sets, such as self-care, dexterity, or work skills. *Adaptive* rehabilitation works to *compensate* for lost or absent capacity or ability. It focuses on providing alternative or supplementary methods to perform a task or activity to optimize the performance. Adaptive rehabilitation includes the following methods:

- Providing equipment that substitutes for lost capacities
- Teaching new methods of performing tasks that incorporate existing capacities
- Altering the environment to facilitate performance
- Changing the requirements of the task

Most rehabilitation therapists use a combination of remedial and adaptive rehabilitation methods to obtain optimal function.

We hope at this point that the reader understands that the rehabilitation process is multifactorial, that a variety of factors and issues must be addressed to achieve the goal of obtaining optimal function and participation in life for the individual patient with arthritis. Thus, it is logical that the rehabilitation process would require a multidisciplinary approach to achieve these goals. The following discussion is presented mainly from the perspective of two of these disciplines: physical therapy and occupational therapy. However, it should be recognized that depending on the specific problems and needs of the individual patient, services of other health care professionals, such as clinical psychologists, vocational rehabilitation counselors, rehabilitation engineers, or recreational therapists should be employed to provide the most comprehensive care for each patient.

Although it would make things easier if we were to have a clear line of distinction between the roles and responsibilities of the physical and occupational therapies, in reality, this is not the case. In fact, there are many areas in the rehabilitation process in which the roles and responsibilities of physical and occupational therapies overlap. For example, both disciplines use methods to address a variety of impairments related to functional deficits. Both disciplines also employ methods of functional retraining, education in joint protection techniques, and the use of assistive devices in their treatment programs. Because of the significant overlap in roles and responsibilities between these two disciplines, we will not differentiate between them in this chapter in the presentation of methods and issues related to the rehabilitation of people with arthritis.

REMEDIAL REHABILITATION APPROACHES

Pain control

Pain is a major cause of disability in people with arthritis. Physical agents, including thermal agents and electrical stimulation, have been included in recommendations for the treatment of pain in people with arthritis.[2,3] Thermal agents include hot or cold packs, paraffin, short-wave diathermy (SWD), ultrasound (US), and low-level laser modalities. The evidence supporting the use of these interventions for pain control is not particularly strong at present and seems to support selective rather than global use of these modalities. Low-level laser therapy has been shown to provide some relief of pain and stiffness in the feet, knees, and hands of patients with rheumatoid arthritis (RA) and also of knee pain in patients with knee osteoarthritis (OA).[3,4] Ultrasound used in water at 0.5 W/cm^2 has shown to demonstrate some small benefits in relief of hand pain in patients with RA but was not effective for relieving knee pain in patients with knee OA or in patients with back pain.[3,5,6] Paraffin applied to the hand in combination with an exercise program seems helpful in reducing pain and stiffness and improving range of motion in patients with RA and in those with scleroderma, but the use of paraffin alone does not seem to be beneficial.[7,8]

A recent randomized clinical trial compared the combined use of exercise with either hot packs, hot packs and US, hot packs and SWD, or hot packs and transcutaneous electrical nerve stimulation (TENS) to exercise alone in women with knee OA.[9] The researchers reported greater improvements in pain relief when exercise was combined with the thermal agent interventions. There were, however, no clinically meaningful differences in pain relief between any of the thermal agent groups, suggesting that a hot pack alone with exercise may be adequate in achieving the beneficial effects. A recent, non-randomized pilot study was conducted to examine changes in synovial pouch thickness and pain between the use of coiled SWD, SWD combined with a non-steroidal anti-inflammatory drug, and a control group in patients with knee OA.[10] There were significant reductions in synovial pouch thickness and pain in both intervention groups compared with the control group; however, the treatment effects were not different between groups, suggesting that SWD alone was adequate in obtaining the effects. Further study is needed to determine the effectiveness of SWD in relieving pain in patients with arthritis.

TENS, the process of providing an electrical stimulus through the skin using surface electrodes for the purpose of reducing pain, has been shown to be effective in the treatment of pain. There are many different applications of TENS that combine various stimulus parameters (pulse frequency, pulse duration, pulse amplitude) and various treatment durations. Low-frequency, high-amplitude TENS (sometimes referred to as acupuncture-like TENS) was shown to be effective for relieving hand and wrist pain in patients with RA, whereas higher-frequency TENS was not.[3] In patients with knee OA, greater pain relief was observed when high-intensity burst modes and acupuncture-like TENS

were used than when high-frequency TENS was used. Repeated use of TENS was more effective than a single treatment, and TENS was more effective than placebo when it was used for a duration of 4 weeks or more.[11] Use of TENS for less than 4 weeks was no more effective than placebo.[11] Use of TENS has been advocated as a stand-alone treatment for pain in published treatment guidelines for arthritis.[2,3,12] TENS has not been found to be effective for treatment of low back pain.[6]

In summary, although there is a place for the use of thermal agents and TENS for pain control in people with arthritis, their use should be limited to selective cases rather than global applications across all people with arthritis. When considering rising costs of health care, many patients may be better served by instructing them in the home use of hot packs, warm baths, paraffin, or TENS for pain control, rather than having them make frequent visits to therapy to receive these treatments. An alternative to the use of physical agents for pain control is the use of exercise and physical activity. A number of different types of exercise activities including aerobics and strengthening exercises may have a systemic effect on modulating pain. Studies have shown a reduction in pain thresholds to different types of pain stimuli at areas remote from the exercised limb segments, suggesting a centralized, systemic response.[13,14] Splinting has also been shown to reduce pain. We will address the use of various exercise applications for improving pain and function in subsequent sections of this chapter.

Range of motion

Loss of joint motion is a common impairment associated with arthritis. Limitations in joint motion or joint stiffness can increase the difficulty of performing activities of daily living, resulting in greater disability. It is also conceivable that with reduced joint motion, there is less available joint surface area for distributing compression and shear loads across the joint surface. This could result in a more concentrated loading in smaller areas of the joint surface, leading to increased joint stress and potentially accelerating the progression of arthritis. Therefore, addressing limitations in joint motion is an important element of rehabilitation for people with arthritis. Published guidelines for the treatment of hip and knee OA recommend the use of treatments designed to maintain or improve joint mobility.[2] Such interventions may include stretching exercise (sometimes referred to as flexibility exercise), joint mobilization, muscle-strengthening exercise, and splinting to improve pain, function, and joint motion.[2,15,16] In this section, we will discuss stretching exercise and joint mobilization interventions designed to improve joint motion. Strengthening exercise and splinting are discussed in subsequent sections of this chapter.

Stretching exercises are designed to increase the length of soft tissue structures, such as the joint capsule and musculotendinous units, that may be limiting joint motion. Stretching exercise involves moving the joint to the end of the available range of motion and then applying some manual overpressure to increase the passive tension in the target soft tissue structures. The stretch position should induce enough passive tension in the target structure to elicit a "slight stretch discomfort" but not to the extent that joint or soft tissue pain is elicited. This position is then held for a period of time. Although few studies have specifically studied stretching exercise dosage in people with arthritis, there are studies that have examined dosage in elderly subjects.

In a small randomized trial of 19 female subjects between the ages of 65 to 89 years with limited ankle dorsiflexion motion, subjects who received an 8-week calf-stretching program, consisting of 10 repetitions of a 15-second hold at the end of the available range of ankle dorsiflexion, had improved ankle dorsiflexion, higher agility test scores, and faster walking speeds compared with control subjects.[17] Hamstring stretching for a duration of 60 seconds, five times per week in subjects who are 65 years and older with limited hamstring length, yielded the best improvements in knee extension motion with longer lasting effects, compared with stretches performed at 15 and 30 seconds of duration.[18] Although the most effective dosage for stretching may vary from muscle to muscle, it appears from these studies that improvements in muscle length and joint motion may be obtained from moderate-intensity stretching exercise. Patients who can hold a position for longer durations may not need to do as many repetitions. Likewise, if they cannot tolerate holding the stretch position for longer periods, benefits may still be obtained by performing more repetitions at shorter durations. Adding a modest weight (0.45 to 1.35 kg) to assist in holding the stretch position during exercise also seems to enhance the effects of a stretching exercise on improving joint motion in elderly subjects.[19]

Joint mobilization techniques are frequently used to improve joint motion, by improving accessory joint motions (i.e., sliding or distractions between joint surfaces) that accompany normal joint motion. For example, during knee flexion, the tibia slides posteriorly on the femur during the flexion motion of the joint. If this posterior sliding is limited, there will be limited knee flexion motion. The therapist performs joint mobilization techniques designed to restore the normal posterior slide, which, in turn, improves the knee flexion motion. Joint mobilization techniques vary, depending on the joint motions being targeted and the accessory motions that accompany the targeted motions. Higher-intensity mobilizations (oscillations of the accessory motions near the end of the available range) are used to improve joint motion, but lower-intensity mobilizations (oscillations of the accessory motions in the middle of the available range) can be used to induce relaxation and perhaps pain modulation.

There have been only a few studies examining the effects of joint mobilization in patients with arthritis. In a randomized clinical trial in patients with knee OA, the combined use of joint mobilization with a supervised stretching and strengthening exercise program for all impaired lower extremity joints and the spine resulted in greater improvements in self-reported and performance-based measures of function than when only a home exercise program without joint mobilization was employed.[20] Changes in knee motion were not reported in this study. Similarly, in a randomized trial in patients with hip OA, subjects receiving a distraction joint manipulation technique combined with lower extremity stretching and strengthening had greater improvements in pain, self-reported hip function, hip range of motion, and walking speed than subjects randomized to exercise without hip manipulation.[21] In these studies, groups receiving exercise only did not appear to receive equivalent exercise programs to the groups receiving the joint mobilization/manipulation techniques. Therefore, the exact contribution of these techniques to the outcomes is not clear. At any rate, the combined use of the joint mobilization techniques with other exercises appeared helpful. Furthermore, it should be noted that the interventions were designed to address limitations in joint mobility of all joints in the lower extremity and not just in the knee or hip. This underscores the need to examine and address all existing impaired joint motions to maximize the effects of rehabilitation.

Muscle strength

Muscle strengthening is recognized as an important element of rehabilitation for people with arthritis.[2,15,22,23] Muscle weakness is frequently associated with greater disability in patients with arthritis and, in some cases, such as knee osteoarthritis, there is debate as to whether muscle weakness may be a precursor to arthritis. In addition, muscles can play a significant role in absorbing and dissipating loads across joints, which may help to reduce pain and prevent damage to the joint structures. Muscle-strengthening programs have resulted in reduced pain, increased muscle force output, and improvements in performance-based and self-reported function measures for some people with various forms of arthritis.[2,15,22,23]

There are several alternative types of strengthening exercises. Isometric exercises involve contracting the muscle against a resistance without allowing joint motion to occur. These types of exercises are usually performed at multiple angles throughout the joint range of motion. Isotonic exercise involves moving a constant amount of resistance through the joint range of motion. Weight-lifting exercises are a type of isotonic exercise. In some clinic settings, computerized dynamometers are available to allow for isokinetic exercise, in which resisted muscle contractions can be performed through a range of motion at constant velocity. There have been few studies performed comparing the effectiveness of isometric, isotonic, and isokinetic exercise. Recent studies indicate that all three types can improve pain, walking speed, muscle strength, and self-reported disability.[24,25] In one study, isotonic exercise resulted in the best results for pain control and isokinetic exercise resulted in the best results for walking speed.[24] More

subjects in the isokinetic group terminated the study earlier, presumably owing to increased pain symptoms.[24]

Both isotonic and isokinetic exercise involve moving the joint against resistance through a range of motion. These types of exercise may expose the joint to greater shearing forces compared with isometric exercise. We have found in our experience that when patients with arthritis have difficulty performing resisted motions, isometric exercises seem to be a more tolerable alternative. The reason for this may be that because there is no joint motion during the muscle contraction, there is less shearing applied to the joint, which may make the exercise more tolerable.

Strengthening exercises can be designed to use concentric or eccentric contractions. During concentric contractions the limb is accelerated against an external resistance (e.g., gravity, weights), resulting in an overall shortening of muscle length during the movement. During eccentric contractions the limb is decelerated against an external resistance, resulting in an overall lengthening of the muscle.

Functional activities involve combinations of isometric, isotonic, concentric, and eccentric muscle contractions. Therefore, a well-rounded strengthening program should include activities that involve each of these types of muscle contractions. Recently, some investigators have explored the use of functional task-specific strengthening in elderly subjects.[26,27] In this type of training, the therapist and the patient identify which functional tasks are most problematic. The therapist then breaks the task up into segments that can be used as strengthening exercises. In this manner, patients train their weak muscles exactly as they will need to use them to perform tasks. As the patient gets stronger, the therapist adjusts how the patient performs the task-specific exercise, demanding more effort from the target muscles as they get stronger. There is some evidence to suggest that this approach may be more effective in improving overall function than standard exercise approaches.[26,27]

No matter what type of exercise is used in the strengthening program, adequate training dosage is an important consideration to obtain beneficial effects. The approach must provide enough loading to the muscle to induce a strength-training effect without exacerbating pain and inflammation of the joints. Recent studies indicate that using a graded progression of exercise resistance and adjusting training volume to match the level of resistance allows people with either fibromyalgia or rheumatoid arthritis to train intensely enough to obtain improvements in pain, strength, muscle hypertrophy, and performance-based and self-reported measures of function without exacerbating symptoms at their joints.[28-30] The amount or resistance used in these studies was based on a percentage of a one-repetition-maximum (1-RM), which is the maximum load a person can lift for a given exercise in one repetition. For the first few weeks, subjects exercise at 40% to 60% of 1-RM and perform 15 to 20 repetitions (lower loads, more repetitions.) In the next few weeks, the load was increased to 60% to 70% of 1-RM and the repetitions reduced to 8 to 12 repetitions. In the final few weeks of the program, the load was progressed to 70% to 80% of 1-RM and the repetitions were reduced to 5 to 10 repetitions. Subjects were gradually exposed to higher loads over the course of training; and as the load increased, the number of repetitions were reduced to keep the overall intensity of exercise tolerable. A new 1-RM was re-established every few weeks, so that as subjects became stronger, the exercise load could be increased accordingly.

In many forms of arthritis, such as RA, the hands are particularly affected, with significant decreases in strength and range of motion secondary to the development of deformities. Therapy often focuses on remediating hand function by providing a home program of hand-specific resistive exercises, such as Thera-Putty, and full-range passive or active range of motion exercises. Although it is common practice to provide these exercises, the evidence to support this practice is minimal and conflicting.[31] There are no guidelines as to which exercises are most effective or to the frequency and duration of the exercises.[32] Wessel[31] comments that although much further research needs to be completed to determine the effectiveness of hand-specific exercises, clinicians should continue to recommend these programs.

Aerobic capacity

Aerobic exercises are typically moderate-intensity exercises, involving larger muscle groups, that are performed over extended periods of time

(30-60 minutes or longer) to improve cardiovascular function. Examples of aerobic exercise include walking, cycling, and pool exercises. For the activity to be considered aerobic, the intensity of the exercise should typically range between 50% to 70% of the individual's heart rate reserve (heart rate reserve = 220 − age − resting heart rate × (% intensity) + resting heart rate). For example, for 60-year-old individuals with a resting heart rate of 80 who want to exercise at 60% of their heart rate reserve, the calculated target heart rate would be (220 − 60 − 80 × .60) + 80 = 128 beats per minute.

Aerobic exercise has been recommended as part of the management for patients with a variety of rheumatologic disorders in a number of published treatment guidelines.[2,12,15,33,34] Aerobic exercise programs have been shown to reduce pain,[2,34] improve function and quality of life,[2,15,34] improve aerobic capacity and endurance,[35-37] and improve mental health.[36-38]

Walking programs have generally been studied for effectiveness. The type of walking program found to be beneficial typically involves a 10-minute warm-up of muscular stretching and slow walking, followed by 30 to 40 minutes of walking at 50% to 70% of the individual's heart rate reserve, then followed by a 10-minute cool down period.[39] Cycling is another form of aerobic exercise that can be beneficial. Mangione and associates reported that stationary cycling for 25 minutes, three times a week, at either 40% or 70% of the heart rate reserve resulted in reduced pain, improved aerobic capacity, and improved performance on functional tests in subjects with knee OA.[35] Cycling should be considered for subjects with arthritis who may have difficulty with a walking program due to joint pain.

Aquatic exercise programs are an alternative for people with rheumatologic conditions because the buoyancy of the water helps to reduce loading on joints, making it easier for patients with arthritis or fibromyalgia to exercise. These programs can include a combination of limb movements against water resistance and walking or jogging in the pool. Similar to studies of other aerobic exercises, those studies of aquatic programs that maintain an aerobic dose (60% to 75% of heart rate reserve) have reported improvements in variables such as pain, muscle strength, aerobic capacity, self-report and performance-based measures of function, day-time fatigue, anxiety, and depression.[36-38]

Balance and agility

In recent years, more attention has been given to the importance of balance in patients with arthritis. Studies have indicated that people with knee OA have deficits in measures of balance compared with age- and gender-matched controls and that these balance deficits may be associated with limitations in function[40,41] and functional decline.[42] In some cases, balance may be altered, even in the absence of muscular strength deficits.[43] Therefore, rehabilitation programs may need to incorporate interventions specifically designed to challenge balance abilities for people with arthritis.

A variety of activities can be used in balance training for people with arthritis. Some authors have described techniques that use a combination of balance board and roller board activities.[44,45] Single-leg standing and tandem standing activities, as well as agility training techniques that focus on quick stops and starts, sudden changes in direction, and cross-over stepping have also been combined with balance board activities to challenge balance.[44-46] Tai chi activities are also being used more frequently for aging people and people with arthritis.[47] Although strengthening exercise can result in improved balance and function,[45,48] there is some evidence that balance and agility training techniques, when combined with strengthening exercises, can result in greater short-term improvements in function measures compared with strengthening alone.[45] Tai chi programs have also resulted in improvements in balance measures in people with knee OA, but it is not clear at this time whether they are any more effective than other forms of exercise.[47]

Pain-related fear

The patient's perception that physical activity or exercise may harm his or her joints is sometimes referred to as "pain-related fear." Pain-related fear may be a barrier to optimal patient participation in an exercise or physical activity program. Pain-related fear has been shown to be associated with poorer physical function scores in people with arthritis.[49] Strategies have been developed to help patients with low back pain overcome their fear of physical activity during rehabilitation, and these strategies might be helpful for people with arthritis who also have higher degrees of pain-related fear.

An approach that has been found to improve the outcome of rehabilitation for people with low back pain who have pain-related fear is known as "Graded *in-vivo* Exposure" (GivE).[50] In this approach, the therapist and patient identify the types of physical activities or tasks that invoke a fear response and then rank the tasks with respect to the amount of fear. At the beginning of therapy, patients are educated in the concept of fear-avoidance behaviors and how these can limit an individual's ability to function. During therapy, the therapist models task-specific modifications and proper body mechanics for the fear-inducing tasks or activities. The patient then practices these modifications and body mechanic techniques under the supervision of the therapist. The gradual and systematic exposure to the fear-inducing activities is intended to disconfirm the patient's pain- and fear-related expectations associated with the physical activity.

Although the GivE approach has not been formally evaluated in people with arthritis, it would seem that this type of approach could be helpful for those patients with arthritis who fear performing certain physical tasks or activities. This type of approach should also fit with the task-specific strengthening principles described earlier. At any rate, clinicians should assess whether their patients with arthritis are experiencing pain or activity-related fears and pursue approaches that will help diminish the fear so that functional capacity can be optimized.

ADAPTIVE REHABILITATION APPROACHES

Because many arthritic conditions are progressive in nature, teaching compensatory skills to promote independent, safe, and comfortable functioning is a key rehabilitation technique. Many people with arthritis experience limitations in their ability to perform activities of daily living (ADLs) owing to limitations in range of motion, strength, and endurance. ADLs refer to a very large category of tasks and activities: those that involve taking care of oneself and one's immediate environment. They are often broken down into basic ADLs (BADLs), which are tasks related to self-maintenance, such as functional mobility (including transfers), personal hygiene/grooming, bathing, bowel/bladder management/hygiene, dressing, eating, and sexual activity, and instrumental ADLs (IADLs), which are tasks that involve interacting with the immediate environment, such as care of others, communication device use, community mobility, financial management, meal preparation, home care, emergency response, and shopping.[51] There are strong associations between ADL ability and impairments in strength, range of motion, and endurance, which suggests that remediating these impairments can improve ADL performance.[52-54] However, research also suggests that a person's level of impairment does not always predict ADL performance[54-56] because other factors, such as the environment or pain-related fear, can facilitate or prevent function. Providing compensatory techniques is one method to improve ADL ability and is the most responsive to changes in abilities as the disease progresses.

Assistive devices

One method to remediate ADLs is to provide assistive devices. *Assistive device* is a broad term defined according to the Technology-Related Assistance for Individuals with Disabilities Act of 1988 as "any item, piece of equipment, or product system, whether acquired commercially off the shelf, modified or customized, that is used to increase, maintain, or improve functional capabilities of individuals with disabilities." Table 46.1 provides some of the more common assistive devices and their uses during BADL activities.[57] Although the prescription of assistive devices is common in therapy, there is limited high-quality evidence to support their use.[58] Available research suggests that assistive devices can improve performance in people with arthritis[59] and have been associated with improved psychological well-being.[60] Unfortunately, compliance with assistive device use may be limited; estimations suggest that 36% of bathing equipment, 26% of dressing devices, and 19% of mobility devices are not used.[61] Compliance depends on a

TABLE 46.1 COMMONLY PRESCRIBED ASSISTIVE DEVICES FOR BASIC ACTIVITIES OF DAILY LIVING (BADLS)	
Functional mobility	Walker, cane, wheeled mobility (i.e., wheelchair, scooter), orthotic device for hip/knee/ankle
Transfers	Stand assist device, transfer (sliding) boards, pivot discs, transfer poles, push-up bars, grab bars, bed rails, trapeze, lift chairs, seat assists, raised seating (e.g., raised toilet seat, hospital bed, chair)
Grooming/hygiene	Long, easy grip, and/or angled handled tools (e.g., toothbrush, brush, razor, deodorant holder, toenail clippers, tweezers); electric toothbrush; aerosol can adapter; pump toothpaste dispenser; floss sticks; hands-free hair dryer holder; suction cup fingernail cutters/brush/file; toilet paper holder; toilet transfer assists
Bathing	Tub seat, bath transfer assists, non-slip bath mat, hand-held shower; long-handled sponge, soap dispensers, shower caddy
Dressing	Dressing stick, long-handled shoe horn; sock aid; elastic laces, Velcro closures, button hook, zipper pull, adapted bra
Eating	Long, easy grip, swivel, and/or angled handled tools (e.g., spoon, fork); rocker knife; two-handled cups; Dycem/non-slip materials; high-sided or scoop plate; ring pull can opener; bottle opener; packaging opener; kettle/jug tipper
Other devices	Reacher, medication manager, pill bottle opener, phone holder/headset, large-button phone, portable stool, pen/pencil cushions, doorknob turners, lamp switch enlargers, easy grip/high leverage key holders, adapted scissors

variety of factors, such as age, diagnosis, disease severity, and the perception of the utility and attractiveness of the assistive device.[62] The environment in which the device will be used affects compliance: for example, durable medical equipment, such as toilet seats, may be discarded if they do not fit the toilet, if the user cannot access the bathroom due to narrow doorways, or if they do not fit the person.[61] One way to increase compliance is to ensure that assistive devices are prescribed by an experienced person and that patients are properly trained in their use.[61]

Orthotic devices and splints

One type of assistive device that can be either remedial or compensatory is the hand orthotic device, or splint. Hand splints can be used for a variety of reasons—to provide support, align joints, immobilize joints, reduce pain, prevent or correct deformity, assist a weak muscle, or position the hand for functional activities[63]—and are particularly used for patients with RA and carpometacarpal joint OA. Hand splints can be custom made by an occupational therapist or be purchased prefabricated.

Although hand splints are frequently provided for patients with arthritis, there have been few high-quality studies done on their effectiveness. Systematic reviews of the effectiveness of splints for RA reported that the evidence was unclear as to whether splints significantly improved work performance,[63,64] although some reviews have suggested that they have a positive effect on pain.[64] A systematic review on the effectiveness of opponens-type splints (a splint that immobilizes the thumb) in the treatment of carpometacarpal joint OA reported that these splints were effective in both reducing pain and increasing function.[65] One study that examined the effectiveness of splinting on increasing range of motion of the proximal interphalangeal joints of individuals with RA reported that both static splints (i.e., splints that have no moving parts) and dynamic splints (i.e., splints that apply a graded/increasing force on a contracted joint) were effective in

increasing range of motion, increasing hand strength, and improving function.[66] Although the evidence to support hand splints is somewhat equivocal, and more high-quality studies are needed to support or refute their use, Egan and associates suggested that because splints are relatively inexpensive and not harmful, current clinical practice should be to prescribe splints for patients on a case-by-case basis to see if they help.[63]

Lower extremity orthoses, such as knee braces and shoe inserts, can also be used as adjunct interventions to reduce pain, relieve joint stress, or improve joint stability for people with arthritis. Knee orthoses have specially designed axes and straps to reduce compartmental loading of the knee. The most common type is a valgus brace, in which a valgus force is applied to the knee through the brace to unload the medial compartment.[67] These types of braces can also be modified to apply a varus load to the knee for patients with lateral compartment involvement. The evidence for effectiveness of these braces is limited, but it appears they can help some individuals.[68,69] Biomechanical studies have shown that these braces can reduce joint compartmental loading,[67,70] and a recent study suggested that the bracing may improve joint stability.[71] Currently, there are no specific guidelines that identify who will respond to this type of bracing. There is likely a cutoff point with regard to the degree of joint deformity beyond which the brace may no longer be effective, but this cutoff point has not yet been established. The willingness of a patient to wear the brace can also be a limiting factor, because some patients find the brace to be cumbersome. However, newer, lighter-weight designs may help address this problem. Valgus bracing may also be a reasonable option for those patients who are not good candidates for surgical realignment procedures.

Like knee braces, shoe inserts may also be used to reduce lower extremity pain or joint stress. In some cases they are used as cushioning to help dissipate some of the loading transmitted through the lower extremity, relieving some joint stress and discomfort. Recently, the use of laterally wedged inserts has become popular for people with medial compartment knee arthritis. The lateral wedge insert is believed to reduce medial compartment loading indirectly by enhancing foot and ankle pronation, which, in turn, should result in an increased valgus load at the knee. There have been some biomechanical studies to indicate that these inserts can reduce varus moments at the knee.[72,73] The use of a "subtalar" strap, combined with the lateral wedge seems to have a moderately better effect on reducing the knee adduction moment compared with a lateral wedge alone, in people with moderately severe, but not severe radiographic knee OA.[74] The strapping may help by preventing excessive pronation at the foot and ankle, which might otherwise dissipate the effects of the insert on the knee.

The evidence for the effectiveness of the lateral wedge inserts is mixed. Baker and colleagues[75] did not find an overall difference between groups using a lateral wedge insert compared to a neutral insert for people with medial knee OA, although there did appear to be a subgroup of patients in this study with less severe OA and lower BMI who had improvements in pain[75]; a subtalar strap was not used with the lateral wedge in this study. In contrast, Toda and Segal have observed significant improvements in pain and function when using a lateral wedge insert combined with subtalar strapping.[72] Regardless of whether a subtalar strap is used or not, it appears that this intervention is most effective in patients with mild to moderate arthritis and may not be very effective in those with severe knee OA.

Self-management instruction

One common trend in arthritis management is education in self-management techniques.[76] These programs provide people with arthritis with education about aspects of their disease, such as pain management, fitness/exercise, and healthy eating and are often combined with training in effective coping, such as goal setting, action plans, and problem solving.[76,77] The programs can vary tremendously in content and can include disease information, methods of pain management, exercise, training in ADLs, social skills training, and relaxation techniques.[76] Although the quality of the research varies, studies have generally found that education programs have a small effect on pain and a moderate effect on function in the short term,[64] the carryover of these positive outcomes is less apparent.[64,77-80] Self-management

TABLE 46.2 PRINCIPLES OF JOINT PROTECTION TECHNIQUES

Joint protection techniques	Example
Respect pain.	Immediately stop activity if increased pain is experienced.
Maintain muscle strength and range of motion.	Maintain a regular hand exercise program consisting of resistive exercises and full range of motion stretches.
Ensure correct patterns of movement.	Avoid using compensatory motions to substitute for painful joints because this will increase deformity and decrease available range of motion (ex: externally rotating shoulder to supinated palm).
Use each joint in its most stable anatomic and/or functional position.	Position the joint so the muscles, not the ligaments, provide stability during the activity (ex: gripping with the whole hand rather than pinching with the finger/thumb).
Avoid positions of deformity.	Avoid tasks in which the external load encourages the joints to move into the position of deformity (ex: holding up a book by the edges to read pulls the metacarpophalangeal joints into ulnar deviation).
Use the strongest joints available for the job.	Use the largest joint possible to do the job (ex: Carry bags over the shoulder rather than in the fingers).
Reduce forces.	Use the lightest possible object for any task (ex: replace glass or ceramic mugs with plastic mugs).
Avoid staying in one position for long periods of time.	Change positions and take breaks frequently (ex: taking a standing break after 20 minutes of sitting).
Avoid starting an activity that cannot be stopped immediately if proves to be beyond a person's ability.	Plan activities so as to take breaks before becoming fatigued. Know the task and environment so that appropriate breaks can be taken (ex: shop in a mall where there are numerous benches so sitting breaks can be taken when needed).
Balance rest and activity.	Take planned rest breaks; alternate heavier and lighter tasks; plan to complete longer activities in shorter segments.

From Yasuda YL. Rheumatoid arthritis, osteoarthritis, and fibromyalgia. In: Radomsky MV, Trombly Latham CA, eds. Occupational therapy for physical dysfunction, 6th ed. Philadelphia: Lippincott Williams & Wilkins, 2008:1214-1243.

programs have been shown to be effective using a variety of session numbers,[76] group versus individual,[81] as well as delivery systems such as a mail delivery program[82] or the Internet.[83] One common educational program is joint protection. Joint protection techniques are primarily taught to those with RA, although patients with OA have also been trained in joint protection.[84] Joint protection programs focus on teaching techniques thought to reduce the stresses on joints weakened by the disease, thereby reducing the tendency for deformities such as subluxation and ulnar drift (Table 46.2). There are several high-quality systematic reviews that specifically support the effectiveness of joint protection techniques for improving function.[64]

Fatigue

Chronic fatigue is a very common, yet frequently undertreated symptom of many types of arthritis. Chronic fatigue in arthritis has been described as different from the normal tiredness experienced by healthy people. Chronic fatigue is characterized as a profound lack of energy that is not linked to specific overexertion but occurs almost randomly.[85]

Chronic fatigue is reported by patients with arthritis to significantly affect many aspects of their life, including BADLs, work and leisure, family relationships, and emotional responses to situations. Fatigue is reported to limit social contact, and many workers cut back their work due to fatigue.[86,87] Although fatigue is often identified to be as limiting as pain for many people with arthritis, they seldom discuss it with others. The importance of measuring fatigue as an outcome measure was only recently identified during OMERACT 6 in 2002,[88] and, therefore, there has been only limited research to assess effective methods of reducing fatigue in people with arthritis.

Interventions to remediate fatigue can generally be divided into two types: aerobic exercise and behavioral interventions. Aerobic exercise has been shown to be an effective method of reducing fatigue, and research suggests that low-intensity aerobics (e.g., brisk walking) performed at least three times weekly for 15 to 30 minutes can reduce feelings of chronic fatigue.[85,89] Behavioral programs, which provide education in self-management techniques, have been shown to be effective for reducing fatigue.[85] One fatigue self-management program is energy conservation. Energy conservation provides persons with arthritis-specific strategies to address issues related to fatigue, such as valuing rest, budgeting and banking energy, taking planned rest periods, breaking down fatiguing tasks into smaller components, using good body mechanics, using energy efficient appliances, and learning to communicate personal needs to others.[90]

Work adaptations

Work is a valued activity, both for individuals and society. Arthritis is the third leading cause of work disability: 8.2 million working aged U.S. adults (about 1 in 20) report work limitations due to arthritis.[91] *Work disability* refers to limitations in ability to work due to impaired health and is manifested as premature work cessation (prior to normal age of retirement) and, among employed persons, as reduced productivity.

People with RA have identified several job accommodation strategies that reduce work disability. One common accommodation was to make the job more flexible, including controlling work hours, taking rest breaks, or delegating tasks. However, Chorus and colleagues reported that job modifications that resulted in loss of productivity, such as working fewer hours or delegating, were associated with a greater risk of eventual work disability.[92] Modifications developed with the assistance of a health care provider, such as work-specific self-management programs and ergonomic assessments to modify the work environment or work task methods to better fit the needs of the worker with arthritis have been reported to be effective ways to adapt the job.[93-98] Workers who report having received work interventions by health care professionals were less likely to report work disability.[95,96]

One method to obtain work modifications is the Americans with Disability Act (ADA), Title I. The ADA was enacted in 1990 to prevent discrimination against workers with disabilities in the workplace. An important aspect of the ADA was to ensure that employers provide workers with any requested "reasonable accommodation," a modification or adjustment to a job or work environment that enables a qualified person with a disability to perform essential job tasks. Reasonable accommodations can include physical changes to the environment (e.g., raising or lowering work heights), adaptive equipment (e.g., special chairs, power-assisted lifting devices), or changes to the work organization (e.g., telecommuting, altered hours, changes in nonessential job function). The U.S. Department of Labor's Office of Disability Employment Policy (ODEP) has created the Job Accommodation Network (JAN) (http://www.jan.wvu.edu/) to provide employers, people with disabilities, and other interested parties with information on the ADA and reasonable accommodations. Although the ADA is available for people with arthritis, few use it to remain employed. A recent study reported that whereas 63% of workers with arthritis needed a job accommodation, only 10% had used the ADA. Factors that affected the use of the ADA included not knowing that the ADA was available, the perception that they had a disability that could be addressed through the ADA, lack of skill in requesting reasonable accommodations, and no interaction with a health care professional who suggested using the ADA.[99]

Vocational rehabilitation is another method to prevent work disability. Vocational rehabilitation is a coordinated, multidisciplinary program that addresses work retention, preventing work loss, or return-to-work programs. Vocational rehabilitation assists people to reenter employment in the same or different jobs after a period of sick or disability leave. The actual interventions vary according to the needs of each patient and are developed on a case-by-case basis. The effectiveness of vocational rehabilitation for people with arthritis has been assessed with conflicting results. A systematic review on six uncontrolled studies on vocational rehabilitation for people with arthritis reported some evidence of short-term improvement in employment.[100] More recent controlled studies were equivocal: Allaire and associates reported that vocational rehabilitation had a positive effect on job loss,[101] whereas de Buck and colleagues reported no difference when compared with usual outpatient care.[102] Most states have departments of vocational rehabilitation. Workers who receive federal disability benefits may be able to obtain these services at no cost; others pay on a sliding scale depending on need.

Unfortunately, work disability is rarely addressed in arthritis. A recent qualitative study examining issues experienced by workers with arthritis suggested that work is rarely discussed with physicians or health care practitioners.[95] Studies on workers with arthritis find that they frequently implement coping strategies such as changing jobs, reducing hours, or reconfiguring their workstation[95,98] but rarely have interventions by health care practitioners. Those in these studies that report having had work interventions by health care professionals were more likely to report less work disability.[95,96]

Although ergonomics assessment, work self-management, and potentially vocational rehabilitation may be effective strategies to reduce work disability, most workers with arthritis do not obtain these interventions. They may not know that ergonomic assessments exist, they may not know who to request or pay for an ergonomic assessment, and they may fear disclosing their condition to an employer.[95] An unwillingness to disclose their arthritis condition to an employer and coworkers is fairly common among workers with RA. Many workers with RA report that they fear adverse consequences, such as work loss, discrimination in job promotions, being less valued as a worker, stigmatization, and dealing with negative coworker reactions if they do disclose their arthritis.[95] In addition to the barriers to obtaining ergonomic assessment and intervention through work, many workers with RA do not discuss their problems at work with their rheumatologists who are gatekeepers for these interventions.[98]

CONCLUSION

The purpose of rehabilitation is to assist patients with arthritis in restoring and maintaining an optimal level of function. The patient is the main stakeholder in this endeavor and therefore sets the bar in determining the optimal level of function. Rehabilitation therapists identify the barriers that may limit the ability of people with arthritis to achieve optimal function and then provide interventions to overcome these barriers. Because the barriers are often multifactorial, a successful rehabilitation process will require a multidisciplinary effort, involving not only physical and occupational therapists but also clinical psychologists, vocational rehabilitation counselors, rehabilitation engineers, and recreational therapists.

In this chapter we discussed both remedial and adaptive rehabilitation approaches (Table 46.3). Many patients with arthritis will need a combination of both approaches. Remedial rehabilitation is directed at restoring or establishing physical capacity and ability, focusing on addressing impairments associated with arthritis. We discussed intervention approaches and the degree of evidence supporting interventions to improve pain, joint motion, muscular strength, aerobic capacity, and balance and agility for people with arthritis. The role of pain-induced fear and strategies to overcome fear during rehabilitation was also discussed.

Adaptive rehabilitation is directed at finding ways to compensate for lost or absent physical capacity or ability and focuses on developing alternative or supplementary methods to assist patients in improving their task performance. The use and available evidence for using assistive devices, orthotics, and splinting techniques were discussed.

We also identified the effectiveness of educating patients in self-management procedures such as joint protection techniques, coping strategies for dealing with chronic pain, managing fatigue, and promoting self-efficacy. Because many people with arthritis are still of working age, the importance of ergonomic assessments and work task modifications for these patients was explored. We noted that this is an area of care that does not always receive adequate attention. Physicians and therapists may need to take a more pro-active role in making sure occupational needs are being assessed and addressed for their patients with arthritis.

TABLE 46.3 SUMMARY OF REHABILITATION TECHNIQUES

Intervention	Application	Comments
Remedial approaches		
Physical agents Thermal agents (e.g., heat, cold, ultrasound) Electrical stimulation (e.g., TENS)	Pain control	Most appropriately applied on a case-by-case basis
Stretching/range of motion	Improve joint motion Improve function	
Joint mobilization	Improve joint motion Pain control Improve function	Lower-intensity joint mobilization may be effective in pain control.
Strengthening exercises Isometric Isotonic Isokinetic "Task specific"	Increased muscle force output Pain control (when combined with physical agents) Improve balance Improve function	Patients need a combination of strengthening (e.g., isometric, concentric) to best improve functional ability.
Aerobic exercise	Improve aerobic capacity and endurance Pain control Reduce fatigue Improve function Improve mental health	Walking or cycling programs have been shown to be effective methods to improve aerobic fitness.
Balance training	Improve balance and agility Improve function	Tai chi programs are potentially effective methods to improve balance.
Adaptive approaches		
Assistive devices	Compensate for impairments Improve function Improve mental health	Compliance can be an issue if the devices are improperly prescribed or provided without training in their use.
Splinting	Pain control Improve joint motion Provide support Immobilize joint Correct deformity Assist with weak muscle Improve function	Splints should be considered on a case-by-case basis.
Educational programs Self-management Joint protection Vocational rehabilitation	Pain control Improve function Reduce fatigue	

KEY REFERENCES

2. Zhang W, Moskowitz RW, Nuki G, et al. OARSI recommendations for the management of hip and knee osteoarthritis: II. OARSI evidence-based, expert consensus guidelines. Osteoarthritis Cartilage 2008;16:137-162.

3. Ottawa P. Ottawa Panel evidence-based clinical practice guidelines for electrotherapy and thermotherapy interventions in the management of rheumatoid arthritis in adults. Phys Ther 2004;84:1016-1043.

4. Jamtvedt G, Dahm KT, Christie A, et al. Physical therapy interventions for patients with osteoarthritis of the knee: an overview of systematic reviews. Phys Ther 2008;88:123-136.

5. Welch V, Brosseau L, Peterson J, et al. Therapeutic ultrasound for osteoarthritis of the knee. Cochrane Database Syst Rev 2001;(3): CD003132.

6. Philadelphia Panel evidence-based clinical practice guidelines on selected rehabilitation interventions for low back pain. Phys Ther 2001;81:1641-1674.

9. Cetin N, Aytar A, Atalay A, et al. Comparing hot pack, short-wave diathermy, ultrasound, and TENS on isokinetic strength, pain, and functional status of women with osteoarthritic knees: a single-blind, randomized, controlled trial. Am J Phys Med Rehabil 2008;87:443-451.

11. Osiri M, Welch V, Brosseau L, et al. Transcutaneous electrical nerve stimulation for knee osteoarthritis. Cochrane Database Syst Rev 2000;(4):CD002823.

12. Jordan KM, Arden NK, Doherty M, et al. EULAR Recommendations 2003: an evidence based approach to the management of knee osteoarthritis: Report of a task force of the Standing Committee for International Clinical Studies Including Therapeutic Trials. Ann Rheum Dis 2003;62:1145-1155.

15. Ottawa Panel evidence-based clinical practice guidelines for therapeutic exercises and manual therapy in the management of osteoarthritis. Phys Ther 2005;85:907-971.

16. Philadelphia Panel evidence-based clinical practice guidelines on selected rehabilitation interventions for knee pain. Phys Ther 2001;81:1675-1700.

17. Gajdosik RL, Vander Linden DW, McNair PJ, et al. Effects of an eight-week stretching program on the passive-elastic properties and function of the calf muscles of older women. Clin Biomech 2005;20:973-983.

20. Deyle GD, Allison SC, Matekel RL, et al. Physical therapy treatment effectiveness for osteoarthritis of the knee: a randomized comparison of supervised clinical exercise and manual therapy procedures versus a home exercise program. Phys Ther 2005;85:1301-1317.

21. Hoeksma HL, Dekker J, Ronday HK, et al. Comparison of manual therapy and exercise therapy in osteoarthritis of the hip: a randomized clinical trial. Arthritis Rheum 2004;51:722-729.

22. Ottawa Panel evidence-based clinical practice guidelines for therapeutic exercises in the management of rheumatoid arthritis in adults. Phys Ther 2004;84:934-972.

23. Brosseau L, Wells GA, Tugwell P, et al. Ottawa Panel evidence-based clinical practice guidelines for strengthening exercises in the management of fibromyalgia: II. Phys Ther 2008; 88:873-886.

24. Huang MH, Lin YS, Yang RC, et al. A comparison of various therapeutic exercises on the functional status of patients with knee osteoarthritis. Semin Arthritis Rheum 2003;32:398-406.

26. de Vreede PL, Samson MM, van Meeteren NL, et al. Functional-task exercise versus resistance strength exercise to improve daily function in older women: a randomized, controlled trial. J Am Geriatr Soc 2005;53:2-10.

29. Hakkinen A, Hannonen P, Nyman K, et al. Effects of concurrent strength and endurance training in women with early or longstanding rheumatoid arthritis: comparison with healthy subjects. Arthritis Rheum 2003;49:789-797.

31. Wessel J. The effectiveness of hand exercises for persons with rheumatoid arthritis: a systematic review. J Hand Ther 2004;17:174-180.

32. Chadwick A. A review of the history of hand exercises in rheumatoid arthritis. Musculoskeletal Care 2004;2:29-39.

33. American College of Rheumatology Subcommittee on Osteoarthritis Guidelines. Recommendations for the medical management of osteoarthritis of the hip and knee: 2000 update. Arthritis Rheum 2000;43:1905-1915.

34. Brosseau L, Wells GA, Tugwell P, et al. Ottawa Panel evidence-based clinical practice guidelines for aerobic fitness exercises in the management of fibromyalgia: I. Phys Ther 2008;88:857-871.

47. Lee MS, Pittler MH, Ernst E. Tai chi for osteoarthritis: a systematic review. Clin Rheum 2008;27:211-218.

49. Heuts PHTG, Vlaeyen JWS, Roelofs J, et al. Pain-related fear and daily functioning in patients with osteoarthritis. Pain 2004;110:228-235.

50. Woods MP, Asmundson GJ. Evaluating the efficacy of graded in vivo exposure for the treatment of fear in patients with chronic back pain: a randomized controlled clinical trial. Pain 2008;136:271-280.

54. Keysor JJ. Does late-life physical activity or exercise prevent or minimize disablement? A critical review of the scientific evidence. Am J Prevent Med 2003;25:129-136.

58. Steultjens EM, Dekker J, Bouter LM, et al. Occupational therapy for rheumatoid arthritis. Cochrane Database Syst Rev 2004;(1):CD003114.

61. Rogers JC, Holm MB. Assistive technology device use in patients with rheumatic disease: a literature review. Am J Occup Ther 1992;46:120-127.

63. Egan M, Brosseau L, Farmer M, et al. Splints/orthoses in the treatment of rheumatoid arthritis. Cochrane Database Syst Rev 2003;(1):CD004018.

64. Christie A, Jamtvedt G, Dahm KT, et al. Effectiveness of nonpharmacological and nonsurgical interventions for patients with rheumatoid arthritis: an overview of systematic reviews. Phys Ther 2007;87:1697-1715.

65. Egan MY, Brousseau L. Splinting for osteoarthritis of the carpometacarpal joint: a review of the evidence. Am J Occup Ther 2007;61:70-78.

68. Kirkley A, Webster-Bogaert S, Litchfield R, et al. The effect of bracing on varus gonarthrosis. J Bone Joint Surg Am 1999;81:539-548.

72. Toda Y, Segal N. Usefulness of an insole with subtalar strapping for analgesia in patients with medial compartment osteoarthritis of the knee. Arthritis Care Res 2002;47:468-473.

76. Newman S, Mulligan K, Steed L. What is meant by self-management and how can its efficacy be established? Rheumatology 2001;40:1-4.

77. Riemsma RP, Taal E, Kirwan JR, et al. Systematic review of rheumatoid arthritis patient education. Arthritis Rheum 2004;51:1045-1059.

78. Brady TJ, Kruger J, Helmick CG, et al. Intervention programs for arthritis and other rheumatic diseases. Health Ed Behav 2003;30:44-63.

80. Warsi A, LaValley MP, Wang PS, et al. Arthritis self-management education programs: a meta-analysis of the effect on pain and disability. Arthritis Rheum 2003;48:2207-2213.

85. Neill J, Belan I, Ried K. Effectiveness of non-pharmacological interventions for fatigue in adults with multiple sclerosis, rheumatoid arthritis, or systemic lupus erythematosus: a systematic review. J Adv Nurs 2006;56:617-635.

86. Power JD, Badley EM, French MR, et al. Fatigue in osteoarthritis: a qualitative study. BMC Musculoskelet Disord 2008;9:63.

87. Repping-Wuts H, Uitterhoeve R, van Riel P, et al. Fatigue as experienced by patients with rheumatoid arthritis (RA): a qualitative study. Int J Nurs Studies 2008;45:995-1002.

92. Chorus AM, Miedema HS, Wevers CW, et al. Work factors and behavioural coping in relation to withdrawal from the labour force in patients with rheumatoid arthritis. Ann Rheum Dis 2001;60:1025-1032.

93. Allaire SH, Li W, LaValley M. Work barriers experienced and job accommodations used by persons with arthritis and other rheumatic diseases. Rehabil Couns Bull 2003;46:147-156.

95. Lacaille D, White MA, Backman CL, et al. Problems faced at work due to inflammatory arthritis: new insights gained from understanding patients' perspective. Arthritis Rheum 2007;57:1269-1279.

96. Lacaille D, Sheps S, Spinelli JJ, et al. Identification of modifiable work-related factors that influence the risk of work disability in rheumatoid arthritis. Arthritis Rheum 2004;51:843-852.

98. Mancuso CA, Paget SA, Charlson ME. Adaptations made by rheumatoid arthritis patients to continue working: a pilot study of workplace challenges and successful adaptations. Arthritis Care Res 2000;13:89-99.

99. Allaire SH, Evans SR, LaValley MP, et al. Use of the Americans with Disabilities Act by persons with rheumatic diseases and factors associated with use. Arthritis Care Res 2001;45:174-182.

100. de Buck PDM, Schoones JW, Allaire SH, et al. Vocational rehabilitation in patients with chronic rheumatic diseases: a systematic literature review. Semin Arthritis Rheum 2002;32:196-203.

101. Allaire SH, Li W, LaValley MP. Reduction of job loss in persons with rheumatic diseases receiving vocational rehabilitation: a randomized controlled trial. Arthritis Rheum 2003;48:3212-3218.

102. de Buck PD, le Cessie S, van den Hout WB, et al. Randomized comparison of a multidisciplinary job-retention vocational rehabilitation program with usual outpatient care in patients with chronic arthritis at risk for job loss. Arthritis Rheum 2005;53:682-690.

REFERENCES

Full references for this chapter can be found on www.expertconsult.com.

Complementary and alternative medicine

47

Brian M. Berman, Elena Gournelos, George T. Lewith, and Brooke Seidelmann

- The majority of rheumatology patients use some form of complementary and alternative medicine (CAM).
- Acupuncture, herbal medicine, nutriceuticals, and homeopathy are among the most commonly used CAM treatments.
- The evidence for the efficacy of these therapies is limited.
- The majority of research on traditional Chinese medicine in the West has focused on acupuncture.
- Studies have shown acupuncture to be effective for specific types of pain reduction.
- Some herbal therapies may be as effective as analgesic and anti-inflammatory drugs for rheumatic and musculoskeletal conditions.
- Nutriceuticals, in particular glucosamine and chondroitin, have variable results in the treatment of osteoarthritis and in preventing long-term joint damage.
- Homeopathy has not been definitively proven to work for rheumatologic conditions.
- Moderate evidence exists for the effectiveness of mind-body therapies as adjuncts in the treatment of rheumatoid arthritis and osteoarthritis.
- Physicians should consider that CAM can be integrated into the conventional management of rheumatologic conditions in a thoughtful, professional, and cooperative manner.

INTRODUCTION

Complementary, alternative, and *integrative medicine* are blanket terms that comprise a large variety of health treatments clustered together because they exist outside the parameters of conventional treatment (i.e., neither taught widely in medical schools nor generally available in hospitals[1]). They include whole systems of medicine as well as individual treatment options. The terms *complementary, alternative,* and *integrative* refer not to the particular modalities used but to the manner in which health care is obtained; in other words, people can obtain health care from a non-conventional practitioner in conjunction with conventional care (complementary), instead of conventional care (alternative), or from a provider or group of providers who have blended conventional and non-conventional care in their practice (integrative). Moreover, the status of any therapeutic practice is in constant flux; many therapies once considered complementary or alternative may gain acceptance and be slowly incorporated into mainstream practice, whereas others may prove ineffective or dangerous.

Although it is commonly known that the traditional medical systems of Asia have been practiced for thousands of years, the history of complementary and alternative medicine (CAM) in the West, although well documented,[2] is not always discussed. CAM use in the West is not a recent phenomenon; rather, many of the alternative systems of medicine being used today (e.g., herbalism, chiropractic, naturopathy, and homeopathy) have evolved alongside allopathic medicine. Although the medicinal use of Western herbs predates history, herbalism as it is practiced today was first developed in the late 18th century. Homeopathy was developed during the same time period, whereas chiropractic, osteopathy, and naturopathy followed in the late 19th century. In addition, Asian systems of medicine were formally introduced to the West as early as 1683, when the first European text on acupuncture and arthritis was written; the first journal articles on acupuncture appeared in the 1820s.[3] Over time, as these medical systems developed and the needs of the population continuously changed, the popularity of CAM ebbed and flowed accordingly.[4]

In recent years, CAM use has been on the rise. In the United States, a 2008 Centers for Disease Control and Prevention (CDC) National Health Interview Survey reported from 23,393 interviews that 38% of adults and 12% of children had used some form of CAM therapy during the past 12 months.[1] Although there is no compelling evidence to suggest that the use of CAM among rheumatology patients has increased dramatically over the past 15 years,[5] usage rates among this subpopulation are still higher than average. Studies have reported usage rates as high as 94%, but recent surveys report that, on average, 44% to 66% of rheumatology patients use CAM.[6,7] However, the usage rate of fibromyalgia patients is particularly high, at 91%.[8]

Because of the chronic nature of rheumatic disease, as well as the palliative nature and adverse effects associated with conventional care for this condition, it is not surprising that so many rheumatology patients are using CAM. Eisenberg and colleagues[9] found that 4 of 10 CAM users do so to treat chronic disease. The 2002 CDC survey found that patients turned to CAM for various reasons:

1. Fifty-four percent believed CAM combined with conventional treatment would help.
2. Fifty percent utilized CAM because they thought it might be interesting to try.
3. Twenty-six percent used CAM because a conventional medical professional suggested they try it.
4. Twenty-eight percent of CAM users believed it would be more effective than conventional treatment.[1]
5. Thirteen percent believed conventional treatment was too expensive.

Another survey in the United States, however, found that dissatisfaction with conventional medicine was no more prevalent among CAM users than among nonusers; rather, the study found that people were more likely to choose CAM if it was congruent with their own values, beliefs, and philosophical orientations toward health and life.[10] Still, this study reported that chronic problems such as low back pain, chronic pain, anxiety, and generally poor health status were predictors of CAM use.

WIDELY USED COMPLEMENTARY AND ALTERNATIVE MEDICINE SYSTEMS AND THERAPIES

Surveys indicate that chiropractic, copper bracelets, magnets, herbs, topical treatments, electrical stimulators, nutriceuticals, homeopathy, massage, acupuncture, diet therapies, relaxation, and spiritual healing are all therapies used by rheumatology patients.[5,7] This section aims to give a brief introduction to the philosophy and practice of a few main, commonly used modalities; in particular, therapies that are supported by evidence are discussed. Moreover, these examples have been chosen to illustrate the complexity of CAM systems as well as to introduce the reader to some of the main clinical, philosophical, and research issues that must be confronted if integration of these therapies into mainstream medical practice is to occur. Table 47.1 provides a glossary of CAM therapies. A recent report by the Arthritis Research

TABLE 47.1 GLOSSARY OF COMMON COMPLEMENTARY AND ALTERNATIVE MEDICINE THERAPIES

	Description
Alternative medical systems	Complete systems of diagnosis and practice that are based on a unique theoretical framework and are developed independently of biomedicine
Traditional Chinese medicine	Originating in China over 2000 years ago, this system uses acupuncture, herbs, massage, and meditative exercise (qi gong) to restore balance within the body and with nature. It is based on the eight principles of yin, yang, hot, cold, external, internal, deficiency, and excess.
Ayurveda	In this traditional medical system of India, herbs, massage, yoga, and therapeutic elimination are used to restore balance within the body and with nature. It is based on balancing the three doshas: vata, pitta, and kapha.
Homeopathy	A system of medicine developed in Germany in the late 1700s, homeopathy is based on the law of similars, in which compounds that cause a set of symptoms in large doses can purportedly cure the same symptoms when given in minute doses.
Naturopathy	A system of medicine founded on the healing power of nature, naturopathy uses a combination of therapies from the sciences of clinical nutrition, herbal medicine, homeopathy, physical medicine, exercise therapy, counseling, stress management, acupuncture, natural childbirth, and hydrotherapy.
Mind-body interventions	Therapies that employ techniques designed to facilitate the mind's capacity to affect bodily function and symptoms.
Meditation	Intentional self-regulation of attention or a systematic mental focus is used on particular aspects of inner or outer experience. Most meditation practices were developed within a religious/spiritual context and held as their ultimate goal some type of spiritual growth, personal transformation, and/or transcendental experience. However, it has been argued that, as a health care intervention, meditation can be effective regardless of an individual's cultural or religious background.
Relaxation techniques	Techniques are specifically designed to elicit a psychophysiologic state of hypoarousal. They may be aimed at reducing sympathetic nervous system activity and blood pressure, easing muscle tension, slowing metabolic processes, or altering brain wave activity.
Guided imagery	Mental images are used to promote relaxation and wellness or to facilitate healing of a particular ailment (e.g., cancer, psychological trauma). The images can involve any of the senses and may be self-directed or guided by a practitioner.
Hypnosis	This describes a state of attentive and focused concentration in which people can be relatively unaware of, but not entirely unconscious of, their surroundings. Hypnotized individuals become absorbed in the images presented by the hypnotherapist and tend not to register experiences as a part of their conscious awareness.
Biofeedback	Mechanical devices that amplify physiologic signals (e.g., blood pressure, muscle activity) are used to teach methods of regulating these physiologic processes through intention.
Biologically based therapies	Natural and biologically based practices, interventions, and products
Herbalism	Plants are used to treat disease and promote health.
Orthomolecular therapies	Molecules normally found in the body (e.g., hormones, vitamins, and nutrients) are used to treat disease and promote health.
Diet therapies	Specialized dietary regimens (e.g., Gerson therapy, Kelley regimen, macrobiotic diet, Ornish diet, Pritikin diet) are advised for the treatment or prevention of a specific disease (e.g., cancer, cardiovascular disease) or for the promotion of general health.
Biologic therapies	Substances (e.g., shark cartilage) or molecules (e.g. SAM-e, glucosamine) that are naturally occurring in animal physiology are used to treat specific diseases.
Body-based therapies	Manipulation or movement of the body for healing purposes
Chiropractic	Manipulation of bones and joints based on the relationship between structure (e.g., the spine) and function (i.e., central nervous system) to restore balance to the body
Massage	Manipulation of body tissues to promote wellness and reduce pain and stress
Rolfing	Manipulation and stretching of the fascias to reestablish a healthy alignment of bone and muscle
Reflexology	Application of manual pressure to specific areas of the foot that theoretically correspond to different organs or systems of the body
Postural re-education	The use of movement and touch to help patients relearn healthy posture. The therapies seek to release habitual, harmful ways of holding the body by focusing on awareness through movement.
Energy therapies	Therapeutic practices that focus on energy fields originating either within the body (biofields) or from external sources (electromagnetic fields)
Magnets	Magnets are placed on the body to ease pain.
Pulsed electrical field	Injured body parts are placed in an induced electrical field to facilitate healing.
Reiki	In this technique of Japanese origin a practitioner channels energy through his/her body and into a patient's body to promote healing.
Therapeutic touch	Often referred to as "laying on of hands" even though actual touch is not required, this therapy uses the healing energy of the therapist to identify and repair imbalances in a patient's biofield.
External qi gong	This is a subset of Chinese medical qi gong practice in which a master healer uses the energy of his/her own biofield to bring another person's energy into balance.

Complementary and alternative medicine therapies have been organized into five major groups by the National Center for Complementary and Alternative Medicine: alternative medical systems, mind-body interventions, biologically based interventions, manual therapies, and energy therapies.

Campaign (U.K.) systematically reviewed a wide range of nutritional and herbal products and their likely clinical effects in osteoarthritis (OA), rheumatoid arthritis (RA), and fibromyalgia[1]; it is primarily targeted at patients but provides an important source of unbiased and rigorous information about these approaches.

Traditional Chinese medicine and acupuncture

Philosophy and history

Traditional Chinese medicine (TCM) is the product of thousands of years of philosophical, political, spiritual, and scientific evolution. Although its exact origin remains controversial, it is generally accepted that the first true Chinese medical texts emerged around 200 BC.[11] Today, TCM is an intricate medical system based on ancient philosophies, symptom-based clinical practice, a complicated individualized diagnostic system, and a variety of treatment modalities, including various types of acupuncture, massage (tui na), and herbal medicines.

Like many CAM systems, TCM is based on a belief in the existence of a life force or vital energy that runs through the body and affects its functioning. This energy takes the form of the vital substances: qi, blood, essence, and body fluids. People are healthy when their energy is unobstructed, balanced, and harmonious; it is the practitioner's aim to restore this energetic state through the manipulation of the vital essences. Imbalances are diagnosed into syndrome patterns according to a number of complex yet subtle theories that provide the basis for treatment. Central to this is the theory of yin and yang (Fig. 47.1). The terms and concepts within TCM have no Western equivalents; at best, they are roughly translated and are therefore easily misinterpreted. For example, concepts such as blood or kidney may seem familiar but their meaning in the context of TCM encompasses more and differs

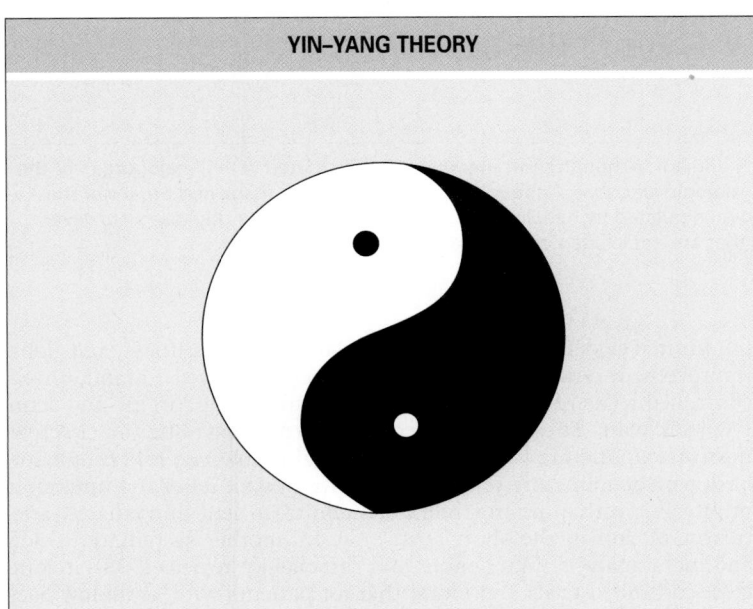

YIN–YANG THEORY

Fig. 47.1 Yin-yang theory. The concept of yin and yang is of utmost importance in traditional Chinese medicine, as well as in other styles of oriental medicine and acupuncture. Yin and yang are two dynamic parts of a whole; they are opposing, interchangeable forces that contain and define each other. They are always in flux and both are always present: one cannot exist without the other. Yin is characteristically cool, heavy, dark, moist, condensing, descending, and still; yang is bright, expansive, creative, hot, light, ascending, and active. Yin is associated with the earth, whereas yang is associated with the sun and the heavens. All people contain a balance of yin and yang; when this balance is disrupted, health may be affected. For example, yin deficiency/yang excess may manifest as hot, dry inflammation with restlessness, whereas yin excess/yang deficiency could manifest as heavy, dull pain that is exacerbated by cold and accompanied by general listlessness. Yin-yang theory is the basis for more detailed diagnostic theories such as the "eight principles" and zhang-fu organ differentiation. According to ancient Chinese philosophy, yin-yang theory is an elegant model for all of nature and the universe.

significantly from the Western biomedical model. Learning TCM without stepping out of a Western framework is like trying to edit a Chinese text with English grammar rules.

Treatment

The TCM system encompasses many different treatment modalities, each used to shift the vital energy of the body. Many of these techniques stimulate specific points on the body to alter the flow of qi; usually, these points are located on meridians (specific channels that carry qi through the body; Fig. 47.2). Acupuncture, the most well known, involves the insertion of thin, stainless steel needles into these points (Fig. 47.3). Similarly, moxibustion (the burning of a specific variety of the herb *Artemisia vulgaris*), cupping (the use of suction), and acupressure (manual stimulation) all stimulate acupuncture points. Internal remedies are a vital component of TCM; a materia medica of over 10,000 herb and animal compounds has been developed. These herbal remedies are always given in combination and are chosen to complement and balance each other. Additionally, TCM incorporates a unique system of massage called tui na and uses meditative exercises such as qi gong.

The TCM approach to rheumatic disease is very different from that of conventional modern medicine. First, the concept of rheumatic disease as it is understood in the West does not exist in TCM. Rather, the majority of rheumatic disorders fall into the general classifications of painful obstructions (bi syndrome). Within this general diagnosis, the particular energetic characteristics that a patient expresses (e.g., hot, cold, yin deficiency, blood stagnation, wind, damp) will determine diagnosis and treatment. Thus, TCM treatment of rheumatic disorders, as with many CAM disciplines, is individualized; patients with the same conventional diagnosis may receive different TCM diagnoses and treatments.

Evidence

Although herbal combinations and other treatments are used in conjunction with acupuncture in clinical practice, the vast majority of research on TCM in the West focuses on acupuncture. A large body of evidence exists for the underlying physiologic mechanisms of acupuncture in the treatment of pain.[12] Most basic research in acupuncture focuses on mechanisms for acupuncture analgesia; these include neural, humoral, and bioelectric components.[13] Numerous studies show that various levels of the nervous system are involved in acupuncture analgesia from the afferent pathways to the thalamus.[14,15] Moreover, the endorphin system is implicated in acupuncture physiology as endorphin levels in cerebrospinal fluid rise after acupuncture.[16] Different needling frequencies have been found to release different substances: for example, 2 to 4 Hz releases β-endorphins and met-enkephalins, whereas 100 to 200 Hz releases serotonin and dynorphins.[13] The serotonergic and cholinergic systems have also been implicated in acupuncture analgesia, which may account for the partial naloxone inhibition.[17] In addition, recent work with positron emission tomography by the Southampton group in conjunction with University College, London, suggests that there may be specific neural substrates for acupuncture over and above the endorphin-rich placebo expectation matrix that has previously been identified as being associated with acupuncture and pain. Defining the underlying mechanisms and substrates through which real acupuncture may operate will provide important insights into not only acupuncture but also the mechanisms of the placebo effect in chronic pain.[18]

However, evidence for the efficacy of acupuncture in the treatment of rheumatic and musculoskeletal disorders is mixed. Different systematic reviews of the clinical effects of acupuncture analyzed many of the same, rather poor-quality, randomized controlled trials and, although agreeing about the paucity of research in this field, have come to different conclusions with respect to its clinical effectiveness.[18-22]

Ezzo and associates[23] reviewed seven trials of acupuncture for OA and found limited evidence that acupuncture is more effective than waiting lists or usual treatment, strong evidence that acupuncture is more effective than sham for pain, and inconclusive evidence for function. However, another study by Ernst and coworkers[19] reviewed 11 OA randomized controlled trials; in 7 trials positive results were reported but were of poor quality. A review of the randomized controlled trials of acupuncture for fibromyalgia[21] (n = 7) found positive

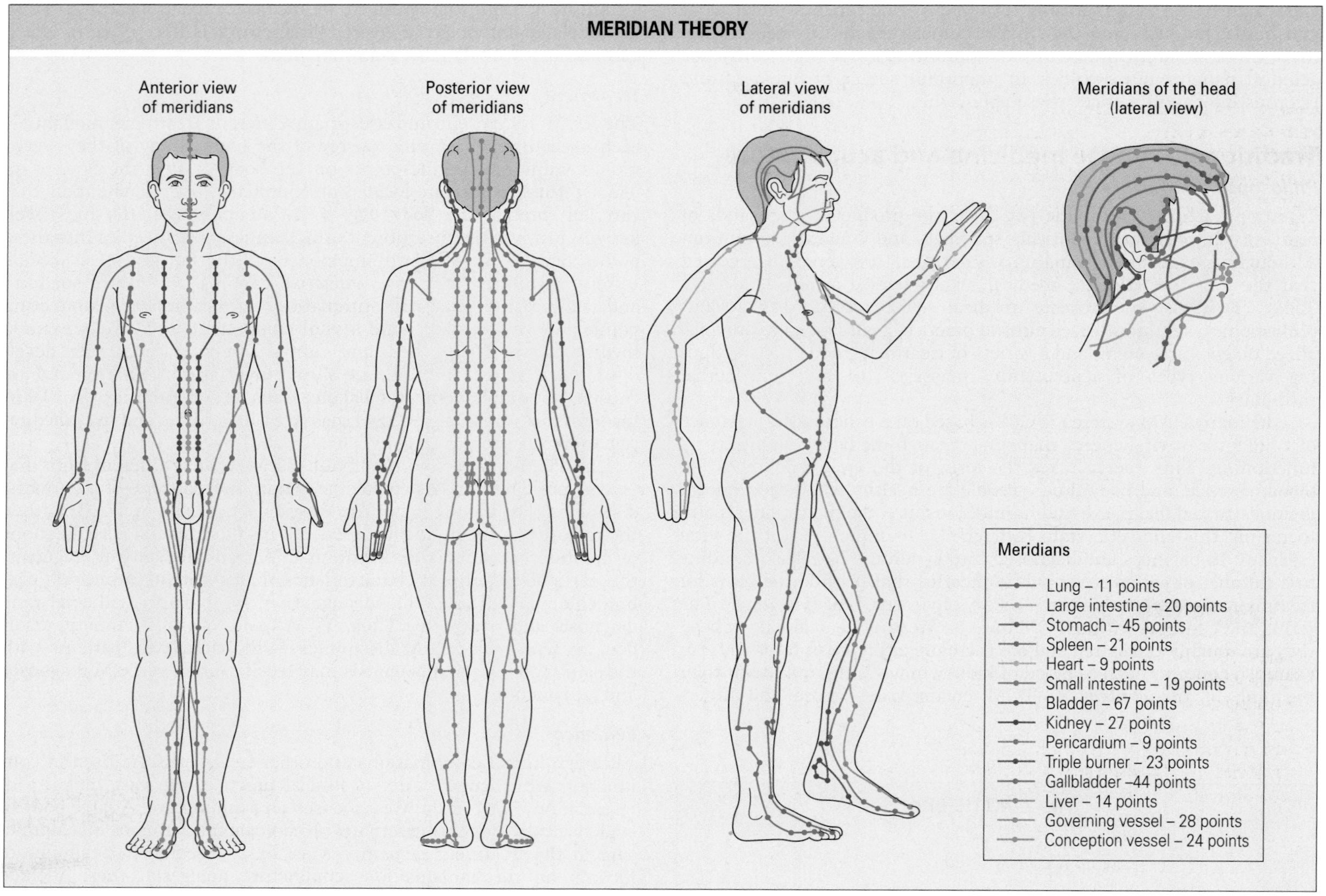

MERIDIAN THEORY

Anterior view of meridians

Posterior view of meridians

Lateral view of meridians

Meridians of the head (lateral view)

Meridians

- Lung – 11 points
- Large intestine – 20 points
- Stomach – 45 points
- Spleen – 21 points
- Heart – 9 points
- Small intestine – 19 points
- Bladder – 67 points
- Kidney – 27 points
- Pericardium – 9 points
- Triple burner – 23 points
- Gallbladder –44 points
- Liver – 14 points
- Governing vessel – 28 points
- Conception vessel – 24 points

Fig. 47.2 Meridian theory. Qi is believed to run through the body in channels called meridians; although most meridians are associated with a major organ of the body (e.g., kidney, spleen), they each govern a much broader range of emotional/physiologic functions. Although they flow inside the tissue and organs of the body, the meridians are accessible from the surface in some areas; thus, the qi can be manipulated by needling acupuncture points on the meridians. However, qi flow is not restricted to specific channels; there are numerous acupuncture points that are not located on meridians.

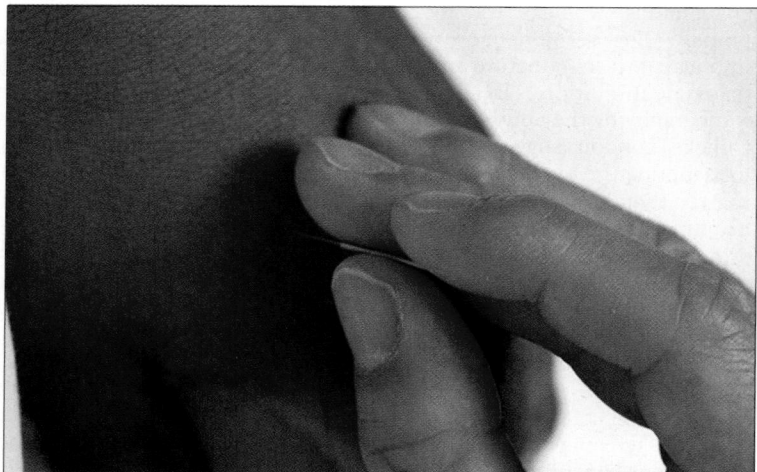

Fig. 47.3 Acupuncture. Acupuncture is one tool a traditional Chinese medical doctor uses to shift a person's vital energy. It involves the insertion of thin, solid, stainless-steel needles into specific points on the body. There are numerous styles of acupuncture, including Japanese, Korean, five-element, and six energetic levels. Acupuncture points can also be stimulated manually without the use of needles; this approach may be better suited for children or the elderly.

but limited evidence that acupuncture affects pain, stiffness, and global improvement ratings. Furlan and colleagues[22] reviewed 35 randomized, controlled trials of acupuncture in the treatment of chronic and acute low back pain. The data provided no evidence regarding the effectiveness of acupuncture for acute low back pain; however, for chronic low back pain acupuncture was more effective in pain relief and functional improvement than no treatment or sham treatment immediately after treatment and in the short term only. In another systematic review and meta-analysis, Manheimer and associates[24] reviewed 33 randomized, controlled trials and found that for patients with acute low back pain, acupuncture proved to be ineffective. However, for patients with chronic low back pain acupuncture was significantly more effective than sham treatment or no treatment but, although the results were significant, further research is still necessary to assess the effect of acupuncture on acute low back pain and the long-term effects on chronic low back pain. A review of acupuncture for chronic pain (n = 51) found limited evidence that acupuncture is more effective than no treatment and inconclusive evidence that it is more effective than placebo, sham acupuncture, or standard care.[20] Cummings has reviewed some of the recent large German studies and showed that acupuncture is both cost-effective and considerably more therapeutically effective than standard conventional care for chronic back pain, OA knee, migraine, tension headache, and neck pain.[2]

There are very few randomized controlled trials investigating acupuncture for RA; preliminary evidence is positive and suggests that more research is warranted.[25]

The differing conclusions from these systematic reviews may in part be caused by the standard rating scales used (e.g., Jadad scale), which strongly favor placebo-controlled trials. Acupuncture has no true placebo, so many valid randomized controlled trials may be given low methodologic scores.[26] Important methodologic improvements must guide further research. First, most acupuncture trials use formulaic acupuncture treatments that are applied to all patients; however, because acupuncture treatments are highly individualized in clinical practice, this study design tests acupuncture outside its therapeutic context.[27] Regardless of whether investigators choose a standardized, individualized, or hybrid design, an appropriate number of treatments must be administered; positive results are significantly correlated with trials that include six or more treatments.[20] Also, appropriate acupuncture points must be chosen: because there is no standard protocol for any given condition, the knowledge and skill of the investigators are of the utmost importance. Furthermore, appropriate controls must be used. Because placebo-controlled trials are difficult, numerous sham procedures have been developed; however, there is no single design that will control for all non-specific effects.[27]

With these questions in mind, in 2004 the University of Maryland conducted a large randomized, controlled trial (n = 570) of acupuncture for OA of the knee.[28] The participants were divided into three groups receiving different therapies. The experimental group received true acupuncture, whereas the two control groups received either sham acupuncture or educational treatment. After 26 weeks the true acupuncture group experienced greater pain relief than the sham or educational groups in the WOMAC function score, WOMAC pain score, and the patient global assessment. Overall, the study showed significant data that acupuncture provides improvement in pain relief and function as a complementary therapy for OA of the knee when compared with sham and educational control groups. This conclusion has now largely been supported with the publication of two positive systematic reviews.[3,4]

In the late 1990s, the evidence for the use of acupuncture in chronic mechanical neck pain was limited.[29] A recent study by the CAM Research Unit in Southampton demonstrated that acupuncture for chronic mechanical neck pain has a similar specific effect size to that reported by Berman and associates.[28,30] Perhaps the most interesting thing about both these large studies is the large and sustained nonspecific effect produced by acupuncture, a particularly relevant observation when its safety is also taken into account.[31,32]

Herbalism

Philosophy and history

Although herbs are the most popular and ancient CAM modality,[9] herbalism is one of the least understood systems of medicine. For example, herbs are commonly used in isolation by patients with expectations that they will treat a particular disease or symptom; however, herbs are very rarely used in isolation by professional herbalists. Also, when a herb is shown to be effective for a specific condition, the herb tends to be narrowly categorized and its other therapeutic properties are ignored. Traditionally, herbs are used in multiple organ systems and are applicable to many different conditions. Furthermore, herbal treatment protocols are highly individualized and indications for herbs may be very specific. Sometimes, herbs are used in an overtly dangerous manner. The majority of herb users self-medicate without informing their doctors,[9] and inappropriate selection or combinations of herbs can cause adverse events that may mimic, magnify, or oppose the effects of pharmaceuticals[33] (Table 47.2). Moreover, serious adverse effects are often the result of intentional and inappropriate marketing of potent herbs, as in the case of ephedra (ma huang) for weight loss and energy. Traditionally used to treat asthma in China, ephedra is a powerful sympathetic nervous system stimulant that has caused cardiovascular and CNS events, such as hypertension and stroke.[34]

The practice of traditional herbalism (TCM or ayurveda) is plant centered and requires the use of whole plant material because it is found naturally. On an energetic level, the whole plant is believed to contain a unique life force that is essential for treatment; on the biochemical level, the whole plant is needed to ensure that all the possible complex and unidentified, synergistic compounds within the plant are included with the known active constituents.

Treatment

Herbs are usually prescribed in combination and treatment is individualized. A herbalist approaches the body as a whole system and formulates treatments that address underlying physiologic problems as well as acute symptoms. Treatments are usually given orally but may be prescribed as external salves. The bulk of a herbal formula is composed of alternatives: antirheumatics and anti-inflammatories such as sarsaparilla, black cohosh, celery, meadowsweet, nettle, turmeric, boswellia, wild yam, devil's claw, and ginger (Fig. 47.4; Table 47.3). Often, blends will contain diuretics, immune stimulants, circulatory stimulants, and digestive tonics as well; only a small portion of the blend addresses symptoms through analgesic action.[35] Nutritional approaches are frequently combined with herbs; ideally, herbs are woven into the daily diet as spices and foods.

Evidence

To date, systematic and meta-analytic reviews of the literature in rheumatology indicate that a number of herbs may be effective treatments for rheumatic and musculoskeletal conditions.[36-39] Randomized controlled trials have shown that devil's claw (*Harpagophytum procumbens*) and bromelain (a pineapple extract) may significantly reduce pain associated with OA[40] and low back pain[41]; two randomized controlled trials indicate that willow bark extract improves WOMAC pain scores in OA patients.[38,42] Six randomized controlled trials of the herbal mixture Phytodolor (golden rod, aspen leaf/bark, and ash bark) showed significantly decreased pain,[38] increased function, and decreased rescue medication for mixed rheumatic disorders, including OA; there was no significant difference between Phytodolor and piroxicam.[38] Randomized controlled trials investigated topical capsaicin (cayenne) for the treatment of OA[43,44]; collectively, meta-analysis of these data indicates that capsaicin is an effective therapy for pain, tenderness, and range of motion.[39,45]

There are also a handful of single studies, but although they were of adequate quality, one study is insufficient to draw conclusions about the efficacy of any intervention. For instance, one small study (n = 27) showed that topical application of nettle leaf reduced pain and disability[46] and another herbal combination, Reumalex, significantly reduced pain in arthritic patients but was not significantly efficacious in OA patients alone.[47] A systematic review by Little and colleagues[48] compared herbal interventions using herbs rich in γ-linolenic acid (GLA) to treat RA. The sources of GLA were borage oil, evening primrose oil, and blackcurrant seed oil. Compared with the placebo oils (olive oil, sunflower oil, cottonseed oil, liquid paraffin, and soybean oil) the oils containing GLA significantly improved joint tenderness, swelling, stiffness, and functionality. However, to date, single studies of ginger[49] and the herbal combinations Eazmov[50] and Gitadyl[51] have not produced evidence of efficacy.

Because of the paucity of quality trials, many herbs traditionally used by professional herbalists have not been adequately investigated (if at all). Further research is clearly needed.

Nutriceuticals

The term *nutriceuticals* is a general classification that refers to the wide array of biologically based products available to health practitioners and consumers; they include vitamins, minerals, neurotransmitters, hormones, animal products such as shark cartilage and glandulars, and other naturally occurring substances such as glucosamine and S-adenosyl-methionine (SAM-e). The sheer number of these products can be overwhelming to both practitioners and consumers; to date, the efficacy and safety of most of these therapies have not been thoroughly investigated. However, there are a few nutriceuticals for which a substantial evidence base is beginning to emerge in the treatment of rheumatic and musculoskeletal diseases, most notably, glucosamine and chondroitin, SAM-e, and essential fatty acids.

Glucosamine and chondroitin

Numerous narrative and meta-analytic reviews suggest that glucosamine, either combined with chondroitin or alone, is effective in reducing pain and improving physical function in treatment for OA.[52-54] Towheed and coworkers[54] reviewed 16 randomized double-blind studies and found glucosamine to be significantly more effective than placebo

TABLE 47.2 REPORTED POTENTIAL HERB-DRUG INTERACTIONS RELEVANT TO RHEUMATOLOGY PRACTICE

Herb	Pharmaceutical	Effect	Mechanism/comment
Asian herbal mixtures:			
Sho-saiko-to	Prednisone	Decreased AUC	Contains *Glycyrrhiza glabra, Bupleurum falcatum, Pinellia ternate, Scutellaria abaicalensis, Zizyphus vulgaris, Panax ginseng, Zingiber officialis*
Saiboku-to		Increased AUC	Same as above, with addition of *Poria cocos, Magnolia officinalis,* and *Perillae frutescens*
Betel nut (*Areca catechu*)	Prednisone, albuterol (salbutamol)	Inadequate control of asthma	Arecoline challenge caused dose-related bronchoconstriction
Cayenne (*Capsicum* spp.)	ACE inhibitors	Cough	Capsaicin depletes substance P
	Theophylline	Increased absorption and bioavailability	
Devil's claw (*Harpagophytum procumbens*)	Warfarin	Purpura	
Dan shen (*Salvia miltlorrhiza*)	Warfarin	Increased INR, prolonged PT/PTT	Decreased elimination of warfarin in rats
	Aspirin	Spontaneous hyphema	Inhibition of platelet adhesion factor
	Warfarin	Intracerebral hemorrhage	
	Paracetamol and ergotamine/caffeine	Bilateral subdural hematoma	May be due to gingko alone
	Thiazide diuretic	Hypertension	Gingko alone is not associated with hypertension.
GLA-rich herbs (evening primrose, blackcurrant, borage)	Drugs that lower seizure threshold	Increased side effects	Decreased seizure threshold
Licorice (*Glycyrrhiza glabra*)	Prednisone	Glycyrrhizin decreases plasma clearance, increases AUC, increases plasma concentrations of prednisolone	Glycyrrhizin and its metabolite, glycyrrhetinic acid, are inhibitors of 5α,5β-reductase and 11β-dehydrogenase (converts endogenous cortisol to cortisone
	Hydrocortisone	Glycyrrhetinic acid potentiates cutaneous vasoconstrictor response	
	MAOIs	Increased side effects	Glycyrrhizin is an MAOI
	Oral contraceptives	Hypertension, edema, hypokalemia	Oral contraceptives may increase sensitivity to glycyrrhizin
Nettles (*Urtica dioica*)	NSAIDs	Increased therapeutic effect	Potentiation of anti-inflammatory activity
Panax ginseng	Warfarin	Decreased INR	
	Phenelzine	Headache and tremor, mania	
	Corticosteroids	Increased side effects	Similar side effects
	Estrogen replacement	Postmenopausal bleeding or mastalgia	
Papaya (*Carica papaya*)	Warfarin	Increased INR	
St. John's wort (*Hypericum perforatum*)	Paroxetine	Lethargy/incontinence	
	Trazodone	Mild serotonin syndrome	Can occur with St. John's wort alone
	Sertraline	Mild serotonin syndrome	
	Nefazodone	Mild serotonin syndrome	
	Theophylline	Decreased theophylline concentrations	
	Digoxin	Decreased AUC, decreased peak and trough concentrations	Most studies indicate that St. John's wort inhibits cytochrome P450 isoenzymes.
	Phenprocoumon	Decreased AUC	
	Cyclosporin	Decreased concentrations in serum	
	Oral contraceptives	Breakthrough bleeding	
Tamarid (*Tamarindus indica*)	Aspirin	Increased bioavailability of aspirin	
Yohimbe (*Pausinystalla yohimbe*)	Tricyclic antidepressants	Hypertension	Yohimbe alone is associated with hypertension; combination with tricyclics lowers active yohimbe dose.

ACE, angiotensin converting enzyme; AUC, area under the curve; INR, international normalized ratio; GLA, γ-linolenic acid; MAOI, monoamine oxidase inhibitor; NSAID, non-steroidal anti-inflammatory drug; PT, dilute prothrombin time; PTT, partial thromboplastin time. It is impossible to summarize all drug-herb interactions. Clinical data are sparse, uncontrolled, and often unreliable; most data are in the form of case reports, and issues of dosage, temporal relations, contamination, and concomitant drug-herb use are often unreported. Moreover, the majority of the herb-drug interactions described in the literature are theoretical in nature and have not been shown to occur in clinical practice; thus, only clinically reported interactions are summarized here. In addition, the effects may depend on mode of ingestion; for example, effects may be stronger if an extract is used (e.g., standardized allicin) as compared with incorporation of herbs into the diet (e.g., garlic cloves in food).

Data from Fugh-Berman A. Herb-drug interactions. Lancet 2000;355:134-138; Deal CL, Schnitzer TJ, Lipstein E, et al. Treatment of arthritis with topical capsaicin: a double-blind trial. Clin Ther 1991;13:383-395; and Hardy M. Herb-drug interactions: an evidence-based table. Alter Med Alert 2000;June:64-69.

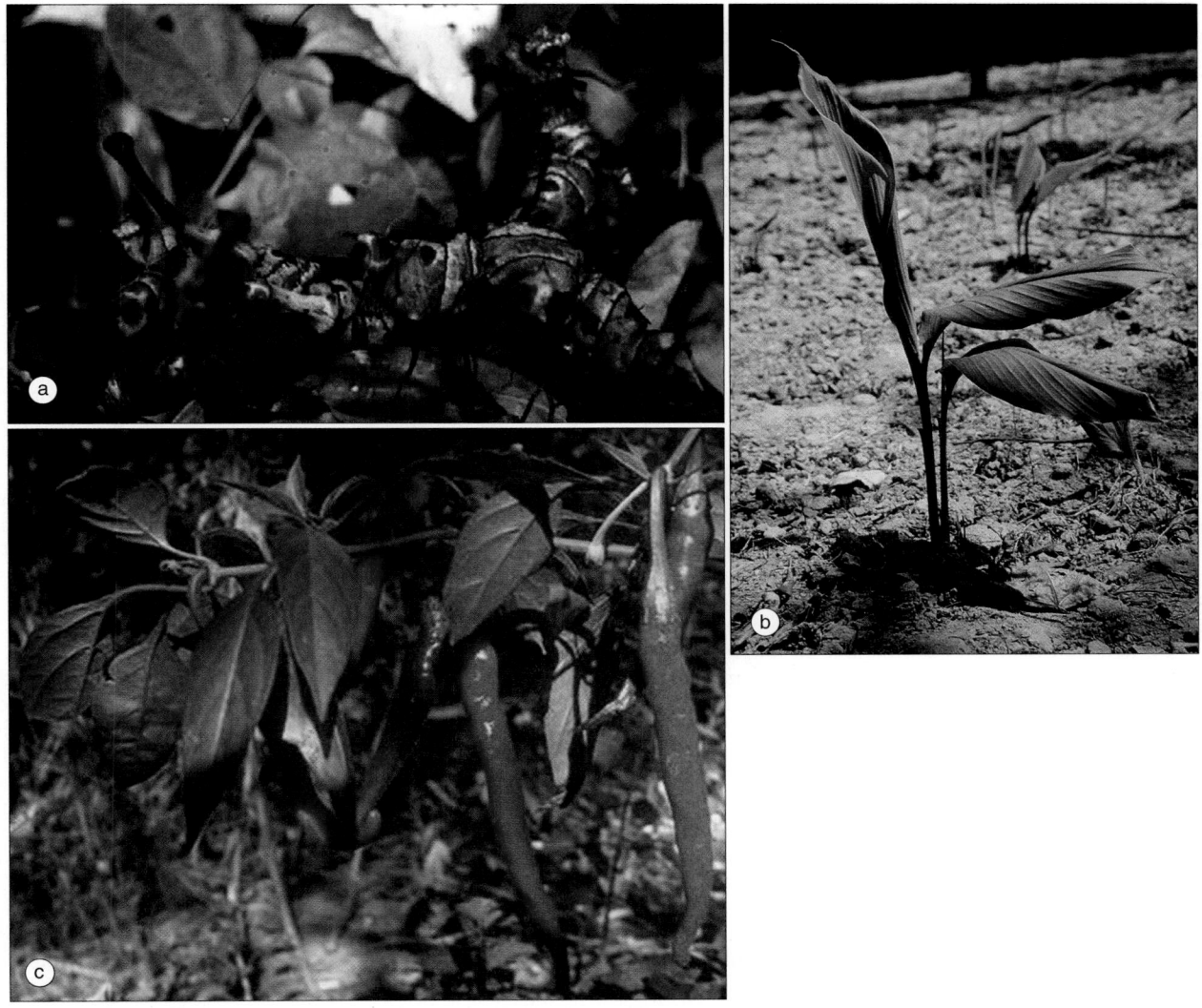

Fig. 47.4 Examples of herbs used in rheumatologic conditions. (a) Sarsaparilla (*Smilax rotundifolia*): the root is used medicinally. (b) Turmeric (*Curcuma longa*): the root is used medicinally. (c) Cayenne (*Capsicum annuum*): the fruit is used medicinally. *(Courtesy of M. Moore, Southwest School of Botanical Medicine.)*

TABLE 47.3 MECHANISMS OF PHYTO ANTI-INFLAMMATORY DRUGS

Herb	Cyclooxygenase	Lipoxygenase	Cytokine release	Antioxidant
Devil's claw	Inhibition	Inhibition	Inhibition	?
Stinging nettle	Inhibition	Inhibition	Inhibition	?
Willow bark	Inhibition	Inhibition	?	Yes
Blackcurrant seed	Inhibition	Inhibition	?	?
Blackcurrant leaf	Inhibition	Inhibition	?	Yes
Evening primrose seed	Inhibition	Inhibition	?	?
Borage seed	Inhibition	Inhibition	?	?
Goldenrod leaf, aspen leaf/bark, and ash bark	Inhibition	Inhibition	?	Yes

Known anti-inflammatory mechanisms of medical plants have been summarized by Chrubasik & Roufogalis.[35]

(effect size [ES] = 1.4) and more effective than or equal to non-steroidal anti-inflammatory drugs (NSAIDs) with minimal adverse effects (approximately 6%). McAlindon and associates[53] reviewed randomized trials of both glucosamine and chondroitin and found moderate to large effect sizes (0.44 and 0.78, respectively); modest yet positive effective sizes (0.3 and 0.4, respectively) were found when methodologically weak studies were excluded and results were recalculated for outcomes at 4 weeks. A narrative review of six trials by Delafuente[52] also supports the use of glucosamine for OA of the knee; although optimal dosage

has not yet been determined, a dose of 500 mg three times daily is generally used.

A randomized controlled trial (n = 212) published since the above reviews[55] has shown that patients taking 1500 mg of oral glucosamine sulfate daily over 3 years experienced no significant joint space loss and minimum joint space narrowing compared with patients on placebo. However, in that study the reliability of the radiographic findings is in question owing to the radiographic method used for determining joint space narrowing. A National Institutes of Health (NIH)-funded, multicenter, double-blind trial studied glucosamine, chondroitin sulfate, the combination, or placebo in 1583 patients with knee OA for 6 months.[56] The primary outcome measurement was 20% reduction in knee pain. Neither solo therapy nor the combination was superior to placebo in reduction in pain.

Glucosamine and chondroitin have been suggested to be chondroprotective agents.[56] Both are constituents of connective tissue and are capable of increasing proteoglycan synthesis in articular cartilage.[57] Moreover, despite controversy in this area, both substances appear to be absorbed intact in the digestive tract.[58] In contrast to NSAIDs, no serious or fatal side effects have been reported for glucosamine and chondroitin.[53]

S-adenosyl-methionine

Originally used to treat depression,[59,60] the effects of SAM-e on joint pain were discovered serendipitously when they were observed as side effects in clinical trials. Produced from L-methionine and adenosine triphosphate, SAM-e is a methyl donor involved in a wide variety of metabolic processes throughout the body.[60] Although the mechanism of action is not completely understood, SAM-e has been shown to have anti-inflammatory and analgesic effects without gastrointestinal damage in animal models[61]; in vitro, SAM-e has exhibited chondroprotective effects via the stimulation of chondrocytes and the subsequent increase in new cartilage production.[62]

A recent meta-analysis of 13 trials investigating SAM-e in the treatment of OA[63] indicated that SAM-e is comparable to ibuprofen (ES = 0.16) and superior to placebo (ES = 0.36); however, demonstrated efficacy was not related to dosage or length of intervention. SAM-e has no known side effects,[59] but the long-term effects are unknown.

Essential fatty acids

Essential fatty acids, including omega-6 fatty acids (linolenic acid [LA]) and γ-linolenic acid [GLA]) and omega-3 fatty acids (α-linolenic acid [ALA], eicosapentaenoic acid [EPA], and docosahexaenoic acid [DHA]) are the first components of a physiologic cascade that results in prostaglandin, leukotriene, and thromboxane production.[64] Specifically, the presence of omega-3 fatty acids can antagonize the cellular biosynthesis of prostaglandins E_2 and LTB_4, interleukin-1β, and tumor necrosis factor[65]; these lipids play an important role in the pathophysiology of RA.[66] Moreover, omega-3 fatty acids may inhibit the platelet-activating factor synthesis pathway, the cyclooxygenase pathway, and the 5-lipoxygenase pathway.[67]

Omega-3 fatty acids have been shown in numerous reviews to improve RA symptoms.[65,68,69] Studies have consistently shown that omega-3 supplementation reduces the number of tender joints and morning stiffness; effects are modest but clear.[65,68,70] In addition, multiple studies indicate that omega-3 supplementation can reduce dependence on NSAIDs and antirheumatic drugs[71-74]; however, additional studies are needed before definitive conclusions can be made.[65] No significant toxicities have been associated with their use.[75]

Omega-3 fatty acids are found in fish oils (EPA, DHA), leafy green vegetables (ALA), and plant oils such as flaxseed, rapeseed, and walnuts (ALA); while all forms are important, EPA and DHA are more easily utilized by the body.[76] To date, most studies have investigated the effects of fish oils; these show that a minimum daily dosage of 3 g of EPA and DHA is required for clinical efficacy; benefits become apparent after a minimum of 12 weeks.[65] Although no serious toxicity has been reported, potential adverse effects associated with EPA and DHA have been increases in low-density lipoprotein levels and bleeding times and a worsening glycemic index in diabetics.[77] However, by monitoring the dosage clinicians may easily prevent such safety concerns.

In addition, there is evidence for the efficacy of certain omega-6 fatty acids[64]; these, however, are generally administered in the form of herbal extracts of evening primrose, borage, or blackcurrant[74,78] (see earlier).

Homeopathy

Homeopathy is probably one of the most widespread, and certainly one of the most controversial, treatments within CAM. It involves the prescription of often very dilute, indeed in some cases ultramolecular, doses of usually herbal products that have been shaken and serially diluted. Homeopathy was developed by Samuel Hahnemann, a German physician, some 200 years ago. The first principle of homeopathy is that of similars: this states that patients who present with particular signs and symptoms can be cured if they are given a homeopathic medication that produces the same signs and symptoms in a healthy individual. In other words, homeopathy is designed around the concept of matching the patient's symptoms with a drug picture produced by a homeopathic remedy and the idea of "like cures like" is derived from this concept. The second principle, and probably the most confusing to orthodox physicians, is that serial dilutions of a medication, often until the medication has no molecules of the original product, will result in the medication still retaining its homeopathic effects even though it is diluted beyond the Avogadro number. Homeopathy therefore confronts conventional science at its core and many believe that homeopathy can have no more than a placebo effect. In spite of the continuing debate concerning the effects of ultramolecular doses of medicine, evidence is beginning to emerge that homeopathy may be of value in fibromyalgia. There are now four positive clinical trials of individualized homeopathy, all of which suggest that it may have something to offer this intractable condition.[5-8] However, our reason for including homeopathy in this chapter is not to provide conclusive evidence that it "works" in arthritic conditions but to illustrate some of the problems that face us within CAM research.[79]

Evidence

Jonas and associates[80] undertook a systematic review of the quality of homeopathic clinical trials. The study contained 59 studies of various homeopathic treatments, ranging from stroke, postoperative complications, arthritis, and fibromyalgia to influenza. The studies in rheumatology indicate an odds ratio that, overall, significantly favors homeopathy but would suggest, as indeed does the whole of Jonas and associates' systematic review, that there is currently inadequate evidence to make specific claims about homeopathy in any particular condition but overall evidence that homeopathy is more than a simple placebo effect.

Of particular interest in the context of these studies is that of Fisher and coworkers, published in the *British Medical Journal* in 1989.[81] In this study, patients with a defined diagnosis (fibromyalgia) were entered with a dual allocation process. Patients were entered if they fulfilled the diagnostic criteria for fibromyalgia but a second inclusion criterion involved them in only being entered into the double-blind, randomized, controlled trial if they also fulfilled the specific requirements for the prescription of a particular homeopathic remedy, *Rhus tox*. Fisher's study indicated that individualized treatment need not be a bar to entry and therefore evaluates a particular homeopathic remedy against placebo in a well-defined, conventional complaint. In a second, more recent study, Bell and colleagues[82] performed a double-blind, randomized trial of homeopathy in the treatment of fibromyalgia. Fifty-three patients were randomized to receive either oral, daily liquid homeopathic remedies or an indistinguishable placebo. After 3 months the participants who received homeopathic treatments showed significantly greater improvements in tender point count and tender point pain, quality of life, global health, and less depression than those who received the placebo.

Homeopathy therefore provides us with excellent examples of both individualized treatment and innovative study methodology as far as CAM is concerned. If homeopathy is effective and can be proved to be so, this must represent an interesting and complex challenge to modern pharmacology.

Mind-body interventions

Mind-body therapies (MBTs) do not constitute a system of medicine in and of themselves. Rather, it is a general classification that encompasses a wide spectrum of interventions from many different medical paradigms; in both traditional and modern practice, MBTs are often used as adjunctive or preventative therapies. They include more conventional Western therapies such as psychotherapy, cognitive-behavioral therapy, and hypnosis as well as techniques native to Asian medical systems and cultures such as yoga, qi gong, and meditation. In addition, MBTs include techniques such as relaxation response, guided imagery, and biofeedback as well as more controversial therapies such as art, music, and dance therapies; prayer; and distant healing.

Although these techniques are all based on their own underlying philosophies and vary widely in their complexity, they are linked together by a fundamental concept. They not only assume that the mind and body are inextricably linked but they are also based on the idea that the mind can be trained to improve the functioning of the body. Common characteristics of MBT include self-regulation of attention, focused concentration, and development of self-awareness and mental equanimity.[83] Sometimes, as in the cases of yoga and qi gong, this process is facilitated by physical movements specifically developed for this purpose. In other therapies, the mind-body connection is developed through external cues. For example, biofeedback uses a mechanical device that amplifies physiologic indicators (e.g., blood pressure) to help patients become "tuned in" to the functioning of their body; when the mind has been "trained" to consciously regulate these physiologic indicators, the device is no longer needed because patients are able to independently alter their physiologic state. Other more traditional MBTs (e.g., meditation and prayer) were developed as a part of religious or spiritual practice. Some controversial therapies, such as distant healing, may even be able to establish a mind-body connection between people who are not in immediate contact.[84]

Evidence

Moderate evidence suggests that MBTs are effective adjuncts in the treatment of RA and OA. A meta-analytic comparison (n = 47) of psychoeducational interventions (i.e., biofeedback, relaxation, coping skills, information, behavioral instruction, social support) and NSAID treatment found that psychoeducational components provided additional benefits over NSAID treatment alone.[85] Although the effect sizes for MBT were not large, they provided an additional 20% to 30% relief of pain in OA and RA, 40% increase in functional ability in RA, and 60% to 80% decrease in joint tenderness in RA over NSAID treatment alone. The Arthritis Self-Management Program (ASMP) may be particularly effective for arthritis (especially OA).[86,87]

In addition, a meta-analysis of similar MBTs for RA found small but significant effect sizes for pain (ES = 0.22), disability (ES = 0.36), and depression (ES = 0.17).[88] Moreover, a meta-analysis of behavioral therapies for chronic low back pain[89] found that there was strong evidence that MBTs have a moderately positive effect on pain (ES = 0.62) and a small positive effect on both functional status (ES = 0.35) and behavioral outcomes (ES = 0.40) as compared with inactive controls; there was moderate evidence, however, that MBTs do not improve outcomes as adjunct treatments for low back pain. The one exception to this is a recent trial of the Alexander technique for low back pain that showed this to be a very effective (and cost-effective) intervention. The Alexander technique involves one-on-one lessons with a trained teacher who provides a combination of a "hands on" approach, exercises, and MBT that relates to an individual's posture and movement.[9,10]

The current evidence for efficacy of MBT for fibromyalgia is equivocal: a review of 13 randomized controlled trials found limited evidence that MBTs are more effective than waiting list, usual care, and placebo for some outcomes; inconclusive evidence for MBTs when compared with education/attention controls; and limited evidence that moderate/high-intensity exercise is more effective than MBTs.[90]

The current evidence indicates that MBTs are particularly suited to improving quality of life by decreasing pain, disability, and depression[88] and improving mood, coping, and social function.[91] However, MBT research is still in its early stages and issues such as the relative efficacy of different MBTs for specific medical conditions, as well as synergistic effects of multiple MBTs, have not been adequately examined. Moreover, although some studies have suggested that MBTs may be cost-effective,[92-94] no definitive data currently exist and conclusions are premature.[87]

TABLE 47.4 LICENSING AND TRAINING OF MAJOR COMPLEMENTARY AND ALTERNATIVE MEDICINE THERAPIES IN THE UNITED STATES

Therapy	Licensure (as of 2006)	Appropriate training	Professional organizations
Acupuncture	All states except Alabama, Delaware, Kansas, Kentucky, Michigan, Mississippi, Nevada, Oklahoma, South Dakota, and Wyoming	Minimum 3-year master's or doctorate degree, variable postgraduate training for medical providers Board exams	American Association of Oriental Medicine American Academy of Medical Acupuncture National Acupuncture Foundation Accreditation Commission for Acupuncture and Oriental Medicine National Certification Commission for Acupuncture and Oriental Medicine
Chiropractic	All 50 states	3- to 4-year doctorate program at an accredited university Board exams	American Chiropractic Organization Foundation for Chiropractic Education and Research
Massage therapy	Alabama, Arkansas, Connecticut, Delaware, District of Columbia, Florida, Hawaii, Iowa, Louisiana, Maine, Maryland, Mississippi, Missouri, Nebraska, Nevada, New Hampshire, New Jersey, New Mexico, New York, North Carolina, Ohio, Oregon, Rhode Island, South Carolina, Tennessee, Texas, Utah, Virginia, Washington, West Virginia, and Wisconsin	Minimum of 500 hours, usually from an accredited program Board exams	American Massage Therapy Association Commission on Massage Training Accreditation National Certification Board for Therapeutic Massage and Bodywork
Herbalism	None; often practiced under another health care license	Apprenticeship program or 3-year degree	American Herbalist's Guild American Botanical Council Herb Research Foundation
Naturopathy	Arkansas, Arizona, Connecticut, Hawaii, Maine, Montana, New Hampshire, Oregon, Utah, Vermont, and Washington	4-year accredited doctorate program Board exams	American Association of Naturopathic Physicians North American Board of Naturopathic Examiners
Homeopathy	Arizona, Connecticut, and Nevada; often practiced under another health care license	Naturopathic program, postgraduate training for medical providers, homeopathic universities abroad	National Center for Homeopathy American Board of Homeotherapeutics Homeopathic Academy of Naturopathic Physicians Council for Homeopathic Certification

Licensing laws vary widely from state to state in terms of eligibility, examination, scope of practice, and autonomy; moreover, many states have introduced statutes that have yet to take effect. Training is highly variable; the minimum training required for professional competency is listed here. Contact the appropriate professional organization for information on qualified practitioners in your area.

REFERRAL AND PROFESSIONAL PRACTICE

Above all, physicians need to initiate an open dialogue with their patients about CAM therapies; more than 70% of patients who use CAM do not inform their physician that they are doing so.[95] When discussing CAM use with patients, it is important to remain neutral, because negative attitudes or labels such as "unorthodox" may discourage the patient from discussing CAM use.[95] Moreover, issues of safety and efficacy (of both conventional and CAM options) should always be reviewed and patient preferences and expectations should be discussed and documented. From here, patients and physicians can make responsible decisions about treatment options and monitor progress together with the CAM provider. Table 47.4 provides information about the licensing and professional training of CAM practitioners in the United States.

It is impossible to provide specific guidelines for the training and practice of CAM on a worldwide basis. As a consequence, we have provided some general questions that should be asked by physicians thinking of referring patients to CAM or patients thinking of seeking CAM treatment.

How do I know the therapist is competent?

1. Do you think that the practitioner is technically competent? This usually means, is he or she a member of an appropriate organization and has adequate training?
2. Might the therapist advise the patient to change his or her conventional medical treatment without seeking the advice of the patient's doctor?
3. Can the proposed treatment be provided safely? If you are discussing referral to a herbalist, are you sure the herbalist is aware of the potential cross reactions between herbal medicine and conventional medications?
4. Will the complementary practitioner set guidelines at the first appointment for how the practitioner thinks the treatment should progress? Should the patient expect a response to treatment after 3 or 4 acupuncture sessions, or would it be more reasonable to assess the treatment after 8 or 10 sessions?
5. Is the therapist a professional?
6. Is the environment in which treatment is provided safe and appropriate?
7. Does the therapist have professional indemnity?
8. Do therapists have a code of ethics, are the data they hold legally protected, and will they treat the information given to them in a confidential manner?
9. Do therapists have an organization that employs a process of self-regulation and will it remove members from their lists if they are not behaving ethically?
10. Are therapists aware of, and do they have a process of reporting, adverse reactions to the treatments they provide?
11. Is CAM treatment appropriate?
12. Has a clear diagnosis of the problem been made? If such a diagnosis cannot be made, have other common problems been excluded? Is the patient missing out on an appropriate conventional medical treatment?
13. If the patient has a chronic condition that is relatively stable, then it may be reasonable to try a CAM approach, either to help symptoms or minimize the use of potentially damaging long-term conventional medications.
14. You may know a competent complementary therapist to whom you regularly refer; are you sure that the therapist is a safe, professional, and competent person?
15. You may wish to refer a patient to another doctor practicing some form of CAM; this kind of referral should be treated in exactly the same manner as referral to any other properly medically qualified specialist.

In general, we have so little information about whether complementary medicine works that it is usually impossible to make an evidence-based decision. In our view, it is reasonable to embark on CAM treatment as long as it is safe and provided in the context of proper professional practice associated with clear clinical guidelines.

KEY REFERENCES

1. Barnes PM, Powell-Griner E, McFann K, Nahin RL. Complementary and alternative medicine use among adults: United States, 2002. Adv Data 2004;343:1-19.
9. Eisenberg DM, Davis RB, Ettner SL, et al. Trends in alternative medicine use in the United States, 1990-1997: results of a follow-up national survey. JAMA 1998;280:1569-1575.
10. Astin JA. Why patients use alternative medicine: results of a national study. JAMA 1998;279:1548-1553.
13. Sims J. The mechanism of acupuncture analgesia: a review. Complement Ther Med 1997;5:102-111.
18. Pariente J, White P, Frackowiak RSJ, Lewith GT. Expectancy and belief modulate the neuronal substrates of pain treated by acupuncture. NeuroImage 2005;25:1161-1167.
19. Ernst E. Acupuncture as a symptomatic treatment of osteoarthritis: a systematic review. Scand J Rheumatol 1997;26:444-447.
21. Berman BM, Ezzo J, Hadhazy V, Swyers JP. Is acupuncture effective in the treatment of fibromyalgia? J Fam Pract 1999;48:213-218.
23. Ezzo J, Hadhazy V, Birch S, et al. Acupuncture for osteoarthritis of the knee: a systematic review. Arthritis Rheum 2001;44:819-825.
24. Manheimer E, White A, Berman B, et al. Meta-analysis: acupuncture for low back pain. Ann Intern Med 2005;142:651-663.
28. Berman BM, Lao L, Langenberg P, et al. Effectiveness of acupuncture as adjunctive therapy in osteoarthritis of the knee: a randomized, controlled trial. Ann Intern Med 2004;141:901-910.
29. White P, Lewith GT, Berman B, Birch S. Reviews of acupuncture for chronic neck pain: pitfalls in conducting systematic reviews. Rheumatology 2002;41:1224-1231.
30. White P, Lewith GT, Prescott P, Conway J. Acupuncture versus placebo for the treatment of chronic mechanical neck pain: a randomized, controlled trial. Ann Intern Med 2004;141:901-910.
31. MacPherson H, Thomas K, Walters S, Fitter M. The York acupuncture safety study: prospective study of 34,000 treatments by traditional acupuncturists. BMJ 2001;323:486-487.
32. White A, Hayhoe S, Hart A, Ernst E. Adverse events following acupuncture: prospective survey of 32,000 consultations with doctors and physiotherapists. BMJ 2001;323:485-486.
33. Fugh-Berman A. Herb-drug interactions. Lancet 2000;355:134-138.
38. Ernst E, Chrubasik S. Phyto-anti-inflammatories: a systematic review of randomized, placebo-controlled, double-blind trials. Rheum Dis Clin North Am 2000;26:13-27.
39. Long L, Soeken K, Ernst E. Herbal medicines for the treatment of osteoarthritis: a systematic review. Rheumatology 2001;40:779-793.
40. Brien SB, Walker A, Hicks SM, Middleton D. Bromelain as a treatment for osteoarthritis: a review of clinical studies. Evidence Based Complement Med 2004;1:251-257.
41. Chrubasik S, Zimpfer C, Schutt U. Effectiveness of Harpagophytum procumbens in treatment of acute low back pain. Phytomedicine 1996;3:1-10.
42. Schaffner W. Antirheumatikum der modernen Phytotherapie? In: Chrubasik S, Wink M, eds. Rheumatherapie mit Phytopharmaka. Stuttgart: Hippokrates-Verlag, 1997:125-127.
45. Zhang WY, Li Wan Po A. The effectiveness of topically applied capsaicin: a meta-analysis. Eur J Clin Pharmacol 1994;46:517-522.
53. McAlindon TE, LaValley MP, Gulin JP, Felson DT. Glucosamine and chondroitin for treatment of osteoarthritis: a systematic quality assessment and meta-analysis. JAMA 2000;283:1469-1475.
54. Towheed T, Anastassiades T, Shea B, et al. Glucosamine therapy for treating arthritis. In: The Cochrane Library, Issue 1. Oxford: Update Software, 2001.
55. Reginster JY, Deroisy R, Rovati LC, et al. Long-term effects of glucosamine sulphate on osteoarthritis progression: a randomised, placebo-controlled clinical trial. Lancet 2001;357:251-256.
56. Clegg DO, Reda DJ, Harris CL, et al. Glucosamine, chondroitin sulfate, and the two in combination for painful knee osteoarthritis. N Engl J Med 2006;354:795-808.
63. Soeken KL, Lee WL, Bausell RB, et al. Safety and efficacy of s-Adenosylmethionine (SAMe) for osteoarthritis: a meta-analysis. J Fam Pract 2002;51:425-430.
64. Belch J, Hill A. Evening primrose oil and borage oil in rheumatological conditions. Am J Clin Nutr 2000;71(Suppl 1):352s-356s.
68. James MJ, Cleland LG. Dietary v-3 fatty acids and therapy for rheumatoid arthritis. Semin Arthritis Rheum 1997;27:85-97.
69. Fortin P, Liang M, Beckett L, et al. A meta-analysis of the efficacy of fish oil in rheumatoid arthritis. Arthritis Rheum 1992;35:S201.
75. Cleland L, James M. Fish oil and rheumatoid arthritis: anti-inflammatory and collateral health benefits. J Rheumatol 2000;27:2305-2307.
77. Oh R. Practical applications of fish oil (omega-3 fatty acids) in primary care. J Am Board Fam Pract 2005;18:28-36.
80. Jonas WB, Anderson RL, Crawford CC, Lyons JS. A systematic review of the quality of homeopathic clinical trials. BMC Complement Altern Med 2001;1:1-12.
81. Fisher P, Greenwood A, Huskisson EC, et al. Effect of homeopathic treatment on fibrositis (primary fibromyalgia). BMJ 1989;299:365-366.
82. Bell IR, Lewis DA 2nd, Brooks AJ, et al. Improved clinical status in fibromyalgia patients treated with individualized homeopathic remedies versus placebo. Rheumatology (Oxford) 2004;43:577-582.
84. Astin JA, Harkness E, Ernst E. The efficacy of 'distant healing': a systematic review of randomized trials. Ann Intern Med 2000;132:903-910.
85. Superio-Cabuslay E, Ward MM, Lorig KR. Patient education interventions in osteoarthritis and rheumatoid arthritis: a meta-analytic comparison with non-steroidal anti-inflammatory drug treatment. Arthritis Care Res 1996;9:292-301.

87. Astin JA, Shapiro SL, Eisenberg DE. Mind-body medicine: state of the science, implications for practice. J Am Board Fam Pract 2003;16:131-147.
88. Astin JA, Beckner W, Soeken K, et al. Psychological interventions for rheumatoid arthritis: a meta-analysis of randomized controlled trials. Arthritis Rheum 2002;47:291-302.
89. Van Tulder MW, Ostelo R, Vlaeyen JW, et al. Behavioral treatment for chronic low back pain: a systematic review within the framework of the Cochrane Back Review Group. Spine 2000;25:2688-2699.
90. Hadhazy VA, Ezzo J, Creamer P, Berman BM. Mind-body therapies for the treatment of fibromyalgia: a systematic review. J Rheumatol 2000;27:2911-2918.
91. Morley S, Eccleston C, Williams A. Systematic review and meta-analysis of randomized controlled trials of cognitive behaviour therapy and behaviour therapy for chronic pain in adults, excluding headache. Pain 1999;80:1-13.
95. Eisenberg DM. Advising patients who seek alternative medical therapies. Ann Intern Med 1997;127:61-69.
96. Complementary and alternative medicines for the treatment of rheumatoid arthritis, osteoarthritis and fibromyalgia. Arthritis Research Campaign, 2009.
97. Cummings M. Modellvorhaben Akupunktur—a summary of the ART, ARC and GERAC trials. Acupuncture Med 2009;27:26-30.
98. Manheimer MS, White A, Berman B, et al. Meta-analysis: acupuncture for low back pain. Ann Intern Med 2005;142:651-663.
99. White A, Foster NE, Cummings M, Barlas P. Acupuncture treatment for chronic knee pain: a systematic review. Rheumatology 2007;46:384-390.
102. Fisher P, Greenwood A, Huskisson EC, et al. Effect of homoeopathic treatment of fibrositis (primary fibromyalgia). BMJ 1989;299:365-366.
103. Bell IR, Lewis DA, Brooks AJ, et al. Improved clinical status in fibromyalgia patients treated with individualized homeopathic remedies versus placebo. Rheumatology 2004;43:577-582.
104. Little P, Lewith G, Webley F, et al. Randomised controlled trial of Alexander Technique lessons, exercise and massage (ATEAM) for chronic and recurrent back pain. BMJ 2008;337:438-441.
106. Barnes PM, Bloom B, Nahin RL. Complementary and alternative medicine use among adults and children: United States, 2007. National Health Statistics Reports No. 12. Hyattsville, MD, National Center for Health Statistics, 2008.

REFERENCES

Full references for this chapter can be found on www.expertconsult.com.

Non-pharmacologic pain management

48

Hayley James and Stanton P. Newman

- Pain is determined by a combination of biological, psychological, and social factors.
- Sixty percent of rheumatology patients report severe pain and irritation.
- Non-pharmacologic interventions include cognitive behavioral therapy, relaxation therapy, biofeedback, patient education, self-management, and social support interventions.
- These types of interventions aim to change behavior, cognitions, and emotions by targeting the psychosocial processes that are implicated in the perceptions and response to pain.
- There is good evidence that these interventions can be effective in changing pain, particularly in relation to the cognitions surrounding pain; this, however, is predominantly in the short term.
- More research is needed to identify who may benefit from non-pharmacologic interventions.

INTRODUCTION

The traditional biomedical model suggests that pain is a direct result of a confirmed organic dysfunction. Treatments are, therefore, aimed at alleviating or curing this damage and/or by blocking these impulses. It is, however, now widely accepted that associations between physical impairment and pain report and disability are modest at best. Purely physiologic explanations for pain symptoms have been unable to explain the reports of pain in the absence of physical damage and why identical conditions lead to large differences in pain severity, intensity, or quality. In response to the shortcomings of the physiologic model, the gate control theory of pain was proposed.[1,2] This incorporates both psychological and physiologic factors, and it offers a biologic basis for the role of psychological factors in pain. The biopsychosocial model is often seen as an extension of the gate control theory and recognizes the role of biology and psychology but also the social determinants of pain regardless of its source or whether it is associated with psychopathology. It proposes that environmental factors such as the responses of significant others, cognitive factors such as beliefs about pain, and coping behaviors all influence the experience of pain.

PREVALENCE OF PAIN IN RHEUMATOLOGIC CONDITIONS

Pain is ranked by rheumatoid arthritis (RA) patients as the most important symptom.[3] In over 11,000 participants with a rheumatic condition, over 60% reported severe pain and irritation. Of these, 45% said the pain limited daily activities, with 37% reporting that the ability to lead a normal life was affected and 22% who said they were always in pain. When the different types of rheumatic disorders were compared, the proportions were highest for those with RA, with half reporting that they were always in pain.[4] The impact of pain goes beyond the sensation; it is associated with frequent use of medication, health services,[5] and time off work.[6] Besides the sensation of pain, its widespread influence results in a significant impact on quality of life.

MEASUREMENT OF PAIN

Pain is a personal experience: it is not amenable to direct clinical measurement and therefore must be inferred from subjective pain reports. There are various aspects of pain to measure and many ways to perform this measurement. Pain intensity is most commonly measured via rating scales, many of which are considered to be reliable, valid, and appropriate to clinical practice.[7] Some may, however, be best suited to individuals suffering from constant daily pain.[8] There are also composite pain scales that are well validated, including that in the Arthritis Impact Measure Scale (AIMS).[9] As well as measures of intensity there are instruments that assess the impact of pain (e.g., Multidimensional Pain Inventory[10] and the different ways in which people respond to pain.

The experience and qualities of pain have been captured in the McGill questionnaire.[11] This instrument has shown similarities and differences between individuals with different rheumatic conditions. Those with RA and fibromyalgia both use the description "aching and exhausting" to describe their pain. They differ in that RA patients use the words "stiff" and "moving" most frequently, whereas fibromyalgia patients use the words "nagging" and "hurting."[12] Pain quality is also dependent on the activity that individuals are engaged in as pain at rest tends to be described differently to pain in movement.[13]

PSYCHOLOGICAL FACTORS AND PAIN

It is understandable that chronic pain that persists for months and years will influence all aspects of a person's functioning. A review by Keefe and colleagues[14] suggests that more severe pain is associated with catastrophizing, pain-related fear, helplessness, and avoidant coping. In contrast, lower levels of pain are linked to higher levels of self-efficacy, a greater perception of control, active coping, readiness to change, and acceptance. *Catastrophizing* is defined as the tendency to focus on pain and negatively evaluate one's ability to deal and control it. Positive relationships have been found between catastrophizing and severity of pain, tenderness, pain-related disability, and potentially inflammatory disease activity.[15] Similarly, feelings of helplessness have been positively related to levels of pain[16,17] and may explain why some patients view pain as inevitable and discontinue treatment as a result of failed coping attempts.

Coping is the cognitive, behavioral, and emotional strategies people use on a day-to-day basis to help them manage the consequences of their disease and has been found to mediate the relationship between pain and physical disability in RA.[18] A person's belief in their ability to control their pain, known as self-efficacy, has been linked to improved adjustment and lower levels of pain.[19,20] There is growing evidence that increasing levels of self-efficacy through psychosocial interventions is related to improved outcomes.[21,22]

Emotions and pain

A number of factors increase the likelihood that in rheumatology clinics a significant proportion of patients may present with depression. Firstly the prevalence of rheumatic diseases is higher in women, as are levels of depression.[23] There is also a vast amount of literature demonstrating that the presence of pain is not only associated with depression[24] but appears to predict future depression in people with RA.[25]

Feelings of anxiety, in particular fear of completing tasks that may exacerbate pain, can lead to avoiding activities and situations that involve movement. Studies suggest that fear of movement and re-injury better predict functional limitations than biologic factors and even pain severity and duration.[26]

PSYCHOSOCIAL INTERVENTIONS FOR PAIN

Non-pharmacologic interventions to address pain aim to change behavior, cognitions, and emotions by targeting the psychosocial processes that are implicated in the perceptions and response to pain. These interventions are often offered after traditional biomedical therapies have failed and increasingly alongside traditional pain interventions. A number of general reviews have been undertaken that reveal that psychosocial interventions for people with rheumatologic conditions in general significantly reduce pain and increase pain self-efficacy after treatment in comparison to control conditions, although the overall effect size is often small.[8,27] Psychosocial interventions include a variety of techniques, often related to each other and presented in combination. Therefore, a description of the main types and their underlying principles is presented prior to an examination of evidence.

Cognitive behavioral therapy

The most widely applied and dominant intervention, cognitive behavioral therapy (CBT), acknowledges that cognitive and affective factors influence behavior and aims to alter maladaptive cognitive and behavioral responses to pain. The aim is to assist patients to understand that they can manage their pain effectively and then provide them with the skills to do so. There are five primary assumptions that underlie all CBT interventions (Box 48.1).[28]

The four essential components of CBT are education, skills acquisition, cognitive behavioral rehearsal, and generalization plus maintenance. Education aims to provide a credible rationale for the intervention by engaging the patients and encouraging them to believe that they are able to learn the skills necessary to cope better with their pain. Skills acquisition allows patients to learn these new behaviors and cognitions and practice them in the real world. Patients are encouraged to formulate a problem, define an achievable goal, and identify strategies to achieve that goal and are rewarded for successful completion. To ensure generalization and maintenance after the completion of the sessions patients are encouraged to anticipate and plan for future events concerning their pain, recognizing that setbacks will occur and that they now have the techniques that will allow them to overcome these problems.

Relaxation therapy

Relaxation is a widely used component of many psychosocial interventions to address pain and aims to reduce the psychophysiologic arousal frequently associated with pain. It involves steady and deep breathing and passively ignoring everyday thoughts and is encouraged as a distraction technique to cope when pain is particularly bad. The various forms of relaxation therapy include progressive muscle relaxation (PMR), meditation, autogenic training, and guided imagery.

Biofeedback

Biofeedback is based on the principle that people learn to perform a particular response by making appropriate behavioral adjustments when they receive feedback about the consequences of that response. Non-invasive electronic biofeedback devices measure the small changes in physiologic functions, mostly via the skin surface. These recordings are presented as a signal to allow patients to consciously monitor their physiologic response. Through this feedback patients learn to regulate the physiologic indicators of their bodily states. The aim is to remove the biofeedback device when patients are able to regulate their physiologic state in the absence of visual or auditory feedback.

Patient education

Patient education refers to a set of planned educational activities designed to reduce pain and its consequences. Pain education activities include topics such as information about the condition, encouragement of feasible activities that promote quality of life, the pacing of activities, coping advice, and information about sources of support. The underlying assumption is that patients who are better informed about their condition, treatment options, and prognosis will be better able to manage their disease and therefore achieve better health.

Self-management

Self-management is in part a combination of CBT and patient education, incorporating the idea of patient empowerment. According to Barlow and colleagues,[29] "self management refers to the individual's ability to manage the symptoms, treatment, physical and psychosocial consequences and life style changes inherent in living with a chronic condition." There are a range of possible components to a self-management intervention, education being one of these. Other widely adopted techniques include self-monitoring, skills training, challenging unhelpful behaviors, managing emotions, enhancing communication skills, social support, promoting readiness to change, enhancing self-efficacy, problem solving, and goal setting. Fundamental to self-management is skills training to assist patients in managing their condition. Information is seen as a necessary but not sufficient factor in behavior change, encouraging adaptation, reducing the consequences of pain.

Self-management interventions can help patients understand how their thoughts influence their behavior and mood and allow people to explore different ways of viewing situations. There are many different psychological theories that have been used to develop self-management interventions (Table 48.1).[30-34] These models all identify the factors that need to be modified to produce a desired change in behavior. By encouraging the routine use of self-management techniques for a particular aspect of a person's disease, such as pain, the hope is they will go on to translate these techniques into other aspects of their condition. Despite the evidence base for these theories, a number of intervention studies that claim to use self-management techniques are not explicitly based on any theory.

Social support interventions

Social isolation has been found to impact upon health; therefore, altering levels of social support have been targeted. The premise is that having others around providing support can encourage appropriate behaviors,[35] provide emotional support and information, and offer alternative ways of dealing with the condition. This can be achieved by creating new social networks relevant to the needs of the patient, such as self-help or support groups. An alternative is to focus on those people already in the patient's life and develop their skills to provide additional and appropriate support.

TABLE 48.1 MODELS OF BEHAVIOR CHANGE

Self-Regulation or Common Sense Model[30]	■ Describes how a patient will come to understand his or her illness and how to develop the coping strategies necessary to manage their disease ■ Relies on an individual's ability to monitor his or her own actions and reflect on them and their associated consequences
Social Cognition Model based on social cognition theory[31,32]	■ Implies that changing illness perceptions may lead to changes in relevant self-management behaviors ■ Suggests that behavior is directly influenced by goals and self-efficacy expectations and indirectly by self-efficacy, outcome expectations, and sociostructural factors. A majority of the empirical applications of this theory focus on self-efficacy.
Theory of Planned Behavior[33]	■ Suggests that behavior is determined by the strength of a person's intention to perform that behavior and the amount of actual control that person has over performing it
Stages of Change or Transtheoretical Model[34]	■ Assumes that behavior change involves movement through a sequence of discrete stages ■ Different factors influence the different stage transitions and therefore interventions should be matched to the stage the person is currently at

EVIDENCE BASE

When putting together the evidence base for these interventions a number of issues need to be acknowledged. Description of the interventions are often not detailed enough to be entirely clear of the content. The labeling of interventions can also be confusing; for instance, an intervention could be called CBT and another one, patient education or self-management when, in fact, they involve similar components. In addition, interventions may have similar content but may differ significantly in duration and the way in which they were delivered. These problems are common in attempting to integrate findings from complex interventions and make it difficult not only to group interventions by type and compare them but also to draw distinct conclusions about what makes them effective and efficacious. An additional important caveat is that some interventions are not primarily aimed to address pain, but it is measured as one of many secondary outcomes.

Unlike pharmacology, non-pharmacologic interventions are delivered over a discrete period and are assessed at various time points post intervention. The duration of follow-up to determine efficacy has characteristically been immediately after or relatively soon after the intervention has ceased. The determination of enduring effects of non-pharmacologic interventions has infrequently been performed. For example, in the review by Dixon and associates,[8] only 10% assessed the impact of the intervention beyond the immediate post-treatment period. The way in which pain is measured rather than the intervention *per se* can result in different final conclusions. Finally, a number of studies have compared an intervention to "standard care." Any conclusion about an intervention's effectiveness requires an appreciation of "standard care," which differs vastly and cannot be considered a constant.

CBT

In a recent review of psychological interventions for pain management in arthritis, 80% were labeled as CBT[8] and of these only two indicated significant effects. In practice, interventions in the rheumatic diseases have used CBT in a variety of ways and in combination with a range of other techniques. General reviews have offered contradictory results regarding CBT and pain. A narrative review by Bradley and associates[36] concluded that CBT is a well-established treatment for RA pain and is probably efficacious for patients with knee osteoarthritis. However, the authors of a recent Cochrane review, who had a more restrictive selection criteria for studies, examined the effectiveness of psychological therapies for non-malignant chronic pain, including a number of

rheumatic conditions, and concluded that the evidence for its effectiveness was weak.[37]

Key to understanding the impact of CBT is to establish for whom the intervention works and what techniques are related to success. Keefe and Van Horn[38] attribute the variability in the success of CBT intervention to differences in psychological variables such as self-efficacy, pain coping strategies, and feelings of control over pain, as previously discussed. Similarly, when looking at the mediating and moderating factors that predict therapeutic change in CBT, pre- to post-test treatment changes in pain beliefs, catastrophizing, and self-efficacy for managing pain were found to mediate the effects of CBT.[39] Importantly, but often taken for granted, other studies have demonstrated that those who adhere to a CBT program are more likely to show gains.[40]

Although some studies fail to find differences in self-reported pain, changes in other associated pain measures have been affected. When comparing CBT to an education intervention and standard care for patients with RA, Parker and coworkers[40] found no significant difference on self-reported pain but significant changes in pain-related coping strategies, such as control over pain at 6 months and 12 months post intervention. In addition, when occupational therapy and a standard care control group are compared with CBT, Kraaimaat and associates[41] found that CBT resulted in significant changes in the pain coping behavior of distraction by pleasant activities for people with RA after treatment but in no other pain-related measures.

The long-term effectiveness of CBT has been extensively debated. When CBT is compared with standard care,[42] patient education,[43] and symptom monitoring interventions,[44] CBT was found to significantly improve various aspects of pain; however, these significant changes were not maintained in the long term. Similarly, Greco and colleagues[45] compared biofeedback-assisted CBT including relaxation to a symptom-monitoring support intervention and usual care for people with lupus. CBT resulted in statistically significant reductions in pain frequency, severity, and the impact of pain on the patient's family, social activities, and work. However, these improvements were not maintained at the 9-month follow-up.

Conversely, Keefe and coworkers[22] found CBT skills training resulted in higher levels of pain self-efficacy at 6 and 12 months compared with education and spousal support for osteoarthritis patients with knee pain. However, no significant changes were found in self-reported pain or pain behavior. More recently, Redondo and colleagues[46] compared CBT including relaxation with physical exercise for fibromyalgia patients and found that CBT showed significant improvements in the ability to cope with chronic pain at 12 months that were significantly greater than exercise. There were, however, no significant differences between the groups on any other variables, including self-reported pain or pain management.

These studies suggest that CBT interventions show some evidence of a small effect on pain. However, they result in greater improvements in the cognitive and behavioral aspects of pain, such as pain behavior and pain self-efficacy rather than on self-reported measures of pain intensity. These benefits tend to be found immediately after interventions, but there are mixed findings regarding whether they are maintained at long-term follow-up. Overall, the need to examine individual differences to identify in whom these interventions are effective and determining which variables influence outcome is vital.

Relaxation training

A number of systematic reviews have been published looking at the efficacy of specific relaxation techniques on chronic pain. Carroll and Seers[47] looked at nine randomized controlled trials that reported the use of only a relaxation strategy as an active treatment when compared with at least one other active or control treatment in a variety of conditions. The most common form of relaxation was progressive muscle relaxation (PMR) with audiotapes and regular home practice. Little evidence was found to support the effectiveness of relaxation in the relief of all forms of chronic pain. The two studies on rheumatology patients produced contradictory results. One with RA patients found a significant benefit on at least one pain outcome in favor of relaxation,[48] whereas hydrogalvanic baths were found to be more beneficial than relaxation therapy for fibromyalgia patients.[49]

In a more recent systematic review, Kwekkeboom and Gretarsdottir[50] included studies in which relaxation training has been used in combination with other interventions, such as guided imagery or CBT. They conclude, when looking across conditions, that a majority of studies found a significant effect for relaxation on pain. However, they report that PMR, autogenic training, jaw relaxation, and systematic relaxation were effective, whereas rhythmic breathing and other relaxation interventions were not. Despite significant reductions in pain being reported from baseline to follow-up for PMR, when compared with exercise therapy[51] and hypnosis[52] no significant effects on pain were found.

These interventions reveal a somewhat mixed picture in terms of the efficacy of relaxation training for pain management. Those studies that utilize relaxation techniques in combination with other psychological interventions appear to be more successful than those that use relaxation alone, suggesting that it may be other components of the programs that result in the significant changes in pain.

Biofeedback

The available literature on biofeedback for chronic pain in general is so extensive that a comprehensive discussion of studies is beyond the scope of this chapter. Biofeedback has been evaluated for use in a number of rheumatic conditions, but a systematic review or meta-analysis is yet to be undertaken.

Many studies of biofeedback in rheumatic diseases have concentrated on fibromyalgia. Of the studies using a control group for comparison, Ferraccioli and colleagues[53] found that electromyographic (EMG) biofeedback resulted in improvements in the number of tender points, pain intensity, and morning stiffness that were maintained at 6 months for 56% of patients. Babu and associates[54] found that pain scores as determined by a visual analog scale (VAS) had significantly decreased after an EMG biofeedback intervention compared with a sham biofeedback group.

Some studies have combined biofeedback with other interventions. Buckelew and coworkers[55] compared a combination biofeedback and relaxation training program for fibromyalgia patients with exercise, a combination biofeedback and exercise group, and a control group. Self-reported pain scores were found to improve significantly in all three intervention groups; some long-term improvements were seen in the combined exercise and biofeedback group, but they were also seen in the other intervention groups at 3 months, and 1 and 2 years. As mentioned earlier, auditory EMG biofeedback combined with CBT, in contrast to self-monitoring support and usual care, revealed greater short-term changes in pain severity and frequency and the impact of pain but these were not maintained long term.[45]

These studies suggest that biofeedback interventions alone when not combined with other interventions are more successful and do have some immediate and long-term effects on pain, both in terms of self-reported pain levels and pain behavior. However, very few studies have actually compared true biofeedback with so-called sham biofeedback to establish the true efficacy of this type of intervention and most studies have focused on fibromyalgia patients and not those with other rheumatic conditions.

Self-management and education interventions

Self-management interventions have received much attention over the past decade. These interventions do not tend to focus on pain per se but frequently assess pain as an outcome in studies of arthritis. The most well-established self-management intervention is the Arthritis Self-Management Program (ASMP). This 6-week program is open to all people with rheumatic conditions and involves peer-led sessions. The sessions include information about arthritis, an overview of self-management principles, exercise, cognitive symptom management, dealing with depression, nutrition, communication with family and health professionals, and contracting. Weekly goal setting is encouraged as a means of practicing the skills taught in class and as a way of increasing self-efficacy. There have been numerous studies looking at the efficacy of this training program in various populations. The large U.K. evaluation of this intervention in a mixed group of individuals with chronic conditions showed disappointing results,[56] and the

effectiveness of the ASMP has not been replicated in the primary care setting.[57]

A number of systematic reviews have been undertaken to summarize the effectiveness of both patient education and self-management interventions. In a meta-analysis of the effect of the ASMP on pain, 17 studies were identified from 1964 to 1998 and the findings suggest a small effect.[58] In addition, Chodosh and colleagues[59] in a meta-analysis of chronic disease self-management programs for older adults found a statistically significant difference between intervention and control groups for osteoarthritis pain. However, the effect size equates to an improvement of only 2 mm on a 100-mm VAS; whether this is clinically significant is debatable.

Hirano and associates[60] reviewed 45 arthritis patient education studies, many of which included biofeedback, exercise, and social support interventions, and found that 12 of 14 that measured pain reported a positive change in pain, with 50% of studies showing statistically significant positive effects. Importantly, in a meta-analysis conducted by Superio-Cabuslay and colleagues,[61] the estimated effects of patient education interventions in osteoarthritis and RA were on average 20% to 30% as great as the effects of non-steroidal anti-inflammatory drug treatment for pain relief. In addition, education interventions that attempt to modify behavior have been found to be more efficacious than those that provide information alone for pain relief.

In a systematic review of RA patient education, Riemsma and associates[62] found a 4% reduction in self-reported pain using a VAS. However, the long-term effects of these patient education programs particularly for patients with RA have been questioned.[63] Seven of the 11 studies identified measured pain, but 3 found no significant difference in pain scores for the intervention group and 1 did no analysis comparing groups over time. The other 3 found significant reductions in pain, knowledge of pain relief, pain self-efficacy, pain behavior, and pain intensity, but these changes did not persist over time. Riemsma and colleagues' Cochrane review[64] of patient education for adults with RA identified 50 studies from 1966 to 2002 and found only a trend toward significance for the effects of patient education at first follow-up on pain scores and no significant effects at final follow-up. Sensitivity analysis, however, found that there was much variation in the way in which pain was assessed and the time frame in which patients were asked to comment varied significantly (i.e., over the past day, week, month). When looking at the studies utilizing a VAS scale to measure pain there was a significant effect for the intervention at first follow-up but no effect when using validated measures such as the AIMS. No long-term effects were found when using different types of measures, nor were there any significant differences when looking at information, counseling, and behavioral treatments separately.

In summary, these reviews have produced somewhat mixed results. The short-term effects of these interventions seem to be fairly well established even though many are not specifically directed to pain. There is, however, little evidence to suggest that these benefits remain long term. These mixed results are probably due to the inclusion of heterogeneous interventions, different pain assessment methods, and different groups of participants. It should also be noted that in a majority of cases these interventions are provided in addition to standard care; therefore, the effects are always supplementary to the benefits of standard practice. The consideration of booster sessions has received little attention in the literature and may be an approach to reinforce the early gains seen in some studies.

CONCLUSION

Overall there is evidence that psychologically based interventions can be effective in changing pain, particularly in relation to pain cognitions. The findings tend to be clearer for the short term, but the evidence is less persuasive that these results persist in the longer term. To maintain improvements after the interventions, special attention needs to be paid to the generalization and maintenance of what has been learned and to the integration of these techniques into everyday life.

There is a distinct lack of research when looking at which individuals benefit from different types of interventions and by which mechanisms these interventions work. In chronic rheumatic pain, attention needs to be devoted to the crucial beliefs and coping strategies that have the capacity to explain the effect on pain of psychological interventions. An effective approach may be to identify the important psychological factors so that future interventions can be tailored.

A common critique of these studies is the distinct lack of detail in terms of the way in which the interventions are developed and implemented, the theory behind which the interventions are based, and the use of multimodal components that thus make it extremely difficult to make firm conclusions regarding effective components.

KEY REFERENCES

1. Melzack R, Casey KL. Sensory, motivational and central control determinants of pain: a new conceptual model. In Kenshalo DZ, ed. The skin senses. Springfield, IL, Charles C Thomas, 1969;423-443.
2. Melzack R, Wall PD. Pain mechanisms: a new theory. Science 1965;150:971-979.
3. Gibson T, Clark B. Use of simple analgesics in rheumatoid arthritis. Ann Rheum Dis 1985;44:27-29.
4. Badley EM, Tennant A. Impact of disablement due to rheumatic disorders in a British population: estimates of severity and prevalence from the Calderdale Rheumatic Disablement Survey. Ann Rheum Dis 1993;52:6-13.
6. Bowsher D, Rigge M, Sopp L. Prevalence of chronic pain in the British population: a telephone survey of 1037 households. Pain Clin 1991;4:223-230.
8. Dixon KE, Keefe FJ, Scipio CD, et al. Psychological interventions for arthritis pain management in adults: a meta-analysis. Health Psychol 2007;26:241-250.
9. Meenan RF, Mason JH, Anderson JJ, et al. AIMS2: the content and properties of a revised and expanded arthritis impact measurement scales health status questionnaire. Arthritis Rheum 1992;35:l-10.
10. Kerns RD, Turk DC, Ruddy TE. The West Haven-Yale Multidimensional Pain Inventory (WHYMPI). Pain 1985;23:345-356.
11. Melzack R. The McGill Pain Questionnaire: major properties and scoring methods. Pain 1975;1:277-299.
12. Leavitt F, Katz RS, Golden HE, et al. Comparison of pain properties in fibromyalgia patients and rheumatoid arthritis patients. Arthritis Rheum 1986;29:775-782.
13. Papageorgiou AC, Badley EM. The quality of pain in arthritis: the words patients use to describe overall pain and pain in individual joints at rest and on movement. J Rheumatol 1989;16:106-112.
14. Keefe FJ, Rumble ME, Scipio CD, et al. Psychological aspects of persistent pain: current state of the science. J Pain 2004;5:195-211.
15. Edwards RR, Bingham CO, Bathon J, et al. Catastrophizing and pain in arthritis, fibromyalgia, and other rheumatic diseases. Arthritis Rheum 2006;55:325-332.
16. Nicassio PM, Schuman C, Radojevic V, et al. Helplessness as a mediator of health status in fibromyalgia. Cognitive Ther Res 1999;23:181-196.
17. Palomino R, Nicassio P, Greenberg M, et al. Helplessness and loss as mediators between pain and depressive symptoms in fibromyalgia. Pain 2007;129:185-194.
18. Covic T, Adamson B, Hough M. The impact of passive coping on rheumatoid arthritis pain. Rheumatology 2000;39:1027-1030.
19. Lefebvre JC, Keefe FJ, Affleck G, et al. The relationship of arthritis self-efficacy to daily pain, daily mood, and daily pain coping in rheumatoid arthritis patients. Pain 1999;80:425-435.
20. Brekke M, Hjortdahl P, Kvien TK. Changes in self-efficacy and health status over 5 years: a longitudinal observational study of 306 patients with rheumatoid arthritis. Arthritis Rheum 2003;49;342-348.

21. Keefe JK, Caldwell DS, Baucom D, et al. Spouse-assisted coping skills training in the management of osteoarthritic knee pain. Arthritis Care Res 1996;9:279-291.
22. Keefe FJ, Caldwell DS, Baucom D, et al. Spouse-assisted coping skills training in the management of knee pain in osteoarthritis: long-term follow-up results. Arthritis Rheum 1999;12:101-111.
23. Geenen R, Mulligan K, Shipley M, et al. Psychosocial dimensions of the rheumatic diseases. In Bilsma J, ed. EULAR: Compendium on rheumatic diseases. London: BMJ Publishing Group, 2009:635-650.
24. Dickens C, McGowan L, Clark-Carter D, et al. Depression in rheumatoid arthritis: a systematic review of the literature with meta-analysis. Psychosom Med 2002;64:52-60.
26. Crombez G, Vlaeyen JW, Heuts PH, et al. Pain-related fear is more disabling than pain itself: evidence on the role of pain-related fear in chronic back pain disability. Pain 1999;80:329-339.
27. Astin JA, Beckner W, Soeken K, et al. Psychological interventions for rheumatoid arthritis: a meta-analysis of randomized controlled trials. Arthritis Rheum 2002;47:291-302.
29. Barlow J, Wright C, Sheasby J, et al. Self-management approaches for people with chronic conditions: a review. Patient Educ Couns 2002;48:177-187.
30. Leventhal H, Nerenz DR, Steele DF. Illness representations and coping with health threats. In Baum A, Singer J, eds. A handbook of psychology and health. Hillsdale, NJ, Erlbaum, 1984:219-252.
31. Bandura A. Social foundations of thought and action: a social cognitive theory. Englewood Cliffs, NJ: Prentice-Hall, 1986.
32. Bandura A. Self-efficacy: the exercise of control. Worth Publishers, 1997.
33. Ajzen I. The theory of planned behavior. Organ Behav Hum Dev 1991;50:179-211.
35. Di Matteo MR. Social support and patient adherence to medical treatment: a meta-analysis. Health Psychol 2004;23;207-218.
36. Bradley LA, McKendree-Smith NL, Cianfrini LR. Cognitive-behavioural therapy interventions for pain associated with chronic illness. Semin Pain Med 2003;1:44-54.
37. Eccleston C, Williams AC, Morley S. Psychological therapies for the management of chronic pain (excluding headache) in adults. Cochrane Database Syst Rev 2009;(2):CD007407.
38. Keefe FJ, Van Horn Y. Cognitive-behavioural treatment of rheumatoid arthritis pain: maintaining treatment gains. Arthritis Care Res 1993;6:213-222.
40. Parker JC, Frank RG, Beck NC, et al. Pain management in rheumatoid arthritis patients: a cognitive behavioral approach. Arthritis Rheum 1988;31:593-601.
41. Kraaimaat FW, Brons MR, Geenen R, Bijlsma JWJ. The effect of cognitive behavior therapy in patients with rheumatoid arthritis. Behav Res Ther 1995;33:487-495.

43. O'Leary A, Shoor S, Lorig K, et al. A cognitive behavioral treatment for rheumatoid arthritis. Health Psychol 1988;7:527-544.
44. Appelbaum KA, Blanchard EB, Hickling EJ, et al. Cognitive behavioural treatment of a veteran population with moderate to severe rheumatoid arthritis. Behav Ther 1988;19:489-502.
45. Greco CM, Rudy TE, Manzi S. Effects of a stress-reduction program on psychological function, pain, and physical function of systemic lupus erythematosus patients: a randomized controlled trial. Arthritis Care Res 2004;51:625-634.
47. Carroll D, Seers K. Relaxation for the relief of chronic pain: a systematic review. J Adv Nurs 1998;27:476-487.
48. Dulski TP, Newman AM. The effectiveness of relaxation in relieving pain of women with rheumatoid arthritis. In Funks SG, Tornquist EM, Champagne MJ, et al, eds. Key aspects of comfort: management of pain, fatigue and nausea. New York: Springer, 1989:150-154.
49. Gunther V, Mur E, Kinigadner U, et al. Fibromyalgia: the effect of relaxation and hydrogalvanic bath therapy on the subjective pain experience. Clin Rheumatol 1994;13:573-578.
50. Kwekkeboom KL, Gretarsdottir E. Systematic review of relaxation interventions for pain. J Nurs Scholarship 2006;38:269-277.
52. Gay MC, Philippot P, Luminet O. Differential effectiveness of psychobiological interventions for reducing osteoarthritis pain: a comparison of Erickson hypnosis and Jacobsen relaxation. Eur J Pain 2002;6:1-16.
53. Ferraccioli G, Ghirelli L, Scita F, et al. EMG-biofeedback training in fibromyalgia syndrome. J Rheumatol 1987;14:820-825.
54. Babu AS, Mathew E, Danda D, et al. Management of patients with fibromyalgia using biofeedback: a randomized control trial. Indian J Med Sci 2007;61:455-461.
55. Buckelew SP, Conway R, Parker J, et al. Biofeedback/relaxation training and exercise interventions for fibromyalgia. Arthritis Care Res 1998;11:196-209.
56. Barlow JH, Turner AP, Wright CC. A randomized controlled study of the Arthritis Self-Management Programme in the UK. Health Educ Res 2002;15:665-680.
59. Chodosh J, Moprton SC, Mojica W, et al. Meta-analysis: chronic disease self-management programs for older adults. Ann Intern Med 2005;143:427-438.
60. Hirano PC, Laurent DD, Lorig K. Arthritis patient education studies, 1987-1991: a review of the literature. Patient Educ Couns 1994;24:9-54.
63. Neidermann K, Fransen J, Knols R, et al. Gap between short- and long-term effects of patient education in rheumatoid arthritis patients: a systematic review. Arthritis Rheum 2004;51:338-398.

REFERENCES

Full references for this chapter can be found on www.expertconsult.com.

Principles of opioid treatment of chronic musculoskeletal pain

49

Maren Lawson Mahowald and Hollis Elaine Krug

- Musculoskeletal pain reduces the quality of life and increases health care utilization. Many patients with rheumatic diseases have acute and chronic pain that is not effectively treated.
- Opioids are an important component of a pain control program and are safe without major organ toxicity. Side effects are generally manageable.
- Opioids have short- and long-term pharmacologic activity and combining them may lead to more effective pain control.
- Dose titration is an important component of a pain control program.
- Opioids vary in half-life, potency, side effect profile, and cost.

INTRODUCTION

Moderate to severe persistent musculoskeletal pain represents an important unmet medical need because it reduces the quality of life and increases health care costs. The two most common causes of disability in the United States continue to be arthritis or rheumatism and back or spine problems. The pain survey of 46,394 individuals in 15 European countries and Israel revealed nearly 1 in 5 had chronic pain of greater than 5 of 10 on the numerical rating scale (NRS).[1] In-depth interviews of 4839 individuals in the survey indicated two thirds had moderate pain (5-7 on NRS), one third had severe pain (8-10 on NRS); 48% reported impaired social activities; and 61% reported impaired work ability. Non-prescription analgesics were used by almost half, 55% used non-steroidal anti-inflammatory drugs (NSAIDs), 43% used paracetamol, and 13% used weak opioids. Two thirds were taking prescription analgesics: 44% NSAIDs, 23% weak opioids (range from 5% to 50% in different countries), 18% paracetamol, and 1% to 16% cyclooxygenase (COX)-2 inhibitors; and only 5% reported taking strong opioids. The pain was caused by rheumatoid arthritis and osteoarthritis in 42% of the respondents. Non-cancer pain was much more common than cancer pain because only 1% reported their pain was due to cancer. Seventy-seven percent were being treated by a family practitioner or internist, 27% by an orthopedist, 9% by a rheumatologist, and 10% by a neurologist or neurosurgeon. Overall, 40% were not satisfied with their pain control and 38% were less than satisfied with the doctor who was treating their pain. Forty percent said they believed their doctor would rather treat their illness than their pain, 20% believed their doctor did not see their pain as a problem, and 30% believed their doctor did not know how to control their pain.[1]

Much has been learned from experience treating cancer pain, especially the World Health Organization (WHO) treatment "ladder" for cancer pain that has been adapted for current guidelines for non-cancer pain. The WHO 3-step pain ladder recommends the order of drugs to be prescribed according to pain intensity[2]:

Step 1. Non-opioids: aspirin and paracetamol with or without adjuvant medications.
Step 2. If pain is persisting or increasing (i.e., non-opioids insufficient) or for mild to moderate pain: use mild opioids such as codeine with or without a non-opioid analgesic.
Step 3. If pain is persisting or increasing: use strong opioids such as morphine, oxycodone, or fentanyl, increasing the dose until the patient is free of pain.

However, concerns have been raised about a progressive step-wise increase in strength of medications that is acceptable for gradually progressive pain but not for pain that is severe to begin with.[3] Step 2 is too restrictive because some patients with pain of 6-8/10 will only get paracetamol and/or an NSAID to start with. In terminal cancer pain, strong opioids were more effective than step 1 and step 2 medications. Therefore, it is not advisable to prescribe short-acting "weak opioids" in step 2 rather than a low dose of strong opioids that are long acting to facilitate activity. "Weak opioids" have not been proven to be superior to NSAIDs in clinical trials of moderate cancer pain. The strength of opioid prescribed should be selected according to the current severity of pain. Based on studies that suggested the efficacy of weak opioids is limited in cancer pain, the International Association for the Study of Pain (IASP) recommended non-opioids for mild pain, low-dose strong opioids for moderate pain, and immediate use of strong opioids for severe pain. Adjuvant medications and neurolytic procedures should be used as needed at any time.

New guidelines for opioid therapy in chronic non-cancer pain from the American Pain Society and American Academy of Pain Medicine were based on expert opinion, review of the literature up to November 2007, and external peer review. A multistage Delphi process resulted in recommendations for chronic opioid therapy that are presented in this chapter. It should be acknowledged that the expert panel made strong recommendations but none of the supporting evidence was high quality (see http://www.ampainsoc.org/pub/opioid.htm, accessed June 15, 2009).[4]

Physician knowledge deficit is probably the most important reason for undertreatment of pain. Physicians may not be able to prescribe opioids skillfully enough because of inadequate training and experience. Providers are often unsure about which opioid preparations to select and how to titrate the dose to an acceptable balance of adequate analgesia and tolerable/manageable side effects. They may not know how to anticipate and manage opioid side effects successfully. Resistance to prescribing chronic opioids also relates to both patient's and provider's unrealistic fears about the risk of opioid addiction from treating musculoskeletal pain compared with cancer pain.[5] Over the past 20 years provider concerns about prescribing opioids has changed little despite the accumulating evidence that long-term opioids are effective, side effects are manageable, and few problems of tolerance, dependence, abuse, or addiction develop. Opioids are safe, without major organ toxicity, and side effects are manageable when anticipated and treated expectantly.[6-9]

HISTORY OF OPIOID TREATMENT OF CHRONIC JOINT PAIN

Opioids in the form of opium have been used for thousands of years. Pharmacologic manufacture began in the 19th century after the morphine alkaloid was identified. Opioids diverted from medical use by forgery, theft, and fraud support the illicit drug trade. Federal and state regulation of opioid medications for the past 100 years has failed to prevent abuse. Legal controls attempting to limit drug abuse resulted in the undertreatment of pain because opioids were so tightly restricted by the end of the 19th century.[10] Medical attitudes against prescribing opioids for chronic pain were also shaped by clinical studies from addiction treatment centers because addicts attributed their opioid addiction to being prescribed opioids for pain. By the end of the 20th century opioids were fully accepted as treatment for acute pain, cancer pain, and end-of-life pain but not as accepted for non-malignant osteoarticular pain or pain after cancer remission. At the beginning of the 21st century, provider bias against opioid treatment of non-malignant pain instilled during medical school and residency training continues to limit provider knowledge, experience, and skill for appropriate opioid prescribing.[11,12] Providers are uncertain about opioid selection and methods of titration to an acceptable balance of pain relief and tolerable/manageable side effects. They have an unwarranted fear about the true risks of tolerance, dependence, abuse, and addiction.[13] The WHO is committed to promote maximal pain relief to every patient in pain by the legitimate use of opioids through the *Access to Controlled Medications Program* and is currently revising the "analgesic ladder" according to new pharmacology, cost restrictions, adjuvant medications, and criticisms of its rigidity as described earlier.

Despite published evidence,[7-9,14] and clinical guidelines from key organizations advocating appropriate opioid treatment of chronic pain,[2-5] many providers remain reluctant to prescribe long-term opioids.[11] Attitudes may be changing as clinical research demonstrates the efficacy and safety of long-term opioid use. Studies of opioid use in patients with persistent pain due to medical disorders published during the past 2 decades suggested there was a very low rate of abuse and addiction in these patients.[6-9,12] In the majority of patients, requirement for increased opioid dose indicates unrelieved pain rather than opioid tolerance or abuse. Unfortunately, recent reports of abuse and diversion of opioids have once again produced political pressures to limit access to these medications and rekindled provider fears of disciplinary sanctions.[15]

MECHANISMS INVOLVED IN ARTICULAR PAIN

A high-intensity noxious stimulus from tissue injury produces acute pain that is proportional to the severity of tissue injury and subsides as the tissue heals. Acute pain provokes an autonomic nervous system response of tachycardia, increased blood pressure, anxiety, and stereotypical behaviors of withdrawal, splinting, rubbing, and or grimacing. Persistent pain due to a chronic underlying condition does not have autonomic overactivity but rather causes physical dysfunction, anxiety, depression, and personality changes. Disorders such as rheumatoid arthritis, osteoarthritis, degenerative disc disease, osteoporotic fractures, chronic gout, and spondyloarthritis cause persistent pain that has intermittent acute exacerbations due to: movement (incident pain), pressure (hyperalgesia or tenderness to palpation), and light touch or temperature changes (allodynia). Persistent neurogenic pain arises from damaged primary afferent neurons and from central nervous system (CNS) pathology in the spinal cord, brain stem, thalamus, or cortex.[16] Painful musculoskeletal disorders often have both pathogenic

nociceptive and neurogenic pain mechanisms. For example, intervertebral disc disease may have both mechanical nociceptive pain in the posterior elements of the spine and neuropathic radicular pain from nerve rootlet compression. Psychogenic factors in chronic pain are very complex. Patients with pain due to underlying chronic musculoskeletal disorders often develop anxiety and depression that may be difficult to detect. Patients with depression may present with pain symptoms that are medically unexplained. Pure psychogenic causes for chronic pain are rare but very difficult to detect and manage. Pain that is out of proportion to underlying disease or without identifiable tissue pathology is referred to as a pain syndrome (previously termed a *pain disorder*) that has *DSM-IV TR* diagnostic criteria[17] for somatoform disorders, malingering, factitious disorder, substance abuse disorder, or personality disorders. It is important to recognize a pain disorder in which psychological factors are significant in the pain onset and severity and distinguish it from conditions of nociceptive and neuropathic pain with associated depression or anxiety.

EVIDENCE SUPPORTING THE USE OF OPIOIDS FOR PERSISTENT OSTEOARTICULAR PAIN

Prior to the mid 1990s many rheumatologists advised against long-term use of opioids, claiming the risk of addiction was greater than the chance of benefit for patients with arthritis pain. Recent contrary opinions, based on evidence, concluded that "patients with chronic pain can achieve satisfactory analgesia with a stable dose of opioids that has minimal risk of addiction."[6-9] Sustained efficacy of opioids for persistent osteoarticular pain has been debated for decades. A systematic review of 11 placebo-controlled oral opioid trials conducted for 4 days to 8 weeks with 1145 total patients who had painful nociceptive and/or neuropathic conditions revealed that mean pain relief with opioids was at least 30% for both nociceptive and neuropathic pain. A few patients may have developed tolerance as opioid doses increased over time; however, no addictive behaviors were reported.[14]

There are few studies of opioid use for longer than 8 to 12 weeks. We performed studies that used patient interviews, analysis of computerized pharmacy records to measure drug dose changes over time, and a standardized review of medical records to examine changes in the clinical condition and occurrences of drug abuse/addiction behaviors.[7,9] In rheumatology clinics and orthopedic spine clinics 442 of 874 patients were prescribed opioids during a 3-year period. There was a significant decrease in pain from 8.2 to 3.6 (on the 0-10 NRS) in rheumatology clinic patients and from 8.3 to 4.5 in orthopedic spine clinic patients. Figure 49.1 illustrates the important observation that opioids were just as effective in those treated with long-term opioids as in those

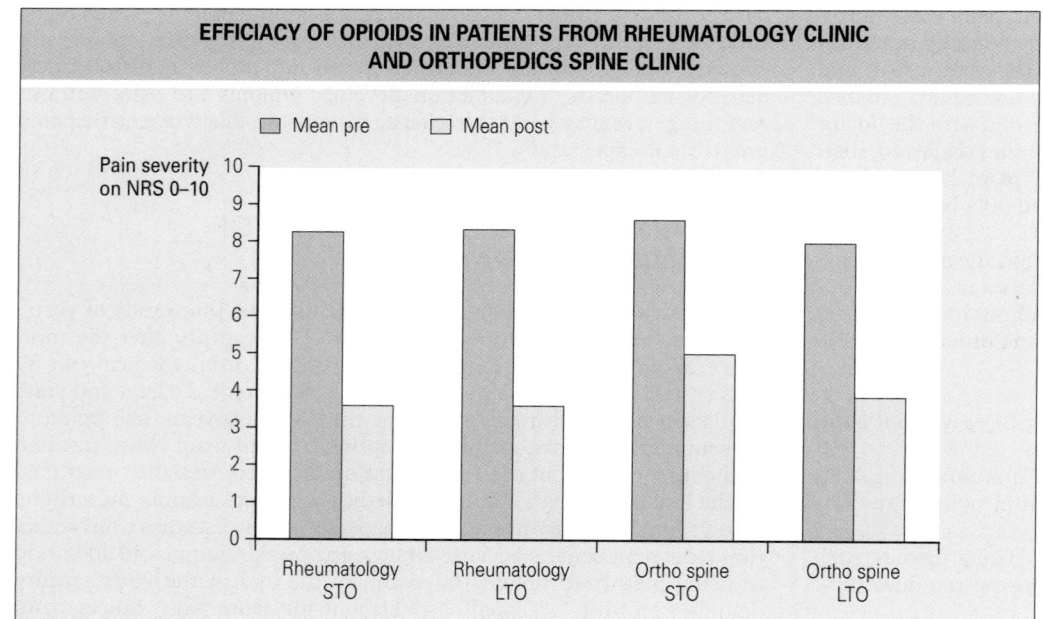

Fig. 49.1 Efficacy of opioids in patients from rheumatology clinic and orthopedics spine clinic. Change in pain severity with opioid treatment. STO, short-term opioid therapy less than 3 months; LTO, long-term opioid therapy more than 3 months; NRS, numerical rating scale of pain severity of 0-10 in which 0 is no pain and 10 is worst imaginable pain.

treated with short-term opioids, suggesting that clinically significant tolerance did not develop in these patients. The average daily dose of opioid increased by more than 60 mg codeine equivalents per day during the 3-year study period in 25% of those prescribed long-term opioids (32/137 rheumatology clinic patients and 17/58 orthopedic spine clinic patients). The increased opioid dose was attributable to progression or complications of the underlying painful condition or a new painful condition such as compression fracture, herpes zoster, or trauma. Unexplained increases in average opioid dose occurred in 4 rheumatology clinic patients and in 3 orthopedic spine clinic patients, representing only 3.6% "problem patients" on long-term opioids who may have developed tolerance and/or abuse behaviors. The rheumatology clinic patients were monitored prospectively for 5 more years after the interviews.[8] Opioid efficacy was sustained, and no opioid tolerance was seen in these patients. These studies support the concept that opioids are effective long term, tolerance was not inevitable, no serious organ toxicity occurred, side effects were manageable, and the incidence of substance abuse was not greater than the general population.

Neuropathic pain is often a component of persistent pain due to rheumatologic disorders. Contrary to previous opinions that opioids were ineffective for neuropathic pain, opioids can reduce neuropathic pain.[18] Many challenging questions about chronic opioid treatment of musculoskeletal disorders remain to be studied. Treatment of chronic pain in the elderly is difficult because of altered drug metabolism, polypharmacy issues, complex drug-drug interaction, and potentially enhanced adverse side effects in those with co-morbid conditions, especially dementia. Expression of pain and response to treatment by patients with dementia may need to be interpreted by a caregiver.[19] Published studies to date do not provide conclusive evidence about mechanisms responsible for failed opioid analgesia, opioid-induced immune modulation, the true risk and clinical impact of opioid tolerance and dependence, magnitude of change in functional status and activity that occurs with adequate pain relief, and what is the best practice for managing opioid treatment of pain in the patient with an addiction disorder.

OPIOID PHARMACOLOGY: MECHANISM OF ACTION AND PHARMAKOKINETICS

Opioids are categorized as endogenous or exogenous. The endogenous opioids are endomorphins and endorphins (bind MOP receptors), enkephalins and deltorphins (bind DOP receptors), dynorphins (bind KOP receptors), and the recently described nociceptin (binds NOP receptors). Opioid receptors are a superfamily (rhodopsin) of seven transmembrane-spanning G protein–coupled membrane receptors that are synthesized in the dorsal root ganglion cell bodies.[20] The terminology of the receptors has recently undergone revision.[21] The classes of opioid receptors mu, delta, kappa, and opioid receptor-like (aka, orphanin FQ or nociceptin) are identified as MOP receptor, DOP receptor, KOP receptor, and NOP receptor. Opioid receptors are expressed within sensory neurons—on dorsal root ganglion cell bodies, peripheral terminals of primary afferent neurons, in the spinal cord, and in the brain. Evidence is conflicting about opioid receptors on sympathetic terminals. The number of nerve terminals is increased in sites of inflamed tissues ("sprouting"), and opioid receptors in the nerve terminals of sensory articular nerves are upregulated during inflammation.[22]

Endogenous opioids are released from monocyte/macrophages and lymphocytes stimulated by corticotropin-releasing factor or interleukin (IL)-1. Opioid receptors have also been found on immunocytes and can modulate cell proliferation, chemotaxis, superoxide and cytokine production, and mast cell degranulation. The clinical impact of these immunomodulatory effects is not clear and has not been correlated with pain transmission. Activation of MOP receptor produces analgesia, meiosis, respiratory depression, reduced gastrointestinal motility, and feelings of well-being. The DOP receptor has high affinity for endogenous enkephalins; however, effects of activation with exogenous opioids in humans are not clear.[23] The KOP receptor has high affinity for the endogenous dynorphin A; its activation produces analgesia, dysphoria, and psychotomimetic effects (disorientation and/or depersonalized feelings). The NOP receptor[20] has low-affinity

binding to opioids and has its own ligand, a small peptide similar to dynorphin A.

The opioid receptor coupled to G-proteins transduces the binding signal to the cell. The receptors inhibit adenylate cyclase, which decreases cyclic adenosine monophosphate (AMP) and increases influx of potassium currents and inactivation of voltage-gated calcium channels. Activation of potassium channels and inhibition of calcium channels hyperpolarizes (inhibits excitation of) neurons and inhibits the release of neurotransmitters acetylcholine, substance P, calcitonin gene–related peptide (CGRP), norepinephrine, glutamate, γ-aminobutyric acid (GABA), and glycine.[21,24]

The MOP receptor has multiple mRNA splice variants (MOP receptor subtypes), multiple polymorphisms, and variability of receptor density in different tissues. Variability in receptor density together with constitutive and genetic variability in cytochrome P450 enzymes produces high variability in individual responses to the opioids. Codeine, a prodrug, is converted to morphine by CYP2D6. Patients who are deficient in this enzyme or who are taking inhibitors of CYP2D6 would not get analgesia from oral codeine. The pharmacology of various opioid receptor subtypes is not yet fully clarified. The different opioid receptor types do not evoke different cellular responses, but different behaviors are produced because of different anatomic distributions of the receptor types. Compounds that activate MOP and DOP receptors produce analgesia and rewarding feelings. Those that activate the KOP receptor produced analgesia, dysphoria, and hallucinations. Most opioids used in clinical practice bind the MOP receptor selectively. Some drug actions are not mediated only by opioid receptors.[25] Methadone and tramadol inhibit serotonin and norepinephrine reuptake and are antagonists of the N-methyl-D-aspartate (NMDA) amino acid excitatory pathway.[25] The intrinsic efficacy of an opioid refers to the degree to which maximal efficacy is produced without full receptor occupancy, that is, the reserve of spare receptors. High-efficacy opioid ligands, such as fentanyl, have many spare receptors, and low-efficacy opioid ligands, such as morphine, have few spare receptors. The proportion of spare receptors might be involved in the development of tolerance; however, experimental data are conflicting.

Opioid tolerance

Increased opioid dose requirement to sustain pain relief is called tolerance, a form of tachyphylaxis. Current concepts of opioid tolerance are controversial and include processes of receptor "desensitization" and/or trafficking. Experience over the past 30 years with the long-term effects of opioids in patients with cancer pain demonstrated that tolerance develops for both analgesic effects and adverse side effects.[26,27] Tolerance to respiratory depression occurs rapidly, whereas the analgesic effects last for a long time in most patients unless the underlying disease progresses. Tolerance to most side effects except constipation occurs over 2 to 3 weeks. In reality, analgesic tolerance is a rare cause of opioid therapy failure. Switching from one opioid to another can improve analgesia and/or decrease adverse effects because there is an incomplete cross-tolerance among different opioid preparations. Calculation of equianalgesic doses is difficult because cross-tolerance cannot be predicted in the individual patient.

Opioid dependence

Opioid dependence is the expected result of prolonged exposure to opioids and refers to the abstinence syndrome of opioid withdrawal symptoms that occurs after abrupt withdrawal of opioids or administration of an opioid antagonist. There is an abrupt increase in cyclic AMP on withdrawal of an opioid that activates protein kinase A and causes neurotransmitter release at many synapses, thereby inducing hyperexcitability at CNS sites such as the periaqueductal gray areas.[21] The opioid abstinence syndrome is characterized by chills alternating with hot flashes, hypertension, tachycardia, lacrimation, rhinorrhea, yawning, coughing, sneezing, mydriasis, diaphoresis and piloerection, salivation, anxiety, irritability, twitching, myoclonus, nausea, vomiting, abdominal cramps and diarrhea, and insomnia. The dose and/or duration of opioid administration needed to produce dependence have not been established for patients being treated with moderate to severe pain. The time course of withdrawal symptoms is related to the

TABLE 49.1 "RED FLAGS" FOR ABUSE BEHAVIOR AND OPIOID ADDICTION

Potential abuse/addiction behaviors*

1. Patient displays an overwhelming focus on opioid issues during clinic visits that occupy a significant proportion of the clinic visit and impedes progress with other pain issues or medical problems.
2. Patient has a pattern of early refills (three or more) or escalating drug use in the absence of acute change or progression of his or her medical condition.
3. The patient generates multiple telephone calls or unscheduled visits to request more opioids, early refills, or problems associated with the opioid prescription that often creates a disturbance of the clinic staff.
4. There is a pattern of prescription problems with reports of medications lost, spilled, or stolen.
5. The patient has supplemental sources of opioids from multiple providers, emergency departments, or illegal sources.

Additional "red flag" abuse behavior

1. Selling prescribed opioid drugs
2. Prescription forgery
3. Stealing another patient's drugs
4. Injecting oral medication
5. Concurrent use of illicit drug
6. Appears intoxicated or oversedated
7. Insists on obtaining a specific opioid medication

Adapted from Chabal criteria for opioid abuse.

TABLE 49.2 CYTOCHROME P450 ENZYMES AND IMPORTANT DRUG INTERACTIONS

Interactions	Examples
Low CYP2D6 activity in 6% of whites, 3% of blacks, and 1% of Asians	"Poor metabolizers"—see increased sensitivity to methadone effects.
CYP2D6 inhibitors—increase methadone levels; increase analgesia and toxicity	Antidepressants: fluoxetine, paroxetine, fluvoxamine, sertraline, bupropion, amitriptyline Miscellaneous: haloperidol, amiodarone, cimetidine, quinidine, quinine, hydroxychloroquine, ritonavir, efavirenz, ciprofloxacin, ketoconazole, fluconazole, ethanol Methadone itself can inhibit CYP2D6.
CYP2D6 inducers—reduce methadone levels, reduce analgesia, and may precipitate opioid withdrawal	Isoniazid and rifampin Gene duplication for CYP2D6 produces "ultra rapid" metabolizers and reduced methadone effects.
CYP3A3/4 inhibitors—may increase methadone levels; may also increase effects of fentanyl, hydrocodone, and oxycodone	Antidepressants: fluoxetine, fluvoxamine, amitriptyline, sertraline, nefazadone, paroxetine Ciprofloxacin, clarithromycin, erythromycin and toxicity Azoles: itraconazole, fluconazole, ketoconazole, metronidazole Antivirals: ritonavir, indonavir Miscellaneous: grapefruit, cimetidine, diltiazem, omeprazole, quinidine, quinine, tacrolimus, valproic acid, ethinyl estradiol
CYP3A3/4 inducers—reduce methadone levels, reduce analgesia, and may precipitate opioid withdrawal	Isoniazid and rifampin Anticonvulsants (phenobarbital, phenytoin, primidone, carbamazepine) Antidepressants (risperidone and St. John's wort) Antivirals (nevirapine, amprenavir, abacavir, nelfinavir, efavirenz, ritonavir) Miscellaneous: clotrimazole, dexamethasone
	Spironolactone: reduces methadone levels
	Cocaine: increases elimination, reduces methadone effects
	Benzodiazepines, alcohol: additive effects of increased sedation with methadone and other opioids
	Opioid antagonists: pentazocine (Talwin) and tramadol: precipitate opioid withdrawal symptoms while taking buprenorphine and butorphanol, methadone, and other mu agonists

Modified from VA/DOD. VA/DOD clinical practice guideline for the management of opioid therapy for chronic pain. Office of Quality and Performance Clinical Practice Guidelines 2005. Available at http://www.oqp.med.va.gov/cpg/cpg.htm Volume, 0-111 DOI: http://www.oqp.med.va.gov/cpg/cpg.htm.

half-life of the opioid. With short-acting opioids withdrawal begins within 12 to 24 hours of the last dose and peaks at 48 to 72 hours. A secondary phase of abstinence syndrome occurs thereafter with insomnia, irritability, and muscle aches for 2 to 6 months. With long-acting opioids such as methadone, withdrawal symptoms may not begin for several days, are less florid but may last for several weeks or a month. Withdrawal symptoms usually can be avoided by a slow taper of opioids—first cut the daily dose in half for several days then reduce by 25% every few days until down to a morphine equivalent dose of 30 mg/day, at which time the opioid may be discontinued. Autonomic withdrawal symptoms may be lessened by using a transdermal clonidine patch, 0.1 to 0.2 mg/day. Opioid withdrawal syndrome is not fatal, unlike alcohol withdrawal syndrome. A patient should not be labeled as an opioid abuser or addict because he or she has developed tolerance or dependence.

Opioid abuse and addiction

Opioid tolerance and dependence are not indicative of addiction. Opioid addiction is a psychological and behavioral syndrome characterized by self-destructive behavior, drug craving, compulsive use, the need to use the drug for psychic effects rather than pain relief, and continued use of opioids in spite of harm.[17,28] Abuse behaviors include theft, diversion for sale of drugs, hoarding of drugs, obtaining drugs from multiple physicians, and unsanctioned use of higher doses than prescribed. The addict exhibits drug-seeking behavior and becomes focused on using and procuring the drug. "Red flags" for abuse behavior are listed in Table 49.1.[29] The fear of producing iatrogenic addiction is an important reason for the undertreatment of pain. In reality, the risk of addiction in patients being treated for pain is very low.[7-10] An interesting phenomenon, "pseudoaddiction," is an iatrogenic condition produced by inadequate treatment of persistent pain. Inadequate pain relief drives the patient to display "abuse behaviors" as he or she seeks more medication for adequate pain treatment. Their behaviors resemble the addict's but they resolve when the pain is treated adequately.

PHARMACOKINETICS AND OPIOID METABOLISM

Opioid drugs are metabolized primarily by three systems: oxidation, reduction, and glucuronidation. Active metabolites of morphine, codeine, oxycodone, and hydromorphone can accumulate with chronic administration, dehydration, and dose escalation and with renal failure, producing enhanced analgesia and/or increased adverse side effects.

Methadone does not have active metabolites and does not undergo significant renal excretion.

Variation in the cytochrome P450 system influences response to many drugs (Table 49.2). The CYP2D6 and CYP3A4 enzymes are responsible for opioid biotransformation to active metabolite and metabolic clearance. Ethnic variability exists in the P450 enzyme system. CYP2D6 is absent in 6% of whites (poor metabolizers) and is inhibited by other drugs such as selective serotonin reuptake inhibitors (SSRIs), antiepileptic agents, and antihistamines.[30] CYP2D6 catalyzes O-dealkylation of codeine, hydrocodone, oxycodone, and tramadol. CYP3A4 catalyzes N-demethylation of morphine, codeine, oxycodone, and tramadol. Morphine, hydromorphone, and codeine are glucuronidated on free hydroxy groups.[31] For example, codeine is biotransformed to morphine, the active metabolite, by CYP2D6. Absence of the enzyme or interference by other drugs would inhibit analgesic response to codeine. Conversely, gene duplication for CYP2D6 results in enhanced activity and increased effects of codeine (ultra-rapid metabolizer

TABLE 49.3 GUIDELINES FOR OPIOID DOSE SELECTION, CONSERVATIVE INITIAL STARTING DOSES FOR OPIOID-NAIVE INDIVIDUALS, AND CONVERSION RATIOS FOR OPIOID ROTATION IN PATIENTS ON CHRONIC OPIOIDS

Opioid naive	Morphine SR	Codeine	Oxycodone	Hydrocodone	Hydromorphone	Methadone	Fentanyl	Oxymorphone
Initial dose and range in opioid-naive patient (starting dose range for repeated dosing)*	15 mg (15-30 mg q 8-12h)	30 mg (15-60 mg q 4-6h)	5 mg (5-15 mg q 4-6h)	5 mg (5-10 mg q 4-6h)	2 mg (2-4 mg q 4-6h)	2.5 mg q 6-12h	NA	5 mg q 4-6h
Opioid tolerant converting from:	**Morphine PO**	**Codeine**	**Oxycodone**	**Hydrocodone**	**Hydromorphone**	**Methadone**	**Fentanyl**	**Oxymorphone**
Morphine IM 10 mg (the gold standard for opioid comparisons)	20-30 mg	60-90 mg†	5 mg	5-10 mg q 4-6h	2 mg	2.5 mg	25-µg patch/72 hr	5 mg (the gold standard for opioid comparisons)
Morphine SR 30 mg PO q 8-12h, 60-90 mg/24hr		30-90 mg q 4h	3-45 mg/24 hr Oxycodone, approx 50% of morphine dose	30-45 mg/24 hr	12-18 mg/24 hr	24-hr dose morphine 30-90 mg 4:1 conversion 90-300 mg 8:1 conversion >300 mg 12:1	25 mcg patch/72 hr	5 mg q 12h ER
Codeine 30-60 mg q 4h	15-30 mg q 3-4h		5-7.5 mg q 4h	5-10 mg q 4h	12 mg/24 hr	2.5 mg q 8-12h	12.5-µg patch/72 hr	2.5-5 mg q 4-6h IR
Oxycodone 5 mg q 3-4h	10 mg	30-60 mg q 3-4h		5-10 mg q 4h	12 mg/24 hr	2.5 mg q 8-12h	25-µg patch/72 hr	5 mg q 4-6h IR
Hydrocodone 10 mg q 3-4h	15 mg	30-60 mg q 3-4h	5 mg q 3-4h		12 mg/24 hr		12.5-µg patch/72 hr	2.5-5 mg q 4-6h IR
Hydromorphone 2 mg q 4h	10 mg		5 mg	5-10 mg q 4h		2.5 mg q 8-12h	25-µg patch/72 hr	5 mg q 4-6h IR
Methadone 5 mg q 8h	20 mg SR q 8h		10 mg q 3-4h		4 mg q 4-6h		25-µg patch/72 hr	5 mg q 12h ER
Fentanyl 25 µg/hr patch	90 mg morphine per 24-hr (1 µg to 4 mg morphine)					5 mg q 8-12h		5 mg q12 h ER
Oxymorphone ER 5 mg q 12h	15 mg SR q 12h		5 mg q 8-12h	10 mg q 4-6h	12 mg/24 hr	5 mg q 8-12 h	25-µg patch/72 hr	

Note: Recommended starting doses are low and should be titrated upward slowly to minimize adverse effects. Limitations of equianalgesic tables exist because they are based on single-dose studies in opioid-naive individuals. Convert opioid 1 to morphine equivalents and calculate dose of opioid 2 according to conversion ratio then reduce the calculated dose for opioid 2 by ⅓ to ½ to ensure safety of the 24-hr total daily dose. Rescue dose is 10-20% of daily opioid dose given every 3 to 4 hours as needed. Titration upward for unrelieved pain should be by 25% to 30% of the current 24-hr dose, adjusted by daily amount of rescue medications needed over a several-week period.
Equivalent or equianalgesic doses for the different opioid preparations vary in different publications.
*Conservative low equianalgesic starting doses for opioid-naive individuals adapted from published recommendations.[28,33]
†Doses above 1.5 mg/kg not recommended because of increase in side effects.[33]
‡Daily dose above 180 mg has not been validated for treatment of chronic pain.
ER, extended release; IR, immediate release.
Data from references 13, 23, 28, 33, 35, 58, and 59.

phenotype) in 2.6% of whites.[30] Hydrocodone is metabolized by CYP2D6, but analgesic effects are not affected by CYP2D6 inhibitors. Methadone both inhibits CYP2D6 and is metabolized by it so that blood levels gradually increase with prolonged use. Morphine glucuronidation produces morphine-3-glucuronide (inactive metabolite) and morphine-6-glucuronide (an active mu agonist), which are excreted by the kidney so accumulate in renal insufficiency.[30]

OPIOID DOSING AND ROTATION

Individual variability in analgesic responsiveness to the different opioids is considerable, and no individual opioid preparation is more efficacious than another. Published opioid equianalgesic dose charts compare starting doses for opioid preparations that produce approximately the same amount of analgesia in opioid-naive patients.[13] Equianalgesic starting doses are typically determined by single-dose studies

in opioid-naive individuals and are not recommended for selecting conversion doses in patients already taking opioids because of incomplete cross tolerance among the different opioids (Table 49.3). Morphine does not appear to have a "ceiling" effect. As the dose is increased, the analgesic effects increase on a logarithmic scale and adverse side effects increase on a linear scale up to the point of unconsciousness. The side effect profiles of opioid preparations are similar; however, individual patient responses are variable. Opioid rotation/switching can enhance analgesia and reduce side effects because of incomplete cross-tolerance among different opioids.[32] One fourth to one half the calculated equianalgesic conversion dose should be selected for switching to a different opioid preparation followed by cautious upward titration of the dose. Conservative ratios of milligrams of morphine to milligrams of an alternate opioid are 4 to 6:1 of hydromorphone; 2:1 for oxycodone, 90 to 100 mg to 25 µg/hr for the fentanyl patch, and 4:1 for methadone if less than 100 mg morphine per day, 8:1 if 100 to

300 mg morphine per day, and 12 : 1 if more than 300 mg morphine per day.

Conservative recommendations (see Table 49.3) for initial opioid doses to start a titration in opioid-naive individuals and cautious conversion doses to an alternate opioid preparation in those already on opioids have been adapted from published studies.[4,13,33] The initial opioid dose and the calculated conversions dose for a different opioid should be titrated upward slowly to avoid intolerable adverse effects. Sequential trials of different opioids may be required to determine which preparation has the most favorable balance of analgesia and side effects in the individual patient.[34] Mechanisms underlying the variability in responsiveness to opioids are unknown. Elderly patients (>70 years) have reduced metabolism and prolonged elimination time for opioids so that starting doses should be reduced by 25% to 50%.

The first opioid should be titrated upward to limiting side effects before rotating to an alternate opioid. Dosing for stable persistent pain should be on a scheduled basis with rescue doses only as needed for breakthrough pain (10% to 15% of scheduled daily dose). Dosing for intermittent or incident pain should be on an as-needed basis. Tolerance to opioid analgesia and opioid side effects seems to be related to genetic factors, duration of opioid treatment, and dose of the current opioid. Dehydration and renal insufficiency cause accumulation of active metabolites that contribute to variability in opioid responses and toxicity.[35] If pain relief is not adequate without intolerable side effects, opioid preparation should be switched or rotated to take advantage of incomplete cross-tolerance (see Table 49.3). Receptor diversity due to splice variants may reduce the amount of cross-tolerance between the current and new opioid preparation. A conservative recommendation to ensure safety is to reduce the equianalgesic conversion dose calculated for the new opioid by 25% to 50% and slowly titrate upward the dose of the new opioid to achieve adequate analgesia without intolerable side effects.[35]

Weaker opioids such as codeine or hydrocodone formulated with aspirin, acetaminophen, or non-steroidal anti-inflammatory agents are often selected first because they are schedule III drugs and the prescription can be written with five refills (plain codeine sulfate prescriptions must be rewritten monthly). Opioids with acetaminophen should be limited to a maximum daily dose of less than 4 g of acetaminophen because of potential hepatotoxicity (see later). It is important to remember that codeine and hydrocodone must be metabolized to their active metabolite, morphine, to exert an analgesic effect. Methadone has no active metabolites, and its metabolism and elimination are independent of renal function.[35]

OPIOID PREPARATIONS

Opium is an extract of the poppy plant that contains two classes of alkaloids: phenanthrenes and benzyl-isoquinolones. The term *opioid* refers to natural, semi-synthetic derivatives, and synthetic chemicals that have opium-like effects.[23,25] A phenanthrene such as thebaine is toxic and not an analgesic but can be transformed into analgesic drugs. Most opioid analgesics are MOP receptor agonists.[21] The pure mu agonist opioids are morphine, hydromorphone, methadone, and fentanyl and have no ceiling effect. Doses above 180 mg of morphine per day have not been validated in clinical trials with chronic pain patients. Benzomorphan opioids (pentazocine) should not be used long term in those with persistent pain because they bind the KOP receptor to produce psychotomimetic effects and dysphoria with minimal analgesia. The DOP receptor agonists are antinociceptive, antidepressant, and proconvulsive in animal models.[21] Methadone is also an NMDA receptor antagonist and is a selective norepinephrine reuptake inhibitor (SNRI), thus providing multimodal analgesia.

Opioid selection and dosing should be based on the temporal characteristics and severity of pain. Patients with constant persistent pain of moderate intensity (4 to 6 on a 0-10 pain scale) often do well on around-the clock dosing with codeine, dihydrocodeine, hydrocodone, sustained-release oxycodone, or low-dose morphine. Hydromorphone, higher dose morphine, methadone, and transdermal fentanyl are typically used for severe pain (7 to 10 on the 0-10 pain scale). Patients with intermittent severe pain and "breakthrough" pain require additional rapid-onset/short-acting preparations on an as needed (PRN) schedule. Patients with waxing and waning pain intensity do well with

an "as needed" dosing schedule. In general, oral short-acting opioids (morphine, oxycodone, hydrocodone, hydromorphone) have a slower onset of effect (20 to 60 minutes) because they are hydrophilic and have both slow absorption and slow crossing of the blood-brain barrier. Long-acting morphine and oxycodone (e.g., Oxycontin) and fentanyl patches are long acting because the sustained-release formulation produces prolonged absorption. Methadone is long acting because it has an intrinsically long elimination half-life. Lipophilic opioids such as transdermal and transmucosal fentanyl rapidly cross the blood-brain barrier and have a more rapid onset of action in 5 to 10 minutes. Liver disease and renal disease may prolong elimination half-life and increase cumulative drug effects to cause symptoms of overdose and an increase in adverse side effects.

Meperidine should not be used for long-term opioid treatment because the meperidine metabolite, normeperidine, is a CNS excitotoxin that produces anxiety, myoclonus, tremulousness, and seizures, especially in patients with renal insufficiency.[23] Accumulation of the propoxyphene metabolite norpropoxyphene may cause cardiac toxicity.[23] Patients who are hypovolemic may be more susceptible to hypotensive effects of morphine.[23] Do not use controlled-release or long-acting opioids for upward titration. Begin titration with a short-acting preparation to determine total daily dose of opioid needed. Then switch to a long-acting preparation at 50% or less of the calculated equianalgesic converting dose followed by a slow upward titration to adequate pain relief. Starting and converting doses should be reduced to 25% to 33% of the calculated dose in those older than age 65 and with impaired liver or renal function. "Rescue doses" for breakthrough pain are provided at 10% to 15% of the total daily dose as a short-acting preparation. The daily scheduled dose is gradually adjusted by adding the average rescue dose per day until the total daily dose that produces adequate pain relief is reached.

Morphine

Morphine is one of 20 alkaloids isolated from opium 200 years ago and is still the gold standard against which all analgesics are judged.[23] Morphine is a naturally occurring opioid alkaloid (phenanthrene) that is hydrophilic and does not cross the blood-brain barrier well. It has poor oral bioavailability of 20% to 30% and is metabolized in the liver by microsomal mixed-function oxygenases using the P450 system. Three metabolites are morphine-6-glucuronide (M6G), a potent analgesic; morphine-3-glucuronide (M3G), which is not analgesic but is neuroexcitotoxic and can actually cause hyperalgesia and allodynia; and normorphine, which is also analgesic. Morphine metabolites are excreted in urine and bile. M6G is a more potent analgesic than morphine and accumulates to a higher serum concentration with chronic administration. Elimination half-life is normally 2 to 4 hours. However, the metabolism of morphine is reduced in liver failure, resulting in a prolonged half-life that can be almost double that in normal individuals so that the dosing interval should be increased to avoid excessive blood levels. Morphine, M6G, and M3G clearance is reduced in renal failure so these metabolites accumulate causing increasing toxicity, especially neurotoxicity (i.e., reduce morphine dose or avoid morphine). Morphine induces histamine release causing itching and vasodilatation with hypotension in hypovolemic patients and problems in patients with asthma and atopy. In general, duration of analgesia increases with aging and plasma levels were 15% higher in those older than 65 years. Long-acting morphine preparations are MS-Contin, morphine SR, Oramorph SR (q 8-12h), Kadian, and Avinza (24-hour dosing interval). The onset of action is within 30 minutes, and elimination half-life is 2 to 4 hours. Steady-state levels are achieved in approximately 24 hours. Long-acting preparations may have to be given more often than every 12 hours. Sustained-release tablets must not be split, crushed, or chewed. Intramuscular injection of 10 mg of morphine is equivalent to 60 mg of oral morphine in single-dose studies of postoperative pain but equivalent to 30 mg of oral morphine for repeated dosing. For chronic musculoskeletal pain, the daily dose of oral morphine is usually up to 180 mg/day, but rarely up to 300 mg/day is required. The potential for incomplete cross-tolerance between opioids, especially at high doses, suggests two approaches for switching to a new opioid preparation. First, switch to one third to one half the equianalgesic dose and use a short-acting preparation for rescue doses for breakthrough pain as needed until the dose needed is established. Alternatively, one can reduce the current opioid dose to one half and add half the calculated equianalgesic dose of the new opioid for several days and monitor analgesic level before completing the switch (a taper/titrate conversion).

Codeine

Codeine, the methyl ether of morphine, was isolated in 1832 as an impurity in morphine extracted from opium.[36] It is widely used as a safe antitussive and analgesic for mild to moderate pain because it has little respiratory suppression effects and minimal tolerance, dependence, or abuse and addiction problems. Up to 10% of the codeine dose is demethylated to morphine by CYP2D6 and CYP3A3/4 enzymes; therefore, individuals with low levels of P450 enzyme activity may have no analgesic effects from codeine. Codeine analgesic effects as well as side effects can be reduced by inhibitors of these enzymes (see Table 49.2). The elimination half-life ranges from 2.5 to 3 hours. Codeine doses should be decreased by 25% to 50% with renal insufficiency and failure. It has been shown to be effective for osteoarthritis pain in a randomized placebo-controlled 4-week trial of a controlled-release formulation (dihydrocodeine) in a dose range of 100 to 400 mg/day (mean dose, 320 mg/24 hr). The frequency of side effects in this study was 82% for codeine and 58% for placebo, leading to discontinuation in nearly 40% of those treated with codeine.[6] Individual doses of codeine above 60 mg prolong but do not increase analgesia and tend to produce more side effects. Plain codeine is a schedule II drug, and prescriptions must be rewritten each month. Codeine compounded with a non-opioid analgesic (acetaminophen with codeine) is a schedule III medication and prescriptions may have five refills. A controlled-release formulation available outside the United States, dihydrocodeine (Codeine Contin), was significantly more effective for osteoarthritis hip or knee pain than placebo.[6]

Hydrocodone

Hydrocodone is a semi-synthetic derivative of morphine that is a schedule III medication and only available compounded with acetaminophen (Vicodin, Lortab, Lorcet, Maxidone, Norco, and Zydone) and with ibuprofen (Vicoprofen). Hydrocodone, 10 mg, is equianalgesic to 60 mg codeine. Hydrocodone has a complex metabolism involving two P450 enzymes, CYP2D6 and CYP3A4, that produce several hydroxymetabolites, including hydromorphone, which is an active mu receptor agonist. It has a half-life of 3.8 to 4.5 hours and should be used with caution in the elderly and those with renal or hepatic dysfunction. Low CYP2D6 activity may decrease conversion to the active metabolite, but the clinical effects on analgesia are unknown.

Hydromorphone

Hydromorphone (Dilaudid, Hydromorph Contin) is more potent than morphine (2 mg of hydromorphone is approximately equianalgesic to 10 mg morphine). It is a semi-synthetic hydrogenated ketone of morphine developed in the 1920s and is a schedule II drug. Immediate-release 2- and 4-mg tablets have an onset of action within 30 minutes and duration of action about 4 hours (half-life of 2 to 3 hours). A slow-release preparation has a duration of action of 12 to 24 hours. It does not have a 6-glucuronide metabolite; however, a 3-glucuronide is not analgesic but is neuroexcitotoxic[30] and can cause increased pain, allodynia, myoclonus, and seizures. The usual starting dose is 2 to 4 mg every 4 to 8 hours. High-dose hydromorphone may be associated with severe nausea and delirium. The hydromorphone/3-glucuronide plasma level is 30-fold greater than the parent drug with chronic dosing and up to 100-fold higher with renal failure. If there is associated myoclonus and/or confusion the patient should be rotated to a different opioid.[37] It has partial lipid solubility with delayed penetration of the blood-brain barrier. It is faster acting than morphine (more lipid soluble) and not as fast acting as fentanyl (less lipid solubility). There are no randomized controlled trials of hydromorphone for musculoskeletal pain. The morphine to hydromorphone conversion ratio is about 5:1. Caution should be used in prescribing hydromorphone to the elderly and those with hepatic and renal dysfunction.

Oxycodone

Oxycodone is a semi-synthetic derivative of thebaine (a phenanthrene opioid alkaloid) that has been in clinical use since 1917.[38] Randomized controlled trials of oxycodone for musculoskeletal pain[39-42] and two trials for neuropathic pain[43,44] demonstrated significant pain reduction in osteoarthritis and neuropathic pain. Adverse events were common and caused drug discontinuation in 10% to 36% of patients. Oxycodone is 6 to 9.5 times as potent as codeine (5 mg oxycodone = 30 to 50 mg codeine) and 1.5 to 2 times as potent as morphine (5 mg oxycodone = 10 mg morphine). Oxycodone metabolism is catalyzed by the liver enzyme CYP2D6 for O-demethylation to oxymorphone (an active metabolite with 10-fold greater analgesic potency) and by N-demethylation to noroxycodone then noroxymorphone. Low levels of CYP2D6 and inhibitors of CYP2D6 may reduce levels of oxymorphone, but the clinical impact on analgesia is not known.

Oxycodone is a schedule II medication (prescriptions must be rewritten monthly). Short-acting oxycodone is available as plain oxycodone and compounded with acetaminophen (Percocet, Roxicet, or Tylox) or aspirin (Percodan). Controlled-release oxycodone (OxyContin and generic oxycodone-CR) has an initial brief rapid absorption followed by prolonged absorption. Chewing or breaking the tablets results in rapid release and potential for opioid overdose. Oxycodone and metabolites are excreted free or in glucuronidated form. Elimination half-life is approximately 3.2 hours for immediate-release oxycodone and 4.5 hours for controlled-release oxycodone so that steady-state levels are achieved in 24 to 36 hours.

Dosing interval ranges from 8 hours (in up to a third of patients) to 12 hours (in two thirds of patients). In clinical trials two thirds of patients had effective pain control on 40 mg or less per day. Titration of oxycodone dose to adequate analgesia can be made by increasing the daily dose by 25% to 50% every 1 to 2 days (time to reach steady state) or by reducing dose interval from every 12 hours to every 8 hours. The oxycodone dose should be a third to a half lower in those older than age 65 years because they have a 15% higher serum concentration. In kidney failure (creatinine clearance < 60 mL/min), oxycodone-CR has 50% higher plasma concentration because the half-life is longer.[38] The plasma level was 40% to 50% higher, and the half-life was 2 hours longer in patients with mild to moderate hepatic impairment. In patients with cirrhosis, the half-life was 13.9 hours before liver transplantation and 3.4 hours after transplantation.[38] Interestingly, women had 25% higher plasma concentration than men when adjusted for body weight. The oxycodone dose should be reduced in those taking sedatives, hypnotics, tranquilizers, and alcohol. Interaction with SSRIs can cause increased serotonin levels and the serotonin syndrome with visual hallucinations and tremors.[38]

Acetaminophen warning

In 2009, the U.S. Food and Drug Administration (FDA) issued a ruling that required revised labeling to include warnings about potential safety risks with acetaminophen. This new labeling requirement applies to acetaminophen and to any medication that contains acetaminophen. Manufacturers must ensure that the active ingredients of these drugs are prominently displayed on the labels of both packages and bottles and must warn about the risk of severe liver damage and unintentional overdose. New labeling instructs patients to consult with their physician prior to using acetaminophen if they are taking warfarin and warns against the combined use of acetaminophen and alcohol. This new labeling requirement is effective as of April 28, 2010. Patients must be warned not to consume alcohol while taking these medications to avoid unintentional liver toxicity and to be aware of other over-the-counter medications that might contain acetaminophen. They should be advised to limit their total daily acetaminophen dose to below 4000 mg/day.

Methadone

Methadone is a synthetic opioid that has been used for the past 40 years primarily as a maintenance treatment for heroin addiction because it can control cravings, prevent withdrawal symptoms, is long acting, and is legal. Recently it has been used to treat cancer and non-cancer persistent pain.[32,45] A systematic literature review reported that 59% of methadone-treated patients had "meaningful effects," that is, more than 30% reduction of pain and/or statistically significant improvement with tolerable or manageable side effects supporting the use of methadone for chronic pain.[45] Methadone is very inexpensive and has a relatively low street value. It has no active metabolites, is not eliminated by the kidney, and has minimal neuroexcitotoxicity. Methadone is comparable to morphine for analgesia and side effect profile and has less severe withdrawal symptoms.[21] It can mitigate opioid tolerance because of incomplete cross-tolerance with other opioids and its multiple-receptor activity.[45]

Methadone produces analgesia through opioid and non-opioid mechanisms.[26] The *l*-isomer is a MOP and DOP receptor agonist. The DOP activity may account for methadone's ability to counteract opioid tolerance and dependence.[32] Both isomers are moderate-affinity NMDA receptor blockers in the brain and spinal cord and may attenuate opioid tolerance. NMDA is an excitatory neurotransmitter responsible for the pain amplification of "wind up." The NMDA receptor blocker action also decreases neuropathic pain. Additionally, the *l*-isomer inhibits serotonin and norepinephrine neuronal reuptake.[23,46,47]

The pharmacokinetics of methadone are very complex. Methadone is well absorbed with up to 85% bioavailability.[48] It is highly lipophilic, and the onset of action begins in 1 to 2 hours with peak plasma level by 4 hours.[48] Duration of analgesia is 4 to 8 hours after each dose. The usual dosing for pain is two to three times per day, but some patients may require a dose every 4 to 6 hours initially. The dosing interval can be lengthened after repeated administration. Methadone has a long elimination half-life that carries with it the risk of delayed overdose. Methadone metabolism occurs in the gut, kidney, and liver by P450 enzymes, CYP3A4 (the main methadone demethylator), CYP2D6, and possibly CYP2B6; however, no active metabolites are produced.[32] Slow elimination results in a long and variable half-life with daily administration (range: 12 to over 100 hours with an average of about 24 hours).[27] Four to five half-lives are required to reach steady state. During this period of slow drug accumulation there is an increased risk for delayed toxicity. Methadone administration is also complicated by important drug interactions. Buprenorphine, pentazocine, naltrexone, naloxone, and tramadol are contraindicated in patients taking methadone because they may precipitate withdrawal symptoms.[45]

Agents that induce CYP3A4 enzyme activity increase the metabolism of methadone and thereby reduce blood levels so that analgesia is less and withdrawal symptoms may occur (see Table 49.2). Agents that inhibit CYP3A4 and inhibit CYP2D6 reduce the metabolism of methadone and may increase methadone levels and cause increased opioid effects. Spironolactone may increase methadone clearance. Benzodiazepines, tramadol, and alcohol increase adverse effects of methadone. There is minimal elimination of methadone by the kidney and gut so that methadone clearance is minimally affected by age and renal insufficiency; however, in end-stage renal failure the dose should be reduced by 50%.[46] Hemodialysis and peritoneal dialysis remove less than 1% of the daily dose of methadone and are not useful to manage overdoses. Clearance is normal in patients with stable alcoholic liver disease; however, CYP enzymes may be induced during active hepatitis C infection so that much higher doses of methadone may be required. Side effects are similar to those of other opioids (Table 49.4). Nausea, vomiting, constipation, and drowsiness may be less with methadone; however, dry mouth, myoclonus, sweating, and confusion do still occur.[11,49] Some patients may develop QTc prolongation by more than 60 ms, increasing the risk of developing arrhythmias such as torsades des pointes. Prolongation of the QTc is usually dose related above 30 mg/day, and arrhythmias occur with doses above 70 to 100 mg methadone per day.

There are several methadone prescribing strategies:"start low, go slow," "stop and go," and "taper titrate." Methadone titration can be difficult because of the long and unpredictable half-life that can also be affected by the important drug interactions just described[23,32,45,49,50] and in Table 49.2. Additional details on methadone dosing recommendations for treatment of chronic pain are available at www.atforum.com, www.vapbm.org, or vaww.pbm.med.va.gov.[11] Recommendations in Table 49.5 were modified for a more conservative approach to methadone prescribing based on our experience and recent reports.[47,49,50,52] Titration of methadone should begin with small doses and/or doses adjusted according to current opioid dose. The onset of analgesia is within 30 to 60 minutes, and duration of analgesia may be 4 to 8 hours when starting this drug. Drug tissue accumulation with repetitive dosing increases the duration of analgesic action up to 12 hours and reduces dosing to one to three times a day. Elimination half-life ranges from 4.2 to 130 hours and may result in drug accumulation and toxicity. The long duration of action at steady state reduces instances of breakthrough pain and end-of-dose abstinence symptoms.[47] Abstinence withdrawal symptoms are protracted after methadone discontinuation.

Methadone dosing must be cautiously individualized. The methadone dose used to treat heroin addiction is 20 to 60 mg administered once every 24 hours. It would be toxic for an individual who is not tolerant to opioids.[46] Conversion to methadone to treat chronic pain requires conversion dose ratios that vary with the daily morphine equivalent dose (see Table 49.5).[49] It is important to remember that equianalgesic dose charts are usually based on single-dose analgesic studies and are only approximate comparisons that tend to underestimate the potency of methadone and grossly overestimate the steady-state dose level of methadone that will be required for adequate analgesia.[4,51]

The first step is to calculate the morphine equivalent dose of the current opioid. The morphine equivalent dose is 3.7 times the daily hydromorphone dose and 2 times the Oxycontin daily dose. The second step is to convert the daily dose of morphine equivalent into the starting methadone dose:

- Less than 200 mg morphine equivalent per day: use 10% for conversion methadone dose
- 200 to 500 mg morphine equivalent per day: use 7% for conversion methadone dose

The third step is to select a dosing strategy for the methadone titration that is based on current analgesic regimen (see Table 49.5). Conservative calculations of the conversion dose for methadone are based on the morphine equivalent dose per day.

Strategy 1—The "start low, go slow" strategy

This strategy is recommended for opioid-naive patients to avoid side effects during upward titration to effective analgesia. Start the titration with 2.5 to 5 mg methadone every 8 to 12 hours plus a short-acting opioid for breakthrough pain. Slowly increase the methadone dose by 2.5 mg at 2- to 4-weekly intervals based on the clinical response (i.e., analgesia and adverse effects).

Strategy 2—The "stop and start" strategy

This strategy is recommended for those taking codeine and hydrocodone (weak opioids) or those on less than 200 mg morphine equivalent per day of other opioids. Calculate 10% of the morphine equivalent dose per day for the starting methadone dose per day in two to three divided doses per day. Use a short-acting opioid only for breakthrough pain and increase the methadone dose by 2.5 mg every 8 hours every 2 to 4 weeks. Do not increase the methadone dose more often than every 2 weeks.

Strategy 3—The "taper titrate" strategy

This strategy is recommended for patients on more than 200 to 500 mg of morphine equivalent per day.

Calculate 7% of the morphine equivalent dose for the target conversion methadone dose per day divided into three every 8 hourly doses per day. Start with 50% of the calculated target methadone dose per day (divided into three every 8 hourly doses) and reduce the current opioid by 50%. Slowly upward titrate the methadone dose by increasing the daily dose by 2.5 to 5.0 mg per day every 2 to 4 weeks and taper the current opioid by half each time the methadone is increased.

If the patient develops sedation or respiratory suppression during methadone titration, hold the next dose of methadone, decrease subsequent doses, and make increments less frequently. Short-acting opioids (codeine, hydrocodone, or oxycodone) for breakthrough pain will avoid excessive methadone accumulation. Methadone dose reduction will be required as methadone accumulates over several weeks. The maintenance dose of methadone will be less than the equianalgesic chart starting dose,[4] and disproportionately smaller doses

TABLE 49.4 ADVERSE SIDE EFFECTS OF OPIOIDS

Side effects 50% overall incidence	Opioid effect and impact	Recommendations
Constipation (40% to 70% incidence)	Reduces secretions and peristalsis in small and large intestine Increases tone in pyloric sphincter, ileocecal valve, anal sphincter Does not decrease over time	Prophylactic treatment with laxatives that are gut stimulants, not stool softeners Docusate, senna (2-6 tabs bid), bisacodyl Lactulose PO and enemas Oral naloxone 0.8 mg bid
Nausea and vomiting (15% to 30% incidence)	Binds receptors in brain stem, stimulates chemoreceptor trigger zone plus slows gastrointestinal motility	Ondansetron, prochlorperazine, thiethylperazine, or haloperidol Hydroxyzine, transdermal scopolamine Metoclopramide if caused by reduced motility Corticosteroids (dexamethasone) may help Rotate to alternative opioid
Sedation/somnolence (20% to 60%)	In early treatment decreases rapidly but may be persistent If appears later in treatment may indicate accumulation	Methylphenidate (5-10 mg), pemoline dextroamphetamine (2.5-10 mg), caffeine (65-200 mg/d) Increase dose interval
Dizziness (14%)	Unclear mechanism	Meclizine or scopolamine
Cognitive impairment	Distinguish from slowed cognition due to sedation	Reduce dose or increase dosing interval
Delirium with confusion, agitation, hallucinations Dysphoria or euphoria	Uncertain mechanisms	Haloperidol for delirium, benzodiazepine for agitation, opioid rotation
Headache	Unclear mechanism	Lower dose, rotate opioid
Skin effects; pruritus and urticaria, flushing, rashes, and sweating (2% to 10%)	Histamine release from mast cells also causes vasodilatation, sweating	Antihistamines, paroxetine Opioid rotation
Myoclonus (increases with higher doses)	Neuroexcitotoxic side effect (is dose related)	Diazepam, clonazepam, midazolam, baclofen, valproic acid, and dantrolene Opioid rotation if dose reduction not possible
Dry mouth	Autonomic effects	
Respiratory depression	Depression of mu2 receptor mediated brain stem respiratory centers Depresses response to CO_2 and respiratory rate, cough suppression Increases obstructive sleep apnea, respiratory arrest	Naloxone 0.4 mg/10 mL saline: infuse 5 mL q 2 min until respiratory depression reversed
Urinary retention and hesitancy	Increases the tone of urinary tract smooth muscle Can cause ureteral spasm, sphincter spasm, bladder spasm with urinary urgency, and difficulty passing urine Inhibits voiding reflex so decreased tone in bladder detrusor muscle can cause urinary retention	Opioid rotation catheterization
Circulatory depression (lightheadedness)	Vagal stimulation causes bradycardia Reduced sympathetic output resulting in vasodilation and venodilation can cause hypotension especially if patient is hypovolemic or septic	Give intravenous fluids
Antitussive effects	Depression of cough center in the medulla	
Meiosis	Parasympathetic stimulation at the Edinger-Westphal nucleus of the oculomotor nerve	No symptoms
Hormonal effects: hypothalamic-pituitary-adrenal axis	Loss of libido, impotence, aggression, amenorrhea, galactorrhea	Due to reduced cortisol, increased prolactin, and decreased luteinizing hormone, follicle-stimulating hormone, testosterone, and estrogen
Immune effects	Evidence of immune modulation in humans is limited (pain itself can modulate the immune system). Decreases function of T cells, B cells, NK cells, and macrophages	Opioid-like receptors on immune cells More pronounced effects in immunosuppressed HIV-infected persons
Overdose with opioids	Respiratory depression, somnolence to coma, skeletal muscle flaccidity, cold and clammy skin, constricted pupils, bradycardia, hypotension, death	Control airway and provide ventilatory assist Give naloxone 0.4 to 2 mg IV to maintain alertness and respiratory function (can use continuous infusion); can precipitate abstinence syndrome. If no response after 10 mg it is probably not opioid overdose.

Data from references 13, 28, and 58.

of methadone are needed with higher morphine equivalent doses. Dosing intervals may be increased to every 12 hours when the analgesic dose is stable (producing adequate pain relief and manageable side effects). Patients should be monitored every 1 to 2 weeks during titration and monthly thereafter. Significant toxicity may occur if dose increments are made too frequently, dose conversion ratio is too high, or dose intervals too close. Educate patients about the slow onset of analgesia as the medication accumulates, about side effects to anticipate, the dangerous drug interactions with methadone, and about withdrawal symptoms if they stop the medication abruptly. The conservative dose calculation proposed may result in an initial undertreatment of pain. Rescue medication for breakthrough pain should be

TABLE 49.5 DOSING STRATEGIES FOR CONVERSION TO METHADONE

Current opioid dose	Oral daily dose example	Methadone conversion ratio and dosing strategy depends on current opioid daily
Patient on no opioid	NA	**'Start Low, Go Slow' gradual titration in the clinic** Start methadone at 2.5 mg q8h then increase by 2.5 mg q8h every 2 to 4 weeks
Morphine equivalent dose < 200 mg/day	150 mg/day	**'Stop and Start'** Calculate 10% of 150 mg = conversion dose of 15 mg methadone/day Start methadone at half this conversion dose with 2.5 mg q 8h and increase by 2.5 mg q8h every 2 to 4 weeks
Morphine equivalent dose = 200-500 mg/day	500 mg/day	**'Taper Titrate'** Calculate 7% of 500 mg = conversion dose of 35 mg methadone/day, start with about ⅓ of this dose = 5 mg q8h. Decrease current opioid to ⅔ of daily opioid dose. Increase methadone by thirds and taper current opioid by thirds every 2 to 4 weeks.

Data from references 13 and 50.

TABLE 49.6 COST COMPARISONS OF LONG-ACTING OPIOIDS

Drug (manufacturer)	Dose	VA cost per dose in July 2009	Monthly cost
Transdermal fentanyl (Janssen Duragesic)	25 µg/hr*	$2.06 each patch	$20.60/mo q 3 days
	50 mg/hr	$3.84	$38.40
	75 mg/hr	$5.72	$57.20
	100 mg/hr	$7.66$5	$76.60
Generic transdermal fentanyl patch (Mylan) (½ the cost of Duragesic)	25 µg/h*	$1.25 each patch	$12.50
	50 µg/h	$2.29	$22.90
	75 µg/h	$3.51	$35.10
	100 µg/h	$7.23	$72.30
Oxycodone controlled release (Purdue Pharma)	10 mg	$92.00 per #100 tablets	$55.20/mo (bid dosing) $105.60/mo
	40 mg*	$176.00/100 tablets	$105.60
Morphine SA (generic Mallinckrodt)	20 mg	$312.00	$187.20/mo
	15 mg	$7.34 per #100 tablets	$ 4.40/mo (bid dosing)
	30 mg*	$11.27	$6.76
	60 mg	$23.20	$13.92
Methadone (Mallinckrodt)	2.5 mg* (½ tab)		$1.49/mo (tid dosing)
	5 mg*		$1.98 (bid dosing)
	10 mg	$5.00/100	$3.00 (bid dosing)

*Approximate equianalgesic doses per American Pain Society.
VA, U.S. Department of Veteran's Affairs.

TABLE 49.7 COST COMPARISONS OF SHORT-ACTING OPIOIDS (VA, JULY 2009)

Opioid	Cost per #100	Cost per month for 2 tabs qid (#240)
Codeine 30 mg with acetaminophen	$4.70	$11.28
Hydrocodone 5 mg with acetaminophen	$2.49	$5.98
Oxycodone 5 mg	$5.90	$14.16
Oxycodone 5 mg with acetaminophen	$3.60	$8.74
Morphine sulfate 15 mg	$3.40	$8.16
Hydromorphone 2 mg	$6.29	$15.10
Oxymorphone 5 mg	$143.60	$344.64

VA, U.S. Department of Veteran's Affairs.

placebo for osteoarthritis pain, but only 50% completed the 6-week study.[52] It is 100 times as potent as morphine and has no active metabolites. A transdermal patch produces 72 hours of systemic drug delivery through the skin. Transdermal fentanyl should not be started in opioid-naive patients because of possible respiratory depression and should not be used for initial opioid titration. Patients must be warned not to chew or swallow the patch and not to place a hot pack on the patch or wear it during magnetic resonance imaging (MRI). Pain relief does not begin for 6 to 8 hours after applying the patch. Fentanyl patches should be reserved for those patients who cannot swallow or are unable to tolerate morphine SR and methadone. The elimination half-life after removing the patch is at least 17 hours because of drug sequestration in adipose tissue. Metabolites are excreted in the urine.

Initial dose calculation for switching from another opioid should be based on the calculated 24-hour morphine equivalent dose. Approximate equianalgesic conversion doses are 25 mcg/hr, 72-hour patch for 90 mg of oral morphine per 24 hours; for 45 mg of oxycodone per 24 hours; and for 12 mg of hydromorphone per 24 hours (see Table 49.3). Drug conversion ratios and recommended doses for transdermal fentanyl published by the manufacturer are conservative so that upward dose titration will likely be needed. Fentanyl dose should not be increased in less than 6 days. Dose increases should be based on the amount of rescue medication (supplemental short-acting opioid) required per 24 hours. A 90-mg/24 hr oral morphine equivalent dose of rescue medication warrants a 25-µg/hr increase in the fentanyl patch dose. A recent drug warning from the manufacturer warns concomitant use of CYP3A4 inhibitors (ritonavir, ketoconazole, diltiazem, itraconazole, troleandomycin, clarithromycin, nelfinavir, and nefazadone) may result in high plasma fentanyl concentrations and increased adverse drug effects, especially potentially fatal respiratory depression. It is important to remember that 17 or more hours are required for the blood level to decrease by 50% after the patch is removed. Concomitant use with other opioids, sedatives, hypnotics, tranquilizers (e.g., benzodiazepines), general anesthetics, phenothiazines, skeletal muscle relaxants, and alcohol may cause respiratory

provided at 10% to 15% of the daily methadone dose with a short-acting opioid such as oxycodone, hydrocodone, or codeine.[34]

A strong case can be made to use methadone for chronic musculoskeletal pain and chronic neuropathic pain because it has a comparable efficacy and side effect profile to morphine. Methadone has no active metabolites, so it can be used in renal insufficiency (reduce dose by 50% in patients in end-stage renal failure or on dialysis) and stable chronic liver disease (with mild to moderate dysfunction). Methadone is the least expensive opioid (Tables 49.6 and 49.7).

Transdermal fentanyl

Fentanyl (Duragesic, generic) is a short-acting, highly lipophilic opioid derivative of meperidine.[52] It was significantly more effective than depression, hypotension, profound sedation, or coma. Increased body temperature may increase transdermal diffusion, and MRI procedures can heat the patches.

Buprenorphine

Buprenorphine is a semi-synthetic, highly lipophilic opioid that is derived from the morphine alkaloid thebaine.[23] It is a partial agonist with very high affinity at the MOP and is an antagonist at the KOP. It is 30 to 40 times more potent than morphine, but because of the antagonist activity the analgesic effects plateau at higher doses. It is used for narcotic addiction therapy because of its antagonist properties. Because of its high affinity for MOP, buprenorphine may block the effect of other opioids. It is dosed once daily for treatment of addiction disorders but three or four times daily for analgesia. Individuals on daily buprenorphine for addiction treatment who need analgesia for acute or chronic pain may increase the dose frequency to four times a day, with a maximal daily dose of 32 mg. At higher doses, buprenorphine behaves more like an antagonist. If this is not effective, other high-affinity opioids such as fentanyl or hydromorphone can be used. Buprenorphine is contraindicated for pain treatment in opioid-dependent patients because it may precipitate severe withdrawal symptoms. Oral buprenorphine is extensively (80%-90%) metabolized in the liver by first-pass metabolism; therefore, oral bioavailability is poor. Sublingual absorption has better (55%-70%) bioavailability, with peak plasma concentrations at 90 minutes and a half-life of 4 to 5 hours. A transdermal formulation with similar bioavailability is available in Europe. Interestingly, opioid-induced hyperalgesia, which can be seen after exposure to higher doses of pure mu agonist opioids, does not appear with buprenorphine. Buprenorphine has anti-hyperalgesic effects that may be due to its antagonist effect on the KOP receptor that are thought to promote the hyperalgesic pain state and antinociceptive tolerance. The combination drug buprenorphine plus naloxone (Suboxone) is FDA approved for use only in the treatment of opioid dependence. This indication is strictly adhered to by the manufacturer and its federal co-sponsor (Center for Substance Abuse Treatment). The off-label use of this drug for pain management is not supported. The risk of precipitation of severe opioid withdrawal with improper use is not insignificant. Ten hours of training toward supplemental Drug Enforcement Agency licensure is required to prescribe it safely and effectively (Scott McNairy, director of Addiction Psychiatry, University of Minnesota, personal communication).[53]

Oxymorphone

Oxymorphone is a new semi-synthetic opioid agonist available in both immediate-release (IR) and extended-release (ER) as a schedule II controlled substance and is very expensive.[54] Oxymorphone is only about 10% bioavailable when taken orally. This is increased by hepatic or renal dysfunction. Food increases the concentration of oral oxymorphone by 38% to 50%; therefore, it must be given at least 1 hour before or 2 hours after meals. If the ER formulation is taken with 20% alcohol the concentration may be increased by as much as 260%. There is a black box warning for patients taking oxymorphone ER against consuming alcohol. Oxymorphone is not metabolized by and does not inhibit or induce the CYP450 enzymes. It is 10 times more potent than morphine when given by injection. A 10-mg tablet, if crushed and injected, will deliver a potentially lethal dose equivalent to 100 mg morphine. The starting dose in opioid-naive patients is recommended at 5, 10, or 20 mg every 4 to 6 hours. The ER formulation is recommended at 5 mg every 12 hours. Caution should be exercised in patients with moderate to severe renal disease or mild hepatic impairment. It should not be given to patients with moderate to severe liver disease.

Other mu agonist analgesics

Several common mild mu agonist analgesics are used for mild persistent pain but are generally not recommended for persistent moderate to severe pain. Tramadol (Ultram or Ultracet compounded with acetaminophen) is an unscheduled analgesic with weak MOP receptor affinity and inhibition of norepinephrine and serotonin reuptake. It is 10-fold less potent in binding mu receptors than codeine and is similar to other weak opioids but is more expensive. Tramadol should not be used long term because safer, more effective, and less expensive medications are available. Side effects include headache, constipation and nausea, dizziness, sedation, and CNS stimulation with spasticity, agitation, anxiety, euphoria, hallucinations, and seizures. Seizures have been reported especially in those using tricyclic antidepressants (TCAs), cyclobenzaprine, promethazine, SSRIs, monoamine oxidase inhibitors, and neuroleptics. The risk of tramadol-induced seizures may be increased in those with epilepsy, brain injury, metabolic disorders, alcohol withdrawal, or CNS infection.

The recommended doses are 25 to 100 mg every to 6 hours not to exceed 400 mg/day.[13] Dose interval and maximum dose should be reduced to less than 200 mg every 12 hours when creatinine clearance is less than 30 mL/min. Daily dose should not exceed 300 mg/day in those older than age 75 or 50 mg every 12 hours in those with hepatic dysfunction. The manufacturer's information sheet recommends tramadol not be used with hepatic impairment. Drug interactions with tramadol are significant. Tramadol is subject to both metabolic induction and inhibition so that analgesia may be reduced by low CYP2D6 activity (inherent or drug-induced reduction of conversion to active metabolite) as well as by induction of CYP2D6 (e.g., carbamazepine increases metabolism), which reduces analgesic efficacy and the half-life up to 50% (see Table 49.2). Tramadol may produce a serotonin-like syndrome if administered with an SSRI (citalopram, sertraline, fluoxetine, fluvoxamine, or paroxetine). In a tramadol overdose, naloxone may increase the risk of seizure and it is minimally removed by hemodialysis. Opioid-like withdrawal symptoms may occur after abrupt discontinuation.

Propoxyphene napsylate (100 mg [Darvon-N] and with acetaminophen [Darvocet-N]) and propoxyphene hydrochloride (65 mg [Darvon] and with aspirin and caffeine [Darvon Compound 65]) are weak opioid agonists with a chemical structure similar to methadone. This drug is regarded as a dangerous pain killer because toxicity develops at only slightly above the recommended daily dose, and it was withdrawn from the market in Great Britain in 2007, where it is viewed as a poor pain killer with a narrow therapeutic window and toxicity in overdose that is unacceptable. It is not scheduled as a controlled substance but can produce opioid-like dependence with withdrawal symptoms after abrupt discontinuation. It is only one half to two thirds as potent as codeine. The half-life is highly variable and ranges from 6 to 12 hours.[23] N-demethylation produces norpropoxyphene, which has a long half-life of 30 to 36 hours so that accumulation and toxicity occur with repeated dosing (CNS and respiratory depression, seizures, delusions, hallucinations, confusion, cardiotoxicity, prolonged conduction time, and pulmonary edema). Deliberate and accidental overdose alone or in combination with tranquilizers, antidepressants, and alcohol has a high risk of serious toxicity and death. Ingestion of 6 to 20 capsules with alcohol can produce serious toxicity/death. Naloxone can antagonize the respiratory depression and cause seizures and cardiotoxicity and arrhythmias.[13,23] Propoxyphene should not be prescribed for long-term use and should not be used in those with renal and hepatic insufficiency. Propoxyphene is inappropriate for use in those older than age 65 years because the metabolism is reduced and the half-life prolonged. Propoxyphene may also interfere with the metabolism of antidepressants, anticonvulsants (especially carbamazepine), and Coumadin. The FDA recently required stricter labeling of drugs containing propoxyphene after an expert advisory panel recommended the drug be withdrawn. The FDA concluded that propoxyphene is useful enough to remain on the market but required a "boxed warning" regarding the risk of death at higher than prescribed doses. Propoxyphene overdose frequently produces death within the first hour. This is thought possibly due to prolonged QT interval causing fatal arrhythmia.

CLINICAL APPROACH TO LONG-TERM OPIOID PRESCRIBING

Making the decision to prescribe long-term opioid therapy must be preceded by a thorough investigation of the medical, psychological, and socioeconomic complexities of the persistent pain problem. The arrival of a patient on opioids prescribed by another provider is never sufficient justification to conclude opioids are appropriate for that patient. The initial opioid titration phase must demonstrate effectiveness in the individual patient before deciding to prescribe long-term opioids.

Standardized assessment of the patient

Six steps of a standardized assessment are needed to arrive at the clinical decision that opioids are appropriate for this patient.

The *first step* is a comprehensive standard medical history to include medical and psychiatric disorders and to identify important co-morbidities. The comprehensive pain history should be taken with a standardized format to avoid missing important information and to minimize patient leading the interview. Avoid the mistake of recommending a prior failed treatment. Detailed family history, current social history, education and vocational history, functional status, current medications, and current legal or disability issues are essential for the assessment. Define the cardinal features of the pain at its onset, progression since onset, and current condition. Determine whether the pain is spontaneous and persistent at rest or intermittent and produced by movement (incident pain), pressure, touch, and change in temperature. Ask the patient to describe the character of the pain (i.e., burning, lancinating, sharp, dull, aching), and the radiation pattern. Determine what factors worsen the pain and what tends to relieve the pain. Ask the patient to quantitate the pain severity on a 0 to 10 scale, with 0 being no pain and 10 the worst possible pain.

Inquire about early family dynamics and any history of abuse, alcoholism, and psychiatric disorders in the immediate family and spouse. Inquire about interpersonal problems to reveal indicators suggestive of additional psychopathology.

The *second step* is a thorough physical examination that includes a meticulous detailed neurologic and musculoskeletal examination. The physical examination process serves to identify objective abnormalities that reasonably explain the patient's pain and to define functional status.

The *third step* is to make a deliberate effort to identify psychiatric co-morbidities early in the decision-making process. It is very important to identify personality disorders because their history may not be accurate, and these patients have problems with impulsivity and impaired judgment as well as substance abuse. Expression of rage toward family members, employers, insurance adjustors, and every physician is seen as a "red flag" for a personality disorder diagnosis. Detection of malingering and deception in patients with chronic pain is crucial because correct assessment and treatment depends on accurate patient self-report. Refusal to permit access to old medical records, history of multiple hospitalizations, and compensation claims are also "red flags" for deception.

Assessment for risk of opioid abuse and addiction should be clearly documented.[57] Several assessment instruments are recommended because they are easy to score and have been validated in populations with medical illnesses. The Screener and Opioid Assessment for Patients with Pain (SOAPP) is a validated self-administered screening tool to predict future medication misuse (available for download at www.painedu.org). The D.I.R.E. score can be used to select patients for chronic opioid therapy based on clinician rating of factors that predict efficacy of and compliance with long-term opioid treatment.[55]

The *fourth step* is to formulate a working diagnostic impression of the predominant or most likely underlying pathogenic mechanism(s) causing the pain:

- Active or progressive structural disease of the musculoskeletal system (i.e., nociceptive)
- A disorder of the nervous system (i.e., neurogenic or neuropathic)
- A psychiatric disorder producing or accentuating complaints of pain (i.e., somatization disorder) *or*
- Some combination of these mechanisms

The *fifth step* is to ask the patient what he or she expects from your evaluation and recommendations. The patient may be seeking a second opinion to validate another physician's evaluation and treatment recommendations, may be seeking a different diagnosis and treatment plan, may be applying for disability and need a medical statement, or may be looking for a physician willing to prescribe opioids.

The *final step* before prescribing opioids is to establish at the outset that you expect it is unlikely the pain will be eliminated completely but some improvement can be anticipated. It is important to discuss realistic treatment outcome goals for pain relief and the specific functional improvements. Determine whether your assessment does or does not match the patient's goals before starting opioid treatment. Discuss the patient's responsibility in working to improve function and to abide by the clinic's rules. For patients determined to be at high risk for abuse or addiction, explain the need for more careful monitoring and more frequent urine toxicology screens. It may be useful to use a pain diary or a patient pain treatment satisfaction questionnaire to monitor the patient's progress over time. Set a clear expectation of regular assessment of whether goals are being met, agreement to follow the clinic rules for opioid prescribing (see later for details), and willingness to discontinue opioid therapy if goals are not met.

Prescribing opioids

Opioid treatment of persistent osteoarticular pain must be individualized because this pain is often due to a variable combination of mechanical mechanisms, inflammatory mechanisms, and neuropathic injury mechanisms. Pain that persists despite specific therapy for the underlying mechanical or inflammatory disorders or inadequate response to non-opioid analgesics warrants treatment with opioids. Most patients with chronic musculoskeletal pain have become physically deconditioned and will need a directed rehabilitation program when pain has been decreased enough to permit an increase in physical activity. Analgesic selection, route, dosage, and scheduling should be individualized. It is the obligation of providers and patients to search for the best cost/benefit ratio for treatment of patients in pain. Tables 49.6 and 49.7 present cost data for medications in the U.S. Department of Veterans Affairs (VA) system. Despite marketing efforts to influence physician prescribing practices for analgesics, there are no data to prove superior efficacy or side effect profile for any individual opioid preparation. Patient response should direct medication selections. If pain is present for most of the day, the drug should be scheduled regularly rather than on an as-needed basis. The majority of patients with defined musculoskeletal disease will have pain incident to movement and should be taught how to schedule analgesic doses to permit as high a level of physical activity as possible. Rational polypharmacy with adjuvant therapies helps to reduce pain severity, minimize opioid side effects, and treat psychosocial consequences of persistent pain such as anxiety and depression and is well established in the field of pain management. Non-opioid analgesics are only useful for mild to moderate pain (2 to 4 on the 0-10 scale) regardless of the underlying joint disease. Opioids are warranted for moderate to severe pain or in those with less severe pain who have contraindications to the non-opioid analgesics. Treating patients who have chronic musculoskeletal pain and an active addiction disorder is very difficult and should be done in collaboration with ongoing addiction treatment and/or 12-step programs. Opioid treatment in patients with dementia is challenging and requires input from the primary caregiver to assess response to treatment.

Opioid titration trial

A weak opioid such as codeine or hydrocodone with acetaminophen should be tried first (see Table 49.3). Opioids do not have a ceiling effect for analgesia but, if compounded with acetaminophen, care should be taken to keep the daily dose of acetaminophen to less than 4 g. Side effects are less if dose titration is slow and adjuvant medications can be used to diminish nausea, prevent constipation with a gut stimulant, or reduce sedation (see Table 49.4). When starting a new opioid medication patients should be advised to take the first dose at home to determine whether sedation, dizziness, or confusion occurs. Caution patients about taking an opioid with other sedating medications or after drinking alcohol. Explain to the patient that more frequent monitoring may be necessary if there is a history of substance abuse. The comprehensive evaluation, decision-making process for recommendation of opioid treatment, conduct of the informed consent process, explanation of the rules of opioid prescribing, and the expectations set with patient preferred goals must be thoroughly documented in the medical record.

Published charts on usual starting dose for moderate to severe pain are not all the same. Table 49.3 presents our more cautious recommendations for starting doses in opioid-naive patients especially if older than age 65 and for those with liver dysfunction, renal insufficiency, or cognitive impairment. Most opioid trials for non-malignant pain used moderate opioid doses (up to 180 mg morphine equivalents per day). The initial opioid dose should be titrated upward every 2 to 4 weeks depending on pain relief and adverse side effects. There is large variability in individual responses to opioids. Increases in dose above 180 mg morphine equivalents per day should be done with caution because there are no long-term high-dose trials of opioids for non-malignant pain that examined efficacy and adverse events. In general, it will require a 3- to 4-month titration period to determine the dose needed to reduce pain severity to approximately 4 on the 0 to 10 scale without intolerable side effects. It is recommended that the physician who initiates the opioid trial be responsible for an informed consent discussion regarding the risk of side effects and addiction, the clinic rules for participating in the opioid renewal clinics, realistic expectations of attaining adequate pain relief to a level of 4 of 10 (not total elimination of all pain), and expectation of participation in rehabilitation activities to increase function. The patient is informed the opioids will be continued after the titration period if opioids are effective in reducing pain severity and if function has improved.

Decision to prescribe long-term opioid therapy

At the end of the 12- to 16-week opioid titration trial a decision should be made with the patient whether the opioid reduced the pain sufficiently, whether side effects were manageable, and whether the patient is ready to begin a program to increase function or is able to perform some activity he or she was unable to do before the opioids. Most patients will have a good response to opioids and maintain a stable dose for long periods of time. If pain relief was only "minimally improved," further dose titration upward or trial of a stronger/different opioid should be recommended. Increased function should be an objective outcome of the treatment plan. It is usually more convenient for the patient to take a long-acting opioid preparation (sustained-release morphine, sustained-release oxycodone, methadone, or fentanyl patches) with planned short-acting opioids for breakthrough pain. It is not advisable to prescribe two long-acting preparations simultaneously.

When the decision for long-term opioid treatment has been made, the "rules" for long-term opioids must be clearly explained in a patient–provider agreement that may or may not be signed by the patient and physician (Fig. 49.2). The patient must agree to keep all scheduled appointments, have random urine toxicology screens, seek opioid prescriptions only from a single provider, and agree not to go to the emergency department or come in to clinic unscheduled for an early prescription refill. With rare exceptions there should be no excuses for early refills or "lost" medications (emphasize it is the patient's responsibility to secure his or her medications). When the opioid dose has been selected, a trained nurse can take over the monthly monitoring for efficacy, side effects, signs of abuse or drug diversion, and the timely refilling of prescriptions (Fig. 49.3). It is important to get all physicians in the clinic to agree to write only prescriptions prepared by the nurse managing opioid monitoring and prescription refills in the clinic. The medical record should detail the opioid prescribed, dose, and administration schedule with number of pills to be dispensed per month. Opioid refills should be made by the initial prescribing physician or a designated nurse if an opioid refill system is established. The patient is given the responsibility of calling in to request medication refills in a timely manner. The nurse is the key link for assessment of pain relief and medication side effects, general status, monitoring for new problems, and indicators warning of possible abuse. Increase in opioid dose should not be made without re-examining the patient. Management becomes more complicated and time consuming with those few patients who do not have a good response. Having a documented clear opioid policy with the patient–provider agreement will avoid acquiescing to unexpected demands for more opioids when treatment goals are not met or if the patient is not taking medications according to instructions. A defined opioid prescription renewal policy, a patient–provider agreement, and a clinical protocol for a nurse-managed opioid renewal clinic can prevent many problems and reduce the stress and effort when problems do emerge (see later).[57]

Opioid rotation

There is incomplete cross-tolerance among the various opioid preparations so that switching to a different opioid can increase efficacy and/or reduce intolerable opioid side effects. There are problems with published "equianalgesic" charts and "conversion ratio charts" for patients on chronic opioids because they are usually based on single-dose studies in opioid-naive subjects. They should not be used for switching opioids in patients on long-term opioid therapy or in patients with renal and hepatic insufficiency.[4] Incomplete cross-tolerance of the first opioid can lead to greater opioid potency than anticipated with the second opioid. Large inter-individual variability in responses to opioids also makes the outcome of opioid rotation more unpredictable.[58] Table 49.3 is based on multiple published recommendations for cautious initial dosing in an opioid-naive patient and for patients on long-term opioids. Conversion ratio charts for switching from first opioid to second opioid that are provided by drug manufacturers have conservative low estimates for the dose of a new opioid to avoid these problems with incomplete cross-tolerance. The calculated dose of the second opioid should be reduced initially by 30% to 50% to accommodate variability in response and possible incomplete cross-tolerance.[51] Do not use conversion drug ratios to switch in the opposite direction because a reverse calculation may result in an overestimation of the "equivalent" dose and excessive toxicity can occur.[35] Rescue doses of a short-acting opioid should be provided during the conversion period at 10% to 20% of the daily dose of the long-acting opioid every 3 to 4 hours.[59]

Both analgesia and side effects increase with increasing opioid dose and produce confusion, agitation, myoclonus, dry mouth, nausea and constipation, itching, and sedation. When opioid titration/escalation fails, reconsider whether opioids are appropriate treatment for a particular patient's pain. Gradually wean off the opioids and reassess after a "detoxification" period of 2 to 3 months. Some patients will actually have a reduction of pain and overcome the fear of living without opioids. In those who still have pain, restart a different opioid formulation at a lower dose with slow upward titration. Apparent failed opioid titration may represent aberrant drug-seeking behavior due to inadequate analgesia ("pseudoaddiction"), a manifestation of non-compliance such as drug diversion to others, or a true addiction disorder with compulsive uncontrolled use.[14] It should be remembered that the rate of addiction in the general population is no different than the rate of addiction in chronic pain patients: 3.8% to 18%.[7-9]

Managing breakthrough pain

Breakthrough pain refers to sudden increases in pain severity with certain movements, activities, or postures, spontaneous idiopathic acute flares of pain severity, and return of pain with decrease in the serum drug concentration before the next medication dose (end-of-dose failures). Breakthrough pain can be managed preemptively by prescribing a rescue dose of opioid before activities known to increase pain severity, such as a physical therapy session. End-of-dose failure can be eliminated by reducing the intervals between doses of a long-acting preparation and/or scheduled addition of a rescue dose of the opioid.

Opioid hyperalgesia

Some patients develop generalized hyperesthesia or an increased sensitivity to pain. This paradoxical opioid-induced increased pain is termed *opioid-induced hyperalgesia* (OIH).[60,61] It appears that not all opioids induce this syndrome. The phenanthrene opioid morphine has produced OIH in both animals and humans, but piperidine derivatives such as fentanyl or sufentanil have not. Similar diffuse pain and hyperalgesia is also a component of opioid withdrawal syndrome. There are case reports of other opioids producing OIH in humans, but the distinction between OIH and withdrawal or other causes of hyperalgesia was not always clear. There are several proposed mechanisms of OIH,

Patient–Provider Agreement for Long-term Opioid Therapy between:

Patient Name	and Dr.	At the Minneapolis VAMC

Chronic Opioid Therapy for Intractable Pain will be Prescribed under the following Conditions:
1. If (drug prescribed) is effective for adequate pain control with tolerable side effects
2. If Scheduled appointments are kept: if appointment is failed the prescription will not be renewed
3. If the Patient agrees to obtain pain medications only from Dr: And NOT to go to the ER or Urgent Care for more meds
4. If the patient agrees NOT to request "early" or "partial" prescription refills from the MVAMC Pharmacy
5. If the patient agrees NOT to come to the Rheumatology clinic without an appointment to request more Pain Medications
6. There will be no acceptable excuses for "lost medications"
7. If the Patient agrees to be responsible for taking medications as directed. If the Pain medication supply is used up before the end of the prescription period, the patient has the option of admission for opioid withdrawal under supervision or will "tough it out" at home. NO additional pain medications will be prescribed.
8. Pain Severity and function will be re-evaluated after _____ months of an Opioid Trial to determine whether continued use of chronic opioids is justified by clinical improvement
9. I understand that urine samples will be randomly tested for drugs
PATIENT AND PHYSICIAN ARE TO SIGN BELOW:
PATIENT SIGNATURE: PHYSICIAN SIGNATURE:

DATE				NAME SSN		

MEDICINE SERVICE   RHEUMATOLOGY CLINIC

Fig. 49.2 Patient provider agreement for long-term opioid treatment.

including (1) inhibition of the central glutaminergic system which increases the amount of glutamate available to activate the excitatory NMDA receptors; (2) increased spinal dynorphin in response to MOP agonists activates KOP receptors, leading to release of spinal excitatory neuropeptides such as calcitonin gene-related peptide; and (3) direct facilitation of spinal nociceptive processing by the action of opioids on the on and off cells of the rostral ventromedial medulla (RVM)—descending facilitation. NMDA antagonists such as ketamine can reverse OIH. Methadone is a pure MOP agonist but occurs in a racemic mixture in which the *d*-isomer is an NMDA receptor antagonist. These properties of methadone may make it a good choice for treating or avoiding OIH. KOP receptors are also thought to play a role in OIH. KOP receptor agonists consistently produce hyperalgesia. Buprenorphine, a partial opioid agonist with antagonist properties, is also a KOP receptor antagonist and has been shown to be effective in treating experimentally induced hyperalgesia.

Managing opioid side effects

Success of opioid treatment depends on successful management of side effects, which is a major clinical challenge. Adverse effects that appear in the setting of stable opioid dose are probably not due to the opioid but rather a complication of the underlying disorder or a new co-morbid condition (e.g., dehydration, hypercalcemia, hypoxemia, sepsis, bowel obstruction) or adverse reaction from a concomitant medication such as benzodiazepines, TCAs, corticosteroids, or NSAIDs.[1] Side effects will occur in most patients treated with opioids (see Table 49.4). Approximately 50% of 5546 patients in 34 trials had at least one side effect and 20% of those with an opioid adverse effect discontinued the medication.[62] There is no strong evidence that one opioid preparation has fewer adverse effects than another, excluding meperidine.[58] Nausea (21%), constipation (15%), dizziness (14%), sedation (14%), and vomiting (10%) were the most common side effects identified in this systematic literature review.[62] There is a striking, unexplained inter-individual variability in the occurrence and tolerability of opioid side effects. Aging and co-morbid renal and hepatic dysfunction, drug interactions that alter absorption, metabolism, and clearance may enhance toxicity in some patients. Side effects during initial opioid initiation and dose escalation will abate spontaneously except for constipation.[58] Driving and ability to operate machinery are not impaired with stable, moderate opioid doses; however, cognitive function may be impaired for up to a week after opioid doses are increased.

3D Narcotic Telephone Renewal Clinic

Renewal For	Last Filled on:	#pills dispensed	DATE STARTED
How many pills are you using per day? LEAST	MOST		
Are you using any other pain medications? NO YES If yes, what? ?OTC from another MD?			
Does the medication help? A LOT SOME A LITTLE NOT AT ALL			
Rate your pain from 0 to 10 BEFORE you take the pain medication _____ and AFTER taking it _____			
Have you had any side effects from the pain medication, such as: FEEL SLEEPY OR SEDATED CONFUSION DIZZINESS CONSTIPATION NAUSEA OTHER:			
How do you feel your pain control is? Residual pain Amount of time with no pain			
How many days per week do you take the pain medications?: How many pills per day do you take on those days?			
Do you feel the pain medication has lost its effectiveness? NO YES If yes, have you increased the dose? NO YES COMMENTS:			
Do you receive pain medication from doctors not at the MVAMC NO YES If yes, what medication by whom: Reason it was prescribed?			
Have you become addicted to the opioid? NO YES If yes, describe:			
Are you afraid of becoming addicted? NO YES If yes, comment:			
Do you have a history of addiction to alcohol or other drugs? NO YES If yes, describe			
PRESCRIPTION WRITTEN FOR SCHEDULED NARCOTIC TELEPHONE RENEWAL CLINIC ON (DATE) _____	#PILLS/MO	RENEWED	MD
DATE	NAME:		SSN

MEDICINE SERVICE   3D   RHEUMATOLOGY CLINIC

Fig. 49.3 Questionnaire for nurse-managed narcotic renewal clinic program.

The key to managing opioid side effects is to recognize the symptoms as such. The first response to opioid toxicity should be to reduce the dose and give it more frequently or as a sustained-release preparation.[58] Adverse effects can also be managed with symptom-specific treatment (see Table 49.4). If symptoms persist, rotate to a different opioid preparation that may be better tolerated, as described earlier.

Trouble-shooting problems with long-term opioid therapy

Problems do arise managing patients long term with opioids for persistent osteoarticular pain. Providers who prescribe opioids must monitor for patient behaviors that suggest opioid misuse and/or diversion and document the absence of evidence of misuse or diversion in the medical record (see Fig. 49.3). The most common problem is patient report of loss of analgesia. This complaint has a differential diagnosis that includes (1) progression of underlying disease with increased peripheral nociception or a new problem with increased inflammation, tumor, neuropathic process, osteoporotic fracture; (2) development of anxiety or depression; (3) cognitive change altering pain perception or reporting such as dementia or delirium; (4) opioid tolerance (rare); or (5) development of abuse, addiction problem, or criminal intent.

Some patient behaviors are those of misuse and diversion, and other behaviors are "red flags" for loss of control with excessive opioid intake or suggest diversion of the prescribed medication. The dilemma in the clinical setting is differentiating the patient with chronic pain who is misusing opioids from the drug addict whose use of opioids is unrelated to chronic pain, that is, differentiating pain relief–seeking behavior from abusive drug-seeking behavior. Repeated requests for early refills indicate the patient's pain severity has increased or the patient has lost control of taking the prescription as directed or is diverting his or her pills. The term *drug-seeking behavior* is a pejorative term suggesting an abuse behavior; however, it may (and usually does) indicate inadequate pain relief, driving the patient's attempt to get more medication and is referred to as "pseudoaddiction." The provider's first response should be to discuss the situation face to face with the patient and examine the patient to determine what has changed. If there is no explanation for increased pain severity and no progression of the underlying problem/disorder and the patient has not followed prescription directions, limit further prescriptions to a 1- or 2-week supply of medications until he or she can control taking medications according to directions. Remind the patient of his or her responsibility for taking medications as prescribed. Review and have the patient sign the patient–provider agreement that details the patient's rights and responsibilities. At times it may be necessary to shorten prescriptions to only a 3-day supply until compliance is regained (see Fig. 49.2). If these behavior modification techniques are not successful, the patient should have an addiction evaluation and possibly co-management with a mental health provider. There are certain aberrant behaviors that raise the question about abuse or addiction behaviors (see Table 49.1).

Patients with three or more abuse criteria were highly likely to progress to drug treatment program, psychiatric treatment, or legal problems or fail to return to the clinic within a year. These behaviors should prompt urine toxicology screen.

The goals of urine drug testing in the setting of chronic opioid analgesic therapy are to ensure that the patient is taking the medications that have been prescribed and not taking illegal drugs.

A negative urine toxicology screen could indicate the patient is not taking the opioid prescribed (suggests hoarding or selling medication). A positive urine toxicology screen will have to be followed by a confirmatory test that identifies the specific drug. Urine screens may not identify oxycodone unless specifically requested. On-site dipstick testing can produce false-positive and false-negative results and may not differentiate between different opioids and may not be able to detect low levels of drug. Decisions about non-compliance or drug abuse should await confirmatory urine testing that accurately identifies individual opioids and is sensitive enough to detect low levels of illegal street drugs.[63]

Measurement of analgesic blood levels 1 to 2 hours after a usual dose together with clinical assessment of pain level, alertness, ambulation, blood pressure, pulse rate, and pupil reaction identify opioid tolerance or detect malabsorption or rapid metabolism indicating the need for a higher dose or alternate route of administration to reach analgesic blood levels. In addition, confusing urine test results can be clarified by blood testing.[64]

The opioid provider must have an exit strategy for patients who do not benefit from opioid treatment or display unacceptable behavior. It is not appropriate or ethical to abruptly discontinue opioid prescriptions without formulating an alternative treatment plan and making referral to an appropriate provider or treatment program. If the decision to discontinue chronic opioids is made, patients must be warned about opioid withdrawal symptoms if medication is stopped abruptly. Opioid withdrawal is a "flu-like" syndrome with rhinorrhea, lacrimation, coughing, sneezing, coryza, hypertension, tachycardia, chills, sweating, piloerection, yawning, aching muscles, abdominal cramps and diarrhea, restlessness, and irritability that lasts 3 to 7 days (longer after methadone). These symptoms can be avoided by reducing opioid dose by 10% to 15% every 2 to 3 days over a 2- to 3-week period. Clonidine 0.2 to 0.4 mg may reduce withdrawal symptoms.

Legal aspects of chronic opioid prescribing

Physicians have an ethical obligation to relieve suffering and to promote the dignity and autonomy of their patients. Drugs should be administered in whatever dose is necessary to relieve suffering even if doing so causes foreseeable side effects if the patient has been so advised. A written patient–provider agreement (see Fig. 49.2) detailing the conditions required for ongoing opioid prescribing should be discussed with the patient. An informed consent process regarding the risk of inducing side effects and addiction with a realistic estimate of how much pain relief is expected should be done before starting opioids. The medical record must document the diagnosis and assessment of risk for abuse and addiction and delineate these decision-making steps and the process of informed consent. Progress toward treatment goals, adverse effects, and absence of abuse behaviors must be documented. The treatment plan should be reviewed periodically. Those with a significant history of drug abuse may have an increased risk for opioid abuse and benefit from consultation and/or ongoing co-management with an addiction specialist. Actively addicted patients with chronic pain present a major therapeutic challenge because they pose a significant risk to themselves and the provider who may lack the expertise to manage their mental illness and opioid treatment. The detection of illicit drug use should trigger assessment for possible substance abuse disorder, and, if refused, the patient should not continue to be treated with a controlled substance.

Adjunctive medications for chronic pain

Evidence is emerging that neurogenic mechanisms often are involved in the pain of osteoarticular disorders, suggesting that medications typically used for neuropathic pain may provide added benefit. Advances in the treatment of neuropathic pain are being applied to rational polypharmacy in the treatment of chronic pain of diverse origin.[65] Antidepressant drugs have long been used for chronic pain. TCAs and antiepileptic drugs are useful adjuncts to analgesic therapy in patients with low back pain, radiculopathy, postherpetic neuralgia, and neuropathic pain even in the absence of depression.[66] There is strong evidence that TCAs decrease neuropathic pain and weaker evidence that anticonvulsants, antiarrhythmics, and topical agents are effective.[67] Antidepressants inhibit reuptake of biogenic amines serotonin and norepinephrine, modulate sodium channels, and inhibit excitatory neurotransmitters. The tertiary amines block uptake of both norepinephrine and serotonin (amitriptyline, imipramine, clomipramine, and doxepin); the secondary amines block only norepinephrine uptake (nortriptyline and desipramine) and have less sedation and anticholinergic side effects. TCAs have adverse effects of sedation, weight gain, orthostatic hypotension, and anticholinergic symptoms of dry mouth, urinary retention, constipation, and delirium, which are worse in the elderly. TCAs must be used with caution in those with heart disease (especially conduction disturbances), glaucoma, and prostatism. Venlafaxine (an SNRI) was effective in diabetic neuropathy pain, had fewer side effects than TCAs, and had few anticholinergic effects. The SSRIs are generally not very effective analgesics but are better tolerated than the TCAs. Fluoxetine was not an effective analgesic, and paroxetine and citalopram had only modest effects.[68] TCAs are often effective at low doses, and analgesic effects occur in a week.

Opioids were previously considered ineffective for neuropathic pain; however, recent studies have demonstrated that controlled-release oxycodone, 20 to 99 mg/day,[43,69] morphine, methadone,[65] and tramadol[68] were effective for neuropathic pain.

Antiepileptic drugs that inhibit sodium channel activation can modulate peripheral sensitization by decreasing action potential propagation, membrane depolarization, and neurotransmitter release.[68] First-generation antiepileptic drugs, carbamazepine (Tegretol) and phenytoin (Dilantin), are not used very often because of adverse effects and because safer drugs are available. Carbamazepine is structurally similar to the TCAs and can enhance sodium channel inactivation, reduce excitatory neurotransmitter release, and modulate L-type calcium channels. It has been shown to be effective in diabetic neuropathy and postherpetic neuralgia pain.[70] Phenytoin has had variable efficacy in neuropathic pain.

The second-generation antiepileptic drugs include gabapentin (Neurontin), tiagabine (Gabitril), topiramate (Topamax), levetiramate (Keppra), oxacarbazepine (Trileptal), and lamotrigine and act via multiple mechanisms and have shown promise in clinical trials of painful neuropathy. Gabapentin, titrated up to 3200 mg/day, produced significant pain relief but dose titration was limited by sedating side effects and dizziness. Doses must be reduced in renal failure. Oxcarbazepine acts on sodium channels and N-type calcium channels and may modulate both peripheral and central sensitization. It is less toxic than carbamazepine. Lamotrigine acts on sodium channels, inhibits release of excitatory neurotransmitters, and modulates N-type calcium channels. It has had variable efficacy for peripheral neuropathic pain, and common side effects include rash. In one trial, in 44% of patients with central post-stroke pain the pain decreased with 200 mg/day of lamotrigine.[70] Topiramate has multiple mechanisms of action, inhibits voltage-gated sodium and calcium channels, has GABAergic and glutaminergic effects, and has shown modest effects in diabetic neuropathy. Modulators of central sensitization such as gabapentin[67,70] and pregabalin, GABA analogs, may act on calcium channels within the spinal cord, modulate GABA release, inhibit sodium channels, and alter monoamine neurotransmitter release. Zonisamide, a sodium and T-type calcium channel blocker, increases GABA release but had marginal benefit and a high occurrence of adverse events.[70] However, some patients who had failed multiple prior medications did obtain pain relief. Mexiletine is a sodium channel blocker structurally similar to lidocaine. It improved night-time pain and sleep in patients with diabetic neuropathy but had minimal daytime benefit, and its use is limited by side effects of tremors, confusion, agitation, and nausea and vomiting.

Blocking NMDA channels to decrease central sensitization has been limited by drug side effects.[71] Intravenous and subcutaneous ketamine at subanesthetic doses was an effective analgesic but caused severe dysphoria, sedation, and dissociative episodes. Dextromethorphan, an over-the-counter cough suppressant is a low-affinity NMDA channel blocker. The antitussive dose of 120 mg/day is not sufficient for neuropathic analgesia. In a National Institutes of Health clinical trial of up to 960 mg/day, 7 of 13 patients with diabetic neuropathy reported moderate or greater relief; however, it was ineffective in postherpetic neuralgia.[71] Side effects were substantial, including sedation, dizziness, and ataxia.

Lidocaine patches may give local pain relief. Topical capsaicin, an alkaloid in hot chili peppers that binds to the vanilloid receptor on C and Aδ fibers, depletes substance P from sensory nerve endings and may actually cause degeneration of nerve endings. It effectively reduced pain of diabetic neuropathy when used over 8 weeks.

Muscle relaxants

Muscle relaxants are reviewed herein to emphasize they should not be used for long-term persistent pain. Drugs such as carisoprodol (Soma) and cyclobenzaprine (Flexeril) are useful adjuncts to opioid therapy of acute pain but are not indicated for the treatment of chronic musculoskeletal pain. As a group the "muscle relaxants" may have some effects secondary to sedating side effects and are categorized as "Do Not Use" because of minimal effectiveness and potentially dangerous side effects. Carisoprodol is metabolized to meprobamate, which has abuse potential. Chlorzoxazone (Parafon Forte DSC) is approved for acute painful musculoskeletal conditions but does not relieve muscle spasm. It may cause serious liver toxicity and has an additive sedating effect if taken with alcohol. Cyclobenzaprine's structure is similar to amitriptyline and is approved for acute pain and muscle spasm. There is a risk of seizure if administered with tramadol. Methocarbamol (Robaxin) is approved for relief of acute painful conditions, but it does not relax tense muscles. Side effects include sedation, dizziness, nausea, vomiting, abdominal distress, and lightheadedness. Orthenadrine (Norflex) has anticholinergic effects that may cause confusion, delirium, disorientation, dry mouth, urinary retention, and constipation. It is approved to treat acute painful conditions but does not relax tense muscles.

When to refer a patient to a pain specialist or a multidisciplinary pain program

Patients with a chronic pain disorder have persistent pain when the presumptive cause of the pain has been eliminated. This chronic pain disorder consists of the physical, psychological, and social degeneration of the patient with chronic pain. Patients who have prominent psychological and socioeconomic/occupational features in their chronic pain experience are better cared for by a multidisciplinary pain team rather than a single office-based provider. The individual clinician does not possess the multiple skills and specialized knowledge to fully assess all the dimensions of the pain experience in patients with the chronic pain disorder. Physicians who are unaware of the psychosocial dimensions of chronic psychophysiologic pain syndromes will usually fail to identify such patients and become frustrated and suspicious of the lack of response to "standard" treatments. Therefore, these patients need physical, psychological, and social rehabilitation in concert with medical management. Such a biopsychosocial model of chronic pain syndrome requires a multidisciplinary pain management program in which pain reduction has lower priority to pain acceptance and restoration of function. In specialty pain treatment programs, behavior not focused on pain is rewarded and pain-focused behavior is ignored to redirect the patient's efforts away from seeking pain relief to changing behavior and reducing disability. The program includes intensive exercise therapy, management of depression and anxiety, supportive psychotherapy, and patient education. The primary criteria for selection of a patient for a multidisciplinary pain program are the definitive diagnosis of non-reversible pain (no planned surgery) and readiness to change (i.e., patient is motivated toward rehabilitation goals). The patient must not have active substance abuse, suicidal ideation, cognitive impairment, and personality or thought disorder that would interfere with the group milieu, learning, or communication. Chronic pain programs vary in quality and should be carefully evaluated before referring patients. A pain specialty center should have multidisciplinary groups of medical specialists for intensive medical, neurologic, psychological, and physical therapy, not simply personnel to perform nerve blocks.

KEY REFERENCES

1. Breivik H, et al. Survey of chronic pain in Europe: prevalence, impact on daily life, and treatment. Eur J Pain 2005;11:47.
2. World Health Organization. Cancer pain relief, 2nd ed. Geneva: WHO, 1996.
3. International Association for the Study of Pain. Time to modify the WHO analgesic ladder? IASP Pain Clin Updates 2005;XIII(no. 5):1-4. Available at pdf/opiods_doc_2004.pdf.
4. Chou R, Fanciullos GJ, Fine PG, et al. Opioid treatment guidelines: clinical guidelines for the use of chronic opioid therapy in chronic noncancer pain. J Pain 2009;10:113-130.
5. Roth CS, Burgess, DJ, Mahowald M. Medical residents' beliefs and concerns about using opioids to treat chronic cancer and noncancer pain: a pilot study. J Rehab Res Devel 2007;44:263-270.
6. Peloso PM, et al. Double blind randomized placebo control trial of controlled release codeine in the treatment of osteoarthritis of the hip or knee. J Rheumatol 2000;27:764-771.
7. Ytterberg SR, Mahowald ML, Woods SR. Codeine and oxycodone use in patients with chronic rheumatic disease pain. Arthritis Rheum 1998;41:1603-1612.
8. Lazovskis J, Mahowald ML, Singh J. Lack of evidence for opioid tolerance in patients with rheumatic disease. Arthritis Rheum 2003;46:S102.
9. Mahowald M. Opioid use by patients in an orthopedics spine clinic. Arthritis Rheum 2005;52:312-321.
11. Turk DC, Brody MC, Okifuji EA. Physicians' attitudes and practices regarding the long-term prescribing of opioids for non-cancer pain. Pain 1994;59:201-208.
12. Jensen M, Thomsen A, Hojsted J. Ten-year follow-up of chronic non-malignant pain patients: opioid use, health related quality of life and health care utilization. Eur J Pain 2006;10:423-433.
13. VA/DOD. VA/DOD clinical practice guideline for the management of opioid therapy for chronic pain. Office of Quality and Performance Clinical Practice Guidelines

2005. Available at http://www.oqp.med.va.gov/cpg/cpg. htm Volume, 0-111 DOI: http://www.oqp med.va.gov/cpg/cpg.htm.
14. Kalso E, et al. Opioids in chronic non-cancer pain: systematic review of efficacy and safety. Pain 2004;112:372-380.
16. Bolay H, Moskowitz MA. Mechanisms of pain modulation in chronic pain syndromes. Neurology 2002;59(Suppl 2):S2-S7.
17. American Psychiatric Association. Diagnostic and statistical manual of mental disorders, 4th ed. Text revision, 4th TR ed. Washington, DC: American Psychiatric Association, 2000:1-942.
18. Eisenberg E, McNicol E, Carr D. Efficacy and safety of opioid agonists in the treatment of neuropathic pain of nonmalignant origin. JAMA 2005;293:3043-3052.
19. Scherder E, Herr K, Pickering G, et al. Pain in dementia. Pain 2009;145:276-278.
20. Waldhoer M, Bartlett S, Whistler J. Opioid receptors. Annu Rev Biochem 2004;73:953-990.
22. Stein C, et al. Analgesic effect of intraarticular morphine after arthroscopic knee surgery. N Engl J Med 1991;325:1123-1126.
25. Ballantyne J, Fishman M, Abdi S, eds. The Massachusetts General Hospital handbook of pain, 2nd ed. Philadelphia: Lippincott Williams & Wilkins, 2002: 1-587.
28. American Pain Society. Principles of analgesic use in the treatment of acute pain and cancer pain, 4th ed. Glenville, IL: American Pain Society, 1999:1-64.
29. Chabal C, et al. Prescription opiate abuse in chronic pain patients: clinical criteria, incidence and predictors. Clin J Pain 1997;13:150-155.
32. Fishman S, et al. Methadone reincarnated: novel clinical applications with related concerns. Pain Med 2002;3:339-348.
34. Indelicato RA, Portenoy RK. Opioid rotation in the management of refractory cancer pain. J Clin Oncol 2002;20:348-352.

35. Pereira J, et al. Equianalgesic dose ratios for opioids: a critical review and proposals for long-term dosing. J Pain Symptom Mgmt 2001;22:672-687.
37. Murray A. Hydromorphone. J Pain Sympt Mgmt 2005;29:S57-S66.
38. Kalso E. Oxycodone. J Pain Sympt Mgmt 2005;29:S47-S56.
39. Markenson J, et al. Treatment of persistent pain associated with osteoarthritis with controlled release oxycodone tablets in a randomized controlled clinical trial. Clin J Pain 2005;21:524-535.
40. Caldwell J, Hale ME, Boyd RE, et al. Treatment of osteoarthritis pain with controlled release oxycodone or fixed combination oxycodone plus acetaminophen added to non-steroidal antiinflammatory drugs: a double blind, randomized, multicenter, placebo controlled trial. J Rheumatol 1999;26:862-869.
43. Watson CP, Babul N. Efficacy of oxycodone in neuropathic pain: a randomized trial in postherpetic neuralgia. Neurology 1998;50:1837-1841.
44. Watson C, et al. Controlled release oxycodone relieves neuropathic pain: a randomized controlled trial in painful diabetic neuropathy. Pain 2003;105:421-428.
45. Sandoval J, Furlan A, Mailis-Gagnon A. Oral methadone for chronic noncancer pain: a systematic literature review of reasons for administration prescription patterns, effectiveness, and side effects. Clin J Pain 2005;21:503-512.
47. Rhodin A, et al. Methadone treatment of chronic nonmalignant pain and opioid dependence—a long tern follow-up. Eur J Pain 2006;10:271-278.
49. Bruera E, et al. Opioid rotation in patients with cancer pain: a retrospective comparison of dose ratios between methadone, hydromorphone and morphine. Cancer 1996;78:852-857.
50. Mercadante S, et al. Switching from morphine to methadone to improve analgesia and tolerability in cancer patients: a prospective study. J Clin Oncol 2001;19:2898-2904.

51. Ripamonti C, et al. Switching from morphine to oral methadone in treating cancer pain: what is the equianalgesic dose ration? J Clin Oncol 1998;16:3216-3221.

52. Langford R, et al. Transdermal fentanyl for improvement of pain and functioning in osteoarthritis. Arth Rheum 2006;54:1829-1837.

55. Belgrade MJ, Schamber CD, Lindgren BR. The DIRE Score: predicting outcomes of opioid prescribing for chronic pain. J Pain 2006;7:671-681.

56. Passik SD, Kirsh KL. The interface between pain and drug abuse and the evolution of strategies to optimize pain management while minimizing drug abuse. Exp Clin Psychopharmacol 2008;16:400-404.

57. Goldberg K, Simel D, Oddone E. Effect of an opioid management system on opioid prescribing and unscheduled visits in a large primary care clinic. JCOM 2005;12:621-628.

58. Cherny N, et al. Strategies to manage the adverse effects of oral morphine: an evidence-based report. J Clin Oncol 2001;19:2542-2554.

59. Gammaitoni A, et al. Clinical application of opioid equianalgesic data. Clin J Pain 2003;19:286-297.

60. Silverman SM. Opioid induced hyperalgesia: clinical implications for the pain practitioner. Pain Physician 2009;12:679-684.

62. Moore R, McQuay H. Prevalence of opioid adverse events in chronic non-malignant pain: systematic review of randomized trials of oral opioids. Arthritis Res Ther 2005;7:R1046-R1051.

63. Kozma AJ. Urine drug screening in everyday practice. Pract Pain Management 2007;2007:18.

64. Tennant F. Urine and blood tests: why and when to use each test in pain treatment. Practical Pain Manage 2007;18.

65. Perrot S, et al. Guidelines for the use of antidepressants in painful rheumatic conditions. Eur J Pain 2006;10:185-192.

67. Backonja M, et al. Gabapentin for the symptomatic treatment of painful neuropathy in patients with diabetes mellitus: a randomized controlled trial. JAMA 1998;280:1831-1836.

69. Gimbel JS, Richards P, Portenoy RK. Controlled-release oxycodone for pain in diabetic neuropathy: a randomized controlled trial. Neurology 2003;60:927-934.

REFERENCES

Full references for this chapter can be found on www.expertconsult.com.

Non-steroidal anti-inflammatory drugs

50

Carlo Patrono

- Non-steroidal anti-inflammatory drugs (NSAIDs) continue to provide "background" anti-inflammatory therapy for rheumatic diseases.
- Variability in response to NSAIDs is seen both in terms of anti-inflammatory activity and adverse events.
- Newer NSAIDs with selective inhibition of cyclooxygenase (COX)-2 (inducible) enzyme are associated with a lower incidence of gastrointestinal adverse events.
- The vast majority of COX-2 inhibitors, regardless of selectivity, are associated with increased risk of myocardial infarction.

INTRODUCTION

Non-steroidal anti-inflammatory drugs (NSAIDs) constitute a chemically heterogeneous group of compounds that provide symptomatic relief of pain and inflammation associated with a variety of human disorders, including the rheumatic diseases. Their shared therapeutic actions (i.e., analgesic, anti-inflammatory, and antipyretic) are usually accompanied by mechanism-based adverse effects that can, at least in part, be attenuated as a function of individual pharmacokinetic and/or pharmacodynamic properties.[1] The main chemical classes of NSAIDs are detailed in Table 50.1.

MECHANISM OF ACTION

The best characterized mechanism of action of NSAIDs is inhibition of the cyclooxygenase (COX) activity of prostaglandin (PG) H synthase 1 and 2 (PGHS-1 and -2, also referred to as COX-1 and COX-2) (Fig. 50.1). Given the role that prostanoids, such as PGE_2, PGI_2, and thromboxane $(TX)A_2$, play in the local modulation of many important cellular functions, this mechanism of action is probably sufficient to explain the clinical effects of NSAIDs.

The administration of PGE_2 and PGI_2 causes erythema, an increase in local blood flow, and, in concert with other inflammatory mediators (e.g., bradykinin), hyperalgesia and enhanced vascular permeability.[1] Moreover, PGE_2 interacting with its EP_3 receptor can produce fever. Thus, prostanoids reproduce the main signs and symptoms of the inflammatory response. Because of the redundancy of mediators of this response, it is not surprising that NSAIDs only exert a moderate anti-inflammatory effect, are effective only against pain of low-to-moderate intensity, and reduce fever but do not interfere with the physiologic control of body temperature.[1]

The production of prostanoids involved in these responses appears to be triggered by the immediate availability of constitutively expressed COX-1 and to be amplified and sustained by the local induction of COX-2 in response to inflammatory and mitogenic stimuli.[2] Although the analgesic, anti-inflammatory, and antipyretic actions of traditional NSAIDs are largely reproduced by coxibs (a class of selective inhibitors of COX-2), this finding does not exclude a potential role for COX-1 in mediating, at least in some individuals, the PG-dependent contribution to pain and inflammation.[3]

Although the clinical effects of NSAIDs can be adequately explained in terms of inhibition of prostanoid synthesis and action, at high concentrations these drugs can also produce COX-independent effects.

These include inhibition of the expression of adhesion molecules and reduced production of superoxide radicals and proinflammatory cytokines. However, none of these COX-independent effects has been characterized *in vitro* or *ex vivo* at therapeutic concentrations achieved in humans after oral dosing of conventional doses of NSAIDs.[1]

The ability of acetaminophen to inhibit COX-1 and COX-2 is importantly conditioned by the peroxide tone of the environment.[4] This may explain, at least in part, the clinical observation that, while sharing the analgesic and antipyretic effects of NSAIDs, acetaminophen has relatively poor anti-inflammatory activity at conventional doses. High concentrations of leukocyte-derived peroxides accumulate at sites of inflammation and may impair the ability of acetaminophen to inhibit COX-2.[4] However, circulating plasma levels of the drug after the administration of 1000 mg inhibit systemically COX-2 activity to a comparable degree as traditional NSAIDs and coxibs.[5]

COX-ISOZYME SELECTIVITY

PG G/H-synthase is found in two isoforms that are products of two different genes (see Fig. 50.1): PGHS-1 or COX-1, which is expressed constitutively in all cells but is inducible under appropriate conditions, and PGHS-2 or COX-2, which is inducible in response to inflammatory, mitogenic or hemodynamic stimuli but is also constitutively expressed in some tissues, for example, certain areas of the human kidney and brain.[2,3] Splice variants of COX-1 that retain some enzymatic activity have been described, one of which has been called "COX-3." The pathophysiologic significance of the latter is largely unknown.

The COX-isozyme selectivity of a particular drug is critically dependent on its concentration.[3] One can describe the selectivity profile of different COX-2 inhibitors by plotting the drug concentrations required to inhibit the activity of human platelet COX-1 against those required to inhibit human monocyte COX-2 by 50% (IC_{50}) in whole-blood assays (Fig. 50.2). This type of analysis establishes two important facts:

1. COX-2 selectivity is a continuous variable that does not justify a dichotomous definition of selective and non-selective inhibitors.
2. There is substantial overlap in COX-2 selectivity between some coxib (e.g., celecoxib) and some traditional NSAIDs (e.g., nimesulide and diclofenac).[3]

Because there is substantial variability between patients in plasma concentrations of the COX-2 inhibitor after oral administration of a standard therapeutic dose as well as in the extent of inhibition of each COX-isoform corresponding to any given concentration of the inhibitor, one can pragmatically characterize three levels of COX-2 selectivity in terms of the probability of sparing COX-1 at therapeutic plasma levels: low (e.g., acetaminophen), intermediate (e.g., celecoxib, nimesulide, and diclofenac), and high (e.g., rofecoxib, etoricoxib, and lumiracoxib).

PHARMACOKINETICS AND DRUG INTERACTIONS

The vast majority of NSAIDs are organic acids that are well absorbed orally, highly bound (i.e., 95%-99%) to plasma proteins, metabolized by the liver, and excreted by either glomerular filtration or tubular secretion.[1] Lumiracoxib (which is structurally related to diclofenac) is the only coxib sharing these acidic properties of traditional NSAIDs. Most NSAIDs are rapidly and completely absorbed from the gastrointestinal tract, with peak plasma concentrations occurring within 1 to 4 hours. Food tends to delay absorption without affecting peak plasma levels.[1]

TABLE 50.1 MAIN CHEMICAL CLASSES AND REPRESENTATIVE NSAIDs, WITH SELECTED PHARMACOKINETIC AND PHARMACODYNAMIC PROPERTIES

Chemical class and representative drugs	Time to peak plasma concentration (hr)	Half-life (hr)	Dosing regimen	COX-isozyme selectivity
Salicylates				
Aspirin	0.5-1	0.3	q 4-6 hr	COX-1=COX-2
Diflunisal	2-3	12	q 8-12 hr	NA
Para-aminophenol				
Acetaminophen	0.5-1	2	q 4 hr	COX-2>COX-1
Acetic acid				
Indomethacin	1.5	2.5	q 12 hr	COX-1>COX-2
Sulindac	8 (active metabolite)	13 (active metabolite)	q 12 hr	NA
Etodolac	1	7	q 6-8 hr	COX-2>COX-1
Anthranilic acid				
Mefenamic acid	2-4	3-4	q 6 hr	NA
Sulfonanilides				
Nimesulide	1-3	2-5	q 12 hr	COX-2>>COX-1
Heteroaryl acetic acid				
Diclofenac	2-3	1-2	q 8-12 hr	COX-2>>COX-1
Ketorolac	0.5-1	5	q 4-6 hr	NA
Arylpropionic acid				
Ibuprofen	1-2	2	q 6-8 hr	COX-1>COX-2
Naproxen	2	14	q 12 hr	COX-1>COX-2
Ketoprofen	1-2	2	q 6-8 hr	NA
Enolic acid				
Piroxicam	3-5	45-50	qd	COX-1>COX-2
Meloxicam	5-10	15-20	qd	COX-2>COX-1
Alkanones				
Nabumetone	4-5	24	q 12-24 hr	COX-1=COX-2
Coxib				
Celecoxib	2-3	11	q 12-24 hr	COX-2>>COX-1
Etoricoxib	2-3	15-22	qd	COX-2>>>COX-1

NSAIDs tend to accumulate at sites of inflammation, potentially confounding the relationship between plasma concentrations and duration of the anti-inflammatory/analgesic effects. Some pharmacokinetic features of representative NSAIDs are listed in Table 50.1. Several traditional NSAIDs (e.g., ibuprofen and diclofenac) are characterized by very short half-lives (1-2 hours) that would hardly justify thrice- or twice-daily regimens of administration. To prolong duration of action, some of these older NSAIDs (e.g., diclofenac) have been developed with formulations and doses that achieve high-grade and sustained inhibition of COX-2 in the systemic circulation. Although this may improve clinical efficacy, it may also influence COX-2–dependent untoward effects, such as cardiovascular toxicity (see later). Some NSAIDs, such as sulindac and nabumetone, are administered as inactive prodrugs that are converted by the large intestine and/or the liver into active metabolites that are largely responsible for COX inhibition. Some of these redox reactions are reversible. Enterohepatic recycling of indomethacin and sulindac can occur and contribute to sustained plasma concentrations of the NSAID.[1]

The pharmacokinetics of most NSAIDs can be affected to some extent by liver disease, renal disease, or old age. NSAIDs should either be avoided or used with caution under these circumstances and daily dose adjusted accordingly.[1]

NSAIDs can modify the pharmacokinetics or pharmacodynamics of other drugs given concurrently, resulting in clinically important drug interactions (Table 50.2). Pharmacokinetic interactions are related to the capacity of NSAIDs to modify the metabolism (e.g., warfarin), protein binding (e.g., sulfonylurea hypoglycemic drugs), or renal excretion (e.g., lithium) of other drugs, often resulting in supratherapeutic plasma levels of the latter; the dosage of such agents may require adjustment to prevent toxicity.[1]

A pharmacodynamic interaction may occur between most NSAIDs and several classes of antihypertensive drugs. Reduced production of vasodilator PGI_2 in the renal cortex and of natriuretic PGE_2 in the medulla, as a consequence of COX-2 inhibition, results in vasoconstriction and sodium and water retention that, in turn, tend to elevate blood pressure, regardless of the mechanism of action of antihypertensive drugs.[1] This pharmacodynamic interaction has been described with most traditional NSAIDs (including acetaminophen)[6] and coxibs[3] but not with low-dose aspirin.[7]

The pharmacokinetic interaction between NSAIDs and warfarin that may result in supratherapeutic plasma concentrations of the latter, because of its displacement from plasma protein binding and reduced metabolism, is further complicated by the fact that NSAIDs may transiently inhibit platelet function in some patients, thus amplifying the impairment of primary hemostasis induced by warfarin.

Some NSAIDs favoring COX-1 versus COX-2 inhibition, such as ibuprofen and naproxen (see Fig. 50.2), may interfere with the antiplatelet effect of low-dose aspirin by competing with acetylsalicylic acid for a common docking site (arginine-120) within the COX-1 channel.[8] Prior occupancy of Arg-120 by an NSAID will prevent aspirin from

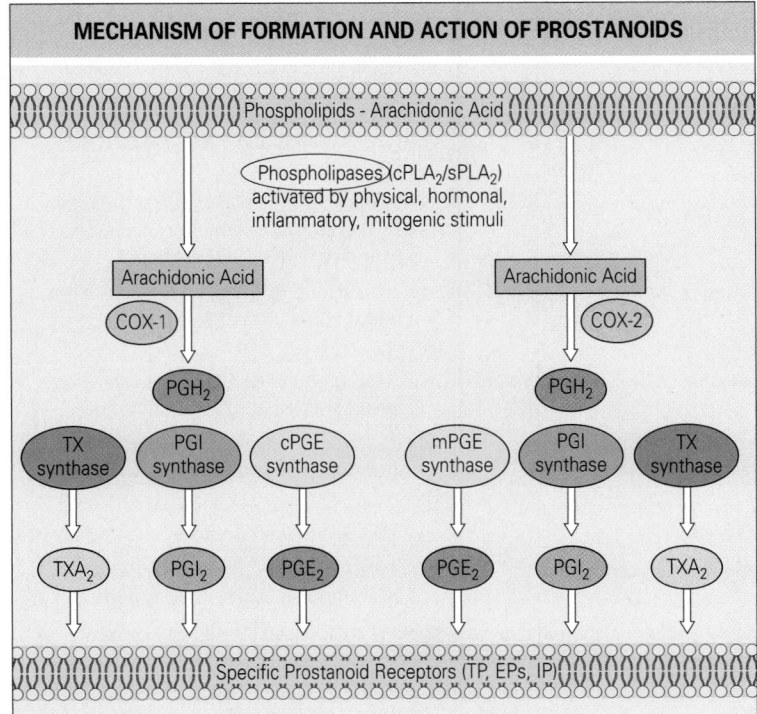

MECHANISM OF FORMATION AND ACTION OF PROSTANOIDS

Fig. 50.1 Mechanism of formation and action of prostanoids. Arachidonic acid, a 20-carbon fatty acid containing four double bonds, is liberated from the sn2 position in membrane phospholipids by phospholipases, which are activated by diverse stimuli. Arachidonic acid is converted by cytosolic prostaglandin (PG) G/H synthases, which have both cyclooxygenase (COX) and hydroperoxidase activity, to the unstable intermediate PGH_2. The synthases are colloquially termed *cyclooxygenases* and exist in two forms: COX-1 and COX-2. PGH_2 is converted by tissue-specific isomerases to multiple prostanoids. These bioactive lipids activate specific cell membrane receptors of the superfamily of G protein–coupled receptors.

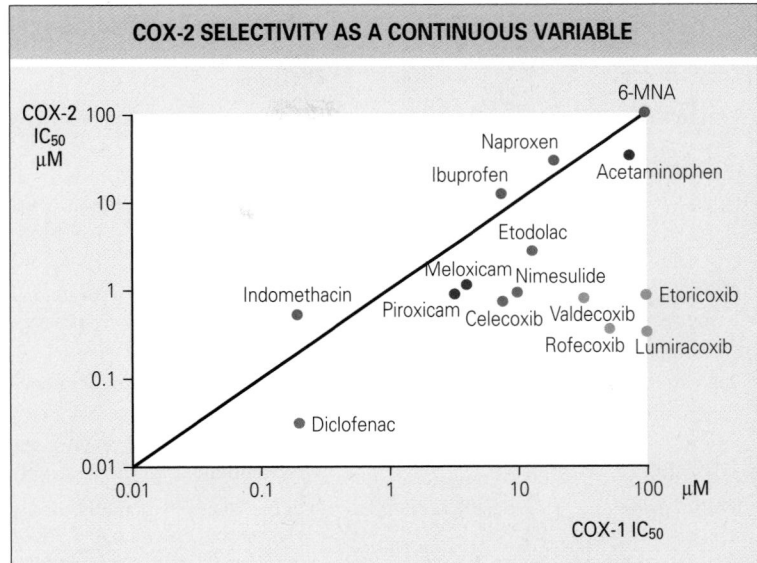

COX-2 SELECTIVITY AS A CONTINUOUS VARIABLE

Fig. 50.2 COX-2 selectivity as a continuous variable. Concentrations of various COX-2 inhibitors to inhibit the activity of platelet COX-1 and monocyte COX-2 by 50% (IC_{50}) are plotted on the abscissa and ordinate scales, respectively. The solid line describes equipotent inhibition of both COX-1 and COX-2. Symbols to the left of this line denote greater inhibition of COX-1 than COX-2. Symbols to the right of this line indicate progressively greater inhibition of COX-2 than COX-1, that is, increasing degrees of COX-2 selectivity. 6-MNA denotes 6-methoxy-2-naphthylacetic acid, the active metabolite of nabumetone. *(Data from references 3 and 27.)*

acetylating a serine residue (Ser-529) just below the COX catalytic site of the enzyme, which forms the basis of the unique mechanism of action of aspirin, resulting in permanent inactivation of platelet COX-1.[7] Drugs favoring COX-2 versus COX-1 inhibition, such as acetaminophen and diclofenac, do not interfere with the pharmacodynamic effect of low-dose aspirin, similar to celecoxib and rofecoxib (Fig. 50.3).[8] Based on current analysis of available data, the U.S. Food and Drug Administration (FDA) has issued a statement informing patients and health care professionals that ibuprofen can interfere with the antiplatelet effect of low-dose aspirin (81 mg/day), potentially rendering aspirin less effective when used for cardioprotection and stroke prevention (http://www.fda.gov/cder/drug/infopage/ibuprofen/default.htm).

Low-dose aspirin can cause upper gastrointestinal bleeding.[7] In two large outcome trials, subgroup analyses suggested that aspirin may attenuate the gastrointestinal safety of coxibs as compared with traditional NSAIDs.[9,10]

CLINICAL EFFICACY

NSAIDs are most widely used as analgesic and anti-inflammatory agents in the management of osteoarthritis, rheumatoid arthritis, and ankylosing spondylitis. The clinical efficacy of these drugs is related to symptomatic relief of pain and inflammation associated with these musculoskeletal disorders. However, NSAIDs are not disease-modifying agents and do not arrest the progression of tissue injury.[1]

The results of phase 3 efficacy studies in osteoarthritis, rheumatoid arthritis, and various models of acute pain have established that the analgesic and anti-inflammatory effects of coxibs are indistinguishable from those of several NSAID comparators (often, diclofenac, ibuprofen, or naproxen), consistently with similar COX-2 inhibition at comparable doses.[3]

Potential variables contributing to different COX-2–dependent effects include the daily dose of the inhibitor determining the extent of COX-2 inhibition; the half-life and dosing interval of the inhibitor determining the duration of COX-2 inhibition; and the patient's substrate, inasmuch as the importance of COX-2 dependent prostanoids is likely to vary in different clinical settings.[3]

NSAIDs are particularly effective when inflammation has caused sensitization of pain receptors to normally painless mechanical or chemical stimuli. Pain that accompanies inflammation and tissue injury probably results from local stimulation of pain fibers and enhanced pain sensitivity (hyperalgesia), in part as a consequence of increased excitability of central neurons in the spinal cord.[1]

The choice among different NSAIDs for the treatment of osteoarthritis and rheumatoid arthritis remains largely empirical, based on efficacy, but may be rationally guided by safety considerations (see later). Substantial differences in clinical response have been noted among individuals treated with the same NSAID and within an individual treated with different NSAIDs. This may be related to the quite substantial interindividual variability in the pharmacokinetic/pharmacodynamic relationship, as noted earlier.

If the patient does not achieve therapeutic benefit from a 2-week trial with one particular NSAID, another should be tried. There is no scientific rationale for combination therapy with more than one NSAID, and the risk of adverse effects is at least additive.

ADVERSE EFFECTS

Shared adverse effects of NSAID therapy are listed in Table 50.3. The list includes minor symptomatic disturbances as well as serious and life-threatening complications. The latter represent a growing safety concern, particularly in elderly patients, because age is associated with an increased probability of developing serious adverse reactions to NSAIDs.[11] When assessing clinically relevant outcomes of NSAID therapy, one should consider the variable incidence rate of these outcomes in the general population (Table 50.4). No placebo-controlled trials of adequate size and duration have been performed with traditional NSAIDs to evaluate reliably the excess of these serious outcomes attributable to NSAID therapy. Thus, we have to rely almost entirely on the results of observational studies that give a quantitative assessment of the risk of important outcomes (see Table 50.4). If the associations found in epidemiologic studies were causal, then approximately 300 upper gastrointestinal bleeding or perforation events, a similar

TABLE 50.2 INTERACTIONS BETWEEN NSAIDs AND OTHER DRUGS

Drug affected	NSAID implicated	Effect	Approach to management
Oral anticoagulants	Phenylbutazone Oxyphenbutazone Azapropazone	Inhibition of metabolism of S-warfarin, increasing anticoagulant effect	Avoid NSAIDs if possible. Use careful monitoring when use is unavoidable.
Lithium	Probably all NSAIDs	Inhibition of renal excretion of lithium, increasing lithium serum concentrations, and risk of toxicity	Use sulindac or aspirin if NSAID unavoidable. Careful monitoring of lithium concentration and appropriate dose reduction
Oral hypoglycemic agents	Phenylbutazone Oxyphenbutazone Azapropazone	Inhibition of metabolism of sulfonylurea drugs, prolonging half-life and increasing risk of hypoglycemia	Avoid this group of NSAIDs if possible; if not, monitor blood glucose level closely.
Phenytoin	Phenylbutazone Oxyphenbutazone	Inhibition of metabolism of phenytoin, increasing plasma concentration, and risk of toxicity	Avoid this group of NSAIDs if possible; if not, intensify therapeutic drug monitoring.
	Other NSAIDs	Displacement of phenytoin from plasma protein, reducing total concentrations for the same unbound (active) concentration	Avoid aspirin; closely monitor plasma concentration if other NSAID is used.
Methotrexate	Probably all NSAIDs	Reduced clearance of methotrexate (mechanism unclear) increasing plasma concentration and risk of severe toxicity	This is only relevant to high-dose methotrexate used in cancer chemotherapy.
Sodium valproate	Aspirin	Inhibition of valproate metabolism, increasing plasma concentration	Avoid aspirin; closely monitor plasma concentration if other NSAID is used.
Digoxin	All NSAIDs	Potential reduction in renal function (particularly in very young and very old) reducing digoxin clearance and increasing plasma concentration	Avoid NSAIDs if possible; if not, perform frequent checks of digoxin plasma concentration and plasma creatinine level.
Aminoglycosides	All NSAIDs	Reduction in renal function in susceptible individuals, reducing aminoglycoside clearance and increasing plasma concentration	Close plasma concentration monitoring and dose adjustment
Antihypertensive agents: β-blockers, diuretics ACE inhibitors, vasodilators	Indomethacin Other NSAIDs	Reduction in hypotensive effect, probably related to inhibition of renal prostaglandin synthesis (producing salt and water retention) and vascular prostaglandin synthesis (producing increased vasoconstriction)	Avoid all NSAIDs in patients with cardiac failure; monitor clinical signs of fluid retention.
Diuretics	Indomethacin Other NSAIDs	Reduction in natriuretic and diuretic effects; may exacerbate congestive cardiac failure	Avoid NSAIDs in patients with cardiac failure; monitor clinical signs of fluid retention.
Anticoagulants	All NSAIDs	Gastrointestinal tract mucosal damage, together with inhibition of platelet aggregation, increasing risk of gastrointestinal bleeding in patients on anticoagulants	Avoid all NSAIDs if possible.
Low-dose aspirin	Ibuprofen and naproxen	Prevention of irreversible inactivation of platelet COX-1	Use NSAIDs with some degree of COX-2 selectivity

ACE, angiotensin-converting enzyme.

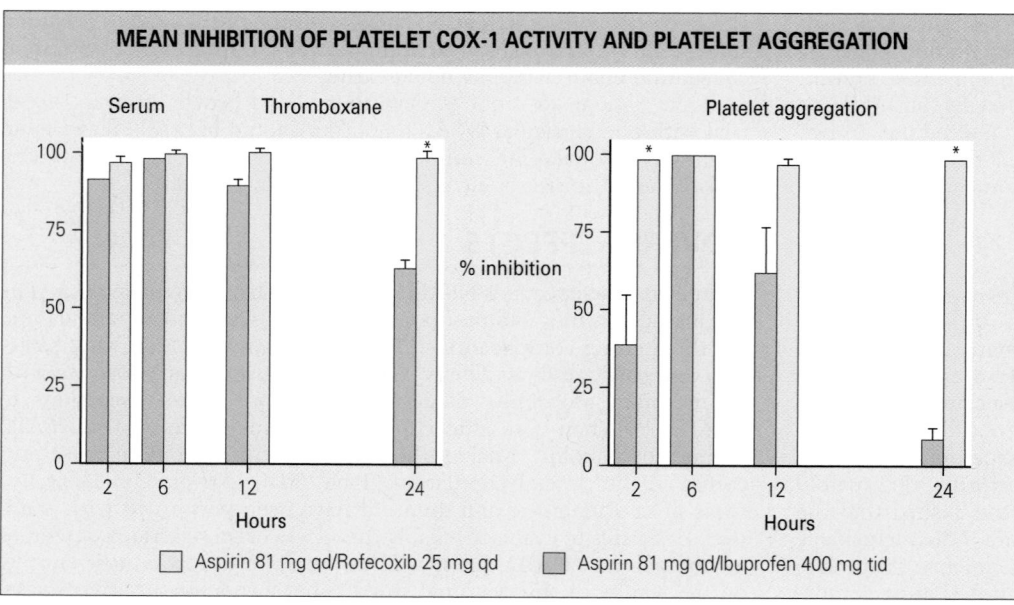

MEAN INHIBITION OF PLATELET COX-1 ACTIVITY AND PLATELET AGGREGATION

Serum   Thromboxane

Platelet aggregation

% inhibition

Hours

Hours

☐ Aspirin 81 mg qd/Rofecoxib 25 mg qd   ▨ Aspirin 81 mg qd/Ibuprofen 400 mg tid

Fig. 50.3 Mean inhibition of platelet COX-1 activity (left panel) and platelet aggregation (right panel) in healthy subjects taking enteric-coated aspirin (81 mg) 2 hours before either ibuprofen (400 mg tid) or rofecoxib (25 mg qd) on day 6 of daily dosing. *(Adapted from Catella-Lawson F, Reilly MP, Kapoor SC, et al. Cyclooxygenase inhibitors and the antiplatelet effects of aspirin. N Engl J Med 2001;345:1809-1817.)*

TABLE 50.3 SHARED SIDE-EFFECTS OF NSAIDs

System	Manifestations
Gastrointestinal	Abdominal pain Nausea Anorexia Erosions/ulcers in small and large bowel Anemia Gastrointestinal hemorrhage and perforation Diarrhea
Renal	Salt and water retention Edema, worsening of renal function in renal/cardiac and cirrhotic patients Acute renal failure Hyperkalemia
Central nervous system	Headache Vertigo Dizziness Confusion Depression Lowering of seizure threshold
Blood platelets	Inhibited platelet activation Propensity for bruising Increased risk of hemorrhage
Uterus	Prolongation of gestation Inhibition of labor
Hypersensitivity	Vasomotor rhinitis Angioneurotic edema Asthma Flushing Hypotension Shock
Cardiovascular	Closure of ductus arteriosus Precipitation or worsening of heart failure Myocardial infarction Hemorrhagic stroke
Liver	Transient rise in enzymes Cholestasis Acute liver injury
Skin	Photosensitivity Erythema multiforme Urticaria Toxic epidermal necrolysis

TABLE 50.4 INCIDENCE RATES OF MAJOR EVENTS POSSIBLY CAUSED BY TRADITIONAL NSAIDs, AS ASSESSED IN OBSERVATIONAL STUDIES IN THE GENERAL POPULATION

Event	Incidence rate per 1000 patient-years	Increased risk	Hospitalizations per 100,000 NSAID users
Heart failure	2-4	2-fold	300
Myocardial infarction	1-4	2-fold	300
Upper gastrointestinal bleeding	0.6-1.7	4-fold	300
Acute renal failure	0.02-0.08	2-4-fold	4-8
Acute liver injury	0.02-0.04	2-fold	5

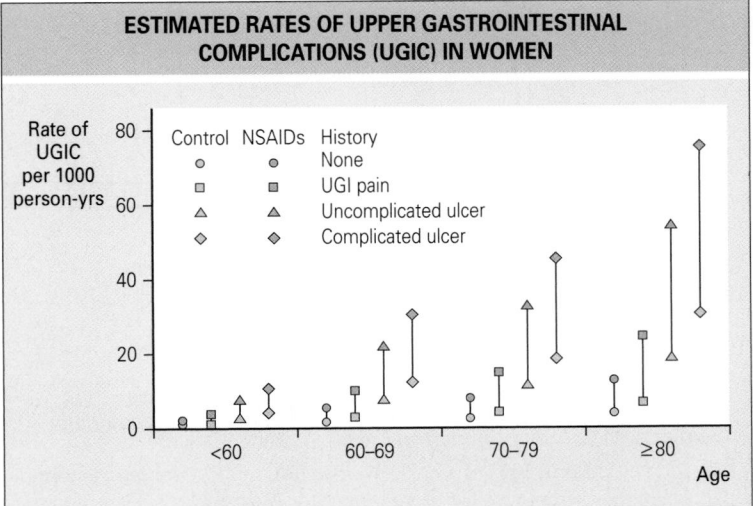

ESTIMATED RATES OF UPPER GASTROINTESTINAL COMPLICATIONS (UGIC) IN WOMEN

Fig. 50.4 Estimated rates of upper gastrointestinal complications (UGIC) in women, according to age and the presence or absence of a history of such complications and regular use of traditional NSAIDS. The solid lines connecting each pair of blue and red symbols depict the excess risk of complications related to NSAID therapy. *(Data from Hernandez-Díaz S, García Rodríguez LA. Epidemiologic assessment of the safety of conventional nonsteroidal anti-inflammatory drugs. Am J Med 2001;110[Suppl]:20S-27S and from unpublished results of S. Hernández-Díaz and L.A. García Rodríguez.)*

number of hospitalizations for congestive heart failure and nonfatal myocardial infarction, five acute liver injuries, and four to eight hospitalizations for acute renal failure per 100,000 persons per year would be attributable to NSAID therapy.[11]

Gastrointestinal

The most common symptoms associated with NSAID therapy are gastrointestinal, including nausea, abdominal pain, and diarrhea. These symptoms do not necessarily reflect NSAID-induced mucosal lesions or ulcers, because they commonly occur in placebo-treated patients. Gastroduodenal ulcers, as assessed by endoscopy, are detectable in 30% to 50% of NSAID-treated patients and develop in a dose- and time-dependent fashion. However, less than 10% of NSAID-treated patients have symptomatic ulcers, thus emphasizing the poor correlation between upper gastrointestinal symptoms and lesions. Gastroduodenal ulcers may be single or multiple and can be accompanied by gradual blood loss, leading to anemia, or by life-threatening bleeding. The risk of NSAID-induced ulceration is increased in patients infected with *Helicobacter pylori,* heavy alcohol drinkers, or those taking concomitant low-dose aspirin, clopidogrel, warfarin, or glucocorticoids.[1]

Coxibs have been shown to be associated with a lower incidence of endoscopic gastroduodenal ulcers than equally effective doses of traditional NSAIDs.[3] Prophylaxis with a proton pump inhibitor, such as

omeprazole, or a prostaglandin analog, such as misoprostol, has been shown to reduce the risk of NSAID-induced endoscopic ulcers.[1]

Upper gastrointestinal complications (hemorrhages, perforations, and obstructions) occur in 1% to 2% of NSAID-treated patients. The mortality rate associated with hospitalization due to major gastrointestinal events is 5% to 6% in recent studies.[12] Mortality rates associated with upper or lower gastrointestinal complications due to NSAIDs are similar.[12] The major risk factors for upper gastrointestinal bleeding are represented by age and a prior history of gastrointestinal disorders (Fig. 50.4).[11] Male gender, cigarette smoking, and heavy alcohol intake increase this risk by less than twofold, as do oral glucocorticoids. Oral anticoagulants, thienopyridines, and low-dose aspirin increase the risk of NSAID-induced bleeding complications by twofold to threefold.[11] The excess of these complications due to traditional NSAIDs has been estimated to range between 3 and 30 events per 1000 patients treated per year,[11] depending on the absence or presence of risk factors.

Because of the low event rate of ulcer complications, very large sample sizes or prolonged drug exposure is needed to detect differences between drugs. Four large (8000-35,000 patients) randomized trials of 6 to 18 months' treatment have compared the gastrointestinal safety of coxibs with traditional NSAIDs: CLASS[9] (celecoxib vs. ibuprofen and diclofenac), VIGOR[13] (rofecoxib vs. naproxen), TARGET[10] (lumiracoxib vs. ibuprofen and naproxen), and MEDAL[14] (etoricoxib vs. diclofenac). The main characteristics of the 69,000 patients enrolled in these studies are detailed in Table 50.5. The rate of ulcer complications

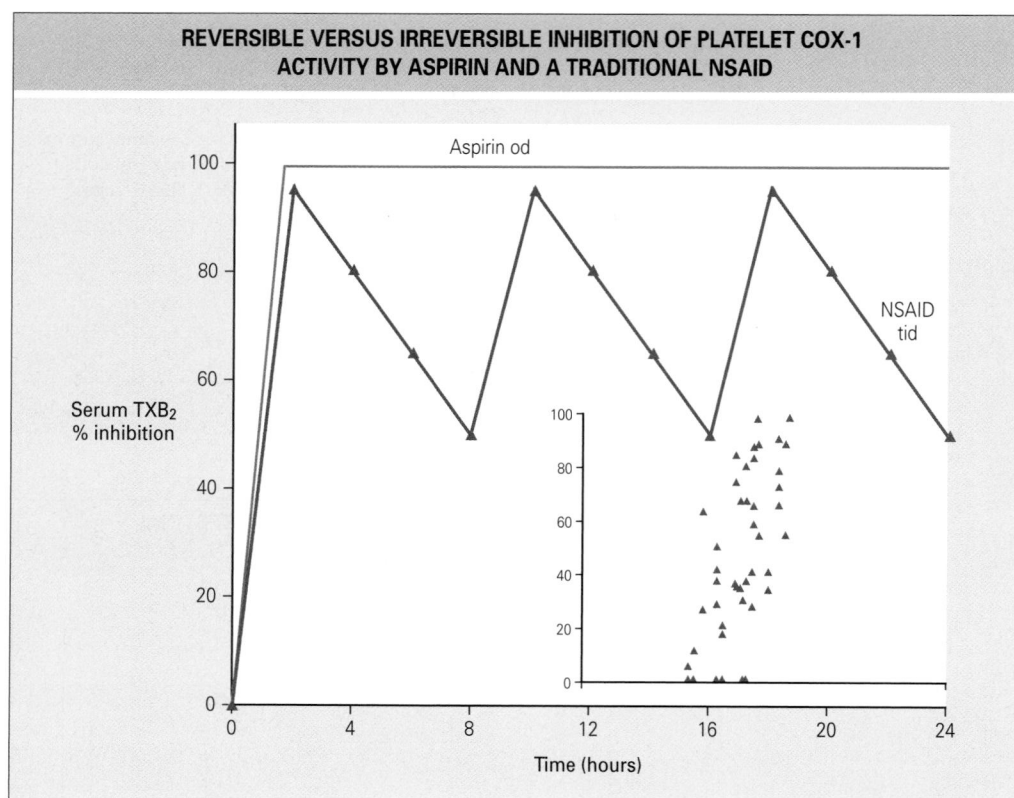

REVERSIBLE VERSUS IRREVERSIBLE INHIBITION OF PLATELET COX-1 ACTIVITY BY ASPIRIN AND A TRADITIONAL NSAID

Fig. 50.5 Reversible vs. irreversible inhibition of platelet COX-1 activity by aspirin and a traditional NSAID, respectively. The average time course of inhibition of serum TXB_2, an *ex-vivo* index of platelet COX-1 activity, is depicted over 24 hours after the administration of low-dose aspirin once daily and a traditional NSAID with short half-life given every 8 hours. The inset depicts the interindividual variability in the relationship between NSAID plasma levels plotted on the abscissa log scale and the corresponding level of inhibition of platelet COX-1 plotted on the ordinate. Only 2 of 44 individual blood samples achieved greater than 95% inhibition of platelet COX-1 activity.

Trial	Mean age (yr)	Women (%)	Prior gastrointestinal history (%)	Aspirin use (%)	NSAID UGIC rates per 1000 patient-years
CLASS	60	69	9.6	20	15
VIGOR	58	80	7.8	0	14
TARGET	63	76	0	24	9.1
MEDAL	63	74	7	35	4.7

TABLE 50.5 BASELINE CHARACTERISTICS OF OA/RA PATIENTS AND RATES OF ULCER COMPLICATIONS ASSOCIATED WITH 6- to 12-MONTH TREATMENT WITH NSAIDs IN COXIB GASTROINTESTINAL OUTCOME TRIALS

UGIC, upper gastrointestinal complications.

associated with traditional NSAIDs in these trials ranged between 5 and 15 per 1000. As can be appreciated in Figure 50.4, these values are consistent with the rates of upper gastrointestinal complications predicted by an analysis of epidemiologic data for a comparable low-risk population (i.e., women aged 60 with largely negative prior gastrointestinal history).[11] Both in VIGOR and TARGET, a highly selective COX-2 inhibitor was associated with a statistically significant 50% to 66% relative risk reduction in ulcer complications as compared with naproxen or ibuprofen.[10,13]

When contrasting the options of using a highly selective COX-2 inhibitor or a traditional NSAID plus a proton pump inhibitor, the following points should be borne in mind:

1. In contrast to coxibs, proton pump inhibitors have not been demonstrated to reduce the risk of NSAID-induced ulcer complications in adequately sized randomized trials.
2. Whereas coxibs have been shown to reduce the risk of both upper and lower gastrointestinal events, proton pump inhibitors would not be expected to protect against the latter.

Finally, it should be emphasized that any COX-2 inhibitor may eventually inhibit COX-1 in some patients (because of interindividual variability in pharmacokinetics and/or pharmacodynamics) and that there may be untoward COX-2–dependent effects (e.g., interference with ulcer healing) that are shared by all COX-2 inhibitors regardless of selectivity.

Cardiovascular

Persistent (throughout the dosing interval and beyond) and virtually complete (i.e., greater than 97%) inhibition of platelet COX-1 by any commercially available dose of aspirin is associated with a 20% to 30% reduction in major vascular events (non-fatal myocardial infarction, non-fatal stroke, or vascular death), as demonstrated by over 50 placebo-controlled randomized trials in approximately 100,000 subjects at high cardiovascular risk.[7] Traditional NSAIDs have long been thought to pose no cardiovascular hazard or to be somewhat cardio-protective, in the absence of any randomized study supporting this widely held assumption. Because of their reversible mechanism of action in inhibiting platelet COX-1 and their short half-lives (see Table 50.1), most traditional NSAIDs inhibit TXA_2-dependent platelet activation only transiently and incompletely in the vast majority of users (Fig. 50.5). A notable exception is provided by naproxen, which has been shown to inhibit TXA_2 biosynthesis *in vivo* to the same extent as low-dose aspirin, when administered regularly at 500 mg twice daily,[15] consistent with its relative COX-1 selectivity and longer half-life than other commonly used NSAIDs.

Three placebo-controlled trials have now revealed a twofold to three-fold increased risk of vascular events in approximately 6000 patients treated short term (10 days) with valdecoxib[16] or long term (up to 3 years) with celecoxib[17] or rofecoxib,[18] both with and without concomitant aspirin treatment. These findings are consistent with a mechanism-based cardiovascular hazard for the class.[19] In fact, coxibs

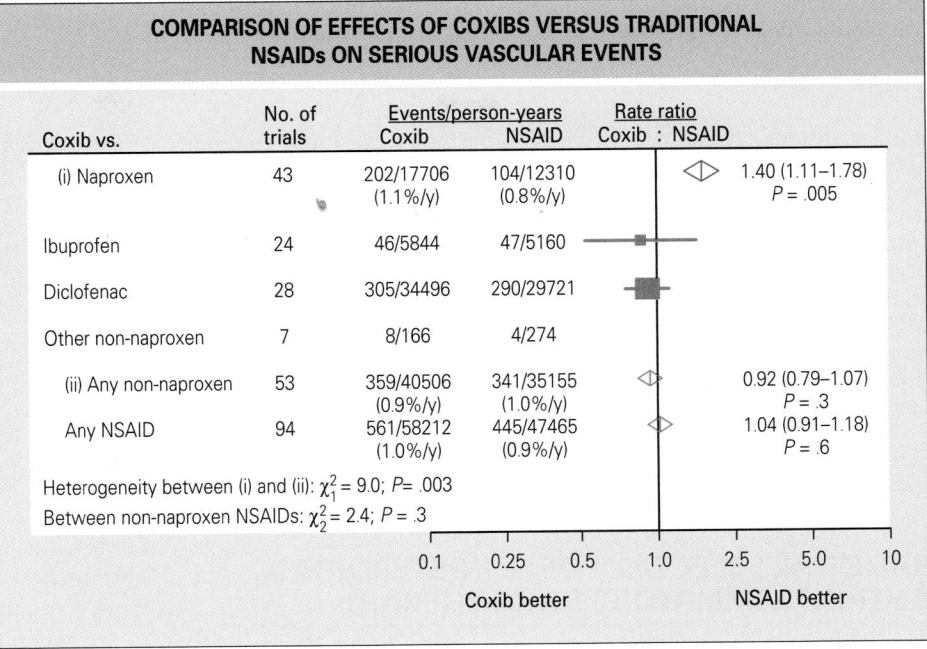

COMPARISON OF EFFECTS OF COXIBS VERSUS TRADITIONAL NSAIDs ON SERIOUS VASCULAR EVENTS

Coxib vs.	No. of trials	Events/person-years Coxib	Events/person-years NSAID	Rate ratio Coxib : NSAID	
(i) Naproxen	43	202/17706 (1.1%/y)	104/12310 (0.8%/y)	◇	1.40 (1.11–1.78) P = .005
Ibuprofen	24	46/5844	47/5160	■	
Diclofenac	28	305/34496	290/29721	■	
Other non-naproxen	7	8/166	4/274		
(ii) Any non-naproxen	53	359/40506 (0.9%/y)	341/35155 (1.0%/y)	◁	0.92 (0.79–1.07) P = .3
Any NSAID	94	561/58212 (1.0%/y)	445/47465 (0.9%/y)	◇	1.04 (0.91–1.18) P = .6

Heterogeneity between (i) and (ii): $\chi^2_1 = 9.0$; $P = .003$
Between non-naproxen NSAIDs: $\chi^2_2 = 2.4$; $P = .3$

0.1   0.25   0.5   1.0   2.5   5.0   10

Coxib better   NSAID better

Fig. 50.6 Comparison of effects of coxibs versus traditional NSAIDs on serious vascular events. Event numbers and person-years of exposure, with corresponding mean annual event rates in parenthesis, are presented for patients allocated to coxib and NSAID. Event rate ratios, with 95% confidence intervals, are indicated by a diamond; rate ratios for individual non-naproxen NSAIDs, with 99% confidence intervals, are indicated by a square and horizontal line. Diamonds to the right of the solid line indicate hazard with coxib compared with NSAID, but this is conventionally significant only if the diamond does not overlap the solid line. (Adapted from Patrono C, Baigent C. Low-dose aspirin, coxibs, and other NSAIDs: a clinical mosaic emerges. Mol Interv 2009;9:31-39.).

depress atheroprotective PGI_2 formation *in vivo* without concomitant inhibition of platelet activation.[20] A meta-analysis of tabular data from 138 randomized trials of five different coxibs in approximately 145,000 patients has revealed that, in placebo comparisons, allocation to a coxib was associated with a 42% increased incidence of vascular events with no statistically significant heterogeneity among the different coxibs.[21] This excess risk of vascular events was derived primarily from a twofold increased risk of myocardial infarction. Overall, there was no significant difference in the incidence of vascular events between a coxib and any traditional NSAID, but there was evidence of a significant heterogeneity between naproxen and the other traditional NSAIDs (largely represented by ibuprofen and diclofenac).[21] The apparent lack of a significant difference in the rate of vascular events between patients treated with any coxib and those treated with non-naproxen NSAIDs, as reported in this meta-analysis, is confirmed by the cardiovascular findings of the MEDAL program.[22] In this prespecified pooled analysis of data from three trials in 34,701 patients with osteoarthritis or rheumatoid arthritis, treated on average for 18 months, the hazard ratio for thrombotic cardiovascular events was 0.95 (95% confidence interval, 0.81-1.11) for etoricoxib compared with diclofenac. The results of an updated meta-analysis of coxib trials[23] that includes the MEDAL[22] and ADAPT[24] studies confirm the statistical heterogeneity between coxib versus naproxen and coxib versus non-naproxen NSAID comparisons (Fig. 50.6).

Given the non-linear relationship between inhibition of platelet COX-1 activity and inhibition of platelet activation *in vivo*,[25] it is perhaps not surprising that the cardiovascular safety profiles of coxibs and some non-naproxen NSAIDs appear similar, because they both fail to inhibit platelet activation adequately irrespective of their COX-2 selectivity. Whether the variable level and duration of COX-1 inhibition by different NSAIDs modulate the cardiovascular consequences of COX-2 inhibition is presently unknown, given the limited utilization of NSAIDs other than ibuprofen, diclofenac, and naproxen in coxib trials.

Thus, coxibs and some traditional NSAIDs moderately increase the risk of vascular events, particularly myocardial infarction, but there remains considerable uncertainty about the magnitude of this hazard for particular drug regimens and patient subgroups. Although early appearance,[26] dose dependence,[27] and slow dissipation[26] of risk appear as important features of COX-2-related cardiotoxicity, additional data are required to properly assess the relative contribution of these factors.[23]

Use of NSAIDs can lead to the development of congestive heart failure in susceptible individuals.[28] Based on epidemiologic studies,[11,28] current users of NSAIDs are estimated to have a twofold increase in risk of hospitalization for congestive heart failure. The effect is greater among patients with preexisting heart disease. The risk appears to be dose dependent and somewhat higher during the first month of therapy.[11,28]

Renal

Both traditional NSAIDs and coxibs have been associated with renal and renovascular adverse events, consistently with the important role of constitutively expressed COX-2 in sustaining the physiologic production of vasodilator and natriuretic prostanoids in the human kidney.[1,3]

COX-2 inhibitors have little effect on renal function or blood pressure control in healthy subjects. However, in patients with chronic glomerular disease, hepatic cirrhosis, congestive heart failure, hypovolemia, and other states of activation of the sympathoadrenal or renin-angiotensin systems, maintenance of renal blood flow and glomerular filtration rate is critically dependent on renal prostaglandin synthesis.[1,3]

Some studies evaluating the risk of chronic renal conditions (e.g., analgesic nephropathy) associated with traditional NSAIDs, including aspirin and acetaminophen, have found that NSAID users have a twofold increase in the risk of these conditions. The risk increases with age and is related to dose and duration of NSAID intake.[11,29]

The incidence rate of hospitalization for acute renal failure among non-users is approximately 2 per 100,000 persons per year. Current users of NSAIDs are estimated to experience a twofold to fourfold increase in the risk of hospitalization for acute renal failure. The risk is dose dependent and is considerably higher during the first month of therapy.[11,29]

Other risk factors for acute renal failure are male gender, increasing age, cardiovascular co-morbidity, renal diseases, concomitant use of other nephrotoxic drugs, and recent hospitalization for disorders other than renal disease.[11,29]

Respiratory

Asthma is most common with salicylates but may be precipitated or exacerbated by NSAIDs. Symptoms may be mild or severe, and fatal attacks of bronchospasm have been precipitated by a single dose of NSAID. If aspirin-sensitive asthmatic patients require an NSAID, then a low dose should be administered in a controlled environment equipped with facilities to reverse bronchospasm. Pulmonary alveolitis has also been reported with NSAID therapy and, although rare, should be considered when an illness suggestive of pulmonary infection but failing to respond to antibiotic therapy develops in a patient on an

NSAID. Limited data suggest that coxibs can be used safely in asthmatics. Non-acetylated salicylates are often used in this situation.

Liver

Both traditional NSAIDs and coxibs are among the most common agents associated with drug-induced liver injury, ranging from asymptomatic elevations in aminotransferase levels to serious liver injury with acute hepatic failure. Observational studies have reported nimesulide, sulindac, and diclofenac to be associated with the highest risk of liver injury, and the only risk factor consistently identified in these analyses is the concomitant use of other hepatotoxic drugs.[11,30] In the MEDAL program,[22] diclofenac caused elevations of aminotransferase levels more frequently than etoricoxib, generally during the first 4 to 6 months of therapy, although clinical liver events requiring hospitalization were relatively rare.

Nimesulide has been withdrawn in Finland and Spain, because of hepatotoxicity, while it continues to be the most prescribed NSAID in Italy and Portugal.

RATIONAL SELECTION OF NON-STEROIDAL ANTI-INFLAMMATORY DRUG THERAPY

Patients with rheumatic disease show quite substantial interindividual variability in their response to NSAIDs. The therapeutic challenge in each case is to find the right NSAID and appropriate dosing regimen to provide an acceptable level of pain relief while minimizing the risk of serious adverse events.

Because gastrointestinal and cardiovascular adverse events contribute the largest share of NSAID-induced toxicity, careful consideration should be given to the assessment of risk factors for these complications in the individual patient.

Because of the nature of serious complications that could be caused or prevented by one particular NSAID versus another, patients' values and preferences should be considered in the choice of NSAID therapy. Moreover, patients should be adequately informed about the balance

TABLE 50.6 ELEMENTS OF A HETEROGENEOUS AND EVOLVING SCENARIO CONCERNING NSAID THERAPY IN USA AND EUROPE

Variable	USA	Europe
Marketing scenario	Celecoxib is the only marketed coxib. Some COX-2 selective NSAIDs (e.g., nimesulide) are not marketed.	Celecoxib and etoricoxib are marketed in most countries. Nimesulide is marketed in some countries, but has been withdrawn in others.
Regulatory scenario	Etoricoxib and lumiracoxib have not been approved. Celecoxib is not contraindicated in patients at high cardiovascular risk. Cardiovascular warning on celecoxib and all traditional NSAIDs, except aspirin.	Celecoxib and etoricoxib are contraindicated in patients at high cardiovascular risk. No such contraindication in the label of traditional NSAIDs

of benefits and risks to obtain their cooperation in achieving the following goals:

- Minimizing the level and duration of drug exposure
- Avoiding concomitant over-the-counter analgesic medications
- Complying with prescribed dietary, physical, and pharmacologic means to manage modifiable cardiovascular risk factors (i.e., cigarette smoking and higher than optimal blood pressure, cholesterol, and body weight)

In light of the heterogeneous regulatory and marketing environment in the United States versus Europe (Table 50.6), uniform treatment recommendations are difficult to make. Although some preferred treatment options have been suggested[31-34] according to the level of cardiovascular and gastrointestinal risk, these are largely based on expert opinion. Efforts should be made through a multidisciplinary consensus conference to provide evidence-based treatment guidelines on NSAID therapy.

REFERENCES

1. Burke A, Smyth E, FitzGerald GA. Analgesic-antipyretic and anti-inflammatory agents and drugs employed in the treatment of gout. In: Brunton LL, Lazo JS, Parker KL, eds. Goodman & Gilman's the pharmacological basis of therapeutics. New York: McGraw-Hill, 2006:673-715.
2. Smith WL, Langenbach R. Why there are two cyclooxygenase isozymes. J Clin Invest 2001;107:1491-1495.
3. FitzGerald GA, Patrono C. The coxibs, selective inhibitors of cyclooxygenase-2. N Engl J Med 2001;345:433-442.
4. Boutaud O, Aronoff DM, Richardson JH, et al. Determinants of the cellular specificity of acetaminophen as an inhibitor of prostaglandin H2 synthases. Proc Natl Acad Sci U S A 2002;99:7130-7135.
5. Hinz B, Cheremina O, Brune K. Acetaminophen (paracetamol) is a selective cyclooxygenase-2 inhibitor in man. FASEB J 2008;22:383-390.
6. Forman JP, Stampfer MJ, Curhan GC. Non-narcotic analgesic dose and risk of incident hypertension in US women. Hypertension 2005;46:500-507.
7. Patrono C, García Rodríguez LA, Landolfi R, Baigent C. Low-dose aspirin for the prevention of atherothrombosis. N Engl J Med 2005;353:2373-2383.
8. Catella-Lawson F, Reilly MP, Kapoor SC, et al. Cyclooxygenase inhibitors and the antiplatelet effects of aspirin. N Engl J Med 2001;345:1809-1817.
9. Silverstein FE, Faich G, Goldstein JL, et al. Gastrointestinal toxicity with celecoxib vs nonsteroidal anti-inflammatory drugs for osteoarthritis and rheumatoid arthritis. The CLASS Study: a randomized controlled trial. JAMA 2000;284:1247-1255.
10. Schnitzer TJ, Burmester GR, Mysler E, et al. Comparison of lumiracoxib with naproxen and ibuprofen in the Therapeutic Arthritis Research and Gastrointestinal Event Trial (TARGET), reduction in ulcer complications: randomised controlled trial. Lancet 2004;364:665-674.
11. Hernandez-Díaz S, García Rodríguez LA. Epidemiologic assessment of the safety of conventional nonsteroidal anti-inflammatory drugs. Am J Med 2001;110(Suppl):20S-27S.
12. Lanas A, Perez-Aisa MA, Feu F, et al. A nationwide study of mortality associated with hospital admission due to severe gastrointestinal events and those associated with nonsteroidal anti-inflammatory drug use. Am J Gastroenterol 2005;100:1685-1693.
13. Bombardier C, Laine L, Reicin A, et al. Comparison of upper gastrointestinal toxicity of rofecoxib and naproxen in patients with rheumatoid arthritis. VIGOR Study Group. N Engl J Med 2000;343:1520-1528.
14. Laine L, Curtis SP, Cryer B, et al, for the MEDAL Steering Committee. Assessment of upper gastrointestinal safety of etoricoxib and diclofenac in patients with osteoarthritis and rheumatoid arthritis in the Multinational Etoricoxib and Diclofenac Arthritis Long-term (MEDAL) programme: a randomised comparison. Lancet 2007;369:465-473.
15. Capone ML, Tacconelli S, Sciulli MG, et al. Clinical pharmacology of platelet, monocyte and vascular cyclooxygenase inhibition by naproxen and low-dose aspirin in healthy subjects. Circulation 2004;109:1468-1471.
16. Nussmeier NA, Whelton AA, Brown MT, et al. Complications of the COX-2 inhibitors parecoxib and valdecoxib after cardiac surgery. N Engl J Med 2005;352:1081-1091.
17. Solomon SD, McMurray JJ, Pfeffer MA, et al. Cardiovascular risk associated with celecoxib in a clinical trial for colorectal adenoma prevention. N Engl J Med 2005;352:1071-1080.
18. Bresalier RS, Sandler RS, Quan H, et al. Cardiovascular events associated with rofecoxib in a colorectal adenoma chemoprevention trial. N Engl J Med 2005;352:1092-1102.
19. Grosser T, Fries S, FitzGerald GA. Biological basis for the cardiovascular consequences of COX-2 inhibition: therapeutic challenges and opportunities. J Clin Invest 2006;116:4-15.
20. McAdam BF, Catella-Lawson F, Mardini IA, et al. Systemic biosynthesis of prostacyclin by cyclooxygenase (COX)-2: the human pharmacology of a selective inhibitor of COX-2. Proc Natl Acad Sci U S A 1999;96:272-277.
21. Kearney PM, Baigent C, Godwin J, et al. Do selective cyclooxygenase-2 inhibitors and traditional non-steroidal anti-inflammatory drugs increase the risk of atherothrombosis? Meta-analysis of randomised trials. BMJ 2006;332:1302-1308.
22. Cannon CP, Curtis SP, FitzGerald GA, et al. Cardiovascular outcomes with etoricoxib and diclofenac in patients with osteoarthritis and rheumatoid arthritis in the Multinational Etoricoxib and Diclofenac Arthritis Long-term (MEDAL) programme: a randomised comparison. Lancet 2006;368:1771-1781.
23. Patrono C, Baigent C. Low-dose aspirin, coxibs, and other NSAIDs: a clinical mosaic emerges. Mol Interv 2009;9:31-39.
24. ADAPT Research Group. Cardiovascular and cerebrovascular events in the randomized, controlled Alzheimer's Disease Anti-Inflammatory Prevention Trial (ADAPT). PLoS Clin Trials 2006;1:e33.
25. Santilli F, Rocca B, De Cristofaro R, et al. Platelet cyclooxygenase inhibition by low-dose aspirin is not reflected consistently by platelet function assays. J Am Coll Cardiol 2009;53:667-677.
26. Baron JA, Sandler RS, Bresalier RS, et al. Cardiovascular events associated with rofecoxib: final analysis of the APPROVe trial. Lancet 2008;372:1756-1764.
27. García Rodríguez LA, Tacconelli S, Patrignani P. Role of dose potency in the prediction of risk of myocardial infarction associated with nonsteroidal anti-inflammatory drugs in the general population. J Am Coll Cardiol 2008;52:1628-1636.
28. García Rodríguez LA, Hernández-Diaz S. Non-steroidal anti-inflammatory drugs as a trigger of clinical heart failure. Epidemiology 2003;14:240-246.
29. Huerta C, Castellsague J, Varas-Lorenzo C, García Rodríguez LA. Nonsteroidal anti-inflammatory drugs

and risk of ARF in the general population. Am J Kidney Dis 2005;45:531-539.

30. de Abajo FJ, Montero D, Madurga M, García Rodríguez LA. Acute and clinically relevant drug-induced liver injury: a population based case-control study. Br J Clin Pharmacol 2004;58:71-80.

31. Antman EM, Bennett JS, Daugherty A, et al. Use of nonsteroidal antiinflammatory drugs: an update for clinicians: a scientific statement from the American Heart Association. Circulation 2007;115:1634-1642.

32. Strand V. Are COX-2 inhibitors preferable to non-selective non-steroidal anti-inflammatory drugs in patients with risk of cardiovascular events taking low-dose aspirin? Lancet 2007;370:2138-2151.

33. American College of Rheumatology ad hoc group on use of selective and nonselective nonsteroidal antiinflammatory drugs. Recommendations for use of selective and nonselective nonsteroidal anti-inflammatory drugs: an American College of Rheumatology white paper. Arthritis Rheum 2008;59:1058-1073.

34. Chan FK, Abraham NS, Scheiman JM, Laine L; First International Working Party on Gastrointestinal and Cardiovascular Effects of Nonsteroidal Anti-inflammatory Drugs and Anti-platelet Agents. Management of patients on nonsteroidal anti-inflammatory drugs: a clinical practice recommendation from the First International Working Party on Gastrointestinal and Cardiovascular Effects of Nonsteroidal Anti-inflammatory Drugs and Anti-platelet Agents. Am J Gastroenterol 2008;103:2908-2918.

Systemic glucocorticoids in rheumatology

51

Kenneth G. Saag

- Glucocorticoids act via a number of pathways including inhibition of transcription factors NF-κb and AP-1.
- Glucocorticoids decrease synthesis of proinflammatory cytokines and proinflammatory enzymes, T-cell function, and Fc receptor expression.
- Short-term use of low-dose glucocorticoids in rheumatoid arthritis decreases clinical disease activity. These agents also have a beneficial effect on radiographic activity.
- Adverse events are common with these drugs, and many of the side effects are dose dependent. Careful titration of dose and strategies to minimize toxicity is essential when using glucocorticoids.

INTRODUCTION

Discovered more than 50 years ago, synthetic cortisone was first shown to be remarkably effective in relieving the inflammation associated with rheumatoid arthritis (RA).[1] This pioneering work by Hench, Kendall, and colleagues subsequently resulted in their award of a Nobel Prize in Medicine. Despite the advent of many disease-specific therapies, the use of synthetic glucocorticoids in rheumatology remains a common, albeit controversial, therapy for many inflammatory disorders.

NOMENCLATURE AND PHARMACOLOGY

Preparations and structure

The term *corticosteroid* is often used synonymously with glucocorticoid, although glucocorticoid is the preferred designation when using exogenous agents therapeutically because corticosteroids encompass both glucocorticoid and mineralocorticoid hormones.[2] A variety of synthetic glucocorticoid preparations are commercially available and have variable chemical structure (Fig. 51.1), potency, and half-life (Table 51.1). The 11β- and 17α-hydroxyl groups are important for glucocorticoid activity; and prednisone, a synthetic analog of cortisone, is also hydroxylated before becoming biologically active. The additional double bond in ring A of the resultant prednisolone enhances glucocorticoid activity without increasing mineralocorticoid activity, an effect that is increased by 6α-methylation (to produce methylprednisolone) or 9α-fluorination (triamcinolone) or both (dexamethasone). In rheumatology, the most commonly used oral glucocorticoids are prednisone and prednisolone whereas methylprednisolone is the predominant preparation used parenterally.

Dosing

Thresholds for low, medium, and high doses are not well defined. Some rheumatologists consider 10 mg/day of prednisone equivalent as the upper threshold of "low dose"; others use 7.5 mg/day,[3] which is actually somewhat above the daily endogenous production of cortisol (hydrocortisone) by the adrenal glands, which averages 5.7 mg/m^2/day.[4] A European Union League Against Rheumatism (EULAR) standing committee defined low dose as up to 7.5 mg/day, medium dose as greater than 7.5 but less than or equal to 30 mg/day, high dose as greater than 30 but less than or equal to 100 mg/day, and very high dose as greater than 100 mg/day prednisolone equivalent.[2] Dosing designations were considered based on the percent binding of the glucocorticoid receptors and the risk of perceived adverse effects. These dosing conventions will be used in this discussion.

Bioequivalence and bioavailability

The different preparations of glucocorticoids have the same rate of gastrointestinal absorption. Most commercially available prednisone tablets are bioequivalent, independent of tablet strength[5]; and the systemic bioavailability of prednisone and prednisolone are similar. Glucocorticoid bioavailability does not appear to be affected by pregnancy.

Metabolism and drug interactions

In contrast to endogenous cortisol, which is 80% bound, synthetic glucocorticoids bind poorly to cortisol-binding globulin (CBG, transcortin). Prednisolone has about 60%, prednisone has about 5%, and methylprednisolone, dexamethasone, betamethasone, and triamcinolone have less than 1% of the affinity of cortisol for CBG. Half-life ranges from about 1 hour for prednisone to more than 4 hours for dexamethasone. Prednisone is rapidly metabolized in the liver by CYP3A4 (a cytochrome P450 isoform) to prednisolone; the elimination of prednisone is approximately 13 times faster than prednisolone.[6] Hyperthyroidism and nephrotic syndrome increase clearance whereas aging and liver disease impair clearance. Prednisolone is preferred to prednisone in patients with significant hepatic dysfunction.

Enhancement of the rate of metabolism of some glucocorticoids has been noted with concurrent administration of phenobarbital, phenytoin, and rifampin (rifampicin). Concurrent use of aspirin and glucocorticoids concurrently decreases salicylate levels by causing an increased rate of salicylate metabolism.

Clearance and dose timing

The elimination half-life of prednisolone is approximately 3 hours.[7] Total prednisolone clearance increases by 75% as the intravenous dose increased from 5 to 40 mg.[8] Clearances also vary with the time of day. Both prednisolone and methylprednisolone clearance is up to 25% lower in the morning than in the evening.[9] This property, in combination with the disruption of the usual cortisol diurnal rhythm with exogenous glucocorticoids, results in variations in efficacy when glucocorticoids are administered at different times during the day.[10] Administration of short-acting glucocorticoids very early in the morning, in contrast to later in the day, better complements the normal diurnal variation in endogenous hormones and further blocks pro-inflammatory cytokine production such as IL-6[11] and inflammatory symptoms.[12] For example, a low-dose prednisone compound with a delayed-release mechanism (drug released 4 hours after ingestion) when taken in the evening reduced rheumatoid arthritis morning stiffness more than placebo at 12 weeks.[13] Timing of administration of the glucocorticoid dose also influences toxicity. For example, daily "split-dose" therapy is more immunosuppressive and should be used for shorter duration owing to its more profound disruption of the normal hypothalamic-pituitary-adrenal (HPA) axis function.

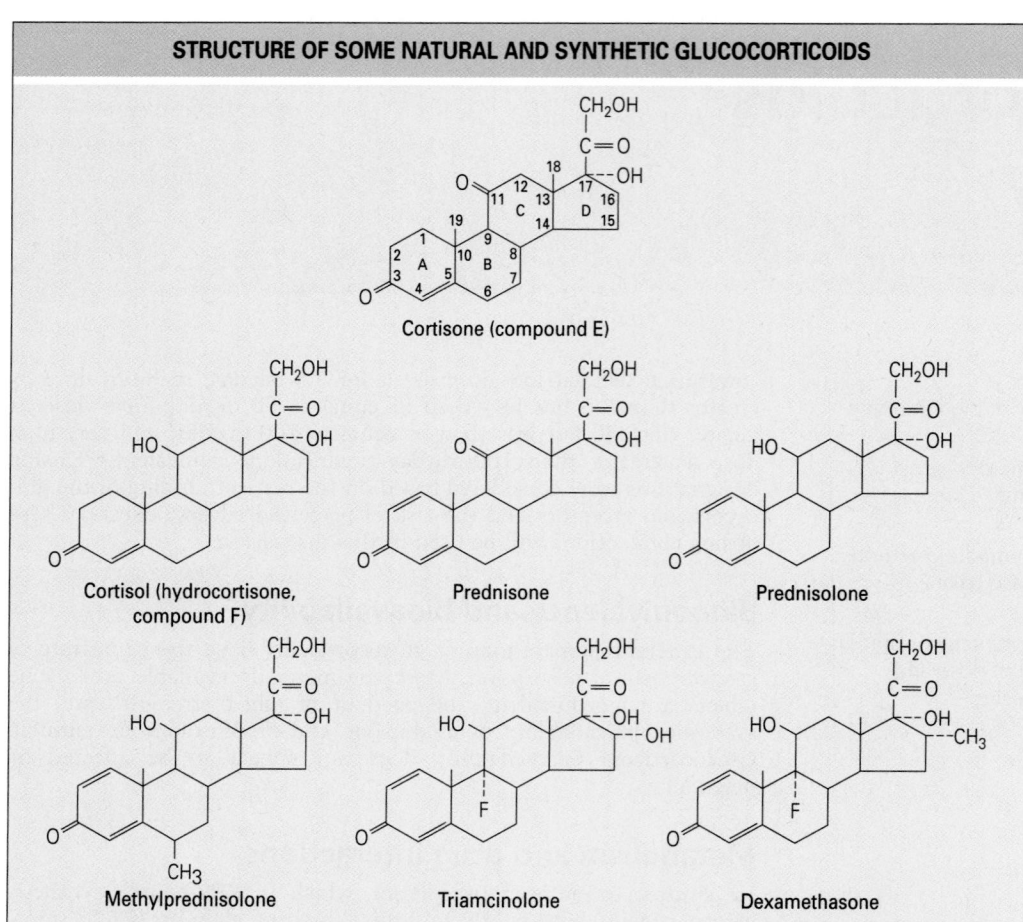

STRUCTURE OF SOME NATURAL AND SYNTHETIC GLUCOCORTICOIDS

Cortisone (compound E)

Cortisol (hydrocortisone, compound F)

Prednisone

Prednisolone

Methylprednisolone

Triamcinolone

Dexamethasone

Fig. 51.1 Structure of some natural and synthetic glucocorticoids.

TABLE 51.1 SOME COMMONLY USED GLUCOCORTICOIDS				
Glucocorticoid	Equivalent oral dose (mg)	Plasma half-life (mg)	Relative anti-inflammatory effect	Relative mineralocorticoid effect
Cortisol	20	90	1	1
Prednisolone	5	200	4	0.8
Methylprednisolone	4	200	5	0.5
Triamcinolone	4	200	5	0
Dexamethasone	0.75	300	25	0

MECHANISMS OF GLUCOCORTICOID ACTION

Glucocorticoids act as anti-inflammatory mediators via a number of pathways that continue to be further elucidated.[14-19] Oral glucocorticoids at doses less than 30 mg/day of prednisone equivalent circulate in the plasma and diffuse through the plasma membrane where they bind to the cytosolic glucocorticoid receptor, a 95-kDa phosphorylated protein. Diversity in the function of the glucocorticoid receptor is influenced by variations in genetic transcription mediated by alternate splice sites. The relative levels of either the α or β receptor influence the sensitivity or resistance of cells to glucocorticoids. Glucocorticoid resistance is reported in patients with severe RA and has been associated with higher levels of glucocorticoid receptor β, activation of mitogen-activated protein kinases (MAPKs) that inhibit glucocorticoid signaling, or antibodies to lipocortin-1.[20-23] Persons with glucocorticoid receptor polymorphisms have higher sensitivity to exogenously administered glucocorticoids.[24] Persons with relative glucocorticoid resistance may have diminished *in-vitro* response of their peripheral blood mononuclear cells to glucocorticoid stimulation.[25] Imbalances in the two isoforms of 11β-hydroxysteroid dehydrogenase may play a central role in glucocorticoid resistance.[26]

Glucocorticoids act on the cell through genomic and non-genomic ways in several ways (Fig. 51.2).[18]

- Heat-shock protein chaperones the glucocorticoid-glucocorticoid receptor complex to the nucleus where it binds reversibly and exerts potent effects on transcription via binding to positive and negative glucocorticoid response elements in promoter or suppressor sites of target genes.
- The glucocorticoid/glucocorticoid receptor complex inhibits transcription factors such as nuclear factor—κB (NF-κB) and activator protein-1 (AP-1). Most anti-inflammatory effects are believed to occur as a result of inhibited gene transcription via these effects on NF-κB (transrepression), whereas the adverse effects of glucocorticoids, such as metabolic side effects, are mediated in large part via activation of transcription of certain genes (transactivation) (Fig. 51.3).
- Glucocorticoid signaling occurs through membrane-associated receptors and second messengers (non-genomic pathways). At high glucocorticoid doses (>100 mg/day prednisolone equivalent), glucocorticoid receptors become saturated, and these non-genomic effects emerge. These are mediated by incorporation of glucocorticoid molecules into cell membranes.[16]

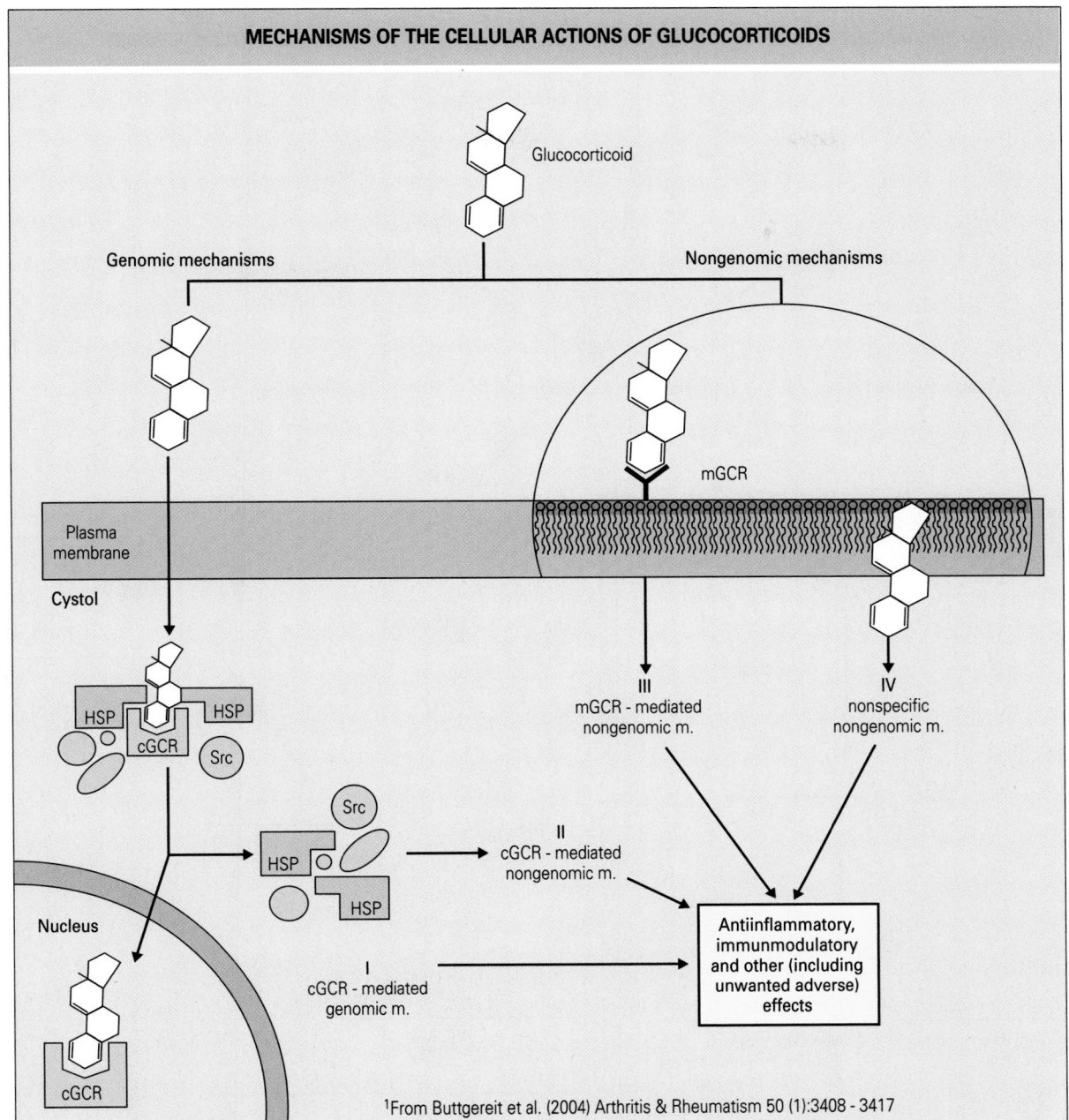

MECHANISMS OF THE CELLULAR ACTIONS OF GLUCOCORTICOIDS

[1]From Buttgereit et al. (2004) Arthritis & Rheumatism 50 (1):3408 - 3417

Fig. 51.2 Mechanisms of the cellular actions of glucocorticoids. As lipophilic substances, glucocorticoids pass very easily through the cell membrane into the cell, where they bind to ubiquitously expressed cytosolic glucocorticoid receptors (cGCRs). This is followed either by the classic cGCR-mediated genomic effects (I) or by cGCR-mediated non-genomic effects (II). Moreover, the glucocorticoid is very likely to interact with cell membranes either specifically via membrane bound glucocorticoid receptors (mGCR) (III) or via non-specific interactions with cell membranes (IV). HSP, heat-shock protein; m, mechanism. *(From Buttgereit F, Straub RH, Wehling M, Burmester GR. Glucocorticoids in the treatment of rheumatic diseases: an update on the mechanisms of action. Arthritis Rheum 2004;50:3408-3417.)*

The relative contributions of these three mechanisms are not yet fully understood, but in combination they result in the decreased synthesis of proinflammatory cytokines such as interleukin (IL)-1, IL-2, IL-2 receptor, interferon (IFN)-α, IL-6, and tumor necrosis factor (TNF) α.[14,15,27] Glucocorticoids increase the rate of synthesis of lipocortin (annexin I), which inhibits phospholipase A_2. Phospholipase A_2 converts membrane-bound phospholipids into arachidonic acid with the subsequent intracellular production of prostaglandins, leukotrienes, and oxygen radicals.[28] Glucocorticoids also induce MAPK phosphatase 1 (which inactivates all proteins of the MAPK family including Jun N-terminal kinase), and glucocorticoids repress transcription of cyclooxygenase 2 (COX-2).[29] Independent of change in gene expression, glucocorticoids exert rapid effects via activation of endothelial nitric oxide as well as activation of β-adrenoreceptors, endonucleases, and

neutral endopeptidases explains other observed effects.[30] Glucocorticoids, even in very low concentrations, inhibit the synthesis of a variety of proinflammatory enzymes, including the macrophage products collagenase, elastase, and plasminogen activator.[31] Glucocorticoids have a direct effect on lymphocytes by decreasing T-cell function and circulating number. They further inhibit Fc receptor expression (reducing clearance of antibody coated blood cells), increase the number of circulating neutrophils, and affect leukocyte adhesion to endothelial cells.[32]

Drug development efforts are attempting to exploit an improved knowledge of molecular biology of glucocorticoids. Considerable effort has been directed to developing selective glucocorticoid receptor agonists (SEGRAs) that differentially affect levels of some of these transactivation and transrepression.[33,34] In preliminary experiments

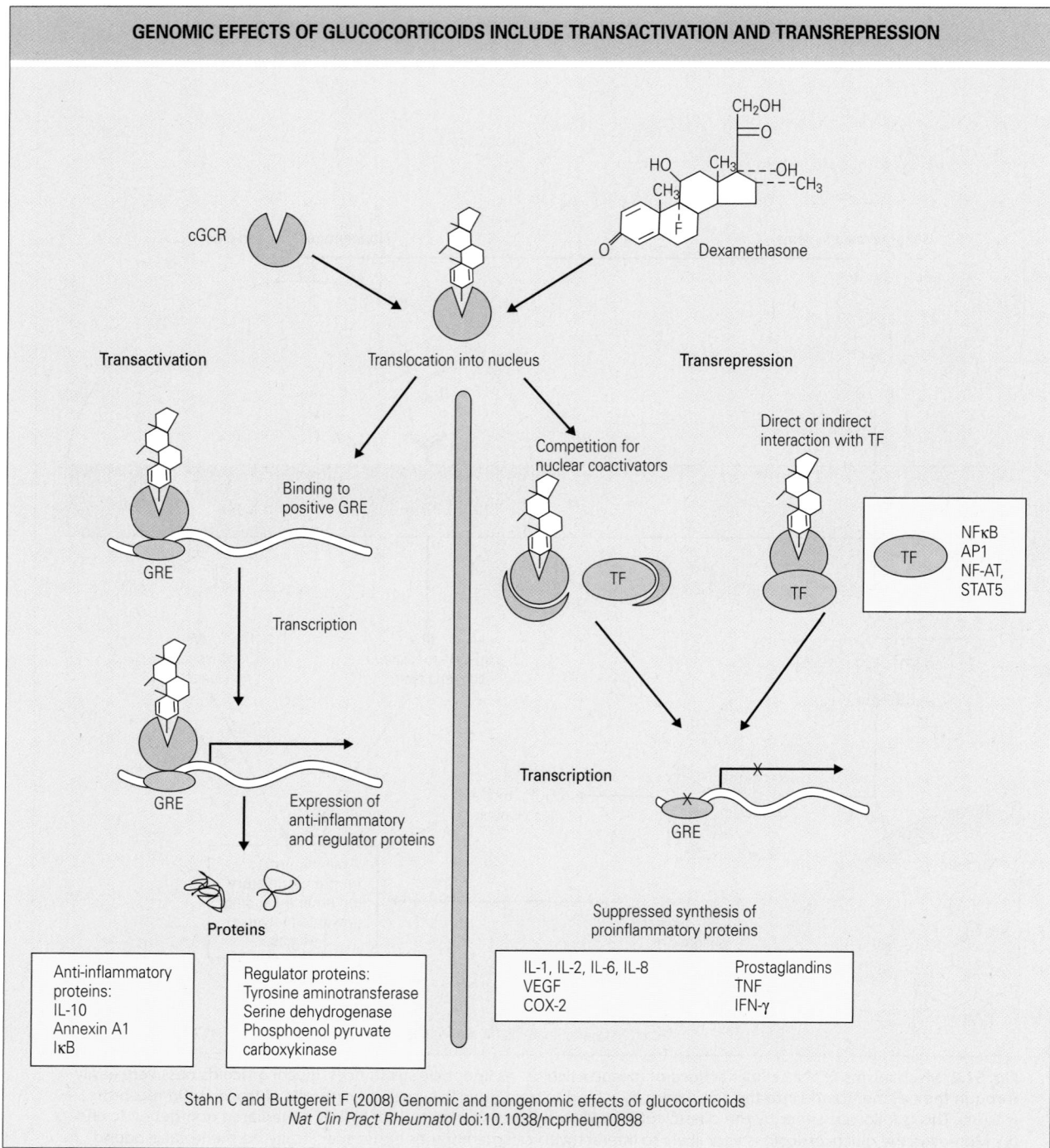

GENOMIC EFFECTS OF GLUCOCORTICOIDS INCLUDE TRANSACTIVATION AND TRANSREPRESSION

cGCR

Dexamethasone

Transactivation

Translocation into nucleus

Transrepression

Binding to positive GRE

GRE

Transcription

Competition for nuclear coactivators

Direct or indirect interaction with TF

TF

NFκB
AP1
NF-AT,
STAT5

TF

TF

GRE

Expression of anti-inflammatory and regulator proteins

Transcription

Proteins

GRE

Suppressed synthesis of proinflammatory proteins

| Anti-inflammatory proteins:
IL-10
Annexin A1
IκB | Regulator proteins:
Tyrosine aminotransferase
Serine dehydrogenase
Phosphoenol pyruvate
carboxykinase |

| IL-1, IL-2, IL-6, IL-8
VEGF
COX-2 | Prostaglandins
TNF
IFN-γ |

Stahn C and Buttgereit F (2008) Genomic and nongenomic effects of glucocorticoids
Nat Clin Pract Rheumatol doi:10.1038/ncprheum0898

Fig. 51.3 Genomic effects of glucocorticoids include transactivation and transrepression. Binding of the glucocorticoid-cGCR complex to GREs leads to expression of anti-inflammatory and regulatory proteins such as IL-10 or IκB (transactivation). A suppressed synthesis of proinflammatory proteins (transrepression) is caused by competition for nuclear co-activators or direct or indirect interaction with transcription factors. AP1, activator protein 1; cGCR, cytosolic glucocorticoid receptor; COX-2, cyclooxygenase 2; GRE, glucocorticoid response element; IκB, inhibitor of NFκB; IFN-γ, interferon γ; IL, interleukin; NF-AT, nuclear factor of activated T cells; NFκB, nuclear factor κB; STAT5, signal transducer and activator of transcription 5; TF, transcription factor; TNF, tumor necrosis factor; VEGF, vascular endothelial growth factor. *(From Stahn C, Buttgereit F. Genomic and nongenomic effects of glucocorticoids. Nat Clin Pract Rheumatol 2008;4:525-533.)*

compounds appear to exhibit similar anti-inflammatory effects as traditional glucocorticoids but may have fewer adverse effects, such as blood glucose elevation or skin thinning.[35,36] Liposomal glucocorticoids are being developed with the aim of providing more prolonged concentrations of glucocorticoids at the site of inflammation and lower plasma levels. Part of their mechanism of action may be via insertion of higher concentrations of glucocorticoids into cell membranes.[37] Lastly, early phase attempts have been made to link nitric oxide to prednisolone in an effort to increase anti-inflammatory effects but with lower toxicity to bone.[38]

EFFICACY

Efficacy in rheumatoid arthritis

Short- to moderate-term glucocorticoid studies reveal improved disease activity and functional status when compared with control therapy.[39,40] Long-term anti-inflammatory benefits of glucocorticoids on disease activity are not as well supported by the literature. Anti-inflammatory benefits of glucocorticoids appear to decline after the first year[41-43] and are often not seen even beyond 5 months.[44,45] In contrast to earlier reports, two randomized controlled trials showed that at 2 years either

TABLE 51.2 STUDIES OF ORAL GLUCOCORTICOIDS AND RADIOGRAPHIC PROGRESSION IN RHEUMATOID ARTHRITIS

Study (year)	Experimental group	Control group	Study type (no. of subjects)	Effect on radiologic progression	Comments
MRC[133] 1955	Cortisone (69 mg/day)	ASA	CT (100)	No difference	Trend toward protective effect
MRC[134] 1959	Prednisolone (Initial 20 mg, 12 mg/day by yr 1, 10 mg/day by yr 2)	ASA	CT (77)	Reduction after 2 yr, less after 3 yr	Control patients offered prednisolone in year 3
Bernsten[135] 1961	Various glucocorticoids, dose not reported	IM gold, analgesics	Retrospective (388)	Deterioration in all groups	Many patients had already failed other Rx
Harris[136] 1983	Prednisone (5 mg/day) & DMARD	PBO & DMARD	DB RCT (34)	No significant difference	Trend toward reduction
Million[137] 1984	Prednisolone (10.3 mg/day) & DMARD	No prednisolone	RCT (103)	Significant reduction	10-year study
Kirwan[41] 1995	Prednisolone (7.5 mg/day) & DMARD	PBO & DMARD	DB RCT (106)	Significant reduction	
Boers[44] 1997	Prednisolone (60 mg/day with taper) & MTX, SSZ	PBO & SSZ	DB RCT (102)	Significant reduction	
Hansen[45] 1999	Prednisolone (6 mg/day) & DMARD	DMARD	RCT (102)	No significant difference	Trend toward reduction
Van Everdingen[89] 2002	Prednisolone (10 mg/day) & SSZ as rescue	PBO & SSZ as rescue	DB RCT (81)	Significant reduction	Only study since the MRC to not allow background DMARDs. SSA allowed after 6 months
Capell[88] 2004	Prednisolone (7 mg/day) & SSZ	PBO & SSZ	DB RCT (167)	No significant difference	Discordance in radiographic interpretations between readers
Wassenberg[47] 2005	Prednisolone (5 mg/day) & either AU or MTX	PBO & either AU or MTX	DB RCT (166)	Significant reduction	Relatively new-onset RA. One of the lowest doses to show radiographic protection
Svensson[46] 2005	Prednisolone (7.5 mg/day) & DMARD	No prednisone & DMARD	Open RT (225)	Significant reduction	Early RA

MRC, Medical Research Council; R, randomized; CT, controlled trial; DB, double blind; IM, intramuscular; ASA, high-dose aspirin; MTX, methotrexate; SSZ, sulfasalazine; AU, auranofin; DMARD, disease-modifying antirheumatic drug; PBO, placebo; NA, not assessed; NS, not significant.

5.0 or 7.5 mg of prednisolone resulted in variable levels of improvement in joint indices, functional status, and remission criteria compared with patients taking placebo.[46,47]

Beyond disease activity, joint damage as assessed by radiographic criteria (bony erosions and joint space narrowing) is a critical efficacy outcome. Although it is known that methotrexate, the anti-TNF agents, and newer biologic response modifiers are disease-modifying antirheumatic drugs (DMARDs) in RA, there is now consensus that glucocorticoids function similarly. A synopsis of many of the RA studies evaluating the effects of glucocorticoids on radiographic progression is summarized in Table 51.2. Many of these investigations allowed concomitant use of DMARDs, making it difficult to discern the independent effects of glucocorticoids. Although many of the earlier investigations failed to demonstrate a benefit of low-dose glucocorticoids on radiographic progression, an increasing number of placebo-controlled randomized or open-label clinical trials have now demonstrated that low dose glucocorticoids prevent radiographic joint destruction in RA. Although the vast majority of glucocorticoid use internationally in RA is via lower-dose oral therapy,[3,48] a few RA studies have examined other routes of administration such as pulsed-dose and intramuscular depot approaches.[49,50]

Efficacy in systemic connective tissue disorders and vasculitis

Medium- to high-dose glucocorticoids are the therapeutic mainstay in rheumatology for managing serious inflammatory disorders with life- or organ-threatening manifestations. Glucocorticoids have been used for serious extra-articular manifestation of RA, including interstitial lung disease, bronchiolitis obliterans with organizing pneumonia, pericarditis, scleritis, and vasculitis.[51]

For these serious sequelae of RA and in other major inflammatory disorders such as systemic lupus erythematosus, inflammatory myopathy, and systemic vasculitis, glucocorticoids are typically started at dose range of 1 mg/kg/day of prednisone equivalent. Although highly effective in causing remission or improving control of these disorders,

glucocorticoids do not inhibit the generation of platelet-derived thromboxane; and in certain forms of vasculitis, patients can develop progressive ischemia despite glucocorticoids.[52]

For life- or organ-threatening complications, intravenous pulse therapy is used at doses of 250 to 1000 mg/day of methylprednisolone for a typical period of 3 days. The intent of pulse therapy is to rapidly and aggressively suppress severe systemic inflammation while minimizing exposure to prolonged very-high-dose therapy. Rapidly progressive glomerulonephritis and pulmonary and central nervous system vasculitis are among the disorders in which very-high-dose pulse therapy has been advocated.[53,54] Compared with prednisolone, methylprednisolone has more than threefold more non-genomic effects at equivalent doses, contributing to its preference over prednisone in this setting.[55]

Efficacy in polymyalgia rheumatica and large-vessel vasculitis

Glucocorticoids are the mainstay for therapy in polymyalgia rheumatica, giant cell (temporal) arteritis, and Takayasu's arteritis.[56,57] Because of the older age of most persons with polymyalgia rheumatica and giant cell arteritis, glucocorticoids need to be used cautiously and monitored more closely in this population. Although a variety of other immunosuppressive agents have been tested as possible glucocorticoid-sparing agents, there are little compelling data that these agents are effective alternatives to glucocorticoid in these disorders. A typical prednisone starting dose in giant cell arteritis is 60 mg/day whereas 15 to 20 mg/day is usually adequate for polymyalgia rheumatica. Although efforts to taper glucocorticoids are initiated early in the disease course, it can require more than 6 months to reach a low dose in persons with giant cell arteritis.[58] It is not uncommon for persons with giant cell arteritis to require in excess of 2 years of glucocorticoid therapy. Glucocorticoid-tapering regimens for polymyalgia rheumatica are not well standardized, and symptoms often wax and wane over many years remaining partially responsive to low-dose prednisone therapy. Guidance from a meta-analysis suggests that once a prednisone dose of

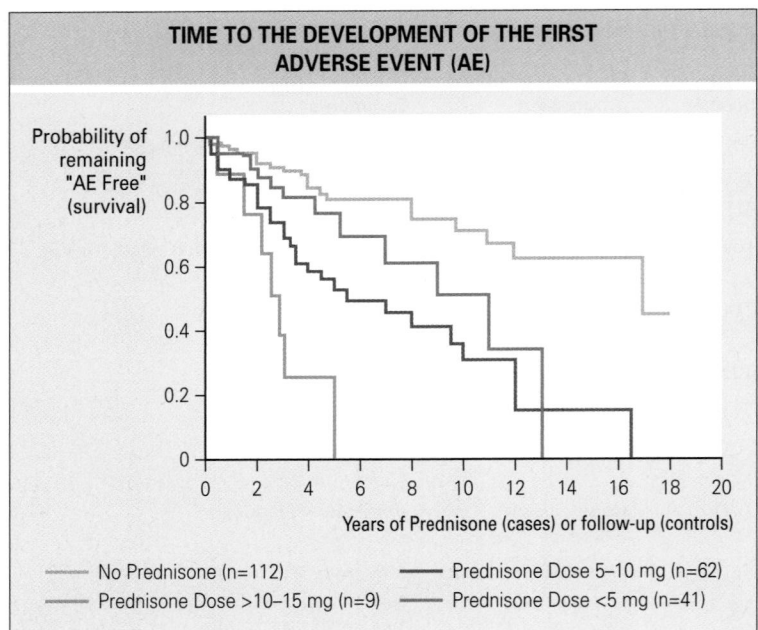

Fig. 51.4 Probability of remaining free from adverse events (adverse events) over time while on low-dose (<5 mg), intermediate dose (5-10 mg), or high-dose (>10-15 mg) prednisone compared with a control group. *(Adapted with permission from Saag KG, Koehnke R, Caldwell JR, et al. Low dose long-term corticosteroid therapy in rheumatoid arthritis: an analysis of serious adverse events. Am J Med 1994;96:115-123.)*

10 mg/day is reached, tapering by 1 mg/month or less results in fewer relapses.[59]

ADVERSE EFFECTS

Despite the considerable benefits of glucocorticoids in controlling serious inflammation and improving functional status in a plethora of disorders, serious adverse effects dampen enthusiasm, particularly for long-term use. Most studies of glucocorticoid toxicity tend to be retrospective and observational. The ability to differentiate bad outcomes attributable to glucocorticoids from those occurring owing to the underlying diseases or other comorbidities confounds potential associations. A strong physician selection bias for glucocorticoid use exists because physicians are inclined to treat patients with more severe disease with glucocorticoids (i.e., confounding by indication). The use of glucocorticoids at variable points in the disease course, limited data defining the "threshold" dose for particular adverse events,[60] and toxicity reports in a heterogeneous group of glucocorticoid-treated diseases all further hinder interpretation of these data.

Several large retrospective reviews indicate that long-term, relatively low-dose glucocorticoid use is a significant independent predictor of numerous potentially serious adverse events.[52,61-63] Lending further credibility to causality, a glucocorticoid-adverse event association was both dose and time dependent (Fig. 51.4). Both cumulative and mean glucocorticoid dose are independently associated with adverse events.

Less serious adverse effects (e.g., skin thinning, cushingoid appearance) are often of great concern to patients, whereas more debilitating toxicities, such as vertebral fractures and cataracts, may be initially unrecognized or asymptomatic.[64] Compared with other anti-rheumatic agents, glucocorticoids have a low incidence of short-term symptomatic toxicity and patients uncommonly discontinue therapy for these reasons. What follows is an overview of the most common adverse effects that have been associated with glucocorticoids. Recent international recommendations provide guidance on how to most safely use glucocorticoids.[65]

Bone and muscle

Glucocorticoid-induced osteoporosis (GIOP) is the most potentially devastating complication of protracted glucocorticoid therapy, and it is estimated from observational studies that as many as 40% of glucocorticoid users will develop bone loss leading to fracture.[66] Although glucocorticoids diminish sex hormone production and decrease circulating levels of receptor of activator of NF-κB (RANK) ligand, all of which lead to enhanced osteoclast-mediated bone resorption, a direct glucocorticoid-induced defect in bone formation is believed to be the predominant pathway of importance.[67,68] Glucocorticoid-induced osteoporosis initially affects trabecular bone. However, with chronic glucocorticoid use, cortical bone at sites such as the femoral neck is also affected.[66] Comparison of studies examining bone effects of glucocorticoids is made difficult by the differential timing of glucocorticoid initiation, variable dosing regimens, use of different bone mass measurement techniques, and disparities between the sites of measurement.

Observational studies of RA and other glucocorticoid-requiring diseases show a mean first-year loss of bone ranging from 1.5% to 20% at the dose range less than or equal to 10 mg/day of prednisone.[33] With continued use, bone loss remains greater than normal and is estimated at 1.5% to 3.0% per year, dependent on dose, in subsequent years. Although a decline in bone mineral density is strongly correlated with fracture risk and bone mineral density is considered the best overall predictor, the rate of bone turnover, bone quality, and other factors also play important roles.[69] At very low doses, some data suggest that glucocorticoids prevent bone loss in RA because of their inhibitory effects on proinflammatory cytokines that modulate osteoclast activity as well as their beneficial effects on functional status, which promotes more weight-bearing activities.[70,71] Several studies including a meta-analysis have failed to demonstrate an association of low-dose glucocorticoid use with low axial bone mineral density, even in the setting of an increased fracture rate.[71-74] The presence of biochemical changes in bone remodeling with very low dose oral[75] or even intra-articular use[76] argues against a "safe" glucocorticoid dose from the standpoint of bone.[77]

Thus, the confounding effects in trying to identify an association between glucocorticoid treatment and osteoporosis in RA relate to two principal issues: the heightened risk of osteoporosis caused by the RA disease process itself[78-80] and a higher rate of osteoporosis in postmenopausal women, the demographic group with the highest prevalence of RA.[81]

Given the inconsistencies in bone mineral density studies and the knowledge that fractures in glucocorticoid-treated patients occur at a higher bone mineral density and are dependent on other factors,[82,83] it is necessary to examine long-term studies that evaluate actual fracture incidence. In a large cohort of RA patients,[84] 34% of more than 300 women on a mean dose of prednisone of 8.6 mg/day had a self-reported fracture within 5 years of follow-up. Two case-control studies of hip fractures in patients both with and without RA showed a twofold increased risk even after adjusting for the presence of RA.[78,85] Cohort studies identify fractures as one of the most commonly documented complications of supraphysiologic glucocorticoid use.[61,62,86] Hip and other non-vertebral fractures occur with glucocorticoids in both a dose- and time-dependent fashion.[77,87] Randomized controlled trials in the most common glucocorticoid-requiring illness, RA, have not confirmed an increased rate of fracture.[41,46,47,88,89] However, none of these trials has been large or long enough to fully clarify the magnitude of the fracture risk, some have not systematically assessed fractures outcomes in all patients, and in at least one[88] patients were allowed to use bone protective medications.

Considerable advancement has occurred in the development of anti-osteoporotic therapies, and numerous clinical trials have specifically tested anti-osteoporosis therapies for patients newly initiating and chronically using glucocorticoids. All RA patients with or at risk of GIOP should receive initial therapy with adequate calcium and vitamin D,[90,91] with strong evidence-based consideration given to the addition of a bisphosphonate.[92-96] Teriparitide, which may directly inhibit glucocorticoid-mediated deleterious effects on bone formation, is another treatment option for glucocorticoid users at high risk for fracture.[97] Internationally, a variety of specialty societies have promulgated recommendations on appropriate testing and treatment to prevent GIOP.[98-102]

Osteonecrosis of bone is a significant problem in patients receiving high-dose glucocorticoid doses, particularly for treatment of systemic lupus erythematosus. Osteonecrosis is more strongly associated with peak dose of glucocorticoid rather than cumulative dose,[103] perhaps owing to osteocyte and osteoblast apoptosis.[68] The presence of antiphospholipid antibodies contributes to osteonecrosis independent of glucocorticoid use. Osteonecrosis is seldom seen when the prednisone dose is maintained at less than 20 mg/day.[104]

Similar to osteonecrosis, the occurrence of myopathy in patients receiving glucocorticoids is very rare at a low dose. In patients with inflammatory myopathy it is often difficult to disentangle ongoing muscle inflammation from glucocorticoid myopathy. Gradual muscle improvement with dose reduction is often a diagnostic clue because electromyography and muscle biopsy findings are often insufficiently specific to differentiate these two entities. Based on small studies, fluorinated glucocorticoid preparations, such as triamcinolone, are more strongly associated with myopathy than prednisone.[105] Myopathy has been reported to occur at a dose as low as 8 mg/day of triamcinolone after only 3 months of treatment. In general, myopathy attributable to prednisone requires a higher dose and longer duration of treatment.

Cardiovascular effects

Glucocorticoids at medium to high dose promote fluid retention based in some[106] but not all studies.[107,108] This can be problematic for patients with underlying heart or kidney disease, although susceptibility is modified by both glucocorticoid dose and dietary factors. Patients with essential hypertension require closer surveillance of blood pressure and may need modification of their antihypertensive regimens while on glucocorticoid therapy. In some studies glucocorticoids at even low or moderate dose have been associated with hypertension, but this may be a reflection of channeling bias due to RA disease severity.[109] Glucocorticoids can cause sodium retention and can potentiate vasopressive response to catecholamines and angiotensin II. In patients receiving less than 10 mg/day, age and elevated pre-treatment blood pressure likely better explains significant hypertension than the use of glucocorticoids.[110]

Although several observational studies suggest that glucocorticoids at doses of greater than 10 mg/day adversely affect serum lipid profiles, a national sample from the United States was unable to confirm this association.[111] Moderate- to low-dose glucocorticoids (20 mg tapered to 5 mg over 3 months) had no significant adverse effect on lipoprotein levels if other risk factors were controlled.[112] Some studies even have suggested that glucocorticoids reverse an unfavorable lipid profile.[113]

Another difficult-to-study potential toxicity of low-dose glucocorticoids is the development of premature atherosclerotic vascular disease. Increasing attention to the importance of accelerated atherosclerotic disease in RA and other inflammatory conditions has raised interesting questions about the role of chronic inflammation on the vascular endothelium.[114] Although atherosclerotic vascular disease is known to be accelerated in patients with Cushing's disease and at least one study shows increased carotid plaque and decreased arterial compressibility in RA patients on glucocorticoids,[115] there are insufficient data to confirm an independent risk in patients on low-dose glucocorticoids, in particular. In contrast, there is also evidence that glucocorticoids may trend toward a protective vascular effect in persons with polymyalgia rheumatica.[116] On the other hand, high-dose glucocorticoid therapy has been associated with a greater than 2.5-fold increased risk of cardiovascular events, even after adjustment for known covariates.[117]

Cardiac arrhythmias have been described during pulsed-dose glucocorticoid therapy. This rare occurrence, reported mostly in patients with renal disease, predicates a pre-infusion check of serum electrolytes and strong consideration for cardiac monitoring during infusion. Slower infusion rates (administration over 1 to 2 hours) may attenuate this concern.

Dermatologic effects and appearance

Even at the low dose, skin thinning and ecchymoses represent one of the most common glucocorticoid adverse events. A cushingoid appearance that manifests as moon facies, truncal obesity, and "buffalo hump" is very troubling to patients but is uncommon at doses below the physiologic glucocorticoid replacement range. Moon facies develop in slightly more than 10% of patients receiving even short-term low-dose therapy. Alternate-day therapy decreases the incidence of cushingoid appearance. Steroid acne and, to a lesser extent, hirsutism and stria are other undesirable dermatologic side effects that can occur even at lower doses. Glucocorticoids also impair wound healing by inhibiting the synthesis of matrix metalloproteinases and collagen.[118] Weight gain and fat redistribution occur at moderate to high doses, in particular. The effects of hyperinsulinemia on leptin, increased adipocyte conversion of cortisone to cortisol, and increased appetite all contribute to weight gain and fat redistribution.

Gastrointestinal effects

Although glucocorticoids are considerably less toxic to the upper gastrointestinal tract than non-steroidal anti-inflammatory drugs (NSAIDs), glucocorticoids slightly increase the risk of adverse gastrointestinal events such as gastritis, ulcers, and gastrointestinal bleeding. The increased risk of glucocorticoids on gastrointestinal events is very small, with estimated relative risks varying from 1.1 (not significant) to 1.5 (marginally significant).[119,120] In addition to reports of upper gastrointestinal morbidity there are case reports of intestinal rupture, diverticular perforation, and pancreatitis believed to be caused by glucocorticoids. Glucocorticoids are frequently used concurrently with NSAIDs in rheumatology, and the combination synergistically results in a higher risk of gastrointestinal adverse events. Glucocorticoids cause a nearly twofold increased risk of gastrointestinal adverse events among NSAID users[121]; and the combined use of NSAIDs and glucocorticoids results in more than a fourfold increased risk of gastrointestinal adverse events when compared with nonusers.[120]

Infectious diseases

Moderate- to very high-dose glucocorticoid therapy leads to an increased risk of serious infections. However, no studies have adequately explored the risk of infection in patients treated with low-dose glucocorticoids. The risk of infection appears to be lessened by initiating alternate-day therapy. The association of glucocorticoids with infectious adverse events becomes an even greater concern if glucocorticoids are used in combination with biologic anti-rheumatic agents.[122] At higher dose exposure, glucocorticoids appear to be a risk factor for tuberculosis.[123]

Metabolic and endocrine effects

Glucocorticoid users with diabetes mellitus will commonly have higher blood glucose levels while taking glucocorticoids. Moreover, in patients with early diabetes or glucose intolerance, new-onset hyperglycemia or, rarely, a nonketotic hyperosmolar state can develop *de novo*. Ketosis in glucocorticoid-associated diabetes is very rare, because the gluconeogenic and glycogenic effects of glucocorticoids offer protection against this complication. It is uncommon for frank diabetes to develop as a result of glucocorticoid therapy.

A significant concern of chronic glucocorticoid use is hypothalamic-pituitary-adrenal (HPA) insufficiency. HPA insufficiency is both dose and duration specific. High-dose therapy results in protracted suppression of adrenocorticotropic hormone (ACTH) release and adrenal hyporesponsiveness in as little as 5 days. More typically, adrenal suppression can be detected in 6 weeks at 10 mg/day or 15 mg/day in 4 weeks.[60] Spontaneous recovery of the HPA axis is normal in patients on less than or equal to 5 mg of prednisone; however, even subphysiologic doses (<7.5 mg/day) given for long-term periods may lead to HPA blunting.[124] HPA suppression is worsened if glucocorticoids are given twice daily.

Neuropsychiatric effects

Patients on even low-dose glucocorticoid therapy report a slight increase in their overall sense of well-being, which appears to be independent of improvement in disease activity. Symptoms of akathisia, insomnia, and depression are also occasionally observed in patients taking low-dose therapy. Memory impairment, particularly in older patients, can occur even at low doses. Daily split-dose therapy, in particular, tends to be troublesome because the evening dose promotes sleep disturbances. True glucocorticoid psychosis is distinctly uncommon at doses less than 20 mg/day of prednisone.

Ophthalmologic effects

Posterior subcapsular cataracts are a well-described complication of prolonged glucocorticoid use. There is no minimal safe dose with respect to this complication, and reports exist of cataract formation even with inhaled glucocorticoid preparations.[125] However, cataracts rarely occur in patients taking less than 10 mg/day for less than 1 year.[126,127] Nearly a third of RA patients taking a mean dose of 8 mg/day for an average of 7 years developed cataracts.[61] Cortical cataracts also have also been associated with glucocorticoid use.[128]

In addition to cataracts, glucocorticoid-treated patients can develop increased intraocular pressure, which can lead to visual disturbances. The development of frank glaucoma, particularly with low-dose therapy, is rare and tends to appear in patients who are otherwise genetically predisposed.

Use in pregnancy

Glucocorticoids are often used in pregnant patients to control peripartum inflammatory disease activity. Although safer than many other antirheumatic agents during pregnancy, glucocorticoid use can cause fetal growth retardation and low birth weight of offspring. It is difficult, however, to fully discern whether these adverse fetal outcomes are due to the glucocorticoids or the underlying chronic inflammatory disorder. Prednisone or prednisolone is preferred over other glucocorticoids if the aim is to treat a pregnant mother because the placenta will convert active prednisolone back to prednisone and thereby limit fetal exposure. The American Academy of Pediatrics considers prednisone and its active metabolite prednisolone to be compatible with breast-feeding. Even at doses above 1 mg/kg/day, the amount of glucocorticoid secreted into the breast milk is less than 10% of a nursing infant's endogenous cortisol production.

PRACTICAL RECOMMENDATIONS
Evidence-based treatment guidelines

In an era of internationally rising health care costs and highly efficacious but very expensive biologic disease-modifying agents, glucocorticoids provide an apparent inexpensive approach to management of inflammatory and autoimmune disorders. While the cost per pill of oral glucocorticoid is low, other costs such as those associated with adverse effects must also be considered.[129]

Once the decision is made to initiate glucocorticoids, every effort should be made to use these agents as safely and effectively as possible. Increasing data have shown that more aggressive use of glucocorticoids earlier rather than later in the course of RA might be best. However, practitioners skeptical of the disease-modifying benefits of glucocorticoid therapy or excessively concerned about glucocorticoid adverse effects should strive to achieve the lowest effective dose. Despite this evidence and an international call to action to prevent GIOP among even chronic glucocorticoid users, fewer than half of all chronic glucocorticoid users are receiving adequate bone prophylaxis or evaluation.[130]

Perioperative and stress-dose considerations

Chronic glucocorticoid users preparing for major surgeries or undergoing considerable physiologic stress associated with severe illness should receive prophylactic stress-dose glucocorticoids commonly in conjunction with a mineralocorticoid. Hydrocortisone at a dose of 100 mg three times per day is empirically recommended, but for patients on low-dose glucocorticoids or undergoing less significant physiologic insult, half this dose is often sufficient. Identifying which patients require stress-dose glucocorticoids requires consideration of both dose and duration of glucocorticoids. Guidelines for low dose use were discussed earlier. Any person who has received more than 20 mg/day of prednisone equivalent for more than 3 weeks or who has developed clinical Cushing's syndrome should undergo prophylaxis. If clinically feasible, the need for stress-dose glucocorticoids can be determined by testing for the responsiveness of the HPA axis with a low-dose synthetic ACTH (cosyntropin) stimulation test.

Glucocorticoids in children

Growth retardation can occur in children receiving glucocorticoids because these agents inhibit linear bone growth and delay epiphyseal closure. Regular daily administration of more than 7.5 mg of prednisolone is associated with inhibition of linear growth. The mechanism of action is unknown, although suppression of growth hormone secretion and other metabolic effects can contribute. Alternate-day administration of the same total dose reduces this effect[131] and is preferred, if clinically practical.

Glucocorticoid withdrawal regimens and alternate-day therapy

There is little science to guide the necessary but challenging process of glucocorticoid dose reduction. For conditions such as RA, a very subtle dose reduction is most effective in promoting eventual glucocorticoid discontinuation. In systemic lupus erythematosus and other diseases in which immune complexes play a significant role in pathogenic consequences, alternate-day therapy is a consideration once disease control is achieved. Alternate-day therapy serves to minimize HPA axis suppression and, in turn, certain adverse effects, and it affords a reduction in cumulative glucocorticoid dose. However, in RA, alternate-day therapy is often not well tolerated owing to an increase in joint symptoms in days off therapy.

Steroid withdrawal syndrome is not clearly associated with HPA insufficiency but presents as extreme weakness and arthralgias. Glucocorticoid tapering from 20 mg/day by increments of 2.5 mg/day every 2 weeks resulted in rebound deterioration in over half of RA patients.[42] While accommodating convenience and individual patient disease response, a relatively stable decrement of 10% to 20% of glucocorticoid dose every 1 to 2 weeks is recommended until the dose reaches 10 mg, and than tapering should proceed more slowly for long-term users. Indeed, difficulty withdrawing patients from glucocorticoids is sometimes cited as a compelling reason for not initiating them.[132] Many rheumatologists report significant difficulties in tapering glucocorticoids for most RA patients, and abrupt withdrawal can result in dramatic flares in disease activity. Thus, it is recommended that patients on long-term low-dose glucocorticoid therapy for inflammatory arthritis or polymyalgia rheumatica lower their dose in increments as small as 1 mg/month (sometimes facilitated by cutting the dose on alternate days) to maximize their prospects for successful withdrawal. However, further research on appropriate tapering regimens is greatly needed.

KEY REFERENCES

1. Hench PS, Kendall EC, Slocumb CH, et al. Effects of cortisone acetate and pituitary ACTH on rheumatoid arthritis, rheumatic fever and certain other conditions. Arch Intern Med 1950;85:545-666.
2. Buttgereit F, da Silva JAP, Boers M, et al. Standardised nomenclature for glucocorticoid dosages and glucocorticoid treatment regimens: current questions and tentative answers in rheumatology. Ann Rheum Dis 2002;61:718-722.
3. Saag KG. Low-dose corticosteroid therapy in rheumatoid arthritis: balancing the evidence. Am J Med 1997;103:31S-39S.
4. Esteban NV, Loughlin T, Yergey AL, et al. Daily cortisol production rate in man determined by stable isotope dilution/mass spectrometry. J Clin Endocrinol Metab 1991;72:39-45.
5. Francisco GE, Honigberg II, Stewart JT. In vitro and in vivo bioequivalence of commercial prednisone tablets. Biopharm Drug Dispos 1984;5:335.
6. Hale V, Aizawa K, Sheimer LB, et al. Disposition of prednisone and prednisolone in the perfused rabbit liver: modeling hepatic metabolic processes. J Pharmacokinet Biopharm 1991;19:597.
7. Hill M, Szefler SJ, Ball BD, et al. Monitoring glucocorticoid therapy: a pharmacokinetic approach. Clin Pharmacol Ther 1990;48:390.

8. Legler U, Frey FJ, Benet LZ. Prednisolone clearance at steady state in man. J Clin Endocrinol Metab 1982;55:762.
9. Miffin PJ, Brooks PM, Sallustio BC. Alterations in prednisolone disposition as a result of time of administration, gender and dose. Br J Clin Pharmacol 1984;17:395.
10. Theissen JJ. Bioavailability monograph: prednisolone. J Am Pharm Assoc 1976;NS16:143.
11. Arvidson NG, Gudbjornsson B, Larsson A, Hallgren R. The timing of glucocorticoid administration in rheumatoid arthritis. Ann Rheum Dis 1997;56:27-31.
12. Reinberg A, Gervais P, Chaussade M, et al. Circadian changes in effectiveness of corticosteroids in eight patients with allergic asthma. J Allergy Clin Immunol 1983;71:425.
13. Buttgereit F, Doering G, Schaeffler A, et al. Efficacy of modified-release versus standard prednisone to reduce duration of morning stiffness of the joints in rheumatoid arthritis (CAPRA-1): a double-blind, randomised controlled trial. Lancet 2008;371:205-214.
14. Boumpas DT, Chrousos GP, Wilder RL, et al. Glucocorticoid therapy for immune-mediated diseases: basic and clinical correlates. Ann Intern Med 1993;119:1198-1208.
15. Barnes PJ, Adcock I. Anti-inflammatory actions of steroids: molecular mechanisms. TiPS. 1993;14:436-441.
16. Buttgereit F, Wheling M, Burmester GR. A new hypothesis of modular glucocorticoid actions—steroid treatment of rheumatic diseases revisited. Arthritis Rheum 1998;41:761-767.
17. Gustafsson J-A, Carlstedt-Duke J, Poellinger L, et al. Biochemistry, molecular biology, and physiology of the glucocorticoid receptor. Endocr Rev 1987;8:185-234.
18. Rhen T, Cidlowski JA. Antiinflammatory action of glucocorticoids—new mechanisms for old drugs. N Engl J Med 2005;353:1711-1723.
19. Stahn C, Buttgereit F. Genomic and nongenomic effects of glucocorticoids. Nat Clin Pract Rheumatol 2008;4:525-533.
20. Chikanza IC. Mechanisms of corticosteroid resistance in rheumatoid arthritis: a putative role for the corticosteroid receptor beta isoform. Ann N Y Acad Sci 2002;966:39-48.
21. Taitoura DC, Rothman PB. Enhancement of MEK/ERK signaling promotes glucocorticoid resistance in CD4+ T cells. J Clin Invest 2004;113:619-627.
22. Podgorski MR, Goulding NJ, Hall ND, et al. Autoantibodies to recombinant lipocorrin in RA and SLE. Br J Rheumatol 1987;26(Suppl 2):54-55.
23. Goulding NJ, Podgorski MR, Hall ND, et al. Autoantibodies to recombinant lipocortin-1 in rheumatoid arthritis and systemic lupus erythematosus. Ann Rheum Dis 1989;48:843-850.
24. Huizenga NA, Koper JW, De Lange P, et al. A polymorphism in the glucocorticoid receptor gene may be associated with an increased sensitivity to glucocorticoids in vivo. J Clin Endocrinol Metab 1998;83:144-151.
25. Sliwinska-Stanczyk P, Pazdur J, Ziolkowska M, et al. The effect of methylprednisolone on proliferation of PBMCs obtained from steroid-sensitive and steroid-resistant rheumatoid arthritis patients. Scand J Rheumatol 2007;36:167-171.
26. Bartholome B, Spies CM, Gaber T, et al. Membrane glucocorticoid receptors (mGCR) are expressed in normal human peripheral blood mononuclear cells and up-regulated after in vitro stimulation and in patients with rheumatoid arthritis. FASEB J 2004;18:70-80.
27. Kern JA, Laumb RT, Reed JC, et al. Dexamethasone inhibition of interleukin-1beta production by human monocytes: post-transcriptional mechanisms. J Clin Invest 1988;81:237-244.
28. Vishwanath BS, Frey FJ, Bradtury MJ, et al. Glucocorticoid deficiency increases phospholipase A2 activity in rats. J Clin Invest 1993;92:1974-1980.
29. Szczepanski A, Moatter T, Carley WW, Gerritsen ME. Induction of cyclooxygenase II in human synovial microvessel endothelial cells by interleukin-1: inhibition by glucocorticoids. Arthritis Rheum 1994;37:495-503.
30. Palmer RM, Bridge L, Foxwell NA, Moncada S. The role of nitric oxide in endothelial cell damage and its inhibition by glucocorticoids. Br J Pharmacol 1992;105:11-12.
31. Werb Z. Biochemical actions of glucocorticoids on macrophages in culture-specific inhibition of elastase, collagenase and plasminogen activator secretion and effects on other metabolic functions. J Exp Med 1978;147:1695-1712.
32. Cronstein BN, Kimmel SC, Levin RI, et al. A mechanism for the anti-inflammatory effects of corticosteroids: the glucocorticoid receptor regulates leukocyte adhesion to endothelial cells and expression of endothelial-leukocyte adhesion molecule-1 and intercellular adhesion molecule 1. Proc Natl Acad Sci U S A 1992;89:9991-9995.
33. Bijlsma JWJ, Saag KG, Buttgereit F, da Silva JAP. Developments in glucocorticoid therapy. Rheum Dis Clin North Am 2005;31:1-17.
34. Stahn C, Lowenberg M, Hommes DW, Buttgereit F. Molecular mechanisms of glucocorticoid action and selective glucocorticoid receptor agonists. Mol Cell Endocrinol 2007;275:71-78.
35. Coghlan MJ, Jacobson PB, Lane B, et al. A novel antiinflammatory maintains glucocorticoid efficacy with reduced side effects. Mol Endocrinol 2003;17:860-869.
36. Schacke H, Schottelius A, Docke WD, et al. Dissociation of transactivation from transrepression by a selective glucocorticoid receptor agonist leads to separation of therapeutic effects from side effects. Proc Natl Acad Sci U S A 2004;101:227-232.
37. Schmidt J, Metselaar JM, Wauben MH, et al. Drug targeting by long-circulating liposomal glucocorticosteroids increases therapeutic efficacy in a model of multiple sclerosis. Brain 2003;126:1895-1904.
38. Paul-Clark MJ, Roviezzo F, Flower RJ, et al. Glucocorticoid receptor nitration leads to enhanced anti-inflammatory effects of novel steroid ligands. J Immunol 2003;171:3245-3252.
39. Gotzsche PC, Johansen HK. Meta-analysis of short term low dose prednisolone versus placebo and non-steroidal anti-inflammatory drugs in rheumatoid arthritis. BMJ 1998;316:811-818.
40. Saag KG, Criswell LA, Sems KM, et al. Low-dose corticosteroids in rheumatoid arthritis: a meta-analysis of their moderate-term effectiveness. Arthritis Rheum 1996;39:1818-1825.
41. Kirwan JR, Arthritis and Rheumatism Council Low Dose Glucocorticoid Study Group. The effect of glucocorticoids on joint destruction in rheumatoid arthritis. N Engl J Med 1995;333:142-146.
42. Van Gestel AM, Laan RFJM, Haagsma CJ, et al. Low-dose oral steroids as bridge therapy in rheumatoid arthritis patients starting with parenteral gold: a randomized double-blind placebo-controlled trial (and personal correspondence). Br J Rheumatol 1995;34:347-351.
43. Van Schaardenburg D, Valkema R, Dijkmans BAC, et al. Prednisone for elderly-onset rheumatoid arthritis: outcome and bone mass in comparison to treatment with chloroquine. Arthritis Rheum 1995;38:334-342.
44. Boers M, Verhoven AC, Markusse HM, et al. Randomised comparison of combined step-down prednisolone, methotrexate and sulphasalazine with sulphasalazine alone in early rheumatoid arthritis. Lancet 1997;350:309-318.
45. Hansen M, Podenphant J, Florescu A, et al. A randomised trial of differentiated prednisolone treatment in active rheumatoid arthritis: clinical benefits and skeletal side effects. Ann Rheum Dis 1999;58:713-718.
46. Svensson B, Boonen A, Albertsson K, et al., for the BARFOT Study Group. Low-dose prednisolone in addition to the initial disease-modifying antirheumatic drug in patients with early active rheumatoid arthritis reduces joint destruction and increases the remission rate: a two-year randomized trial. Arthritis Rheum 2005;52:3360-3370.
47. Wassenberg S, Rau R, Steinfeld P, Zeidler H, for the Low-Dose Prednisolone Therapy Study Group. Very low-dose prednisolone in early rheumatoid arthritis retards radiographic progression over two years: a multicenter, double-blind, placebo-controlled trial. Arthritis Rheum 2005;52:3371-3380.
48. Thiele K, Buttgereit F, Huscher D, Zink A, for the German Collaborative Arthritis Centres. Current use of glucocorticoids in patients with rheumatoid arthritis in Germany. Arthritis Rheum (Arthritis Care Res) 2005;53:740-747.
49. Choy EHS, Kingsley G, Corkhill MM, Panayi GS. Intramuscular methylprednisolone is superior to pulse oral methylprednisolone during the induction phase of chrysotherapy. Br J Rheumatol 1993;32:734-739.
50. Weusten BLAM, Jacobs JWG, Bijlsma JWJ. Corticosteroid pulse therapy in active rheumatoid arthritis. Semin Arthritis Rheum 1993;23:183-192.

REFERENCES

Full references for this chapter can be found on www.expertconsult.com.

Parenteral gold, antimalarials, and sulfasalazine

Floris A. van Gaalen and Cornelia F. Allaart

52

- Sulfasalazine, hydroxychloroquine and gold are disease-modifying antirheumatic drugs (DMARDs) that can still have a useful role in the management of inflammatory joint disease.
- There are limited data on efficacy of sulfasalazine, hydroxychloroquine and gold in terms of achieving low disease activity or remission and suppression of joint damage progression.
- Hydroxychloroquine has been shown to have an additive effect when used in conjunction with methotrexate and sulfasalazine.
- Gold requires careful monitoring; serious side-effects can occur in patients on established treatment.
- Interactions with drugs used for co-morbid conditions are important with this group of DMARDs.

INTRODUCTION

Gold, antimalarials, and sulfasalazine are what are called disease-modifying antirheumatic drugs (DMARDs), a category of otherwise unrelated drugs used to suppress inflammation and possibly progression of radiologic damage in patients with rheumatoid arthritis (RA). Unlike the newer biologic antirheumatic drugs, and unlike corticosteroids, DMARDs have a slow onset of action, making the patient wait at least 4 weeks before an effect on signs and symptoms can be noticed. Despite often evident symptom reduction, in many patients the response is insufficient, or there may be side effects that prevent continuation of treatment. Rapid achievement of clinical remission or at least low disease activity is the most important determinant of optimal daily functioning and quality of life and of prevention or progression of joint damage.[1-4] In severe RA, because of a delayed action, an insufficient suppression of disease activity, the uncertain effect on prevention of joint damage progression, and the risk of adverse events, gold, antimalarials, and sulfasalazine are not the first choice of treatment. If therapies with more favorable profiles have failed, or if other therapies cannot be used, these "golden oldies," alone or in combination with other drugs, may still be tried.

PARENTERAL GOLD

Introduced by Jacques Forestier in the 1920s, parenteral gold therapy was shown to have beneficial effects in later placebo-controlled trials in the second half of the 20th century. Sodium and disodium aurothiomalate, with a 50% gold by weight, are still in use today.

Pharmacology

After intramuscular injection, gold is rapidly absorbed into the circulation, where most of it is bound to albumin.[5] The peak serum concentration is reached within 2 to 4 hours after injection.[6] Gold is slowly eliminated from the body mostly via the kidney and the remainder in the feces. It can be found in tissues up to 20 years after the last dose.[7]

Mode of action

Various cellular and enzymatic effects are ascribed to gold, but it is not clear which mechanisms are responsible for the therapeutic effects.

In synovium, gold therapy reduces the number of monocytes and macrophages and decreases production of proinflammatory cytokines, interleukin (IL)-1α, IL-1β, IL-6, and tumor necrosis factor (TNF)-α, produced by T cells, macrophages, monocytes, or dendritic cells.[8,9]

Efficacy

Compared with placebo, parenteral gold reduces the number of inflamed joint and laboratory measures of inflammation. Observational studies and short-term trials suggest that gold slows radiologic progression.[10] In one comparative study with methotrexate (MTX), 15 mg/wk, parenteral gold appeared to be as effective.[11]

Gold treatment, however, has a higher dropout rate owing to side effects than other DMARDs, including MTX.[12]

Toxicity

Side effects of gold affect many different organ systems and frequently result in discontinuation of therapy.[13] The most common complications are dermatitis (rash, pruritus) and stomatitis. These can mostly be managed by temporarily stopping the drug and continuing at a lower dose.[14] Proteinuria occurred in clinical trials in 3% to 4% of patients. Mild proteinuria may resolve spontaneously even with continuation of the drug or after decreasing the dose, but nephrotic syndrome has been described and it is recommended to stop treatment when severe proteinuria occurs.[15] Approximately 5% of patients treated with aurothiomalate experience nitritoid reactions: transient symptoms of flushing, sweating, dizziness, nausea, hypotension, and malaise that occur within minutes of drug administration.[16] Patients who use angiotensin-converting enzyme inhibitors appear especially to be at risk and should receive gold therapy while in the recumbent position.

Aplastic anemia is the most serious, but rare, complication of gold treatment. Between 1965 and 1971 the British Committee on Safety of Medicines reported on nine fatal episodes of aplastic anemia in patients treated with injectable gold. Thrombocytopenia is the most frequent blood dyscrasia associated with gold therapy, with the incidence ranging from 0% to 5%. It tends to occur in the first 6 months of treatment and is usually due to immune-mediated destruction with an active bone marrow.[17]

Other rare complications that have been described are enterocolitis, hepatotoxicity, pancreatitis, peripheral neuropathy, cranial nerve palsies, and a Guillain-Barré–like syndrome. Chrysiasis is a slate-gray skin pigmentation of the sun-exposed skin after long-term parenteral gold therapy. There is limited published information on the safety of gold in pregnancy, but gold may be a treatment option in women planning pregnancy.[18]

Dosage

An initial dose of 10 mg is usually given to test for possible hypersensitivity. Thereafter, 50 mg/wk is given until the disease activity is sufficiently reduced. A clinical effect can be delayed by many weeks. Once a good clinical response is achieved, the dose may be reduced, by increasing the interval between the injections up to once per 6 weeks. Regular blood tests to detect thrombocytopenia and leukopenia and urinalysis to check for proteinuria are recommended.

ANTIMALARIALS

In the early 1950s, several case series reported substantial efficacy of various antimalarials in the treatment of RA but the first clinical trials with antimalarials showed disappointing results. Two antimalarials, chloroquine (CQ) and hydroxychloroquine (HCQ), are in clinical use in RA. HCQ comprises the vast majority of prescriptions for RA. The fact that these compounds are 4-aminoquinoline derivates is far less important than the fact that almost everybody uses HCQ.

Pharmacology

After oral absorption (~70% both for HCQ and CQ),[19] the drugs are rapidly cleared from plasma and distributed in tissues, including muscle, liver, spleen, kidney, lung, and hematopoietic cells. Steady-state concentrations are not achieved for at least 3 months.[20] Higher loading dosages are associated with more rapid beneficial clinical effects, but also with more frequent adverse gastrointestinal side effects. Excretion of HCQ and CQ is mostly by renal clearance of the drugs or of their hepatic compounds and for a small part via feces. The elimination half-life is approximately 40 days.[21] Small amounts of CQ were found in plasma and red blood cells and urine several years after the last dose. Hydroxychloroquine may lead to increased plasma digoxin levels[22] and can increase the bioavailability of β-blockers.[23]

Mode of action

Antimalarials have a wide variety of action, but the precise mode of action in RA is not known. Perhaps because antimalarials are weak bases they interfere with functions that depend on an acidic pH, such as antigen presentation.[24] Non-lysosomotropic mechanisms play a role in the reported inhibition of release of IL-1β, IL-6, and TNF from lipopolysaccharide-stimulated monocytes by CQ.[25]

Efficacy

Antimalarials have limited efficacy when used alone.[26] A combination with MTX or with MTX and sulfasalazine appears to be more effective than MTX alone,[27-29] but a combination with just sulfasalazine probably is not useful.[30]

Toxicity

Antimalarials are considered to be among the safest of drugs used for RA.[13] The most common side effects are related to the gastrointestinal tract (nausea, anorexia, muscle-related abdominal cramps in 7.1%), the skin (3.5%, especially a pruritic rash), and the eyes (7.4%, mainly due to corneal deposits in patients using CQ, which are usually reversible on discontinuation and do not affect vision.[31] Retinopathy, which can lead to blindness, appears to be extremely rare, especially in the first 5 years of therapy.[32] Screening guidelines tailored to different ages and risk groups have been published.[33] An uncommon but important side effect is neuromyotoxicity with proximal lower extremity weakness, normal creatine phosphokinase, and abnormal muscle and nerve biopsy results.[34] Therapy with HCQ is thought to be safe during pregnancy and lactation.[35]

SULFASALAZINE

In 1938 the Swedish professor Nanna Svartz synthesized what is now called sulfasalazine (SSZ). SSZ was truly introduced as a drug for arthritis in the late 1970s when McConkey and colleagues reported beneficial effects of SSZ in RA with fewer side effects compared with the then-standard drugs gold and penicillamine.

Pharmacology

After ingestion, most of SSZ is split in the large intestine by bacterial enzymes into sulfapyridine (SP), which is then absorbed, and 5-aminosalicylic acid (5-ASA), which is nearly all excreted via the feces. The SSZ that is absorbed intact is highly protein bound and excreted unchanged in the urine with an elimination half-life of 5 hours.[36] Both SP and intact SSZ are found in synovial fluid at concentrations related to but slightly lower than that of plasma.[37]

Mode of action

The mode of action of SSZ is unclear. Intact SSZ, SP, and 5-ASA are all biologically active but SP seems the most relevant component in RA treatment.

Efficacy

Several placebo-controlled trials of 24 to 48 weeks' duration have shown a benefit of 2 g/day of SSZ on the inflammatory activity of patients with RA.[38] A meta-analysis suggests that SSZ is also effective in decreasing the progression of radiologic damage on cartilage and bone.[10] Direct comparisons between different DMARDs as initial treatment are rare and show that, in achieving short-term clinical improvement, SSZ does not appear to be less effective than low to medium doses of MTX.[39,40] However, current recommendations favor MTX over SSZ because of a more favorable long-term clinical and radiologic efficacy and toxicity profile.[41,42]

Initial combination therapy of SSZ with MTX does not appear to be more effective as initial treatment than therapy with either monotherapy. In the BeSt study, a comparison study of four treatment strategies, SSZ was tested as the second option after failure on MTX monotherapy, either add-on or as a single DMARD.[4] The percentage of patients who achieved prolonged low disease activity (DAS44 ≤ 2.4) on SSZ after failure on MTX monotherapy was the same with or without MTX and disappointing (only 20%).[43]

A combination of SSZ with MTX and a tapered high dose of prednisone was proven very effective in patients with recent-onset RA.[4,44] The initial and follow-up data suggest that prednisone is the most important component in establishing an early reduction in disease activity and suppression of damage progression.[44,45] Similar results came from the FIN-RACo study,[3] in which recent-onset patients were treated with SSZ, 1 g/day, MTX, 7.5 mg/wk, and HCQ, 300 mg/day plus prednisolone, 5 mg/day, or SSZ, 2 g/day, with or without prednisolone.

Toxicity

The most common adverse effects of SSZ are minor gastrointestinal, central nervous system, and cutaneous side effects. The withdrawal rate because of side effects is approximately 25%.[46] Symptoms include anorexia, headache, vomiting, diarrhea, gastric distress, and nausea. Pruritic rash occurs in about 5% of patients. Leukopenia occurs in less than 3% of patients and is usually mild and transient, but serious agranulocytosis has been observed, usually in the first 6 weeks of treatment.[47] Less frequently reported problems include a decrease in immunoglobulins, megaloblastic anemia, hepatotoxicity (usually mild), eosinophilic pneumonia, and anaphylactic reactions.[48,49] Temporary oligospermia may occur in men taking SSZ. SSZ is generally thought to be safe during pregnancy. As such, it may be an alternative to MTX in women who want to become pregnant during treatment. It should be used cautiously in women who are breast-feeding, because SP concentrations in breast milk are 40% to 50% of those in maternal serum.[50]

Dosage

The standard dose of SSZ is 2 g/day, but the dose may be increased to 3 g/day. Nausea is usually transient during the first few days of treatment or when the dosage is increased and can be prevented by using a protocol of gradually increasing the dosage (e.g., start with 0.5 g/day and increase to 2 g/day over a period of 3 weeks). Patients who start SSZ should be instructed to consult a physician if they have a fever with or without sore throat, because this could be a manifestation of underlying agranulocytosis. Routine laboratory tests are recommended once a month in the initial phase and once every 3 months during chronic use.

REFERENCES

1. Grigor C, Capell H, Stirling A, et al. Effect of a treatment strategy of tight control for rheumatoid arthritis (the TICORA study): a single-blind randomised controlled trial. Lancet 2004;364:263-269.
2. Verstappen SM, Jacobs JW, van der Veen MJ, et al. Intensive treatment with methotrexate in early rheumatoid arthritis: aiming for remission. Computer Assisted Management in Early Rheumatoid Arthritis (CAMERA, an open-label strategy trial). Ann Rheum Dis 2007;66:1443-1449.
3. Möttönen T, Hannönen P, Leirisalo-Repo M, et al. Comparison of combination therapy with single-drug therapy in early rheumatoid arthritis: a randomised trial. FIN-RACo trial group. Lancet 1999;353:1568-1573.
4. Goekoop-Ruiterman YP, de Vries-Bouwstra JK, Allaart CF, et al. Clinical and radiographic outcomes of four different treatment strategies in patients with early rheumatoid arthritis (the BeSt study): a randomized, controlled trial. Arthritis Rheum 2005;52:3381-3390.
5. Herrlinger JD, Weikert W. [Protein binding of gold in serum of patients treated with different gold preparations]. Z Rheumatol 1982;41:230-234.
6. Gottlieb NL, Smith PM, Smith EM. Pharmacodynamics of ^{197}Au and ^{195}Au labeled aurothiomalate in blood: correlation with course of rheumatoid arthritis, gold toxicity and gold excretion. Arthritis Rheum 1974;17:171-183.
7. Vernon-Roberts B, Dore JL, Jessop JD, Henderson WJ. Selective concentration and localization of gold in macrophages of synovial and other tissues during and after chrysotherapy in rheumatoid patients. Ann Rheum Dis 1976;35:477-486.
8. Kirkham BW, Navarro FJ, Corkill MM, Panayi GS. In-vivo analysis of disease modifying drug therapy activity in rheumatoid arthritis by sequential immunohistologic analysis of synovial membrane interleukin 1 beta. J Rheumatol 1994;21:1615-1619.
9. Yanni G, Nabil M, Farahat MR, et al. Intramuscular gold decreases cytokine expression and macrophage numbers in the rheumatoid synovial membrane. Ann Rheum Dis 1994;53:315-322.
10. Jones G, Halbert J, Crotty M, et al. The effect of treatment on radiological progression in rheumatoid arthritis: a systematic review of randomized placebo-controlled trials. Rheumatology (Oxford) 2003;42:6-13.
11. Rau R, Herborn G, Menninger H, Sangha O. Radiographic outcome after three years of patients with early erosive rheumatoid arthritis treated with intramuscular methotrexate or parenteral gold: extension of a one-year double-blind study in 174 patients. Rheumatology (Oxford) 2002;41:196-204.
12. Clark P, Tugwell P, Bennet K, et al. Injectable gold for rheumatoid arthritis. Cochrane Database Syst Rev 2000;(2):CD000520.
13. Felson DT, Anderson JJ, Meenan RF. The comparative efficacy and toxicity of second-line drugs in rheumatoid arthritis: results of two meta-analyses. Arthritis Rheum 1990;33:1449-1461.
14. Klinkhoff AV, Teufel A. How low can you go? Use of very low dosage of gold in patients with mucocutaneous reactions. J Rheumatol 1995;22:1657-1659.
15. Hall CL. The natural course of gold and penicillamine nephropathy: a long-term study of 54 patients. Adv Exp Med Biol 1989;252:247-256.
16. Ho M, Pullar T. Vasomotor reactions with gold. Br J Rheumatol 1997;36:154-156.
17. Adachi JD, Bensen WG, Kassam Y, et al. Gold induced thrombocytopenia: 12 cases and a review of the literature. Semin Arthritis Rheum 1987;16:287-293.
18. Almarzouqi M, Scarsbrook D, Klinkhoff A. Gold therapy in women planning pregnancy: outcomes in one center. J Rheumatol 2007;34:1827-1831.
19. Furst DE. Pharmacokinetics of hydroxychloroquine and chloroquine during treatment of rheumatic diseases. Lupus 1996;5(Suppl 1):S11-S15.
20. Tett SE, Cutler DJ, Day RO, Brown KF. Bioavailability of hydroxychloroquine tablets in healthy volunteers. Br J Clin Pharmacol 1989;27:771-779.
21. Furst DE, Lindsley H, Baethge B, et al. Dose-loading with hydroxychloroquine improves the rate of response in early, active rheumatoid arthritis: a randomized, double-blind six-week trial with eighteen-week extension. Arthritis Rheum 1999;42:357-365.
22. Leden I. Digoxin-hydroxychloroquine interaction? Acta Med Scand 1982;211:411-412.
23. Somer M, Kallio J, Pesonen U, et al. Influence of hydroxychloroquine on the bioavailability of oral metoprolol. Br J Clin Pharmacol 2000;49:549-554.
24. Fox RI, Kang HI. Mechanism of action of antimalarial drugs: inhibition of antigen processing and presentation. Lupus 1993;2(Suppl 1):S9-S12.
25. Weber SM, Levitz SM. Chloroquine interferes with lipopolysaccharide-induced TNF-alpha gene expression by a nonlysosomotropic mechanism. J Immunol 2000;165:1534-1540.
26. Suarez-Almazor ME, Belseck E, Shea B, et al. Antimalarials for treating rheumatoid arthritis. Cochrane Database Syst Rev 2000;(4):CD000959.
27. Ferraz MB, Pinheiro GR, Helfenstein M, et al. Combination therapy with methotrexate and chloroquine in rheumatoid arthritis: a multicenter randomized placebo-controlled trial. Scand J Rheumatol 1994;23:231-236.
28. Clegg DO, Dietz F, Duffy J, et al. Safety and efficacy of hydroxychloroquine as maintenance therapy for rheumatoid arthritis after combination therapy with methotrexate and hydroxychloroquine. J Rheumatol 1997;24:1896-1902.
29. O'Dell JR, Haire CE, Erikson N, et al. Treatment of rheumatoid arthritis with methotrexate alone, sulfasalazine and hydroxychloroquine, or a combination of all three medications. N Engl J Med 1996;334:1287-1291.
30. Faarvang KL, Egsmose C, Kryger P, et al. Hydroxychloroquine and sulphasalazine alone and in combination in rheumatoid arthritis: a randomised double blind trial. Ann Rheum Dis 1993;52:711-715.
31. Avina-Zubieta JA, Galindo-Rodriguez G, Newman S, et al. Long-term effectiveness of antimalarial drugs in rheumatic diseases. Ann Rheum Dis 1998;57:582-587.
32. Block JA. Hydroxychloroquine and retinal safety. Lancet 1998;351:771.
33. Marmor MF. New American Academy of Ophthalmology recommendations on screening for hydroxychloroquine retinopathy. Arthritis Rheum 2003;48:1764.
34. Stein M, Bell MJ, Ang LC. Hydroxychloroquine neuromyotoxicity. J Rheumatol 2000;27:2927-2931.
35. Costedoat-Chalumeau N, Amoura Z, Huong DL, et al. Safety of hydroxychloroquine in pregnant patients with connective tissue diseases: review of the literature. Autoimmun Rev 2005;4:111-115.
36. Box SA, Pullar T. Sulphasalazine in the treatment of rheumatoid arthritis. Br J Rheumatol 1997;36:382-386.
37. Farr M, Brodrick A, Bacon PA. Plasma and synovial fluid concentrations of sulphasalazine and two of its metabolites in rheumatoid arthritis. Rheumatol Int 1985;5:247-251.
38. Suarez-Almazor ME, Belseck E, Shea B, et al. Sulfasalazine for rheumatoid arthritis. Cochrane Database Syst Rev 2000;(2):CD000958.
39. Haagsma CJ, van Riel PL, de Jong AJ, van de Putte LB. Combination of sulphasalazine and methotrexate versus the single components in early rheumatoid arthritis: a randomized, controlled, double-blind, 52 week clinical trial. Br J Rheumatol 1997;36:1082-1088.
40. Dougados M, Combe B, Cantagrel A, et al. Combination therapy in early rheumatoid arthritis: a randomised, controlled, double blind 52 week clinical trial of sulphasalazine and methotrexate compared with the single components. Ann Rheum Dis 1999;58:220-225.
41. American College of Radiology. Guidelines for the management of rheumatoid arthritis: 2002 update. Arthritis Rheum 2002;46:328-346.
42. Combe B, Landewe R, Lukas C, et al. EULAR recommendations for the management of early arthritis: report of a task force of the European Standing Committee for International Clinical Studies Including Therapeutics (ESCISIT). Ann Rheum Dis 2007;66:34-45.
43. van der Kooij SM, de Vries-Bouwstra JK, Goekoop-Ruiterman YP, et al. Limited efficacy of conventional DMARDs after initial methotrexate failure in patients with recent onset rheumatoid arthritis treated according to the disease activity score. Ann Rheum Dis 2007;66:1356-1362.
44. Boers M, Verhoeven AC, Markusse HM, et al. Randomised comparison of combined step-down prednisolone, methotrexate and sulphasalazine with sulphasalazine alone in early rheumatoid arthritis. Lancet 1997;350:309-318.
45. Landewe RB, Boers M, Verhoeven AC, et al. COBRA combination therapy in patients with early rheumatoid arthritis: long-term structural benefits of a brief intervention. Arthritis Rheum 2002;46:347-356.
46. Donovan S, Hawley S, MacCarthy J, Scott DL. Tolerability of enteric-coated sulphasalazine in rheumatoid arthritis: results of a co-operating clinics study. Br J Rheumatol 1990;29:201-204.
47. Amos RS, Pullar T, Bax DE, et al. Sulphasalazine for rheumatoid arthritis: toxicity in 774 patients monitored for one to 11 years. BMJ 1986;293:420-423.
48. Aletaha D, Kapral T, Smolen JS. Toxicity profiles of traditional disease modifying antirheumatic drugs for rheumatoid arthritis. Ann Rheum Dis 2003;62:482-486.
49. Jobanputra P, Amarasena R, Maggs F, et al. Hepatotoxicity associated with sulfasalazine in inflammatory arthritis: a case series from a local surveillance of serious adverse events. BMC Musculoskelet Disord 2008;9:48.
50. Janssen NM, Genta MS. The effects of immunosuppressive and anti-inflammatory medications on fertility, pregnancy, and lactation. Arch Intern Med 2000;160:610-619.

Methotrexate*

Alyssa K. Johnsen and Michael E. Weinblatt

- Methotrexate, a structural analog of folic acid, can be administered orally or parenterally to treat a variety of rheumatic diseases.
- Although the exact mechanism responsible for the therapeutic action of methotrexate is unknown, suppression of inflammation mediated by increases in adenosine, may play a central role.
- The effectiveness of methotrexate in treating rheumatoid arthritis was established by randomized controlled trials.
- Careful monitoring of methotrexate therapy is required, although most adverse events are mild and do not require discontinuation of the drug.
- Serious liver disease and idiosyncratic pulmonary hypersensitivity are rare potential adverse effects.
- Methotrexate is a known teratogen and effective contraception should be considered in women with the potential for pregnancy.

INTRODUCTION

Methotrexate (MTX), first used to treat malignant disease more than 50 years ago, has since become the cornerstone of therapy of rheumatoid arthritis (RA), being administered to at least 500,000 patients with RA worldwide.[2] Low-dose MTX has been shown to be highly efficacious and, when monitored appropriately, has an excellent safety profile. For these reasons, it has become the most commonly prescribed disease-modifying anti-rheumatic drug (DMARD) in the treatment of RA.[2]

PHARMACOLOGY

MTX is structurally similar to folic acid, differing only by the substitution of an amine for a hydroxyl group in the pteridine ring and the addition of a methyl group on the 10(th) nitrogen of para-amino-benzoic acid.

The bioavailability of MTX is relatively high but can vary among individuals. The bioavailability of intramuscular versus subcutaneous injection is equivalent.[3] At 7.5 mg/week, oral and parenteral absorption is the same, but at doses of 15 mg/week or more, oral absorption may decrease by as much as 30% compared with parenteral dosing.[2] For example, at doses of 25 mg or more each week, the bioavailability of oral MTX ranged from 0.21 to 0.96 when compared with subcutaneous administration.[4] A prospective, randomized, controlled trial showed that subcutaneous administration was significantly more effective than oral delivery at a dose of 15 mg each week, with 24-week American College of Rheumatology (ACR)-20 percentages of 78% versus 70%, respectively, and no difference in tolerability.[5] Oral absorption is limited because MTX is absorbed from the gastrointestinal tract primarily from a saturable active transport system. Although oral absorption is not affected by food intake, it can be reduced in the setting of intestinal pathology. After absorption, 10% of MTX is converted to 7-hydroxymethotrexate in the liver. Approximately 50% of MTX is albumin-bound, whereas 90% to 95% of 7-hydroxymethotrexate is albumin-bound.[6] The half-life of MTX in the serum ranges from 6 to 8 hours after administration, and MTX is undetectable in the serum by 24 hours.[7] The majority of both MTX and 7-hydroxymethotrexate

is excreted in the urine, although a small portion is also excreted in the bile.[7] Renal clearance is likely due to a combination of filtration and secretion in the proximal tubule with subsequent reabsorption in the distal tubule. Renal insufficiency can therefore lead to toxicity caused by impaired clearance of MTX. The drug is generally not cleared in dialysis and therefore dialysis is an absolute contraindication to MTX use. Excretion of MTX is inhibited by weak organic acids such as aspirin, non-steroidal anti-inflammatory drugs, piperacillin, penicillin G, probenecid, and perhaps cephalosporins. This interaction is generally only clinically relevant with higher-dose MTX.[2] Sulfonamides may also decrease renal tubular secretion and therefore increase levels of MTX. In addition, trimethoprim/sulfamethoxazole (Bactrim) interferes with folic acid metabolism and therefore may increase the risk of bone marrow suppression with concomitant MTX.

Folates and antifolates enter cells via two separate mechanisms. The reduced folate carrier (RFC) is a bidirectional anion exchanger that demonstrates a higher affinity for MTX than for folic acid. MTX may also bind to folate receptors (FR-α and FR-β) and then be transported inside the cell by endocytosis, but this mechanism has higher affinity for folic acid than MTX and is therefore thought to be less important for the action of the drug.[8] Sulfasalazine is a non-competitive inhibitor of the RFC that has been shown to decrease MTX effects in cultured cells.[9] In fact, no increased efficacy was found when the combination of MTX and sulfasalazine was compared with monotherapy with either agent,[10] although triple therapy with MTX, sulfasalazine, and hydroxychloroquine was more efficacious than dual therapy with hydroxychloroquine and sulfasalazine (see "Efficacy in Rheumatoid Arthritis" later).[11]

Inside cells, one to four glutamyl residues are added to MTX. These polyglutamated forms are not readily transported across the cell membrane and therefore can accumulate intracellularly. This modification is particularly important because the polyglutamated forms demonstrate significantly increased affinity for certain folate-dependent enzymes, including thymidylate synthase (TS), 5-aminoimidazole carboxamide ribonucleotide transformylase (AICAR transformylase), and glycinamide ribonucleotide transformylase (GAR transformylase).[12] MTX in its ingested form is therefore essentially a prodrug, with its polyglutamated form being the active compound.

The dose required for efficacy is variable among individuals, but the concentration of polyglutamated MTX within red blood cells has been correlated with disease activity.[13-15] The median half-life of accumulation for polyglutamated MTX within red blood cells was determined to range from 1.9 to 45.2 weeks, suggesting that significant time may be required to reach a steady state after a dose change.[16]

Mechanism of action

MTX is an analog of folic acid (Fig. 53.1) and therefore can interfere with its ability to serve as a co-factor for a variety of enzymes that are essential for purine and pyrimidine synthesis and cell replication. One of the first mechanisms proposed for MTX, therefore, was inhibition of proliferation of cells responsible for synovial inflammation, such as lymphocytes. MTX and its polyglutamate derivatives bind to dihydrofolate reductase (DHFR) with high affinity and inhibit its action, thereby depriving the cell of tetrahydrofolate (Fig. 53.2).[17] MTX and its derivatives also antagonize thymidylate synthase (TS), a critical enzyme in the *de novo* production of dTMP from dUMP.[18] In addition, MTX has been shown to block amidophosphoribosyltransferase, the first step of *de novo* purine synthesis.[19] In support of MTX's action on nucleotide synthesis, the drug was able to block activation-induced cell division of human peripheral blood lymphocytes (PBLs) *in vitro*, and this was reversible if thymidine was added to cultures.[20] In addition, *in vitro*

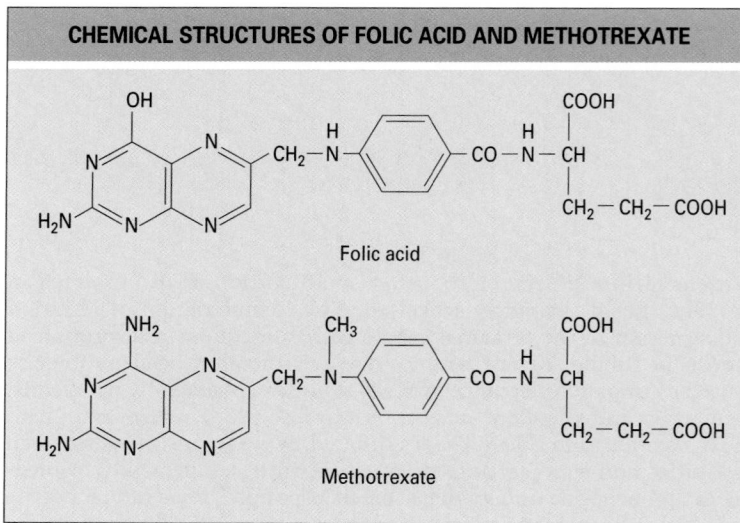

CHEMICAL STRUCTURES OF FOLIC ACID AND METHOTREXATE

Folic acid

Methotrexate

Fig. 53.1 Chemical structures of folic acid and methotrexate. *(From Battistone MJ, Williams HJ. DMARDs 3: methotrexate. In: Hochberg M, Silman AJ, Smolen JS, et al, eds. Rheumatology. Philadelphia: Elsevier, 2008:449-460.)*[152]

activation of PBLs from RA patients 24 hours after a weekly intramuscular MTX injection resulted in apoptosis that could be inhibited by folic and folinic acid.[21] However, the fact that folic acid supplementation generally does not reverse the anti-inflammatory effects of MTX has encouraged the exploration of other potential mechanisms.[22,23]

In addition to being a critical co-factor in pyrimidine synthesis, tetrahydrofolate is responsible for donating a methyl group for the conversion of homocysteine to methionine (see Fig 53.2). Methionine is then converted to S-adenosylmethionine, which donates a methyl group to the synthesis of the polyamines spermine and spermidine.[17] This is of interest because these polyamines are scavengers of reactive oxygen species that can be toxic to lymphocytes.[24] Thus MTX, by decreasing levels of tetrahydrofolate, is hypothesized to indirectly increase reactive oxygen species, which will lead to apoptosis of activated lymphocytes.[24] A related mechanism derives from the fact that MTX increases homocysteine levels and therefore S-adenosylhomocysteine, which can inhibit the methylation of the Ras G-protein. In cultured cell lines, MTX treatment leads to Ras mis-localization to the cytosol.[25] These proposed mechanisms for MTX function led to the trial of 3-deazaadenosine, an inhibitor of S-adenosylhomocysteine hydrolase, in the treatment of RA. Unfortunately, the drug did not diminish RA disease activity.[17]

An alternative mechanism for the anti-inflammatory actions of MTX has recently gained favor. MTX-polyglutamates bind 5-amino-imidazole-4-carboxamide ribonucleotide (AICAR) transformylase, which leads to increased levels of AICAR, an inhibitor of AMP deaminase, and AICA riboside, an inhibitor of adenosine deaminase (see Fig. 53.2).[17] This inhibition would be expected to increase the levels of intracellular AMP and adenosine and to increase levels of extracellular adenosine that will bind to cell surface receptors (as reviewed in reference 26).[17] Adenosine A_{2A} receptors are expressed on T cells, NK cells, monocytes, macrophages, and neutrophils and receptor ligation has been shown to dampen inflammation by a variety of mechanisms, including suppression of T-cell activation and cell-mediated cytotoxicity, inhibition of neutrophil oxidative burst, and suppression of NF-κB and its downstream effects.[27]

Major support for the adenosine hypothesis comes from animal models of inflammation. Mice treated with MTX demonstrated decreased leukocyte accumulation in carrageenan-inflamed air pouches but with increased adenosine in the inflamed tissue.[28,29] This effect was abrogated in mice deficient in adenosine receptors A_{2A} or A_3,[29] as well as in mice lacking ecto-5'-nucleotidase, an enzyme responsible for the extracellular conversion of adenine to adenosine.[30] In a rat adjuvant-induced arthritis model, the beneficial effect of MTX could be reversed by treatment with the non-selective adenosine antagonists theophylline or caffeine, but not by selective antagonists of adenosine receptors A_1, A_{2A}, or A_{2B}.[31] The *in vivo* data in humans has been less definitive.

TABLE 53.1 EFFECTS OF METHOTREXATE TREATMENT

Cytokines	
T cells	Decreased IL-4, IL-6, IL-13, TNF-α, IFN-γ, GM-CSF (as reviewed[24])
Whole peripheral blood mononuclear cells	Increased IL-4 and IL-10 and decrease in IL-2 and IFN-γ[153,154] Reduction in 34 genes regulated by NFκB[155]
Co-culture of synovial fibroblasts and T cells	Decreased IL-15, IL-6, IL-8, CD69, CD25, IFN-γ, and IL-17[24]
Monocytes	Increased in IL-1Ra and decrease of IL-1β[156] Decreased zymosan-stimulated IL-1 activity[157]
Sera	Reduction of IL-6, sIL-2R, TNFR p55[158,159]
Fc Receptors	
Monocytes	Decreased FcγRI and FcγRIIA on monocytes[160]
Adhesion molecules	
T cells	Decreased ICAM-1, CLA[161]
Synovium	Reduced ICAM-1, VCAM-1[162]
Bone formation	
Co-culture of PBMCs and fibroblast-like synoviocytes	Decreased RANKL, increased OPG[163]
Osteoblasts	Decreased stimulated IL-6 production (as reviewed [24])
Angiogenesis	
Human umbilical vein endothelial cells	Inhibition of endothelial cell proliferation[164]
Degradative enzymes	
Sera	Decreased MMP-3[165]
Synovium	Decreased collagenase RNA expression[166] Decreased MMP-1–to–TIMP-1 ratio[162]
Neutrophil function	
Synovial fluid	Decrease in neutrophil chemotaxis[167]
	Inhibition of leukotriene B4 synthesis[168,169]
Lymphocyte function	
B cells	Decrease in IgM-RF and IgA-RF[170]
T cells	Decreased survival of primary mouse T cells[20]
Prostaglandins	
Synovium	Decrease in IL-1β stimulated production of prostaglandin E_2[171]

GM-CSF, granulocyte-macrophage colony-stimulating factor.

Patients taking low-dose MTX for psoriasis excrete increased amino-imidazole carboxamide in their urine,[32] but caffeine intake does not influence the dose of MTX required to treat psoriasis or psoriatic arthritis.[33] Although initial studies in RA showed diminished effects of MTX in patients with high caffeine intake,[34] a larger prospective trial did not show any association between caffeine intake and MTX efficacy.[35] Further support for the effect of MTX on adenosine was illustrated when patients with inflammatory arthritis treated with MTX 15 mg/week showed enhancement in dipyridamole-induced vasodilation, an effect dependent on extracellular adenosine levels.[36]

Regardless of the specific molecular mechanism whereby low-dose MTX interferes with cellular metabolism, it is clear that it produces a myriad of dampening effects on the immune system and inflammation, some examples of which are summarized in Table 53.1.

Efficacy in rheumatoid arthritis

The efficacy of aminopterin, the parent compound of MTX, in RA was first reported in 1951 when five of six patients treated with the drug

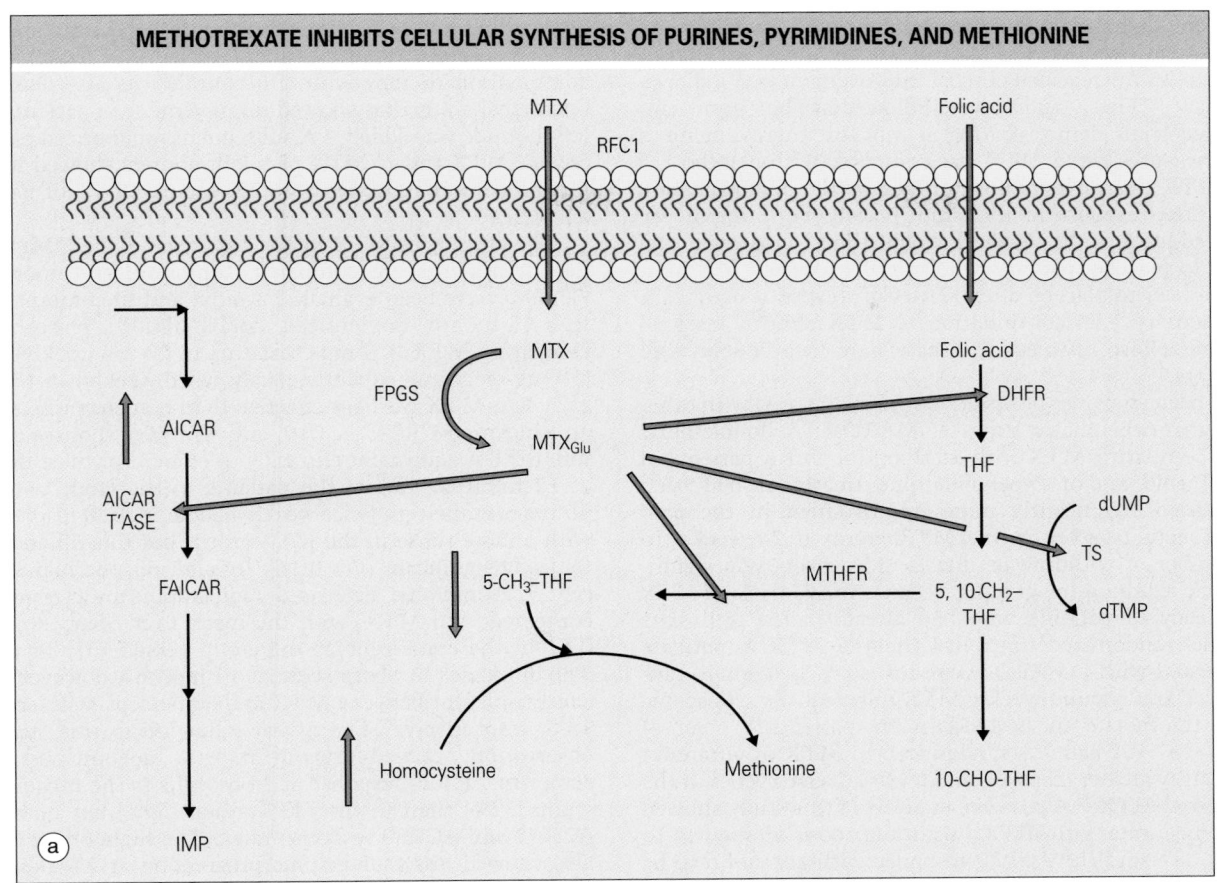

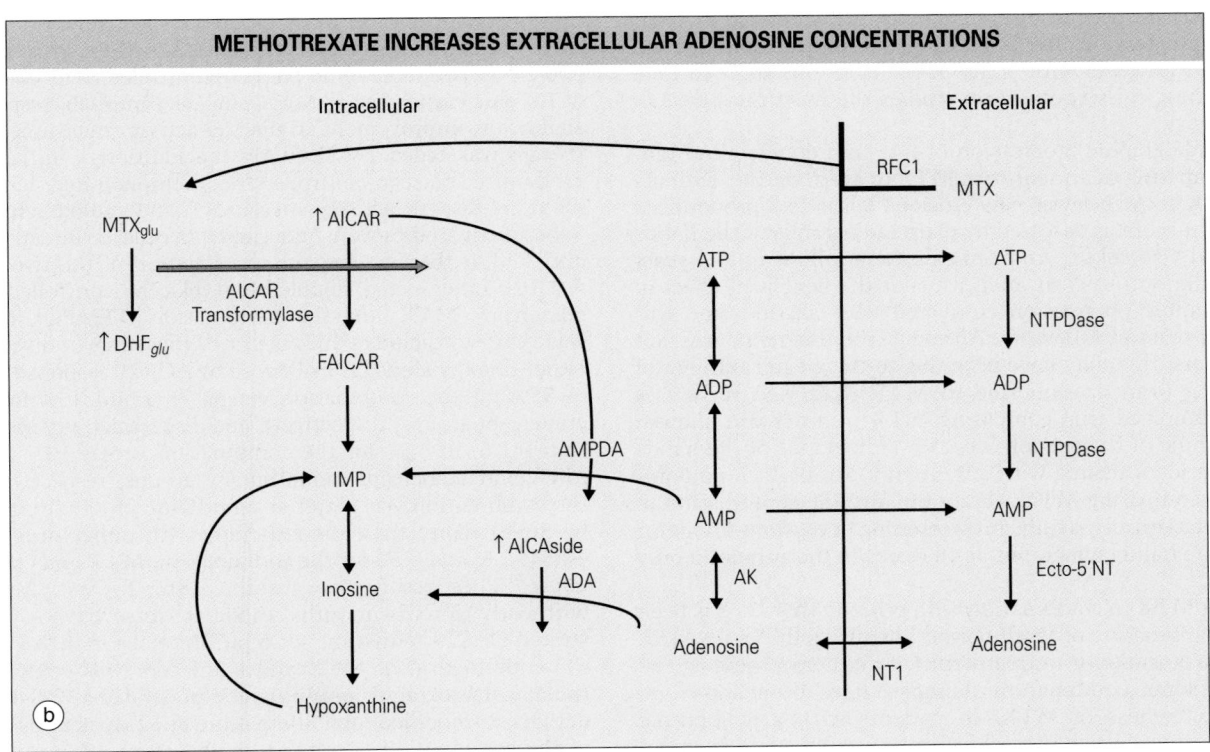

Fig. 53.2 (a) Methotrexate inhibits cellular synthesis of purines, pyrimidines, and methionine. AICAR, 5-aminoimidazole-4-carboxamide ribonucleotide; AICAR T'ASE, AICAR transformylase; DHFR, dihydrofolate reductase; FPGS, folyl polyglutamate synthase; MTHFR, methylene tetrahydrofolate reductase; MTX, methotrexate; MTX_{Glu}, methotrexate polyglutamate; RFC1, reduced folate carrier 1; THF, tetrahydrofolate; TS, thymidylate synthase. (b) Methotrexate increases extracellular adenosine concentrations. ADA, adenosine deaminase; AICAside, aminoimidazole carboxamidoribonucleoside; AK, adenosine kinase; AMPDA, AMP deaminase; DHF_{Glu}, dihydrofolate polyglutamate; FAICAR, formyl AICAR; MTX, methotrexate; MTX_{Glu}, methotrexate polyglutamate; NTPDase, nucleoside triphosphate dephosphorylase; Ecto-5'NT, ecto-5'-nucleotidase; NT1, nucleoside transporter 1; RFC1, reduced folate carrier 1. (*Adapted from Cronstein BN. Low-dose methotrexate: a mainstay in the treatment of rheumatoid arthritis. Pharmacol Rev 2005;57:163-172.*)

at 1 to 2 mg per day demonstrated decreased joint pain, swelling, and stiffness.[37] Subsequent open-label studies of weekly MTX with doses ranging from 7.5 to 25 mg revealed clinical improvement in a majority of treated patients.[38-46] These studies were followed by short-term randomized controlled trials demonstrating significant improvement in disease activity measures when MTX was compared with placebo.[47-50] The efficacy of MTX was further substantiated by the demonstration of a clear linear dose-response relationship (placebo vs. 5 mg/m² vs. 10 mg/m²).[51] In addition, in a 24-week double-blind crossover trial comparing MTX to placebo, patients who initially received MTX but were then crossed over to placebo after 12 weeks showed a significant flare in disease activity.[48] Discontinuation of MTX after at least 36 months of treatment also resulted in disease flare in a double-blind study of 10 patients.[52]

MTX has also been shown to be effective when compared with other disease-modifying antirheumatic drugs (DMARDs). A double-blind randomized trial comparing MTX with azathioprine in RA patients in whom parenteral gold and/or D-penicillamine treatment had been unsuccessful revealed significantly more improvement in the pain score and disease activity score in the MTX group at 24 weeks. In addition, the number of withdrawals due to side effects was significantly higher in the azathioprine group.[53] Because initial trials of MTX evaluated its efficacy in patients who had already failed gold salts or D-penicillamine, randomized controlled trials of MTX in patients not previously treated with DMARDs were initiated. Two small, randomized, controlled trials found weekly MTX to be equally efficacious to gold sodium thiomalate in DMARD-naïve patients.[54,55] Subsequently, a trial of 281 RA patients randomized to MTX or auranofin showed a significantly greater response and fewer adverse events in the patients who received MTX.[56] A *post hoc* analysis of this study showed the ACR 20 response rate with MTX (maximum dose 15 mg/wk) to be approximately 68% and the ACR20 response with auranofin to be approximately 30%.[57] More recently, MTX was shown to be superior to leflunomide with respect to disease activity measures after 1 year and radiographic progression after 2 years in a randomized double-blind trial involving 999 patients with active RA.[58] It is important to note that in most of these early comparison studies the maximum dose of MTX was 15 mg/wk.

MTX slows radiographic progression of RA. In a double-blind randomized trial comparing treatment with MTX to azathioprine, patients treated with MTX showed fewer new erosions and a less pronounced change in the joint score as assessed by plain radiographs of the hands and feet at 24 and 48 weeks.[53] An open extension follow-up to 4 years showed, in an intention-to-treat analysis, that the beneficial effect of MTX on radiographic progression compared with azathioprine was sustained after 2 years of follow-up. Although the difference was not sustained at 4 years, this may have been due to the greater number of patients switching from azathioprine to MTX than vice versa.[59] A double-blind randomized trial comparing MTX to auranofin showed significant worsening of the erosion score on radiographs of the hands and feet in the patients treated with auranofin.[60] Similarly, a randomized clinical trial comparing MTX, auranofin, and the combination of the two showed statistically significant worsening of erosions and joint space narrowing on hand radiographs at 48 weeks in the auranofin only group.[61]

The efficacy of MTX in combination with other DMARDs has been evaluated. The combination of azathioprine[62] or auranofin[63] with MTX was not shown to be superior to treatment with either of these agents alone. However, some combination therapies have been shown to increase the effectiveness of MTX. In patients with a suboptimal response to MTX, the addition of weekly intramuscular gold[64] or cyclosporine[65] resulted in increased efficacy. In addition, DMARD-naïve patients treated with the combination of MTX, intra-articular betamethasone, and cyclosporine were more likely to achieve an ACR20 than those treated with MTX and intra-articular betamethasone alone.[66] Although no significant difference was found comparing patients treated with a combination of MTX and sulfasalazine to patients on monotherapy with these agents,[10] a study of triple therapy with MTX, hydroxychloroquine, and sulfasalazine showed that patients treated with the combination of all three were more likely to sustain clinical improvement than those treated with either MTX alone or dual therapy with hydroxychloroquine and sulfasalazine.[11] Therapy with

doxycycline and MTX was also found to be superior at achieving an ACR50 response than treatment with MTX alone.[67] The efficacy of combination therapy with leflunomide was also demonstrated in an open-label study that showed improvement in patients on MTX when leflunomide was added.[68] A subsequent randomized placebo-controlled trial of MTX versus MTX plus leflunomide showed increased efficacy for the combination, with 46.2% versus 19.5% of patients achieving an ACR20.[69]

The efficacy of MTX in RA has made it the DMARD to which all new treatments are compared. Inhibitors of tumor necrosis factor (TNF)-α have been evaluated against and in combination with MTX. In a 12-month, randomized, double-blinded, placebo-controlled trial comparing MTX (7.5 mg escalating to 20 mg weekly) with etanercept (10 mg or 25 mg subcutaneously twice weekly) in 652 patients with early RA, MTX was less effective than etanercept 25 mg twice weekly at achieving ACR20, ACR50, and ACR70 responses during the first 4 months but equivalent clinically to etanercept thereafter. For example, at 12 months, 72% of the patients in the group assigned to receive 25 mg of etanercept twice weekly had an ACR20 response, as compared with 65% of those in the MTX group, but this difference was not statistically significant ($P = 0.16$). In addition, the higher dose of etanercept demonstrated decreased radiographic progression at 6 months compared with MTX, with the mean total Sharp score increasing by 0.57 in the etanercept 25-mg group versus 1.06 in the MTX group. The difference in Sharp score at 12 months, however, was not significantly different between MTX and etanercept, with scores of 1.59 and 1.00, respectively.[70] The 2-year follow-up to this study using a last-observation, carried-forward analysis documented more patients achieving ACR20 response at 24 months in the higher-dose etanercept group (72%) than in the MTX group (59%) but no difference in the ACR50 and ACR70 response rates. The higher-dose etanercept group also showed less radiographic progression at 24 months, with mean changes from baseline in the Sharp scores of 1.3 and 3.2 units in the 25-mg etanercept and MTX groups, respectively.[71]

In order to evaluate the combination of MTX with anti-TNF therapy, two 24-week double-blind placebo-controlled trials comparing MTX to MTX plus etanercept or MTX plus adalimumab, respectively, showed significant improvement in disease activity measures when anti-TNF therapy was added.[72,73] Similarly, the addition of infliximab to MTX in randomized placebo-controlled trials demonstrated significant improvement in disease activity measures[74] and radiographic progression.[75] Subsequent studies were undertaken in order to directly compare MTX, anti-TNF-α therapy, and the combination of the two in treatment of RA. In a randomized, double-blind, placebo-controlled trial comparing etanercept, MTX, and the combination (TEMPO), the combination was more efficacious with respect to measures of disease activity than either therapy alone, as evidenced by ACR20 response rates at week 52 of 85% for the combination versus 75% and 76% for the MTX and etanercept groups, respectively, and disease activity score (DAS) remission (<1.6) in 35% for the combination versus 13% and 16% for the MTX and etanercept monotherapy groups, respectively. In addition, the combination was better at retardation of joint damage, as assessed by Sharp score, than monotherapy with either drug, with scores of −0.54, 2.8, and 0.52 for the combination, MTX and etanercept, respectively.[76] These results were sustained after 2 years.[77] A study in patients with early (3 to 24 months) moderate-to-severe RA (Comet) demonstrated DAS28 remission (<2.6) at 52 weeks in 50% versus 28% when the combination of MTX and etanercept was compared with MTX therapy. Radiographic non-progression defined as 0.5 or less on the van der Heijde-modified total Sharp score at 52 weeks was achieved in 80% of the combination treatment group versus 59% in the MTX monotherapy group.[78] Similar results were found for the combination of adalimumab and MTX when compared with either drug alone (PREMIER).[79] The combination of infliximab and MTX was also found to be more efficacious than treatment with MTX plus placebo (ASPIRE).[80] These studies have been useful not only in demonstrating the efficacy of anti-TNF-α therapy and MTX in combination but also in providing excellent data on the efficacy of MTX therapy as a single agent, with ACR20 percentages ranging from 54 to 73 (Table 53.2).

Efficacy of MTX in combination with two newer therapies for RA, anti-CD20 antibody (rituximab) and CTLA4-Ig (abatacept), has also been demonstrated. Patients with an incomplete response to MTX

TABLE 53.2 METHOTREXATE EFFICACY AS MONOTHERAPY IN STUDIES OF ANTI-TNF EFFICACY

	TEMPO*	PREMIER†	ASPIRE‡
ACR20 (%)	75	63	54
ACR50 (%)	43	46	32
ACR70 (%)	19	28	21
DAS (%)	13	21	15

*Study comparing methotrexate, etanercept, and the combination of both drugs.[76]
†Study comparing methotrexate, adalimumab, and the combination of both drugs.[79]
‡Study comparing methotrexate to methotrexate plus infliximab.[80]

showed significant improvement at 24 weeks when rituximab was added to their regimen, with ACR20 scores of 54% versus 28% and change in DAS28 scores of −2.05 versus −0.67 for two 1000-mg infusions of rituximab plus MTX versus MTX alone, respectively (Dancer).[81] In a study of rituximab in patients with active disease on MTX who had failed anti-TNF therapy (Reflex), the combination of rituximab and MTX again showed enhanced efficacy compared with MTX alone, as measured by the ACR20, ACR50, ACR70, and DAS28 scores at 24 weeks; however, no significant difference in the total Genant-modified Sharp radiographic scores was demonstrated.[82] It is interesting to note that MTX as monotherapy was less efficacious in these studies, as measured by the ACR and DAS28 scores, in comparison with the anti-TNF trials, in spite of therapeutic doses of MTX (mean doses of ≈15 mg each week). When the combination of abatacept and MTX was compared with MTX monotherapy, the ACR20 was 67.9% versus 39.7%, respectively, at 24 weeks, and 73.1% versus 39.7%, respectively, at 1 year. In addition, the mean change from baseline total Genant-modified Sharp scores at 1 year was 1.21 versus 2.32 in the combination therapy versus MTX monotherapy groups, respectively.[83]

Although many of the studies documenting the efficacy of MTX were of relatively short duration, long-term prospective studies have demonstrated sustained effects on disease activity and radiographic progression. Weinblatt and colleagues[84] prospectively followed a cohort of 26 RA patients and reported on their status after 36, 84, and 132 months of MTX therapy. For the 10 patients who completed the study to 132 months, significant improvement compared with baseline (P < 0.001) was noted in the number of painful joints, swollen joints, and physician and patient global assessments. There was 50% improvement in the joint pain index and joint swelling index in more than 65% of the patients. There was no significant difference, however, in the improvement in clinical variables between 12 and 132 months. From the original cohort, withdrawal caused by MTX toxicity occurred in three patients, including two for pneumonitis and one for alopecia. Only one withdrawal occurred because of lack of efficacy.[84] In a study by Kremer and colleagues,[85] an original cohort of 29 patients was reported on after 29, 53, and 90 months of MTX therapy. For the 18 patients who were still being followed at 90 months, a significant improvement from baseline was maintained in all clinical parameters except the number of tender joints. In addition, a significant improvement compared with 53 months of treatment was found for the number of tender joints, grip strength, and functional class. In spite of continued MTX therapy, 9 of the 17 patients in whom sequential radiographs were obtained showed radiographic progression. From the original cohort, four patients withdrew due to MTX toxicity, including two for MTX pneumonitis and two for nausea. Two patients withdrew because of decreased efficacy.[85] An additional report after 13.3 years on 5 patients from this cohort still on MTX continued to show clinical benefit compared with baseline.[86] A larger multicenter prospective trial including 123 patients who were followed for 5 years showed significant improvement compared with baseline in all clinical disease variables, functional status, and erythrocyte sedimentation rate. Sixty-four percent of patients completed this study and were still taking MTX. Seven percent of patients withdrew because of lack of efficacy and 7% because of adverse events.[87]

In addition to demonstrating clinical efficacy, many clinical trials have shown that MTX decreases markers of inflammation, including the erythrocyte sedimentation rate and C-reactive protein (CRP). The decrement in CRP is rapid, with the minimum value being noted on day 3 after once-weekly dosing.[88,89]

Treatment with MTX was associated with reduced mortality in a retrospective study of 1240 patients with RA, but only after adjustment for confounding by indication.[90] MTX was prescribed to 588 patients, and these patients were more likely to have higher disease activity. The unadjusted mortality hazard ratio of MTX compared with no MTX use was 0.8 with 95% confidence intervals of 0.6 to 1.0. However, when a weighted Cox proportional hazards model was used to adjust for potential confounders, including measures of disease activity, the adjusted mortality hazard ratio was 0.4 (0.2 to 0.8). Forty-four percent of the 191 deaths were due to cardiovascular causes. The hazard ratio for cardiovascular mortality was 0.3 (0.2 to 0.7) versus 0.6 (0.2 to 1.2) for non-cardiovascular death.

In addition to systemic treatment with MTX, localized intra-articular administration has been evaluated. Although studies on a small number of patients initially demonstrated improvement of persistent knee synovitis after treatment with intra-articular MTX,[91,92] a subsequent study showed inferiority in comparison with intra-articular triamcinolone.[93] In addition, no advantage of adding intra-articular MTX to intra-articular hydrocortisone or triamcinolone could be demonstrated.[94,95]

Adverse effects

Although MTX has clearly shown substantial benefit in the treatment of RA, an understanding of the potential adverse effects is critical for safe long-term maintenance of therapy. The most common reactions associated with low-dose, weekly MTX are anorexia, nausea, vomiting, and diarrhea, reported in 10% of patients studied in early short-term controlled trials and small long-term, open-label studies. Most of these reactions occurred shortly after the drug was administered and were mild, although in 2.5% of patients led to discontinuation. In this same group of patients, stomatitis occurred in 6% and alopecia in 1%.[96]

Hematologic abnormalities were found in 3% of the patients in this study and included leukopenia (most common), anemia, and thrombocytopenia.[96] A review of the literature was conducted to identify published cases of pancytopenia in response to low-dose MTX for RA. Seventy patients with pancytopenia were identified from 1980 to 1995 and 12 of these patients died. Toxicity data from long-term prospective studies showed an incidence of pancytopenia of 1.4%.[97] In a study of 481 patients followed for an average of 58 months of MTX therapy, 2 patients had thrombocytopenia and 13 patients had leukopenia, with 2 of 2 of the thrombocytopenic patients and 3 of 13 of the leukopenic patients discontinuing the drug. Hypoalbuminemia correlated independently with an increased percentage of abnormal platelet counts.[98] Other risk factors for MTX hematologic toxicity include drug overdoses, incorrect dosing such as daily dosing, renal insufficiency, dialysis, and concomitant drugs such as trimethoprim/sulfa.

In this same population, 74 patients were noted to have an elevated aspartate aminotransferase (AST), and this resulted in permanent discontinuation of MTX in 17. Independent predictors of a significantly higher percentage of abnormal AST values were lack of folate supplementation and untreated hyperlipidemia.[98] In order to determine the risk of serious liver disease in patients with RA taking MTX, members of the American College of Rheumatology were surveyed to identify cases of cirrhosis and liver failure. A case-control study was then conducted by reviewing medical records to determine prognostic factors. Twenty-four cases of cirrhosis and liver failure were identified, giving a 5-year cumulative incidence of approximately 1 per 1000 treated patients. Six of the 24 patients died, including 4 who died from the initial liver disease. Late age at first use of MTX and duration of therapy with MTX were independent predictors of serious liver disease.[99] The frequency of liver disease is less in RA than in psoriasis. Some reasons for the higher rates in psoriasis could include higher alcohol consumption, higher mean body index with fatty liver disease, and higher doses of MTX.

Although the possible hepatic toxicity of MTX is well known, a potentially serious complication of MTX treatment in patients infected with hepatitis B and C virus is less appreciated. The usual picture is the development of fulminant hepatitis with MTX withdrawal.

TABLE 53.3 ADVERSE EFFECTS OF METHOTREXATE IN RHEUMATOID ARTHRITIS

Adverse effect	Estimated incidence in rheumatoid arthritis
Gastrointestinal: Anorexia, nausea, vomiting, diarrhea	10%[96]
Hematologic: Leukopenia, anemia, thrombocytopenia	3%[96,98]
Hepatic: Elevated transaminases Cirrhosis/liver failure	15%[98] 0.1% 5-yr cumulative incidence[99]
Pulmonary: Acute interstitial pneumonitis	3.3%[172]
Epstein-Barr virus–associated lymphomas	Unknown
Accelerated nodulosis	Unknown
Central nervous system: Dizziness, headache, mood alteration, memory impairment	25%[106]

Reactivation of immune system by discontinuation of the MTX is postulated as the cause.[100]

MTX can also cause lung injury, which is generally acute interstitial pneumonitis. A retrospective combined cohort review and abstraction from the literature identified 29 cases from 1981 to 1993 who had probable or definite MTX lung injury. Predominant clinical features included shortness of breath in 93.1%, cough in 82.8%, and fever in 69.0%. Five of these patients died, and four of six patients retreated with MTX developed recurrent lung toxicity.[101] A case-control study of patients treated with MTX with and without lung injury was undertaken to identify risk factors for lung toxicity. The strongest predictors of lung injury were older age, diabetes, rheumatoid pleuropulmonary involvement, previous use of DMARDs, and hypoalbuminemia.[102]

Other potential adverse effects of MTX include an increased risk of Epstein-Barr virus–associated lymphomas[103] that may regress on discontinuation of MTX,[104] accelerated nodulosis,[105] and non-specific central nervous system effects such as dizziness, headache, mood alteration, or memory impairment[106] (Table 53.3).

The clear risk of MTX therapy during pregnancy deserves special mention. MTX is a known teratogen and can be used to induce abortion. An unfortunate case in which a fetus was exposed during the first trimester to low-dose weekly MTX resulted in multiple congenital abnormalities consistent with the "aminopterin syndrome."[107]

Folic acid supplementation

To prevent adverse effects of MTX, folic acid or folinic acid (leucovorin) is given concomitantly. Folinic acid is the reduced active form of folic acid. Support for this practice comes from a prospective trial in which 92 RA patients were given folinic acid or placebo 24 hours after the MTX dose (up to 30 mg each week). The patients treated with folinic acid reported fewer adverse effects but had no difference in disease activity compared with placebo,[22] in contrast to an earlier placebo-controlled trial on 27 patients in which clinical and laboratory indices of disease worsened only in the patients treated with leucovorin.[108] Folic acid has also been shown in a randomized placebo-controlled trial to decrease the toxicity without influencing efficacy of MTX, given as 5 mg or 27.5 mg each week.[23] In a larger study of 434 patients randomly assigned to receive placebo, folic acid 1 mg/day or folinic acid 2.5 mg/week in addition to MTX (dose escalation to 25 mg/week), both regimens reduced the incidence of elevated liver enzyme levels and decreased toxicity-related discontinuation but had no effect on other adverse effects, including gastrointestinal and mucosal side effects. The mean dosages of MTX at the end of the 48-week study were higher in the folic acid and folinic acid groups, suggesting that a higher dose of MTX might be necessary for the same clinical effect.[109]

Pharmacogenomics

Although MTX is generally well tolerated, some patients experience adverse effects and occasionally these are serious. In addition, while MTX is efficacious for many patients, some patients do not respond. Therefore, ideally we would like to treat only those patients who will safely tolerate MTX and for whom it will have some benefit. Because the critical players in the function and metabolism of MTX are known, it has been possible to study polymorphisms in some of these proteins to determine if they influence the drug's effects.

The best-studied protein polymorphisms are in methylene tetrahydrofolate reductase (MTHFR). MTHFR is a critical enzyme associated with the regeneration of 5-methyl-tetrahydrofolate from 5,10-methylene-tetrahydrofolate. 5-Methyl-tetrahydrofolate contributes a methyl group to homocysteine for regeneration of methionine, and deficiency can lead to hyperhomocysteinemia and methionine deficiency. A mutation exists in the population (C677T), such that the CC genotype provides normal function, whereas the CT and TT provide 40% and 70% decrement in enzyme function, respectively.[110] In RA patients, the CT and TT genotypes have been associated with increased toxicity and MTX discontinuation.[111-113] In addition, the C allele at A1298C was shown to be associated with receiving a lower dose of MTX[112] and toxicity.[114,115] MTHFR 677TT, as well as serine hydroxymethyltransferase (SHMT1) 1420CC, AICAR transformylase 347GG, and thymidylate synthase (TSER) VNTR *2/*2, have been associated with adverse effects.[116]

Polymorphisms in several other enzymes affected by or affecting MTX activity have also been analyzed. Dervieux and colleagues[13] found that homozygous variant genotypes in the reduced folate carrier (RFC-1), AICAR transformylase (ATIC), and thymidylate synthase were associated with decreased disease activity on MTX. In addition, an association of an intron polymorphism in ATIC and decreased disease activity on MTX was found by Lee and colleagues.[117] MTHFR 1298AA and 677CC, AMPD1 34C, ITPA 94C, and ATIC 347C have been associated with clinical improvement.[115,118] The TT genotype at 3435 in ABCB1 (ATP-binding cassette protein B1), one of the transporters responsible for MTX efflux from cells, was found to be enriched in poor responders to MTX.[119] Finally, a haplotype of GGH (gamma-glutamyl hydrolase), an enzyme that removes polyglutamates from MTX, has been associated with improved DAS scores at 3 months.[120] These studies suggest that in the near future we may be able to screen patients to determine risk and benefit of MTX before initiating therapy. However, the small number of patients examined thus far and the lack of large prospectively controlled studies limits our current use of genetic screening for MTX efficacy and safety.

Methotrexate use in rheumatoid arthritis: recommendations

The American College of Rheumatology issued a consensus statement in 1994 providing guidelines for monitoring liver toxicity (Box 53.1).[121] Before starting MTX, the guidelines recommend obtaining liver blood tests and hepatitis B and C serologies in addition to other standard tests, including the complete blood count and serum creatinine. Although the 1994 statement recommends that the AST, alanine aminotransferase, and albumin levels should be monitored at intervals of every 4 to 8 weeks, a recent consensus statement recommends monitoring every 8 to 12 weeks after 3 months and every 12 weeks after 6 months of therapy.[122] Routine surveillance liver biopsies are not recommended for RA patients receiving traditional doses of MTX. However, a biopsy should be performed if a patient develops persistent abnormalities on liver blood tests, defined as elevations in the AST of 5 of 9 determinations within a 12-month interval (6 of 12 if tests are performed monthly) or a decrease in serum albumin below the normal range.[121]

MTX is usually started at a dose of 7.5 to 10 mg weekly, and the dose is escalated every 4 to 8 weeks until disease activity is under control. The therapeutic dose is generally between 15 and 25 mg per week. Generally it takes 4 to 6 weeks after the therapeutic dose is reached for a clinical effect to be noted. We generally start at 7.5 mg per week and then 4 weeks later, if there has been no adverse event, the dose is increased to 15 mg and then 4 weeks later to 20 mg per week. After another 4 weeks, if there is no clinical effect, we would add another DMARD. It is important to maximize the MTX dose in order to achieve the maximum efficacy with this drug. If there is an impressive clinical response the MTX dose may be decreased, but most patients require persistent therapy to control the arthritis. Discontinuation of MTX is generally associated with a flare of arthritis 4 to 6 weeks after stopping the drug. The maximum dose of oral MTX is generally considered to be 20 to 25 mg/week. MTX can be delivered subcutaneously in patients with gastrointestinal intolerance or in non-responders with a predicted higher bioavailability than the oral dose. Folic acid 1 mg each day is recommended in all patients who are on MTX. If adverse effects occur, the folic acid should be increased to 2 mg per day. Outside the United States the folic acid dose is usually 5 mg 5 to 6 days per week. If side effects continue despite folic acid, leucovorin starting at 5 mg/week should be used. The dose of leucovorin can be escalated to block side effects and should be given 8 to 24 hours after the MTX. If administered within 8 hours of the MTX, it might block the efficacy of MTX.

Patients should be aware of the adverse event profile of this drug. Generally the drug should be held during infections. We also hold it the week of surgery and the first postoperative week. Laboratory monitoring should be done on a regular basis, and we continue to monitor the liver function tests, creatinine, and complete blood count every 4 to 8 weeks, which is more conservative than the most recent recommendations.[122] Patients should receive routine vaccinations including influenza vaccine but should not receive live vaccines while on MTX. We also recommend restricting alcohol use. Women of child-bearing potential must use birth control while on the drug.

Methotrexate in other rheumatic diseases

Psoriatic arthritis

Although MTX is commonly used as a first-line agent for psoriatic arthritis, the data supporting its efficacy in this disease are minimal, including two underpowered, double-blind, placebo-controlled trials and several retrospective and observational studies.[123] Of note, in studies of liver biopsies among patients with psoriasis receiving MTX, significant fibrosis occurred in 2% to 33.3% and cirrhosis in 0% to

25.6% of patients. The current guidelines for monitoring MTX in psoriasis therefore include recommendations for a pretreatment liver biopsy in patients with risk factors for liver disease (previous or current excessive alcohol, persistent abnormal liver chemistry studies, history of liver disease, family history of inheritable liver disease, diabetes mellitus, obesity, or history of exposure to hepatotoxins) and a monitoring liver biopsy for all patients after each cumulative 1- to 1.5-g dosage.[124] Some authors have suggested a relaxation of these recommendations, recommending a liver biopsy after a 4-g cumulative dose in patients with no known risk factors receiving long-term, oral, low-dose, once-weekly MTX.[125]

Juvenile rheumatoid arthritis

MTX efficacy was demonstrated in a study including various forms of juvenile polyarthritis[126] and subsequently in extended oligoarticular and systemic juvenile idiopathic arthritis.[127] Among non-responders to the standard dosage of MTX (8 to 12.5 mg/m²/week), 62.5% of those who received a subcutaneous or intramuscular dose of 15 mg/m²/week achieved an ACR Pediatric 30 response rate. However, no significant additional improvement was observed at a dose of 30 mg/m²/week.[128] The safety of MTX in juvenile arthritis has also been investigated. A retrospective review of adverse events in patients with polyarticular juvenile RA treated with weekly MTX demonstrated transient liver test abnormalities in 9 of 62. However, none of the 12 patients that underwent liver biopsies for assessment of occult liver disease after cumulative doses of 815 to 2980 mg showed fibrosis or cirrhosis. Two patients required hospitalization for bacterial infections. There were no cases of MTX-induced pneumonitis and there was no reduction in pulmonary function in 26 patients who were tested serially.[129]

Ankylosing spondylitis

One double-blind, randomized, placebo-controlled trial of MTX 7.5 mg weekly in patients with active ankylosing spondylitis (AS) showed a higher response rate at 24 weeks in the MTX group on the basis of a composite index of improvement in five of the following scales: severity of morning stiffness, physical well-being, the Bath Ankylosing Spondylitis Disease Activity Index (BASDAI), the Bath Ankylosing Spondylitis Functional Index (BASFI), the Health Assessment Questionnaire for Spondyloarthropathies (HAQ-S), and physician and patient global assessment of the disease activity.[130] In contrast, a double-blind, placebo-controlled study using disease activity (BASDAI) and metrology (BASMI) as primary outcomes found no significant difference between AS patients who received MTX 10 mg weekly versus placebo, even in the subgroup of patients with peripheral arthritis.[131] In a comparison of MTX 7.5 mg weekly plus naproxen versus naproxen alone, only the "global evaluation of the physician" was significantly improved in the MTX group, in contrast to all other objective and subjective measurements, leading the authors to conclude that the combination of MTX and naproxen did not provide any advantage over treatment with naproxen alone.[132]

Felty syndrome

Case reports[133-135] and one small retrospective study[136] have demonstrated reversal of neutropenia with MTX treatment in patients with Felty syndrome.

ANCA-associated vasculitis

An unblended, prospective, randomized, controlled trial in patients with newly diagnosed antineutrophil cytoplasmic antibody (ANCA)-associated vasculitis without critical organ manifestations showed that MTX plus prednisolone was not inferior to oral cyclophosphamide plus prednisolone for induction of remission. However, in the MTX group, the remission was delayed and these patients experienced more relapses. The MTX regimen was also less effective for induction of remission in patients with extensive disease and pulmonary involvement.[137] With respect to maintenance therapy, in patients who had achieved a remission with intravenous cyclophosphamide and corticosteroids, MTX and azathioprine provided similar rates of adverse events and relapse.[138] Although azathioprine has been shown to have similar safety and efficacy to oral cyclophosphamide for maintenance of remission in non-life-threatening Wegener granulomatosis and microscopic polyangiitis,[139] MTX has not been directly compared with oral cyclophosphamide for maintenance therapy in a randomized controlled trial.

Polymyalgia rheumatic/giant cell arteritis

Randomized controlled trials of adjunctive MTX in giant cell arteritis (GCA) have yielded discrepant results.[140,141] However, an individual patient data meta-analysis concluded that the addition of MTX lowers the risk of relapse and reduces exposure to corticosteroids in GCA.[142] Similarly, the randomized double-blind placebo-controlled trials of adjunctive MTX in patients with polymyalgia rheumatic have yielded different results. In the study by van der Veen and colleagues,[143] there was no difference in time to remission, duration of remission, number of relapses, or cumulative prednisone dose. In contrast, Caporali and colleagues[144] found that adjunctive MTX was associated with a shorter duration of prednisone treatment.

Inflammatory myopathy

Although there are no randomized, placebo-controlled trials of adjunctive MTX in the treatment of inflammatory myopathies, observational studies and retrospective reviews have supported its use in corticosteroid-resistant disease. For example, in a retrospective review of 22 patients with polymyositis or dermatomyositis who had failed corticosteroid therapy alone, 17 of these patients normalized muscle enzyme levels and demonstrated improved strength when intravenous MTX was added to their regimen.[145] Similarly, in a review that included 55 patients with idiopathic inflammatory myopathy (dermatomyositis, polymyositis, and inclusion body myositis) who received MTX after failing to respond to prednisone, 31 responded, with 9 showing a complete response. These authors also showed that patients receiving MTX were more likely to respond completely than those receiving a second trial of prednisone.[146] Of note, in a retrospective review of dermatomyositis cases treated with 7.5 to 14.2 mg of adjunctive MTX weekly, 4 of 10 patients underwent liver biopsies with two patients showing mild hepatic fibrosis.[147] Although using MTX as a first-line therapy in adult myositis has not been carefully studied, a retrospective cohort study of childhood dermatomyositis showed that using adjunctive MTX as a first-line therapy halved the cumulative exposure to corticosteroids with similar improvement in strength and physical function.[148]

Systemic lupus erythematosus

Only two randomized, double-blind, placebo-controlled trials of MTX in lupus have been performed. The first demonstrated in patients with mild disease activity that MTX 15 to 20 mg weekly was effective in controlling cutaneous and articular manifestations and facilitating a decrease in the prednisone dose.[149] A double-blind, randomized, placebo-controlled trial in patients with moderately active lupus subsequently showed that weekly MTX was associated with a lower prednisone dose and a slightly decreased Systemic Lupus Activity Measure (SLAM).[150]

In an exploratory study, five patients with chronic calcium pyrophosphate deposition disease treated with MTX (5 to 10 mg/week) reported a significant decrease in pain, tender and swollen joint counts, and the frequency of attacks.[151]

CONCLUSIONS

MTX is currently considered a first-line agent in the treatment of RA and the "anchor drug" for combination therapy with other DMARDs. It has become the standard of care and the most widely used drug in the treatment of RA. When used appropriately, it has excellent efficacy and tolerability in the treatment of the signs and symptoms of RA and is the DMARD to which all new therapies should be compared. The effectiveness of MTX in other rheumatic diseases still requires further study, but existing results suggest that MTX is a useful tool in the treatment of a variety of systemic rheumatic diseases.

KEY REFERENCES

2. Kremer J. Toward a better understanding of methotrexate. Arthritis Rheum 2004;50:1370-1382.

5. Braun J, Kastner P, Flaxenberg P, et al. Comparison of the clinical efficacy and safety of subcutaneous versus oral administration of methotrexate in patients with active rheumatoid arthritis: results of a six-month, multicenter, randomized, double-blind, controlled, phase IV trial. Arthritis Rheum 2008;58:73-81. A.

14. Dervieux T, Furst D, Lein Do, et al. Pharmacogenetic and metabolite measurements are associated with clinical status in patients with rheumatoid arthritis treated with methotrexate: results of a multicentred cross sectional observational study. Ann Rheum Dis 2005;64:1180-1185. B.

16. Dalrymple JM, Stamp LK, O'Donnell JL, et al. Pharmacokinetics of oral methotrexate in patients with rheumatoid arthritis. Arthritis Rheum 2008;58:3299-3308. B.

22. Shiroky JB, Neville C, Esdaile JM, et al. Low-dose methotrexate with leucovorin (folinic acid) in the management of rheumatoid arthritis: results of a multicenter randomized, double-blind, placebo-controlled trial. Arthritis Rheum 1993;36:795-803. A.

23. Morgan SL, Baggott JE, Vaughn WH, et al. Supplementation with folic acid during methotrexate therapy for rheumatoid arthritis. A double-blind, placebo-controlled trial. Ann Intern Med 1994;121:833-841. A.

28. Cronstein BN, Naime D, Ostad E. The antiinflammatory mechanism of methotrexate. Increased adenosine release at inflamed sites diminishes leukocyte accumulation in an in vivo model of inflammation. J Clin Invest 1993;92:2675-2682.

30. Montesinos MC, Takedachi M, Thompson LF, et al. The antiinflammatory mechanism of methotrexate depends on extracellular conversion of adenine nucleotides to adenosine by ecto-5'-nucleotidase—findings in a study of ecto-5'-nucleotidase gene-deficient mice. Arthritis Rheum 2007;56:1440-1445.

37. Gubner R, August S, Ginsberg V. Therapeutic suppression of tissue reactivity. Ii. Effect of aminopterin in rheumatoid arthritis and psoriasis. Am J Med Sci 1951;22:176-182.

43. Hoffmeister RT. Methotrexate therapy in rheumatoid arthritis: 15 years experience. Am J Med 1983; 75:69-73. C.

48. Weinblatt ME, Coblyn JS, Fox DA, et al. Efficacy of low-dose methotrexate in rheumatoid arthritis. N Engl J Med 1985;312:818-822. A.

49. Williams HJ, Willkens RF, Samuelson Co Jr, et al. Comparison of low-dose oral pulse methotrexate and placebo in the treatment of rheumatoid arthritis. A controlled clinical trial. Arthritis Rheum 1985;28:721-730. A.

51. Furst DE, Koehnke R, Burmeister LF, et al. Increasing methotrexate effect with increasing dose in the treatment of resistant rheumatoid arthritis. J Rheumatol 1989;16:313-320. A.

52. Kremer JM, Rynes RI, Bartholomew LE. Severe flare of rheumatoid arthritis after discontinuation of long-term methotrexate therapy. Double-blind study. Am J Med 1987;82:781-786. A.

53. Jeurissen ME, Boerbooms AM, Van De Putte LB, et al. Methotrexate versus azathioprine in the treatment of rheumatoid arthritis. A forty-eight-week randomized, double-blind trial. Arthritis Rheum 1991;34:961-972. A.

56. Weinblatt ME, Kaplan H, Germain BF, et al. Low-dose methotrexate compared with auranofin in adult rheumatoid arthritis. A thirty-six-week, double-blind trial. Arthritis Rheum 1990;33:330-338. A.

60. Weinblatt ME, Polisson R, Blotner SD, et al. The effects of drug therapy on radiographic progression of rheumatoid arthritis: results of a 36-week randomized trial comparing methotrexate and auranofin. Arthritis Rheum 1993;36:613-619. A.

64. Lehman AJ, Esdaile JM, Klinkhoff AV, et al. A 48-week, randomized, double-blind, double-observer, placebo-controlled multicenter trial of combination methotrexate and intramuscular gold therapy in rheumatoid arthritis—results of The METGO Study. Arthritis Rheum 2005;52:1360-1370. A.

69. Kremer JM, Genovese MC, Cannon GW, et al. Concomitant leflunomide therapy in patients with active rheumatoid arthritis despite stable doses of methotrexate—A randomized, double-blind, placebo-controlled trial. Ann Intern Med 2002;137:726-733. A.

70. Bathon JM, Martin RW, Fleischmann RM, et al. A comparison of etanercept and methotrexate in patients with early rheumatoid arthritis. N Engl J Med 2000;343:1586-1593. A.

72. Weinblatt ME, Kremer JM, Bankhurst AD, et al. A trial of etanercept, a recombinant tumor necrosis factor receptor:Fc fusion protein, in patients with rheumatoid arthritis receiving methotrexate. N Engl J Med 1999;340:253-259. A.

73. Weinblatt ME, Keystone EC, Furst DE, et al. Adalimumab, a fully human anti-tumor necrosis factor a monoclonal antibody, for the treatment of rheumatoid arthritis in patients taking concomitant methotrexate—The ARMADA trial. Arthritis Rheum 2003;48:35-45. A.

76. Klareskog L, Van der Heijde D, De Jager JP, et al. Therapeutic effect of the combination of etanercept and methotrexate compared with each treatment alone in patients with rheumatoid arthritis: double-blind randomised controlled trial. Lancet 2004; 363:675-681. A.

80. St Clair EW, van der Heijde DM, Smolen JS, et al. Combination of infliximab and methotrexate therapy for early rheumatoid arthritis: a randomized, controlled trial. Arthritis Rheum 2004;50: 3432-3443. A.

84. Weinblatt ME, Trentham DE, Fraser PA, et al. Long-term prospective trial of low-dose methotrexate in rheumatoid arthritis. Arthritis Rheum 1988;31: 167-175. B.

85. Kremer JM, Phelps CT. Long-term prospective study of the use of methotrexate in rheumatoid arthritis: update after a mean of 90 months. Arthritis Rheum 1992;35:138-145. B.

90. Choi HK, Hernán MA, Seeger JD, et al. Methotrexate and mortality in patients with rheumatoid arthritis: a prospective study. Lancet 2002;359:1173-1177. B.

97. Gutierrez-Ureña S, Molina JF, García CO, et al. Pancytopenia secondary to methotrexate therapy in rheumatoid arthritis. Arthritis Rheum 1996;39:272-276. C.

99. Walker AM, Funch D, Dreyer NA, et al. Determinants of serious liver disease among patients receiving low-dose methotrexate for rheumatoid arthritis. Arthritis Rheum 1993;36:329-335. B.

101. Kremer JM, Alarcón GS, Weinblatt ME, et al. Clinical, laboratory, radiographic, and histopathologic features of methotrexate-associated lung injury in patients with rheumatoid arthritis—a multicenter study with literature review. Arthritis Rheum 1997;40: 1829-1837. B.

102. Alarcón GS, Kremer JM, Macaluso M, et al. Risk factors for methotrexate-induced lung injury in patients with rheumatoid arthritis—a multicenter, case-control study. Ann Intern Med 1997;127:356-364. B.

104. Kamel OW, Van de Rijn M, Weiss LM, et al. Reversible lymphomas associated with Epstein-Barr virus occurring during methotrexate therapy for rheumatoid arthritis and dermatomyositis. N Engl J Med 1993;328:1317-1321. C.

107. Buckley LM, Bullaboy CA, Leichtman L, Marquez M. Multiple congenital anomalies associated with weekly low-dose methotrexate treatment of the mother. Arthritis Rheum 1997;40:971-973. C.

108. Joyce DA, Will RK, Hoffman DM, et al. Exacerbation of rheumatoid arthritis in patients treated with methotrexate after administration of folinic acid. Ann Rheum Dis 1991;50:913-914. A.

109. Van Ede AE, Laan RF, Rood MJ, et al. Effect of folic or folinic acid supplementation on the toxicity and efficacy of methotrexate in rheumatoid arthritis: a forty-eight week, multicenter, randomized, double-blind, placebo-controlled study. Arthritis Rheum 2001;44:1515-1524. A.

110. Kremer JM. Methotrexate pharmacogenomics. Ann Rheum Dis 2006;65:1121-1123.

116. Weisman MH, Furst DE, Park GS, et al. Risk genotypes in folate-dependent enzymes and their association with methotrexate-related side effects in rheumatoid arthritis. Arthritis Rheum 2006;54:607-612.

121. Kremer JM, Alarcon GS, Lightfoot RW Jr, et al. Methotrexate for rheumatoid arthritis. Suggested guidelines for monitoring liver toxicity. American College of Rheumatology. Arthritis Rheum 1994;37:316-328.

126. Giannini EH, Brewer EJ, Kuzmina N, et al. Methotrexate in resistant juvenile rheumatoid arthritis. Results of the U.S.A.-U.S.S.R. double-blind, placebo-controlled trial. The Pediatric Rheumatology Collaborative Study Group and The Cooperative Children's Study Group. N Engl J Med 1992;326:1043-1049.

140. Hoffman GS, Cid MC, Hellman DB, et al. A multicenter, randomized, double-blind, placebo-controlled trial of adjuvant methotrexate treatment for giant cell arteritis. Arthritis Rheum 2002;46:1309-1318. A.

REFERENCES

Full references for this chapter can be found on www.expertconsult.com.

Leflunomide

Edward Keystone and Boulos Haraoui

54

- Leflunomide inhibits pyrimidine synthesis, resulting in blockade of T-cell proliferation.
- Leflunomide is used in patients with moderate to severe active rheumatoid arthritis with early or late disease.
- Monotherapy with leflunomide has been shown to be equally as effective as methotrexate and sulfasalazine in improving symptoms and signs of rheumatoid arthritis.
- Leflunomide as monotherapy results in substantial inhibition of joint damage, as assessed radiologically.
- Leflunomide provides additional benefit in patients partially responsive to methotrexate.
- The most common side effects of leflunomide are gastrointestinal symptoms and hepatotoxicity.
- Combination of leflunomide with methotrexate results in a significant increase in liver enzyme abnormalities.
- Leflunomide is teratogenic in animals and is therefore contraindicated in women who may become pregnant.

CHEMICAL STRUCTURE AND MODE OF ACTION

Leflunomide, N-(4-trifluoromethylphenyl)-5-methylisoxazole-4-carbox-amide $(C_{12}H_9F_3N_2O_2)$, is an isoxazole derivative with immunomodulatory and disease-modifying properties in rheumatoid arthritis (RA). It is a prodrug that is rapidly converted in the submucosal wall of the intestinal tract and after first passage in the liver into its active metabolite A77 1726, a manolonitrilamide.

A77 1726 inhibits dihydroorotate dehydrogenase (DHODH), a mitochondrial enzyme that is critical for the *de novo* synthesis of pyrimidines (Fig. 54.1).[1] It is thought that this property effectively blocks the proliferation of human lymphocytes, which are highly dependent on this pathway for nucleotide synthesis.[2] This leads to an arrest in the G1/S phase of the cell cycle. The concentration of A77 1726 needed to block T-cell proliferation after mitogen stimulation varies greatly between species and can be reversed *in vitro* by the exogenous addition of uridine in a dose-dependent fashion.[3,4] Pyrimidines are also needed by proliferating cells to form the lipids and macromolecules essential to several cell functions such as cell-cell contact, diapedesis, and intracellular signaling (Fig. 54.2).

Furthermore, DHODH may be involved in other cellular mechanisms such as B-cell proliferation and immunoglobulin synthesis.[5,6]

In several *in-vitro* stimulated and unstimulated cell lines, A77 1726 was demonstrated to inhibit two important transcriptional factors critical to the function of cells of the immune system and inflammation[7,8]: tyrosine kinase activity and nuclear factor (NF)-κB activation and gene expression. A77 1726 was also shown to suppress more efficiently than dexamethasone, interleukin (IL)-1β expression, and matrix metalloproteinase (MMP)-1 production.[9] On the other hand, it did not have any effect on IL-4 production or IL-2 receptor expression.[10] After 1 year of treatment of RA patients with leflunomide there was a reduction in the levels of IFN-γ but not of IL-6, suggesting a preferential effect on T cells.[11,12]

Leflunomide has also been shown to inhibit chemotaxis of peripheral blood neutrophils in RA patients.[12] Studies of synovial tissues in RA patients receiving leflunomide revealed a reduction in synovial macrophages as well as intracellular adhesion molecule (ICAM)-1 and vascular cell adhesion molecule (VCAM)-1 expression.[13] A decreased ratio of MMP-1 to tissue inhibitor of metalloproteinases (TIMP)-1 was also demonstrated.

In vitro, the active metabolite A77 1726 was shown to directly inhibit both the generation and the activity of osteoclasts.[14] This activity seems to be independent of its inhibition of uridine synthesis or the blockade of NF-κB.

HUMAN CLINICAL PHARMACOKINETICS

Absorption and bioavailability

After oral absorption, leflunomide is rapidly metabolized to A77 1726 within the gut wall, plasma, and the liver. The active metabolite is very highly bound to plasma protein (>99%) and, correspondingly, has a low apparent volume of distribution. At a dose of 20 mg/day, steady state is reached in 7 weeks and the average plasma concentration of A77 1726 is approximately 35 mg/mL. Trough plasma concentrations are linearly related to the maintenance dose of leflunomide, indicating linear pharmacokinetics.

A77 1726 undergoes enterohepatic circulation and biliary recycling, which contributes to its long elimination half-life of approximately 2 weeks. Therefore, to obtain a rapid steady state, a loading dose followed by a lower maintenance dose has been used.

Metabolism and elimination

Almost half of the administered dose is excreted as unmetabolized A77 1726 in the feces. Glucuronide conjugates and oxanilic acid derivatives are the principal metabolites recovered in the urine. A77 1726 is still detectable in the urine 36 days after administration of a single dose. A77 1726 readily binds to orally administered activated charcoal and even more so to cholestyramine, thus enhancing its elimination; these characteristics are used in clinical situations whenever toxicity is present or rapid reduction of blood levels is required.

Drug interactions

In a clinical trial with RA patients, the pharmacokinetics of A77 1726 and methotrexate were not altered by concomitant coadministration.[15] The maximum concentration of A77 1726 after the loading and maintenance doses remained within the range seen in patients treated with leflunomide alone.

In vitro, A77 1726 is an inhibitor of the isoenzyme 2C9 of cytochrome P450 (CYP2C9), through which warfarin, tolbutamide, phenytoin, and several non-steroidal anti-inflammatory drugs are metabolized. However, in human *in-vivo* situations the free unbound drug is below the half maximal inhibitory concentration (IC_{50}) for this enzyme and no clinically significant drug interactions have been reported.

Based on recent pharmacokinetics studies in a pediatric population, the recommended daily dose of leflunomide is 20 mg for subjects weighing more than 40 kg, 15 mg for those between 20 and 40 kg, and 10 mg in patients weighing less than 20 kg.[16]

EFFICACY

Monotherapy

Evidence from four multicenter double-blind randomized controlled trials shows that leflunomide monotherapy is effective in the treatment of RA, significantly superior to placebo, and similar in efficacy to sulfasalazine as well as moderate-dose methotrexate.

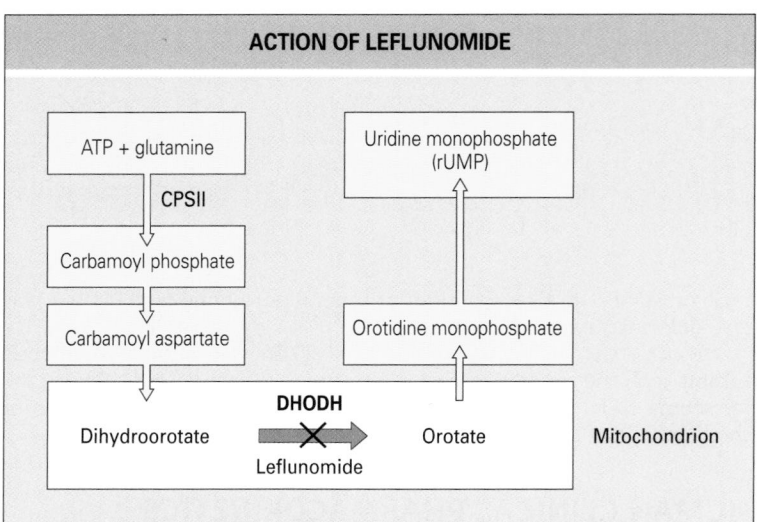

Fig. 54.1 Leflunomide blocks dihydroorotate dehydrogenase (DHODH), a key enzyme in the *de novo* synthesis of uridine. ATP, adenosine triphosphate; CPSII, carbamoyl phosphate synthetase II.

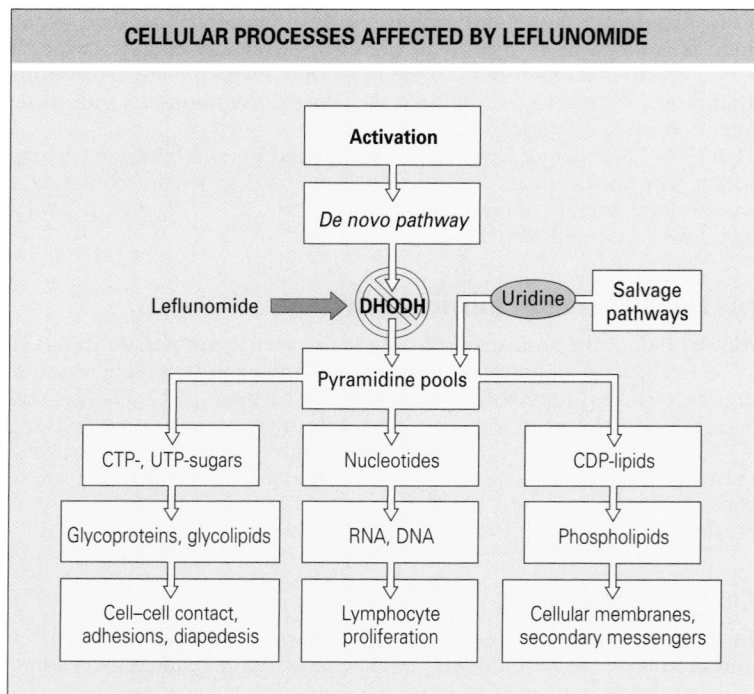

Fig. 54.2 Cellular processes affected by leflunomide. Effect of leflunomide on cellular processes through inhibition of *de novo* pyrimidine biosynthesis. CDP, cytosine diphosphate; CTP, cytosine triphosphate; DHODH, dihydroorotate dehydrogenase; UTP, uridine triphosphate.

In the initial 6-month placebo-controlled dose-ranging study of 402 patients (with a disease duration of 8.3 years), leflunomide was evaluated in doses of 5, 10, and 25 mg preceded by a single loading dose. In this study the two highest doses proved to be most efficacious, with American College of Rheumatology (ACR) 20% (ACR20) response rates of 52% and 60%, respectively.[17] Swollen joint counts improved by approximately 40%.

In a subsequent 12-month study of leflunomide in 482 patients (with disease duration of 7 years), leflunomide was evaluated at a dose of 20 mg/day (after 100-mg loading doses on days 1-3) in comparison with methotrexate (mean dose, 13.5 mg/wk) and placebo.[18] Using the less stringent ACR20 last observation carried forward analysis, leflunomide demonstrated a response rate of 52% compared with 46% for methotrexate. Both agents exhibited higher responses than the placebo group (26%) (Fig. 54-3). Clinically meaningful and statistically significant improvement in measures of function and health-related quality

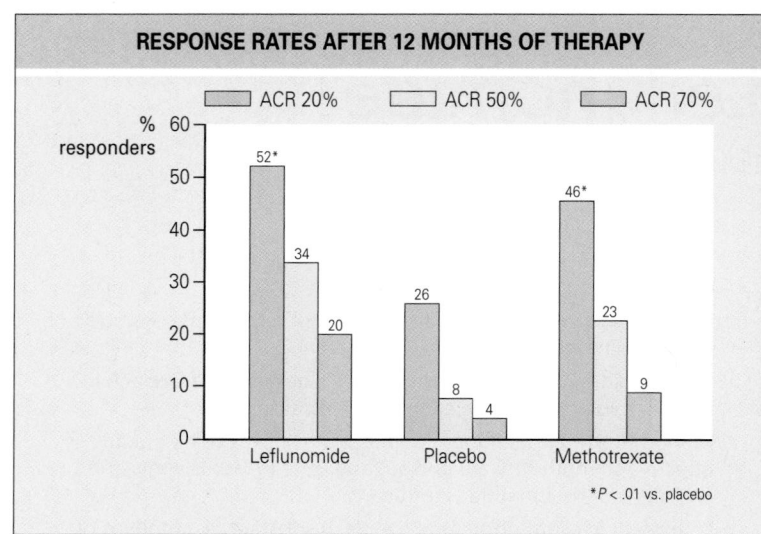

Fig. 54.3 Response rates after 12 months of therapy. Percentage of patients treated with leflunomide, methotrexate, or placebo who met the American College of Rheumatology's (ACR) response criteria for improvement of 20%, 50%, 70%, or more at 12 months. (*Data from Strand V, Cohen S, Schiff M, et al. Treatment of active rheumatoid with leflunomide compared with placebo and methotrexate. Arch Intern Med 1999;159:2542-2550.*)

of life and work productivity was seen during treatment with leflunomide compared with placebo (Fig. 54.4). Leflunomide resulted in significantly more improvement in a number of the disability and quality of life measures.[19] It is notable that leflunomide exhibited a more rapid onset of action than methotrexate, as evidenced by the higher proportion of patients achieving an ACR20 response after 4 weeks of therapy. Leflunomide and methotrexate inhibited disease progression in approximately half the patients as measured by radiographic analysis (Fig. 54.5). Both leflunomide and methotrexate resulted in statistically significantly less radiographic progression compared with placebo at 12 months.[20]

Longer-term efficacy was evaluated in a 12-month extension study in which completers at 52 weeks were given the option of continuing therapy for an additional year.[21] Both leflunomide and methotrexate showed consistent improvement in signs and symptoms in the year 2 cohort with significantly more leflunomide- than methotrexate-treated patients achieving a clinically relevant (ACR20) response. Improvement in measures of function and health-related quality of life were maintained over the second year and were significantly better than the improvement with methotrexate. The withdrawal rate in both groups in the year 2 cohort was low (<5%).

Leflunomide was also compared with methotrexate in a head-to-head study involving 999 patients with earlier disease (3.7 years in duration).[22] In this study, leflunomide was evaluated in a dose of 20 mg/day after three 100-mg loading doses, whereas the methotrexate dose was 10 to 15 mg/wk. At 52 weeks, patients were given the option of continuing double-blind therapy for an additional 52 weeks. At the end of the first year more methotrexate-treated patients met ACR20 criteria (64.3%) than leflunomide-treated patients (50.5%) (Fig. 54.6). Improvement in signs and symptoms was also greater in the methotrexate-treated group after 1 year of therapy. As in the previous study, leflunomide elicited a more rapid response to therapy. Whether the higher methotrexate response rate in this study was a result of not including a folate supplement is unclear. In the subset of patients who elected to continue therapy for a second year, the ACR20 response rates were comparable with both drugs after 2 years of therapy. Disease modification as measured radiographically at 52 weeks was similar with both drugs but was more effective with methotrexate compared with leflunomide after 2 years of therapy.

Leflunomide was also compared with sulfasalazine in a 6-month placebo-controlled study of 358 patients with a disease duration of 7 years.[23] At 6 months, the ACR20 response was comparable for the groups treated with leflunomide (55%) and sulfasalazine (56%) and superior to the placebo group (29%) (Fig. 54.7). Improvement in tender and swollen joints was similar with both drugs. Leflunomide

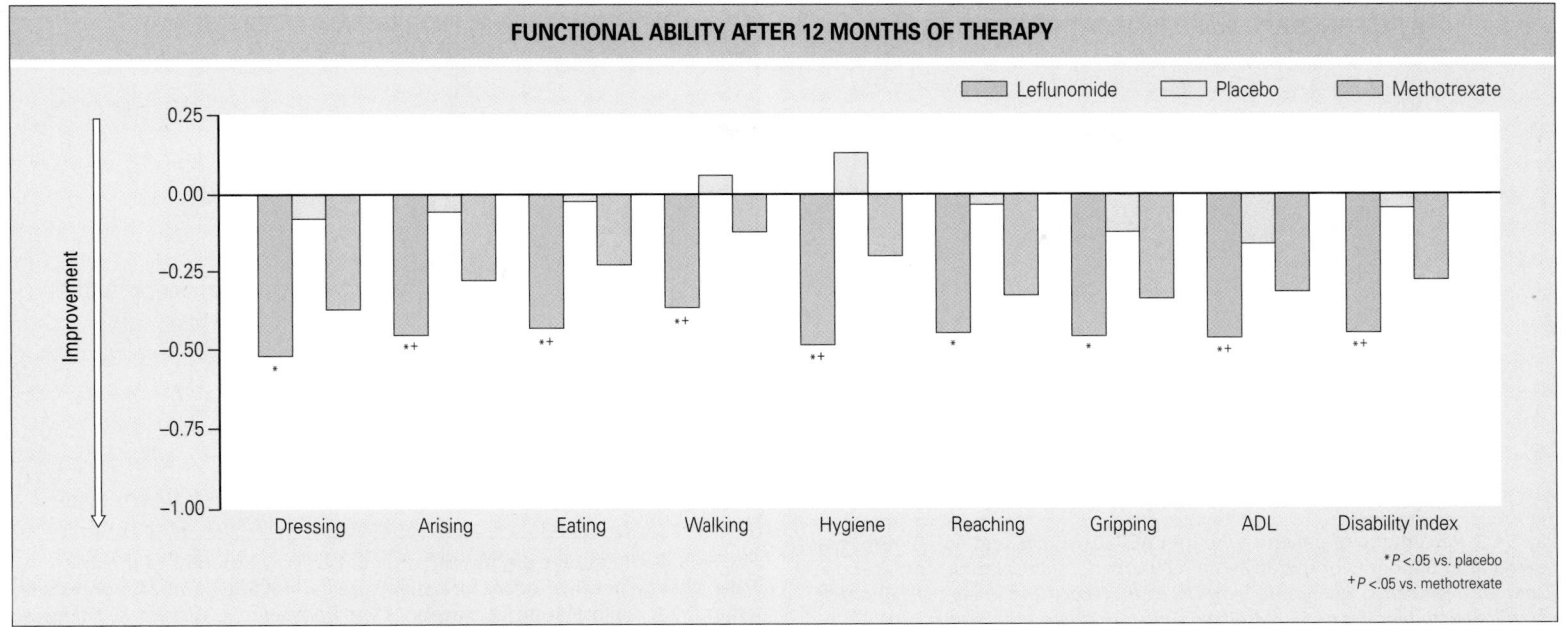

Fig. 54.4 Functional ability after 12 months of therapy. Individual subcategories of the Health Assessment Questionnaire score after 12 months of therapy with leflunomide, methotrexate, or placebo. *(Data from Strand V, Tugwel P, Bombardier C, et al. Function and health-related quality of life: results from a randomized controlled trial of leflunomide versus methotrexate or placebo in patients with active rheumatoid arthritis. Arthritis Rheum 1999;42:1870-1878.)*

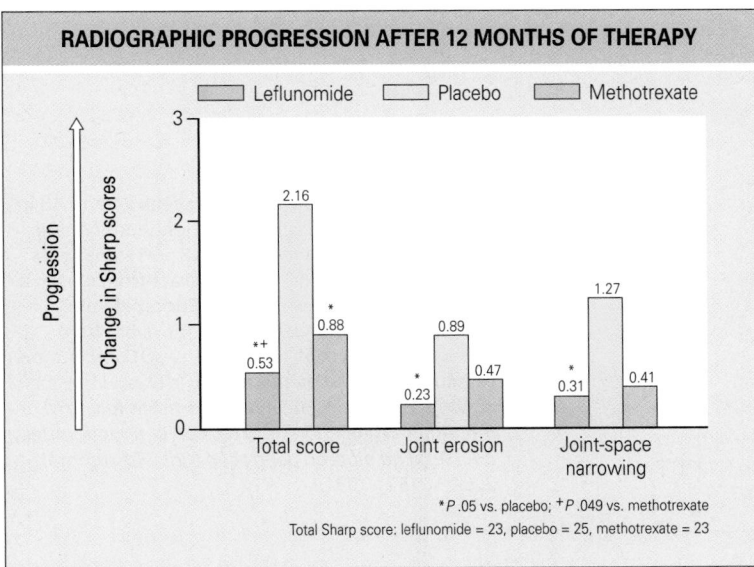

Fig. 54.5 Radiographic progression after 12 months of therapy. Mean changes from baseline in total Sharp scores and erosion and joint-space narrowing subscores for the intent-to-treat population. *(Data from Strand V, Tugwel P, Bombardier C, et al. Function and health-related quality of life: results from a randomized controlled trial of leflunomide versus methotrexate or placebo in patients with active rheumatoid arthritis. Arthritis Rheum 1999;42:1870-1878.)*

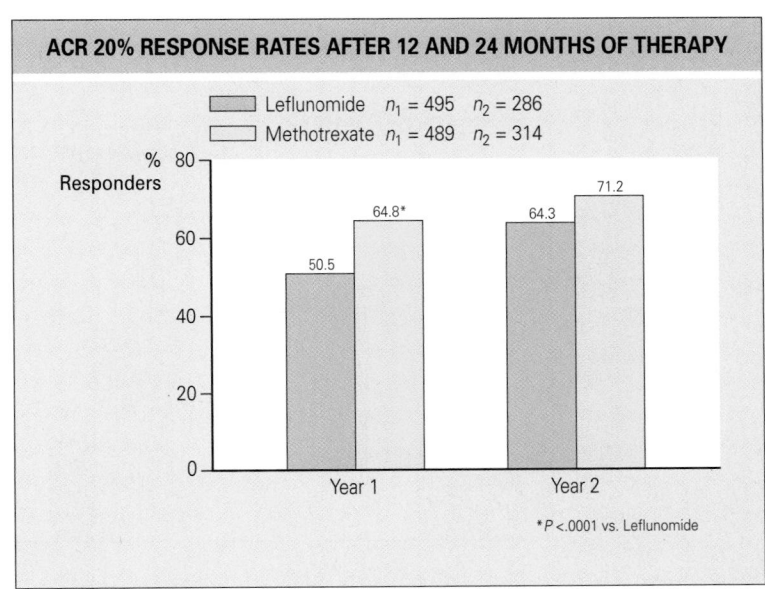

Fig. 54.6 Percentage of patients who met ACR20 response criteria after 12 and 24 months of therapy with leflunomide or methotrexate. *(Data from Emery P, Breedveld FC, Lemmel EM, et al, and the Multinational Leflunomide Study Group. A comparison of the efficacy and safety of leflunomide and methotrexate for the treatment of rheumatoid arthritis. Rheumatology 2000:39:655-665.)*

demonstrated a more rapid onset of action, particularly evident after 1 month of therapy. At 6 months, both drugs inhibited radiographic progression to a similar extent. Patients completing the initial 6-month phase were given the option of continuing in a double-blind fashion in 12- and 24-month extension studies, with the placebo group switching to sulfasalazine. Leflunomide- and sulfasalazine-treated patients demonstrated a sustained response out to 12 months, with the leflunomide cohort demonstrating a significantly greater ACR20 response rate compared with sulfasalazine at 24 months. Little disease progression as determined radiographically was observed at 1 year and 2 years in the cohort of leflunomide and sulfasalazine patients remaining on therapy (Fig. 54.8). Taken together, the data demonstrated consistent reduction of radiographic progression in three separate studies of leflunomide, comparable at 12 months to both methotrexate and sulfasalazine.

Combination therapy

Because methotrexate is thought to act primarily on the purine pathways of cellular metabolism whereas leflunomide inhibits pyrimidine pathways, the combination of leflunomide and methotrexate has the potential for synergy in inhibiting the proliferation of cells involved in the immune inflammatory response.

The safety and efficacy pharmacokinetics of combination therapy with leflunomide and methotrexate were initially evaluated in an open-label 52-week study of 30 patients who exhibited active disease despite 17 mg/wk of methotrexate.[15] After a loading dose of 100 mg/day for 2 days, leflunomide was given in a dose of 10 mg/day for 3 months and then increased as required to 20 mg in patients with persistently active disease.

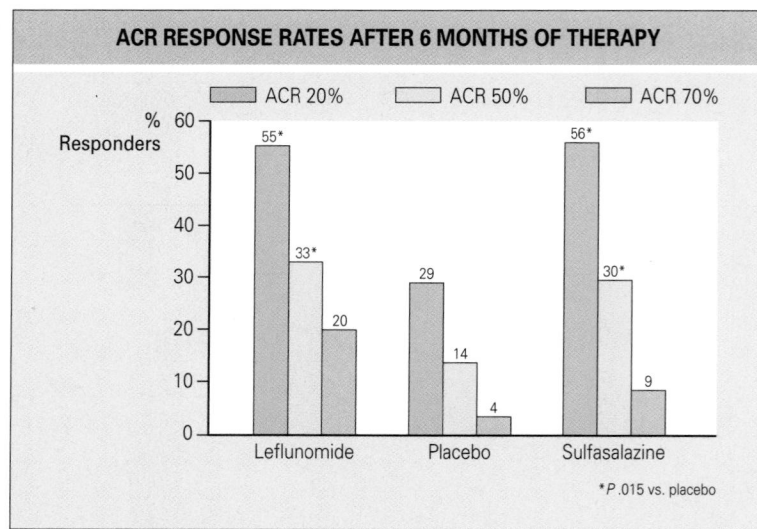

Fig. 54.7 Percentage of patients who met ACR20, ACR50, and ACR70 response criteria after 6 months of therapy with leflunomide, sulfasalazine, or placebo. *(Data from Smolen JS, Kalden JR, Scott DL, et al. Efficacy and safety of leflunomide compared with placebo and sulfasalazine in active rheumatoid arthritis: a double-blind randomized multicentre trial. Lancet 1999;353:259-266.)*

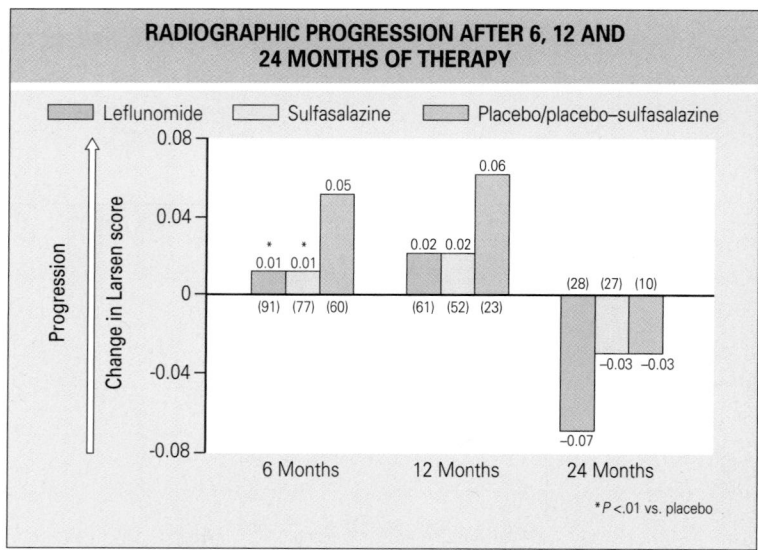

Fig. 54.8 Radiographic progression after 6, 12, and 24 months of therapy. Mean change in Larsen score for patients treated for 6, 12, and 24 months with leflunomide, sulfasalazine, or placebo. *(Data from Scott DL, Smolen JS, Kalden JR, et al. Treatment of active rheumatoid arthritis with leflunomide: two-year follow-up of a double-blind, placebo-controlled trial versus sulfasalazine. Ann Rheum Dis 2001;60:913-923.)*

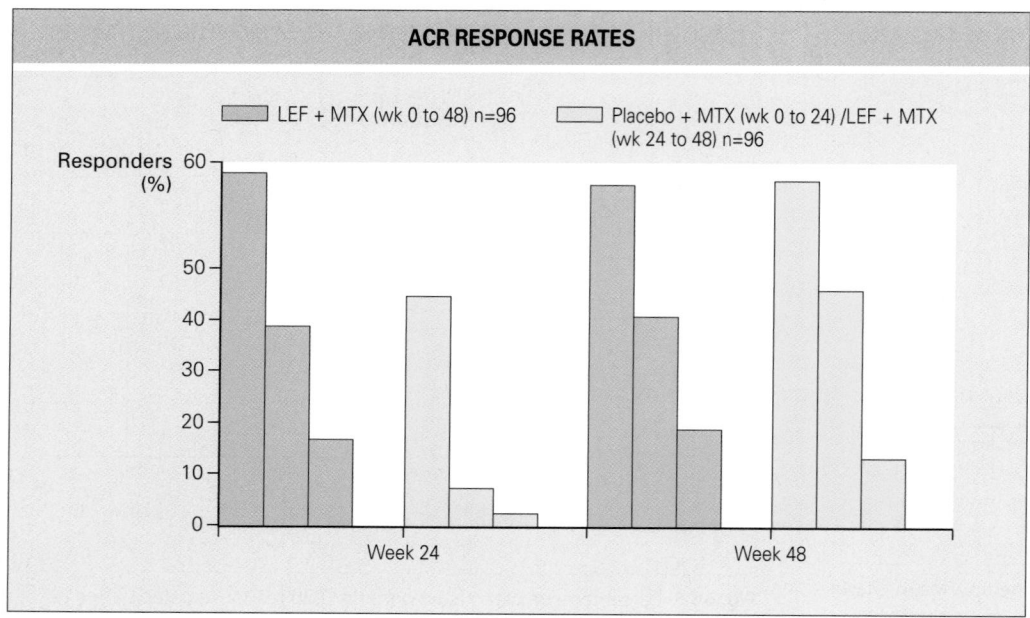

Fig. 54.9 ACR response rates at week 24 and 48 in patients receiving double-blind leflunomide and methotrexate from weeks 0 to 48 versus patients receiving placebo and methotrexate from weeks 0 to 24 followed by open-label leflunomide and methotrexate from weeks 24 to 48. *(Data from Kremer J, Genovese M, Cannon G, et al. Combination of leflunomide and methotrexate (MTX) therapy for patients with active rheumatoid arthritis failing MTX monotherapy: open-label extension of a randomized, double-blind placebo controlled trial. J Rheumatol 2004;31:1521-1531.)*

There was no significant pharmacokinetic interaction between leflunomide and methotrexate. The combination was generally well tolerated; however, liver enzyme elevations were seen in the majority of patients (63%). Efficacy measures revealed a good response, with 53% of patients achieving ACR20 criteria. Liver biopsies in three patients with elevated liver enzymes revealed mild (not clinically significant) hepatic fibrosis in two patients and a normal biopsy in one patient.

The combination of leflunomide and methotrexate was subsequently evaluated in a 24-week double-blind, placebo-controlled study of 263 patients with RA who exhibited an inadequate response to methotrexate.[24] Leflunomide was given in a dose of 10 mg (after 2 × 100-mg loading doses) for 2 months, after which the dose could be increased to 20 mg/day. The results showed that leflunomide provided additional benefit in 51.5% of patients partially responding to methotrexate alone. Elevated liver function test results were observed in 28% of patients receiving combination therapy. These data suggest that the leflunomide-methotrexate combination can be used with appropriate

liver enzyme monitoring. A 6-month open-label extension was carried out in which patients continued treatment with the combination of leflunomide and methotrexate, whereas patients previously on methotrexate alone now received leflunomide (in combination with methotrexate) in a dose of 10 mg/day without a loading dose, with subsequent dose adjustment based on the patient's response.[25] The combination of leflunomide and methotrexate continued to provide significant therapeutic benefit, whereas patients switching from placebo to leflunomide obtained the same magnitude of response after 6 months despite the lack of a loading dose (Fig. 54.9). These data suggest that, in patients with an inadequate response to methotrexate, leflunomide is effective without the use of a loading dose. A recent randomized controlled trial supported the concept that the combination of sulfasalazine with leflunomide was ineffective by demonstrating no significant difference in the Disease Activity Score (DAS) response when sulfasalazine was added on to leflunomide or used alone in leflunomide inadequate responders.[26] A trend to a higher response was seen and the ACR70 of the combination was superior to monotherapy. A subsequent analysis of 968 patients with RA demonstrated that adding leflunomide or sulfasalazine to methotrexate versus switching to monotherapy did not result in significantly different retention rates for leflunomide or sulfasalazine. In a recent study in a large observational database of 1214 RA patients the clinical outcomes of two potential strategies were evaluated in patients discontinuing DMARDs for ineffectiveness: switching to another DMARD or step-up combination therapy, with methotrexate or sulfasalazine or leflunomide was evaluated. Retention rates for leflunomide and sulfasalazine were similar for adding or switching.[27]

The increasing use of biologic agents in RA coupled with the concept of combination therapy has resulted in an increased use of a combination of leflunomide and biologic agents.[28,29] Combination of leflunomide with infliximab has been evaluated in eight retrospective and open-label prospective studies.[29] Approximately 460 patients have been evaluated in these studies with efficacy comparable to that of open-label studies of an infliximab/methotrexate combination. No new safety signals have been seen. In one prospective study of 162 RA patients, 57 patients took infliximab combined with leflunomide while 105 patients used other DMARDs.[30] No difference in drug survival, disease activity, or adverse events was observed. In the safety trial of adalimumab plus standard DMARD therapy a higher rate of adverse events was reported in patients receiving leflunomide and adalimumab. Taken together, preliminary results of the leflunomide/biologic agent combination studies suggest that the combination is efficacious and relatively safe. Whether efficacy is comparable to combinations of methotrexate and other biologic agents remains to be addressed.

Long-term efficacy

A 5-year open-label uncontrolled extension study demonstrated that the early efficacy of leflunomide based on ACR response rates and HAQ scores seen at 1 year was maintained for up to 5 years.[31] The long-term safety profile was similar to previous studies. The sustainability of improvement in physical function and health-related quality of life (HRQOL) was examined in the three phase-3 randomized controlled trials comparing leflunomide, sulfasalazine, and methotrexate. Over 24 months, improvements in physical function were shown to be sustained and reflected improvements in mental as well as physical domains of HRQOL.[32]

Recently, the effectiveness of leflunomide was compared with infliximab and etanercept using survival on drug as an evaluation tool. Patients in a standardized clinical protocol were evaluated over 12 months. Patients not responding to DMARDs, including methotrexate, were treated with etanercept (n = 184), infliximab (n = 223), or leflunomide (n = 114). Survival on drug as a percentage of the number followed revealed rates of 82%, 55%, and 32% at 12 months for etanercept, infliximab, and leflunomide, respectively. However, differences in patient selection and drug efficacy may influence the comparison between the tumor necrosis factor blockers and leflunomide.[33] Similar data regarding sustainability of leflunomide were obtained in a prospective case series study in 136 patients initiating therapy with the drug. After a median follow-up of 317 days, 56% of patients receiving leflunomide withdrew, mainly because of adverse drug reactions (29%) or lack of efficacy (13%).[34]

The effect of long-term (>2 years) leflunomide treatment on radiographic progression was evaluated in 128 of the original 824 patients involved in one of three phase-3 trials. Patients for whom paired evaluable radiographs at baseline and study endpoint were available were included. Mean leflunomide treatment was 4.3 years to final radiograph. After leflunomide treatment the predicted yearly progression rate improved in 72% of patients and deteriorated in 16%. In 33% of patients who had erosions at baseline no progression occurred with leflunomide.[35]

Dosing studies

The efficacy and safety profiles of 10-mg versus 20-mg dose of leflunomide were evaluated in a 24-week multinational randomized double-blind parallel group study of 402 RA patients.[36] Patients receiving 10 mg of leflunomide received one 100-mg loading dose on day 3 while

the 20-mg group received a 100-mg loading dose on days 1 to 3. The results demonstrated superiority of the 20-mg dose.

Leflunomide has also been examined in daily practice in large observational databases.[37] Analysis of one cohort of 285 patients in terms of the percentage of patients discontinuing treatment over time compared with other conventional DMARDs including methotrexate and sulfasalazine demonstrated higher discontinuation rates for toxicity but similar discontinuation for efficacy.

Leflunomide has been evaluated in a large multicenter international study of psoriatic arthritis.[38] In a 24-week controlled study of 188 patients with psoriatic arthritis, a modified ACR20 result was achieved in 36% of patients at 24 weeks compared with 20% in placebo.[38] Fifty-nine percent of the leflunomide-treated patients as compared with 30% of the placebo-treated patients achieved a psoriatic arthritis response (PsARC). The effect on psoriasis was also mild, with 17% of patients on leflunomide and 7% of those on placebo achieving a significant clearing of skin disease (the PASI-75). Leflunomide has also been compared with methotrexate in a 16-week study in 94 patients with polyarticular juvenile rheumatoid arthritis. There was a more positive response as defined by the ACR Pedi30 response criteria in patients receiving methotrexate than in those who had received leflunomide (89% vs. 68%).[39] Encouraging results have been observed with leflunomide therapy in ANCA-associated granulomatous vasculitis, dermatomyositis, scleroderma, and sarcoidosis.[29] It was found to be ineffective in a pilot study of primary Sjögren's syndrome and a randomized controlled trial of ankylosing spondylitis.

SAFETY AND TOLERABILITY

In clinical trials involving a total of 1339 patients treated with leflunomide monotherapy, the frequency of side effects and the safety profile are in general similar to those of moderate-dose methotrexate and sulfasalazine (Table 54.1). However, the side effects tend to persist longer with leflunomide, even with dose reduction or discontinuation of therapy, because of the long half-life of the drug. The most common reported side effects are gastrointestinal symptoms such as diarrhea, dyspepsia, nausea, vomiting, and abdominal pain. Diarrhea is generally mild to moderate and usually occurs within the first 3 months. In approximately 30% of patients, diarrhea resolved within 1 week, but in about 35% the symptoms persisted for more than 1 month. Nausea and vomiting are usually transient. Significant weight loss has also been reported in 7% of 70 patients beginning leflunomide therapy.[40] A large retrospective chart study of 108 patients with inflammatory arthritis treated at U.K. centers with a combination of leflunomide and methotrexate was carried out to evaluate tolerability of the combination.[41] At a median of 24.5 months, 51% of patients remained on the combination. The most common reasons for discontinuation were nausea, vomiting, diarrhea, as well as abnormal liver function test results.

Nervous system effects of leflunomide include headache, dizziness, and paresthesia. The central nervous system side effects are usually mild to moderate and are uncommonly a cause for stopping the drug. Case reports of peripheral neuropathy submitted to the U.S. Food and Drug Administration (FDA) in association with leflunomide were reviewed.[42] Of 80 reported patients, symptoms began after a mean of 6 months of treatment. Electrodiagnosis was consistent with distal axonal, sensory, or sensorimotor polyneuropathy in most patients. Patients withdrawing from leflunomide within 30 days were more likely to have improvement. In a recent study to monitor the potential clinical neurotoxicity in 113 leflunomide-treated patients, eight incident cases of peripheral neuropathy and two cases of worsening of preexisting neuropathy were diagnosed by nerve conduction (incidence, 9.8%).[42] Compared with patients not receiving leflunomide, patients receiving leflunomide were older (mean age, 69), more often diabetic (30%), and more often treated with potentially neurotoxic drugs (20%). At least one risk factor was found in 50% of patients with neuropathy (56% positive predictive value; 96% negative predictive value). The results suggest careful monitoring of the patient's neurologic status during leflunomide treatment. Patients have been reported to stabilize symptomatically and electrophysiologically on cessation of the drug.

TABLE 54.1 ADVERSE EVENTS IN CLINICAL TRIALS OF LEFLUNOMIDE

Adverse event	All RA studies (%)	Placebo-controlled trials (%) MN 301 and US 301				Active-controlled trials (%) MN 302*	
	LEF N = 1339	LEF N = 315	PBO N = 210	SSZ N = 133	MTX N = 182	LEF N = 501	MTX N = 498
Body as a whole							
Allergic reaction	—	5	2	0	6	—	2
Worsening RA	8	5	11	20	4	17	19
Asthenia	3	6	4	5	6	3	3
Flu syndrome	—	4	2	0	7	—	0
Infection	4	—	0	0	0	—	0
Injury, accident	5	7	5	3	11	6	7
Pain	—	4	2	2	5	—	<1
Abdominal pain	6	5	4	4	8	6	4
Back pain	5	6	3	4	9	8	7
Cardiovascular							
Hypertension	10	9	4	4	3	10	4
Chest pain	—	4	2	2	4	—	2
Gastrointestinal							
Anorexia	3	3	2	5	2	3	3
Diarrhea	17	27	12	10	20	22	10
Dyspepsia	5	10	10	9	13	6	7
Gastroenteritis	3	—	1	0	6	3	3
Abnormal LFTs	5	10	2	4	10	6	17
Nausea	9	13	11	19	18	13	18
GI/abdominal pain	5	6	4	7	8	8	8
Mouth ulcer	3	5	4	3	10	3	6
Vomiting	3	5	4	4	3	3	3
Hematic and lymphatic							
Leukopenia (<200 g/L)	3	—	0	2	1	4	3
Metabolic and nutritional							
Hypokalemia	—	3	1	1	1	—	<1
Weight decrease	4	—	1	2	0	—	2
Musculoskeletal system							
Leg cramps	—	4	2	2	6	—	0
Joint disorder	4	—	2	2	2	8	6
Synovitis	—	—	1	0	2	4	2
Tenosynovitis	3	—	0	1	2	5	1
Nervous system							
Dizziness	4	5	3	6	5	7	6
Headache	7	13	11	12	21	10	8
Paresthesia	—	3	1	1	2	4	3
Respiratory system							
Bronchitis	7	5	2	4	7	8	7
Increased cough	3	4	5	3	6	5	7
Respiratory infection	15	21	21	20	32	27	25
Pharyngitis	3	—	1	2	1	3	3
Pneumonia	—	3	0	0	1	—	2
Rhinitis	—	5	2	4	3	—	2
Sinusitis	—	5	5	0	10	—	1
Skin and appendages							
Alopecia	10	9	1	6	6	17	10

TABLE 54.1 ADVERSE EVENTS IN CLINICAL TRIALS OF LEFLUNOMIDE—cont'd

Adverse event	All RA studies (%) LEF N = 1339	Placebo-controlled trials (%) MN 301 and US 301				Active-controlled trials (%) MN 302*	
		LEF N = 315	PBO N = 210	SSZ N = 133	MTX N = 182	LEF N = 501	MTX N = 498
Eczema	—	—	1	1	1	3	2
Pruritus	4	5	2	3	2	6	2
Rash	10	12	7	11	9	11	10
Dry skin	—	3	2	2	0	3	1
Urogenital system							
Urinary tract infection	5	5	7	4	2	5	6

*Study MN 302, an active controlled study, treated a total of 999 subjects using 1 : 1 randomization to either leflunomide, 20 mg/day after a loading dose of 100 mg/day for 3 days, or methotrexate, 10 mg/wk or escalation to 15 mg/wk.
The table lists the percentage of patients with adverse events occurring in more than 3% in any leflunomide-treated group. Treatment duration was 52 weeks.
GI, gastrointestinal; LEF, leflunomide; LFTs, liver function tests; MTX, methotrexate; PBO, placebo; SSZ, sulfasalazine.

Hypertension is the most common cardiovascular effect of leflunomide. Data from clinical trials suggest that aggravation of hypertension is more likely to be a problem with leflunomide than new-onset hypertension.

Clinical trials did not show a higher incidence of infection in patients receiving leflunomide than in patients receiving the placebo. As a consequence of the potential for immunomodulation, leflunomide is not recommended for patients with some immunodeficiency, substantial impairment of bone marrow function, or serious infections (i.e., requiring intravenous antibiotics or hospitalization). If infection occurs in patients receiving combination therapy with another immunosuppressant such as methotrexate or corticosteroids, early and vigorous treatment should be considered. Leflunomide should be discontinued in the event of a serious infection and a wash-out procedure should be initiated. No cases of disseminated fungal or viral disease or opportunistic infections have been reported during clinical trials with leflunomide. Patients with a reactive purified protein derivative skin test or a history of *Mycobacterium tuberculosis* exposure or who come from an area where tuberculosis is endemic should be carefully monitored for reactivation of the disease. A recent retrospective study of 201 patients revealed an increased risk of postoperative wound-healing complications of elective orthopedic surgery in patients receiving leflunomide therapy (40.6%) compared with patients receiving methotrexate (13.6%) (*P* = .01).[43] Although it was recommended to interrupt leflunomide treatment preoperatively in this group of patients, the long half-life of leflunomide makes it impractical.

Leflunomide exhibited a higher rate of skin reactions than placebo in clinical trials, with an overall incidence of rash of 9.9%, as well as pruritus and a maculopapular rash. Most rashes occurred between the second and fifth months and resulted in discontinuation of therapy in 1.3% of patients. Rare cases of Stevens-Johnson syndrome and toxic epidermal necrolysis have been reported. In all cases, patients were receiving other co-medication known to be associated with these skin lesions. Several cases of severe cutaneous reactions associated with fever and generalized weakness occurring 4 to 6 weeks after onset of leflunomide have been reported recently.[44] Any suspicion of either of these conditions necessitates discontinuation of leflunomide and initiation of a cholestyramine wash-out procedure; this involves administration of 24 g/day for 11 days. Under these circumstances, re-exposure to leflunomide is contraindicated. Alopecia was observed with low frequency and was reversible on discontinuing the drug. A small percentage of patients (<1.0%) withdrew on the basis of alopecia. Mouth ulcers occurred with the same frequency as with placebo in the trials.

Interstitial lung disease (ILD) has been reported in patients receiving leflunomide.[45] Baseline pulmonary disease and/or abnormal chest radiograph or computed tomographic scans were observed in 69% of 29 patients before initiating leflunomide. Prior methotrexate therapy was reported in 42% of patients. Concurrent use of corticosteroids was observed in 62%. Forty-one percent of patients died.[43] Most patients initially present with acute pneumonitis, but a number of patients present with slowly progressive ILD. In one report the mean duration of leflunomide treatment was 14.5 months before the onset of ILD. In another report, pneumonitis occurred 12 to 20 weeks after the addition of leflunomide to methotrexate. A significant mortality rate, as high as 30%, has been associated with this pulmonary complication. Histologic findings include a mosaic pattern of acute and organizing diffuse alveolar damage. Treatment has been shown to be effective with early withdrawal of leflunomide, high-dose corticosteroids, and cholestyramine in some patients.[46] A recent population-based epidemiology study using a claims database of 62,734 RA patients demonstrated that the increased risk of ILD was associated with leflunomide in patients with a history of methotrexate use or preexisting ILD with a relative risk of 2.6 (95% CI, 1.2-5.6).[47] The risk of ILD was not elevated (RR 1.2; 95% CI, 0.4-3.1) with no previous methotrexate or history of ILD. The results were thought to be a consequence of channeling high-risk patients to leflunomide. Recently post-marketing surveillance for leflunomide was reported in 5043 consecutive Japanese patients. Sixty-one patients were reported to have lung injury with one third dying of it. Risk factors included preexisting ILD, loading dose, smoking history, and low body weight (40 kg or less).

Rare cases of pancytopenia have been observed in post-marketing experience, primarily in patients with known risk factors for blood dyscrasias; many cases were confounded by concomitant medications. Significantly, leflunomide was not associated with an increased risk of lymphoproliferative disorders, with a frequency of 0.2% in around 2077 patient-years of exposure. The frequency was in line with the expected rate of lymphoproliferative disorders in RA of 0.2%. No increase in the incidence of malignancies has been demonstrated, with a reported rate of 1.3% compared with 1.2% for placebo.

Laboratory tests

The incidence of elevated liver enzymes—alanine aminotransferase (ALT) and aspartate aminotransferase (AST)—with leflunomide is similar to that observed with moderate-dose methotrexate therapy in patients receiving folate supplementation. ALT elevations less than three times normal levels are usually reversed without discontinuation of leflunomide and may decrease with continued therapy or with dose reduction. Elevations greater than three times normal also reverse with dose reduction or discontinuation. Persistently elevated liver function test results should not be tolerated and should prompt drug withdrawal. Cholestyramine should be administered in patients with persistent elevation above three times normal despite withdrawal. A cholestyramine wash-out of 4 g three times daily for 5 days is generally adequate. Liver function abnormalities are generally asymptomatic and are not associated with decreased serum albumin or prolonged prothrombin time. Because the active metabolite is cleared by the liver and biliary system, leflunomide is contraindicated in patients with impaired liver function. Leflunomide should be monitored on a regular basis.

Hepatotoxicity has been increased in studies of combination therapy with leflunomide and methotrexate. In the larger study by Kremer and colleagues,[24] nearly 30% of patients exhibited an increase in AST or ALT at any time during the 6-month study but only 1.5% and 3.8% demonstrated a threefold elevation of AST and ALT, respectively. The substantial proportion of patients exhibiting liver function abnormalities with the leflunomide-methotrexate combination suggests careful monitoring of liver function with the combination. The data concerning serious liver toxicity reported to date with the combination (see earlier) have emphasized this requirement. A post-marketing report from the European Agency for the Evaluation of Medicinal Products detailed the experiences in leflunomide-treated RA patients with a total drug exposure of 104,000 patient-years. The report described 296 cases of hepatic abnormality, including 129 cases of serious liver disease. The 296 case reports included 232 patients with liver function abnormalities, 2 with cirrhosis, 15 with liver failure, and a total of 15 deaths. Most of the liver abnormalities occurred within the first 6 months without predilection for age or gender. Most of the patients with serious hepatotoxicity were taking another potentially hepatotoxic drug (i.e., concomitant non-steroidal anti-inflammatory drugs and/or methotrexate) and had one or several co-morbidities (including alcohol abuse, hepatitis A, B, and C, interstitial lung disease, renal insufficiency, autoimmune liver disease, and pancreatitis).

After an extensive review of available clinical trials and several medical databases and post-marketing surveillance, the FDA Advisory Committee concluded that serious hepatotoxicity such as hepatocellular jaundice and acute liver failure is rare.[48] Post-marketing surveillance spontaneous reporting by the FDA revealed that hepatic failure occurred with an incidence of 14 per 100,000 patient-years, similar to that observed with other DMARDs.[49] A large claims database studies demonstrated comparable results.

Treatment-related anemia was not observed with leflunomide. Some patients experienced transient reductions in white blood cell count without sustained leukopenia, as well as transient thrombocytopenia. In patients with recent or concurrent treatment with immunosuppressive drugs or with bone marrow toxicity potential or hematological abnormalities, frequent hematologic monitoring should be performed. No clinically significant effect of leflunomide on plasma electrolytes, total protein, creatinine, bilirubin, alkaline phosphatase, glucose, cholesterol, or triglycerides has been noted. A reduction in serum uric acid was observed in 30% of treated patients with an average reduction of 60 mm/L during therapy, not associated with reduced calcium phosphate or bicarbonate limbs. Uricosuria was related to inhibition of uric acid reabsorption. Renal function as determined by serum creatinine and urea levels was unaffected. However, given that leflunomide is partially eliminated by the kidney, it should be used with caution in patients with mild renal insufficiency. Leflunomide is contraindicated in patients with moderately severe renal impairment. Several case reports have addressed a potential interaction between leflunomide and warfarin. Such an interaction was at least partially responsible for an increase in a patient with a previously stable international normalized ratio. Clinicians should increase their frequency of monitoring of the international normalized ratio and adjust the warfarin dosage accordingly.

PRESCRIBING TIPS

Leflunomide is indicated in patients with moderate to severe active RA, in both early and late disease. Because of its long half-life, leflunomide therapy has been initiated with a loading dose of one 100-mg tablet per day for 3 days. However, because of toxicity concerns, many rheumatologists have stopped using the loading dose. Generally, a daily maintenance dose of 10 to 20 mg/day is used. If dosing at 20 mg/day is not well tolerated clinically, the dose may be decreased to 10 mg/day. In patients in whom the risk of toxicity is greater (i.e., those who are taking leflunomide in combination with methotrexate or those who are elderly) the maintenance dose may be initiated at 10 mg/day for 2 months with a dose escalation to 20 mg if there is an inadequate response. As noted earlier, for patients not requiring a rapid response to therapy, consideration should be given to initiating therapy without a loading dose.

Before initiation of the drug a complete blood cell count, including a differential white blood count and platelets, and liver function tests, including an AST and ALT, must be performed. According to the product monograph, a complete blood cell count and liver blood tests should also be performed every 2 weeks for the first 6 months and then every 8 weeks thereafter. More frequent early monitoring might be done if used in combination with methotrexate.

Patients experiencing a serious side effect of leflunomide should undergo a wash-out with cholestyramine (8 g three times daily) or activated charcoal (50 g four times daily) for 11 days. The metabolite of leflunomide, A77 1726, is not removed with peritoneal dialysis, although with hemodialysis A77 1726 is cleared somewhat more rapidly and with a shorter half-life. These data suggest that dialysis is not an effective wash-out procedure.

Leflunomide is contraindicated in patients with impaired liver function, severe renal impairment, severe hypoproteinemia (e.g., in nephrotic syndrome, serious infections, known immunodeficiency, bone marrow dysfunction, anemia, leukopenia, neutropenia, thrombocytopenia) due to causes other than RA, or known hypersensitivity to the drug. Leflunomide should be used with caution in combination with methotrexate. It is contraindicated in serious infection, and patients should be advised to seek medical advice if they note potentially worsening fatigue, bruising, sore throat, increased susceptibility to infection, and skin or mucous membrane lesions.

Leflunomide is teratogenic in animals and therefore should be used with caution in women of child-bearing age. It should not be used in women who are, or may become, pregnant or those who are breastfeeding. Women should wait for 2 years after stopping leflunomide to ensure clearance of the metabolite and have their plasma A77 1726 level checked to ensure that it is below 0.02 mg/L, which the manufacturer deems to present minimal teratogenic risk. In women wishing to become pregnant before the 2-year wash-out, accelerated removal using cholestyramine (8 g three times daily for 11 days) or activated charcoal should be carried out, shortening the clearance time to 3 months. After the wash-out, plasma levels of the active metabolite must be evaluated and be less than 0.02 mg/L (0.02 mg/mL). This plasma level must be verified by a second test at least 14 days after the first plasma level (<0.02 mg/L) is achieved. Women should be advised to be sure they are not pregnant before starting leflunomide and, while receiving the drug, use reliable contraception. Although no data exist, it is suggested by the manufacturer that men wishing to father a child should discontinue leflunomide and undergo an accelerated removal procedure.

REFERENCES

1. Davis JP, Cain GA, Pitts WJ, et al. The immunosuppressive metabolite of leflunomide is a potent inhibitor of human dihydroorotate dehydrogenase. Biochemistry 1996;35:1270-1273.
2. Fairbanks LD, Bofil M, Ruckemann K, et al. Importance of ribonucleotide availability to proliferating T-lymphocytes from healthy humans. J Biol Chem 1995;270:29682-29691.
3. Cao WW, Kao PN, Chao AC, et al. Mechanism of the antiproliferative action of leflunomide. J Heart Lung Transplant 1995;14:1016-1030.
4. Cherwinski HM, McCarley D, Schatzman R, et al. The immunosuppressant leflunomide inhibits lymphocyte progression through cell cycle by a novel mechanism. J Pharmacol Exp Ther 1995;272:460-468.
5. Siemasko K, Chong A-SF, Williams JW, et al. Regulation of B cell function by the immunosuppressive agent leflunomide. Transplantation 1996;61:635-642.
6. Siemasko K, Chong A-SF, Jäck H-M, et al. Inhibition of JAK3 and STAT6 tyrosine phosphorylation by the immunosuppressive drug leflunomide leads to a block in IgG1 production. J Immunol 1998;160:1581-1588.
7. Xu XL, Williams JW, Bremmer EG, et al. Inhibition of protein tyrosine phosphorylation in T cells by a novel immunosuppressive agent, leflunomide. J Biol Chem 1995;270:12398-12403.
8. Manna SK, Aggarwal BB. Immunosuppressive leflunomide metabolite (A77 1726) blocks TNF-dependent nuclear factor-κB activation and gene expression. J Immunol 1999;161:2095-2102.
9. Déage V, Burger D, Dayer JM. Exposure of T-lymphocytes to leflunomide but not to dexamethasone favors the production by monocytic cells of interleukin-1 receptor

antagonist and tissue inhibitor of metalloproteinases-1 over that of interleukin-1β and metalloproteinase. Eur Cytokine Netw 1998;9:663-668.

10. Lang R, Wagner H, Heeg K. Differential effects of the immunosuppressive agents cyclosporine and leflunomide in vivo: leflunomide blocks clonal T cell expansion yet allows production of lymphokines and manifestations of T cell-mediated shock. Transplantation 1995;59:382-389.

11. Kraan MC, Smeets TJ, Van Loon MJ, et al. Differential effects of leflunomide and methotrexate on cytokine production in rheumatoid arthritis. Ann Rheum Dis 2004;63:1056-1061.

12. Kraan MC, Reece RJ, Barg EC. Modulation of inflammatory and metalloproteinase expression in synovial tissue by leflunomide and methotrexate in patients with active rheumatoid arthritis: findings in a prospective, randomized, double-blind, parallel design clinical trial in thirty-nine patients at two centers. Arthritis Rheum 2000;43:1820-1830.

13. Kraan MC, DeKoster BM, Elferinde JGR, et al. Inhibition of neutrophil migration in patients with rheumatoid arthritis: findings of a prospective, randomized, double-blind clinical trial in fifteen patients. Arthritis Rheum 2000;43:1488-1498.

14. Kobayashi Y, Ueyama S, Arai Y, et al. The activity of leflunomide, A771726, inhibits both the generation of and the bone resorbing activity of osteoclasts by acting directly on cells of the osteoclast lineage. J Bone Miner Metab 2004;22:318-328.

15. Weinblatt ME, Kremer JM, Coblyn JS, et al. Pharmacokinetics, safety and efficacy of the combination of methotrexate and leflunomide in patients with active rheumatoid arthritis. Arthritis Rheum 1999;42:1322-1328.

16. Shi J, Kovacs SJ, Ludden TM, et al. Population pharmacokinetics analysis of A771726 after oral administration of leflunomide in pediatric subjects with polyarticular course juvenile rheumatoid arthritis. Clin Pharmacol Ther 2004;75:5(abstract I-7).

17. Mladenovic V, Domljan Z, Rozinan B, et al. Safety and effectiveness of leflunomide in the treatment of patients with active rheumatoid arthritis. Arthritis Rheum 1995;38:1595-1603.

18. Strand V, Cohen S, Schiff M, et al. Treatment of active rheumatoid arthritis with leflunomide compared with placebo and methotrexate. Arch Intern Med 1999;159:2542-2550.

19. Strand V, Tugwel P, Bombardier C, et al. Function and health-related quality of life: results from a randomized controlled trial of leflunomide versus methotrexate or placebo in patients with active rheumatoid arthritis. Arthritis Rheum 1999;42:1870-1878.

20. Sharp JT, Strand V, Leung H, et al. Treatment with leflunomide slows radiographic progression of rheumatoid arthritis: results from three randomized controlled trials of leflunomide in patients with active rheumatoid arthritis. Arthritis Rheum 2000;43:495-505.

21. Cohen S, Cannon GW, Schiff M, et al. Two-year, blinded, randomized, controlled trial of treatment of active rheumatoid arthritis with leflunomide compared with methotrexate. Arthritis Rheum 2001;44:1984-1992.

22. Emery P, Breedveld FC, Lemmel EM, et al, and the Multinational Leflunomide Study Group. A comparison of the efficacy and safety of leflunomide and methotrexate for the treatment of rheumatoid arthritis. Rheumatology 2000:39:655-665.

23. Smolen JS, Kalden JR, Scott DL, et al. Efficacy and safety of leflunomide compared with placebo and sulfasalazine in active rheumatoid arthritis: a double blind randomized multicentre trial. Lancet 1999;353:259-266.

24. Kremer JM, Genovese MC, Cannon GW, et al. Concomitant leflunomide therapy in patients with active rheumatoid arthritis despite stable doses of methotrexate: a randomized, double-blind, placebo-controlled trial. Ann Intern Med 2002;137:726-733.

25. Kremer J, Genovese M, Cannon G, et al. Combination of leflunomide and methotrexate (MTX) therapy for patients with active rheumatoid arthritis failing MTX monotherapy: open-label extension of a randomized, double-blind placebo controlled trial. J Rheumatol 2004;31:1521-1531.

26. Dougados P, Emery E, Lemmel E, et al. When a DMARD fails, should patients switch to sulfasalazine or add sulfasalazine to continuing leflunomide. Ann Rheum Dis 2005;64:44-51.

27. Schoels M, Kaprat T, Stamm T, et al. Step up combination versus switching of non-biologic disease modifying antirheumatic drugs in rheumatoid arthritis: results from a retrospective observational study. Ann Rheum Dis 2007;66:1059-1065.

28. Combe B. Leflunomide combined with conventional disease-modifying antirheumatic drugs or biologics in patients with rheumatoid arthritis. Joint Bone Spine 2006;73:587-590.

29. Pinto P, Dougados M. Leflunomide in clinical practice. Acta Reumatol Port 2006;31:215-224.

30. Flendie M, Creemers MC, Welsing PM, et al. The influence of previous and concomitant leflunomide on the efficacy and safety of infliximab therapy in patients with rheumatoid arthritis; a longitudinal observational study. Rheumatology (Oxford) 2005;44:472-478.

31. Kalden JR, Schattenkirchner M, Sorensen H, et al. The efficacy and safety of leflunomide in patients with active rheumatoid arthritis. Arthritis Rheum 2003;48:1513-1520.

32. Strand V, Scott DL, Emery P, et al. Physical function and health related quality of life: analysis of 2-year data from randomized, controlled studies of leflunomide, sulfasalazine, or methotrexate in patients with active rheumatoid arthritis. J Rheumatol 2005;32:590-601.

33. Geborek P, Crnkic M, Telemeen A, et al. Tolerability using survival on drug evaluation tool: experience of etanercept, infliximab and leflunomide in rheumatoid arthritis. Ann Rheum Dis 2002;61:793-798.

34. Van Roon EN, Jansen TL, Mourad L, et al. Leflunomide in active rheumatoid arthritis: a prospective study in daily practice. Br J Clin Pharmacol 2004;58:201-208.

35. Van Der Heijde D, Kalden J, Scott D, et al. Long term evaluation of radiographic disease progression in a subset of patients with rheumatoid arthritis treated with leflunomide beyond 2 years. Ann Rheum Dis 2004;63:737-739.

36. Poór G, Strand V, for the Leflunomide Multinational Study Group. Efficacy and safety of leflunomide 10 mg versus 20 mg once daily in patients with active rheumatoid arthritis: multinational double-blind, randomized trial. Rheumatology 2004;43:744-749.

37. Bettembourg-Brault I, Gossec L, Pham T, et al. Leflunomide in rheumatoid arthritis in daily practice: treatment discontinuation rates in comparison with other DMARDs. Clin Exp Rheumatol 2006;24:168-171.

38. Kaltwasser JP, Nash P, Gladman D, et al. Efficacy and safety of leflunomide in the treatment of psoriatic arthritis and psoriasis: a multinational, double-blind, randomized, placebo-controlled clinical trial. Arthritis Rheum 2004;50:1939-1950.

39. Silverman E, Mouy R, Spigel L, et al. Leflunomide or methotrexate for juvenile rheumatoid arthritis. N Engl J Med 2005;342:1655-1666.

40. Coblyn JS, Shadick N, Helfgott S. Leflunomide-associated weight loss in rheumatoid arthritis. Arthritis Rheum 2001;44:1048-1051.

41. Kaul A, O'Reilly DT, Slack RK, et al. Tolerability of methotrexate and leflunomide combination therapy for inflammatory arthritis in routine clinical practice: results of a four-centre study. Rheumatology 2008;47:1430-1431.

42. Bonnel RA, Graham DJ. Peripheral neuropathy in patients treated with leflunomide. Clin Pharmacol Ther 2004;75:580-585.

43. Fuerst M, Mohl H, Baumacgtel K, et al. Leflunomide increases risk of early healing complications in patients with rheumatoid arthritis undergoing elective, orthopedic surgery. Rheumatol Int 2006;26:1138-1142.

44. Shastri V, Betkerur J, Kushalappa P, et al. Severe cutaneous adverse drug reaction to leflunomide: a report of five cases. Indian J Dermatol Venereol Lepereol 2006;72:286-289.

45. Cannon G, Strand V, Simon L, et al. Interstitial lung disease in rheumatoid arthritis patients receiving leflunomide. Arthritis Rheuma 2004;40(Suppl):S561.

46. Inokuma S, Sata T, Sagaiva A, et al. Proposals for leflunomide use to avoid lung injury in patients with rheumatoid arthritis. Mod Rheumatol 2008;18:442-446.

47. Suissa S, Ernst P, Hudson M, et al. Newer disease-modifying antirheumatic drugs and the risk of serious hepatic adverse events in patients with rheumatoid arthritis. Am J Med 2004;117:87-91.

48. Goldkind L, Simon LS. FDA Meeting March 2003; updating the safety of new drugs for rheumatoid arthritis: III. Safety and efficacy update on leflunomide (Arava). Available online at www.rheumatology.org/publications/hotline/0503leffda.asp?and=mem.

49. Food and Drug Administration Arthritis Advisory Committee. Briefing information. Arava (leflunomide) 2003. Available online at: www.fda.gov/ohrms/dockets/ac/03/briefing/3930b2.htm.

Immunosuppressives (chlorambucil, cyclosporine, cyclophosphamide [Cytoxan], azathioprine [Imuran], mofetil, tacrolimus)

Daniel E. Furst, Eresha Markalanda, and Philip J. Clements

55

- There is some evidence that cyclophosphamide (CYC) and cyclosporine inhibit bony damage resulting from rheumatoid arthritis (RA).
- CYC and cyclosporine are associated with the most serious toxicity of the disease-modifying antirheumatic drugs (DMARDs).
- Combination DMARD therapy may be effective in aggressive RA.

INTRODUCTION

This chapter reviews the use of disease-modifying antirheumatic drugs (DMARDs) that are not covered in other chapters, namely azathioprine, chlorambucil, cyclophosphamide (CYC), cyclosporine, tacrolimus, mycophenolate mofetil, and combination therapy.

Because the mechanisms of action of these drugs demonstrate some similarities (as well as differences), their mechanisms of action are addressed together (Table 55.1). Likewise, the pertinent pharmacokinetics of these medications are discussed in a single section. Thereafter, the evidence that these drugs are effective, their toxicities, and tips on their use are addressed, each separately. The suggestions regarding therapeutic use represent generally accepted approaches but are often not fully tested.

MECHANISMS OF ACTION

Azathioprine

Azathioprine (AZA) interferes with adenine and guanine ribonucleotide via suppression of inosinic acid synthesis. Its main active metabolite is 6-thioguanine. This, in turn, is a metabolic product of azathioprine's principal metabolic product, 6-mercaptopurine (6-MP).[1] In rheumatoid arthritis (RA), azathioprine reduces the numbers of circulating B and T lymphocytes (particularly suppressor, or CD8+, cells), mixed lymphocyte reactivity, immunoglobulin (Ig) M and IgG synthesis, and interleukin (IL)-2 secretion.

Chlorambucil

Chlorambucil's mechanism of action is similar to that of cyclophosphamide: it cross-links DNA and proteins, thereby preventing cell replication.[2] Chlorambucil itself is not cytotoxic but is rapidly and almost completely metabolized to phenylacetic acid mustard, its principal and most active metabolite.

Cyclophosphamide

Active metabolites of CYC (principally phosphoramide mustard) cross-link DNA so that it cannot replicate. CYC is cytotoxic to both resting and dividing lymphocytes.[3] In RA patients cyclophosphamide (intravenous [IV] or oral) suppresses helper cell functions, decreases the number of activated T cells by 30% to 40% (which correlates with clinical improvement), and dramatically decreases B cells for months.[4]

CYC suppresses primary cellular and humoral immune responses, especially if administered immediately after an antigen challenge, but it can also inhibit an established humoral or immune response. It effectively suppresses many cell-mediated immune responses such as the delayed hypersensitivity skin test and graft-versus-host reactivity, and it is anti-inflammatory.[3]

IL-2 inhibitors (cyclosporine, sirolimus, tacrolimus)

All calcineurin inhibitors

Cyclosporine complexes with cyclophilin (a cytoplasmic protein), which then binds calcineurin, an intracellular phosphatase. Tacrolimus complexes with a different binding protein (FKBP-12) but also interacts with calcineurin. This in turn regulates gene transcription coding for IL-2 and other cytokines.[3,5] Thus cyclosporine and tacrolimus inhibit IL-2 and IL-1 receptor production and inhibit macrophage–T-cell interactions and T-cell responsiveness. Further recent data demonstrate that cyclosporine inhibits IL-17 production by Th17 cells.[6] Additionally, cyclosporine is antiangiogenic in rheumatoid synovial fibroblasts via inhibition of AP-1–mediated vascular endothelial growth factor (VEGF) expression,[6] demonstrating a possible mechanism to reduce synovial proliferation.

Cyclosporine and tacrolimus block the amplification of cellular immune responses and the generation of T-cell effectors and other functions dependent on IL-2. They inhibit the B-cell production of antibody to T-cell–dependent antigens, gamma-interferon (IFN) production, and natural killer cell (NK) activity. Growth of bone marrow–derived myeloid, erythroid, or B-lymphocyte cell line responses to T-cell–independent antigens are not affected. Although cyclosporine and tacrolimus are strong inhibitors of delayed hypersensitivity, they do not impair macrophage responses to lymphokines.[3]

Sirolimus also inhibits IL-2 function but does so by blocking mammalian target of rapamycin (TOR), thereby blocking B- and T-cell activation and many of the same downstream events as outlined for cyclosporine and tacrolimus, including both calcium-dependent and calcium-independent pathways such as IL-2, IL-3, IL-5, IL-6, and IL-15.[7]

Mycophenolate mofetil

Mycophenolate mofetil breaks down rapidly to mycophenolic acid (MPA), the active form of this drug. MPA inhibits inosine monophosphate dehydrogenase. Cyclin-dependent kinase activity is inhibited and cyclin-dependent kinase inhibitor P27 elimination is blocked. This inhibits T-cell lymphocyte proliferation and downstream effects, such as intercellular adhesion to endothelial cells. *In vitro*, the expression of E-selectin, P-selectin, and intercellular adhesion molecule (I CAM)-1 on endothelial cells is markedly reduced. The complementary T-cell ligands LFA, VLA-4, and P-selection glycoprotein ligand 1 are functionally impaired, thus reducing T-cell adhesion to and penetration through the endothelium and reducing lymphocyte recruitment to sites of inflammation.[8]

Enteric-coated mycophenolate sodium (EC-MPA) was designed as an alternative to mycophenolate mofetil (MMF). EC-MPA releases a different formulation of MPA. MPA dissolves slowly after reaching the small intestine, thus delaying the release of MPA. EC-MPA 720 mg twice daily is therapeutically equivalent to MMF 1000 mg twice daily in renal transplant patients and apparently decreases the side effects relative to the non-EC compound.

PHARMACOKINETICS

Table 55.2 summarizes the most pertinent pharmacokinetics of these drugs. Additional comments regarding the pharmacokinetics of each drug are outlined as follows.

Azathioprine

Azathioprine is chemically cleaved to 6-mercaptopurine (6-MP), which is catalyzed to the inactive metabolite, 6-methylmercaptopurine (6-MMP), or is methylated to the active metabolites, 6-thioguanine nucleotides (6-TGNs) and 6 methyl mercaptopurine ribonucleotides (6-MMPRs). The methylation of 6-MP to active 6-TGNs and 6-MMPRs is catalyzed by thiopurine methyltransferase (TPMT), an enzyme that exhibits a threefold difference in 6-TGN alleles and helps explain the large interindividual variations seen in efficacy and toxicity when using azathioprine.

Eighty-nine percent of subjects have normal to high levels of TPMT activity, 11% have intermediate activity, and 0.3% have low or absent TPMT activity.[9-11] Subjects with low or absent TPMT levels are at high risk of myelosuppression,[11,12] whereas patients with normal or high levels have a lower frequency of toxicity.[10,11] Patients with intermediate levels of TPMT activity have a relative risk of 3.1 for development of severe side effects (predominantly gastrointestinal) compared with patients with high levels of TPMT activity.[10,11] Because secondary intracellular metabolites are the source of azathioprine activity, measuring plasma levels of azathioprine is not useful.[13] Despite some inherent problems regarding measuring erythrocyte TPMT levels, this method may provide a useful guide to how patients are likely to handle azathioprine and thus may help to guide dosing of the drug (both initial and escalation).[10,14]

Thiopurine has a narrow therapeutic index. Increased serum concentration can cause life-threatening toxicity. Thiopurine has exhibited a genetic polymorphism[15] across ethnic groups with 1 out of 300 Caucasians being markedly deficient in TPMT. Heterozygous or homozygous deficiency leads to marked and toxic myelosuppression.[16]

In chronic inflammatory disease, patients with TPMT activity below 11.9 nmol/mL RBC × h experienced more side effects (rash, cholestasis, and bone marrow toxicity).[17]

An approximate doubling of the 6-TGN level 1 to 3 weeks after infliximab therapy in Crohn disease has been observed, but its clinical significance is unclear.[18]

Chlorambucil

The oral bioavailability of chlorambucil is adequate (0.70). It is rapidly and almost completely metabolized at unknown sites to phenylacetic acid mustard and several other poorly characterized metabolites.[19] Each dose of chlorambucil is almost completely metabolized and excreted within 24 hours.[15] Renal excretion of drug and metabolites is the main disposition pathway.

Cyclophosphamide

CYC itself is not cytotoxic, but it is enzymatically converted by hepatic microsomal enzymes (cytochrome p 450) to multiple metabolites, of which phosphoramide mustard is probably the most active cytotoxic agent.[2,20] CYC and its metabolites are excreted largely by the kidney. The drug is extensively metabolized before excretion, with less than 25% of the administered dose appearing in the urine unchanged. Of the urinary metabolites, about 50% consists of carboxyphosphamide and about 15% is 4-ketophosphamide.[20] Acrolein, a metabolite excreted in the urine, is thought to be responsible for urologic toxicity. The concurrent use of 2-mercaptoethane sulfonate (Mesna) may detoxify acrolein, reducing bladder toxicity.[21] Only small amounts of radioactive label appear in stool, expired air, spinal fluid, sweat, breast milk, saliva, and synovial fluid.[2,22]

TABLE 55.1 MECHANISMS OF ACTION

Drug	Active agent(s)	Mechanism
Azathioprine	6-thioguanylic acid, 6-methyl-mercaptopurine ribonucleosides	Interfere with adenine and guanine ribonucleotides
Chlorambucil	Phenylacetic acid mustard (metabolite)	Cross-links DNA
Cyclophosphamide	Phosphoramide mustard (metabolite)	Cross-links DNA
Cyclosporine and other IL-2 inhibitors	Parent compound and up to 15 metabolites	Suppresses IL-2 synthesis and release Suppresses T-cell response and interaction
Mycophenolate mofetil	Mycophenolic acid	Interferes with inosine monophosphate Dehydrogenase inhibits T-cell and endothelial function

TABLE 55.2 PHARMACOKINETICS OF DMARDs

	Bioavailability	Clearance (mL/min/kg)	Serum elimination half-life (hr)	Unbound fraction	Routes of elimination	Site of metabolism
Azathioprine	0.8 (6-MP)	21-200 (AZA) 114 (6-MP)	1.7 (AZA) 1.2-1.5 (6-MP)	0.30 0.80 (6-MP)	Renal (20%-45%)	Liver renal
Chlorambucil	0.7	20	1.3-1.7 1.9-2.6 (mustard)	0.01	Renal (20%-70%)	?
Cyclophosphamide	0.97	1.2	2-8 8.7 (mustard)	0.87 0.45 (mustard)	Renal (cyclophosphamide 50% metabolites 8%-35%)	Liver
Cyclosporine	0.2-0.5	2-32	10-30	0.10	Renal (6%) Bile (94%)	Liver
Mycophenolic mofetil	94	1.0	11.6	3	GI	Liver, GI
Sirolimus	14	3.17 variable	62	8	GI	Liver, GI
Tacrolimus	17-23	0.7-1.4	11-34	1	GI	Liver, GI

DMARDs, disease-modifying antirheumatic drugs; GI, gastrointestinal.

TABLE 55.3 DRUG INTERACTIONS WITH CYCLOSPORINE, RAPAMYCIN, AND TACROLIMUS

Drugs that increase IL-2 inhibitor concentrations (inhibit CYP3A4)	Drugs that decrease IL-2 inhibitor concentrations (induce CYP3A4)
Antiacids: metoclopramide, cisapride	**Anticonvulsants:** phenytoin, carbamazepine, phenobarbital
Antifungals (azoles): ketoconazole, itraconazole	**Antituberculosis:** rifampin
Antituberculosis: isoniazid	**Antibiotic:** nafcillin, aminoglutethimide
Calcium-channel blockers: diltiazem (cyclosporine, rapamycin only), nicardipine, verapamil	**Miscellaneous:** St. John's wort
Antibiotics: ciprofloxacin, clarithromycin, erythromycin, doxycycline, protease inhibitors	
Miscellaneous: grapefruit juice, quinidine, diclofenac	

Because dialysis removes 72% of CYC, the drug should be administered after dialysis[20] and the dose should be reduced when administered to patients with renal failure. Allopurinol and cimetidine (but not ranitidine) inhibit hepatic microsomal enzymes, resulting in increased CYC alkylating metabolite levels.[20]

When undergoing total body irradiation (TBI), patients on CYC showed[23] lower postirradiation peak serum levels. This needs to be confirmed in further controlled studies before recommending an increase in the dose in TBI patients.

Cyclosporine

Absorption of the usual cyclosporine formulation is erratic and incomplete.[24-26] A cyclosporine microemulsion is associated with a significant increase in the rate, extent, and consistency of absorption.[26-28] On a milligram-for-milligram basis, this has resulted in a 20% to 30% increase in exposure to cyclosporine.[27,28] Tacrolimus, too, has low and variable bioavailability.[29] Both cyclosporine and tacrolimus are strong substrates for CYP3A4, so drugs that induce CYP3A4 (e.g., rifampin, phenobarbital, phenytoin) decrease these drug levels, whereas drugs that inhibit CYP3A4 (ketoconazole, diltiazem) increase these drug levels (Table 55.3). Grapefruit juice also increases drug levels (by 62% in one study) because of its effect on inhibiting CYP3A4 activity.[30] Cyclosporine and tacrolimus are largely distributed outside the blood volume (body fat, liver, pancreas, lungs, kidneys, adrenal glands, spleen, and lymph nodes have higher concentrations than serum). They are highly bound to plasma proteins, erythrocytes, and lipoproteins.[24,25] About 11% of a cyclosporine dose is found in infant cord blood.[31] Cyclosporine is metabolized in the liver by the cytochrome P450 mixed function oxidase to at least 15 known metabolites, some of which have immunosuppressive properties.[24,25,29] CYP3A (hepatic metabolizing enzyme) activity correlates with cyclosporine dosing requirement after renal transplant ($r = 0.55$).[32] At steady state, colonic tissue cyclosporine concentrations are 50 to 250 times blood levels, indicating significant tissue concentration of cyclosporine. Elimination of cyclosporine and tacrolimus are primarily via the biliary system, with only small amounts appearing in the urine.[24,25,29]

Administration of cyclosporine with other nephrotoxic agents such as amino glycosides and nonsteroidal anti-inflammatory drugs (NSAIDs) may increase cyclosporine's or tacrolimus's nephrotoxic potential.[24,25] Cyclosporine may potentiate methotrexate (MTX) by inhibiting metabolism of MTX to less active forms.[33]

Mycophenolate mofetil

MMF is rapidly changed to MPA, the active moiety. MPA is 93% bioavailable with a clearance of 11 liters/hr and an elimination half-life of 11 to 16 hours.[34,35] Although 90% is renally excreted, there is an enterohepatic recirculation that can supply a safety valve if renal insufficiency supervenes.[35]

The concentration of MPA correlates with serum bilirubin, creatinine, and albumin concentrations, thus being affected by both renal and liver disease.[34] Areas under the curve of MPA, rather than a single level, correlate best with efficacy and toxicity, and a limited sample model over 6 hours is sufficiently accurate to predict the total area under the curve.[36] Although monitoring MPA concentrations in transplantation therapy is recommended, monitoring MPA concentrations in rheumatologic disease is not common practice.

Besides the degree of renal and hepatic disease (mentioned earlier), other factors such as bowel decontamination and enterohepatic recirculation (contributing to a mean of 29% to MPA bioavailability) affect MPA concentrations.[37] Tacrolimus and cyclosporine increase MPA concentrations, possibly by augmenting the bioavailability of mycophenolate by inhibiting MPA glucuronidation.[38] *In vitro*, diflunisal and mefenamic acid and its congeners significantly inhibit MPA glucuronidation as well.[39] Although these interactions again speak to the need for monitoring MPA concentrations in transplant patients, monitoring of MPA levels in rheumatology practice still needs to be evaluated.

EFFICACY, TOXICITY, AND THERAPEUTIC USES

Azathioprine

Efficacy

Azathioprine 1.25 to 3.0 mg/kg/day is more effective than placebo in RA.[1,2] There appears to be a dose-response relationship in RA, comparing placebo, azathioprine 1.0 mg/kg/day, and azathioprine 2.5 mg/kg/day (although the data are not completely consistent).[1] A meta-analysis of three trials that included 81 RA patients who were treated with azathioprine reported that azathioprine was more effective than placebo (odds ratio of 1.45 to 10.50), although adverse reactions were also statistically more frequent in the azathioprine group.[40]

In controlled trials comparing azathioprine with other DMARDs, results are too inconsistent to reach any conclusion regarding clinically significant differences comparing the efficacy of azathioprine versus cyclosporine, CYC, and chloroquine. However, azathioprine was not as effective as MTX in the treatment of RA.[41,42]

A small placebo-controlled trial in reactive arthritis (eight patients in a crossover trial) showed positive results over 4 to 6 months.[43] A 16-patient controlled trial comparing azathioprine plus prednisone to prednisone alone in polymyositis/dermatomyositis showed only the superiority of azathioprine after 3 years of follow-up; at 3 months no differences between the two regimens were discernible.[1] A placebo-controlled, 2-year study of 73 patients with Behçet syndrome (37 of whom received azathioprine) concluded that azathioprine was effective in controlling the progression of Behçet syndrome, especially in its most serious manifestation, eye disease.[44] A meta-analysis of azathioprine in renal systemic lupus eruthematosus (SLE) reported that azathioprine plus steroids decreased renal SLE all-cause mortality (relative risk of 0.60; 95% confidence interval (CI), 0.36 to 0.99) but did not alter renal outcomes, nor was it associated with increased infections compared with steroids.[45] An open 2-year study in 75 SLE patients demonstrated that AZA was equivalent to cyclosporine in preventing lupus nephritis flares.[46]

Anecdotal case series suggest possible azathioprine efficacy in scleroderma lung disease and pediatric renal lupus.[47,48] In small studies of antineutrophil cytoplasmic antibody (ANCA)-associated vasculitis[49] and scleroderma,[50] AZA was used after cyclophosphamide induction and demonstrated that AZA was well tolerated and tended to maintain disease control, although deteriorations and relapses did occur.

Toxicity

The most common adverse events seen with azathioprine are gastrointestinal intolerance, including nausea and diarrhea. Other toxicities include rash, pancreatitis, cholestatic hepatitis, and stomatitis (Table 55.4). More viral infections in RA patients using azathioprine have been observed by some investigators.[2] A 50-fold increase in relative risk of malignant disease has been documented in azathioprine-treated renal transplant patients (particularly non-Hodgkin lymphoma).[1] In

RA, the azathioprine-related risk of lymphoma (and non-Hodgkin lymphoma) is confounded by an increased relative risk secondary to RA per se.[1] Overall, there is probably a small added risk of developing some malignancy when using AZA in RA of 1.3 and a relative risk of between 2.2 and 8.7 for developing a lymphoproliferative disorder.[1,2] This increased risk was not found, however, among 626 patients with inflammatory bowel disease using azathioprine for 27 months.[51] Reversible lymphoma associated with Epstein-Barr virus has also been observed after azathioprine therapy.[52] Bone marrow toxicity has been associated with intermediate or reduced (especially low or absent) levels of TPMT in RA patients (see Pharmacokinetics earlier).[9-12]

In different chronic inflammatory diseases, the patients have suffered with minor and severe adverse effects such as serum sickness, rash, cholestatic jaundice, and bone marrow suppression.

Therapeutic use

Before using azathioprine, a discussion of risks and treatment goals should be conducted and a good history and physical examination and laboratory testing should be conducted. TPMT levels should be tested to help determine sensitivity to azathioprine toxicity before the drug is started. TPMT activity is useful to determine the likelihood of bone marrow toxicity.[53] However, TPMT levels are higher in new RBCs, so the levels should not be determined shortly after bone marrow depression or with the post-transplant response of increased erythropoiesis.

An alternative to testing TPMT levels for predicting azathioprine sensitivity is to institute a daily dose of 25- to 50-mg doses for the first week followed by a complete blood count. Thereafter, doses are increased regularly by 0.5 mg/kg/day every month, aiming for 2 to 3 mg/kg/day. The dose may then be adjusted to the minimum effective dose.

Monitoring includes hemoglobin, white blood cells (WBCs), and platelet counts every 2 weeks while dosing regimens are being changed and every 4 to 6 weeks during stable regimens. Liver function tests can be performed every 6 to 8 weeks. Monitoring for lymphoproliferative disease and other malignancy is appropriate but undefined, as is monitoring for pregnancy.

Most pertinent pharmacokinetics are outlined in Table 55.3, but the pharmacokinetics of AZA in breast milk bears mentioning. Peak breast milk concentrations of azathioprine are about 10% of blood[54] levels with small total amounts of azathioprine actually being absorbed (0.008 mg/kg infant weight/24 hr). The data suggest that mothers receiving azathioprine can breastfeed[55] (Table 55.5).

Chlorambucil

Efficacy

Only one double-blind, placebo-controlled study of chlorambucil (CHL) has been reported in RA (25 patients received chlorambucil and 23 received placebo over 3 months).[2,56] Multiple clinical and serologic parameters improved significantly in the chlorambucil-treated group compared with the placebo-treated group. In uncontrolled series, the overall response rate in RA was about 70%.[2,57]

A controlled trial of chlorambucil versus cyclosporine was reported in 40 patients with Behçet disease. Chlorambucil was more effective for extraocular disease (skin, arthritis), whereas cyclosporine was more effective for ocular Behçet disease.[58]

Although chlorambucil has been used in SLE, polyarteritis nodosa, ANCA-associated granulomatous vasculitis, multiple sclerosis, sarcoidosis, scleroderma, dermatomyositis, and amyloidosis, no controlled studies have substantiated its effectiveness in these disorders.[56,59]

TABLE 55.4 TOXICITY OF DMARDs				
	AZA (%)	CHL (%)	CYC (%)	CSA (%)
Shared				
Dose-related marrow suppression	4-27	14-50	6-32	2-6
Leukopenia/ thrombocytopenia	0-5	8-37	0-4	≤2
Susceptibility to infection				
Overall	0-9	18-27	0-22	0-6
Herpes zoster	0-6	4-27	5-30	0-3
Gastrointestinal intolerance				
Nausea, vomiting	9-23	4	19-45	4-40
Diarrhea	≤1	—	3-18	2-18
Rash	1-6	0-18	0-2	0-2
Not shared				
Hair				
Alopecia	—	2	7-80	—
Hypertrichosis	—	—	—	7-49
Stomatitis	0-5	—	—	0-8
Gum hyperplasia	—	—	—	4-12
Hepatic				
Abnormal liver function	0-5	—	—	0-8
Fibrosis/cirrhosis	—	—	—	—
Azoospermia/oligospermia	—	≤100	60-100	—
Amenorrhea	—	2-8	0-53	—
Cystitis	—	—	4-45	—
Teratogenesis	±	—	—	±
Neoplasia	—	—	—	—
Decreased GFR	—	—	—	50-87
Hypertension	—	—	—	33
Neurotoxicity	—	—	—	10-40
Pneumonitis	—	—	—	—

DMARDs, disease-modifying antirheumatic drugs; GFR, glomerular filtration rate.

TABLE 55.5 EFFICACY OF DMARDs IN RHEUMATOID ARTHRITIS						
Drug	Placebo	AZA	CYC	DPA	Gold	HCQ/CQ*
Azathioprine (AZA)	AZA > placebo	—	AZA = CYC	AZA = DPA	AZA = gold	AZA = CQ
Chlorambucil (CHL)	CHL > placebo	—	—	—	—	—
Cyclophosphamide (CYC)	CTX > placebo	CYC = AZA	—	—	CYC = gold	—
Cyclosporine (CSA)	CSA > placebo	—	—	CSA = DPA	—	—
Tacrolimus	TAC > plac	—	—	—	—	—

*Hydroxychloroquine (HCQ) or chloroquine (CQ)—controlled trials only.
DMARDs, disease-modifying antirheumatic drugs.

Toxicity

The most common toxicities with chlorambucil use are dose-related bone marrow suppression (usually granulocytopenia or thrombocytopenia) and infertility (see Table 55.4). Cumulative bone marrow toxicity occurs regularly with chlorambucil and often requires drug discontinuation. In one study only 1 of the 28 subjects was able to continue the drug for longer than 21 months.[57]

The risk of infertility, azoospermia, and amenorrhea rises by increasing the duration and doses. Spermatogenesis has returned 15 to 17 years after discontinuation of chlorambucil.[2] Irreversible azoospermia was regularly produced in adult males who received more than 400 mg chlorambucil, although hormonal function was maintained.[60] In postpubertal females, both gametogenesis and hormonal function are altered adversely and menopause occurs. Although the frequency of infertility in males is quite high, it is lower in females.

In subjects receiving chlorambucil, the risk of neoplasia is increased, particularly of the skin and hematologic systems.[2,61] An acute leukemia incidence of 0.93% was reported in a group of 1711 RA patients treated with chlorambucil for 1 to 13 years.[61]

Therapeutic use

As a general rule, there is little indication for the use of this drug in the modern era of managing patients with RA. When used, chlorambucil can be instituted orally in doses between 0.1 and 0.2 mg/kg/day.[28,31] Once response or toxicity has occurred (often within 3 to 4 months of instituting therapy), the drug can be continued at a lower dose that maintains the white blood cell count (WBC) between 3000 and 4000/mm[1] (usually a dose between 3 and 4 mg daily). Because oral contraceptives and inhibitors of gonadotropin-releasing hormone protect ovarian function from cytotoxic damage in animal models, consideration might be given with the use of one or the other agent in female subjects interested in preserving fertility. Their use in humans remains purely exploratory.

Regular monitoring includes hemoglobin, WBC, and platelet counts every 1 to 2 weeks while dosing regimens are being changed and every 2 to 4 weeks during stable regimens. Pregnancy should be avoided.

Cyclophosphamide

Efficacy

In five placebo-controlled trials in RA, oral CYC was consistently better than placebo when used in doses of more than 1.5 mg/kg/day, both clinically and in terms of erythrocyte sedimentation rate (ESR) and rheumatoid factor.[21] It has not been consistently effective in doses less than 1.0 mg/kg/day. CYC reached its peak effectiveness after approximately 16 weeks. In small studies, CYC retarded bone destruction.[21]

When compared with other DMARDs, CYC is equal to azathioprine and is equal, or superior, to intramuscular gold for both clinical and radiologic endpoints.[21] Due to toxicity issues and better newer agents, cyclophosphamide is principally used now only for the extra-articular manifestations of RA (i.e., vasculitis or interstitial lung disease).

For 2 decades, cyclophosphamide (oral and IV) has been the treatment of first choice for diffuse proliferative SLE nephritis, rapidly progressive pauci-immune crescentic glomerulonephritis, and severe and progressive organ involvement of the systemic vasculitides (ANCA-associated granulomatous vasculitis, microscopic polyarteritis, Behçet syndrome).

The management of these conditions has recently taken on a peculiarly oncologic flavor. Terms such as "induction" and "maintenance" (continuation with less aggressive/toxic medications such as azathioprine or MTX) are now commonly used when referring to therapy with CYC, both in the clinic and in the conduct of therapeutic research trials. Until recently, for example, the treatment of choice for lupus nephritis (particularly World Health Organization [WHO] class III focal proliferative nephritis [(FPGN] and class IV diffuse proliferative nephritis [DPGN]) was cyclophosphamide, using 14 IV infusions of 0.5 to 0.75 g/m[2]) over 30 months.[62,63] In that protocol, the induction phase included the first 6 monthly cyclophosphamide infusions, followed by a maintenance phase that included 8 quarterly cyclophosphamide infusions.[64] Since the publication of six randomized trials comparing MMF and cyclophosphamide, which resulted in conflicting results, the place of cyclophosphamide as the drug of choice for SLE nephritis has been questioned. The ultimate place of cyclophosphamide in this situation will require further research.

High-dose IV CYC (50 mg/kg for 4 days, 200 mg/kg overall) was compared with IV cyclophosphamide 750 mg/mo for 12 months in a randomized clinical trial of renal and central nervous system (CNS) SLE.[65] For the first 12 months the high-dose CYC group fared significantly better than the monthly lower-dose CYC group, although these differences disappeared by 30 months.[65]

An interesting registry study examined the effect of CYC[66] on pulmonary catastrophic antiphospholipid syndrome (p-CAPS) versus SLE-CAPS. CYC in p-CAPS was associated with increased mortality, while cyclophosphamide improved survival in SLE-CAPS. These data need to be repeated prospectively because selection bias may have skewed the results.

The treatment of the systemic vasculitides (ANCA-associated granulomatous vasculitis, microscopic polyarteritis [MPA], and crescentic glomerulonephritis) has been divided into phases of "remission induction" and "maintenance therapy."[67] The induction phase has usually included cyclophosphamide, azathioprine, or MTX.[68-71] The rate of relapse was lower and the event-free survival was greater (P < 0.05) in patients receiving 12 monthly pulses of IV cyclophosphamide versus 6 monthly pulses.[68] Remission induced by cyclophosphamide could be successfully maintained by therapy with azathioprine over 18 months. Remission could be induced equally by cyclophosphamide and MTX, but the rate of relapse by 18 months was significantly higher when using methotrexate for maintenance[70] rather than continued cyclophosphamide.

IV CYC 65 (up to 900 mg/m[2]) without maintenance has real but limited usefulness in ANCA-associated granulomatous vasculitis because 52% of patients relapse despite good initial response.[72]

A 1-year placebo-controlled trial of oral CYC for SSc interstitial lung disease showed a modest effect on FVC and more robust effects on activities of daily living, quality of life, and skin thickening.[73] A study in a small group of patients given 6 monthly IV CYC, followed by 6 months of oral azathioprine, generally supported these results.[50]

Toxicity

Cyclophosphamide's significant toxicity is the major factor limiting its clinical use in the rheumatic diseases. Major toxicities include carcinogenicity (especially bladder cancer), propensity to cause infertility, frequent cumulative bone marrow toxicity, and hemorrhagic cystitis. Kinlen's experience with 643 RA patients suggests a relative risk of 12.8 for all cancers combined, a relative risk of 10.9 for non-Hodgkin lymphoma, and a 10-fold increase in bladder cancer.[74]

Irreversible azoospermia was regularly produced in adult males receiving a total dose of more than 18 g of cyclophosphamide. In men, plasma testosterone levels tend to remain normal, as does the histologic appearance of Leydig and Sertoli cells, suggesting sparing of hormonal function. The risk of infertility, azoospermia, and amenorrhea with CYC increases with increasing duration of therapy, doses, and increasing age in women. In postpubertal females, both gametogenesis and hormonal function are altered adversely and menopause occurs.

A study of 17 women demonstrated amenorrhea in all the patients on cyclosphosphamide. In those given luteinizing hormone releasing agent, menstruation returned and ovarian function reversed when cyclophosphamide was stopped. When not given the agonist, ovarian function did not return.[75] Somers and coworkers also reported that ovarian function could be protected by a depot leuprolide acetate injection in SLE patients given cyclosphosphamide.[76]

The urologic adverse effects of CYC are thought to be related to its urinary metabolite, acrolein. Hemorrhagic cystitis has been reported in about one third of subjects receiving oral CYC daily and there was a significant but much lower incidence of bladder fibrosis and bladder carcinoma.[77] In a cohort study of 119 RA patients, nine developed bladder cancer during an average 13.1 years of follow-up, although three bladder cancers occurred after 14, 16, and 17 years.[78] Cystitis and bladder carcinoma are markedly reduced when CYC is used on an intermittent IV basis. Bladder toxicity can also be reduced by the concomitant administration of 2-mercatopurine sulfate (Mesna).[79] Because Mesna is administered intravenously, it is useful primarily when cyclophosphamide is used intravenously.

Other side effects include infections, gastrointestinal side effects, and even death.

Therapeutic use

Because CYC has significant toxicity, its use in RA should be limited to patients with extra-articular manifestations suggestive of polyarteritis-like disease and those who have failed all other DMARDs, including biologics, but still have severe active RA. In these cases, oral CYC doses of 2 mg/kg/day might be considered. An IV regimen of CYC has been suggested for management of rheumatoid vasculitis. In this regimen, 500 to 1000 mg of CYC and 500 to 1000 mg of methylprednisolone are given intravenously on days 1, 8, 29, and 58. Patients were continued on oral DMARDs. In either case, once the disease is under control, switching to a less toxic drug over a longer period should be considered.

Whenever using CYC, the IV form is preferred in managing SLE-associated diffuse proliferative glomerulonephritis. It is usually started at 0.50 to 0.75 g/m^2 when glomerular filtration rate (GFR) is greater than one third of predicted normal. When renal function is less than one third of normal, the starting dose is 0.5 g/m.^{2} CYC can be administered in 150 mL of a 5% glucose solution over 30 to 60 minutes. There are no established regimens for giving 2-mercaptopurine sulfate (Mesna) with IV CYC to reduce bladder toxicity. The general rule, however, has been that its dose should be equivalent to the CYC dose and that it should be given in two to three divided doses over several hours. The IV and oral doses of CYC are equally bioavailable and the drug can be given either way.

Diuresis should be ensured by increased IV and oral fluids and possibly diuretics. Nausea and vomiting are common and may require antiemetic therapy (prophylactically and as needed). IV pulse methylprednisolone (10 to 100 mg) or dexamethasone (10 mg) may also be given. This may help decrease nausea and is also part of the treatment for glomerulonephritis.

IV pulse cyclophosphamide (with or without IV methylprednisolone) may be given once every 1 to 3 months thereafter for up to 2 to 5 years' total therapy. This drug is also given as "induction" therapy for 6 months followed by "maintenance" therapy with either azathioprine or mycophenolate mofetil.

CYC given orally is usually the preferred method for managing polyarteritis and ANCA-associated granulomatous vasculitis.[56] The dose should be instituted at 2 mg/kg/day (75 to 125 mg/day) and altered to maintain the WBC between 3000 and 3500/mm.

Laboratory evaluation for toxicity is important with CYC. Complete blood count, platelet count/estimate, and urinalysis with microscopic examination should be obtained every 7 to 14 days initially and can be reduced to every 2 to 4 weeks once the disease and dose have been stabilized for 2 to 3 months.

Avoidance of pregnancy is strongly recommended. Consideration might be given to using oral contraceptives or gonadotropin-releasing hormone inhibitors if the patient is interested in preserving fertility, although the use of these medications in this context is still exploratory.[80,81]

Cyclosporine

Efficacy

Placebo-controlled trials, including one trial in which a medium dose was compared with a low dose of cyclosporine (CSA), have been performed and show that cyclosporine is efficacious in RA.[82-84] In these studies, nearly 400 subjects with RA received cyclosporine in initial doses of 1 to 10 mg/kg/day. The studies continued for 4 to 6 months, at which time the final cyclosporine dose ranged from 3.8 to 7.4 mg/kg/day. Cyclosporine improved clinical symptoms and signs; however, no significant improvement was noted in laboratory parameters such as ESR or rheumatoid factor titers. Nephrotoxicity has been the major limiting factor preventing the use of higher doses. On the basis of these studies and a meta-analysis,[84] patients treated with 2.5 to 4.0 mg/kg/day of cyclosporine should show a substantial response within the first month.

Double-blind controlled trials showed cyclosporine (up to 5 mg/kg) was as effective as D-penicillamine, chloroquine, or azathioprine in RA.[5,85] In other studies, patients who were randomized to MTX plus cyclosporine after failing MTX fared better than those randomized to MTX plus placebo.[86] Two blinded trials found that cyclosporine was superior to conventional therapy (colchicine or prednisone/chlorambucil) in the management of Behçet disease, particularly for its ocular complications.[5,85] Cyclosporine has been successfully used in open trials and anecdotal series in dermatomyositis, ANCA-associated granulomatous vasculitis, and systemic sclerosis. In psoriasis, cyclosporine appeared to be as effective as mycophenolate mofetil.[87,88] Cyclosporine seems to be effective in clearing cutaneous lesions in psoriasis[5,85] and as a possible choice for psoriatic arthritis.[89,90]

Toxicity

When cyclosporine is used to treat rheumatic disease, side effects are generally mild and reversible at low doses.[5,24] Dose-related decreases in GFR often occur with corresponding increases in serum creatinine (the principal adverse effect). In patients using more than 5 mg/kg/day, cyclosporine renal biopsies sometimes showed focal interstitial fibrosis, tubular atrophy, and/or arteriolar lesions. However, these did not occur if the dose of cyclosporine remained 5 mg/kg/day or less and if serum creatinine did not rise more than 50% above baseline.[91] In Tugwell and colleagues' study (average dose 3.8 mg/kg/day), serum creatinine rose over the first 4 months but then stabilized; after discontinuation of cyclosporine, serum creatinine returned to within 15% of baseline in all except two patients.[85]

In a secondary analysis of registry data, cyclosporine was associated with osteoporosis, although well-controlled trials will be necessary to prove these early data.[92] In a large randomized study, an increase in insulin-like growth factor (somatomedin C) and insulin-requiring diabetes[93] was seen in RA patients during long-term cyclosporine therapy.[94] This, too, will need more studies.

Elevation of blood pressure is another common side effect of cyclosporine therapy. New-onset hypertension has been reported in about one third of rheumatoid and psoriatic arthritis patients. Although antihypertensive therapy may be required, potassium-sparing diuretics should be avoided because cyclosporine may cause hyperkalemia. Because diltiazem (but not isradipine or nifedipine) may increase cyclosporine levels by decreasing its metabolism, changes in cyclosporine dosage may be required when using diltiazem.

Significant hepatotoxicity manifested as elevated hepatic enzymes and bilirubin may be seen, but usually only with higher cyclosporine doses. In RA patients treated for up to 12 months, creatinine increased greater than 30% at some point in 48%, hypertrichosis occurred in 35%, paresthesias were seen in 29%, gum hyperplasia was demonstrated in 14%, and gastrointestinal complaints (mostly nausea) occurred in 47% of patients.[95] Lymphomas have been observed with this drug, including reversible Epstein-Barr virus–associated lymphomas.

Therapeutic use

Consensus guidelines for the use of cyclosporine (for both conventional and microemulsion formulations) in RA have been published and should be reviewed by any practitioner using cyclosporine.[96] Cyclosporine therapy may be instituted after a discussion of the risks (particularly nephrotoxicity and hypertension) and treatment goals, following a good history, physical examination, and laboratory testing. Cyclosporine use should be avoided in patients with preexisting renal disease (creatinine clearance <60 mL/min).

Both conventional and microemulsion formulations may be instituted at 2.5 mg/kg/day in two divided doses every 12 hours. The dose may be cautiously increased by 0.5 to 0.75/kg/day every 4 to 8 weeks until a maximum dose of 5 mg/kg/day for the conventional formulation (or 4 mg/kg/day for the microemulsion) is reached, unless this is prevented by a rise in serum creatinine of 30% or greater. Dosage reductions of 0.5 to 0.75 mg/kg/day are warranted if serum creatinine increases above baseline by 30% or if uncontrolled hypertension appears (systolic >140 mm Hg and/or diastolic >90 mm Hg). Hypertension can usually be managed with calcium-channel blockers (especially isradipine or nifedipine) and β-blockers and with reduction of the cyclosporine dose.

Mycophenolic acid delays cyclosporine absorption, showing a potentially important drug-drug interaction. Thus the institution of cyclosporine therapy may require dose adjustment of mycophenolic acid when mycophenolic acid and cyclosporine are to be used together.

Mycophenolate mofetil

Efficacy

Data using MMF to treat RA are limited, but in one study (abstract only) there was no difference between 2 g and 4 g MMF daily for the treatment of RA.[97] The American College of Rheumatology (ACR)-20 response rate was 29% for 2 g and 4 g MMF daily and 47% for 5 g daily. Double-blind studies using MMF in lupus proliferative and membranous glomerulonephritis have shown this drug to be effective for these patients. Response was noted in 92% using MMF plus prednisone compared with 90% of patients treated with cyclophosphamide plus prednisolone, while the toxicity of MMF was less than that of cyclophosphamide.[98,99] In addition, case series point to the possibility that MMF may be useful in ANCA-positive vasculitides, including microscopic polyangiitis and ANCA-associated granulomatous vasculitis.[98,99]

Although controversial, a meta-analysis of five studies stated that MMF is preferred over CYC in SLE nephritis.[100] Bullous pemphigoid[101] may also respond to MMF.

Toxicity

Comparisons with azathioprine in the renal transplantation literature show that azathioprine and MMF have similar gastrointestinal, hematopoietic, and hepatic toxicity profiles, with possibly a somewhat decreased incidence of fungal infections among patients treated with MMF.[102] Diarrhea is the most common side effect observed. Nausea, leukopenia, anemia, thrombocytopenia, thinning of scalp hair, pancreatitis, and bacterial and viral infections have also been seen. Regular monitoring for hepatic and hematologic toxicity is required. Careful observation for infections (particularly for latent viral infections such as progressive multifocal leukoencephalopathy and BK virus nephropathy) is appropriate. MMF is contraindicated in pregnancy (pregnancy category D).[103]

Therapeutic use

MMF is a relatively new drug. It has been introduced as an immunosuppressive drug, but it also has effects on non-immune cells (e.g., vascular smooth muscle cells, fibrocytes). It has therapeutic value in SLE-associated kidney disease.[104] Systolic and diastolic blood pressure does not seem to be increased when using MMF.[105] Long-term controlled clinical trials are necessary to define the role of MMF in the management of lupus nephritis.

The drug can be instituted at a dose of 0.5 g twice daily for 1 week. The dose can then be increased to 1.0 g twice daily for 1 week and then to 1.5 g twice daily, if one wishes. MMF can be taken before or with food.

In renal transplant patients, a dose of 720 mg of enteric-coated mycophenolic acid has been therapeutically demonstrated to be equivalent to a 1000-mg dose of MMF. Enteric-coated mycophenolic acid is safe and effective in maintenance and *de novo* therapy in renal transplant patients. To date, MMF therapeutic drug monitoring is highly variable[106] and not yet considered useful. In renal transplantation the data suggest that both enteric-coated mycophenolic acid and mycophenolate mofetil result in equivalent mycophenolate exposure.[107]

Tacrolimus

Efficacy

There have been only limited well-controlled trials of tacrolimus in RA.[108,109] In these trials, the patients were those who had insufficient response to other DMARDs. A dose-response trial in 268 patients showed a small response rate compared with placebo over 24 weeks.[108] Compared with a 15.5% ACR20 response rate in the placebo group, only the 3-mg and 5-mg daily treatment groups separated statistically from placebo (34.4% and 50% ACR20 responses, respectively). However, the 5-mg group had more creatinine elevations (discontinuation in 10.9%). This degree of toxicity effectively ruled out the higher dose in future trials. A second trial, in 464 patients, compared 2 mg and 3 mg daily dosing versus placebo over 6 months.[109] Compared with a 10.2% placebo response, the 2-mg and 3-mg daily tacrolimus groups demonstrated an 18.8% and 26.8% response, respectively ($P \leq 0.01$ for both versus placebo). While real, these response rates would not make this drug one of the first choices in treating RA. The addition of tacrolimus (1 to 3 mg/day) to low-dose MTX (up to 7.5 mg/day) was effective in a small retrospective publication.[110] Tacrolimus has also been used after other DMARDs with some success.[111]

No trials have compared tacrolimus directly with MTX or other DMARDs.

Other topical forms of tacrolimus (0.03% and 0.1% ointments) have been used in moderate to severe atopic dermatitis and have been useful for the skin lesions of SLE or dermatomyositis.[112]

Toxicity

The toxicity in the double-blind trials[108,109] and the open-label, long-term safety experience[113] were similar: drop-out for tacrolimus-related toxicity was 16.2% over 1 year. In the open-label experience, the most common adverse events among 896 patients with RA were diarrhea (14.6%), nausea (10.3%), tremor (9.0%) , headache (8.75%), abdominal pain (7.9%), dyspepsia (7.6%), increased creatinine (6.8%), and hypertension (5.4%). Overall, 20.3% had a greater than or equal to 30% increase in serum creatinine from baseline, although only 3.2% withdrew from the study for that reason. Serious adverse events occurred in 2.7% of the patients, with the most common serious adverse events being pneumonia (0.6%), hyperglycemia (0.3%), gastroenteritis (0.2%), pancreatitis (0.2%), and diabetes mellitus (0.2%). CNS symptoms such as agitation, anxiety, confusion, and somnolence have been reported in the transplant literature at a rate of 3% to 15%, but only rarely in RA. Hypertriglyceridemia, partially related to inhibition of lipoprotein lipase, occurs in 3% to 15% of patients. Instances of cancer have been reported in the transplant literature.

The Food and Drug Administration (FDA) has issued an advisory with respect to the use of tacrolimus and pimecrolimus (another topically applied calcineurin inhibitor) (FDA advisory concerning tacrolimus—March 11, 2005). The FDA stated that the risk of skin cancer and lymphoma is increased when these drugs are used to treat eczema. The risk was believed to be related to the dose and duration of exposure. The FDA also stated that "this risk is uncertain," particularly with respect to the drugs' use for atopic dermatitis. No statements were issued regarding their use in SLE.

The concomitant or staggered uses of tacrolimus or cyclosporine in patients using sirolimus results in a 40% to 80% increase in the area under the curve for sirolimus.[114,115] No kinetic interactions between tacrolimus and MMF exist.

COMBINATION DISEASE-MODIFYING ANTIRHEUMATIC DRUG THERAPY

DMARDs can be combined rationally on the basis of complementary mechanisms of action, non-overlapping pharmacokinetics, and non-overlapping toxicities.[116]

Two general designs have been published for the use of combination DMARD therapy. One is a "complete design" in which each drug is examined individually and tested versus the combination: This design most clearly defines additive and synergistic effects. An example would be a trial comparing MTX, sulfasalazine, or their combination. Unfortunately, the results of "complete-design," double-blind trials of DMARDs have been disappointing and no combination of synthetic DMARDs has been shown to be better than at least one of the single drugs alone in these studies (Table 55.6). In the previous design ACR20 response criteria were met by 59% of the patients using sulfasalazine (SSZ), 59% of those using MTX, and 65% of those using the combination (results were not statistically different).[117] However, biologics (anti-TNF therapy) and MTX combinations have proven to be better statistically than either anti-TNF therapy or MTX alone (see Chapter 49).[118,119]

Another design might be called "additive design" studies. In these studies, partial responders to one of the DMARDs (most often MTX) are entered into a double-blind trial using patients in whom the first DMARD is already partially effective and well tolerated. For example, this design would take partial responders to MTX and add cyclosporine or placebo. These trials are more likely to be positive as one is adding an effective DMARD or placebo to the management of a patient who has already partially responded to another DMARD.

TABLE 55.6 DOUBLE-BLIND, RANDOMIZED CLINICAL TRIALS OF DMARD COMBINATION THERAPY

Authors	Parallel	Outcome	Rationale	RA Type
Haagsma et al	MTX vs. SSZ	=MTX + SSZ	±	Early
Dougador et al	MTX vs. SSZ	<MTX + SSZ + HCQ	±	Early
O'Dell et al	MTX vs. SSZ + HCQ	<MTX + SSZ + HCQ	+	Later
Wilkens et al	MTX ≥ AZA	≤MTX + AZA	±	Later
Ferraz et al	MTX	<MTX + chloroquine	+	Later
Calguneri et al	MTX to SSZ to HCQ vs. MTX + SSZ to MTX + HCQ	<MTX + SSZ + HCQ	+	Later
Williams et al	MTX ≥ auranofin	≤MTX + auranofin	−	Later
Tranavsky et al	MTX + HCQ	=HCQ	+	Later
Gerards et al	MTX + CSA	>CSA	+	Early
Marchesoni et al	MTX	<MTX + CSA	+	Early
Faarvang et al	SSZ vs. HCQ	=SSZ + HCQ	+	Late
Scott et al	HCQ + gold	≥Gold	+	Late
Gibson et al	HCQ vs. D-pen	=HCQ + D-pen	+	Late
Miranda et al	CSA	<CSA + chloroquine		Early
Step-up or add-on design				
Tugwell et al	MTX	<TX + CSA	±	Late
Kremer et al	MTX	<MTX + leflunomide	−	Late
Vanden Borne et al	HCQ	<HCQ + CSA	+	Early
Porter et al	HCQ + gold	>Gold	+	Late
Bendix et al	CSA + gold	>Gold	−	Late
Yasuda et al	Gold + bucillamine	>Gold	−	Late
Step-down (all with corticosteroids)				
Van der Veen et al	MTX + MP/P	>MTX	+	Late
Gough et al	SSZ + MP	>SSZ	+	Early
Ciconelli et al	SSZ + MP	>SSZ	+	Late
Boers et al	SSZ + MTZ + P	>SSZ	±	Early
Wong et al	Gold + MP	>Gold	+	Late
Corkill et al	Gold + MP	>Gold	+	Late
Van Gestel et al	Gold + P	>Gold	+	Late

AZA, azathioprine; CSA, cyclosporine; D-pen, D-penicillamine; DMARD, disease-modifying antirheumatic drug; HCQ, hydroxychloroquine; MP, methylprednisolone; MTX, methotrexate; P, prednisone; RA, rheumatoid arthritis; SSZ, sulfasalazine.
Modified from Choy EH, Smith C, Dore CJ, Scott DL. A meta-analysis of the efficacy and toxicity of combining disease-modifying anti-rheumatic drugs in rheumatoid arthritis based on patient withdrawal. Rheumatology 2005;44:1414-1421.

Although somewhat biased toward a positive response, this approach is frequently used in actual practice. For example, the addition of cyclosporine to background MTX in one study resulted in an additional 29% ACR20 response when cyclosporine was added to MTX compared with when placebo was added to MTX. The results of such "additive-design," double-blind trials of DMARDs are seen in the lower half of Table 55.6.

In one study the use of leflunomide (LEF) and MTX for the treatment of 74 patients with active RA proved they were effective and well tolerated in the treatment of active RA. LEF and MTX treatment achieved ACR20 criteria at the 20th week of treatment. This combination may be a useful initial treatment to be considered for early active RA.

Information in Table 55.6 is generally clear, although a few additional general comments may be helpful to understand this table. There may be pharmacokinetic reasons for the added benefits. For example, when cyclosporine is used in combination with MTX, cyclosporine elevates the MTX levels while lowering 7-OH MTX. This was the first combination DMARD therapy to show such an effect.[120] There may be pharmacodynamic reasons for the interactions, or lack thereof.[116] For example, sulfasalazine induces the multidrug resistance–related drug efflux pump in a prolonged manner in certain T cells. In the presence of sulfasalazine, MTX, once taken into the cell, is rapidly pumped out of the cell by the induced efflux pump, decreasing the effect of the MTX. This results in relative resistance to MTX, so it is not surprising that the combination of sulfasalazine and MTX is not always better than monotherapy.[120] In contrast, cyclosporine A and chloroquine inhibit the efflux pumps, thus possibly helping explain their efficacy in combination with MTX.[121]

In another realm the step-down combination using prednisolone, MTX, and sulfasalazine was the first combination therapy to clearly show cost effectiveness and cost utility compared with monotherapy.[122] Finally, the combinations of adalimumab, etanercept, or infliximab plus MTX show clear added benefit and are more fully examined in Chapter 49 (Table 55.7).

RECENT TRIALS OF COMBINATION THERAPY
Double-blind trial

In the placebo-controlled, randomized MASCOT study,[123] patients were started on sulfasalazine and those who did not achieve Disease Activity Score (DAS) remission were offered MTX, sulfasalazine, or their combination. The combination group achieved better results in

TABLE 55.7 SUBANALYSES OF COMBINATION THERAPY (EXCLUDING TNF-α BLOCKING AGENTS)

	Studies	No. patients	RR (95% CI)	P value
Established rheumatoid arthritis	21	2728	0.4 (0.28-0.56)	0.00001
Early	9	1031	0.56 (0.35-0.91)	0.02
Combinations excluding corticosteroids as bridging therapy	29	4934	0.35 (0.27, 0.44)	0.00001
Excluding studies that are done poorly	30	4858	0.31 (0.25, 0.4)	0.00001

Modified from Choy EH, Smith C, Dore CJ, Scott DL. A meta-analysis of the efficacy and toxicity of combining disease-modifying anti-rheumatic drugs in rheumatoid arthritis based on patient withdrawal. Rheumatology 2005;44:1414-1421.

ACR20/50/70 and EULAR Good responses than either monotherapy, but the monotherapy groups did not differ. This study contradicts a previous study of this combination and further analyses or studies may be necessary.

Open randomized trials of DMARD combinations

These designs yield usable results despite their unavoidable biases. Among 195 RA patients, sulfasalazine or MTX in sequence was compared with their combination in a randomized trial, aiming for remission. Prednisone was allowed in both groups. At 2 years, 36 of 97 (37%) in the combination group were in remission, compared with 18 of 98 (18%) in the single-therapy group (P = 0.003).[124]

A 2-year study examined the benefits of glucocorticoids and cyclosporine[125] added to MTX in early RA patients who were MTX-inadequate responders. Outcomes included new erosions, disability, and quality of life. The use of corticosteroids and cyclosporine on a MTX background reduced disability and improved quality of life compared with MTX alone. Radiographs, however, progressed equally in all groups. The authors felt that although the combination of MTX and prednisolone used in this trial reduced erosive damage, two DMARDs with prednisolone were needed to improve quality of life.

Another randomized trial compared single DMARDs versus one or more combination DMARDs. Patients in group I were treated with a single DMARD (MTX 7.5 to 15 mg/week or sulfasalazine 1 to 2 g/day or hydroxychloroquine 200 mg/day), group II used MTX and sulfasalazine or MTX and hydroxychloroquine, while group III used the triple combination of MTX, sulfasalazine, and hydroxychloroquine. All three

groups improved both clinically and by laboratory parameters, but all combination groups improved significantly more than the monotherapy group. Further, the triple combination was more effective than either monotherapy or the two-drug combinations. These data need confirmation because the groups were small and the trial was open.

The BEST study was of 508 early RA patients aiming for DAS remission less than 1.6 (this is one of several DAS remission criteria). Patients were randomized to one of four groups: (1) sequential, which sequentially used MTX, sulfasalazine or leflunomide; (2) add on, which started with MTX, then sequentially added sulfasalazine, hydroxychloroquine and prednisone; (3) combination therapy which started with a combination of MTX, sulfasalazine, hydroxychlorozine and prednisone; or (4) MTX plus infliximab. Only the non-biologic groups are compared here. The combination of MTX/sulfasalazine/hydroxychloroquine/prednisone resulted in remission in approximately 25% of patients at 6 months, compared with about 15% in the monotherapy or sequential addition groups. Because switching was mandated if treatment was not successful and all therapies eventually devolved to combination therapy with a biologic, the results at 6 months were used before too much switching occurred.[126]

In the randomized, open controlled study called the Tight Control of RA Study (TICORA), the patients were either treated "conventionally" or were treated aiming for tight control (DAS < 2.4). Treatment consisted of the following sequence: (1) sulfasalazine; (2) triple therapy with MTX, sulfasalazine, and hydroxychloroquine; (3) escalating doses of MTX and sulfasalazine; (4) the addition of prednisone; and (5) finally, switching to MTX and cyclosporine. At 18 months, ACR70 responses were 67% for the tight control group and 18% among the conventionally treated group (P < 0.001).

Overall, the weight of these recent data lends support for the use of the following combinations:

1. MTX plus sulfasalazine (±prednisone)
2. MTX plus cyclosporine plus prednisone
3. MTX plus hydroxychloroquine
4. MTX plus sulfasalazine plus hydroxychloroquine

Recommendations for use and monitoring

The ACR Ad Hoc Committee on Clinical Guidelines has produced recommendations for use and monitoring of DMARDs.

The specific recommendations are complex and it is advisable to consult these recommendations. In brief, they suggest evaluating patients in terms of disease activity, duration, and prognosis. Less aggressive, milder disease may be treated with monotherapy, whereas disease that is of longer duration, is more active, and has a poor prognosis needs combination DMARDs. Monitoring must take into account the specific toxicities associated with specific drugs, although most require appropriate blood and urine monitoring.[128]

KEY REFERENCES

1. McKendry RJR. Purine analogs. In: Dixon J, Furst DE, eds. Second-line agents in the treatment of rheumatic diseases. New York: Marcel Dekker, 1991:223-237.

3. Tsokos GC. Immunomodulatory treatment in patients with rheumatic disease: mechanisms of action. Semin Arthritis Rheum 1987;17:24-38.

5. Furst DE. Cyclosporine, leflunomide and nitrogen mustard. Innovative treatment approaches for rheumatoid arthritis, 9th ed. London: Bailliere Tindall, 1995:711-729.

8. Furst DE. Leflunomide, mycophenolic acid and matrix metalloproteinase inhibitors. Rheumatology (Oxford) 1999;38(suppl 2):14-18.

9. Black AJ, McLeod HL, Capell HA, et al. Thiopurine methyltransferase genotype predicts therapy-limiting severe toxicity from azathioprine. Ann Intern Med 1998;129:716-718.

12. Escousse A, Mousson C, Santona L, et al. Azathioprine-induced pancytopenias in homozygous thiopurine methyltranferase-deficient renal transplant recipients: a family study. Transplant Proc 1995;27:1739-1742.

16. Zhou S. Clinical pharmacogenomics of thiopurine S-methyltransferase. Curr Clin Pharmacol 2006;1:119-128.

20. Moore MJ. Clinical pharmacokinetics of cyclophosphamide. Clin Pharmacokinet 1991;20:194-208.

24. Kowal A, Carstens JH Jr, Schnitzer T. Cyclosporin in rheumatoid arthritis. In: Furst DE, Weinblatt M, eds. Immunomodulators in the rheumatoid diseases. New York: Marcel Dekker, 1990:61-98.

27. Anderson IF, Helve T, Hannonen P, et al. Conversion of patients with rheumatoid arthritis from the conventional to a microemulsion formulation of cyclosporine: a double blind comparison to screen for differences in safety, efficacy, and pharmacokinetics. J Rheumatol 1999;26:556-562.

29. Curran MP, Perry CM. Tacrolimus in patients with RA. Drugs 2005;65:993-1003.

30. Ducharme MP, Warbasse LH, Edwards DJ. Disposition of intravenous and oral cyclosporine after administration with grapefruit juice. Clin Pharmacol Ther 1995;57:485-491.

33. Fox RI. Combined oral CsA and MTX therapy in patients with rheumatoid arthritis. Rheumatology 2003;42:989-994.

35. Bullingham RE, Nicholls AJ, Kamm BR. Clinical pharmacokinetics of mycophenolate mofetil. Clin Pharmacokinet 1998;34:429-455.

40. Suarez-Almazor ME, Spooner C, Belseck E. Azathioprine for treating RA. Cochrane Database Syst Rev 2000;(4):CD001461.

41. Jeurissen ME, Boerbooms AM, van de Putte LB, et al. Ifluence of MTX and azathioprine on radiologic progression in rheumatoid arthritis. A randomized, double-blind study. Ann Intern Med 1991;114:999-1004.

42. Wilkens RF, Urowitz MB, Stablein DM, et al. Comparison of azathioprine, methotrexate, and the combination of both in the treatment of rheumatoid arthritis. A controlled clinical trial. Arthritis Rheum 1992;35:849-856.

45. Flanc RS, Roberts MA, Strippoli GF, et al. Treatment for lupus nephritis. Cochrane Database Syst Rev 2004;(1):CD002922.

46. Moroni G, Doria A, Mosca M, et al. A randomized pilot trial comparing cyclosporine and azathioprine for maintenance therapy in diffuse lupus nephritis over four years. Clin J Am Soc Nephrol 2006;1:925-932. Epub 2006 Jun 28.

56. Clements PJ, Davis J. Cytotoxic drugs: their clinical application to the rheumatic diseases. Semin Arthritis Rheum 1986;15:231-254.

57. Cannon GW, Jackson CG, Samuelson CO Jr, et al. Chlorambucil therapy in rheumatoid arthritis: clinical

experience in 28 patients and literature review. Semin Arthritis Rheum 1985;15:106-118.

60. Chapman RM, Sutcliffe SB. Protection of ovarian function by oral contraceptives in women receiving chemotherapy for Hodgkin's disease. Blood 1981;58:849-851.

61. Kahn MF, Arlet J, Bloch-Michel H, et al. Acute leukemias after treatment using cytotoxic agents for rheumatological purposes: 19 cases among 2006 patients. Nouv Presse Med 1979;8:1393-1397.

62. Boumpas DT, Austin HA 3rd, Vaughn EM, et al. Control trial of pulse methylprednisolone versus two regimens of pulse cyclophosphamide in severe lupus nephritis. Lancet 1992;340(8822):741-745.

63. Flanc RS, Roberts MA, Strippoli GFM, et al. Treatment for lupus nephritis. Cochrane Database System Rev 2004;(1):CD002922.

64. Moore RA, Derry S. Systematic review and meta-analysis of randomised trials and cohort studies of mycophenolate mofetil in lupus nephritis. Arthritis Res Ther 2006;8:R182.

68. Guillevin L, Cohen P, Mahr A, et al. Treatment of polyarteritis nodosa and microscopic polyangiitis with poor prognosis factors: a prospective trial comparing glucocorticoids and six or twelve cyclophosphamide pulses in sixty-five patients. Arthritis Rheum 2003;49:93-100.

70. de Groot K, Rasmussen N, Bacon P, et al. A randomized trial of cyclophosphamide versus methotrexate for induction of remission in early systematic antineutrophil cytoplasmic antibody- associated vasculitis. Arthritis Rheum 2005;52:2461-2469.

71. Langford CA, Talar-Williams C, Barron KS, Sneller MC. A staged approach to the treatment of ANCA-associated granulomatous vasculitis: induction of remission with glucocorticoids and daily cyclophosphamide switching to methotrexate for remission maintenance. Arthritis Rheum 1999;42:2666-2673.

73. Tashkin DP, Elashoff R, Clements PJ, et al. Effects of 1-year treatment with cyclophosphamide on outcomes at 2 years in scleroderma lung disease. Am J Respir Crit Care Med 2007;176:1026-1034. Epub 2007 Aug 23.

77. Calguneri M, Ozbalkan Z, Ozturk MA, et al. Intensified, intermittent, low-dose intravenous cyclophosphamide together with oral alternate-day steroid therapy in lupus nephritis (long-term outcome). Clin Rheumatol 2006;25:782-788. Epub 2006 Mar 18.

81. Tugwell P, Bombardier C, Gent M, et al. Low-dose cyclosporine versus placebo in patients with rheumatoid arthritis. Lancet 1990;335:1051-1055.

83. Wells G, Haguenauer D, Shea B, et al. Cyclosporine for rheumatoid arthritis. In: Cochrane Database of Systematic Reviews. Oxford: Update software, 2001.

85. Tugwell P, Pincus T, Yocum D, et al. Combination therapy with cyclosporine and methotrexate in severe rheumatoid arthritis. The Methotrexate-Cyclosporine Combination Study Group. N Engl J Med 1995;333:137-141.

96. Schiff M, Stein G, Leishman B. CellCept (mycophenolate mofetil, MMF), a new treatment for RA: A 9 month randomized, double blind trial comparing 1 gm bid and 2 gm bid. Arthritis Rheum 1990;40:S980(abstract).

98. Chan TM, Li FK, Colin SO, et al. Efficacy of mycophenolate in patients with diffuse proliferative lupus nephritis. N Engl J Med 2000;343:1156-1162.

100. Hu W, Liu Z, Chen H, et al. Mycophenolate mofetil vs. cyclophosphamide therapy for patients with diffuse proliferative lupus nephritis. Chin Med J (Engl) 2002;115:705-709.

102. Furst DE, Saag K, Fleischmann MR, et al. Efficacy of tacrolimus in rheumatoid arthritis patients who have been unsuccessfully treated with methotrexate: a six months, double-blind, randomized, dose ranging study. Arthritis Rheum 2002;46:2020-2028.

103. Ostensen M, Lockshin M, Doria A, et al. Update on safety during pregnancy of biological agents and some immunosuppressive antirheumatic drugs. Rheumatology (Oxford) 2008;47(suppl 3):iii28-31.

110. Morita Y, Sasae Y, Sakuta T, et al. Efficacy of low-dose tacrolimus added to methotrexate in patients with rheumatoid arthritis in Japan: a retrospective study. Mod Rheumatol 2008;18:379-384.

113. Wu FI, Tsai MK, Chen RR, et al. Effects of calcineurin inhibitors on sirolimus pharmacokinetics during staggered administration in renal transplant patients. Pharmacotherapy 2005;25:646-653.

115. Fathy N, Furst DE. Combination therapy for autoimmune disease: the rheumatoid arthritis model. Springer Semin Immunopathol 2001;23:5-26.

116. Douglas M, Combe B, Cantagrel A, et al. Combination therapy in early rheumatoid arthritis: a randomized, controlled, double blind 52 week clinical trial of sulphasalazine and methotrexate compared with the single components. Ann Rheum Dis 1999;58:220-225.

120. Verhoeven AC, Bibo JC, Boers M, et al. Cost-effectiveness and cost-utility of combination therapy in early rheumatoid arthritis: randomized comparison of combined step-down prednisolone, methotrexate and sulphasalazine with sulphaslazine alone. COBRA trial group. Combinatietherapie Bij Reumatoide Artritis. Br J Rheumatol 1998;37:1102-1109.

122. Choy EH, Smith C, Dore CJ, Scott DL. A meta-analysis of the efficacy and toxicity of combining disease-modifying anti-rheumatic drugs in rheumatic arthritis based on patient withdrawal. Rheumatology 2005; July 19 (e-publication).

123. Capell HA, Madhok R, Porter DR, et al. Combination therapy with sulfasalazine and methotrexate is more effective than either drug alone in patients with rheumatoid arthritis with a suboptimal response to sulfasalazine: results from the double-blind placebo-controlled MASCOT study. Ann Rheum Dis 2007;66:235-241.

124. Moottonen TT, Hannmen PJ, Leirisalirepo M, et al. Comparison of combination therapy with single drug treatment in early RA; a randomized trial, FINRACO trial group. Lancet 1999;353:1565-1573.

125. Choy EH, Smith CM, Farewell V, et al. Factorial randomized controlled trial of glucocorticoids and combination disease-modifying drugs in early rheumatoid arthritis. Ann Rheum Dis 2008;67:656-663.

126. Goekoop-Riuterman YP, de Vries-Boustra JK, Allaart CF, et al. Clinical and radiographic outcomes of four different treatment strategies in patients with early RA (the BEST study): a randomized, controlled trial. Arthritis Rheum 2005;52:3381-3390.

128. Saag KG, Teng GG, Patkar NM, et al. American College of Rheumatology 2008 recommendations for the use of nonbiologic and biologic disease-modifying antirheumatic drugs in rheumatoid administration. J Clin Pharmacol 1993;33:522-526.

REFERENCES

Full references for this chapter can be found on www.expertconsult.com.

Dapsone, penicillamine, thalidomide, bucillamine, and the tetracyclines

56

Mohamed M. Thabet and Tom W. J. Huizinga

- Dapsone is a sulfone with anti-infective and anti-inflammatory properties; it has efficacy in rheumatoid arthritis and its toxicity includes hematologic and dermatologic effects.

- D-Pencillamine is a disease-modifying therapy in RA but rarely used now; its toxicity includes autoimmune syndromes and hematologic toxicity.

- Thalidomide has immunomodulatory properties and is used in Behçet's syndrome and cutaneous lupus erythematosus; its major toxicity is teratogenesis, and peripheral neuropathy and somnolence are common adverse events.

- The (doubtful) antirheumatic effects of minocycline relate to its anti-inflammatory and immunomodulatory properties rather than to its antimicrobial properties. Patients who request treatment with minocycline, however, still believe its antirheumatic effects are mediated by its antimicrobial activity. Minocycline can be used in patients who have failed other DMARDs and in whom an anti-TNF-α compound is not an option or in patients with early RA in whom hydroxychloroquine is being considered.

INTRODUCTION

During the past decade it has become clear that reduction of disease activity is the goal in the proper treatment of rheumatoid arthritis (RA). To this end a large armamentarium of pharmacologic agents is available that is discussed in other chapters. There are, however, still patients who either cannot tolerate current drugs, do not respond to current drugs, or for whom current drugs are not available. In such cases a number of other agents have been used, such as dapsone, penicillamine, thalidomide, bucillamine, as well as the tetracycline antibiotics.

DAPSONE

Dapsone (4,4′-diaminodiphenylsulfone [DDS]), a synthetic sulfone with chemical similarities to sulfapyridine, has been used for a number of years to treat leprosy and dermatitis herpetiformis.[1] Although dapsone was first synthesized in 1908 by Fromm and Wittmann,[2] it was not established as an agent to treat leprosy until the late 1940s and early 1950s.[3] Its anti-inflammatory and antimalarial properties were discovered soon after and are now well documented.[4]

In 1976 McConkey and colleagues[5] studied the therapeutic effect of dapsone in RA in a non-randomized, unblinded open study, in which 71 patients with consistently active RA were given dapsone, 50 mg daily, for 1 week, then 100 mg daily. There was a significant improvement in subjective clinical state, and there were significant falls in serum C-reactive protein (CRP) and the erythrocyte sedimentation rate (ESR); the Rose-Waaler titer did not fall. The results were compared with those in another group of 78 patients who had gold therapy. Subjective clinical improvement was slower with gold, but from 6 weeks the pattern of changes in clinical score, CRP, and ESR was similar for both drugs. The titers of rheumatoid factor fell during gold treatment. The results suggest dapsone is effective in RA; overall these data indicated a slightly less effectiveness than gold but associated with much more toxicity.[5] From that time on, a number of prospective, randomized, double-blind trials have shown effectiveness of dapsone in the management of RA, with dapsone being superior to placebo and comparable to chloroquine and hydroxychloroquine (Table 56.1).[6-8] Its mode of anti-inflammatory actions in RA is not clearly understood, but modulation of neutrophil activity or inhibition of neutrophil inflammatory product formation or release has been suggested as the possible mode of action.[1]

Ujiie and associates recently published a case report of lupus erythematosus profundus (LEP) successfully treated with dapsone with remission of pain, limitation of expansion of the indurated area, and rapid re-epithelialization of skin ulcers within 6 weeks.[9] They also reviewed the literature investigating the use of dapsone in treating LEP, and in summary there were 10 different case reports including theirs of successful treatment of LEP with dapsone.[9] The mode of action in cutaneous lupus erythematosus was investigated by Abe and coworkers where, *in vitro*, dapsone was found to significantly decrease levels of tumor necrosis factor (TNF)-α in the culture supernatant of activated mononuclear cells.[10]

Pharmacology

Dapsone is absorbed rapidly and nearly completely from the gastrointestinal tract. Peak concentrations of dapsone in plasma are reached within 2 to 8 hours after administration. The mean half-life of elimination is 20 to 30 hours. Twenty-four hours after oral ingestion of 100 mg, plasma concentrations range from 0.4 to 1.2 μm/mL, and a dose of 100 mg/day produces steady-state plasma concentrations of free dapsone of 2 to 6 mmol/L. About 70% of the drug is bound to plasma protein. Dapsone is distributed throughout total body water and is present in all tissues. However, it tends to be retained in skin and muscle and especially in the liver and kidney: traces of the drug are present in these organs up to 3 weeks after therapy cessation.[4]

After absorption from the gastrointestinal tract, dapsone is transported through the portal circulation to the liver, where it is metabolized by two distinct routes, *N*-acetylation and *N*-hydroxylation. Dapsone toxicity, in particular, methemoglobin formation, is putatively initiated by *N*-oxidation, resulting in the formation of a hydroxylamine metabolite by cytochrome P450.[11] A single dose of disulfiram, a slowly reversing inhibitor of CYP2E1 *in vivo*, inhibited dapsone hydroxylamine formation clearance by 73% and inhibited methemoglobin formation by 78% in a group of healthy volunteers. Dapsone-induced methemoglobin formation in healthy volunteers was also diminished by 61% after the administration of cimetidine, a relatively non-selective cytochrome P450 inhibitor, and thus the treatment-limiting toxicities of dapsone might be diminished by co-administration of a suitable inhibitor of hydroxylamine formation.[12] The adverse effects of dapsone are listed in Table 56.2.

Effective clinical use of dapsone is limited because of dose-dependent adverse hematologic reactions, even at the low daily dosages of 100 mg. Patients with a genetic deficiency of certain enzymes (i.e., glucose-6-phosphate dehydrogenase or glutathione reductase) are more susceptible to the hematologic effects.[13] The hemotoxicity of dapsone is not caused by the drug itself but by its hydroxylamine metabolites. Methemoglobinemia occurs to some extent in all patients receiving dapsone and becomes less pronounced as treatment is continued, owing to an adaptive increase in the activity of NADH-dependent reductase in the erythrocytes. Methemoglobin levels of less than 20% are not usually associated with symptoms. Dyspnea, nausea, and tachycardia usually occur at levels of 30% or higher, whereas lethargy, stupor, and deteriorating consciousness occur as methemoglobin levels approach 55%. Levels of 70% are usually fatal.[14]

TABLE 56.1 DOUBLE-BLIND RANDOMIZED STUDIES OF DAPSONE IN RHEUMATOID ARTHRITIS

Study	Duration (wk)	No. of patients*	Comparison groups	Conclusions
Swinson et al (1981)[6]	14	41	Dapsone (100 mg/day); placebo	Dapsone significantly superior to placebo
Fowler et al (1984)[7]	12	60	Dapsone (100 mg/day) Chloroquine (250 mg/day)	Equal improvement with both drugs
Haar et al (1993)[8]	24	80	Dapsone (100 mg/day) HCQ (250 mg/day) Dapsone (100 mg/day) + HCQ (250 mg/day)	Similar improvement in all three groups, but dapsone groups had significant ESR and CRP reductions over the HCQ group.

HCQ, hydroxychloroquine; ESR, erythrocyte sedimentation rate; CRP, C-reactive protein.
*Number in all groups on entry.

TABLE 56.2 SIDE EFFECTS OF DAPSONE

Side effects	Frequency
Hematologic	
Hemolytic anemia (dose-related)	Very common
Methemoglobinemia (dose-related)	Very common, but usually asymptomatic
Leukopenia	<5%
Agranulocytosis	<1%
Dermatologic	
Exfoliative dermatitis, toxic erythema, erythema multiforme, toxic epidermal necrolysis, morbilliform and scarlatiniform eruptions, urticaria, erythema nodosum, phototoxicity	10%
Neurologic	
Peripheral neuropathy (motor)	Rare
Psychosis	Rare
Gastrointestinal	
Toxic hepatitis	Rare
Cholestatic jaundice	Rare
Renal	
Nephrotic syndrome	Rare
Renal papillary necrosis	Rare
Miscellaneous	
Nausea, vomiting, abdominal pain, headache, vertigo, nervousness, insomnia, fatigue, weakness, tinnitus, blurred vision (dose related)	20%
Hypoalbuminemia without proteinuria	Rare
Dapsone hypersensitivity syndrome	Rare

Agranulocytosis is a rare hematologic adverse effect of dapsone, which occurs in less than 1% of cases.[1] Unlike methemoglobinemia, this severe adverse effect is due to an unpredictable idiosyncratic reaction. For unknown reasons, the risk of agranulocytosis in patients with dermatitis herpetiformis is more than 25-fold compared with other patients. Factors such as drug dosage, immune status, degree of malnutrition, and ethnic origin have been suggested to be determinants of the risk of developing agranulocytosis.[15]

Another very rare serious idiosyncratic adverse effect is the dapsone hypersensitivity syndrome. The unpredictability and potential severity of this reaction make it a major concern in clinical practice. It usually appears 4 or more weeks after initiation of therapy. Symptoms include a mononucleosis-like rash with fever and lymphadenopathy. Involvement of other organs varies and includes liver disease (hepatomegaly, icterus, hepatitis, and hepatic encephalopathy), eosinophilia, and other disorders. The course of the disease is variable, but it may last 4 weeks or more, and fatalities have been reported. Exanthematous skin eruptions usually resolve within 2 weeks of stopping dapsone, although patients in whom Stevens-Johnson syndrome or toxic epidermal necrolysis develops have increased morbidity and mortality. The use of dapsone in RA patients during pregnancy is contraindicated owing to a low risk of congenital malformations in patients receiving dapsone during pregnancy. In lactating mothers, it is recommended that if dapsone is required, breast-feeding should be discontinued because dapsone diffuses into breast milk and there are reports of hemolytic anemia induced by this drug transmitted through breast milk.

Monitoring guidelines

Dapsone is considered unsafe and should not be used in the following conditions: severe anemia, porphyria, deficiency of glucose-6-phosphate dehydrogenase, glutathione reductase or methemoglobin reductase, allergy to sulfonamides, or significant liver disease. It should not be paired with other hemolytics or dideoxyinosine. Before starting therapy, a complete blood cell count, reticulocyte count, glucose-6-phosphate dehydrogenase level, liver function studies, urinalysis, and renal function tests are recommended. During therapy, a complete blood cell count, reticulocyte count, platelet count, and leukocyte count with differential should be obtained weekly for the first month, then twice per month during the next 2 months and every 3 months thereafter. Liver and renal functions should be tested every 3 months. Methemoglobin levels are indicated in patients who become symptomatic for methemoglobinemia. As for other antirheumatic drugs, no data are available whether such monitoring policies are cost-effective.

Increasing patient tolerance

A number of attempts have been made to increase the tolerance of patients to dapsone, including the co-administration with dapsone of vitamins E and C either alone or in combination.[16] These antioxidant studies demonstrated little impact on the methemoglobinemia caused by the drug. An alternative approach is the use of metabolic inhibitors of cytochrome P450, to attenuate the methemoglobin. Cimetidine is probably the most practical inhibitor for use in humans. Studies showed that co-administration of cimetidine (3 × 400 mg/day) and a single dose of dapsone in human volunteers resulted in a significant reduction in methemoglobin formation, as well as a fall in hydroxylamine excretion as its N-glucuronide.[17] More potent and less toxic derivatives of dapsone have been synthesized and tested but have not been registered for clinical use. In the meantime, the use of a metabolic inhibitor such as cimetidine can be considered when methemoglobin formation prohibits effective dosage regimens.

PENICILLAMINE

Penicillamine has been used in the treatment of RA for more than 40 years.[18] Over this period of time, most texts considered penicillamine as an effective disease-modifying agent, improving many of the clinical and laboratory indices of disease activity. Given the availability of much more effective second-line agents, the place of penicillamine in the current therapeutic repertoire has become less clear.[19]

Pharmacology

Structurally penicillamine is an amino acid with a thiol side chain (Fig. 56.1). It can exist as two enantiomers: D and L. However only the D type is clinically useful owing to excessive toxicity of the L type. Oral absorption is good in fasting subjects with a bioavailability of 40% to 70%[20]; however, availability is severely reduced if penicillamine is taken in conjunction with iron preparations, antacids, or food.[21]

Within the body, penicillamine is rapidly oxidized to form various disulfides. The most important of these are with the proteins cysteine, homocysteine, and penicillamine itself. The serum half-life of a single dose of penicillamine is 2 to 4 hours. In patients on long-term therapy, the half-life rises to 4 to 6 days, although traces of penicillamine can be detected in the serum weeks after cessation of therapy, presumably owing to mobilization of a tissue-bound pool. Clearance of the disulfides is mainly in the urine, although a substantial proportion is excreted in the feces.[22]

Mode of action

The method by which penicillamine acts as a disease-modifying agent in the treatment of RA is unclear. The thiol group on penicillamine and the oxidative reactions involved in the metabolism of penicillamine appear to be central to all the proposed modes of action. *In-vitro* studies have shown a potential immunomodulatory effect as well as direct actions at sites of inflammation.[19]

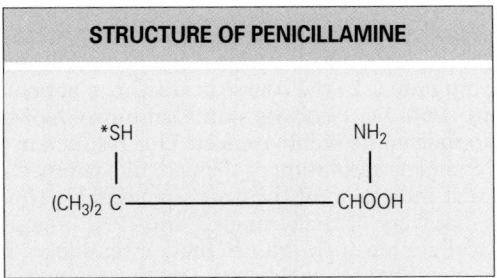

STRUCTURE OF PENICILLAMINE

Fig. 56.1 Structure of penicillamine (*denotes thiol side chain).

Initially it was thought that penicillamine acted by dissociating the bonds binding the macromolecules of IgM that made up rheumatoid factor.[23] This theory can be discounted because the concentration of penicillamine required is not achieved *in vivo* using conventional doses and there is no correlation with reduction in rheumatoid factor and clinical efficacy.[24] The reduction in globulins is probably due to penicillamine having an inhibitory action on T-helper cell–mediated B-cell expansion and activation rather than a direct action on B cells.[25] In the presence of copper, penicillamine undergoes oxidation of its thiol group to form H_2O_2; this molecule has a direct inhibitory effect on T-helper cell function and possibly also natural killer T cells.[26] Penicillamine may also act at the site of inflammation by impairing fibroblast proliferation and, thus, pannus formation. Again this occurs due to H_2O_2 production in the presence of copper. Studies have also shown that penicillamine may scavenge some of the free radicals released by activated neutrophils and inhibit the granular enzyme myeloperoxidase, thus reducing local tissue damage.[27]

Benefits

Versus placebo

It was found that moderate-dose (500-1000 mg/day) and high-dose (≥1000 mg/day) penicillamine versus placebo significantly reduced the number of swollen joints and ESR and improved the global physician score at 4 to 6 months.[28] There have been a number of placebo-controlled studies, which in the aggregate document the efficacy of penicillamine in the treatment of RA; these are summarized in Table 56-3.[29-32]

Versus other disease-modifying antirheumatic drugs (DMARDs)

In 1992, a systematic review compared the effectiveness of penicillamine versus other DMARDs. No consistent differences in effectiveness between penicillamine and other drugs were identified, although some trials found penicillamine to be superior to antimalarial agents.[33] Another 5-year open randomized controlled study done in 1998 that compared the effect of penicillamine to other DMARDs in 541 patients showed that patients on penicillamine had the smallest amount of improvement in CRP, ESR, Ritchie index, pain scores, and combined grip strength, but the differences were small.[34] Table 56.4 summarizes

TABLE 56.3 PENICILLAMINE PLACEBO-CONTROLLED STUDIES				
	Multicenter trial group[29]	**Dixon et al**[30]	**Shiokawa et al**[31]	**Williams et al**[32]
Year	1973	1975	1977	1983
No. of patients	105	121	179	225
Maximum dose (mg)	1500	600/1200	600	125/500
Duration of study (weeks)	52	24	24	30
Withdrawal rate (%)	42	29/45	34	20/29
Randomized and double blind	Yes	Yes	Yes	Yes
Comment at 12 weeks	High dose with high dropout rate	No difference in efficacy between high and low doses	Response rate: 44% at 12 weeks and 65% at 24 weeks	Lower dose no better than placebo

TABLE 56.4 PENICILLAMINE COMPARATIVE STUDIES					
Author	**Year**	**Drugs**	**No. of patients**	**Double blind and randomized**	**Comment**
Hochberg et al[35]	1986	D-Pen/Auranofin	88	Yes	Penicillamine more effective and toxic
Gibson et al[36]	1976	D-Pen/Myocrisin	87	Not blinded	No difference
Thomas et al[37]	1984	D-Pen/Myocrisin	50	Yes	No difference
Bunch et al[38]	1984	D-Pen/HCQ/combination	54	Yes	Penicillamine more effective
Capell et al[39]	1990	D-Pen/sulfasalazine	200	Yes	No difference
Paulus et al[40]	1984	D-Pen/azathioprine	206	Yes	No difference
Berry et al[41]	1976	D-Pen/azathioprine	65	Single blind	No difference

D-Pen, D-penicillamine; HCQ, hydroxychloroquine.

comparative studies, comparing D-penicillamine to other DMARDs.[35-41]

Use in combination therapy

Taggart and colleagues[42] studied 29 patients over 5 months and found that there was a slightly better response rate with sulfasalazine/D-penicillamine compared with sulfasalazine alone at the expense of greater toxicity. A different approach to the use of combination therapy is to add a second agent to patients tolerating but not responding to therapeutic doses of penicillamine.[43] Combination therapy with intramuscular gold had been more promising despite the obvious concerns regarding its similar toxicity profile. Bitter[44] reported the results of two trials looking at combination therapy in patients who had responded inadequately to gold or penicillamine alone after 1 to 2 years of treatment. It was found that 75% of patients staying on combination therapy improved significantly compared with 7% of those who stayed on monotherapy. The minor effect sizes reported in these trials are reflected by common practice in which no combination therapy that includes penicillamine has become part of mainstream rheumatologic practice. Despite the modest effect on group level in individual cases, D-penicillamine can be considered as a therapeutic option.[19]

Side effects

Adverse effects of penicillamine are common and sometimes serious. Reactions include mucocutaneous reactions, altered taste, gastrointestinal reactions, proteinuria, hematologic effects, myositis, and other autoimmune diseases, such as drug-induced lupus, systemic lupus erythematosus, and myasthenia gravis. The most frequent adverse effects responsible for D-penicillamine discontinuation were hematologic, mucocutaneous, impaired/loss of taste, renal, and gastrointestinal.[28] Another rare side effect of penicillamine is mammary hyperplasia; identification of the problem and immediate cessation of penicillamine in such cases is mandatory.[45] The most important side effects are detailed in Table 56.5.

Drug interactions

The most common drug interactions with penicillamine are due to its chelating properties. In particular, iron preparations and antacids containing either magnesium or aluminum can reduce the absorption of penicillamine by as much as 66%. If these medications are necessary, then they should be taken 12 hours before or after penicillamine.[20]

Dosage

Because side effects are more common at higher doses, it is customary to start with a dose of penicillamine of 125 mg daily and increase the dose every 4 weeks by 125 mg, aiming for a target daily dose of 500 mg. Patients are advised that it can take 3 to 6 months before the full benefit may be apparent. If there is inadequate clinical response at 18 to 24 weeks, the dose can be increased up to 750 mg and maintained at this for a further 12 weeks. Again, if the response is inadequate, but the patient is tolerating the drug well, further increments up to 1 g can be made before treatment is abandoned. It has been recommended that initially the hemoglobin value, white blood cell count, platelet count, and urinalysis should be monitored every 2 weeks until a stable dose is achieved; thereafter monitoring can be reduced to every 4 weeks. No cost-effectiveness studies for such monitor guidelines have been performed; thus no definitive guidelines can be made.

THALIDOMIDE

Thalidomide was first introduced in West Germany in 1956 and in the rest of Europe, Australia, Canada, and South Africa in 1957. Fortuitously, the U.S. Food and Drug Administration delayed its release pending clarification of concerns regarding the results of neurotoxicologic studies in animals. It was initially marketed as a sedative, with its rapid speed of onset, lack of hangover effect, and apparent safety after overdose making it an attractive alternative to barbiturates. In addition, it was a powerful antiemetic and was widely taken by pregnant women for the treatment of morning sickness. However, soon after its release, there followed a rapid rise in reported cases of a previously rare birth defect, phocomelia (congenital limb foreshortening). In 1961, after reports linking this to in-utero thalidomide exposure, the drug was withdrawn, leaving a legacy of between 6000 and 10,000 affected children.[46] However, a few years later, the serendipitous discovery of thalidomide's anti-inflammatory potential ensured it was never entirely forgotten. In the course of treating a patient with mania and leprosy, in 1964, Dr. Jacob Sheskin,[47] administered some old supplies of thalidomide for its sedative effect. This resulted in the dramatic and virtually complete resolution of the patient's cutaneous symptoms and was the first indication of the drug's potential.[47] However, it was not until the discovery of thalidomide's anti–TNF-α activity in 1991 that interest really intensified.[48] Since then, a significant body of work has now been published to elucidate the mode of action and potential uses of this unique drug.[49]

Pharmacology

Thalidomide, a derivative of glutamic acid, is administered clinically as a 1 : 1 racemic mixture of its S and R isomers. It is well absorbed after oral administration with maximal plasma levels of 1 to 4 mg/mL reached within 2 to 4 hours. There is some evidence to suggest that individual isomers have different biologic properties with the S-isomer responsible for the immunomodulatory effects while the R-isomer accounts for the sedative effects.[50,51] In animal studies, both isomers caused fetal malformations when administered to the New Zealand rabbit (a species known to be sensitive to its teratogenic effects), whereas in rodents (a less sensitive species), malformations were only observed in those who received the S-isomer.[52] However, in humans, the rapid chiral interconversion that occurs between the two isomers in vivo limits any potential benefit from administering a specific isomer.[53] Thalidomide is eliminated by pH-dependent spontaneous hydrolysis to multiple chemically inactive metabolites and has a half-life of approximately 5 hours. Because there is virtually no excretion via the liver or renal pathways the risk of drug interactions is low.[37] Thalidomide has been shown to be present in the semen after oral dosing.[54] The structure of thalidomide is shown in Figure 56.2.[49]

Immunologic properties

Thalidomide's immunomodulatory properties are complex and incompletely understood. Multiple mechanisms of action have been reported, with the best recognized being its ability to inhibit the production of TNF-α.[49] Another potentially important property of thalidomide is its antiangiogenic effects. In-vitro studies have shown thalidomide to be capable of inhibiting angiogenesis induced by vascular endothelial-derived growth factor and basic fibroblast growth factor.[55,56] A subsequent study has also shown this effect to be independent of TNF-α

System	Occurrence rate (%)	Side effects
TABLE 56.5 SIDE EFFECTS OF PENICILLAMINE		
Mucocutaneous	10-20	Mouth ulcers, urticarial rashes, pruritus, lichen planus, and pemphigus
Gastrointestinal	10-20	Dysgeusia and nausea, rarely abnormal liver function
Renal	10-15	Proteinuria, glomerulonephritis, and Goodpasture's syndrome
Hematologic	5-10	Thrombocytopenia, leukopenia, and aplastic anemia
Autoimmune	Uncommon	Myasthenia gravis, polymyositis, pemphigus, systemic lupus erythematosus, and Goodpasture's syndrome
Lungs	Rare	Bronchiolitis obliterans
Pregnancy	Rare	Fetal connective tissue abnormalities

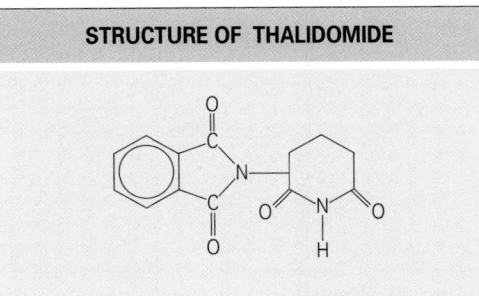

STRUCTURE OF THALIDOMIDE

Fig. 56.2 Structure of thalidomide.

TABLE 56.6 IMMUNOLOGIC EFFECTS OF THALIDOMIDE

- Switch cytokine production from Th1 to Th2 profile
- Inhibit TNF-α synthesis
- Inhibit IL-6 synthesis
- Inhibit IL-12 synthesis
- Inhibit IFN-γ synthesis
- Augment IL-4 production
- Augment IL-10 production
- Act as a T-cell co-stimulant
- Augment IFN-γ synthesis
- Augment IL-2 synthesis
- Augment IL-10 synthesis
- Reduce expression of intracellular adhesion molecule-1
- Reduce expression of vascular cell adhesion molecule-1
- Reduce synthesis of basic fibroblast growth factor
- Reduce synthesis of vascular endothelial-derived growth factor

suppression.[57] The immunologic effects of thalidomide in *in-vitro* studies are summarized in Table 56.6.[49]

Derivatives

Over the past few years the re-emergence of thalidomide has awakened interest in developing structural analogs that possess its immuno-modulatory properties without the associated side effects. Several such compounds have recently been developed that are up to 50,000-fold more potent than thalidomide at inhibiting TNF-α on a molar basis.[58] They are broadly split into two main groups, dependent on their bio-logic effects. The first class, immunomodulatory drugs, strongly inhibit TNF-α along with interleukin (IL)-1β, IL-6, and IL-12 while augment-ing IL-10 production. These compounds are also potent co-stimulators of T cells when activated through the T-cell receptor, increase T-cell proliferation, and do not inhibit phosphodiesterase-4. The second class, selective cytokine inhibitory drugs, again potently inhibit TNF-α, although much more selectively, having considerably less effect on other inflammatory cytokines. They have little effect on T-cell activa-tion, causing only a slight inhibition in T-cell proliferation. These compounds do markedly inhibit phosphodiesterase-4, although it is currently unclear how much this contributes to their biologic effects.[59] Importantly, preliminary results from animal studies have shown at least some of these compounds to be clinically effective and non-toxic and non-mutagenic.[60,61] Several are now undergoing phase 1 and phase 2 clinical trials of which no reports are yet available.

Clinical applications

Currently, thalidomide has a wide scale of therapeutic potential. The conditions for which thalidomide has shown a therapeutic potential are summarized in Table 56.7. From this list of conditions only the rheumatologic disorders are discussed here.

Results from animal studies indicate that thalidomide and its deriv-atives are effective in inhibiting the development of arthritis in specific mouse models.[62] In 1989 a study showed that 12 of 17 patients with refractory RA responded to treatment with thalidomide.[63] Results from more recent clinical studies have shown little or no benefit.[64,65] Huiz-inga and associates in 1996,[64] performed an open study in RA patients to assess toxicity, the effect on TNF production, and the antiarthritic effects of thalidomide and pentoxifylline. In this study, 12 patients with active RA were treated with 1200 mg of pentoxifylline and 100 mg of thalidomide a day for 12 weeks. In addition, TNF production was assessed by *ex-vivo* whole blood cultures stimulated with endotoxin. Adverse events such as xerostomia, drowsiness, and constipation occurred in almost all patients, which led to discontinuation in 3 patients. The drugs halved the TNF production capacity during treat-ment, whereas production capacity of IL-6, IL-10, and IL-12 was not affected. Of the 9 patients who completed the study, 5 fulfilled the American College of Rheumatology 20% (ACR20) response criteria after 12 weeks of treatment. Thus, although pentoxifylline/thalidomide reduced the production capacity of TNF, the benefit/side effects ratio was poor owing to multiple adverse effects, whereas clinical observation suggests limited efficacy.

There have been several small case series of patients with refractory sarcoidosis,[66,67] scleroderma,[68] cutaneous lupus,[67,69] systemic lupus ery-thematosus,[67] and systemic-onset juvenile RA[70] who responded to

TABLE 56.7 CONDITIONS FOR WHICH THALIDOMIDE HAS BEEN SUGGESTED TO HAVE THERAPEUTIC POTENTIAL

Gastrointestinal	Behçet's disease Recurrent aphthous oral ulceration HIV-associated oral and esophageal ulceration Crohn's disease
Rheumatologic	Rheumatoid arthritis Systemic lupus erythematosus Discoid lupus erythematosis Sjögren's syndrome Sarcoidosis
Dermatologic	Leprosy Actinic prurigo Prurigo nodularis Uremic pruritus Pyoderma gangrenosum
Hematologic malignancy	Multiple myeloma Myelodysplasia Acute myeloid leukemia/chronic myeloid leukemia
Solid tumors	Malignant glioma Kaposi's sarcoma Prostatic carcinoma Colorectal carcinoma Renal cell carcinoma
Cachexia and weight loss	HIV-associated wasting Cancer cachexia Tuberculosis-associated wasting
Miscellaneous	Graft-versus-host disease Intractable insomnia Neuropathic pain

thalidomide. However, no convincing large case series or randomized controlled trials have yet been published, and currently there is not enough reliable evidence to report efficacy.[49]

Adverse effects

Many adverse effects of thalidomide have been reported (Table 56.8). The most relevant adverse effects are teratogenicity and peripheral neuropathy.

Teratogenicity

Phocomelia is the best-known congenital abnormality associated with thalidomide, but duodenal stenosis, esophageal fistulas, neural tube abnormalities, microphthalmia, deformities of the ears, and midline hemangiomas have also been reported.[71]

TABLE 56.8 ADVERSE EFFECTS OF THALIDOMIDE

Teratogenicity	One 50-mg dose can produce severe defects
Peripheral neuropathy	Predominantly sensory Axonal degeneration Occasionally permanent
Somnolence	Virtually universal Administer at bedtime to reduce effect Tolerance develops
Constipation	Laxatives commonly needed Occasionally severe
Macular rash	Self-limiting on stopping treatment More common in HIV-positive patients
Neutropenia	Rare More common in HIV-positive patients

Peripheral neuropathy

Peripheral neuropathy associated with thalidomide typically includes symmetric, painful paresthesias of the hands and feet, often accompanied by sensory loss in the lower limbs. A recent review of 42 patients found that neurologic symptoms did not correlate with either the duration of treatment or the daily dose and confirmed that women and older persons are at greater risk.[72] Published estimates of the incidence of peripheral neuropathy range from 1% to 70%.[73] Symptoms and signs of peripheral neuropathy have been reported to resolve slowly or to be irreversible.[74] To reduce the risk of neuropathy, patients should be educated about its earliest symptoms, such as pricking or paresthesias of the lower limbs, and instructed to contact the physician immediately if they occur. Examinations for signs of neuropathy should be performed monthly for the first 3 months after starting treatment and periodically thereafter. The exact place of measurement of sensory nerve action potentials is unclear. Once signs of neuropathy are suspected and there is clinical need to continue thalidomide, electrophysiologic testing should be performed frequently if the amplitude decreases by more than 30%; a decrease of 50% warrants stopping therapy. Thalidomide therapy may be restarted cautiously once symptoms of peripheral neuropathy symptoms resolve.[75]

BUCILLAMINE

Bucillamine [N-(2-mercapto-2-methylpropionyl)-L-cysteine] is a DMARD. Oral bucillamine is only approved in Asia for treatment of RA. The beneficial effects of bucillamine in the treatment of RA have been well appreciated in several clinical trials, and its effect sizes were found comparable to those of methotrexate.[76-79] Bucillamine is a thiol compound that differs from D-penicillamine by the presence of two free sulfhydryl groups (Fig. 56.3). As a result, a considerable fraction of bucillamine can form an intramolecular disulfide that appears to have unique immunosuppressive activities. Thus, bucillamine exerts immunosuppressive effects that are similar to those of D-penicillamine, as well as unique inhibitory effects that depend on the capacity of bucillamine to form an intramolecular disulfide.[80] Moreover, at pharmacologically attainable concentrations, bucillamine directly suppresses B-cell IgM production but not T-cell interferon-γ production, whereas D-penicillamine inhibits the latter but not the former, suggesting that, as a result of the formation of the internal disulfide, bucillamine and D-penicillamine have different targets of immunosuppressive action in vivo.[81] The hallmarks of the pathologic changes in the RA synovium include hyperplasia of synovial lining cells and follicle-like aggregation of lymphocytes and plasma cells.[82] A number of studies have indicated that angiogenesis as well as activation of endothelial cells to express adhesion molecules play a crucial role in recruiting inflammatory cells and immunocompetent cells into the synovium.[83-85] Of note, bucillamine has been shown to inhibit the production of vascular endothelial growth factor, a potent inducer of angiogenesis, by cultured rheumatoid synovial cells[86] and bovine retinal microcapillary endothelial cells.[87]

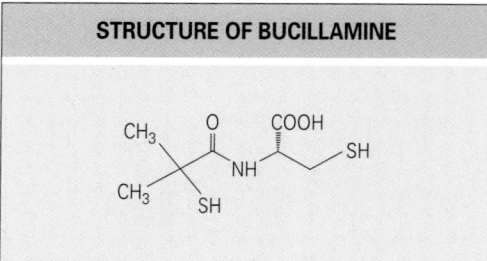

STRUCTURE OF BUCILLAMINE

Fig. 56.3 Structure of bucillamine.

Side effects

Proteinuria is reported to be the most frequent adverse effect of bucillamine.[88] In patients with bucillamine-induced proteinuria, membranous nephropathy is the most common disorder. Immediate withdrawal of bucillamine results in prompt and complete resolution of the proteinuria without deterioration of renal function. It is recommended that urinary protein excretion should be monitored during treatment with bucillamine.[89] Other rare side effects include skin disorders including rash, vesicles, eruption, swollen lips,[88,90] and yellow nails[91] and, less frequently, gastrointestinal disorders, respiratory disorder, renal dysfunction, and bone marrow suppression.[88]

ANTIBIOTICS

The interest in antibiotic therapy for RA, particularly tetracyclines, dates back to 1960s[92] when RA was hypothesized to be possibly caused by infection with *Mycoplasma* or similar organisms.[93] During the 1970s and 1980s, Brown and his colleagues continued to use antibiotics (not only tetracyclines) for the treatment of RA, but the data gathered by Brown and colleagues were never published in a peer-reviewed publication.[94] This fact, plus a negative study published by Skinner and associates[95] in the early 1970s, contributed to the skepticism about the benefits of this treatment modality. The Skinner paper was, however, underpowered to be able to detect differences between the two treatment groups (30 patients total, with only 27 patients finishing the treatment protocol), and the dose of tetracycline used was relatively small (250 mg/day).[96]

Interest in the use of tetracyclines for the treatment of RA resurfaced in the 1980s. This interest came about not only because the possible microbial etiology of RA had not vanished (the discovery of *Borrelia burgdorferi* as the organism responsible for Lyme disease and arthritis heightened this possibility) but also because tetracyclines were discovered to have non-antimicrobial properties (anti-inflammatory, immunomodulatory, and chondroprotective).[96] Moreover, synthetic tetracyclines, devoid of antimicrobial activity, were found to have antirheumatic properties in experimental animal models of arthritis.[97,98]

Properties of tetracyclines and their derivatives
Anti-inflammatory properties

Tetracycline derivatives have been shown to inhibit phospholipase A2 and consequently to affect the production of lipooxygenase and cyclo-oxygenase derivatives, both in vivo and in vitro.[99-101] Other proinflammatory mediators, including nitric oxide (NO) and oxygen radicals, have been shown in in-vitro studies either to be released less efficiently or to be scavenged in the presence of tetracycline derivatives by down-regulating NO synthetase, an important mediator of collagen degradation.[102] Minocycline, but not other tetracyclines, has been shown to reduce NO production by inhibition of the NO synthetase at the level of mRNA expression and protein synthesis in a dose-dependent manner[100,103] and also to upregulate IL-10, a potent inhibitory cytokine in the synovial tissue.[104]

The anti-inflammatory properties of minocycline have also been evident in clinical double-blind studies, with a significant decrease in ESR and CRP and an increase in hemoglobin levels.[104,105]

Immunomodulatory properties

Sera from patients receiving tetracyclines impair leukotaxis and phagocytosis; and in animal models, tetracyclines can arrest lymphocyte proliferation, induce lymphocyte apoptosis (Fas/fas ligand mediated),[106-109] and inhibit calcium influx during T-cell activation.[110] Tetracyclines impair the proliferation and activation of human lymphocytes and synovial tissue cells, resulting in the abrogation of the local production of proinflammatory cytokines in a comparable manner to chloroquine.[111,112] Furthermore, the combination of minocycline and chloroquine results in an additive anti-inflammatory effect, supporting their possible concomitant use in the clinical setting.[112]

Chondroprotective properties

Tetracyclines can reduce matrix metalloproteinases (MMPs) or collagenase enzyme activity, resulting in decreasing cartilage breakdown by several different mechanisms; it is important to note that not all tetracyclines produce their chondroprotective effect by the same mechanism. Doxycycline and minocycline directly inhibit the enzymatic activity of MMPs, although the concentrations required are higher than the concentrations achievable *in vivo*; thus, this effect is not adequate to explain the chondroprotective effects of these tetracycline derivatives.[113] Doxycycline downregulates the production of MMPs at the levels of mRNA expression and protein systhesis[114] and upregulates tissue inhibitors of MMPs (TIMPs) with the consequent decreased activity of the different mammalian MMPs.[115] Doxycycline also regulates the balance of chondrocyte autocrine production by decreasing the proinflammatory cytokines (IL-1, IL-6, and TNF-α) and increasing an anti-inflammatory cytokine (tumor growth factor [TGF]-β), which results in decreased production of MMPs.[94,100,114] Tetracyclines inhibit MMPs and collagenase activities both *in vitro* and *in vivo*,[115-122] leading investigators to study these agents in osteoarthritis.[115]

In summary, the antirheumatic effects of tetracyclines and their derivatives could result from the inhibition of MMPs and of different proinflammatory mediators. Whether their action could also result from their antimicrobial activity has not been satisfactorily demonstrated. Patients with RA who are seeking treatment with minocycline or other tetracycline derivatives do so with the absolute conviction that RA is an infectious process and that they need these drugs for their antimicrobial properties. Such patients are, unfortunately, not open to the idea that such treatment may fail; they therefore continue to request antibiotics, beyond what a reasonable therapeutic trial (e.g., 6-9 months) would suggest.[123] We have had the opportunity to witness what appear to be "antibiotic-sensitive" RA patients; these are patients with RA who are prescribed an antibiotic for either a urinary tract or a respiratory infection and who experience significant improvement of their articular manifestations. Subsequently, these patients continue to request antibiotics and, in fact, in some patients the drugs seem to remain efficacious. There is no published literature supporting this experience.

Pharmacology and drug interactions

Tetracyclines are readily absorbed from the gastrointestinal tract; they circulate bound to plasma proteins. They are concentrated in the liver in the bile and excreted in both the urine and feces in their active form. Minocycline and doxycycline (the tetracyclines used in RA and osteoarthritis [OA] studies) have a serum half-life of 11 to 22 hours in individuals with normal renal function. In subjects with impaired renal or hepatic function, the half-life has been shown to vary from 11 to 69 hours. The absorption is not affected by most food, but it is impaired by antacids containing aluminum, calcium, or magnesium and by iron preparations; food containing calcium (dairy products) can, therefore, affect their absorption.[124] A similar effect is seen with quinolones. Tetracyclines form a stable calcium complex in any bone-forming tissue; since they cross the placenta, they may negatively affect the development of the fetal skeleton.[125] They may also produce permanent yellow/gray/brown tooth discoloration and should not be administered to children or pregnant women.[125]

Tetracyclines have been shown to depress plasma prothrombin activity. Patients taking anticoagulants may, therefore, require a decrement in the dose of warfarin. For reasons that are unclear, oral contraceptives have been shown to be less effective in patients treated with tetracyclines; additional contraceptive measures should be recommended in patients taking both compounds (this is particularly important in view of the possible negative effects of tetracyclines on fetal development).[126]

TABLE 56.9 BASELINE DEMOGRAPHIC AND CLINICAL FEATURES OF RA PATIENTS IN MINOCYCLINE TRIALS

Variables	Kloppenburg et al[127] n = 80	MIRA[123] n = 219	O'Dell et al[128] n = 46	O'Dell et al[130] n = 60
Age (yr)	56	54	45	60
Gender, women (%)	68	78	72	73
Ethnicity:				
White (%)	100*	66	100*	100*
Non-white (%)	0	34	0	0
Disease duration (yr)	13.0	8.6	0.4	0.5
Previous DMARD† use (%)	69	46	0	0
Corticosteroid use (%)	11	31	0	100‡
Rheumatoid factor positivity (%)	89	56	100	100
ESR (mm/hr)	50	34	32	32
Functional assessment, 0-3, mean	1.7	0.9	ND§	ND§

*Probably.
†Disease-modifying antirheumatic drug.
‡Require at study initiation.
§Not done.
ESR, erythrocyte sedimentation rate.

Tetracyclines for the treatment of rheumatoid arthritis

Efficacy data

Minocycline randomized controlled trials

To date, there have been four large double-blind, randomized, clinical trials using minocycline in RA.[123,127-130] Three of these trials were conducted in the United States and one in Europe (Tables 56.9 and 56.10). In addition, there are now some smaller non-randomized studies relating experience with the use of minocycline in different parts of the world (China, Japan, Israel).[131-133]

The first published trial came from The Netherlands; this was a 6-month, multicenter study involving 80 patients with long-standing RA (disease duration > 10 years), who had already failed more than one DMARD and who were randomized to receive either minocycline (200 mg/day) or placebo in addition to their background medication, which could include a DMARD.[127] The second published study came from the MIRA Group; sponsored by the National Institute of Arthritis, Musculoskeletal and Skin (NIAMS) Diseases, this was a 1-year study and included 219 patients with established, yet not very severe, RA who had failed one or more DMARDs.[123] Patients were not continued on a DMARD during the actual trial.

The other two studies have been conducted by the RAIN (RA Investigational Network) group.[128,130] In both studies, patients were DMARD naive, seropositive for IgM rheumatoid factor (RF) and had disease of less than 1 year in duration. In the first study from this group, 46 RA patients were randomized to receive either minocycline or placebo for a total of 6 months.[128] In the second study, 60 RA patients were enrolled; the control group received an active compound (hydroxychloroquine).[130] Another important feature of these studies is the fact that in addition to the initial trial data, O'Dell and colleagues have been able to gather longitudinal data on their patients.[129,130,134]

With the exception of the second study from the RAIN group,[129,130,134] the other three studies were planned prior to the formulation of the ACR definition of clinical improvement (ACR20, ACR50, etc.); therefore, they do not include the same outcome parameters. Nevertheless, the

TABLE 56.10 OUTCOME DATA FOR MINOCYCLINE IN RA CLINICAL TRIALS

Outcome	Kloppenburg et al[127]	MIRA[123]	O'Dell et al[128]	O'Dell et al[130]
Trial design	Placebo controlled	Placebo controlled	Placebo controlled	Active comparator (hydroxychloroquine)
Primary*	25% or greater improvement in Ritchie index and swollen joints	50% or greater improvement in joint tenderness and swelling	50% or greater improvement in Paulus criteria[†]	ACR50 response The steroid dosage
Secondary, favored minocycline				
Yes	ESR, CRP, IgM-RF, hemoglobin, hematocrit, platelets	Grip strength, ESR, IgM-RF, platelets	Patient and physician globals	Patient global, WBC, hemoglobin
No	Pain at rest and motion, fatigue, morning stiffness, grip strength, functional assessment	Patient and physician globals, morning stiffness, functional assessment	Tender and swollen joint counts	Tender and swollen joint counts, ESR, physician global, pain, functional assessment
Indirect	None	More protocol violations: ↑ dose corticosteroids, initiation of DMARDs, IACS injections, changes in NSAIDs in placebo-treated than minocycline-treated patients	At 1 and 4 years, more minocycline patients still on and/or not receiving other DMARDS	Significant reduction in prednisone dose among minocycline-treated patients
Not ascertained	Patient and physician globals	CRP	IgM-RF, CRP, functional assessment	

Favored minocycline in all the studies.
†*50% or greater improvement in three of the following: joint tenderness, joint swelling, morning stiffness, and ESR.*
ESR, erythrocyte sedimentation rate; CRP, C-reactive protein; IgM-RF, IgM rheumatoid factor; DMARD, disease-modifying antirheumatic drug; IACS, intra-articular corticosteroids.

overall results are consistent within the four studies and favor the use of minocycline in the treatment of RA; in particular, the second study from O'Dell and colleagues demonstrated a better response to minocycline than to hydroxychloroquine. Genetic studies were performed only in the MIRA study; white subjects having the shared epitope were more likely to respond to minocycline treatment than those not having it.[135]

Doxycycline randomized controlled trials

To date, there have been four double-blind, randomized, clinical trials using doxycycline in RA. The first published study was a 16-week trial in which a 3-week course of intravenous (IV) doxycycline (200 mg/day) was followed by 200 mg IV weekly, compared with either oral azithromycin or placebo in RA patients with active and erosive disease. DMARDs were not allowed in this trial. The primary endpoints were a decrease in the tender joint count, in ESR, and in urine pyridinolines (products of collagen degradation) at day 28 as compared with the baseline values. This trial was, however, stopped prematurely owing to both lack of efficacy and infusion-related events, although none of them was serious.[136]

The second trial was a pilot study of a 12-week course of doxycycline (300 mg given intravenously over 2 hours for 14 days) or placebo in 23 RA patients with active disease (10 received doxycycline and 13 received placebo).[137] Stable doses of DMARDs were allowed in this study. Only one patient in the doxycycline group and none in the placebo group achieved response criteria. Difficulties with patient recruitment and intravenous access as well as lack of efficacy prompted the termination of this trial. The authors concluded that given the very small proportion of responders, it is unlikely that the potential efficacy of intravenous administration of doxycycline in the treatment of RA would outweigh the risk and inconvenience of intravenous administration.[137]

The third trial was a 36-week, crossover trial in which oral doxycycline 50 mg twice a day (or placebo) was used in 66 RA patients with active disease.[138] Stable doses of DMARDs were permitted in this trial. Doxycycline failed to reduce either disease activity or joint destruction in this trial.[138]

The data from these three trials have failed to demonstrate the efficacy of doxycycline in RA patients with active and erosive disease.[136-138] Although the efficacy of doxycycline cannot be ruled out because of the small number of patients or relatively short follow-up time in these trials, the difficulties with patient recruitment and with the intravenous administration of doxycycline make it unlikely that further studies of doxycycline for treatment of RA will be undertaken.

The fourth trial in contrast to the first three studies was conducted in early seropositive RA patients who were DMARD naive. Sixty-six patients were randomized to three groups: (1) oral methotrexate alone; (2) oral doxycycline, 20 mg twice daily with oral methotrexate; and (3) oral doxycycline, 100 mg twice daily with oral methotrexate. The patients were followed for 2 years. Initial therapy with methotrexate plus doxycycline was superior (based on an ACR50 response) to treatment with methotrexate alone. The therapeutic responses to low-dose and high-dose doxycycline were similar, suggesting that the antimetalloproteinase effects were more important than the antibacterial effects.[139]

Minocycline and doxycycline meta-analysis

A meta-analysis of the treatment of RA with antibiotics has been conducted recently.[140] Although the authors referred to 10 randomized controlled trials (1 tetracycline study, 6 minocycline studies, and 3 doxycycline studies), 2 studies were counted twice (using different outcomes). Thus, the analyses included 535 patients from 9 different trials[95,123,127,128,130,136,141-143]; only 3 trials were considered to be of high quality by the authors.[127,136,141] In addition, because not all outcomes had been ascertained in all 9 trials, not all patients were included in all the analyses.

A small but clinically meaningful reduction in disease activity as measured by tender and swollen joint counts was found in the active treatment group as compared with the placebo group. In contrast, there was a marked reduction in ESR in the active treatment group. It should be noted that the treatment effect was more evident in the subgroup of patients with early seropositive disease (disease duration < 1 year); furthermore, minocycline was found to be more effective than doxycycline in reducing disease activity.[140] There was no difference in terms of radiologic progression (erosions and joint space narrowing) between both treatment groups, which could be due to the true lack of efficacy or the result of patient selection (milder disease activity). Moreover, the radiographic outcome was not the primary endpoint and thus these studies could have been underpowered to detect an effect. These data are depicted in Tables 56.11 and 56.12.

In summary, this meta-analysis modestly favored the use of minocycline and doxycycline over the control treatment groups.

Long-term data

The long-term efficacy data have been systematically assessed only in the studies of O'Dell and colleagues.[129,134] Four years later, more patients randomized to minocycline in the first study were still

TABLE 56.11 META-ANALYSIS OF TENDER JOINT COUNT, SWOLLEN JOINT COUNT, AND EROSIONS IN PATIENTS WITH RA RANDOMIZED TO RECEIVE A TETRACYCLINE DERIVATIVE OR A CONTROL TREATMENT

Outcomes	Treatment (n)	Control (n)	SMD* (95% CI)	SMD* (95% CI)
Tender joint counts[†]	246	248		−0.39 (−0.74, −0.05)
Swollen joint counts[†]	246	248		−0.23 (−0.41, −0.05)
Erosions[‡]	143	150		0.17 (−0.29, 0.64)

−1.0   −0.5   0.0   0.5   1.0
Favor treatment   Favor control

*Standardized mean difference.
[†]Data from references 123, 127, 128, 136, 142, and 143.
[‡]Data from references 123 and 141.
Modified from Stone M, et al. Should tetracycline treatment be used more extensively for rheumatoid arthritis? Meta-analysis demonstrates clinical benefit with reduction in disease activity. J Rheumatol 2003;30:2112-2122.

TABLE 56.12 META-ANALYSIS OF ERYTHROCYTE SEDIMENTATION RATE IN PATIENTS WITH RA RANDOMIZED TO RECEIVE A TETRACYCLINE DERIVATIVE OR A CONTROL TREATMENT

Outcome	Treatment (n)	Control (n)	WMD* (95% CI)	WMD* (95% CI)
Erythrocyte sedimentation rate	246	248		−8.96 (−14.51, −3.42)

50   25   0   25   50
Favor treatment   Favor control

*Weighted mean difference.
Modified from Stone M, et al. Should tetracycline treatment be used more extensively for rheumatoid arthritis? Meta-analysis demonstrates clinical benefit with reduction in disease activity. J Rheumatol 2003;30:2112-2122.

TABLE 56.13 TOXICITY DATA FOR MINOCYCLINE IN RA CLINICAL TRIALS

Manifestation (%)	Kloppenburg et al[127]		MIRA[123]		O'Dell[128*]		O'Dell[130]	
	Minocycline n = 40	Placebo n = 40	Minocycline n = 109	Placebo n = 110	Minocycline n = 20	Placebo n = 18	Minocycline n = 30	HCQ n = 30
Gastrointestinal	58	15	24	0	0	0	0	3
Dizziness	40	15	19	0	0	0	3	0
Cutaneous								
Rash	0	3	5	0	0	0	3	3
Hyperpigmentation	0	0	0	0	0	0	3	0
Pneumonitis	3	0	0	0	0	0	0	0
Others (infection)	0	8	0	0	0	0	0	0

*After 4 years of follow-up four patients (20%) had developed integument changes.[141]

receiving this compound and/or were in remission as compared with the ones randomized to placebo.[134] Efficacy was still observed in the second study 2 years later.[129]

Toxicity data

In terms of toxicity, the data are also quite different. In the MIRA study there were some adverse reactions but they were comparable in frequency and severity in the placebo and minocycline-treated patients.[123] In contrast, in the study from The Netherlands some patients in the minocycline group experienced vestibular manifestations, which led to falls and even some fractures.[127] Rare manifestations that have been described associated with the use of minocycline, particularly in the younger patient, include a lupus-like syndrome or "autoimmune" hepatitis, nephritis, pneumonitis, and/or central nervous system involvement.[144-154]

The studies from O'Dell's group demonstrated an impressive tolerability to minocycline; in fact, only 3 patients (9%) withdrew from these studies, either because of integument changes (fingernail discoloration and an erythematous rash) or dizziness.[128,130] Of interest, after

4 years of follow-up from the first study, pigmentary changes were observed in 4 patients (20%); 1 patient chose to continue treatment with minocycline (Table 56.13).[134]

In the meta-analysis, 381 patients were included; there were no statistical differences in the risk of adverse events between both treatment groups.[140]

Minocycline use is well documented to cause cutaneous hyperpigmentation, although not frequently observed in initial clinical trials in RA.[123,127,128,130] There are four classic types of minocycline-induced hyperpigmentation:

- Type I is a blue-black macular pigmentation confined to previous scars or inflammatory tissue on the face.
- Type II includes blue-black, brown, or slate gray macules seen on healthy skin, mainly of the shins, forearms, or legs.
- Type III is described as symmetric muddy-brown pigmentation of sun-exposed skin.[155]
- Type IV was recently described as blue-gray discoloration within scar tissue on the back.[156]

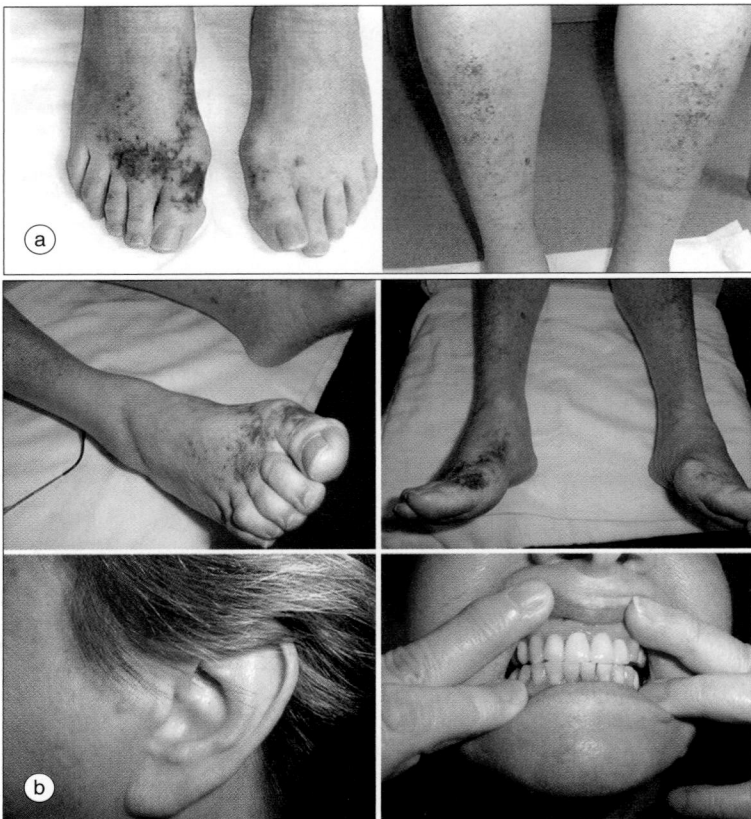

Fig. 56.4 Pigmentary changes in a patient with RA treated with minocycline for more than 5 years. (a) Pigmentation observed around a bunionectomy scar and on the shins after 4 years of treatment (02/2004). (b) Pigmentation over the bunionectomy scar has worsened. Pigmentation around the pinna's superior crux and concha and oral mucosa is evident after 5 years of treatment (02/2005). *(Courtesy of Dr. Graciela S. Alarcón.)*

Figure 56.4 shows an example of these pigmentary changes in a patient with RA treated with minocycline for more than 5 years.

Dose-related toxicities associated with the use of tetracycline derivatives include vestibular dysfunction (dizziness, tinnitus, vertigo), gastrointestinal upset, integument pigmentation, pancreatitis, and hepatitis, whereas systemic lupus erythematosus, headaches, benign intracranial hypertension, and Stevens-Johnson syndrome are more likely to be idiosyncratic.

Monitoring

Complete blood cell counts and chemistry profile should be monitored every 3 months while treatment is continued.

Tetracyclines for the treatment of osteoarthritis

Efficacy data

In-vivo studies have shown that oral doxycycline administration decreases the progression of OA in animal models. A NIAMS-sponsored, multicentric, double-blind study comparing oral doxycycline (100 mg twice a day) and placebo for 30 months has been conducted.

This trial included 431 obese women with unilateral knee OA confirmed by conventional standing views of knee radiographs (Kellgren's grade II-III in the OA knee and 0-I in the other).[157,158] The primary outcome was changes in the joint space width of the medial tibiofemoral compartment. Adherence and subject retention to dosing regimen were remarkably high, at 92% and 71%, respectively.[157] Patients in the doxycycline group experienced 33% less joint space narrowing in the OA knee (0.30 ± 0.60 mm versus 0.45 ± 0.70 mm, adjusted $P = .017$) but not in the contralateral knee, as compared with the placebo group. There were no differences in terms of pain score (Western Ontario and McMaster Universities Osteoarthritis Index (WOMAC) and 50-foot walk pain), WOMAC function, and median scores of patient's and physician's global assessment of disease activity between doxycycline and placebo groups. Nonetheless, the frequency with which subjects reported 20% or more increase in knee pain (WOMAC pain score) in the following visits was reduced in the doxycycline group as compared with those in the placebo group (23.8 ± 22.7 vs. 30.2 ± 21.1, $P = .004$). However, this effect was not observed in the contralateral knee. Overall, doxycycline treatment did not fulfill the proposed Outcome Measures in Rheumatology Clinical Trials (OMERACT) OA responder criteria[159]; however, these criteria have been developed in patients with advanced OA and whether they can be used in patients with milder disease has not been determined.

Toxicity data

In terms of adverse events, photosensitivity, non-specific gastrointestinal manifestations, and candidal vaginitis were reported more frequently in the doxycycline group than in the placebo group, but only a few patients discontinued the study prematurely because of these untoward events. Of interest, patients in the doxycycline group reported fewer urinary tract infections and a trend toward fewer upper respiratory tract infections.[158]

CONCLUSION

The data reviewed clearly demonstrate the adequate benefit/toxicity ratio of oral minocycline in the treatment of RA. Supporting additional evidence has come from smaller open studies conducted in different parts of the world, including China, Japan, and Israel.[131-133] In contrast, the benefit of intravenous doxycycline (or azithromycin), a regimen comparable to the one prescribed by Brown's followers, has not been proven. However, high-dose oral doxycycline in combination with methotrexate might be beneficial in patients with early RA.[139] Finally, the benefits of intra-articular minocycline have not been demonstrated.[160]

Minocycline may be a reasonable treatment alternative in RA under the following circumstances:

- As an adjunctive treatment in patients who are not responding to standard therapy and are unable to afford or tolerate other DMARDs or in whom anti–TNF-α agents are not an option because of increased risk of infections, such as in patients with bronchiectasis
- For the treatment of patients with early RA whose disease course is believed to be not too aggressive and in whom hydroxychloroquine may have been considered.

The benefit of using doxycycline for the treatment of knee OA has now been demonstrated in terms of slowing the radiographic progression and perhaps diminishing pain, and it thus may be a reasonable treatment option for patients with mild-to-moderate knee OA.

SUGGESTED READING

Trapnell CB, Donahue SR, Collins JM, et al. Thalidomide does not alter the pharmacokinetics of ethinyl estradiol and norethindrone. Clin Pharmacol Ther 1998; 64:597-602.

KEY REFERENCES

4. Zuidema J, Hilbers-Modderman ES, Merkus FW. Clinical pharmacokinetics of dapsone. Clin Pharmacokinet 1986;11:299-315.

5. McConkey B, Davies P, Crockson RA, et al. Dapsone in rheumatoid arthritis. Rheumatol Rehabil 1976;15:230-234.

6. Swinson DR, Zlosnick J, Jackson L. Double-blind trial of dapsone against placebo in the treatment of rheumatoid arthritis. Ann Rheum Dis 1981;40:235-239.

7. Fowler PD, Shadforth MF, Crook PR, Lawton A. Report on chloroquine and dapsone in the treatment of rheumatoid arthritis: a 6-month comparative study. Ann Rheum Dis 1984;43:200-204.

8. Haar D, Solvkjaer M, Unger B, et al. A double-blind comparative study of hydroxychloroquine and dapsone, alone and in combination, in rheumatoid arthritis. Scand J Rheumatol 1993;22:113-118.

15. Coleman MD. Dapsone-mediated agranulocytosis: risks, possible mechanisms and prevention. Toxicology 2001;162:53-60.

19. Munro R, Capell HA. Penicillamine. Br J Rheumatol 1997;36:104-109.

22. Perrett D. The metabolism and pharmacology of D-penicillamine in man. J Rheumatol 1981;7:S41-S50.

24. Wernick R, Merryman P, Jaffe I, Ziff M. IgG and IgM rheumatoid factors in rheumatoid arthritis: quantitative response to penicillamine therapy and relationship to disease activity. Arthritis Rheum 1983;26:593-598.

27. Ledson MJ, Bucknall RC, Edwards SW. Inhibition of neutrophil oxidant secretion by D-penicillamine: scavenging of H_2O_2 and HOCl. Ann Rheum Dis 1992;51:321-325.

29. Controlled trial of D-penicillamine in severe rheumatoid arthritis. Lancet 1973;1:275-280.

30. Dixon AS, Davis J, Dormandy TL, Synthetic D. D-penicillamine in rheumatoid arthritis. Ann Rheum Dis 1975;34:416-421.

31. Shiokawa Y, Horiuchi Y, Honma M, et al. Clinical evaluation of D-penicillamine by multicentric double-blind controlled study in chronic rheumatoid arthritis. Arthritis Rheum 1977;20:1464-1472.

32. Williams HJ, Ward JR, Reading JC, et al. Low-dose D-penicillamine therapy in rheumatoid arthritis: a controlled, double-blind clinical trial. Arthritis Rheum 1983;26:581-592.

33. Felson DT, Anderson JJ, Meenan RF. Use of short-term efficacy/toxicity trade-offs to select second-line drugs in rheumatoid arthritis: a meta-analysis of published clinical trials. Arthritis Rheum 1992;35:1117-1125.

34. Jessop JD, O'Sullivan MM, Lewis PA, et al. A long-term five-year randomized controlled trial of hydroxychloroquine, sodium aurothiomalate, auranofin and penicillamine in the treatment of patients with rheumatoid arthritis. Br J Rheumatol 1998;37:992-1002.

35. Hochberg MC. Auranofin or D-penicillamine in the treatment of rheumatoid arthritis. Ann Intern Med 1986;105:528-535.

36. Gibson T, Huskisson EC, Wojtulewski JA, et al. Evidence that D-penicillamine alters the course of rheumatoid arthritis. Rheumatol Rehabil 1976;15:211-215.

37. Thomas MH, Rothermich NO, Philps VK, et al. Gold vs D-penicillamine double blind and follow-up. J Rheumatol 1984;11:764-767.

38. Bunch TW, O'Duffy JD, Tompkins RB, O'Fallon WM. Controlled trial of hydroxychloroquine and D-penicillamine singly and in combination in the treatment of rheumatoid arthritis. Arthritis Rheum 1984;27:267-276.

39. Capell HA, Marabani M, Madhok R, et al. Degree and extent of response to sulphasalazine or penicillamine therapy for rheumatoid arthritis: results from a routine clinical environment over a two-year period. Q J Med 1990;75:335-344.

40. Paulus HE, Williams HJ, Ward JR, et al. Azathioprine versus D-penicillamine in rheumatoid arthritis patients who have been treated unsuccessfully with gold. Arthritis Rheum 1984;27:721-727.

41. Berry H, Liyanage SP, Durance RA, et al. Azathioprine and penicillamine in treatment of rheumatoid arthritis: a controlled trial. BMJ 1976;1:1052-1054.

42. Taggart AJ, Hill J, Astbury C, et al. Sulphasalazine alone or in combination with D-penicillamine in rheumatoid arthritis. Br J Rheumatol 1987;26:32-36.

49. Gordon JN, Goggin PM. Thalidomide and its derivatives: emerging from the wilderness. Postgrad Med J 2003;79:127-132.

57. Kenyon BM, Browne F, D'Amato RJ. Effects of thalidomide and related metabolites in a mouse corneal model of neovascularization. Exp Eye Res 1997;64:971-978.

64. Huizinga TW, Dijkmans BA, van der Velde EA, et al. An open study of pentoxyfylline and thalidomide as adjuvant therapy in the treatment of rheumatoid arthritis. Ann Rheum Dis 1996;55:833-836.

72. Barlogie B, Desikan R, Munshi N. Single course D.T. PACE anti-angiochemotherapy effects CR in plasma cell leukemia and fulminant multiple myeloma. Blood 1998;92(Suppl 1, pt 2):273b.

78. Ichikawa Y, Saito T, Yamanaka H, et al. Therapeutic effects of the combination of methotrexate and bucillamine in early rheumatoid arthritis: a multicenter, double-blind, randomized controlled study. Mod Rheumatol 2005;15:323-328.

88. Yokota N, Kuga Y, Kanazawa T, et al. Ten years results of bucillamine in the treatment of rheumatoid arthritis. Mod Rheumatol 2007;17:33-36.

93. Ford DK. The microbiological causes of rheumatoid arthritis. J Rheumatol 1991;18:1441-1442.

96. Alarcón GS, Mikhail IS. Antimicrobials in the treatment of rheumatoid arthritis and other arthritides: a clinical perspective. Am J Med Sci 1994;308:201-209.

104. Alarcón GS. Tetracyclines for the treatment of rheumatoid arthritis. Exp Opin Invest Drugs 2000;9:1491-1498.

123. Tilley BC, Alarcón GS, Heyse SP, et al. Minocycline in rheumatoid arthritis: a 48-week, double-blind, placebo-controlled trial. MIRA Trial Group. Ann Intern Med 1995;122:81-89.

125. Demers P, Fraser D, Goldbloom RB, et al. Effects of tetracyclines on skeletal growth and dentition. A report by the Nutrition Committee of the Canadian Paediatric Society. Can Med Assoc J 1968;99:849-854.

126. Helms SE, Bredle DL, Zajic J, et al. Oral contraceptive failure rates and oral antibiotics. J Am Acad Dermatol 1997;36:705-710.

127. Kloppenburg M, Breedveld FC, Terwiel JP, et al. Minocycline in active rheumatoid arthritis: a double-blind, placebo-controlled trial. Arthritis Rheum 1994;37:629-636.

128. O'Dell JR, Haire CE, Palmer W. Treatment of early rheumatoid arthritis with minocycline or placebo: results of a randomized, double-blind, placebo-controlled trial. Arthritis Rheum 1997;40:842-848.

129. O'Dell JR, Blakely KW, Mallek JA. Early sero-positive rheumatoid arthritis treatment: a 2-year, double-blind comparison of minocycline and hydroxychloroquine. Arthritis Rheum 2000;43:S382.

130. O'Dell JR, Blakely KW, Mallek JA. Treatment of early seropositive rheumatoid arthritis: a two-year, double-blind comparison of minocycline and hydroxychloroquine. Arthritis Rheum 2001;44:2235-2241.

134. O'Dell JR, Paulsen G, Haire CE. Treatment of early seropositive rheumatoid arthritis with minocyline: four-year followup of a double-blind, placebo-controlled trial. Arthritis Rheum 1999;42:1691-1695.

135. Reveille JD, Alarcon GS, Fowler SE. HLA-DRB1 genes and disease severity in rheumatoid arthritis. Arthritis Rheum 1996;39:1802-1807.

136. St. Clair EW, Wilkinson WE, Pisetsky DS. The effects of intravenous doxycycline therapy for rheumatoid arthritis: a randomized, double-blind, placebo-controlled trial. Arthritis Rheum 2001;44:1043-1047.

137. Pillemer S, Gulko P, Ligier S. Pilot clinical trial of intravenous doxycycline versus placebo for rheumatoid arthritis. J Rheumatol 2001;30:41-43.

138. van der Laan W, Molenaar E, Ronday K, et al. Lack of effect of doxycycline on disease activity and damage in patients with rheumatoid arthritis. J Rheumatol 2001;28:1967-1974.

139. O'Dell JR, Elliott JR, Mallek JA, et al. Treatment of early seropositive rheumatoid arthritis: doxycycline plus methotrexate versus methotrexate alone. Arthritis Rheum 2006;54:621-627.

140. Stone M, Fortin PR, Pacheco-Tena C, Inman RD. Should tetracycline treatment be used more extensively for rheumatoid arthritis? Meta-analysis demonstrates clinical benefit with reduction in disease activity. J Rheumatol 2003;30:2112-2122.

157. Mazzuca SA, Brandt KD, Katz BP, et al. Subject retention and adherence in a randomized placebo-controlled trial of a disease-modifying osteoarthritis drug. Arthritis Rheum 2004;51:933-940.

158. Brandt KD, Mazzuca SA, Katz BP. Effect of doxycycline on progression of osteoarthritis: results of a randomized placebo-controlled double blind trial. Arthritis Rheum 2005;52:2015-2025.

160. Weinberger A, Ben-Gal T, Roizman P, Abramovici A. Intraarticular minocycline injection in experimental synovitis. Clin Rheumatol 1996;15:290-294.

REFERENCES

Full references for this chapter can be found on www.expertconsult.com.

Immunotherapies: T cell and complement

57

Ernest H. S. Choy

- Immunotherapeutic agents, unlike previous drugs for rheumatoid arthritis, have been developed rationally by targeting processes important in disease pathogenesis.
- Immunotherapy usually involves the use of biologic agents such as monoclonal antibodies, soluble receptors, or peptides, although immunoactive drugs are increasingly being developed.
- Anti–T-cell therapy shows a limited short-term effect but may have the potential to effect a more fundamental alteration in the disease process.
- Preliminary evidence in animal models suggests anti-complement therapies may be effective in RA but large randomized controlled trials are required to confirm these findings.

A BRIEF OVERVIEW OF PATHOGENESIS

Rheumatoid arthritis (RA) is a chronic immune-mediated inflammatory disease primarily affecting joints. The disease-modifying effects of drugs in current use were discovered empirically; potential benefits for the joint are often indivisible from unwanted effects on a host of other systems. The concept behind immunotherapy is that treatments based on a clear understanding of disease pathogenesis will be more efficacious, more specific, and, it is hoped, less toxic.

Although the cause of RA remains unknown, a considerable amount is now known about the pathologic processes involved in the disease. Because this has been addressed in detail elsewhere in this book, only a brief summary is given here. RA may be initiated by an unknown antigenic peptide derived either from an exogenous antigen (e.g., an infectious agent) or an autoantigen. The putative arthritogenic peptide is presented by the RA-associated MHC class II antigens, such as HLA-DRB1*0404 or HLA-DRB1*0401, to arthritogenic CD4+ T cells. These become activated, release interleukin (IL)-2, and induce clonal expansion of other CD4+ T cells. Their production of various other cytokines and growth factors activates other cell types, including B cells, monocyte/macrophages, and synoviocytes, and enhances leukocyte recruitment into the joint. These processes together generate the immune-inflammatory cascade of synovitis. Binding of T-cell receptor to antigenic peptide in the HLA-DR groove is insufficient for full T-cell activation. A second signal provided by co-stimulatory molecules such as CD28 on T cells binding to CD80 and CD86 on antigen-presenting cells is necessary. In the absence of co-stimulatory signal, T cells will not only fail to activate but also become refractory to activation. Some researchers have suggested that, in the late stages of RA, synovitis and joint destruction are due to a monocyte-synoviocyte–driven process independent of T-cell mechanisms. However, the beneficial effect of the anti–T-cell drugs, cyclosporine, tacrolimus,[1] and, recently, the biologic agent abatacept, which inhibits T-cell activation by blocking co-stimulatory signals, even in long-standing disease, argues strongly in favor of a continuing role for T cells. In this chapter the focus is on therapies against T cells, except abatacept (see Chapter 58), and on the complement cascade.

THERAPIES AGAINST T CELLS

The "holy grail" for those interested in T cells as therapeutic targets in RA is to develop a treatment that affects, primarily or exclusively, the arthritogenic T cells. Clearly, such specific therapy will be less toxic than a general anti–T-cell therapy. However, it is more difficult to achieve especially in established disease because the arthritogenic peptide and disease-specific T cells in RA remain unknown. Therapies against T cells can be broadly divided into those that deplete T cells or those that modulate their function.

T-cell depletion

Early T-cell depletion therapies included thoracic duct drainage, total lymphoid irradiation, and lymphocytopheresis. These have been abandoned because of side effects and impracticability for clinical use, although some studies suggested efficacy.

Based on these successes, a number of depleting anti–T-cell monoclonal antibodies (mAbs) targeting different T-cell subsets were tested in RA. The first anti–T-cell mAb used in a clinical trial was anti-CD7. Both murine and chimeric antibodies were used, but they were ineffective[2] because they targeted a subset of T cells now thought to be unimportant in RA.[3]

CD5+ is an immunoconjugate of the murine anti-CD5 mAb and the plant toxin ricin, which deletes CD5+ T and B cells. Although the results from open studies were promising, the placebo-controlled trial was negative.[4] This lack of effect may have resulted both from an unexpectedly high placebo response rate and from the use of a lower dose than was used in the open study so as to avoid profound lymphopenia.

IL-2-DAB is another immunotoxin in which IL-2 is joined to a diphtheria toxin A chain. Because high-affinity IL-2 receptors are only found on activated T cells, IL-2-DAB was thought to be potentially a more specific agent. Placebo-controlled trials[5] showed that it was superior to placebo, but the percentage of patients who responded was only 18% compared with 0% in the placebo group. Furthermore, in the treatment group, the withdrawal rate was high (12 of 45 patients) and half the patients showed an abnormal rise in liver transaminase levels after treatment.

Campath-1H (anti-CDw52) is a complement-fixing humanized mAb used in RA.[6] Clinical improvement was observed after intravenous therapy with Campath-1H.[7] One of the major side effects associated with Campath-1H was a cytokine release syndrome, which developed in all patients on the first day of treatment. It was characterized by high fever, rigors, chills, diarrhea, and, most seriously, significant hypotension. Campath-1H led to profound and protracted peripheral blood lymphopenia lasting many months. However, disease improvement did not correlate with peripheral blood lymphopenia. Indeed, disease often relapsed long before the lymphocyte count returned to normal. When synovia from treated patients were examined, a large number of lymphocytes still persisted[8]; possible explanations for these findings are that either synovial lymphocytes are more resistant to lysis or that the antibody did not adequately penetrate into the joint.

As a result of the murine work, the chimeric anti-CD4 mAb cM-T412 (Centocor) was tested in a number of clinical trials in RA. Neither single nor repeated weekly treatments with cM-T412 produced any clinical improvement. However, there was a dose-related peripheral blood CD4 lymphopenia lasting between 1 and 12 weeks. Although an open study of cM-T412 produced promising results,[9] a placebo-controlled trial of the agent in early RA did not show any significant benefit.[10] However, the dose of cM-T412 used in this study was less than the previous study because of concerns about CD4 lymphopenia.

As a result of these problems, anti-CD7, CD5+, IL-2-DAB, Campath-1H, and cM-T412 have been abandoned as treatments for RA. One possible explanation for these negative results is the effect of lymphocyte depletion on CD4+ regulatory T cells (Treg) whose phenotype type and function have only been discovered over the past decade. Sakaguchi and colleagues have shown that CD4+ Treg cells express high level of CD25[11] and the transcription factor Foxp3.[12] They express α-β T-cell receptors and, similar to other T cells, can only be activated by antigenic peptide bound by class II MHC molecules. In addition, they also express CTLA-4, which binds to CD80 and CD86 molecules on antigen-presenting cells. Indeed, enhancing Treg cell number or function has been used as a therapeutic strategy to develop treatments with sustained efficacy in many autoimmune diseases as well as to prevent transplant rejection. The conflicting results of T-cell depletion may be the result of removal of Treg cells. Hence, T-cell depletion has largely been abandoned for the treatment of RA in favor of immunomodulation.

Semi-specific T-cell immunomodulation

Non-depleting anti-CD4 monoclonal antibodies

The rationale for using non-depleting anti-CD4 mAb in RA was developed initially in animal models in which such treatments induced "immunologic tolerance."[13] In streptococcal cell wall arthritis, a single course of a non-depleting anti-CD4 mAb, given at the time of disease induction, prevented the development of arthritis. Moreover, the treated animals acquired a resistance to further attempts at disease induction. This phenomenon is known as immunologic tolerance. In non-obese diabetic mice, an animal model of type I diabetes, anti-CD4 mAb can induce tolerance even in established disease.[14] Interestingly, CD4 lymphocyte depletion was not necessary to produce tolerance.[15] On the contrary, established anti-CD4 mAb–mediated tolerance could be broken by lymphocyte depletion, suggesting tolerance is an active lymphocyte-mediated process[16] probably mediated through CD4+ Treg cells. If anti-CD4 mAbs could induce tolerance in established human autoimmune diseases, such as RA, it is hypothesized that this could result in "re-programming" of the immune response and, hence, long-term disease improvement.[17] Four non-depleting anti-CD4 mAbs have been tested in RA.

IDEC-CE9.1/SB-210396 (Smith Kline and Beecham) is a primatized non-depleting anti-CD4 mAb. It is known as a primatized mAb because it was raised initially in macaques. In a randomized placebo-controlled trial,[18] patients with refractory RA were treated with either placebo or three different doses (40, 80, and 140 mg) of IDEC-CE9.1/SB-210396 twice weekly for 4 weeks. In the two high-dose groups, there were statistically significant clinical improvements, although some patients in the 140-mg group developed leukocytoclastic vasculitis that necessitated termination of treatment.

4162W94 (Glaxo Wellcome) is a humanized non-depleting anti-CD4 mAb. In an open-labeled dose-escalating study, 24 RA patients in four cohorts were treated with five daily doses of 10 mg, 30 mg, 100 mg, or 300 mg of mAb, respectively. Clinical improvement with reduction in erythrocyte sedimentation rate and C-reactive protein was seen in patients treated with either 100- or 300-mg doses.[19] A subsequent placebo-controlled trial was done in 48 patients with RA who were dosed with one (cohort 1), two (cohort 2), or three (cohort 3) cycles of 5 × 300 mg 4162W94 or placebo (12 and 4 patients, respectively, per cohort) at monthly intervals.[20] Sixteen patients were dosed in each of the first two cohorts; however, the dose was reduced in cohort 3 after 5 patients received greater than or equal to two dose cycles owing to accumulating evidence of a high frequency of rash. These patients were analyzed according to the number of cycles received. A further 8 patients received 5 × 100 mg for one to three cycles before stopping the study for administrative reasons. An American College of Rheumatology 20% response (ACR20) was observed in 4/13 ($P = .119$ vs. placebo) and 7/13 ($P = .015$ vs. placebo) in cohorts 1 and 2, respectively. None of the 5 × 100-mg/day or placebo patients achieved ACR20. Four patients were still responding at the end of the 3-month follow-up period. CD4 lymphocyte suppression (<0.2 ×109/L on ≥two successive occasions) occurred in 11/34 patients who received 4162W94 versus none on placebo. Rash occurred in 21/34 mAb-treated patients,

including 1 patient with biopsy-confirmed cutaneous vasculitis. Thus, 4162W94 demonstrated significant clinical efficacy in this study. However, because of unacceptable CD4 lymphopenia and rash, the original hypothesis of prolonged CD4 "blockade" to give lasting clinical benefit could not be tested.

Humax-CD4/HM6G (Genmab) is a fully human anti-CD4 IgG1 monoclonal antibody. A single dose of Humax-CD4 of 0.005, 0.05, 0.15, 0.5, or 1.0 mg/kg was given by subcutaneous injection to cohorts of 5 patients, with 4 patients randomized to active treatment and 1 patient to placebo.[21] Between days 1 and 7 CD4+ lymphocyte counts transiently decreased after treatment but recovered by day 7. Improvements in the disease during the follow-up period were reported in the highest dose groups. For most patients the maximal improvement occurred 28 days after treatment. A phase 2 randomized placebo-controlled trial has been completed, but the result has not been reported.

The results of a placebo-controlled trial using the humanized non-depleting anti-CD4 mAb OKT4-cdr4a (Johnson & Johnson) have not been published in full, but a preliminary communication suggested that it might be efficacious.[22]

Development of IDEC-CE9.1/SB-210396 and 4162W94 has been stopped because of lymphocyte depletion and side effects. Although short-term clinical trials suggest non-depleting anti-CD4 mAbs suppress inflammation, long-term studies are necessary to assess whether they could achieve the "holy grail" of immunotherapy, the induction of prolonged disease remission without the need for ongoing long-term treatment.

T-cell vaccination

In animal models, it is fairly easy to identify the arthritogenic clones that induce disease because they can be transferred from one animal to another. This has led to the development of the technique of T-cell vaccination,[23] analogous to bacterial vaccination, in which animals are immunized with pathogenic T cells, attenuated by chemicals or radiation such that they no longer induce disease. The animals develop an anti-vaccine immune response that also inhibits the non-attenuated but otherwise immunologically identical pathogenic T cells responsible for the disease. T-cell vaccination in animal models is able both to prevent and to treat established disease. Attempts have been made to apply this technique to humans, using synovial T cells that are postulated to contain a higher proportion of pathogenic T cells than those in the blood. A recent open-label clinical study recruited 15 patients in whom autologous synovial T cells were used as vaccines.[24] A total of six subcutaneous injections were administered over 12 months. Ten of 15 patients (67%) achieved an ACR50 improvement at 12 months. This was associated with an increase in CD4+ Tregs and CD8+ cytotoxic T cells specific for the vaccine. Although the clinical benefit of this treatment was promising, its clinical efficacy will require confirmation by randomized control trials.

T-cell receptor vaccination

An alternative approach to the identification of pathogenic T cells examined whether T cells with particular T-cell receptor Vα or Vβ chains were expanded in lesional sites, such as the synovium, compared with blood. It was proposed that such expansions would be pathogenetically relevant; it was further suggested, by analogy with experiments in animals, that vaccination with unique peptides, derived from the sequence of the T-cell receptors found on the surface of the pathogenic T cells, would inhibit disease.[23] Sadly, T-cell populations expressing many different Vα and Vβ chains were reported as expanded by various groups of investigators. However, one group looked at Vβ usage by recently activated T cells, defined as T cells expressing the IL-2 receptor; they believed these recently activated cells were more relevant to disease pathogenesis. On the basis of results showing an increase of Vβ17+ usage by IL-2 receptor positive (IL-2R+) T cells in the synovium, these investigators embarked on a clinical trial of a Vβ17-derived peptide in RA.[25] This was an uncontrolled open dose-finding study, so evidence of clinical and biologic efficacy must be treated cautiously. However, the investigators noted that patients' joint scores decreased at all follow-up visits as did the frequency of Vβ17+ IL-2R+ T cells in the blood. Indeed, approximately 40% of patients developed a T-cell response to the vaccinated peptide. No toxicity was observed. Subsequently, these investigators have used a combination of three T-cell receptor peptides (Vβ3, Vβ14, Vβ17) in incomplete Freund's adjuvant as a vaccine (IR501, Immune Response Corp) in a placebo-controlled trial of 99 RA patients.[26] The vaccine (90 μg or 300 μg) or placebo was administered as intramuscular injections at weeks 0, 4, 8, and 20. In the 90-μg group there was a statistically significant improvement when compared with placebo, although only a third of the patients showed a response to the vaccine. A subsequent randomized placebo-controlled trial assessed the effect of IR501 and IR703 in 340 RA patients.[27] IR703 consists of three, 40-amino acid peptides, which encompass the IR501 peptides. Patients were randomized into five groups and received IR501 (30 μg, 90 μg), IR703 (30 μg, 90 μg), or placebo. Four intramuscular injections were given at weeks 0, 4, 8, and 20. Thirty-four percent of the patients in the IR501 30-μg group showed a statistically significant ACR20 improvement compared with 18% in the placebo group. The IR501 90-μg and IR703 90-μg groups also showed improvement, but these did not reach statistical significance. Patients not receiving concomitant corticosteroids and those with disease for less than 3 years showed greater clinical improvement.[27]

MHC and MHC-peptide vaccines

Because RA is linked with the HLA-DRB1*0404 and DRB1*0401 in Northern Europeans and North Americans, vaccination using the disease-associated MHC or MHC-peptide may be efficacious. In RA, three doses (1.3 mg, 4 mg, and 13 mg) of HLA-DRB1*0404/B1*0401-peptide (Anergen) were administered to 52 RA patients who were heterozygous for the shared epitope as an adjunct to methotrexate.[28] Treatment was well tolerated, and no significant immunosuppression was seen. However, only 33% and 31% of the patients developed antibody response to the vaccine.

A further study investigated the use of HLA-DRB1*0404/B1*0401 conjugated with the putative cartilage-derived RA autoantigen HC-gp39 as a vaccine. AG4263 is HLA-DRB1*0404/CDP263 (13mer peptide from HC gp-39). It was given to 31 HLA-DRB1*0404-positive RA patients in a randomized placebo-controlled trial as an adjunct to methotrexate.[29] Seven intravenous doses of either placebo or 0.5 to 150 mg/kg of AG4263 were infused over 6 weeks. Eighty-nine percent of all AG4263-treated patients compared with 57% of placebo patients achieved Paulus 20 improvement criteria at any time point. Response was greatest among patients receiving the highest doses of CDP263, with 85.7%, 28.6%, and 0% in the 150-μg, 60-μg, and placebo groups responding, respectively, at day 28. Interestingly, T-cell response to tetanus toxoid and tuberculin purified protein derivative was unaffected by treatment.

Oral tolerance

Oral tolerance was initially defined as the capacity to decrease immunologic reactivity to an antigen by administering that same antigen via the gut. However, more detailed study has shown that, in certain systems, oral antigens may induce tolerance not only to themselves but also to other antigens from the same tissue. This phenomenon, known as "bystander suppression," is critical to therapy for human diseases because the pathogenic antigen is usually unknown. Also crucially for treating humans, tolerance can be induced where an immune reaction is ongoing. One interesting recent development is that highly effective tolerance can also be induced by inhalation of a very low dose of antigen, so-called nasal tolerance.

Immunologic tolerance can potentially involve three main processes: deletion of specific T-cell clones, clonal anergy, and active suppression.[30] Both the two latter mechanisms have been shown to operate in different oral tolerance systems. A currently popular model suggests that exposure to low-dose oral antigen, for example, type II collagen, induces antigen-specific regulatory (Th2) T cells in the gut lymphoid tissue to produce immunosuppressive cytokines. These cells then migrate from the gut to the target organ. In the case of T cells specific for type II collagen this would be the joint. There they would encounter their cognate antigen, again leading to the local release of immunosuppressive cytokines, which would suppress any ongoing immune process in the target tissue whether triggered by the original cognate antigen or any other antigen present in the diseased tissue, hence the induction of bystander tolerance. In contrast, higher doses of oral antigen, perhaps because they are partially absorbed systemically, directly induce unresponsiveness (anergy) of pathogenic T cells. Such clonal anergy is antigen specific and thus of less use in treating human disease due to ignorance of all the relevant pathogenic antigens.

In animal models of arthritis, oral administration of type II collagen before or after disease onset has been shown to be effective at preventing or ameliorating collagen-induced arthritis. Bystander suppression has also been demonstrated because adjuvant arthritis, induced by mycobacterial proteins, can be suppressed by feeding with type II collagen.

Native type II collagen has been used to induce mucosal tolerance in RA. The initial study[31] showed a clinical improvement in patients treated with chicken-derived type II collagen compared with placebo. Disappointingly, a study from a different group, using bovine type II collagen,[32] failed to demonstrate any significant effect. Both studies were underpowered and the former had serious trial design faults. The results of a large placebo-controlled trial of 274 RA patients treated with oral chicken type II collagen have been published recently.[33] In this study, patients were treated with placebo or 20, 100, 500, or 2500 μg/day of chicken type II collagen for 24 weeks. Three response criteria were used: Paulus, ACR, and greater than or equal to 30% reduction in both tender and swollen joint counts. Statistically significant improvement was detected only in the 20-μg/day group when compared with placebo (39% vs. 19%) using Paulus criteria.

Hitherto, the collagen in these studies has been administered in orange juice. However, this liquid formulation is unlikely to deliver a precise dose. A recent double-blind, randomized, placebo-controlled trial in RA examined the therapeutic effect of bovine type II collagen tablets with a lactose base that may deliver a more consistent dose of collagen.[34] Fifty-five patients with established disease for more than 2 years who had failed at least one disease-modifying antirheumatic drug were studied. They were randomly assigned to receive placebo, 0.05 mg, 0.5 mg, or 5.0 mg daily of bovine type II collagen for 3 months. There was no significant difference in disease activity score between the placebo, 0.05-mg, and 5.0-mg groups. However, in the 0.5-mg group, disease activity scores were reduced by approximately 15% from week 8 to 24, which was statistically significant when compared with the placebo-treated group.

Current evidence suggests that oral tolerance may be efficacious, although the clinical effect is small and the therapeutic window is narrow. New strategies to enhance the immunomodulatory effect of mucosal tolerance, such as nasal tolerance or conjugation with cholera toxin,[35] may lead to more effective treatment.

CD28 superagonists

Enhancing CD4+ Treg cell number or function has been suggested as a therapeutic strategy to develop treatments with sustained efficacy in many autoimmune diseases.

One strategy based on research conducted in animal models is to target a special region of the co-stimulatory molecule CD28. CD28 "superagonists" target a specific epitope on the CD28 molecule that can activate T cells without a requirement for signal 1. In animal models, CD28 superagonists expand Treg cells with beneficial results.[36] Unfortunately, when the CD28 superagonist TGN1412 was administered to normal healthy individuals it caused multiple-organ failure due to a cytokine storm.[37]

As a result of this catastrophic episode, this strategy of using CD28 superantigen to induce tolerance has been abandoned.

Summary of anti-T cell therapy in RA

Current evidence suggests that T cells are pathogenic in RA and have an important role in sustaining synovitis even in established disease. Inhibiting T-cell activity may suppress inflammation and improve disease. In animal models of RA, immunomodulation of T cells can indeed produce prolonged disease remission. This has yet to be demonstrated in human disease. Most of our current attempts are relatively non-specific. Increased understanding of T-cell activation in RA may lead to more specific therapy in the future.

THERAPIES AGAINST COMPLEMENT

Complement in RA

Complement activation has been implicated in the pathogenesis of many chronic inflammatory and autoimmune diseases. Immune complexes are thought to be responsible for complement activation in RA. There are large amounts of immunoglobulin aggregates in the rheumatoid joints; consequently, activation of complement could be demonstrated in the rheumatoid synovium and articular cartilage, especially those with vasculitis.[38,39] In support of these possibilities, studies have shown the entire complement cascade is activated in the rheumatoid synovial joint[40]; levels of C4 and C2 are reduced in the joints of patients with active RA[40]; early components of the complement system are made by rheumatoid lining cells[41]; C3 and C2 are present throughout the synovial vessels, interstitium, and lining layers[41]; and the level of C3a in the synovial fluid correlates with disease activity.[42] Terminal complement activation is known to lead to leukocyte activation, cytokine release, protease production, and adhesion molecule upregulation,[43] all of which occur in RA synovitis.

Anti-complement therapy in animal models of RA

In antigen-induced arthritis, intra-articular injection of membrane-targeting complement regulatory protein, derived from human complement receptor 1 (CR-1), APT070, led to a dose-dependent reduction in the severity of arthritis with minimal evidence of erosive disease in the active treatment group.[44] In collagen-induced arthritis, injection of fibroblasts engineered to express CR1 using retrovirus-mediated gene transfer inhibited arthritis development, reduced anti–type II collagen antibody levels, and inhibited T-cell response to type II collagen.[45] Similar results were obtained when naked DNA containing tsCR1 and tsCR1-Ig genes was injected intramuscularly into the immunized animals.[45]

The effect of two different variable fragments, anti-C5 single-chain Fv (scFv) was evaluated in antigen-induced arthritis.[46] One anti-C5 scFv (TS-A 12/22) inhibits both release of C5a and assembly of the terminal complement complex. The other, TS-A 8, is a selective blocker of the terminal complement complex. Both were equally effective in reducing disease severity, suggesting that this complex is mainly responsible for disease.

Orally active C5a receptor antagonist, the cyclic peptide PMX53, reduces the severity of pathology in methylated bovine serum albumin–induced arthritis.[47] Animals treated with PMX53 had significantly greater reductions in knee swelling with reduced synovitis as assessed by immunohistology.

The success of complement inhibition in the experimental models of RA suggests a novel therapeutic approach to the treatment of human inflammatory arthritis.

Anti-complement therapy in RA

Jain and colleagues examined the effect of eculizumab, a humanized anti-C5 antibody (h5G1.1, Alexion Pharmaceuticals) in RA.[48] h5G1.1 is a high-affinity humanized monoclonal antibody to C5 that inhibits the cleavage of C5 to the proinflammatory products C5a and C5b-9. Forty RA patients with active disease were given a single intravenous injection of 0.1, 0.3, 0.75, 2.0, 4.0, and 8.0 mg/kg of h5G1.1 or placebo.[48] In the 8.0-mg/kg group, inhibition of C5 lasted 10 days. Mean C-reactive protein was significantly reduced at day 7 compared with baseline and returned to baseline by day 14. Tender and swollen joint counts and patient disease assessment and pain scores also improved on day 7, but the differences were not statistically significant. Subsequently, a large 6-month double-blind, randomized, placebo-controlled trial recruited 368 RA patients treated with methotrexate or leflunomide. Monthly administration of eculizumab after an induction period was associated with a modest ACR20 score of 34% versus placebo (22%) at 6 months that was statistically significant ($P = .04$).[49]

A double-blind, placebo-controlled trial of PMX53 was conducted in RA.[50] Twenty-one patients were randomized 2 : 1 to treatment with PMX53 or placebo for 28 days. However, PMX53 did not improve disease or reduce synovial inflammation despite the serum levels of PMX53 that were adequate to block C5aR-mediated cell activation *in vitro*, suggesting that C5aR blockade does not result in reduced synovial inflammation in RA patients.

Summary of anti-complement therapy in RA

Although animal studies suggest complement inhibition may have efficacy, clinical trials in RA have not produced convincing results. Further studies are needed to determine the ideal complement targets and the best tools to inhibit them.

CONCLUSION

Immunotherapies against T cells undoubtedly improve symptoms and signs in RA, but current treatments have limited efficacy especially in the medium and long term. Better understanding of T-cell immunology and immunomodulation in RA could lead to more effective treatment in the future. Preliminary scientific evidence suggests that treatments with complement may be efficacious in RA but so far the results of early clinical trials have been negative. Further research is needed to identify the optimum complement targets in RA.

REFERENCES

1. Yocum DE, Furst DE, Kaine JL, et al. Efficacy and safety of tacrolimus in patients with rheumatoid arthritis—a double-blind trial. Arthritis Rheum 2003;48:3328-3337.
2. Kirkham BW, Pitzalis C, Kingsley GH, et al. Monoclonal antibody treatment in rheumatoid arthritis: clinical and immunological effects of a CD7 monoclonal antibody. Br J Rheumatol 1991;30:459-463.
3. Lazarovits AI, White MJ, Karsh J. CD7– T cells in rheumatoid arthritis. Arthritis Rheum 1992;35:615-624.
4. Olsen NJ, Brooks RH, Cush JJ, et al. A double-blind, placebo-controlled study of anti-CD5 immunoconjugate in patients with rheumatoid arthritis. Arthritis Rheum 1996;39:1102-1108.
5. Moreland LW, Sewell KL, Trentham DE, et al. Interleukin-2 diphtheria fusion protein (DAB486IL-2) in refractory rheumatoid arthritis: a double-blind, placebo-controlled trial with open-label extension. Arthritis Rheum 1995;38:1177-1186.
6. Isaacs JD, Watts RA, Hazelman BL, et al. Humanised monoclonal antibody therapy for rheumatoid arthritis. Lancet 1992;340:748-752.
7. Isaacs JD, Manna VK, Rapson N, et al. Campath-1H in rheumatoid arthritis—an intravenous dose-ranging study. Br J Rheumatol 1996;35:231-240.
8. Ruderman EM, Weinblatt ME, Thurmond LM, et al. Synovial tissue response to treatment with Campath-1H. Arthritis Rheum 1995;38:254-258.

9. Choy EH, Pitzalis C, Cauli A, et al. Percentage of anti-CD4 monoclonal antibody-coated lymphocytes in the rheumatoid joint is associated with clinical improvement: implications for the development of immunotherapeutic dosing regimens. Arthritis Rheum 1996;39:52-56.
10. van der Lubbe PA, Dijkmans BA, Markusse HM, et al. A randomized, double-blind, placebo-controlled study of CD4 monoclonal antibody therapy in early rheumatoid arthritis. Arthritis Rheum 1995;38:1097-1106.
11. Sakaguchi S, Sakaguchi N, Asano M, et al. Immunological self-tolerance maintained by activated T-cells expressing IL-2 receptor alpha-chains (Cd25)—breakdown of a single mechanism of self-tolerance causes various autoimmune diseases. J Immunol 1995;155:1151-1164.
12. Hori S, Nomura T, Sakaguchi S. Control of regulatory T cell development by the transcription factor Foxp3. Science 2003;299:1057-1061.
13. Van den Broek MF, Van de Langerijt LG, Van Bruggen MC, et al. Treatment of rats with monoclonal anti-CD4 induces long-term resistance to streptococcal cell wall-induced arthritis. Eur J Immunol 1992;22:57-61.
14. Hutchings P, O'Reilly L, Parish NM, et al. The use of a non-depleting anti-CD4 monoclonal antibody to re-establish tolerance to beta cells in NOD mice. Eur J Immunol 1992;22:1913-1918.

15. Carteron NL, Wofsy D, Seaman WE. Induction of immune tolerance during administration of monoclonal antibody to L3T4 does not depend on depletion of L3T4+ cells. J Immunol 1988;140:713-716.
16. Parish NM, Hutchings PR, Waldmann H, Cooke A. Tolerance to IDDM induced by CD4 antibodies in nonobese diabetic mice is reversed by cyclophosphamide. Diabetes 1993;42:1601-1605.
17. Cobbold SP, Qin SX, Waldmann H. Reprogramming the immune system for tolerance with monoclonal antibodies. Semin Immunol 1990;2:377-387.
18. Levy R, Weisman M, Wiesenhutter C, et al. Results of a placebo-controlled, multicenter trial using a primatized, non-depleting, anti-CD4 monoclonal antibody in the treatment of rheumatoid arthritis. Arthritis Rheum 1996;39(Suppl):S122.
19. Choy EH, Connolly DJA, Rapson N, et al. Pharmacokinetic, pharmacodynamic and clinical effects of a humanised IgG1 anti-CD4 monoclonal antibody in the peripheral blood and synovial fluid of rheumatoid arthritis patients. Rheumatology 2000;39:1139-1146.
20. Choy EHS, Panayi GS, Emery P, et al. Repeat-cycle study of high-dose intravenous (iv) 4162w94 anti-CD4 monoclonal antibody (mAb) in rheumatoid arthritis (RA). Rheumatology 2002;41:1142-1148.
21. Choy EH. Oral tolerogens in rheumatoid arthritis. Curr Opin Invest Drugs 2000;1:58-62.

22. Schulze-Koops H, Davis LS, Haverty P, et al. Reduction of Th1 cell activity in patients with rheumatoid arthritis after treatment with a non-depleting monoclonal antibody to CD4. Arthritis Rheum 1997;40(Suppl):S191.

23. Choy EHS, Kingsley GH, Panayi GS. T-cell regulation. In: Brooks PM, Furst DE, eds. Innovative treatment approaches for rheumatoid arthritis. London: Bailliere Tindall, 1995:653-671.

24. Chen GJ, Li NL, Zang YCQ, et al. Vaccination with selected synovial T cells in rheumatoid arthritis. Arthritis Rheum 2007;56:453-463.

25. Moreland LW, Heck LW Jr, Koopman WJ, et al. Vb17 T cell receptor peptide vaccination in rheumatoid arthritis: results of phase I dose escalation study. J Rheumatol 1996;23:1353-1362.

26. Moreland L, Koopman WJ, Adamson T, et al. Results of phase II rheumatoid arthritis clinical trial using T cell receptor peptides. Arthritis Rheum 1997;40:S223.

27. Matsumoto AK, Moreland LW, Strand V, et al. Results of phase IIb rheumatoid arthritis clinical trial using T-cell receptor peptides. Arthritis Rheum 1999;42:281.

28. St. Clair EW, Cohen SB, Fleischmann RM, et al. Vaccination of rheumatoid arthritis patients with DR4/1-peptide. Arthritis Rheum 1997;40:S96.

29. From the NCHTC: Evaluation of therapeutic apheresis for rheumatoid arthritis. JAMA 1981;246:1053.

30. Weiner HL, Friedman A, Miller A, et al. Oral tolerance: immunologic mechanisms and treatment of animal and human organ-specific autoimmune disease by oral administration of autoantigens. Annu Rev Immunol 1994;12:809-837.

31. Trentham DE, Dynesius-Trentham RA, Orav EJ, et al. Effects of oral administration of type II collagen on rheumatoid arthritis. Science 1993;261:1727-1730.

32. Sieper J, Kary S, Sorensen H, et al. Oral type II collagen treatment in early rheumatoid arthritis: a double-blind, placebo-controlled, randomized trial. Arthritis Rheum 1996;39:41-51.

33. Barnett ML, Kremer JM, St. Clair EW, et al. Treatment of rheumatoid arthritis with oral type II collagen: results of a multicenter, double-blind, placebo-controlled trial. Arthritis Rheum 1998;41:290-297.

34. Choy EHS, Scott DL, Kingsley GH, et al. Control of rheumatoid arthritis (RA) by oral tolerance with bovine type II collagen (CII). Ann Rheum Dis 1999;58(Suppl):5.

35. Sun JB, Rask C, Olsson T, et al. Treatment of experimental autoimmune encephalomyelitis by feeding myelin basic protein conjugated to cholera toxin B subunit. Proc Natl Acad Sci U S A 1996;93:7196-7201.

36. Beyersdorf N, Gaupp S, Balbach K, et al. Selective targeting of regulatory T cells with CD28 superagonists allows effective therapy of experimental autoimmune encephalomyelitis. J Exp Med 2005;202:445-455.

37. Suntharalingam G, Perry MR, Ward S, et al. Cytokine storm in a phase 1 trial of the anti-CD28 monoclonal antibody TGN1412. N Engl J Med 2006;355:1018-1028.

38. Elson CJ, Carter SD, Cottrell BJ, et al. Complement activating properties of complexes containing rheumatoid factor in synovial fluids and sera from patients with rheumatoid arthritis. Clin Exp Immunol 1985;59:285-292.

39. Scott DGI, Bacon PA, Allen C, et al. IgG rheumatoid-factor, complement and immune-complexes in rheumatoid synovitis and vasculitis—comparative and serial studies during cytotoxic therapy. Clin Exp Immunol 1981;43:54-63.

40. Ruddy S, Austen KF. Activation of complement and properdin systems in rheumatoid-arthritis. Ann N Y Acad Sci 1975;256:96-104.

41. Firestein GS, Paine MM, Littman BH. Gene-expression (collagenase, tissue inhibitor of metalloproteinases, complement, and HLA Dr) in rheumatoid-arthritis and osteoarthritis synovium—quantitative analysis and effect of intraarticular corticosteroids. Arthritis Rheum 1991;34:1094-1105.

42. Moxley G, Ruddy S. Elevated Plasma C-3 anaphylatoxin levels in rheumatoid-arthritis patients. Arthritis Rheum 1987;30:1097-1104.

43. Elson CJ, Thompson SJ, Westacott CI, Bhoola KD. Mediators of joint swelling and damage in rheumatoid arthritis and pristane-induced arthritis. Autoimmunity 1992;13:327-331.

44. Linton SM, Williams AS, Dodd I, et al. Therapeutic efficacy of a novel membrane-targeted complement regulator in antigen-induced arthritis in the rat. Arthritis Rheum 2000;43:2590-2597.

45. Dreja H, Annenkov A, Chernajovsky Y. Soluble complement receptor 1 (CD35) delivered by retrovirally infected syngeneic cells or by naked DNA injection prevents the progression of collagen-induced arthritis. Arthritis Rheum 2000;43:1698-1709.

46. Fischetti F, Durigutto P, Macor P, et al. Selective therapeutic control of C5a and the terminal complement complex by anti-C5 single-chain Fv in an experimental model of antigen-induced arthritis in rats. Arthritis Rheum 2007;56:1187-1197.

47. Woodruff TM, Strachan AJ, Dryburgh N, et al. Antiarthritic activity of an orally active C5a receptor antagonist against antigen-induced monarticular arthritis in the rat. Arthritis Rheum 2002;46:2476-2485.

48. Jain RI, Moreland LW, Caldwell JR, et al. A single dose, placebo controlled, double blind, phase I study of the humanized anti-C5 antibody h5G1.1 in patients with rheumatoid arthritis. Arthritis Rheum 1999;42:42.

49. Mojcik CF, Kremer J, Bingham C, et al. Results of a phase 2B study of the humanized anti-C5 antibody eculizumab in patients with rheumatoid arthritis. Ann Rheum Dis 2004;63:301.

50. Vergunst CE, Gerlag DM, Dinant H, et al. Blocking the receptor for C5a in patients with rheumatoid arthritis does not reduce synovial inflammation. Rheumatology 2007;46:1773-1778.

T-cell co-stimulation

Roshan Dhawale and Larry W. Moreland

58

INTRODUCTION

Rheumatoid arthritis (RA) is the most common inflammatory arthritis, affecting 0.5% to 1% of the general population worldwide.[1] The management of patients with RA is based on an emerging understanding of the biology and natural history of the disease.[2] Abatacept is the first in a new class of biologic agents in development called co-stimulation modulators. It is a recombinant receptor-IgG Fc fusion protein consisting of the extracellular domain of human cytotoxic T-cell–associated antigen-4 (CTLA4 fusion protein) linked to the hinge, CH2, and CH3 domains of human IgG1. Abatacept (CTLA4-Ig) became the first co-stimulatory blocker to be approved by the U.S. Food and Drug Administration (FDA) in December 2005 for the treatment of patients with RA who have had an inadequate response to other drugs. Subsequently, the European Commission licensed it for use in the United Kingdom in May 2007. At this time, abatacept is positioned in our armamentarium as a useful alternative for individuals with RA who have failed to respond to methotrexate and/or the tumor necrosis factor (TNF)-blocking biologic agents. A discussion is provided here of its role in the immunologic interaction between T cells and antigen-presenting cells (APCs) and of clinical trials looking at effectiveness and safety of abatacept in the treatment of RA.

T-CELL CO-STIMULATION

Activated T cells have a central role in the orchestration of the immune pathways that contribute to the inflammation and joint destruction characteristic of RA.[3,4] Differentiation of naïve CD4+ T lymphocytes into effector cells for cell-mediated immunity (CMI) requires antigen recognition and co-stimulation. When T cells become activated, they differentiate, migrate, and penetrate into inflamed tissues, proliferate, produce cytokines, initiate T-cell effector functions, and regulate downstream immune responses. In patients with RA, the activated T cells subsequently stimulate a variety of other cell types and induce cellular activities that propagate immunopathogenic disease mechanisms, including the release of proinflammatory cytokines, activation of the autoantibody-producing B cells, macrophage activation, release of the matrix metalloproteinases, and activation of osteoclasts that facilitate bone loss.[5-8]

Like the induction and propagation of other cellular pathways, specific signaling mechanisms are required for activation of T cells.[3] However, in contrast to many of these pathways that require a single ligand receptor-mediated signal, T-cell activation has been found to require multiple signaling mechanisms (Figs. 58.1 and 58.2). The first of these signals is presentation of a major histocompatibility peptide-antigen complex by an APC to an antigen-specific receptor on the T cells. So-called co-stimulatory signals, of which there are several, consist of an interaction between a cell-surface ligand on the APC and a cognate cell-surface receptor molecule on the T cell.[8,9] The absence of co-stimulatory signaling in the presence of the major histocompatibility complex (MHC)-antigen presentation induces a state of T-cell anergy, in which the T cells remain in a functionally inactivated or hyporesponsive state.[10]

Best known of these co-stimulation pathways is an interaction between CD28 on T cells and CD80 and CD86, also known as B7-1 and B7-2, which are expressed only on professional APCs. CD28 is constitutively expressed on the naive T-cell surface. CD80/86 binds with CD28, providing a second signal for induction of endogenous interleukin (IL)-2 mRNA accumulation and IL-2 production, resulting in T-cell activation and proliferation (see Figs. 58-1 and 58-2).[11,12] Cytotoxic T-lymphocyte–associated antigen (CTLA4), an important endogenous downregulator of T-cell activation, is expressed on Th2

cells 48 to 72 hours after onset of stimulation, based on *in-vitro* data.[13] Activated T cells upregulate the cell surface expression of CTLA4. This ligates CD80 or CD86 with greater avidity than CD28 and exerts its inhibitory effects at two stages.[14] First, CTLA4 interrupts CD28-mediated co-stimulation, thereby attenuating CD28-induced IL-2 gene transcription and production, which is essential for T-cell proliferation and clonal expansion.[14,15] Second, CTLA4 directly inhibits the expression of key components of cell cycle machinery, such as cyclin D3 and cyclin-dependent kinases cdk4 and cdk6.[15] These antigen-specific effector T cells, in turn, generate proinflammatory cytokines, including TNF-α and interferon-γ (IFN-γ).[16] CTLA4 binds to CD80 and CD86 with 2500-fold and 570-fold greater affinity, respectively, than does CD28 (Fig. 58.3).[14] The greater affinity of CTLA4 for the ligand results in competition with CD28 for binding sites and may, in part, regulate the magnitude of the immune response. Engagement of CTLA4 results in downmodulation of the immune response and can prevent CD28-dependent T-cell activation.[17,18]

Abatacept was designed as a therapeutic molecule developed to modulate the T-cell co-stimulatory signal that is mediated by the CD28-CD80/86 pathway. It consists of the extracellular binding domain of CTLA4 fused to the heavy chain constant region of human Ig1 (Fig. 58.4). As well as preventing this positive co-stimulation, the intracellular domain of endogenous CTLA4 provides a negative co-stimulatory signal, suppressing further T-cell activation, thus preventing the formation of subsequent components of the inflammatory cascade (Fig. 58.5).[17] The binding of abatacept to CD80/86 may provide an inhibitory signal to the APC itself, further dampening the immune response.[19] A second-generation CTLA4Ig, belatacept, also known as LEA29Y, is a modified version of abatacept that carries two amino acid mutations, which increases its avidity for CD86, thereby resulting in a 10-fold increase in potency.[20] Belatacept is being evaluated as an alternative immunosuppressant in patients with renal transplantation. Selective inhibition of T-cell co-stimulation by CTLA4-Ig early in the immune cascade could downmodulate T-cell effector functions and inflammatory cytokine production and impact a variety of downstream cell types, including autoantibodies producing B cells, APCs, macrophages, and osteoclasts. The specificity of this mechanism of action allows other immune pathways to remain largely intact. Therefore, utilizing such intrinsic properties of our immune system to curtail and perhaps reverse the pathogenic derangement is a rational strategy for RA.[21]

Molecules other than CD28 that can deliver activating or co-activating signals to T cells include CD2, CD11a/ CD18, lymphocyte function-associated antigen-1 (LFA-1), CD6, and CD60.[22] These molecules are expressed on the great majority of T cells found in RA synovial fluid and tissue. With the exception of CD60, which is present on a minority of peripheral blood T cells in both normal individuals and patients with RA,[23,24] all of these structures are also expressed on most circulating T cells. A role for these structures (and other structures) in T-cell activation is suggested by mitogenic effects of monoclonal antibodies against such molecules.[23-26] Except for CD60, whose ligand is unknown, each of these molecules has well-characterized ligands that are expressed by various APCs, including cells in RA synovial tissue.[27] Another molecule of significant importance in the interaction of T cells with APCs is the CD40 ligand (CD154), which appears on the cell surface early in the course of T-cell activation. This molecule binds to CD40, a cell membrane protein expressed by virtually all APCs, and activates a variety of functional programs in such cells, including expression of ligands for CD28. Both CD40 and its ligands are expressed by cells within RA synovium, and this molecular interaction may have an important role in the formation of germinal center–like structures in synovial tissue.[28] Certain co-stimulatory

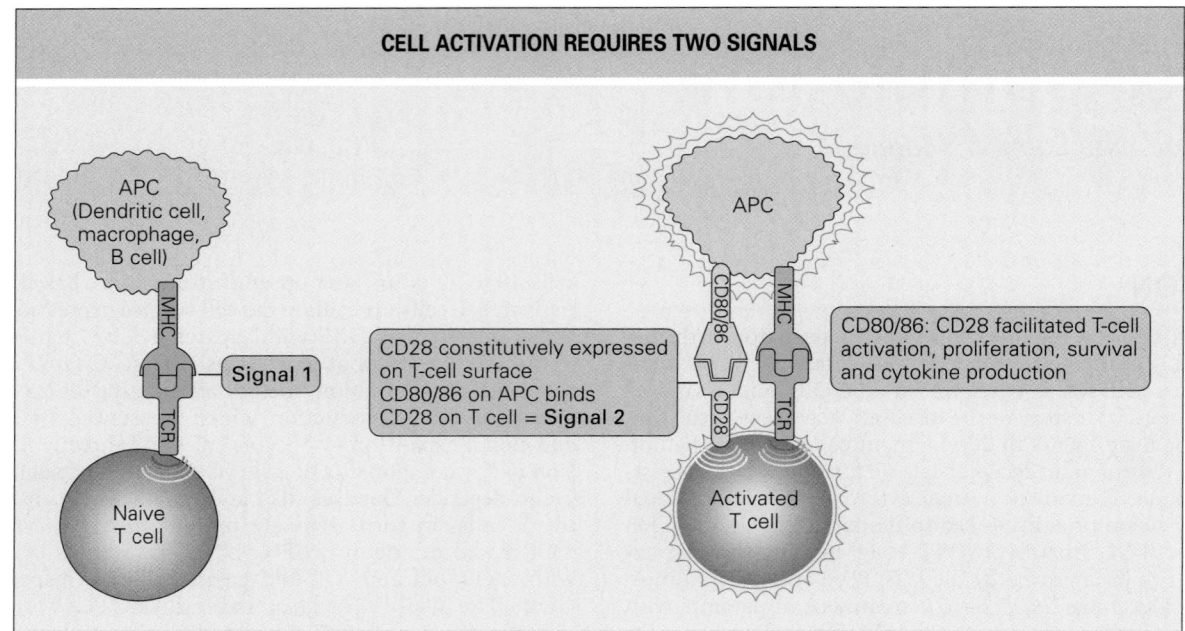

CELL ACTIVATION REQUIRES TWO SIGNALS

Fig. 58.1 T-cell activation requires two signals. After engagement of the T-cell receptor with the MHC antigen complex processes by antigen-presenting cells (APCs) (first signal), a second signal is transmitted by CD28 that interacts with either CD80 and CD86 ligands on APCs, leading to T-cell activation and proliferation. *(Reproduced with permission from Teng GG, Turkiewicz AM, Moreland LW. Abatacept: a co-stimulatory inhibitor for treatment of rheumatoid arthritis. Expert Opin Biol Ther 2005;5:1245-1254.)*

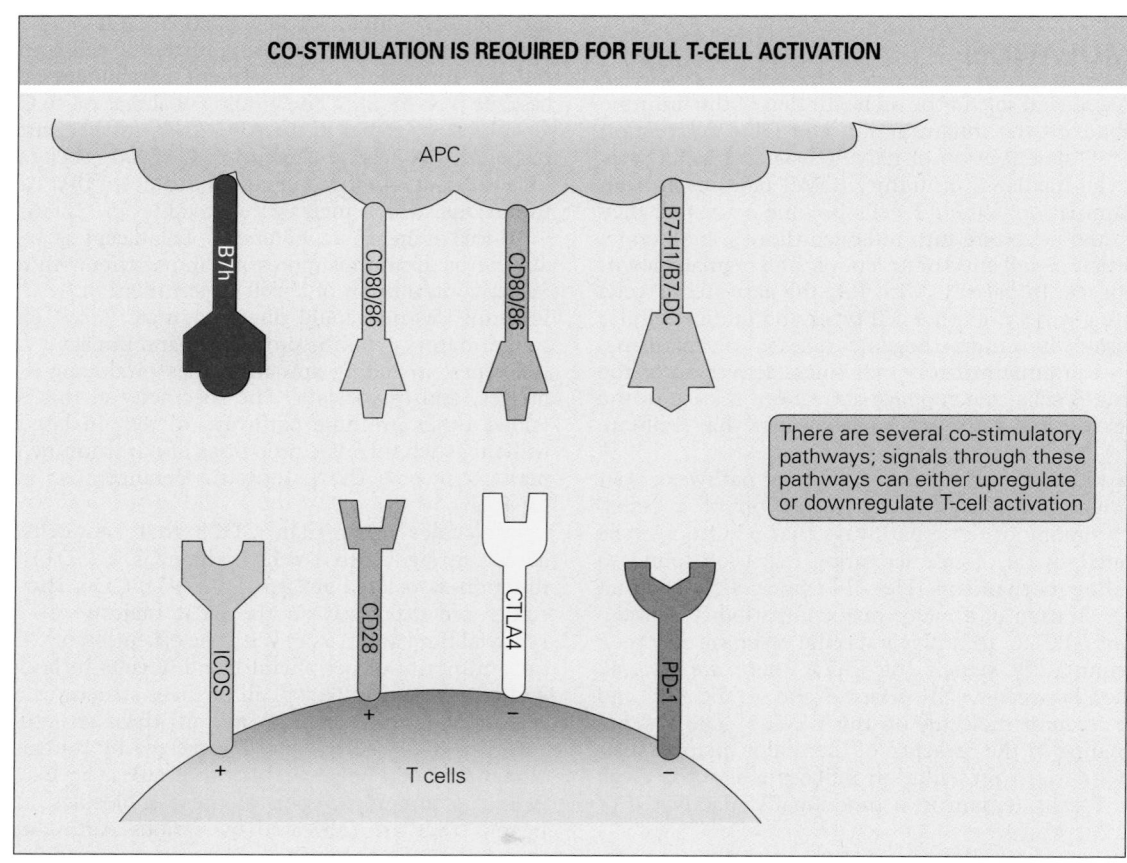

CO-STIMULATION IS REQUIRED FOR FULL T-CELL ACTIVATION

Fig. 58.2 Co-stimulation is required for full T-cell activation. There are several co-stimulatory pathways; signals through these pathways can either upregulate or downregulate T-cell activation. APC, antigen-presenting cell; CTLA, cytotoxic T-lymphocyte antigen; DC, dendritic cell; ICOS, inducible co-stimulator. *(Reproduced with permission from Teng GG, Turkiewicz AM, Moreland LW. Abatacept: a co-stimulatory inhibitor for treatment of rheumatoid arthritis. Expert Opin Biol Ther 2005;5:1245-1254.)*

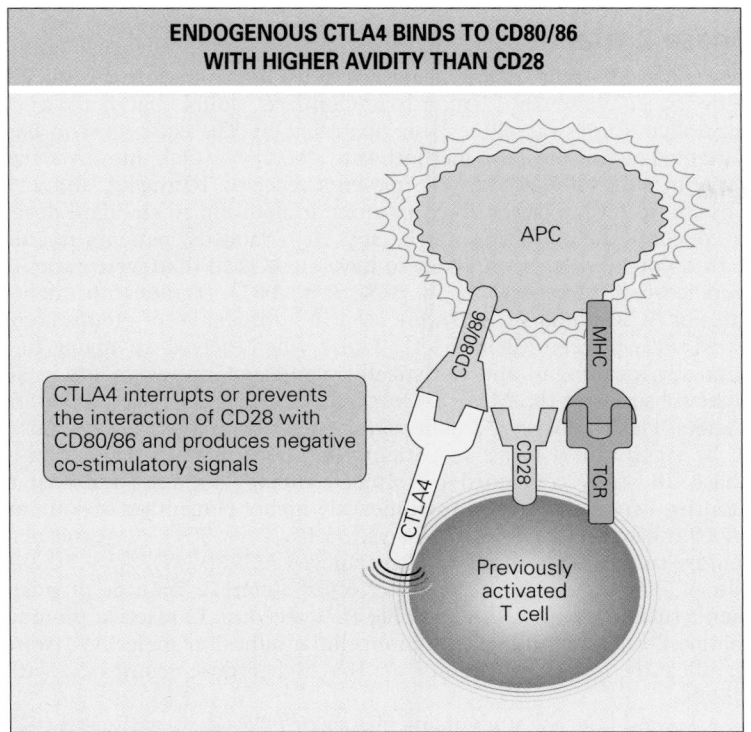

ENDOGENOUS CTLA4 BINDS TO CD80/86 WITH HIGHER AVIDITY THAN CD28

CTLA4 interrupts or prevents the interaction of CD28 with CD80/86 and produces negative co-stimulatory signals

Fig. 58.3 Endogenous CTLA4 binds to CD80/86 with higher avidity than CD28 and downregulates CD28-mediated T-cell activation. APC, antigen-presenting cell; CTLA, cytotoxic T-lymphocyte antigen; TCR, T-cell receptor. *(Reproduced with permission from Teng GG, Turkiewicz AM, Moreland LW. Abatacept: a co-stimulatory inhibitor for treatment of rheumatoid arthritis. Expert Opin Biol Ther 2005;5:1245-1254.)*

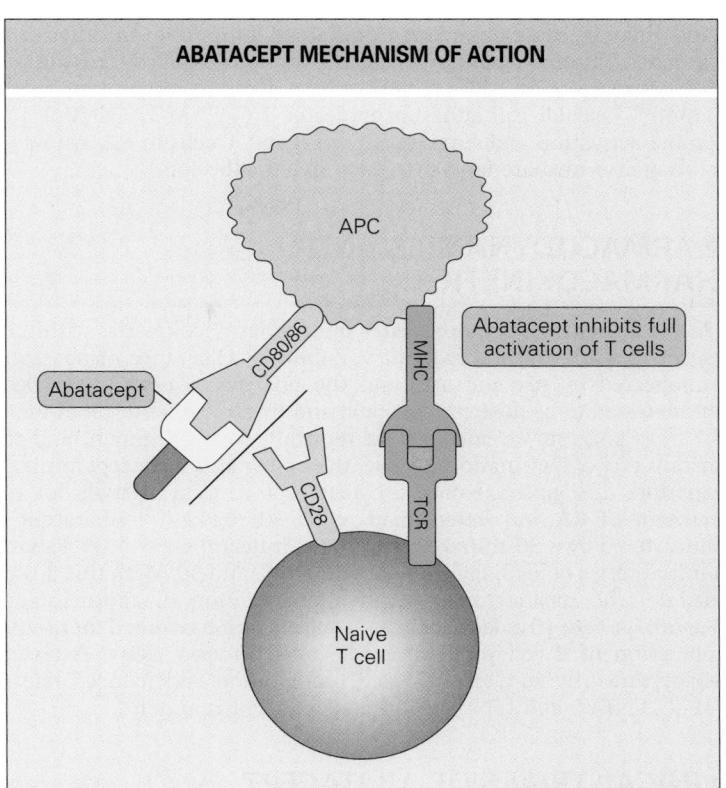

ABATACEPT MECHANISM OF ACTION

Abatacept inhibits full activation of T cells

Fig. 58.5 Abatacept: mechanism of action. Abatacept binds to CD80/86 and inhibits T-cell co-stimulation. APC, antigen-presenting cell; MHC, major histocompatibility complex; TCR, T-cell receptor. *(Reproduced with permission from Teng GG, Turkiewicz AM, Moreland LW. Abatacept: a co-stimulatory inhibitor for treatment of rheumatoid arthritis. Expert Opin Biol Ther 2005;5:1245-1254.)*

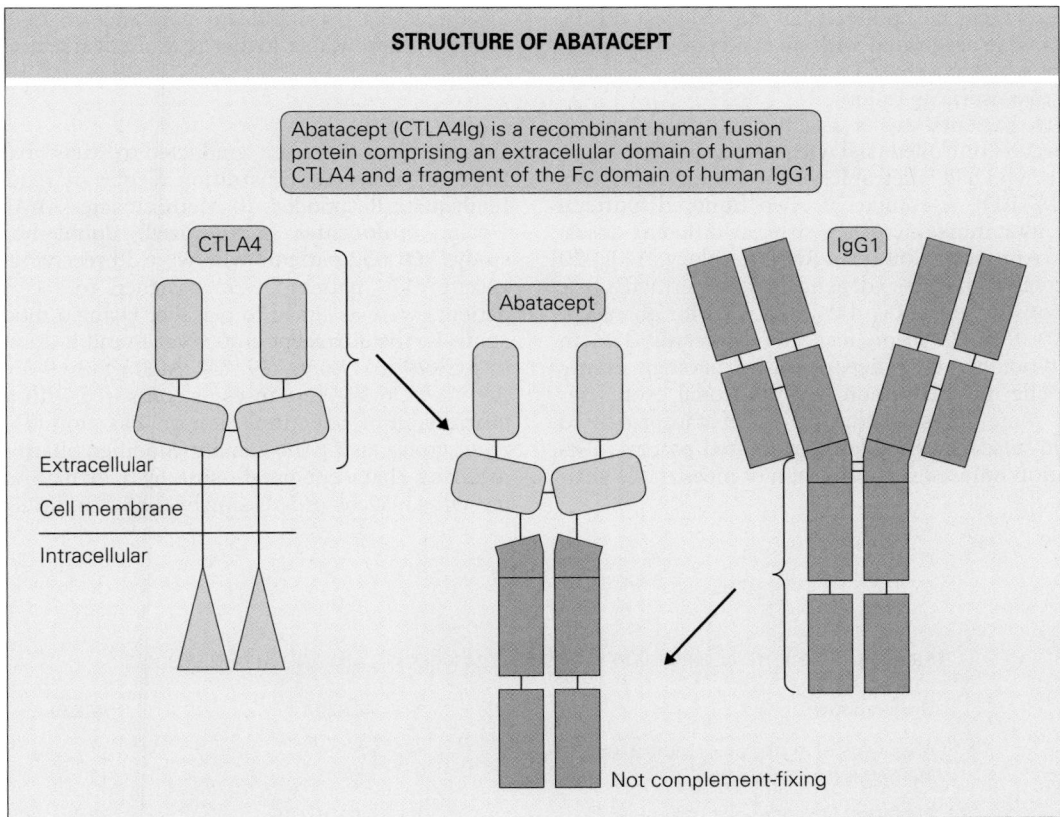

STRUCTURE OF ABATACEPT

Abatacept (CTLA4Ig) is a recombinant human fusion protein comprising an extracellular domain of human CTLA4 and a fragment of the Fc domain of human IgG1

Fig. 58.4 Structure of abatacept. Abatacept consists of an extracellular domain of human CTLA4 fused to the heavy-chain constant region of human IgG1. CTLA, cytotoxic T-lymphocyte antigen. *(Reproduced with permission from Teng GG, Turkiewicz AM, Moreland LW. Abatacept: a co-stimulatory inhibitor for treatment of rheumatoid arthritis. Expert Opin Biol Ther 2005;5:1245-1254.)*

ligands may be more abundant in inflamed joints than in other compartments. Thrombospondin-1 can co-stimulate T cells by crosslinking a distinct receptor on APCs (CD47) with a different receptor on T cells (CD36).[29] Vascular cell adhesion molecule-1 (VCAM-1, CD106) may promote activation and survival of both B and T cells in RA synovium and may also mediate leukocyte-endothelial adhesion.[30]

PHARMACODYNAMICS AND PHARMACOKINETICS

In humans, abatacept demonstrates linear pharmacokinetics within its dose range with low interpatient variability.[31] Clearance of abatacept is unaffected by sex and age, and the pharmacokinetics have been demonstrated to be dose proportional and linear.[31] A serum half-life of 14.7 days suggests an adequacy of monthly dosing regimen, and the constant rate of elimination is indicative of low anti-abatacept antibody formation. The optimal dose for abatacept in clinical trials for the treatment of RA was determined to be 10 mg/kg.[32,33] Abatacept is administered by a 30-minute intravenous infusion every 4 weeks after an initial series of loading doses on days 1, 15, and 30. With this dosing schedule, the mean trough serum concentration of approximately 30 µg/mL is 7- to 10-fold higher than concentration required for *in-vitro* suppression of T-cell proliferation.[34] In an *in-vitro* assay, abatacept dose-dependently suppressed T-cell proliferation and reduced release of IL-2, TNF-α, and IFN-γ in a time-dependent manner.[34]

CLINICAL TRIALS OF ABATACEPT

Phase 1 trials

Abatacept was first studied in human subjects with psoriasis.[31] In a 26-week open-label dose escalation study involving 43 patients who received four infusions of abatacept at doses ranging from 0.5 mg/kg to 50 mg/kg, 46% of patients achieved a 50% or greater sustained improvement (physician global assessment) in clinical disease activity, with progressively greater effects observed at the highest-dosing cohorts.[31] Improvements were associated with quantitative reductions in epidermal hyperplasia, which correlated with quantitative reduction in T cells infiltrating active psoriasis lesions.[31]

The first study in RA patients was a small, double-blind, dose-finding, multicenter, placebo-controlled trial with abatacept and belatacept (LEA29Y) in patients who had failed at least one disease-modifying antirheumatic drug (DMARD) or etanercept. Two hundred fourteen RA patients were given four infusions of the drug at different doses: 0.5, 2.0, and 10 mg/kg.[32] American College of Rheumatology (ACR)-20 responses at day 85 increased in a dose-dependent manner; with 0.5, 2.0, and 10 mg/kg, responses were 23%, 44%, and 53% for abatacept and 34%, 45%, and 61% for belatacept, respectively, versus 31% in placebo.[32] There were no notable renal, hepatic, or hematologic events noted during the trial. The most common peri-infusional events for the drug (vs. placebo) were nausea/vomiting in abatacept-treated patients (7% vs. 3%) and headache in belatacept-treated patients (8% vs. 3%). Neither medication induced the formation of measurable anti-drug antibodies.[32]

Phase 2 trials

Two phase-2 trials using abatacept have been performed in RA patients. A phase 2b 12-month randomized, double-blind, placebo-controlled study was done using abatacept in 339 patients who had remained active despite methotrexate therapy.[33] One hundred five patients received 2 mg/kg, 115 patients received 10 mg/kg, and 119 patients received placebo for 6 months, in addition to standard doses of concomitant methotrexate therapy. At 6 months, patients treated with 10 mg/kg were more likely to have an ACR20 than were patients who received placebo (60% vs. 35%, $P < .001$). Significantly higher rates of ACR50 and ACR70 were seen in both abatacept groups compared with placebo (Table 58.1). Those who received 10 mg/kg had clinically meaningful and statistically significant improvements in all eight subscales of the Medical Outcomes 36-Item Short-Form (SF-36) General Health Survey.[33] Inflammatory markers of disease were found to be significantly lower in patients on the drug.[34] Patients in this phase 2b study continued on blinded therapy for an additional 6 months. After 12 months, a significantly higher percentage of patients on 10 mg/kg met ACR20 (62.6% vs. 36.1%, $P < .001$). A greater percentage treated with 10 mg/kg also achieved ACR50 (41.7% vs. 20.2%) and ACR70 responses (20.9% vs. 7.6%).[35] After 12 months of treatment, serum levels of IL-6, soluble IL-2 receptor, C-reactive protein, soluble E-selectin, and soluble intercellular adhesion molecule-1 were significantly lower in patients on the higher dose, compared with placebo.[34,36]

A second phase 2 study using abatacept in patients with active RA on stable doses of etanercept was performed; 121 patients receiving etanercept were randomized to receive 2 mg/kg abatacept (a low dose that was minimally clinically effective) or placebo.[37,38] At 6 and 12 months, ACR20 response was not significantly different at 48.2% vs. 30.6% ($P = .072$).[23,24] The primary goal of this trial was to explore the potential combination of two biologic agents that had different mechanisms of action. Thus, the low dose was used initially to assess any potential adverse effects of the combination. At 1 year, 80 patients entered an open-label extension and all received abatacept at 10 mg/kg; there was no significant difference in ACR20 after an additional year, but there was a higher risk of adverse events in the combination group.[37,38]

Phase 3 trials

Two phase 3 trials were conducted to study abatacept in order to fulfill Food and Drug Administration regulatory requirements. Abatacept in Inadequate Responders to Methotrexate (AIM) was a phase 3 trial, a 1-year, multicenter, randomized, double-blind, placebo-controlled study.[39] Of 652 patients who were all receiving stable doses of methotrexate, 433 patients were assigned to receive 10 mg/kg and 219 patients were assigned to placebo. Using a modified intention-to-treat analysis, the abatacept group was found to have significant differences in ACR20 (67.9% vs. 39.7%), ACR50 (39.9% vs. 16.8%), and ACR70 (19.8% vs. 6.5%) responses as compared with placebo.[39] At 1 year, the progression of structural damage was around 50% lower in the treatment group, using the Genant-modified Sharp score, with the patients receiving abatacept progressing by a median score of 0.25 and those receiving placebo progressing by 0.53.[39] In findings similar to the phase

TABLE 58.1 PATIENTS ACHIEVING RESPONSES AT 24 WEEKS IN AIM AND ATTAIN STUDIES				
Study	Drug regimen	ACR20	ACR50	ACR70
Phase 2b[33]	Abatacept 10 mg/kg plus methotrexate Methotrexate plus placebo	60 35	37 12	17 2
Phase 3 AIM[39]	Abatacept 10 mg/kg plus methotrexate Methotrexate plus placebo	67.9 39.7	39.9 16.8	19.8 6.5
Phase 3 ATTAIN[41]	Abatacept 10 mg/kg plus methotrexate Methotrexate plus placebo	50.4 19.5	20.3 3.8	10.2 1.5

ACR, American College of Rheumatology; AIM, Abatacept in Inadequate Responders to Methotrexate; ATTAIN, Abatacept Trial in Treatment of Anti-TNF Inadequate Responders.

2b study, abatacept plus methotrexate induced disease activity score (DAS28) remission (<2.6) in 14.8% of patients at 6 months and in 23.8% at 12 months, compared with 2.8% and 1.9% of patients receiving methotrexate plus placebo at the corresponding time points (P < .001). Physical function significantly improved in 63.7% of the abatacept plus methotrexate group, versus 39.3% of the placebo plus methotrexate group (P < .001).[39] Patients completing the double-blind phase of the AIM study over 12 months were eligible to enter a long-term extension phase in which all participants received methotrexate plus abatacept at a fixed dose approximating 10 mg/kg every 4 weeks.[40] Clinically meaningful reductions in disease activity were maintained through 2 years, accompanied by an improved sense of subjective well-being assessed by patient-reported outcomes. Abatacept was considered safe and efficacious in the open-label extension.

The Abatacept Trial in Treatment of Anti-TNF inadequate responders (ATTAIN) compared abatacept with placebo in patients whose disease was refractory to either etanercept or infliximab. All patients at baseline were on at least one DMARD (but no TNF blocker).[41] After 6 months, the proportion of patients with an ACR20, ACR50, or ACR70 response was higher in the abatacept group (see Table 58.1). Patients taking abatacept also had an improvement in physical function on Health Assessment Questionnaire (HAQ) scores.[41] Rates of remission (DAS28 < 2.6) were significantly higher in the abatacept group as compared with the placebo group (10% vs. 0.8%, P < .001).[41] All patients who completed the 6-month double-blind phase of the ATTAIN study were eligible to enter a 1-year, long-term extension phase during which all patients received a once-monthly fixed dose of abatacept in addition to at least one conventional DMARD.[42] Of a total of 258 patients randomized to abatacept, 223 completed 6 months of treatment and 218 entered the extension. Of these, 168 completed 18 months' treatment. The rate of serious adverse effects was similar in the two groups. No unique safety observations were reported during the open-label extension. Improvements in signs and symptoms of RA, physical function, and health-related quality of life observed after 6 months were maintained throughout the 2 years in patients with difficult-to-treat disease.[43]

COMPARISON WITH INFLIXIMAB

A trial comparing abatacept with infliximab was performed in RA patients who had an inadequate response to methotrexate.[44] The patients had a mean baseline DAS28 of 6.8. They were randomized to receive abatacept at a dose of 10 mg/kg every 4 weeks (156 patients), infliximab 3 mg/kg every 8 weeks (165 patients), or placebo every 4 weeks (110 patients).[44] Patients randomized to placebo were switched to abatacept after 6 months but were not included in the 1-year analyses. With respect to efficacy through 6 months, ACR response rates, changes in DAS28, HAQ, and SF-36 were similar after treatment with either abatacept or infliximab.[44] However, as noted in other studies, abatacept was observed to have increasing efficacy beyond 6 months in contrast to the infliximab group; in the latter, measures apparently reached a plateau or diminished over time. The mean change from baseline in DAS28 for abatacept was –2.3 at 6 months and –2.9 at 1 year; for infliximab, it was –2.3 at both 6 and 12 months.[44] A weakness of this study is the fixed dose of infliximab used. In clinical practice, many RA patients require higher doses of infliximab to achieve maximal clinical response.

SAFETY OF ABATACEPT

Overall, abatacept is considered to have an acceptable safety and tolerability profile. It can be safely combined with other DMARDS but not with TNF or IL-1 blockers. The Abatacept Study of Safety in Use with Other RA Therapies (ASSURE) trial was a 1-year, multicenter, randomized, double-blind, placebo-controlled trial designed to assess the safety of abatacept at 10 mg/kg compared with placebo in 1441 patients with active RA concurrently on one or more traditional non-biologic and/or biologic DMARD(s) for a minimum of 3 months before entry, with a stable dose over 28 days.[37] Of the 1441 patients, 1231 completed 1 year. Results were presented according to the DMARD group: biologic versus non-biologic agent. Overall,

the abatacept group was similar to the placebo group in terms of incidence of adverse events (AEs) (90% vs. 87%), serious adverse events (SAEs) (13% vs. 12%), and severe or very severe AEs (16% vs. 15%).[37] Discontinuations of the drug were similar in both groups (5% vs. 4%). Regardless of the treatment arm, patients receiving background non-biologic therapy had similar rates of AEs and SAEs. However, in the biologic group, those who received abatacept had more AEs (95.1% vs. 89.1%) and more SAEs (22.3% vs. 12.5%) as compared with those receiving a placebo.[37] Less than 4% of patients in each group had a severe or very severe infection, but life-threatening infections, those resulting in hospitalization or death, were more likely to be seen in the abatacept group (2.9% vs. 1.9%). Interestingly, the abatacept-treated patients with background biologic therapy had more serious infections than the placebo group (5.8% vs. 1.6%), whereas the abatacept-treated group on non-biologic therapy showed a similar trend (2.6% vs. 1.7%).[37]

The ASSURE trial findings mirrored those of a smaller randomized, placebo-controlled, double-blind pilot study. This phase 2b trial investigated the efficacy and safety of the addition of abatacept infusions at 2 mg/kg over 1 year in patients who had inadequate response on etanercept. The biologic combination had limited clinical benefit over etanercept and placebo infusions but was associated with an increase in the proportion of patients experiencing SAEs (16.5% vs. 2.8%) and serious infections (3.5% vs. 0%).[37,38]

In the pivotal phase 2 and phase 3 clinical trials, the overall safety profile of abatacept was similar to that of placebo. The most commonly reported AEs in 10% or more of patients on abatacept included headaches, upper respiratory tract infections, nasopharyngitis, and nausea.[45] No clinically significant antibody response to abatacept was detected in active treatment groups.[32,37,39] In placebo-controlled trials, infection occurred more often in abatacept-treated patients. Infection was the adverse event frequently requiring clinical intervention. Serious infection occurred in 1.9% of placebo-treated patients and 3% of abatacept-treated patients, with pneumonia being the most serious infection.[45] Notably, the risk of serious infections rose to 4.4% (vs. 1.5% in controls), when combined with TNF-α blockers, and their combined use is not recommended.[46] Abatacept should be used with caution in patients with chronic obstructive airway disease, because adverse respiratory events occurred more frequently in these patients.[37] Patients should not receive a live vaccine during treatment or within 3 months of stopping abatacept.[45] There are no adequate and well-controlled studies in pregnant women, and it should be used in pregnancy only if absolutely indicated.[45]

With respect to tuberculosis risk and activation of latent tuberculosis, it has been shown that abatacept does not exacerbate chronic Mycobacterium tuberculosis infection in mice. Chronic M. tuberculosis infection was established in C57BL/6 mice.[47] Four months after infection, mice were treated for up to 16 weeks with abatacept, antimurine TNF, or vehicle. Abatacept and vehicle both maintained control of M. tuberculosis infection, with 100% survival after 16 weeks of treatment. In contrast, 100% mortality was seen in the anti-TNF antibody-treated group by week 9 along with increased pathology, consistent with exacerbation of M. tuberculosis infection.[47] In clinical practice, patients should be screened for latent tuberculosis with a tuberculin test before initiating abatacept. Patients testing positive should be treated with standard medical practice before initiating abatacept.[45]

In the ATTEST trial, when compared with infliximab, at the end of the first 6 months, the frequency of serious adverse events was 5.1%, 11.5%, and 11.8% for abatacept, infliximab, and placebo, respectively. In the same order, the frequency of acute infusion-related adverse events was 5.1%, 18.2%, and 10%. Over the 1-year period, infections reported as serious adverse events were more frequent with infliximab (8.5%) than with abatacept (1.9%). These included two cases of tuberculosis, both in infliximab-treated patients.[44]

To assess the effects of abatacept on malignancies, an abatacept clinical development program (CDP) was established for comparison with similar RA patients and the general population. Patients identified from five data sources—the population-based British Columbia RA Cohort, the Norfolk Arthritis Register, the National Data Bank for Rheumatic Diseases, the Sweden Early RA Register, and the General Practice Research Database—comprised a total of 4134 RA patients treated with abatacept in 7 trials and 41,529 DMARD-treated RA patients.[48] In the abatacept-treated patients, of the 51 malignancies (excluding non-melanoma skin cancer [NMSC]), the 7 cases of breast cancer, 2 cases of colorectal cancer, 13 cases of lung cancer, and 5 cases of lymphoma observed were not greater than the range of expected cases from the five RA cohorts. The age and sex-adjusted standardized incidence ratios comparing RA patients to the general population were consistent with those reported in the literature. The age and sex-adjusted incidence ratios of total malignancy (excluding NMSC), breast, colorectal, and lung cancers and lymphoma in the abatacept clinical development program were consistent with those in a comparable RA population. These data suggest no new safety signals with respect to malignancies, which will continue to be monitored.[48]

CONCLUSION

Abatacept may be used as monotherapy or concomitantly with DMARDs other than TNF antagonists. It is not recommended for use concomitantly with TNF antagonists. Not only is the combination associated with an increased risk of serious infections, but also it does not add significant clinical benefit. Based on the clinical data, we know that abatacept represents a new addition to the therapeutic options for treatment of RA patients who have not responded adequately to methotrexate and TNF blocking agents. The data so far emphasize the relatively slow time to peak clinical response with abatacept in comparison with TNF blockade, with increasing efficacy beyond short-term benefits. It will be important to see whether these early safety data are maintained over the long term. The comparative effects of abatacept, rituximab, and TNF blockade on structural damage are still unknown. For RA patients with an inadequate response to a DMARD and TNF inhibitor, abatacept offers an excellent alternative agent. Abatacept is being evaluated in other conditions such as lupus nephritis and various vasculitides. It remains to be seen if there is a potential role for abatacept in other autoimmune diseases. Long-term safety data, comparative cost-effectiveness analyses, and the route of administration may help determine the relative positioning of the biologic agents in the future.

REFERENCES

1. Firestein GS, Budd RC, Harris Ed Jr, et al. Etiology and pathogenesis of rheumatoid arthritis. In: Kelley's textbook of rheumatology, 8th ed. Elsevier Saunders, 2008.
2. Lee DM, Weinblatt ME. Rheumatoid arthritis. Lancet 2001;358:903.
3. Kremer JM. Selective costimulation modulators. J Clin Rheumatol 2005;11:S55-S62.
4. Salomom B, Bluestone JA. Complexities of CD 28/B7: CTLA-4 co-stimulatory pathways in autoimmunity and transplantation. Annu Rev Immunol 2001;19:225-252.
5. Panayi GS, Corrigall V, Pitzalis C. Pathogenesis of rheumatoid arthritis: the role of T cells and other beasts. Rheum Dis Clin North Am 2001;27:317-334.
6. Choy EH, Panayi GS. Cytokine pathways and joint inflammation in RA. N Engl J Med 2001;344:907-916.
7. Udagawa N, Kotake S, Kamatani N, et al. The molecular mechanisms of osteoclastogenesis in RA. Arthritis Res 2002;4:281-289.
8. Carreno BM, Collins M. The B7 family of ligands and its receptors: new pathways for costimulation and inhibition of immune responses. Annu Rev Immunol 2002;20:29-53.
9. Stuart RW, Racke MK. Targeting T cell costimulation in autoimmune disease. Exp Opin Ther Targets 2002;6:275-289.
10. Schwartz RH. T cell anergy. Annu Rev Immunol 2003;21:305-334.
11. Lindsley PS, Ledbatter JA: The role of CD28 receptor during T cell responses to antigen. Ann Rev Immunol 1993;11:191-212.
12. Koulava L, Clark EA, Shu G, Dupont B. The CD28 ligand B7/BB1 provides costimulatory signal for alloactivation of CD4+ T cells. J Exp Med 1991;173:759-762.
13. Alegre ML, Shiels H, Thompson CB, Gajewski TF. Expression and function of CTLA-4 in Th1 and Th2 cells. J Immunol 1998;161:3347-3356.
14. Greene JL, Leytze GM, Emswiler J, et al. Covalent dimerization of CD28/CTLA-4 and oligomerization of CD80/CD86 regulate T-cell costimulatory interactions. J Biol Chem 1996;271:26762-26771.
15. Brunner MC, Chambers CA, Chan RK, et al. CLTA-4 mediated inhibition of early events of T cell proliferation. J Immunol 1999;162:5813-5820.
16. Weyand CM, Goronzy JJ. T-cell targeted therapies in rheumatoid arthritis. Nat Clin Pract 2006;2:201-210.
17. Linsley PS, Brady W, Urnes M, et al. CTLA-4 is a second receptor for the B cell activation antigen B7. J Exp Med 1991;174:561-569.
18. Walunas TL, Lenschow DJ, Bakker CY, et al. CTLA-4 can function as a negative regulator of T cell activation. Immunity 1994;1:405-413.
19. Grohmann U, Orabona C, Fallarino F, et al. CTLA-4Ig regulates tryptophan catabolism in vivo. Nat Immunol 2002;3:1097-1101.
20. Larsen CP, Pearson TC, Adams AB, et al. Rational development of LEA29Y, a high affinity variant of CTLA4-Ig with potent immunosuppressive properties. Am J Transplant 2005;5:443-453.

21. Teng GG, Turkiewicz AM, Moreland LW. Abatacept: a co-stimulatory inhibitor for treatment of rheumatoid arthritis. Expert Opin Biol Ther 2005;5:1245-1254.
22. Weinblatt M, Combe B, Covucci A, et al. Safety of the selective costimulation modulator abatacept in rheumatoid arthritis patients receiving background biologic and nonbiologic disease-modifying antirheumatic drugs: A one-year randomized, placebo-controlled study. Arthritis and Rheum 2006;54(9):2807-2816.
23. Fox D, Millard J, Kan L, et al. Activation pathways of synovial T lymphocytes. Expression and function of the UM4D4/CDw60 antigen. J Clin Invest 1990; 86:1124-1136.
24. Higgs J, Zeldes W, Kozarsky K, et al. A novel pathway of human T lymphocyte activation: identification by a monoclonal antibody generated against a rheumatoid synovial T cell line. J Immunol 1988;140:3758-3765.
25. Meuer S, Hussey R, Fabbi M, et al. An alternative pathway of T cell activation: a functional role for the 50 kd T11 sheep erythrocyte receptor protein. Cell 1984;36:897-906.
26. Bott C, Doshi J, Morimoto C, et al. Activation of human T cells through CD6; functional effects of a novel anti-CD6 monoclonal antibody and definition of four epitopes of the CD6 glycoprotein. Int Immunol 1993;5:783-792.
27. Levesque M, Heinly C, Whichard L, et al. Cytokine-regulated expression of activated leukocyte cell adhesion molecule (CD166) on monocyte-lineage cells and in rheumatoid arthritis synovium. Arthritis Rheum 1998;41:2221-2229.
28. Wagner U, Kurtin P, Wahner A, et al. The role of CD8+ CD40L+ T cells in the formation of germinal centers in rheumatoid synovitis. J Immunol 1998;161:6390-6397.
29. Vallejo A, Mugge L, Klimiuk P, et al. Central role of thrombospondin-1 in the activation and clonal expansion of inflammatory T cells. J Immunol 2000;164:2947-2954.
30. Carter R, Wicks I. Vascular cell adhesion molecule 1 (CD106): a multifaceted regulator of joint inflammation. Arthritis Rheum 2001;44:985-994.
31. Abrams JR, Lebwohl MG, Guzzo CA, et al. CTLA4-Ig mediated block of T cell co-stimulation in patients with psoriasis vulgaris. J Clin Invest 1999;103:1243-1252.
32. Moreland LW, Alten R, Van den Bosch F, et al. Costimulatory blockade in patients with rheumatoid arthritis; a pilot, dose-finding, double-blind, placebo-controlled clinical trial evaluating CTLA4-Ig and LEA29Y eighty-five days after first infusion. Arthritis Rheum 2002; 46:1470-1479.
33. Kremer JM, Westhovens R, Leon M, et al. Treatment of rheumatoid arthritis by selective inhibition of T-cell activation with fusion protein CTLA4-Ig. N Engl J Med 2003;349:1907-1915.
34. Nadler S, Townsend R, Mikesell G, et al. Abatacept inhibits T cell activation and subsequent activation of inflammatory cell types, as demonstrated by sustained reductions in multiple inflammatory biomarkers. Ann Rheum Dis 2004;63(Suppl 1):138, abstract THU008.

35. Kremer JM, Dougados M, Emery P, et al. Treatment of RA with the selective costimulation modulator abatacept. Arthritis Rheum 2005;52:2263-2271.
36. Weisman MH, Durez P, Hallegua D, et al. Reduction of inflammatory biomarker response by abatacept in treatment of RA. J Rheumatol 2006;33:11.
37. Weinblatt M, Combe B, Covucci A, et al. Safety of the selective costimulation modulator abatacept in RA patients receiving background biologic and non-biologic DMARDs. Arthritis Rheum 2006;54:2807-2816.
38. Weinblatt M, Schiff M, Goldman A, et al. Selective costimulation modulation using abatacept in patients with active RA while receiving etanercept: a randomized controlled trial. Ann Rheum Dis 2007;66:228-234.
39. Kremer JM, Genant HK, Moreland LW, et al. Effects of abatacept in patients with methotrexate-resistant active RA. Ann Intern Med 2006;144:865-876.
40. Kremer JM, Emery P, Becker JC, et al. Abatacept provides significant and sustained benefits in clinical and patient-reported outcomes through 2 years in rheumatoid arthritis and an inadequate response to methotrexate: the long-term extension (LTE) of the AIM trial. Ann Rheum Dis 2006;65(Suppl 2):327.
41. Genovese MC, Becker JC, Schiff M, et al. Abatacept for rheumatoid arthritis refractory to TNF alpha inhibition. N Engl J Med 2003;353:1114-1123.
42. Genovese MC, Schiff M, Luggen M, et al. Efficacy and safety of the co-stimulation modulator abatacept following two years of treatment in patients with rheumatoid arthritis and an inadequate response to anti-TNF therapy. Ann Rheum Dis 2008;67:547-554.
43. Siblia J, Schiff M, Genovese MC, et al. Sustained improvement in disease activity score 28 (DAS28) and patient reported outcomes (PRO) with abatacept in rheumatoid arthritis patients with an inadequate response to anti-TNF therapy: the long-term extension of the ATTAIN trial. Ann Rheum Dis 2006;65(Suppl 2):501.
44. Schiff M, Keiserman M, Codding C, et al: The efficacy and safety of abatacept or infliximab versus placebo in ATTEST: a phase III, multicenter, randomized, double-blind, placebo-controlled study in patients with rheumatoid arthritis and an inadequate response to methotrexate. Ann Rheum Dis 2008;67:1096-1103.
45. Orencia (package insert). Bristol Myers Squib Company, 2007.
46. Furst DE, Breedveld FC, Kalden JR, et al. Updated consensus statement on biological agents for treatment of rheumatic diseases 2007. Ann Rheum Dis 2007;66(Suppl 3):2-22.
47. Bigbee CL, Gonchoroff DG, Vratsanos G, et al. Abatacept treatment does not exacerbate chronic Mycobacterium tuberculosis in mice. Arthritis Rheum 2007;56:2557-2565.
48. Simon TA, Smitten AL, Franklin J, et al. Malignancies in rheumatoid arthritis abatacept clinical development program: an epidemiological assessment. Ann Rheum Dis 2008; Dec 3 [Epub ahead of print].

Rituximab

Shouvik Dass, Edward M. Vital, and Paul Emery

59

INTRODUCTION

The treatment of rheumatic diseases has advanced significantly in the past decade with the advent of targeted therapies. Such targets have included specific lymphocyte subsets, often T cell related, cell-surface receptors, adhesion molecules, and a variety of cytokines. These targets were often identified on the basis of theoretical work and as such *in vivo* have yielded variable clinical results. Most successful of all in rheumatoid arthritis (RA) have been anti–tumor necrosis factor (TNF) agents. Experience of the safety and efficacy of these agents is now widespread. However, such experience has also shown that there are significant numbers of patients who either do not respond to such agents or lose their response or develop toxicity, which prevents continuation of therapy.

B cells were originally regarded as playing key roles in pathogenesis in RA,[1] but research interest in this area was eventually surpassed by that into T cells and anticytokine therapies.[2] However, the development of agents targeting B cells in hematologic malignancies—in particular the anti-CD20 agent rituximab—allowed a practical method by which investigation of B cells' potentially key roles in RA could be taken forward.[3] After an initial case report of improvement of RA in a patient treated with combination rituximab and other chemotherapeutic agents,[4] the promising results in a small case series of patients[5] led to the conduct of key multicenter, randomized, controlled trials.

The issues of debate at the outset of B-cell depletion therapy are still extant, to varying degrees. To a certain extent these remain driven by the dosing strategies of the agents. As with previous therapies for RA, the use of rituximab was associated in significant proportions of patients with clinical responses—and even a period of remission in some—but it soon became clear that in most patients the disease would eventually relapse. Furthermore, the anxieties of using a cell-depleting therapy were perhaps alleviated by the discovery that B-cell depletion was temporary, although this very phenomenon might be implicated in the equally temporary nature of the effect of one "cycle" of therapy in most patients.

Use of rituximab therefore established a different therapeutic paradigm than for other RA therapies, one initially clearly drawn from experience of treating malignancy. This was an agent that would not be used on a regularly repeated basis but rather would be used to induce a response and then would be used again to regain response once relapse had occurred. The immediate clinical question of importance has been focused on the efficacy and safety of repeated cycles of therapy. Beyond that, however, this question leads to issues regarding the best dosing intervals for such an agent and the challenges of maintaining stable disease control and possibly predicting relapse.

The marked effect on structural progression of RA observed with anti-TNF agents over conventional disease-modifying antirheumatic drug (DMARD) therapy[6] has raised the bar for the expected benefits of novel therapies in RA. Therefore, although initial clinical trials with rituximab concentrated on clinical outcomes, effect on radiographic progression was also included in some studies as secondary outcome measures and more recently has been the primary study outcome.

The fact that rituximab is the first approved biologic agent to act by a completely different mechanism to those currently in widespread use has led to a specific question as to where it should be positioned in the biologic hierarchy. This has been part of a general debate as to the comparative merits of different biologic modes of action, as well as a practical discussion of when it may be appropriate to switch patients from one therapy to another and in what order.[7] Ultimately, the presence of different agents are driving the search to identify distinct groups of patients who will respond to different therapies.

Aside from clinical considerations, the use of rituximab has inevitably led to greater interest in the roles and effects of B cells in RA pathogenesis. It is of course widely understood that RA is the result of multiple pathologic processes, arising from abnormalities of the immune system and dysregulation of inflammatory responses. The use of an agent with such a specific target has allowed for closer investigation of the levels at which B cells are involved in the pathogenesis of RA. Furthermore, although rituximab only appears to have one biologic effect—to lead to the destruction of B cells—it is only relatively recently that data have emerged as to the variability of this biologic effect between patients. This in turn has led to further investigation of methods of enhancing the effect of rituximab, both during its initial use and with repeated cycles of therapy.

Rituximab is distinctive in that it has been shown to have therapeutic effects across a wide range of autoimmune rheumatic disorders. As yet, this has not been consistently demonstrated by other biologic agents. In some regards, the unmet need for therapy in diseases such as systemic lupus erythematosus and antineutrophil cytoplasmic antibody (ANCA)-associated vasculitis could be argued to be even greater than that in RA. Although the experience of some clinicians and patients with rituximab has been encouraging, the availability of a targeted biologic therapy—and in particular, the expense associated with such therapies—has led to the challenges of designing and undertaking robust clinical studies in these disease areas.

B CELLS IN RHEUMATOID ARTHRITIS

B lymphocytes are generated in bone marrow with specific antigen reactivity and released into the circulation as transitional cells, ultimately becoming mature naïve B cells. They become activated on meeting their cognate antigen and then participate in germinal center reactions. These involve interaction of B and T cells arising from B-cell presentation of the antigen, along with other co-stimulatory molecules. This process leads to a number of effector mechanisms. Memory B cells are generated, as well as short-lived and long-lived plasma cells that secrete antibody.[8] Memory B cells contribute to immune memory by requiring a lower threshold for reactivation on re-encountering their cognate antigen and thereafter rapidly differentiating into plasma cells. Short-lived plasma cells provide an immediate antibody response, and in the case of IgM, plasma cells may arise without T-cell help. Long-lived plasma cells persist for many years after migrating to the bone marrow and hence contribute to immune memory and maintenance of normal immunoglobulin levels. Lastly, T-cell activation following interaction with B cells may activate other effector mechanisms besides B and plasma cells, such as release of inflammatory cytokines. It is not known whether the B or T cell is primarily responsible for loss of self-tolerance in RA, but during germinal center reactions antibodies are modified by affinity maturation and epitope spreading. This may provide the opportunity for autoreactive antibodies to arise.

In RA the autoantibodies rheumatoid factors (RFs) and anticyclic citrullinated protein antibodies (CCPs) are produced. RFs may be pathogenic by self-associating and self-generating immune complexes,[9] which then cause inflammation in sites where their receptor FcγRIIIa is expressed (the synovium, serosal surfaces, and sites of rheumatoid nodule formation). In addition, RF-producing B cells, which could arise by chance during germinal center reactions, have been shown to be capable of eliciting help from non-autoreactive T cells, thereby bypassing T cell self-tolerance and proliferating. Anti-citrullinated protein antibody (ACPA) is highly specific to RA and its target is expressed in the synovium. Both of these antibodies may be expressed years

563

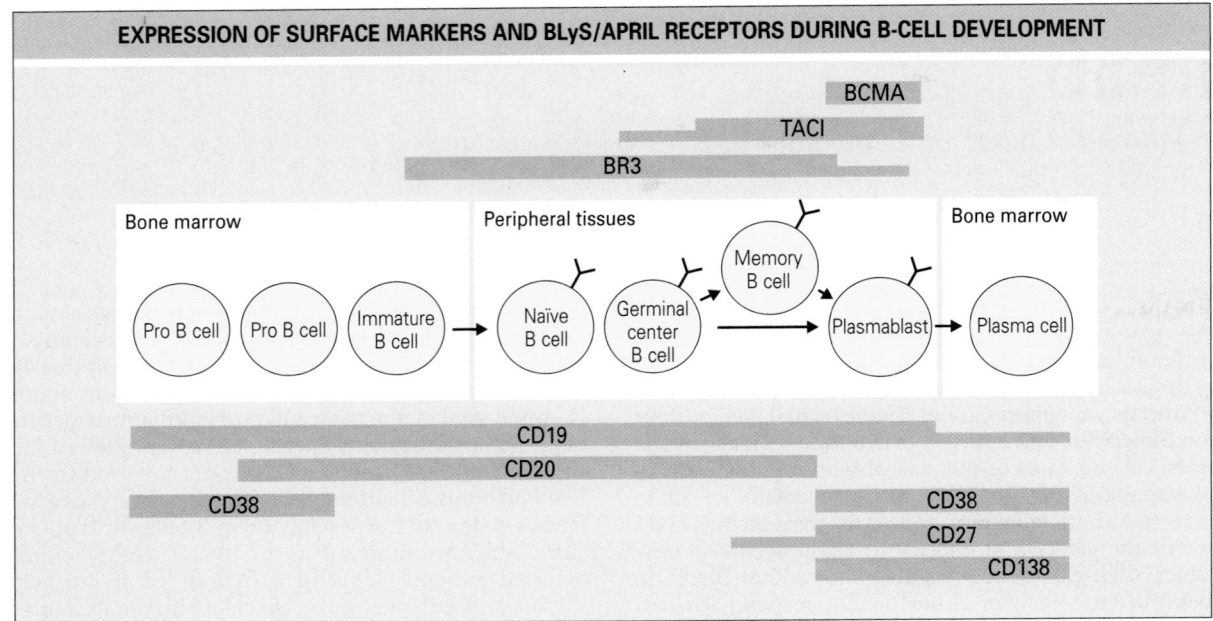

Fig. 59.1 Expression of surface markers and BLyS/APRIL receptors during B-cell development.

before clinical features of RA develop,[10] also supporting the primacy of the B cell in disease initiation.

TARGETING CD20

Recent advances in understanding the central role of B cells in RA pathogenesis have been accompanied by novel therapeutic approaches. The most widely used has been that of selective B-cell depletion using antibodies directed against anti-CD20. Rituximab, which was already available for use in non-Hodgkin lymphoma, was the first of these agents to be used in RA.

CD20 is a 33- to 37-kDa, non-glycosylated phosphoprotein expressed on the surface of mature naïve B cells that have exited the bone marrow to enter blood; it is neither expressed on stem cells nor on plasma cells that have returned to the bone marrow (Fig. 59.1). This selective expression on mature B cells but not on precursors such as stem cells or on antibody-secreting plasma cells makes it an attractive target, particularly from the point of view of theoretical safety concerns. Depletion via CD20 would be expected to permit B-cell regeneration and prevent reduction of immunoglobulin levels, at least with initial therapy. Furthermore, on binding antibody, CD20 was not thought to be shed from the cell surface or detectable in the serum and is not internalized.[11] However, evidence from hematology patients has shown that targeted epitope expression may decline after infusion of monoclonal antibodies. It has been demonstrated *in vitro* that rituximab/CD20 complexes may be removed from B cells by THP-1 monocytes. This is a reaction mediated by FcγR.[12]

The biology of CD20 and the mechanisms by which it may be targeted are not completely understood. CD20 appears to have no natural ligand and CD20 knockout mice display an almost normal phenotype.[13,14] Various anti-CD20 monoclonal antibodies have been used in experimental settings and have induced a range of different calcium flux responses, supporting the theory that CD20 may be involved in the generation and regulation of calcium transport triggered by other receptors.[15]

Rituximab is a high-affinity chimeric monoclonal antibody specific to CD20, consisting of fusion of light and heavy chain variable regions of a murine antihuman monoclonal anti-CD20 antibody with human immunoglobulin κ light chain and γ1 heavy chain constant regions.[16] This was originally developed for the treatment of refractory CD20+ B cell non-Hodgkin lymphoma, in which it has shown substantial evidence of efficacy and has now been used in more than 700,000 patients.[17] Its mechanism of B-cell depletion *in vivo* is not fully understood, but there is evidence for antibody-dependent, cell-mediated cytotoxicity by effector cells, complement-dependent cytotoxicity, and

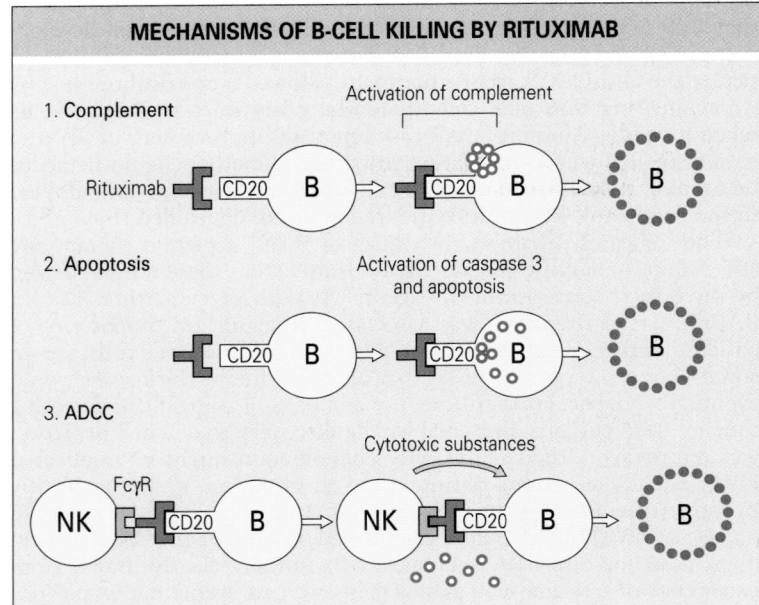

Fig. 59.2 Mechanisms of B-cell killing by rituximab.

apoptosis (Fig. 59.2).[18] From a clinical perspective, rituximab has been used to successfully target CD20 in a variety of hematologic malignancies[19] and rheumatic autoimmune diseases.[20]

Rituximab is formulated for intravenous administration. It should be diluted to a concentration of 1 to 4 mg/mL in either 0.9% sodium chloride or 5% dextrose. If a prepared infusion is not used immediately, the solution is stable at 2° C to 8° C for 24 hours and for a further 24 hours at room temperature. Clinical pharmacokinetic data are available for two consecutive doses of 500 mg and two doses of 1000 mg given on days 1 and 15. Mean terminal elimination half-life ranged from 16 to 16.5 days (after the second infusion) for the former dose and 18 to 21 days for the latter. There was no difference in pharmacokinetics between the first and second cycles of treatment. Due to risk of infusion-related reactions (discussed in more detail later), it is recommended that rituximab should be administered in clinical environments where full resuscitation facilities are available. Prophylaxis with paracetamol (1 g) and diphenhydramine HCl (25 to 50 mg, or equivalent dose of similar agent) should be given 30 to 60 minutes before infusion of rituximab.[21]

Efficacy of rituximab in rheumatoid arthritis: pivotal clinical trial data

Most clinical data leading to the licensing of rituximab for use in RA are drawn from three double-blind, randomized, placebo-controlled studies that have subsequently entered extension phases and preceding smaller studies. It should be noted that in these "placebo"-controlled studies, there was never any arm that received no treatment but rather all investigative agents were compared with treatment with methotrexate alone, the latter representing the control arm. Rituximab was given as two infusions, 2 weeks apart. Primary outcomes were at 6 months, with clinical outcomes measured by American College of Rheumatology (ACR) improvement criteria and Disease Activity Score 28 joint assessment (DAS28) in order to determine the European League Against Rheumatism (EULAR) response.

The first of these was a phase 2a study with four arms comparing placebo, rituximab monotherapy, rituximab with cyclophosphamide, and rituximab with methotrexate.[22] The DANCER study aimed to compare two different doses of rituximab (two infusions of 500 mg vs. two infusions of 1000 mg), as well varying concomitant steroid regimens.[23] The phase 3 REFLEX trial compared the latter dose of rituximab with placebo and included only patients who had had inadequate response or toxicity following anti-TNF therapy.[24] These studies are considered in more detail later.

Clinical features and responses of patients entered into pivotal trials of rituximab

As would be expected for a novel biologic agent, patients entered into these studies often had relatively severe disease. Patients in the phase 2a study had active disease despite treatment with methotrexate; patients had also failed between one and five DMARDs other than methotrexate. In the DANCER study, the mean duration of disease was 9.3 to 11.1 years and the mean number of previous DMARDs other than methotrexate was 2.2 to 2.5. Overall, 29% of patients had received prior biologic agents. For the REFLEX study, comprising patients who had all previously received anti-TNF therapy, median disease duration was approximately 12 years; swollen joint count was 23; and DAS28 was 6.9. More than 90% of patients had previously taken either one or two anti-TNF agents and 9% had received three anti-TNF agents. Ninety-one percent of patients had demonstrated an inadequate response to anti-TNF therapy because of lack of efficacy.

The eventual licensed dose of two infusions of rituximab of 1000 mg each (given 14 days apart) preceded by 100 mg methylprednisolone with concomitant ongoing methotrexate therapy demonstrated significant benefit over placebo in all these studies (the effect of other doses and regimens is discussed later). In the phase 2a study, in terms of ACR20 response, all groups treated with rituximab had a significantly higher proportion of responders (65% to 76% vs. 38%, $P = 0.025$). With regard to EULAR response criteria, patients receiving rituximab had a significantly higher proportion of responders compared with those receiving methotrexate alone (83% to 85% vs. 50%, $P = 0.004$). In the DANCER study, the proportion of patients achieving ACR20 response was significantly higher in patients receiving rituximab than placebo (54.1% rituximab vs. 27.9% placebo, $P < 0.001$). ACR50 and ACR70 responses were consistent with those observed for ACR20. In the REFLEX study, at 24 weeks, there was a significant difference between the two arms in the proportion of patients reaching the primary endpoint of ACR20 response: 51% versus 18% for the rituximab and placebo arms, respectively ($P < 0.0001$). With regard to ACR50 and ACR70 responses, these were also significantly increased in rituximab-treated patients (27% vs. 5% and 12% vs. 1% for ACR50 and 70, respectively). Similarly, when moderate to good EULAR responses were considered, the proportion of responders was significantly higher in those who had received rituximab (65% vs. 22%, $P < 0.0001$). At week 24, 12% of patients receiving rituximab had withdrawn due to lack of efficacy in comparison with 40% of those receiving placebo. There were also significant improvements in patient-based outcomes such as pain and fatigue.

On the basis of these results, rituximab was licensed by the Food and Drug Administration and European Medicines Agency (EMEA) for the treatment of severe active RA in patients with an inadequate response to anti-TNF therapy.

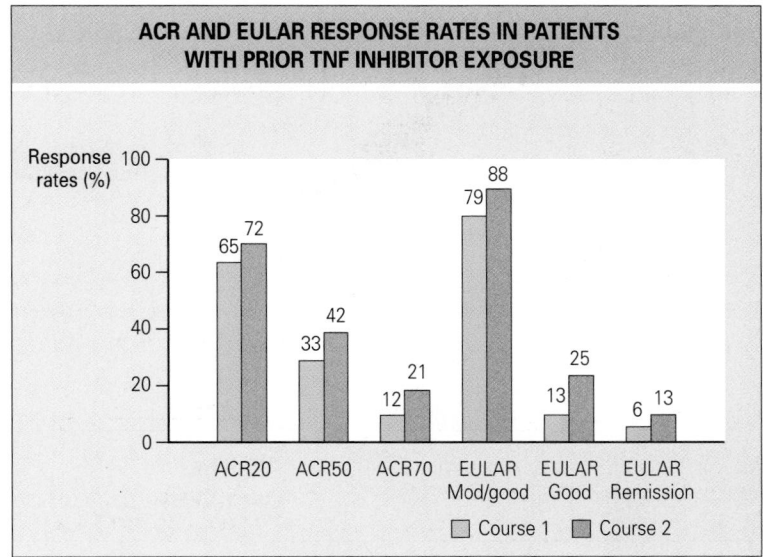

ACR AND EULAR RESPONSE RATES IN PATIENTS WITH PRIOR TNF INHIBITOR EXPOSURE

Fig. 59.3 American College of Rheumatology (ACR) and European League Against Rheumatism (EULAR) response rates in patients with prior tumor necrosis factor inhibitor exposure who received at least two cycles of rituximab in long-term extensions of phase 2 DANCER and REFLEX studies ($n = 155$). (*From Keystone E, Fleischmann R, Emery P, et al. Safety and efficacy of additional courses of rituximab in patients with active rheumatoid arthritis: an open-label extension analysis. Arthritis Rheum 2007;56:3896-3908.*) Note that in order to qualify for retreatment, patients had to have demonstrated a 20% improvement in tender and swollen joint counts during the previous cycle (even if not showing improvement in the other criteria needed to attain an ACR20 response) and have eight tender and swollen joints at the time of retreatment.

Repeat treatment: efficacy

Patients from the original large randomized studies were followed up in open-label extension studies.[25] Patients who were deemed to be responders (by predefined criteria) were eligible for retreatment with a further cycle of two infusions of 1000 mg rituximab with preceding methylprednisolone if they subsequently had deterioration in disease activity (Fig. 59.3). It is worth noting that the thresholds in studies determining both response and relapse are higher than would generally be seen in clinical practice, as reflected in the EULAR consensus statement, which defines response as a minimum improvement in DAS28 of 1.2.[26] Due to the potentially slow onset of action of rituximab, response should not be determined earlier than 16 weeks after treatment. A subsequent increase in DAS28 of greater than 0.6 is regarded as a clinically relevant deterioration, warranting retreatment. This is only recommended after 6 months have passed since the previous course.

Data are available from these open-label extension studies for up to four courses of therapy[27] and further courses are reported in case series and reports.[28] The median treatment interval between first, second, and third courses in patients with previous anti-TNF exposure remained stable at approximately 30 weeks (Fig. 59.4). Clinical responses were also sustained. ACR and DAS responses were similar after first and second courses and the proportions of patients achieving ACR70, DAS28 low disease activity (DAS28 < 3.2), and DAS28 remission (DAS28 < 2.6) increased after the second course. The change in DAS28 after each course from baseline was consistent, implying cumulative progressive reduction in disease activity with repeated treatment.

The most commonly used paradigm of rituximab therapy therefore is one of repeated therapy if a patient deteriorates after initially improving. Inherent in this is a degree of instability, with potential clinical implications such as more short-term steroid use, and this may also be potentially detrimental to long-term outcomes; there is evidence to suggest that the less that patients' disease activity rises before retreatment, the better the outcome.[29] Predictors of relapse are currently being studied; B-cell measurement by conventional sensitivity flow cytometry has not been especially informative; the vast majority of patients

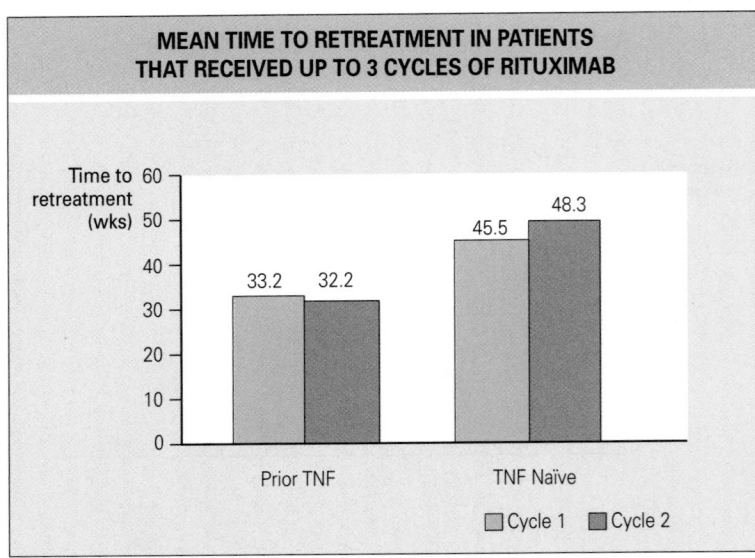

Fig. 59.4 Mean time to retreatment in patients that received up to 3 cycles of rituximab in long-term extensions of phase 2 DANCER and REFLEX studies according to prior TNF exposure. Error bars represent 95% confidence intervals. *(From Keystone E, Fleischmann R, Emery P, et al. Safety and efficacy of additional courses of rituximab in patients with active rheumatoid arthritis: an open-label extension analysis. Arthritis Rheum 2007;56:3896-3908.)*

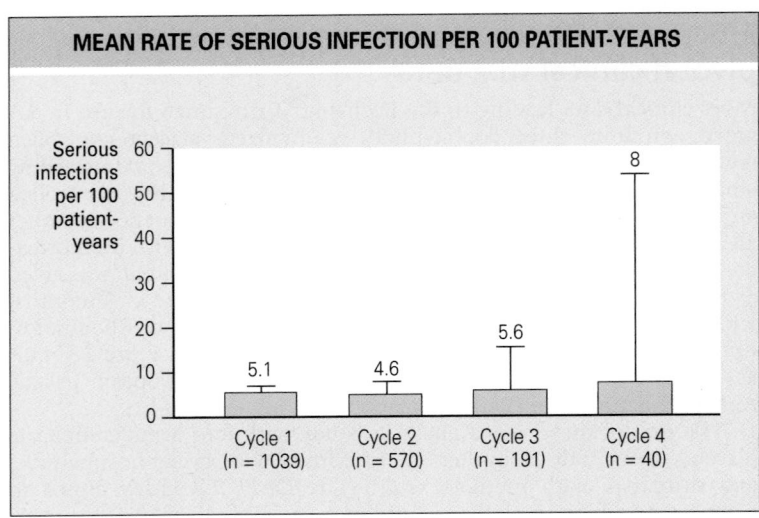

Fig. 59.5 Mean rate of serious infection per 100 patient-years in patients who received up to four cycles of rituximab in long-term extensions of phase 2 DANCER and REFLEX studies according to prior TNF exposure. Error bars represent 95% confidence intervals. *(From Keystone E, Fleischmann R, Emery P, et al. Safety and efficacy of additional courses of rituximab in patients with active rheumatoid arthritis: an open-label extension analysis. Arthritis Rheum 2007;56:3896-3908.)*

have B-cell return at some point before or with relapse, but a more specific temporal relationship has not been established.[30] It has been suggested that the specific subsets of B cells at the time of repopulation may be important, with those patients who repopulate with a predominantly naïve phenotype displaying longer responses.[31]

In order to address the issue of unstable clinical disease control, studies have been designed with fixed retreatment intervals and there have been attempts to compare fixed versus on-demand retreatment. Results from these studies are considered later.

Safety

No new safety signals have emerged from the use of rituximab in RA when compared with the extensive data available from hematology and oncology practice.[32] Pertinent issues regarding rheumatologic practice are addressed later.

Screening before therapy

It is recommended that potential patients be screened with history for chronic or concomitant co-morbidity—focusing on cardiovascular and pulmonary disease, as well as infections—and a full physical examination. A chest radiograph may not be required in all cases. No increased risk of tuberculosis has been observed in lymphoma patients treated with rituximab,[32] so routine screening for this is not recommended. Screening for hepatitis B is recommended because of cases of reactivation of infection with fulminant hepatitis.[33] From the oncology literature, patients with hepatitis B have been successfully treated with antiviral prophylaxis (with lamivudine)[34] and patients with hepatitis C have been treated without any prophylaxis. Close monitoring for reactivation of hepatitis B is recommended in patients with evidence of previous infection.

Infusion reactions

Infusion reactions are the most frequent adverse events observed with rituximab therapy. These include pruritus, urticaria, pyrexia, throat irritation, hypotension, and hypertension and are usually mild to moderate in severity. In rituximab-treated patients it has been suggested that these reactions are due to cytokine release following B-cell lysis.[35] Such symptoms affect up to 30% of patients, but it should be noted that the incidence following the second infusion is much lower.[23] This could be because B-cell numbers are already significantly reduced by the first infusion. The lower rate of infusion reactions in RA patients compared with non-Hodgkin lymphoma patients may also be related to this because the latter group often has a heavier B-cell load before

therapy. A small number of patients (<1%) experienced a serious infusion reaction (anaphylaxis and bronchospasm).

Use of intravenous steroid before infusion of rituximab reduced infusion reactions from 37% to 29% in patients receiving a first infusion of 1000 mg rituximab.[23] Repeated courses of therapy are associated with fewer infusion reactions.[27] Infusion reactions can be managed with additional paracetamol, antihistamines, and, if required, bronchodilators and steroids.

Infections

Rituximab should be delayed until active infections have resolved. Most infections after rituximab that have been reported in RA patients were minor and were largely upper respiratory or urinary tract infections. There was a slight increase in serious infections (5.2 vs. 3.7/100 patient-years) over placebo in REFLEX. No data suggest an increased risk of opportunistic infections, including tuberculosis. A small number of patients with previous tuberculosis or positive Mantoux test have been treated without reactivation of disease. It has been observed that there is a cumulative reduction in immunoglobulin levels with repeated cycles of therapy. After a third course of rituximab, 23.5% of patients have lower than normal level of IgM (Fig. 59.5).[27] However, there appears to be no change in the rate of incidence of infections in these patients before and after IgM fell below the normal limit. After cycles 3 and 4, approximately 5% of patients have low levels of IgG at any time. The incidence of infections is increased in patients within the lowest quartile of IgG levels versus those in the highest quartile.[36] However, no statistically significant difference in serious infections (i.e., those requiring hospitalization and/or intravenous antibiotics) between these two groups has been observed.

There is an increase in infection rates after anti-TNF is administered in the relatively small numbers of patients who have received rituximab previously, although this has not reached statistical significance.[37]

Vaccination responses and immunization following rituximab

A randomized, controlled study (SIERRA) was undertaken to compare immunization responses between patients treated with combination rituximab and methotrexate and those receiving methotrexate alone.[38] All patients had similar effective responses to recall antigen (tetanus) and the ability to mount a cutaneous delayed-type hypersensitivity response to *Candida albicans* was similarly preserved but responsiveness to pneumococcal vaccine (a polysaccharide antigen response) and a neoantigen (keyhole limpet hemocyanin) was diminished among rituximab-treated patients. It is recommended that vaccination be completed 4 weeks before rituximab therapy.

Progressive multifocal leukoencephalopathy

Four cases of progressive multifocal leukoencephalopathy (PML) have been reported in patients receiving rituximab for autoimmune diseases.[39] One patient had RA, two had systemic lupus erythematosus (SLE), and one had vasculitis. All patients had previously received extensive immunosuppression, in some cases with cytotoxic drugs. The patient with RA had features of overlap with connective tissue disease and had also been treated with chemotherapy for oropharyngeal carcinoma after receiving rituximab. This is the only reported case of PML in RA patients treated with rituximab. It is recommended that PML be considered in the differential diagnosis of any patient treated with rituximab who presents with change in neurologic status.[40]

PRACTICAL CLINICAL CONSIDERATIONS IN USING RITUXIMAB

Which patient groups benefit from use of rituximab?

Position in biologic hierarchy

As would be expected for a novel biologic agent, patients entered into these studies often had relatively severe disease. Patients in the phase 2a study had active disease despite treatment with methotrexate and between one and five other DMARDs. The DANCER study included patients who had active disease despite DMARDs and some who had already received anti-TNF agents, and the patient population in the REFLEX study was exclusively composed of those who had "failed" anti-TNF therapy. Patients treated with an anti-TNF agent may either demonstrate complete lack of response (primary non-response) or initial response that is subsequently lost (secondary non-response). It is not clear which is the most appropriate therapeutic strategy to follow subsequently in such patients. Some evidence suggests that switching to an alternative anti-TNF agent is beneficial in some patients[41] but may not be in all cases. In the REFLEX study, better outcomes were obtained in those patients who had only received one anti-TNF agent prior to rituximab in comparison with those who had received two or three. However, this may simply reflect less severe baseline disease activity and shorter disease duration in the former group. One observational cohort study[42] has suggested that there is greater reduction in DAS28 in patients with an inadequate response to anti-TNF therapy who then received rituximab rather than an alternative anti-TNF agent. However, other groups have shown equivalent responses to rituximab and a second anti-TNF agent in patients who are switching from their first anti-TNF agent.[43] Formal, randomized, controlled studies that might be stratified according to the pattern of non-response to anti-TNF are required before the place of rituximab in the hierarchy of biologic therapies can be more precisely identified.

Since initial studies were performed for licensing purposes, rituximab has also been used in populations with earlier disease. The SERENE study entirely comprised patients who were all inadequate responders to methotrexate but had not been exposed to anti-TNF therapy.[44] Two doses of rituximab—500 mg × 2 and 1000 mg × 2—were compared with methotrexate alone. Both treatment arms had significantly better clinical outcomes at week 24 (ACR 20, 1000 mg × 2 vs. 500 mg × 2 vs. placebo, 50.6% vs. 54.5% vs. 23.3%). The IMAGE study enrolled patients who were methotrexate naïve, with median disease duration of 11 months.[45] The same dosing regimen as the SERENE study was employed, but imaging outcomes were defined as the primary outcome measure (discussed later). Clinical outcomes consistent with an early RA population treated with biologic therapy were seen—ACR20 responses at 6 months for 1000 mg × 2 vs. 500 mg × 2 vs. placebo were 80% vs. 76.7% vs. 64.3, significantly in favor of rituximab-treated arms.

Effect of antibody status on clinical efficacy

Because autoantibody production by B cells is pivotal to their role in RA pathogenesis, the question of whether patients' autoantibody status affects clinical outcome following rituximab is potentially of key importance. The phase 2a study included only patients who were positive for rheumatoid factor; in DANCER, 380 patients were RF positive and 85 were RF negative; in REFLEX both RF positive (81%) and negative patients were also included. The last of these found that baseline RF status had no significant effect on ACR response, although fewer RF-negative patients achieved ACR20 (41%) than RF-positive patients (54%). When patients who were negative for both RF and anti-CCP antibody were considered, the EULAR response rate dropped to 44% (compared with 75% in seropositive patients).[46] In the DANCER study, there was a high placebo response rate (52% achieved ACR20), which was greater than the response rate for rituximab (48%) in seronegative patients.

What is the role of concomitant corticosteroids and DMARDs?

The DANCER study also investigated the role of concomitant steroid therapy, both intravenous (100 mg methylprednisolone prior to each infusion on days 1 and 15) and oral (prednisolone, 60 mg on days 2 to 7 and 30 mg on days 8 to 14). These were compared with placebo. Use of intravenous steroid as premedication appeared to reduce acute infusion-related reactions and is therefore recommended. However, use of oral corticosteroids appeared unnecessary in terms of improving long-term outcomes and had no effect on infusion reactions after the second infusion. Steroids did improve the initial clinical response at 4 weeks after therapy; subsequently, the clinical improvement (ACR20 response) continued before reaching a plateau at 12 weeks. The EULAR consensus statement regarding rituximab[26] recommends advising patients that they may experience an immediate but transient benefit after therapy followed by slower response, which may take up to 12 weeks to become apparent.

The role of concomitant DMARDs has also been investigated. Although patients who received rituximab monotherapy (i.e., without concomitant methotrexate) in the phase 2a study had significant improvement over placebo for ACR20 at 24 weeks post therapy, this benefit was lost by 48 weeks. In contrast, patients who received rituximab in combination with methotrexate were the only ones to demonstrate significant benefits at all ACR response thresholds and at both 24 and 48 weeks. However, by week 48, responses were declining; with the refinement of retreatment strategies (discussed further later), it may be that with lower thresholds for retreatment than in the original studies, the apparent prolongation of response with combination therapy may no longer be relevant. The duration of B-cell depletion after rituximab appears unrelated to the use of concomitant methotrexate.[30] In fact, data provided by highly sensitive flow cytometry to measure very low levels of B cells after rituximab (discussed in more detail later) indicate that initial B-cell depletion is greater in patients who are on concomitant methotrexate. In a study of more than 100 patients, patients who had received concomitant methotrexate had almost twice the rate of complete B-cell depletion than those receiving rituximab monotherapy (proportion of patients with complete B-cell depletion, rituximab and methotrexate vs. rituximab monotherapy, 47.7% vs. 25.1%, $P = 0.05$).[47] Use of concomitant DMARDs other than methotrexate—in particular, leflunomide—has been reported to be safe and effective in small numbers of patients. Prolonged responses have been reported with leflunomide in particular.[48]

Effect of dose of rituximab

The DANCER study compared two doses of rituximab (2 × 500 mg vs. 2 × 1000 mg). ACR20 (55.3%, lower-dose rituximab and 54.1%, higher-dose rituximab) and ACR50 (33% lower dose and 34% higher dose) responses were similar for both doses, but ACR70 responses were slightly higher in the higher-dose group (20% vs. 13%), although this did not reach significance. The ACR70 response rose during the course of the study with higher-dose rituximab, suggesting that there may be a time-related cumulative effect of this dose. With regard to EULAR responses, rituximab treatment significantly improved responses when compared with placebo ($P < 0.001$). There was no statistically significant difference between different doses of rituximab with respect to EULAR response, although a higher proportion of patients treated with the higher dose of rituximab achieved a "good" EULAR response (27.9%, 13.8%, and 4.1% for higher-dose, lower-dose, and placebo, respectively). No significant differences in safety and tolerability were identified between the two doses. The REFLEX study used only one dosing regimen of rituximab (2 × 1000 mg), so this became the licensed dose in this population.

Two further multicenter trials (MIRROR and IMAGE)[45,49] have studied different dose regimens. In the former, three regimens were compared—a "standard" regimen (rituximab 1000 mg × 2, repeated at 6 months), a reduced-dose regimen (2 × 500 mg, repeated at 6 months), and an escalating dose regimen (rituximab 1000 mg × 2, with 500 mg × 2 at 6 months). ACR20, 50, and 70 clinical responses at 48 weeks were equivalent for all three arms, but overall EULAR response rates were significantly higher for the "standard" regimen, 89% versus 71% versus 72% ("standard" vs. "reduced" vs. "escalating" regimens, $P < 0.03$). The IMAGE study enrolled a cohort of patients with earlier disease who had not been treated with methotrexate. Patients were randomized to placebo with methotrexate, rituximab 2 × 500 mg with methotrexate, or rituximab 2 × 1000 mg with methotrexate. Retreatment was given with the same dose after 6 months to all patients with DAS28 greater than 2.6 and later to patients in remission at 6 months when the DAS28 increased above 2.6. Clinical outcomes were significantly better for patients receiving either dose of rituximab than those on methotrexate alone; ACR outcomes were numerically higher for those on the higher-dose rituximab, but this difference did not reach statistical significance. The primary outcome of this study was on radiographic progression (discussed later).

Imaging outcomes after rituximab

Data on radiographic progression following rituximab are available from the REFLEX and IMAGE studies. The patient populations in these studies were quite different. The former enrolled patients with relatively long disease duration (approximately 12 years) and who had already had an inadequate response to anti-TNF therapy. In the latter, patients had much shorter disease duration (mean disease duration, 0.9 month) and had not yet received methotrexate. In the REFLEX study, described in detail earlier, patients were already on methotrexate and then randomized to either rituximab (1000 mg × 2) or placebo. Retreatment with the same dose was given when patients flared after initial response; patients randomized to placebo could be given rescue treatment with rituximab but for the purposes of analysis, such patients were still considered part of the "placebo" group. Radiographs of hands and feet were obtained at baseline, week 24, and week 56 and scored using the Genant-modified Sharp method. Patients who received rituximab had significantly less radiographic disease progression than those who received placebo. The mean change from baseline in the total Genant-modified Sharp score at week 56 was significantly lower for patients treated with rituximab (1.00 vs. 2.31, rituximab vs. placebo, $P = 0.005$); changes in erosion scores (0.59 vs. 1.32, rituximab vs. placebo, $P = 0.011$) and joint space narrowing (0.41 vs. 0.99, $P < 0.001$) were significantly in favor of rituximab. Those patients treated with rituximab whose clinical outcomes were no better than those receiving placebo still had less radiographic progression.

The IMAGE study measured similar outcomes in 715 patients randomized equally to three arms as described earlier. At 52 weeks, patient who received higher-dose rituximab (i.e., 2 × 1000 mg, repeated at 6 months in patients not in remission and given to patients in remission at 6 months if and when DAS later worsened) had significantly lower changes in mean Total Sharp Score (mTSS) (0.359 vs. 1.079, $P < 0.001$) and more patients had no progression in mTSS when treated with that dose of rituximab (63.5 vs. 53.4, $P < 0.05$). Significant differences were not observed between patients receiving methotrexate alone and those treated with the lower dose of rituximab.

Rituximab has demonstrated safety and efficacy in the treatment of various RA populations, including those with severe disease, which has proved refractory to all previously available therapies. However, as a relatively new agent, it continues to be evaluated in wider groups of patients and a number of issues arise, which may inform future practice.

The most significant of these relates to predictors of response and relapse. These may revolve around greater understanding of B-cell depletion and repletion, as well the fundamentals of rituximab's mechanism of action. For the former, conventional sensitivity flow cytometry (with a typical lower limit of detection of 0.1×10^9 cells/L) suggests that all patients deplete peripheral B cells completely and hence this offers no correlation with response. However, more sensitive assays (with a lower limit of detection 100 times lower, at 0.0001×10^9/L) have revealed considerable variation in peripheral depletion. Many patients have incomplete depletion, with particular variability in the rate of depletion. Most persistent B cells are preplasma cells, whose rate of depletion or persistence in the circulation is thought to correlate with B-cell activity in other tissues. Some patients have completely undetectable B cells after the first infusion of rituximab—almost all of these patients subsequently respond clinically—while poorer initial depletion has correlated with shorter duration of clinical response.[50] This may inform strategies designed to enhance B-cell depletion. With regard to repletion, it has been suggested that patients who display a predominantly naïve B-cell phenotype at repletion tend to have longer responses. How far these peripheral changes at depletion and repletion reflect B cells in compartments elsewhere in the body is also unclear. B cells exist in greater numbers in compartments such as spleen, bone marrow, lymph nodes, and synovium than in peripheral blood. It is not yet known whether B cells in a certain location need to be depleted to achieve optimal clinical response or whether a pathogenic subset of B cells can be identified and targeted.

From a clinical perspective, the need to observe clinical deterioration before administering repeat courses of therapy may be an approach that can be improved. Another approach might entail fixed-interval retreatment, in order to maintain stable responses. However, the safety aspects of this would need to be closely studied, particularly as this might lead to overtreatment of some patients. Ultimately combination therapy with other targeted biologic agents might be used to enhance the effect of rituximab. The use of biomarkers to inform clinical strategies might eventually allow stable responses to be achieved using individually tailored therapy to provide patients with the smallest required dose.

Rituximab: effect on synovium

The importance of B cells in the site of inflammation (i.e., the RA synovium) is not fully understood. B cells are usually present in the RA synovium and in some patients organize with T and follicular dendritic cells into germinal center–like structures surrounded by plasma cells—a process sometimes known as *ectopic lymphoid neogenesis*. However, because the development of autoantibodies is known to precede the onset of synovitis sometimes by years, it seems that the autoimmune process begins distant from the joint such as in other lymphoid tissues or bone marrow. Highly sensitive flow cytometry indicates that circulating preplasma cells in the absence of circulating naïve and memory B cells is predictive of clinical response. These findings suggest that depletion of other tissues may be a determinant of clinical response to rituximab and led to several studies examining synovial biopsy before and after rituximab therapy.

These studies varied in methodology and findings but several identified differences in number or depletion of B-lineage cells between clinical responders and non-responders. These included higher CD79a+ B cells at baseline,[51] reduced depletion of CD19+ B cells at 6 months,[52] and persistence of CD138+ plasma cells at 16 weeks.[53] One study included biopsy at both 4 and 16 weeks after rituximab and demonstrated that there is a specific depletion of B cells that preceded the more generalized reduction in synovial cellularity that accompanies clinical response.[53]

Rituximab: use in connective tissue diseases

Rituximab has also been increasingly widely used in the treatment of connective tissue diseases. Because many of these conditions are regarded as autoantibody driven, B-cell depletion could theoretically be considered a rational approach. This theory has to some extent been supported by clinical data, although rituximab is not licensed for use in any of these conditions. Randomized studies have been conducted in SLE and primary Sjögren syndrome (pSS), but the majority of the data is drawn from open-label series in these conditions, as well as vasculitis (ANCA-associated granulomatous vasculitis and other vasculitides) and myositis.

TABLE 59.1 CASE SERIES OF RITUXIMAB IN SYSTEMIC LUPUS ERYTHEMATOSUS

Authors	n	Disease manifestations	Outcome
Ng et al, 2007 [56]	32	Systemic, renal, hematologic, arthritis, cutaneous, cerebral, cardiac, respiratory, serositis, vasculitis	28/30 responded. 1 lost to follow-up, 1 failed to deplete. 12 had sustained response (no relapse 12-60 mo). 10 relapsed but responded to re-treatment.
Vital et al, 2008 [57]	27	Systemic, renal, hematologic, arthritis, cutaneous, cerebral, cardiac, respiratory, serositis, vasculitis	23/27 complete response, 4 partial/non-response. Significant reduction in global BILAG, autoantibodies, and inflammatory markers.
Leandro et al, 2005 [61]	24	Systemic, renal, hematologic, arthritis, cutaneous, cerebral, cardiac, respiratory, serositis, vasculitis	23/24 response. Significant reduction in global BILAG, autoantibodies, and inflammatory markers.
Looney et al, 2004 [55]	18	Arthritis, rash, renal, hematologic, serositis	Dose-ranging study—all 11 patients with adequate depletion responded. 3 serious adverse events considered unrelated to rituximab.
Tanaka et al, 2007 [62]	15	Systemic, renal, hematologic, arthritis, cutaneous, cerebral, cardiac, respiratory, serositis, vasculitis	Variable doses and combinations. 9 responses, 5 non-responses, 1 without follow-up.
Gomard-Mennesson et al, 2006 [63]	26	Primary indication AIHA	25/26 responded. Recurrence rate 3 per 100 patient-years. Other manifestations also improved.
Leandro et al, 2002 [64]	6	Systemic, mucocutaneous, renal, hematologic, serositis, cerebral	5/5 patients with follow-up responded. 10 infections, none serious.
Ng et al, 2006 [65]	7	Repeat cycles of treatment	Good efficacy and safety maintained with each cycle.
Gunnarsson et al, 2007 [66]	7	Proliferative glomerulonephritis	Renal study with repeat biopsies. All patients improved clinically, 3 were in complete remission. All biopsies improved.
Tokunaga et al, 2007 [67]	10	Neuropsychiatric	All 10 patients improved, response ≥12 mo in 5.
Gillis et al, 2007 [68]	6	Systemic, renal, hematologic, arthritis, cutaneous, cerebral, cardiac, respiratory, serositis, vasculitis	5/6 responded.
Chehab et al, 2007 [69]	9	Renal, neurologic, hematologic, cutaneous, systemic	6 had good responses. 1 had serious adverse event considered unrelated to rituximab.

BILAG, British Isles Lupus Assessment Group's Index.

Systemic lupus erythematosus

Open-label series have reported efficacy of rituximab in a range of disease manifestations.[54] These include lupus nephritis, arthritis, hematologic disease (immune thrombocytopenia [ITP] and autoimmune hemolytic anemia [AIHA]), cutaneous involvement, serositis, and cardiac, respiratory, and cerebral organ involvement. The largest series have reported data from approximately 30 patients each, by Looney and colleagues,[55] Ng and colleagues,[56] and Vital and colleagues.[57] Most patients had received immunosuppression with DMARDs, including cyclophosphamide, before treatment with rituximab. Various doses—usually either two infusions of 1 g rituximab or four infusions of 375 mg/m^2—were used, as were a different combination of DMARDs and rituximab monotherapy. Clinical outcome measures including the British Isles Lupus Assessment Group's Index (BILAG) and Systemic Lupus Erythematosus Disease Activity Index (SLEDAI) were endpoints in the majority of series. There has also been some evidence of histologic improvement in renal biopsies after rituximab for lupus nephritis.[66] The results of the larger case series are summarized in Table 59.1.

Two randomized, controlled trials have been carried out with rituximab in SLE: EXPLORER and LUNAR. The former enrolled patients with disease manifestations of SLE other than cerebral and renal disease, while the latter enrolled patients with grade III or IV lupus nephritis (with or without grade V changes). The study results have been reported in abstract form. In EXPLORER, patients were randomized to either rituximab or continuing previous immunosuppressive agents with a reducing course of oral steroid (starting dose 1 mg/kg). Improvement in BILAG was used as primary outcome measure. No significant difference was observed between either arm at 6 months. Patients in LUNAR were randomized either to rituximab with mycophenolate or mycophenolate alone (high-dose steroids were used in both arms). No significant difference in primary outcome (achievement of "complete renal response," defined as specific percentage improvement in proteinuria and normalization of serum creatinine) was observed between the two groups. Full assessment of these studies has yet to be undertaken, but comments have been raised regarding the

patient populations enrolled—which tended to have failed fewer therapies than those cases in open-label series and in the EXPLORER study were generally cases of arthritis and mucocutaneous disease—and the effect of high-dose therapy with steroids may have masked the clinical benefit of rituximab.

Sjögren syndrome

Sjögren syndrome can be regarded as a disorder of B-cell hyperactivity with autoantibody-driven disease and hypergammaglobulinemia. Open-label studies have indicated improvements in sicca symptoms and objective measures, as well as in histologic changes associated with MALT lymphoma.[58] A pilot randomized, double-blind, placebo-controlled trial of rituximab in pSS did show greater improvement in fatigue scores with rituximab over placebo.[59] Larger randomized studies are currently being designed.

Vasculitis

Following open-label reports of efficacy of rituximab in ANCA-associated vasculitis, a randomized study has now been reported in abstract form (RAVE).[60] This was designed as a non-inferiority study comparing rituximab (375 mg/m^2 intravenous × 4) with cyclophosphamide (2 mg/kg/day by mouth) for 3 months followed by azathioprine. Intravenous and oral steroids were used in both groups. The primary outcome was remission, defined as BVAS score of 0 without any concomitant steroid therapy at 6 months. Patients had either ANCA-associated granulomatous vasculitis or microscopic polyangiitis. The results demonstrated that rituximab was not inferior to cyclophosphamide/azathioprine and, in fact, more patients treated with rituximab were in remission (64% vs. 55%, $P = 0.21$). Significantly fewer patients treated with rituximab had one or more adverse events in comparison with those receiving cyclophosphamide/azathioprine.

SUMMARY

B-cell depletion therapy with rituximab has proven to be a promising area in terms of both clinical management and research into disease pathogenesis. In RA, the clinical benefits have been important for the significant numbers of patients who have active progressive disease despite conventional and biologic DMARDs; evidence is now accruing of its benefit in earlier disease populations. Data regarding structural benefit are also increasing. Questions remain regarding the most appropriate dose and the frequency of repeat treatments. The safety profile has been reassuring, with the treatment being suitable for some patients who may have contraindications to anti-TNF for safety reasons. Immunoglobulin levels—particularly IgG after several cycles—must be monitored carefully. The current research agenda is focusing on the mechanisms and effects of B-cell depletion in different compartments,

and this may shed light on targeting the therapy by predicting responders and subsequent flare. It may also allow for different dosing strategies to be used in different patients, including initial non-responders.

In connective tissue diseases, the open-label data show that many patients with severe, resistant disease have had good outcomes following therapy. Rituximab may also be a better alternative in terms of toxicity than cyclophosphamide, although careful surveillance for infection, especially PML, will be required. In SLE, further work is required in designing robust clinical trials with appropriate patient populations and outcome measures to demonstrate similar results.

KEY REFERENCES

1. Zvaifler NJ. The immunopathology of joint inflammation in rheumatoid arthritis. Adv Immunol 1973;16:265-336.
2. Firestein GS. Evolving concepts of rheumatoid arthritis. Nature 2003;423:356-361.
3. Buske C, Feuring-Buske M, Unterhalt M, Hiddemann W. Monoclonal antibody therapy for B cell non-Hodgkin's lymphomas: emerging concepts of a tumour-targeted strategy. Eur J Cancer 1999;35:549-557.
4. Protheroe A, Edwards JC, Simmons A, et al. Remission of inflammatory arthropathy in association with anti-CD20 therapy for non-Hodgkin's lymphoma. Rheumatology (Oxford) 1999;38:1150-1152.
5. Edwards JC, Cambridge G. Sustained improvement in rheumatoid arthritis following a protocol designed to deplete B lymphocytes. Rheumatology (Oxford) 2001;40:205-211.
6. Jones G, Halbert J, Crotty M, et al. The effect of treatment on radiological progression in rheumatoid arthritis: a systematic review of randomized placebo-controlled trials. Rheumatology (Oxford) 2003;42:6-13.
7. Rubbert-Roth A, Finckh A. Treatment options in patients with rheumatoid arthritis failing initial TNF inhibitor therapy: a critical review. Arthritis Res Ther 2009;11(suppl 1):S1.
8. Hoyer BF, Manz RA, Radbruch A, Hiepe F. Long-lived plasma cells and their contribution to autoimmunity. Ann N Y Acad Sci 2005;1050:124-133.
9. Edwards JC, Cambridge G. Rheumatoid arthritis: the predictable effect of small immune complexes in which antibody is also antigen. Br J Rheumatol 1998;37:126-130.
10. Rantapaa-Dahlqvist S, de Jong BA, Berglin E, et al. Antibodies against cyclic citrullinated peptide and IgA rheumatoid factor predict the development of rheumatoid arthritis. Arthritis Rheum 2003;48:2741-2749.
11. Glennie MJ, French RR, Cragg MS, Taylor RP. Mechanisms of killing by anti-CD20 monoclonal antibodies. Mol Immunol 2007;44:3823-3837.
12. Beum PV, Kennedy AD, Williams ME, et al. The shaving reaction: rituximab/CD20 complexes are removed from mantle cell lymphoma and chronic lymphocytic leukemia cells by THP-1 monocytes. J Immunol 2006;176:2600-2609.
13. Uchida J, Lee Y, Hasegawa M, et al. Mouse CD20 expression and function. Int Immunol 2004;16:119-129.
14. O'Keefe TL, Williams GT, Davies SL, Neuberger MS. Mice carrying a CD20 gene disruption. Immunogenetics 1998;48:125-132.
15. Bubien JK, Zhou LJ, Bell PD, et al. Transfection of the CD20 cell surface molecule into ectopic cell types generates a Ca^{2+} conductance found constitutively in B lymphocytes. J Cell Biol 1993;121:1121-1132.
16. Reff ME, Carner K, Chambers KS, et al. Depletion of B cells in vivo by a chimeric mouse human monoclonal antibody to CD20. Blood 1994;83:435-445.
17. Solal-Celigny P. Safety of rituximab maintenance therapy in follicular lymphomas. Leuk Res 2006;30(suppl 1):S16-S21.
18. Cragg MS, Walshe CA, Ivanov AO, Glennie MJ. The biology of CD20 and its potential as a target for mAb therapy. Curr Dir Autoimmun 2005;8:140-174.
19. Collins-Burow B, Santos ES. Rituximab and its role as maintenance therapy in non-Hodgkin lymphoma. Expert Rev Anticancer Ther 2007;7:257-273.

20. Edwards JC, Cambridge G, Leandro MJ. B cell depletion therapy in rheumatic disease. Best Pract Res Clin Rheumatol 2006;20:915-928.
21. Roche. Investigators Brochure, Rituximab. In press, 2009.
22. Edwards JC, Szczepanski L, Szechinski J, et al. Efficacy of B-cell-targeted therapy with rituximab in patients with rheumatoid arthritis. N Engl J Med 2004;350:2572-2581.
23. Emery P, Fleischmann R, Filipowicz-Sosnowska A, et al. The efficacy and safety of rituximab in patients with active rheumatoid arthritis despite methotrexate treatment: results of a phase IIB randomized, double-blind, placebo-controlled, dose-ranging trial. Arthritis Rheum 2006;54:1390-1400.
24. Cohen SB, Emery P, Greenwald MW, et al. Rituximab for rheumatoid arthritis refractory to anti-tumor necrosis factor therapy: results of a multicenter, randomized, double-blind, placebo-controlled, phase III trial evaluating primary efficacy and safety at twenty-four weeks. Arthritis Rheum 2006;54:2793-2806.
26. Smolen JS, Keystone EC, Emery P, et al. Consensus statement on the use of rituximab in patients with rheumatoid arthritis. Ann Rheum Dis 2007;66:143-150.
27. Keystone E, Fleischmann R, Emery P, et al. Safety and efficacy of additional courses of rituximab in patients with active rheumatoid arthritis: an open-label extension analysis. Arthritis Rheum 2007;56:3896-3908.
28. Popa C, Leandro MJ, Cambridge G, Edwards JC. Repeated B lymphocyte depletion with rituximab in rheumatoid arthritis over 7 yrs. Rheumatology (Oxford) 2007;46:626-630.
29. Mease PJ, Kaell A. Predicting outcome of a second course of rituximab for rheumatoid arthritis. Ann Rheum Dis 2007;66(suppl II):434.
30. Emery P, Breedfeld F, Martin-Mola E, et al. Relationship between peripheral B cell levels and loss of EULAR response in rheumatoid arthritis patients treated with rituximab. Ann Rheum Dis 2007;66(suppl II):124.
31. Leandro MJ, Cambridge G, Ehrenstein MR, Edwards JC. Reconstitution of peripheral blood B cells after depletion with rituximab in patients with rheumatoid arthritis. Arthritis Rheum 2006;54:613-620.
32. Kimby E. Tolerability and safety of rituximab (MabThera). Cancer Treat Rev 2005;31:456-473.
34. He YF, Li YH, Wang FH, et al. The effectiveness of lamivudine in preventing hepatitis B viral reactivation in rituximab-containing regimen for lymphoma. Ann Hematol 2008;87:481-485.
35. Hainsworth JD. Safety of rituximab in the treatment of B cell malignancies: implications for rheumatoid arthritis. Arthritis Res Ther 2003;5(suppl 4):S12-S16.
36. Emery P, van Vollenhoven, Bingham CO, et al. Extended follow up of the long term safety of rituximab in rheumatoid arthritis. Rheumatology 2008;47(suppl II):ii16.
37. Genovese MC, Breedveld FC, Emery P, et al. Safety of biologic therapies following rituximab treatment in rheumatoid arthritis patients. Ann Rheum Dis 2009;68:1894-1897.
38. Bingham III CO, Looney RJ, Deodhar A, et al. Immunization responses in rheumatoid arthritis patients treated with rituximab: results from a controlled clinical trial (SIERRA). Ann Rheum Dis 2009;68(suppl III):75.
39. Carson KR, Evens AM, Richey EA, et al. Progressive multifocal leukoencephalopathy after rituximab therapy

in HIV-negative patients: a report of 57 cases from the Research on Adverse Drug Events and Reports project. Blood 2009;113:4834-4840.
40. Calabrese LH, Molloy ES. Therapy: rituximab and PML risk-informed decisions needed! Nat Rev Rheumatol 2009;5:528-529.
41. Buch MH, Bingham SJ, Bejarano V, et al. Therapy of patients with rheumatoid arthritis: outcome of infliximab failures switched to etanercept. Arthritis Rheum 2007;57:448-453.
42. Finckh A, Ciurea A, Brulhart L, et al. B cell depletion may be more effective than switching to an alternative anti-tumor necrosis factor agent in rheumatoid arthritis patients with inadequate response to anti-tumor necrosis factor agents. Arthritis Rheum 2007;56:1417-1423.
43. Buch MH, Dass S, Vital EM, et al. Is switching to rituximab more effective than switching to an alternative tumour necrosis factor blocking therapy (TNF-BT) in patients with rheumatoid arthritis (RA) who have failed previous TNF-BT? Single centre cohort experience. Ann Rheum Dis 2009;68(suppl III):574.
44. Emery P, Rigby W, Combe B, et al. Efficacy and safety of rituximab (RTX) as a first-line biologic therapy in patients (pts) with active rheumatoid arthritis (RA): results of a phase III randomised controlled study (SERENE). Arthritis Rheum 2008;58(9 suppl):S302.
45. Tak PP, Rigby W, Rubbert A, et al. Inhibition of joint damage and improved clinical outcomes with a combination of rituximab (RTX) and methotrexate (MTX) in patients (pts) with early active rheumatoid arthritis (RA) who are naive to MTX: a randomised active comparator placebo-controlled trial. Ann Rheum Dis 2009;68(suppl III):75.
46. Tak PP, Cohen SB, Emery P, et al. Baseline autoantibody status (RF, Anti-CCP) and clinical response following the first treatment course with rituximab. Arthritis Rheum 2006;54(9 suppl):S368.
47. Dass S, Vital EM, Buch MH, et al. Effect of concomitant DMARD on B cell depletion with rituximab in rheumatoid arthritis. Ann Rheum Dis 2009;68(suppl III):579.
48. Vital EM, Dass S, Rawston AC, et al. Combination rituximab and leflunomide produces lasting responses in rheumatoid arthritis. Ann Rheum Dis 2008;67(suppl II):90.
49. Rubbert-Roth A, Tak PP, Bombardieri S, et al. Efficacy and safety of various dosing regimens of rituximab in patients with active RA: results of a phase III randomised study (MIRROR). Arthritis Rheum 2008;58(9 suppl):S301.
50. Dass S, Rawston AC, Vital EM, et al. Highly sensitive B cell analysis predicts response to rituximab therapy in rheumatoid arthritis. Arthritis Rheum 2008;58:2993-2999.
54. Ramos-Casals M, Soto MJ, Cuadrado MJ, Khamashta MA. Rituximab in systemic lupus erythematosus: a systematic review of off-label use in 188 cases. Lupus 2009;18:767-776.
59. Dass S, Bowman SJ, Vital EM, et al. Reduction of fatigue in Sjögren syndrome with rituximab: results of a randomised, double-blind, placebo-controlled pilot study. Ann Rheum Dis 2008;67:1541-1544.

REFERENCES

Full references for this chapter can be found on www.expertconsult.com.

Cytokine neutralizers: IL-1 inhibitors

Cem Gabay

60

- IL-1α and IL-1β (also termed IL-1) are prototypical proinflammatory cytokines that activate effector cells by binding to IL-1 receptors.

- IL-1 is a very potent cytokine, the activities of which are tightly regulated by natural inhibitors such as IL-1 receptor antagonist (IL-1Ra), type 2 IL-1R, and soluble receptors. The balance between IL-1 and its natural inhibitor, IL-1Ra, has been shown to play a major role in the regulation of inflammatory responses.

- The production of mature and bioactive IL-1β is regulated by two signals: signal 1 induces the production of pro-IL-1β, a non-active 31-kDa propeptide. Activation of the inflammasome, a cytosolic complex of proteins, leads to the activation of caspase-1, causing pro-IL-1β processing into mature 17-kDa IL-1β and its release outside the cells.

- Exogenous microbial components and endogenous agents (monosodium urate and calcium dihydrate pyrophosphate crystals) can activate the NALP3 inflammasome. In addition, some mutations of *NALP3* lead to spontaneous inflammasome and caspase-1 activation and overproduction of IL-1β, causing recurrent episodes of fever with inflammatory systemic manifestations.

- Strategies aiming to block IL-1 bioactivity were shown to be modestly effective in the treatment of rheumatoid arthritis. In contrast, IL-1 inhibitors have been reported to be markedly effective in the management of systemic-onset juvenile idiopathic arthritis, adult-onset Still's disease, crystal-induced arthritis, and periodic fever syndromes associated with *NALP3* mutations and overproduction of IL-1β.

INTERLEUKIN (IL)-1 FAMILY

Ligands and receptors

The IL-1 family includes three ligands: IL-1α, IL-1β, and IL-1 receptor antagonist (IL-1Ra).[1] The amino acid identities between these human proteins are IL-1α and IL-1β, 22%; IL-1α and IL-1Ra, 18%; and IL-1β and IL-1Ra, 26%. Moreover, human IL-1α is approximately 55% identical to the murine and rat forms of this molecule, with IL-1β being approximately 78% identical and IL-1Ra approximately 76% identical. The genes for IL-1α, IL-1β, and IL-1Ra are located close to each other in the human chromosome 2q14 region.[2,3] IL-1α and IL-1β exert agonist activities and play critical roles in inflammatory responses. IL-1α and IL-1β are the products of two different genes and are synthesized by multiple cells, including monocytes, macrophages, neutrophils, and epithelial cells. IL-1α and IL-1β are produced as 31-kDa propeptides, lack leader sequences, and are not secreted from cells by the usual mechanism from the Golgi apparatus. Pro-IL-1α can be cleaved by calpain protease, and pro-IL-1β is processed by caspase-1 (also termed IL-1β–converting enzyme [ICE])[4] to generate 17-kDa mature peptides. Both pro-IL-1α and mature IL-1α are biologically active, whereas pro-IL-1β is biologically inactive and must be converted into mature IL-1β to acquire the ability to bind to receptors and activate cells. The majority of IL-1α remains cell associated either bound to the plasma membrane or inside the cell. The amino-terminal region of pro-IL-1α possesses a nuclear localization sequence, which allows its translocation to the nucleus where pro-IL-1α exerts different effects on cell growth, tumor transformation, apoptosis, pro-collagen-I, and cytokine production.

The IL-1 receptor family includes three receptors: type 1 IL-1 receptor (IL-1RI), type 2 IL-1 receptor (IL-1RII), and IL-1 receptor accessory protein (IL-1RAcP) (Fig. 60.1). The IL-1 receptor accessory protein is also the co-receptor of other cytokines that belong to the IL-1 superfamily, such as IL-1F6, IL-1F8, IL-1F9, and IL-1F11 (IL-33). IL-1RI, IL-1RII, and IL-1RAcP belong to the immunoglobulin (Ig) gene superfamily with their extracellular segment containing three Ig-like domains. IL-1RI and IL-1RAcP, but not IL-1RII, have cytoplasmic domains that are related to the Toll-like receptor (TLR) superfamily, the Toll-like/IL-1R (TIR) domains. The most striking structural difference between IL-1RI and IL-1RII is the short cytoplasmic domain of IL-1RII (29 amino acids), whereas IL-1RI possesses a cytoplasmic tail of 213 residues.[5] IL-1 binding to IL-1RI leads to the recruitment of IL-1RAcP. The formation of the trimeric IL-1/IL-1RI/IL-1RAcP complex leads to the recruitment of a number of intracellular adaptor molecules, including MyD88, IRAK, and TRAF6, to activate signal transduction pathways such as NF-κB, AP-1, JNK, and p38 MAP kinase. IL-1RII has a short intracytoplasmic domain and is unable to transduce any intracellular signal and, thus, functions as a decoy receptor.[6] IL-1RII can be cleaved from the cell surface. Both membrane-bound and soluble IL-1RII can bind to IL-1β and exert inhibitory functions (see Fig. 60.1).

IL-1 receptor antagonist is structurally closely related to the other IL-1 ligands but has undergone mutations, rendering it incapable of interacting with IL-1RAcP. IL-1Ra binds avidly to IL-1RI but fails to activate cells, functioning as a specific competitive inhibitor of IL-1 (Fig. 60.2). Because the binding of only a few IL-1 molecules is sufficient to activate cells, a large excess of IL-1Ra is necessary (100- to 1000-fold) to block the effect of IL-1. Several different isoforms of IL-1Ra are produced from the same gene through the use of different first exons, messenger RNA splicing, and alternative translation. Secreted IL-1Ra (sIL-1Ra) has a leader sequence and is glycosylated and released through the classical secretory pathway largely from the same cells that release IL-1β. Three other IL-1Ra isoforms lack a leader sequence and remain intracellular. The function of these intracellular isoforms remains unclear.[7]

IL-1 plays a critical role in inflammation

In healthy human subjects, IL-1β, contrary to other cytokines, is barely detectable in the bloodstream, suggesting that its circulating levels are below 10 pg/mL. Such low levels have to be maintained because of the tremendous potency of IL-1β to induce inflammatory responses.[8] Indeed, intravenous injections of IL-1β in human subjects at doses as low as 1 ng/kg were associated with chills and fever, with increase in febrile response magnitude as a function of IL-1β doses. A prominent neutrophilia was noted within several hours, to be followed by a more sustained thrombocytosis. Administration of 100 ng/kg IL-1β or higher resulted in a severe drop of the systolic blood pressure in almost all the subjects.[9-11] These dramatic effects of IL-1β illustrate why its production is tightly controlled at several levels. These include the regulation of gene transcription, mRNA turnover (presence of AU-rich elements), translation, and secretion.

There is some evidence to indicate that IL-1 controls immune responses and exerts proinflammatory activities (Fig. 60.3) through:

- Stimulation of T cells
- Expression of adhesion molecules on endothelial cells
- Cytokine and chemokine expression (IL-6, IL-8, etc.)
- Acute-phase protein production
- Production of inflammatory mediators (prostaglandins, nitric oxide, platelet-activating factor)
- Matrix metalloproteinase production
- Release of RANK ligand and osteoclast activation

Several experimental studies indicate that IL-1 is involved in the development of arthritis. Gene knockout animals deficient in IL-1β or

THE FAMILY OF IL-1 RECEPTORS

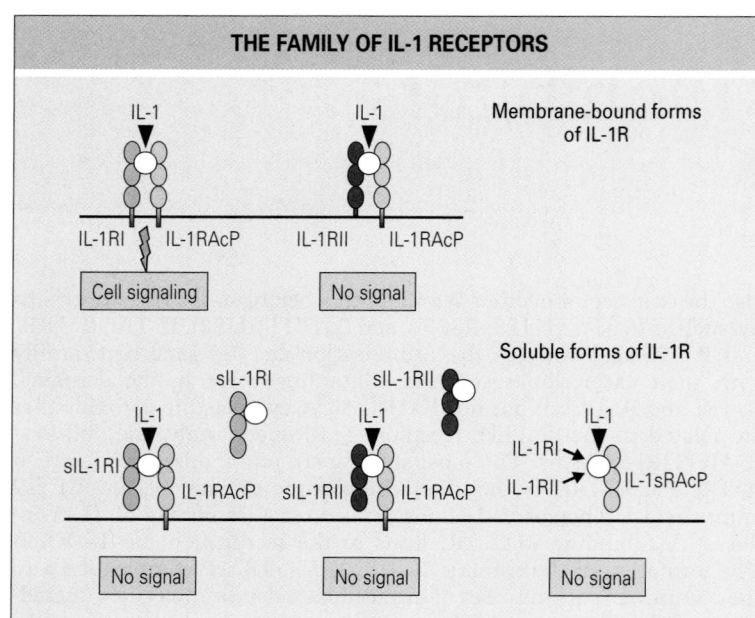

Fig. 60.1 The family of IL-1 receptors (membrane-bound and soluble forms) and their role in IL-1 signal transduction regulation. Interleukin-1 signals into the cell on binding to IL-1 receptor type I (IL-1RI), which subsequently recruits IL-1 receptor accessory protein (IL-1RAcP). IL-1 signaling is regulated by different combinations between membrane-bound and soluble IL1 receptor type II (IL-1RII) and soluble forms of IL-1RI and sIL-1RAcP. IL-1RII lacks a long cytoplasmic domain and does not exert any signaling activity on IL-1 binding (decoy receptor). Proteolytic cleavage of the extracellular domain of IL-1RII plays an additional role in the control of IL-1 activities by preventing the interaction between IL-1 and cell surface receptors. Additionally, sIL-1RAcP competes with membrane-bound IL-1RAcP for interacting with IL-1RI and therefore neutralizes the effect of IL-1. *(Redrawn with permission from Jacques C, Gosset M, Berenbaum F, Gabay C. The role of IL-1 and IL-1Ra in joint inflammation and cartilage degradation. Vitam Horm 2006;74:371-403.)*

POTENTIAL STRATEGIES TO BLOCK THE EFFECT OF IL-1

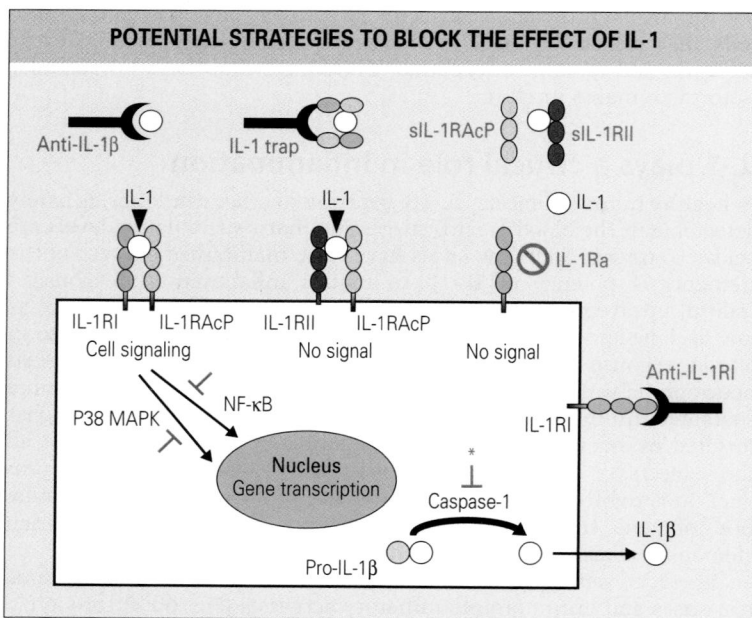

Fig. 60.2 Potential strategies to block the effect of IL-1. The maturation and release of IL-1β can be inhibited by caspase-1 inhibitors. Extracellular free IL-1 can be blocked by specific antibodies (e.g., anti-IL-1β), fusion molecules containing binding motifs of IL-1 receptors (IL-1 trap), and soluble receptors (sIL-1RII, sIL-1RAcP). Binding to cell surface receptors can be inhibited by IL-1Ra and antibodies directed against IL-1RI (anti–IL-1RI). Postreceptor signaling inhibitors targeting p38 MAPK and NF-κB pathways can block the biologic effect of IL-1 and of other cytokines. *refers to caspase-1 inhibitors. *(Redrawn with permission from Jacques C, Gosset M, Berenbaum F, Gabay C. The role of IL-1 and IL-1Ra in joint inflammation and cartilage degradation. Vitam Horm 2006;74:371-403.)*

SYSTEMATIC MANIFESTATIONS OF IL-1β

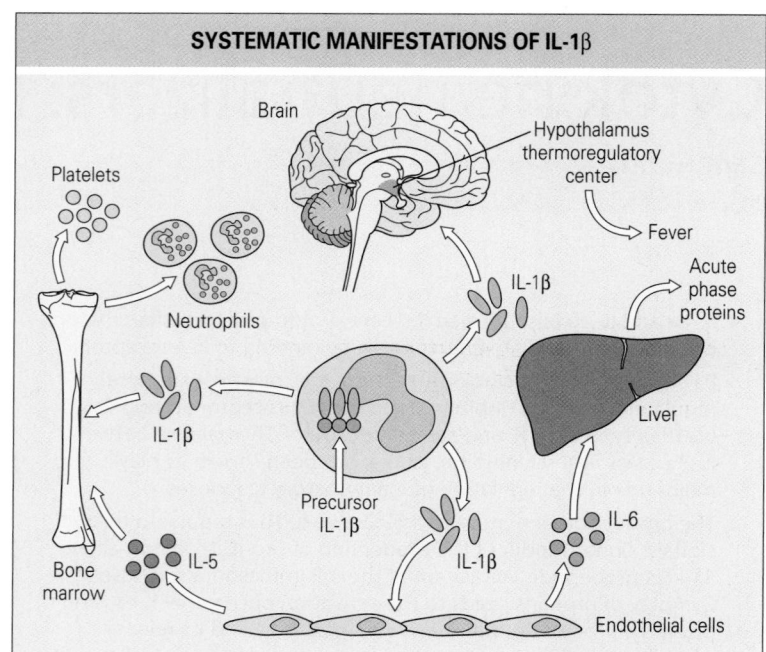

Fig. 60.3 Systemic manifestations of IL-1β. Active IL-1β is secreted by many cell types, including monocytes and macrophages (center). IL-1β enters in the circulation and binds to IL-1R on hypothalamic vascular network, resulting in the synthesis of COX-2, which causes a rise in prostaglandin E_2 levels, thus activating the thermoregulatory center for fever production. In the periphery, IL-1β activates endothelial cells, resulting in increased expression of adhesion molecules, chemokines, and IL-6 production. IL-6 stimulates the production of acute-phase proteins by the hepatocytes. IL-1β also acts on bone marrow to increase the mobilization of granulocyte progenitors and mature neutrophils, resulting in neutrophilia. IL-1β–induced IL-6 increases platelet production, resulting in thrombocytosis. IL-6 also stimulates hepcidin production by hepatocytes, resulting in increased iron storage in macrophages and decreased intestinal iron absorption. IL-1β also causes decreased erythropoietin response, thus causing anemia. *(Redrawn from Dinarello CA. Blocking IL-1 in systemic inflammation. J Exp Med 2005;201:1355-1359, copyright Rockefeller Experimental University Press.)*

IL-1RI are protected from the occurrence of collagen-induced arthritis, and the administration of blocking anti-IL-1β antibodies or recombinant IL-1Ra attenuated the severity of several experimental models of arthritis.[12]

The importance of IL-1Ra as an endogenous modulator of inflammatory responses has been demonstrated by the use of gene knockout mice. IL-1Ra–deficient mice bred into the BALB/c background present a spontaneous form of polyarthritis and exhibit elevated levels of autoantibodies such as rheumatoid factors, antibodies to double-stranded DNA, and collagen type II.[13] The mRNAs for proinflammatory cytokines such as IL-1β, IL-6, and tumor necrosis factor-α (TNF-α) are elevated in the joints of these arthritic mice, indicating an important regulatory role for IL-1Ra in the cytokine network. Subsequent studies indicated that TNF-α, IL-23, and IL-17 are required for the development of arthritis. In addition, arthritis does not develop in germ-free conditions and TLR4-deficient mice have an attenuated form of arthritis indicating the dependence of the microbial flora. TLR4 enhanced the disease by activating Th17 cells and increasing IL-17 production.[14] These results suggest that uncontrolled IL-1 activities in response to microbial products may induce the spontaneous development of arthritis through an imbalance in the cytokine network and alterations in T-cell function. Accordingly, the contribution of innate immune cells is particularly important to the equilibrium between IL-1 and IL-1Ra and the subsequent immune responses. Conditional knockout mice in which myeloid cells including macrophages and dendritic cells are selectively deficient in IL-1Ra exhibit an earlier onset and more severe form of collagen-induced arthritis with increased Th1 and Th17 responses.[15] The recent description of children with genetic deficiency in IL-1Ra exhibiting early and severe systemic autoinflammatory clinical manifestations and a rapid favorable response after the administration of recombinant IL-1Ra further supports the fundamental role of this cytokine in the regulation of inflammatory responses.[16]

The regulation of IL-1β maturation by the inflammasome

The mechanisms leading to the processing and release of mature IL-1β have great relevance to many acute and chronic inflammatory diseases. It is currently hypothesized that two signals are required for IL-1β release from normal human monocytes. Toll-like receptors and NOD-like receptors (NLRs), two major recognition systems of the innate immune system, are involved in signal 1 and signal 2, respectively. First, Pro-IL-1β synthesis is stimulated on binding of bacterial or endogenous components to TLR; that is, lipopolysaccharide, a typical gram-negative bacteria component, is a common stimulus for signal 1 through binding to TLR4. The second signal is NLR-induced IL-1β processing and release through a caspase-1–dependent mechanism involving the cell surface nucleotide receptor $P2X_7$. ATP binding to $P2X_7$ receptor induces potassium efflux from the cell. The mechanism whereby loss of potassium from the cell leads to activation of caspase-1 is not completely known, but it requires NALP3/cryopyrin, an NLR family member, and the adaptor protein ASC (apoptosis-associated speck-like protein CARD domain).[17,18] The inflammasome is a caspase-activating complex in the cytosol containing caspase-1 and caspase-5, an adaptor protein ASC, and the sensor protein of the NLR family. The interaction of microbial molecules or of endogenous factors such as monosodium urate crystals to the inflammasome leads to the activation of caspase-1 from a pro-molecule. Studies in NALP3/cryopyrin-deficient mice indicate a requirement for NALP3/cryopyrin in TLR- and ATP-induced assembly of the inflammasome.[17,18] Thus, stimulation through both TLRs and NLRs as well as an intact NALP3/cryopyrin inflammasome are all required for processing and release of IL-1β (as well as IL-18) from monocytes.[19] Interestingly, the activation of the NALP3/cryopyrin inflammasome has proven particularly important for many diseases characterized by an overproduction of IL-1β, such as some periodic fever syndromes and crystal-induced arthritis.[20-23]

THERAPEUTIC INHIBITORS OF IL-1 IN RHEUMATIC DISEASES

Figure 60.2 depicts the different strategies that have been developed to inhibit the biologic effects of IL-1. The subsequent paragraphs describe the effect of IL-1 antagonists in the different rheumatic diseases (Table 60-1).

Rheumatoid arthritis

Anakinra (Kineret)

A 24-week randomized double-blind, placebo-controlled multicenter trial including 472 patients with rheumatoid arthritis (RA), as well as the 24-week extension of this study, demonstrated that anakinra, at a daily dose of 150 mg, was more efficacious than placebo according to the American College of Rheumatology (ACR) response criteria.[24,25] In addition, a significantly greater retardation of radiologic joint damage was observed at 48 weeks in comparison with 24 weeks in patients treated with IL-1Ra alone.[26] In two further trials in RA, anakinra was

TABLE 60.1 IL-1 INHIBITORS IN THE TREATMENT OF RHEUMATIC DISEASES

Disease	Biologic agent	Type of study	Primary outcome	Results
RA	Anakinra	RCT	ACR20 response criteria	Significant improvement[24,25]
RA	Anakinra	RCT	Genant and Larsen scores	Limits structural damage[26]
RA	Anakinra + MTX	RCT	ACR20 response criteria	Significant improvement[27,28]
		RCT	HAQ-DI	Significant improvement[29]
RA	Anakinra + etanercept vs. etanercept	RCT	ACR50 response criteria	No difference but increased frequency of SIE[34]
RA	Rilonacept + MTX	RCT	ACR20 response criteria	Non-significant effect[†]
RA	Canakinumab + MTX	RCT	ACR20 response criteria	Non-significant effect[46]
RA	AMG 108 + MTX	RCT	ACR20 response criteria	Significant improvement[47]
RA	Pralnacasan + DMARDs	RCT	ACR20 response criteria	Non-significant effect[48]
AS	Anakinra	Case series	Multiple outcomes	Improvement[49]
AS	Anakinra	Case series	ASAS response criteria	ASAS20 in 5/20 patients[50]
PsA	Anakinra	Case series	Multiple outcomes	Improvement of arthritis but no effect on skin psoriasis[51]
SLE	Anakinra	Case series	Multiple outcomes	Improvement in two thirds of patients[52]
SLE	Anakinra	Case series	Multiple outcomes	Some improvement[53]
Knee OA	Anakinra vs. placebo	RCT	WOMAC questionnaire	No improvement[54]
Gout	Anakinra	Case series	Multiple outcomes	Improvements in all[57]
Gout	Rilonacept	Placebo-controlled*	Pain visual analog score	Improvement[60]
Gout	Rilonacept	RCT	Prophylaxis of gout flares	Significant preventive effect[†]
Pseudogout	Anakinra	Case reports	Multiple outcomes	Improvement and prevention[58,59]
SOJIA	Anakinra	Case series	Multiple outcomes	Remission in some cases[61,62]
AOSD	Anakinra	Case series	Multiple outcomes	Improvement[64]
FCAS, MWS	Anakinra	Case series	Multiple outcomes	Improvement[65,66]
FCAS	Rilonacept	Case series	Multiple outcomes	Improvement[67]
FCAS and MWS	Rilonacept	RCT	Composite score	Significant improvement[68]

AOSD, adult-onset Still's disease; AS, ankylosing spondylitis; FCAS, familial cold autoinflammatory syndrome; HAQ-DI, Health Assessment Questionnaire-Disability Index; MWS, Muckle-Wells syndrome; OA, osteoarthritis; PsA, psoriatic arthritis; RA, rheumatoid arthritis; RCT, randomized placebo-controlled clinical trial; SOJIA, systemic-onset juvenile idiopathic arthritis.
*Non-randomized, single-blind study.
†Unpublished study.

administrated in combination with methotrexate in patients with active RA despite treatment by methotrexate for 6 consecutive months. The combination of methotrexate with anakinra (1 mg/kg and 2 mg/kg) resulted in a significantly higher rate of ACR responses (ACR20 to ACR70) than in those treated with methotrexate alone.[27,28] Anakinra also improved the functional status of responding RA patients and led to greater improvements in patient-reported than physician-reported outcomes.[29,30]

Safety data of larger population indicate that anakinra in combination with methotrexate as well as other disease-modifying antirheumatic drugs (DMARDs) is safe with a rate of serious infections slightly higher in the anakinra than in the placebo group (2.1% vs. 0.4%). The safety profile of anakinra was high even in patients with multiple comorbid conditions.[31-33]

In preclinical studies, it was demonstrated that the administration of IL-1Ra in combination with PEGylated soluble TNF receptor type I was superior to either therapy alone. In a randomized clinical trial the combination of anakinra and etanercept versus etanercept alone in RA patients did not show any advantage of the combination treatment regimen. Moreover, the incidence of serious infections was significantly higher in patients receiving the combination, indicating that blockade of two cytokines involved in innate immune responses may result in increased susceptibility to infections.[34] The use of anakinra in patients who had a previous incomplete response to TNF-α inhibitors did not show any advantage in a recent study.[35]

Soluble IL-1 receptors

The administration of soluble IL-1RI resulted in significant attenuation of joint inflammation and tissue damage in an experimental model of arthritis.[36] In contrast, treatment with soluble IL-1RI administered either by intra-articular or subcutaneous injection was devoid of significant effect in patients with RA.[37] The administration of soluble IL-1RI may have inhibited the binding of IL-1Ra to cell surface IL-1 receptors, thus further enhancing the inflammatory effects of IL-1 on target cells. Soluble IL-1RII binds to IL-1β with higher affinity than IL-1Ra and could thus constitute a promising IL-1 inhibitor. The administration of soluble IL-1RII in experimental models resulted in a marked inhibition of joint swelling and joint damage and exerted a chondroprotective effect in vitro.[38-40] Despite these interesting effects, clinical trials with soluble IL-1RII have been abandoned. A soluble form of the IL-1 receptor accessory protein (sIL-1RAcP) is also present in the circulation of healthy individuals. sIL-1RAcP increases the binding affinity of IL-1α or IL-1β to soluble IL-1RII by 100-fold, while leaving unaltered the low binding affinity of IL-1Ra.[41] Local production of sIL-1RAcP by injection of transduced fibroblasts into knee joints led to a marked reduction in inflammation and in cartilage and bone destruction.[42] Systemic delivery of either IL-1Ra or sIL-1RAcP using adenoviral vectors prevented the development of collagen-induced arthritis in mice; in contrast to IL-1Ra, IL-1RAcP ameliorated the arthritis without affecting T-cell immunity.[43] Currently, no data are available on the use of sIL-1RAcP in patients with RA.

IL-1 trap (rilonacept [Arcalyst]) is a fusion protein containing some of the extracellular binding motifs of IL-1RI and IL-1RAcP coupled to the Fc fraction of the human immunoglobulin IgG1. IL-1 trap binds IL-1β with a much stronger affinity than IL-1Ra and, thus, should not affect the anti-inflammatory effect of endogenous IL-1Ra. IL-1 trap has a prolonged circulating half-life ranging from 128 to 214 hours that permits once-weekly subcutaneous dosing. Administration of a murine form of IL-1 trap almost completely blocked the development of mouse collagen-induced arthritis.[44] In a phase I randomized, dose escalating, double-blind, placebo-controlled trial, an average ACR20 was achieved by 74% of patients receiving the highest dose of IL-1 trap as compared with 36% of placebo-treated patients.[45] A multicenter, randomized, double-blind, placebo-controlled phase II clinical trial including 200 RA patients failed to show a significant effect even in patients receiving the highest dose of IL-1 trap (100 mg weekly), but these results have not been published so far.

Monoclonal antibodies

The safety and efficacy of ACZ885 (canakinumab [Ilaris]), an intravenously or subcutaneously infused, fully human monoclonal antibody that neutralizes the bioactivity of human IL-1β, was recently examined in a 6-week randomized, placebo-controlled, dose-escalating, clinical trial including 32 RA patients with incomplete response to methotrexate. In comparison with methotrexate alone, a higher number of patients achieved an ACR20 response with the combination of methotrexate and the highest dose of ACZ885 (10 mg/kg), although the difference was not statistically significant.[46]

Neutralizing antibodies against IL-1RI have the theoretical advantage to block the bioactivity of both IL-1α and IL-1β. The safety and efficacy of AMG-108, a fully human anti-IL-1RI monoclonal antibody was examined in 813 RA patients who had an inadequate response to methotrexate in a 24-week randomized, double-blind, placebo-controlled, parallel-dosing clinical trial. AMG-108 was administered subcutaneously monthly at doses of 50, 125, or 250 mg in combination with methotrexate. After 24 weeks, 40.4% and 20.2% of patients receiving the highest dose of AMG-108 achieved ACR20 and ACR50 responses as compared with 29.1% and 8.4% in those treated with methotrexate alone ($P = .022$ and $P < .001$, respectively). No difference was detected between the different groups regarding the ACR70 response. There were no notable differences in either the frequency or type of adverse events.[47]

Inhibition of IL-1β production

Caspase-1 cleaves pro-IL-1β (and pro-IL-18) to generate mature active cytokines, and is therefore a potential target in the treatment of arthritis. Consistent with this hypothesis, the administration of a caspase-1 inhibitor blocked the progression of collagen-induced arthritis in mice. The efficacy and safety of pralnacasan, a synthetic orally administered caspase-1 inhibitor, was examined in a 12-week phase 2 placebo-controlled multicenter study in RA patients receiving concurrent DMARDs. ACR20 response rate was not significantly higher in patients treated with pralnacasan than in the placebo group.[48] This disappointing result can be partly explained by the fact that other enzymes are also able to cleave pro-IL-1β. In addition, caspase-1 does not influence the biologic effects of IL-1α.

Taken together, the results of clinical trials using anakinra as well as other IL-1 inhibitors showed only modest effects in the treatment of RA patients. Despite the absence of controlled trials, these results as well as those of clinical practice suggest that the effects of IL-1 blockade on disease activity are weaker than those obtained with anti-TNF agents. These findings indicate that, although some patients showed a clear benefit of this therapeutic strategy, IL-1 may not be an important target in the treatment of RA.

Ankylosing spondylitis

Anakinra treatment was moderately successful in a subset of patients with ankylosing spondylitis (AS). In a 3-month open-label study, 9 patients received daily subcutaneous injections of anakinra. The results showed significant improvement in the Bath AS functional index (BASFI), Bath AS disease activity index (BASDAI), AS Quality of Life, and biologic markers of inflammation (C-reactive protein [CRP] and erythrocyte sedimentation rate). Sixty-one percent of enthesitis and osteitis lesions improved, as assessed by magnetic resonance imaging (MRI).[49] In another open-label clinical trial, 100 mg of anakinra was administered daily by subcutaneous injections to 20 AS patients refractory to non-steroidal anti-inflammatory drugs. After 24 weeks, ASAS20, ASAS40, and ASAS70 responses were achieved by 5, 4, and 2 patients, respectively. There was no change in serum levels of CRP or MRI scores.[50]

Psoriatic arthritis

An open-label, proof-of-concept, single-center study of 12 patients with psoriatic arthritis demonstrated significant clinical benefits. After 12 weeks, 50% met the psoriatic arthritis response criteria. In this study, anakinra had no effect on the cutaneous manifestations of psoriasis.[51]

Systemic lupus erythematosus

Anakinra led to interesting results in a few patients with lupus arthritis.[52,53]

Osteoarthritis

In patients with osteoarthritis, a good effect was observed in an open-label trial when anakinra was administered as a single intra-articular injection. However, the results of a subsequent randomized, double-blind, placebo-controlled study failed to show positive effects of a single intra-articular injection of 50 mg or 150 mg anakinra in knee OA at the 12-week evaluation.[54] This result is not unexpected considering the short half-life of IL-1Ra. Of note, there was a positive trend ($P = .051$) regarding the Western Ontario McMaster Universities Osteoarthritis Index (WOMAC) pain score at day 4 in the 150-mg anakinra group as compared with placebo. These findings suggest that continuous treatment with anakinra or another IL-1 antagonist may have beneficial effects on pain. In addition, further studies should investigate the rationale of IL-1 targeting in the prevention of cartilage damage.

Crystal-induced arthritis

Monosodium urate (MSU) and calcium pyrophosphate dihydrate (CPPD) crystals are the agents responsible for gout and pseudogout, respectively. Both MSU and CPPD crystals are able to stimulate the production of IL-1β by monocytes and macrophages through mechanisms similar to those induced by microbial components. MSU crystals bind to TLRs and activate the synthesis of pro-IL-1β. In addition, MSU and CPPD crystals can stimulate the NALP3 inflammasome leading to an increased IL-1β production.[23] The results of experimental studies indicate that monocytes and macrophages are the cellular sources of IL-1β and that endothelial and stromal cells respond to IL-1β.[55] The hypothesis was proposed that IL-1β induction of adhesion molecules and chemokines is critical for the migration of polymorphonuclear neutrophils, resulting in the occurrence of acute arthritis.[56]

A first open-label clinical trial including 10 patients with gout refractory to classical therapy showed that administration of a 3-day course of anakinra (100 mg/day) led to a rapid resolution of inflammatory signs within 2 days without any adverse event.[57] More recently, anakinra was shown to be efficacious in the treatment of an acute episode of severe pseudogout refractory to non-steroidal anti-inflammatory drugs and glucocorticoids.[58] Chronic administration of anakinra, 100 mg, to a patient with frequent pseudogout episodes and end-stage renal failure prevented the occurrence of acute attacks for more than 8 months of observation.[59]

Other IL-1 antagonists have been examined in the treatment of gout. The use of rilonacept (IL-1 trap) in a clinical trial on acute gout has provided interesting preliminary results.[60] In addition, a recent 12-week, multicenter, randomized, double-blind, placebo-controlled, clinical trial examined the efficacy and safety of rilonacept in the prophylaxis of gout flares during urate-lowering therapy. The results showed that patients receiving an initial dose of 320 mg rilonacept followed by weekly doses of 160 mg rilonacept in combination with allopurinol experienced significantly fewer gout attacks than those treated with allopurinol and placebo (unpublished data). The effect of canakinumab (anti-IL-1β) in gout is currently under investigation in clinical trials.

Systemic-onset juvenile idiopathic arthritis and adult Still's disease

Recently, some elegant studies suggested that IL-1β is involved in the pathophysiology of systemic-onset juvenile idiopathic arthritis (SOJIA). Incubation of peripheral blood mononuclear cells of healthy donors in the serum of patients with SOJIA induced an increased production of IL-1β. Treatment with anakinra was reported to be dramatically successful in 9 patients with SOJIA. These patients had failed treatment with numerous other agents, including corticosteroids, methotrexate, and TNF-α inhibitors.[61] A recent observational study indicates that patients with SOJIA can be divided as good responders, partial responders, or non-responders. Of note, only 40% of patients had a dramatic and persistent response leading to the reduction or discontinuation of co-medications, including corticosteroids. Higher neutrophil count and lower number of active joints was associated with a good response to anakinra. In vitro the production of IL-1β or IL-18 by monocytes from SOJIA patients in response to various stimuli was not increased and was independent of treatment efficacy. Likewise, IL-1Ra production

was not impaired in SOJIA. Surprisingly, the release of IL-1β production in response to exogenous ATP was decreased without any relation with treatment response.[62] Anakinra may also be useful in the treatment of macrophage activation syndrome, a severe complication occurring in some cases of SOJIA.[63] Anakinra has been reported to be effective in adult Still's disease, with responses that could be even better than in SOJIA.[64]

Canakinumab has also been examined in patients with SOJIA. Currently in phase 3 clinical development, canakinumab was recently granted European Union and U.S. orphan drug status for this condition as well as for cryopyrin-associated periodic syndromes (see later). Early clinical trials have shown that administration of canakinumab every 2 weeks is safe and effective, offering thus a considerable advantage over anakinra.

IL-1 inhibition in periodic fever syndromes

The term *cryopyrinopathies* or *cryopyrin-associated periodic syndromes (CAPS)* was coined for a group of inherited disorders, including neonatal-onset multisystem inflammatory disease (NOMID) (also known as chronic infantile neurologic, cutaneous, articular syndrome [CINCA]), Muckle-Wells syndrome (MWS), and familial cold autoinflammatory syndrome (FCAS), characterized by recurrent episodes of fever and inflammatory responses in multiple organs such as the joints, skin, eyes, ears, and central nervous system. All these diseases have been associated with mutations of the CIAS1 or NLRP3 gene, encoding for cryopyrin or NALP3, leading to the spontaneous assembly of the inflammasome with increased caspase-1 activation and IL-1β secretion. The administration of anakinra to patients with MWS and FCAS resulted in the cessation of symptoms within hours of the first injection, with a concomitant decrease in serum amyloid A, an acute-phase protein, that reached normal levels after 3 days of treatment.[65,66] Significant improvement in NOMID/CINCA with anakinra has also been reported. Taken together, these marked beneficial effects of anakinra and the identification of the mandatory role of the inflammasome complex in IL-1β secretion opened the way for clinical trials aiming at blocking IL-1β activity in autoinflammatory diseases belonging to the family of CAPS. Rilonacept has also been tested with success in these diseases. In an initial open-label clinical trial including 5 patients with FCAS, rilonacept was administered subcutaneously at a loading dose of 300 mg, followed by weekly injections. The clinical symptoms subsided within hours after the initial injection of rilonacept. In the extension study, dosage escalation to 160 mg to 320 mg resulted in better control of rash and arthralgia as well as to lower levels of acute-phase proteins. Of note, 3 patients with hearing loss demonstrated no further hearing deterioration during the following 2 years.[67] These favorable results were confirmed by two consecutive randomized, placebo-controlled phase 3 clinical trials including 47 adults with CAPS. The treatment was well tolerated besides injection site reactions and upper respiratory tract infections.[68] These results led to the approval of rilonacept by the U.S. Food and Drug Administration for the treatment of FCAS and MWS in adults or children age 12 years or older. Early reports suggest that canakinumab is also efficacious in the treatment of patients with CAPS.

Several other disorders featuring periodic fever, joint symptoms, and systemic manifestations are also classified as "autoinflammatory diseases." These conditions include familial Mediterranean fever (FMF), TNF receptor–associated periodic syndrome (TRAPS), hyperimmunoglobulinemia D with periodic fever syndrome, and Blau syndrome. With the exception of hyperimmunoglobulinemia D with periodic fever syndrome and TRAPS, these diseases are linked with mutations in proteins participating in the inflammasome complex.[69] The spectacular effect of anakinra treatment in MWS inspired several clinical trials in other autoinflammatory syndromes. Symptom regression after anakinra treatment was observed in pyogenic arthritis, pyoderma gangrenosum acne (PAPA) syndrome, and FMF patients who did not respond to colchicine.[70] Interestingly, anakinra had also a beneficial effect in TRAPS, an inherited disease due to a mutation modifying the control of TNF signaling but not IL-1 regulation.[71] In addition to systemic autoinflammatory diseases associated with mutations in proteins related to inflammasome, anakinra also displays efficacy in Schnitzler's syndrome.[72]

KEY REFERENCES

1. Dinarello CA. Biologic basis for interleukin-1 in disease. Blood 1996;87:2095-2147.

4. Black RA, Kronheim SR, Cantrell M, et al. Generation of biologically active interleukin-1 beta by proteolytic cleavage of the inactive precursor. J Biol Chem 1988;263:9437-9442.

5. Sims JE, Giri JG, Dower SK. The two interleukin-1 receptors play different roles in IL-1 actions. Clin Immunol Immunopathol 1994;72:9-14.

6. Colotta F, Dower SK, Sims JE, Mantovani A. The type II "decoy" receptor: a novel regulatory pathway for interleukin 1. Immunol Today 1994;15:562-566.

7. Arend WP, Malyak M, Guthridge CJ, Gabay C. Interleukin-1 receptor antagonist: role in biology. Annu Rev Immunol 1998;16:27-55.

11. Ogilvie AC, Hack CE, Wagstaff J, et al. IL-1 beta does not cause neutrophil degranulation but does lead to IL-6, IL-8, and nitrite/nitrate release when used in patients with cancer. J Immunol 1996;156:389-394.

13. Horai R, Saijo S, Tanioka H, et al. Development of chronic inflammatory arthropathy resembling rheumatoid arthritis in interleukin 1 receptor antagonist-deficient mice. J Exp Med 2000;191:313-320.

14. Abdollahi-Roodsaz S, Joosten LA, Roelofs MF, et al. Inhibition of Toll-like receptor 4 breaks the inflammatory loop in autoimmune destructive arthritis. Arthritis Rheum 2007;56:2957-2967.

15. Lamacchia C, Palmer G, Seemayer CA, et al. Myeloid cell specific interleukin-1 receptor antagonist deficiency enhances Th1 and Th17 responses and the severity of arthritis. Arthritis Rheum 2010;62:452-462.

16. Aksentijevich I, Masters S, Ferguson PJ, et al. An autoinflammatory disease with deficiency of the interleukin-1 receptor antagonist. N Engl J Med 2009;360:2426-2437.

18. Mariathasan S, Weiss DS, Newton K, et al. Cryopyrin activates the inflammasome in response to toxins and ATP. Nature 2006;440:228-232.

21. Hoffman HM, Mueller JL, Broide DH, et al. Mutation of a new gene encoding a putative pyrin-like protein causes familial cold autoinflammatory syndrome and Muckle-Wells syndrome. Nat Genet 2001;29:301-305.

22. Agostini L, Martinon F, Burns K, et al. NALP3 forms an IL-1beta-processing inflammasome with increased activity in Muckle-Wells autoinflammatory disorder. Immunity 2004;20:319-325.

23. Martinon F, Petrilli V, Mayor A, et al. Gout-associated uric acid crystals activate the NALP3 inflammasome. Nature 2006;440:237-241.

24. Bresnihan B, Alvaro-Gracia JM, Cobby M, et al. Treatment of rheumatoid arthritis with recombinant human interleukin-1 receptor antagonist. Arthritis Rheum 1998;41:2196-2204.

25. Nuki G, Bresnihan B, Bear MB, McCabe D. Long-term safety and maintenance of clinical improvement following treatment with anakinra (recombinant human interleukin-1 receptor antagonist) in patients with rheumatoid arthritis: extension phase of a randomized, double-blind, placebo-controlled trial. Arthritis Rheum 2002;46:2838-2846.

26. Jiang Y, Genant HK, Watt I, et al. A multicenter, double-blind, dose-ranging, randomized, placebo-controlled study of recombinant human interleukin-1 receptor antagonist in patients with rheumatoid arthritis: radiologic progression and correlation of Genant and Larsen scores. Arthritis Rheum 2000;43:1001-1009.

28. Cohen SB, Moreland LW, Cush JJ, et al. A multicentre, double blind, randomised, placebo controlled trial of anakinra (Kineret), a recombinant interleukin 1 receptor antagonist, in patients with rheumatoid arthritis treated with background methotrexate. Ann Rheum Dis 2004;63:1062-1068.

29. Cohen SB, Woolley JM, Chan W. Interleukin 1 receptor antagonist anakinra improves functional status in patients with rheumatoid arthritis. J Rheumatol 2003;30:225-231.

31. Fleischmann RM, Schechtman J, Bennett R, et al. Anakinra, a recombinant human interleukin-1 receptor antagonist (r-metHuIL-1ra), in patients with rheumatoid arthritis: a large, international, multicenter, placebo-controlled trial. Arthritis Rheum 2003;48:927-934.

32. Schiff MH, DiVittorio G, Tesser J, et al. The safety of anakinra in high-risk patients with active rheumatoid arthritis: six-month observations of patients with comorbid conditions. Arthritis Rheum 2004;50:1752-1760.

34. Genovese MC, Cohen S, Moreland L, et al. Combination therapy with etanercept and anakinra in the treatment of patients with rheumatoid arthritis who have been treated unsuccessfully with methotrexate. Arthritis Rheum 2004;50:1412-1419.

35. Buch MH, Bingham SJ, Seto Y, et al. Lack of response to anakinra in rheumatoid arthritis following failure of tumor necrosis factor alpha blockade. Arthritis Rheum 2004;50:725-728.

37. Drevlow BE, Lovis R, Haag MA, et al. Recombinant human interleukin-1 receptor type I in the treatment of patients with active rheumatoid arthritis. Arthritis Rheum 1996;39:257-265.

39. Bessis N, Guery L, Mantovani A, et al. The type II decoy receptor of IL-1 inhibits murine collagen-induced arthritis. Eur J Immunol 2000;30:867-875.

40. Attur MG, Dave MN, Leung MY, et al. Functional genomic analysis of type II IL-1beta decoy receptor: potential for gene therapy in human arthritis and inflammation. J Immunol 2002;168:2001-2010.

41. Smith DE, Hanna R, Della F, et al. The soluble form of IL-1 receptor accessory protein enhances the ability of soluble type II IL-1 receptor to inhibit IL-1 action. Immunity 2003;18:87-96.

43. Smeets RL, Joosten LA, Arntz OJ, et al. Soluble interleukin-1 receptor accessory protein ameliorates collagen-induced arthritis by a different mode of action from that of interleukin-1 receptor antagonist. Arthritis Rheum 2005;52:2202-2211.

44. Economides AN, Carpenter LR, Rudge JS, et al. Cytokine traps: multi-component, high-affinity blockers of cytokine action. Nat Med 2003;9:47-52.

45. Guler HP, Caldwell J, Littlejohn T, et al. A phase 1, single dose escalation study of IL-1 Trap in patients with rheumatoid arthritis. Arthritis Rheum 2001;44:S370.

46. Alten R, Gram H, Joosten LA, et al. The human anti-IL-1 beta monoclonal antibody ACZ885 is effective in joint inflammation models in mice and in a proof-of-concept study in patients with rheumatoid arthritis. Arthritis Res Ther 2008;10:R67.

47. Bensen WG, Cardiel MH, Forejtova S, et al. Results of a phase 2 randomized, double-blind study of AMG 108 (a fully human monoclonal antibody to IL-1R type I) in patients with rheumatoid arthritis. Arthritis Rheum 2008;58:S535.

48. Pavelka K, Rasmussen MJ, Mikkelsen K, et al. Clinical effects of pralnacasan (PRAL), an orally-active

interleukin-1 beta converting enzyme (ICE) inhibitor, in a 285 patient Phase II trial in rheumatoid arthritis. Arthritis Rheum 2002;46:LB02.

49. Tan AL, Marzo-Ortega H, O'Connor P, et al. Efficacy of anakinra in active ankylosing spondylitis: a clinical and magnetic resonance imaging study. Ann Rheum Dis 2004;63:1041-1045.

50. Haibel H, Rudwaleit M, Listing J, Sieper J. Open label trial of anakinra in active ankylosing spondylitis over 24 weeks. Ann Rheum Dis 2005;64:296-298.

51. Gibbs A, Markham T, Walsh C, et al. Anakinra (Kineret) in psoriasis and psoriatic arthritis: a single-center, open-label, pilot study. Arthritis Res Ther 2005;7:68.

53. Ostendorf B, Iking-Konert C, Kurz K, et al. Preliminary results of safety and efficacy of the interleukin 1 receptor antagonist anakinra in patients with severe lupus arthritis. Ann Rheum Dis 2005;64:630-633.

54. Chevalier X, Goupille P, Beaulieu AD, et al. Intraarticular injection of anakinra in osteoarthritis of the knee: a multicenter, randomized, double-blind, placebo-controlled study. Arthritis Rheum 2009;61:344-352.

57. So A, De Smedt T, Revaz S, Tschopp J. A pilot study of IL-1 inhibition by anakinra in acute gout. Arthritis Res Ther 2007;9:R28.

58. McGonagle D, Tan AL, Madden J, et al. Successful treatment of resistant pseudogout with anakinra. Arthritis Rheum 2008;58:631-633.

59. Announ N, Palmer G, Guerne PA, Gabay C. Anakinra is a possible alternative in the treatment and prevention of acute attacks of pseudogout in end-stage renal failure. Joint Bone Spine 2009;76:424-426.

61. Pascual V, Allantaz F, Arce E, et al. Role of interleukin-1 (IL-1) in the pathogenesis of systemic onset juvenile idiopathic arthritis and clinical response to IL-1 blockade. J Exp Med 2005;201:1479-1486.

62. Gattorno M, Piccini A, Lasiglie D, et al. The pattern of response to anti-interleukin-1 treatment distinguishes two subsets of patients with systemic-onset juvenile idiopathic arthritis. Arthritis Rheum 2008;58:1505-1515.

64. Lequerre T, Quartier P, Rosellini D, et al. Interleukin-1 receptor antagonist (anakinra) treatment in patients with systemic-onset juvenile idiopathic arthritis or adult onset Still disease: preliminary experience in France. Ann Rheum Dis 2008;67:302-308.

65. Hoffman HM, Rosengren S, Boyle DL, et al. Prevention of cold-associated acute inflammation in familial cold autoinflammatory syndrome by interleukin-1 receptor antagonist. Lancet 2004;364:1779-1785.

66. Hawkins PN, Lachmann HJ, McDermott MF. Interleukin-1-receptor antagonist in the Muckle-Wells syndrome. N Engl J Med 2003;348:2583-2584.

68. Hoffman HM, Throne ML, Amar NJ, et al. Efficacy and safety of rilonacept (interleukin-1 Trap) in patients with cryopyrin-associated periodic syndromes: results from two sequential placebo-controlled studies. Arthritis Rheum 2008;58:2443-2452.

69. Burger D, Dayer JM, Palmer G, Gabay C. Is IL-1 a good therapeutic target in the treatment of arthritis? Best Pract Res Clin Rheumatol 2006;20:879-896.

70. Dierselhuis MP, Frenkel J, Wulffraat NM, Boelens JJ. Anakinra for flares of pyogenic arthritis in PAPA syndrome. Rheumatology (Oxford) 2005;44:406-408.

72. Martinez-Taboada VM, Fontalba A, Blanco R, Fernandez-Luna JL. Successful treatment of refractory Schnitzler syndrome with anakinra: comment on the article by Hawkins et al. Arthritis Rheum 2005;52:2226-2227.

REFERENCES

Full references for this chapter can be found on www.expertconsult.com.

Tumor necrosis factor blocking therapies

61

John J. Cush and Arthur Kavanaugh
Edited and revised by Peter C. Taylor

- Tumor necrosis factor (TNF) has multiple proinflammatory effects and plays a key role in rheumatoid arthritis.
- Inhibition of TNF with monoclonal antibodies or the p75 soluble receptor leads to a rapid and significant improvement in rheumatoid arthritis activity. Clinical effect is observed within weeks of starting therapy, with ACR 20 responses observed in 50% to 70% of patients. Improvement in quality of life, functional status, and structural progression is observed with these therapies.
- Anti-TNF therapy appears more effective in combination with methotrexate than as a monotherapy.
- Anti-TNF therapy also significantly benefits those with juvenile arthritis, psoriatic arthritis, psoriasis, and ankylosing spondylitis.
- Serious adverse events are rare but include serious infection, tuberculosis, demyelinating syndromes, increased risk of certain malignancies, and drug-induced lupus.

INTRODUCTION

The introduction of biologic agents targeting tumor necrosis factor (TNF) has significantly modified the treatment paradigm for numerous inflammatory disorders and unequivocally validated TNF as a molecular target for therapy. The clinical success and impact of TNF inhibitors has fostered the development of other biologic and small molecule modulators of proinflammatory cytokines. Monoclonal antibodies or Fv antibody fragments have specificity for TNF-α. In contrast, the fusion protein etanercept acts as a competitive inhibitor of TNF-α and can also bind lymphotoxin (TNF-β). TNF inhibition appears to be safe, well tolerated, and capable of ameliorating a variety of inflammatory disorders, although the range of disease phenotypes responding appears to differ with the two biologic approaches to TNF inhibition currently available such that doses of etanercept effective in rheumatoid and other forms of inflammatory arthritis are not effective in granulomatous diseases such as inflammatory bowel disease, in distinction to the antibodies, which are. As such, therapeutic TNF inhibition has expanded our understanding of the pathogenesis of these diseases, the role of TNF in health and inflammation, and the proper use of parenterally administered biologic agents.

Although TNF plays an important regulatory role in host defense, the amplified and dysregulated production of this cytokine mediates the inflammatory response that characterizes disorders such as rheumatoid arthritis (RA), ankylosing spondylitis, Crohn disease, psoriatic arthritis, psoriasis, and other inflammatory disorders. Numerous studies have documented the excess production of local and systemic TNF and a reciprocal rise in TNF receptors (TNF-Rs) in these disorders. Byproducts of TNF-mediated proinflammatory events are also evident. Excessive levels of other proinflammatory cytokines, increased nitric oxide, collagenase, prostaglandins, increased adhesion molecule expression, and evidence of spontaneous erosive synovitis are all found in both human inflammatory diseases and transgenic mice overexpressing TNF.[1-3] TNF is therefore an attractive molecular target for therapy. Definitive verification of a primary role for TNF in these disorders comes from clinical trials demonstrating the impressive amelioration of disease with TNF blockade.

Clinical studies have shown that TNF blockade in RA, psoriatic arthritis (PsA), and ankylosing spondylitis (AS) consistently improves disease activity and quality of life, and it lessens radiographic progression of peripheral joint damage. Three biologic agents that inhibit TNF have been approved for RA and prescribed to more than a million patients worldwide: the soluble dimeric p75 TNF-receptor IgG1-Fc fusion construct (etanercept), a chimeric anti-TNF-α IgG1 monoclonal antibody (mAb) (infliximab), and a human IgG1 anti-TNF-α mAb (adalimumab).[4-6] On the basis of the success of these agents, other biologics targeting TNF are being developed for clinical use. For example, certolizumab pegol was approved by the U.S. Food and Drug Administration for use in Crohn disease in 2008 and both this agent and golimumab are in advanced stages of clinical development for use in a number of potential indications. Numerous advances in RA therapeutics alone have been realized with the development of this class of therapy. Box 61.1 lists the several benefits seen with TNF blockade, including wide approval in many inflammatory disorders, higher remission rates, protection against structural/radiographic deterioration, and possibly a reduced rate of cardiovascular events in RA patients.[7,8]

MECHANISM OF ACTION

TNF and TNF receptors are members of a family of molecules (including Fas-ligand/Fas, CD40 ligand/CD40) possessing crucial regulatory functions that include cellular activation and apoptosis. TNF is an attractive therapeutic target owing to its abundant expression in the rheumatoid joint and plethora of proinflammatory effects that include regulation of other proinflammatory mediators.

TNF-α is made intracellularly and the 26-kDa precursor transmembrane form is cleaved off by a specific metalloproteinase, TNF-α converting enzyme (TACE) to produce soluble biologically active TNF. This molecule aggregates as a homotrimer in its active form. TNF-α and the closely related TNF-β (also known as lymphotoxin-α) equally bind the p55 (CD120a) or p75 (CD120b) receptors (also known as TNF-RI and TNF-RII, respectively) present on many cell types. The TNF receptor has an extracellular domain that can also be cleaved and released as a soluble TNF receptor (sTNF-R) and functions as a naturally occurring inhibitor.

The TNF receptors differ in their binding abilities and signaling properties; these differences also reflect the differences in their primary functions.[9] The presence of both receptors on nearly all cell types (except erythrocytes) underscores the wide-ranging biologic effects of TNF. Whereas TNF-RI (p55) is constitutively expressed on all cell types, TNF-RII (p75) is induced and expressed in larger amounts on hematopoietic and endothelial cells. Although binding of TNF to its receptor initiates a cascade of biologically profound events, both cell-bound and circulating TNF-α may also be bound to soluble TNF receptors serving as natural, counterregulatory TNF antagonists. The extracellular domain of cell-bound TNF receptors may be cleaved off (especially in an inflammatory milieu) to circulate in soluble form, where they bind TNF and will ultimately be excreted by the kidney. The binding of TNF-RI and TNF-RII to TNF-α appears to be similar, with the main difference lying in the dissociation kinetics. Thus although the binding of the p55 TNF-RI is static and almost irreversible (due to slow off-rate), the binding of the p75 TNF-RII is more dynamic owing to a more rapid off-rate. It appears that the physiologic activities of soluble TNF are largely mediated through the TNF-RI receptor, whereas TNF-RII is involved in ligand passing. The binding

SIMPLIFIED DIAGRAM OF THE MOLECULAR STRUCTURES OF 5 BIOLOGIC TNF INHIBITORS

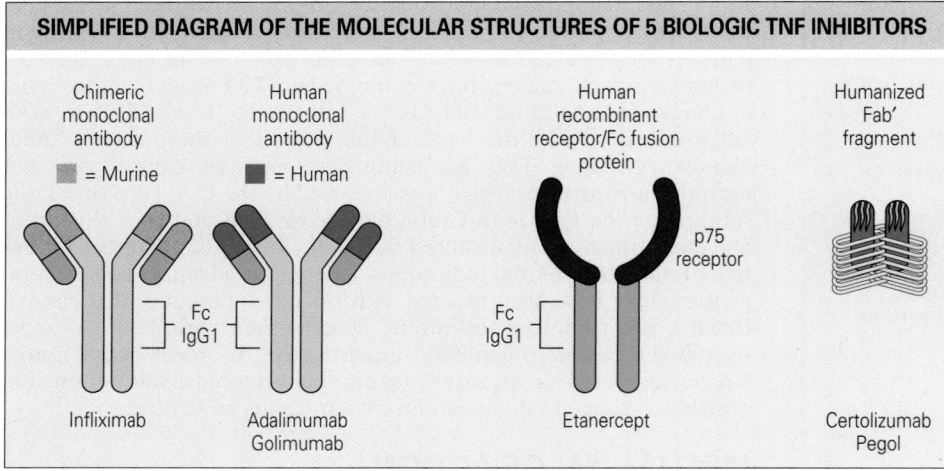

Fig. 61.1 Simplified diagram of the molecular structures of five biologic TNF inhibitors. Infliximab is a mouse/human chimeric monoclonal anti-TNF antibody of IgG1 isotype. Adalimumab and golimumab are fully human IgG1 monoclonal anti-TNF antibodies. Etanercept is a fusion protein of the p75 (TNFR2) and the Fc portion of IgG1. Certolizumab is a PEGylated Fab' fragment of a humanized IgG1 monoclonal anti-TNF antibody.

of TNF-α to its receptor can initiate several signaling pathways, including the activation of transcription factors (e.g., nuclear factor-κB [NF-κB]), protein kinases (e.g., c-Jun N-terminal kinase [JNK], p38 MAP kinase), and proteases (e.g., caspases) that markedly impact immune and inflammatory responses.

TNF-α primarily mediates inflammation by promoting cellular activation and trafficking of leukocytes to inflammatory sites. The biologic properties affected by TNF are listed in Box 61.2. TNF-α is produced primarily by monocytes and macrophages but may also be produced by other cell types (e.g., B cells, T cells, mast cells, fibroblasts). TNF-α may further contribute to the pathogenesis of RA by induction of proinflammatory cytokines such as interleukin (IL)-1 and IL-6, enhancement of leukocyte migration by increasing endothelial layer permeability and expression of adhesion molecules by endothelial cells and leukocytes, activation of neutrophils and eosinophils, induction of the synthesis of acute-phase reactants, and the induction of tissue-degrading enzymes (matrix metalloproteinase enzymes) produced by synoviocytes and/or chondrocytes.

Although all biologic TNF inhibitors share many biologic, clinical, and adverse effects, there are differences among them beyond their pharmacokinetics. The monoclonal antibodies infliximab, adalimumab, golimumab, and certolizumab are specific for TNF-α; etanercept binds both TNF-α and LT-α. Infliximab, adalimumab, and golimumab are IgG1 antibodies and etanercept contains an IgG1 portion; certolizumab is a PEGylated Fv fragment lacking an Fc portion. In addition to sharing the ability to inhibit TNF, all five agents bind to TNF with high affinity, and all three are virtually the same in their ability to neutralize soluble and transmembrane TNF. The induction of cell lysis in a cell line overexpressing TNF-α has been demonstrated by *in vitro* studies with infliximab and adalimumab (Fig. 61.1).

The first formal proof that TNF-α regulates other proinflammatory cytokines *in vivo* was the observation that there is a rapid reduction in serum IL-6 concentrations, closely followed by falling serum C-reactive protein (CRP), following administration of infliximab.[10,11]

Although IL-1 concentrations are often below the limit of detection in the peripheral blood of rheumatoid arthritis patients, where it is detectable, downregulation has been reported in a proportion of patients.[12] Similarly, in a small study of repeat synovial biopsies obtained before and 2 weeks after a single infusion of 10 mg per kg of infliximab, computerized image analysis of sections stained for cytokine-producing cells demonstrated a reduction in synovial IL-1α and IL-1β in a subgroup.[13] It is clear that the benefits of anti-TNF therapy are not mediated by upregulation of endogenous proinflammatory cytokine inhibitors because circulating IL-1ra and soluble TNF receptor levels fall after infliximab infusion.[11]

It is thought that a major mechanism of action of TNF inhibitors is likely to be mediated by modulation of inflammatory cell traffic. A dose-dependent rise in peripheral blood lymphocyte counts is observed following infliximab infusion, with a maximum rise within 24 hours of treatment.[14] This is mediated by modulation of both arms of the inflammatory cell recruitment cascade. Thus there is reduced histologic expression of synovial cytokine–induced vascular adhesion molecules, such as E-selectin and VCAM-1, following anti-TNF treatment[15] and a significant dose-dependent reduction in soluble serum E-selectin and ICAM-1 concentrations,[14] as well as significantly diminished immunohistologic expression of the chemokines IL-8 and MCP-1, with a trend to reduction in a number of other chemokines.[16]

Further indirect evidence to suggest TNF blockade reduces inflammatory cell recruitment to the joint is based on the observation that infliximab therapy is associated with a reduction in numbers of synovial tissue macrophages and lymphocytes.[15,16] However, the definitive confirmation that TNF blockade reduces leukocyte traffic to inflamed joints was obtained in an open-label clinical trial demonstrating a 40% to 50% decrease in retention of autologous indium-111 labeled granulocytes in the hands, wrists, and knees 2 weeks after infliximab treatment.[16] There is a reduction in the marginating granulocyte pool after infliximab treatment, an observation that would normally be associated with a rise in peripheral blood granulocyte counts.[17] However, in contrast to peripheral blood lymphocyte counts, numbers of peripheral blood granulocytes decrease after infliximab with maximal changes within 24 hours. The reason for this is that myeloid cell production is reduced secondary to downregulation of granulocyte macrophage colony stimulating factor (GM-CSF) as a consequence of TNF blockade. Because of the short circulating half-life of the granulocyte, of approximately 8 hours, a diminished rate of cell production dominates the peripheral blood picture.

One factor contributing to the rapid reduction in joint swelling observed by both patients and physicians after anti-TNF therapy is likely to be a reduction in tissue edema and capillary leak, mediated by vascular endothelial growth factor (VEGF), a cytokine implicated in new blood vessel formation and found to be elevated in the serum of rheumatoid arthritis patients.[18] Serum concentrations of VEGF show a dose-dependent reduction following infliximab infusions, but without normalization. There is also reduction in synovial vascular density and in particular a reduction in angiogenesis, as assessed by diminished number of vessels expressing the $\alpha V\beta 3$ integrin.[19] Further evidence for a reduction in synovial vascularity following TNF blockade is the observation that the vascular signal on quantitative power Doppler imaging is significantly reduced following infliximab therapy.[20,21]

Relatively early in the history of clinical trials of TNF blockade, marked reduction in circulating concentrations of the precursors of the matrix metalloproteinase enzymes MMP-1 and MMP-3 were reported,[22] as well as a significant reduction in synovial tissue expression of matrix metalloproteinases.[23] Similarly, serum levels of osteoprotegerin (OPG) and soluble receptor activator of nuclear factor κB ligands (sRANKL), both of which are elevated in rheumatoid compared with normal sera, are normalized following infliximab therapy without influencing the OPG:sRankL ratio.[24] These observations predicted the disease-modifying capability of anti-TNF inhibitors, which is now established.

One hypothesis for the failure of etanercept to give clinical benefits in trials of Crohn disease, in contrast to the marked benefits demonstrated with monoclonal antibodies to TNF-α, is that the antibodies may cause an increase in apoptosis of lamina propria and peripheral T cells through caspase-dependent mechanisms.[25] However, this topic remains controversial and the relevance of modulation of apoptosis as the mechanism of action of TNF inhibitors in rheumatoid arthritis is unclear. In one study, decreased synovial cellularity was reported as early as 48 hours after infliximab administration, but with no corresponding evidence of apoptosis.[26] In another study, however, apoptosis in synovial macrophages has been reported to be induced by both etanercept and infliximab, with a corresponding increase in active caspase-3 expression. No increase in lymphocyte apoptosis was observed, however.[27] The relevance of these interesting observations to the mode of action of TNF inhibitors in rheumatoid arthritis is not clear.

Approved indications and practical use

Table 61.1 details the 2007 Food and Drug Administration (FDA)-approved indications for the use of anti-TNF therapy. TNF blockers were initially approved in RA, juvenile arthritis, and psoriatic arthritis for patients with moderately to severely active disease who had failed an adequate trial of methotrexate (MTX) or other disease-modifying anti-rheumatic drugs (DMARDs). They were also indicated for the control of signs and symptoms and the prevention of functional or radiographic deterioration in RA and psoriatic arthritis. These recommendations have recently been modified because large controlled trials in early RA patients now allow their use as the initial DMARD in RA and thus the provision to fail MTX (or other DMARD) was removed (see Table 61.1). Thus while MTX and TNF inhibitors appear to be equally effective in clinical trials, TNF inhibitor therapy has been established as yielding better radiographic outcomes (alone or in combination with MTX). Despite the clinical and radiographic potency of TNF blockade, particularly with concomitant MTX therapy, the circumstances in which this combination should be initiated as a first-line therapy have not been firmly established because a variety of other factors determine these choices.

Beyond the FDA-approved indications for the use of TNF inhibitors, there are no collectively agreed upon guidelines for their use in practice. There are, however, situations wherein TNF inhibitor use is not advisable (Box 61.3). These relative contraindications include lupus, overlap

TABLE 61.1 U.S. FOOD AND DRUG ADMINISTRATION–APPROVED INDICATIONS FOR TNF-α INHIBITORS

Indication	Etanercept	Infliximab	Adalimumab
Rheumatoid arthritis (RA)	Yes[1]	Yes[1R]	Yes[1]
Early RA	Yes	Yes	Yes
Polyarticular juvenile arthritis (JA)	Yes[2]	—	—
Psoriatic arthritis	Yes[3E]	Yes[3]	Yes[3]
Ankylosing spondylitis	Yes[4]	Yes[4]	Yes[4]
Psoriasis	Yes[5]	Yes	—
Crohn disease	—	Yes[6]	Yes[6]
Ulcerative colitis	—	Yes[7]	—

[1]Indicated for reducing signs and symptoms, inhibiting the progression of structural damage, and improving physical function for patients with moderately to severely active rheumatoid arthritis. It can be initiated alone or in combination with methotrexate.
[1R]Infliximab is approved for use in combination with methotrexate only.
[2]Indicated for reducing signs and symptoms of moderately to severely active polyarticular course juvenile rheumatoid arthritis patients who have had an inadequate response to one or more DMARDs.
[3]Indicated for reducing signs and symptoms of active arthritis in patients with psoriatic arthritis.
[3E]Only etanercept is indicated to inhibit the progression of structural damage and improve physical function for patients with moderately to severely active psoriatic arthritis. It can be used in combination with methotrexate in patients who do not respond adequately to methotrexate alone.
[4]Indicated for reducing signs and symptoms in patients with active ankylosing spondylitis.
[5]Indicated for the treatment of adult patients (>18 years) with chronic moderate to severe plaque psoriasis who are candidates for systemic therapy or phototherapy.
[6]Indicated for reducing signs and symptoms and inducing or maintaining clinical remission in patients with moderately to severely active Crohn disease who have had an inadequate response to conventional therapy. Infliximab is also indicated for reducing the number of enterocutaneous and rectovaginal fistulas and maintaining fistula closure in fistulizing Crohn disease.
[7]Only infliximab is indicated for reducing signs and symptoms, achieving clinical remission and mucosal healing, and eliminating corticosteroid use in patients with moderately to severely active ulcerative colitis who have had an inadequate response to conventional therapy.

BOX 61.3 RELATIVE CONTRAINDICATIONS TO THE USE OF TUMOR NECROSIS FACTOR INHIBITORS

■ Systemic lupus erythematosus, lupus overlap syndrome
■ Multiple sclerosis, optic neuritis, demyelinating disorders
■ Current, active, serious infections
■ Recurrent or chronic infections
■ Untreated latent or active mycobacterial infection
■ Hepatitis B infection
■ Congestive heart failure
■ Pregnancy

syndromes, a history of demyelinating disorders (MS, optic neuritis), untreated active or latent tuberculosis, congestive heart failure, and pregnancy. The use of a TNF inhibitor in these situations is currently experimental in terms of risks and benefits, and the clinician should carefully consider the anticipated hazards versus potential benefits before proceeding.

The optimal candidate for TNF inhibition has not been defined. To date, there are no studies demonstrating a clinical phenotype or serologic, genomic and proteomic profile to ensure the appropriateness and safety of such an expensive intervention. Thus current use of these agents in RA, psoriatic arthritis, and ankylosing spondylitis varies widely. Guidance regarding use may be gleaned from several resources. A 2005 survey of 1023 practicing rheumatologists disclosed the top five indications for TNF inhibitor use in RA to be (1) failure of methotrexate, (2) failure of multiple DMARDs, (3) physician assessment of active disease, (4) radiographic erosions, and (5) functional disability.[28] Hence most rheumatologists currently assess the level of clinical RA activity, response to prior DMARD therapy, and radiographic findings when considering TNF inhibitor therapy in RA.

Wolfe and colleagues[29] proposed the elimination of synovitis and disease activity as the goal for RA treatment paradigms and proposed a revision of current RA treatment paradigms on the basis of the growing knowledge of the disease and the introduction of novel treatment alternatives. In general, their consensus guidelines insist on (1) early and appropriately aggressive therapy, (2) use of the best available therapies from the outset, (3) treatment of all RA patients with either DMARDs or biologics, (4) treatments tailored to the presence of poor prognostic factors, (5) biologic use based on disease activity and response to DMARDs, and (6) warning against withholding cytokine therapies for only those with advanced or DMARD-resistant disease.

The British Society of Rheumatology (BSR) and the National Institute for Health and Clinical Excellence (NICE) have established guidelines for TNF inhibitor use that require (1) active RA (defined by a Disease Activity Score [DAS] >5.1 on two occasions, at least 1 month apart); (2) failure of at least two DMARDs; and (3) withdrawal of TNF inhibitory therapy if there is not a reduction in DAS greater than 1.2 after 3 months of treatment. Patients receiving TNF inhibitors in the United Kingdom (U.K.) must meet these criteria and be enrolled in a registry that will allow for the periodic examination of both these guidelines and their clinical utility.[30]

Even with the introduction of several new and potent TNF inhibitors, MTX remains the gold standard against which all new drugs are judged. Hence unless there is a contraindication to its use, MTX should be considered the front-line DMARD of choice in RA and should be carefully considered for use in all RA patients and those with persistent inflammatory polyarthritis. Although other oral DMARD compounds may subsequently be considered as a monotherapy replacement, TNF inhibitors are among the most effective second-line therapies available, especially in patients with active RA, not controlled by an adequate duration and dose of MTX. TNF inhibitors are an effective and expensive alternative to an inadequate trial of MTX or DMARD therapy. It is currently unclear whether TNF inhibitors are a more effective option than step-up combination DMARDs (e.g., MTX plus leflunomide), although limited data from the BeST trial suggest that MTX plus TNF inhibitor is superior to add-on or sequential combination DMARD regimens.[31]

The employment of TNF inhibitor therapy with or without concomitant MTX as an appropriate initial treatment choice is currently being debated. Such patients must manifest a weighty combination of risk factors that portends a severe outcome. These "high-risk" RA patients may be identified as those with active polysynovitis and radiographic erosions or damage and either (1) be seropositive for RF and/or cyclic citrullinated peptide (CCP) antibodies, (2) have functional impairment, or (3) have sustained elevations of the erythrocyte sedimentation rate (ESR) or CRP. The identification of such high-risk patients mandates the combined use of MTX and TNF inhibition because studies have repeatedly shown the best clinical and radiographic outcomes when this combination is used instead of TNF inhibitor or MTX alone.

Another compelling reason for the use of TNF inhibitors is the rapid onset of effect and enhanced well-being reported by patients receiving TNF blockade. The brisk mitigation of stiffness and malaise and subsequent resumption of physical or pleasurable activities previously forfeited commonly follow TNF inhibitor initiation. Whether this represents a central nervous system or systemic effect of TNF inhibition is unknown. However, Andersson and colleagues[32] have shown infliximab to decrease cerebrospinal fluid (CSF) prostaglandin levels, while having no effect on CSF TNF, interferon-γ, IL-10, or nitric oxide.

The popularity of these agents is evident from their growth worldwide. Practice surveys suggest that nearly one in five RA patients has received a TNF inhibitor. Conversely, most RA, AS, PsA, and psoriasis patients have yet to receive these agents. Several factors have limited their widespread use, including patient or physician reluctance, high cost, limited or variable coverage by third-party insurance carriers, and toxicity concerns. Although clinicians reluctant to use these agents frequently point to limited long-term safety data, it should be noted that these agents have been employed in more than 1 million patients worldwide with greater than a decade of clinical trial and postmarketing experience. Hence safety concerns have been reduced since their introduction by time, expanded use, and ongoing safety reports from regulatory agencies, registries, and databases. Nonetheless, barriers to their use exist and include physician reluctance or lack of experience, need for time-consuming attempts to obtain prior authorization, requirements for one or more DMARD failures, unacceptably high co-

payments for some, and patient aversion to new drugs or parenteral drug administration.[28]

PHARMACOECONOMIC CONSIDERATIONS

Although the addition of TNF inhibitors has significantly impacted the lives of hundreds of thousands of patients worldwide, their addition to the arsenal of standard antirheumatic therapy has dramatically augmented the cost of care in RA for those requiring such therapies. It is prudent to note that the cost of having a chronic inflammatory disease (e.g., RA, psoriatic arthritis, ankylosing spondylitis) is often overlooked in these deliberations. For example, in reaching their conclusions about the cost-effectiveness of biologic anti-TNFs in the United Kingdom, NICE does not take into account the broader societal implications of the underlying condition such as loss of employment, loss of productivity for those in work, the need for state benefits, the cost of careers, and other indirect costs. The relatively higher acquisition cost of novel biologic agents has brought pharmacoeconomic considerations to the forefront in rheumatology. Beginning with RA and now expanding into other conditions, there is a growing body of data confirming the substantial cost implications of autoimmune rheumatic diseases. For the TNF inhibitors, the notable clinical efficacy observed needs to be factored into a comprehensive assessment of their value. Results from a number of studies have begun to make a compelling case that these agents may have an incremental cost-effectiveness within the range of currently accepted medical interventions. Given the current health care environment, pharmacoeconomic considerations are likely to remain a central factor affecting the use of novel therapies in rheumatology and in other disciplines.

ADALIMUMAB (HUMIRA)

Adalimumab became commercially available in December 2002. At the time of FDA approval, over 2468 RA patients in 17 different clinical trials had received this drug.

Pharmacology

Adalimumab is a fully human IgG1 anti-TNF-α monoclonal antibody. This recombinant human monoclonal antibody is produced by phage display and has a terminal half-life of 10 to 20 days (mean 14 days), thereby permitting every-other-week dosing. After a single 40-mg subcutaneous dose, the maximum serum concentration is achieved within 131 (±56) hours. The antibody binds circulating and cell-bound TNF-α and blocks its interaction with p55 and p75 receptors but does not interact with lymphotoxin (TNF-β). The drug induces cell lysis of TNF-expressing cells (in the presence of complement). Although concomitant MTX use reduces the clearance of adalimumab by 29% to 44%, it is unknown if adalimumab pharmacokinetics are altered in the setting of renal or hepatic impairment.

Indications and use

Adalimumab is indicated to reduce signs and symptoms, inhibit the radiographic damage or progression, and improve physical function in moderate to severe RA that is unresponsive to an adequate trial of one or more DMARDs. It is also indicated to reduce signs and symptoms of patients with psoriatic arthritis, ankylosing spondylitis, and Crohn disease. Adalimumab may be used as monotherapy or in combination with methotrexate and the usual recommended dose is 40 mg administered subcutaneously every other week (EOW). Higher doses (e.g., 80 mg EOW) were used during drug development but were not shown to be more effective in short-term trials. A minority of patients may require dose escalation (e.g., 40 mg weekly); however, observational studies in RA patients showed that few patients (<5%) will need to escalate adalimumab dosing.[33] In the PREMIER early RA trial, dose escalation was permitted for those not achieving an ACR20 response. Patients receiving adalimumab alone were more likely to escalate to weekly dosing compared with those on combined adalimumab and methotrexate (25% vs. 11%, respectively).[34] However, these patients seldom improved their efficacy parameters with dose escalation.

TABLE 61.2 SUMMARY OF PIVOTAL ADALIMUMAB CLINICAL TRIALS IN RHEUMATOID ARTHRITIS (RA)*

Trial	Van De Putte[35]	ARMADA[26]	DE019[37]	PREMIER[34]
Trial intervention	Adalimumab[†] monotherapy	MTX/adalimumab[†] combination	MTX/adalimumab[†] combination	Early RA MTX/adalimumab[†] combination
Trial duration	26 wk	24 wk	52 wk	24 mo
No. enrolled	544	271	619	799
Disease duration	12 yr	11-13 yr	11 yr	0.7 yr
ACR20	46%	67%	59%	73%
ACR50	22%	55%	42%	62%
ACR70	12%	27%	23%	46%
Rx effect	27%	53%	35%	NA
DAS remission	ND	ND	ND	49%
Change HAQ	−0.4	0.6	−0.7	−1.3
Mean TSS Δ	ND	ND	+0.1	+1.9
No Δ in TSS	ND	ND	62%	61%
Withdrawal	ND	ND	22%	24%
ISR %	ND	15%	26%	
URI	ND	ND	19%	ND
SIE rate	ND	ND	0.06/patient-year	0.03/patient-year

*Multicenter, randomized, controlled trials.
†Reporting rates for 40-mg adalimumab every-other-week group.
ACR, American College of Rheumatology; DAS, Disease Activity Score; HAQ, health assessment questionnaire; ISR, injection site reaction; MTX, methotrexate; ND, no data; SIE, serious infections event; TSS, total Sharp score; URI, upper respiratory infection.

Adalimumab in rheumatoid arthritis pivotal trials

Early studies showed that a single dose of adalimumab produced significant and rapid clinical improvement, reduced acute-phase reactants, increased circulating lymphocyte counts, and significantly reduced systemic IL-6 and IL-1ra levels for at least 2 weeks. In controlled dose-ranging monotherapy studies, American College of Rheumatology (ACR)-20 response rates ranged from 46% to 73% (Table 61.2). In a large placebo-controlled monotherapy trial of 544 RA patients, a dose-dependent rise in ACR response rates was seen, with 46% of those receiving 40 mg EOW achieving an ACR20 response.[35]

The ARMADA trial examined the efficacy of adalimumab in 271 RA patients with an inadequate response to methotrexate.[36] In this 6-month, multicenter, randomized controlled trial, patients remained on stable doses (mean of 16 to 17 mg/week) of MTX and received placebo or 20 mg, 40 mg, or 80 mg adalimumab every 2 weeks. These patients with active and uncontrolled RA had mean disease duration of 11 to 13 years and received an average of three prior DMARDs. ACR20 response rates were 14%, 48%, 66%, and 66% for those taking placebo, 20 mg, 40 mg, or 80 mg, respectively. Similarly, the ACR70 responses were 3%, 11%, 24%, and 19% for those taking placebo, 20 mg, 40 mg, or 80 mg, respectively. Injection site reactions occurred in 15% of patients and no increase in unusual or serious adverse events was noted.

Another pivotal trial (DE019) examined the efficacy and radiographic outcomes in a 619-patient, 52-week trial where adalimumab or placebo was given to methotrexate partial responders.[37] Patients remained on MTX and were given either placebo or adalimumab 20 mg or 40 mg every other week. With a mean age of 56 years and disease duration of 11 years, these patients had failed an average of 1.9 DMARDs at entry. Although 77% of adalimumab 40-mg patients completed the 12-month trial, only 70% of placebo patients did the same. ACR20 response rates after 52 weeks were 24%, 55%, and 59% in the placebo, adalimumab 20-mg, and 40-mg groups, respectively. Responses were sustained in the 457 patients who went on to receive open-label adalimumab for a second year. Radiographic deterioration, as measured by modified Sharp scores, was significantly worse in the placebo group (+2.7 Sharp units) compared with the 20-mg/wk (+0.7 Sharp units) or 40-mg EOW (+0.1 Sharp units) groups.

The role of adalimumab in the treatment of early RA was first examined in a subanalysis of the DE019 study, wherein 27 patients with early disease (mean of 1.2 years) were compared with 180 patients with long-standing (mean of 12.5 years) RA and showed a trend toward better ACR20 (70% vs. 62%) and ACR70 responses (41% vs. 18%) and Health Assessment Questionnaire (HAQ) improvement (0.79 vs. 0.57) in early versus late RA patients, respectively.[38] The PREMIER trial further established the efficacy of adalimumab in early RA (see Table 61.2). In this 2-year, early RA (<3 years' duration) trial, 799 DMARD-naïve patients were randomized to receive either adalimumab, methotrexate (MTX), or the combination of MTX and adalimumab.[34] Although this study demonstrated adalimumab and MTX to be equipotent with regard to clinical outcomes (ACR20/50/70 responses, DAS remission), the combined use of MTX and adalimumab was significantly better. ACR70 responses (47% vs. 27%) and 6 months' sustained, major clinical response rates (49% vs. 25%) were twofold higher when combined MTX/adalimumab was compared with adalimumab alone. Primary outcome measures included a 62% ACR50 response rate and a minimal change (+1.3 Sharp unit) in total Sharp score (TSS) for those on MTX plus adalimumab for 12 months (Fig. 61.2).

ETANERCEPT (ENBREL)

Etanercept was commercially approved for use in RA in late 1999.

Pharmacology

Etanercept is a dimeric fusion construct that links two p75 (type II) TNF receptors to the Fc portion of IgG, containing domains CH2 and CH3 and the hinge region. Etanercept is produced by recombinant DNA technology in Chinese hamster ovary cells and has a molecular weight of 150 kDa. It is capable of binding two circulating or cell-bound TNF-α molecules and will inhibit the binding of TNF-α and TNF-β (lymphotoxin) to TNF receptors. In contrast to the monoclonal antibodies, etanercept does not induce cell lysis or apoptosis of TNF-expressing cells. The half-life of etanercept in adult RA patients is 102 hours (±30 hours) with a range of 4.1 to 12.5 days. Pharmacokinetics in children are assumed to be similar, although drug clearance may be reduced in children between the ages of 4 and 8 years.

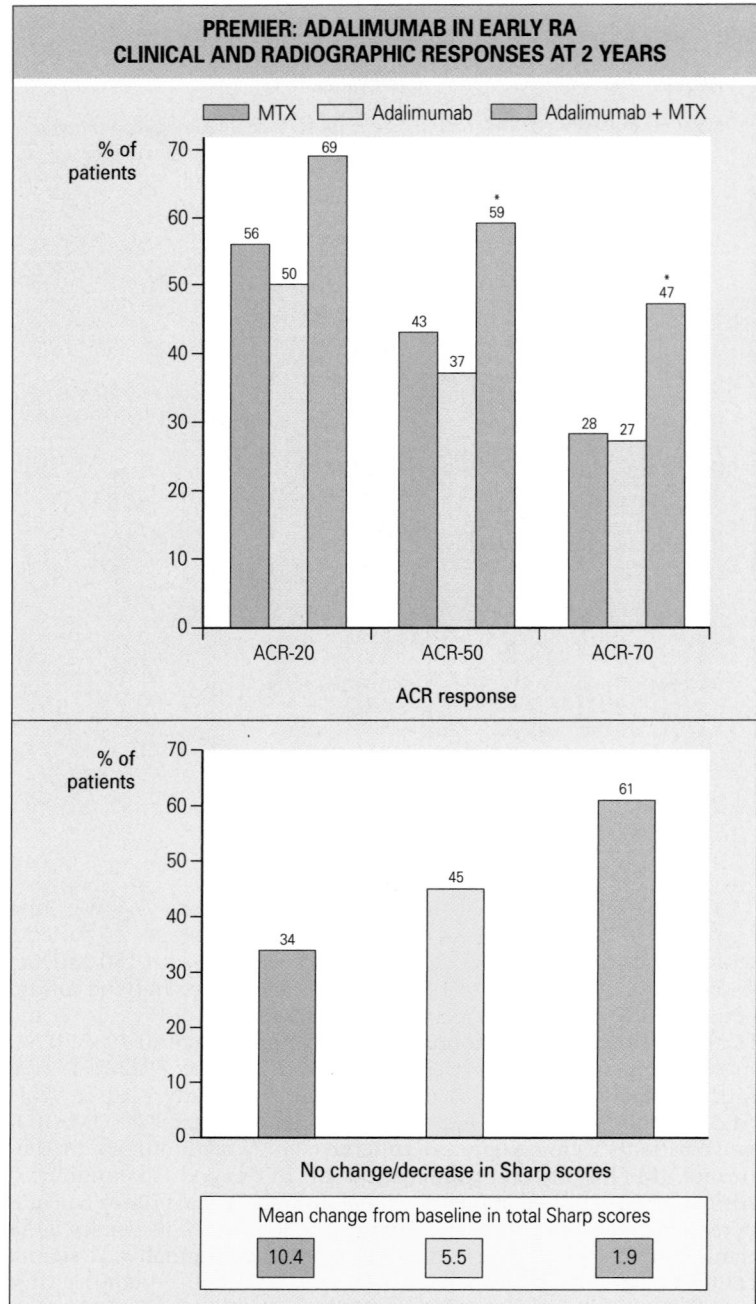

**PREMIER: ADALIMUMAB IN EARLY RA
CLINICAL AND RADIOGRAPHIC RESPONSES AT 2 YEARS**

Fig. 61.2 PREMIER: adalimumab in early rheumatoid arthritis. *(From Breedveld FC, Weisman MH, Kavanaugh AF, et al. The PREMIER study: a multicenter, randomized, double-blind clinical trial of combination therapy with adalimumab plus methotrexate versus methotrexate alone or adalimumab alone in patients with early, aggressive rheumatoid arthritis who had not had previous methotrexate treatment. Arthritis Rheum 2006;54:26-37.)*

Pharmacokinetics has not been well studied in children younger than 4 years old. Serum concentration profiles at steady state were comparable among patients with RA treated with 50 mg once weekly or 25 mg twice weekly. The route of clearance from the circulation is unclear, although it is thought to be mediated through Fc binding by the reticuloendothelial system. Methotrexate has no effect on the pharmacokinetics of etanercept.

Indications and use

Etanercept is indicated in patients with established or early RA to reduce signs and symptoms, inhibit structural damage, and improve physical function in those with moderate to severe disease. Etanercept may be used alone or in conjunction with methotrexate. In adult RA

patients, etanercept is given by self-administered subcutaneous injection at 50 mg once a week (or 25 mg twice weekly). In a controlled clinical trial, higher doses (50 mg twice weekly) were not associated with increased efficacy but were associated with more adverse events.[39]

Etanercept is also approved for use in patients with active, moderate-to-severe polyarticular juvenile arthritis, PsA, and AS (see Table 61.1). It is approved for moderate to severe plaque psoriasis at a higher dose of 50 mg twice weekly for 3 months followed by a maintenance dose of 50 mg once weekly.

Etanercept in rheumatoid arthritis pivotal trials

The efficacy of etanercept has been established in four pivotal clinical trials of 1637 RA patients (Table 61.3). Collectively these trials consistently demonstrate impressive clinical outcomes, with ACR20 responses ranging from 59% to 75% and ACR70 response rates of 15% to 40% after 6 to 12 months of therapy.

A 6-month randomized controlled study compared placebo and etanercept (10 mg or 25 mg) subcutaneously twice weekly.[40] This was the first of several studies revealing the inferior efficacy of the 10-mg dose. Nonetheless, 59% ACR20 and 15% ACR70 response rates were seen in patients taking etanercept 25 mg twice weekly. When etanercept was given to RA patients with an insufficient response to methotrexate therapy, patients receiving etanercept and methotrexate achieved a 71% ACR20 response compared with 27% placebo/MTX response.[41] Many of these patients were enrolled in a long-term, open-label observational study and exhibited static ACR20, ACR50, and ACR70 response rates over 3 years. Importantly, sustained efficacy allowed for a 68% to 85% decrease or discontinuation of methotrexate or prednisone and 39% to 59% of patients were able to discontinue methotrexate and prednisone use after 3 years.[42]

Etanercept was the first biologic therapy tested head to head against methotrexate in an early RA (ERA) trial. In the ERA study, 632 active, early-RA patients (mean disease duration 11 months) were enrolled in a 12-month trial of etanercept versus methotrexate.[43] Patients were randomized to receive MTX 20 mg/week or etanercept (10 or 25 mg twice weekly). After 12 months, both methotrexate and 25-mg etanercept–treated groups fared equally well with ACR20 response rates of 65% and 72%, respectively. The only significant group difference was the more rapid onset of effect in those treated with etanercept in the first 4 months. Both drugs were well tolerated but etanercept-treated patients had fewer adverse events and nonrespiratory infections and more injection site reactions compared with methotrexate patients. Serious infectious events were infrequent in both groups (<3%). In the second year, a trend toward greater ACR20 response rates was seen in the etanercept group (72%) compared with the MTX group (59%).[44]

The ERA trial showed that radiographic progression was diminished by both agents when assessed after 6, 12, and 24 months of therapy (Fig. 61.3). In the first year, modified Sharp scores showed little change in MTX (1.3 units) and etanercept (0.8 units) groups, yet both were significantly better than their projected rates of x-ray deterioration (estimated to be ≈9 Sharp units per year). In the second year of the trial, significant differences were seen, with etanercept patients increasing only 1.3 Sharp units (no progression in 63%) and MTX patients increasing 3.2 Sharp units (no progression in 51%). The ERA trial was pivotal in demonstrating the potency of both MTX and etanercept in patients with early, aggressive RA. The additional radiographic advantage of TNF inhibition over methotrexate in early disease was largely seen in those with erosions at entry to the study.

The TEMPO trial reported the comparative efficacy of methotrexate, etanercept, and the combination of etanercept plus methotrexate in 682 patients with active RA and a mean disease duration of 7 years.[45] At both 12 and 24 months the combination of etanercept and MTX was significantly more effective than either monotherapy MTX or etanercept alone (see Table 61.3). At 24 months the combination group demonstrated impressive ACR20 (86%) and ACR70 (49%) responders and DAS remissions (38%). These results may have been enriched by the inclusion of prior MTX responders, although comparison of MTX-naïve and previously treated MTX patients failed to show significant differences in outcomes. The mean total Sharp score was decreased by 0.56 units in patients receiving combination etanercept plus methotrexate and 78% had no radiographic worsening. By

TABLE 61.3 SUMMARY OF PIVOTAL ETANERCEPT CLINICAL TRIALS IN RA*

Trial	Moreland[40]	Weinblatt[41]	ERA[43]	TEMPO[45]	COMET[46]
Description	Monotherapy	MTX/etanercept combination	Early RA (monotherapy)	MTX/etanercept combination	Early RA MTX/etanercept combination
Trial duration	6 mo	6 mo	12 mo	<24 mo	Reported to 12 mo 24 mo study
No. enrolled	234	89	632	682	542
Disease duration	12 yr	13 yr	0.99 yr	7 yr	0.75 yr
ACR20[†]	59%	71%	72%	86%	86%
ACR50[†]	40%	39%	49%	71%	71%
ACR70[†]	15%	15%	25%	49%	48%
Rx effect	48%	44%	NA	NA	NA
DAS remission	ND	ND	ND	38%	50%
Change HAQ	−0.6	−0.6	−0.7	−1.1	−1.0
Mean TSS Δ	ND	ND	Etanercept −1.3	−0.56	0.27
No Δ in TSS	ND	ND	72% No Δ Erosion score	78%	75%
Withdrawal rate (etanercept)	28%	3%	7%	29%	19%
ISR %	49%	42%	37%	11%	ND
URI	33%	22%	35%	ND	ND
SIE rate	ND	ND	<3%	6%	12%

*Multicenter, randomized, controlled trials (results shown for patients receiving etanercept 25 mg biweekly).
[†]At study end.
ACR20, placebo ACR20; ERA, early RA trial (Bathon); HAQ, health assessment questionnaire; ISR, injection site reactions; MTX, methotrexate; NA, not applicable; ND, no data; RA, rheumatoid arthritis; Rx effect, active drug; SIE, serious infectious event; TSS, total Sharp score; URI, upper respiratory infection.

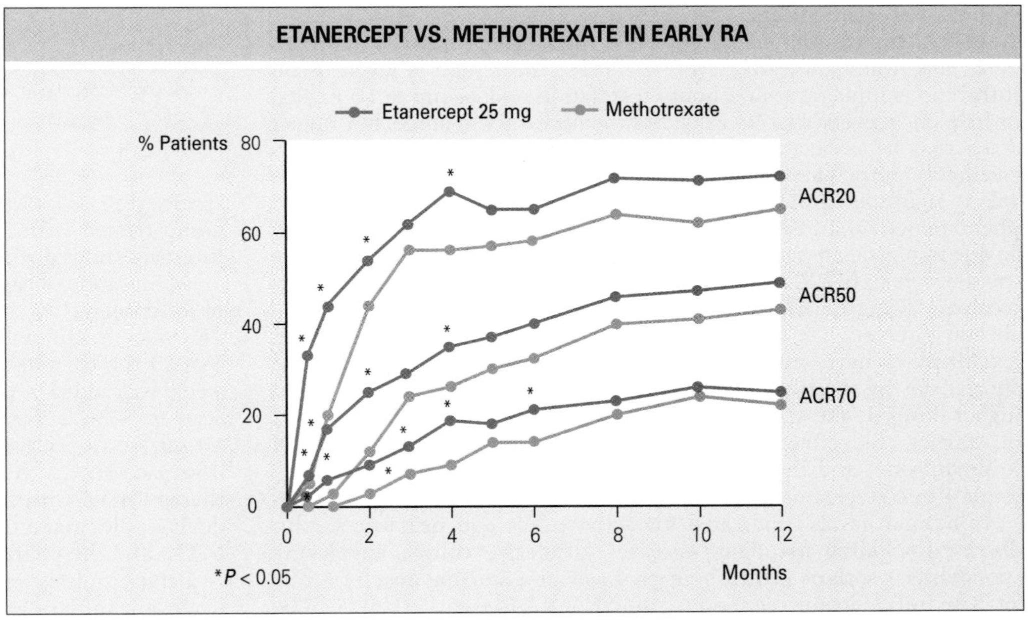

Fig. 61.3 ERA: etanercept in early RA. (From Genovese MC, Bathon JM, Martin RW, et al. Etanercept versus methotrexate in patients with early rheumatoid arthritis: two year radiographic and clinical outcomes. Arthritis Rheum 2002;46:1443-1450.)

comparison, total Sharp scores were increased in those taking etanercept (+0.5 units) or methotrexate (+2.8 units) and 60% to 68% showed no radiographic progression while on MTX or etanercept, respectively. This study underscores the potential additive clinical and radiographic protection afforded by the combination of MTX and TNF therapy, especially in patients with aggressive disease.

With growing experience of anti-TNF use and greater expectations for efficacy, the primary outcome measures for clinical trials have become more ambitious. The COMET trial[46] compared the effects of a combination of etanercept and methotrexate with MTX alone in 542 MTX-naïve patients with early RA (≥3 months and ≤2 years). The co-primary endpoints were DAS28 remission (<2.6) at week 52 and radiographic non-progression measured by modified Sharp scores from baseline to week 52. Half of the patients who took combined treatment achieved clinical remission and 80% achieved radiographic

non-progression compared with 28% and 59%, respectively taking methotrexate alone. This study further confirms that for a majority of patients with early, severe RA, clinical remission and radiographic non-progression are achievable goals within 1 year of combined treatment with etanercept plus methotrexate.[46]

INFLIXIMAB (REMICADE)

Remicade was first approved for use in moderate to severe Crohn disease in 1998 and was shortly thereafter marketed for use in RA.

Pharmacology

Infliximab is a chimeric anti-TNF monoclonal antibody that combines human IgG1κ (constant region) to a murine Fv (variable) region. The antibody is produced in a murine myeloma cell line transfected with cloned DNA coding for cA2 and subsequently purified. Infliximab has been shown to bind with high affinity to both soluble and membrane-bound TNF and is capable of neutralizing TNF *in vitro* and *in vivo*. This antibody can mediate cytotoxicity of TNF-expressing cells *in vitro* and is capable of inducing cell lysis of TNF-expressing cells via antibody-dependent cellular cytotoxicity (ADCC) *in vitro*. Infliximab binds TNF-α but not lymphotoxin (TNF-β). The median terminal half-life in RA and Crohn patients is 8 to 9.5 days (mean 210 hours) using doses of 3 to 10 mg/kg. Infliximab exhibits a linear dose-related pharmacokinetic profile at doses ranging from 3 to 20 mg/kg. Pharmacokinetic studies in the elderly and patients with renal or hepatic dysfunction have not been done. Infliximab serum concentrations tended to be slightly higher when used along with MTX (7.5 mg once a week). The development of human antichimeric antibodies (HACA) has been shown to increase clearance and reduce serum levels of infliximab.

Indications and dosing

In established and early RA, infliximab (with methotrexate) is indicated to reduce signs and symptoms, inhibit the radiographic progression, and improve physical function in patients with moderately to severely active RA. Concurrent use of methotrexate (7.5 mg/week) with infliximab has been shown to limit the immunogenic response to the construct (e.g., HACA formation). This is particularly relevant at lower doses (e.g., infliximab 3 mg/kg), where immunogenicity is more likely than at higher doses (e.g., 10 mg/kg). Infliximab monotherapy (without MTX) is customary in Crohn disease, ankylosing spondylitis, and psoriasis, where higher doses are usually employed. Nevertheless, one RA registry claims that 14% of more than 1400 RA patients have received infliximab monotherapy (without MTX or other DMARDs)[47] without untoward effects.

In RA, the recommended dose is 3 mg/kg given initially at weeks 0, 2, and 6 and thereafter every 8 weeks. Infliximab is given as an intravenous infusion over 2 hours. Escalation of dose (up to 10 mg/kg) or frequency (every 4 to 6 weeks) may be necessary in some, but higher doses may be associated with a higher frequency of serious infections (see later). Some patients will require changes in dosing or dose intervals to maintain clinical efficacy. The loss of efficacy and "dose creep" phenomenon are most common after the first year of therapy and may be due to physician/patient efforts to reduce the use of other adjunctive therapies (e.g., MTX, NSAIDs, prednisone). Although 26% of patients receiving 3 mg/kg have undetectable infliximab levels at 8 weeks, shorter intervals (i.e., 4 weeks) and higher doses (i.e., 10 mg/kg) were less likely to have undetectable levels.[48,49] This study suggested that shorter dosing intervals would yield higher trough levels than would higher doses at the same intervals. For patients demonstrating a loss of efficacy, the clinician should first optimize the dose of MTX (+ prednisone) and then, if necessary, decrease dosing intervals (e.g., every 4 to 6 weeks) or employ higher doses (up to 10 mg/kg).

Infliximab is also indicated for active adult and pediatric Crohn disease (including fistulizing disease), ulcerative colitis, ankylosing spondylitis, psoriatic arthritis, or psoriasis at a starting dose of 5 mg/kg. The initial dosing regimen is similar to RA (see earlier) and can be given every 8 weeks (or every 6 weeks in ankylosing spondylitis) thereafter.

Clinical efficacy of infliximab in rheumatoid arthritis

The efficacy and safety of infliximab in RA were initially established in monotherapy trials, after a DMARD washout. An 8-week open-label trial[50] demonstrated equivalent efficacy when infliximab was given as (1) two infusions of 10 mg/kg 2 weeks apart or (2) four monthly infusions of 5 mg/kg. Clinical benefits were noted after week 3 and were maximal by week 6 with normalization of CRP levels in nearly 90% of patients. Following the last infusion, clinical responses lasted a median of 14 weeks (range of 8 to 25 weeks). Another placebo-controlled, monotherapy trial with a single infusion of 1 mg/kg or 10 mg/kg demonstrated significant improvement by week 4, with Paulus 20% responses in 44% and 79%, respectively.[51] Eight responders went on to

TABLE 61.4 SUMMARY OF PIVOTAL INFLIXIMAB CLINICAL TRIALS IN RA*

Trial	ATTRACT[53]		ASPIRE[55]	
Description	MTX*/infliximab combination		Early RA, MTX/ infliximab combination	
Trial duration	54 wk		52 wk	
No. enrolled	428		1049	
Duration	8.4 yr		0.8 yr	
Dose (every 8 wks)	3 mg/kg	10 mg/kg	3 mg/kg	6 mg/kg
ACR20%	42	59	62	66
ACR50%	21	39	46	50
ACR70%	10	25	33	37
Rx effect %	25	42	NA	NA
DAS remission %	ND		21	31
Change HAQ	−0.4		−0.8	−0.9
Mean TSS Δ	1.3	0.2	0.4	0.5
No Δ in TSS (%)	54		58	59
Withdrawal %	21		18	20
Infusion reactions	25% (2.3% withdrew)		21% (0.5% serious)	15%
URI	34%		25%	28%
SIE	6%		5.6%	5.0%
ANA/DNA positive	61%	10	40%	24%
HACA	8%		14.5%	6.7%

*Results at week 54 presented for 3 mg and 10 mg administered every 8 weeks IV; mean MTX dose, 16 mg/wk.
DAS, Disease Activity Score; HACA, Human Anti-Chimeric Antibody; HAQ, health assessment questionnaire; SIE, serious infectious event; TSS, total Sharp score; URI, upper respiratory infection.

receive repeated infusions when clinical relapse became evident. In this group treated with infliximab alone, a trend toward shorter response intervals showed some correlation with the presence of HACA.

Maini and colleagues[52] reported on the safety and immunogenicity of infliximab (1, 3, or 10 mg/kg) when given with or without MTX for 26 weeks. A Paulus 20% response was seen in 60% of patients receiving 3 or 10 mg/kg. Additive responses were seen when MTX (7.5 to 15 mg/ week) was added to the regimen. After 26 weeks, HACA responses were seen in 53%, 21%, and 7% of those receiving 1 mg/kg, 3 mg/kg, and 10 mg/kg, respectively. The concurrent use of low-dose MTX further decreased HACA to 15%, 7%, and 0%, respectively. These early monotherapy trials with infliximab were important in establishing optimal dosing, the magnitude of efficacy, the importance of concomitant MTX, and the pharmacokinetics of infliximab use.

Larger multicenter trials further established the efficacy and safety of chronic infliximab with background MTX in patients with RA (Table 61.4). The ATTRACT trial was a 428-patient randomized, placebo-controlled trial of infliximab (3 mg/kg or 10 mg/kg) given every 4 or 8 weeks in active RA patients with a prior inadequate response to weekly methotrexate.[53] The addition of infliximab (3 or 10 mg/kg) to background MTX showed significantly higher ACR20 responses (50% to 58%) compared with methotrexate alone (20%) at 30 weeks. After 54 weeks ACR20 responses were 42% to 59% in the 3 mg and 10 mg/kg groups.[53] Radiographic damage was progressive in the MTX/placebo group, increasing by a mean of 7 Sharp units at 1 year. By contrast, all the infliximab-treated groups (3 or 10 mg/kg) showed little change (1.3 and 0.2 units) after 12 months. In long-term extension studies, 22% of placebo patients showed no evidence of radiographic progression and 43% to 47% of the 3 mg/kg group and 64% of the 10 mg/kg group showed no evidence of radiographic change over 2 years. Further analysis of the ATTRACT study patients without erosions at entry revealed infliximab plus MTX to be superior to MTX alone in halting further radiographic progression.[54]

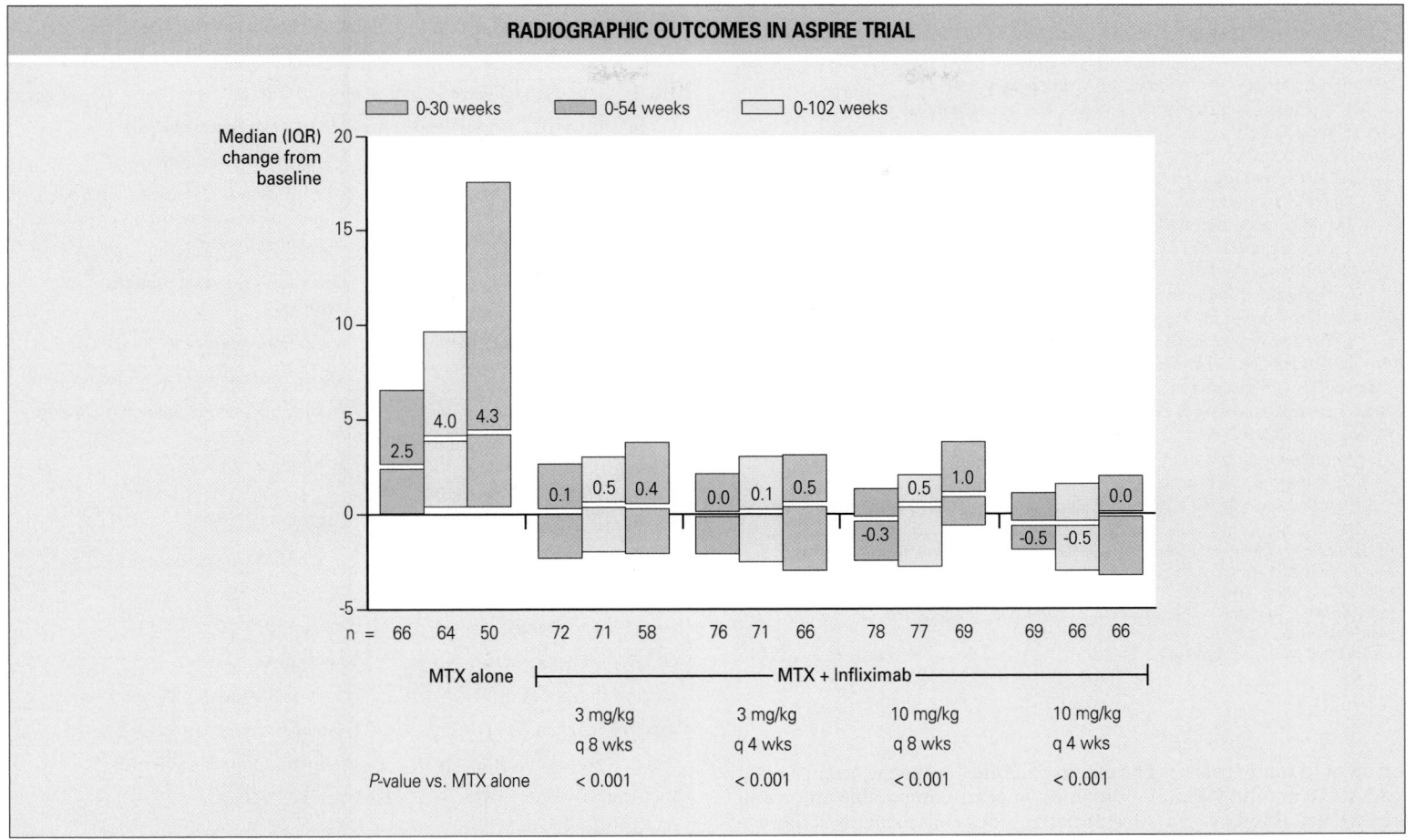

RADIOGRAPHIC OUTCOMES IN ASPIRE TRIAL

Fig. 61.4 ASPIRE: infliximab in early RA. *(From St Clair EW, Van Der Heijde DM, Smolen JS, et al. Active-Controlled Study of Patients Receiving Infliximab for the Treatment of Rheumatoid Arthritis of Early Onset Study Group. Combination of infliximab and methotrexate therapy for early rheumatoid arthritis: a randomized, controlled trial. Arthritis Rheum 2004;50:3432-3443.)*

The ASPIRE trial examined the effects of MTX and infliximab in patients with early RA.[55] This 12-month, 1049-patient trial enrolled patients with a mean disease duration of 7 months. All patients received weekly MTX (20 mg/week) and also received placebo or infliximab (3 mg/kg or 6 mg/kg). Although MTX/placebo-treated patients exhibited good ACR20 (54%) and ACR70 (21%) responses and DAS remissions (15%), patients treated with MTX/infliximab showed significantly higher ACR20 (62% to 66%) and ACR70 (33% to 37%) responses and DAS remissions (21% to 33%) at 54 weeks (Fig. 61.4). Radiographic progression was primarily observed in patients treated only with methotrexate alone in the ASPIRE trial (see Fig. 61.4). Although 45% of the MTX/placebo patients showed no progression, those on infliximab demonstrated greater protection (58% to 59%) from progression in x-ray scores.

Two recent trials have suggested that the early use of infliximab in patients with new-onset RA may allow for its subsequent discontinuation with maintenance of efficacy on MTX alone.[31,56] A pilot study of 12 months of MTX and infliximab therapy in 20 high-risk early RA patients resulted in clinical and magnetic resonance imaging (MRI) benefits that were sustained for a year after infliximab was withdrawn.[56] The BeST trial was a large multicenter trial that compared four treatment strategies for DMARD and biologic use in patients with early RA.[31] DMARD switch or add-on monotherapy was compared with a COBRA-like combination DMARD regimen and combined MTX/infliximab. The protocol called for the cessation of infliximab if remission was achieved after 9 months of therapy. Observation of this cohort revealed that after 4 years, more than half of infliximab/MTX-treated patients discontinued infliximab while maintaining a DAS less than 2.4 and 18% of patients stopped both MTX and infliximab (drug-free remission) without recurrence or radiographic progression.[57] A *post hoc* analysis of patients in the four strategy limbs suggests that using MTX plus infliximab as initial treatment for recent-onset RA patients

is more effective than reserving MTX plus infliximab for patients who failed on traditional DMARDs, with more HAQ improvement over time, more infliximab discontinuation, and less progression of joint damage.[58] Initial combination therapy led to significantly faster improvement in all patient-reported measures.[59] Although high rates of substantial improvement on infliximab are to be expected in early RA, the observation that drug-free or MTX-maintained remission may be maintained without ongoing TNF inhibition is an exciting development that will require further study and confirmation.

EXPANDED INDICATIONS

Neutralization of TNF-α has proven to be a highly effective intervention for a variety of inflammatory disorders. TNF-α inhibitors have been successfully studied and approved for use in juvenile arthritis, moderate-to-severe RA, early RA, psoriatic arthritis, psoriasis, ankylosing spondylitis, Crohn disease, pediatric Crohn disease, and ulcerative colitis (see relevant chapters). With clinical success in these disorders comes the anticipation that such therapies may be equally beneficial in other inflammatory diseases. Although exploratory clinical trial results in some disorders thought to be TNF mediated (e.g., multiple sclerosis, congestive heart failure, sarcoidosis, ANCA-associated granulomatous vasculitis) have been disappointing, others have been encouraging while fulfilling a large unmet clinical need. This is particularly true in PsA, spondyloarthritis (SpA), and AS (Box 61.4, Table 61.5) where traditional DMARDs have been proven ineffective or potentially toxic.

Ankylosing spondylitis

TNF inhibitors reproducibly induce substantial improvements in the signs and symptoms of AS and are significantly superior to placebo

TABLE 61.5 USE OF TUMOR NECROSIS FACTOR (TNF) INHIBITION IN ORPHAN DISORDERS

TNF Inhibitor Use: Unapproved Indications and Orphan Use	
Large prospective randomized controlled trials or meta-analysis	
Benefits shown	Ineffective/equivocal findings
Anterior uveitis	Etanercept in ANCA-associated granulomatous vasculitis Sjögren syndrome
Limited reports of clinical benefits*	**Uncertain/equivocal benefits reported†**
Reactive/undifferentiated arthritis	Autoimmune inner ear disease
Pustular psoriasis	Sarcoidosis: pulmonary, ocular, resistant
Acrodermatitis continua of Hallopeau	Chronic obstructive pulmonary disease
Psoriatic onychopachydermoperiostitis	Asthma
Pyoderma gangrenosum	Aphthous stomatitis
Pemphigus	Sneddon-Wilkinson disease
SAPHO syndrome	Eosinophilic fasciitis
Hepatitis C virus infection	Panniculitis
Constrictive pericarditis	Eosinophilic fasciitis
Multicentric reticulohistiocytosis	Necrobiosis lipoidica diabeticorum
Recurrent ovarian cancer	Hidradenitis suppurativa
Graft-versus-host disease	Idiopathic pulmonary fibrosis
Polyarteritis nodosa	Inclusion body myositis
Takayasu arteritis	Dermatomyositis
Behçet disease (ocular > skin)	Polymyositis
Adult-onset Still disease	Scleroderma
Systemic juvenile idiopathic arthritis	Recalcitrant hand pompholyx
TNF receptor-associated periodic	Myelodysplastic syndrome (TRAPS)
Hyper-IgD syndrome	Sciatica
PAPA syndrome	Discogenic spinal pain
Orbital myositis	Infertility
Amyloidosis	Endometriosis
ANCA-associated granulomatous vasculitis	Pulmonary tuberculosis
	Systemic lupus erythematosus

*Limited benefit results: implies >1 positive, anecdotal, or uncontrolled report of benefit.
†Uncertain/equivocal benefit: implies single, limited and uncontrolled report of benefit or several negative or several conflicting reports.

treatment in many trials.[60] The extent of clinical response, as measured by ASAS 20 and BASDAI 50 outcomes, appears comparable among all three agents. Moreover, a substantial minority of patients achieve a high-level response, defined as "partial remission." In addition, all TNF inhibitors have been shown to improve spinal mobility measures, with the greatest changes noted in the cervical spine (occiput to wall measurement) and the least noted in the lumbar spine (Schober test).

Nonetheless, all AS patients appear to flare on discontinuation of therapy, with the mean time to flare ranging from 6 weeks with etanercept to 17.5 weeks with infliximab. This suggests that continuous therapy with TNF inhibitors will likely be necessary to maintain clinical benefit in patients with AS. TNF inhibitors have also been shown to improve the quality of life among treated AS patients. There are also data suggesting that therapy may improve extra-articular inflammatory involvement in AS. In a systematic review that included data from randomized controlled trials and open-label experience, it was observed that flares of anterior uveitis occurred less frequently under TNF inhibitor therapy (6.8/100 patient-years) compared with placebo (15.6/100 patient-years).[61]

Several MRI studies of AS patients treated with TNF inhibitors have shown attenuation of spinal inflammation.[60] Although suppression of inflammation was maintained for up to 2 years, it was not completely eliminated in most. The extent to which changes shown by MRI will correlate with and predict attenuation of subsequent radiographic structural damage remains to be elucidated. Data presented from a recent study examining x-ray progression in etanercept-treated patients (compared with historical controls) over 2 years did not reveal inhibition of radiographic progression.[62] However, a variety of methodologic considerations may have influenced these results. TNF inhibitor use in AS can follow guidelines that have been developed by an international group of rheumatologists (see Box 61.4).

Psoriatic arthritis

TNF inhibitor therapy has proven effective in controlling both the skin and joint disease. There has been a progression of TNF inhibitor use in PsA, starting with early open-label trials and followed by large randomized, placebo-controlled trials of patients with established joint and skin disease, to recent trials of psoriatic spondylitis and psoriasis subsets. All three TNF inhibitors reproducibly induce substantial improvements (as measured by ACR20/50/70 responses) in the signs and symptoms of peripheral arthritis in PsA. Interestingly, placebo responses among PsA patients in general seem lower than those in comparable studies of RA. TNF inhibitor therapy in PsA has also improved functional status, quality of life, dactylitis, and enthesitis.[60] Treatment with TNF inhibitors has also been shown to diminish the progression of radiographic peripheral joint damage in PsA patients to the same degree as that seen in RA.[60]

Although improvement in cutaneous disease was seen in most TNF inhibitor PsA trials, such patients often had less baseline cutaneous involvement (as measured by the Psoriasis Activity Severity Index [PASI]) compared with the psoriasis trials. Although cutaneous disease and peripheral arthritis improved with all TNF inhibitors, the extent of improvement in the skin disease appears to be greater with the monoclonal antibodies (infliximab and adalimumab) than with the soluble receptor construct (etanercept). Whether this difference relates to dosing, different mechanisms of action, or other factors remains to be defined.

Other orphan disorders

The use of TNF inhibitors has rapidly spread to a growing list of uncommonly encountered inflammatory disorders (see Table 61.5).[63,64] Reports of their utility in these "orphan" disorders are limited to investigator-initiated, single-center, open-label, and uncontrolled trials with few treated patients. Many of these reports have only been presented in abstract form, without appearing in peer-reviewed publications. Moreover, assessment of outcomes suffers from the lack of standardized and validated measures. Table 61.5 lists those conditions where TNF blockade has been attempted, has succeeded, or has failed.

Granulomatous disease

Inhibition of TNF has been proposed as a potential means of controlling granulomatous inflammation. TNF has been shown to be crucial in the containment of tuberculosis and other latent opportunistic infections (e.g., fungal). TNF-α plays a pivotal role in granuloma formation and stabilization, by promoting the differentiation of epithelioid macrophages to form granulomas capable of sequestering infected cells. Therapeutic inhibition of TNF in animal models has consistently led to breakdown of granulomas with lethal spread of opportunistic organisms. Similar events have been observed in patients treated with TNF blockade. For these reasons, anti-TNF therapy was expected to be effective in diseases characterized by granulomatous inflammation. Although early uncontrolled reports have shown some therapeutic success in these disorders, subsequent research has undermined these as potential indications.

ANCA-associated granulomatous vasculitis

Uncontrolled exploratory trials have shown that the addition of infliximab or etanercept lowers Birmingham Vasculitis Activity Scores (BVAS) or induces remission.[65] Nonetheless, reports of efficacy in anti-neutrophil cytoplasmic antibody (ANCA)-associated granulomatous vasculitis were questioned when a large ($n = 180$ patients), 9-month trial of etanercept versus placebo in patients with active ANCA-associated granulomatous vasculitis failed to show any benefit of adding etanercept to background therapy.[66] This trial failed to show a change in response rates or vasculitis flares, and etanercept was associated with an increased number of malignancies compared with placebo treatment. Although many subjects on both arms of the study had received prior cyclophosphamide treatment, the increase in solid tumor malignancies was limited to the etanercept group.[67]

Giant cell arteritis

Anecdotal case reports have suggested benefit when TNF inhibition is used in GCA.[63,64,68] However, an interim analysis of a controlled trial failed to show any benefit in 44 corticosteroid-treated patients who received either infliximab (5 mg/kg) or placebo. Relapse rates and steroid reduction were the same in both groups after 54 weeks of observation.[69]

Polymyalgia rheumatica

Open-label reports have suggested that infliximab may be effective in polymyalgia rheumatica (PMR). However, a 22-week, placebo-controlled trial of 51 consecutive PMR patients from seven centers in Italy failed to show any benefit of infliximab over placebo.[70]

Sarcoidosis

A number of anecdotal reports suggested the efficacy of infliximab, etanercept, and adalimumab in sarcoidosis.[63,64,71–74] Most responders were treated with infliximab and had extrapulmonary manifestations (skin [lupus pernio], ocular [uveitis], joint or bone) of sarcoidosis. A small placebo-controlled trial in ocular sarcoid failed to show any benefit of infliximab over placebo controls.[74] Although few reports of improved pulmonary sarcoid exist, a 30-patient, prospective, open-label trial of etanercept in stage II was negative.[75] Recently a large placebo-controlled trial showed modest but significant improvement in chronic pulmonary sarcoidosis patients treated with infliximab.[76]

Pyoderma gangrenosum

Numerous reports have demonstrated rapid resolution of pyoderma gangrenosum lesions using single or multiple doses of infliximab 5 mg/kg (given at weeks 0, 2, and 6). Continued therapy and occasional dose escalation were necessary to maintain control or remission in some of these patients.

Takayasu arteritis

There are limited reports of favorable outcomes when TNF blockade was used in patients with this large vessel vasculitis.[63,64] Four open-label, uncontrolled reports claimed efficacy in patients who were active despite treatment with corticosteroids and methotrexate. All uniformly claimed amelioration of disease and a corticosteroid-sparing effect. Limited numbers and potential positive reporting bias should temper enthusiasm until better controlled trials are done.

Inflammatory eye disease/uveitis

Inflammatory ocular outcomes have often been seen in clinical trials in patients with juvenile arthritis (JRA) or spondyloarthritis, wherein joint indices have responded well but variable ocular benefits were seen. A recent meta-analysis of AS trials using TNF inhibitors studied the pretreatment prevalence and post-treatment flares of anterior uveitis.[61] The frequency of uveitis flares in placebo patients was 15.6/100 patient-years and 6.8/100 patient-years for those receiving etanercept or infliximab. Nonetheless, these trials showed several instances of new-onset anterior uveitis while receiving etanercept or infliximab. Uncontrolled reports have claimed TNF inhibition to also be effective in the management of non-infectious, refractory posterior uveitis.[77,78]

Behçet syndrome

Anecdotal reports of TNF inhibitor use in Behçet disease have suggested therapeutic benefits in difficult cases.[63,79,80] Although most of these reports used infliximab therapy, all three agents have been successfully used in uncontrolled reports. In a 40-patient, placebo-controlled, 4-week trial, etanercept has been shown to lessen the frequency of mucocutaneous manifestations in Behçet patients.[81]

Sjögren syndrome

A double-blind, randomized, placebo-controlled trial of infliximab failed to show any improvement in dryness, joint pain, fatigue, salivary flow rate, Schirmer test, or CRP levels.[82] Similar negative results were seen in a placebo-controlled study of etanercept in Sjögren patients.[83] Collectively, these data suggest that TNF inhibition is not an effective treatment for Sjögren syndrome.

Chronic lung disease

Although there have been uncontrolled reports of TNF blockade in interstitial pneumonitis patients, a placebo-controlled study showed a lack of efficacy in chronic obstructive pulmonary disease (COPD) patients treated with infliximab.[84] What is disturbing is the report that infliximab treatment of COPD patients was associated with an increased number of lung and head/neck cancers in this population of patients in spite of lack of therapeutic benefit.[6] There is still hope that TNF blockade may be beneficial in patients with refractory asthma; however, these trials have yet to be published. Somewhat disturbing are rare reports of new-onset asthmatic flares, pulmonary infiltrates, granulomas, and fibrosing alveolitis after receiving etanercept, infliximab, or adalimumab. Whether the latter related to the particular TNF inhibitor or the underlying inflammatory disorder is unknown. Larger, controlled trials are necessary to establish the efficacy of TNF inhibition in these chronic inflammatory pulmonary disorders.

Hepatitis B and C

Elevated TNF levels have been demonstrated in patients with hepatitis C. Hence a pathogenic role for TNF in HCV infection has been suggested but not clarified. Open-label, retrospective, and prospective studies have not demonstrated worsening of hepatic enzymes or viral load titers with TNF inhibition.[85,86] The potential adjuvant effect of etanercept therapy, combined with interferon and ribavirin, was studied in 50 non-arthritic, chronic HCV patients.[87] This 6-month, double-blind, placebo-controlled trial showed lower viral loads, normal hepatic enzymes, and fewer adverse events when etanercept was combined with this antiviral regimen. These data suggest TNF inhibition may be cautiously used in HCV-infected patients with markedly limited treatment alternatives.

A recent rise in reports of HBV reactivation following TNF inhibition has led some to suggest that TNF blockade patients should be screened for HBV infection prior to use.[86] Reports of worsening, reactivation, and occasional fatalities have provided strong caution for the use of these agents in patients with HBV infection; however, this is tempered by few reports of improvement on TNF inhibitors. Moreover, several HBV patients have successfully received TNF inhibitors while receiving lamivudine prophylaxis. It appears prudent to test for HBV infection before TNF initiation, especially in those at risk.

BASELESS USE OF TUMOR NECROSIS FACTOR INHIBITORS

The popularity of TNF blockade has often led to its application in a variety of conditions presumed to have an underlying inflammatory or immune-mediated pathogenesis. Table 61.5 lists many conditions where the benefits of TNF inhibition are uncertain and unproven. We believe there is no current objective evidence to support the use of these agents in patients with autoimmune hearing loss, infertility, or non-inflammatory spinal disorders. Two small, uncontrolled clinical trials have shown that patients with autoimmune hearing loss or immune-mediated cochleovestibular disorders have no discernible benefit from treatment with etanercept.[88,89] The clinical use of TNF inhibitors in patients with refractory infertility is unfortunate, anecdotal, and currently without scientific merit.

Several anecdotal reports suggest that discogenic spinal pain and pain from spinal metastases or sciatica may be mitigated with TNF blockade.[90] The prevalence and complexity of these spinal conditions mandate that well-designed, controlled trials be performed before one can consider the use of a TNF inhibitor.

P55 TNF inhibitors

Three different p55-directed TNF inhibitors (lenercept, onercept, pegsunercept) have been developed for clinical use, but none is currently approved or actively under investigation for inflammatory indications. Onercept is a recombinant, monomeric soluble TNF-RI (p55). Despite favorable early safety studies in normal volunteers and RA patients, future development was halted. Lenercept is a recombinant fusion protein with two p55 soluble TNF receptors fused to the Fc portion of IgG1. It was originally developed for use in RA and sepsis, but its development was halted when clinical trials did not meet their stated objective of superiority of lenercept over methotrexate due to the development of non-neutralizing antibodies. In a 12-week trial of 247 RA patients, ACR20 response rates were similar between lenercept (53%), methotrexate (50%), and combined lenercept and methotrexate (64%).[91] Pegsunercept is a recombinant monomeric p55 soluble TNF receptor with polyethylene glycol (PEG) linked to enhance its half-life. Several placebo-controlled trials in RA patients showed an encouraging dose-dependent ACR20 response rate.[28,92] Reasons underlying the deferment of development of these p55 inhibitors are unclear but may relate to clinical trial results, toxicity concerns, or pharmacokinetic issues.

TNF inhibitors in early rheumatoid arthritis

Numerous studies have confirmed the efficacy and safety of TNF inhibition in patients with new-onset RA. On the basis of the results of the ERA,[43] ASPIRE,[55] and PREMIER[34] trials, etanercept, infliximab, and adalimumab have been FDA approved for use (as the initial DMARD) in patients with new-onset RA. Although entry into these early RA trials was limited to disease duration of less than 3 years, patients had a mean duration of disease of 6 to 12 months. Hence several large, randomized, controlled trials in early RA (ERA, ASPIRE,

PREMIER, BeST) have taught us that (1) ACR20 responses with TNF inhibitors are equivalent to, or in some cases better than, methotrexate; (2) the best responses (DAS remission, ACR70) are achieved when TNF inhibitors are combined with MTX; (3) TNF inhibitors are superior to MTX in halting radiographic progression (especially when combined with MTX); and (4) the safety of TNF inhibition in early RA appears to be equal to, or better than, that seen with established or severe RA. Nonetheless, it is generally accepted that patients with new-onset RA should receive MTX as their primary DMARD. TNF inhibition should be employed early when MTX cannot be used and/or when the patient is at high risk for severe RA and when more aggressive therapies are indicated.

TNF inhibitors in children

The use of TNF inhibition in children with juvenile arthritis has been limited by few studies. The safety and efficacy of adalimumab or infliximab in children have not been established in clinical trials. Currently, only etanercept is approved for use in patients with active, polyarticular juvenile arthritis after an inadequate response to MTX or other DMARD therapy. The safety and efficacy of etanercept have been studied in 69 patients with polyarticular juvenile arthritis unresponsive to MTX.[93] Patients (4 to 17 years of age) received 0.4 mg/kg twice weekly for 90 days and showed a 74% response rate. After 90 days, responders were randomized to receive placebo or etanercept for 4 months and flare rates were assessed. The time to flare was much shorter for placebo patients (28 days) than for those on etanercept (>116 days). Etanercept has not been studied in children with psoriasis, psoriatic arthritis, or ankylosing spondylitis.

Although a small pilot study of infliximab in pediatric (11 to 17 years) Crohn disease has shown no pharmacokinetic differences between children and adults,[5] the safety and efficacy of infliximab and adalimumab in children with juvenile arthritis, psoriasis, Crohn disease, or ulcerative colitis have not yet been established. There is, however, limited experience with infliximab in juvenile arthritis to suggest it may be helpful in treating the articular, and possibly the systemic, manifestations in systemic-onset juvenile arthritis.[94]

TNF inhibitors in the elderly

There have been few studies that specifically address the use of TNF blockade in an elderly population. Drug development pharmacokinetic studies of all three agents failed to show any influence of age or gender. During infliximab clinical trials in RA, 181 geriatric (>65 years) patients demonstrated efficacy and safety similar to younger patients; however, both infliximab and control patients exhibited more serious adverse events than did younger patients. Etanercept has been studied in older patients with RA and psoriatic arthritis patients in clinical trials demonstrating no difference in efficacy or safety between elderly and younger patients.[95]

Because advancing age appears to be a risk for serious infection, TNF inhibitors should be used with caution in a geriatric patient, especially if co-morbidities, debility, and a past history of serious infection exist.

OTHER BIOLOGIC TUMOR NECROSIS FACTOR BLOCKERS UNDER INVESTIGATION

A variety of other strategies are being tested with the ultimate goal of inhibiting the function of TNF. Some of these are macromolecules, including the PEGylated human anti-TNF-α mAb Fab fragment CDP870 (certolizumab pegol) and golimumab. PEG has been shown to increase the half-life of compounds to which it is bound.

In phase 2 studies, subcutaneous injections of increasing doses of certolizumab pegol were well tolerated in active RA with rapid improvement in ACR responses.[96] The efficacy and safety of certolizumab pegol in active rheumatoid arthritis have now been assessed in three phase 3, multicenter, randomized, double-blind, placebo-controlled clinical trials. The RAPID 1[97] and RAPID 2[98] studies evaluated the efficacy and safety of lyophilized and liquid formulations, respectively, of subcutaneous certolizumab pegol versus placebo, plus methotrexate

(MTX), in patients with active RA. Patients randomized to receive active drug were given a dose of 400 mg at weeks 0, 2, and 4 followed by 200 mg or 400 mg plus MTX, or placebo plus MTX, every 2 weeks for 24 weeks. Among the 982 patients enrolled to RAPID 1, at week 24, ACR20 response rates using non-responder imputation for the certolizumab pegol 200-mg and 400-mg groups were 58.8% and 60.8%, respectively, as compared with 13.6% for the placebo group. Differences in ACR20 response rates versus placebo were significant at week 1 and were sustained to week 52 ($P < 0.001$). The trial also showed that the drug improved physical function as early as week 1 and slowed mean radiographic progression from baseline by week 52; certolizumab pegol 200 mg (0.4 Sharp units) or 400 mg (0.2 Sharp units) as compared with that in placebo-treated patients (2.8 Sharp units) ($P < 0.001$). Neither RAPID 1 nor RAPID 2 showed any advantage of 400 mg over 200 mg certolizumab pegol over 52 weeks, after induction with 400 mg.

FAST4WARD was a 24-week, randomized, double-blind, placebo-controlled study evaluating certolizumab as monotherapy in 220 patients who had previously failed one or more DMARDs.[99] They were randomized to receive subcutaneous certolizumab 400 mg ($n = 111$) or placebo ($n = 109$) every 4 weeks. The primary endpoint of ACR20 response at week 24 was 45.5% for the certolizumab group and 9.3% for the placebo group ($p < 0.001$). Differences for certolizumab pegol versus placebo in the ACR20 response were statistically significant as early as week 1 through to week 24 ($P < 0.001$). Significant improvements in ACR50, ACR components, DAS28(ESR)-3, and all patient-reported outcomes were also observed early with certolizumab pegol and were sustained throughout the study.

Golimumab is a fully human anti-TNF monoclonal antibody currently in a comprehensive phase 3 development program of studies for the treatment of RA, Crohn disease, psoriatic arthritis, and ankylosing spondylitis. It can be administered intravenously or subcutaneously. Findings from two multicenter, randomized, double-blind, placebo-controlled phase 3 RA studies have been reported in three important populations—MTX-naïve patients (GO-BEFORE), patients with active RA despite ongoing treatment with MTX (GO-FORWARD), and prior anti-TNF refractory patients (GO-AFTER). These studies showed that patients receiving every 4-week subcutaneous injections of golimumab 50 mg and 100 mg and weekly methotrexate (MTX) experienced significant improvements in the signs and symptoms, as well as in physical function and disease activity, with some patients achieving remission as measured by DAS28.

The GO-BEFORE study investigated the efficacy and safety of golimumab delivered once every 4 weeks by subcutaneous injection at a dose of either 100 mg alone, 50 mg, or 100 mg or in combination with MTX versus MTX alone in MTX-naïve patients with active RA. When three patients did not receive the study drug but were included in the analysis as non-responders, the primary endpoint, ACR50 by intent-to-treat (ITT) analysis, was not achieved. However, when the three patients who did not receive golimumab were excluded, a modified ITT analysis showed that the proportion of patients achieving ACR50 was statistically higher in the 4 weekly 50-mg golimumab plus MTX than in those receiving MTX alone.[100] In the GO-FORWARD study, in subjects with active RA despite MTX, both the 50-mg and 100-mg doses of golimumab were studied in patients whose disease was active despite ongoing treatment with MTX.[101] At week 14, 55% of patients receiving golimumab 50 mg plus MTX and 56% receiving golimumab 100 mg plus MTX achieved at least 20% improvement in signs and symptoms of RA (ACR20), compared with 33% of patients receiving placebo and MTX ($P < 0.01$ and $P < 0.001$, respectively). Improvements were seen as early as first clinical assessment, which was 4 weeks after the first golimumab injection, and generally continued to improve over time. At 24 weeks, 68% of patients in the golimumab 50-mg dosing group and 72% of patients receiving golimumab 100 mg experienced clinically relevant improvement in physical function (improvement in HAQ score of at least 0.25 from baseline), compared with 39% of patients receiving placebo plus MTX ($P < 0.0001$). GO-AFTER is the first large, phase 3, double-blind, placebo-controlled trial to test the efficacy of anti-TNF switching in patients failing on a first anti-TNF agent.[102] It included 461 patients with active RA of 8.65 years' mean duration. All patients had previously received at least one anti-TNF agent, with 25% ($n = 115$) having been treated

with two therapies and 9% ($n = 43$) with three. Discontinuation of previous anti-TNF therapy was due to lack of efficacy (58%), intolerance (17%), and other reasons (40%). Patients were randomized to one of three treatment groups: subcutaneous placebo, golimumab 50 mg, or golimumab 100 mg every 4 weeks. At baseline, 66% of patients were receiving methotrexate; 5% and 7% of patients were receiving sulfasalazine and hydroxychloroquine, respectively. Patients continued to receive stable doses of methotrexate, sulfasalazine, and/or hydroxychloroquine if receiving them at baseline. Among patients who discontinued previous anti-TNF because of lack of efficacy, 35.7% and 42.7% of patients in the golimumab 50-mg and 100-mg groups, respectively, had ACR20 responses at week 14 compared with 17.7% in the placebo group.

SAFETY OF ANTI-TUMOR NECROSIS FACTOR THERAPY

Advances in treatment afforded by TNF blockade have been tempered by safety concerns, many of which have been disclosed by controlled clinical trials with large numbers of patients treated with etanercept (3094 patients), infliximab (3263 patients), and adalimumab (2468 patients). These clinical trials established the most common adverse events among thousands of patients enrolled for having low or no co-morbidities, with limitations on age, disease status, and background therapies. A real-world spectrum of TNF inhibitor-related safety concerns depends on a variety of pharmacovigilance efforts (e.g., open-label extension trials, phase 4 trials, postmarketing surveillance, passive physician and patient reports, disease databases and registries) performed in less select populations, with co-morbidities and variable drug dosing and background medications. In the postmarketing era, the safety of TNF inhibitors has accumulated with more than 8 years of experience and over 1.2 million patients treated worldwide. Although pharmacovigilance data may be limited by event underreporting, unverified diagnoses, duplicate reports, confounding co-morbidities or medications, and uncertain temporal associations or causality, they offer our most comprehensive view of TNF inhibitor safety.[103]

Ongoing reviews of comprehensive safety data have important implications with regard to how, when, and in whom such therapies may be used. The duration and dose of TNF inhibitor use should be considered when choosing such therapy for a chronic, active, and difficult-to-control inflammatory disorder. New and developing indications require the re-establishment of long-term safety in these new indications. The greater the experience with long-term drug use, the more certain the safety profile of that agent in that indication. Lastly, the realization that TNF blockade may impact immunosurveillance or host resistance to infection mandates the need for ongoing, population-based safety research and guidance regarding proper patient selection.

Safety is best ensured by awareness of safety issues and avoidance of unnecessary risk. Box 61.3 details the relative contraindications to the use of TNF inhibitors. Moreover, the use of these agents in unapproved, rare, or orphan conditions may be associated with unexpected or unsatisfactory outcomes. Although many safety issues (e.g., tuberculosis, opportunistic infection, lupus) might have been predicted on the basis of preclinical studies, the development of unanticipated adverse events in newly exposed patient populations (e.g., demyelinating disease, heart failure, cytopenia) should temper inappropriate and widespread use of TNF inhibitors.

One indication of both efficacy and safety is the durability of an agent (e.g., how long a patient remains on such therapy). In randomized, placebo-controlled clinical trials, patients receiving TNF inhibitor consistently demonstrated higher study completion rates and lower dropout rates compared with placebo or matched controls.[4-6] Real-world observational studies have shown that the durability of the TNF inhibitors compares favorably with MTX, such that 65% to 80% of RA patients are still taking their TNF inhibitors 1 year after drug initiation.[42,104] Dropouts for safety account for approximately 30% to 50% of those who discontinue TNF inhibitor therapy. Several studies consistently show the dropout rate of these agents to be nearly 10% to 15% per year in the first 2 years and roughly 10% per annum thereafter.

Infusion reactions

Reactions to these parenterally administered agents are among the most common of side effects. Clinical trials have shown that 20% of infliximab-treated patients have experienced an infusion reaction. However, less than 1% of infliximab-treated patients develop serious infusion-related reactions, and only 2.5% of reactions are the cause of drug cessation. Most infliximab infusion reactions occur during infusion or within 2 hours postinfusion. Common complaints include headache (20%), nausea (15%), urticaria, pruritus, rash, flushing, fever, chills, tachycardia, or dyspnea. In many, infusion reactions are the result of a rapid infusion rate (i.e., <2 hours). These reactions are usually transient, are rarely severe, and can typically be controlled by slowing the rate of infusion or treating with acetaminophen, nonsedating antihistamines, or short-acting corticosteroids. Premedication with the aforementioned agents is not routinely required but may be necessary in those who exhibit infusion reactions.

Rarely, severe or anaphylactic reactions occur wherein findings of chest tightness, bronchospasm, hypotension, diaphoresis, anaphylaxis, or "feeling of impending doom" may occur. In these individuals, infliximab therapy should be halted, and supportive or emergent care administered until the patient is stabilized. For these reasons infliximab infusions should only be delivered with appropriately trained medical personnel in attendance with ready access to parenteral corticosteroids, diphenhydramine, and epinephrine.

Infusion reactions are twofold to threefold more likely if HACA are present. The immunogenicity of infliximab can be mitigated by concomitant MTX use or higher doses. Experience with intermittent treatment of Crohn disease has shown reactions to be more likely when infliximab therapy is intermittent and suspended for more than 2 years. In these patients, 25% developed delayed (3 to 12 days postinfusion) reactions with symptoms of myalgia, arthralgia, fever, chills, rash, urticaria, edema, dysphagia, and sore throat.[5]

Injection site reactions

During the RA adalimumab and etanercept clinical trials, cutaneous injection site reactions (ISRs) were seen in 20% and 37% of patients. However, these are less frequent in practice and rarely require drug discontinuation. ISRs are usually mild or moderate and resolve within 7 days, and they are most common during the first 4 to 8 weeks of use. Patients may describe dysesthesia, bruising, erythema, pruritus, or urticaria at administration sites. Lastly, ISRs are not correlated with drug dose, frequency of administration, or the presence of neutralizing antibodies. Interestingly, in the TEMPO (etanercept) trial, fewer ISRs were observed in the MTX plus TNF inhibitor group when compared with the TNF inhibitor alone.[45]

Other cutaneous reactions

Rarely, other cutaneous reactions have been ascribed to these TNF inhibitors, including lupus-like rashes (see Autoimmune responses later), hypersensitivity vasculitis, palpable purpura, urticaria, folliculitis, new-onset psoriasis, pernio, granuloma annulare, interstitial granulomatous dermatitis, lichenoid eruptions, bullous lesions, erythema multiforme, chilblains, opportunistic skin infections, and cutaneous T-cell lymphoma (Box 61.5).[105-107]

Infectious risk

In otherwise healthy individuals, TNF plays an important role in defense against infections, especially intracellular organisms. In the context of infection, TNF enhances endothelial cell activation at the site of involvement, promotes inflammatory cell recruitment, and has a procoagulant role in limiting the spread of infection. It also increases the ability of activated macrophages to phagocytose and kill mycobacteria. Concerns that modulation of physiologic or excess TNF levels by specific inhibitors might promote infectious complications were heightened on the basis of animal studies demonstrating the fatal effects of TNF inhibition in models of sepsis or endotoxic shock and the protective role of TNF with respect to opportunistic infections such

---

BOX 61.5 CUTANEOUS DISORDERS AND TUMOR NECROSIS FACTOR (TNF) INHIBITOR THERAPY

Anecdotal improvements with TNF	TNF inhibitor-induced cutaneous inhibitor therapy disorders
Pustular psoriasis	Lupus-like rashes
Acrodermatitis continua of Hallopeau	Hypersensitivity vasculitis, palpable
Psoriatic onychopachydermoperiostitis	Purpura
Pyoderma gangrenosum	Urticaria, angioedema
Pemphigus	Folliculitis
SAPHO syndrome	Interstitial granulomatous dermatitis
Graft-versus-host disease	Eosinophilic cellulitis
PAPA syndrome	Alopecia areata
Sarcoidosis	Pernio
Aphthous stomatitis	New-onset psoriasis
Sneddon-Wilkinson disease	Bullous lesions
Eosinophilic fasciitis	Granuloma annulare
Panniculitis	Lichenoid eruptions
Necrobiosis lipoidica diabeticorum	Erythema multiforme
Hidradenitis suppurativa	Chilblain
Scleroderma	Scleredema
	Subcutaneous fat atrophy
	Opportunistic skin infections
	Cutaneous T-cell lymphoma
	Oral epithelial dysplasia

---

as *Mycobacterium tuberculosis*, *Candida*, *Histoplasma*, *Leishmania*, and malaria.[108] Several early trials of TNF inhibition in sepsis, undertaken in an attempt to treat shock, failed to show any consistent benefit or hazard to TNF neutralization.[109,110] Whereas sepsis was not pursued as an indication for TNF blockade, inflammatory disorders were subsequently studied.

RA patients have approximately twice the mortality rate of the general population, and serious infection (leading to hospital admission, intravenous antibiotics, or death) is a major contributing factor. When considering whether anti-TNF biologics raise infection risks, the higher background infection rates in RA need to be considered. Similarly, the influence of concomitantly administered drugs must also be taken into account. For example, Wolfe and colleagues[111] reviewed the national databank for rheumatic diseases in the United States following over 16,000 patients for 3.5 years. They observed the risk of hospitalized pneumonia to be 1.7 times higher in patients receiving corticosteroids. Prednisolone at doses of only 5 mg/day or less gave a hazard ratio of 1.4 (95% confidence interval (CI): 1.1 to 1.6).[111]

Data on the magnitude of infection risk on anti-TNF drugs come either from clinical trials or observational studies. Controlled trials have produced conflicting messages with respect to the risk of serious infectious complications. Some studies have suggested increased serious infection rates, and others have found no difference from controls.

In the etanercept, infliximab, and adalimumab clinical trials, common, non-serious infections (e.g., upper respiratory tract infections [URI], bronchitis, sinusitis, pharyngitis, urinary tract infections) were seen in 20% to 37% of patients. During these trials, anti-TNF therapy was not suspended or stopped for these non-serious infections and all responded well to either observation or symptomatic therapy.

Serious infectious events (e.g., pneumonia, cellulitis, joint infections) or death from infection were infrequently reported in clinical trials before FDA approval and, overall, were not observed at a rate greater than that seen in placebo-treated controls. In the randomized placebo-controlled trials of all three TNF target agents (n = 6303 patients followed for 6 to 12 months), the rate of serious infectious events ranged from three to four events per 100 patient-years of therapy compared with two events per 100 patient-years in placebo-treated

TABLE 61.6 FREQUENCY OF SERIOUS ADVERSE EVENTS WITH TUMOR NECROSIS FACTOR INHIBITORS

	Infliximab*	Etanercept	Adalimumab
Pneumonia	1.7%*	<1%*	0.92%[†]
Tuberculosis	0.4%*	0.03%[‡]	0.23%[†]
Cytopenia[§]	0.9-1.4%[†]	ND	0.08/100 pt-yr[†]
Lymphoma	0.31%[‡]	0.26%[‡]	0.41%[‡]
Demyelinating disorders	ND	ND	0.08%[†]
Drug-induced lupus	0.2%[4]		0.05%[†]
Congestive heart failure	0.2%[‡]	0.06%[‡]	0.1%[‡]
Transaminitis (<3-fold)	34%[†]	ND	ND
Hepatic failure	0.006[†]	ND	ND

*Package insert data from pivotal randomized clinical trial results.[4-6]
[†]2004 Postmarketing data reported (data provided by manufacturer).
[‡]Data from 2003 FDA Arthritis Advisory Committee review of TNF safety.[97,101]
[§]Cytopenia includes leukopenia, neutropenia, thrombocytopenia.[4] De Bant and colleagues estimate the frequency to be 0.19%.[99]

patients.[4-6] Although many trials have shown no increase in serious infections (compared with placebo or active controls), several trials have shown higher rates of serious infections. For example, serious infections in the ATTRACT and ASPIRE trials were seen in 5.4% of infliximab/MTX patients and 3.4% of patients on MTX alone.[52,55] Pneumonia was seen in 1.7% of infliximab patents and 0.3% of placebo patients (Table 61.6). Similarly, the DE019 trial found more serious infections among the adalimumab/MTX group (3.8%) compared with MTX/placebo group (0.5%).[36] Lastly, the PREMIER trial revealed different serious infection rates (1.6, 0.7, and 2.9 events per 100 patient-years) in patients treated with MTX, adalimumab, or the combination of MTX/adalimumab, respectively.[34] Postmarketing studies have also shown mixed results with either equal and increased infection rates seen between TNF inhibitors and DMARD controls.[112-114] Reported serious infections include pneumonia, cellulitis, septic arthritis, prosthetic joint infections, postsurgical or wound infection, diverticulitis, pyelonephritis, abscess, and sepsis.

A recent meta-analysis was performed because analysis of sparse event data from individual trials is typically too brief or not powered to detect these differences between active and placebo groups. This analysis revealed a pooled odds ratio of 2.0 for serious infections in patients taking anti-TNF antibodies compared with the control groups,[113] thus confirming some of the studies referred to earlier.

As in the case of controlled trials, observational studies have produced conflicting messages with respect to the risk of serious infectious complications, some studies suggesting increased serious infection rates, and others no difference from comparator groups. These apparent discrepancies may depend on many factors including the variation in background rate of infection in different populations and locations, the duration of exposure to TNF inhibition[114,115] in addition to confounders with respect to concomitant therapy, and differences in disease severity between anti-TNF treated and comparator cohorts. Another factor may relate to the biology of TNF inhibition. Evidence suggests that normalization of immune disequilibrium in RA may restore physiologic immune responses. For example, infliximab treatment in RA results in significant increases in circulating T regulatory cells and reversal of their anergic phenotype.[116] Thus it is possible that patients with well-controlled inflammation become less susceptible to infection than those with partially controlled inflammation or oversuppression of TNF.[117]

At first sight, a review of infectious risk data emerging from observational studies and the various national registries suggests a variable level of risk. But when the incidence rate ratios are plotted against the duration of follow-up, a clear and consistent pattern emerges,

suggesting that risk of infectious complications is highest during the initial period of exposure to an anti-TNF, tending to decline after 6 months of therapy.[115] In patients enrolled onto the German biologics register (RABBIT; etanercept $n = 512$, infliximab $n = 346$, DMARD control $n = 601$), the reported relative risk of serious infections was 2.2 (95% CI: 0.9 to 5.4) for etanercept (64/1000 patient-years) and 2.1 (0.8 to 5.5) for infliximab (62/1000 patient-years) compared with patients on DMARDs only (23/1000 patient-years).[118] Despite the lower confidence intervals overlapping with 1.0, these findings suggest a trend to increased risk of serious infection. This was independent of RA severity or duration, rheumatoid factor seropositivity, concomitant steroid use, diabetes, or lung disease.

A retrospective U.S. study by Curtis and colleagues[119] studied 3894 person-years of anti-TNF therapy and 4846 person-years of methotrexate over a median of 17 months. They demonstrated an adjusted risk of hospitalization caused by bacterial infection, which was 1.9-fold higher in the anti-TNF patients (4.2-fold higher in the first 6 months). The Spanish registry showed a 1.6-fold increase in rate of serious infection of 2868 patient-years on anti-TNF drugs compared with 2433 patient-years of controls.[120] Bernatsky and colleagues[121] carried out a case-control cohort study of 23,733 RA patients, suggesting a twofold increase in risk of all infections in patients on TNF blockers (infliximab and etanercept). However, because of the limited number of patients on anti-TNF ($n = 261$), the confidence interval was wide. In a retrospective study of 709 RA patients, Salliot and colleagues[122] found the incidence of serious infections before anti-TNF was 3.4 per 100 patient-years, and 10.5 afterwards.

The British Society for Rheumatology Biologics Register (BSRBR) reported findings on a national prospective observational study of 7664 anti-TNF and 1354 DMARD-treated RA patients. No increase in serious infections in total was observed in anti-TNF–treated patients compared with conventional DMARD-treated patients.[123] The incidence of serious infections in the anti-TNF group was 53.2 per 1000 person-years versus 41.2 in the control group. However, serious skin and soft tissue infections were more frequent in anti-TNF–treated patients (incidence risk ratio of 4.2). A total of 19 serious bacterial intracellular infections occurred, all in patients in the anti-TNF-treated cohort. Moreover, after extended analysis, Dixon and colleagues[114] have found an increased adjusted incidence rate of serious infection (ratio 4.6; 95% CI: 1.8 to 11.9) over the first 90 days after starting on anti-TNF drugs compared with DMARD therapy.

Klareskog and colleagues[124] followed 686 patients for 52 weeks and found no difference in the prevalence of serious infections in those receiving methotrexate and etanercept in combination versus either drug alone (about 4% for all groups). In a large cohort of 16,788 patients followed up over 3.5 years, Wolfe and colleagues[111] found no increase in the pneumonia risk for anti-TNF treatment. Schneeweiss and colleagues[125] performed a retrospective study of patients older than 65 years of age, with 1900 patients on methotrexate compared with 469 on anti-TNF drugs, followed up for 0.2 to 1.3 years. No increase was reported in infection rate in the anti-TNF group.

In conclusion, despite apparently contradictory findings with respect to the risk of infectious complications of anti-TNF therapy arising from observational studies and registry data, a more detailed analysis of available data suggests a more or less coherent pattern of an increased risk shortly after treatment starts.[115]

Current prescribing guidelines caution against the use of TNF inhibitors in patients with active serious infections or in those with chronic or recurrent infections and that patients should be monitored for signs and symptoms of infection while receiving TNF inhibitors. Although these therapies may be indicated as inflammation and disease severity increase, there may be a point at which TNF blockade provides no benefit and may instead increase the risk of infection.[3] Moreover, the infectious risk may be heightened in the presence of well-known risk factors, such as advanced age, debility, extreme inflammatory activity, corticosteroid use (especially higher doses), co-morbidities, skin breakdown, and planned major surgery (e.g., joint replacement). Increasing data suggest that higher-dose TNF blockade may also increase the risk of infection.[52,117] Serious bacterial infections may therefore be averted by proper patient selection, proper dosing, or TNF inhibitor avoidance if numerous infectious risk factors are present.

Lastly, the combination of anakinra and a TNF inhibitor should be avoided as both open-label and controlled trials showed no clinical benefit but yielded an increased risk of serious infections (7%) and neutropenia (2%).[126] Similarly, the biologic co-stimulation blocker abatacept (CTLA4-Ig) should not be combined with TNF inhibitor therapy because this combination also yielded higher rates of serious infections (5.8% vs. 1.9%) in a randomized clinical trial.[127]

Guidelines for the prevention and management of infections, especially serious infection, are currently lacking. Patients experiencing mild to moderate URI, bronchitis, or sinusitis can be symptomatically managed or closely observed without drug cessation. However, patients demonstrating high fevers or other suspicious symptomatology may benefit from drug suspension and further evaluation. TNF inhibitors should be stopped when patients have a serious infection, hospitalizable infection, or opportunistic infection and should not be restarted until adequate control has been achieved. Patients undergoing elective major surgery (e.g., joint replacement surgery) may also benefit from suspending the TNF inhibitor for at least one dosing cycle (e.g., etanercept 7 days, adalimumab 14 days, infliximab 6 to 8 weeks) before surgery, provided such cessation does not induce a major inflammatory flare. Although one study showed that RA patients receiving TNF inhibitors had a fivefold increased risk in postoperative serious infections following joint arthroplasty,[128] further research is necessary into how to best manage these patients.

Tuberculosis

TNF antagonist therapy can interfere with the host's ability to protect itself from mycobacterial infection. TNF plays an important role in the formation and maintenance of granulomas. Tuberculosis (TB) and other opportunistic infections have been associated with all three currently marketed TNF blocking agents (see Table 61.6). Hence therapeutic inhibition of TNF augments the risk of reactivation of latent mycobacterial (or fungal) infection. Interestingly, 30% to 50% of such patients present with extrapulmonary, miliary, or disseminated and non-pulmonary presentations of TB.[3] Although the risk of TB is increased by TNF inhibition, even greater rates are seen in populations from geographic regions where TB is endemic.[129] Although current product labeling calls for TB screening with adalimumab and infliximab initiation (but not etanercept), TB infections have occurred with all three agents.

Although no cases of TB emerged in the etanercept clinical trials, postmarketing analyses demonstrated 38 confirmed cases of etanercept-associated TB worldwide in the first 150,000 patients treated through December 2002.[3] For infliximab, 441 cases of infliximab-related TB were reported among 492,874 treated patients worldwide, whereas there were only six infliximab-related TB cases reported in the clinical trials.[130] Ninety-seven percent of the infliximab-related cases occurred within 7 months, with a median time to onset of 12 weeks. The incidence of TB in clinical trials with adalimumab was higher in early clinical trials when the dose of adalimumab was higher and no screening procedures were used or enforced. The incidence of TB dropped 85% when adalimumab dose was reduced and screening measures for latent TB infection (purified protein derivative [PPD], chest x-ray) were required before therapy.[129,130] To date, a greater number of cases have been seen among patients receiving infliximab than the other TNF inhibitors, but this may in part relate to greater worldwide use (especially endemic regions), older patient population (influenced by Medicare reimbursement), different screening procedures between the United States and Europe, slower off-rate (sustained TNF binding), induction of apoptosis or cell lysis, and the need for dose escalation over time ("dose creep") in a minority of patients. Because TB and opportunistic infections have been reported with all three TNF inhibitors, this should be considered a class-related risk.

The increased risk and extrapulmonary presentations of TB with TNF blockade mandate screening, close follow-up, and ongoing clinical suspicion. The risk of developing TB with TNF antagonists is significantly reduced with screening and appropriate monitoring. Two different data sets have shown the preventive value of screening prior to drug initiation. In the adalimumab clinical trials, a TB infection rate of 1.3 per 100 patient-years was decreased to less than 0.11 per 100 patient-years with mandated screening (PPD in North America and chest radiographs in Europe).[6,130] Carmona and colleagues[129] have also shown a nearly 80% reduction in active TB cases once screening and treatment of latent TB became an official recommendation in Spain.

Current guidelines from the Centers for Disease Control and Prevention (CDC) and the American Thoracic Society recommend PPD skin testing before TNF antagonist therapy. The tuberculin skin test (PPD) must be read within 48 to 72 hours by a health care professional and is considered positive if induration is greater than 5 mm. Patients previously vaccinated with bacille Calmette-Guérin (BCG) should also be screened with a tuberculin skin test. The use of controls is not recommended because up to one third of RA patients may be anergic. Chest radiographs are not routinely performed but should be done in those with a positive tuberculin skin test, recent or past exposure to TB, signs or symptoms of TB, or travel to high-risk endemic areas.[131] If the PPD test is positive and the patient is without signs, symptoms, or chest radiographic evidence of active infection, treatment for latent TB should commence before or with anti-TNF therapy. CDC guidelines suggest that 9 months of isoniazid (INH) therapy are optimal, although 6 months of INH or other alternative regimens also have proven efficacy.

The PPD test is of limited benefit in immunosuppressed individuals who often fail to mount a delayed-type hypersensitivity reaction. In such patients, newer interferon-gamma–releasing assays may be a more robust method for diagnosing tuberculosis and assessment of latent TB. M. tuberculosis expresses the antigens Early Secretory Antigenic Target-6 (ESAT-6) and Culture Filtrate Protein-10 (CFP-10). These antigens are used in the ELISpot to stimulate peripheral blood mononuclear cells (PBMCs). In patients with active or latent tuberculosis, the PBMCs have been exposed to ESAT-6 and CFP-10 and on restimulation with these antigens produce interferon-gamma (IFN-γ). The numbers of PBMCs producing IFN-γ are quantified. ESAT-6 and CFP-10 are not present in the Mycobacterium bovis BCG vaccine and certain mycobacterial strains including M. fortuitum. The ELISpot is therefore not confounded by prior BCG vaccination or exposure to environmental mycobacteria. However, it should be noted that a negative ELISpot does not exclude non-tuberculous mycobacterial species, usually considered benign contaminants, that are nonetheless increasingly recognized to be associated with pulmonary disease in immunocompromised hosts.

Patients taking TNF inhibitors should be considered at risk for opportunistic infection. Those exhibiting signs and symptoms of active mycobacterial or opportunistic infections merit evaluation, suspension of anti-TNF therapy, and appropriate therapy. TNF therapy should be avoided until the infection is controlled. Common sites of extrapulmonary infection include the joint, bone, vertebra, bladder, meninges, peritoneum, and lymph nodes.

Other opportunistic infections have also been reported. Atypical mycobacterial infections were reported, including reports of Mycobacterium avium intracellulare, Mycobacterium kansasii, and Mycobacterium marinarum. Fungal and opportunistic pathogens have been observed with all three TNF inhibitors, including histoplasmosis, pneumocystis, aspergillosis, coccidioidomycosis, sporotrichosis, nocardia, listeriosis, and cytomegalovirus. Because no reliable skin or serologic testing exists to screen for these infections, clinicians must closely monitor patients for symptoms or signs of opportunistic infections, especially in endemic regions (e.g., Europe, South America, Ohio River Valley, San Joaquin Valley). It should be noted that chronic prednisone therapy may also predispose to such infections. Lastly, although there are reports of herpes zoster in patients receiving TNF inhibitors, it is unknown if this is related to the TNF inhibitor, underlying diagnosis, or background therapies.

Neoplasia and lymphoma

Numerous population-based studies have generally shown that RA patients have an increased risk of lymphoma but are not at risk for other malignancies (e.g., solid tumors) and may in fact be at a lower risk of adenocarcinoma of the colon, presumably from the use of nonsteroidal anti-inflammatory drugs or cyclooxygenase-2 inhibitors. An overall twofold to threefold increase in lymphoma (primarily non-Hodgkin) has been shown in RA population studies. The lymphoma risk appears to increase with age and increasing inflammatory disease activity. In a 2003 FDA analysis of this issue, six lymphomas were found among 6303 RA patients treated with TNF inhibitors in controlled clinical trials, but none were observed in placebo-treated patients. A total of 23 lymphomas was observed (9 etanercept, 4 infliximab, 10 adalimumab) during drug development, with an increased standardized incidence ratio (SIR, relative risk) of 3.47, 6.35, and 5.42, respectively. However, the 95% confidence intervals for these SIRs were particularly wide and overlapping, thus not permitting any separation of lymphoma risk due to drug or active RA alone.

Thus lymphoma rates in RA patients taking TNF inhibitors are elevated, but it is not yet known if this merely reflects an excess risk above that incurred by active disease alone. Data from safety registries suggest that it is disease activity rather than TNF inhibition that accounts for the observed increase in lymphoma rates associated with TNF blockade.[132,133] However, there are also reports indicating an increased lymphoma risk related to anti-TNF treatment.[134] The lag time from TNF blocker exposure to the onset of lymphoma varied, but most occurred after 6 to 24 months of TNF therapy. Hodgkin lymphoma occurred in 15%, with the remaining being non-Hodgkin lymphomas usually of the diffuse, large, B-cell class. Follicular, mantle, MALT, and T-cell lymphomas were uncommonly observed.[6,35] These issues merit continued scrutiny in long-term population-based surveillance registries of RA patients on biologic and non-biologic DMARD therapy to provide a clearer understanding of the risk for lymphoma. There have been rare and fatal reports of hepatosplenic T-cell lymphoma in pediatric Crohn disease patients receiving infliximab.[6] These events have not been observed with adalimumab or etanercept. At present, any risk of lymphoma is considered sufficiently limited such that it does not exert a major influence in the decision to initiate or continue anti-TNF treatment in patients with RA and high disease activity or rapidly progressive joint damage.

Rates of solid tumors were not increased when TNF-associated malignancies were compared with population expectations at an FDA meeting in 2003.[135] Similarly, in registry studies, no overall increase in risk has been reported in RA patients whether or not exposed to TNF inhibitors.[136] However, a recent meta-analysis of patients on TNF inhibitors (limited to the monoclonal antibodies) showed more malignancies (0.8%) compared with the placebo-matched population (0.2%), with a pooled odds ratio (OR) of 3.3 compared with placebo-treated patients. The risks appear to be dose dependent, with those on high-dose therapy (defined as ≥6 mg/kg infliximab every 8 weeks or ≥40 mg adalimumab every other week) having the greatest risk (OR: 4.3; 95% CI: 1.6 to 11.8), with no important increased risk below these doses.[113] The lower than expected rate of neoplasia in the placebo group has been questioned and may relate to the inaccuracies of a shorter duration of placebo and TNF inhibitor exposure. Nonetheless, there have been other studies demonstrating a higher rate of solid tumors. A 9-month, 180-patient trial of etanercept in ANCA-associated granulomatous vasculitis revealed six solid tumors in the etanercept group and none among the placebo controls.[66] Although all six of these patients had received cyclophosphamide, it appears that the addition of cyclophosphamide to etanercept may increase the risk of malignancy. Additionally, a trial of infliximab in patients with severe COPD demonstrated an excess of solid tumors among patients receiving the TNF inhibitor.[6] Thus these analyses suggest the rates of solid tumors may be increased in certain at-risk populations and that more research is necessary on this issue.

Antibiologic antibody responses

Antibodies against these agents, which are large foreign proteins, are inevitable. Although the clinical relevance of such antibodies is presently unclear, it is nonetheless possible that they may lead to immune complex formation, hypersensitivity reactions, or even impaired drug efficacy. Approximately 3% of the etanercept-treated patients developed antibodies to etanercept.[5] In one study, antibodies to infliximab developed in 53%, 21%, and 7% of patients receiving 1, 3, or 10 mg per kilogram of drug, respectively.[52] RA trials of infliximab with or without concomitant methotrexate treatment revealed that immunogenicity was decreased by concomitant MTX, due perhaps in part to the increase in the half-life of infliximab associated with MTX use.[6] A multicenter trial of infliximab therapy in Crohn disease revealed that the induction

of these anti-infliximab antibodies might have contributed to hypersensitivity reaction in some patients who had been treated with this drug. Although antibodies to adalimumab develop in about 12% of patients, the rate is reduced to 1% with concurrent methotrexate treatment.[130] Routine testing for antibodies to these anti-TNF constructs is not currently recommended because the assays have not been standardized and the results would be of questionable clinical value.

Autoimmune responses

Although nearly 40% of RA patients have serum antinuclear antibodies (ANA), the prevalence of ANA positivity increases with the use of anti-TNF agents. The mechanism(s) underlying autoantibody induction are uncertain but may relate to a compensatory increase in IL-10 or interferon-α, both of which are inhibited by TNF.[135] Both can increase B-cell activity and are increased in patients treated with anti-TNF therapy. Antibodies to double-stranded DNA (ds-DNA) have also been reported to develop in about 5% to 10% of RA patients treated with all anti-TNF therapies.[4-6] However, few (0.2% to 0.4%) develop symptoms consistent with drug-induced lupus.[135,137,138] Findings of ANA or dsDNA seropositivity are poorly predictive of subsequent toxicity and thus pretreatment or routine monitoring of autoantibodies is not recommended.

The occurrence of drug-induced lupus has been ascribed to all three TNF inhibitors. Such patients need not meet criteria for lupus but must manifest a lupus-specific feature with evidence of ANA or dsDNA positivity and resolution with drug cessation. During drug development, there were few reports of TNF inhibitor-related rashes (discoid lupus, subacute cutaneous lupus, hypersensitivity vasculitis), serositis, cytopenias, and polyarthritis. Review of the literature reveals more than 100 cases of drug-induced lupus.[135] Several points about drug-induced lupus related to the TNF inhibitors are worth summarizing:

- Common skin findings include malar rash, palpable purpura, or a "sun-burnt" rash.
- The new onset of an acute large and small joint polyarthritis in a previously stable RA patient treated with a TNF inhibitor may be an indication of drug-induced lupus.
- Fever, serositis, and cytopenias are common.
- ANA or dsDNA positivity is required to consider the diagnosis.
- Diagnostic confirmation rests with resolution of symptoms upon drug cessation.

Demyelinating syndromes

Multiple sclerosis (MS), optic neuritis, and other forms of demyelinating neurologic dysfunction have been described when using etanercept, infliximab, and adalimumab. This includes reports of new-onset optic neuritis, de novo MS, recurrence or flare of MS, encephalitis, myelitis, Guillain-Barré syndrome,[139] chronic inflammatory demyelinating polyneuropathy, neuropathy, transverse myelitis, seizures, and leukoencephalopathy. Nearly all of these cases improved or resolved with discontinuation of TNF inhibitor therapy. It is unclear if these rare events exceed those seen in the general or rheumatoid populations, and the epidemiology of demyelinating disorders in RA is also unknown. TNF antagonists may exacerbate existing demyelinating disease.[4-6] A randomized study of the p55 receptor lenercept in MS reported more flares in the patients receiving lenercept as compared with placebo.[140] It is recommended that clinicians should exercise caution when considering a TNF antagonist for a patient with a preexisting or recent-onset optic neuritis, MS, or other demyelination disorder. There are no reports of progressive multifocal leukoencephalopathy in patients receiving TNF inhibitors, as has been reported with other biologics such as natalizumab and rituximab.

Congestive heart failure

TNF has been implicated in the pathogenesis of heart failure and cardiac cachexia. TNF levels are found to be consistently elevated in patients with congestive heart failure (CHF), and TNF has been shown to have negative inotropic effects on the myocardium and cause myocyte dysfunction. Lastly, RA patients are known to have increased risk of CHF, presumably reflecting the effects of systemic TNF and inflammation on the heart.[3,130]

For these reasons it was anticipated that TNF inhibition would improve cardiac outcomes in patients with CHF. However, clinical trials with high-dose infliximab (10 mg/kg) in patients with CHF were discontinued early because of increase in death and worsening of CHF in patients with New York Heart Association (NYHA) class III-IV CHF.[141,142] Two large etanercept trials in CHF were also terminated due to lack of efficacy and the observation that a high dose (25 mg, three times weekly) was associated with worse cardiac outcomes.[102] The etiopathogenesis of these hazardous outcomes is unknown. Despite the negative reported outcomes in CHF patients,[143] TNF antagonists in RA clinical trials were not associated with an increase in new-onset CHF and they might actually reduce risk.[142] Nevertheless, increased caution is recommended when using anti-TNF agents in patients with CHF, especially with NYHA class III and IV disease.

Cytopenias

Rare reports of pancytopenia and aplastic anemia have been described with etanercept, infliximab, and adalimumab, and a minority of these resulted in death. Cytopenias developed in the first few weeks (median, 4 weeks) after initiating TNF inhibitors. Reasons for this sporadic association are unclear but may be attributed to co-morbidities or other myelosuppressive drugs in use. Periodic monitoring (every 3 to 6 months) of blood cell counts should be considered. Patients with features of blood dyscrasias (fever, pallor, bleeding, sore throat) should be evaluated for this complication.

Hepatotoxicity

Elevations in aminotransferases and reports of hepatic failure have been reported with anti-TNF usage (see Table 61.6). A 2003 FDA review of TNF safety revealed an unexpected 134 spontaneous reports of TNF inhibitor-related liver failure.[102] When 50 cases were reviewed, confounding diagnoses or hepatotoxin exposure was seen in 43 cases (e.g., sepsis, TB, isoniazid use, alcohol, viral hepatitis, GVHD, hepatotoxic drugs). However, in seven cases (14%) no other cause could be identified, suggesting that TNF inhibitor use may have led to hepatic failure. In the clinical trials with infliximab and adalimumab, sporadic twofold to threefold elevations in liver function tests may have been attributed to the TNF inhibitor. Clinicians should be aware of these rare events and monitor hepatic enzymes every 3 to 6 months. Nonetheless, there are rare reports of hepatic failure with infliximab.[11] Reactivation of chronic HBV infection has been reported following TNF inhibitor use. Hence patients at risk should be tested for HBV before drug initiation.

Pregnancy and lactation

There are no controlled trials of TNF inhibitors in pregnant women and there is a dearth of information on the use of TNF inhibitors in women who are or may become pregnant. Infliximab, adalimumab, and etanercept are a category B pregnancy risk because there are no controlled studies in pregnant women. We surveyed more than 1200 U.S. and Canadian rheumatologists and identified 463 pregnancies conceived while taking a TNF inhibitor.[28,144] Moreover, nearly 30% (n = 142) of these continued to take the drug throughout the pregnancy. Outcomes were quite favorable, with nearly 85% reporting full-term live births and few premature births, miscarriages, or therapeutic/elective abortions. There were two reported fetal malformations, a meromelia and VATER syndrome, but no neonatal deaths. Although this malformation rate (3%) approximates that expected in the normal population, there are insufficient data to advise continuation or starting of anti-TNF therapy if a patient becomes pregnant. The BSRBR described 22 pregnancies in patients with rheumatic diseases and exposed to anti-TNF at conception (16 etanercept, three infliximab, three adalimumab). They resulted in 6 first-trimester miscarriages (three in patients also receiving methotrexate and one receiving leflunomide at conception), 3 elective terminations, and 13 live births. One patient treated with adalimumab reported recurrent cystitis during pregnancy.[145] The TREAT Registry reported pregnancies in 66 Crohn disease patients, 36 of whom were exposed to infliximab. No fetal

malformations occurred, and the rates of miscarriage (P = 0.53) and neonatal complications (P = 0.78) did not differ between infliximab-treated and untreated patients.[146]

It is not known if TNF-blocking agents are secreted in human milk, and the safety of these agents during lactation has not been established. Although it appears that the risk to the fetus and mother is negligible, further research is necessary.

Unusual toxicities reported

One of the more unusual toxicities associated with TNF inhibitors is accidental injuries (e.g., falls, fractures) (Box 61.6). Several studies have shown higher rates of accidental injury in the TNF inhibitor-treated cohort.[4-6] Improved well-being and resumption of physically aggressive activities appear to account for this unexpected occurrence. Also surprising are occasional reports of weight gain with TNF inhibition. It is not clear if this is related to increased leptin levels or resolution of the anorectic effects of TNF.[147] Numerous cutaneous adverse events have been reported with TNF blockade (see Box 61.5). In a study of new-onset psoriasis reported as an adverse event from among 9826 anti-TNF–treated and 2880 DMARD-treated patients with severe RA from BSRBR, 25 incident cases of psoriasis were reported in patients receiving anti-TNF therapy and none in the comparison cohort between January 2001 and July 2007. Furthermore, patients treated with adalimumab had a significantly higher rate of incident psoriasis compared with patients treated with etanercept and infliximab.[148] Box 61.6 also lists other unusual events reported with TNF inhibitor therapy including fibrosing alveolitis, adult respiratory distress syndrome, granulomatous lung disease, colonic perforations, vesicocolic fistula, paresthesia, neuropathy, seizures, foot drop, azoospermia, and glomerulonephritis (with and without lupus).[149-158]

Monitoring

Before initiating anti-TNF therapy, the clinician must weigh the potential clinical benefits of TNF-α inhibition against potential adverse

---

BOX 61.6 ADVERSE EVENTS ASSOCIATED WITH USE OF TUMOR NECROSIS FACTOR INHIBITORS

Common
- Injection site reactions
- Infusion reactions
- Upper respiratory tract infections

Uncommon
- Serious infectious events
- Mycobacterial infection
- Fungal infections
- Opportunistic infections
- Viral infection (herpes zoster, hepatitis B virus)
- Lymphoma and malignancy
- Autoimmunity, autoantibodies, and lupus-like disease
- Heart failure
- Cytopenias
- Demyelinating disorders
- Hepatotoxicity

Rare/uncertain relationship
- Accidental injury
- Weight gain
- Pulmonary fibrosis
- Asthma
- Adult respiratory distress syndrome
- Granulomatous lung disease
- Colonic perforations
- Vesicocolic fistula
- Paresthesia
- Neuropathy
- Seizures
- Foot drop
- Asthenozoospermia
- Glomerulonephritis
- Proliferative lupus nephritis

effects. Although specific laboratory monitoring is not mandated by current package labeling, physicians are strongly advised to obtain complete blood count and liver function tests every 3 months (for the first 6 to 12 months) in patients treated with anti-TNF agents.[159] Although autoimmune disorders (e.g., drug-induced lupus, multiple sclerosis) have arisen in anti-TNF–treated patients, there is no value in employing pretreatment or periodic serologic testing because these have no predictive value. By contrast, patients exhibiting signs of autoimmune disease should undergo serologic testing to help establish a diagnosis. If the patient has risk factors for hepatitis B, then testing before drug initiation is advised.

At each visit the patient should be carefully evaluated for the risk or presence of infection, malignancy, demyelinating disorders, cytopenia, or any other co-morbidities that may alter the patient's risk-to-benefit ratio. Physicians should suspend anti-TNF therapy and exercise caution when patients develop a serious infection. Tuberculin skin testing using PPD is recommended before starting treatment with all TNF inhibitors. If the PPD skin test is positive, chest radiography is recommended to establish latent versus active disease. Appropriate antituberculous treatment should be started if latent or active tuberculosis is discovered.

CONCLUSION

Although currently available TNF blockers have undoubtedly constituted a considerable advance in the management of RA, future challenges remain. For example, further research is necessary to identify the ideal patient to receive TNF inhibition or the patient in whom TNF inhibition should be avoided. Moreover, the identification of demographic, clinical, laboratory, or genetic factors that would predict clinical response or toxicity to these agents is highly desirable. If it turns out to be true that there is an increased incidence (albeit small) of malignancy in patients receiving these drugs, the risk factors for this increase need to be identified and the tradeoffs in the use of these agents should be clarified for each individual patient.

In all, anti-TNF therapy has given much hope and needed relief of pain with reduction in disability in our patients; the future employment of these agents is an evolving story.

KEY REFERENCES

1. Feldmann M, Brennan FM, Foxwell BM, et al. The role of TNF alpha and IL-1 in rheumatoid arthritis. Curr Dir Autoimmun 2001;3:188-199.
2. Firestein GS, Alvaro-Gracia JM, Maki R. Quantitative analysis of cytokine gene expression in rheumatoid arthritis. J Immunol 1990;144:3347-3353.
3. Cush JJ. Cytokine inhibitors. In: Hochberg M, Silman A, Smolen A, et al, eds. Rheumatology, 3rd ed. Edinburgh: Mosby, 2003:461-484.
4. www.fda.gov/medwatch/SAFETY/2005/Oct_PI/Humira_PI.pdf
5. www.fda.gov/medwatch/SAFETY/2005/jul_PI/Enbrel_PI.pdf
6. www.fda.gov/medwatch/SAFETY/2004/Remicade_12-22-04_PI.pdf
7. Wolfe F, Michaud K. Heart failure in rheumatoid arthritis: rates, predictors, and the effect of anti-tumor necrosis factor therapy. Am J Med 2004;116:305-311.
8. Jacobsson LT, Turesson C, Gulfe A, et al. Treatment with tumor necrosis factor blockers is associated with a lower incidence of first cardiovascular events in patients with rheumatoid arthritis. J Rheumatol 2005;32:1213-1218.
9. Cush JJ. p55 TNF receptor therapy. In: Moreland L, Emery P, eds. TNF-α inhibition in the treatment of rheumatoid arthritis. London: Martin Dunitz, 2003:95-104.
10. Elliott MJ, Maini RN, Feldmann M, et al. Repeated therapy with monoclonal antibody to tumour necrosis factor alpha (cA2) in patients with rheumatoid arthritis. Lancet 1994;344:1125-1127.
11. Charles P, Elliott MJ, Davis D, et al. Regulation of cytokines, cytokine inhibitors, and acute-phase proteins following anti-TNF-alpha therapy in rheumatoid arthritis. J Immunol 1999;163:1521-1528.
12. Lorenz HM, Antoni C, Valerius T, et al. In vivo blockade of TNF-alpha by intravenous infusion of a chimeric monoclonal TNF-alpha antibody in patients with rheumatoid arthritis. Short term cellular and molecular effects. J Immunol 1996;156:1646-1653.
13. Ulfgren AK, Andersson U, Engstrom M, et al. Systemic anti-tumor necrosis factor alpha therapy in rheumatoid arthritis down-regulates synovial tumor necrosis factor alpha synthesis. Arthritis Rheum 2000;43:2391-2396.
14. Paleolog EM, Hunt M, Elliott MJ, et al. Deactivation of vascular endothelium by monoclonal anti-tumor necrosis factor alpha antibody in rheumatoid arthritis. Arthritis Rheum 1996;39:1082-1091.
15. Tak PP, Taylor PC, Breedveld FC, et al. Decrease in cellularity and expression of adhesion molecules by anti-tumor necrosis factor alpha monoclonal antibody treatment in patients with rheumatoid arthritis. Arthritis Rheum 1996;39:1077-1081.
16 Taylor PC, Peters AM, Paleolog E, et al. Reduction of chemokine levels and leukocyte traffic to joints by tumor necrosis factor alpha blockade in patients with rheumatoid arthritis. Arthritis Rheum 2000;43:38-47.
17. Taylor PC, Peters AM, Glass DM, Maini RN. Effects of treatment of rheumatoid arthritis patients with an antibody against tumour necrosis factor alpha on reticuloendothelial and intrapulmonary granulocyte traffic. Clin Sci (Lond) 1999;97:85-89.

18. Paleolog EM, Young S, Stark AC, et al. Modulation of angiogenic vascular endothelial growth factor by tumor necrosis factor alpha and interleukin-1 in rheumatoid arthritis. Arthritis Rheum 1998;4:1258-1265.
19. Taylor PC. Serum vascular markers and vascular imaging in assessment of rheumatoid arthritis disease activity and response to therapy. Rheumatology (Oxford) 2005;44:721-728.
20. Taylor PC, Steuer A, Gruber J, et al. Comparison of ultrasonographic assessment of synovitis and joint vascularity with radiographic evaluation in a randomized, placebo-controlled study of infliximab therapy in early rheumatoid arthritis. Arthritis Rheum 2004;50:1107-1116.
21. Taylor PC, Steuer A, Gruber J, et al. Ultrasonographic and radiographic results from a two-year controlled trial of immediate versus one-year-delayed addition of infliximab to ongoing methotrexate therapy in patients with erosive early rheumatoid arthritis. Arthritis Rheum 2006;54:47-53.
22. Brennan FM, Browne KA, Green PA, et al. Reduction of serum matrix metalloproteinase 1 and matrix metalloproteinase 3 in rheumatoid arthritis patients following anti-tumour necrosis factor-alpha (cA2) therapy. Br J Rheumatol 1997;36:643-650.
23. Catrina AI, Lampa J, Ernestam S, et al. Anti-tumour necrosis factor (TNF)-alpha therapy (etanercept) down-regulates serum matrix metalloproteinase (MMP)-3 and MMP-1 in rheumatoid arthritis. Rheumatology (Oxford) 2002;41:484-489.
24. Ziolkowska M, Kurowska M, Radzikowska A, et al. High levels of osteoprotegerin and soluble receptor activator of nuclear factor kappa B ligand in serum of rheumatoid arthritis patients and their normalization after anti-tumor necrosis factor alpha treatment. Arthritis Rheum 2002;46:1744-1753.
25. Van den Brande JM, Braat H, van den Brink GR, et al. Infliximab but not etanercept induces apoptosis in lamina propria T-lymphocytes from patients with Crohn's disease. Gastroenterology 2003;124:1774-1785.
26. Smeets TJ, Kraan MC, van Loon ME, Tak PP. Tumor necrosis factor alpha blockade reduces the synovial cell infiltrate early after initiation of treatment, but apparently not by induction of apoptosis in synovial tissue. Arthritis Rheum 2003;48:2155-2162.
27. Catrina AI, Trollmo C, af Klint E, et al. Evidence that anti-tumor necrosis factor therapy with both etanercept and infliximab induces apoptosis in macrophages, but not lymphocytes, in rheumatoid arthritis joints: extended report. Arthritis Rheum 2005;52:61-72.
28. Cush JJ. Biological drug use: US perspectives on indications and monitoring. Ann Rheum Dis 2005;64(suppl 4):iv18-iv23.
29. Wolfe F, Cush JJ, O'Dell JR, et al. Consensus recommendations for the assessment and treatment of rheumatoid arthritis. J Rheumatol 2001;28:1423-1430.
30. Deighton CM, George E, Kiely PD, et al. Updating the British Society for Rheumatology guidelines for anti-tumour necrosis factor therapy in adult rheumatoid arthritis (again). Rheumatology 2006;45:649-652.

31. Goekoop-Ruiterman YP, De Vries-Bouwstra JK, Allaart CF, et al. Clinical and radiographic outcomes of four different treatment strategies in patients with early rheumatoid arthritis (the BeSt study): a randomized, controlled trial. Arthritis Rheum 2005;52:3381-3390.
32. Andersson M, Svenungsson E, Khademi M, et al. No signs of immunoactivation in the cerebrospinal fluid during infliximab treatment. Ann Rheum Dis 2006;65:1237-1240.
33. Finckh A, Simard JF, Gabay C, et al. Evidence for differential acquired drug resistance to anti-tumour necrosis factor agents in rheumatoid arthritis. Ann Rheum Dis 2006;65:746-752.
34. Breedveld FC, Weisman MH, Kavanaugh AF, et al. The PREMIER study: a multicenter, randomized, double-blind clinical trial of combination therapy with adalimumab plus methotrexate versus methotrexate alone or adalimumab alone in patients with early, aggressive rheumatoid arthritis who had not had previous methotrexate treatment. Arthritis Rheum 2006;54:26-37.
35. Van De Putte LB, Atkins C, Malaise M, et al. Efficacy and safety of adalimumab as monotherapy in patients with rheumatoid arthritis for whom previous disease modifying antirheumatic drug treatment has failed. Ann Rheum Dis 2004;63:508-516.
36. Weinblatt ME, Keystone EC, Furst DE, et al. Adalimumab, a fully human anti-tumor necrosis factor alpha monoclonal antibody, for the treatment of rheumatoid arthritis in patients taking concomitant methotrexate: the ARMADA trial. Arthritis Rheum 2003;48:35-45.
37. Keystone EC, Kavanaugh AF, Sharp JT, et al. Radiographic, clinical, and functional outcomes of treatment with adalimumab (a human anti-tumor necrosis factor monoclonal antibody) in patients with active rheumatoid arthritis receiving concomitant methotrexate therapy: a randomized, placebo-controlled, 52-week trial. Arthritis Rheum 2004;50:1400-1411.
38. Keystone EC, Haraoui B, Bykerk VP. Role of adalimumab in the treatment of early rheumatoid arthritis. Clin Exp Rheumatol 2003;21(5 suppl 31):S198-S199.
39. Johnsen AK, Schiff MH, Mease PJ, et al. Comparison of 2 doses of etanercept (50 vs 100 mg) in active rheumatoid arthritis: a randomized double blind study. J Rheumatol 2006;33:659-664.
40. Moreland LW, Baumgartner SW, Schiff MH, et al. Treatment of rheumatoid arthritis with a recombinant human tumor necrosis factor receptor (p75)-Fc fusion protein. N Engl J Med 1997;337:141-147.
41. Weinblatt ME, Kremer JM, Bankhurst AD, et al. A trial of etanercept, a recombinant tumor necrosis factor receptor:Fc fusion protein in patients with rheumatoid arthritis receiving methotrexate. N Engl J Med 1999;340:253-259.
42. Kremer JM, Weinblatt ME, Bankhurst AD, et al. Etanercept added to background methotrexate therapy in patients with rheumatoid arthritis: continued observations. Arthritis Rheum 2003;48:1493-1499.
43. Bathon JM, Martin RW, Fleischmann RM, et al. A comparison of etanercept and methotrexate in patients

with early rheumatoid arthritis. N Engl J Med 2000;343:1586-1593.

44. Genovese MC, Bathon JM, Martin RW, et al. Etanercept versus methotrexate in patients with early rheumatoid arthritis: two year radiographic and clinical outcomes. Arthritis Rheum 2002;46:1443-1450.

45. van der Heijde D, Klareskog L, Rodriguez-Valverde V, et al. Comparison of etanercept and methotrexate, alone and combined, in the treatment of rheumatoid arthritis. Arthritis Rheum 2006;54:1063-1074.

46. Emery P, Breedveld FC, Hall S, et al. Comparison of methotrexate monotherapy with a combination of methotrexate and etanercept in active, early, moderate

to severe rheumatoid arthritis (COMET): a randomised, double-blind, parallel treatment trial. Lancet 2008;372:375-382.

47. Weaver AL, Lautzenheiser RL, Schiff MH, et al, RADIUS Investigators. Real-world effectiveness of select biologic and DMARD monotherapy and combination therapy in the treatment of rheumatoid arthritis: results from the RADIUS observational registry. Curr Med Res Opin 2006;22:185-198.

48. St Clair E, Wagner C, Fasanmade A, et al. Relationship of serum infliximab concentrations to clinical improvement in rheumatoid arthritis. Arthritis Rheum 2002;46:1451-1459.

49. Edrees AF, Misra SN, Abdou NI. Anti-tumor necrosis factor (TNF) therapy in rheumatoid arthritis: correlation of TNF-alpha serum level with clinical response and benefit from changing dose or frequency of infliximab infusions. Clin Exp Rheumatol 2005;23:469-474.

50. Elliott MJ, Maini RN, Feldman M, et al. Treatment of rheumatoid arthritis with chimeric monoclonal antibodies to tumor necrosis factor α. Arthritis Rheum 1993;36:1681-1690.

REFERENCES

Full references for this chapter can be found on www.expertconsult.com.

Tyrosine kinase inhibition

Ferdinand Breedveld

62

- Small molecules, usually orally administered, that inhibit the production or reduce the effects of TNF or IL-1 have not been found so far to be effective antirheumatic drugs.

- Nuclear factor-kB, involved in the production of proinflammatory cytokines, adhesion molecules and metallo-proteinases, is an attractive target in the development of antirheumatic drugs.

- Inhibitors of p38MAP kinase can reduce the production of proinflammtory cytokines by synoviocytes and reduce the severity of animal models of arthritis. Clinical trials are in progress in rheumatoid arthritis.

- Inhibitors of matrix metalloproteinases, despite impressive efficacy in animal models of arthritis, have shown toxic side effects or low efficacy in preliminary clinical studies in rheumatoid arthritis.

Tyrosine kinases are divided into two groups. Cytoplasmic kinases transduce signals from a separate surface receptor while receptor tyrosine kinases have intrinsic tyrosine phosphorylation activity. The four Janus kinases (JAKs) are cytoplasmic tyrosine kinases that pair in several combinations to integrate signaling in various cytokines and growth factors. JAK-3 is critical for signal transduction from the common γ-chain of the receptors for interleukin (IL)-2, IL-4, IL-7, IL-15, and IL-21 on the plasma membrane to the nuclei of immune cells.[1] These interleukins are integral to lymphocyte activation, function, and proliferation. JAK-3 is predominantly expressed in cells of the immune system.[2] Expression has been reported in other cell types on rare occasions; however, the functional significance of this is not fully understood at present. JAK-3 knockout mice have defects in T lymphocytes, B lymphocytes, and natural killer (NK) cells, with no other defects reported; and mutations in JAK-3 have been identified as a cause of autosomal-recessive severe combined immunodeficiency disorder. Therefore, agents that selectively inhibit JAK-3 have the potential to mediate potent immune modulation, affecting T lymphocytes, B lymphocytes, macrophages, and NK cells, without significantly affecting other organ systems.

CP-690,550 is an oral JAK antagonist in development for the treatment of rheumatoid arthritis (RA) and other autoimmune conditions, as well as for the prevention of renal allograft rejection. It is a potent, selective inhibitor of the JAK family of kinases with an approximately 1000-fold selectivity over 82 other kinases tested in a selectivity panel compared with the potency of JAK-3. In cell-based assays, CP-690,500 potently inhibited JAK-$\frac{1}{3}$- and JAK-1-dependent STAT activities with 50% inhibition concentration (IC_{50}) values in the 26- to 63-nM range, whereas IC_{50} values for JAK-2-mediated pathways ranged from 129 to 501 nM.

The pharmacokinetic profile of CP-690,550 in RA patients is linear and is characterized by rapid absorption and rapid elimination, with a half-life of about 3 hours. CP-690,550 produced dose-dependent decreased clinical scores in collagen-induced arthritis and

adjuvant-induced arthritis in mice and rats, with more than 90% disease reduction observed with the 15-mg/kg/day dosage. The 24-hour area under the curve of this dosage in rodents (1,680-6,216 ng/hr/mL) was within twofold of that observed with dosages of 15 mg twice daily in humans. Histologic evidence of inflammation was reduced in both models, with histologic parameters equivalent to those in naive mice at the 15-mg/kg/day dosage in the collagen-induced arthritis model.

Recently, the first randomized, double-blind, placebo-controlled trial of three dosage levels of CP-690,550 revealed American College of Radiology (ACR) 20% (ACR20) response rates at week 6 of 70%, 81%, and 77% in the 5-mg, 15-mg, and 30-mg twice-daily groups, respectively, compared with 29% in the placebo group ($P < .001$).[2] Side effects observed included headache and nausea. Furthermore, increases in mean low-density lipoprotein cholesterol and high-density lipoprotein cholesterol levels and increases in mean serum creatinine level were seen in all CP-690,550 treatment arms of the trial. The side effects were reversible with drug discontinuation. Subsequently a 24-week double-blind, placebo-controlled study investigating doses of 1 to 15 mg twice a day showed statistically significant efficacy (ACR20 up to 66%) in patients receiving 3 mg or higher twice a day.[3] In another study these observations were confirmed.[4]

CP-690,550 is about 20-fold more selective for JAK-3 than for JAK-2. JAK-2 is essential for signaling by many hematopoietic growth factors, with mutations in JAK-2 causing embryonic death in mice due to the absence of erythropoiesis. Significant inhibition of JAK-2 could, therefore, cause anemia, leukopenia, and thrombocytopenia. The observed hematologic adverse events, particularly the complex changes in hemoglobin level, may be due to a combination of competitive factors, including inhibition of disease activity as well as measure of JAK-2 inhibition. However, despite the potentially additive risks of infectious adverse events from neutropenia and immunosuppression, the incidence of infections typically associated with neutropenia was not increased relative to placebo, nor was the incidence of infection increased. These data suggest that CP-690,550 is efficacious in the treatment of RA.

Spleen tyrosine kinase (Syk) also belongs to the intracellular tyrosine kinase family. Syk is expressed in B cells and macrophages and binds to the immune receptors. In synovial fibroblasts Syk regulates the MAP kinase cascade, including IL-6 and metalloproteinase-3.[5] Syk inhibition was able to suppress inflammation and destruction in a rat arthritis model.[6] Treatment with tamatinib fosdium (R788), an oral Syk inhibitor, suggested significant improvement in RA patients.[7]

R788 also demonstrated clinical efficacy in a 3-month trial in RA patients treated with methotrexate. Patients received either 100 mg of R788 twice a day or placebo. Although a significant decrease in the acute-phase response was observed, there were no significant differences in the ACR responses between the groups.[8] In a 6-month placebo-controlled study including 457 patients with active RA on methotrexate, two R788 doses (100 mg twice daily and 150 mg once daily) showed ACR20 responses of 57% and 66%, respectively, significantly higher than the 35% observed with placebo. The most common adverse event was diarrhea. These data suggest that Syk inhibition may be another useful target in the treatment of RA.[9]

REFERENCES

1. Kawamura M, McVicar DW, Johnston JA, et al. Molecular cloning of L-JAK, a Janus family protein-tyrosine kinase expressed in natural killer cells and activated leukocytes. Proc Natl Acad Sci U S A 1994;91:6374-6378.
2. Kremer JM, Bloom BJ, Breedveld FC, et al. The safety and efficacy of a JAK inhibitor in patients with active rheumatoid arthritis. Arthritis Rheum 2009;60: 1895-1905.
3. Kremer J, Cohen S, Wilkinson B, et al. Safety and efficacy after 24 week (wk) dosing of the oral JAK inhibitor CP-690,550 (CP) in combination with methotrexate (MTX) in patients with active rheumatoid arthritis (RA). Arthritis Rheum 2009;60 (Suppl 10):S719.
4. Fleischmann RM, Genovese MC, Gruben D, et al. Safety and efficacy after 24 week (wk) dosing of the oral JAK inhibitor CP-690,550 (CP) as monotherapy in patients (pts) with active rheumatoid

arthritis (Ra). Arthritis Rheum 2009;60(Suppl 10): S718.

5. Cha HS, Boyle DL, Inoue T, et al. A novel spleen tyrosine kinase inhibitor blocks c-Jun N-terminal kinase-mediated gene expression in synoviocytes. J Pharmacol Exp Ther 2006;317:571-578.

6. Pine PR, Chang B, Schoettler N, et al. Inflammation and bone erosions are suppressed in models of rheumatoid arthritis following treatment with a novel Syk inhibitor. Clin Immunol 2007;124:244-257.

7. Weinblatt ME, Kavanaugh A, Burgos-Vargas R, et al. Treatment of rheumatoid arthritis with a Syk kinase inhibitor: a twelve-week, randomized, placebo-controlled trial. Arthritis Rheum 2008;58:3309-3318.

8. Genovese MC. An oral Syk kinase inhibitor in the treatment of rheumatoid arthritis (RA): a 3-month randomized placebo controlled phase 2 study in patients with active RA who had failed biologic agents. Arthritis Rheum 2009;60:3860.

9. Weinblatt M, Kavanaugh A, Genovese M, et al. Treatment of rheumatoid arthritis (RA) with an oral Syk kinase inhibitor: a 6-month randomized placebo controlled phase 2b study in patients with active RA on chronic methotrexate. Arthritis Rheum 2009;60:3859.

REFERENCES

Full references for this chapter can be found on www.expertconsult.com.

Emerging therapeutic targets: IL-15, IL-17, IL-18, and IL-23

63

Alison M. Gizinski and David A. Fox

- IL-15, IL-17, IL-18 and IL-23 are all proinflammatory cytokines found in the synovial compartment in rheumatoid arthritis.
- IL-17 is produced primarily by T cells. IL-15, IL-18 and IL-23 are produced by antigen presenting cells and tissue cells.
- Unique features of the biology and regulation of each cytokine point to specific strategies for either neutralization or down regulation by therapeutic biologics.
- In autoimmune diseases, cytokines function within a complex matrix of stimulatory and feedback loops such that perturbation of one cytokine is likely to influence the production and function of many others.

POTENTIAL CYTOKINE TARGETS IN RHEUMATIC DISEASES

There are multiple potential strategies that can be employed to inhibit the biologic effects of cytokines in rheumatic diseases. These include monoclonal antibodies to cytokines or to their receptors, soluble receptors, or receptor antagonists. Additionally, cytokines can be inhibited by targeting their processing, intracellular signaling pathways, or synthesis.

Intelligent design of inhibitors involves an understanding of their unique biologic activities, receptors, and signaling pathways while being mindful of potential complications that could result from their specific inhibition. Ideally, inhibitors of cytokines would be designed to alter the underlying immune dysfunction specific to a rheumatic disease while protecting the targeted tissues and allowing for preservation of a host's immune defenses. As our understanding of the role of specific cytokines in rheumatic diseases evolves, more targets are being identified and potential new therapies are being tested for their safety and tolerability profiles.

IL-15

Description, receptor, function

Interleukin (IL)-15 is a 14- to 15-kDa four α-helix cytokine. IL-15 exists in two isoforms, one that is anchored to the plasma membrane or alternatively processed and secreted from the cell and another that remains within the cytoplasm and nucleus.[1] IL-15 is produced by monocytes, macrophages, dendritic cells, osteoclasts, fibroblasts, and epithelial cells. It enhances natural killer (NK) cell survival, proliferation, cytotoxicity, and cytokine production. IL-15 activates memory T cells, is a T-cell growth factor, and inhibits T-cell apoptosis.[1] IL-15 signals through a heterotrimeric receptor comprised of three subunits: IL-15Rα, IL-15Rβ (also known as IL-2/15Rβ), and the common γ-chain that is also a subunit of other cytokine receptors. The IL-15Rα subunit exclusively binds IL-15. IL-15Rβ can also bind to IL-2, and the common γ-chain can be bind several cytokines. IL-15 binds to the IL-15β/γ-chain complex with intermediate affinity and binds the heterotrimeric complex with higher affinity.[1] The IL-15R complex is present on monocytes, dendritic cells, NK cells, T cells, and fibroblasts.[1] IL-15Rα has a

unique signaling property that allows it to signal in either a *cis* or *trans* distribution on adjacent cells (Fig. 63.1).[2] For example, IL-15 bound to IL-15α on the surface of antigen-presenting cells can be presented in *trans* to T cells, NK cells, and non-lymphoid cells expressing the IL-15Rβ/γ complex.[1] IL-15Rα can mediate the *trans*-endosomal recycling of IL-15, allowing IL-15 function to persist despite local depletion of IL-15.[2] A soluble form of IL-15Rα has been identified, and there is evidence to suggest that the biologic activity of IL-15 is enhanced when bound to this soluble form of IL-15Rα. Thus, use of a soluble decoy IL-15Rα is an attractive strategy for IL-15 suppression.[3] IL-15R signals through AKT, ras MAP kinase, and Jak pathways, activating transcription of genes that are induced by phosphorylated STAT3 and STAT5 (Table 63-1).[1]

IL-15 in rheumatic disease

The mRNA and protein levels of IL-15 are elevated in the synovium and serum of patients with rheumatoid arthritis and psoriatic arthritis.[1] IL-15 activates synovial neutrophils to produce IL-18 and promotes synovial T-cell proliferation.[4] IL-15 and IL-15Rα are expressed by psoriatic keratinocytes; this co-expression suggests a feedback loop could exist in psoriatic plaques.[5] Patients with systemic lupus erythematosus have increased serum levels of IL-15 and increased IL-15Rα expression on peripheral leukocytes.[6]

Clinical trials

A proof of concept study was performed in rheumatoid arthritis patients using a monoclonal neutralizing human IgG1 antibody that binds and neutralizes the activity of soluble and membrane-bound IL-15 by blocking the site required for interaction with the γ-chain. This phase 1/2 study demonstrated that the monoclonal antibody was well tolerated, and improvements in disease activity were seen 8 weeks after a single dose, with an American College of Rheumatology 20% response (ACR20) in 63% of patients, ACR50 response in 38% of patients, and ACR70 response in 25% of patients receiving active drug. Placebo response was not reported. There were no striking infectious complications, but the limited duration of the study did not allow for extensive safety evaluation. There were no alterations observed in circulating levels of leukocyte subsets including NK cells and CD8+ memory T cells.[7]

IL-17

Description, receptor, function

To date, the IL-17 family has six identified members, designated A to F, of which IL-17A and IL-17F are the most studied. IL-17A and IL-17F are homodimeric cytokines, but human CD4+ T cells can also produce an IL-17A/F heterodimer that has inflammatory effects.[8] IL-17A and IL-17F are produced by activated CD4+ and CD8+ T cells. IL-17B and IL-17D are expressed in resting CD4+ T cells and can induce the secretion of IL-6, IL-8, and granulocyte-macrophage colony-stimulating factor (GM-CSF) in fibroblasts, epithelial cells, and endothelial cells.[9,10]

The IL-17 family members bind to a distinct class of cytokine receptors. IL-17RA is a subunit of a multimeric preformed receptor complex with IL-17RC. This complex undergoes a conformation change when bound.[11] IL-17 receptor is expressed on monocytes, macrophages, chondrocytes, osteoblasts, and fibroblasts.[12]

TABLE 63.1 CYTOKINES, THEIR SOURCES, RECEPTORS, SIGNALING PATHWAYS, AND MAJOR FUNCTIONS

Cytokine	Cellular source	Receptor	Signaling pathway	Function
IL-15	Monocytes, macrophages, FLS, endothelial cells, DC, osteoclasts, fibroblasts, epithelial cells	IL-15Rα, IL-15Rβ, γ-chain	Ras MAPK, AKT, Jak1, Jak3, STAT3, STAT5	NK cell survival, proliferation, cytotoxicity, activate memory T cells, inhibits T-cell apoptosis, T-cell proliferation
IL-17A, IL-17F	T cells, γδ T cells, NK T cells, neutrophils, eosinophils	IL-17RA/IL-17RC	TRAF6, MAPK, TAK1, NF-κB	IL-6, IL-8, and GM-CSF production by epithelial cells and fibroblasts, production of IL-1β and TNF-α from monocytes, MMPs synthesis
IL-18	Monocytes, macrophages, DC, FLS, osteoblasts, Kupffer cells, adrenal cortex cells, intestinal epithelial cells, microglial cells	IL-18Rα/Rβ	MyD88, IRAK, TRAF6, NF-κB	IFNγ production by Th1 cells, cytotoxic T cells, NK cells and macrophages, angiogenesis
IL-23	Macrophages, DC, T cells, B cells, endothelial cells	IL-12Rβ1/IL-23R	Jak2, Tyk2, STAT3, STAT4, (? STAT1, STAT5)	Maintains Th17 cells, induces memory T cells to proliferate and produce IFNγ and IL-17

FLS, Fibroblast-like synoviocyte; DC, dendritic cell; MAPK, mitogen-activated protein kinase; Jak, Janus kinase; STAT, signal transducer and activator of transcription; NK, natural killer; γδ, gamma delta; TRAF, TNF receptor associated factor; TAK, TGF-β–activated kinase; NF-κB, nuclear factor-kappa B; MMPs, matrix metalloproteinases; MyD88, myeloid differentiation primary response gene 8; IRAK, IL-1 receptor-associated kinase; Tyk, tyrosine kinase.

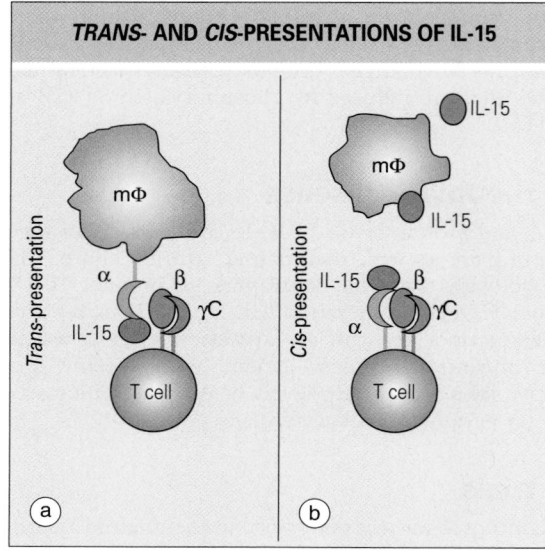

Fig. 63.1 (a) *Trans*-presentation of IL-15 bound to the surface IL-15Rα of a macrophage to the IL-15Rβ/γ complex on a T cell. (b) *Cis*-presentation of IL-15 bound to the IL-15Rαβ/γ complex on a T cell. mφ, macrophage; α, IL-15Rα; β, IL-15Rβ; γc, common gamma chain.

IL-17 is a proinflammatory cytokine that induces epithelial cells to produce IL-8, which is a chemoattractant for neutrophils, and IL-17 also induces the production of IL-1β and tumor necrosis factor-α (TNF-α) from monocytic cells.[13] The production of antimicrobial peptides is induced by IL-17 in epithelial cells, suggesting a role for IL-17 in host defense.[14]

IL-17 in rheumatic disease

High levels of IL-17A have been found in the sera, synovial fluid, and synovial biopsy specimens of patients with rheumatoid arthritis.[12] Additionally, increased levels of IL-17 expression in the synovium were predictive of more severe joint damage in a prospective study of patients with rheumatoid arthritis.[15] IL-17 contributes to cartilage and bone destruction in the joint. It inhibits chondrocyte metabolism, causes proteoglycan breakdown, and induces production of metalloproteinases associated with cartilage destruction.[12] IL-17 can trigger osteoclastogenesis by upregulating RANKL on osteoblasts, allowing interaction with RANK on osteoclasts responsible for bone erosion.[12] IL-17A can act synergistically with TNF-α and IL-1β to induce inflammatory mediators in synoviocytes, osteoblasts, myoblasts, and chondrocytes.[11] IL-17RA and IL-17RC are overexpressed in rheumatoid arthritis.[11] Taken together, these findings make IL-17 and its receptor promising targets in treatment of rheumatoid arthritis.

IL-17A and IL-17F have been found in the cutaneous plaques of patients with psoriasis.[16] IL-17 can induce the production of IL-6 by human keratinocytes and may initiate a positive feedback loop, because IL-6 can enhance the differentiation of Th17 cells, resulting in amplification of IL-17 and IL-22 responses in the skin.[12,17]

IL-17 has been detected in the sera and tissues of patients with systemic lupus erythematosus and systemic sclerosis.[18,19] IL-17 protein has been identified in synovial fluid of patients with reactive arthritis and is induced in T cells by bacteria-infected dendritic cells that produce IL-23.[13] IL-17–producing Th17 cells have been found to be elevated in patients with seronegative spondylarthritides.[20] IL-17–producing T cells have been shown to be enriched in number in the peripheral blood of juvenile inflammatory arthritis patients compared with healthy controls.[21]

Clinical trials

A proof of concept trial is currently enrolling to test a monoclonal antibody to IL-17 in rheumatoid arthritis patients.[22] A phase 1b/2a trial of an antibody directed against IL-17R is currently enrolling rheumatoid arthritis patients.[23]

IL-18

Description, receptor, function

IL-18 is a member of the IL-1 superfamily and was originally described as the interferon-γ (IFN-γ)-inducing factor. IL-18 is synthesized as a biologically inactive 24-kDa precursor that is cleaved by caspase-1 to the biologically active 18-kDa protein. It is expressed in monocytes, macrophages, dendritic cells, Kupffer cells, keratinocytes, osteoblasts, adrenal cortex cells, intestinal epithelial cells, microglial cells, and synovial fibroblasts.[1] IL-18 binds a heterodimeric receptor consisting of IL-18Rα, to which IL-18 binds, and IL-18Rβ, which does not directly bind IL-18 but is recruited to form a heterotrimeric complex with IL-18 and IL-18Rα and is responsible for transducing the signal. This heterotrimeric complex recruits MyD88 and IRAK. Autophosphorylation of IRAK enables its disassociation from the receptor to bind TRAF-6 with further signaling through NF-κB.[1] The ligand binding IL-18Rα receptor is expressed on naive T cells, mature T-helper-1 (Th1) lymphocytes, macrophages, neutrophils, B cells, basophils, mast cells, NK cells, chondrocytes, endothelial cells, smooth muscle cells, keratinocytes, and dendritic cells.[1]

IL-18 is closely regulated. Cleavage of the 24-kDa precursor by caspase-1 limits the generation of the active 18-kDa form. Control of IL-18 biologic activity is mediated through regulation of caspase-1 activity, because inflammatory stimuli do not appear to impact IL-18 precursor production.[24] Extracellular IL-18 is antagonized by IL-18BP, a unique soluble protein that binds to the active form of IL-18 with high affinity and prevents its interaction with cell surface receptors.[25] IFN-γ appears to upregulate IL-18BP production, and thus IL-18 indirectly increases the production of its own inhibitor.[24]

IL-18 is further regulated by IL-1F7, a member of the IL-1 family of cytokines. IL-18Rα does not recruit IL-18Rβ and no signal is transduced when bound by IL-1F7. In addition, IL-1F7 can enhance the activity of IL-18BP. IL-1F7, when bound to IL-18BP, can then bind to IL-18Rβ, preventing the β chain from forming a signaling complex with IL-18Rα.[26]

IL-18, in synergy with IL-12, promotes Th1 differentiation and the production of IFN-γ by Th1, cytotoxic T cells, NK cells, and macrophages. Maturation and acquisition of cytotoxic function by T and NK cells is accelerated by IL-18. IL-18 plays a vital role in the clearance of intracellular pathogens through induction of IFN-γ as well as the induction of cytotoxic T cells required for clearing viral infection.[24]

IL-18 in rheumatic disease

Levels of IL-18 are elevated in synovial tissue, synovial fluid, and sera of patients with rheumatoid arthritis. IL-18 found in the synovial membrane of rheumatoid arthritis patients promotes the release of TNF-α, GM-CSF, and IFN-γ reduces chondrocyte proliferation and cartilage anabolism and enhances angiogenesis by up-regulation of vascular endothelial growth factor (VEGF) and vascular cellular adhesion molecule-1 (VCAM-1) production by synovial fibroblasts.[27,28] IL-18 expression in the rheumatoid synovium was found to correlate with IL-1β expression, macrophage infiltration, and inflammation. Rheumatoid arthritis disease severity correlated with the bioactivity of IL-18; and after DMARD therapy there was decreased tissue expression of IL-18, serum IL-18, and C-reactive protein.[29] IL-18BP levels are also elevated in rheumatoid arthritis, suggesting a possible altered balance between IL-18 and its inhibitor IL-18BP.[29] Anti-TNF therapy has also been shown to reduce IL-18 production.[30] IL-18 and IL-23 together amplify IL-17 production, which, in rheumatoid arthritis, could promote cartilage destruction and osteoclastogenesis.[31]

IL-18 expression is elevated in the synovium and serum of patients with psoriatic arthritis.[32,33] Keratinocytes in the skin are able to produce IL-18 in response to inflammatory stimuli, and increased levels of IL-18 are present in active and progressive psoriatic skin plaques.[34,35]

Serum and synovial fluid levels of IL-18 are elevated in patients with juvenile idiopathic arthritis and correlate with measures of disease including C-reactive protein, number of active joints, and radiographic score.[36] Serum levels of IL-18 are elevated in adult-onset Still's disease compared with patients with rheumatoid arthritis, systemic lupus erythematosus, systemic sclerosis, polymyositis/dermatomyositis, Sjögren's syndrome, or healthy individuals and correlate with serum ferritin values and disease severity.[37]

Targeting

Potential strategies for blocking the biologic effects of IL-18 include developing neutralizing antibodies or soluble receptors or blocking the processing or release of IL-18. Antibodies specific for IL-18 are in development.[1] A fusion protein of IL-18BP coupled to the Fc fragment of human IgG1 has been developed. This fusion protein binds to IL-18, neutralizing its effects.[24]

Clinical trials

IL-18 was targeted in a phase 2 randomized, placebo-controlled trial in rheumatoid arthritis patients with an inhibitor of caspase-1, pralnacasan, but the results were not promising and the trial was stopped owing to an animal toxicity study that observed liver abnormalities.[38] An antagonist of the P2X$_7$ receptor, a receptor that may be involved in the release and maturation of IL-1 and IL-18, is being tested in a phase 2a study in rheumatoid arthritis patients.[39] A recombinant IL-18BP fusion protein has been tested in animal models of arthritis and phase 1 trials have been completed in healthy volunteers, patients with stable plaque psoriasis, and patients with rheumatoid arthritis with a favorable safety profile.[1,40]

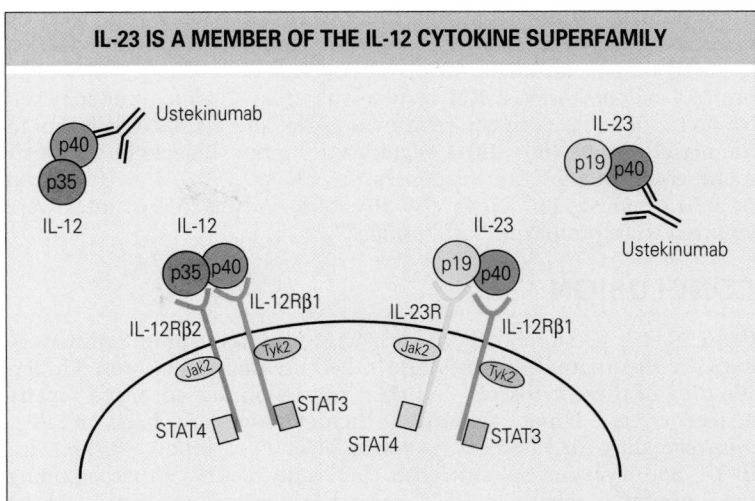

IL-23 IS A MEMBER OF THE IL-12 CYTOKINE SUPERFAMILY

Fig. 63.2 IL-23 is a member of the IL-12 cytokine superfamily and is composed of two subunits, the p40 and p19. IL-23 binds to a heterodimeric receptor composed of the IL-12Rβ (shared with IL-12R) and IL-23R. Ustekinumab is a monoclonal antibody that binds to the shared p40 subunit of the interleukins 12 and 23. Jak2 = Janus kinase 2; Tyk = Tyrosine kinase 2; STAT4 = Signal Transducer and Activator of Transcription 4.

IL-23

Description, receptor, function

IL-23 is a member of the IL-12 cytokine superfamily and is composed of two subunits, the p40 and p19 peptides. IL-23 is produced by dendritic cells and binds to a heterodimeric receptor composed of the IL-12Rβ1 (shared with IL-12R) and IL-23R (Fig. 63-2).[41] T cells, NK cells, monocytes and dendritic cells express the IL-23 receptor.[42] IL-23 induces memory T cells to proliferate and produce IFN-γ. IL-23 mediates the development and proliferation of IL-17, producing CD4+ Th17 cells.[42] IL-23 signals through the JAK-STAT pathway, leading to activation of JAK2, Tyk2, STAT1, STAT3, STAT4, and STAT5.[1,41] The association of a *STAT4* polymorphism marked by rs7574865 has been described in rheumatoid arthritis, systemic lupus erythematosus, Crohn's disease, and ulcerative colitis.[43] Additionally, a polymorphism in the *IL23R* gene has been linked to susceptibility to Crohn's disease.[44]

IL-23 in rheumatic diseases

IL-23 has been identified in the sera and synovial fluid of rheumatoid arthritis patients, and expression of the p19 subunit is increased in the synovial fibroblasts of patients with rheumatoid arthritis.[45]

Monocytes and dendritic cells in psoriatic skin plaques express high levels of IL-23 p19 and p40 subunits.[46] Elevated serum levels of the IL-23 p40 subunit were found to distinguish between patients with psoriatic arthritis and healthy individuals.[47]

Infections due to *Salmonella* and *Mycobacterium* have been described in individuals with homozygous mutations of either the *IL12B* gene, which encodes for the p40 subunit common to IL-12 and IL-23, or the *IL12BR1* gene, which encodes a subunit of the IL-12 and IL-23 receptors.[48] This suggests that IL-23 may play an important role in defense against pathogens and may have implications for safety issues in blockade of IL-23.

Clinical trials

An oral IL-12/23 inhibitor, STA-5326 mesylate, is being tested in patients with rheumatoid arthritis to determine safety, pharmacokinetic, and synovial tissue outcomes.[49]

A phase 2 trial of ustekinumab, a human monoclonal antibody that binds to the shared p40 subunit of IL-12 and IL-23, blocking their signaling, was performed in psoriatic arthritis. Study subjects received ustekinumab, 90 mg or 63 mg, every week for 4 weeks, followed by placebo at weeks 12 and 16 (n = 76) or placebo weekly for 4 weeks, followed by ustekinumab, 63 mg, at weeks 12 and 16 (n = 70). The primary endpoint was ACR20 response at week 12, which was achieved by 42.1% of subjects in the treatment group and 14.3% of subjects in the placebo group ($P < .001$). Significantly more subjects in the treatment group had ACR50 responses (25.0% vs. 7.1%, $P = .004$) and ACR70 responses (10.5% vs. 0%, $P = .005$). Adverse event rates were reported to be similar in both groups.[50]

CONCLUSION

IL-15, IL-17, IL-18, and IL-23 each have important proinflammatory roles in rheumatoid arthritis and other rheumatic diseases. Understanding of these cytokines and their regulation has advanced rapidly in recent years. Unique features of each cytokine have been revealed: *trans*-signaling for IL-15, six isoforms of IL-17, a binding protein for IL-18, and a shared subunit with IL-23 and IL-12. Notwithstanding some potential safety concerns, careful therapeutic trials of blocking strategies directed against each of these molecules are justified by available animal data, *in-vitro* studies, and measurements performed in patients with rheumatic diseases (Table 63.2).

TABLE 63.2 CYTOKINES, POTENTIAL INHIBITORS AND RHEUMATIC DISEASE TARGETS

Cytokine	Method of inhibition	Disease targets
IL-15	Monoclonal antibody to IL-15 Neutralizing IL-15Rα antibody Jak/STAT inhibitor	Rheumatoid arthritis Psoriatic arthritis Systemic lupus erythematosus
IL-17A, IL-17F	Monoclonal antibody to IL-17 Monoclonal antibody to the IL-17R IL-17R fusion protein	Rheumatoid arthritis Psoriatic arthritis Spondyloarthropathies
IL-18	Inhibition of caspase 1 Blocking secretion by P2X$_7$ receptor inhibition Monoclonal antibody to IL-18 IL-18BP isoform	Rheumatoid arthritis Juvenile idiopathic arthritis Systemic lupus erythematosus Adult-onset Still's disease
IL-23	Monoclonal antibody to IL-23 Monoclonal antibody to p40 subunit of IL-12 and IL-23 Jak/STAT inhibitor	Rheumatoid arthritis Psoriatic arthritis Spondyloarthropathies

Jak, Janus kinase; STAT, signal transducer and activator of transcription; P2X7, purinergic receptor P2X ligand-gated ion channel 7.

REFERENCES

1. Anderson EJ, McGrath MA, Thalhamer T, McInnes IB: Interleukin-12 to interleukin "infinity": the rationale for future therapeutic cytokine targeting. Springer Semin Immunopathol 2006;27:425-442.
2. Dubois S, Mariner J, Waldmann TA, Tagaya Y: IL-15Ralpha recycles and presents IL-15 In trans to neighboring cells. Immunity 2002;17:537-547.
3. Rubinstein MP, Kovar M, Purton JF, et al: Converting IL-15 to a superagonist by binding to soluble IL-15Rα. Proc Natl Acad Sci U S A 2006;103:9166-9171.
4. Verri WA Jr, Cunha TM, Ferreira SH, et al: IL-15 mediates antigen-induced neutrophil migration by triggering IL-18 production. Eur J Immunol 2007;37:3373-3380.
5. Ruckert R, Asadullah K, Seifert M, et al: Inhibition of keratinocyte apoptosis by IL-15: a new parameter in the pathogenesis of psoriasis? J Immunol 2000;165:2240-2250.
6. Baranda L, de la Fuente H, Layseca-Espinosa E, et al: IL-15 and IL-15R in leucocytes from patients with systemic lupus erythematosus. Rheumatology (Oxford) 2005;44:1507-1513.
7. Baslund B, Tvede N, Danneskiold-Samsoe B, et al: Targeting interleukin-15 in patients with rheumatoid arthritis: a proof-of-concept study. Arthritis Rheum 2005;52:2686-2692.
8. Wright JF, Guo Y, Quazi A, et al: Identification of an interleukin 17F/17A heterodimer in activated human CD4+ T cells. J Biol Chem 2007;282:13447-13455.
9. Fossiez F, Djossou O, Chomarat P, et al: T cell interleukin-17 induces stromal cells to produce proinflammatory and hematopoietic cytokines. J Exp Med 1996;183:2593-2603.
10. Starnes T, Broxmeyer HE, Robertson MJ, Hromas R: Cutting edge: IL-17D, a novel member of the IL-17 family, stimulates cytokine production and inhibits hemopoiesis. J Immunol 2002;169:642-646.
11. Zrioual S, Toh ML, Tournadre A, et al: IL-17RA and IL-17RC receptors are essential for IL-17A-induced ELR+ CXC chemokine expression in synoviocytes and are overexpressed in rheumatoid blood. J Immunol 2008;180:655-663.
12. Tesmer LA, Lundy SK, Sarkar S, Fox DA: Th17 cells in human disease. Immunol Rev 2008;223:87-113.
13. Gaston JS: Cytokines in arthritis—the "big numbers" move centre stage. Rheumatology (Oxford) 2008;47:8-12.
14. Liang SC, Tan XY, Luxenberg DP, et al: Interleukin (IL)-22 and IL-17 are coexpressed by Th17 cells and cooperatively enhance expression of antimicrobial peptides. J Exp Med 2006;203:2271-2279.
15. Kirkham BW, Lassere MN, Edmonds JP, et al: Synovial membrane cytokine expression is predictive of joint damage progression in rheumatoid arthritis: a two-year prospective study (the DAMAGE study cohort). Arthritis Rheum 2006;54:1122-1131.

16. van Beelen AJ, Teunissen MB, Kapsenberg ML, de Jong EC: Interleukin-17 in inflammatory skin disorders. Curr Opin Allergy Clin Immunol 2007;7:374-381.
17. Albanesi C, Scarponi C, Cavani A, et al. Interleukin-17 is produced by both Th1 and Th2 lymphocytes, and modulates interferon-gamma- and interleukin-4-induced activation of human keratinocytes. J Invest Dermatol 2000;115:81-87.
18. Wong CK, Ho CY, Li EK, Lam CW: Elevation of proinflammatory cytokine (IL-18, IL-17, IL-12) and Th2 cytokine (IL-4) concentrations in patients with systemic lupus erythematosus. Lupus 2000;9:589-593.
19. Kurasawa K, Hirose K, Sano H, et al: Increased interleukin-17 production in patients with systemic sclerosis. Arthritis Rheum 2000;43:2455-2463.
20. Jandus C, Bioley G, Rivals JP, et al. Increased numbers of circulating polyfunctional Th17 memory cells in patients with seronegative spondylarthritides. Arthritis Rheum 2008;58:2307-2317.
21. Nistala K, Moncrieffe H, Newton KR, et al. Interleukin-17–producing T cells are enriched in the joints of children with arthritis, but have a reciprocal relationship to regulatory T cell numbers. Arthritis Rheum 2008;58:875-887.
22. Double blind, placebo-controlled study of the safety, tolerability and pharmacokinetics of AIN457 in rheumatoid arthritis patients. Available at http://clinicaltrials.gov/ct2/show/NCT00669942. Accessed March 31, 2009.
23. Multiple-dose study to evaluate the safety, tolerability, pharmacokinetics, pharmacodynamics and efficacy of AMG 827 in subjects with rheumatoid arthritis. Available at http://clinicaltrials.gov/ct2/show/NCT00771030?term=NCT00771030&rank=1. Accessed March 31, 2009.
24. Arend WP, Palmer G, Gabay C: IL-1, IL-18, and IL-33 families of cytokines. Immunol Rev 2008;223:20-38.
25. Kim SH, Eisenstein M, Reznikov L, et al. Structural requirements of six naturally occurring isoforms of the IL-18 binding protein to inhibit IL-18. Proc Natl Acad Sci U S A 2000;97:1190-1195.
26. Bufler P, Azam T, Gamboni-Robertson F, et al. A complex of the IL-1 homologue IL-1F7b and IL-18-binding protein reduces IL-18 activity. Proc Natl Acad Sci U S A 2002;99:13723-13728.
27. McInnes IB, Liew FY, Gracie JA: Interleukin-18: a therapeutic target in rheumatoid arthritis? Arthritis Res Ther 2005;7:38-41.
28. Amin MA, Mansfield PJ, Pakozdi A, et al. Interleukin-18 induces angiogenic factors in rheumatoid arthritis synovial tissue fibroblasts via distinct signaling pathways. Arthritis Rheum 2007;56:1787-1797.
29. Bresnihan B, Roux-Lombard P, Murphy E, et al. Serum interleukin 18 and interleukin 18 binding protein in rheumatoid arthritis. Ann Rheum Dis 2002;61:726-729.

30. Pittoni V, Bombardieri M, Spinelli FR, et al. Anti-tumour necrosis factor (TNF) alpha treatment of rheumatoid arthritis (infliximab) selectively down regulates the production of interleukin (IL) 18 but not of IL12 and IL13. Ann Rheum Dis 2002;61:723-725.
31. Yago T, Nanke Y, Kawamoto M, et al. IL-23 induces human osteoclastogenesis via IL-17 in vitro, and anti-IL-23 antibody attenuates collagen-induced arthritis in rats. Arthritis Res Ther 2007;9:R96.
32. van Kuijk AW, Reinders-Blankert P, Smeets TJ, et al. Detailed analysis of the cell infiltrate and the expression of mediators of synovial inflammation and joint destruction in the synovium of patients with psoriatic arthritis: implications for treatment. Ann Rheum Dis 2006;65:1551-1557.
33. Arican O, Aral M, Sasmaz S, Ciragil P: Serum levels of TNF-alpha, IFN-gamma, IL-6, IL-8, IL-12, IL-17, and IL-18 in patients with active psoriasis and correlation with disease severity. Mediators Inflamm 2005;2005:273-279.
34. Naik SM, Cannon G, Burbach GJ, et al. Human keratinocytes constitutively express interleukin-18 and secrete biologically active interleukin-18 after treatment with pro-inflammatory mediators and dinitrochlorobenzene. J Invest Dermatol 1999;113:766-772.
35. Companjen A, van der Wel L, van der Fits L, et al. Elevated interleukin-18 protein expression in early active and progressive plaque-type psoriatic lesions. Eur Cytokine Netw 2004;15:210-216.
36. Lotito AP, Campa A, Silva CA, et al. Interleukin 18 as a marker of disease activity and severity in patients with juvenile idiopathic arthritis. J Rheumatol 2007;34:823-830.
37. Kawashima M, Yamamura M, Taniai M, et al. Levels of interleukin-18 and its binding inhibitors in the blood circulation of patients with adult-onset Still's disease. Arthritis Rheum 2001;44:550-560.
38. Pavelka K, Kuba V, Rasmussen J, et al. Clinical effects of pralnacasan (PRAL), an orally-active interleukin-1beta converting enzyme (ICE) inhibitor, in a 285 patient PhII trial in rheumatoid arthritis (RA). Presented before the American College of Rheumatology 66th annual scientific meeting. New Orleans, 2002.
39. Ferrari D, Pizzirani C, Adinolfi E, et al. The P2X7 receptor: a key player in IL-1 processing and release. J Immunol 2006;176:3877-3883.
40. Tak PP, Bacchi M, Bertolino M: Pharmacokinetics of IL-18 binding protein in healthy volunteers and subjects with rheumatoid arthritis or plaque psoriasis. Eur J Drug Metab Pharmacokinet 2006;31:109-116.
41. Parham C, Chirica M, Timans J, et al. A receptor for the heterodimeric cytokine IL-23 is composed of IL-12Rbeta1 and a novel cytokine receptor subunit, IL-23R. J Immunol 2002;168:5699-5708.

42. Boniface K, Blom B, Liu YJ, de Waal Malefyt R: From interleukin-23 to T-helper 17 cells: human T-helper cell differentiation revisited. Immunol Rev 2008;226:132-146.

43. Martinez A, Varade J, Marquez A, et al. Association of the STAT4 gene with increased susceptibility for some immune-mediated diseases. Arthritis Rheum 2008;58:2598-2602.

44. Duerr RH, Taylor KD, Brant SR, et al. A genome-wide association study identifies IL23R as an inflammatory bowel disease gene. Science 2006;314:1461-1463.

45. Kim HR, Kim HS, Park MK, et al. The clinical role of IL-23p19 in patients with rheumatoid arthritis. Scand J Rheumatol 2007;36:259-264.

46. Lee E, Trepicchio WL, Oestreicher JL, et al. Increased expression of interleukin 23 p19 and p40 in lesional skin of patients with psoriasis vulgaris. J Exp Med 2004;199:125-130.

47. Szodoray P, Alex P, Chappell-Woodward CM, et al. Circulating cytokines in Norwegian patients with psoriatic arthritis determined by a multiplex cytokine array system. Rheumatology (Oxford) 2007;46:417-425.

48. Filipe-Santos O, Bustamante J, Chapgier A, et al. Inborn errors of IL-12/23- and IFN-gamma-mediated immunity: molecular, cellular, and clinical features. Semin Immunol 2006;18:347-361.

49. A randomized, double-blind, placebo-controlled clinical study of the oral IL-12/23 inhibitor, STA-5326 mesylate, administered to patients with rheumatoid arthritis to determine safety, tolerability, pharmacokinetic and synovial tissue outcomes. Available at http://clinicaltrials.gov/ct2/show/NCT00642629?term=NCT00642629&rank=1. Accessed on March 31, 2009.

50. Gottlieb A, Menter A, Mendelsohn A, et al. Ustekinumab, a human interleukin 12/23 monoclonal antibody, for psoriatic arthritis: randomised, double-blind, placebo-controlled, crossover trial. Lancet 2009;373:633-640.

Infections and biologic therapy in rheumatoid arthritis

Kevin L. Winthrop

64

INTRODUCTION

Rheumatoid arthritis (RA) patients are at increased risk for infectious disease–related morbidity and mortality. This risk is due in part to the underlying immune cell dysfunction associated with RA and the immunosuppressive therapies directed against it. In the past decade, a number of newly developed biologic therapies have delivered tremendous clinical benefits to RA patients. With these therapies, however, come new challenges to patients and their physicians regarding the prevention and management of serious bacterial and opportunistic infections. These drugs include those that inhibit tumor necrosis factor-α (TNF-α), for which there exists a large amount of pre- and post-marketing data suggesting an elevated serious infection risk. For the more recently approved biologic drugs that target B and T lymphocytes, the risk of infection is less clear. In this chapter the infectious diseases typical of RA and biologic therapy are reviewed and the treating rheumatologist is provided with tools to prevent their associated infectious morbidity.

INCREASED INFECTIOUS RISK IN RHEUMATOID ARTHRITIS

Patients with RA have long been recognized to suffer a greater burden of serious infection. Case reports from the 20th century attest to increased numbers of bone and joint, pulmonary, and skin and soft tissue infections.[1] Later studies documented that RA patients suffer earlier death than healthy counterparts, with some of this excess mortality attributable to infection.[2,3] In one of the first large epidemiologic studies in the United States to address this issue, Wolfe and associates showed that RA patients were five times more likely to die of pneumonia than the general population.[2] This increased infectious risk was postulated to be due to corticosteroid use, surgery, as well as other traditional disease-modifying antirheumatic drugs (DMARDs) used against RA. In 2002 and before the widespread use of biologic therapy, Doran and colleagues conducted a cohort study among RA patients within Minnesota's Mayo Clinic patient population. With over 600 RA patients and a similar number of matched non-RA controls, the investigators found culture and/or radiographic proven serious infections (i.e., those requiring hospitalization) were significantly more common in RA patients and occurred at a rate of 9/100 patients per year, a rate nearly double their non-RA counterparts, even after controlling for the effects of important co-morbidities and other infectious risks.[4] Consistent with historical reports, they found that RA patients frequently suffered from serious pulmonary and skin infections (Table 64.1), and whereas bone and joint infections occurred much less frequently, they were most strongly associated with RA and occurred 10 to 15 times more frequently than in healthy controls.

Doran and colleagues went beyond documenting the increased infectious risk due to the RA disease state itself. They, and subsequently others, documented a significant 1.5- to 2.0-fold increase in risk with corticosteroid therapy, even at "low dose" (e.g., <15 mg/day).[5] In 2006, Wolfe and associates reviewed the national databank for rheumatic diseases in the United States and found a dose-response relationship with risk at doses less than or equal to 5 mg/day (hazard ratio [HR], 1.4; 95% confidence interval [CI], 1.1-1.6) increasing with higher doses of 10 to 15 mg/day (HR, 2.3; 95% CI, 1.6-3.2).[6] Similar risks were more recently documented in prospective fashion in a U.K.

cohort of inflammatory arthritis patients, in whom corticosteroids doubled the risk of serious infection.[7] Despite these infectious risks and the advent of newer biologic therapies, corticosteroid use in RA remains common.[8]

IMMUNE DYSFUNCTION OF RA AND PREDISPOSITION TO INFECTION

The immunopathology of RA is complex, and the precise immune derangements that decrease the host's response to infection are not clearly known. After time, RA patients can develop an overabundance of CD28 null T lymphocytes and a lack of CD28+ T lymphocytes, a process driven by overproduction of TNF-α.[9] CD28 null T lymphocytes, in distinction to their CD28+ counterparts, have lost their capacity to stimulate B cells and instead can downregulate antigen-presenting dendritic cells. Given CD28's known co-stimulatory role in the activation and proliferation of T lymphocytes, this suggests that RA patients can develop diminished T-lymphocyte responses in the presence of antigen presentation. RA patients are known to have a reduced capacity to generate new T lymphocytes, and their T-lymphocyte repertoire becomes severely contracted over time.[10] This T-lymphocyte senescence is similar to that seen in the normal aging host and could explain why elderly patients are more prone to infectious diseases in general.[11] Other studies suggest a genetic predisposition toward infection among RA patients, with patients exhibiting certain polymorphisms in either Fc receptor, tumor necrosis factor, or lymphotoxin-α genes more likely to suffer respiratory and urinary tract infections.[12] It is likely that a variety of RA-associated host factors predispose patients toward infection, including physical derangements (e.g., destruction of articular surfaces) that might also impair local immunity or provide a respite for circulating pathogens.

Anti-tumor necrosis factor-α (anti-TNF) therapy in RA

In the past 10 years, three anti-TNF compounds with remarkable clinical efficacy have gained U.S. Food and Drug Administration (FDA) approval for use against RA in the United States: infliximab, etanercept, and adalimumab.[13] As a group, these drugs inhibit TNF-α, a proinflammatory cytokine involved in the pathogenesis of RA and other autoimmune diseases but also essential to the host's innate immune system. TNF is expressed by activated macrophages, T lymphocytes, and other immune cells and plays a crucial role in the host response against a variety of infections, in particular *Mycobacterium tuberculosis* and other intracellular pathogens.[14] It is essential in the control and containment of intracellular pathogens by stimulating inflammatory cell recruitment to the area of infection and by stimulating the formation and maintenance of granulomas that contain infection. In murine models of tuberculosis (TB), mice deficient in either TNF or its p55 signaling receptors fail to recruit inflammatory cells to the site of infection and fail to form functioning granulomas.[15-17] Similarly, in mice already infected with *M. tuberculosis*, neutralization of TNF causes lysis of already formed granulomas, leading to mycobacterial spread and death.[18,19] In addition, TNF directly activates macrophages to phagocytose and kill mycobacteria and a variety of other pathogens.[20] Mice deficient in the TNF/p55 signaling pathway are highly susceptible to *Listeria*, *Histoplasma*, and parasitic and even extracellular bacterial organisms such as *Klebsiella pneumoniae* and *Streptococcus pneumoniae*, both frequent causes of pneumonia in humans.[21-24]

TABLE 64.1 THE PRE-BIOLOGIC ERA: FREQUENCY OF INFECTIONS AMONG RA PATIENTS AND HEALTHY CONTROLS FROM A MINNESOTA COHORT

Infection type	Incidence per 100 patient-years RA	Incidence per 100 patient-years Non-RA	RR (95% CI)
Pneumonia	4.0	2.4	1.7 (1.5-1.9)
Skin	3.0	0.9	3.3 (2.7-4.1)
Sepsis	0.78	0.51	1.5 (1.1-2.1)
Septic joint	0.40	0.02	14.9 (6.1-73.7)
Intra-abdominal	0.22	0.08	2.8 (1.4-6.2)
Osteomyelitis	0.17	0.01	10.6 (3.4-126.8)

Adapted from Doran MF, Crowson CS, Pond GR, et al. Frequency of infection in patients with rheumatoid arthritis compared with controls: a population-based study. Arthritis Rheum 2002;46:2287-2293.

TABLE 64.2 THE BIOLOGIC ERA: RATES AND RELATIVE RISKS OF SERIOUS INFECTIONS IN RA PATIENTS USING ANTI-TNF THERAPY FROM EUROPEAN AND NORTH AMERICAN OBSERVATIONAL COHORT STUDIES

Country	Incidence per 100 patient-years Anti-TNF treated	Incidence per 100 patient-years Non-biologic comparator	Adjusted RR* (95% CI)
Germany	6.4, ETN	2.3	2.2 (0.9-5.4) ETN
	6.2, INF		2.1 (0.8-5.5) INF
United Kingdom	5.5	3.9	1.3 (0.9-1.8)[‡]
			4.6 (1.8-11.9)[†]
United States	2.9[§]	1.4[§]	4.2 (2.0-8.8)[§]
			1.9 (1.3-2.8)
Sweden	5.4	Not published	1.43 (1.2-1.7)[¶]

*Relative rate using non-biologic users as the referent.
[†]When restricted to the first 90 days of therapy, and adjusted for age, sex, disease duration and severity, extra-articular rheumatoid arthritis, baseline steroid use, diabetes, chronic obstructive pulmonary disease, pulmonary disease, and smoking history.
[‡]Adjusted relative rate when not restricted to the first 90 days of therapy.
[§]Analysis restricted to the first 6 months after initiation of anti-TNF therapy
[¶]Rate calculated at 1 year after starting treatment and adjusted for RA severity and co-morbidities associated with infections.

Currently used anti-TNF drugs and their differential properties

Infliximab and adalimumab are monoclonal antibodies, and etanercept is a soluble construct of the p75 receptor. Infliximab is delivered as an infusion dosed every 4 to 8 weeks. Adalimumab (given every 2 weeks) and etanercept (given weekly) are delivered by subcutaneous injection.[13] All three agents bind TNF, but important differences exist between these drug types with regard to their modulation of TNF activity. Infliximab binds TNF with greater avidity than does etanercept, and it binds to it for longer.[25] The half-life of infliximab is approximately 10.5 days, and its biologic effect can persist for up to 2 months.[26,27] Etanercept's half-life is 3 days, and its effect on TNF is much shorter-lived.[28] It binds TNF in a reversible manner, with disassociation of nearly 50% after only 10 minutes.[25] These differences, coupled with differences in dosing, suggest that infliximab usage results in a greater, more sustained inhibition of TNF activity. Pharmacokinetically, adalimumab behaves more similarly to infliximab.[29] The monoclonal antibodies infliximab and adalimumab might also result in a greater downregulation of host interferon-γ responses, which has been shown *in vitro* with lymphocytes activated by TB antigens; interferon-γ is noted to be important in the immune response to mycobacterial and other infections.[30] Additional studies modeling anti-TNF effects on murine TB granuloma suggest that the monoclonal antibodies penetrate, and remain within, TB granulomas to a greater extent than etanercept.[31] Mathematical models based on such differential penetration suggest this could result in an increased disassociation rate of TNF from etanercept, which hypothetically could allow for greater TNF signaling within the granuloma.[32] These and potentially other factors could explain why the activation of latent TB infection and other granulomatous diseases are reported more frequently among those treated with the monoclonal antibodies.

Risk of serious infections in the anti-TNF setting

Infectious signals first emerged in infliximab randomized clinical trials (RCTs) in which an increased risk of pneumonia was noted, including cases of TB.[33,34] Although etanercept RCTs did not necessarily show elevated infectious risk, like most RCTs, these studies were not well powered to detect small increases in adverse events. In at least one adalimumab RCT an elevated serious infection risk was suggested when adalimumab was combined with methotrexate as compared with adalimumab alone, and a high rate of TB was eventually reported in North American RCTs.[35,36]

With the epidemiologic luxury of national health care databases, and with the advent of biologic registries, European and other investigators have conducted observational studies encompassing large numbers of biologic-treated and naive RA patients. To date, most of the registries have reported similar and elevated rates of serious infections in patients using anti-TNF therapies (Table 64.2). German investigators found that the rate of serious infection in RA patients taking anti-TNF drugs was 6/100 patient-years and more than 2.5-fold higher than the rate seen in unexposed patients.[37] The U.K. registry examined rates of site-specific infections and found similar rates of serious infections overall in anti-TNF treated patients (5.3/100 patient-years), including a statistically significant fourfold increase in osteomyelitis (as compared with RA patients not receiving anti-TNF drugs).[38] With other site-specific infections, however, they did not find elevated risk associated with anti-TNF therapy. However, when the U.K. registry reanalyzed its data and restricted its definition of "time-at-risk" for patients using anti-TNF therapy to the first 90 days after initiation, they demonstrated a fourfold increase in all types of serious infections with no significant differences in risk noted between the three anti-TNF agents.[39] In the United States, Curtis and coworkers used administrative claims data to evaluate outcomes in over 5000 RA patients and found the rates of serious infections in anti-TNF users were elevated twofold over non-biologic users and were highest (relative risk, 4.2) in the 6 months after initiation of anti-TNF therapy.[40]

Tuberculosis, endemic mycosis, and other intracellular pathogens

A number of opportunistic infections have been reported in patients taking anti-TNF therapy. Some of these reports came from clinical trials, but most were spontaneously reported in the post-approval period. These include severe and sometimes lethal infections with *Histoplasma, Coccidioides, Listeria, Salmonella, Aspergillus, Nocardia,* nontuberculous mycobacteria, and others.[41] Perhaps the most frequently reported opportunistic complication and one of the most serious public health concerns is the development of active TB in some patients receiving these drugs.[42] Cases of TB were reported in clinical trials with infliximab,[33] and soon after infliximab approval in the United States. Wolfe and associates documented an annual rate for TB of 52.5/100,000 among RA patients treated with infliximab versus 6.2/100,000 in a non-biologic RA cohort several years earlier (the rate difference did not reach statistical significance).[43] Population-based studies from Sweden subsequently reported a fourfold increase in TB among RA patients using anti-TNF drugs versus non-biologic exposed RA comparators. Of the 15 TB cases found in this study (conducted before adalimumab approval), 10 patients had exposure to infliximab and 5 had exposure to etanercept, and the overall crude rate of TB in those with anti-TNF therapy was 118/100,000, well above the background rate of 5/100,000 of Sweden.[44] Spanish investigators reported rates near 1900/100,000, which were 10- to 20-fold higher among RA anti-TNF users as compared with biologic-naive RA patients. These rates have since decreased dramatically with institution of widespread screening for latent TB infection before anti-TNF use.[45] Recent population-based studies from France affirm that the monoclonal antibodies confer at least a several fold higher risk of TB than etanercept.[45a] In the United States, little population-level data exist on which to estimate the risk of TB associated with anti-TNF therapy. The risk is presumably less than in countries like Spain where the background prevalence of TB is higher.

For rates of intracellular infections in general, much less data exist. U.K. researchers found a strong and significant association of such infections with anti-TNF agents. During their study, they documented 19 cases of intracellular infection (incidence of 2/1000 patient-years), and all occurred exclusively in anti-TNF users, including 10 cases of TB (rate varied between 50 and 150 per 100,000 person-years depending on the anti-TNF compound, with higher, but not statistically significant rates seen with the monoclonal antibodies). Other intracellular infections captured in this study included nontuberculous mycobacteria (n = 3), *Salmonella* (n = 3), and *Listeria* (n = 3).[38] In the United States, a recent nationwide survey of infectious diseases consultants suggested that nontuberculous mycobacteria (most frequently *M. avium*) and histoplasmosis both occurred more frequently than TB in this setting, perhaps not surprising given the United States' relatively low background TB prevalence.[46] A registry of anti-TNF–treated RA patients in France followed patients for 1 year and documented 10 cases of legionellosis (adalimumab, n = 6; etanercept, n = 2; infliximab, n = 2) with a rate estimated to be 16 to 21 times higher than the general French population.[47] At the time of this writing, there is a great need for population-based studies to ascertain the risk of intracellular infections other than TB and their association with biologic therapy. Invariably their risks will vary regionally according to environmental and population factors.

Prevention of serious bacterial infections in anti-TNF–treated patients

It is presumed that the serious bacterial infections common in this setting are caused by the same types of organisms seen in the general public, with many skin and soft tissue infections likely due to *Staphylococcus aureus* and *Streptococcus* species and with most septic arthritis in RA patients due to *S. aureus*.[48] Colonization with *S. aureus* might predispose RA patients to subsequent staphylococcal infection. Some studies report rates of colonization as high as 50% for RA patients as compared with 30% for the general public,[49,50] with one small study suggesting rates to be higher in patients concurrently receiving anti-TNF therapy and methotrexate.[51] The risk of colonization on subsequent infection has not been evaluated in RA, but an increased risk is plausible based on data from intensive care unit, presurgical, and hemodialysis settings.[52] Of particular concern is the rise of methicillin-resistant *S. aureus* (MRSA) within the general public. Emergency department–based surveillance from across the United States suggests that nearly 60% of presenting soft tissue infections are now caused by MRSA.[53] Infection with MRSA should be high in the differential diagnosis for any RA patient presenting with signs of skin infection, particularly when accompanied by furuncles or abscess formation. Patients who suffer such recurrent infections could potentially be screened for *S. aureus* and decolonized with antibiotic therapy and chlorhexidine scrubs before anti-TNF therapy.[54]

A significant number of RA patients are also hospitalized each year with community-acquired pneumonia, where, similar to the case with soft tissue infections, organism-level data are lacking.[4,6,37] It is likely the same organisms that cause pneumonia in general populations are frequent: *Streptococcus pneumoniae*, *Haemophilus influenzae*, *S. aureus*, and gram-negative bacilli are some of the most common causes.[55] For *S. pneumoniae*, it is widely recommended that patients receive 23-valent pneumococcal vaccine before initiating anti-TNF and other long-term immunosuppressive therapies, primarily because it protects against invasive pneumococcal disease and not pneumonia.[56] Immunogenicity to this vaccine is poor and diminished by methotrexate, and rituximab, so if possible, patients should be vaccinated while unexposed to methotrexate.[57] A booster vaccination 3 to 5 years after the initial vaccine is not unreasonable. RA patients are known to have some reduction in their response to influenza vaccine, although this appears not related to methotrexate, prednisone, or anti-TNF therapy. Despite this, most achieve protective levels of antibodies and therefore should be immunized annually before the onset of influenza season.[58]

Prevention of tuberculosis before long-term immunosuppressive therapy

TNF antagonists should be used with caution in any person with risk factors for TB, and screening for latent TB should be undertaken before starting anti-TNF, prednisone, or other forms of long-term immunosuppressive therapy.[42] Recommendations for TB screening have been issued by various public health authorities and professional societies.[42,59,60] In general, these recommendations vary according to regional differences in background TB prevalence as well as bacille Calmette-Guérin (BCG) vaccine usage, which can interfere with interpretation of the tuberculin skin test. Recently, interferon-γ release assays (IGRAs) have been developed in response to the latter concern: the Quanti-FERON Gold In-Tube (Cellestis, Australia) and T-SPOT.TB (Oxford Immunotec, United Kingdom). These assays measure lymphocyte interferon-γ response to antigens highly specific to TB and absent from strains of BCG and subsequently offer a highly specific test for TB. In some areas, particularly those with high BCG penetrance, these assays have replaced the tuberculin skin test in initial screening.[59] In addition, in the past 2 years, several studies have suggested that IGRAs offer similar or better sensitivity in detecting latent TB among RA and other immunosuppressed populations and that they might be less likely to give false-negative results in patients using prednisone.[61] Other studies, however, reiterate that even IGRAs, like the tuberculin skin test, can yield false-negative results due to immunosuppression, including concurrent anti-TNF use, and negative results should be considered with suspicion in any patient with a history of TB exposure.[62]

Screening for and treatment of latent TB

Given the regional and national differences in background TB prevalence and BCG usage around the world, the negative and positive predictive values of tuberculin skin tests and IGRAs vary, and not surprisingly so does the screening guidance.[42,59,60] Using one or both of these screening tests in combination with taking a close history for TB risk factors is recommended (Fig. 64.1); and for patients thought to have latent TB, treatment with isoniazid or other preferred therapies should be initiated before anti-TNF therapy.[42] Such a screening strategy is supported by observational data from Spanish investigators who adopted such a protocol and subsequently saw an 85% reduction in TB cases associated with infliximab.[45] A 4-month course of rifampin-based therapy could be considered an alternative in patients who cannot tolerate 9 months of isoniazid.[63] Although isoniazid-related hepatotoxicity is not common in the general population, a large proportion of anti-TNF candidates will be on methotrexate or other hepatotoxic drugs such that liver function testing should be performed at baseline and then monthly in all such patients.[63]

Presentation and treatment of TB in patients already using anti-TNF therapy

In patients using anti-TNF therapy, extrapulmonary and disseminated manifestations of TB are more common with chest radiographs normal in a large proportion of these cases.[42] The diagnosis should be pursued in any such patient presenting with a prolonged febrile or respiratory illness with or without constitutional symptoms. For patients diagnosed with TB in this setting, most recommend discontinuing anti-TNF or other biologic therapy and starting standard four-drug therapy for TB.[42] There are case reports of immune reconstitution inflammatory syndrome occurring in TB patients in whom anti-TNF therapy was stopped,[64] although one recent study suggested this phenomenon is probably not frequent.[46] Clinicians should delay resumption of anti-TNF therapy until after the patient has completed TB therapy or, at the least, has demonstrated clinical improvement while adhering to an appropriate anti-TB regimen.[42]

Nontuberculous Mycobacterium, *Histoplasma*, and other intracellular infections

Non-tuberculous mycobacteria are a large and diverse group of environmental organisms that cause serious pulmonary and extrapulmonary infections. Patients with underlying structural lung disease from rheumatoid arthritis, chronic obstructive pulmonary disease,

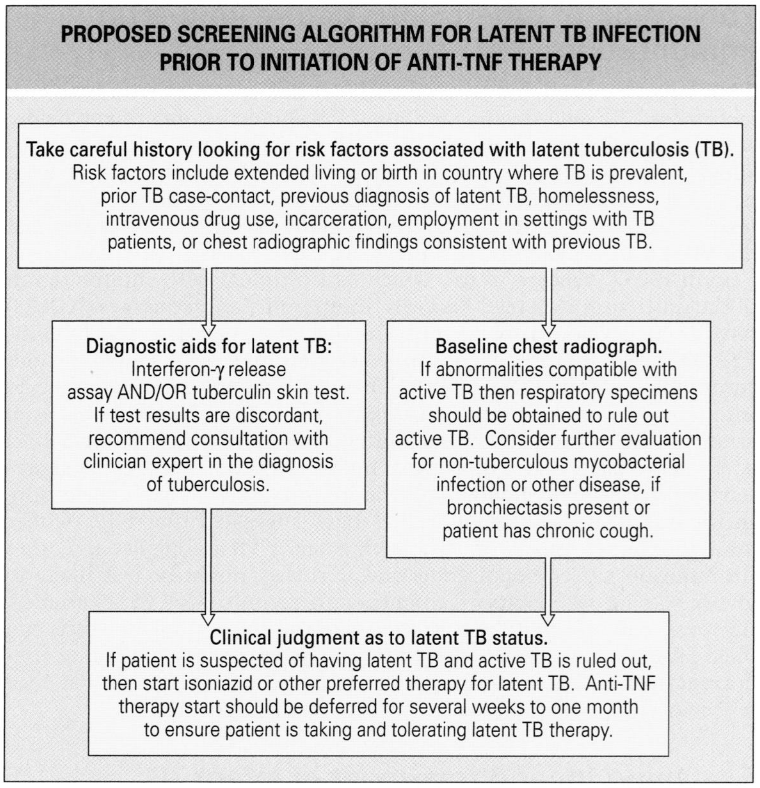

PROPOSED SCREENING ALGORITHM FOR LATENT TB INFECTION PRIOR TO INITIATION OF ANTI-TNF THERAPY

Take careful history looking for risk factors associated with latent tuberculosis (TB).
Risk factors include extended living or birth in country where TB is prevalent, prior TB case-contact, previous diagnosis of latent TB, homelessness, intravenous drug use, incarceration, employment in settings with TB patients, or chest radiographic findings consistent with previous TB.

Diagnostic aids for latent TB:
Interferon-γ release assay AND/OR tuberculin skin test. If test results are discordant, recommend consultation with clinician expert in the diagnosis of tuberculosis.

Baseline chest radiograph.
If abnormalities compatible with active TB then respiratory specimens should be obtained to rule out active TB. Consider further evaluation for non-tuberculous mycobacterial infection or other disease, if bronchiectasis present or patient has chronic cough.

Clinical judgment as to latent TB status.
If patient is suspected of having latent TB and active TB is ruled out, then start isoniazid or other preferred therapy for latent TB. Anti-TNF therapy start should be deferred for several weeks to one month to ensure patient is taking and tolerating latent TB therapy.

Fig. 64.1 Proposed screening algorithm for latent TB before initiation of anti-TNF therapy. A careful history for the risk factors of TB is of upmost importance and helps to categorize the patient's *a priori* probability of having been previously exposed to *M. tuberculosis*. Note that a screening strategy that employs both tuberculin skin testing and interferon-γ release assays could be considered in an effort to maximize sensitivity in the detection of latent TB in this setting.

bronchiectasis, and other conditions are at higher risk.[65] A small number of biologic therapy–associated cases have been reported in the literature, although a recent survey of practicing infectious disease physicians in the United States suggested these infections might be more common than TB in the anti-TNF setting.[46] Pulmonary and disseminated cases of *M. avium*, *M. marinum*, *M. kansasii*, *M. abscessus*, and others have been reported. It is unclear whether the risk of such infections is elevated by anti-TNF therapy, but it is clear that such cases are occurring and that they can cause severe morbidity and death.[46,66] Screening for non-tuberculous mycobacterial disease before anti-TNF treatment is largely theoretical but could be considered in any patients with abnormalities on their baseline radiograph or in those with chronic cough. Such workup could include chest computed tomography and culture of respiratory specimens.[66] Whether it is safe to pursue anti-TNF therapy in patients with active non-tuberculous mycobacterial infections, treated or untreated, is unknown.

Histoplasma capsulatum is a dimorphic fungus with a worldwide distribution, although it is most commonly found in tropical areas and in the Tennessee/Ohio/Mississippi river basins. Histoplasmosis appears to be the most common fungal infection associated with anti-TNF therapy in the United States.[41,42] Similar to TB, *Histoplasma* is a pulmonary pathogen that can cause primary disease within the lungs or disseminate to involve other organ systems. It can remain latent or slowly progressive for years and can progress to "active" disease during immunosuppression. Screening for such infection before TNF blockade is largely theoretical. Evidence of previous infection by serologic testing could be obtained before drug start; however, it is unclear how useful these tests are and whether positive results would indicate a need for prophylaxis or avoidance of TNF blockade. Currently, serologic testing for histoplasmosis is not routinely recommended in HIV-infected persons.[67] Prophylaxis with itraconazole (200 mg daily) can be considered in severely immunosuppressed HIV patients (CD4 counts > 150 cells/µL) who live in highly endemic areas, although this has not

been shown to reduce mortality in such settings,[68] and a recent study of over 500 transplant patients living in a hyperendemic area failed to show any benefit for itraconazole prophylaxis.[69]

For patients currently prescribed anti-TNF medications who present with symptoms consistent with pulmonary or disseminated histoplasmosis, their anti-TNF therapy should be stopped and empirical therapy with intravenous amphotericin of hospitalized patients considered. Diagnosis of disseminated disease is facilitated by the use of a urinary antigen test, although this test is poorly sensitive in patients with pulmonary histoplasmosis. Similar to guidelines for other immunosuppressive settings, patients who have finished treatment for histoplasmosis and are considering starting immunosuppression with anti-TNF therapy should get a urinary antigen level before initiation and then every 2 to 3 months during the course of therapy, with an increase in urinary antigen levels triggering cessation of anti-TNF therapy and diagnostic investigation for active histoplasmosis.[67]

Coccidioides immitis and *C. posadasii* are dimorphic fungi endemic to the southwestern United States and Central and South America. A recent study from the highly endemic area of Arizona suggests that up to 29% of community-acquired pneumonia in that region may be due to coccidioidomycosis.[70] Like histoplasmosis and TB, it can exist in a latent or subclinical infectious state after exposure and can later progress to disease, particularly during immunosuppression. In this setting, disease generally disseminates from the lung to involve other viscera, including skin, bone, lymph, and central nervous system and is associated with higher mortality rates, particularly in patients of Asian and African descent.[71] Consideration could be given to screening patients in endemic areas with serology before initiation of TNF blockade, although many of the coccidioidomycosis cases reported in association with TNF blockade appear to be acute infection and not reactivation, making the utility of this approach unknown.[72] Furthermore, HIV-infected individuals living in endemic areas are not routinely screened for coccidioidomycosis; and given the paucity of reported coccidioidomycosis cases in association with TNF blockade, it is unclear whether there exists a need for screening before initiation of such therapy. Similar to histoplasmosis, patients currently prescribed anti-TNF medications who are diagnosed with coccidioidomycosis should have their anti-TNF therapy stopped. After appropriate antifungal treatment, it is unclear if it is safe to ever resume anti-TNF therapy because of the potential for reactivation, particularly in those with disseminated forms of disease. *Blastomyces dermatitidis* is another dimorphic fungus endemic in the southeastern and south central states of the United States, along the Mississippi and Ohio Rivers. There have been reports of blastomycosis in patients taking anti-TNF[46] but no published details of these cases. The recommendations for patients on immunosuppressive therapy who develop blastomycosis are similar to those described for histoplasmosis.[73]

Intracellular bacterial pathogens

Fatal cases of listeriosis have occurred in persons taking TNF-blocking agents.[41,74] *Listeria monocytogenes* is an intracellular pathogen acquired via the ingestion of contaminated meats and dairy products. Accordingly, patients under TNF blockade should be wary of undercooked meat, delicatessen meat, and unpasteurized milk products. *Salmonella* species are also known to cause serious infections in those receiving anti-TNF therapy.[38,41] They are typically transmitted by contaminated raw or undercooked foods, including fresh produce, cheese made from raw milk, and even reptiles sold as pets. Patients should be advised to wash produce, cook meat thoroughly, and practice good hand hygiene in general.

RITUXIMAB AND ABATACEPT

In addition to the anti-TNF compounds, rheumatologists have recently gained access to two additional biologic therapies: rituximab and abatacept. Rituximab, approved for RA in 2006, is an anti-CD20 B-lymphocyte depletion agent; and abatacept, approved in late 2005, is a CTLA-4 fusion protein that modulates T-lymphocyte activation and proliferation. Because of the more recent approval of these agents, less is known regarding their infectious risks and the clinical manifestations of serious infections in patients using these compounds. Clinical trials with rituximab among RA patients did not suggest a significantly increased risk of infection.[75] There are case reports of both TB and non-tuberculous mycobacterial disease in patients on rituximab, although these patients also have been on methotrexate and prednisone, and to date there are no data to suggest a need to screen for these infections in patients using rituximab.[46,76] Because most patients using rituximab will already have been screened for TB before anti-TNF therapy, this is likely not of practical significance.

In many areas of the world, chronic hepatitis B and C are prevalent. Although the anti-TNF compounds appear relatively safe in patients with hepatitis C, at least in the short term, this is less clear for hepatitis B. For rituximab, there are reports of patients who reactivated hepatitis B infections, and, similar to patients beginning anti-TNF therapy, all patients should be screened for viral hepatitis before using rituximab.[13] In addition, rare cases of progressive multifocal leukoencephalopathy, a disease generally seen in the HIV setting, have been reported in lupus and lymphoma patients using rituximab concurrent with other immunosuppressive or cytotoxic agents. It is unclear if rituximab poses a risk for this infection in these or other disease settings such as RA.[13]

For abatacept, some clinical trials suggested a small increased risk of serious infection, particularly respiratory infections and exacerbations in patients with chronic obstructive pulmonary disease.[77,78] The risk of serious infections was significantly elevated when abatacept was combined with anti-TNF therapy.[79,80] For TB and other opportunistic infections, there is no known increased risk documented to date, although patients were screened for latent TB in abatacept clinical trials and therefore should also be screened in clinical practice until further data are known. In animal studies, abatacept does not appear to negatively affect the immune system of mice who are exposed to tuberculosis.[81] In humans, Schiff and associates recently conducted a randomized trial to compare the efficacy and safety of abatacept with infliximab. At 12 months of follow-up, patients using abatacept suffered significantly fewer serious infections than infliximab-treated patients (1.9% vs. 8.5%), with a rate similar to that seen in the placebo group at 6-month follow-up (2.7%). No cases of opportunistic infections were seen in the abatacept-treated group, whereas five such cases were seen in the infliximab group, including two cases of TB in patients who had negative tuberculin skin test results at baseline and one case of *Pneumocystic jiroveci* pneumonia.[82] As for other RA patients, vaccination for influenza should take place yearly and pneumovax given to decrease the risk of invasive pneumococcal disease as appropriate. If possible, vaccinations should be given before the use of rituximab as it is associated with reduced immunogenecity to both pneumococcal and influenza vaccines.[83,84]

ANAKINRA

Although used less frequently for RA, this recombinant interleukin (IL)-1 receptor antagonist has also been shown to significantly increase the risk of infection, particularly when combined with prednisone or anti-TNF therapy. Fleischmann and coworkers evaluated a 3-year open-label extension study with anakinra and documented the rate of serious infection to be 5.4/100 patient-years as compared with 1.65/100 patient-years in unexposed patients during the placebo-controlled portion of the trial. This increased risk was substantially driven by baseline concurrent prednisone use, such that anakinra-treated patients without baseline corticosteroid usage had an elevated, but lower, risk of infection of 2.9/100 patient-years.[85] In a 6-month RCT, Genovese and colleagues documented a significantly increased risk of serious infection in background methotrexate-treated patients receiving concurrent anakinra and etanercept (5.5%) compared with etanercept alone (0%), leading to clear warnings that such concurrent anti-TNF therapy should be avoided.[86]

CONCLUSION

Patients with RA are at higher risk for serious infections and death from infection than the general public. Anti-TNF agents and prednisone further raise this risk, particularly with regard to skin and soft tissue, bone, joint, lung, and opportunistic infections. Clinicians should remain vigilant for these infections in any RA patient undergoing long-term immunosuppressive therapy of any kind. Some of these infections are preventable with screening (i.e., TB), vaccination, and patient education. As newer biologic-targeted therapies are developed, new infectious challenges will arise with established and emerging pathogens. Future post-marketing surveillance efforts will remain key to detecting these infectious signals early, so that physicians and patients can minimize the infectious risks of such therapy.

KEY REFERENCES

2. Wolfe F, Mitchell DM, Sibley JT, et al. The mortality of rheumatoid arthritis. Arthritis Rheum 1994;37:481-494.

4. Doran MF, Crowson CS, Pond GR, et al. Frequency of infection in patients with rheumatoid arthritis compared with controls: a population-based study. Arthritis Rheum 2002;46:2287-2293.

5. Doran MF, Crowson CS, Pond GR, et al. Predictors of infection in rheumatoid arthritis. Arthritis Rheum 2002;46:2294-2300.

6. Wolfe F, Caplan L, Michaeud K. Treatment for rheumatoid arthritis and the risk of hospitalization for pneumonia. Arthritis Rheum 2006;54:628-634.

14. Ehlers S. Tumor necrosis factor and its blockade in granulomatous infections: differential modes of action of infliximab and etanercept? Clin Infect Dis 2005;41(Suppl 3):S199-S203.

15. Flynn JL, Goldstein MM, Chan J, et al. Tumor necrosis factor-alpha is required in the protective immune response against *Mycobacterium tuberculosis* in mice. Immunity 1995;2:561-572.

16. Algood HM, Lin PL, Flynn JL. Tumor necrosis factor and chemokine interactions in the formation and maintenance of granulomas in tuberculosis. Clin Infect Dis 2005;41(Suppl 3):S189-S193.

17. Roach RR, Bean AGD, Demangel C, et al. TNF regulates chemokine induction essential for cell recruitment, granuloma formation, and clearance of mycobacterial infection. J Immunol 2002;168:4620-4627.

22. Deepe GS Jr. Modulation of infection with *Histoplasma capsulatum* by inhibition of tumor necrosis factor-alpha activity. Clin Infect Dis 2005;41(Suppl 3):S204-S207.

23. O'Brien DP, Briles DE, Szalai AJ, et al. Tumor necrosis factor alpha receptor I is important for survival from *Streptococcus pneumoniae* infections. Infect Immun 1999;67:595-601.

25. Scallon B, Cai A, Solowski N, et al. Binding and functional comparisons of two types of tumor necrosis factor antagonists. J Pharmacol Exp Ther 2002;301:418-426.

26. Long R, Gardam MA. Tumor necrosis factor-α inhibitors and the reactivation of latent tuberculosis infection. Can Med Assoc J 2003;168:1153-1156.

30. Saliu OY, Crismale C, Schwander SK, Wallis RS. Tumor-necrosis-factor blockers: differential effects on mycobacterial immunity. J Antimicrob Chemother 2007;60:994-998.

31. Plessner HL, Lin PL, Kohno T, et al. Neutralization of tumor necrosis factor (TNF) by antibody but not TNF receptor fusion molecule exacerbates chronic murine tuberculosis. J Infect Dis 2007;195:1643-1650.

32. Marino S, Sud D, Plessner H, et al. Differences in reactivation of tuberculosis induced from anti-TNF treatments are based on bioavailability in granulomatous tissue. PLoS Comput Biol 2007;3:1909-1924.

33. St Clair EW, van der Heijde DM, Smolen JS, et al. Active-controlled study of patients receiving infliximab for the treatment of rheumatoid arthritis of early onset study group. Arthritis Rheum 2004;50:3432-3443.

34. Westhovens R, Yocum D, Han J, et al. The safety of infliximab, combined with background treatments, among patients with rheumatoid arthritis and various comorbidities: a large, randomized, placebo-controlled trial. Arthritis Rheum 2006;54:1075-1086.

35. Breedveld FC, Weisman MH, Kavanaugh AF, et al. The PREMIER study: A multicenter, randomized, double-blind clinical trial of combination therapy with adalimumab plus methotrexate versus methotrexate alone or adalimumab alone in patients with early, aggressive rheumatoid arthritis who had not had previous methotrexate treatment. Arthritis Rheum 2006;54:26-37.

36. Schiff MH, Burmester GR, Kent JM, et al. Safety analysis of adalimumab in global clinical trials and US postmarketing surveillance of patients with rheumatoid arthritis. Ann Rheum Dis 2006;65:889-894.

37. Listing J, Strangfeld A, Kary S, et al. Infections in patients with rheumatoid arthritis treated with biologic agents. Arthritis Rheum 2005;52:3403-3412.

38. Dixon WG, Watson K, Lunt M, et al. Rates of serious infection, including site-specific and bacterial intracellular infection, in rheumatoid arthritis patients receiving anti-tumor necrosis factor therapy: results from the British Society for Rheumatology Biologics Register. Arthritis Rheum 2006;54:2368-2376.

39. Dixon WG, Symmons DP, Lunt M, et al. Serious infection following anti-tumor necrosis factor alpha therapy in patients with rheumatoid arthritis: lessons from interpreting data from observational studies. Arthritis Rheum 2007;56:2896-2904.

40. Curtis J, Patkar N, Xie A, et al. Risk of serious bacterial infections among rheumatoid arthritis patients exposed to tumor necrosis factor alpha antagonists. Arthritis Rheum 2007;56:1125-1133.

41. Wallis RS, Broder MS, Wong JY, et al. Granulomatous infectious diseases associated with tumor necrosis factor antagonists. Clin Infect Dis 2004;38:1261-1265; correction, Clin Infect Dis 2004;39:1254-1255.

42. Winthrop KL, Seigel JN, Jereb J, et al. Tuberculosis associated with therapy against tumor necrosis factor-alpha. Arthritis Rheum 2005;52:2968-2974.

44. Askling J, Fored CM, Brandt L, et al. Risk and case characteristics of tuberculosis in rheumatoid arthritis associated with tumor necrosis factor antagonists in Sweden. Arthritis Rheum 2005;52:1986-1992.

45. Carmona L, Gomez-Reino JJ, Rodriguez-Valverde V, et al. Effectiveness of recommendations to prevent

reactivation of latent tuberculosis infection in patients treated with tumor necrosis factor antagonists. Arthritis Rheum 2005;52:1766-1772.

46. Winthrop KL, Yamashita S, Beekman SE, Polgreen PM. Mycobacterial and other serious infections in patients receiving anti-TNF and other newly approved biologic therapies; case-finding via the Emerging Infections Network. Clin Infect Dis 2008;46:1738-1740.

47. Tubach F, Ravaud P, Salmon-Céron D, et al. Emergence of *Legionella pneumophila* pneumonia in patients receiving tumor necrosis factor-alpha antagonists. Clin Infect Dis 2006;43:e95-e100.

48. Dubost JJ, Soubrier M, De Champs C, et al. No changes in the distribution of organisms responsible for septic arthritis over a 20 year period. Ann Rheum Dis 2002;61:267-269.

51. Bassetti S, Wasmer S, Hasler P, et al. Staphylococcus aureus in patients with rheumatoid arthritis under conventional and anti-tumor necrosis factor-alpha treatment. J Rheumatol 2005;32:2125-2129.

53. Moran GJ, Krishnadasan A, Gorwitz RJ, et al. Methicillin-resistant *S. aureus* infections among patients in the emergency department. N Engl J Med 2006;355:666-674.

54. Gorwitz RJ, Jernigan DB, Powers JH, et al. Strategies for clinical management of MRSA in the community: summary of an experts meeting convened by the Centers for Disease Control and Prevention, 2006 (accessed electronically 3/12/09). http://www.cdc.gov/ncidod/dhqp/pdf/ar/CAMRSA_ExpMtgStrategies.pdf.

55. Kollef MH, Shorr A, Tabak YP, et al. Epidemiology and outcomes of health-care-associated pneumonia: results from a large US database of culture-positive pneumonia. Chest 2005;128:3854-3862. Erratum in Chest 2006;129:831.

57. Kapetanovic MC, Saxne T, Sjoholm A, et al. Influence of methotrexate, TNF blockers and prednisolone on antibody responses to pneumococcal polysaccharide vaccine in patients with rheumatoid arthritis. Rheumatology (Oxford) 2006;45:106-111.

58. Fomin I, Caspi D, Levy V, et al. Vaccination against influenza in rheumatoid arthritis: the effect of disease modifying drugs, including TNFα blockers. Ann Rheum Diseases 2006;65:191-194.

59. Beglinger C, Dudler J, Mottet C, et al. Screening for tuberculosis infection before the initiation of an anti-TNF-alpha therapy. Swiss Med Wkly 2007;137:620-622.

60. British Thoracic Society Standards for Care Committee. BTS recommendations for assessing risk and for managing *Mycobacterium tuberculosis* infection and disease in patients due to start anti-TNF-alpha treatment. Thorax 2005;60:800-805.

61. Winthrop KL, Daley CD. A novel assay for screening patients for latent tuberculosis infection prior to anti-tumor necrosis factor therapy. Nat Clin Prac Rheum 2008;4:456-457.

62. Lalvani A, Millington KA. Screening for tuberculosis infection prior to initiation of anti-TNF therapy. Autoimmun Rev 2008;8:147-152.

63. American Thoracic Society. Targeted tuberculin testing and treatment of latent tuberculosis infection. Am J Respir Crit Care Med 2000;161:S221-S247.

65. Griffith DE, Aksamit T, Brown-Elliott BA, et al. An official ATS/IDSA statement: Diagnosis, treatment, and prevention of nontuberculous mycobacterial diseases. Am J Respir Crit Care Med 2007;175:367-416.

67. Wheat LJ, Freifeld AG, Kleiman MB, et al. Infectious Diseases Society of America. Clinical practice guidelines for the management of patients with histoplasmosis: 2007 update by the Infectious Diseases Society of America. Clin Infect Dis 2007;45:807-825.

72. Bergstrom L, Yocum DE, Ampel NM, et al. Increased risk of coccidioidomycosis in patients treated with tumor necrosis factor alpha antagonists. Arthritis Rheum 2004;50:1959-1966.

74. Slifman NR, Gershon SK, Lee JH, et al. *Listeria monocytogenes* infection as a complication of treatment with tumor necrosis factor-alpha–neutralizing agents. Arthritis Rheum 2003;48:319-324.

75. Salliot C, Gossec L, Dougados M. Rituximab, abatacept, and anakinra do not increase the risk of serious infections: a meta-analysis of published randomized clinical trials. Ann Rheum Dis 2007;66(Suppl II):436.

76. Lutt JR, Pisculli ML, Weinblatt M, et al. Severe nontuberculous mycobacterial infection in 2 patients receiving rituximab for refractory myositis. J Rheumatol 2008;35:1683-1685.

77. Furst DE. The risk of infections with biologic therapies for rheumatoid arthritis. Semin Arthritis Rheum 2008; Dec 29. [Epub ahead of print].

80. Weinblatt M, Schiff M, Goldman A, et al. Selective co-stimulation modulation using abatacept in patients with active rheumatoid arthritis while receiving etanercept: a randomised clinical trial. Ann Rheum Dis 2007;66:228-234.

82. Schiff M, Keiserman M, Codding C, et al. Efficacy and safety of abatacept or infliximab vs placebo in ATTEST: a phase II, multi-centre, randomized, double-blind, placebo-controlled study in patients with rheumatoid arthritis and an inadequate response to methotrexate. Ann Rheum Dis 2008;67:1096-1103.

85. Fleischmann RM, Tesser J, Schiff MH, et al. Safety of extended treatment with anakinra in patients with rheumatoid arthritis. Ann Rheum Dis 2006;65:1006-1012.

REFERENCES

Full references for this chapter can be found on www.expertconsult.com.

Drugs and pregnancy

Bonnie Lee Bermas

65

- Pregnancy induces immunologic changes that may differentially impact rheumatic disorders.
- If possible, patients with inflammatory arthritis and systemic rheumatic diseases should have their disease under good control prior to conception.
- Patients who have preexisting renal disease in the context of either systemic lupus erythematosus or another collagen vascular disease should be in remission for 6 months prior to conception.
- Clinicians should treat symptoms and signs of active disease and not necessarily a diagnosis or a laboratory test.
- Aspirin, nonsteroidal anti-inflammatory drugs, and cyclo-oxygenase-2 inhibitors can be used after the time of implantation up until the last trimester.
- Glucocorticoids may be used during pregnancy for disease flares. There is a slight increased risk of cleft palate formation. Maternal risks include glucose intolerance, hypertension, and osteoporosis.
- Antimalarials, sulfasalazine, azathioprine, and cyclosporine may be used during pregnancy when appropriate.
- Gold, penicillamine, cyclophosphamide, methotrexate, leflunomide, and chlorambucil must be avoided during pregnancy and women should not conceive while on leflunomide or methotrexate.
- Data on anti–tumor necrosis factor (TNF) therapy use during pregnancy are limited. There have been case reports of congenital anomalies. Our current recommendations are to discontinue this medication at the time of conception.
- Clinicians should review the potential toxicities of medications prior to initiating therapy during pregnancy.

Rheumatologic disorders occur commonly in women of childbearing years. Thus some women, who are under treatment for their rheumatologic condition, may desire pregnancy. A pregnancy's impact on the mother's disease activity, coupled with the potential toxicity to both mother and fetus of many antirheumatic medications, make disease management challenging. Data on a particular pharmacologic agent's potential toxicity are often limited or incomplete. We commonly rely on animal studies that use super pharmacologic dosing to assess for drug teratogenicity and toxicity during pregnancy. Alternatively, we refer to case reports that profile a single pregnancy. Neither of these sources may adequately reflect the true risk of a particular therapy during pregnancy. The U.S. Food and Drug Administration (FDA) use-in-pregnancy ratings are likewise based on limited information (Table 65.1). In 1996 the American College of Rheumatology published its own guidelines for the use of antirheumatic drug therapy in pregnancy and lactation.[1] However, since these guidelines were published, there has been more clinical experience with the use of some of these medications during pregnancy. This chapter discusses the treatment of the pregnant patient with a rheumatic disease. The safety of antirheumatic therapies during pregnancy and nursing is reviewed. Medications discussed include aspirin and the non-steroidal anti-inflammatory drugs, the glucocorticoids, the antimalarials, gold salts, penicillamine, the immunosuppressive agents, the antimetabolites, the cytotoxic agents, intravenous immune globulin (IVIG), and the biologics (Table 65.2). Treatment recommendations and approaches to patients are described wherever possible.

PREGNANCY

In order for a pregnancy to be successful, the mother must tolerate the fetus, which is a hemi-allograft. There have been many hypotheses on what allows this tolerance to the fetus to occur, but almost all support the notion that some degree of immunosuppression is necessary. Theories of what happens to the immune system include variations in cytokine levels, alterations in levels of expressed adhesion molecules, and attenuation of natural killer cell activity.[2] These changes in the immune system during pregnancy may modify disease activity of some rheumatologic conditions.

Rheumatic diseases and pregnancy

Rheumatic diseases are affected differently by pregnancy (Table 65.3). Conventional wisdom is that in patients with rheumatoid arthritis (RA), 70% to 80% will go into remission when pregnant.[3] However, more recent evidence suggests that the actual number of patients who improve during pregnancy may be closer to 50%.[4] This improvement appears to be mediated by the degree of Human Leukocyte Antigen (HLA) disparity between the mother and the fetus.[5] Thus the more genetically different the mother and fetus are, the more likely RA will remit. Why this occurs is unclear but may be related to some of the alterations in inflammatory cytokine levels that are observed during pregnancy. For example, tumor necrosis factor (TNF)-α and other cytokines are downregulated during pregnancy.[6] We know that therapy aimed at blocking TNF-α is successful in improving RA. Thus if circulating TNF-α is lowered by pregnancy, this can have a positive impact on disease activity in RA.[7]

In contrast, the data on systemic lupus erythematosus (SLE) are murkier. Some studies suggest that SLE is not impacted by pregnancy, whereas other studies suggest that SLE is exacerbated by pregnancy.[8,9] There is even more limited information regarding other rheumatologic disorders. Therefore the clinician may not be able to predict which patient with a rheumatic condition will flare during pregnancy.

One can adhere to several principles when approaching the patient with rheumatic disease who desires pregnancy (Table 65.4). First, the provider should aim for the patient to be in clinical remission or under good control at the time of conception. Specifically, in patients who have lupus nephritis or another rheumatologic disorder with renal involvement, the kidney disease should be in remission for at least 6 months before conception. I apply this same paradigm to those patients with other rheumatologic disorders with significant organ involvement. One should try to minimize or discontinue medications, or maintain patients on a therapeutic regimen that can be continued during pregnancy. For example, in patients with RA that is under good control, I often discontinue their medications before conception because there is a high likelihood that these patients will go into remission during pregnancy. On the other hand, if the patient has very active RA, it may be advantageous to keep her on some of her medications that are considered compatible with pregnancy until a positive pregnancy test is confirmed. Finally, just because a patient carries a diagnosis of a rheumatic disease does not necessarily mean that she needs to be treated during pregnancy unless she has active clinical issues. The clinician should treat active disease symptoms and signs and not a clinical diagnosis. Thus there is no role for empiric immunosuppression in pregnant patients with a stable systemic rheumatologic disorder.

ASPIRIN, NON-STEROIDAL ANTI-INFLAMMATORY DRUGS, AND COX-2 INHIBITORS

Aspirin, the non-steroidal anti-inflammatory drugs (NSAIDs), and the cyclooxygenase-2 (COX-2) inhibitors are the cornerstones of treatment

TABLE 65.1 FOOD AND DRUG ADMINISTRATION USE-IN-PREGNANCY RATINGS

A	Controlled studies show no risk. Adequate, well-controlled studies in pregnant women have failed to demonstrate risk to the fetus.
B	No evidence of risk in humans. Either animal findings show risk but human findings do not, or, if no adequate human studies have been performed, animal findings are negative.
C	Risk cannot be ruled out. Human studies are lacking and results of animal studies are either positive for fetal risk or lacking as well. However, potential benefits may justify the potential risk.
D	Positive evidence of risk. Investigational or postmarketing data show risk to the fetus. Nevertheless, potential benefits may outweigh the potential risk.
X	Contraindicated in pregnancy. Studies in animals or humans, or investigational or postmarketing reports, have shown fetal risk that clearly outweighs any possible benefit to the patient.

for the pain and joint inflammation in arthritic conditions. In animals, high doses of aspirin are found to be teratogenic.[10] However, in humans, a series of 5128 pregnancies in which fetuses were exposed to high-dose aspirin did not show an increased rate of fetal malformation.[11] Furthermore, low-dose aspirin is currently the standard of care for the treatment of pregnant women with the antiphospholipid antibody syndrome and obstetric complications.[12] The American Academy of Pediatrics concludes that aspirin is compatible with breastfeeding.[13]

In animals, high doses of some non-steroidals are teratogenic.[14] In humans, non-steroidals do not cause fetal malformations but can cause premature closure of the ductus arteriosus when used during the third trimester.[15] One can use these medications during the first two trimesters but they need to be discontinued at the beginning of the third trimester. The American Academy of Pediatrics considers most non-steroidals to be compatible with breastfeeding.[13]

Data on the use of the newer COX-2 inhibitors during pregnancy are limited. Thus far, there are no reports of fetal malformations after exposure *in utero*. In animal studies COX-2 inhibitors can interfere with implantation.[16] Because non-steroidals have both COX-1 and COX-2 inhibitory effects, patients should discontinue both non-steroidals and COX-2 inhibitors at the beginning of a menstrual cycle in which they plan to conceive. No data are available on the safety of the COX-2 inhibitors in breastfeeding mothers.

Aspirin, NSAIDs, and COX-2 inhibitors can be used during the pregnancy. The NSAIDs and COX-2 inhibitors should be discontinued during the third trimester and during a conception cycle.

GLUCOCORTICOIDS

Glucocorticoids are used to treat many disorders. There is now substantial clinical experience using these medications during pregnancy. Prednisone and prednisolone are not readily metabolized by the placenta and reach the fetus at eightfold lower concentrations than seen maternally. In contrast, betamethasone and dexamethasone, the fluorinated glucocorticoids, reach the fetus at higher concentrations and can be used for treating fetal conditions such as lung immaturity.[17] In animals, glucocorticoids have been shown to increase aggressive behavior in the mother and increase the incidence of cleft palate formation in the fetus.[18,19] In humans, there have been case reports of cleft palate occurring in infants exposed to glucocorticoids during pregnancy.[20] However, a large series of pregnant asthma patients who were treated with glucocorticoids (mean dose 8 mg a day) failed to show an increased incidence of fetal abnormalities in offspring of these women.[21]

In contrast, a meta-analysis of the use of glucocorticoids during pregnancy found a 3.4-fold increase in risk of cleft palate formation in offspring who are exposed to glucocorticoids during pregnancy. Nonetheless, in the authors' prospective analysis of 184 pregnancies in which there was an exposure to glucocorticoids, no fetal anomalies were noted.[22]

In addition to the risks outlined earlier, glucocorticoids can cause premature rupture of the membranes and small-for-gestational-age babies. Mothers are at increased risk for the development of gestational diabetes, hypertension, and osteoporosis.

Glucocorticoids can be used in pregnant patients who have failed NSAIDs or who require immunosuppression. Patients should be informed that there is a slight increased risk of cleft palate formation in children exposed to glucocorticoids *in utero* during the first trimester. Clinicians should use the lowest possible dose of glucocorticoids that will control clinical symptoms. In patients who have been treated with glucocorticoids during pregnancy and who have a prolonged labor or require a cesarean section, stress doses of steroids (50-100 mg hydrocortisone sodium succinate, intravenously every 8 hours) should be administered during labor and delivery.

Five percent of the glucocorticoid dose is secreted in breast milk. This is not a problem for patients who are taking less than 20 mg a day. In patients who are taking greater than 20 mg a day, the recommendation is to pump and discard breast milk in the 4 hours following the steroid dose.[23]

ANTIMALARIALS

In rheumatology practices, the 4-aminoquinoloine antimalarial agents, hydroxychloroquine and chloroquine, are used for the treatment of mild inflammatory arthritis, SLE, and connective tissue disorders. In animals, use of these medications during pregnancy can cause chorioretinotoxicity.[24] The FDA considers these medications to be a category C for use during pregnancy. This rating is predominantly based on a single case report in which a mother took 250 mg of chloroquine phosphate two times a day during four pregnancies. Three of the pregnancies resulted in congenital defects (pigment deposition in the retina, cochleovestibular paresis, and mental retardation) and one pregnancy ended in a spontaneous abortion.[25] In lower doses, the antimalarials have been safely used in pregnancy for malarial prophylaxis.[26] In higher doses, these medications have been given to pregnant patients with SLE with no increased reports of fetal malformations. Khamashta and colleagues[27] reported on 33 women who safely took antimalarials during pregnancy and Parke and Rothfield[28] reported on 16 lupus patients who took antimalarials during pregnancy with no adverse effects. A survey of North American rheumatologists revealed that 69% of these physicians maintain patients on this medication during pregnancy.[29] In a recent study, ophthalmic examinations were performed in 21 children whose mothers were taking either hydroxychloroquine or chloroquine during pregnancy (average dose 317 mg and 332 mg, respectively, each day). There were no ophthalmic abnormalities detected.[30] Furthermore, there is some evidence that keeping patients with SLE on hydroxychloroquine during pregnancy may improve outcome. Current evidence and practice suggest that antimalarials are compatible with pregnancy and may be used. One approach is to discontinue antimalarials in patients with an inflammatory arthritis such as RA because these patients are likely to go into remission during pregnancy. Nonetheless, the half-life of these medications is so long that this does not guarantee that exposure is eliminated. In patients whose lupus or connective tissue disease is well controlled with antimalarials, one should consider continuing these medications during pregnancy.

The American College of Rheumatology believes that this medication is incompatible with breastfeeding despite the American Academy of Pediatrics' opposing view that this medication can be used in nursing mothers.[1,13] The higher doses used in treating rheumatologic disorders support the American College of Rheumatology's recommendations that this medication should not be used in nursing mothers.

GOLD

Although gold salts were among the first effective treatments of RA and inflammatory arthritic conditions, their use has been curtailed by the advent of other disease-modifying agents. In animals, the gold salts cross the placenta and can cause congenital abnormalities including hydrocephaly and hydronephrosis.[31] In humans the data are limited on pregnancies in which gold therapy was continued. There is one case report of congenital anomalies occurring in an infant in which the mother was treated with gold salts.[32] Gold therapy should be stopped during pregnancy, although the long half-life of this medication means that there are usually significant body stores of this medication at the time of pregnancy. This medication is considered to be compatible with breastfeeding.

TABLE 65.2 TOXICITIES OF ANTIRHEUMATIC THERAPIES IN ANIMALS AND HUMANS

Drug	Animals		Humans		
	Embryotoxic	Fetal	Maternal	Fetal	Breastfeeding
Aspirin and NSAIDs	No	In high doses—teratogenic	No	Premature closure of the ductus arteriosus	Compatible
Glucocorticoids	No	Cleft palate Aggressive behavior	PROM Hypertension Glucose intolerance Osteoporosis Osteonecrosis	SGA Adrenal hypoplasia Promotes lung maturity Cleft palate* Stillbirth*	Crosses into breast milk at low concentration, well tolerated
Antimalarials	No	Chorioretinotoxicity	No	Case reports of pigment deposition in the retina, cochleovestibular paresis, dorsal column disease, and mental retardation	Crosses into breast milk, contraindicated
Gold	No		No		Compatible
Penicillamine			No	Cutis laxa, connective tissue abnormalities	Contraindicated
Sulfasalazine	†	Teratogenic in rats	No	Cleft palate VSD Coarctation of the aorta Macrocephaly Oligospermia	Crosses the placenta, contraindicated
Azathioprine	Yes	Skeletal abnormalities Cleft palate Decreased thymic development and hematopoiesis	†	Diminished fertility in offspring*	Contraindicated†
6-Mercaptopurine	Yes	Cleft palate	†	SGA Prematurity Intrauterine growth retardation Cleft palate	†
Cyclosporine A	Yes	Renal tubular cell damage	Renal insufficiency	Spontaneous abortions	Contraindicated
Mycophenolate mofetil	†	†	†	Case reports: Shortened digits and hypoplastic nails Auditory canal atresia Cleft lip and palate Micrognathia Hypertelorism Ocular coloboma	†
Methotrexate	Yes	Skeletal abnormalities Cleft palate	†	Embryotoxic Skeletal abnormalities Facial abnormalities	Contraindicated†
Cyclophosphamide	Yes	SGA Skeletal abnormalities Cleft palate Exophthalmos Decreased fertility	Decreased fertility in males and females	SGA Limb abnormalities Coronary artery agenesis Tumors in offspring*	Contraindicated
Leflunomide				Multiple congenital anomalies	Contraindicated
Chlorambucil	Yes	SGA Skeletal abnormalities Renal agenesis	†	SGA Skeletal abnormalities Renal agenesis	Contraindicated*
Intravenous immunoglobulin	†	†	†	SGA Autoantibodies	†
Etanercept Adalimumab Infliximab	†	†	†	VACTERL anomalies?	‡
Rituximab	†	†	†	†	†
Abatacept	†	†	†	†	†

*Theoretical risk or case reports only.
†No information available.
‡Conflicting information.
PROM, premature rupture of the membranes; SGA, small-for-gestational age offspring; VSD, ventricular septal defect.

TABLE 65.3 RHEUMATIC DISEASES DURING PREGNANCY

Disease	Activity during pregnancy
Rheumatoid arthritis	Remits in 70%-80% of cases
Systemic lupus erythematosus	Stable or worsens. Active renal disease is particularly problematic
Psoriatic arthritis	Generally improves
Scleroderma	Limited data
Dermatomyositis	Limited data

TABLE 65.4 TREATMENT PRINCIPLES OF PATIENTS WITH RHEUMATIC DISEASES DURING PREGNANCY

1. Disease should be in remission or under good control at the time of conception.
2. Minimize medications or discontinue medications as appropriate.
3. Treat the disease symptoms, not the diagnosis (e.g., patient with systemic lupus erythematosus does not empirically need steroids during pregnancy unless the disease is active).

PENCILLAMINE

Penicillamine is occasionally used in the treatment of progressive systemic sclerosis. It is less commonly used in the treatment of inflammatory arthritic conditions such as RA. In mice, penicillamine can interfere with collagen biosynthesis and cause malformations.[33] In humans, cases of cutis laxa and connective tissue disorders have been reported following exposure to this medication in utero.[34] Given its potential for fetal toxicity and the many alternative therapies, penicillamine should not be administered during pregnancy.

The American Academy of Pediatrics advises against giving this medication to lactating women.

SULFASALAZINE

Sulfasalazine was initially developed in the 1930s to treat RA. However, until the past decade, its biggest application has been in the treatment of inflammatory bowel disease. Thus most of the data regarding the use of this medication in pregnancy is found in the inflammatory bowel disease literature. Sulfasalazine crosses the placenta with its metabolite sulfapyridine. The latter can displace bilirubin from albumin, but this is not thought to be clinically relevant.[35] Although there have been case reports of fetal malformations in humans, large case series have failed to show an increased risk of teratogenicity.[36,37] Sulfasalazine inhibits the absorption of folic acid. Some clinicians recommend additional folic acid in pregnant women on this medication.[38] This medication may be used during pregnancy and is a good option for women who have active inflammatory arthritis.

Sulfasalazine interferes with both spermatogenesis and sperm motility. Therefore we recommend discontinuing this medication for 3 months before attempting conception.[39,40] There has been one report of bloody diarrhea in a breastfed infant whose mother was ingesting sulfasalazine. Therefore the American Academy of Pediatrics warns against using this medication in nursing mothers.[13,41]

IMMUNOSUPPRESSIVE AGENTS

Immunosuppressive agents are used in the treatment of rheumatic diseases, transplant recipients, and other disorders. Fortunately we have a plethora of information on the use of these medications during pregnancy because of the well-published transplant registries. Azathioprine, cyclosporine, and mycophenolate mofetil are the major immunosuppressive agents used in the treatment of rheumatic diseases. This section will also discuss 6-mercaptopurine because it is the major metabolite of azathioprine.

Azathioprine and 6-mercaptopurine

The purine analogs, azathioprine and its major metabolite 6-mercaptopurine have been used for treatment of SLE, RA, and spondylitic variants.

In rats treated with azathioprine during pregnancy, reduced fetal and placental size was observed. In rats that were injected with high doses of medication (20 mg/kg/day), trophoblastic damage was observed.[42] In humans, azathioprine is metabolized in vivo to 6-mercaptopurine. The metabolites of 6-mercaptopurine are thiouric acid, an inactive metabolite, and inorganic sulfate. In one study, radioactive-labeled azathioprine was given to three pregnant women. Only thiouric acid, the inactive metabolite, was found in fetal blood in significant concentration. Minute levels of 6-mercaptopurine were found.[43] The authors concluded that azathioprine was not effectively metabolized to 6-mercaptopurine by the fetus and hence may explain the low teratogenicity of this medication.

There have been case reports of a child born with pancytopenia and combined immunodeficiency, as well as chromosomal abnormalities and craniofacial malformations after exposure to azathioprine in utero.[44,45] Larger case series have failed to substantiate an increased risk of congenital anomalies in offspring of women who are treated with azathioprine during pregnancy. In one series where 14 inflammatory bowel disease patients were treated with azathioprine during 16 pregnancies, the only adverse outcome was a case of hepatitis B virus infection in one woman.[46] In seven lupus patients who were taking azathioprine during pregnancy, no adverse outcomes were seen in the offspring.[47] In 142 transplant recipients who were given azathioprine during pregnancy, there were some anomalies seen including metatarsus adductus, kidney malformation, ventricular septal defect, patent ductus arteriosus, and a hearing deficit. But this was thought not to be above the background rate of congenital anomalies.[48] In all of these studies, patients were receiving other medications such as glucocorticoids and cyclosporine, so attributing risk to any particular medication is difficult. In all studies small-for-gestational-age infants and premature rupture of the membranes, as well as intrauterine growth retardation, have been reported. Although the FDA considers this medication a class D, the literature suggests that azathioprine may be used in pregnant patients who require immunosuppression.

Six-mercaptopurine is teratogenic in animals inducing cleft palate formation, microcephaly, and dilatation of the cerebral ventricles.[49,50] In humans, there are few case series available for review. In one review of 79 pregnancies in which the offspring was exposed to 6-mercaptopurine, there was one case of anomalies that included cleft palate, microphthalmia, hypoplasia of the thyroid and ovaries, corneal opacity, and cytomegaly.[39] One series of 15 infants of inflammatory bowel disease patients who were exposed to this medication while in utero showed no malformations (D.H. Present, personal communication). Despite this reassuring report, the data do not support the use of this medication during pregnancy.

The washout period for this medication in male patients is a significant issue. In one series of 13 male patients who had taken this medication in the 3 months preceding conception, there were two spontaneous abortions and two offspring born with skeletal congenital anomalies.[51] Therefore this medication should be discontinued in men for 3 months before conception.

Both azathioprine and 6-mercaptopurine can cause immunosuppression in the newborn and should not be used in nursing mothers.

Cyclosporine

In rodents cyclosporine crosses the placenta in very low concentrations.[52] Pregnant rodents administered high doses (25 mg/kg/day) of cyclosporine have increased fetal mortality and renal abnormalities, although other studies have not shown any impact on organogenesis.[53,54] In humans, there are differing opinions on whether or not cyclosporine A crosses the placenta in significant concentrations.[55,56] Regardless, there seems to be no increased risk of teratogenicity over background rates. In one study of 154 pregnancies in renal transplant patients in which the mothers were taking cyclosporine A, 22% of the children had complications including respiratory distress syndrome, kidney malformation, ventricular septal defect, and patent ductus arteriosus. This rate was not higher than those patients who were not taking cyclosporine.[48] However, the babies were smaller and more often premature, and the mothers had an increased incidence of maternal diabetes and hypertension. Other transplant series and registries have confirmed these findings.[57] In the U.S. National Transplantation Pregnancy Registry, 500 pregnancies have been reported. There is no increased risk of congenital anomalies, although the live birth rate is lower in those patients who have received cyclosporine. However, the sicker patients tend to be on cyclosporine, which may explain this observation.[58] Finally, a recent meta-analysis concluded that cyclosporine does not appear to be a major teratogen, although it may be associated with increased rates of prematurity.[59] There is some concern that *in utero* exposure to cyclosporine may impair T, B, and natural killer-cell development. Whether this will have long-term impact and whether immunization schedules in these infants should be modified are unclear.[60] The literature suggests that cyclosporine may be used for immunosuppression during pregnancy. Cyclosporine A is not compatible with nursing because of the risk of immunosuppression in the offspring.

Mycophenolate mofetil (CellCept)

Mycophenolate mofetil is a purine synthesis inhibitor that has been used to prevent organ rejection. More recently, it has been used in the treatment of lupus nephritis.[61] In animals, this agent may cause premature meiotic maturation.[62] In humans, there is one case report of this medication being used during pregnancy in a renal transplant patient. The baby was born prematurely and was noted to have hypoplastic nails and short fifth fingers. No other abnormalities were noted.[63] This medication is considered a category C by the FDA. Due to the paucity of available information, this medication should be avoided during pregnancy and nursing.

Methotrexate

Methotrexate is a folate antagonist that has been used widely over the past 2 decades for the treatment of RA and other inflammatory conditions. Current practice suggests that this medication should be the building block for the treatment of RA.[64] In pregnant rodents, this agent causes skeletal abnormalities in the offspring and increased fetal resorption rate.[65,66] In humans this medication is profoundly abortigenic and is now commonly used for the non-surgical treatment of ectopic pregnancies.[67] It can also cause severe teratogenicity including craniofacial abnormalities and mental retardation.[68] Most of the toxicity appears to occur during the sixth through eighth week of gestation and at doses greater than 10 mg a week. There have been a few case reports of offspring in whom there was no teratogenicity when exposed to this medication before 6 weeks of gestation and at doses less than 10 mg a week.[69,70] However, the FDA considers this medication a category X. Furthermore, in a recent review of this topic, Lloyd and colleagues suggest that there is no safe window and that there is a 10/42 chance of abnormality in a fetus exposed to methotrexate during the first trimester. They suggest that the washout period before conception in both men and women should be 6 months.[71] Donnenfeld and associates suggest that the medication should be discontinued 12 weeks before conception because of the high spontaneous abortion rate.[72] Patients who are on this medication should use a reliable form of birth control. The American College of Rheumatology recommends that men discontinue this medication 3 months before attempting conception. They suggest that women wait at least one ovulatory cycle after stopping methotrexate before trying to get pregnant. This medication is not compatible with breastfeeding.

Cyclophosphamide

Cyclophosphamide is a cytotoxic agent that is the backbone of many cancer chemotherapy regimens. In lupus patients, this medication has greatly reduced the morbidity and mortality of renal disease.[73] It is also used for the treatment of vasculitis and organ involvement in a variety of rheumatic diseases. In pregnant mice, cyclophosphamide causes chromosomal rearrangements and impairs blastocyst development in embryos.[74] This medication can also cause glomerular sclerosis in the kidneys of mice exposed to cyclophosphamide *in utero*.[75] In

humans, cyclophosphamide exposure during pregnancy can lead to problems with digit development and limb formation, iris development, and coronary artery abnormalities.[76,77] There have been case reports of individuals being treated for Wegener granulomatosis from the 17th week of gestation on and being treated for Hodgkin lymphoma in the third trimester with no adverse effects in the offspring.[78,79] Cyclophosphamide should be avoided during pregnancy except in life-threatening situations when no alternative treatment is available. Patients who need to be treated with this medication during the first trimester and early second trimester of pregnancy should be counseled about the high risk of congenital anomalies in the fetus. Cyclophosphamide is transferred to breast milk and should not be used in nursing mothers.

Prolonged use of cyclophosphamide can also induce infertility in women. Risk factors for cyclophosphamide-induced infertility include age greater than 30, more than 15 pulses of therapy, and a cumulative dose of greater than 10 g.[80] Concomitant use of leuprolide acetate (Lupron) or oral contraceptives may offset this effect.[81]

CHLORAMBUCIL

Chlorambucil is an alkylating agent that is occasionally used in the treatment of rheumatic disorders. In rats, this medication can cause skeletal and renal malformations in offspring exposed to this medication *in utero*.[82,83] In humans, there have likewise been reports of renal agenesis in an infant exposed to chlorambucil during the first trimester.[84] Given the many alternative medications available, this medication should be avoided during pregnancy and nursing.

INTRAVENOUS IMMUNE GLOBULIN

IVIG is used for the treatment of dermatomyositis and other rheumatic conditions. Data on the use of this medication during pregnancy are limited. In one case report of an individual with steroid-resistant idiopathic thrombocytopenic purpura, this medication was used with no adverse effects on the offspring.[85] This medication has also been used to manage the obstetric complications of the antiphospholipid antibody syndrome without inducing congenital malformations.[86]

TUMOR NECROSIS FACTOR-α BLOCKADE AND INHIBITORS

Biologics that are directed against the tumor necrosis factor-α receptor or inhibit this cytokine are successful in treating RA.[7] These medications are rated category B for use during pregnancy. Recently, there have been two reports to the FDA of potential congenital anomalies consistent with the VACTERL syndrome.[87] Because the true number of exposed pregnancies is unknown, the significance of this finding has been questioned.[88] Nonetheless, we are recommending that patients discontinue these medications during pregnancy (at least at the time of a confirmed pregnancy test) until further information is available.

LEFLUNOMIDE

Leflunomide is used to treat inflammatory arthritis, Behçet disease, and other disorders. This medication is extremely teratogenic (risk category is X) and is absolutely contraindicated in pregnancy. Because of its extremely long half-life, drug elimination with cholestyramine is recommended for women who desire pregnancy. The manufacturer recommends that cholestyramine, 8 g three times a day be given for 11 days. Subsequently, drug levels should be obtained. Without cholestyramine, it can take up to 2 years to eliminate this drug.

RITUXIMAB AND OTHER EXPERIMENTAL THERAPY

Data on the safety of rituximab, abatacept, and other depleting therapy during pregnancy are limited. Current recommendations would be to avoid these medications during pregnancy. How long after therapy with rituximab conception can be attempted is also unknown and the timing is left to the discretion of the practitioner.

TABLE 65.5 TREATMENT RECOMMENDATIONS*	
Symptoms/conditions	**Treatment options**
Mild arthralgias, arthritis, pleuritis, skin rashes	NSAIDs (first two trimesters only) Low-dose glucocorticoids (5-10 mg prednisone a day)
Inflammatory arthritis	Consider sulfasalazine in addition to above
Systemic lupus erythematosus or connective tissue disease	Consider antimalarials
Moderate disease	Glucocorticoids (higher doses), azathioprine, cyclosporine
Severe disease	Pulse steroids, IVIG, azathioprine, cyclosporine
Life threatening	Cyclophosphamide—only in life-threatening circumstances

Methotrexate, 6-mercaptopurine, penicillamine, and chlorambucil should be avoided.

CONCLUSION

Treating the pregnant patient with an underlying rheumatologic disorder is a clinical challenge. The toxicities of the medications must be weighed against the patient's need for disease control. Often there is no ideal therapy for a given situation. One approach (Table 65.5) is to treat mild symptoms with non-steroidals or low doses of glucocorticoids. In the third trimester, non-steroidals should be stopped. If inflammatory arthritis is the major complaint, sulfasalazine can be used. In patients with SLE and mixed connective tissue disease who are well controlled with antimalarials, the patients can remain on these medications during pregnancy. For moderate disease, higher doses of glucocorticoids, azathioprine, and cyclosporine can be used. For severe diseases, pulse steroid therapy, IVIG, azathioprine, and cyclosporine can be used. Cytotoxic agents should be avoided in all but life-threatening situations. At this point, the data suggest that biologics ought to be discontinued during pregnancy. In all cases, the treating clinician and the patient should discuss the potential hazard to either the mother and/or the fetus of any therapy.

KEY REFERENCES

1. American College of Rheumatology Ad Hoc Committee on Clinical Guidelines. Guidelines for monitoring drug therapy in rheumatoid arthritis. Arthritis Rheum 1996;5:723-731.
2. Branch DW. Physiologic adaptations of pregnancy. Am J Reprod Immunol 1992;28:120-122.
3. Smith WD, West HF. Pregnancy in rheumatoid arthritis. Acta Rheumatol Scand 1960;6:189-201.
4. De Man YA, Dolhain RJEM, Van de Giejn FE, et al. Disease activity of rheumatoid arthritis during pregnancy: results from a nationwide prospective study. Arthritis Rheum 2008;59:1241-1248.
5. Nelson JL, Hughes KA, Smith AG, et al. Fetal-maternal disparity in HLA class II alloantigens and the pregnancy induced remission of rheumatoid arthritis. N Engl J Med 1993;329:466-471.
6. Raghupathy R. TH-1-type immunity is incompatible with successful pregnancy. Immunol Today 1997;18:478-482.
7. Moreland LW, Baumgartner SW, Schiff MH, et al. Treatment of rheumatoid arthritis with a recombinant human tumor necrosis factor receptor (p75)-Fc fusion protein. N Engl J Med 1997;337:141-147.
8. Meng C, Lockshin M: Pregnancy in lupus. Curr Opin Rheumatol 1999;11:348-351.
9. Petri M, Howard D, Repke J, et al. The Hopkins Lupus Pregnancy Center: 1987-1991 update. Am J Reprod Immunol 1992;28:188-191.
10. Warkary J, Takacs E: Experimental production of congenital malformations in rats by salicylate poisoning. Am J Pathol 1959;35:315-319.
11. Slone D, Heinonen OP, Kaufman DW, et al. Aspirin and congenital malformations. Lancet 1976;1:1373-1375.
12. Cowchuck FS, Reece EA, Balaban D, et al. Repeated fetal losses associated with antiphospholipid antibodies: a collaborative randomized trial comparing prednisone with low-dose heparin treatment. Am J Obstet Gynecol 1992;166:1318-1323.
13. American Academy of Pediatrics Committee on Drugs: Transfer of drugs and other chemicals into human milk. Pediatrics 1989;84:924-936.
14. Klein KL, Scott WJ, Clark KE, et al. Placental transfer, cytotoxicity, and teratology in the rat. Am J Obstet Gynecol 1981;141:448-452.
15. Schoenfeld A, Bar Y, Merlob P, et al. NSAIDs: Maternal and fetal considerations. Am J Reprod Immunol 1992;28:141-147.
16. Lim H, Paria BC, Das SK, et al. Multiple female reproductive failures in cyclooxygenase 2-deficient mice. Cell 1997;91:197-208.
17. Blanford AT, Murphy BE. In vitro metabolism of prednisolone, dexamethasone, betamethasone, and cortisol by the human placenta. Am J Obstet Gynecol 1977;127:264-267.

18. Reinisch JM, Simon NG, Grandelman R. Prenatal exposure to prednisone permanently alters fighting behavior of female mice. Pharmacol Biochem Behav 1980;12:213-216.
19. Pinsky L, DiGeorge AM. Cleft palate in the mouse: a teratogenic index of glucocorticoid potency. Science 1965;147:402-403.
20. Harris JWS, Ross IP. Cortisone therapy in early pregnancy: relation to cleft palate. Lancet 1956;1:1045-1047.
21. Schatz M, Patterson R, Zeitz S, et al. Corticosteroid therapy for the pregnant asthmatic patient. JAMA 1975;233:804-807.
22. Park-Wyllie L, Mazzotta P, Pastuszak A, et al. Birth defects after maternal exposure to corticosteroids: prospective cohort study and meta-analysis of epidemiological studies. Teratology 2000;62:385-392.
23. Ost L, Wettrell G, Bjorkhem I, et al. Prednisolone excretion in human milk. J Pediatr 1985;106:1008-1011.
24. Ullberg S, Lindquist NG, Sjostrand SE. Accumulation of chorioretinotoxic drugs in the foetal eye. Nature 1970;2227:1257-1258.
25. Hart C, Naunton R. The ototoxicity of chloroquine phosphate. Arch Otolaryngol 1964;80:407-412.
26. Steketee R, Wirima J, Slutsker L, et al. Malaria treatment and prevention in pregnancy: indications for use and adverse events associated with use of chloroquine or mefloquine. Am J Trop Med Hyg 1996;55:50-56.
27. Khamashta M, Buchanan M, Hughes G. The use of hydroxychloroquine in lupus pregnancy: the British experience. Lupus 1996;5(suppl 1):S65-S66.
28. Parke A, Rothfield N. Antimalarial drugs in pregnancy: the North American experience. Lupus 1996;5(suppl 1):S67-S69.
29. Al-Herz A, Shulzer M, Esdaile JM. Survey of antimalarial use in lupus pregnancy and lactation. J Rheumatol 2002;29:700-706.
30. Klinger G, Morad Y, Westall CA, et al. Ocular toxicity and antenatal exposure to chloroquine or hydroxychloroquine for rheumatic diseases. Lancet 2001;358:813-814.
31. Szabo KT, Di Febbo ME, Phelan DG. The effects of gold-containing compounds on pregnant rabbits and their fetuses. Vet Path 1978;15(suppl 5):97.
32. Fuchs U, Lippert T. Gold therapy and pregnancy. Dtsch Med Wochenschr 1986;111:31-34.
33. Uitto J. Effect of D-penicillamine on collagen biosynthesis in culture. Biochem Biophys Acta 1969;144:498-503.
34. Scheinberg I, Sternlieb I. Pregnancy in penicillamine-treated patients with Wilson's disease. N Engl J Med 1975;65:273-285.

35. Jarnerot G, Into-Malmberg MB, Esbjorner E. Placental transfer of sulfasalazine and sulfapyridine and some of its metabolites. Scand J Gastroenterol 1981;16:693-697.
36. Korelitz BI. Pregnancy, fertility and inflammatory bowel disease. Am J Gastroenterol 1981;16:693-697.
37. Mogadam M, Dobbins WOI, Korelitz BI, et al. Pregnancy in inflammatory bowel disease: effect of sulfasalazine and corticosteroids on fetal outcome. Gastroenterology 1981;80:72-76.
38. Levy N, Roisman I, Teodor I. Ulcerative colitis in pregnancy in Israel. Dis Colon Rectum 1981;24:351-354.
39. Donaldson RM. Current concepts: management of medical problems in pregnancy—inflammatory bowel disease. N Engl J Med 1985;312:1616-1619.
40. Chatzinoff M, Guarino JM, Corson SK, et al. Sulfasalazine induced abnormal sperm penetration assay reversed on changing to 5-aminosalicylic acid enemas. Dig Dis Sci 1988;33:108-110.
41. Briggs GG, Freeman RK, Yaffe SJ. Drugs in pregnancy and lactation. Baltimore: Williams & Wilkins, 1998.
42. Gross A, Fein A, Serr DM, et al. The effect of Imuran on implantation and early embryonic development in rats. Obstet Gynecol 1977;50:713-718.
43. Saarikoski S, Seppala M. Immunosuppression during pregnancy: transmission of azathioprine and its metabolites from the mother to the fetus. Am J Obstet Gynecol 1973;115:1100-1106.
44. DeWitte DB, Buick MK, Cyran SE, et al. Neonatal pancytopenia and severe combined immunodeficiency associated with antenatal administration of azathioprine and prednisone. J Pediatr 1984;105:625-628.
45. Oster H, Tamberg J, Perinchief P. Two chromosome aberrations in the child of a woman with systemic lupus erythematosus treated with azathioprine and prednisone. Am J Med Genet 1984;17:627-632.
46. Alstead EM, Ritchie JK, Lennard-Jones JE, et al. Safety of azathioprine in pregnancy in inflammatory bowel disease. Gastroenterology 1990;99:443-446.
47. Meehan RT, Dorsey JK. Pregnancy among patients with systemic lupus erythematosus receiving immunosuppressive therapy. J Rheumatol 1987;14:252-258.
48. Armenti VT, Ahlswede KM, Ahlswede BA, et al. National transplantation pregnancy registry—outcomes of 154 pregnancies in cyclosporine-treated female kidney transplant recipients. Transplantation 1994;57:502-506.
49. Burdett DN, Waterfield JD, Shah RM. Vertical development of the secondary palate in hamster embryos following exposure to 6-mercaptopurine. Teratology 1988;37:591-597.
50. Arakawa T, Fujii M, Hayashai T. Dilatation of cerebral ventricles of rat offspring induced by 6-mercaptopurine administration to dams. J Exp Med 1967;91:143-148.

REFERENCES

Full references for this chapter can be found on www.expertconsult.com.

Aspiration and injection of joints and periarticular tissues and intralesional therapy

66

Juan J. Canoso and Esperanza Naredo

- Synovial aspiration is a basic diagnostic tool in rheumatology.
- Major diagnostic errors can be made by simply assuming the nature of an effusion.
- Corticosteroid injections and infiltrations and viscosupplementation are basic treatment tools in rheumatology, orthopedics, physiatry, and general medicine. These procedures carry minimal risk to the patient when properly performed.
- Synoviorthesis, or medical synovectomy, may be achieved by the intra-articular injection of sclerosing agents or radioactive materials.
- Some of these procedures are within the realm of general medicine, whereas others involving joints and soft tissue sites difficult to approach, viscosupplementation, and synoviorthesis require specialized knowledge.
- Rheumatologists trained in musculoskeletal ultrasonography are able to perform, at low cost and minimal risk to the patients, procedures that in the past required expensive and even risky techniques.

INDICATIONS FOR ASPIRATING OR INJECTING MUSCULOSKELETAL TISSUES

Aspirating fluid for diagnostic or therapeutic purposes

In patients in whom sepsis, crystal synovitis, or bleeding is the suspected cause of a joint, bursal, or tendon sheath lesion, aspiration and analysis of the fluid are essential for diagnosis.[1,2] In addition, knowledge of the nature of the synovial fluid, particularly the inflammatory cell content and the presence or absence of crystals, even when an effusion is not clinically detectable,[3] will complement findings from the history and physical examination and help provide the basic framework for diagnosis and treatment. In patients with tense joint effusions, aspiration of synovial fluid provides prompt relief of pain and permits the patient to move or bear weight on the affected joint. Finally, in hemarthrosis or septic arthritis, the blood and pus within a synovial cavity may be damaging to the joint cartilage and synovial membrane, so evacuation of the fluid is necessary to avoid permanent joint damage. Large articular effusions should be drained as fully as possible to decrease pressure, improve synovial circulation, and prevent muscle atrophy. Synovial fluid analysis is discussed in Chapter 30.

Practical procedure and aftercare

Procedure

Aspiration or injection of joints or soft tissues is an outpatient procedure that does not require specialized equipment (Table 66.1) unless performed under ultrasound (US) guidance. The procedure must be explained fully to the patient. Universal precautions must be followed during the procedure including the use of gloves.

(a) Blind aspiration or injection. The patient should be in a supine position in lower extremity procedures and in the sitting position in a chair with armrests in upper extremity procedures. Anatomic landmarks need to be identified by palpation and the needle site marked in some way, such as with a thumbnail imprint in the skin. The skin must then be carefully cleaned with antiseptic agents. For local anesthesia, the skin and subcutaneous tissues can be infiltrated down to the level of the periarticular lesion or joint capsule using 1% or 2% lidocaine without epinephrine (adrenaline) and a small-bore needle. However, experienced physicians may use topical ethyl chloride or no anesthetic at all. With the proper technique, the needle passes freely through the extra-articular tissues and a "pop" may be felt as the needle enters the joint. The ease with which fluid can be withdrawn depends on the needle size used, viscosity of the fluid, and presence of any fibrin clots or "rice bodies" in the joint fluid. Free flow of fluid is often suddenly interrupted because of clogging of the needle end by the synovial membrane or debris. Rotating the needle, withdrawing it slightly, or even reinjecting a little of the fluid will often help unclog the needle. If corticosteroids or other substances are to be injected, this should be done through the same needle.

(b) US-guided aspiration or injection.[4-6]
Two methods of musculoskeletal needle placement guided by US are used.

- Skin marking or indirect method (Fig. 66.1a and b). With this method, US is used to select the potentially most successful puncture site over the target but not to guide the progression of the needle. After scanning the pathologic area, the target is imaged in two perpendicular planes. The midpoint of the transducer corresponds to the midpoint of the US image on the screen. When the target is imaged in the center of the screen in both longitudinal and transverse plane, the edges of the probe are drawn on the skin with a skin-marking indelible pen. The depth of the target is measured perpendicularly to the skin. Then, the probe is removed and a mark is drawn on the skin in the center of the previously drawn rectangle. After sterilization of the skin, the needle is inserted in the central skin mark and directed perpendicularly toward the known depth of the target.
- Needle guidance under direct ultrasonographic control (Fig. 66.2a and 66.2b). Continuous monitoring of the needle progression under direct US visualization, although requiring more experience and hand-eye coordination, provides a more accurate control of the progression of the needle from the skin to the target during the procedure. The authors prefer this method.

At the end of any procedure, the needle should be swiftly withdrawn, and light pressure should be put on the needle site in the skin. The application of a simple adhesive plaster (tape) for a few hours is all that is usually required thereafter.

Aftercare

In most cases, it is sensible for patients to rest the affected joint for 24 to 48 hours after a therapeutic injection, to minimize leakage of the therapeutic agent and improve the anti-inflammatory response.

 Whenever you see this icon, please go to **www.expertconsult.com** to view the corresponding chapter figure.

TABLE 66.1 EQUIPMENT REQUIRED FOR JOINT AND SOFT TISSUE INJECTIONS

Procedure	Details
Skin preparation	Antiseptic solution (povidone-iodine), alcohol swabs, 4 × 4 gauze pads
Local anesthetic	1% or 2% lidocaine without epinephrine
Needles	23-27 gauge for local anesthetic, 18 gauge for large to moderate-sized joints (knees, shoulders, ankles, etc.), 23-27 gauge for small joints (wrists, metacarpophalangeal joints, etc.)
Syringes	3 mL or 5 mL for anesthetic-steroid injection and 10-50 mL for joint aspiration (sterile steroid-prefilled syringes are preferable where available)
Miscellaneous	Gloves; forceps for removing needles from syringe; specimen tubes/plates for cultures and fluid studies

All the required supplies should be assembled in advance. Importantly, the needle must be long enough to reach the intended place and have a caliber adequate to the nature of the fluid. Although standard needle lengths work well in thin patients, longer needles and even a spinal needle may be required in obese patients. On the other hand, a 1-mL syringe with a half-inch no. 27 needle is particularly useful to infiltrate superficial structures such as the interphalangeal, metacarpophalangeal, and metatarsophalangeal joints; digital flexor tendon sheaths; the carpal tunnel; de Quervain tenovaginosis; and the elbow joint through the lateral approach. Purulent effusions require no. 18 or no. 16 needles. A failure to fully drain a septic joint indicates large debris or loculation and calls for tidal lavage, arthroscopy, or arthrotomy.

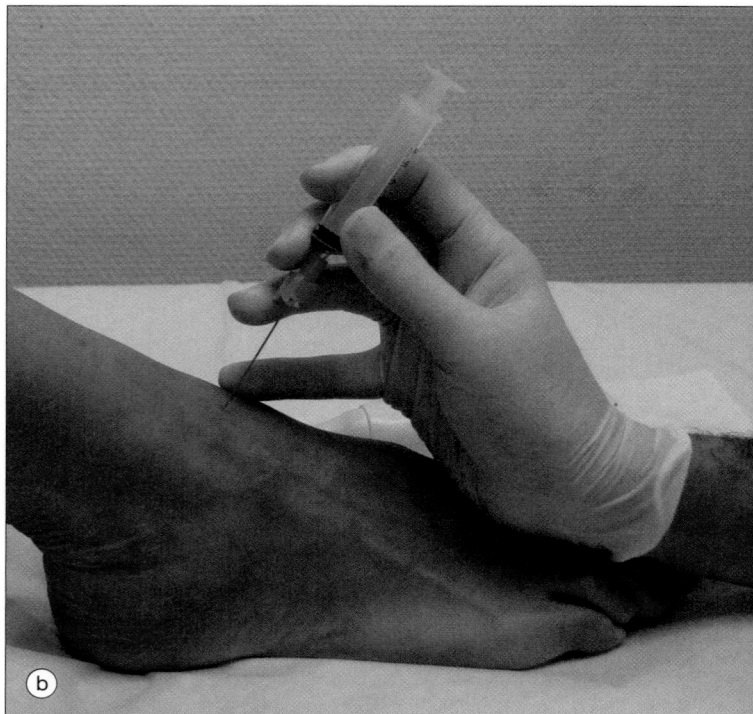

Fig. 66.1b The needle is inserted perpendicular to the skin.

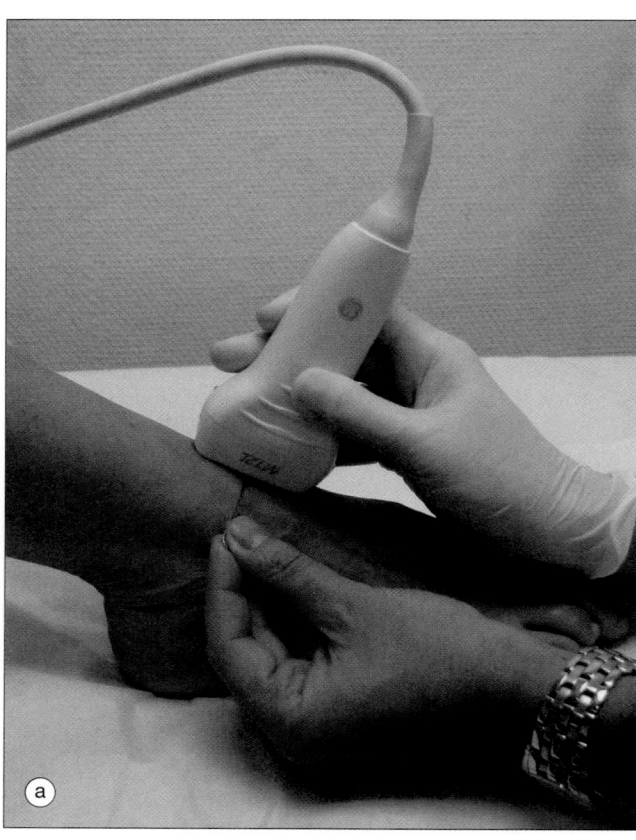

Fig. 66.1a Ultrasound-guided indirect method of injection of the right tibiotalar joint. An extended paperclip is displaced between the probe and the skin until its tip is imaged at the center of the target. The puncture point is marked in the patient's skin with the clip.

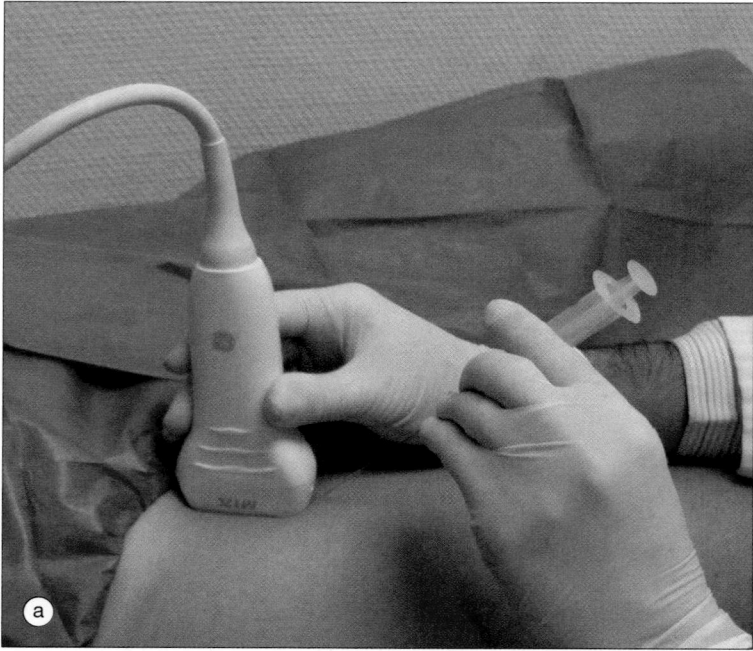

Fig. 66.2a Ultrasound-guided direct method of injection of the right hip joint. The needle is inserted adjacent to the transducer and directed to the anterior recess of the hip.

CONTRAINDICATIONS AND COMPLICATIONS

Contraindications

There are few absolute contraindications to joint or soft tissue aspirations and injections; if infection is suspected, fluid should always be aspirated from a joint. In other indications, the procedures should probably be avoided if there is infection of the overlying skin or subcutaneous tissues or if bacteremia is suspected. The presence of a significant bleeding disorder or diathesis or a severe thrombocytopenia may also preclude joint aspiration. However, if it is deemed necessary for diagnosis or therapy, the procedure may be carried out after appropriate cover for the bleeding disorder. Warfarin anticoagulation with international normalization ratio values in the therapeutic range is not a contraindication to joint or soft tissue aspiration or injection.[7] Aspiration of a joint with a prosthesis in it is often best left to surgeons using full aseptic techniques.

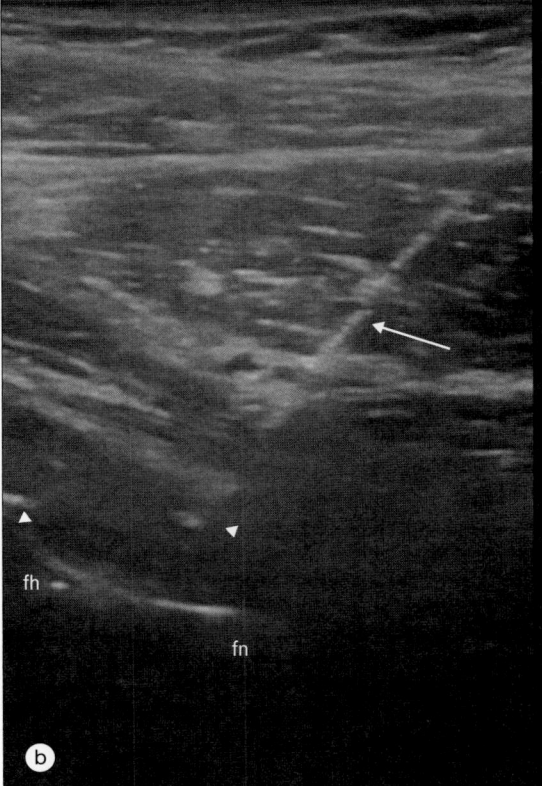

Fig. 66.2b In the ultrasound image, the needle tip (arrowhead) is seen hyperechogenic inside the hip effusion. The needle (arrow) appears hyperechoic into the iliopsoas muscle. fn, femoral neck; fh, femoral head.

CORTICOSTEROID INJECTIONS

Corticosteroid injections are frequently used to achieve local anti-inflammatory activity. The indications for their use include the presence of persistent inflammation at a single site. Synovial joints and other cavities should generally be injected with a long-acting crystalline form of corticosteroid such as triamcinolone hexacetonide or methylprednisolone acetate. These crystals persist longer in the fluid than mixtures of depot and soluble betamethasone,[8] allowing continued local release into the targeted area. Only a relatively small proportion escapes into the general circulation, but, during the first 24 hours after injection, patients may experience flushing or other evidence of a corticosteroid "pulse." For periarticular injections, particularly subcutaneous bursae and de Quervain tenovaginosis, methylprednisolone acetate should be used because the less soluble (and therefore more potent) triamcinolone hexacetonide is likely to induce skin atrophy.

Local anesthetic is sometimes mixed with corticosteroids for such injections. In the case of some periarticular lesions (e.g., rotator cuff lesions around the shoulder), this can have the advantage of confirming the correct placement of the injection because the local anesthetic should result in almost immediate relief of the pain if the injection is correctly placed.

Corticosteroid doses vary with the structure injected. For each of the following procedures, a dose range based on the use of methylprednisolone acetate 40 mg/mL is shown. If the more potent triamcinolone hexacetonide 20 mg/mL is used, the lower figure of the range should be chosen. Intracavitary position of the needle can be ascertained by withdrawing some articular fluid or checking to see if the cavity distends as fluid is injected. In the soft tissues, correct positioning may be ascertained by elimination of pain by a preceding lidocaine infiltration. However, if available and in procedures in which needle misplacement is common, ultrasound guidance gives best results.[9] Rest of the injected site for 48 hours following the procedure is generally recommended.

Complications of corticosteroid injections and infiltrations

- Local bleeding. In patients without a bleeding diathesis, pressing the puncture site with a sterile gauze for about a minute, or a longer time in those taking prophylactic aspirin, stops the bleeding. In procedures in the upper extremity, arm elevation prevents venous bleeding.
- Facial flushing. Occurs in perhaps 40% of cases. Transient and inconsequential, it may nevertheless worry unwarned patients.
- Postinjection flare. Corticosteroid crystal–induced synovitis occurs in about 5% of intra-articular injections. Pain appears several hours following the procedure and may last from a few hours to 1 day. Persisting pain and mounting swelling may indicate infection; these joints should be re-aspirated for Gram stain and aerobic and anaerobic cultures.
- Skin atrophy. This is a frequent complication, particularly in elderly individuals, of superficial infiltrations and olecranon bursa injections. The condition is characterized by cigarette-paper-like skin, recurrent ecchymosis, and chronic pressure pain.
- Fat atrophy. This complication may occur when repeated fatty tissue infiltrations are given such as in Morton neuroma and proximal plantar enthesopathy (fasciitis).
- Skin hypopigmentation. Superficial corticosteroid infiltrations such as in de Quervain tenosynovitis often cause a hypopigmented patch, which may be quite disfiguring in people with dark skin.
- Infection. The rate of a septic arthritis following corticosteroid injection is on the order of 4.6 to 4.8 cases per 100,000 procedures when the corticosteroid is aspirated from a vial and around 0.6 cases per 100,000 procedures when prefilled syringes are used.[10] Patients who have severe immunodeficiency problems, as well as those with implants, may be at greater risk. Postinjection septic bursitis may occur from exacerbation of a missed infection or may be caused by contamination of a sterile bursa through the needle track.
- Tendon rupture. A ruptured tendon following a corticosteroid injection may indicate abuse of the procedure, intratendinous injection, or coincidental rupture caused by the very condition that led to the injection. Conditions that lead to spontaneous tendon rupture include dorsal wrist tenosynovitis and posterior tibialis tenosynovitis in rheumatoid arthritis (RA), degenerative changes in the supraspinatus or long biceps tendon, chronic corticosteroid use, overuse Achilles tendinopathy, fluoroquinolone-induced Achilles tendinopathy, uremia, hyperparathyroidism, and systemic lupus erythematosus.
- Corticosteroid arthropathy. Abuse of intra-articular injections may result in a Charcot-like arthropathy similar to the one described in calcium pyrophosphate crystal deposition disease (see Chapter 186).
- Nerve damage. Knowledge of regional anatomy should largely avoid this complication. However, because anatomic variations are frequent, the needle insertion should always be cautious.
- Osteonecrosis. This is a reported complication of abused articular or soft tissue corticosteroid infiltrations.
- Systemic complications. Corticosteroid injections cause pituitary inhibition that recovers in 1 to 2 weeks[11] and in diabetics, transient hyperglycemia that lasts 2 to 3 days; anaphylactic shock, albeit exceedingly rare, may also occur.[12]

WRIST AND HAND

Finger and metacarpophalangeal joints

Indications. Active Bouchard nodes, RA,[13] psoriatic arthritis. US guidance is not required.

Corticosteroid dose. 10 to 15 mg methylprednisone acetate (no. 25 or no. 27 needle).

Approach. Dorsolateral with the digit in semiflexion (Fig. 66.3, online Figs. 66.4 and 66.5). **Note:** In this and other clinical pictures the skin had been sterilized with alcohol, and the needle seen in place was for local anesthesia before injecting the steroid. Multiple joints may be injected in the same session.

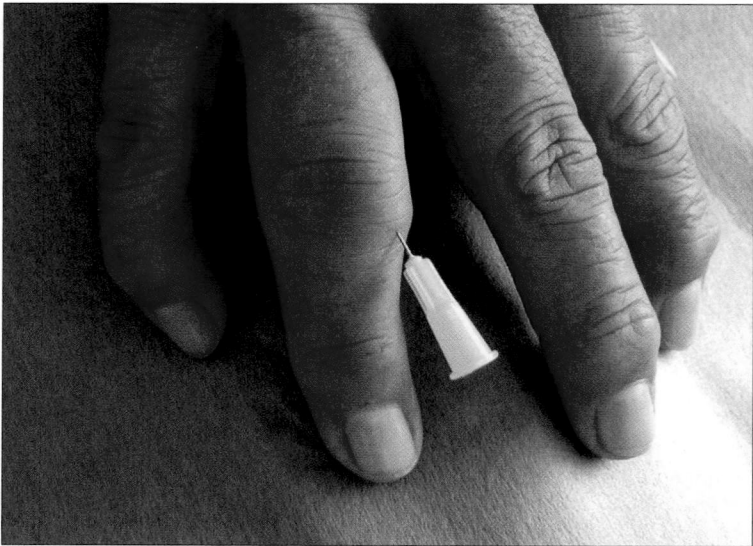

Fig. 66.3 Injection of right fourth proximal interphalangeal joint in osteoarthritis.

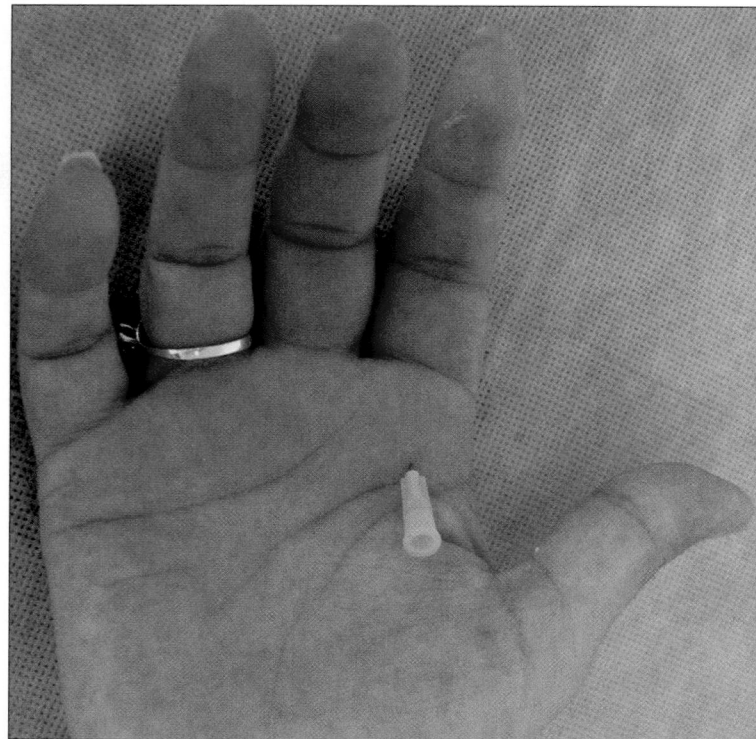

Fig. 66.9 Injection of trigger finger, right index finger.

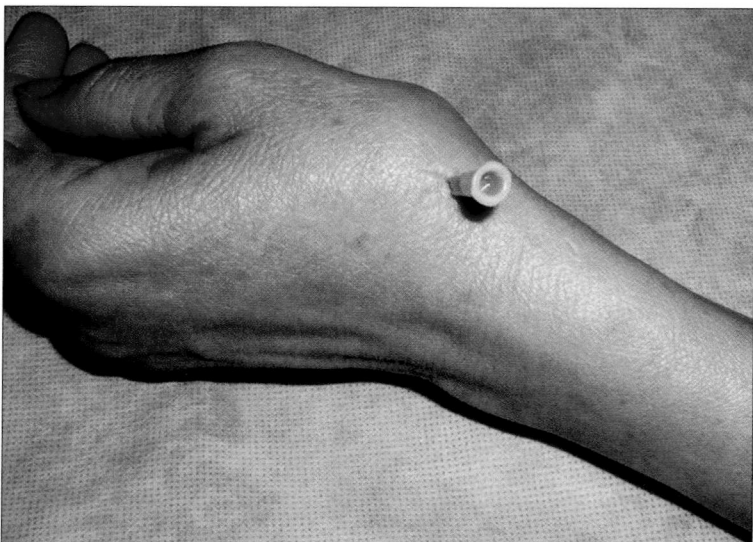

Fig. 66.6 Injection of the left trapeziometacarpal joint in osteoarthritis.

Precautions. Do not overdistend joint(s). Fluid tends to back up; keep firm pressure with a sterile gauze for at least 2 minutes following the procedure.

Complications. Joint hyperlaxity, capsular calcification (frequent but inconsequential).

First carpometacarpal joint

Indications. Painful osteoarthritis (OA). The efficacy of steroid injection has been disputed.[14] Viscosupplementation may be useful as an alternative to surgery.[15] US guidance is not required.

Corticosteroid dose. 15 to 30 mg methylprednisone acetate (no. 25 or no. 27 needle).

Approach. A common entry site is at the anatomic snuffbox while flexing the thumb across the palm, which optimally exposes the joint just proximal to the protruding base of the first metacarpal (Fig. 66.6).

Precautions. Avoid the radial artery as it traverses the anatomic snuffbox.

Complications. None.

Wrist

Indications. For diagnosis in acute arthritis. Most cases of acute wrist arthritis are due to calcium pyrophosphate dihydrate pseudogout, gout, and septic arthritis. For injection in RA, other sterile synovitides, and OA such as is associated with chondrocalcinosis and hemochromatosis. US guidance is preferred.

Corticosteroid dose. 30 to 40 mg methylprednisone acetate (no. 25 or no. 27 needle). Aspiration should be attempted before injection. For aspiration alone, use a no. 20 or no. 18 needle.

Approach in blind injections. The radiocarpal joint is approached dorsally just distal to Lister tubercle (a bony prominence in the dorsal distal radius) or at the midcarpal joint 1 cm ulnar and 5 mm distal to Lister tubercle (online Figs. 66.7 and 66.8). The wrist should be slightly palmar flexed to assist the procedure.

Precautions. There are no neurovascular structures of concern at this site.

Complications. None.

Trigger finger and trigger thumb

Indications. Only 30% of trigger fingers resolve spontaneously and injections are highly efficacious.[16] A lesser success rate of injections is seen in diabetics. US guidance is not required.

Approach. Just distal to proximal palmar crease (index) (Fig. 66.9), between the proximal and distal creases in the long finger (online Fig. 66.10) and just distal to the distal crease in the ring and little fingers (online Fig. 66.11) with needle held at a 45-degree distal inclination; just proximal to digital crease and aiming to sesamoids of thumb (Fig. 66.12).

Corticosteroid dose. 15 to 20 mg methylprednisone acetate mixed with 1 to 2 mL lidocaine (no. 25 or no. 27 needle).

Precautions. Avoid intratendinous injection. Intrasheath injection is not a requirement for success.[17] Up to three injections given 3 weeks apart are allowed.

Complications. Focal palmar fat atrophy. Large published series comment on a lack of tendon rupture and iatrogenic infection.

Digital flexor tenosynovitis

Indications. RA, psoriatic arthritis, etc. In flexor tenosynovitis, injection must be intrasheath and therefore US guidance is preferred (Fig. 66.14, online Fig. 66.13).

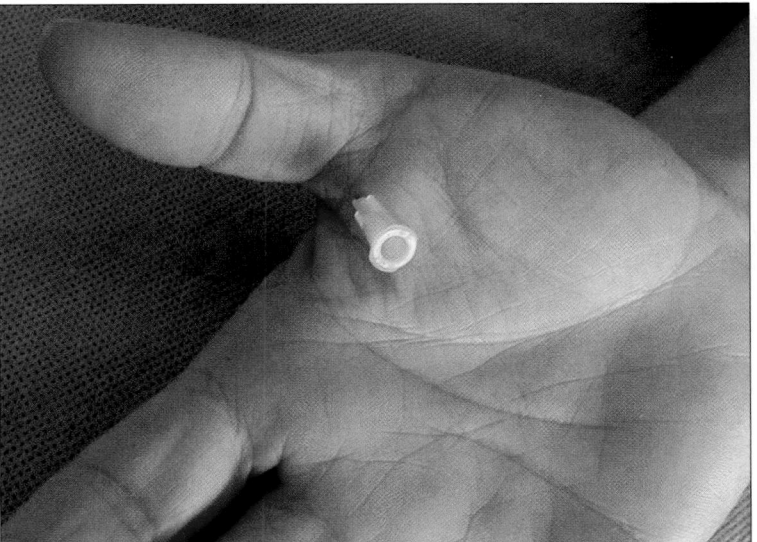

Fig. 66.12 Injection of right trigger thumb.

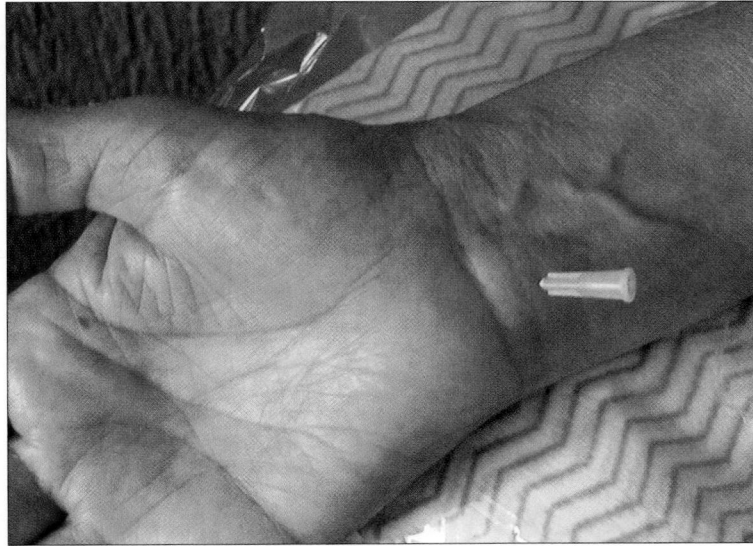

Fig. 66.15 Injection of right carpal tunnel syndrome.

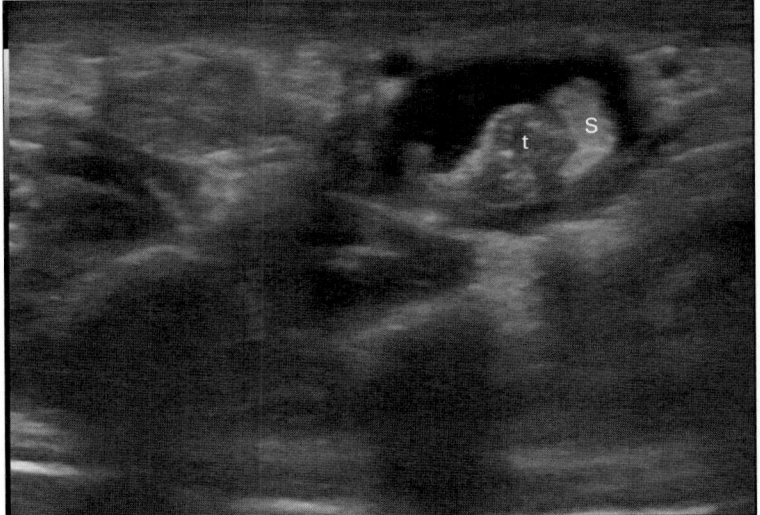

Fig. 66.14 Same patient as in online Fig. 66.13. After the injection the steroid suspension (S) is seen hyperechogenic within the tendon sheath and adjacent to the flexor tendon (t).

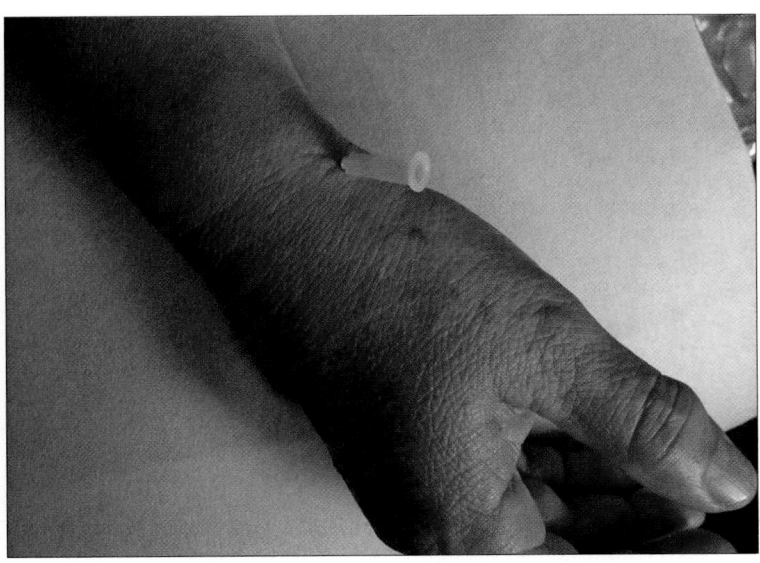

Fig. 66.17 Injection of right de Quervain tenovaginosis.

Corticosteroid dose. 15 to 20 mg methylprednisone acetate mixed with 1 to 2 mL lidocaine (no. 25 or no. 27 needle).

Approach. If US is unavailable, inject as in trigger finger.

Precautions. Avoid intratendinous injection.

Complications. As in trigger finger; tendon rupture occasionally occurs.

Carpal tunnel syndrome[18]

Indications. Injection treatment is indicated in all etiologies of carpal tunnel syndrome except acute cases (hypoesthesia, severe pain, and tense bulging) due to synovitis, fracture, hemorrhage, infection, and carpal tunnel syndrome of late pregnancy. US guidance is optional in routine cases but is a must in unilateral cases to rule a mass lesion.[19]

Corticosteroid dose. 30 to 40 mg methylprednisolone acetate, straight or mixed with 2 to 3 mL lidocaine (no. 25 or no. 27 needle).

Approach. About 10 mm proximal to the distal wrist crease and just medial to palmaris longus tendon (Fig. 66.15, online Fig. 66.16). If palmaris longus is absent (14% of people), replace by midline. The needle is inserted to a depth of 0.8 to 1 cm with a 45-degree distal inclination and a 45-degree lateral inclination. The steroid is placed in the proximal extension of the ulnar bursa.

Precautions. Paresthesias indicate median nerve engagement; reposition needle. Reciprocal needle motion on gentle finger motion indicates tendon engagement; reposition needle. A wrist splint in neutral is a useful adjunct to the injection.

Complications. Pain, which may last 1 to 3 days; transient increase of paresthesias. The patient should be instructed to use an ice pack intermittently, 5 minutes on and 5 off, at the first hint of pain.

De Quervain tenovaginosis[20-22]

Indications. Steroid injection is the treatment of choice in this condition. US guidance is optional.

Corticosteroid dose. 15 to 20 mg methylprednisolone acetate (no. 25 or no. 27 needle).

Approach. The needle is aimed toward the radial styloid, which underlies the sheath (Fig. 66-17). The needle is then pulled back by the millimeter and injection is attempted. Successful injections distend the sheaths of both abductor pollicis longus and extensor pollicis brevis. Separate injections may be required. Do not overdistend. Up to three injections given 3 weeks apart are allowed.

Precautions. The corticosteroid must remain within the sheath. Do not infiltrate grossly thickened sheaths because mycobacterial infection may be present.

Complications. Skin hypopigmentation and skin atrophy.

Wrist extensor tenosynovitis

Indications. Sustained tenosynovitis in RA and psoriatic arthritis. Failure of one injection is an indication for tenosynovectomy.

Corticosteroid dose. 15 to 20 mg methylprednisolone acetate.

Approach. A direct US-guided injection is preferred (online Figs. 66.18 and 66.19).

Complications. The extensor digital tendons are prone to spontaneous rupture in RA. An intratendinous injection probably enhances this tendency. Whether to inject an extensor tendon sheath or proceed to tenosynovectomy should be discussed with a hand surgeon.

ELBOW REGION

Elbow

Indications. Aspiration in acute arthritis, injection in RA, and psoriatic arthritis.

Corticosteroid dose. 30 to 40 mg methylprednisone acetate (no. 22, no. 25, or no. 27 needle). Aspiration should be attempted before injection. For aspiration alone, use a no. 20 or no. 18 needle, depending on the suspected diagnosis. US guidance is optional.

Approach for blind injections. There are two commonly used entries; for both entries the elbow is held flexed at 90 degrees.

- Inferolateral approach. The midpoint cleft between the olecranon tip and the lateral epicondyle is palpated. The needle is then inserted perpendicularly, aiming at the center of the joint.
- Lateral approach. The radiocapitellar joint may be entered from the side just proximal to the radial head. The needle is passed perpendicular to the skin between the two bones (Fig. 66.20).

Precautions. There are no neurovascular structures in the vicinity.

Complications. None.

Olecranon bursa

Indications. For diagnosis of effusion and for treatment of refractory aseptic bursitis (traumatic or idiopathic).[23] A negative bursal fluid culture is required prior to the steroid injection. US guidance is not necessary.

Corticosteroid dose. 20 mg methylprednisolone acetate (no. 20 or no. 22 needle). Empty the bursa before injection.

Approach. Lateral through normal skin, aiming at the center of the bursa (online Fig. 66.21).

Precautions. Taps at the tip of the bursa may create a chronic leak. Medial entries may damage the ulnar nerve.

Complications. The injection of 20 mg of methylprednisolone acetate has not caused complications.[23]

Lateral epicondylar syndrome or tennis elbow[24]

Indications. Failure of conservative treatment. To shorten symptomatic period (with the caveat that long-term outcome may be worse in injected than uninjected patients). US guidance is not necessary.

Corticosteroid dose. 10 to 20 mg methylprednisone acetate (no. 25 or no. 27 needle).

Approach. At the most tender point (Fig. 66.22). Pass the needle to periosteal contact and infiltrate with 1 mL lidocaine. Failure to eradicate pain on resisted wrist dorsiflexion indicates the wrong injection site; reposition needle and reinfiltrate with lidocaine. The corticosteroid should be infiltrated deeply at the enthesis and radially within the proximal tendon.

Precautions. Avoid injecting too superficially.

Complications. Transient increase in pain in 20% to 40% of patients. Repeated corticosteroid infiltrations may result in chronic pain.

Medial epicondylar syndrome or golfer's elbow[25]

Indications. Medial epicondylar syndrome that has not resolved with conservative measures. Also used to shorten the symptomatic period. US guidance is not necessary.

Corticosteroid dose. As in lateral epicondylar syndrome.

Approach. Aim needle to distal portion of medial epicondyle where the wrist flexor muscles insert. Avoid injecting the posterior surface of the epicondyle to stay away from the ulnar nerve (online Fig. 66.23).

Complications. None.

SHOULDER REGION

Shoulder (glenohumeral joint)

Indications. Aspiration in acute arthritis; injection in RA, spondyloarthritis, the initial stages of frozen shoulder,[26] viscosupplementation in OA. US guidance is necessary in the latter indication.

Corticosteroid dose. 40 to 80 mg methylprednisone acetate (no. 22 needle). Aspiration should be attempted before injection. In the frozen shoulder, injection into the joint may be difficult on account of the capsular restriction. For aspiration alone, use a no. 20 or larger needle.

Approach for blind injections. Two entries are described: the posterior approach, which is preferred by the authors, and the anterior approach.

- Posterior approach (Fig. 66.24, online Figs. 66.25 and 66.26). The patient should be sitting. The posterior margin of the acromion is palpated. The needle is then inserted posteroanteriorly 1 cm

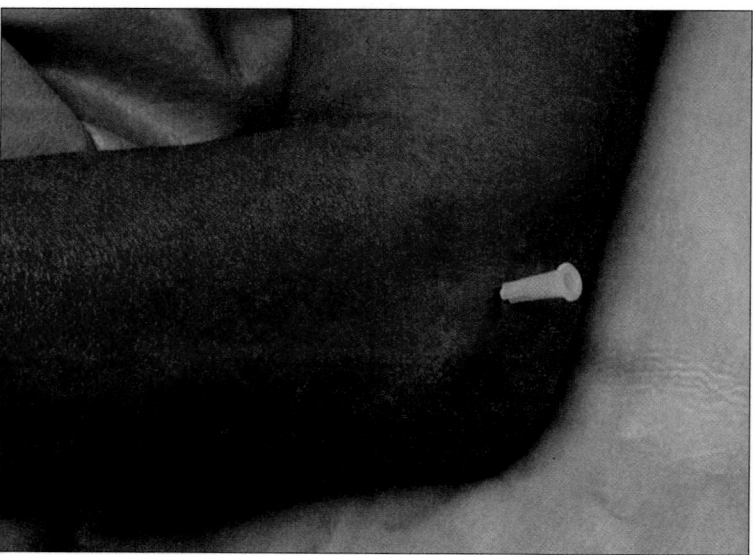

Fig. 66.20 Lateral (radiocapitellar) injection of the left elbow in rheumatoid arthritis.

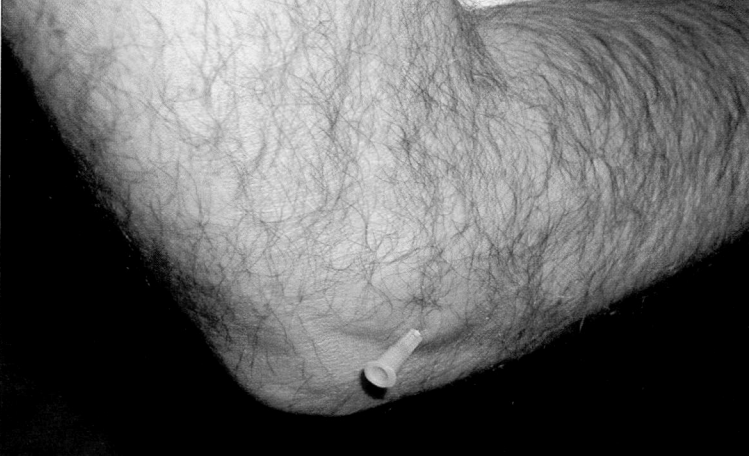

Fig. 66.22 Injection in right tennis elbow (lateral epicondylar syndrome).

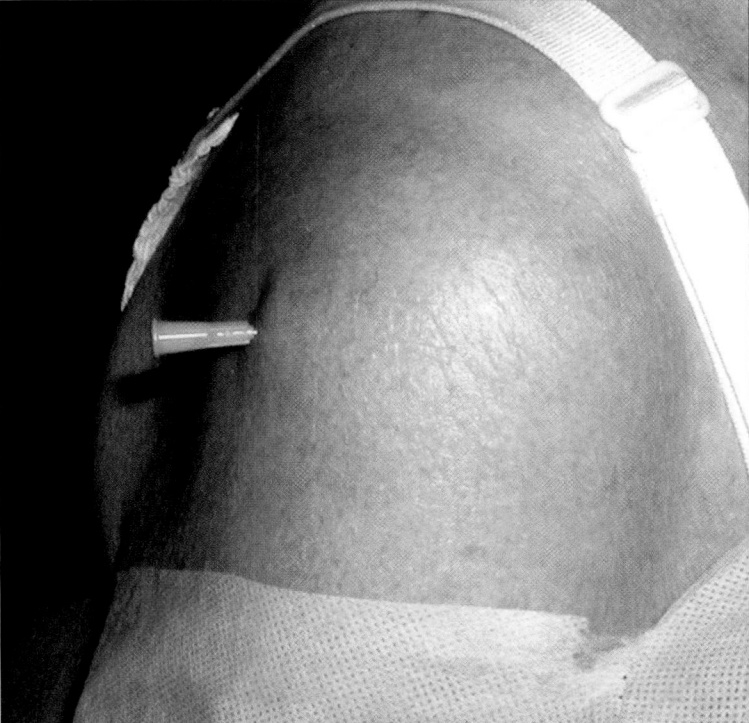

Fig. 66.24 Posterior approach to the right shoulder in frozen shoulder.

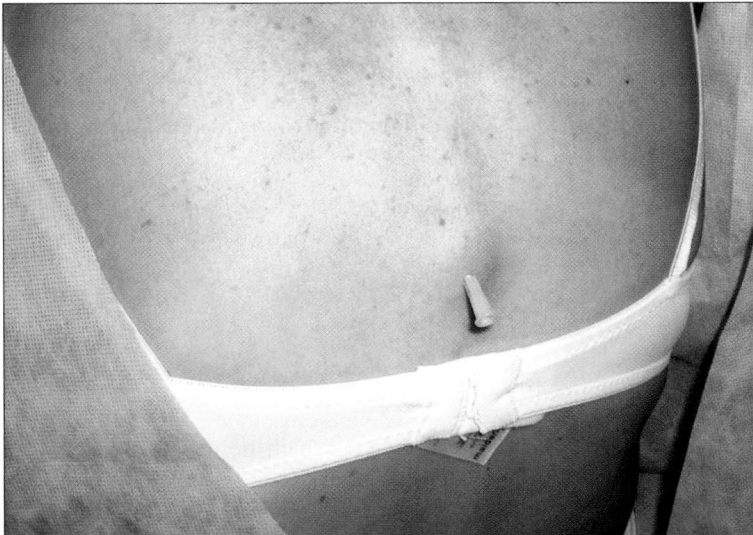

Fig. 66.31 Injection in interspinous ligament enthesitis.

below and 1 cm medial to posterior corner of the acromion, aiming toward the coracoid process until bone is touched at the articular space.

- Anterior approach. Again, the patient should be sitting with the arm hanging at the side of the body, elbow flexed 90 degrees, and forearm in the sagittal plane. The needle is entered anteroposteriorly 1 cm distal and 1 cm lateral to the coracoid process. Once the bone is touched, the forearm is very gently and passively brought into internal rotation as the needle is pushed into the articular space.

Precautions. Use a chair with armrests; watch for fainting.

Complications. Vasovagal syndrome. Misplaced anterior injections may encounter neurovascular structures.

Acromioclavicular joint

Indications. Aspiration in acute arthritis, injection in OA, RA, and spondyloarthritis. US guidance is not required.

Corticosteroid dose. 10 to 20 mg methylprednisone acetate (no. 25 or no. 27 needle). Aspiration should be attempted before injection. For aspiration alone use a no. 20 needle.

Approach. Aim the needle perpendicular to the skin into the articular cleft; aspirate or inject to distend joint (online Fig. 66.27).

Precautions. The procedure is difficult because the acromioclavicular joint is narrow and has a partial meniscus.

Complications. None.

Subacromial bursa[9,27]

Indications. Injection may be indicated in rotator cuff tendinopathy and some cases of calcific tendinitis. US guidance is highly desirable (online Figs. 66.28 and 66.29).

Corticosteroid dose. 30 to 40 mg methylprednisone acetate (no. 22 or no. 25 needle).

Approach for blind injection. The needle is inserted laterally near the posterior angle of the acromion and aimed anteromedially, ensuring that it passes under the anterior half of the acromion. Easy flow and bulging outlining the bursa indicate bursal injection.

Precautions. None.

Complications. None.

Note: Only about 50% of blind subacromial bursa injections fall on target.

Bicipital tendinosis

Indications. This is a tenuous indication because most cases of bicipital tendinosis are caused by subacromial impingement. US guidance is highly desirable.

Corticosteroid dose. 15 to 20 mg methylprednisone acetate (no. 22, no. 25, or no. 27 needle).

Approach. The bicipital tendon should be palpated and a mark made on the skin. The needle is then directed somewhat superiorly, tangentially to the tendon (online Fig. 66.30).

Precautions. Inject under low pressure.

Complications. The relatively common postinjection rupture may reflect the underlying impingement as much as a direct effect of the corticosteroid on the tendon.

SPINE

Interspinous ligaments

Indications. Spondyloarthritis with supraspinous and interspinous ligament enthesis. US guidance is not necessary.

Corticosteroid dose. 15 to 20 mg methylprednisone acetate (no. 25 or no. 27 needle).

Approach. Posteroanterior at the midline between the vertebral spinous processes (Fig. 66.31); infiltrate ligament and its attachments. Several levels may have to be treated.

Precautions. This is an intraligamentous infiltration and a fair amount of pressure is required to make the steroid flow. There is no need to infiltrate deeper than 1.5 cm.

Complications. None.

HIP REGION

Hip[28]

Indications. Diagnosis of septic arthritis including the differential diagnosis of septic arthritis versus aseptic loosening in a prosthetic hip; viscosupplementation. US guidance is required.

Corticosteroid dose. Although the procedure is generally performed for diagnosis, there are proponents of steroid injection or preferably viscosupplementation in advanced hip osteoarthritis. 40 to 60 mg methylprednisone acetate mixed with 3 mL of 1% lidocaine (no. 22 needle). Aspiration should be attempted before injection.

Approach. US guidance is required (see Fig. 66.2a and b).

Precautions. The danger of injuring the femoral neurovascular bundle is averted by using US.

Complications. None.

Iliopsoas bursa

Indications. Painful iliopsoas bursitis[29] and bursal distention causing neurovascular compression.

Corticosteroid dose. 30 to 40 mg methylprednisone acetate mixed with 3 mL of 1% lidocaine (no. 22 needle). Aspiration should be attempted before injection.

Approach. US guidance, as in hip.

Precautions. As in hip.

Complications. None.

Trochanteric syndrome

Indications. Lateral hip pain with trochanteric tenderness.[30] US guidance is not required.

Corticosteroid dose. 40 mg methylprednisolone acetate mixed with 5 mL of 1% lidocaine (no. 22 1.5-inch needle; a longer needle may be required in obese patients).

Approach. With the patient lying on his or her opposite side, the greater trochanter is identified by distal to proximal palpation along the femur. The point of maximal tenderness is usually located at the posterior corner of the trochanter. The needle is inserted vertically to periosteal contact. The mixture of corticosteroid and lidocaine should then be infiltrated radially to cover the base of a cone 3 cm in diameter, half on bone and half in the proximal soft tissues (online Fig. 66.32).

Precautions. The needle should be of sufficient length to reach bone.

Complications. None.

KNEE REGION

Knee

Indications. For diagnosis in any joint effusion. For corticosteroid injection in RA, spondyloarthritis, OA, occasionally in crystal-induced synovitis. For viscosupplementation, US guidance is not required.

Corticosteroid dose. 40 to 80 mg methylprednisone acetate (no. 22 needle). The authors' impression is that the larger dose is far more effective. Aspiration should be attempted before injection. For aspiration alone use a no. 20 or no. 18 needle depending on the clinical suspicion.

Approach. Lateral, aiming needle to the patellar undersurface mid-distance between the upper and lower poles of the patella (Fig. 66.33). A lateral approach, theoretically better because a thick medial intra-articular fat pad may result in a "dry tap" in some patients,[31] may indeed be associated with frequent injection misplacements.[32] This has not been the experience of the authors.

Precautions. Beware of superimposed septic arthritis in RA patients. Postpone the injection of an acutely inflamed joint until a negative synovial fluid culture result becomes available.

Complications. None.

Baker cyst

In very large cysts direct aspiration through a large-bore needle followed by instillation of a corticosteroid is appropriate. Although the content of some cysts is liquid, in others debris is abundant and may intermittently occlude the needle. US guidance is highly desirable (Fig. 66.34).

Pes anserinus syndrome

Indications. The syndrome of pes anserinus.[33,34] US guidance is not required.

Corticosteroid dose. 20 to 40 mg methylprednisone acetate mixed with 2 to 3 mL of lidocaine (no. 22 needle).

Approach. The injection site is best determined by following the medial tendinous border of the thigh (semitendinosus tendon), with the knee in semiflexion, to the tibia, where a mark is placed. The knee is then brought to extension and the needle is entered perpendicularly to tibial contact (Fig. 66.35). An area 3 cm in diameter is infiltrated adjacent to the periosteum.

Precautions. Paresthesias extending along the medial leg indicate engagement of the saphenous nerve; reposition needle.

Complications. None.

ANKLE AND FOOT

Ankle

Indications. As for the knee. US guidance is preferable (see Figs. 66.1a and b).

Corticosteroid dose. 40 to 60 mg methylprednisone acetate (no. 22 or no. 25 needle). Aspiration should be attempted before injection. For aspiration alone use a no. 20 needle.

Approach for blind injection. With the patient supine on the examination table, seek the cleft between tibia and talus by gently flexing and extending the foot. Insert the needle vertically medial to the anterior tibialis tendon (online Fig. 66.36).

Precautions. Avoid the dorsalis pedis artery.

Complications. None.

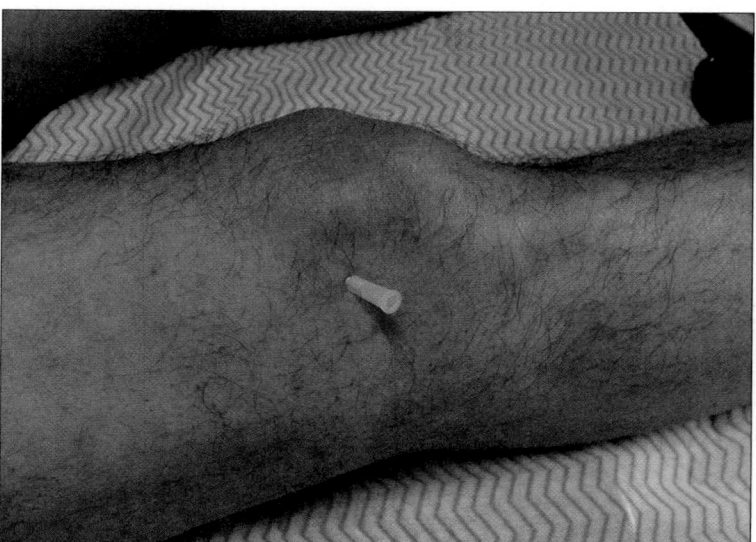

Fig. 66.33 Knee injection, lateral approach, right knee osteoarthritis.

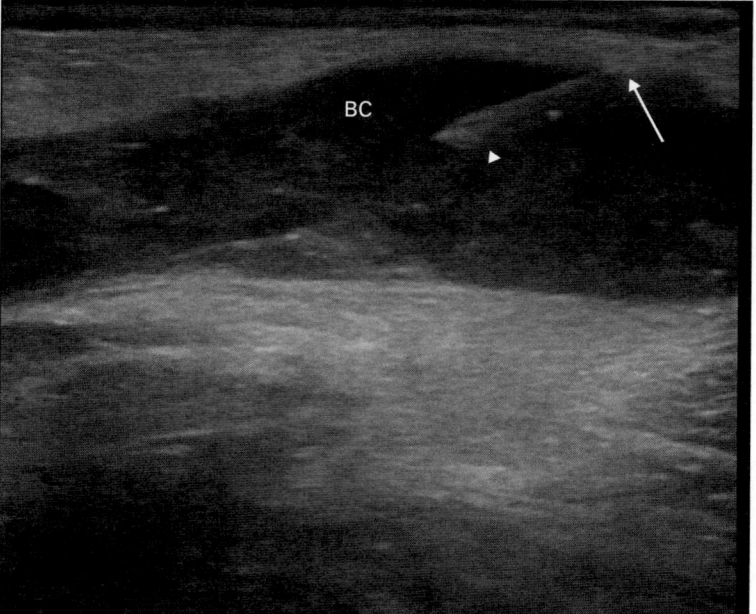

Fig. 66.34 Ultrasound-guided injection of a Baker cyst. The needle (arrow) and the needle tip (arrowhead) are seen hyperechoic inside the Baker cyst (BC).

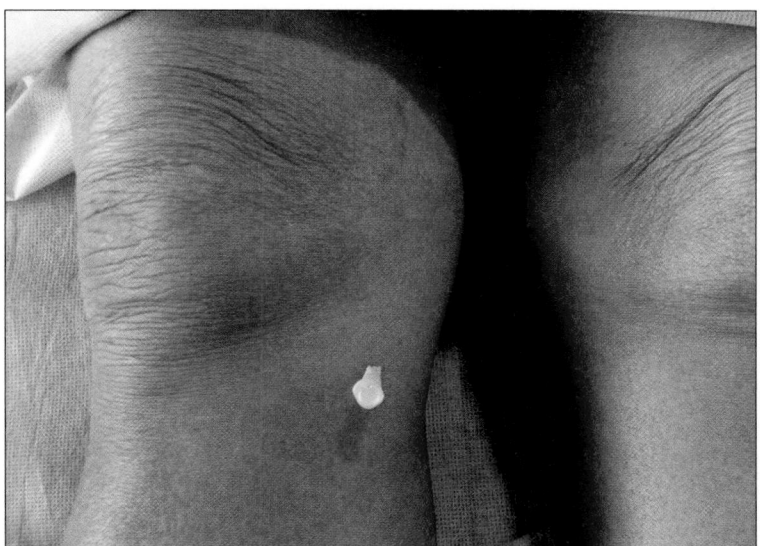

Fig. 66.35 Injection in right pes anserinus syndrome.

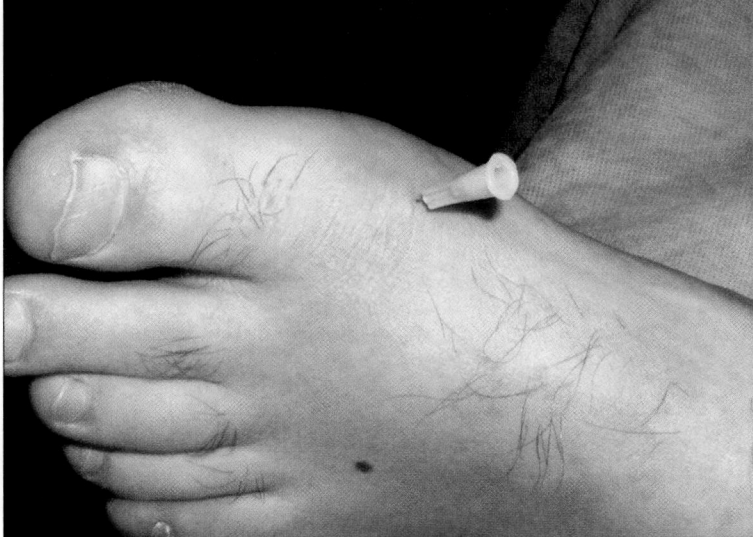

Fig. 66.38 Aspiration of left first metatarsophalangeal joint in gout.

Subtalar joint

Indications. As for the knee. US guidance is optional.

Corticosteroid dose: 20 to 30 mg methylprednisone acetate (no. 22 needle). Aspiration should be attempted before injection. For aspiration alone use a no. 20 needle.

Approach. By gently inverting and everting the foot, find the soft cleft (sinus tarsi) anterior to the lateral malleolus. Insert the needle perpendicularly toward the tip of the medial malleolus. Aspiration of fluid proves an articular insertion. Inject under low pressure (online Fig. 66.37).

Precautions. This procedure should only be performed by health professionals with a thorough knowledge of anatomy.

Complications. None.

Metatarsophalangeal joints

Indications. Aspiration for the diagnosis of gout (usually the first metatarsophalangeal). Injection in hallux rigidus, RA, and the spondyloarthropathies. US guidance is optional.

Corticosteroid dose. 10 to 20 mg methylprednisolone acetate (no. 22, no. 25, or no. 27 needle). Attempt aspiration before injection. For aspiration alone use a no. 22 needle.

Approach for blind injection. Dorsal, lateral, or medial to extensor tendon. Slight passive plantar flexion facilitates the procedure (Fig. 66-38, online Figs. 66.39 and 66.40).

Precautions. None.

Complications. None.

Retrocalcaneal bursa

Indications. Refractory Achilles tendon enthesis organ inflammation in spondyloarthritis; RA. Whenever possible this procedure should be performed under US guidance (Fig. 66.41a and b).

Corticosteroid dose. 15 to 20 mg methylprednisone acetate (no. 22, no. 25, or no. 27 needle or butterfly). Aspiration should be attempted before injection. Presence of fluid (usually a trace) proves intrabursal location.

Approach for blind injection. Posterior approach.[35] Patient lies prone on examination table with foot outside mattress. Allow calf relaxation. A 13-mm no. 27 insulin needle may be best suited for this procedure. The needle is advanced vertical to the skin, transtendinously, aiming at the posterior superior calcaneal angle.

Precautions. Do not inject large volumes because high pressures produce back flow as the needle is removed. This procedure should only be performed by health professionals with a thorough knowledge of anatomy.

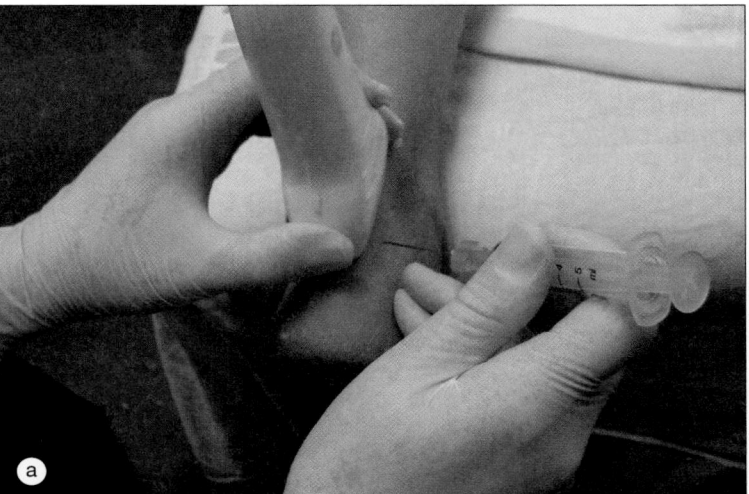

Fig. 66.41a Ultrasound-guided direct injection of the retrocalcaneal bursa. The needle is inserted adjacent to the transducer and perpendicular to its long axis.

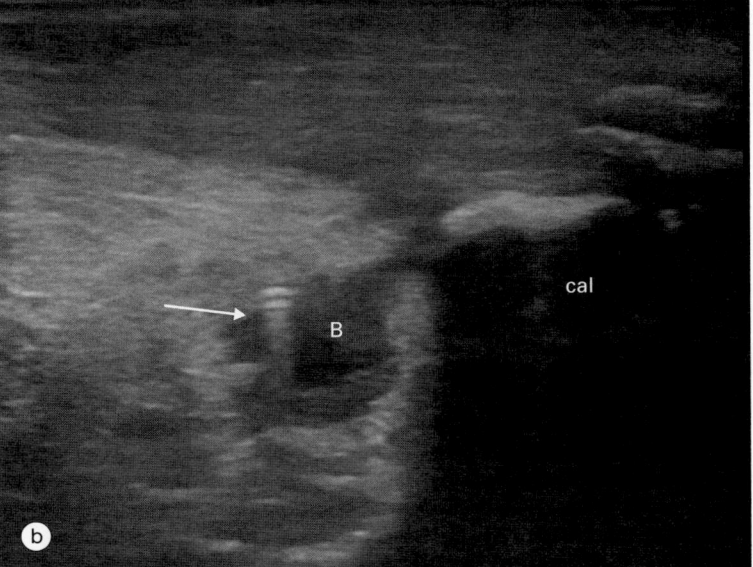

Fig. 66.41b In the ultrasound image, the tip of the needle (arrow) is seen hyperechogenic inside the retrocalcaneal bursitis.

Complications. Tendon rupture is possible and more than one reinjection is discouraged.

Posterior tibialis tendon sheath

Indications. Posterior tibialis tenosynovitis in RA and spondyloarthritis; tarsal tunnel syndrome. US guidance is highly desirable (Fig. 66.42).

Corticosteroid dose. 20 to 30 mg methylprednisolone acetate (no. 22 or no. 25 needle).

Approach for blind injection. Patient lies supine with the injected leg resting on the contralateral knee. Have patient invert the foot to identify the posterior tibialis tendon, which tents the skin. The needle is inserted tangentially, three finger breadths proximal to the tip of the medial malleolus. Inject under low pressure. Fluid may be seen and felt distending the sheath.

Precautions. Aspirate first to make sure that the posterior tibial artery has not been punctured. Plantar paresthesias indicate engagement of the posterior tibial nerve. This procedure should only be performed by health professionals with a thorough knowledge of anatomy.

Complications. The posterior tibialis tendon is prone to spontaneous rupture in RA. A misplaced (intratendinous) injection probably enhances this tendency.

Plantar fascia calcaneal enthesis[36,37]

Indications. Refractory plantar fasciitis in spondyloarthritis. US guidance is optional.

Corticosteroid dose. 20 to 30 mg methylprednisone acetate diluted with 2 mL of lidocaine (no. 22 needle).

Approach for blind procedure. Medial, needle parallel to the plantar skin 2 cm deep to plantar surface. Aim the needle into the medial plantar tubercle of the calcaneus. Resilience indicates a fascial location. Relocate the needle and inject deeply and superficially to the fibrous fascia (online Fig. 66.43).

Precautions. This procedure should only be performed by health professionals with a thorough knowledge of anatomy.

Complications. Repeated infiltrations result in fat atrophy and pressure plantar heel pain. Plantar fascia rupture may also occur. Discourage more than one reinjection (2 to 3 weeks after the initial injection).

Intermetatarsal bursae

Indications. Intermetatarsal bursitis in RA (two or more toes spread apart). US guidance is optional.

Corticosteroid dose. 20 to 30 mg methylprednisone acetate (no. 25 or no. 27 needle).

Approach. Dorsal to plantar aiming the needle to the space in between metatarsal heads (online Figs. 66.44 and 66.45).

Precautions. Plantar fat atrophy is minimized by using an insulin needle.

Complications. None.

Morton neuroma[38]

Indications. Morton neuroma. US guidance is optional.

Corticosteroid dose. 20 to 30 mg methylprednisolone acetate mixed with 1 mL lidocaine (no. 22 or no. 25 needle).

Approach for blind procedure. Through web space in the plantar side (Fig. 66.46). The needle is advanced distal to proximal aimed at the neuroma (technique taught to one of the authors by Lilia Andrade-Ortega, M.D., Mexico City).

Precautions. Inject under low pressure. This procedure should be performed by health professionals with a thorough knowledge of anatomy.

Complications. None are expected; up to two reinjections 2 to 3 weeks apart are allowed.

Ganglia

Indications. Local corticosteroids are highly effective in the treatment of routine dorsal ganglia. Ganglia within the carpal tunnel, those that impinge on neurovascular structures, and those larger than 3 cm in diameter should be injected under US guidance[39] or treated surgically.

Corticosteroid dose. Depends on the lesion; usually 15 to 20 mg methylprednisone acetate (no. 20 or no. 18 needle; thinner needles may be clogged).

Approach. The needle is aimed to the center of the lesion, which is aspirated before injection. Ganglia contain a viscous, translucent fluid. Fluids with other characteristics indicate that the lesion is not a ganglion; they should therefore be cultured and inspected for crystals (online Fig. 66.47).

Precautions. In wrist and anatomic snuffbox ganglia, rule out radial artery aneurysm, which mimics a ganglion. These lesions are expansile with the pulse, as opposed to the focal pulsation caused by a normal adjacent radial artery.

Complications. None.

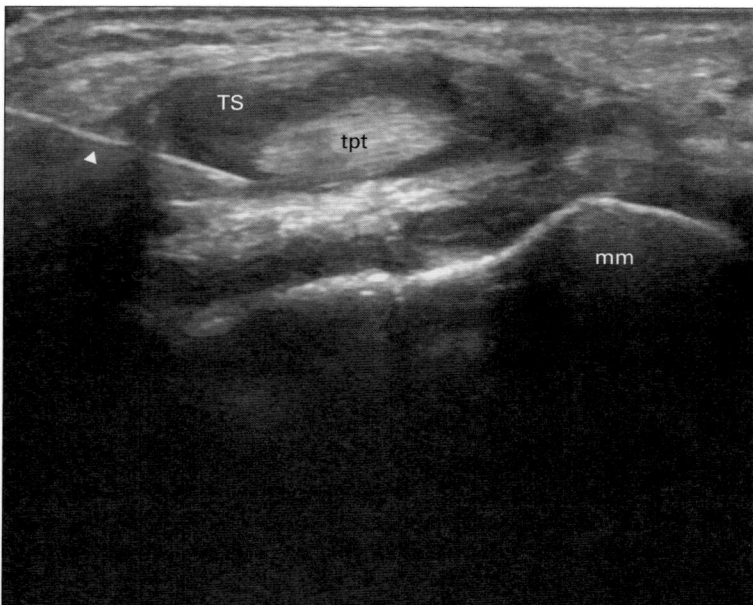

Fig. 66.42 Ultrasound-guided direct injection of a tenosynovitis of the tibialis posterior tendon. The needle (arrowhead) is inserted within the distended tendon sheath (TS). mm, medial malleolus; tpt, tibialis posterior tendon.

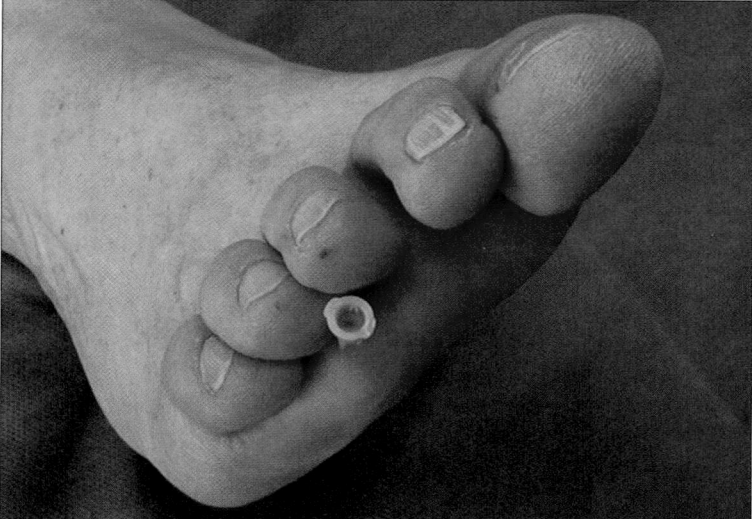

Fig. 66.46 Injection in Morton neuroma, right foot, third web space.

Trigger points in the myofascial syndromes

Indications. Acute cases if pressure on a point or nodule consistently reproduces pain. US guidance is not required.

Corticosteroid dose. 3 to 5 mL of lidocaine or bupivacaine (no. 22 needle). Twenty to 30 mg of methylprednisolone acetate may be mixed with the local anesthetic.

Approach. Aim at a tender point or the center of a nodule, which should be infiltrated radially throughout the indurated area.

Precautions. None.

Complications. None.

INTRALESIONAL CORTICOSTEROID TREATMENT

Intralesional corticosteroid treatment is sometimes used in discoid lupus,[40] the medical treatment of rheumatoid nodules[41] (online Fig. 66.48), nodular fasciitis,[42] occasionally in Sweet syndrome,[43] granulomatous disease including Crohn disease affecting the oral cavity,[44] tracheal granulomas in Wegener granulomatosis,[45] eosinophilic granuloma of the skin,[46] and inflammatory eye conditions unresponsive to oral or parenteral agents.[47]

VISCOSUPPLEMENTATION

Viscosupplementation is the term that describes the use of intra-articular hyaluronates for the treatment of pain in osteoarthritic joints. Two types of agents are in use. One is hylan G-F 20, a high-molecular-weight preparation (MW 6,000,000). The other type includes lower-molecular-weight hyaluronan preparations in the range of MW 800,000 to 2,000,000. Viscosupplementation is often effective in relieving pain in osteoarthritis.[48,49] As compared with intra-articular corticosteroids, the beneficial effect of viscosupplementation has a delayed action but lasts longer.[50] The relative merits of hylan G-F 20 and the lower MW compounds are still in dispute.[51,52] Although the initial use of these agents was in the knee, other joints such as the trapeziometacarpal joint, the shoulder, the hip, and the ankle have all been treated with benefit. Three weekly intra-articular injections are customarily used. Viscosupplementation is associated with several risks. Postinjection pain, not necessarily associated with a significant effusion, has been common in the authors' experience. Another complication is a pseudo septic effusion associated with pyrexia.[53] These reactions require hospital admission and intravenous antibiotics pending culture results. A granulomatous reaction has also been reported.[54] A further risk of viscosupplementation is an allergic reaction in patients with avian protein allergy (egg products, feathers). Usual indications of viscosupplementation include (1) patients who cannot tolerate anti-inflammatory medications and whose pain is unrelieved with analgesics and (2) patients with advanced osteoarthritis who refuse, or are not suitable candidates for, surgery. Medication and administration costs of viscosupplementation are considerable. However, a Canadian cost analysis has shown superiority of viscosupplementation over appropriate care without viscosupplementation.[55]

SYNOVIORTHESIS

Synoviorthesis, or medical synovectomy, may be achieved with the intra-articular injection of chemicals such as osmic acid, rifampicin, and rifamycin or radioactive colloids such as yttrium-90 (^{90}Y), erbium-169 (^{169}Er), dysprosium-165 (^{165}Dy), and gold-198 (^{198}Au), among others. The procedure may be used in RA, osteoarthritis, pigmented villonodular synovitis,[56] and other chronic effusive conditions, as well as in hemophilia to terminate recurrent hemarthrosis.[57] Chemical agents are believed to be less efficacious than radioactive colloids and among these, beta-emitting radioisotopes such as ^{90}Y, ^{169}Er, and ^{165}Dy are preferred over gamma-emitting radioisotopes such as ^{198}Au that cause total body irradiation. There are few randomized controlled trials of radioactive and chemical synoviorthesis.[58] Adverse effects of radioactive synoviorthesis are uncommon. A possible untoward local effect is a burn at the needle tract. This may be prevented by injecting a corticosteroid suspension while slowly removing the injecting needle. A greater concern has been a possible oncogenic effect of the radioactive colloid. However, although chromosomal damage has been found rather frequently in peripheral blood following these procedures, a 30-year Finnish follow-up study of ^{90}Y synoviorthesis in more than a thousand patients failed to show excess cancer deaths.[59] Thus, radioactive synoviorthesis, a low-risk, relatively low-cost outpatient procedure that disrupts minimally the patient's activities is a plausible alternative to surgical synovectomy in carefully selected patients. In hemophilia, according to experts, failure of three consecutive radioactive synoviortheses is an indication for open or arthroscopic synovectomy.

ACKNOWLEDGEMENT

We thank our patients for generously allowing us to take pictures during aspiration or injection procedures for the benefit of others. We also thank Ana Cruz, MD, and Félix Cabero, MD, from the Department of Rheumatology of the Hospital Severo Ochoa for their help in obtaining the pictures of the US-guided injection methods.

KEY REFERENCES

1. Schumacher HR Jr, Reginato AJ. Atlas of synovial fluid analysis and crystal identification. Philadelphia: Lea & Febiger, 1991:1-257.
2. Courtney P, Doherty M. Joint aspiration and injection. Baillieres Best Pract Res Clin Rheumatol 2005;19:345-369.
3. Pascual E, Doherty M. Aspiration of normal or asymptomatic pathological joints for diagnosis and research: indications, technique and success rate. Ann Rheum Dis 2009;68:3-7.
4. Koski JM. Ultrasound-guided injections in rheumatology. J Rheumatol 2000;27:2131-2138.
5. Grassi W, Farina A, Filippucci E, et al. Sonographically guided procedures in rheumatology. Semin Arthritis Rheum 2001;30:347-353.
6. Del Cura JL. Ultrasound-guided therapeutic procedures in the musculoskeletal system. Curr Probl Diagn Radiol 2008;37:203-218.
7. Thumboo J, O'Duffy JD. A prospective study of the safety of joint and soft tissue aspirations and injections in patients taking warfarin sodium. Arthritis Rheum 1998;41:736-739.
8. Rull M, Clayburne G, Sieck M, et al. Intra-articular corticosteroid preparations: different characteristics and their effect on inflammation induced by monosodium urate crystals in the rat subcutaneous air pouch. Rheumatology 2003;42:1093-1100.
9. Naredo E, Cabero F, Beneyto P, et al. A randomized comparative study of short term response to blind

injection versus sonographic-guided injection of local corticosteroids in patients with painful shoulder. J Rheumatol 2004;31:308-314.
10. Seror P, Pluvinage P, d'Andre FL, et al. Frequency of sepsis after local corticosteroid injection (an inquiry on 1,160,000 injections in rheumatological private practice in France). Rheumatology 1999;38:1272-1274.
11. Mader R, Lavi I, Luboshitzky R. Evaluation of the pituitary-adrenal axis function following single intraarticular injection of methylprednisolone. Arthritis Rheum 2005;52:924-928.
12. Mace S, Vadas P, Pruzanski W. Anaphylactic shock induced by intraarticular injection of methylprednisolone acetate. J Rheumatol 1997;24:1191-1194.
14. Meenagh GK, Patton J, Kynes C, Wright GD. A randomised controlled trial of intra-articular corticosteroid injection of the carpometacarpal joint of the thumb in osteoarthritis. Ann Rheum Dis 2004;63:1260-1263.
15. Stahl S, Karsh-Zafrir I, Ratzon N, et al. Comparison of intraarticular injection of depot corticosteroid and hyaluronic acid for treatment of degenerative trapeziometacarpal joints. J Clin Rheumatol 2005;11:299-302.
16. Peters-Veluthamaningal C, Winters JC, Groenier KH, et al. Corticosteroid injections effective for trigger finger in adults in general practice: a double-blinded randomised placebo controlled trial. Ann Rheum Dis 2008;67:1262-1266.

17. Kazuki K, Egi T, Okada M, et al. Clinical outcome of extrasynovial steroid injection for trigger finger. Hand Surgery 2006;11:1-4.
18. Piazzini DB, Aprile I, Ferrara PE, et al. A systematic review of conservative treatment of carpal tunnel syndrome. Clin Rehab 2007;21:299-314.
19. Grassi W, Farina A, Filippucci E, et al. Intralesional therapy in carpal tunnel syndrome: a sonographic guided approach. Clin Exp Rheumatol 2002;20:73-76.
20. Sawaizumi T, Nanno M, Ito H. De Quervain's disease: efficacy of intra-sheath triamcinolone injection. Int Orthop 2007;31:265-268.
22. Richie CA 3rd, Briner WW Jr. Corticosteroid injection for treatment of de Quervain's tenosynovitis: a pooled quantitative literature evaluation. J Am Board Fam Pract 2003;16:102-106.
23. Smith DL, McAfee JH, Lucas LM, et al. Treatment of nonspecific olecranon bursitis. A controlled, blinded prospective trial. Arch Intern Med 1989;149:2527-2530.
24. Bisset L, Smidt N, Van der Windt DA, et al. Conservative treatments for tennis elbow: do subgroups of patients respond differently? Rheumatology 2007;46:1601-1605.
25. Stahl S, Kaufman T. The efficacy of an injection of steroids for medial epicondylitis. A prospective study of sixty elbows. J Bone Joint Surg 1997;79-A:1648-1652.
26. Carette S, Moffet H, Tardif J, et al. Intraarticular corticosteroids, supervised physiotherapy, or a combination of the two in the treatment of adhesive

capsulitis of the shoulder: a placebo-controlled trial. Arthritis Rheum 2003;48:829-838.

27. Akgun K, Birtane M, Akarirmak U. Is local subacromial corticosteroid injection beneficial in subacromial impingement syndrome? Clin Rheumatol 2004;23:496-500.

28. Robinson P, Keenan AM, Conaghan PG. Clinical effectiveness and dose response of image-guided intra-articular corticosteroid injection in hip osteoarthritis. Rheumatology 2007;46:285-291.

30. Shbeeb MI, O'Duffy JD, Michet CJ Jr, et al. Evaluation of glucocorticosteroid injection for the treatment of trochanteric bursitis. J Rheumatol 1996;23:2104-2106.

31. Roberts WN. Primer: pitfalls of aspiration and injection. Nat Clin Pract Rheumatol 2007;3:464-472.

33. Calvo-Alén, J, Rua-Figueroa I, Erausquin C. Treatment of anserine bursitis. Local corticosteroid injection vs. a NSAID. A prospective study. [Spanish] Rev Esp Reumatol 1993;20:13-15.

34. Uson J, Aguado P, Bernad M, et al. Pes anserinus tendino-bursitis: what are we talking about? Scand J Rheumatol 2000;29:184-186.

35. Canoso JJ, Wohlgethan JR, Newberg AH, Goldsmith MR. Aspiration of the retrocalcaneal bursa. Ann Rheum Dis 1984;43:308-312.

36. Crawford F. Plantar heel pain and fasciitis. Clin Evid 2004;11:1589-1602.

37. Genc H, Saracoglu M, Nacir B, et al. Long-term ultrasonographic follow-up of plantar fasciitis patients treated with steroid injection. Joint Bone Spine 2005;72:61-65.

38. Markovic M, Crichton K, Read JW, et al. Effectiveness of ultrasound-guided corticosteroid injection in the treatment of Morton neuroma. Foot Ankle Int 2008;29:483-487.

39. Breidahl WH, Adler RS. Ultrasound-guided injection of ganglia with corticosteroids. Skeletal Radiol 1996;25:615-638.

40. Ting WW, Sontheimer RD. Local therapy for cutaneous and systemic lupus erythematosus: practical and theoretical considerations. Lupus 2001;10:171-184.

41. Baan H, Haagsma CJ, van de Laar MA. Corticosteroid injections reduce size of rheumatoid nodules. Clin Rheumatol 2006;25:21-23.

43. Cohen PR, Kurzrock R. Sweet's syndrome: a review of current treatment options. Am J Clin Dermatol 2002;3:117-131.

45. Solans-Laqué R, Bosch-Gil J, Canela M, et al. Clinical features and therapeutic management of subglottic stenosis in patients with ANCA-associated granulomatous vasculitis. Lupus 2008;17:832-836.

47. Ozkiris A, Erkilic K. Complications of intravitreal injection of triamcinolone acetonide. Can J Ophthalmol 2005;40:63-68.

48. Bellamy N, Campbell J, Robinson V. Viscosupplementation for the treatment of osteoarthritis of the knee. Cochrane Database Syst Rev 2005;(2):CD005321.

49. Aggarwal A, Sempowski IP. Hyaluronic acid injections for knee osteoarthritis. Systematic review of the literature. Can Fam Physician 2004;50:249-256.

50. Caborn D, Rush J, Lanzer W, et al. Synvisc 901 Study Group. A randomized, single-blind comparison of the efficacy and tolerability of hylan G-F 20 and triamcinolone hexacetonide in patients with osteoarthritis of the knee. J Rheumatol 2004;31:333-343.

51. Raman R, Dutta A, Day N, et al. Efficacy of hylan G-F 20 and sodium hyaluronate in the treatment of osteoarthritis of the knee—a prospective randomized clinical trial. Knee 2008;15:318-324.

52. Juni P, Reichenbach S, Trelle S, et al. Efficacy and safety of intraarticular hylan or hyaluronic acids for osteoarthritis of the knee: a randomized controlled trial. Arthritis Rheum 2007;56:3610-3619.

55. Torrance GW, Raynauld JP, Walker V. Canadian Knee OA Study Group. A prospective, randomized, pragmatic, health outcomes trial evaluating the incorporation of hylan G-F 20 into the treatment paradigm for patients with knee osteoarthritis (Part 2 of 2): economic results. Osteoarthr Cartil 2002;10:518-527.

56. Ward WG Sr, Boles CA, Ball JD, et al. Diffuse pigmented villonodular synovitis: preliminary results with intralesional resection and p32 synoviorthesis. Clin Orthop Rel Res 2007;454:186-191.

57. Bossard D, Carrillon Y, Stieltjes N, et al. Management of haemophilic arthropathy. Haemophilia 2008;14(Suppl 4):11-19.

58. Kahan A, Modder G, Menkes CJ, et al. (169)Erbium-citrate synoviorthesis after failure of local corticosteroid injections to treat rheumatoid arthritis-affected finger joints. Clin Exp Rheumatol 2004;22:722-726.

59. Vuorela J, Sokka T, Pukkala E. Does yttrium radiosynovectomy increase the risk of cancer in patients with rheumatoid arthritis? Ann Rheum Dis 2003;62:251-253.

REFERENCES

Full references for this chapter can be found on www.expertconsult.com.

Perioperative care of the rheumatic disease patient

67

C. Ronald MacKenzie and Stephen A. Paget

- Careful preoperative evaluation, patient selection, and postoperative care are essential; coordination between the surgeon and rheumatologist is necessary.
- Orthopedic surgery can relieve pain and improve function.
- Joint replacement including hip, knee, shoulder, elbow, and wrist has been successful.
- Arthroscopy, osteotomy, and fusion might be indicated and helpful in selected instances.

Patients with rheumatologic disease often require surgery for problems that arise in the course of their condition. Although such surgery is frequently of an orthopedic nature, the protean clinical manifestations of the chronic rheumatic diseases result in challenges that span the entire breadth of surgical expertise and practice. Consequently, rheumatologists may be asked to evaluate and provide care for their patients in the perioperative context. As such, a familiarity with the extensive literature pertaining to medical care in the surgical setting is required.[1-5]

This chapter reviews the clinical domain and literature pertaining to perioperative medicine. Beginning with a general consideration of the indications for orthopedic surgery, this chapter develops a stepwise approach to the preoperative medical evaluation, the assessment of surgical risk, and reviews the literature pertaining to perioperative evaluation and care emphasizing problems relevant to patients who suffer from chronic rheumatic conditions.

INDICATIONS FOR ORTHOPEDIC SURGERY

Elective surgery

The ultimate indications for elective orthopedic surgery are refractory pain and disability due to a well-defined and significant pathologic state that is intolerable to the patient. The final decision to go ahead with such surgery reflects the outcome of a partnership among the patient, orthopedist, and primary care physician. A rheumatologist is often consulted as well. As noted later, many facts must be incorporated into the final equation *before* surgery is scheduled and performed, and each part of the co-management team has specific questions that must be asked and answered. Ultimately the patient and his or her physician must agree that the positive effects of the surgery outweigh the potentially negative consequences. This balance is often complicated, especially in older patients with significant co-morbidities.

Joint replacement surgery

The indication for such surgery, whether it involves the hip, knee, shoulder, ankle, or other joint, is severe pain and functional limitation that cannot be ameliorated by conservative treatment.

Spine surgery

This, too, is commonly performed to decrease pain and improve function, but the patient may also have a progressive or incapacitating neurologic problem that demands immediate treatment, such as a severe radiculopathy or a myelopathy. For example, acute foot drop is a common precipitant of lumbar spine surgery.

Decision-making in the preoperative context can be viewed from the perspective and viewpoints of the significant decision-makers.

Patient

- Have I seen the right doctors to define the cause of my pains and disability, its extent, and severity and have I failed all the therapies recommended? Should I seek a second opinion?
- Are my pain and functional limitation sufficient to warrant thinking about and undergoing surgery?
- Does my overall medical status enable me to safely undergo surgery? What does my internist/rheumatologist think about this important question? If there is a high risk, can that risk be ameliorated in a timely and safe manner?
- If I have systemic lupus erythematosus, rheumatoid arthritis, psoriatic arthritis, or another type of systemic arthritis or autoimmune disorder, do I have specific needs and problems that must be addressed prior to, during, and after surgery? Do these problems increase the chance that I will have a medical or surgical complication? If so, what can I do to avoid them? If I am on steroids, what type of steroid preparation is needed preoperatively and postoperatively? What should be done with my other rheumatic disease medications?
- Does my surgeon have a lot of experience in performing this exact surgery (i.e., numbers of surgery per year) and what are his or her outcomes? Do I trust and am I able to communicate appropriately with the surgeon? Can I speak to a patient on whom he or she has recently performed surgery? Is the hospital a good one with an exceptional track record and medical and rehabilitation support?
- Do I have optimal support at home after the surgery to assure the best of care, safety, and comfort?

Surgeon

- Am I sure about the type and extent of the musculoskeletal problem that is causing the patient's pain and disability? Have I ruled out referred pain, infection, or fracture?
- Has the patient received the proper conservative care for this problem? If not, what needs to be done before considering surgery?
- Is the problem of such severity that surgery is the only way to improve pain and function and get the patient back to the life that he or she desires?
- Are the patient's expectations appropriate?
- Is this patient medically and psychologically prepared for this planned surgery? Is he or she at an increased risk for thromboembolic disease and, if so, what is the optimal type of prophylaxis that is necessary and fits well with his or her medical status?
- Which consulting physicians are required on the preoperative team to assure the best outcome?
- Is the patient's vascular status normal and, if not, what can be done to improve it?
- What type of antibiotic prophylaxis is necessary? Does this patient have allergies to antibiotics and, if so, which antibiotic is appropriate?
- Does the patient need to be sent to a rehabilitation center before discharge home? Is the home setting and social support sufficient to ensure an optimal outcome?

Rheumatologist/internist

- Has the patient had a proper assessment of the musculoskeletal problem causing their pain and disability?
- Is the patient medically and psychologically prepared for the planned surgery? If not, what do I need to do to assure the best

possible outcome? Do I need to simplify or change the medication regimen in preparation for the surgery?

- Which preoperative assessments should I do? Does the patient have an increased risk of a cardiovascular problem intraoperatively and postoperatively such as experienced by patients with diabetes, rheumatoid arthritis, and systemic lupus erythematosus? If so, does the patient need a stress test or echocardiography? Does her or she need preoperative β-blockers?
- If the patient has diabetes or is on steroids, what needs to be done to assure the best outcome?
- What type of thromboembolic prophylaxis is both necessary and conforms best to the patient's medical status?
- How do I keep in touch with the hospital team preoperatively and postoperatively to assure the best continuity of care and communication about problems that arose in the hospital and medication changes that were made?

Anesthesiologist

- Have I spoken to or communicated with the patient's internist, rheumatologist, other pertinent consultants, and surgeon to assure that I am up to date on the patient's medical status and potential complications of this surgical procedure?
- Have I discussed the type of anesthesia that I will be giving with the patient, medical, and surgical team and explained why I chose it in this specific patient?
- Which of the patient's current medications has he or she taken or not taken on the day before or the day of surgery?
- If the patient is on steroids or has diabetes, have the appropriate medications or monitoring been given/instituted to optimize the patient's medical status?
- If the patient has cardiac, pulmonary, neurologic, or other medical problems, what specific monitoring is necessary perioperatively?

NON-ELECTIVE (EMERGENCY) ORTHOPAEDIC SURGERY

There are times when the careful and thoughtful deliberations noted earlier are not possible because of the life-threatening and compelling nature of the clinical problem such as a hip fracture, a myelopathy, or a septic patient with an infected native or prosthetic joint. In these settings, when time is usually of the essence and the patient's overall health is at risk, the medical and surgical team must stabilize the patient as much as possible to optimize the outcome, but time is of the essence.

Preoperative evaluation

The purposes of the preoperative medical and subsequent perioperative management are as follows:

- Identification of the nature, severity, and degree of control of all co-morbid conditions that may affect perioperative clinical decision-making and medical care;
- Optimization of the treatment of all active medical problems;
- Assessment of anesthesia and surgery-associated risk (both in magnitude and type);
- Anticipation and subsequent identification and management of postoperative complications, the risk and severity of which might be reduced if considered preoperatively;
- Education of patients and families concerning the perioperative experience;
- Motivation of the patient to commit to preoperative preventive practices (i.e., smoking cessation, weight loss, medication compliance, and adherence to care plans preoperatively and postoperatively).

As a consequence of medical advances, as well as financial and resource constraints and their impact on the medical system at large, there has been a substantial trend toward the performance of surgery in the ambulatory, outpatient setting. Indeed, the percentage of all surgical procedures performed on an outpatient basis in the United States rose from 20% in 1982 to 60% in 1995, a trend particularly relevant to the arthroscopic techniques of orthopedic surgery.[6,7] Among

a number of benefits of these developments has been one highly positive consequence, the opportunity to move the preoperative medical evaluation to the outpatient arena as well, often weeks before the surgical date. This change in practice allows time for discourse with the other physicians involved in the patient's care, for supplementary consultation and investigation, and when necessary for the institution of therapy directed at optimizing the patient's medical status before the contemplated surgery. Practiced in this manner, the preoperative evaluation becomes a focal point of communication between all members of the medical team caring for the patient, enhancing the deliberative and collaborative nature of the consultative process and ultimately the patient's care.

Although the efficacy of preoperative assessment has not been definitively established,[8,9] the aging and increasing complexity of modern-day surgical patients justifies the enduring support for this clinical practice. Published observations from the Australian Incident Monitoring Study (AIMS) shed light on preoperative assessments.[10] In this study 11% of preoperative assessments were considered either inadequate or incorrect, with 3.1% of all adverse postoperative events directly resulting from these flawed practices. Indeed, among those patients experiencing postoperative complications, the morbidity was considered major. Only 5% of such events were considered unpreventable. In another study of anesthetic-related deaths, 39% (53/135) of deaths involved suboptimal preoperative assessment and management.[11] Delays in surgery, subsequent complications, and unexpected postoperative admissions to higher levels of care have been shown to be reduced by preoperative evaluation.[12] Further anxiety, pain, length of stay, and patient satisfaction are favorably influenced by the preoperative evaluation. In one study patients rated meeting with the anesthesiologist preoperatively a higher priority than that of obtaining information on pain relief, methods of anesthesia, and discussion concerning potential complications of surgery.[13]

Although no consensus exists regarding what constitutes the optimal preoperative medical evaluation, a growing literature pertaining to perioperative medicine supports various core principles that underlie effective medical consultation. Depending on the setting and institutional approach to perioperative care, the preoperative consultation may be conducted by an MD (internist, medical subspecialist, hospitalist, or anesthesiologist) or by physician extenders (nurse practitioners, physician assistants) under supervision. Although the manner in which consultation takes place also varies as a result of how and in what discipline one was trained, the role played by the medical consultant may also be changing when compared with historical practices. Because the complexity of medicine, especially the growth in pharmacology, the challenges of the elderly with their co-morbidities and restricted physiologic reserve, and productivity and reimbursement pressures that keep surgeons in the operating room (as opposed to rounding on the floors), surgeons are desirous of a more involved consultant.[14] This may take the form of a more active participation in the patient's care (ordering rather than recommending medications), adopting a co-management strategy for the patient's postoperative care, or in some instances assuming full responsibility for the patient after completion of the surgery. No matter which of the paradigms is agreed on, communication between the referring and consulting physicians remains essential to the provision of optimal care. Evolving from earlier guidelines (Ten Commandments for Effective Consultation),[15] a recent revision stressed such considerations as (1) determine the customer; (2) establish the urgency; (3) gather your own information; (4) be brief, specific, but talk to the referring physician; (5) establish contingency plans; (6) establish one's turf and don't stray; (7) teach with tact; and (8) follow up.[12]

HISTORY AND PHYSICAL EXAMINATION

The needs of the patient in the perioperative context depend on a number of considerations, notably age, functional capacity, co-morbidity, and the type of anesthesia and surgery to be performed. A complete history and physical examination constitute the bedrock preoperative evaluation providing the clinical context on which informed decisions concerning the value of additional ancillary testing can be premised. The focus and content of the preoperative history do differ from general medical practice, however. The reason the patient is having the surgery should be ascertained because the risks vary with the magnitude and urgency of the procedure. Patients should be asked about their prior experience with surgery and anesthesia, and the presence, severity, and stability of all co-morbid conditions should be established. All prescription and over-the-counter medications, including the use of herbs and supplements, should be recorded with their dosages and dosing schedules. The use of tobacco, alcohol, and other drugs should also be documented, as should the patient's allergic history.

The physical examination is more than a supplement, confirming and often amplifying information obtained from the medical history. In the preoperative context, not only should the examination be thorough, it should also focus on patient characteristics that might adversely affect the patient's postoperative course. In addition to the vital signs, body mass index (BMI) should be calculated (weight/height) because this parameter is associated with the development of various chronic diseases. Obesity is a risk factor for surgery. Careful auscultation of the heart is important because the presence of third and fourth heart sounds may indicate congestive heart failure and, depending on their nature and severity, valvular heart disease may compromise cardiac function at times of physiologic stress such as surgery. Obesity, large neck circumference, and hypertension predict obstructive sleep apnea, an important but underappreciated problem in the postoperative setting.

LABORATORY STUDIES

The benefit of preoperative laboratory testing has been examined in many studies, and its benefit (or lack thereof) continues to be widely debated. Should such testing be procedure or disease driven or is the practice of screening laboratory panels justified in the preoperative setting? Regarding testing when there are no clinical indications, less than 1% has been shown to provide useful information[16]; indeed, there is evidence to suggest that overall, such testing may actually be harmful.[17] Not surprisingly, preoperative diagnostic tests ordered as a consequence of a finding uncovered on history and physical examination are more likely to be abnormal[18]; of particular importance is the previously abnormal result that is associated with new or persistent abnormalities.[19]

Recent practice in perioperative medicine has resulted in a marked diminution in the ordering of ancillary testing before surgery. Encompassing an array of preoperative investigations, an extensive literature has failed to demonstrate that such testing improves surgical outcome.[20] The establishment of guidelines, the effect of which was to reduce preoperative testing, has been shown to not result in untoward perioperative events or test ordering.[21] In studies involving healthy patients who underwent minor procedures, routine preoperative laboratory testing appears unnecessary.[22-24] Nonetheless, depending on the patient and the nature and magnitude of the surgery to be performed, a number of investigations may be considered appropriate and are commonly performed on patients before major surgical procedures (Table 67.1).

Assessment of operative risk

A primary purpose of the preoperative medical evaluation is the identification of patients who are at higher risk for postoperative complications. Although the standard history and physical examination remain the principal screening method for the detection of conditions likely to affect surgical outcome, rating systems have been developed to identify patients who are most likely to develop postoperative complications.

The best known and most widely used is the American Society of Anesthesiologists (ASA) Physical Status Scale, which has a high correlation with the patient's postoperative course. The ASA scale consists of five levels of risk (associated surgical mortality in parentheses) based on the presence of a systemic disturbance: I, absent (0.2%); II, mild (0.5%); III, severe/non-incapacitating (1.9%); IV, incapacitating/threat to life (4.9%); and V, moribund/survival less than 24 hours without surgery (NA); the subdesignation E denotes emergency surgery, which doubles the risk.[25] Having been first proposed in 1941,[26] a revision of the scale became the ASA Physical Status Scale.[27] Although criticized for the vagueness of its criteria, it has proven an extraordinarily durable and useful assessment tool. Nonetheless, the search for more robust prediction methodologies has continued and considerable success has been achieved in the assessment of cardiac risk specifically.

The landmark work of Goldman on the cardiac risk assessment of patients undergoing noncardiac surgery can now be seen as having

TABLE 67.1 RECOMMENDATIONS FOR LABORATORY TESTING BEFORE ELECTIVE SURGERY

Test	Incidence of abnormalities that influence management	LR+	LR−	Indications
Hemoglobin	0.1%	3.3	0.90	Anticipated major blood loss or symptoms of anemia
While blood cell count	0.0%	0.0	1.00	Symptoms suggest infection, myeloproliferative disorder, or myelotoxic medications
Platelet count	0.0%	0.0	1.00	History of bleeding diathesis, myeloproliferative disorder, or myelotoxic medications
Prothrombin time	0.0%	0.0	1.01	History of bleeding diathesis, chronic liver disease, malnutrition, recent or long-term antibiotic use
Partial thromboplastin time	0.1%	1.7	0.86	History of bleeding diathesis
Electrolytes	1.8%	4.3	0.80	Known renal insufficiency, congestive heart failure, medications that affect electrolytes
Renal function	2.6%	3.3	0.81	Age >50 yr, hypertension, cardiac disease, major surgery, medications that may affect renal function
Glucose	0.5%	1.6	0.85	Obesity or known diabetes
Liver function tests	0.1%			No indication. Consider albumin measurement for major surgery or chronic illness
Urinalysis	1.4%	1.7	0.97	No indication
Electrocardiogram	2.6%	1.6	0.96	Men >40 yr, women >50 yr, known CAD, diabetes, or hypertension
Chest radiograph	3.0%	2.5	0.72	Age >50 yr, known cardiac or pulmonary disease, symptom or examination suggests cardiac or pulmonary disease

CAD, coronary artery disease.
From Smetana GW, MacPherson DS. The case against routine preoperative laboratory testing. Med Clin N Am 2003;87:7-40.

TABLE 67.2 REVISED CARDIAC RISK INDEX

High-risk surgery	Intraperitoneal, intrathoracic, suprainguinal vascular
History of ischemic heart disease	Myocardial infarction, positive stress test, angina, nitrate therapy, pathologic Q waves
History of congestive heart failure	Congestive heart failure, pulmonary edema, paroxysmal nocturnal dyspnea, rales or S3 gallop, vascular redistribution on chest radiograph
History of cerebrovascular disease	TIA or stroke
Preoperative treatment with insulin	
Preoperative serum creatinine >2.0 mg/dL	

From Lee HT, Marcantonio ER, Mangione CM, et al. Derivation and prospective validation of a simple index for prediction of cardiac risk of major noncardiac surgery. Circ 1999;100:1043-1049.

ushered in the field of perioperative medicine.[28] The Goldman Cardiac Risk Index has undergone extensive study and subsequent revision.[29-31] The Revised Cardiac Risk Index is the most widely employed scoring system today (Table 67.2). One point is assigned for each of the six independent risk factors for major cardiac complications in patients undergoing emergency surgery. The incidence of such complications in patients with zero, one, two, or three risk factors was 0.4%, 0.9%, 7%, and 11% in a validation cohort.[31]

The search continues, however, to develop more global indicators of risk. Holt and Silverman have proposed a *resilience* score for organ systems compromised by an underlying disease process.[32] An overall resilience score for a given organ system is derived by adding the standard ASA score to a surgical complexity score (rated 1 to 5). A maximal score would therefore be 10 and the higher the score, the more likely that a given organ system will suffer injury or fail in the setting of a surgical stress. The individual scores for each organ system assigned a score of greater than 3 can be added and reflect the impact of multisystem disease. Although of interest, more work needs to be done using this approach in order to determine its utility in diverse surgical populations.

Recent epidemiologic studies by Memtsoudis and colleagues[33-34] provide an interesting context from which to examine trends in the performance and outcomes of orthopedic surgery and provide useful information relevant to perioperative risk assessment. In an ongoing series of studies, observations concerning the outcome of specific orthopedic procedures are drawn from two large national datasets. These include the National Hospital Discharge survey (NHDS), which is composed of medical information collected annually since 1965 by the National Center for Health Statistics (a database of inpatient utilization) and the National Inpatient Sample (NIS), the largest annual all-payer database in the United States. The power of these studies is derived from the enormous size of the database, which in the case of one study involved nearly 7 million patient discharges.[36]

Thus far this work has focused on lower extremity arthroplasty, specifically the outcomes, complications, and mortality after total knee replacement (unilateral, bilateral, revision). The preoperative characteristics, specifically co-morbidities of these patients, the postoperative outcomes, and data pertaining to discharge considerations are well described in these studies. Several broad themes relevant to perioperative care can be derived from the analysis. First, the use of total joint arthroplasty has increased over time and trends in the prevalence of co-morbidities confirm an increase in the frequency of hypertension, diabetes mellitus, hypercholesterolemia, obesity, pulmonary disease, and coronary artery disease over time.[33,35] Overall complication rates have decreased in spite of a decreasing length of stay except in the case of bilateral procedures. Indeed, among the population undergoing bilateral total joint arthroplasty, procedure-related complication rates were higher as compared with unilateral procedures despite a

younger average age and lower co-morbidity burden.[34] Mortality after total joint arthroplasty of the hip and knee was most strongly correlated with postoperative pulmonary embolism and stroke.[34] Preoperative risk factors for in-hospital mortality were revision total joint arthroplasty, advanced age (>85 years), and the presence of specific co-morbidities, predominately dementia, renal, and cerebrovascular disease. There was a steady decrease in the risk of death over the time period of the study (1990-2004).

ANESTHESIA IN PATIENTS WITH RHEUMATIC DISEASE

A variety of issues, including airway considerations, the site and anticipated duration of surgery, existing co-morbidity, and the patient's emotional state, are important determinants of the type of anesthesia to be used, whether invasive monitoring will be necessary, and the length of time the patient will spend in the recovery room after surgery.

Type of anesthesia

General and regional anesthesia is commonly used in the surgical treatment of patients with rheumatic disease. General anesthesia with endotracheal intubation may present a particular danger in patients with rheumatoid arthritis or ankylosing spondylitis (see Section V). In patients with cervical spine instability or a rigid airway, fiberoptic intubation may be required. Regional anesthesia may take the form of local anesthesia for minor procedures, peripheral nerve block for surgery of the upper and lower extremity, and epidural/spinal anesthesia for arthroplasty in the lower extremity.

Although the debate concerning the relative superiority of regional versus general anesthesia remains unresolved, many surgical procedures, particularly orthopedic surgery, are well suited for regional anesthetic techniques.[35] Evidence does exist, however, suggesting that regional anesthesia does reduce the incidence of major perioperative complications. These include a reduction in the following: blood loss,[36,37] deep venous thrombosis and pulmonary embolism, postoperative respiratory events, and death.[38,39] Further, postoperative pain management, a significant problem for patients with a painful rheumatic disease, may be best managed with regional anesthetic approaches.[40] Peripheral nerve blocks using longer-acting anesthetics and infusion methodologies are another consideration because they provide both excellent intraoperative anesthesia and postoperative pain relief.[41,42]

Monitoring techniques

Patients undergoing major surgical procedures should have continuous electrocardiographic and pulse oximeter monitoring intraoperatively. At the discretion of the anesthesiologist, arterial and Swan-Ganz catheter monitoring may be helpful in selected patients. Such monitoring is often employed in patients undergoing bilateral joint replacement surgery and in those with a history of prior cardiac disease.

Postoperative analgesia

A number of options exist for the control of postoperative pain, including the traditional intravenous or intramuscular routes (systemic) versus the administration of epidural analgesia. Patient-controlled analgesia via an epidural route of administration is an effective method of pain control postoperatively and often facilitates postoperative physical therapy, which is important in the restoration of range of motion in patients undergoing orthopedic surgery. This technique also reduces the systemic absorption of analgesics, thereby minimizing the problem of narcotic-induced respiratory depression. Parenterally administered nonsteroidal anti-inflammatory agents are a useful alternative to traditional analgesia after surgery and can be used to reduce narcotic requirements after major surgery. These drugs should not be given to patients with the common contraindications to nonsteroidal anti-inflammatory agents such as peptic ulcer disease, renal disease, and ischemic heart disease with the concomitant use of anticoagulants.

PERIOPERATIVE MANAGEMENT OF CO-MORBID MEDICAL CONDITIONS

In the following section the important co-morbidities encountered in the perioperative setting are reviewed, emphasizing possible problems relevant to the rheumatic disease patient.

Ischemic heart disease

The contribution of cardiovascular disease to the risk of noncardiac surgery cannot be overstated. From epidemiologic evidence it is predicted that the number of persons older than 65 years in the United States will increase by 25% to 35% over the next 30 years,[43] coinciding with the demographic group on which the majority of surgery is performed.[44] On this basis it has been estimated that the annual number of noncardiac surgical procedures performed in this age group could increase from 6 to 12 million per year during this time period. Because many of these are major surgical procedures (intra-abdominal, thoracic, vascular, and orthopedic), it can be anticipated that postoperative cardiovascular morbidity and mortality will remain a primary focus of those interested in the practice of medicine in the perioperative setting. Fortunately, cardiovascular disease is the most investigated and well documented arena of perioperative medicine. Practical guidelines intended to guide physicians involved in the assessment and care of patients with cardiac disease are widely recognized and are updated regularly as evidence accrues.[45] As discussed earlier, prediction rules predicated on readily available clinical data have been extensively studied and validated and disseminated to the practicing community.

With respect to the identification of the presence of preexisting cardiac disease, the predictive value of the routine clinical assessment, the history and physical examination, electrocardiogram, and chest radiograph, supplemented by other non-invasive methodologies, are well established. Also important is the definition of disease **severity and stability** and **prior treatment** because these factors working in concert with other clinical characteristics such as age, functional capacity, co-morbidity, and type of surgery to be performed ultimately define postoperative risk. A series of factors may predict postoperative myocardial infarction, congestive heart failure, and death after orthopedic surgery (Table 67.3).

The American College of Cardiology (ACC)/American Heart Association (AHA) Guidelines for the Perioperative Cardiovascular Evaluation for Noncardiac Surgery[43] is the most extensive and current discussion of the approach to the preoperative cardiac evaluation. This document provides algorithms with respect to every level of decision making in this clinical setting including the indications for preoperative **exercise stress testing and coronary angiography.** Multiple modalities for the noninvasive cardiac evaluation are available, some of which assess cardiac function under resting conditions while others "stress" the patient either with exercise or passively using pharmacologic induction of physiologic stress. In patients who by history report high exercise tolerance in the routine course of their lives, little useful information is likely to be gained from such testing. In others (e.g., chronically ill rheumatic disease patients), the evaluation of cardiac function preoperatively may be useful because the illness may limit the natural physical "stress." Such decisions should be made on an individual basis, tempered by literature concerning the utility of the available testing modalities.

On the basis of the belief that impairment in left ventricular function would predict postoperative cardiac complications, multiple studies have examined this correlation. The conclusion reached from these investigations, however, is that the incidence of postoperative complications occurred in patients with a left ventricular ejection fracture (LVEF) of less than 35%. While linking such cardiac phenomena as ischemia, congestive heart failure, and death to impaired cardiac function, a resting echocardiogram has never been demonstrated to be a reliable predictor of postoperative ischemic events.[46,47] Other noninvasive methods for the detection of coronary artery disease that employ exercise to improve sensitivity and specificity are widely available and have spawned an extensive literature. Exercise stress testing, with or without nuclear imaging or echocardiography, is extensively used in the assessment and detection of coronary artery disease in general practice. Whether the method employs formal exercise (e.g., treadmill or bicycle) or pharmacologic (dipyridamole, adenosine) means for its stress simulation, the goal of such testing is the provocation of myocardial ischemia by increasing myocardial oxygen demand relative to supply. In these studies fixed defects, which do not change after exercise-induced redistribution of blood flow, represent myocardial scar from prior infarction and have less predictive value for postoperative ischemic events. In patients with reversible abnormalities, cardiac risk increases with increasing size and number of reperfusion abnormalities.[44] The superiority of one test over another has not been established. A meta-analysis of 68 studies involving 10,278 patients undergoing noncardiac surgery compared the predictive value of stress echocardiography versus thallium imaging.[48] In this study the stress echocardiogram had superior predictive capability for postoperative cardiac events. Nonetheless, more than one third of the complications occurred in patients with negative tests. Currently it remains unclear whether one approach to stress testing is definitively superior to another. Indeed, they may all be reasonably good for preoperative risk assessment and which is chosen may be related more to the patient's physical capacity to participate in the stress induction and the local availability of such testing. The former is particularly true in the disabled rheumatic disease or orthopedic patient. Further, the important question is not which test should be performed, but rather which patients will benefit from such assessments?

Strategies to reduce cardiac risk in noncardiac surgery may involve medical therapy or invasive cardiac interventions performed preoperatively, alterations in anesthetic technique, and aggressive management of adverse hemodynamic developments intraoperatively and postoperatively. For the internist-rheumatologist who evaluates the patient preoperatively, the relevant approaches include medical management, specifically the use of β-blockers, antiplatelet agents, and statin therapy. The widespread use of cardiac stents has become an important management problem in the preoperative setting. On occasion, coronary revascularization prior to the noncardiac surgery is considered.

Recognition of the protective role of β-**blockade** in the perioperative setting has been considered the most significant advance in perioperative medical care. β-Blockers protect the heart by improving myocardial oxygen balance by slowing heart rate and reducing contractility. The slowing of the heart rate has additional benefits through an improvement of diastolic filling while decreasing myocardial oxygen consumption. Although widely employed in the treatment of coronary artery disease for decades, it was not until 1996 that a potential role for this class of medication in the prevention of postoperative cardiac

TABLE 67.3 SERIES OF FACTORS THAT MAY PREDICT POSTOPERATIVE MYOCARDIAL INFARCTION, CONGESTIVE HEART FAILURE, AND DEATH AFTER ORTHOPEDIC SURGERY

Major predictors of increased perioperative cardiac risk include:	Intermediate predictors of increased perioperative cardiac risk include:	Minor predictors of increased perioperative risk include:
■ recent myocardial infarction (<30 days) ■ unstable or severe angina ■ poorly compensated congestive heart failure ■ significant arrhythmias ■ severe valvular disease	■ mild angina ■ prior myocardial infarction by history or pathologic Q waves ■ compensated or prior congestive heart failure ■ diabetes mellitus	■ advanced age ■ abnormal electrocardiogram ■ rhythm other than sinus ■ low functional capacity ■ prior stroke ■ poorly controlled hypertension ■ prior cardiac revascularization, currently asymptomatic

complications was shown. In the first study examining the role of perioperative β-blockade, by Mangano and colleagues,[49] patients with known coronary artery disease or a significant risk factor profile were randomized to receive atenolol or placebo starting 7 days before surgery and continuing for 1 month after surgery. A significant reduction in cardiac events was noted postoperatively, a benefit that remained significant for a 2-year period.[50,47] Subsequent work from the Dutch[51] appeared to have confirmed the benefit of the preoperative and postoperative administration of β-blockers in the noncardiac surgical setting. The practice was subsequently widely promulgated. However, another large-scale randomized controlled trial has thrown this practice into question.[52] This study, involving 8351 patients at 190 centers across the globe, confirmed the findings of numerous previous clinical trials, that prophylactic β-blockade significantly decreased the incidence of postoperative myocardial infarction. However, this benefit was negated by the higher incidence of death (3.1% vs. 2.3%), stroke (1.0% vs. 0.5%), clinically significant hypotension (15% vs. 9.7%), and bradycardia (6.6% vs. 2.4%), raising concern about the overall net safety of this practice. This, the major current controversy in perioperative medicine, is under active debate. The most prudent approach to the use of perioperative β-blockers is to employ them only in selected circumstances: for high-risk patients not already on β-blockers, start therapy early (days to weeks before surgery), aim for a lower heart rate (60 beats per minute), and continue therapy for at least 1 week postoperatively.[53]

Chronic aspirin (acetylsalicylic acid, ASA) therapy for both the primary and secondary prevention of atherosclerotic cardiovascular disease is highly prevalent; indeed, the use of such therapy in the rheumatic diseases is also significant. As such, the use of ASA and other antiplatelet agents in the perioperative setting is commonplace. Due to its perceived bleeding risk, such agents were, until recently, usually discontinued 5 days before surgery when possible. Nonetheless, as the protective role of such therapy has been better appreciated, the practice of discontinuing ASA before surgery has been called into question. A meta-analysis evaluating this issue has demonstrated that ASA withdrawal preceded up to 10% of all acute cardiovascular events, and that while aspirin-related bleeding complications increased, the bleeds tended to be mild and of little significance (except in intracranial surgery and transurethral resection of the prostate).[54] Other antiplatelet drugs (thienopyridines, clopidogrel, ticlopidine) are also in common usage, though guidelines for application in the perioperative setting have not been established. Owing to their longer half-life, the general practice is to discontinue these agents at least 10 days before the surgical procedure.

A related problem of increasing prevalence is the management of antiplatelet therapy in noncardiac surgery in patients with intracoronary stents. Reports of stent thrombosis in the perioperative period in patients who have had such therapy discontinued preoperatively have raised concern about the attendant risks.[55-57] Such thrombosis is associated with high rates of myocardial infarction (up to 50%). Two major classes of stents are currently employed, bare metal (BMS) and drug-eluting stents (DES). The latter contain drugs that prevent endothelialization of the stent and hence restenosis. Because the use of antiplatelet agents (usually dual antiplatelet therapy) significantly reduces the incidence of stent thrombosis, the protective influence of such medication is important. Further, the risk of stent thrombosis varies with the type of stent employed, with the BMS resulting in a lower risk in the setting of the discontinuation of antiplatelet therapy. The heightened risk of thrombosis after DESs is believed to persist for up to a year. According to a recent advisory statement, for patients who require surgery and have had a DES placed in the preceding 12-month period, ASA alone should be maintained with the other antiplatelet agents being stopped 7 to 10 days before surgery.[58]

Last there are the statins, medications known to have both lipid-lowering and anti-inflammatory activity, the latter of which stabilizes coronary plaque, improves endothelial function, and inhibits platelet aggregation. As a consequence of these theoretical benefits and a number of clinical trials suggesting a cardioprotective effect in the perioperative setting,[59-61] it is recommended that statin therapy be continued in the perioperative period despite the well-known potential complications of such therapy (hepatotoxicity, myositis, rhabdomyolysis) that need to be kept in mind.

Although fewer patients with rheumatoid arthritis and spondyloarthropathies are undergoing orthopedic surgery due to the early and effective treatment strategies employed today, some will still require surgical intervention and their particular cardiovascular risks need to be appreciated. Rheumatoid arthritis results in premature development of atherosclerosis, myocardial infarction, and arterial stiffening. Congestive heart failure is likewise independently related to rheumatoid arthritis, possibly because of impaired LV diastolic filling. Though effective control of disease activity may be beneficial in ameliorating vascular and myocardial disease, those patients with severe disease are the most likely to have subclinical coronary disease. Like rheumatoid arthritis, systemic lupus erythematosus (SLE) results in premature development of atherosclerosis, myocardial infarction, and arterial stiffening. Left ventricular hypertrophy develops in SLE unrelated to traditional stimuli to hypertrophy and may be due to inflammation-related arterial stiffening.[62] All COX-2 selective and traditional nonsteroidal anti-inflammatory drugs increase the risk for ischemic heart disease and should be factored into the perioperative risk assessment.

OTHER CARDIOVASCULAR DISEASES

Hypertension

The prevalence of hypertension in the perioperative setting is 20%. Its association with coronary artery disease secures it as a risk factor for adverse outcome after surgery. Indeed, it has been shown to be one of five independent predictors of postoperative myocardial ischemia and one of three predictors of postoperative mortality.[63] Despite these associations, clinical experience suggests that the magnitude of risk conferred by blood pressure elevations alone appears small and current practice supports that surgery should not be postponed in patients with mild to moderate elevations in blood pressure. One large study of patients with chronically elevated blood pressure demonstrated no significantly different outcome based on whether or not surgery was cancelled for patients with diastolic blood pressures in the 110- to 130-mm Hg range.[64] Patients with greater elevations in blood pressure or those with major end organ (cardiac, neurologic, renal) complications of the disorder should probably be cancelled until their pressure is under better control.

Valvular heart disease

Dysfunction of the cardiac valves is a common manifestation of the connective tissue diseases.[65] Beginning with the classic descriptions of the Libman-Sacks vegetations of SLE, regurgitation of the mitral valve has also been well described in rheumatoid arthritis.[66] Aortic valve disease, particularly aortic insufficiency, has been well described in the HLA-B27–associated spondyloarthropathies.[67] In these conditions the aortic regurgitation has been shown to result from aortitis and subsequent dilatation of the aorta.[68] In addition to these associations, there is the high prevalence of aortic and aortic valve involvement in the systemic vasculitides including granulomatous disorders, systemic vasculitis, giant cell arteritis, and Takayasu arteritis.[63] In these conditions, the inflammatory involvement of the great vessels results in aneurysmal dilatation of the aorta, aortic root dilatation and insufficiency, and ultimately in some instances aortic dissection. Along with perioperative prothrombotic issues, antiphospholipid antibodies in SLE are associated with mitral valve nodules and significant mitral regurgitation, possibly due to valvular endothelial cell activation.[69]

Surgical risks in patients with valvular heart disease depend on the valve affected, as well as the nature and severity of the valvular lesion. The lesion conferring the highest perioperative risk is hemodynamically significant aortic stenosis, fortunately a relatively uncommon valvular lesion in the connective tissue diseases (although relatively prevalent in an aging surgical population). Mitral valve disease and aortic insufficiency, if not severe, are usually well tolerated, although any valvular disease associated with significant left ventricular dysfunction (New York Heart Association (NYHA) Class 3 or 4) increases the risk of surgery. Therefore, patients with a significant cardiac murmur, accompanied by signs or symptoms of left ventricular dysfunction, should undergo an echocardiographic assessment preoperatively, particularly if a major procedure is planned. Invasive hemodynamic monitoring perioperatively may be indicated in patients at higher risk.

Conduction abnormalities and arrhythmias

Although cardiac conduction system disease and arrhythmias are frequently a marker for underlying cardiac or pulmonary disease, metabolic abnormalities, or drug toxicity, they are more frequently seen in patients with the connective tissue diseases. This is especially true in scleroderma where myocardial fibrosis is believed to compromise the cardiac conduction system leading to heart block and a wide range of electrocardiographic abnormalities and arrhythmias.[62] Therefore when patients with this and other connective tissue diseases present preoperatively with apparent conduction problems, the clinician should search for such conditions and institute corrective action, if possible, before surgery.

A problem that arises with some frequency is **the patient with chronic atrial fibrillation on long-term anticoagulation.** Because the risk of embolic stroke in such patients who are not anticoagulated is low, it is safe to temporarily discontinue warfarin (Coumadin) for a sufficient period of time preoperatively to allow for normalization of the prothrombin time and international normalized rate (INR). Five days before surgery is generally sufficient and reinstitution on the night of surgery is safe and appropriate.

Pulmonary disease

Although the prevention and management of cardiac complications after surgery have received the most attention in the medical literature, postoperative pulmonary complications are frequent and important adverse events in the postoperative period.[70-73] One large study (1055 patients) has reported a 2.7% incidence of pulmonary complications in patients thought to be at low to moderate risk; patients developing such problems had a significantly longer length of stay (27.9 vs. 4.5 days).[74] Indeed, such problems as atelectasis, pneumonia, aspiration pneumonia, respiratory failure, and the exacerbation of chronic obstructive pulmonary disease (COPD) may have more severe consequences than cardiac disease and have been shown to be more predictive of long-term mortality.[75,76] Smokers have a 1.4- to 4.3-fold risk of postoperative pulmonary complications.[77] Chronic obstructive pulmonary disease is the most important patient-related factor predicting postoperative complications. Such patients have a 6% to 28% risk for the development of pulmonary complications after surgery.[68] Asthmatics are also at increased risk if their disease is not well controlled preoperatively. The implications of chronic pulmonary disease in the perioperative setting is further underscored by the increased prevalence of cardiovascular disease in these patients.

Chronic pulmonary disease can be divided into three categories: asthma, obstructive lung disease, and restrictive lung disease. Chronic obstructive lung disease (chronic bronchitis, emphysema) and asthma are the two most prevalent forms of chronic pulmonary disease and, as such, are the pulmonary problems seen most frequently in the preoperative setting. Characterized by a reduced forced expiratory volume in 1 second (FEV_1) coupled with a normal to increased lung capacity, these conditions are important predictors of postoperative pulmonary complications, which may be pulmonary or non-pulmonary. Minor pulmonary complications (atelectasis, bronchitis) are increased in patients who smoke, have a chronic cough, or have abnormal spirometry. The risk of severe postoperative pulmonary complications (pneumonia, respiratory failure) is increased mainly in those patients with marked impairment in lung function ($FEV_1 < 1.5$ liters).

Restrictive lung disease, although generally less common, deserves special mention owing to its prevalence in the connective tissue diseases. Defined by a symmetric decrease in FEV_1 and forced vital capacity (FVC), with a reduction in the total lung capacity (TLC), such restrictive patterns of lung spirometry are characteristic of the functional abnormality seen in such conditions as rheumatoid arthritis, polymyositis/dermatomyositis, and SLE.[78]

Risk factors for the development of postoperative pulmonary complications are divided into two categories: patient and procedure related.[72,79] Patient-related risk factors include such characteristics as age, existing chronic obstructive lung disease (COPD), cigarette use,

congestive heart failure (CHF), co-morbidities, functional capacity, obesity, sleep apnea, and cognitive impairment. In contrast, procedure-related risk factors include surgical site (increased complication rate in procedures near the diaphragm), duration of surgery, anesthetic technique, and emergency surgery. Although attempts to develop an overall pulmonary predictive risk index similar to the Goldman Cardiac Risk index (or its variants) have thus far been unsuccessful, two separate pulmonary risk indices have been published, one for the prediction of postoperative pneumonia[80] and another for respiratory failure occurring after surgery.[81]

Two other pulmonary-related conditions are increasingly recognized for their contribution to postoperative complications, sleep apnea and chronic pulmonary arterial hypertension. Sleep apnea syndrome is defined as greater than five apneic events (airflow stops for > 10 seconds despite continued respiratory effort) or more than 15 hypopneic events per hour (airflow lessens >50% for > 10 seconds) during a 7-hour sleep study. Although three types are recognized—obstructive (OSA), central, and mixed—it is usually the obstructive form that comes to light in the postoperative period.[82] Typically, morbidly obese patients with no documented history of the condition are observed in the recovery room to experience upper airway obstruction, suggesting the presence of the condition. Other physical characteristics associated with OSA include a neck circumference of 17 inches, craniofacial abnormalities affecting the airway, anatomic nasal obstruction, and tonsils touching in the midline. A preoperative interview is an efficient means of screening patients. The Berlin questionnaire, composed of 10 questions that pertain to risk factors for sleep apnea (snoring, wake time sleepiness/fatigue, hypertension), has been shown to be predictive of the condition.[83] These patients present a number of management difficulties, beginning with an often challenging airway and intubation and after surgery with such problems as hypoxemia, hypertension, atrial fibrillation, and heart failure. Pulmonary arterial hypertension (PAH) also may arise as a consequence of long-standing, untreated OSA.

An increasingly recognized challenge in the perioperative setting, PAH is also seen in association with connective tissue diseases, most often arising as a consequence of the pulmonary disease accompanying these conditions. Its association with such conditions as scleroderma and mixed connective tissue disease is well known to the rheumatologist. In the surgical setting PAH is an especially treacherous problem, challenging the medical and anesthesiologic management, and it is associated with substantial mortality.[84] A pathophysiologic state characterized by elevated right heart afterload, decreased venous return, reduced cardiac output, and deficient oxygen saturation,[85] PAH is categorized according to its underlying etiology: Primary pulmonary hypertension, or PAH, arises as a consequence of left heart disease, hypoxic pulmonary disorders (for instance, OSA), or chronic thromboembolic phenomenon.[86] The sustained elevations in pulmonary vascular resistance and pulmonary arterial pressure, coupled with impaired vascular reactivity, may result in significant systemic hypotension in the setting of anesthesia. The negative inotropic effects of some anesthetic agents may exacerbate this tendency and precipitate right heart failure. The adverse consequences arising on the left side of the circulation (systemic hypotension) are further exacerbated by concomitant right-sided responses, where the pulmonary vessels constrict in response to the resultant hypoxia promoting the development of hypercarbia, acidosis, hypothermia, and the release of catecholamines. If allowed to progress too far, this cascade of events may result in further hemodynamic deterioration and frank circulatory collapse.[81] Although new and effective vasodilator medications such as endothelin receptor antagonists and prostaglandins can significantly decrease the pulmonary artery pressures,[87] PAH no matter its underlying etiology is a potent risk factor for adverse outcomes after surgery. It demands a knowledgeable and collaborative group of physicians to make the correct cost-benefit decision with the patient.

The general risk of perioperative lung dysfunction depends, in large part, on the type of surgery performed. Patients with severe lung impairment can tolerate minor procedures, even under general anesthesia. The risk of pneumonia following major peripheral limb surgery (such as hip or knee surgery) is low, even in the patients with chronic lung disease. This is in marked contrast to intra-abdominal or intra-thoracic surgery, which is associated with a high risk of atelectasis or pneumonia in patients, particularly in patients with severe COPD.

Regional anesthesia for surgery on the extremities circumvents many of these problems. However, interscalene block may transiently paralyze the ipsilateral diaphragm and reduce the FVC by 30% to 40%.[14] Therefore patients with COPD undergoing shoulder surgery, in which interscalene block is frequently employed, should have pulmonary function studies performed preoperatively. In patients with severely impaired pulmonary function ($FEV_1 < 1$ liter), interscalene block should be avoided altogether. Patients with COPD fare well with this anesthesia, especially in the sitting position.

Patients who have been using **bronchodilators** on a chronic basis before surgery should be given their standard dosage the night before surgery; bronchodilator therapy should be administered postoperatively either systemically or by nebulizer. Incentive spirometry 10 times daily and early mobilization are helpful in the prevention of postoperative atelectasis.

Endocrine problems

Diabetes mellitus

Diabetes is the most important endocrine disorder encountered in surgical patients and in the postoperative setting should be regarded as placing the patient at higher risk for such complications as myocardial infarction, stroke, infection, and death.[88] Further, diabetics with autonomic insufficiency (manifested by postural hypotension, impotence, nocturnal diarrhea) may be at risk for sudden cardiopulmonary arrest postoperatively.[89] The importance of this chronic disease is underscored by its inclusion as one of the risk factors comprising the Revised Cardiac Risk Index. Given the high prevalence of coronary artery disease in diabetics, cardiovascular risk assessment is a focal point of the preoperative evaluation of these patients and should be approached as outlined in the section dealing with patients with established cardiac disease or those deemed at risk due to their clinical profile. Otherwise, the principal perioperative consideration is the management of the underlying metabolic disease (i.e., *glycemic* control).

The achievement and maintenance of good glycemic control in the surgical setting is often challenging. Owing to a complex interplay of factors, the stimulatory effects of anesthesia and surgery enhance the production of counter-regulatory hormones such as glucagon, epinephrine, cortisol, and corticotrophin while decreasing the endogenous production of insulin. These responses, coupled with an increase in lipolysis and ketogenesis and the often poor caloric intake after surgery, result in significant derangements of overall glycemic control, the net tendency of which is to drive the blood sugars higher. Although the value of tight glucose control in the surgical setting has not been definitively established, an important clinical trial on this problem has been reported. In this study, Van den Berghe and colleagues have shown that, in critically ill surgical patients, tight glucose control may reduce postoperative mortality by one third.[90] Nonetheless, a recently published meta-analysis concerning tight glucose control in the critically ill patient failed to show benefit (reduced mortality, new dialysis), while such treatment increased the risk of hypoglycemia.[91] Thus although some controversy persists about the advantages of good control in the perioperative setting, three primary observations lend support to this practice. First, many diabetics are at high risk in the surgical setting and efforts to reduce these risks are justified. Second, it is a common clinical problem—an estimated 25% of diabetics will require surgery in the course of their lifetime. Third, in the perioperative setting good glycemic control may reduce the rate of wound infection, vascular complications, and death. Nonetheless, clinical trials report that 40% to 80% of blood sugar determinations fall outside the target range,[92-94] so achieving good control is hard to do.[95]

The clinical considerations important to perioperative decision-making in the diabetic are protean.[96] Added to the routine assessments employed in the non-diabetic are such considerations as the long-term (end-organ) complications of this disorder (micro- and macrovascular, neuropathic) with particular attention to cardiovascular and renal disease. Although the importance of optimal preoperative glycemic control has not been clarified, it is important to characterize the type of diabetes (types 1 and 2), determine the specifics of the patient's treatment (medications, timing of and adherence to therapy), and determine the degree of glycemic control. The occurrence and frequency of hypoglycemia should also be ascertained. A clear understanding of the nature and magnitude of the type of surgery to be performed is also important.

In general the goal of therapy is the maintenance of the glucose level between 150 and 200 mg/dL during surgery in order to protect against hypoglycemia. Numerous regimens have been recommended for the management of the diabetic in the perioperative setting[91] and the approach employed is influenced significantly by the type and severity of the patient's diabetes. Regardless of the severity of the disease, however, management should be proactive as opposed to reactive. Whenever possible, diabetics should be scheduled as one of the early cases of the day in order to avoid prolonged periods of fast on the day of surgery. For patients treated with oral agents, these medications are usually given on the day before surgery and then held postoperatively until the patient is tolerating oral intake postoperatively. For insulin-dependent patients, the patient's usual insulin regimen should be continued. Type 1 diabetics should take a fractional amount (1/3 to 1/2 their usual dosage) of their long-acting insulin on the morning of surgery. Type 2 diabetics should take none to one third of their dosage, whereas those patients managed with an insulin pump should continue at their basal rate of insulin infusion.

During the immediate postoperative period, blood sugars may be unstable and difficult to control. As such, divided doses of intermediate-acting (twice daily) or short-acting insulin (usually four to six daily) can be supplemented by the subcutaneous administration according to a predetermined algorithm. Such an approach is maintained until the patient's oral intake is fully re-established. A different regimen is indicated for patients taking **oral hypoglycemic agents:** these medications can be taken the day before surgery and resumed when the patient is eating. Continuous insulin infusions are occasionally employed postoperatively in the patient with severe, brittle disease.

Chronic corticosteroid therapy

Because many rheumatic disease patients take corticosteroids, prophylaxis against adrenal insufficiency and management of the patient's

---

BOX 67.1 PREOPERATIVE ASSESSMENT OF THE SURGICAL CANDIDATE WITH DIABETES MELLITUS

Operative risk assessment
   Routine risk factors
      Cardiac
      Pulmonary
      Renal
      Hematologic
   Diabetes-related risk factors
      Macrovascular complications
      Microvascular complications
      Neuropathic complications
Diabetes therapeutic regimen
   Reestablish correct diagnostic classification of diabetes
   Pharmacologic regimen
      Medication type
      Dosage
      Timing
   Meal plan
      Carbohydrate content
      Timing of meals
   Activity level
   Hypoglycemia
      Frequency
      Awareness
      Severity
Anticipated surgery
   Type of surgical procedure
   Inpatient or outpatient
   Type of anesthesia
   Start time
   Duration of procedure

From Jacober SJ, Sowers JR. An update on perioperative management of diabetes. Arch Int Med 1999;159:2405-2411.

TABLE 67.4 RECOMMENDATIONS FOR PERIOPERATIVE GLUCOCORTICOID COVERAGE

Surgical stress	Target hydrocortisone equivalent	Preoperative steroid dose	Intraoperative steroid dose	Postoperative steroid dose*	Postoperative steroid dose day 1*	Postoperative steroid dose day 2*
Minor (e.g., inguinal herniorrhaphy)	25 mg/day for 1 day	Usual daily dose of steroid	None[†]	None[†]	Usual daily dose[†]	
Moderate (e.g., colon resection, total joint replacement, lower extremity revascularization)	50-75 mg/day for 1-2 days	Usual daily dose of steroid	50 mg hydrocortisone	20 mg hydrocortisone every 8 hr	20 mg hydrocortisone every 8 hr	
Major (e.g., pancreatoduodenectomy, esophagectomy)	100-150 mg/day for 2-3 days	Usual daily dose of steroid	50 mg hydrocortisone	50 mg hydrocortisone every 8 hr	50 mg hydrocortisone every 8 hr	50 mg hydrocortisone every 8 hr

*If postoperative complications occur, continued glucocorticoid administration will be necessary commensurate with the level of stress. From Salem M, Tainsh RE, Bromberg J, et al. Perioperative glucocorticoid coverage. A reassessment 42 years after emergence of a problem. Ann Surg 1994;219:416-425.
[†]If the postoperative course is uncomplicated, patients can resume their usual steroid dose on postoperative day 1.
From Sweitzer BJ. Preoperative assessment and management. Philadelphia: Wolters Kluwer Lippincott Williams & Wilkins, 2008, p 409.

corticosteroid therapy in the perioperative setting are critically important. Five to 7.5 mg daily of prednisone approximates the normal daily adrenal output of cortisol (30 mg). Patients believed to be at increased risk for adrenal insufficiency include those currently taking more than 20 mg prednisone daily for longer than 3 weeks, those who have taken such doses for more than 2 weeks in the preceding year, and those who are receiving replacement corticosteroid therapy for known adrenal insufficiency. Although surgery may produce sufficient "stress" to provoke adrenal insufficiency, surgeries vary in the amount of stress they produce and the circulating cortisol concentration usually normalizes within 24 to 48 hours in most patients after surgery.[97] Thus the amount of supplementation should depend on the anticipated degree of stress (a function of the duration and severity of the surgical procedure) and the chronic daily steroid dose. Table 67.4 provides recommendations for perioperative glucocorticoid coverage according to the magnitude of the surgery to be performed.

Gastrointestinal disease

Gastrointestinal problems, both exacerbations of chronic conditions or problems arising *de novo*, may complicate the postoperative period and produce significant morbidity. Among the most common of these is the development of postoperative nausea and vomiting (PONV), a problem that arises in 20% to 30% of patients after surgery.[98] An outcome rated by patients to be among the 10 most undesirable consequences of surgery,[99] PONV is believed to be multifactorial in etiology with an array of patient, surgical, and anesthetic factors contributing to the development of this problem.[100] Patient factors most often cited as risk factors include female sex, need for opioids for postoperative pain, and a history of motion sickness or PONV with prior surgery. The presence of none, one, two, three, or four such risk factors is associated with an incidence of 10%, 21%, 39%, 61%, or 79%, respectively.[101] Such difficulties often herald the onset of more significant problems, specifically that of postoperative abdominal ileus.

The impairment of gastrointestinal (GI) motility after surgery is a relatively common postoperative complication, albeit not one restricted to patients with chronic gastroenterologic problems. Characterized by constipation, the accumulation of gas and fluids in the bowel with the development of abdominal distention, and intolerance to enteral feeding, postoperative ileus is generally a self-limited condition lasting 3 to 5 days.[102] Perturbations in GI motility after surgery arise from a number of adverse influences arising in the postoperative period. Some of these are external such as narcotic analgesia and anesthesia, the fasting state, and the reintroduction of oral feeding. Others can be considered internal or physiologic responses to surgery. Such influences include surgery-related increases in sympathetic nervous system tone, the hypothalamic release of corticotrophin-releasing factor, and the release of nitric oxide, all of which have a negative influence on the motility of the GI tract. As a preventive maneuver, careful consideration should be given to the optimal timing for the resumption of oral intake of both liquids and solids, and **potent narcotic therapy should be weaned down as quickly as possible,** particularly in patients with chronic GI complaints and conditions. Early mobilization is also believed to be an effective preventive strategy.[97] A number of pharmacologic approaches are also commonly required in order to resolve such problems. These include the use of agents acting on the autonomic nervous system (bethanechol, carbachol, methacholine) and more recently the role of cholinesterase inhibitors such as neostigmine.[103] The latter is generally reserved for severe cases of adynamic ileus with massive dilatation of the colon in the absence of mechanical obstruction (Ogilvie syndrome), a highly threatening complication with an attendant mortality of 50%.[104,105] For motility problems that are more directly a consequence of postoperative narcotic therapy, the μ-opioid-receptor antagonist methylnaltrexone (Relistor) has recently been approved and may be useful in the postoperative setting.[106] A simple and novel preventive approach is the use of chewing gum as a stimulant of GI motility in the postoperative setting.[107]

Other GI conditions may also present in the postoperative period. Intestinal volvulus is usually seen in patients with a history of abdominal surgery, chronic diverticular disease that may flare in the postoperative setting, and even colon cancer, which may declare itself at this time. Indeed, all three may mimic and present as abdominal ileus. A fourth and important consideration is the development of *Clostridium difficile*–induced colitis.[108] Owing to an increasing prevalence of this organism in the population and the subsequent colonization of hospitals (a direct consequence of the widespread use of antibiotics), severe infectious colitis has been increasingly seen in the postoperative period, a setting in which patients are potentially debilitated and highly vulnerable. *C. difficile*–induced colitis may be asymptomatic, present with diarrhea alone (without colitis), or as acute pseudomembranous colitis progressing to life-threatening toxic megacolon. Treatment requires aggressive fluid support and the institution of oral antibiotic therapy, either metronidazole (250 mg qid) or vancomycin (125 mg qid). More resistant cases have been recently described[109] and new antibiotics are available for those patients unresponsive to the previously mentioned medical therapy. Rarely, in the most severe of cases, surgery including total colectomy may be required. As simple a prevention measure as handwashing can significantly decrease the transfer of this organism from patient to patient.

Peptic ulcer disease, a reasonably common problem in the orthopedic/rheumatic disease population due to the high usage of non-steroidal anti-inflammatory agents and steroids, may become active after surgery; it is particularly problematic in patients who require anticoagulation prophylaxis such as those who have undergone total joint arthroplasty. Therefore, **patients with a history of peptic ulcer disease, GI bleeding, or active dyspepsia should receive a prophylactic proton pump inhibitor or H₂ blocker throughout the postoperative period.** In the presence of a strong clinical suspicion that an active peptic process is ongoing, the surgery should be canceled, a work-up performed, and treatment instituted before proceeding. In patients at risk for the development of GI bleeding after surgery, serial stool guaiacs are a good surveillance approach.

Genitourinary conditions

As a consequence of bed rest, the use of narcotics and epidural anesthesia, and the presence of prostate disease, urinary catheters are frequently placed in patients after major surgery. In general, such **catheters should be removed as early as possible and a surveillance urine culture performed to rule out the development of a urinary tract infection.** If urinary catheters are removed within 48 hours of surgery and urinary retention is avoided, the risk of urinary tract infection is small.

Prostatic hypertrophy leading to urinary outflow obstruction is a common problem in men after surgery. In patients with significant chronic symptomatology, urologic consultation should be obtained before surgery and therapy (including transurethral resection of the prostate) performed, if deemed necessary. In patients with a propensity to urinary retention and those with enlarged prostate glands who report obstructive symptomatology, therapy with agents such as terazosin (Hytrin) and tamsulosin (Flomax) could be instituted before or at the time of surgery. In patients with a history of nephrolithiasis, dehydration should be rigorously avoided to help prevent development of acute renal colic.

Prevention of postoperative infection

The risk of infection in a prosthetic joint is of great concern in patients undergoing total joint arthroplasty. Efforts to prevent and detect any infectious processes preoperatively and postoperatively are of utmost importance. The skin and urinary tract are sites of specific concern, and infection can be ruled out by a careful physical examination and routine preoperative urine culture. In addition, formal dental consultation may be appropriate in patients with poor oral hygiene and dentition.

Prophylactic antibiotic therapy for total joint arthroplasty patients should begin less than 2 hours before surgery and continue for 24 hours. The recommended protocol at Hospital for Special Surgery involves cefazolin (Ancef) 1 g every 8 hours (total of three doses) or, in penicillin-allergic patients, vancomycin 1 g every 12 hours (total of two doses).

Neurologic problems

Postoperative delirium

Delirium, an acute confusional state most often seen in the setting of systemic illness, may arise in the postoperative period, particularly in the elderly.[110] Characterized by an alteration in the level of consciousness, a diminished ability to maintain and focus attention, often with hallucinations, delusions, and agitation, it may have a diurnal variation (onset of and more severe at night) and an unpredictable duration.[111] Patients are at increased risk for the development of delirium after surgery due to a confluence of factors arising in this clinical setting. These risk factors include acute infections, drug (psychoactive, analgesia, anesthetic) and alcohol toxicity or withdrawal, dehydration, fluid/electrolyte/metabolic disturbances, and states of low perfusion (heart failure and shock). The incidence of this problem is high in some postoperative settings. For example, in patients undergoing emergent surgical repair of a fractured hip, 37% of the nondemented patients have been reported to develop postoperative delirium.[112] The significance of this finding is underscored by the observation that among those who experienced delirium after surgery, 69% developed frank dementia over a subsequent 5-year period of follow-up (as compared with a 20% incidence in those without postoperative delirium). Further, Monk and colleagues have recently reported that patients with postoperative cognitive dysfunction at discharge were more likely to die within the first year after surgery.[113]

Although acute delirium is usually a transient phenomenon, clinicians should focus on the detection and treatment of correctable causes that may present in this fashion, particularly in the geriatric patient population. Such causes include metabolic disturbances (hyponatremia, hypoxemia); medications (which might be discontinued); infection; and various acute conditions (e.g., respiratory failure, myocardial infarction, cardiac arrhythmias, congestive heart failure, pulmonary embolism and fat embolism syndrome). Likewise, elderly patients and patients with underlying neurologic dysfunction (e.g., alcoholism, Parkinsonism) are at increased risk for postoperative delirium. Formal neurologic consultation and workup is occasionally necessary though generally unrevealing. Specific alcohol withdrawal protocols should be developed and employed because the overall mortality is higher in these patients. A significant reduction in the incidence of postoperative delirium through proactive geriatric consultation has also been reported.[114]

Peripheral nerve injuries

Peripheral nerve injuries arise more often after upper and lower extremity surgery because they are generally a result of excessive traction on the nerve. Alternatively, they arise as a consequence of nerve compression resulting from prolonged positioning of the extremity during surgery or as a result of a cast. Early detection and intervention are critical to the ultimate outcome in these circumstances. Patients with antecedent neurologic disease like neuropathies in diabetics or spinal stenosis are at increased risk of nerve injury.

Emotional/psychiatric problems

Patients who live with the consequences of chronic rheumatic diseases or disabling orthopedic conditions may suffer emotional difficulties due to chronic pain, disability, impaired social interactions and personal relationships, and constrained career opportunities. Because surgery is a significant life stress, such individuals may require additional emotional support perioperatively. Further, some patients may be taking or require antidepressant or antianxiolytic medication. In the relatively rare patient who is being treated with monoamine oxidase inhibitors, it is recommended that the medication be discontinued 10 to 14 days before surgery and the anesthesiologist alerted to the situation. Patients on these agents are at risk of marked circulatory instability with general anesthesia and certain narcotics, especially meperidine.

Management of specific clinical problems

Specific clinical problems that may be encountered and benefit from perioperative management are discussed here roughly in order of how often they are encountered.

Venous thromboembolism

Prevention of venous thromboembolic phenomenon after orthopedic surgery is the most thoroughly studied of potential postoperative complications.[115-117] Pulmonary embolism, perhaps the most dreaded complication of orthopedic surgery, remains an important cause of postoperative mortality.[118] Although most of the prodigious literature on this problem in the orthopedic surgery literature has concentrated on lower extremity arthroplasty, a recent study suggests that these treatment paradigms should also be considered after total shoulder arthroplasty, in which the risk of thromboembolism may be higher than generally appreciated.[119]

Every surgery sets up some degree of a prothrombotic state and thus it is not *whether* prophylaxis is considered, but *which one*. In the setting of orthopedic surgery, a complicated balance exists between a possible life-threatening pulmonary embolus and potential bleeding of such a degree as to compromise the surgical outcome. Numerous protocols have documented efficiency in minimizing this risk. Prevention begins at the time of the procedure. Expeditious surgery reduces the risk of deep venous thrombosis following operations such as total hip replacement. The type of anesthesia employed is also important; epidural anesthesia reduces the risk of proximal deep venous thrombosis following total hip replacement by twofold to threefold and also reduces the overall risk of deep venous thrombosis by at least 20%.[120] Other intraoperative interventions, such as hypotensive anesthesia and intraoperative heparin administration, further reduce thrombogenesis.[121]

Mechanical methods of reducing the risk of thromboembolism also have proven efficacy and include pneumatic compression boots, foot pumps, compression stockings, foot flexion/extension exercises, and early ambulation. These maneuvers are safe and effective and do not increase the risk of bleeding.[122] However, the mainstay of treatment is some form of anticoagulation. Prophylactic anticoagulation is begun immediately following surgery. Regimens include aspirin, Coumadin with a target INR of 2.0 to 2.5, low-molecular-weight (LMW) heparin, and even newer medications on the horizon.[123-125] Aspirin is also effective when combined with other modalities and continues to have its proponents, particularly in low-risk patients. A multimodal approach, relying on a combination of intraoperative modalities, postoperative mechanical devices, early ambulation, and low-intensity postoperative anticoagulation, is preferred for the majority of patients by most experts and clinicians.[126,127]

Fat embolism syndrome

The embolization of fat in the circulation is a well-described complication of skeletal trauma and surgery, as well as procedures involving instrumentation of the femoral medullary canal.[128] Although the embolization of fat occurs in almost all patients who sustain hip or femoral fractures, the development of frank fat embolism syndrome (FES) occurs in relatively few. One to 3% of patients undergoing joint replacement surgery (particularly simultaneous bilateral procedures in which it is presumably a "dose" effect) and 5% to 10% of patients who have sustained multiple long bone fractures[129] develop FES.

The signs and symptoms of FES involve the respiratory, neurologic, hematologic, and cutaneous systems. **Time of onset is variable;** hemodynamic instability may develop **almost immediately** (presaged by a rise in pulmonary artery pressure when the prosthesis is cemented) **or more insidiously over the first 2 to 3 postoperative days.** In the latter group, it is often unclear what is happening early on because patients gradually become moderately to severely hypoxemic after surgery, may be hypotensive, and, in the case of the elderly, often become confused. Hematologic abnormalities such as transient thrombocytopenia are commonly seen. Respiratory signs are the most common manifestation of FES. The majority of patients develop mild to moderate hypoxemia, some radiographic changes (mainly bilateral alveolar infiltrates), and only a minority will develop a life-threatening adult respiratory distress syndrome (ARDS) and require aggressive supportive measures and intubation. Neurologic manifestations range from mild drowsiness to an acute confusional state to severe obtundation and coma, all consequences of the associated hypoxemia and the direct effect of the embolization of fat on the brain.[130] The skin eruption, which is rare in the total joint arthroplasty patient, takes the form of a petechial rash involving the conjunctiva and oral mucosa and distributed over the folds of the neck and axillae. Retinal edema and hemorrhage are common.

The pathophysiology of FES remains unclear, although it is thought to involve mechanical and/or biochemical factors. The mechanical theory states that in circumstances in which intramedullary pressure exceeds venous pressure, fat globules will be embolized, ultimately logging in the pulmonary capillary bed. As a consequence of these events, pulmonary hypertension develops, opening the foramen ovale and allowing for the passage of the fat globules into the arterial circulation. These globules then lodge in the cerebral, retinal, and dermal capillaries, producing their end-organ effects. Alternatively, the biochemical theory states that the embolized fat globules initiate an inflammatory response producing the adverse clinical phenomenon associated with this condition. These theories are not mutually exclusive. Indeed, these pathophysiologic mechanisms may be acting in concert.[109,131] Further interesting observations concerning age-related factors and specifically marrow fat also have pathophysiologic implications. Owing to differences in the lipid composition of the adult bone marrow (olein), FES is less common in children whose primary marrow-derived lipids of palmitin and stearin are less likely to produce emboli.[132]

Although patients suspected to have developed FES need to be closely monitored, in most instances such embolic events are generally clinically benign. Treatment is supportive and includes the administration of increased concentrations of inspired oxygen (possibly via ventilator), the prevention of pulmonary hypertension by fluid restriction and the use of diuretics and venodilators, and the control of pain. **Corticosteroid therapy has not been demonstrated to be of benefit and is not recommended.** In the majority of patients, the condition resolves within 3 to 7 days, although in severe cases the mortality rate has remained in the 5% to 15% range even with modern aggressive therapy.[133]

Antiphospholipid syndrome

Antiphospholipid syndrome (APS) is a condition consisting of vascular thrombosis (and/or pregnancy-related morbidity) arising as a conse-

quence of the presence of antiphospholipid antibodies (aPL), most often the lupus anticoagulant or anticardiolipin antibodies.[134] This syndrome may exist in a primary form, unassociated with an underlying connective tissue disease. It is considered secondary when it arises in the setting of such conditions as systemic lupus erythematosus. As a consequence of their general hypercoagulability, patients with APS who require surgery are at increased risk of postoperative thrombosis. Their need for long-term anticoagulation results in challenges in perioperative management, specifically managing the often delicate balance between the patient's propensity to thrombosis against the risk of postoperative bleeding due to the need for anticoagulation.

Although fraught with potential risk, surgery may be necessary in patients with APS and recommendations have been published from which to guide medical management.[135] First, the important, adjunctive role of physical methods in the prevention of venous thrombosis should not be forgotten. Therefore such methods as intermittent venous compression should be aggressively employed preoperatively and postoperatively. Second, the perioperative period without anticoagulation should be kept to a minimum. Thus for patients on chronic Coumadin therapy, the medication should be stopped 3 to 4 days before surgery to allow for normalization of the INR, while concomitant therapy with LMW heparin instituted at therapeutic dosages (1 mg per kg, every 12 hours) and continued until the night before surgery, when it should be stopped. For many surgical procedures, particularly orthopedic surgery, Coumadin can be restarted the night of the surgical procedure. If there is no contraindication, LMW heparin in prophylactic dosages (30 mg, every 12 hours) can be restarted simultaneously with Coumadin and maintained until a therapeutic INR has been achieved. It should be remembered that conventional dosages of these agents may result in "undercoagulation" of patients with APS and larger dosages, if feasible, may be considered necessary postoperatively, irrespective of the bleeding risk such therapy confers.

Given the frequent use of epidural and spinal anesthesia in patients undergoing orthopedic surgery, the risk of epidural and spinal hematoma as a complication of such anesthesia should be noted. The avoidance of this serious complication is, in part, the rationale for the omitting of the heparin dose the night before surgery. In addition, at our institution heparin is not restarted until at least 4 hours after the removal of the epidural/spinal needle.

Hip fracture

Hundreds of thousands of patients are admitted to hospital in the United States annually for treatment of a fractured hip, resulting in major costs to society, patients, and their families.[136-138] Within the first year of fracture, 20% of elderly hip fracture patients die, compared with 9% of age-matched, non-fracture patients. Further, one sixth of patients who survive 1 year after fracture are confined to long-term care facilities, while another one third continue to require assistive devices or the help of others to manage their daily activities. Therefore after a fracture of the hip, most patients experience permanent impairment in functional capacity and the rates of permanent institutionalization are high. Risk factors thought to increase the need for nursing home placement include living alone before the fracture, having no children, and female gender.

The majority of hip fractures occur in frail, elderly women with osteoporosis who have sustained a fall. Indeed, falls are the most common antecedent event in these circumstances, and fractures are the most common serious fall-related injury. Risk factors for hip fracture include increasing age, poor general health, maternal history of hip fracture, a history of thyroid disease, poor depth perception, the use of psychoactive medication, sedentary lifestyle, and major life events.[139]

Femoral neck and intertrochanteric fractures occur at approximately equal frequencies and, in order to restore patient mobility and functional status, most will require surgical intervention.[124] Although a matter of ongoing debate, more severe (i.e., displaced) intracapsular femoral neck fractures are often treated with joint replacement because they may result in a serious compromise to the blood supply of the femoral head leading to osteonecrosis, collapse of the femoral head, and secondary osteoarthritis.[140-143] Internal fixation is the usual surgical approach to displaced femoral neck fractures. However, in the frail, elderly patient with lower anticipated functional requirements and life expectancy, such fractures may be treated with total joint arthroplasty as well.

The preoperative medical assessment and care of the patient with a fractured hip is challenging. Owing to the patient's age, frailty and functional compromise, existing co-morbidities, and the poorer outcome when surgery is delayed,[144,145] the opportunity to optimally evaluate and prepare such patients before surgery is constrained and by necessity relies more on general principles of perioperative care. Published evidence suggests that preoperative cardiac stress testing results in very low rates of formal cardiac intervention and is not helpful in this setting.[146] Given the perioperative care demands such patients impose, clinical pathways[124,147] and other integrated co-management (medical-surgical) approaches have been reported both for hip fracture[148] and total joint arthroplasty.[149] The experience with such approaches has been variable, although improvement in outcomes have been observed with such strategies in terms of length of stay, postoperative complications and mortality, late readmission to hospital, and with respect to functional recovery. One study employing proactive geriatric consultation reports a significant reduction in the incidence of postoperative delirium.[116]

Difficult neck

Some patients with rheumatoid arthritis, generally those with advanced and aggressive disease, may manifest significant cervical spine involvement with instability arising from atlantoaxial or subaxial subluxation. This complication presents both important risks to the patient undergoing surgery and significant challenges for the anesthesiologist, particularly if endotracheal intubation is required. These patients have an increased risk for cord compression during intubation or from uncontrolled neck movement during positioning for surgery.

Cervical spine instability should be ruled out before surgery with flexion/extension films in those patients with neck pain or crepitus on range-of-motion testing, radicular symptoms, and arm or leg weakness. Affected patients should wear a soft cervical collar to the operating room, both for neck immobilization and as a warning to all involved not to overmanipulate the neck. When possible, epidural or spinal anesthesia should be employed.

Additional problems arising from the rheumatoid disease process include involvement of the temporomandibular joint, which may limit jaw opening, and arthritis of the cricoarytenoid joints. Because these problems may also influence the choice of airway management, the anesthesiologist should be informed preoperatively about these manifestations of the disease process as well.

The converse situation arises in patients with ankylosing spondylitis, in whom their rigid cervical spine may also present technical challenges for the anesthesiologist during intubation. In this setting a fiberoptic method is often employed in this clinical context.

Immunosuppressive/anti-inflammatory therapy

The potential contribution of corticosteroids and other disease-modifying antirheumatic drugs (DMARDS) to the genesis of postoperative infection and wound dehiscence have been long recognized by clinicians, although a consensus regarding how to manage these medications in the perioperative setting has proven elusive.[150,151] The primary challenge in this context is to achieve an optimal balance between the maintenance of control of the underlying disease while minimizing the risk of postoperative wound infection and/or wound breakdown.[152-154] Animal studies on wound healing[155-158] and clinical investigation concerning postoperative infection[159-161] have produced conflicting data. Nonetheless, a number of studies and opinion papers have recently been published and two international groups have formulated recommendations on the basis of their accrued experience. These include the guidelines of the Club Rhumatismes et Inflammations (CRI) in France[162,163] and the recommendations of the British Society for Rheumatology (BSR).[164] Both groups recommend the discontinuation of anti–tumor necrosis factor agents for short periods of time before surgery, generally in the range of 2 to 4 weeks. The French favor the longer 4-week interval for infliximab and adalimumab due to the longer half-lives of these agents. There is virtually no information concerning postoperative infection and wound healing with the newer agents such as anakinra, rituximab, and abatacept.[117] Recommendations similar to those of the other biologics will therefore have to suffice until more data can be gathered. Further, patient-related considerations should also be taken into account and influence decision-making. For example, in patients undergoing minor surgical procedures with an associated low risk of infection, the continuation of treatment through the perioperative period might be reasonable. However, even in these surgical settings, other patient-specific characteristics such as diabetes or chronic corticosteroid use would argue for an adherence to the previously mentioned guidelines.

Integument

As a result of chronic therapy (i.e., corticosteroids, immunosuppressive agents) or as a manifestation (i.e., decubitus ulceration) of the debilitating consequences of underlying rheumatic disease or orthopedic condition, skin integrity may be compromised before and after procedures in patients undergoing orthopedic surgery. In addition, delayed wound healing and a propensity to infection may result from these influences. The early institution of preventive measures to combat the development of decubitus ulcers (particularly of the heels and buttock region) is vital to an uncomplicated postoperative course.

Eye

Patients taking chronic optic medication should have their eye drops instilled before surgery, especially if a prolonged procedure is anticipated. The one exception to this recommendation involves the use of phosphodiesterase inhibitors in the treatment of glaucoma. These agents may prolong the action of the neuromuscular blocker succinylcholine. This is particularly pertinent in patients with Sjögren syndrome who require artificial tears to prevent perioperative conjunctival injury.

Patients in the prone position are at risk for ocular injury secondary to external pressure. Patients with underlying vasculitis of the optic vessels are at particular risk of ischemic injury to the eye. Thus the anesthesiologist must take particular care to position the patient carefully, avoiding excessive pressure on the eye, and provide appropriate eye protection.

KEY REFERENCES

1. Newman MF, Fleisher LA, Fink MP. Perioperative medicine: managing for outcome. Philadelphia: Saunders Elsevier, 2008.

3. Sweitzer BJ. Preoperative assessment and management. Philadelphia: Wolters Kluwer Lippincott Williams & Wilkins, 2008.

4. MacKenzie CR, Sharrock N. Perioperative care of the patient with rheumatic disease. In: Paget S, Gibofsky A, Beary JF, et al, eds. Manual of rheumatology and outpatient orthopedic disorders: diagnosis and treatment, 5th ed. Philadelphia: Lippincott Williams & Wilkins, 2006.

5. MacKenzie CR, Sharrock NE. Perioperative medical considerations in patients with rheumatoid arthritis. Rheum Clin N Am 1998;24:1-17.

19. Macpherson DS, Snow R, Logren RP. Preoperative screening: value of previous tests. Ann Intern Med 1990;113:969-973.

20. Smetana GW, Macpherson DS. The case against routine preoperative laboratory testing. Med Clin N Am 2003;87:7-40.

25. Prause G, Ratzenhofer-Comenda B, Pierer G, et al. Can ASA grade or Goldman's cardiac risk index predict peri-operative mortality? A study of 16,227 patients. Anaesthesia 1997;52:203-206.

26. Saklad M. Grading of patients for surgical procedures. Anesthesiology 1941;2:73-89.

27. Keats AS. The ASA Classification of physical status-a recapitulation. Anesthesiology 1978; 49:233.

28. Goldman L, Caldera DL, Nussbaum SR, et al. Multifactorial index of cardiac risk in noncardiac surgical procedures. N Engl J Med 1977;297:845-850.

29. Detsky A, Abrams H, McLaughlin J, et al. Predicting cardiac complications in patients undergoing non-cardiac surgery. J Gen Intern Med 1986;1:211-219.

31. Lee HT, Marcantonio ER, Mangione CM, et al. Derivation and prospective validation of a simple index for prediction of cardiac risk of major noncardiac surgery. Circulation 1999;100:1043-1049.

32. Holt N, Silverman DG. Modeling perioperative risk: can numbers speak louder than words? Anesthesiol Clin N Am 2006;24:427-459.

33. Memtsoudis SG, Besculides MC, Reid S, et al. Trends in bilateral total knee arthroplasties. 153,259 Discharges

34. Memtsoudis SG, Yan M, Gonzalez Della Valle A, et al. Perioperative outcomes after unilateral and bilateral total knee arthroplasty. Anesthesiology 2009. Accepted for publication.

35. Urban MK. Anesthesia for Orthopedic Surgery. In: Miller RD, Eriksson LI, Fleisher LA, et al, eds. Miller's Anesthesia, 7th edition. Philadelphia: Elsevier, 2009.

39. Rodgers A, Walker N, Schug S, et al. Reduction in postoperative mortality and morbidity with epidural or spinal anesthesia: results from overview of randomized trials. BMJ 2000;321:1-12.

45. Fleisher LA, Beckman JA, Brown KA, et al. ACC/AHA 2007 guidelines on perioperative cardiovascular evaluation and care for noncardiac surgery: a report of the American College of Cardiology/American Heart Association Task Force on Practice Guidelines. J Am Coll Cardiol 2007;50:e159-e242.

48. Beattie WS, Abelnaem E, Wijeysundera DN, et al. A meta-analytic comparison of preoperative stress echocardiography and nuclear scintigraphy imaging. Anesth Anal 2006;102:8-16.

49. Mangano DT, Layug B, Tateo I, et al. Effect of atenolol on mortality and cardiovascular morbidity after noncardiac surgery. Multicenter Study of Perioperative Ischemia Research Group. N Engl J Med 1996;335:1713-1720.

51. Poldermans D, Boersma E, Bax JJ, et al. The effect of bisoprolol on perioperative mortality and myocardial infarction in high-risk patients undergoing vascular surgery. Dutch Echocardiographic Cardiac Risk Evaluation. Applying Stress Echocardiography Study Group. N Engl J Med 1999;341:1789-1794.

52. Devereaux PJ, Yang H, Yusuf S, et al. POISE Study Group. Effects of extended-release metoprolol succinate in patients undergoing non-cardiac surgery (POISE trial): a randomized controlled trial. Lancet 2008;371:1839-1847.

55. Kaluza GL, Joseph J, Lee JR, et al. Catastrophic outcomes of non-cardiac surgery soon after coronary stenting. J Am Coll Cardiol 2000;35:1288-1294.

57. Schouten O, van Domburg RT, Bax JJ, et al. Noncardiac surgery after coronary stenting: early surgery and the interruption of antiplatelet therapy are associated with an increase in major adverse cardiac events. J Am Coll Cardiol 2007;49:122-124.

59. Hindler K, Shaw AD, Samuels J, et al. Improved postoperative outcomes associated with preoperative statin therapy. Anesthesiology 2006;105:1260-1272.

60. Durazzo AE, Machada FS, Ikeoka DT, et al. Reduction in cardiovascular events after vascular surgery with atorvastatin: a randomized trial. J Vasc Surg 2004;39:967-975.

62. Roman MH, Salmon J. Cardiovascular manifestations of rheumatologic disease. Circulation 2007;116:2346-2355.

63. Hollenberg M, Mangano DT, Browner WS, et al. Predictors of post-operative myocardial ischemia in patients undergoing noncardiac surgery. The Study of Perioperative Ischemia Research Group. JAMA 1992;268:205-209.

65. Coblyn J, O'Gara PT. The heart in rheumatic disease, 3rd ed. In: Hochberg MC, Silman AJ, Smolen JS, et al, eds. Rheumatology. St Louis: Mosby Elsevier.

66. Guedes C, Bianchi-Flor P, Cormier B, et al. Cardiac manifestation of rheumatoid arthritis: a case-controlled transesophageal echocardiography study in 30 patients. Arthritis Care Res 2001;45:129-135.

67. Bergfeldt L. HLA-B27 associated cardiac disease. Ann Intern Med 1997;127:621-629.

69. Farzaneh-Far A, Roman MJ, Lockshin MD, Devereux RB, et al. Relationship of antiphospholipid antibodies to cardiovascular manifestations of systemic lupus erythematosus. Arthritis Rheum 2006;54:3918-3925.

70. Smetana GW, Lawrence MD, Cornell JE. Preoperative pulmonary risk stratification for noncardiothoracic surgery: systematic review for the American College of Physicians. Ann Intern Med 2006;144:581-595.

77. Smetana GW. Preoperative pulmonary evaluation. N Engl J Med 1999;340:937-944.

80. Arozullah AM, Khuri SF, Henderson WG, Daley J. Development and validation of a multifactorial risk index for predicting postoperative pneumonia after major noncardiac surgery. Ann Intern Med 2001;135:847-857.

81. Arozullah AM, Daley J, Henderson WG, Khuri SF. Multifactorial risk index for prediction postoperative respiratory failure in men after major noncardiac surgery. Ann Surg 2000;232:242-253.

82. Cartagena R. Preoperative evaluation of patients with obesity and obstructive sleep apnea. Anesth Clin North Am 2005;23:463-478.

84. Ramakrishna G, Sprung J, Ravi BS, et al. Impact of pulmonary hypertension on the outcome of noncardiac surgery. Predictors of perioperative morbidity and mortality. J Am Coll Card 2005;45:1691-1699.

96. Jacober SJ, Sowers JR. An update on perioperative management of diabetes. Arch Intern Med 1999;159:2405-2411.

100. Fund D, Gan TJ. Gastrointestinal system: prevention and treatment of gastrointestinal morbidity. In: Newman MF, Fleisher LA, Fink MP. Perioperative medicine: managing for outcome. Philadelphia: Saunders Elsevier, 2008:383-396.

113. Monk TG, Weldon BC, Garvan CW, et al. Predictors of cognitive dysfunction after major noncardiac surgery. Anesthesiology 2008;108:18-30.

116. Geerts WH, Pineo GF, Heti JA, et al. Prevention of venous thromboembolism. Chest 2004;126:228S-400S.

126. Della Valle AG, Serota A, Go G, et al. VTE is rare with a multimodal prophylaxis protocol after THA. Clin Ortho Rel Res 2006;444:146-153.

135. Erkan D, Leibowitz E, Berman J, Lockshin M. Perioperative medical management of antiphospholipid syndrome: hospital for special surgery experience, review of literature, and recommendations. J Rheum 2002;294:843-849.

145. Novack V, Jotkowitz A, Etzion O, Porath A. Does delay in surgery after hip fracture lead to worse outcome? A multicenter survey. Int J Quality in Health Care 2007;19:170-176.

148. Fisher AA, Davis MW, Rubenach SE, et al. Outcomes for older patients with hip fractures: the impact of orthopedic and geriatric medicine cocare. J Orthop Trauma 2006;20:172-180.

149. Huddleston H, Long KH, Naessens JM, et al. Medical and surgical comanagement after elective hip and knee arthroplasty. A randomized, controlled trial. Ann Intern Med 2004;141:28-39.

150. Scanzello C, Figgie M, Nestor BJ, Goodman SM. Perioperative management of medications used in the treatment of rheumatoid arthritis. HSS J 2006;2:141-147.

153. Pieringer H, Stuby U, Biesenbach G. Patients with rheumatoid arthritis undergoing surgery: how should we deal with antirheumatic treatment? Semin Arthritis Rheum 2007;36:278-286.

154. Goupille P, Pham T, Sibilia J, Mariette X. Perioperative management of patients with rheumatoid arthritis treated with TNF-Alpha blocking agents. Semin Arthritis Rheum 2007;37:202-203.

REFERENCES

Full references for this chapter can be found on www.expertconsult.com.

REGIONAL AND WIDESPREAD PAIN

Neck pain

Les Barnsley

68

- Neck pain is a common regional pain syndrome usually arising from undefined mechanical or musculoskeletal disturbance.
- It occurs acutely with marked hypomobility. Chronic symptoms are poorly understood.
- Neck pain may rarely be a feature of a serious underlying malignant, infective, or inflammatory disorder and can occur in association with neurologic involvement (myelopathy and radiculopathy).
- No examination or imaging findings are known that reliably identify the source of pain, although it may be investigated with techniques targeting the pain.

INTRODUCTION

The neck provides a link of great flexibility between the sensory platform of the head and the trunk. Simultaneously it provides vital conduits for neural and vascular tissue between the brain and the rest of the body. These conflicting priorities are achieved through the structure of the cervical spine, which combines strength with an extraordinary range of movement. The strength is achieved through a bony tube made up of the individual vertebrae. The range of movement is achieved through a complex articular system involving ligamentous intervertebral discs and paired posterior zygapophyseal joints in the lower neck and loosely constrained synovial joints at the upper levels. The discs fissure posteriorly as part of the normal aging process,[1] permitting rotatory movements through an oblique axis.[2] The posterior zygapophyseal joints have no bony constraint and facilitate a broad range of movement through having flat surfaces that glide in concert to permit flexion and extension and in opposite directions to produce rotation. This complex is the subject of almost constant activity, with the neck being reported to move over 600 times per hour or once every 6 seconds.[1]

Pain perceived in the region of the neck arises as a result of noxious stimulation of any of the structures innervated by the cervical spinal nerves. These encompass local sources of pain among the intrinsic structures of the cervical spine and distant sources that refer pain to the neck by virtue of being supplied by nerves that arise in the neck but leave the cervical region and enter the head or thoracic region. The majority of neck pain is acute and self-limiting and can be attributed to unspecified mechanical problems; but a small percentage of neck pain becomes chronic, and it is this pain that is the focus of this chapter. Most instances of chronic neck pain will prove to be musculoskeletal in origin and are usually recognizable as such, but it is incumbent on the physician to exclude other serious and potentially treatable pathologic processes. Fortunately, the history and physical examination typically permit ready differentiation of musculoskeletal causes from other causes of neck pain. Once non-mechanical conditions have been excluded, the second responsibility is to provide a diagnosis as to the structure and pathology producing the neck pain. Only with a sound anatomic diagnosis can therapy be targeted and rational.

Frequently discussed in association with neck pain, but really a separate problem, is the question of cervical nerve root or cervical cord compression. These problems warrant assessment on their own merits, independent of any associated neck pain, and are considered later.

EPIDEMIOLOGY

Although less common than low back pain, neck pain represents a common human experience: its universality and unpleasantness is reflected by the colloquial use of the words "pain in the neck" to describe a particularly disagreeable circumstance or individual. A comprehensive review of the burden of neck pain revealed a 12-month prevalence of any pain of between 30% and 50% and a prevalence of activity-limiting pain of 1.75% to 11.5%.[3] The high prevalence of neck pain persists into old age, with centenarians still experiencing a 1-month prevalence of 23% in women and 19% in men.[4]

Acute neck pain and stiffness is a common problem. Prevalence data indicate a frequency of 18% in a randomly sampled population.[5] Australian data indicate that 18% of people wake with some neck pain or stiffness and 4% experience neck pain for all of the day.[6] The determinants of chronic, mechanical neck pain are still incompletely studied. There is no doubt that trauma, particularly whiplash injury, is an important contributor to the burden of chronic neck pain. A clear relationship has been demonstrated between the nature of occupation and neck pain, with manual workers having higher frequencies of neck pain than those with sedentary jobs.[7] More recent studies have shown that the chance of being symptom free years after an initial episode of neck pain is less in manual workers than sedentary workers.[8] Other positive associations with neck pain include self-reported heavy workload, level of education[9] (probably a confounding factor with heavy workload), and depression.[10] A longitudinal study of adolescents has demonstrated that dynamic loading sports of the upper limbs during adolescence were associated with a risk reduction of 40% in the development of neck and shoulder pain 7 years later, but psychosomatic symptoms were associated with up to 10% increase in risk. Increased flexibility in adolescent males has been shown to be protective of later neck symptoms in males, whereas in females good endurance strength confers similar benefits.[11] One of the strongest predictors of future neck and shoulder pain was frequent symptoms of neck and shoulder pain during adolescence.[12] Neck pain also has substantial genetic components, with a twin study suggesting heritability of 35% to 58%.[13]

NATURAL HISTORY

Neck pain is divided arbitrarily into acute pain, lasting less than 3 months, and chronic pain, lasting more than 3 months. For a given episode of acute neck pain, approximately 40% of patients will either recover fully or have mild symptoms. Moderate or severe symptoms will persist in a further 30%.[14] For patients presenting to a general practitioner with neck pain for less than 6 weeks, after 12 months over three fourths will be fully recovered or much improved.[15]

In the setting of whiplash, 56% of patients with neck pain will recover in 3 months and 80% within 12 months.[16] The main physical risk factor for chronic neck pain after whiplash is the severity of the initial symptoms.[17] A recent best evidence synthesis highlights the role of psychological factors such as passive coping style, depressed mood, and fear of movement in slowing recovery.[18]

Chronic neck pain is weakly predicted by the presence of concomitant low back pain, older age, previous episodes of neck pain, and stable symptoms for the 2 weeks before assessment.[19]

CLINICAL FEATURES

Neck pain may be classified as being referred from distant (non-cervical structures), as arising through involvement of cervical structures by neoplastic, inflammatory, or infectious disease, or as being mechanical or musculoskeletal in origin. Diseases that may refer pain to the neck are outlined in Table 68.1. Fortunately, these conditions are usually readily recognized through their other clinical characteristics, such as exertion-induced pain in angina, but the need for a complete history, including features other than those symptoms referable to the neck, is highlighted. A cross tabulation of those conditions that can affect the components of the cervical spine is shown in Table 68.2. The clinical history should cover those characteristics of the pain listed in Box 68.1. Each category reveals features that enable serious and distinctive conditions to be identified or, at least, strongly suspected.

Onset of pain

The setting in which the complaint of pain starts is most helpful in raising the suspicion of a diagnosis of non-mechanical neck pain. The patient's age and a past history of malignancy, particularly of the lung, breast, prostate, thyroid, or kidney, should raise the possibility of metastatic bone disease. Previous surgery, immunosuppression, and past infections increase the risk of hematogenous osteomyelitis or septic arthritis. Inflammatory conditions such as ankylosing spondylitis, rheumatoid arthritis, and polymyalgia rheumatica are suggested by involvement of areas other than the cervical spine, a history of pain and stiffness on first rising and after immobility ("gelling"), and systemic features such as weight loss or sweats.

Musculoskeletal pain typically arises after trauma or unaccustomed activity.[20] Whiplash injuries in motor vehicle accidents are probably the most common cause of traumatic neck pain (see later), although sports injuries and industrial accidents lead to similar symptoms. Intrinsic disease processes, such as osteoarthritis, may be responsible for the development of pain.

Details of any trauma should be documented when possible so that the direction and magnitude of the forces applied to the neck can be estimated. Flexion imparts compressive forces to the vertebral bodies and discs and distractive forces on posterior spinal elements such as the zygapophyseal joint capsules and posterior neck muscles. Conversely, extension injuries compress posterior cervical structures such as the articular pillars and zygapophyseal joints while distracting anterior components such as the anterior annulus fibrosus of the disc, the vertebral endplates, and anterior longitudinal ligament.[21]

Quality of pain

The pain of mechanical, musculoskeletal derangement is typically dull, deep, and aching. Exacerbations are usually short-lived, with sharp pains superimposed on the chronic symptoms. Pain that does not follow this pattern, for instance, pain that is shooting or electrical, should raise suspicion that neural structures are involved. Deep, unremitting pain with no periods of relief is a sinister sign implying ongoing distention, deformation, or invasion of pain-sensitive structures that may occur in malignancy.

Frequency and duration of episodes of pain

Mechanical or non-inflammatory musculoskeletal pain is typically experienced in episodes that are related to movement and exertion. The pain is made worse by particular postures or exercises and is characteristically improved by rest and immobility. Pain that does not follow this pattern, that is not altered by movement, and that worsens spontaneously suggests a more sinister underlying cause.

Site and radiation of pain

Musculoskeletal cervical pain is typically perceived over the posterior aspect of the neck and rarely radiates past the anterior border of the sternomastoid muscle. Pain in the anterior part of the neck usually indicates disease of one of the anterior structures (see Table 68.1). Intrinsic neck pain can radiate into the head and down onto the shoulders. Headache is particularly common in those patients with upper cervical pathology, particularly at C3 and above. Pain from structures at these levels is often perceived in the distribution of the first division

TABLE 68.1 NON-MUSCULOSKELETAL SOURCES OF NECK PAIN

Structure	Condition
Pharynx	Pharyngitis
Larynx	Laryngitis Carcinoma
Trachea	Tracheitis
Thyroid	Thyroiditis
Lymph nodes	Lymphadenitis
Carotid arteries	Carotidynia Dissection Inflammation
Aorta	Aneurysm Dissection
Heart	Angina Infarction
Pericardium	Pericarditis
Diaphragm	Inflammation by blood, infection

BOX 68.1 FEATURES OF PAIN TO BE ELICITED FROM THE CLINICAL HISTORY

- Mode and time of onset
- Site of pain
- Quality of pain
- Radiation of pain
- Frequency and duration of episodes of pain
- Pattern of episodes
- If periodic, mode of onset and time of onset
- Aggravating factors
- Relieving factors
- Associated features

TABLE 68.2 MUSCULOSKELETAL STRUCTURES AND PATHOLOGIC PROCESSES

	Muscles	Joints	Discs	Bone	Dura	Ligament	Other
Infectious		Septic arthritis	Discitis	Osteomyelitis	Abscess Meningitis		Epidural abscess
Neoplastic				Primary	Neurofibroma		Spinal cord tumor
				Secondary	Meningioma		
Inflammatory	Polymyositis/dermatomyositis, polymyalgia rheumatica	Rheumatoid arthritis	Discitis? Ankylosing spondylitis				
Metabolic				Paget's disease Osteoporosis Osteomalacia			

of the trigeminal nerve or the back of the head and neck and is most likely mediated through the trigeminocervical nucleus in the upper spinal cord.[22] Pain from lower cervical levels can be referred to the shoulder girdle, arm, interscapular region, and chest wall.[23] It has been observed that the more severe the pain, the larger the area of referral.

Significance of site and radiation of neck pain

There are no means by which a single structure such as the dura, cervical zygapophyseal joints, or intervertebral discs can be singled out as the source of pain on the basis of clinical history and examination. However, studies of normal individuals have demonstrated the patterns of pain referral stemming from the noxious stimulation of cervical structures. Probing the anterior part of the cervical discs in awake patients produced pain in the posterior neck, several segments below the level stimulated (Fig. 68.1a).[24] Classic studies by Feinstein revealed that injections of hypertonic saline into deep cervical muscles produced distinct patterns of pain, again over the posterior neck (see Fig. 68.1b).[25] Dwyer and associates distended the capsules of the cervical zygapophyseal joints (C2-3 to C6-7) of normal volunteers.[26] Each joint had a reproducible and characteristic pattern of pain referral (see Fig. 68.1c). The sclerotome of C6-7 involved the posterior lower neck extending well across the scapula, so that pain arising from this joint could be mistakenly considered to be arising from the shoulder. Stimulation of C5-6 resulted in pain over the crook of the neck but above the spine of the scapula, and C4-5 and C3-4 referred pain to the mid neck with biases to the lower and upper neck, respectively. Pain from C2-3 was located in the suboccipital region, extending up onto the occipital part of the skull and down to the upper half of the neck. Similar methodology was used by Dreyfuss and colleagues to investigate referral patterns of pain from the atlantoaxial joint (AAJ) and atlanto-occipital joint (AOJ).[27] Injecting these joints in normal volunteers produced pain in the suboccipital region (see Fig. 68.1d). There is extensive overlap between different structures, so that "disc pain" may occur in an identical distribution to zygapophyseal joint pain or deep muscle pain. Moreover, adjacent structures have extensive overlap in the area to which they refer pain. In particular, the upper cervical zygapophyseal joints and the AAJ and AOJ all refer pain to the suboccipital region.

The clinical consequence of this information is that it is impossible to determine the site of origin of neck pain on the basis of the site of pain alone. At best, the approximate level of involvement may be determined, but in practice this may be up to two or even three segments out and may reflect pain from a number of different structures. To complicate the issue further, a single source of pain may produce pain over a wide area through enhanced receptive fields of spinal neurons, so that pain may appear diffuse and unfocused. It is incumbent on the physician to carefully assess the "core" of such pain in considering where to start further investigation. Pain maps and diagrams of the affected body part that are completed by the patient may be useful in this regard.

Other musculoskeletal structures referring pain to the neck

Two structures have been shown to refer pain proximally to the neck, potentially drawing attention away from the true source of pain. In similar experiments on normal volunteers, injection of hypertonic saline solution into the acromioclavicular joint[28] and sternoclavicular joints[29] frequently produced pain in the neck, sometimes with little local discomfort over the target joint.

Associated features

Infections are typically accompanied by fevers and malaise as well as specific features reflecting the tissues involved. Pain arising from malignant disease may be accompanied by paraneoplastic conditions such as peripheral neuropathy, hypercalcemia, or features of metastatic disease elsewhere. Symptoms that may accompany primary neck pain are dizziness and visual disturbances, which may be unaccompanied by abnormalities on conventional, neurologic examination. The exact pathophysiologic basis for these symptoms has not been elucidated, but a variety of hypotheses and increasing volumes of experimental data suggest an organic basis.[21] These symptoms should not be interpreted as indicating a neurotic basis for the neck pain.

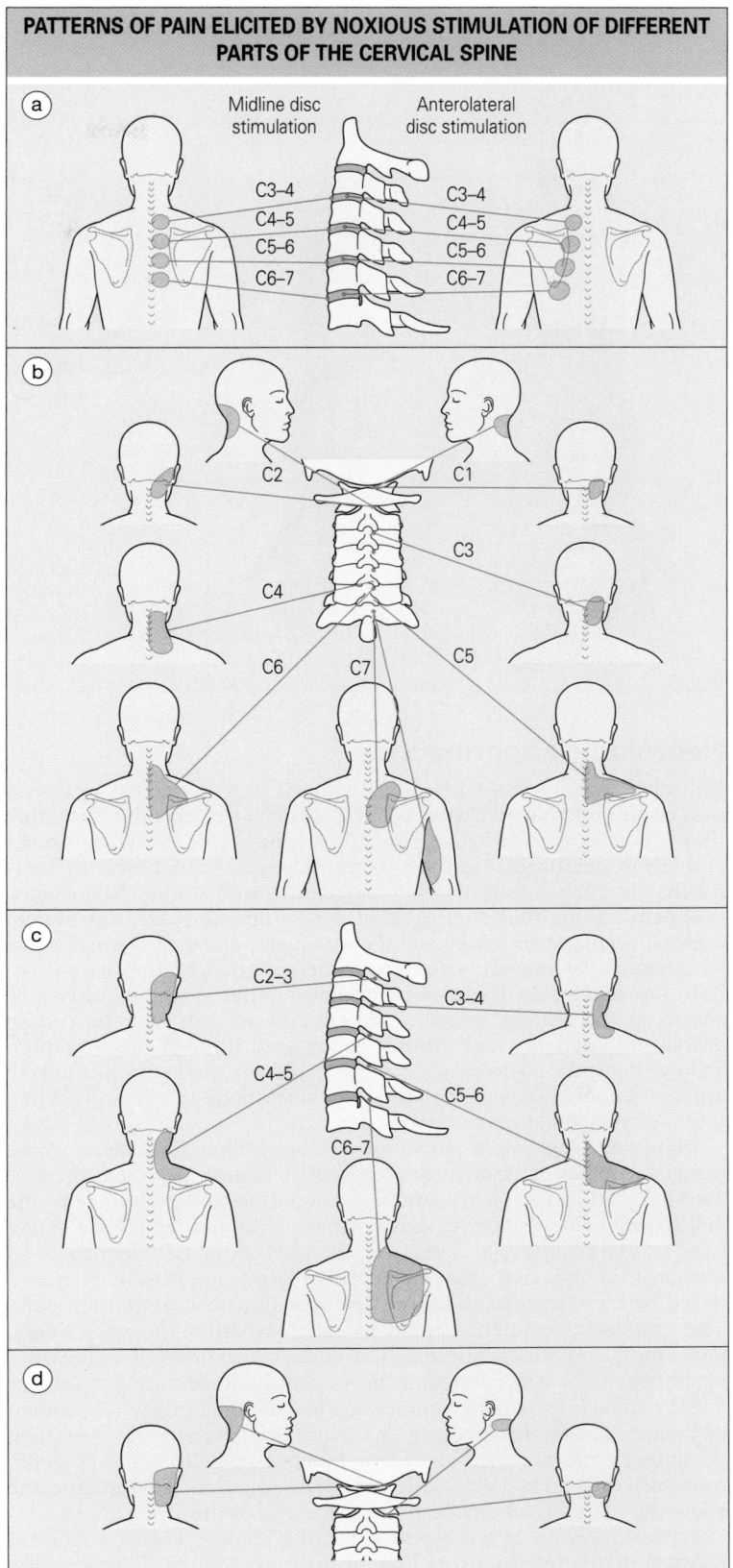

PATTERNS OF PAIN ELICITED BY NOXIOUS STIMULATION OF DIFFERENT PARTS OF THE CERVICAL SPINE

Fig. 68.1 Patterns of pain elicited by noxious stimulation of different parts of the cervical spine. The red represents the site stimulated to produce the pain pattern represented by the shaded area. (a) Intervertebral discs: probing of the discs in the midline anteriorly and lateral to the midline anteriorly (modified from Cloward[24]). (b) Deep musculoligamentous tissue: site of pain consistently produced by the injection of 6% saline into the interspinous region, just to the right of the midline, at cervical levels from C1 to C8 (modified from Feinstein et al[25]). (c) Zygapophyseal joints: sites of pain consistently produced by distention of the cervical zygapophyseal joints from C2-3 to C6-7 through intra-articular injections of contrast medium (modified from Dwyer et al[26]). (d) Upper cervical synovial joints: sites of pain consistently produced by distention of the atlanto-occipital (AOJ) and atlantoaxial (AAJ) joints through intra-articular injections of contrast medium (modified from Dreyfuss et al[27]).

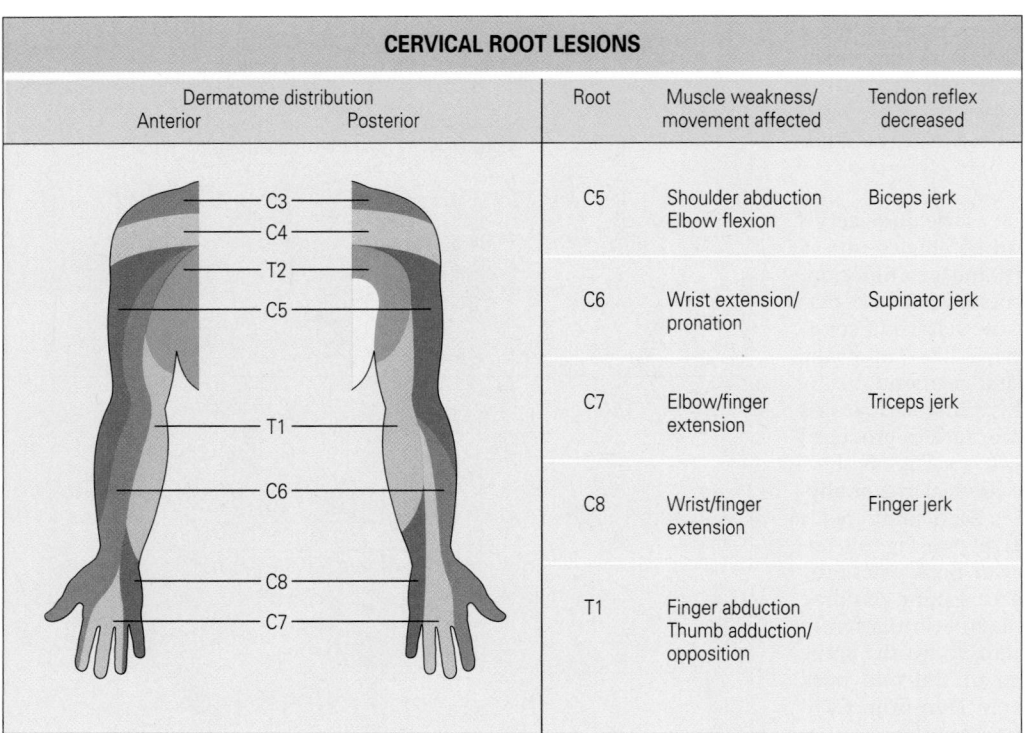

CERVICAL ROOT LESIONS

Dermatome distribution		Root	Muscle weakness/ movement affected	Tendon reflex decreased
Anterior	Posterior			
		C5	Shoulder abduction Elbow flexion	Biceps jerk
		C6	Wrist extension/ pronation	Supinator jerk
		C7	Elbow/finger extension	Triceps jerk
		C8	Wrist/finger extension	Finger jerk
		T1	Finger abduction Thumb adduction/ opposition	

Fig. 68.2 Cervical root lesions. Sensory and motor distribution of the cervical roots.

Neurologic abnormalities

Neurologic symptoms such as paresthesia and subjective weakness may occur in neck pain patients. Their significance depends on whether they are accompanied by definite neurologic signs. Weakness in the absence of neurologic signs may seem to suggest a non-organic basis for the complaints, but a variety of experimental studies have shown that pain has an inhibitory effect on motor neuron pools, resulting in a greater demand for effort and a consequent, subjective sensation of weakness.[30] Paresthesia suggestive of nerve root irritation may arise, however, as a result of functional thoracic outlet syndrome caused by spasm of the scalene muscle.[31] Alterations in sensation have been described in patients with chronic pain states, through complex interactions between nociceptive and other sensory pathways leading to reports of altered sensation that do not correspond to classical dermatomal or peripheral nerve distributions.

Hard neurologic signs are an uncommon finding in patients whose primary complaint is of neck pain, but if neurologic impairment is detected, the thrust of investigation should be to determine the site and nature of the lesion. Coexistent neck pain and neurologic deficit may be due to intrinsic disease of the cord, dura, or nerve roots by neoplasia or infection (see Table 68.2) or by compression of neural tissue by bone or discs that are themselves intrinsic sources of pain. The clinical assessment should establish whether the spinal cord, nerve roots, or both are affected. The unexplained onset of, or presence of, impaired sphincter function, lower limb weakness, and a sensory level are indicative of cord compression and demand urgent assessment by magnetic resonance imaging (MRI) or myelography (with or without computed tomography [CT]). These imaging modalities should determine whether a reversible cause of cord compression is present and allow the planning of any decompressive procedures.

Signs suggestive of a nerve root disorder, such as loss of a reflex or reflexes, dermatomal sensory loss, or myotomal motor weakness (Fig. 68.2) should be investigated with cross-sectional imaging, specifically MRI where available or with CT, to demonstrate the site and nature of the lesion and whether the problem is intrinsic or extrinsic compression. Nerve conduction studies and electromyography may help characterise equivocal or unexplained neurological symptoms or signs. These investigations are not justified in the absence of neurologic signs, where neck pain alone is the clinical problem.

Cervical nerve root compression

Pain arising from overt compression or disease of the nerve root typically follows the appropriate dermatome and is therefore felt in the arm and not the neck. This pain will typically be radicular in quality, that is, pain that is perceived in a narrow band on the skin of the arm and that has electrical, radiating, or shooting properties. However, more somatic (i.e., deep, diffuse aching) pain in proximal structures can be produced by nerve root compression.[32] At the same time, pain that is perceived in the forearm or hand is unlikely to be somatic referred pain and is more likely to be radicular in origin. Pain may be accompanied by neurologic symptoms such as numbness, paresthesia, altered sensation, and motor weakness. Pain may be perceived across the top of the shoulder from C4 and in the the face and head from lesions affecting C2 and C3. However, these are uncommon levels to be affected, so much so that isolated lesions at these levels should prompt a systematic search for sinister, space-occupying pathologic process. The overwhelming majority of cervical root lesions occur at C6 to C8, and all tend to produce symptoms referable to the forearm and hand and have distinctive clinical features (see Fig. 68.2). Because of the extensive overlap of dermatomes in the arm and the complex central representation of the upper limb, the pain referred to the arm through root irritation may be far more diffuse than the traditional diagrams of dermatomes would suggest. Unlike the lumbar spine, disc prolapse itself is not the predominant cause of cervical nerve root irritation. This is because the nerve root in the lower cervical spine lies in the lower part of the foramen, at or below the level of the disc.[33] More typically, this part of the foramen is compromised by osteophytic involvement from the adjacent uncinate process or through hypertrophic changes in the adjacent zygapophyseal joint.[1] Discogenic neural encroachment in the cervical spine is typically due to discrete fragments of the disc that herniate into the foramen to cause neural compromise.

CLINICAL EXAMINATION

The principal role of the clinical examination in the setting of neck pain is to exclude other conditions that may be present and contributing to the pain, such as infection, malignancy, or inflammatory arthropathy, or to exclude neurologic involvement. Once the diagnosis is that of isolated or mechanical neck pain, the diagnostic utility of a clinical examination of the neck is extremely limited.

General examination

The general examination is performed to exclude non-mechanical causes of neck pain. This should be particularly focused on any system(s) where abnormalities have been suggested by history. In addition, examination of temperature, skin, joints, lymph nodes, abdomen, and breasts should be performed. The yield from such assessment in the setting of neck pain is not known and is probably low, but the serious consequences of missing a potentially treatable systemic illness, malignancy, or infection make the performance of such an examination most important.

Neurologic examination

The aims of a neurologic examination in the presence of neck pain are to exclude cervical nerve root lesions or spinal cord lesions. The former requires a detailed examination of the arms. The muscles should be examined for wasting and fasciculation indicative of lower motor neuron lesions. Tone and power should then be assessed, before testing the biceps (C5-6), triceps (C6-7), supinator (C5-6), and finger (C8) jerks. Sensation to light touch and pain (pinprick) should then be checked for any dermatomal sensory loss. The lower limbs should be similarly examined, with the principal aim being the exclusion of any upper motor neuron signs (spasticity, clonus, positive Babinski sign, hyperreflexia, and weakness) indicative of cord compression due to the painful lesion in the neck.

Local examination

The neck examination again requires that non-mechanical causes such as local infection, bruising, lymphadenitis, and so on, are excluded. This is readily accomplished with routine inspection and palpation. The other cervical structures, such as the larynx, thyroid, lymph nodes, and carotid arteries, should be carefully palpated for evidence of swelling or tenderness. However, in the absence of suggestive history, the yield from such examination is likely to be small. The neck should be examined for tenderness. This is best achieved by exerting pressure first on a control area such as the occipital protuberance. This pressure should then be applied along the spinous processes and then the articular pillars as well as the trapezii. This provides some standardization of the stimulus and permits some grading of response. Unfortunately, the localization of tenderness contributes little in the way of diagnostic information. There has been no demonstrated correlation between tenderness in a particular area and a specific anatomic diagnosis. At most, examination for tenderness permits the approximate level of any causative pathologic process to be estimated. Tenderness is also a subjective finding, so that it is subject to reporting biases from patients keen to either exaggerate or diminish their problems.

Neck movement

Examination of the neck traditionally incorporates the documentation of active and passive ranges of movement. However, basic research casts grave doubts on the diagnostic utility and reliability of such assessments. Detailed cineradiographic techniques employed by Van Mameren and associates to assess flexion and extension have revealed that even normal individuals display marked variation in the pattern and amplitude of both segmental and total ranges of neck movement.[34] Such variability in controlled laboratory situations is likely to translate to a much larger error in clinical situations with the added variability of many observers and different measurement environments. Therefore, only gross abnormalities of range of motion, such as reproducible asymmetry of movement, are likely to be assessed reliably. Furthermore, the clinical utility of neck movement assessment is open to serious question. Biomechanical studies have shown that 50% of cervical rotation takes place at the atlantoaxial joints.[35] The remaining rotation occurs in approximately equal proportions below C2, so that each segment contributes less than 7 degrees of movement. Therefore, even complete fusion of a segment below C1-2 may be clinically undetectable and will most likely fall within measurement error. At the same time, it is conceivable that a painful lesion of the neck may produce marked loss of movement, in excess of 50% of range, owing to reflex inhibition of muscle pain, fear of pain being produced, or local muscle spasm due to pain. This is readily appreciated in patients with acute hypomobility, whose site of pain (typically in the lower neck) would be inconsistent with AAJ pain but whose range of movement is markedly reduced. Despite these observations, some have advocated

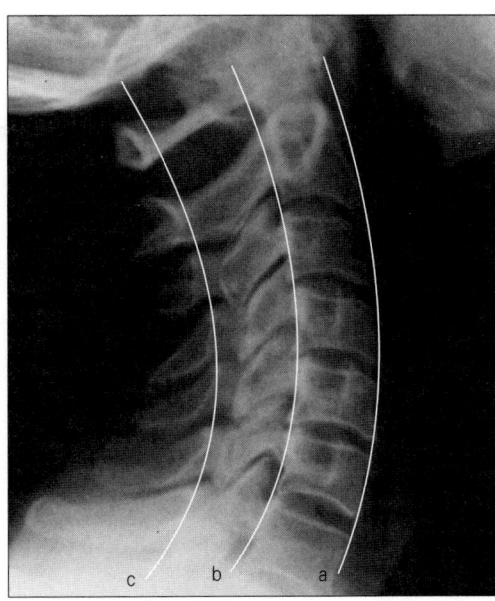

Fig. 68.3 Plain lateral radiograph of a normal cervical spine. Lines joining the anterior part of the vertebral body (a), the posterior aspect of the vertebral body (b), and the anterior border of the laminae (c) should describe a smooth arc.

that reduction of range of movement in the neck of greater than 50% is a "non-organic" sign, suggestive of abnormal illness behavior[36]; this is a potentially dangerous assumption. An even more fundamental issue is the diagnostic significance of any observed motion restriction. No correlations have been established between motion abnormalities and any specific anatomic diagnoses. Therefore, the measurement of ranges of motion in the neck provides no reliable or discriminatory diagnostic information. At best, restriction of movement in the neck indicates that there is one or more of disturbance of the neuromuscular control of the neck, a painful lesion aggravated by movement, or a mechanical restriction anywhere in the complex articular arrangements between two or more vertebrae.

Test for nerve root entrapment

The most specific test for nerve root entrapment is the compression, or Spurling's, test. The patient's neck is moved passively into extension and rotated to the symptomatic side. Axial pressure is then applied to the neck by the examiner. This series of movements has been shown to narrow the intervertebral foramina. If the patient's radicular symptoms are reproduced, then the test is positive.[37] This test has good inter-rater reliability and is highly specific but relatively insensitive. The combination of a positive compression test and abnormal neurologic signs in the arm is strongly predictive of nerve root compression on CT myelography.

INVESTIGATIONS

Radiography

Plain radiographs of the cervical spine are ordered almost universally for patients presenting with neck pain. This may be appropriate when there is a history suggestive of severe trauma likely to produce fracture or severe subluxation or when major instability is suspected. The most useful views in these circumstances are lateral flexion and extension views, open-mouth views, and, to a lesser extent, the anteroposterior view. To assess for subluxation, lines linking the anterior vertebral bodies, posterior vertebral bodies, and posterior border of the intervertebral canal in a lateral projection are constructed. These should describe a smooth arc (Fig. 68.3). The presence of a "step" in this arc is a sign of subluxation, either through retrolisthesis or spondylolisthesis. Gross abnormalities of motion may be detected through comparing flexion and extension views, and instability is demonstrated by comparing the construction lines just described on flexion and extension views. Of particular note is the issue of atlantoaxial instability. This occurs almost exclusively in rheumatoid arthritis but can occur in the presence of other destructive lesions affecting the odontoid peg or transverse or alar ligament complex. This is assessed by comparing the gap between the anterior part of the odontoid peg and the posterior margin of the anterior arch of the atlas as seen on lateral flexion and extension views. This should normally be less than 5 mm.

Alert patients with acute neck pain and a history of trauma should be evaluated according to the Canadian C-Spine rule, which uses a combination of historical and clinical features to determine those patients requiring radiographs.[38] They can be summarized that the patients meeting all the following criteria do not need radiographs:

- Minor trauma
- Age younger than 65 years
- No peripheral paresthesias
- Sitting in the emergency department
- Ambulant at any time after the trauma
- No immediate neck pain
- No midline tenderness
- Active neck rotation greater than 45 degrees

Plain radiographs may also be useful in excluding primary bone disorders such as Paget's disease, significant sclerotic malignant infiltration of bone, and destructive lesions such as osteomyelitis. However, standard views of the cervical spine are complex pictures with many structures being superimposed on all views, in contrast to a radiograph of a long bone. This means that radiographs tend to be insensitive in the detection of small abnormalities, such as purely lytic lesions without significant cortical bone destruction. When such lesions are suspected but not detected on plain films, further imaging with CT, MRI, or nuclear medicine techniques is desirable.

For those patients with mechanical pain, the value of plain radiographs is much more limited. It has been repeatedly demonstrated that the presence of degenerative or spondylitic changes in the spine does not correlate with symptoms of neck pain. Friedenburg and Miller studied the plain radiographs of 92 pairs of age- and sex-matched patients with and without neck pain.[39] The incidence of degenerative changes rose with age, was most common at the C5-6 level, both at the intervertebral disc and the zygapophyseal joints, but bore no relationship to the presence of neck pain.

Computed tomography

The principal value of CT in the assessment of cervical lesions is the visualization of the bony conduits through which neural tissue must pass. This ability can be enhanced by the introduction of radiopaque contrast medium into the thecal sac (CT myelography), which permits direct visualization of the nerve roots and sheaths and the spinal cord itself. CT is of less value in assessing soft tissues. The selection of these investigations would therefore be dictated by the clinical suspicion of a neurologic abnormality, either cervical myelopathy, cord compression, or cervical nerve root compression. For neck pain alone, without neurologic symptoms or signs and without clinical or plain radiographic evidence of non-mechanical disorder, the role of CT remains to be determined.

Magnetic resonance imaging

Similar comments pertain to the use of MRI, which is highly specific and sensitive for disc herniations when compared with surgical findings and has results comparable to CT myelography (Fig. 68.4).[40] MRI is particularly helpful in visualizing neural and soft tissue structures and intra-cord pathologic processes in the cervical region (e.g., demyelination, intra-axial tumors, and spinal cord infarction) and enables accurate appraisal of developmental defects such as the Arnold-Chiari malformation. However, for the assessment of neck pain of mechanical origin, MRI, like CT, has not been validated. It has been shown that nearly one fifth of all asymptomatic patients had abnormalities on MR images, with 60% of older patients having abnormalities of their intervertebral discs.[41] Surface coil MR images of isolated cervical spines have revealed that, even with optimal imaging parameters, the soft tissue components of the zygapophyseal joints are seen poorly, if at all.[42] MRI

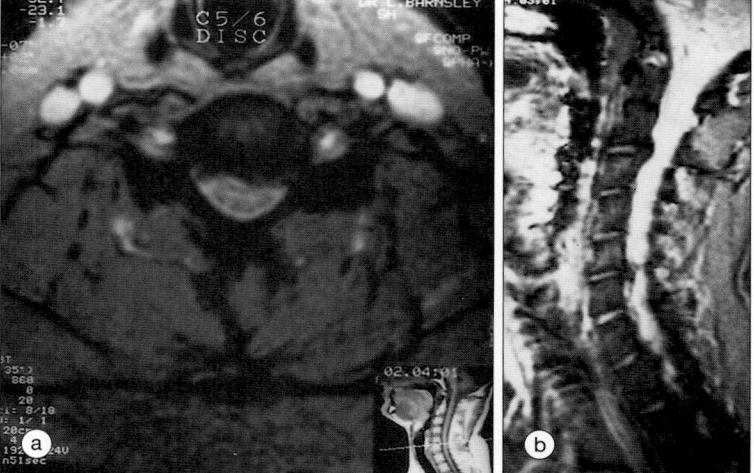

Fig. 68.4 Disc herniation on MRI. Axial (a) and sagittal (b) MR images of a 47-year-old man with neck pain and decreased left biceps jerk with numbness over his thumb after a motor vehicle accident. The scans demonstrate a significant left posterolateral disc protrusion at C5-6, which significantly compromises the exiting C6 nerve root.

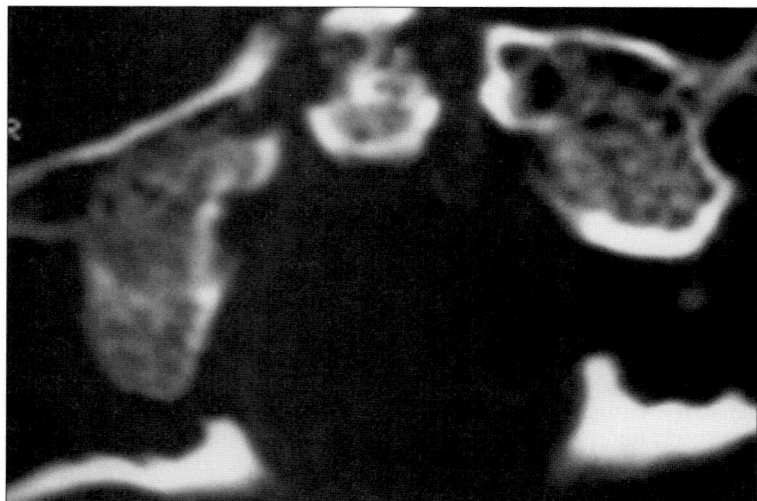

Fig. 68.5 Detection of myeloma. CT scan of a 63-year-old man with known multiple myeloma who developed neck pain. Plain radiographs and bone scan failed to demonstrate the osteolytic lesions affecting the odontoid peg.

should be reserved for those patients in whom there is a clinical suspicion of intraspinal pathology, neural compromise, or other neurologic disorder.

Scintigraphy

Bone scintigraphy using technetium-labeled methylenediphosphonate (^{99m}Tc-MDP) is highly sensitive for the detection of bony pathology with the notable exception of those lesions that have a purely lytic pathology, particularly multiple myeloma (Fig. 68.5). However, for the tumors that most commonly metastasize to bone—lung, breast, prostate, thyroid, and kidney—the technique is the investigation of choice for the early detection of metastases. Bone scintigraphy may also be useful in the detection of infection, showing avid uptake in the affected region. Using an early, angiographic assessment during the injection of the radiopharmaceutical and a blood pool image a short time later, increased vascularity can be assessed that can help differentiate infection or inflammation from degenerative change. Areas of increased radiopharmaceutical uptake in the cervical spine must be assessed with knowledge of the usual pattern of uptake. Notable in the cervical spine is the normal, physiologic increase in uptake over the C2 spinous process compared with lower cervical vertebrae.

Bone scintiscans have an important role in the assessment of patients where tumor or infection are suspected, but plain radiographs are normal or equivocal. In this setting their superior sensitivity to early disturbances in osteoblastic activity may reveal important pathologic processes well before plain radiographic changes emerge. A difficult area is differentiating increased uptake from degenerative changes in the neck from other, more sinister, pathologic processes. This may require further imaging of the region of interest with co-registered CT scanning, separate CT, or MRI where significant doubt exists. However, in the cervical spine, degenerative changes typically affect the intervertebral joints so that increased uptake in these regions should arouse less suspicion than uptake localized to, for example, the vertebral body.

Blood tests

Blood tests have no role in the assessment of pain that is mechanical on the basis of history and clinical examination. When other problems such as tumor or infection are suspected they may provide supportive evidence. The most useful investigations would be a complete blood cell count (CBC) and determination of erythrocyte sedimentation rate (ESR) and/or C-reactive protein value and serum alkaline phosphatase level. Infection and tumor are typically associated with an elevated ESR, infection with an elevated white blood cell count, and Paget's disease with an increased alkaline phosphatase level.

Myelography

Myelography is the introduction of radiographic contrast medium into the cerebrospinal fluid in the subarachnoid space with images then being collected as the contrast agent spreads or is guided to the area of interest. The primary value of myelography is not the elucidation of a source of neck pain but the demonstration of the outline of the subarachnoid space, in particular the spinal cord and nerve root sheaths. This is of value in revealing intrusions on the cervical spinal canal and intervertebral foramina and compression of the cord or nerve roots by discs and disc fragments, infection, or tumors. However, all of these lesions would need to be suspected on the basis of neurologic symptoms and signs and would rarely, if ever, present as neck pain alone. MRI is largely replacing myelography in the investigation of patients with suspected spinal neurologic disturbance.

Investigations targeting pain

In the absence of reliable morphologic correlates of mechanical neck pain on imaging, it is necessary to target the pain itself to identify the painful structure. This can be accomplished either by stimulating a potentially painful structure and determining whether pain is produced or by anesthetizing a structure and determining whether pain is relieved, thereby implicating that structure as a source of pain.

Zygapophyseal joint blocks

The techniques for the diagnosis of cervical zygapophyseal joint pain rely on the simple principle that if a given joint is a source of pain, anesthetizing that joint will relieve the pain. Cervical zygapophyseal joints can be anesthetized by injecting local anesthetic into the joint or, alternatively, the nerves that convey pain from the joint can be anesthetized.

Intra-articular joint blocks

Intra-articular blocks of the cervical zygapophyseal joints are performed under fluoroscopic control. The procedure has been described using either a posterior or a lateral approach. In either case, a narrow-gauge spinal needle is directed toward the center of the target joint. Once the needle is believed to have pierced the joint capsule, a minimal volume of contrast medium must be injected to confirm intra-articular placement (Fig. 68.6). Thereafter, 0.7 to 1.0 mL of local anesthetic can be injected to anesthetize the joint.

The total injected volume should not exceed the joint capacity (generally accepted to be less than 1.0 mL) because distention beyond this volume may cause capsular rupture or extra-articular leakage,

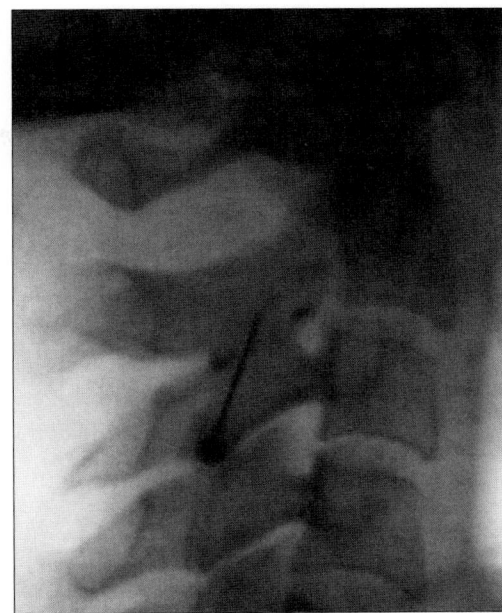

Fig. 68.6 Arthrogram of the C2-3 zygapophyseal joint. A needle has been placed into the center of the joint, and injected contrast medium has filled the loose anterior and posterior recesses.

including epidural spread. The direction of spread, after extra-articular leakage, is typically posteriorly. Extra-articular spread may compromise the specificity of an intra-articular block by anesthetizing structures other than the target joint. The disposition of the injected contrast medium should be noted. Any significant spread to the epidural space or spinal nerve would result in numbness or other neurologic signs. A post-procedural, neurologic examination should be performed to detect these effects.

Medial branch blocks

Cervical medial branch blocks are a more expedient way to anesthetize a cervical zygapophyseal joint. They are easier to perform, are less painful to the patient, and appear to provide the same diagnostic information.[43] They are performed under fluoroscopic control using either a posterior or a lateral approach. These blocks take advantage of the anatomy of the nerve supply to the cervical zygapophyseal joints.

Innervation of the cervical zygapophyseal joints

The cervical zygapophyseal joints are innervated by articular branches derived from the medial branches of the cervical dorsal rami. The C4-C8 dorsal rami arise from their respective spinal nerves just outside the intervertebral foramina and pass dorsally over the roots of the transverse processes. The medial branches of the typical cervical dorsal rami course posteriorly, hugging the waists of their ipsi-segmental articular pillars. They are covered by the tendinous slips of origin of the semispinalis capitis (Fig. 68.7). Articular branches arise as the nerve approaches the posterior aspect of the articular pillar. An ascending branch innervates the zygapophyseal joint above, and a descending branch innervates the joint below (see Fig. 68.7). Consequently, each typical cervical zygapophyseal joint receives a dual innervation, from the medial branch above and from the medial branch below its location. Beyond the zygapophyseal joints the medial branches of the cervical dorsal rami supply the semispinalis and multifidus muscles.

The medial branches of the C3 dorsal ramus comprise a deep medial branch that passes around the waist of the C3 articular pillar and participates in the innervation of the C3-4 zygapophyseal joint. The superficial medial branch of C3 is larger and is known as the third occipital nerve. It winds around the lateral aspect and then the posterior aspect of the C2-3 zygapophyseal joint. As it does so, it furnishes articular branches to the C2-3 zygapophyseal joint.[44] Articular branches may also arise from a communicating loop that crosses the back of the joint between the third occipital nerve and the C2 dorsal ramus. Beyond the C2-3 zygapophyseal joint, the third occipital nerve furnishes muscle branches to the semispinalis capitis and becomes

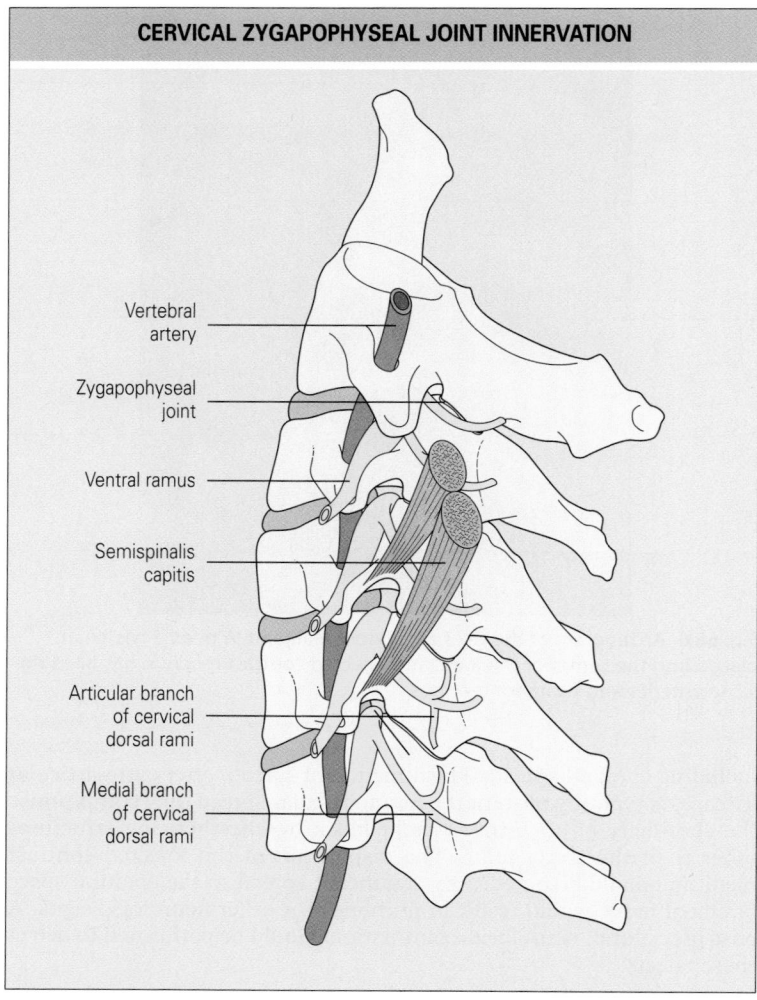

CERVICAL ZYGAPOPHYSEAL JOINT INNERVATION

Vertebral artery

Zygapophyseal joint

Ventral ramus

Semispinalis capitis

Articular branch of cervical dorsal rami

Medial branch of cervical dorsal rami

Fig. 68.7 Cervical zygapophyseal joint innervation. A posterolateral view of the cervical spine illustrating the course of the medial branches of the cervical dorsal rami. All muscles except the origins of the semispinalis capitis at C4 and C5 have been removed. The medial branches of the cervical dorsal rami are seen to course across the waist of the articular pillars. At C4 and C5, they are shown covered by the tendinous origins of the semispinalis capitis. Articular branches arise from each medial branch, on the posterior aspect of the articular pillar, to innervate the zygapophyseal joints above and below. The medial branches are well away from the ventral rami of the spinal nerves and the vertebral artery.

cutaneous over the suboccipital region. The C3 dorsal ramus is the lowest cervical dorsal ramus that regularly has a cutaneous distribution. The dorsal rami of C4 and C5 may have cutaneous branches, whereas those from C6 to C8 rarely do.

The cervical medial branches below the third occipital nerve (i.e., C3-7) can be anesthetized by placing a small amount (0.5 mL) of local anesthetic onto the nerve as it passes across the waist of the articular pillar. This is accomplished by placing a needle under image intensifier guidance onto the centrode of the articular pillar, usually from a lateral approach (Fig. 68.8). It has been shown that injections so placed do not spread laterally, posteriorly, or inferiorly to affect any other diagnostically important structure.[45] The third occipital nerve is anesthetized by placing local anesthetic onto the nerve as it passes across the C2-3 joint, which it ultimately innervates. Because of the more variable course of this nerve, lying on the convex aspect of the joint rather than the concavity at the waist of the lower articular pillars, three injections are placed to bracket its less consistent course (Fig. 68.9).

To fully anesthetize a given zygapophyseal joint at typical cervical levels, both medial branches that supply it must be blocked. In the case of the C2-3 zygapophyseal joint, the third occipital nerve must be blocked. Adequate blockade of this nerve is indicated by the onset of numbness in its cutaneous territory.

The value of blocks as a diagnostic tool hangs on the correct interpretation of the patient's responses. This involves both the patient's reporting and the physician's interpretation of that report, which are necessarily subjective. Formal appraisal of the value of single blocks finds them wanting in accuracy, with a false-positive rate between 27% and 45%.[46,47] To circumvent this, two blocks should be used, administered on different occasions, using anesthetics with different durations of action, in random order under double-blind conditions. The veracity of the patient's response is then adjudicated through their report of the duration of pain relief afforded by the anesthetic given. Because the medial branches below the third occipital nerve do not have reliable cutaneous representation, the only way that a patient can tell which anesthetic was used is through the duration of pain relief. It is therefore axiomatic that only a patient with pain can correctly identify the longer acting local anesthetic. This approach has been formally tested and found to be a valid means of identifying cervical zygapophyseal joint pain.[48]

A further refinement to this process is the addition of a third, placebo injection using normal saline as the injectant. Using a criterion standard of failure to respond to a double-blind administered placebo and any positive response to the local anesthetics reveals that simply using the two anesthetics results in high specificity but poor sensitivity.[49] Whichever approach is adopted depends on the aim of the investigation. Where aggressive neurolytic therapy is being considered, the extra accuracy afforded by triple, saline-controlled blocks may be warranted. Other situations, in which less invasive therapy is being considered, may require only double blocks.

In summary, medial branch blocks are a useful tool for the diagnosis of cervical zygapophyseal joint pain. They are valid techniques that, when correctly and thoughtfully applied, provide a syndromic, anatomic diagnosis in many patients with otherwise undiagnosable neck pain. Studies using these techniques attest to a prevalence of cervical zygapophyseal joint pain of 54% in patients with chronic neck pain (whiplash) after motor vehicle accidents[50] and between 36% and 55% in less selected patients.[51,52]

Other anesthetic blocks

Anesthetic blocks of other structures, such as the greater occipital nerve and ventral rami of the spinal nerves, can occasionally be useful in confirming or eliminating structures in their territories as causes of pain; however, in contrast to zygapophyseal joint blocks these procedures do not have documented reliability and specificity and do not currently have a place in the routine assessment of the neck pain patient.

Provocation discography

The only regularly used provocative test in the neck is provocation cervical discography, in which a disc is punctured by a needle and distended by injecting contrast media. A positive discogram occurs when the procedure reproduces the patient's usual pain and implicates that disc as the source of pain.[53] The response can occasionally be confirmed by injecting local anesthetic to try to abolish the pain.[54] In practice the procedure itself can be quite painful and it is often difficult for patients to judge whether it is their usual pain that is being reproduced.

The reliability of discography has been called into question by the observation that, in a significant proportion of patients, pain reproduced by discography can be completely eliminated by subsequent zygapophyseal joint blocks at that level.[55] Because zygapophyseal joint blocks do not have any effect on pain perception from the disc, these observations must indicate that discograms are liable to false-positive interpretations, wrongly incriminating the disc as a cause of pain when the true problem resides in the zygapophyseal joint. Furthermore, if zygapophyseal joint pain can be reproduced by stressing the disc at that segment, other structures with the same segmental nerve supply or mechanical relationships to the disc may be being falsely incriminated by seemingly positive discograms. On the basis of current evidence, discograms should only be considered as true positives if zygapophyseal joint blocks at that level are negative (i.e., no pain relief). The side effects of discography have been assessed in a audit study in a single practice that revealed the rate of discitis to be 0.16% per injection.[56]

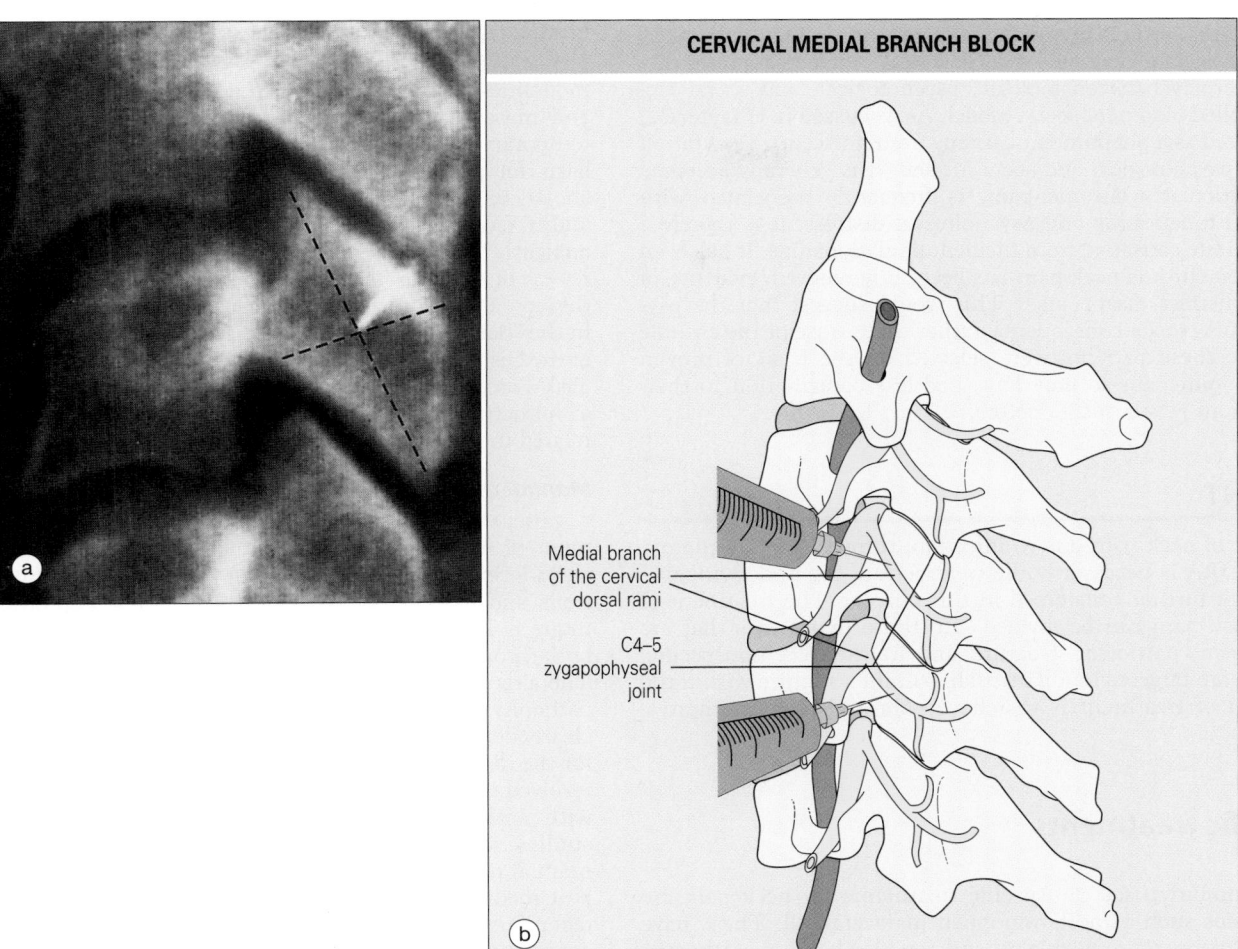

CERVICAL MEDIAL BRANCH BLOCK

(a)

(b)

Medial branch
of the cervical
dorsal rami

C4–5
zygapophyseal
joint

Fig. 68.8 Cervical medial branch block. (a) Radiograph illustrating a needle correctly placed for an injection onto the medial branch of the C5 dorsal ramus. The target point is the centrode of the articular pillar as seen on a true lateral view. (b) A schematic diagram of medial branch blocks of the C4 and C5 dorsal rami to anesthetize the C4-5 zygapophyseal joint. Needles inserted from a lateral approach are positioned for infiltration of the medial branches of the cervical dorsal rami of C4 and C5. Note that the needle tips are proximal to the origins of the ascending and descending articular branches.

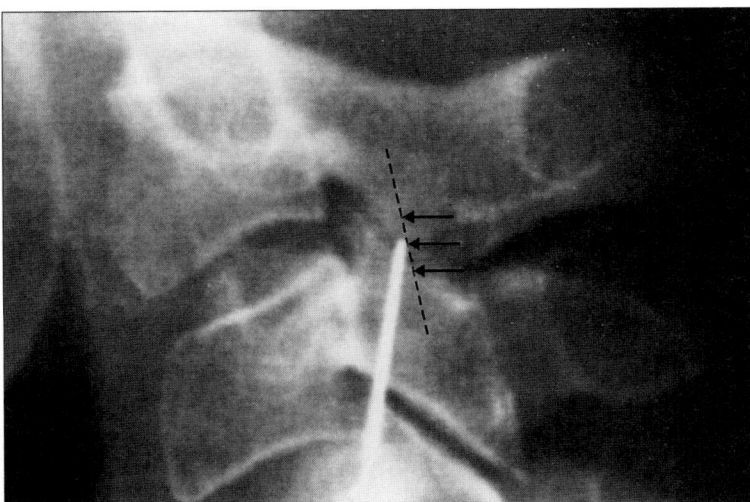

Fig. 68.9 Injecting the third occipital nerve. Lateral radiograph of the cervical spine with arrows indicating the target points for injections to anesthetize the third occipital nerve and thus the C2-3 zygapophyseal joint. The points lie along a line that vertically bisects the articular pillar of C3 seen on a lateral projection. The middle point lies over the joint line, the upper point over the subchondral plate of the C2 inferior articular surface, and the lower point over the subchondral plate of the superior articular surface of C3.

PATHOGENESIS

The exact cause of most mechanical neck pain remains elusive. Because it is not a life-threatening problem there is a paucity of pertinent pathologic data, and currently available imaging modalities provide morphologic information that does not necessarily correlate with pain. In the case of acute neck pain, it has been suggested that the pain and hypomobility may stem from entrapment of the intra-articular menisci of the cervical zygapophyseal joint in the large capsular recesses of these joints, with inflammation, pain, and stiffness ensuing before the meniscus is "reduced."[57] This may account for the rapid response of such acute hypomobility to mobilizing therapy. The source of more chronic neck pain remains arcane. The pathologic data concerning necks focuses on those problems that lead to neurologic compromise. The use of the techniques such as zygapophyseal joint blocks enables, at least, the anatomic source of pain to be impuned in a significant proportion of cases. In the case of the disc, annular tears extending into the innervated outer third of the disc may well be the source of pain,[58] but why the normal age-related changes, including extensive posterolateral fissuring, fail to cause pain in a significant proportion of patients is not understood.[59] A variety of lesions resulting from trauma to the neck could affect the cervical zygapophyseal joints (see later). Many of these could result in premature osteoarthritic change, which can be expected to be painful. Alternatively, intra-articular adhesions, capsulitis (analogous to frozen shoulder), or ongoing synovitis may be responsible for chronic zygapophyseal joint pain. A broader view of neck pain should also incorporate the possibility that some chronic neck pain is mediated within the spinal cord through "wind up" of

653

neuronal networks, principally in the posterior horn, There are views that chronic neck pain may be a multifactorial problem, representing a complex interplay between biologic, psychological, and social factors—the so-called biopsychosocial model. As discussed in Chapter 22, pain is recognized as a phenomenon arising from nociceptive excitation perceived in a psychological and social milieu. It is generally accepted that pain, particularly chronic pain, is frequently associated with impaired social functioning and psychological distress. It is therefore difficult to separate causative from incidental relationships. It has been noted that when chronic neck pain has been fully relieved, evidence of psychological distress disappears.[60] This would suggest that the psychological distress was a consequence rather than cause of the chronic pain. However, these patients were selected on the basis of proven zygapophyseal joint pain so may have had less contribution to their chronic pain from psychosocial factors.

TREATMENT

The treatment of neck pain due to infection, tumor, or inflammatory disease such as RA is necessarily the treatment of the underlying disorder and is not further considered in this chapter. The treatment of mechanical neck pain can be divided into those treatments that are not targeted at any particular structure, and are therefore nonspecific, and those that are targeted at a particular, painful structure within the neck. The aim of treatment is to relieve pain and thereby improve function.

Non-specific treatments

Analgesics

The most commonly used nonspecific treatments for neck pain are simple analgesics such as acetaminophen (paracetamol). These have an important role in acute neck pain and can also be used safely over long periods of time in more chronic problems where other treatment is ineffective. In patients with more severe pain, synthetic and non-synthetic opioids, such as dextropropoxyphene or codeine, can be used, but the potential for abuse and dependency needs to be considered before they are prescribed. These concerns should not prevent the physician from treating severe, refractory and incapacitating pain appropriately. Sustained-release oxycodone taken for 4 weeks has been shown to be superior to placebo in patients with flare of chronic neck pain with a decrease in pain and improvement in quality of life scales.[61] Tricyclic antidepressants, in doses considerably less than those used in depression, can be used as co-analgesics. They are particularly useful when nocturnal sedation is desirable and when depression is present. Other newer agents such as gabapentin, pregabalin, and duloxetine have not yet been formally studied for neck pain.

Exercises

Neck exercises have two principal aims. The first is to restore a normal range of motion. The second is to strengthen the neck musculature. The rationale for the latter is strengthened by observations that women with chronic neck pain have lower cross-sectional area of the cervical multifidus muscles than people without neck pain.[62] In women with chronic neck pain, high-intensity strength training has been demonstrated to be superior to range-of-motion exercises and stretching in the control of pain.[63] This suggestion is supported by observations from a study that compared exercise therapy to manipulative therapy. It concluded that for chronic neck pain, the use of strengthening exercise, whether in combination with spinal manipulation or in the form of a machine assisted program, appears to be more beneficial to patients with chronic neck pain than the use of spinal manipulation alone.[64] Expert panel recommendations derived from comprehensive literature reviews advocate a useful role for exercise-based therapy.[65] A systematic review of exercise therapy for chronic mechanical neck disorders sought to garner the evidence for exercise therapy alone.[66] This review, although limited to a relatively short publication period (1985-2001), found strong evidence supporting the effectiveness of strengthening and proprioceptive training exercises for frequent (i.e., recurrent acute) and chronic neck disorders.

Physical therapy

Physical therapy incorporates a number of potentially therapeutic modalities such as heat, cold, interferential, laser, ultrasound, traction, and massage. The undoubted fact that patients report modest and temporary benefit from these approaches has provided a pragmatic basis for pursuing formal studies. Low-level laser therapy has been shown to have short-term benefit in a randomized controlled trial,[67] and a recent systematic review of acupuncture attests to a limited analgesic benefit over no treatment.[68] The most recent systematic review of massage finds little data to support massage as an individual therapy and highlights the difficulties in standardizing interventions in the "hands on" therapies. These findings are reflected in the findings of the best evidence synthesis of the Bone and Joint Decade 2000-2010 Task Force on Neck Pain and Its Associated Disorders that supports acupuncture and low-level laser therapy for patients with neck pain not related to trauma.[69]

Manual therapy/manipulation

A variety of "hands on" techniques have been described in the treatment of neck pain. The best studied and most widely practiced are short-lever high-velocity "adjustments," usually described as manipulations and used principally by chiropractors. The other leading technique is known as mobilization and involves oscillatory movements both through the physiologic and accessory movements of spinal joints. The aim is to stretch tight joint capsules of symptomatic joints. The pathophysiologic basis for either of these approaches remains to be clearly demonstrated. Key issues of inter-rater and intra-rater reliability for the diagnosis of vertebral subluxation or tight joints have yet to be resolved. Studies to date have therefore grouped together all patients with neck pain and have also often included lumbar pain. These studies show small benefit, of uncertain clinical significance, for manual techniques over conventional physical therapy modalities and best medical care.[70] The application of mobilization or manipulative techniques in acute pain may be expected to have a modest effect.[71] A comprehensive meta-analysis of manual techniques for cervical pain and headache has concluded that mobilization was probably of benefit for acute neck pain and that manipulation is slightly better than mobilization or physical therapy for chronic neck pain.[72] A more recent review notes that manipulation and/or mobilization, when combined with exercises, may be useful in patients with chronic neck pain.[73] Attempts to quantify the risks of cervical manipulation have concluded on the basis of a number of assumptions that the risk of death or serious injury was in the order of less than 1 per 500,000 to 1 million manipulations..

Pillows and posture correction

There is a paucity of reliable data to show that either "posture correction" or the use of variously profiled pillows helps patients with chronic neck pain. However, these are benign interventions and in the absence of proven efficacious treatment their use may be justified. Although again lacking empirical clinical trial evidence, the modification of workplace environments and practices to decrease extreme movements of the neck and decrease the amount of time that a fixed cervical posture is maintained are sensible adjuncts to other therapy and have some basis in that extreme cervical postures have been shown to be associated with neck pain in normal individuals. Water-based pillows have been shown to decrease waking pain in patients with chronic neck pain.[74]

Specific treatments

Zygapophyseal joints

When a definitive diagnosis of cervical zygapophyseal joint pain has been made, therapy can be targeted at the specific joint. A randomized controlled trial of corticosteroid injected into painful cervical zygapophyseal joints after whiplash injury has shown no benefit over injections of local anesthetic, with neither group obtaining useful relief.[75] It is not known whether patients whose pain arises spontaneously also fail to respond to intra-articular corticosteroids.

The other treatment modality proposed for cervical zygapophyseal joint pain is denervation of the joint through percutaneous radiofrequency neurotomy of the medial branches of the cervical dorsal rami. A randomized controlled trial of this technique has demonstrated prolonged relief of zygapophyseal joint pain. The active treatment group had a median duration of pain relief of 263 days, compared with 8 in the control group.[76] Similar results have been reproduced by other groups[77] and have been found in published audits of this author's experience. The long-term effects of denervating a cervical zygapophyseal joint are not known, but clinical experience on limited numbers of patients has indicated no lasting adverse effects, with the procedure being safely repeated at such time as the pain recurs over periods up to 3 years. Surgical intervention for proven cervical zygapophyseal joint pain has not yet been described.

Discs

The treatment options for proven disc pain are limited. By virtue of their diffuse innervation, they cannot be denervated to control pain in a manner analogous to that for the cervical zygapophyseal joints. Moreover, the exact site of pain production within a painful disc cannot yet be determined so that sclerosing or excising particular disc components is not currently a viable option. The current practice for the treatment of suspected or proven cervical disc pain is cervical disc excision, usually with fusion, carried out from an anterior approach. The rationale for this approach is simple—remove the part that hurts—but empirical efficacy studies on the effects of cervical spine surgery on neck pain are not available. The only studies available are open and non-randomized and constitute retrospective reviews of individual practitioners' experiences.[78,79] Randomized, controlled studies of this operation on patients with proven disc pain are needed. For the time being, physicians contemplating such invasive intervention should ensure that the diagnosis of cervical disc pain is sound and that the patient is made aware of the potential risks of such operations, as well as the uncertainty of response.

CERVICAL NERVE ROOT COMPRESSION

Natural history

Fundamental to any consideration of treatment of cervical nerve root irritation is a clear understanding of the natural history. This has been reviewed in detail.[80] The majority of patients with cervical radicular pain will have resolution of their pain over a few weeks or months. Over prolonged periods of observation, less than 10% of patients have persisting moderate or severe disability.[81]

Treatment

There are very few interventions that have been shown, unequivocally, to be any better than others in the treatment of cervical nerve root pain. In particular, a three-armed, randomized study failed to show any long-term differences between a cervical collar physiotherapy or surgery.[82] However, it would appear that any reasonable treatment is better than no intervention, with patients in the treated arms of trials reporting better satisfaction than those in placebo arms. Typical treatments that can be expected to increase patients' perceptions of improvement include physiotherapy, traction, transcutaneous electrical nerve stimulation (TENS), analgesics, and isometric exercises. These types of interventions can be applied with the understanding that there is a generally favorable natural history and that there is no evidence for the superiority of any one intervention over any other. The choice therefore hinges on minimizing harm.

Corticosteroid injections

Corticosteroid injections into the epidural space, either through an interlaminar route or into the root sleeve, have been advocated for radicular pain. The rationale is to decrease inflammation around the nerve root. No randomized trials of transforaminal corticosteroid injections have been performed, and the generally favorable natural history makes the sensible interpretation of benefits noted in cohort studies nearly impossible. Any enthusiasm for the technique needs to be tempered with the knowledge that serious, fatal and disabling outcomes have been reported from such injections, thought to be due to occlusion of radicular vessels supplying the spinal cord.[83,84] The frequency of

these events is not known, but in a series of over 500 injections no serious adverse events were reported.[85] Notwithstanding this, the procedure is clearly accompanied by a material risk that anybody considering administering or receiving such treatment should consider. The key issue is how cervical transforaminal corticosteroid injections perform compared with surgical decompression in terms of efficacy and safety.

Surgery

Surgery has the potential to relieve the compression on the affected nerve root and should therefore be able to "cure" cervical radiculopathy and pain from cervical nerve root entrapment. However, this does not seem to always be the case. Marshaling the available empirical evidence suggests that, in the acute setting, surgery is likely to improve symptoms faster than conservative measures, without making any long-term difference when compared with conservative treatment. In the chronic arena, surgery is likely to improve symptoms in the majority of patients but is unlikely to effect a "cure."[80] In the absence of serious underlying cause of radiculopathy (e.g., tumor, infection), reasonable indications for surgery would include progressive neurologic deficit or refractory and disabling pain.

WHIPLASH

Whiplash injuries warrant particular mention in any discussion of neck pain. Whereas there is no doubt that whiplash injuries are a common cause of acute neck pain, there remains vigorous debate about the frequency with which they cause chronic pain.

Biomechanics

Biomechanical studies have demonstrated that the traditional view of hyperextension being the primary event in whiplash is incomplete and is a simplistic explanation for the behavior of the cervical spine in rear end vehicular accidents. In particular, it has been found that axial compression and unnatural, double curvatures of the cervical spine are important and potentially damaging components of the cervical spine's response to inertial loading. Cadaver experiments have demonstrated that after rear end impact, the lower cervical spine is thrust upward and forward.[86] The neck is, therefore, compressed from below. The lower cervical segments are extended while the upper segments are relatively flexed. As a result, the cervical spine assumes an S-shape during the first 50 to 75 ms. Thereafter, all segments are progressively extended until the head is thrown forward into extension. Similar observations were reported in experiments in which normal volunteers were studied using high-speed cineradiography during simulated collisions of approximately 5 kph.[87] The authors again emphasized the compression imparted to the cervical spine. A more detailed cineradiographic study of normal volunteers described the motion of individual cervical segments during the extension phase of whiplash.[88] After an 8-kph impact that resulted in 4-g acceleration, the C6 vertebra was driven upward. As it moved, the C6 vertebra extended underneath the rest of the cervical spine, causing the higher segments to undergo a small initial flexion, of some 2 to 5 degrees in amplitude, before undergoing extension. The net result was that the cervical spine assumed an S-shape at about 100 ms, as lower segments began extension while higher segments were still undergoing initial flexion (Fig. 68.10). These movements took place around abnormal axes of rotation, with the pathologic axes being higher than normal. As a result, the anterior end of the vertebra separated from the vertebral body below and, posteriorly, the tip of the inferior articular process chiseled into the supporting superior articular process. Subsequently, the cervical spine underwent extension, as described in the classical model. These observations provide a biomechanical substrate for injuries to several structures in the spine, most notably the cervical zygapophyseal joints, which seem to be particularly susceptible to damage through uncontrolled rotation through abnormal axes.[89]

Pathology

Our understanding of the pathology of whiplash has languished behind that of other spheres of rheumatology, primarily because of the paucity

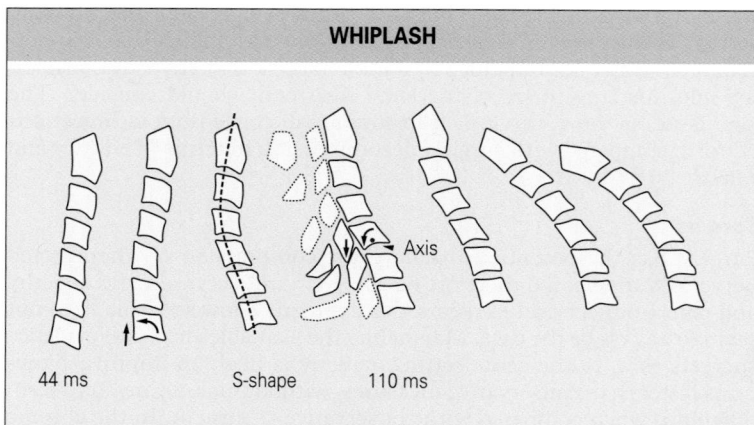

WHIPLASH

44 ms   S-shape   110 ms

Axis

Fig. 68.10 Whiplash. The appearance of sequential radiographs of the cervical spine during the extension phase of whiplash. At 110 ms the C5 vertebra rotates about an abnormally high axis of rotation, causing the vertebral body to separate anteriorly from C6, and the inferior articular process of C5 to chisel into the superior articular process of C6. (*Redrawn from Barnsley et al,[21] based on Kaneoka et al[88].*)

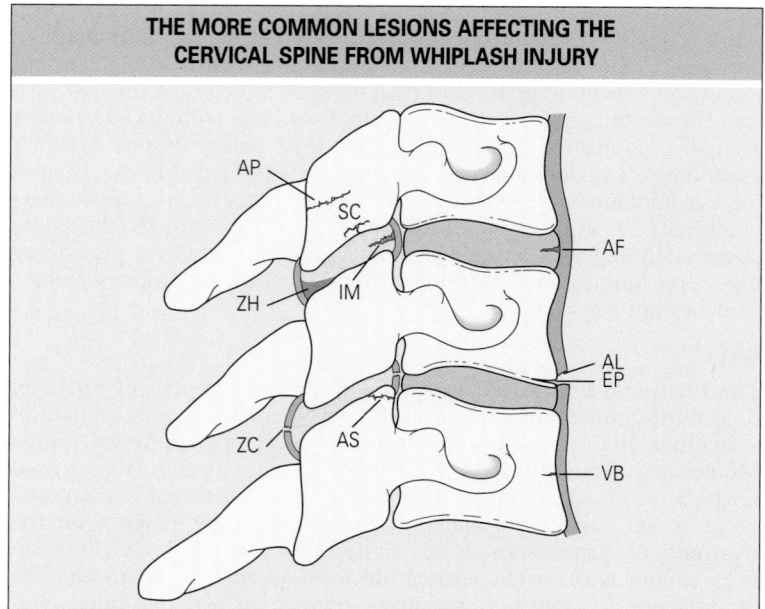

THE MORE COMMON LESIONS AFFECTING THE CERVICAL SPINE FROM WHIPLASH INJURY

AP
SC
ZH
IM
AF
ZC
AS
AL
EP
VB

Fig. 68.11 The more common lesions affecting the cervical spine from whiplash injury. AF, tear of the annulus fibrosus of the intervertebral disc; AL, tear of the anterior longitudinal ligament; AP, articular pillar fracture; AS, fracture involving the articular surface; EP, endplate avulsion and/or fracture; IM, contusion of the intra-articular meniscus of the zygapophyseal joint; SC, fracture of the subchondral plate; VB, vertebral body fracture; ZC, rupture of tear of the zygapophyseal joint capsule; ZH, hemarthrosis of the zygapophyseal joint. (*Adapted from Barnsley et al[21].*)

of pathologic material and the generally benign nature of the condition. However, there are a number of pathologic entities whose existence has been determined through clinical, animal, cadaveric, and postmortem studies.[21] These are summarized in Figure 68.11. Notwithstanding the extent and variety of lesions possible after whiplash, plain radiographs have been shown to be profoundly insensitive to the detection to all but the most severe bony injuries of the cervical spine. Twenty-two cervical spines were harvested from patients who had died of head injuries.[90] The specimens were then x-rayed under optimal conditions. Subsequent photographs of submillimeter slices revealed 245 injuries to various structures. Only four were detected on plain radiographs, even on second look.

Natural history

The natural history of whiplash is, for the most part, benign. Most patients recover within a few weeks of injury and have no residual symptoms. It has been argued that apparent differences in the rates of chronicity in whiplash in different countries are evidence that chronic whiplash is a socially programmed phenomena pivoting on the presence of a compensation system.[91] However, a careful analysis of the data reveals that many of the studies proffered to support this view were compromised by small sample size, poor study design, and inappropriate end points such as insurance claims rather than clinical information.[92,93] A series of follow-up studies of an inception cohort of patients assembled in the United Kingdom in the early 1980s has demonstrated that most patients destined to improve do so within a few months, with very little improvement after 2 years. The frequency of chronic symptoms classified as intrusive or severe at 15 years (presumably well after the settlement of any compensation claim) was in the order of 25%.[94]

Treatment

Treatment in the acute phase of whiplash is aimed at preventing chronicity, minimizing symptoms, and improving function. A review of the

conservative treatment of acute whiplash found that treatments such as cervical collars, rest, and passive physical modalities were generally inferior to programs involving activation, multimodal interventions emphasizing improved function, and simple reassurance and encouragement to resume normal activities.[95] Subsequent studies have supported the principle of early activation and exercise, rather than rest, improving the long-term outcome,[96,97] and this approach is endorsed by recent best evidence synthesis.[69]

There are very few controlled studies of the treatment of chronic neck pain after whiplash injury. The single most promising avenue has been that of percutaneous radiofrequency neurotomy for chronic cervical zygapophyseal joint pain (see earlier).[76] This remains a palliative treatment but one that can be highly valuable for patients with constant and debilitating pain. Otherwise, the rather unsatisfactory options for the management of any chronic neck pain, as discussed earlier, can be applied.

CONCLUSION

Neck pain is a common and usually self-limiting disorder, but it is important to exclude serious underlying illness and neurologic involvement. Future progress in the field of chronic and refractory pain will depend on reliably identifying the source of pain, typically through invasive analgesic or provocation techniques, and testing potential treatments in methodologically sound studies in selected patients. Increasing sophistication of trials has enhanced the evidence base for some existing therapies, particularly activation in acute whiplash and exercise therapy in chronic neck pain.

KEY REFERENCES

1. Bland JH, Boushey DR. Anatomy and physiology of the cervical spine. Semin Arthritis Rheum 1990;20:1-20.
3. Hogg-Johnson S, van der Velde G, Carroll LJ, et al. The burden and determinants of neck pain in the general population: results of the Bone and Joint Decade 2000-2010 Task Force on Neck Pain and Its Associated Disorders. Spine 2008;33(4 Suppl):S39-S51.
8. Grooten WJ, Mulder M, Josephson M, et al. The influence of work-related exposures on the prognosis of neck/shoulder pain. Eur Spine J 2007;16:2083-2091.
12. Siivola SM, Levoska S, Latvala K, et al. Predictive factors for neck and shoulder pain: a longitudinal study in young adults. Spine 2004;29:1662-1669.
13. MacGregor AJ, Andrew T, Sambrook PN, Spector TD. Structural, psychological, and genetic influences on low back and neck pain: a study of adult female twins. Arthritis Rheum 2004;51:160-167.
15. Vos CJ, Verhagen AP, Passchier J, Koes BW. Clinical course and prognostic factors in acute neck pain: an

16. Radanov BP, Sturzenegger M, Di Stefano G. Long-term outcome after whiplash injury: a 2-year follow-up considering features of injury mechanism and somatic, radiologic, and psychosocial findings. Medicine 1995;74:281-297.

17. Scholten-Peeters GG, Verhagen AP, Bekkering GE, et al. Prognostic factors of whiplash-associated disorders: a systematic review of prospective cohort studies. Pain 2003;104:303-322.

18. Carroll LJ, Holm LW, Hogg-Johnson S, et al. Course and prognostic factors for neck pain in whiplash-associated disorders (WAD): results of the Bone and Joint Decade 2000-2010 Task Force on Neck Pain and Its Associated Disorders. Spine 2008;33(4 Suppl):S83-S92.

19. Hoving JL, de Vet HC, Twisk JW, et al. Prognostic factors for neck pain in general practice. Pain 2004;110:639-645.

21. Barnsley L, Lord SM, Bogduk N. The pathophysiology of whiplash. In: Teasell RW, Shapiro A, eds. Spine state of the art reviews: cervical flexion-extension/whiplash injuries. Philadelphia: Hanley and Belfus, 1998:209-242.

24. Cloward RB. Cervical diskography: a contribution to the etiology and mechanism of neck, shoulder and arm pain. Ann Surg 1959;150:1052-1064.

25. Feinstein B, Langton NJK, Jameson RM, Schiller F. Experiments on pain referred from deep somatic tissues. J Bone Joint Surg Am 1954;36:981-997.

26. Dwyer A, Aprill C, Bogduk N. Cervical zygapophyseal joint pain patterns. I: a study in normal volunteers. Spine 1990;15:453-457.

27. Dreyfuss P, Michaelsen M, Fletcher D. Atlanto-occipital and atlanto-axial joint pain patterns. Spine 1994;19:1125-1131.

32. Slipman CW, Plastaras CT, Palmitier RA, et al. Symptom provocation of fluoroscopically guided cervical nerve root stimulation: are dynatomal maps identical to dermatomal maps? Spine 1998;23:2235-2242.

34. Van Mameren H, Drukker J, Sanches H, Beursgens J. Cervical spine motion in the sagittal plane (I) range of motion of actually performed movements, an X-ray cinematographic study. Eur J Morphol 1990;28:47-68.

37. Viikari Juntura E, Porras M, Laasonen EM. Validity of clinical tests in the diagnosis of root compression in cervical disc disease. Spine 1989;14:253-257.

39. Friedenberg ZB, Miller WT. Degenerative disc disease of the cervical spine: a comparative study of symptomatic and asymptomatic patients. J Bone Joint Surg Am 1963;45:1171-1178.

41. Boden SD, McCowin PR, Davis DO, et al. Abnormal magnetic-resonance scans of the cervical spine in asymptomatic subjects. J Bone Joint Surg Am 1990;72:1178-1184.

42. Fletcher G, Haughton VM, Khang-Cheng Ho, Shiwei Yu. Age-related changes in the cervical facet joints: studies with cryomicrotomy, MR, and CT. AJNR Am J Neuroradiol 1990;11:27-30.

45. Barnsley L, Bogduk N. Medial branch blocks are specific for the diagnosis of cervical zygapophysial joint pain. Reg Anesth 1993;18:343-350.

47. Manchukonda R, Manchikanti KN, Cash KA, et al. Facet joint pain in chronic spinal pain: an evaluation of prevalence and false-positive rate of diagnostic blocks. J Spinal Disord Tech 2007;20:539-545.

48. Barnsley L, Lord SM, Bogduk N. Comparative local anaesthetic blocks in the diagnosis of cervical zygapophysial joint pain. Pain 1993;55:99-106.

49. Lord SM, Barnsley L, Bogduk N. The utility of comparative local anaesthetic blocks versus placebo-controlled blocks for the diagnosis of cervical zygapophysial joint pain. Clin J Pain 1995;11:208-213.

50. Barnsley L, Lord SM, Wallis BJ, Bogduk N. The prevalence of chronic cervical zygapophysial joint pain after whiplash. Spine 1995;20:20-26.

51. Speldewinde GC, Bashford GM, Davidson IR. Diagnostic cervical zygapophyseal joint blocks for chronic cervical pain. Med J Aust 2001;174:174-176.

55. Bogduk N, Aprill C. On the nature of neck pain, discography, and cervical zygapophysial joint blocks. Pain 1993;54:213-217.

57. Mercer S, Bogduk N. Intra-articular inclusions of the cervical synovial joints. Br J Rheumatol 1993;32:705-710.

60. Wallis BJ, Lord SM, Bogduk N. Resolution of psychological distress of whiplash patients following treatment by radiofrequency neurotomy: a randomised double-blind placebo controlled trial. Pain 1997;73:15-22.

65. Philadelphia panel evidence-based clinical practice guidelines on selected rehabilitation interventions for neck pain. Phys Ther 2001;81:1701-1717.

66. Sarig-Bahat H. Evidence for exercise therapy in mechanical neck disorders. Man Ther 2003;8:10-20.

67. Chow RT, Heller GZ, Barnsley L. The effect of 300 mW, 830 nm laser on chronic neck pain: a double-blind, randomized, placebo-controlled study. Pain 2006;124:201-210.

68. Trinh KV, Graham N, Gross AR, et al. Acupuncture for neck disorders. Cochrane Database Syst Rev 2006;3:CD004870.

69. Hurwitz EL, Carragee EJ, van der Velde G, et al. Treatment of neck pain: noninvasive interventions: results of the Bone and Joint Decade 2000-2010 Task Force on Neck Pain and Its Associated Disorders. Spine 2008;33(4 Suppl):S123-S152.

72. Hurwitz EL, Aker PD, Adams AH, et al. Manipulation and mobilization of the cervical spine: a systematic review of the literature. Spine 1996;21:1746-1760.

73. Gross AR, Hoving JL, Haines TA, et al. A Cochrane review of manipulation and mobilization for mechanical neck disorders. Spine 2004;29:1541-1548.

75. Barnsley L, Lord SM, Wallis BJ, Bogduk N. Lack of effect of intra-articular corticosteroids for chronic cervical zygapophysial joint pain. N Engl J Med 1994;330:1047-1050.

76. Lord SM, Barnsley L, Wallis BJ, et al. Percutaneous radio-frequency neurotomy for chronic cervical zygapophyseal-joint pain. N Engl J Med 1996;335:1721-1726.

77. Sapir DA, Gorup JM. Radiofrequency medial branch neurotomy in litigant and nonlitigant patients with cervical whiplash: a prospective study. Spine 2001;26:E268-E273.

80. Bogduk N. Medical management of acute cervical radicular pain: an evidence based approach. Newcastle, Australia: Newcastle Bone and Joint Institute, 1999.

81. Radhakrishnan K, Litchy WJ, O'Fallon WM, Kurland LT. Epidemiology of cervical radiculopathy: a population-based study from Rochester, Minnesota, 1976 through 1990. Brain 1994;117:325-335.

82. Persson LC, Carlsson CA, Carlsson JY. Long-lasting cervical radicular pain managed with surgery, physiotherapy, or a cervical collar: a prospective, randomized study. Spine 1997;22:751-758.

84. Rathmell JP, Aprill C, Bogduk N. Cervical transforaminal injection of steroids. Anesthesiology 2004;100:1595-1600.

89. Cusick JF, Pintar FA, Yoganandan N. Whiplash syndrome: kinematic factors influencing pain patterns. Spine 2001;26:1252-1258.

90. Jónsson H Jr, Bring G, Rauschning W, Sahlstedt B. Hidden cervical spine injuries in traffic accident victims with skull fractures. J Spinal Disord 1991;4:251-263.

93. Teasell RW, Merskey H. The Quebec Task Force on whiplash-associated disorders and the British Columbia Whiplash Initiative: a study of insurance company initiatives. Pain Res Manage 1999;4:141-149.

94. Squires B, Gargan MF, Bannister GC. Soft-tissue injuries of the cervical spine: 15-year follow-up. J Bone Joint Surg Br 1996;78:955-957.

95. Peeters GG, Verhagen AP, De Bie RA, Oostendorp RA. The efficacy of conservative treatment in patients with whiplash injury: a systematic review of clinical trials. Spine 2001;26:E64-E73.

REFERENCES

Full references for this chapter can be found on www.expertconsult.com.

Lumbar spine disorders

Zacharia Isaac and Jeffrey N. Katz

69

- Mechanical low back pain is the most common presenting lumbar syndrome and is a general category of pain that in severe refractory cases requires methodical evaluation.
- One of the most important roles of the physician is to recognize non-mechanical causes.
- Investigation is indicated in patients with persistent or progressive pain and those in whom a non-mechanical cause is suspected.

EPIDEMIOLOGY

Occurrence

Low back pain is the most frequent disorder of mankind after the common cold.[1,2] Between 65% and 80% of the world's population develop back pain at some point during their lives. More than 60 million adults in the United States report having back pain at some point in the past 3 months.[3] The most prevalent impairments in people aged up to 65 years are musculoskeletal, with back and spine impairments the most frequently reported subcategory at 51.7%.[4] In the United States, mechanical low back pain is the fifth most common reason (2.8%) for physician office visits. Of these visits, non-specific low back pain was the most frequent diagnostic group at 56.8%.[5] Impairments of the back and spine are the chronic conditions that most frequently cause activity limitation among people aged 45 years or younger and they represent the third most common reason for impairment in people aged 45 to 64 years.[6] More than 7 million adults in the United States report activity limitation due to low back pain.[3]

Impact

More than 50% of all patients with back pain improve after 1 week, and more than 90% are better at 8 weeks.[7] The remaining 7% to 10% continue to experience symptoms for longer than 6 months. However, as many as 75% of individuals who improve are at risk of having a relapse of back pain in the next 12 months.[8] The high costs associated with low back pain are related to these individuals with chronic pain. For example, in the United States the estimated cost of industrial claims for low back pain in 1995 was $8.8 billion despite a decrease in the number of claims.[9] Frymoyer[10] has estimated that the direct cost of back pain in the United States in 1990 was more than $27.6 billion.

Risk factors

Recent twin studies indicate that heredity plays a more important role than environmental factors in disc degeneration, explaining 74% of the variance in adult populations. Genetic influences have been confirmed by the identification of several genes associated with disc degeneration.[11-13]

Many of the environmental risk factors described for back pain involve occupational or psychological characteristics. Workers involved in heavy-duty labor who are older than 45 years of age have a 2.5 times greater risk of absence from work secondary to back pain than workers aged 24 years or younger.[14] Those individuals with an initial episode of back pain lasting 3 months or more have a 50% higher risk for recurrence in the following year than those with an initial episode of only 1 day's duration.[15]

A number of psychological conditions are associated with back pain. Neurosis, hysteria, and conversion reaction are more frequently associated with acute back pain than depression.[16] Depression is a frequent complication of patients who develop chronic low back pain, although psychological distress predisposes to both a new episode and chronicity. Although psychiatric co-morbidities complicate treatment and can affect pain perception, true psychogenic pain is rare. Cigarette smoking is associated with an increased risk of back pain, although the data are inconsistent.[17] Although obesity is a minor factor in the causation of back pain, excessive weight assists perpetuation of episodes.[18]

CLINICAL EVALUATION

Introduction

Lumbar spine disorders can be categorized broadly as being mechanical, neuropathic, or medical in origin (Table 69.1). Up to 90% of patients with back pain have a mechanical or neuropathic reason for their pain.[19] Mechanical implies that pain is secondary to overuse of a normal anatomic structure, to trauma, or to deformity of an anatomic structure. Examples include discogenic pain, lumbar radiculopathy, spinal stenosis, facet syndrome, sacroiliac joint syndrome, and musculoskeletal sprain and strain. Neuropathic pain includes involvement of the peripheral or central nervous system either via direct compression of the spinal cord or spinal nerve roots, or via changes in the function of the neurologic system due to chronic pain. Given the difficulty in separating purely mechanical from purely neuropathic symptoms, many advocate the term *low back pain*. Patients with referred limb symptoms manifesting as weakness, pain, sensory disturbance, or reflex change caused by involvement of the spinal nerve are classified as having *radicular pain*. Defining a diagnosis is difficult because of the overlap of history, examination, and pain referral patterns of various pain generators and the high incidence of asymptomatic radiologic imaging findings.[20-24] Frequently, however, no trauma or deformity can be identified with certainty in patients with low back pain. For the overwhelming majority of patients with pain that responds to time, medications, and physical therapy, no specific diagnosis needs to be sought. Diagnostic functional testing with interventional spinal injection procedures is helpful in delineating the pain generator in refractory cases but requires thoughtful consideration of technical adequacy, placebo effect, and psychological pain behavior. Systemic illness accounts for the other 10% of adults with back pain.[25] More than 70 non-mechanical illnesses may be associated with back pain.[26] Careful clinical evaluation helps separate patients with low back pain from those with systemic illness.

The evaluation of a patient with low back pain thus requires an organized approach that should be tailored to the specific complaints of the patient. Understanding the mechanism of pain generation helps determine what types of therapeutic exercise, activity modifications, pharmacologic measures, spinal interventional procedures, and surgical options can be considered in the treatment algorithm.

History

Certain disorders occur more commonly in younger individuals, whereas others are associated with older patients. Familial predisposition does occur in certain medical illnesses associated with back pain. Of particular importance is the group of illnesses that cause spondyloarthropathy. A full occupational and social history is important for identifying those patients at risk of developing low back pain. The association of work and the onset of pain are important in regard to compensation. The patient's opinion about the association of the pain and his or her work must be determined, as well as the expectation of work-related sickness payments for injury and return to work.[27] Previ-

TABLE 69.1 CATEGORIES OF LOW BACK PAIN

Category	Source/pathologic entity	Quality
Superficial somatic	Skin, subcutaneous tissues (cellulitis)	Sharp, burning
Deep somatic	Muscles, fascia, periosteum, ligaments, joints, vessels, dura (arthritis)	Sharp, dull ache, boring
Radicular	Spinal nerves (herniated disc, spinal stenosis)	Radiating, shooting, tingling
Neurogenic	Mixed motor sensory nerves (femoral neuropathy)	Burning
Visceral referred	Abdominal viscera, pelvic viscera, aorta (autonomic sensory nerves)	Boring, colicky, tearing
Psychogenic	Cerebral cortex (conversion reaction, malingering)	Variable

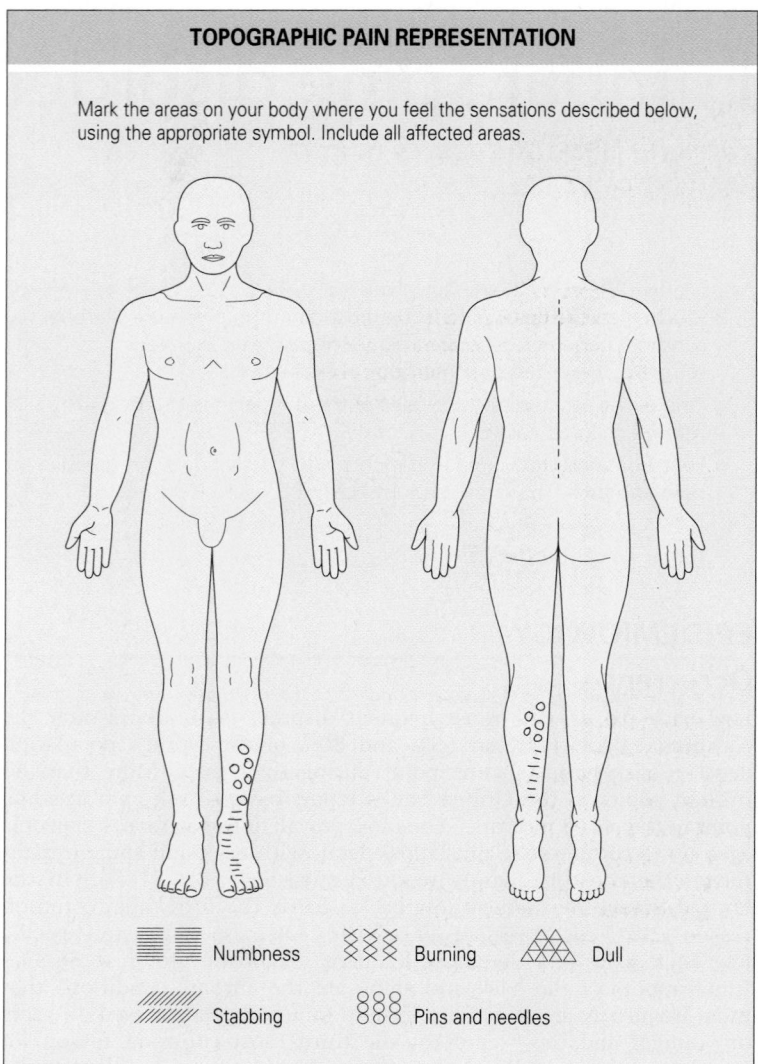

Fig. 69.1 Topographic pain representation. Pain distribution diagram of a patient with radiculopathy secondary to a lumbar intervertebral disc herniation.

ous history of malignancy, arthritis, or metabolic bone disease may influence the differential diagnosis. A history of coronary artery or cerebrovascular disease raises concern for peripheral vascular disease in the lower extremity, which can mimic lumbar stenosis symptoms. History of diabetes mellitus is important in that diabetic neuropathic pain syndrome can mimic lumbar radiculopathies. Review of systems should target questions about disordered sleep, which can compound pain; skin lesions, which can be of importance in spondyloarthropathy; and weight loss or nocturnal pain, which can be seen with malignancy.

Site of pain

It is helpful to ask the patient whether symptoms are predominantly axial (defined as the lumbosacral junction) or in the extremity (thigh, calf, or foot). The buttock region is often difficult to categorize because this can be affected with both axial low back pain and radicular pain due to irritation of spinal nerve roots. Most back pain is limited to the lumbosacral area. Radiation of pain in the thighs or to the knees may be referred from elements of the spine, such as intervertebral disc, zygapophyseal joints, sacroiliac joint, muscle, or ligaments, by somatic referral, previously known as *sclerotomal referral*. Pain that radiates from the low back to below the knees is usually radicular in origin and suggests a pathologic process affecting spinal nerve roots. In these cases, extremity symptoms in the thigh, calf, or foot are typically greater than axial low back symptoms.

Aggravating and relieving factors

Elucidating factors that aggravate and alleviate pain is helpful in defining potential sources for the symptom. Typically, disorders such as discogenic axial low back pain worsen with activity, including prolonged sitting and standing and bending forward, and improve with recumbency initially. Patients with disc herniations typically experience back and leg symptoms with sitting, driving, and slouching. The symptoms are typically relieved with walking and shifting positions. Patients with spinal stenosis typically experience gluteal, thigh, and calf pain with standing, walking, and lumbar extension. Patients with degenerative causes to their complaints typically have a variable severity with some good days and some bad.

Some patients with medical disorders that affect the spine, such as osteoporotic compression fractures, traumatic fractures, pathologic fractures or acute infection, may find relief of their pain with recumbency and even complete immobility, though some find no association with body position. Patients with a spondyloarthropathy classically report increased pain and stiffness when they remain in bed for a few hours and relief with movement and exercise. Patients with tumors that involve the structures of the lumbar spine may often experience worsening pain with recumbency and nocturnal exacerbation of pain. Patients with viscerogenic pain may have symptoms that are worsened or exacerbated with meals or bowel movements, abdominal tenderness,

perimenstrual exacerbation, or a history of excess alcohol or non-steroidal anti-inflammatory drugs (NSAID) consumption. Patients may move around with a forward flexed posture to avoid tension on the abdominal muscles, trying to achieve a comfortable position.

Measurement of pain severity

The severity of pain may be measured by a number of means. Patients may fill in a diagram with the location, quality, and severity of pain (Fig. 69.1). On a 100-mm visual analog scale, where a horizontal line is marked with 0 as no pain and 100 as the worst imaginable pain, the patient is asked to draw an intersecting line to indicate the pain. The Wong-Baker Faces scale combined with a 0 to 10-point numeric rating scale is often easily understood by patients. Questions about functional impairment such as dressing, with attention to donning shoes and socks, toileting, driving, light cleaning, shopping, and work assess how patients function in daily activities.

Physical examination

General examination

When a medical or systemic cause of low back pain is suspected, a general physical examination should be completed in addition to the examination of the spine. Changes in various organ systems (e.g., skin, ocular, gastrointestinal) may be noted in patients with medical low back pain. The objective of the physical examination of the lumbosacral spine is to demonstrate those static and dynamic abnormalities

TABLE 69.2 ANCILLARY TESTS FOR EVALUATION OF LOW BACK PAIN

Test	Tests for
Schober test	Lumbosacral motion
Contralateral straight-leg-raising test	Nerve root compression
Bow string sign	Nerve root compression (L5, S1)
Straight-leg raise	Nerve root compression (L5, S1)
Femoral stretch test or hip extension	Nerve root compression (L2, L3, L4)
FABER test	Sacroiliac joint dysfunction, hip range of motion
Hoover test	Patient effort
Vertebral percussion	Osseous pain/fracture

TABLE 69.3 LUMBAR ROOT LESIONS

Root	Muscle weakness/movement affected	Tendon reflex decreased
L2	Hip flexion/adduction	
L3	Hip adduction	Knee jerk
	Knee extension	
L4	Knee extension	Knee jerk
	Foot inversion/dorsiflexion	
L5	Hip extension/abduction	
	Knee flexion	
	Foot/toe dorsiflexion	
S1	Knee flexion	Ankle jerk
	Foot/toe plantarflexion	
	Foot eversion	

Cutaneous, motor, and reflex functions of the lower extremity.

that can help sort out the disease entities that may be responsible for low back pain.

Genital and rectal examinations should be performed in patients who have symptoms and signs suggestive of medical low back pain or cauda equina syndrome. These examinations are helpful in detecting patients with prostatic abnormalities, rectal cancer, or endometriosis. Low or absent rectal tone and absent voluntary anal contraction can be seen in patients with cauda equina syndrome. A number of ancillary physical examination tests may be used to confirm abnormalities discovered during the routine examination (Table 69.2).

Spinal examination

The spine is viewed for curvatures and postural deformities. A list is present if the first thoracic vertebra is not centered over the sacrum. Hyperlordosis or a flattened lumbosacral curve may be identified, whereas marked kyphosis is noted best from the lateral position. The spinous processes and sacrum can be palpated and percussed or pressure applied to determine if there is any osseous injury. The ischial tuberosity can be palpated to determine if proximal hamstring tenderness or bursitis is present. The paraspinal muscles can be palpated for any areas of spasm, taut bands, or trigger points. In the supine position, leg lengths should be measured to document discrepancies.

Lumbar range of motion

Spinal motion is important in terms of symmetry, rhythm, and range of motion. The patient is asked to flex, extend, and laterally bend the lumbosacral spine. Patients with localized mechanical disorders maintain the lordosis while bending from the hips when asked to flex forward. Patients with injuries in musculoskeletal structures at the L4/5 and L5/S1 interspaces will experience abnormal motion secondary to protective muscle contraction. Range of motion can be more precisely measured using an inclinometer.

Patients with spondyloarthropathy may have an abnormal Schober test. This is performed by having the patient stand erect and marking the distance between the midpoint of the posterior superior iliac spines ("dimples of Venus") and 10 cm above that point. The patient is then asked to maximally forward flex while the more caudal spot is kept stationary, and the more cephalad point on the tape measure should normally demonstrate at least 5 cm of excursion. This abnormality can also be seen in lumbar degenerative disc disease.

After full flexion, it is helpful to observe how the patient regains the erect posture. Patients with back lesions return to the erect position using a fixed lordosis and rotating the pelvis with the help of knee and hip flexion. Classic teaching is that an increase in pain with forward flexion suggests an abnormality in the anterior elements of the spine, including discogenic disease. This is likely mediated by increases in intradiscal pressure with forward flexion. Pain that is increased by extension suggests disease in the posterior elements of the spinal column, including the zygapophyseal joints.

Manual muscle testing

Of the possible neurologic abnormalities, persistent muscle weakness is the most reliable indicator of nerve compression.[28] It is useful to measure muscle strength on the Medical Research Council six-point scale (0 to 5 muscle grade scores). Routinely tested muscle groups may include knee extension and flexion; hip abduction and adduction; foot eversion and inversion; and ankle dorsiflexion and plantarflexion. When testing muscle power, the intervening joints should be in neither full flexion nor extension and the examiner should be in a position of mechanical advantage. Broad variability exists as to how much strength is normal, and the examiner's experience is required to determine expected strength for a patient. Examiner's judgment is required to distinguish true weakness from pain inhibited, apprehension inhibited, of effort-dependent strength deficits. At a minimum, function of the three most commonly affected nerve roots should be tested (Table 69.3). Additional muscle groups are often tested to exclude a broader neurologic problem.

The L5 myotome includes the ankle dorsiflexors, great toe extensors, hip abductors, and ankle evertors. Dorsiflexion power of the foot is tested by asking the patient to dorsiflex the foot while the examiner applies steady downward pressure with the palm of the hand on the dorsal aspect of the foot while cupping the heel with the other hand. Resisted great toe extension tests the extensor hallucis longus and the L5 myotome. Asking the patient to heel walk provides a good screening test for the L5 nerve root. Severe weakness of the L5 myotome may be detected by the Trendelenburg test. The patient is asked to stand on one leg. Weakness of hip abduction is highlighted by the sagging of the pelvis on the side opposite the affected leg. Patients may also have a Trendelenburg sign with hip osteoarthritis or history of a neuromuscular disorder.

The S1 myotome includes the gastrocnemius and hip extensors. Gluteus maximus strength is tested by having the patient lie prone and extend the hip against resistance with the knee bent. Asymmetry of strength or presence of atrophy suggests an abnormality of S1. The gastrocnemius is not readily overcome with manual muscle testing even when weak and a more sensitive screen for S1 weakness is completing more than 10 single-leg calf raises on each side.

The L4 myotome includes the quadriceps and ankle dorsiflexors. The L3 myotome includes the quadriceps but not ankle dorsiflexors. Single-leg squatting is a good test to challenge the quadriceps muscle, which is often too strong to be overcome by the examiner's upper limb musculature.

The L1 and L2 myotomes include the hip flexors, which are tested by asking the supine patient to lift the thigh off the examining table. Having the hip externally rotated minimizes the substitution of the rectus femoris of the quadriceps, which receives L2 through L4 contributions.

Neurologic examination

Upper motor neuron and peripheral nerve abnormalities may also cause neurologic dysfunction. Patients with upper motor neuron dysfunction develop muscle spasticity, hyperreflexia, and Babinski and Hoffman signs. The distinction among upper motor neuron, nerve root, and peripheral nerve lesions is essential for the differential diagnosis of back pain. Different disease processes preferentially affect upper motor (e.g., multiple sclerosis), nerve root (disc herniation), or peripheral nerve (diabetes).

Sensory examination

Sensory findings are less reliable because they are affected by the state of fatigue and emotional state of the patient. A given area of skin also receives innervation by two dermatomes, making sensory testing less specific for defining the affected nerve root. However, if a peripheral nerve is injured, a specific muscle may become paralyzed or specific skin areas become anesthetic (Figs. 69.2 and 69.3). The L5 dermatome involves the buttock, lateral thigh, lateral calf, dorsal foot, and great toe. The S1 dermatome involves the buttock, posterior thigh, posterior calf, and lateral foot. The L4 dermatome involves the anterior thigh, anterior knee, and pretibial region of the shin.

Deep tendon reflexes

Testing deep tendon reflexes, especially the patellar reflex (L4) and Achilles reflex (S1), can be useful. However, there is no reliable reflex to test for L5. Older individuals may lose reflex function, particularly at the Achilles (which is likely to be symmetrical), and previous episodes of nerve compression may have caused a loss of reflexes, which may not return even with recovery of motor and sensory function.[29]

Excessively brisk reflexes can be indicative of an upper motor neuron process such as cervical myelopathy.

Provocative maneuvers

The hip joints should be moved through their range of motion. Differentiation of hip pain from sacroiliac joint pain may be determined by the Patrick or "FABER" (flexion, abduction, external rotation) test. A Patrick maneuver producing low back pain suggests sacroiliac joint pain but can be non-specific and seen with spondylolisthesis, spinal stenosis, facet syndrome, and acute discogenic pain due to annular tear. A Patrick maneuver producing groin or anterior thigh discomfort suggests hip disease. The greater trochanter can be palpated to determine the presence of bursitis. Sustained lumbar extension precipitating thigh or calf discomfort suggests lumbar stenosis.

Root tension signs

The straight-leg-raising test detects irritation of the sciatic nerve (L5, S1). The passive raising of the leg by the foot with the knee extended stretches the sciatic nerve, its nerve roots, and dural attachments (Fig. 69.4). When the dura is inflamed and stretched, the patient will experience pain along its anatomic course to the lower leg, ankle, and foot. Dural movement starts at 20 degrees of elevation. Pain of dural origin should not be felt below that degree of elevation. Pain is maximal between 20 and 70 degrees of elevation. Symptoms at greater degrees of elevation may be of nerve root origin but may also be related to mechanical low back pain secondary to muscle strain or joint disease.[30] Dorsi-

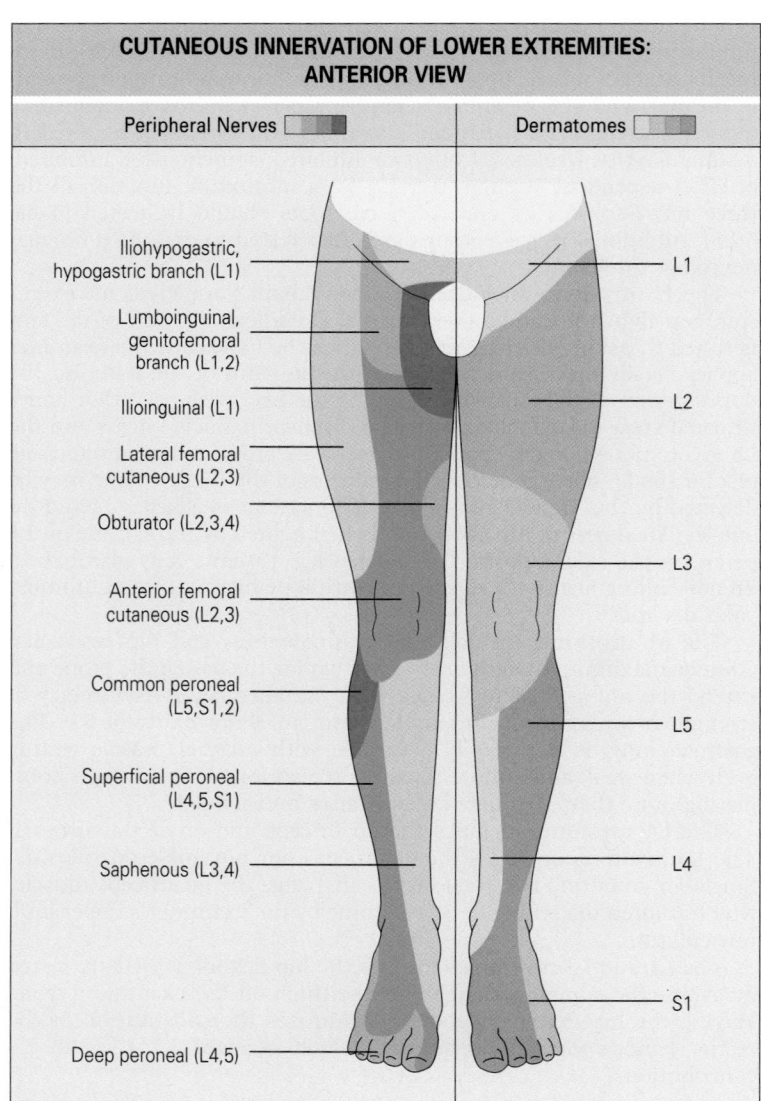

Fig. 69.2 Cutaneous sensory innervation. Anterior view of lower extremities illustrating skin areas supplied by nerve roots (right) and peripheral nerves (left).

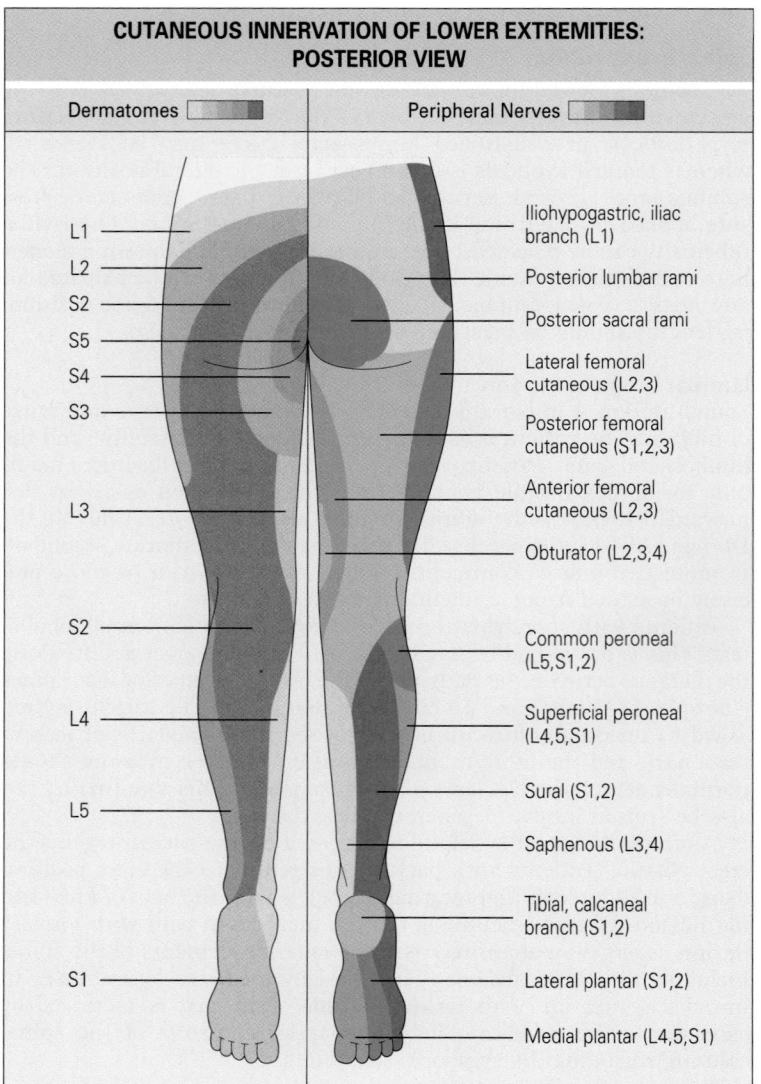

Fig. 69.3 Cutaneous sensory innervation. Posterior view of lower extremities illustrating skin areas supplied by nerve roots (left) and peripheral nerves (right).

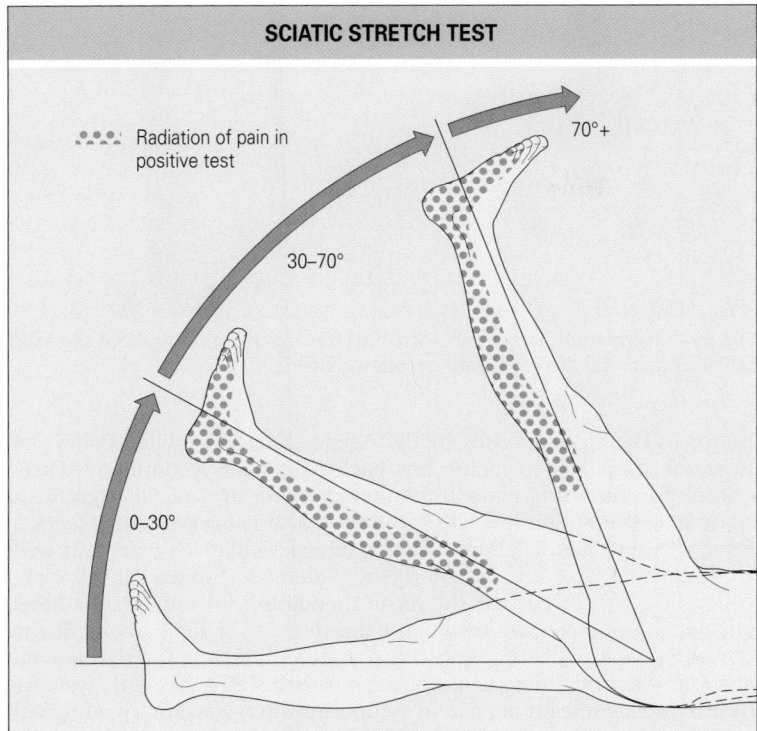

SCIATIC STRETCH TEST

Radiation of pain in positive test

70°+

30–70°

0–30°

Fig. 69.4 Sciatic stretch test. In the straight-leg-raising test, the leg is lifted with the knee extended. Sciatic roots are tightened over a herniated disc between 30 and 70 degrees. Dorsiflexion of the foot increases pain with nerve impingement.

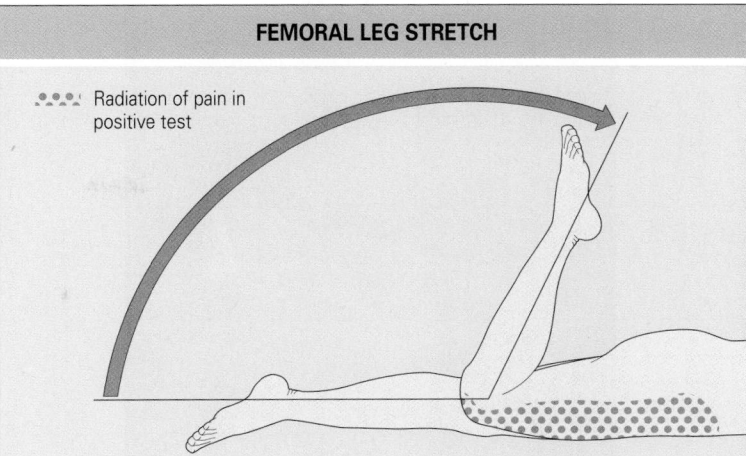

FEMORAL LEG STRETCH

Radiation of pain in positive test

Fig. 69.5 Femoral leg stretch. In the femoral stretch test, the knee is flexed and lifted superiorly. Sharp pain generated in the anterior thigh is considered to constitute a positive test.

flexion of the foot will exacerbate the radicular pain, also known as *Braggard maneuver*. Pain may also be experienced in the leg below the knee when the contralateral normal leg is raised, known as the *crossed straight-leg raise*. The presence of contralateral pain suggests a large herniation causing traction on the opposite nerve root when the normal leg is raised. The crossed straight-leg-raising test is insensitive but highly specific.[31] Patients with L5 or S1 radicular pain will classically experience pain down the leg below the knee to the ankle or foot. Patients with hamstring tightness will experience symmetrical posterior thigh or posterior knee discomfort but no pain radiation below the knee.

In the positive sitting root sign, where the knee is passively extended, familiar symptoms in the calf and foot are reproduced. This is analogous to the supine straight-leg raise. Patients will also lean backward to minimize the traction on neural elements (tripod sign or flip sign). In lumbar radiculopathy, upper motor neuron signs such as a Babinski reflex (extension of the large toe and spreading of the other toes) should be absent because the spinal cord conus is situated at L1/2 level. If present, an upper motor neuron abnormality should be sought.

The neurologic examination is completed by testing for higher lumbar and sacral nerve root function. Dural irritation of nerve roots from L2 to L4 are tested by the femoral stretch test or reverse straight-leg raise (Fig. 69.5). With the knee bent, the thigh is elevated from the examining table. The test is positive if pain is reproduced in the front of the thigh or the medial aspect of the leg.

Gait analysis

The patient's gait should be analyzed for heel walking and toe walking to screen for L5 and S1 myotomal deficits, respectively. Antalgia may be indicative of sacral, hip, knee, or foot and ankle injuries but can also be seen in acute radicular pain and with pain behavior. A forward stooped posture can be seen in patients with spinal stenosis and in patients with ankylosing spondylitis. A mechanical gait can be seen as part of cervical or thoracic myelopathy.

Reproducibility of physical signs

McCombe and colleagues[32] evaluated the reproducibility between three observers of 54 physical signs used for back pain evaluation. The signs that were adequately reproducible included the following:

- measurements of lordosis (by tape measure from the maximum kyphosis of the thoracic spine to that of the sacrum)
- flexion range (Schober test)
- determination of pain location on flexion and lateral bend
- straight-leg-raising test (pendulum goniometer measurement of the angle at which pain was first experienced and angle of maximum tolerance)
- determination of pain location in the thigh and legs
- sensory changes in the legs

Nerve root tension signs were reliable if the location of pain was described. Reproducibility of bone tenderness over the sacroiliac joints, spinous processes, and iliac crests was greater than that associated with soft tissue structures.

The diagnostic value of disturbed sensory and motor function was tested prospectively by Jensen in 52 patients with lumbar disc herniations confirmed at surgery.[33] The positive predictive value of disturbed sensation in the L5 dermatome and weakness of foot dorsiflexion was 76% for herniation from the L4/5 lumbar disc. The positive predictive value of altered sensation in the S1 dermatome was only 50%.

Non-organic physical signs

Patients with psychological pain behavior often have subjective complaints that are much greater than their objective findings.[34] Waddell has described five tests that identify individuals with "functional" or "exaggerated" symptoms (Table 69.4).[35] A finding of three or more of the five signs is clinically significant. Isolated positive signs are ignored. Patients who feign weakness during manual muscle testing may resist pressure for a few seconds and then release the muscle suddenly or in a manner resulting in a "cogwheel" or "giveway" effect. The significance of these findings is often overstated and generally does not indicate willful malingering. Symptoms of psychological pain behavior do not exclude concomitant nociceptive pain and tissue injury. Patients with psychological pain behavior warrant comprehensive treatment.

INVESTIGATIONS

Imaging

Plain radiographs

The Quebec Task Force on Spinal Disorders suggested that in patients without neurologic dysfunction, plain radiographs should not be done during the first week of an acute episode of back pain.[36]

Patients with back pain of a mechanical origin frequently have radiographs that are normal. In adults younger than the age of 50, the yield of unexpected important findings can be as low as 1 in 2500.[18] By contrast, many individuals with radiographic abnormalities may be entirely asymptomatic.[37] Thus congenital abnormalities, including spina bifida, transitional vertebrae, Schmorl nodes and mild scoliosis, are only rarely causes of back pain.[38] In normal persons older than 50,

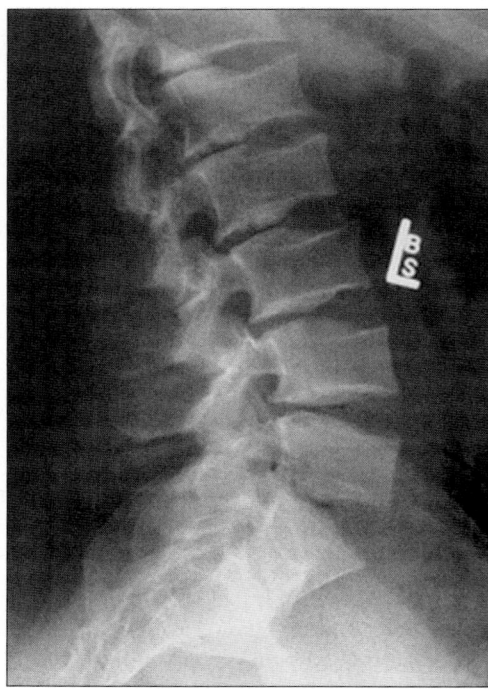

Fig. 69.6 Spondyloepiphyseal dysplasia. Plain radiograph, lateral view, demonstrating elongation of vertebral bodies at multiple levels of the spine.

TABLE 69.4 WADDELL TESTS FOR FUNCTIONAL LOW BACK PAIN	
Tenderness to superficial touch	
Simulation tests	Axial loading
	Spinal rotation in one plane
Distraction tests	Inconsistent results on confirmatory testing
Regional disturbances	Abnormalities not following neuroanatomic structures
Overreaction	Disproportionate verbalization

the prevalence of radiographic change is high: 67% have evidence of intervertebral disc degeneration, of whom two thirds are asymptomatic. In addition, osteoarthritis of zygapophyseal joints noted on radiographs is not strongly correlated with symptoms.[39] Further, abnormalities confirmed at operation are not identified by plain radiographs. In one study, plain radiographs failed to identify two thirds of those who at surgery were found to have disc protrusion.[40]

Some radiologic abnormalities may not be clinically meaningful.[41] A review of 35 studies reported a wide range in the strength of associations between non-specific low back pain and radiographic abnormalities on plain radiographs, including disc space narrowing, sclerosis, and osteophytes.[42] The findings of spondylolysis, spondylolisthesis, and spina bifida were not associated with back pain. Plain radiographs do expose the patient to radiation and add a significant cost to the initial evaluation of patients.[43]

When lumbar radiographs are obtained, a single lateral film may be adequate (Fig. 69.6) and may offer the highest yield view to detect vertebral compression fractures. Padley and colleagues[44] reviewed lumbosacral spine radiographs of 200 patients with back pain and no neurologic signs. Others have suggested that anteroposterior and lateral views are adequate for evaluation.[45,46] The coned lateral view of the lumbosacral junction and oblique views do not identify therapeutically important lesions that cannot be seen on the other views.[47] The anteroposterior views and lateral views offer important information of scoliotic curvature and sagittal balance, which can often help specialists with interpreting biomechanics. Flexion and extension views can demonstrate segmental instability, which can be a potential cause of unexplained back and radicular symptoms. The clinical practice guidelines

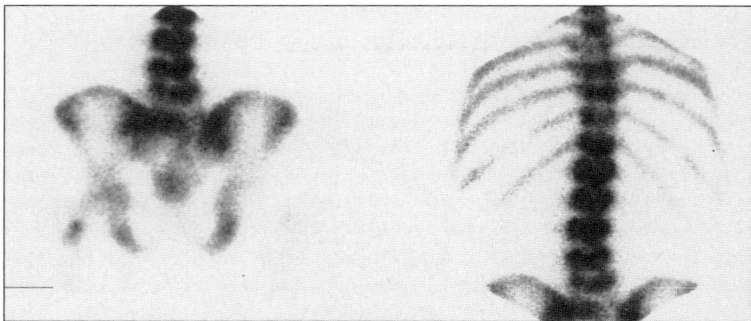

Fig. 69.7 Technetium bone scan. Increased tracer activity throughout the axial skeleton secondary to metastatic prostate cancer.

issued in the United States by the Agency for Health Care Policy and Research (AHCPR) for acute low back pain have recommended that criteria for obtaining plain films include older age, recent significant trauma, history of prolonged steroid use, prior cancer, recent infection, fever, intravenous drug abuse, unexplained weight loss, or pain with recumbency.[48] In a review of these guidelines, Suarez-Almazor and colleagues[48a] reported that the recommendation for radiographs based on older age alone may result in excessive use of radiographs during the initial visit. The use of criteria of failure to respond to therapy and signs of systemic illness is more cost-effective.[49] Patients with systemic illness and significant persistent symptoms often warrant imaging with magnetic resonance imaging (MRI) or computed tomography (CT) scan, and negative plain radiographs do not provide sufficient reassurance of absence of malignancy.

Radionuclide bone scintigraphy

Technetium-99m diphosphonate scans are useful in screening for infection, tumors, inflammatory arthritis, and fractures.[50,51] The sensitivity of bone scan is generally equal to MRI (90% vs. 96%) but it is less specific, for example, in detecting vertebral osteomyelitis (78% vs. 92%).[49] Gallium and indium scans increase the specificity when used with a technetium scan but are less sensitive when used alone.[52] Bone scintigraphy is better than MRI when evaluation of the whole skeleton is required,[53] such as in patients with metastatic disease who may have unsuspected bone lesions in other parts of the skeleton (Fig. 69.7). Increased activity in appendicular joints, as well as in axial joints, is suggestive of polyarthritis, usually associated with a spondyloarthropathy. The addition of bone single photon emission computed tomography (SPECT) imaging can be useful for identifying facet pathology and predicting patients who respond to intra-articular facet injection.[54]

Computed tomography

CT is useful for evaluating abnormalities of the lumbosacral spine, where the spatial anatomy is complex.[55] The CT scan is the best technique for assessing the bony architecture of the spinal column, including the sacroiliac joints, before changes are noted on plain radiographs.[56] In addition, the structural relationships of soft tissues (ligaments, nerve roots, fat, intervertebral discs) can be evaluated as they relate to their bony environment. CT is an excellent technique for identifying mechanical disorders, including spinal stenosis, spondylosis, spondylolysis, spondylolisthesis, trauma, and congenital anomalies (Fig. 69.8).[57-60] CT can visualize cortical bone destruction, calcified tumor matrix, and soft tissue extension of tumors affecting the spine and is superior to MRI in this regard (Fig. 69.9).[61] CT can also be used in an outpatient setting for percutaneous needle biopsy guidance of bony lesions.[62]

The clinical significance of CT abnormalities must be evaluated in the setting of the patient's clinical findings. In a study of 53 asymptomatic patients with lumbar CT scans, abnormal findings were described in 34.5% of individuals.[63] In patients younger than age 40, 19.5% had a CT diagnosis of an intervertebral disc herniation. In patients older than 40, 50% had abnormal findings, including disc herniation, spinal stenosis, and apophyseal joint degeneration. In addition, there was agreement among the three neuroradiologists in only 11% of the cases. The implication is that a patient with no historical or physical findings indicative of spinal pathology has a one in three

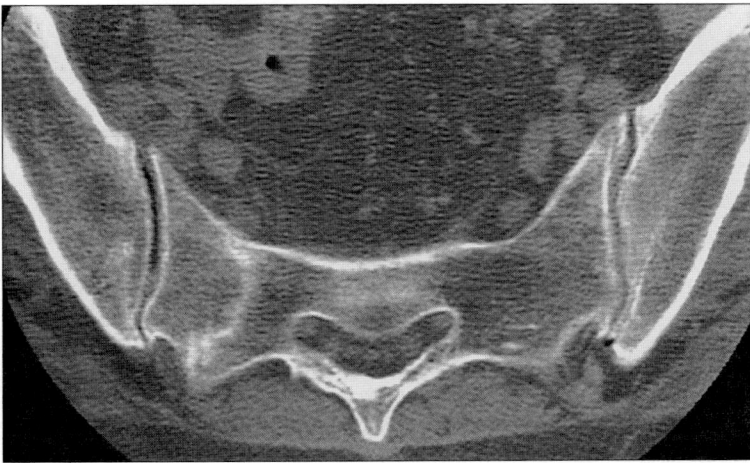

Fig. 69.8 Fracture. Computed tomography study of sacral spine demonstrating sacral fracture not visualized with plain radiographs.

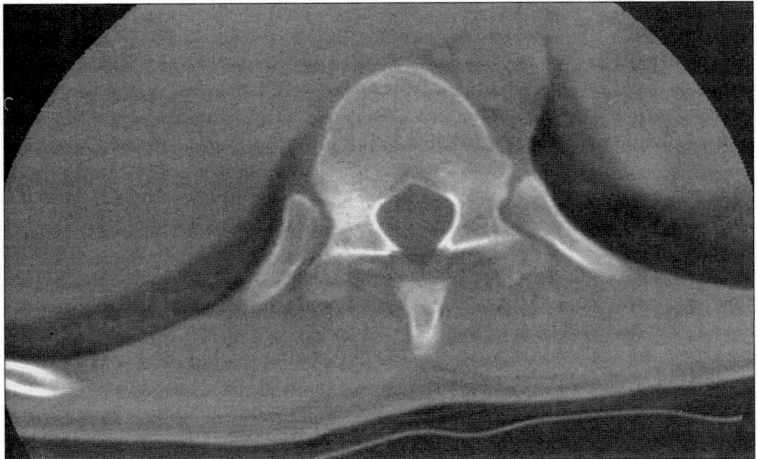

Fig. 69.9 Osteoid osteoma. Computed tomographic study of thoracic spine demonstrating increased sclerosis associated with an osteoid osteoma.

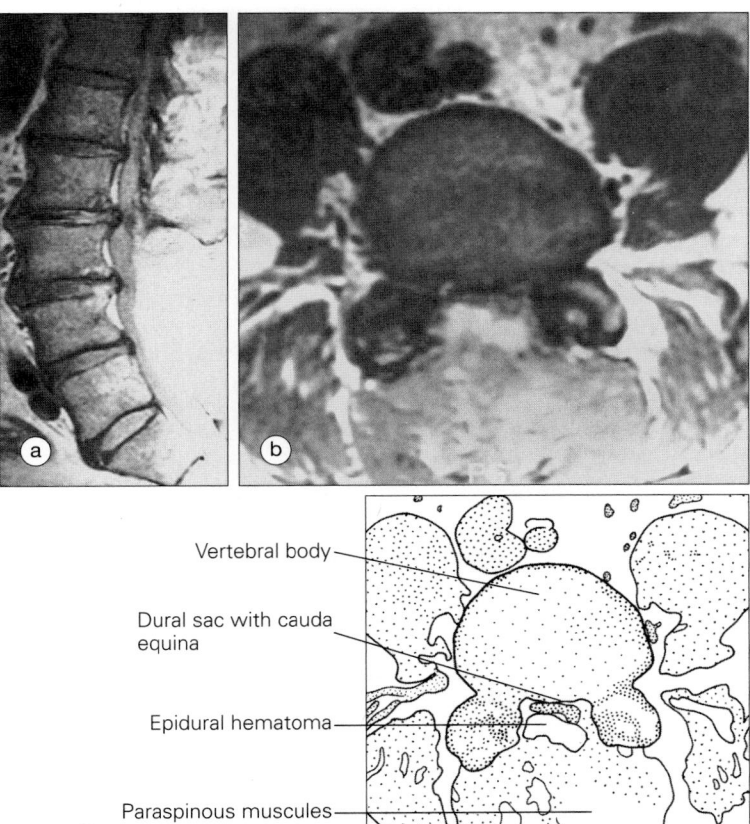

Fig. 69.10 Epidural hematoma. Postoperative sagittal and axial magnetic resonance imaging studies showing an epidural hematoma compressing the cauda equina.

chance of having an abnormal CT scan. Surgical intervention cannot be based on anatomic abnormalities without clinical symptoms and physical signs that correlate with radiographic findings. CT should be used as a confirmatory test and not solely as a diagnostic test.

Myelography

Myelography is an invasive procedure requiring the injection of contrast media through a spinal needle. All the complications associated with a lumbar puncture may occur with a myelogram (headache, hematoma, infection, back pain, and seizures).[64] In combination with CT, myelography is helpful in detecting cord compression caused by fracture and soft tissue impingement associated with tumors. Cerebrospinal fluid may be removed for laboratory evaluation.[65] CT enhanced with contrast (CT myelogram) improves the accuracy of postoperative assessment of epidural fibrosis versus recurrent disc.[66] Arachnoiditis may also be evaluated by CT myelography. CT myelography is most helpful for these conditions when patients are unable to undergo MRI evaluation.[67]

Like the CT scan, the myelogram should be employed as a confirmatory study. An abnormal iophendylate myelogram may be identified in 24% of individuals without back pain.[68] The myelogram should be reserved for the preoperative situation to confirm the presence of a herniated disc, a congenitally anomalous nerve root, or a tumor. Myelography is not as accurate as CT or MRI for the diagnosis of herniated nucleus pulposus.[69]

Magnetic resonance imaging

MRI has become the imaging modality of choice to evaluate lumbar spine disorders.[70] The procedure is well tolerated by most patients except for claustrophobic individuals, who may require sedation. The entire length of the spinal cord and canal may be evaluated in multiple planes. MRI is able to define bony and soft tissue structures without intrathecal contrast. Patients who are not candidates for MRI evaluation include those on life support systems and those who have a cardiac pacemaker or ferromagnetic clips in the abdomen or brain or on blood vessels.

MRI is an excellent technique to view the spinal cord. It identifies syringomyelia, atrophy, cord infarction, cord injury, multiple sclerosis, and intramedullary tumors (Fig. 69.10).[71] The development of contrast media (gadopentetate dimeglumine) for MRI has improved the characterization of spinal cord tumors.[72,73] Contrast-enhanced MRI is able to identify spinal cord pial metastases not visible by other radiographic techniques.[74] MRI delineates the extent of extradural tumor invasion of the spinal canal and compression or displacement of the spinal cord. It can identify the vertebral bodies in which bone marrow has been replaced with tumor (Fig. 69.11).[75,76]

MRI is an excellent technique for detecting infection of the spine, including discitis, osteomyelitis, epidural abscess, paraspinal abscess, and myelitis.[77] It is more sensitive in the detection of vertebral osteomyelitis than plain radiographs or CT.[78] Changes in the vertebral bodies and adjacent intervertebral disc spaces are visualized on T1-weighted images as areas of low signal intensity. On T2-weighted images, high signal intensity is seen crossing the involved bone and disc space.

MRI is also a useful technique for evaluating mechanical disorders of the lumbosacral spine. Disorders of the intervertebral disc are readily detected. Herniations can be identified in the sagittal plane and confirmed on the axial images.[79] Early degenerative changes are revealed by the loss of water, indicated by the darkening of the disc on the T2-weighted image. MRI is also useful in the assessment of traumatic and non-traumatic fractures of vertebral bodies.[80] MRI can identify degenerative vertebral endplate changes and categorize them as edema, fatty, or sclerotic. MRI can identify high-intensity zone lesions, representing annular tears and neovascularization.

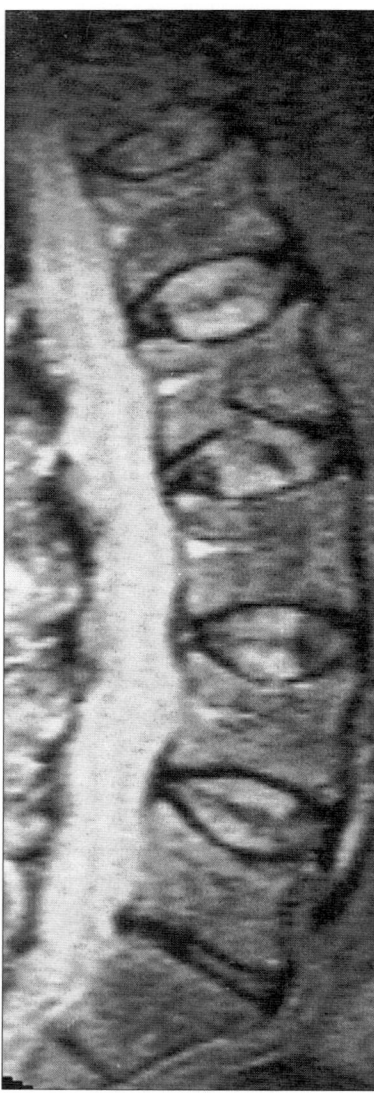

Fig. 69.11 Spinal cord tumor. Lumbar spine magnetic resonance imaging study of a multiple myeloma patient with abnormal bone marrow signal throughout the vertebral bodies, associated with remodeling and pathologic fractures.

The addition of gadolinium contrast can help in the evaluation of spinal tumors, infection, and epidural fibrosis. Use of gadolinium contrast in patients with renal failure has been associated with a scleroderma-like disorder called *nephrogenic systemic fibrosis* (see Chapter 166).[81,82]

Correlation between MRI and clinical findings

As with CT and myelography, the interpretation of MRI findings must take account of the clinical presentation. Boden and colleagues[20] reported on a total of 104 MRI scans of 67 asymptomatic and 37 symptomatic individuals interpreted by three neuroradiologists for abnormalities. The radiologists read 19 of 67 (28%) of the asymptomatic people as having substantial abnormalities. Herniated discs (24%) and spinal stenosis (4%) were the most common findings. Older persons (aged 60 to 80 years) had the majority of the abnormal findings. Jensen and colleagues[83] completed an MRI study on 98 asymptomatic individuals. Only 36% of these individuals (mean age 42.3 years) had normal results. Some 52% had a disc bulge at one level, 27% had a protrusion, and 1% had an extrusion. An abnormality at two levels or more was noted in 38%.[83] Other investigators have reported similar results in different asymptomatic populations.[84,85]

Comparison between MRI and other modalities

In the diagnosis of herniated discs and spinal stenosis, MRI has a sensitivity equal to or greater than that of CT or myelography.[86] In a

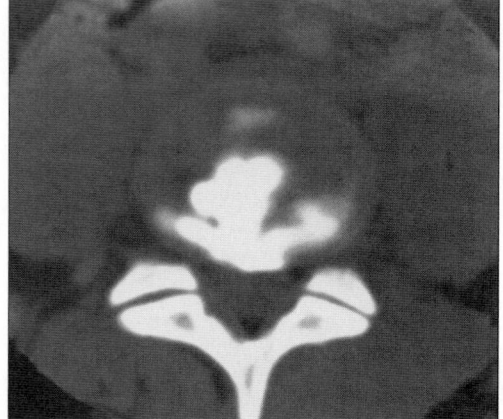

Fig. 69.12 Postdiscography computed tomography scan. A scan demonstrating a painful grade 4 disruption of an anulus fibrosus.

study comparing MRI with contrast CT for the diagnosis of herniated disc confirmed at surgery, MRI had 90% accuracy, whereas CT had an accuracy rate of only 77%.[87] MRI had greater sensitivity (88%) than myelography (75%) for the diagnosis of herniated discs.[88] It is also accurate in the diagnosis of spinal stenosis: a 97% agreement between MRI and contrast CT was identified for 41 patients evaluated for spinal stenosis in the central canal, lateral recess, and foramina.[89]

In addition, MRI was able to identify disc degeneration in 74 of 123 interspaces, whereas CT identified only 27. Currently, MRI is the technique of choice for investigation of spinal stenosis and disc degeneration. The major limitation of MRI is the cost.

Other imaging techniques

A number of other radiographic techniques are available for the evaluation of the lumbosacral spine. They are used infrequently compared with the techniques already discussed.

Spinal angiography permits the identification of the arterial origins and the venous drainage of vascular lesions of the spinal cord and column.[90] Arteriovenous malformations are characterized by arteriovenous communication without an intervening capillary network.

Abnormalities of disc integrity may be missed on plain radiographs and CT scans. Lumbar discography is a procedure associated with the injection of contrast material through a percutaneous needle into the nucleus pulposus suspected of causing back pain. The reproduction of the patient's pain is considered a positive test (Fig. 69.12). The test is used for patients with a degenerative disc who may be considered for spinal fusion, disc replacement, or intradiscal therapy because of persistent pain.[91] Its clinical significance remains controversial.[92]

The prevalence and significance of discographic abnormalities continue to be investigated.[23] MRI is equally sensitive in detecting disc degeneration by identifying high-intensity zones in an intervertebral disc (Fig. 69.13).[93] However, MRI is unable to reproduce patient symptoms. The role of discography will be decided on its relevance to patient symptoms and the development of better, non-surgical therapies.

CLINICAL LABORATORY TESTS

The vast majority of individuals with low back pain do not require laboratory studies with their initial evaluation. However, patients who are elderly, who have constitutional symptoms, or who have failed conservative therapy may benefit from a laboratory evaluation. The most useful test in helping to differentiate medical from mechanical low back pain is measurement of the erythrocyte sedimentation rate (ESR), which can suggest the presence of systemic inflammation. In one study, an ESR greater than 25 mm/hr had a false-positive rate of only 6%.[94] C-reactive protein (CRP) is increasingly used along with the ESR as a serum biomarker of inflammation.

Abnormalities in the complete blood count (hematocrit, leukocyte, or platelet count) may be indicative of an inflammatory disorder, including neoplasms. Alterations of calcium concentration and alkaline phosphatase activity suggest diffuse bone disease. Elevated acid

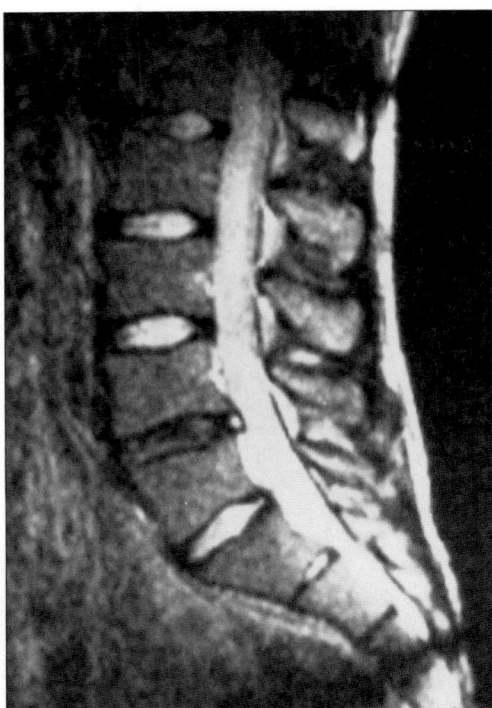

Fig. 69.13 Disc degeneration. Magnetic resonance imaging demonstrating a high-intensity zone lesion (arrow) in the L4/5 intervertebral disc.

phosphatase activity may mirror the extent of metastases from prostatic cancer. Urinalysis can identify the individual with renal abnormalities (nephrolithiasis). Detection of occult blood in the stool is a screening test for ulcers or gastrointestinal tumors.

ELECTRODIAGNOSTIC STUDIES

Electrodiagnostic studies are extensions of the neurologic examination and provide a means to identify nerve and muscle damage. These tests can confirm the clinical suspicion of nerve root compression, define the distribution and severity of involvement, and document or exclude other disorders of nerves or muscles that contribute to the patient's symptoms and signs. This tool is most helpful in cases where a peripheral entrapment, plexitis, anterior horn cell disease, or myopathy may be present. It is in the diagnosis of these non-spine–related conditions where electrodiagnostic studies are most useful.

Electrodiagnostic tests can be helpful in identifying neurophysiologic abnormalities in a patient in whom clinical examination (pain radiation, sensory changes, muscular weakness) does not necessarily indicate nerve root dysfunction.[95] Neurophysiologic tests can also document normal function where radiographic techniques have revealed anatomic abnormalities.

Electromyography

Electromyography (EMG) is the test most commonly ordered to document the presence of a radiculopathy.[96] The needle EMG is the most sensitive tool for the diagnosis of electrophysiologically identifiable radiculopathy. Electromyography measures the action potentials of muscle fibers. As the nerve supplying a muscle becomes compressed, fibers to that muscle are lost and are eventually replaced with regenerated fibers. This process of denervation and reinnervation occurs over time. Electromyography may not be able to document abnormalities until 3 to 4 weeks after the initial insult.

Abnormalities associated with radiculopathy can include increased duration and amplitude of motor unit potentials, fibrillation potentials, and prolonged insertional activity, which occur in the affected myotome or myotomes. A negative EMG does not invalidate a patient's pain and sensory complaints but does make complaints of weakness and motor deficit much less likely to be based on spinal nerve injury.

Nerve conduction tests

In contrast to EMG, nerve conduction tests become abnormal as soon as nerve damage occurs.[97] Nerve conduction tests include evaluation of the conduction velocity and amplitude along a segment of a peripheral nerve. They are helpful in distinguishing peripheral entrapment and neuropathy from a radiculopathy. The limitations of electrodiagnostic studies must be considered when evaluating patients with low back pain without radicular features. An abnormal EMG is corroborative evidence of organic disease and helps the physician determine who is a potential candidate for surgical intervention. Electromyography changes may recede with resolution of the nerve impingement. However, patients undergoing operative decompression with relief of symptoms may have persistent EMG abnormalities 1 year after surgery.[98] In patients without neurologic dysfunction, EMG and nerve conduction tests are normal.

NON-MECHANICAL CAUSES OF LUMBAR SPINE PAIN

Most patients with low back pain have a mechanical cause for their symptoms and do not require any diagnostic tests (Table 69.5). However, there are a number of serious and potentially life-threatening disorders that must be considered. These include cauda equina compression, abdominal aneurysm, infection, and neoplasms of various types. The first two are local disorders, but the latter often have systemic consequences. Clues to a potentially serious cause of back pain include the following:

- constitutional symptoms: fever and/or weight loss or increased pain on recumbency (e.g., sleeping in a chair) or nocturnally
- morning stiffness lasting hours
- acute, localized lumbosacral bone pain
- visceral pain associated with alterations in gastrointestinal or genitourinary function

Cauda equina compression

Patients with cauda equina compression have a symptom complex that may include low back pain, bilateral sciatica, saddle anesthesia, or bladder and bowel incontinence. The most common mechanical causes of cauda equina compression are large central herniations of intervertebral discs, whereas epidural abscesses or hematomas and tumor masses constitute the most frequent non-mechanical causes. Once the diagnosis is suspected, the patient should undergo a radiographic procedure to visualize the affected anatomic area of the lumbosacral spine. MRI is the most sensitive radiographic technique for detecting these lesions. Patients with cauda equina syndrome have the best opportunity for return of neurologic function if the cause of the compression can be eliminated within 48 hours.[99]

Abdominal aortic aneurysm

A patient with "tearing" or "throbbing" back pain who has experienced acute dizziness may have an expanding abdominal aneurysm. Any change in the frequency, intensity, or location of the pain suggests expansion in the size of the aneurysm. Patients with an abdominal aneurysm are usually older individuals who have had a history of lower extremity claudication. If patients complain of syncope or are hypotensive, they must be evaluated for an aneurysm on an emergency basis. Physical examination of the abdomen may reveal a pulsatile mass, abdominal bruits, and decreased pulsations in the lower extremities. Patients with expanding aneurysms may be evaluated with CT or ultrasonography, depending on the patient's hemodynamic status. Patients with an expanding aneurysm require surgical correction of the aneurysmal defect.

Infections

Patients with fever and/or weight loss may have an infection (or tumor) as a cause of their pain. The clinical presentation of the patient with a spinal infection depends on the infecting organism (Table 69.6). Bacterial infections cause acute, toxic symptoms, whereas tuberculosis

TABLE 69.5 COMMON DEGENERATIVE CAUSES OF LOW BACK PAIN

	Muscle strain	Spondylolisthesis	Herniated disc	Osteoarthritis	Spinal stenosis
Age (yr)	20-60	20-40	20-60	Over 40	Over 50
Pain pattern					
Initial location	Back	Back	Leg > back	Back > leg	Leg > back
Onset	Acute	Insidious	Acute	Insidious	Insidious
Standing	+	+	–	+	+
Sitting	–	–	+	–	–
Flexion	+		+	–	–
Extension	–	+	–	+	+
Straight-leg raise	–	–	+	–	–
Plain radiograph	–	+	–	+	+

TABLE 69.6 INFECTIOUS DISORDERS AFFECTING THE LUMBOSACRAL SPINE*

Vertebral osteomyelitis	Bacterial
	Tuberculous
	Fungal
	Spirochetal
	Parasitic
Discitis	
Pyogenic sacroiliitis	

All of these may cause localized low back pain.

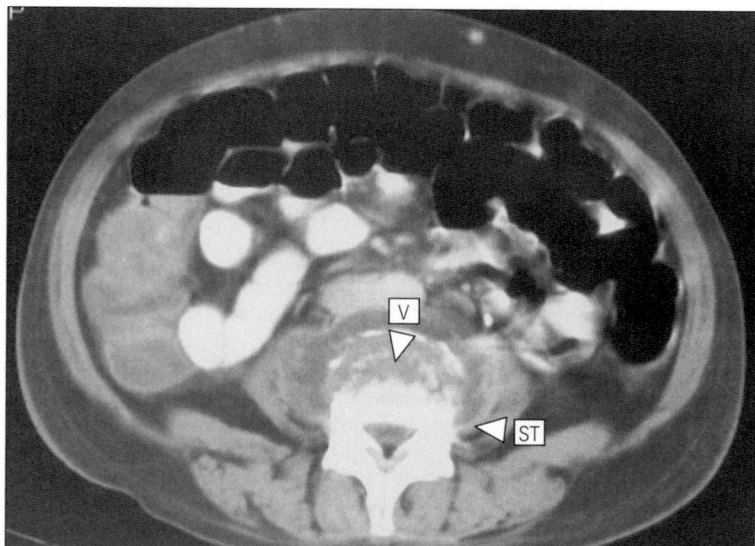

Fig. 69.14 Vertebral osteomyelitis. Computed tomography scan, axial view, demonstrating destruction of vertebral body (V) with soft tissue extension (ST) into the paravertebral space.

and fungal infections are indolent. The pain in bacterial infections is persistent, present at rest, and exacerbated by motion. Pain radiating to the abdomen or both legs and the presence of abdominal discomfort may confuse the diagnosis. Paraplegia is more closely associated with lesions in the cervical or thoracic spine but can occur with lumbar infections. Physical findings include decreased range of motion, muscle spasm, and percussion tenderness over the involved bone. Plain radiographs may reveal localized areas of osteopenia. If radiographs are normal, technetium bone scintigraphy or MRI can be used to investigate the entire lumbosacral spine for the presence of local infection. MRI also detects soft tissue extension of lesions beyond the bony confines of the vertebral column. CT should take place after MRI evaluation to delineate the bony architecture of lesions not visualized adequately by MRI (Fig. 69.14).

The definitive diagnosis of infection is based on the recovery and identification of the causative organism from blood cultures or from aspirated material or biopsy of the lesion. Antibiotic therapy is adequate to cure most spinal infections. Surgical intervention for drainage is necessary if neurologic dysfunction has occurred or appears imminent secondary to the infection.

Vertebral osteomyelitis

Vertebral osteomyelitis follows hematogenous spread from an extraosseous source.[100] Organisms may enter bone from nutrient arteries or from the venous plexus of Batson, a valveless system of veins that supplies the spinal column. Organisms that cause osteomyelitis include bacteria, mycobacteria, fungi, spirochetes, and parasites. The primary sources for spinal infections include the genitourinary tract, respiratory tract, and skin. The most frequently encountered organism causing infection in 60% of cases is *Staphylococcus aureus*.[101] Gram-negative organisms are often grown from samples from the elderly and from parenteral drug abusers (*Escherichia coli* and *Pseudomonas aeruginosa*,[102] respectively). In patients who have undergone surgery or trauma to the spine, non-pathogenic organisms (diphtheroids, *Staphylococcus epidermidis*) may be associated with an indolent infection of the vertebral column.[103] Workers in the meat-processing industry may

acquire a brucellosis infection.[104] Tuberculous and fungal infections of the vertebral column occur most often in the elderly and other immunocompromised individuals. The clinical presentation of a patient with tuberculous spondylitis is pain over the involved vertebrae, low-grade fever, and weight loss. The process is indolent and may be present for years before diagnosis (Fig. 69.15).[105]

Disc infection

Spondylodiscitis occurs in the setting of concurrent extraspinal infection[106] and in adults is also associated with lumbar disc surgery.[107] The ESR is almost universally elevated in the case of established disc space infections, often exceeding 100 mm/hr along with a leukocytosis.[108] Plain radiographs may be normal at the onset of infection but will demonstrate increasing destruction with prolonged duration of infection (Fig. 69.16). Radiographic evidence of established disc infection includes the following:

- symmetric destruction of adjacent endplate surfaces of two vertebrae
- loss of disc height
- reactive new bone formation
- sclerosis of bone endplates, with or without evidence of bone destruction or bone formation
- soft tissue abscesses
- kyphosis or subluxations after there has been significant bone destruction

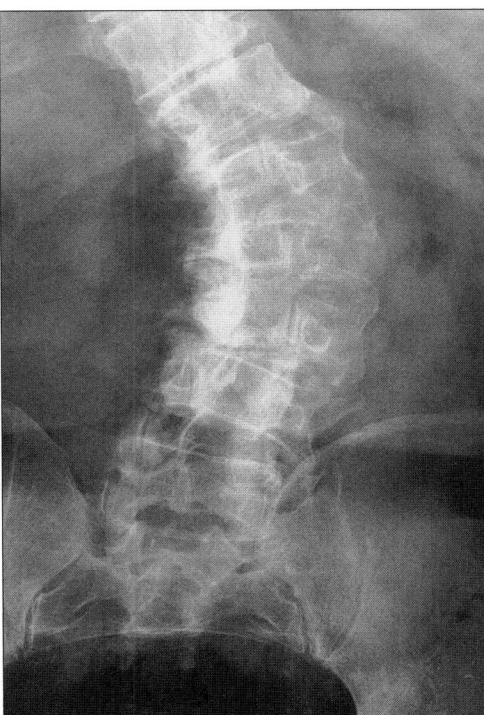

Fig. 69.15 Lumbosacral spine involvement. Pott disease affecting the lumbosacral spine at L3, resulting in rotatory scoliosis and lateral calcification.

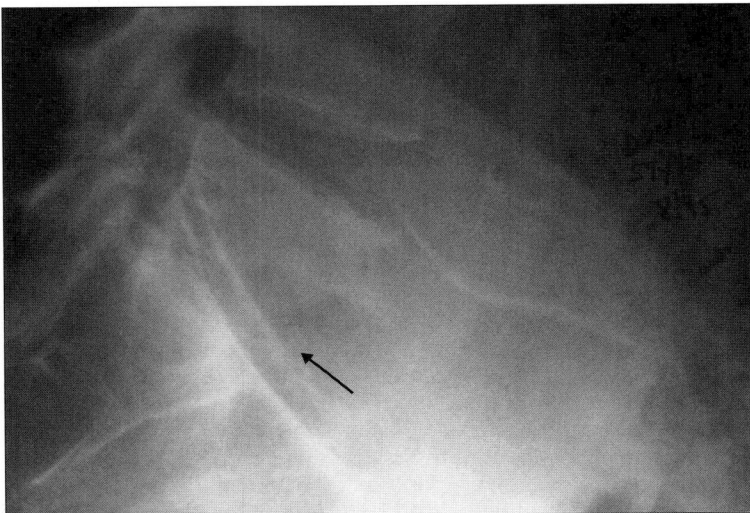

Fig. 69.16 Infection of the intervertebral disc space. Plain lateral radiograph of the lumbar spine showing narrowing of the L5/S1 disc space with new bone formation at the L5 endplate (arrow) and a soft tissue mass pushing the great vessels anteriorly. This finding of narrowing of the disc space and new bone formation with displacement of the great vessels strongly suggests the diagnosis of spinal infection with a soft tissue abscess.

On CT, changes in disc space and vertebral endplates can be seen, as can soft tissue abscesses (Fig. 69.17). Diagnosis is confirmed by identifying the causative organism from blood cultures, aspirated disc material, or biopsy of infected adjacent bone. Six weeks of parenteral antibiotics and possibly additional oral antibiotic therapy usually provides adequate treatment for patients with radiologic evidence of disc space infection and a positive culture. The ESR provides a method of assessing the efficacy of therapy in these patients.

Surgical intervention, including drainage and débridement of spinal infections, is indicated in patients who develop paraparesis or paraplegia. The following factors appear to increase the risk of neurologic deficits:

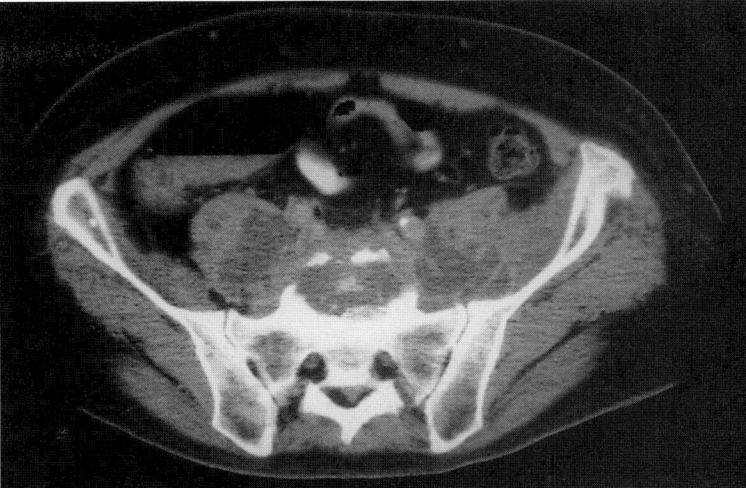

Fig. 69.17 Spinal infection imaged by computed tomography of the lumbar spine. At the L5/S1 level lucent areas in both psoas muscles and destructive changes in the intervertebral disc space suggest the presence of spinal infection with bilateral abscesses.

- older age
- cervical or thoracic infection
- staphylococcal infection as opposed to other organisms
- coexisting diabetes or rheumatoid arthritis

When surgical treatment is selected, controversy exists involving the use of bone grafts to achieve bony fusion. The experience of the spinal surgeon at the time of surgical débridement can help to determine the appropriate course of action.

Pyogenic sacroiliitis

Pyogenic sacroiliitis is an unusual form of septic arthritis.[109] The disease is associated with acute symptoms, severe sacroiliac joint pain, and fever. Diagnosis of the causative organism may be obtained by blood cultures, fluoroscopic fine-needle aspiration, or open biopsy. Antibiotic therapy for 6 weeks is usually adequate to eradicate the infection without the need for surgical drainage.

Neoplasms

Tumors of the spinal column or spinal cord may cause pain at night or with recumbency. Both benign and malignant neoplasms cause these symptoms. Nocturnal pain may be caused by swelling of neoplastic tissues associated with inactivity in the supine position or by stretching the neural tissues over the neoplastic mass. A number of benign and malignant tumors are associated with involvement of the lumbosacral spine (Table 69.7). Benign lesions tend to cause local pain and involve the posterior elements of vertebrae. Malignant lesions cause more diffuse pain and systemic symptoms and involve the anterior elements of vertebrae.

Patients with malignancies have pain that is gradual in onset but persistent and increasing in intensity. Physical examination shows localized tenderness over the lesion along with neurologic dysfunction if neural elements are compressed. Radiographic evaluation is useful in detecting the location and characteristics of the neoplastic lesion.

Osteoid osteoma

Osteoid osteoma is a benign tumor of bone that affects the lumbar spine. The tumor is most frequently found in young adults aged 20 to 30 years. Approximately 7% of osteoid osteomas occur in the spine, most frequently in the lumbar area.[110] The pain associated with this lesion is intermittent and vague initially but with time becomes constant and aching, with a boring quality. The pain is frequently worse at night and disturbs sleep. In the spine, osteoid osteomas are associated with non-structural scoliosis. The appearance of marked paravertebral muscle spasm and the sudden onset of scoliosis in a young adult require an evaluation for the presence of this lesion. The lesion is on the concave side of the scoliosis. The symptoms of osteoid osteoma

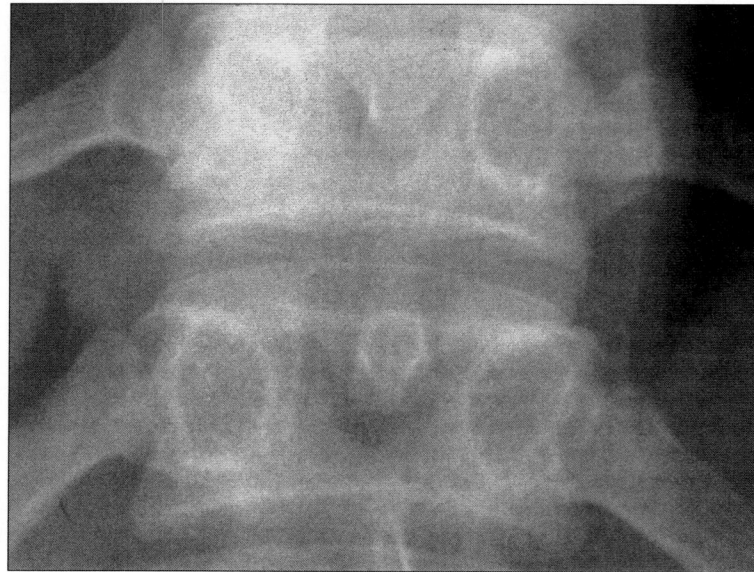

Fig. 69.18 Osteoid osteoma. Plain radiograph of the thoracic spine demonstrating sclerosis affecting the right pedicle of T11.

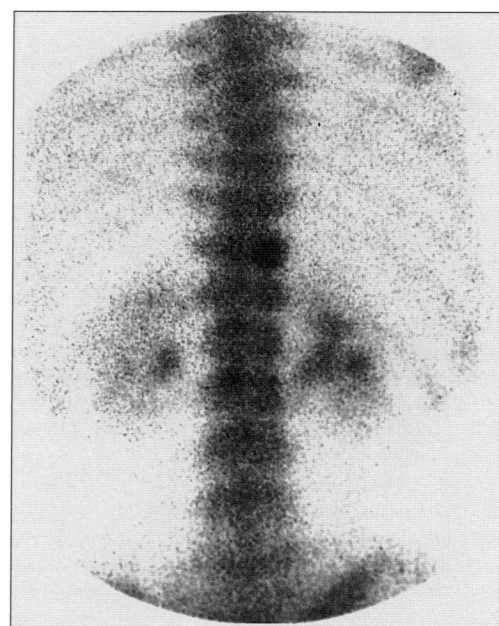

Fig. 69.19 Osteoid osteoma. Bone scintigraphy (posterior view) demonstrating increased uptake in T11. There is no other area of increased uptake in the skeleton.

TABLE 69.7 NEOPLASTIC LESIONS OF THE LUMBOSACRAL SPINE*		
Benign	**Malignant**	**Spinal cord tumors**
Osteoid osteoma	Multiple myeloma	Extradural metastases
Osteoblastoma	Chondrosarcoma	Intradural-extramedullary
Osteochondroma	Chordoma	Neurofibroma
Giant cell tumor	Lymphoma	Meningioma
Aneurysmal bone cyst	Skeletal metastases	Intramedullary
Hemangioma		Ependymoma
Eosinophilic granuloma		Astrocytoma
Sacroiliac lipoma		

All of these may cause localized low back pain.

may be present for a considerable time before plain radiographic findings become evident. The pain is often relieved by low doses of NSAIDs. Physical examination reveals local tenderness. Scoliosis is reversible early in the course of the lesion. With prolonged spasm, muscle atrophy may occur. Vertebral deformity may occur in young individuals who are growing. Hyperemia of the tumor may cause swelling and erythema of the skin if the lesion is superficial in location.

The radiographic finding of a lucent nidus with a diameter of 1.5 cm and a surrounding well-defined area of dense sclerotic bone is virtually pathognomonic of osteoid osteoma. The lesions are in the neural arch in 75% of affected vertebrae, articular facets in 18%, and vertebral bodies in 7% (Fig. 69.18). Bone scans or CT scans should be employed if an osteoma is suspected and not found on plain radiographs (Fig. 69.19).[111,112]

The treatment for an osteoid osteoma is simple excision of the nidus and surrounding sclerotic bone. If the nidus is not entirely removed, recurrence of the lesion is possible and symptoms may persist. On occasion, osteoid osteomas may undergo spontaneous healing.

Other primary spinal tumors

Neoplastic lesions may also occur inside the central spinal canal. These intraspinal neoplasms may be extradural, between bone and the outermost covering of the spinal cord (the dura); intradural-extramedullary, between the dura and the spinal cord; and intramedullary, in the spinal cord proper. Extradural tumors are most commonly metastatic in origin. Intradural-extramedullary tumors are primarily meningiomas, neurofibromas, or lipomas (Fig. 69.20). Intramedullary tumors

are ependymomas or gliomas. MRI, by its ability to define the exact location, size, and character of the lesions, has revolutionized the visualization of intraspinal lesions.[73]

Multiple myeloma

Multiple myeloma is the most common primary malignancy of bone in adults, accounting for 27% of biopsied bone tumors in one series.[113] Patients typically range in age from 50 to 70 years. Low back pain is the initial complaint in 35% of patients. The pain is aching and intermittent at onset, aggravated by weight bearing and improved with bed rest. Some patients may have radicular symptoms that mimic those of sciatica and arthritis.[114] Significant neurologic dysfunction, including paraplegia, occurs more commonly with solitary plasmacytoma than with multiple myeloma.[115] Physical examination may demonstrate diffuse bone tenderness, fever, pallor, and purpura in the later stages of the illness. Signs of spinal cord compression are present if vertebral body collapse has progressed to a significant degree. Abnormal laboratory results may include anemia, leukocytosis, thrombocytopenia, elevated ESR, hypercalcemia, hyperuricemia, elevated creatinine, and a positive Coombs test. An increase in serum proteins is secondary to the presence of abnormal immunoglobulins in any of the five classes. Urinalysis may detect Bence Jones protein formed by the production of excess immunoglobulin light chains. Bone marrow aspirate or biopsy reveals an excess number of plasma cells of varied histologic grades.

Plain radiographs demonstrate osteolysis without reactive sclerosis and sparing of the posterior elements of the spine (Fig. 69.21).[116] Solitary plasmacytomas in the spine have variable radiographic appearances. They may be expansile, with or without reactive bone. They may invade an intervertebral disc space and mimic discitis. Bone scintigraphy does not detect myeloma because there is no reactive component of osteoblasts to the myeloma cells. MRI and CT are better techniques for identifying the presence and extent of myeloma lesions in the bone and soft tissues. MRI is able to detect spinal bone marrow involvement in asymptomatic myeloma patients.[117]

The diagnosis of multiple myeloma is based on clinical data, along with the detection of abnormal plasma cells on biopsy. Myeloma is treated with the use of chemotherapeutic agents to control the growth of the malignant plasma cells. In patients with cord compression, decompression laminectomy is indicated, with or without local radiotherapy.

Skeletal metastases

Skeletal metastases are 25 times more common than primary tumors as the cause of neoplastic lesions in the spine. Autopsy results dem-

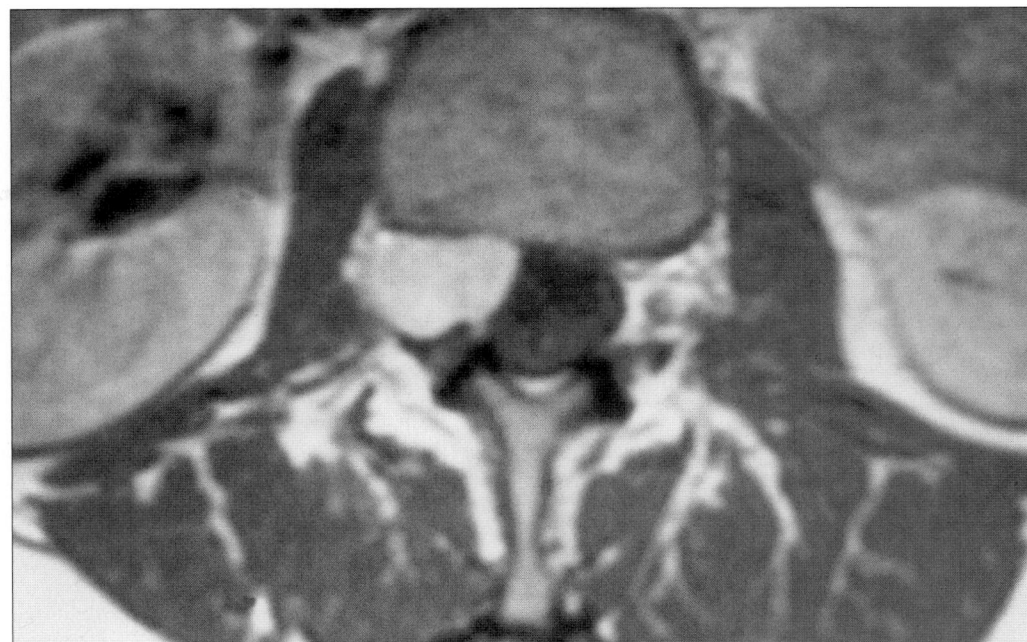

Fig. 69.20 Caudal neurofibroma. Transverse T1-weighted MRI following intravenous gadolinium shows an enhancing mass occluding the right neural foramen of L2. Note how local bone erosion has widened the neural foramen.

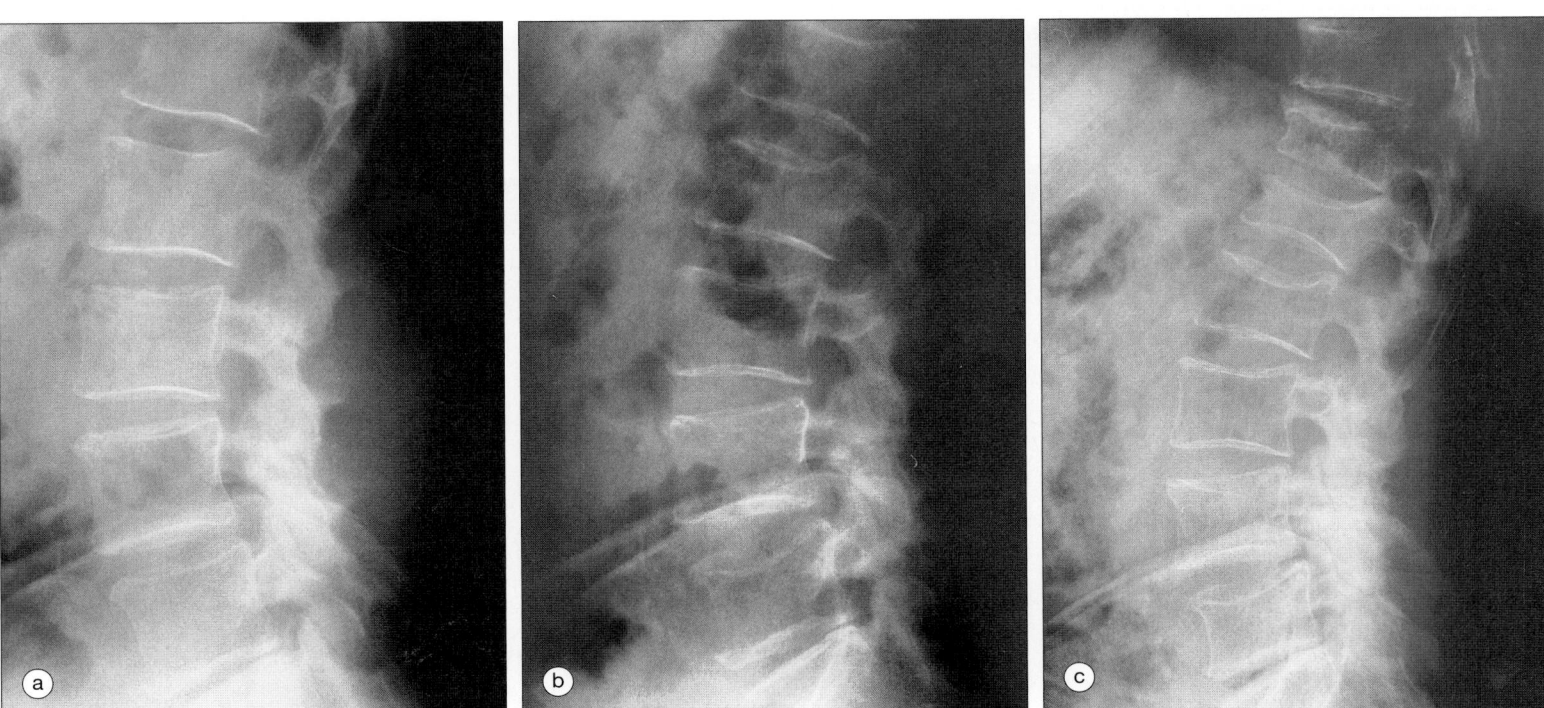

Fig. 69.21 Multiple myeloma. A series of plain radiographs taken over a 3-month period. Progressive osteopenia and pathologic compression fractures are noted. (a) Initial evaluation. (b) At 12 weeks. (c) At 14 weeks. Diagnosis was made at 12 weeks after initial presentation.

onstrate that 70% of patients with primary tumors develop metastases to the thoracolumbar spine.[118] The common primary sources for skeletal metastases include tumors of the breast, prostate, lung, kidney, thyroid, colon, uterine cervix, and bladder. Lumbar pain is typically of gradual onset and increasing intensity and is provoked by motion, sneezing, or coughing. The pain is local at the onset but may become radicular in character. Neurologic abnormalities may occur abruptly over a 4- to 6-month period. Physical examination may demonstrate pain on palpation over the affected bone. Muscle spasm and limitation of motion are associated findings. Neurologic abnormalities are indicative of nerve root or spinal cord impingement. Laboratory findings may include anemia, elevated ESR, abnormal urinalysis, increased alkaline phosphatase, and, in metastatic prostate cancer, increased prostatic acid phosphatase. Histologic features of biopsy specimens may suggest

the identity of the primary tumor, but some lesions are too undifferentiated for identification.

Radiographic abnormalities depend on the character of the underlying malignancy. Kidney and thyroid metastases are typically osteolytic, whereas colon lesions are osteoblastic. Mixed lytic and blastic lesions are noted with breast, lung, prostate, or bladder tumors (Fig. 69.22). Plain radiographs may not show any abnormalities until 30% to 50% of bone calcium is lost.[119] Bone scans are positive in more than 85% of patients with metastases. MRI is able to show tumor in the spinal cord, extraosseous extension, and bone marrow replacement, whereas CT is more helpful for detecting cortical bone involvement and bone mineralization.[120]

Treatment of metastatic disease of the spine is directed toward pain palliation. A cure is rarely possible because few metastatic lesions are

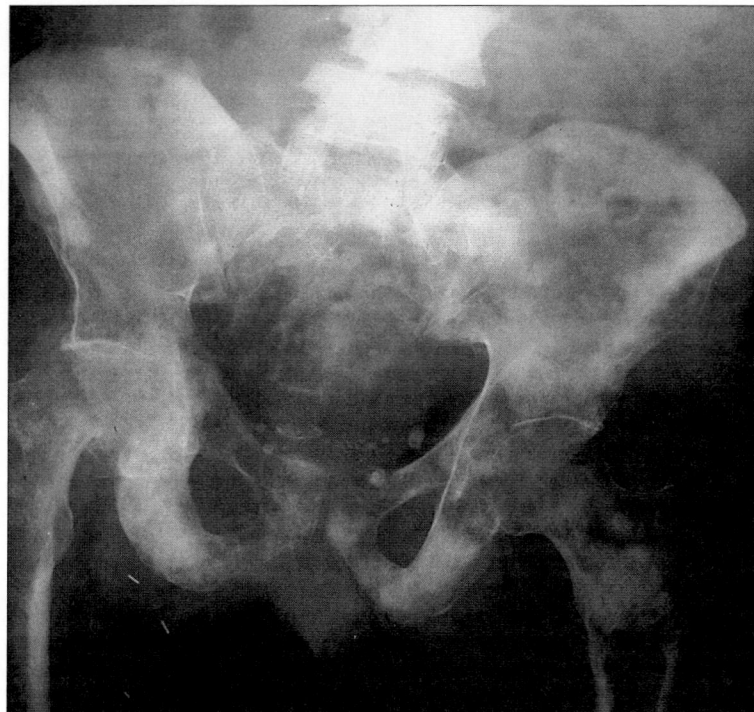

Fig. 69.22 Metastatic prostate cancer. Plain radiograph demonstrating osteoblastic lesions replacing lower lumbar vertebral bodies and most of the bony pelvis.

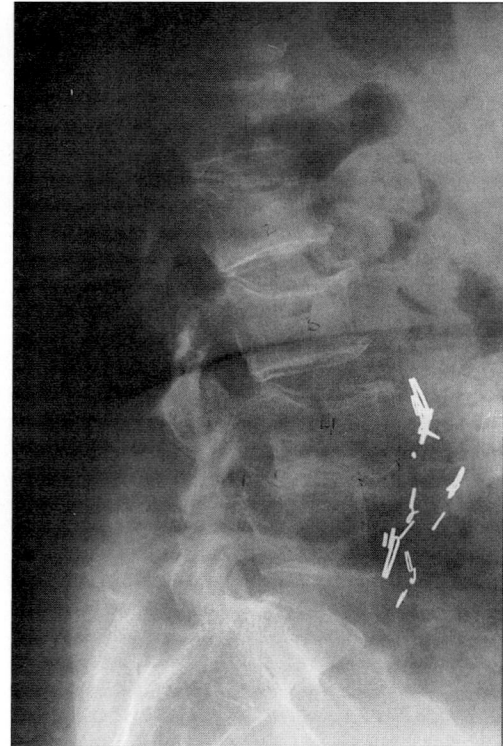

Fig. 69.23 Osteoporosis. Plain radiograph, lateral view, demonstrating diffuse osteopenia and multiple compression fractures.

TABLE 69.8 ENDOCRINOLOGIC, HEMATOLOGIC, AND MISCELLANEOUS DISORDERS AFFECTING THE LUMBOSACRAL SPINE*	
Endocrinologic/metabolic	Osteoporosis
	Osteomalacia
	Hyperparathyroidism
Hematologic	Hemoglobinopathy
	Myelofibrosis
	Mastocytosis
Miscellaneous	Paget disease
	Subacute endocarditis
	Sarcoidosis
	Retroperitoneal fibrosis

All of these may cause acute localized bone pain.

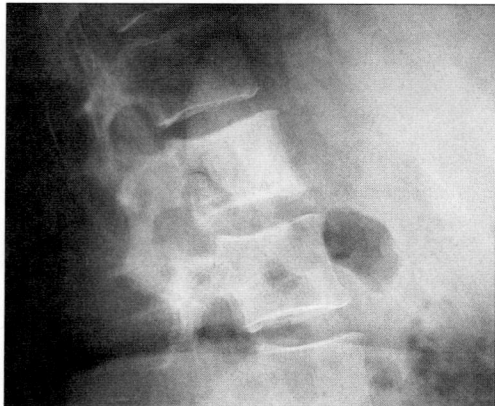

Fig. 69.24 Paget disease. Plain radiograph demonstrating osteosclerotic alterations of bony trabeculae in L2 vertebral body. The body is slightly increased in size. This patient had elevation of serum alkaline phosphatase.

solitary. Radiotherapy is useful to control spinal pain. Decompressive laminectomy is recommended for patients who have recently developed neurologic dysfunction.

Rheumatologic causes

There are a number of rheumatologic causes of back pain that are discussed in detail elsewhere in this volume including polymyalgia rheumatica (Chapter 152), fibromyalgia (Chapter 77), and ankylosing spondylitis (Chapter 112).

Primary bone disorders

Acute localized bone pain is usually caused by a fracture or expansion of bone (Table 69.8). Bone pain may be the initial manifestation of disease or may occur in the setting of associated symptoms. A medical history, including the review of systems, may elicit responses that suggest the underlying cause of the patient's back pain (kidney stones—hyperparathyroidism, chronic cough—sarcoidosis). Physical examination often shows localized tenderness, typically with surrounding muscle spasm. Anemia or an increased ESR should raise the suspicion of an inflammatory process. Serum chemistry may detect abnormalities of calcium metabolism associated with vitamin D deficiency (osteomalacia) or elevated parathyroid hormone level (hyperparathyroidism). Elevations in alkaline phosphatase may suggest increased bone activity associated with neoplasms or Paget disease.

Plain radiographs may show osteopenia only when more than 30% to 50% of the bone calcium has been lost (Fig. 69.23). Areas of sclerosis related to healed fractures or Paget disease may be identified (Fig. 69.24). Microfractures cause significant pain and may not be detected with plain films. Bone scintigraphy is useful in this context for detection of increased bone activity associated with fractures. CT scans may identify the location of a fracture or an area of bone that has been replaced by inflammatory tissue. A magnetic resonance scan can detect abnormalities of bone marrow that are associated with alterations in bone mineral density (Figs. 69.25 and 69.26).[121]

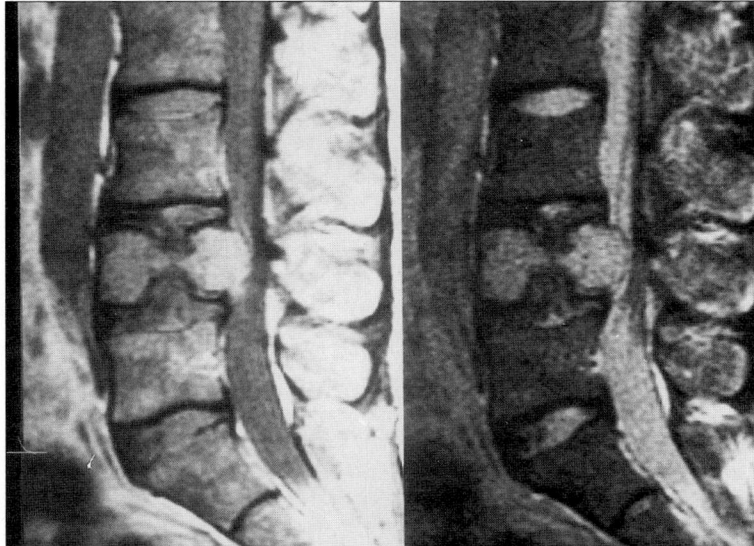

Fig. 69.25 Plasmacytoma. Magnetic resonance imaging scan, sagittal view, demonstrating replacement of the vertebral body with a mass lesion extending into the spinal canal.

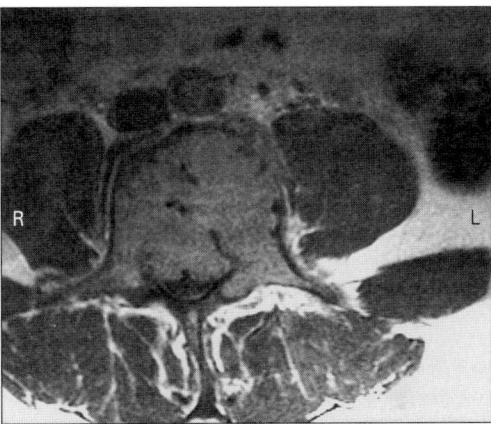

Fig. 69.26 Plasmacytoma. Magnetic resonance imaging scan, axial view, revealing replacement of the vertebral body and pedicles with a homogeneous mass. The mass has extended into the spinal canal, compressing the cauda equina.

Therapy for patients with acute localized bone pain must be tailored to the specific disease process causing their illness. In the instance of severe bony compromise, stabilization of the spine may require bone graft and/or rod placement (Fig. 69.27). Vertebroplasty can be used to treat vertebral compression fractures that remain painful and disabling after 6 weeks.[121] In this procedure, methylmethacrylate is injected through a cannula into the collapsed vertebral body. The cement stabilizes the fracture and may result in rapid pain relief. In rare circumstances the cement will escape from the vertebral body. Kyphoplasty uses an inflatable bone tamp to reduce kyphotic fractures.[122] These procedures may also be associated with rapid relief of spinal pain in individuals with acute and subacute osteoporotic compression fractures. The efficacy of vertebroplasty is debated and a high quality randomized controlled trial is necessary.

Herpetic neuralgia

Herpes zoster, also known as *shingles*, results from reactivation of latent varicella zoster infection within the dorsal root ganglia. It is characterized by a painful, unilateral vesicular eruption, which usually occurs in a dermatomal distribution. The thoracic and lumbar dermatomes are the most commonly involved sites of herpes zoster. Approximately 75% of patients have prodromal pain in the dermatome, where the rash subsequently appears, leaving a time frame during which the

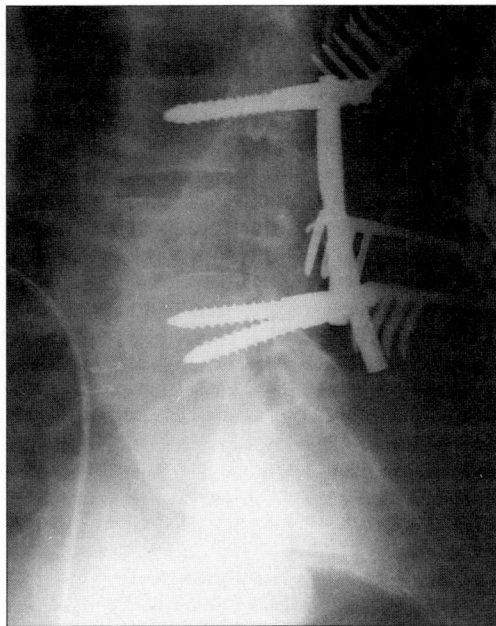

Fig. 69.27 Plasmacytoma. Postoperative plain radiograph, lateral view, demonstrating placement of rods to stabilize the spine and prevent neurologic damage.

source of the acute back pain can be misconstrued as a sprain or strain. A common consequence of herpes zoster is postherpetic neuralgia.[123]

Pain referred from other visceral organs

Disorders of the vascular, genitourinary, and gastrointestinal systems can cause stimulation of sensory nerves that results in the perception of pain both in the damaged area and in superficial tissues supplied by the same segments of the spinal cord (Table 69.9). Colicky pain occurs in peristaltic waves and is associated with a hollow viscus, such as the ureter, uterus, gallbladder, or colon. Throbbing pain is associated with vascular structures.

MECHANICAL CAUSES OF LOW BACK PAIN

Although the majority of patients with radicular symptoms improve with time, patients with axial low back pain make up the largest group of patients with chronic persistent pain.

Spondylolysis and spondylolisthesis

Spondylolysis is a break in the pars interarticularis. If the defect permits displacement of one vertebra on another, it is termed a *spondylolisthesis* (Fig. 69.28). Evaluation of the lumbar spine with plain radiographs is indicated, with flexion and extension views if spinal instability is suspected. Spondylolysis, with or without spondylolisthesis, is a commonly identified structural abnormality; however, only 5% of patients with it become symptomatic. Most patients with symptomatic spondylolisthesis complain of pain when their spine is placed in extension (increased displacement) as opposed to flexion (which tends to normalize vertebral body position). Most patients have a good response to non-operative measures, including patient education, flexion exercises, and a flexion back support. The development of progressive intervertebral disc degeneration associated with vacuum phenomenon and vertebral osteophytes at the listhetic level in the third decade of life coincides with the development of increasing back pain. These individuals may benefit from spinal fusion.[126]

Intervertebral disc disorder

Mechanisms of pain

Degenerative disc disease can be associated with back pain by several mechanisms. The outer third of the lumbar disc anulus receives

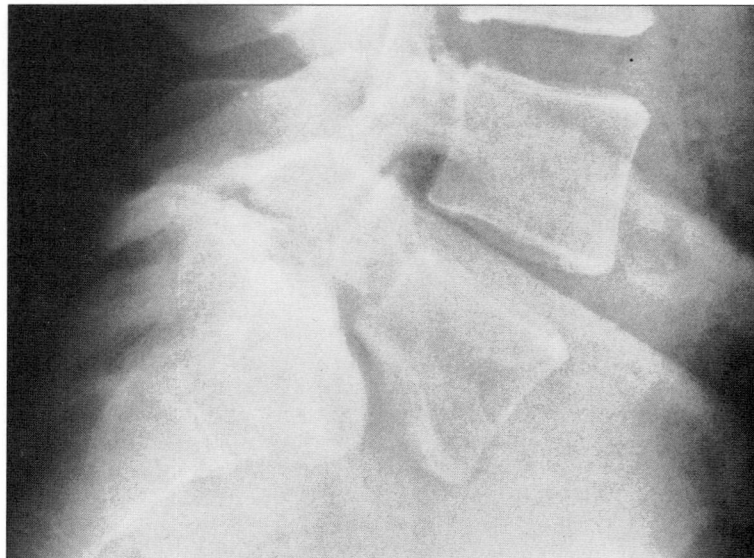

Fig. 69.28 Grade II developmental spondylolisthesis. At the L5/S1 level.

TABLE 69.9 VISCEROGENIC PAIN REFERRED TO THE LUMBAR SPINE*	
Vascular	Expanding aortic aneurysm
Genitourinary	Endometriosis
	Tubal pregnancy
	Kidney stone
	Prostatitis
Gastrointestinal	Pancreatitis
	Peptic ulcers
	Colon cancer

All of these disorders can cause referred pain to the lower back.

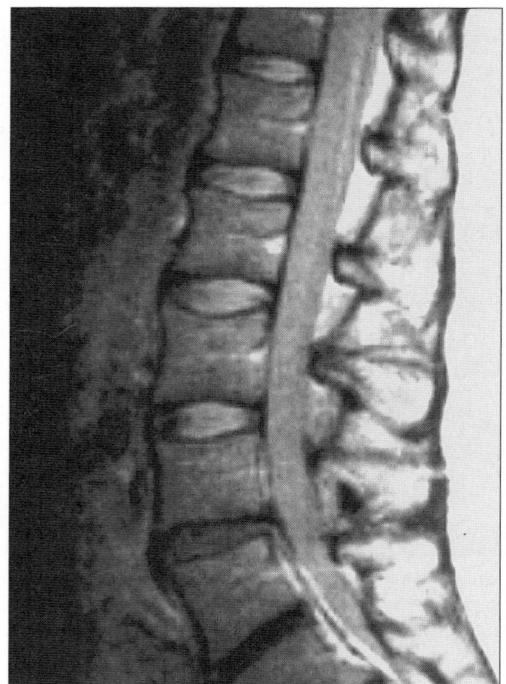

Fig. 69.29 Herniated intervertebral lumbar disc. Sagittal magnetic resonance imaging demonstrates a herniated disc with caudal migration of the disc at the L4/5 interspace.

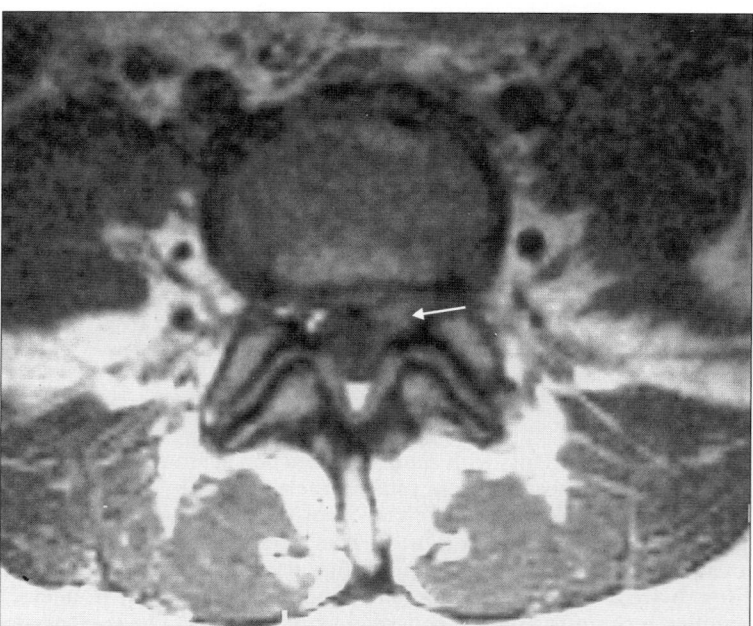

Fig. 69.30 Herniated intervertebral lumbar disc. Axial magnetic resonance imaging demonstrates a herniated disc (arrow) blocking the left neural foramen.

innervation from the sinuvertebral nerve or recurrent nerve of Lushcka.[127-129] Injury to the annular fibers, in the form of either an annular tear or a herniation of nucleus pulposus, can cause local inflammation and thus both chemical and mechanical sensitization of these annular fibers. Disc herniations can put tension on and sensitize the posterior longitudinal ligament and cause pain. Neural and vascular ingrowth into regions of the annular tear can create a chronic nociceptor. Because of noxious stimuli, the vertebral segment may attempt to splint itself, resulting in limited range of motion, regional areas of tenderness in the back, muscle spasm, taut bands, and trigger points. Spasms, taut bands, and trigger points can be painful in and of themselves but often stem from injury to the deeper spinal structures.

Clinical presentation

Symptoms are often first seen in the 20- to 50-year-old age group. They are typically worse with prolonged sitting, standing, and forward bending and are often relieved with walking and frequent positional shift. Symptoms can radiate to the limb without nerve compression via somatic referral. Herniated nucleus pulposus is associated with leg pain exacerbated with flexion of the lumbar spine or with prolonged sitting. Individuals may experience sensory and/or motor deficits. Bedrest does not accelerate recovery.[130]

Investigations

When pain persists, further diagnostic tests are indicated to document the anatomic abnormalities. Depending on the circumstances, the patient should undergo MRI or CT evaluation (Figs. 69.29 and 69.30). MRI can demonstrate disc desiccation, focal protrusions, high-intensity zone lesions, and vertebral endplate changes. Degenerative disc disease can also be an asymptomatic finding that needs to be taken into account in interpreting the imaging results.

Treatment

In patients with axial symptoms only, those who fail to respond to conservative management and who have no specific radiographic abnormalities may improve with a local injection of an anesthetic agent into the area of maximal tenderness. A fluoroscopically guided spinal epidural corticosteroid injection can be helpful in refractory patients and in patients who cannot tolerate their exercise regimen. There is currently no definitive proof of efficacy for trigger point injections or epidural steroid injections for the treatment of axial low back pain.

For patients with disc herniation, additional therapy in the form of fluoroscopically guided epidural corticosteroid injections may be given if pain persists and is functionally limiting.[131] Long-acting corticosteroid is injected into the epidural space transforaminally, close to the location of nerve root compression. Approximately 66% to 84% of patients will have a benefit that is sustained even at 1-year follow-up.[132,133] The maximum benefit is typically noted after 4 weeks. Leg symptoms typically respond better than axial symptoms.

If injections are effective in alleviating the patient's leg pain, the patient should be encouraged to increase physical activity, although limiting activities that increase intradiscal pressure, such as heavy lifting or sitting for long periods of time. Preliminary studies report that sequestrated intervertebral discs that are highlighted by the gadolinium contrast material are more likely to resorb spontaneously than protruded discs that do not absorb contrast.[134] If conservative measures have not been effective, the patient may consider surgical intervention. The choice of surgical procedure (laminectomy with discectomy versus microdiscectomy) is beyond the scope of this chapter. Some studies showed that discectomy produces better pain relief than non-surgical treatment over a 4-year period, but outcomes of operative and non-operative therapy are similar at 10-year follow-up.[135] The Spine Patient Outcomes Research Trial (SPORT) demonstrated that surgery may offer more rapid relief of radicular symptoms; however, long-term symptoms at 1 and 2 years appear to be comparable in surgically and nonsurgically treated groups. Of note, the intention-to-treat analyses in SPORT are not readily interpretable because of high rates of cross-over from operative to non-operative and from non-operative to operative therapy. Thus the conclusions of the study are based on the more interpretable "as-treated" analyses, which afford less protection against bias.[136,137] Needless to say, the success of any of these surgical procedures is dependent on choosing the patient who requires surgery. Surgery for radicular symptoms is helpful in relieving leg pain, but it has not been shown to improve back pain.

Zygapophyseal (facet) joint syndrome

The zygapophyseal joint can also cause low back pain. Articular degeneration with zygapophyseal joint sclerosis may be associated with back pain.[138] Patients with facet joint syndrome can often experience back and buttock pain that is worse with standing and walking or lumbar extension and alleviated with forward flexion. Diagnosis of symptomatic facet syndrome requires anesthetization of the joint via an intra-articular block or anesthetization of the joint's innervation. At least two blocks are required to be confident the facet joint is mediating pain due to the high incidence of non-specific/placebo effect.[139,140]

Lumbar spinal stenosis

Spinal stenosis can be defined as narrowing of the spinal canal secondary to degenerative changes that occur in the spinal canal with time (Fig. 69.31). Other forms of spinal stenosis occur secondary to congenital abnormalities, traumatic, postsurgical, or metabolic disorders. Patients with spinal stenosis experience leg pain with standing or walking: the classic syndrome of neurogenic claudication.

Epidemiology

The prevalence of narrowing of the lumbar spinal canal increases with age. A midsagittal narrowing to less than 10 mm is abnormal.[141] Myelographic,[68] CT,[63] and MRI studies[20] have all shown that 20% to 25% of asymptomatic populations older than 40 years have marked narrowing of the lumbar spinal canal. These *in vivo* measurements support the conclusion drawn from postmortem morphometry studies that many cases of "morphologic" lumbar spinal stenosis have no recognizable clinical expression.

Etiology and pathogenesis

The lumbar spinal canal is bounded anteriorly by lumbar discs, vertebral bodies, and the posterior longitudinal ligament, laterally by the laminae and facet joints, and posteriorly by the ligamentum flavum

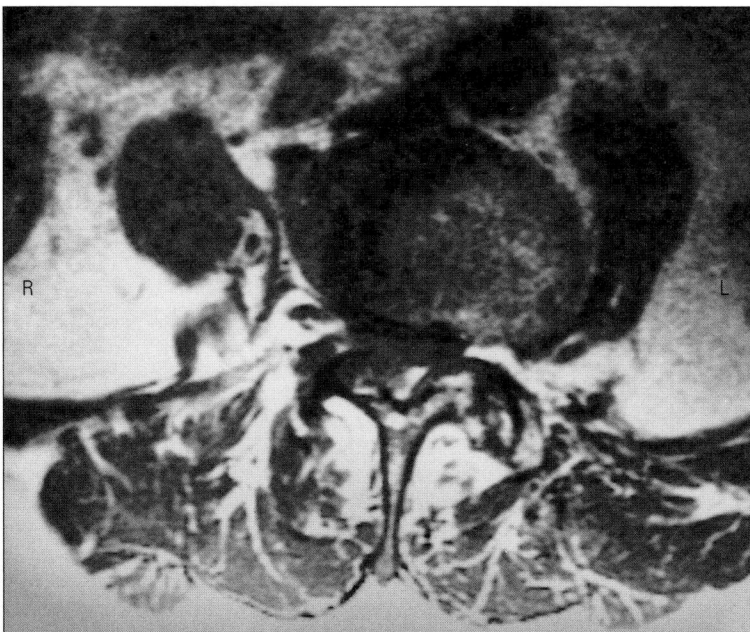

Fig. 69.31 Spinal stenosis. Magnetic resonance imaging, axial view, of the L3/4 disc level demonstrating osteophytic overgrowth, disc degeneration, and ligamentous hypertrophy. The cauda equina is compressed in the central area of the canal.

(Fig. 69.32). The nerve root canals through which spinal nerves exit the spinal canal are bounded anteriorly by the posterior surface of discs and vertebral body, posteriorly by facet joints and pars interarticularis, and medially by the central vertebral canal.[142] Stenosis develops when there is a relative narrowing of the dimensions of the lumbar spinal canal due to either congenital or acquired factors. Many cases of lumbar spinal stenosis syndrome are the result of both congenital and acquired narrowing of the lumbar spinal canal, thus limiting the utility of any rigid etiologic classification.[143]

Pathologic studies of the lumbar nerve root canal show that lumbar spondylosis is associated with reduction in the vertical dimension due to disc space narrowing, posterior bulging of the intervertebral discs, retropulsion of anulus fibrosus remnants, and the formation of sclerotic ridges around the vertebral endplates (see Fig. 69.32). Osteoarthritic facet joints project osteophytes anteriorly from the superior articular processes and there are often synovial effusions, hemarthroses, and derangements of meniscal synovial folds. In extension and rotation there is significant encroachment on the nerve root complex (see Fig. 69.32).[144] Flexion-extension myelography has shown consistent anterior displacement of the entire lumbar dural sac on extension, caused by shortening and thickening of the ligamentum flavum.[145] Furthermore, the discs bulge posteriorly, particularly at the L3/4 and L4/5 levels, and with spinal extension there is also facet joint subluxation anteriorly, further compromising the dimensions of the lumbar spinal canal.

The precise mechanisms that produce neurogenic claudication are poorly understood. The neuropathology of patients has shown chronic segmental compression of nerves at regular intervals corresponding to the site of myelographic obstruction, with confirmatory histologic features of nerve fiber damage.[146] Abnormalities of the pial vessels have been reported,[147] and some patients have high cauda equina cerebrospinal fluid pressures.[148] Any or all of these factors may play a role in the genesis of pseudoclaudication.

Clinical features

The most characteristic symptom is neurogenic claudication, defined as discomfort in the buttock, thigh, or leg on standing or walking that is relieved by rest and is not produced by peripheral vascular insufficiency. Such discomfort is generally described as pain but is occasionally appreciated as numbness, weakness, or various combinations of these symptoms.[146]

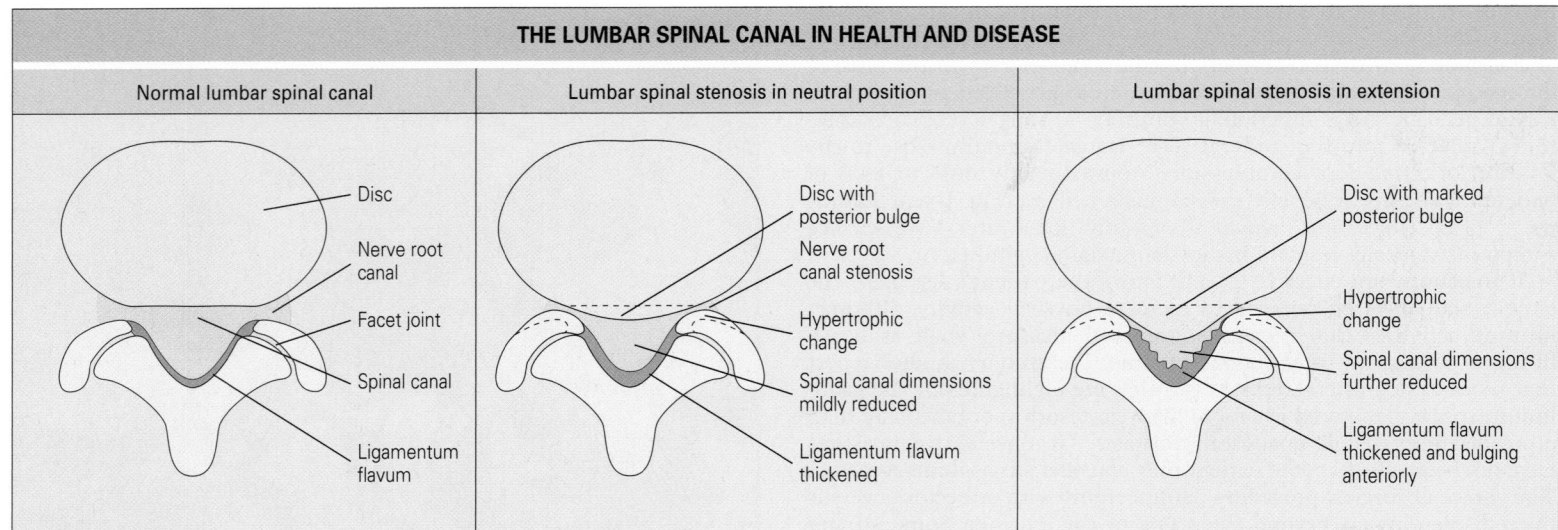

THE LUMBAR SPINAL CANAL IN HEALTH AND DISEASE

| Normal lumbar spinal canal | Lumbar spinal stenosis in neutral position | Lumbar spinal stenosis in extension |

Fig. 69.32 The lumbar spinal canal in health and disease. (Left) The normal spinal canal. (Center) The spinal canal in central spinal and nerve root canal stenosis in the neutral position. (Right) The effect of lumbar extension on the spinal canal.

Neurogenic claudication is generally relieved by lying down, sitting, leaning forward on a shopping cart, leaning on a church pew, or adopting a bent forward position while walking (simian stance). Symptoms and signs typically affect multiple dermatomes. Some 40% of cases have bilateral symptoms.[146] Restriction of straight-leg raising (Lasègue sign) is present in only 10% of cases of lumbar spinal stenosis. Ankle jerks are absent in 40%, knee jerks are absent in 10%, and a small percentage have sensory loss or weakness.[146,149] A condition identical to meralgia paresthetica can be produced by stenosis at the upper lumbar levels.[150]

Bowel and bladder sphincter disturbances can develop but are relatively uncommon. Their presence constitutes an absolute indication for surgery to stabilize the deficit and allow some potential for recovery of bladder function.[151] Rarely, intermittent priapism has been reported as a manifestation of lumbar spinal stenosis.[152] Men have been described as unable to void in the standing position but able to do so while sitting, a cauda equina equivalent of pseudoclaudication.

Restriction of lumbar spinal motion is common in this condition because most cases have significant and often severe spondylotic changes. It has been estimated that 65% of patients who undergo lumbar spinal surgery for lumbar spinal stenosis have significant mechanical lumbar pain.[146] This probably represents a substantial underestimate of the extent of lumbar pain in this context because the more mechanical lumbar pain a patient has, the less likely he or she is to be offered lumbar spinal surgery.

Investigations

The purpose of investigation is to confirm the diagnosis in patients with a clinically defined lumbar stenosis syndrome and, if necessary, to exclude other diseases. Imaging techniques and neurophysiologic investigations allow demonstration of the defined anatomy so that appropriate therapy can be planned. The imaging techniques are complementary, and in most cases a combination of techniques is necessary.

Plain film changes are insensitive for the diagnosis of spinal stenosis. Arthritic changes that may be associated with stenosis include narrowing of disc spaces, zygapophyseal joint osteoarthritis, and degenerative spondylolisthesis, particularly at L4/5.[146] Spondylolysis with spondylolisthesis frequently causes distortion of the nerve root exit foramen, which may lead to compromise of the exiting nerve in the foramen and the descending spinal nerve root in the lateral recess. If severe listhesis exists, it can compromise the central canal.

CT can demonstrate articular facet hypertrophy, enlargement of laminae, hyperplasia, and ossification of the ligamentum flavum and disc prolapse (Fig. 69.33). The technique allows definition of the osseous margins and shape of the lumbar spinal canal. A trefoil shape of the lumbar canal is typical of severe lumbar spinal stenosis.

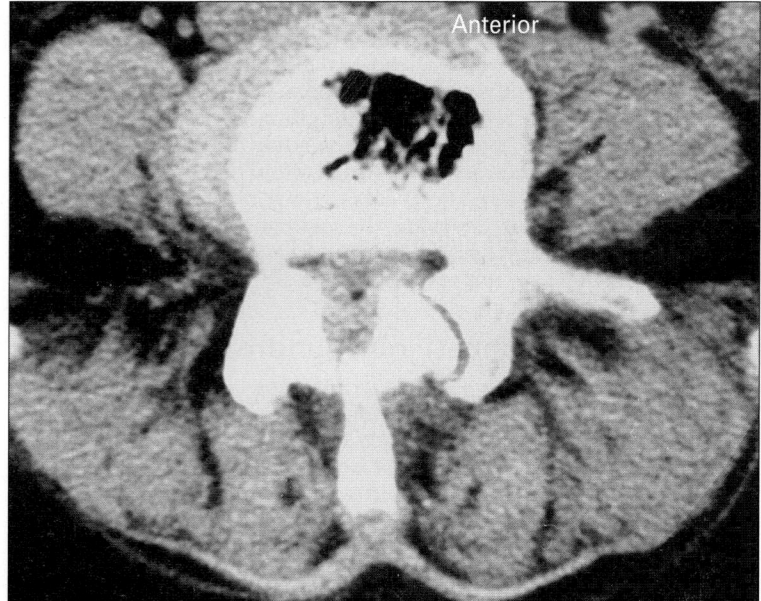

Fig. 69.33 Lumbar spine stenosis. Computed tomography showing thickened ligamentum flavum, facet joint hypertrophy, and posterior disc bulging. Note absence of epidural fat with trefoil deformity of lumbar spinal canal.

Contrast myelography can be helpful for surgical planning. Demonstration of obstruction to dye flow can be dependent on posture, with compression of the dural sac by the ligamentum flavum and disc being more severe in extension (Fig. 69.34). The combination of contrast myelography and CT directed at specific levels can demonstrate lateral recess and/or nerve root canal with greater definition than CT or myelography alone.

MRI is the non-invasive study of choice. However, asymptomatic changes of stenosis occur in 21% of asymptomatic subjects older than the age of 60.[91] MRI and contrast CT are comparable in demonstrating spinal stenosis at any one segment.[152] Few adequate studies have compared these various imaging modalities.[153] On balance, MRI and CT myelography are comparable in establishing the radiologic (in contrast to clinical) diagnosis of lumbar spinal stenosis.[154]

Electrodiagnostic studies can be confirmatory of the diagnosis of spinal stenosis. Of 37 patients with surgically proven lumbar spinal stenosis, 34 had an abnormality on electromyogram with evidence of one or more radiculopathies.[146] These abnormalities can be difficult to interpret, with one study demonstrating that 11 of 36 patients with stenosis had electromyographic abnormalities at levels higher than

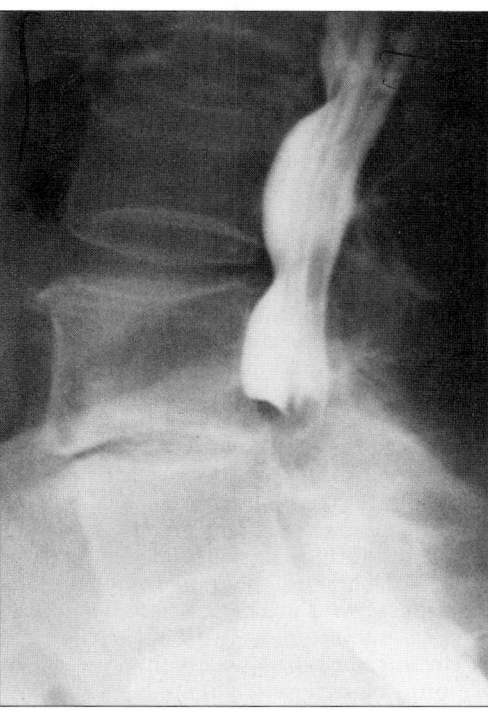

Fig. 69.34 Lumbar spine stenosis: myelogram in extension. Note increased block with marked posterior indentation due to the ligamentum flavum.

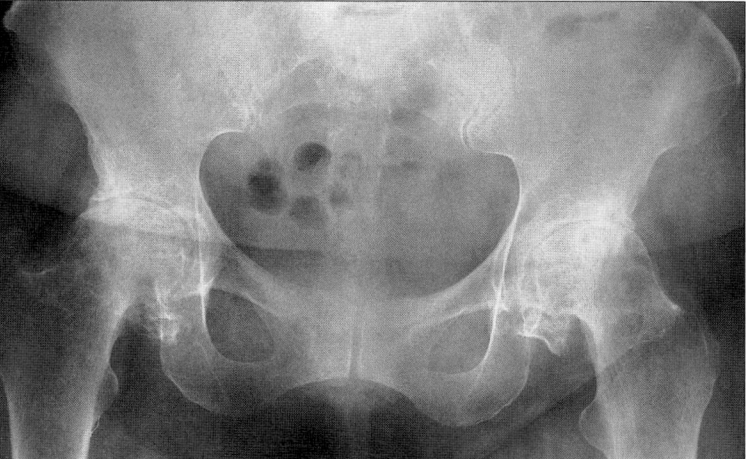

Fig. 69.35 Hip arthritis. Plain radiograph of pelvis demonstrating severe osteoarthritis of both hips. The patient had presented with back and knee pain. Hip examination revealed no motion of the joint. Back pain was reduced with joint replacement.

BOX 69.1 **DIFFERENTIAL DIAGNOSIS OF LUMBAR SPINAL STENOSIS SYNDROME**

Lumbar spondylosis without spinal stenosis
Herniated nucleus pulposus
Atherosclerotic occlusive peripheral vascular disease
Spinal tumors
Restless legs syndrome
Peripheral nerve entrapment
Cervical and thoracic spinal stenosis
Peripheral neuropathy
Anterior tibial compartment syndrome

---

those expected on the basis of myelography.[155] Much of the usefulness of electromyography lies in excluding peripheral neuropathy and peripheral nerve entrapment syndromes.[156] Cortical somatosensory-evoked potentials provide a sensitive test of neurologic compromise and have been used in assessing the adequacy of neural decompression intraoperatively.[157] The specificity of this test is uncertain and it is expensive; it is currently more of a research tool than a routine clinical procedure.

Differential diagnosis

A number of conditions must be distinguished from lumbar spinal stenosis syndrome (Box 69.1). Peripheral vascular disease can be diagnosed on the basis of history, examination, exercise, ankle brachial indexes, and vascular surgical consultation.[158] The possibility of a herniated nucleus pulposus causing sciatica is associated with abrupt onset. Hip osteoarthritis can cause thigh discomfort exacerbated by standing and walking but often has significant pain with transitioning from sit to stand and has diminished range of motion and pain production with examination. The possibility of two pain generators is common in this aging population. Trochanteric bursitis can cause regional thigh pain and can mimic radicular pain. Peripheral nerve entrapment may produce extremity pain. Electromyography with nerve conduction studies is usually required for diagnosis.[156] Lumbar spinal stenosis may be associated with stenosis in the cervical and thoracic areas. Some cases of thoracic spinal stenosis produce a pure pseudo-claudication syndrome.[159] Furthermore, myelopathy due to more

rostral narrowing of the spinal canal will result in difficulty in walking and sphincter disturbance.[160]

Back pain with regional radiation

Anterior thigh pain

Back pain with anterior thigh pain has a number of possible sources. Pain in the anterior thigh may be related to hip disease, a hernia, kidney disorders, femoral neuropathy, lateral femoral cutaneous nerve entrapment (meralgia paresthetica), or retroperitoneal process. Hip arthritis causes pain that is primarily in the groin and exacerbated by hip motion, especially internal rotation. However, hip disease may present as lateral low back and anterior thigh pain. The patient's pain should be recreated by putting tension on the hip joint. Plain films of the hips can document the presence of joint disease (Fig. 69.35). For patients in whom a diagnosis remains unclear because of degenerative changes in both the spine and hip, a diagnostic anesthetization of the hip with fluoroscopic guidance and preprocedural and postprocedural pain diagrams and visual analog scales can make the diagnosis.

Disorders of the femoral nerve may be associated with anterior thigh pain. The anterior femoral cutaneous nerve (L2, L3) supplies the anterior thigh. Neuropathies, such as diabetic polyradiculopathy or plexopathy (diabetic amyotrophy) or a focal mononeuropathy involving the femoral nerve, can occur in diabetes. Any retroperitoneal process may refer pain to the anterior thigh. Retroperitoneal structures that may cause pain include the aorta, kidneys, tumor or infiltrative process. If a retroperitoneal process is suspected, CT evaluation is appropriate to determine the status of the aorta, kidney, and lymph nodes.

Posterior or lateral thigh pain

Posterior or lateral thigh discomfort can have a broad differential. These patients may have referred or radicular pain. Patients with referred pain have it on the basis of somatic (sclerotomal) referral because of injury to the bone, muscle, zygapophyseal joint, intervertebral disc, or sacroiliac joint. The muscles of the posterior thigh and buttocks have the same embryologic origin as those of the lumbar spine. An injury to these structures in the lumbar spine may be referred to the posterior thigh. Posterior thigh discomfort can also be commonly due to radicular pain involving the S1, and lateral thigh discomfort is commonly caused by the L5 nerve root. However, referral between these two spinal nerve roots can have significant overlap. A complementary therapeutic exercise regimen is important to maximize outcome.

Other non-spinal causes of pain

Sacral fractures can entrap or irritate sacral nerve roots in the foramen and cause radicular pain referring to the buttock or thigh. Hip arthritis and vascular disease can also refer to the buttock and posterior thigh. Hamstring injuries and ischial bursitis are soft tissue disorders that can refer symptoms to the posterior thigh, whereas trochanteric bursitis and iliotibial band tightness can be associated with pain in the lateral thigh.

MANAGEMENT OF LUMBAR SPINE DISORDERS

No single form of therapy is effective for all forms of back pain. Patients with systemic causes must be treated with specific therapies effective for their underlying disease as discussed earlier. The following section provides guidelines for the management of non-specific back pain.

The recommendations of a panel of spine experts in relation to the general management of back pain remain useful, despite being published more than a decade ago.[48]

- Bedrest for more than 2 days is not helpful and may debilitate the patient. During the acute phase, patients are encouraged to ambulate as tolerated.
- Relief of pain may be accomplished most safely with non-prescription analgesics or non-steroidal medication. Spinal manipulation by an osteopathic physician or trained physical therapist is helpful during the first 4 weeks in patients without radiculopathy.
- Low-stress aerobic activities can be safely started in the first 2 weeks of symptoms. Trunk muscle exercises should be delayed for at least 2 weeks.
- Patients should be encouraged to return to usual activities, both vocational and recreational, as soon as possible.

Frequently the ability of patients to cope with their symptoms can be helped by careful explanation of the cause of the symptoms. The key to conservative management lies in the patient's acceptance of mild disability because most continue to be symptomatic in the longer term.

Conservative approaches

Components of a conservative management program for low back pain patients include patient education, controlled physical activity, bedrest, exercise, and drug therapy in the form of NSAIDs and muscle relaxants. Bedrest should be kept to a minimum or eliminated completely by encouraging the patient to avoid extremes of activity or inactivity. Scientific data support regular activity as being as effective as a short course of bedrest.[161-163] The best outcome for low back pain is associated with resuming normal activity as opposed to extension exercises or bedrest.[162]

Physical modalities

Physical modalities may be used to diminish symptoms for short periods of time. These forms of therapy include ice massage, hot packs, diathermy, ultrasound, and transcutaneous electrical nerve stimulation (TENS). These therapies may be applied by the patients themselves or by a therapist.

Patients with acute low back pain may experience analgesia with ice massage or cold packs. Cold temperatures decrease swelling, pain, and muscle spasm during the acute phase of an injury. Cold reduces metabolic activity locally, decreases muscle spindle activity, and slows nerve conduction. Patients may experience at least 33% reduction in pain following ice massage.[164]

Heat also has utility in the treatment of low back pain patients. Heat should not be used in patients with back pain arising from acute trauma because it causes vasodilation and increased blood flow, which can increase damage to an area recently traumatized. However, heat increases the elastic properties of connective tissues and may be of particular utility in patients who complain of stiffness associated with their back pain. Heat also decreases γ-fiber activity, muscle spindle excitability, and resting muscle tension. Heat has been shown to be helpful for reducing pain in hospitalized patients with low back discomfort.[165]

Transcutaneous electrical nerve stimulation

TENS therapy is based on the gate control theory of pain, which suggests that counterstimulation of the sensory system will modify pain perception in the cerebral cortex. TENS preferentially stimulates low-threshold αA fibers. The stimulation of these fibers is thought to inhibit the nociceptive impulses of the small C unmyelinated and αD fibers. The effect of TENS on pain is not mediated through opiate receptors. The electrical stimulation is produced by an electrical pulse generator, which delivers current that can be varied in form, intensity, and frequency to superficial electrodes. The optimal placement of the electrodes is proximal to the painful area. The average time for the onset of analgesia is approximately 20 minutes. Therapy should be given for at least 30 minutes. The pain relief from TENS may be present only during stimulation or may last for a considerable period of time. TENS is not indicated for patients with acute low back pain.[48] TENS has been shown to be superior to massage and equivalent to cold therapy.[164] However, a large, randomized, placebo-controlled study found no benefit of TENS for chronic low back pain.[166] The role of TENS in the therapy of low back pain is in question and it should not be considered as sole therapy.

Exercise

Physical therapy, particularly in the form of therapeutic exercises, may be particularly helpful in controlling mechanical low back pain.[167] A number of different exercise programs are available for patients with low back pain. These include flexion exercises, extension exercises, core stabilization, stretching regimens, and aerobic conditioning. As a generalization, patients with mechanical disorders of the discs prefer extension exercises, whereas those with stenosis prefer flexion exercises. In most circumstances patients eventually take part in a combination of both forms of exercise.

Patients may feel worse before they feel better following an exercise program. In one study of patients with chronic low back pain,[168] 2 months were required before a benefit was noted. The treating physician should find a physical therapist who is interested in taking care of back patients and communicate his or her concerns about patients to the therapist.

Exercises may also play a significant role in preventing back pain in asymptomatic individuals. In a comparison with educational strategies, mechanical supports, and risk modification, exercises that strengthen back and abdominal muscles were the only intervention associated with decreased frequency and duration of low back pain.[169]

Oral drug therapy

The types of medication used for low back pain include analgesics, NSAIDs, muscle relaxants, and neuropathic pain medications. The potential toxicities must also be considered when choosing an agent for a patient.

Analgesics

Patients may benefit from acetaminophen. A slow-release form of the drug may allow for a more prolonged analgesic effect in back pain patients. The drug has a synergistic effect with NSAIDs and may be used in combination to increase analgesia without increasing toxicity.

Tramadol, a synthetic analgesic that binds opiate μ-receptors, is a useful agent that can be given independently or in combination with non-steroidal drugs for the relief of chronic low back pain. This agent is most helpful for individuals with back pain who are unable to tolerate NSAIDS and narcotic analgesics.

Narcotic analgesia should be reserved for patients with severe functionally limiting pain and used along with NSAIDs, other adjuvant analgesics, and a bowel regimen. This form of therapy may be used in an outpatient setting along with controlled physical activity and modalities. Stronger narcotic analgesia should be reserved for patients who are unable to perform activities of daily living because of persistent pain. The continuation of narcotic analgesics in the outpatient setting should be discouraged unless the patient is committed to maximizing physical function through increased activity.[170]

Non-steroidal anti-inflammatory drugs

Non-steroidal anti-inflammatory drugs have analgesic properties in low doses and anti-inflammatory properties at higher doses. The onset of action of the agents is important. In acute back pain, a rapid onset of action is important to control symptoms quickly. In chronic pain, the onset of action is not as important as efficacy and safety over extended periods of time.

Naproxen, piroxicam, and diflunisal have been reported to be more effective than placebo in relieving low back pain.[171,172] NSAIDs as a class of agents are effective in low back pain therapy.[173] There are no specific selection criteria for the choice of a single agent. The drug is given for a period of 2 to 4 weeks as a therapeutic trial and is continued if it is efficacious and well tolerated. Cyclo-oxygenase (COX)-2-selective inhibitors are indicated for low back pain treatment in individuals with a history of peptic ulcer disease or gastrointestinal intolerance to dual COX-1/COX-2 inhibitors. They are associated with increased risk of cardiovascular thrombotic events and consequently they are being used less often, and their role in the management of acute and chronic back pain syndromes is being reassessed. Chronic use in the elderly is discouraged, and careful use of opiates may be safer.

Muscle relaxants

The use of muscle relaxants in low back pain remains controversial.[174] The muscle relaxants used for low back pain patients work centrally to affect the activity of muscle stretch reflexes. Drugs including cyclobenzaprine, carisoprodol, and chlorzoxazone have been shown to be more effective than placebo in treating patients with muscle spasm.[175] In appropriately selected patients with acute muscle spasm, the combination of an NSAID and a muscle relaxant is more effective than the same NSAID alone.[176] The combination of an NSAID and a muscle relaxant offers significant relief of pain compared with other combinations of therapies, including those with narcotics.[177] The major side effects of muscle relaxants are drowsiness, headache, dizziness, and dry mouth.

Neuropathic pain agents

Tricyclic antidepressants have been used for the treatment of chronic pain for patients with or without depression. A number of mechanisms have been suggested to explain the pain relief associated with the tricyclics. Double-blind studies have documented the role of tricyclics for relieving chronic pain. Low doses in the range of 10 to 25 mg may be adequate to control symptoms.[178] Rare patients may require up to 150 mg per day. The drug does not work immediately and may need to be continued for a number of weeks before decreased symptoms are noted. Selective serotonin reuptake inhibitors (sertraline, fluoxetine) are not as effective as tricyclics for chronic pain relief.[179] Mixed norepinephrine and serotonin reuptake inhibitors (venlafaxine and duloxetine) seem to have a more effective role in the management of chronic pain.

The second major class of neuropathic pain agents includes antiepileptic medications, such as pregabalin, gabapentin, and carbamazepine (Tegretol). Neuropathic pain medications have a potential role where pain is mediated via both peripheral and central mechanisms. Examples of peripheral nerve–mediated pain include spinal stenosis, herniated nucleus pulposus, and epidural fibrosis. Chronic axial low back pain, although believed to be in part mediated by central sensitization and other chronic changes occurring in the brain and spinal cord, may also benefit from a trial of these agents. Strong evidence for the use of these agents is lacking, but judicious use can improve patient pain and quality of life and help restore sleep.

Injection therapy

Local or regional anesthesia given by injection is part of the therapeutic regimen for some patients with low back pain. By blocking peripheral pain input, the local area of pain can be eased, as well as areas of referred pain and increased muscle tension. Patients who describe localized areas of muscle or ligamentous tenderness are candidates for local anesthetic therapy. The area injected may be an area of local trauma or a myofascial trigger point.[180] Trigger points are areas of the muscle that are painful at rest, prevent full lengthening of the muscle, weaken the muscle, refer pain in the muscle group on direct palpation, and cause a local contraction when palpated. Trigger points may be found in the paraspinous muscles, the quadratus lumborum, and the gluteal muscles. A study by Garvey and colleagues suggests that needling the area with or without medication may have a beneficial effect.[181] Injections may be given on a weekly basis for 3 to 4 additional

weeks. Controlled studies designed to evaluate the efficacy of this treatment modality have yet to be carried out.

Epidural injections

Epidural corticosteroid injections are used for patients with radicular pain who do not respond to less invasive management. The efficacy of these injections for the therapy of herniated discs and spinal stenosis with radiculopathy has been questioned, though they have been found to be effective in some patients.[182-186] The benefits include decreased pain and more rapid return of sensory function.[131] Epidural steroids may be administered via the interlaminar, transforaminal, and caudal routes. Fluoroscopic guidance improves the likelihood of administration of medication to the intended target, decreases the risk of vascular penetration, and enhances safety. Whenever possible, injections should be offered that are most specific to the suspected predominant pain generator. Transforaminal epidural steroid injections place medication around the specifically involved nerve root and in experienced hands can offer effective treatment of radicular pain due to herniated disc.[132,133]

Facet joint injection

Facet syndrome can mimic radicular pain. The diagnosis of facet syndrome is based on diagnostic anesthetization of the joint or its innervation. Steroid injections can be performed to decrease pain.[187] The injections are done under fluoroscopic control to document the appropriate placement of the needle. A facet joint receives innervation by the medial branches of the dorsal rami from the same level and the level above. Injections of steroid and anesthetic can also be offered intra-articularly at the suspect joint or joints. If facet syndrome is confirmed on the basis of time-dependent medial branch anesthetic block or a placebo-controlled intra-articular block, the medial branches can be denervated with radiofrequency ablation.[188,189] The efficacy of facet injections and medial branch blocks has been questioned[190] and presents an area for further study.

Calcitonin

Calcitonin dispensed by injections or nasal spray is useful in cases of lumbar spinal stenosis associated with Paget disease.[191] Open studies have suggested that calcitonin may be effective in treating patients with neurogenic claudication without Paget disease. A subsequent double-blind study yielded less impressive results,[192] and further studies indicate that such treatment is helpful but unlikely to be effective in severe neurogenic claudication with walking distances of less than 200 meters.[193]

Complementary therapies

Complementary therapies are used for a variety of medical problems, including low back pain.[194] Therapies promoted for the treatment of low back pain include spinal manipulation, massage, acupuncture, and magnets.

Spinal manipulation is recommended by the AHCPR guidelines. Osteopathic physicians and experienced physical therapists may offer manipulation as a therapy for low back pain. In a study of 215 patients who visited a physician and 242 who visited a chiropractor, overall satisfaction with care was three times greater with the chiropractors than with the physicians.[195] Patient satisfaction with chiropractors is related to the chiropractor's willingness to listen to a patient's concerns. On the other hand, chiropractic care is associated with the greatest number of visits per episode and the highest outpatient cost compared with other health care providers.[196] We discuss both the greater satisfaction with chiropractic care and the higher cost and utilization with patients and encourage them to make up their own minds about chiropractic care.

Therapeutic massage has benefit for individuals with chronic low back pain. This therapy given once a week over 10 weeks has demonstrated benefit months after the last treatment. The efficacy of this form of treatment is limited to the availability of massage therapists.[197]

The use of magnets for individuals with chronic back pain was reported in a double-blind placebo-controlled trial. This study demonstrated no significant difference between the study groups. Magnets did not decrease back pain in this trial.[198]

Acupuncture is also commonly used for low back pain. A meta-analysis reported that for the primary outcome of short-term relief of chronic pain, acupuncture is significantly more effective than sham treatment and no additional treatment. For patients with acute low back pain, data are sparse and inconclusive. Data are also insufficient for drawing conclusions about acupuncture's short-term effectiveness compared with most other therapies.[199] Another systematic review done according to the guidelines established by the criteria recommended by the Cochrane Back Review Group concluded that the data do not allow firm conclusions regarding the effectiveness of acupuncture for acute low back pain. For chronic low back pain, acupuncture is more effective for pain relief and functional improvement than no treatment or sham treatment immediately after treatment and in the short term only. Acupuncture is not more effective than other conventional and "alternative" treatments. The data suggest that acupuncture and dry-needling may be useful adjuncts to other therapies for chronic low back pain. Because most of the studies were of lower methodologic quality, there is a clear need for higher-quality trials in this area.[200]

Surgical treatment

A thorough treatment of surgery is beyond the scope of this chapter. A small percentage of individuals with low back pain require surgical intervention to improve their condition. Indications for surgery vary according to the patient characteristics but include sphincter and sexual dysfunction due to compression of the conus medullaris or cauda equina; severe radicular symptoms, particularly if there are progressive neurologic motor deficits; and radicular symptoms failing to respond to conservative management. The operative procedure is determined by the characteristics of the lesions and the skill of the surgeon with the specific technique.

With spinal stenosis, the success of surgical approaches depends on adequate decompression of areas of absolute stenosis and good judgment with respect to adequacy of decompression of areas of relative stenosis. Preoperative assessment and planning are essential. Before surgery there must be demonstration of compression of spinal nerve structures that correspond to the patient's clinical symptoms and signs. Surgery should not be carried out for clinically asymptomatic spinal stenosis.

Most patients require multiple-level procedures and in one study 72% of patients had three or more laminae removed. In the follow-up of those patients 4 years after surgery, 64% reported that surgery had yielded good to excellent results but 36% still had more than half of their preoperative disability.[146] Similar results are reported for community-based cohort studies and from pooled series.[201,202]

An analysis of laminectomy failure in 45 stenosis patients found that only half had the clinical picture of neurogenic claudication and only 10 had radiologic evidence of severe lumbar canal stenosis. The most common technical problem was inadequate neural decompression.[203] Co-morbidities, including hip arthritis, osteoporosis, and cardiovascular disease, are associated with persistent pain after surgical correction.[204] Surgery is most effective when patients have a clinical picture dominated by manifestations of nerve compression.

Surgery for patients with radicular pain due to herniated disc primarily involves decompression. Removal of the protruded, extruded, or sequestered disc material and inspection and release of the tethered nerve root are performed. Before closure, subcutaneous fat soaked in steroid is placed over the spinal nerve to minimize adherence of muscle to the exposed dura overlying the spinal nerve and scar formation. Indications for concomitant spinal fusion remain controversial. Patients with spondylolisthesis, degenerative scoliosis, history of prior surgery, segmental instability, or predominantly axial pain with concordant discography are possible candidates for concomitant fusion.

Patients with lumbar spondylolisthesis with symptoms of low back pain with or without neurologic symptoms from irritation of the spinal nerve roots may benefit from surgical fusion. In contrast, among patients with axial low back pain with non-specific degenerative changes, spinal fusion should only be considered after exhaustive attempts at non-operative care and psychological counseling. In this small subpopulation, spinal fusion may be considered for patients with two or fewer adjacent degenerated discs demonstrated to be concordant for reproducing the patient's symptoms on non-sedated lumbar discography with at least one asymptomatic level. Even in this highly selected population, concerns about adjacent-level degeneration and subsequent return of pain can occur. Artificial discs hold some promise in terms of reducing adjacent-level degeneration; the efficacy has been reported to be comparable with fusion.[205]

The SPORT studies shed additional light on the role of surgery in patients with back pain. The SPORT investigators performed three parallel studies involving patients with herniated nucleus pulposus and sciatica; patients with lumbar spinal stenosis and neurogenic claudication; and patients with degenerative spondylolisthesis. Each trial was compromised by high rates of crossover from one randomized group to the other. Essentially, about half of SPORT subjects did not receive the intervention to which they were randomly assigned. Consequently, the investigators presented sophisticated as-treated analyses that take advantage of the unique SPORT data. These analyses consistently show that in the first 2 years of follow-up, outcomes are better following surgery than following non-operative therapy. Longer follow-up will determine whether these differences persist.[206,207]

Unfortunately, in spite of adequate conservative and operative management, some patients are left with ongoing severe back pain and limitation. Multidisciplinary pain management and functional restoration techniques should be considered for these patients and the management involves both physical and psychological assessment and treatment.[208]

KEY REFERENCES

1. Lawrence RC, Felson DT, Helmick CG, et al. Estimates of the prevalence of arthritis and other rheumatic conditions in the United States. Part II. Arthritis Rheum 2008;58:26-35.
2. Andersson GB. Epidemiological features of chronic low-back pain. Lancet 1999;354:581-585.
3. Hart LG, Deyo RA, Cherkin DC. Physician office visits for low back pain. Frequency, clinical evaluation, and treatment patterns from a U.S. national survey. Spine 1995;20:11-19.
4. Frymoyer JW, Cats-Baril WL. An overview of the incidences and costs of low back pain. Orthop Clin North Am 1991;22:263-271.
5. Battie MC, Videman T, Parent E. Lumbar disc degeneration: epidemiology and genetic influences. Spine 2004;29:2679-2690.
6. MacGregor AJ, Andrew T, Sambrook PN, Spector TD. Structural, psychological, and genetic influences on low back and neck pain: a study of adult female twins. Arthritis Rheum 2004;51:160-167.
7. Deyo RA, Weinstein JN. Low back pain. N Engl J Med 2001;344:363-370.
8. Atlas SJ, Chang Y, Kammann E, et al. Long-term disability and return to work among patients who have a herniated lumbar disc: the effect of disability compensation. J Bone Joint Surg Am 2000;82:4-15.
9. Emad Y, Ragab Y, Zeinhom F, et al. Hippocampus dysfunction may explain symptoms of fibromyalgia syndrome. A study with single-voxel magnetic resonance spectroscopy. J Rheumatol 2008;35:1371-1377.
10. Vroomen PC, de Krom MC, Knottnerus JA. Diagnostic value of history and physical examination in patients suspected of sciatica due to disc herniation: a systematic review. J Neurol 1999;246:899-906.
11. McCombe PF, Fairbank JC, Cockersole BC, Pynsent PB. 1989 Volvo Award in clinical sciences. Reproducibility of physical signs in low-back pain. Spine 1989;14:908-918.
12. Waddell G, McCulloch JA, Kummel E, Venner RM. Nonorganic physical signs in low-back pain. Spine 1980;5:117-125.
13. Devo RA, Rainville J, Kent DL. What can the history and physical examination tell us about low back pain? JAMA 1992;268:760-765.
14. Wiesel SW, Feffer HL, Rothman RH. Industrial low-back pain. A prospective evaluation of a standardized diagnostic and treatment protocol. Spine 1984;9:199-203.
15. Rossignol M, Suissa S, Abenhaim L. The evolution of compensated occupational spinal injuries. A three-year follow-up study. Spine 1992;17:1043-1047.
16. Merskey H. The characteristics of persistent pain in psychological illness. J Psychosom Res 1965;9:291-298.
17. Deyo RA, Bass JE. Lifestyle and low-back pain. The influence of smoking and obesity. Spine 1989;14:501-506.
18. Leboeuf-Yde C, Kyvik KO, Bruun NH. Low back pain and lifestyle. Part II—Obesity. Information from a population-based sample of 29,424 twin subjects. Spine 1999;24:779-783; discussion 83-84.
19. Nachemson A. The lumbar spine: an orthopaedic challenge. Spine 1976:59-71.
20. Boden SD, Davis DO, Dina TS, et al. Abnormal magnetic-resonance scans of the lumbar spine in asymptomatic subjects. A prospective investigation. J Bone Joint Surg Am 1990;72:403-408.
21. Dreyfuss P, Michaelsen M, Pauza K, et al. The value of medical history and physical examination in diagnosing sacroiliac joint pain. Spine 1996;21:2594-2602.
22. Fukui S, Ohseto K, Shiotani M, et al. Distribution of referred pain from the lumbar zygapophyseal joints and dorsal rami. Clin J Pain 1997;13:303-307.

23. Schwarzer AC, Aprill CN, Derby R, et al. The prevalence and clinical features of internal disc disruption in patients with chronic low back pain. Spine 1995;20:1878-1883.
24. Slipman CW, Jackson HB, Lipetz JS, et al. Sacroiliac joint pain referral zones. Arch Phys Med Rehabil 2000;81:334-338.
25. Deyo RA, Weinstein JN. Low back pain. N Engl J Med 2001;344:363-370.
26. Borenstein DG, Wiesel S, Boden S, eds. Low back pain: medical diagnosis and comprehensive management, 2nd ed. Philadelphia: WB Saunders, 1995.
27. Atlas SJ, Chang Y, Kammann E, et al. Long-term disability and return to work among patients who have a herniated lumbar disc: the effect of disability compensation. J Bone Joint Surg Am 2000;82:4-15.
28. Spengler DM, Freeman CW. Patient selection for lumbar discectomy. An objective approach. Spine 1979;4:129-134.
29. Blower PW. Neurologic patterns in unilateral sciatica. A prospective study of 100 new cases. Spine 1981;6:175-179.
30. Fahmi W. Observation on straight leg raising with special reference to nerve root adhesions. Can J Surg 1966;9:44-48.
31. Vroomen PC, de Krom MC, Knottnerus JA. Diagnostic value of history and physical examination in patients suspected of sciatica due to disc herniation: a systematic review. J Neurol 1999;246:899-906.
32. McCombe PF, Fairbank JC, Cockersole BC, Pynsent PB. 1989 Volvo Award in clinical sciences. Reproducibility of physical signs in low-back pain. Spine 1989;14:908-918.
33. Jensen OH. The level-diagnosis of a lower lumbar disc herniation: the value of sensibility and motor testing. Clin Rheumatol 1987;6:564-569.
34. Vallfors B. Acute, subacute and chronic low back pain: clinical symptoms, absenteeism and working environment. Scand J Rehabil Med Suppl 1985;11:1-98.
35. Waddell G, McCulloch JA, Kummel E, Venner RM. Nonorganic physical signs in low-back pain. Spine 1980;5:117-125.
36. Devo RA, Rainville J, Kent DL. What can the history and physical examination tell us about low back pain? JAMA 1992;268:760-765.
37. Witt I, Vestergaard A, Rosenklint A. A comparative analysis of x-ray findings of the lumbar spine in patients with and without lumbar pain. Spine 1984;9:298-300.
38. Deyo RA, Bigos SJ, Maravilla KR. Diagnostic imaging procedures for the lumbar spine. Ann Intern Med 1989;111:865-867.
39. Lawrence JS, Bremner JM, Brier F. Osteo-arthrosis. Prevalence in the population and relationship between symptoms and x-ray changes. Ann Rheum Dis 1966;25:1-24.
40. Hakelius A, Hindmarsh J. The comparative reliability of preoperative diagnostic methods in lumbar disc surgery. Acta Orthop Scand 1972;43:234-238.
41. Devo RA, McNeish LM, Cone RO III. Observer variability in the interpretation of lumbar spine radiographs. Arthritis Rheum 1985;28:1066-1070.
42. van Tulder MW, Assendelft WJ, Koes BW, Bouter LM. Spinal radiographic findings and nonspecific low back pain. A systematic review of observational studies. Spine 1997;22:427-434.
43. Liang M, Komaroff AL. Roentgenograms in primary care patients with acute low back pain: a cost-effectiveness analysis. Arch Intern Med 1982;142:1108-1112.
44. Padley S, Gleeson F, Chisholm R, Baldwin J. Assessment of a single lumbar spine radiograph in low back pain. Br J Radiol 1990;63:535-536.
45. Eisenberg RL, Hedgcock MW, Williams EA, et al. Optimum radiographic examination for consideration of compensation awards: II. Cervical and lumbar spines. AJR Am J Roentgenol 1980;135:1071-1074.
46. Gehweiler JA Jr, Daffner RH. Low back pain: the controversy of radiologic evaluation. AJR Am J Roentgenol 1983;140:109-112.
47. Scavone JG, Latshaw RF, Weidner WA. Anteroposterior and lateral radiographs: an adequate lumbar spine examination. AJR Am J Roentgenol 1981;136:715-717.
48. Braen SBOBG. Acute low back problems in adults. In: Agency for Health Care Policy and Research PHS, US Department of Health and Human Services, ed. Rockville, Md: AHCPR Publications, 1994.
49. Russell MS-AEBA. Use of lumbar radiographs for the early diagnosis of low back pain. JAMA 1997;277:1782-1786.
50. Pomeranz SJ, Pretorius HT, Ramsingh PS. Bone scintigraphy and multimodality imaging in bone neoplasia: strategies for imaging in the new health care climate. Semin Nucl Med 1994;24:188-207.

REFERENCES

Full references for this chapter can be found on www.expertconsult.com.

The shoulder

Seamus E. Dalton

- Shoulder motion involves four articulations: the glenohumeral, acromioclavicular, sternoclavicular, and scapulothoracic.
- The stability of the shoulder depends on static and dynamic restraints.
- Common shoulder disorders include rotator cuff tendinopathies, capsulitis (frozen shoulder), glenohumeral arthritis, and acromioclavicular syndromes.
- Most shoulder conditions can be diagnosed clinically by a careful history and physical examination.
- In tendinopathies there is pain on active and resisted motion but passive range of motion tends to be normal. Degenerative tendinopathies are common, age-related, and often asymptomatic.
- In capsulitis and glenohumeral arthritis, active and passive motions are painful, there is no pain on resisted motion, and passive motion is decreased.

FUNCTIONAL ANATOMY

The clavicle, scapula, and humerus make up the bony skeleton of the shoulder girdle. The relationship of these bones with the axial skeleton is maintained largely through muscular attachments and also through the articulation of the clavicle with the thoracic cage at the sternoclavicular joint. Shoulder movement occurs through many planes and is achieved through motion at four articulations: the glenohumeral, acromioclavicular, sternoclavicular, and scapulothoracic. The scapula acts as a mobile platform on which glenohumeral motion can take place. The glenohumeral joint is a multiaxial joint that allows the greatest freedom of movement of any joint of the body, although this is at the expense of stability. Ligamentous support is important in maintaining the static stability of the joints of the shoulder and allowing synchronous movements to take place. Some constraint is also afforded to the head of the humerus through the subacromial joint by the overlying acromion and coracoacromial ligament. Muscles act as prime movers at the shoulder as well as providing dynamic stability to the glenohumeral joint. The shoulder girdle also acts as a conduit for the brachial plexus and major vessels supplying the upper limb.

Glenohumeral joint

The glenohumeral joint is not a true ball-and-socket joint and allows a certain amount of translation, which is increased when there is laxity of the musculoligamentous support to the joint. Inherent bony stability is poor because of the shallow glenoid fossa and larger humeral head, although it is enhanced through a process of joint adhesion and negative intra-articular pressure. The glenoid labrum is a rim of fibrocartilage at the periphery of the glenoid that effectively deepens the glenoid fossa and increases its diameter and contact with the humeral head, thereby affording some increased stability.

The joint capsule is thin and lax, especially inferiorly, which allows rotation and elevation but becomes taut at the extremes of motion with tensile load in one region of the capsule associated with laxity in the contralateral region. In conditions in which the capsule contracts there is restriction of glenohumeral motion. Restriction in this capsule posteriorly results in increased superior and anterior translation with forward flexion, which can lead to subacromial impingement.

Glenohumeral ligaments

The joint capsule is thickened anteriorly to form separate components known as the glenohumeral ligaments, which act to strengthen the anterior and inferior capsule. The superior glenohumeral ligament runs from the anterosuperior aspect of the glenoid to the proximal edge of the lesser tuberosity of the humerus, with the middle glenohumeral ligament running just below this. The inferior glenohumeral ligament runs from the anteromedial aspect of the glenoid to the distal edge of the lesser tuberosity and proximal shaft of the humerus and has three components enabling it to sustain loading in multiple directions (Fig. 70.1).[1,2] It is important in the provision of anteroinferior stability to the joint, particularly with the arm in abduction and external rotation, and is the major restraint of external rotation in the neutral and abducted position.[3] It has also been shown to provide some posterior stability, especially in flexion and internal rotation. The joint capsule functions like a hammock or cylinder, with many regions acting as a restraint to external rotation.

Anatomic variants in glenohumeral ligaments

Deficiencies in this ligament complex are important in the development of instability. Several studies have described a number of anatomic variations in the glenohumeral ligaments and capsulolabral attachments that need to be differentiated from truly pathologic conditions.[4] With the advent of magnetic resonance imaging (MRI) and arthroscopy, these variants have been demonstrated in the normal and symptomatic population (Fig. 70.2). An example is the variable development of the middle glenohumeral ligament and anterosuperior labrum, with normal variants such as the Buford complex (absent anterior superior labrum and cord-like middle glenohumeral ligament) and sublabral hole (or window) often being mistakenly identified as a pathologic lesion, that is, Bankart's defect (isolated tear in the anterior inferior glenoid labrum).[5]

Coracohumeral and coracoacromial ligaments

The coracohumeral ligament originates from the coracoid process with a variable insertion into the rotator interval or anterior rotator cuff, and in conjunction with the superior glenohumeral ligament it limits inferior translation and external rotation of the adducted shoulder. The coracoacromial ligament extends from the undersurface of the medial acromion to the superolateral border of the coracoid process, although several types have been described.[6] It acts as a tension band supporting the acromion and coracoid and has an important role in transmitting force from the surrounding muscles. Along with the acromion, it acts as a roof over the subacromial space under which the rotator cuff tendons slide, with the subacromial bursa lying between. This structure has been implicated in the pathology of impingement of the shoulder. The transverse humeral ligament runs between the greater and lesser tuberosities, covering the long head of the biceps tendon (Fig. 70.3).

Stabilizers of the shoulder

The stabilizers of the shoulder can be divided into two groups: static and dynamic (i.e., passive and active restraints). The capsule, labrum, glenohumeral, and, to a lesser extent, coracohumeral ligaments can be thought of as static stabilizers of the glenohumeral joint. There are two sleeves of muscles about the shoulder: superficial and deep. The deep group comprises the rotator cuff muscles (supraspinatus, subscapularis, infraspinatus, and teres minor) and the tendon of the long head of biceps. This layer acts dynamically to stabilize the humeral head in the glenoid fossa during shoulder movement while simultaneously providing rotation (through subscapularis, teres minor, and infraspinatus) and abduction (through supraspinatus).

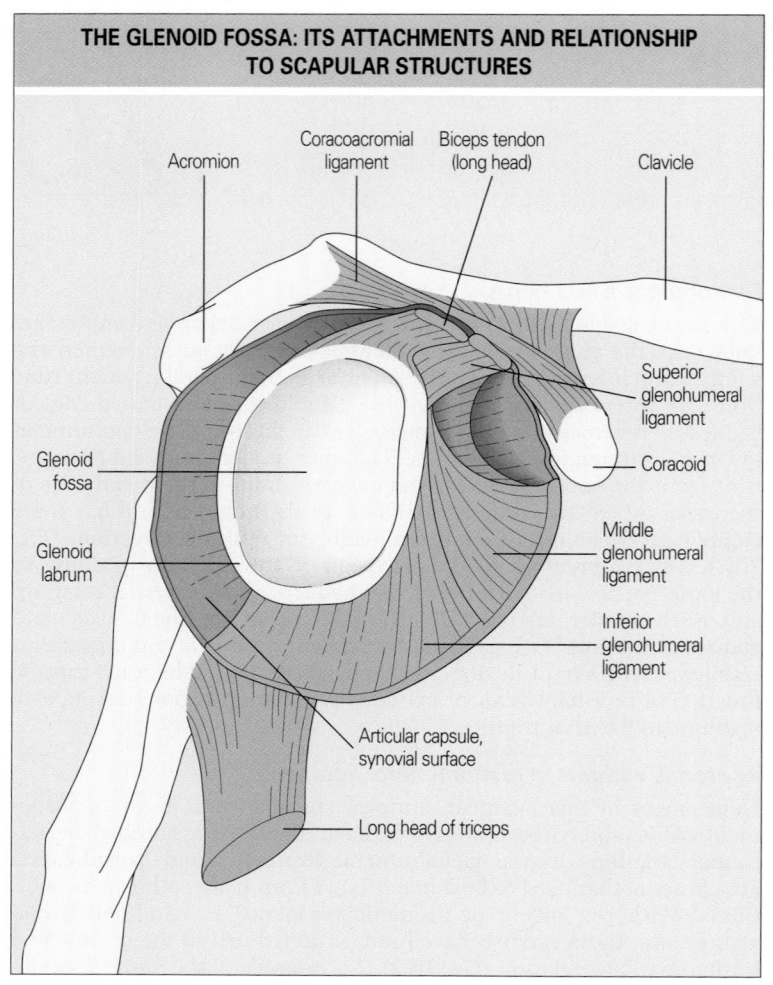

THE GLENOID FOSSA: ITS ATTACHMENTS AND RELATIONSHIP TO SCAPULAR STRUCTURES

Acromion

Coracoacromial ligament

Biceps tendon (long head)

Clavicle

Superior glenohumeral ligament

Coracoid

Glenoid fossa

Glenoid labrum

Middle glenohumeral ligament

Inferior glenohumeral ligament

Articular capsule, synovial surface

Long head of triceps

Fig. 70.1 The glenoid fossa: its attachments and relationship to scapular structures.

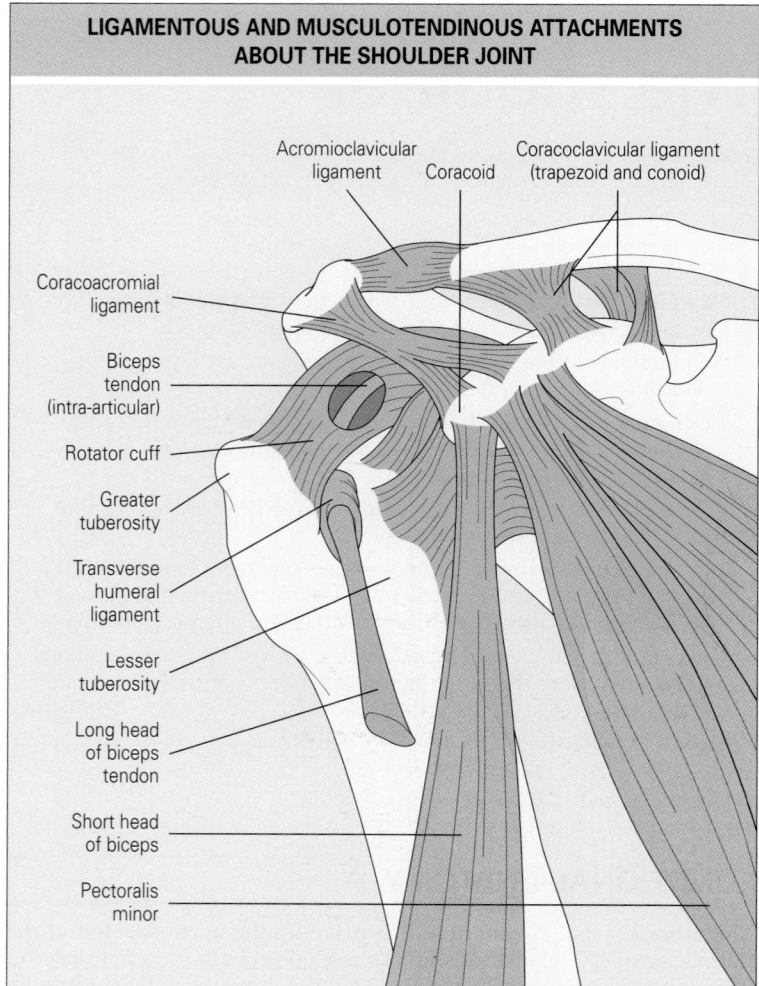

LIGAMENTOUS AND MUSCULOTENDINOUS ATTACHMENTS ABOUT THE SHOULDER JOINT

Acromioclavicular ligament

Coracoid

Coracoclavicular ligament (trapezoid and conoid)

Coracoacromial ligament

Biceps tendon (intra-articular)

Rotator cuff

Greater tuberosity

Transverse humeral ligament

Lesser tuberosity

Long head of biceps tendon

Short head of biceps

Pectoralis minor

Fig. 70.3 Ligamentous and musculotendinous attachments about the shoulder joint.

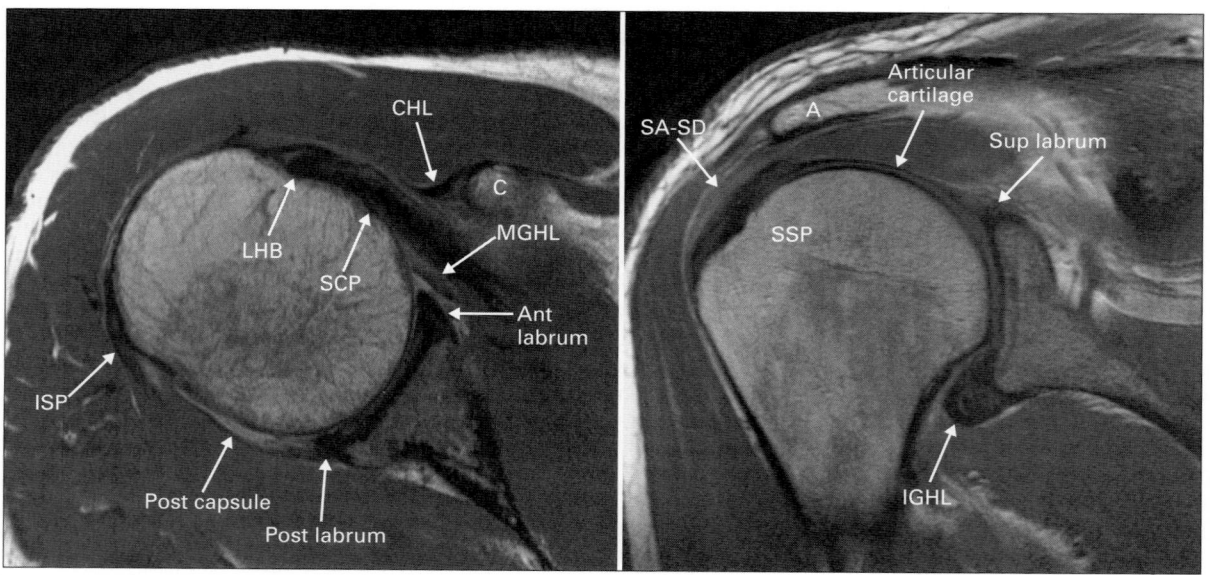

CHL

C

LHB

SCP

MGHL

Ant labrum

ISP

Post capsule

Post labrum

SA-SD

A

Articular cartilage

Sup labrum

SSP

IGHL

Fig. 70.2 MRI of the shoulder showing anatomic features of the glenohumeral joint.

Rotator cuff

The rotator cuff has also been shown to provide some passive restraint to glenohumeral joint translation, especially posteriorly.[7] During the initiation of shoulder abduction or elevation, the larger, more powerful deltoid muscle, if unopposed, would pull the humeral head superiorly toward the acromion. The rotator cuff muscles and the biceps tendon act as humeral head depressors to prevent this translational movement superiorly. This is known as the "force-couple." The subscapularis also acts to resist the tendency of the humeral head to sublux anteriorly in the upper ranges of abduction, although its role is less important than

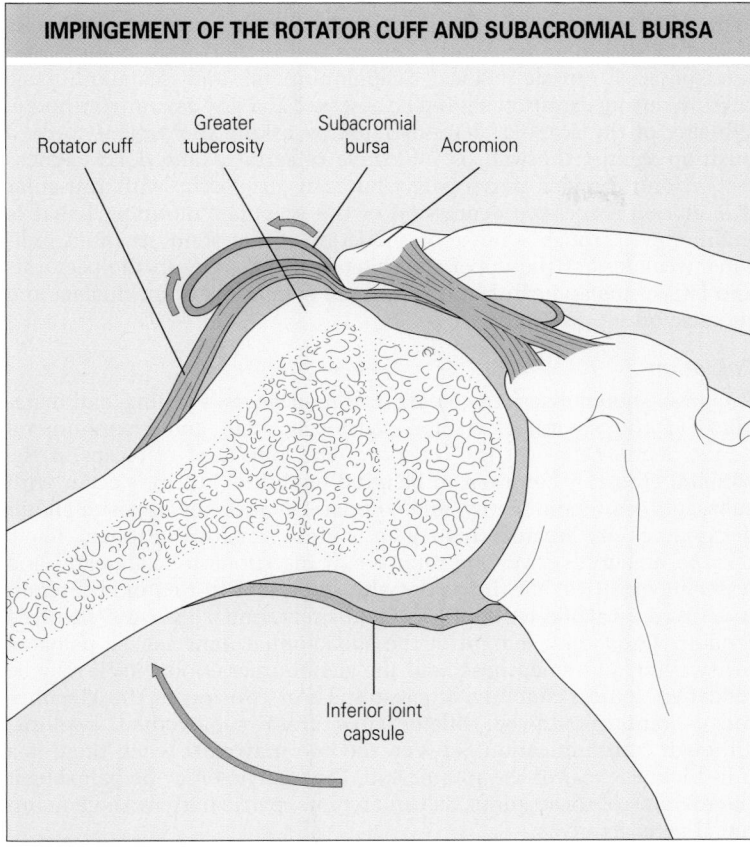

IMPINGEMENT OF THE ROTATOR CUFF AND SUBACROMIAL BURSA

Rotator cuff — Greater tuberosity — Subacromial bursa — Acromion

Inferior joint capsule

Fig. 70.4 Impingement of the rotator cuff and subacromial bursa. Mechanism of impingement of the rotator cuff and subacromial bursa between the humeral head and overlying coracoacromial arch.

was previously thought and it has been found to be less effective at the extremes of motion.[8,9] Dysfunction of the rotator cuff muscles, either through weakness or a tear, results in diminished stabilization of the humeral head. This leads to weakness of the arm in elevation as well as superior migration of the humeral head, increasing the likelihood of subacromial compression or impingement (Fig. 70.4).[10] Therefore, the four tendons of the rotator cuff grip and the humeral head act as guy ropes to stabilize it during shoulder movement, resisting this sliding tendency within the joint.

Furthermore, there is a gap or thinning of the cuff, between the supraspinatus and subscapularis tendons, known as the "rotator interval," which is composed of the coracohumeral ligament, the superior glenohumeral ligament, and part of the joint capsule.[11] The rotator interval is of variable size, has a role in the prevention of inferior translation of the humeral head, and may be implicated in some patients with anterior glenohumeral instability. Two functionally different parts of the rotator cuff have been identified, and it has been reported that the coracohumeral ligament is an important structure in the rotator interval that, in conjunction with the superior glenohumeral ligament, has a role in the control of external rotation as well as inferior translation in the adducted shoulder.[3]

Biceps tendon

The biceps tendon arises from the superior labrum or directly from the supraglenoid tubercle, although a number of variations in this attachment have been reported. The long head of the biceps has been described as a humeral head depressor in full abduction and has also been shown to contribute to anterior stability of the shoulder.[12] It has been reported as a significant dynamic restraint in the abducted shoulder near end-range rotation. However, one study suggests that its role as a stabilizer of the glenohumeral joint is either a passive one or dependent on tension associated with elbow and forearm activity.[13]

Outer muscle sleeve

The outer sleeve of muscles comprises the deltoid, teres major, pectoralis major, latissimus dorsi, and trapezius muscles. They act as prime movers of the humerus, although the trapezius acts through movement of the scapula and clavicle. The combination of these large muscles (which provide abduction, flexion, extension, adduction, and a degree of rotation) with the deep layer of rotator cuff muscles (which provide more rotation of the humeral head and act as a stabilizing force) allows the expansive movement of the arm in actions such as reaching behind one's back or behind the head. However, in certain positions overactivity in these muscles, notably the deltoid and pectoralis major, may actually reduce glenohumeral stability.[14]

Deltoid

The deltoid muscle has three bellies—anterior, middle and posterior—producing, respectively, flexion, abduction, and extension of the shoulder. All three muscles converge to an insertion on the deltoid tubercle on the lateral aspect of the humeral shaft. The rotator cuff muscles originate from the scapula and attach to the greater (supraspinatus, infraspinatus, and teres minor) and lesser (subscapularis) tuberosities of the humerus.

Nerve supply

Nerve supply to the glenohumeral joint is provided by those peripheral nerves supplying muscles acting on the joint: the axillary, suprascapular, subscapular, and musculocutaneous nerves. Innervation is via the fifth, sixth, and seventh cervical roots; and the brachial plexus passes anterior and inferior to the glenohumeral joint.

Other joints

Acromioclavicular joint

A fibrous disc separates the non-congruous surfaces of the distal end of the clavicle and the acromion and allows movement at this joint. During abduction and elevation the clavicle rotates through 30 to 40 degrees, which largely occurs at the sternoclavicular joint.[15] There is a small amount of movement at the acromioclavicular joint, and compressive force is applied to the joint in full elevation and horizontal adduction, which is the basis of stress tests applied to this joint. The joint is stabilized posteriorly by the posterior transverse ligament and inferiorly by the inferior ligament; and the deltoid and trapezius muscles act to provide some anterior and superior stability through their fascial layer. Of particular importance are the conoid and trapezoid, or coracoclavicular, ligaments, which maintain the close relationship between the scapula and clavicle during shoulder movement.

Scapulothoracic joint

The scapula lies against the posterolateral aspect of the thoracic wall, rotating and sliding laterally in abduction, elevation, and flexion. It provides the origin for the rotator cuff muscles as well as the deltoid muscle, and the trapezius inserts along its superior aspect. The scapulothoracic joint represents that articulation between the scapula and thoracic cage, and motion here is important for normal functioning of the shoulder.

Elevation and abduction of the arm involve synchronous motion at the glenohumeral and scapulothoracic joints. As elevation increases above 90 degrees, so does the proportion of scapulothoracic motion relative to glenohumeral motion. Scapulohumeral rhythm is representative of the ratio between movement at these two joints and is important in several shoulder disorders. Disturbance of the normal scapulohumeral rhythm affects the biomechanics of the shoulder joint and may result in secondary impingement or tendinitis of the shoulder. This is well demonstrated in elite swimmers or participants in overhead sports, in whom muscle imbalances such as serratus anterior fatigue can give rise to tendinitis or impingement in this manner. Several muscles (levator scapulae, serratus anterior, trapezius, rhomboids) act to stabilize and control movement of the scapula, and the balance between scapula elevators, rotators, depressors, retractors, and protractors provides scapular control and determines scapulothoracic movement. Scapular control by these muscles is becoming better understood as an important factor in glenohumeral instability and rotator cuff dysfunction. Muscle imbalance about the scapula also particularly can lead to fatigue and overactivity in the levator and upper trapezius muscles.

Sternoclavicular joint

Like the acromioclavicular joint, the sternoclavicular joint contains an intra-articular fibrous disc, which allows rotation of the clavicle during abduction and elevation. Strong ligaments stabilize this joint anteriorly and posteriorly.

Bursae

Significant variation exists in regard to the number and extent of bursae around the shoulder. The subacromial bursa lies between the rotator cuff (mainly supraspinatus tendon) and overlying acromion. This bursa does not consist of a distinct sac, and its synovial layers blend in with and are firmly attached to the acromion and rotator cuff. In subacromial impingement and rotator cuff tendinitis there is reactive inflammation of this bursa. The subscapularis bursa communicates with the synovial joint cavity between the superior and middle glenohumeral ligaments, and the synovial membrane of the joint invests the tendon of the long head of biceps. Other bursae include the subdeltoid, coracoid, infraserratus, and bursae at the insertion of the tendon of trapezius and at the tendon insertions on the humerus.

HISTORY AND PHYSICAL EXAMINATION

History

Shoulder pain may be seen in association with several medical conditions and may be referred from cervical, thoracic, or abdominal sources. Any history suggestive of such a secondary cause (e.g., diabetes or Raynaud's phenomenon) may be crucial in diagnosis. Similarly, the mechanism of any precipitating injury is of value. A fall on an outstretched arm can give rise to instability in the younger patient or a rotator cuff tear in the elderly. A fall on the point of the shoulder may result in injury to the rotator cuff or acromioclavicular joint. Throwing injuries tend to stress the capsulolabral complex and ligament attachments of the glenohumeral joint and can also give rise to rotator cuff or bicipital tendinitis.

A thorough history is essential, because the location and type of pain vary between conditions. Pain referred from the cervical spine is often maximal over the suprascapular region with associated paresthesia or pain referred into the upper limb. Although acromioclavicular and sternoclavicular pain is usually localized to the involved joint, it often radiates proximally, even into the neck. Pain from rotator cuff pathology is usually felt at the outer aspect of the upper arm or deltoid region. Adhesive capsulitis tends to give rise to an intense aching deep in the shoulder, although features similar to rotator cuff disease are common in the early stages. Radiating pain into the arm may indicate a cervical pathologic process, thoracic outlet syndrome, compressive neuropathy, brachial neuritis, or a neuropathic pain syndrome. Night pain tends to be either sharp pain associated with movement, indicative of rotator cuff tendinitis or an acromioclavicular pathologic process, or pain of a deep, constant aching nature more suggestive of capsulitis or a chronic tear of the rotator cuff.

Examination

Inspection

Inspection should be performed from anterior, posterior, and lateral aspects. The patient's ability to undress should be observed, because difficulty may indicate functional limitations. Areas of erythema and bruising should be noted. Although uncommon, swelling of the shoulder joint may be seen anteriorly in the projection of the subscapularis bursa. Deformity of the shoulder girdle exists with acromioclavicular joint separation or fractures of the clavicle or humerus. It is important to look for positioning of the shoulder such as asymmetric elevation or overprotraction. Neck positioning should also be recorded. Rupture of the long head of biceps tendon is readily seen with anterior bulging

in the upper arm. Muscle wasting may be present in cases of cervical or brachial neuropathy (e.g., suprascapular nerve entrapment) but is also seen with chronic rotator cuff disease in the supraspinatus and infraspinatus muscle bellies. Scapulohumeral and scapulothoracic rhythm during elevation should be assessed and any asymmetry noted. Winging of the scapula, demonstrated by asking the patient to do a push-up against the wall, is indicative of serratus anterior weakness (as in long thoracic nerve palsy) but can also occur with muscular dysfunction. Excessive depression of the scapula ("dumping") that is maintained through a range of abduction of the shoulder often indicates weakness of the upper trapezius or overactivity in the pectorals and latissimus and can lead to pain and symptoms of brachialgia and thoracic outlet syndrome.

Palpation

Palpation should assess the presence of tenderness, swelling, and instability of the acromioclavicular, sternoclavicular, and glenohumeral joints. Tenderness over the tendon of the long head of biceps at the bicipital groove is common in bicipital tendinitis but may occur with subscapularis tendinopathy, and comparison with the opposite shoulder is necessary because this region is often sensitive to touch. There may be tenderness over the rotator cuff insertions to the greater and lesser tuberosities, but this is not always present in rotator cuff tendinitis. Acute calcific tendinitis is exquisitely tender over the involved tendon. The lateral margin of the subacromial joint can be palpated for swelling and tenderness, and the glenohumeral joint itself may be tender in acute instability or capsulitis. An effusion of the glenohumeral joint should be differentiated from subacromial swelling, although communication between the two may exist when there is a full-thickness tear of the rotator cuff. Osteophytes may be palpable at the margins of these joints, as can crepitus, particularly with glenohumeral osteoarthrosis.

Instability of the acromioclavicular and sternoclavicular joints is readily demonstrable, but glenohumeral instability requires a more detailed examination combining assessment of laxity in anterior, posterior, and inferior directions with stress and apprehension tests to determine the presence of symptomatic instability. This assessment must be carried out in the young adult presenting with shoulder pain, because underlying instability is a frequent cause of tendinitis around the shoulder. Muscles of the shoulder girdle and neck region should be palpated for trigger points and tender points, typically present with myofascial syndromes and fibromyalgia, respectively.

Range of movement

Active and passive ranges of motion of both shoulders should be assessed in the planes of abduction, forward flexion, and external rotation, both with the arm by the side and at 90 degrees of abduction. Internal rotation is frequently assessed as a combined maneuver with extension in bringing the arm up behind the back. This is limited in many periarticular conditions, and a better assessment of true glenohumeral joint restriction can be done by measuring internal rotation with the arm by the side and the elbow extended. Internal rotation should also be assessed with the arm in abduction. Any limitation of movement should be noted as well as any discrepancy between active and passive motion. Glenohumeral joint pathology is unlikely in the presence of a normal range of passive motion.

Further assessment should include passive adduction of the flexed and internally rotated shoulder to look for tightness of the posterior capsule and external rotators, because this is often seen in a chronic pathologic process of the rotator cuff. Resisted shoulder movements are performed to assess involvement of muscles and tendons. The patient is asked to resist a specific movement so as to elicit an isolated, isometric contraction in the particular muscle group. The supraspinatus is tested with the arm abducted to 90 degrees, flexed to 30 degrees, and internally rotated (i.e., thumb downward). The examiner then resists abduction from this position. However, in symptomatic cases this is often very painful and resisted flexion (at 30 degrees of flexion) with the arm internally rotated is often a sensitive and less aggravating test of rotator cuff (particularly supraspinatus) function. Resisted internal rotation tests the subscapularis (best done with the hand behind the back or placed across the abdomen, known as the lift-off and belly press tests, respectively), and resisted external rotation tests

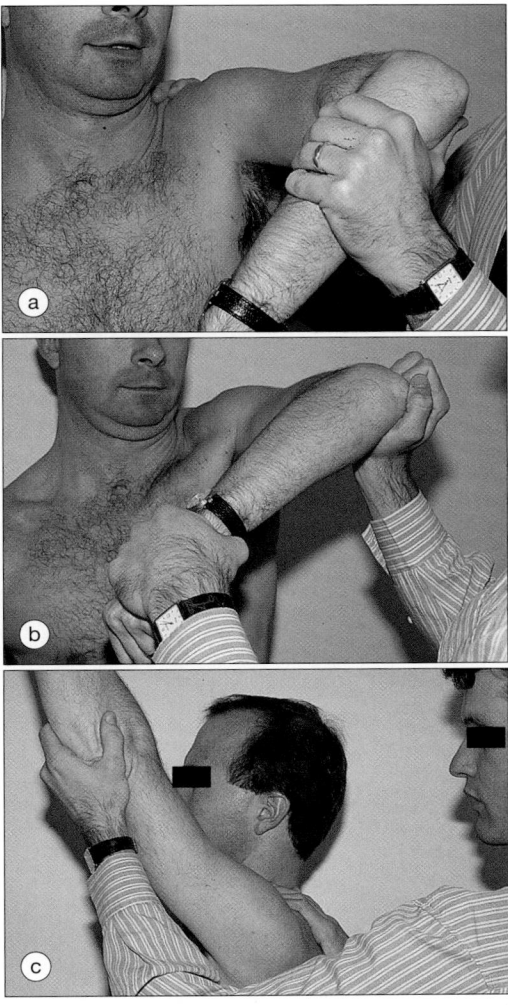

Fig. 70.5 Impingement tests. (a) Forced passive internal rotation. (b) Resisted external rotation. (c) Forced passive full forward flexion.

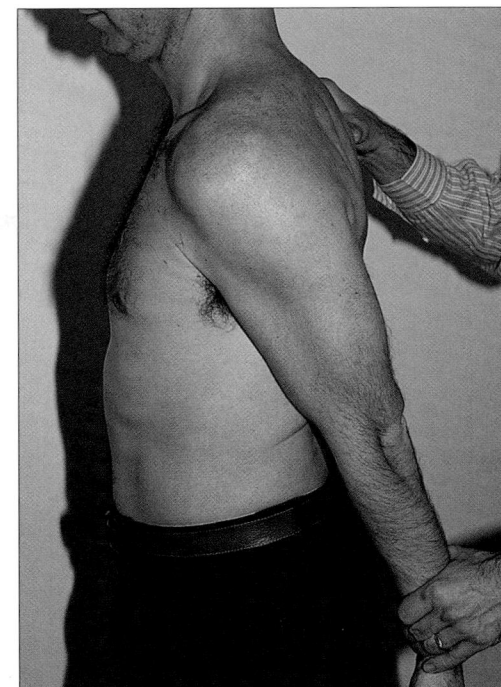

Fig. 70.6 An adduction stress test of the acromioclavicular joint.

the infraspinatus and teres minor (although 22% to 33% of external rotation force can be attributed to the supraspinatus[16]). Resisted abduction should also be carried out with the arm by the side. Biceps function can also be tested by resisting shoulder flexion with the elbow extended (Speed's test) or resisting supination with the elbow flexed to 90 degrees (Yergason's test), although the sensitivity and specificity of these tests are questionable. Any assessment must include an examination of the cervical spine to assess range of motion and the presence of any referred upper limb pain (see Chapter 68).

Special movements

Specific examination techniques can be employed to further localize the source of pain in the shoulder region.[17] Various tests for impingement have been described. In one the arm is flexed to 90 degrees, adducted, and then forcefully internally rotated and slightly elevated by the examiner, with the scapula stabilized by the examiner's other hand (Fig. 70.5a). In another variation the arm is placed in the adducted, flexed, internally rotated position and the patient is asked to externally rotate the arm against resistance (see Fig. 70.5b). A further impingement test is carried out by passively forcing the arm into full forward flexion while the examiner stabilizes the top of the scapula with the other hand (see Fig. 70.5c). In all situations a positive test is recorded if pain is felt as the subacromial bursa and the rotator cuff are forced against the undersurface of the acromion, although it appears likely that these tests also provoke contact between anatomic structures associated with internal impingement.

A number of clinical tests for superior labral and biceps anchor pathologic processes (SLAP lesions) and for labral and biceps pathologic processes have been described, but their diagnostic validity remains uncertain. O'Brien's test has been described as a provocation test for SLAP lesions, but it also elicits pain in acromioclavicular joint disorders.

Pain at the acromioclavicular joint can be localized by performing various stress tests. In one, the arm is held with the elbow and shoulder extended and then passively adducted across behind the back (Fig. 70.6). In another less-specific maneuver the arm is abducted to 90 degrees and then adducted across the patient's chest under the chin. In both tests pain is felt over an inflamed acromioclavicular joint at the limits of these movements. Assessment for a thoracic outlet syndrome is always difficult, and several maneuvers are described that may provoke the symptoms of neurovascular compression (see Chapter 78). A number of upper limb neural tension tests have also been described and are useful when assessing the etiology of diffuse or non-specific upper limb pain.

Joint hypermobility

The patient should be assessed for the presence of joint hypermobility. Laxity of the glenohumeral joint in anterior and posterior directions is determined by carrying out draw tests in which the humeral head is gripped firmly and moved backward and forward in the glenoid fossa. This is best performed with the patient lying supine and the abducted arm supported by the examiner's hand (Fig. 70.7). Inferior laxity is assessed by applying distal retraction to the arm while palpating the gap between the humeral head and acromion. The presence of a distinct gap can be felt and even seen and is referred to as a positive sulcus sign, which is indicative of multidirectional laxity of the joint. Anterior apprehension and stress tests are carried out with the examiner slowly extending and externally rotating the abducted arm with the patient supine. A positive test occurs when the patient experiences pain or apprehension during this maneuver and is confirmed when these symptoms disappear as the examiner's free hand applies a downward, (i.e., stabilizing) force to the anterior aspect of the upper humerus. This often allows further external rotation of the arm (Fig. 70.8). Symptoms return as this stabilizing force is slowly withdrawn. It is important to differentiate between a positive test eliciting pain alone, as opposed to apprehension, because this may simply indicate internal impingement as opposed to true instability. The posterior stress test is carried out by applying gentle axial pressure to the humerus with the arm in the forward flexed, internally rotated, and slightly adducted position, again in an attempt to reproduce pain and apprehension.

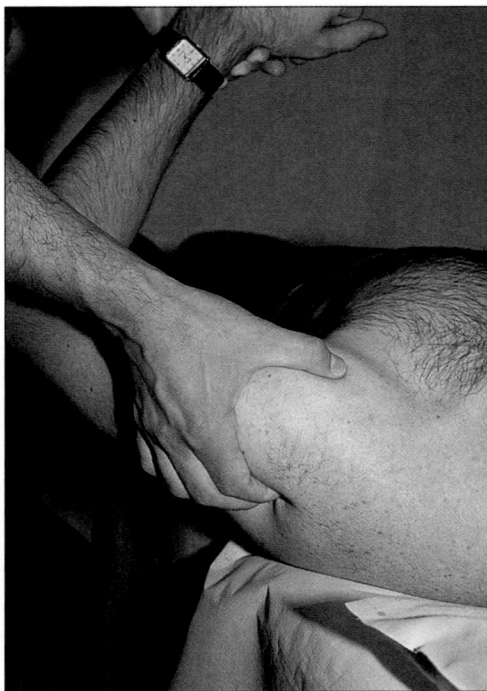

Fig. 70.7 The anterior draw test.

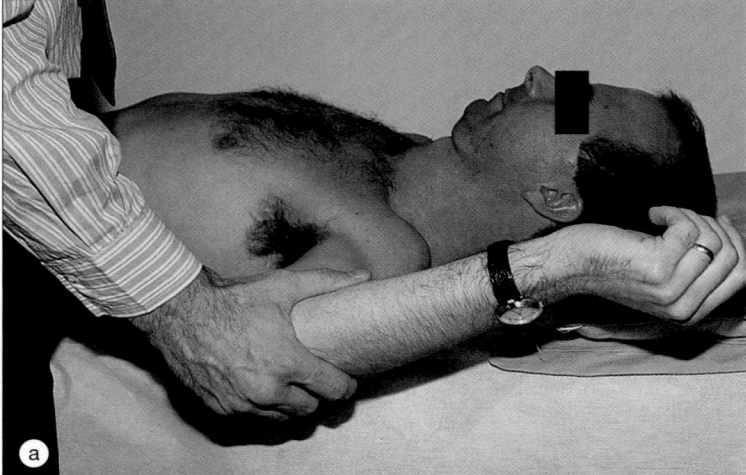

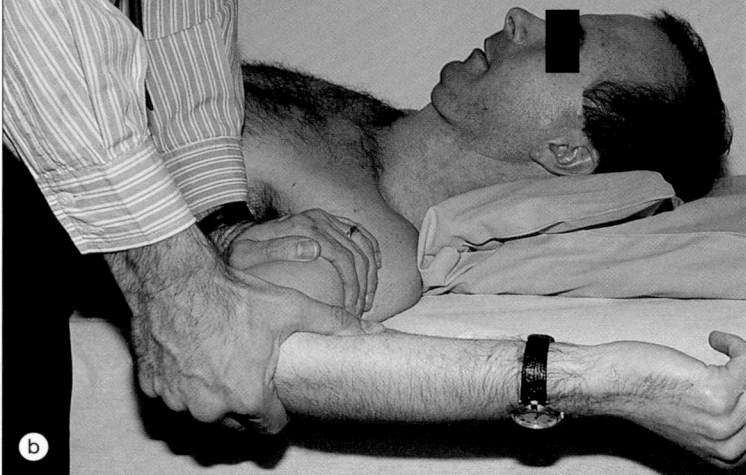

Fig. 70.8 A stress test for anterior glenohumeral instability. (a) The examiner slowly extends and externally rotates the abducted arm. (b) Containment sign: applying pressure anteriorly relieves the symptoms and allows further external rotation.

DIFFERENTIAL DIAGNOSIS OF SHOULDER PAIN

Shoulder pain typically arises from disorders affecting the shoulder joint or from those affecting the periarticular structures. Pain can also be referred from other structures.

The glenohumeral joint may be affected as part of widespread joint disease or polyarthropathy such as rheumatoid arthritis or in isolation by conditions such as septic arthritis, neuropathic (Charcot's) arthritis, osteonecrosis, and idiopathic destructive arthritis. In articular disorders of the shoulder there may be swelling and invariably there is an effect on passive and active motion of the glenohumeral joint with pain, restriction of motion, and often crepitus.

Periarticular conditions affecting the shoulder can be loosely grouped into those with and without capsulitis. If there is no capsular involvement, then passive joint motion is largely unaffected, whereas active movement may be limited by pain and/or weakness (e.g., rotator cuff disorders). With capsulitis there is multidirectional restriction of passive motion, and differentiation from articular conditions of the shoulder is made from clinical and radiologic findings.

Referred pain to the shoulder can occur with cervical disorders, Pancoast's tumor of the lung, subphrenic pathology, entrapment neuropathies, and brachial neuritis. In these conditions passive and often active movements of the shoulder are largely unaffected and there is usually little or no pain when testing rotator cuff function. However, cervicobrachial pain is often associated with painful restriction of passive and active shoulder motion and may be confused with adhesive capsulitis. Again, differentiation from disorders of the shoulder is possible with an adequate history and examination (Table 70-1).

ROTATOR CUFF DISORDERS

The spectrum of disorders affecting the rotator cuff ranges from the mild transient tendinitis that follows an episode of glenohumeral instability in the young patient to a complete tear in the degenerative rotator cuff of the older patient.

Etiology

The anatomic configuration of the shoulder joint is such that the cuff is subjected to stresses when the arm is in the elevated position. Impingement can occur as the supraspinatus tendon is compressed between the humeral head and the overlying anterior acromion, coracoacromial ligament, and even the inferior border of the acromioclavicular joint.[18] Impingement may be structural, owing to the presence of an acromial spur or degenerative acromioclavicular joint, but it may also be functional, owing to superior migration of the humeral head during abduction and elevation.[9] Mechanical impingement by the coracoid process on the rotator cuff or rotator interval has also been recognized as a clinical entity, although the diagnosis can only be confidently confirmed at the time of surgery.[19] Underlying glenohumeral instability is a frequent cause of rotator cuff tendinitis, particularly in the younger patient, as is eccentric overload in the throwing athlete, where the rotator cuff muscles act as decelerators of the throwing arm.

Pathology

As the rotator cuff becomes inflamed, thinned, or torn, its function as a humeral head depressor is compromised and superior migration of the humeral head can occur through the unopposed action of the deltoid, giving rise to further impingement. In the degenerative cuff with a complete tear this can eventually result in a cuff arthropathy with osteoarthritis at the subacromial and glenohumeral joints. The subacromial bursa lies between the rotator cuff tendons and the overlying coracoacromial arch and becomes inflamed with this impingement. This is a reactive process and is usually a secondary phenomenon, although primary subacromial bursitis can result from trauma.

TABLE 70-1 DIFFERENTIAL DIAGNOSIS OF SHOULDER PAIN: CLINICAL AND RADIOGRAPHIC FEATURES OF COMMON CAUSES OF SHOULDER PAIN

Diagnosis	Age	Type of onset	Location of pain	Night pain	Active range of motion	Passive range of motion	Impingement signs	Radiation of pain	Paresthesia	Weakness	Instability	Radiographic changes	Special features
Rotator cuff tendinitis	Any	Acute or chronic	Deltoid region	+	↓↓ guarding	Normal	+++	–	–	Only due to pain	Look for	In chronic cases	Painful arc of abduction
Rotator cuff tears (chronic)	>40 yr	Often chronic	Deltoid region	++	↓↓↓	Normal (may ↓ later)	++	–	–	++	–	+	Wasting of cuff muscles
Bicipital tendinitis	Any	Overuse	Anterior	–	↓ guarding	Normal	+	Occasionally into biceps	–	Only due to pain	Look for	None	Special examination tests
Calcific tendinitis	30–60 yr	Acute	Point of shoulder	++	↓↓↓ guarding	Normal except for pain	+++	–	–	Only due to pain	–	++	Tenderness ++
Capsulitis "frozen shoulder"	>40 yr	Insidious	Deep in shoulder	++	↓↓	↓↓	+	–	–	–	–	–	Global range of motion ↓
Acromioclavicular joint	Any	Acute or chronic	Over joint	Lying on side	Ø full elevation	Normal	–	–	–	–	–	In chronic cases	Local tenderness
Osteoarthrosis of glenohumeral joint	>40 yr	Insidious	Deep in shoulder	++	↓↓	↓↓	–	–	–	May have mild	–	+++	Crepitus
Glenohumeral instability	Usually < 25 yr	Episodic	Anterior or posterior	–	Only apprehension	Only apprehension	Possible	–	+ with acute episodes	+ with acute episodes	+++	Often	Stress tests
Cervical spondylosis	>40 yr	Insidious	Suprascapular	Often	Normal	Normal	–	++	+++	+	–	In cervical spine	Pain with neck movement
Thoracic outlet syndrome	Any	Usually with activity	Neck, shoulder, arm	–	Normal	Normal	–	++	++	++	–	–	Special examination tests

Rotator cuff tendinitis

Pathology

Impingement has been shown to occur in forward flexion when the anterior margin of the acromion impinges on the supraspinatus tendon. Vascular studies have demonstrated that there is a constant area of avascularity or "critical zone" extending from a point approximately 1 cm proximal to the point of insertion of the tendon into the greater tuberosity, and this compromise in microvascularity is seen with the arm in the adducted (neutral) position.[20] However, Iannotti and associates detected substantial blood flow in this critical zone using laser Doppler imaging.[21] It has long been supposed that this region of relative hypovascularity is compromised in elevation and abduction, thereby producing an inflammatory response and subsequent tendinitis. The pathology of this impingement syndrome was classified by Neer into three stages:

- Stage I: edema and hemorrhage of the tendon
- Stage II: fibrosis of the subacromial bursa and tendinitis of the rotator cuff
- Stage III: tendon degeneration, bony changes at the acromion and humeral head, and eventual tendon rupture

The bicipital tendon is frequently involved as part of this condition but is not usually the primary pathologic site. Neer's initial proposal that rotator cuff tendinopathy resulted from subacromial impingement has been found to be an oversimplification of the pathogenesis of rotator cuff disease because there are clearly both extrinsic and intrinsic mechanisms involved.[22]

Histologic studies have shown that degenerative changes are more prominent on the articular surface of the rotator cuff insertions,[23] and a number of radiologic studies have confirmed the relative incidence of bursal, articular surface, intrasubstance, and lamination tears of the rotator cuff.

There appears to be progressive tendon failure leading to cuff rupture, with the prevalence of cuff tears increasing with age in the asymptomatic population.[24] Full-thickness tears have been reported in 20% to 30%, and partial thickness tears have been found in an additional 20% to 30% of people aged over 60 years of age, with the prevalence of full-thickness tears rising to 50% in those older than age 70 years. Possible etiologic factors include trauma, attrition, ischemia, and impingement. A number of studies have looked at biochemical changes within the tendon matrix that may predispose to tendon rupture.[25-28]

History

Presentation depends to a degree on the age of the patient and the likely etiology. Tendinitis resulting from eccentric overload or glenohumeral instability in the young adult usually presents acutely after an activity such as throwing. In the middle-aged individual, onset may be more gradual, reflecting the underlying chronic changes seen in the involved tendon. The patient may present with aching and discomfort in the shoulder, pain on movement, and a history of repetitive or strenuous upper limb activity. The elderly patient may present with no history of antecedent trauma or repetitive activity, and there is usually a gradual onset of increasing shoulder discomfort, night pain, pain with movement, and weakness if a degenerative tear is present. Except in the young patient with a history of explosive arm activity or trauma, onset tends to be gradual and aggravated by movements such as abduction and elevation or sustained overhead activity, which are commonly sports or occupation related. Patients frequently complain that they have difficulty reaching up behind their back when dressing. The pain at night usually occurs when rolling onto the affected side and is typically felt in the deltoid region rather than the point of the shoulder, although this can occur. Active movements may be restricted by pain and in the more severe or chronic cases a secondary capsulitis can develop, further restricting movement at the shoulder.

Examination

Findings on examination include a painful arc of abduction usually occurring between 70 and 120 degrees. When lowering from full abduction there is often a "catch" of pain, usually at mid range as impingement occurs, particularly when there is associated scapular dyskinesia. Passive motion tends to be full and pain free if adequate muscle relaxation can be achieved. Point tenderness over the greater tuberosity and distal rotator cuff can occur but is not always present. The diagnosis is confirmed by reproducing pain when resisting movement of the affected tendon and with impingement testing. In the older patient, acromioclavicular joint arthritis is often present and there may be early joint stiffness. The probability that there is an underlying cuff tear increases with age.

Investigations

Plain radiographs may show evidence of rotator cuff degeneration, that is, cystic and sclerotic changes at the greater tuberosity insertion, and there may be calcification in the rotator cuff tendons in chronic cases. Ultrasonography and MRI can be used to identify changes of rotator cuff tendinitis and partial tears, but in the case of ultrasonography interpretation is fairly observer dependent. Dynamic ultrasonography can also demonstrate thickening of the subacromial bursa and impingement.

Differential diagnosis

Pain felt in the deltoid may suggest referred cervical pain, although this is more likely to present as suprascapular pain being felt into the arm. Pain on active arm movement and impingement testing will assist in differentiation, and preservation of passive range of movement will differentiate rotator cuff tendinitis from a capsulitis. In cases of tendinitis due to underlying instability—and this must be suspected in patients younger than 25 years of age—examination should confirm symptomatic instability.

Management

The treatment of rotator cuff tendinitis is made difficult by continued participation in aggravating activities. Rest and activity modification are necessary to prevent the problem becoming chronic. Initial treatment should be directed at reducing inflammation by means of nonsteroidal anti-inflammatory drugs (NSAIDs) if required. There is little evidence to support the use of modalities such as ultrasound or laser.[29] When there is failure to settle symptoms by these means, a subacromial injection of corticosteroid can be used (see Chapter 66), taking care not to inject the rotator cuff directly. In a Cochrane review it was concluded that although such injections may be beneficial their effect may be small and not well maintained.[30]

As well as reducing pain, treatment should be directed at restoring range of motion and the normal biomechanics of shoulder movement, paying particular attention to scapulohumeral rhythm. This is especially important in cases in which such a disturbance in biomechanics has aggravated or even precipitated the problem. Proprioceptive taping can be used to assess the role of scapular dyskinesia in the genesis of dynamic subacromial impingement and is a useful tool in the early rehabilitation of shoulder dysfunction. Once the pain has lessened and normal shoulder movement patterns have been restored, a strengthening program should be instituted concentrating on rotator cuff exercises to restore its function as a humeral head stabilizer and depressor, thereby reducing the likelihood of further injury. A review of level 1 and 2 studies in the literature has found that exercise is effective as a treatment for the reduction of pain in rotator cuff tendinitis and impingement syndromes and its effect may be augmented with manual therapy.[31] The younger patient with instability needs a comprehensive rehabilitation program and rarely requires injection to the shoulder. The older patient with a degenerative rotator cuff and an associated pathologic process of the acromioclavicular joint may be resistant to conservative treatment.

Indications for surgery vary according to the age of the patient, stage of impingement or tendinitis, and the symptoms. The major indication for surgical intervention is pain; and, in the presence of an intact rotator cuff, failure to respond to a conservative program within 1 year is a reasonable indication for surgery. This involves subacromial decompression and may consist of an anterior acromioplasty and resection of the coracoacromial ligament, both of which can be performed arthroscopically. Any impingement due to an acromioclavicular joint pathologic process must also be addressed at operation. The results of subacromial decompression have generally been reported as good or excellent.[32] However, there is a significant body of opinion that impingement usually results from a disturbance of normal glenohumeral kinematics attributable to capsular tightness, glenohumeral instability, scapulohumeral dysfunction, or loss of rotator cuff function as a humeral head stabilizer. Also, in some cases preservation of the coracoacromial arch is considered important in maintaining humeral head stability. Therefore, an accurate clinical diagnosis and evidence of impingement at surgery are important in determining outcome after subacromial decompression.[33] In some patients a capsular release or stabilization procedure may be more appropriate. In other words, subacromial impingement is frequently the result rather than the cause of shoulder dysfunction.

Prevention

In the young patient or athlete, attention to proper preparation for exercise and correct technique is important. Many athletes develop muscular imbalances about the shoulder, through either tightness or weakness, and secondary impingement and tendinitis can result if these are not corrected. Serratus anterior fatigue results in loss of scapular stability and can lead to subacromial or internal impingement. In the older patient, avoidance of sustained above-shoulder activities or explosive lifting will help prevent this condition from worsening or perhaps even developing.

Rotator cuff tears

Pathology

The incidence of degenerative cuff tears increases with age, as does the size of the tear.[34] Superior migration of the humeral head against the undersurface of the acromion occurs as the incompetent rotator cuff fails to stabilize and depress the humeral head and therefore counteract the pull of the deltoid. This leads to degenerative change both at the subacromial joint and secondarily at the glenohumeral joint, known as rotator cuff arthropathy. Neer estimated that 4% of cuff tears ultimately progress to a cuff arthropathy,[35] although the true figure is probably greater.

Clinical presentation and features

Rotator cuff tears may be acute or chronic and partial or full thickness. Partial-thickness tears may occur in any age group after trauma, but a full-thickness (or complete) tear is unusual in the patient younger than 40 years of age. In the young adult a partial tear can result from a fall or explosive shoulder movement and presents very much as a rotator cuff tendinitis, although onset is acute. Also, full active range of motion may be preserved. The acute complete rupture after trauma should be readily diagnosed. The mechanism of injury is usually a fall onto the outstretched arm, a hyperabduction injury, or a fall onto the side of the shoulder. Bruising is often delayed and occurs in the upper arm, and there is usually an immediate loss of active abduction with weakness of abduction and external rotation. There is a close association between dislocation of the shoulder in the patient older than 40 years of age and partial or complete tears of the rotator cuff. In one review of 40 patients the prevalence of full-thickness tears was 90%.[36]

Previous studies have recorded the incidence of chronic full-thickness tears found at autopsy,[37] although more recent MRI studies have reported a greater prevalence in the asymptomatic population and many patients with a documented complete tear of the supraspinatus tendon have full active abduction, often in the absence of pain, even in the presence of abnormal glenohumeral kinematics and superior humeral head migration.[38] There may be no history of trauma, and symptoms frequently become apparent with increased activity, although the clinical expression of rotator cuff tears is variable.[39] The usual picture is one of pain on abduction and flexion with varying degrees of loss of active movement, depending on the size of the tear. The patient may complain of weakness of abduction, flexion, and internal or external rotation, depending on the tendon involved.

Night pain is common and often severe. Examination reveals many of the features of rotator cuff tendinitis, but there is often an inability to maintain the arm in abduction when lowering from the elevated position, that is, a positive "drop-off" sign. Subacromial crepitus and pain on impingement testing are usually present. A common clinical finding is wasting of the infraspinatus and, to a lesser extent, supraspinatus muscle bellies, together with weakness of abduction, but more often weakness of external rotation reflects the size of the tear.

Isometric measurement of rotation strength correlates well with the functional integrity of the rotator cuff, along with the patient's function and quality of life.[40] Rupture of the long head of the biceps tendon is frequently associated with a chronic rotator cuff pathologic process.

Investigations

Features of chronic rotator cuff degeneration can be seen on plain radiography with sclerosis and cystic changes at the greater tuberosity. Osteophyte formation may be present along the anterior inferior acromion, with possible acromioclavicular joint osteoarthritis. With a complete tear there may be superior migration of the humeral head and narrowing of the subacromial space (<6 mm indicates a tear). This finding, along with degenerative change, is seen in cuff arthropathy.

Full-thickness tears are readily demonstrated with single- or double-contrast arthrography, and sensitivity approaches 90%. Partial tears can occasionally be seen (Fig. 70.9). However, estimation of the size of the defect using this technique is unreliable. Ultrasonography can identify and size tears, both full and, to a lesser extent, partial thickness (Fig. 70.10).[41] MRI compares favorably with arthrography in the diagnosis of complete tears (Fig. 70.11). It is less consistent in the assessment of partial and lamination tears[42] (Fig. 70.12) but allows assessment of tear retraction, muscle atrophy, and fatty degeneration in the rotator cuff muscles, which is important in the selection of patients for surgery. Arthroscopy may be used to establish the diagnosis in the patient with shoulder pain who requires further assessment. It is particularly useful

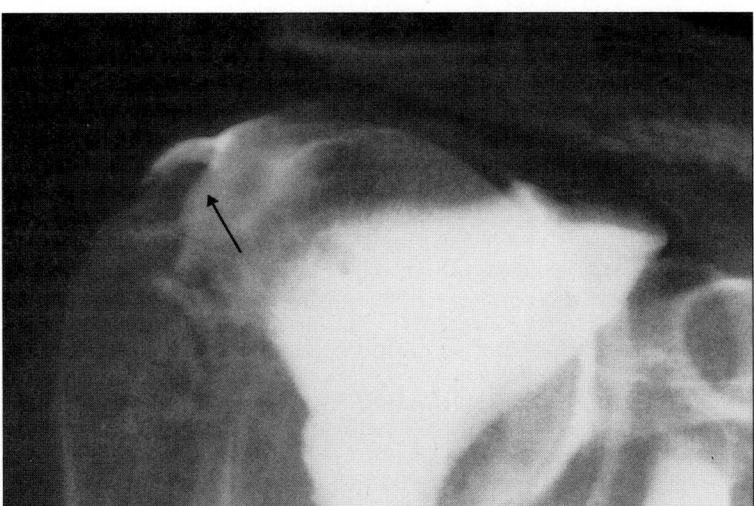

Fig. 70.9 Arthrogram of the shoulder showing leakage of dye into the supraspinatus tendon confirming a partial tear (arrow). This investigation is more accurate in the assessment of full-thickness tears of the rotator cuff.

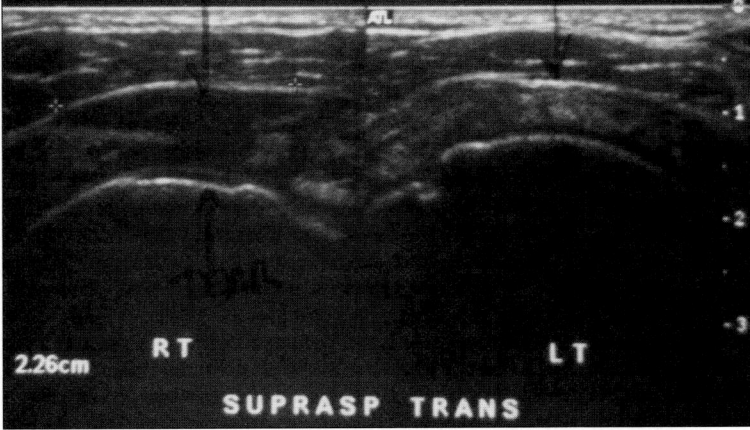

Fig. 70.10 Ultrasound image of acute full-thickness rotator cuff tear.

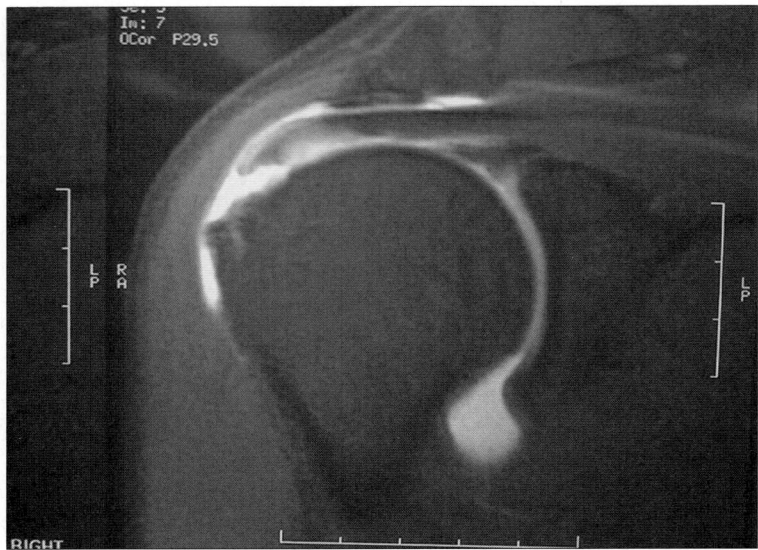

Fig. 70.11 MR image shows a full-thickness tear of the distal supraspinatus tendon with early retraction of the articular side of the tendon.

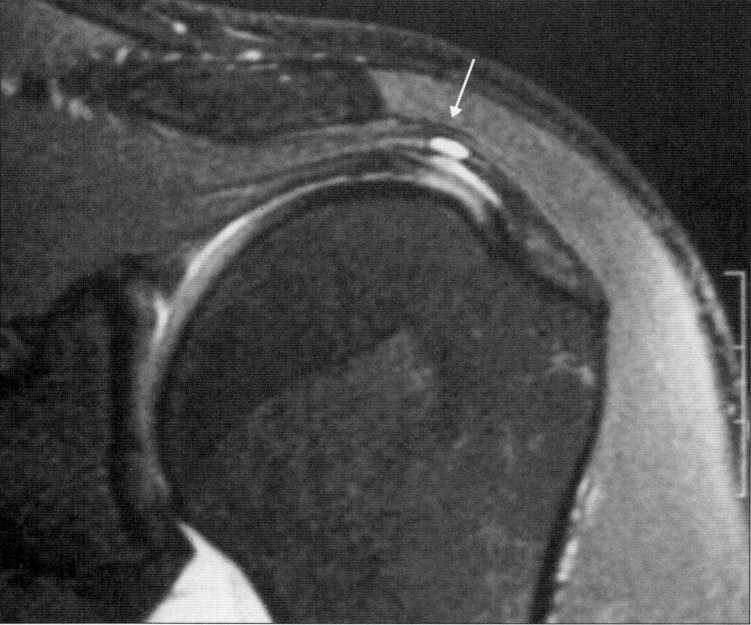

Fig. 70.12 MR image shows a partial articular surface rotator cuff tear along with a laminar defect and small cyst in the distal supraspinatus tendon.

in the assessment of instability while at the same time allowing visualization of the rotator cuff, subacromial bursa, intra-articular bicipital tendon, and glenoid labrum. It also has a role in the estimation of the size of a cuff tear before more definitive surgery.

Management

Initially, partial rotator cuff tears should all be managed conservatively, as for rotator cuff tendinitis, although corticosteroid injection is not advisable within 4 to 6 weeks of an acute injury. Bursal and articular surface tears may be amenable to arthroscopic débridement, decompression, and possibly repair, but intrasubstance and laminar tears are best treated non-operatively unless there is associated subacromial impingement. The surgical management of complete tears is somewhat controversial. Acute ruptures in the young or active patient should be managed surgically earlier rather than later. In the older or less active patient it is reasonable to have a trial of conservative

management, but if there is no substantial improvement within 3 months then subacromial decompression and repair is advisable.[43]

Chronic complete tears should all be treated with an adequate conservative program in the first instance. Failure to achieve pain relief is a major indication for surgical intervention. Any operative procedure should be directed primarily at relief of impingement, débridement of the cuff tear, and usually repair of the defect.[44] Surgery should also be considered when there is an associated rupture of the biceps tendon because these cases appear more likely to develop a cuff arthropathy.

The results of surgical repair of rotator cuff tears are usually good but depend on the age of the patient and on the size and age of the tear. Pain relief is usually achieved, but recovery of strength is less predictable and restoration of joint motion may depend on the amount of postoperative stiffness that develops. A major predictor of outcome after cuff repair is the degree of rotator cuff muscle atrophy and fatty infiltration present, which can be assessed preoperatively with computed tomography or MRI.[45] Therefore, a number of factors must be taken into account when deciding whether to proceed to surgery. These include the patient's age and occupation, the size and type of tear (repair of lamination and complex tears can be difficult), and the presence of tendon retraction and muscle atrophy. Surgery should be delayed if there is an associated capsulitis, and a capsular release may be required beforehand. Full-thickness tears of the subscapularis are best repaired early, because delayed closure may not be possible once the torn tendon has retracted. In large or massive retracted tears a latissimus dorsi or pectoralis major muscle transfer may be required to close the defect and improve function, but other surgical options include simple débridement and decompression or partial repair leaving a residual defect.

OTHER PERIARTICULAR DISORDERS

Bicipital tendinitis

Pathology

The tendon of the long head of biceps may be involved at several sites: (1) its attachment to the superior glenoid labrum, which may be injured in a fall or throwing action (SLAP lesion[46]); (2) as it runs across the glenohumeral joint (intra-articular) where it is stabilized by a pulley system made up of the coracohumeral ligament, superior glenohumeral ligament, and fibers of the supraspinatus and subscapularis tendons; or (3) as it runs in the bicipital groove (extra-articular). The transverse humeral ligament stabilizes the tendon in the bicipital groove; and if this mechanism is disrupted, subluxation or dislocation of the tendon can result. This tends to occur as the arm is rotated in the abducted position. The tendon can become inflamed, thickened, and fibrotic in chronic cases; and it has been shown that bicipital groove anatomy correlates with biceps tendon disease.[47] In the older patient there may be attenuation and thinning of the tendon and eventual rupture. This latter presentation is almost always indicative of underlying rotator cuff degeneration because the bicipital tendon appears to become stressed in its attempt to act as a humeral head depressor in cases of rotator cuff incompetence. Also, the presence of a complete rotator cuff tear exposes the intra-articular portion of the bicipital tendon to the overlying acromion and further impingement.

Clinical presentation and features

Although frequently diagnosed, bicipital tendinitis is not often seen in isolation and usually occurs in association with rotator cuff tendinitis or impingement or with glenohumeral instability. Primary involvement of the tendon is seen as an overuse injury in sports such as weight lifting in which there is a repetitive stress placed on the tendon or after prolonged and repetitive carrying (e.g., of small children). The bicipital tendon acts as a secondary stabilizer of the humeral head, and the translational movement seen with glenohumeral laxity can place increased stress on the tendon, leading to tendinitis. As with rotator cuff tendinitis, the young patient with bicipital tendinitis should be assessed for instability. With chronic impingement or rotator cuff degeneration the biceps tendon may become fibrotic and attenuated and eventually rupture. Acute ruptures are also seen in young power-lifters, and the diagnosis is made easily in the acute presentation.

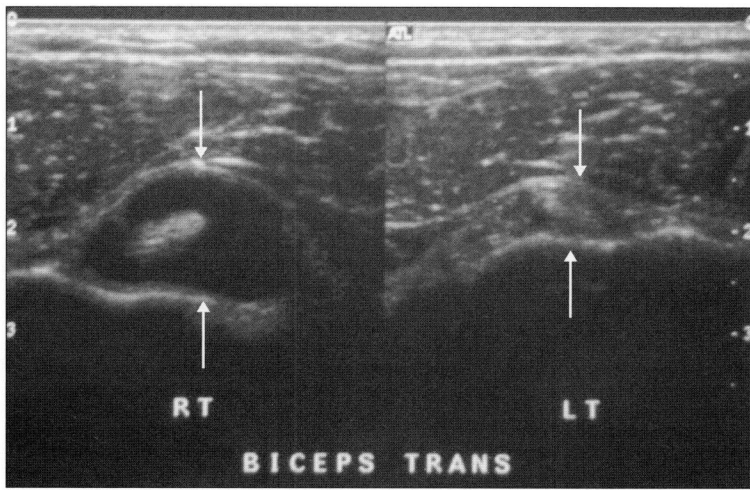

Fig. 70.13 Ultrasound image of bicipital tendinitis. Transverse image shows large effusion in the long head of biceps tendon sheath.

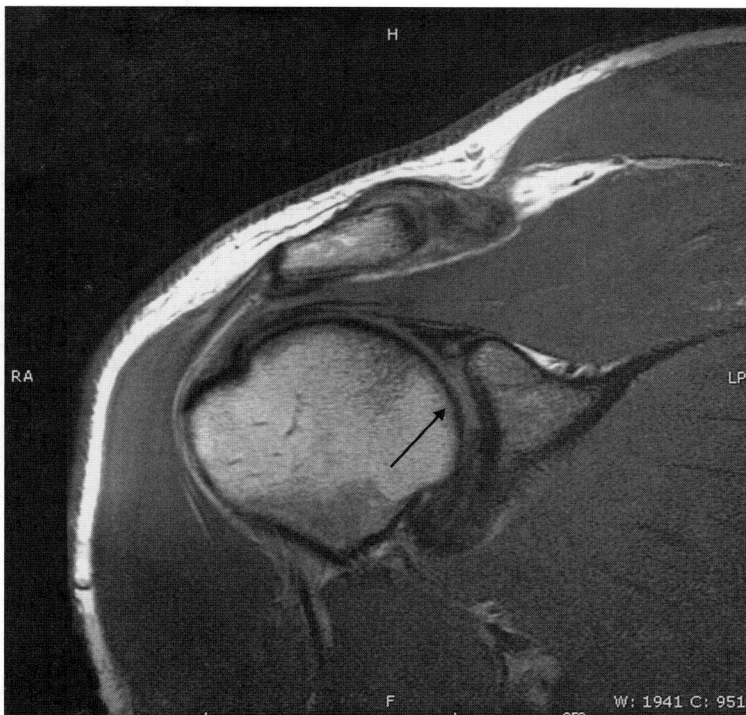

Fig. 70.14 SLAP type 2: Non-arthrographic coronal proton density MR image demonstrating tear (arrow) at the base of the superior labrum, involving the biceps anchor.

Pain is usually felt over the anterior aspect of the shoulder, often radiating into the biceps muscle, with tenderness over the tendon as it runs in the bicipital groove. Pain is felt with overhead activities and often with shoulder extension and elbow flexion. Examination may reveal features of impingement, rotator cuff tendinitis, and instability, all of which are important in the etiology of bicipital tendinitis. Pain may be reproduced with resisted elbow flexion, supination, and shoulder flexion; and various provocation tests are described, although none appears to be consistently positive. Passive shoulder extension stretches the biceps and may be painful. Rupture of the tendon is characterized by deformity of the upper arm with bunching up of the lateral muscle belly of the biceps, best seen with resisted elbow flexion and supination.

Acute rupture of the transverse humeral ligament can result in subluxation or dislocation of the tendon. This can present as symptoms similar to bicipital tendinitis, but often a more specific complaint is made of "catching" and a clicking sensation at the shoulder. Clinical examination may demonstrate subluxation of the tendon, which is felt as the arm is passively moved through internal and external rotation while in the 90-degree abducted position. Medial dislocation of the tendon is usually associated with tears of the subscapularis tendon.

Investigations

Special radiographic views demonstrate the bicipital groove, allowing assessment of its depth and the presence of any hypertrophic spurring. Filling of the synovial extension around the tendon is seen on arthrography and may be reduced in cases of chronic fibrosis. The tendon and any surrounding fluid can be seen well with ultrasonography (Fig. 70.13), and this assists in the diagnosis of tears, both partial and complete, as well as tendinitis. It can also be used to demonstrate subluxation/dislocation of the tendon. MRI or arthroscopy allows visualization of the intra-articular portion of the tendon and its labral attachment (Fig. 70.14).

Management

It is necessary to establish whether the tendinitis is primary or secondary, because a failure to address any underlying rotator cuff pathology or instability will lead to a recurrence of symptoms. The principles of management are rest, physical modalities, and use of NSAIDs as required. Low-power laser therapy has been reported to have a beneficial effect, although this has been disputed.[48] Corticosteroid injection is helpful in chronic cases, but care should be taken not to inject the tendon itself. An intra-articular injection or injection to the bicipital groove may be given, but both are best done under ultrasound guidance. Because most cases of bicipital tendinitis are secondary, they usually settle as the primary condition is treated. The primary cases due to lifting or other activities respond to rest and simple anti-inflammatory measures. Surgery can be considered in chronic resistant cases; this may involve subacromial decompression in cases of impingement or

tenodesis when there is chronic thickening of the tendon in the groove. Rupture of the tendon is normally treated conservatively except in the occasional young patient in whom upper arm strength is critical to a sport or profession. Usually, weakness after this injury is not significant. Subluxation of the tendon is usually treated conservatively, although occasionally surgery is necessary and medial subluxation/dislocation of the tendon out of the groove usually indicates the presence of a tear in the subscapularis tendon, which may not be apparent with ultrasonography.

Any conservative program must include range of motion exercises, stretches, and, once symptoms have settled, a graduated eccentric and concentric biceps and rotator cuff strengthening program.

Subacromial bursitis

The close relationship between the subacromial bursa and the rotator cuff, specifically the supraspinatus tendon, is such that the term *subacromial bursitis* is frequently used when describing the pathology of impingement. In most cases, inflammation of the bursa arises as part of the impingement process and coexists with an underlying rotator cuff tendinitis. This bursitis is therefore a reactive phenomenon. In chronic cases the bursa becomes thickened and fibrotic and surgical excision or débridement may be necessary. Treatment of rotator cuff tendinitis is directed at reducing the inflammation in the subacromial space or bursa as well as reducing the impingement.

Acute traumatic bursitis in the form of hemorrhage and edema can occur as a result of a fall or a direct blow to the point of the shoulder. Pain on abduction is present, but differentiation from rotator cuff tendinitis is possible on the basis of increased tenderness and fluid at the subacromial space. A period of rest combined with simple measures, such as ice, usually allows resumption of normal activities, but occasionally persistent impingement develops, requiring further treatment.

Capsulitis

Capsulitis of the shoulder remains a condition both difficult to define and universally awkward to manage. Many labels have been given to the situation in which there is a painful restriction of shoulder movement apparently of soft tissue origin. These include frozen shoulder, periarthritis or pericapsulitis of the shoulder, adhesive capsulitis, and adherent or obliterative bursitis. There has been an attempt to classify patients with a painful stiff shoulder according to the presence or absence of capsular joint restriction as seen at arthrography.[49] Perhaps incorrectly, the term *frozen shoulder* is applied to many conditions in which restriction of movement is largely due to pain from an underlying condition, such as rotator cuff tendinitis, rather than to the classic global restriction of glenohumeral joint motion seen with a true adhesive capsulitis.

Primary capsulitis of the shoulder can be defined as a condition of unknown etiology in which there is a painful restriction of glenohumeral movement in all planes of motion, both active and passive, in the absence of joint degeneration sufficient to explain this restriction. A similar condition, known as *secondary capsulitis*, exists when the condition is associated with a clearly defined clinical disorder or precipitating event.

Pathology

The etiology of adhesive capsulitis is not known. There is some evidence for its association with a number of conditions, including diabetes mellitus, thyroid disease, hyperlipidemia, pulmonary disorders such as tuberculosis or carcinoma, and cardiac disease or surgery, cerebrovascular accident, and, particularly, shoulder trauma. The evidence for such associations, however, is generally unconvincing. Dupuytren's disease is often seen in association with adhesive capsulitis, and it has been suggested that the two conditions may have similar biochemical and histologic characteristics.[50] After traction or hyperabduction injuries to the shoulder, a mixed clinical picture of capsulitis and cervicobrachialgia may develop, further complicating diagnosis and treatment.

Capsulitis is more prevalent in diabetics (prevalence, 10%-20%), usually occurring at a younger age and often associated with prolonged duration of the diabetes, insulin dependence, the development of limited joint mobility syndrome, and widespread microvascular disease. Bilateral involvement is also more common in diabetes. The links between diabetes and capsulitis may revolve around microvascular disease, abnormalities of collagen repair, or predisposition to infection.[51] An association between capsulitis and thyroid disease and pulmonary conditions has been noted but provides little information regarding its pathogenesis. Histologic studies have failed to demonstrate the presence of inflammatory cell infiltrates, granulomas, or vasculitis in the joint capsule or synovium. Also, there is nothing to implicate infection, crystal arthropathy, or trauma.

Histologic studies of the joint capsule early in the disease are difficult to perform, and the heterogeneity of patients loosely labeled as having capsulitis makes study of this condition problematic. Lundberg noted an increase in fibrous tissue, fibroblast numbers, and vascularity with no change in the synovial lining and no inflammatory cell infiltrate.[52] Bunker and Anthony have reported that fibroblasts and myofibroblasts lay down a dense type III collagen matrix in the shoulder joint capsule, leading to joint contracture.[53] Cytokine, matrix metalloproteinase (MMP), and MMP inhibitor abnormalities have been reported, and it has been proposed that increased production of growth factors is the central precursor to capsular fibrosis.[54] Several studies have looked at a variety of immunologic factors, and no immunologic disturbance has been demonstrated.[55]

Clinical presentation

Estimation of the prevalence of adhesive capsulitis is difficult owing to variation in populations studied and diagnostic criteria used, but it appears to be 2% to 3% in non-diabetics. Onset when younger than the age of 40 years is rare, with the mean age at onset being in the sixth decade. Women are affected more often than men. Involvement of the contralateral shoulder occurs in 6% to 17% of patients over the subsequent 5 years.[56] It is commonly stated that recurrence in the same shoulder does not occur. There is a frequent history of minor shoulder strain or injury before the onset of symptoms, but whether this represents a true strain of the shoulder or simply the earliest awareness of pain is unclear.

The natural history of this condition has been assessed, and it appears that there are three phases in its development and progression.

The shoulder moves from being simply painful to being painful and stiff and eventually to being less painful but profoundly stiff. This last stage appears to be self-limiting, and recovery is gradual and spontaneous. These phases have been termed painful, adhesive, and resolution. The duration of each stage in the overall condition varies considerably, but approximate durations are 3 to 8 months for the painful phase, 4 to 6 months for the adhesive phase, and 1 to 3 years for the resolution phase. The extent of recovery is variable, with quoted figures of 33% to 61% of patients having a clinically detectable limitation of shoulder movement; and, although many remain asymptomatic, 7% to 15% of patients may have a persisting functional disability.[51,57] The extent to which the duration of the painful and adhesive phases determines the degree of residual disability remains controversial. It does appear that capsulitis in a diabetic patient runs a more protracted course with marked stiffness and less complete recovery.

Painful phase

The painful phase is characterized by the insidious onset of symptoms, usually in the form of pain on shoulder movement and background ache in the shoulder region, often in the upper trapezius muscle. As the condition becomes established there is the development of increasing pain at rest and at night, the latter becoming quite disturbing and frequently waking the patient in the absence of a history of precipitative movement. Muscle spasm may develop, further limiting shoulder movement, which becomes restricted with the increase in pain and stiffness at the shoulder. Toward the end of this phase stiffness becomes a major complaint.

Adhesive phase

Usually after several months the character of pain alters and becomes less severe. There is a reduction in pain at rest and at night, but discomfort and a more severe pain at the limits of movement persist. Shoulder movement becomes more restricted during this phase, and this can lead to periscapular pain owing to the increase in scapulothoracic motion.

Resolution phase

The pain is less evident, and the dominant symptom is restriction of shoulder movement, which often appears less distressing for the patient now that the pain has eased. There is a slow and gradual improvement in range of motion, although this is frequently incomplete. The onset and rate of recovery are variable and unpredictable.

Clinical examination

The physical signs alter to a degree as the condition progresses, with pain, often severe, present in the earlier stages. Differentiation from rotator cuff tendinitis is possible on the basis of a global restriction of passive movement rather than simply the loss of abduction and flexion that is seen with chronic rotator cuff conditions. A useful early clinical indicator of developing capsulitis is pain at the limit of passive external rotation of the shoulder with the arm by the side. In the painful phase there is painful restriction of active and passive motion (often mild in the earlier stages). There may be pain on impingement testing and resisted movement, although this is less common than in rotator cuff tendinitis. Associated findings are tenderness in the upper trapezius muscle and early scapular hitching in elevation. In some patients pain can be severe, necessitating opioid analgesia, and the clinician may feel the need to exclude other causes such as avascular necrosis or neoplastic disease. In the latter phases the important finding is significant restriction of glenohumeral movement with a compensatory increase in scapulothoracic motion during flexion and abduction. Pain may be present, but there is less discrepancy between active and passive ranges. Disuse atrophy of the rotator cuff and deltoid muscles may exist. Joint line tenderness may be present in the painful phase.

Investigations

Diagnosis is made largely on clinical grounds because there are few abnormalities found on investigation. Plain radiographs are not helpful in making the diagnosis except to exclude widespread osteoarthritic changes, calcific tendinitis, or neoplasm. In the younger patient presenting with clinical features of adhesive capsulitis, avascular necrosis should be suspected and must be excluded before considering intra-articular corticosteroid injection.

Classic features at arthrography are limitation of joint volume with a loss of the normal dependent axillary fold or pouch and irregularity of the capsular insertion to the anatomic neck of the humerus. Between 10% and 30% of patients who undergo arthrography have a demonstrable complete tear of the rotator cuff.[51,52] Other studies have suggested that a significant number of patients with a clinical diagnosis of adhesive capsulitis have normal findings at arthrography.[58] Arthroscopy allows further evaluation of these patients, and different stages of synovitis and contracture have been described.[49]

Bone scintigraphy may demonstrate increased isotope uptake in the affected shoulder region, but this appears to have no predictive value in terms of outcome or response to treatment and is therefore of limited diagnostic value.[58] An average reduction in bone mineral content of 50% in the affected humeral head has been demonstrated, although again this is of little diagnostic or therapeutic value. Ultrasonography has been used, and typical findings are a biceps sheath effusion, restriction of movement, and subacromial impingement resulting from the capsular contracture; but these features are not diagnostic, and patients are often mistakenly treated for impingement tendinitis. Indeed, a failure to respond to treatment and the early loss of joint motion should alert the clinician to the possibility of a developing capsulitis.

Management

Many therapies have been tried in an attempt to modify the natural history of capsulitis, and clinical studies of the efficacy of various treatment methods have been compromised by difficulties with patient selection, diagnostic criteria, and the variability in the natural resolution of the condition. The emphasis of treatment in the early stages should be on pain reduction and minimization of joint restriction. Analgesics and anti-inflammatory drugs provide limited relief of pain but do little to alter the course of the disorder. Physiotherapy utilizes physical modalities to modify pain and reduce protective muscle spasm while attempting to encourage range of motion exercises early on to maintain joint mobility. Shoulder immobilization should be discouraged if at all possible, although in the painful phase the patient tends to minimize shoulder movement.

Few treatments have been shown to consistently affect rate of recovery or limit restriction of movement. Intra-articular corticosteroid injections are commonly used and have been shown to reduce pain and disability for 3 months or more, although no long-term benefit has been demonstrated.[59] The addition of supervised physiotherapy appears to provide faster improvement in range of joint motion. Intra-articular injection is best done under ultrasound guidance or fluoroscopy, and failure to do so in previous studies may account for the variable response to corticosteroid injection in the past. It still remains a useful and often effective means of relieving pain and hastening recovery. Oral corticosteroids have also been shown to improve pain but not to affect the rate of recovery.[60] Careful utilization of analgesic or anti-inflammatory drugs with physiotherapy may be of benefit, although this may be due to a reduction in the protective spasm seen in the untreated patient.

Hydrodistention of the joint capsule has been used as a treatment in various stages of this condition, usually in conjunction with corticosteroid injection, but it is still unclear whether it offers any additional benefit to corticosteroid injection alone. Manipulation under anesthetic has been used to restore joint motion but may involve rupture of the inferior capsule and possibly the subscapularis tendon at its insertion. Care should be taken when carrying out this procedure, especially in the elderly patient, to avoid humeral fracture, shoulder dislocation, or a significant rotator cuff rupture. Aggressive early rehabilitation in the immediate post-manipulation period is needed to maintain joint mobility, and patient cooperation and tolerance of this treatment are essential. Manipulation during the painful phase is not recommended because painful re-contraction of the capsule may occur; and this treatment method is usually reserved for the adhesive phase once the pain has eased.

Non-operative treatment is effective in the vast majority of cases, but arthroscopic capsulotomy can be used to treat recalcitrant cases of frozen shoulder.[61,62] Some authors do not restrict the use of this treatment to those patients who no longer have significant pain and advocate arthroscopic capsular release rather than manipulation, given that it allows direct visualization of the joint capsule and therefore less risk of tendon rupture. For many patients, however, once the painful phase of their condition has subsided, the prospect of this painful procedure is not appealing. Improvement in range of movement after manipulation or capsulotomy is variable and is perhaps dependent on patient selection. Long-term recovery appears unchanged, although resolution may be accelerated immediately after manipulation.

ACROMIOCLAVICULAR SYNDROMES

Pain localized to the acromioclavicular joint is commonly seen as either an acute or a chronic condition. In the younger patient this joint is frequently subjected to trauma as a result of falls or contact sports, which may result in an acute injury and also predispose the joint to further problems, such as instability or secondary osteoarthritis. Non-traumatic acromioclavicular joint pain is common and may be difficult to distinguish from other causes of shoulder pain. Infection of this joint is rare, but septic arthritis has been described.[63]

Trauma

Disruption of the acromioclavicular joint may be seen in association with fractures of the outer end of the clavicle and often leads to the development of secondary osteoarthritis. More common are injuries to the joint itself, which are graded according to the degree of disruption of the joint capsule and supporting ligaments.[64] Grade I injury involves minor sprain to the joint capsule without ligament disruption. Grade II injury involves subluxation of the joint with downward displacement of the acromion relative to the distal end of the clavicle. There is stretching of the inferior acromioclavicular ligaments and stretching and possibly a partial tear, but not complete rupture, of the coracoclavicular ligaments. In a grade III injury, complete dislocation of the joint occurs through rupture of the coracoclavicular ligaments. Grade III injuries can be further classified (often as grades IV, V, and VI) according to the extent (and direction) of disruption or perforation of the overlying deltotrapezius fascial or muscle layer by the displaced outer end of the clavicle.

Clinical features

The mechanism of injury usually involves a fall directly onto the point of the shoulder. Pain is localized to the top of the shoulder in the region of the involved joint, which is tender and often swollen to palpation. Abduction is often limited, both actively and passively, according to the degree of joint disruption. With a minor injury in which there is good preservation of movement, acromioclavicular joint stress tests can be carried out to localize symptoms. In complete dislocation of the joint a visible step deformity is seen and examination will determine whether this dislocation can be reduced. This is important in the differentiation of grade III to VI injuries. The patient often describes a feeling of the shoulder having dropped, owing to the downward displacement of the acromion.

Management

For the grade I or II injury, treatment is largely symptomatic, with analgesics and provision of a sling for days to weeks depending on the symptoms. Shoulder movements should be encouraged as pain settles and functional recovery is excellent.

Controversy exists over the management of grade III injuries. Provided perforation of the overlying muscle or fascial layer has not occurred, most patients settle with conservative treatment over a period of 6 to 10 weeks. Strapping of the joint has no effect on long-term stability and is not indicated in these patients. Surgical stabilization by means of internal fixation is associated with significant complication and failure rates, but several procedures involving reconstruction of the coracoclavicular ligaments have been shown to be effective, although long-term results are not demonstrably better than for non-operative treatment. Surgical advances have lowered the complication rate and thus the threshold for considering surgical repair or reconstruction of the acromioclavicular joint, particularly in manual

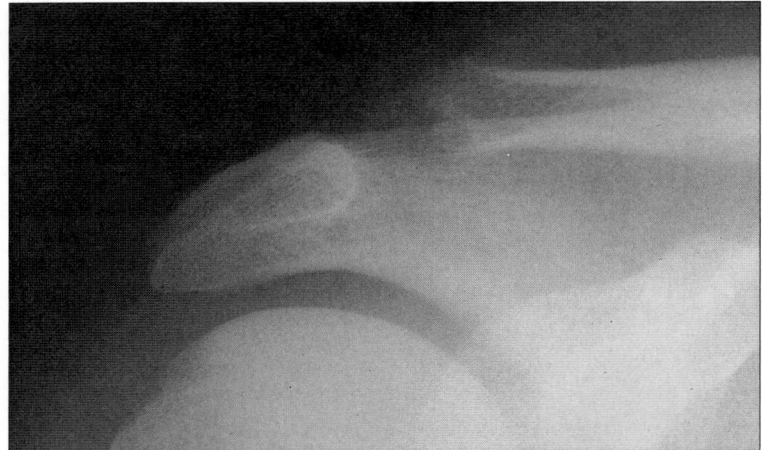

Fig. 70.15 Radiographic changes of osteolysis of the clavicle.

workers or people dependent on overhead function. However, surgery is usually reserved for severe grade III disruptions or when an individual's occupation may be compromised by persistent deformity or instability at that joint.

Late sequelae

Patients may present with persistent pain at the acromioclavicular joint. This represents low-grade joint inflammation and may be associated with an underlying instability, early development of secondary osteoarthritis, or osteolysis of the distal end of the clavicle. Persistent pain after joint injury may also result from damage to the intra-articular fibrocartilage sustained at the time of injury. Treatment is symptomatic, with anti-inflammatory medication or injection of intra-articular corticosteroid for resistant cases. Delayed surgical stabilization may be carried out in cases of gross instability, and tears of the fibrocartilage can be débrided arthroscopically. Long-term treatment is as for osteoarthritis of the joint.

Osteolysis of the clavicle

Osteolysis of the distal clavicle is a condition that may follow an acute injury or repetitive stress to the shoulder.[65]

Symptoms are usually similar to those of acromioclavicular inflammation, with aching and pain at the limits of flexion and abduction. Radiographic changes typically show resorption of the distal clavicle, often with osteophyte formation, osteoporosis, or tapering (Fig. 70.15). Response to activity modification and conservative treatment is usually satisfactory, but excision of the distal clavicle may be necessary. There may even be reconstitution of the distal clavicle with rest.

Osteoarthritis

Acromioclavicular joint morphology appears to be associated with the development of osteoarthritis, although cadaveric studies have shown that degenerative changes occur in this joint with normal aging after age 40 years.[66] A previous history of joint injury is common when osteoarthritis of this joint occurs in isolation, but the joint may also be involved as part of generalized osteoarthritis. Acromioclavicular osteoarthrosis is common and frequently asymptomatic.

Clinical features

Pain and tenderness are localized to the joint, which is often prominent because of osteophyte formation. Pain exists on full abduction or horizontal adduction and can also be reproduced with adduction of the extended arm. Crepitus is frequently localized to the joint. It is important to note that osteoarthritis of the joint is often seen in association with rotator cuff degeneration and that inferior osteophytes at the acromioclavicular joint may contribute to the development of a rotator cuff tear. Clinical features of both conditions frequently coexist, especially in the older patient.

Investigations

Osteoarthritis can be diagnosed on plain radiography. Traction or weight-bearing views can be taken to demonstrate joint instability.

Management

Initial management consists of local modalities and the use of analgesic or anti-inflammatory drugs. A suitable exercise program should be provided to restore normal scapulohumeral rhythm, glenohumeral range of motion, and deltoid and rotator cuff strength once symptoms have settled. Intra-articular corticosteroid injection usually provides good symptom relief but often needs to be repeated. Cases resistant to conservative treatment may require surgery, which usually consists of excision arthroplasty of the joint while ensuring that instability is minimized. Careful assessment of rotator cuff function is important and, in the presence of a significant tear, rotator cuff repair or an acromioplasty may be indicated. Excision arthroplasty may also be indicated in the younger patient with chronic symptoms, whether due to degenerative change, osteolysis, or instability.

CALCIFIC TENDINITIS

The prevalence of radiologically detectable calcification in the rotator cuff tendons is reported to be 2.7% to 7.5%, occurring in both symptomatic and asymptomatic shoulders.[67,68] It often involves the supraspinatus tendon and has been reported as being more common in women and sedentary individuals. Bosworth[69] estimated that 35% to 45% of individuals with calcification seen on radiography developed symptoms. Frequently bilateral, it usually occurs between the ages of 40 and 60 years but can present as an acute condition in the younger patient. Patients may present with chronic symptoms of "catching" pain with movement due to impingement.

Acute calcific tendinitis has a quite different presentation, with acute severe pain limiting passive or active shoulder movement almost completely and with exquisite point tenderness and occasionally erythema over the involved tendon. The onset of symptoms can be rapid with no history of injury or overuse, and this occurs during the resorptive phase of calcification.

Patients can therefore be divided into two groups: (1) those patients with an acute onset of severe pain and limitation of movement, often in the absence of any previous shoulder symptoms, and (2) patients who have a more chronic catching pain associated with movement presenting as an impingement problem.

Pathophysiology

It has been argued by various authors that calcification occurs as part of a degenerative process involving the rotator cuff tendons, largely because it is rarely seen in people before the fourth decade. Also, complete cuff tears have been found in 21% of patients with calcific tendinitis.[70] Histologic studies have confirmed that calcification follows as a result of tendon fibrosis and subsequent necrosis.

Uhthoff and colleagues[68] have proposed a model for the pathogenesis of calcific tendinitis based on its clinical presentation as a self-healing condition in which the calcific process is actively mediated by cells in a viable environment. They classify the disease in three stages: precalcific, calcific, and postcalcific. In the precalcific stage it is thought that there is fibrocartilaginous transformation in the avascular or "critical" zone of the supraspinatus tendon. In the calcific stage, calcium crystals are deposited in matrix vehicles to form large deposits (known as the formative phase). After a variable period of inactivity (resting period) there is spontaneous resorption of the calcium by means of peripheral vascularization and phagocytosis of the deposit (resorptive phase). After removal of the calcium the space is filled with granulation tissue (postcalcific stage). Occasionally, a deposit can rupture into the overlying subacromial bursa. There has been a reported association between this condition and HLA-A1.[68]

Investigations

A plain radiograph will identify and localize the calcific deposit to a particular tendon, usually the supraspinatus. In the formative phase of

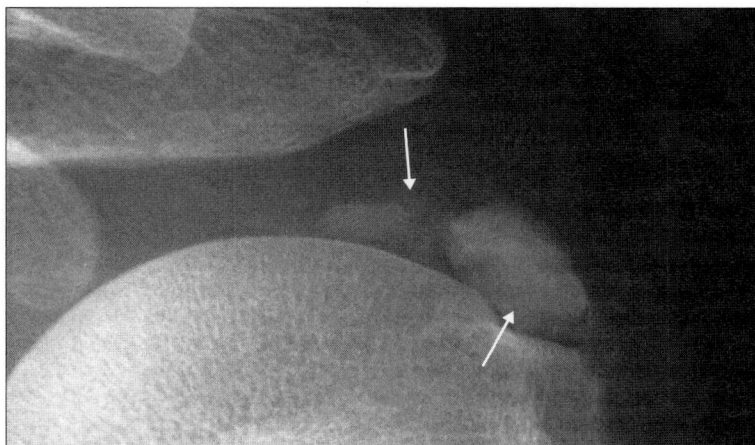

Fig. 70.16 Calcific tendinitis: formative phase (large arrow) and resorptive phase (small arrow).

calcification the deposit is well defined and homogeneously dense. In the resorptive phase, usually presenting as the acute condition, the deposit is less well defined, is irregular, and has a fluffy, less dense appearance (Fig. 70.16). In patients in whom the deposit is in contact with bone there is cortical erosion, and some authors consider that there is a subset of patients with osteolytic lesions of the tuberosities in whom the disease runs a more protracted course.[71] Degenerative rotator cuff disease and arthropathy may have radiologically detectable calcification, but this is usually associated with other features of these conditions and the areas of calcification are usually small, stippled, and close to the tendon insertion at the greater tuberosity.

Laboratory investigation usually does not reveal any abnormality of calcium or phosphate metabolism. There is no associated leukocytosis, raised erythrocyte sedimentation rate, or change in serum alkaline phosphatase activity.

Management

Asymptomatic patients require no specific treatment. In patients with chronic symptoms, conservative management should consist of mobility and strengthening exercises about the glenohumeral joint, physical modalities, and NSAIDs for symptom relief if required. An injection of a corticosteroid should only be given if there are clear-cut features of impingement and subacromial inflammation and should only be repeated with caution. Extracorporeal shock wave therapy has been reported as being effective in selected patients. In the acute stages treatment should include resting the arm in a sling, analgesics, anti-inflammatory medication, and local application of ice. Injection of a corticosteroid should be avoided because this may inhibit the resorption of calcium; however, needling and aspiration of the deposit under ultrasound control may result in a subsequent reduction in pain. Injection of subacromial lidocaine should also be given for temporary relief of pain. Some authors, however, advocate corticosteroid injection in the acute phase.

Surgical intervention is indicated when conservative management of the chronic condition has failed and there are persistent features of impingement. The deposit can be removed arthroscopically or at an open procedure and may be followed by resection of the coracoacromial ligament and anterior acromioplasty, although there is some evidence that these additional procedures are unnecessary and in some cases associated with a poorer outcome.

SCAPULOTHORACIC BURSITIS

Scapulothoracic crepitus should by no means always be considered a pathologic symptom because it is frequently found in the normal population. Rarely, it may represent changes in the bony structure of the deep surface of the scapula or underlying ribs, such as an osteochondroma of the scapula or a rib exostosis. These lesions tend to give rise to a more pronounced snapping sound and may result in deviation of the scapula away from the chest wall. Soft tissue causes are more common, and frequently a diagnosis of scapulothoracic bursitis is made, although the exact pathologic process, if present, is difficult to define. Crepitus is frequently found in association with muscular complaints and probably represents a frictional sound as the scapula glides across the underlying muscle layers. Treatment is probably best directed at relief of symptoms and postural exercises, although subscapular injections have been given with variable results and at considerable risk of pneumothorax. Arthroscopic débridement has also been described and usually involves bursectomy with or without resection of the superomedial border of the scapula.

GLENOHUMERAL INSTABILITY AND INTERNAL IMPINGEMENT

Glenohumeral instability is a major cause of symptoms and pathology around the shoulder joint. The more traditional orthopedic model of shoulder dislocation, whether acute or recurrent, has been expanded to encompass the more subtle but equally important subluxations and occult instabilities that can play an important role in the development of shoulder pain, especially in a young active population. Glenohumeral instability can be classified according to the etiology, direction, type, and circumstance of the instability, although in reality this represents a spectrum of disorders ranging from traumatic unidirectional dislocation with a Bankart lesion to the atraumatic multidirectional instability resulting from bilateral glenohumeral laxity.[72] Symptomatic subluxation or instability often presents as a painful shoulder with all the signs and features of a rotator cuff or bicipital tendinitis, but a careful history and examination coupled with a high index of suspicion in the young adult should confirm the presence of instability. Patients with glenohumeral instability may also present with symptoms of a labral tear, such as painful clicking and catching. A ganglion cyst arising from the posterior glenoid labrum in patients with an underlying posterior instability may lead to compression of the suprascapular nerve at the spinoglenoid notch, causing such patients to occasionally present with significant weakness of external rotation (Fig. 70.17).

In the throwing athlete there are adaptive changes, with stretching of the anterior capsule and contraction of the posterior capsule giving an increased range of external rotation and reduced internal rotation that allows higher throwing velocities. There is also some evidence of adaptive change in the humerus and glenoid (increased retroversion).[73] As a result of such changes or in those athletes with occult instability where there is increased glenohumeral rotation, angulation, and anterior translation of the humeral head, the undersurface of the posterosuperior aspect of the rotator cuff impinges against the posterosuperior glenoid rim. This is known as "internal impingement."[74] A number of potential pathologic sites of pain exist, namely, the rotator cuff, capsule, labrum, glenoid, or greater tuberosity; and differentiation between internal impingement and symptoms of instability can be difficult.[75,76] It is, however, important to distinguish between internal as opposed to external (subacromial) impingement because the etiology, treatment, and rehabilitation differ considerably in the two conditions.

Management of tendinitis in the young patient with instability should be directed at the resolution of symptoms, restoration of normal flexibility and scapular control, and correction of faulty technique in athletes and then a suitable strengthening program for the dynamic stabilizers of the shoulder joint, notably, the rotator cuff muscles. Also, correction of any muscle imbalance about the shoulder girdle is important (i.e., weakness of serratus anterior). Arthroscopy allows closer evaluation of shoulder pathology and has an important role in the treatment of symptomatic instability, even to the extent of performing stabilization procedures to the biceps anchor or glenoid labrum as well as formal reconstruction.

PRINCIPLES OF REHABILITATION

Effective rehabilitation of shoulder disorders requires a good understanding of the functional anatomy and biomechanical properties of the shoulder girdle. Pathologic processes cannot be treated in isolation

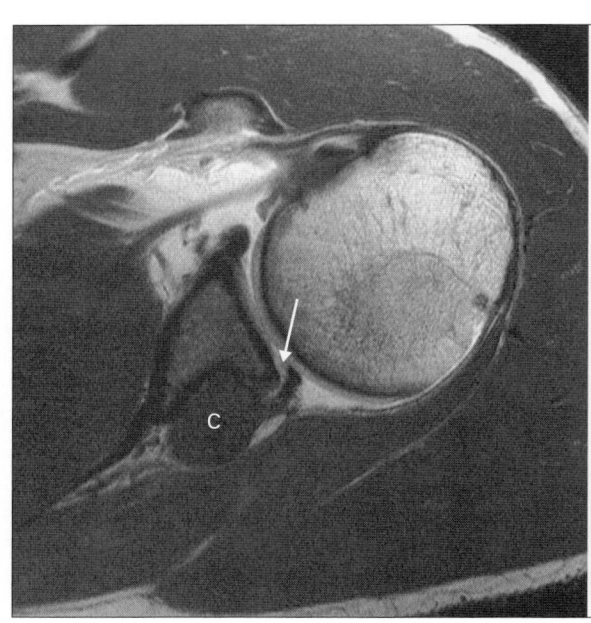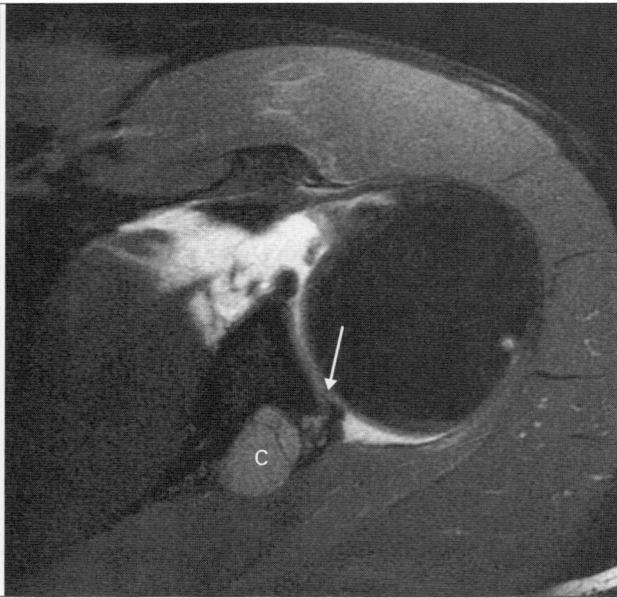

Fig. 70.17 MRI showing a ganglion cyst (arrow) arising from a tear in the posterior glenoid labrum.

because of the complex relationship between the cervicothoracic spine, thoracic cage, scapula, and glenohumeral joint. The clinician and physical therapist need to understand this relationship to design an exercise program to restore normal shoulder kinematics. A simple range of motion and strengthening exercise program will not suffice, especially in those conditions in which there has been a disturbance of scapulothoracic and scapulohumeral rhythm. In a significant number of patients with shoulder pain it is this scapular dysfunction that has precipitated or aggravated the underlying pathologic process.

KEY REFERENCES

1. Turkel SJ, Panio MW, Marshall JL, Girgis FG. Stabilizing mechanisms preventing anterior dislocation of the glenohumeral joint. J Bone Joint Surg Am 1981;63:1208-1217.
2. Wang VM, Flatow EL. Pathomechanics of acquired shoulder instability: a basic science perspective. J Shoulder Elbow Surg 2005;14S:2-11.
3. Kuhn JE, Huston LJ, Soslowsky LJ, et al. External rotation of the glenohumeral joint: ligament restraints and muscle effects in the neutral and abducted position. J Shoulder Elbow Surg 2005;14S:39-48.
5. Williams MM, Snyder SJ, Buford D Jr. The Buford complex, the cord-like middle glenohumeral ligament and absent anterosuperior labrum complex: a normal anatomical capsulolabral variant. Arthroscopy 1994;10:2417.
6. Kesmezacaar H, Akgun I, Ogut T, et al. The coracoacromial ligament: The morphology and relation to rotator cuff pathology. J Shoulder Elbow Surg 2008;17:182-188.
9. Alpert SW, Pink MM, Jobe FW, et al. Electromyographic analysis of deltoid and rotator cuff function under varying loads and speeds. J Shoulder Elbow Surg 2000;9:47-58.
13. Levy AS, Kelly BT, Lintner SA, et al. Function of the long head of the biceps at the shoulder: electromyographic analysis. J Shoulder Elbow Surg 2001;10:250-255.
14. Labriola JE, Lee TQ, Debski RE, McMahon PJ. Stability and instability of the glenohumeral joint: the role of shoulder muscles. J Shoulder Elbow Surg 2005;14S:32-38.
15. Inman VT, Saunders JB de CM, Abbott LC. Observations on the function of the shoulder joint. J Bone Joint Surg 1944;26:1-30.
16. Itoi E, Minagawa H, Sato T, et al. Isokinetic strength after tears of the supraspinatus tendon. J Bone Joint Surg Br 1997;79:77-82.
17. Dalton SE. Clinical examination of the painful shoulder. In: Hazleman BL, Dieppe PA, eds. The shoulder joint. Baillière's Clinical Rheumatology. London: Baillière Tindall, 1989:453-474.
20. Rathbun JB, MacNab I. The microvascular pattern of the rotator cuff. J Bone Joint Surg Br 1970;52:540-553.
21. Iannotti JP, Swiontkowski M, Esterhafi J, Boulas HJ. Intraoperative assessment of rotator cuff vascularity

using laser Doppler flowmetry. Abstract presented to AAOS Meeting, Las Vegas, NV, 1989.
23. Sano H, Ishii H, Trudel G, Uhthoff HK. Histologic evidence of degeneration at the insertion of 3 rotator cuff tendons: a comparative study with human cadaveric shoulders. J Shoulder Elbow Surg 1999;8:574-579.
24. Tempelhof S, Rupp S, Seil R. Age-related prevalence of rotator cuff tears in asymptomatic shoulders. J Shoulder Elbow Surg 1999;8:296-299.
25. Riley GP, Harrall RL, Constant CR, et al. Tendon degeneration and chronic shoulder pain: changes in the collagen composition of the human rotator cuff tendons in rotator cuff tendinitis. Ann Rheum Dis 1994;53:359-366.
26. Riley GP, Harrall RL, Constant CR, et al. Glycosaminoglycans of human rotator cuff tendons: changes with age and in chronic rotator cuff tendinitis. Ann Rheum Dis 1994;53:367-376.
27. Dalton S, Cawston TE, Riley GP, et al. Human shoulder tendon biopsy samples in organ culture produce procollagenase and tissue inhibitor of metalloproteinases. Ann Rheum Dis 1995;54:571-577.
28. Gigante A, Marinelli M, Chillemi C, Greco F. Fibrous cartilage in the rotator cuff: a pathogenetic mechanism of tendon tear? J Shoulder Elbow Surg 2004;13:329-332.
30. Buchbinder R, Green S, Youd JM. Corticosteroid injections for shoulder pain (Cochrane Review). The Cochrane Library, Issue 3. Chichester: John Wiley, 2005.
31. Kuhn JE. Exercise in the treatment of rotator cuff impingement: A systematic review and a synthesized evidence-based rehabilitation protocol. J Shoulder Elbow Surg 2009;18:138-160.
34. Sher JS, Uribe JW, Posada A, et al. Abnormal findings on magnetic resonance images of asymptomatic shoulders. J Bone Joint Surg Am 1995;77:10-15.
35. Neer CS. Rotator cuff arthropathy. J Bone Joint Surg Am 1983;65:1232-1244.
36. Berbig R, Weishaupt D, Prim J, Shahin O. Primary anterior shoulder dislocation and rotator cuff tears. J Shoulder Elbow Surg 1999;8:220-225.
37. Hijioka A, Suzuki K, Nakamura T, Hojo T. Degenerative change and rotator cuff tears: an anatomical study in 160 shoulders of 80 cadavers. Arch Orthop Trauma Surg 1993;112:61-64.

38. Yamaguchi K, Sher JS, Andersen WK, et al. Glenohumeral motion in patients with rotator cuff tears: a comparison of asymptomatic and symptomatic shoulders. J Shoulder Elbow Surg 2000;9:6-11.
39. Duckworth DG, Smith KL, Campbell B, Matsen FA. Self-assessment questionnaires document substantial variability in the clinical expression of rotator cuff tears. J Shoulder Elbow Surg 1999;8:330-333.
40. MacDermid JC, Ramos J, Drosdowech D, et al. The impact of rotator cuff pathology on isometric and isokinetic strength, function and quality of life. J Shoulder Elbow Surg 2004;13:593-598.
45. Fuchs B, Weishaupt D, Zanetti M, et al. Fatty degeneration of the muscles of the rotator cuff: assessment by computed tomography versus magnetic resonance imaging. J Shoulder Elbow Surg 1999;8:599-605.
46. Snyder SJ, Karzel RP, Del Pizzo W. SLAP lesions of the shoulder. Arthroscopy 1990;6:274-279.
47. Pfahler M, Branner S, Refior HJ. The role of the bicipital groove in tendopathy of the long biceps tendon. J Shoulder Elbow Surg 1999;8:419-424.
48. Gam AN, Thorsen H, Lonnberg F. The effect of low-level laser therapy on musculoskeletal pain: a meta-analysis. Pain 1993;52:63-66.
50. Smith SP, Devaraj WS, Bunker TD. The association between frozen shoulder and Dupuytren's disease. J Shoulder Elbow Surg 2001;10:149-151.
51. Nash P, Hazleman BL. Frozen shoulder. In: Hazleman BL, Dieppe PA, eds. The shoulder joint. Baillière's Clinical Rheumatology. London: Baillière Tindall, 1989: 551-566.
52. Lundberg BJ. The frozen shoulder. Acta Orthop Scand 1969;119(Suppl):1-59.
53. Bunker TD, Anthony PP. The pathology of frozen shoulder. J Bone Joint Surg Br 1995;77:677-683.
54. Mullett H, Byrne D, Colville J. Adhesive capsulitis: human fibroblast response to shoulder joint aspirate from patients with stage II disease. J Shoulder Elbow Surg 2007;16:290-294.
59. Carette S, Moffet H, Tardiff J, et al. Intraarticular corticosteroids, supervised physiotherapy or a combination of the two in the treatment of adhesive capsulitis of the shoulder. Arthritis Rheum 2003;48:829-838.

61. Levine WN, Kashyap CP, Bak SF, et al. Nonoperative management of idiopathic adhesive capsulitis. J Shoulder Elbow Surg 2007:16:569-573.
62. Omari A, Bunker TD. Open surgical release for frozen shoulder: surgical findings and results of the release. J Shoulder Elbow Surg 2001;10:353-357.
64. Rockwood CA, Young DC. Disorders of the acromioclavicular joint. In: Rockwood CA, Matsen FA, eds. The shoulder, vol 2. Philadelphia: WB Saunders, 1990:413-476.
67. Bosworth BM. Calcium deposits in the shoulder and subacromial bursitis: a survey of 12,122 shoulders. JAMA 1941;116:2477-2482.
68. Uhthoff HK, Sarkar K. Calcifying tendinitis. In: Hazleman BL, Dieppe PA, eds. The shoulder joint. Baillière's Clinical Rheumatology. London: Baillière Tindall, 1989:567-581.
70. Hsu HC, Wu JJ, Jim YF, et al. Calcific tendinitis and rotator cuff tearing: a clinical and radiographic study. J Shoulder Elbow Surg 1994;3:159-164.
71. Porcellini G, Paladini P, Campi F, Pegreffi F. Osteolytic lesion of greater tuberosity in calcific tendinitis of the shoulder. J Shoulder Elbow Surg 2009;18:210-215.
72. Dalton SE, Snyder SJ. Glenohumeral instability. In: Hazleman BL, Dieppe PA, eds. The shoulder joint. Baillière's Clinical Rheumatology. London: Baillière Tindall, 1989:2477-2482.
73. Fitzpatrick MJ, Tibone JE, Grossman M, et al. Development of cadaveric models of a thrower's shoulder. J Shoulder Elbow Surg 2005;14S:49-57.
74. Davidson PA, Elattrache NS, Jobe CM, Jobe FW. Rotator cuff and posterior-superior glenoid labrum injury associated with increased glenohumeral motion: a new site of impingement. J Shoulder Elbow Surg 1995;4:384-390.
75. McFarland EG, Hsu C-Y, Neira C, O'Neil O. Internal impingement of the shoulder: a clinical and arthroscopic analysis. J Shoulder Elbow Surg 1999;8:458-460.
76. Edelson G, Teitz C. Internal impingement in the shoulder. J Shoulder Elbow Surg 2000;9:308-315.

REFERENCES

Full references for this chapter can be found on www.expertconsult.com.

The elbow

Michael Denis Chard

- The elbow is a complex hinge joint essential for the positioning and full use of the hand.
- Relevant anatomy includes the radiohumeral and ulnohumeral hinge, the connecting proximal radioulnar joint, the radial head, the medial and lateral epicondyles, the ulnar nerve groove, the muscles spanning the elbow, and the olecranon bursa.
- Soft tissue lesions such as lateral epicondylitis and olecranon bursitis are far more frequent than many common joint diseases.
- Diagnosis of elbow conditions is largely based on pain characteristics, location of swelling, presence of point tenderness, and the results of passive, active and resisted motion.

FUNCTIONAL ANATOMY

Bony components

The elbow is considered to be a hinge joint but is more accurately classified as a trochoginglymus joint because it is a hinged joint about a trochlea or pulley. This allows for the motions of pronation and supination of the forearm. The combination of flexion and rotation at the elbow enables the hands to be brought into view and provides a steady but adjustable base for the hands to make best use of the highly mobile fingers and opposable thumb. It is a compound synovial joint because it is composed of articulation between the ulnar notch and trochlea of the humerus and between the radial head and humeral capitellum (Fig. 71.1). In continuity with these is the proximal radioulnar joint.[1]

Humerus

At its distal end the humerus is expanded to form a modified condyle, widest transversely, and consists of articular and non-articular parts. The capitellum on the lateral aspect is curved, forms less than half a sphere, and contributes anterior and inferior surfaces. A shallow groove separates the capitellum from the medial trochlea, which has anterior, inferior, and posterior surfaces. The medial flange is larger, and so the medial margin projects inferiorly, which results in the plane of the joint being tilted inferomedially. This is the main determinant of the angulation between the long axis of the radius and ulna in an extended supinated position. Medial and lateral bony projections of the lower humerus form the epicondyles, which, along with olecranon and coronoid and radial fossae, make up the non-articular part of the condyle. The fossae accept the relevant parts of the ulna and radius during extremes of extension and flexion movements. Above the larger medial and less prominent lateral epicondyle formed by the flaring of the distal humerus are the supracondylar ridges. The medial epicondyle provides a groove for the ulnar nerve as it crosses the elbow to enter the forearm.

Radius

At its proximal end the radius has a head, neck, and tuberosity. The head is discoid, with a proximal shallow cup for the humeral capitellum and an articular periphery that is deepest medially where it contacts the ulnar radial notch. Distal to this is the constriction of the neck, which leads on medially to the bony prominence of the tuberosity. The large proximal ulna has large olecranon and coronoid processes, with a large trochlear and smaller radial notches to articulate with humerus and radius. The deep trochlear notch articulating with the humeral trochlea is a major contributor in making the elbow joint one of the most congruous and inherently stable. Together, the ulnohumeral and radiohumeral joints provide approximately 50% of the joint stability, the rest being due to soft tissue constraint.

Soft tissue components

Ligaments

Varus-valgus stability of the elbow is largely due to the collateral ligaments (Fig. 71.2).[2] The medial (ulnar) collateral ligament has anterior, posterior, and inferior (oblique) parts. It forms a triangular band with its apex attached around the medial epicondyle and extending in a fan-shaped fashion to insert into a proximal tubercle on the medial coronoid margin (anteriorly) and the medial margin of olecranon (posteriorly). The anterior portion is the most important elbow stabilizer. The lateral (radial) collateral ligament is attached low on the lateral epicondyle and extends to the annular ligament. Its superficial fibers are blended with those of the attachment of supinator and extensor carpi radialis brevis.

The annular ligament is a strong band that encircles the radial head, holding it against the radial notch of the ulna. It attaches to the edge of the notch anteriorly and on a ridge at, or just behind, the edge posteriorly. The proximal annular border is continuous with the cubital capsule, except posteriorly where the capsule passes deep to it at the radial notch. The distal annular border attaches loosely to the radial neck after passing over a synovial reflection. Posterior to the ligament are the anconeus and the interosseus recurrent artery. Where the ligament internally is in contact with the radial head it is lined with a thin layer of cartilage, but distally it is covered by a reflected fold of synovium on the radial neck.

Mechanoreceptors have been found in the elbow ligaments, which suggests they may provide significant sensory function to the elbow joint, as well as being its major mechanical restraints.[3]

Articular capsule

The articular capsule of the elbow joint is a thin structure. Anteriorly it is broad, attaching proximally to the front of the humerus, medial epicondyle (above the coronoid), and radial fossa (in continuity on its sides with the collateral ligaments) and distally attaching to the edge of the ulna, coronoid process, and annular ligament. It receives fibers from the brachialis. Posteriorly it attaches to the humerus behind the capitellum, goes around the olecranon fossa (except inferiorly) and the back of the medial epicondyle, and extends to the superior and lateral margins of the olecranon. Laterally it is continuous with the superior radioulnar joint capsule deep to the annular ligament. The anconeus and triceps are related to it posteriorly.

Synovium

The synovial membrane extends from the articular margins of the humerus, lines the articular components of the joint, and descends below the border of the annular ligament. Sometimes there is irregularity of the synovial lining of the joint in the coronoid process on flexion, usually occurring adjacent to the medial collateral ligament, but otherwise it is smooth. There are four fat pads between synovium and capsule: one in the synovial fold, which partly divides the joint into humeroradial and humeroulnar parts, and the others in relation to the fossae of the lower end of the humerus.

Muscles

Muscles that are related to the elbow joint are the brachialis (in front), the triceps and anconeus (behind), the supinator and common extensor tendon of extensor digitorum communis and extensor digitorum brevis (laterally), and the common flexor tendon and flexor carpi ulnaris (medially) (Fig. 71.3). Anterior to the brachialis, the biceps tendon passes on its way to insertion into the radial tuberosity. The common superficial flexor tendon is attached to the medial epicondyle and the common superficial extensor tendon to the lateral epicondyle, both

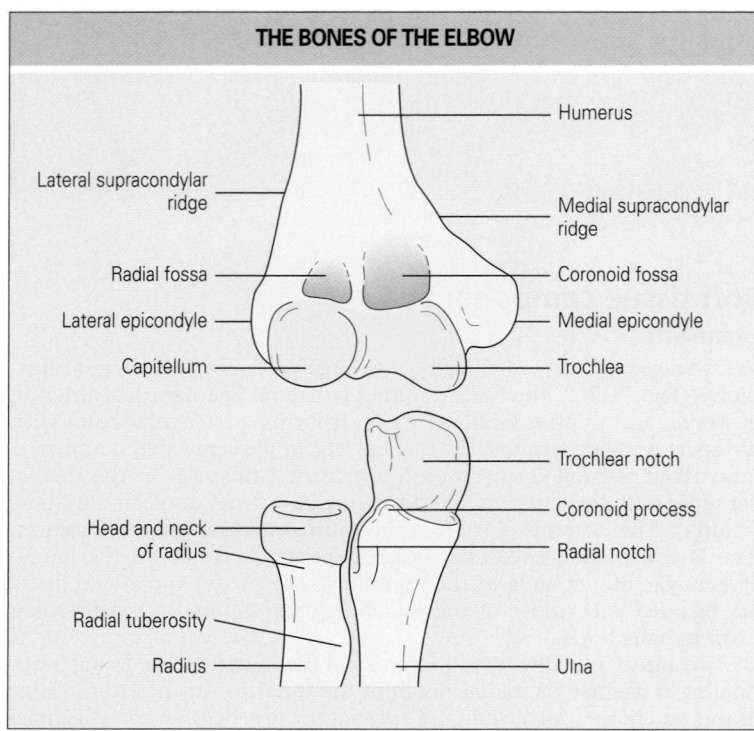

Fig. 71.1 The bones of the elbow. Expanded view of the elbow joint showing the bony features.

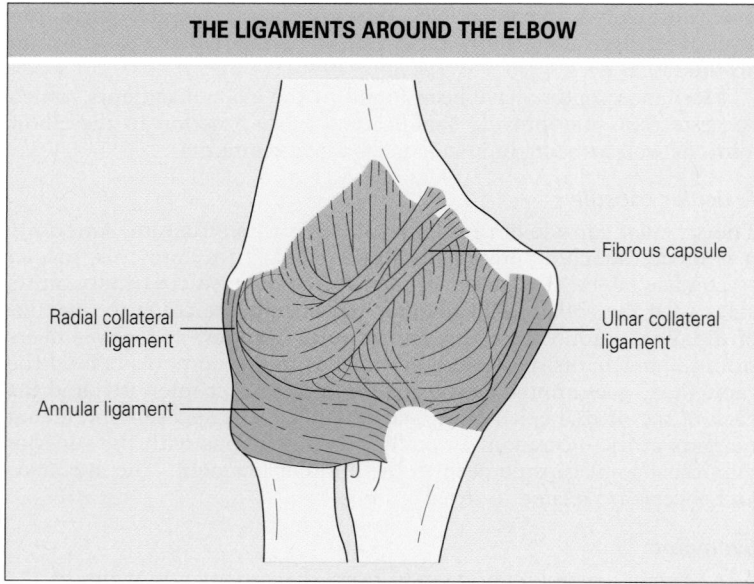

Fig. 71.2 The ligaments around the elbow. Anterior view of the elbow joint showing the ligaments and capsule.

exterior to the joint capsule. The anconeus attaches to the posterior aspect of the lateral epicondyle. Above the medial epicondyle on the supracondylar ridge is attached the humeral head of the pronator teres, while the lateral supracondylar ridge gives attachment to the extensor carpi radialis longus. The triceps passes posteriorly over the elbow joint to insert into the olecranon.

Bursae

The main bursa around the elbow is the superficial olecranon bursa, which separates the olecranon from the overlying skin. This forms in late childhood.[4] A small bicipitoradial bursa is found close to where the biceps tendon inserts into the posterior aspect of the radial tuberosity. Superficial epicondylar and radiohumeral bursae are sometimes found.

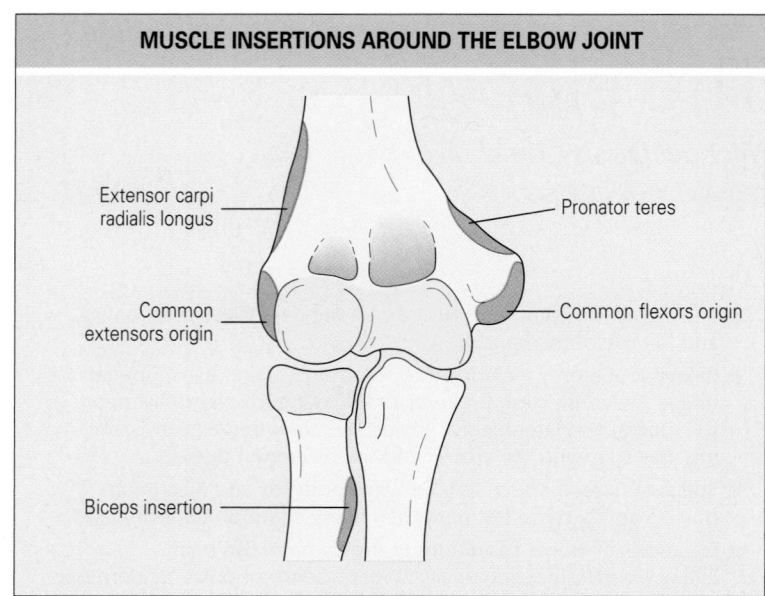

Fig. 71.3 Muscle insertions around the elbow joint. Anterior view of the elbow joint showing the muscle insertions.

Movement

Consideration of movement at the elbow functionally includes the cubital joint itself and the proximal radioulnar joint. The cubital hinge joint traverses an area of flexion of around 150 degrees. Pronation of 75 to 80 degrees and supination of 85 to 90 degrees are achievable but require an intact distal radioulnar joint as well as the proximal one.[5] The combination leads to the large variety of movements possible at this articulation. Because of the shape of the trochlea, extension results in valgus positioning of the forearm to the arm of 10 to 15 degrees (more in women), the "carrying angle." In flexion, a similar degree of varus positioning helps when bringing the hand in close proximity to the mouth. Flexion at the elbow is carried out by the brachialis and biceps, the latter also acting as a supinator of the forearm. The brachioradialis muscle assists their action. Extension is carried out by the triceps and aided by the anconeus.

Neurovascular relationships

The elbow joint receives articular arteries from numerous periarticular anastomoses that are supplied mainly by the brachial artery. Articular nerves are derived principally from the radial and musculocutaneous nerves, but the median, ulnar, and sometimes the anterior interosseous nerves contribute. These nerves follow the supply of blood vessels and probably contain vasomotor fibers as well as pain and proprioception afferents. The neurovascular structures of the arm have an intimate relationship with the joint capsule. The brachial artery traverses the joint anteriorly, just medial to the biceps tendon in the antecubital space. The musculocutaneous nerve innervates the biceps and brachialis above the level of the elbow and terminates distally to form the lateral cutaneous nerve of the forearm. The course of the median nerve takes it anterior to the joint capsule and medial to the biceps tendon and brachial artery. The radial nerve passes anterior to the lateral epicondyle, descending beneath the brachialis and brachioradialis muscles. The ulnar nerve traverses the elbow in the ulnar groove behind the medial epicondyle.

CLINICAL EVALUATION

History

The examination of the elbow must be preceded by a precise history to allow emphasis to be placed on particular areas. Complaints usually consist of pain, loss of movement, weakness, clicking, or locking. There may be sharply localized pain, typical of an extra-articular pathologic process, deep joint pain, or the poorly localized pain of ulnar

TABLE 71.1 EXAMINATION OF THE ELBOW

Inspection	Swelling—joint, bursa
	Deformity
	Carrying angle
Palpation	Synovium
	Joint line, epicondyles/soft tissues
	Ulnar nerve
Movement	Active
	Passive
	Resisted
Other	Upper limb neurologic examination
	Neck and shoulder

TABLE 71.2 DIFFERENTIAL DIAGNOSIS OF ELBOW PAIN

Local	
Articular	Arthritis, osteochondritis, loose bodies, subluxation
Periarticular	Lateral and medial epicondylitis, olecranon bursitis, ligamentous lesions, entrapment neuropathy
Referred	Cervical and shoulder disease

neuropathy with or without typical paresthesia extending to the hand. The functional interplay between elbow, shoulder, and wrist means that examination of all these joints may be necessary. Referred pain in the elbow, especially from the neck or shoulder, is usually diffuse.

Physical examination

Examination must include comparison of right and left arms (Table 71.1).

Inspection

Inspection is very important because much of the elbow joint is subcutaneous and so alterations in soft tissue or bony anatomy are easily seen. Anteriorly viewing of the elbow in the extended, supinated position allows assessment of the carrying angle. It is increased in certain congenital conditions, such as Turner syndrome, and may be altered by fractures around the elbow. Synovial proliferation and effusion are each detected as a fullness in the region of the lateral infracondylar recess. The swelling may be obliterated by pressure in the case of effusion. A hard bony swelling is detected where there is a radial head pathologic process, such as a previous fracture. Posteriorly, swelling of the subcutaneous olecranon bursa may be detected, and in rheumatoid arthritis nodules often occur extending distally along the border of the ulna. Occasionally, ulnar neuritis may result in enlargement of the ulnar nerve, which is seen medially.

Palpation

Palpation of the subcutaneous lateral and medial epicondyles and olecranon tip is easily undertaken. Tenderness over the lateral epicondyle is typical of lateral epicondylitis. The radial head is palpated by gentle pressure over the radiocapitellar joint and assessed during pronation and supination movements. Loose bodies may be detected in the infracondylar recess. Medially the ulnar nerve may be palpated to detect thickening, and assessment with the elbow in flexion and extension detects ulnar nerve subluxation. The nerve may displace anteriorly during flexion, sometimes with an obvious snap, and be associated with ulnar nerve paresthesia. Posteriorly, the tip of the olecranon and the olecranon fossa above can be felt if the elbow is not in full extension. Flexion to around 15 degrees also enables assessment of the collateral ligaments. These may be palpated. Varus stress with the humerus in full internal rotation and valgus stress in full external rotation test for lateral and medial instability, respectively, but abnormality is often subtle and requires experience to detect.

Movement

Active and passive ranges of movement should be measured, including flexion, extension, and rotation. Most frequently, a reduced range of movement is due to pain. After injury, elbow joint extension is both the first movement to be lost and the last to recover. The normal range of flexion/extension, 0 to 150 degrees, is in excess of that needed for everyday activity, which is of the order of 30 to 130 degrees; hence,

patients may be unaware of a small fixed flexion deformity. Forcibly moving the joint beyond the pain-free range helps to identify the predominant cause of the restriction. In extension, posterior pain indicates a posterior impingement problem, whereas anterior pain indicates tightness of the anterior capsule. The reverse is true for loss of flexion. Early in arthritis, flexion and extension are limited but rotational movements are often spared. Motion is best assessed with the elbow flexed to 90 degrees and held to the side of the body, with supination often greater than 85 degrees and a little less for pronation.

Pain should be sought on resisted active movements, particularly where there is no major intra-articular pathologic process. These are carried out with the elbow held at 90 degrees. Flexion and supination strength is normally greater than extension and pronation. Passive, but not resisted, movements producing pain indicate an intra-articular pathologic process, whereas pain on resisted movement alone indicates a musculotendinous pathologic process associated with that movement. To complete the assessment of muscles around the elbow, resisted flexion and extension of the wrist must be performed. Neurologic examination must not be omitted, with particular attention paid to structures supplied by the C5, C6, and C7 nerve roots. Biceps jerk (C5), brachioradialis reflex (C6), and triceps jerk (C7) should also be assessed.

Differential diagnosis of elbow pain

Pain felt at the elbow may be due to either a local pathologic process or referred pain (Table 71.2). As indicated earlier, shoulder and cervical problems frequently produce pain referred to the elbow. In the case of cervical spine lesions the pain is often associated with frank neurologic symptoms. Although referred pain is usually part of more generalized arm pain symptoms, it may be localized. Examination of the neck and shoulder is therefore important in the assessment of elbow pain. Intrathoracic pathologic processes can give rise to arm pain but is rarely localized to the elbow.

True elbow pain may be related to joint disease but is more commonly due to lesions of the soft periarticular tissues. These causes can usually be distinguished by history and appropriate examination. Primary osteoarthritis is not common; elbow involvement frequently occurs in more generalized inflammatory arthritis. The joint can be inflamed in gout or affected by septic arthritis. Traumatic effusions occur, and the joint may be involved by a fracture of the bones, with minor fractures sometimes being missed and only presenting as an effusion. A traumatic/overuse form of osteochondritis of the radial head can occur in some throwing sports, especially in the teenage child. The joint may be affected by loose bodies and synovial osteochondromatosis. Traumatic partial subluxation of the radial head through the annular ligament occurs in children, especially if they have a hypermobile tendency.

Investigations

Plain anteroposterior and lateral radiographs are useful in assessing joint pathologic processes. Further investigation by arthroscopy[6] is very useful, but magnetic resonance imaging (MRI) is a better, non-invasive alternative. MRI may be combined with arthrography. MRI and MR arthrography are better than computed tomographic arthrography except for assessment of the cartilage of the elbow when CT arthrography is better.[7] High-resolution ultrasonography is a less costly alternative, particularly useful for assessment of periarticular soft tissues.[8] This is especially so with the development of color (power) Doppler

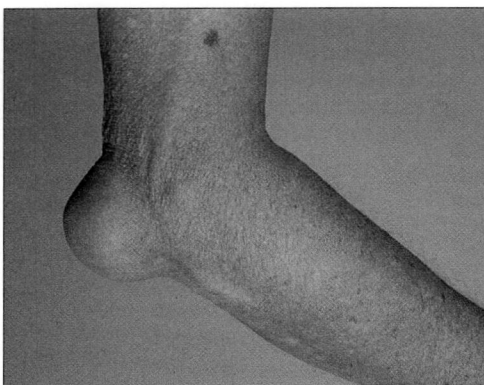

Fig. 71.4 A case of olecranon bursitis in early rheumatoid arthritis.

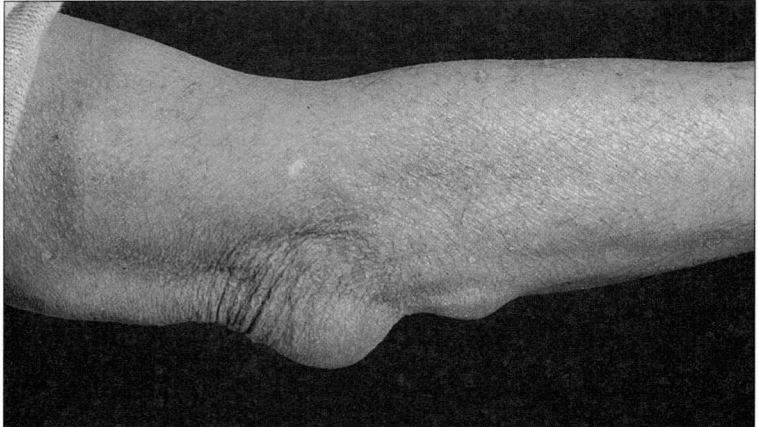

Fig. 71.5 A case of olecranon bursitis in later rheumatoid arthritis; a rheumatoid nodule is also shown.

imaging, allowing detection of abnormalities of blood flow and new vessel formation (angiogenesis), in addition to standard gray-scale ultrasonography. Ultrasonography is very dependent on operator skill, although precision of the latest equipment is enabling some clinicians to use it as an office investigation.

SOFT TISSUE ELBOW LESIONS

Apart from lateral epicondylitis ("tennis elbow"), medial epicondylitis ("golfer's elbow"), and olecranon bursitis, soft tissue lesions at the elbow are relatively rare.

Olecranon bursitis

Bursal inflammation around the elbow can occur and principally affects the olecranon bursa. Both epicondylar and radiohumeral bursitis have been reported but are rare, producing vague symptoms around the elbow with swelling. They have in the past been suggested as causes of tennis elbow but rarely, if ever, have the same clinical features. The condition is most commonly seen in younger men as a consequence of recurrent elbow trauma either due to work (e.g., automobile mechanics, miners) or related to leisure activities (throwing darts, gymnastics, gardening). There is often no obvious precipitating cause of olecranon bursitis. It rarely occurs in childhood for developmental reasons.[4]

Etiology

The olecranon bursa is a subcutaneous synovial pouch located on the extensor aspect of the elbow. It allows the skin to glide freely over the olecranon process, preventing tissue tears. Because of its superficial position over the olecranon, with little soft tissue padding, the olecranon bursa is vulnerable to trauma by friction or a blow and to infection through abrasions, puncture wounds, or cellulitis. Olecranon bursitis occurs when the bursa swells because of trauma, inflammation, or infection (Fig. 71.4). Such swelling occurs easily and is readily visible. The swelling may be the result of fluid accumulation but may be due to synovial tissue hypertrophy or fibrosis. In addition to trauma, the bursa may also be involved in crystal arthropathies (gout or, rarely, calcium pyrophosphate arthritis) or in generalized inflammatory arthritis, especially rheumatoid arthritis. Swelling of the olecranon bursa may be seen in association with rheumatoid nodules on the ulnar border of the forearm (Fig. 71.5). Rheumatoid nodules may form within the bursa, but intrabursal nodules may also form as a consequence of traumatic fibrosis or gouty tophi.

Clinical aspects

Olecranon bursitis can be classified clinically into three general categories (Table 71.3):

- Traumatic (or idiopathic) non-inflammatory
- Aseptic inflammatory
- Septic inflammatory

Appropriate therapy depends on the bursitis category. Therefore, it is important for the cause to be defined as soon as possible through history, examination, and, when appropriate, bursal aspiration. The main diagnostic challenge is to distinguish septic and non-septic bursitis as the septic bursitis has the greatest potential for morbidity and must be diagnosed as soon as possible. A clinician must also be aware there is a potential for a rapid change in the cause of the bursitis, that is, a change from non-septic to septic. This should be considered at each follow-up visit.

Questions regarding occupation, duration of symptoms, and possible trauma or skin injury are important aspects of the history. Information on other causes of bursitis such as rheumatoid arthritis, gout, or uremia should be sought. Diabetes or conditions associated with immunosuppression can increase the risk of sepsis. During the physical examination the size and turgor of the bursa should be noted (and size change at follow-up visits). Warmth and erythema of the bursa or skin along with the presence of nodules or lymphadenopathy provide important clues. An effusion in the adjacent elbow joint may occur, especially with inflammatory arthritis. Evidence of trauma, particularly with skin breakage, should be sought. General physical status should be assessed, particularly looking for fever. Key features in the differential diagnosis are provided in Table 71.3.

In traumatic or idiopathic olecranon bursitis, pain is usually localized and typically does not occur on passive or resisted movement. It is usually provoked by leaning on the elbow or flexion with a constriction around the elbow such as a coat sleeve. Tenderness should be sought about the tip of the olecranon and will be present, sometimes with palpable thickening of the bursal wall, even in the absence of significant effusion; the area is generally very sensitive to pressure. Septic olecranon bursitis occurs less frequently but should not be missed. Usually it occurs after an abrasion or may be associated with an initial cellulitis of the skin. Septic olecranon bursitis usually causes pain with elbow flexion and sometimes with resisted extension, but it is different from acute arthritis because gentle passive extension is unimpaired.[9]

When inflammation or infection is suggested, percutaneous diagnostic aspiration of the bursa is indicated. Aspiration of the bursa both reduces symptoms and allows assessment of the fluid. Along with gross visualization of blood staining, or turbidity of the fluid, white blood cell count and differential and Gram stain with culture of the fluid should be undertaken to exclude infection. Polarized light microscopy should be performed to reveal any crystals. Elbow radiographs are rarely necessary and should only be used to exclude traumatic fracture or preexisting joint injury. Ultrasonography can be used to define the characteristics of the bursitis and may assist needle placement for aspiration and injection in some cases. MRI gives even greater soft tissue definition but cannot usually be reliably used to distinguish septic from non-septic bursitis.

Management

Non-inflammatory, traumatic (or idiopathic) bursitis usually responds to simple conservative therapy, including rest, elbow protection, and anti-inflammatory drug treatment. Padded elbow support may help to prevent further trauma and skin abrasion. Percutaneous needle

TABLE 71.3 DIFFERENTIAL DIAGNOSIS OF OLECRANON BURSITIS

| | Traumatic (idiopathic) non-inflammatory | Aseptic inflammatory | | | Septic inflammatory |
		Rheumatoid arthritis	Crystalline	Uremia	
Symptoms					
Trauma	+++	+	+	0/+	+++
Tenderness	+	+	++	+	+++
Skin breakage	+	0	0	0	+++
Signs					
Fever	0	0	0	0	++
Warmth	+	+	++	+	+++
Erythema	+	+	++	+	+++
Cellulitis	0	0	+	+	+++
Lymphadenopathy	0	0/+	0/+	0	++
Edema	0/+	0/+	0/+	0	++
Bursal fluid					
Color	C, S, H	C, S	S, H	S	S, H, P
White blood cells per mm³	50-10,000 (mean 1100)	1000-60,000 (mean 3000)	1000-20,000 (mean 2900)	1200	350,000-450,000 (mean 75,000)
Gram stain	Negative	Negative	Negative	Negative	Positive (70%)
Crystals	Negative	Rare cholesterol	Monosodium urate or pyrophosphate	Rare	Negative
Culture	Negative	Negative	Negative	Negative	Positive

Differential diagnosis: 0, usually absent; +, rare; ++, occasional; +++, common. Bursal fluid color: C, clear; H, hemorrhagic; P, purulent; S, serosanguineous.

aspiration should be considered for patients having significant symptoms. The aspiration itself reduces symptoms and, in addition, a compressive elastic bandage may be used to prevent recurrence of swelling. If infection has been satisfactorily excluded by culture, local corticosteroid injection may be performed, which is effective in speeding recovery.[10] However, this can lead to complications (infection, skin atrophy, chronic pain) and should only be used sparingly for traumatic bursitis. In inflammatory olecranon bursitis, related to rheumatoid arthritis or crystalline arthropathy, intrabursal corticosteroid injection is useful. In such cases it should be preceded by aspiration and investigation to exclude infection. An injection of 20 mg of methylprednisolone acetate usually leads to rapid recovery.

The finding of infection requires appropriate antibiotic therapy and re-aspiration of pus as necessary. *Staphylococcus aureus* is the most frequently found organism, although a group A β-hemolytic streptococcus or *Streptococcus epidermidis* is less commonly found.[9,11] Rarely *Hemophilus influenzae* and *Pseudomonas* species may be the cause. In immunocompromised patients (malignancy, HIV-positive status, or systemic corticosteroid therapy), special cultures for mycobacteria, fungi, or anaerobic bacteria may be necessary.

Patients who fail to respond to outpatient therapy or who at the outset have more severe initial infection need to be hospitalized for intravenous antibiotic therapy. This includes patients with high fever, chills, prolonged duration of symptoms, and cellulitis. Hospitalization also needs to be considered for those with complicating medical conditions (diabetes, uremia, rheumatoid arthritis) and immunosuppression.

Repeated aspiration of the infected bursa is essential and may initially need to be carried out on a daily basis. This can be done percutaneously or if necessary with the placement of a suction-irrigation system. Measuring the cell counts and repeated culture should be used to monitor the response to therapy. Patients requiring initial intravenous antibiotic therapy can be switched to oral medication as soon as signs and symptoms show consistent improvement. In general, antibiotic therapy should be continued for 10 to 14 days, although there is evidence that patients beginning treatment within a week of onset actually require only half this duration to sterilize the bursa.

Surgical drainage or bursectomy is occasionally required in the management of olecranon bursitis. If repeated traumatic bursitis occurs, then surgical removal of the bursa should be considered, either arthroscopically or by open resection. Persistent aseptic inflammatory bursitis may require open resection. Bursectomy may be required for septic bursitis if the acute infection fails to resolve or if, after repeated infection, a fibrotic, chronically inflamed bursa is left.[12]

Lateral epicondylitis
Epidemiology

Used synonymously with the term *tennis elbow*, this condition is one of the most common lesions of the arm. The first description is attributed to Runge in 1873,[13] but the name "tennis elbow" is derived from Morris's description of "lawn tennis arm" in *The Lancet* in 1882.[14] One to 3 percent of the population are affected by it,[15] mostly those aged between 40 and 60 years, the dominant arm being affected most frequently. Forty to 50 percent of tennis players suffer with it, mainly older players,[16] but in clinical practice fewer than 5% of cases are due to the game.[17] It is found most often in non-athletes, and the majority are not manual workers. Many patients cannot describe any specific precipitating factors.[18] The onset of symptoms may be brought on by overuse, and hence lateral epicondylitis is more often seen in the active middle-aged population than the less active elderly population. In manual workers, relative overuse of wrist and finger extensors may precipitate the condition, which most often affects the dominant arm. Sometimes there may be bilateral involvement, either due to increased stress placed on the unaffected arm or resulting from a general tendency to soft tissue lesions that occurs in some individuals.[17,18]

Etiopathology

There have been more than 25 suggested causes of the condition,[19] and this reflects the use of the diagnosis non-specifically for lateral elbow pain. Pathologic material for study is relatively rare because most cases do not come to surgery. Reported operative findings in relatively few chronic cases have included periostitis,[13] infection,[19] radiohumeral joint disease,[20] radial nerve entrapment,[21] and a lesion of the orbicular (annular) ligament.[22] It is believed, however, that the majority of cases are due to a musculotendinous lesion of the common extensor tendon at the attachment to the lateral epicondyle or nearby, especially that portion derived from the extensor carpi radialis brevis.[17] The anatomic

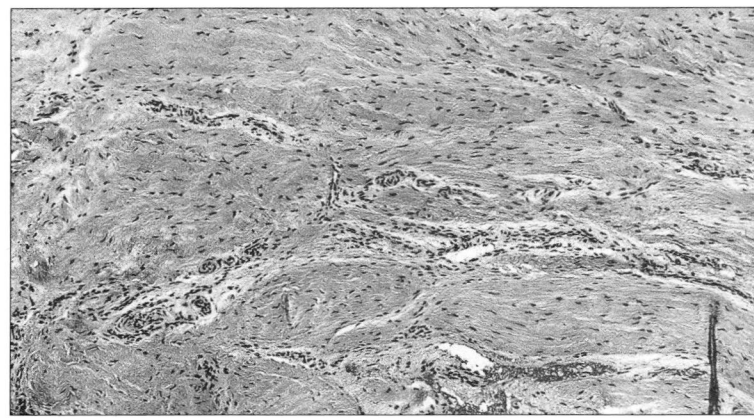

Fig. 71.6 Angiofibroblastic hyperplasia.

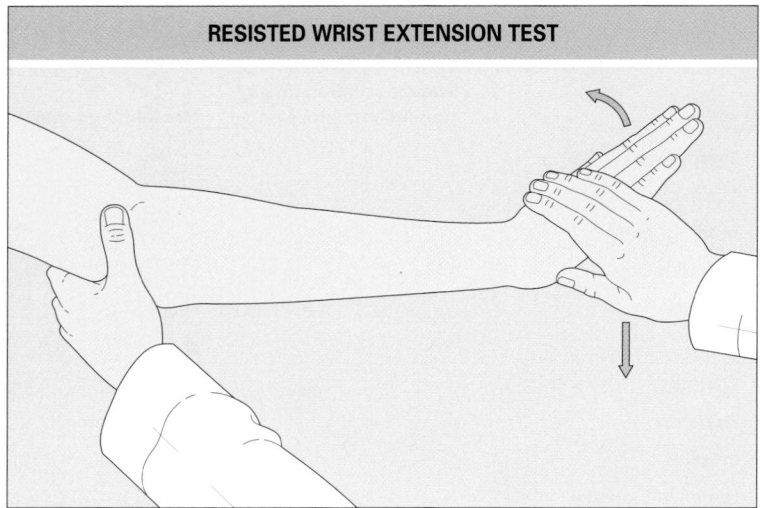

Fig. 71.7 Resisted wrist extension test.

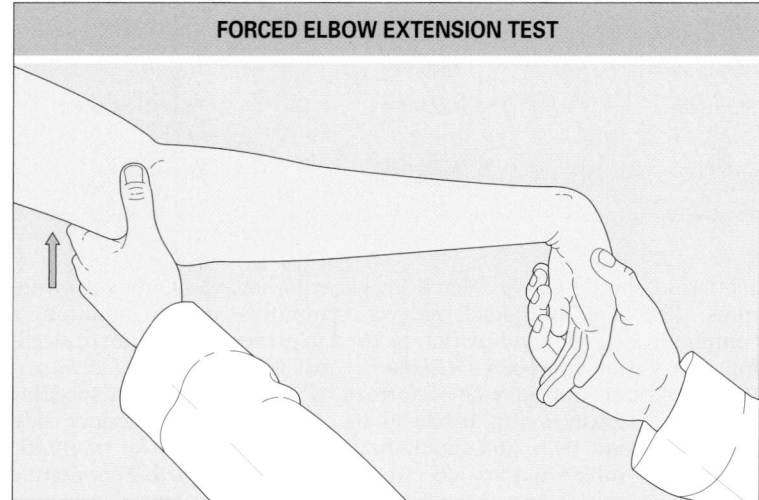

Fig. 71.8 Forced elbow extension test.

location of the extensor carpi radialis brevis makes this undersurface vulnerable to contact and abrasion against the lateral edge of the capitulum with the elbow in motion.[23]

Macroscopic tears in the common extensor tendon are sometimes found at operation,[17] but repeated high-dose local corticosteroid injections may have affected findings. Microfractures, cystic and fibrinoid degeneration and round cell infiltrations, immature fibrous tissue, hyaline degeneration and vascular plus fibroblastic proliferation ("angiofibroblastic tendinosis"; Fig. 71.6), sometimes with calcific debris, and attempts at repair have been described.[16,17,24,25] Some cases show a chronic traction effect. The angiogenesis as part of the process is consistent with vascular changes seen on color (power) Doppler imaging.[8,26] Histologic evidence of inflammation has not been found. The changes seen are similar to those seen in the rotator cuff with advancing age, where tendon vascular factors are believed to be important.[27] There is some evidence that neurogenic changes of the enthesis may be part of the pathophysiology.[28] The relationship of such findings to the acute lesion is uncertain. Ischemic stress may be important because the tenoperiosteal junction (enthesis) and nearby tendon are relatively avascular, because the blood supply is a watershed of that derived from muscle and bone and working muscle takes up the blood supply at the expense of tendon.

Age is an important factor, because lateral epicondylitis rarely occurs before the age of 30 years. Adult maturity is associated with alterations in the enthesis, including changes in collagen content, reduction in cells and ground substance, and increase in lipids, which then probably predispose it to injury.[29] Other possible changes that may be important, including those due to tendon elasticity, have yet to be elucidated. Basic science biochemical investigation of tendon turnover in relation to age and disease may, in the future, lead to further insights into the pathophysiology and possibly novel therapies.

Clinical findings

Lateral epicondylitis usually arises slowly and apparently spontaneously; a blow or acute traumatic strain is relatively rarely remembered. Pain is localized to the lateral epicondyle but may spread up and down the upper limb. Grip is impaired because of pain, and this may result in restricted daily activities. Tenderness over the epicondyle is usual, although maximum tenderness is sometimes found at nearby sites.[22] The other cardinal sign is increase in pain on resisting wrist dorsiflexion with the elbow in extension (Fig. 71.7). Symptoms may also be precipitated by extending the elbow with the wrist flexed (Fig. 71.8) and by resisted middle finger extension. Resisted supination may also be painful. The range of movement of the elbow is usually normal, but a few degrees of extension may be lost in some severe and chronic cases.

Differential diagnosis

It is important to exclude other conditions producing elbow pain, especially that referred from the cervical spine or shoulder, as well as arthritis of the elbow, although this is usually obvious.

A nerve entrapment around the elbow may produce diagnostic confusion. Radial tunnel syndrome or compression of the posterior

interosseous nerve[21] can produce lateral elbow and upper forearm pain. It can be the cause of apparent lateral epicondylitis that is unresponsive to conservative treatment but is believed to be a rare cause of resistant cases.[30] These entrapments have been found to be due to compressive lesions caused by abnormal fibrous bands in front of the radial head, a sharp tendinous origin of extensor carpi radialis brevis, or a radial recurrent fan of vessels. More rarely, a lipoma or ganglion has been found to be the cause. Compression of the posterior interosseous nerve may occur where it passes through the supinator muscle just below the elbow joint. A well-defined arcade of Frohse is present in 30% of subjects[31] and makes a compression neuropathy more likely. Diffuse pain, symptoms distal to the lateral epicondyle, and the presence of muscle weakness may be useful distinguishing features.

Investigations

Investigations are not usually required, but radiographs of the elbow may be helpful in excluding joint disease and may occasionally show lateral soft tissue calcification. Electromyography may be helpful in excluding a nerve entrapment. Quantitative assessment of severity and response to treatment is difficult, but grading pain, tenderness, and pain on resisted wrist extension can be helpful, and lifting graded weights and grip strength measurement aid objectivity.[32] A truly objective measurement is that of infrared thermography of the affected elbow, which shows a discrete localized area of increased heat near the lateral epicondyle in 98% of affected elbows (Fig. 71.9). Analysis of the gradient across the abnormal area reveals a correlation with clinical severity. Lack of general availability of this technique means it is

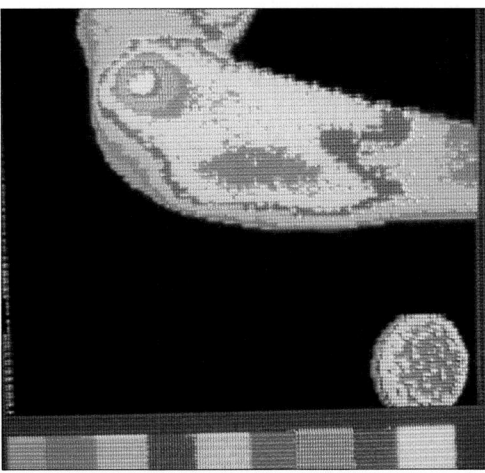

Fig.71.9 Lateral epicondylitis. An infrared thermographic pattern in lateral epicondylitis showing a localized "hot spot."

TABLE 71.4 MANAGEMENT OF LATERAL EPICONDYLITIS		
		Evidence grade
Early/mild	Rest, splinting, NSAID	A/B A (short-term)
Established	Local corticosteroid injection	A (short term)
	Physical therapy	A (weak)
Resistant	Manipulation?	B/C
	Surgery—lateral release	B/C

mainly a research tool. MRI has been used to identify tissue abnormalities before surgery in chronic cases.[33] High-resolution ultrasonography, often with color (power) Doppler imaging, is increasingly used to assess the tissue lesion at an earlier stage and may be used to guide treatment including therapeutic injections and in the future may help to predict resistant cases that will require surgical intervention.[8,26]

Management

More than 40 treatment regimens for lateral epicondylitis have been described in the literature, ranging from extremes of "prolonged observation" to x-ray therapy. Reduced activity may result in resolution of symptoms in some cases, especially early on and in conjunction with splinting (Table 71.4). The efficacy of orthotic devices has been the subject of a systematic review, and no definite conclusion could be drawn on their effectiveness.[34] Oral non-steroidal anti-inflammatory drugs (NSAIDs) or NSAID gels are often used. They have some benefit but are only shown to be effective in the short term, especially in early cases. Long-term benefit is uncertain.[35]

Numerous physical modalities of treatment have been used to treat lateral epicondylitis, but the efficacy of most of them remains unproven. Lack of evidence may relate to quality of trials rather than lack of efficacy. An eccentric exercise program may be of greater benefit than standard stretching and strengthening.[36] Studies of ultrasound therapy have given conflicting results.[37] Benefit has not been shown for low-level laser light therapy but may relate to not using optimal doses and wavelengths.[38] Extracorporeal shock wave therapy has been advocated for persistent cases, but with conflicting results, and is not generally recommended. However, there is some evidence of possible benefit under well-defined, restrictive conditions.[39] Acupuncture has also been used in treatment but only been shown, so far, to have short-term benefit.[40]

Local injections of corticosteroids have been widely used and are efficacious and cost effective, with around 90% of subjects responding. But the injection frequently causes transient increased pain. Although producing a rapid response of good benefit for 6 weeks, the improvement may not last due to a significant relapse rate. Whether this is a

true failure of the corticosteroid or the rapid improvement in the pain leading to increased activity too soon is unknown.[37,41] The injection may be repeated after 2 to 4 weeks, in the event of failure to respond or relapse, but should not be repeated more than twice because it is unlikely to be effective, increasing the risk of side effects (loss of subcutaneous fat, with dimpling and depigmentation) and predisposition to chronic pain. Indeed, there is evidence to suggest that those who experience relapse may have a worse long-term prognosis at 1 year than when just a wait-and-see modified activity approach is used.[37,42]

In recent years a number of other modalities of treatment have been advocated. Topical nitric oxide, using a glyceryl trinitrate patch, appears beneficial but has to be applied daily for up to 6 months.[43] Sclerosant treatment using policodanol has been used and ultrasonography and color (power) Doppler imaging have guided injection, but there is uncertainty about the long-term consequences for the tendon tissue; and a randomized controlled trial did not show greater benefit than lidocaine plus epinephrine.[44] Autologous blood injection using ultrasound guidance has been claimed to be of benefit, but there have been no randomized controlled trials to date. Also there is uncertainty about the contributory effects of the dry needling of the tendon carried out before the blood injection. There also have been conflicting results of the use of botulinum toxin A injection into the origin of the extensor forearm muscles. The idea is to temporarily, partially paralyze the muscles with the aim of interrupting repetitive microtrauma and allow recovery, albeit at the expense of some weakness. Preliminary study of the use of injections of the matrix metalloproteinase inhibitor aprotinin to treat tendinopathy shows that this agent has promise, but it has yet to be used for lateral epicondylitis.[45]

The problem with assessing the benefits of active conservative treatment is that the natural history of lateral epicondylitis is for resolution in around 80% of cases after about 1 year. Therefore, the aim of treatment is mainly to achieve recovery sooner. But there is concern that the failure of some treatments or relapse after improvement may adversely affect outcome and be worse than a wait-and-see approach.[42] A low percentage of patients are resistant to conservative management, but to date it is not possible to reliably identify early on those patients who will not do well.

Role of surgery

Surgical intervention is considered for the 10% of patients whose disorder fails to respond to conservative treatments. The value of manipulation as a means of avoiding surgery is controversial. It may be effective when performed under general anesthesia, in conjunction with a local corticosteroid injection, but surgery is more effective.[46] There is no evidence-based consensus on the best surgical management. Most reported experience is of an open procedure, with there being two main types. One involves resection or débridement of damaged tissue and tendon repair, with or without decortication or drilling of the lateral epicondyle.[17,24] The alternative is a simple "lateral release" by division of the origin of the common extensor tendon. Advocates of the removal of abnormal tendon and repair claim a more reliable response and are concerned about weakness caused by the "lateral release." Others believe that the "lateral release" gives long-term results of 90% and may be done using a simple percutaneous procedure that can be performed under local anesthesia.[47] It may be done as ambulatory surgery or possibly even as an office procedure. A randomized controlled study comparing standard open débridement and repair surgery with percutaneous "lateral release" showed recovery and return to work were significantly quicker after the simpler technique.[48] Arthroscopic release, although more technically challenging and time consuming, has been shown in a comparative study to be as good as the standard open technique but with a quicker return to work.[49] Also, advocates of arthroscopy point to the fact that the joint can be examined at the same time and may reveal abnormalities contributing to symptoms and allow their correction. There is general agreement that extensive lateral release with resection of the proximal third of the annular ligament is best avoided because of the risk of subsequent elbow instability.

Most described treatments for lateral epicondylitis, conservative or operative, are not supported by robust scientific evidence.[50] Until there is greater proof, clinicians have to be guided by the available evidence, a pragmatic, if subjective, viewpoint, and clinical experience.

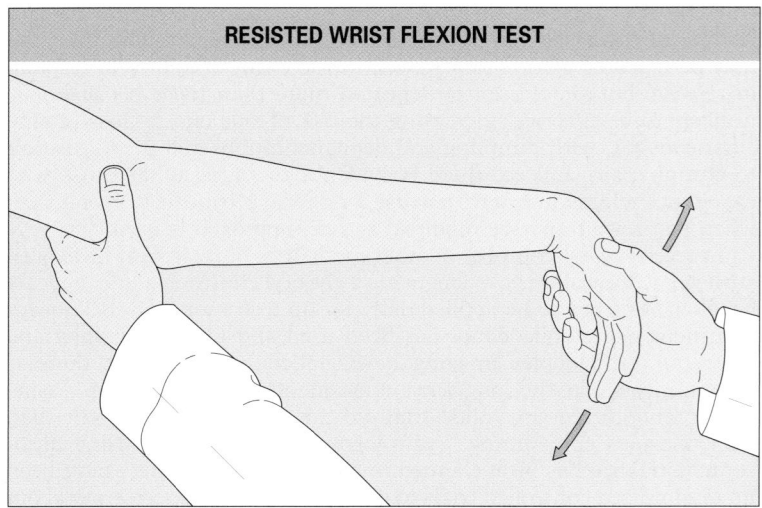

RESISTED WRIST FLEXION TEST

Fig. 71.10 Resisted wrist flexion test.

Prognosis

Lateral epicondylitis has been considered to be a self-limiting disorder with patients improving with or without treatment within 1 year. However, in one study, 40% of patients had prolonged minor discomfort, which in some persisted for 5 years. Manual workers, especially mechanics, builders, and domestic workers are most susceptible to recurrence on resumption of the activity that induced the initial pain.[18] Early treatment may improve prognosis. Firm strapping of the forearm muscles just distal to the elbow joint, or the use of one of the commercial elbow splints, may be helpful. Although emphasis is on rest, graded exercise, with stretching, may be prescribed, especially in a patient wishing to return to a sport. In a few cases, persistence of lateral elbow pain despite local treatment is due to a cervical lesion that was not originally clinically apparent, and re-examination may be

necessary. Up to 10% of patients fail to respond to physical therapy and injections.

Medial epicondylitis

Otherwise known as "golfer's elbow," this condition is around 15 times less commonly seen than lateral epicondylitis.[17] It is a lesion of the common flexor tendon at the medial epicondyle. As with "tennis elbow," a sporting cause is relatively rare. The condition is usually milder, and often pain and tenderness are less well localized to the medial epicondyle, being felt a little distal to the flexor origin. Pain on resisted wrist flexion with the elbow in extension is the most reliable sign (Fig. 71.10), although rarely flexion of the fingers rather than of the wrist best elicits symptoms. The pathology and management are essentially the same as those for lateral epicondylitis.

Other disorders of the elbow

Biceps tendinitis is characterized by local pain and tenderness in the region of the bicipital tuberosity of the radius, with pain on resisted flexion and supination. Pain on resisted flexion alone indicates the rarer brachialis muscle lesion, with pain and tenderness that is less well localized and is found behind the biceps tendon. Although uncommon, such a tear is particularly prone to develop myositis ossificans, which in the early phases produces a warm, firm mass that can be mistaken for a tumor. Pain on resisted supination alone is said to indicate a supinator lesion, but this very rarely, if ever, occurs and pain would be felt farther down the forearm. It is unusual to have a lesion at the site of triceps insertion into the olecranon (triceps tendinitis), but instead these occur higher in the arm at the musculotendinous junction. Ligamentous lesions do not usually occur in isolation, most often being associated with traumatic joint synovitis or effusion if not frank joint derangement or fracture. Medially, a ligamentous lesion may form at least part of the elbow injury caused by some throwing sports, such as the javelin event, and may, if an overuse injury, need to be distinguished from medial epicondylitis.

REFERENCES

1. Standing S, editor in chief. Gray's anatomy, 40th ed. Edinburgh: Churchill Livingstone, 2008.
2. Morrey BF, An KN. Articular and ligamentous contributions to stability of the elbow joint. Am J Sports Med 1983;11:315-319.
3. Petri S, Collins JG, Solomonow M, et al. Mechanoreceptors in the human elbow ligaments. J Hand Surg [Am] 1998;23:512-518.
4. Chen J, Alk D, Eventov I, Wientroub S. Development of the olecranon bursa: an anatomic cadaveric study. Acta Orthop Scand 1987;58:408-409.
5. Boone DC, Azen SP. Normal range of motion of joints in male subjects. J Bone Joint Surg Am 1979;61:756-759.
6. Baker CL, Brooks AA. Arthroscopy of the elbow. Clin Sports Med 1996;15:261-281.
7. Shahabpour M, Kichouh M, Laridon E, et al. The effectiveness of diagnostic imaging methods for the assessment of soft tissue and articular disorders of the shoulder and elbow. Eur J Radiol 2008;65:194-200.
8. Tran N, Chow K. Ultrasonography of the elbow. Semin Musculoskel Radiol 2007;11:105-116.
9. Canoso JJ, Barza M. Soft tissue infections. Clin Rheum Dis 1993;19:293-309.
10. Smith DL, McAfee JH, Lucas LM, et al. Treatment of nonseptic olecranon bursitis: a controlled blinded prospective trial. Arch Intern Med 1989;149:2527-2530.
11. Ho G, Su EY. Antibiotic therapy of septic bursitis: its implication in the treatment of septic arthritis. Arthritis Rheum 1981;24:905-910.
12. Stewart NJ, Manzanares JB, Morrey BF. Surgical treatment of a septic olecranon bursitis. J Shoulder Elbow Surg 1997;6:49-54.
13. Runge F. Zur Genese und Behandlung des Schreiberkrampfes. Berl Klin Wochenschr 1873;10:245-248.
14. Morris H. Rider's sprain. Lancet 1882;2:557.
15. Allander E. Prevalence, incidence and remission rates of some common rheumatic diseases and syndromes. Scand J Rheumatol 1974;3:145-153.
16. Nirschl RP, Pettrone FA. Tennis elbow. J Bone Joint Surg Am 1973;61:832-839.

17. Coonrad RW, Hooper WR. Tennis elbow: course, natural history, conservative and surgical management. J Bone Joint Surg Am 1973;55:1177-1187.
18. Binder AI, Hazleman BL. Lateral humeral epicondylitis—a study of natural history and the effect of conservative therapy. Br J Rheumatol 1983;22:73-76.
19. Cyriax JH. The pathology and treatment of tennis elbow. J Bone Joint Surg 1936;18:921-940.
20. Newman JH, Goodfellow JW. Fibrillation of the radial head as one cause for tennis elbow. BMJ 1975;2:328-330.
21. Roles NC, Maudsley RH. Radial tunnel syndrome: resistant tennis elbow as a nerve entrapment. J Bone Joint Surg Br 1972;54:499-508.
22. Bosworth DM. The role of the orbicular ligament in tennis elbow. J Bone Joint Surg Am 1955;37:527-533.
23. Burata R, Brown D, Capelo R. Anatomic factors related to the cause of tennis elbow. J Bone Joint Surg Am 2007;89:1955-1963.
24. Nirschl RP, Pettrone FA. Tennis elbow: the surgical treatment of lateral epicondylitis. J Bone Joint Surg Am 1979;61:832-839.
25. Regan W, Lester E, Coonrad R, Morrey BF. Microscopic histopathology of chronic refractory lateral epicondylitis. Am J Sports Med 1992;20:746-749.
26. Du Toit C, Stieler M, Saunders R, et al. Diagnostic accuracy of power Doppler ultrasound in patients with chronic tennis elbow. Br J Sports Med 2008;42:872-876.
27. Chard MD, Cawston TE, Riley GP, et al. Rotator cuff degeneration and lateral epicondylitis: a comparative histological study. Ann Rheum Dis 1994;53:30-34.
28. Ljung BO, Alfredson H, Forsgren S. Neurokinin 1: receptors and sensory neuropeptides in tendon insertions at the medial and lateral epicondyles of the humerus: studies on tennis elbow and medial epicondylalgia. J Orthop Res 2004;22:321-327.
29. Neipal GA, Sitaj S. Enthesopathy. Clin Rheum Dis 1979;5:857-862.
30. Van Rossum J, Buruma OJS, Kamphrisen HAC, Onvlee GJ. Tennis elbow—a radial tunnel syndrome? J Bone Joint Surg Am 1978;60:197-208.

31. Spinner M. The arcade of Frohse and its relationship to posterior interosseous nerve paralysis. J Bone Joint Surg Br 1968;50:809-812.
32. Binder A, Parr G, Thomas PP, Hazleman B. A clinical and thermographic study of lateral epicondylitis. Br J Rheumatol 1983;22:77-81.
33. Potter HG, Hannefin JA, Morwessel RM, et al. Lateral epicondylitis: correlation of MR imaging, surgical and histopathological findings. Radiology 1995;196:43-46.
34. Struijs PA, Smidt N, Arola H, van Dijk CN; Orthotic devices for the treatment of tennis elbow. Cochrane Database Syst Rev 2002;(2):CD001821.
35. Green SE, Assendelft WJJ, Barnsley L, et al. Non-steroidal anti-inflammatory drugs (NSAIDs) for treating lateral elbow pain in adults. Cochrane Database Syst Rev 2002;(2):CD003686.
36. Croisier JL, Foidart-Dessalle M, Tinant F, et al. An isokinetic eccentric programme for the management of chronic lateral epicondylar tendinopathy. Br J Sports Med 2007;41:269-275.
37. Nimgrade A, Sullivan M, Goldman R. Physiotherapy, steroid injections or rest for lateral epicondylosis: what the evidence suggests. Pain Practice 2005;5:203-215.
38. Bjordil JM, Lopes-Martins RAB, Joensen J, et al. A systematic review of low level laser therapy in lateral elbow tendinopathy (tennis elbow). BMC Musculoskeletal Dis 2008;9:75.
39. Rompe JD, Maffulli N. Repetitive shock wave therapy for lateral elbow tendinopathy (tennis elbow): a systematic and qualitative analysis. Br Med Bull 2007;83:355-378.
40. Trinh KV, Phillips SD, Hoe E, et al; Acupuncture for the alleviation of lateral epicondyle pain: a systematic review. Rheumatology 2004;43:1085-1090.
41. Smidt N, Assendelft WJJ, van der Windt D, et al. Corticosteroid injections for lateral epicondylitis: a systematic review. Pain 2002;96:23-40.
42. Bisset L, Beller E, Jull G, et al. Mobilization with movement and exercise, corticosteroid injection or wait and see for tennis elbow: a randomized trial. BMJ 2006;333:939-941.

43. Paoloni JA, Appleyard RC, Nelson J, Murrell GAC. Topical nitric oxide application in the treatment of chronic extensor tendinosis at the elbow. Am J Sports Med 2003;31:915-920.

44. Zersig E, Fahlstrom M, Ohberg L, Alfredson H. Pain relief after intratendinous injections in patients with tennis elbow: results of a randomized trial. Br J Sports Med 2008;42:267-271.

45. Orchard J, Massey A, Brown R, et al. Successful management of tendinopathy with injections of the MMP-inhibitor aprotinin. Clin Orthop Relat Res 2008;466:1625-1632.

46. Maden S, Jowett RL. Lateral epicondylagia: treatment by manipulation under anaesthetic and steroid injection and operative release. Acta Orthop Belg 2000;66:449-454.

47. Verhaar J, Walenkamp G, van Mameren H, van der Linden T. Lateral extensor release for tennis elbow: a prospective long term follow-up study. J Bone Joint Surg Am 1993;75:1034-1043.

48. Dunkow PD, Jatti M, Muddu BN. A comparison of open and percutaneous techniques in the surgical treatment of tennis elbow. J Bone Joint Surg Br 2004;86:701-704.

49. Peart RE, Strickler SS, Schweitzer KM. Lateral epicondylitis: a comparative study of open and arthroscopic lateral release. Am J Orthop 2004;33:565-567.

50. Assendorf W, Green S, Buchbinder R, et al. Tennis elbow. Clin Evid 2004;12:1753-1764.

The wrist and hand

George S. M. Dyer, Brandon E. Earp, Philip E. Blazar, and Barry P. Simmons

72

- Pain or loss of function in the wrist and hand may originate in the bones and joints, periarticular soft tissues, or peripheral neurovascular structures or may be referred from the cervical spine, thoracic outlet, shoulder, or elbow.
- Precise diagnosis depends on a meticulous history, a thorough physical examination, and appropriately selected diagnostic studies.

INTRODUCTION

The hand is the main tactile sensory organ and is uniquely designed for fine motor activities. Any deviation from the normal architecture or limitation from a painful condition may lead to disability. Understanding this anatomy in detail will help in diagnosis and treatment (Figs. 72.1 to 72.4).[1-7] The focus of this chapter is on the common localized disorders of the hand and wrist.

CLINICAL EVALUATION

History

The evaluation should begin with a complete history, including details about the start of symptoms; the location, nature, and duration of these symptoms; and factors that aggravate or alleviate them. Particularly important is any history of an inciting event, including trauma, to which the patient attributes the symptoms. Often chronic conditions have simply worsened over time, and the patient may relate a long-standing history of repetitive or strenuous activity that now is painful or difficult to accomplish.

Physical examination

Inspection should include observing resting posture, swelling, deformity, ecchymosis, atrophy, or skin and nail changes.[2,5,6] An excellent understanding of the surface anatomy of the hand and wrist is very important for appropriate evaluation of injuries (Fig. 72.5).

Resting posture

A normal resting posture will have the metacarpophalangeal (MCP) joints flexed 45 to 70 degrees and each of the interphalangeal (IP) joints slightly flexed up to 10 degrees.[8] Rheumatoid arthritis (RA) and other chronic inflammatory diseases can cause volar subluxation of the carpus, carpal collapse, and radial deviation of the carpus. Chronic arthritis of the distal radioulnar joint may result in instability with dorsal subluxation of the ulnar head that displays a "piano key" movement on downward pressure.[4]

Swelling and deformity

The fingers and thumb may demonstrate swelling and deformity of the joints, clubbing, subcutaneous nodules, gouty tophi, Heberden's (distal IP [DIP] joint) or Bouchard's (proximal IP [PIP] joint) nodes, sclerodactyly, telangiectasia, ischemic digital ulcers, pitting of the skin, nailfold abnormalities, periungual erythema, or psoriatic skin and nail lesions.[4,5] Swelling due to MCP synovitis may obliterate the normal concavity seen between the metacarpal heads. Digital flexor tenosynovitis produces a diffuse swelling (sausage finger) with tenderness over the volar aspect of the finger along the tendon sheath. MCP joint deformities include ulnar drift, volar subluxation, and flexion deformities. A boutonnière deformity is flexion of the PIP joint and hyperextension of the DIP joint (Fig. 72.6a). A swan-neck deformity describes hyperextension of the PIP joint and flexion of the DIP joint (see Fig. 72.6b). A Z-shaped deformity of the thumb (commonly seen in RA) involves flexion of the MCP joint and hyperextension of the IP joint (see Fig. 72.6c).[4] Telescoped shortening of the digits, produced by partial resorption of the phalanges with loss of the articulations secondary to psoriatic arthritis, RA (arthritis mutilans), or inflammatory arthritis conditions, may demonstrate concentric wrinkling of the skin (opera-glass hand).[4]

Differential diagnosis of joint swelling

It is important to try to distinguish between swelling related to the joint versus tenosynovial inflammation versus a localized mass. In tenosynovitis there is more passive than active range of motion. Arthritis of a joint usually produces a diffuse circumferential swelling. Extensor tenosynovitis usually demonstrates a longitudinal or oval dorsal swelling localized to the region of the tendon sheath at the wrist level. When the fingers are actively extended the distal margin of the swelling moves proximally and folds in, like a sheet being tucked under a mattress ("tuck" sign).[2,4] Tenosynovitis of the common flexor tendons will present as swelling on the volar aspect of the wrist just proximal to the carpal tunnel (volar "hot dog" sign).[4] The wrist is also a relatively common site for benign masses; ganglions may mimic the just-mentioned inflammatory processes (Fig. 72.7).

General examination

Dryness or cracking of fingertips can indicate nerve injury. Normal capillary refill is less than 2 seconds. Allen's test evaluates the vascular arches of the hand. Sensory function is evaluated in the fingertips by light touch and two-point discrimination using a paper clip or calipers. Normal two-point discrimination is less than 5 mm.[9]

Palpation can often localize a specific region with an underlying pathologic process. The wrist is best examined in slight flexion by palpating the dorsal surface of the wrist with the thumbs while supporting the wrist with the fingers of both hands.[2,3] This technique can gently identify and often distinguish an effusion, inflamed tenosynovium, or other dorsal wrist pathologic process. A similar technique is suited to the carpometacarpal (CMC) and MCP joints as well, where thick volar skin, subcutaneous tissue, and flexor tendons may make volar palpation less helpful. Dorsal fluctuance may indicate an effusion: pressure from one hand on one side of the joint will produce a fluid wave that will be transmitted to the second hand placed on the opposite side of the joint.[4]

The PIP and DIP joints are palpated for nodules, tenderness, capsular irregularities, or effusion using the thumbs and forefingers of both hands placed on opposite sides of the joint.[3] Although synovitis and other inflammatory processes may be tender, dorsal knuckle pads demonstrate non-tender skin thickening localized to the dorsal surface of the PIP joints.

Tendon nodules usually occur at the level of the metacarpal heads opposite the A1 pulleys. These can be palpated in the palm while the patient slowly flexes and extends the affected finger and may result in a "triggering" sensation.

Range of motion

Active motion should be assessed before passive manipulation. Lack of ability to flex or extend across a joint or malalignment with motion may indicate either underlying tendon disruption or displacement or joint subluxation/dislocation. As the digits are flexed, the fingertips should point toward the scaphoid. The distal nail tips should be aligned when the fingers are in a partially flexed position.

BONES AND JOINTS OF THE WRIST AND HAND

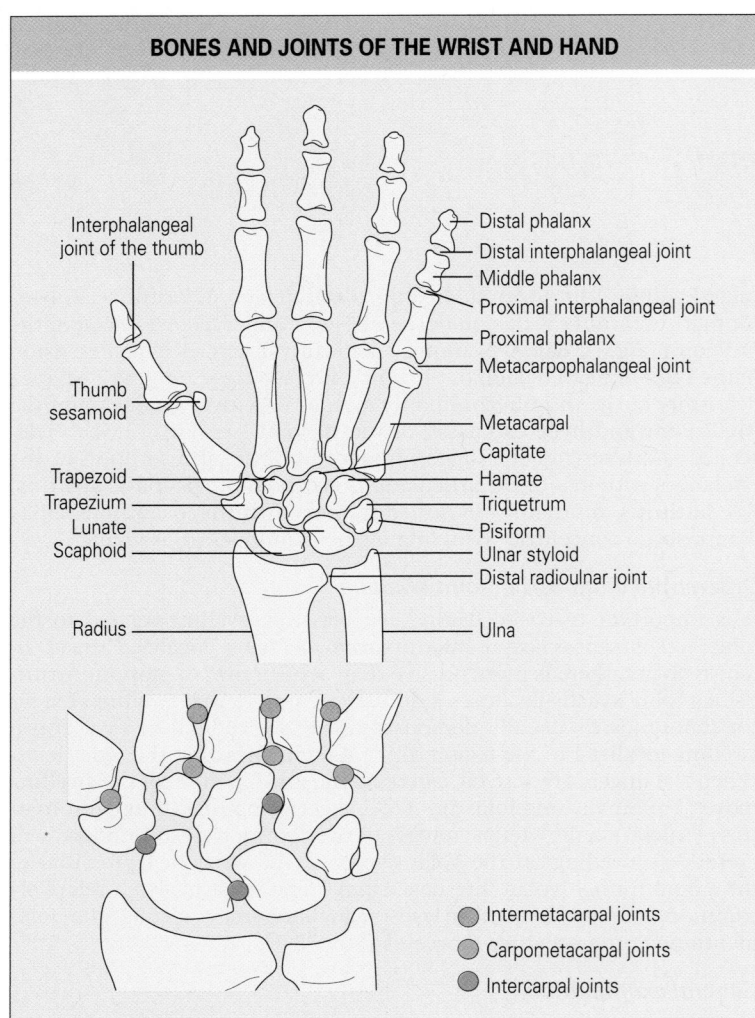

- Intermetacarpal joints
- Carpometacarpal joints
- Intercarpal joints

Fig. 72.1 Bones of the wrist and hand. *(Used with permission from Fam AG. The wrist and hand. In: Hochberg M, Silman A, et al, eds. Rheumatology, 3rd ed. St. Louis: Mosby, 2003:641-650.)*

FLEXOR TENDON SHEATHS OF THE WRIST AND FINGERS

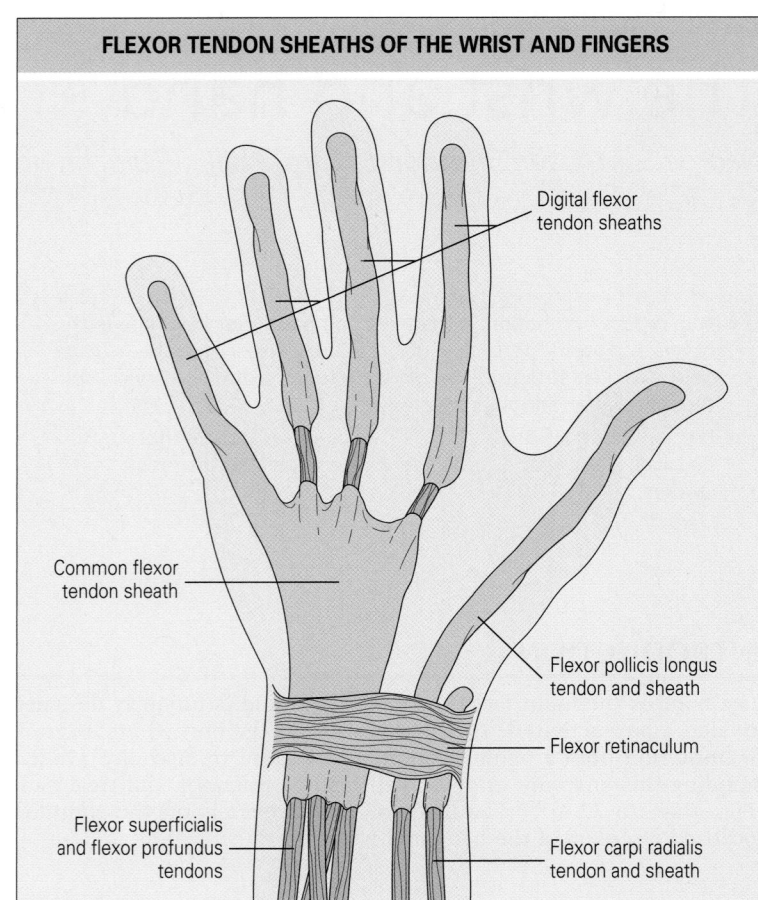

Fig. 72.2 Flexor tendon sheaths of the wrist and fingers. *(Used with permission from Fam AG. The wrist and hand. In: Hochberg M, Silman A, et al, eds. Rheumatology, 3rd ed. St. Louis: Mosby, 2003:641-650.)*

TENDON INSERTIONS OF THE FINGER

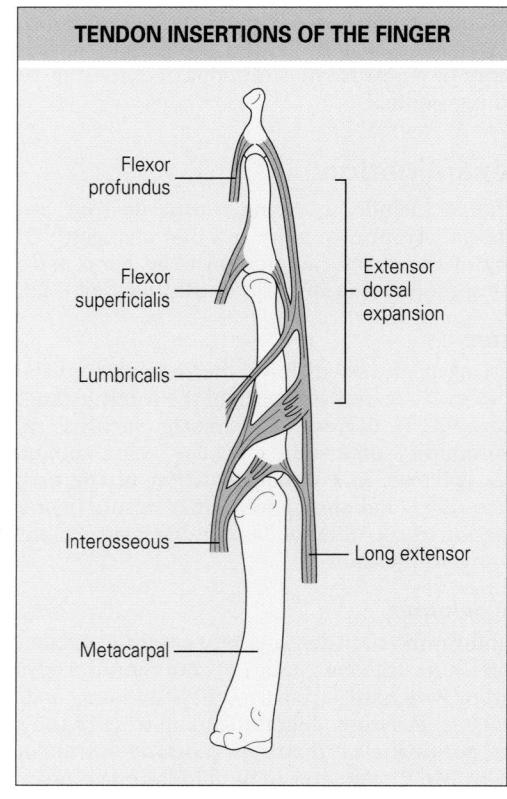

Fig. 72.3 Tendon insertions of the finger. *(Used with permission from Fam AG. The wrist and hand. In: Hochberg M, Silman A, et al, eds. Rheumatology, 3rd ed. St. Louis: Mosby, 2003:641-650.)*

Wrist motion should be assessed for flexion, extension, pronation, supination, and radial and ulnar deviation. The normal range is 65 to 80 degrees of flexion, 55 to 75 degrees of extension, 30 to 45 degrees of ulnar deviation, and 15 to 25 degrees of radial deviation.[10] The intercarpal joints and radiocarpal joint allow for wrist flexion and extension. Pronation and supination of the hand and forearm occur at the proximal and distal radioulnar joints. Full composite digital flexion should allow the fingertips to touch the palm opposite the MCP joints at the level of the distal palmar crease (see Fig. 72.5). Motion at the thumb CMC joint is variable within the population. The sum of thumb CMC + thumb MCP + thumb IP motion is about 180 degrees in most healthy people, but the proportion of motion at each joint is distributed differently so some people have stiffer CMC joints but looser MCP and IP joints, or vice versa. Disease may change these proportions. Patients with arthritis of the thumb CMC joint may compensate for lost CMC motion by hyperextending the thumb MCP joint to preserve the span of the first web space to encompass large objects.

Strength testing should include resisted motion across each joint. Resisted DIP flexion will test the strength of the flexor digitorum profundus, and individual digit testing of resisted PIP flexion while maintaining the other digits extended will evaluate flexor digitorum superficialis function. Isolated extension across the MCP, PIP, and DIP joints is important in patients with rheumatic disease to separate extrinsic and intrinsic extensor capabilities.

Joint stability of the MCP joint is evaluated by flexing to 90 degrees to place the radial and ulnar collateral ligaments on stretch and then attempting lateral motion while stabilizing the metacarpal joint. The

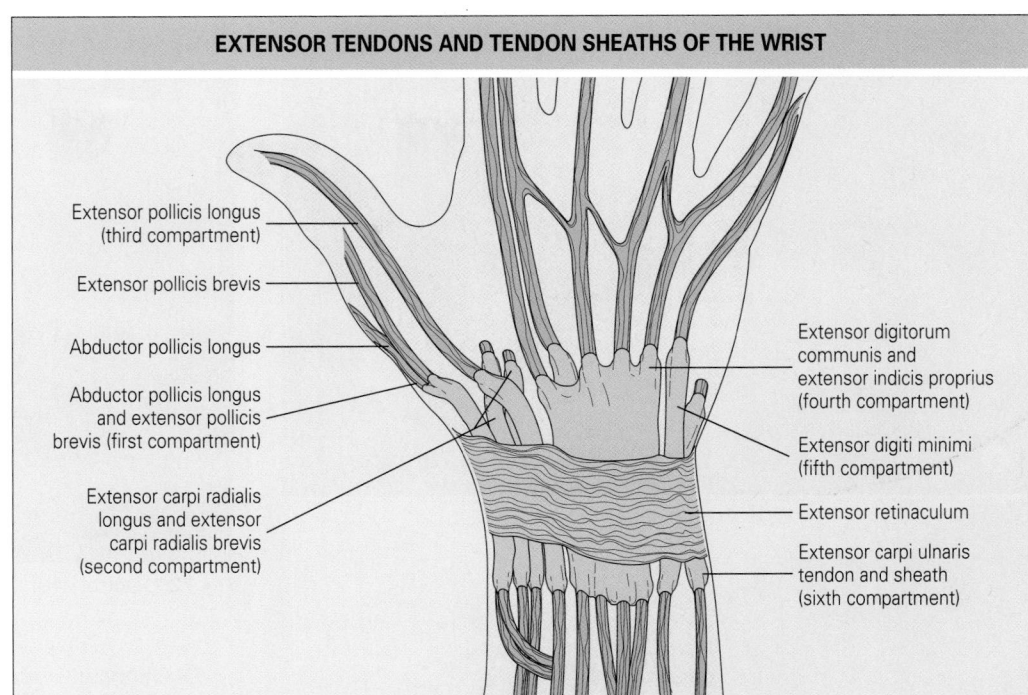

EXTENSOR TENDONS AND TENDON SHEATHS OF THE WRIST

Extensor pollicis longus (third compartment)

Extensor pollicis brevis

Abductor pollicis longus

Abductor pollicis longus and extensor pollicis brevis (first compartment)

Extensor carpi radialis longus and extensor carpi radialis brevis (second compartment)

Extensor digitorum communis and extensor indicis proprius (fourth compartment)

Extensor digiti minimi (fifth compartment)

Extensor retinaculum

Extensor carpi ulnaris tendon and sheath (sixth compartment)

Fig. 72.4 Extensor tendons and tendon sheaths of the wrist. *(Used with permission from Fam AG. The wrist and hand. In: Hochberg M, Silman A, et al, eds. Rheumatology, 3rd ed. St. Louis: Mosby, 2003:641-650.)*

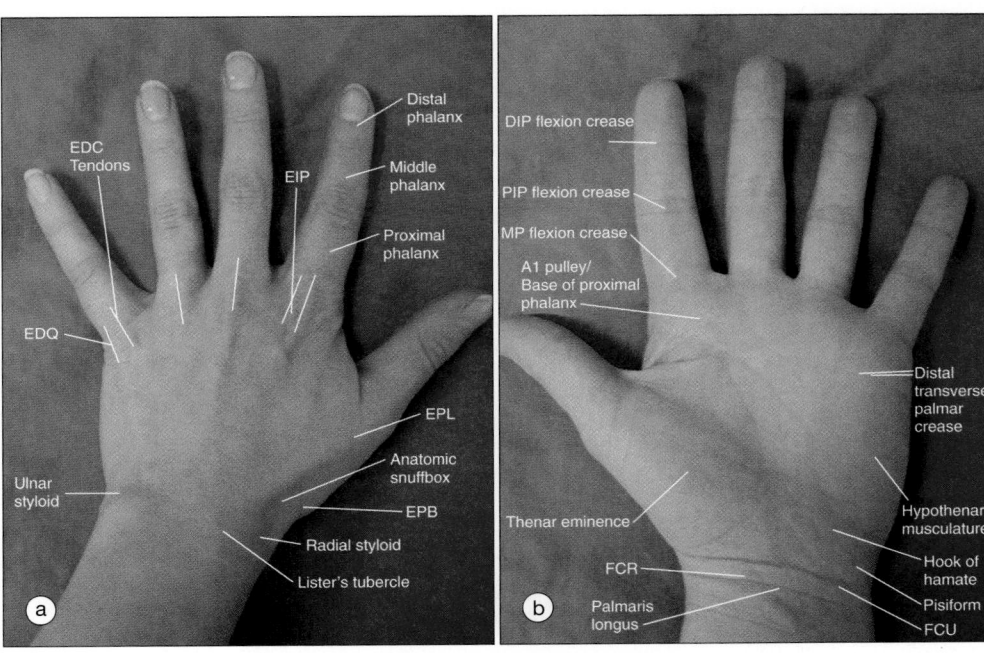

Fig. 72.5 Surface anatomy of the dorsal (a) and volar (b) wrist and hand. EPB, extensor pollicis brevis; EPL, extensor pollicis longus; EIP, extensor indicis proprius; EDC, extensor digitorum communis; EDQ, extensor digiti quinti; FCR, flexor carpi radialis; FCU, flexor carpi ulnaris; DIP, distal interphalangeal; PIP, proximal interphalangeal; MP, metacarpophalangeal. *(Used with permission from Earp BE, Waters PM. The wrist and hand. In: Frontera W, et al, eds. Clinical sports medicine—medical and rehabilitation aspects. Philadelphia: Elsevier Saunders, 2006.)*

stability of the radial and ulnar collateral ligaments of the PIP and DIP joints can be assessed by applying lateral stresses with the joint at 0 and 30 degrees of flexion.

Differential diagnosis of wrist and hand pain

Pain and functional disability in the wrist and hand may demonstrate common symptoms but actually relate to a wide range of underlying causes, including pathologic processes of the bones and joints of the wrist and hand, periarticular soft tissues, tendons, and peripheral neurovascular structures, or may be referred from the more proximal structures of the cervical spine, thoracic outlet, shoulder, or elbow. Table 72.1 details many disorders of the wrist and hand based on the site of origin of symptoms and the primary location. Precise diagnosis rests on a thorough history and physical examination and a few rationally selected diagnostic studies.

SPECIFIC DISORDERS OF THE WRIST AND HAND

Tenosynovitis

As the extrinsic tendons cross the wrist, they provide both power and dexterity to the hand. Each tendon passes through a tendon sheath, which is lined by an inner (visceral) synovial layer that adheres closely to the tendon and an outer (parietal) synovium that covers the inside of the fibrous tendon sheath.[4] The visceral and parietal synovial sheaths are attached by the mesotendon, through which pass the vessels and nerves to the tendon. The mesotendon may be less substantial in some tendon sheaths, represented by only threads or vinculae.[11] With aging, tendons become less elastic and less able to tolerate stresses without injury.[4]

Stenosing tenosynovitis is a usually idiopathic condition that results from inflammatory changes, with fibrosis and thickening of the tendon

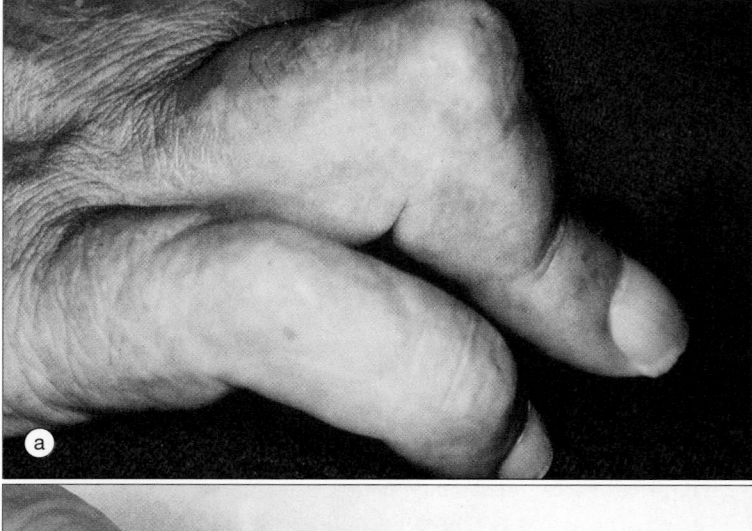

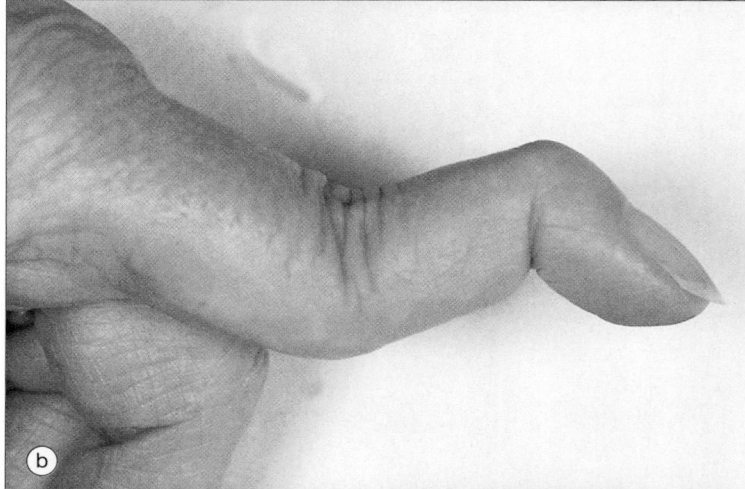

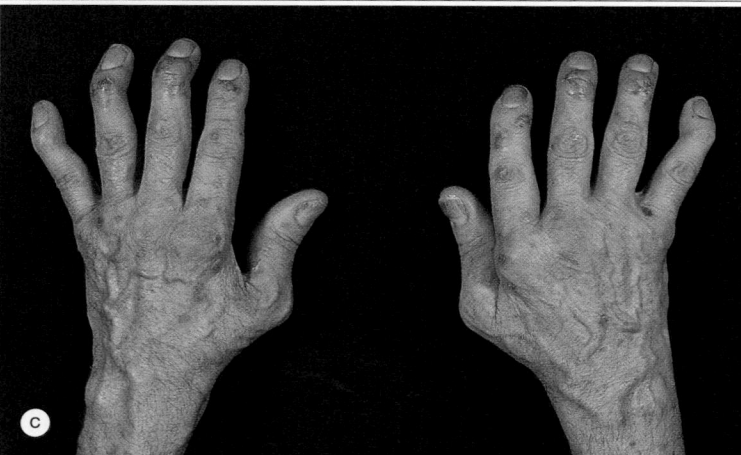

Fig. 72.6 Deformities of the fingers and thumb. (a) Boutonnière deformity. (b) Swan-neck deformity. (c) Z-shaped deformity of the thumb. *(Used with permission from Fam AG. The wrist and hand. In: Hochberg M, Silman A, et al, eds. Rheumatology, 3rd ed. St. Louis: Mosby, 2003:641-650.)*

sheath, and "fibrillar creep" of the tendon, in which the fibers become edematous and bunched.[11,12] The result is that tendon gliding is impaired and the patient may experience "catching," "triggering," or "locking" on either side of the retinacular ligament or pulley. Tenosynovitis is uncommonly related to a single traumatic event.

Patients with tenosynovitis most frequently describe symptoms of discomfort along the tendon, stiffness or lack of motion of the digit, and swelling. On examination, there will be tenderness along the affected tendon longitudinally and crepitus may be palpated, especially with motion. Provocative testing includes placing the tendon under tension, either by resisted muscular contraction or by passive stretching, which will result in an exacerbation of symptoms.

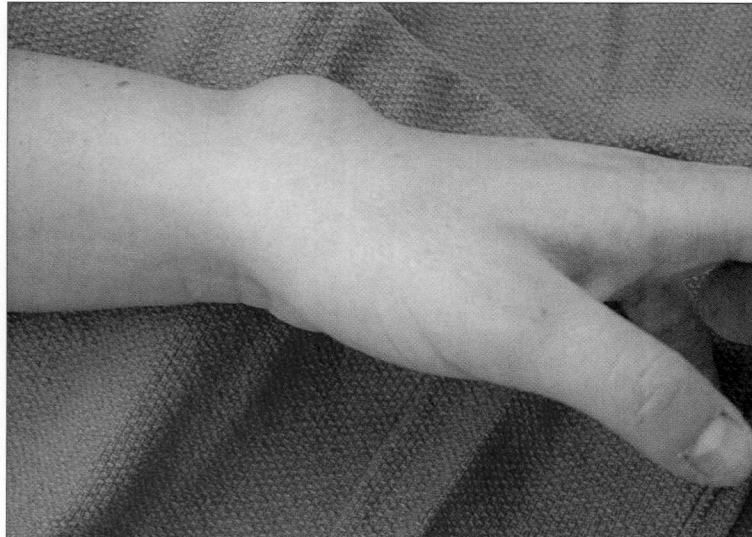

Fig. 72.7 Dorsal wrist ganglion.

DeQuervain's tenosynovitis, intersection syndrome, and trigger finger/thumb are all common conditions caused by "primary" tenosynovitis unrelated to an underlying medical condition.

Secondary causes of tenosynovitis are less common. These include RA, systemic lupus erythematosus, scleroderma, psoriatic arthritis, reactive arthritis, infection (bacterial, mycobacterial, fungal, and viral), microcrystalline disease (gout and calcium pyrophosphate and hydroxyapatite or calcific tenosynovitis), amyloid deposition, sarcoidosis, and pigmented villonodular tenosynovitis.[4]

De Quervain's syndrome

De Quervain's syndrome describes tenosynovitis of the first dorsal compartment tendons: the abductor pollicis longus (APL) and the extensor pollicis brevis (EPB) (see Fig. 72.4). It is most common in women between 30 and 50 years of age[4,11,13,14] and may occur in association with rheumatoid, psoriatic, or other inflammatory arthritis conditions, localized trauma, and pregnancy or during the postpartum period.[15,16] Repetitive activity that involves active thumb flexion while radially and ulnarly deviating the wrist may result in inflammation and subsequent thickening and stenosis of the tendon sheath as it passes over the radial styloid beneath the extensor retinaculum.[17] This may lead to significant radial-sided wrist pain with focal swelling and tenderness and crepitus 1 to 2 cm proximal to the radial styloid over these tendons (Fig. 72.8).[13] In Finklestein's test the thumb is flexed into the palm and then the wrist is gently ulnarly deviated, reproducing the focal discomfort.[18]

Symptoms of de Quervain's tenosynovitis may be similar to those of osteoarthritis of the first CMC joint or from intersection syndrome.

Treatment of patients with milder symptoms is usually with activity modification, rest, use of a long opponens splint with the IP joint free, and anti-inflammatory medication, if indicated.[19] In patients with more severe or persistent pain, corticosteroid injection may be beneficial, giving complete and lasting relief in about 70% of patients.[20-22] If conservative management fails to alleviate symptoms, surgical release of the first dorsal compartment, with or without tenosynovectomy, may be appropriate.[21] Multiple slips of the APL tendon and an interposed septum between the APL and EPB may exist, and these should be identified and released if found, because there is significant variability in anatomy in this region, with up to 76% of patients having more than one slip of the APL tendon and 60% having a dividing septum in the compartment.[23]

Intersection syndrome

Intersection syndrome is a similar condition related to tenosynovitis at the "intersection" between the first and second dorsal extensor

TABLE 72.1 DIFFERENTIAL DIAGNOSIS OF WRIST AND HAND PAIN

Articular	
Arthritis of the wrist, MCP, PIP and/or DIP due to:	Trauma, hypermobility, sprain RA (wrist, MCP, PIP joints) Osteoarthritis (first CMC, PIP and DIP joints) Other forms of arthritis: gout, psoriatic arthritis, infection Joint neoplasm
Periarticular	
Subcutaneous	RA nodules, gouty tophi, painful subcutaneous calcific nodules in scleroderma, glomus tumor of nail bed
Palmar fascia	Dupuytren's contracture
Tendon sheath	Wrist extensor tenosynovitis, including de Quervain's tenosynovitis and extensor carpi radialis tenosynovitis Wrist volar flexor tenosynovitis (including carpal tunnel syndrome) Thumb flexor tenosynovitis (trigger or snapping thumb) Finger flexor tenosynovitis (trigger finger) Pigmented villonodular tenosynovitis (giant cell tumor of the tendon sheath)
Acute calcific periarthritis Ganglion	Wrist, MCP, and rarely PIP and DIP
Osseous	
Bone lesions	Fractures, neoplasm, infection, osteonecrosis including Kienböck's disease (lunate) and Preiser's disease (scaphoid)
Neurologic	
Nerve entrapment syndromes	
Median nerve	Carpal tunnel syndrome (at wrist) Pronator teres syndrome (at pronator teres) Anterior interosseous nerve syndrome
Ulnar nerve	Cubital tunnel syndrome (at elbow) Guyon's canal (at wrist)
Posterior interosseous nerve syndrome	Radial nerve palsy (spiral groove syndrome)
Lower brachial plexus	Thoracic outlet syndrome, Pancoast's tumor
Cervical nerve roots	Herniated cervical disc, tumors
Spinal cord lesion	
Spinal tumors, syringomyelia	
Vascular	
Vasoplastic disorders with Raynaud's phenomenon Small- or large-vessel vasculitis	Scleroderma, occupational vibration syndrome, etc. With digital ischemia, ischemic ulcers, e.g., systemic lupus erythematosus, RA, and Takayasu's arthritis
Referred pain	
Cervical spine disorders Reflex sympathetic dystrophy syndrome (RSDS)	Shoulder-hand syndrome and causalgia
Cardiac	Angina pectoris

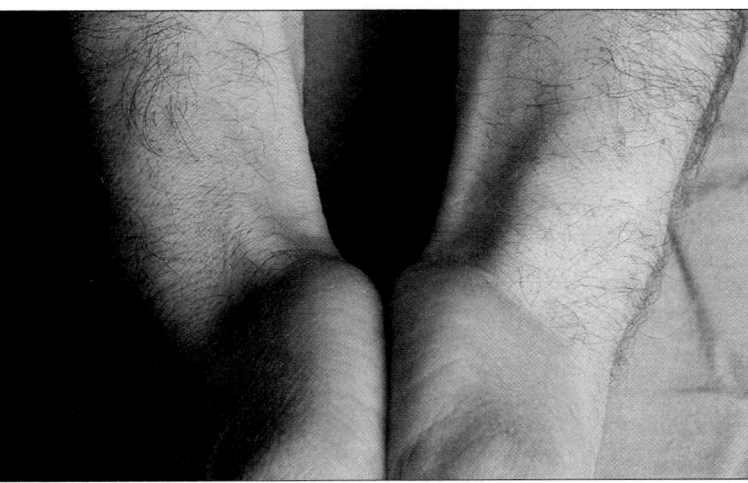

Fig. 72.8 DeQuervain's tenosynovitis of the wrist. *(Used with permission from Fam AG. The wrist and hand. In: Hochberg M, Silman A, et al, eds. Rheumatology, 3rd ed. St. Louis: Mosby, 2003:641-650.)*

respond well to splinting, rest, use of anti-inflammatory agents, and possibly an injection, depending on the severity and duration of symptoms. Surgical release can be performed in refractory cases, which entails release of the tendon sheaths of both compartments and excising the interposed bursal tissue.[25]

Trigger finger/thumb (stenosing digital tenosynovitis)

Trigger finger/thumb is one of the most common causes of pain and disability in the hand and can be found more frequently in patients with RA, diabetes mellitus, gout, and other disease entities that are associated with connective tissue disorders.[26] The disorder is commonly limited to one digit but may be seen in multiple digits over time.

The pathologic condition is a tenosynovitis that leads to fibrosis with constriction of the first annular pulley (A1) that overlies the MCP joint.[27-29] A tendon nodule may develop and can be felt as a palpable mass in the palm that moves with the tendon as the digit flexes and extends. The nodule and/or tendon sheath constriction interfere mechanically with normal tendon gliding. Intermittent locking of the digit in flexion may also develop, most frequently noted on awakening. Over time, not moving the joint can lead to flexion deformity.[4]

Early management may consist of modification of hand activities, heat therapy, gentle exercises, and anti-inflammatory medications as required.[27,28] Extension splinting of the affected digit at night prevents the painful locking of the digit most often found in the morning.

Sometimes, trigger fingers or thumbs may resolve spontaneously. Treatment with corticosteroid injection is often curative, with success rates up to 85%.[26,30-31] Insulin-dependent diabetes has been identified as a significant independent predictor for failure of relief from an injection alone.[32] If this fails, surgical release of the A1 pulley is indicated.[29,33]

Ganglions of the wrist and hand

Ganglions are cystic masses arising from a nearby joint capsule, tendon, or tendon sheath. They are the most common soft tissue tumor in the hand, comprising 50% to 75% of all masses, and they commonly occur in women in their 20s and 30s.[4] They are lined with synovial tissue and contain a clear, gelatinous fluid. They typically are thin-walled and may be unilocular or multilocular. Some may be quite large; others are occult, only seen on magnetic resonance imaging (see Fig. 72.7).

Ganglion cysts most commonly arise on the dorsal wrist (60%-70%) and can typically be traced by their stalk to the capsule overlying the scapholunate ligament.[34] The second most common location is the volar radiocarpal joint (20%).[4] Ganglions can also be found arising as cysts of tendon sheath in the region of the A1 pulley, as mucinous cysts typically related to DIP joint arthrosis, or along any of the extensor and flexor tendons. Ganglions can also be discovered within the

compartments. The APL and EPB cross over the second compartment tendons (extensor carpi radialis longus and brevis—ECRL and ECRB) at this point, located approximately 4 cm proximal to the wrist joint.[24,25] This syndrome, which results from frequent repetitive wrist movements most commonly seen in athletes (rowers, canoeists, weight lifters),[4] is associated with localized tenderness and swelling in that region and palpable or audible crepitus noted with wrist flexion and extension. Similar to de Quervain's tenosynovitis, most patients carpal tunnel and Guyon's canal, where they may cause symptoms of nerve compression.[35] Intraosseous ganglions may be difficult to diagnose based on plain radiography and physical examination alone, and further imaging studies such as computed tomography or magnetic resonance imaging may be helpful.[35]

Ganglions typically present as painless, well-circumscribed swellings on the dorsum of the wrist. They may cause mild to moderate discomfort when doing activities such as push-ups or other motions that load the wrist in an extended position. Most patients present because of the appearance of the ganglion rather than its functional limitation. They may note that the mass has changed in size over time, becoming larger for a while and then regressing. The mass may be palpably firm or soft, depending on how tense the cyst is when examined. Patients with symptoms of ulnar or median nerve compression should be closely evaluated because a space-occupying mass such as a ganglion in Guyon's canal or the carpal tunnel can elicit these symptoms.[35,36]

Radiographs of the affected region may demonstrate soft tissue swelling, but ultrasonography or MRI may be required to better delineate the ganglion and trace its origin back to a joint capsule or tendon sheath.[35]

Histologically, the ganglion comprises compressed collagen fibers partially lined by fibroblast-like cells, simulating synovium.[35] There is typically minimal inflammatory tissue. The stalk of the ganglion may take a quite circuitous path as it connects from the joint or tendon sheath to the main body of the cyst. The liquid inside a cyst is a clear, viscous, gelatinous-type fluid containing high levels of hyaluronic acid, glucosamine, albumin, and globulin.[4]

The etiology of ganglion cysts is poorly understood. There has been some association with trauma, although most patients cannot recall a specific traumatic event. It is thought that mild repetitive trauma may thin or tear the joint capsule or tendon sheath and allow for egress of fluid into a subcutaneous location. Arthrography has shown that intra-articular fluid will enter the cyst, but cystograms typically show that the cystic fluid does not re-enter the joint, indicating that the stalk must include a type of one-way valve.[37] The valvular mechanism may explain why aspiration or simple excision of the ganglion without removal of the stalk can result in a recurrence rate of 50%.[38]

Treatment of dorsal wrist ganglions begins with reassuring the patient that the condition does not require treatment unless it is causing the patient difficulties. Home remedies such as hitting the cyst with a large book are not recommended. Ganglion cysts may change size over time and can spontaneously disappear. Aspiration may lead to complete resolution but, as noted earlier, recurrence is quite common. Aspiration of cysts in some areas may be less indicated owing to the risk of damaging neurovascular structures. Surgery is indicated when symptomatic ganglions fail to respond to more conservative methods. After surgical excision, including eradication of the capsular stalk, recurrence is less than 5%.[38] Wrist ganglions have also been treated successfully with arthroscopic elimination of the stalk from within the joint.[39]

Carpal tunnel syndrome

Carpal tunnel syndrome usually presents as burning/tingling sensations and/or numbness over the volar aspect of the radial three digits. Pain at night and difficulty sleeping are commonly noted.

Uncommon in the young, carpal tunnel syndrome is most often an idiopathic disease of aging. There is an increase in the pressure on the nerve as it passes through the relatively restrictive carpal tunnel along with nine flexor tendons. Any swelling in this area due to tenosynovitis, fluid retention, trauma, or arthritis may decrease the space available for the nerve and can cause symptoms. Pregnancy, thyroid disease, rheumatoid and other inflammatory arthritis conditions, and diabetes are also associated with carpal tunnel syndrome.

On physical examination, patients may have decreased two-point discrimination in the median nerve distribution, and in later stages there may be weakness of the thenar musculature. Testing of the abductor pollicis brevis (APB) by resisted palmar abduction is important. Many patients may not be able to exactly articulate or distinguish the regions of sensory deficit, and some will have objective decreased two-point discrimination in the ulnar two digits as well, possibly related to pressure increases in Guyon's canal related to the underlying

carpal tunnel syndrome. Tenosynovitis of the digital flexors may be noted especially in inflammatory arthropathies. Provocative testing includes eliciting Tinel's sign (distally radiating altered sensibility with percussion of the median nerve just radial to the palmaris longus at the level of the volar wrist crease), Phalen's test (reproduction of symptoms with the wrist held in gravity-assisted flexion with the elbows extended for 60 seconds), and Durkin's test (reproduction of symptoms with continuous applied pressure over the carpal tunnel). Atrophy is a late finding associated with long-standing compression. Many patients respond to non-operative management with modification of activity, night-time splints, anti-inflammatory medications, and possibly corticosteroid injection. If this fails, nerve conduction testing should be undertaken to confirm the diagnosis. Surgical release of the carpal tunnel, with tenosynovectomy as indicated, may be indicated for symptom relief and to prevent further nerve damage. Surgery is the definitive treatment in older patients with chronic numbness, muscle weakness, and symptoms lasting for longer than 6 to 12 months. In patients with co-morbidities such as mucopolysaccharidoses, dysplasias, endocrine disorders, inflammatory conditions, and connective tissue abnormalities, a surgical procedure is more commonly necessary for treatment.[40]

Dupuytren's disease

Dupuytren's disease or contracture is a usually painless hereditary condition in which the palmar fascia (aponeurosis) becomes markedly thickened. It may cause small lumps or nodules to form deep to the skin at the base of the digits or in the palm, and pitting of the skin may be noticed.[41,42] The ring finger is most commonly affected, followed by the small and long fingers. Bilateral disease is not uncommon. The myofibroblast is the cell type associated with this condition. Contraction of the myofibroblasts in the palmar fascia leads to the early nodular findings. The skin may become involved through local invasion by fibroblastic cells, resulting in the aforementioned pitting (Fig. 72.9). Despite being called "local invasion," Dupuytren's disease is non-cancerous. In some patients the disorder may never progress from the nodular stage and thus may not require further medical treatment. Most patients will gradually, over months to many years, develop increasing thickening with extension into the digits, leading to restriction of motion and flexion contracture. The tendons and joints are not involved with the Dupuytren's tissue.

Many patients will not notice or complain of the condition until bands or cords have formed that gradually contract, causing the affected digits to become flexed toward the palm. Most patients present to the physician when they are unable to flatten their hand against a tabletop or other smooth surface or when it becomes difficult to put the hand into a pocket or glove (see Fig. 72.9).

The cause of Dupuytren's contracture is not well understood, and there is no definitive cure.[41,42] It is seen most frequently in white patients of Northern European descent. Men are affected seven times more often than women, and it is rarely seen in patients younger than 40.[4] Patients frequently can identify another family member who has had similar findings, indicating an autosomal dominant condition with variable penetrance. It has also been associated with smoking, alcohol abuse, vascular conditions, epilepsy, and diabetes.[41,42] Trauma has not been proven to be an associated cause.

Some patients are affected by Dupuytren's diathesis, a more severe and aggressive condition that can affect other parts of the body, including the soles of the feet, the popliteal fascia, knuckle pads, and the penis. These patients frequently develop symptoms at an earlier age than otherwise seen.

Treatment depends on how much contracture exists, how rapidly the contracture is progressing, and the functional disability the patient experiences. With mild disease, local heat, stretching exercises, and use of protective gloves may be helpful.[4,41-43] Splinting does not appear to alter the progression of the disease. In patients with a painful nodule, intralesional corticosteroid injections may provide symptomatic aid.[41-43] Newer studies on localized injections of collagenase, to break down the abnormal collagen, and intralesional infiltrations of interferon-γ, a cytokine produced by T-helper lymphocytes that inhibits fibroblastic proliferation and collagen formation, appear promising but are not yet considered proven treatment.[43,44] For patients with progressive

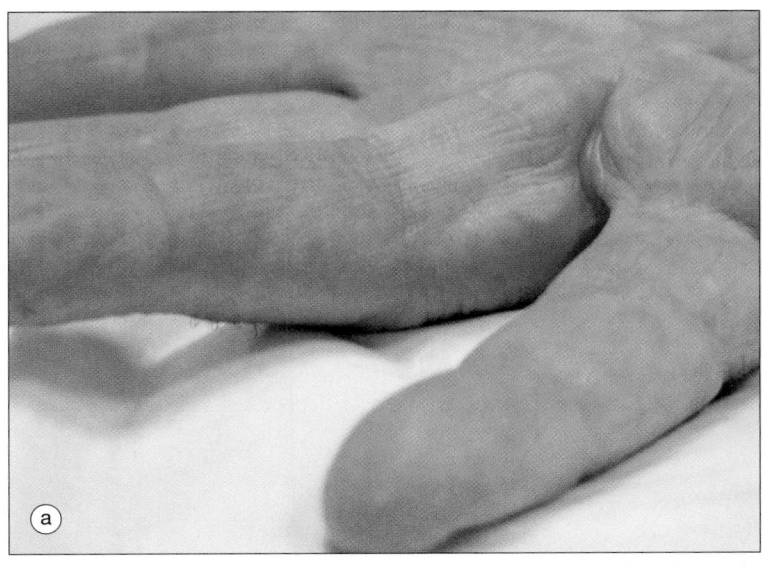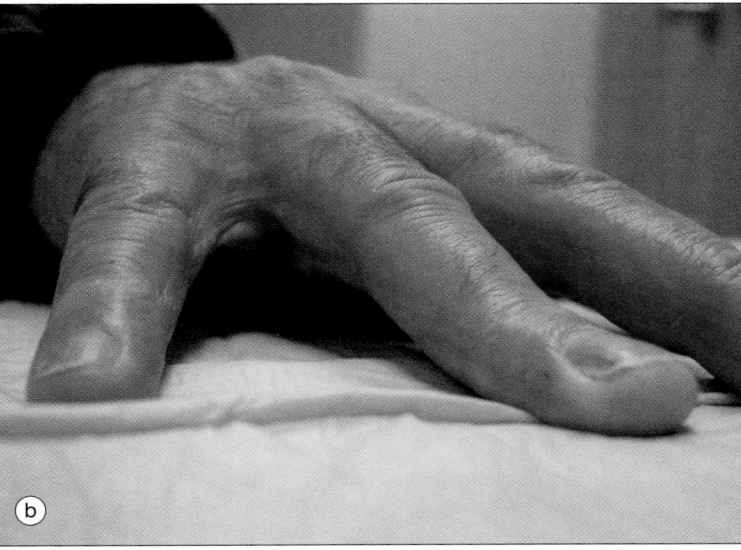

Fig. 72.9 Dupuytren's contracture of the ring finger. (a) Pitting of the skin and a longitudinal cord can be seen causing metacarpophalangeal (MCP) joint flexion. (b) Contracture/flexion deformity at the MCP joint keeps this patient from flattening his hand against a flat surface.

deformity or static contracture greater than 30 degrees at the MCP and/or PIP joints, or those with functional impairment, surgical treatment is indicated. This entails a limited or total palmar fasciectomy with or without skin grafting.[45] Despite successful surgical excision, the risk of recurrence in the same digits or new formation of disease in other digits is significant. This risk is increased in younger patients with aggressive bilateral disease, in those with a strong family history, and in patients with fibrotic lesions elsewhere in their bodies.[4,44] Sometimes the disease has progressed to the point that the MCP or PIP joint capsules have become significantly contracted, and, in these cases, full digital extension may not be possible without extensive joint release and neurovascular risk.

REFERENCES

1. Markison RE, Kilgore ES. Hand. In: Davis JH, ed. Clinical surgery. St. Louis: CV Mosby, 1987:2292-2353.
2. McMurtry RY, Little AH. The wrist. In: Little AH, ed. The rheumatological physical examination. Orlando, FL: Grune & Stratton, 1986:83-89.
3. Kauer JMG. Functional anatomy of the wrist. Clin Orthop 1980;149:9-20.
4. Fam AG. The wrist and hand. In: Hochberg MC, Silman AJ, Smolen JS, et al, eds. Rheumatology, 3rd ed. Philadelphia: Mosby, 2003:641-650.
5. McMurtry RY. The hand. In: Little AH, ed. The rheumatological physical examination. Orlando, FL: Grune & Stratton, 1986:91-100.
6. Williams PL, Warwick R, Dyson M, Bannister LH. Joints of the upper limb. In: Williams JL, Warwick, R, Dyson M, et al, eds. Gray's anatomy, 37th ed. Edinburgh: Churchill Livingstone, 1989:499-516.
7. Strauch B, de Moura W. Digital flexor tendon sheath: an anatomic study. J Hand Surg 1985;10:785-810.
8. American Society for Surgery of the Hand. The physical examination. In: The hand: primary care of common problems. New York: Churchill Livingstone, 1985:3-7.
9. American Society for Surgery of the Hand. History and general examination. In: The hand, examination and diagnosis, 2nd ed. New York: Churchill Livingstone, 1983:3-10.
10. Li ZM. The influence of wrist position on individual finger forces during forceful grip. J Hand Surg Am 2002;27:886-896.
11. Fam AG. Bursitis and tendinitis: a practical approach to diagnosis. Geriatrics 1992;8:35-42.
12. Thorson E, Szabo RM. Common tendinitis problems in the hand and forearm. Orthop Clin North Am 1992;23:65-74.
13. Canoso JJ. Bursitis, tenosynovitis, ganglions, and painful lesions of the wrist, elbow and hand. Curr Opin Rheumatol 1990;2:276-281.
14. Field JH. De Quervain's disease. Am Fam Physician 1979;20:103-104.
15. Gray RG, Gottlieb NL. Hand flexor tenosynovitis in rheumatoid arthritis: prevalence, distribution, and associated rheumatic features. Arthritis Rheum 1977;20:1003-1008.
16. Nygaard IE, Saltzman CL, Whitehouse MB, Hankin FM. Hand problems in pregnancy. Am Fam Physician 1989;39:123-126.
17. Clarke MT, Lyall HA, Grant JW, Matthewson MH. The histopathology of de Quervain's disease. J Hand Surg [Br] 1998;23:732-734.
18. Finkelstein H. Stenosing tendovaginitis at the radial styloid process. J Bone Joint Surg Am 1930;12:509-540.
19. Resnik CS. Wrist and hand injuries. Semin Musculoskelet Radiol 2000;4:193-204.
20. Witt J, Pess G, Gelberman RH. Treatment of de Quervain's tenosynovitis: a prospective study of the results of injection of steroids and immobilization in a splint. J Bone Joint Surg Am 1991;73:219-222.
21. Weiss A-PC, Akelman E, Tabatabai M. Treatment of de Quervain's disease. J Hand Surg [Am] 1994;19:595-598.
22. Lane LB, Boretz RS, Stuchin SA. Treatment of de Quervain's disease: role of conservative management. J Hand Surg [Br] 2001;26:258-260.
23. Bahm J, Szabo Z, Foucher G. The anatomy of de Quervain's disease: a study of operative findings. Int Orthop 1995;19:209-211.
24. Cooney WP. Sports injuries to the upper extremity. Postgrad Med 1984;76:45-50.
25. Grundberg AB, Keagan DS. Pathologic anatomy of the forearm: intersection syndrome. J Hand Surg [Am] 1985;10:299-302.
26. Saldana MJ. Trigger digits: diagnosis and treatment. J Am Acad Orthop Surg 2001;9:246-252.
27. Freiberg A, Mulholland RS, Levine R. Nonoperative treatment of trigger fingers and thumbs. J Hand Surg [Am] 1989;14:553-558.
28. Kraemer BA, Young VL, Arfken C. Stenosing flexor tenosynovitis. South Med J 1990;83:806-811.
29. Sampson SP, Badalamente MA, Hurst LC, Seidman J. Pathobiology of the human A1 pulley in trigger finger. J Hand Surg [Am] 1991;16:714-721.
30. Rhoades CE, Gelberman RH, Manjarris JF. Stenosing tenosynovitis of the fingers and thumb: results of a prospective trial of steroid injection and splinting. Clin Orthop 1984;190:236-238.
31. Anderson B, Kaye S. Treatment of flexor tenosynovitis of the hand "trigger finger" with corticosteroids: a prospective study of the response to local injection. Arch Intern Med 1991;151:153-156.
32. Rozental TD, Zurakowski D, Blazar PE. Trigger finger: prognostic indicators of recurrence following corticosteroid injection. J Bone Joint Surg Am 2008;90:1665-1672.
33. Patel MR, Bassini L. Trigger fingers and thumb: when to splint, inject or operate. J Hand Surg [Am] 1992;17:110-113.
34. Nelson CL, Sawmiller S, Phalen GS. Ganglions of the wrist and hand. J Bone Joint Surg Am 1972;54:1459-1464.
35. Subin GD, Mallon WJ, Urbaniak JR. Diagnosis of ganglion in Guyon's canal by magnetic resonance imaging. J Hand Surg [Am] 1989;14:640-643.
36. Kerrigan JJ, Bertoni JM, Jaeger SH. Ganglion cysts and carpal tunnel syndrome. J Hand Surg [Am] 1988;13:763-765.
37. Andreu L, Eiken O. Arthrographic studies of wrist ganglions. J Bone Joint Surg Am 1971;53:299-302.
38. Thornburg LE. Ganglions of the hand and wrist. J Am Acad Orthop Surg 1999;7:231-238.
39. Kang L, Akelman E, Weiss AP. Arthroscopic versus open dorsal ganglion excision: a prospective, randomized comparison of rates of recurrence and of residual pain. J Hand Surg [Am] 2008;33:471-475.
40. Van Meir N, De Smet L. Carpal tunnel syndrome in children. Acta Orthop Belg 2003;69:387-395.
41. Benson LS, Williams CS, Kahle M. Dupuytren's contracture. J Am Acad Orthop Surg 1998;6:24-35.
42. Rayan GM. Clinical presentations and types of Dupuytren's disease. Hand Clin 1999;15:87-96.
43. Hurst LC, Badalamente MA. Non-operative treatment of Dupuytren's disease. Hand Clin 1999;15:97-107.
44. Badalamente MA, Hurst LC. Efficacy and safety of injectable mixed collagenase subtypes in the treatment of Dupuytren's contracture. J Hand Surg [Am] 2007;32:767-774.
45. Armstrong JR, Hurren JS, Logan AM. Dermofasciectomy in the management of Dupuytren's disease. J Bone Joint Surg Br 2000;82:90-94.

The hip

Simon Görtz, Kevin B. Fricka, and William D. Bugbee

- Hip pain is a common symptom with diverse causes, but most cases can be diagnosed based on a careful history, a thorough physical examination, and appropriate radiologic studies.
- Although radiographic findings often lag behind actual pathologic changes, most intra-articular hip disorders can be effectively diagnosed radiographically and standard hip and pelvis views should be routinely obtained.
- The role of MRI in the diagnosis of hip pathology is evolving and increasingly reliable.
- Hip pain in a young, active individual should raise a high index of suspicion for a labral pathologic process.
- The differential diagnosis of unexplained hip pain should include osteonecrosis, even in lieu of apparent risk factors.
- Hip dysplasia describes bony dysmorphisms affecting either component of the hip joint owing to developmental anomalies, leading to decreased coverage of the femoral head.
- The concept of femoroacetabular impingement describes the situation of mechanical conflict between a morphologically abnormal proximal femur and/or acetabular rim.

FUNCTIONAL ANATOMY

Bony structures

The hip joint is a ball-and-socket synovial joint in which the round head of the femur articulates with the cup-shaped acetabulum (Figs. 73.1 and 73.2). Despite the resulting degree of stability, the hip joint possesses multiaxial mobility in the sagittal, transverse (rotational), and frontal planes, with the greatest freedom sagittally. The motion required for performing activities of daily living is flexion of at least 120 degrees, abduction of 20 degrees, and rotation of 20 degrees, although sports activities often necessitate a greater range of motion.[1]

The acetabular cup is approximately 45 degrees abducted and 15 degrees anteverted, encompassing the femoral head. This bony socket is augmented by the fibrocartilaginous labrum, which extends femoral coverage circumferentially around the perimeter of the acetabulum except at its base, where it continues as the transverse acetabular ligament. The articular cartilage surface of the acetabulum resembles a horseshoe, the central cavity of which is occupied by the pulvinar, a fat pad covered by synovium. The concave opening or acetabular fossa lies inferomedially and gives rise to the ligamentum teres, which inserts at the fovea capitis, a small divot in the medial femoral head. Although the fovea itself is devoid of cartilage, the remaining articulating two thirds of the femoral head possesses cartilage varying in thickness from 3 mm in the posterosuperior segment to 1 mm peripherally, reflecting varying degrees of weight-bearing demand (Fig. 73.3).

The proximal femur comprises the head/neck and intertrochanteric segments. In most hips the center of the femoral head lies at the level of the tip of the greater trochanter, the bony prominence where the gluteal muscles insert laterally. The smaller lesser trochanter is situated medially and serves as an insertion point for the hip flexors (iliopsoas). The head/neck segment lies about 15 degrees anteverted in relationship to the shaft of the femur. The normal neck shaft angle is between 125 and 140 degrees. *Coxa valga* is the term referred to when this angle increases above this range, and *coxa vara* is used when the angle decreases below this range (Fig. 73.4).

Joint capsule

Contributing to the stability of the hip joint is the strong and dense fibrous capsule. It attaches around the periphery of the acetabulum just outside the labrum and inferiorly along the transverse acetabular ligament, respectively. On the femur, the capsule inserts along the intertrochanteric line anteriorly and continues posteriorly just proximal to the intertrochanteric crest, resulting in more than 95% of the femoral neck being intracapsular. The capsule is reinforced by three prominent structures: the iliofemoral, the pubofemoral, and the ischiofemoral ligaments. The iliofemoral ligament, also referred to as the Y ligament of Bigelow, is the strongest and most important. It resembles the inverted letter "Y," originating at the anterior inferior iliac spine, with its diverging fibers fanning out over the anterior hip joint to insert distally along the intertrochanteric line. This ligament prevents excessive extension and helps maintain an erect posture because it is taut in extension and relaxed in flexion. The pubofemoral ligament strengthens the capsule inferiorly, whereas the ischiofemoral ligament reinforces the posterior capsule. These ligaments all coil and tighten in extension, making this the position of maximum stability for the hip joint.

Hip musculature

The hip joint and its surrounding musculature function to meet the requirements of efficient walking. To accomplish this, the hip girdle must maintain stability of the weight-bearing limb despite changes in limb and body position as it propels the body forward. The origins and insertions of the surrounding hip musculature are shown in Figures 73.1 and 73.2. The primary hip flexors are the iliopsoas, rectus femoris, and sartorius. The gluteus maximus and the hamstring muscles (long head of biceps femoris, semimembranosus, and semitendinosus) are the primary hip extensors. Abduction of the hip joint is accomplished by the gluteus medius and gluteus minimus. The adductor group consists of the adductor longus, adductor magnus, adductor brevis, gracilis, and pectineus. The short external rotators, which extend across the posterior aspect of the hip capsule, include the obturator internus and externus, the superior and inferior gemellus, the quadratus femoris, and the piriformis muscles. There are no primary internal rotators of the hip, but many muscles do so secondarily, such as the anterior fibers of the gluteus medius.

Bursae

Along with the many muscle groups surrounding the hip joint there are several prominent bursae to facilitate gliding of soft tissues over areas of potential friction. Because they are lined with synovial tissue, they may be affected by any of the inflammatory diseases that can affect the hip joint, such as rheumatoid arthritis and infectious or crystal-induced synovitis. Most commonly, however, bursitis and tendinitis around the hip are induced by trauma or repetitive microtrauma.

The trochanteric bursa lies between the gluteus maximus and the posterior lateral aspect of the greater trochanter, the iliopsoas bursa lies anteriorly between the hip capsule and the iliopsoas tendon, and the ischiogluteal lies posteriorly between the gluteus maximus and the ischial tuberosity.

Blood supply

Although the hip joint itself is well perfused, the tenuous vascular anatomy of the femoral head makes it highly susceptible to avascular necrosis resulting from dislocation, injury, or fracture to the femoral

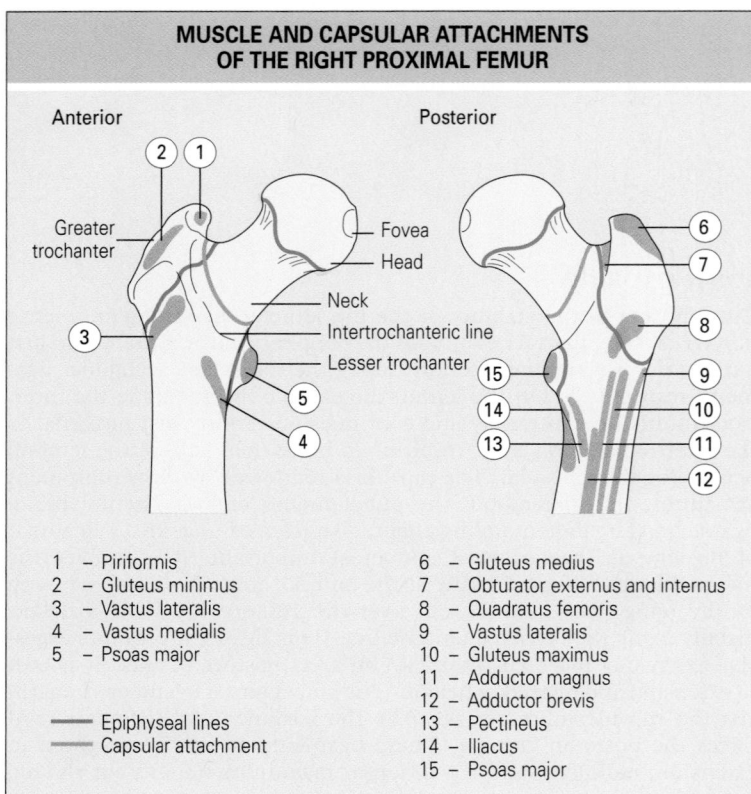

MUSCLE AND CAPSULAR ATTACHMENTS OF THE RIGHT PROXIMAL FEMUR

Anterior   Posterior

Greater trochanter
Fovea
Head
Neck
Intertrochanteric line
Lesser trochanter

1 – Piriformis
2 – Gluteus minimus
3 – Vastus lateralis
4 – Vastus medialis
5 – Psoas major

6 – Gluteus medius
7 – Obturator externus and internus
8 – Quadratus femoris
9 – Vastus lateralis
10 – Gluteus maximus
11 – Adductor magnus
12 – Adductor brevis
13 – Pectineus
14 – Iliacus
15 – Psoas major

——— Epiphyseal lines
——— Capsular attachment

Fig. 73.1 Anterior and posterior aspects of the proximal right femur, showing the attachments of the muscles and hip capsule.

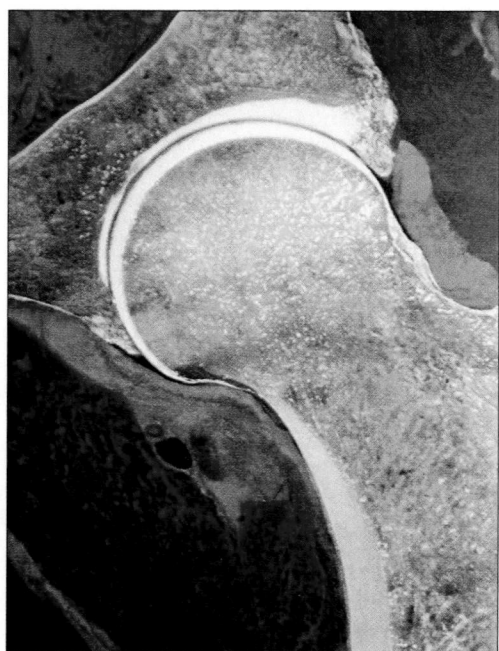

Fig. 73.3 Thickness variations of acetabular and femoral head cartilages.

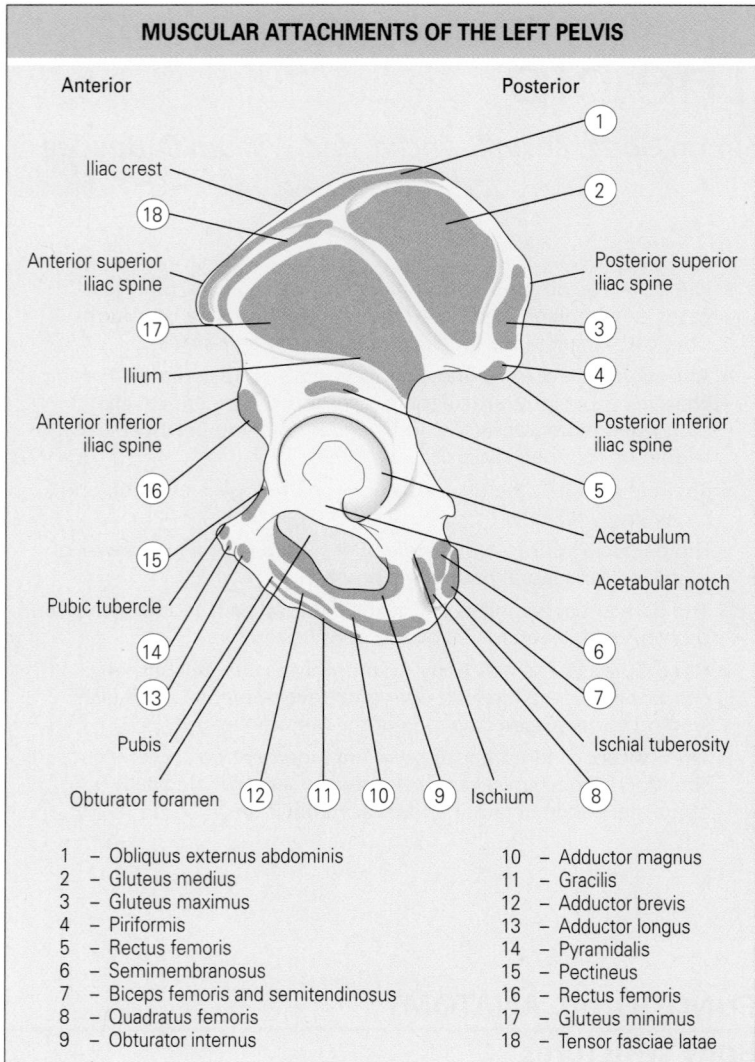

MUSCULAR ATTACHMENTS OF THE LEFT PELVIS

Anterior   Posterior

Iliac crest
Anterior superior iliac spine
Ilium
Anterior inferior iliac spine
Pubic tubercle
Pubis
Obturator foramen   Ischium

Posterior superior iliac spine
Posterior inferior iliac spine
Acetabulum
Acetabular notch
Ischial tuberosity

1 – Obliquus externus abdominis
2 – Gluteus medius
3 – Gluteus maximus
4 – Piriformis
5 – Rectus femoris
6 – Semimembranosus
7 – Biceps femoris and semitendinosus
8 – Quadratus femoris
9 – Obturator internus

10 – Adductor magnus
11 – Gracilis
12 – Adductor brevis
13 – Adductor longus
14 – Pyramidalis
15 – Pectineus
16 – Rectus femoris
17 – Gluteus minimus
18 – Tensor fasciae latae

Fig. 73.2 Muscular attachments of the left pelvis—lateral view.

CLINICAL EVALUATION

Hip pain is a common symptom with diverse causes, but most cases can be diagnosed based on a careful history, a thorough physical examination, and appropriate radiologic studies.

History

Elucidating the characteristics of the pain—including location, severity, and frequency—is paramount. Onset, alleviating or aggravating factors, and radiation of the pain up or down the leg should also be noted.

Location of pain

In the general sense, "hip pain" is often considered to include locations from the lower back, pelvic girdle, and proximal thigh. A classification of hip pain, based on the tissues primarily involved in specific disorders, is outlined in Table 73.1. Of these, osteoarthritis of the hip, trochanteric bursitis, and spinal disorders account for the vast majority of conditions seen in clinical practice. True intra-articular hip pathology will most often cause groin pain with occasional radiation to the knee, with the pain being referred along the continuation of the obturator and femoral nerves via their respective sensory articular branches in the hip capsule. Radiation to the anterior, medial, or lateral thigh is quite common. The most common cause of lateral pain is usually related to trochanteric bursitis. Lumbar pathologic processes most

neck. The femoral head is supplied by the terminal ascending branches of the medial femoral circumflex artery, a branch of the profunda femoris artery.[2,3] These small, delicate branches run along the posterior superior neck and perforate the femoral head near its base. In developing children, the metaphyseal and epiphyseal blood supplies are separate until physeal closure.[3]

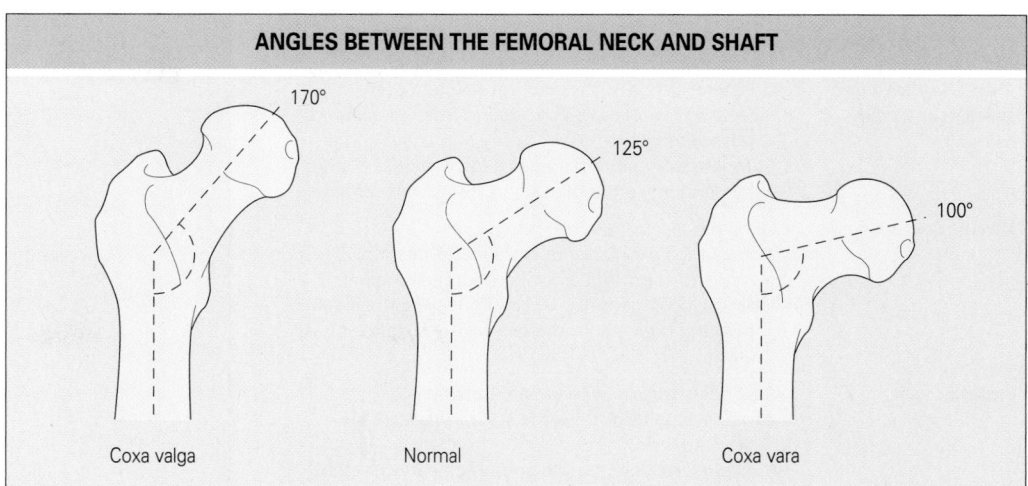

ANGLES BETWEEN THE FEMORAL NECK AND SHAFT

170°   125°   100°

Coxa valga   Normal   Coxa vara

Fig. 73.4 Neck-shaft angle of the proximal femur.

TABLE 73.1 DIFFERENTIAL DIAGNOSIS OF HIP PAIN	
Articular	**Periarticular**
Inflammatory joint diseases	Bursitis
Rheumatoid arthritis	Trochanteric
Spondyloarthropathies	Iliopsoas
Polymyalgia rheumatica	Ischiogluteal
Degenerative joint disease	Tendinitis
Primary osteoarthritis	Trochanteric
Secondary osteoarthritis	Adductor
Metabolic joint diseases	Acute calcific periarthritis
Gout	Heterotopic ossification
Pseudogout	**Osseous**
Ochronosis	Bone lesions
Hemochromatosis	Fractures
Wilson's disease	Neoplasms
Acromegaly	Infection
Femoroacetabular impingement	Osteonecrosis of the femoral head
Acetabular labral tear	Paget's disease
Infections	Metabolic bone disease
Tumors	Stress fracture
Benign	Transient osteoporosis
Pigmented villonodular sclerosis	In children:
Osteochondromatosis	Congenital dislocation of the hip
Malignant	Acetabular dysplasia
Synovial sarcoma	Coxa vara
Synovial metastasis	Slipped capital femoral epiphysis
Hemarthrosis	Legg-Calvé-Perthes disease
In children:	Rickets
Toxic synovitis	**Neurologic**
Juvenile chronic arthritis	Entrapment neuropathies
	Lateral femoral cutaneous nerve
	(meralgia paresthetica)
Referred pain	Lumbar nerve root compression
	L2, L3, and L4
Thoracolumbar spine	**Vascular**
Intra-abdominal structures	Atherosclerosis of aorta, iliac vessels
Retroperitoneal structures	

often refer pain to the posterior aspect of the hip area, and radicular symptoms usually radiate pain posteriorly along the buttock and below the knee. Posterior hip/buttock pain can also be referred from the sacroiliac joints. If associated with an insidious onset and severe morning stiffness that is relieved by activity, the diagnosis of sacroiliitis is usually considered. In those cases in which findings of the history and examination are inconclusive in distinguishing the source of pain, therapeutic corticosteroid injections into the lumbar epidural space or the sacroiliac joint can be helpful in differentiating lumbar disease, sacroiliitis, and hip pain.

Non-rheumatologic causes of hip pain

Somatic pain can be referred to the pelvic region from visceral pathologic processes, vascular ischemic conditions, and malignancies. Various intra-abdominal and retroperitoneal conditions can refer pain to the inguinal and anterior thigh region, and hernias can cause anterior groin pain. Iliopsoas abscess or other inflammatory processes can refer pain to the hip region. Episodic pain of the lower abdomen and flank region along with a characteristic history raises suspicion of nephrolithiasis. Underlying gynecologic conditions should be ruled out in female patients with unexplained hip pain.

Assessing characteristics and impact

The severity of the pain is best assessed in terms of the patient's ability to perform functional activities such as getting in and out of the car, climbing stairs, taking care of foot hygiene, or sitting comfortably in low chairs. The patient's recreational and occupational functions should be discussed, and any alterations in these activities should be sought. Prior treatments to include forms of self-treatment, physical therapy, and medications along with responses to these modalities must also be explored.

The onset and character of pain is worth noting in efforts to distinguish pain at rest, indicating an underlying more advanced degenerative process, from mechanical activity-related pain, suggesting soft tissue injury or early degenerative disease.

Further questioning to characterize the alleviating or aggravating factors can help differentiate certain disorders. Degenerative joint symptoms usually are exacerbated by activity and subside with rest. If the pain persists with rest, an infectious or inflammatory process should be suspected. Prolonged morning stiffness relieved by activity is typical of an inflammatory arthropathy. Pain aggravated by lying on the affected side is highly suggestive of trochanteric bursitis, whereas buttock pain aggravated by sitting suggests ischiogluteal bursitis. Posterior buttock pain with radiation can be associated with a lumbar pathologic process if symptoms arise with the spine in an upright or extended position, flexion or leaning forward alleviates the pain, and symptoms are not immediately resolved upon rest. A vascular cause should be suspected if the pain is aggravated with any muscular activity and relieved within minutes of rest. A careful history may reveal a previous catheterization or other trauma to the femoral vessels.

General inquiry

The history should also include questions about childhood hip disorders (sepsis, developmental dysplasia, Perthes' disease, slipped capital femoral epiphysis), previous problems/injuries regarding the hip, and previous treatment and/or surgery. A history of recent increase in activity should be questioned to rule out stress or overuse injuries. Significant medical factors potentially relating to hip disorders should be sought. These include prior history of trauma, corticosteroid use, alcohol use, coagulopathies, immune-mediated or inflammatory disorders, and prior malignancies. These can provide insight into conditions

TABLE 73.2 GAIT PATTERNS IN HIP PATHOLOGY	
Trendelenburg gait (abductor lurch)	Unilateral deficient abductor muscle function Individual compensates by leaning trunk over stance-phase limb Compensatory pattern, reduces forces across the hip by bringing center of gravity close to hip center
Circumduction gait	Weak hip flexor muscle function Normal hip flexor function accelerates the limb forward, important as swing phase initiated Individual compensates by circumducting the leg and pivoting body about the contralateral stance-phase limb
Antalgic gait	Secondary to pain with weight bearing Avoidance gait, shortens the stance phase of the affected limb Individual reduces motion and time bearing weight on painful limb.
Waddling gait	Bilateral abductor muscle weakness Rolling gait, the hips are not stabilized Individual shifts upper body laterally from side to side; these lateral shifts result from the hip bulging out laterally during stance phase with the opposite pelvis drooping secondary to abductor weakness.

such as avascular necrosis, pathologic fracture, or the inflammatory arthritides. General medical factors, including concurrent illnesses, medications, allergies, previous surgery, family history, and social history will provide the physician with a complete and thorough history.

Physical examination

Apart from a detailed examination of the hip, a thorough physical examination requires a detailed assessment of the relevant neurologic, muscular, and vascular systems. Neurologic examination, in addition to manual muscle testing, should include assessment of normal sensation to light touch and palpation. Vital signs including temperature should be recorded because septic arthritis should be ruled out in patients presenting with hip pain and fever.

Gait examination

Inspection is the first tenet of a thorough physical examination and begins with watching the patient walk into the examination room. The physician should evaluate the patient's gait and foot progression angle, how he or she rises from a chair, what type of posture is assumed, and how much disability is exhibited. Gait analysis is a complex science; nonetheless, a physician evaluating hip disorders should be able to assess and classify slight, moderate, and severe limps. There are two phases to the normal walking cycle: the weight-bearing stance phase, which begins with heel strike and ends with toe off, and the non–weight-bearing swing phase between toe off and heel strike. During the stance phase, the hip joint loads three times the body weight and the length of time spent in single-leg stance by the patient will provide insight into what type of limp is present. The various gait patterns with hip pathology are described in Table 73.2.

With the patient still standing, it is easy to assess for abductor weakness with Trendelenburg's test (Fig. 73.5). This is performed by having the patient stand on one leg. When the abductors are functioning well, they will contract on the stance limb and cause the contralateral pelvis to rise. However, with gluteus medius/abductor weakness or any condition that interferes with gluteus medius action (e.g., that caused by dislocation of the hip, coxa vara, or arthritis), the contralateral pelvis will not rise during one-legged stance and potentially will drop toward the stance side. The upper body will also shift over the stance limb to reduce muscular demand on the hip. This is described as a Trendelenburg sign, and most patients with this sign will exhibit a Trendelenburg gait (see Table 73.2).

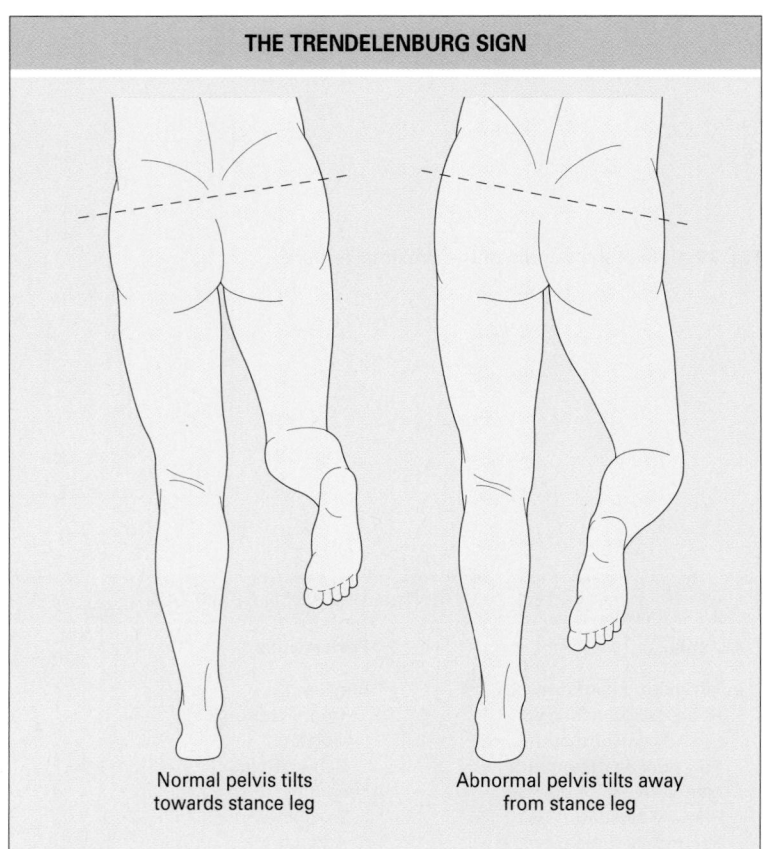

THE TRENDELENBURG SIGN

Normal pelvis tilts towards stance leg

Abnormal pelvis tilts away from stance leg

Fig. 73.5 The Trendelenburg sign. In a negative test, the pelvis tilts toward the stance leg because of adequate abductor contraction. In a positive test, the pelvis tilts away from the stance leg due to abductor weakness.

Inspection

The patient should be standing up and adequately disrobed for a proper examination. Any atrophy or asymmetry and previous surgical scars are noted. Assessment for pelvic obliquity is done by placing a finger above both iliac crests and checking if they are level. Pelvic obliquity suggests a leg-length discrepancy or a contracture of the hip causing compensatory obliquity. The resting posture of the hip that causes the least pressure within the joint is the flexed, abducted, and externally rotated posture. Patients with acute synovitis or inflammatory effusions may be resting in this position to help splint the pain.

Palpation

Palpation should begin in the standing position as well, because this makes it easier to access and feel all bony landmarks to include the iliac crest, the greater trochanter, ischial tuberosity, pubic symphysis, posterior superior iliac spine, and anterior superior iliac spine. Tenderness of some of these areas is suggestive of certain pathologic processes. Pain with palpation over the greater trochanter is very likely consistent with bursitis, and pain over the pubic symphysis can signal osteitis pubis or athletic pubalgia. The inguinal region should be examined as well for adenopathy, inguinal or femoral hernias, and the femoral artery pulse. Tenderness to palpation, pulsations, and/or a bruit may alert the clinician to a vascular cause arising from thrombosis or aneurysm formation of the iliac vessels and its branches.

Range of motion

The supine position is best to assess passive and active range of motion of the hip, both of which should be tested in all planes: flexion, extension, adduction, abduction, external rotation, and internal rotation. In the general population there is considerable variability in normal range of motion, so the examiner should always measure both sides for comparison,[4] keeping in mind that the comparison side can also exhibit bilateral pathologic processes. Normal flexion should reach between 100 and 135 degrees. Similarly, extension of the hip should reach from

PATRICK'S TEST (FABER TEST)

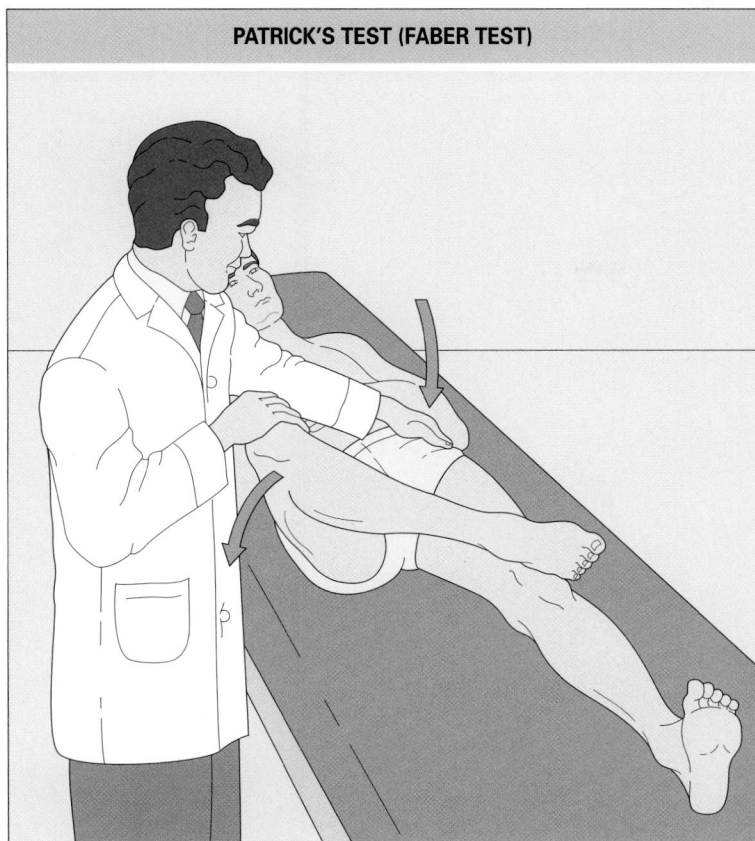

Fig. 73.6 Patrick's test (FABER test). The contralateral iliac crest is stabilized with downward pressure while lowering the ipsilateral flexed, abducted, and rotated leg. Groin pain suggests hip disease, whereas posterior pain suggests sacroiliac disease.

THE THOMAS TEST

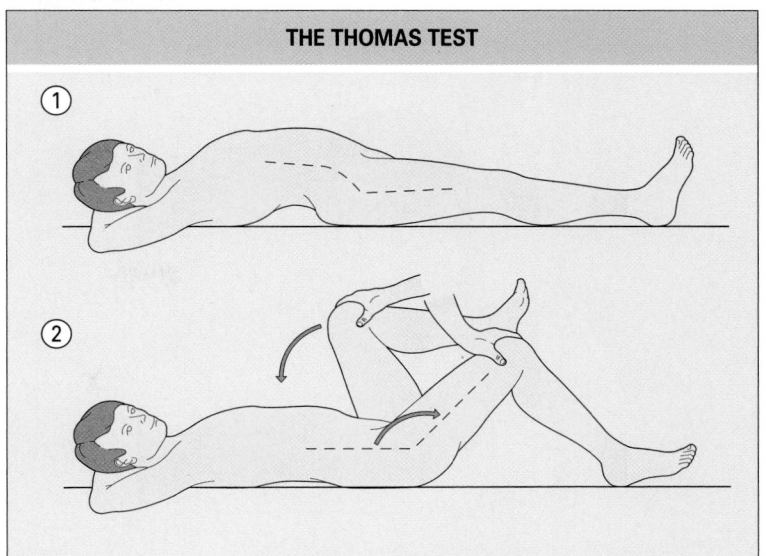

Fig. 73.7 The Thomas test. A flexion deformity of the hip is masked by an increased lumbar lordosis (1). Flexion of the contralateral hip flattens the lordosis and reveals the flexion deformity of the hip (2).

0 to between 15 and 30 degrees. Abduction and adduction testing is done with the patient supine, and stabilization of the pelvis must be performed to record accurate values. With testing, the patient's pelvis should be level and balanced and there should be no pelvic motion. Normal hip abduction should achieve 40 degrees, and adduction should be 30 degrees from neutral. Rotational motions of the hip are best measured with the hip flexed but also can be done with the hip extended using the log-roll maneuver, which is less sensitive but more specific when assessing for an intra-articular pathologic process. From the neutral position, internal rotation normally reaches between 30 and 40 degrees. External rotation is usually greater, reaching between 40 and 60 degrees. The first motions typically diminished in patients with hip arthrosis are internal rotation and abduction. An increase in internal rotation greater than normal is usually indicative of rotational deformities about the proximal femur, such as seen with increased femoral anteversion and dysplasia.

Special tests

The Patrick test (FABER test)
Patrick's test is helpful in detecting limited hip motion and distinguishing hip pain from sacroiliac disease. The test is sometimes referred to by the acronym FABER, derived from the initial letters of the movements that it evaluates (*f*lexion, *ab*duction, *e*xternal *r*otation) (Fig. 73.6).

With the patient lying supine, the knee and hip are flexed to 90 degrees and the foot of the examined extremity is placed on top of the opposite knee ("figure-4 position"). The thigh is then slowly fully abducted and externally rotated toward the examining table. The presence of groin pain, spasm, or limitation of movement is suggestive of a hip pathologic process. Patrick's test can also be used to stress the sacroiliac joints. To do so, one hand is placed on the abducted knee and the other on the opposite anterior superior iliac spine. Pain localized to the back when sudden pressure is applied simultaneously on each of these points suggests sacroiliac disease.[5]

The Stinchfield test
This test is performed from a supine position with the knee extended. The patient is asked to actively elevate the leg while gentle manual resistance is applied by the examiner. A positive response suggesting hip disease would be reproduction of pain in the groin, thigh, buttock, and occasionally the knee, a typical pattern related to the sensory innervation of the hip. Sometimes associated weakness is present.

The Thomas test
The Thomas test quantifies flexion contracture of the hip by stabilizing the pelvis and eliminating compensatory lumbar lordosis. With the patient lying supine, the thigh opposite the side to be tested is fully flexed on the abdomen to flatten the spine and stabilize the pelvis. This leg is then held in position, and the examined limb is allowed to extend to neutral. Failure of the hip under observation to lie flat on the examining table allows for easy measurement of the degree of fixed flexion (Fig. 73.7).

The Ober test
Ober's test evaluates the presence of contracture of the iliotibial band. With the patient lying on the unaffected side, the lower knee and hip are flexed to eliminate lumbar lordosis and then the upper leg is extended and abducted and slowly released from abduction to neutral. Failure of the extremity to fall on the table when the supporting hand is withdrawn suggests the presence of contracture of the iliotibial band (Fig. 73.8).

The Ely test
This test assesses for contracture of the rectus femoris muscle. The maneuver is performed with the patient prone. The knee is passively flexed, and if contractures are present the hip will spontaneously flex. Normally, the thigh will remain flat against the examination table. Both sides should be tested to allow a comparison between a normal and tight rectus femoris.

Apprehension tests
These sets of dynamic maneuvers are provocative tests that evaluate for the presence of labral pathologic processes. With the patient lying supine on the examination table, the examiner moves the patient's hip from a flexed, externally rotated and abducted position to an extended, internally rotated and adducted position. This set of motions tests for anterior labral disease, whereas reversing the maneuver will test for posterior disease. The presence of a labral disorder will usually produce a painful click or a searing sensation in the groin or deep anterolateral symptoms.[6] This should be compared with the contralateral side,

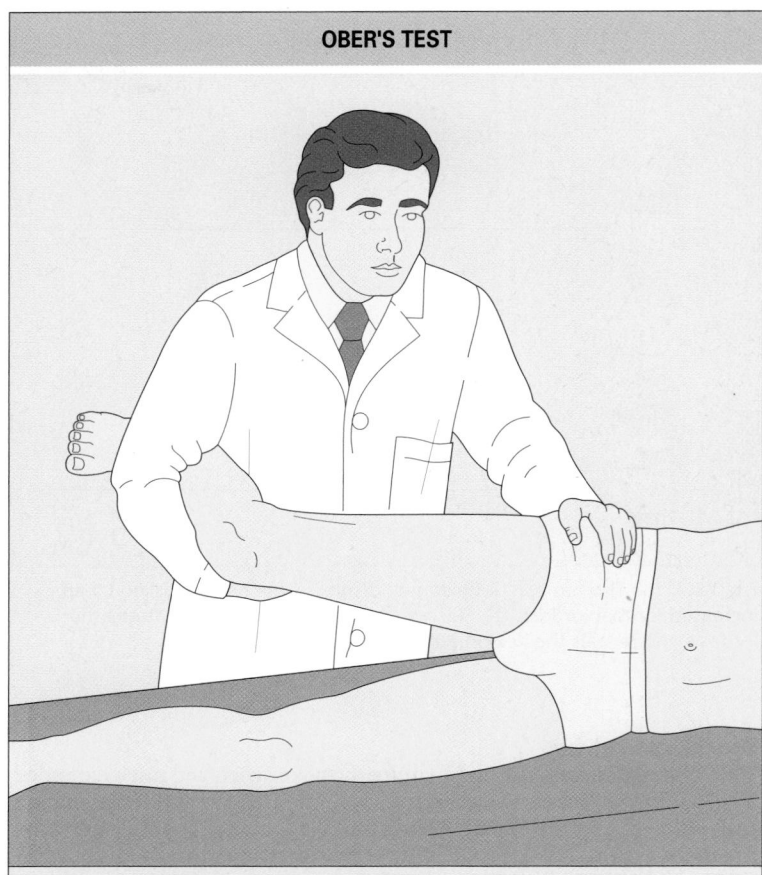

OBER'S TEST

Fig. 73.8 Ober's test. In the presence of contraction of the iliotibial band, the uppermost hip remains abducted and does not drop back toward the table when the leg is released.

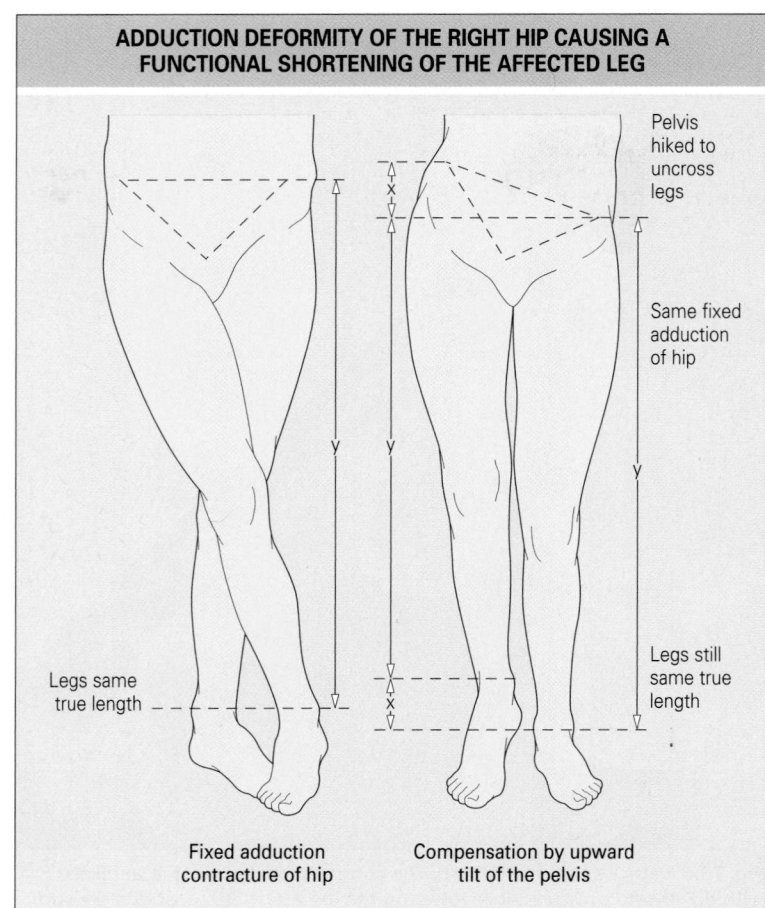

ADDUCTION DEFORMITY OF THE RIGHT HIP CAUSING A FUNCTIONAL SHORTENING OF THE AFFECTED LEG

Pelvis hiked to uncross legs

Same fixed adduction of hip

Legs still same true length

Legs same true length

Fixed adduction contracture of hip

Compensation by upward tilt of the pelvis

Fig. 73.9 Adduction deformity of the right hip causing a functional shortening of the affected leg.

because this set of motions may cause minor discomfort even in a healthy hip. The impingement test is a subset of apprehension maneuvers useful for assessing both femoroacetabular impingement (FAI) as well as hip dysplasia. With the hip in varying degrees of flexion (between 45 and 120 degrees), the hip is maximally adducted and internally rotated. Contact between the femoral neck and acetabular rim causes a shearing force at the labrum or chondral surface, eliciting symptoms that generally worsen with higher degrees of flexion.[6] Reversing this maneuver (hyperextension, external rotation, abduction in prone position) tests for posterior FAI, acetabular retroversion, and cartilage damage or contrecoup lesions.

Leg-length measurement

Measurements of leg length are best performed with the patient lying supine with the legs fully extended and placed 15 to 20 cm apart. Measurements are made for both true and apparent leg-length inequality. True leg-length measurements are made between fixed bony landmarks, from the anterior superior iliac spine to the middle of the lateral and medial malleolus. Apparent leg-length inequality is measured from a fixed point in the center of the body, usually the umbilicus, to the middle of the medial and lateral malleolus. Standing radiographs of the pelvis can be used to detect leg-length discrepancy as well. In the absence of contracture and pelvic obliquity, a difference in the height of the femoral heads indicates leg-length inequality.[7] A difference in length between the two legs of 1 cm or less usually is not clinically significant. An apparent (or functional) leg-length discrepancy on inspection may result from a pelvic tilt due to a scoliosis or contractures of the hip (Fig. 73.9). In these situations, measurements from the umbilicus will show an apparent shortening of the leg on the side with the higher pelvis. However, when measured from the anterior superior iliac spine, the legs will have the same length.

True leg-length discrepancy can be due to various congenital or acquired disorders. The most common of these include congenital

dislocation of the hip, acetabular dysplasia, Legg-Perthes disease, slipped capital femoral epiphysis, and congenital coxa vara. Leg-length discrepancy is associated with an increased incidence of trochanteric bursitis on the longer leg, which is typically held in adduction under a tilted pelvis. This results in decreased acetabular covering of the femoral head. The increased localized stress on the remaining weight-bearing area of the femoral head may contribute to the development of osteoarthritis.[8]

RADIOGRAPHIC EVALUATION

Plain radiography

Most intra-articular hip disorders can be effectively diagnosed radiographically. Thus, a complete evaluation of a patient with hip pain should include an anteroposterior view of the pelvis and either true cross-table or frog lateral views of the hip. Obtaining the pelvis view to include both the right and left hip makes a built-in comparison readily available (Fig. 73.10). The clinician should use these radiographs to assess for fractures, leg-length discrepancy, extent of degenerative/inflammatory arthropathy, evidence of dysplasia or other deformities, and the occurrence of abnormal calcification/ossification as seen with calcific bursitis or sacroiliitis, respectively. Although plain radiographs cannot be used to diagnose fluid in the hip joint, labral disease, chondral defects, unmineralized loose bodies, or tendon disorders, they may demonstrate clues to sources of referred pain, such as ureteral stones, lumbar disease, or severe calcific vascular disease.

Other imaging studies

Depending on what is learned from these initial radiographs, further imaging studies may be warranted. If the clinician is concerned about fluid in the hip joint, ultrasound evaluation is most efficient and cost

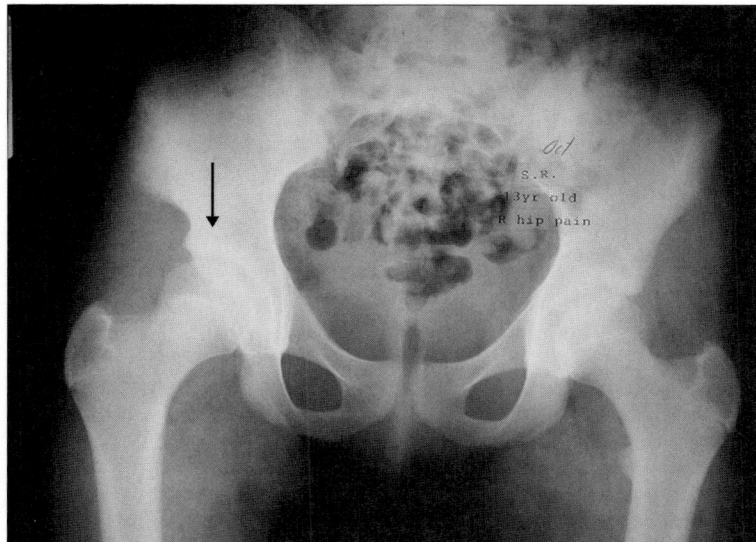

Fig. 73.10 Anteroposterior view of the pelvis demonstrating right hip dysplasia (arrow) and the normal contralateral hip. This view allows for a built-in comparison.

effective in determining the amount of fluid and the possible need for joint aspiration. Bone scans can be useful for evaluation of bone metabolism and osseous pathologic processes, such as occult femoral neck fractures. However, magnetic resonance imaging (MRI) has been shown to be more cost effective when evaluating for occult femoral neck fractures because of earlier detection.[9] The role of MRI in the diagnosis of hip disease is evolving and increasingly reliable, with the development of specialized protocols and high-resolution scanners employing bigger magnets. Although cost is an issue, MRI is most valuable in assessing for the presence of avascular necrosis of the femoral head but can also be used for detecting fluid in the hip joint or extra-articular soft tissue abnormalities. The addition of gadolinium arthrography has increased sensitivity in detecting intra-articular disorders, such as articular cartilage delamination or fragmentation and labral changes, including hypertrophy, tears, and associated paralabral cyst formation. Although computed tomography (CT) does not visualize soft tissue pathologic processes as well as MRI, it is superior when imaging bony architecture, alignment, and abnormalities. Three-dimensional rendered CT surface models especially are useful when assessing acetabular version, femoral alignment, and femoral head coverage.

Role of imaging in clinical practice

Although radiographic findings often lag behind actual pathologic changes and are unimpressive in early stages of disease, they will usually show characteristic changes over time and the diagnosis should pose little difficulty. For instance, it is easy to diagnose Paget's disease (abnormal bone remodeling showing coarsened trabeculae, a blastic appearance, and remodeled cortices) involving the femur and hip joint. Similarly, primary hip osteoarthritis is readily diagnosed in the presence of subchondral sclerosis, marginal osteophytes, and superolateral joint space narrowing. The same applies to late stages of osteonecrosis when flattening of the femoral head has occurred or to chondrocalcinosis when calcific deposits are visible in the hyaline cartilage and/or acetabular labrum. Inflammatory arthritis may be suspected when subchondral erosions, osteopenia, and minimal joint space narrowing without osteophytes or sclerosis are present. In other more difficult cases, radiographs are abnormal but are not characteristic of a specific disorder. A pathologic process of bone may be suspected by localized or diffuse osteopenia or sclerosis of the femoral head, neck, or acetabulum. Diagnosis and management are even less obvious when patients present with hip pain and normal radiographs. In those circumstances, further diagnostic modalities should be guided by a careful history and physical examination. A clinical suspicion of early osteonecrosis may require MRI for confirmation. An arthrogram may be helpful in documenting chondromatosis, synovial tumors, and labrum tears as well

as local thinning, cystic changes, delamination, or fragmentation of the cartilage in the weight-bearing areas of an early osteoarthritic joint. The suspicion of a chronic septic or crystal-induced synovitis would require joint aspiration for synovial fluid analysis. Limitation of hip movements in all directions in a diabetic patient suggests an adhesive capsulitis of the hip joint. The presence of systemic symptoms, such as fatigue, fever, weight loss, or worsening of pain at night suggests infection or malignancy.

SPECIFIC HIP DISORDERS

Hip disorders that occur as part of a generalized rheumatologic problem such as osteoarthritis, RA, and ankylosing spondylitis are discussed elsewhere in this volume. The focus here is on other conditions of the hip and hip region.

Hip dysplasia

Developmental dysplasia of the hip (DDH) describes bony dysmorphisms affecting either component of the hip joint owing to developmental anomalies, leading to decreased coverage of the femoral head (see Fig. 73.10).[10] Excessive vertical slope of the acetabulum with according valgus angulation of the femoral neck is generally considered a hallmark of classic dysplasia and can be associated with excessive anteversion or retroversion of the acetabulum. The femoral head is commonly aspherical and situated laterally in the acetabulum, comprising the labrum part of the weight-bearing surface of the acetabulum.[11] The vertical center edge (CE) angle of Wiberg can be determined from an anteroposterior radiograph to assess the amount of femoral head coverage. The CE angle is measured between a line connecting the lateral edge to the center of the femoral head and the vertical line extending from the center of the head. A normal CE angle is more than 25 degrees, while it is less than 20 degrees in the dysplastic hip. Values between 20 and 25 degrees should be considered borderline dysplastic. Likewise, a vertical center anterior angle can be derived from a "false profile" lateral view to measure sagittal version and assess anterior coverage of the head.[10] Labral tears are a common feature in hips with subtle or severe dysplasia.[11] Thus, any patient with a known labral tear should be carefully evaluated for underlying hip dysplasia.

Femoroacetabular impingement

The concept of femoroacetabular impingement (FAI) describes the situation of mechanical conflict between a morphologically abnormal proximal femur and/or acetabular rim. The condition occurs when the proximal femur repeatedly comes into contact with the native acetabular rim during normal hip range of motion. Repetitive abutment, especially during terminal flexion and internal rotation, leads to cumulative damage to the labrum and, subsequently, delamination or ulceration of the articular cartilage overlying the adjacent acetabular rim and, occasionally, contrecoup lesions on the opposite, usually posterior, side of the acetabulum.[12]

As a distinct entity, FAI has been suggested to be a preosteoarthritic mechanism. Early diagnosis and surgical management are imperative to delay degenerative changes associated with these conditions. FAI is most prevalent in young, active patients. Physical examination should include evaluation of gait and foot progression angle, as well as leg-length measurement, hip range of motion, and abductor strength. Imaging studies, including plain radiographs and magnetic resonance arthrography, aid in accurate diagnosis. Surgical treatment options include surgical hip dislocation, periacetabular osteotomy, and hip arthroscopy.[12]

Subtypes

Although two types of FAI, cam and pincer, are recognized and defined by their cause, a combination of both types is commonly seen: In cam-type FAI, the primary site of malformation is the femur, whereas in pincer-type FAI it is the acetabular component that is dysmorphologic. The cam type is characterized by an increased radius of the neck/head junction with a loss of sphericity, either primarily due to lack of head offset or due to bony buildup secondary to pincer type FAI. Repetitive trauma to the labrum due to impingement by the neck segment in flexion and internal rotation results in damage to cartilage and

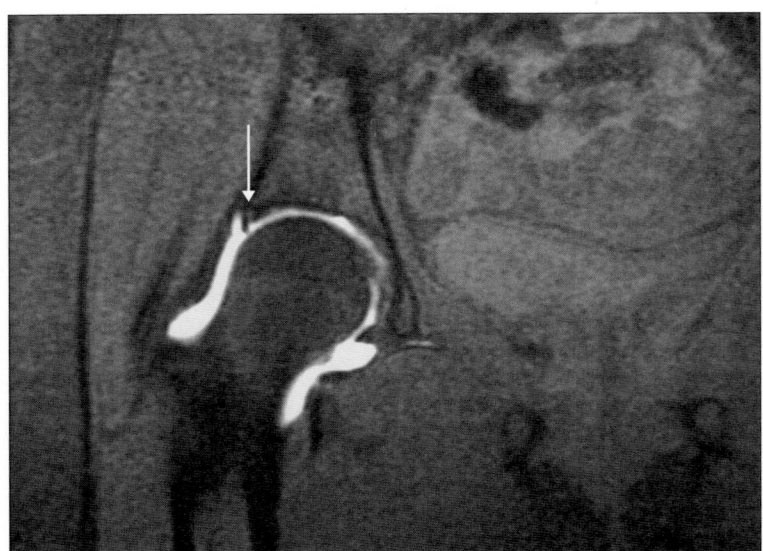

Fig. 73.11 MRI arthrogram of the hip demonstrating slight effusion and superior labral tear (arrow).

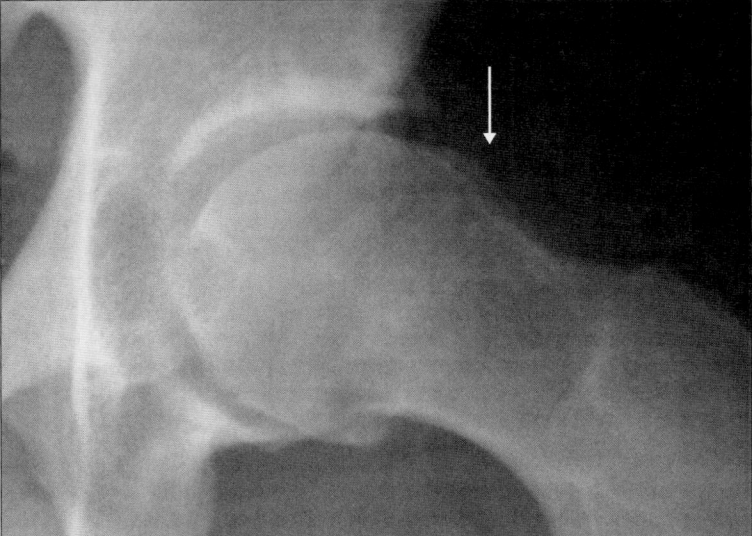

Fig. 73.12 Lateral view of the left hip demonstrating bony buildup (arrow) with loss of sphericity at the femoral head/neck junction.

ultimately labral-osseous separation, mostly in the anterosuperior region (Fig. 73.11). Conditions associated with development of cam-type impingement include femoral neck retroversion and a history of slipped capital femoral epiphysis (SCFE) or Perthes' disease.[13] Pincer-type FAI results from lack of acetabular clearance, leading to linear contact between the anterior acetabular rim and head/neck junction. The resulting relative overcoverage of the femoral head causes increased impaction and, ultimately, failure of the labrum and, with subsequent rim ossification, worsening overcoverage and abutment, which can lead to kissing lesions on the femoral neck. Associated conditions include coxa profunda, protrusion, acetabular retroversion, and a history of acetabular fracture.[12] Demographically, cam impingement typically presents in young athletic males with labral tears, whereas pincer impingement is more common in middle-aged active women and usually has a more benign course.

Clinical features

Typically, patients will experience intermittent, progressive, activity-related groin pain with occasional mechanical symptoms. Pain in the position of impingement (flexion, internal rotation, adduction), especially after prolonged sitting, is commonly present. Physical examination findings include decreased motion in internal rotation and adduction in flexion, generally with a positive impingement test.

Imaging

Radiographic evidence is usually subtle, but close scrutiny may reveal bony prominence of the femoral head/neck segment (Fig. 73.12) as well as flattening and reduced offset of the anterolateral neck (pistol grip deformity). Rim ossification/os acetabuli and herniation pits can also be assessed and allow conclusions as to the acetabular cartilage status at the impingement site.[12] Suspicion of FAI in the presence of inconclusive screening radiographs should be followed up by special lateral views and/or three-dimensional tomography with surface rendering, which usually is accurate in diagnosing an underlying pathologic process.

Treatment

Non-arthroplasty surgical options include arthroscopy with débridement of the affected soft tissues and/or surgical hip dislocation with osteoplasty of a femoral neck bump or hypertrophic acetabular lip to restore the clearance mechanism of the hip.

Transient osteoporosis

Transient osteoporosis of the hip is a rare condition that affects young and middle-aged men and women in the third trimester of pregnancy.[14] Patients will usually walk with a limp and complain of limited range

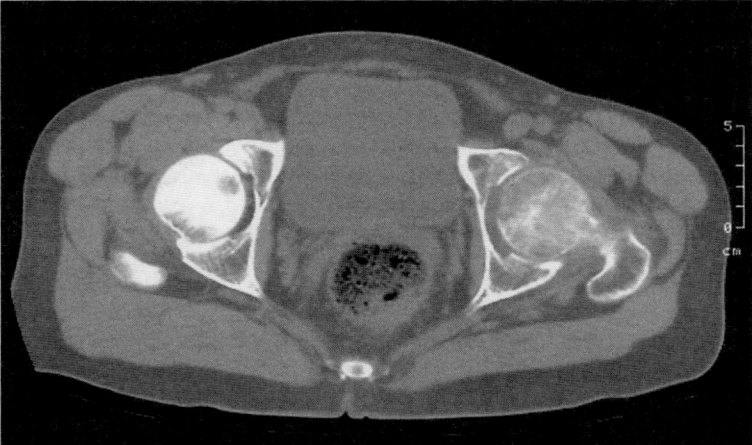

Fig. 73.13 Marked osteoporosis of the head of the left femur in a case of transient painful osteoporosis of the hip.

of motion, functional disability, and groin pain, sometimes referred to the anterior knee on weight bearing. The erythrocyte sedimentation rate (ESR) is occasionally raised, but this can be non-specific during pregnancy. Differentiating transient osteoporosis from avascular necrosis is important to prevent unnecessary surgery and to ensure appropriate treatment.[15] Most patients with avascular necrosis will have classic risk factors associated with this entity. The cause of transient osteoporosis is unknown, but vascular and neurologic disturbances have been proposed as possible pathogenic mechanisms.[16] The diagnosis is usually one of exclusion of more common entities and remains dependent on clinical recognition and radiographic evidence.

Imaging

Plain radiographs demonstrate pronounced osteopenia of the proximal femur with attenuation of the subchondral cortex without evidence of joint space narrowing or destruction. Isotope scans may be positive much earlier in revealing demineralization of the femoral head. MRI also demonstrates characteristic changes, including low signal on T1-weighted sequences in the proximal femur without localization to the femoral head (Fig. 73.13).[17] Short tau inversion recovery sequences will show very high signal in the affected areas, and often a joint effusion is present. Diffuse MRI signal changes throughout the proximal femur without focal changes isolated to the femoral head are suggestive of a transient process rather than a chronic process such as avascular necrosis.

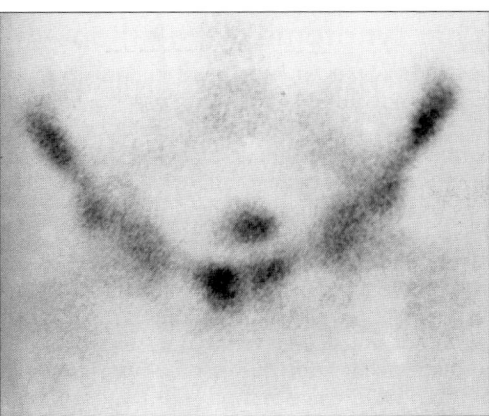

Fig. 73.14 Osteitis pubis. This bone scan demonstrates increased retention of isotope at the symphysis pubis, suggesting osteitis pubis.

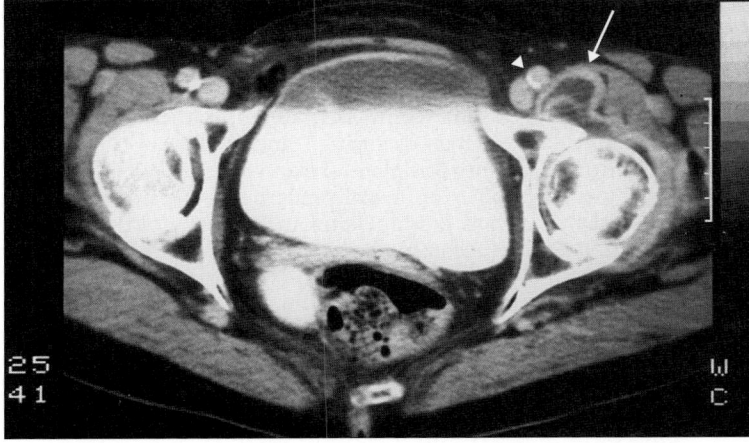

Fig. 73.15 CT scan of a patient with rheumatoid arthritis. The scan shows an enlarged fluid-filled iliopsoas bursa (arrow) communicating with the hip joint and displacing the neurovascular bundle (arrowhead). *(Used with permission from Letourneau L, Dessureault M, Carette S. Rheumatoid iliopsoas bursitis presenting as unilateral femoral nerve palsy. J Rheumatol 1991;18:462-463.)*

Course and treatment

Transient osteoporosis may present as severe symptoms, but spontaneous resolution in 2 to 9 months is usually the case with gradual disappearance of radiographic osteopenia paralleling clinical improvement.

Patients should be prescribed limited weight bearing, range of motion exercises, progressive ambulation, and analgesics. In pregnant patients, radiographs and non-steroidal anti-inflammatory agents (NSAIDs) should also be avoided if possible. Anti-resorptive agents may shorten the disease course; calcitonin has shown promise in decreasing the duration of the disease and in one study demonstrated complete resolution of symptoms within 6 to 9 weeks.[18] Surgery, involving core decompression of the hip, has also been shown to provide symptom relief and shorten the duration of the disease.[19]

Osteitis pubis

Osteitis pubis is considered the most common inflammatory disease of the pubic symphysis and typically is a self-limiting condition. Although its pathogenesis is unknown, many authors believe that periosteal trauma is the initiating event.[20] The condition is seen more frequently in men, but with a greater number of women participating in athletics the incidence in females is rising. The typical symptom of osteitis pubis is pain in the groin/lower abdomen region, with major differential diagnoses including osteomyelitis and sports hernia. Patients may have difficulty ambulating, sometimes presenting with a characteristic "waddling gait."[20] The pain is exacerbated by athletic activity or even Valsalva maneuvers and is partially relieved by rest. On examination, there is marked tenderness over the symphysis pubis, rectus insertion, and adductor longus, with painful and decreased bilateral hip abduction and pain on lateral compression of the pelvis. A history of recent (within 3 weeks) athletic injury, childbirth, or pelvis surgery should provide the clinician with a high index of suspicion.

A low-grade fever and elevated ESR are quite common. Plain radiographic findings such as reactive sclerosis, osteolysis, and rarefaction lag behind clinical symptoms by about 4 weeks. Therefore, initial radiographs are usually normal. Bone scintigraphy is always positive with enhanced uptake of the pubic bone and is probably the single most useful test (Fig. 73.14). MRI demonstrates bone marrow lesions within the os pubis, joint surface irregularity, and, occasionally, inflammation within the rectus insertion or the adductor longus musculature.

Most cases are self-limiting and the prognosis for recovery is good, although it can be lengthy. Initial management should consist of rest, ice, compression, physical therapy, and a trial of NSAIDs. Physical therapy should involve strengthening the core musculature as well as improving hip range of motion. Systemic oral corticosteroids and corticosteroid injections have been used with variable success in patients with prolonged symptoms.[21] Refractory cases of over 6 months' duration may respond to surgical intervention when all conservative measures have been exhausted.[22] For recalcitrant cases, further non-operative management could consist of intravenous pamidronate given over 3 to 6 months. Clinical remission can be accomplished, and this has been shown to be a safe and effective treatment option.[23]

Periarticular soft tissue problems

Several problems of the hip are related to the soft tissue structures around the joint and its surrounding muscles. Although relatively common, many of these problems are poorly defined, misdiagnosed, or both.[24]

Bursitis

Trochanteric bursitis

Trochanteric bursitis is the most common cause of pain about the hip region. Patients with trochanteric bursitis present with a deep, aching pain sometimes associated with a burning sensation on the lateral aspect of the hip and thigh that increases with activity and can be associated with a limp.[25] Typically, the pain decreases at rest, although it is frequently worse at night, especially when the patient is lying on the affected side. Tenderness can be elicited on palpation of the area around the greater trochanter. The trochanteric bursa is usually not palpable unless it is distended or inflamed. Resisted abduction of the hip when the patient is lying on the opposite side may accentuate the discomfort. The hip range of motion is usually preserved, but in severe cases the discomfort can limit motion. Slight irregularities of the greater trochanter or peritrochanteric calcifications of the bursa are sometimes seen on plain radiographs. The course of trochanteric bursitis is varied: an acute phase may last several days, followed by the gradual abatement of symptoms, although low-grade discomfort may persist for weeks or months.

Treatment includes rest as well as physical therapy for abductor and iliotibial band conditioning and stretching. NSAIDs can be used, but results are often mixed. Infiltration of a local anesthetic and of a long-acting corticosteroid preparation has been shown to be helpful in confirming the diagnosis and bringing long-term relief.[24,25] It is considered by many to be the most effective treatment modality. Various surgical procedures including bursectomy have been proposed for refractory cases, but these are rarely needed.

Iliopsoas bursitis

The iliopsoas bursa can communicate with the hip joint in approximately 15% of adults. Thus, iliopsoas bursitis can manifest in association with a variety of hip disorders, including osteoarthritis, rheumatoid arthritis, synovial chondromatosis, pigmented villonodular synovitis, osteonecrosis, and septic arthritis.[26] The direction and degree of bursal enlargement will dictate symptoms, and patients may present with a painful inguinal mass, groin pain, varicosities secondary to femoral vein compression, or paresthesias secondary to femoral nerve compression.[27,28] CT has been proposed as the best diagnostic test to document iliopsoas bursitis (Fig. 73.15). Treatment with bursography with the instillation of corticosteroids is an effective diagnostic and therapeutic modality. Occasionally, symptoms persist after non-operative measures such as physical therapy and NSAIDs. In these cases, surgical excision of the bursa is sometimes necessary.

Ischiogluteal bursitis

Ischiogluteal bursitis is most commonly seen in patients engaged in jobs that require long periods of sitting[29] and is thus also known as "weaver's bottom." Patients complain of exquisite pain over the ischia, aggravated by sitting and lying. Local tenderness on palpation of the ischial tuberosity is always found. Using an 8- to 10-cm thick rubber cushion with holes to accommodate the ischial prominences may alleviate symptoms. Trunk and knee-to-chest stretching exercises while lying on the cushion should also be encouraged. A local injection of corticosteroid may be used in refractory cases, avoiding the sciatic nerve that passes just laterally to the bursa.

Adductor tendinitis

Adductor tendinitis tends to occur in patients engaged in sports activities involving straddling. The pain is typically located in the groin and inner aspect of the thigh and is increased by passive abduction of the thighs and active adduction against resistance. Tenderness may also be elicited by local palpation of the adductor muscles, especially near their insertion on the front of the pubis. The differential diagnosis includes hernias, genitourinary afflictions, osteitis pubis, and arthritis of the hip. Treatment consists of rest, ice, and NSAIDs during the acute phase, with ultrasound treatment and progressive stretching exercises added in the subacute phase. Local corticosteroid injections are reserved for patients resistant to these conservative modalities.

Snapping hip syndrome (coxa saltans)

Snapping hip syndrome is an uncommon entity reported most frequently in young individuals. It encompasses a collection of extra-articular and intra-articular pathologic processes associated with an audible and sometimes palpable clicking or snapping sensation in the hip region[30] and can be a diagnostic dilemma for the clinician. Extra-articular causes include the iliopsoas tendon snapping over the iliopectineal eminence or the lesser trochanter, the iliofemoral ligaments snapping over the femoral head, the long head of the biceps snapping over the ischial tuberosity, and, the most common, the iliotibial band snapping over the greater trochanter. These can be very difficult to distinguish from intra-articular pathologic processes such as labral tears or loose bodies that can cause a snapping or clicking sensation within the hip joint. On examination, the patient can usually reproduce the snapping sensation, which often can be felt by the examiner. Attempting to block the snapping sensation in the area of the greater or lesser trochanter may help corroborate the entity that is causing the snapping. MRI, CT, and ultrasonography have all been used to evaluate the cause of the snapping hip. Treatment is aimed at the cause of the snapping. Iliotibial band stretching exercises may help alleviate snapping over the greater trochanter, iliopsoas bursography with corticosteroid may relieve snapping over the lesser trochanter, and hip arthroscopy will treat clicking sensations caused by labral tears or intra-articular loose bodies.[30]

REFERENCES

1. Busconi BD. Anatomy. In: McCarthy JC, ed. Early hip disorders. New York: Springer, 2003:51-55.
2. Gautier E, Ganz K, Krügel N, et al. Anatomy of the medial femoral artery and its surgical implications. J Bone Joint Surg Br 2000;82:679-683.
3. Chung SMK. The arterial supply of the developing end of the human femur. J Bone Joint Surg Am 1976;58:961-970.
4. Lea RD, Gerhardt JJ. Range-of-motion measurements. J Bone Joint Surg Am 1995;77:784-798.
5. Russell AS, Maksymowych W, LeClercq S. Clinical examination of the sacroiliac joints: a prospective study. Arthritis Rheum 1981;24:1575-1577.
6. Fitzgerald RH Jr. Acetabular labrum tears: diagnosis and treatment. Clin Orthop Relat Res 1995;60-68.
7. Clarke GR. Unequal leg length: an accurate method of detection and some clinical results. Rheum Phys Med 1982;11:385-390.
8. Bjerkreim I. Secondary dysplasia and osteoarthritis of the hip joint in functional and in fixed obliquity of the pelvis. Acta Orthop Scand 1974;45:873-882.
9. Rubin SJ, Marquardt JD, Gottlieb RH, et al. Magnetic resonance imaging: a cost-effective alternative to bone scintigraphy in the evaluation of patients with suspected hip fractures. Skeletal Radiol 1998;27:199-204.
10. Lequesne M, Morvan G. Description of the potential of an arthrometer for standard and reduced radiographs suitable to measurement of angles and segments of hip, knee, foot and joint space widths. Joint Bone Spine 2002; 69:282-292.

11. McCarthy JC, Lee J. Acetabular dysplasia: a paradigm of arthroscopic examination of chondral injuries. Clin Orthop 2002;405:122-128.
12. Sierra RJ, Trousdale RT, Ganz R, Leunig M. Hip disease in the young, active patient: evaluation and nonarthroplasty surgical options. J Am Acad Orthop Surg 2008;16:689-703.
13. Siebenrock KA, Wahab KHA, Werlen S, et al. Abnormal epiphyseal extension of the femoral head as a cause of femoro-acetabular impingement. Clin Orthop 2004;418:54-60.
14. Schapira D. Transient osteoporosis of the hip. Semin Arthritis Rheum 1992;22:98-105.
15. Balakrishnan A, Schemitsch EH, Pearce D, McKee MD. Distinguishing transient osteoporosis of the hip from avascular necrosis. Can J Surg 2003;46:187-192.
16. Bijl M, van Leeuwen MA, van Rijswijk MH. Transient osteoporosis of the hip: presentation of (a)typical cases and a review of the literature. Clin Exp Rheumatol 1999;17:601-604.
17. Alarcon GS, Sanders C, Daniel WW. Transient osteoporosis of the hip: magnetic resonance imaging. J Rheumatol 1987;14:1184-1189.
18. Arayssi TK, Tawbi HA, Usta IM, Hourani MH. Calcitonin in the treatment of transient osteoporosis of the hip. Semin Arthritis Rheum 2003;32:388-397.
19. Radke S, Rader C, Kenn W, et al. Transient marrow edema syndrome of the hip: results after core decompression: a prospective MRI-controlled study in 22 patients. Arch Orthop Trauma Surg 2003;123:223-227.

20. Lentz SS. Osteitis pubis: a review. Obstet Gynecol Surv 1995;50:310-315.
21. O'Connell MJ, Powell T, McCaffrey NM, et al. Symphyseal cleft injection in the diagnosis and treatment of osteitis pubis in athletes. AJR Am J Roentgenol 2002;179:955-959.
22. Williams PR, Thomas DP, Downes EM. Osteitis pubis and instability of the pubic symphysis: when nonoperative measures fail. Am J Sports Med 2000;28:350-355.
23. Maksymowych WP, Aaron SL, Russell AS. Treatment of refractory symphysitis pubis with intravenous pamidronate. J Rheumatol 2001;28:2754-2757.
24. Lotke PA. Soft tissue afflictions. In: Steinberg ME, ed. The hip and its disorders. Philadelphia: WB Saunders, 1991:669-682.
25. Schapira D, Nahir M, Scharf Y. Trochanteric bursitis: a common clinical problem. Arch Phys Med Rehabil 1986;67:815-817.
26. Toohey AK, LaSalle TL, Martinez S, Polisson RP. Iliopsoas bursitis: clinical features, radiographic findings, and disease associations. Semin Arthritis Rheum 1990;10:41-47.
27. Helfgott SM. Unusual features of iliopsoas bursitis. Arthritis Rheum 1988;31:1331-1333.
28. Letourneau L, Dessureault M, Carette S. Rheumatoid iliopsoas bursitis presenting as unilateral femoral nerve palsy. J Rheumatol 1991;18:462-463.
29. Swartout R, Compere EL. Ischio-gluteal bursitis. JAMA 1974;227:551-552.
30. Allen WC, Cope R. Coxa saltans: the snapping hip revisited. J Am Acad Orthop Surg 1995;3:303-308.

The knee

Lewis L. Shi and John Wright

74

- The knee is a complex diarthrodial joint that forms a highly modified hinge between the distal femur and proximal tibia.

- Knee stability is provided by congruent osseous anatomy, four major ligaments, the anterior and posterior cruciate and medial and lateral collateral ligaments, the medial and lateral menisci, and the adjacent musculature that together provide static and dynamic stability to the joint.

- Several bursae are distributed around the knee where soft tissues move against bony prominences or in fascial planes. Inflammation, or bursitis, may occur in any of the bursae, and concomitant swelling may mimic knee effusion.

- Knee pain may arise from the joint itself or from periarticular tissues such as tendons and bursae, or it may be referred from distant sites such as the hip or femur.

- Accurate diagnosis of knee conditions can usually be made on the basis of the history and physical examination. Standard investigations include synovial fluid analysis, conventional radiography, magnetic resonance imaging, and arthroscopy.

SKELETAL ANATOMY

The knee is a complex diarthrodial joint that forms a highly modified hinge between the distal femur and proximal tibia. Articular surfaces comprising the knee joint include the medial and lateral femoral condyles, the medial and lateral condyles of the tibial plateau, the trochlea of the distal femur, and the patella. These comprise three disparate articulations or compartments: the medial tibiofemoral, the lateral tibiofemoral, and the patellofemoral (Fig. 74.1). The femur and tibia are the largest long bones in the body, and they perform the principal structural, weight-bearing, and locomotive functions of the lower extremity.

Distal femur

The distal femur is bicondylar; the medial femoral condyle is larger in anteroposterior dimension, is less convex, and extends farther distally. The lateral femoral condyle is smaller and more spherical (Fig. 74.2). The domed intercondylar notch located between the medial and lateral condyles contains the femoral origins of the anterior cruciate ligament (ACL) and the posterior cruciate ligament (PCL).

Proximal tibial plateau

The proximal tibial plateau contains two condyles that articulate with the distal femur to form the medial and lateral tibiofemoral compartments (Fig. 74.3). The medial condyle is concave and longer in the anteroposterior plane to accommodate the medial femoral condyle. The lateral condyle is smaller, mildly convex, and slightly more distally sloped from anterior to posterior. A bony intercondylar eminence including the tibial spines separates the condyles and is the distal insertion of the ACL.[1]

Patella

The patella, located within the quadriceps tendon, is the largest sesamoid bone in the body. The trochlea of the distal femur, an intercondylar groove measuring approximately 140 degrees, articulates with the underside of the patella to form the patellofemoral joint. In contrast to the tibiofemoral joint, which is in constant apposition through the knee's full flexion and extension arc, the patella engages the trochlea when the knee is flexed more than 30 degrees. The patella enhances knee biomechanics during active extension by increasing the moment arm of the quadriceps, and it is therefore subject to magnified contact forces that can reach eight times body weight with high impact activities. Reflecting these high contact stresses, patellar articular cartilage is the thickest in the body, and it may reach 7 mm in thickness.[2,3]

SOFT TISSUE ANATOMY

Ligaments

Ligamentous structures statically stabilize and dynamically constrain knee motion. Through sensory innervations, connective tissue structures also provide proprioceptive feedback. There are four major ligamentous structures in the knee: the medial collateral ligament (MCL), the lateral collateral ligament (LCL), the ACL, and the PCL (Figs. 74.4 and 74.5).[4,5]

The MCL is a broad ligament composed of a superficial layer arising from the medial epicondyle and fanning out over the medial side of the tibia where its posterior border blends with the capsule of the knee joint.[6,7] The deep layer originates with the superficial layer, and it inserts into the medial meniscus just above the joint line, acting to stabilize the fibrocartilage. The deep layer blends with the superficial layer distally, and both insert into the tibia in an oblique manner approximately 10 cm below the joint line. Functionally, the MCL resists valgus stress across the knee and provides secondary rotational stability.

The LCL is smaller and shorter, arising from the lateral femoral condyle and inserting into the posterior aspect of the fibular head. Because of its relatively posterior position, the LCL is taut when the knee is in extension, and, in combination with the posterolateral capsule, it is the primary restraint to varus knee stresses.[8]

The two cruciate ligaments, the ACL and PCL, are intra-articular but extrasynovial. Together, they resist excessive anterior and posterior translation of the tibia through the full range of knee flexion and extension by creating a four-bar linkage system.[9,10] The ACL is composed of two bundles, an anteromedial bundle that traverses the anterior aspect of the femoral origin to the medial side of the tibial insertion and a posterolateral bundle that travels from the posterior femoral attachment to the lateral side of the tibial insertion. The bundles spiral around each other as they travel from femoral origin to tibial insertion, allowing for constant tension throughout knee movement. The anteromedial bundle is taut in knee flexion, and the posterolateral bundle is taut when the knee is extended.[10,11] The ACL resists excessive anterior translation and internal rotation of the tibia relative to the femur.

The PCL originates from the lateral surface of the medial femoral condyle and inserts on the posterior tibia approximately 1 cm distal to the articular surface. The PCL is also composed of two distinct bundles, the anterolateral and posteromedial. The posteromedial bundle of the PCL is taut when the knee is extended and the anterolateral bundle is taut when the knee is flexed, resulting in functional stability through the complete arc of knee motion. The PCL primarily functions to prevent excessive posterior translation of the tibia.[12,13]

The posterolateral corner of the knee contains a collection of muscular and ligamentous structures that prevent excessive external rotation, varus angulation, and posterior translation of the tibia. These include the iliotibial (IT) band, biceps femoris tendon, LCL, popliteus, popliteofibular ligament, arcuate ligament, and posterolateral joint capsule (Fig. 74.6).[14-16]

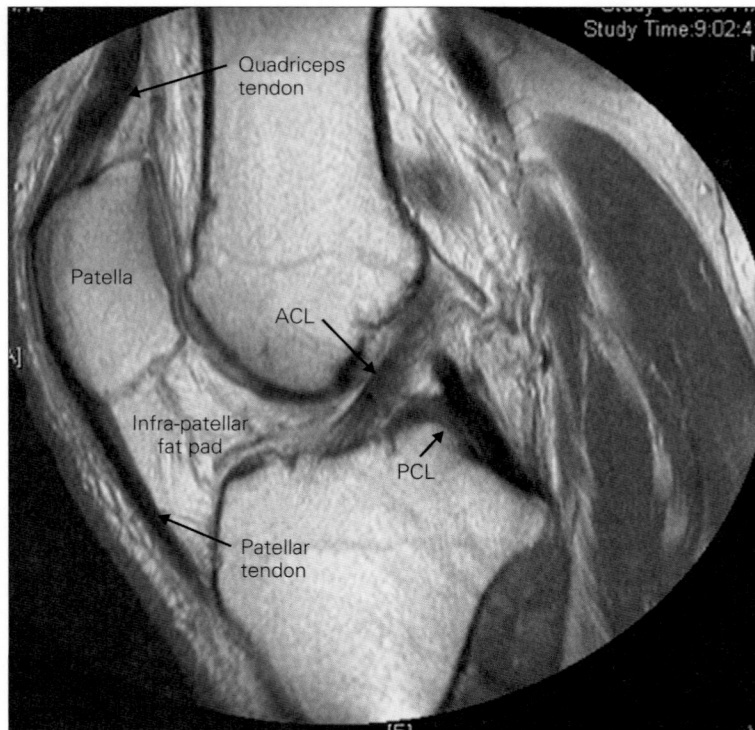

Fig. 74.1 Sagittal section of the knee joint.

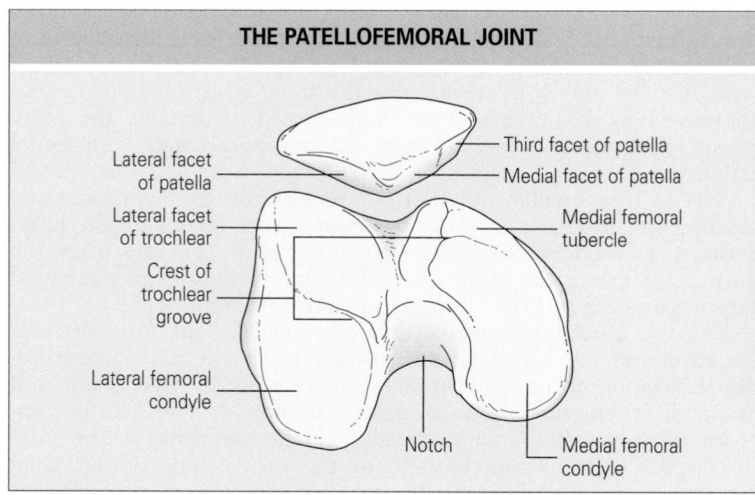

Fig. 74.2 Diagram of the distal femur.

THE PATELLOFEMORAL JOINT

Lateral facet of patella
Third facet of patella
Medial facet of patella
Lateral facet of trochlear
Medial femoral tubercle
Crest of trochlear groove
Lateral femoral condyle
Notch
Medial femoral condyle

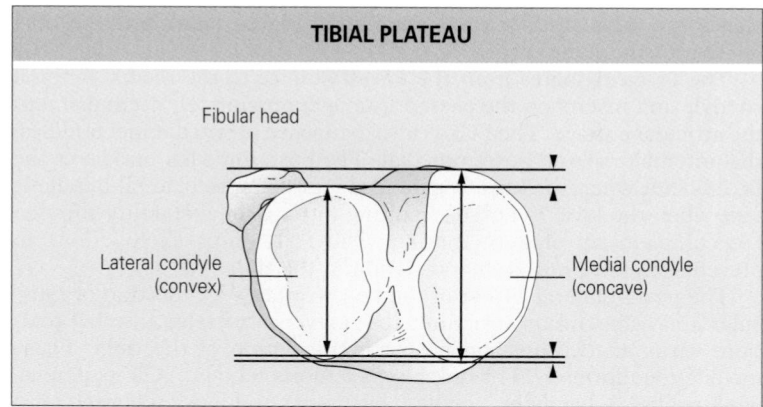

Fig. 74.3 Diagram of the tibial plateau.

TIBIAL PLATEAU

Fibular head
Lateral condyle (convex)
Medial condyle (concave)

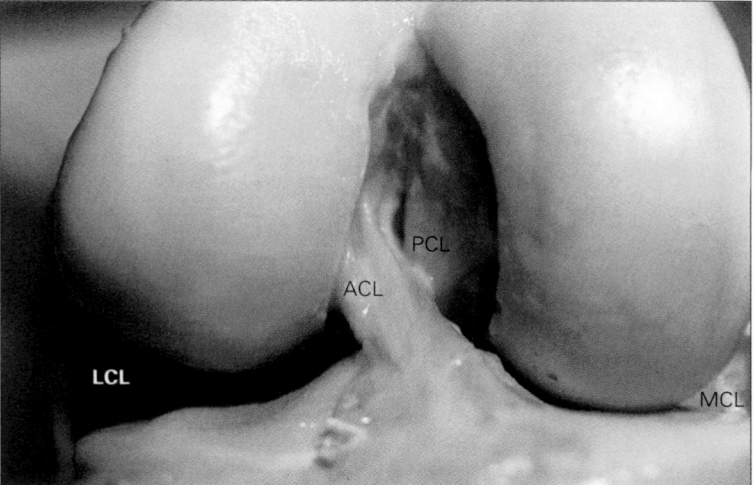

Fig. 74.4 Gross appearance of a right knee.

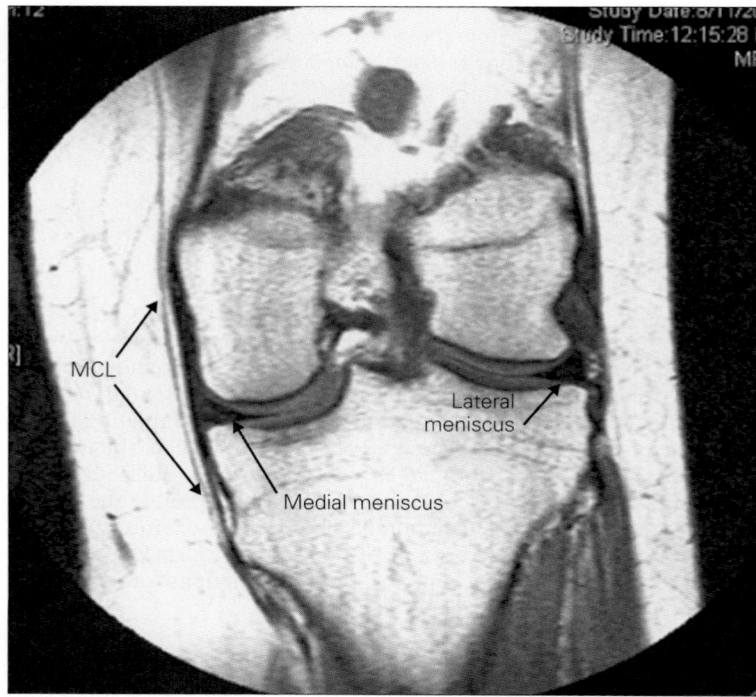

Fig. 74.5 Coronal MR image demonstrating MCL and menisci ligaments.

Menisci

The menisci are crescentic discs of fibrocartilage interposed between the articular surfaces of the femur and tibia that deepen and stabilize the tibiofemoral articulations and distribute the weight-bearing load across a greater articular surface area. In cross section, the menisci are triangular with a thick periphery and thin, concave center. The central two thirds of the meniscus contain collagen bundles predominantly arrayed in a radial pattern to dissipate compressive forces across the knee joint while the outer third contains circumferential collagen fibers that absorb hoop stresses. Biomechanical studies suggest that the lateral meniscus transmits and dissipates approximately 70% of the compressive load in the lateral compartment while the medial meniscus and medial tibiofemoral articular cartilage share forces across the medial compartment equally (Fig. 74.7).[17,18]

The peripheral third of the menisci, the "red zone," is vascularized through capsular attachments arising from the medial and lateral geniculate vessels and therefore has the potential to heal if it is injured. The central third of the menisci, the "white zone," in contrast, is avascular and has minimal healing potential. The intermediate "red/white zone" has limited healing potential.[18]

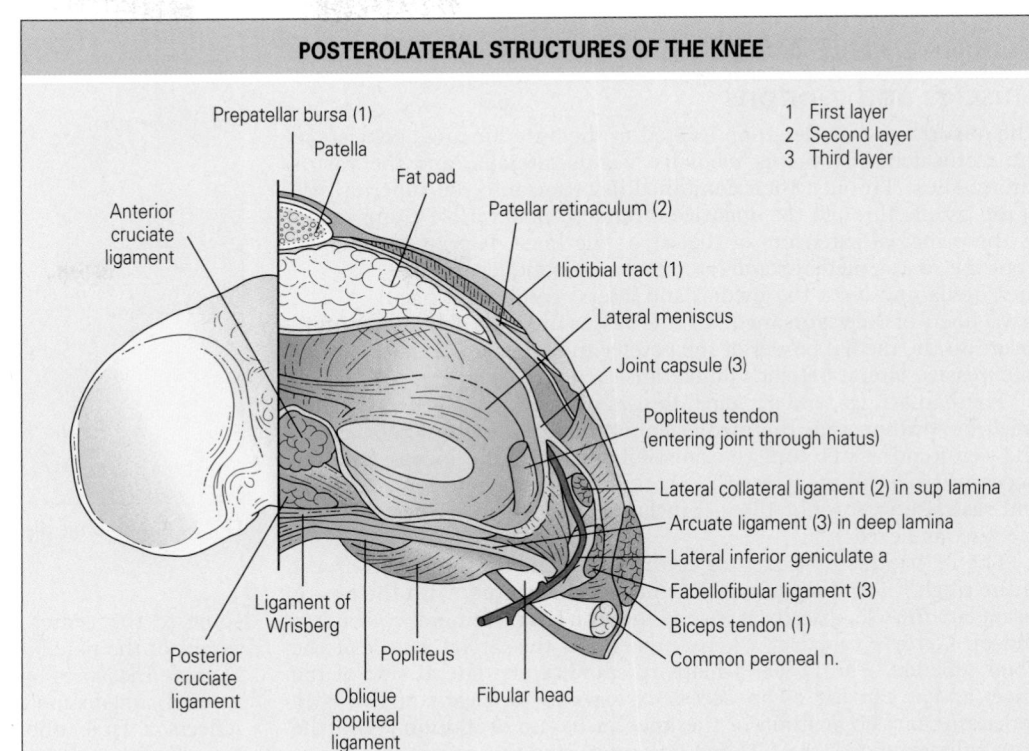

POSTEROLATERAL STRUCTURES OF THE KNEE

1	First layer
2	Second layer
3	Third layer

Prepatellar bursa (1)
Patella
Fat pad
Patellar retinaculum (2)
Anterior cruciate ligament
Iliotibial tract (1)
Lateral meniscus
Joint capsule (3)
Popliteus tendon (entering joint through hiatus)
Lateral collateral ligament (2) in sup lamina
Arcuate ligament (3) in deep lamina
Lateral inferior geniculate a
Fabellofibular ligament (3)
Biceps tendon (1)
Common peroneal n.
Ligament of Wrisberg
Posterior cruciate ligament
Oblique popliteal ligament
Popliteus
Fibular head

Fig. 74.6 Posterolateral structures of the knee. The drawing shows the complexity of the layers and attachments controlling the posterior rotation of the tibial plateau. *(Redrawn with permission from Seebacher JR, Ingilis AE, Marshal JL, et al. The structure of the posterolateral aspect of the knee. J Bone Joint Surg Am 1982;64:536-541.)*

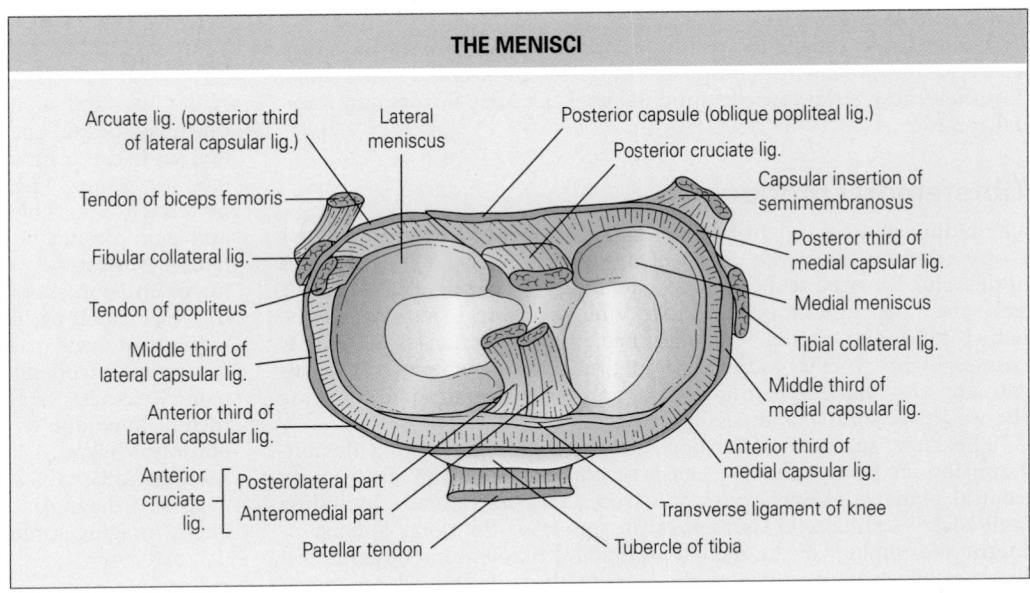

THE MENISCI

Arcuate lig. (posterior third of lateral capsular lig.)
Lateral meniscus
Posterior capsule (oblique popliteal lig.)
Posterior cruciate lig.
Tendon of biceps femoris
Capsular insertion of semimembranosus
Fibular collateral lig.
Posteror third of medial capsular lig.
Tendon of popliteus
Medial meniscus
Middle third of lateral capsular lig.
Tibial collateral lig.
Anterior third of lateral capsular lig.
Middle third of medial capsular lig.
Anterior cruciate lig. — Posterolateral part / Anteromedial part
Anterior third of medial capsular lig.
Transverse ligament of knee
Patellar tendon
Tubercle of tibia

Fig. 74.7 The menisci. The superior surface of the tibial plateau, demonstrating the anatomic position, size, and attachments of the menisci.

The medial meniscus is semi-circular, and its anterior and posterior horns are attached to the tibial intercondylar eminence. The periphery of the medial meniscus is closely attached to the medial capsule and deep MCL by the coronary ligaments. In contrast, the lateral meniscus is nearly circular, and it has looser peripheral attachments. A hiatus in the posterolateral capsule where the popliteus tendon enters the joint contains no attachment to the lateral meniscus.[17,19] Posteriorly, the meniscofemoral ligaments of Humphrey and Wrisberg attach the posterior horn of the lateral meniscus to the lateral aspect of the medial femoral condyle.[17] Greater motion of the lateral meniscus allowed by looser capsular and bony attachments enables the lateral meniscus to translate during physiologic knee roll-back and screw-home rotation.

Bursae

Several bursae are distributed around the knee where soft tissues move against bony prominences or in fascial planes. Anteriorly, the prepatellar bursa is located in the subcutaneous layer between the lower half of the patella and the skin. Deeper, the infrapatellar bursa lies between the patellar tendon and tibial tubercle. On the medial side, the anserine bursa is superficial to the medial collateral ligament and separates it from the tendons of the pes anserinus (sartorius, gracilis, and semitendinosus). Accessory bursae may be present either medially or laterally in fascial layers separating ligaments, tendons, and bone.[20] When distended, the gastrocnemius-semimembranosus bursa, which communicates with the knee joint in 50% of adults, causes a Baker cyst. Any of the knee bursae may become swollen and inflamed, and this appearance can mimic an effusion within the knee joint capsule.

An understanding of the location of knee bursae and careful palpation to assess the tissue depth of a fluid collection is essential before attempted aspiration around the knee. Needle penetration traversing a superficial cellulitis or infected bursitis into a sterile knee joint should be avoided, because it may result in iatrogenic septic knee arthritis requiring surgical irrigation and débridement and a prolonged course of intravenous antibiotics.

NORMAL KNEE MOVEMENT

Muscles and tendons

The quadriceps muscle group located in the anterior thigh consists of the rectus femoris, vastus medialis, vastus lateralis, and the vastus intermedius. Through their conjoined insertion into the superior pole of the patella through the quadriceps tendon, this muscle group serves as the principal extensors of the leg at the knee. Fibrous expansions from the vastus medialis and lateralis insert obliquely into the sides of the patella and form the medial and lateral patellar retinacula.[21] The distal fibers of the vastus medialis, the vastus medialis obliquus (VMO), insert on the medial border of the patella and are a key active restraint to excessive lateral patella subluxation.

The hamstrings, the principal flexors of the knee, are usually classified by location into the medial hamstrings, the semimembranosus and semitendinosus, and the lateral hamstring, the biceps femoris. Accessory roles for the hamstrings include providing rotational stability and restraining anterior tibial translation relative to the femur when the knee is flexed.

The IT band is a thickening of the fascia lata on the lateral aspect of the thigh.[22] Proximally, the IT band is in continuity with the tensor fascia lata muscle; distally, it inserts into the lateral femoral epicondyle and on Gerdy's tubercle, a bony process on the lateral aspect of the tibial tubercle. The IT band helps to stabilize the lateral side of the knee, and it can act as an accessory extensor or flexor of the knee depending on the position of the knee in its arc of motion. With the knee fully extended, the IT band lies anterior to the axis of rotation of the knee, and it acts as a knee extensor; as the knee is flexed the IT band translates posteriorly behind the center of rotation of the knee and it acts as a flexor.[23]

The pes anserinus is the common tendinous insertion of the sartorius, gracilis, and semitendinosus into the proximal medial tibia. Together, these strap muscles function as weak knee flexors and internal rotators.

Tibiofemoral motion

The biomechanical weight-bearing axis of the lower extremity follows a line extending from the center of the femoral head to the midpoint of the talus. Located at the approximate midpoint of the weight-bearing axis, the knee functions to transfer and dissipate loads among the femur, tibia, and patella.[24] At the knee, the mechanical axis usually crosses slightly medial to the anatomic midline. Degenerative changes can alter the relative positions of the femur and tibia thereby shifting the weight-bearing axis medially or laterally.

The knee, in simplest terms, is a hinge joint enabling a flexion-extension arc from 0 to 135 degrees or greater. Motion in the primary sagittal plane is closely coupled to secondary movements including "roll-back," sliding, and rotation of the femur on the tibia. The asymmetric morphology of the medial and lateral tibiofemoral osseous and ligamentous structures guides the complex kinematics of knee movement. As the knee flexes, the lateral femoral condyle translates posteriorly by rolling or sliding twice as far as the medial condyle. The differential motion between the medial and lateral condyles results in tibial internal rotation with flexion and tibial external rotation with extension.[23,25]

Patellofemoral motion

The patella functions to augment the moment arm of the extensor mechanism. As the knee flexes past 30 degrees, the articular surface of the patella engages the trochlear groove of the distal femur. The stability of patellofemoral movement, called "tracking," is a result of the congruent osseous anatomy of the patella and trochlea augmented by soft tissue constraints including the vastus lateralis and lateral retinaculum that pull the patella laterally and the vastus medialis obliquus and medial patellofemoral ligament that stabilize the patella medially.[2,3]

The Q angle is a measurement that reflects the balance of medial and lateral forces on the patella exerted by the extensor mechanism. The angle is subtended by a line drawn from the anterior superior iliac

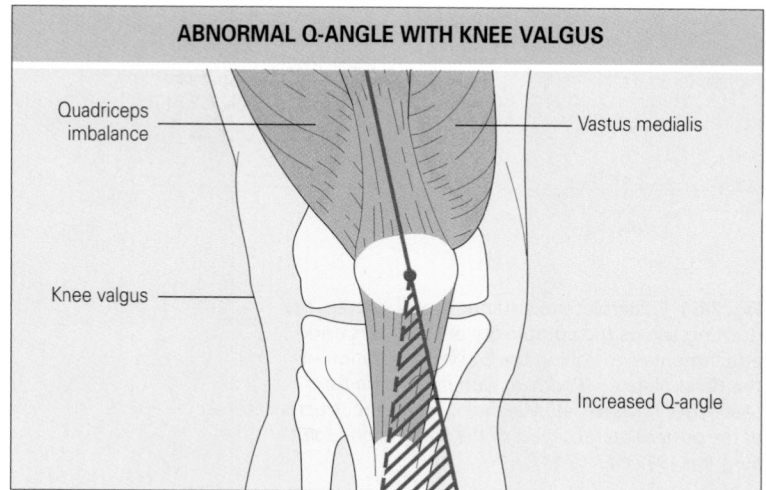

Fig. 74.8 Anatomic diagram of quadriceps musculature with onlay of Q angle.

spine to the center of the patella and another line drawn from the center of the patella to the tibial tubercle (Fig. 74.8).[26] A normal knee Q angle measures approximately 13 degrees in men and 18 degrees in women, and an angle exceeding 20 degrees is abnormal. A high Q angle reflects a large unbalanced force vector tending to pull the patella laterally.[26]

HISTORY AND EXAMINATION

History

A detailed and anatomically precise history is essential to accurate diagnosis of knee pathology. The patient's age is a key initial consideration because most knee diagnoses characteristically occur in a specific age group. The onset or exacerbation of knee symptoms should be related if possible to specific traumatic events, sports, or activities, and pain should be localized when possible to the anterior, medial, lateral, or posterior aspect of the knee. A relevant history of knee swelling or effusion should be sought, and "mechanical" symptoms including knee catching, clicking, locking, or giving way should be elicited. Significant back pain symptoms may be relevant because radicular symptoms involving the L3 or L4 nerve roots may cause referred knee pain, weakness, or hypoesthesia. Hip pain may also be referred to the medial knee due to shared sensory innervation of both areas by the obturator nerve. A history of inflammatory arthritis or crystal deposition arthropathy is also important to investigate. A careful history will suggest a diagnosis that a targeted physical examination and subsequent imaging studies will confirm.

Examination

Observation and palpation

The knee examination begins with observation of the patient's gait. Use of a cane (stick) and which hand is used to hold the cane should be noted, because this may reflect knee pain or subjective instability. Signs of varus or valgus thrust while walking or evidence of an antalgic gait, which refers to a cadence designed to minimize weight bearing on a painful knee, should also be noted.

With the patient positioned supine on the examination table, the whole lower limb is exposed, and a visual assessment of lower extremity alignment is made. Skin lacerations, ecchymoses, erythema, or previous surgical incisions should prompt further inquiry. Areas of muscle atrophy, especially of the vastus medialis obliquus, should also be noted. If quadriceps atrophy is suspected, thigh circumference measured four fingerbreadths above the proximal pole of the patella can be compared with the contralateral side.

The normal knee is aligned at approximately 7 degrees of valgus; and although variations in alignment may be constitutional, varus alignment or excessive valgus may reflect underlying knee pathology. The magnitude of varus deformity may be clinically assessed as the distance between the knees with the ankle medial malleoli together, and the amount of valgus may be measured as the distance between the ankles with the knees held together.

The knee is next examined for evidence of swelling or effusion. It is frequently difficult to distinguish swelling within a bursa from fluid within the knee joint itself by observation alone. Fluid collections that are more superficial by palpation and limited to one quadrant around the knee, especially distal to the patella, are more suggestive of bursitis than joint effusion. The "patellar ballottement test," in which the examiner presses the patella down onto an extended knee may be helpful to demonstrate moderate-sized joint effusions. Subtle joint effusions may be detected by milking fluid out of the suprapatellar pouch with one hand while gently squeezing the sulci on either side of the patellar tendon.

Palpation of the knee extensor mechanism is performed next, with the examiner identifying the patella, quadriceps tendon, patellar tendon, and tibial tubercle. A palpable defect in the quadriceps tendon, patella, or patellar tendon may represent a disruption in the extensor mechanism requiring surgery, so further evaluation of the finding is warranted. The initial step is to flex the patient's knee 90 degrees over the side of the examination table and to ask the patient to actively extend the knee. Because the IT band functions as an accessory knee extensor with the knee in an extended position, a patient with a disrupted extensor mechanism may be able to maintain knee extension from an initially extended position. Active knee extension from a flexed starting position must therefore be assessed. This examination may be facilitated by aspirating an existing knee effusion or hemarthrosis under sterile conditions and injecting the knee joint with local anesthetic.

Further palpation of the knee should include the femoral epicondyles, collateral ligaments, hamstrings, pes anserinus, and IT band. Tenderness, swelling, or ecchymosis along these structures may indicate traumatic injury or rupture. Posterior palpation should include the popliteal pulse and any masses. If a popliteal mass is pulsatile, auscultation should be performed to assess for a bruit that would suggest a popliteal aneurysm. Palpation of the medial and lateral joint line may reveal areas of tenderness or masses suggestive of meniscal injury or meniscal cyst.

Range of motion

Active and passive knee range of motion should be assessed. The normal passive and active flexion-extension arc of the knee is from 0 to 135 degrees, although considerable variation occurs.[27] Up to 10 degrees of hyperextension, or "recurvatum," may be normal, especially in younger patients (Fig. 74.9). Among older patients with advanced osteoarthritis, a progressively worsening flexion contracture is common. Asymmetry between active and passive extension of the knee, termed extensor lag, suggests weakness or disruption of the extensor mechanism and should prompt further evaluation.

The Q angle may be assessed with the patient supine and the knee flexed 15 degrees. One line is measured from the anterior superior iliac spine to the center of the patella, and another is drawn from the center of the patella to the tibial tubercle. These bony landmarks are subcutaneous and should be easily palpable. The angle subtended by these lines is measured and recorded.

Patellofemoral movement is assessed through the entire flexion-extension arc. With one hand resting lightly on the patella, the knee is flexed and extended to ascertain patellofemoral crepitus. Patellar tracking refers to the ability of the patella to smoothly engage and stably articulate with the distal femoral trochlea. In patients with a high Q angle or other causes of lateral patellar subluxation, the patella may translate laterally during the terminal 30 degrees of knee extension causing a "J-sign."

Ligamentous stability

The position and function of the principal ligamentous stabilizers of the knee make them accessible to provocative testing. Because there is considerable physiologic variation in overall soft tissue laxity, all examinations should be performed on both legs and results should be compared between affected and unaffected sides.

The MCL is tested with the patient supine. With the knee fully extended and the thigh stabilized, a valgus stress is placed across the

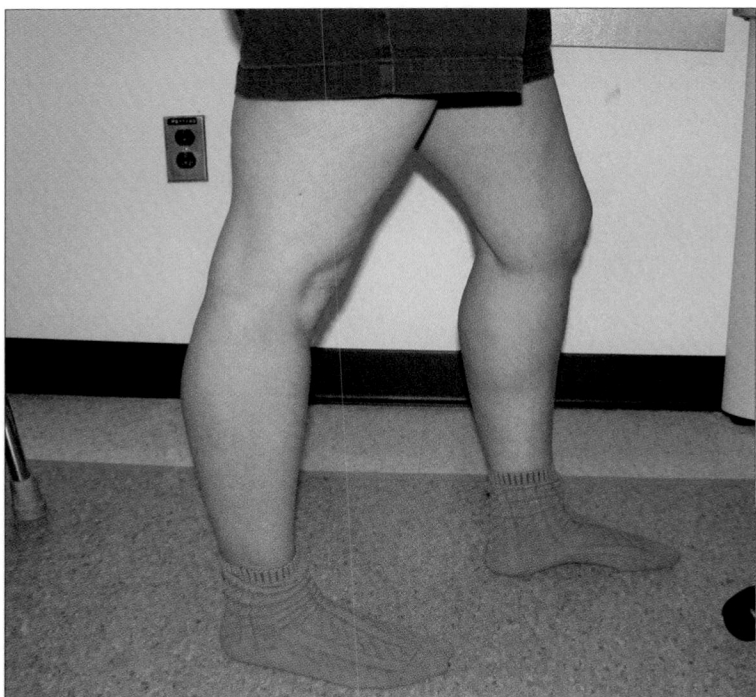

Fig. 74.9 Physiologic recurvatum.

knee. If laxity is present or if this maneuver elicits pain, a tear of the MCL, medial capsule, posteromedial corner, and the PCL may be present.[28] The test is repeated with the knee at 30 degrees of flexion; laxity suggests sprain or rupture of the MCL and the posteromedial capsule. Analogous testing using varus stress is used to identify injury to the LCL and possible combined injuries to posterolateral structures and PCL.[29]

Competence of the ACL may be tested using three distinct physical examination maneuvers:

1. The Lachman test has a high positive predictive value for detecting ACL rupture.[30] It is performed with the patient supine and the knee flexed approximately 20 degrees. The examiner stabilizes the patient's thigh with one hand and grasps the proximal tibia just below the joint line with the other hand. Anterior translation stress is then applied across the knee, and laxity is measured (Fig. 74.10).
2. The anterior drawer test is similar to the Lachman test, but it is performed with the knee flexed 90 degrees. The examiner grasps the proximal tibia with both hands and applies a firm anterior translation stress.
3. The pivot-shift test can be performed with the patient either supine or in a lateral decubitus position. With the patient supine and the knee extended, the examiner grasps and internally rotates the patient's leg with one hand and applies a valgus stress across the knee with the other hand. The examiner then applies a moderate axial load to the knee and gradually flexes it. A positive test yields a palpable clunk in the knee at approximately 30 degrees of flexion.

More apprehensive patients may be placed in a lateral decubitus position for the pivot-shift test. In this position, the patient's knee is extended and the tibia is placed in an internally rotated position. The examiner then applies a valgus stress to the knee while flexing it, again producing a clunk at 30 degrees of flexion with a positive test.[31]

An important consideration while performing tests for ACL competence is that the hamstrings may act as an active restraint to anterior tibial translation when the knee is flexed. In the context of acute injury or an apprehensive patient, the hamstrings may be in spasm, leading to false-negative findings by physical examination. Provocative tests may therefore be of limited value in the context of acute trauma, and in many cases the tests may be deferred for later evaluation 1 to 2 weeks after initial presentation. While performing the Lachman and

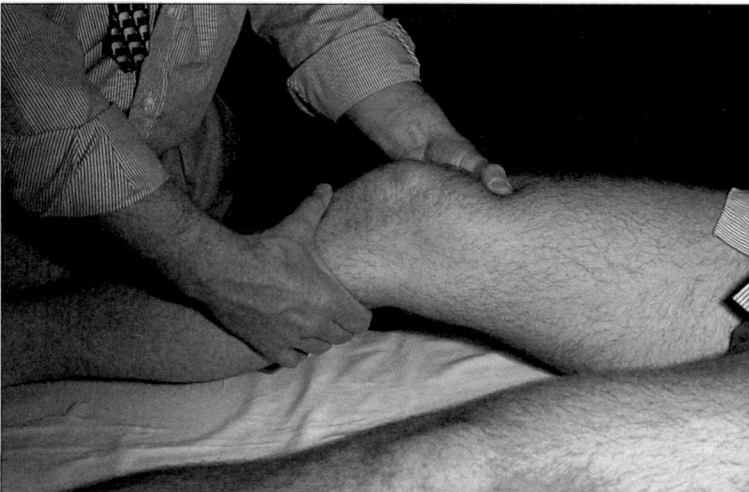

Fig. 74.10 Lachman test for anterior translation.

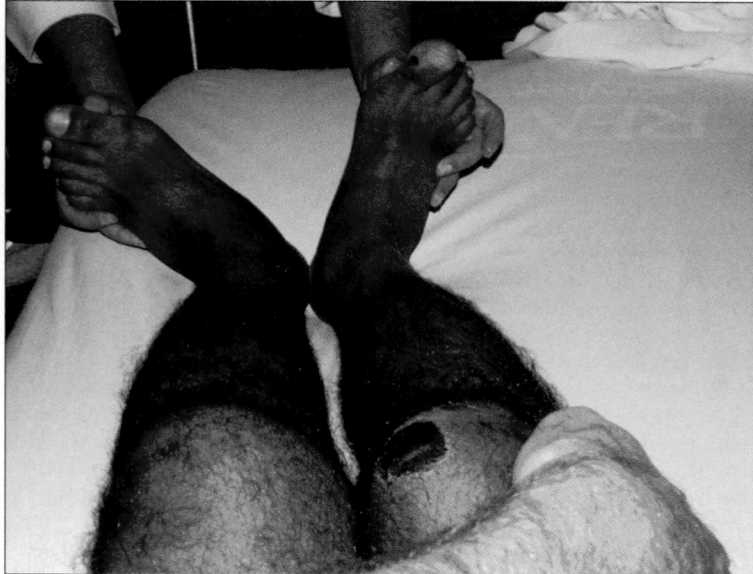

Fig. 74.12 Dial test.

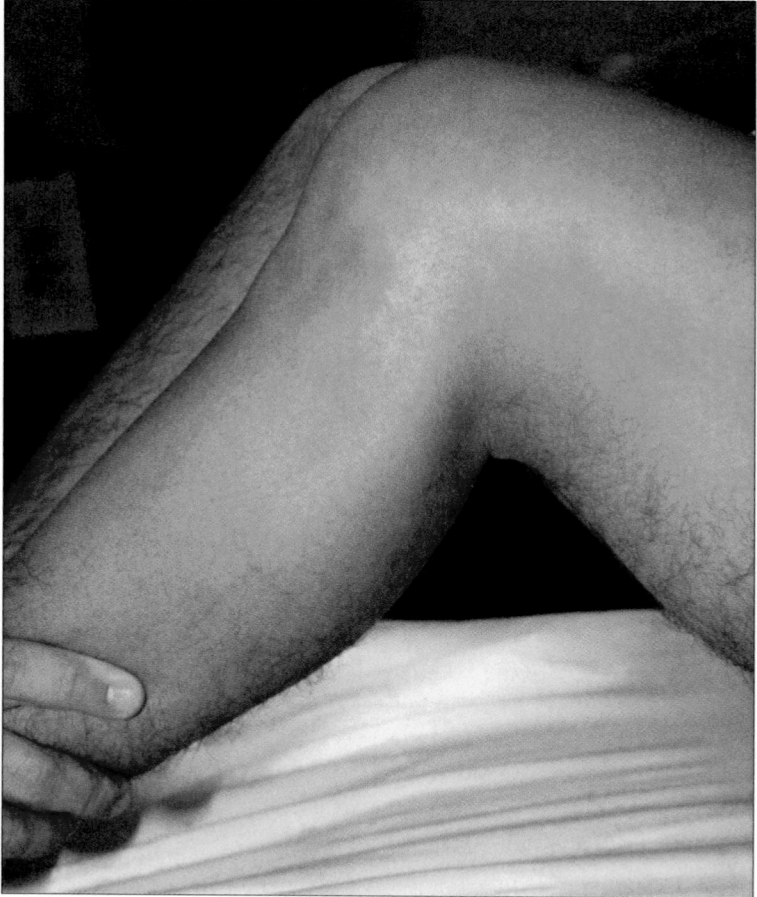

Fig. 74.11 Posterior drawer test for PCL tear.

anterior drawer tests, the examiner's hand on the proximal tibia is in a suitable position to assess hamstring tone when exerting anterior translation stress.

PCL laxity is assessed using the posterior drawer test. With the patient supine and the knee flexed to 90 degrees, the proximal tibia is grasped and a firm posterior translation force is applied. A positive posterior drawer test, indicating disruption of the PCL, is present when the anterior tibia displaces posteriorly until it is flush with the distal femoral condyle (Fig. 74.11). The posterior sag test also signals PCL injury. The patient is seated upright in a chair with hips and knees flexed to 90 degrees. The examiner then extends the patient's knee and

supports the leg under the ankle. A positive test is present when the proximal tibia sags posteriorly under the level of the patella.

The complex of structures located in the knee posterolateral corner including the IT band, biceps femoris tendon, LCL, popliteus, popliteo-fibular ligament, arcuate ligament, and posterolateral joint capsule may be disrupted alone or in combination with other ligamentous injuries. Specific tests have been devised to distinguish combined injuries from more common, isolated patterns. The tibial external rotation test or "dial test" is performed with the patient prone or supine. With the knees flexed 30 degrees, an external rotation stress is exerted. A difference of greater than 10 degrees of laxity is considered significant. The maneuver is repeated with the knees flexed to 90 degrees. Increased rotational laxity with the knees flexed 30 degrees but not at 90 degrees suggests an isolated posterolateral corner injury whereas laxity at 30 degrees and 90 degrees indicates combined PCL and posterolateral corner disruption (Fig. 74.12).[32]

SPECIFIC DISORDERS OF THE KNEE

A key to accurate diagnosis of knee disorders is knowledge of characteristic diagnoses relevant to each patient age group (Table 74.1). Here, we discuss the most common knee disorders and briefly summarize diagnostic pearls, characteristic radiographic findings, and therapeutic options.

Infancy and early childhood

Knee pain in an infant or young child is uncommon, but it is always significant. The limping child must be treated with a degree of urgency, and a cause for the symptoms must be confirmed because overlooked causes may lead to serious sequelae and permanent disability. Diagnosis of pediatric knee disorders may be hindered by a child's inability to communicate an accurate history of trauma, the difficulty of performing a systematic physical examination on an uncooperative subject, the fact that physeal injuries to the growth plate are not visible on plain radiographs, and the possibility that the knee pain is actually referred from the hip.

Referred hip pain

Knee pain may be caused by disorders of the hip because of the common sensory innervation of both territories by branches of the obturator nerve. Children with hip abnormalities including fracture, dislocation, Legg-Calvé-Perthes disease, slipped capital femoral epiphysis (SCFE), hip joint transient synovitis, or septic arthritis may therefore present primarily with medial-sided knee pain. Differentiating

TABLE 74.1 COMMON CAUSES OF KNEE PAIN IN DIFFERENT AGE GROUPS

Age group	Intra-articular	Periarticular	Cause Referred
Childhood (2-10 yr)	Juvenile chronic arthritis	Osteomyelitis	Perthes disease
	Osteochondritis dissecans		Transient synovitis of the hip
	Septic arthritis		Septic hip arthritis
	Torn discoid lateral meniscus		Slipped capital femoral epiphysis
Adolescence (10-18 yr)	Osteochondritis dissecans	Osgood-Schlatter disease	Slipped capital femoral epiphysis
	Torn meniscus	Sinding-Larsen-Johansson syndrome	
	Anterior knee pain syndrome	Osteomyelitis	
	Patellar malalignment	Tumors	
Early adulthood (18-30 yr)	Torn meniscus Instability Anterior knee pain syndrome Inflammatory conditions	Overuse syndromes Bursitis	Rare
Adulthood (30-50 yr)	Degenerate meniscal tears Early degeneration after injury or meniscectomy Inflammatory arthropathies	Bursitis Tendinitis	Degenerative hip disease secondary to hip dysplasia or injury Lumbar herniated disc
Older age (>50 yr)	Osteoarthritis Inflammatory arthropathies	Bursitis Tendinitis	Osteoarthritis of the hip Lumber spondylosis, stenosis

among these diagnoses may be facilitated by a complete history and laboratory studies, including the erythrocyte sedimentation rate (ESR) and C-reactive protein (CRP) value.[33] Plain radiography, hip ultrasonography, and magnetic resonance imaging (MRI) are frequently useful imaging studies.

Septic arthritis

Septic arthritis of the knee in children is usually the result of hematogenous spread, although a local penetrating wound should also raise concern. Examination of the infected joint reveals a warm, tense effusion, sometimes with overlying erythema or induration. The knee is held in a slightly flexed position to maximize the intracapsular volume and thereby reduce pain generated by capsular stretch receptors. Passive flexion and extension is severely limited by pain.

Knee joint aspiration should be performed in every case where septic arthritis is suspected because missed diagnosis may lead to osteonecrosis, growth arrest, and sepsis. If there is skin erythema over the proposed aspiration location, alternative sites should be considered to avoid any possibility of spreading cellulitis into deeper tissue. Synovial fluid obtained should be submitted to the laboratory for immediate cell count and differential, Gram stain, and culture. Where tests suggest infection, urgent arthroscopic irrigation and débridement should be performed to minimize chondrolysis and other damaging consequences of septic arthritis. Antibiotics should be started after adequate synovial fluid has been submitted for culture and sensitivity.

Osteomyelitis

Acute hematogenous osteomyelitis commonly affects the lower femoral and upper tibial metaphyses. The diagnosis should be suspected in a child with a temperature of more than 38° C (100.4° F) and pain over the distal femoral or proximal tibial metaphysis. The diagnosis is further supported by an elevated white blood cell count, ESR, and CRP value. Aspiration using a bone marrow biopsy needle may be helpful in obtaining a sample to be submitted for culture, speciation, and sensitivity analysis. Radiographic changes on plain radiographs including sequestra or involucra may take weeks to appear, but MRI reveals changes typical of bone marrow infection including hypointense signal on T1-weighted images and increased signal on T2-weighted series. Occasionally, acute osteomyelitis is contained by host defenses, and it becomes a sterile cavity surrounded by a rim of scar called Brodie's abscess. In other cases, prolonged intravenous antibiotics and even surgical débridement may be necessary. Septic knee arthritis may be

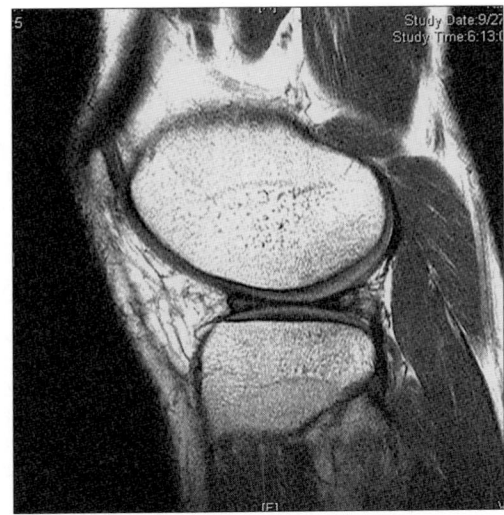

Fig. 74.13 MR image of discoid meniscus showing degeneration in young adult.

present adjacent to tibial or femoral osteomyelitis, especially in infants where blood vessels cross the physis and enable local spread of infection. In other patients, a sterile sympathetic effusion may exist in the knee.

Discoid meniscus

In a child younger than 10 years of age, degenerative tears of the knee menisci are very uncommon. When a young child complains of mechanical knee symptoms including pain, effusion, catching, clicking, and locking, the cause may be discoid meniscus. A discoid meniscus results when usually the lateral meniscus does not differentiate into a semilunar shape and instead forms a thick wafer of fibrocartilaginous tissue. Discoid menisci are classified as stable or unstable depending on the presence or absence of the usual capsular and bony attachments of the meniscus. Where the discoid meniscus has preserved tibial attachments, symptomatic tears may be treated with arthroscopic débridement and saucerization. When the discoid meniscus is unstable due to incompetent attachments, stabilization and partial meniscectomy may be necessary (Fig. 74.13).[34,35]

Malignancy and hematologic conditions

Malignancies can first present as arthritis caused by malignant cell infiltration of the structures surrounding the joint. Patients are typically ill and may have difficulty using the affected limb. One or many joints can be affected. Pathologic fractures associated with benign or malignant lesions may present as sudden disability and severe pain. A complete blood cell count, ESR, and radiographs are often the first step toward a diagnosis.

Hematologic conditions can cause limb pain around the knee. Hemophilia most commonly manifests as joint swelling secondary to hemorrhage. Knee hemarthrosis is most common, followed by elbow hemarthrosis. Acutely, the joint may become warm, distended, and tender. Chronically an effusion with thickening of the capsule may develop with loss of range of motion as a result of the erosion of the cartilage, resulting in chronic arthropathy.

Children with sickle cell anemia may experience knee pain in the context of vaso-occlusive sickle cell crises. Knee pain may be accompanied by warmth, erythema, swelling, and local tenderness. Pain is caused by bone marrow ischemia, which can lead to avascular necrosis of the distal femur or proximal tibia. Other frequently affected sites are the spine, shoulder, and elbow. In some cases ischemia can lead to avascular necrosis with an acute inflammatory infiltrate. Areas of inadequate perfusion are predisposed to infection, and hematogenous osteomyelitis or septic arthritis may develop. Although *Salmonella* infections are more common in this context than in normal hosts, *Staphylococcus* species are the predominant organisms.[36]

Inflammatory disease of the knee and Lyme disease

Inflammatory conditions include juvenile rheumatoid arthritis (JRA) and pediatric spondyloarthropathies. School-aged children and adolescents are most affected by polyarticular-onset JRA and type 2 pauciarticular arthritis.[37] There is a wide spectrum of symptom severity in JRA, ranging from mild pain and swelling with minimal limitation in activity to deforming and incapacitating symptoms. Long-term medical treatment may be required depending on the type and severity of the arthritis. Early diagnosis and intervention are important to allow for normal growth and development.

Juvenile-onset spondyloarthropathies (JSPAs) often affect boys at approximately 10 years of age and occur at an estimated rate of 2 per 100,000 in the United States. JSPAs include the gastrointestinal-associated arthropathies, reactive arthritis, and psoriatic arthritis. JSPA may present as an isolated arthritis, enthesitis, tendonitis, or dactylitis or as a clinical syndrome called seronegative enthesopathy and arthropathy. The majority of children with these syndromes will evolve into ankylosing spondylitis or another spondyloarthropathy over the subsequent decades. These children often will present with an asymmetric arthritis commonly involving the knee, midtarsal joint, and ankle. Spondyloarthropathy should be suspected if there is a history of enthesitis affecting the Achilles tendon or insertion site of the plantar fascia to the os calcis.

Lyme disease is transmitted by deer ticks (*Ixodes dammini*) that carry the spirochete *Borrelia burgdorferi*. The disease can have several manifestations. A common symptom is knee pain or inability to bear weight that may present acutely, similar to septic arthritis, but may also be less painful and more insidious in onset. As with JRA, multiple joints may be involved. Often there is a history of malaise, headache, fever, myalgia, and/or erythema migrans. There may be neurologic symptoms (including peripheral neuropathy and seventh cranial nerve palsy) and/or cardiac symptoms (myocarditis, atrioventricular block). The ESR is elevated in Lyme disease, as may be the white blood cell count. *B. burgdorferi* may be detected by enzyme-linked immunosorbent assay and Western blot analysis. Treatment generally is with amoxicillin or doxycycline. Intravenous ceftriaxone may be used when the response to oral agents is inadequate.[38]

Early adolescence

In young children, musculoskeletal tissues are generally more pliable and absorb much of the impact from external forces. In older children,
the skeletally immature knee is subject to adult-type forces and stresses. Through adolescence, bone stiffness increases and bone becomes less resilient to impact. Overuse injuries have become much more common in concert with earlier and more intense youth participation in organized, competitive sports.

Pediatric sports-related knee injuries

In recent years, the huge investments into promoting active lifestyles in children have significantly increased the number of sports-related knee injuries. Sports injuries have been reported to account for 41% of all musculoskeletal injuries in patients aged 5 to 21 years presenting to pediatric emergency departments.[39] It is estimated that a fourth of all American children are injured per year.[40]

Pediatric knee injuries differ from the adult knee in that growth can be affected after injuries to the growth plates around the knee joint. The distal femoral physis represents the most active growth plate in the body, approximately 0.9 cm per year of growth, providing 70% of the longitudinal growth of the femur. Proximal tibial physis contributes approximately 0.6 cm per year, accounting for 55% of the longitudinal growth of the tibia. Injuries to these areas can result in leg-length discrepancies or angular deformities.

In general, children's more flexible tissues are protective against sports-related injuries. Several intrinsic risk factors have been identified. Specific to anterior knee pain and patellar tracking problems is the influence of the Q angle, that is, the angle of lateral traction of the quadriceps muscle complex on the patella. Pronated hindfeet, limb-length discrepancy, and a flat foot arch have also been advocated as risk factors. Hypermobility of the patella has a positive correlation with patellofemoral pain. Poor quadriceps and gastrocnemius muscle flexibility impaired reflex response time, especially of vastus medialis obliquus and vastus lateralis muscles. Developmental knee problems such as genu valgum and genu varum have also been implicated in making children's knees more prone to injury. Extrinsic risk factors influencing sports injuries include poor training techniques, improper use of equipment, and poor child supervision and coaching.

Osgood-Schlatter disease

Osgood-Schlatter disease is a juvenile traction apophysitis of the tibial tuberosity.[41,42] It occurs most commonly in boys aged 10 to 14 years, and it results from excessive repetitive stresses on the skeletally immature tibial tubercle apophysis due to jumping activities. Patients classically present complaining of pain and tenderness over the tibial tuberosity that is exacerbated by jumping activities.[41,42] Inspection of the knee reveals tender swelling over the tibial prominence (Fig. 74.14). Resisted knee extension may replicate symptoms. Early in the course of the condition, radiographs are usually normal. Later, osseous fragments may become visible anterior to the tibial tubercle within the distal insertion of the patellar tendon on the lateral knee radiograph

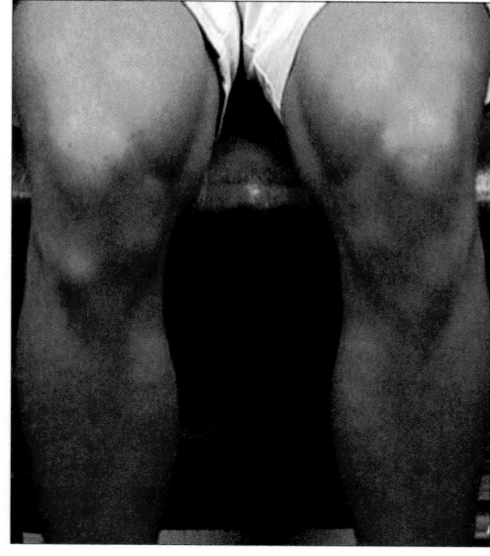

Fig. 74.14 Osgood-Schlatter disease of right knee. Enlarged tibial tubercle.

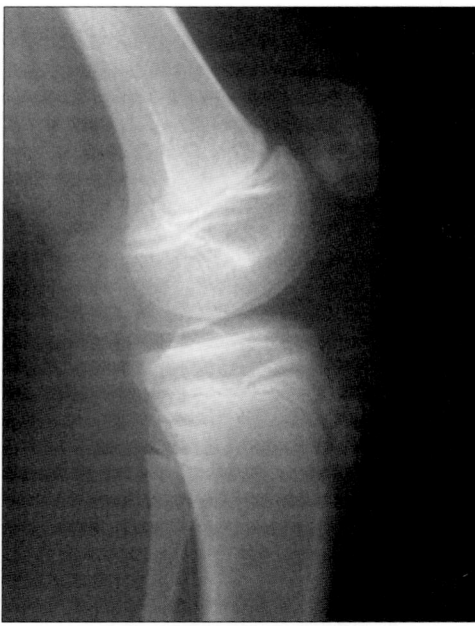

Fig. 74.15 Osgood-Schlatter disease. Loose ossicles in the patellar tendon.

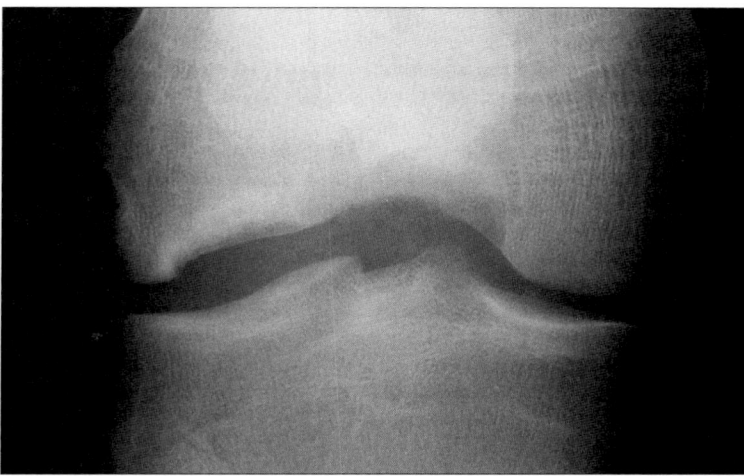

Fig. 74.16 Notch radiograph showing MFC lesion. The radiograph shows an osteochondral defect in a 17-year old with a defect over the weight-bearing area of the lateral femoral condyle.

(Fig. 74.15). Treatment of Osgood-Schlatter disease is generally non-operative, and symptoms resolve as a rule after skeletal maturity. Patients are advised to avoid strenuous jumping activities, and a removable knee brace may ameliorate acute symptoms. Surgery is rarely necessary, but it may be indicated when osteochondral fragments cause persistent pain with kneeling or when a complete avulsion of the tibial tubercle develops.

Sinding-Larsen-Johansson syndrome

Sinding-Larsen-Johansson (SLJ) syndrome is another juvenile traction apophysitis involving the extensor mechanism but, unlike Osgood-Schlatter syndrome, it affects the distal pole of the patella.[43] The pathognomonic findings in SLJ syndrome are pain and tenderness at the distal pole of the patella. As with Osgood-Schlatter disease, the mainstay of treatment is moderate activity limitation, and the condition generally improves spontaneously after skeletal maturity. Physical therapy consisting of quadriceps strengthening and closed-chain exercises may be helpful.

Osteochondritis dissecans

Juvenile osteochondritis dissecans (OCD) is avascular necrosis of bone affecting the osteochondral junction of the epiphysis. Boys are affected three times more commonly than girls, with peak incidence occurring during the second decade of life. The knee joint is by far the most common anatomic site, although the dome of the talus and elbow may also be affected. Within the knee, the most common OCD location is the lateral border of the medial femoral condyle. Less common areas of involvement are the posterior aspect of the lateral femoral condyle, the trochlea and the patella.

The etiology of OCD is multifactorial, with hereditary factors, mechanical stress, and repetitive microtrauma contributing to the development of lesions. Patients present with a history of participation in athletics, presumably leading to recurrent trauma, or with a history of a single, direct trauma to the knee. Symptoms include knee pain and effusion; when an osteochondral fragment is unstable or loose, mechanical symptoms including locking or catching may be present. Examination of the knee reveals effusion and local tenderness over the OCD lesion. Wilson's test may be positive. The test involves straightening the internally rotated knee from a flexed position. Pain at 30 degrees of flexion that is relieved by externally rotating the tibia is suggestive of an OCD lesion of the medial femoral condyle.[44]

Several imaging modalities are useful in delineating the size and severity of OCD lesions. Plain knee radiographs may delineate the OCD lesion or identify osteochondral free bodies. The tunnel view—with the knee flexed 30 degrees and the x-ray beam aimed through the intercondylar notch—is especially good for identifying classic OCD lesions on the lateral aspect of the medial femoral condyle (Fig. 74.16). Computed tomography (CT) provides precise spatial rendering of the osseous extent of the lesion, but, like plain radiographs, it cannot show whether the overlying hyaline cartilage is intact. MRI, especially MR arthrography, provides slightly less osseous detail, but it can help differentiate stable from unstable lesions by revealing the integrity of the overlying cartilage and the condition of the bone/lesion interface (Fig. 74.17).[45,46] Bone scintigraphy distinguishes active lesions from those that have already healed.

Treatment of OCD depends on the age of the patient and the severity of the lesion. There are four stages of OCD lesions, based on severity and arthroscopic appearance (Fig. 74.18):

Stage 1 lesions show softening and irregularity of the articular cartilage without fissuring.
Stage 2 lesions are non-displaced, but the articular cartilage is breached.
Stage 3 lesions are displaced but remain attached *in situ* by intact fibrocartilage.
Stage 4 lesions have a completely displaced osteochondral fragment.

Generally, younger, skeletally immature patients with non-displaced stage 1 or 2 lesions have a more favorable prognosis. Asymptomatic patients do not require treatment. Symptomatic patients may initially be treated with limitation of activities, protected weight-bearing, and physical therapy. Conservative treatment may be attempted for up to 6 months before surgery is considered.

In older children or young adults with a stable OCD lesion, conservative therapy may be attempted, although the prognosis for spontaneous healing is less favorable. Operative management is indicated when conservative measures have failed to result in healing or where the lesion becomes unstable and detaches. Stable lesions are treated with arthroscopic débridement and retrograde drilling to stimulate fibrocartilage formation. Unstable lesions require removal of small loose bodies and fixation of larger unstable osteochondral fragments using Kirschner wires, cannulated screws, Herbert screws, or bioabsorbable devices implanted arthroscopically or after open arthrotomy.

A variety of surgical techniques have been developed to address the difficult problem of large cartilage defects in young patients.[47] Procedures such as microfracture and abrasion, where the bony bed of the defect is débrided and drilled, are designed to stimulate fibrocartilage production by provoking an inflammatory reaction by local marrow cells. The resulting fibrocartilage lacks the tensile properties of hyaline cartilage, and it degenerates over time.[48] Osteochondral allograft or autograft transfer (OAT) procedures involve the harvesting of osteochondral plugs from non–weight-bearing joint surfaces and reimplantation of the plugs into an osteochondral defect in a weight-bearing

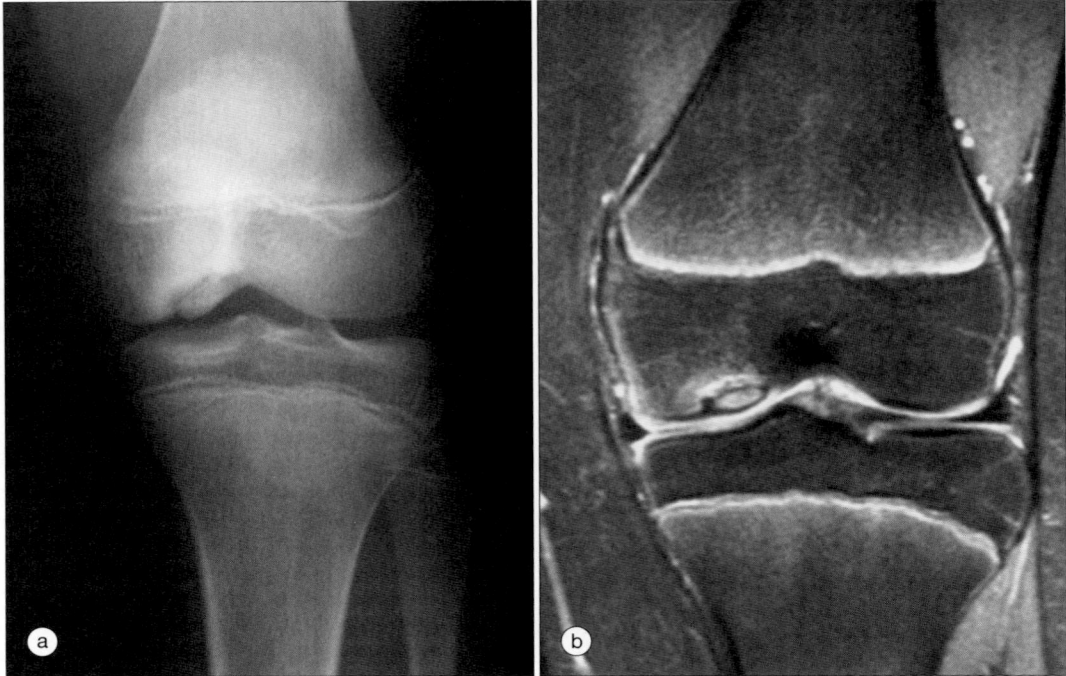

Fig. 74.17 Radiograph (a) and MR image (b) of an OCD lesion.

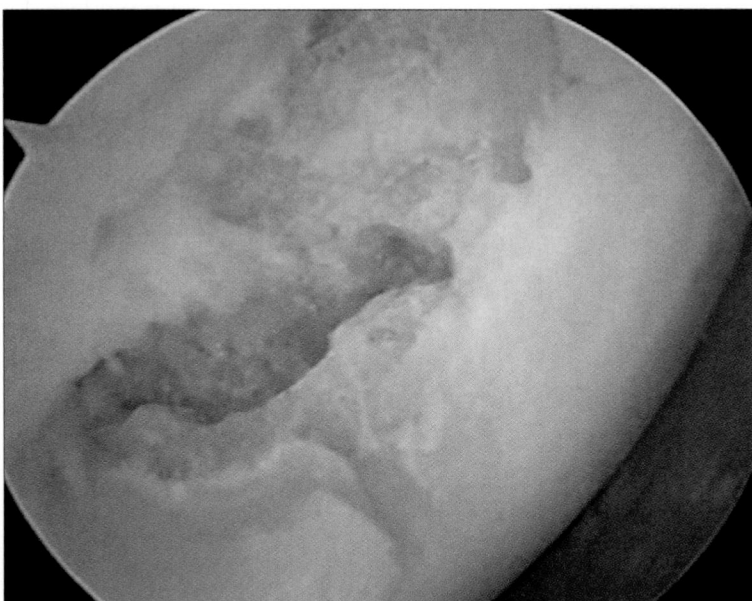

Fig. 74.18 Arthroscopic view of a knee OCD lesion.

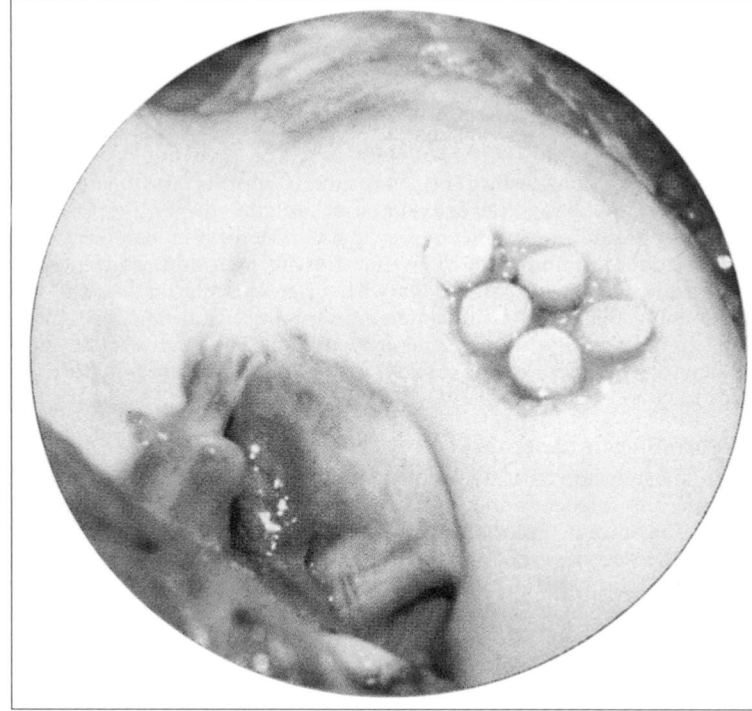

Fig. 74.19 OAT procedure. Note multiple osteochondral plugs.

area (Fig. 74.19). Although good results have been demonstrated using this technique, the area that can be grafted is limited by the availability of donor site cartilage and by donor site morbidity.[49] Where allograft is used, a small risk of disease transmission is recognized.

A more recent development in cartilage repair surgery is autologous cartilage implantation (ACI). In this technique, a patient first undergoes a diagnostic knee arthroscopy in which the size and location of the osteochondral defect is noted and a small, full-thickness sample of articular cartilage is harvested. From this sample, chondrocytes are isolated and cultured *ex vivo*. At least 6 weeks later, the patient returns to the operating room and cultured chondrocytes are implanted into the cartilage defect and sealed there using a periosteal patch, sutures, and fibrin glue. Early results from this procedure show encouraging clinical outcomes and histology that shows regrowth and integration of hyaline cartilage (Fig. 74.20).[50]

Physeal injuries and fractures

Injuries of the pediatric knee most commonly result in physeal injuries because the ligaments are stronger than the growth plates. Mechanically, the growth plate has only one third the strength of the surrounding ligaments. With fractures around the knee, the biggest concern is growth disturbance.

Distal femoral physeal fracture

In skeletally immature patients, the distal femoral physis is susceptible to fracture from direct trauma. Diagnosis may be based primarily on an accurate history and physical examination, because non-displaced

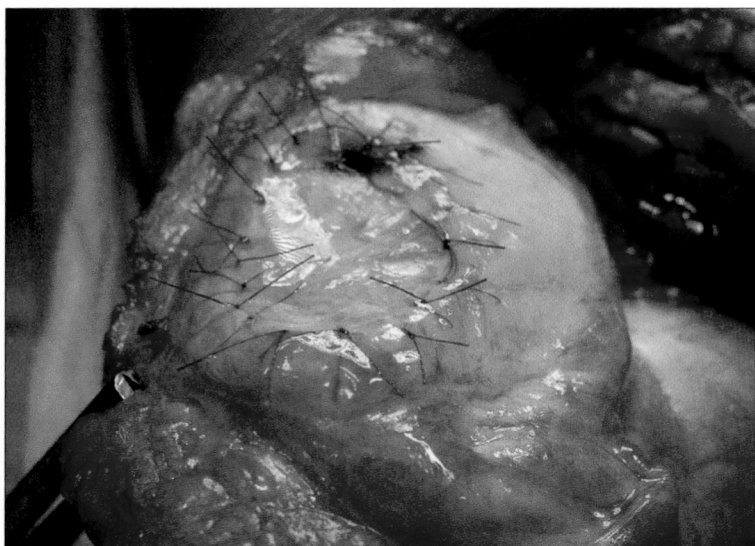

Fig. 74.20 Patellar autologous chondrocyte implantation.

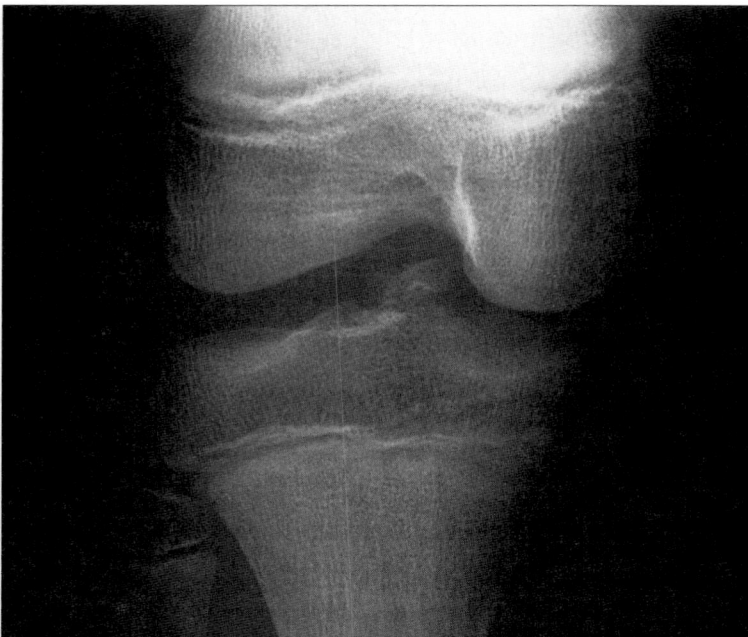

Fig. 74.22 Radiograph showing tibial spine fracture.

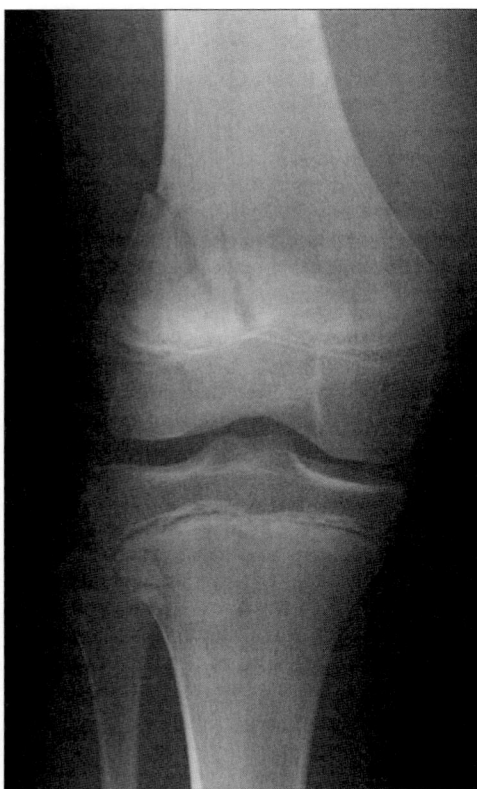

Fig. 74.21 Radiograph showing a Salter-Harris II distal femoral physeal fracture.

fractures through the cartilaginous physis are not visible on plain radiographs. A history of a direct trauma to the knee and tenderness and hemarthrosis on physical examination are consistent with physeal fracture. In select cases, stress radiographs may be obtained to demonstrate instability across the physis, but in most cases a fracture is presumptively treated with a long-leg cast or hip spica cast for 6 weeks. Displaced fractures that cannot be reduced by closed means may require open reduction and internal fixation (Fig. 74.21). Growth arrest may result from physeal injury.

Tibial spine fracture and ACL rupture

Avulsion fractures of the anterior tibial spine are the pediatric equivalent of ACL rupture. The mechanism of injury usually involves falling from a bike or twisting injuries during sports. Physical examination reveals hemarthrosis and reluctance to bear weight. Specific provocative tests including the Lachman, anterior drawer, and pivot shift test may be positive. Plain radiographs show the avulsed tibial spine and the degree of displacement (Fig. 74.22). For McKeever type 1 tibial spine nondisplaced fractures, closed treatment with a long-leg cast in extension is warranted. For type 2 fractures, where the avulsed fragment is elevated but still attached by a posterior hinge, closed reduction by knee extension is attempted. If this is successful, closed treatment with a long-leg cast is possible. Irreducible fractures require open or arthroscopic reduction of the fragment and fixation using suture, wire, or a screw. Type 3 fractures, completely displaced, require surgical reduction and fixation.[51] Isolated ACL rupture is much less common in children than fracture of the tibial spine. Even with anatomic reduction and complete healing of a tibial spine fracture, however, concomitant severe sprains or partial tears of the ACL that do not heal spontaneously may lead to functional incompetence of the ACL. Patients with an isolated ACL rupture present with a palpable hemarthrosis and a history consistent with a twisting fall or valgus or rotational trauma to the knee. Surgical treatment of ACL tears in skeletally immature patients is controversial because techniques employed for replacing the damaged ligament in adults would damage the physis and cause growth disturbance. For this reason, extraphyseal methods of reconstruction have been developed for use in young children who require a stabilizing surgery to return to sports. When a child has no specific sports requirement and is not disabled by ACL laxity, surgery can be delayed until skeletal maturity, when a standard transphyseal technique can be used.[52,53]

Other proximal tibial fractures

Complete fracture of the proximal tibial physes is rare because of the stabilization of the collateral ligaments. There is an association with arterial injury and compartment syndromes. Malreduction or growth arrest may cause genu valgum and varus.

Proximal tibial tuberosity fracture is often an avulsion injury sustained with a sudden quadriceps contraction associated with jumping. This injury may be intra-articular or extra-articular. Intra-articular injuries present with hemarthrosis and often require internal fixation. Extra-articular fractures that are minimally displaced may be treated with immobilization for 4 to 6 weeks.

Late teens/early adulthood

Between early skeletal maturity and adulthood, the most common knee diagnoses are anterior knee pain and traumatic knee injuries.

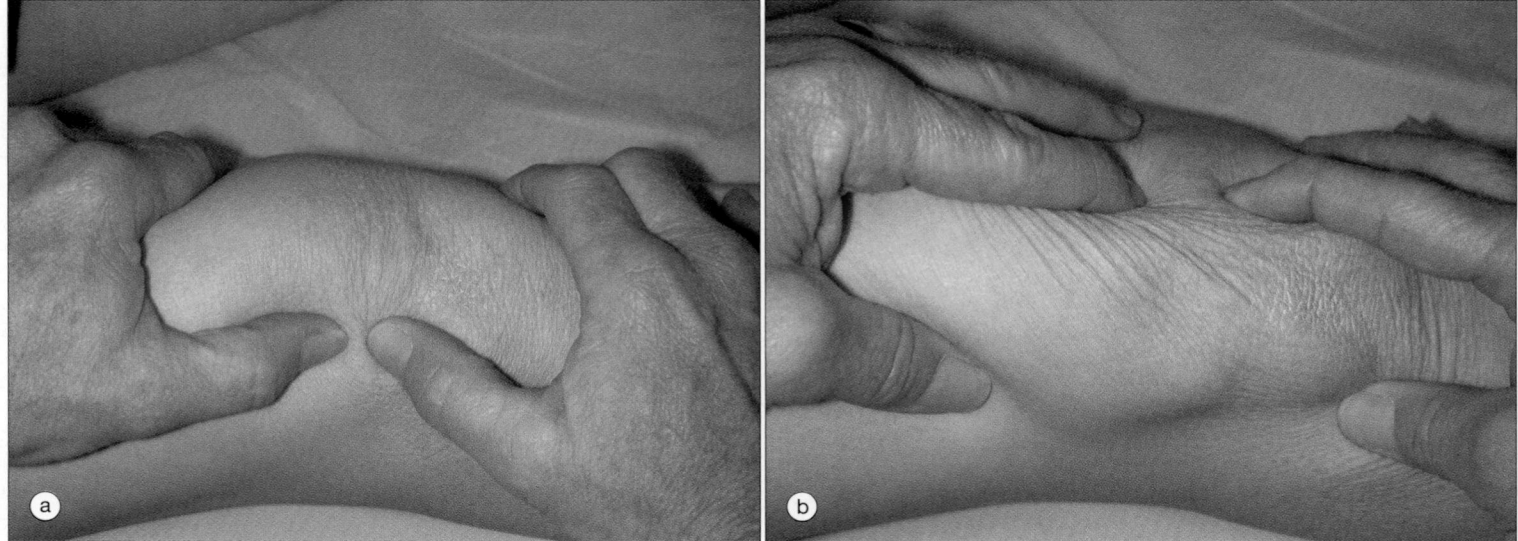

Fig. 74.23 (a and b) The patella apprehension test.

Anterior knee pain

Anterior knee pain can present a difficult diagnostic challenge due to the broad spectrum of possible causes, including patellofemoral maltracking, chondromalacia patellae, and medial plica syndrome. To narrow the list of potential diagnoses, a careful history should elicit the precise anatomic location of the pain and what activities exacerbate or relieve knee pain.[54]

Patellofemoral maltracking, subluxation, and dislocation

Instability of the patellofemoral articulation results from imbalance between medial and lateral forces on the patella. This may be the result of static malalignment in patients with an abnormally high Q angle or dynamic imbalance from atrophy of the principal medial stabilizers of the knee—the medial patellofemoral ligament (MPFL) and the vastus medialis obliquus (VMO)—or contracture of lateral structures—the lateral retinaculum and the IT band.[55,56] A high Q angle may be caused by genu valgum, a laterally positioned tibial tuberosity, persistent femoral anteversion, external tibial torsion, or excessive foot pronation. Patella alta, an abnormally proximal position of the patella relative to the femur, may exacerbate patellofemoral instability by shifting the point where the undersurface of the patella engages the distal femoral trochlea to a later point in the knee flexion arc.[57]

Patellofemoral instability may be characterized by habitual subluxation (when the patella subluxes laterally during every cycle of knee flexion and extension) or recurrent subluxation (when the patella displaces in response to episodic stresses, especially during athletic activity) or by acute dislocation. In patients with habitual subluxation, tight lateral structures may prevent knee flexion if the patella is held in a reduced position. Acute patellofemoral dislocation may result from a direct blow to the medial aspect of the patella. Examination reveals a painful swollen knee with obvious lateral dislocation of the patella. If the patella has spontaneously reduced, the principal finding is tenderness over the torn medial retinaculum and associated knee swelling. Acute dislocation may be associated with an osteochondral fracture of the lateral femoral condyle.

Patients with chronic patellofemoral maltracking present with symptoms ranging from anterior knee pain, caused by excessive lateral stresses on the patellofemoral articular cartilage and stretching of the medial soft tissues, to recurrent episodes of knee "giving way," owing to patella lateral subluxation or frank dislocation. Physical examination may demonstrate a positive "J sign" and tenderness over the medial border of the patella. Other specific tests include the apprehension test, where the knee is held in 20 degrees of flexion and the patella is manually subluxed laterally to reproduce symptoms of instability (Fig. 74.23) and the patella tilt test, where the knee is flexed to 20 degrees and the lateral margin of the patella is flipped upward. A positive patella tilt test, denoting a tight lateral retinaculum, is present when the patella cannot be tilted upward past horizontal.

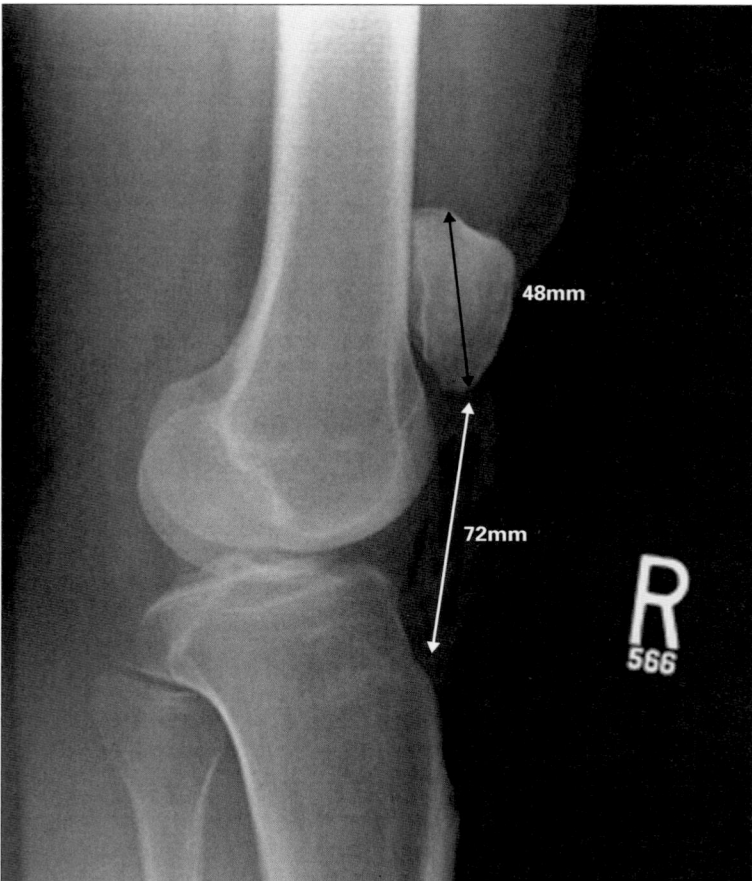

Fig. 74.24 Lateral knee radiograph with Insall-Salvati ratio measurement.

Plain knee radiographs in patients with patellofemoral maltracking may reveal lateral placement of the patella, patella alta, hypoplasia of the distal femoral trochlea, or incongruity of the patellofemoral osseous anatomy. Patella alta is recognized on the lateral view by comparing the length of the patella to the length of the patellar tendon. The average ratio is approximately 1:1 (Fig. 74.24).[57] Skyline views of the patellofemoral joint, taken with the knee flexed at 30 degrees, may show the patella to be tilted laterally and translated toward the lateral femoral condyle (Fig. 74.25). Sclerosis may be seen in the subchondral bone of the lateral facet indicating arthrosis from stress concentrated across the articulation. CT and MRI are rarely necessary, but they may add further spatial information regarding the osseous and ligamentous structures. Patellar subluxation should be distinguished from patellar dislocation (Fig. 74.26).

Treatment of patellofemoral maltracking varies according to the severity of symptoms. For acute dislocation or mild recurrent patellar subluxation, a brief period of knee immobilization with subsequent physical therapy for VMO strengthening and IT band stretching is indicated.[58] Use of a patellar stabilizing brace may also be helpful. Recurrent dislocation may increase patients' risk of chondral injury; and surgeries including repair and imbrication of the MPFL, VMO advancement, lateral retinacular release, quadriceps Z-lengthening, and tibial tubercle osteotomy have been described.

Chondromalacia patellae

Chondromalacia patellae is a descriptive term used to identify pathologic softening and fragmentation of the articular cartilage of the patella due to impact loading and excessive shear stresses. Severity of cartilage involvement is classified in four stages.

Stage 1 denotes softening and swelling of the articular cartilage.
Stage 2 involves deep fissures extending to the subchondral bone.
Stage 3 indicates fibrillation of the articular surface.
Stage 4 constitutes loss of articular cartilage with exposed subchondral bone.

Clinical symptoms associated with these findings include retropatellar pain, especially with ascending or descending stairs or with prolonged sitting. Physical examination is significant for patellofemoral crepitus. When chondromalacia patellae is associated with patellofemoral

malalignment, correction of the underlying abnormality ameliorates clinical symptoms. In idiopathic cases, physical therapy including isometric quadriceps exercises and hamstring stretching is the mainstay of treatment. Arthroscopic débridement chondroplasty with removal of loose chondral fragments may be indicated in severe cases.

Medial plica syndrome

During embryonic development, the knee is divided into three synovial compartments, which break down in the fourth intrauterine month. Failure of complete breakdown results in synovial shelves or plicae. The medial plica lies above the medial femoral condyle, and it may cause irritation and abrasion to the adjacent medical femoral condyle articular cartilage when the knee is flexed. Repeated irritation of the plica leads to fibrosis, which can cause impingement of the plica on the medial femoral condyle or patella.

Clinical manifestations of medial plica syndrome may mimic medial meniscal tear, including snapping, catching, and medial joint line tenderness. A fibrotic, hypertrophic medial plica can sometimes be palpated just above the medial joint line. Treatment is generally non-operative and includes anti-inflammatory medications and rest followed by physical therapy. Rarely, a symptomatic plica may be resected arthroscopically.[59]

Traumatic ligamentous injuries

Ligamentous injuries are common in young athletes. A ligament sprain is an injury in which the fibers are stretched or torn. In a first-degree sprain there are torn fibers but unimpaired function. In a second-degree sprain more fibers are torn, with stretching of the ligament, causing abnormal joint laxity. A third-degree sprain involves a complete ligament rupture, with marked instability.[60] The degree of instability after ligament injury is assessed by specific provocative maneuvers and quantified using a three-point scale: 1+ laxity is up to 5 mm; 2+ is 5 to 10 mm, and 3+ is 10 to 15 mm.

Anterior cruciate ligament injuries

ACL injuries are common among athletes in sports requiring cutting, twisting, or jumping. Injuries are significantly more common among women, with female athletes being eight times more likely to experience ACL injuries than male athletes.[61,62] Potential risk factors include Q angle, femoral anteversion, genu valgum, external tibial torsion, femoral intercondylar notch shape and size, ACL thickness, hormonal influences, and training techniques. Specific mechanisms of injury

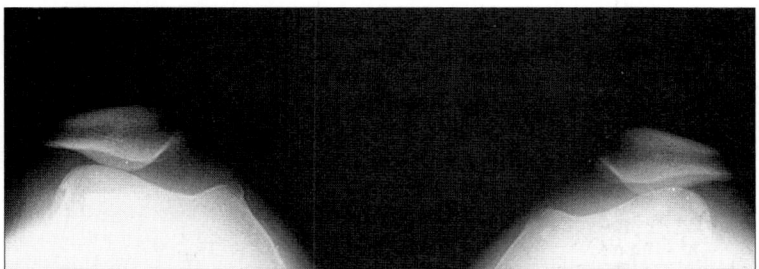

Fig. 74.25 Skyline radiograph showing patellar lateral subluxation.

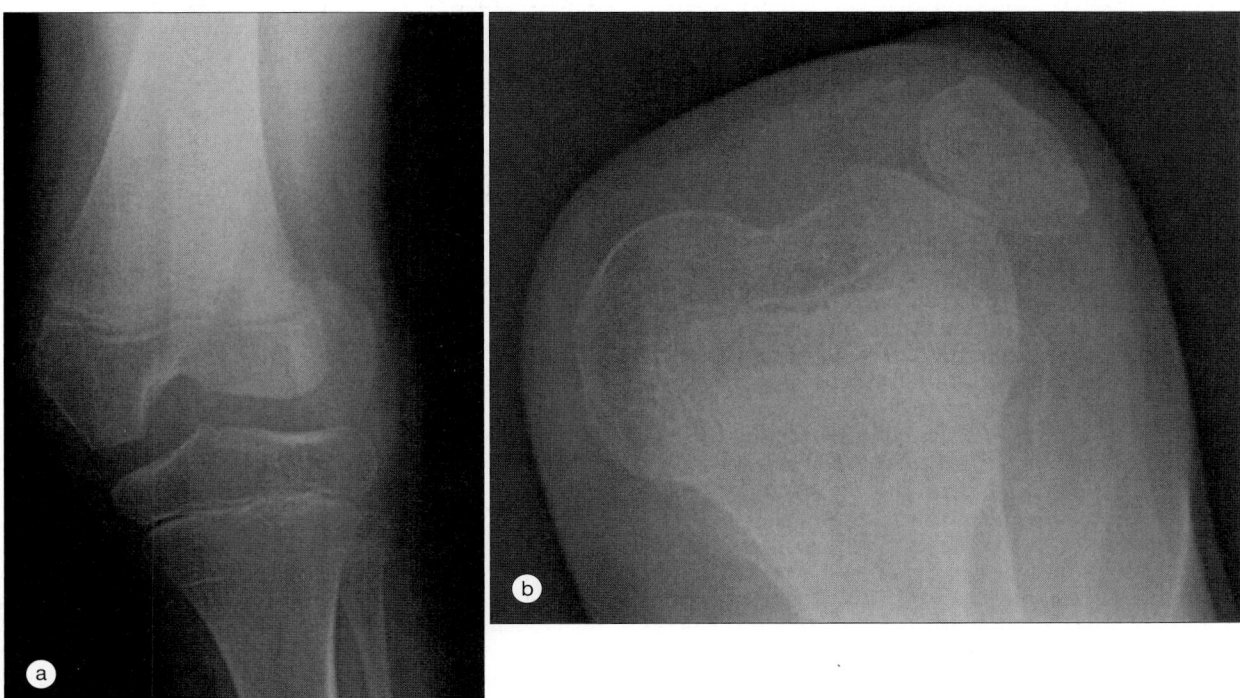

Fig. 74.26 Anteroposterior (a) and skyline (b) radiographs showing patellar dislocation.

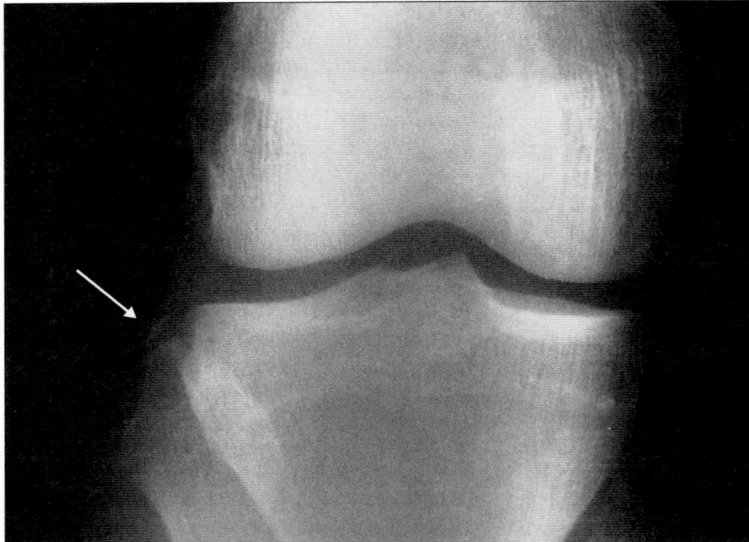

Fig. 74.27 Anteroposterior radiograph of Segond fracture. The figure demonstrates the flake of bone (arrow), showing the avulsion of the anterolateral capsule in the region of Gerdy's tubercle, frequently associated with ACL rupture.

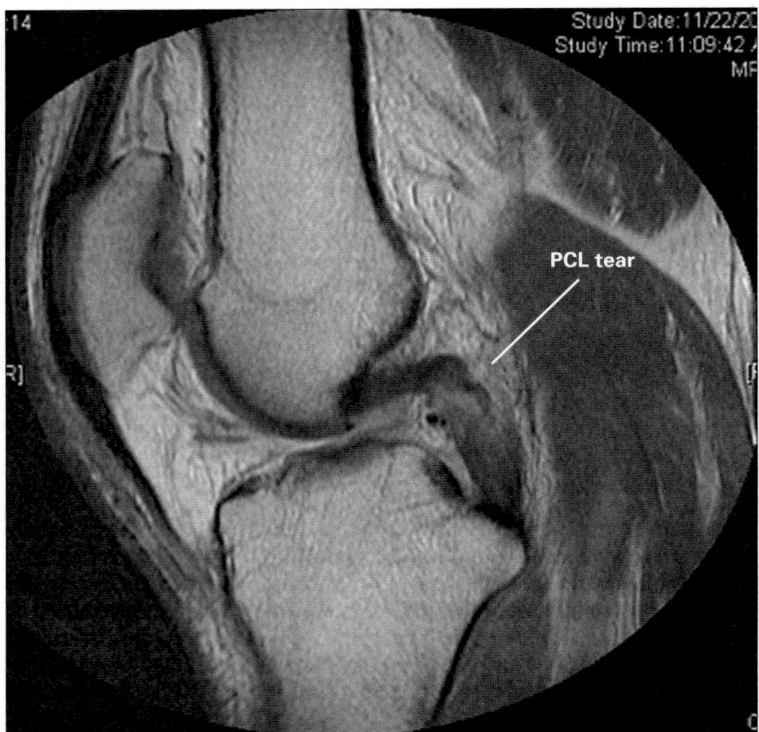

Fig. 74.28 MR image showing PCL rupture.

include direct valgus trauma to a flexed knee and knee hyperextension with concomitant tibial internal rotation.[62] Meniscal tears accompany ACL injuries in up to 70% of cases.[63] Rupture of the ACL, medial meniscus tear, and rupture of the MCL constitute a severe combined injury termed the *O'Donoghue unhappy triad.*

Patients with ACL rupture frequently describe a twisting, backward fall with a palpable "pop" followed by knee pain and swelling.[64] Physical examination of the ACL is described earlier. Especially in the context of acute tear, hamstring spasm may complicate provocative testing including the Lachman, anterior drawer, and pivot shift tests. Radiographs should be taken to look for avulsion injuries of the tibial spines and other associated fractures. A small avulsion fracture of the lateral tibial plateau called a Segond fracture (Fig. 74.27) strongly suggests ACL rupture, especially in the context of a consistent history and physical examination.[65] MRI is a valuable tool for establishing ACL injury and screening for associated meniscal tears.

Many patients with an ACL-deficient knee are asymptomatic, especially if their lifestyle does not require abrupt cutting or jumping activities. Among cutting or jumping athletes, symptoms of an ACL-deficient knee are giving way, swelling, and pain. In general, symptoms are due to rotational instability rather than anteroposterior laxity. Mechanical symptoms of locking or catching may occur in conjunction with a coexisting meniscal tear. Even where initial trauma does not result in meniscal pathology, degenerative tears may result from ACL instability.[64]

Treatment of ACL tears parallels the activity demands and symptoms of the patient. For low demand, asymptomatic patients, no treatment is necessary. Moderate demand athletes or young adults may respond well to physical therapy consisting of hamstring strengthening and fitting with a hinged knee brace. Surgical management involves replacement of the torn ligament with allograft or autograft anchored through bony tunnels in the femur and proximal tibia. Superior functional results are achieved when surgery is delayed until after the initial inflammatory reaction to trauma has subsided and knee range of motion is restored: this allows for immediate rehabilitation postoperatively.[66,67]

Posterior cruciate ligament injuries

PCL injuries are much less common than ACL tears, because the ligament is biomechanically twice as strong as the ACL.[68] Typical mechanisms of injury include a fall onto a flexed knee with the foot in plantarflexion or a direct blow to the anterior tibia with the knee in flexion (dashboard injury). Physical examination reveals a positive posterior drawer sign and posterior sag test. Despite these positive provocative test findings, isolated rupture of the PCL does not result

in significant functional knee instability unless other structures, especially the posterolateral corner, have also been damaged.[68-70] Routine plain radiographs are usually normal, although a small avulsion fracture of the tibial insertion of the PCL is sometimes visible on the lateral knee radiograph. MRI is the imaging gold standard for detecting PCL injury. Nonoperative treatment of isolated PCL injuries consists of short-term immobilization and protected weight bearing followed by quadriceps strengthening and range of motion exercises (Fig. 74.28).

Medial collateral ligament injuries

The MCL is usually injured as a result of a valgus force, often associated with external rotation of the tibia. As with most extracapsular ligamentous injuries, acute-phase findings include swelling and bruising over the course of the ligament with tenderness over the joint line or femoral insertion. Loss of full extension may be present in an incomplete tear due to pain as the ligament comes under tension in the last 20 degrees of extension. Treatment of isolated MCL tears is conservative, consisting of a few weeks in a knee immobilizer followed by progressive physical therapy.[71]

Pellegrini-Stieda disease is an infrequent chronic sequela of MCL injury in which a patient presents with persistent pain over the MCL femoral insertion due to local calcification. The area is tender to palpation, and pain is elicited on stressing of the ligament. Radiographs reveal characteristic calcification at the ligament insertion (Fig. 74.29).[72] Treatment consists of rest and NSAIDs, since the condition is usually self-limiting. Occasionally, a targeted corticosteroid injection helps to ameliorate symptoms.

Lateral collateral ligament injuries

The LCL is the least common knee ligament to be injured in isolation; LCL rupture is usually associated with damage to the posterolateral ligament complex (lateral capsule, arcuate ligament, and popliteus tendon). The cruciate ligaments may also be damaged. The mechanism of injury is usually a varus stress on an extended knee. The ligament usually ruptures at its fibular insertion, or it may avulse off the fibular styloid. A peroneal nerve palsy may be associated with an LCL tear, so distal sensory and motor function should be assessed. LCL rupture leads to greater functional disability than MCL rupture, so conservative management should be attempted only for low-grade instability. Severe disruptions or combined posterolateral corner injuries should be repaired acutely in active young athletes.[68]

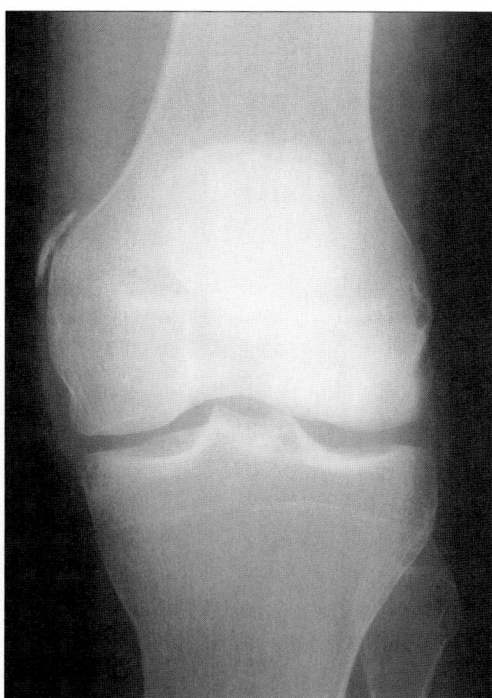

Fig. 74.29 Pellegrini-Stieda disease. Radiograph showing calcification of the insertion of the medial collateral ligament.

Adult

Bursitis

Bursitis refers to inflammation of a synovial-lined bursa. Causes of bursitis include direct trauma, recurrent minor injury, infection, or crystal deposition diseases. The prepatellar bursa is the most frequent site of knee bursitis. Specific causes linked to prepatellar bursitis include direct trauma to the anterior aspect of the knee or recurrent trauma from prolonged kneeling, especially among carpet layers, roofers, and floor cleaners, giving rise to the eponym "housemaid's knee." Symptoms including anterior knee erythema, swelling, and tenderness over the patella may be difficult to distinguish from septic or inflammatory arthritis, although the history may be suggestive and the effusion is more superficial in prepatellar bursitis. Knee range of motion may also be somewhat less painful in cases of prepatellar bursitis than in knee septic arthritis.

Most cases of prepatellar bursitis are caused by trauma or gout rather than infection. Distinguishing between these causes is facilitated most directly by aspiration of the bursa fluid and subsequent analysis by Gram stain, culture, cell count, and microscopy for crystals. The examiner should exercise care when aspirating bursa fluid so as to not enter the knee capsule, because this risks seeding of bacteria from a septic bursitis to a sterile knee joint. Treatment of prepatellar bursitis depends on the underlying etiology. Traumatic bursitis may respond well to bursa aspiration and injection with corticosteroid, rest, and avoidance of kneeling. Crystal deposition bursitis is treated with systemic anti-inflammatory medications. Septic bursitis is treated with rest, serial aspirations, and parenteral, followed by oral, antibiotics. Surgical drainage may be indicated for loculated bursitis, and recurrent bursitis may require open bursectomy.

Patellar tendonitis

Patellar tendonitis is an overuse syndrome precipitated by repetitive running and jumping sports such as soccer, volleyball, and basketball. Also called "jumper's knee," patellar tendonitis results from cumulative microtears of the deep fibers of the patellar tendon, especially near the insertion at the inferior pole of the patella.[73] In older patients, the superior pole of the patella may be affected by analogous quadriceps tendonitis. Symptoms of patellar tendonitis including pain at the inferior pole of the patella are exacerbated by bent knee activities such as squatting, climbing stairs, and jumping. Puddu's test, performed with the knee in extension by pushing the patella distally and palpating the lower pole of the patella, may help to localize the point of maximal tenderness. Standard radiographs are usually normal, and MRI or CT is not generally necessary to make the clinical diagnosis.

The first therapeutic option for patellar tendonitis is always non-operative, with the majority of patients responding well to activity modification, hamstring and quadriceps stretching, and non-steroidal anti-inflammatory drugs. A variety of braces and straps that stabilize the patella and compress the tendon may be added to the physical therapy program. Occasionally, operative treatment to excise the involved portion of tendon is necessary.

Iliotibial band syndrome

Iliotibial band syndrome is another overuse syndrome associated with long distance running, leading to the eponym "runner's knee."[74,75] Distance runners with genu varum and planovalgus foot alignment are biomechanically predisposed to increased friction between the IT band and lateral femur, especially during the swing phase of gait when there is a physiologic varus moment. Increased contact stresses lead to inflammation of the IT band and its underlying bursa, resulting in lateral knee pain that worsens with activity. Physical examination reveals tenderness over the lateral epicondyle. Treatment of IT band syndrome is usually conservative, with activity restriction and IT band stretching being most important. For acute exacerbations, local injection of corticosteroid may provide lasting relief.

Popliteal cysts

Posterior knee pain is frequently caused by popliteal Baker cysts.[76,77] Cysts originate from a communication between the knee joint and the gastrocnemius-semimembranosus bursa, usually where the tendon of the medial head of gastrocnemius leaves the joint capsule.[78,79] With increasing age, degeneration and loss of elasticity of the joint capsule coupled with elevated intracapsular pressure from persistent effusions due to degenerative osteoarthritis result in more frequent cyst formation.

Cysts enlarge due to a one-way valve phenomenon in which pressurized synovial fluid flows into the cyst with knee extension and is trapped in the cyst during knee flexion. As with other synovial cysts, Baker cysts may enlarge or regress gradually over time or they may rupture acutely. Cyst rupture is typically accompanied by a sensation of water running down the posterior calf.

Patients with Baker cysts complain of achy posterior knee pain, frequently with a palpable popliteal mass. Physical examination may reveal a palpable posterior knee mass in the context of a moderately sized knee effusion. If the mass is pulsatile and a bruit is heard over it, a popliteal artery aneurysm is possible and further evaluation with ultrasonography or MRI is indicated. Other rare posterior knee masses are nerve sheath tumors and sarcoma.

Treatment in adults is initially tailored to address the cause of the knee effusion.[77] Knee aspiration and corticosteroid injection may be performed to reduce synovial fluid volume and to reduce fluid production. Arthroscopic knee synovectomy with ablation of the communication between the cyst and the joint is reserved for painful cysts that have failed more conservative management.

Synovial chondromatosis

Synovial chondromatosis is a rare condition of unknown etiology in which multiple metaplastic foci of cartilage develop in joints, tendon sheaths, and bursae. It occurs as a result of metaplasia in the subsynovial connective tissue. The cartilaginous bodies may become pedunculated or loose within the joint. The knee is by far the most common joint affected by both intra-articular and extra-articular disease. Milgram classified the disease into three phases: early, with active intrasynovial disease but no loose bodies; transitional, with active intrasynovial disease and loose bodies; and late, with multiple loose bodies but no synovial disease (Fig. 74.30).[80]

The condition tends to occur in middle age but may present as early as the late teens.[81] Knee pain and swelling are characteristic early symptoms, with mechanical locking developing when chondral lesions become pedunculated or loose bodies. Examination reveals a swollen knee with thickened synovium, crepitus on movement, and palpable loose bodies. In later stages of disease, knee range of motion may be decreased.

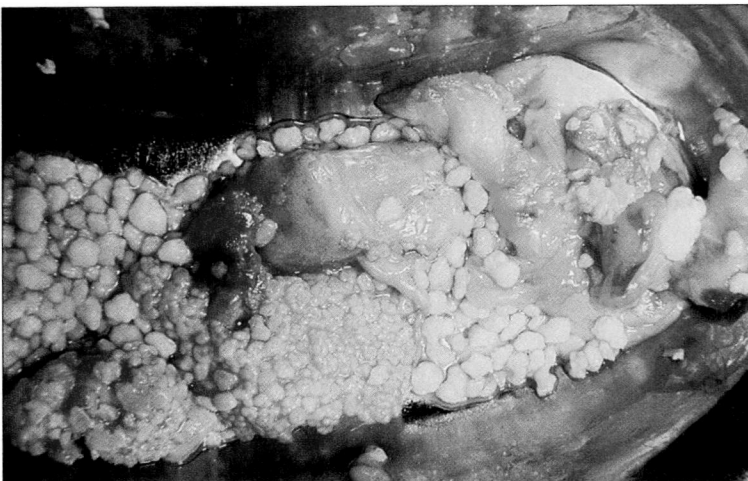

Fig. 74.30 Synovial chondromatosis.

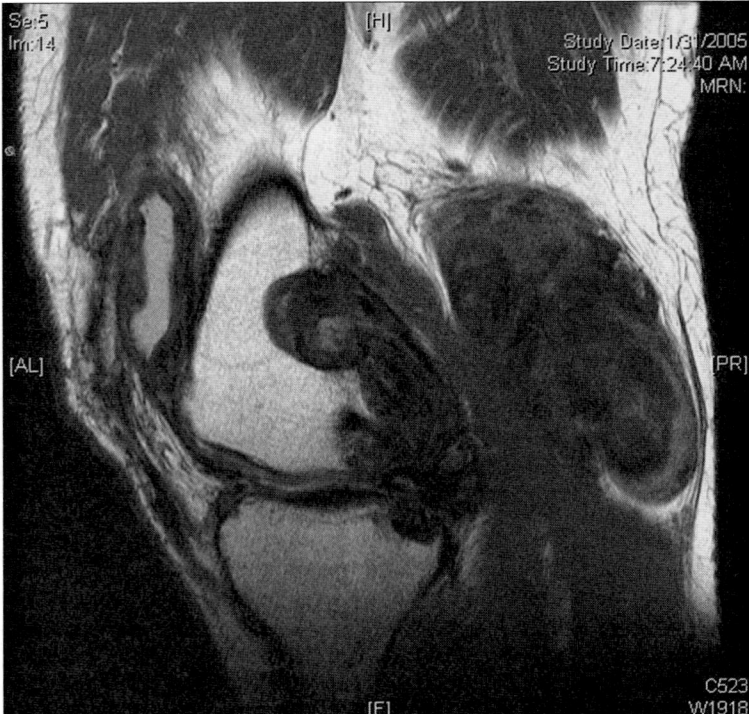

Fig. 74.31 MR image of a knee with PVNS showing bony erosion.

Radiographs in early synovial chondromatosis show multiple, stippled cartilaginous bodies, which are visible in greater resolution using double-contrast arthrography. In later stages of the disease, calcified lesions are clearly visible on plain radiographs. Treatment of symptomatic synovial chondromatosis involves arthroscopic removal of symptomatic loose bodies. In the first and second phases of disease, active synovium should be excised. Total synovectomy is impractical and unnecessary. Recurrence is uncommon, and it may be treated with repeat arthroscopic débridement.

Pigmented villonodular synovitis

Pigmented villonodular synovitis (PVNS) is an uncommon proliferative tumor of synovial tissue that most frequently affects the knee. The presenting complaint is typically episodic knee pain and swelling, although mechanical locking may occur if the proliferative synovium becomes trapped between the joint surfaces. A history of recurrent atraumatic knee hemarthrosis with no underlying coagulopathy may also suggest PVNS. Physical examination reveals a tender, swollen joint with limited range of motion. MRI is the mainstay for imaging of PVNS, with characteristic findings including synovial hypertrophy with T1 and T2 signal changes consistent with hemosiderin deposition (Fig. 74.31). Aspiration of brown synovial fluid in the absence of recent trauma is characteristic and may often be the first indication of the disease. On arthroscopy, thickened nodular synovium that is reddish brown is seen. Histologic examination shows a stroma of reticulum and collagen fibers with multinucleated giant cells, foam cells, and hemosiderin deposits.

Treatment of PVNS depends on the extent and intracapsular or extracapsular location of the disease. Limited, intracapsular nodular PVNS may successfully be treated with arthroscopic débridement, but extensive, extracapsular synovial proliferation may require open anterior and posterior synovectomy and adjuvant radiation therapy to reduce the likelihood of recurrent disease.[82,83]

Meniscal injuries

Meniscal injuries are common in young adults, usually occurring as sports-related injuries and often in combination with ligamentous injury, particularly rupture of the ACL. Meniscal injuries are also associated with chronic ligamentous instability. Acute meniscal tears result from a twisting force applied to the weight-bearing knee, causing entrapment of the meniscus between the tibial and femoral condyles. Hemarthrosis developing within 1 hour after a meniscal tear may signal a concomitant ligamentous or osteochondral injury or it may indicate extension of the tear into the vascularized peripheral red zone. Delayed hemarthrosis, in contrast, usually signifies meniscal injury within the avascular red-white or white zones.

Among older patients, the meniscal fibrocartilage is less elastic and degenerative tears can occur without a specific traumatic event.[84] Degenerative tears are usually horizontal cleavage tears or radial tears.

Patients with an acute meniscal tear characteristically report a twisting injury that causes immediate, severe pain at the joint line. The knee may be locked in flexion or extension if a torn fragment of the meniscus is interposed between the articular surfaces. Physical examination classically demonstrates a knee effusion, joint line tenderness adjacent to the meniscal tear, pain with knee hyperflexion, or pain with knee hyperextension. A locked knee will exhibit a springy block to extension with pain on forced extension. Unlocking of the knee is accompanied by a characteristic clunk. A complete ligamentous examination should be performed on a patient with a suspected meniscus tear to assess for possible concomitant injuries.

McMurray's test, a provocative test for meniscal injury, is performed with the patient supine. While the knee is slowly extended from a flexed position a valgus and external rotation force is applied across the knee to test the lateral compartment. The knee is then flexed, and the maneuver is repeated with varus and internal rotation force to test the medial knee compartment. A positive test elicits a palpable click during knee extension accompanied by reproduction of pain symptoms.[85] Apley's grinding test is performed with the patient prone and the knee flexed. The tibia is loaded axially while it is internally and externally rotated. Pain or a clicking sensation is said to be suggestive of a meniscal tear.[86]

Plain radiographs of patients with a meniscal tear are generally normal unless there is an associated osseous injury. MRI is the study of choice to confirm a meniscal tear, with diagnostic accuracy greater than 90% (Fig. 74.32).[87]

Treatment of meniscal tears depends on a complex synthesis of factors, including the location, length, stability, and pattern of the tear and patient factors such as age, chronicity of the tear, concurrent injuries, and general condition of the knee joint. Conservative management of meniscus tears is generally appropriate in older patients with low functional demand and with chronic, central meniscus tears in the context of significant degenerative joint disease. Short, radial tears less than 5 mm in length, stable longitudinal tears of the peripheral two thirds, and partial thickness tears in various patterns and locations may also be treated conservatively, because many will become asymptomatic.[88] A standard regimen includes activity modification, nonsteroidal anti-inflammatory drugs, and, in some cases, periodic intra-articular corticosteroid injection.

Meniscal tear is the most common surgical lesion in the knee. For young patients with symptomatic meniscal tears involving the central

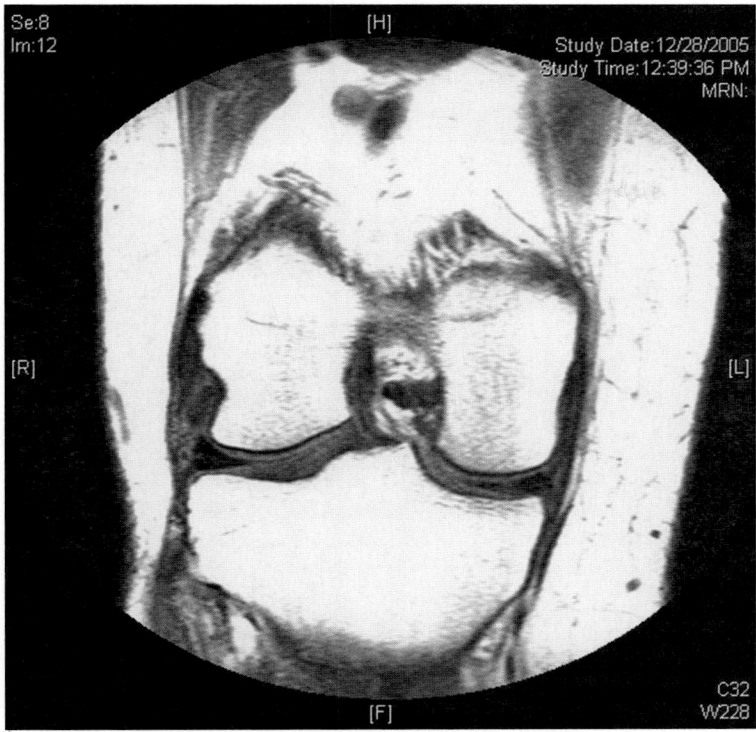

Fig. 74.32 MR image of medial meniscus tear.

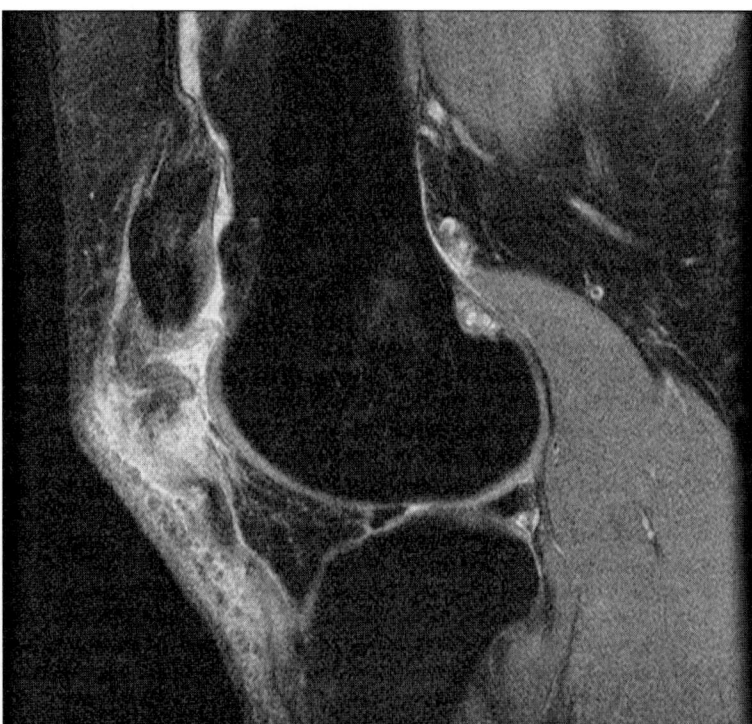

Fig. 74.34 MR image showing patellar tendon rupture.

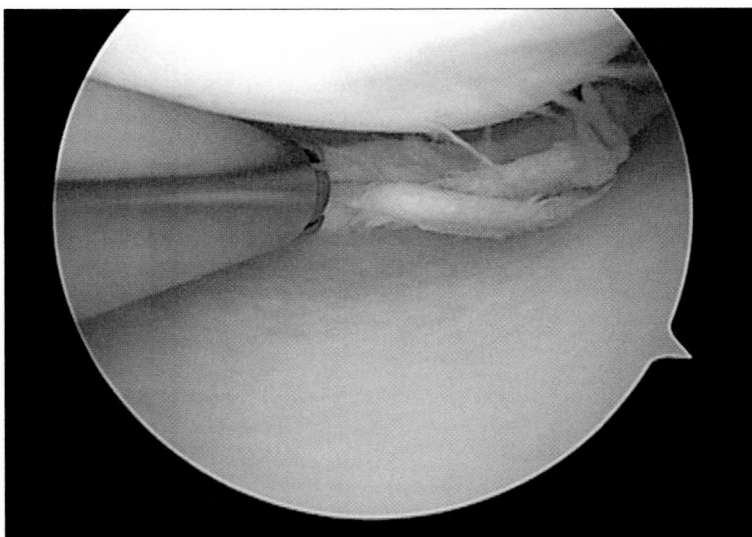

Fig. 74.33 Arthroscopic partial medial meniscectomy.

two thirds of the meniscus, the treatment is arthroscopic partial meniscectomy (Fig. 74.33). For peripheral tears within the red vascular zone of the meniscus, repair by arthroscopic or open techniques may be attempted. Where there is a co-existent ACL rupture, meniscus repair in conjunction with ACL reconstruction is associated with improved results.[89]

Extensor mechanism injuries

The most common knee tendinous injury among elderly patients is rupture of the patellar or quadriceps tendon. Common mechanisms include a forward fall, in which the quadriceps muscles contract forcefully and eccentrically against a flexed knee. This force, acting on an already degenerate patellar or quadriceps tendon, leads to tendon rupture. Patients present with acute anterior knee pain and inability actively to extend the knee. As noted earlier, the IT band may act as an accessory knee extensor when the knee is fully extended, so the ability to straight-leg raise does not exclude tendon rupture. A more specific test is to assess active knee extension from a flexed position. Patella alta may be apparent on physical examination or on the lateral knee radiograph where the patellar tendon is ruptured. A defect may also be palpable in the substance of the ruptured quadriceps or patellar tendon.

Fracture of the patella may also lead to disruption of the extensor mechanism. It can be distinguished from tendon rupture by tenderness localizing over the patella, palpation of a bony diastasis, and findings on lateral knee radiography.

Diagnosis of a patellar or quadriceps tendon injury can usually be established from a complete history, physical examination, and plain radiographs. Where further confirmation is necessary, or where anatomic delineation of the injury is necessary for operative planning, MRI is the study of choice (Fig. 74.34).

Treatment of complete patella or quadriceps tendon rupture requires surgery.

KNEE PAIN SYNDROMES

Fibromyalgia syndrome is most common in midlife but may be seen at all ages. Its symptoms may overlap with chronic fatigue syndrome. Symptoms include polymyalgias, polyarthralgias, non-restorative sleep, difficulty concentrating, and fatigue. Examination shows typical tender points, absence of joint swelling, and neurologic findings. Patients with fibromyalgia generally do not respond to salicylate or other anti-inflammatory medications. Reassurance, medications (especially tricyclic antidepressants), moderate exercise, and proper sleep are the mainstays of therapy (see Chapter 77).

Complex regional pain syndromes (CRPS) involve persistent pain, allodynia (pain evoked by light touch), and autonomic dysfunction. The two types of CRPS are classified based on absence or presence of overt nerve injury, respectively: CRPS type 1, reflex sympathetic dystrophy (RSD), and type 2, causalgia. RSD usually follows a relatively minor trauma, such as knee sprain, often as part of sports injuries.[90] There is a heavy female-to-male predilection, and 80% of cases involve the lower extremity. Treatment of RSD patients involves a multidisciplinary approach. A physiotherapy program is important to desensitize patients and help them overcome fear of touch and movement. Psychological management is necessary, with continued reassurance for the patient. Pharmacotherapy treatments include anti-inflammatory agents, antidepressants, gabapentin, and nerve blocks.

THE RELATIONSHIP OF INJURY TO DEGENERATION

Any injury that alters the alignment, stability, or osseous congruence of the knee joint will accelerate the development of degenerative (osteo-) arthrosis. Intra-articular fractures alter the loading pressures across hyaline cartilage, so anatomic reduction of the joint surface is essential. Metaphyseal fractures that alter the weight-bearing axis of the lower extremity also unbalance the forces across the knee, leading to excessive selective loading of one knee compartment.

Surgery can also lead to altered knee joint biomechanics. It is well recognized that total meniscectomy increases the risk of degenerative change.[91] Jackson found a 21% incidence of degeneration after total meniscectomy compared with a 5% incidence on the contralateral side.[92] Partial meniscectomy also increases load transmission across articular cartilage and thereby accelerates degenerative changes. Because of this, surgeons retain as much of the meniscus as possible to leave a "balanced" stable rim.

The role of ligamentous injury in accelerating degenerate changes in the knee is also well established. Instability associated with ACL-deficient knees increases the likelihood of meniscus tears and early degenerative joint disease. Despite this, there is little evidence to suggest that surgical ACL reconstruction restores the knee to a normal timeline of degenerative change.[93] ACL stabilization therefore can reduce symptoms of instability, allow return to athletics, and reduce the risk of consequential meniscal tears, but early knee arthrosis still occurs. One explanation for these findings is that the traumatic event causing the ACL rupture also injured the knee articular cartilage or subchondral bone sufficiently to accelerate cartilage degeneration.

ASPIRATION AND INJECTION OF THE KNEE

Although the knee is a large superficial joint, access to the joint cavity for aspiration or injection may be difficult, especially in patients without an effusion or with a large body habitus. The capsule of the knee is large and extends several centimeters above the superior pole of the patella. Absent a knee effusion, this large cavity contains only a few milliliters of synovial fluid.

With the patient lying supine, the upper and lateral borders of the patella are palpated. The patella is pushed medially to widen the interval between the lateral patellar border and the lateral femoral condyle. The decision to use preliminary local anesthetic depends on patient factors and practitioner experience, but in general, 2 mL of 1% lidocaine injected at the aspiration site into the subcutaneous tissue using a 22-gauge needle enables injection or aspiration of fluid from the knee with minimal discomfort. A large-bore needle is inserted just lateral to the patella through the skin, lateral retinaculum, joint capsule, and into the knee joint. Once the needle tip is inside the joint, fluid should inject freely with little resistance. Aspiration of even a large effusion may be hindered if it consists mostly of coagulated blood, a loculated fluid collection, or many loose bodies. The appropriate dose of corticosteroid, 40 mg of methylprednisolone, is usually mixed with 2 to 3 mL of 1% lidocaine before injection.

The most reliable technique for knee injection or aspiration is lateral to the patella, as described earlier, or medial to the patella, after pushing the patella laterally. The medial approach may be favored in patients with chronic lateral patellar subluxation, where the lateral patellofemoral articulation may be degenerative and narrowed. Efforts to enter the knee joint through areas mimicking the medial and lateral arthroscopy portals with the knee in 90 degrees of flexion are commonly thwarted by the infrapatellar fat pad that lies behind the patellofemoral joint and fits snugly against the condylar surface. Injection of corticosteroid into the fat pad may also exacerbate knee pain.

KEY REFERENCES

1. Last RJ. Some anatomical details of the knee joint. J Bone Joint Surg Br 1948;30:683-688.
2. Grelsamer RP, Weinstein CH. Applied biomechanics of the patella. Clin Orthop Relat Res 2001;389:9-14.
3. Goodfellow J, Hungerford DS, Zindel M. Patellofemoral mechanics and pathology: I. Functional anatomy of the patellofemoral joint. J Bone Joint Surg Br 1976;58:287-290.
4. Blankevoort L, Huiskes R, de Lange A. The envelope of passive knee joint motion. J Biomech 1988;21:705-720.
5. Fu FH, Harner CD, Johnson DL, Woo SL. Biomechanics of knee ligaments: basic concepts and clinical application. Instr Course Lect 1994;43:137-148.
6. Brantigan OC, Voshell AF. The tibial collateral ligament: its function, its bursae and its relation to the medial meniscus. J Bone Joint Surg 1943;25:121-131.
7. Warren LF, Marshall JL, Girgis FG. The prime static stabiliser of the medial side of the knee. J Bone Joint Surg Am 1974;56A:665-674.
8. Fulkerson JP, Gossling HR. Anatomy of the knee joint lateral retinaculum. Clin Orthop 1980;153:183-188.
9. Girgis FG, Marshall JL, Al Monajem ARS. The cruciate ligaments of the knee joint. Clin Orthop Relat Res 1975;106:216-231.
10. Muller M, de Ruijter M. The derivation of knee joint types from the geometry of the cruciate ligament four-bar system. J Theoret Biol 1998;193:507-518.
11. Arnoczky SP. Anatomy of the anterior cruciate ligament. Clin Orthop Relat Res 1983;172:19-25.
12. Gollehon DL, Torzilli PA, Warren RJ. The role of the posterolateral and cruciate ligaments in the stability of the human knee: a biomechanical study. J Bone Joint Surg 1987;69:233-242.
13. Butler DL, Noyes FR, Grood ES. Ligamentous restraints to anterior-posterior drawer in the human knee: a biomechanical study. J Bone Joint Surg 1980;62:259-270.
14. Seebacher JR, Inglis AE, Marshal JL, et al. The structure of the posterolateral aspect of the knee. J Bone Joint Surg Am 1982;64:536-541.
15. Covey DC. Injuries of the posterolateral corner of the knee. J Bone Joint Surg 2001;83:106-118.
16. Terry GC, Laprade RF. The posterolateral aspect of the knee: anatomy and surgical approach. Am J Sports Med 1996;24:732-739.
17. Rath E, Richmond JC. The menisci: basic science and advances in treatment. Br J Sports Med 2000;34:252-257.
18. Arnoczky SP, Warren RF. Microvasculature of the human meniscus. Am J Sports Med 1982;10:90-95.
19. Last RJ. The popliteus muscle and the lateral meniscus. J Bone Joint Surg Br 1950;32:93-99.
20. Henigan SP, Schneck CD, Mesgarzadeh M, Clancy M. The semimembranosus-tibial collateral ligament bursa. J Bone Joint Surg Am 1994;76:1322-1327.
21. Chhabra A, Elliot C, Miller MD. Normal anatomy and biomechanics of the knee. Sports Med Arthroscop Rev 2002;9:166-177.
22. Kaplan EB. The iliotibial tract: clinical and morphological significance. J Bone Joint Surg Am 1985;40:817-832.
23. Hollister AM, Jatana S, Singh AK, et al. The axes of rotation of the knee. Clin Orthop Relat Res 1993;290:259-268.
24. Dye SF. The knee as a biologic transmission with an envelope of function: a theory. Clin Orthop Relat Res 1996;325:10-18.
25. Piazza SJ, Cavanagh PR. Measurement of the screw-home of the knee is sensitive to errors in axis management. J Biomech 2000;33:1029-1034.
26. Fulkerson JP, Shea KP. Disorders of patellofemoral alignment: current concepts review. J Bone Joint Surg Am 1990;72:1424-1429.
27. Grood ES, Stowers SF, Noyes FR. Limits of movement of in the human knee: effects of sectioning the PCL and posterolateral structures. J Bone Joint Surg Am 1988;70:88-97.
28. Hughston JC, Andrews JR, Cross MJ. Classification of knee ligament instabilities: I. The medial compartment and cruciate ligaments. J Bone Joint Surg Am 1976;58:159-172.
29. Hughston JC, Andrews JR, Cross MJ, Moschi A. Classification of knee ligament instabilities: II. The lateral compartment. J Bone Joint Surg Am 1976;58:173-179.
30. Solomon DH, Simel DL, Bates DW, et al. The rational clinical examination: does this patient have a torn meniscus or ligament of the knee? Value of the physical examination. JAMA 2001;286:1610-1620.
31. Galway RD, Beaupre A, MacIntosh DL. Pivot shift. J Bone Joint Surg Br 1972;54:763.
32. Garrett WE, Speer KP, Kirkendall DT. Orthopaedic Sports Medicine. Philadelphia: Lippincott Williams & Wilkins, 2000:675-685.
33. Kocher M, Zurakowski D, Kasser J. Differentiating between septic arthritis and transient synovitis of the hip in children: an evidence-based clinical prediction algorithm. J Bone Joint Surg Am 1999;81:1662-1670.
34. Jordan MR. Lateral meniscus variants: evaluation and treatment. J Am Acad Orthop Surg 1996;4:191-200.
35. Kaplan EB. Discoid lateral meniscus of the knee joint: nature, mechanism and operative treatment. J Bone Joint Surg Am 1957;39:77-87.
36. Epps CH, Bryant D, Coles-Maxime JM, et al. Osteomyelitis in patients who have sickle-cell disease: diagnosis and management. J Bone Joint Surg Am 1991;73:1281-1294.
37. Green M: Limb and musculoskeletal pain. In: Pediatric diagnosis: interpretation of symptoms and signs in children and adolescents, 6th ed. Philadelphia: WB Saunders, 1998:152.
38. Feder HM, Hunt MS: Pitfalls in the diagnosis and treatment of Lyme disease in children. JAMA 1995:274:66-68.
39. Damore DT, Metzl JD, Ramundo M, et al: Patterns in childhood sports injury. Acad Emerg Med 2001:8:458.
40. Hosalkar H, Lou J, Flynn J: Pediatric musculoskeletal trauma. Curr Opin Orthop 2002:13:413-418.
41. Osgood RB. Lesions of the tibial tubercle occurring during adolescence. Boston Med Surg J 1903;148:114.
42. Ogden JA, Southwick WO. Osgood-Schlatter's disease and tibial tuberosity development. Clin Orthop 1976;116:180-189.
43. Sinding-Larsen C. A hitherto unknown affection of the patella in children. Acta Radiol 1921;1:171.

44. Wilson JN. A diagnostic sign in osteochondritis dissecans of the knee. J Bone Joint Surg Br 1967;49:440-447.
45. DeSmet AA, Fisher DR, Burnstein MI, et al. Value of MR imaging in staging osteochondral lesions of the talus (osteochondritis dissecans): results in 14 patients. Am J Roentgenol 1990;154:555-558.
46. Dipaola JD, Nelson DW, Colville MR. Characterizing osteochondral lesions by magnetic resonance imaging. Arthroscopy 1991;7:101-104.

47. Cain EL, Clancy WG. Treatment algorithm for osteochondral injuries of the knee. Clin Sports Med 2001;20:321-342.
48. Nehrer S, Spector M, Minas T. Histologic analysis of tissue after failed cartilage repair procedures. Clin Orthop Relat Res 1999;365:149-162.

49. Cahill B. The treatment of juvenile osteochondritis dissecans and osteochondritis dissecans of the knee. Clin Sports Med 1985;4:367.
50. Minas T. Autologous chondrocyte implantation for focal chondral defects of the knee. Clin Orthop Relat Res 2001;391(Suppl):S349-S361.

REFERENCES

Full references for this chapter can be found on www.expertconsult.com.

The ankle and foot

Pamela G. Allen and Lew C. Schon

75

- Pain in the ankle and foot may arise from the bones and joints, periarticular soft tissues (cutaneous and subcutaneous tissues, plantar fascia, tendon sheaths, and bursae), nerve roots, and peripheral nerves or vascular structures or be referred from the lumbar spine or knee joint.
- Static disorders, due to inappropriate footwear, foot deformities, and/or weak intrinsic muscles, account for the vast majority of painful foot conditions.
- Precise diagnosis of ankle and foot pain requires a careful history, a thorough examination, and a few rationally selected diagnostic studies.

FUNCTIONAL ANATOMY

The foot and ankle are our interface between our musculoskeletal system and the earth's surface. The numerous structures that make up this distal appendage synergistically are well suited for a vast array of weight-bearing and non–weight-bearing functions that involve movement, stability, and force transmission. These functions include locomotion, balance, climbing, elevating, dancing, jumping, ascending and descending, kneeling, squatting, kicking, applying focal impact, operating pedals, shock absorption, and flexibility on uneven surfaces.

Ankle

The ankle is a hinge joint composed of the distal end of the tibia and fibula and the talar dome (Fig. 75.1). The talus, a bone whose total surface area is 75% covered with cartilage, is stabilized by the distal extensions of the fibula and the medial tibia, known as the lateral and medial malleolus. The strength of the ankle joint is augmented by the deltoid ligament medially and three ligaments laterally: the posterior talofibular, calcaneofibular, and anterior talofibular ligaments, which are often injured in ankle sprains. The less commonly strained syndesmotic ligaments stabilize the fibula to the tibia, permitting a few degrees of rotation and a few millimeters of translation. Extensor tendons cross the anterior aspect of the ankle extending from the anterior compartment of the leg distally to their insertion on the foot (Fig. 75.2). They are covered in a tenosynovial sheath for part of their course. These tendons include the tibialis anterior, extensor hallucis, extensor digitorum longus, and peroneus tertius from medial to lateral. The tendons are stabilized by a superior and an inferior retinaculum. Their main function is to dorsiflex the ankle and toes.

The peroneus longus and brevis are located in the lateral compartment of the lower leg, and their tendons travel posterior to the fibular and lateral malleolus (see Fig. 75.2). They are found in a single tenosynovial sheath. They are also stabilized by the superior and inferior retinacula. Their primary role is as invertors of the foot and ankle. They also function as plantarflexors.

Located on the medial side of the ankle posterior to the medial malleolus are tendons as well as the neurovascular bundle extending from the posterior compartment of the leg (Fig. 75.3). Hugging the medial malleolus, the posterior tibial tendon is the most medial and anterior, followed in the posterior direction by the flexor digitorum longus, posterior tibial artery/veins, posterior tibial nerve, and flexor hallucis longus (FHL). The low-lying muscle of the FHL is closely apposed to the posterior tibia, and its tendon runs in a tight sheath directly behind the talus and between the posterior lateral and posterior medial tubercles. The relationship is so close that often subtalar or ankle synovitis will track along the FHL tendon sheath on magnetic

resonance imaging (MRI). A flexor retinaculum, the "roof" of the tarsal tunnel, encases the posterior medial tendons and is anchored from the medial malleolus to the calcaneus. Perhaps the most structurally critical of the medial tendons, the posterior tibial tendon provides support for a neutral heel position, prevents arch collapse secondary to gravity (the main result being the adult acquired flatfoot), provides critical pushoff during ambulation, and controls inversion of the subtalar joint through its insertion on the navicular.

On the posterior aspect of the ankle, the gastrocnemius and soleus tendon complex (Achilles tendon) inserts into the posterior surface of the calcaneus (Fig. 75.4). There is no specific tenosynovial sheath encasing the tendon, but it is surrounded by a paratenon as well as superficial and deep bursae. The deep, retrocalcaneal bursa is found between the Achilles tendon insertion and the posterior calcaneus and serves to decrease friction between the tendon and bone. The superficial bursa is the adventitial bursa, which is located between the skin and the paratenon to provide protection. The gastrocnemius/soleus complex through the Achilles tendon provides powerful plantarflexion, resistance to gravity during standing, transition from a seated position to upright, forward propulsion of the legs during gait, stair climbing, and jumping.

The movements of the ankle include dorsiflexion and plantarflexion with the axis of movement generated approximately between the tips of the malleoli. Normal passive range of motion of the ankle is 15 to 25 degrees of dorsiflexion and 40 to 50 degrees of plantarflexion (Fig. 75.5).

Foot

The foot can be divided into three separate units: hindfoot, midfoot, forefoot. The bones of the hindfoot include the talus and calcaneus (Fig. 75.6). The articulations of the hindfoot include the subtalar (talus and calcaneus), talonavicular, and the calcaneocuboid joints. The subtalar joint provides hindfoot inversion and eversion and is assisted by the remaining hindfoot articulations. The normal passive motion of the hindfoot is 5 to 15 degrees of inversion and 20 to 35 degrees of eversion (Fig. 75.7). The motion of the hindfoot is guided by the peroneal tendons, allowing eversion, and the posterior tibial tendon and tibialis anterior tendons, which contribute to inversion. The gastrocnemius/soleus complex also contributes to hindfoot inversion.

The midfoot bones consist of the navicular, cuboid, and three cuneiforms and functionally include the tarsometatarsal (TMT) joints (see Fig. 75.6). The motion of the midfoot is small relative to the hindfoot and ankle. These joints permit plantarflexion/dorsiflexion and rotation. They serve to decrease stresses during gait or impact loading. Their ability to perform fine adjustments to uneven terrain and transition forces generated at the forefoot through the midfoot into the transverse tarsal joints (talonavicular and calcaneo-cuboid) are useful for balance and fluid ambulation.

The forefoot extends from distal to the TMT joints and includes the metatarsals and phalanges (see Fig. 75.6). Each metatarsophalangeal (MTP) joint has its own synovium-lined capsule supported by medial and lateral collateral and plantar ligaments. Forefoot motion includes dorsiflexion and plantarflexion as well as pronation and supination as directed by the hindfoot. The first MTP joint accommodates 70 to 80 degrees of dorsiflexion and 40 to 50 degrees of plantarflexion. The interphalangeal (IP) joints in the toes are hinge joints that allow strictly plantarflexion and dorsiflexion. There is only one IP joint in the great toe, whereas there are typically two in each of the other toes (proximal IP joint and distal IP joints). These joints are curled or plantarflexed by the FHL and flexor digitorum longus (FDL) muscles through their plantar-based tendons and straightened through the extensor hallucis longus (EHL) and extensor digitorum longus (EDL) through their dorsally based tendons. The toes help with proprioception, balance, rising up on the ball of the foot during gait, and assisting with ascending/descending stairs.

CLINICAL EVALUATION

Physical examination

The physical examination of the foot and ankle should begin with a thorough visual inspection in the sitting and standing position. When evaluating from the front, attention should be directed to any varus or valgus deformity about the ankle and foot as well as the location of any swelling. Angular deformities of the great toe (hallux valgus or hallux varus) and lesser toes (deviated toes and claw/hammer toes) are also noted (Fig. 75.8). The side views will reveal arch height abnormalities known as pes planus (flat) or cavus (high arch) and flexion or extension deformities of the toe joints (Fig. 75.9). The posterior view allows one to evaluate hindfoot varus (inversion) and valgus (eversion), forefoot/midfoot abduction ("too many toes sign"—indicative of posterior tibial tendon dysfunction) and adduction, and Achilles tendon pathology (e.g., an enlarged retrocalcaneal bursae or thickened Achilles tendon). As the patient is visualized from all sides, skin abnormalities such as subcutaneous nodules, callus formation, ulcers, vascular compromise, skin irritation from shoe pressure, tophi, and psoriatic changes should be noted.

A gait analysis should be performed first without shoes, walking for a distance in the hallway. There are two phases of the gait cycle (stance and swing), which are further subdivided into four segments (heel-strike, foot flat, toe-off, and swing). The stance phase extends from heel strike to toe off and consists of 60% of the cycle, which is the weight-bearing portion. The swing phase is from toe-off to heel-strike and forms 40% of the gait cycle. Ambulating with a painful limb leads to an antalgic gait in which the stance phase is shortened for the affected limb. Foot placement on the ground during ambulation should be viewed for dynamic changes in the foot structure, such as medial arch collapse, as well as avoiding contact with certain areas of the foot with the hard surface to prevent discomfort. Evaluation of the patient's shoes to assess the wear patterns can also be instructive. Watching the patient walk in the shoes further elucidates pathologic mechanics and may lead to useful solutions with modification of the shoes and or addition of foot and ankle braces. Palpation of the ankle joint is performed in slight plantarflexion and should be directed just distal to the tibia and medial to the tibialis anterior tendon as well as just anterior to the fibula on the lateral aspect of the ankle (Fig. 75.10). Effusions and synovial thickening can be palpated at these sites. More superficial central palpation will permit encounter with the extensor tendons traversing the ankle joint. Palpation posterior to the lateral malleolus will reveal the peroneal tendons. The posterior compartment tendons are located behind the medial malleolus, specifically the posterior tibialis tendon. Pain with deep palpation over the course of the tendon, especially if the tendon is tensioned by the patient activation of the muscle, is often seen with tenosynovitis and tendinopathy. Distinguishing between tendon tenderness and joint tenderness can be difficult. If there is no extension of the tenderness beyond the zone of the joint, it is more commonly synovitis. Also with synovitis the anteromedial and anterolateral corners of the joints are both tender.

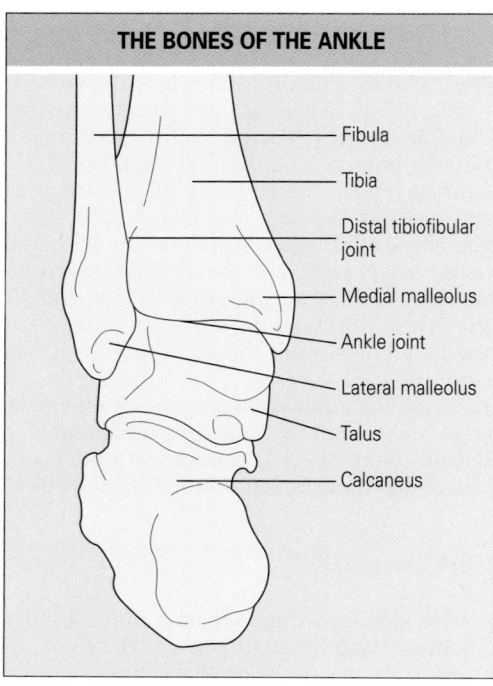

THE BONES OF THE ANKLE

- Fibula
- Tibia
- Distal tibiofibular joint
- Medial malleolus
- Ankle joint
- Lateral malleolus
- Talus
- Calcaneus

Fig. 75.1 The bones of the ankle: posterior view.

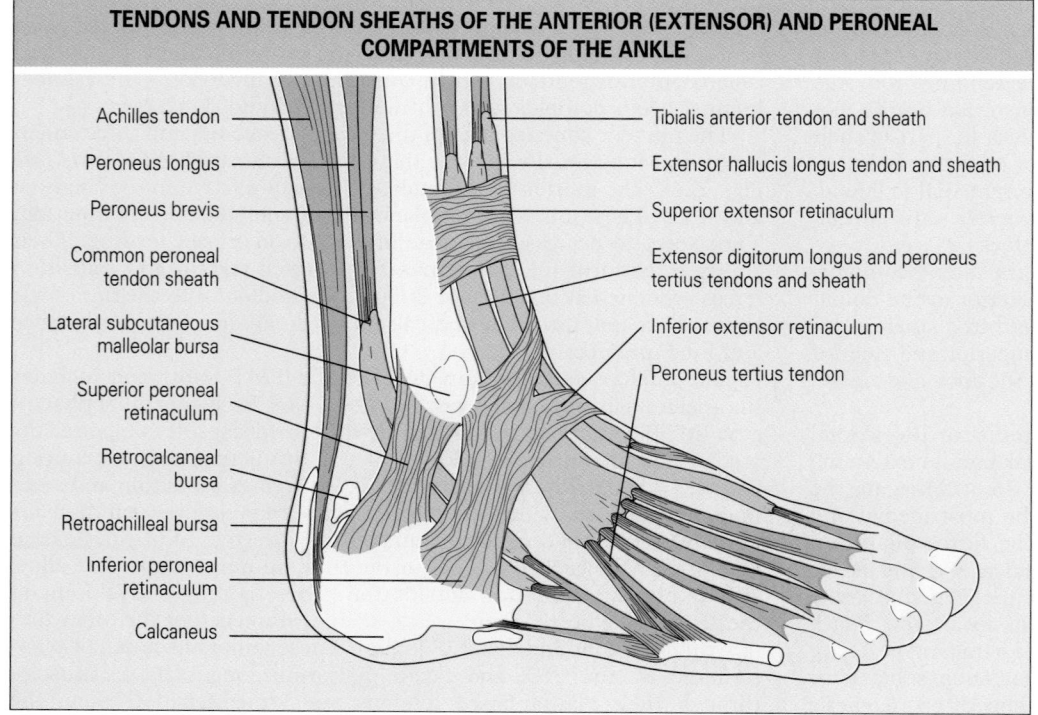

TENDONS AND TENDON SHEATHS OF THE ANTERIOR (EXTENSOR) AND PERONEAL COMPARTMENTS OF THE ANKLE

- Achilles tendon
- Peroneus longus
- Peroneus brevis
- Common peroneal tendon sheath
- Lateral subcutaneous malleolar bursa
- Superior peroneal retinaculum
- Retrocalcaneal bursa
- Retroachilleal bursa
- Inferior peroneal retinaculum
- Calcaneus

- Tibialis anterior tendon and sheath
- Extensor hallucis longus tendon and sheath
- Superior extensor retinaculum
- Extensor digitorum longus and peroneus tertius tendons and sheath
- Inferior extensor retinaculum
- Peroneus tertius tendon

Fig. 75.2 Tendons and tendon sheaths of the anterior (extensor) and lateral (peroneal) compartments of the ankle.

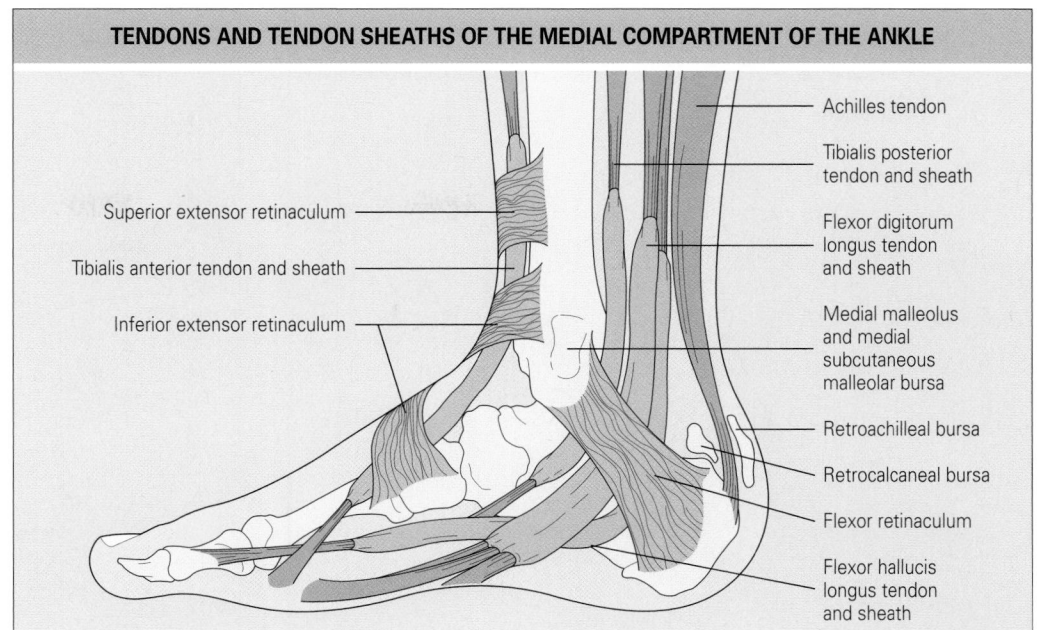

Fig. 75.3 Tendons and tendon sheaths of the medial (flexor) compartment of the ankle.

TENDONS AND TENDON SHEATHS OF THE MEDIAL COMPARTMENT OF THE ANKLE

- Achilles tendon
- Tibialis posterior tendon and sheath
- Flexor digitorum longus tendon and sheath
- Medial malleolus and medial subcutaneous malleolar bursa
- Retroachilleal bursa
- Retrocalcaneal bursa
- Flexor retinaculum
- Flexor hallucis longus tendon and sheath
- Superior extensor retinaculum
- Tibialis anterior tendon and sheath
- Inferior extensor retinaculum

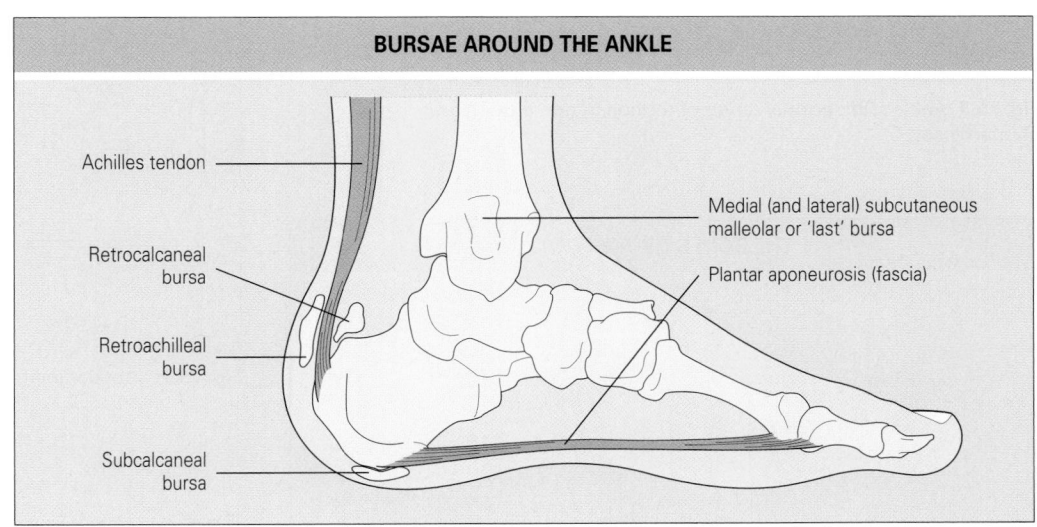

Fig. 75.4 Anatomy of the plantar fascia, Achilles tendon, and related bursae.

BURSAE AROUND THE ANKLE

- Achilles tendon
- Retrocalcaneal bursa
- Retroachilleal bursa
- Subcalcaneal bursa
- Medial (and lateral) subcutaneous malleolar or 'last' bursa
- Plantar aponeurosis (fascia)

Palpation of the hindfoot will identify the calcaneus with the insertion of the Achilles tendon on the posterior aspect. Tenderness along the posterior aspect of the bone may indicate insertional Achilles tendinopathy or bursitis, whereas tenderness more proximal may be tendinopathy at the area where the Achilles tendon has a diminished blood supply 2 to 6 cm above the dorsal aspect of the calcaneus (the watershed area). Palpation on the plantar aspect of the calcaneus at the medial tubercle will evaluate the origin of the plantar fascia. Tenderness at this site may indicate plantar fasciitis. The subtalar joint is not directly palpable, but tenderness in the sinus tarsi region located laterally below the tip of the fibula and slightly anterior may indicate intra-articular pathology. Pain with compression of the medial and lateral aspects of the calcaneus may be a sign of a calcaneal stress fracture.

Along the dorsal surface of the foot, the articulations of the midfoot as well as the extensor tendons traveling to their sites of insertion can be palpated. Medial palpation reveals the navicular, and tenderness at this location may indicate insertional tendinopathy of the posterior tibial tendon or a symptomatic accessory navicular (an extra bone at the medial pole of the navicular). Tenderness along the plantar surface of the midfoot may reveal pathology within the plantar ligaments supporting the arch such as the spring ligament or within the plantar fascia (see Fig. 75.4). Nodules may also be present on the sole of the foot.

Rheumatoid nodules are firm and somewhat mobile and are located over bony prominences, particularly the metatarsal heads or heels. They are often inflamed and boggy, deforming on compression like a soft rubber ball (Fig. 75.11). Plantar fibromas, which occur within the plantar fascia, are firm like a "superball," relatively immobile, and rarely inflamed.

Palpation of the forefoot should be performed in a medial to lateral progression. The first metatarsal is palpated along the shaft of the bone medially or dorsally, which can be significant for a metatarsal stress fracture. The first MTP joint is identified and palpated dorsally as well as plantarly, with specific attention paid to the fibular and tibial sesamoids under the first metatarsal head. The lesser rays should undergo similar examination. Discomfort with dorsal and plantar palpation at the MTP joints and signs of fullness of the joints may represent synovitis. When chronic, the fullness is often accompanied by deviations of the MTP joints or hammer toe deformities. The fat pad under the metatarsal heads should be assessed for thinning consistent with atrophy of chronic disease and/or corticosteroid use. The fat pad may undergo distal migration in conjunction with MTP deformities, which leaves the metatarsal head vulnerable to pressure calluses, bursal or nodule formation, or ulceration. The IP joints should also be palpated for signs of synovitis and for bony prominences related to deformity that may impact shoe wear.

ANKLE JOINT: NORMAL RANGE OF DORSIFLEXION AND PLANTARFLEXION

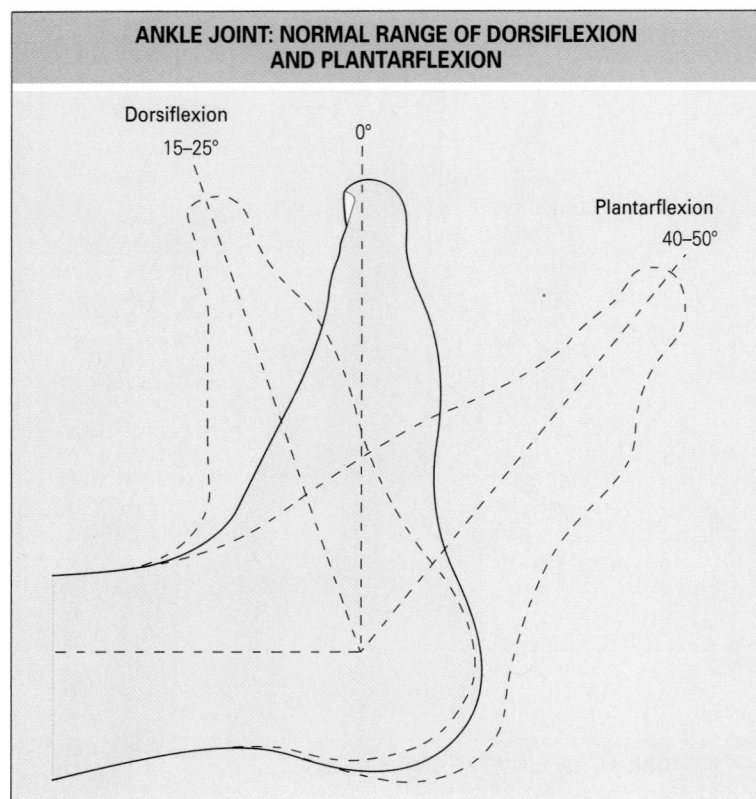

Dorsiflexion
15–25°

0°

Plantarflexion
40–50°

Fig. 75.5 Ankle joint: normal range of motion in dorsiflexion and plantarflexion.

THE BONES OF THE FOOT

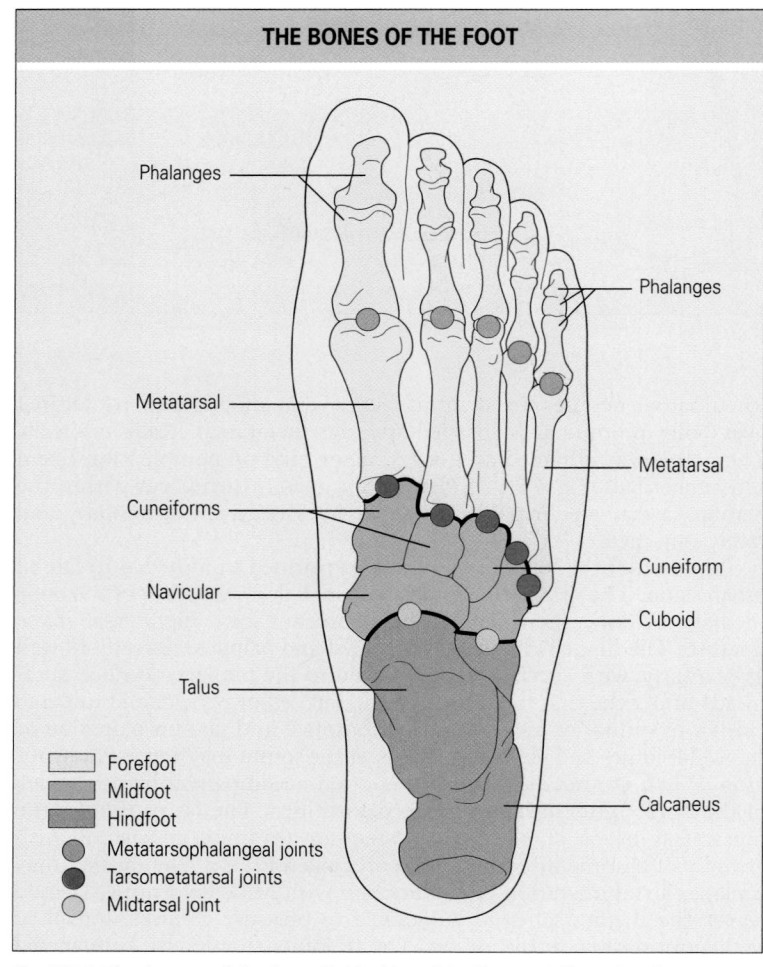

Phalanges

Phalanges

Metatarsal

Metatarsal

Cuneiforms

Cuneiform

Navicular

Cuboid

Talus

Calcaneus

☐ Forefoot
■ Midfoot
■ Hindfoot
● Metatarsophalangeal joints
● Tarsometatarsal joints
○ Midtarsal joint

Fig. 75.6 The bones of the foot divided into hindfoot, midfoot, forefoot: superior view.

SUBTALAR JOINT: EXAMINATION AND RANGE OF MOVEMENTS

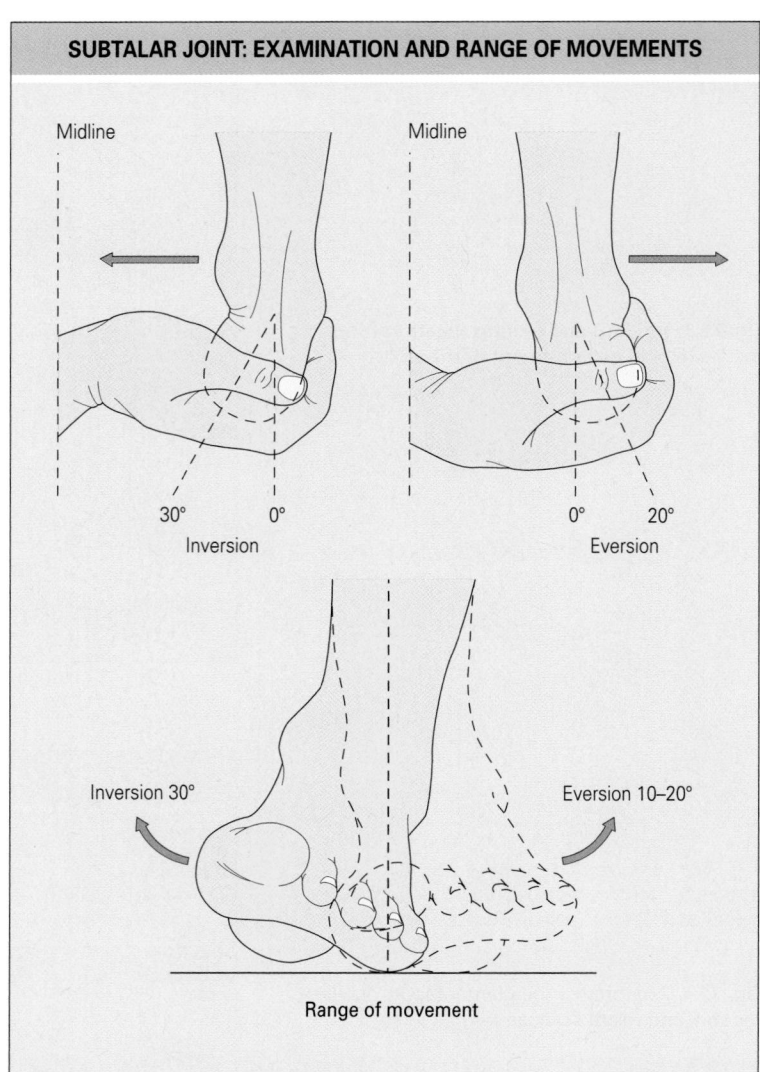

Midline

Midline

30°   0°
Inversion

0°   20°
Eversion

Inversion 30°

Eversion 10–20°

Range of movement

Fig. 75.7 Subtalar joint: normal range of motion in inversion and eversion.

Radiographic evaluation

As part of the full evaluation for a foot or ankle complaint, weight-bearing radiographs of the affected area should be obtained. For a foot complaint, anteroposterior, oblique, and lateral views should be taken. If an ankle complaint is identified, then anteroposterior, mortise, and lateral views should be taken. Computed tomography (CT) is utilized when there is a need to evaluate the extent of arthritis at a particular joint and also the success of an intra-articular fusion. MRI is chosen when evaluation of soft tissues is necessary, such as in infection, tumor, tendinopathy, bursitis, ligament damage, or cartilage injury.

Diagnostic injections

The anatomy of the foot and ankle comprises many structures in a confined space. At times, it is difficult to isolate which articulation is symptomatic or whether multiple joints are involved. To help sort out these difficult situations, diagnostic/therapeutic injections can be performed in the clinic. A combination of anesthetic and corticosteroid can be injected into a specific joint when the articulation is easily identified to evaluate symptomatic relief. For more challenging articulations, an arthrogram can be performed using an anesthetic, corticosteroid, and contrast agent with fluoroscopy to guide the injection. Ultrasonography can also be beneficial. These injections will assist in better identification of the locus of a specific pain emanating from one joint and help to guide treatment decisions.

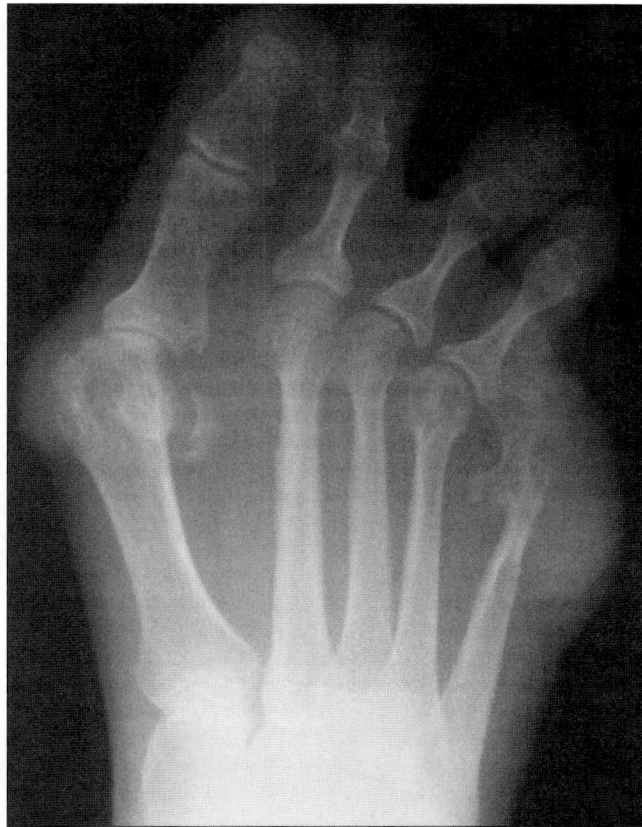

Fig. 75.8 Hallux valgus. Anteroposterior view of the forefoot reveals severe lateral deviation of the proximal phalanx on the first metatarsal head, known as hallux valgus. The lesser toes show variable amounts of deviation owing to weight-bearing force changes and weakening of the restraining structures.

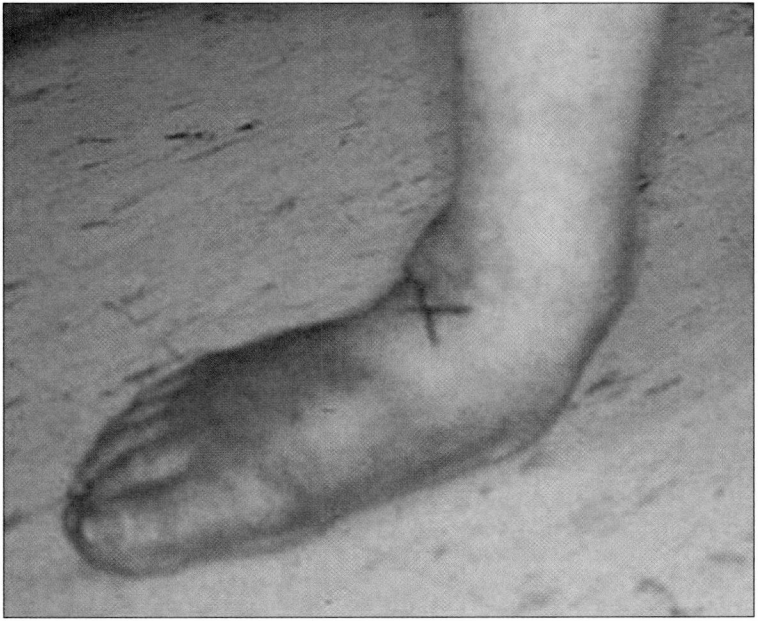

Fig. 75.9 Planovalgus foot deformity. Anterior view reveals the hindfoot in valgus, collapse of the midfoot, and abduction of the forefoot.

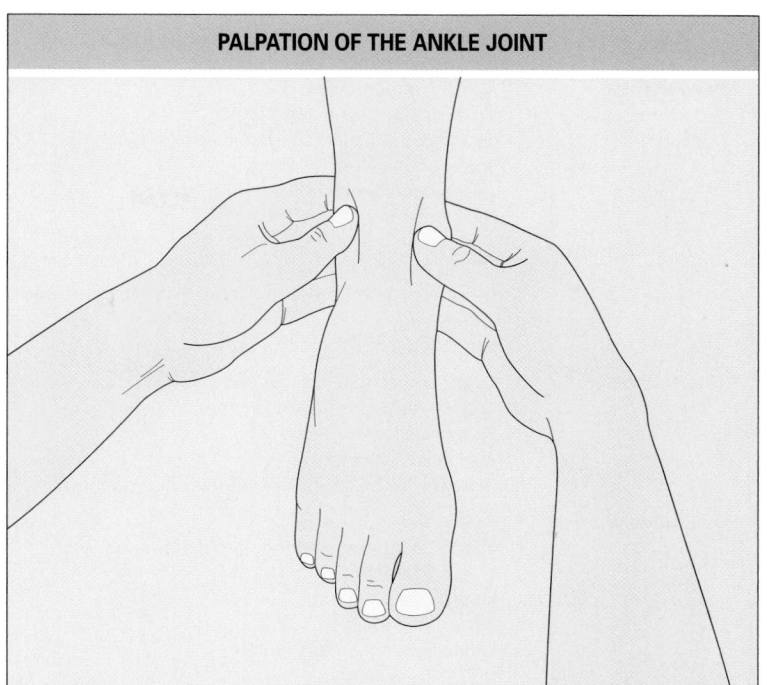

PALPATION OF THE ANKLE JOINT

Fig. 75.10 Palpation of the ankle joint at the distal aspect of the tibia medial to the tibialis anterior tendon and lateral to the extensor tendons.

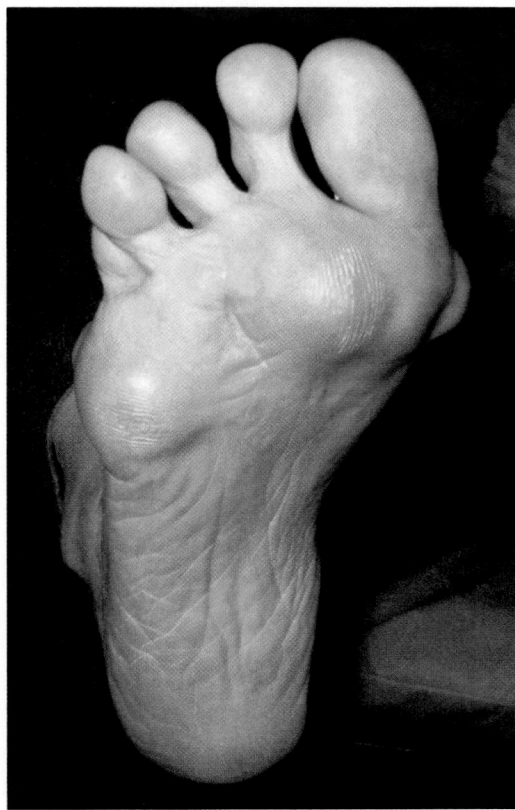

Fig. 75.11 Rheumatoid nodules. View of the plantar surface of the foot in a rheumatoid patient with rheumatoid nodules along the first MTP, fifth MTP, and under the second metatarsal head.

DIFFERENTIAL DIAGNOSIS

Evaluation of a foot and ankle complaint should be approached from an anatomic perspective. Pain in the foot and ankle can stem from bone and joint pathology, soft tissue structures, or referred pain from local (e.g., neuromas) or more proximal (e.g., radiculopathies) nerve disorders. Peripheral vascular disease may also produce foot and ankle pain due to ischemia or venous insufficiency. A classification of painful foot and ankle disorders based on anatomic location is outlined in Table 75.1.

Ankle pain

In a study of rheumatologic patients, a minority had significant ankle pain but a much larger number identified it as a problem in daily life.[1] The patient may complain of decreased range of motion impacting

TABLE 75.1 DIFFERENTIAL DIAGNOSIS OF ANKLE AND FOOT PAIN

Anterior ankle	Anterior impingement Ankle arthritis/synovitis Osteochondral defect/lesion (cartilage injury) Loose body within the joint Talar avascular necrosis Talar stress fracture Tenosynovitis of the EHL, EDL Tibialis anterior ligament injury (sprain) Deep (central) or superficial (anterolateral) peroneal nerve injury Saphenous (anteromedial) nerve injury
Posterior ankle	Os trigonum (accessory ossicle involving the posterior lateral tubercle of talus) Retrocalcaneal bursitis Achilles tendinopathy Flexor hallucis longus (FHL) tendinopathy or stenosis
Posterolateral ankle	Peroneal tendinopathy Subfibular impingement due to flatfoot and impingement Fibular stress fracture Sural nerve injury Lateral ligament injury (sprain)
Posteromedial ankle	Posterior tibial tendinopathy FDL/FHL tendinopathy Tibial stress fracture Medial malleolar stress fracture Tarsal tunnel syndrome Tibial nerve injury Deltoid ligament injury
Heel	Achilles insertional tendinopathy Plantar fasciitis Calcaneal stress fracture

Hindfoot	Subtalar, talonavicular, or calcaneocuboid arthritis/
	   synovitis
	Posterior tibial tendon dysfunction/tendinopathy
	   (medial) or peroneal tendon dysfunction (lateral)
	Occult fracture of talus, calcaneus cuboid, or
	   navicular
	Accessory navicular

Midfoot	Insertional tendinopathy (peroneal, posterior tibial,
	   tibialis anterior)
	Arthritis/synovitis (navicular-cuneiform, cuneiform-
	   metatarsal, cuboid-metatarsal)

Forefoot: first ray, first MTP joint, hallux	Arthritis/synovitis MTP (hallux rigidus) and interphalangeal (IP) joints Hallux valgus Hallux varus Sesamoiditis
Forefoot: second to fifth rays, MTP joints, lesser toes	Arthritis/synovitis (MTP, proximal and distal IP joints) Lesser toe deformities (hammer and claw toes) Metatarsalgia MTP instability MTP dislocations Morton's neuroma (interdigital neuralgia) Stress fracture of the metatarsals Bunionette (fifth metatarsal phalangeal deviation) Rheumatoid nodules Bursitis Ulcers Infections

activities of daily living. Discomfort about the ankle is best approached by creating a differential diagnosis based on the anatomic location of the pain. Anterior ankle pain is often related to an intra-articular problem (synovitis, arthritis, osteochondral defects/lesions, loose bodies), which can often be palpable due to the superficial nature of the joint at this location. Arthritic changes within the ankle often lead

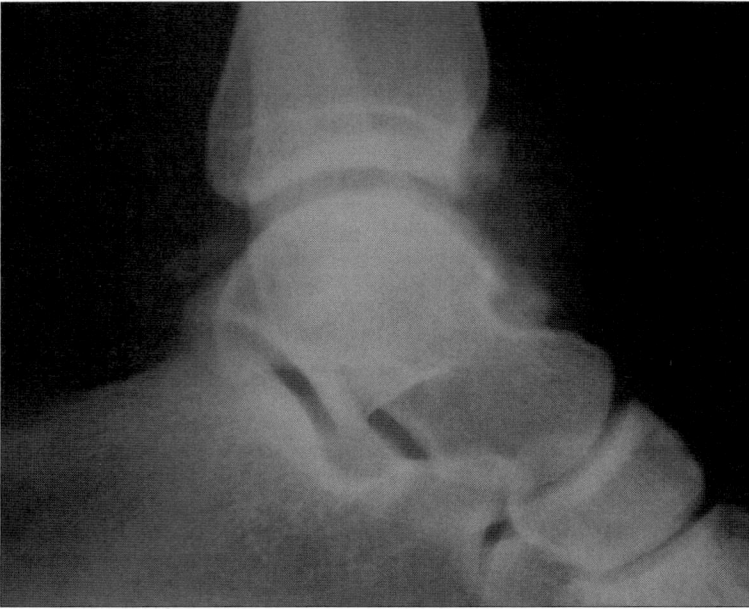

Fig. 75.12 Anterior tibial spur. Osteophyte formation due to arthritis leads to impingement with dorsiflexion of the ankle.

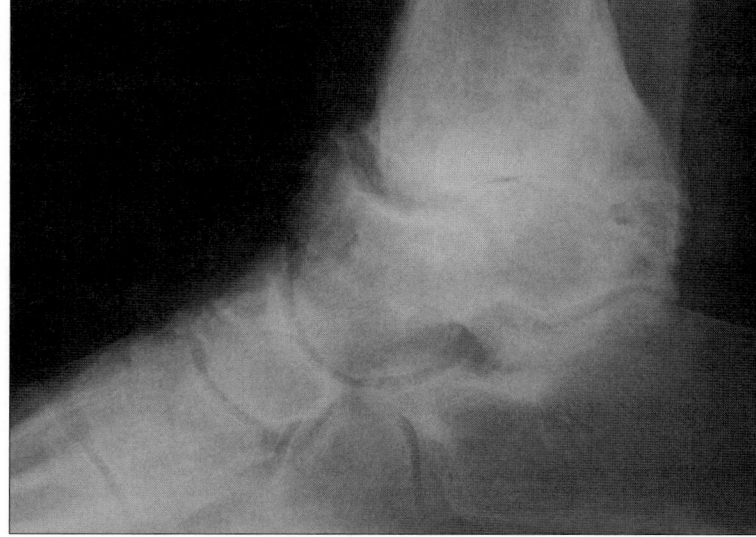

Fig. 75.13 Diffuse ankle arthritis. Lateral view of the ankle reveals significant joint space narrowing of the tibiotalar joint with osteophyte formation along the anterior and posterior joint lines.

to osteophyte formation on the anterior lip of the distal tibia and on the dorsal talar neck (Fig. 75.12). When this occurs, dorsiflexion of the ankle leads to impingement of the protruding surfaces, causing tenderness, warmth, and edema at the anterior ankle. The patient complains about difficulty with inclines or stair climbing. Diffuse ankle arthritis will also present as decreased range of motion, particularly dorsiflexion and anterior ankle pain (Fig. 75.13). Intra-articular pain can also be confused with tenosynovitis of the extensor compartment, most commonly the tibialis anterior tendon. Physical examination would reveal bogginess along the course of a painful tendon.

An injury to the cartilage such as an osteochondral defect, which can also extend to the subchondral bone, may present as anterior ankle pain (Fig. 75.14). Although this is usually seen in the sports setting with younger patients, ankle sprains or repetitive overuse can lead to this disorder. Distal tibia and talar stress fractures and talar avascular necrosis are also sources of anterior ankle pain and are often associated with inflammatory arthritis owing to the periarticular osteopenia (Fig. 75.15). Progressive inflammatory arthropathy can lead to deformities of the foot and ankle, which predisposes the tibia and fibula to stress fractures based on the direction of alignment.[2]

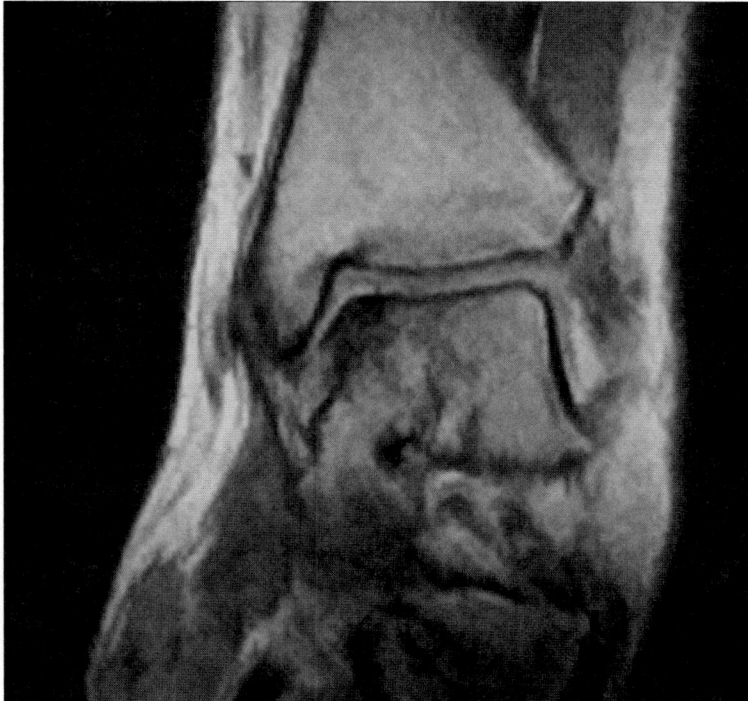

Fig. 75.14 Osteochondral defect of the talus. Coronal MR image shows decreased signal intensity at the medial shoulder of the talus representing an injury to the cartilage and underlying subchondral bone.

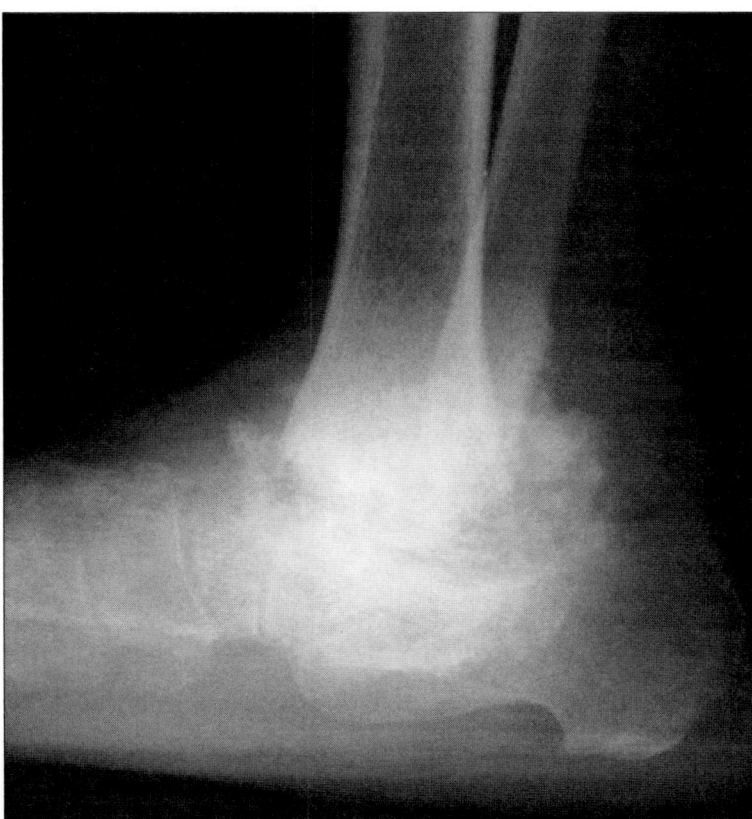

Fig. 75.15 Avascular necrosis of the talus. Lateral radiograph of the ankle shows collapse of the talus and arthritic disease at the tibiotalar and subtalar joints.

Pain at the posterior aspect of the ankle is most commonly due to Achilles tendon pathology. There are several causes associated with the Achilles tendon that can cause discomfort. The tendon itself does not have a synovial lining, unlike the other tendons in the foot and ankle, and therefore the pain here is typical for tendinopathy. In the literature,

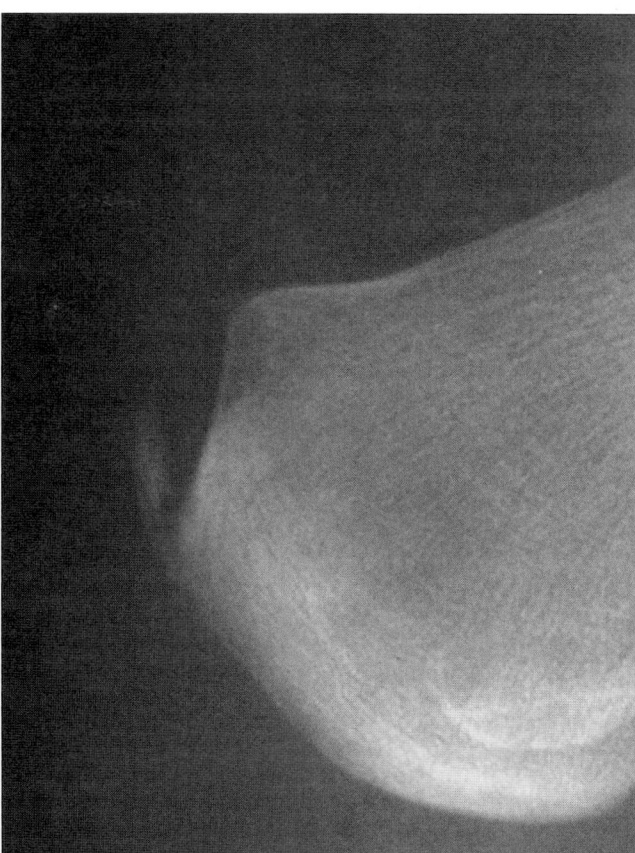

Fig. 75.16 Posterior calcaneal spur at the insertion of the Achilles tendon seen in chronic Achilles tendinopathy.

intrasubstance degeneration has been known as tendinosis. Currently the term *tendinopathy* is preferred. Tendinopathy can occur at the insertion of the Achilles on the posterior calcaneus and proximal to the insertion in the watershed area. Partial or complete rupture of the tendon can occur at either site of tendinopathy. Plain films often reveal calcifications within the tendon and spur formation along the posterior calcaneus (Fig. 75.16). The two bursae can also become inflamed, causing pain and swelling along the posterior aspect of the ankle. Retrocalcaneal (deep) bursitis is usually associated with Achilles tendinopathy and can be further aggravated by a large posterosuperior calcaneal process known as Haglund's deformity. The superficial bursa posterior to the tendon can be irritated by shoe wear. Os trigonum, or the accessory ossicle off the posterior talus (the posterior lateral tubercle of the talus), can also cause symptoms at the posterior ankle. With a symptomatic os trigonum, forcing the foot into plantarflexion will elicit an impingement type pain as the ossicle pinches between the tibia and the calcaneus. The tenderness with this condition is usually located laterally and is deep to the peroneal tendons. The FHL tendon can also cause symptoms in this location separate from or associated with an os trigonum. Flexion and extension of the hallux will isolate the FHL tendon. Palpation of the posteromedial aspect of the ankle is typically positive. A lateral radiograph of the ankle will reveal the presence of this accessory ossicle or a large protruding posterior trigonal process. The coexistence of the FHL tendinopathy and trigonal impingement leads to both findings.

Lateral ankle pain

Pain along the lateral aspect of the ankle in front of the fibula often reflects intra-articular pathology if it is located at the joint line. More distally based discomfort along the anterior fibula may reflect a ligamentous injury to the anterior talofibular ligament, often injured with inversion (sprain) injuries. The patient may also complain of feeling that the ankle is unstable, especially on uneven ground. An anterior drawer maneuver performed by stabilizing the distal leg with one hand

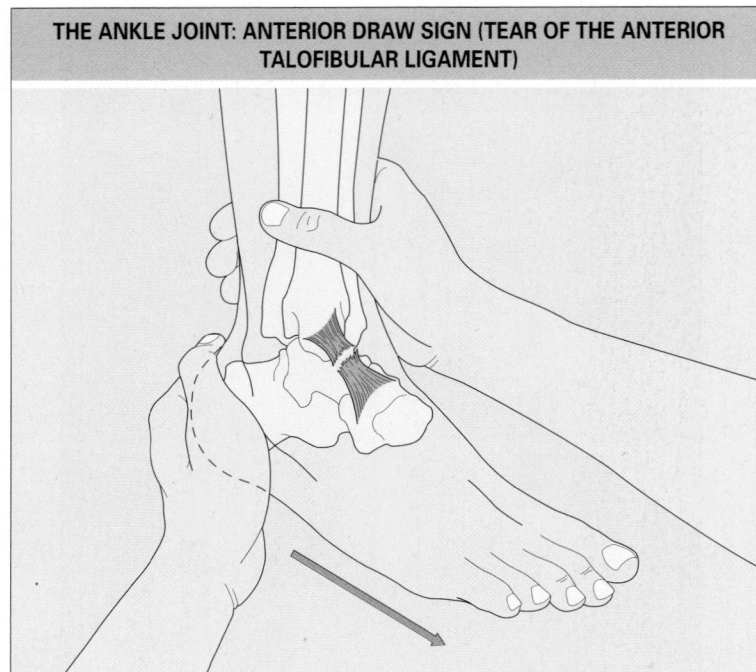

THE ANKLE JOINT: ANTERIOR DRAW SIGN (TEAR OF THE ANTERIOR TALOFIBULAR LIGAMENT)

Fig. 75.17 The ankle joint anterior drawer test to assess ligamentous injury (anterior talofibular ligament) contributing to ankle instability.

and translating the talus anteriorly by pulling forward on the heel held by the other hand will allow assessment of the integrity of the ligaments (Fig. 75.17). When the talus slides anteriorly out of the joint, a complete tear of the ligaments is established. Tenderness, boggy edema, and warmth located directly over the fibula may indicate a fibular stress fracture. The peroneal tendons are located posterior to the fibula and are subject to tenosynovitis and tendinopathy, which can cause significant pain in this region. Instability of these tendons can also cause discomfort as they "snap" anteriorly out of the fibular groove. With chronicity, this can lead to degeneration and tearing. Weakness of the peroneal tendons with lack of full eversion motion is consistent with a rupture. Chronic rupture of the peroneals will lead to a varus deformity of the hindfoot and ankle.

Anteromedial ankle pain in front of the malleolus is usually articular in origin. Tenderness here over the tibialis anterior is distinguished by being more superficial than the deeper joint. The tendon should bow out tautly as it passes to the medial cuneiform where it inserts. Thickening and focal warmth are evident in addition to the weakness of dorsiflexion. In advanced cases, the patient will exhibit a footdrop during gait. This slapping gait may occur from tendon attenuation, rupture, radiculopathy, or common peroneal nerve compression, so a more thorough evaluation is warranted. Discomfort directly over the medial malleolus is worrisome for a stress fracture, whereas pain posterior to the malleolus can stem from multiple sources. Tenosynovitis and degeneration of the tendons posterior to the medial malleolus are important causes of pain at this location. The posterior tibial tendon (PTT) is located closest to the malleolus and is the largest of the medial tendons. The normal function of this tendon is to invert the hindfoot while also supporting the longitudinal arch. A painful flatfoot can come from chronic inflammation and overuse of this powerful tendon. This is known as posterior tibial tendon dysfunction (PTTD) or the adult acquired flatfoot deformity (see Fig. 75.9). The neurovascular bundle, residing between the posteromedial flexor tendons, can be entrapped and cause symptoms posterior to the malleolus. Tinel's sign may be present with paresthesias produced by percussion over the tibial nerve along its course into the sole of the foot. This finding is consistent with the diagnosis of a tarsal tunnel syndrome that can be caused by anything that decreases the volume within the tunnel (ganglion, tumor, ankle synovitis, flexor tenosynovitis, tendinopathy). In a study of rheumatoid disease by McGuigan and associates, 13.3% of patients had evidence of tarsal tunnel syndrome on examination.[3]

Hindfoot pain

Hindfoot involvement is found in 58% to 72% of chronic rheumatoid patients, but the hindfoot is rarely abnormal in early disease. Hindfoot pain is associated with involvement of the subtalar and midtarsal joints.[4,5] Inflammation of these joints leads to changes in the integrity of the bone and capsules, particularly the subtalar and talonavicular joints.[5-8] As these joints and the calcaneocuboid joint become unstable, pronation forces at the subtalar joint ultimately result in ligamentous incompetence and the development of a pes planovalgus. The talar head shifts medial and plantarly, and the calcaneus rotates laterally, creating a valgus deformity with loss of the longitudinal arch. This deformity leads to significant pain in the hindfoot, PTT, midfoot, and forefoot. An Achilles tendon contracture may be observed in longstanding deformity. The role of the PTT in the pathophysiology of acquired pes planovalgus deformity is controversial because the deformity is similar to that seen in non-rheumatoid PTTD.[9] A study by Keenan and coworkers compared quantitated electromyographic values in valgus deformity versus no deformity in rheumatoid patients and found that only patients with deformity had increased activity in the PTT. This increased activity represents the PTT working harder to maintain inversion and the longitudinal arch.[5] PTTD likely occurs after tenosynovitis and overworking to save the normal foot structure that failed secondary to instability of the hindfoot. Our observation clinically is that there is hindfoot synovitis with or without subtle posterior tibial tendon attenuation, which leads to ligamentous failure involving the spring ligament, deltoid, talonavicular capsule, interosseous, and cervical (talocalcaneal) ligaments. These findings are confirmed at times by MRI and observed during surgery. More study on this issue is warranted.

Midfoot pain

Arthritic change at the TMT joints is often the main cause of pain in the midfoot (Fig. 75.18). The most common location within the midfoot is the first TMT joint, which causes pain on the medial column of the foot and along the first ray. The first TMT joint can also become unstable, like the hindfoot, leading to excessive load on the neighboring metatarsals and joints. The naviculocuneiform and first TMT joints contribute to the acquired pes planovalgus deformity by flattening of the longitudinal arch and abduction of the foot seen on a radiograph as midfoot sag. If there is primary failure of the TMT or the naviculocuneiform, the arch height drops, causing a pes planus without the valgus of the hindfoot.[10] Interestingly, the lateral TMT joints are less symptomatic unless the medial joints begin to create a plantar medial prominence or rocker-bottom deformity. Occasionally the naviculocuneiform joints will collapse, and this is associated with lateral TMT instability, which manifests as a plantar lateral prominence or lateral rocker-bottom deformity.[11] Other causes for midfoot pain along the medial column include an accessory navicular, insertional posterior tibial tendinopathy, and tibialis anterior tendinopathy. Dorsal and lateral midfoot pain is often related to extensor tenosynovitis, and peroneal tendinopathy can occur at the insertion of the tendon on the fifth metatarsal.

Forefoot pain

Ninety percent of adults with chronic rheumatoid disease have forefoot pathology leading to pain and deformity.[4] Evaluation of the hallux in patients with and without rheumatoid arthritis can reveal a bunion (the prominent medial eminence of the progressively exposed metatarsal head) or hallux valgus deformity. In patients with rheumatoid arthritis the incidence of hallux valgus has been quoted to be between 60% and 90%, and the rate increases with the chronicity of the disease.[1] A painful rheumatoid hallux valgus may require more aggressive surgical reconstruction due to the loss of soft tissue integrity around the joint and its secondary effects on the lesser MTPs and toes. These structures will sublux, dislocate, or develop severe erosions as they are subjected to more load from the failure of the first MTP. A painful first MTP joint without the deformity can be due to degenerative arthritis called hallux rigidus (Fig. 75.19). The patient will have decreased range of motion that is painful at the extremes of dorsiflexion and

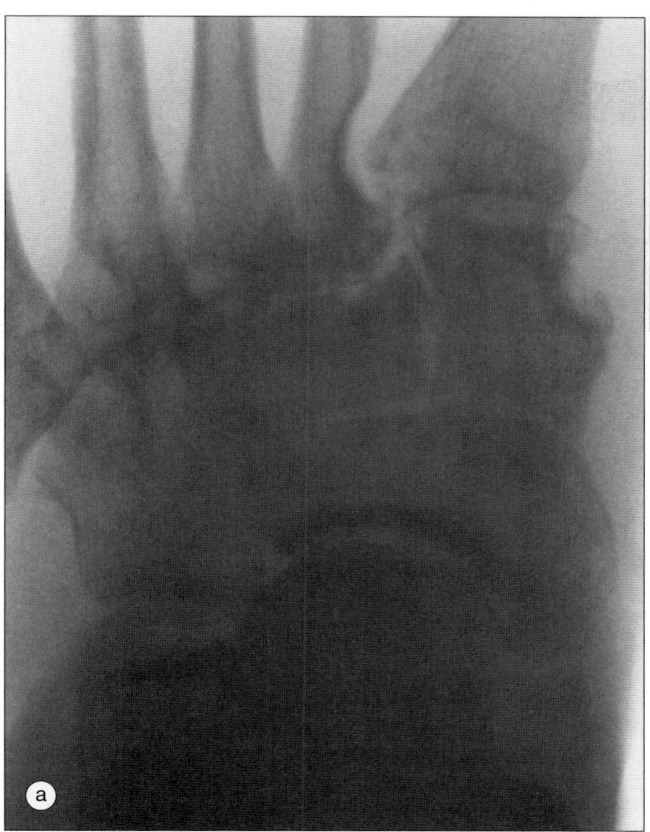
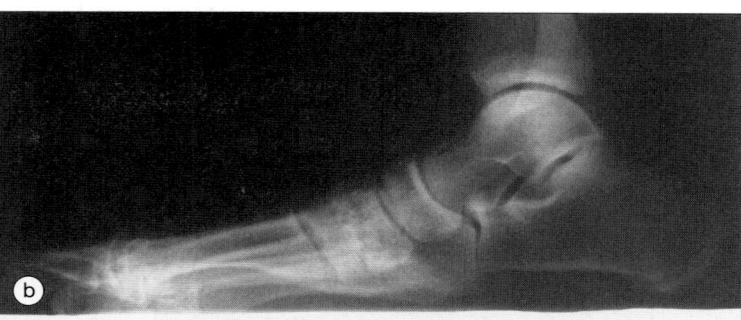

Fig. 75.18 Midfoot arthritis. (a) Anteroposterior view of the midfoot reveals arthritic changes at the tarsometatarsal joints. (b) Lateral view of the foot shows joint space narrowing of the tarsometatarsal joints. Midfoot collapse is noted due to the degenerative changes.

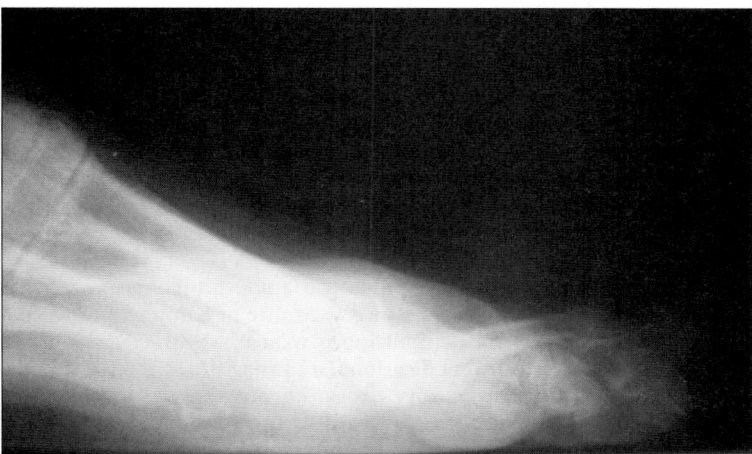

Fig. 75.19 Hallux rigidus. Lateral view of the foot reveals advanced disease of the first MTP joint with narrowing of the joint space and dorsal osteophytes.

plantarflexion. Dorsally, there are large osteophytes that are visible and palpable. These painful prominences will cause the skin to be irritated as they rub against the inside of the toe box of the shoe. Other sources of pain around the hallux include a metatarsal stress fracture and osteonecrosis of the first metatarsal head. Sesamoiditis associated with plantar pain underneath the first MTP joint occurs in osteoarthritis, rheumatoid arthritis, and gouty arthritis.

Involvement of the lesser toes in rheumatologic disease is seen in more than 90% of patients with chronic disease. The basic pathophysiology of forefoot pain and deformity in the setting of inflammatory arthritis begins with synovial inflammation leading to distention of the MTP capsules. As chronic distention occurs, the collateral ligaments and capsule integrity fail. The loss of structural support with continued ambulation leads to MTP dorsal subluxation with distal migration of the fat pad, leaving the metatarsal heads uncovered.

Continued ambulation leads to painful plantar keratotic lesions under the metatarsal heads and may result in ulcerations. The intrinsic and extrinsic muscle groups become unbalanced with the dorsal subluxation, and a hammer toe (hyperextended MTP joint, hyperflexed proximal IP joint) and/or claw toe (adding a hyperflexed distal IP joint) (Fig. 75.20) result. Usually lateral instability is noted with the lesser toes deviating and is greatly influenced by medial pressure from a hallux valgus deformity. Within the first 1 to 3 years of rheumatoid arthritis, 65% of patients will have MTP synovitis.[1] In chronic rheumatoid arthritis, two thirds of patients will experience subluxation or dislocation of the lesser MTP joints.[10] Patients will complain that they can no longer walk barefoot because of the prominent metatarsal heads with keratoses, yet wearing shoes is difficult because of the lesser MTP subluxation and resultant hammer toe, which exhibits signs of painful wear from the dorsum of the shoe. Gait becomes unstable owing to the loss of the normal tripod structure of the foot weight-bearing surface. It is important to pay attention to the hindfoot when evaluating the forefoot. Disease in the hindfoot, as discussed earlier, can lead to progressive changes in the forefoot due to redistribution of the weight-bearing forces.[12] In this situation, the hindfoot will need to be addressed or correction of the forefoot will fail. In general with the advent of disease-modifying medications and earlier conservative treatment (thicker less-flexible soled shoes with higher wider toe boxes) the incidence of the forefoot deformities from all the arthropathies has dramatically been reduced.

There are other causes of forefoot pain without concomitant deformity. Metatarsalgia, or pain on the plantar surface of the foot under the metatarsal heads, can occur with long second metatarsal, hammer toes, Achilles tendon tightness causing forefoot load, and fat pad atrophy seen in inflammatory arthritis and with age. A shooting pain into the lesser toes associated with burning and numbness may be associated with Morton's neuroma. Morton's neuroma often results from entrapment of the digital nerve in the web space under the intermetatarsal ligament, which leads to perineural fibrosis and compression. It typically occurs in the third web space. An anesthetic injection can often be diagnostic if the symptoms improve after injection. Pain at the fifth MTP joint with an associated angular deformity is known

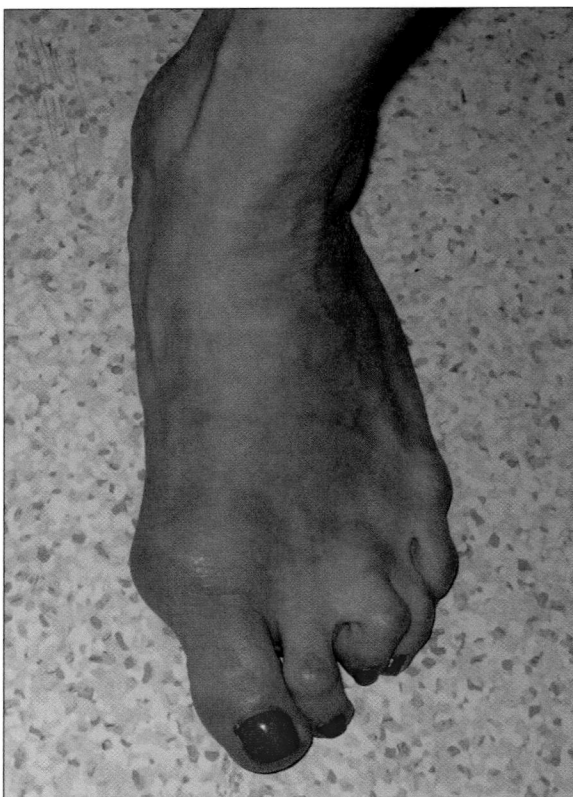

Fig. 75.20 Lesser toe deformities. Dorsal view of the forefoot reveals hammertoe deformity of the lesser toes, most severe at the second and third toes.

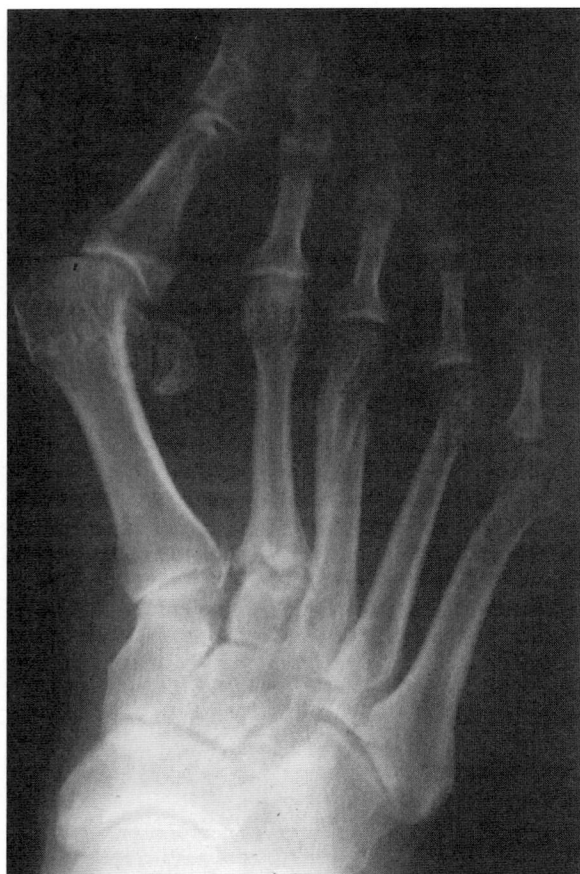

Fig. 75.21 Metatarsal stress fracture. Anteroposterior radiograph of the foot reveals a hallux valgus deformity of the first MTP joint and second and third metatarsal stress fractures at different stages of healing.

as a bunionette. Plantar and lateral skin irritation or hyperkeratosis may be present, as well as a palpable bursa. Dorsal metatarsal neck and shaft pain with edema is often indicative of a stress fracture. It can be associated with a recent increase in activity in patients with inflammatory arthritides and osteoporosis. Radiograph findings can be subtle (Fig. 75.21). Bone scintigraphy, CT, or MRI may be needed for further investigation.

Heel pain

There are several causes of heel pain, one of which was discussed previously in the ankle section—Achilles tendinopathy. Plantar fasciitis is a common cause of heel pain seen in both rheumatologic and non-rheumatologic patients. It is caused by repetitive microtrauma to the plantar fascia at its origin on the medial calcaneal tuberosity and along its course through the arch. The patient will describe pain that is typically worse when first getting up in the morning and when attempting to ambulate after a period of rest. This pain can be associated with Achilles tightness (thus the often effective treatment with Achilles stretching and night splints). A calcaneal stress fracture can present as diffuse heel pain that is worsened with activity. On examination, the heel should be compressed medially and laterally at the same time to try to illicit pain; this is known as a positive "squeeze test." The medial or lateral calcaneal wall tenderness found with stress fractures is uncommon in plantar fasciitis. Further radiologic workup with an MRI, CT, or bone scintigraphy is helpful to confirm the diagnosis.

TREATMENT

The goals of treatment should include pain relief, prevention of deformity and loss of function, and correction of deformity. Grondal and colleagues evaluated the effects of new medications on the treatment of rheumatoid disease and found that patients complained of 3 affected joints versus 13 joints in the 1990s.[13] It was believed that the total number of surgical procedures in the rheumatoid patient for foot and ankle correction is decreasing secondary to new medication regimens.[14] These studies emphasize the point that conservative management will

likely play a larger role than it has previously in the care of patients with inflammatory arthritis. The treating physician will need to evaluate the functional demands of the patient and the anticipated severity of the disease. By approaching a treatment plan in this manner and involving a pedorthist early, the progression of foot and ankle deformity can be predicted and a plan can be created for prevention of further problems.[1,6]

When planning treatment of foot and ankle problems in patients with inflammatory arthritis, the increased rate of complications must be considered. The risk of complications increases with severity of the systemic disease, types of medications, and magnitude of deformities. Non-steroidal anti-inflammatory drugs, corticosteroids, and disease-modifying anti-rheumatic drugs such as methotrexate and the biologic response modifiers have had an important impact on improving quality of life, but the side-effects can influence surgical decision-making and outcome. Increased rate of infection, wound complications, non-union, and implant failure are a few common complications related to the disease and medications. One study found that more than 12.5 mg of prednisone increased the risk of complication with ankle fusions used to treat end-stage arthritis.[15]

Ankle

Conservative management plays a significant role in the treatment of symptoms around the ankle. Shoe wear adjustments such as adding a rocker bottom to the sole of the shoe help decrease the motion required of the ankle for normal gait. Over-the-counter ankle braces may be useful in early disease with synovitis. As symptoms increase, custom bracing such as a plastic or composite (leather and plastic) ankle-foot orthosis (AFO) can provide stability to the ankle joint and minimize motion through the tibiotalar and subtalar joints. Prudent use of intra-articular corticosteroids and anesthetic agents can be used to alleviate symptoms in painful joints but should be avoided in and around tendons because it can alter the biomechanical properties of the tendon,

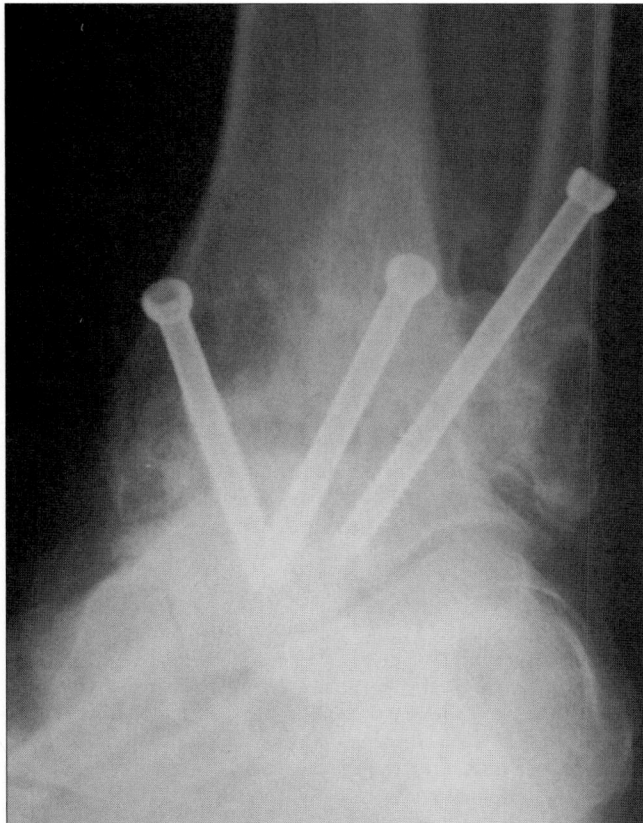

Fig. 75.22 Ankle fusion. Fusion of the tibiotalar joint for severe arthritic disease.

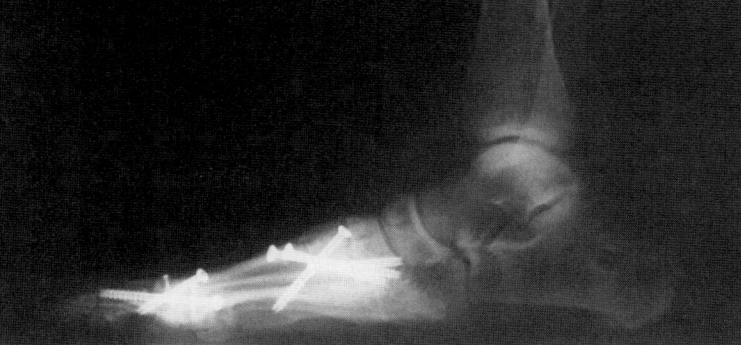

Fig. 75.23 Triple arthrodesis. Fusion of the subtalar, talonavicular, and calcaneocuboid joints.

leading to tearing or rupture. Tendon pathology around the ankle should be treated with immobilization and an anti-inflammatory agent initially. As symptoms improve, athletic braces can be used to support the tendon as activity is increased. Physical therapy also plays a role in non-operative management by maintaining range of motion and maintaining strength.[16] Extracorporeal shock wave treatment has been studied for tendinopathy and found to be helpful.[17] Its role in specific rheumatologic diseases is still being assessed. The role of platelet-rich plasma injections from either peripheral blood or bone marrow aspiration for diseased but not ruptured ligament or tendons is under study. Preliminary research indicates that the growth factors within the platelets have beneficial effect on collagen production, fibroblast proliferation, and tenocyte function.

Surgical options after failure of conservative management in the ankle are based on the severity of the disease and the level of function of the patient. Chronic synovitis with minimal radiographic changes may be treated with arthroscopic synovectomy. Anterior osteophytes causing impingement with dorsiflexion can be resected to improve range of motion. As intra-articular pathology progresses, surgical options become more aggressive. Ankle fusion (arthrodesis) is the standard surgical treatment of refractory end-stage ankle arthritis (Fig. 75.22).[2] It is an effective method of treating the painful rheumatoid ankle but, as discussed previously, the morbidity rate is high. Another surgical option for end-stage arthritis gaining popularity is total-ankle arthroplasty (replacement). The advantage of arthroplasty over arthrodesis is preservation of motion, but this method is limited by technical challenges, bone quality to prevent migration of the prosthesis, and the amount of bone resected, which can limit revision procedures if failure occurs.[16]

Tendon pathology can also be resistant to non-operative care. MRI should be performed to better evaluate tendon integrity. Isolated tenosynovitis without degenerative changes can be treated with a tenosynovectomy. As degeneration occurs, reconstruction with allograft or a tendon transfer can be performed with resection or débridement/repair of the diseased tendon, as with PTTD and peroneal tendon tears. After failed extended immobilization, Achilles tendinopathy may require débridement with resection of Haglund's deformity of the calcaneus and possible FHL tendon transfer to augment the remaining Achilles tendon. Treatment of tarsal tunnel syndrome after failed immobilization may benefit from surgical decompression of the tibial nerve.

Hindfoot

Pain in the hindfoot and flexible mild valgus deformity of the heel can be treated non-operatively with shoe modification or bracing. A custom full-length orthotic can be created with a medial heel posting. As the valgus progresses but remains flexible, a University of California Biomechanics Laboratory (UCBL) insert can help in maintaining the position of the foot.[16] A stirrup brace is designed to treat a collapsed foot from PTTD. The brace not only has medial and lateral vertical struts but also has a strap that runs from underneath the arch to the vertical upright to support the midfoot and an inflatable adjustable pneumatic chamber to further lift the arch. As deformity and pain progress, more aggressive bracing may be needed, such as a rigid custom AFO, to prevent any instability.

The goal of surgery in the hindfoot is to create a plantigrade foot with the heel in 5 degrees of valgus.[2] Before the advancement of medical management in rheumatoid disease, arthrodesis was the mainstay to correct hindfoot deformity. The approach to surgical treatment has become more focused on joint preservation, using osteotomies to correct the deformity around the joint rather than fusing the joint. Calcaneal osteotomy is an excellent example of a corrective osteotomy to bring the heel out of excessive valgus by sliding the bone cut and fixing it with screws in a stable position. An osteotomy through the medial cuneiform can help correct midfoot collapse and forefoot pronation using a bone graft wedge. In addition, transferring the FDL tendon to the navicular can re-create the inversion force of the diseased PTT. Joint preservation works only if the joints are relatively disease free before surgery. When arthritic changes have occurred at the subtalar, talonavicular, or calcaneocuboid joints in the setting of a hindfoot deformity, a single, double, or triple arthrodesis should be considered (Fig. 75.23).[16]

Midfoot

The approach to midfoot symptoms is similar to what has been discussed previously. In an acute flare, immobilization, an anti-inflammatory, and limited weight bearing should be attempted first. In more chronic cases with arthritic changes in the midfoot, a rocker-bottom shoe will provide relief by decreasing compressive forces across midfoot joints. Custom orthotics or over-the-counter bracing can also assist when the deformity is flexible.

Arthritis in the midfoot can cause symptomatic spurring that affects shoe wear. If there is minimal joint change, a cheilectomy (osteophyte excision) may be performed. For degenerative midfoot joints, surgical treatment of midfoot arthritis is arthrodesis of the affected joints (Fig. 75.24). Most commonly, the medial joints are involved (naviculocuneiform, first to third TMT joints) and disease in the lateral TMT joints often remains asymptomatic. Fusion of the lateral joints should be avoided because they are important in accommodating foot contact with the ground. In advanced deformities a rocker-bottom reconstruction is warranted with use of plantar plating and possible transpedal osteotomies.[11]

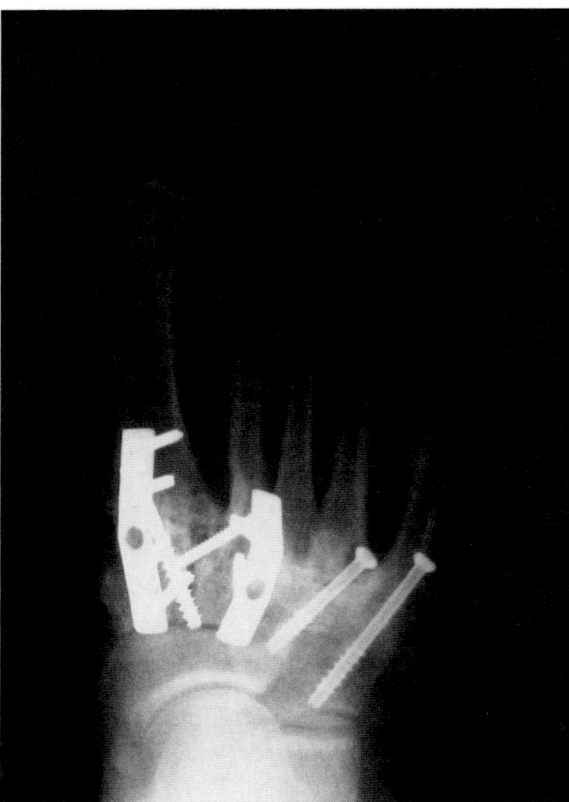

Fig. 75.24 Midfoot fusion. Anteroposterior radiograph reveals tarsometatarsal joint fusions to correct arthritic pain and deformity.

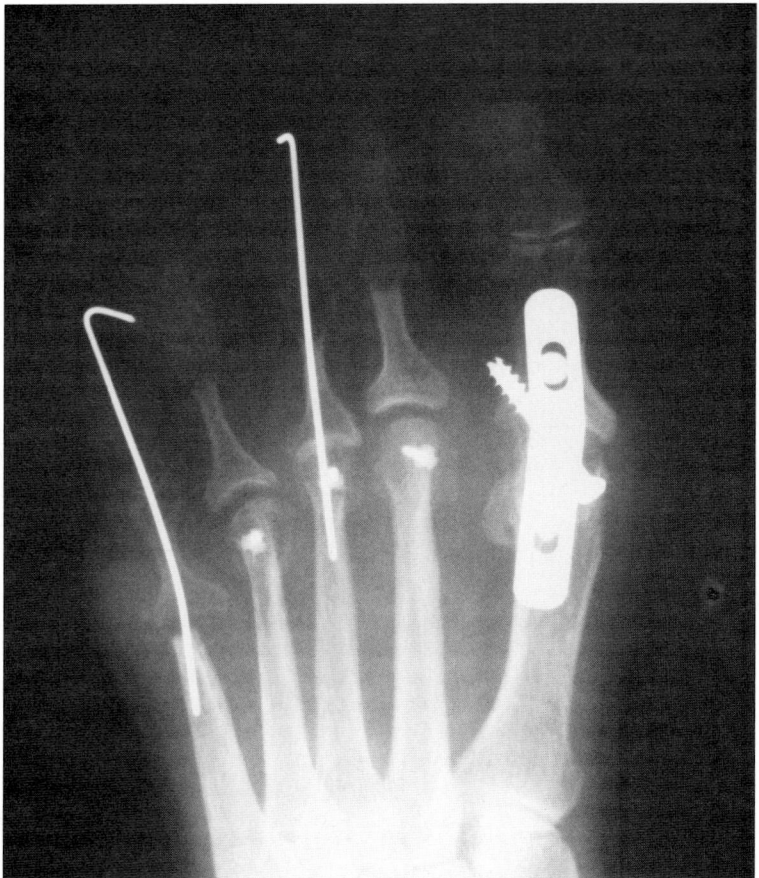

Fig. 75.25 First metatarsophalangeal joint fusion and lesser toe correction. Anteroposterior radiograph reveals fusion of the first MTP joint, shortening osteotomies of the second through fourth toes, PIP fusion of the third toe, and resection arthroplasty of the fifth toe.

Forefoot

Footwear alterations are the mainstay in non-operative management of forefoot pathology. For metatarsalgia and painful keratoses, a metatarsal pad can be placed proximal to the metatarsal heads or specific cutouts can be made in a custom orthotic under the affected area to provide relief. A Plastazote or viscoelastic insole may be helpful with fat pad atrophy but should be replaced every 3 months.[2] In mild to moderate disease, a broad, soft-soled shoe should be sufficient. As the disease progresses, a custom extra-depth shoe may be necessary to prevent dorsal wear on the lesser toes and medial wear due to the hallux valgus deformity. Often, a combination of all these modifications is used as the disease progresses. Physical therapy is also of assistance early in the disease with heel cord stretching, MTP motion, and intrinsic muscle strengthening. Caution should be used with intra-articular steroid injections because joint laxity can be worsened.

Fixed deformities and severe pain resistant to non-operative care require surgical intervention. In hallux deformity, the major consequence is the shift of the weight-bearing force laterally to the lesser metatarsal heads. The goal of surgical treatment is to regain weight-bearing function of the great toe. In mild disease with good soft tissue and flexible deformity, joint preservation with a corrective osteotomy of the first metatarsal can be performed to correct the valgus deformity. As the disease advances, arthrodesis of the first MTP joint is necessary to eliminate pain and prevent recurrence (Fig. 75.25). Arthroplasty of the first MTP joint using a metal or plastic implant is controversial. Some investigators have reported excellent results, whereas others have had significant complications such as pain, recurrence, metatarsalgia, synovitis, and osteolysis.[18] Arthrodesis of the first MTP is the current treatment of choice.

Surgical reconstruction of the lesser toes is performed to realign the MTP joints, relocate the plantar fat pad, and improve footwear options. The more traditional surgery in the forefoot has been metatarsal head excision of the second through fifth metatarsals in a gentle cascade of decreasing length to address the MTP joint pathology.[18] Recently, shortening osteotomies of the lesser metatarsals (second, third, and sometimes fourth) called Weil osteotomies are gaining popularity over resection of the metatarsal heads. Hammer toes and claw toes are best addressed by fusion of the proximal IP joint with temporary pinning of the lesser toes (see Fig. 75.25).[18] Amputation of a single symptomatic hammer toe is another option for patients with significant co-morbidities.

Heel

Plantar fasciitis is a frustrating problem for patients because of pain and prolonged recovery. Achilles stretches, plantar fascia massage, heel cups, an anti-inflammatory agent, and night splinting to hold the foot in a plantigrade position are all reasonable methods that can be combined to treat this problem. The patient should be reassured that it can take several months for the symptoms to improve but that the condition can recur. A calcaneal stress fracture should be treated with immobilization and restricted weight bearing. One or two corticosteroid shots administered at the plantar fascia origin can be helpful. Extracorporeal shock wave treatment and/or platelet-rich plasma injections have been found by the authors to be helpful for resistant cases.

REFERENCES

1. Michelson J, Easley M, Wigley FM, Hellma D. Foot and ankle problems in rheumatoid arthritis. Foot Ankle Int 1994;15:608-613.
2. Coughlin MJ, Mann RA, Saltzman CL. Surgery of the foot and ankle, 8th ed. Philadelphia: Elsevier, 2007.
3. McGuigan L, Burke D, Fleming A. Tarsal tunnel syndrome and peripheral neuropathy in rheumatoid disease. Ann Rheum Dis 1983;42:128-131.
4. Nassar J, Cracchiolo A. Complications in surgery of the foot and ankle in patients with rheumatoid
   arthritis. Clin Orthop Relat Res 2001;391: 140-152.
5. Keenan M, Peabody T, Gronley J, Perry J. Valgus deformities of the feet and characteristics of gait in patients who have rheumatoid

arthritis. J Bone Joint Surg Am 1991;73: 237-247.

6. Shi K, Tomita T, Hayashida K, et al. Foot deformities in rheumatoid arthritis and relevance of disease severity. J Rheumatol 2000;27:84-89.

7. Dimonte P, Light H. Pathomechanics, gait deviations, and treatment of the rheumatoid foot. Phys Ther 1982;62:1148-1156.

8. Tillman K. The pathomechanics of rheumatic foot deformities. In: The rheumatoid foot: diagnosis, pathomechanics, and treatment. Stuttgart: Georg Thieme, 1979:44-49.

9. Michelson J, Easley M, Wigley F, Hellman D. Posterior tibial tendon dysfunction in rheumatoid arthritis. Foot Ankle 1995;16:156-161.

10. Vidigal E, Jacoby R, Dixon A, et al. The foot in chronic rheumatoid arthritis. Ann Rheum Dis 1975;34:292-297.

11. Schon LC, Weinfeld SB, Horton GA, Resch S. Radiographic and clinical classification of acquired midtarsus deformities. Foot Ankle Int 1998;19:394-404.

12. Platto M, O'Connell P, Hicks J, Gerber L. The relationship of pain and deformity of the rheumatoid foot to gait and an index of functional ambulation. J Rheumatol 1991;18:38-43.

13. Grondal L, Tengstrand B, Nordmark B, et al. The foot: still the most important reason for walking incapacity in rheumatoid patients. Acta Orthop 2008;79:257-261.

14. Weiss R, Stark A, Wick M, et al. Orthopaedic surgery of the lower limbs in 49802 rheumatoid arthritis patients:

results from the Swedish National Inpatient Registry during 1987 to 2001. Ann Rheum Dis 2006;65:335-341.

15. Cracchiolo A, Cimino W, Lian G. Arthrodesis of the ankle in patients who have rheumatoid arthritis. J Bone Joint Surg Am 1992;74:903-909.

16. Cimino W, O'Malley M. Rheumatoid arthritis of the ankle and hindfoot. Rheum Dis Clin North Am 1998;24:157-172.

17. Han S, Lee J, Guyton G, et al. Effect of extracorporeal shock wave therapy on cultured tenocytes. Foot Ankle Int 2009;30:93-98.

18. Burra G, Katchis S. Rheumatoid arthritis of the forefoot. Rheum Dis Clin North Am 1998;24:173-180.

The temporomandibular joint

David M. Adlam

■ The temporomandibular joint (TMJ) is a synovial joint with a meniscus and lined by connective tissue, not hyaline cartilage.

■ TMJ pain is common, usually presenting as a functional and self-limiting disorder with pain in the masticatory muscles.

■ The diagnosis of TMJ pain can usually be made from the history and physical examination. The specific and generalized joint diseases require plain radiographs, computed tomography, magnetic resonance imaging, and hematologic investigations.

CLASSIFICATION

The temporomandibular joint (TMJ) disorders are a group of conditions often with overlapping signs, symptoms, and etiology. TMJ pain is a subgroup of craniofacial pain problems. There is no simple classification, but the major clinical subgroups are as follows[1-5]:

1. Myofascial pain disorder (MPD) is the most common disorder and was previously called temporomandibular pain dysfunction syndrome, facial arthromyalgia, and originally Costen's syndrome. It also has some features of fibromyalgia (see Chapter 77). The characteristics are pain in the masticatory muscles often with neck shoulder and back pain. Jaw dysfunction with limited movements, joint noises, and a jaw swing to the affected side may occur. Headaches, depression, somatization, psychosocial factors, and chronic pain syndrome are all features of this multifactorial condition. Precipitating factors include trauma, wisdom tooth removal, and a bruxism habit.
2. TMJ internal derangement. Displacement of the meniscus is anterior and medial and may be reducible or irreducible (closed lock) (Fig. 76.1). There is limited mouth opening. Meniscal displacement may be the end result of chronic muscle dysfunction.
3. Joint disease. Inflammatory conditions include rheumatoid arthritis and psoriatic arthritis and non-inflammatory conditions, including osteoarthritis.
4. Specific TMJ disease. Congenital and developmental conditions include hemifacial microsomia and condylar hyperplasia. Other specific conditions are fracture, dislocation, infection, ankylosis, joint mobility problems, and neoplasia.

Identifying the subgroup and the specific cause can be difficult but important in treatment planning.

FUNCTIONAL ANATOMY

Each TMJ is formed from membranous bone from the first branchial arch and cranium. The craniomandibular articulation is a synovial joint with an intracapsular meniscus dividing the joint into upper and lower joint compartments (Fig. 76.2).[6] The articulating joint surfaces are unusual in that they are lined by fibrous connective tissue and not by hyaline cartilage.

The TMJs are unique in that, first, they are the only joints for which the movement is limited and guided by the dental occlusion, and, second, the mandible connects the two joints, which can only move in unison; one joint cannot move alone. Each joint is supported laterally by the temporomandibular ligament and medially by the sphenomandibular ligament (Fig. 76.3). The main muscles of mastication—the masseter, temporalis, and medial and lateral pterygoid muscles—are the primary muscles moving these joints. They allow opening and closing of the mouth as well as lateral and protrusive movements of

the mandible. The temporalis muscle plays a major role in the limitation of joint loading, and the lateral pterygoid muscle helps to stabilize each joint by controlling both the meniscus (upper head of the lateral pterygoid) and the condylar position (lower head of the lateral pterygoid muscle).

Mouth opening involves an initial hinge (rotation) in the lower jaw space to some 24 mm. On wider opening, the movement is a forward translation in the upper joint space as the condyle moves down the articular eminence to open 34 to 44 mm (Fig. 76.4). In normal active opening there is a combination of hinge and translation movements. Functional problems usually affect the translating movement as the meniscus is displaced anteriorly; internal derangement such as a closed lock with limited opening and a stretching of the bilaminar zone is shown in Figure 76.1.

The meniscus is composed of avascular fibrous tissue and cartilage. There is an anterior thick band and a thicker and larger posterior band, the narrowest area of the meniscus being between the condyle and the posterior surface of the articular eminence.

Anteriorly, the meniscus is attached to the condyle and the upper head of the lateral pterygoid muscle. Posteriorly, the meniscus does not normally articulate and is attached to the bilaminar zone. In the bilaminar zone posteriorly, the superior surface is mostly composed of elastic tissue with vessels and nerves, the inferior portion being cartilaginous. The TMJ is innervated by the auriculotemporal nerve and also small components from the posterior deep temporal and masseteric nerves. The capsule, lateral ligament, and posterior fat pads are innervated. However, the central part of the meniscus and the synovium do not appear to be innervated, an important consideration when diagnosing pain related to the joint.

There is much controversy as to whether the joint is load bearing. It is mostly non–load bearing but appears to be load bearing in some instances. This may be important in parafunction and a cause of pain. The aim of conservative management of the joint is to reduce joint loading and keep the meniscus in the correct relationship to the condyle.

Physical examination

The findings on physical examination must be carefully recorded, because this is not only helpful in reaching a diagnosis and the formulation of a treatment plan but also invaluable in the monitoring of treatment success.[2] The physical examination of the joint and associated structures may reproduce the symptoms.

General examination

On examination, look for any visible swelling. Palpation of the joint may reveal tenderness overlying the joint. A finger is placed in both external auditory meatus and the patient is asked to open, close, and protrude the mandible (Fig. 76.5). Clicking or joint noises during these movements should be noted, along with any deviation of movement. Biting on a wooden spatula, either unilaterally or bilaterally, may stop the click or relieve the pain. Auscultation of the joint may confirm any clicking. The ear should be examined with an otoscope, if indicated.

Muscles

The following muscles should then be examined:
- The masseter can be palpated bilaterally, with the fingers over the angle of the mandible (Fig. 76.6). Tenderness may be detected at rest or when the jaw is clenched. In addition, a gloved finger may be placed inside the mouth to bimanually palpate the muscle at rest or under tension (Fig. 76.7). Differences may be detected between the two sides.

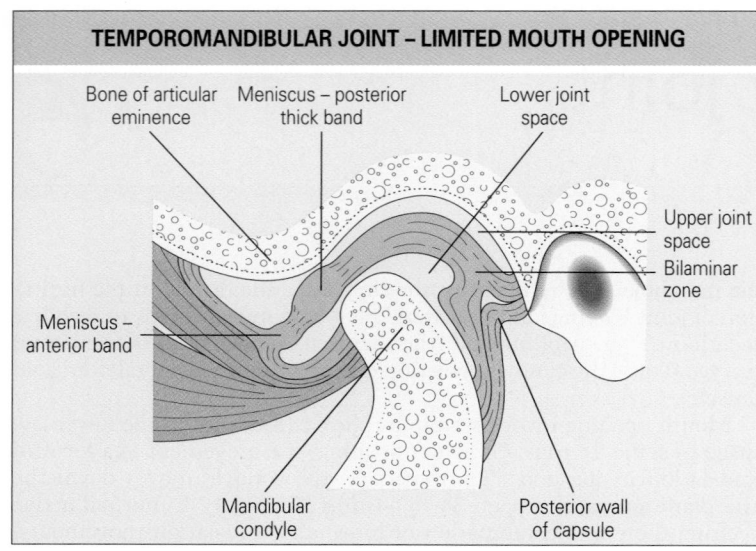

Fig. 76.1 Limited opening of the temporomandibular joint showing anterior displacement of the meniscus (internal derangement).

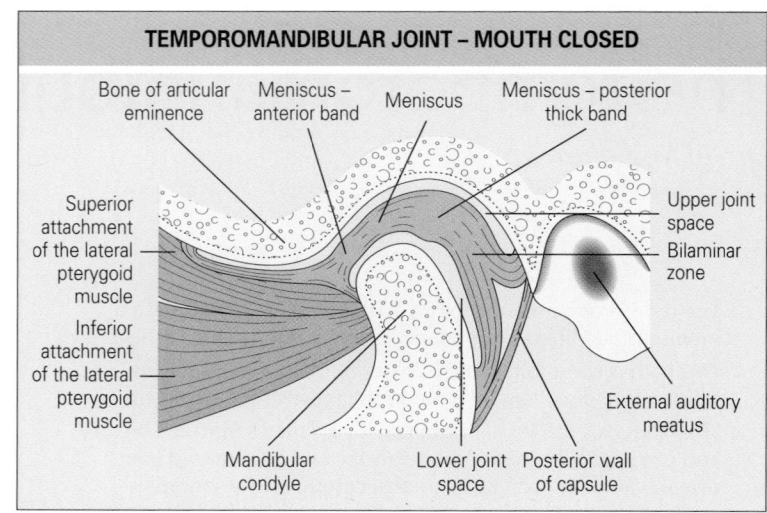

Fig. 76.2 Anatomy of the temporomandibular joint in the closed position (sagittal section).

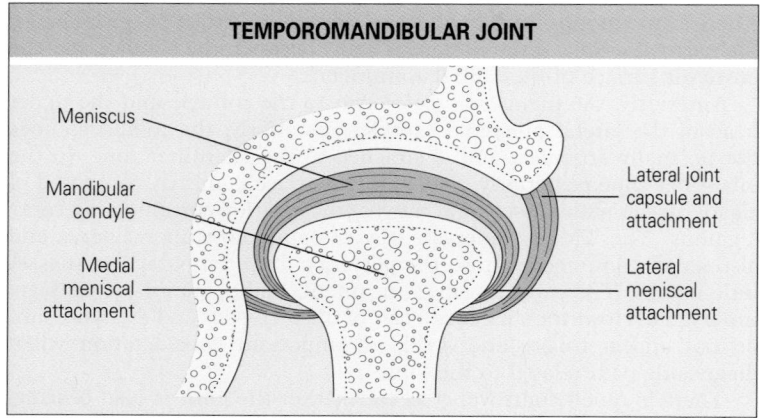

Fig. 76.3 Anatomy of the temporomandibular joint (coronal section).

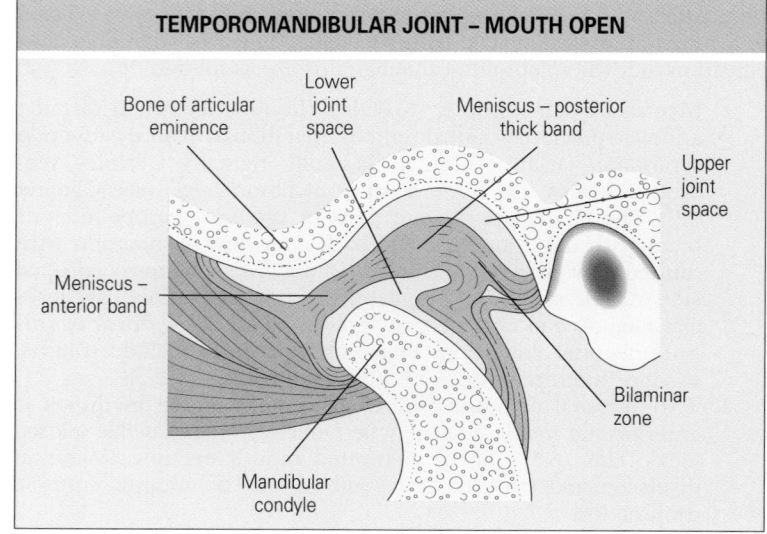

Fig. 76.4 The temporomandibular joint in the open position.

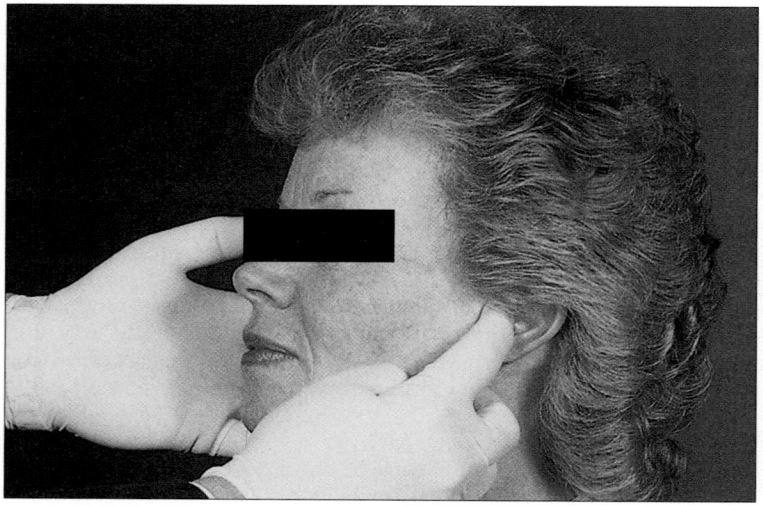

Fig. 76.5 Extraoral examination.

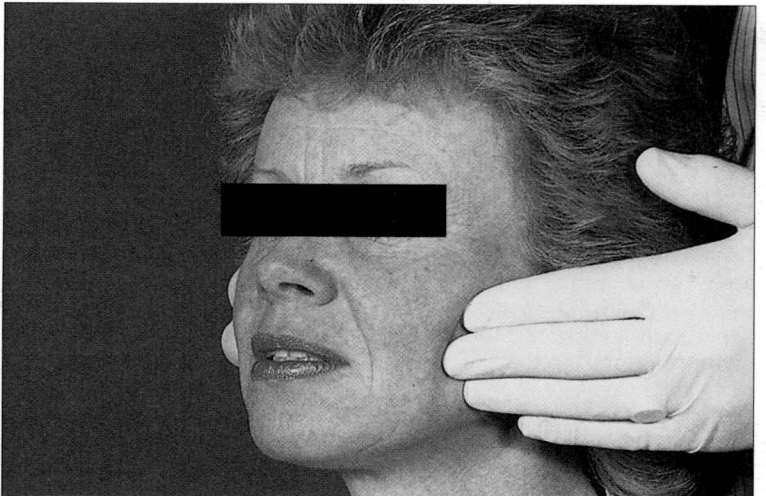

Fig. 76.6 Bilateral palpation of masseters.

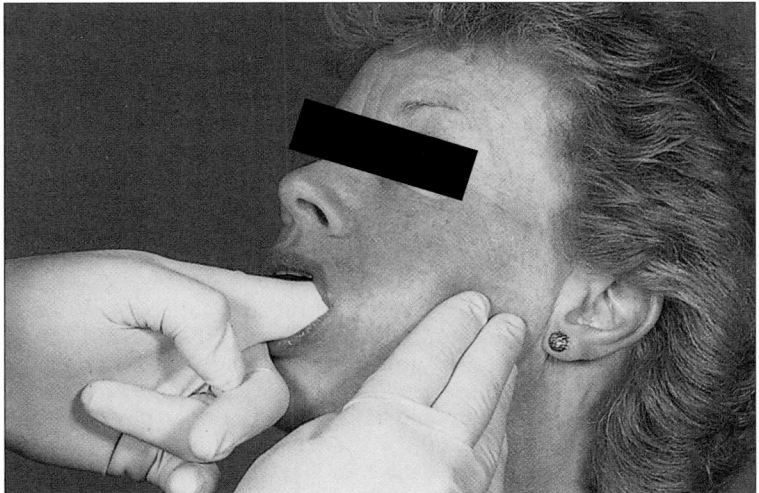

Fig. 76.7 Bimanual palpation of masseter.

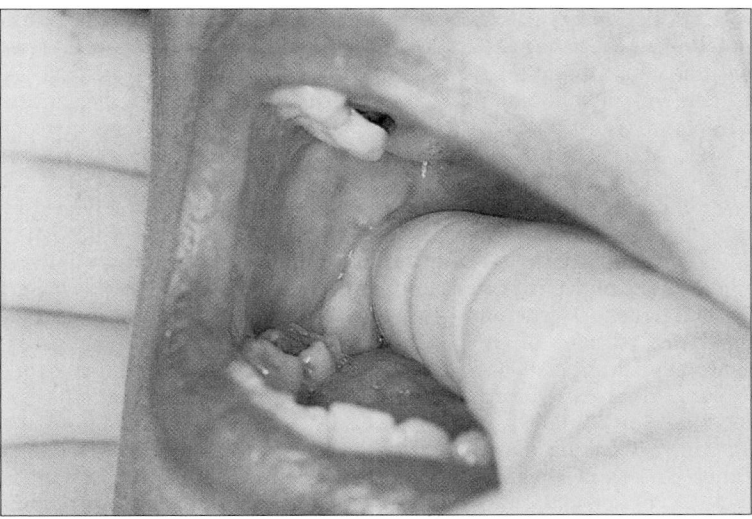

Fig. 76.9 Intraoral examination of medial pterygoid.

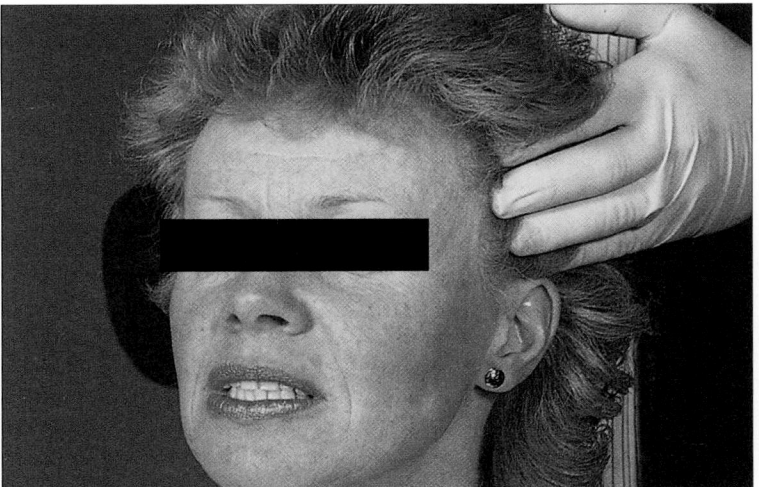

Fig. 76.8 Palpation of temporalis.

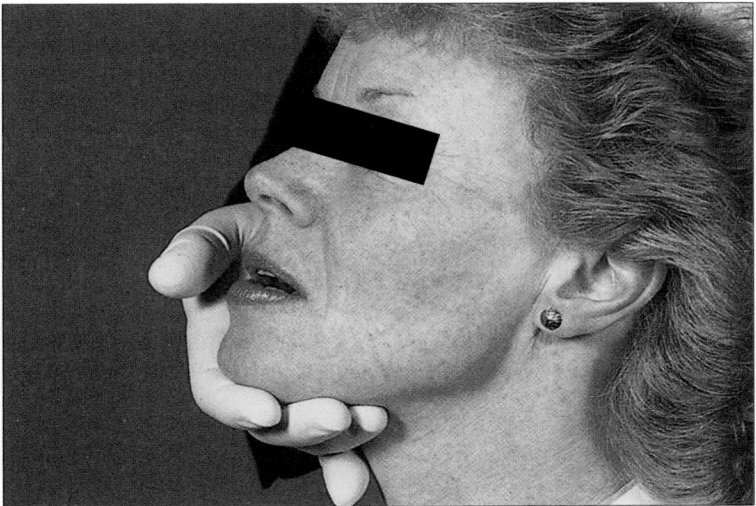

Fig. 76.10 Examination of lateral pterygoid.

- The temporalis muscle covers a wide area over the temple. The entire area of the muscle should be palpated with the jaw relaxed and then clenched (Fig. 76.8). The patient may help to locate the area of tenderness.
- The medial pterygoid is difficult to examine because it lies medial to the ramus of the mandible. The posterior border may be palpated extraorally by placing the fingers around the posterior border of the ramus of the mandible. It can also be examined intraorally by placing a finger on the medial ramus of the mandible (Fig. 76.9), but this often produces a gag reflex, making interpretation difficult.
- The lateral pterygoid may be examined by standing behind the patient and placing the palm of the hand over the chin. The patient is then asked to open the mouth gently, against resistance (Fig. 76.10) and to move the jaw laterally. The muscle can also be palpated intraorally in a cooperative patient. In addition, the muscles of the neck and shoulder may require examination.

Intraoral examination

The movement of the jaw can be measured actively, with the patient opening the mouth, or passively, with the jaw being manipulated by the examiner. The degrees of opening and deviation are recorded for subsequent monitoring of treatment. The interincisor opening is normally 34 to 44 mm. Opening of less than 20 mm indicates a closed lock.

Active protrusion of the mandible should be measured; this is normally up to 10 mm. Lateral movements of the mandible should be equidistant from the midline. This can be measured by asking the patient to move the jaw from side to side, with the teeth held lightly together. Lateral movement is normally in the region of 10 mm to each side.

A simple examination of the teeth and occlusion is helpful, noting any carious teeth, premature contacts, restorations, and dentures. The attrition of the teeth may be an indication of a grinding habit. Cheek biting and scalloping of the lateral border of the tongue as a result of pressure against the teeth are often seen in bruxism.

MYOFASCIAL PAIN DISORDER

Epidemiology

TMJ disorders are common but not always reported by the patient.[2] Surveys suggest that physical signs of TMJ disorders are very frequent in the population, with a prevalence of 50% to 75%. The prevalence of symptomatic disorder is lower, at 20% to 25%, but only 3% to 4% seek treatment. The overall prevalence of symptoms in both sexes is similar, although there is a fivefold excess of females among those who present for treatment.

Clinical features

History

The first consultation is particularly important, not only to establish a thorough history and physical examination but also to gain a good rapport with the patient. It has been shown that a good doctor-patient relationship affects the success of treatment of myofascial pain.[7,8] It is not unusual for the patient to have been seen by several specialists, with no cause found for the pain, before reaching a diagnosis of MPD.

Pain on mandibular movement is the most common presenting complaint in MPD. The pain is usually chronic but may present acutely. It is described as a constant dull ache, which is worse on chewing, especially hard foods. The side of the face and the cheek are often localized as the site of pain, rarely the TMJ itself. The pain may radiate, usually to the muscle groups affected by muscle spasm. MPD is more often unilateral, with the associated muscle spasm resulting in deviation of the mandible to the affected side.

The patient is generally aware of a limitation of movement, associated with stiffness of the joint. This is often worse in the morning, especially with a history of nocturnal clenching of the teeth (bruxism). Noises from the TMJ are common and described as clicking, popping, or grinding. These noises may be easily audible and palpable to the examiner. Clicking may vary from day to day and even be absent at times. A loss of clicking and subsequent limitation of movement is called a "closed lock" and indicates displacement of the meniscus with internal derangement (see Fig. 76.1).

Locking may be a confusing term for the patient: it is not a joint dislocation but rather a result of the disc displacement, allowing only very limited opening. The patient may describe this as a jamming or dislocation of the joint. It usually occurs when the teeth are slightly apart during opening or closing of the mouth. Inability to overcome the lock is very distressing to the patient. It may last a few seconds, resolving spontaneously or being overcome by the patient. It can, however, be a persistent problem requiring intervention.

There are numerous associated symptoms occurring in patients with MPD that are rarely volunteered by the patient and must be specifically elicited (Box 76.1). Habits such as bruxism, nail biting, and cheek biting exacerbate both the pain and the muscle spasm. Stress-related problems are invariably present. Tension headaches, with a pressure sensation over the top of the head and down the neck, may be a daily occurrence. The headache may respond to simple analgesia, but the dull ache in the jaw is persistent. Simple analgesia rarely controls the constant dull ache.

There is often a history of recent dental and otolaryngologic consultations that revealed no abnormalities. The wisdom teeth may be suspected as the origin of pain but are rarely a contributing factor. However, wisdom tooth removal and trauma may be a trigger.[1] Emotional and stress-related problems may coincide with the onset of the pain. Problems at school, with friendships, and with sibling rivalry are factors in school-age patients, whereas problems related to housing, work, family, and marriage, in addition to chronic ill health, post-traumatic stress disorder, bereavement, depression, and loneliness are associated factors in adults.

BOX 76.1 DEFINITION AND CLINICAL FEATURES OF MYOFASCIAL PAIN DISORDER

Definition

- Acute or chronic musculoskeletal pain with dysfunction of the masticatory system
- Pain aggravated by jaw movements
- Pain localized to the temporomandibular joint and masticatory muscles but may be associated with other joint pains
- Independent of local oral, dental, and ear disease

Clinical features

- Unilateral or bilateral joint pain that is worse with movement
- Joint stiffness and trismus
- Jaw may swing to the affected side on opening, with reduced lateral movements
- Joint noises: clicking or popping with dysfunction or crepitus with degenerative disease
- Intermittent or persistent locking with internal derangement
- Parafunctional habit (e.g., bruxism, nail biting)
- Masticatory muscle and joint tenderness
- Headache (tension)
- Dental bite that feels altered

Investigations

Investigations of MPD may be divided into those aiming to examine a cause outside the joint complex and those specific to the TMJ. Laboratory investigation is not indicated in internal derangement or osteoarthritis but is helpful in systemic disease and rheumatoid arthritis. A number of imaging modalities are available. A plain radiograph may reveal gross bone and/or dental pathology. An orthopantogram is useful to screen the teeth and jaws but should be interpreted with caution. Either conventional tomograms or computed tomography (CT) may be useful in detecting either osteoarthritis or ankylosis, although, for the latter, CT with three-dimensional reconstruction is the most helpful.

Magnetic resonance imaging (MRI), and now dynamic MRI, is the investigation of choice for the accurate assessment of position of the meniscus in the joint to make a diagnosis of internal derangement. The availability of this technique has replaced arthrography and diagnostic arthroscopy. Arthroscopy of the TMJ may be combined with arthrocentesis and may have a place in diagnosis and treatment with lysis of adhesions.[5]

Electromyographic studies of masticatory muscles can show abnormal muscle activity but have a research rather than a clinical application. There is no specific test or investigation to confirm a diagnosis of MPD, which is a clinical diagnosis.

Differential diagnosis

Facial pain is frequently complex and from more than one source. The causes of facial pain are varied, some being very specific, such as giant cell arteritis and trigeminal neuralgia, others less so, such as MPD. Indeed, two types of facial pain, such as MPD and atypical facial pain, may coexist.

The following should be considered in the differential diagnosis of facial pain and MPD.

Atypical facial pain

This is a dull aching pain or, occasionally, a sharp pain, most commonly felt over the cheeks. It affects the non-muscular parts of the face and may occur unilaterally or bilaterally. It is chronic, with no provoking or relieving factors. Analgesia has little effect. The pain may be worse at times of stress. A history of otolaryngologic and dental treatment is often given, with no subsequent relief from the pain. Anxiety and depression are often associated. Management is non-surgical.

Trigeminal neuralgia

Trigeminal neuralgia is a severe lancinating pain in the face that lasts only a few seconds. It is characteristically provoked by stimulating a trigger zone and may be provoked by jaw movements. The pain is localized to a branch of the trigeminal nerve, most commonly in the mandibular or maxillary branches. Improvement in pain with carbamazepine may be considered diagnostic.

Giant cell arteritis

Giant cell arteritis causes a severe throbbing pain, usually in the temporal region, but may involve any branch of the external carotid artery. The area is painful and tender to touch and may affect the jaw joint with painful mastication and claudication. There may be associated visual symptoms. The condition is predominantly restricted to the elderly. A finding of a raised erythrocyte sedimentation rate aids in the diagnosis (see Chapter 152).

Osteoarthritis

The pain in osteoarthritis is localized to the joint and is worse on movement, with grinding noises or crepitus. It is more commonly found after the fourth decade. The onset may be sudden, producing a constant dull, aching pain with limitation in the range of jaw movements. However, unlike MPD, the pain is localized to the joint, which is tender, and there is rarely associated muscle spasm. Pain from degenerative disease of the cervical spine and, in particular, the facet joints may also present as facial pain. Management is non-surgical, but in severe cases surgery is needed.

Inflammatory arthropathies

The TMJ, although often affected by rheumatoid arthritis, causes symptoms in only a minority of patients. Joint tenderness and stiffness are most frequently seen. In severe disease there is destruction of the joint surface, with pain, stiffness, crepitations, and anterior open bite; the latter is the inability to bite the front teeth together because of loss of the height of the mandibular condyle. Management is principally non-surgical, but occasionally joint replacement is required. The TMJ is affected in approximately 50% of cases of juvenile idiopathic arthritis (see Section 7: Pediatric rheumatology). When present, it is very destructive, producing secondary effects in the dental occlusion, particularly an anterior open bite and loss of condylar height.

Salivary gland disorders

The pain of these disorders is localized to the affected parotid gland and is worse with eating, particularly if the gland is obstructed. Tenderness and swelling of the gland are normally evident but may have resolved by the time the patient is seen. Malignancy or infection of the salivary glands may present as pain in the TMJ.

ENT causes of facial pain

Pain from the sinuses may be unilateral or bilateral and associated with infection or tumor. In maxillary sinus infections the maxillary teeth are often tender and hypersensitive. The pain may be exacerbated by changes in head position. There is associated nasal congestion and discharge. The ear may be a source of pain, and expert help is advised to differentiate this from joint pain.

Central and vascular causes of facial pain

Cerebral tumors are a rare cause of facial pain but must be considered. CT or MRI should be arranged when more common causes of pain have been excluded. Psychogenic pain is particularly difficult to diagnose, and psychiatric assessment may be required.

Dental causes

Odontogenic causes of pain are generally specific but may be referred to the TMJ. Acute pulpitis is severe and throbbing, with the pain being exacerbated by hot or cold but poorly localized. Chronic pulpitis and dental abscess produce pain localized to a tender tooth. Dental treatments requiring prolonged mouth opening such as surgical procedures may precipitate MPD.

Management

The management of patients with MPD requires a careful history and examination.[1-5] It is important to reassure the patient that this is a common condition that is usually self-limiting and resolves over time. The pain mostly emanates from the muscles rather than the joint itself, presenting the complex problem of pain without a pathologic process. Only a minority of patients may progress to persistent internal derangement and degenerative joint disease. Many patients only require an explanation and reassurance, while a minority need great perseverance and support. The aim of treatment is to reduce pain, improve dysfunction, and prevent progression.

The overriding principle is conservative management and to avoid any irreversible treatment. Permanent changes to the dental occlusion, oral rehabilitation, and orthognathic surgery are not recommended. The evidence base for treatment is grade B[1-5,8] with no clear evidence of a single most effective treatment. A positive, warm, and reassuring rapport between patient and clinician is essential for success.[9]

Initial management is always non-surgical, with education, reassurance, and a soft diet. This may progress to exercises, physical therapy, and pharmacologic pain control with non-steroidal anti-inflammatory drugs (NSAIDs), which are the mainstay of treatment. Because anxiety and depression are often associated, a psychological assessment may be helpful.[7,10] This may progress to relaxation, psychotherapy (behavior modification), and antidepressants. The tricyclic antidepressants have proved the most helpful pharmacologic agents. The injection of tender muscle and trigger joints with local anesthetic or botulinum toxin (Botox) is helpful in some patients. Intra-articular corticosteroids should be reserved for patients with osteoarthritis or inflammatory arthropathies. The use of occlusal appliances (splint therapy) is the most widely employed non-surgical management and is discussed later.[10]

Non-surgical management is recommended for at least 6 months before considering a surgical intervention. This may be a simple arthrocentesis of the joint with lavage and corticosteroids. Manipulation and arthroscopy may be considered with MRI evidence of meniscal displacement. Open joint surgery is rarely indicated and needs to be supported by continued non-surgical management, especially if MPD is associated with other causes of facial pain.

Non-surgical management

Non-surgical management consists of explanation, reassurance, and soft diet. It may help to explain that the pain is from tender muscles resulting from clenching and the muscle spasms lead to jaw stiffness and clicking because the meniscus may be displaced by constant muscle pull. The patient should be reassured that this is a self-limiting condition and can be helped by stopping clenching and grinding of teeth, taking a soft diet, and avoiding excessive jaw movements, together with relaxation. Some clinicians recommend gentle jaw exercises especially to correct any jaw deviation. Cognitive behavior therapy, acupuncture, ultrasound therapy, and soft laser therapy have all been used to some relief, but there is no confirmed evidence base.

Drug treatment

Analgesia in the form of NSAIDs is advised for pain and inflammation. Occasionally, in patients with acute muscle spasm, the very short-term use of anxiolytics is recommended. Psychological problems[11] are present in approximately one third of patients, and 10% have clinical depression. Anxiety and psychosocial problems are common in MPD. Psychological and psychiatric management may be needed as well as the use of antidepressants; the tricyclic antidepressants in particular have some limited evidence of success. Opioid analgesia is not recommended and rarely helpful.

Injections

Muscular trigger areas may respond to local anesthetic or Botox injections; Botox reduces muscle spasm and may prevent some meniscal displacement. Corticosteroids around the joint capsule or intra-articular corticosteroids appear to have short-term benefits.

Intraoral appliances (occlusal splints)

Occlusal splints are a frequently used treatment, but their effectiveness is not proven.[10] Any splint that permanently changes the occlusion should be avoided. The most widely used splint is the stabilizing splint that opens the occlusion. An example of a soft splint is shown (Fig. 76.11). The splint reduces joint loading and is usually worn at night. It can be effective in treating bruxism. The anterior repositioning splint brings the mandible forward with the aim of repositioning the displaced meniscus, but there is no evidence this is better than a simple stabilization splint.

Surgical management

Manipulation

Therapeutic manipulation[12] under general anesthesia for MPD with or without meniscal displacement is helpful in almost one third of patients. There is improved opening and reduction in muscle tenderness but not always a loss of clicking.

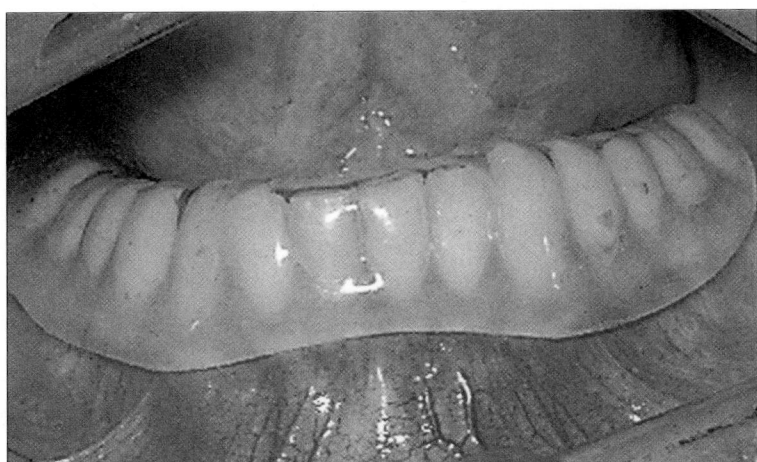

Fig. 76.11 Occlusal splint.

Arthroscopy and arthrocentesis

Arthroscopy may be used for diagnosis and therapeutic purposes in internal derangement.[13] Lysis and lavage of the joint in MPD have been helpful in some series. However, the results of arthroscopic surgery are yet to be proven. Arthrocentesis with lavage and corticosteroids is helpful in degenerative conditions.

Open TMJ surgery

Surgery is reserved for patients with internal joint derangements or degenerative disease who fail to respond to the conservative treatments. Careful case selection is important, because long-term results are often poor, with continued need for conservative management. Sound radiologic or arthroscopic evidence is needed before surgery. Indications for surgery include meniscal displacement with failed conservative treatment, osteoarthritis, adhesions, and meniscal perforations. Eminectomy (excision of bony articular eminence) and meniscal plication in the bilaminar zone have been successful in several series.[14] Menisectomy (disectomy) has also had promising results for an apparently destructive procedure.[15] TMJ surgery is rarely indicated in MPD because the outcome is disappointing. However, surgery for other conditions such as ankylosis, hyperplasia, and tumor is often successful.

REFERENCES

1. Scrivani SJ, Keith DA, Kaban LB. Temporomandibular disorders. N Engl J Med 2008;359;25:2693-2705.
2. Gray RJM, Davies SJ, Quayle AA. A clinical guide to temporomandibular disorders. London, British Dental Journal Books, 1995.
3. National Institutes of Health. Technology assessment conference statement. 29 April-1 May 1996. Available at www.consensus.nih.gov/ta/018/018-statement.htm.
4. National Institute of Dental and Craniofacial Research, National Institutes of Health. TMD: temporomandibular disorders. Available at www.nider.nih.gov.
5. American Society of Temporomandibular Joint Surgeons. Guidelines for diagnosis and management of disorders involving the temporomandibular joint and related musculoskeletal structures. Available at www.astmjs.org/guidelines.html.
6. Drangsholt MT. Risk factors for diagnostic subgroups of painful temporomandibular disorders (TMD). J Dent Res 2002;81:284-288.
7. Laskin D, Greenfield W, Gale F, eds. The president's conference on the examination, diagnosis and management of temporomandibular joint disorders. Am Dent Assoc 1983;106:75-79.
8. Harris M, Feinmann C, Wise M, Treasure F. Temporomandibular joint and orofacial pain: clinical and medicolegal management problem. Br Dent J 1993;174:129-136.
9. Norman JDP, Bramley P, eds. A textbook and colour atlas of the temporomandibular joint. London: Wolfe, 1990.
10. Evidence-based dentistry. 2004;5:65-66. Available at www.nature.com/ebd
11. Hunter S. The management of "psychogenic" orofacial pain. BMJ 1992;304:329.
12. Foster ME, Gray RJM, Davies SJ, Macfarlane TV. Therapeutic manipulation of the temporomandibular joint. Br J Oral Maxillofac Surg 2000;38:641-644.
13. Miyamoto H, Sakashita H, Miyata M, Goss AM. Arthroscopic surgery of the temporomandibular joint: a comparison of two successful techniques. Br J Oral Maxillofac Surg 1999;37:397-400.
14. Baldwin AJ, Cooper JC. Eminectomy and plication of the posterior disc attachment following arthrotomy for temporomandibular joint internal derangement. J Craniomaxillofac Surg 2004;32:354-359.
15. Nyberg J, Adell R, Svensson B. Temporomandibular joint disectomy for the treatment of unilateral internal derangement—a 5-year follow-up evaluation. Int J Oral Maxillofacial Surg 2004;33:8-12.

Fibromyalgia and related syndromes

Daniel J. Clauw

77

- Fibromyalgia is one of many "central pain syndromes" that occur commonly in the population.
- Fibromyalgia is strongly familial, and specific genes that might confer an increased risk of developing disease have been identified.
- Susceptible individuals seem to be more likely to develop fibromyalgia following exposure to one or more biologic stressors.
- The hallmark mechanism is augmented central pain processing with an increased "gain" or "volume control" in sensory processing systems.
- Pain and other symptoms of fibromyalgia are not primarily occurring because of damage or inflammation in peripheral tissues.
- The most effective drugs for this condition are neuroactive compounds that downregulate sensory processing.
- Tricyclic drugs, mixed reuptake inhibitors, and anti-epileptics have the best established efficacy.
- Non-pharmacologic therapies such as exercise and cognitive behavioral therapy are extremely beneficial in fibromyalgia.

INTRODUCTION

Clinical practitioners commonly see patients with pain and other somatic symptoms that they cannot adequately explain on the basis of the degree of damage or inflammation noted in peripheral tissues. In fact, this may be among the most common predicaments for which individuals seek medical attention.[1] Fibromyalgia (FM) is merely the current term for individuals with chronic widespread musculoskeletal pain, for which no alternative cause can be identified.

Until recently, unexplained pain syndromes perplexed researchers, clinicians, and patients. However, the following facts are now clear:

- Individuals will sometimes only have one of these "idiopathic" pain syndromes over the course of their lifetime. But more often, individuals with one of these entities, as well as their family members, are likely to have several of these conditions.[2-4] This is not surprising because recent studies have shown that a variety of chronic pain conditions are familial, and specific genetic polymorphisms that increase or decrease pain processing are rapidly being identified.[5-7] Many terms have been used to describe these co-aggregating syndromes and symptoms, including functional somatic syndromes, somatization disorders, allied spectrum conditions, chronic multi-symptom illnesses, and medically unexplained symptoms.[3,8-10]
- Some of these individuals have co-morbid psychiatric conditions, but at any given time, most do not. A number of different types of studies, including recent elegant twin studies, make it clear that these pain syndromes are clearly different and separable from depression and anxiety, and have strong genetic underpinnings (Figs. 77.1 and 77.2).[11-13]
- Women are more likely to have these disorders than men, but the sex difference is much more apparent in clinical samples (especially tertiary care) than in population-based samples.[14,15]
- A hallmark of these conditions (e.g., FM, irritable bowel syndrome [IBS], headache, temporomandibular disorder [TMD]) is that individuals display diffuse hyperalgesia (increased pain to normally painful stimuli) and/or allodynia (pain to normally non-painful

stimuli).[16-20] This suggests that these individuals have a fundamental problem with pain or sensory processing rather than an abnormality confined to the region of the body where the person is currently experiencing pain. These findings can be corroborated by the presence of these same phenomena on functional neuroimaging studies and appear to be in part due to imbalances in neurotransmitters that affect pain and sensory transmission.

- Similar types of therapies are efficacious for all of these conditions, including both pharmacologic (e.g., drugs that raise anti-nociceptive neurotransmitters such as serotonin and norepinephrine, lower pro-nociceptive neurotransmitters such as glutamate and substance P) and non-pharmacologic treatments (e.g., exercise, cognitive behavioral therapy). Conversely, individuals with these conditions typically do not respond to therapies that are effective when pain is due to damage or inflammation of tissues (e.g., non-steroidal anti-inflammatory drugs [NSAIDs], opioids, injections, surgical procedures).
- A significant unmet medical need is not being addressed because these individuals display high levels of disability, as well as direct and indirect medical costs as they go untreated or poorly treated, and traverse health systems seeking care. Current studies suggest that diagnosing and labeling individuals with one of these syndromes actually reduces health care utilization, largely because they get fewer medical tests and subspecialty visits in subsequent years.[21]
- The review regarding FM below focuses on our current understanding of this disorder as one of the prototypical "central pain syndromes."

HISTORIC PERSPECTIVE

Although the term *fibromyalgia* is relatively new, this condition has been described in the medical literature for centuries. Sir William Gowers coined the term *fibrositis* in 1904. During the next half century, fibrositis was considered by some to be a common cause of muscular pain, by others to be a manifestation of "tension" or "psychogenic rheumatism," and by the rheumatology community in general to be a non-entity.

The current concept of FM was established by Smythe and Moldofsky[22] in the mid-1970s. The name change reflected the fact that there was increasing evidence that there was no *-itis* (inflammation) in the connective tissues of individuals with this condition, but instead *-algia* (pain). These authors characterized the most common tender points (regions of extreme tenderness in these individuals) and reported that patients with FM had disturbances in deep and restorative sleep and that selective stage 4 interruptions induced the symptoms of FM.[23] Yunus and colleagues[24] then reported on the major clinical manifestations of patients with FM seen in rheumatology clinics.

The next advance in FM was the development of the American College of Rheumatology (ACR) criteria for FM, which were published in 1990.[25] These classification criteria require that an individual have both a history of chronic widespread pain (CWP) and 11 or more of 18 possible tender points on examination. These ACR classification criteria were intended for research use to standardize definitions of FM. In this regard, the criteria have been extremely valuable. Unfortunately, many practitioners use these criteria in routine clinical practice to diagnose individual patients, and this unintended use has led to many of the current misconceptions regarding FM, which are discussed later.

The finding of diffusely increased tenderness, as well as a lack of finding "-itis" in the muscles or other tissues of FM patients, caused the name of this entity to be changed from fibrositis to FM. The diffuse

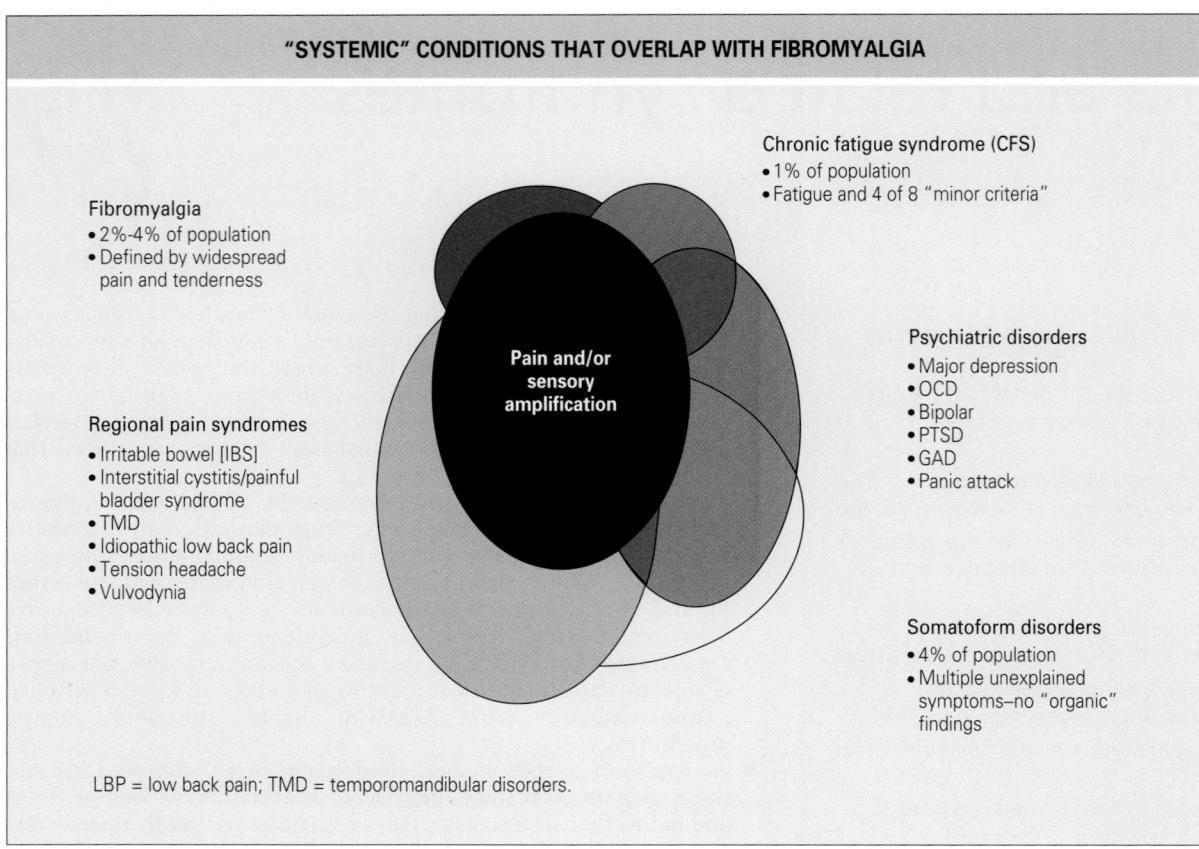

"SYSTEMIC" CONDITIONS THAT OVERLAP WITH FIBROMYALGIA

Fibromyalgia
• 2%-4% of population
• Defined by widespread pain and tenderness

Regional pain syndromes
• Irritable bowel [IBS]
• Interstitial cystitis/painful bladder syndrome
• TMD
• Idiopathic low back pain
• Tension headache
• Vulvodynia

Pain and/or sensory amplification

Chronic fatigue syndrome (CFS)
• 1% of population
• Fatigue and 4 of 8 "minor criteria"

Psychiatric disorders
• Major depression
• OCD
• Bipolar
• PTSD
• GAD
• Panic attack

Somatoform disorders
• 4% of population
• Multiple unexplained symptoms–no "organic" findings

LBP = low back pain; TMD = temporomandibular disorders.

Fig. 77.1 The "systemic" conditions that overlap with fibromyalgia.

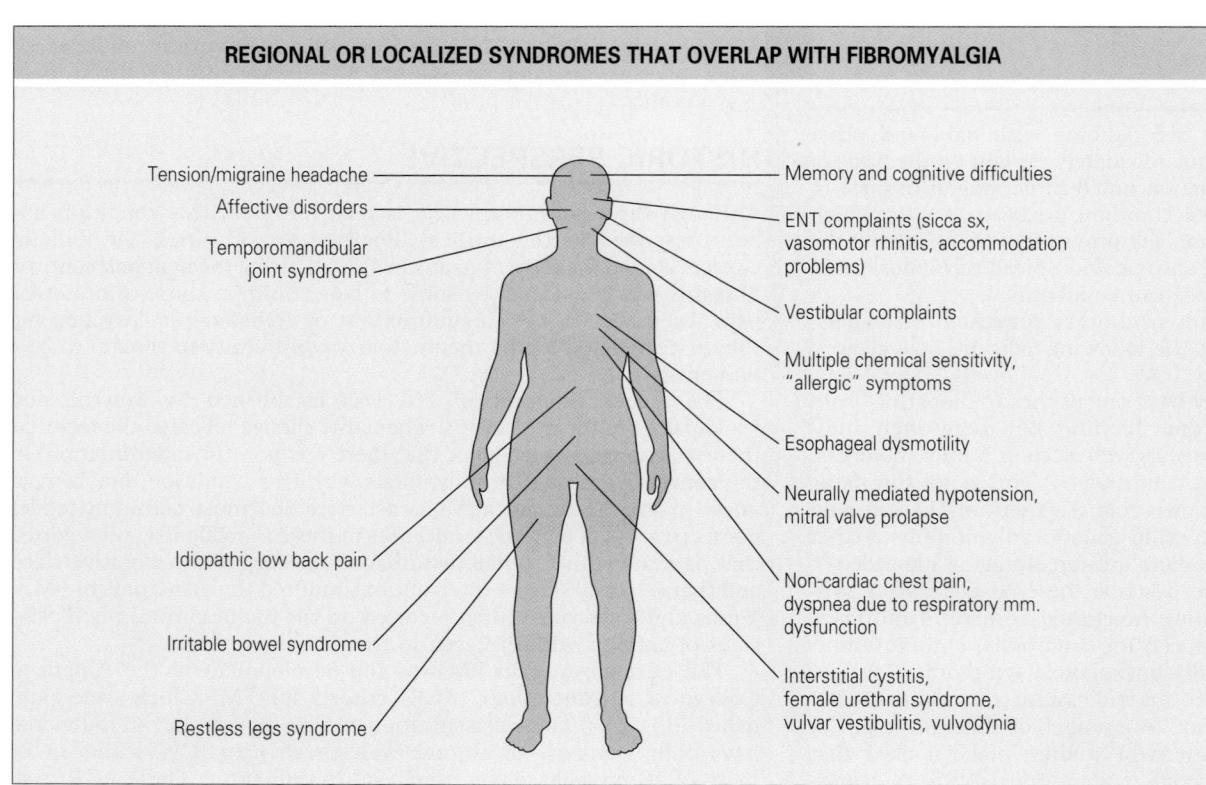

REGIONAL OR LOCALIZED SYNDROMES THAT OVERLAP WITH FIBROMYALGIA

Tension/migraine headache

Affective disorders

Temporomandibular joint syndrome

Idiopathic low back pain

Irritable bowel syndrome

Restless legs syndrome

Memory and cognitive difficulties

ENT complaints (sicca sx, vasomotor rhinitis, accommodation problems)

Vestibular complaints

Multiple chemical sensitivity, "allergic" symptoms

Esophageal dysmotility

Neurally mediated hypotension, mitral valve prolapse

Non-cardiac chest pain, dyspnea due to respiratory mm. dysfunction

Interstitial cystitis, female urethral syndrome, vulvar vestibulitis, vulvodynia

Fig. 77.2 Regional or localized syndromes that overlap with fibromyalgia in prevalence, mechanisms, and treatment.

nature of the pain and tenderness also led many groups of investigators to explore neural mechanisms to explain the underlying pathogenesis of these disorders.[26,27] In fact, major advances have only occurred in understanding individual syndromes within this spectrum once investigators concluded that this was not a condition caused by peripheral damage or inflammation and began to explore central, neural mecha-

nisms of these diseases. Thus the conditions we now understand best within this spectrum include FM, IBS (previously termed *spastic colitis* until the recognition that there was little "-itis" and that motility changes were not the major pathologic feature), and temporomandibular disorder (previously termed *temporomandibular joint disorder* until it was recognized the problem was not largely within the joint).

EPIDEMIOLOGY

Chronic widespread pain

Epidemiologic studies of the historical component of the ACR criteria for FM, chronic widespread pain (CWP), have been extremely instructive. CWP is typically operationalized as pain above and below the waist, involving the left and right sides of the body, and also involving the axial skeleton. Population-based studies of CWP suggest that 5% to 15% of the population has this symptom at any given point in time.[28-30] Chronic regional pain is found in 20% to 25% of the population. Both chronic widespread and regional pain occur about 1.5 times as commonly in women than men.

Fibromyalgia

The ACR criteria for FM require that an individual has both a history of CWP and the finding of 11 or more of 18 possible tender points on examination. Tender points represent nine paired predefined regions of the body, often over musculotendinous insertions.[25] If an individual reports pain when a region is palpated with 4 kg of pressure, this is considered a positive tender point. Between 25% and 50% of individuals who have CWP will also have 11 or more tender points and thus meet criteria for FM.[30,31] The prevalence of FM is just as high in rural or non-industrialized societies as it is in countries such as the United States.[32,33]

Significance of tender points

When the ACR criteria were published, it was thought that there may be some unique significance to the locations of tender points. In fact, the term *control points* was coined to describe areas of the body that should not be tender in FM, and individuals were assumed to have a psychological cause for their pain if they were tender in these regions. Since then, we have learned that the tenderness in FM extends throughout the entire body. Thus relative to the pain threshold that a normal non-FM patient would experience at the same points, "control" regions of the body such as the thumbnail and forehead are just as tender as in FM tender points.[34-36] Thus to assess tenderness in clinical practice, the practitioner can apply pressure wherever he or she wishes, and as long as the examination is performed with the same pressure in a series of patients, the practitioner can get a good sense of the overall pain threshold of any individual patient.

The tender point requirement in the ACR criteria not only misrepresents the nature of the tenderness in this condition (i.e., local rather than widespread) but also strongly influences the demographic and psychological characteristics of FM. Women are only 1.5 times more likely than men to experience CWP but are 10 times more likely than men to have 11 or more tender points.[28] Because of this, women are approximately 10 times as likely to meet ACR criteria for FM than men. Yet most of the men in the population who have CWP but are not tender enough to meet criteria for FM likely have the same underlying problem as the women who meet the ACR criteria for FM.

Another unintended consequence of requiring both CWP and at least 11 tender points to be diagnosed with FM is that many individuals with FM have high levels of distress. Wolfe[37] has described tender points as a "sedimentation rate for distress" because of population-based studies showing that tender points are more common in distressed individuals. Distress is usually considered as a combination of somatic symptoms and symptoms of anxiety and/or depression.[37] Until recently, many assumed that because *tender points* were associated with distress, that *tenderness* (an individual's sensitivity to mechanical pressure) was associated with distress. However, recent evidence suggests that this latter association is probably due to the standard tender point technique, which consists of applying steadily increasing pressure until reaching 4 kg. In this situation, individuals who are anxious or "expectant" tend to "bail out" and report tenderness. Recently, more sophisticated measures of tenderness that give stimuli in a random, unpredictable fashion have been developed, and the results of these tests are independent of psychological status.[38,39] Because tender points are associated with high levels of distress, requiring 11 or greater tender points in order to diagnose someone with CWP with FM dramatically increases the likelihood that these individuals will be female and/or distressed, compared with individuals with CWP and fewer than 11 tender points.[30]

In fact, population-based studies suggest that the primary symptom of FM, CWP, is only modestly associated with distress, and distress is only weakly associated with the subsequent development of CWP.[40,41] Far more psychologically "normal" individuals develop CWP than distressed or depressed people, and most individuals with CWP do not have or subsequently develop distress or depression.

In summary, although many clinicians uniquely associate FM with women who display high levels of distress, much of this is an artifact of (1) the ACR criteria that require 11 tender points and (2) the fact that most studies of FM have originated from clinical samples from tertiary care centers, where health care–seeking behaviors lead to the fact that psychological and psychiatric co-morbidities are much higher.[15] When all these biases are eliminated by examining CWP in population-based studies, a clearer picture of FM can be gleamed and chronic widespread pain becomes much like chronic musculoskeletal pain in any other region of the body.

ETIOLOGY

Genetic factors

Research has indicated a strong familial component to the development of FM. First-degree relatives of individuals with FM display an eightfold greater risk of developing FM than those in the general population.[4] These studies also show that family members of individuals with FM are much more tender than the family members of controls, regardless of whether they have pain or not. Family members of FM patients are also much more likely to have IBS, TMD, headaches, and a host of other regional pain syndromes.[3,42,43] This familial and personal co-aggregation of conditions that includes FM was originally collectively termed *affective spectrum disorder*,[44] and more recently *central sensitivity syndromes* and chronic multisymptom illnesses.[10,45] In population-based studies, the key symptoms that often co-aggregate besides pain are fatigue, memory difficulties, and mood disturbances.[10,46]

Recent twin studies have been particularly helpful in establishing that these somatic syndromes strongly co-aggregate with each other and are strongly genetic, and they are clearly separable from anxiety and depression.[11,12,47] These studies also suggest that approximately half of the risk of developing these conditions is due to genetic factors, and half environmental.[11]

Recent studies have begun to identify specific genetic polymorphisms that are associated with a higher risk of developing FM. To date, the serotonin 5-HT2A receptor polymorphism T/T phenotype, serotonin transporter, dopamine 4 receptor, and COMT (catecholamine *O*-methyl transferase) polymorphisms have all been seen in higher frequency in FM.[48-51] Of note, all of the polymorphisms identified to date involve the metabolism or transport of monoamines, compounds that play a critical role in activity of the human stress response. It is likely that there are scores of genetic polymorphisms, involving other neuromodulators and monoamines, which in part determine an individual's "set point" for pain and sensory processing.

Environmental factors

As with most illnesses that may have a genetic underpinning, environmental factors may play a prominent role in triggering the development of FM and related conditions. Environmental "stressors" temporally associated with the development of either FM or chronic fatigue syndrome include physical trauma (especially involving the trunk), certain infections such as hepatitis C, Epstein-Barr virus, parvovirus, Lyme disease, and emotional stress (Box 77.1). The disorder is also associated with other regional pain conditions or autoimmune disorders.[27,52,53] Of note, each of these stressors only leads to CWP or FM in approximately 5% to 10% of individuals who are exposed; the overwhelming majority of individuals who experience these same infections or other stressful events regain their baseline state of health.

- Peripheral pain syndromes
- Infections (e.g., parvovirus, Epstein-Barr virus, Lyme disease, Q fever; not common upper respiratory infections)
- Physical trauma (automobile accidents)
- Psychological stress/distress
- Hormonal alterations (e.g., hypothyroidism)
- Drugs
- Vaccines
- Certain catastrophic events (war, but not natural disasters)

PATHOGENESIS

Role of stressors

Once FM develops, the mechanisms responsible for ongoing symptom expression are likely complex and multifactorial. Because disparate "stressors" can trigger the development of these conditions, the human stress response has been closely examined for a causative role. These systems are mediated primarily by the activity of the corticotropin-releasing hormone (CRH) nervous system located in the hypothalamus and locus-ceruleus-norepinephrine/autonomic (sympathetic/LC-NE) nervous system in the brain stem. Recent research suggests that although this system in humans has been highly adaptive throughout history, the stress response may be inappropriately triggered by a wide assortment of everyday occurrences that do not pose a real threat to survival, thus initiating the cascade of physiologic responses more frequently than can be tolerated.[54]

The type of stress and the environment in which it occurs also affect how the stress response is expressed. Victims of accidents experience a higher frequency of FM and myofascial pain than those who cause them, which is congruent with animal studies showing that the strongest physiologic responses are triggered by events that are accompanied by a lack of control or support and thus perceived as inescapable or unavoidable.[55] In humans, daily "hassles" and personally relevant stressors seem to be more capable of causing symptoms than major catastrophic events that do not personally affect the individual.[56]

Two studies performed in the United States just before and after the terrorist attacks of 9/11 point out that not all psychological stress is capable of triggering or exacerbating FM or somatic symptoms. In one study performed by Raphael and colleagues,[57] no difference in pain complaints or other somatic symptoms was seen in residents of New York and New Jersey who had been surveyed before and then just following the terrorist attacks on the World Trade Center. In another study performed in the Washington, D.C. region (near the Pentagon—the other site of attack) during the same time period, patients with FM had no worsening of pain or other somatic symptoms following the attacks, compared with just before the attack.[58]

Recent reviews regarding the role that "stressors" (e.g., infections, physical trauma, emotional stress) or catastrophic events may have in triggering the development of FM or related conditions have identified a number of factors that may be much more important than the intensity of the "stressor" in predicting adverse health outcomes. Female gender, worry or expectation of chronicity, lack of control of the stressor, intensity of the initial symptoms, and inactivity or time off work following the stressor make it more likely to trigger the development of pain or other somatic symptoms.[53] Naturally occurring catastrophic events such as earthquakes, floods, or fires are much less likely to lead to chronic somatic symptoms than similarly stressful events that are "man made" such as chemical spills or war.[59] Being exposed to a multitude of stressors simultaneously, or over a period of time, may also be a significant risk for later somatic symptoms and or psychological sequelae. Intensely stressful events can lead to permanent changes in the activity of both mouse and human stress response systems.[54,60]

To complete this vicious circle, these changes in baseline function of the stress response (i.e., of the autonomic and neuroendocrine systems, discussed later) that may occur following a stressor earlier in life have been shown to predict which symptom-free individuals without chronic pain or other somatic symptoms are more likely to develop these somatic symptoms. This has been noted both in population-based studies and in experiments where healthy young adults are deprived of regular sleep or exercise.[61,62]

This theoretical link between stress, changes in stress axis activity, and subsequent susceptibility to develop somatic symptoms or syndromes is also supported by studies showing that patients with FM and related conditions may be more likely than non-affected individuals to have experienced physical or sexual abuse in childhood.[63-66] Twin studies have recently supported a link between post-traumatic stress disorder (PTSD)/trauma and CWP.[67] Just as a lack of or cessation of exercise following trauma seems to be associated with a higher likelihood of developing pain or other somatic symptoms, a recent study of Israeli war veterans with PTSD showed that those who exercised regularly were much less likely to develop CWP or FM.[68]

Role of neuroendocrine abnormalities

Because of this link between exposure to "stressors" and the subsequent development of FM, the human stress systems have been extensively studied in this condition. These studies have generally shown alterations of the hypothalamic-pituitary-adrenal (HPA) axis and the sympathetic nervous system in FM and related conditions.[69-72] Although these studies often note either hypoactivity or hyperactivity of both the HPA axis and sympathetic nervous system in individuals with FM and related conditions, the precise abnormality varies from study to study. Moreover, these studies only find "abnormal" HPA or autonomic function in a small percentage of patients, and there is tremendous overlap between patients and controls in any of these studies.

The inconsistency of these findings should not be surprising because nearly all of these studies were cross-sectional studies assuming that if HPA or autonomic dysfunction or both were found in FM, they must have *caused* the pain and other symptoms. Data now suggest the opposite. As noted earlier, better data suggest that especially HPA abnormalities might represent a diathesis or be *due to* the pain or early life stress, rather than causing it. In fact, in two recent studies examining HPA function in FM, McLean showed that salivary cortisol levels co-varied with pain levels and that cerebrospinal fluid (CSF) levels of CRH were more closely related to an individual's pain level or a history of early life trauma than whether they were a FM patient or control.[73,74] Because most previous studies of HPA and autonomic function in FM failed to control for pain levels, a previous history of trauma, and PTSD or other co-morbid disorders that could affect HPA or autonomic dysfunction, it is not surprising for these inconsistencies.

Heart rate variability at baseline and in response to tilt table testing has been evaluated in patients with FM as a surrogate measure of autonomic function. The consistent and reproducible finding of lower baseline heart rate variability in FM compared with controls (in three cross-sectional studies by two different groups) makes it a more useful measure than tilt table testing.[72,75,76] An abnormal drop in blood pressure or excessive rate of syncope during tilt table testing has been noted in two of three cross-sectional studies completed by three different groups.[77,78] One study noted no difference between normals and controls using univariate analysis.[79] Moreover, recent findings also suggest that aberrations in heart rate variability may predispose to FM symptoms,[61,62,80] possibly identifying patients at risk. Also, a recent study showed that heart rate variability was normalized following exercise therapy, suggesting that this finding might also be an epiphenomenon due in part to deconditioning.[81,82]

These neurobiologic alterations are likely shared with other syndromes known to be associated with HPA and/or autonomic function such as depression or PTSD. In fact, some researchers who have superficially reviewed the neurobiologic data regarding FM have erroneously concluded that this condition shares many biologic underpinnings with depression.[83] A model of susceptibility and development of these disorders that takes into account both genetics and personality as risk factors is illustrated in Figure 77.3. This recognizes the critical importance of stressors in "re-setting stress response systems," as well as other factors including (i) the role of behavioral adaptations to these stressors such as cessation of routine exercise and (ii) whether an individual is in an environment characterized by control or support.

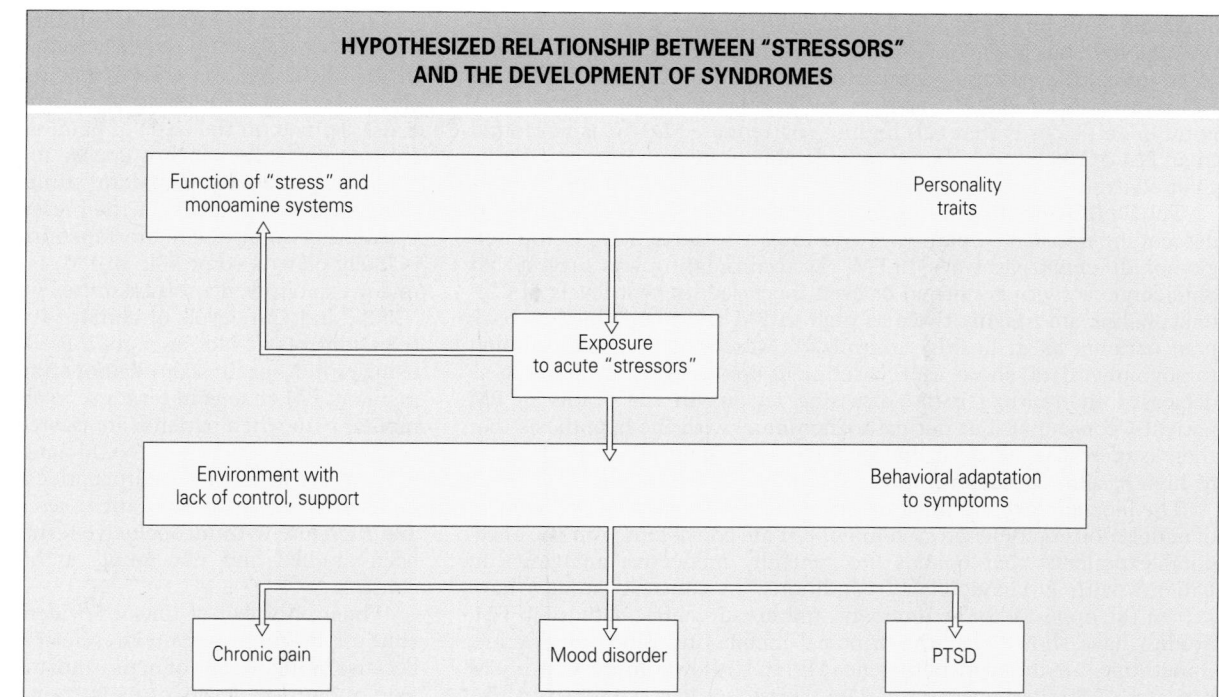

HYPOTHESIZED RELATIONSHIP BETWEEN "STRESSORS" AND THE DEVELOPMENT OF SYNDROMES

Fig. 77.3 The hypothesized relationship between "stressors" and the development of syndromes such as fibromyalgia, posttraumatic stress disorder, and depression.

Augmented pain and sensory processing as a hallmark of fibromyalgia and related syndromes

Once FM is established, by far the most consistently detected objective abnormalities involve pain and sensory processing systems. Because FM is defined in part by tenderness, considerable work has been performed exploring the potential reason for this phenomenon. The results of 2 decades of psychophysical pressure pain testing in FM have been instructive.[84]

One of the earliest findings in this regard was that the tenderness in FM is not confined to tender points but instead extends throughout the entire body.[28,35] Theoretically, such diffuse tenderness could be due to either primarily psychological (e.g., hypervigilance, where individuals are too attentive to their surroundings) or neurobiologic (e.g., the plethora of factors that can lead to temporary or permanent amplification of sensory input) factors.

Early studies typically used dolorimetry to assess pressure pain threshold and concluded that tenderness was in large part related to psychological factors because these measures of pain threshold were correlated with levels of distress.[28,37,85] Also, nuances such as the rate of increase of stimulus pressure, control by the operator versus by the patient, and patient distress have been shown to influence pain threshold when it is measured in this manner.[86,87]

To minimize the biases associated with "ascending" (i.e., the individual knows that the pressure will be predictably increased) measures of pressure pain threshold, a series of studies were performed that presented stimuli in a random rather than predictable manner. Studies showed that (1) the random measures of pressure pain threshold were not influenced by levels of distress of the individual, whereas tender point count and dolorimetry examinations were, (2) FM patients were much more sensitive to pressure even when these more sophisticated paradigms were used, (3) FM patients were not any more "expectant" or "hypervigilant" than controls, and (4) pressure pain thresholds at any four points in the body are highly correlated with the average tenderness at all 18 tender points and 4 "control points" (the thumbnail and forehead).[34,39,88,89]

Because of this close link between tenderness and FM, the phenomenon has also been well studied as a potential relevant outcome in clinical trials of new FM therapies. In a number of longitudinal, randomized, placebo-controlled trials in FM, improvements in clinical pain have corresponded with a significant change in tender point counts or tender point index.[90] In contrast, other studies did not show a correspondence between improvements in clinical pain and tender point counts.[91-96] These discrepancies between previous studies could

be because these therapies did not improve tenderness or because tender points are not a good measure of tenderness. Two recent studies suggest the latter because when individuals with FM were simultaneously assessed using tender point counts, dolorimetry, and random pressure paradigms, the random pressure paradigms showed the most responsiveness to change.[97,98]

Heat, cold, and electrical stimuli

In addition to the heightened sensitivity to pressure noted in FM, other types of stimuli applied to the skin are also judged as more painful or noxious by these patients. FM patients also display a decreased threshold to heat,[88,99-101] cold,[100,102] and electrical stimuli.[103] Similar but somewhat attenuated decreases in pain threshold have also been noted in individuals with CWP without 11 or more tender points.[104]

Responses to other sensory stimuli

FM patients also display a low noxious threshold to auditory tones, and this finding has been replicated.[105,106] However, both of these studies used ascending measures of auditory threshold, so these findings could theoretically be due to expectancy or hypervigilance. A recent study used an identical random staircase paradigm to test FM patients' threshold to the loudness of auditory tones and to pressure.[98] This study found that FM patients displayed low thresholds to both types of stimuli. The correlation between the results of auditory and pressure pain threshold testing suggested that some of these low sensory thresholds were due to shared variance, whereas others were unique to one stimulus or the other. The notion that FM and related syndromes might represent biologic amplification of all sensory stimuli has significant support from functional imaging studies that suggest that the insula is the most consistently hyperactive region (see later). This region has been noted to play a critical role in sensory integration, with the posterior insula serving a purer sensory role and the anterior insula being associated with the emotional processing of sensations.[107,108]

Specific mechanisms that may lead to a low pain threshold in fibromyalgia

Two different specific pathogenic mechanisms in FM have been identified using experimental pain testing: (1) an absence of descending analgesic activity and (2) increased wind-up or temporal summation.

Attenuated diffuse noxious inhibitory controls in fibromyalgia

In healthy humans and laboratory animals, application of an intense painful stimulus for 2 to 5 minutes produces generalized whole-body analgesia. This analgesic effect, termed *diffuse noxious inhibitory controls* (DNIC), has been consistently observed to be attenuated or absent in groups of FM patients, compared with healthy controls.[100,109-111] In IBS there is a similar decrease in descending analgesic activity.[112] A point of emphasis is that this finding of attenuated DNIC is not found in all FM or IBS patients but is considerably more common in patients than controls.

The DNIC response in humans is believed to be partly mediated by descending opioidergic pathways and in part by descending serotonergic-noradrenergic pathways. In FM, the accumulating data suggest that opioidergic activity is normal or even increased, in that levels of CSF enkephalins are roughly twice as high in FM and idiopathic low back pain patients as in healthy controls.[113] Moreover, positron emission tomography data show that baseline μ-opioid receptor binding is decreased in multiple pain processing regions in the brains of FM patients, consistent (but not pathognomonic) with the hypothesis that there is increased release of endogenous μ-opioid ligands in FM leading to high baseline occupancy of the receptors.[114]

The biochemical and imaging findings suggesting increased activity of endogenous opioidergic systems in FM are consistent with the anecdotal experience that opioids are generally ineffective analgesics in patients with FM and related conditions. In contrast, studies have shown the opposite for serotonergic and noradrenergic activity in FM. Studies have shown that the principal metabolite of norepinephrine, 3-methoxy-4-hydroxyphenethylene (MPHG), is lower in the CSF of FM patients.[115] Similarly, there are data suggesting low serotonin in this syndrome. Patients with FM were shown to have reduced serum levels of serotonin and its precursor, L-tryptophan, as well as reduced levels of the principal serotonin metabolite, 5-HIAA, in their CSF.[115,116] Further evidence for this mechanism comes from treatment studies, where nearly any type of compound that simultaneously raises both serotonin and norepinephrine (tricyclics, duloxetine, milnacipran, tramadol) has been shown to be efficacious in treating FM and related conditions.[96,117-119]

Increased wind-up in fibromyalgia

Experimental pain testing studies have also suggested that some individuals with FM may have evidence of wind-up, indicative of evidence of central sensitization.[120,121] In animal models, this finding is associated with excitatory amino acid and substance P hyperactivity.[122,123] Just as with the findings regarding DNIC earlier, these results of psychophysical pain testing are congruent with both levels of neurotransmitters in the CSF, as well as clinical trials of drugs. Four independent studies have shown that patients with FM have approximately three-

fold higher concentrations of substance P in CSF, when compared with normal controls.[124-127] Other chronic pain syndromes such as osteoarthritis of the hip and chronic low back pain, are also associated with elevated substance P levels, although chronic fatigue syndrome (which is not defined on the basis of pain) is not. Interestingly, once elevated, substance P levels do not appear to change dramatically and do not rise in response to acute painful stimuli. Thus high substance P appears to be a biologic marker for the presence of chronic pain.

Another important neurotransmitter in pain processing, and one that is likely playing some role in FM, is glutamate. Glutamate (Glu) is a major excitatory neurotransmitter within the central nervous system (CNS), and CSF levels of glutamate are twice as high in FM patients than controls.[128] Not only are these levels elevated, but a recent study using proton spectroscopy demonstrated that the glutamate levels in the insula in FM change in response to changes in both clinical and experimental pain when patients are treated with acupuncture.[129]

Nerve growth factor (NGF) and calcitonin gene-related peptide (CGRP) are additional neuropeptides that have been evaluated in FM. NGF was shown to have increased levels in FM and not in FM/RA and therefore with inconclusive results.[130] CSF and serum CGRP have been studied and not found to be different in FM patients and controls.[131,132]

Thus a number of lines of evidence point to the fact that FM is a state of heightened pain or sensory processing, and it might occur because of high levels of neurotransmitters that increase pain transmission and/or low levels of neurotransmitters that decrease pain transmission (Fig. 77.4).

Abnormalities on functional neuroimaging

Functional neural imaging enables investigators to visualize how the brain processes the sensory experience of pain. The primary modes of functional imaging that have been used in FM include functional magnetic resonance imaging (fMRI), single photon emission computed tomography (SPECT), positron emission tomography (PET), and proton spectroscopy (H-MRS).

SPECT was the first functional neuroimaging technique to be used in FM. The first trial using SPECT imaging in FM patients,[133] in 10 FM patients and 7 age- and education-matched healthy controls, indicated that both the caudate and thalamus of FM patients had decreased blood flow. These were largely replicated in a second SPECT study.[134] In a third SPECT trial, using a more sensitive radioligand (99mTc-ECD) in FM patients and pain-free controls,[135,136] Guedj and colleagues[135,136] found hyperperfusion in FM patients within the

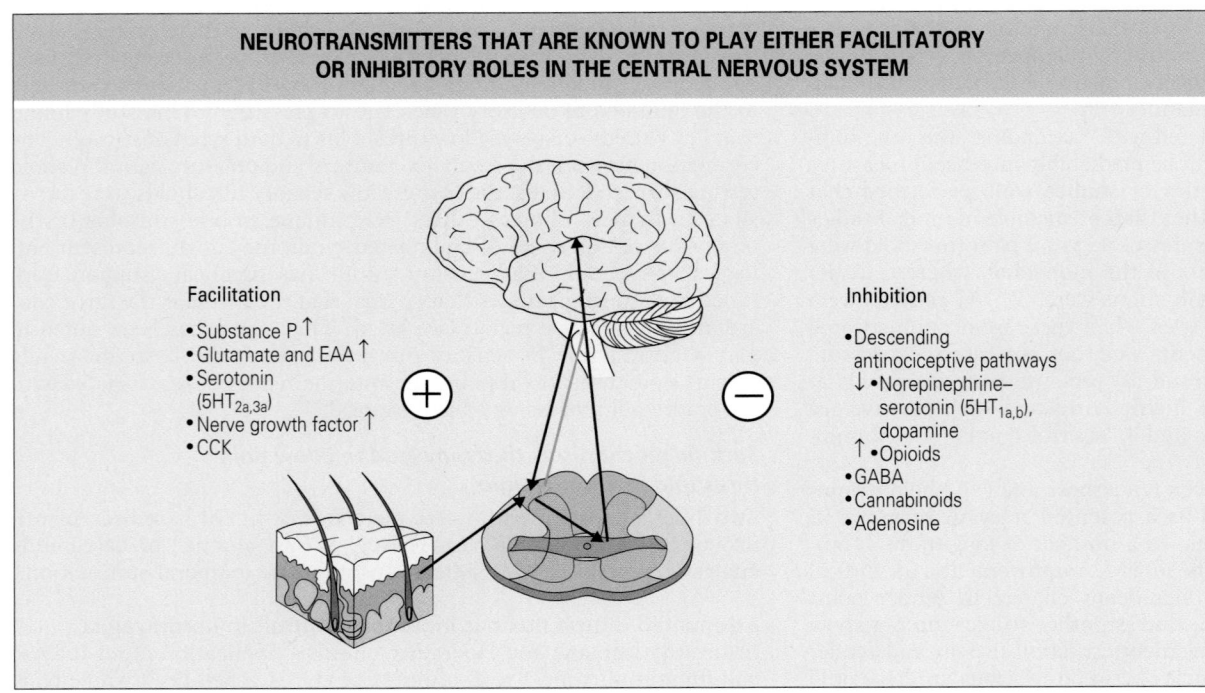

NEUROTRANSMITTERS THAT ARE KNOWN TO PLAY EITHER FACILITATORY OR INHIBITORY ROLES IN THE CENTRAL NERVOUS SYSTEM

Facilitation
- Substance P ↑
- Glutamate and EAA ↑
- Serotonin (5HT$_{2a,3a}$)
- Nerve growth factor ↑
- CCK

Inhibition
- Descending antinociceptive pathways ↓
  - Norepinephrine–serotonin (5HT$_{1a,b}$), dopamine ↑
  - Opioids
- GABA
- Cannabinoids
- Adenosine

Fig. 77.4 Neurotransmitters that are known to play either facilitatory (indicated in red, and generally increasing pain transmission in the spinal cord) or inhibitory (indicated in blue, and decreasing pain transmission) roles in the CNS. The arrows indicate the direction of the abnormality that has been identified in fibromyalgia (FM), (arrows are only present on neurotransmitter systems that have been studied in FM). The only neurotransmitter system that has been studied in FM that has not been found to be abnormal in a direction that would cause hyperalgesia/allodynia is the opioidergic system, which may explain why this class of drugs is not efficacious in FM.

somatosensory cortex and hypoperfusion in the anterior and posterior cingulate, the amygdala, medial frontal and parahippocampal gyrus, and the cerebellum. Finally, if these regional cerebral blood flow (rCBF) differences are relevant for FM pathology, one could hypothesize that changes in rCBF should track with changes in pain symptoms over time. One longitudinal treatment trial used SPECT imaging to assess changes in rCBF following administration of amitriptyline to 14 FM patients.[137] After 3 months of treatment with amitriptyline, increases in rCBF in the bilateral thalamus and the basal ganglia were observed. Because the same two regions had been implicated previously, these data suggest that amitriptyline may normalize the altered blood flow, thereby reducing pain symptoms.

Functional magnetic resonance imaging

fMRI is a non-invasive brain imaging technique that relies on changes in the relative concentration of oxygenated to deoxygenated hemoglobin within the brain. In response to neural activity, oxygenated blood flow is increased within the local brain area. This causes a decrease in the concentration of deoxygenated hemoglobin. Because deoxygenated hemoglobin is paramagnetic, this in turn causes a change in the magnetic property of the tissue. Unlike SPECT and PET, which can measure baseline levels of blood flow, the fMRI BOLD signal originates from a difference between experimental conditions and does not assess baseline blood flow. Typically in FM trials involving fMRI, evoked pain sensations are compared with "off" conditions that have either no pain or involve an innocuous sensation.

In one study 16 FM patients and 16 matched controls were exposed to painful pressures during the fMRI experiment.[138] The authors found increased neural activations (i.e., increases in the BOLD signal) in patients compared with pain-free controls when stimuli of equal pressure magnitude were administered. Regions of increased activity included the primary and secondary somatosensory cortex, the insula, and the anterior cingulate, all regions commonly observed in fMRI studies of healthy normal subjects during painful stimuli (Fig. 77.5). Interestingly, when the pain-free controls were subjected to pressures that evoked equivalent pain ratings in the FM patients, similar activation patterns were observed. These findings were entirely consistent with the "left-shift" in stimulus-response function noted with experimental pain testing and suggest that FM patients experience an increased gain or "volume setting" in brain sensory processing systems. In a similar experiment, with painful heat stimuli during fMRI, a

significant increase in the pain ratings of patients and augmented pain processing within the contralateral insula was seen.

fMRI has also proved useful in determining how co-morbid psychological factors influence pain processing in FM. The anterior insula and amygdala activations correlated with depressive symptoms, consistent with these regions being involved with affective or motivational aspects of pain processing in 30 patients with FM.[140] However, the degree of neuronal activation in areas of the brain thought to be associated with the "sensory" processing of pain (i.e., where the pain is localized and how intense it is) were not associated with levels of depressive symptoms or the presence or absence of major depression. These data are consistent with a plethora of evidence in the pain field that different regions of the brain are responsible for pain processing devoted to sensory intensity versus affective aspects of pain sensation, and they suggest that the former and latter are largely independent of each other. In contrast, this same group showed that the presence of catastrophizing, a patient's negative or pessimistic appraisal of their pain, influences both the sensory and affective dimensions of pain on fMRI in FM.[141]

PET has been used in several studies in FM. In the one study, there were no differences in regional cerebral blood flow between FM patients and controls.[142] However, another study showed that attenuated dopaminergic activity may be playing a role in pain transmission in FM.

Other serologic and biochemical abnormalities
Autoantibodies

The search for representative autoantibodies was a predictable step for a disease like FM, often evaluated by rheumatologists and co-existing with autoimmune diseases. Antiserotonin antibody, antiganglioside antibody, and antiphospholipid antibody have been shown to be different in patients and controls, but the applicability of these findings is not yet clear.[143] Antinuclear antibodies (ANA), antithyroid antibodies, antisilicone antibodies, and antiglutamic acid decarboxylase are not informative in FM.

This inconsistent increase in antibodies to a number of antigens may be a non-specific finding that arises from a subtle shift in immune function in this spectrum of illness. In the closely related chronic fatigue syndrome and Gulf War illnesses, investigators have noted a shift from a TH1 to TH2 immune response, which would be expected to lead to increased production of non-specific antibodies. Thus any antibody or autoantibody proposed as either a diagnostic test or bio-

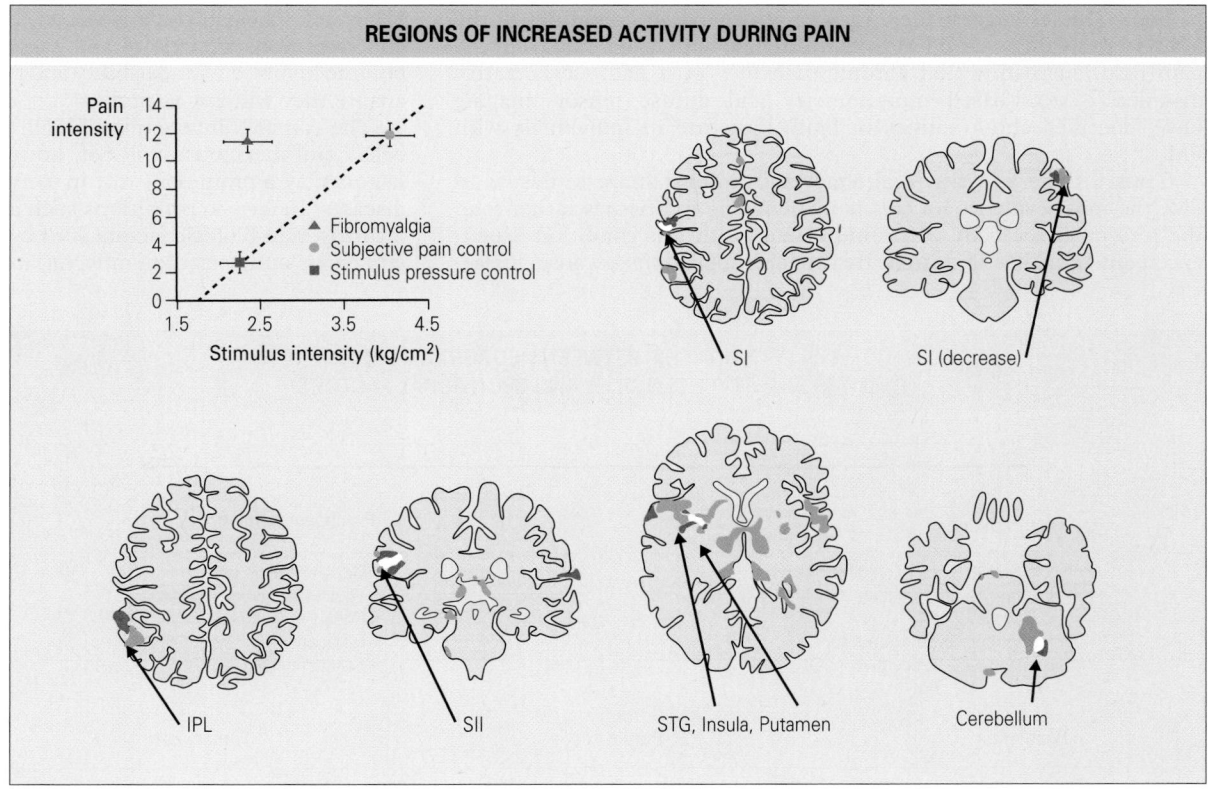

Fig. 77.5 In top left panel, individuals with fibromyalgia (red) given a low-pressure stimulus have similar levels of pain, and of neuronal activation in areas of the brain known to be involved in pain processing (ends of arrows) as controls given nearly twice as much pressure. Controls given the same low pressure that causes pain in fibromyalgia rate their pain as 2/20 instead of 12/20 and have no neuronal activation in pain processing regions with this amount of pressure.

marker of FM must be carefully tested using stringent controls to ensure its authenticity.

Other biochemical and cytokine abnormalities

Although all these conditions were originally believed to be autoimmune or inflammatory diseases and then later believed not to be, recent findings are leading to a re-consideration of whether subtle inflammatory changes may be responsible for some of the symptoms seen. Immunologic cascades have a role in the maintenance of central sensitivity and chronic pain, which is enhanced through release of proinflammatory cytokines by CNS glial cells; thus, the traditional paradigm regarding inflammatory versus non-inflammatory pain may gradually become less dichotomic. As may be expected in any complex biologic system, a delicate apparatus of checks and balances is at work in the spinal transmission of pain. Multiple inhibitory transmitters act at the spinal level to reduce the "volume" of pain transmission. Serotonin, norepinephrine, enkephalins, dopamine, and gamma-aminobutyric acid (GABA)[144] are among the better known players in this balance.

The amino acid tryptophan and the cytokine interleukin (IL)-8 have both been shown to be different in patients compared with controls in several studies, but none have been evaluated in longitudinal studies.[145,146] IL-8 has been consistently demonstrated in three studies by two different groups. Moreover, IL-8 has been shown to correlate with symptoms and not to be associated with depressed FM. IL-8 levels are closely tied to autonomic function, and the findings of these increased levels could be due to the dysautonomia seen in FM and related conditions. Serum IL-6 was evaluated and found to be normal in FM.

Low tryptophan, a precursor for serotonin, has been found in two of three studies.[116,147,148]

Structural abnormalities in fibromyalgia

Although a few studies have found mild abnormalities in the *skeletal muscles* of FM patients (these findings have been inconsistent and may be due to deconditioning rather than the illness itself),[149-152] a few studies suggest there may be subsets of FM patients with damage to *neural* structures. [31]P spectroscopy has been used to examine muscle metabolism in FM and the results are conflicting, with one study comparing sedentary controls with FM patients finding no differences, and the other finding lower adenosine triphosphate levels among FM patients.[152,153] Studies suggest that the tenderness in FM is not confined to just the muscle, so in aggregate most investigators have concluded that primary muscle disease is not a likely cause of the pain associated with FM.

Some studies suggest there may be structural abnormalities of the brain in individuals with FM that are aligned with other studies in the pain field, suggesting that chronic pain may be a neurodegenerative disorder.[154] Voxel-based morphometry and diffuse tensor imaging have identified abnormalities in brain structure in individuals with FM.[155-159]

Thus if there are structural abnormalities or damage to tissues in FM, the most evidence for this is involving neural tissues rather than the regions of the body where individuals with this condition experience pain. This has important treatment implications because analgesic drugs that primarily act peripherally to reduce pain (e.g., NSAIDs) are not effective in these central or neuropathic pain states.

Sleep and activity in fibromyalgia

In addition to pain, other symptoms commonly seen in FM include disturbed sleep and poor physical function. One of the first biologic findings in FM was that selective sleep deprivation led to symptoms of FM in healthy individuals, and these findings have subsequently been replicated by several groups.[23,160] However, the electroencephalographic abnormalities that were noted in this first study and initially thought to be a marker for FM, so-called *alpha intrusions*, have subsequently been found in normals and in individuals with other conditions.[161,162]

More recent findings on polysomnography that occur more commonly in FM include demonstration of fewer sleep spindles, an increase in cyclic alternating pattern rate, upper airway resistance syndrome, and/or poor sleep efficiency.[163,164] However, sleep abnormalities are rarely shown to correlate with symptoms in FM, and many investigators anecdotally believe that even identifying and treating specific sleep disorders often seen in FM patients (e.g., obstructive sleep apnea, upper airway resistance, restless legs or periodic limb movement syndromes) do not necessarily lead to improvements in the core symptoms of FM.

Behavioral and psychological factors

In addition to neurobiologic mechanisms, behavioral and psychological factors also play a role in symptom expression in many FM patients. The rate of current psychiatric co-morbidity in patients with FM may be as high as 30% to 60% in tertiary care settings, and the rate of lifetime psychiatric disorders even higher.[3,165,166] Depression and anxiety disorders are the most commonly seen. However, these rates may be artifactually elevated by virtue of the fact that most of these studies have been performed in tertiary care centers. Individuals who meet ACR criteria for FM who are identified in the general population do not have nearly this high a rate of identifiable psychiatric conditions (Fig. 77.6).[15,167]

As already noted, population-based studies have demonstrated that the relationship between pain and distress is complex and that distress is both a cause and consequence of pain. In this latter instance, a typical pattern is that as a result of pain and other symptoms of FM, individuals begin to function less well in their various roles. They may have difficulties with spouses, children, and work inside or outside the home, which exacerbate symptoms and lead to maladaptive illness behaviors. These include isolation, cessation of pleasurable activities, and reductions in activity and exercise. In the worst cases, patients become involved with disability and compensation systems that almost ensure they will not improve.[168]

The complex interaction of biologic, behavioral, psychological, and behavioral mechanisms is not, however, unique to FM. Non-biologic factors play a prominent role in symptom expression in all rheumatic diseases. In fact, in conditions such as rheumatoid arthritis and osteoarthritis, non-biologic factors such as level of formal education, coping strategies, and socioeconomic variables account for more of the vari-

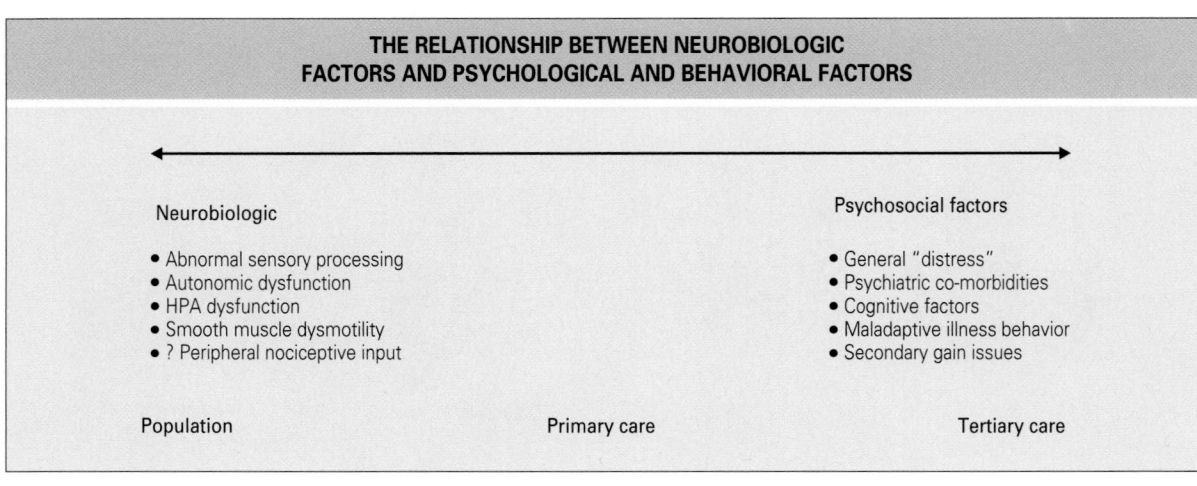

THE RELATIONSHIP BETWEEN NEUROBIOLOGIC FACTORS AND PSYCHOLOGICAL AND BEHAVIORAL FACTORS

Neurobiologic
- Abnormal sensory processing
- Autonomic dysfunction
- HPA dysfunction
- Smooth muscle dysmotility
- ? Peripheral nociceptive input

Psychosocial factors
- General "distress"
- Psychiatric co-morbidities
- Cognitive factors
- Maladaptive illness behavior
- Secondary gain issues

Population   Primary care   Tertiary care

Fig. 77.6 The relationship between neurobiologic factors that initiate or cause pain and other symptoms, and psychological and behavioral factors that either preexist or develop as a result of pain, and can perpetuate or worsen symptoms. These latter factors increase in frequency as one moves from examining pain patients in the population to those seen in tertiary care centers.

ance in pain report and disability than biologic factors, such as the joint space width or sedimentation rate.[169,170]

Because of the biopsychosocial nature of FM, several groups have attempted to identify subgroups of individuals with this condition that may present differently or respond differentially to treatment.[171,172] One of these studies examined how differential degrees of depression, maladaptive cognitions, and hyperalgesia might interact to lead to different subgroups of patients. Three identified subgroups can be usefully identified (Fig. 77.7). The first comprises approximately half of the patients who have low levels of depression and anxiety, have normal cognition regarding pain, and are mildly tender (although tender enough to meet the ACR criteria). The second subgroup, representative of a "tertiary care" FM patient, is slightly tenderer and also displays high levels of depression. These patients also have cognitions associated with a poor prognosis in many pain conditions. These include an external locus of pain control, defined as feeling that they can do nothing about their pain, and catastrophizing, defined as having a negative and pessimistic view of their pain. The third subgroup, perhaps the most interesting,

is the most tender but has no negative psychological or cognitive factors. This suggests that in some "resilient" individuals, positive psychological and cognitive factors may actually "buffer" neurobiologic factors leading to pain and other symptoms in FM. Similar results have been noted in several other studies of pressure pain in FM, as well as in another study using thermal pain.[139]

Functional imaging studies have been instructive with regard to how these co-morbid mood disorders or cognitions may be influencing pain processing in FM. fMRI undertaken on 30 FM patients with variable levels of depression, with additional experimental pain testing, investigated how the presence or absence of depression influenced pain report.[140] This study found that the level of depressive symptomatology did not influence the degree of neuronal activation in brain regions responsible for coding for the sensory intensity of pain, the primary and secondary somatosensory cortices. As expected, the depressed individuals did display greater activations in brain regions known to be responsible for the affective or cognitive processing of pain, such as the amygdala and insula. Another study with similar methodology examined how the presence or absence of catastrophizing might influence pain report in FM.[141] In contrast to the results mentioned earlier, the presence of catastrophizing was associated with increased neuronal activations in the sensory coding regions. These studies thus provide empirical evidence for the value of treatments such as cognitive behavioral therapy. This is especially the case if individuals exhibit cognitions such as catastrophizing, which, independent of other factors, may be capable of increasing pain intensity.

EVALUATION OF INDIVIDUALS WITH CHRONIC WIDESPREAD PAIN

The evaluation of an individual with chronic pain is a complex process. In contrast to most other medical problems, simply arriving at a "diagnosis" is typically insufficient to guide treatment. This is because within any given pain diagnosis, there is tremendous heterogeneity with respect to the underlying causes and contributors to symptoms and the most effective treatments. In particular, individuals with chronic pain can have greater or lesser peripheral nociceptive (i.e., tissue damage, inflammation) and central non-nociceptive (i.e., pain amplification, psychological factors) contributions to their pain (Fig. 77.8). Therefore, the differential diagnosis of chronic pain involves identifying which of these factors are present in which individuals so that the appropriate pharmacologic, procedural, and psychological therapies can be administered.

A suggested diagnostic and therapeutic paradigm for individuals suspected of having FM is outlined in Figure 77.9. A careful musculo-

---

SUBGROUPS OF FIBROMYALGIA PATIENTS

Group 1 (n = 50)
- Low depression/anxiety
- Not very tender
- Low catastrophizing
- Moderate control over pain

Psychological factors neutral

Group 2 (n = 31)
- Tender
- High expression/anxiety
- Very high catastrophizing
- No control over pain

Psychological factors *worsening* symptoms

Group 3 (n = 16)
- Extremely tender
- Low depression/anxiety
- Very low catastrophizing
- High control over pain

Psychological factors improving symptoms

Fig. 77.7 Subgroups of fibromyalgia patients based on grouping by psychological, cognitive, and neurobiologic (degree of hyperalgesia) factors.

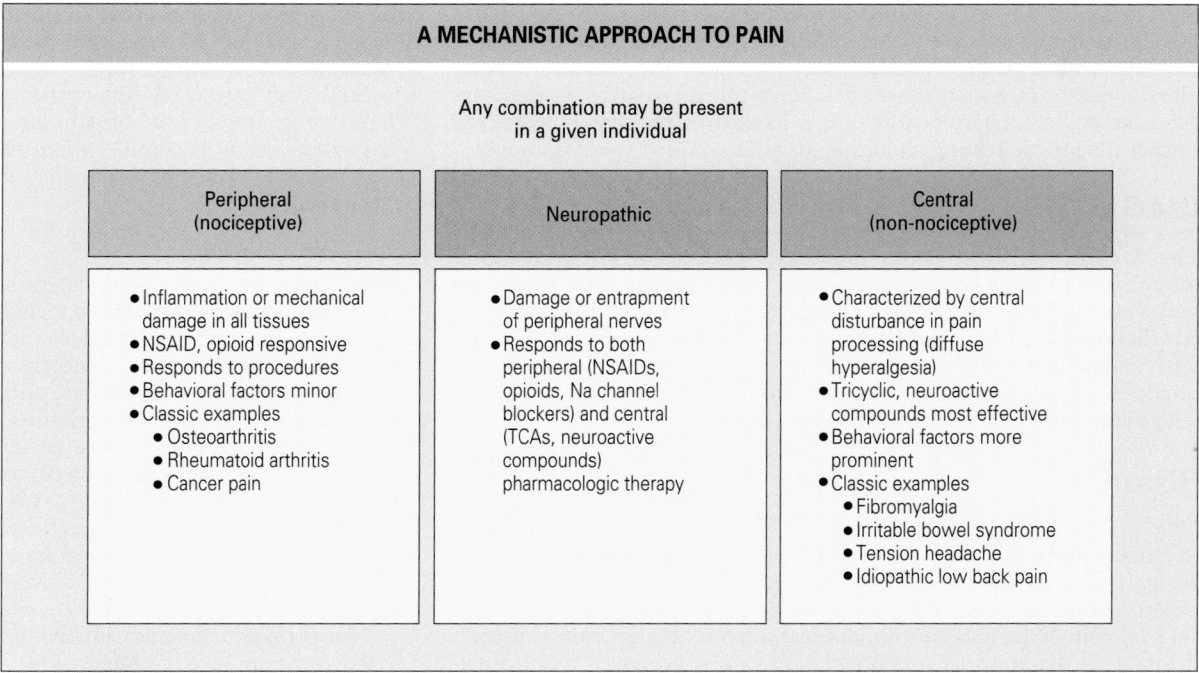

A MECHANISTIC APPROACH TO PAIN

Any combination may be present in a given individual

Peripheral (nociceptive)	Neuropathic	Central (non-nociceptive)

• Inflammation or mechanical damage in all tissues
• NSAID, opioid responsive
• Responds to procedures
• Behavioral factors minor
• Classic examples
  • Osteoarthritis
  • Rheumatoid arthritis
  • Cancer pain
	• Damage or entrapment of peripheral nerves
	• Responds to both peripheral (NSAIDs, opioids, Na channel blockers) and central (TCAs, neuroactive compounds) pharmacologic therapy
		• Characterized by central disturbance in pain processing (diffuse hyperalgesia)
		• Tricyclic, neuroactive compounds most effective
		• Behavioral factors more prominent
		• Classic examples
		  • Fibromyalgia
		  • Irritable bowel syndrome
		  • Tension headache
		  • Idiopathic low back pain

Fig. 77.8 A mechanistic approach to pain requires that for any chronic pain patient, clinicians assess whether an individual has nociceptive (peripheral inflammation or damage), neuropathic pain (due to nerve damage), and/or central pain (due to disturbance in spinal or supraspinal mechanisms) and base treatment on this characterization rather than the typical type of pain experienced by most individuals with that condition (e.g., peripheral for OA and central for FM).

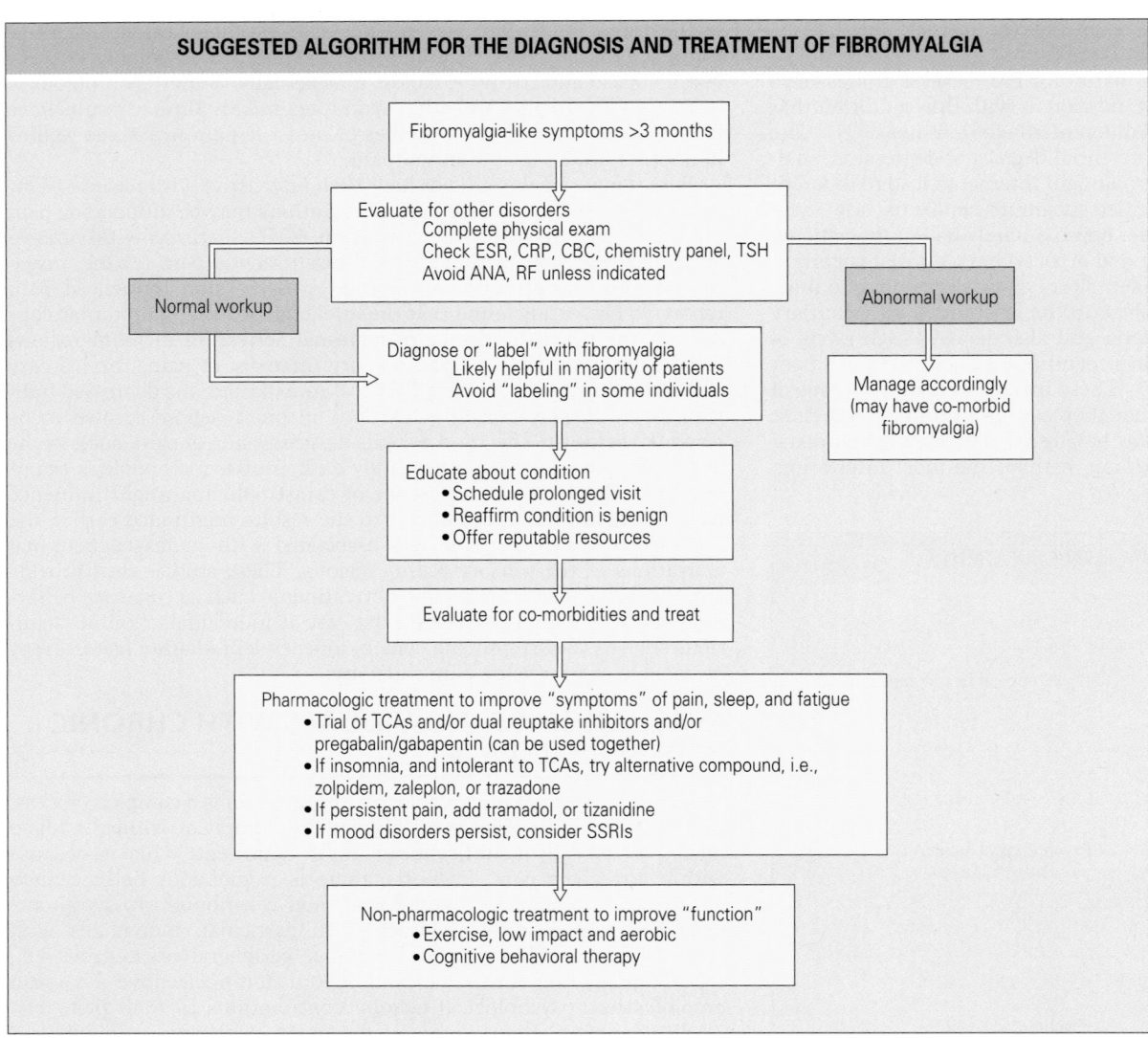

SUGGESTED ALGORITHM FOR THE DIAGNOSIS AND TREATMENT OF FIBROMYALGIA

Fibromyalgia-like symptoms >3 months

Evaluate for other disorders
Complete physical exam
Check ESR, CRP, CBC, chemistry panel, TSH
Avoid ANA, RF unless indicated

Normal workup

Abnormal workup

Diagnose or "label" with fibromyalgia
Likely helpful in majority of patients
Avoid "labeling" in some individuals

Manage accordingly
(may have co-morbid
fibromyalgia)

Educate about condition
• Schedule prolonged visit
• Reaffirm condition is benign
• Offer reputable resources

Evaluate for co-morbidities and treat

Pharmacologic treatment to improve "symptoms" of pain, sleep, and fatigue
• Trial of TCAs and/or dual reuptake inhibitors and/or
  pregabalin/gabapentin (can be used together)
• If insomnia, and intolerant to TCAs, try alternative compound, i.e.,
  zolpidem, zaleplon, or trazadone
• If persistent pain, add tramadol, or tizanidine
• If mood disorders persist, consider SSRIs

Non-pharmacologic treatment to improve "function"
• Exercise, low impact and aerobic
• Cognitive behavioral therapy

Fig. 77.9 Suggested algorithm for the diagnosis and treatment of fibromyalgia.

skeletal history and examination remains the most important diagnostic test for musculoskeletal pain. A high proportion of the healthy, asymptomatic population has a positive antinuclear antibody, positive rheumatoid factor, or abnormal results of imaging studies.[173-175] Worse yet, these diagnostic tests rarely tell us how "severe" the pain is because there is typically a significant discordance between the results of laboratory or imaging studies and the severity of pain and other symptoms that the individual is experiencing. Therefore the musculoskeletal history and examination must allow the clinician to arrive at the diagnosis (or at worst a narrow differential diagnosis), and then if necessary, further diagnostic testing should be used to confirm these findings.

DIAGNOSIS

The American College of Rheumatology criteria for FM were never intended to be used as strict diagnostic criteria for use in clinical practice. Many individuals who clearly have FM will not have pain throughout their entire body or not have 11 tender points. Moreover, pain and tenderness occur across a continuum in the population, and it is impossible to know where to "draw the line" between an individual with symptoms and someone with an "illness."[176]

History

Pain

In clinical practice, one should suspect FM in individuals with multifocal pain that cannot be fully explained on the basis of damage or inflammation in those regions of the body. In most cases musculoskeletal pain is the most prominent feature, but because pain pathways throughout the body are amplified, pain can be perceived more gener-

ally. Thus chronic headaches, sore throats, chest pain, abdominal pain, and pelvic pain are common in individuals with FM, and patients with chronic regional pain in any of these locations are more likely to have FM.

Because pain is a defining feature of FM, it is helpful to focus on the features of the pain that can help distinguish it from other disorders. The pain of FM is typically diffuse or multifocal, often waxes and wanes, and is frequently migratory in nature. These characteristics of "central pain" are quite different from "peripheral" pain, where both the location and severity of pain are typically more constant. Patients may complain of discomfort when they are touched or when wearing tight clothing and may experience dysesthesias or paresthesias that accompany the pain.

Non-pain symptoms

Aside from the pain, a number of seemingly non-related symptoms may develop and persist. These include fatigue, sleep difficulties, weakness, problems with attention or memory, unexplainable weight fluctuations, and heat and cold intolerance. "Allergies" are reported much more commonly in FM patients, although these excess symptoms are better considered hypersensitivities rather than true IgE-mediated immunologic reactions. These patients are also more prone to non-allergic rhinitis, sinus and nasal congestion, and lower respiratory symptoms, all of which again may be primarily attributable to neural mechanisms. Distortions in hearing, vision, and vestibular symptoms are often reported, as are sicca symptoms (sometimes so prominent that these individuals will overlap with those with Sjögren syndrome).

"Functional disorders" involving visceral organs have long been noted to be more common in FM. These include non-cardiac chest pain, heartburn and palpitations, and the frequent co-morbidity of irritable bowel syndrome. Mitral valve prolapse, esophageal dysmotility, and reduced static inspiratory and expiratory pressure on pulmonary function tests have been seen in patients with FM. Syncope and hypotension are symptoms that may occur in FM, and in some cases they are accompanied by neurally mediated hypotension or postural orthostatic tachycardia. Pelvic complaints are common, including not only pain but also urinary frequency and urgency. In females the frequent co-morbid diagnoses are dysmenorrhea, interstitial cystitis, endometriosis, and sensitivity disorders like vulvar vestibulitis and vulvodynia, whereas in males these same symptoms are sometimes diagnosed as chronic or non-bacterial prostatitis.

Physical examination and laboratory investigations

Physical examination is often unremarkable, except for the presence of tenderness. Tenderness may be generalized and thus present anywhere in the body. Laboratory testing is generally not useful, except for the purpose of differential diagnosis. One factor that can help guide the intensity of the diagnostic work-up is the length of time the patient has had symptoms. If the patient's symptoms have persisted for several years, minimal testing is required, whereas a more aggressive strategy should be employed for acute or subacute onset of symptoms. Simple testing should be limited to complete blood count and routine serum chemistries, along with thyroid-stimulating hormone (TSH) and erythrocyte sedimentation rate (ESR) and/or C-reactive protein.

Serologic studies such as ANA and rheumatoid factor assays should generally be avoided unless there are historic features not seen in FM, or abnormalities on physical examination. This represents a problem in clinical practice because several autoimmune disorders share overlapping symptomatology with FM. These include not only fatigue, arthralgias, and myalgias, but also such symptoms as morning stiffness and subjective swelling of the hands and feet. Certain dermatologic features commonly seen in FM, including malar flushing, livedo reticularis, and Raynaud-like reddening of the hands, also mimic symptoms of autoimmune disorders. This sometimes results in patients with FM being misdiagnosed as having an autoimmune disorder such as systemic lupus erythematosus.

Aside from the many co-morbid conditions already discussed, FM may present similarly to a number of disorders or concurrently with other disorders that may confuse the diagnosis. Box 77.2 shows conditions that often mimic or present concurrently with FM. Hypothyroidism and polymyalgia rheumatica can be differentiated from FM by results of TSH and ESR. Sleep apnea and hepatitis C also simulate FM and tend to present more often in men than women.

TREATMENT

Progress in the understanding of FM has led to more therapeutic options for patients with this condition. Investigators are examining the utility of newer medications, as well as non-pharmacologic interventions in controlled trials (Fig. 77.10). It is important to use symptom-based pharmacologic therapy together with non-pharmacologic therapies because medications typically target symptoms, whereas non-pharmacologic therapies target dysfunction/functional decline.[177]

BOX 77.2 **CONDITIONS THAT SIMULATE FIBROMYALGIA**

Common
Hypothyroidism
Polymyalgia rheumatica
Early in course of autoimmune disorders (e.g., rheumatoid arthritis or systemic lupus erythematosus)
Sjögren syndrome

Less common
Hepatitis C
Sleep apnea
Chiari malformation
Celiac sprue

Diagnostic labeling

Once a physician rules out other potential disorders, an important and at times controversial step in the management of FM is asserting the diagnosis. Despite some assumptions that being "labeled" with FM may adversely affect patients, one study indicated that patients had significant improvement in health satisfaction and symptoms after being "labeled."[167] Nonetheless, in certain select individuals (i.e., adolescents or young adults, or overtly anxious persons), the preferred route may still be not to label. Regardless, diagnosis confirmation should be ideally coupled to patient education, an intervention shown to be effective in randomized controlled trials.[177]

Pharmacologic therapy

The majority of FM clinical trials have involved antidepressants of one class or another (Box 77.3). Trials studying the oldest class of agents, tricyclic antidepressants (TCAs), are most abundant, though several recent studies have focused on selective serotonin reuptake inhibitors and "atypical antidepressants"—a class that includes dual-reuptake inhibitors and monoamine oxidase inhibitors (MAOIs).

Tricyclic antidepressants

The most frequently studied pharmacologic therapy for FM is low doses of tricyclic compounds. Most TCAs increase the concentrations of serotonin and/or norepinephrine (noradrenaline) by directly blocking their respective reuptake. The effectiveness of TCAs, particularly amitriptyline and cyclobenzaprine, in treating the symptoms of pain, poor sleep, and fatigue associated with FM is supported by several randomized, controlled trials.[96] Tolerability is a problem but can be improved by beginning at low doses (e.g., 10 mg amitriptyline or 5 mg cyclobenzaprine), giving the dose a few hours before bedtime, and slowly escalating the dose.

BOX 77.3 **PHARMACOLOGIC THERAPIES**

- **Strong evidence:** tricyclics (amitriptyline, cyclobenzaprine); dual-reuptake inhibitors (SNRI/NSRI—duloxetine, milnacipran); alpha-2-delta ligands (pregabalin, gabapentin)
- **Modest evidence:** tramadol; selective serotonin reuptake inhibitors (SSRIs); dopamine agonists; gamma hydroxybutyrate (GHB)
- **Weak evidence:** growth hormone, 5-hydroxytryptamine, tropisetron, S-adenosyl-L-methionine (SAMe)
- **Not shown to be effective:** opioids, NSAIDs, corticosteroids, benzodiazepine and nonbenzodiazepine hypnotics, melatonin, guaifenesin, dehydroepiandrosterone

---

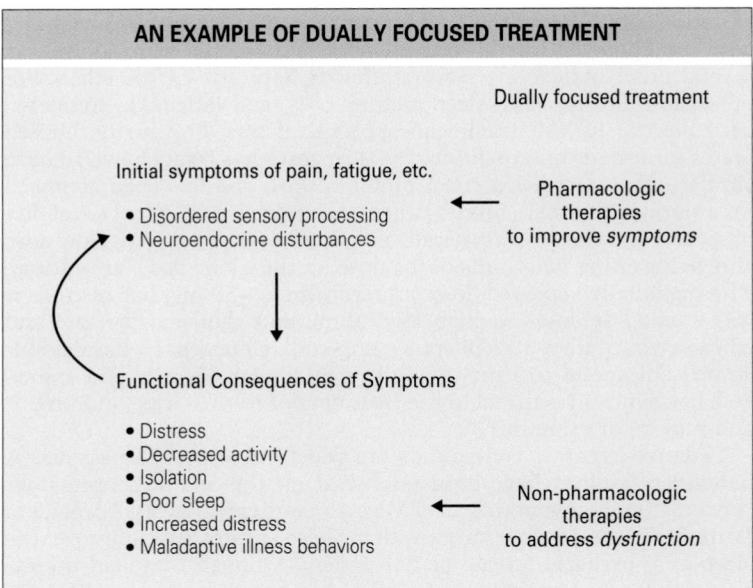

AN EXAMPLE OF DUALLY FOCUSED TREATMENT

Dually focused treatment

Initial symptoms of pain, fatigue, etc.
- Disordered sensory processing
- Neuroendocrine disturbances

Pharmacologic therapies to improve *symptoms*

Functional Consequences of Symptoms
- Distress
- Decreased activity
- Isolation
- Poor sleep
- Increased distress
- Maladaptive illness behaviors

Non-pharmacologic therapies to address *dysfunction*

Fig. 77.10 An example of dually focused treatment.

Selective serotonin reuptake inhibitors

Because of a better side effect profile, newer antidepressants (i.e., selective serotonin reuptake inhibitors [SSRIs]) are frequently used in FM. The SSRIs fluoxetine, citalopram, and paroxetine have each been evaluated in randomized, placebo-controlled trials.[177-180] In general, the results of studies of SSRIs in FM have paralleled the experience in other pain conditions. The newer "highly selective" serotonin reuptake inhibitors (e.g., citalopram) seem to be less efficacious than the older SSRIs, which have some noradrenergic activity at higher doses.[181]

Because TCAs and high doses of certain "SSRIs" such as fluoxetine and sertraline that have the most balanced reuptake inhibition are the most effective analgesics, many have concluded that dual-receptor inhibitors such as serotonin-NE and NE-serotonin reuptake inhibitors (SNRIs and NSRIs) may be of more benefit than pure serotonergic drugs.[181] These drugs are pharmacologically similar to some TCAs in their ability to inhibit the reuptake of both serotonin and NE but differ from TCAs in being generally devoid of significant activity at other receptor systems. This selectivity results in diminished side effects and enhanced tolerability. The first available SNRI, venlafaxine, has data to support its use in the management of neuropathic pain, and retrospective trial data demonstrate that this compound is also effective in the prophylaxis of migraine and tension headaches.[182] Two studies in FM have had conflicting results, with the one using a higher dose showing efficacy.[177]

Two new SNRIs, milnacipran and duloxetine, have undergone recent multicenter trials and were shown to be effective in a number of outcome variables. Both are now approved in the United States for the treatment of FM.[117,183] In the study evaluating milnacipran, statistically significant differences were noted in overall improvement, physical functioning, level of fatigue, and degree of reported physical impairment. In the trial of duloxetine compared with placebo, participants treated with duloxetine had decreased self-reported pain and stiffness and a reduced number of tender points. In both studies, benefits were shown to be independent of the drug effect on mood, thus suggesting that the analgesic and other positive effects of this class of drugs in FM are not simply due to their antidepressant effects. Both drugs are better tolerated if taken with food and patients are warned about initial nausea. Patients should be counseled that nausea typically resolves in a week or so, but if not, they should discontinue the drug. The maximum approved dose of duloxetine is 60 mg per day, but it was studied in trials at doses up to 120 mg and shown to be safe. Similarly, the initial dose of milnacipran is 100 mg, but some patients will benefit from increasing the dose as high as 200 mg.

Other central nervous system–acting drugs

Antiepileptic drugs are widely used in the treatment of various chronic pain conditions, including postherpetic neuralgia and painful diabetic neuropathy.[184] Pregabalin and gabapentin have the same mechanism of action and bind to the α_2-delta subunit of calcium channels, and both are approved for the treatment of neuropathic pain, as well as several other indications. Several studies have shown the efficacy of pregabalin against pain, sleep disturbances, and fatigue as compared with placebo in FM, leading to approval of this drug in the United States for use in this condition.[185] Gabapentin has been shown to have similar efficacy and side effect profile in FM, and has been approved for a number of other chronic pain states as well.[184,186] The tolerability of these drugs can be dramatically enhanced by beginning at a low dose and giving either two thirds of the dose, or the entire dose, at bedtime. The maximally approved dose of pregabalin is 450 mg, but in trials it was studied at doses as high as 600 mg and shown to be safe and efficacious. Another antiepileptic compound, clonazepam, has demonstrated efficacy in treating temporal mandibular disorder and associated jaw pain and is useful in the treatment of restless legs syndrome[184] and may be of value in FM.

Sedative-hypnotic compounds are widely used by FM patients. A handful of studies have been published on the use of certain non-benzodiazepine hypnotics in FM such as zopiclone and zolpidem tartrate. These reports suggest that these agents can improve the sleep and, perhaps, fatigue of FM patients, though they had no significant effects on pain. On the other hand, gamma-hydroxybutyrate (also known as *sodium oxabate*), a precursor of GABA with powerful sedative properties, was recently shown to be useful in improving fatigue, pain, and sleep architecture in patients with FM.[187] Note, however, that this agent is a scheduled substance due to its abuse potential.

Pramipexole is a dopamine agonist indicated for Parkinson disease that has shown utility in the treatment of periodic leg movement disorder.[188] Recent studies suggest that this compound may improve both pain and sleep in FM patients.[189]

Tizanidine is a centrally acting α_2-adrenergic agonist approved by the U.S. Food and Drug Administration for the treatment of muscle spasticity associated with multiple sclerosis and stroke. Literature suggests that this agent is a useful adjunct in treating several chronic pain conditions, including chronic daily headaches and low back pain. A recent trial reported significant improvements in several parameters in FM, including sleep, pain, and measures of quality of life.[190] Of particular interest was the demonstration that treatment with tizanidine resulted in a reduction in substance P levels within the CSF of patients with FM.

Analgesics

No adequate, randomized, controlled clinical trials of opiates in FM have occurred, and many in the field (including the author) have not found this class of compounds to be effective in anecdotal experience. Tramadol is a compound that has some opioid activity (weak μ-agonist activity) combined with serotonin/NE reuptake inhibition. This compound does appear to be somewhat efficacious in the management of FM, as both an isolated compound and as a fixed-dose combination with acetaminophen.[188]

A large number of FM patients use NSAIDs and acetaminophen. Although numerous studies have failed to confirm their effectiveness as analgesics in FM, there is limited evidence that patients may experience enhanced analgesia when treated with combinations of NSAIDs and other agents. This phenomenon may be a result of concurrent "peripheral" pain (i.e., due to damage or inflammation of tissues such as osteoarthritis and rheumatoid arthritis) conditions that may be present and/or co-morbid peripheral pain generators that might lead to worsening of "central" pain.

Non-pharmacologic therapies

The two best-studied non-pharmacologic therapies are cognitive behavioral therapy and exercise (Box 77.4). Both therapies have been shown to be efficacious in the treatment of FM, as well as a plethora of other medical conditions.[177,191] Both treatments can lead to sustained (e.g., longer than 1 year) improvements and be effective when an individual complies with therapy.

Alternative therapies have been explored by patients managing their own illness, as well as health care providers. As with other diseases, there are few controlled trials to advocate their general use. Trigger-point injections, chiropractic manipulation, acupuncture, and myofascial release therapy are among the more commonly used modalities, which achieve varying levels of success. Two randomized, sham-controlled trials of acupuncture showed no difference between the two groups.[97,192] A usual-care comparison group was not studied. Some evidence indicates that the use of alternative therapies gives patients a greater sense of control over their illness. In instances where this sense of control is accompanied by an improved clinical state, the decision to use these therapies is between physicians and patients themselves.

BOX 77.4 NON-PHARMACOLOGIC THERAPIES

- **Strong evidence:** cardiovascular exercise, cognitive behavior therapy, patient education, multidisciplinary therapy
- **Modest evidence:** strength training, acupuncture, hypnotherapy, biofeedback, balneotherapy
- **Weak evidence:** acupuncture, chiropractic, manual and massage therapy, electrotherapy, ultrasound
- **No evidence:** tender (trigger) point injections, flexibility exercise

PROGNOSIS

The prognosis of FM depends largely on where the individual falls on a continuum. One end of the continuum comprises individuals with chronic widespread pain, or individuals with FM who are seen in primary care, with the prognosis being quite good.[193,194] On the other hand, individuals with FM seen in tertiary care settings do quite poorly.[195] In this latter study, there was little change in symptoms over time and no significant change in health satisfaction, symptoms, or functional disability.

With regard to function in FM, studies have reported varying disability rates from 9% to 44%.[194,196,197] Disability has been most strongly associated with functional and work status, pain, mood disturbances, coping ability, depression, pending litigation, and educational background.

SUMMARY

Much has been learned about chronic pain by studying FM. It is now viewed as the prototypical "central pain syndrome" that occurs primarily because of spinal and supraspinal mechanisms involved in pain transmission, rather than due to peripheral inflammation or damage or due to nerve damage. The same mechanisms that lead to centrally mediated pain also lead to other somatic symptoms such as fatigue and insomnia, likely because similar neurotransmitter imbalances can also cause these symptoms. Because of this, any patient with chronic pain, especially if he or she has widespread multifocal pain and the pain is accompanied by other somatic symptoms and syndromes, should be considered to possibly have a co-morbid FM or an element of FM.

Wolfe and colleagues[176] have clearly demonstrated that FM is **both** a discrete illness (i.e., an individual with FM) **and** the end of a continuum of pain processing. Wolfe[198] has reported that the degree of "fibromyalgia-ness" an individual with any rheumatic disorder has (including individuals with osteoarthritis, rheumatoid arthritis, regional pain syndromes) as measured by his symptom inventory is closely correlated with his or her level of pain and/or disability, even if there is a "peripheral" cause for pain. The symptom inventory (or other measures of the current or lifetime level of somatic symptoms or "somatization") is a good measure for whether an individual has this spectrum of illness or an element of central sensitivity, no matter if he or she also has a peripheral cause for pain or not. A better understanding of the underlying mechanisms and most effective treatment for this spectrum of illness is critical to rheumatologists because many patients with rheumatic disorders have a little, or a lot, of "fibromyalgia-ness."

KEY REFERENCES

3. Hudson JI, Hudson MS, Pliner LF, et al. Fibromyalgia and major affective disorder: a controlled phenomenology and family history study. Am J Psychiatry 1985;142:441-446.
4. Arnold LM, Hudson JI, Hess EV, et al. Family study of fibromyalgia. Arthritis Rheum 2004;50:944-952.
5. Mogil JS, Yu L, Basbaum AI. Pain genes? natural variation and transgenic mutants. Annu Rev Neurosci 2000;23:777-811.
6. Diatchenko L, Nackley AG, Tchivileva IE, et al. Genetic architecture of human pain perception. Trends Genet 2007;23:605-613.
7. Tegeder I, Costigan M, Griffin RS, et al. GTP cyclohydrolase and tetrahydrobiopterin regulate pain sensitivity and persistence. Nat Med 2006;12:1269-1277.
11. Kato K, Sullivan PF, Evengard B, Pedersen NL. Importance of genetic influences on chronic widespread pain. Arthritis Rheum 2006;54:1682-1686.
12. Kato K, Sullivan PF, Evengard B, Pedersen NL. A population-based twin study of functional somatic syndromes. Psychol Med 2008;26:1-9.
15. Aaron LA, Bradley LA, Alarcon GS, et al. Psychiatric diagnoses in patients with fibromyalgia are related to health care-seeking behavior rather than to illness [see comments]. Arthritis Rheum 1996;39:436-445.
18. Giesecke T, Gracely RH, Grant MA, et al. Evidence of augmented central pain processing in idiopathic chronic low back pain. Arthritis Rheum 2004;50:613-623.
22. Smythe HA, Moldofsky H. Two contributions to understanding of the "fibrositis" syndrome. Bull Rheum Dis 1977;28:928-931.
23. Moldofsky H, Scarisbrick P, England R, Smythe H. Musculosketal symptoms and non-REM sleep disturbance in patients with "fibrositis syndrome" and healthy subjects. Psychosom Med 1975;37:341-351.
24. Yunus M, Masi AT, Calabro JJ, et al. Primary fibromyalgia (fibrositis): clinical study of 50 patients with matched normal controls. Semin Arthritis Rheum 1981;11:151-171.
25. Wolfe F, Smythe HA, Yunus MB, et al. The American College of Rheumatology 1990 Criteria for the Classification of Fibromyalgia. Report of the Multicenter Criteria Committee. Arthritis Rheum 1990;33:160-172.
26. Yunus MB. Towards a model of pathophysiology of fibromyalgia: aberrant central pain mechanisms with peripheral modulation. J Rheumatol 1992;19:846-850.
27. Clauw DJ, Chrousos GP. Chronic pain and fatigue syndromes: overlapping clinical and neuroendocrine features and potential pathogenic mechanisms. Neuroimmunomodulation 1997;4:134-153.
28. Wolfe F, Ross K, Anderson J, Russell IJ. Aspects of fibromyalgia in the general population: sex, pain threshold, and fibromyalgia symptoms. J Rheumatol 1995;22:151-156.
34. Petzke F, Khine A, Williams D, et al. Dolorimetry performed at three paired tender points highly predicts overall tenderness. J Rheumatol 2001;28:2568-2569.
37. Wolfe F. The relation between tender points and fibromyalgia symptom variables: evidence that fibromyalgia is not a discrete disorder in the clinic. Ann Rheum Dis 1997;56:268-271.
42. Buskila D, Neumann L, Hazanov I, Carmi R. Familial aggregation in the fibromyalgia syndrome. Semin Arthritis Rheum 1996;26:605-611.
44. Hudson JI, Goldenberg DL, Pope HGJ, et al. Comorbidity of fibromyalgia with medical and psychiatric disorders. Am J Med 1993;92:363-367.
45. Yunus MB. Central sensitivity syndromes: a new paradigm and group nosology for fibromyalgia and overlapping conditions, and the related issue of disease versus illness. Semin Arthritis Rheum 2008;37:339-352.
52. Buskila D, Neumann L, Vaisberg G, et al. Increased rates of fibromyalgia following cervical spine injury. A controlled study of 161 cases of traumatic injury [see comments]. Arthritis Rheum 1997;40:446-452.
57. Raphael KG, Natelson BH, Janal MN, Nayak S. A community-based survey of fibromyalgia-like pain complaints following the World Trade Center terrorist attacks. Pain 2002;100:131-139.
58. Williams DA, Brown SC, Clauw DJ, Gendreau RM. Self-reported symptoms before and after September 11 in patients with fibromyalgia. JAMA 2003;289:1637-1638.
59. Clauw DJ, Engel CC Jr, Aronowitz R, et al. Unexplained symptoms after terrorism and war: an expert consensus statement. J Occup Environ Med 2003;45:1040-1048.
61. Glass JM, Lyden A, Petzke F, Clauw D. The effect of brief exercise cessation on pain, fatigue, and mood symptom development in healthy, fit individuals. J Psychosom Res 2004;57:391-398.
69. Crofford LJ, Pillemer SR, Kalogeras KT, et al. Hypothalamic-pituitary-adrenal axis perturbations in patients with fibromyalgia. Arthritis Rheum 1994;37:1583-1592.
85. Gracely RH, Grant MA, Giesecke T. Evoked pain measures in fibromyalgia. Best Pract Res Clin Rheumatol 2003;17:593-609.
91. Arnold LM, Hess EV, Hudson JI, et al. A randomized, placebo-controlled, double-blind, flexible-dose study of fluoxetine in the treatment of women with fibromyalgia. Am J Med 2002;112:191-197.
92. Goldenberg D, Mayskiy M, Mossey C, et al. A randomized, double-blind crossover trial of fluoxetine and amitriptyline in the treatment of fibromyalgia. Arthritis Rheum 1996;39:1852-1859.
99. Gibson SJ, Littlejohn GO, Gorman MM, et al. Altered heat pain thresholds and cerebral event-related potentials following painful CO_2 laser stimulation in subjects with fibromyalgia syndrome. Pain 1994;58:185-193.
102. Kosek E, Ekholm J, Hansson P. Sensory dysfunction in fibromyalgia patients with implications for pathogenic mechanisms. Pain 1996;68:375-383.
107. Tracey I, Mantyh PW. The cerebral signature for pain perception and its modulation. Neuron 2007;55:377-391.
108. Craig AD. Human feelings: why are some more aware than others? Trends Cogn Sci 2004;8:239-241.
109. Lautenbacher S, Rollman GB. Possible deficiencies of pain modulation in fibromyalgia. Clin J Pain 1997;13:189-196.
114. Harris RE, Clauw DJ, Scott DJ, et al. Decreased central μ-opioid receptor availability in fibromyalgia. J Neurosci 2007;27:10000-10006.
115. Russell IJ, Vaeroy H, Javors M, Nyberg F. Cerebrospinal fluid biogenic amine metabolites in fibromyalgia/fibrositis syndrome and rheumatoid arthritis. Arthritis Rheum 1992;35:550-556.
117. Arnold LM, Lu Y, Crofford LJ, et al. A double-blind, multicenter trial comparing duloxetine with placebo in the treatment of fibromyalgia patients with or without major depressive disorder. Arthritis Rheum 2004;50:2974-2984.
118. Bennett RM, Kamin M, Karim R, Rosenthal N. Tramadol and acetaminophen combination tablets in the treatment of fibromyalgia pain: a double-blind, randomized, placebo-controlled study. Am J Med 2003;114:537-545.
119. Gendreau RM, Thorn MD, Gendreau JF, et al. The efficacy of milnacipran in fibromyalgia. J Rheumatol 2005;32:1975-1985.
122. Woolf CJ, Thompson SW. The induction and maintenance of central sensitization is dependent on N-methyl-D-aspartic acid receptor activation; implications for the treatment of post-injury pain hypersensitivity states. Pain 1991;44:293-299.
126. Russell IJ, Orr MD, Littman B, et al. Elevated cerebrospinal fluid levels of substance P in patients with the fibromyalgia syndrome. Arthritis Rheum 1994;37:1593-1601.
127. Bradley LA, Alberts KR, Alarcon GS, et al. Abnormal brain regional cerebral blood flow and cerebrospinal fluid levels of substance P in patients and non-patients with fibromyalgia. Arthritis Rheum 1996;39[9S]:1109.
129. Harris RE, Clauw DJ. How do we know that the pain in fibromyalgia is "real"? Curr Pain Headache Rep 2006;10:403-407.
130. Giovengo SL, Russell IJ, Larson AA. Increased concentrations of nerve growth factor in cerebrospinal fluid of patients with fibromyalgia. J Rheumatol 1999;26:1564-1569.

133. Mountz JM, Bradley LA, Modell JG, et al. Fibromyalgia in women. Abnormalities of regional cerebral blood flow in the thalamus and the caudate nucleus are associated with low pain threshold levels. Arthritis Rheum 1995;38:926-938.
138. Gracely RH, Petzke F, Wolf JM, Clauw DJ. Functional magnetic resonance imaging evidence of augmented pain processing in fibromyalgia. Arthritis Rheum 2002;46:1333-1343.
140. Giesecke T, Gracely RH, Williams DA, et al. The relationship between depression, clinical pain, and experimental pain in a chronic pain cohort. Arthritis Rheum 2005;52:1577-1584.
172. Giesecke T, Williams DA, Harris RE, et al. Subgrouping of fibromyalgia patients on the basis of pressure-pain thresholds and psychological factors. Arthritis Rheum 2003;48:2916-2922.
181. Fishbain D. Evidence-based data on pain relief with antidepressants. Ann Med 2000;32:305-316.

REFERENCES

Full references for this chapter can be found on www.expertconsult.com.

Entrapment neuropathies and compartment syndromes

78

*Stephany A. McGann, Raymond H. Flores, and David J. Nashel**

- An entrapment neuropathy results from increased pressure on a nerve as it passes through an enclosed space.
- Knowledge of the anatomy of each potential site of entrapment is essential for an understanding of the clinical manifestations of these syndromes.
- Conservative measures such as splinting, non-steroidal anti-inflammatory drugs, and local corticosteroid injections usually suffice when symptoms are mild and of short duration. Surgical procedures to decompress the nerve are indicated in more severe cases.

INTRODUCTION

Entrapment neuropathy results from increased pressure on a nerve as it passes through an enclosed space. A nerve is most vulnerable to compression as it traverses a fibro-osseous canal, where there is a disproportion of contents and capacity. Nerves that have previously been affected by a neuropathic process, as with diabetes or alcoholism, appear to be even more vulnerable to entrapment. For the clinician to fathom fully the manifestations of each syndrome, familiarity with the anatomy of each site is essential.

Mechanisms for nerve injury by compression are not fully understood. Mild amounts of pressure can lead to physiologic dysfunction, and friction and ischemia may also play a role in this process.[1] Surgical exposure often reveals nerve swelling proximal to the site of entrapment.

The signs and symptoms that accompany nerve entrapment may at times be subtle and easily confused with rheumatic disorders. In addition, rheumatic diseases that manifest synovitis or tenosynovitis are capable of causing compression neuropathy. Because entrapment neuropathies produce focal neurologic deficits, other conditions that can present with similar patterns (e.g., vasculitis, radiculopathy, reflex sympathetic dystrophy) must be included in the differential diagnosis.

There are many recognized sites of neural entrapment (Table 78.1). In this chapter the focus is on those compressive neuropathies that are most often encountered in clinical practice.

THORACIC OUTLET SYNDROME

Thoracic outlet syndrome (TOS) results from compression of one or more of the neurovascular elements that pass through the superior thoracic aperture. In the majority of cases, it is neurogenic entrapment that accounts for the symptoms and rarely is there an isolated vascular lesion. In those relatively rare cases in which there is clear-cut involvement of the brachial plexus, the disorder is referred to as true neurogenic TOS. Non-specific or disputed TOS refers to those patients with more poorly defined pain syndromes.[2]

Anatomy

The thoracic outlet consists of several narrow channels through which the subclavian vessels and the lower trunk of the brachial plexus (eighth cervical and first thoracic fibers) pass from the thoracocervical region to the axilla (Fig. 78.1). The first area of narrowing, and

*The authors would like to acknowledge the contributions of Dr. David J. Nashel who was the author of this chapter in the previous edition.

potential entrapment, is between the scalenus anterior and scalenus medius muscles as they attach to the first rib. Next is the costoclavicular space, which is bordered by the clavicle anteriorly, the first rib posteromedially, and the superior margin of the scapula posterolaterally. Lastly, the neurovascular bundle travels under the coracoid process and beneath the pectoralis minor tendon.

Etiology

Because the thoracic outlet has three well-defined areas of narrowing, traditional teaching has ascribed specific clinical syndromes to each area. Thus, a fairly rigid classification has evolved that includes the anterior scalene, costoclavicular, and hyperabduction syndromes. However, it is more likely that anatomic abnormalities and trauma to the shoulder girdle region have a far more pivotal role in causing this syndrome.

Cervical ribs, some incomplete and having fibrous attachments to the first rib, are an anomaly often associated with true neurogenic TOS. Some have suggested that too much significance has been placed on this finding, because cervical ribs may be noted in up to 0.5% of routine radiographs. Furthermore, abnormal anatomy of the thoracic outlet, and in particular the presence of fibrous bands, is a common finding in the general population.[3] The congenital bands may arise from a cervical rib or from the transverse process of the seventh cervical vertebra, or they may be associated with the scalene muscles. These cervical bands and certain scalene muscle abnormalities appear to play an important part in the pathogenesis of neurogenic TOS.[4]

Clinical presentation

Patients usually experience sensory symptoms as the first manifestation of TOS. Paresthesias are common and follow the ulnar nerve distribution along the medial aspect of the arm and forearm and then to the fourth and fifth fingers. Aching pain, radiating to the neck, shoulder, and arm, is a frequent complaint, often being more diffuse than the paresthesias. Carrying heavy objects, persistent abduction of the shoulder, and work that requires using the arms over the head may exacerbate these symptoms. TOS is also more likely to occur in individuals with poor posture and drooping shoulders.

Signs of motor weakness, if they appear, usually follow the sensory complaints. The patients may describe a feeling of weakness or clumsiness in using the hand. Wasting of the thenar, hypothenar, and intrinsic muscles of the hand is indicative of true neuropathic TOS.

A small number of patients have vasomotor disturbances. These may take the form of coldness, blanching, or cyanosis. In more extreme cases, trophic changes and even infarction of tissues at the fingertips may appear.[5]

Diagnosis

The most useful diagnostic approach to TOS is a careful neurologic examination, which may reveal tenderness over the brachial plexus, sensory deficits, motor weakness, or signs of muscle atrophy. Certain clinical stress tests have traditionally been used to diagnose TOS. The Adson, costoclavicular, and hyperabduction maneuvers (Figs. 78.2 to 78.4) are used. However, because these maneuvers are positive in the majority of normal individuals (there is a reduction in the radial pulse), they have diagnostic utility only when the patient's sensory symptoms are reproduced.

TABLE 78.1 PERIPHERAL ENTRAPMENT NEUROPATHIES

	Nerve	Location/syndrome
Upper extremity and thorax	Brachial plexus	Thoracic outlet
	Dorsal scapular	Scalenus medius
	Suprascapular	Scapular notch
	Musculocutaneous	Elbow
	Radial	Posterior interosseous nerve syndrome
	Median	
	At elbow	Ligament of Struthers
	At forearm	Pronator teres
	At wrist	Carpal tunnel syndrome
	Anterior interosseous	Forearm
	Ulnar	
	At elbow	Cubital tunnel syndrome
	At wrist	Ulnar tunnel syndrome
Lower extremity	Obturator	Pelvis
	Sciatic	Piriformis syndrome
	Ilioinguinal	Lower abdomen
	Lateral femoral cutaneous	Meralgia paresthetica
	Femoral	Hip
	Peroneal	Fibular tunnel
	Saphenous	Hunter's canal
	Sural	Lower leg
	Posterior tibial	Tarsal tunnel syndrome
	Interdigital plantar	Morton's metatarsalgia

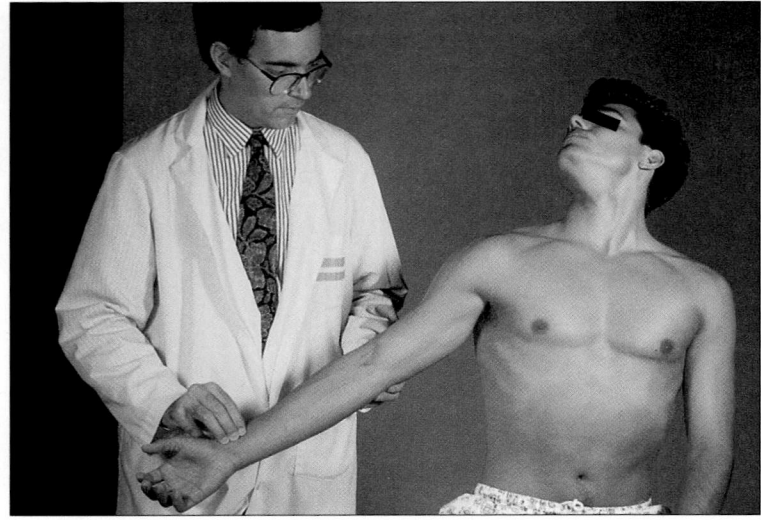

Fig. 78.2 The Adson maneuver. The patient inhales deeply, extends the neck fully, and turns the head to the side being examined. This tests for compression in the scalene triangle and is positive if there is a diminution in the radial pulse and reproduction of the patient's symptoms.

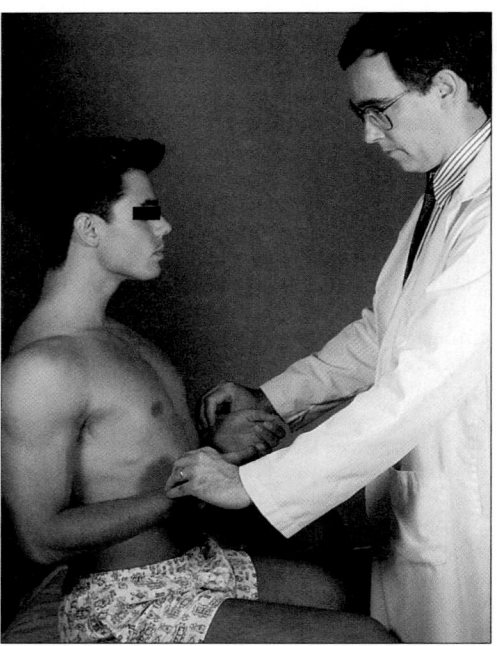

Fig. 78.3 The costoclavicular maneuver. The patient takes an exaggerated military position of attention with the shoulders thrust backward and downward. Decreased radial pulse and reproduction of symptoms suggest neurovascular compression between the clavicle and first rib.

A radiograph of the cervicothoracic region may reveal a cervical rib or an elongated transverse process of C7, a clue to the presence of a fibrous band. The anatomy of the thoracic outlet can be well visualized by magnetic resonance imaging (MRI). Functional imaging can now be obtained with open-magnet MRI.[6] Using this technology, one can assess compression of the brachial plexus by measurement of the distance between the clavicle and first rib while the arm is in abduction.

Nerve conduction studies may be helpful in diagnosing true TOS.[7] Although electrophysiologic studies are unrevealing in disputed TOS, they may be useful in diagnosing other conditions that might be confused with TOS, such as cervical radiculopathy, cubital tunnel syndrome, or carpal tunnel syndrome. The differential diagnosis of disputed TOS should include other cervical lesions (tumors, disc disease, spondylosis) and reflex sympathetic dystrophy; in patients with vascular signs, other disorders of vessels should be considered (e.g., vasculitis and atherosclerosis).

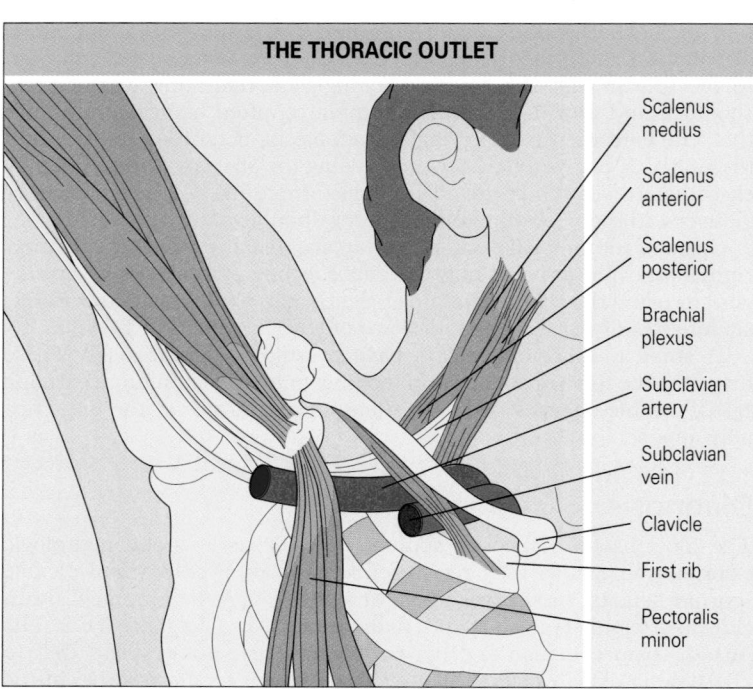

THE THORACIC OUTLET

- Scalenus medius
- Scalenus anterior
- Scalenus posterior
- Brachial plexus
- Subclavian artery
- Subclavian vein
- Clavicle
- First rib
- Pectoralis minor

Fig. 78.1 The thoracic outlet. Three narrow channels of the outlet include the scalene triangle, the costoclavicular passage, and the pectoralis minor attachment at the coracoid process.

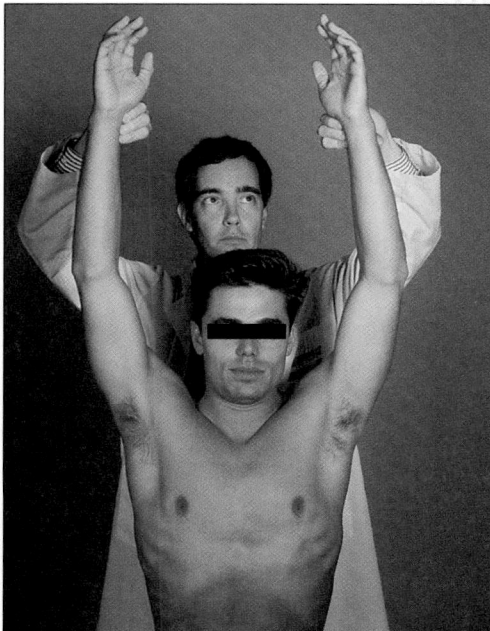

Fig. 78.4 The hyperabduction maneuver. The patient lifts the hands above the head with the elbows somewhat flexed and extending out laterally from the body. This maneuver tests compression by the pectoralis minor at the coracoid process.

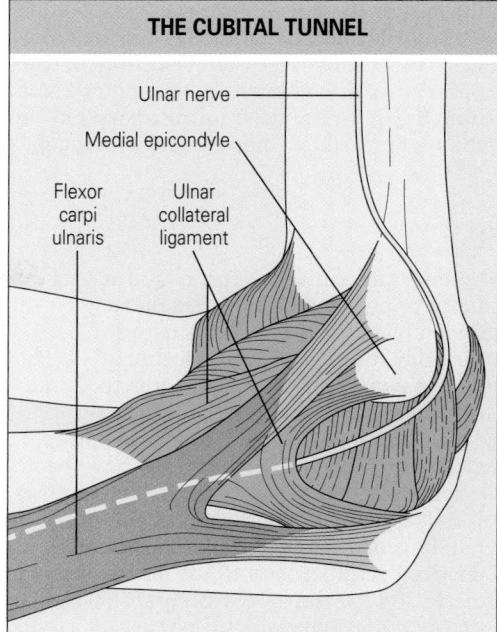

THE CUBITAL TUNNEL

Fig. 78.5 The cubital tunnel. The fibro-osseous canal is formed by the medial epicondyle, ulnar collateral ligament, and flexor carpi ulnaris muscle. Elbow flexion decreases the volume of the channel.

Treatment

Conservative management of TOS is the course that should be pursued initially. This consists of appropriate exercises designed to improve posture by strengthening the rhomboid and trapezius muscles. Avoidance of hyperabduction is important, and patients may have to consider changing occupation if their job requires prolonged use of the arms above the head.

It must be remembered, however, that carpal tunnel syndrome may present as pain radiating to the shoulder region and may thus be confused with TOS.[8] Accordingly, distal nerve entrapment should be excluded before definitive therapy for TOS is considered.

"Caution" must be the watchword when surgical treatment of TOS is under consideration. The large number of treatment failures reported by some authors suggests that many of these patients may have had the more common or disputed form of neurogenic TOS, which does not generally respond to surgical intervention. Thus, careful screening of patients is mandatory before surgery. In addition, there is considerable risk of injury to the brachial plexus during surgery.[9] Conservative treatment should be continued as long as the neurologic symptoms are only subjective. When there is evidence for true neurogenic TOS, namely, an abnormal nerve conduction study, intrinsic hand muscle atrophy, and presence of a fibrous band or cervical rib, then surgery should be considered. Other indications for surgery are intermittent fleeting paresthesias replaced by continuous sensory loss, incapacitating pain, or worsening circulatory impairment (if present).[4]

Because it is often difficult to define an exact anatomic area of compression preoperatively, success rates of particular surgical procedures are, not surprisingly, quite variable. The transaxillary approach with first rib resection has many proponents. This method is useful for costoclavicular compression. Others prefer supraclavicular exploration with division of the scalenus anterior muscle and resection of the first rib.[10] In either case, the surgeon must also search for constricting fibrous bands.

ULNAR NERVE COMPRESSION SYNDROMES

Cubital tunnel syndrome

Compression neuropathy of the ulnar nerve as it traverses the elbow has long been recognized as a complication of local trauma, particularly as a result of fractures of the humerus. Only in recent years has the concept of constriction of the nerve in a fibro-osseous tunnel been suggested.[11]

Anatomy

The osseous portion of the cubital tunnel is formed anteriorly by the medial epicondyle, the fibrous portion by the ulnohumeral ligaments laterally, and the aponeurosis of the two heads of the flexor carpi ulnaris posteromedially (Fig. 78.5). The size of the tunnel is reduced when the elbow is placed in flexion.

Etiology

Without a history of trauma, it may be difficult to give a precise cause for cubital tunnel syndrome. However, chronic pressure over the ulnar groove, which may be exerted by occupational stress or from unusual elbow positioning, appears to play an etiologic role. Arthritic conditions that result in synovitis at the elbow, or osteophyte production, may also cause compression of the nerve.

Clinical presentation

Paresthesias are noted in the distribution of the ulnar nerve, and in many instances the neuropathy is bilateral. Symptoms are often aggravated by prolonged use of the elbow in a flexed position. Tinel's sign may be positive over the ulnar groove, and pain may be provoked by putting pressure directly on the nerve, which may be noticeably swollen. A majority of patients will demonstrate atrophy of intrinsic muscles and weakness in pinch and grasp. There may be wasting of the hypothenar muscles and slight clawing of the fourth and fifth fingers. A positive Wartenberg sign indicates weakness in adduction of the fifth finger.

Diagnosis

Consideration must be given to compression of the ulnar nerve at other locations, including the cervical spine, thoracic outlet, and Guyon's canal (see later). Also, cubital tunnel syndrome must be differentiated from tardy ulnar palsy, in which neuropathy develops years after an injury.

Radiographs may be helpful in defining the cubital tunnel area and may reveal lesions such as osteophytes, which may impinge on the nerve. Electrodiagnostic studies are useful in establishing that the site of ulnar compression is indeed the elbow and in following recovery after treatment. The readily accessible location of the entrapment area allows for direct testing of sensory and motor conduction across the cubital tunnel. High-resolution ultrasonography and MRI can accurately demonstrate ulnar nerve thickening as a result of entrapment.[12,13]

Treatment

When the symptoms are primarily sensory and motor weakness is not marked, avoidance of prolonged elbow flexion may be sufficient treatment. Compression resulting from inflammatory lesions, such as rheumatoid synovitis, may respond to local injection of corticosteroid along the ulnar groove, paying particular attention to avoid direct needle contact with the nerve.

In more advanced cases of cubital tunnel syndrome, a number of surgical procedures to decompress the nerve have been used. These include simple release of flexor carpi ulnaris aponeurosis, medial epicondylectomy, and anterior transposition of the nerve, the last being the most demanding operation. Simple decompression of the ulnar nerve is as effective as transposition and has fewer complications.[14] Because re-innervation of the nerve occurs slowly, in severe cases postsurgical recovery may take up to a year after a decompression procedure.

ULNAR TUNNEL SYNDROME

Ulnar tunnel syndrome results from entrapment of the ulnar nerve in Guyon's canal at the wrist.[15] Many factors that affect the carpal tunnel can also influence the ulnar tunnel, which is in close proximity; at times, both areas are simultaneously involved.

Anatomy

The ulnar tunnel is bounded on the sides by the hook of the hamate and the pisiform bone. Above and below the tunnel are the volar and transverse carpal ligaments, respectively (Fig. 78.6). Inside the tunnel, the ulnar nerve divides into sensory and motor branches.

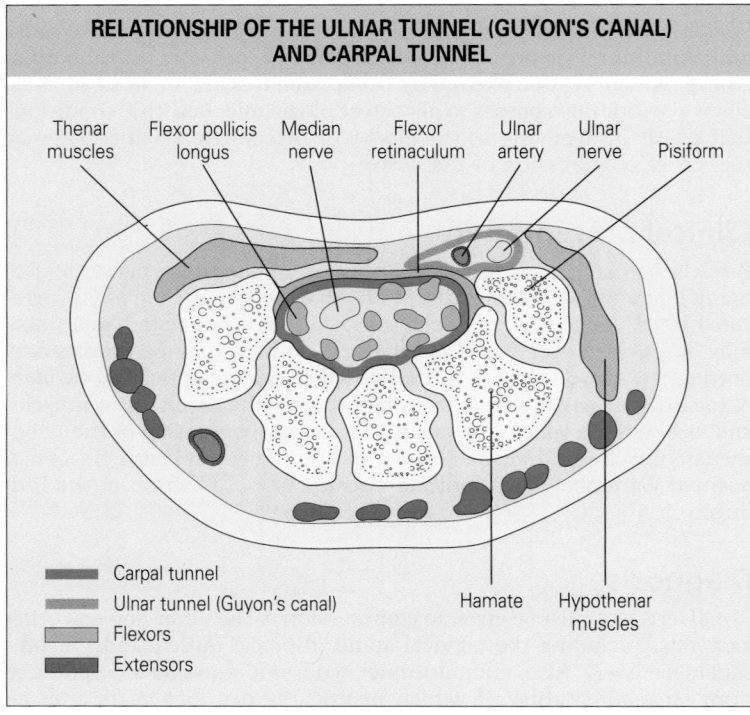

RELATIONSHIP OF THE ULNAR TUNNEL (GUYON'S CANAL) AND CARPAL TUNNEL

Thenar muscles — Flexor pollicis longus — Median nerve — Flexor retinaculum — Ulnar artery — Ulnar nerve — Pisiform

Carpal tunnel
Ulnar tunnel (Guyon's canal)
Flexors
Extensors

Hamate — Hypothenar muscles

Fig. 78.6 Relationship of the ulnar tunnel (Guyon's canal) and carpal tunnel. Because of the close relationship of the ulnar tunnel to the carpal tunnel, pathologic processes affecting one may simultaneously affect the other.

Etiology

The most common cause of nerve compression in Guyon's canal is ganglia. Aberrant muscles, Dupuytren's disease, rheumatoid arthritis (RA), and osteoarthritis may also cause impingement. Chronic trauma from use of certain tools and occupations that require blows to the palm also predispose to ulnar tunnel syndrome.

Clinical presentation

When compression of the nerve occurs in the proximal portion of the ulnar tunnel, the patient will have combined sensory and motor deficits, hypoesthesia in the hypothenar region and fourth and fifth fingers (see Fig. 78.10), and weakness of the intrinsic muscles of the hand. More distal lesions may present as either motor or sensory impairment.

Diagnosis

Electrodiagnostic studies are helpful in determining the site of entrapment and in defining which branches are involved. Ulnar tunnel syndrome must be differentiated from TOS and cubital tunnel syndrome.

Treatment

If conservative measures, such as avoidance of trauma to the palm, do not result in improvement, then surgical decompression may be necessary. When entrapment is caused by ganglia, synovitis, or fibrosis, offending tissue is excised.

MEDIAN NERVE COMPRESSION SYNDROMES

Forearm entrapments

Anterior interosseous nerve syndrome

The anterior interosseous nerve is a purely motor branch of the median nerve (Fig. 78.7). It innervates the pronator quadratus, the flexor pollicis longus, and the flexor digitorum profundus to the index finger. The nerve branches off from the median nerve about 6 cm below the lateral epicondyle. Entrapment may result from compression by aberrant or accessory muscles or fibrous bands beneath the pronator teres or by pressure from an enlarged bicipital bursa.

Because there are no sensory fibers in the nerve, the patient has no sensory complaints and experiences only motor weakness. The typical pattern is loss of distal flexion of the thumb and index finger, giving a characteristic pinch sign (Fig. 78.8). The pronator quadratus is tested with the elbow fully flexed. There is decreased resistance to forced supination of the forearm. The patient may also note a dull, aching pain in the volar aspect of the proximal forearm.

Confirmation of anterior interosseous nerve entrapment depends on electromyography of the forearm muscles. Findings on MRI include increased signal intensity on T2-weighted or short tau inversion recovery sequences and/or atrophy of the innervated muscles. Differential diagnosis for this syndrome should include rupture of the flexor pollicis longus tendon, which may occur in RA, and more proximal lesions such as brachial neuritis.

Because the condition improves with time in most patients, initial management is conservative, unless the condition has been brought about by a wound. The patient is advised to avoid repetitive forearm motions (pronation-supination). If the weakness does not resolve after 2 or 3 months, surgery is usually recommended.[16]

Pronator teres syndrome

There are several potential sites of median nerve entrapment in the forearm (see Fig. 78.7). It may occur at the lacertus fibrosus, at the proximal edge of the flexor digitorum superficialis, or, most commonly, by the pronator teres muscle itself or fibrous bands at the superficial head of this muscle.

The most consistent symptom in pronator teres syndrome is an aching pain in the proximal forearm, which often begins insidiously. This may be exacerbated by activities that require intensive use of the

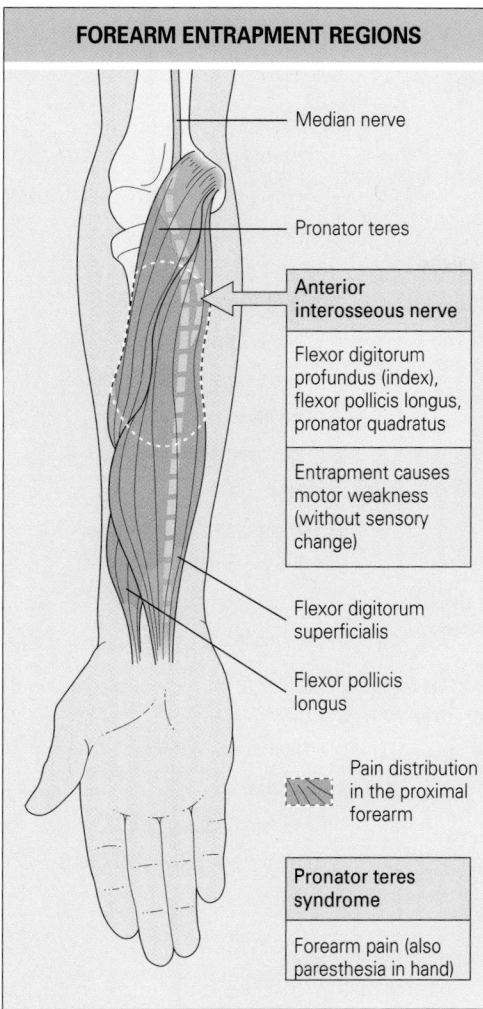

Fig. 78.7 Forearm entrapment regions. The median nerve may be compressed at several locations in the forearm, most commonly as it traverses the pronator teres muscle. The anterior interosseous branch of the median nerve is solely motor; thus entrapment produces no sensory deficit.

FOREARM ENTRAPMENT REGIONS

- Median nerve
- Pronator teres
- Anterior interosseous nerve
- Flexor digitorum profundus (index), flexor pollicis longus, pronator quadratus
- Entrapment causes motor weakness (without sensory change)
- Flexor digitorum superficialis
- Flexor pollicis longus
- Pain distribution in the proximal forearm

Pronator teres syndrome

Forearm pain (also paresthesia in hand)

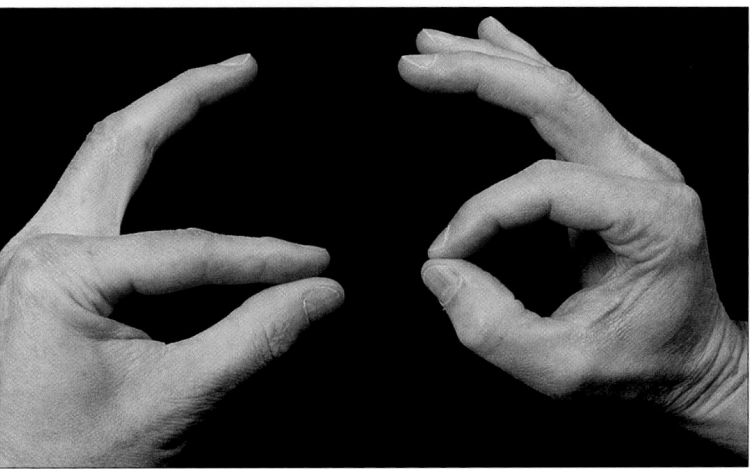

Fig. 78.8 Anterior interosseous nerve paralysis. The hand on the left demonstrates loss of function of flexor pollicis longus and flexor digitorum profundus muscles, resulting in a characteristic flattened pinch pattern.

elbow including pronation and grasping. Paresthesias are common and follow the median nerve distribution into the hand (see Fig. 78-10). Because sensory findings are similar to those of carpal tunnel syndrome (CTS), the two conditions may be confused. However, unlike in CTS, in pronator teres syndrome the nocturnal paresthesias are less frequent.

Physical examination may reveal local tenderness on palpation over the pronator teres muscle. In addition, percussion in this area may elicit a positive Tinel sign with radiation of pain into the hand. A provocation test that may reproduce the pain consists of pronation of the forearm and flexion of the wrist, performed against resistance. Some thenar atrophy may be noted, but profound muscle weakness is rare.

In a study by Hartz and colleagues,[17] electrophysiologic testing was often inconclusive and could not be relied on to exclude pronator teres syndrome. Differential diagnosis of pronator teres syndrome should include CTS and more proximal nerve lesions at the cervical spine or thoracic outlet. However, with thoracic outlet lesions the pain usually radiates into the ulnar rather than radial portion of the hand. There are few reports of effective imaging in this syndrome.

For some patients, sufficient treatment may be abstention from activities that aggravate the condition. Surgical decompression is performed when symptoms become chronic.

CARPAL TUNNEL SYNDROME

Carpal tunnel syndrome is the most common entrapment neuropathy. The syndrome has gained increased recognition in recent years because of the prominent attention it has received in certain industrial settings, and it is now one of the most commonly reported occupational illnesses.

Anatomy

The carpal tunnel is bound on its dorsal and lateral surfaces by the carpal bones with their connecting ligaments and on the volar or anterior aspect by the transverse carpal ligament (Fig. 78.9). Nine flexor tendons and the median nerve pass through the tunnel. There are two ways in which the median nerve may be entrapped: pressure may be exerted on the nerve as a result of reduction in capacity of the carpal tunnel, as with swelling or lesions of surrounding tissues, or there may be an increase in volume of the contents of the tunnel, an example being flexor tenosynovitis. Increased intracarpal canal pressures in patients with CTS have been confirmed by use of a wick catheter measuring device.[18]

Etiology

There are many causes of CTS (Table 78.2), but in some patients an underlying disease process cannot be identified and the designation "idiopathic CTS" is used. Because there is an increased awareness that certain occupational activities predispose to this disorder, and because more sophisticated diagnostic techniques have been developed, an attributable cause for CTS can now often be found.

Carpal tunnel syndrome is noted most commonly in persons whose occupation or avocation requires substantial use of the hands. The fact that CTS is found to occur more often in the dominant hand of both right- and left-handed individuals supports the concept that aggregate activity of the hand plays an important part in the genesis of this disorder.

Crystal-induced rheumatic disorders have been known to cause CTS. In the case of gout, tophaceous deposits or tenosynovitis may result in nerve entrapment. Both calcium pyrophosphate dihydrate and apatite crystals have been found in biopsy material taken from tendon sheaths during surgery for CTS.

CTS is reported as a complication of several connective tissue diseases, including systemic sclerosis, polymyositis, polymyalgia rheumatica, and, most commonly, RA. There are widely varying estimations of CTS frequency in RA, but it is the experience of many practitioners that it occurs commonly. Indeed, prolonged median nerve sensory conduction velocities have been noted in up to 50% of all RA patients tested.[19] Generally, CTS is a result of rheumatoid flexor tenosynovitis. When the symptoms are mild, it may be difficult to differentiate the muscle atrophy noted in CTS from that associated with severe rheumatoid disease. Interestingly, when CTS complicates juvenile arthritis, sensory abnormalities are rare, whereas thenar atrophy is more commonly noted than in adult CTS.[20]

THE CARPAL TUNNEL AND COURSE OF THE MEDIAN NERVE

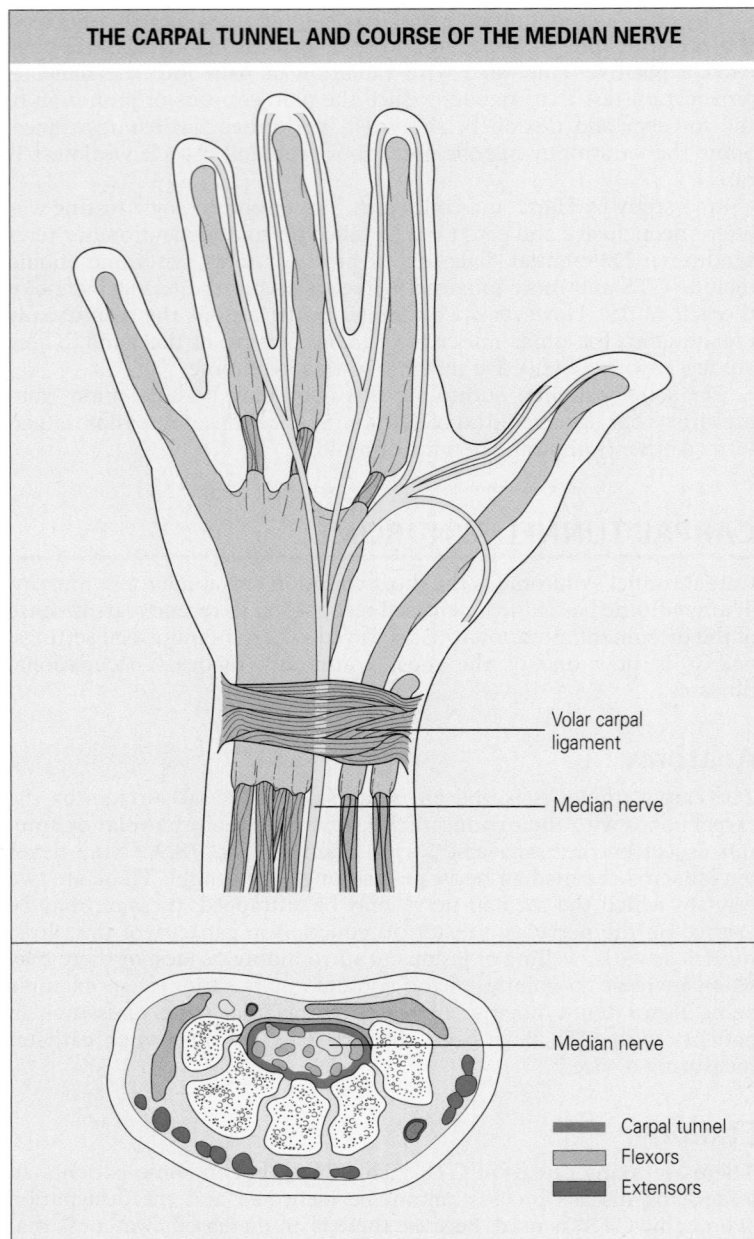

Volar carpal ligament

Median nerve

Median nerve

| Carpal tunnel |
| Flexors |
| Extensors |

Fig. 78.9 The carpal tunnel and course of the median nerve. The space for the median nerve and flexor tendons is very confined. The median nerve courses under the region occupied by the palmaris longus and flexor carpi radialis tendons.

TABLE 78.2 CONDITIONS ASSOCIATED WITH CARPAL TUNNEL SYNDROME

Space-occupying lesions	Ganglia
	Hemangioma
	Osteoid osteoma
	Thickened transverse carpal ligament (familial)
	Anomalous muscles
	Tenosynovitis (nonspecific)
Connective tissue disease	Rheumatoid arthritis
	Osteoarthritis
	Progressive systemic sclerosis
	Polymyositis
	Polymyalgia rheumatica
Crystal-induced rheumatic disease	Gout
	Calcium pyrophosphate dihydrate disease
	Hydroxyapatite disease
Occupational disease (repetitive motion disorders)	Meat cutters
	Musicians
	Keyboard workers
Metabolic and endocrine disease	Diabetes
	Thyroid (myxedema)
	Acromegaly
	Mucopolysaccharidosis
Infection	Osteomyelitis (carpal bones)
	Tenosynovitis
	Tuberculosis
	Atypical mycobacterial infection
	Histoplasmosis
	Coccidioidomycosis
Iatrogenic	Hematoma
	Phlebitis
Miscellaneous conditions	Pregnancy
	Amyloidosis
	Dialysis
	Fractures

Uremia, which is often complicated by peripheral neuropathy, also predisposes patients to entrapment neuropathy. CTS is particularly common in patients receiving hemodialysis[21]; and in many of these cases it is the result of β_2-microglobulin amyloid deposition. The erosive arthropathy associated with this variety of amyloid may also cause CTS when the wrist is affected.[22]

A number of metabolic and endocrine diseases may have CTS as one of their manifestations. These include diabetes, myxedema, mucopolysaccharidosis, and acromegaly. There is also an interesting, but as yet unexplained, association between idiopathic CTS and lateral humeral epicondylitis.

Infections involving carpal bones or flexor tendons at the wrist may result in CTS. These include chronic granulomatous infections caused by *Coccidioides, Histoplasma, Mycobacterium tuberculosis,* and atypical mycobacteria.

Familial occurrence of CTS has also been reported. Amyloid deposition has not been identified in these individuals, but in some cases thickening of the transverse carpal ligament has been noted at surgery. This condition might be an important factor in compression of the median nerve. In one family, the mean age at onset of CTS was 24 years and flexor tenosynovitis was the dominant finding.[23] The onset of symptoms in familial CTS may even occur in early childhood.

All varieties of amyloidosis—primary, secondary, hereditary and associated with myeloma—may cause CTS. Some hereditary forms of amyloidosis predispose to development of peripheral neuropathy, whereas others are more likely to cause CTS. Lambird and Hartmann[24] have shown that the transverse carpal ligament may appear grossly normal at the time of surgery but, unless histologic stains for amyloid are performed, the diagnosis of hereditary amyloidosis may be missed. In myelomatosis, there may be significant amyloid deposition along the flexor tendons, resulting in tethering of the tendons in the carpal tunnel.

Although the occurrence of CTS in pregnancy has been well documented, the high incidence of this disorder has not been appreciated. It has been attributed, by some, to fluid retention. In one series, 21% of pregnant women described paresthesias or hypoesthesia quite typical of CTS.[25] For the majority of patients, symptoms begin in the third trimester, usually resolve spontaneously after delivery, and do not require surgery.

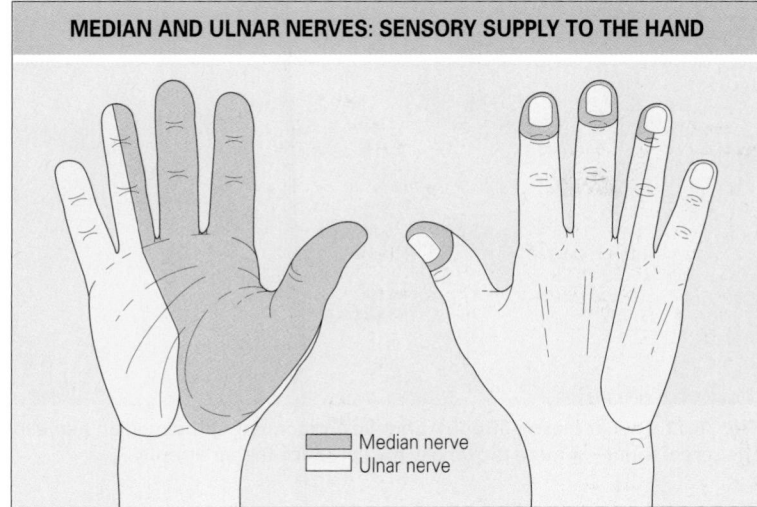

MEDIAN AND ULNAR NERVES: SENSORY SUPPLY TO THE HAND

Median nerve
Ulnar nerve

Fig. 78.10 Median and ulnar nerves: sensory supply to the hand. The radial three digits and half of the ring finger are supplied by sensory branches of the median nerve. The fifth finger and half of the ring finger are supplied by sensory branches of the ulnar nerve.

TABLE 78.3 SYMPTOMS AND SIGNS OF CARPAL TUNNEL SYNDROME	
Symptom or sign	Percentage of patients*
Median paresthesias	100
Nocturnal paresthesias	71
Proximal extension of pain	38
Tinel's sign	
Positive	55
Negative	29
Unknown	17
Phalen's test	
Positive	53
Negative	23
Unknown	24
Sensation on sensory examination	
Decreased	28
Normal	36
Unknown	36
Thenar muscle strength	
Decreased	18
Normal	42
Unknown	41
Thenar muscle bulk	
Wasted	18
Normal	31
Unknown	50

*Data from 1016 patients.
Data from Spinner RJ, Bachman JW, Amadio PC. The many faces of carpal tunnel syndrome. Mayo Clin Proc 1989;64:829-836.

In addition, CTS may also be a manifestation of repetitive strain syndrome. Workers who spend long hours using a keyboard, musicians who keep the wrist in a flexed position, and meat cutters are all especially susceptible to developing CTS.

A number of local space-occupying lesions may impinge on the contents of the carpal tunnel. These include an anomalous median artery, ganglia, hemangiomas, osteoid osteomas, and lipomas. Anomalous muscles may also compromise the carpal tunnel space. Most often this is caused by abnormalities of the palmaris longus, an extremely variable muscle, which inserts on the transverse carpal ligament.[26]

Clinical presentation

Because the median nerve supplies sensory branches to the radial three fingers and one half of the ring finger, these digits may have sensory loss in CTS (Fig. 78.10). Typically, patients complain of burning, pins-and-needles sensations, numbness, and tingling in the fingers (Table 78.3). When they are questioned about the location of paresthesias, many will indicate that the entire hand is involved. Only after careful examination does it become clear that the sensory abnormalities are limited to the area of median nerve distribution.

In some cases, pain may not follow the usual pattern of radiation in the median nerve distribution of the hand. Silver and colleagues[27] found that 34% of patients with CTS also had signs of ulnar nerve compression. Proximal pain, often with a dull or aching quality, is also a common feature of CTS.[8] Pain may radiate to the antecubital region or to the lateral shoulder area. Although the possibility of more proximal entrapment should be kept in mind, the majority of patients experience symptom improvement after nerve decompression at the carpal tunnel.

Perhaps the archetypal complaint of patients with CTS is that they are awakened at night by abnormal sensations. Often it is this interruption of sleep that is the most troublesome aspect of CTS. Commonly, the patient will shake the hand in an attempt to relieve the numbness and may run it under warm water to improve the circulation.

Activities that result in persistent or repeated flexion or extension of the wrists are more likely to intensify symptoms. These include holding a newspaper or book, grasping a steering wheel, and occupations such as meat cutting, in which a utensil is grasped with the wrist in flexion. Some patients report that they are more likely to drop objects, and they attribute this to hand weakness. However, these individuals rarely have profound weakness on grip testing and it is more likely that the problem stems from sensory deficit at the fingertips.

Tests

Testing for Tinel's sign consists of tapping lightly over the median nerve and is positive if the patient perceives paresthesia that radiates distally. The diagnostic value depends largely on how the test is conducted. Mossman and Blau[28] found that, to be effective, percussion must be performed with the patient's wrist in extension so that the carpal tunnel is compressed. They also noted that using a fingertip or small neurology hammer is less effective than using a broad-head hammer that can percuss over the entire transverse carpal ligament and somewhat more proximally (Fig. 78.11). The wrist flexion (Phalen's) test (Fig. 78.12) is performed by having the patient hold the wrists in extreme but unforced flexion for 1 minute. It is positive if paresthesias are reproduced. As with Tinel's sign, the wrist flexion test in CTS is not invariably positive, but when it is it helps substantiate the diagnosis.

Another provocative test for CTS is the carpal compression test, in which pressure is applied directly over the carpal tunnel and underlying median nerve. Opinions are conflicting as to whether it is more sensitive or specific than Tinel's or Phalen's tests. When compared with the gold standard of electrophysiologic testing, the carpal compression test appears to have only marginal predictive value.[29]

To determine motor loss, the strength of the thenar muscles should be tested. The easiest muscle to test is the abductor pollicis brevis. With the thumb first adducted toward the fifth finger, the patient is then asked to abduct against resistance to the distal phalanx. The opponens pollicis muscle is tested by having the patient touch the tip of the thumb to the tip of the fifth finger, then the examiner attempts to break the pinch. Inspection of the hand may reveal atrophy of the thenar muscles (Fig. 78.13).

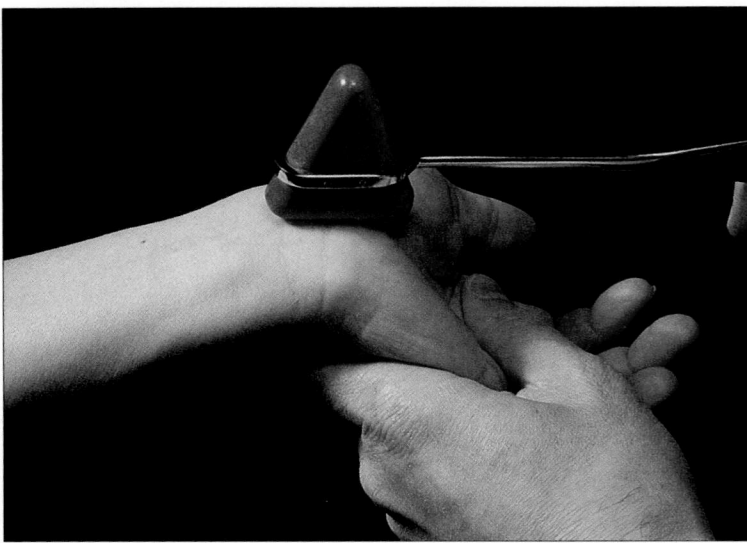

Fig. 78.11 Tinel's sign. The wrist is held in extension while gentle percussion is performed over and just proximal to the transverse carpal ligament.

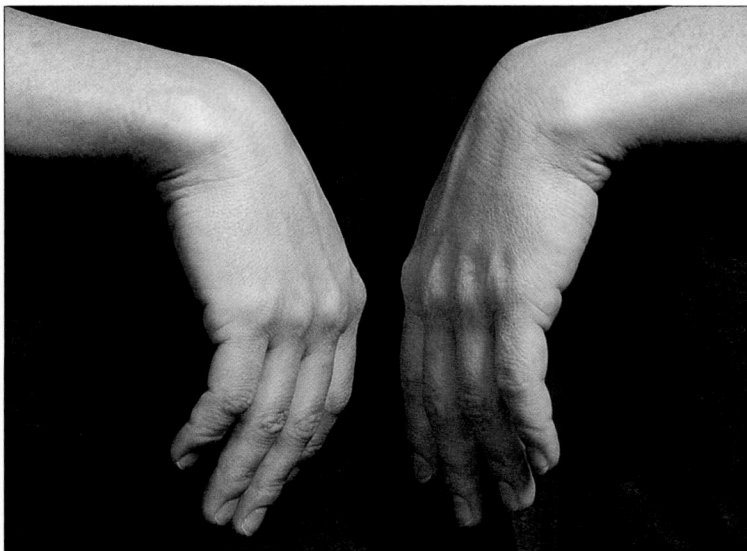

Fig. 78.12 Phalen's (wrist flexion) test. With the wrists held in unforced flexion for 30 to 60 seconds, a positive test reproduces or worsens the patient's symptoms.

Diagnosis

Carpal tunnel syndrome is diagnosed on the basis of the patient's history and clinical examination, but imaging and electrodiagnostic studies may be useful in confirming the diagnostic impression. Conventional radiographs using a carpal tunnel projection can help to delineate the soft tissues and the carpal bones. Increasingly, ultrasonography has been found to be very effective in diagnosing CTS.[30] Typically, it reveals swelling of the median nerve in the proximal tunnel and flattening more distally. Some have even suggested that it should be the study of first choice even before electodiagnostic testing.[31] However, the anatomy of the carpal tunnel, thickening of flexor tendon sheaths, or presence of space-occupying lesions or aberrant muscle can be better visualized by MRI.[32]

The most important electrodiagnostic study is the measurement of sensory nerve conduction velocity across the carpal tunnel. A slowed conduction velocity, along with prolongation of distal motor latency, lends support to the diagnosis of CTS.

In about 15% of the population, fibers from the median nerve travel via the ulnar nerve to the thenar muscles: the Martin Gruber anastomosis. It is important to recognize this entity, because it may result in the sparing of the thenar muscles in CTS. A clue to the presence of

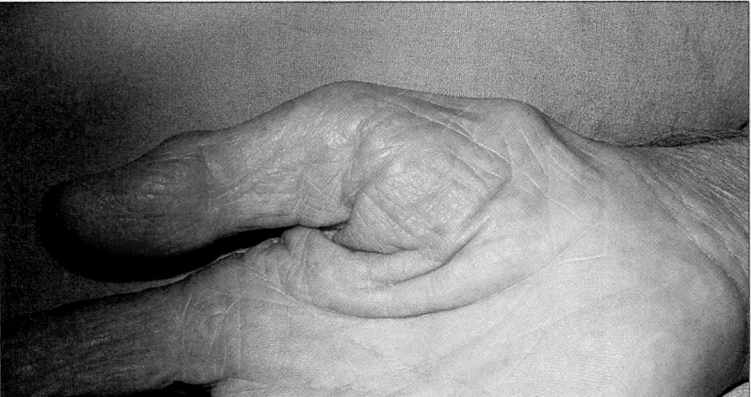

Fig. 78.13 Thenar muscle atrophy. Chronic entrapment of the median nerve in the carpal tunnel or more proximally may produce thenar atrophy.

this anatomic variation is the finding of normal proximal latency but a prolonged distal latency.

Differential diagnosis of CTS must include median nerve entrapment proximal to the carpal tunnel.[5] As noted earlier, compression of the median nerve near the elbow, as found in pronator teres syndrome, may give similar sensory findings.

Treatment

The specific treatment of CTS depends, to a large degree, on whether there is an identifiable cause of the entrapment. Conservative measures may suffice when symptoms are of short duration. Repeated electromyographic determinations, performed over time, may help the clinician determine the correct therapeutic approach. Patients with progressive increases in distal motor latency times should be considered for surgery.

Splinting

Splinting is a simple and cost-effective modality that, if successful in relieving symptoms, helps to confirm the diagnosis of CTS. Because wrist motion often worsens CTS, splinting is an important treatment element. A volar wrist splint that keeps the wrist in a neutral position is particularly helpful during the night, when the wrist often falls into a position of flexion. Splinting alone may be sufficient to relieve CTS, primarily in cases in which symptoms are of recent onset.

Local injection of corticosteroid

Injection of the carpal tunnel is another effective treatment in individuals whose disease is of shorter duration and in whom there is no significant muscle wasting. The best response to injection is in patients whose symptoms have been present for less than 1 year and in whom there is no significant muscle atrophy or weakness. A recent randomized, controlled trial comparing local corticosteroid injection to surgical decompression found that, over the short term, injection provided better relief and was equal to surgery in alleviating symptoms at 1 year.[33]

Before injection is attempted, certain landmarks should be identified, including the tendons of the palmaris longus and flexor carpi radialis muscles (Fig. 78.14). This is most easily accomplished by asking the patient to flex against resistance. Injection can be facilitated if the wrist is placed in slight extension (the wrist draped over a small rolled up towel). The needle is inserted ulnar (medial) to the palmaris longus tendon and proximal to the wrist crease (Fig. 78.15). Local anesthetic may be used, but deep infiltration is unwise, because the patient will not be responsive to needle contact with the median nerve and a neuritis might result. If the patient notes median nerve paresthesia during injection, the needle should be withdrawn and repositioned. Methylprednisolone or triamcinolone may be used to treat CTS and, if improvement is not complete, consideration may be given to a second injection. Frequent injections are proscribed because there is danger of tendon rupture.

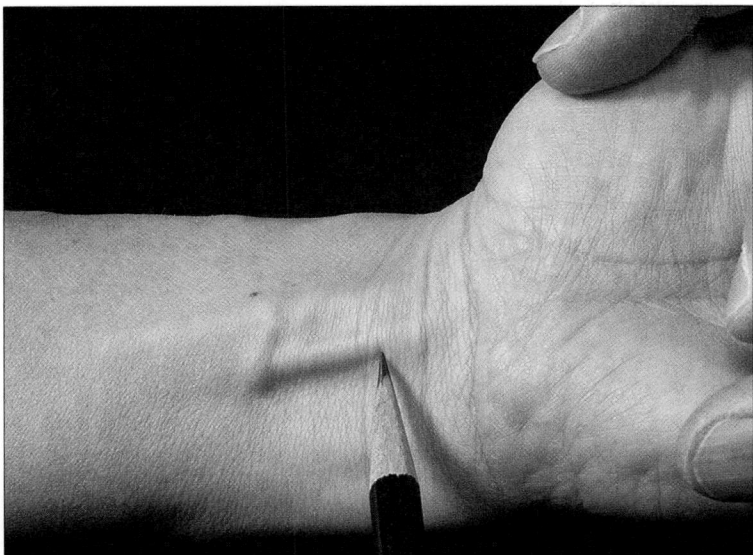

Fig. 78.14 Palmaris longus tendon. The pencil point identifies the tendon of the palmaris longus muscle, an important landmark in determining the site of injection for carpal tunnel syndrome. The tendon of the flexor carpi radialis can be seen just to the radial side of the palmaris longus tendon.

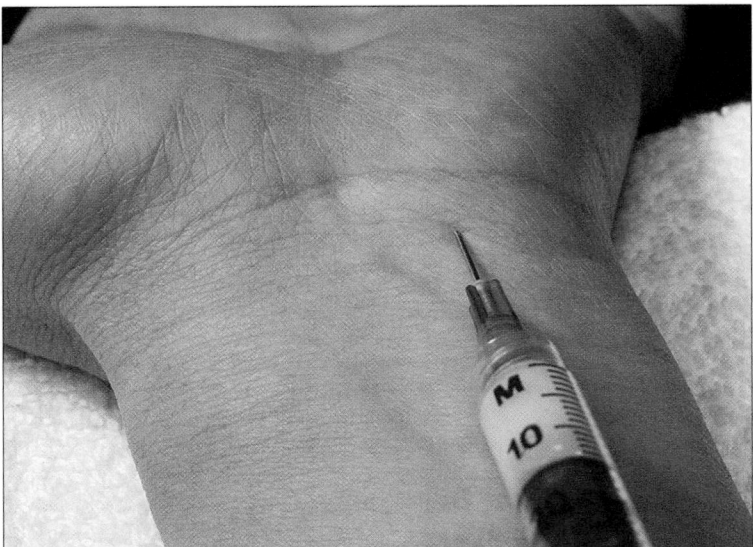

Fig. 78.15 Carpal tunnel injection. The needle is inserted just proximal to the wrist crease and to the ulnar side of the palmaris longus tendon.

Non-steroidal anti-inflammatory drugs and other agents

Use of non-steroidal anti-inflammatory drugs (NSAIDs) is generally limited to instances in which there is an underlying inflammatory lesion, such as tenosynovitis. Oral corticosteroids also appear to be an effective treatment in mild to moderate cases of CTS.

Surgery

Surgical release of the transverse carpal ligament is the definitive treatment for more severe cases of CTS. Surgery is indicated when response to conservative measures is inadequate, when there are progressive or persistent neurologic changes, or when there is muscle atrophy. In those circumstances in which there is marked tenosynovitis, as with RA or granulomatous disease, simple decompression of the carpal tunnel may not be sufficient; additional tenosynovectomy with lysis of adhesions may be necessary. Furthermore, when there are infiltrating processes, such as amyloid deposits, attached to tendons, the more complicated procedure of tenolysis may be necessary. Because tuberculosis and fungal infections are sometimes a cause of CTS,

appropriate cultures and histologic studies should be undertaken at the time of surgery, particularly if tenosynovitis is noted. The traditional surgical approach of ligament sectioning using a palmar incision is increasingly being replaced by endoscopic release. However, there is controversy among hand surgeons because there is no strong evidence supporting this newer technique.[34] Although equally effective, it must be performed with great care to avoid injury to the superficial palmar arterial arch or to the median or ulnar nerves.[35]

Failure of surgery to relieve symptoms is often the result of incomplete release of the ligament. Postoperative improvement depends in part on the severity of initial nerve deficit. Although most patients' symptoms are ameliorated by surgery, those individuals whose occupations require repetitive motions may need to be retrained for less hand-intensive work.

RADIAL NERVE COMPRESSION SYNDROME

Posterior interosseous nerve syndrome

Posterior interosseous nerve syndrome is a well recognized, but uncommon entity. It is caused by the compression of the radial nerve. The most common site of compression is at the level of the supinator muscle.[36]

Anatomy

The radial nerve comes off the posterior branch of the brachial plexus (C5 through C8, T1), and it branches proximal to the lateral epicondyle into a superficial sensory branch and a deep motor branch. The deep motor branch pierces the supinator muscle and courses along the dorsal aspect of the interosseous membrane. The deep motor branch is called the posterior interosseous nerve.[37]

Etiology

Posterior interosseous nerve syndrome can be caused by intrinsic as well as extrinsic lesions. Trauma, inflammatory processes such as rheumatoid arthritis, and space-occupying lesions may be causative.[37]

Clinical presentation

The patient with posterior interosseous syndrome usually presents with forearm pain. Other patients describe weakness of the extensor muscles. If entrapment occurs at the level of the supinator, the radial wrist extensors innervated at this level will be spared because they branch off proximal to the posterior interosseous nerve. Complete sparing of the extensor carpi radialis longus and frequent sparing of the extensor carpi radialis brevis occurs because they, too, branch off proximal to the posterior interosseous nerve. As a result, the ulnar wrist extensors and extensors of the metacarpophalangeal joints will be compromised. With attempted wrist extension, the wrist deviates radially in the posterior interosseous nerve syndrome. The extensor muscles of the fingers are affected, which makes it difficult to maintain the fingers in extension. There is no reflex or sensory loss in this syndrome.

Diagnosis

The differential diagnosis of posterior interosseous nerve syndrome includes lateral epicondylitis and other chronic pain syndromes in the region of the elbow and forearm. Other diagnoses to consider in patients with wristdrop and fingerdrop include a central lesion or a lesion in the posterior cord of the brachial plexus. Electrodiagnostic studies are useful in confirming the diagnosis of posterior interosseous nerve syndrome from other causes.[38]

Treatment

The treatment of posterior interosseous nerve syndrome is usually via conservative methods. Modalities such as splinting can be used. For those patients who do not have a resolution of their symptoms through

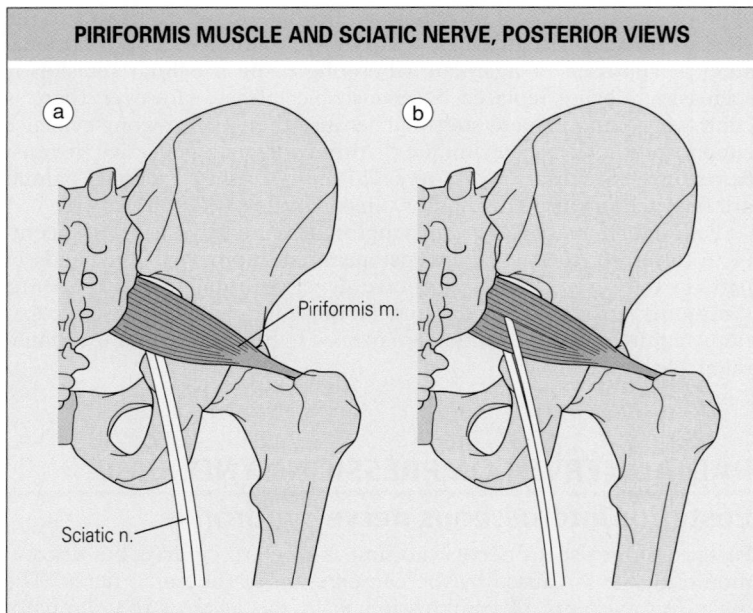

PIRIFORMIS MUSCLE AND SCIATIC NERVE, POSTERIOR VIEWS

(a) (b)

Piriformis m.

Sciatic n.

Fig. 78.16 Piriformis muscle and sciatic nerve, posterior views. The piriformis muscle arises from the anterior surface of the sacrum and the gluteal surface of the ilium and crosses the greater sciatic foramen to insert onto the superior border of the greater trochanter. (a) In most instances, the sciatic nerve passes along the anterior surface of the piriformis muscle and exits the pelvis below the piriformis muscle, passing posteriorly along its inferior border. (b) In some individuals, a portion of the sciatic nerve passes through the piriformis muscle. Other anatomic variants have been described.

conservative management, surgery is an option. Posterior interosseous nerve syndrome that results from compression by a tumor should be treated surgically.[37]

PIRIFORMIS SYNDROME

Piriformis syndrome results from compression of the sciatic nerve by the piriformis muscle. This syndrome, although relatively uncommon and underdiagnosed, nevertheless accounts for a discrete portion of patients who present with buttock and sciatic-type pain.

Anatomy

As the sciatic nerve passes through the greater sciatic foramen, it is in close proximity to the piriformis muscle (Fig. 78.16). The muscle originates from the anterior surface of the sacrum and the gluteal surface of the ilium. After passing through the sciatic foramen, it inserts on the medial aspect of the greater trochanter. Usually the sciatic nerve passes below the piriformis muscle, but in some cases a segment of the nerve or the whole nerve passes through the muscle.

Etiology

The leading cause of piriformis syndrome is believed to be trauma to the gluteal region with resultant inflammation and spasm of the muscle. This, in turn, leads to irritation of the sciatic nerve. When the nerve, or a portion of the nerve, passes through the muscle, nerve compression can occur with stretching of the muscle on internal hip rotation.

Clinical presentation

Typically, patients with piriformis syndrome complain of pain in the buttock region with radiation to the posterior thigh. However, discomfort and paresthesias may occur along the whole course of the sciatic nerve. Pain may be brought on by prolonged sitting or by stooping and lifting.

On physical examination, pain may be elicited by direct pressure applied over the gluteal region. Also, piriformis muscle tenderness or spasm may be noted on rectal or pelvic examination. Maneuvers that internally rotate, flex, and adduct the hip often cause aggravation of

the pain because this stretches the piriformis muscle. With the patient seated, resisted abduction of the hip (the Pace sign) may also elicit pain.

Diagnosis

Included in the differential diagnosis of piriformis syndrome are conditions that result in sciatic nerve irritation, such as herniated lumbar disc, spinal stenosis, or pelvic lesion, but it is unusual for the patient with piriformis syndrome to have neurologic defects. Thus, the diagnosis is often one of exclusion.

MRI is useful in detecting changes in the piriformis muscle and in defining its relationship to the sciatic nerve.[39] It is also a means of excluding mass lesions in the pelvic area as well as spinal stenosis and disc herniation.

Treatment

Initial management of piriformis syndrome consists of conservative measures, including physical therapy, analgesics, and non-steroidal anti-inflammatory drugs (NSAIDs). Direct injection of corticosteroids or botulinum toxin into the piriformis muscle appears to benefit some patients.[40] Patients who do not respond to conservative therapy may be candidates for surgical intervention. The piriformis is released from its insertion on the femur to allow for reattachment in a shortened position.[41]

MERALGIA PARESTHETICA

The term *meralgia* has it roots in the Greek words for thigh (*meros*) and a painful condition (*algia*). Meralgia paresthetica is caused by entrapment of the lateral femoral cutaneous nerve. One of the earliest descriptions of this entity was by Sigmund Freud, in which he related the typical symptoms of meralgia paresthetica that he experienced.[42] Although meralgia paresthetica occurs primarily in adults, children may be affected; and often there is a significant delay in diagnosis.[43]

Anatomy

The lateral femoral cutaneous nerve is entirely sensory and arises from the second and third lumbar roots. It proceeds from the lateral border of the psoas muscle, along the ilium, to pass under or through the lateral aspect of the inguinal ligament just medial to the anterior superior iliac spine, the most common site of entrapment (Fig. 78.17). The nerve travels down the anterior thigh, where it divides into anterior and posterior branches. These supply sensation to the anterolateral portion of the thigh.

Etiology

Direct pressure from belts and other tight-fitting garments may contribute to the entrapment of the lateral femoral cutaneous nerve as it passes under the inguinal ligament. Workers who support heavy bundles on their thigh are also at risk. Several clinical conditions have been associated with the development of meralgia paresthetica, including obesity, pregnancy, diabetes, ascites, and trauma to the thigh or inguinal region. The neuropathy may also occur as a consequence of direct injury to the nerve during surgery in the pelvic region (e.g., appendectomy, inguinal herniorrhaphy, iliac bone procurement, bariatric surgery).

Clinical presentation

Patients with meralgia paresthetica typically complain of burning pain and dysesthesia in the sensory distribution of the nerve. However, a smaller area of sensory deficit is common. The patient may volunteer that certain positions seem to exacerbate the discomfort, such as sitting with the legs crossed, prolonged standing, or extending the leg posteriorly.

Diagnosis

In the differential diagnosis of meralgia paresthetica it is important to consider the possibility that there may be radiculopathy of the L2 or L3 nerve roots or spinal stenosis causing the symptoms. Some patients will report direct tenderness over the inguinal ligament.

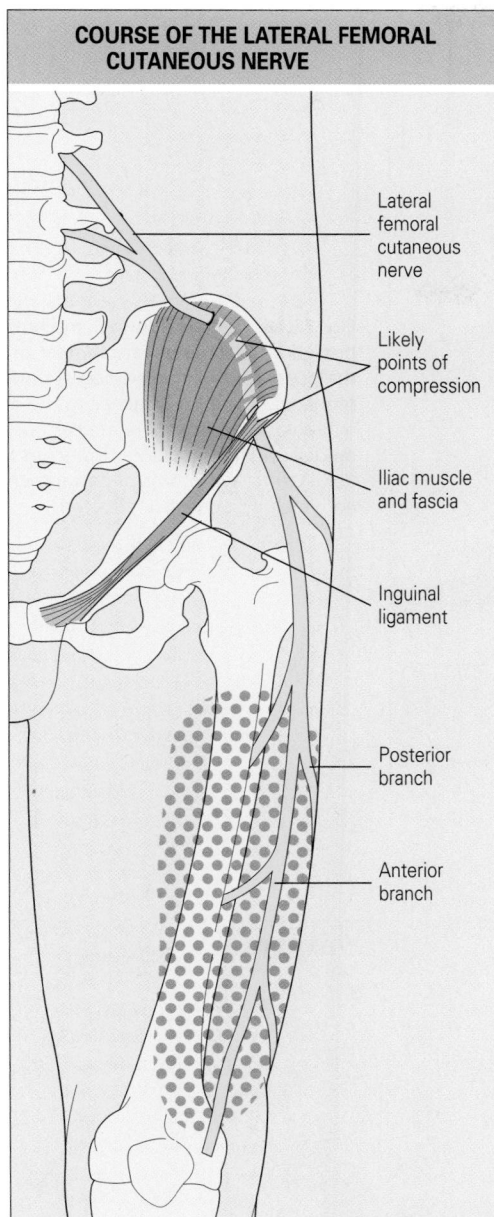

COURSE OF THE LATERAL FEMORAL CUTANEOUS NERVE

Lateral femoral cutaneous nerve

Likely points of compression

Iliac muscle and fascia

Inguinal ligament

Posterior branch

Anterior branch

Fig. 78.17 Course of the lateral femoral cutaneous nerve. The potential for entrapment of the lateral femoral cutaneous nerve can be seen by its course just under the inguinal ligament and medial to the anterior superior iliac spine.

Electrodiagnosis, using superficial electrodes to measure the conduction velocity of the nerve, may be useful in confirming the diagnosis. Nerve block may also affirm the diagnosis in addition to offering pain relief.

Treatment

Because meralgia paresthetica is often self-limiting, conservative measures should be used. These might include weight reduction, elimination of occupational trauma, and avoidance of external mechanical pressure over the inguinal ligament. Local injection of anesthetic and corticosteroids may be useful, as may be NSAIDs.

If meralgia paresthetica becomes chronic and the pain unremitting, surgical decompression (neurolysis) or transection of the nerve may be considered.[44] When it is of spinal origin, epidural injection of a corticosteroid may be helpful.

TARSAL TUNNEL SYNDROME

The occurrence of tarsal tunnel syndrome is undoubtedly more frequent than is suggested by isolated reports in the literature.[45] It is often mistaken for other disorders of the foot, and clinicians are less likely to include this entrapment neuropathy in the differential diagnosis of foot pain (see Chapter 75).

Anatomy

The tarsal tunnel is a fibro-osseous canal formed by the flexor retinaculum (laciniate ligament) as it extends from the medial malleolus down onto the calcaneus (Fig. 78.18). The posterior tibial nerve passes through the tunnel, along with vascular structures, tendons of the flexor hallucis longus, and the flexor digitorum longus muscles. Along its course, the tibial nerve gives off calcaneal branches and then lateral and medial plantar branches (see Fig. 78.18). The calcaneal branches are solely sensory, but the plantar nerves have mixed motor and sensory functions. Because the narrowest aspect of the tunnel is the distal or anteroinferior portion, this is where the plantar nerve branches are most likely to be entrapped.

Etiology

A number of abnormalities have been described as causing tarsal tunnel syndrome. These include bone deformity after fractures, pressure from casts, hypertrophy of the laciniate ligament or of the abductor hallucis muscle, flexor tenosynovitis, synovial cysts, ganglia, and diabetes mellitus. Proliferative synovitis accompanying RA is also causative.

Clinical presentation

Signs and symptoms of tarsal tunnel syndrome depend on the level of stenosis and consequently on which branches of the posterior tibial nerve are involved. The patient usually complains of burning pain or paresthesias in the toes, sole, or heel of the foot. As in CTS, pain may awaken the patient at night and may move in a retrograde fashion to the calf. Relief may be obtained by walking. Commonly, there is tenderness to direct palpation over the nerve posterior to the medial malleolus and there may be a fusiform swelling in this region. Other findings can include a positive Tinel sign over the tarsal tunnel, vasomotor changes, and weakness of toe flexion and of the intrinsic muscles of the foot.

Diagnosis

In the differential diagnosis of tarsal tunnel syndrome, one must consider arthritis of the tarsal bones, plantar fasciitis, vascular insufficiency, and systemic peripheral neuropathy. Tarsal tunnel syndrome may also be confused with lumbosacral nerve root radiculopathy. Another differential condition, particularly in runners, is hypertrophy of the abductor hallucis muscle; however, in this case, the compression of the plantar nerve occurs distal to the laciniate ligament.

Electrodiagnostic studies are useful in confirming the diagnosis of tarsal tunnel syndrome. Nerve conduction velocities are often diminished, and there may be abnormalities of distal motor latencies. Prolonged distal motor latencies of plantar nerves may occur in 25% of patients with RA. MRI is the best method for demonstrating the anatomy of the tarsal tunnel and thus for detecting space-occupying lesions.[38]

Treatment

A number of conservative therapies have been used in tarsal tunnel syndrome, including local injection of corticosteroid, NSAIDs, and orthotics. None of these has been consistently effective. The standard treatment is surgical decompression, which gives excellent results in the majority of patients.[46] If the patient's symptoms are the result of pressure on the nerve from the abductor hallucis muscle, release of the muscle at its origin is performed, rather than sectioning of the flexor retinaculum.

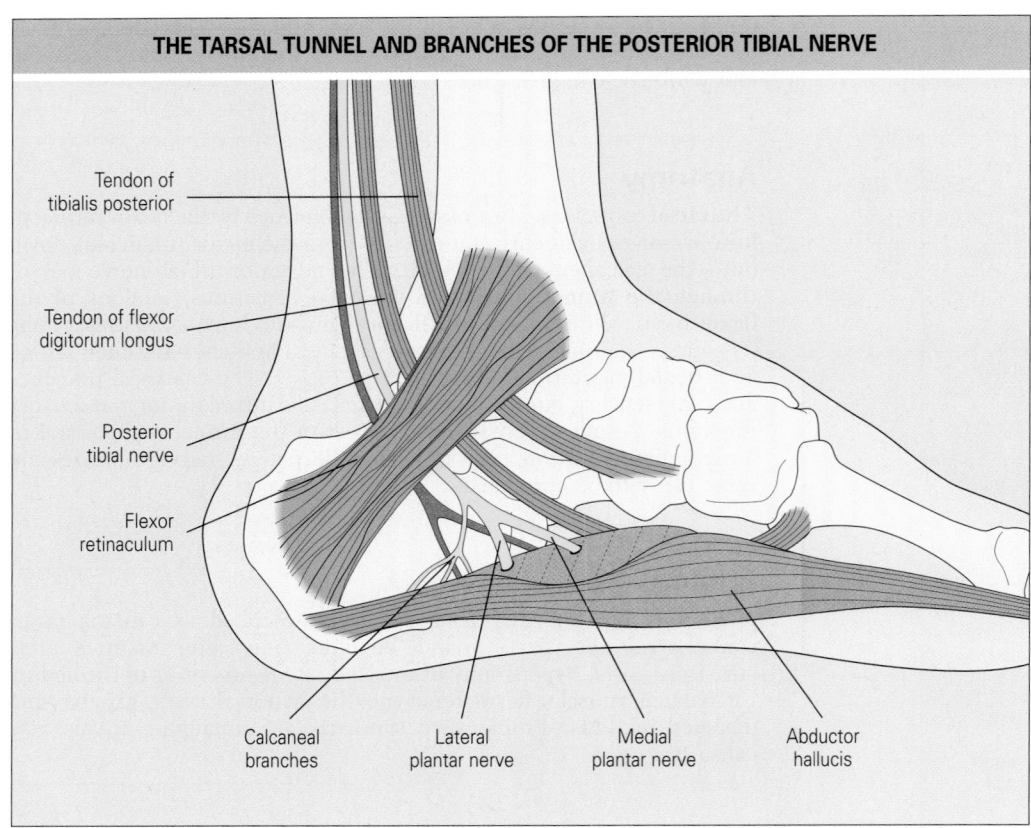

THE TARSAL TUNNEL AND BRANCHES OF THE POSTERIOR TIBIAL NERVE

Tendon of tibialis posterior

Tendon of flexor digitorum longus

Posterior tibial nerve

Flexor retinaculum

Calcaneal branches

Lateral plantar nerve

Medial plantar nerve

Abductor hallucis

Fig. 78.18 The tarsal tunnel and branches of the posterior tibial nerve. Entrapment of branches of the posterior tibial nerve occurs under the flexor retinaculum, which attaches to the medial malleolus. Because there are calcaneal as well as medial and lateral plantar branches of the posterior tibial nerve, symptoms of entrapment will depend on which branches are affected.

MORTON'S METATARSALGIA (MORTON'S NEUROMA, INTERDIGITAL NEURITIS)

Entrapment neuropathy of the interdigital plantar nerves occurs most commonly in the web space between the third and fourth toes but may affect other interspaces also. Chronic irritation of the nerve may lead to the development of a neuroma (see Chapter 75).

Anatomy

The medial and lateral plantar nerves of the foot divide into digital nerves in the web spaces between the toes. These interdigital nerves lie on the plantar side of the transverse metatarsal ligament (Fig. 78.19). Between the metatarsal joints are bursae that project distally and are close to the neurovascular bundle.

Etiology

Because the interdigital nerves are on the plantar side of the transverse metatarsal ligament, entrapment as a result of compression between the metatarsal heads, as originally proposed by Morton, is highly unlikely. It is more probable that the taut ligament itself is the cause of entrapment. In addition, there is evidence that the intermetatarsal bursae may also impinge on the nerve directly or, when inflamed, cause metatarsalgia. Wearing tight-fitting shoes or high heels also tends to aggravate the condition, and this may explain why women are more often affected.

Clinical presentation

Typically, patients complain of an aching or burning pain that radiates from the web space distally to the affected toes. Activities such as jogging or long periods of standing may worsen the metatarsalgia, as does walking on hard surfaces. There is often tenderness when direct pressure is applied over the interspace between the metatarsal bones, and occasionally a painful nodule may be palpated.

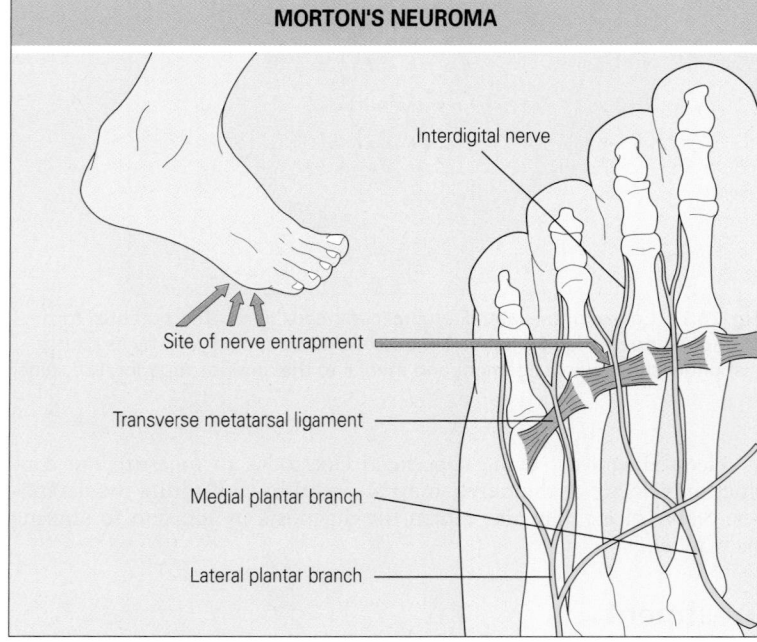

MORTON'S NEUROMA

Interdigital nerve

Site of nerve entrapment

Transverse metatarsal ligament

Medial plantar branch

Lateral plantar branch

Fig. 78.19 Morton's neuroma. On the plantar surface of the foot, the interdigital nerve is compressed below the transverse metatarsal ligament and not between the metatarsal heads (plantar view).

Diagnosis

Morton's metatarsalgia must be differentiated from inflammatory conditions affecting the forefoot. RA may present as metatarsalgia, but in most cases examination reveals synovitis, and neuritic pain is uncommon. Conventional radiographs are of little value in diagnosing Morton's neuroma but may demonstrate other causes of forefoot pain such as exostosis or fracture. Ultrasonography can identify neuromas, which appear as ovoid, hypoechoic lesions. MRI is very effective in identifying and localizing the neuroma. Interestingly, lesions consistent with neuroma may be found in 33% of asymptomatic individuals.[47]

Treatment

Initial treatment should include conservative measures such as padding the metatarsal area and use of broad-toed shoes. There are also reports of benefit derived from injection of a local anesthetic and corticosteroids.

When conservative treatment fails, the traditional approach has been surgical resection of the neuroma. The clear drawback to this procedure is that the patient is left with a sensory deficit. Another strategy is release of the transverse metatarsal ligament and epineural neurolysis of the interdigital nerve.[48] This method avoids neurectomy, while decompressing the nerve.

Compartmental syndromes

Compartmental syndromes can be defined as an increase in tissue pressure, within a confined space or muscle compartment, that compromises local circulation and neurologic function.

Acute compartment syndrome

Acute compartment syndrome is a surgical emergency and may result from a direct blow to the muscle, from the trauma associated with a fracture, or from prolonged pressure over a muscle compartment. It also occurs rarely after prolonged exertion. Acute compartment syndromes can lead to rapid and complete muscle necrosis due to vascular compromise. Early surgical decompression of the compartment may allow restoration of circulation to the muscle and preserve function. The clinical diagnosis of acute compartment syndrome is suspected in patients who have pain that is out of proportion to the injury or history of injury, swelling and firmness of the muscle compartment, and pain on passive stretch. Later in the evolution of acute compartment syndrome, patients develop signs of decreased perfusion, including decreased pulses, decreased capillary refill, and skin pallor. Neurologic symptoms may also appear.

Chronic compartment syndrome

This is the typical form seen in athletes and is characterized by a return to normal function between episodes of exercise-induced pain. It is most commonly seen in the lower leg.

The muscles of the leg are contained within four compartments separated by deep transverse fascia (Fig. 78.20). The athlete describes aching or cramping of the leg, roughly in the distribution of the involved compartment. The period from commencement of exercise to the onset of symptoms is variable and depends on the type and intensity of exercise but is usually within 10 to 30 minutes. Return to normal is

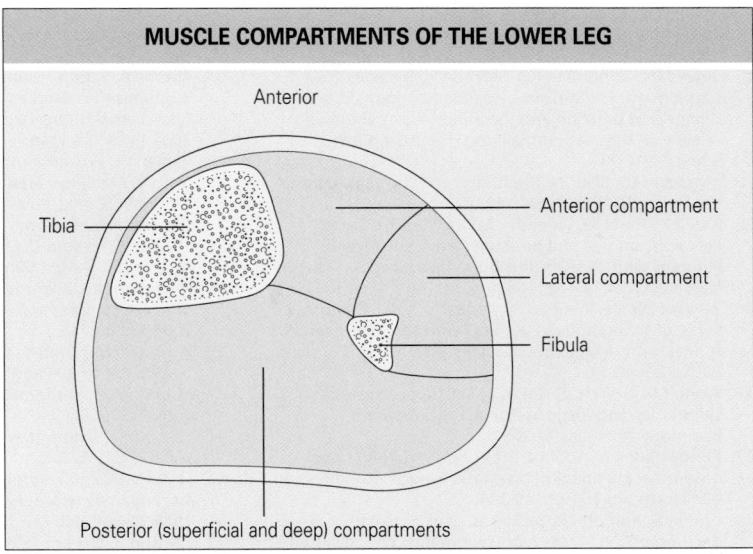

MUSCLE COMPARTMENTS OF THE LOWER LEG

Anterior

Tibia

Anterior compartment

Lateral compartment

Fibula

Posterior (superficial and deep) compartments

Fig. 78.20 Muscle compartments of the lower leg.

also variable, taking minutes in most cases but in more severe cases occasionally taking hours for complete resolution. Neurologic symptoms may occur because of ischemia of nerves, particularly in the anterior tibial syndrome.

There are no diagnostic signs at rest, making the diagnosis difficult and dependent on a good history. However, fascial defects may be found in up to 40% of cases with MRI. After sufficient exercise, tenderness and fullness will be found in the muscle compartment involved, most commonly the anterolateral compartment.

Slit catheter measurement of intracompartmental pressure before and after exercise can be used to select patients suitable for surgical decompression, provided it is performed in a specialized center with reliable standardization.[49] However, there remains controversy about the significance of mild elevation of pressure in some patients. It is likely that MRI will prove of increasing importance in diagnosis, with the development of more sophisticated imaging techniques looking at biochemical shifts or pH changes.[50]

Compartmental syndrome of the forearm is much less common but may be seen in weight lifters[51] and rowers, particularly. The deep fascia of the forearm encloses both the flexor and extensor muscles, which are separated by the radius, ulna, and interosseus membrane. The deep flexor compartment of the forearm is the more common site of involvement.

REFERENCES

1. Dawson DM, Hallett M, Millender LH. Pathology of nerve entrapment. In: Entrapment neuropathies, 2nd ed. Boston: Little & Brown, 1990:5-23.
2. Huang JH, Zager EL. Thoracic outlet syndrome. Neurosurgery 2004;55:897-903.
3. Juvonen T, Satta J, Laitala P, et al. Anomalies at the thoracic outlet are frequent in the general population. Am J Surg 1995;170:33-37.
4. Liu JE, Tahmoush AJ, Roos DB, Schwartzman RJ. Shoulder-arm pain from cervical bands and scalene muscle anomalies. J Neurol Sci 1995;128:175-180.
5. Sunderland S. In: Nerve and nerve injuries, 2nd ed. Edinburgh: Churchill Livingstone, 1978:905-919.
6. Smedby O, Rostad H, Klaastad O, et al. Functional imaging of the thoracic outlet syndrome in an open MR scanner. Eur Radiol 2000;10:597-600.
7. Naidu SH, Kothari MJ. Thoracic outlet syndrome: does fiction outweigh facts? Curr Opin Orthop 2003;14:209-214.
8. Cherington M. Proximal pain in carpal tunnel syndrome. Arch Surg 1974;108:69.
9. Dale WA. Thoracic outlet compression syndrome. Arch Surg 1982;117:1437-1445.
10. Maxey TS, Reece TB, Ellman PI, et al. Safety and efficacy of the supraclavicular approach to thoracic outlet

decompression. Ann Thorac Surg 2003;76:396-399.
11. Folberg CR, Weiss AP, Akelman E. Cubital tunnel syndrome: I. Presentation and diagnosis. Orthop Rev 1994;23:136-144.
12. Beekman R, Schoemaker MC, van der Plas JPL, et al. The diagnostic value of high-resolution sonography in ulnar neuropathy at the elbow. Neurology 2004;62:767-773.
13. Bordalo-Rodrigues M, Rosenberg ZS. MR imaging of entrapment neuropathies at the elbow. Magn Reson Imaging Clin North Am 2004;12:247-263.
14. Bartels RHMA, Verhagen WIM, van der Wilt GJ. Prospective randomized controlled study comparing simple decompression versus anterior subcutaneous transposition for idiopathic neuropathy of the ulnar nerve at the elbow: I. Neurosurgery 2005;56:522-530.
15. Moneim MS. Ulnar nerve compression at the wrist: ulnar tunnel syndrome. Hand Clin 1992;8:337-344.
16. Chan KM, Lamb DW. The anterior interosseous nerve syndrome. J R Coll Surg Edin 1984;29:350-353.
17. Hartz CR, Linscheid RL, Gramse RR, Daube JR. The pronator teres syndrome: compressive neuropathy of the median nerve. J Bone Joint Surg 1981;63A:885-890

18. Gelberman RH, Hergenroeder PT, Hargens AR, et al. The carpal tunnel syndrome: a study of carpal canal pressures. J Bone Joint Surg Am 1981;63:380-383.
19. Barnes CG, Currey HLF. Carpal tunnel syndrome in rheumatoid arthritis. Ann Rheum Dis 1967;26:226-233.
20. Ishikawa K, Patiala H, Raunio P, Vainio K. Carpal tunnel syndrome in juvenile rheumatoid arthritis. Arch Orthop Trauma Surg 1975;82:85-91.
21. Halter SK, DeLisa JA, Stolov WC, et al. Carpal tunnel syndrome in chronic renal dialysis patients. Arch Phys Med Rehabil 1981;62:197-201.
22. Kessler M, Hestin D, Aymard B, et al. Carpal-tunnel syndrome with beta$_2$-microglobulin amyloid deposits and erosive arthropathy of the wrist and spine in a uraemic patient before chronic haemodialysis. Nephrol Dial Transplant 1995;10:298-299.
23. Gray RG, Poppo MJ, Gottlieb NL. Primary familial bilateral carpal tunnel syndrome. Ann Intern Med 1979;91:37-40.
24. Lambird PA, Hartmann WH. Hereditary amyloidosis, the flexor retinaculum, and the carpal tunnel syndrome. Am J Clin Pathol 1969;52:714-719.
25. Gould JS, Wissinger A. Carpal tunnel syndrome in pregnancy. South Med J 1978;71:144-146.

26. Spinner RJ, Bachman JW, Amadio PC. The many faces of carpal tunnel syndrome. Mayo Clin Proc 1989;64:829-836.

27. Silver MA, Gelberman RH, Gellman H, Rhoades CE. Carpal tunnel syndrome: associated abnormalities in ulnar nerve function and the effect of carpal tunnel release on these abnormalities. J Hand Surg Am 1985;10:710-713.

28. Mossman SS, Blau JN. Tinel's sign and the carpal tunnel syndrome. BMJ 1987;294:680.

29. Kaul MP, Pagel KJ, Wheatley MJ, Dryden JD. Carpal compression test and pressure provocative test in veterans with median-distribution paresthesias. Muscle Nerve 2001;24:107-111.

30. Ziswiler HR, Reichenbach S, Vogelin E, et al. Diagnostic value of sonography in patients with suspected carpal tunnel syndrome: a prospective study. Arthritis Rheum 2005;52:304-311.

31. Wong SM, Griffith JF, Hui AC, et al. Carpal tunnel syndrome: diagnostic usefulness of sonography. Radiology 2004;232:93-99.

32. Mesgarzadeh M, Triolo J, Schneck CD. Carpal tunnel syndrome: MR imaging diagnosis. Magn Reson Imaging Clin North Am 1995;3:249-264.

33. Ly-Pen D, Andréu J-L, de Blas G, et al. Surgical decompression versus local steroid injection in carpal tunnel syndrome. Arthritis Rheum 2005;52:612-619.

34. Scholten RJ, Gerritsen AA, Uitdehaag BM, et al. Surgical treatment options for carpal tunnel syndrome. Cochrane Database Syst Rev 2004;(4):CD003905.

35. Thoma A, Veltri K, Haines T, et al. A meta-analysis of randomized controlled trials comparing endoscopic and open carpal tunnel decompression. Plast Reconstr Surg 2004;114:1137-1146.

36. Kaplan PE. Posterior interosseous neuropathies: natural history. Arch Phys Med Rehabil 1984;65:399-400.

37. Goldman S, et al. Posterior interosseous nerve palsy in the absence of trauma. Arch Neurol 1969;21:435-441.

38. Shapiro B, Preston D. Entrapment and compressive neuropathies. Med Clin North Am 2009;93:285-315.

39. Hochman MG, Zilberfarb JL. Nerves in a pinch: imaging of nerve compression syndromes. Radiol Clin North Am 2004;42:221-245.

40. Fishman LM, Konnoth C, Rozner B. Botulinum neurotoxin type B and physical therapy in the treatment of piriformis syndrome. Am J Phys Med Rehabil 2004;83:42-50.

41. Foster MR. Piriformis syndrome. Orthopedics 2002;25:821-825.

42. Freud S. Uber die Bernhardtische Sensibilitats-storungam Oberschenkel. Neurol Zentralbl 1985;14:491-492.

43. Edelson R, Stevens P. Meralgia paresthetica in children. J Bone Joint Surg Am 1994;76:993-999.

44. Siu TL, Chandran KN. Neurolysis for meralgia paresthetica: an operative series of 45 cases. Surg Neurol 2005;63:19-23.

45. Oh SJ, Meyer RD. Entrapment neuropathies of the tibial (posterior tibial) nerve. Neurol Clin 1999;17:593-615.

46. Sammarco GJ, Chang L. Outcome of surgical treatment of tarsal tunnel syndrome. Foot Ankle Int 2003;24:125-131.

47. Bencardino J, Rosenberg ZS, Beltran J, et al. Morton's neuroma: is it always symptomatic? AJR Am J Roentgenol 2000;175:649-653.

48. Weinfeld SB, Myerson MS. Interdigital neuritis: diagnosis and treatment. J Am Acad Orthop Surg 1996;4:328-335.

49. Pedowitz RA, Hargens AR, Mubarak SJ, et al. Modified criteria for the objective diagnosis of chronic compartment syndrome of the leg. Am J Sports Med 1990;18:35.

50. Amendola A, Rorabeck CH, Vellett D, et al. The use of magnetic imaging in exertional compartment syndromes. Am J Sports Med 1990;18:29.

51. Fricker PA, Taunton JE, Ammann W. Osteitis pubis in athletes. Infection, inflammation or injury? Sports Med 1991;12:266-279.

Complex regional pain syndrome (reflex sympathetic dystrophy)

Rachel Gorodkin and Ariane L. Herrick

79

DEFINITION

- *Complex regional pain syndrome (CRPS) type I* is now considered preferable to the term *reflex sympathetic dystrophy (RSD)*, although the latter remains in common usage.
- There are no diagnostic tests for CRPS type I/RSD: the diagnosis is made on the basis of specific symptoms and signs.

CLINICAL FEATURES

- There is usually a preceding noxious event or period of immobilization.
- The most characteristic feature is spontaneous pain, usually beginning in an extremity and then extending proximally and disproportionate to the initiating event.
- Edema and vasomotor and sudomotor abnormalities (with color, temperature, and sweating changes) are common but variable features.
- Patients who progress to late-stage disease can develop tremor, weakness, dystrophic changes, and contractures.
- Radiographs of the affected extremity show patchy osteoporosis, which is most marked in the juxta-articular region but can frequently be diffuse.

HISTORY AND TERMINOLOGY

In 1864, Mitchell and colleagues[1] described what we now recognize as complex regional pain syndrome (CRPS, previously termed *reflex sympathetic dystrophy* [RSD]) when reporting the complications of peripheral nerve injuries caused by gunshot wounds sustained by soldiers during the American Civil War. The term *RSD* was first used by Evans in the mid 1940s.[2] Since then, many terms, some of which are listed in Box 79.1, have been used to describe the painful swelling of an extremity that is usually associated with a preceding injury. This multiplicity of terms has been confusing, and in recent years considerable effort has been invested in clarifying the definition and terminology of CRPS/RSD. At the VIth World Congress on Pain, the following definition for RSD was suggested[3]:

RSD is a descriptive term meaning a complex disorder or group of disorders that may develop as a consequence of trauma affecting the limbs, with or without an obvious nerve lesion. RSD may also develop after visceral diseases and central nervous system lesions or, rarely, without an obvious antecedent event. It consists of pain and related sensory abnormalities, abnormal blood flow and sweating, abnormalities in the motor system and changes in structure of both superficial and deep tissues ('trophic' changes). It is not necessary that all components are present. It is agreed that the name 'reflex sympathetic dystrophy' is used in a descriptive sense and does not imply specific underlying mechanisms.

This definition was an important milestone because it emphasized that CRPS/RSD is not a single entity with a specific pathophysiology but rather a descriptive term.

Complex regional pain syndrome

CRPS type I (without preceding nerve injury) equates to what was previously termed RSD and CRPS type II is what was previously termed *causalgia* (severe burning pain after a major peripheral nerve injury, usually traumatic). Therefore, the problems that Mitchell and colleagues[1] described in soldiers would now more accurately be called CRPS type II.

A patient diagnosed as having CRPS type I must satisfy criteria 2 to 4 of those listed in Box 79.2.[4] A preceding noxious event is not strictly necessary. It has, however, been suggested that these criteria are not specific for CRPS, and for research purposes another set of diagnostic criteria, with increased specificity (but lower sensitivity), has been proposed.[5] These criteria stipulate that, in addition to continuing pain, a patient must report at least one symptom in each of the four categories of sensory, vasomotor, sudomotor/edema, and motor/atrophic. The patient must also display at least one sign in two or more of the same four categories.[5] Further work on diagnostic criteria is ongoing.[6]

One of the reasons why the term *RSD* fell from favor was the implication that the sympathetic nervous system has an important role in its pathophysiology. This may not always be true.[7] If the pain were sympathetically maintained, then it could be relieved by a local anesthetic block of the sympathetic ganglia that serve the painful area (always with the caveat that some patients will demonstrate a placebo response). However, although some patients with CRPS type I/RSD have sympathetically maintained pain, others do not. Conversely, many patients with sympathetically maintained pain do not have CRPS (e.g., patients with phantom limb pain or with herpes zoster). To complicate the matter further, the pain in a patient with CRPS type I may be maintained only partly sympathetically and partly independently of the sympathetic nervous system. This balance may vary over time within an individual.

Henceforth in this chapter the term *CRPS* will be used, although usually meaning CRPS type I.

EPIDEMIOLOGY

The problems with definition described earlier make it difficult to obtain accurate data on either the prevalence or incidence of CRPS after injury. However, it is clear that minor forms are not rare. Some investigators have reported, in prospective studies, a cumulative incidence of around 30% after Colles' or tibial fractures,[8] although others reported an incidence as low as 1%.[9] Fortunately, only a minority of patients progress to late-stage disease (see later). A recent study from the Netherlands estimated the overall incidence rate to be 26.2/100,000 person-years, with the highest incidence rate in the 61- to 70-year age group.[10] However, CRPS can occur in persons of any age and is now well recognized in children.[11] It has been reported more frequently in women than in men.[10,12,13]

Triggers

A variety of triggers can precipitate CRPS (Table 79.1). The most common causes are peripheral trauma (fracture or soft tissue injury) and orthopedic surgery. CRPS can also develop after central nervous system or spinal disorders and rarely after visceral lesions such as myocardial infarction. Up to 10% of patients have no identifiable causative event.[12,13] Immobilizing a limb (for any reason) is likely to be a significant predisposing factor: in one large study, 47% of subjects had

TABLE 79.1 TYPICAL TRIGGERING EVENTS FOR CRPS	
Trauma	Wrist fractures
	Tibial fractures
	Soft tissue injuries
Surgery	Carpal tunnel decompression
	Arthroscopy
	Lumbar spine surgery
Central nervous system or spinal disorders	Head injury
	Hemiplegia
Visceral lesions	Myocardial infarction

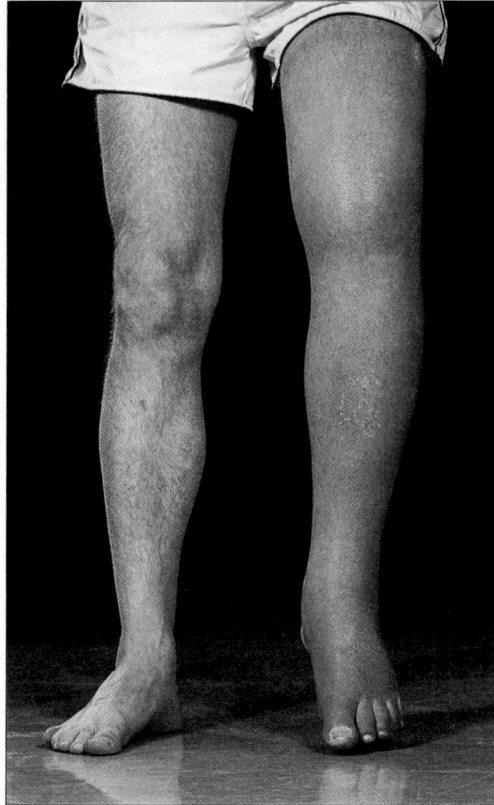

Fig. 79.1 CRPS affecting the lower limb, showing marked swelling and color change. *(Reproduced with permission from Salford Royal NHS Foundation Trust.)*

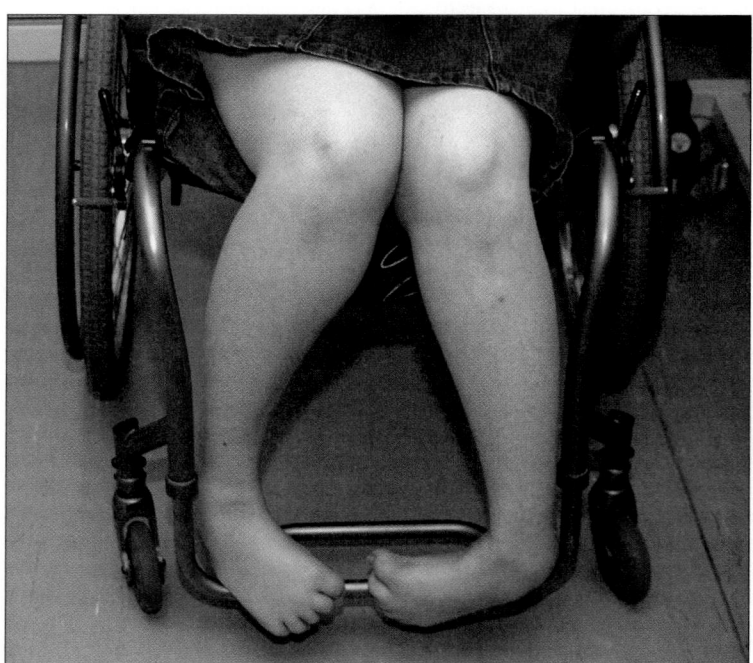

Fig. 79.2 Bilateral CRPS with contractures. *(Reproduced with permission from Salford Royal NHS Foundation Trust.)*

undergone a period of limb immobilization before diagnosis.[12] Recent studies have examined whether there might be a genetic disposition to CRPS, but at present there is no clear consensus of opinion on this.

Personality traits

Patients with CRPS are often extremely distressed by their pain; and it has been suggested that certain personality traits are associated with CRPS, but there is no convincing evidence to support this hypothesis.[14] It seems likely that the pain behavior that undoubtedly develops in a proportion of patients is a consequence of, rather than a predisposing factor for, their CRPS.

CLINICAL FEATURES

CRPS is primarily a clinical diagnosis and is often difficult to make. The diagnostic criteria for CRPS rely purely on symptoms and signs, and so the clinician needs to be familiar with these. In addition to varying between patients, clinical features vary within an individual patient over time. Almost invariably, it is an extremity that is affected. Hand and wrist, knee, or foot and ankle are most commonly involved, although an entire limb can become affected, as shown in Figure 79.1. The term *shoulder-hand syndrome* described a variant of CRPS in which the entire upper limb was affected. Usually only one limb is affected, but the condition may be bilateral or another limb might become affected at a later date (Fig. 79-2).[15] Rarely, the face or trunk may be affected.

Both symptoms and signs can be grouped under four headings, which will be considered in turn: pain and related sensory abnormalities, vasomotor, sudomotor/edema, and motor/trophic. These features are summarized in Table 79.2.

TABLE 79.2 CLINICAL FEATURES OF CRPS

Pain and related sensory abnormalities	Pain, often burning, extending beyond the area of the original injury Allodynia Hyperalgesia/hyperpathia Disturbed body perception
Vasomotor	Color change* Temperature change*
Sudomotor/edema	Edema Increased sweating
Motor/trophic	Weakness/inability to initiate movement Tremor Muscle spasms Dystonic features Contractures Skin, hair, and nail changes

As compared with the unaffected side.

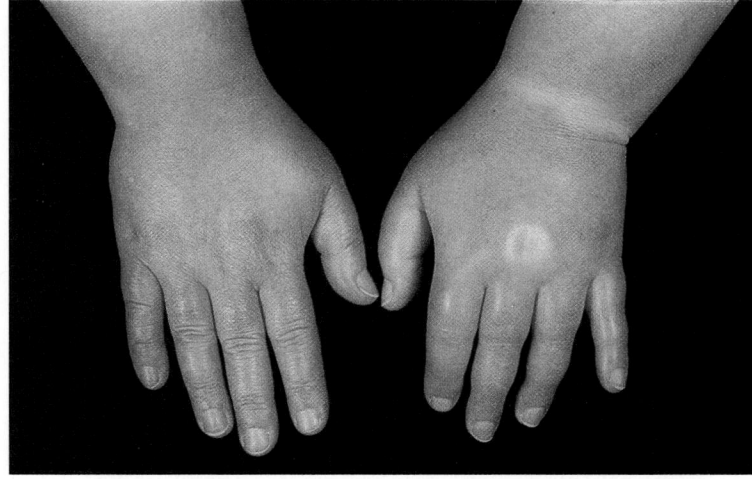

Fig. 79.3 Early CRPS of the left hand and wrist, showing edema. *(Reproduced with permission from Salford Royal NHS Foundation Trust.)*

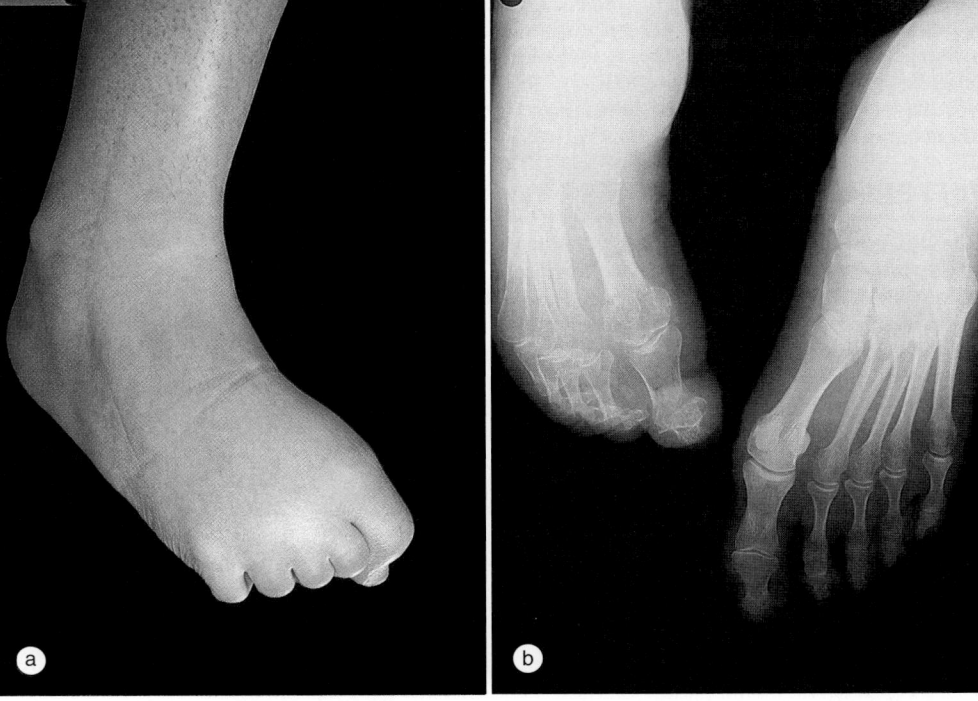

Fig. 79.4 CRPS of the ankle and foot. (a) Well-established CRPS of the right ankle and foot, showing contracture. (b) The extent of deformity associated with CRPS is well demonstrated radiographically. The affected foot is osteoporotic. *(Reproduced with permission from Salford Royal NHS Foundation Trust.)*

Pain and related sensory abnormalities

The most characteristic feature of CRPS is severe, persistent pain, which often has a burning quality. The pain is different in character from that of the injury that precipitated the CRPS and, although usually beginning in the extremity, frequently extends proximally in a non-dermatomal pattern. On examination, the affected site is diffusely tender, often with allodynia and hyperalgesia. These are separate phenomena: *allodynia* is pain that is provoked by a stimulus that is not normally painful, whereas *hyperalgesia* is an exaggerated response to a painful stimulus. *Hyperpathia* is also observed in patients with CRPS (especially those with later disease) and can be defined as an increased response to a stimulus, particularly repetitive. It is being increasingly recognized that patients with CRPS may experience disturbances in body perception.[16]

Vasomotor

The patient may complain of changes in skin color or temperature in the affected extremity, which are revealed on clinical examination by comparison with the unaffected side. Typically, the affected limb is initially warm and red and may then become mottled and intermittently warm and cool before becoming more permanently cold and cyanotic. However, not all patients pass through these three phases (see later). It has been suggested that patients who report early coldness are at high risk of going on to develop severe, late-stage disease, with infection, ulcers, chronic edema, dystonia, and myoclonus.[17]

Sudomotor/edema

Swelling of the affected extremity is common, especially in the early phase (Fig. 79.3), and may be associated with increased or reduced sweating.

Motor/trophic

Patients who develop motor or trophic changes, or both, tend to have a poor prognosis, in that they have progressed beyond the early stages of CRPS. The patient may complain of inability to initiate movement, weakness (although this is difficult to assess in the presence of severe pain), tremor, or muscle spasms. Sometimes there are dystonic features.[18] Hair growth and nail changes are all commonly seen, and the skin may become atrophic and shiny. Contractures can occur in late-stage disease (Fig. 79.4).

NATURAL HISTORY

The clinical course of CRPS has been divided into three stages; and although there is some doubt as to the clinical usefulness of this subdivision, it may be of help when considering studies of pathophysiology and treatment. For example, it seems unlikely that a patient with late-stage disease, as shown in Figure 79.4, has the same prospect of responding to treatment as the patient shown in Figure 79.3, with earlier disease. The three stages are as follows:

Stage 1: acute. The limb may be either warm or cool, with edema. In at least a proportion of patients, the clinical features of acute disease may be inflammatory.[12] The pain is exacerbated by dependency.

Stage 2: dystrophic. The limb continues to be painful but now it becomes cooler, and either mottled or cyanotic, with early dystrophic changes of the skin and nails.

Stage 3: atrophic. During this stage, the pain spreads proximally (in some patients the limb may become less painful) and disability is increased as a result of irreversible atrophic changes and contracture. In some patients ankylosis can occur.

The duration of each of these three stages is highly variable, and patients may exhibit features of more than one stage simultaneously. A period of 6 to 12 months has been quoted for stage 1, 1 to 2 years for stage 2, and up to several years for stage 3.[19] Many patients never progress beyond stage 1.

A myofascial pain syndrome, with trigger points, has been reported to occur in a proportion of patients with CRPS.

DIFFERENTIAL DIAGNOSIS

The differential diagnosis, at least in the early stages of CRPS, is that of the causes of a tender, often swollen limb. Inflammatory arthritis, cellulitis, osteomyelitis, deep venous thrombosis, malignancy, and fracture might all be suspected, but a careful history should point to the diagnosis, especially when there is a preceding history of trauma. Neuropathic pain disorders also enter into the differential diagnosis. Chronic vascular insufficiency must be considered in the differential diagnosis of late-stage CRPS.

INVESTIGATIONS

There is no diagnostic test for CRPS. However, certain investigations may give supportive evidence. The full blood cell count and erythrocyte sedimentation rate should be normal.

Plain radiographs

The characteristic radiographic findings of CRPS are well described. The typical appearance is of patchy osteoporosis of the affected extremity. This is most marked in the juxta-articular region (Fig. 79.5) but is frequently diffuse, occasionally with erosive changes.[20] Soft tissue swelling is often present, at least in early disease. The joint space is usually preserved, although in patients who progress to late-stage disease there may be loss of joint space and ankylosis.

Isotope bone scanning

Traditionally, isotope bone scanning (especially three-phase imaging) was considered useful in the diagnosis of CRPS, as one sought asymmetry between affected and non-affected limbs, although the actual abnormality is dependent on disease stage. Thus, there is increased uptake in early disease (Fig. 79.6) and reduced uptake in later disease.[21] However, there has been some skepticism as to the true usefulness of isotope bone scanning.[13]

Magnetic resonance imaging

Appearances on magnetic resonance imaging tend to be non-specific and include soft tissue changes and bone marrow edema.[22] At present, magnetic resonance imaging is not considered part of the routine diagnostic evaluation of CRPS but may be useful if the diagnosis is unclear.

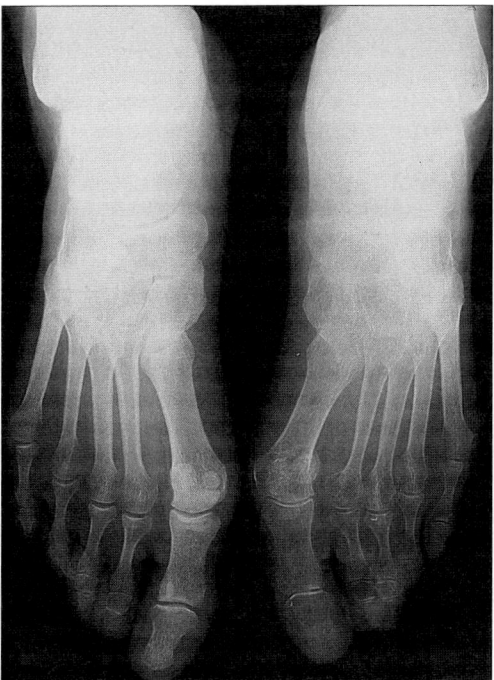

Fig. 79.5 Rarefaction of bone in a patient with CRPS affecting the left ankle and foot. The changes are most marked in the midfoot. *(Reproduced with permission from Salford Royal NHS Foundation Trust.)*

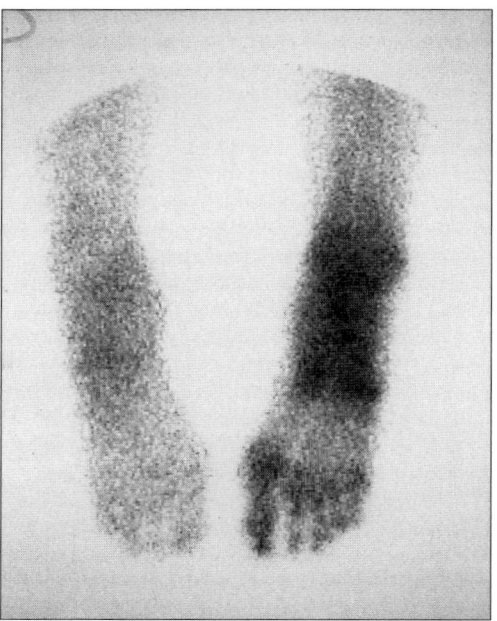

Fig. 79.6 Isotope bone scan showing diffuse increased uptake in the distal tibia, talus, and navicular in a patient with CRPS of the left ankle and foot. *(Reproduced with permission from Salford Royal NHS Foundation Trust.)*

Thermography

Thermography measures surface temperature. It therefore detects asymmetry in limb temperature (Fig. 79.7) and so may aid in the diagnosis of CRPS.[23] However, the technique is not widely available and is mainly a research tool.

Other investigations

A number of other investigations have been used primarily on a research basis.[24] These include quantitative sweat testing (using the quantitative sudomotor axon reflex test), quantitative sensory testing

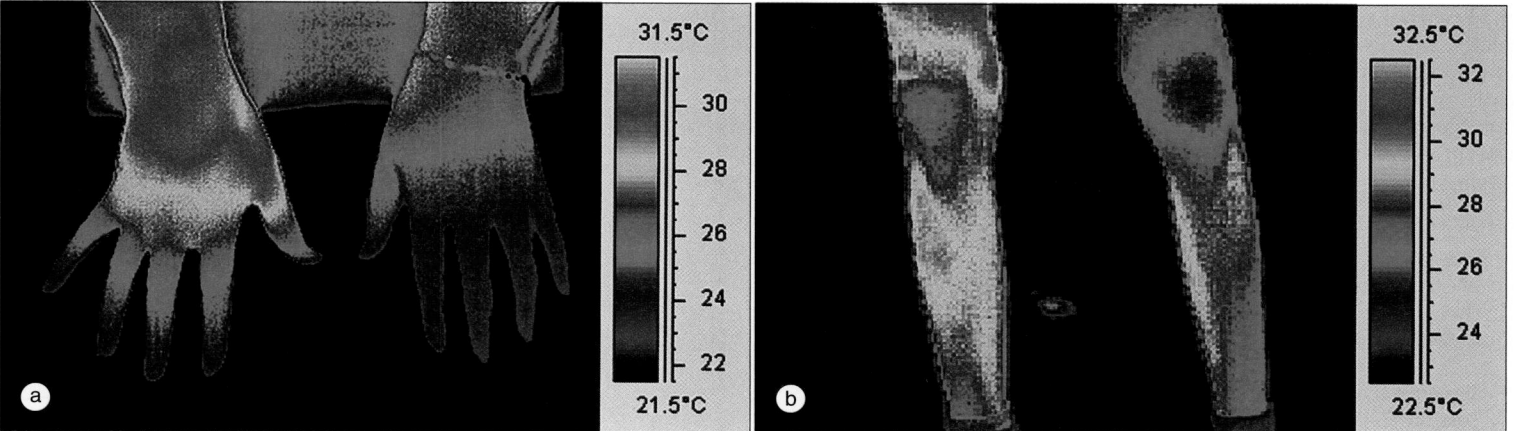

Fig. 79.7 Thermographic images. (a) A patient with CRPS of the left hand (same patient as in Fig. 79.3). The affected hand is cooler: the temperature difference between the dorsum of the left hand and the dorsum of the right hand is 3.4°C. (b) A patient with CRPS of the left knee. The affected knee is cooler: the temperature difference between the left and right knees is 1.9°C. *(Reproduced with permission from Salford Royal NHS Foundation Trust.)*

(testing small fiber function), sympathetic skin response (which measures skin conductance), and psychological tests.

PATHOLOGY

The pathology of CRPS is not well described, reflecting the reluctance to subject affected limbs to biopsy, for fear of exacerbating the clinical problem. A pathologic study of skeletal muscle and peripheral nerve tissue from lower limb amputations from eight patients revealed muscle changes consisting of type I fiber atrophy, an increase in lipofuscin (suggestive of free radical–mediated injury) and capillary abnormalities, with thickening/duplication of the basement membrane.[25] In contrast, there were no consistent abnormalities in peripheral nerves. The authors postulated that a microangiopathy was central to pathophysiology.[25] A study of skin biopsies from 18 patients with CRPS demonstrated subtle small fiber axonal damage: the authors speculated that CRPS is a neurologic condition.[26]

PATHOPHYSIOLOGY

The pathophysiology of CRPS is not fully understood. It is unknown why some patients, after only a minor injury, go on to develop CRPS, whereas most go on to make an uncomplicated recovery. Many different theories have been suggested.[19,24,27-29] It seems most likely that both peripheral and central mechanisms are involved, interacting to maintain a vicious cycle of events the end result of which is the persisting pain of CRPS, with its accompanying vasomotor, sudomotor, and trophic changes. Neurogenic inflammation and microcirculatory dysfunction, possibly resulting in oxidant stress, have also been proposed as important mechanisms of tissue injury. It seems probable that these different aspects of pathophysiology are all interrelated (Fig. 79.8).

Peripheral mechanisms

It is likely that trauma to type C nerve fibers and Aδ afferents is an initiating event in the CRPS process, and at least some patients go on to demonstrate sensitization of their C or Aδ nociceptors in the context of thermal and mechanical hyperalgesia.[19] It was originally believed that the sympathetic nervous system was invariably important in the pathogenesis of CRPS. Although this is no longer accepted at all stages of the disease process, there is no doubt that many patients have sympathetically maintained pain,[27] as demonstrated by their response to sympathetic blockade.

It has been suggested that enhanced vasoconstrictor activity in CRPS contributes to hyperalgesia.[30] Sympathetic activity may activate both mechanoreceptors and nociceptors and could therefore contribute to the vicious cycle involving central mechanisms referred to earlier. Considerable attention has been paid to the hypothesis that the α-adrenoreceptor is a key player in the pathogenesis of CRPS; these receptors may be overexpressed in hyperalgesic skin of patients with

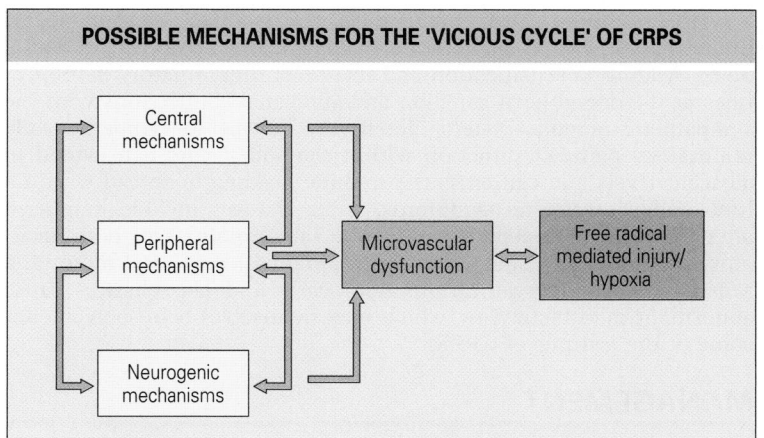

Fig. 79.8 Possible mechanisms for the "vicious cycle" of CRPS.

CRPS and may then be activated through sympathetic discharge.[27] The fact that at least some patients experience pain relief from α-adrenergic blockade with intravenous phentolamine is supportive of this hypothesis. However, the situation is highly complex, with several studies suggesting a reduction in sympathetic efferent activity, leading to supersensitivity to catecholamines.[31,32] Catecholamine supersensitivity would be consistent with increased α-adrenoceptor responsiveness.[33]

Central mechanisms

It has been suggested that, in CRPS, an initial activation of nociceptors for some reason leads to alteration of central information processes, resulting in central sensitization. This disordered processing of nociceptor impulses may be the most important mechanism of persisting pain in late-stage CRPS. As a result of this disordered processing, activation of low-threshold mechanoreceptors is subsequently interpreted as noxious. This would explain the phenomenon of allodynia. A role for the *N*-methyl-D-aspartate (NMDA) receptor has been suggested.[19] Inhibitory neurons using γ-aminobutyric acid (GABAergic) may also play a part, as indicated by improvement in dystonia in response to baclofen (a GABA receptor agonist).[34] There is increasing interest in the role that abnormal cortical processing plays in CRPS, with motor and sensory cortical reorganization demonstrated via various techniques including magnetoencephalography and functional magnetic resonance imaging.[35]

Neurogenic inflammation

There is considerable evidence to suggest that neurogenic inflammation contributes to the pathogenesis of CRPS.[29] This might explain why some of the early clinical features of CRPS are inflammatory.[12] Release of vasoactive peptides, including substance P and calcitonin gene–related peptide, from afferent nerve fibers causes vasodilation, with increased vascular permeability and protein leakage. It is likely that these neuropeptides also increase the excitability of primary sensory nerve fibers, leading to changes in the dorsal horn.

Microvascular dysfunction

It is not known whether the vascular changes of CRPS drive the disease process by causing hypoxia and free radical–mediated damage or whether they are secondary. A number of investigators have confirmed microvascular dysfunction in CRPS,[31,32] and hypoxia has been directly demonstrated in CRPS-affected limbs.[36] Relevant to this is that vitamin C, a powerful antioxidant, may prevent the development of CRPS[37] and free radical scavengers may have a beneficial effect in the treatment of CRPS.[38]

Summary

Our current state of knowledge regarding the pathophysiology of CRPS can be summed up as follows: the condition is most likely initiated by a peripheral injury causing subclinical nerve damage and neurogenic inflammation. Initial changes are mediated by nociceptive Aδ and C fibers, leading to sensitization and release of inflammatory neuropeptides at the dorsal horn ganglion and abnormal connections with the sympathetic nervous system, potentially leading to sympathetically maintained pain. Dysfunction within the spinal cord can extend to adjacent levels and can cross the midline, leading to spread within a limb and contralateral symptoms. Later changes include long-term alterations in neuropeptide production, abnormalities of both excitatory and inhibitory spinal and supraspinal pathways, and motor and sensory cortical reorganization. Both early and late changes cause abnormalities of blood flow, which may themselves be responsible for some of the features of CRPS.

MANAGEMENT

There are a number of treatment options in CRPS, which are summarized in Table 79.3.

Although many patients with mild forms of CRPS may experience spontaneous improvement, those who go on to a late stage with atrophy and contracture are very unlikely to recover. These patients are left with pain and major functional disability. Therefore, early diagnosis is a key principle of management.

In addition to being a condition that is difficult to diagnose and treat, CRPS is difficult to study, because of its heterogeneity, the problems in definition earlier referred to, a lack of outcome measures,[39] and the incomplete understanding of its pathophysiology. As a result, until very recently there have been very few controlled clinical trials[40] and those that do exist tend to be in small numbers of patients, with subjective endpoints. Many of the recommendations about treatment (including those considered here) are based on anecdotal observations or small series of patients. The frequency of the disorder does mean that there is considerable anecdotal experience in its management. The main aims are to reduce pain and to restore function.

The treatment of CRPS should be multidisciplinary. Many of the patients demonstrate marked pain behavior, and their distress may be compounded by the fact that, before diagnosis, their pain was believed to be "non-organic." Patient education and an approach based on pain management are integral to management. A proportion of patients benefit from psychological counseling.

Prevention

Ideally, the development of CRPS should be prevented by early mobilization of patients with predisposing conditions and careful attention to surgical technique. A recent study (albeit not a randomized trial) of 300 patients undergoing surgery for Dupuytren's contracture suggested that anesthetic technique was also likely to influence outcome: patients who had an axillary block or intravenous regional anesthesia with lidocaine and clonidine were less likely to develop postoperative CRPS

TABLE 79.3 APPROACHES TO THE TREATMENT OF CRPS	
Prevention	Early mobilization
Physiotherapy	Desensitization techniques
	Mirror therapy
	Graded motor imagery
Sympathetic blocks	Paravertebral
	Regional intravenous
Other regional blocks	Epidural
	Brachial or lumbar plexus
Drug treatment	Analgesics
	Non-steroidal anti-inflammatory drugs
	Antidepressants
	Anticonvulsants
	Bisphosphonates
	Free radical scavengers (dimethyl sulfoxide [topical] and acetylcysteine)
	α-Blockers and other vasodilators
	Corticosteroids
	Calcitonin
	Intrathecal baclofen
	Ketamine (intravenous)
	Capsaicin (topical)
	Lidocaine patches
Transcutaneous nerve stimulation	
Acupuncture	
Dorsal column stimulation	
Surgery (very rarely indicated)	Surgical sympathectomy
	Amputation

than those who had a general anesthetic or intravenous regional anesthesia with lidocaine alone.[41] As stated earlier, it has been suggested that vitamin C, a powerful antioxidant, may prevent the development of CRPS[37] (grade A evidence), the rationale being that oxidant stress contributes to pathophysiology. Although potentially very exciting, this observation requires confirmation in further studies.

Physiotherapy and occupational therapy

Physiotherapy alone may correct mild cases of CRPS. In more advanced disease, physiotherapy is used in combination with other treatment modalities, which should facilitate the physiotherapy (grade B evidence). Both physiotherapy and occupational therapy, in a randomized trial of upper limb CRPS, conferred benefit in terms of pain reduction and functional improvement.[42] The emphasis is on mobilization, although this can be very difficult in patients with severe pain and tenderness. An algorithm for therapy, with an emphasis on the rehabilitative aspects, has been put forward by Stanton-Hicks and coworkers.[43] This begins cautiously, with approaches such as heat, massage, and gentle movement to help restore normal sensory processing. This is then followed with isometric strengthening and electrode stimulation, treatment of any secondary myofascial pain syndrome, and general aerobic conditioning until complete functional rehabilitation. In many patients, severe pain proves a barrier to this approach to functional restoration and medical and psychological interventions must be applied in parallel. Mirror therapy/graded motor imagery has recently been advocated, with a small randomized trial suggesting benefit in early disease, but further studies are required (grade B evidence).[44]

Nerve blockade

Sympathetic blockade

In the past, sympathetic blockade has been recommended as a treatment for CRPS, and a good response to this has been considered an aid to diagnosis. However, as discussed earlier, a response to sympathetic blockade does not mean that the pain is caused by CRPS per se but rather that a significant component of the pain is sympathetically maintained.

There are two main methods of temporarily blocking the sympathetic nervous system: paravertebral blockade and regional intravenous blockade. With paravertebral blockade, usually a series of local anesthetic blocks is given, the frequency depending on the patient's response. The stellate ganglion is blocked for upper limb CRPS and the lumbar sympathetic chain for the lower limb. Intravenous blockade, usually with guanethidine, essentially produces a noradrenergic neuron block by applying a high concentration of guanethidine directly to the nerve endings in the treated extremity. As with the sympathetic ganglion blocks, these intravenous blocks can be repeated as necessary. Despite their widespread use, there is very little evidence base from controlled clinical trials for either paravertebral[45] or regional blocks (grade A evidence): many clinicians, however, believe that they have a place particularly in patients with sensory and vasomotor changes, in whom a nerve block might facilitate a rehabilitation program.

Other regional blocks

Epidural blocks (cervical or lumbar) have also been used but have the disadvantage of blocking not only the sympathetic nervous system but also somatic nerves. Continuous blockade of the brachial or lumbar plexus has also been advocated, the rationale being that, as long as the catheter is in place, the patient can maximize his or her benefit from a graded program of physiotherapy. These blocks are likely to be of benefit early on in the disease process, to facilitate the rehabilitative approach.

Drug treatment

A very large number of drugs have been suggested for the treatment of CRPS (see Table 79.3), but few have been proven to be effective in randomized clinical trials.[40] Usually the first line of pharmacologic intervention is with analgesics and non-steroidal anti-inflammatory drugs (grade C evidence). The latter might be expected to confer benefit early on, when there may be an inflammatory component to the CRPS. Low-dose antidepressants may be helpful, as may carbamazepine, phenytoin, sodium valproate, or gabapentin (grade C evidence). These recommendations are based on clinical impressions and not on strong clinical trial evidence.

Recently there has been considerable interest in bisphosphonates. For example, alendronate has been shown to reduce pain and improve function (grade A evidence).[44,46] Results from studies on calcitonin (grade A evidence) have given conflicting results.[44] Another recent target for therapy, as mentioned earlier, is based on the pathologic role of free radial scavengers. Both dimethyl sulfoxide and N-acetylcysteine were reported to confer benefit in a double-blind study, although there was no placebo control.[38]

Other drugs that have been advocated for CRPS include α-blockers and other vasodilators and corticosteroids. In a randomized, crossover trial (grade A evidence) intrathecal baclofen was shown to improve upper limb dystonia in six of seven patients with CRPS.[47] Ketamine at subanesthetic doses blocks NMDA receptors and therefore reduces the excitatory effect of glutamate on the central nervous system; benefit has been reported[48] (grade C evidence), but further studies are required. Topical treatments suggested include capsaicin,[40] although patients often struggle to tolerate it. Lidocaine 5% patches show promise[49] (grade C evidence), and in addition to their local anesthetic effect they also protect allodynic skin from contact with clothing.

Other treatments

Other treatments include transcutaneous nerve stimulation and acupuncture. Spinal cord stimulation has been shown to be effective in

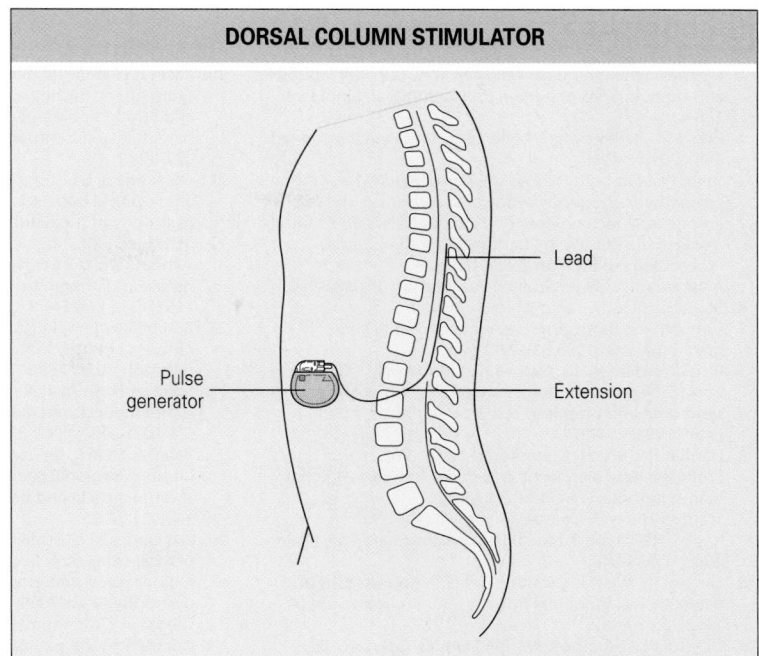

DORSAL COLUMN STIMULATOR

Lead

Pulse generator

Extension

Fig. 79.9 Dorsal column stimulator. The schematic representation shows a fully implanted system with an internal power source.

reducing pain (but not in improving function) in patients with well-established CRPS (grade A evidence), although its effectiveness decreases over time.[50] The procedure involves placement of an electrode in the epidural space on the dorsal aspect of the spinal cord (Fig. 79.9), at the level of the nerve roots subserving the painful area. The rationale is that the electrical current thus produced induces paresthesias that suppress the pain. Because the procedure is not without risk, patients must be carefully selected. The related technologies are continuing to evolve.

A small proportion of patients come to surgical treatment. Rarely, surgical sympathectomy has been advocated if a patient gains benefit from temporary sympathetic blocks. Amputation is not recommended for pain alone, because phantom limb pain at the amputation stump may result, but it may be indicated, for example, if a limb is chronically infected.

Future therapies

Recent years have seen a huge expansion in research interest in CRPS, with the result that classification criteria (a major stumbling block to earlier research) are being improved and thus will facilitate clinical trials of new treatments. Development of new therapies will, in turn, be directed by advances in understanding of pathophysiology and will include vasoactive and antioxidant treatments in addition to different forms of analgesia. However, to evaluate new treatments, it is imperative that objective outcome measures are developed or refined and, as recently discussed, outcome measures are needed that will evaluate handicap and disability, in addition to impairment.[39]

CONCLUSION

CRPS remains a condition that is difficult to diagnose, to treat, and to study. However, it is a major source of pain and disability to that subgroup of patients who go on to develop severe, late disease. The rheumatologist's task is to maintain a high index of suspicion of CRPS in a patient with a painful extremity and to institute treatment, including mobilization, early, in an attempt to prevent progression to late disease. Ideally, patients with CRPS should be cared for by an experienced multidisciplinary team.

REFERENCES

1. Mitchell SW, Morehouse GR, Keen WW. Gunshot wounds and other injuries of nerves. Philadelphia: JB Lippincott, 1864.

2. Evans JA. Reflex sympathetic dystrophy. Ann Intern Med 1947;26:417-426.

3. Janig W, Blumberg H, Boas RA, Campbell JN. The reflex sympathetic dystrophy syndrome: consensus statement and general recommendations for diagnosis and clinical research. In: Bond MR, Charlton JE, Woofe CJ, eds. Proceedings of the VIth World Congress on Pain. Amsterdam: Elsevier Science Publishers, 1991:373-376.

4. Stanton-Hicks M, Janig W, Hassenbusch S, et al. Reflex sympathetic dystrophy: changing concepts and taxonomy. Pain 1995;63:127-133.

5. Bruehl S, Harden RN, Galer BS, et al. External validation of IASP diagnostic criteria for complex regional pain syndrome and proposed research diagnostic criteria. Pain 1999;81:147-154.

6. Harden RN, Bruehl S, Stanton-Hicks M, Wilson PR. Proposed new diagnostic criteria for complex regional pain syndrome. Pain Med 2007;8:326-331.

7. Stanton-Hicks M. Complex regional pain syndrome (type I, RSD; type II, causalgia): controversies. Clin J Pain 2000;16:S33-S40.

8. Sarangi PP, Ward AJ, Smith EJ, et al. Algodystrophy and osteoporosis after tibial fractures. J Bone Joint Surg Br 1993;75:450-452.

9. Dijkstra PU, Groothoff JW, Ten Duis HJ, Geertzen JHB. Incidence of complex regional pain syndrome type I after fractures of the distal radius. Eur J Pain 2003;7:457-462.

10. De Mos M, Bruijn AGJ, Huygen FJPM, et al. The incidence of complex regional pain syndrome: a population-based study. Pain 2007;129:12-20.

11. Wilder RT, Berde CB, Wolohan M, et al. Reflex sympathetic dystrophy in children. J Bone Joint Surg Am 1992;74:910-919.

12. Veldman PHJM, Reynen HM, Arntz IE, Goris RJA. Signs and symptoms of reflex sympathetic dystrophy: prospective study of 829 patients. Lancet 1993;342:1012-1016.

13. Allen G, Galer BS, Schwartz L. Epidemiology of complex regional pain syndrome: a retrospective chart review of 134 patients. Pain 1999;80:539-544.

14. Ciccone DS, Bandilla EB, Wu W. Psychological dysfunction in patients with reflex sympathetic dystrophy. Pain 1997;71:323-333.

15. Maleki J, LeBel AA, Bennett GJ, Schwartzman RJ. Patterns of spread in complex regional pain syndrome, type I (reflex sympathetic dystrophy syndrome). Pain 2000;88:259-266.

16. Lewis JS, Kersten P, McCabe CS, et al. Body perception disturbance: a contribution to pain in complex regional pain syndrome (CRPS). Pain 2007;133:111-119.

17. Van Der Laan L, Veldman PHJM, Goris JA. Severe complications of reflex sympathetic dystrophy: infections, ulcers, chronic edema, dystonia, and myoclonus. Arch Phys Med Rehabil 1998;79:424-429.

18. Van Rijn MA, Marinus J, Putter H, van Hilten JJ. Onset and progression of dystonia in complex regional pain syndrome. Pain 2007;130:287-293.

19. Schwartzman RJ. The autonomic nervous system and pain. Handbook Clin Neurol 2000;75:309-347.

20. Kozin F, Genant HK, Bekerman C, McCarty DJ. The reflex sympathetic dystrophy syndrome: II. Roentgenographic and scintigraphic evidence of bilaterality and of periarticular accentuation. Am J Med 1976;60:322-328.

21. Demangeat J, Constantinesco A, Brunot B, et al. Three-phase bone scanning in reflex sympathetic dystrophy of the hand. J Nucl Med 1988;29:26-32.

22. Schweitzer ME, Mandel S, Schwartzman RJ, et al. Reflex sympathetic dystrophy revisited: MR imaging findings before and after infusion of contrast material. Radiology 1995;195:211-214.

23. Bruehl S, Lubenow TR, Nath H, Ivankovich O. Validation of thermography in the diagnosis of reflex sympathetic dystrophy. Clin J Pain 1996;12:316-325.

24. Stanton-Hicks M. Reflex sympathetic dystrophy: a sympathetically mediated pain syndrome or not? Curr Rev Pain 2000;4:268-275.

25. Van Der Laan L, ter Laak HJ, Gabreels-Festen A, et al. Complex regional pain syndrome I (RSD): pathology of skeletal muscle and peripheral nerve. Neurology 1998;51:20-25.

26. Oaklander AL, Rissmiller JG, Gelman LB, et al. Evidence of focal small-fiber axonal degeneration in complex regional pain syndrome-I (reflex sympathetic dystrophy). Pain 2006;120:235-243.

27. Gibbs GF, Drummond PD, Finch PM, Phillips JK. Unravelling the pathophysiology of complex regional pain syndrome: focus on sympathetically maintained pain. Clin Exp Pharmacol Physiol 2008;35:717-724.

28. Janig W. The puzzle of reflex sympathetic dystrophy: mechanisms, hypotheses, open questions. In: Janig W, Stanton-Hicks M, eds. Reflex sympathetic dystrophy: a reappraisal. Progress in pain research and management, vol 6. Seattle: IASP Press, 1996:1-24.

29. Birklein F, Schmelz M. Neuropeptides, neurogenic inflammation and complex regional pain syndrome (CRPS). Neurosci Lett 2008;437:199-202.

30. Baron R, Schattschneider J, Binder A, et al. Relation between sympathetic vasoconstrictor activity and pain and hyperalgesia in complex regional pain syndromes: a case control study. Lancet 2002;359:1655-1660.

31. Kurvers HAJM, Jacobs MJHM, Beuk RJ, et al. Reflex sympathetic dystrophy: result of autonomic denervation? Clin Sci 1994;87:663-669.

32. Wasner G, Schattschneider J, Heckmann K, et al. Vascular abnormalities in reflex sympathetic dystrophy (CRPS I): mechanisms and diagnostic value. Brain 2001;124:587-599.

33. Arnold JMO, Teasell RW, MacLeod AP, et al. Increased venous alpha-adrenoceptor responsiveness in patients with reflex sympathetic dystrophy. Ann Intern Med 1993;118:619-621.

34. Schwartzman RJ. New treatments for reflex sympathetic dystrophy. N Engl J Med 2000;343:654-656.

35. Swart CMA, Stins JF, Beek PJ. Cortical changes in complex regional pain syndrome (CRPS). Eur J Pain 2009;13(9):902-907.

36. Koban M, Leis S, Schultze-Mosgau S, Birklein F. Tissue hypoxia in complex regional pain syndrome. Pain 2003;104:149-157.

37. Zollinger PE, Tuinebreijer WE, Breederveld RS, Kries RW. Can vitamin C prevent complex regional pain syndrome in patients with wrist fractures. J Bone Joint Surg Am 2007;89:1424-1431.

38. Perez RSGM, Zuurmond WWA, Bezemer PD, et al. The treatment of complex regional pain syndrome type I with free radical scavengers: a randomized controlled study. Pain 2003;102:297-307.

39. Schasfoort FC, Bussman JB, Stam HJ. Outcome measures for complex regional pain syndrome type I: an overview in the context of the international classification of impairments, disabilities and handicaps. Disabil Rehabil 2000;22:387-398.

40. Harden RN. Pharmacotherapy of complex regional pain syndrome. Am J Phys Med Rehab 2005;84(Suppl):S17-S28.

41. Reuben SS, Pristas R, Dixon D, et al. The incidence of complex regional pain syndrome after fasciectomy for Dupuytren's contracture: a prospective observational study of four anesthetic techniques. Anesth Analg 2006;102:499-503.

42. Oerlemans HM, Oostendorp RAB, de Boo T, Goris RJA. Pain and reduced mobility in complex regional pain syndrome I: outcome of a prospective randomised controlled clinical trial of adjuvant physical therapy versus occupational therapy. Pain 1999;83:77-83.

43. Stanton-Hicks M, Baron R, Boas R, et al. Complex regional pain syndromes: guidelines for therapy. Clin J Pain 1998;14:155-166.

44. Sharma A, Williams K, Raja SN. Advances in treatment of complex regional pain syndrome: recent insights on a perplexing disease. Curr Opin Anaesthesiol 2006;19:566-572.

45. Cepeda MS, Carr DB, Lau J. Local anaesthetic sympathetic blockade for complex regional pain syndrome. Cochrane Database Syst Rev 2005;(4):CD004598.

46. Manicourt D-H, Brasseur J-P, Boutsen Y, et al. Role of alendronate for posttraumatic complex regional pain syndrome type I of the lower extremity. Arthritis Rheum 2004;50:3690-3697.

47. Van Hilten BJ, Van De Beek WT, Hoff JI, et al. Intrathecal baclofen for the treatment of dystonia in patients with reflex sympathetic dystrophy. N Engl J Med 2000;343:625-630.

48. Correll GE, Maleki J, Gracely EJ, et al. Subanesthetic ketamine infusion therapy: a retrospective analysis of a novel therapeutic approach to complex regional pain syndrome. Pain Med 2004;5:263-275.

49. Oaklander A. Evidence-based pharmacotherapy for CRPS and related conditions. In: Wilson P, Stanton-Hicks M, Harden RN, eds. CRPS: Current diagnosis and therapy, progress in pain research and management, vol 32. Seattle: IASP Press, 2005.

50. Taylor RS, van Buyten J, Buchser E. Spinal cord stimulation for complex regional pain syndrome: a systematic review of the clinical and cost-effectiveness literature and assessment of prognostic factors. Eur J Pain 2006;10:91-101.

Sports medicine: clinical spectrum of injury

80

Patrick Ellender, Adam Harder, Benjamin Sanofsky, and Laurence D. Higgins

- Sports medicine encompasses the science as well as the clinical evaluation and treatment of acute and chronic injuries to the musculoskeletal system during sporting and work related activities.
- The dynamics and stability of the shoulder joint rely heavily on its soft tissue components which are subjected to a tremendous amount of force especially in overhead athletes.
- The key to diagnosing shoulder injuries correctly is to understand the surrounding functional anatomy and also being able to perform a good history and physical examination.
- Most inflammatory conditions involving tendon and muscular origins/insertions can be treated with activity modification, NSAIDs, and physical therapy.
- A thorough history and physical exam prior to advanced imaging can help in the accurate diagnosis of sports related injuries.
- Many sports related orthopaedic injuries can initially be managed with rest, activity modification, anti-inflammatory medication, and physical therapy.
- It is important to recognize the subset of injuries that may warrant more urgent surgical intervention such as ACL tears, quadriceps, patella, and Achilles tendon ruptures.

INTRODUCTION

In this chapter, clinical injuries resulting from both acute trauma and chronic repetition during the engagement of sports-related activities are discussed and a variety of treatment options are presented for ensuring pain relief, functional range of motion, and an overall improved quality of life.

INJURIES AND DISORDERS OF THE UPPER EXTREMITIES

Injuries and disorders of the shoulder

The shoulder comprises three joints (glenohumeral, sternoclavicular, and acromioclavicular) and one articulation (scapulothoracic).

The main static stabilizers include the glenoid labrum, the glenohumeral ligaments and capsular complex, the coracoacromial and coracohumeral ligaments, and the negative intracapsular pressure. The superior, middle, and inferior glenohumeral ligaments are intimate with the joint capsule and act as checkreins at the extremes of motion (Fig. 80.1). Along with the optimal positioning of the glenoid by the scapulothoracic articulation, the rotator cuff muscles act as the main dynamic stabilizers through concavity/compression forces during the arc of motion. If any of these components are disrupted either through acute injury or by overuse, the normal biomechanics are altered, which can then result in pain, dysfunction, and further injury to the rotator cuff, proximal biceps tendon, labrum, and articular cartilage.

Careful history taking, along with a systematic physical examination, is the key to accurately diagnosing patients with shoulder injuries. If the patient is an athlete who uses overhead movements, the nature and timing of the pain should be elicited, focusing on the exact phase of throwing or athletic motion that precipitates the pain. If rotator cuff involvement is present, the patient may complain of night pain

and difficulty with overhead activity through a painful arc near 90 degrees. Anterior instability can be subtle and may present as symptoms of a "dead arm" or a feeling of coming apart, especially with the late cocking or early acceleration phase of throwing (Fig. 80.2). If posterior instability is a component, the symptoms will usually be present during the follow-through phase.

The physical examination should always include a complete cervical spine and neurologic examination to ensure the lack of a C5 radicular component. Palpation examination should focus on the sternoclavicular and acromioclavicular joints, proximal biceps tendon, posterior joint line, and over the greater tuberosity. Range of motion should be tested and compared with the contralateral shoulder. Throwers will often have increased external rotation and compensatory decreased internal rotation in their pitching arm. Whether this is adaptive or a result of a posterior capsular contracture is still a matter of debate. Glenohumeral internal rotation deficit can result from contracture of the posterior band of the inferior glenohumeral ligament and posterior capsule and can cause excessive anterior/superior translation of the humeral head. This can cause internal impingement of the humeral head against the posterosuperior labrum in late cocking and be a source of posterior joint-line pain as well as a risk factor for the development of a SLAP (superior labral anterior/posterior) lesion. The remainder of the examination should focus on testing of the rotator cuff strength, assessing the degree of normal laxity or presence of instability, and performing certain provocative maneuvers to elicit specific disorders (Table 80.1). It is important to keep in mind that laxity is a normal finding in patients, in contrast to instability, which is defined as symptomatic glenohumeral laxity. Also, accurate assessment of the symptomatic shoulder is highly dependent on the ability to compare the findings to the asymptomatic, contralateral shoulder.

Glenohumeral instability

The normal degree of laxity among patients varies. Instability ranges from subtle subluxation episodes to acute, frank dislocations, which require sedation and reduction in an emergency department setting. Proper classification of shoulder instability is important in establishing a correct diagnosis and in planning a successful treatment plan. Table 80.2 outlines the classification scheme, which focuses on establishing the degree, frequency, etiology, and direction of instability. The direction of instability can be classified as unidirectional, bidirectional, or multidirectional. Patients with multidirectional instability will often lack a history of trauma or microtrauma and usually have signs of generalized ligamentous laxity, such as the ability to hyperextend their knees, elbows, and metacarpal joints and hyperabduct their thumbs.

Acute anterior shoulder dislocations

Traumatic anterior shoulder dislocations are the most common pattern of instability affecting the glenohumeral joint. This pattern constitutes over 90% of shoulder instability cases and is more common in athletes participating in contact and collision sports such as football, hockey, and rugby.[1] The mechanism of injury is a forced external rotation and extension force to an abducted and externally rotated arm. Patients with an acute anterior dislocation hold the arm fixed in a slightly externally rotated and abducted position and have a loss of the normal contour of the deltoid. An axillary view (Fig. 80.3) of the shoulder is required to definitively make the diagnosis because the anteroposterior and scapular-Y views may give false-negative impressions. The essential lesion of traumatic anterior shoulder dislocations (Bankart lesion)

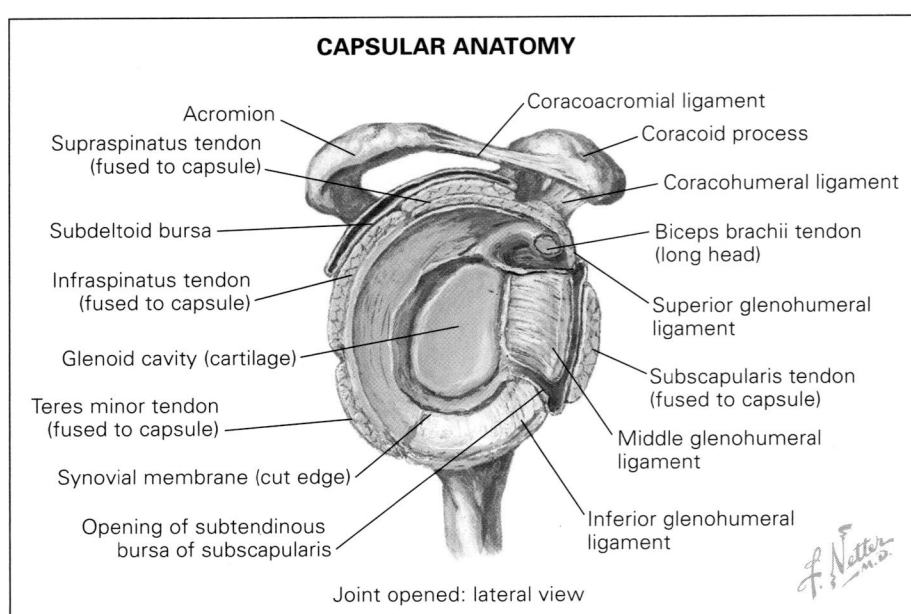

CAPSULAR ANATOMY

Acromion

Supraspinatus tendon (fused to capsule)

Coracoacromial ligament

Coracoid process

Coracohumeral ligament

Subdeltoid bursa

Infraspinatus tendon (fused to capsule)

Glenoid cavity (cartilage)

Teres minor tendon (fused to capsule)

Synovial membrane (cut edge)

Opening of subtendinous bursa of subscapularis

Biceps brachii tendon (long head)

Superior glenohumeral ligament

Subscapularis tendon (fused to capsule)

Middle glenohumeral ligament

Inferior glenohumeral ligament

Joint opened: lateral view

Fig. 80.1 Capsular anatomy.

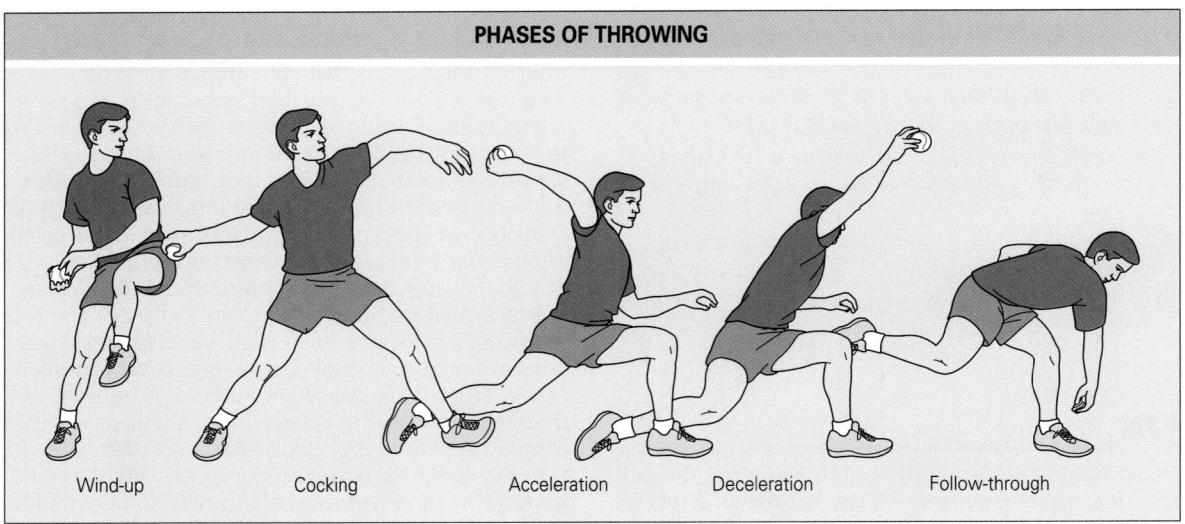

PHASES OF THROWING

Wind-up   Cocking   Acceleration   Deceleration   Follow-through

Fig. 80.2 Phases of throwing. *(From Miller MD, Cooper DE, Warner JJP. Review of sports medicine and arthroscopy. Philadelphia: WB Saunders, 1995:123.)*

is an avulsion with or without bone of the anteroinferior glenoid labrum with the capsular/ligament complex.[2] Additional pathologic processes surrounding anterior shoulder dislocations include anterior capsular attenuation and insufficiency, rotator cuff tears, Hill-Sachs lesions, glenoid rim fractures, SLAP lesions, and humeral avulsion of the glenohumeral ligament (HAGL) lesions.

Recurrence rates have been shown to be as high as 90% in young athletes who were treated conservatively.[3] Several other studies have verified the high risk of recurrence in the younger patient population (50%-66%) but found a benefit from refraining from early return to sports activities.[4] Recent data have shown that immobilizing the shoulder in external rotation more closely approximates the anteroinferior labral/capsular complex to its normal position on the glenoid and may reduce recurrence rates.[4]

Treatment of acute dislocations requires a pre-reduction neurologic examination especially to assess the function of the axillary nerve, which can be injured in 9% to 18% of acute dislocations. There are numerous reduction techniques described, and this can be accomplished with either conscious sedation or an intra-articular lidocaine injection. Regardless of what technique is used, the most important aspect is to ensure a successful reduction is adequate patient and muscular relaxation. Once the reduction is performed, radiographs must be obtained to confirm the reduction; we prefer an external sling immobilizer for a period of 3 to 6 weeks. Because of the high recurrence rates in young active patients, some have advocated acute surgical

stabilization for first-time acute dislocations. Prospective randomized trials show a significant decrease in the recurrence rates with improved function for the operative patients, but the decision to proceed with acute stabilization is still controversial and largely depends on patient-specific factors, such as age, activity level, and desire to return to preinjury status.[5]

Recurrent anterior shoulder instability

Recurrent anterior shoulder instability is disabling and ranges from pain with apprehension during specific activities to episodic subluxations and recurrent dislocation. Clinical assessment can be difficult mainly owing to patient apprehension and compliance with physical examination. Anterior instability tests are both objective and subjective and best when compared with the contralateral shoulder. The anterior apprehension and relocation test is specific for anterior instability and is best done with the patient supine with the shoulder at the edge of the table. In addition to standard radiographs, specific radiographs can be obtained looking for specific lesions. For further investigation of bony lesions, a computed tomography (CT) scan is recommended; and for soft tissue pathologic processes such as capsular redundancy or labral tears (Bankart lesion), a magnetic resonance (MR) arthrogram is the tool of choice. Open stabilization procedures have stood the test of time, with recurrence rates ranging from 3% to 5%. However, many of these procedures involved non-anatomic reconstructions; and although they prevented recurrent instability, lack of motion (mainly external

TABLE 80.1 MUSCLE TESTING FOR SHOULDER INJURIES

Examination	Technique	Significance
Impingement/RTC		
Impingement sign	Passive FF > 90°	Pain = impingement syndrome
Impingement test	Same after subacromial injection	Relief of pain = impingement syndrome
Hawkins test	Passive FF 90° and lift	Pain = impingement syndrome
Jobe test	Resisted pronation/FF 90°	Pain = supraspinatus lesion
Drop arm test	Maintain FF in plane of scapula	Instability = supraspinatus lesion
Hornblower test	Resisted max ER/abd 90°	Pain = infraspinatus/(post) supraspinatus lesion
Rubber band sign	Resisted max ER/slight abd	Pain = infraspinatus lesion
Lift-off test	Arm IR behind back	Inability to elevate from back = subscapularis lesion
Modified lift-off test	Resisted arm held off back	Inability to keep elevated off back = subscapularis lesion
Belly-push test	Elbow held anterior with abd pressure	Inability to hold elbow forward = subscapularis lesion
Instability		
Apprehension test	Supine abd 90° and ER	Apprehension = ant instability
Relocation test	Apprehension with posterior force	Relief of apprehension = ant instability
Load and shift test	Ant/post force on humeral head	Degree of translation = laxity vs. instability
Modified load and shift test	Supine load/shift with elbow bending	Degree of translation = laxity vs. instability
Jerk test	Post force w/ arm add and FF	"Clunk" = posterior subluxation
Sulcus sign	Inferior force w/ arm at side	Increased acromiohumeral interval = int laxity vs. instability
Labrum/Biceps		
Active compression test	10° add, 90° FF, max pronation	Pain with resistance = SLAP lesion
Anterior slide test	Hand on hip, joint loading	Pain with resistance = SLAP lesion
Crank test	Full abd, humeral loading, rotation	Pain = SLAP lesion
Speed test	Resisted FF in scapular plane	Pain = bicipital tendinitis
Yerguson test	Resisted supination	Pain = bicipital tendinitis
Miscellaneous		
Spurling maneuver	Lat flexion, rotation, cervical loading	Cervical spine pathology
Wright test	Ext-abd-ER of arm w/ neck rotated away	Loss of pulse and reproduction of symptoms = thoracic outlet syndrome

RTC, rotator cuff; FF, forward flexion; IR, internal rotation; ER, external rotation; abd, abductor; ant, anterior; post, posterior; add, adduction; ext, extension; inf, inferior; max, maximum; SLAP, superior labrum from anterior to posterior; lat, lateral.

TABLE 80.2 CLASSIFICATION OF SHOULDER INSTABILITY

Degree

Dislocation
Subluxation
Microinstability

Frequency

Acute (primary)
Chronic
    Recurrent
    Fixed

Etiology

Traumatic (macrotrauma)
Atraumatic
    Voluntary (muscular)
    Involuntary
Acquired (microtrauma)

Direction

Unidirectional
    Anterior
    Posterior
    Inferior
Bidirectional
    Anteroinferior
    Posteroinferior
Multidirectional

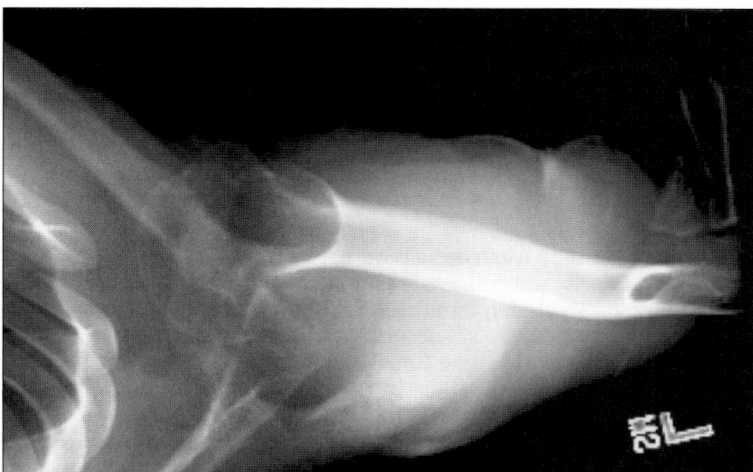

Fig. 80.3 Axillary radiograph of anterior shoulder showing dislocation with Hill-Sachs lesion.

components of instability and any other pathologic processes that may be present. Arthroscopic surgery also allows for a quicker recovery, less postoperative pain, and less morbidity and can be performed as an outpatient procedure.

Posterior shoulder instability

Posterior instability is much less common than anterior instability, accounting for only a small percentage of instability cases. Acute, frank dislocations are uncommon and are often missed (50%) on their initial presentation. The more common presentation of posterior instability includes pain localized to the posterior joint line and subtle subluxations during the provocative position of flexion, adduction, and internal rotation. In athletes, a direct blow to the anterior shoulder or, more commonly, a posteriorly directed force to the shoulder while held in the provocative position is the typical mechanism of injury. Football linemen, overhead throwers, and swimmers are subjected to repetitive microtrauma during sports that can cause injury to the posterior labrum and associated capsular/ligament complex. Patients who present with an acute dislocation typically hold their arm in an

rotation) and subsequent arthritis were problems with some of these reconstructions.[6] Arthroscopic shoulder stabilizations have results that are now matching those of open repairs.[7] Arthroscopic procedures allow surgeons to better visualize the capsular/ligament complex as well as the entire glenohumeral joint, which affords the ability to address all

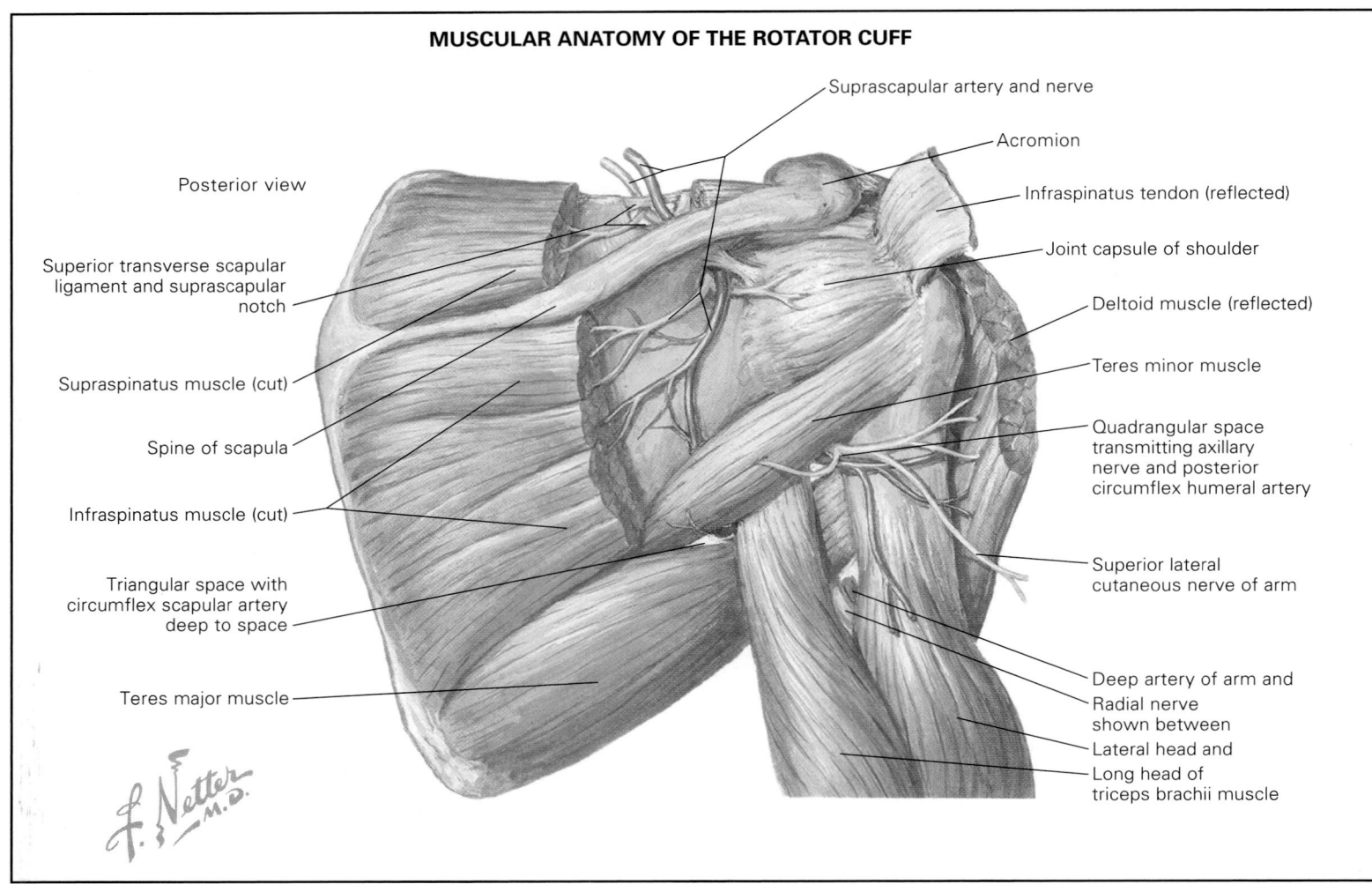

MUSCULAR ANATOMY OF THE ROTATOR CUFF

Posterior view

Superior transverse scapular ligament and suprascapular notch

Supraspinatus muscle (cut)

Spine of scapula

Infraspinatus muscle (cut)

Triangular space with circumflex scapular artery deep to space

Teres major muscle

Suprascapular artery and nerve

Acromion

Infraspinatus tendon (reflected)

Joint capsule of shoulder

Deltoid muscle (reflected)

Teres minor muscle

Quadrangular space transmitting axillary nerve and posterior circumflex humeral artery

Superior lateral cutaneous nerve of arm

Deep artery of arm and Radial nerve shown between Lateral head and Long head of triceps brachii muscle

Fig. 80.4 Muscular anatomy of the rotator cuff.

adducted, internally rotated position with prominence of the coracoid process anteriorly and fullness posteriorly. A trauma series including the axillary view will demonstrate an empty glenoid with a posteriorly displaced humeral head. Reduction should be performed, but caution should be used because these injuries sometimes present late and can be extremely difficult to reduce in the emergency department setting and may require anesthesia and an open reduction.

For recurrent posterior shoulder instability, some patients will be able to demonstrate their instability pattern by positioning and selective muscle activation. The medical professional should be alerted to the patient who habitually and willfully dislocates his or her shoulder for secondary gain. Physical examination should include tests for all types of instability, including the jerk test, load and shift, and sulcus test, which are specific for posterior and inferior instability. Often, these tests will elicit symptoms of pain and grinding rather than discernible translation. Testing for generalized ligamentous laxity is important because it has implications for potential treatment options. After acute reductions, immobilization in the neutral position for 4 to 6 weeks, followed by physical therapy for periscapular and rotator cuff strengthening is the initial treatment of choice. The incidence of recurrence after acute dislocations is much less than with acute anterior dislocations; patients with an atraumatic or microtraumatic onset have a high rate of success with conservative treatment.[8] Those patients who fail conservative treatment may require surgical stabilization, which ranges from open, bone-block, and muscle-tendon transfers to arthroscopic anatomic repair and capsular plications. Arthroscopic posterior instability surgery has results that are now as good as open procedures, with success rates ranging from 90% to 97%.[9]

Multidirectional shoulder instability

Multidirectional instability of the shoulder is a complex entity that warrants careful investigation to avoid unnecessary surgery that may fail. Affected patients have global (anterior, posterior, and inferior) excessive laxity of the glenohumeral joint and usually will have signs of generalized ligamentous laxity. Onset is frequently atraumatic, and the chief complaint is normally pain through the mid ranges of motion; terminal ranges of motion are normally avoided. The contralateral shoulder often displays equal laxity but may be asymptomatic, which leads investigators to search for other pathologic causes besides excessive and redundant capsular/ligament tissue. These factors may include subtle losses of strength and/or neuromotor coordination of the rotator cuff and scapular stabilizing muscles, as well as defective proprioceptive responses. An aggressive and prolonged course of physical therapy (at least 6 months) focusing on periscapular and rotator cuff strengthening and conditioning with modalities to increase proprioception and coordination has been shown to be successful in 80% to 90% of cases.[8] Surgery is an option for patients who were compliant with a specific exercise program but who remain symptomatic. Surgery is not offered to voluntary dislocators with emotional problems or to behaviorally immature teenagers. An open inferior capsular shift remains the gold standard for surgical treatment of multidirectional instability of the shoulder with results yielding greater than 90% success with recurrent instability and/or persistent pain being defined as failure.[10]

Rotator cuff pathology and impingement syndrome
Pathology of the rotator cuff

The rotator cuff is a tendinous confluence of the supraspinatus, infraspinatus, subscapularis, and teres minor muscles (Fig. 80.4). It has an intimate association with the proximal biceps tendon, which runs through the rotator interval (the space between the superior border of the subscapularis and the anterior leading edge of the supraspinatus) from its variable insertion on the superior glenoid and labrum. The main function of the rotator cuff is to maintain the humeral head through compressive forces in the center of the glenoid throughout the arc of glenohumeral motion. In addition to being dynamic stabilizers, the individual muscles based on their force vectors allow for shoulder rotation. The infraspinatus and teres minor are primarily external rotators, whereas the subscapularis internally rotates the humeral head. Without their compressive forces, the humeral head would migrate superiorly into the subacromial space and lead to impingement with a loss of the fulcrum, which the powerful deltoid muscle relies on for its action. The cuff acts to fine tune these powerful movements and is subjected to a tremendous amount of force during overhead and throwing motions, which have been shown to be the greatest with eccentric muscle contraction during the follow-through and deceleration phases.

Rotator cuff disease is commonly seen in clinical practice, and the incidence of rotator cuff tears has been reported to be between 39% and 60% based on cadaveric specimens, which may not accurately reflect the incidence in the general population or in athletes. Tears may be present in asymptomatic patients, which make it difficult to know the true incidence of rotator cuff tears; however, the incidence increases with patient age.

The pathogenesis of rotator cuff tears is complex. The bursal side of the tendon displays greater deformation and tensile strength, which is a possible explanation for the increased incidence of articular-sided tears. In young patients and overhead throwers, most tears are found on the articular side of the cuff; similarly, most degenerative tears are also found on the articular side. No one factor can be attributed to rotator cuff tears, and with intrinsic weakness leading to superior humeral head migration and subsequent impingement a vicious cycle can arise, resulting in further impingement and possible bursal-sided cuff injury.[11]

Patients with rotator cuff tears present with symptoms of pain especially at night and with overhead activity. The amount of pain can vary depending on the amount of impingement, status of the biceps tendon, and the size of the tear. Partial tears are often more painful than full-thickness tears, and patients who present with stiffness usually have more pain. The onset and duration of pain should be elicited to determine if the tear is acute, chronic, or acute on chronic. The location of pain is typically anterolateral owing to the supraspinatus being the most commonly involved tendon; however, involvement of the subscapularis and biceps tendon may cause more anterior-based pain. Weakness may or may not be present depending on the amount of associated pain, integrity of the intact cuff, and compensation from the deltoid and surrounding muscles. The examination should be comprehensive, starting with inspection looking for any muscular atrophy or scapular winging. A complete neurologic and cervical spine examination should be performed to rule out radiculopathy or suprascapular nerve entrapment. In addition to instability tests, impingement signs, and range of motion assessment, specific tests looking for weakness of the individual rotator cuff muscles should be performed. Patients with massive tears may have specific signs such as the external rotation lag sign or hornblower's sign.

Plain radiographs are usually normal; and for patients who fail conservative treatment, further imaging is required, such as conventional arthrography, ultrasonography, CT arthrography, and magnetic resonance imaging (MRI). Ultrasonography is advantageous because it is non-invasive and inexpensive; however, it is highly user dependent and not as sensitive for partial-thickness tears. MRI is the preferred modality because it more clearly defines the nature of the tear and allows for assessment of tissue quality. The presence of muscle atrophy and fatty degeneration within the muscle belly can be detected, indicating a chronic tear. Chronic tears of the rotator cuff may have implications on surgical options, and advanced muscular atrophy may make the rotator cuff unable to be repaired.

Conservative treatment for patients who present with signs and symptoms of impingement and rotator cuff pathology should be initiated. This consists of rest, activity modification, and non-steroidal anti-inflammatory drugs (NSAIDs) followed by physical therapy for range of motion, rotator cuff, and periscapular strengthening exercises. There is no well-accepted timeline for the duration of conservative treatment, and some patients will continue to improve up to 18 months. Successful conservative management for partial- and full-thickness rotator cuff tears has been documented to be 50% to 80%.[12] For patients who give a history of an acute traumatic injury or for patients who report a recent exacerbation of a chronic problem, further

imaging should be done earlier to rule out a complete, full-thickness tear. The natural history of partial-thickness tears is incompletely understood, but there is some evidence that few heal on their own and there is potential for progression over a short period of time. Surgical intervention generally is considered for patients with symptoms of sufficient duration and intensity. The timing of surgery has ranged from a few months to 5 years, but it should be based on the patient's symptoms, improvement, and rate of improvement with non-surgical therapy as well as on the goals of the patient. The decision on whether to débride or repair partial-thickness tears should be made based on intraoperative findings, and tears with greater than 50% thickness should be repaired with the use of suture anchors or osseous bone tunnels. In general, surgical management with decompression and rotator cuff repair has yielded satisfactory results (>90% in most series) with mini-open and arthroscopic techniques.

Subacromial impingement syndrome

The diagnosis of impingement syndrome has been increasingly used for patients with shoulder pain and dysfunction. Impingement can be described as primary or secondary. Primary impingement can be caused from intrinsic (intratendinous) or extrinsic (extratendinous) factors, whereas secondary impingement is a result of another process such as glenohumeral instability or neurologic injury. Disruption in the dynamic function of the rotator cuff or periscapular muscles can lead to encroachment of the subacromial structures between the greater tuberosity and the anterior acromion, acromial or distal clavicle spur, or coracoacromial ligament. Extrinsic factors that may aid in the development of impingement include abnormal acromial morphology, calcified or hypertrophied coracoacromial ligament, degenerative acromioclavicular joint with spurring, and an unfused distal acromial epiphysis (os acromiale). Three stages of impingement have been described: stage I involves hemorrhage and edema within the bursa, stage II is characterized by fibrosis and tendinitis of the rotator cuff, and stage III entails more chronic changes represented by partial- and full-thickness tears of the rotator cuff tendons.[13]

Patients who present with impingement syndrome mainly complain of pain, which can often be accompanied by stiffness and weakness. Onset is usually insidious, but patients may offer a history of a minor event that may have started the process. For athletes, a change in their normal routine or recent overuse may precipitate the onset. Primary impingement is more common in patients older than age 40 years, whereas secondary impingement is usually found in younger patients and athletes; therefore, an underlying cause such as glenohumeral instability or a labral pathologic process (SLAP lesion) must be sought in this population. Physical examination should focus on range of motion, rotator cuff strength, instability testing, and various provocative maneuvers in a search for impingement and acromioclavicular joint arthrosis. Shoulder pain can cause weakness during physical examination, which may cloud the clinical picture. The impingement test is performed by injecting a local anesthetic such as lidocaine into the subacromial space and then repeating the rotator cuff strength examination. If weakness persists, further investigation is warranted to check for the integrity of the rotator cuff and rule out cervical spine disease or suprascapular nerve entrapment. In addition to standard shoulder radiographs, a special view called the supraspinatus outlet radiograph (Fig. 80.5), a lateral radiograph that is made in the plane of the scapula with the x-ray beam directed 10 degrees caudad, can be used to better view the subacromial space and classify the acromial morphology.

Treatment of impingement syndrome is centered on minimizing patient discomfort with activity modification, NSAIDs, and physical therapy to restore the strength and normal biomechanics of the shoulder joint. The use of subacromial corticosteroid injections is still widely used as an adjunct to physical therapy despite the lack of efficacy in recent randomized controlled trials.[14] Variability exists on the length of conservative treatment for impingement given the association with a concomitant pathologic process. For certain etiologic factors such as a hooked acromion (which may impinge on the rotator cuff), a labral pathologic process, or a full-thickness rotator cuff tear, surgery may be indicated sooner than later to address these issues. The current procedure of choice is an arthroscopic subacromial decompression with bursectomy and anterior acromioplasty. The results vary depending on the status of the rotator cuff and glenohumeral joint, but overall satisfactory results are achieved 80% to 90% of the time when the joint is intact and the rotator cuff cannot be repaired.

Injuries to the sternoclavicular joint, acromioclavicular joint, and scapula

Injuries to the sternoclavicular joint

Injuries to the sternoclavicular joint are rare and can be the result of direct or indirect forces. The joint is unique in that it has the least amount of bony stability of all the major joints in the body but is supported by the surrounding soft tissue envelope. The spectrum of injury can range from a mild sprain to a complete dislocation. Radiographs can be difficult to interpret, and CT has been found to be the best imaging modality to characterize the injury. The majority of injuries are anterior dislocations, which are usually unstable even after attempted reduction. These injuries typically cause little to no functional limitations, but a persistent anterior prominence of the dislocated clavicle is to be expected. Operative treatment for these injuries is fraught with complications and should be avoided. The less frequent posterior dislocation should be carefully evaluated owing to the surrounding structures, which can result in the following injuries: brachial plexus compression, pneumothorax, respiratory distress, vascular compromise, dysphagia, hoarseness, and death. A review of the literature found a 25% incidence (16 of 60) of complications associated with this injury and noted that most were present at the time of injury. Prompt attention should be given to these injuries, and treatment should consist of closed reduction in the operating room with a vascular or cardiothoracic surgeon available. If closed reduction fails, operative intervention is warranted because of persistent problems associated with a posteriorly protruding medial clavicle.

Injuries to the acromioclavicular joint

The acromioclavicular (AC) joint is one of the most vulnerable and commonly injured joints in athletics. The mechanism of injury can be direct or indirect and most often is the result of a fall onto the acromion with the humerus in an adducted position. Subluxation or dislocation can result, depending on the status of the supporting ligaments, which are the capsular ligaments (AC ligaments) and the coracoclavicular (CC) ligaments. Patients will present with acute pain, swelling, ecchymosis, and sometimes deformity over the joint. Radiographs should include an anteroposterior view of both AC joints for comparison, an axillary view to determine anteroposterior translation, and a Zanca view (10°-15° cephalic tilt), which isolates the AC joint. Rockwood's classification is used to describe these injuries (Fig. 80.6). Treatment of types I and II are generally conservative with rest, ice, and gradual return to activities. In a small number of these patients, chronic symptoms of pain and fatigue may persist that can be successfully managed with a distal clavicle excision. For types IV, V, and VI, surgery is normally the treatment of choice owing to the morbidity associated with the marked displacement of the distal clavicle and concomitant effect it has on shoulder function. Controversy still exists on the most optimal treatment of type III injuries. There are no clear data that patients who receive surgery for type III injuries do better than those treated conservatively; in a meta-analysis, 88% of the operatively

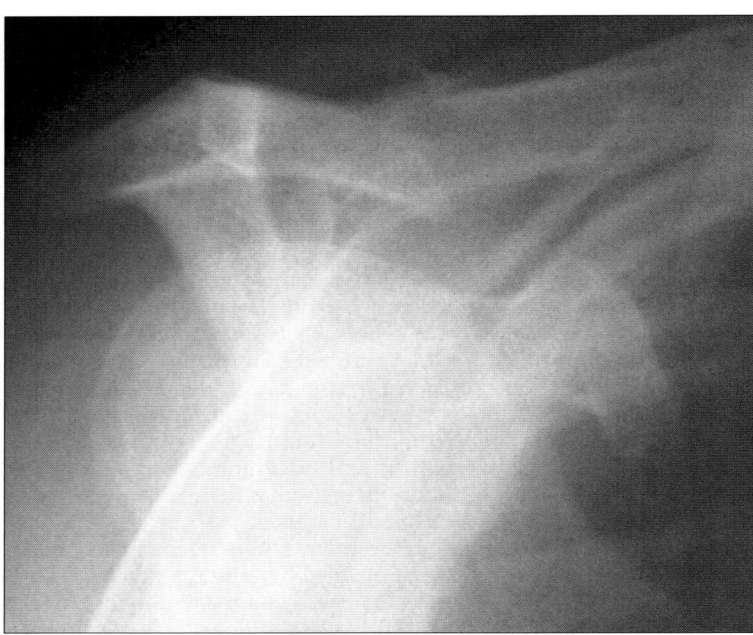

Fig. 80.5 Supraspinatus outlet radiograph showing stage III acromion impingement.

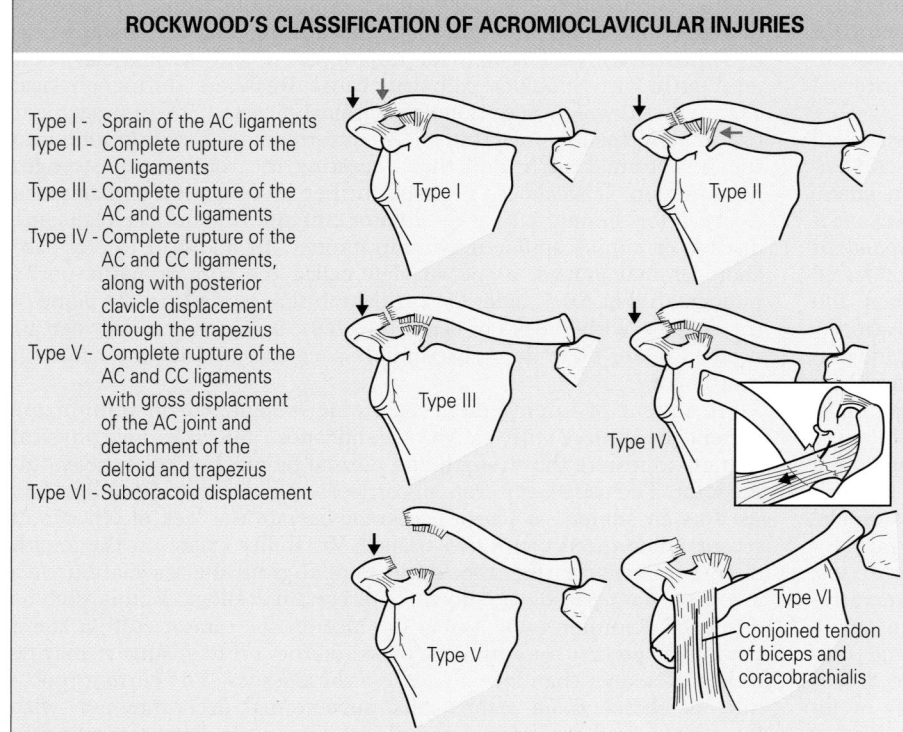

ROCKWOOD'S CLASSIFICATION OF ACROMIOCLAVICULAR INJURIES

Type I - Sprain of the AC ligaments
Type II - Complete rupture of the AC ligaments
Type III - Complete rupture of the AC and CC ligaments
Type IV - Complete rupture of the AC and CC ligaments, along with posterior clavicle displacement through the trapezius
Type V - Complete rupture of the AC and CC ligaments with gross displacment of the AC joint and detachment of the deltoid and trapezius
Type VI - Subcoracoid displacement

Type I
Type II
Type III
Type IV
Type V
Type VI
Conjoined tendon of biceps and coracobrachialis

Fig. 80.6 Rockwood's classification of acromioclavicular injuries. Type I: Sprain of the AC ligaments. Type II: Complete rupture of the AC ligaments. Type III: Complete rupture of the AC and CC ligaments. Type IV: Complete rupture of the AC and CC ligaments, along with posterior clavicle displacement through the trapezius. Type V: Complete rupture of the AC and CC ligaments with gross displacement of the AC joint and detachment of the deltoid and trapezius. Type VI: Subcoracoid displacement.

treated and 87% of the non-operatively treated patients had satisfactory outcomes.[15] Surgery should not be performed for cosmetic reasons. If symptoms persist for more than 6 months, surgery can be considered for pain relief and return of function. Surgical procedures are geared toward stabilizing the joint and resecting the distal clavicle. Anatomic based repairs of the coracoclavicular ligaments are in favor.[16] Newer arthroscopic techniques have also been developed for stabilizing AC joint dislocations, but no data exist on whether this offers any advantage for acute stabilization of type III injuries.

Disorders of the scapulothoracic articulation

The scapulothoracic articulation is an integral link in the kinetic chain that together with the glenohumeral, elbow, and wrist joint ultimately places the hand in space to perform routine activities of daily living. In the case of athletes, the scapula performs highly coordinated movements that produce controlled, precise actions, such as pitching a baseball. Snapping scapula syndrome is characterized by pain and crepitation usually located at the superior and medial border of the scapula. The etiology of this condition includes osseous deformity from an osteochondroma, postural changes from kyphosis and scoliosis, and soft tissue abnormalities resulting in inflammation and resultant bursitis. The mainstay of treatment is rest, NSAIDs, and physical therapy for conditioning and strengthening of the periscapular muscles. Recalcitrant cases can be addressed with surgery, including open partial scapulectomies and arthroscopic débridement of the subscapular space.

Tendinopathy in the shoulder and elbow

Disorders of the proximal biceps tendon and superior labrum

The proximal biceps tendon has a considerable amount of variation in regard to its origin from the superior glenoid and labrum, and its mechanical function is not completely understood but it is thought to act as a glenohumeral joint stabilizer. The tendon and its origin are placed under a great deal of tension and force during activities such as throwing and are subjected to injury that can result in degeneration,

instability, and even complete rupture. Disorders of the proximal biceps tendon can be a considerable source of pain and disability for overhead throwers and laborers. Biceps degeneration and tendinosis can be associated with impingement and injury to the rotator cuff. Like the bursal side of the rotator cuff, the proximal biceps tendon can be subjected to mechanical irritation by the coracoacromial arch. A SLAP lesion describes an injury to the superior labrum at the biceps origin with a classification system that includes four injury patterns (Fig. 80.7).[17] Most SLAP lesions consist of degeneration with fraying (type I) and, in more severe cases, detachment of the tendon anchor (type II). In addition, intra-articular lesions often accompany these lesions, particularly in rotator cuff pathology.

Presenting complaints vary from pain located at the bicipital groove to a deep-seated pain with mechanical symptoms, such as grinding or a catching sensation. The history may reveal an acute injury or repetitive overhead activity. For patients with tendinosis and instability, tenderness can usually be elicited by palpating the tendon at the bicipital groove. Patients with chronic disease may describe a spontaneous rupture with sudden relief of symptoms with a residual fullness in the anterior brachium (Popeye sign). Specific tests for the biceps tendon and SLAP lesions include the Speed, Yergason, and O'Brien active compression tests. The most sensitive test for identifying SLAP lesions and other disorders of the proximal biceps tendon is an MR arthrogram. Conservative treatment is usually initiated first, with surgery reserved for those patients whose condition does not improve.

Injuries to the pectoralis major tendon

Rupture of the pectoralis major tendon is uncommon but usually occurs in males at the humeral insertion site. Most ruptures are complete and involve an eccentric contraction, whereas the arm is in abduction, extension, and external rotation. Diagnosis may be difficult initially owing to swelling and ecchymosis, but the anterior axillary fold may reveal abnormal contour and medial retraction of the tendon may create a bulging in the anterior chest wall. MRI may aid in the

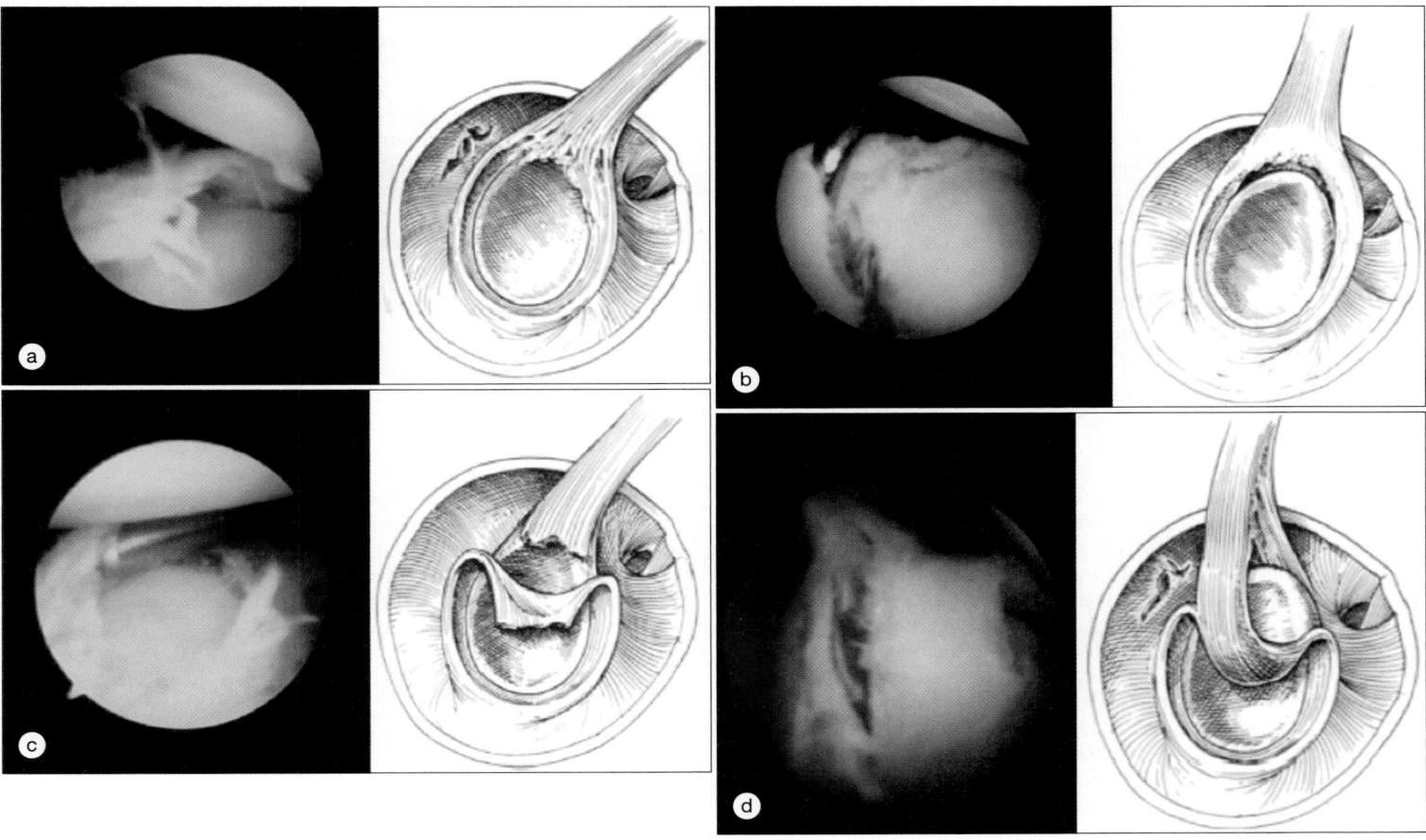

Fig. 80.7 Classification of SLAP lesions. (a) Type I. (b) Type II. (c) Type III. (d) Type 4. *(From Snyder SJ, Karzel RP, Del Pizzo W, et al. SLAP lesions of the shoulder. Arthroscopy 1990;6:274-279.)*

diagnosis. Non-surgical treatment is reserved for partial-thickness tears and the muscle belly injury. Surgical repair, indicated for pectoralis tendon avulsions, has shown superior results to conservative treatment with a good return of strength and resumption of preinjury activities.

Ruptures of the distal biceps tendon

Rupture of the distal biceps tendon from its insertion on the radial tuberosity is usually seen in the dominant arm in males who are between 40 and 60 years of age. Preexisting tendon degeneration is thought to play a role in the pathogenesis, with a forced eccentric contraction being the most common mechanism of injury. Patients usually report feeling a tearing or ripping sensation at the time of injury. Initial presentation demonstrates pain, swelling, and ecchymosis in the antecubital region with a visible and palpable defect for complete ruptures. Patients who present with chronic ruptures will normally complain about weakness and early fatigue with elbow flexion and especially supination maneuvers, such as using a screwdriver or wrench. Surgery is recommended for these injuries, and results are best when treated early.

Lateral epicondylitis

Lateral epicondylitis, often referred to as "tennis elbow," is a common diagnosis and affects mostly the origin of the extensor carpi radialis brevis muscle. The key examination finding is point tenderness located 2 mm anterior to the lateral epicondyle with pain on resisted wrist and finger extension. Treatment is mostly conservative, consisting of rest, activity modification, NSAIDs, wrist/forearm extension counterforce braces, and corticosteroid injections. Iontophoresis with the application of a topical corticosteroid cream has been used with some success along with gentle strengthening exercises once the pain has subsided. Although most patients do well with conservative measures, open, arthroscopic, and percutaneous releases of the extensor origin have been described with good success for recalcitrant cases.[18]

Medial epicondylitis

Medial epicondylitis is not as common as its lateral counterpart and usually affects laborers and athletes who undergo repetitive wrist flexion and pronation such as golfers, bowlers, and tennis players. These maneuvers stress the origin of the flexor/pronator muscles and are characterized by pain and tenderness located at the anterior aspect of the medial epicondyle. Non-surgical treatment is similar to that of lateral epicondylitis, and results are favorable. Ulnar neuritis is in the differential diagnosis and must be ruled out; care must be taken when administering corticosteroid injections so as not to injure the nerve. For cases that do not respond to a prolonged course of conservative therapy, open débridement and repair can be performed with good results.[19]

Athletic injuries to the elbow

Medial ulnar collateral ligament injuries, valgus extension overload, and posterior medial impingement

The thrower's elbow is subjected to a tremendous amount of valgus stress during the late cocking and early acceleration phases of throwing. The anterior band of the medial ulnar collateral ligament (MUCL) is the primary restraint to valgus stress with contributions from the flexor/pronator mass and the congruous articular geometry. Injury to the MUCL can occur from chronic attenuation or from an acute injury. Patients with injury to the MUCL rely on the dynamic stability from the flexor/pronator muscle group, which can be inhibited by pain or by alterations in the coordinated muscle firing pattern. This can predispose the MUCL to further injury as well as overload the articular constraints, which consist of the olecranon and its fossa and the radiocapitellar joint. With valgus stress and combined extension forces during the throwing motion, repetitive forceful shearing of the olecranon within its fossa can cause posteromedial impingement, with the development of chondromalacia and eventual osteophyte formation. This constellation of valgus instability and posteromedial impingement is referred to as valgus extension overload.

Athletes with valgus instability experience medial elbow pain during the acceleration phase of throwing. If the injury is chronic, patients will note the gradual onset of pain even during low-velocity attempts

and complain of decreased pitching velocity. Acute injuries create a sudden, sharp pop with pain and inability to continue throwing. Concomitant ulnar nerve symptoms are common in chronic injuries and include paresthesias radiating into the fourth and fifth digits. Complaints of catching, grinding, or locking may indicate loose bodies or impingement secondary to osteophytes. Range of motion should be checked for the presence of full extension, because pain with terminal extension and/or the lack of terminal extension may be a sign of posteromedial impingement. Tenderness along the medial joint line and medial epicondyle may be related to flexor/pronator strain, MUCL injury, or ulnar neuritis. The ulnar nerve should be assessed for subluxation, and the Tinel sign should be elicited. The milking maneuver, which also tests for valgus instability, is done by pulling on the patient's thumb while the forearm is supinated and the elbow flexed beyond 90 degrees. The subjective feeling of apprehension, instability, or pain is indicative of an MUCL injury.

Valgus stress radiographs may be obtained to assess the amount of medial opening; more than 3 mm when compared with the other side is diagnostic of valgus instability. MRI is extremely sensitive for complete tears of the MUCL, but the sensitivity significantly decreases for partial-thickness tears. Saline- or gadolinium-enhanced MR arthrography can be used and has been shown to increase the sensitivity for the diagnosis of partial-thickness tears when compared with standard MRI. Partial-thickness injuries can be managed conservatively with rest (3-6 weeks), NSAIDs, and physical therapy modalities, followed by a supervised return to throwing through a regulated, interval throwing program. For complete ruptures, it is less likely that conservative management will lead to favorable results in the overhead thrower. Partial-thickness tears that do not respond to conservative measures and full-thickness tears can be treated with a variety of techniques that reconstruct the anterior band of the MUCL. In high school, collegiate, and professional baseball players, a return to previous or higher level of competition can be expected 68% to 86% of the time.[20]

Osteochondritis dissecans of the capitellum

The capitellum ossific nucleus is the first to ossify and appear in the pediatric elbow and can begin to fuse with the trochlea and lateral epicondyle as early as 10 years of age. The lateral elbow compartment is subjected to high forces especially in the athletic adolescent, which can predispose the capitellum to injury. The exact etiology of osteochondritis dissecans (OCD) is not well understood, but repetitive microtrauma has been proposed to disrupt the subchondral blood supply, which is the hallmark of OCD lesions. Subchondral bone necrosis with loss of structural support may lead to fragmentation and articular cartilage delamination. OCD involving the capitellum occurs in adolescents (>13 years of age) and is characterized by the insidious onset of dull, poorly localized pain that is worst with activity and relieved with rest. The presence of locking and catching may indicate a loose fragment. Plain radiographs may be normal or show rarefaction and irregular ossification of the capitellum. With disease progression, a demarcated island of subchondral bone may be observed and MRI is indicated to determine the size of the lesion as well as to determine the presence of separation or displacement. Treatment depends on the stage of the lesion, and results are better for younger patients with non-displaced lesions. Non-displaced lesions can be treated conservatively, whereas displaced, loose fragments are treated with a variety of surgical procedures with variable results. If a loose fragment has just cartilage without any subchondral bone, fixation of this piece is not possible and removal of the loose piece with débridement of the bed is performed. If the piece has subchondral bone remaining, then internal fixation can be performed in hopes of achieving bony union with resultant salvage of the articular cartilage.

INJURIES TO THE LOWER EXTREMITIES

Injuries to the hip, thigh, and pelvis

History and diagnosis

Hip and pelvic injuries can result from an acute event or from a chronic overuse mechanism. Often, hip or pelvic pain can be difficult for the patient to localize but determining the exact location of the pain can be quite helpful in narrowing the differential diagnosis. In addition, evaluating whether the symptoms began after a discrete injury versus the insidious onset of discomfort over a period of time can aid in narrowing the likely source of pain. The examination begins when the patient enters the room with careful observation of the patient's gait pattern. Pain that is difficult for the patient to clearly localize with their history may be better appreciated with reproduction of their symptoms on examination. Range of motion should be evaluated and compared with the normal contralateral extremity. A thorough neurovascular examination including strength and sensory testing should always be undertaken because lumbar spine injuries can often be confused with thigh, hip, and pelvis pathologic processes.

Plain radiographs of the affected area should be obtained to evaluate for fracture. Advanced imaging with CT or MRI is sometimes indicated depending on the findings of the examination and radiographs. In general, a bony pathologic process is best evaluated with CT scan, whereas soft tissue structures are better visualized with MRI. The addition of intra-articular contrast in combination with CT or MRI can improve the sensitivity and specificity of these examinations and is sometimes indicated when evaluating certain soft tissue injuries in and around the hip and pelvis.

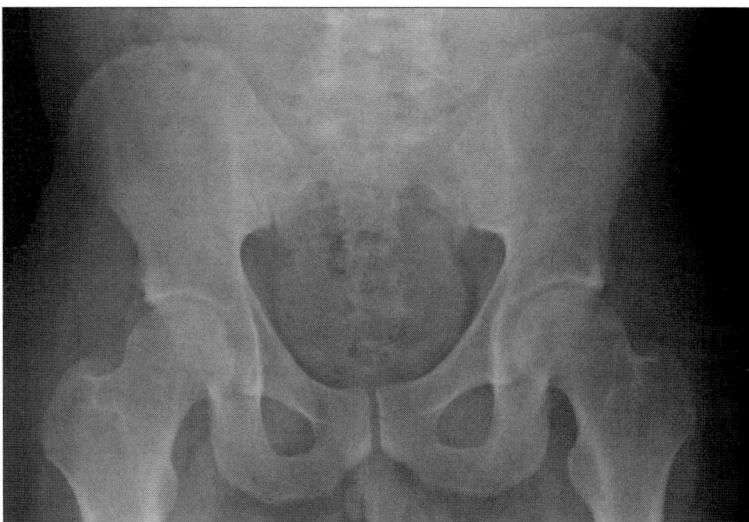

Fig. 80.8 Anteroposterior radiograph showing decreased offset at the femoral head/neck junction.

Acute injuries to the hip, thigh, and pelvis
Iliac crest contusions
Iliac crest contusions are also commonly referred to as hip pointers. They result from direct trauma to the area, usually during a contact sport. They present as localized pain directly over the iliac crest as well as ecchymosis and tenderness. Radiographs should be obtained to rule out an iliac wing fracture or possibly an avulsion fracture in the pediatric population. Otherwise, treatment is conservative, consisting of ice, compression, and analgesia with NSAIDs. Additional padding over the affected area can be helpful with providing some additional protection in the acute phase and allowing an earlier return to sport.

Quadriceps contusions
A quadriceps contusion results from a direct blow mechanism and presents as swelling, localized tenderness, and ecchymosis. Management consists of compression, ice, and NSAIDs. In addition, placing and holding the knee in 120 degrees of flexion immediately after a quadriceps contusion shortens the time to return to unrestricted activities.[21] With severe injuries that produce a large hematoma, evaluation for compartment syndrome is required. Myositis ossificans can sometimes be appreciated in follow-up radiographs but is rarely symptomatic.

Labral tears
Advances in clinical examination, diagnostic imaging, and surgical techniques have led to an improvement in the diagnosis as well as the management of labral tears of the hip. Labral tears are now the most commonly diagnosed hip joint lesions in athletes. They commonly occur after a twisting or pivoting injury with the acute onset of groin pain and mechanical symptoms. The onset may also be insidious with no history of a well-defined injury. Diagnosis can be complicated by a number of causes of referred hip pain involving the lumbar spine, the sacroiliac joint, and the pelvis. Patients with labral tears will often localize the discomfort to the groin region anteriorly. Mechanical symptoms such as clicking or catching can also be reported. The most common physical examination findings include increased groin pain or mechanical symptoms with flexion, adduction, and internal rotation of the hip. A resisted straight-leg raise or axial loading of the hip with forced internal rotation can reproduce symptoms as well. The "C" sign is also characteristic of hip joint pathology and refers to the patient cupping the hand above the greater trochanter with the thumb over the posterior aspect and the fingers in the groin region.

Imaging begins with plain radiographs of the pelvis and dedicated views of the involved hip; 87% of patients with labral tears demonstrated at least one abnormal finding on plain radiographs, including acetabular dysplasia, decreased offset at the femoral head/neck junction, and retroversion of the acetabulum (Fig. 80.8).[22] Fluoroscopically guided injection of the hip joint with an anesthetic and corticosteroid can be quite helpful in localizing the cause of the hip discomfort to the hip joint itself as opposed to some other extra-articular cause. Improvement in symptoms after an anesthetic arthrogram of the hip is 90%

reliable as an indicator of an intra-articular pathologic process.[23] MRI and MR arthrography can also be quite helpful in evaluation of the soft tissue structures around the hip, including the labrum. One complicating factor, however, is that labral pathology as visualized on MRI has been documented among asymptomatic volunteers.[24] Conservative management is the first line of treatment for hip labral tears and consists of physical therapy, activity modification, NSAIDs, as well as anesthetic injection. In cases of failed conservative management, surgical intervention, either open or arthroscopic, is a treatment option. Arthroscopic treatment of labral tears can be quite effective, with reported satisfactory outcomes ranging from 67% to 93%.[25]

Apophyseal avulsion injuries
Avulsion fractures occur almost exclusively in the athletic adolescent population. The mechanism of injury typically consists of a sudden and forceful concentric or eccentric contraction of a muscle group that attaches to an apophysis. A variety of different apophyseal fractures can occur around the hip and pelvis. Fractures of the anterior superior iliac spine result from contractions of the sartorius and tensor fascia lata. Anterior inferior iliac spine fractures are caused by contraction of the rectus femoris. Fractures at the ischial tuberosity are the most common and result from contraction of the semitendinosus, semimembranosus, and adductor muscles. These fractures often present as acute onset of hip or groin pain with decreased range of motion and difficulty bearing weight. Swelling, ecchymosis, and tenderness are often appreciated at the site of the fracture. Plain radiographs often reveal the injury, but more subtle fractures may only be appreciated on CT or MRI evaluations. Treatment is conservative, consisting of rest and protected weight bearing, with the majority of patients returning to sporting activities by 4 months.[26] Indications for surgical management of these fractures with internal fixation include fractures with more than 3 cm of displacement, painful non-unions, and high-level athletes who require a more rapid return to their sport.

Chronic injuries to the hip, thigh, and pelvis
Bursitis
Trochanteric bursitis presents as localized tenderness over the greater trochanter laterally. Patients will often complain of an inability to lie on the affected side, particularly at night. It is most commonly seen in female long distance runners, particularly those who commonly train on banked surfaces. Treatment consists of rest, NSAIDs, and stretching exercises. Corticosteroid injections can also be helpful in alleviating symptoms. Patients treated with corticosteroid injection have often been shown to experience rapid and prolonged improvement of their pain.[27] Iliopsoas bursitis can be a common cause of anterior hip pain, whereas ischial bursitis presents as posterior discomfort, particularly with prolonged sitting. Hamstring injuries can often be confused with ischial bursitis.

Athletic pubalgia

Athletic pubalgia is often referred to as a sports hernia. In athletic pubalgia, injury to the muscles of the abdominal wall or adductor longus produce anterior pelvis or groin pain. It can result from an acute or chronic injury pattern, although more commonly it is a result of a chronic overuse injury. It is most commonly seen in sports such as hockey, soccer, rugby, and sprinting where there is repetitive, sudden, forceful contracture and rotation of the hip and lower abdomen. Athletes will present with recurrent exertional pain in the region of the pubic symphysis; however, the pain can often be difficult to localize. Patients will typically display tenderness over the symphysis region, and provocative maneuvers such as sit-ups or resisted hip adduction will often re-create the discomfort. Imaging studies, including MRI, are often negative, making athletic pubalgia a diagnosis of exclusion that is based largely on history and findings of physical examination. Treatment consists of rest, physical therapy, NSAIDs, and a gradual return to sports. Rarely, surgical intervention is warranted in the presence of failed conservative treatment.[28]

Snapping hip

Two distinct forms of snapping hip syndrome are commonly recognized. The more common type, external snapping hip, refers to the condition in which the iliotibial band catches on the greater trochanter and can be reproduced with passive hip flexion from an adducted position. It is most commonly seen in females and is once again strongly associated with running on banked surfaces. Internal snapping hip is less common and refers to the condition in which the iliopsoas tendon catches on the hip capsule. This version can be diagnosed by extending and internally rotating the hip from a flexed and externally rotated position. It is most commonly seen in ballet dancers. Both types result in audible snapping with certain motions of the hip joint. The snapping may not always be associated with pain, but repetitive snapping often results in mechanical irritation, bursitis, and pain. Imaging studies are uniformly unremarkable. Treatment is conservative, consisting of rest, activity modification, NSAIDs, stretching and strengthening exercises targeting the iliopsoas and iliotibial band, and modalities such as ultrasound to alleviate swelling. Occasionally, surgical release is warranted in patients with refractory symptoms that fail to respond to a prolonged course of conservative management. A variety of surgical procedures have been described depending on the underlying cause, with excellent results, including a return to the preoperative level of activity.[29] Many cases requiring surgical intervention can now be managed successfully with arthroscopic surgery through less invasive means with a more rapid return to sporting activities.[30]

Injuries to the knee

History and diagnosis

Evaluation of a patient with a knee injury begins with a thorough history. Pertinent questions include whether there was a discrete injury or whether the onset of discomfort was insidious. If an injury did occur, a careful determination of the mechanism can aid in diagnosis. Determining which activities exacerbate the discomfort can also be helpful. It also can be useful to obtain an understanding of how significant the injury is by determining whether it causes discomfort only with aggressive sporting activities or with simple daily activities. Having the patient carefully and specifically localize the area of discomfort can aid tremendously with narrowing the differential diagnosis. A careful history before any physical examination or imaging studies can often greatly narrow the potential diagnoses.

The physical examination begins by simply observing the patient's gait. Attention is then turned to the uninjured extremity because this can be used as a baseline for comparison to the injured side. The range of motion in the uninjured extremity should be carefully noted. Ligamentous stability should be checked for subsequent comparison to the injured side. Examination of the injured knee begins with observation to appreciate any skin lesions or effusion that may be present. A large effusion is often indicative of a significant intra-articular injury. Range of motion is then checked and compared with the uninjured side. The knee is then carefully and systematically palpated to determine areas of maximal tenderness. The extensor mechanism should be palpated

for defects as well as for areas of tenderness. A straight-leg raise should be performed to ensure that there is not a disruption of the extensor mechanism itself.

A ligamentous examination is next performed and is fundamental to the overall knee examination. Varus and valgus stability of the knee is checked with one hand on the knee and one hand placed on the foot to provide the stress (Fig. 80.9). This test should be performed both in full extension as well as at 30 degrees of flexion. Comparison can then be made to the unaffected knee. Increased laxity in full extension is indicative of a combined injury to a cruciate ligament as well as a collateral ligament, whereas laxity at 30 degrees alone indicates an isolated collateral ligament injury. The Lachman examination is critical to evaluate the competence of the anterior cruciate ligament. With the knee flexed to 20 degrees, the distal femur is stabilized with one hand and the proximal tibia is pulled forward with the other (Fig. 80.10). If there is increased anterior translation in comparison to the uninjured side with a soft endpoint, this is highly suggestive of an anterior cruciate ligament rupture. Evaluation of the posterior cruciate ligament is best performed with the posterior drawer test (Fig. 80.11). With the knee flexed to 90 degrees and the foot stabilized, a posterior force is directed on to the proximal tibia. Increased laxity with this maneuver compared with the uninjured side is indicative of an injury to the posterior cruciate ligament. A meniscal pathologic process is best evaluated by noting any tenderness to palpation along the medial or lateral joint lines. McMurray test can be performed to further evaluate the menisci. The test is performed with the patient lying supine and the hip and knee flexed to approximately 90 degrees. One hand is placed on the knee to apply compression, and the other hand holds the foot, repeatedly moving it from external rotation to internal rotation. The maneuver can trap the torn meniscus, producing a pop or click that may be appreciated by the examiner as well as causing discomfort that is localized to either the medial or lateral joint line by the patient. Any injury to the knee should initially be evaluated with radiographs in orthogonal planes to rule out a bony injury. If there is concern for a soft tissue injury based on history and findings on physical examination, MRI can be a powerful tool for further evaluation. Bony lesions or injuries not sufficiently appreciated on plain radiographs can be further evaluated with CT.

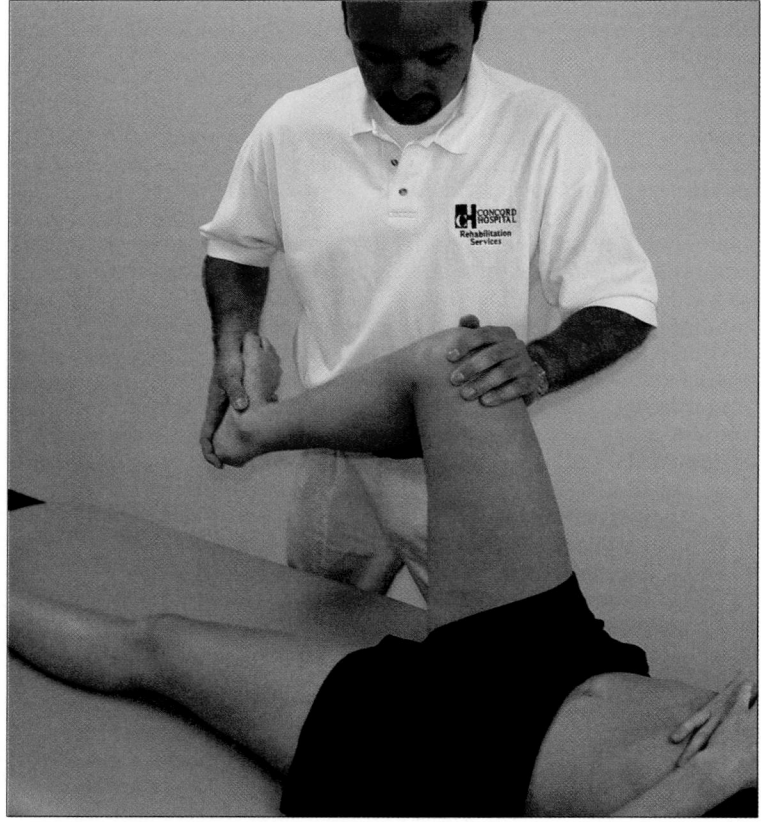

Fig. 80.9 Demonstration of ligamentous stress test.

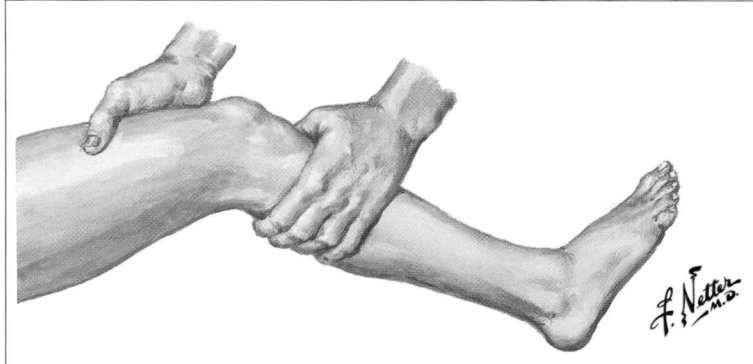

Fig. 80.10 Demonstration of Lachman test.

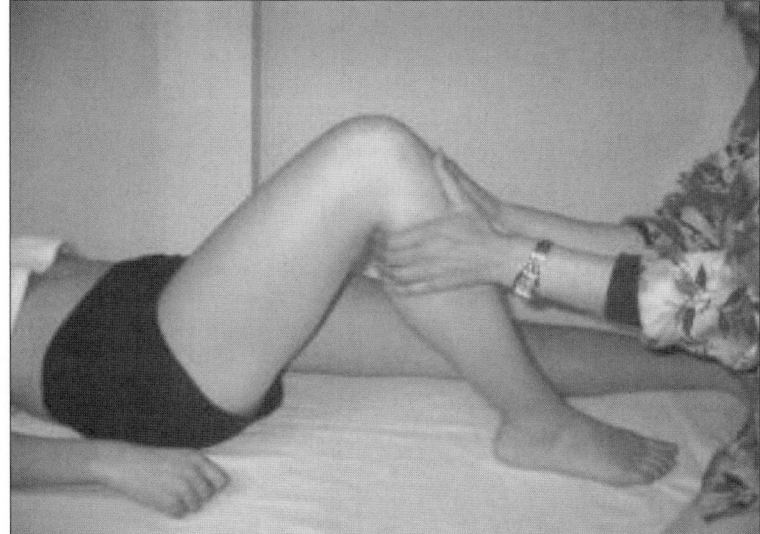

Fig. 80.11 Demonstration of posterior drawer test.

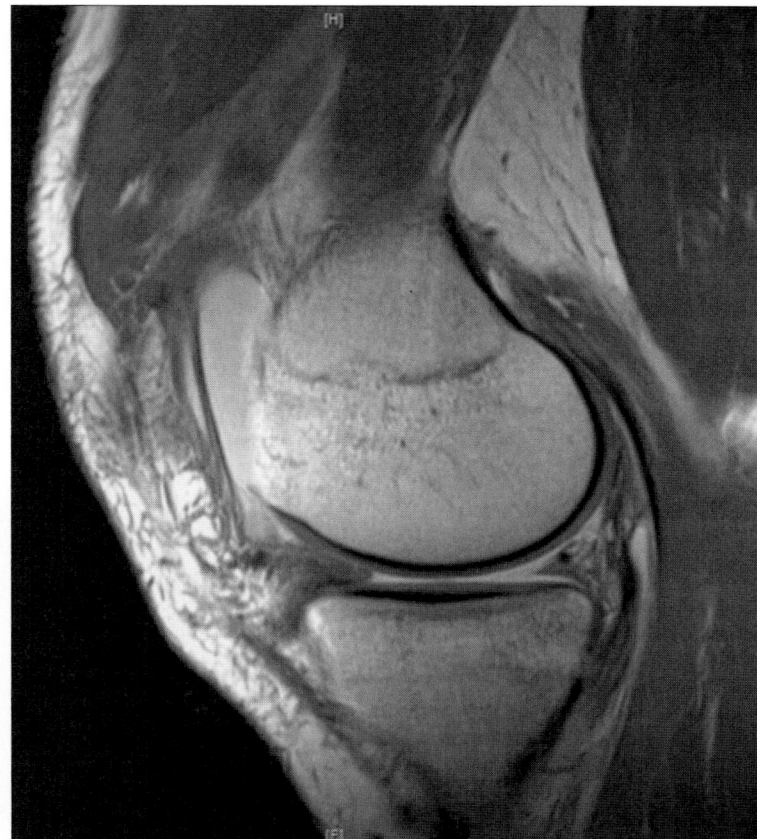

Fig. 80.12 Sagittal MRI of the knee showing missing medial meniscus with bucket-handle tear.

Acute injuries to the knee

Meniscal injuries

Injuries to the meniscus are quite common and increase in prevalence with increasing age, with a peak in the fourth and fifth decades. The incidence of acute meniscal tears in the United States has been reported to be as high as 60 to 70 cases per 100,000 persons per year. They are often associated with underlying arthritis in older individuals. In younger individuals, the onset of pain can be acute, commonly caused by rotation and axial loading of the flexed knee. In older individuals with some component of underlying arthritis, the onset of symptoms is more often insidious with no discrete injury. Pain is often localized to either the medial or lateral joint lines. Joint line tenderness is the best clinical sign of a meniscal tear, with a 74% sensitivity and 50% positive predictive value. A small effusion or intermittent swelling may be noted. Discomfort is improved with rest and exacerbated by weight-bearing activities, particularly those that involve pivoting or twisting. Mechanical symptoms such as painful clicking or catching are highly specific for a meniscal pathologic process. Patients may also present with or describe intermittent locking of their knee, which is highly suggestive of a displaced meniscal tear. Joint line tenderness, an effusion, and discomfort with McMurray testing is often noted.

Definitive diagnosis of a meniscal tear is often made with MRI (Fig. 80.12). The accuracy of MRI in the detection of meniscal tears is between 80% and 90%.[31] Previous studies have reported a 5% to 6% rate of false-positive MRI findings in asymptomatic patients between the ages of 18 and 39 with normal findings on clinical examination.[32] With increasing age there is an increased prevalence of asymptomatic meniscal tears. In one study of asymptomatic patients, 13% younger than 45 years old had meniscal tears on MRI, whereas 36% older than 45 had a tear.[33] It is critical to rely on the entire clinical picture and not simply the MRI findings.

Conservative management consists of rest, ice, elevation, NSAIDs, and physical therapy. A trial of conservative care is often warranted in older patients with underlying osteoarthritis and no discrete mechanical symptoms. In a young patient with a well-preserved joint, meniscal type symptoms, and a meniscal tear on MRI, surgical intervention is often indicated. Older patients with mild degenerative changes on radiographs who have failed conservative management are also surgical candidates. Mechanical symptoms with locking of the knee warrant immediate surgical intervention. Surgery to treat meniscal tears can be accomplished through arthroscopic techniques with high rates of successful outcomes. Treatment can range from partial meniscectomy to meniscal repair, depending on the location and characterization of the meniscal tear.[34]

Ligament injuries

Knee stability is very dependent on ligamentous support provided by the cruciate and collateral ligaments. With increased participation in aggressive athletic activities as well as improvements in diagnostic abilities, ligamentous injuries have become increasingly common. Both contact and non-contact injuries can lead to ligamentous disruption. The history almost always involves a discrete injury with immediate onset of significant pain and the development of an acute effusion. Evaluation includes a detailed history as well as a careful ligamentous examination with comparison made to the uninjured contralateral knee. The Lachman, posterior drawer, and varus and valgus stability testing can provide the examiner with a good sense of which ligaments may be involved. Examination can sometimes be limited secondary to pain as well as a large effusion. MRI is warranted when there is concern based on the history and physical examination for a possible ligamentous injury (Fig. 80.13). There is a role for both operative and non-operative management of ligamentous injuries depending on the patient as well as which ligaments are involved. In general, any functional instability in the knee is an indication for surgical intervention.

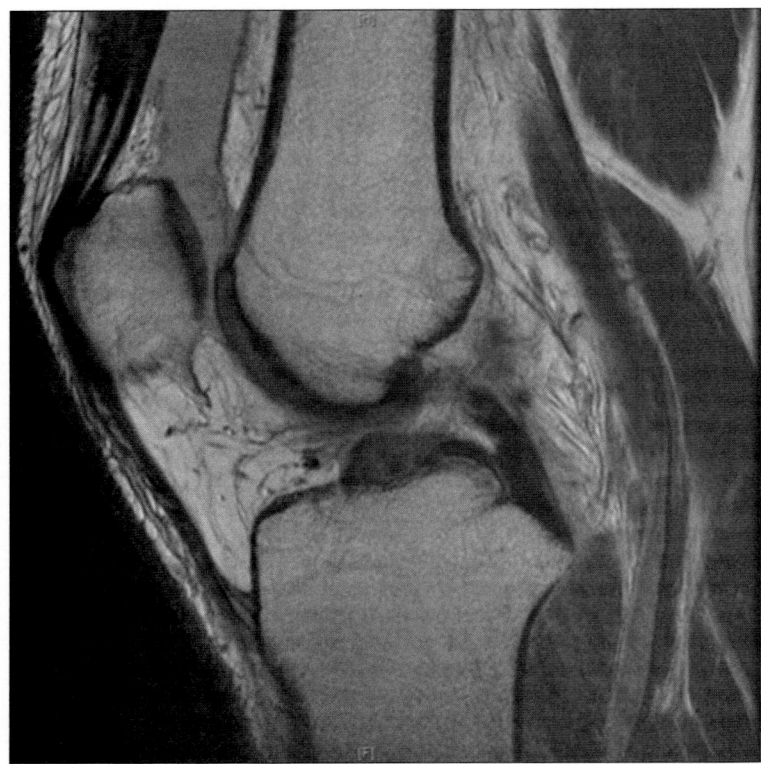

Fig. 80.13 Sagittal MRI showing rupture of the anterior cruciate ligament.

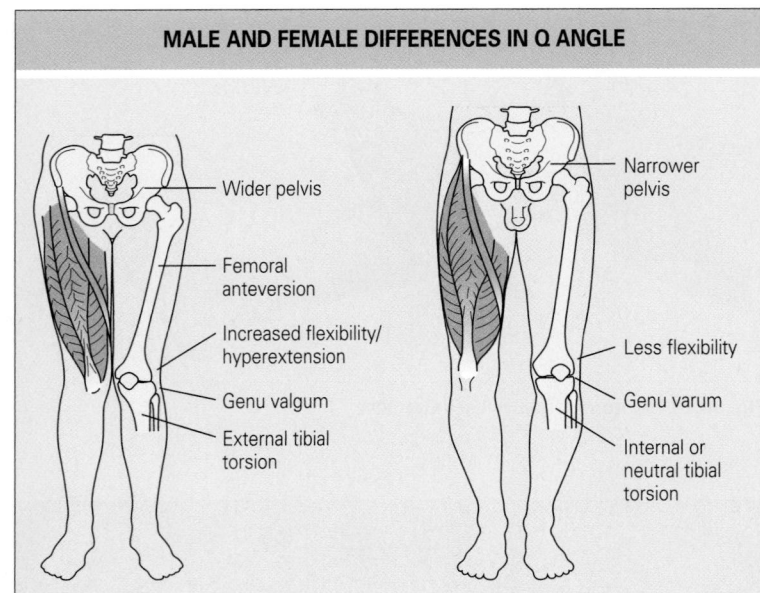

MALE AND FEMALE DIFFERENCES IN Q ANGLE

Wider pelvis

Femoral anteversion

Increased flexibility/ hyperextension

Genu valgum

External tibial torsion

Narrower pelvis

Less flexibility

Genu varum

Internal or neutral tibial torsion

Fig. 80.14 Male and female differences in Q angle. *(From Griffin LY. Rehabilitation of the injured knee. St. Louis: Mosby–Year Book, 1995.)*

In the case of a ligamentous injury, further evaluation and consultation with an orthopedic surgeon is warranted.[35]

Patellar dislocation

Dislocation of the patella typically occurs when the knee is slightly bent and absorbs a valgus force. The injury is more common in women due to differences in their alignment. An increased Q angle is a risk factor for patellar subluxation and dislocation, and women typically have larger Q angles than men. The Q angle is measured by drawing a line from the anterior superior iliac spine to the center of the patella and a second line from the center of the patella to the tibial tubercle (Fig. 80.14). Other risk factors for patellar dislocation include patella alta, a dysplastic trochlea, genu recurvatum, and patellar hypermobility. Patella alta refers to a high-riding patella and is determined by the Insall-Salvati ratio, which represents the length of the patellar tendon divided by the length of the patella. After a patellar dislocation, patients typically present acutely with the patella dislocated laterally. Commonly there is a significant hemarthrosis. The reduction maneuver is performed with the knee in extension. Lateral dislocation of the patella often results in injury to the medial patellofemoral ligament, and therefore patients will often be tender over the medial femoral condyle or at the site of ligament rupture on the patella. Radiographs should be obtained to evaluate for an osteochondral injury or avulsion fracture (Figs. 80.15 and 80.16). MRI can also be helpful to evaluate the articular surfaces. Rehabilitation is typically considered the treatment of choice for acute dislocations, although recurrence rates may approach 50%.[36] Non-operative treatment typically includes physical therapy, focusing on strengthening of the gluteal muscles and the vastus medialis obliquus and patellar taping or bracing. Indications for surgical intervention include a loose body after acute dislocation or recurrent dislocations that fail to resolve with a prolonged course of conservative management.[37]

Quadriceps tendon rupture

Rupture of the quadriceps tendon occurs most commonly in patients older than 40 years of age. Patients typically describe an acute event

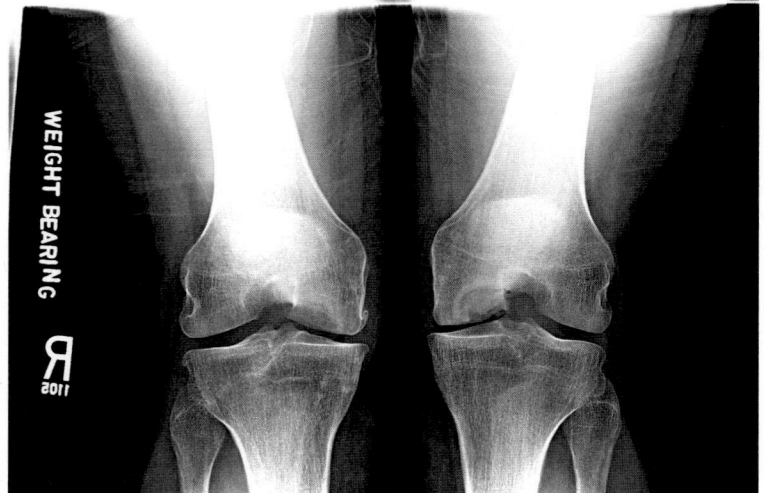

WEIGHT BEARING

Fig. 80.15 This weight bearing radiograph reveals bilateral osteochondral defects with some associated spurring and degenerative changes of the medial compartment of the right knee. The lesion in the left knee appears larger in size and both are located in the classic position involving the lateral aspect of the medial femoral condyle.

during which they felt a sharp and painful pop anteriorly on their knee. Commonly, patients will present acutely with a hemarthrosis and significant swelling of the knee. There is tenderness at the superior pole of the patella, and often a palpable defect can be appreciated. An inability to perform a straight-leg raise without a significant extensor lag should raise concern for an injury to the extensor mechanism. Radiographs should be obtained to rule out fracture, and MRI can be helpful (Fig. 80.17). Ruptures are almost universally treated with surgery, and delay can complicate the repair.

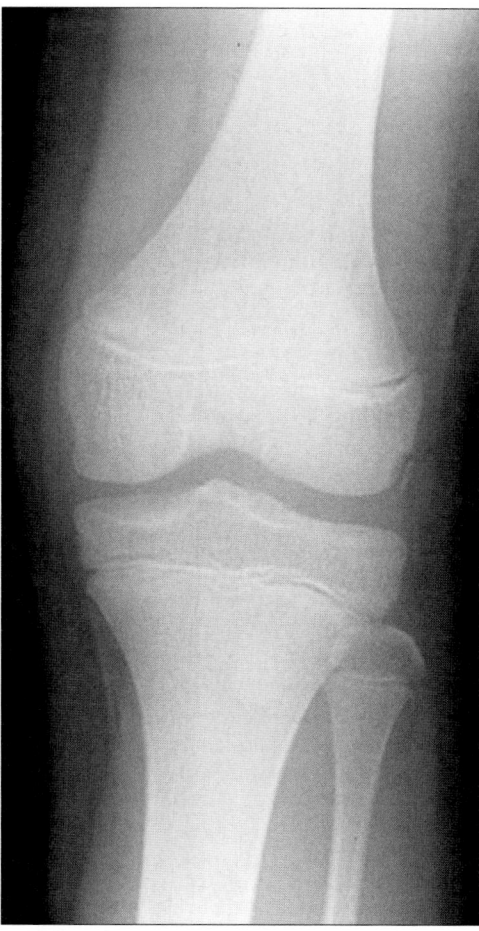

Fig. 80.16 Anteroposterior radiograph showing avulsion fracture. *(Courtesy of Heidi Gable and Norfolk and Norwich University Hospital NHS Foundation Trust.)*

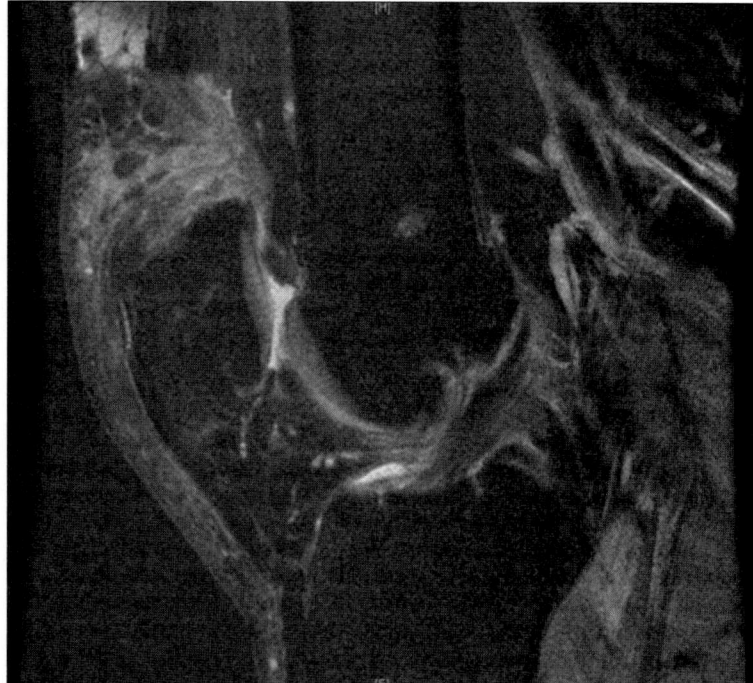

Fig. 80.17 Sagittal MR image showing quadriceps tendon rupture. *(Courtesy of Heidi Gable and Norfolk and Norwich University Hospital NHS Foundation Trust.)*

Patellar tendon rupture

Rupture of the patellar tendon is more common in patients younger than 40 years of age. It presents very similarly to a quadriceps rupture as inability to perform a straight-leg raise and tenderness at the inferior pole of the patella. Radiography and MRI are once again helpful as part of the evaluation, and surgical intervention is warranted. Expeditious repair can help avoid complications that can often occur when dealing with chronic injuries.[38]

Osteochondral fracture

An osteochondral fracture involves an articular cartilage surface and the underlying subchondral bone. They are commonly seen in children and adolescents, often involving the knee. They typically result from a twisting injury to the knee and present as immediate onset of pain and swelling. Radiographs are important to obtain, and CT and MRI can further assist in diagnosis. Treatment options vary depending on the location of the fracture, the age of the patient, the size of the bony fragment, and the amount of displacement. Non-displaced fractures are commonly treated conservatively with immobilization and protected weight bearing, whereas larger displaced fractures often warrant surgical intervention.[39]

Plica synoviales

A plica is a fold of synovial tissue that is commonly found in up to 20% of normal knees. Plicae occur commonly in the suprapatellar pouch both on the medial and lateral sides. On rare occasion, a plica may become thickened and symptomatic, more commonly on the medial side. As the knee moves from extension into flexion, the plica can rub against the medial femoral condyle, producing pain. It also can become pinched between the patella and the condyle, leading to discomfort as well as a slight loss of motion. On examination, the plica can sometimes be palpated between the patella and the medial femoral condyle with the knee flexed to 45 degrees. Patients will often experience tenderness during the examination. To avoid overtreatment, it is essential to note that a plica is a normal variant that is often not symptomatic. Conservative management is often indicated, consisting of rest, ice, NSAIDs, physical therapy, and corticosteroid injections. If symptoms persist and are refractory to conservative care, arthroscopy with excision of the plica is warranted.[40]

Chronic injuries to the knee
Iliotibial band syndrome

Iliotibial band syndrome is a common source of lateral knee pain and is seen in cyclists and runners, particularly those running regularly on hills. Pain at the lateral aspect of the knee results from repetitive abrasion of the iliotibial band on the lateral femoral condyle. Patients will typically display localized tenderness over the lateral femoral condyle, particularly with the knee flexed to 30 degrees. The Ober test can be performed to evaluate for tightness in the iliotibial band, which is associated with iliotibial band syndrome. The Ober test is performed by having the patient lie in the lateral decubitus position, with the unaffected side down. The hip is placed into hyperextension, and the leg is brought from abduction to adduction. The perception of tightness with this maneuver is indicative of a tight iliotibial band. Physical therapy consisting of stretching of the iliotibial band as well as rest and activity modification is usually successful in alleviating symptoms, although it may take a significant amount of time. Occasionally, surgical intervention is warranted in chronic cases that fail to respond to conservative management.

Patellar tendinitis

Patellar tendinitis is often referred to as jumper's knee and is commonly seen in athletes participating in jumping sports such as basketball or volleyball. Patients typically describe an insidious onset with no discrete injury because it commonly is a result of overuse. Pain is localized to the patellar tendon, most commonly at the inferior pole of the patella. The extensor mechanism remains intact, but resisted knee extension may be uncomfortable. Diagnosis is usually based on history and findings of the physical examination, although ultrasonography and MRI are sometimes useful (Fig. 80.18). Treatment is most commonly non-operative, consisting of rest, ice, NSAIDs, and avoidance of jumping activities. Very rarely in chronic cases is surgical intervention warranted, with successful outcomes typically achieved in 70% to 90% of cases.[41]

817

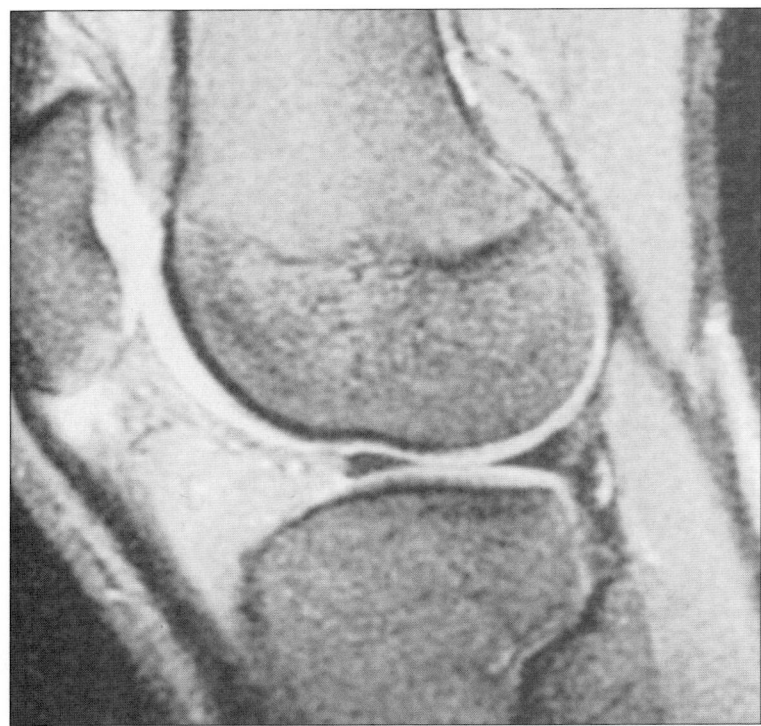

Fig. 80.18 Sagittal MR image showing patellar tendinitis.

Patellofemoral pain syndrome

Patellofemoral pain syndrome is a common cause of anterior knee pain in athletes and non-athletes and is frequently a bilateral complaint with an insidious onset. It is significantly more common in females and most often presents in the second decade of life. Risk factors include a shortened quadriceps muscle, abnormal vastus medialis obliquus muscle reflex response time, decreased explosive strength, and hypermobile patella.[42] Patients often describe poorly localized anterior knee pain that cannot be reproduced by palpation on examination. Discomfort is often most pronounced with repetitive activities requiring knee flexion and extension such as stair climbing and descent, lunges, squatting, and running. Prolonged sitting with the knees in a flexed position can also lead to discomfort. Patellofemoral crepitus is sometimes appreciated on examination in addition to quadriceps atrophy. Radiographs will occasionally reveal lateral patellar tilt in the trochlear groove. Physical examination and radiographic findings are often normal. Treatment of patellofemoral pain syndrome is almost entirely non-operative. Physical therapy focusing on quadriceps and vastus medialis obliquus strengthening is the mainstay of treatment. Patellar taping techniques can be effective as well. A long, dedicated course of physical therapy is often necessary to achieve a good outcome. Avoidance of inciting activities is also helpful in treatment as are NSAIDs. Patients should exhaust all conservative measures before surgical intervention is considered.

Injuries to the leg, foot, and ankle

History and diagnosis

A detailed information about the history and nature of the injury can significantly narrow the differential diagnosis before any physical examination or advanced imaging techniques. Careful observation of the patient's gait pattern followed by inspection of the foot and ankle itself looking for any areas of swelling, ecchymosis, or malalignment should be done first. The area should then be carefully and systematically palpated for areas of tenderness. Ankle range of motion should be evaluated and compared with the unaffected side, and a neurovascular examination is also required. Ankle stability is checked with specialized tests, including the anterior drawer test and varus stress test. The anterior drawer test is designed to test the anterior talofibular ligament. With the ankle in 20 degrees of plantarflexion, the tibia is stabilized with one hand, and the other hand is used to grasp the

hindfoot and pull anteriorly. Findings should be compared with the uninjured side, and an increase in anterior translation is representative of an injury to the anterior talofibular ligament. A varus stress test is utilized to assess the competence of the calcaneofibular ligament. The tibia is stabilized with one hand with the ankle in neutral dorsiflexion. The other hand is then used to grasp the calcaneus and invert the hindfoot. Increased inversion compared with the uninjured sign is indicative of an injury to the calcaneofibular ligament.

Evaluation should begin with plain radiographs to assess for fracture, degenerative changes, or malalignment. When possible, weight-bearing views are preferred. MRI and scintigraphy can aid in the diagnosis of stress fracture and in evaluation of soft tissue injuries, whereas CT can aid in the diagnosis of subtle bony injuries.

Acute injuries to the leg, foot, and ankle

Ankle sprains

Ankle sprains are one of the most common injuries occurring in athletes, accounting for 20% of all sports injuries in the United States.[43] The mechanism of injury is most commonly an inversion injury to a plantarflexed foot. Patients present acutely with pain and swelling around the ankle, and there may be significant ecchymosis. The Ottawa ankle and foot rules can aid in determining whether radiographic evaluation is warranted. Initial treatment is with rest, ice, compression, elevation, protected weight bearing, and NSAIDs. Once swelling and discomfort from the acute injury has subsided, physical therapy focusing on peroneal muscle strengthening and proprioceptive training before returning to sports activities can be useful in preventing recurrence. Functional bracing can also aid in avoiding repeat injury. Patients who sustain multiple recurrent sprains with chronic lateral ankle instability are potential surgical candidates. Over 90% of patients should respond to conservative measures, however. High ankle sprains are slightly different than traditional lateral ankle injuries and can result in syndesmotic injury (1%-10% of all ankle sprains). They typically occur with dorsiflexion and eversion of the ankle combined with internal rotation of the tibia. This injury results in a protracted recovery with resolution of symptoms between 8 and 12 weeks. In cases in which diastasis is evident on radiographic evaluation, surgical intervention is warranted.[44,45]

Achilles tendon rupture

Achilles tendon rupture is most commonly seen in males between 30 and 50 years of age. Most commonly during participation in a jumping sport, a sudden forceful contraction of the Achilles will result in a rupture. Patients will report a feeling of being shot in the back of the leg with immediate pain. Swelling and ecchymosis typically follow. A palpable defect is often appreciated at the level of the tear, and weakness with plantarflexion is evident. The Thompson test can be quite helpful in confirming the diagnosis. With the patient in the supine position, the knee is flexed and the calf is squeezed. If there is no plantarflexion of the foot with this maneuver, this is reported as a positive Thompson test and is indicative of an Achilles tendon rupture. Most ruptures are treated surgically, although sedentary patients or those with significant medical co-morbidities may be treated non-operatively with immobilization in plantarflexion. A re-rupture rate of 2.8% with surgery versus 11.7% in patients managed non-operatively has been reported; however, a significant complication rate does exist with surgical intervention.[46]

Turf toe

The term *turf toe* refers to a soft tissue hyperextension injury to the hallux metatarsophalangeal joint (Fig. 80.19). It is most commonly seen in football players, particularly those playing on artificial turf. The mechanism of injury is typically an axial load applied to the heel of a plantarflexed foot, which results in injury to the plantar complex. Patients will present with variable amounts of swelling and ecchymosis at the hallux metatarsophalangeal joint with potential instability and tenderness on the plantar aspect of the joint. Radiographic evaluation is required to rule out a possible avulsion fracture, and MRI can be useful for evaluation of the extent of the soft tissue injury. Non-operative management consists of rest, ice, elevation, and use of NSAIDs. Taping and shoe wear modifications to limit hallux metatarsophalangeal motion can be helpful with achieving an earlier return to

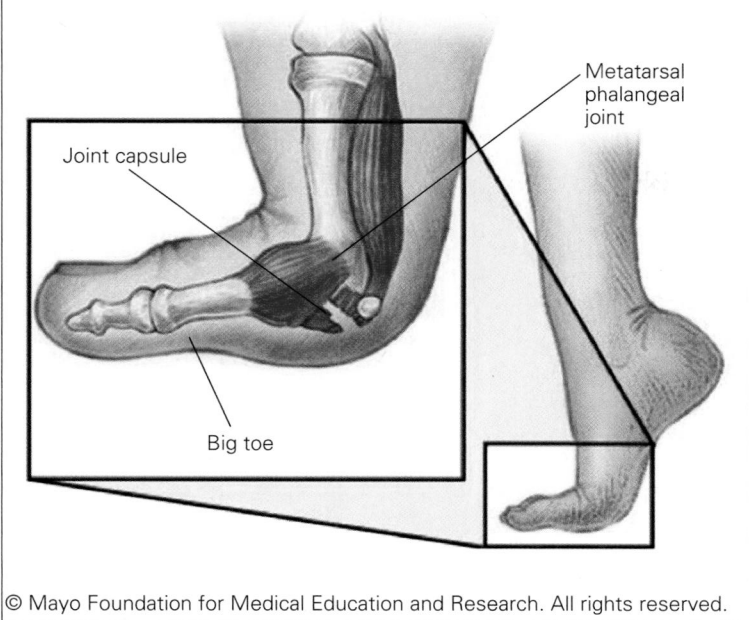

Joint capsule

Metatarsal phalangeal joint

Big toe

Fig. 80.19 Representation of turf toe, resulting from hyperextension of the metatarsophalangeal joint. (*© Mayo Foundation for Medical Education and Research.*)

sport. Surgery is rarely indicated except in the case of significant instability or an associated fracture.[47]

Chronic injuries to the leg, foot, and ankle

Achilles tendinitis

Achilles tendinitis is a chronic overuse injury commonly seen in runners. Patients will typically present initially with pain only after strenuous activities. With time and disease progression, pain will occur with daily activities and sometimes even at rest. Examination can reveal swelling, tenderness, thickening, and warmth around the tendon. Despite the discomfort, plantarflexion ability should be intact with good strength. Radiographic evaluation may reveal bony exostoses that may be irritating the tendon. MRI can assist in visualizing chronic degenerative changes of the tendon. Conservative care is the first line of treatment, consisting of rest, activity modification, shoe wear modification, and use of NSAIDs. Corticosteroid injections into the region should be avoided secondary to the risk of subsequent tendon rupture. Surgical intervention is warranted in cases in which conservative management fails to alleviate symptoms.[48]

Peroneal tendon pathology

Peroneal tendon pathology can result from direct trauma to the tendons, ankle sprains, and calcaneal fractures. Simple tenosynovitis may present as pain and swelling posterior to the lateral malleolus with underlying tenderness. Reproduction of the pain is seen with resisted foot eversion. Conservative management is the mainstay of treatment consisting of rest, ice, elevation, activity modification, orthotics, and NSAIDs. In chronic situations that fail to respond to a prolonged course of conservative treatment, surgical intervention is an option. Subluxation and dislocation of the peroneal tendons can also occur. With acute injuries, non-operative management with cast immobilization has a 50% success rate. In chronic situations or those that recur after conservative management, surgical intervention with reconstruction of the retinaculum is warranted.[49]

Plantar fasciitis

Plantar fasciitis is a common entity seen in runners, accounting for approximately 10% of running injuries. Repetitive running or other activities are thought to cause inflammation and microtears of the plantar fascia, most commonly at its origin on the medial calcaneus. Patients typically present with plantar medial heel pain, which is insidious in onset. Patients will report discomfort that is most significant when first rising from bed and standing. Patients are often tender directly over the medial calcaneal tuberosity. Tightness in the gastrocsoleus complex is often appreciated.[50] Conservative care is the first line of treatment, consisting of rest, stretching of the Achilles tendon, and NSAIDs. In addition, night splinting in dorsiflexion can alleviate symptoms in 80% of cases. Corticosteroid injection is typically avoided because this can result in an increased rate of plantar fascial rupture. Iontophoresis as well as extracorporeal shock wave treatment are other modalities that have shown promise. Conservative management is typically successful in 80% to 90% of cases, although surgical release of the fascia is an option in recalcitrant cases.

REFERENCES

1. Wang RY, Arciero RA. Treating the athlete with anterior shoulder instability. Clin Sports Med. 2008;27:631-648.
2. Bankart A. The pathology and treatment of recurrent dislocation of the shoulder joint. Br J Surg 1938;26:23-29.
3. Rowe CR. Prognosis in dislocations of the shoulder. J Bone Joint Surg Am 1956;38:957-977.
4. Itoi E, Hatakeyama Y, Kido T, et al. A new method of immobilization after traumatic anterior dislocation of the shoulder: a preliminary study. J Shoulder Elbow Surg 2003;12:413-415.
5. Kirkley A, Griffin S, Richards C, et al. Prospective randomized clinical trial comparing the effectiveness of immediate arthroscopic stabilization versus immobilization and rehabilitation in first traumatic anterior dislocations of the shoulder. Arthroscopy 1999;15:507-514.
6. Rowe CR, Patel D, Southmayd WW. The Bankart procedure: a long-term end-result study. J Bone Joint Surg Am 1978;60:1-16.
7. Cole BJ, L'Insalata J, Irrgang J, Warner JJ. Comparison of arthroscopic and open anterior shoulder stabilization: a two to six-year follow-up study. J Bone Joint Surg Am 2000;82:1108-1114.
8. Burkhead WZ Jr, Rockwood CA Jr. Treatment of instability of the shoulder with an exercise program. J Bone Joint Surg Am 1992;74:890-896.
9. Kim SH, Ha KI, Park JH, et al. Arthroscopic posterior labral repair and capsular shift for traumatic unidirectional recurrent posterior subluxation of the shoulder. J Bone Joint Surg Am 2003;85:1479-1487.
10. Neer CS 2nd, Foster CR. Inferior capsular shift for involuntary inferior and multidirectional instability of the shoulder: a preliminary report. J Bone Joint Surg Am 1980;62:897-908.

11. Luo ZP, Hsu HC, Grabowski JJ, et al. Mechanical environment associated with rotator cuff tears. J Shoulder Elbow Surg 1998;7:616-620.
12. Bokor DJ, Hawkins RJ, Huckell GH, et al. Results of nonoperative management of full-thickness tears of the rotator cuff. Clin Orthop Relat Res 1993;(294):103-110.
13. Neer CS 2nd. Anterior acromioplasty for the chronic impingement syndrome in the shoulder: a preliminary report. J Bone Joint Surg Am 1972;54:41-50.
14. Alvarez CM, Litchfield R, Jackowski D, et al. A prospective, double-blind, randomized clinical trial comparing subacromial injection of betamethasone and xylocaine to xylocaine alone in chronic rotator cuff tendinosis. Am J Sports Med 2005;33:255-262.
15. Phillips AM, Smart C, Groom AF. Acromioclavicular dislocation: conservative or surgical therapy. Clin Orthop Relat Res 1998;(353):10-17.
16. Mazzocca AD, Santangelo SA, Johnson ST, et al. A biomechanical evaluation of an anatomical coracoclavicular ligament reconstruction. Am J Sports Med 2006;34:236-246.
17. Snyder SJ, Karzel RP, Del Pizzo W, et al. SLAP lesions of the shoulder. Arthroscopy 1990;6:274-279.
18. Szabo SJ, Savoie FH 3rd, Field LD, et al. Tendinosis of the extensor carpi radialis brevis: an evaluation of three methods of operative treatment. J Shoulder Elbow Surg 2006;15:721-727.
19. Gabel GT, Morrey BF. Operative treatment of medial epicondylitis: influence of concomitant ulnar neuropathy at the elbow. J Bone Joint Surg Am 1995;77:1065-1069.
20. Conway JE, Jobe FW, Glousman RE, Pink M. Medial instability of the elbow in throwing athletes: treatment by repair or reconstruction of the ulnar collateral ligament. J Bone Joint Surg Am 1992;74:67-83.

21. Aronen JG, Garrick JG, Chronister RD, McDevitt ER. Quadriceps contusions: clinical results of immediate immobilization in 120 degrees of knee flexion. Clin J Sport Med 2006;16:383-387.
22. Wenger DE, Kendell KR, Miner MR, Trousdale RT. Acetabular labral tears rarely occur in the absence of bony abnormalities. Clin Orthop Relat Res 2004;(426):145-150.
23. Byrd JW, Jones KS. Diagnostic accuracy of clinical assessment, magnetic resonance imaging, magnetic resonance arthrography, and intra-articular injection in hip arthroscopy patients. Am J Sports Med 2004;32:1668-1674.
24. Lecouvet FE, Vande Berg BC, Malghem J, et al. MR imaging of the acetabular labrum: variations in 200 asymptomatic hips. AJR Am J Roentgenol 1996;167:1025-1028.
25. Shindle MK, Voos JE, Nho SJ, et al. Arthroscopic management of labral tears in the hip. J Bone Joint Surg Am 2008;90(Suppl 4):2-19.
26. Metzmaker JN, Pappas AM. Avulsion fractures of the pelvis. Am J Sports Med 1985;13:349-358.
27. Shbeeb MI, O'Duffy JD, Michet CJ Jr, et al. Evaluation of glucocorticosteroid injection for the treatment of trochanteric bursitis. J Rheumatol 1996;23:2104-2106.
28. Tibor LM, Sekiya JK. Differential diagnosis of pain around the hip joint. Arthroscopy 2008;24:1407-1421.
29. Dobbs MB, Gordon JE, Luhmann SJ, et al. Surgical correction of the snapping iliopsoas tendon in adolescents. J Bone Joint Surg Am 2002;84:420-424.
30. Kelly BT, Williams RJ 3rd, Philippon MJ. Hip arthroscopy: current indications, treatment options, and management issues. Am J Sports Med 2003;31:1020-1037.

31. Muellner T, Weinstabl R, Schabus R, et al. The diagnosis of meniscal tears in athletes: a comparison of clinical and magnetic resonance imaging investigations. Am J Sports Med 1997;25:7-12.

32. LaPrade RF, Burnett QM 2nd, Veenstra MA, Hodgman CG. The prevalence of abnormal magnetic resonance imaging findings in asymptomatic knees: with correlation of magnetic resonance imaging to arthroscopic findings in symptomatic knees. Am J Sports Med 1994;22:739-745.

33. Boden SD, Davis DO, Dina TS, et al. A prospective and blinded investigation of magnetic resonance imaging of the knee: abnormal findings in asymptomatic subjects. Clin Orthop Relat Res 1992;(282):177-185.

34. Greis PE, Bardana DD, Holmstrom MC, Burks RT. Meniscal injury: I. Basic science and evaluation. J Am Acad Orthop Surg 2002;10:168-176.

35. Woo SL, Vogrin TM, Abramowitch SD. Healing and repair of ligament injuries in the knee. J Am Acad Orthop Surg 2000;8:364-372.

36. Hawkins RJ, Bell RH, Anisette G. Acute patellar dislocations: the natural history. Am J Sports Med 1986;14:117-120.

37. Colvin AC, West RV. Patellar instability. J Bone Joint Surg Am 2008;90:2751-2762.

38. Maffulli N, Wong J. Rupture of the Achilles and patellar tendons. Clin Sports Med 2003;22:761-776.

39. Cain EL, Clancy WG. Treatment algorithm for osteochondral injuries of the knee. Clin Sports Med 2001;20:321-342.

40. Calmbach WL, Hutchens M. Evaluation of patients presenting with knee pain: II. Differential diagnosis. Am Fam Physician 2003;68:917-922.

41. Kaeding CC, Pedroza AD, Powers BC. Surgical treatment of chronic patellar tendinosis: a systematic review. Clin Orthop Relat Res 2007;455:102-106.

42. Witvrouw E, Lysens R, Bellemans J, et al. Intrinsic risk factors for the development of anterior knee pain in an athletic population: a two-year prospective study. Am J Sports Med 2000;28:480-489.

43. Beynnon BD, Renstrom PA, Alosa DM, et al. Ankle ligament injury risk factors: a prospective study of college athletes. J Orthop Res 2001;19:213-220.

44. Zalavras C, Thordarson D. Ankle syndesmotic injury. J Am Acad Orthop Surg 2007;15:330-339.

45. Williams GN, Jones MH, Amendola A. Syndesmotic ankle sprains in athletes. Am J Sports Med 2007;35:1197-1207.

46. Lo IK, Kirkley A, Nonweiler B, Kumbhare DA. Operative versus nonoperative treatment of acute Achilles tendon ruptures: a quantitative review. Clin J Sport Med 1997;7:207-211.

47. Anderson R. Turf toe injuries to hallux metatarsal phalangeal joint. Tech Foot Ankle Surg 2002;(1):102-111.

48. McShane JM, Ostick B, McCabe F. Noninsertional Achilles tendinopathy: pathology and management. Curr Sports Med Rep 2007;6:288-292.

49. Mason RB, Henderson JP. Traumatic peroneal tendon instability. Am J Sports Med 1996;24:652-658.

50. Riddle DL, Pulisic M, Pidcoe P, Johnson RE. Risk factors for plantar fasciitis: a matched case-control study. J Bone Joint Surg Am 2003;85:872-877.

6

RHEUMATOID ARTHRITIS AND OTHER SYNOVIAL DISORDERS

Classification and epidemiology of rheumatoid arthritis

81

Katherine P. Liao and Elizabeth W. Karlson

- Rheumatoid arthritis (RA) has an annual incidence of approximately 0.4 per 1000 in females and 0.2 per 1000 in males.

- A prevalence of 0.4% to 1% is reported in diverse populations worldwide.

- Twin and family studies demonstrate a heritability of 60%; approximately 30% of genetic risk is attributed to the shared epitope encoded on the human leukocyte antigen molecules.

- Hormonal and reproductive factors contribute to the female excess and parity, breast feeding, and exogenous hormones are modifiers of risk.

- Smoking is the strongest known environmental risk factor for RA; other lifestyle factors and exposures such as alcohol, antioxidant intake, and traffic pollution may also play a role.

CLASSIFICATION OF RHEUMATOID ARTHRITIS

The 1987 American College of Rheumatology (ACR), formerly the American Rheumatism Association (ARA), criteria for the classification of rheumatoid arthritis (RA) is the current standard for identifying subjects with RA for research studies.[1] These criteria were initially developed in 1957 by a committee of expert rheumatologists who compiled components of the physical examination and diagnostic testing that they considered important for the diagnosis of RA.[2,3] Subjects were classified into four groups: possible RA, probable RA, definite RA, and, then classic RA (added in 1958).[3] In 1987 the criteria were revised, simplifying the classification to identify individuals with definite RA (Table 81.1).[1]

The 1987 ACR criteria for the classification of rheumatoid arthritis were developed from a cohort of subjects with long-standing RA (mean duration of symptoms, 7.7 years).[1] Validation studies conducted in the outpatient clinics confirmed that the criteria were an accurate method of classifying RA with a sensitivity in the range of 77% to 95% and specificity in the range of 85% to 98%.[4] Because of the nature of the cohort for which the criteria were developed, the criteria performs best at distinguishing subjects with long duration and active RA from those with other arthritides.

Recent studies have demonstrated that early aggressive treatment for RA can halt or slow the progression of synovitis and bone erosions, decreasing disease-related disability and increasing the rate of disease remission.[5-10] This has led to strong interest in identifying the disease earlier in the clinical setting and for research studies. However, the current classification criteria do not perform as well for early RA (in studies defined as arthritis symptoms ranging from 4 weeks to 2 years) compared with long-duration RA. Criteria such as joint erosions and rheumatoid nodules are often absent early in the disease, thus decreasing the sensitivity of the classification criteria.

Studies assessing the performance of the 1987 ACR criteria on patients with early RA found a wide range of sensitivities from 25% to 90% and a specificity ranging from 60% to 90%.[11-15]

Impact on classification of antibodies to citrullinated peptides

Since 1987, there have been several advances in our approach to diagnosing RA, most notably, the use of anti-citrullinated protein antibodies (ACPA). ACPA may be involved in the pathogenesis of the disease[16,17] and have been shown to be a more specific marker for RA than rheumatoid factor (RF), particularly for subjects with early disease. In early RA, the specificity of ACPA ranges from 94% to 100% compared with RF, in which the specificity ranges from 23% to 96%; the sensitivity of RF and ACPA are equivalent in both early and long-duration RA.[18-24] The impact of the addition of ACPA to the existing 1987 ACR criteria to classify early RA, in which 4 of 8 rather than 4 of 7 criteria are required, results in an increase in the sensitivity for detecting early RA (defined as disease duration ≥ 6 weeks) in one study from 25% to 44%; there was no change in the specificity of 86%.[15]

Although the added utility of ACPA in the diagnosis of RA is now established, its utility as an added criterion in the current classification criteria for definite RA for use in research studies is undergoing further investigation. Methods to add ACPA as a criterion to a new classification criteria set for RA are under development by an international committee of experts (a joint effort by the ACR and the European League Against Rheumatism [EULAR]).

ACPA has also played an important role in our understanding of genetic and environmental risk factors for RA and will be discussed in context in the relevant sections.

DISEASE OCCURRENCE

The measurement of both disease incidence and prevalence in RA presents methodologic problems. The ideal study of RA incidence would be conducted by continual surveillance of a stable population over time. Because of the low incidence of the condition, only a few studies have been conducted with sample sizes and follow-up adequate to provide estimates that are statistically precise. Studies of prevalence would ideally include all past and inactive cases of disease in a population (and hence provide a measure of "lifetime cumulative prevalence"). For a study to recognize remitted disease requires the use of criteria specifically designed for this purpose. It is often difficult to establish the extent to which remitted disease has been included in published reports.

Direct comparisons of published data of RA occurrence are problematic because of the need to take into account the differences in the sensitivity and specificity of criteria sets used at the time of the study, such as the 1958 ARA criteria or the 1987 ACR criteria. In addition, the incidence and severity of RA may be declining and the disease may be entering remission earlier after treatment. Hence, older prevalence estimates may be less relevant to the contemporary pattern of disease occurrence.

Incidence

Overall, incidence rates are higher in northern Europe and North America compared with southern Europe (Table 81.2) based on a review of studies using the 1987 ACR criteria.[25] Per 100,000 population, the median observed incidence was 29 cases (range, 24-36), in northern Europe, 38 cases (range, 31-45) in North America, and 16.5 cases (range, 9-24) in southern Europe.[25]

Prevalence

There have been a number of contemporary studies of the prevalence of RA based on large-scale cross-sectional population samples.

TABLE 81.1 THE 1987 ACR CRITERIA (TRADITIONAL FORMAT)

1. Morning stiffness	Morning stiffness in and around the joints, lasting at least 1 hour before maximal improvement
2. Arthritis in three or more joint areas*	Soft tissue swelling or fluid (not bony overgrowth) observed by a physician presenting simultaneously for at least 6 weeks
3. Arthritis of hand joints	Swelling of wrist and metacarpophalangeal or proximal interphalangeal joints for at least 6 weeks
4. Symmetric arthritis	Simultaneous involvement of the same joint areas (defined in 2, above) on both sides of the body (bilateral involvement of proximal interphalangeal, metacarpophalangeal, or metatarsophalangeal joints is acceptable without absolute symmetry) for at least 6 weeks
5. Rheumatoid nodules	Subcutaneous nodules over bony prominences, extensor surfaces, or in juxta-articular regions, observed by a physician
6. Rheumatoid factor	Detected by a method that is positive in fewer than 5% of normal controls
7. Radiographic changes	Typical of RA on posteroanterior hand and wrist radiographs; they must include erosions or unequivocal bony decalcification localized in or most marked adjacent to the involved joints (OA changes alone do not qualify)

*Possible areas: right or left proximal interphalangeal, metacarpophalangeal, wrist, elbow, knee, ankle, metatarsophalangeal joints.
NOTE: At least four criteria must be fulfilled for classification of RA; patients with two clinical diagnoses are not excluded.

TABLE 81.2 INCIDENCE RATES OF RA WORLDWIDE IN STUDIES BASED ON THE 1987 ACR CRITERIA

Reference	Population/country	Incidence (cases/1000 inhabitants)		
		Female	Male	Total
Doran et al, 2002[29]	United States	0.6	0.3	0.5
Savolainen et al, 2003[99]	Finland	0.5	0.3	0.4
Chan et al, 1993[100]	United States	0.5	0.2	0.3
Kaipiainen-Seppanen et al, 2001[28]	Finland	0.4	0.2	0.3
Riise et al, 2000[101]	Norway	0.4	0.2	0.3
Uhlig et al, 1998[102]	Norway	0.4	0.1	0.3
Drosos et al, 1997[103]	Greece	0.4	0.1	0.2
Symmons et al, 1994[104]	England	0.3	0.1	0.2
Soderlin et al, 2002[105]	Sweden	0.3	0.2	0.2
Guillemin et al, 1994[106]	France	0.1	0.1	0.1

Adapted from Alamanos Y, Voulgari PV, Drosos AA. Incidence and prevalence of rheumatoid arthritis, based on the 1987 American College of Rheumatology criteria: a systematic review. Semin Arthritis Rheum 2006;36:182-188.

Estimates using the 1987 ACR criteria conducted in various populations worldwide are listed in Table 81.3.[25] Estimates using past criteria sets are listed in Table 81.4. Most studies show a female to-male excess of between two and three times. In all studies, age-specific prevalence rates increase with age.

Geographic variation

Overall, the majority of estimates for RA prevalence worldwide range between 0.4% and 1% (see Tables 81.3 and 81.4). Northern Europe and North America had higher prevalence rates, ranging from 0.4% to 1% compared with the rest of the world. Southern Europe had lower prevalence rates, ranging from 0.3% to 0.7%. The two studies from the Middle East suggest that prevalence rates in that region are similar to those of the northern countries. Prevalence rates in Africa and Asia tended to be lower, with the majority ranging between 0.2% and 0.3%, with higher rates in urban areas. Notably, the majority of the studies conducted in these two continents either predated or did not have information pertaining to the 1987 ACR criteria. Particularly high prevalence rates of RA have been found in certain Native American groups, including the Pima, Yakima, and Chippewa. This excess is not seen in other Native Americans, such as the Blackfoot and Haida tribes.

Time trends

Several studies over the past 4 decades have documented a declining incidence of RA with time. This trend was seen between 1976 and 1987 in females in the United Kingdom.[26] In the Pima Indian population, the incidence of RA was observed to have halved in both males and females in the 25 years between 1965 and 1990.[27] Declining age-specific incidence has also been reported in the Finnish population.[28] Data from a study in the United States, in which similar methods of case ascertainment have been in place for 40 years, confirm a decline in incidence from 0.61 per 1000 in 1955-1964 to 0.33 per 1000 in 1985-1994.[29] The decrease was greatest in females. The declining incidence was also seen through successive birth cohorts. The data show a striking cyclical variation in the rate from year to year, suggesting the possibility of specific risk factors acting at different points in time (Fig. 81.1).

The severity of RA may also be declining over time. In an analysis of the features of disease severity in successive birth cohorts of patients, one study showed that there was a peak in erosive, seropositive, and nodular disease in individuals presenting with RA in the 1960s but a decline in the severity of disease in subsequent generations.[30] A decline in prevalence of RF seropositivity has also been reported among younger birth cohorts in the Pima Indian population, suggesting that early environmental influences contribute to disease.[31] However, this trend has not been seen in the Rochester data,[29] which show no evidence that the proportion of patients with RF seropositivity or erosive change has diminished over time. The mortality from RA also remained constant over the 40-year period of observation.

GENETIC FACTORS

Twin and family studies

Siblings of individuals affected with RA have a twofold to fourfold risk of developing disease when compared with unrelated individuals.[32] This increased risk could be the result of either their shared genetic background or factors in their shared family environment. These two influences can be distinguished by comparing disease recurrence risks (disease concordance) in co-twins of affected monozygotic and dizygotic twins. Because both types of twins are assumed to share their common environment to a similar extent, a greater concordance in monozygotic than in dizygotic twins suggests a genetic influence. Two studies of twins from groups in Finland and in the United Kingdom have included sufficiently large sample sizes to provide adequate power to detect genetic effects and rigorous methods of case ascertainment to avoid potential biases in recruitment. In Finland the concordance for RA in monozygotic twins was 12%, compared with 4% in dizygotic pairs.[14] The U.K. study showed a similar trend, with concordance for RA of 15% in monozygotic twins compared with 4% in dizygotic twins.[15]

The elevated risk among family members was demonstrated in a Swedish study based on a multiple-generation register. The relative risk of developing RA for an offspring of an affected parent was three times that of the normal population. The risk was almost five times higher

TABLE 81.3 PREVALENCE ESTIMATES OF RA WORLDWIDE FROM STUDIES BASED ON THE 1987 ACR CRITERIA

Reference	Population/Country	Prevalence of definite RA (%)		
		Female	Male	Combined
Asia				
Lau et al, 1993[107]	China			0.4
Dai et al, 2003[108]	China	0.4	0.1	0.3
European and North American whites				
Symmons et al, 2002[109]	England	1.1	0.4	0.9
Hakala et al, 1993[110]	Finland	1.0	0.6	0.8
Guillemin et al, 2005[111]	France	0.5	0.1	0.3
Saraux et al, 1999[112]	France	0.8	0.2	0.5
Andrianakos et al, 2003[113]	Greece	1.9		0.7
Drosos et al, 1997[103]	Greece	0.5	0.2	0.4
Power et al, 1999[114]	Ireland			0.5
Cimmino et al, 1998[115]	Italy	0.5	0.1	0.3
Kvien et al, 1997[116]	Norway	0.7	0.2	0.4
Riise et al, 2000[101]	Norway	0.7	0.2	0.4
Carmona et al, 2002[117]	Spain	0.8	0.2	0.5
Simonson et al, 1999[118]	Sweden	2.0-7.4		0.5
Gabriel et al, 1999[119]	United States	1.4	0.7	1.1
Stojanovic et al, 1998[120]	Yugoslavia	0.3	0.1	0.2
Middle East				
Akar et al, 2004[121]	Turkey	0.7	0.2	0.4
South America				
Spindler et al, 2002[122]	Argentina	0.3	0.1	0.2

Adapted from Alamanos Y, Voulgari PV, Drosos AA. Incidence and prevalence of rheumatoid arthritis, based on the 1987 American College of Rheumatology criteria: a systematic review. Semin Arthritis Rheum 2006;36:182-188.

TABLE 81.4 PREVALENCE ESTIMATES OF RA WORLDWIDE FROM POPULATIONS NOT REPRESENTED IN TABLE 81-3 WHERE INFORMATION ON 1987 ACR CRITERIA WAS UNAVAILABLE

Reference	Population/Country	Prevalence of definite RA (%)		
		Female	Male	Combined
Africa				
Moolenburgh et al, 1986[123]	Lesotho	0.4	0	0.3
Silman et al, 1993[124]	Nigeria	0	0	0
Beighton et al, 1975[94]	Rural South Africa	0.1		
Solomon et al, 1975[95]	Urban South Africa	1.4	0	0.9
Asia				
Shichikawa et al, 1981[125]	Japan	0.3		
Darmawan et al, 1993[126]	Rural Indonesia			0.2
Darmawan et al, 1993[126]	Urban Indonesia			0.3
Chou et al, 1994[96]	Rural Taiwan	0.4	0.2	0.3
Chou et al, 1994[96]	Urban Taiwan	1.2	0.6	0.9
Minh Hoa et al, 2003[127]	Urban Vietnam			0.3
Europe				
Sorensen, 1973[128]	Denmark	1.2	0.3	0.8
Middle East				
Al-Rawi et al, 1978[129]	Iraq			1
Pountain, 1991[130]	Oman			0.8
Native American				
Oen et al, 1986[131]	Inuit Eskimos, Canada	1.8		
Boyer et al, 1998[132]	Inupiat, Alaska	2.3	0.6	1.4
Jacobsson et al, 1994[27]	Pima Indians, USA	3.1	1	
Boyer et al, 1991[133]	Southeast Alaskan Indians	3.5	1.3	2.4
Boyer et al, 1998[132]	Yupik, Alaska	1	0.1	0.6

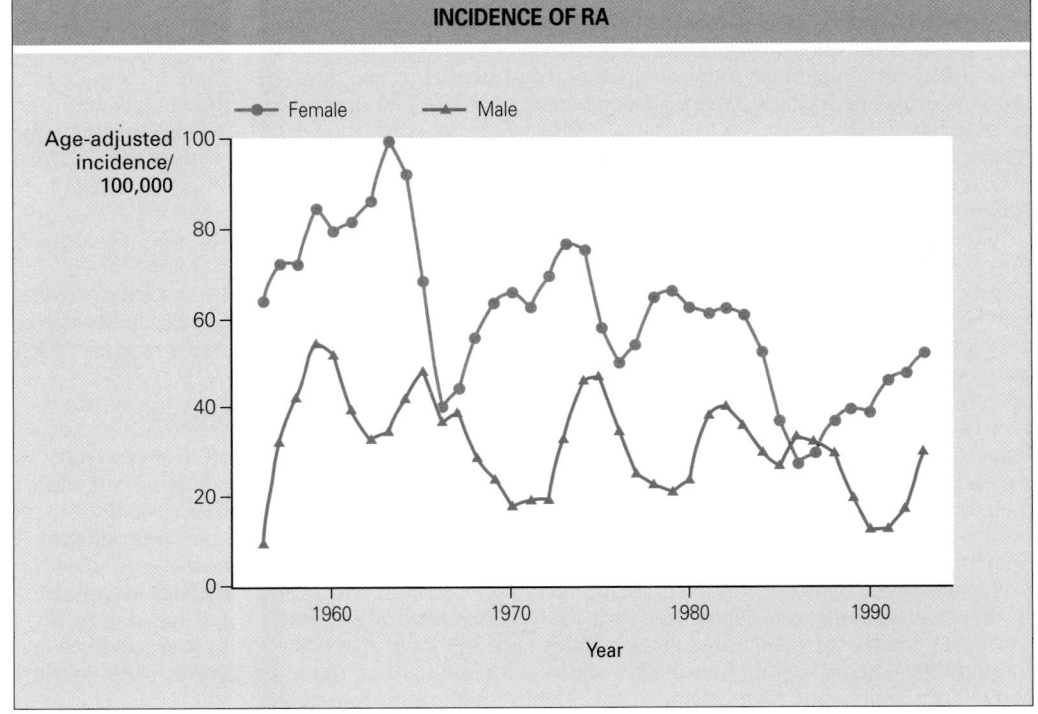

INCIDENCE OF RA

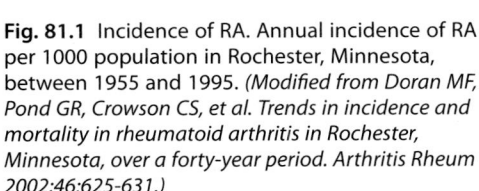

Fig. 81.1 Incidence of RA. Annual incidence of RA per 1000 population in Rochester, Minnesota, between 1955 and 1995. *(Modified from Doran MF, Pond GR, Crowson CS, et al. Trends in incidence and mortality in rheumatoid arthritis in Rochester, Minnesota, over a forty-year period. Arthritis Rheum 2002;46:625-631.)*

if an individual has an affected sibling. If both a parent and a sibling have RA, an individual's risk of developing the disease was approximately nine times higher than those who do not have family members with RA.[33]

These twin concordance and familial studies show convincingly that the risk of disease in relatives of affected persons is conferred by shared genetic factors. When interpreted against the background prevalence of RA of 1% in unrelated individuals, they stress the predominant importance of genetic factors in conferring risk of RA.

Disease-specific genes

The nature of much of the genetic risk in RA is becoming increasingly clear. The contribution of genetic variation in the human leukocyte antigen (HLA) region was first recognized in 1978 by Stastny, who reported an increased frequency of HLA-DR4 among patients with severe RA.[34] The association has since been refined to alleles encoding a "shared epitope" on the HLA-DRB1 molecule (the HLA association is discussed in detail in Chapter 86).

Genetic variation in the HLA region may explain only 30% of the population's genetic susceptibility to disease.[32,35] In the past few years, researchers have identified non-HLA risk alleles for RA through genetic linkage and association using both genome-wide and candidate gene approaches. These findings have been facilitated by the assimilation of family data in several large-scale studies as well as through the establishment of large, well-characterized cohorts of unrelated cases and controls.

At the time of publication, there are more than 20 risk alleles that explain an estimated one third of the genetic burden of seropositive RA risk.[36] Much of the risk is derived from 8 alleles that reside within the major histocompatibility complex (MHC) region,[35] with up to 5% of risk explained by 15 alleles outside the MHC.[36] Genetic risk factors for RA are discussed in more detail in Chapter 86.

HOST FACTORS

Reproductive and endocrine

The greater incidence of RA among females, which is most apparent before menopause, suggests an influence of reproductive and hormonal factors. Epidemiologic interest has focused on the influence of pregnancy itself, on risk factors such as breastfeeding in the postpartum period, and on the contribution of endogenous and exogenous hormones.

Nulliparity has been suggested as a risk factor for RA from the results of several case-control studies. However, the association is inconsistent and has not been confirmed in two prospective cohort studies.[37,38] It is difficult to determine whether any putative association with nulliparity reflects an increased risk of infertility before the development of RA or a protective effect of pregnancy itself. The observations that the frequency of RA is no greater in unmarried than in married women and that family size is similar for patients with RA and for controls suggest that pregnancy does not have a protective influence overall.[39]

There is evidence that pregnancy influences the timing of disease onset. One study showed that the risk of new-onset RA is reduced during pregnancy itself but is increased in the 12 months after delivery.[40] This effect was most apparent after the first pregnancy.

Recent data show that overall women who breastfeed their infants have a decreased risk for RA. One prospective U.S. study observed that breastfeeding for more than 12 months was associated with decreased risk of RA and that the risk decreases with increasing duration of breastfeeding.[41] A subsequent case-control study in Sweden confirmed this association.[42] In contrast to the small group of women who report a postpartum onset of RA, breastfeeding, especially after the first pregnancy, increased the risk of RA fivefold.[43]

The importance of the timing of pregnancy to the onset and severity of RA suggests a contribution from hormonal factors. Women with RA have a relative androgen deficiency, with lower concentrations of testosterone and dehydroepiandrosterone. Males with RA have also been found to have low testosterone concentrations. The finding that androgen concentrations are lower than expected before the onset of disease

in females suggests a possible causal link[44]; however, this association has not been confirmed in a larger study.[45]

Exogenous hormones have also been extensively studied. Overall, the studies of association between oral contraceptive use and risk of RA have been conflicting. In most studies, oral contraceptive use has been shown to decrease risk of RA[46-52]; however, others show no association.[53-57] A meta-analysis of these data concluded that use of the oral contraceptive pill had no influence on RA risk overall but may postpone the onset of disease.[58] There have been fewer studies of the effect of hormone replacement on RA, and a similarly conflicting picture has emerged.

Birth weight

In a case-control study in Sweden, higher weight at birth (>4 kg) was found to be associated with as high as a threefold increase in risk of RA.[59] This finding was confirmed by a subsequent U.S. study that showed that infants weighing greater than 4.5 kg at birth compared with those who were 3.2 to 3.9 kg, had a twofold risk of developing RA.[60] Although the pathophysiology behind this association is unknown, it is hypothesized that the common pathology between the two processes is hypothalamic pituitary axis (HPA) dysfunction, which is associated with both RA and individuals with high birth weight.[61,62]

ENVIRONMENTAL FACTORS

Lifestyle factors

Cigarette smoking is the strongest known environmental risk factor for RA and was identified over a decade ago.[63] Subsequent studies have further characterized the nature of this association. Smoking is most strongly associated with ACPA-positive and RF-positive RA.[64,65] The risk of RA increases with the intensity (pack per day) and duration of cigarette use.[66,67] An individual's risk can remain elevated for up to 20 years after smoking cessation.[66]

The number of copies of the shared epitope that an individual carries can modify the risk of RA in smokers, suggesting a gene-environment interaction. Smokers who carry the shared epitope have a 1.5-fold elevated risk of developing ACPA-positive RA over non-smokers who do not carry copies of the shared epitope. Smokers who have two copies of the shared epitope have a 21-fold higher risk of developing RA than non-smokers who do not carry the shared epitope.[68,69]

This gene-environment interaction between smoking, the shared epitope, and the increased risk of ACPA+ RA forms a potential model for the etiology of RA. Smoking increases the proportion of citrulline-positive cells in the lungs (demonstrated to occur via bronchoalveolar lavage in smokers and absent in non-smokers).[68] Individuals with the shared epitope may be genetically predisposed to develop ACPA, thereby placing them at higher risk to develop RA.

Alcohol consumption may also lower the risk for developing RA, particularly ACPA-positive RA.[65] A dose-dependent effect was also observed whereby individuals with the highest consumption (≥5 drinks or 80 g ethanol per week) had a decreased risk of RA on the order of 40% to 50% compared with those with low to no consumption (<0.5 g ethanol per week).[70] Coffee consumption has also been implicated as a risk factor for seropositive RA in longitudinal data from Finland[63] as has decaffeinated coffee in the United States,[71] but neither of these associations was replicated in a subsequent study.[72]

Nutrition

Studies of dietary influences on the risk of RA have been conflicting, reflecting the difficulty in both undertaking and interpreting such studies. Olive oil and fish oil have been reported to protect against the risk of developing RA. Protein and red meat intake were found to increase the risk of inflammatory arthropathy,[73] but a subsequent study showed no association with protein, red meat, and fish consumption and the risk of developing RA.[74]

Vitamin D is an important modulator of the inflammatory response through the vitamin D receptor (VDR)[75] in addition to its role in bone and mineral homeostasis. Despite its importance in other autoimmune diseases such as type 1 diabetes and multiple sclerosis, its role in the risk of RA is equivocal.[76-78] Lower intake of vitamin D was associated with an increased risk of RA in one study,[79] whereas no association was observed in another prospective study.[80] In a study measuring vitamin D levels before RA diagnosis, there was no difference in vitamin D levels at any time point, 1 year, 2 years, or 5 years or more before diagnosis.[81] Diets high in vitamin C were associated with a reduced risk of inflammatory polyarthritis in the United Kingdom, suggesting that antioxidants may protect against development of RA.[82] There is also some evidence that copper and selenium deficiency are linked with RA.[83]

Infectious agents

Classic epidemiologic evidence of an infectious etiology for RA has not been forthcoming. Incident cases of RA do not cluster in space or time.[84] Concordant monozygotic twins, sibling pairs, and spouse couples show very little similarity in the timing of disease onset. Overcrowding as assessed by sibship size has also not been found to be a risk factor. Furthermore, cases of new-onset RA do not report an increased number of infections before disease onset.[85]

However, these observations cannot rule out infection as a potential cause. It is conceivable that a ubiquitous infectious agent may be responsible for the disease in a genetically susceptible host. Plausible biologic mechanisms for the action of several specific infectious agents in inducing RA have been suggested from the results of animal models, from the isolation of specific agents from human synovium, and from the existence of homology between the antigenic components of infectious organisms, synovium, and cartilage.[86]

Attempts to confirm these observations epidemiologically have focused on examining serologic evidence for past infection. A number of potential associations with infectious agents have been found. Increased titers of antibodies to the Epstein-Barr virus have been demonstrated in RA; titers were also shown to be increased before disease onset in a small group of patients in one longitudinal study.[87] Antibodies to human parvovirus B19 were also found to be increased in females with RA in one case-control study.[88] However, the association with Epstein-Barr virus has not been reported consistently across studies and it is conceivable that increased antibody concentrations may be a reflection of the disease process itself. Similarly, with parvovirus the observations are not reported consistently and the agent is unlikely to cause disease in the majority of patients with RA. Serologic data have yielded no conclusive evidence of association with a number of other putative infectious triggers, including *Proteus*, cytomegalovirus, retroviruses, *Mycoplasma*, and mycobacteria.[89]

Socioeconomic status and occupation

The data regarding the association between socioeconomic status and RA are varied. Socioeconomic status may be a proxy for social or environmental factors in RA susceptibility. The most recent studies demonstrate an inverse association between socioeconomic status measured by education and occupational class and risk of RA.[90] Furthermore, this risk was highly associated with RF-positive RA and not RF-negative RA in a Finnish cohort.[91] There was a twofold lower risk of RA when comparing individuals with the longest education compared with those with the lowest level of education. These results concur with a previous population-based study in Sweden where the risk of RA in subjects without university degrees was 40% higher compared with those with university degrees. For subjects whose occupation required manual labor, the risk was 20% higher than for non-manual workers.[90] These associations were not seen in a study conducted in the United Kingdom.[92]

Urban and industrialized environments

A more general association between RA and urban industrialized environments has been suggested. In the 1970s, Lawrence proposed that the declining incidence of RF in successive birth cohorts may be related to the decline in atmospheric pollution after the Clean Air acts in 1956.[93] The influence of urbanization on increased risk of RA is suggested in studies of RA prevalence in urban environments compared with rural environments in both South Africa[94,95] and in Taiwan.[96] However, this association is not seen all population groups. With the development of reliable methods to study geographic location, there is evidence that location of residence is associated with differential risk of RA in the United States. Women living in the northeastern United States had the overall highest risk compared with other regions of the country,[97] and exposure to traffic pollution is associated with an increased risk for RA.[98]

KEY REFERENCES

1. Arnett FC, Edworthy SM, Bloch DA, et al. The American Rheumatism Association 1987 revised criteria for the classification of rheumatoid arthritis. Arthritis Rheum 1988;31:315-324.

5. Korpela M, Laasonen L, Hannonen P, et al. Retardation of joint damage in patients with early rheumatoid arthritis by initial aggressive treatment with disease modifying antirheumatic drugs. Arthritis Rheum 2004;50:2072-2081.

15. Liao KP, Batra KL, Chibnik L, et al. Anti-CCP revised criteria for the classification of rheumatoid arthritis. Ann Rheum Dis 2008;67:1557-1561.

16. Kuhn KA, Kulik L, Tomooka B, et al. Antibodies against citrullinated proteins enhance tissue injury in experimental autoimmune arthritis. J Clin Invest 2006;116:961-973.

17. Rantapaa-Dahlqvist S, de Jong BA, Berglin E, et al. Antibodies against cyclic citrullinated peptide and IgA rheumatoid factor predict the development of rheumatoid arthritis. Arthritis Rheum 2003;48:2741-2749.

21. Nielen MM, van der Horst AR, van Schaardenburg D, et al. Antibodies to citrullinated human fibrinogen (ACF) have diagnostic and prognostic value in early arthritis. Ann Rheum Dis 2005;64:1199-1204.

25. Alamanos Y, Voulgari PV, Drosos AA. Incidence and prevalence of rheumatoid arthritis, based on the 1987 American College of Rheumatology criteria: a systematic review. Semin Arthritis Rheum 2006;36:182-188.

26. Silman AJ. Has the incidence of rheumatoid arthritis declined in the United Kingdom? Br J Rheumatol 1988;27:77-79.

27. Jacobsson LT, Hanson RL, Knowler WC, et al. Decreasing incidence and prevalence of rheumatoid arthritis in Pima Indians over a twenty-five-year period. Arthritis Rheum 1994;37:1158-1165.

29. Doran MF, Pond GR, Crowson CS, et al. Trends in incidence and mortality in rheumatoid arthritis in Rochester, Minnesota, over a forty-year period. Arthritis Rheum 2002;46:625-631.

31. Enzer I, Dunn G, Jacobsson L, et al. An epidemiologic study of trends in prevalence of rheumatoid factor seropositivity in Pima Indians: evidence of a decline due to both secular and birth-cohort influences. Arthritis Rheum 2002;46:1729-1734.

33. Hemminki K, Li X, Sundquist J, Sundquist K. Familial associations of rheumatoid arthritis with autoimmune diseases and related conditions. Arthritis Rheum 2009;60:661-668.

34. Stastny P. Association of the B-cell alloantigen DRw4 with rheumatoid arthritis. N Engl J Med 1978;298:869-871.

35. Gregersen PK, Silver J, Winchester RJ. The shared epitope hypothesis: an approach to understanding the molecular genetics of susceptibility to rheumatoid arthritis. Arthritis Rheum 1987;30:1205-1213.

36. Raychaudhuri S, Remmers EF, Lee AT, et al. Common variants at CD40 and other loci confer risk of rheumatoid arthritis. Nat Genet 2008;40:1216-1223.

38. Heliovaara M, Aho K, Reunanen A, et al. Parity and risk of rheumatoid arthritis in Finnish women. Br J Rheumatol 1995;34:625-628.

40. Silman AJ. Parity status and the development of rheumatoid arthritis. Am J Reprod Immunol 1992;28:228-230.

41. Karlson EW, Mandl LA, Hankinson SE, Grodstein F. Do breast-feeding and other reproductive factors influence future risk of rheumatoid arthritis? Results from the Nurses' Health Study. Arthritis Rheum 2004;50:3458-3467.

42. Pikwer M, Bergstrom U, Nilsson JA, et al. Breast-feeding, but not oral contraceptives, is associated with a reduced risk of rheumatoid arthritis. Ann Rheum Dis 2009;68:526-530.

43. Brennan P, Silman A. Breast-feeding and the onset of rheumatoid arthritis. Arthritis Rheum 1994;37:808-813.

44. Masi AT, Chatterton RT, Aldag JC. Perturbations of hypothalamic-pituitary-gonadal axis and adrenal androgen functions in rheumatoid arthritis: an odyssey of hormonal relationships to the disease. Ann N Y Acad Sci 1999;876:53-62; discussion 62-63.

45. Karlson EW, Chibnik LB, McGrath M, et al. A prospective study of androgen levels, hormone-related genes and risk of rheumatoid arthritis. Arthritis Res Ther 2009;11:R97.

47. Doran MF, Crowson CS, O'Fallon WM, Gabriel SE. The effect of oral contraceptives and estrogen replacement therapy on the risk of rheumatoid arthritis: a population-based study. J Rheumatol 2004;31:207-213.

58. Spector TD, Hochberg MC. The protective effect of the oral contraceptive pill on rheumatoid arthritis: an overview of the analytic epidemiological studies using meta-analysis. J Clin Epidemiol 1990;43:1221-1230.

59. Jacobsson LT, Jacobsson ME, Askling J, Knowler WC. Perinatal characteristics and risk of rheumatoid arthritis. BMJ 2003;326:1068-1069.

60. Mandl LA, Costenbader KH, Simard J, Karlson EW. Is birthweight associated with risk of rheumatoid

arthritis? Data from a large prospective cohort study. Ann Rheum Dis 2009;68:514-518.

65. Pedersen M, Jacobsen S, Klarlund M, et al. Environmental risk factors differ between rheumatoid arthritis with and without auto-antibodies against cyclic citrullinated peptides. Arthritis Res Ther 2006;8:R133.

66. Costenbader KH, Feskanich D, Mandl LA, Karlson EW. Smoking intensity, duration, and cessation, and the risk of rheumatoid arthritis in women. Am J Med 2006;119:503:e1-e9.

67. Stolt P, Bengtsson C, Nordmark B, et al. Quantification of the influence of cigarette smoking on rheumatoid arthritis: results from a population based case-control study, using incident cases. Ann Rheum Dis 2003;62:835-841.

68. Klareskog L, Stolt P, Lundberg K, et al. A new model for an etiology of rheumatoid arthritis: Smoking may trigger HLA-DR (shared epitope)-restricted immune reactions to autoantigens modified by citrullination. Arthritis Rheum 2006;54:38-46.

69. Karlson EW, Chang S, Cui J, et al. Gene-environment interaction between HLA-DRB1 shared epitope and heavy cigarette smoking in predicting incident RA. Ann Rheum Dis 2009; Jan 16. [Epub ahead of print].

70. Kallberg H, Jacobsen S, Bengtsson C, et al. Alcohol consumption is associated with decreased risk of rheumatoid arthritis: results from two Scandinavian case-control studies. Ann Rheum Dis 2009;68:222-227.

71. Mikuls TR, Cerhan JR, Criswell LA, et al. Coffee, tea, and caffeine consumption and risk of rheumatoid arthritis: results from the Iowa Women's Health Study. Arthritis Rheum 2002;46:83-91.

72. Karlson EW, Mandl LA, Aweh GN, Grodstein F. Coffee consumption and risk of rheumatoid arthritis. Arthritis Rheum 2003;48:3055-3060.

73. Pattison DJ, Symmons DP, Lunt M, et al. Dietary risk factors for the development of inflammatory polyarthritis: evidence for a role of high level of red meat consumption. Arthritis Rheum 2004;50:3804-3812.

74. Benito-Garcia E, Feskanich D, Hu FB, et al. Protein, iron, and meat consumption and risk for rheumatoid arthritis: a prospective cohort study. Arthritis Res Ther 2007;9:R16.

79. Merlino LA, Curtis J, Mikuls TR, et al. Vitamin D intake is inversely associated with rheumatoid arthritis: results from the Iowa Women's Health Study. Arthritis Rheum 2004;50:72-77.

80. Costenbader KH, Feskanich D, Holmes M, et al. Vitamin D intake and risks of systemic lupus erythematosus and rheumatoid arthritis in women. Ann Rheum Dis 2008;67:530-535.

81. Nielen MM, van Schaardenburg D, Lems WF, et al. Vitamin D deficiency does not increase the risk of rheumatoid arthritis: comment on the article by Merlino et al. Arthritis Rheum 2006;54:3719-3720.

82. Pattison DJ, Silman AJ, Goodson NJ, et al. Vitamin C and the risk of developing inflammatory polyarthritis: prospective nested case-control study. Ann Rheum Dis 2004;63:843-847.

83. Pattison DJ, Symmons DP, Lunt M, et al. Dietary beta-cryptoxanthin and inflammatory polyarthritis: results from a population-based prospective study. Am J Clin Nutr 2005;82:451-455.

84. Silman A, Bankhead C, Rowlingson B, et al. Do new cases of rheumatoid arthritis cluster in time or in space? Int J Epidemiol 1997;26:628-634.

85. Symmons DP, Bankhead CR, Harrison BJ, et al. Blood transfusion, smoking, and obesity as risk factors for the development of rheumatoid arthritis: results from a primary care-based incident case-control study in Norfolk, England. Arthritis Rheum 1997;40:1955-1961.

87. Kouri T, Petersen J, Rhodes G, et al. Antibodies to synthetic peptides from Epstein-Barr nuclear antigen-1 in sera of patients with early rheumatoid arthritis and in preillness sera. J Rheumatol 1990;17:1442-1449.

88. Hajeer AH, MacGregor AJ, Rigby AS, et al. Influence of previous exposure to human parvovirus B19 infection in explaining susceptibility to rheumatoid arthritis: an analysis of disease discordant twin pairs. Ann Rheum Dis 1994;53:137-139.

90. Bengtsson C, Nordmark B, Klareskog L, et al. Socioeconomic status and the risk of developing rheumatoid arthritis: results from the Swedish EIRA study. Ann Rheum Dis 2005;64:1588-1594.

91. Pedersen M, Jacobsen S, Klarlund M, Frisch M. Socioeconomic status and risk of rheumatoid arthritis: a Danish case-control study. J Rheumatol 2006;33:1069-1074.

92. Bankhead C, Silman A, Barrett B, et al. Incidence of rheumatoid arthritis is not related to indicators of socioeconomic deprivation. J Rheumatol 1996;23:2039-2042.

97. Costenbader KH, Chang SC, Laden F, et al. Geographic variation in rheumatoid arthritis incidence among women in the United States. Arch Intern Med 2008;168:1664-1670.

98. Hart JE, Laden F, Puett RC, et al. Exposure to traffic pollution and increased risk of rheumatoid arthritis. Environ Health Perspect 2009;117:1065-1069.

REFERENCES

Full references for this chapter can be found on www.expertconsult.com.

Clinical features of rheumatoid arthritis

Richard D. Brasington, Jr.

- Morning stiffness and symmetric swelling in the wrists and proximal interphalangeal and metacarpophalangeal joints are the typical features of rheumatoid arthritis (RA).

- Early diagnosis of RA is critical, but many cases of "early arthritis" are not RA.

- Anti-citrullinated peptide antibodies (ACPAs) occur earlier than rheumatoid factor and are more specific for RA.

- The Health Assessment Questionnaire, Disease Activity Score, acute-phase reactants, and radiographs of the hands and feet are important for prognosis and for following a patient's disease.

- Aggressive early administration of disease-modifying antirheumatic drugs is critical to a good outcome.

INTRODUCTION

Rheumatoid arthritis (RA) is the paradigm of a systemic autoimmune disease characterized by inflammatory polyarthritis. The hallmark of RA is symmetric synovial proliferation and tenderness of multiple joints, particularly the small joints of the hands and feet. Most patients experience joint stiffness or gelling for more than an hour in the morning. The blood of approximately 80% of RA patients contains rheumatoid factor (RF), an immunoglobulin binding the Fc region of the IgG molecule. Rheumatoid nodules are seen in about 20% of patients. Thus, an individual with a several-week history of symmetric swelling and tenderness of the small joints of the hands, morning stiffness, and a positive RF likely has the diagnosis of RA.

These clinical features are reflected in the 1987 criteria for the classification of RA developed by the American College of Rheumatology (ACR) (Fig. 82.1).[1] These criteria were developed for classification of patients with RA for inclusion in research studies, not to make the clinical diagnosis of RA. Although these criteria are quite specific for the diagnosis if applied over a several-year period, they have several significant limitations because our understanding and approach to RA have changed dramatically since the criteria were composed in 1987. First, these criteria were developed using patients with well-established disease and are not necessarily valid for RA in the first few months of disease.[2,3] Second, the study of "early arthritis" in Europe has shown that a substantial portion of such patients do not have RA.[4,5] Despite these limitations, the 1987 ACR criteria have provided a useful framework in which to consider the major clinical manifestations of RA. However, ACR and the European League against Rheumatism (EULAR) have recently commonly developed new RA classification criteria which allow one to discern RA among patients with early arthritis (REF), thus overcoming the mentioned limitations of the 1987 criteria. These 2010 ACR/EULAR classification criteria for RA are discussed in Chapter 90.

Perhaps the most important concept in our contemporary approach to RA is the recognition that prognosis and outcome are improved when disease-modifying antirheumatic drug (DMARD) therapy is started within a few weeks or months of disease onset.[6] We now believe that it is critical to identify RA within a few weeks or months of its onset, because the immediate institution of DMARDs results in better outcomes than when DMARD administration is delayed for even several months.[7] It is well established that erosive damage on radiographs of the hands and feet develops early in the course of RA.[8] Progression of radiographic damage occurs to a lesser degree in patients receiving early therapy than in those for whom therapy is delayed.[5]

Because there appears to be a general correlation between radiographic damage and disability over time,[9] it is hypothesized that preventing radiographic damage will reduce the extent of disability over the years. Patients have a greater likelihood of attaining remission with early treatment. Thus, it is axiomatic that the diagnosis of rheumatoid arthritis be made as soon as possible so that DMARD treatment can be started without delay.

CLINICAL EVALUATION

History

The patient's history typically is strongly suggestive of the development of inflammatory arthritis. Commonly, patients will present with polyarthritis of the small joints of the hands, but monoarticular involvement can occur initially. The development of joint symptoms may occur almost overnight or may evolve slowly over several months. RF and anti-citrullinated peptide antibodies (ACPAs) have been found in up to half of patients with RA up to 5 years before their development of clinical disease, suggesting the insidious development of disease over time.[10] Stiffness or gelling in the joints is present on arising, often taking several hours to abate. The inability to "wring out a washcloth" is common, as is the need to hold a coffee cup with both hands. Patients will typically report soft tissue swelling over the knuckles and describe markedly reduced grip strength. Discomfort in the feet is generally most prominent in the metatarsal area; patients may complain of the sensation of having a "stone in my shoe." Profound fatigue often accompanies the joint complaints, and anorexia and mild weight loss may occur. Typically, patients with RA do not present with rash, fever, headache, visual disturbance, or pleuropericardial symptoms.

Pain in the joints is universal in patients with RA. The pattern of joint involvement in RA is quite typical in most cases. Affected joints include the proximal interphalangeal joints (PIPs), metacarpophalangeal joints (MCPs), wrists, elbows, shoulders, hips, knees, ankles, and metatarsophalangeal (MTP) joints. However, the quality of the pain may vary depending on the type of joint involvement. For example, the pain associated with chronic inflammatory synovial proliferation may be experienced as a dull ache with little fluctuation in intensity. By contrast, the mechanical pain associated with bone and cartilage damage in the knee or hip, in the absence of inflammation, may be more sharp and acute, associated with activity and relieved with rest.

Patients with musculoskeletal distress commonly complain of joint "swelling," even in the absence of detectable abnormality on physical examination. However, the patient with RA will probably notice swelling in the hands, particularly the MCP joints. Rings may need to be resized or cut off the swollen finger. "Trigger finger" due to flexor tenosynovitis may occur.

Examination and clinical features of specific joints

The key to recognition of the physical findings of RA is the ability to recognize the manifestations of synovial proliferation. Unlike the normal synovial lining, which is only one or two cell layers thick, the RA synovium proliferates out of control. As it grows thicker and covers a greater surface area, the rheumatoid *pannus* (L. for "cloth") becomes palpable between the patient's skin and the underlying bone and cartilage. This proliferating synovium has a "doughy" or "squishy" feel on palpation, quite distinct from bony enlargement or synovial fluid. This finding is often referred to as "synovitis"; however, the classic

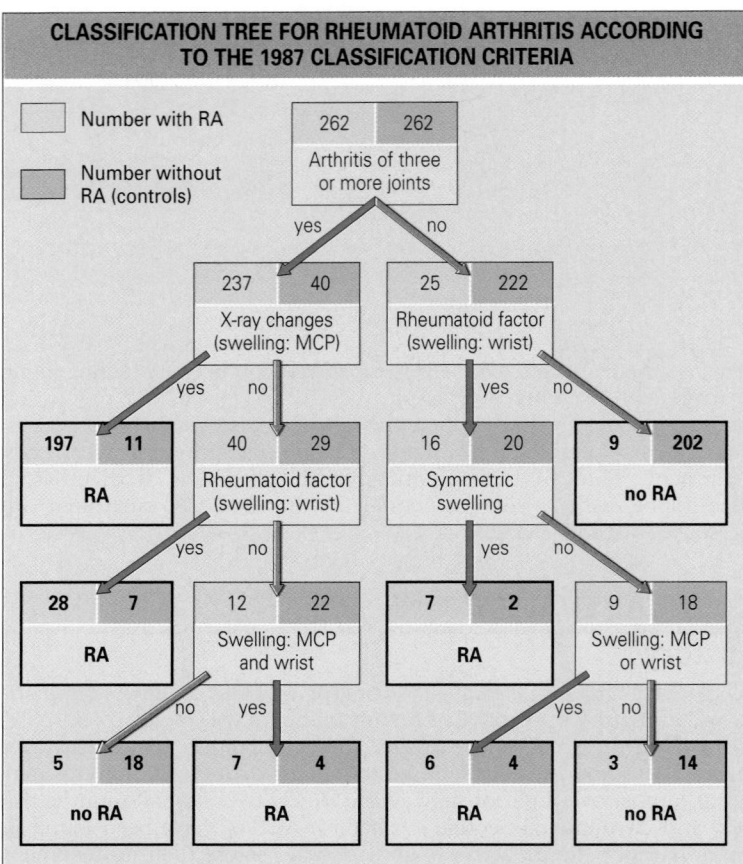

CLASSIFICATION TREE FOR RHEUMATOID ARTHRITIS ACCORDING TO THE 1987 CLASSIFICATION CRITERIA

Fig. 82.1 A modified classification tree for rheumatoid arthritis. The clinical criteria must have been observed by a physician and present for at least 6 weeks. Individuals can be classified as having or as not having RA (no RA). In parentheses are indicated surrogate variables that can be used when another variable (radiograph or RF test result) is not available. Note that this tree is based on the 1987 ACR classification criteria and that new criteria have been developed by ACR and EULAR in 2010 (see Chapter 90).

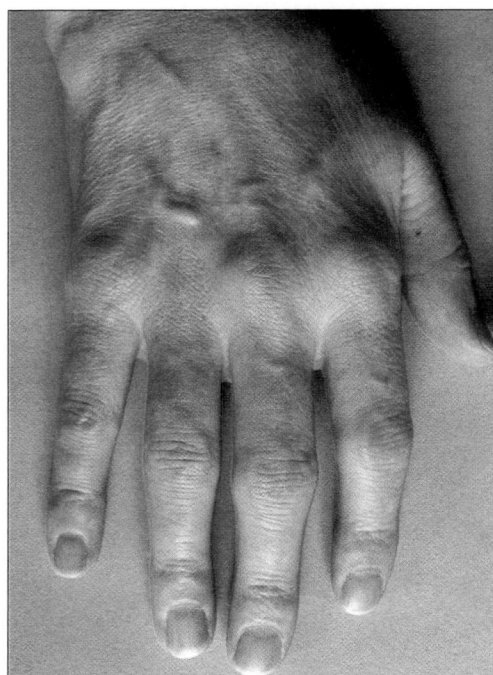

Fig. 82.2 The hand in early RA. View of the right hand, showing swelling of the MCP and PIP joints. Swelling of the PIP joints is typical of RA and associated with morning stiffness, difficulty making a fist, reduced grip strength, and tenderness of the affected joints. The left hand showed similar changes. *(Reproduced with permission from Dieppe P, et al. Slide atlas of clinical rheumatology. London: Gower Medical Publishing, 1983.)*

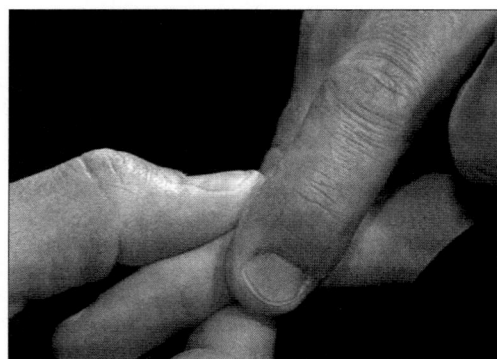

Fig. 82.3 "Four-point" technique for palpating the small joints of the hands. *(From Lawry G. The general musculoskeletal examination. Iowa City, IA: University of Iowa Press, 2002.)*

inflammatory signs of heat and redness are usually absent and external examination cannot determine the functional characteristics of the enlarged synovial tissue. Some prefer to use the term *synovial thickening* to describe palpable synovial proliferation. Because *synovitis* is the most commonly used term, we will subsequently refer to palpable synovial tissue as synovitis, recognizing that acute inflammation is not necessarily present.

Rheumatoid nodules are quite specific for RA and occur in about 20% of patients, generally those with more severe disease and high-titer RF. It is uncommon for nodules to be present within the first year. The nodule is a mass of inflammatory tissue with a central focus of necrosis, presumably the consequence of vascular inflammation, surrounded by chronic inflammatory cells. They occur over extensor surfaces and joints, at sites of chronic mechanical irritation (elbow, toe, and heel), and in the subcutaneous tissues of the fingers. Nodule formation sometimes progresses during methotrexate treatment. Rheumatoid nodules may be confused with gouty tophi, and aspiration for crystals or biopsy is sometimes necessary.

In the hands the MCPs and PIPs are almost always involved (Fig. 82.2), and typically the index and long fingers are more involved than the others. A "four-point" technique, in which the examiner uses both index fingers and thumbs, is preferred for palpating the small joints of the hands (Fig. 82.3). With the patient's hand in pronation, the examiner palpates the dorsal and volar aspect of the MCP and PIP joints (Fig. 82.4). Particular attention should be paid to the second MCP, because synovitis may be especially prominent there. The joint line between the distal metacarpal and proximal phalanx, which is easy to palpate in the normal joint, becomes effaced by the synovitis. The "valleys" between the MCPs are filled in by synovitis. PIP joint synovitis is more easily recognized by lateral palpation of the joint. In RA, the involvement is clearly localized to the PIP joint, unlike the

dactylitis ("sausage" digit) of the spondyloarthropathies. The distal interphalangeal joints (DIPs) are rarely involved in RA, perhaps because they have less synovium than the MCPs and PIPs. Rheumatoid nodules may occur on the extensor aspect of the fingers.

Flexor tenosynovitis is common and may lead to a "trigger finger." The flexor tendons for the fingers pass through a pulley near the palmar surface of the MCP joint. Thickening or nodularity may prevent the flexor tendon from sliding smoothly through the pulley, resulting in a snapping sensation with flexion and extension, or flexion, as if pulling the trigger of a gun. Often a palpable nodularity of the tendon can be felt by palpating this area with the index finger as the patient flexes and extends the finger.

Signs of late disease with irreversible damage include "swan-neck" and "boutonnière" deformities and subluxation at the MCPs with "ulnar drift" (Fig. 82.5), often accompanied by atrophy of the intrinsic muscles of the hand. The boutonnière deformity entails flexion of the PIP and extension of the DIP (see Fig. 82.5). As the central extensor tendon is damaged by tenosynovitis, the PIP joint ruptures dorsally through it, resulting in the lateral and volar displacement of the lateral bands of the tendon. Paradoxically, the lateral bands of the central extensor tendons now function as flexors of the PIP joint and, with tendon shortening, hyperextension of the DIP develops. By contrast, the swan-neck deformity is basically the opposite of the boutonnière deformity, with hyperextension of the PIP and flexion of the DIP (see Fig. 82.5). The lateral bands of the central extensor tendon sublux dorsally as the PIP herniates in a volar direction. Alternatively, the DIP can rupture dorsally through the central extensor tendon (like the PIP in the boutonnière deformity). In either case, progressive shortening of the tendon maintains the DIP flexion and the PIP extension. Early on, both the boutonnière and swan-neck deformities may be reducible. However, as the disease progresses and the tendons shorten, fixed joint contractures develop.

The thumb can be affected by several deformities. Arguably the most common has been described as the flail interphalangeal (IP) joint (Fig. 82.6), in which case the patient loses the ability to flex that joint. This results in significant functional impairment due to loss of pinch strength, whereby the patient pinches the index finger against the proximal phalanx. Surgical fixation of the IP joint in flexion may be required to maintain function. A boutonnière deformity at the thumb develops due to MCP synovitis, resulting in MCP flexion and IP hyperextension. (Imagine the boutonnière deformity described earlier moved back one joint proximally.) The equivalent swan-neck deformity of the thumb develops with dislocation of the first carpometacarpal joint (CMC), MCP hyperextension, and IP flexion.

At the wrist, synovial proliferation around the ulnar styloid occurs (see Fig. 82.6); and as the disease progresses, laxity of the radioulnar ligament gives rise to the "piano key" sign, as the ulnar styloid moves up and down in response to dorsal pressure from the examiner's thumb. Carpal tunnel syndrome from compression of the median nerve is quite common and often responds to treatment of the disease. Subluxation of the wrist can result in severe disease (Fig. 82.7). Extensor tenosynovitis of the extensor carpi ulnaris and extensor digitorum communis sheaths in the dorsal wrist produces a characteristic pattern that is virtually unique to RA (Fig. 82.8); the tubular swelling of the common extensor tendon sheath ends abruptly just distal to the wrist joint. This often obscures swelling at the dorsal wrist (radiocarpal) joint itself. Damage from the chronic tensosynovial inflammation and friction where the extensor tendons of the third, fourth, and fifth fingers cross the jagged and eroded ulnar styloid can lead to tendon rupture with inability to actively extend those fingers (see Fig. 82.7).

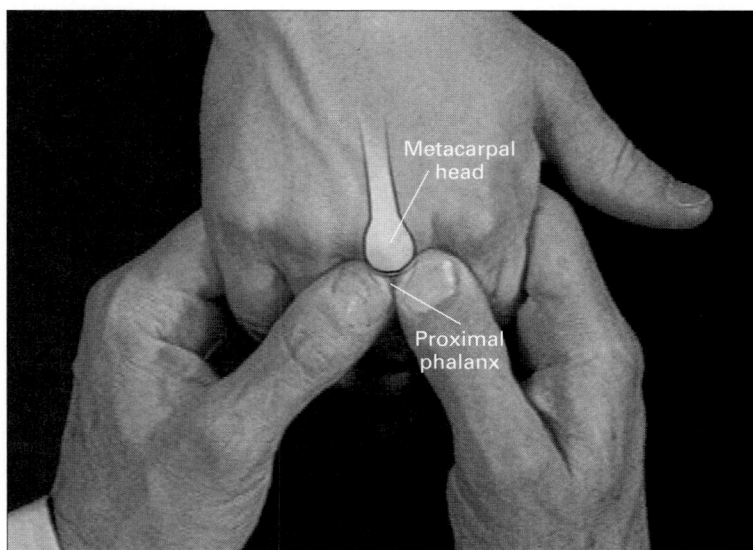

Fig. 82.4 Palpation of the dorsal and volar aspects of the MCP and PIP joints to detect synovial proliferation. *(From Lawry G. The general musculoskeletal examination. Iowa City, IA: University of Iowa Press, 2002.)*

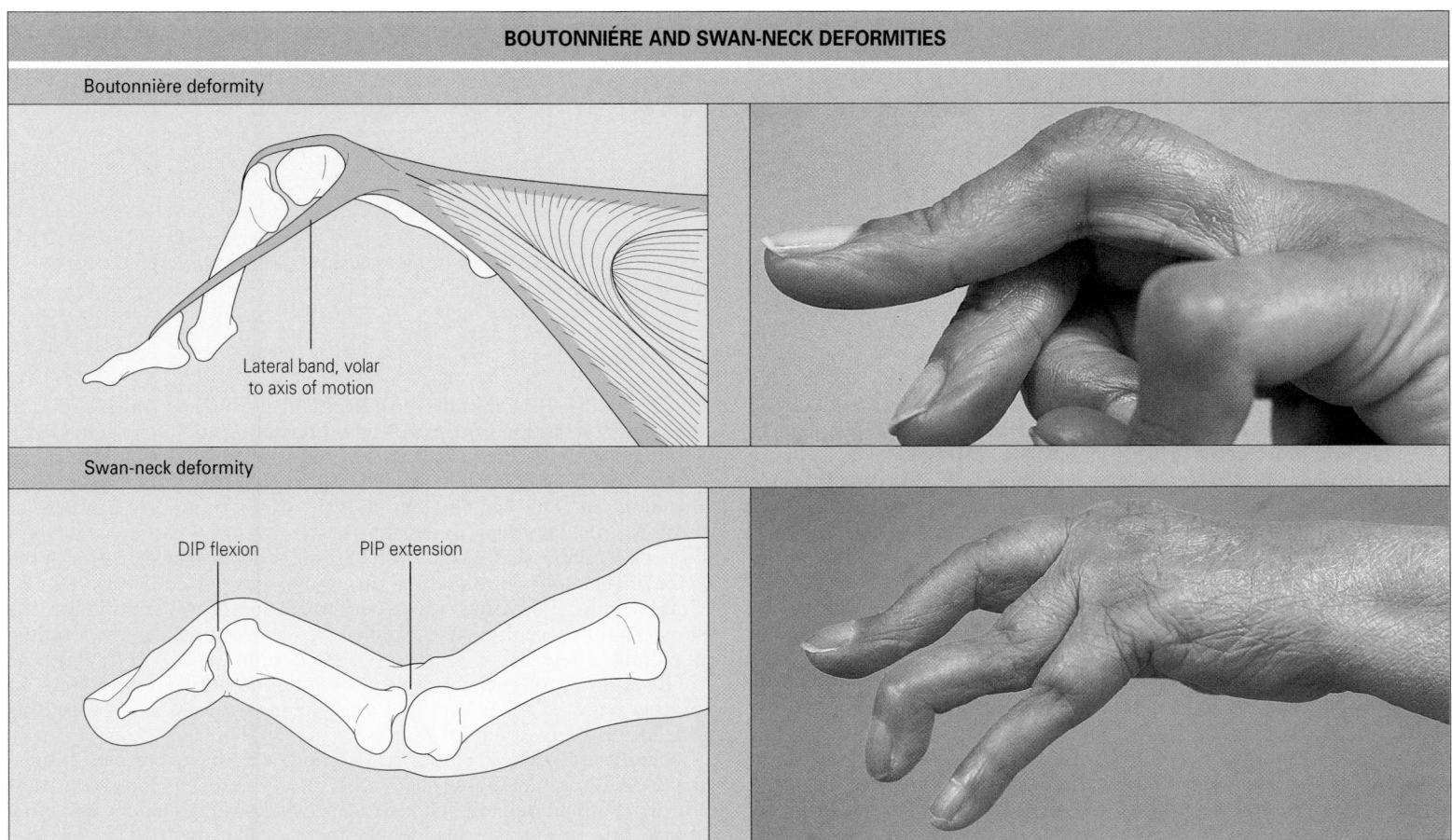

BOUTONNIÉRE AND SWAN-NECK DEFORMITIES

Boutonnière deformity

Lateral band, volar to axis of motion

Swan-neck deformity

DIP flexion   PIP extension

Fig. 82.5 Boutonnière and swan-neck deformities. The boutonnière deformity—PIP flexion and DIP hyperextension—results from relaxation of the central slip, with "buttonholing" of the PIP joint between the lateral bands. The swan-neck deformity—MCP flexion, PIP hyperextension, and DIP flexion—may be mobile, snapping, or fixed. Its pathogenesis may be related primarily to PIP or MCP involvement. Combinations of MCP and PIP involvement are less frequent. *(Adapted with permission from Hastings DE, Welsh RP. Surgical reconstruction of the rheumatoid hand. Toronto: Orthopaedic Medical Management Corporation, 1979.)*

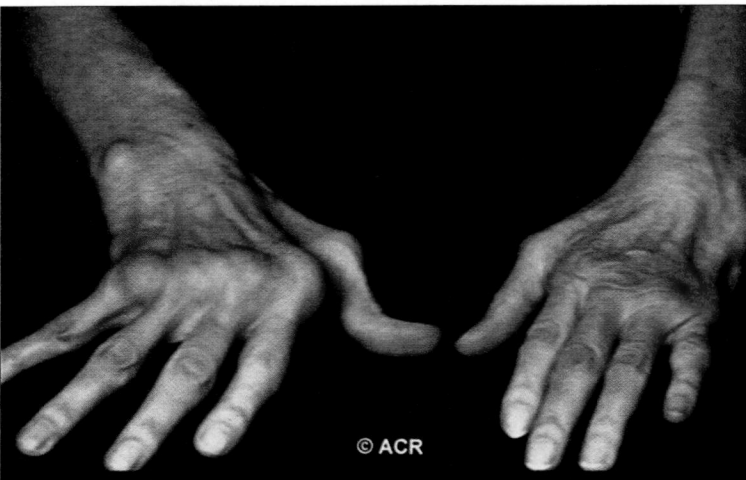

Fig. 82.6 The hyperextension of the IP joint of the right hand illustrates the "flail thumb." Note also the subluxation of the right fifth MCP, the prominent ulnar styloid, and ulnar drift. *(From Clinical Slide Collection on the Rheumatic Diseases, American College of Rheumatology.)*

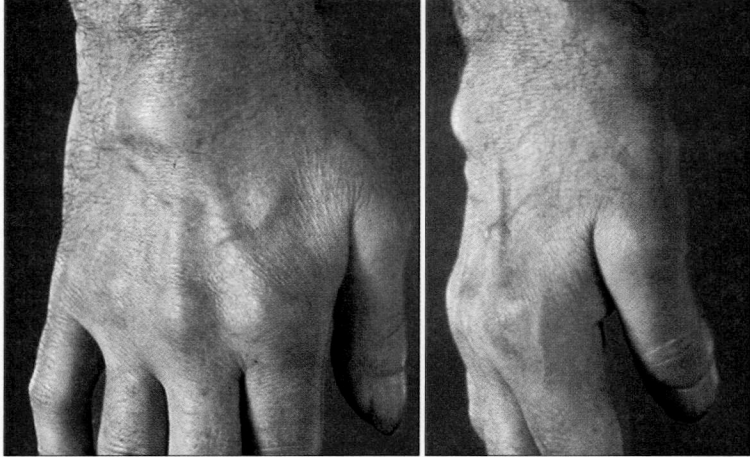

Fig. 82.8 Tenosynovial swelling from tenosynovitis—the "tuck" sign. Tenosynovial swelling overlies the metacarpals of the right hand. Bulging becomes accentuated with full extension of all the fingers of the hand. Persistent tenosynovitis over the dorsal wrist may lead to extensor tendon erosion and rupture, particularly of the tendons of the fourth and fifth fingers.

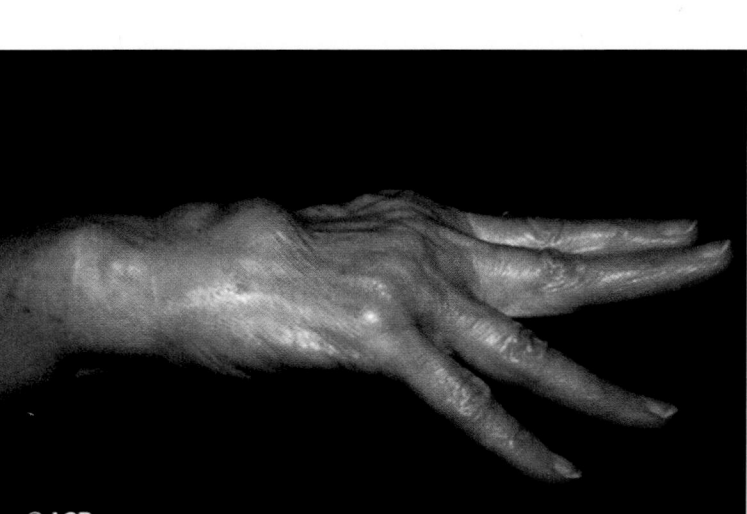
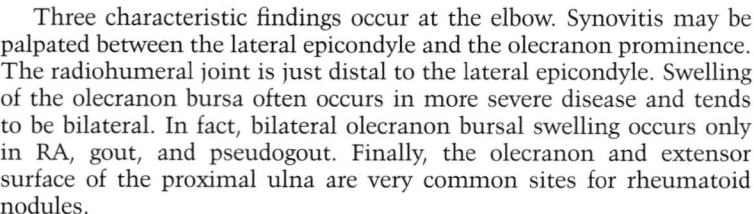

Fig. 82.7 Subluxation of the wrist in severe disease, associated with extensor tenosynovitis and extensor tendon rupture. *(From Clinical Slide Collection on the Rheumatic Diseases, American College of Rheumatology.)*

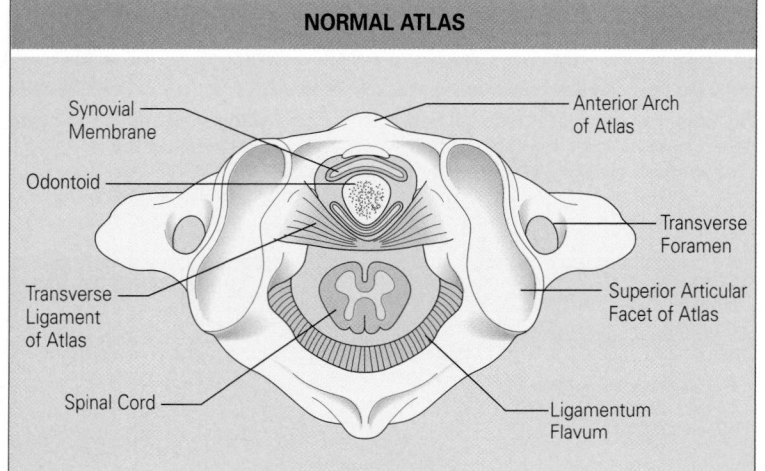

NORMAL ATLAS

Synovial Membrane

Odontoid

Transverse Ligament of Atlas

Spinal Cord

Anterior Arch of Atlas

Transverse Foramen

Superior Articular Facet of Atlas

Ligamentum Flavum

Fig. 82.9 Relationship between the peg of the odontoid and the arch of C1. *(From Clinical Slide Collection on the Rheumatic Diseases, American College of Rheumatology.)*

Three characteristic findings occur at the elbow. Synovitis may be palpated between the lateral epicondyle and the olecranon prominence. The radiohumeral joint is just distal to the lateral epicondyle. Swelling of the olecranon bursa often occurs in more severe disease and tends to be bilateral. In fact, bilateral olecranon bursal swelling occurs only in RA, gout, and pseudogout. Finally, the olecranon and extensor surface of the proximal ulna are very common sites for rheumatoid nodules.

Shoulder involvement typically produces significant limitation of motion in all planes. A visible effusion of the glenohumeral joint is unusual but can produce a "shoulder pad" sign. On examination, the patient will elevate the scapula to improve range of motion for abduction and elevation. Shoulder pain is often referred to the proximal deltoid region. Evidence of impingement of the supraspinatus and biceps tendons is often present. Owing to ongoing synovitis, rupture (either partial or complete) of the rotator cuff group of muscles may occur. Tenderness and swelling may also be seen at the sternoclavicular joint.

Spine involvement in RA is mostly limited to the cervical spine, particularly the upper portion. On examination, one notices decreased range of motion in all planes. The most critical involvement occurs at the atlantoaxial joint, where the ring of C1 pivots on the odontoid peg of C2 (Fig. 82.9). The transverse ligament of the axis courses around the posterior portion of the odontoid, preventing subluxation of C1 on C2. Tenosynovitis here can decrease the space available for the upper cervical cord, as it passes through the bony spinal canal posterior to the odontoid. This can also lead to laxity of the transverse ligament or erosion of the odontoid, in which case the ring of C1 can move forward on neck flexion (atlantoaxial subluxation), reducing the diameter of the spinal canal and compressing the upper cervical cord (Fig. 82.10). Cranial settling describes the caudal migration of the cranium on the spinal column, resulting in movement of the odontoid into the foramen magnum, where it compresses vital structures (Fig. 82.11). Subaxial subluxation represents unstable movement of one vertebral body on another below C1-C2. Vertebral artery compromise can also occur as a result of these structural defects.

Significant cervical spine involvement can have protean clinical manifestations, including headache, neck pain, a sensation that the head might fall off, paresthesias, weakness, transient ischemic attack, and bowel and bladder sphincter impairment. The development of any of these symptoms in a patient with severe RA calls for immediate neurologic examination. Magnetic resonance imaging provides the best information regarding anatomic derangements in the area.

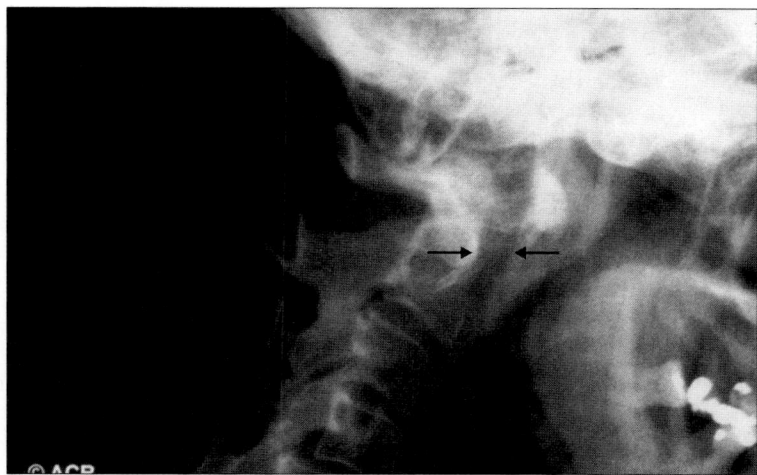

Fig. 82.10 This radiograph of the rheumatoid cervical spine in flexion demonstrates atlantoaxial subluxation as the arch of C1 slides forward (arrows). *(From Clinical Slide Collection on the Rheumatic Diseases, American College of Rheumatology.)*

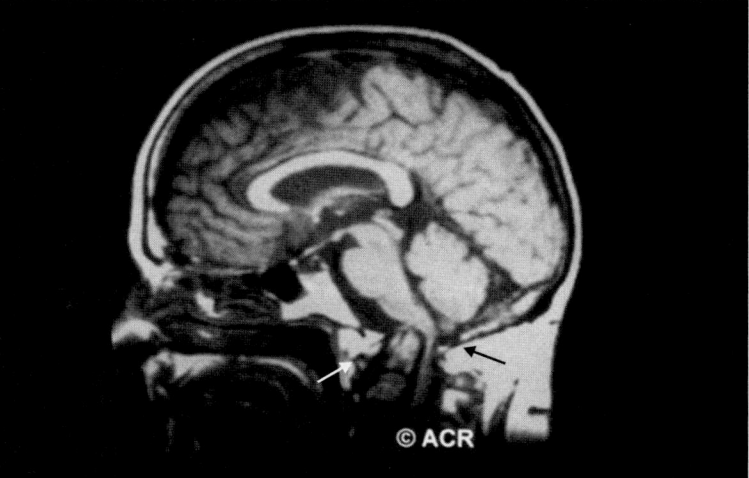

Fig. 82.11 Cranial settling occurs when the cranium migrates caudally onto the odontoid, which impinges on the brain stem above the foramen magnum. The odontoid should not extend much above a line drawn between the white and black arrows. *(From Clinical Slide Collection on the Rheumatic Diseases, American College of Rheumatology.)*

The hip is frequently affected in RA, and progressive disease can lead to severe secondary osteoarthritis requiring total joint replacement. Pain from the hip joint itself is experienced in the groin and medial thigh, sometimes radiating to the buttock. Pain over the greater trochanter, which most patients refer to as the "hip," is more likely due to bursitis. Patrick's test (also known by the acronym FABER for *f*lexion-*ab*duction-*e*xternal *r*otation) puts the hip through passive motion in all major planes and produces groin pain in the presence of true hip disorders. In later disease, it is essential to distinguish symptoms of ongoing synovitis from mechanical pain related to joint damage. Sudden development of hip pain suggests avascular necrosis or fracture in patients taking long-term corticosteroids.

Rheumatoid involvement of the knee joints is easy to detect by physical examination and is often a good indicator of disease activity. Anterior swelling is detectable by the "bulge" sign, in which the examiner strokes the medial knee to move the synovial fluid cephalad and then presses on the lateral knee to produce a visible fluid wave, or "bulge," on the medial knee. With a large tense effusion, it may be impossible to move enough fluid to produce a bulge, in which case ballottement of the patella with the index finger produces downward movement of the patella in the fluid. Distention of the posterior compartment of the knee capsule produces a tense Baker's cyst in the popliteal region. Rupture of such a popliteal cyst can produce swelling, heat, and pain in the posterior calf, resembling a deep venous thrombosis. A hemorrhagic "crescent" sign below the malleoli (Fig. 82.12) may result. Musculoskeletal ultrasound examination can be useful in detecting a popliteal cyst before rupture. Progressive synovitis can lead to loss of articular cartilage, secondary osteoarthritis, and the need for total knee arthroplasty. Examining the synovial fluid can be very helpful in distinguishing between persistent disease activity and mechanical damage. In chronic disease, quadriceps atrophy and flexion contracture are common.

The ankle is another large weight-bearing joint in which active RA can be directly visualized. The capsule of the tibiotalar joint distends anteriorly, effacing the normal contour of the tibialis anterior tendon. The joint line itself can be palpated between that tendon and the medial malleolus, where synovial proliferation can be identified. Progressive joint damage to the tibiotalar, subtalar, and talonavicular joints can result in ankle and midfoot pronation and loss of the transverse arch, producing mechanical symptoms that can be quite challenging to manage. Tendinitis of the posterior tibialis develops posterior and medial to the medial malleolus. In the same area, the posterior tibial nerve can be compressed in the tarsal tunnel, leading to paresthesias on the sole of the foot. "Pump bumps" and rheumatoid nodules commonly develop at the site of shoe friction on the posterior heel.

The forefoot is an area of major rheumatoid involvement. Early in disease, examination will reveal tenderness to palpation of the

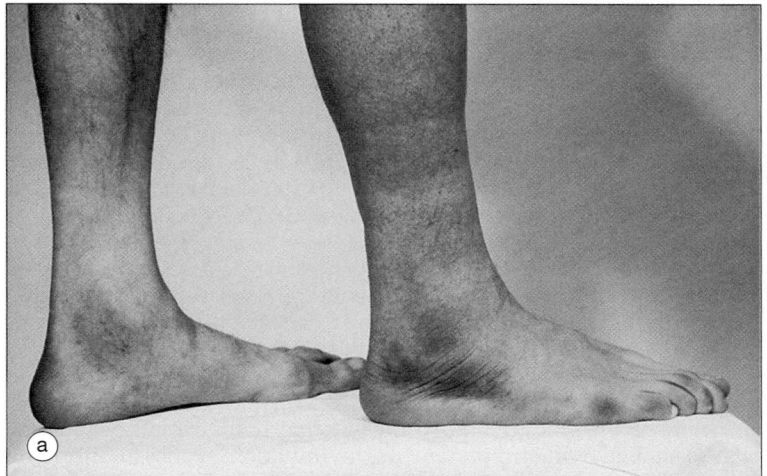

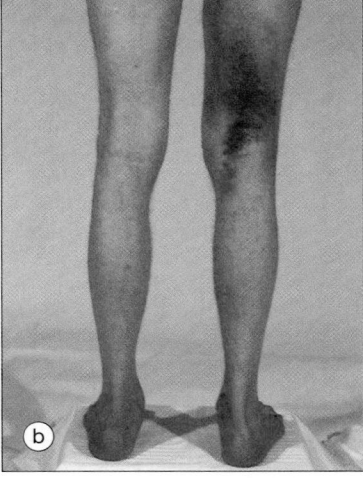

Fig. 82.12 Acute synovial rupture. A 51-year-old man with RA of 3 years' duration developed a right knee effusion after an evening of square dancing. Two days later he noted progressive pain and swelling of the right calf. (a) Six days later there was bluish discoloration of both sides of the ankle. (b) A few weeks later, after more dancing, he noted posterior thigh pain and swelling that soon became associated with purple discoloration of his right posterior thigh.

individual MTP joint or to squeezing the forefoot. Swelling can be seen in the dorsum of the foot just proximal to the toes. As disease progresses, the metatarsals sublux on the plantar aspect of the proximal phalanges, displacing the soft tissue fat pads that normally underlie the metatarsal heads. Furthermore, the forefoot broadens and the transverse arch of forefoot disappears, so that the patient's metatarsal heads are now directly bearing the weight of the entire body. Calluses develop under the metatarsal heads; and in advanced cases of RA, ulcerations occur at this location. Hammertoes (resembling piano key hammers) develop from increased tension on the flexor tendons from the MTP subluxation.

DIAGNOSIS

Rheumatoid arthritis is a clinical diagnosis for which there is no one single physical finding or laboratory test that is pathognomonic. As a practical matter, a patient older than the age of 18 who has symmetric joint pain and swelling in the hands and feet and morning stiffness is likely to have RA, especially if the RF and/or the ACPA findings are positive. Its early presentation can be quite similar to several other conditions, which must be excluded, so one must be cautious to avoid overdiagnosis of RA. On the other hand, early diagnosis is critical so that appropriate treatment can be administered and so irreversible damage does not occur. Some data suggest that definitive treatment should be administered within 3 months of the onset of disease.[2] Therein lies the advantage for the 2010 ACR/EULAR classification criteria for the contemporary clinician: they provide diagnostic support for recognition of early RA, allowing the doctor to make a definitive diagnosis without delay and thus to make a decision to administer DMARD therapy timely and before joint destruction occurs.

The ACR/EULAR criteria provide a useful starting point for one to become familiar with the key clinical features of RA (see Chapter 90). The ability to recognize early synovitis in the joints of the hands and feet is critical (see Fig. 82.2). Radiographs of the hands and feet are sometimes diagnostic at presentation, and musculoskeletal ultrasound and magnetic resonance imaging can detect early evidence of synovitis and erosions not seen on radiographs (see Chapter 85), although the aim today is to prevent joint damage from occurring. The RF test is readily available and positive in about 80% of patients with RA. However, RF may be negative early in RA and positive RF may be seen in many other conditions, especially hepatitis C infection.

The advent of detection of ACPAs has been a major advance in the diagnosis of early RA. Citrullination (conversion of peptidyl-arginine to peptidyl-citrulline) is a post-translational modification of proteins that is thought to be important in the initiation of the autoimmune response that leads to the development of RA. ACPAs are highly specific for RA and can be detected very early in disease.[11] The combination of a positive ACPA test with a positive RF test further increases the specificity for RA.[12] A Swedish study of blood bank samples showed that each of these tests had about a 70% sensitivity for detecting the individuals who ultimately developed RA and the combination of these two tests resulted in 99% specificity.[13] Thus, seropositivity for either of these tests, in a patient with polyarthritis in the hands and feet, makes the diagnosis of RA quite likely. The 2010 ACR/EULAR classification criteria recognize the importance of the number of involved joints as well as of RF and ACPA.

Differential diagnosis

A number of disorders can closely resemble RA and must be considered and excluded when the diagnosis of RA is being made.

Several viral infections can mimic RA. Parvovirus B19 infection is the cause of fifth disease in preschool children, in whom a febrile illness with a characteristic "slapped cheeks" rash occurs. Its presentation in adults is quite different, namely, a symmetric inflammatory polyarthritis resembling RA. The diagnosis can be established by detecting a transient IgM antibody response to the virus, which is present between about 2 and 6 weeks after the onset of arthritis. Parvovirus arthritis typically resolves spontaneously within 2 months; chronic disease is rare.[14] Inflammatory small joint arthritis can also occur after rubella infection or immunization. As with parvovirus, the presentation generally resolves in a matter of weeks, although chronic arthritis has been

described.[15] Both hepatitis B and C infection can cause inflammatory arthritis, which is generally transient. Chronic arthritis has been described with hepatitis C. The immune complex formation associated with these infections may result in a positive RF.

Polymyalgia rheumatica (see Chapter 152) can sometimes be quite difficult to distinguish from early RA in the elderly. Although the diagnosis can be considered as early as the age of 50, it becomes progressively more common with advancing age. Patients typically have profound morning stiffness and often complain of difficulty rolling over in bed at night. The distribution of symptoms classically includes the neck, shoulders, and hip girdle regions; palpable synovitis of the joints is unusual. Both polymyalgia rheumatica and RA respond dramatically to low-dose corticosteroid treatment and the former will often remit after 1 to 2 years. In patients initially diagnosed as having polymyalgia rheumatica, the persistence of disease and the ultimate development of small joint synovitis may lead to the diagnosis of RA.[16]

Remitting seronegative symmetric synovitis with pitting edema (RSSSPE) resembles seronegative RA in the elderly. The onset is typically abrupt and severe. Examination shows profound swelling of the hands (and sometimes the feet) with pitting edema. Response to low-dose corticosteroids is dramatic, and the disease runs a self-limited course.[17]

Palindromic rheumatism is another clinical syndrome that can mimic RA. A palindrome is a word that is spelled the same backward as forward (e.g., the name "Anna"); in palindromic rheumatism, symptoms occur suddenly and resolve just as quickly. Patients typically experience sudden attacks of inflammatory polyarthritis in a distribution similar to RA that last for a number of days before remitting spontaneously. Over time, the duration of the episodes lengthens and the symptom-free intervals shorten, leading to a chronic presentation compatible with RA in up to half of patients.[18]

Adult Still's disease refers to its similarity to the systemic-onset variant of juvenile chronic polyarthritis characterized by fever, arthritis, lymphadenopathy, and rash.[19] The adult presentation is often that of fever of unknown origin. The characteristic quotidian fever spikes once daily (less commonly, twice), usually in the afternoon or evening, then returns to normal; the name "picket fence" fever describes the appearance of the fever curve expressed graphically. In addition to inflammatory arthritis, sore throat, lymphadenopathy, hepatosplenomegaly, and rash often occur. The characteristic rash of Still's disease is a subtle salmon color and evanescent, occurring primarily during the episodes of fever. It may be enhanced by manually stroking the skin or appear where the skin has been creased by the sheets (Koebner's phenomenon). Typically the erythrocyte sedimentation rate (ESR), C-reactive protein (CRP), and serum ferritin values are extremely elevated, whereas antinuclear antibodies and RF are usually negative. The evolution of adult Still's disease to RA has been described.

Systemic lupus erythematosus (SLE) is usually easy to distinguish from RA because of its systemic nature and associated rash, pleuropericarditis, nephritis, nervous system involvement, and hematologic abnormalities. However, SLE primarily with articular involvement can easily be confused with RA. The arthritis in SLE is described as non-erosive and non-deforming. However, hand involvement with ulnar drift can resemble deforming RA. Jaccoud's arthropathy is typically reducible, rather than fixed, because it results from tendon laxity, rather than cartilage and tendon destruction. An overlap syndrome dubbed "rhupus" has been described.[20] The rare development of SLE in RA patients treated with tumor necrosis factor antagonists can add complexity to the diagnosis.[21]

Multicentric reticulohistiocytosis is a very rare syndrome that may mimic RA.[22] Systemic proliferation of multinucleated lipid-laden histiocytes causes swelling in the small joints of the hands and a characteristic erosive pattern on radiographs. A typical "string of pearls" may be seen around the cuticle in some patients.

NATURAL HISTORY

Disease onset

The clinical course of RA follows an onset of disease that may be abrupt and acute, or gradual and insidious, or subacute between these extremes.[23] A gradual onset is most common (at least 50% of cases), whereas a sudden onset is much less common (10% to 25%).[23]

Rheumatoid arthritis begins predominantly as an articular disease, and one or many joints may be affected. It may also start with an extra-articular or non-articular presentation, such as a local bursitis, tenosynovitis, carpal tunnel syndrome, or as a systemic presentation with diffuse polyarthralgia or polymyalgia. Although the onset is predominantly articular, it is frequently associated with a variety of extra-articular features, including generalized weakness, anorexia, weight loss, or fever. In some cases, fatigue alone or diffuse non-specific aching with other extra-articular features, such as pulmonary disease, may herald—by weeks or months—the onset of polyarthritis.

Pattern of presentation

Gradual onset

The most common early presentation is a gradual or insidious one affecting small peripheral joints such as the wrists, MCPs, PIPs, ankles, or MTPs. It is defined as one that the patient can date only to the nearest month. It is usually symmetric, with considerable morning stiffness and the patient complaining of difficulty making a fist and poor grip strength. The morning stiffness may last minutes to hours.

Slow, monarticular presentation

Less common is a slow monarticular presentation affecting larger joints such as shoulders or knees. The symptoms may remain confined to one or two joints but frequently spread over the ensuing days and weeks additively, to affect wrists, fingers, ankles, or feet in a widespread fashion.

Abrupt, acute polyarthritis

Less frequently, RA presents as an abrupt acute polyarthritis of the shoulders, elbows, wrists, fingers, hips, knees, ankles, and feet, with intense joint pain, diffuse swelling, and limitation leading to incapacitation. A sudden onset is defined as one for which the patient can give a specific date. This type of onset may affect patients at any age but has particular significance in the elderly.

Acute monarthritis

An acute monarthritis of a knee, shoulder, or hip can present a picture suggesting a septic, pseudogout, or gouty process, although this presentation is rare. Joint pain more severe than that found in RA is characteristic of pseudogout or gout, which may resemble or even complicate RA. The results of synovial fluid analysis should settle any diagnostic confusion in these cases. An acute monarticular presentation may proceed to more widespread involvement with any of the preceding patterns.

Tenosynovitis or bursitis may also be associated with monarthritis or polyarthritis and subcutaneous nodules over extensor surfaces, such as the elbow, sacrum, or tendo Achilles.

Local extra-articular features

As noted, bursitis and tenosynovitis may be associated with RA. Sometimes, however, the earliest manifestation and presentation of RA may be a median nerve compression (carpal tunnel syndrome) from volar wrist tenosynovitis.[24] Similarly, other local extra-articular features may be the presenting feature.

Systemic extra-articular features

Elderly patients, in particular, may present with polyarthralgias and polymyalgias affecting the neck and shoulders or hips and knees and profound fatigue. Although these features, especially in association with fever and high ESR lasting several weeks, suggest a diagnosis of polymyalgia rheumatica, this picture may be a forerunner of full-blown RA.

Pattern of progression

No matter what the onset or presentation, the patient's subsequent progress may follow several different patterns. It may be a course that is brief and self-limited, episodic (palindromic) or prolonged and progressive, or something intermediate. The severity may vary from mild to intense. Attacks may be prolonged and smoldering or prolonged and progressive.

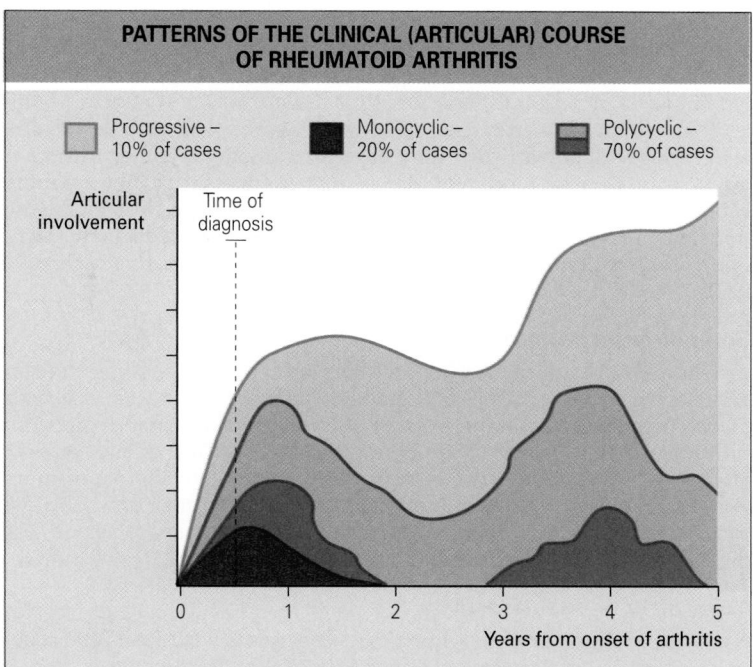

Fig. 82.13 Patterns of the clinical (articular) course of rheumatoid arthritis. Articular patterns in 50 patients with RA. *(Data from Masi AT, Feigenbaum SL, Kaplan SB. Articular patterns in the early course of rheumatoid arthritis. Am J Med 1983;75[Suppl 6A]:16-26.)*

With continuing disease activity, the patient's daily activities and functional capacity are affected to a greater or lesser extent. Although disability is usually proportional to the amount of painful joint involvement, in men who do physically hard work there is sometimes progressive joint dysfunction and disability without much pain. The physical abilities of patients who have this "neuropathic" picture may dwindle insidiously before the work impairment or daily activities decline and the seriousness of the situation becomes apparent. This highlights the importance of careful evaluation and re-evaluation of the patient's condition. For this reason, good records are essential, to document the patient's progress and response to treatment.

Few studies have examined the natural history of a group of patients with well-defined RA over a long period of time. One such representative study is that by Masi and colleagues,[25] who followed 50 patients with early RA for almost 6 years and described three articular patterns (Fig. 82.13):

1. *Monocyclic pattern:* a single cycle with remission for at least 1 year seen in 20% of patients
2. *Polycyclic pattern:* occurred in 70% of patients with either intermittent or continuing subtypes. The latter group showed smoldering activity with incomplete remission or progression.
3. *Progressive pattern:* with increasing joint involvement seen in about 10% of patients

Patients with malignant RA would be in the last category. Most authorities would agree with these general observations, but many current ideas on the natural history of RA must remain speculative until the results of more longitudinal population-based studies become available.

Clinical course—morbidity and mortality

Studies of the natural history of RA could provide insights into outcome variables and prognosis. Understanding prognosis helps us to evaluate better the psychosocial and compensation implications for estimating work disability in RA. It is worthwhile considering whether the type of disease onset and patterns of presentation previously outlined can be used to predict the subsequent course of RA.

Acute-onset pattern

In a series of 102 early cases of adult RA, Fleming and associates[23] reported that 11 patients with sudden disease onset showed, after 5 years, a better functional outcome than did 69 patients with a slow onset of disease. However, in a later series of 100 patients, Jacoby and coworkers[26] observed that, after an 11-year follow-up, there was no difference in functional class whether disease onset was acute, sub-acute, or gradual. In the past, cases with acute onset as a result of a reactive or viral polyarthritis may have been mistaken for RA. Another explanation for a better outcome in acute patients is that they are more likely to seek prompt medical attention. The favorable course of mild, transient, or self-limited RA, however, has not attracted much attention, because rheumatologists are mostly concerned with progressive RA.

Gradual-onset pattern

In Fleming and colleagues' report,[23] a worse prognosis was found in patients with disease that was gradual in onset and associated with involvement of large joints (e.g., shoulders, elbows, wrists, knees) in addition to involvement of the first and second MTPs. In the series of Jacoby and coworkers,[26] the type of onset was not predictive of functional status after 11 years; moreover, in a later Finnish study of 235 patients with RA,[27] radiographically evident damage after 7 years was the same whether the onset had been acute,[28] subacute,[29] or gradual.

Assessment of disease activity

A critical component of providing care to patients with RA is the accurate assessment of disease activity and the extent to which the patient's daily functioning is impaired. To some degree this is intuitive and readily evident from the history and physical examination at each visit. However, more quantitative outcome measures are available and can be applied at selected outpatient visits.

Recording a tender joint count (TJC) and swollen joint count (SJC) is simple and straightforward. Controversy exists regarding the ideal number of joints to be counted: 28, 44, 66, etc. The 28-joint count (PIPs, MCPs, wrists, elbows, shoulders, knees) can be accomplished quickly and efficiently in the office setting,[30] although some argue that the 44-joint count is more representative of the patient's clinical situation. Assuming that the same examiner performs the count on each visit, this is an accurate and reproducible record of the patient's status. Another objective and quantifiable tool is measurement of an acute-phase reactant, either the ESR or the CRP. The ESR can easily be performed in the outpatient setting by office staff, whereas the CRP is a more complex measurement. A more subjective method is marking a 100-mm visual analog scale (VAS) by the patient and/or health care provider. Patients can indicate a VAS measurement for pain, global assessment of arthritis activity, or general sense of health. The most common VAS for the physician to mark is global assessment of arthritis activity.

Two composite scores have been extensively used and validated: the EULAR Disease Activity Score (DAS) and the ACR Core Data Set. Whereas both are used to measure outcome in clinical trials of medications for treatment of RA, the DAS-28 is readily adaptable to repeat visits in the outpatient setting. The DAS-28 is a discrete variable calculated from the TJC and SJC for 28 joints, the ESR or CRP, and the patient's VAS for general health. A rather complicated calculation including logarithmic transformation produces a discrete numeric value between 0 and 10.[30] A DAS calculator is available online[31] to easily generate this number. Some investigators have proposed making specific treatment decisions at each visit based on escalating medication treatment to achieve a DAS below a certain threshold level indicating "remission."[32] Further details on disease activity and outcome assessment are provided in Chapter 93.

The ACR Core Data Set expresses a degree of improvement compared with baseline, rather than a discrete number. For example, a 20% or greater improvement (ACR20) has been proposed as distinguishing a clinical response from a placebo response.[33] The ACR20 requires at least a 20% improvement in both the TJC and SJC and in at least three of the following: physician global VAS, patient global VAS, patient pain VAS, Health Assessment Questionnaire (HAQ) score, and ESR or CRP. Likewise, an ACR50 improvement would indicate at least 50% improvement and the ACR70 at least 70% improvement, and so on. Whereas this outcome measure has become standard in evaluating new anti-rheumatic agents in clinical trials, it has not been widely applied to evaluating the activity of patients seen in clinical practice.

TABLE 82.1 SELF-REPORT QUESTIONNAIRE FOR RHEUMATOID ARTHRITIS

Please check (√) the ONE best answer for your abilities.

At this moment, are you able to	Without any difficulty	With some difficulty	With much difficulty	Unable to do
1. Dress yourself, including tying shoelaces and doing buttons?				
2. Get in and out of bed?				
3. Lift a full cup or glass to your mouth?				
4. Walk outdoors on flat ground?				
5. Wash and dry your entire body?				
6. Bend down to pick up clothing from the floor?				
7. Turn regular faucets (taps) on and off?				
8. Get in and out of a car?				

The questionnaire is used to make a quantitative assessment of the functional capacity of the patient to carry out the tasks of daily living.[34]

The HAQ has become an established outcome measure that is easily self-administered by the patient in a short amount of time.[34] Initially developed at Stanford University, the HAQ has undergone many iterations, each of which has its proponents. In its simplest form, the questionnaire addresses the patient's ability to perform activities of daily living in eight domains (Table 82.1): for example, getting in and out of bed, bending down to pick up clothing from the floor, and so on. The patient indicates the level of difficulty for performing each activity (0 = "without any difficulty" to 3 = "unable to do") and the highest value for each of the eight domains is indicated. These eight values are summed and divided by 8, yielding an HAQ score. As the score increases, so does the level of disability. The HAQ scores can be compared from visit to visit, a change of 0.22 representing a significant difference. Early in disease the HAQ score tends to reflect disease activity, whereas in later disease it tends to indicate level of disability.

The regular application of such outcome measures allows the clinician to make a quantitative determination of how the patient is doing, and this can be especially valuable when assessing a patient's response to a change in treatment. In some situations, documentation of response to treatment is required by health insurance providers as a condition of continuing to provide expensive medications such as monoclonal antibodies or recombinant fusion proteins.

PROGNOSIS

It is critically important for the clinician to make the best possible assessment of prognosis for an individual patient with RA. Although there is consensus that all patients with RA should receive DMARDs, the choice of medications individually or in combination for a particular patient depends greatly on the clinician's judgment as to the severity of illness and the likelihood that joint destruction will occur. For example, there is evidence from several trials that some patients have a better outcome if they are started on a combination regimen immediately, as opposed to an approach in which individual agents are added sequentially.[35,36] Trials are in progress to determine whether some patients with early disease might do better if immediately started on anti–tumor necrosis factor agents, rather than using such medications only after "first-line" drugs such as methotrexate have failed to produce an adequate response. Approaches to treatment are in rapid evolution, and it is unlikely that there will be agreement regarding a single best algorithm for choosing therapeutic agents in the foreseeable future. Nonetheless, a prediction of prognosis at the time of diagnosis or at the time of assuming care is essential.

The literature on prognostic factors for RA is voluminous, and there is no clear consensus regarding which factor or combination of factors is most important. Several factors reported to influence prognosis are discussed below.

The HAQ is a simple self-administered questionnaire that is widely used to assess disease activity early and disability late in disease.[34] A recent study from France attempted to correlate HAQ scores with subsequent radiographic presentation.[37] The authors found, as did other studies, that the HAQ score at baseline is an excellent predictor of outcome.[38] Furthermore, the HAQ score has also been shown to predict the risk of future loss of productivity on the part of the RA patient.[39]

Radiographic damage at onset has been shown to be an important predictor of clinical outcome and radiographic progression. Gossec and colleagues found that a Sharp score (Van Der Heijde modification) of less than 4 points at baseline was predictive of remission (DAS-28 < 1.6) 3 and 5 years later.[40] Not surprisingly, radiographic erosions at baseline are predictive of further radiographic damage 2 to 3 years later.[41]

Acute-phase reactants also have predictive value regarding the development of radiographic damage over time. The ESR at the start of the study was the best predictor of radiographic outcome in the first 5 years in a Swedish study,[42] and the prognostic value of ESR has been demonstrated in other studies.[43,44] Likewise, the baseline CRP is predictive of subsequent radiographic damage.[44]

Serologic markers may predict prognosis. The presence of RF has been consistently associated with radiographic progression.[42,44] Data are emerging that the presence of ACPAs is an independent predictor of radiographic damage.[44-46]

The shared epitope refers to a sequence of amino acids in the hypervariable region of the binding pocket of the HLA-DR molecule. This sequence of QKRAA confers a substantial increase in risk for the development of RA. Furthermore, the presence of the shared epitope is predictive of disease severity in a dose-dependent fashion: an individual with a copy of the gene encoding this sequence from both parents tends to have more severe disease than a patient with only one copy. Although there is abundant evidence of its significance as a predictor, this is not readily available to clinicians and is available only through research laboratories. However, studies are divided with regard to whether a shared epitope is[41,43,47,48] or is not[44] an unfavorable prognostic factor, and recent data suggest that the shared epitope is associated with the antibody response or better with autoantibody (RF, ACPA) positive RA.

In summary, the clinician has a number of readily available tools that can be useful in predicting the prognosis of the RA patient several years later: ESR, CRP, RF, ACPA, HAQ, and baseline radiographs of the hands and feet. Although it is not possible at present to assign the relative importance of these factors in combination, because the presence of each of them has negative implications for prognosis, the presence or absence of these factors can help the clinician make a rational assessment when making treatment decisions for individual patients.

REFERENCES

1. Arnett FC, Edworthy SM, Bloch DA, et al. The American Rheumatism Association 1987 revised criteria for the classification of rheumatoid arthritis. Arthritis Rheum 1988;30:315-324.
2. Paget S. The no man's land of undifferentiated inflammatory polyarthritis. J Rheumatol 2004;31:1673-1676.
3. Symmons DPM, Hazes JM, Silman AF. Cases of early inflammatory polyarthritis should not be classified as having rheumatoid arthritis. J Rheumatol 2003;30:902-904.
4. Harrison BJ, Symmons DPM, Barrett EM, et al. The performance of the 1987 ARA classification criteria for rheumatoid arthritis in a population-based cohort of patients with early inflammatory polyarthritis. J Rheumatol 1998;25:2324-2330.
5. Van Aiken J, Van Bilsen JHM, Allaart CF, et al. The Leiden Early Arthritis Clinic. Clin Exp Rheumatol 2003;21(Suppl 31):S100-S105.
5a. Aletaha D, Neogi T, Silman AJ, Funovits J, Felson DT, Bingham CO 3rd et al. The 2010 American College of Rheumatology/European League Against Rheumatism Classification Criteria for Rheumatoid Arthritis. Arthritis Rheum 2010 …; Ann Rheum Dis. 2010 (details to follow upon acceptance)
6. American College of Rheumatology Subcommittee on Rheumatoid Arthritis Guidelines. Guidelines for the management of rheumatoid arthritis: 2002 update. Arthritis Rheum 2002;46:328-346.
7. Mottonen TP, Hannonen P, Korpela M, et al. Finnish rheumatoid arthritis combination therapy: delay to institution of therapy and induction of remission using single-drug or combination-disease-modifying antirheumatic drug therapy in early rheumatoid arthritis. Arthritis Rheum 2002;46:894-898.
8. Bukhari M, Harrison B, Lunt M, et al. Time to first occurrence of erosions in inflammatory polyarthritis: results from a prospective community-based study. Arthritis Rheum 2001;44:1248-1253.
9. Aletaha D, Funovits J, Breedveld FC, et al. Rheumatoid arthritis joint progression in sustained remission is determined by disease activity levels preceding the period of radiographic assessment. Arthritis Rheum 2009;60:1242-1249.
10. Nielen MMJ, Van Schaqardenburg D, Reesink HW, et al. Specific autoantibodies precede the symptoms of rheumatoid arthritis: a study of serial measurements in blood donors. Arthritis Rheum 2004;50:380-386.
11. Visser H, Le Cessie S, Vos K, et al. How to diagnose rheumatoid arthritis early: a prediction model for persistent (erosive) arthritis. Arthritis Rheum 2002;46:357-365.

12. Schellekens FA, Visser H, De Jong BAW, et al. The diagnostic properties of rheumatoid arthritis antibodies recognizing a cyclic citrullinated peptide. Arthritis Rheum 2000;43:155-163.
13. Rantapaa-Dahlquvist S, De Jong SAW, Beglin E, et al. Antibodies against cyclic citrullinated peptide and IgA rheumatoid factor predict the development of rheumatoid arthritis. Arthritis Rheum 2003;48:2741-2749.
14. Sabella C, Goldfarb J. Parvovirus B19 infections. Am Fam Physician 1999;60:1455-1460.
15. Weibel RE, Benor DE. Chronic arthropathy and musculoskeletal symptoms associated with rubella vaccines: a review of 124 claims submitted to the national vaccine injury compensation program. Arthritis Rheum 2005;39:1529.
16. Pease CT, Haugeberg G, Morgan AW, et al. Diagnosing late onset rheumatoid arthritis, polymyalgia rheumatica, and temporal arteritis in patients presenting with polymyalgic symptoms: a prospective long-term evaluation. J Rheumatol 2005;32:1043-1046.
17. Russell EB. Remitting seronegative symmetrical synovitis with pitting edema syndrome: follow-up for neoplasia. J Rheumatol 2005;32:1760-1761.
18. Gonzales-Lopez L, Gamez-Nava JI, Jhangri GS, et al. Prognostic factors for the development of rheumatoid arthritis and other connective tissue disease in patients with palindromic rheumatism. J Rheumatol 1999;26:540-545.
19. Yamaguci M, Ohtaq A, Tsnematsu T, et al. Preliminary criteria for classification of adult Still's disease. J Rheumatol 1992;19:424-430.
20. Brand CA, Rowley VJ, Tait BD, et al. Coexistent rheumatoid arthritis and systemic lupus erythematosus: clinical, serological and phenotypic features. Ann Rheum Dis 1992;51:173-176.
21. Mohan AK, Edwards ET, Cote TR, et al. Drug-induced systemic lupus erythematosus and TNF-α blockers. Lancet 2002;360:646.
22. Santilli D, Lo Monaco A, Cavazzini PL, et al. Multicentric reticulohistiocytosis: a rare cause of erosive arthropathy of the distal interphalangeal finger joints. Ann Rheum Dis 2002;61:485-487.
23. Fleming A, Crown JM, Corbett M. Early rheumatoid disease: I. Onset. II. Patterns of joint involvement. Ann Rheum Dis 1976;35:357-363.
24. Jacob J, Sartorius D, Kursunoglu S, et al. Distal interphalangeal joint involvement in rheumatoid arthritis. Arthritis Rheum 1986;29:10-15.
25. Masi AT, Feigenbaum SL, Kaplan SB. Articular patterns in the early course of rheumatoid arthritis. Am J Med 1983;75(Suppl 6A):16-26.

26. Jacoby RK, Jayson MIV, Cosh JA. Onset, early stages and prognosis of rheumatoid arthritis: a clinical study of 100 patients with 11-year follow-up. BMJ 1973;2:96-100.
27. Luukkainen R, Isomaki H, Kajander A. Prognostic value of the type of onset of rheumatoid arthritis. Ann Rheum Dis 1983;42:274-275.
28. Wolfe F, Cathey MA. The assessment and prediction of functional disability in rheumatoid arthritis. J Rheumatol 1991;18:1298-1306.
29. Thevenon A, Hardouin P, Duquesnoy B. Popliteal cyst presenting as an anterior tibial mass. Arthritis Rheum 1985;28:477-478.
30. Inoue E, Yamanaka H, Hara M, et al. Comparison of disease activity score DAS28 erythrocyte sedimentation rate and DAS 8 C-reactive protein threshold values. Ann Rheum Dis 2007;66:407-409.
31. DAS calculator. Available at www.das-score.nl/www. das-score.nl/DAS28calc.htm.
32. Grigor C, Capell HA, Stirling A, et al. Effect of a treatment strategy of tight control for rheumatoid arthritis (the TICORA study): a single-blind randomized controlled trial. Lancet 2004;364:263-269.
33. Felson DT, Anderson JJ, Boers M, et al. American College of Rheumatology preliminary definition of improvement in rheumatoid arthritis. Arthritis Rheum 1995;38:727-735.
34. Wolfe F. A reappraisal of HAQ disability in rheumatoid arthritis. Arthritis Rheum 2000;43:2751-2761.
35. Landewé RBM, Boers M, Verhoeven AC, et al. COBRA combination therapy in patients with early rheumatoid arthritis: long-term structural benefits of a brief intervention. Arthritis Rheum 2002;46:347-356.
36. Goekoop-Ruiterman YPM, de Vries-Bouwstra JK, Allaart CF, et al. Comparison of treatment strategies in early rheumatoid arthritis: a randomized trial. Ann Intern Med 2007;146:406-415.
37. Combe B, Cantagrel A, Boupille P, et al. Predictive factors of 5-year Health Assessment Questionnaire disability in early rheumatoid arthritis. J Rheumatol 2003;30:2344-2348.
38. Uhlig T, Smedstad LM, Vaglum P, et al. The course of rheumatoid arthritis and predictors of psychological, physical and radiograph outcome after 5 years of follow-up. Rheumatology 2000;39:732-741.
39. Puokakka K, Kautiainen H, Mottonen T, et al. Predictors of productivity loss in early rheumatoid arthritis: a 5-year follow-up study. Ann Rheum Dis 2005;64:130-133.
40. Gossec L, Dougados M, Goupille P, et al. Prognostic factors for remission in early rheumatoid arthritis: a multiparameter prospective study. Ann Rheum Dis 2004;63:675-680.

41. Combe B, Dougados M, Goupille P, et al. Prognostic factors for radiographic damage in early rheumatoid arthritis. Arthritis Rheum 2001;44:1736-1743.

42. Lindqvist E, Jonsson K, Saxne T, et al. Course of radiographic damage over 10 years in a cohort with early rheumatoid arthritis. Ann Rheum Dis 2003;62:611-616.

43. Lindqvist E, Saxne T, Geborek P, et al. Ten year outcome in a cohort of patients with early rheumatoid arthritis: health status, disease process and damage. Ann Rheum Dis 2002;61:1055-1059.

44. Lindqvist E, Eberhardt K, Bendtzen K, et al. Prognostic laboratory markers of joint damage in rheumatoid arthritis. Ann Rheum Dis 2005;64:196-201.

45. Forslind K, Ahlmen M, Eberhardt K, et al. Prediction of radiological outcome in early rheumatoid arthritis in clinical practice: role of antibodies to citrullinated peptides (anti-CCP). Ann Rheum Dis 2004;63:1090-1095.

46. Vencovsky J, Machacek S, Sedova L, et al. Autoantibodies can be prognostic markers of an erosive disease in early rheumatoid arthritis. Ann Rheum Dis 2003;62:427-430.

47. Mottonen T, Hannonnen P, Nissila M, et al. Delay to institution of therapy and induction of remission using single-drug or combination-disease-modifying antirheumatic drug therapy in early rheumatoid arthritis. Arthritis Rheum 2003;46:8984-8988.

48. Goronzy JJ, Matteson EL, Fulbright JW, et al. Prognostic markers of radiographic progression in early rheumatoid arthritis. Arthritis Rheum 2004;50:43-54.

Extra-articular features of rheumatoid arthritis and systemic involvement

83

Carl Turesson and Eric L. Matteson

- Rheumatoid arthritis may be associated with inflammation in extra-articular organs.
- Features of systemic involvement in rheumatoid arthritis include constitutional symptoms, distinct organ manifestations, and severe multiorgan disease.
- Systemic features may be associated with a poor prognosis, especially vasculitis and rheumatoid lung disease.

INTRODUCTION

Constitutional features of rheumatoid arthritis (RA), such as fatigue and weight loss, may occur early in the course of the disease and may predominate, overshadowing the joint manifestations.

At times, inflammation may extend beyond the joints (Table 83.1). These systemic manifestations occur equally in men and women and may appear at any age.[1,2]

Extra-articular disease manifestations (excepting laboratory abnormalities) occur in about 40% of patients at some time during the course of their disease.[2] The incidence of severe extra-articular disease (vasculitis, vasculitis-related neuropathy, pericarditis, pleuritis, glomerulonephritis, scleritis/episcleritis, or Felty syndrome) has been estimated to be 1/100 person-years in a well-defined population.[2] A decrease in the incidence of rheumatoid vasculitis in recent years has been reported,[3] but there is no clear change in the occurrence of other extra-articular manifestations.[4]

The systemic inflammatory process is a major predictor of mortality in patients with RA. Extra-articular disease confers a mortality risk ratio five times that of patients without these manifestations, even after such co-morbidities as heart and lung disease, malignancy, and dementia are accounted for.[2] Some extra-articular disease manifestations, especially vasculitis, pericarditis, pleuritis, amyloidosis, and Felty syndrome, are associated with a diminished lifespan compared with patients without extra-articular disease (Fig. 83.1).[1,2,5] Smoking,[6] presence of rheumatoid factor, and RA-associated HLA-DRB1*04 genes[7,8] predict extra-articular disease. Other genetic markers such as HLA-C*03 and genes regulating killer immunoglobulin-like receptor expression on T-cell subsets, may have a particular impact on the risk of vasculitis.[9,10] Probably due to interactions between these and other risk factors, extra-articular manifestations tend to cluster in individual patients.[11]

The nature of the specific organ involved and the severity of the involvement guide treatment of the extra-articular manifestations of RA. Often, the therapeutic strategies designed to control the joint involvement, including disease-modifying antirheumatic drugs (DMARDs) and glucocorticoids, are effective in treating systemic disease. Although glucocorticosteroids are the mainstay of treatment of systemic disease, cytotoxic agents such as cyclophosphamide are sometimes necessary for severe disease, including organ-threatening eye disease and systemic vasculitis.[12] Anti–tumor necrosis factor (anti-TNF) antagonists, B cell–depleting therapies, and other specific immunomodulating agents may be particularly useful in managing these manifestations,[13] although extra-articular manifestations sometimes also develop in patients treated with TNF blockers and other biologics.

NODULES

Subcutaneous nodules occur mainly in RA patients who are rheumatoid factor positive and rarely in seronegative patients. Patients with rheumatoid nodules in early RA are at an increased risk of developing severe extra-articular manifestations. Rheumatoid nodulosis (numerous, widespread nodules) occasionally presents as a separate condition, usually in men, with a low-grade and sometimes barely detectable synovitis.[14]

Nodules develop most commonly on pressure areas, including the elbows, finger joints, ischial and sacral prominences, occipital scalp, and Achilles tendon. Rheumatoid nodules are firm and frequently adherent to the underlying periosteum (Fig. 83.2). Histologically, there is a focal central fibrinoid necrosis with surrounding fibroblasts (Fig. 83.3). This is believed to occur as a result of small vessel vasculitis with fibrinoid necrosis, which forms the center of the nodule and surrounding fibroblastic proliferation.

Subcutaneous nodules may regress during treatment with disease-modifying drugs, usually as the RA improves. Paradoxically, methotrexate may increase nodules, particularly over finger tendons (Fig. 83.4), despite improvements in the overall disease activity.

HEMATOLOGIC ABNORMALITIES

The cause of anemia in RA is multifactorial. Iron utilization is impaired, partly due to cytokine-induced upregulation of hepcidin leading to abnormal retention of iron from senescent red blood cells by the reticuloendothelial system and increased lactoferrin, which contributes to the binding and decreasing of serum iron. The ferritin concentration may be low as a result of iron deficiency or increased because of increased synthesis in chronic inflammation. In the setting of anemia in RA, a ferritin concentration less than 50 ng/mL is predictive of iron deficiency, whereas a concentration greater than 100 ng/mL is associated with anemia of chronic disease. Proinflammatory cytokines, including TNF, interleukin-1, and interleukin-6, among others, play an important role in the anemia of RA, likely by acting directly on red cell precursors in the bone marrow. Reduced erythropoietin and a blunted response to erythropoietin also contribute to the anemia of RA. Additional factors include an increased phagocytosis of red blood cells in the spleen and even by the synovium.

The degree of anemia in RA usually correlates with the disease activity, particularly the degree of articular inflammation. It is commonly normochromic and normocytic. Anemia caused by rheumatoid inflammation can improve with therapy that treats the disease successfully. Administration of erythropoietin to RA patients improves red blood cell counts.[15] Iron deficiency may complicate the anemia associated with RA.

Thrombocytosis is a frequent finding in active RA. The degree of thrombocytosis may correlate with the number of joints involved with active synovitis and may be associated with extra-articular features. Thrombocytopenia is rare in RA, except when related to drug treatment or Felty syndrome. Coagulation inhibitors may be produced, and a hyperviscosity syndrome in association with high titers of rheumatoid factor and neurologic and vascular occlusive symptoms has rarely been reported.

Lymphadenopathy is frequent in active RA. Histologic examination usually reveals benign follicular hyperplasia. RA is, however, associated with an increased risk of malignant non-Hodgkin lymphoma compared with the general population.[16] High disease activity[17] and concomitant

TABLE 83.1 INCIDENCE OF EXTRA-ARTICULAR DISEASE MANIFESTATIONS IN A COMMUNITY-BASED SAMPLE OF PATIENTS WITH RHEUMATOID ARTHRITIS[6]

Extra-articular manifestation	30-yr cumulative incidence (%)
Pericarditis	10.9
Pleuritis	9.4
Major cutaneous vasculitis	5.1
Vasculitis-related neuropathy	2.8
Felty syndrome	2.7
Scleritis	1.0
Episcleritis	0.8
Glomerulonephritis	2.9
Amyloidosis	1.0
Secondary Sjögren syndrome	17.1
Pulmonary fibrosis	9.4
Bronchiolitis obliterans	1.2
Subcutaneous rheumatoid nodules	39.4

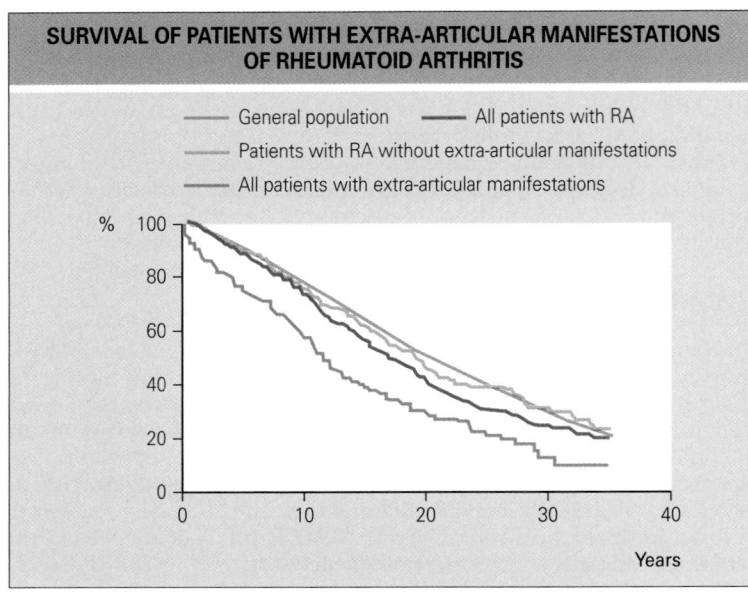

SURVIVAL OF PATIENTS WITH EXTRA-ARTICULAR MANIFESTATIONS OF RHEUMATOID ARTHRITIS

— General population — All patients with RA
— Patients with RA without extra-articular manifestations
— All patients with extra-articular manifestations

Fig. 83.1 Survival of patients with extra-articular manifestations of rheumatoid arthritis.

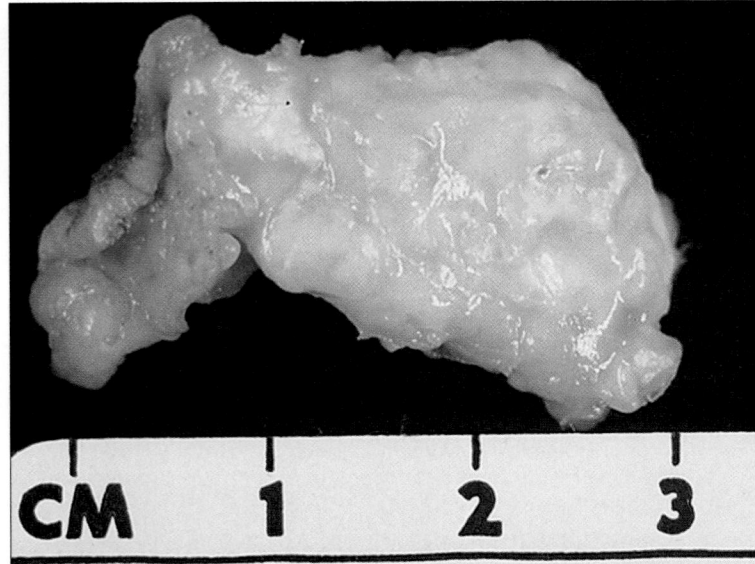

Fig. 83.2 Gross anatomic specimen of a rheumatoid nodule. The yellow tissue is caused by fibrinoid necrosis.

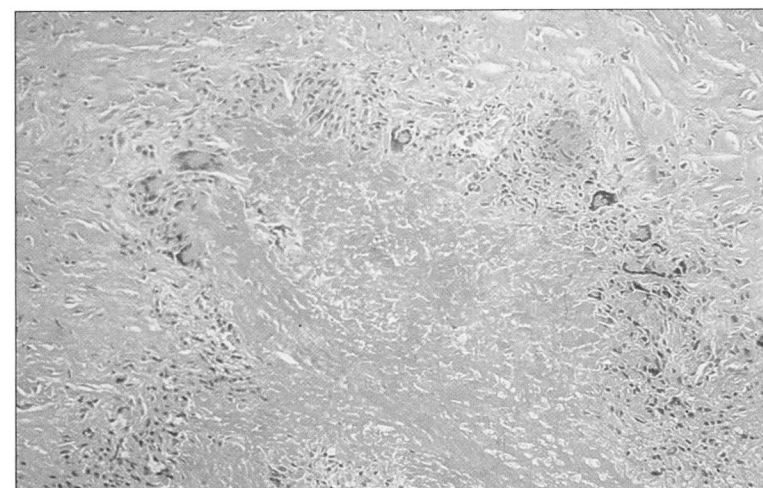

Fig. 83.3 Rheumatoid nodule with granulomatous transformation. There is prominent central fibrinoid necrosis, with surrounding palisading histiocytes and an outer layer of chronic fibrosing connective tissue with inflammatory cells including lymphocytes and fibroblasts (hematoxylin-eosin stain; original magnification ×450).

Sjögren syndrome[18] may confer an increased risk of lymphoma. Lymphadenopathy is sometimes accompanied by splenomegaly, even in the absence of Felty syndrome.

FELTY SYNDROME

Felty syndrome is defined as RA in combination with splenomegaly and leukopenia. The syndrome characteristically occurs in patients with long-standing, seropositive, nodular, deforming RA. In Caucasian patients, the major histocompatibility locus associations with Felty syndrome are due to linkage disequilibrium with HLA-DRB1*0401.[19] Some patients have no active synovitis at the time Felty syndrome develops. Many of these patients have lower extremity ulcerations, hyperpigmentation, and antinuclear antibodies.

Bacterial infections are common in Felty syndrome, correlating with a polymorphonuclear leukocyte count of less than 100/mm³, and account for a substantial mortality in this condition. Other factors associated with an increased incidence of infections are skin ulcers, dose of glucocorticosteroid, hypocomplementemia, and high levels of immune complexes. The bone marrow is usually normal or hyperplastic. In some patients the bone marrow does not respond appropriately

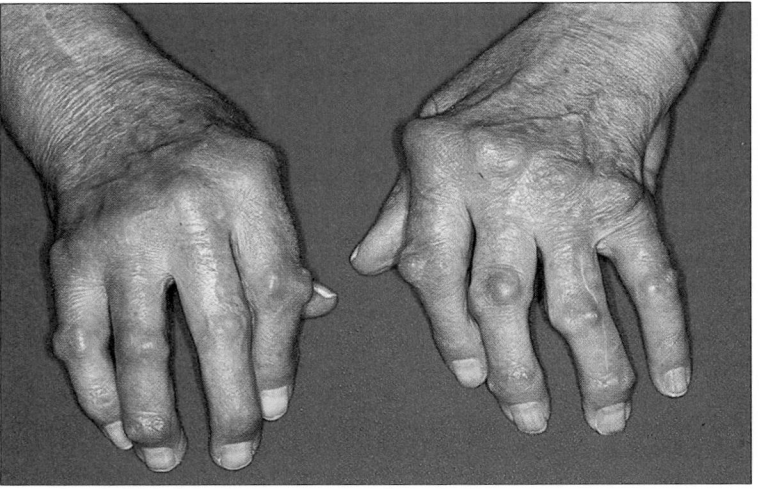

Fig. 83.4 Rheumatoid nodules in a patient with long-standing rheumatoid arthritis treated with low-dose weekly methotrexate.

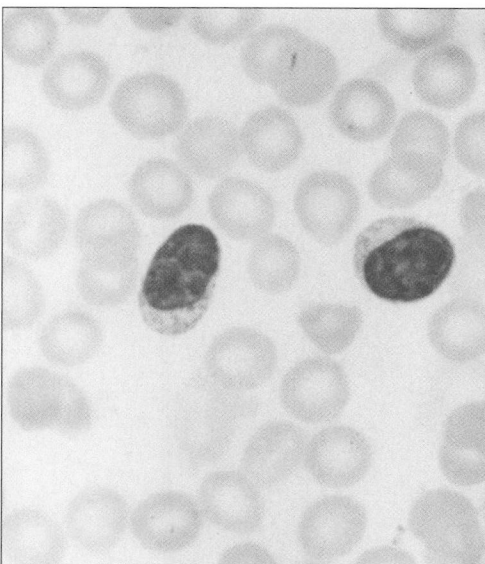

Fig. 83.5 Large granular lymphocytes.

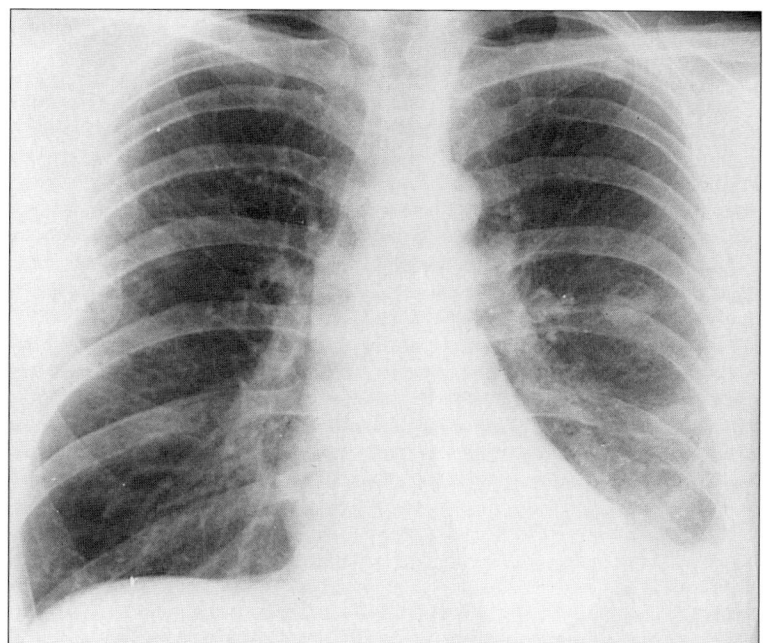

Fig. 83.6 Pleural effusion and rheumatoid nodule in rheumatoid arthritis. Changes associated with diffuse interstitial fibrosis are also present.

to the degree of leukopenia, perhaps because of inhibitors induced by proinflammatory cytokines, which suppress myelopoiesis.[20] Thrombocytopenia also occurs in Felty syndrome.

Treatment with methotrexate[21] or parenteral gold[22] has been shown to improve cytopenias (grade C). Splenectomy may improve the hematologic abnormalities and may be indicated for recurrent serious infections caused by the neutropenia that has been unresponsive to disease-modifying drugs. Splenectomy rarely helps the underlying disease process, although it might improve leg ulcers. Despite splenectomy, granulocytopenia may recur and persist. Glucocorticosteroids transiently improve the granulocytopenia but may predispose to infections. Treatment with granulocyte colony-stimulating factor is indicated in patients with severe neutropenia and recurrent infections but may also lead to a flare of the polyarthritis and even to vasculitis because of an increase in the total load of inflammatory mediators when the neutrophil count is normalized.

There is an increased risk for the development of lymphoproliferative and other malignancies in patients with RA, particularly those with Felty syndrome.[16] A variant of Felty syndrome has been described in which patients have neutropenia and an increase in the number of large granular lymphocytes in blood and bone marrow (Fig. 83.5).[23] The large granular lymphocytes in these patients represent *in vivo* activated cytotoxic T cells and clonality is present. However, rapidly progressive malignancy with decreased survival is unusual. Patients with RA and large granular lymphocytes may also have thrombocytopenia, anemia, and splenomegaly.

HEPATIC ABNORMALITIES

Active RA may be associated with an increase in liver function abnormalities and may parallel the anemia, thrombocytosis, and increased erythrocyte sedimentation rate. With control of the rheumatoid inflammation, the liver function abnormalities return to normal. Examination of liver histology at the time of liver function abnormality reveals only minimal non-specific changes, with some periportal mononuclear cell infiltration.

Liver involvement, including hepatomegaly, may be present in up to 65% of patients with Felty syndrome.[24] There may be histologic abnormalities, even when liver function tests are normal. The liver pathology varies from portal fibrosis and abnormal lobular architecture to nodular regenerative hyperplasia. These patients can develop portal hypertension, esophageal varices, and variceal bleeding.

PULMONARY INVOLVEMENT

Pulmonary involvement in RA is frequent, although not always clinically recognized.[25] Men are affected more often than women. Pleural

disease is common and is usually asymptomatic. In autopsy studies, involvement of the pleura is reported in up to 50% of patients with RA but clinically detected in only about 10% of these cases.[2] Rheumatoid pleural effusions are usually exudates with mixed cell counts, high lactate dehydrogenase concentrations, and high protein concentrations (>4 g/L). The presence of multinucleated giant cells is highly specific for rheumatoid pleuritis, but such cells are seen in less than 50% of these cases. Glucose concentrations are often less than 25 mg/dL (1.4 mmol/L).

Parenchymal pulmonary nodules (Fig. 83.6) are generally asymptomatic and are found in seropositive RA patients who have widespread synovitis and, usually, nodules elsewhere. The pulmonary nodules tend to be peripheral in location and can measure less than 1 cm or up to 6 to 8 cm in diameter. They can cavitate and cause pleural effusions and bronchopleural fistulas. Pathologic examination of the nodules reveals a central necrotic zone surrounded by a cellular area of proliferating fibroblasts. The differential diagnosis of pulmonary rheumatoid nodules includes neoplasms, tuberculosis, and fungal infections. In the case of a solitary rheumatoid nodule in the lung, an excisional biopsy may be necessary to confirm the diagnosis. Treatment of the underlying rheumatoid disease frequently results in improvement of the pulmonary nodules.

Pulmonary nodulosis and pneumoconiosis in patients with RA (Caplan syndrome) is characterized by several nodules greater than 1 cm in diameter, scattered throughout the peripheral lung field (Fig. 83.7). Caplan syndrome is seen in individuals with extensive exposure to coal dust, although exposure to silica and asbestos may also lead to pulmonary nodulosis in these patients.

The cumulative incidence of symptomatic interstitial lung disease (ILD) in a community-based population of patients with RA was 9.4%.[2] The most common radiographic finding is bilateral basilar interstitial abnormalities, which are often asymmetric. Initially, these may appear as patchy alveolar infiltrates; with progressive disease a more reticulonodular pattern is seen. High-resolution computed tomography (CT) and open lung biopsy are considered the gold standard methods for diagnosing interstitial lung disease. Joint disease precedes the interstitial lung involvement in most cases. The clinical presentation and course of pulmonary fibrosis in RA have been reported to be similar to those of idiopathic pulmonary fibrosis, but response to immunosuppression may be better if pulmonary fibrosis occurs in the context of RA or other collagen diseases.[26]

Rheumatoid interstitial pulmonary disease is seen more frequently in men than in women, particularly those who have long-standing

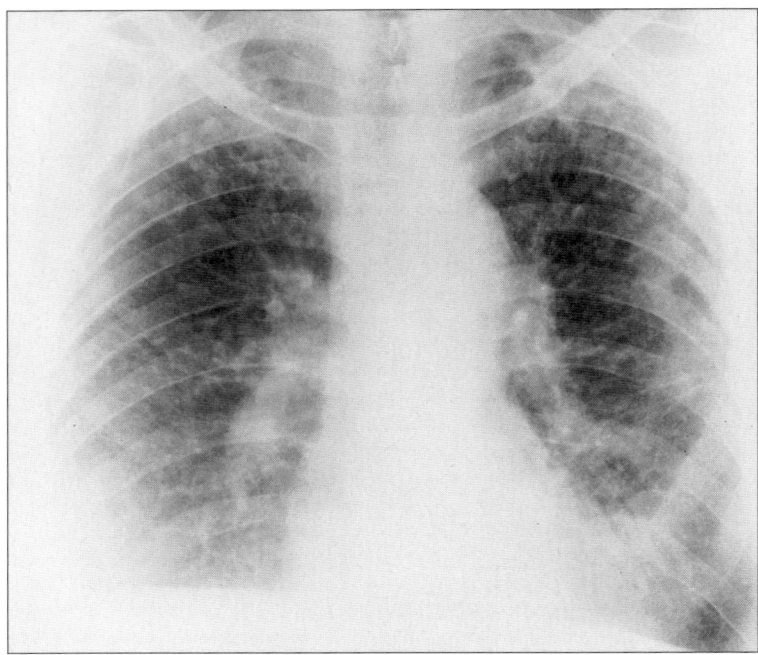

Fig. 83.7 Caplan syndrome.

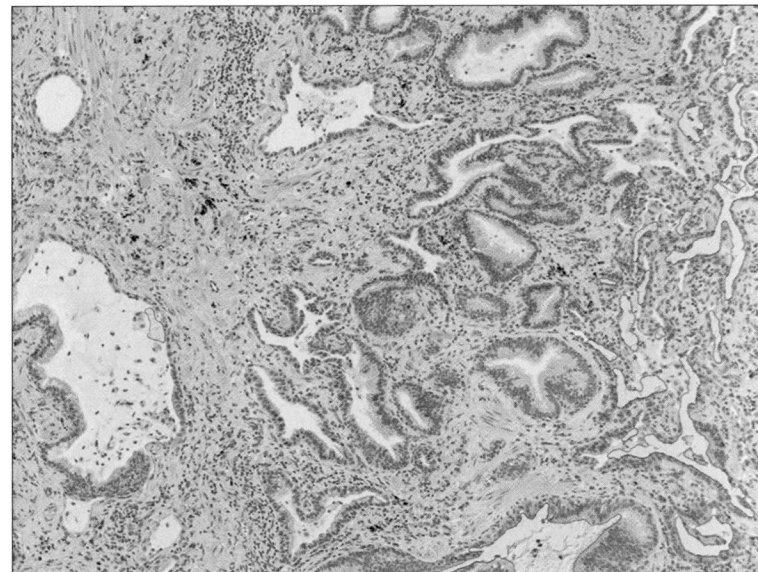

Fig. 83.9 Interstitial pneumonitis with CD4⁺ T cells (red stain) in a patient with RA (original magnification ×100).

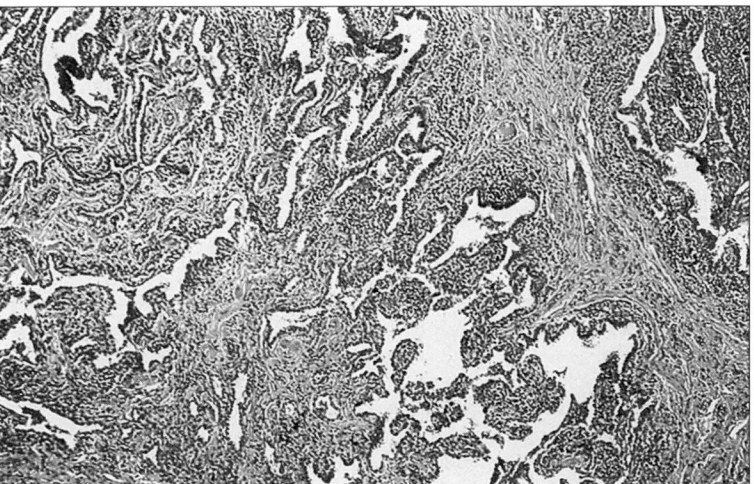

Fig. 83.8 Diffuse interstitial pneumonitis with sclerosing alveolitis. Lymphocytes are prominent (hematoxylin-eosin stain; original magnification ×150).

nodular, seropositive disease and among patients who smoke. Histologic findings and results of bronchoalveolar lavage can be variable, ranging from lymphocytic alveolitis to neutrophilic inflammation. Features on routine histology from lung biopsies are non-specific and include an inflammatory infiltrate with lymphocytes, plasma cells, and histiocytes (Fig. 83.8). Specific stainings have suggested a particular role for B cells and CD4⁺ T cells in patients with RA-associated interstitial pneumonitis (IP) compared with patients with idiopathic interstitial pneumonitis (Fig. 83.9).[27] B cells may be more abundant in lung tissue of patients with RA-associated ILD compared with patients with idiopathic ILD.[28] The greater density of T and B cells observed in RA-related ILD has been linked to high levels of circulating anti–cyclic citrullinated peptide (anti-CCP) antibodies.[29] TNF inhibitors may have a negative effect on RA-associated IP in some cases,[30] possibly due to direct antifibrotic properties of TNF.[31] RA-associated IP needs to be distinguished from methotrexate-induced toxicity, which usually has a subacute onset with rapidly progressive respiratory symptoms, less radiographic evidence of fibrosis, and a histologic pattern dominated by eosinophilia and type 2 pneumocyte hyperplasia.

Cryptogenic obstructive pneumonia (COP; formerly, bronchiolitis obliterans organizing pneumonia) can be associated with RA. This type of pulmonary involvement responds to glucocorticosteroid treatment and has a generally good prognosis. Another distinct type of pulmonary disease in RA, obliterative or constrictive bronchiolitis, responds poorly to treatment and has a poor prognosis. Patients have shortness of breath and a non-productive cough but, unlike COP, there is usually no fever or other constitutional symptoms. Pulmonary biopsy reveals submucosal and peribronchiolar fibrosis, with extrinsic narrowing of the bronchiolar lumen and fibrosis, with scant inflammation.

Obstructive lung disease is more common in patients with RA than age-matched controls, occurring in 9.6% of patients with RA and 6.2% of controls.[32] High-resolution lung CT reveals that up to 50% of patients with RA have bronchiectasis and bronchiolectasis,[33] possibly due to increased susceptibility to airway infections, obstructive airways diseases, and genetic predisposition.

Upper airways obstruction in RA can also be caused by inflammation of the cricoarytenoid joint. Symptoms include sore throat, hoarseness, dysphagia, pain with speech, pain radiating to the ears, a sensation of foreign body in the throat, and difficulty with inspiration. Laryngoscopy and CT scanning are the most sensitive methods for evaluating cricoarytenoid arthritis (Fig. 83.10).

Rare lung complications of RA include pulmonary arteritis, shrinking lung syndrome, and primary pulmonary hypertension. Secondary hypertension is more commonly seen in patients with pulmonary parenchymal disease, especially interstitial lung disease.

CARDIAC DISEASE

The acute and chronic inflammatory disease of RA may lead to cardiac disease by mechanisms of vasculitis, nodule formation, amyloidosis, serositis, valvulitis, and fibrosis. Pericarditis is the most common cardiac manifestation of RA. Although symptomatic pericarditis is relatively uncommon, both random electrocardiographic evaluation of patients with RA and autopsy studies reveal evidence of pericardial inflammation in 50% of patients.[34] An analysis of pericardial fluid reveals changes similar to those found in rheumatoid pleural effusions. Symptomatic patients with mild disease generally respond to glucocorticosteroids. Occasionally pericardiocentesis and intrapericardial glucocorticoid administration and even pericardiectomy may be required if the symptoms are severe or recalcitrant to the usual management (Figs. 83.11 to 83.13).[35]

Myocardial disease resulting from nodular granulomatous lesions or more diffuse fibrosing lesions has been seen in RA. Non-specific myocarditis is usually asymptomatic and rarely affects cardiac size or function. Congestive heart failure may be more frequent than is clinically evident in RA and left ventricular diastolic function is more often

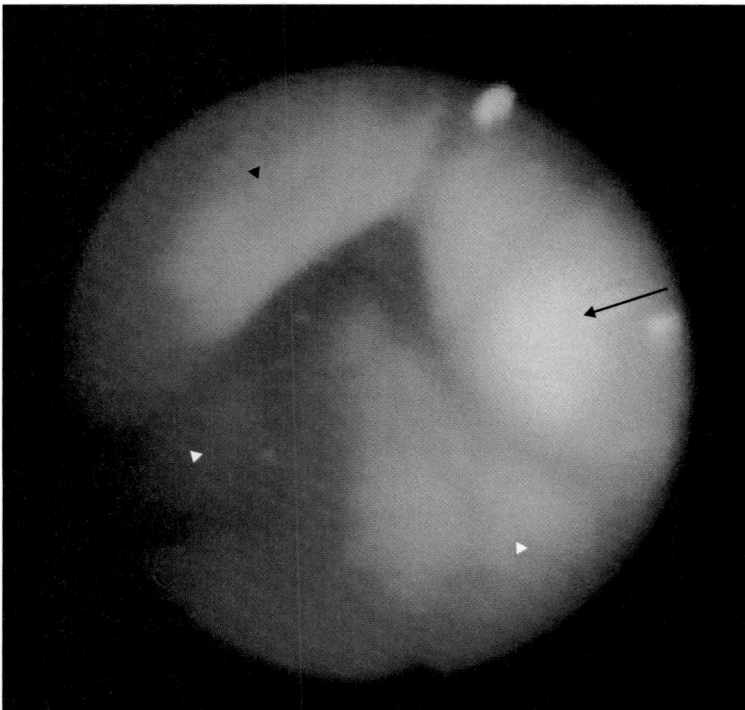

Fig. 83.10 Laryngeal edema with cricoarytenoid arthritis on direct laryngoscopy. Black arrow, left arytenoid; black arrowhead, right arytenoid; white arrowhead, left vocal cord; white arrow, right vocal cord. *(Courtesy Dr. Yuki Nanke.)*

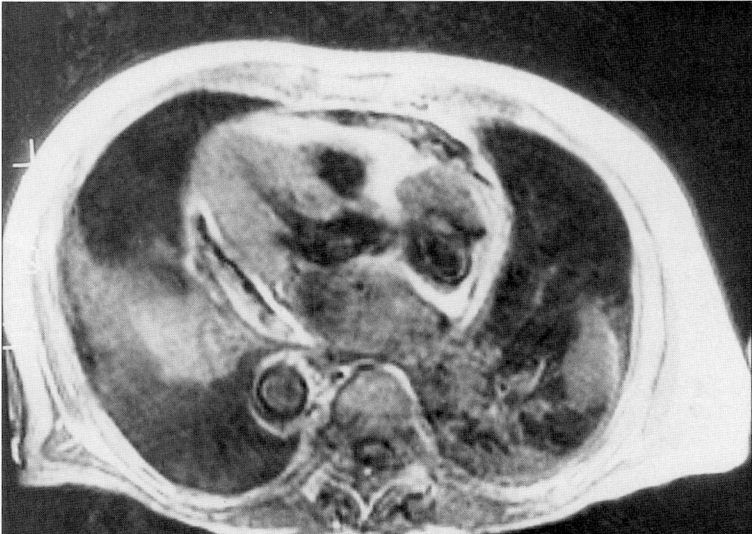

Fig. 83.11 Magnetic resonance imaging of constrictive pericarditis in rheumatoid arthritis. The dense white infiltrate between the pericardium and gray myocardium is pericardial fluid.

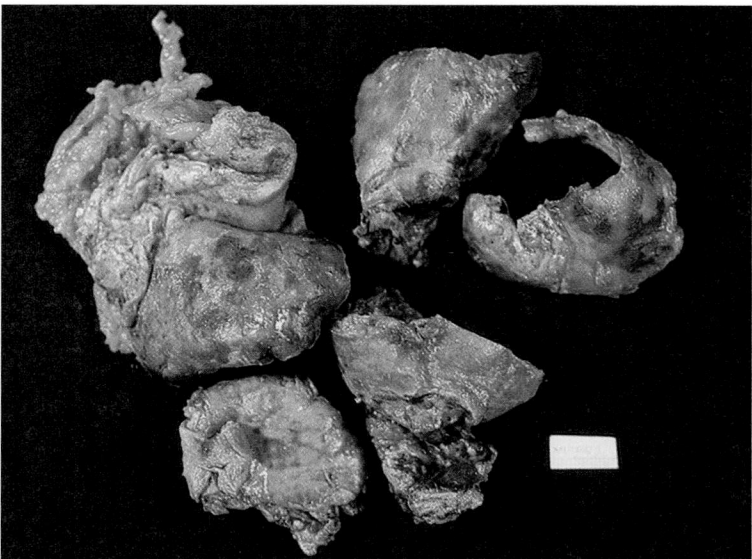

Fig. 83.12 Gross anatomic specimen of constrictive pericarditis obtained at radical pericardiectomy. The fibrotic pericardium is massively thickened, with a diameter of up to 0.5 cm; the outer layer of the pericardium at the top is covered with fat.

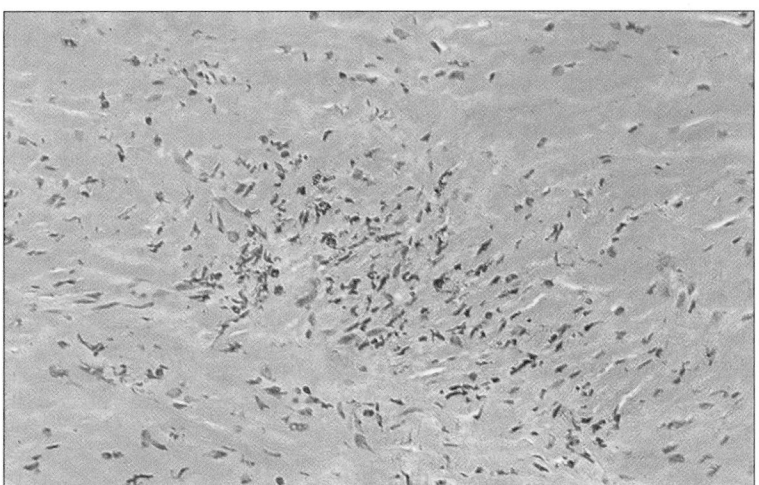

Fig. 83.13 Rheumatoid pericarditis (same patient as Fig. 83.11). There is marked non-calcific dense fibrosis, moderate non-granulomatous lymphoplasmacytic infiltrate, and hemosiderin pigment (hematoxylin-eosin stain; original magnification ×400).

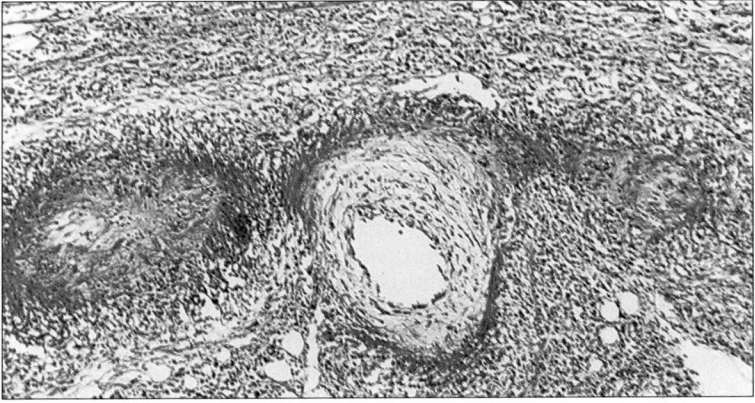

Fig. 83.14 Coronary arteritis. Two arteries are seen. There is a dense inflammatory infiltrate in the adventitia, with some intimal luminal narrowing and destruction of the media of one artery (hematoxylin-eosin stain; original magnification ×250).

impaired than in those without RA in spite of normal left ventricular systolic function.[36]

Echocardiographically detected lesions typical of RA in the absence of symptomatic cardiac disease include posterior pericardial effusion, aortic root abnormalities, and valvular thickening, occasionally with valvular incompetence. Coronary arteritis can occur as part of systemic rheumatoid vasculitis (Fig. 83.14). In addition, RA itself is an independent risk factor for coronary artery disease[37] and patients with severe extra-articular disease are at a particularly increased risk of cardiovascular death.[5] It has been suggested that coronary artery disease may be associated with clonal expansion of CD4$^+$CD28^{null} T cells,[38] which has also been seen in patients with RA, in particular among those with vasculitis. Given this and other suggested shared disease mechanisms,

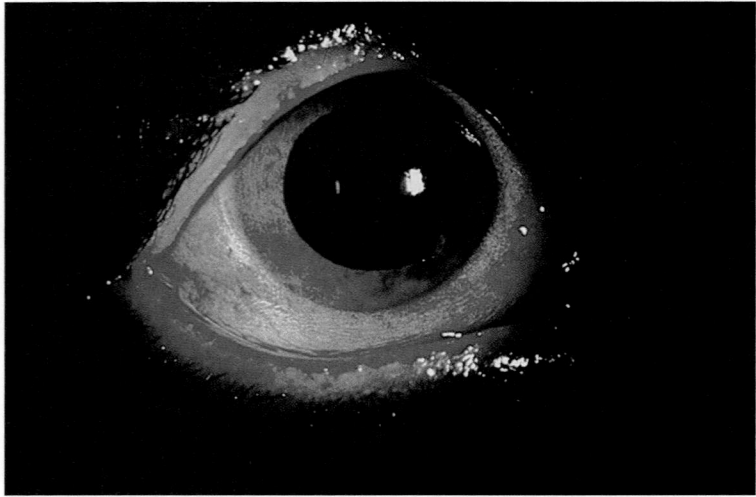

Fig. 83.15 Episcleritis. This usually occurs in the setting of active RA and is associated with the sudden onset of redness and eye pain.

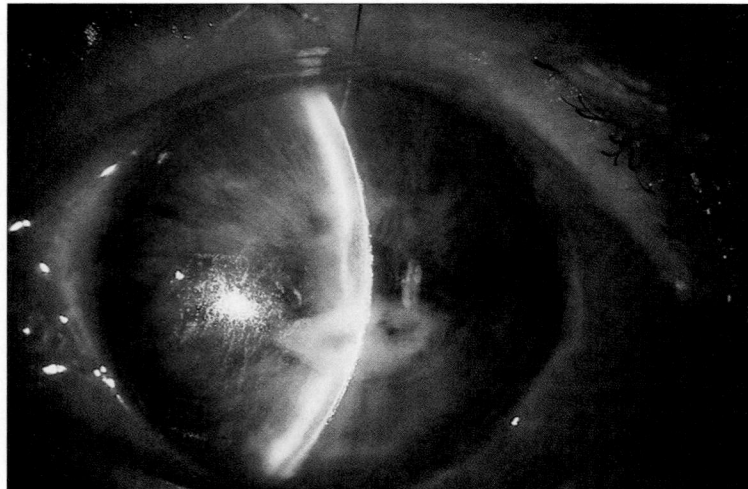

Fig. 83.17 Central keratolysis and corneal perforation. Corneal collagen can degrade in the absence of apparent corneal inflammation in rheumatoid arthritis.

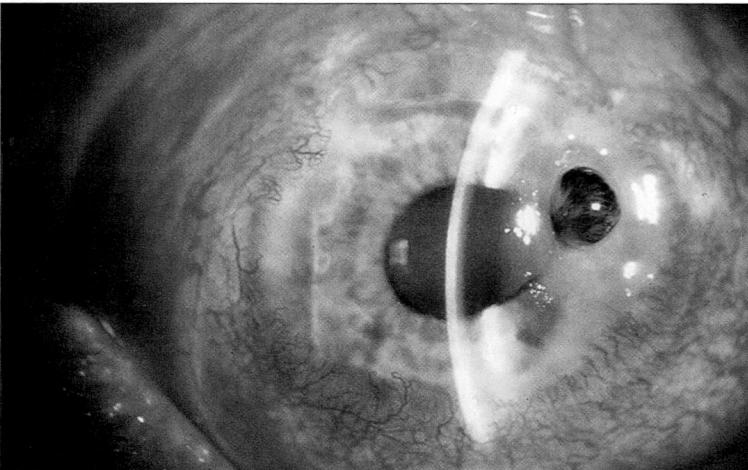

Fig. 83.16 Scleromalacia in a patient with rheumatoid arthritis.

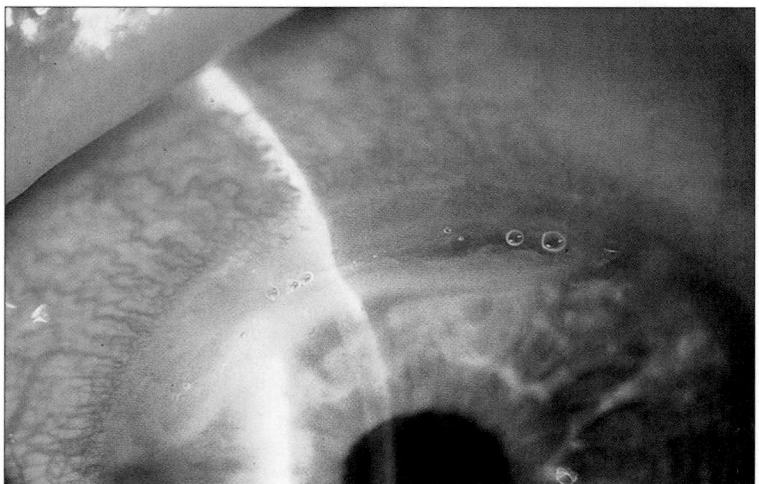

Fig. 83.18 Marginal corneal melt (ulcer) with inflammation.

it has been proposed that atherosclerosis should be regarded as an extra-articular feature of RA.[37] Biomarkers of inflammation predict cardiovascular events in the general population,[39] and patients with RA and a persistently elevated erythrocyte sedimentation rate are more likely to develop vascular disease.[5] Successful DMARD therapy with methotrexate[40] or TNF blockers[41] may substantially reduce the risk of cardiovascular comorbidity.

OCULAR INVOLVEMENT

The most common ocular involvement in RA is keratoconjunctivitis sicca, which affects at least 10% of patients. The severity of the symptoms may not correlate with that of the arthritis.

Episcleritis usually correlates with the activity of RA (Fig. 83.15). This process, which may be either nodular or diffuse, appears acutely and causes eye redness and pain; it causes changes in visual acuity only rarely. Scleritis is less common than episcleritis but is correlated with vasculitis, long-standing arthritis, and active joint inflammation. Untreated scleritis may progress to scleromalacia (Fig. 83.16). Episcleritis or scleritis is sometimes seen in patients whose polyarthritis has responded well to treatment.

Other unusual ocular findings in RA include uveitis, episcleral nodulosis, ulcerative keratitis ("corneal melt," which may be central [Fig. 83.17] or peripheral [Fig. 83.18]), and corneal filamentary keratitis (Fig. 83.19). Peripheral ulcerative keratitis develops as an extension of scleral inflammation, is sometimes bilateral, and may occur in the

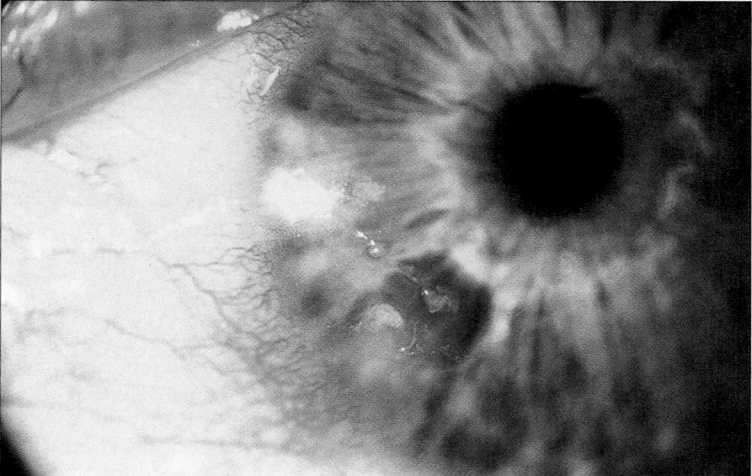

Fig. 83.19 Corneal filamentary keratitis with early corneal stromal activity near the limbus at 8 o'clock and 9:30. Filamentary keratitis concentric to the limbus can be a precursor of marginal corneal ulceration in rheumatoid arthritis.

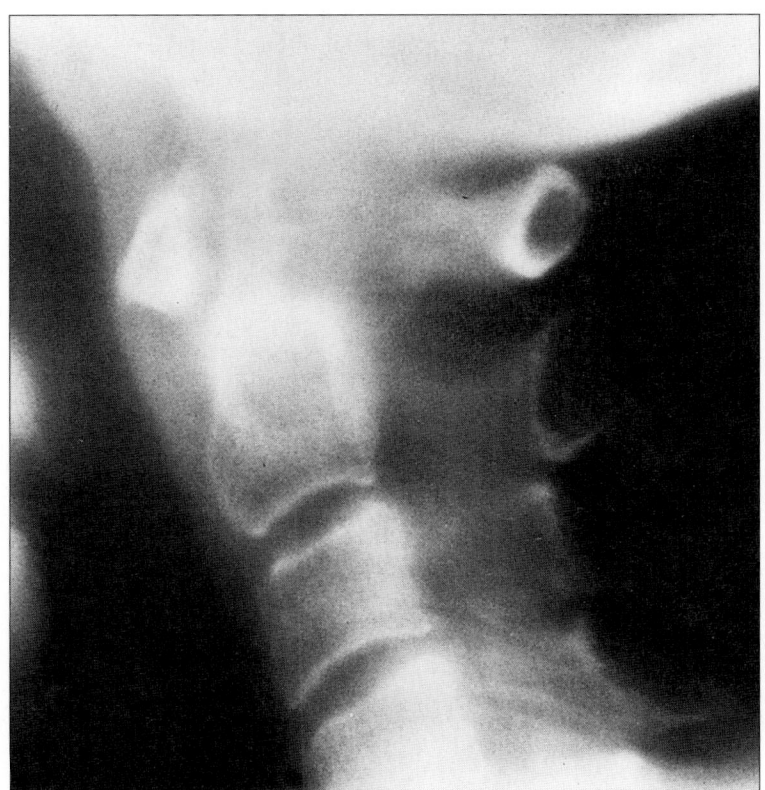

Fig. 83.20 Plain film of cervical spine, showing erosion of the odontoid.

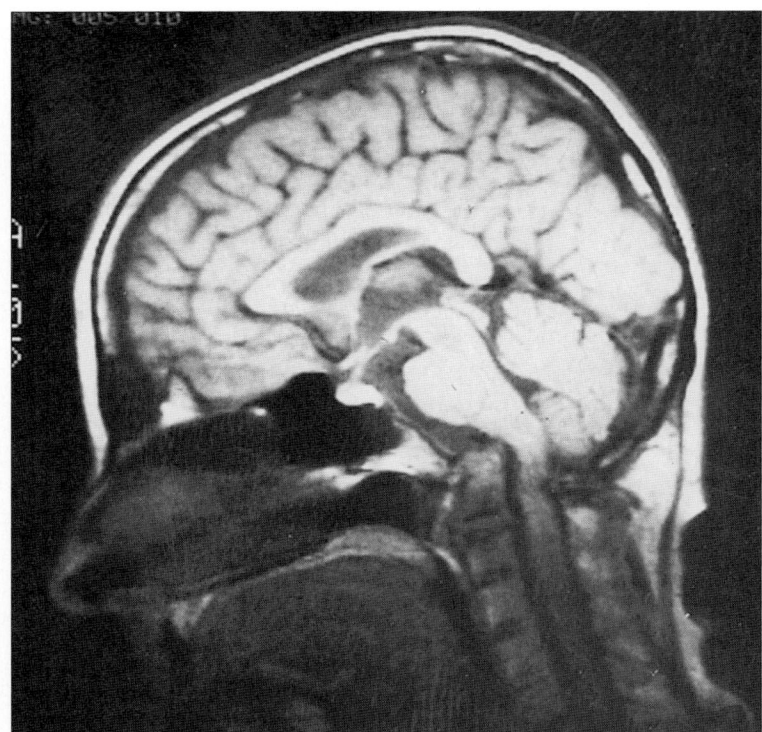

Fig. 83.21 Magnetic resonance imaging of the cervical spine, showing basilar invagination.

absence of scleritis. These conditions are associated with increased mortality and poor outcomes for vision.[42] Treatment may include topical or systemic cytotoxic and glucocorticosteroid therapy or anticytokine agents or both. Lesions resembling vasculitis may be seen in the limbal part of the cornea, and conditions such as scleritis and ulcerative keratitis can herald impending vasculitis.[42] The most common fundus lesions are due to posterior scleritis; exudative retinal detachments and disc and macular edema may also be found in association with RA.

Other uncommon ocular complications of RA include Brown syndrome, which is defined as diplopia on upward and inward gaze and is believed to be the result of inflammation and thickening of the superior tendons, and optic neuritis.

NEUROLOGIC IMPAIRMENT

In addition to systemic involvement, peripheral entrapment neuropathy, which tends to occur when the nerve is compressed by the inflamed synovium against a fixed structure, and atlantoaxial subluxation may cause neurologic impairment in patients with RA. Atlantoaxial subluxation caused by erosion of the odontoid process or the transverse ligament of C1 may allow the odontoid process to slip posteriorly and cause a cervical myelopathy (Fig. 83.20). Basilar invagination, with upward impingement of the odontoid process into the foramen magnum, can also result in cord compression (Fig. 83.21). The presence of cord compression is indicated by a positive Babinski sign, hyperreflexia, and weakness. This may require surgical stabilization.

Peripheral neuropathy, presenting as diffuse sensorimotor neuropathy or mononeuritis multiplex, occurs in a small subset of patients with RA. The underlying mechanism is small vessel vasculitis with ischemic neuropathy. Such lesions are thought to be part of a systemic rheumatoid vasculitis syndrome (see later), although other signs of vasculitis may be absent.

Involvement of the central nervous system in RA is rare. A diffuse, granulomatous pachymeningitis presenting with fever and headache rarely occurs (Figs. 83.22 and 83.23), and vasculitis and amyloidosis may occasionally involve the dura or the choroid plexus in patients with long-standing RA.

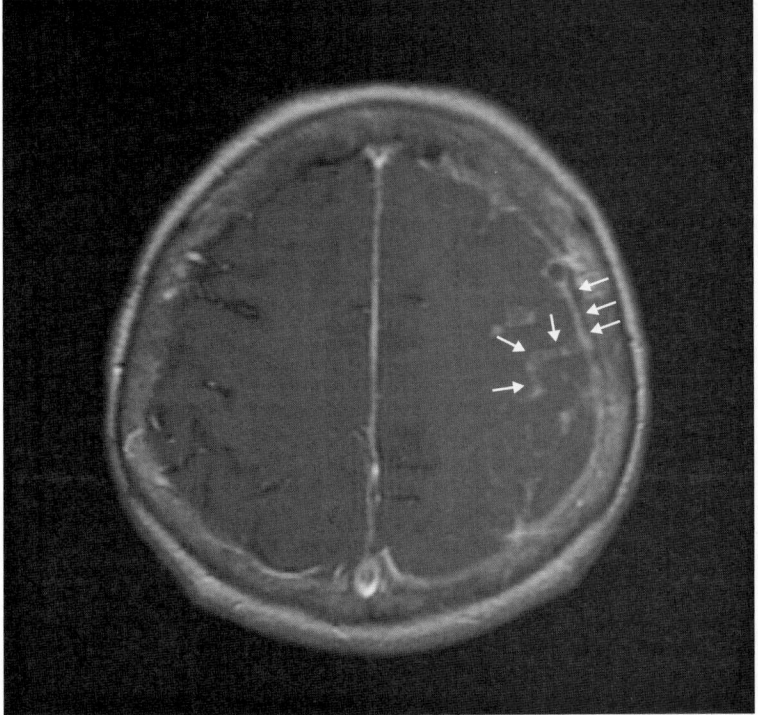

Fig. 83.22 Rheumatoid arthritis–associated meningitis in a patient presenting with headache and fever. Magnetic resonance imaging shows abnormal leptomeningeal enhancement, especially of the left parietal and frontal lobes and temporal dura (arrows).

MUSCULAR INVOLVEMENT

Muscle weakness in RA is usually due to muscle atrophy secondary to joint inflammation. Nutritional problems, medication, and neurologic dysfunction may contribute. A rare inflammatory myopathy has been described with a patchy cellular infiltration in muscle fibers, resulting

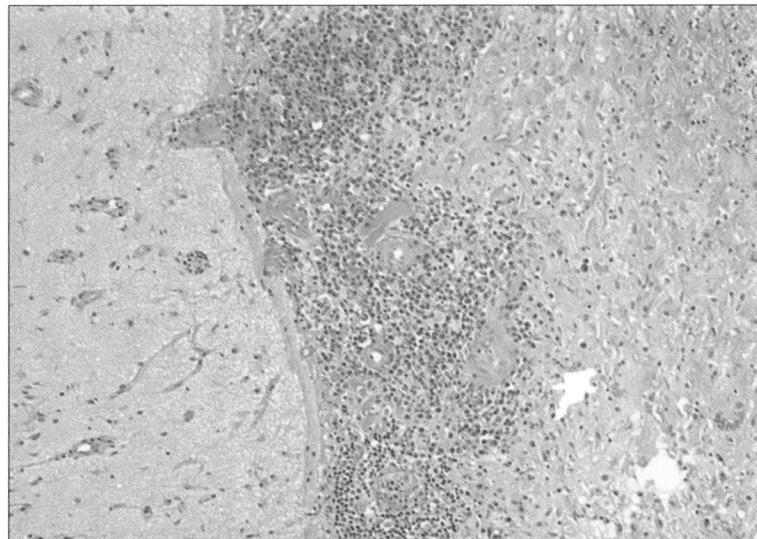

Fig. 83.23 Rheumatoid arthritis–associated meningitis (same patient as Fig. 83.22). Necrotizing granulomatous meningitis. Cultures were negative and the patient improved after immunosuppressive treatment (hematoxylin-eosin stain, original magnification ×200).

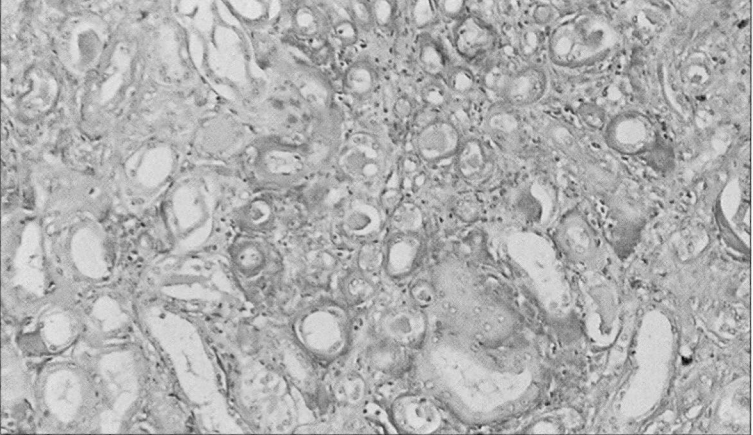

Fig. 83.24 Renal amyloidosis in rheumatoid arthritis (secondary amyloidosis). There is diffuse amyloid deposition throughout the renal parenchyma, with deposition in blood vessel walls. Amyloid deposits are green colored (Sulfated Alcian Blue stain; original magnification ×400).

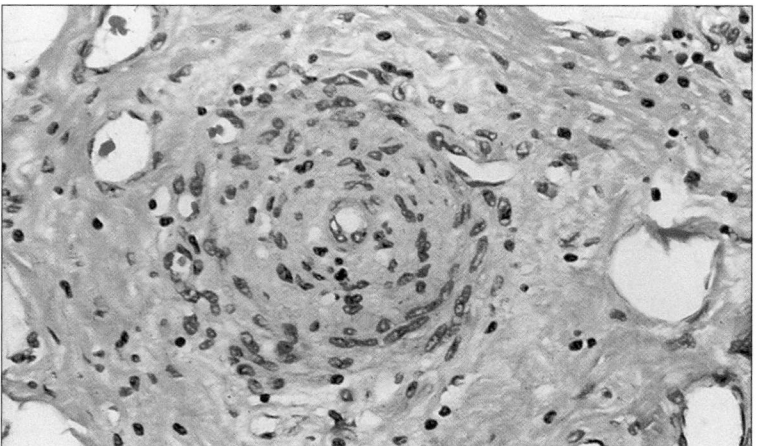

Fig. 83.25 Artery with intimal proliferation and luminal occlusion (hematoxylin-eosin stain; original magnification ×312).

in some fiber degeneration. RA may coexist with idiopathic inflammatory myopathy without other signs of systemic disease.

RENAL ABNORMALITIES

Renal involvement in RA is rare, although a low-grade membranous nephropathy, glomerulitis, vasculitis, and nephrotic syndrome due to secondary reactive amyloidosis have all been described. The perinuclear anticytoplasmic antibody (p-ANCA) has been found in about 20% of patients with RA and renal diseases of various etiologies and may be an independent predictor of nephropathy, even in the absence of systemic vasculitis.[43] Mesangioproliferative glomerulonephritis is considered a sign of systemic organ involvement in a patient with RA.

AMYLOIDOSIS

Amyloidosis may, rarely, complicate long-standing RA. Reports of its occurrence vary widely, but more recent population studies indicate that clinical visceral amyloidosis is detected in 0.7% of patients with RA.[2] In patients with active RA, serum amyloid-A protein concentrations are increased, stimulated by increased cytokine production.

Virtually every organ system may be involved in secondary amyloidosis, including the heart, kidney, liver, spleen, intestines, and skin. The diagnosis is confirmed by biopsy of involved tissue (Fig. 83.24). The presence of secondary amyloidosis in patients with RA portends a poor outcome: 4-year survival rates of about 58% are reported.[44] Cytotoxic drugs may improve the prognosis, but progressive organ failure often occurs in spite of aggressive treatment.

RHEUMATOID VASCULITIS

A small vessel vasculitis is intimately associated with many of the clinical manifestations seen in RA. Subclinical vasculitis is probably common in patients with seropositive RA, and immune deposits have been demonstrated in clinically uninvolved skin and labial salivary glands.[45] The long-term effect of subclinical vasculitis on outcome is unknown.

Systemic endothelial activation has been suggested in patients with severe extra-articular disease, even in the absence of overt signs of vasculitis.[46] Inflammation of the small- and medium-sized arteries in the extremities, peripheral nerves and, occasionally, other organs may complicate RA. There is a greater frequency of HLA-DRB1 alleles and particularly B1*0401 homozygotes in patients with rheumatoid vasculitis than in uncomplicated RA.[7,8]

Study of involved vessels from patients with rheumatoid vasculitis reveals a pathologic picture and distribution similar to that seen in polyarteritis, but renal involvement is rare. Early lesions show fibrinoid necrosis of the vessel wall, with an inflammatory cell infiltrate. Chronic changes, with artery wall fibrosis, occlusion and re-canalization, may be seen (Fig. 83.25). The acute arterial lesions are immune complex mediated, as indicated by the involved arteries (Fig. 83.26). Immune deposits are not detected in the more chronic lesions; rather, fibrinogen is found (Fig. 83.27).

Systemic vasculitis in RA is uncommon and often occurs in rheumatoid patients who have long-standing disease of more than 10 years. Rheumatoid synovitis may not be active when the features of the systemic vasculitis are present. Small vessel vasculitis commonly involves the skin and causes nailfold infarcts (Fig. 83.28), digital gangrene (Fig. 83.29), and leg ulcers. Patients with nailfold infarcts and leg ulcers usually do not develop more widespread vascular involvement. Distal sensory neuropathy is another manifestation seen in small vessel vasculitis that also may occur alone without progression to widespread vascular involvement. The rapid, progressive, and widespread appearance of new areas of involvement, including clinical cutaneous vasculitis and multiple neuropathies, indicates systemic arterial disease and a poorer outcome.[47]

Other factors, in addition to the vasculitis, likely influence the final vascular outcome. In the pathogenesis of leg ulcers, there is usually an underlying vasculitis that initiates the lesions, but ulcer expansion and its chronicity may be influenced by other features, including venous insufficiency, arterial insufficiency, dependent edema, trauma, and chronic use of glucocorticosteroids.

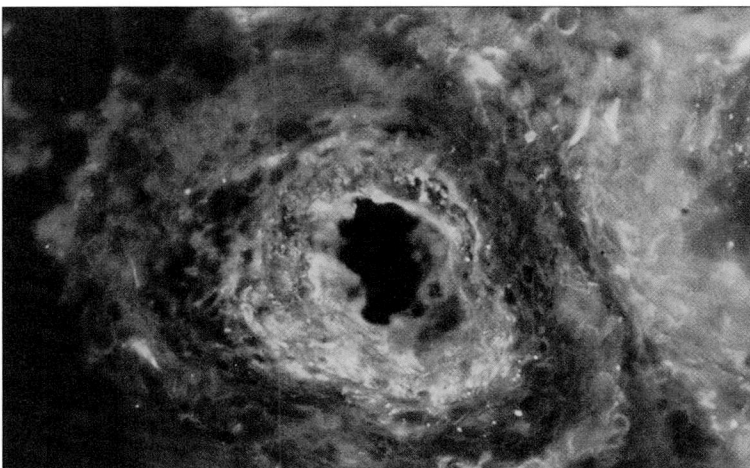

Fig. 83.26 Immunoglobulin M in artery with fibrinoid necrosis (IgM by immunofluorescence; original magnification ×312).

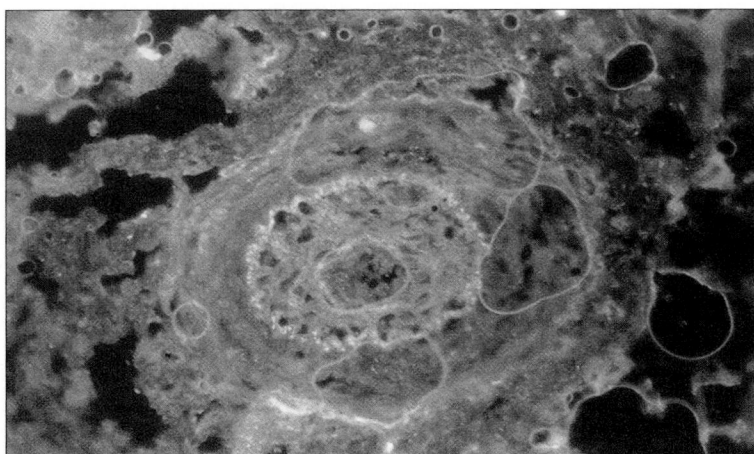

Fig. 83.27 Fibrinogen in artery with intimal proliferation (fibrinogen by immunofluorescence in artery with intimal proliferation; original magnification ×312).

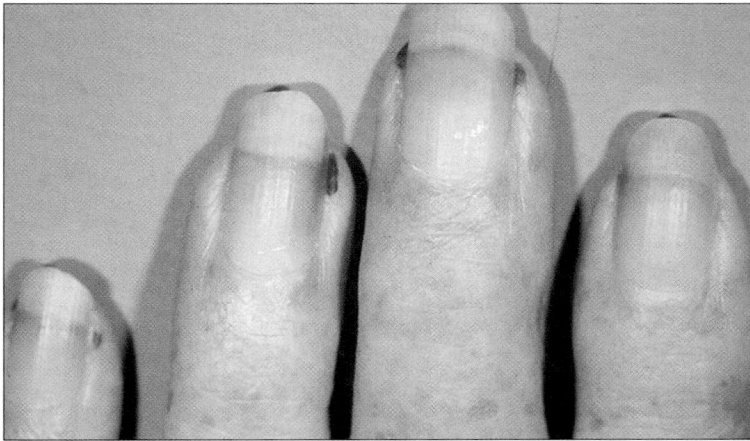

Fig. 83.28 Nailfold infarcts in a patient with rheumatoid arthritis.

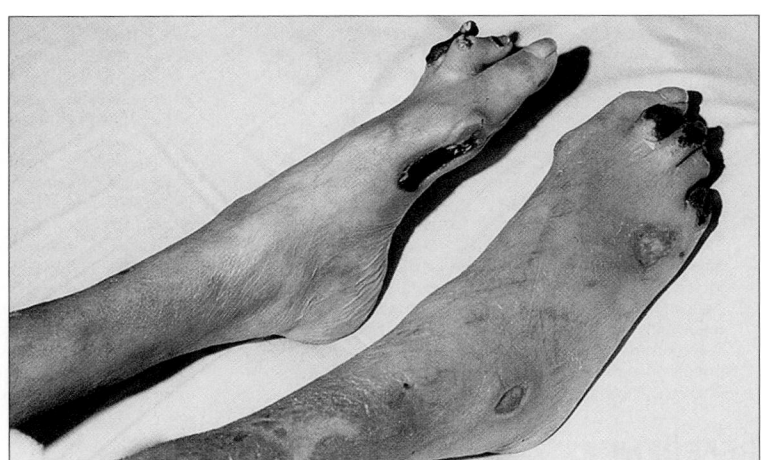

Fig. 83.29 Digital tip and proximal infarcts in a patient with rheumatoid vasculitis.

The treatment of rheumatoid vasculitis must be individualized. In patients with progressive widespread systemic vasculitis involving peripheral nerves, digits, viscera, or the central nervous system, the inflammation must be treated and the resulting vasculopathy anticipated. High doses of prednisone may be necessary initially to control the inflammation. Two controlled trials have demonstrated that pulsed[48] or continuous[42] cyclophosphamide leads to greater clinical benefit than more conservative treatment regimens in patients with

systemic vasculitis (grade B). Anti–B-cell therapy or possibly TNF inhibitors can be effective in patients with rheumatoid vasculitis refractory to cyclophosphamide (grade C).[49] Low doses of aspirin as an antiplatelet agent should also be considered, and prostacyclin infusions may be helpful in patients with threatening peripheral gangrene. Patients with vasculitis and other forms of severe extra-articular manifestations are at an increased risk of cardiovascular events and severe infections and should be adequately monitored for such complications. Preventive measures such as statin therapy should be considered in patients with high cardiovascular risk because patients with RA may benefit from both the anti-inflammatory and lipid-lowering effects of statins.[50,51]

REFERENCES

1. Turesson C, Jacobsson L, Bergstrom U. Extra-articular rheumatoid arthritis: prevalence and mortality. Rheumatology 1999;38:668-741.
2. Turesson C, O'Fallon WM, Crowson CS et al. Occurrence of extra-articular disease manifestations is associated with excess mortality in a population-based cohort of patients with rheumatoid arthritis. J Rheumatol 2002;29:62-67.
3. Watts RA, Mooney J, Lane SE, et al. Rheumatoid vasculitis: becoming extinct? Rheumatology (Oxford) 2004;43:920-923.
4. Turesson C, McClelland RL, Christianson TJ, et al. No decrease over time in the incidence of vasculitis or other extraarticular manifestations in rheumatoid arthritis: results from a community-based study. Arthritis Rheum 2004;50:3729-3731.
5. Maradit-Kremers H, Nicola PJ, Crowson CS, et al. Cardiovascular death in rheumatoid arthritis: a population-based study. Arthritis Rheum 2005;52:722-732.
6. Turesson C, O'Fallon WM, Crowson CS, et al. Extra-articular disease manifestations in rheumatoid arthritis: incidence trends and risk factors over 46 years. Ann Rheum Dis 2003;62:722-727.
7. Weyand CM, Xie C, Goronzy JJ. Homozygosity for the HLA-DRB1 allele selects for extraarticular manifestations in rheumatoid arthritis. J Clin Invest 1992;89:2033-2039.
8. Turesson C, Weyand CM, Matteson EL. Genetics of rheumatoid arthritis: is there a pattern predicting extraarticular manifestations? Arthritis Rheum 2004;51:853-863.
9. Yen JH, Moore BE, Nakajima T, et al. Major histocompatibility complex class I-recognizing receptors are disease risk genes in rheumatoid arthritis. J Exp Med 2001;193:1159-1167.
10. Turesson C, Schaid DJ, Weyand CM, et al. Association of HLA-C3 and smoking with vasculitis in patients with rheumatoid arthritis. Arthritis Rheum 2006;54:2776-2783.
11. Turesson C, McClelland RL, Christianson TJH, et al. Clustering of extra-articular disease manifestations in patients with rheumatoid arthritis. Arthritis Rheum 2004;50:S174.
12. Turesson C, Matteson EL. Management of extra-articular disease manifestations in rheumatoid arthritis. Curr Opin Rheumatol 2004;16:206-211.
13. Unger L, Kayser M, Nusslein HG. Successful treatment of severe rheumatoid vasculitis by infliximab. Ann Rheum Dis 2003;62:587-588.
14. Wisnieski JJ, Askari AD. Rheumatoid nodulosis: a relatively benign rheumatoid variant. Arch Intern Med 1981;141:615-619.
15. Pincus T, Olsen NJ, Russell JI, et al. Multicenter study of recombinant human erythropoietin in correction of anemia in RA. Am J Med 1990;89:161-168.
16. Gridley G, McLaughlin JK, Erbom A, et al. Incidence of cancer among patients with rheumatoid arthritis. J Nat Cancer Inst 1993;85:307-311.

17. Baecklund E, Ekbom A, Sparen P, et al. Disease activity and risk of lymphoma in patients with rheumatoid arthritis: nested case-control study. BMJ 1998;317:180-181.
18. Kassan SS, Chused TL, Moutsopoulos HM, et al. Increased risk of lymphoma in sicca syndrome. Ann Intern Med 1978;89:888-892.
19. Coakley G, Brooks D, Iqbal M, et al. Major histocompatability complex haplotypic associations in Felty's syndrome and large granular lymphocyte syndrome are secondary to allelic association with HLA-DRB1 *0401. Rheumatology 2000;39:393-398.
20. Meliconi R, Uguccioni M, Chieco-Bianchi F, et al. The role of interleukin-8 and other cytokines in the pathogenesis of Felty's syndrome. Clin Exp Rheumatol 1995;13:285-291.
21. Fiechtner JJ, Miller RD, Starkebaum G. Reversal of neutropenia with methotrexate in patients with Felty's syndrome: correlation of response with neutrophil-reactive IgG. Arthritis Rheum 1989;32:194-201.
22. Dillon AM, Luthra HS, Conn DL, et al. Parenteral gold therapy in the Felty syndrome: experience with 20 patients. Medicine 1986;65:107-112.
23. Barton JC, Prasthofer EF, Egan ML. Rheumatoid arthritis associated with expanded populations of granular lymphocytes. Ann Intern Med 1986;104:314-323.
24. Thorne C, Urowitz MB, Wanless I, et al. Liver disease in Felty's syndrome. Am J Med 1982;73:35-40.
25. Nannini C, Ryu JH, Matteson EL. Lung disease in rheumatoid arthritis. Curr Opin Rheumatol 2008;20:340-346.
26. Scott DG, Bacon PA. Response to methotrexate in fibrosing alveolitis associated with connective tissue disease. Thorax 1980;35:725-731.
27. Turesson C, Matteson EL, Colby TV, et al. Increased CD4+ T cell infiltrates in rheumatoid arthritis-associated interstitial pneumonitis compared with idiopathic interstitial pneumonitis. Arthritis Rheum 2005;52:73-79.
28. Atkins SR, Turesson C, Myers JL, et al. Morphologic and quantitative assessment of CD20⁺ B cell infiltrates in rheumatoid arthritis-associated nonspecific interstitial pneumonia and usual interstitial pneumonia. Arthritis Rheum 2006;54:635-641.
29. Bongartz T, Cantaert T, Atkins SA, et al. Citrullination in extra-articular manifestations of rheumatoid arthritis. Rheumatology (Oxford) 2007;46:70-75.
30. Chatterjee S. Severe interstitial pneumonitis associated with infliximab therapy. Scand J Rheumatol. 2004; 33: 276-277.
31. Kuroki M, Noguchi Y, Shimono M, et al. Repression of bleomycin-induced pneumopathy by TNF. J Immunol 2003;170: 567-574.
32. Nannini C. Obstructive lung disease in rheumatoid arthritis. Arthritis Rheum 2008;58:S267-S268.
33. Despaux J, Manzoni P, Toussirot E, et al. Prospective study of the prevalence of bronchiectasis in rheumatoid arthritis using high-resolution computed tomography. Rev Rheum 1998;65:453-461.
34. Bonfiglio T, Atwater EC. Heart disease in patients with seropositive RA. Arch Intern Med 1969;124:714-719.
35. Yurchak PM, Deshpande V. Case record of the Massachusetts General Hospital. Weekly clinicopathological exercises. Case 2-2003. A 60-year-old man with mild congestive heart failure of uncertain cause. N Engl J Med 2003;348:243-249.
36. Mustonen J, Laakso M, Hirvonen T, et al. Abnormalities in left ventricular diastolic function in male patients with RA without clinically evident cardiovascular disease. Eur J Clin Invest 1993;23:246-253.
37. Van Doornum S, McColl G, Wicks IP. Accelerated atherosclerosis: an extraarticular feature of rheumatoid arthritis? Arthritis Rheum 2002;46:862-873.
38. Liuzzo G, Goronzy JJ, Yang H, et al. Monoclonal T-cell proliferation and plaque instability in acute coronary syndromes. Circulation 2000;101:2883-2888.
39. Ridker PM, Hennekens CH, Buring JE, Rifai N. C-reactive protein and other markers of inflammation in the prediction of cardiovascular disease in women. N Engl J Med 2000;342:836-843.
40. Choi HK, Hernan MA, Seeger JD, et al. Methotrexate and mortality in patients with rheumatoid arthritis: a prospective study. Lancet 2002;359:1173-1177.
41. Jacobsson LT, Turesson C, Gülfe A, et al. Treatment with tumor necrosis factor blockers is associated with a lower incidence of first cardiovascular events in patients with rheumatoid arthritis. J Rheumatol 2005;32: 1213-1218.
42. Foster CS, Forstot SL, Wilson LA. Mortality rate in rheumatoid arthritis patients developing necrotizing scleritis or peripheral ulcerative keratitis: effects of systemic immunosuppression. Ophthalmology 1984;91:1253-1263.
43. Mustila A, Korpela M, Mustonen J, et al. Perinuclear antineutrophil cytoplasmic antibody in rheumatoid arthritis: a marker of severe disease with associated nephropathy. Arthritis Rheum 1997;40:710-717.
44. Okuda Y, Takasugi K, Oyama T, et al. Amyloidosis in rheumatoid arthritis—clinical study of 124 histologically proven cases. Ryumachi 1994;34:939-946.
45. Flipo RM, Janin A, Hachulla E, et al. Labial salivary gland biopsy assessment in rheumatoid vasculitis. Ann Rheum Dis 1994;53:648-652.
46. Turesson C, Englund P, Jacobsson LT, et al. Increased endothelial expression of HLA-DQ and interleukin 1alpha in extra-articular rheumatoid arthritis. Results from immunohistochemical studies of skeletal muscle. Rheumatology (Oxford) 2001;40:1346-1354.
47. Puechal X, Said G, Hilliquin P, et al. Peripheral neuropathy with necrotizing vasculitis in RA. Arthritis Rheum 1995;38:1618-1629.
48. Scott DGI, Bacon PA, Allen C, et al. IgG rheumatoid factor, complement and immune complexes in the rheumatoid synovitis and vasculitis: comparative and serial studies during cytotoxic therapy. Clin Exp Immunol 1981;43:54-63.
49. Puéchal X, Miceli-Richard C, Mejjad O, et al. Anti-tumour necrosis factor treatment in patients with refractory systemic vasculitis associated with rheumatoid arthritis. Ann Rheum Dis 2008;67:880-884.
50. McCarey DW, McInnes IB, Madhok R, et al. Trial of atorvastatin in rheumatoid arthritis (TARA): double-blind, randomised placebo-controlled trial. Lancet 2004;363:2015-2021.
51. Bongartz T, Nannini C, Medina-Velasquez YF, et al. Incidence and mortality of interstitial lung disease in rheumatoid arthritis. Arthritis Rheum Febr 12 epub ahead of print 2010.

REFERENCES

Full references for this chapter can be found on www.expertconsult.com.

Adult-onset Still's disease

Johannes C. Nossent

84

- Adult-onset Still's disease is an uncommon autoimmune inflammatory disease, most often seen in young adults.
- It presents as a combination of systemic manifestations typically including spiking fevers, short-lived rashes, and joint symptoms ranging from arthralgia to aggressive arthritis.
- No specific diagnostic test is available; the clinical diagnosis is based on pattern recognition and exclusion.
- The disease remits in a third of patients, whereas a debilitating disease course is mainly seen in those with root joint involvement.
- Modern treatment options include monoclonal antibodies that inhibit cytokine effects; however, there is a striking lack of clinical trials.

INTRODUCTION

George Frederic Still (1868-1941) first reported in 1896 that children may develop a form of joint disease, distinct from the more familiar rheumatoid arthritis (RA)-like syndrome with the occurrence of periods of fever, lymphadenopathy, and splenomegaly as well as pericardial adhesions.[1] Still's disease has thus become an accepted eponym for a subset of idiopathic juvenile arthritis (JIA). In 1944, Wissler described a similar disease named subsepsis allergica, which occasionally occurred in adults.[2] The expression adult-onset Still's disease (AOSD) (also adult-type Still's disease or adult Still's disease) was introduced by Bywaters, who described, in 1971, the occurrence of seronegative polyarthritis, rash, fever, and raised erythrocyte sedimentation rate (ESR) in 14 female patients in their third decade of life with what was considered a good functional outcome at the time (crippling disease in 2 patients after long-term follow-up).[3]

CLASSIFICATION

There is no universally agreed-upon diagnostic test for AOSD. Therefore, the clinical diagnosis is based on the recognition of a specific disease pattern together with the exclusion of other causes of chronic inflammation, such as infection and malignancy.[4] Several criteria sets have been proposed to assist in distinguishing AOSD patients from patients with other febrile and/or joint diseases (Table 84.1).[5-7] The more sensitive criteria of Yamaguchi and colleagues[6] are hampered by a long list of diseases that must be excluded, in contrast to the more specific criteria of Fautrel and associates,[7] which in turn require the not readily available measurement of glycosylated ferritin. Such classification criteria can only indicate a likelihood of disease presence. Misrepresentation of classification schemes as diagnostic criteria can be hazardous and carries the risk that patients fall outside or between categories and do not receive appropriate medical care. The appreciation of this idiosyncrasy, aptly named the Cheshire cat syndrome by Bywaters,[8] is an important feature in the diagnosis of AOSD in particular and in rheumatology in general.

EPIDEMIOLOGY

Based on clinical records maintained by internists and rheumatologists in western France, the annual AOSD incidence was estimated to be 0.16/100,000 between 1987 and 1992.[9] A similar study in 1993 of 125 patients resulted in an estimated crude prevalence of AOSD of 0.73 (males) and 1.47 (females) per 100,000 population. The corresponding crude incidence rate was 0.22 (males) and 0.34 (females).[10] A survey in five districts of Finland estimated the annual AOSD incidence at 1 per million in 1996.[11] A retrospective hospital-based study estimated the annual incidence rate at 0.4/100,000 from 1990 to 2000 in Norway with a point prevalence in 2000 of 6.8/100,000, which doubled over a decade (Table 84.2).[12] Clearly, there is a need for additional data on AOSD epidemiology.

CLINICAL PRESENTATION

The pleiotropic presentation often leads to considerable diagnostic and subsequent treatment delays in AOSD (Table 84.3). AOSD most often affects younger adults, with a higher proportion of female patients in Eastern than in Western countries. In general, a shared constellation of clinical features can be found in most cohort studies reported over the past 5 years from various parts of the world (see Table 84.3).[12-26] The three predominant clinical features are spiking high fevers, arthritis, and transitory rash.

Fever

Fever of unknown origin is the most frequent reason for patients with new-onset AOSD to seek help, and AOSD is the final diagnosis in about 5% of these patients.[27] It is currently defined as febrile illness of more than 3 weeks' duration with body temperature greater than 38.3°C after several determinations and no diagnosis after 1 week of study.[28] High fever (>39°C) is the presenting symptom in more than 95% of AOSD cases in cohort studies (see Table 84.1). The classic fever pattern is one to two daily fever spikes exceeding 39°C, most often occurring late during the day (afternoon or evening) and receding within hours (Fig. 84.1). However, continuous fever or early morning spikes are seen in up to 20%.[20,29] Similar patterns are seen in infectious (malaria, abscesses, bacterial endocarditis) and non-infectious conditions (heat stroke, intracerebral hemorrhage). Increased levels of S100A12, a marker of granulocyte activation, were recently proposed as a diagnostic tool for non-infectious causes of fever of unknown origin.[30]

Arthritis

Musculoskeletal pain is present in virtually all AOSD patients at onset and often worsens during fever periods; it includes myalgia (frequency 20%-90%), arthralgia (27%-100%), and arthritis (18%-82%) (see Table 84.3). Arthritis is most often polyarticular and symmetric, affecting knees, wrists, fingers, and ankles, but asymmetric oligoarthritic and monarthritic presentations involving other joints have been described.[17,31] Early radiographic findings are usually non-specific with periarticular osteopenia and slight joint space narrowing (Fig. 84.2a). Synovial fluid indicative of mild to moderate inflammation is seen in 50% of patients[18] and may even contain rice bodies (mix of fibrinogen and collagen like–structures containing mononuclear cells).[32] The histopathology is non-specific with sublining thickening and monocytic infiltrates of lymphocytes and plasma cells. Intrasynovial follicles as seen in RA have not been described in AOSD.[33] Scintigraphy may disclose additional sites of inflammation,[34] whereas magnetic resonance imaging (MRI) and ultrasonography may prove useful in the detection of low-grade synovitis, early presence of erosions, and soft tissue lesions in patients with musculoskeletal symptoms not otherwise explained (see Fig. 84-2b and c). The prognostic value of these investigations in AOSD remains to be determined. Elevated levels of creatine phosphokinase and electromyographic findings suggestive of myositis are seen in up to 10% of patients.[17,23]

TABLE 84.1 CRITERIA SETS PROPOSED TO ASSIST IN DISTINGUISHING AOSD PATIENTS

	Cush et al (1987)[5]	Yamaguchi et al (1992)[6]	Fautrel et al (2002)[7]
Design	Single center, retrospective	Multicenter, retrospective	Single center, retrospective
Data analysis	Descriptive	Discriminatory statistical analysis	Logistic regression analysis
Cohort size	21	90	72
Disease duration	11.8 years	3.8 years	2.9 years
Case definition	Fever ≥ 39°C and arthralgia/arthritis with any 2 of: leukocytosis, JRA, rash, serositis/RES involvement	Clinical diagnosis upheld after case review by expert committee	Patients undergoing ferritin measurement and clinical diagnosis upheld after prolonged observation and case review by one expert
Excluded from analysis	RF > 1:80 ANA > 1:100	Non-definite cases after review (n = 56)	Non-definite cases after review
Comparator group	None	267 definite non-AOSD cases	130 definite non-AOSD cases
Criteria set	Fever ≥ 39°C and arthralgia/arthritis with any 2 of: leukocytosis, JRA, rash, serositis/RES involvement	*Major:* Fever ≥ 39°C for > 1 week, arthralgia > 2 weeks, maculopapular non-pruritic salmon-pink rash, leukocytosis ≥ 10,000/mm³ with ≥ 80% neutrophils *Minor:* Pharyngitis or sore throat, lymphadenopathy, and/or splenomegaly, abnormal aminotransferases, negative rheumatoid factor or ANA assay	*Major:* Spiking fever ≥ 39°C, arthralgia, transient erythema, pharyngitis, neutrophils > 80%, glycosylated ferritin fraction < 20% *Minor:* Typical rash, leukocytosis ≥ 10,000/mm³
Required	As above	At least 5 criteria, including 2 major	Four major criteria or 3 major and 2 minor criteria
Exclusion needed	None	Infections, malignancies, vasculitides	None
Sensitivity for set	Not analyzed	96%	81%
Specificity for set	Not analyzed	92%	98%

JRA, juvenile rheumatoid arthritis; RES, reticuloendothelial system; RF, rheumatoid factor; ANA, antinuclear antibody.

TABLE 84.2 REPORTED DATA ON THE EPIDEMIOLOGY OF AOSD

Authors	Study period	Method and criteria	No. patients	Population	Incidence per million (95% CI)	Prevalence per million (95% CI)
Magadur-Joly et al[9]	1987-1991	Questionnaire-based identification of patients in regional clinical practices. Fulfilling modified Yamaguchi criteria	62	France	1.6	13 (calculated, not reported)
Wakai et al[10]	1994	Questionnaire-based nationwide identification of hospital-based patients Fulfilling Yamaguchi criteria	125	Japan	NA	M, 7.3 F, 14
Kaipiainen-Seppanen and Aho[11]	1990	Based on diagnostic codes on regional prescriptions. No confirmatory actions	1	Finland	0.9 (CI, 0-5.6)	NA
Evensen and Nossent[12]	1990-2000	Regional; hospital record–based review. Fulfilling Yamaguchi criteria	13	Norway	4 (CI, 1.1-9.1)	34 (8-94 ; in 1990) 70 (27-142; in 2000)

CI, confidence interval; NA, not available.

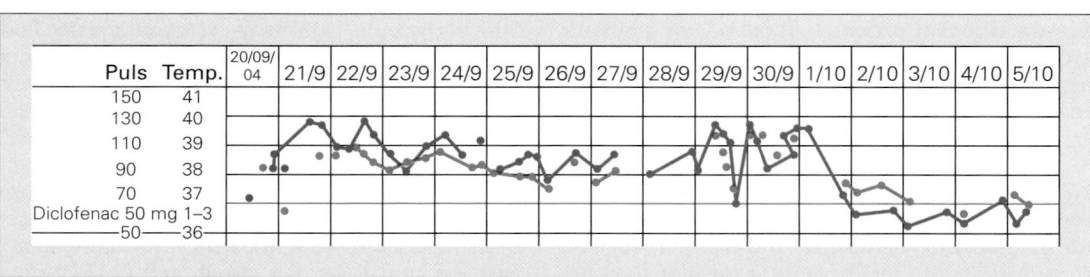

Fig. 84.1 Spiking fever pattern in a patient with active adult-onset Still's disease and reaction to initial NSAID and subsequent treatment with prednisone.

TABLE 84.3 DETAILED OVERVIEW OF FREQUENCY (%) OF CLINICAL DISEASE MANIFESTATIONS AT PRESENTATION IN RECENT (2004 ONWARD) SERIES ON AOSD FROM 14 DIFFERENT COUNTRIES INCLUDING A TOTAL OF 600 PATIENTS

	Zeng	Lee	Merpoor	Mitamura	Singh	Uppal	Cagatay	Alonso	Goumri	Pay	Akridites	Evensen	Crispin	Appenz	Chen
Country	China	Korea	Iran	Japan	India	Kuwait	Turkey	Spain	Tunisia	Turkey	Greece	Norway	Mexico	Brazil	Taiwan
No. in cohort	61	71	28	34	14	28	84	26	11	95	11	13	26	16	82
Age (yr)	38	40	25	41	30	28	33	40	31	27	36	34	29	31	26
Female (%)	74	88	75	65	36	79	70	69	45	53	54	20	42	46	72
Diagnostic delay	NA	4	NA	NA	15	7	NA	NA	NA	3	NA	5	NA	NA	3
Fever > 39°C	100	100	100	94	100	100	95	100	100	99	100	100	100	100	100
Arthralgia	NA	85	27	91	71	100	96	100	100	100	100	NA	92	100	100
Arthritis	82	NA	18	41	NA	64	69	81	90	85	NA	69	88	NA	76
Weight loss > 10%	12	32	NA	24	86	NA	19	NA	NA	17	NA	NA	58	37	NA
Serositis	43	15	8	18	21	25	20	19	NA	30	NA	23	19	18	18
Rash	89	84	25	91	57	85	60	100	73	82	100	77	54	100	87
Lymphadenopathy	53	68	17	58	71	61	33	50	45	37	NA	62	54	50	29
Hepatosplenomegaly	50	30	9	27	57	36	38	81	54	45	NA	23	38	81	20
Myalgia	28	70		50			13	50	69	70	NA	NA	61	50	95
Sore throat	72	57	27	85	36	57	66	56		66	NA	62	65	56	84
Inclusion criteria	Yama	Yama	Yama	Yama	Yama	Yama	Cush	Yama	Yama	Yama	Yama	Yama	Expert	Cush	Yama

Yama, Yamaguchi et al (1992)[6]; Cush, Cush et al (1987).[5]
Data from references 12 to 26.

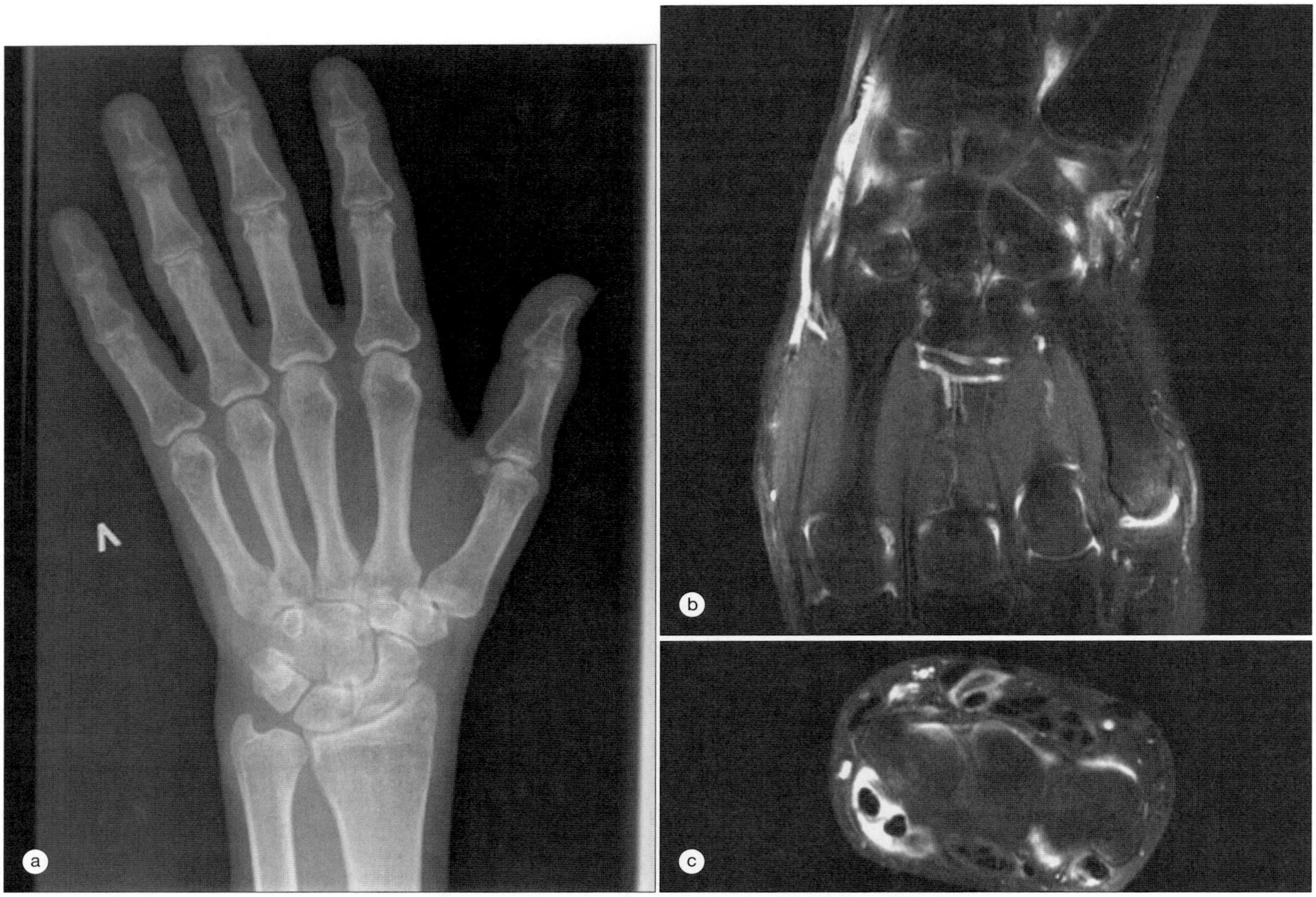

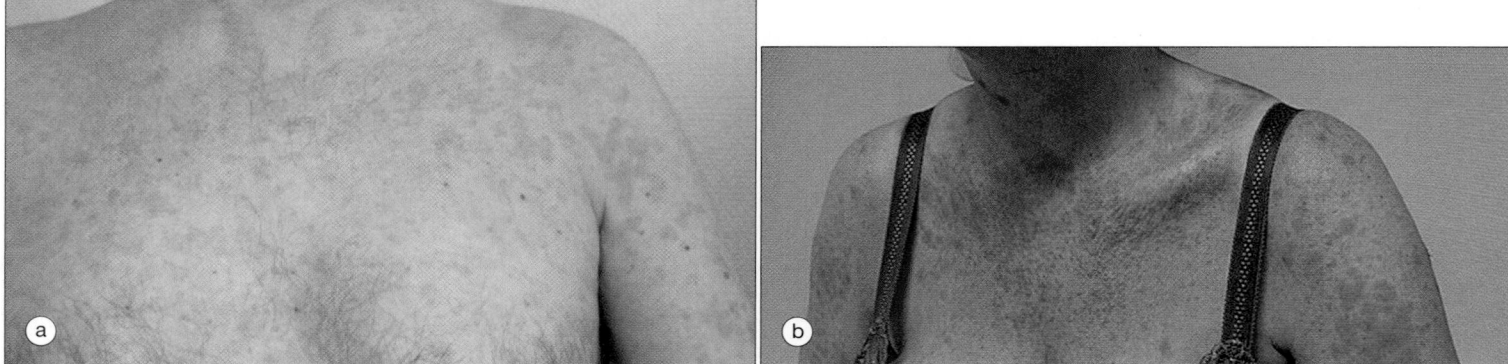

Fig. 84.2 Radiograph and MR image of wrist in patient with new-onset AOSD showing diffuse periarticular osteopenia (a) and carpal synovitis (b and c).

Fig. 84.3 Examples of maculopapular rash that worsened in the early evening hours: salmon pink lesions that (dis)appeared within hours of fever spikes (a) and more intense erythematous lesions that did not regress completely (b).

Rash

The classic skin manifestation is of a maculopapular rash consisting of flat salmon-pink skin areas that have small, confluent bumps. The rash is predominantly seen on the trunk and proximal extremities (Fig. 84.3) and often evanescent (i.e., pronounced during febrile periods and disappearing almost completely in between). Skin biopsies are not diagnostic and show dermal edema and perivascular infiltration by granulocytes and lymphocytes of the superficial dermis (Fig. 84.4)

without deposition of immunoglobulins or complement factors.[35] Dermatographism (Koebner phenomena) is the occurrence of a linear erythematous skin reaction along a line of trauma and, although non-specific, is present in 30% to 60% of AOSD patients and more pronounced during the rash.[22,23] Other skin manifestations of AOSD are palpable purpura (with leukocytoclastic vasculitis on biopsy), folliculitis, erythema nodosum, and urticarial rash. Whether these truly represent disease activity or allergic (drug) reactions is unknown.

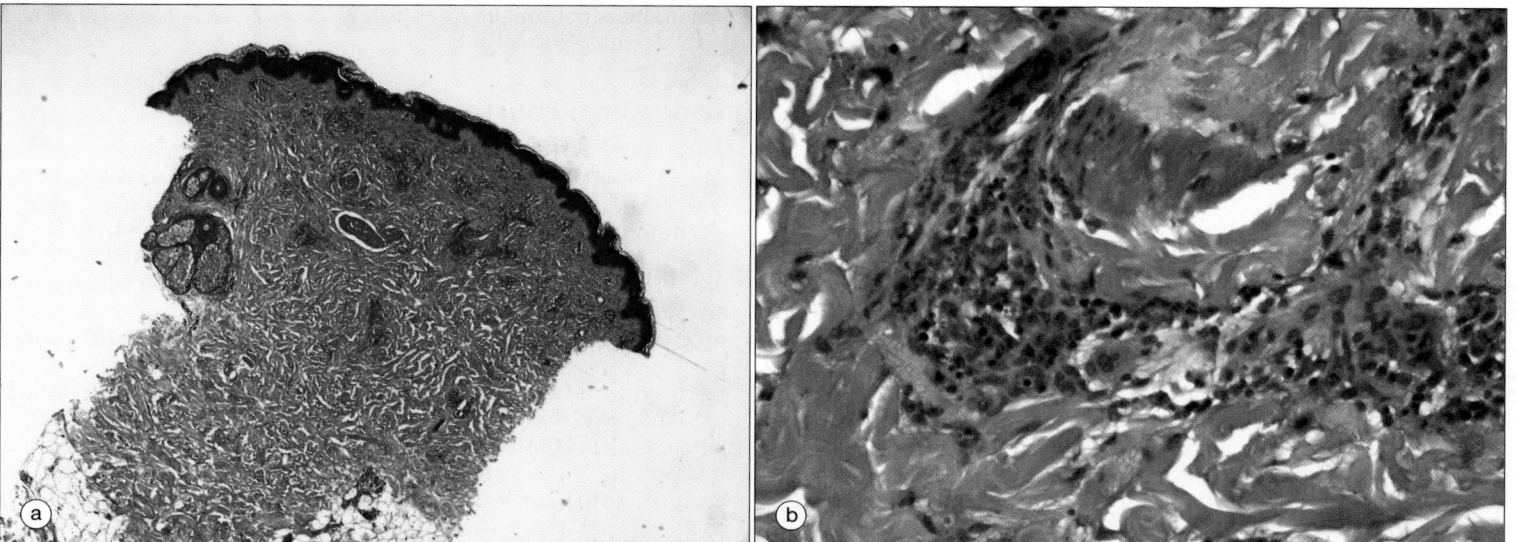

Fig. 84.4 Skin biopsy of maculopapular rash revealing normal appearance of the epidermis. The dermis shows full-thickness, perivascular infiltration of inflammatory cells, mostly lymphocytes and neutrophils. There is no evidence of vasculitis or extravasated red blood cells. Immunofluorescence showed no immunoglobulin deposits. (a, ×4; b, ×40.) *(Courtesy of Dr. Tormod Eggen, Department of Pathology, University Tromsø.)*

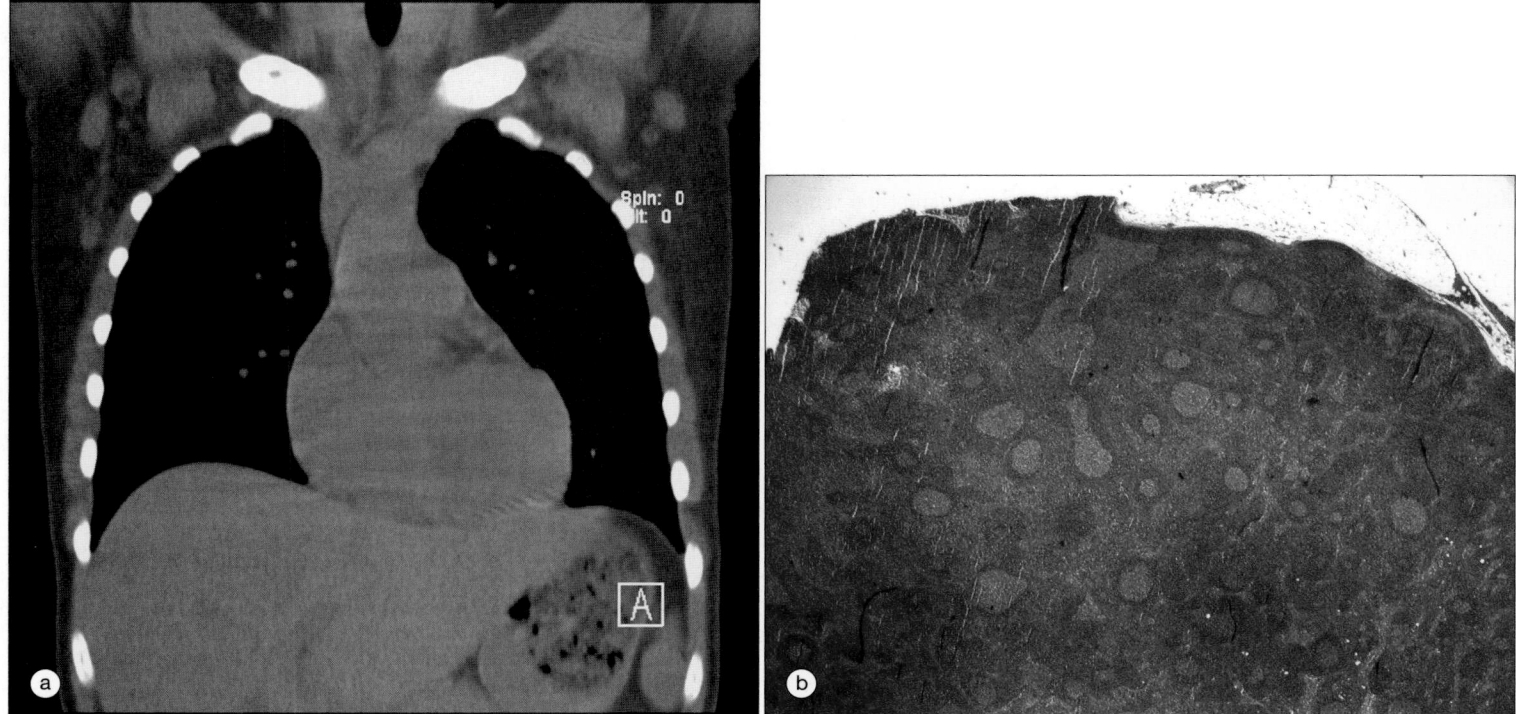

Fig. 84.5 (a) Bilateral axillary lymphadenopathy in AOSD as seen on CT. (b) Left axillary lymph node histology shows a regular node surface surrounded by perinodal fat. The subcapsular and medullary sinus show some histiocytosis. Throughout the lymph node the parenchyma is filled with follicles with well-demarcated germinal centers; no atypical cells are present. Immunohistochemistry revealed a normal distribution of CD3 (T cells) and CD20 (B cells) and negative findings for BCL2 (follicular lymphoma marker). *(Courtesy of Dr. Tormod Eggen, Department of Pathology, University Tromsø.)*

Other frequent findings

The substrate for the throat soreness (in 50%-80% of cases) is unknown. Diffuse pharyngeal erythema can be seen in about 50% of these patients; circumscript mucosal lesions such as aphthae or ulcers are uncommon. Increased MRI signal and contrast enhancement in soft tissue surrounding the cricothyroid cartilage and pharynx is observed.[36]

Lymphadenopathy has no specific distribution and is usually mild with moderately enlarged non-tender nodes detected clinically in 40% to 60% of patients. The precise relationship between lymphadenopathy and other reticuloendothelial system manifestations such as hepatomegaly and/or splenomegaly is unclear; its combined presence with constitutional symptoms (fever, night sweats, weight loss) often leads to diagnostic gland extirpation, which exhibits reactive hyperplasia, sinusoidal histiocytosis, and dermatopathic lymphadenopathy (melanin and fat-laden proliferated histiocytes and macrophages seen in the cortical region of lymph nodes in patients with erythroderma) (Fig. 84.5).[37,38] Lymphadenopathy and concomitant node pathology usually subside after treatment.[38]

Hepatosplenomegaly occurs mainly in the presence of abnormal levels of liver enzymes and is seldom severe.[39] Liver biopsies are not helpful because they may show inflammatory changes in the periportal space, cholestatic changes, or normal liver architecture.[13,40] Pleuritis and/or pericarditis is seen in up to 30% of patients (see Table 84.1), whereas serous peritonitis occurs more seldom. It should be considered, however, as a possible cause of unexplained abdominal pain, reported by up to 30% of patients and which may lead to unhelpful explorative laparotomy.[21,41] Pleuropericardial effusions seldom compromise cardiopulmonary function.[42,43]

Infrequent findings

Over the years, case reports have attributed a range of less common findings to AOSD. These include uveitis, aseptic meningitis and encephalitis, seizures, cerebrovascular ischemia, pulmonary fibrosis, myocarditis, interstitial nephritis, collapsing glomerulopathy, isolated renal and liver failure, as well as multiple organ failure.[44,45]

Laboratory findings

High levels of ESR and C-reactive protein (CRP) together with decreased serum albumin levels testify to the severity of the acute-phase response in AOSD. In addition, leukocytosis (WBC > 10,000/mm^3) due to increased neutrophils (>80%) together with a low-grade normocytic anemia (typically anemia of chronic disease) and thrombocytosis are seen in the majority of patients (Table 84.4). These hematologic abnormalities may sometimes reach extreme levels and mimic primary hematologic diseases. Bone marrow investigations have been reported to show reactive hypercellularity with granulocyte/erythrocyte ratios greater than 6, sporadic increases in plasma cells greater than 10%, and increased numbers of hemophagocytic macrophages and increased iron deposition.[13,18,23,46] Glomerular disease is absent and renal function is rarely compromised in the absence of preexisting disease or drug-induced azotemia.

Abnormal results of liver enzyme studies are most frequent in patients with hepatomegaly and may show a hepatocellular, cholestatic, or a mixed pattern; imaging and histologic examinations fail to reveal a specific substrate. Drug reactions due to often liberal use of antipyretics (acetaminophen [paracetamol] or a non-steroidal anti-inflammatory drug [NSAID]) should always be considered. Liver enzymes tend to normalize with disease remission.[39] Ferritin increases more than five times the normal upper level for increased specificity for AOSD to over 80% and, when associated with a decrease in the proportion of glycosylated ferritin, is the single most discriminative test for AOSD.[47] The presence of low-titer autoantibodies (rheumatoid factor, antinuclear antibody) is not uncommon in AOSD (5%-15%; see Table 84.4), reflects their presence in the general population, and has few clinical implications as long as more specific antibodies are not detected. There are no data on the presence or role of anti-citrullinated peptide antibodies in AOSD. Complement consumption is rare with uncomplicated AOSD, with serum C3 levels in general normal to slightly elevated in the acute phase.[21]

DISEASE COURSE

Mortality

In the initial description of AOSD as a benign disease,[3] all patients remained alive after prolonged follow-up. Later series, however, describe fatality rates up to 12% (see Table 84.5), and 5-year survival has been estimated at 93%.[48] More systematic data of survival rates and predictors as well as causes of death are not available.

Early complications

In the initial phase, uncontrolled activation of T cells, macrophages, and cytokines can lead to a vicious circle of excessive immune responses ("cytokine storm"), culminating in the macrophage activation syndrome (also called reactive hemophagocytic syndrome) and/or disseminated intravascular coagulation. Macrophage activation syndrome has been reported to occur in 5% to 10% of AOSD patients, and the most typical finding is the occurrence of very high serum ferritin levels together with rapidly progressive cytopenias; phagocytosis of hematopoietic cells by macrophages in reticuloendothelial tissue (bone marrow and liver) has been demonstrated in these patients, and the same mechanism is presumably also responsible for the initiation of disseminated intravascular coagulation. Whereas macrophage activation

syndrome is not unique to AOSD, it seems responsible for most of the early deaths reported.[13,14,23,49,50]

Long-term course

Three distinctive patterns are recognized in the disease course of AOSD. In about one third of cases AOSD is a monocyclic disease, in which lasting remission occurs within 1 year of onset, although weaning from drug treatment may take longer (Table 84.5). A remitting-relapsing pattern is seen in 20% to 40% of patients. In 30% to 50% of patients AOSD evolves into a chronic disease, in which progressive inflammatory joint destruction becomes the main concern. The functional outcome is poor in about 25% of these patients owing to erosive destruction and bony fusion of root and hand joints. Baseline risk factors for the development of chronic disease include polyarthritis, root joint (shoulder/hip) involvement, absence of human leukocyte antigen (HLA)-Bw35, moderately elevated serum ferritin levels, high ferritin/CRP ratios, and elevated levels of intracellular adhesion molecule (ICAM)-1 and interleukin (IL)-8.[13,51-53] Other long-term complications include secondary amyloidosis in 2% to 4%, which may be amenable to therapy[12,54]; data on the long-term incidence of cancer and infectious complications are lacking.

ETIOPATHOPHYISOLOGY

Few other patient groups are screened as exhaustively for infectious and neoplastic disease as AOSD patients at disease onset. Although an infectious trigger remains a possibility,[55] the clinical similarities between AOSD and periodic fever syndromes suggest that AOSD belongs to the category of autoimmune inflammatory diseases. These diseases are characterized by the absence of humoral and T-cell–driven autoimmunity and result from defects in the innate immune system, resulting in rapidly waxing and weaning inflammatory responses.[56] Several autoimmune inflammatory diseases have been ascribed to temporary imbalances in danger signaling through cytokines because of alterations in the structure or function of genes involved. Monogenic changes for receptor sites are found in hereditary diseases such as familial Mediterranean fever (FMF), tumor necrosis factor (TNF) receptor–associated periodic fever syndrome (TRAPS), and familial cold urticaria.[57] However, because no familiar disease tendency has been reported in AOSD, it falls within the group of complex autoimmune inflammatory diseases (which also includes Behçet and Crohn disease), in which various genetic imbalances are thought to combine in triggering the cytokine network.[58]

Genetic predisposition

Whereas HLA antigens have been associated with AOSD susceptibility (HLA class II types DRB1*1501 and DRB1*1201)[59] and clinical prognosis (HLA class I B35 to self-limiting disease and DR2 and DR5 to chronic course),[51,52] none has been firmly established as a risk factor.[60] Fcγ receptor polymorphisms are not related to AOSD, indicating that the prominent macrophage activation is unlikely to occur by immune-complex binding.[61] Homozygosity for an IL-18 gene haplotype containing eight single nucleotide polymorphisms was increased in AOSD patients compared with healthy controls.[62]

Acute-phase response

Patients with active AOSD display increased serum levels of CRP and fibrinogen/ESR together with reductions in hemoglobin and albumin levels. The only acute-phase protein (APP) that behaves unpredictably in AOSD is ferritin, which may reach disproportionately high levels in excess of 10,000 ng/mL.[47,53] Ferritin is the highly conserved ubiquitous intracellular protein that stores iron in a non-toxic state within a globular structure, consisting of 24 subunits of heavy (21 kDa; H) or light (19 kDa; L) ferritin. Subunit synthesis is under the control of an iron-responsive element in the 5′ end of the respective genes (chromosome 19 for H-ferritin, chromosome 11 for L-ferritin). Under physiologic conditions only a small amount of ferritin (mainly, glycosylated L-ferritin) is released into the bloodstream[63]; this release decreases with iron deficiency and increases with iron overload. The increased ferritin/

TABLE 84.4 FREQUENCY (%) AND MEAN ESTIMATES OF SELECTED LABORATORY FINDINGS AT AOSD PRESENTATION IN RECENT SERIES (2004 ONWARD) ON AOSD WITH A TOTAL OF 520 PATIENTS

	Zeng 2009	Lee 2008	Merpoor 2008	Mitamura 2008	Singh 2008	Uppal 2007	Cagatay 2007	Alonso 2007	Goumri 2006	Pay 2006	Akridites 2006	Evensen 2006	Crispin 2005	Appenz 2005	Chen 2004
Anemia	15	NA	NA	33	96	54	36	85	NA	75	NA	36	NA	63	71
Leukocytes > 10^4	84	NA	92	74	NA	100	84	88	100	79	100	91	85	100	73
Thrombocytosis	NA	NA	NA	NA	72	82	24	NA	NA	48	NA	46	NA	NA	28
Abnormal liver enzymes	23	NA	89	76	50	55	50	48	80	64	91	62	38	50	40
Hypoalbuminemia	NA	33	NA	70	42	NA	42	NA	NA	43	NA	37	100	NA	NA
Ferritin over ULN	80	NA	71	100	50	89	50	87	73	89	64	62	NA	56	91
ESR (mm/hr)	NA	54	91	NA	98	NA	89	95	NA	NA	NA	90	NA	NA	83
CRP (mg/L)	NA	83	144	NA	NA	NA	116	213	NA	NA	NA	154	NA	NA	104
Ferritin (ng/mL)	NA	12,080	1200	NA	NA	NA	1126	8700	NA	NA	18,350	1266	NA	1100	7224
RF positive	12	12	4	12	10	0	10	0	0	NA	0	0	21	0	3
ANA positive	12	NA	4	23	0	0	0	0	0	NA	0	0	13	0	12

NA, not available; ULN, upper limit of normal; ESR, erythrocyte sedimentation rate; CRP, C-reactive protein; RF, rheumatoid factor; ANA, antinuclear antibody.
Data from references 12 to 26.

TABLE 84.5 DISEASE COURSE IN RECENT SERIES (2004 ONWARD) ON AOSD WITH A TOTAL OF 520 PATIENTS

	Lee 2008	Merpoor 2008	Mitamura 2008	Singh 2008	Uppal 2007	Cagatay 2007	Alonso 2007	Goumri 2006	Pay 2006	Evensen 2006	Akridites	Appenz 2005	Chen 2004
Follow-up (mo)	38	NA	60	19	44	45	88	12	13	69	98	58	52
Disease course													
Monocyclic	42	15	50	71	14	33	54	NA	21	27	81	31	34
Progressive	32	10	15	29	28	27	—	20	41	27	—	15	21
Relapsing	13	75	35	NA	57	33	46	NA	17	46	18	64	45
Crude mortality rate	13	0	3	7	0	NA	0	9	0	7	6	0	4

NA, not available.
Data from references 12 to 26.

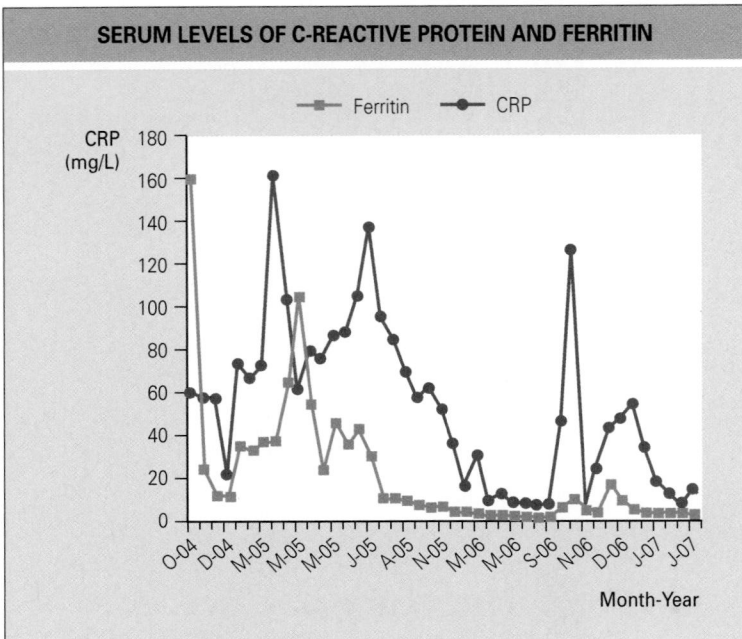

Fig. 84.6 Serum levels of C-reactive protein (normal, < 5 mg/L) and ferritin (normal, 14-295 ng/mL) throughout the disease course of a patient with AOSD diagnosed in 2004, indicating an imbalance in the regulation and secretion of the two proteins.

CRP ratios[53] indicate that CRP and ferritin levels are not closely related in AOSD (Fig. 84.6) and combined with the decrease in glycosylated ferritin indicates an increased synthesis and/or release of H-ferritin. H-ferritin may derive from activated cells in other organ systems than the liver, including fibroblasts, myocytes, endothelial cells, and macrophages; it seems to act in a cytokine manner.[63,64]

Cytokines

Increased levels of several cytokines have been reported in AOSD. Because cytokines are both pleiotropic (have several functions) and redundant (several cytokines can have the same function), the precise role of individual cytokines and especially their interplay in AOSD is not well understood. Overall, a peripheral T-helper cell-1 type response predominates in AOSD, as indicated by increased levels of interferon (IFN)-γ, TNF-α, and sIL-2R in the circulation, in affected skin, and synovial tissue.[33,35,65] Increased IL-6 and IL-8 levels also correlate with disease activity and point to a state of macrophage activation.[50] IL-18 (an inducer of IFN-γ) is upregulated in germinal centers of lymph nodes[66] and associated with enhanced apoptosis of autoreactive immune cells during active AOSD.[67,68]

MANAGEMENT

The often sudden onset with a multitude of symptoms presents patients and physicians with considerable challenges. Multidisciplinary approaches are needed in both the diagnostic and therapeutic phases of the disease. The physical challenges (repeated high fever spikes, severe acute-phase reaction, pain, and limitations due to arthritis) and mental impact (e.g., fear of disability and cancer) may cause severe anxiety in these relatively young patients and their relatives. In addition to a sound medical approach, other health care personnel should be involved early on in the disease course (e.g., physical and occupational therapist, nursing staff, social caretakers) to reduce this anxiety when possible. Existing information on drug management in AOSD is based on data from observational studies (grade B evidence), case series (grade C evidence), as well as evidence-based guidelines (grade D evidence). There are no controlled randomized trials available to guide management and, as a consequence, strategies for the management of other systemic diseases (RA, systemic lupus erythematosus) are being applied to AOSD patients. A systemic score in which 1 point is scored for each of 12 manifestations has been developed to quantify overall disease severity in AOSD and guide treatment but is not helpful as prognostic predictor.[21,23,48]

Acute disease

Symptomatic treatment with pure analgesics without antipyretic effect during the period of diagnostic workup is often insufficient, as indicated by the high number of patients receiving concomitant therapy with empirical antibiotics during the initial phase; in the later phase when infectious disease has become less probable, NSAIDs and systemic corticosteroids are often applied.[4,12,13]

NSAIDs are considered the first-line agents for AOSD and will suffice as monotherapy in about 25% of patients.[69] These patients usually will have a non-chronic disease course and need no further therapy. The response to NSAIDs may, however, be slow, and several agents may have to be used to suppress manifestations. Because of the specific hepatotoxic effects of NSAIDs in AOSD and other side effects in general, some authors have proposed early administration of systemic corticosteroids, which usually provide rapid control over the acute disease manifestations (see Fig. 84.1).[44] The initiation of corticosteroid therapy (starting doses vary from 0.5 to 1 mg/kg/day of prednisolone) is, however, not a trivial matter because long-term corticosteroid therapy is the rule and 20% of patients are still on corticosteroids after 10 years of disease.[31] In patients with life-threatening disease (pericardial tamponade, myocarditis, diffuse intravascular coagulation), corticosteroids are, however, universally applied, often in the form of intravenous pulse therapy.[13] With control of acute disease (clinical and biochemical remission), gradual tapering of corticosteroids over a period from 6 to 12 months should be started under frequent control.[44] As elsewhere, tapering of corticosteroids is an individual matter for both patients and physician because data are mostly lacking.

Not all patients achieve remission with corticosteroid therapy. Given the destructive potential of the arthritis in AOSD and because of its ability to retard this process in RA, several studies have confirmed the efficacy of methotrexate (MTX) in disease remission and as a corticosteroid-sparing agent in AOSD.[70,71] MTX-related liver toxicity is of special concern in AOSD.[44] The efficacy of several other disease-modifying antirheumatic drugs has been reported in small case series. Chloroquine gave similar disease control rates as MTX (75% vs. 83%) when added to corticosteroids,[20] whereas cyclosporine as third-line therapy has been associated with disease remission in 60% to 85% of 13 cases.[14,72] Sulfasalazine therapy has been unsuccessful owing to a high rate of side effects.[15,73,74] Over the past decade the therapeutic use of monoclonal antibodies that inhibit the effects of specific cytokines has proven efficacy and reasonable side-effect profiles in AOSD patients. Thus far, encouraging results have been reported in case histories and small case series for the third-line use of biologic agents in AOSD such as infliximab (an anti-TNF-α agent: 91% remission rate in 44 patients), etanercept (a soluble TNF-α receptor: 72% remission rate in 25 patients), anakinra (an IL-1 receptor antagonist; 91% remission rate in 23 patients), and tocilizumab (an anti-IL-6 receptor): remission in 2 patients.[44]

Relapsing disease

Recurrent disease activity after initial remission is generally classified as relapsing disease, which is associated with a tendency to more future relapses. The timing of relapses is as unpredictable as the disease onset, although most relapses seen within the first year of disease seem related to corticosteroid tapering.[31] Relapses often present as the same manifestations as earlier episodes,[26] and treatment thus follows the same strategy as with initial presentation because relapses are, for the most part, less severe and can be managed less aggressively.[48] This lesser severity may be explained by continued low-dose immunosuppressive therapy and/or closer surveillance.

Chronic disease

Persistent disease activity or recurrent disease activity beyond 1 year of disease is generally classified as chronic disease.[4,5] Chronic disease

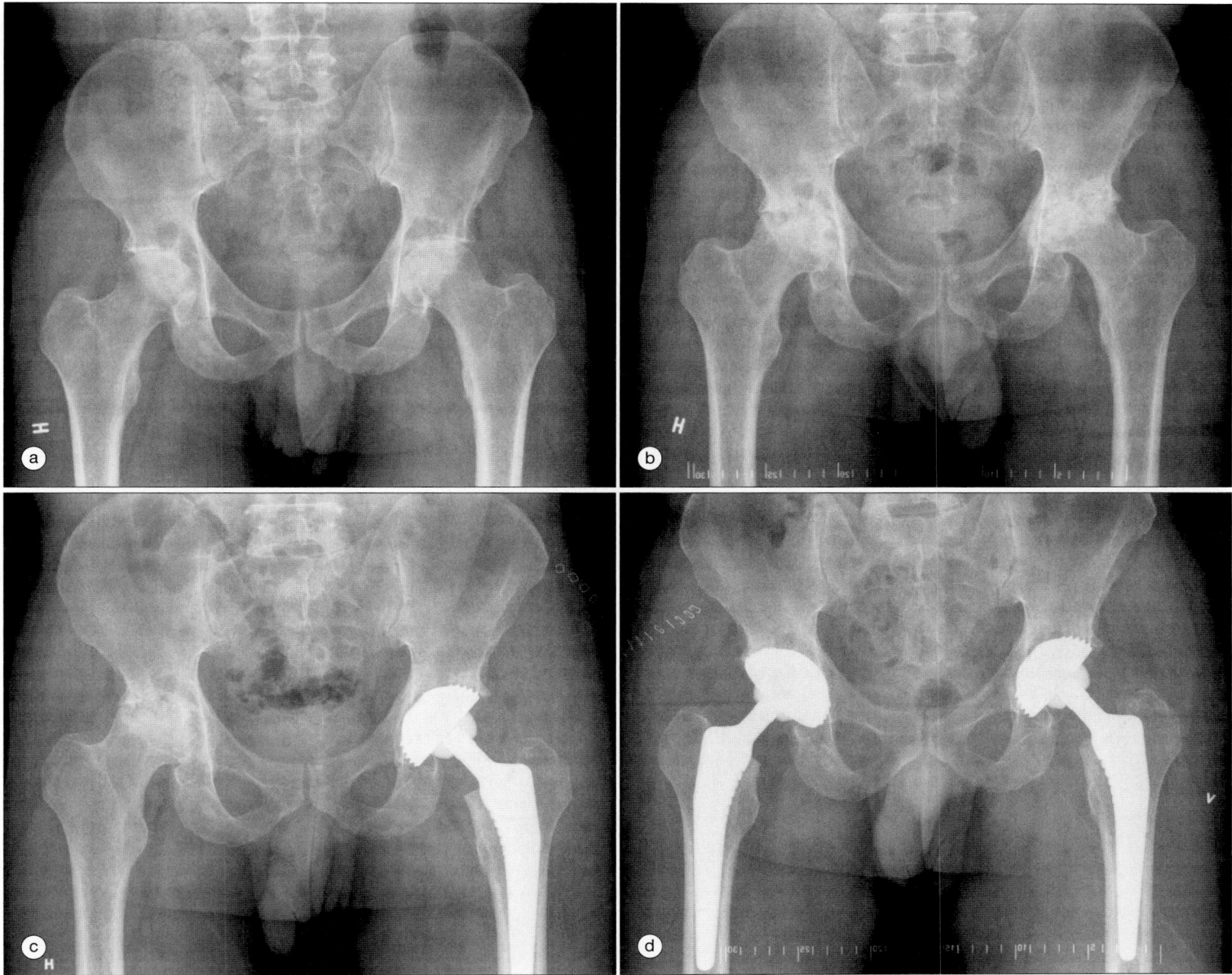

Fig. 84.7 Root joint involvement in AOSD in a 42-year-old man. Erosive disease evolved rapidly in both hips (a to d) and the left shoulder (e to g) despite aggressive cytotoxic therapy.

relates primarily to the development of articular complications because most internal organ complications remit with treatment.[5,31,75] Early studies have drawn particular attention to the development of carpal abnormalities as a diagnostic tool for AOSD because pericapitate abnormalities without radiocarpal alterations were more frequent in AOSD than in RA.[3,76] In these studies, carpal ankylosis developed after 1.5 to 3.5 years of disease with progressive joint space narrowing and only mild osseous erosions; it was more recently detected in 67% of patients after 5 years of disease.[22] The main articular damage associated with poor functional outcome is, however, due to rapidly progressive erosive joint disease in root joints (Fig. 84.7); early risk factors for joint damage include the presence of polyarthritis with shoulder and hip involvement, increased ferritin levels, and increasing ferritin/CRP ratios.[13,31,48,51,53] It would be reasonable to manage such patients in a more aggressive manner in an effort to prevent damage development and subsequent loss of function and income.

KEY REFERENCES

3. Bywaters EG. Still's disease in the adult. Ann Rheum Dis 1971;30:121-133.
4. Kontzias A, Efthimiou P. Adult-onset Still's disease: pathogenesis, clinical manifestations and therapeutic advances. Drugs 2008;68:319-337.
5. Cush JJ, Medsger TA Jr, Christy WC, et al. Adult-onset Still's disease: clinical course and outcome. Arthritis Rheum 1987;30:186-194.
6. Yamaguchi M, Ohta A, Tsunematsu T, et al. Preliminary criteria for classification of adult Still's disease. J Rheumatol 1992;19:424-430.

7. Fautrel B, Zing E, Golmard JL, et al. Proposal for a new set of classification criteria for adult-onset Still disease. Medicine (Baltimore) 2002;81:194-200.
9. Magadur-Joly G, Billaud E, Barrier JH, et al. Epidemiology of adult Still's disease: estimate of the incidence by a retrospective study in west France. Ann Rheum Dis 1995;54:587-590.
10. Wakai K, Ohta A, Tamakoshi A, et al. Estimated prevalence and incidence of adult Still's disease: findings by a nationwide epidemiological survey in Japan. J Epidemiol 1997;7:221-225.

11. Kaipiainen-Seppanen O, Aho K. Incidence of rare systemic rheumatic and connective tissue diseases in Finland. J Intern Med 1996;240:81-84.
12. Evensen KJ, Nossent HC. Epidemiology and outcome of adult-onset Still's disease in Northern Norway. Scand J Rheumatol 2006;35:48-51.
13. Lee SW, Park YB, Song JS, Lee SK. The mid-range of the adjusted level of ferritin can predict the chronic course in patients with adult onset Still's disease. J Rheumatol 2009;36:156-162.

14. Mitamura M, Tada Y, Koarada S, et al. Cyclosporin A treatment for Japanese patients with severe adult-onset Still's disease. Mod Rheumatol 2009;19:57-63.

15. Singh S, Samant R, Joshi VR. Adult onset Still's disease: a study of 14 cases. Clin Rheumatol 2008;27:35-39.

16. Uppal SS, Al Mutairi M, Hayat S, et al. Ten years of clinical experience with adult onset Still's disease: is the outcome improving? Clin Rheumatol 2007;26:1055-1060.

17. Cagatay Y, Gul A, Cagatay A, et al. Adult-onset still's disease. Int J Clin Pract 2009;63:1050-1055.

18. Riera AE, Olive MA, Salles LM, et al. [Adult onset Still's disease: review of 26 cases]. Med Clin (Barcelona) 2007;129:258-261.

19. Goumri S, El Kabli H, Alaoui FZ, et al. [Adult-onset Still disease: 11 cases]. Tunis Med 2006;84:443-449.

20. Pay S, Turkcapar N, Kalyoncu M, et al. A multicenter study of patients with adult-onset Still's disease compared with systemic juvenile idiopathic arthritis. Clin Rheumatol 2006;25:639-644.

21. Crispin JC, Martinez-Banos D, Alcocer-Varela J. Adult-onset Still disease as the cause of fever of unknown origin. Medicine (Baltimore) 2005;84:331-337.

22. Appenzeller S, Castro GR, Costallat LT, et al. Adult-onset Still disease in southeast Brazil. J Clin Rheumatol 2005;11:76-80.

23. Chen DY, Lan JL, Hsieh TY, Chen YH. Clinical manifestations, disease course, and complications of adult-onset Still's disease in Taiwan. J Formos Med Assoc 2004;103:844-852.

24. Mehrpoor G, Owlia MB, Soleimani H, Ayatollahi J. Adult-onset Still's disease: a report of 28 cases and review of the literature. Mod Rheumatol 2008;18:480-485.

25. Akritidis N, Papadopoulos A, Pappas G. Long-term follow-up of patients with adult-onset Still's disease. Scand J Rheumatol 2006;35:395-397.

26. Zeng T, Zou YQ, Wu MF, Yang CD. Clinical features and prognosis of adult-onset Still's Disease: 61 cases from China. J Rheumatol 2009;36:1026-1031.

29. Mert A, Ozaras R, Tabak F, et al. Fever of unknown origin: a review of 20 patients with adult-onset Still's disease. Clin Rheumatol 2003;22:89-93.

30. Wittkowski H, Frosch M, Wulffraat N, et al. S100A12 is a novel molecular marker differentiating systemic-onset juvenile idiopathic arthritis from other causes of fever of unknown origin. Arthritis Rheum 2008;58: 3924-3931.

31. Wouters JM, van de Putte LB. Adult-onset Still's disease; clinical and laboratory features, treatment and progress of 45 cases. Q J Med 1986;61:1055-1065.

33. Chen DY, Lan JL, Lin FJ, et al. Predominance of Th1 cytokine in peripheral blood and pathological tissues of patients with active untreated adult onset Still's disease. Ann Rheum Dis 2004;63:1300-1306.

36. Chen DY, Lan HH, Hsieh TY, et al. Crico-thyroid perichondritis leading to sore throat in patients with active adult-onset Still's disease. Ann Rheum Dis 2007;66:1264-1266.

38. Jeon YK, Paik JH, Park SS, et al. Spectrum of lymph node pathology in adult onset Still's disease; analysis of 12 patients with one follow up biopsy. J Clin Pathol 2004;57:1052-1056.

40. Andres E, Locatelli F, Pflumio F, Marcellin L. Liver biopsy is not useful in the diagnosis of adult Still's disease. Q J Med 2001;94:568-569.

44. Fautrel B. Adult-onset Still disease. Best Pract Res Clin Rheumatol 2008;22:773-792.

45. Efthimiou P, Paik PK, Bielory L. Diagnosis and management of adult onset Still's disease. Ann Rheum Dis 2006;65:564-572.

46. Min JK, Cho CS, Kim HY, Oh EJ. Bone marrow findings in patients with adult Still's disease. Scand J Rheumatol 2003;32:119-121.

47. Fautrel B, Le Moel G, Saint-Marcoux B, et al. Diagnostic value of ferritin and glycosylated ferritin in adult onset Still's disease. J Rheumatol 2001;28: 322-329.

49. Fukaya S, Yasuda S, Hashimoto T, et al. Clinical features of haemophagocytic syndrome in patients with systemic autoimmune diseases: analysis of 30 cases. Rheumatology (Oxford) 2008;47:1686-1691.

51. Wouters JM, Reekers P, van de Putte LB. Adult-onset Still's disease: disease course and HLA associations. Arthritis Rheum 1986;29:415-418.

52. Fujii T, Nojima T, Yasuoka H, et al. Cytokine and immunogenetic profiles in Japanese patients with adult Still's disease: association with chronic articular disease. Rheumatology (Oxford) 2001;40:1398-1404.

53. Evensen KJ, Swaak TJ, Nossent JC. Increased ferritin response in adult Still's disease: specificity and relationship to outcome. Scand J Rheumatol 2007;36:107-110.

55. Valtonen JM, Kosunen TU, Karjalainen J, et al. Serological findings in patients with acute syndromes fulfilling the proposed criteria of adult onset Still's disease. Scand J Rheumatol 1997;26:342-345.

56. Touitou I, Kone-Paut I. Autoinflammatory diseases. Best Pract Res Clin Rheumatol 2008;22:811-829.

57. Galeazzi M, Gasbarrini G, Ghirardello A, et al. Autoinflammatory syndromes. Clin Exp Rheumatol 2006;24(1 Suppl 40):S79-S85.

58. Efthimiou P, Flavell RA, Furlan A, et al. Autoinflammatory syndromes and infections: pathogenetic and clinical implications. Clin Exp Rheumatol 2008;26(1 Suppl 48):S53-S61.

63. Arosio P, Ingrassia R, Cavadini P. Ferritins: a family of molecules for iron storage, antioxidation and more. Biochim Biophys Acta 2009;1790:589-599.

64. Fautrel B. Ferritin levels in adult Still's disease: any sugar? Joint Bone Spine 2002;69:355-357.

66. Conigliaro P, Priori R, Bombardieri M, et al. Lymph node IL-18 expression in adult-onset Still's disease. Ann Rheum Dis 2009;68:442-443.

69. Efthimiou P, Kontzias A, Ward CM, Ogden NS. Adult-onset Still's disease: can recent advances in our understanding of its pathogenesis lead to targeted therapy? Nat Clin Pract Rheumatol 2007;3:328-335.

70. Fautrel B, Borget C, Rozenberg S, et al. Corticosteroid sparing effect of low dose methotrexate treatment in adult Still's disease. J Rheumatol 1999;26:373-378.

72. Marchesoni A, Ceravolo GP, Battafarano N, et al. Cyclosporin A in the treatment of adult onset Still's disease. J Rheumatol 1997;24:1582-1587.

74. Jung JH, Jun JB, Yoo DH, et al. High toxicity of sulfasalazine in adult-onset Still's disease. Clin Exp Rheumatol 2000;18:245-248.

REFERENCES

Full references for this chapter can be found on www.expertconsult.com.

Imaging of rheumatoid arthritis

Thomas J. Learch

85

- Symmetric bilateral rheumatoid arthritis (RA) is commonly seen in the hands and feet, but asymmetric disease is frequently found in large joints.

- Hands and feet show the earliest radiographic changes of RA, which include soft tissue swelling, erosions, and diffuse joint space narrowing.

- Radiographic damage to large joints is seen most frequently in the elbow, shoulder, and knee.

- Sacroiliac joint disease in a patient with RA is relatively insignificant and not common.

- Atlantoaxial subluxation and basilar invagination are frequently present. Lateral cervical spine in flexion is the best way to evaluate atlantoaxial subluxation. Basilar invagination is best appreciated on MRI and CT.

INTRODUCTION

Diagnostic imaging plays an integral role in the diagnosis and follow-up of patients with articular disorders. Patients with unclear and confusing presentations may show specific imaging findings to allow for more accurate and timely diagnosis. For the rheumatologist, diagnostic imaging aids in the clinical diagnosis of rheumatoid arthritis (RA), provides insight into the severity and extent of joint disease, and helps to monitor response to treatment regimens.

With the increasing use of disease-modifying antirheumatic agents (DMARDs) early in the disease, accurate diagnosis, documentation, and staging of disease with imaging studies has become increasingly important. Imaging provides an important tool to aid in the early diagnosis of RA and can also be used to evaluate the extent and severity of disease. Imaging studies provide an objective measure of anatomic damage that defines the course of the disease and the long-term effects of treatment. Imaging studies help monitor disease progression and/or remission and response to therapeutic interventions. Advances in imaging technologies beyond conventional radiography have been dramatic, offering new insights in diagnosis and progression of disease.

APPROACH TO IMAGING AND GENERAL IMAGING FEATURES

The imaging hallmarks of RA are alignment abnormalities, periarticular osteoporosis that progresses to generalized osteoporosis, bony erosions, uniform joint space narrowing, and periarticular soft tissue swelling with synovial cyst and rheumatoid nodule formation. There is generally a bilateral and symmetric distribution, especially of the hands, wrists, and feet, where the earliest changes are seen.

Various imaging modalities can be used to study RA. Each imaging modality has strengths and weaknesses, and some modalities are better at visualizing various pathologic processes than others. A generalized approach to analyzing RA imaging studies has been suggested by Forrester and Brown,[1] who proposed using the mnemonic "the ABC's of arthritis":

    A—Alignment
    B—Bone mineralization
    C—Cartilage and joint space
    D—Distribution
    S—Soft tissues

Alignment changes are searched for in all imaging studies but are particularly common to the wrist and hand, feet, and craniocervical junction. Alignment abnormalities may be reduced and minimized when the patient is positioned for posteroanterior radiographs of the hands but should be readily visualized on oblique and lateral views where the hands are not flattened on the film cassette. Atlantoaxial subluxation is frequently seen only on flexion radiographs, and therefore lateral views of the cervical spine should be obtained with the patient assuming a flexed spine posture.

Bone mineralization is usually normal in all arthropathies except RA. Diffuse osteoporosis is commonly seen in the aging process and with RA. It can also be seen as a side effect of certain medications, such as corticosteroids. Disuse and immobilization also lead to osteoporosis. Conventional radiographs underestimate early osteoporosis but are positive in advanced stages. This is frequently a subjective finding. Periarticular demineralization is subjectively evaluated by a decrease in radiographic density in the osseous structures surrounding a joint space.

Cartilage and joint spaces have the same radiographic density as soft tissues and are therefore not directly visualized on conventional radiographs. Normal joints have a uniform covering of cartilage at their articular ends that correlates to the space seen between the articular surfaces of adjacent bones. Cartilage thinning is inferred on the conventional radiograph by the finding of joint space narrowing. Joint space narrowing in RA is diffuse, unlike in osteoarthritis, in which narrowing occurs along biomechanical vectors of use. As articular cartilage narrows, erosive changes can be seen. Erosions are an important imaging finding that helps to confirm the diagnosis of RA and to demonstrate the severity of disease. Erosions initially appear at the edge of the joint where cartilage is thinnest and where synovium attaches. This is referred to as the "bare area." These erosions are also called marginal erosions.

Distribution of pathology is an important observation because various arthropathies have characteristic areas of occurrence well known to rheumatologists. Symmetric bilateral disease is commonly seen in RA, particularly in the hands and feet. However, asymmetric disease is frequently found in large joints.

Soft tissue changes are easily overlooked on radiographs because the eye is naturally drawn toward the more dense osseous structures. Digital conventional radiographs allow for window/level adjustment on viewing monitors and have led to improved visualization of joint and bursal swelling and effusions. Symmetric swelling about joints in the hands due to a combination of effusion, synovial proliferation, and periarticular soft tissue edema is an early finding on conventional radiography. Advanced imaging modalities such as ultrasonography and MRI optimally resolve any diagnostic difficulties in soft tissue disease.

IMAGING MODALITIES

Conventional radiography

Conventional radiography has long been the mainstay of imaging. It is inexpensive, easily performed, and readily available. Therefore, imaging of articular disorders should start with this modality. Well-performed, high-quality radiographs show osseous and soft tissue changes that document the severity and extent of disease. They often are sufficient, and no further imaging may be required. Follow-up films allow assessment of disease progression or remission.

Hands and wrists

Hands and wrists are commonly involved in RA. The hands (and also the feet) show radiographic changes earliest, and the findings are typical.[2,3] Therefore, these studies are frequently obtained during the

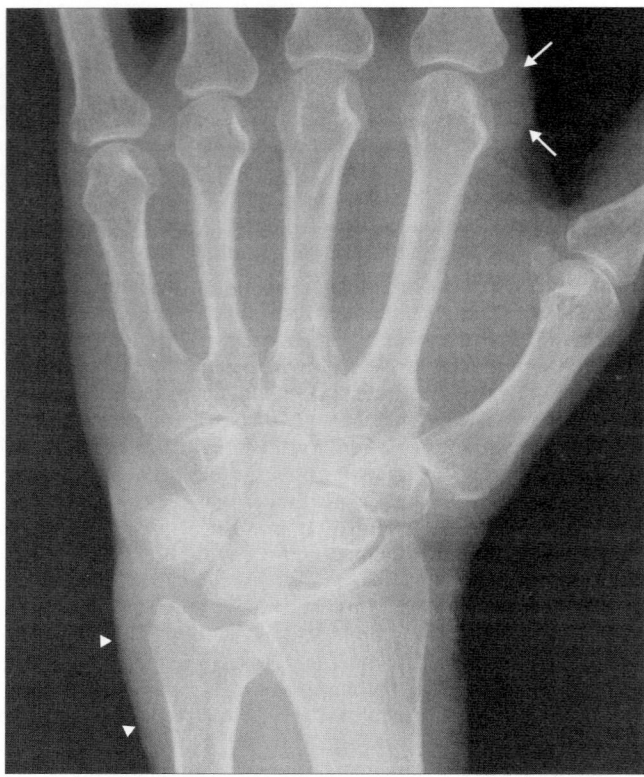

Fig. 85.1 Early rheumatoid arthritis. Mild pancarpal and third through fifth MCP joint space narrowing is present. The second MCP joint is not narrowed, but note the soft tissue fullness (arrows) radial to the joint secondary to pannus and joint fluid. Soft tissue fullness is also present near the distal ulna (arrowheads) secondary to tenosynovitis of the extensor carpi ulnaris.

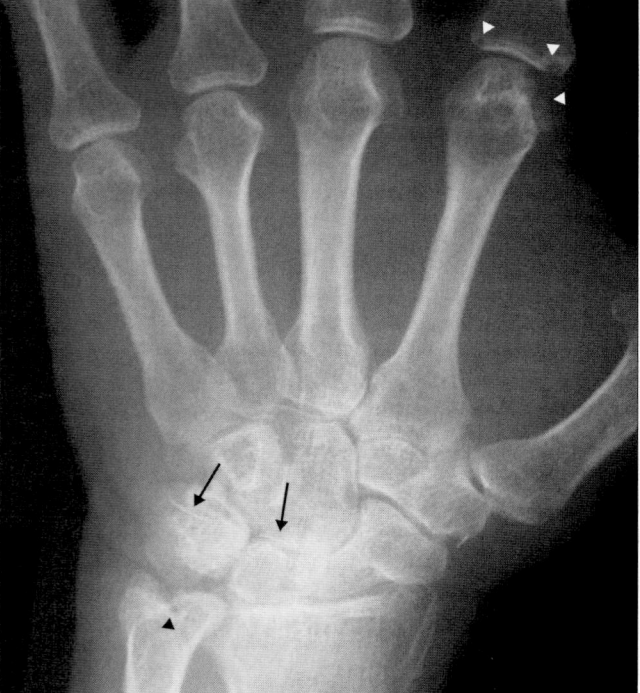

Fig. 85.2 Erosive disease is present at the ulnar styloid and bare areas of the second MCP joint (arrowheads). Note erosive changes of the radial aspect of the second metacarpal head with interruption of the white cortical line compared with the intact third metacarpal head. This is a Korean patient who used acupuncture to treat her RA. Note acupuncture needle tips (arrows) which were left in the patient's soft tissues.

initial workup of the disease. All of the joints of the wrist and hand can be studied on one radiographic study, so in the interest of cost savings, hand films only need be requested. Hand films routinely include the wrist joints.

Soft tissue swelling related to joint effusion, synovitis, and periarticular edema are the earliest radiographic changes and can be seen at the proximal interphalangeal (PIP) and metacarpophalangeal (MCP) joints and at the ulnar styloid (Fig. 85.1). Hyperemia and disuse result in periarticular osteoporosis. Erosions are initially very subtle on conventional radiographs and are seen as irregularity of the white cortical line. Erosions occur earliest about the carpus (usually at the pisiform, triquetrum, and ulnar styloid) and second MCP joint.[3] Initially this may have a dot-dash appearance, progressing to frank defect and irregularity. Bare area erosions at the metacarpal head-neck junction and bases of the phalanges follow. These erosions are more prominent at the radial and volar aspect of the metacarpal head. Inflamed synovial-lined tendons can also lead to erosion. This typically occurs at the ulnar styloid due to tenosynovitis of the adjacent extensor carpi ulnaris tendon (Fig. 85.2).

As cartilage destruction continues, diffuse narrowing of affected joints becomes evident on conventional radiographs. This is well visualized at the carpal and MCP joints. Normally these articulations are uniformly 2 mm wide. Comparison with adjacent or contralateral uninvolved joints or prior studies helps to make this finding more obvious.

Joint ankylosis occurs later in the disease process, typically involving the carpus and rarely the interphalangeal joints.

Alignment abnormalities are most dramatic in the hands and wrists and tend to be symmetric. They are caused by the abnormal kinetic pull of tendons on damaged joints, producing unbalanced forces, resulting in characteristic deformities. The carpus radially deviates and translates toward the ulna. On the posteroanterior view, the lunate normally articulates with the lateral aspect of the radius. When more than half of the lunate articular surface is medial to the ulnar edge of the distal radius, radial deviation and ulnar translation of the carpus has occurred (Fig. 85.3). Characteristic ulnar deviation and

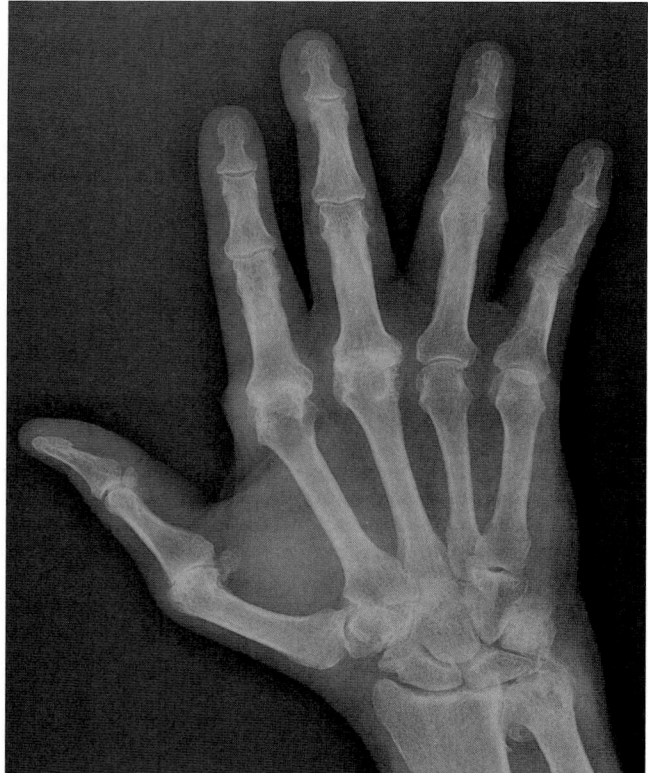

Fig. 85.3 Radial deviation and ulnar translation of the carpus with the majority of the lunate no longer articulating with the radius. There is palmar subluxation and ulnar deviation of the MCP joints with swan neck deformity of the fifth digit.

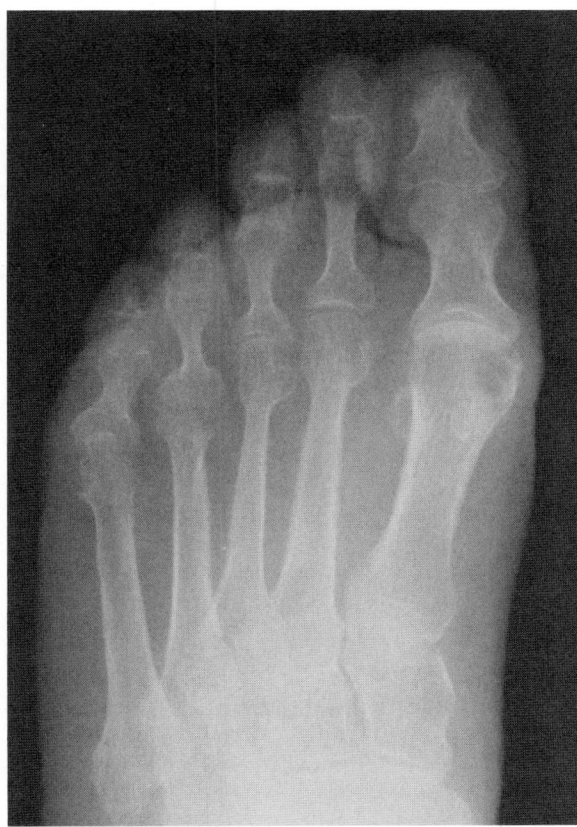

Fig. 85.4 Radiograph of foot demonstrates erosions of the third through fifth metacarpal heads with associated MTP joint space narrowing. There is also joint space narrowing of the first interphalangeal joint with bare area erosions.

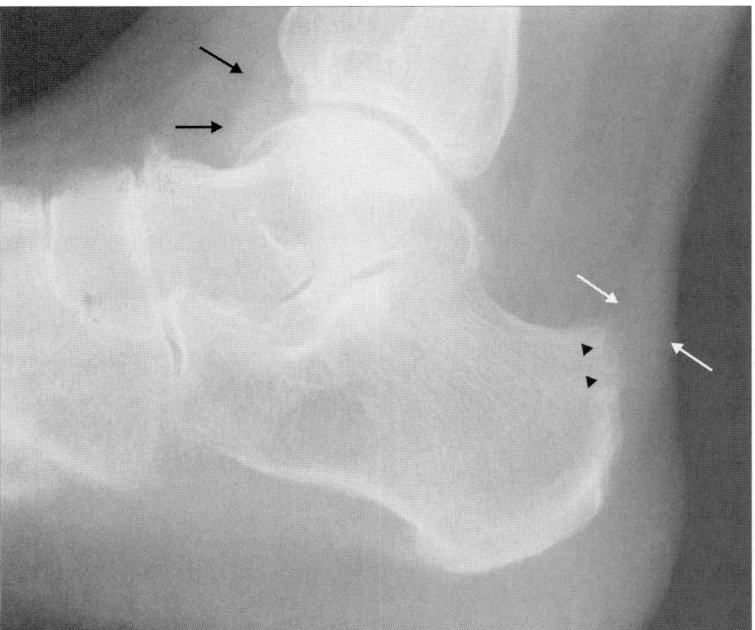

Fig. 85.5 Lateral hindfoot. There is thickening of the Achilles tendon at the insertion of the calcaneus (white arrows) related to retrocalcaneal bursitis. Note associated erosions and irregularity of the posterior calcaneus (black arrowheads). Ankle joint effusion is present (black arrows).

palmar subluxation of the MCP joints, boutonniere and swan neck deformities of the fingers, and Z deformities of the thumb easily assessed clinically are further documented on conventional radiographs (see Fig. 85.3). These alignment changes are also associated with systemic lupus erythematosus and Jaccoud's arthropathy; however, joint space narrowing, erosions, and inflammation are much more prominent in RA.

Feet and ankles

The forefoot has been reported to show the earliest radiographic changes in patients with RA.[3] The lateral fifth metatarsal head is the first area to show erosion. The medial aspect of the first interphalangeal joint is also involved early (Fig. 85.4). Posteroanterior views are best used to assess for early erosions. Oblique views are not necessary and may be overread by inexperienced viewers because the normal facets of the metatarsal heads, exaggerated on this view, may be falsely interpreted as erosions.

Diffuse joint space narrowing of the ankle and tarsal articulations is frequently seen. Ankle joint and retrocalcaneal bursal effusions are readily appreciated on lateral conventional radiographs (Fig. 85.5). As in the carpus, the tarsal joints may become fused in advanced disease.

Alignment abnormalities similar to those seen in the hand occur in the forefoot. Fibular deviation of the toes and dorsolateral subluxation/dislocation of the proximal phalanges at the metatarsal head are common. The fifth toe may be relatively spared.

Large joints

In patients with long-term RA, radiographic damage to the large joints is seen most frequently in the elbow, shoulder, and knee, with rates reported at 32%, 31%, and 27%, respectively. This is followed by the subtalar, ankle, and hip joints, with rates reported at 24%, 22%, and 21%, respectively.[4] Generally, there is a bilateral and symmetric distribution of arthropathy, especially in the small joints of the hands and feet. With large joint involvement, symmetry is less common.

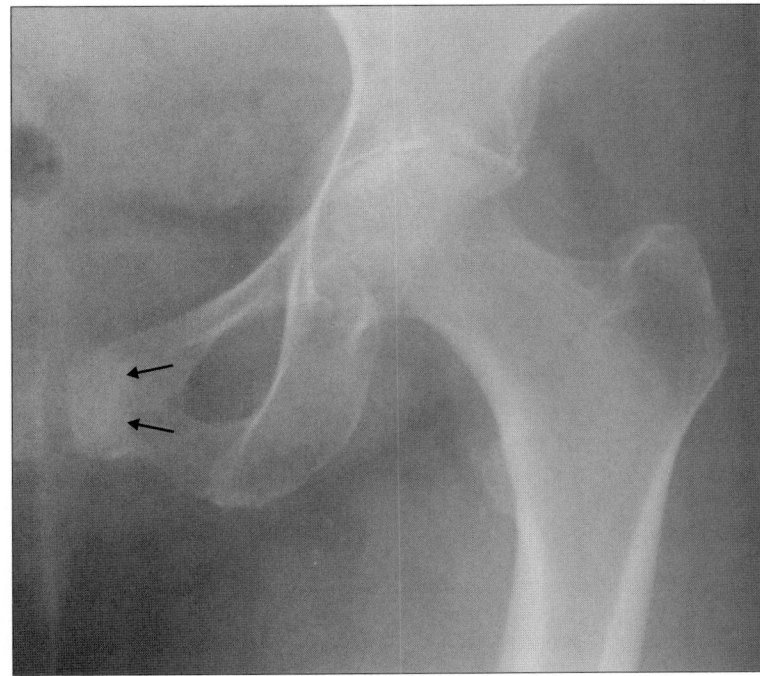

Fig. 85.6 Diffuse left hip joint space narrowing with small erosions of the femoral head. Note linear sclerotic area of pubis (arrows) related to insufficiency fracture.

Pelvis and hips

Soft tissue changes about the hip such as joint effusion, greater trochanteric, and iliopsoas bursitis are not readily appreciated on conventional radiographs. These findings usually require advanced imaging modalities. The hallmark of RA of the hip on conventional radiographs is diffuse joint space narrowing with erosions of the femoral head and neck (Fig. 85.6). Later in the disease process, the erosions may greatly deform and whittle the femoral head. Thinning and erosive disease of the acetabular surface leads to protrusion of the femoral head and acetabulum into the pelvis, called protrusio (Fig. 85.7).

Sacroiliac joint disease in RA is relatively insignificant and is not commonly observed on imaging studies. The SI joints are usually not

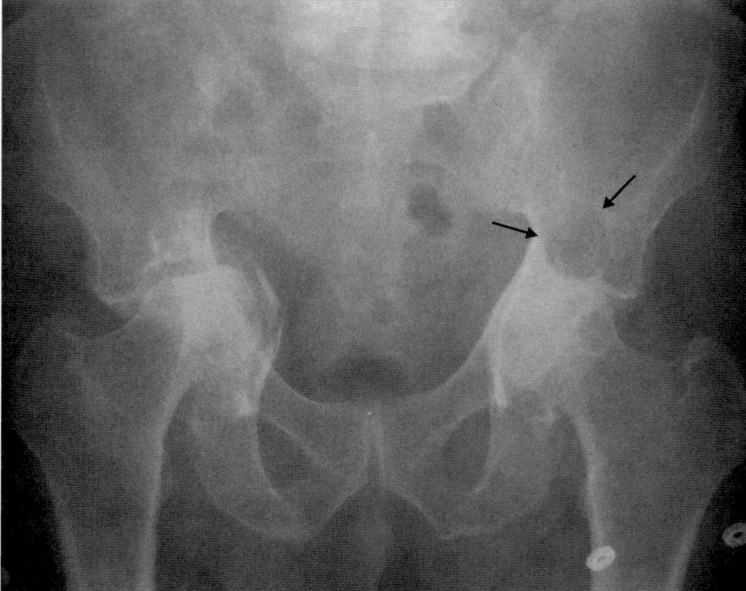

Fig. 85.7 Advanced disease of both hips. The right femoral head is eroded superiorly, and there is acetabular protrusio deformity with marked thinning and resultant fracture. The left hip demonstrates diffuse joint space narrowing with a large subchondral cyst present in the superior acetabulum (arrows).

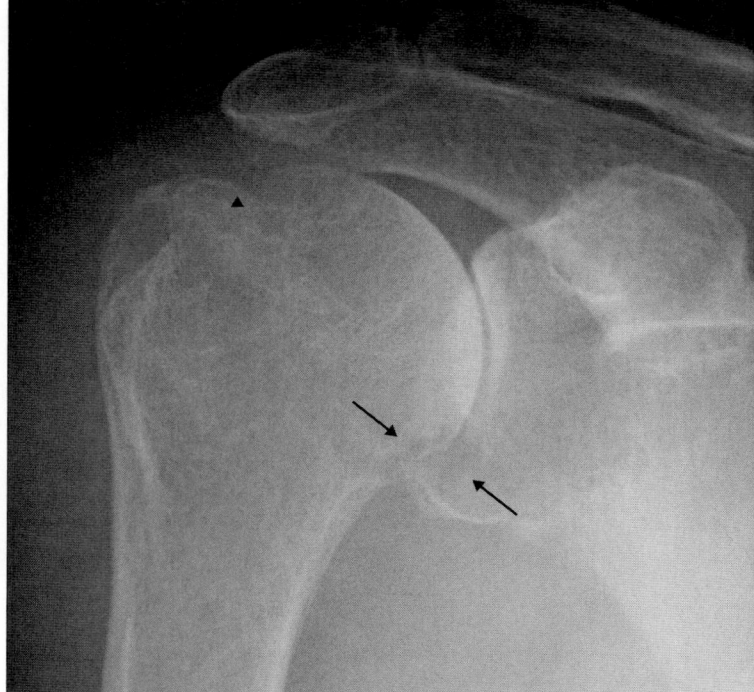

Fig. 85.9 Diffuse glenohumeral joint space narrowing with multiple erosions (arrows). Note large erosion just medial to greater tuberosity (arrowhead). This is the bare area of the shoulder where the earliest erosions are seen.

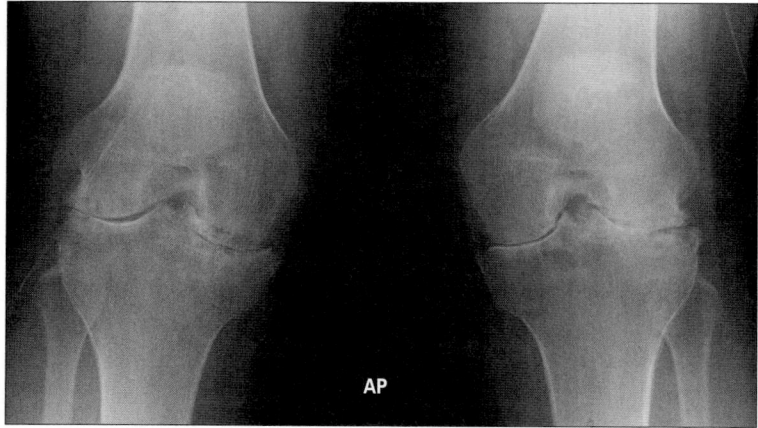

Fig. 85.8 Diffuse joint space narrowing involving both medial and lateral compartments bilaterally. Multiple erosions are present at the articular surface and the bare areas of the knee joint.

radiographically abnormal until late in disease, when asymmetric narrowing, erosions (predominantly on the iliac side due its thinner articular cartilage compared with the sacrum), and possibly areas of fusion may be seen.

Knee

This large synovial joint is frequently affected by RA. Early radiographic findings include joint effusion with engorgement of the suprapatellar bursa seen best on the lateral radiographic, pancompartmental joint space narrowing, and bare area erosions (Fig. 85.8). As ligamentous laxity ensues, varus or valgus deformities are seen. Later in disease, osteophytosis related to secondary osteoarthritis can be seen. Popliteal cysts are commonly seen on advanced imaging studies but are rarely identified on conventional radiography.

Shoulder

Early in disease, marginal erosions are seen at the rotator cuff attachments at the superolateral aspect of the humeral head, where cartilage is thinnest—the bare area of this joint. This is followed by diffuse glenohumeral joint space narrowing as cartilage loss continues (Fig. 85.9). The joint space narrowing may be difficult to appreciate on

routine anteroposterior shoulder radiographs because the glenohumeral joint is not in profile. The Grashey view, obtained in 30 to 40 degrees of posterior oblique torso positioning, provides a perpendicular profiled view of the joint and is more sensitive for joint space narrowing. Glenohumeral joint effusions are not detected on conventional radiographs.

In more chronic disease, rotator cuff atrophy and tearing results in superior migration of the humeral head, narrowing the acromiohumeral distance less than 7 mm, and in eventual mechanical pressure erosion of the uncovered humeral head on the undersurface of the acromion. Erosive changes about the acromioclavicular joint occur with later resorption of the distal clavicle (Fig. 85.10).

Elbow

The elbow is frequently involved by RA; and, indeed, this is the most common arthritis to affect this joint. Soft tissue changes are the early radiographic findings, and they include joint effusion with displacement of the anterior and posterior fat pads away from the humerus and soft tissue swelling posterior to the olecranon corresponding to olecranon bursitis. Diffuse joint space narrowing secondary to cartilage loss and articular erosions occurs in both the radiocapitular and ulnotrochlear compartments (Fig. 85.11). This may become quite severe with marked articular bone loss and subluxation. Other synovial-lined areas about the joint may be involved by synovitis and pannus as well (Fig. 85.12).

Cervical spine

Spinal disease in RA most frequently occurs in the cervical spine, with more than half of all patients with RA having involvement in the course of their disease. Most patients with severe RA will have abnormalities of this area. The most common abnormality is atlantoaxial subluxation, followed by basilar invagination.[5,6]

The most important radiograph in the cervical spine series is the lateral radiograph, with the patient assuming a flexed position. The diagnosis of atlantoaxial subluxation, which is difficult to discern on physical examination, is easily made on this projection (Fig. 85.13). Normally the distance between the anterior arch of C1 and anterior aspect of the dens of C2 measures less than 3 mm in adults and less than 5 mm in children. Subluxation distances greater than 8 mm

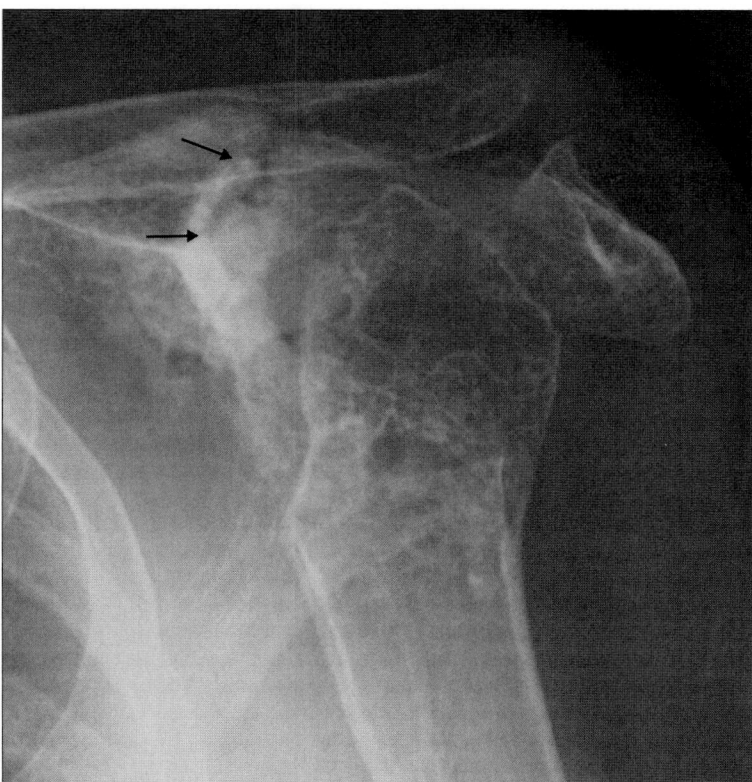

Fig. 85.10 Advanced erosive disease of the glenohumeral joint. Note erosive changes of the distal clavicle. The humerus is high riding secondary to rotator cuff tear and atrophy. The bones are markedly osteopenic with an insufficiency fracture of the acromial spine (arrows).

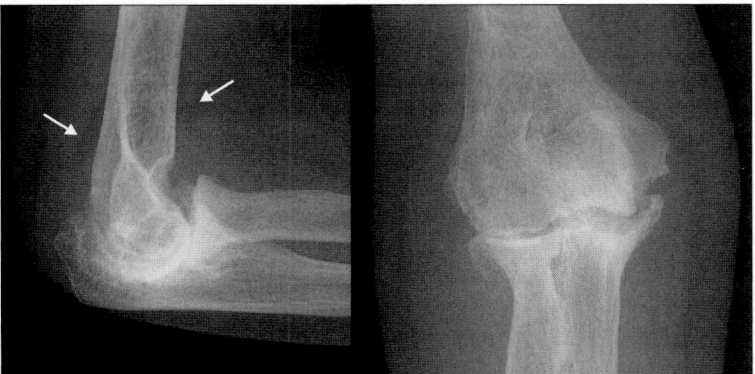

Fig. 85.11 Diffuse elbow joint space narrowing with erosions. The trochlea is much more eroded than the capitulum. Displaced fat pads are present (arrows) secondary to joint effusion.

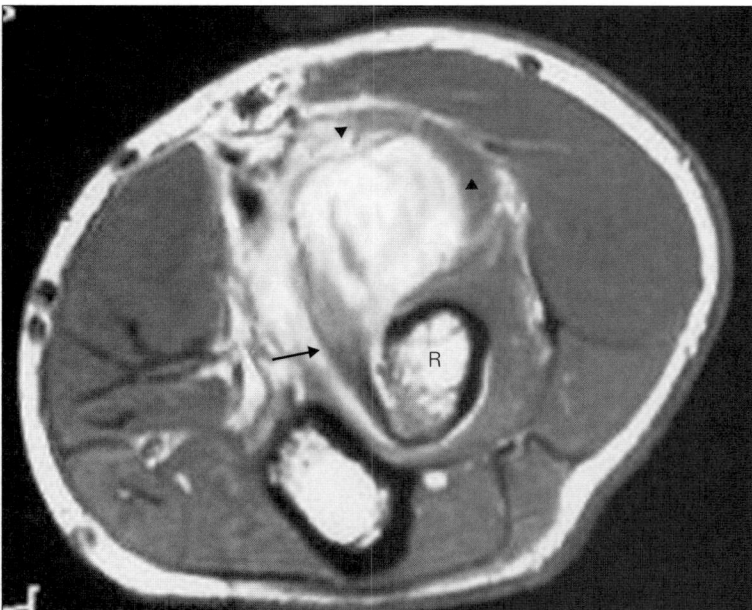

Fig. 85.12 This patient presented with a mass in her elbow. Axial T1-weighted image with fat saturation after intravenous gadolinium enhancement demonstrates enhancing synovium in the bicipitoradial bursa (arrowheads) where the biceps tendon (arrow) inserts on the radius (R). Conventional radiographs of the hands demonstrated changes consistent with RA. This was the patient's initial presentation.

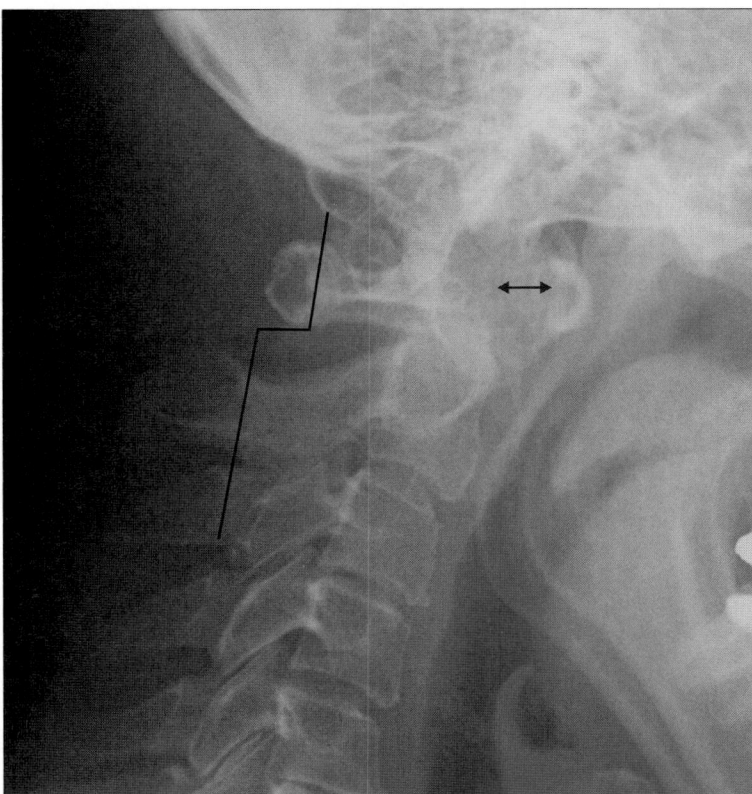

Fig. 85.13 Atlantoaxial subluxation. The anterior arch of C1 is displaced 8 mm anterior to the dens. This is confirmed by the abnormal posterior cervical line.

usually require surgical intervention. The anterior C1/C2 area may be obscured due to cranial settling or basilar invagination. Atlantoaxial subluxation can still be diagnosed by evaluating the posterior cervical line. This is a radiographic line drawn between the spinolamina of C1, C2, and C3 and should be straight. Anterior subluxation of the C1 lamina reflects the same degree of anterior subluxation of the atlantoaxial articulation (see Fig. 85.13). Mid and lower cervical laxity allows for anterior listhesis of the vertebral bodies, resulting in a stepladder appearance on the lateral flexed radiograph. The flexed view also allows for better visualization of the synovial facet joint surfaces as they open. Fusion of the facet joints may occur at some levels, but multilevel posterior ankylosis is rare in adult-onset RA. Basilar invagination may be diagnosed on conventional radiographs but is best studied with MRI or CT.[7,8] This allows for visualization of the adjacent brain stem and spinal cord, which may be impinged by the dens (Fig. 85.14). Advanced imaging also demonstrates associated pannus and erosions about the dens.

Arthrography

Diagnostic arthrography was previously used to evaluate intra-articular structures, the joint capsule, and surrounding ligaments. This has largely been replaced by MRI and ultrasonography. It is rarely used today in the evaluation of patients with RA. Image-guided injection and aspiration of joints, however, still plays an important role for

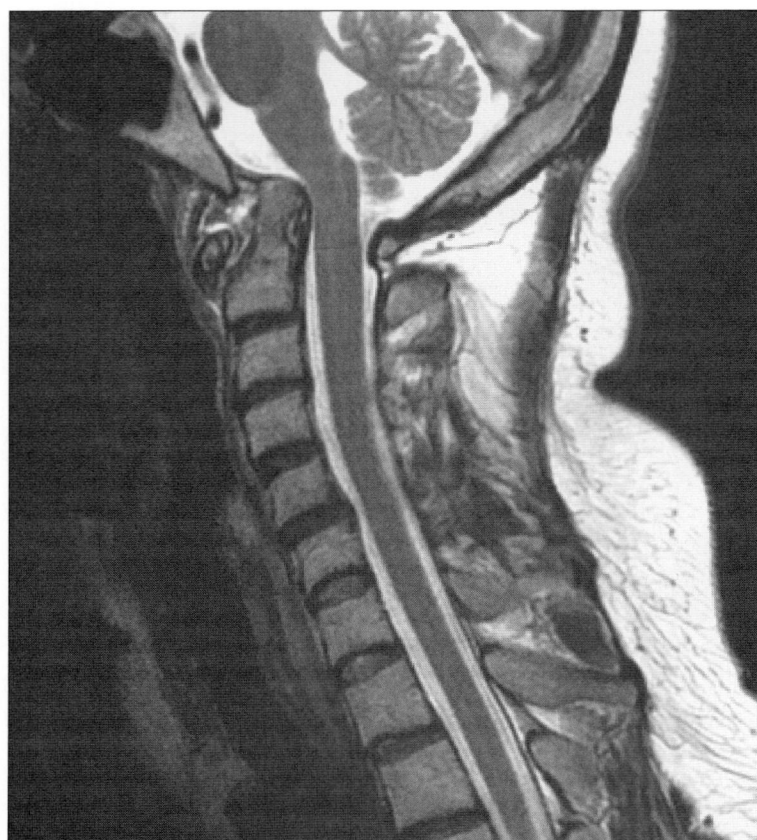

Fig. 85.14 Sagittal T2-weighted image of the craniocervical junction demonstrates basilar invagination with superior migration of the dens through the foramen magnum. The dens indents the medulla.

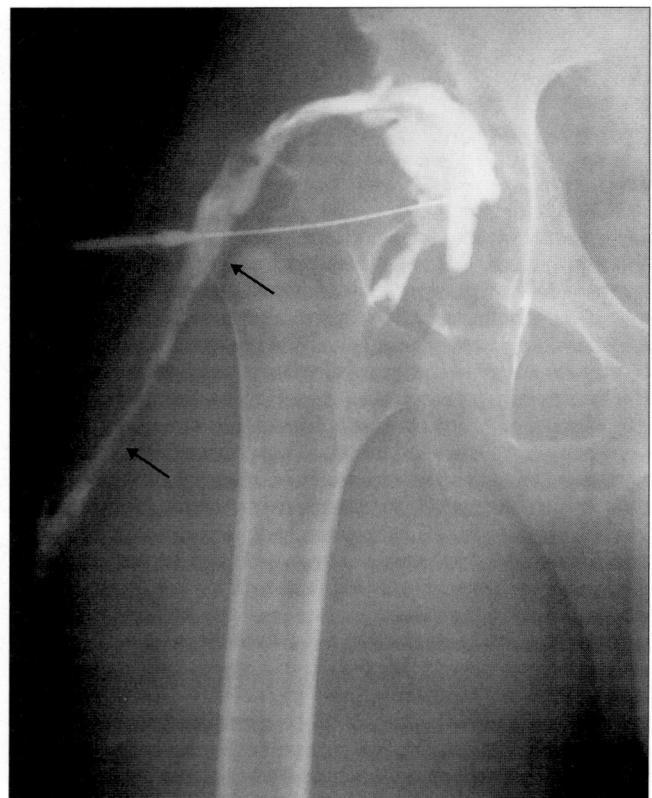

Fig. 85.15 Septic right hip joint with arthrogram demonstrating sinus tract (arrows) exiting the inferolateral thigh.

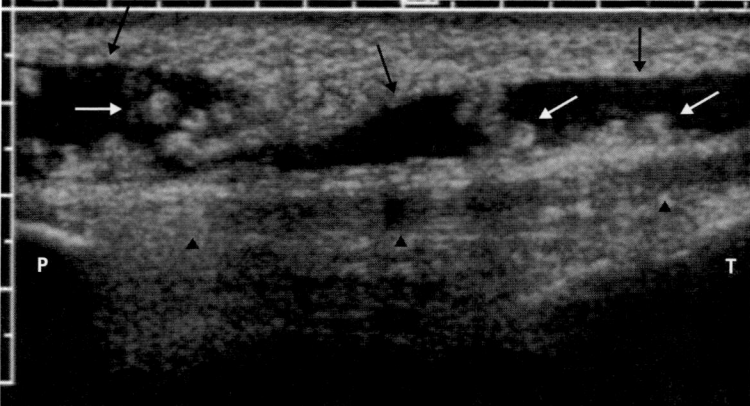

Fig. 85.16 Longitudinal ultrasound image obtained anterior to the knee along the patellar tendon. There is a large fluid collection (black arrows) anterior to the patellar tendon (arrowheads) in the prepatellar and infrapatellar bursae with areas of synovial hypertrophy (white arrows). P, patella; T, tibial tuberosity.

injection of corticosteroids or other medications directly into a specific location and in the diagnosis of rheumatoid joints complicated by infection.

Many of the classic imaging features of RA overlap considerably with septic arthritis, and this differential diagnosis needs to be considered.[9,10] Septic arthritis is usually a monarticular disease. However, it must be kept in mind that patients with RA are at increased risk for septic arthritis due to immune suppression and that previous damage of joints from the disease course places these joints more prone to infection.[11] Because septic arthritis is such a catastrophic illness, prompt aspiration of these joints is essential in the workup and diagnosis of these patients. Cadaveric studies of joint arthrocentesis performed by senior emergency medicine residents have shown success rates of 80% for the accurate positioning of needles in various joints.[12] Because imaging guidance is not routinely used by orthopedic, rheumatology, or emergency physicians, radiologists are frequently requested to aspirate or inject joints. By using fluoroscopic or ultrasound guidance, deep, difficult to palpate joints, such as the hip or shoulder, can easily be accessed. During this procedure, contrast medium is injected into the joint, thus yielding additional information of surrounding synovial cyst formation and the presence of sinus tracks (Fig. 85.15). Image guidance offers the distinct advantage of directed needle placement and imaging proof that the sample obtained did indeed come from the joint itself.

Ultrasonography

Ultrasonography is a readily available and relatively low-cost modality that has increasingly gained wide acceptance in the evaluation of patients with RA, particularly in Europe. In experienced hands, ultrasonography can evaluate soft tissue structures and demonstrate fluid collections and muscle and tendon integrity. It is used for evaluation of muscle/tendon subluxations, dislocations, and tears and tenosynovitis. This can be done in real time with patient movement, and the contralateral side can be quickly imaged for comparison. Fluid collections such as abscesses, popliteal and other synovial cysts, bursae, ganglia, and joint effusions are all well imaged (Fig. 85.16). Under direct ultrasound guidance these collections can be aspirated or injected with medications.

Ultrasound beams cannot penetrate bone, so intraosseous lesions and some intra-articular areas cannot be imaged. Ultrasonography, however, has been increasingly employed to study articular surface cartilage abnormalities, particularly in the evaluation of early erosive disease, and has shown increased sensitivity for detection of erosions compared with conventional radiography.[13] Ultrasonography has been shown to have high sensitivity for assessment of bone destruction and inflammation in finger joints with high correlation to MRI studies done concurrently.[14] The main limitation of ultrasonography, however, remains the steep learning curve in performance of subspecialized examination protocols. Additionally, many hospitals and imaging

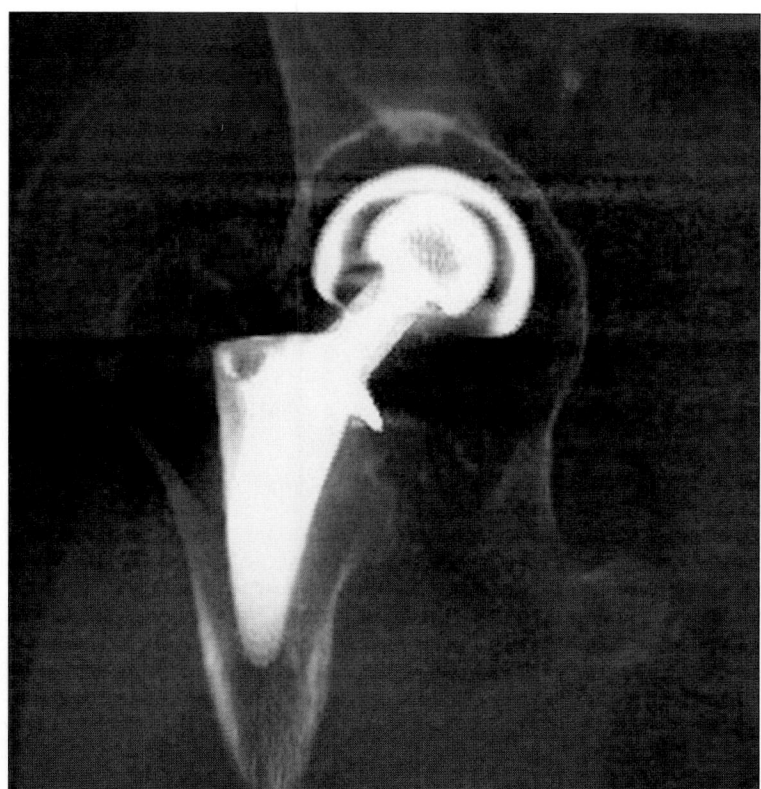

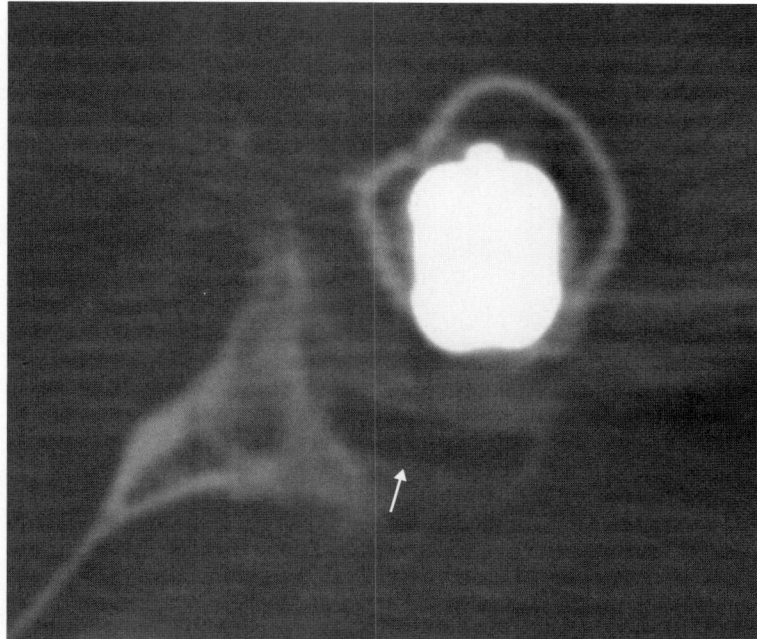

Fig. 85.18 CT arthrogram of total shoulder replacement. Intra-articular contrast medium surrounds the dislocated polyethylene glenoid component (arrow).

Fig. 85.17 Coronal reformatted CT image from a patient with total-hip replacement. There is marked wear of the polyethylene cup superiorly with the femoral head component now in contact with the metal acetabular cup. The interface between the native acetabulum and acetabular cup is markedly widened, resulting in a loose, floating prosthetic cup. Protrusio deformity is present.

facilities, especially in the United States, may not have radiologists familiar with musculoskeletal ultrasonography

Computed tomography

Since the development of CT in the 1970s it has been extensively used to image osseous structures. Most imaging was generally performed in the transverse plane with computer reformatted images in other planes lacking resolution and detail. Imaging of muscle, ligaments, and joint structures was limited and considered insufficient. Imaging of metallic orthopedic hardware and joint replacements caused considerable artifact, limiting CT's usefulness in many musculoskeletal cases.

However, recent developments in multidetector CT technology and computer-enhanced reformatting of image data have revolutionized this modality and broadened its usage. Images are still generally obtained in the transverse plane, but reformatted images in other planes can now be obtained immediately on advanced workstations, allowing for visualization of structures in any linear or even curvilinear plane. Soft tissue resolution in many areas now rivals that of MRI and ultrasonography. With intra-articular injection of a contrast agent, articular structures such as menisci and cartilage are well demonstrated. Decreased streak artifact from metal now permits detailed imaging of joint arthroplasties and other orthopedic hardware.

CT optimally images osseous structures and can easily detect erosions. It is more sensitive than MRI in the detection of early erosions in the hand.[15] CT is often used in the preoperative planning evaluation of patients for joint arthroplasty for optimal evaluation of bone stock, articular surfaces, and version. Postoperative assessment of hardware positioning and complications is also now possible (Figs. 85.17 and 85.18).[16] CT arthrography (done after injection of a contrast agent into the joint) assesses intra-articular structures and cartilage surfaces.[17] This has been increasingly used in patients who cannot tolerate, or have absolute contraindications to, MRI.

Magnetic resonance imaging

MRI is unique in its ability to optimally image bone, articular structures, and soft tissues, with the added advantage of not using ionizing radiation. Initially used to evaluate large joints such as hips, knees, and shoulders, new developments have improved the ability of MRI to resolve smaller joints and structures, furthering its application in the diagnosis and evaluation of patients with RA.

MRI is generally well tolerated by all patients except those with claustrophobia (although open scanner and medications have substantially decreased this problem), the disoriented or confused who may not tolerate the inherent noise the scanner produces or may not be able to stay still during sequence acquisitions, or the morbidly obese where weight limitations may hinder table top movement and positioning. Some relative and absolute contraindications to MRI exist, precluding its usage in some patients. All patients are screened before the procedure to determine any potential contraindications. A common misconception is that patients with joint replacements or other orthopedic hardware cannot have MRI. In fact, MRI has been increasingly used to evaluate painful or infected arthroplasties and newer sequences can minimize metallic artifact. If there is any concern that the patient cannot be in a high field magnetic environment, other imaging strategies such as ultrasonography and CT may be recommended by the radiologist.

MRI has long been advocated for evaluation of joint internal derangement. To this end, it can superbly image ligaments, tendons, menisci, articular cartilage, synovium, and joint fluid (Figs. 85.12, 85.19, and 85.20).

Surrounding articular structures such as musculature and spinal cord are well delineated. MRI is the modality of choice to evaluate the cervicocranial junction for atlantoaxial subluxation and basilar invagination and their effects on the adjacent spinal cord and brain stem (see Fig. 85.14). In patients with symptomatic cervical spine involvement there is a strong correlation between the development of neurologic dysfunction and MRI identification of atlantoaxial spinal canal stenosis, especially in those cases with evidence of upper cervical cord or brain stem compression and subaxial myelopathy changes.[18]

MRI is also the modality of choice in imaging bone marrow abnormalities. In the RA patient, bone infarction, bone marrow edema adjacent to synovial inflammation, and occult traumatic and insufficiency fractures are all optimally imaged with this modality.

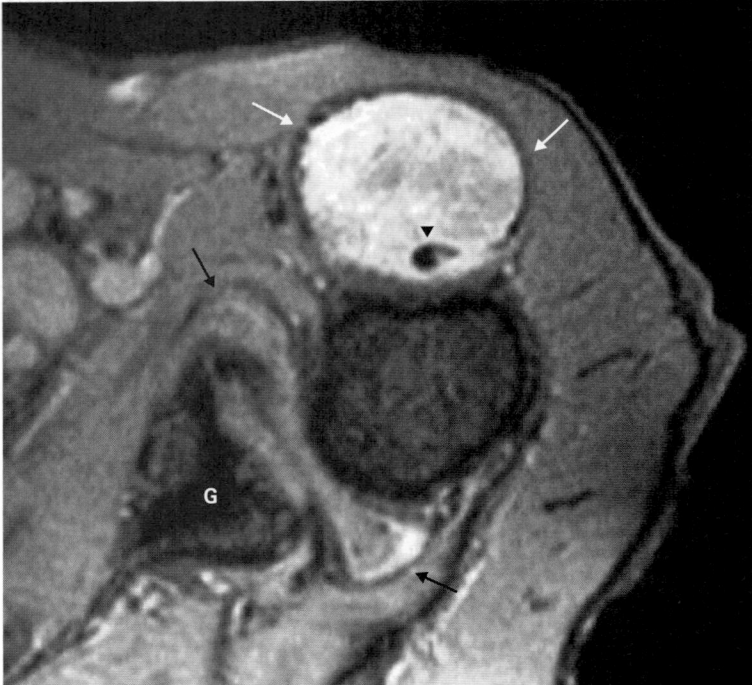

Fig. 85.19 Axial gradient-echo MR image of the shoulder in a patient with RA complaining of a mass. There is a large synovial cyst (arrows) that has dissected along the long head of the biceps tendon (arrowhead). Pannus (black arrows) is present in the glenohumeral joint with marked irregularity erosive change of the glenoid (G).

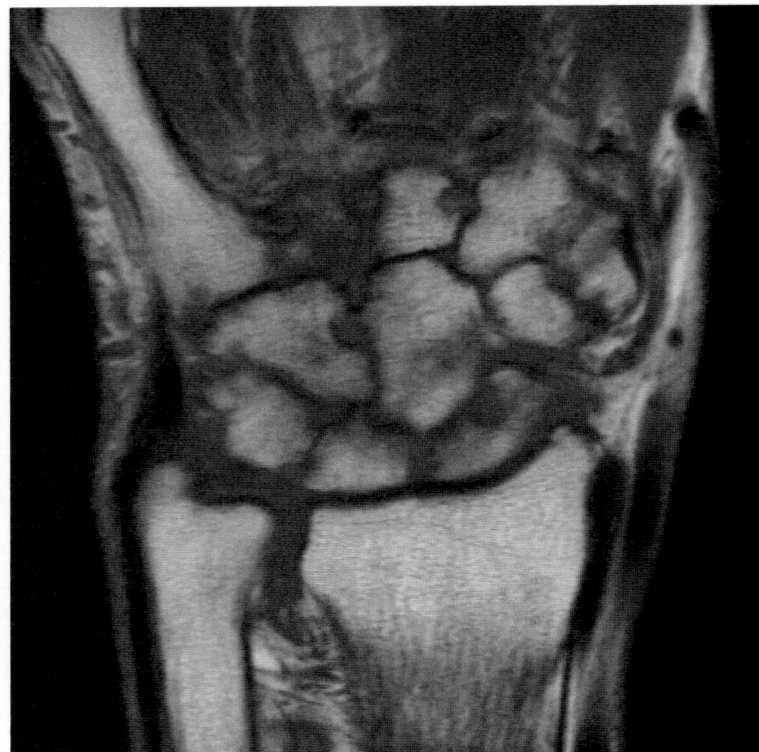

Fig. 85.21 Coronal T1-weighted image of the wrist demonstrates multiple carpal erosions. These were not seen on radiographs.

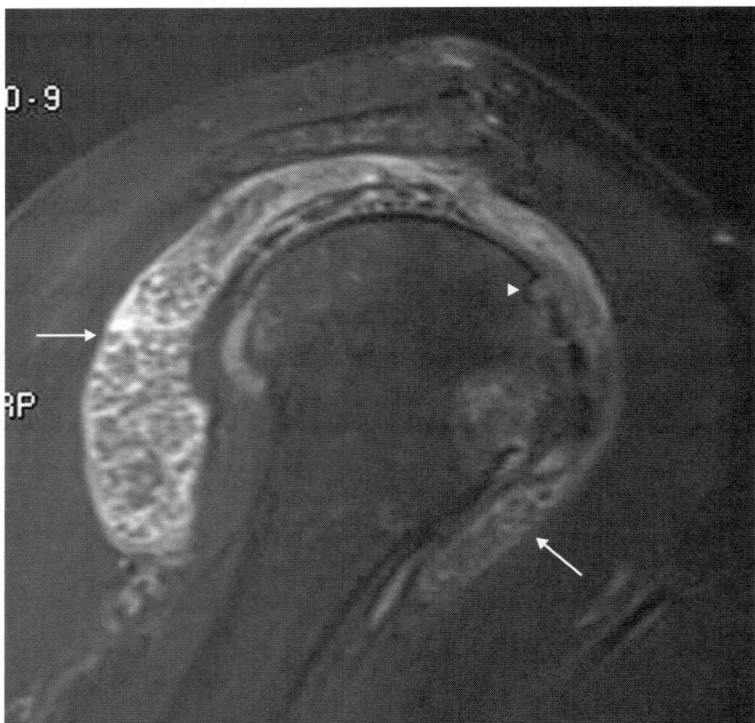

Fig. 85.20 Sagittal fat-saturated proton-density–weighted MR image of the shoulder demonstrates a large chronic subacromial/subdeltoid bursal fluid inflammation and rice body formation (arrows). Erosion (arrowhead) is present in the humeral head.

MRI clearly demonstrates early disease before conventional radiography. As medical therapy for RA has become increasingly more effective, early diagnosis and assessment of disease activity and joint damage is increasingly more important. MRI has also been used to detect early synovitis and to quantify early marginal erosions, joint

effusion, and cartilage disease that are frequently radio-occult (Fig. 85.21).[19] MRI has been shown to detect erosions years before their appearance on conventional radiographs[20] and is more sensitive than ultrasonography.[21]

As such, MRI can play an important role in diagnosis, prognosis, and monitoring the effectiveness of therapies in clinical practice. However, although erosions, synovitis, and tenosynovitis in the hands are frequently encountered in early RA and well demonstrated by MRI, these findings are not specific. They can also be seen in patients with systemic lupus erythematosus and primary Sjögren's syndrome.[22]

MRI's main limitation is expense and availability; however, the modality is now in most hospitals and many outpatient facilities, and its more ubiquitous presence may bring down cost. Its effectiveness in early disease diagnosis has led to increasing usage at disease onset. Cost-saving measures can be employed and advocated by radiologists familiar with early disease. This may include scanning bilateral wrists/hands together in the prayer position, with the patient lying on the side and hands above the head. The right hand can be labeled with a dedicated MR marker to avoid confusion, and simultaneous imaging of both sides can be performed to get a "two for one" study.

As good as 1.5-T MR images are, newer high-field strength 3.0-Tesla imaging can provide even more detailed resolution of smaller structures. 3.0-T imaging is now increasingly available at the university and community level. These magnets produce more detailed image studies, and they are particularly useful in neuroradiology. Although musculoskeletal examinations are generally of higher quality on 3.0-T magnets, improving evaluation of extent of bone edema and synovitis and identification of small bone erosions by 14% to 22%, acceptable image quality is still achieved on 1.5 T.[23]

As further developments in MRI technology, protocols, and research improve our understanding and abilities to image rheumatic diseases, this modality will undoubtedly play an important role in diagnosis, prognosis, and for monitoring effectiveness of therapies in clinical practice.

REFERENCES

1. Forrester DM, Brown JC. The ABC's of arthritis. In: The radiology of joint disease, 3rd ed. Philadelphia: WB Saunders, 1987:1.
2. Pensec VD, Saraux A, Berthelot JM, et al. Ability of foot radiographs to predict rheumatoid arthritis in patients with early arthritis. J Rheumatol 2004;31:66-70.
3. Lindqvist E, Jonsson K, Saxne T, et al. Course of radiographic damage over 10 years in a cohort with early rheumatoid arthritis. Ann Rheum Dis 2003;62:611-616.
4. Drossaers-Bakker KW, Kroon HM, Zwinderman AH, et al. Radiographic damage of large joints in long-term rheumatoid arthritis and its relation to function. Rheumatology 2000;39:998-1003.
5. Bouchaud-Chabot A, Liote F. Cervical spine involvement in rheumatoid arthritis: a review. Joint Bone Spine Rev Rhum 2002;69:141-154.
6. Neva MH, Kaarela K, Kauppi M. Prevalence of radiological changes in the cervical spine—a cross sectional study after 20 years from presentation of rheumatoid arthritis. J Rheumatol 2000;27:90-93.
7. Riew KD, Hilibrand AS, Palumbo MA, et al. Diagnosing basilar invagination in the rheumatoid patient: The reliability of radiographic criteria. J Bone Joint Surg Am 2001;83:194-200.
8. Stiskal MA, Neuhold A, Szolar DH, et al. Rheumatoid arthritis of the craniocervical region by MR imaging: detection and characterization. AJR Am J Roentgenol 1995;165:585-592.
9. Learch TJ, Farooki S. Magnetic resonance imaging of septic arthritis. Clin Imaging 2000;24:236-242.
10. Learch TJ. Imaging of infectious arthritis. Semin Musculoskel Radiol 2003;7:137-142.
11. Pioro MH, Mandell BF. Septic arthritis. Rheum Dis Clin North Am 1997;23:239-259.
12. Learch TJ, Riel J, McCullough M: Joint aspiration: success rates of emergency medicine residents in a cadaver model. Radiology 1999;213:328.
13. Wakefield RJ, Gibbon WW, Conaghan PG, et al. The value of sonography in the detection of bone erosions in patients with rheumatoid arthritis: a comparison with conventional radiography. Arthritis Rheum 2000;43:2762-2770.
14. Szkudlarek M, Klarlund M, Narvestad E, et al. Ultrasonography of the metacarpophalangeal and proximal interphalangeal joints in rheumatoid arthritis: a comparison with magnetic resonance imaging, conventional radiography and clinical examination. Arthritis Res Ther 2006;8:R52.
15. Perry D, Stewart N, Benton N, et al. Detection of erosions in the rheumatoid hand; a comparative study of multidetector computerized tomography versus magnetic resonance scanning. J Rheumatol 2005;32:256-267.
16. Leung S, Naudie D, Kitamura N, et al. Computed tomography in the assessment of periacetabular osteolysis. J Bone Joint Surg Am 2005;87:592-597.
17. Vande Berg BC, Lecouvet FE, Poilvache P, et al. Assessment of knee cartilage in cadavers with dual-detector spiral CT arthrography and MR imaging. Radiology 2002;222:430-436.
18. Narvaez JA, Narvaez J, Serrallonga M, et al. Cervical spine involvement in rheumatoid arthritis: correlation between neurological manifestations and magnetic resonance imaging findings. Rheumatology 2008;47:1814-1819.
19. Conaghan PG, O'Connor P, McGonagle D, et al. Elucidation of the relationship between synovitis and bone damage: a randomized magnetic resonance imaging study of individual joints in patients with early rheumatoid arthritis. Arthritis Rheum 2003;48:64-71.
20. Ostergaard M, Hansen M, Stoltenberg M, et al. New radiographic bone erosions in the wrists of patients with rheumatoid arthritis are detectable with magnetic resonance imaging a median of two years earlier. Arthritis Rheum 2003;48:2128-2131.
21. Hoving JL, Buchbinder R, Hall S, et al. A comparison of magnetic resonance imaging, sonography, and radiography of the hand in patients with early rheumatoid arthritis. J Rheumatol 2004;31:663-675.
22. Bourtry N, Hachulla E, Flipo RM, et al. MR imaging findings in hands in early rheumatoid arthritis: comparison with those in systemic lupus erythematosus and primary Sjögren syndrome. Radiology 2005;236:593-600.
23. Wieners G, Detert J, Streitparth F, et al. High-resolution MRI of the wrist and finger joints in patients with rheumatoid arthritis: comparison of 1.5 Tesla and 3.0 Tesla. Eur Radiol 2007;17:2176-2182.

REFERENCES

Full references for this chapter can be found on www.expertconsult.com.

The contribution of genetic factors to rheumatoid arthritis

86

Robert M. Plenge, Chris Deighton, and Lindsey A. Criswell

- Twin and family studies confirm an important contribution of genetic factors to rheumatoid arthritis.
- Genes encoded within HLA-DRB1 from the major histocompatibility complex (MHC) provide the most consistent evidence of an effect.
- Despite intensive efforts the exact role of MHC genes is still unclear.
- Recent studies, covering the whole genome, have suggested a number of other candidate genes.
- The effect of key genes, including HLA-DRB1, are modified by environmental factors, particularly smoking.

INTRODUCTION

In this chapter we attempt to summarize a wealth of information that has emerged on the contribution of genetic factors to rheumatoid arthritis (RA). Since the first associations of genetic factors with RA that were described more than 4 decades ago, the rate of progress in recent years has been exponential. In this chapter the strength of the evidence suggesting a role for genetics in RA susceptibility is summarized. There is a detailed analysis of the role of both HLA and other loci within the major histocompatibility complex (MHC). Much of the most recent data have come from studies outside the MHC, based on emerging powerful technologies. Finally, there is a brief review of the evidence for gene-environment interactions.

STRENGTH OF A GENETIC CONTRIBUTION

Early evidence for a genetic component to RA was derived from family and twin studies.[1,2] Although the population risk of RA is 0.5% to 1%, the monozygotic twin of a patient with RA has a risk of approximately 15%.[3-5] Moreover, the relative risk to the sibling of a proband with RA (known as λs) is about 5 for RA,[6-8] although the number varies depending on the population studied.[9] A complementary approach to estimate the genetic component is to consider the heritability of a disease, which is the proportion of the variance of the disease that is explained by the inherited genetic variance.[10] Using data on twins, the heritability of RA has been estimated to be about 60%, indicating that genetic factors account for a large proportion of the population's liability to the disease.[11] However, this serves as only an estimate, because measures of heritability may overestimate the genetic component owing to the common environment shared among family members or even underestimate the genetic component owing to complex genetic interactions (e.g., gene-gene or gene-environment interactions).

ROLE OF MAJOR HISTOCOMPATIBILITY COMPLEX GENES

In common with many other autoimmune diseases, much genetic research has revolved around genes within the MHC region on chromosome 6. The MHC region is the most gene-dense region of the mammalian genome, and it plays an important role in the immune system, autoimmunity, and reproductive success. In humans, the 3.6-megabase pair (Mb) MHC region contains over 180 expressed genes, about half of which are of known immunologic function. The genes that have garnered the most attention have been the class II human leukocyte antigen (HLA) genes.

Over the past 4 decades, many genetic studies have demonstrated the importance of the MHC region in susceptibility to RA. In 1969 it was noted that lymphocytes from RA patients were poorly reactive when incubated together in mixed lymphocyte cultures.[12] In the early 1970s, weak and variable associations between RA and HLA class I region genes were described using serologic reagents.[13] More rapid progress was made when techniques became available for testing HLA class II antigens. The earlier mixed lymphocyte cultures (MLC) were further refined in 1976, and an association between RA and MLC type Dw4 was described.[14-16] Hereafter, a serologically defined marker, HLA-DR4, was found to be associated with RA in white populations in the United States. Combining MLC and serologic techniques distilled the RA association to a few specific alleles, namely, DR4 Dw4, DR4 Dw14.1, DR4 Dw14.2, and DR4 Dw15. These techniques were superseded in the 1990s by various DNA-based techniques that provided much greater precision (Fig. 86.1). It was recognized that the MLC and serologic markers just listed represented alleles that changed the amino acid sequence of the HLA-DRB1 gene. These alleles were subsequently renamed HLA-DRB1*0401, *0404, *0408, and *0405, respectively. Overall, it has been estimated that the MHC region accounts for approximately one third of the overall genetic burden of RA.[7,17]

THE SHARED EPITOPE HYPOTHESIS

With the advent of sophisticated DNA typing for HLA-DRB1 alleles, it was noted that not all HLA-DR4 alleles were associated with RA and that different alleles conferred risk of RA in different ethnic populations.[18-29] The most common (>5% population frequency) HLA-DRB1 susceptibility alleles include *0101, *0401, and *0404 in individuals of European ancestry and *0405 and *0901 in individuals of Asian ancestry; less common alleles include *0102, *0104, *0408, *0413, *0416, *1001, and *1402. The classic shared epitope (SE) alleles may not contribute to the risk in African-American and Hispanic-American RA populations,[30,31] and other HLA-DRB1 alleles may be associated with protection against RA (DRB1*0103, *0402, *0802, *1302).[29] (See Table 86-1 for these and other important allelic associations.)

In 1987, Peter Gregersen and coworkers proposed an elegant hypothesis for these complex and diverse associations.[32] They showed that RA risk alleles share similarities in a key sequence of five amino acids at residues 70-74 in the third hypervariable region of the HLA-DRB1 gene: [70]QRRAA[74], [70]QRRAA[74], [70]QRRAA[74]. These residues are important in peptide binding, and thus it is hypothesized that RA-associated alleles bind specific peptides, which in turn facilitates the development of autoreactive T cells. These alleles are now widely known collectively as "shared epitope" alleles (Fig. 86.2). Of note, the *0901 allele observed among Asian populations does not strictly conform to the SE amino acid sequence motif [70]RRRAE[74].

Although SE susceptibility alleles are often considered as a group, the strength of the genetic association to RA susceptibility differs between the individual DRB1 alleles.[33] There are at least two classes of SE risk alleles (high and moderate). In general, DRB1*0401 and *0405 alleles exhibit a high level of risk, with a relative risk (RR) of approximately 3. The DRB1*0101, *0404, *0901, and *1001 alleles exhibit a more moderate relative risk in the range of 1.5.

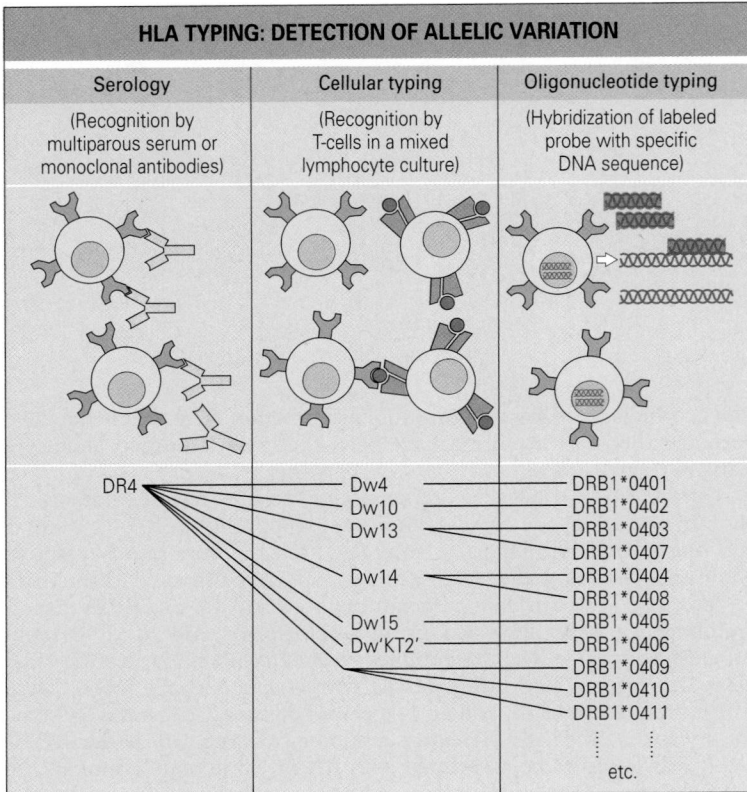

HLA TYPING: DETECTION OF ALLELIC VARIATION

Serology	Cellular typing	Oligonucleotide typing
(Recognition by multiparous serum or monoclonal antibodies)	(Recognition by T-cells in a mixed lymphocyte culture)	(Hybridization of labeled probe with specific DNA sequence)

DR4 — Dw4 — DRB1*0401
Dw10 — DRB1*0402
Dw13 — DRB1*0403
DRB1*0407
Dw14 — DRB1*0404
DRB1*0408
Dw15 — DRB1*0405
Dw'KT2' — DRB1*0406
DRB1*0409
DRB1*0410
DRB1*0411
etc.

Fig. 86.1 HLA typing: detection of allelic variation. The first panel illustrates HLA typing using sera that recognize alloantigens. These sera often recognize broad antigenic specificities, such as DR4, which are epitopes present on a number of different alleles. Finer discrimination is frequently obtained through cellular typing, as diagrammed in the second panel. In this case, mixed lymphocyte culture for T cells of unknown HLA type is used to measure proliferation on responder cells of known HLA type. In this way, "subtypes" of DR4 are defined: Dw4, Dw10, Dw14, etc. Currently, most laboratories utilize oligonucleotide typing, as outlined in the third panel. Based on the known nucleotide sequence of different alleles, synthetic labeled oligonucleotide probes are designed that hybridize specifically to the DNA sequence unique to the gene of interest. In some cases, a series of oligonucleotide probes is required to distinguish among the different alleles and a "matrix" approach can be utilized. In this way even minor differences among alleles can be recognized; for example, this has led to the identification of more than 20 different DR4-positive alleles.

TABLE 86.1 HLA-DRB1 SUSCEPTIBILITY IN RHEUMATOID ARTHRITIS

	DRB1 susceptibility allele	Epitope sequence	Prevalence in RA (%)	Relative risk
Whites	*0401 (DR4, Dw4)	LLEQKRAA	50	6
	*0404 (DR4, Dw14)	LLEQRRAA	30	5
	*0101 (DR1, Dw1)	LLEQRRAA	24	1
Japanese	*0405 (DR4, Dw15)	LLEQRRAA	71	3.5
Yakima	*1402 (DR6, Dw16)	LLEQRRAA	83	3.3
Israeli Jews	*0101 (DR1, Dw1)	LLEQRRAA	28	Unknown

Summary of the important HLA-DRB1 alleles conferring susceptibility to RA in different ethnic populations. Their approximate prevalences in RA patients in each population, along with relative risks, are listed. Each of these alleles includes the shared epitope (or a close variation), even though the sequence of the remainder of the DRB1 gene may be quite varied among these alleles.

It is becoming increasingly clear that HLA-DRB1 SE alleles largely influence the development of seropositive RA and more specifically anti-citrullinated peptide antibody (ACPA)-positive RA.[34,35] Collectively, SE alleles have an odds ratio of over 5 if ACPA-positive RA patients are compared with matched healthy controls. Because these alleles are quite common in the general population (together, allele frequency of approximately 40% in individuals of European ancestry), the attributable risk for SE alleles is quite high.

Biologic function of shared epitope alleles

If the SE is important in predisposing to RA, then how might it work? Despite over 3 decades of research, the answer is not completely clear.

The SE region constitutes a helical domain forming one side of the antigen-binding site, suggesting functional significance and an ability to influence the nature of potentially arthritogenic peptides (Fig. 86.3). In keeping with the hypothesis, those alleles that negatively associate with RA have substitutions of amino acids within the SE that would exert a profound influence on the attributes of any bound antigenic peptide. For example, DRB1*0402 and *0103 alleles have a ^{70}DERAA^{74} motif that would impact markedly on the peptide-binding properties of the molecule.[13] Fascinatingly, canine rheumatoid arthritis (a spontaneous condition affecting dogs that resembles human RA) associates with dog MHC DRB1 alleles that also have the QRRAA sequence in the third hypervariable region.[36] A study from France has suggested that the amino acid sequence RAA at positions 72-74 is the key sequence in increasing susceptibility to RA and that this is modulated by amino acids at positions 70 and 71.[37]

There are three predominant biologic models to explain the association. Each model centers around the interaction between the T-lymphocyte cell receptor (TcR) and class II MHC molecules (Fig. 86.4).

1. HLA molecules are important in the selection and establishment of the antigen-specific T-cell repertoire. Interactions with HLA molecules instruct the T cell to differentiate between self and non-self.[13,38] T cells that show self-reactivity are deleted or inactivated, whereas others are positively selected to establish a repertoire of cells capable of recognizing foreign antigen in the context of self-MHC. It is possible that the SE assists in some way in the positive selection of autoreactive T cells, with a subsequent breakdown in self-tolerance, so that the immune system reacts against the body's own constituent parts.

2. As mentioned earlier, the primary role of HLA molecules is to bind peptide and present it to antigen-specific T cells. The location of the SE in a critical area of the binding site of the HLA-DR molecule would influence the nature and orientation of processed peptides that might bind there and thus exert an impact on the trimolecular complex of HLA-DR molecule, bound peptide, and TcR. Binding with an arthritogenic peptide (e.g., a processed microbial antigen) might initiate and sustain a pathologic immune response. To date, no peptide has been identified that could be recognized by a T-cell clone in the context of all the HLA-DR molecules that associate with RA. However, some mutated variants of naturally occurring peptides approximate to the necessary pattern, suggesting that this model is a possibility.[13,39,40]

3. In a similar fashion to some of the mechanisms that have been proposed for the association between HLA-B27 and spondyloarthropathies, "molecular mimicry" may occur in which similarities between the SE and foreign protein might break self-tolerance and generate autoreactive T-cell clones that eventually lead to RA. Some amino acid sequences from HLA molecules share homology with those from potentially antigenic proteins derived from infectious agents.[41] For example, portions of one of the Epstein-Barr virus glycoproteins share similarity with the SE.[42]

Limitations of the shared epitope hypothesis

However, the veracity of the SE hypothesis has been challenged. There are a number of observations that do not fit comfortably with a straightforward pathogenic association between the SE and RA.

- In all populations that have been studied, a variable but substantial minority of individuals with RA do not possess the SE.[23,43,44]
- Some ethnic populations do not demonstrate significant association with SE alleles and risk of RA, such as African Americans,[45,46]

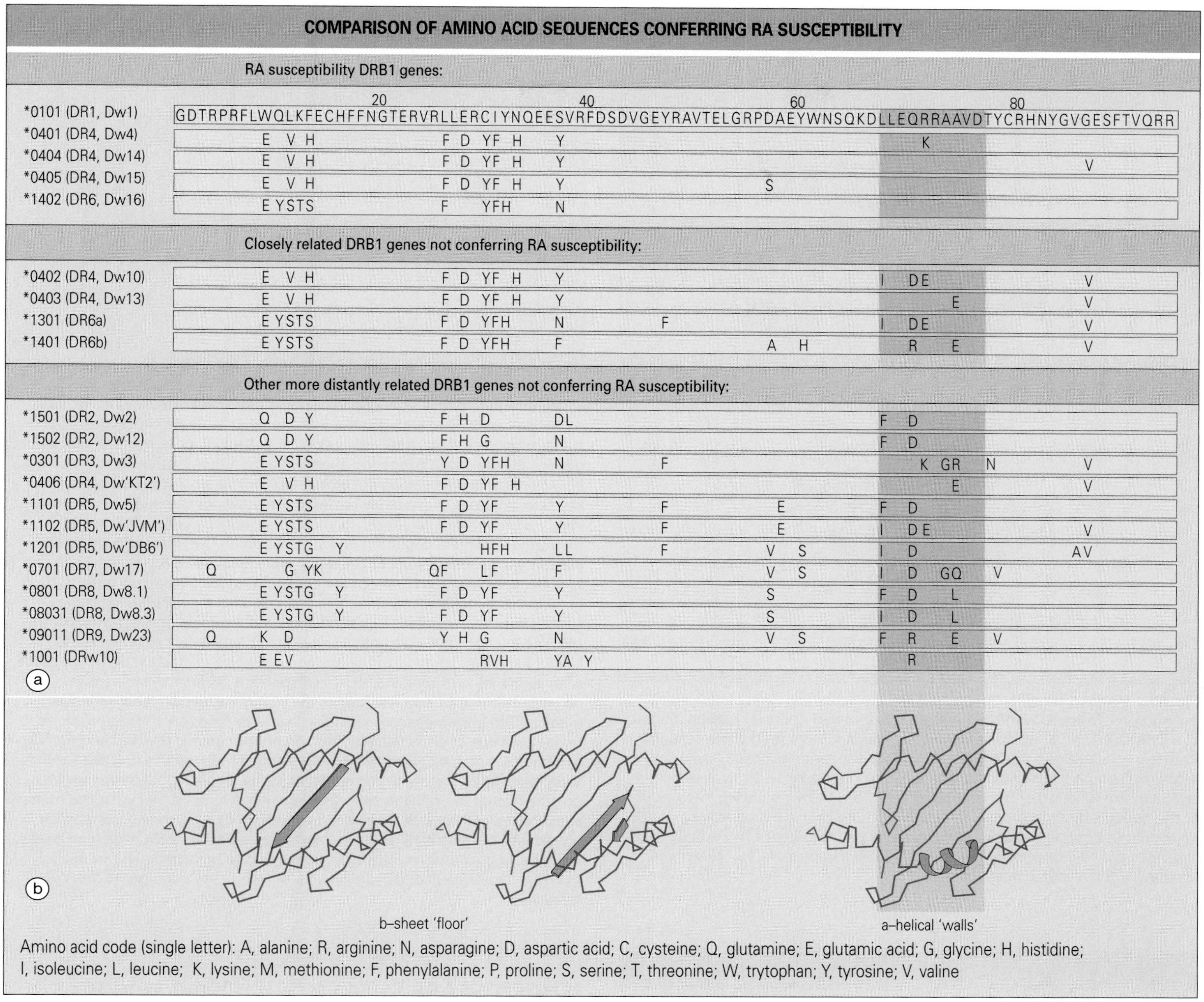

COMPARISON OF AMINO ACID SEQUENCES CONFERRING RA SUSCEPTIBILITY

RA susceptibility DRB1 genes:

*0101 (DR1, Dw1)	GDTRPRFLWQLKFECHFFNGTERVRLLERCIYNQEESVRFDSDVGEYRAVTELGRPDAEYWNSQKDLLEQRRAAVDTYCRHNYGVGESFTVQRR				
*0401 (DR4, Dw4)	E V H	F D YF H	Y	K	
*0404 (DR4, Dw14)	E V H	F D YF H	Y		V
*0405 (DR4, Dw15)	E V H	F D YF H	Y	S	V
*1402 (DR6, Dw16)	E YSTS	F YFH	N		

Closely related DRB1 genes not conferring RA susceptibility:

*0402 (DR4, Dw10)	E V H	F D YF H	Y	I DE	V
*0403 (DR4, Dw13)	E V H	F D YF H	Y	E	V
*1301 (DR6a)	E YSTS	F D YFH	N F	I DE	V
*1401 (DR6b)	E YSTS	F D YFH	F A H	R E	V

Other more distantly related DRB1 genes not conferring RA susceptibility:

*1501 (DR2, Dw2)	Q D Y	F H D DL		F D	
*1502 (DR2, Dw12)	Q D Y	F H G N		F D	
*0301 (DR3, Dw3)	E YSTS	Y D YFH N	F	K GR N	V
*0406 (DR4, Dw'KT2')	E V H	F D YF H		E	V
*1101 (DR5, Dw5)	E YSTS	F D YF Y	F E	F D	
*1102 (DR5, Dw'JVM')	E YSTS	F D YF Y	F E	I DE	V
*1201 (DR5, Dw'DB6')	E YSTG Y	HFH LL	F V S	I D	A V
*0701 (DR7, Dw17)	Q G YK	QF LF F	V S	I D GQ V	
*0801 (DR8, Dw8.1)	E YSTG Y	F D YF Y	S	F D L	
*08031 (DR8, Dw8.3)	E YSTG Y	F D YF Y	S	I D L	
*09011 (DR9, Dw23)	Q K D	Y H G N	V S	F R E V	
*1001 (DRw10)	E EV	RVH YA Y		R	

(a)

(b)

b–sheet 'floor'   a–helical 'walls'

Amino acid code (single letter): A, alanine; R, arginine; N, asparagine; D, aspartic acid; C, cysteine; Q, glutamine; E, glutamic acid; G, glycine; H, histidine; I, isoleucine; L, leucine; K, lysine; M, methionine; F, phenylalanine; P, proline; S, serine; T, threonine; W, trytophan; Y, tyrosine; V, valine

Fig. 86.2 Comparison of amino acid sequences conferring RA susceptibility. Sequences for HLA-DRB1 alleles that do or do not confer susceptibility to RA in different populations. (a) At the top are listed the sequence of the DRB1 alleles known to confer susceptibility to RA, with the shared epitope highlighted. The single-letter amino acid code, defined at the bottom of the figure, is used. Under these sequences are listed very similar sequences from closely related DRB1 alleles that do not confer RA susceptibility. Note the contrast in the sequences of other more distantly related DRB1 alleles that are now known to confer RA susceptibility. The shared epitope occurs only in susceptibility alleles and does not occur in non-susceptibility alleles, even when their "background" sequence is very similar or identical to the susceptibility alleles. (b) Schematic representation of how the amino acid sequence of the first domain of DRB1 relates to the three-dimensional conformation of the final molecule. Red-highlighted arrows correspond to clustered hypervariable sequences in the DRB1 regions shown above, illustrating that the shared epitope constitutes part of the α-helical "wall" of the antigen-binding groove.

whereas others have shown associations with DR markers that do not possess the SE (e.g., HLA-DR3 in Arabs).[47]

- Not all SEs are the same, with a hierarchy of risk attached to the associations with different HLA-DRB molecules. For example, the *0401 allele shows a much greater association with RA than *0101, particularly when *0401 is inherited in combination with *0404 (Table 86.2).[48-51]

- The *0404 and *0405 alleles have the identical SE sequence [70]QRRAA[74], yet have different effect sizes (as measured by the odds ratio [OR]).[33]

- The MHC is an extraordinarily gene-rich area, in which other loci in close proximity to the HLA-DRB1 gene might exert an impact on disease predisposition. This complexity is considered in further detail later.

- If the pathogenic process in RA is a simple presentation of arthritogenic peptide, this would intuitively fit with a dominant mode of inheritance. However, the SE genotype distribution fits better with a multiplicative mode of inheritance.[17,52-54] In keeping with a multiplicative mode of inheritance, concordance rates in siblings sharing two HLA haplotypes are double those of siblings sharing 1 or 0 haplotypes.[55,56] It has been argued that having two copies of the SE could influence downstream T-cell response through earlier effects in modeling the T-cell repertoire.[57]

ANTIGEN-BINDING CLEFT OF HLA-DR MOLECULE

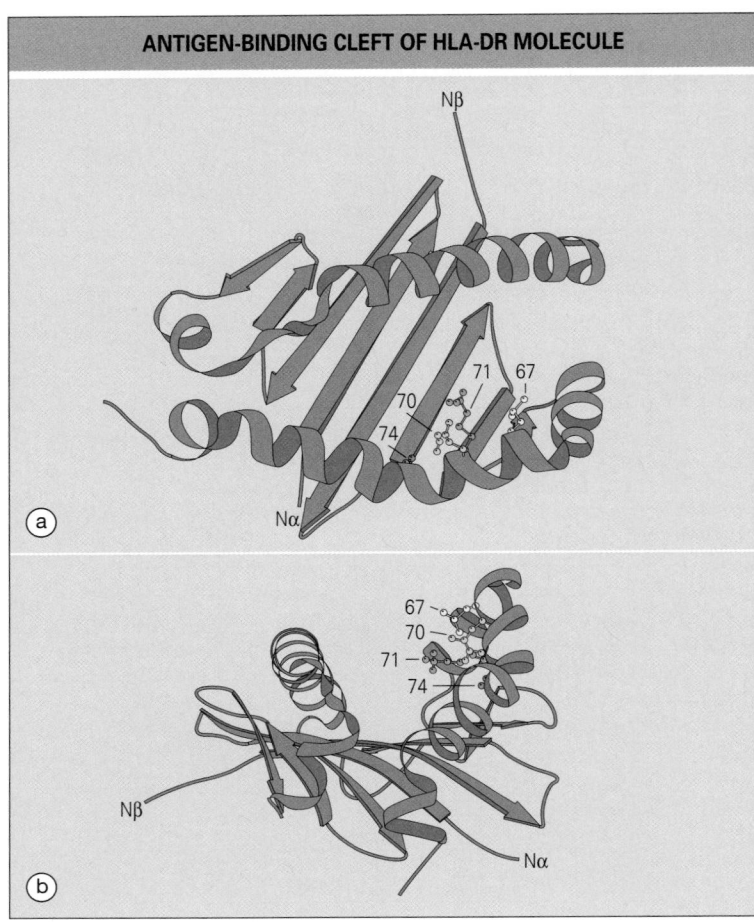

Fig. 86.3 Antigen-binding cleft of HLA-DR molecule. Location of important polymorphic residues with the RA-associated "shared epitope." Ribbon diagram of a DRA/DRB1*0401 molecule viewed (a) looking down from above and (b) from the side. Amino acids 67, 70, 71, and 74, the residues noted from sequence comparisons and from site-directed mutagenesis analysis to be critical in the function of the "shared epitope," are shown pointing into or out of the peptide-binding groove. Residues pointing into the groove are important in binding peptide, whereas those pointing out of the α-helix are hypothesized to interact directly with the T-cell receptor. Na, Nb, N-terminal residues of the α and β chains.

TABLE 86.2 RISK ESTIMATES FOR RHEUMATOID ARTHRITIS IN WHITES

HLA class II allele	Frequency/10,000 population		Approximate risk ratio
	+RA	No RA	
DRB *0401	50	1800	1 in 35
DRB *0404	25	500	1 in 20
DRB *0101	25	2000	1 in 80
0401 or 0404	65	2300	1 in 35
0401, 0404 or 0101	90	4200	1 in 46
0401 and 0404	15	100	1 in 7
Other	10	5800	1 in 580

These numbers represent the "absolute risk" of developing clinical RA among whites. They are based on a disease frequency of 7-10/1000 population and as such represent an upper limit of predictive value.
Adapted with permission from Nepom G. Prediction of susceptibility to rheumatoid arthritis by HLA genotyping. Rheum Dis Clin North Am 1992;18:785-792.

THREE MODELS FOR TcR–HLA MECHANISMS IN AUTOIMMUNITY

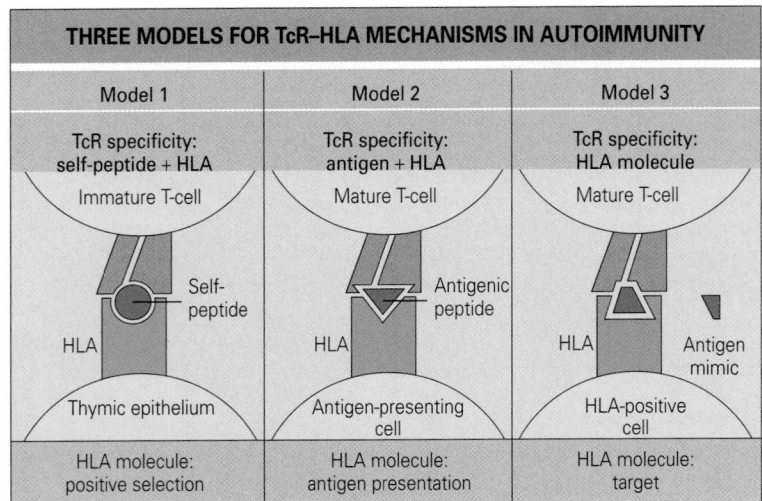

Fig. 86.4 Three models for T-cell receptor TcR-HLA mechanisms in autoimmunity. The key role of polymorphic amino acid residues in the HLA molecules associated with disease indicates that intimate contacts between these amino acids and antigenic peptides or the TcR, or both, are important genetically regulated triggering events in autoimmunity. In model 1, the polymorphic HLA molecule, in combination with a bound self-peptide, has a key selection role, presumably during the thymic development of maturing T cells. An immature T cell "tests" its receptor specificity before leaving the thymus; a suitable recognition and stimulation by the HLA molecule at this point is postulated to lead to the maturation and expansion of the T-cell specificity, which, in an appropriate context, may be potentially autoreactive. In model 2, a similar recognition event occurs in the peripheral immune system between a mature T cell and an HLA-expressing antigen-presenting cell. The polymorphic determinants on the HLA molecule determine the binding and presentation of the antigenic peptide related to the target tissue, such as the joint. In model 3, the T-cell specificity is directed toward the polymorphic amino acid residues of the HLA molecule itself by molecular mimicry. The immune response is postulated to focus on an HLA-positive target by virtue of cross reaction with an antigen mimic that has successfully bypassed normal tolerance mechanisms and stimulated the reactive T cell. A variation of the mimicry hypothesis that partly reconciles all three models postulates that the polymorphic sequence on the HLA molecule is the primary antigenic target but that this is seen by the TcR as a processed self-peptide, bound and presented by another intact HLA molecule. *(MHC structural models were constructed using molecular homology modeling techniques by Carol DeWeese, Department of Bioengineering, University of Washington School of Medicine.)*

MHC: DISEASE SUSCEPTIBILITY OR SEVERITY?

Irrespective of the limitations with the SE hypothesis, the MHC region demonstrates the strongest association with RA and in different family studies is the locus that has most consistently demonstrated genetic linkage.[9,58,59] However, a debate has been generated as to whether the HLA association is more important in predisposing to RA or determining disease severity.

For more than 20 years, studies have shown the HLA-DRB1 alleles are more frequently observed among patients with more severe disease. Clinically, RA is very heterogeneous: some patients have mild, self-limited disease, whereas others have severe multisystem disease. It is entirely plausible that genetic heterogeneity underlies such clinical heterogeneity. Studies in the 1980s suggested that the serologically defined HLA-DR4 association was not observed in community surveys, presumably representing milder RA.[60] Conversely, the HLA-DR4 association was very marked in patients with severe articular disease or extra-articular manifestations, such as Felty syndrome.[61] With the increasing sophistication of molecular typing, it was demonstrated that the SE was not associated with recent-onset inflammatory arthritis.[62] At the opposite end of the clinical spectrum, a meta-analysis of rheumatoid vasculitis[63] and a review of extra-articular manifestations of RA[64] have confirmed the importance of the SE in association with more severe disease. Multivariate analyses have indicated that the presence of the SE predicts erosions at RA presentation as well as erosive outcome at 3 years.[65-68]

The question remains: do SE alleles predict RA risk or RA severity? Genetic association studies alone may not be able to resolve this question. It could be that patients with a greater genetic burden of disease are more likely to develop more severe disease, regardless of which alleles predispose to RA. Or it may be that non-SE genetic factors predispose to risk, whereas SE predisposes to severity. However, all genetic factors are present throughout the life of a patient, and therefore by definition before disease onset. As a consequence, susceptibility and severity are inextricably linked.

ROLE OF NON-HLA GENES WITHIN THE MHC

As discussed briefly earlier, the MHC region encodes more than 180 expressed genes, many of which have immunoregulatory functions (Fig. 86.5).[69-71] Forty percent of the expressed loci have functions related to immune activation and response. Within the MHC, HLA genes are organized into three regions: classes I, II, and III.

1. The class I region, closest to the end of the chromosome (telomeric), contains the class I genes HLA-A, -B and -C.
2. Closer to the center of the chromosome (centromeric), the class II region consists of the HLA-DR, -DP and -DQ loci, encoding the α and β chains of the class II HLA molecules. One of these loci is the HLA-DRB1 gene, alleles of which show the most consistent associations with RA.
3. The class III region sits between the class I and II regions and contains a number of genes whose products are important in immune and inflammatory pathways (e.g., the tumor necrosis factor [TNF]-α locus).

Recombination of genetic material during meiosis in the MHC is rare, such that alleles at different loci within the MHC tend to be inherited as a complete unit, a phenomenon referred to as *linkage disequilibrium*. Consequently, this presents considerable challenges for determining whether alleles at a certain locus that associate with a disease are simply reflecting their close physical proximity to other more important predisposing loci.

Because of the shortcomings of the SE hypothesis, researchers have considered the possibility that other MHC genes might be important in disease predisposition and expression. Furthermore, the MHC has been found to contain multiple independent effects in a variety of complex diseases associated with different HLA-DRB1 alleles, such as multiple sclerosis, type 1 diabetes, and juvenile idiopathic arthritis.[72-74] One model that has been proposed suggests that DQB1*03 and *05 alleles are the true disease susceptibility alleles in RA and that DRB1 associations with RA merely reflect linkage disequilibrium. Some association studies in humans support a direct role for DQ alleles in RA,[75] whereas others have not.[29,76] Studies in severe disease such as Felty syndrome have suggested that the primary RA association is with DRB1*04 alleles.[77] Several studies have demonstrated interactions between the DR and DQ loci in determining disease expression, with HLA-DRB1*0401-DQB1*0301 associated with greater disease severity.[78] The bulk of the evidence supports a primary role for the HLA-DRB1 locus in RA[79] but leaves the door open for interactions between DR and DQ,[80] particularly in disease expression.

An increasing number of studies are addressing other MHC genes outside the class II region. In a Japanese study, four genes including TNF were reported to associate with RA independently from HLA-DRB1.[81] Other studies have supported associations of TNF polymorphisms with RA that are independent of the SE.[82-84] Tuokko and colleagues reported an increase in TNF microsatellites *a6* and *b5* in Finnish RA cases.[85] These alleles are known to be in linkage disequilibrium with DR4. A similar increase in the TNF microsatellite allele *a6* has also been reported in Peruvian RA patients.[86] This is intriguing because RA in this population is not associated with DR4 haplotypes but with DRB1*1402, and this association was found to be independent of the DRB1*1402 haplotype in this population, which suggests that the TNF locus may indeed be a second RA locus in the MHC. A promoter polymorphism in the nuclear factor of κ light polypeptide gene in B cells inhibitor-like 1 gene (*NFKBIL1*) has been suggested to be a further MHC RA susceptibility locus based on associations in a Japanese population.[87] Detailed analysis of a large collection of U.S. RA-affected sibling pairs has revealed at least two genetic effects in addition to DRB1 within the MHC.[88] A U.K. group has provided evidence for the independent effect of lymphotoxin-a (LTA)-TNF haplotypes,[89] consistent with earlier work implicating extended haplotypes stretching from HLA-DRB1 to TNF.[88] A further study has revealed an additional non-DRB1 RA susceptibility locus around the junction of the MHC class III and class I regions, a region rich in immunomodulatory genes.[90] Preliminary data have also implicated a gene known as *DEK*, which is telomeric to the HLA-DRB1 gene, as being independently associated with RA.[91] A study from France has suggested that HLA-DM alleles may represent new markers for RA severity, both independently and through interactions with HLA-DRB1 alleles.[92]

Advances in genomic technology, as described in more detail later, are beginning to unravel the complex genetic relationships within the MHC.[93-95] Several groups have performed high-density genotyping of single nucleotide polymorphism (SNP) across the MHC region in patients with RA. In these studies, thousands of SNPs are genotyped in a single experiment. These SNPs capture a large fraction of common alleles within the MHC region. This approach facilitates conditional analyses to tease apart independent signals. From these studies, at least two independent signals have emerged: alleles found on the conserved A1-B8-DR3 (8.1) haplotype and alleles near the HLA-DPB1 gene. The causal mutations to explain these independent genetic signals have not yet been identified.

In conclusion, the MHC demonstrates an extraordinary complexity of immunomodulatory genes in which researchers have attempted to dissect genetic contributions that are independent of the HLA-DRB1 locus. Further investigation of this rich area of the genome with a denser set of markers, including comparisons across different ethnic populations in order to capitalize on differences in extended HLA region haplotypes, will undoubtedly reveal additional loci that influence the risk and severity of RA.

ROLE OF NON-MHC GENES IN RHEUMATOID ARTHRITIS

Calculations based on monozygotic twin concordance rates and HLA haplotype sharing in affected sibling pairs indicate that HLA genes contribute approximately 30% of the total genetic risk for RA.[7,96] This leaves considerable room for other genes outside the HLA region to contribute to RA risk. It is likely that the remaining genetic risk is distributed among many loci across the human genome, with each locus contributing substantially less to overall RA risk compared to the HLA region.[97]

Genome-wide linkage scans in RA

The human genomes are riddled with DNA variants (alleles) that make each of us unique. There are single base-pair variants (also known as SNPs) and structural variants (including duplications and deletions of many kilobases of DNA). These variants are further classified by the frequency with which they are observed in the general population. As a rule of thumb, those variants present in more than 5% of chromosomes from the general population are considered "common" and those in less than 5% are considered "rare." The rare variants can be further classified as to whether they are "low frequency" (found in multiple families, but generally of a population frequency of more than 0.5%) or "private" (only segregating in a single family due to a recent *de novo* mutation).

A fundamental challenge in human genetics has been: *How do we systematically test human genetic variation for its role in human disease?* The ideal genetic study would re-sequence the entire human genome in a large collection of patients with a disease and controls in which detailed environmental exposures and clinical phenotypic information has been collected. Causal mutations would be recognized by a simple test of association between allele frequency in cases and controls, controlling for potential environmental and clinical confounders. Assuming complete coverage of the human genome, this hypothetical approach would identify all classes of DNA variants (e.g., SNPs, copy number variants) and the entire allele frequency spectrum (e.g., common and rare) in an unbiased manner. Such an approach, however,

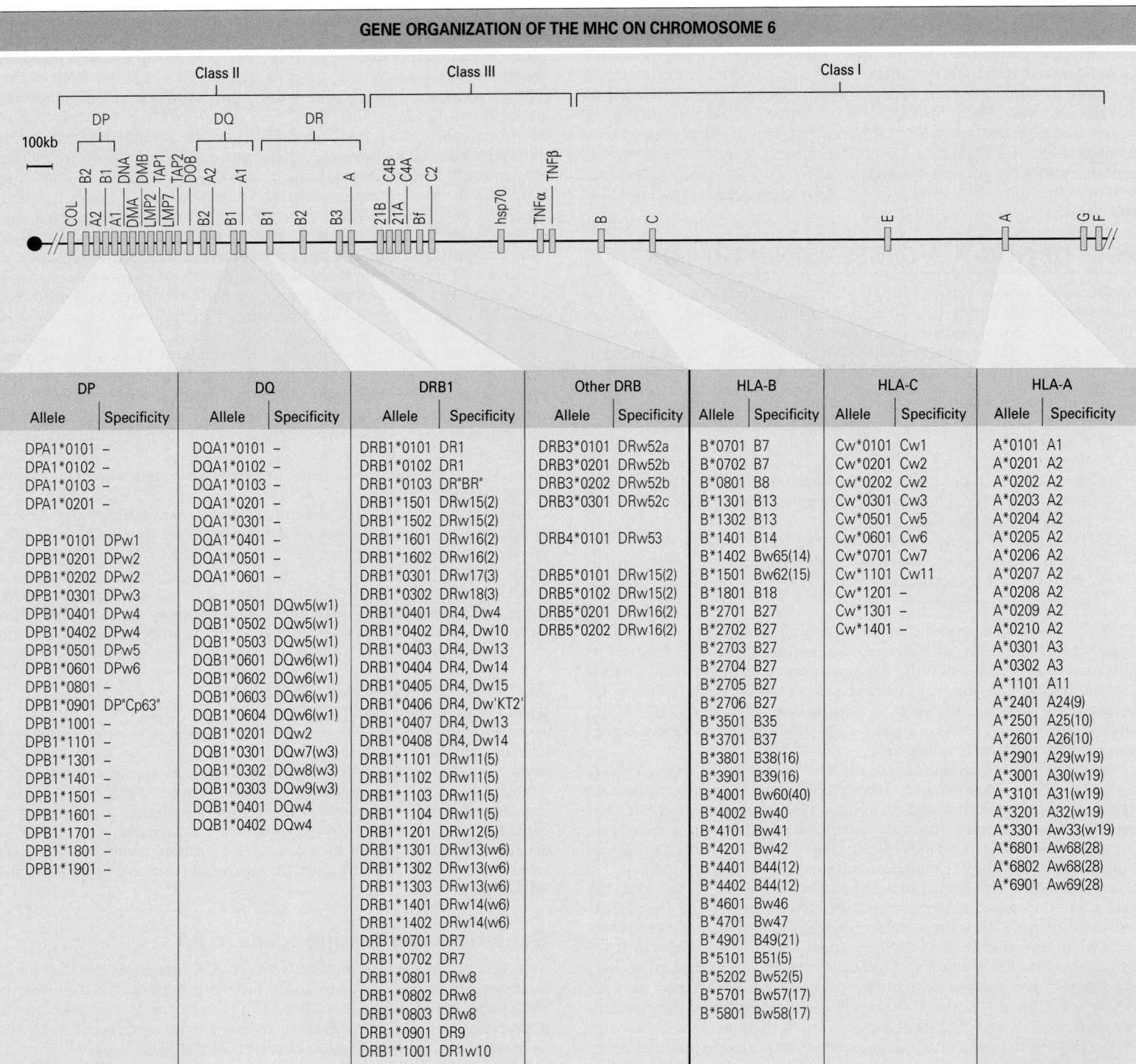

GENE ORGANIZATION OF THE MHC ON CHROMOSOME 6

DP		DQ		DRB1		Other DRB		HLA-B		HLA-C		HLA-A	
Allele	Specificity	Allele	Specificity	Allele	Specificity	Allele	Specificity	Allele	Specificity	Allele	Specificity	Allele	Specificity
DPA1*0101	–	DQA1*0101	–	DRB1*0101	DR1	DRB3*0101	DRw52a	B*0701	B7	Cw*0101	Cw1	A*0101	A1
DPA1*0102	–	DQA1*0102	–	DRB1*0102	DR1	DRB3*0201	DRw52b	B*0702	B7	Cw*0201	Cw2	A*0201	A2
DPA1*0103	–	DQA1*0103	–	DRB1*0103	DR"BR"	DRB3*0202	DRw52b	B*0801	B8	Cw*0202	Cw2	A*0202	A2
DPA1*0201	–	DQA1*0201	–	DRB1*1501	DRw15(2)	DRB3*0301	DRw52c	B*1301	B13	Cw*0301	Cw3	A*0203	A2
		DQA1*0301	–	DRB1*1502	DRw15(2)			B*1302	B13	Cw*0501	Cw5	A*0204	A2
DPB1*0101	DPw1	DQA1*0401	–	DRB1*1601	DRw16(2)	DRB4*0101	DRw53	B*1401	B14	Cw*0601	Cw6	A*0205	A2
DPB1*0201	DPw2	DQA1*0501	–	DRB1*1602	DRw16(2)			B*1402	Bw65(14)	Cw*0701	Cw7	A*0206	A2
DPB1*0202	DPw2	DQA1*0601	–	DRB1*0301	DRw17(3)	DRB5*0101	DRw15(2)	B*1501	Bw62(15)	Cw*1101	Cw11	A*0207	A2
DPB1*0301	DPw3			DRB1*0302	DRw18(3)	DRB5*0102	DRw15(2)	B*1801	B18	Cw*1201	–	A*0208	A2
DPB1*0401	DPw4	DQB1*0501	DQw5(w1)	DRB1*0401	DR4, Dw4	DRB5*0201	DRw16(2)	B*2701	B27	Cw*1301	–	A*0209	A2
DPB1*0402	DPw4	DQB1*0502	DQw5(w1)	DRB1*0402	DR4, Dw10	DRB5*0202	DRw16(2)	B*2702	B27	Cw*1401	–	A*0210	A2
DPB1*0501	DPw5	DQB1*0503	DQw5(w1)	DRB1*0403	DR4, Dw13			B*2703	B27			A*0301	A3
DPB1*0601	DPw6	DQB1*0601	DQw6(w1)	DRB1*0404	DR4, Dw14			B*2704	B27			A*0302	A3
DPB1*0801	–	DQB1*0602	DQw6(w1)	DRB1*0405	DR4, Dw15			B*2705	B27			A*1101	A11
DPB1*0901	DP"Cp63"	DQB1*0603	DQw6(w1)	DRB1*0406	DR4, Dw'KT2'			B*2706	B27			A*2401	A24(9)
DPB1*1001	–	DQB1*0604	DQw6(w1)	DRB1*0407	DR4, Dw13			B*3501	B35			A*2501	A25(10)
DPB1*1101	–	DQB1*0201	DQw2	DRB1*0408	DR4, Dw14			B*3701	B37			A*2601	A26(10)
DPB1*1301	–	DQB1*0301	DQw7(w3)	DRB1*1101	DRw11(5)			B*3801	B38(16)			A*2901	A29(w19)
DPB1*1401	–	DQB1*0302	DQw8(w3)	DRB1*1102	DRw11(5)			B*3901	B39(16)			A*3001	A30(w19)
DPB1*1501	–	DQB1*0303	DQw9(w3)	DRB1*1103	DRw11(5)			B*4001	Bw60(40)			A*3101	A31(w19)
DPB1*1601	–	DQB1*0401	DQw4	DRB1*1104	DRw11(5)			B*4002	Bw40			A*3201	A32(w19)
DPB1*1701	–	DQB1*0402	DQw4	DRB1*1201	DRw12(5)			B*4101	Bw41			A*3301	Aw33(w19)
DPB1*1801	–			DRB1*1301	DRw13(w6)			B*4201	Bw42			A*6801	Aw68(28)
DPB1*1901	–			DRB1*1302	DRw13(w6)			B*4401	B44(12)			A*6802	Aw68(28)
				DRB1*1303	DRw13(w6)			B*4402	B44(12)			A*6901	Aw69(28)
				DRB1*1401	DRw14(w6)			B*4601	Bw46				
				DRB1*1402	DRw14(w6)			B*4701	Bw47				
				DRB1*0701	DR7			B*4901	B49(21)				
				DRB1*0702	DR7			B*5101	B51(5)				
				DRB1*0801	DRw8			B*5202	Bw52(5)				
				DRB1*0802	DRw8			B*5701	Bw57(17)				
				DRB1*0803	DRw8			B*5801	Bw58(17)				
				DRB1*0901	DR9								
				DRB1*1001	DR1w10								

Fig. 86.5 Gene organization of the MHC on chromosome 6. The MHC is located on the short arm of chromosome 6, with the centromere symbolized to the left. HLA genes cluster into two regions, class I and class II. Some of the class II genes are pseudogenes or are not known to be expressed; those transcribed and translated into α and β chains, which dimerize to form the classic class II proteins, are designated with shading (DP, DQ, DRB1, DRB3). The non-HLA class III cluster includes the genes for certain complement components (C4B, C4A, properdin factor B [Bf]), 21-hydroxylase (21B, 21A), a heat-shock protein (hsp70), and tumor necrosis factors (TNF-α, TNF-β). Other non-HLA genes encoded in the MHC that are known or suspected to be relevant for immune function or autoimmune disease include a gene for collagen (COL), peptide transporter molecules (TAP1 and TAP2), HLA-DMA and DMB, and two proteasome components (LMP2 and LMP7). The expressed HLA genes are highly polymorphic. The lower portion of the figure is a partial listing of nomenclature for some of the common polymorphic class I and class II alleles, along with previously used designations.

is impractical because of the limitations of current technology and of cost constraints.

Initial attempts to scan the human genome used hundreds of microsatellite markers and tests of "linkage" in families. These studies rely on meiotic recombination between a microsatellite marker and an unknown mutation that increases risk of disease. This approach has been very successful in identifying rare, highly penetrant alleles that predispose to mendelian forms of disease. However, this strategy has had limited success in patients with more complex patterns of inheritance, such as RA. Several genome-wide linkage studies have been performed in RA.[9,58,59,98] These studies have uniformly identified the MHC region but otherwise no other consistent signal of linkage. Because of the theoretical limitations of linkage scans, researchers in the early 2000s turned their attention to genetic studies of "association."

Candidate gene association studies in RA

An alternative statistical approach to genome-wide linkage was to conduct genome-wide association studies. Instead of mapping disease genes by following transmission in families, association studies compare the frequencies of genetic variants among affected and unaffected individuals. Theoretically, association studies have more power than linkage studies to detect common variants of modest effect size.[99,100] Until recently, genetic association studies were limited to candidate genes. This was simply a matter of practicality: it was prohibitively expensive to genotype more than a handful of SNPs in large patient samples. Furthermore, there was no comprehensive map of common genetic variation, and it was unclear how many SNPs would need to be genotyped to test the majority of common human variation.

One solution in the early 2000s was to select biologically plausible candidate genes and test SNPs that were found in and around these genes. A major limitation of the approach was obvious: there are more than 20,000 genes in the human genome and most candidate gene studies are limited to a small number of candidate genes. There were a handful of successes.

PTPN22

One candidate gene association study selected putative functional SNPs from a set of biologic candidate genes. By this approach, a missense SNP in the intracellular *PTPN22* gene was identified.[101] Outside the MHC region this became the first gene to be widely replicated in multiple independent collections.[102-110] The susceptibility allele is a missense variant that changes an arginine to tryptophan amino acid (R620W). The change results in altered binding of the PTPN22 protein to an intracellular signaling molecule called Csk, which subsequently alters the threshold of T-cell activation.[101,111] The magnitude of the genetic effect, as measured by the odds ratio (OR), is substantially less than for HLA-DRB1*0401 but similar to other SE alleles (*PTPN22*, OR ~1.75). Interestingly, this allele is absent for East Asians and thus not associated with susceptibility in Japanese populations.[112] *PTPN22* only associates with seropositive RA. There is some evidence that *PTPN22* influences age at onset[106] and may have a more significant effect in males compared with females,[106,113] but there is no evidence that it influences disease activity or radiographic erosions.[105,114]

PADI4

PADI4 encodes for an enzyme that post-translationally modifies arginine to citrulline and may therefore be important in generating ACPA autoantibodies. Based on this hypothesis, a Japanese group tested more than 100 SNPs in the region that contains *PADI4* and a cluster of related genes. In the initial report, a common variant (population allele frequency ~35%) was found to increase the risk of RA.[115] Subsequent reports provide support for this allele among individuals of Asian ancestry, with a meta-analysis OR equal to 1.30 per copy of the risk allele.[116] The same allele is either not associated or only modestly associated (OR < 1.10) with the risk of RA among individuals of European ancestry.[106,116,117]

CTLA4

CTLA4 is a negative regulator of T-cell activation. Based on this biology, genetic studies in the early 2000s tested SNPs for association with several autoimmune phenotypes. The association between *CTLA4* and susceptibility to autoimmunity was initially confirmed among patients with type 1 diabetes and autoimmune thyroiditis.[118] An allele in the 3′ untranslated region (UTR) of the gene causes a modest increase in disease risk (OR = 1.2). Several studies extended these findings to RA, where the magnitude of the genetic effect is reproducible but modest (OR = 1.15).[106,119] The association is stronger among autoantibody-positive RA patients.

STAT4

Another strategy for choosing candidate genes is to select those that are biologically plausible *and* localize under suggestive regions of linkage. By this strategy, Remmers and colleagues studied haplotype tagging SNPs within 13 candidate genes under a linkage peak on chromosome 2.[120] In a staged-design of more than 7500 case-control samples, one SNP was reproducibly associated with risk of RA (OR =

1.20). This result has been replicated by others.[121-127] *STAT4* plays a critical role in differentiation of T cells into distinct lineages. It is unclear whether the risk allele alters *STAT4* gene expression. There is no known coding variant that disrupts STAT4 function.

Genome-wide association studies in RA

These four successes notwithstanding, the majority of candidate gene association studies have not led to reproducible genetic associations in RA[106] nor other complex traits.[128,129] Accordingly, a set of resources has been developed to test systematically the majority of common SNPs for their role in disease. The rationale for this approach is rooted in population genetic theory: common SNPs explain much of the genetic diversity in our species. This is a consequence of the historically small size and shared ancestry of the human population.

There are approximately 10 million common SNPs in the human genome, although 9 of 10 of these SNPs are highly correlated ($r2 > 0.80$).[130,131] As a consequence, not every SNP in the human genome needs to be tested directly in a genetic association study. A subset of "tagging" SNPs can adequately capture the majority of common genetic variation across a locus; this is also known as linkage disequilibrium mapping. The International Haplotype Map (HapMap) Project provides a catalog of common SNPs in the human genome,[130,131] which facilitates linkage disequilibrium mapping. The HapMap has genotyped more than 3 million SNPs in four reference groups totaling 270 individuals.

Genetic studies of common variants can now be conducted across the entire human genome. These studies, termed genome-wide association studies (GWAS), are feasible owing to an improved understanding of linkage disequilibrium structure across the human genome,[130,131] technical capacity to genotype hundreds of thousands of SNPs in a cost-effective manner,[132] and methods to analyze large datasets.[133,134] GWAS have a distinct advantage over previous genetic studies in that they are able to test, in an unbiased manner, the majority of common SNPs across the genome in a single experiment. Implementation of GWAS has greatly expanded the number of true-positive loci (i.e., those that have been replicated consistently in more than one study at a high level of statistical confidence) that are associated with complex traits.[129]

In 2007, three GWAS in RA were published that identified two new RA risk loci.[135-137] One GWAS was a collaborative effort between groups in North America; North American Rheumatoid Arthritis Consortium (NARAC), and Sweden; Epidemiological Investigation of Rheumatoid Arthritis (EIRA).[137] A total of approximately 1500 ACPA-positive RA patients and approximately 1800 controls were genotyped for more than 300,000 SNPs, followed by replication of the most significant SNPs in an additional approximately 1000 ACPA-positive RA cases and approximately 1700 controls. The most significant result outside of *PTPN22* and the MHC loci was the *TRAF1-C5* locus. A single SNP on chromosome 9 was strongly associated with susceptibility to ACPA-positive RA (OR = 1.20). An independent group identified the same DNA variant as part of a candidate gene association study.[138] Additional studies have replicated the *TRAF1-C5* association,[124,139,140] including a study of more than 10,000 U.K. samples by the Wellcome Trust Case Control Consortium (WTCCC).[121]

Two other GWAS led to the identification of the *TNFAIP3* locus on chromosome 6q23.[135,136,141] Interestingly, two independent risk alleles were identified, although both were within 5 kb of each other. Both alleles reside approximately 185 kb away from the nearest biologic candidate gene, *TNFAIP3*. The distance of the risk alleles from the nearest candidate gene underscores a limitation of candidate gene association studies: many risk alleles reside some distance from the protein-coding sequence. *TNFAIP3*, also known as A20, is a potent inhibitor of NF-κB signaling and is required for termination of TNF-induced signals.[142] TNF-α levels are increased in patients with RA, and inhibition of TNF-α is a potent treatment of severe RA.[143] Furthermore, mice lacking *Tnfaip3* demonstrate chronic inflammation,[144] consistent with loss of function of this gene playing a role in autoimmunity. Although it may be logical to conclude that the RA risk alleles alter *TNFAIP3* expression, there are no direct data to support this claim. A variety of 6q23/*TNFAIP3* alleles, some of which are different than the RA risk alleles, contribute to the risk of other autoimmune diseases, including systemic lupus erythematosus,[145,146] type 1 diabetes,[147] celiac disease,[148] and psoriasis.[149]

Follow-up studies to these GWAS have identified approximately 10 additional RA risk loci. A meta-analysis of the three largest GWAS (EIRA, NARAC, and WTCCC), followed by independent replication in approximately 9000 RA case-control samples, identified at least five novel RA risk loci.[150] The most significant SNP from the meta-analysis study was located in the first intron of *CD40*. The risk allele has a frequency of 25% among controls and 22% among cases, yielding an OR of 0.86. Further support that this *CD40* variant is important in autoimmunity comes from published genetic studies of autoimmune thyroiditis, in which the same allele is associated with risk of disease.[151] The CD40 protein is a member of the TNF receptor superfamily and is expressed on the surface of developing B cells, monocytes, and T cells. Other genes implicated by this study include *CCL21*, *TNFRSF14*, *PRKCQ*, and *KIF5A-PIP4K2C*. Two of these same gene loci (*PRKCQ* and *KIF5A-PIP4K2C*), plus a third locus containing the *IL2RB* gene, were identified by an independent study from the WTCCC.[152]

Other GWAS follow-up studies have capitalized on the observation that many RA risk loci are associated with other autoimmune diseases. As an example, epidemiologic data suggest an overlap among the risk factors for type 1 diabetes and RA.[153] Consistent with this observation, a locus on 4q27, containing the *IL2* and *IL21* genes, demonstrates a clear association with risk of type 1 diabetes and a highly suggestive association with risk of RA.[154] Approximately half of the validated RA risk loci have strong evidence of association for at least one additional autoimmune disease. Often, the same allele confers risk in both autoimmune diseases (e.g., 4q27/IL2-IL21 and risk of RA/type 1 diabetes). In other instances, different alleles at the same locus confer risk of disease (e.g., *TNFAIP3* and risk of RA/psoriasis). Occasionally, the same allele confers risk in one disease and protection in another (e.g., *PTPN22* and risk of RA/Crohn disease).[155]

Although GWAS and related approaches have greatly expanded the number of RA risk loci, the validated non-MHC alleles explain less than 5% of disease variation.[150] The alleles identified to date are common and of modest effect size. Based on considerations of statistical power, many more RA common risk alleles will be identified in the near future. These discoveries will require continued international collaboration given the large sample sizes needed to achieve statistical significance.

Insight into RA pathogenesis from non-MHC genetic studies

Despite decades of research, the exact cause of RA is unknown.[156] Without knowing the specific pathways that lead to RA, it is very difficult to develop novel therapies and preventative strategies. Because genetic mutations are inherited before disease onset, human genetics provides *prima facie* evidence that a pathway is important in pathogenesis. Moreover, because human genetics can be done without any specific biologic hypothesis (other than the hypothesis that there are alleles that influence risk of RA), human genetics offers an unbiased search of the human genome.

When considering pathways implicated by genetic studies, there are two important caveats to the way in which risk alleles are often described. First, the risk locus is often assigned a gene name (e.g., *TNFAIP3*), even though there may be no direct evidence that the gene itself has been disrupted by the risk allele. Generally, the most-compelling biologic candidate gene from a locus is chosen. Sometimes the choice is clear, as in the case of *TNFAIP3* in which a knock-out mouse model demonstrates severe inflammation, consistent with the phenotype of RA.[144] And second, the reported risk allele most likely represents a highly correlated proxy for the as yet unidentified causal allele. In other words, for most RA risk loci, the exact causal mutation and the exact causal gene have not yet been determined.

Despite these caveats, recent genetic discoveries have identified pathways that are important in RA pathogenesis. One is the NF-κB signaling pathway.[157] NF-κB, a protein complex that acts as a transcription factor, is found in almost all cell types and is involved in a variety of cellular responses to stimuli. Both TNF and CD40 signal through NF-κB to exert their effects on the immune system. Several of the RA risk loci contain genes that are involved in NF-κB signaling, including *CD40*, *TRAF1*, *TNFAIP3*, *PRKCQ*, and *TNFRSF14*.

GENE AND ENVIRONMENT INTERACTIONS

With the heritability of RA approximately 60%,[11] the remainder of the variance in the disease must be accounted for by environmental, non-genetic factors, or complex gene-gene/gene-environment interactions. It seems plausible that interactions occur between genetic and environmental factors or that environmental factors function as "triggers" for promoting and driving the disease process.

Smoking is the known environmental risk factor with strongest risk of developing RA. Over the past 20 years, many studies have convincingly shown that smoking increases risk of developing RA in both males and females by a factor of 1.5 to 2.0.[158,159] Most of these studies demonstrate that the increased risk is in developing autoantibody-positive RA and that the risk is greatest for heavy, current smokers. The risk remains, however, for more than 10 years after smoking cessation.

Other putative environmental risk factors that have not been as widely replicated as smoking include blood transfusions, obesity, occupational silica and mineral oil exposure, and socioeconomic class.[160,161] It is interesting that several of these putative environmental factors are inhaled through the lungs. Silica dust and mineral oil exposure, similar to exposure to cigarette smoke, was a risk factor only for seropositive RA. Mineral oil can also act as an adjuvant capable of inducing experimental arthritis in rodent models.

But although smoking is a clear environmental risk factor, and many MHC and non-MHC genes confer risk of RA, the question remains: *is there an interaction between environmental and genetic risk factors that departs from an expected model?* A challenge in the field is the definition of "expected model." Given that most genetic risk factors conform to a multiplicative (or log-additive) model, the most conservative estimate is to define "interaction" as departure from a multiplicative model. The best example of a gene-environment interaction that appears to depart from a multiplicative model has been the interaction between cigarette smoking and HLA-DRB1 alleles. A study by Padyukov and colleagues using the Swedish EIRA cohort found evidence of an interaction between the presence of the SE and cigarette smoking.[162] Compared with patients who had never smoked and had no copies of the SE, they found an OR of 2.8 for seropositive smokers in SE-positive patients who had never smoked, an OR of 2.4 in current smokers without SE alleles, and an OR of 7.5 in current smokers with SE alleles. Smokers carrying two SE alleles displayed a relative risk of RF-positive RA of 15.7. No influence of smoking or SE alleles was seen for seronegative RA. These data suggest an interaction between smoking, SE alleles, and seropositive RA.

Clearly, additional work will be required to elucidate important interactions between genes and the environment. This will be an important area for future investigation and may empower better clinical prediction models or novel gene discovery.

CONCLUSION

There is considerable evidence that genetic factors are important in the predisposition to RA and contribute to the heterogeneity of the broad spectrum of disease that is currently classified as RA. The contribution of MHC genes and their interactions have yet to be fully elucidated, but recent work indicates that multiple genes within this region influence disease risk. The SE hypothesis alone does not fully explain the complexity of the MHC contribution to RA. Overall, the MHC contributes approximately one third of the total genetic contribution to RA. Advances in genetic technology have enable unbiased scans of the human genome, and, as a consequence, many non-MHC gene loci have been identified. Interactions between genes and environmental factors may be important, but work in this area is quite preliminary. Potential interactions between exposure to tobacco smoke and HLA and non-HLA genes are the best characterized to date. Clearly much progress has been made, although substantial work remains to fully explain the genetic contribution to RA. Progress in this area is likely to translate into greater understanding of disease pathogenesis and the development of improved diagnostic and therapeutic tools for this chronic and disabling illness.

KEY REFERENCES

1. Lawrence JS. Heberden oration, 1969. Rheumatoid arthritis—nature or nurture? Ann Rheum Dis 1970;29:357-379.
2. del Junco D, Luthra HS, Annegers JF, et al. The familial aggregation of rheumatoid arthritis and its relationship to the HLA-DR4 association. Am J Epidemiol 1984;119:813-829.
3. Silman AJ, MacGregor AJ, Thomson W, et al. Twin concordance rates for rheumatoid arthritis: results from a nationwide study. Br J Rheumatol 1993;32:903-907.
4. Aho K, Koskenvuo M, Tuominen J, Kaprio J. Occurrence of rheumatoid arthritis in a nationwide series of twins. J Rheumatol 1986;13:899-902.
7. Deighton CM, Walker DJ, Griffiths ID, Roberts DF. The contribution of HLA to rheumatoid arthritis. Clin Genet 1989;36:178-182.
11. MacGregor AJ, Snieder H, Rigby AS, et al. Characterizing the quantitative genetic contribution to rheumatoid arthritis using data from twins. Arthritis Rheum 2000;43:30-37.
14. Stastny P. Mixed lymphocyte cultures in rheumatoid arthritis. J Clin Invest 1976; 57:1148-1157.
15. Stastny P. Association of the B-cell alloantigen DRw4 with rheumatoid arthritis. N Engl J Med 1978;298:869-871.
18. Wordsworth BP, Lanchbury JS, Sakkas LI, et al. HLA-DR4 subtype frequencies in rheumatoid arthritis indicate that DRB1 is the major susceptibility locus within the HLA class II region. Proc Natl Acad Sci U S A 1989;86:10049-10053.
19. Lee HS, Lee KW, Song GG, et al. Increased susceptibility to rheumatoid arthritis in Koreans heterozygous for HLA-DRB1*0405 and *0901. Arthritis Rheum 2004;50:3468-3475.
32. Gregersen PK, Silver J, Winchester RJ. The shared epitope hypothesis: an approach to understanding the molecular genetics of susceptibility to rheumatoid arthritis. Arthritis Rheum 1987;30:1205-1213.
33. Fernando MM, Stevens CR, Walsh EC, et al. Defining the role of the MHC in autoimmunity: a review and pooled analysis. PLoS Genet 2008;4:e1000024.
34. Huizinga TW, Amos CI, van der Helm-van Mil AH, et al. Refining the complex rheumatoid arthritis phenotype based on specificity of the HLA-DRB1 shared epitope for antibodies to citrullinated proteins. Arthritis Rheum 2005;52:3433-3438.
35. Irigoyen P, Lee AT, Wener MH, et al. Regulation of anti-cyclic citrullinated peptide antibodies in rheumatoid arthritis: contrasting effects of HLA-DR3 and the shared epitope alleles. Arthritis Rheum 2005;52:3813-3818.
55. Deighton CM, Wentzel J, Cavanagh G, et al. Contribution of inherited factors to rheumatoid arthritis. Ann Rheum Dis 1992;51:182-185.
56. Rigby AS, MacGregor AJ, Thomson G. HLA haplotype sharing in rheumatoid arthritis sibships: risk estimates subdivided by proband genotype. Genet Epidemiol 1998;15:403-418.
58. MacKay K, Eyre S, Myerscough A, et al. Whole-genome linkage analysis of rheumatoid arthritis susceptibility loci in 252 affected sibling pairs in the United Kingdom. Arthritis Rheum 2002;46:632-639.

68. Gorman JD, Lum RF, Chen JJ, et al. Impact of shared epitope genotype and ethnicity on erosive disease: a meta-analysis of 3,240 rheumatoid arthritis patients. Arthritis Rheum 2004;50:400-412.
88. Jawaheer D, Li W, Graham RR, et al. Dissecting the genetic complexity of the association between human leukocyte antigens and rheumatoid arthritis. Am J Hum Genet 2002;71:585-594.
93. Lee HS, Lee AT, Criswell LA, et al. Several regions in the major histocompatibility complex confer risk for anti-CCP-antibody positive rheumatoid arthritis, independent of the DRB1 locus. Mol Med 2008;14:293-300.
95. Ding B, Padyukov L, Lundstrom E, et al. Different patterns of associations with anti-citrullinated protein antibody-positive and anti-citrullinated protein antibody-negative rheumatoid arthritis in the extended major histocompatibility complex region. Arthritis Rheum 2008;60:30-38.
101. Begovich AB, Carlton VE, Honigberg LA, et al. A missense single-nucleotide polymorphism in a gene encoding a protein tyrosine phosphatase (PTPN22) is associated with rheumatoid arthritis. Am J Hum Genet 2004;75:330-337.
102. Hinks A, Barton A, John S, et al. Association between the PTPN22 gene and rheumatoid arthritis and juvenile idiopathic arthritis in a UK population: further support that PTPN22 is an autoimmunity gene. Arthritis Rheum 2005;52:1694-1699.
103. Lee AT, Li W, Liew A, et al. The PTPN22 R620W polymorphism associates with RF positive rheumatoid arthritis in a dose-dependent manner but not with HLA-SE status. Genes Immun 2005;6:129-133.
106. Plenge RM, Padyukov L, Remmers EF, et al. Replication of putative candidate-gene associations with rheumatoid arthritis in >4,000 samples from North America and Sweden: association of susceptibility with PTPN22, CTLA4, and PADI4. Am J Hum Genet 2005;77:1044-1060.
115. Suzuki A, Yamada R, Chang X, et al. Functional haplotypes of PADI4, encoding citrullinating enzyme peptidylarginine deiminase 4, are associated with rheumatoid arthritis. Nat Genet 2003;34:395-402.
116. Iwamoto T, Ikari K, Nakamura T, et al. Association between PADI4 and rheumatoid arthritis: a meta-analysis. Rheumatology (Oxford) 2006;45:804-807.
117. Barton A, Bowes J, Eyre S, et al. A functional haplotype of the PADI4 gene associated with rheumatoid arthritis in a Japanese population is not associated in a United Kingdom population. Arthritis Rheum 2004;50:1117-1121.
120. Remmers EF, Plenge RM, Lee AT, et al. STAT4 and the risk of rheumatoid arthritis and systemic lupus erythematosus. N Engl J Med 2007;357:977-986.
121. Barton A, Thomson W, Ke X, et al. Re-evaluation of putative rheumatoid arthritis susceptibility genes in the post-genome wide association study era and hypothesis of a key pathway underlying susceptibility. Hum Mol Genet 2008;17:2274-2279.
122. Kobayashi S, Ikari K, Kaneko H, et al. Association of STAT4 with susceptibility to rheumatoid arthritis and systemic lupus erythematosus in the Japanese population. Arthritis Rheum 2008;58:1940-1946.

123. Lee HS, Remmers EF, Le JM, et al. Association of STAT4 with rheumatoid arthritis in the Korean population. Mol Med 2007;13:455-460.
129. Altshuler D, Daly MJ, Lander ES. Genetic mapping in human disease. Science 2008;322:881-888.
131. Consortium TIHM. A haplotype map of the human genome. Nature 2005;437:1299-1320.
135. Consortium WTCC. Genome-wide association study of 14,000 cases of seven common diseases and 3,000 shared controls. Nature 2007;447:661-678.
136. Plenge RM, Cotsapas C, Davies L, et al. Two independent alleles at 6q23 associated with risk of rheumatoid arthritis. Nat Genet 2007;39:1477-1482.
137. Plenge RM, Seielstad M, Padyukov L, et al. TRAF1-C5 as a risk locus for rheumatoid arthritis—a genome-wide study. N Engl J Med 2007;357:1199-1209.
138. Kurreeman FA, Padyukov L, Marques RB, et al. A candidate gene approach identifies the TRAF1/C5 region as a risk factor for rheumatoid arthritis. PLoS Med 2007;4:e278.
140. Chang M, Rowland CM, Garcia VE, et al. A large-scale rheumatoid arthritis genetic study identifies association at chromosome 9q33.2. PLoS Genet 2008;4:e1000107.
141. Thomson W, Barton A, Ke X, et al. Rheumatoid arthritis association at 6q23. Nat Genet 2007;39:1431-1433.
144. Lee EG, Boone DL, Chai S, et al. Failure to regulate TNF-induced NF-kappaB and cell death responses in A20-deficient mice. Science 2000;289:2350-2354.
145. Musone SL, Taylor KE, Lu TT, et al. Multiple polymorphisms in the TNFAIP3 region are independently associated with systemic lupus erythematosus. Nat Genet 2008;40:1062-1064.
146. Graham RR, Cotsapas C, Davies L, et al. Genetic variants near TNFAIP3 on 6q23 are associated with systemic lupus erythematosus. Nat Genet 2008;40:1059-1061.
147. Fung E, Smyth DJ, Howson JM, et al. Analysis of 17 autoimmune disease-associated variants in type 1 diabetes identifies 6q23/TNFAIP3 as a susceptibility locus. Genes Immun 2009;10:188-191.
150. Raychaudhuri S, Remmers EF, Lee AT, et al. Common variants at CD40 and other loci confer risk of rheumatoid arthritis. Nat Genet 2008;40:1216-1223.
152. Barton A, Thomson W, Ke X, et al. Rheumatoid arthritis susceptibility loci at chromosomes 10p15, 12q13 and 22q13. Nat Genet 2008;40:1156-1159.
154. Zhernakova A, Alizadeh BZ, Bevova M, et al. Novel association in chromosome 4q27 region with rheumatoid arthritis and confirmation of type 1 diabetes point to a general risk locus for autoimmune diseases. Am J Hum Genet 2007;81:1284-1288.
159. Stolt P, Bengtsson C, Nordmark B, et al. Quantification of the influence of cigarette smoking on rheumatoid arthritis: results from a population based case-control study, using incident cases. Ann Rheum Dis 2003;62:835-841.
161. Silman AJ, Pearson JE. Epidemiology and genetics of rheumatoid arthritis. Arthritis Res 2002;4(Suppl 3):S265-S272.
162. Padyukov L, Silva C, Stolt P, et al. A gene-environment interaction between smoking and shared epitope genes in HLA-DR provides a high risk of seropositive rheumatoid arthritis. Arthritis Rheum 2004;50:3085-3092.

REFERENCES

Full references for this chapter can be found on www.expertconsult.com.

Animal models of arthritis

Wim B. van den Berg

87

- Arthritis may be induced in animals by immunization with cartilage components, by non-specific immune stimuli, by bacterial or viral components, or by transgenic manipulation.

- Animal models are tools that mimic various aspects but never fully resemble human RA.

- Models have a defined onset and are useful for kinetic evaluation of arthritis, cell and mediator involvement, and detailed analysis of joint erosion.

- Animal models serve an important role in the evaluation of antirheumatic treatments and provide direction for novel approaches to treatments such as cytokine inhibition.

INTRODUCTION

Experimental animal models of arthritis have contributed to the understanding of basic mechanisms of joint disease. A marked diversity is seen among the numerous models, with arthritis induced by the following:

- Immunization with cartilage components
- Injection of non-specific immune stimuli
- Components of infectious agents
- Immune complexes
- Manipulation of genetic information in transgenic animals

No single animal model of arthritis truly represents the human disease. The wide variety of agents that can induce an experimental arthritis with clinical and histopathologic features close to human arthritides suggests that disparate etiologic pathways could exist in rheumatoid arthritis (RA). Aspects peculiar to individual models are of value but must be interpreted with caution. Much can be learned from general validity of mediator involvement and common concepts. Models provide valuable preclinical data for the development of novel treatments, both pharmacologic and biologic, and insights into relevant mechanisms common to experimental arthritis and RA.

MECHANISMS OF INDUCTION OF EXPERIMENTAL ARTHRITIS

Autoimmunity to cartilage components

Articular cartilage is an intriguing tissue. It is the target of the disease, but it may also function as the trigger, by releasing potential autoantigens and trapping exogenous antigens in its avascular matrix. Destructive forms of RA tend to decline when cartilage is fully destroyed, whereas arthritis also wanes in joints undergoing replacement surgery, both arguments for a crucial role in the arthritic process. Classic arthritis models based on cartilage autoimmunity[1] can be induced by immunization with either of the two major components of hyaline cartilage: type II collagen (CII) and aggrecan proteoglycans (PGs). More recently, similar models have been made identifying other, less abundant cartilage components as potential autoantigens in arthritis.

In principle, any cartilage matrix component can be a potential arthritogen, provided it is released in substantial amounts and natural tolerance is lost. Collagen-induced arthritis (CIA) can be elicited in mice, rats, and primates,[2,3] whereas PG arthritis has only been successfully established in BALB/c mice.[4,5] Both models require induction of a vigorous immune response directed initially against the immunizing (heterologous) cartilage antigen, which subsequently reacts with autologous cartilage antigens. A hypothetic mechanism for the development of collagen-induced and proteoglycan-induced experimental arthritides is shown in Fig. 87.1.

Susceptible strains of animals immunized with either type II collagen or high-density aggrecan proteoglycans in adjuvant recognize specific epitopes presented in the context of major histocompatibility complex (MHC) class II antigens, the equivalent of human leukocyte antigen (HLA)-D region antigens. Autoreactive CD4$^+$ T cells respond against either cross-reactive epitopes (antigens common to both the heterologous and autologous cartilage components) or cryptic epitopes (privileged antigens normally concealed from immune surveillance) and elicit connective tissue antigen-specific Th1 and Th17 cells and autoantibodies. Adoptive and passive transfer experiments suggest that both immunologic elements are required for the generation of chronic arthritis, although transient but destructive forms can be elicited with cocktails of anti-CII autoantibodies only. The localization of antibody and reactive cells in synovial joints causes immune-mediated cartilage damage and the immune response may be perpetuated by the release of cartilage antigens. These damage-associated molecular patterns (DAMPS) may also directly activate cells through toll-like receptors (TLRs), in particular TLR4.

The pathologies of CIA and PG arthritis appear similar and include synovial hypertrophy and hyperplasia, giving rise to pannus formation and severe cartilage erosion. Both models were considered Th1 driven, yet interferon (IFN)-γ deficiency makes Balb/c mice more susceptible to CIA, whereas it prevents proteoglycan arthritis. More recent insight indicated a dominant role of Th17 cells in CIA, whereas Th1 cells are crucial in proteoglycan arthritis,[6] and a role of Th17 in this model is unmasked only under IFN-γ–deficient conditions. The reason for different dominance of Th17 and Th1 in these models is unclear so far. Apparently, immunizations with various cocktails in different substrains of mice can give rise to variable dominance of Th1 and Th17, but both can lead to chronic arthritis. Neutralization of tumor necrosis factor (TNF) was efficacious in early stages of collagen arthritis, whereas IL-1 blocking and IL-17 neutralization suppressed both early and fully established arthritis.[7]

Response to non-specific immunologic stimuli

Injection of non-specific agents with adjuvant activity (the capacity to elicit an indirect immunologic response) can provoke experimental arthritis in certain species. The classic example is adjuvant-induced arthritis (AA) in the Lewis rat.[8] The precise contributions of the oil and the mycobacterial components of Freund complete adjuvant in the pathologic pathway of this experimental disease remain unclear, but both may contribute. A bacterium-specific pathogenesis seems likely in AA because conventionally bred rats are generally resistant to adjuvant arthritis, whereas germ-free Fisher or Wistar rats are susceptible. Germ-free rats lack early contact with bacteria and are therefore not tolerized. This is in striking contrast to suppression of pristane (mineral oil)–induced arthritis in germ-free mice, implying a different pathogenesis.

Adjuvant and pristane arthritis

Incomplete Freund adjuvant, lacking mycobacteria and the mineral oil pristane, can induce arthritis in susceptible rats and mice, identifying that oil can override natural tolerance.[9,10] Arthritogenic consequences appear ultimately to depend on a reaction against either exogenous or autologous antigens. Heat-shock proteins (HSPs) may be regulators in adjuvant-induced arthritis.[11] A hypothetic mechanism for the development of adjuvant-induced arthritis and pristane-induced arthritis is shown in Fig. 87.2. In susceptible strains of animals, macrophages

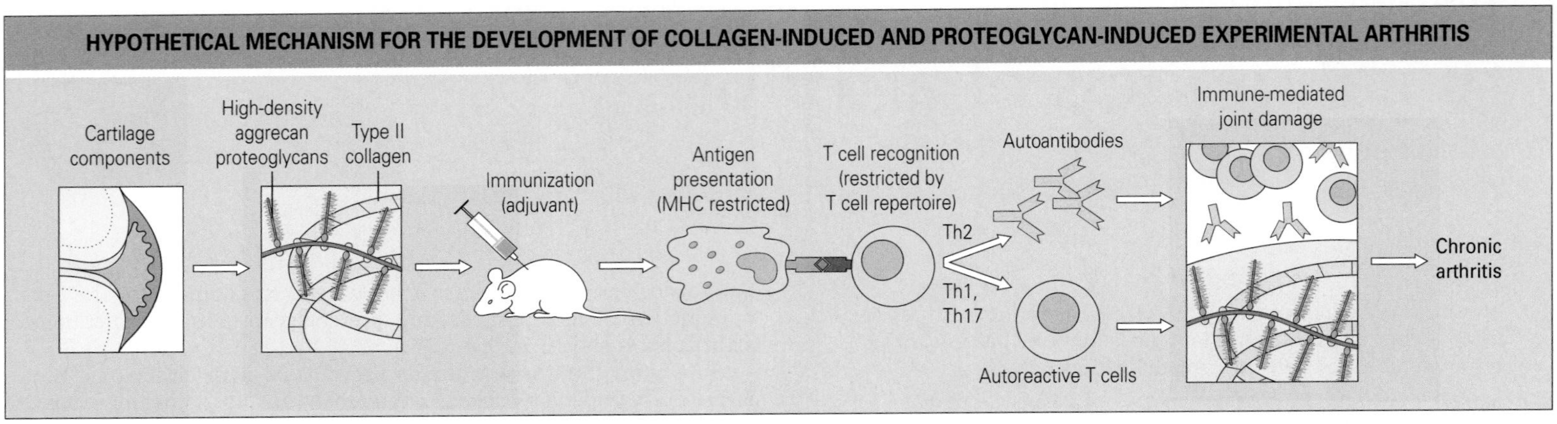

HYPOTHETICAL MECHANISM FOR THE DEVELOPMENT OF COLLAGEN-INDUCED AND PROTEOGLYCAN-INDUCED EXPERIMENTAL ARTHRITIS

Fig. 87.1 Hypothetic mechanism for the development of collagen-induced and proteoglycan-induced experimental arthritis. Animals are immunized with type II collagen or high-density aggrecan proteoglycans, and an autoimmune response results when specific epitopes are presented in the context of MHC class II antigens and recognized by autoreactive CD4+ T cell populations. Autoantibodies and T effector cells reactive against cartilage components develop via T helper pathways (Th1, Th17, and Th2) and localize in synovial joints, causing an immune-mediated inflammatory response. The immune response is perpetuated by the release of cartilage antigens within the damaged joint and chronic arthritis develops.

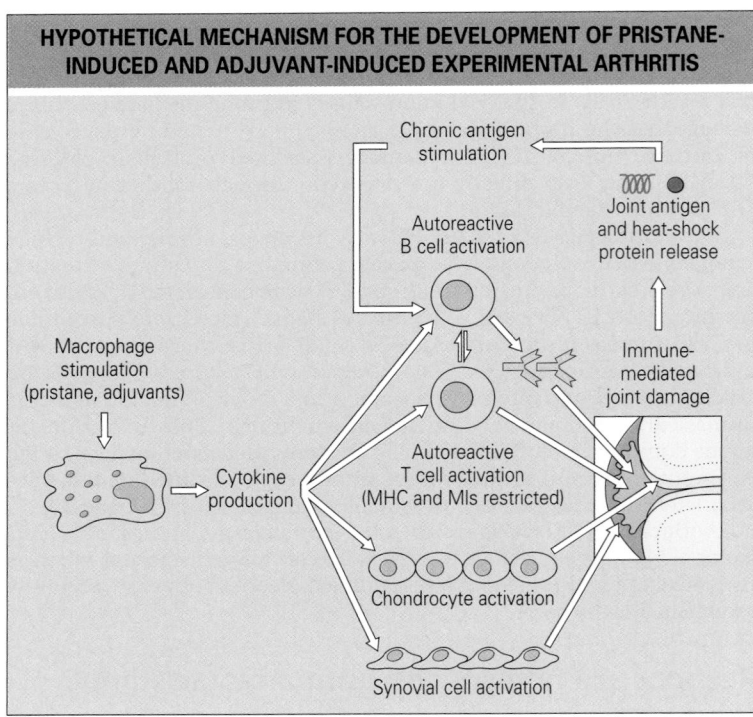

HYPOTHETICAL MECHANISM FOR THE DEVELOPMENT OF PRISTANE-INDUCED AND ADJUVANT-INDUCED EXPERIMENTAL ARTHRITIS

Fig. 87.2 Hypothetic mechanism for the development of pristane-induced and adjuvant-induced experimental arthritis. Circulating macrophages become intensely activated by the non-degradable oil components and produce high levels of proinflammatory cytokines (IL-1 and 6, TNF-α and IFN-γ). Genetic regulation governs the presence of autoreactive T cells and B cells, which become activated and clonally expand. Joint-reactive lymphocytes migrate to the joint, resulting in immune-mediated joint damage. The release of cartilage antigens and heat shock proteins may feed back to the autoreactive lymphocytes, resulting in chronic immune stimulation. Cytokines may also act directly on both synovial cells and chondrocytes, resulting in synovial hypertrophy, abnormal expression of MHC class II antigens, and adhesin molecules and atypical production of matrix components. Arthritis develops as a result of the chronic nature of the inflammatory stimulation.

phagocytose non-degradable oil components, become intensely activated, and produce large concentrations of proinflammatory cytokines (interleukins IL-1 and IL-6, TNF, and IFN-γ). This cytokine-rich environment activates T and B cells. The results of polyclonal activation are apparent in pristane-induced arthritis, in which lymphadenopathy and hypergammaglobulinemia precede the onset of disease.

Expansion of autoreactive T- and B-cell populations can occur as a consequence of the adjuvant activation process, resulting in the migration of cells to the joint and subsequent immune-mediated joint damage and production of a spectrum of autoantibodies against cartilage antigens. Production of rheumatoid factors in pristane-induced arthritis may serve to amplify the autoreactive process. Disease onset is rapid in adjuvant-induced arthritis (2 weeks), often followed by spontaneous remission. Pristane arthritis is slower (months) and shows remissions and relapses, with no indication of B-cell involvement at onset. The pristane model is highly suited to studying genes controlling onset, severity, and chronicity.[12] The spontaneous remission and lack of susceptibility to reinduction make adjuvant arthritis a suitable model for studies on regulation of T-cell tolerance. Histopathology of AA shows major involvement of the bone marrow, bone erosion, extensive bone apposition, and minor direct cartilage damage at early stages (Table 87.1). Indirect cartilage damage occurs later, mainly as a consequence of loss of underlying bone. The latter may explain the cartilage protective effect of treatment with osteoprotegerin (OPG), which is a selective inhibitor of the osteoclast activator RANKL.[13,14] Combination blocking of TNF and IL-1 shows optimal control of arthritis and joint destruction.[15]

Components of infectious agents

The development of arthritis as a consequence of infection is apparent in both natural and induced animal models. Infectious agents may be tropic for the joint as a result of expression of adhesins or other molecules that promote sequestration within synovial tissues. Bacterial cell wall and mycoplasma membrane components may also provide non-specific immune activation through mitogenic activity. Viral infection of synovial cells may elicit novel cell surface antigens or abnormal expression of activation antigens and the overproduction of autoantigens. Viral infection may also disrupt immune regulation, increasing proinflammatory cytokines and immune activity against normally immunologically privileged components of the joint.

Streptococcal cell wall arthritis

Persistence of antigens from micro-organisms within the joint can be critical for the induction of arthritis (Fig. 87.3). This point is emphasized by the model of streptococcal cell wall (SCW) experimental arthritis in rats.[16] It is induced in Lewis rats by the systemic injection of cell wall fragments of group A streptococci, which are highly resistant to biodegradation. A similar disease can be induced with cell wall fragments from other bacteria, such as *Lactobacillus casei* or *Eubacterium aerofaciens*. The underlying principle of this model resides in the poor degradability of the fragments, thereby creating a persistent stimulus.

The lactobacillus and eubacterial models are of particular interest for human disease because these bacteria are part of the normal gastrointestinal flora.[17] Extrapolation of this model to humans suggests that an enormous load of potential arthritogenic stimuli is continuously present in the normal gastrointestinal tract, fragments may

TABLE 87.1 MODELS OF ARTHRITIS

Model	Abbreviation	Species*	Feature	IC	T cell	Refs
Induced models						
Collagen-induced arthritis	CIA	DBA mouse	CII	+	+	2, 3
Proteoglycan arthritis	PG-A	Balb/c mouse	PG	+	+	4, 5
Adjuvant arthritis	AA	Lewis rat	Autoimmune	−	+	7, 10
Oil-induced arthritis	OIA	DA rat	Autoimmune	−	+	8
Pristane-induced arthritis	PIA	DA rat	Autoimmune	−	+	9, 11
Streptococcal cell wall arthritis	SCW-A	Lewis rat	Persistent bacteria	−	+	15, 16
Flare	SCW	Mouse	T IL-17	−	+	18, 19
Antigen-induced arthritis	AIA	Rabbit, mouse	Persistent antigen	+	+	22, 23
Flare	AIA	Mouse	T IL-17	−	+	25
Transgenic models						
KRN arthritis	KRN	K/BxN mouse	GPI	+	+	31, 32
TNF transgenic arthritis	TNFtg	Mouse	TNF overexpression	−	−	39, 40
IL-1 transgenic arthritis	IL-1tg	Mouse	IL-1 overexpression	−	−	43
IL-1ra transgenic arthritis	IL-1ra-/-	Balb/c mouse	Autoimmune T cells	±	+	44, 45
HTLV-induced arthritis	HTLV	Mouse	Viral, transgenic	−	+	34
SKG arthritis	SKG	Mouse	T cell defect	−	+	35, 36
GP130 arthritis	GP130	Mouse	STAT3 defect	−	+	37, 38

Mostly used: IC, immune complexes; GPI, glucose-6-phosphate isomerase.

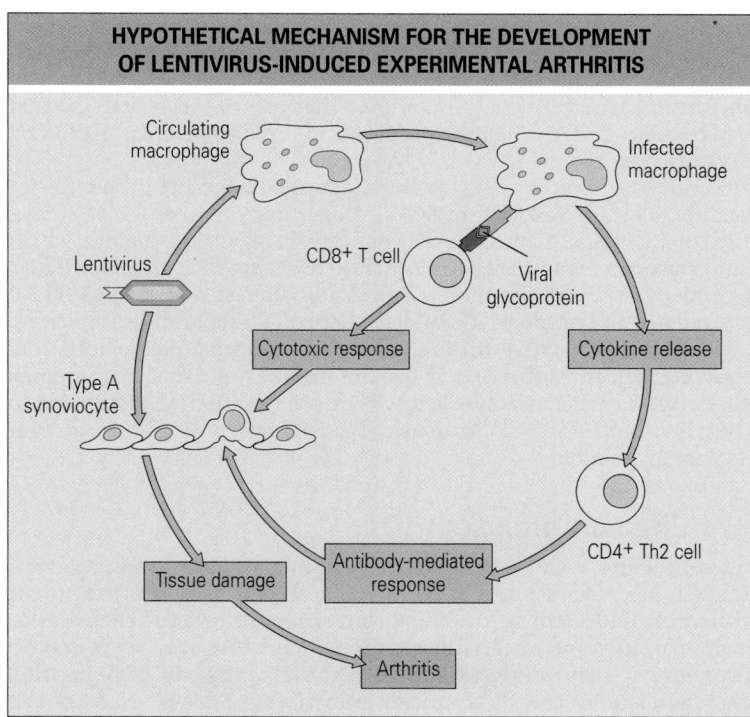

HYPOTHETICAL MECHANISM FOR THE DEVELOPMENT OF LENTIVIRUS-INDUCED EXPERIMENTAL ARTHRITIS

Fig. 87.3 Hypothetic mechanism for the development of lentivirus-induced experimental arthritis. The infection of macrophages and monocytes induces both the expression of cell surface viral antigens and cytokine release. The macrophage activation appears to promote both CD4+ Th2 cell expansion and the development of activated CD8+ T cells. T-cell cytotoxicity directed against infected type A (macrophage lineage) synovial cells may result in a local inflammatory reaction within the joint and cartilage may be damaged concomitantly. The increased Th2 activity may contribute to local immune complex formation, eventually leading to chronic inflammatory activity within the joint and the development of arthritis.

spread in a non-infectious way to other tissues, and this may provoke arthritis when control by immunoregulation is insufficient.

Within 24 hours of administration of cell wall fragments to rats, acute inflammation develops in peripheral joints, coincident with dissemination of cell wall fragments in blood vessels of the synovium and subchondral bone marrow. Acute, complement-dependent inflammation subsides over the next week and is followed within 2 weeks by a chronic, T cell–dependent erosive polyarthritis, involving mainly peripheral joints. In contrast with the acute phase, chronic joint inflammation develops only in susceptible strains, which are unable to maintain tolerance and display SCW-specific T-cell responses. Lewis rats are highly vulnerable to this arthritis. Mouse strains studied so far are not susceptible to the single intraperitoneal injection model, and repeat dosing was needed to break tolerance. It is tempting to speculate that similar loss of tolerance may occur in RA patients with age, combined with costimulatory environmental factors.

In addition to SCW-specific T-cell reactions, cross-reactive autoimmunity ranging from bacterial peptidoglycan to cartilage proteoglycans may contribute to chronicity. However, it is unlikely that the latter cross-reactivity is a major factor at onset because loss of proteoglycan from the articular cartilage is limited at that stage. Only later are marked pannus formation and severe erosions of underlying cartilage and bone frequently observed.

In line with tumor-like behavior of synovial cells in patients with RA, synovial cells from arthritic rats show continued proliferation *ex vivo*, with apparent paracrine and autocrine regulation by growth factors.[18] This observation suggests that sustained macrophage/fibroblast activation by retained bacterial components may be a perpetuating principle, but *in vivo* the T cell is still a critical driving factor. Studies on the involvement of cytokines in SCW arthritis show a combined role of TNF and IL-1, as found in adjuvant arthritis.[15,19] In mice, a chronic relapsing SCW model can be induced by repeated weekly injection of SCW fragments directly into the knee joint, displaying a gradually increasing role of T cell–derived IL-17 and synovial IL-17 receptor-bearing cells with every flare.[20,21]

As an extension of the involvement of bacteria in arthritis, studies have shown that bacterial DNA can induce arthritis. In particular, the CpG motifs in bacterial DNA are arthritogenic and substantial amounts can be found in joint tissues.[22] Macrophages play a major role in this arthritis through TNF production. However, in comparison with cell wall fragments, the cytokine-inducing capacity is weak. Normal joints of individuals contain both bacterial fragments and bacterial CpG (CP61) motifs and it is conceivable that both factors contribute to arthritis.

Antigen-induced arthritis

Antigen-induced arthritis (AIA) provides a designed model of development of chronic erosive arthritis, reflecting a sustained immune reaction to a persistent trigger in joint tissues, in this case a planted protein antigen. It is elicited by local injection of a high dose of antigen in the knee joint of an animal previously hyperimmunized with that antigen in Freund complete adjuvant. Such a model was first developed by Dumonde and Glynn[23] in rabbits. In principle, it can be induced in any species, provided that proper immunity to a particular antigen can be mounted. Applications have since been developed in mice, rats, and guinea pigs.

In contrast to the polyarthritis models described so far, this type of arthritis remains confined to the injected joint. Commonly used antigens are ovalbumin, bovine serum albumin, fibrin or cationic forms such as methylated BSA. Preimmunization with antigen in complete Freund adjuvant induces strong humoral and cell-mediated immunity. Arthritis is usually induced 3 weeks later by a local injection in the knee joint of a large amount of antigen. Initially an immune complex type of reaction dominates, followed by a T cell–mediated chronic inflammation. In the rabbit, chronicity may last for years. Histopathology shows a granulocyte-rich exudate in the joint space, thickening of the synovial lining layer and, at later stages, a predominantly mononuclear infiltrate in the synovium, which later includes numerous T cells and clusters of plasma cells. Interestingly, a large proportion (50%) of these plasma cells are making antibodies to the inciting antigen, suggesting that retained antigen is a driving force in chronic arthritis. Intense immune complex formation is seen in superficial layers of the articular cartilage, which may contribute to localized cartilage destruction. Early loss of proteoglycan, followed by pannus formation and cartilage and bone erosion, is a common finding.

Two important principles emerge from this model: first, chronicity is only found in the presence of sufficient antigen retention in joint tissues, in combination with proper T cell–mediated delayed hypersensitivity; second, joints contain numerous non- and avascular collagenous tissues such as cartilage, ligaments and tendons, which allow for prolonged antigen retention by antibody-mediated trapping and charge-mediated binding.[24,25] Importantly, antigen injected in the skin produces transient inflammation, whereas a similar dose in the joints causes chronic inflammation. Chronicity is caused by generation of local hyperreactivity. Antigen initially trapped in collagenous tissues is slowly released in time to sustain low-grade chronic arthritis. As a consequence, the local T-cell infiltrate gains specificity because retention of specific T cells is shaped by homologous antigen. Small amounts of antigen are sufficient to sustain arthritis, whereas relatively large amounts are necessary for induction. This condition forms the basis for exacerbations (flares) of arthritis with low doses of antigen, described later.

In rabbits, antibody responses are generally high and allow for sufficient immune complex–mediated trapping of antigen in the joint. In mice, antibody levels are lower and cationic antigens are needed as suitable arthritogens, owing to their ability to stick to the negatively charged collagenous structures of the joint and to accumulate immune complex formation at the surface.[25] Of interest, this principle may extend to cationic bacterial or viral components and appears of importance in the more recently developed KRN model of arthritis, where anti-Glucose Phosphate Isomerase (GPI) antibodies stick to GPI antigen trapped at cartilage surfaces.

In antigen-induced arthritis in the rabbit and the mouse, elimination of TNF and IL-1 was poorly effective in suppressing joint inflammation, pointing to substantial "overkill" by other mediators in this severe onset of arthritis. However, elimination of IL-1 did yield impressive protection against cartilage destruction.[26] The model of AIA is most suited to studies into the mechanism of cartilage destruction as induced by a mix of immune complexes and T-cell reactivity. It is assisted by knowledge of exact time of onset, accessibility of the knee joint (as compared with ankles), and the presence of a contralateral control joint. Moreover, the model can be used to evaluate the regulation of local T-cell hyperreactivity against a retained foreign antigen.

Flares of arthritis

In comparison with the chronicity of human RA, most animal models show relatively short duration of a severe and rapidly destructive inflammation. In that respect, models of repeated flares of arthritis, with slower development of lesions, provide a valuable extension.

An arthritic joint bearing retains antigen and a chronic antigen-specific T-cell infiltrate displays a state of local hyperreactivity. This situation is not restricted to retained antigen but also applies to new antigen entering the sensitized joint from the circulation. Flares of smoldering arthritis can be induced with as little as 10 ng of antigen, and T cell–derived IL-17 plays a dominant part in such exacerbations.[27]

In addition to flare models based on protein antigen, similar models have been developed in rats and mice using bacterial cell wall constituents. In contrast to small protein antigens, which are only inflammatory in the context of an immune response, bacterial fragments may function as an antigen but also directly trigger toll-like receptors, in particular TLR2. Ensuing reactions are a mixture of T cell– and macrophage/fibroblast-driven processes. The generation of local hyperreactivity requires large, persistent bacterial peptidoglycan-polysaccharide components, but the recurrence may occur with a variety of components ranging from cell wall fragments, lipopolysaccharide, and CpG motifs to cytokines like IL-1. Strongest flares occur in the presence of T-cell immunity, and a correlation is found between the potential of fragments to induce an exacerbation and to elicit cell wall–specific T-cell proliferation.

In the mouse model of repeat SCW rechallenge, the swelling response of every flare remains TNF dependent. However, the chronic erosive infiltrate in the synovial tissue that occurs after repeat challenges is IL-1 dependent. Cartilage erosion is absent in IL-1–deficient mice but does occur in TNF-deficient mice. The model is more severe and erosive in DBA mice as compared with C57Bl mice, erosion is absent in T/B cell–deficient RAG −/− mice, and IL-17 blocking prevents an erosive phenotype. The repeat rechallenge model becomes Th17 dependent and IL-1 is a major cytokine driving this process of Th17 generation.[21]

Of note, considerable cross-reactivity occurs between cell walls from different bacterial origins, and flares may result from homologous and heterologous fragments.[28] This may extend to cross-reactive autoantigens from cartilage, which underlines that arthritis can start against a particular antigen but may spread to other antigens, including autoantigens.

Recently, toll receptors have been identified as recognition sites for bacteria. TLR2 is involved in SCW recognition, whereas TLR4 is triggered by LPS but also by damaged connective tissue components, which are released in erosive stages. The acute SWC arthritis model is TLR2 dependent, whereas the more chronic rechallenge model loses TLR2 dependence and becomes TLR4 dependent.[29] These principles open up a wide range of putative stimuli involved in exacerbations, simultaneously complicating the search for the driving "antigen" in humans. Flares can be efficiently blocked with a combination of antibodies to TNF, IL-1, and IL-17,[20,27] in particular. Evaluation of efficacy of TLR blockers is warranted.

Immune complex arthritis

Autoantibodies such as rheumatoid factor and anticitrulline antibodies (ACPAs) are a key feature of RA and the recent success of treatment with an anti–B-cell drug (rituximab) enhanced the belief in their pathogenic role. In some of the models discussed earlier such as collagen-, proteoglycan-, and antigen-induced arthritis, immune complex (IC) formation at joint tissues is a major element (see Table 87.1). Although excessive IC formation can cause destructive arthritis, chronicity is limited and much promoted by T cells. The latter may be linked to the need of T cells to sustain antibody production and the greater potential of T cell/macrophage interaction to sustain joint pathology. Minute amounts of antigen suffice to stimulate T cells, whereas considerable amounts of immune complexes are necessary to stimulate inflammatory mediator release from phagocytes. It is likely that IC models mimic part of the RA pathology.

There is growing interest in the use of passive IC models, along with availability of a range of transgenic knockouts, to identify crucial pathways of inflammation and tissue destruction. The advantage of passive systems is the lower dependence of genetic background, avoiding excessive backcrossing to create transgenics in suitable, susceptible mouse strains. Passive transfer of collagen arthritis can be performed with a critical mixture of a number of anticollagen type II (CII) monoclonal antibodies, including complement-binding IgG-2a. Sets are now commercially available, routinely recommending DBA mice as sensitive recipients. Accepted concepts of inflammation pathways include IC-mediated complement activation and Fcγ receptor triggering on phagocytes. Proteoglycan antibodies from the proteoglycan arthritis model can induce transient arthritis upon transfer, with concomitant proteoglycan loss from the cartilage but no erosive damage. IgG-1 seems the critical subclass but the limited destructive potential is yet unclear.

An IC model emerging from the murine AIA model and using the principle of cationic retention is the passive transfer of antilysozyme antibodies to mice that are locally injected in one knee joint with PLL-lysozyme. Poly-l-lysine (PLL)-coupled lysozyme is highly cationic and sufficiently large to be retained in the joint for prolonged periods of time. Both association with synovial tissue and heavy sticking to cartilage surfaces contribute to chronicity and cartilage destruction. An intriguing observation is the more chronic and destructive nature of this arthritis in DBA/1j as compared with Balb/c mice,[30] which seems related to high sustained levels of activating Fcγ receptors on macrophages of DBA/1j. The model shows strong dependence on IL-1, whereas TNF blockade was ineffective.[31] FcγRI rather than III appears crucial in cartilage damage.[32]

A final model to be mentioned here is the passive GPI model, which is addressed following a description of KRN arthritis. Differences between the various IC models lie mainly in the subclasses of antibodies and related complement-binding activity and/or FcγR-mediated activation of granulocytes, macrophages, and mast cells.

KRN-GPI arthritis

An intriguing, novel arthritis model emerged from experiments in transgenic mice overexpressing a self-reactive T-cell receptor (TCR). The cross of K/BxN mice developed arthritis.[33] In principle, many insults or adjuvants that skew regulation of T-cell tolerance have the potential to create autoimmune pathology, including joint inflammation. This holds for adjuvant arthritis and also for the oil-induced models described earlier. The major breakthrough and beauty of the KRN model is the elucidation of the driving antigen and the identification that passive transfer with antibodies induces a protracted arthritis. The TCR recognized the ubiquitous self-antigen glucose-6-phosphate isomerase (GPI) and provoked, through B cell differentiation and proliferation, high levels of anti-GPI antibodies. These antibodies are directly pathogenic on transfer and appear to recognize endogenous GPI, which seems to associate preferentially with the cartilage surface.[34] The latter may underlie the dominance of joint pathology in these mice, although GPI is also abundant at other sites in the body. IgG-1 antibodies are the major subclass and cause a sustained, erosive arthritis after continued transfer, with high sensitivity of Balb/c mice. This pathology brings the model close to passive CIA or IC arthritis, with planted cartilage associated antigen, all having IC formation at the cartilage surface. Differences relate to the IgG subclasses involved.

As an adaptation of this model, Kamradt and colleagues immunized mice with GPI and showed occurrence of arthritis after a few weeks. This direct immunization model is a mix of GPI-specific T cells and anti-GPI antibodies; serum from these mice cannot transfer arthritis.[35] The latter makes the direct immunization model different from classic KRN arthritis.

Strain dependency of passive immune complex arthritis

As mentioned earlier for passive IC models, in general, the severity is dependent on complement factors and Fcγ receptors. Activation of complement through the alternative pathway appears crucial in GPI arthritis, consistent with dominance of IgG-1. Because activity of complement and the level of expression of FcγR on phagocytes are different in various mouse strains, such factors determine to a great extent the variable susceptibility. BALB/c mice are hyperreactive, whereas DBA/1 and C57Bl6 are less susceptible and minor responsiveness is seen in 129/Sv mice, in strong contrast to the low sensitivity of Balb/c mice in

other passive IC arthritis models. GPI antibodies are found in some RA patients but certainly not in all and levels are moderate. Their role in RA remains to be identified.[36]

The involvement of IL-1 and TNF follows earlier observations in similar models. IL-1 is obligatory, with no arthritis in IL-1 deficient mice. TNF is also essential, although less critically than IL-1, because a proportion of TNF-deficient mice develop robust arthritis. When compared with the passive arthritis induced with antibodies to the cationic antigen PLL-lysozyme, a higher TNF sensitivity is apparent, as well as a dependence on mast cells. These findings suggest a role of environmental initiating elements. It is likely that onset of mild GPI arthritis is assisted by local TNF generation and mast cell–dependent histamine release, whereas a model with a planted cationic antigen in the joint generates sufficient non-specific inflammation to initiate arthritis without the need for additional facilitating mediators such as TNF. Once affected, the role of TNF is limited, as in GPI arthritis. T cell IL-17 can accelerate and enhance expression of GPI arthritis,[37] making TNF redundant and illustrating the remarkable potency of the combination of IC and T-cell activation in severity and chronicity of arthritis.

Citrulline arthritis.

Anti-citrullinated protein antibodies (ACPA) are a key feature of RA and in recent years many researchers have attempted to proof the efficacy of such antibodies of RA patients to induce passive arthritis, so far without much success. So the question remained whether the antibodies are pathogenic or just a marker of RA. There is some suggestive evidence for a pathogenic role in the studies of Kuhn and colleagues,[38] demonstrating that such antibodies are present in collagen arthritis and mice tolerized to citrulline responses showed reduced arthritis. However, it cannot be excluded that the immunomodulation process caused innocent bystander effects, not necessarily solely reflecting suppressed anti-citrulline responses.

Very recently, the group of Holmdahl generated a range of monoclonal antibodies specific for citrullinated collagen type II and showed arthritis induction on transfer of the antibodies. In addition, the antibodies could amplify smoldering arthritis.[39] It argues that defined anti-citrulline antibodies can do the job, as was demonstrated earlier for anti-collagen type II and anti-GPI antibodies. Whether similar antibodies occur in significant quantities in RA patients remains to be proven.

Gene manipulation and transgenic models

Transgenic animals, defined as novel strains generated by manipulation of particular genes, have resulted in several new models that prove the importance of certain principles in arthritis and are useful for distinct screening. They do not necessarily provide better translational models for drug targeting in RA. Some recent examples of skewed T cell responses are discussed later.

Mice transgenic for the env-pX region of the human T-cell leukemia virus type 1 genome develop a spontaneous chronic arthritis as a result of expression of the tax gene.[40] Onset occurs at 2 to 3 months of age in female mice but is delayed several months in male animals. Ankle joints are most frequently affected and pannus formation leading to severe erosions of cartilage and bone is observed in transgenic mice after several months of disease. The mice produce autoantibodies and collagen immunization can provoke the onset or exacerbation of arthritis. It is tempting to speculate that a retrovirus could be involved in the pathogenesis of RA, possibly by influencing T-cell responses to cartilage antigens.

Another recent example is the occurrence of chronic autoimmune arthritis in mice with a point mutation of the gene encoding ZAP-70, a key signal transduction molecule in T cells.[41] The aberrant T-cell receptor function leads to positive selection of otherwise negatively selected autoimmune T cells. It is of great interest that these mice fail to develop disease under microbially clean conditions, despite active production of arthritogenic autoimmune cells. A single injection of Zymosan provokes arthritis in a Dectin-1 dependent but TLR-independent manner.[42]

Mice with a homozygous mutation in the gp130 IL-6 receptor subunit show enhanced signal transduction and STAT3 activation and develop a lymphocyte-mediated RA-like joint disease. Increased proliferation of CD4+ T cells is due to elevated production of T-cell activating IL-7 by non-hematopoietic cells.[43,44]

TNF transgenic arthritis

In an elegant series of experiments, Kollias and co-workers provided insight into the possible role of TNF in arthritis induction. By the introduction in mice of a modified human TNF transgene, lacking a TNF 3'UTR region involved in translational repression of TNF, it was shown that pronounced TNF overexpression results in chronic polyarthritis with a 100% incidence.[45] Hyperplasia of the synovium, inflammatory infiltrates in the joint space, pannus formation, and cartilage and bone destruction were observed. Intriguingly, a similar form of arthritis also developed in targeted mutant mice lacking the 3'AU-rich elements, confirming the role of these elements in the maintenance of a physiologic TNF response in the joint.[46] A proposed mechanism is the inability of natural anti-inflammatory signals, such as IL-10, to suppress TNF production under these conditions. These exciting findings stimulated a major search for functional mutations around TNF production in RA patients. However, no clear indications have been found so far.

The model is of great interest in identifying pathways of TNF-induced arthritis and screening the efficacy of various TNF-directed therapies. It is not surprising that anti-TNF treatment blocks the pathology, but it is a remarkable observation that some of the pathology runs through IL-1. Crosses of TNFtg mice with IL-1 deficient mice identified that inflammation is TNF mediated. Bone erosion is 50% dependent of IL-1, whereas cartilage erosion is a fully IL-1 dependent process.[47] The model does not need T or B cells because arthritis occurs in TNF transgenics backcrossed to RAG −/− mice and the pathology can be transferred with selected TNF-producing fibroblasts. Further investigation of TNF receptor involvement showed a crucial role of the p55 type I receptor in mediating the TNF pathology and a suppressive role of the p75 type II receptor.

Apparently, the type II receptor does not have a clear suppressive role in inflammatory bowel disease, which is a pathology also found in TNF transgenic mice. The latter is a T/B cell-dependent disease. It is known that the cytotoxic anti-TNF and the TNF and lymphotoxin scavenging TNF soluble receptor treatments have different efficacy in human RA as compared with Crohn disease, but the reason for this is not fully understood. A dualistic proinflammatory and immunosuppressive role of TNF has been observed and heterogeneity exists in TNF receptor usage in autoimmune suppression versus inflammatory tissue damage.[48] These observations provide a rationale for future treatment of RA with selective anti-TNFR instead of anti-TNF antibodies. However, full understanding of this system is complicated by the finding of cooperative activity of p55 and p75 TNFR in arthritis induced with membrane-bound TNF, in line with the identification of preferential binding of transmembrane as compared with soluble TNF to the p75 receptor. It remains to be elucidated to what extent human RA is driven by soluble or membrane TNF. Of note, soluble TNF is hard to detect in RA synovial fluid and models with dominant overexpression of soluble TNF hamper proper identification of the role of p75 TNFR.

IL-1 transgenic mice and IL-1ra deficient mice

Transgenic IL-1α overexpression was also shown to induce chronic, destructive arthritis.[49] Transgenic mice expressing human IL-1α had high serum levels of IL-1 and developed a severe polyarthritis by 4 weeks of age. Hyperplasia of the synovial lining, pannus formation, and, ultimately, cartilage destruction were evident. T and B cells were scant, but active granulocytes were abundant.

The opposite approach, elimination of IL-1 control by gene targeting of the endogenous IL-1 receptor antagonist (IL-1ra), also yielded a model of arthritis. IL-1ra deficiency in a Balb/ca background resulted in pronounced arthritis at the age of 8 weeks.[50] Marked synovial and periarticular inflammation was noted, with invasion of granulation tissue and articular erosion. Moreover, elevated levels of antibodies against immunoglobulins, type II collagen, and double-stranded DNA were found, suggestive of autoimmune responses. Intriguingly, IL-1ra deficiency in a C57Bl/6J background did not yield arthritis but instead showed arteritis. This genetic variation, although not well understood, underscores an immunologic pathogenetic pathway. Overexpression of a range of cytokines, including IL-1β, TNF, and IL-6, was observed in the joints before onset of arthritis. Interestingly, autoantibody levels did not correlate with disease severity, which may imply that it reflects a reaction to damaged joint tissue.

In sharp contrast to the TNF transgenic model, the arthritis in IL-1ra−/− mice is strongly dependent on T cells, in line with the remarkable genetic restriction. It is consistent with the view that IL-1 is a crucial regulator of T-cell function. Impaired T-cell activation is demonstrated in IL-1–deficient mice, linked to low levels of CD40 ligand and OX40 expression on T cells, and underlies the suppression of collagen arthritis in these mice. Undisturbed IL-1 action, in the absence of IL-1ra, apparently permits activation of IL-17 producing T cells directed against exogenous triggers or endogenous autoantigens. The spontaneous arthritis in IL-1ra−/− mice does not develop under germ-free conditions and is reduced in TLR4-deficient mice.[51] TLR4 blockers are effective in this model.[52] Both TNF and IL-17 deficiency prevent onset of arthritis.[53,54] Features are highlighted in Table 87.2.

CYTOKINES AS TARGETS IN SUSCEPTIBILITY AND DESTRUCTION

Findings on TNF, IL-1, and IL-17 involvement have been addressed partly under the headings of the various models and are further summarized in Table 87.3.

TABLE 87.2 FEATURES OF CLASSIC ARTHRITIS MODELS								
Features	AA	SCW-A	CIA	AIA	KRN	TNFtg	IL-1ra -/-
Impact of bacterial flora*	+	+	−	−	?	?	+
Stimulus	?	Persistent bacteria	CII	Planted Ag	GPI	TNF	Bacteria?
Self-limiting arthritis	+	−	±	−	−	−	−
Flares	Refractory	Spontaneous	Inducible	Inducible	?	−	−
Chronic synovitis	±	++	+	++	+	++	++
Bone marrow inflammation†	++	+	±	±	?	+	+
Main site of expression	Ankle	Ankle	Peripheral	Chosen‡	Peripheral	Ankle	Ankle
Bone erosion	++	+	++	+	++	++	+
Cartilage erosion	±	±	++	++	++	±	+
Dominant feature	Periostitis	Fibrosis	Destructive	Local hyperreactivity	Destructive	IL-1	IL-17

*Impact on susceptibility of strains.
†As an early feature.
‡Chosen by intra-articular injection.

TABLE 87.3 CARTILAGE DESTRUCTION AND CYTOKINE INVOLVEMENT IN MURINE MODELS

Model	Acute inflammation			Cartilage destruction					
	TNF	IL-1	IL-17	PG loss	Surface erosion	Chondrocyte death	TNF*	IL-1	IL-17
SCW	++	−	−	+	±	±	−	+	−
SCW flares	+	+	+	+	+	±	−	++	+
CIA	++	+++	+	++	++	++	+	++	+
AIA	±	±	−	++	±	±	−	++	−
AIA flare	+	+	++	++	++	++	−	++	+++
ICA†	±	++	−	++	++	++	±	++	−
GPI-A‡	+	++	−	++	++	++	+	++	−
TNFtg	++	±	?	+	±	±	++	++	?
IL-1ra −/−	+	++	+	+	+	±	−	+++	

*The role of tumor necrosis factor (TNF) in destruction is mainly indirect, by preventing onset of the arthritic process.
†ICA, passive immune complex arthritis, with poly-L-lysine lysozyme as antigen.
‡Passive arthritis induced with antibodies from the K/BxN arthritic mice.

TNF is a major mediator in the early stages of joint inflammation in every model. Although IL-1 is not a dominant inflammatory cytokine in all models, it is certainly the pivotal cytokine in the inhibition of chondrocyte proteoglycan synthesis in all models studied so far and the blocking of IL-1 has a great beneficial impact on net cartilage destruction.[55] In line with this, chronic destructive arthritis could not be induced in IL-1–deficient mice, using any of the classic arthritis models. In contrast, TNF deficiency reduced the incidence of autoimmune arthritis expression but once joints became afflicted, full progression to erosive arthritis did occur.[56] It is unclear why IL-1 is such a dominant target in IC and T cell–driven models, whereas a crucial role of IL-1 in autoimmune RA is only evident in joint erosion and a role in RA joint inflammation is unlikely. The novel T-cell cytokine IL-17 provides an additional target apart from TNF and IL-1. Local overexpression showed that it can accelerate inflammation and tissue destruction in CIA, independent of IL-1, and IL-17 blocking appeared superior in the T-cell flare of AIA.[27] In addition, the macrophage-derived cytokines IL-15, IL-18, and IL-23 are abundant in RA synovia, can contribute to T-cell maturation and activation, and were shown to promote collagen arthritis. It is now accepted that IL-23 rather than IL-12 stimulates IL-17 T cells and drives arthritis.[57] Its major role is not in generation but in propagation of already differentiated Th17 cells, making this cytokine an attractive therapeutic target.

Cartilage and bone destruction

Animal models are excellent tools for characterizing the kinetics of destructive pathways. Cartilage damage observed in different models ranges from a selective loss of cartilage, underlying pannus tissue to an overall loss of matrix, starting with proteoglycan release and, later, collagen damage. Killing of chondrocytes and complete loss of the superficial and middle cartilage layer are noted in severe forms. This underlines that arthritic processes can be more or less destructive, dependent on the underlying process and cytokine mixture. Enhanced degradation of matrix and inhibited synthesis of proteoglycans by the chondrocyte are general findings in all models. Aggressive overall cartilage loss is predominantly noted in the presence of immune complex deposition, whereas milder, more gradual forms of damage are noted in models driven by macrophage, fibroblast, or T-cell activation. Large variations in progressive destruction are also noted in populations of patients with RA, which may imply separate pathogenetic pathways.

A general lesson that may be deduced from observations in various models is that continuing, irreversible destruction can occur under conditions that will be hardly considered as inflammatory, whereas the opposite occurs as well.[58] Symptomatic relief by anti-inflammatory therapy is promising, but the main challenge of interrupting joint destruction remains. As an example, local gene transfer with IL-4 did not suppress local inflammation yet markedly reduced cartilage and bone destruction in CIA.[59] An intriguing observation was recently made with respect to crucial enzymes involved in cartilage proteoglycan loss. Studies in ADAMTS-4 and 5 knockout mice identified that ADAMTS5 is the crucial enzyme in proteoglycan loss in antigen-induced arthritis, and its absence prevents not only proteoglycan depletion but also collagen damage. As such it opens a novel, indirect way for targeted therapy of cartilage erosion.[60]

It has been demonstrated that RANKL is the crucial activating cytokine of the bone-resorbing osteoclasts. In the absence of RANKL, joint inflammation continues in the passive GPI immune complex arthritis but bone erosion is prevented. Similarly, when TNF transgenic mice were crossed with c-fos deficient mice, joint inflammation continued yet bone erosion was fully absent. C-fos mice lack functional osteoclasts. TNF-driven bone erosion is osteoclast dependent and absence of osteoclasts alters TNF-mediated arthritis from a destructive to a non-destructive phenotype. In line with this, treatment with OPG, which is the natural inhibitor of RANKL, does not reduce inflammation in adjuvant arthritis and TNF transgenic mice, yet bone erosion is reduced.[14,61] Further improvement of therapy and even bone repair can be achieved with combined blocking of cytokines and RANKL, as well as providing an additional anabolic stimulus such as parathyroid hormone.[62,63] These studies indicate that repair of bone is achievable, in line with bone recovery noted in well-treated RA patients.

Repair of cartilage remains a major challenge, probably requiring tissue engineering approaches with stem cells, biodegradable matrices, and supplies of crucial growth factors. A final remark on bone erosion versus bone apposition is in order. Unlike the situation in RA patients, many arthritis models exhibit bone erosion but also pronounced new bone formation. These phenomena occur at distinct sites of the joint. The latter process, bone apposition, is virtually absent in TNF transgenic mice, and a TNF-inducible regulator of bone apposition, DKK-1, was recently identified.[64] It might be argued that most murine arthritis models are relatively devoid of TNF compared with TNFtg mice and human RA, herein providing a possible explanation for excessive bone apposition. Further studies are warranted on factors that regulate the impact of osteoclasts and osteoblasts on bone metabolism under inflammatory conditions and its dependence of local cytokine milieus, including old and novel players like DKKs, TGFb, BMPs, and members of the Wnt family. Proper identification of their involvement and targeting in models may provide new ways of treatment.

- Further insights in the relevance of findings on erosive processes in animal models for human RA are hampered by the paucity of information on progression of cartilage erosion in RA patients. X-rays are a proper tool to evaluate progression of bone erosion, but the joint space narrowing identified with this technique is a non-sensitive measure and overlooks focal erosions occurring in the cartilage. It is recommended that upcoming clinical trials in

RA pay attention to advanced imaging technologies to monitor changes in cartilage damage, which are yet explored and validated in animal models of arthritis.
- Arthritis may be induced in animals by immunization with cartilage components, non-specific immune stimuli, bacterial or viral components, or transgenic manipulation.
- Animal models are tools that mimic various aspects but never fully resemble human RA.

- Models have a defined onset and are useful for kinetic evaluation of arthritis, cell and mediator involvement, and detailed analysis of joint erosion.
- Animal models serve an important role in the evaluation of anti-rheumatic treatments and provide direction for novel approaches to treatments such as cytokine inhibition.

KEY REFERENCES

1. Wooley PH. Animal models of rheumatoid arthritis. Curr Opin Rheumatol 1991;3:407-420.
2. Trentham DE, Townes AS, Kang AH. Autoimmunity to type II collagen: an experimental model of arthritis. J Exp Med 1977;146:857-868.
3. Holmdahl R, Malmstrom V, Vuorio E. Autoimmune recognition of cartilage collagens. Ann Med 1993;25:251-264.
4. Finnegan A, Mikecz K, Tao P, et al. Proteoglycan (aggrecan)-induced arthritis in BALB/c mice is a Th1-type disease regulated by Th2 cytokines. J Immunol 1999;163:5383-5390.
6. Doodes PD, Cao Y, Hamel KM, et al. Development of proteoglycan arthritis is independent of IL-17. J Immunol 2008;181:329-337.
7. Joosten LAB, Helsen MMA, Van De Loo FAJ, et al. Anticytokine treatment of established type II collagen-induced arthritis in DBA/1 mice: a comparative study using anti-TNFa, anti-IL-1a/b and IL-1ra. Arthritis Rheum 1996;39:797-809.
8. Pearson CM. Development of arthritis, periarthritis and periostitis in rats given adjuvants. Proc Soc Exp Biol (New York) 1956;91:95-101.
10. Wooley PH, Seibold JR, Whalen JD, et al. Pristane induced arthritis. The immunologic and genetic features of an experimental murine model of autoimmune disease. Arthritis Rheum 1989;32:1022-1030.
11. Van Eden W, Van Der Zee R, Prakken B. Heat shock proteins induce T cell regulation of chronic inflammation. Nat Rev Immunol Rev 2005;5:318-330.
12. Holmdahl R, Lorentzen JC, Lu S, et al. Arthritis induced in rats with nonimmunogenic adjuvants as models for RA. Immunol Rev 2001;184:184-202.
13. Kong YY, Feige U, Sarosi I, et al. Activated T cells regulate bone loss and joint destruction in adjuvant arthritis through osteoprotegerin ligand. Nature 1999;402:304-309.
14. Pettit AR, Ji H, Von Stechow D, et al. TRANCE/RANKL knockout mice are protected from bone erosion in a serum transfer model of arthritis. Am J Pathol 2001;159:1689-1699.
16. Cromartie WJ, Craddock JG, Schwab JH, et al. Arthritis in rats after systemic injection of streptococcal cell walls. J Exp Med 1977;146:485-602.
18. Lafyatis R, Thompson NL, Remmers EF, et al. Transforming growth factor-β production by synovial tissues from rheumatoid patients and streptococcal cell wall arthritic rats. J Immunol 1989;143:1142-1148.
19. Kuiper S, Joosten LAB, Bendele AM, et al. Different roles of TNFα and IL-1 in murine streptococcal cell wall arthritis. Cytokine 1998;10:690-702.
21. Joosten LAB, Abdollahi-Roodsaz S, Heuvelmans-Jacobs M, et al. T cell dependence of chronic destructive murine arthritis induced by repeated local activation of TLR driven pathways: crucial role of both IL-1 and IL-17. Arthritis Rheum 2008;58:98-108.
22. Deng GM, Tarkowski A. Synovial cytokine mRNA expression during arthritis triggered by CpG motifs of bacterial DNA. Arthritis Res 2001;3:48-53.
23. Dumonde DC, Glynn LE. The production of arthritis in rabbits by an immunological reaction to fibrin. Br J Exp Pathol 1962;43:373-383.

24. Cooke TDV, Hird ER, Ziff M, et al. The pathogenesis of chronic inflammation in experimental antigen induced arthritis. J Exp Med 1972;135:323-338.
25. Van Den Berg WB, Van De Putte LBA, Zwarts WA, et al. Electrical charge of the antigen determines intraarticular antigen handling and chronicity of arthritis in mice. J Clin Invest 1984;74:1850-1859.
27. Koenders MI, Lubberts E, Oppers-Walgreen B, et al. Blocking of IL-17 during reactivation of experimental arthritis prevents joint inflammation and bone erosion by decreasing RANKL and IL-1. Am J Pathol 2005;167:141-149.
29. Abdollahi-Roodsaz S, Joosten LA, Helsen MH, et al. Shift from TLR2 toward TLR4 dependency in the erosive stage of chronic streptococcal cell wall arthritis coincident with TLR4 mediated IL-17 production. Arthritis Rheum 2008;58:3753-3764.
30. Blom AB, Van Lent PL, Van Vuuren H, et al. FcγR expression on macrophages is related to severity and chronicity of synovial inflammation and cartilage destruction during experimental immune-complex-mediated arthritis (ICA). Arthritis Res 2000;2:489-503.
32. Nabbe KC, Boross P, Holthuysen AE, et al. Joint inflammation and chondrocyte death become independent of FcγRIII by local overexpression of IFN-γ during immune complex mediated–arthritis. Arthritis Rheum 2005;52:967-974.
33. Korganow AS, Ji H, Mangialaio S, et al. From systemic T cell self-reactivity to organ-specific autoimmune disease via immunoglobulins. Immunity 1999;10:451-461.
34. Maccioni M, Zeder-Lutz G, Huang H, et al. Arthritogenic monoclonal antibodies from K/BxN mice. J Exp Med 2002;195:1071-1077.
35. Schubert D, Maier B, Morawietz L, et al. Immunization with glucose-6-phosphate isomerase induces T cell dependent peripheral polyarthritis in generally unaltered mice. J Immunol 2004;172:4503-4509.
36. Monach PA, Benoist C, Mathis D. The role of antibodies in mouse models of rheumatoid arthritis and relevance to human disease. Adv Immunol 2004;82:217-248.
37. Koenders MI, Lubberts E, Van De Loo FA, et al. Interleukin-17 acts independently of TNF-α under arthritic conditions. J Immunol 2006;176:6262-6269.
38. Kuhn KA, Kulik L, Tomooka B, et al. Antibodies against citrullinated proteins enhance tissue injury in experimental autoimmune arthritis. J Clin Invest 2006;116:961-973.
39. Uysal H, Bockermann R, Nanadakumar KS, et al. Structure and pathogenicity of antibodies specific for citrullinated collagen type II in experimental arthritis. J Exp Med 2009;206:449-462.
40. Iwakura Y, Tosu M, Yoshida E, et al. Induction of inflammatory arthropathy resembling rheumatoid arthritis in mice transgenic for HTLV-I. Science 1991;253:1026-1028.
41. Hata H, Sakaguchi N, Yoshitomi H, et al. Distinct contribution of IL-6, TNF-alpha, IL-1 and IL-10 to T cell-mediated spontaneous autoimmune arthritis in mice. J Clin Invest 2004;114:582-588.
43. Atsumi T, Ishihara K, Kamimura D, et al. A point mutation of Tyr-759 in IL-6 family cytokine receptor

subunit gp130 causes autoimmune arthritis. J Exp Med 2002;196:979-990.
45. Keffer J, Probert L, Cazlaris H, et al. Transgenic mice expressing human tumor necrosis factor: a predictive genetic model of arthritis. EMBO J 1991;13:4025-4031.
46. Kontoyiannis D, Pasparakis M, Pizarro TT, et al. Impaired on/off regulation of TNF biosynthesis in mice lacking TNF AU-rich elements: implications for joint and gut-associated immunopathologies. Immunity 1999;10:387-398.
47. Zwerina J, Redlich K, Polzer K, et al. TNF induced structural joint damage is mediated by IL-1. Proc Natl Acad Sci U S A 2007;104:11742-11747.
49. Niki Y, Yamada H, Seki S, et al. Macrophage- and neutrophil-dominant arthritis in human IL-1 alpha transgenic mice. J Clin Invest 2001;107:1127-1135.
50. Horai R, Saijo S, Tanioka H, et al. Development of chronic inflammatory arthropathy resembling RA in IL-1ra-deficient mice. J Exp Med 2000;191:313-320.
51. Abdollahi-Roodsaz S, Joosten LA, Koenders MI, et al. Stimulation of TLR2 and TLR4 differentially skews the balance of T cells in a mouse model of arthritis. J Clin Invest 2008;118:205-216.
52. Abdollahi-Roodsaz S, Joosten LA, Roelofs MF, et al. Inhibition of TLR4 breaks the inflammatory loop in autoimmune destructive arthritis. Arthritis Rheum 2007;56:2957-2967.
53. Nakae S, Saijo S, Horai R, et al. IL-17 production from activated T cells is required for the spontaneous development of destructive arthritis in mice deficient in IL-1 receptor antagonist. Proc Natl Acad Sci U S A 2003;100:5986-5990.
55. Van Den Berg WB. What we learn from arthritis models to benefit arthritis patients. Baillière's Clin Rheumatol 2000;14:599-616.
56. Campbell IK, O'Donnell K, Lawlor KE, et al. Severe inflammatory arthritis and lymphadenopathy in the absence of TNF. J Clin Invest 2001;107:1519-1527.
57. Murphy CA, Langrish CL, Chen Y, et al. Divergent pro and anti-inflammatory roles for IL-23 and IL-12 in joint autoimmune inflammation. J Exp Med 2003;198:1951-1957.
59. Lubberts E, Joosten LAB, Chabaud M, et al. IL-4 gene therapy for collagen arthritis suppresses synovial IL-17 and osteoprotegerin ligand and prevents bone erosion. J Clin Invest 2000;105:1697-1710.
60. Stanton H, Rogerson FM, East CJ, et al. ADAMTS5 is the major aggrecanase in mouse cartilage in vivo and in vitro. Nature 2005;434:648-652.
61. Redlich K, Hayer S, Ricci R, et al. Osteoclasts are essential for TNFα-mediated joint destruction. J Clin Invest 2002;110:1419-1427.
63. Redlich K, Gortz B, Hayer S, et al. Repair of local bone erosions and reversal of systemic bone loss upon therapy with anti-TNF in combination with osteoprotegerin or parathyroid hormone in TNF-mediated arthritis. Am J Pathol 2004;164:543-555.
64. Diarra D, Stolina M, Polzer K, et al. Dickkopf-1 is a master regulator of joint remodeling. Nat Med 2007;13:156-163.

REFERENCES

Full references for this chapter can be found on www.expertconsult.com.

Autoantibodies in rheumatoid arthritis

88

Günter Steiner and Markus Hoffmann

- Rheumatoid arthritis (RA) is a systemic autoimmune disease characterized by the presence of autoantibodies and autoreactive T cells in peripheral blood and synovial fluid.
- Autoantibodies are present already in the earliest stages of the disease and may precede disease onset by several years; most autoantibodies are not directed to joint-specific antigens.
- Rheumatoid factors (RF), that is, autoantibodies to the Fc portion of IgG, are the longest-known marker antibodies in RA. High-titer IgM-RF and also IgA-RF are of high diagnostic and prognostic value because they are associated with erosive and more severe disease.
- Autoantibodies to antigens containing the amino acid citrulline (generated by post-translational deimination of arginyl residues) are the most specific marker antibodies for RA. Similar to high-titer RF, they are linked to erosive RA. Citrullinated autoantigens that are also expressed in the inflamed joint include fibrinogen, vimentin, α-enolase, and collagen.
- Among other autoantigens the heterogeneous nuclear ribonucleoprotein-A2 (RA33) may be of pathogenic or pathogenetic relevance because it is also a target of autoreactive T cells and able to stimulate inflammatory cells via Toll-like receptor engagement.
- Autoantibodies may contribute to the pathophysiology of RA by inducing, maintaining, or modulating the disease process. However, for none of the known autoantibodies has a direct pathogenic role been clearly verified and the primary (disease inducing) autoimmune targets remain to be identified.

INTRODUCTION

Autoimmunity, that is, the presence of autoantibodies and autoreactive T cells in blood and joint fluid, is a characteristic feature of rheumatoid arthritis (RA) that distinguishes this disease from other inflammatory or degenerative joint disorders such as psoriatic arthritis, reactive arthritis, or osteoarthritis. As in other systemic autoimmune diseases, most autoantibodies of patients with RA target antigens are widely expressed throughout the body, while joint-specific structures do not seem to be among the primary targets. Thus, the hallmark autoantibody of RA, rheumatoid factor (RF), is directed against immunoglobulin G (IgG), a major serum component, whereas autoantibodies to cartilage proteins such as collagen II occur much less frequently and are not specific for RA. In fact, the most specific autoantibodies are directed to citrullinated proteins such as fibrinogen, vimentin, or α-enolase, and anti-citrullinated protein antibodies (ACPAs) are now generally considered to be the most valuable serologic markers of RA. Other antigens described as targets of autoimmune responses in RA include quite diverse structures, such as nuclear proteins, particularly the heterogeneous nuclear ribonucleoprotein-A2 (hnRNP-A2), heat-shock proteins, some enzymes, or certain cartilage components (Table 88.1). Although most antibodies to these proteins are of limited usefulness for diagnostic purposes, they may nevertheless contribute to the pathologic processes characteristic of RA, such as chronic synovitis and erosion of cartilage and bone, by immune complex formation and subsequent activation of proinflammatory immune responses. In the following sections the major antibody systems are described and their value as diagnostic tools as well as their potential role in the pathogenesis of RA are discussed.

RHEUMATOID FACTORS

Rheumatoid factors are a family of autoantibodies that recognize antigenic determinants on the Fc portion of IgG (Fig. 88.1). This part of the molecule is essential for complement fixation and interaction with the Fc receptor and thus for uptake of immune complexes. In contrast to most other autoantibodies, the major RF species is the IgM isotype, whereas IgG-RF and IgA-RF occur less frequently. RF can be measured by various methods, including agglutination techniques such as the classic Waaler-Rose test, turbidometric techniques such as laser nephelometry, and enzyme-linked immunosorbent assay (ELISA), the latter method being particularly useful for the determination of RF subtypes.

A transient increase of IgM-RF is part of the normal immunoregulatory process occurring during bacterial and viral infections, probably in response to immune complexes containing microbial antigens. Thus, low-titered IgM-RF can be found in 10% to 15% of healthy individuals whereas chronic persistence of high-affinity IgM-RF at elevated titers as well as the presence of IgG and IgA subtypes is a characteristic feature of RA. Interestingly, genes encoding RF from RA patients are often somatically mutated, whereas RF from healthy individuals is predominantly germline encoded and polyreactive. Somatic mutation of immunoglobulin genes and the class switch from IgM to other subtypes are indicators of a T cell–driven process that, however, is still not understood in full detail.[1,2]

Pathogenetic involvement

The physiologic role of RF during a normal immune response is to enhance the avidity and size of immune complexes, thereby improving immune complex clearance. Immune complexes are also present in the joint, and complement fixation by IgG-containing immune complexes is enhanced by IgM-RF binding. This may be particularly important for immune complexes containing antibodies to cartilage antigens and other proteins expressed in the joint, including antigens that are not joint-specific, such as stress proteins, citrullinated proteins, or nuclear antigens. Therefore, it is conceivable that RFs may contribute to the activity and chronicity of the disease via complement-mediated pathways (Fig. 88.2). Furthermore, RF-bearing B cells may act as antigen-presenting cells and efficiently present (foreign or self) antigens to T cells via uptake of immune complexes. Thus, RF in serum and especially the RF-producing B cells in synovial tissue of RA patients may exert such functions and thereby contribute to the pathophysiology of RA. Finally, the association of high-titer RF with more severe disease, particularly with bone erosion and extra-articular manifestations, may be considered further, although indirect, evidence for a pathogenic role of RFs.[1-3]

Role as diagnostic and prognostic markers

IgM-RF can be detected in 60% to 80% of RA patients with established disease, whereas prevalence in patients with early RA usually does not exceed 50%. RFs of all subtypes may be present already in the earliest stages of the disease and can even precede the onset of RA by several years.[4,5] IgM-RF is present in high titers also in the majority of patients with primary Sjögren syndrome or mixed cryoglobulinemia and can

TABLE 88.1 TARGETS OF AUTOANTIBODIES IN RHEUMATOID ARTHRITIS

Antigen	Antibody	Specificity	T cells
Immunoglobulin G	Rheumatoid factors	Moderate-high*	Unknown
Citrullinated proteins	ACPA	High	Yes
HnRNP-A2	Anti-RA33	Moderate	Yes
Collagen II	Anti-collagen	Low	Yes
Stress proteins	Anti-BiP, anti-hsp90	Low	Yes
Glucose-6 phosphate isomerase	Anti-GPI	Low	Unknown
High mobility group box 1 protein	Anti-HMGB1	Low	Unknown
Calpastatin	Anti-calpastatin	Low-high†	Unknown

*Dependent on cut-off value.
†Dependent on the ethnic background.

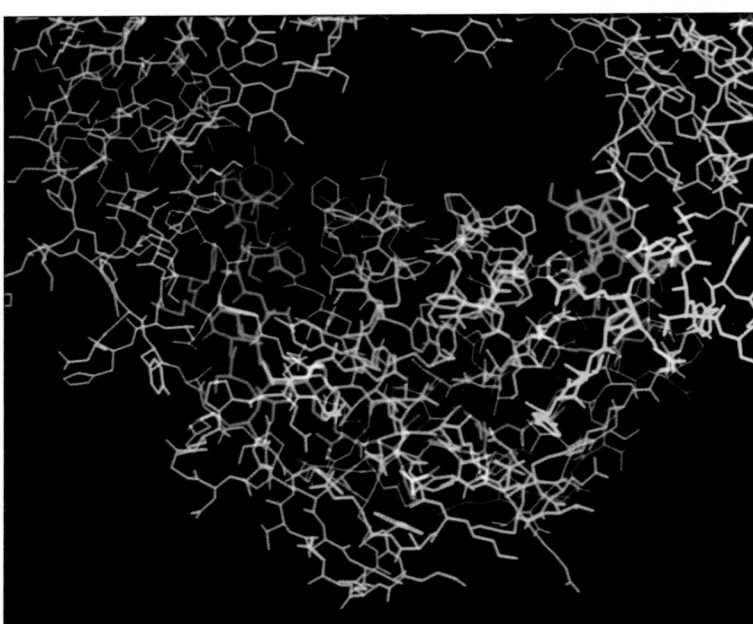

Fig. 88.1 RF epitopes on IgG-Fc. Molecular model of the CH2 and CH3 domains of IgG showing (in yellow) the antigenic sequence around His 435, which can be seen to protrude from the surface. Binding sites are scattered within the Cg2 and Cg3 regions of IgG-Fc. The presence of His 435 is an essential constituent of the Ga determinant and absent in IgG3. *(With permission of Elsevier Science Ltd, reprinted from Peterson C, Malone CC, Williams RC Jr. Rheumatoid factor reactive sites on CH3 established by overlapping 7-mer peptide epitope analysis. Molecular Immunology 1995;35:57-75.)*

be found in lower titers in all other rheumatic autoimmune diseases. At the commonly used cutoff value of 15 or 20 IU/mL, IgM-RF shows only moderate specificity for RA, but specificity is considerably increased at higher titers, and several studies have found RF above 40 or 50 IU/mL (high-titer RF) to be quite specific for RA.[6-10] However, high-titer RF is present in only 50% to 60% of RA patients with established disease and is even less frequent in patients with early RA (Table 88.2). Interestingly, IgA-RF appears to be a more specific marker antibody for RA than IgM- or IgG-RF.[4,11-13] Importantly, high-titer IgM-RF as well as IgA-RF have also considerable prognostic value because they are associated with severity of RA, such as erosiveness (Fig. 88.3), more rapid disease progression, worse outcome, and extra-articular manifestations.[9,12,14-16] Therefore, IgM-RF is still the most widely used serologic marker of RA and one of the seven criteria of the American College of Rheumatology for classification of RA and has recently been included together with ACPAs into the European League Against Rheumatism (EULAR) recommendations for the management of early RA.[17]

SOME ROLES FOR RHEUMATOID FACTOR IN JOINT PATHOLOGY

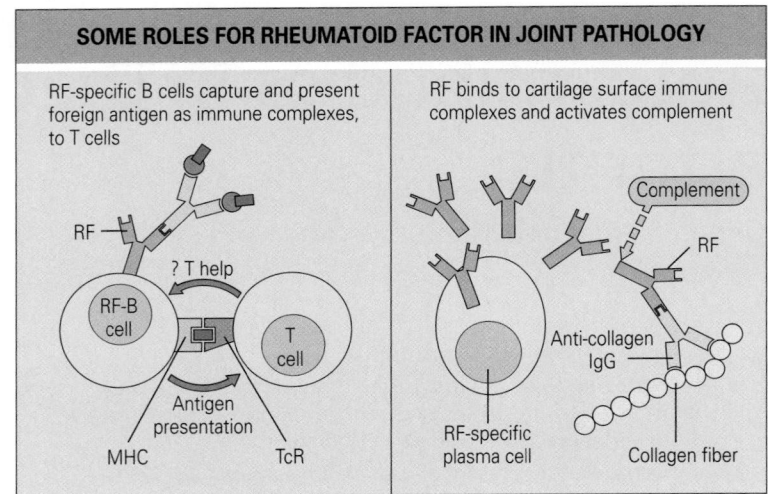

Fig. 88.2 Some roles for rheumatoid factor in joint pathology.

TABLE 88.2 SENSITIVITY AND SPECIFICITY OF IgM-RF FOR RHEUMATOID ARTHRITIS

Diagnosis	RF > 20 U/mL	RF > 50 U/mL
Rheumatoid arthritis (RA)	66%	46%
Sjögren's syndrome	62%	52%
Systemic lupus erythematosus	27%	10%
Scleroderma	44%	8%
Poly/dermatomyositis	18%	0%
Reactive arthritis	10%	4%
Osteoarthritis	25%	4%
Healthy controls	13%	0%
Sensitivity for established RA (%)	66%	46%
Specificity for established RA (%)	78%	88%
Sensitivity for early RA* (%)	56%	46%
Specificity for early RA* (%)	89%	96%

*Data are derived from a prospective early arthritis study including patients with <3 months' disease duration.[9]
RF, rheumatoid factor.

AUTOANTIBODIES TO CITRULLINATED ANTIGENS

The identification of autoantibodies in sera of patients with RA that are directed to epitopes containing the unusual amino acid citrulline has been one of the most exciting contributions to the field of RA research of the past decade.[18,19] Arginyl residues can be post-translationally deiminated by the enzyme peptidyl arginine deiminase (PAD), leading to the generation of citrullinated proteins (Fig. 88.4). Therefore, autoantibodies recognizing citrullinated epitopes are now generally named anti-citrullinated protein antibodies (ACPAs).[19] Five different isoforms of PAD have been described in humans, among which PAD2 is the most widely expressed one, whereas expression of PAD4 is predominantly restricted to white blood cells such as monocytes/macrophages and granulocytes.[20]

Citrullinated epitopes were first identified in filaggrin, a protein that is highly abundant in squamous epithelial cells, where it promotes aggregation of intermediate filaments. Citrullinated filaggrin forms the target of anti-keratin antibodies that were first described in 1979 and shown to be highly specific for RA.[21] Anti-filaggrin antibodies were found to bind to short citrulline-containing peptide epitopes,[22-24] which may also be derived from other proteins or even be of synthetic origin, such as a cyclic citrullinated peptide (CCP), which is now commonly

BOX PLOTS SHOWING THE DIFFERENCE IN LARSEN SCORES IN RA PATIENTS WITH HIGH-TITER RF (>50 U/mL) VERSUS PATIENTS WITH LOW-TITER OR NEGATIVE RF

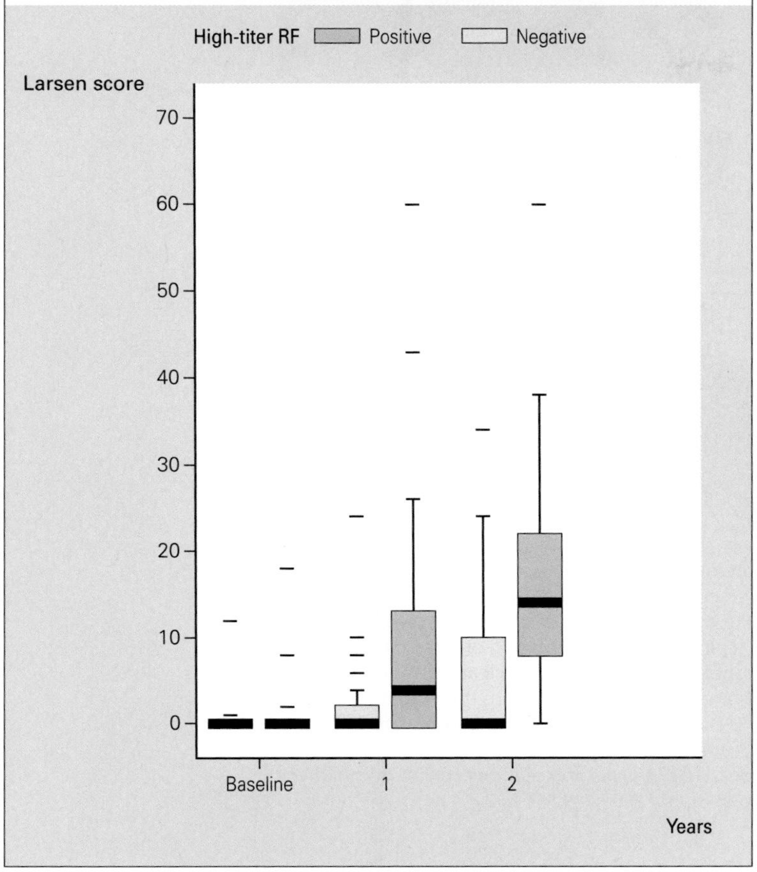

Fig. 88.3 Box plots showing the difference in joint damage defined by radiographic (Larsen) scores in RA patients with high-titer RF (>50 U/mL) versus patients with low-titer or negative RF. The boxes show median values and 25th/75th percentiles. Baseline values were similar in both groups, but Larsen score progression was significantly higher in patients with high-titer RF, both in the overall RA population ($P < .0001$) and also in the subpopulation of ACPA-negative patients ($P = .0014$, not shown). *(Adapted from: Nell V, Machold KP, Stamm TA, et al. Autoantibody profiling as early diagnostic and prognostic tool for rheumatoid arthritis. Ann Rheum Dis 2005;64:1731-1736.)*

employed as an antigen in most commercial assays for determination of ACPAs.[25-27]

Because filaggrin is exclusively expressed in terminally differentiated epithelial cells, it presumably does not represent one of the primary targets of ACPAs but rather seems to be a cross-reacting antigen. A candidate antigen that might be involved in the initiation of the ACPA response is fibrin and its precursor fibrinogen, because citrullinated forms of these proteins are abundantly present in synovial tissue and fluid of patients with RA (Fig. 88.5).[28] Although deimination of fibrin is not specific for RA and can be generally observed in inflamed joints,[29,30] citrullinated fibrin was shown to be recognized almost exclusively by sera of RA patients and also by affinity-purified anti-filaggrin antibodies.[7,28,31,32] Accumulation of fibrin on synovial and cartilage surfaces is a well-known feature of RA; therefore, it is conceivable that deiminated fibrin deposited in the synovial membrane may form a preferred target structure of ACPAs.

Another antigen of interest is the intermediate filament protein vimentin, which has been identified as a target of ACPAs.[33,34] Vimentin is a ubiquitously expressed cytoskeletal protein that occurs in various citrullinated isoforms, and citrullinated forms of vimentin were recently isolated from synovial fluid and tissue of patients with RA.[35,36] Interestingly, some of the citrullinated peptides analyzed were found to carry somatic point mutations,[35] which might contribute to the antigenicity of vimentin. These findings suggest that citrullinated vimentin might indeed form one of the primary initiators of the ACPA response.

DEIMINATION (CITRULLINATION) OF ARGININE BY PEPTIDYLARGININE DEIMINASE (PAD)

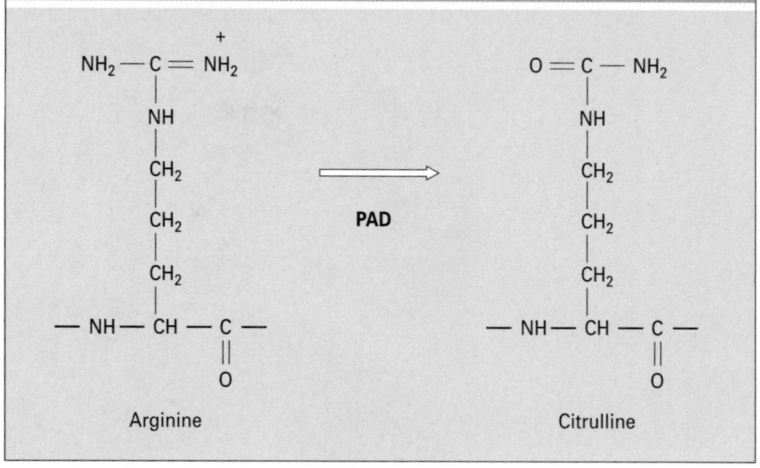

Fig. 88.4 Deimination (citrullination) of an argininyl residue by peptidylarginine deiminase (PAD). Enzymatic arginyl to citrullyl conversion is a post-translational modification that changes the charge and biochemical properties of proteins. Citrullination is predominantly observed in proteins of the cytoskeleton such as cytokeratin, vimentin, or filaggrin and seems to represent a general regulatory mechanism that particularly occurs during apoptosis.

Additional investigations on citrullinated antigens have been performed with α-enolase,[37] Epstein-Barr virus nuclear antigen-1,[38] human papillomavirus,[39] and collagen.[40,41] Although the pathogenic relevance of these antigens is uncertain, evidence is accumulating that some of them may occur in citrullinated form also *in vivo*. This has been recently demonstrated for α-enolase[42] and collagen II.[43]

Pathogenetic involvement

ACPAs are locally produced by synovial B cells and may therefore together with RF contribute to the inflammatory and destructive processes in the rheumatoid joint.[44] Their occurrence shows a strong association with the immunogenetic background, that is, with HLA-DR alleles carrying the "shared epitope,"[45-48] but there is still little known about the autoreactive T cells driving the ACPA response.[49,50] A highly significant association has been found between the occurrence of ACPA, presence of the shared epitope, and smoking, suggesting a link between autoimmunity, genes, and environment.[51-53] Despite these exciting findings, direct experimental evidence for a pathogenetic role of ACPA is scarce and induction of erosive arthritis in experimental animals by immunization with citrullinated fibrinogen has not yet been achieved.[54,55] Surprisingly, however, ACPAs were detected in mice with collagen-induced arthritis and administration of monoclonal antibodies against citrullinated fibrinogen enhanced arthritis, whereas induction of tolerance to a citrullinated peptide led to a significant reduction in disease susceptibility.[56] Furthermore, monoclonal antibodies to citrullinated collagen were recently shown to bind cartilage and induce (mild) arthritis in experimental animals.[43,57] These results seem to provide direct evidence for involvement of the ACPA autoimmune response in the pathogenesis of erosive arthritis, but the role of this response in the initial processes is still far from being fully understood.

Role as diagnostic and prognostic markers

Most commercial assays for the detection of ACPAs use a second-generation CCP (CCP2) as antigen, which was found to correlate highly with antibodies to citrullinated fibrinogen.[7,31] Other assays use third-generation CCP (CCP3), mutated citrullinated vimentin (MCV), filaggrin, or viral peptides. All assays employing CCP2 show similar performance, whereas assays employing citrullinated proteins appear to be somewhat less specific.[27,58] However, antibodies to MCV seem to better correlate with RA disease activity than ACPAs and may therefore

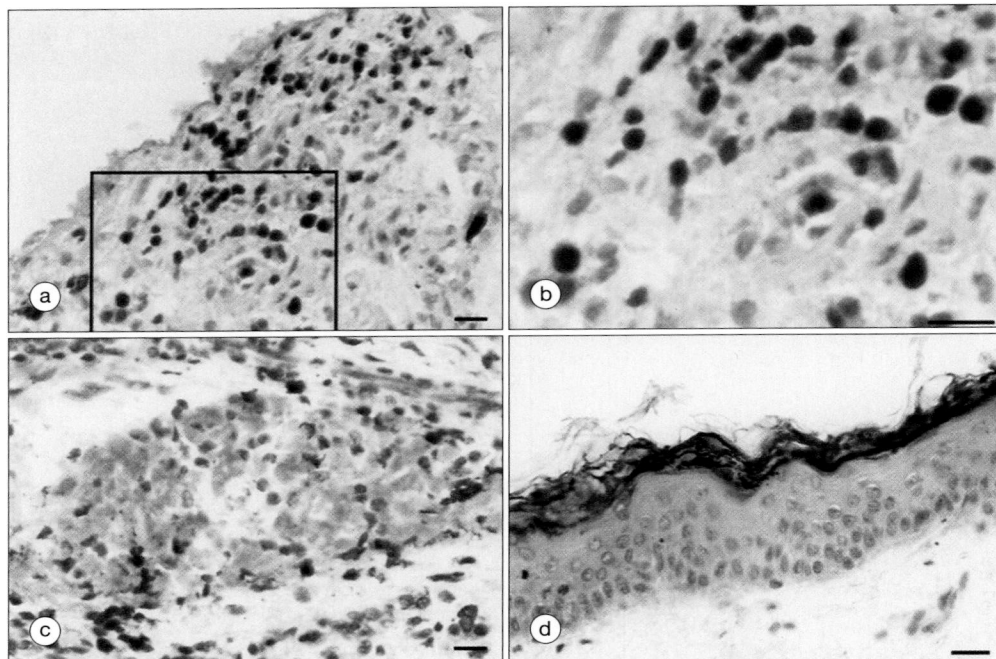

Fig. 88.5 Detection of deiminated (i.e., citrullinated) proteins in RA synovial tissue as demonstrated by immunoperoxidase staining with an antibody to modified citrulline. (a, b) In positive synovial membranes, the cytoplasm of numerous macrophage-like or fibroblast-like mononuclear cells, located in the lining or in the deep synovium, is intensely stained. (c) In addition, the staining of interstitial amorphous deposits located in the vicinity or close periphery of labeled mononuclear cells is observed in the deep synovium. (d) For comparison, a section of human skin is shown, where the whole cornified layer of the epidermis (containing deiminated filaggrin) is stained. Scale bars, 50 μm. *(With permission of the American Association of Immunologists from Masson Bessiere C, Sebbag M, Durieux JJ, et al. In the rheumatoid pannus, anti-filaggrin autoantibodies are produced by local plasma cells and constitute a higher proportion of IgG than in synovial fluid and serum. Clin Exp Immunol 2000;119:544-552.)*

provide additional information for the clinician.[35,59-61] Moreover, even though ACPAs and anti-MCV antibodies are largely overlapping, anti-MCV antibodies may also occur in ACPA (and RF)-negative patients.[59,62,63] However, it is not known whether patients recognizing solely MCV differ clinically from patients recognizing both CCP and MCV, and the disease specificity of isolated anti-MCV antibodies is uncertain.[64]

ACPAs are present early in the course of the disease[6,7,9,65-68] and similar to RF may also precede the clinical onset.[5] ACPAs have at least 95% specificity for RA and a diagnostic sensitivity of approximately 75% in established RA. However, their sensitivity at disease onset was found to be below 50% in patients with very short disease duration and between 55% and 64% in patients with disease of less than 1 year's duration (Table 88.3). The prevalence of ACPAs increases over time, irrespectively of therapy and disease activity, and seroconversion is rarely observed, at least when antibodies are measured by assays employing CCP2 as antigen. Other citrullinated substrates may be more suitable for disease monitoring, an issue requiring further investigation. The positive predictive value of ACPAs is better than 90%, which is comparable or even superior to high-titer IgM-RF.[7,9,68,69] In all studies, ACPA and IgM-RF were found to be highly associated with each other. In patients with early RA, approximately two thirds of ACPA-positive sera are usually also positive for IgM-RF (see Table 88.3); and in patients with long-standing disease the overlap is even higher.

Significant correlations between the presence of ACPA and radiographic disease progression (i.e., erosiveness) have been established in several studies (Fig. 88.6). Most of these studies demonstrated the prognostic value of ACPAs, particularly the correlation with bone damage.[9,12,15,65,68,70,71] Furthermore, ACPA-positive carriers of the shared epitope appear to be at particularly high risk for developing more severe forms of RA[46,72,73] and in a recent retrospective study covering an observation period of 10 years, ACPA and IgM-RF were found to be independent predictors for erosive disease (Fig. 88.7).[74] Thus, it is

TABLE 88.3 ACPA AND RF IN PATIENTS WITH EARLY RHEUMATOID ARTHRITIS

First author, year	Disease duration	Prevalence of ACPA	Specificity of ACPA	Prevalence of RF in ACPA+ patients
Meyer, 2003[70]	<12 mo	59%	—	65%
Kastbom, 2004[71]	<12 mo	64%	—	78%
Forslind, 2004[67]	<12 mo	55%	—	90%
Nielen, 2005[7]	<10 mo	58%	94%	75%
Soderlin, 2004[69]	<3 mo	44%	96%	82%
Nell, 2005[9]	<3 mo	41%	98%	67%

ACPA, anti-citrullinated peptide antibody; RF, rheumatoid factor.
NOTE: In all studies ACPAs were measured by ACPA ELISAs. In patients with very early RA with a disease duration of < 3 months ACPAs were detected in < 50% of the samples whereas prevalence was between 55% and 64% in patients with disease duration < 12 months.

important to measure both IgM-RF and ACPA in patients with early arthritis who do not yet fulfill the diagnostic criteria for classification of RA.[17]

AUTOANTIBODIES TO HETEROGENEOUS NUCLEAR RIBONUCLEOPROTEIN-A2

Autoimmunity to nuclear antigens is less abundant in RA than in most other systemic autoimmune diseases. Thus, antinuclear antibodies are detected by indirect immunofluorescence microscopy in only 20% to 30% of the patients and are of little if any usefulness for diagnostic purposes. An exception are autoantibodies to hnRNP-A2, which appears to have some relevance both for pathogenesis and diagnosis of

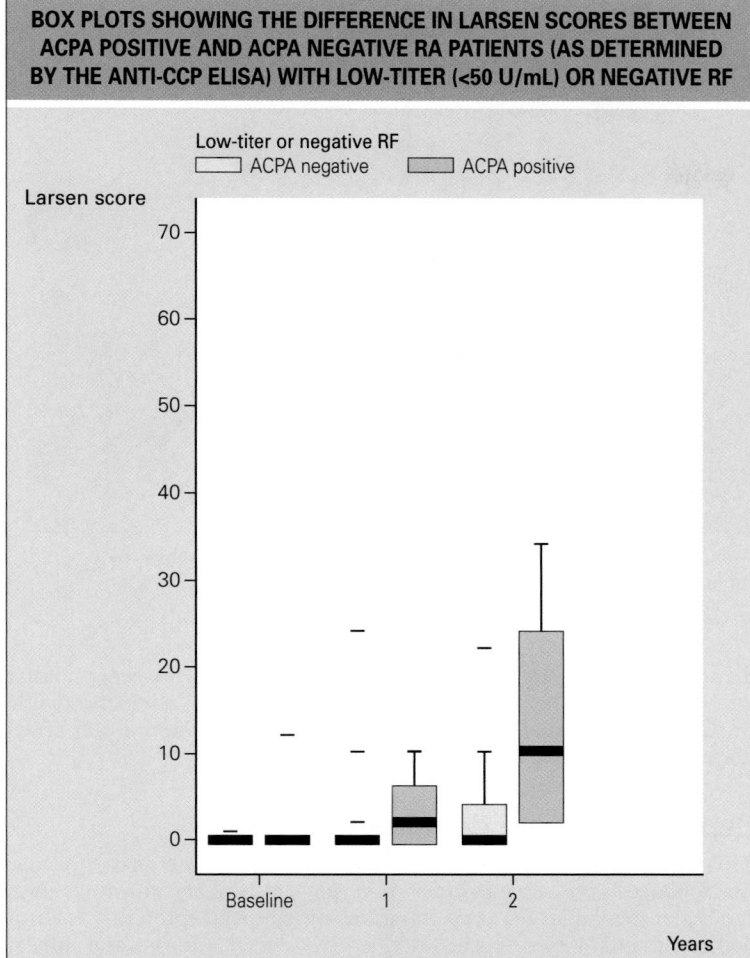

Fig. 88.6 Box plots showing the difference in Larsen scores between ACPA-positive and ACPA-negative RA patients (as determined by the anti-CCP ELISA) with low-titer (<50 U/mL) or negative RF. The boxes show median values and 25th/75th percentiles. Baseline values were similar in both groups, but Larsen score progression was significantly higher in ACPA-positive patients (*P* = .038).

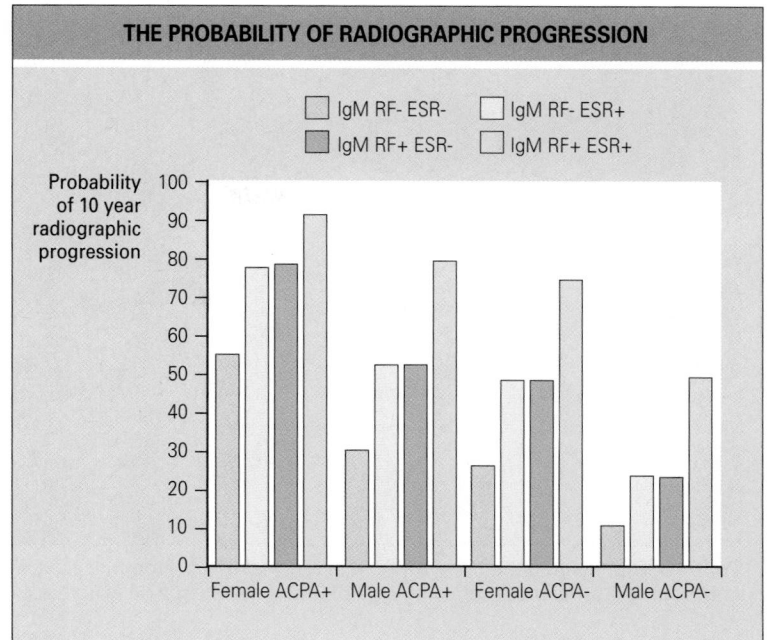

Fig. 88.7 The probability of radiographic progression (change in van der Heijde modified Sharp Score of hands and feet > 10 U/10 years) according to different combinations of the independent predictors IgM-RF, ACPA, and erythrocyte sedimentation rate (ESR) from a logistic regression model. *(From Syversen SW, Gaarder PI, Goll GL, et al. High anti-cyclic citrullinated peptide levels and an algorithm of four variables predict radiographic progression in patients with rheumatoid arthritis: results from a 10-year longitudinal study. Ann Rheum Dis 2008;67:212-217.)*

RA. The antigen, which was initially termed *RA33*,[75] is a 36-kDa protein that is associated with mRNA and involved in regulation of pre-mRNA splicing, mRNA transport, and translation. HnRNP-A2 is more or less ubiquitously expressed, with the highest expression levels observed in skin, lymphoid tissue, brain, and reproductive organs.[76,77]

Pathogenetic involvement

Pronounced T-cell reactivity to hnRNP-A2 has been observed in patients with RA but not in patients with osteoarthritis or psoriatic arthritis, and the antigen was found to be highly overexpressed in inflamed synovial tissue, whereas expression was low in normal joints (Fig. 88.8).[49] Remarkably, antibodies to hnRNP-A2 were also found to spontaneously occur in animal models of arthritis, namely, in tumor necrosis factor (TNF)-α transgenic mice[77] and in rats with pristane-induced arthritis, which also showed pronounced T-cell reactivity to this antigen.[78] Furthermore, immunization of TNF-α transgenic mice with a peptide corresponding to a major hnRNP-A2 B-cell epitope enhanced arthritis significantly.[77] Similar to RA synovial tissue, over-expression of hnRNP-A2 in the affected joints was seen in both animal models. Unexpectedly, hnRNP-A2 also stimulated lymph node cells and monocytes to produce inflammatory cytokines such as TNF-α or interleukin-6. Because this stimulation was dependent on MyD88, a signal transduction adapter molecule that is used by Toll-like receptors (TLRs), it is conceivable that hnRNP-A2 is capable of activating inflammatory cells via this pathway, presumably via its RNA component. Taken together, these findings point to a direct role of hnRNP-A2 in the pathogenesis of experimental arthritis that remains to be confirmed for human disease.

Role as diagnostic and prognostic markers

Autoantibodies to hnRNP-A2, which are also commonly known as anti-RA33 antibodies, occur in approximately one third of RA patients and with similar frequency also in patients with systemic lupus erythematosus (SLE) or mixed connective tissue disease, whereas they are rare in patients with other rheumatic disorders.[79,80] In patients with SLE, their occurrence is significantly associated with the presence of antibodies to spliceosomal antigens (e.g., Sm and U1 snRNP), which are virtually never targeted in RA. Moreover, epitope recognition was found to differ between patients with RA, mixed connective tissue disease, and SLE.[81,82] Because anti-hnRNP-A2 antibodies are rare in arthritides with a non-autoimmune pathogenesis (e.g., osteoarthritis, reactive arthritis, ankylosing spondylitis, or psoriatic arthritis) they can be helpful for differential diagnosis, particularly in patients who are negative for RF and/or ACPA. Anti-hnRNP-A2 antibodies have a specificity of approximately 90% for RA, which is somewhat lower than the specificity of ACPAs or high-titer IgM-RF. Similar to RF and ACPAs, anti-hnRNP-A2 antibodies may be present already in the earliest stages of the disease.[9] Importantly, they do not correlate with IgM-RF or ACPA and are also not associated with radiographic progression but rather seem to characterize patients with a more favorable prognosis.

AUTOANTIBODIES TO OTHER PROTEINS

Additional antigens that have been described to be targeted by autoantibodies from patients with RA include collagen and other cartilage proteins, stress or heat-shock proteins, and proteins with enzymatic properties. However, so far none of these antigens has proven useful for diagnostic or prognostic purposes.

Collagen

Among the 14 different collagens, type II collagen is the major collagen species in the joint and also the major collagen antigen. Antibodies

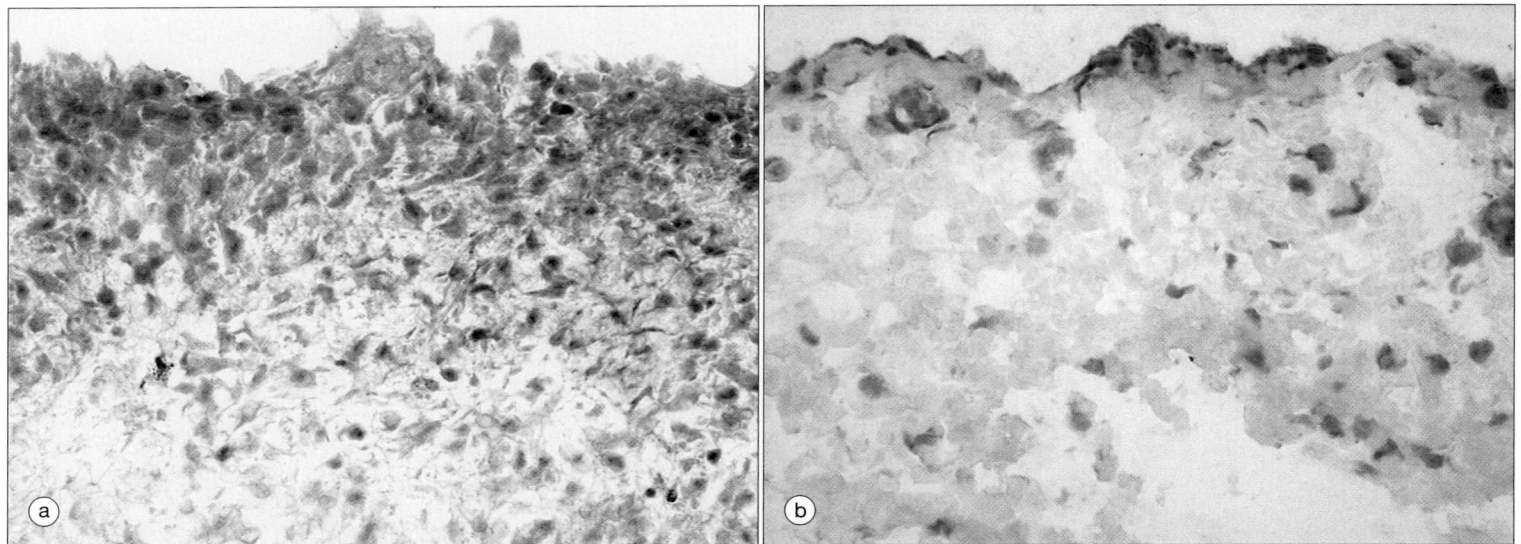

Fig. 88.8 Expression of hnRNP-A2 (RA33) in synovial tissue. Pronounced staining of macrophage-like and fibroblast-like cells overexpressing hnRNP-A2 is seen in the lining layer and the sublining area of RA synovial tissue (a), whereas expression is barely detectable in osteoarthritis synovial tissue (b).

can be directed to both native and denatured forms of collagen II. They are found in numerous pathologic conditions and are therefore not specific for RA. Antibodies to collagen II are present in RA synovial fluids and are presumably locally produced in the joint, as indicated by higher antibody levels in synovial fluid than in serum. Furthermore, autoantibodies to collagen and other cartilage components and immune complexes may be contained within the cartilage, which is ready to absorb and bind these molecules. It is therefore conceivable that immobilized IgG within the cartilage matrix may contribute to local macrophage activation and inflammation in RA. Even though pathogenicity of anti-collagen autoimmunity is obvious in collagen-induced arthritis, there is not much evidence that anti-collagen autoantibodies play a major role in the pathogenesis of human RA. However, recent observations that ACPAs may recognize deiminated forms of collagen may shed some new light on a role of collagen as autoantigen in the pathogenesis of RA.[40,41] Because collagen appears to be deiminated in the joint, it may be among the antigens targeted by ACPAs and thereby contribute to RA pathogenesis. This assumption is supported by recently reported observations that monoclonal antibodies to citrullinated collagen II can bind to cartilage and enhance collagen-induced arthritis.[43]

The prevalence of anti–collagen II antibodies to native collagen in RA is low, but titers may be particularly high in early disease and decline as the disease progresses.[83,84] High levels of serum antibodies to native collagen II are restricted to a small subset of patients with RA, leprosy, and relapsing polychondritis, whereas low-titer antibodies and those to denatured collagen II are found more generally. Most studies do not find a significant correlation between autoantibodies to collagen II and disease duration, activity, and severity of RA. Because of this and their apparent lack of disease specificity, anti-collagen antibodies are generally not considered as useful diagnostic markers.

Stress or heat-shock proteins

Stress or heat-shock proteins are required for correct folding and transport of newly synthesized proteins between cellular compartments. They are upregulated under conditions of cellular stress and protect cells from severe damage and premature death. Stress proteins are evolutionarily highly conserved from bacteria to humans and are among the most immunodominant microbial antigens. This has led to speculations about potentially pathogenic cross-reactivities that might arise in the course of infections.[85] Antibodies to stress proteins can be found in many pathologic conditions, including rheumatic diseases, and may also occur in healthy individuals but do not show specificity for any disease,[86] even though they may be elevated in the sera of RA patients as compared with patients with osteoarthritis as

demonstrated for the 78-kDa stress protein BiP.[87] However, cellular autoimmunity to heat-shock proteins seems to play a beneficial role in RA, involving mostly T-helper 2 (Th2) and regulatory T-cell (Treg) responses and may have therapeutic implications.[88]

Peptidyl arginine deiminase-4 (PAD4)

This enzyme is mainly expressed by immune cells such as monocytes/macrophages and granulocytes and is, presumably together with PAD2, responsible for citrullination of synovial proteins.[20] Antibodies to PAD4 have been described by several authors and appear to be rather specific for RA.[89-92] Because they are mainly detected in ACPA-positive patients their diagnostic value is presumably limited.

Glucose-6-phosphate isomerase

Glucose-6-phosphate isomerase (GPI) is a highly conserved glycolytic enzyme that catalyzes the interconversion of glucose-6-phosphate and fructose-6-phosphate. GPI was identified as the arthritogenic autoantigen in the KRNxNOD mouse model of RA in which a transgenic T-cell receptor induces arthritis closely resembling human RA. In this model, arthritis is dependent on both T and B cells and disease can be transferred by anti-GPI autoantibodies in a complement-dependent manner.[93] Moreover, immunization with GPI has been shown to induce arthritis in susceptible mouse strains.[94] Although anti-GPI antibodies may be present in sera and synovial fluid of RA patients, their incidence is low and they are not specific for RA.[95,96] Interestingly, they were found with increased frequency in RA patients suffering from extra-articular manifestations (Felty syndrome).[97] This, together with the observation of increased GPI levels in serum and synovial fluid of patients with arthritic disorders,[98] may be indicative of a pathogenic involvement of this antigen in human disease.

High mobility group box 1 protein (HMGB1)

HMGB1 is thought to constitute the prototype of a damage-associated molecular pattern or alarmin.[99,100] On tissue damage it is translocated from its homeostatic location in the nucleus to the extracellular milieu by passive release from dying cells and active secretion from monocytes and macrophages.[101] Extracellular HMGB1 exerts strong proinflammatory cytokine and chemoattractant activity and mitogenic activity, promotes angiogenesis, and regulates osteoclastogenesis. Elevated levels of extracellular HMGB1 are thought to contribute to perpetuation of synovitis in animal models of arthritis and patients with RA.[99] Autoantibodies to HMGB1 occur in many autoimmune diseases, among them RA and juvenile RA, and were reported to be associated with erythrocyte sedimentation rate, C-reactive protein, and the presence of RF.[102]

Calpastatin

Calpastatin is a natural inhibitor of the protease calpain, and both proteins can be found in elevated concentrations in RA synovial fluid. Antibodies to calpastatin have been reported to occur in 40% to 60% of RA patients but also have been described in other autoimmune diseases, and it has been suggested that anti-calpastatin antibodies may contribute to RA pathology by inhibiting calpastatin function, thereby aggravating disease.[103] In contrast to white patients, anti-calpastatin antibodies showed higher sensitivity and specificity for RA in Japanese patients and thus might be diagnostically useful at least in the Japanese population.[104] Of note, their occurrence in white RA patients has recently been found to be significantly associated with the shared epitope containing HLA-DR*0404.[105]

THE ROLE OF AUTOANTIBODIES IN THE PATHOGENESIS OF RHEUMATOID ARTHRITIS

Although autoantibodies are commonly present in sera and synovial fluid of most patients with RA, their precise pathogenetic role still has not been fully elucidated. Among the various autoantibodies described, only ACPAs are truly specific for RA, while all other antibody entities may occur also in other rheumatic diseases. The strong association of ACPA with certain HLA-DR alleles and with smoking provides a compelling link between genes, environment, and disease.[45,52,53] Remarkably, upregulation of PAD2 and the presence of citrullinated proteins has been demonstrated in the lungs of cigarette smokers and might represent the first event in the pathogenetic chain of RA.[106] It is currently unknown which citrullinated antigens initiate the ACPA response, but it is presumably not fibrin because fibrin deposition and citrullination occur after the onset of joint inflammation, being a consequence rather than the cause of arthritis. Thus, autoimmunity to citrullinated epitopes, which appears to be strongly dependent on the immunogenetic background, might be induced by ubiquitously expressed antigens such as vimentin or α-enolase. Once set in motion this autoimmune response seems to inevitably lead to development of RA because ACPAs are virtually never seen in healthy subjects and are only rarely observed in other rheumatic diseases. The binding of ACPAs to their targets in the synovial tissue probably has proinflammatory effects, leading to B- and T-cell stimulation and inducing fibrinogen extravasation, fibrin formation, and further deimination. This is most likely a self-maintaining process, which is at least partly responsible for the chronicity of the disease (Fig. 88.9). The recently reported observation that citrullinated forms of collagen may be present in synovial fluid of patients with RA suggests that collagen may become a target of ACPAs as well, even though it is certainly not primarily involved in the generation of the anti-citrulline response.[43,57] The immune complexes consisting of ACPAs and citrullinated antigens may represent the main target for RF, which would also explain the close association of these two antibodies.

The lack of disease specificity of autoantibodies other than ACPAs does not necessarily exclude a pathogenic role for them. Also, in other systemic autoimmune diseases only a few antibodies are truly disease specific. For example, antiphospholipid antibodies are among the pathogenic key players of the antiphospholipid syndrome but are also frequently found in patients with SLE. Another example is hnRNP-A2, which is an autoimmune target in RA, SLE, and mixed connective tissue disease.[107] However, epitope recognition differs between the three disorders[81,82] and differences have also been found at the T-cell level.[49,108] This RNA binding protein is unusual among the antigens targeted in RA because nucleic acid binding proteins are typically recognized by patients with SLE and other connective tissue diseases, where they may play a pivotal pathogenic role. The reason for the specific selection of ubiquitously expressed nucleic acid binding proteins as autoantigens has remained blurred for many years. With the discovery of pattern recognition receptors able to bind RNA or DNA it has become evident that the selection of nucleic acid–containing particles for the autoimmune attack is based on their intrinsic ability to activate those nucleic acid–recognizing receptor

SCHEMATIC VIEW OF THE ROLE PRESUMABLY PLAYED BY THE AUTOIMMUNE RESPONSE TO DEIMINATED FIBRIN IN THE PATHOPHYSIOLOGY OF RA

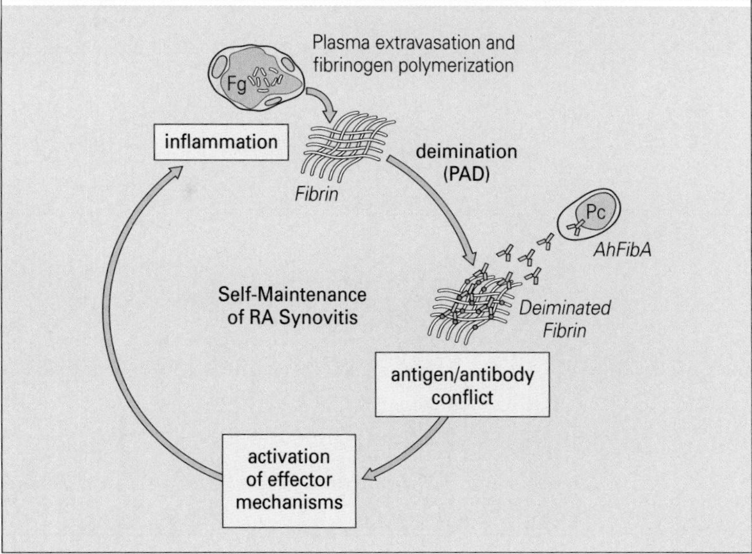

Fig. 88.9 Schematic view of the role presumably played by the autoimmune response to deiminated fibrin in the pathophysiology of RA. In the rheumatoid synovial tissue, fibrin is deiminated by PAD isoforms PAD2 and PAD4, which are abundantly expressed by synovial monocytes/macrophages and granulocytes, and becomes the target of the disease-specific antibodies (AhFibA) locally produced by synovial plasma cells (Pc). This leads to antigen/antibody complexes that, via activation of effector mechanisms probably involving complement and/or Fc receptors, have proinflammatory effects. In turn, these effects lead to plasma extravasation and fibrinogen polymerization and therefore provoke the formation of new fibrin deposits in the tissue, which become the substrate of one or several locally expressed PADs. This closes a vicious circle that could account for the self-maintenance of rheumatoid inflammation. In the synovial tissue of non-RA patients, even if deiminated fibrin is present, the absence of AhFibA prevents establishment of this self-maintenance loop. Fg, fibrinogen.

systems, thereby crucially contributing to disease pathogenesis.[109] Thus, inappropriate activation of nucleic acid–binding TLRs such as TLR7 or TLR9 by self nucleic acid ligands within autoantigenic complexes (e.g., snRNPs, hnRNPs, or nucleosomes) might be an important factor contributing not only to the pathogenesis of SLE but also to that of RA and other (systemic) autoimmune disorders.[110] Recent data obtained in rats with pristane-induced arthritis have provided some evidence that such a mechanism may indeed play a role in the pathogenesis of erosive arthritis.[78] Furthermore, overexpression of TLR3, TLR4, and TLR7 in the synovium of RA patients has been reported, suggesting involvement of their respective ligands in the inflammatory process.[111,112]

Taking all these observations into consideration a general model for the initiation of arthritogenic autoimmune responses is suggested in which an environmental trigger (e.g., a toxic substance or an infectious agent) induces apoptosis in tissues (e.g., the lung) and/or lymphoid organs, leading to extensive modification (e.g., deimination or phosphorylation) and degradation of proteins. Inappropriate uptake of apoptotic materials capable of stimulating TLRs (and other pattern recognition receptor systems) by dendritic cells will lead to activation of autoreactive T and B cells and subsequently to autoantibody production on a susceptible genetic background (Fig. 88.10). Autoreactive lymphocytes will then migrate to the joint, where they set in motion the inflammatory and destructive processes that lead to abundant release of joint-specific antigens. This may give rise to further autoimmunization of the patient via phagocytosing macrophages and dendritic cells and subsequent immune complex formation involving also RFs. Autoimmune reactions to other proteins such as stress proteins, hnRNPs, GPI, or HMGB1 may arise due to overexpression, posttranslational modification(s), and aberrant processing of the antigens

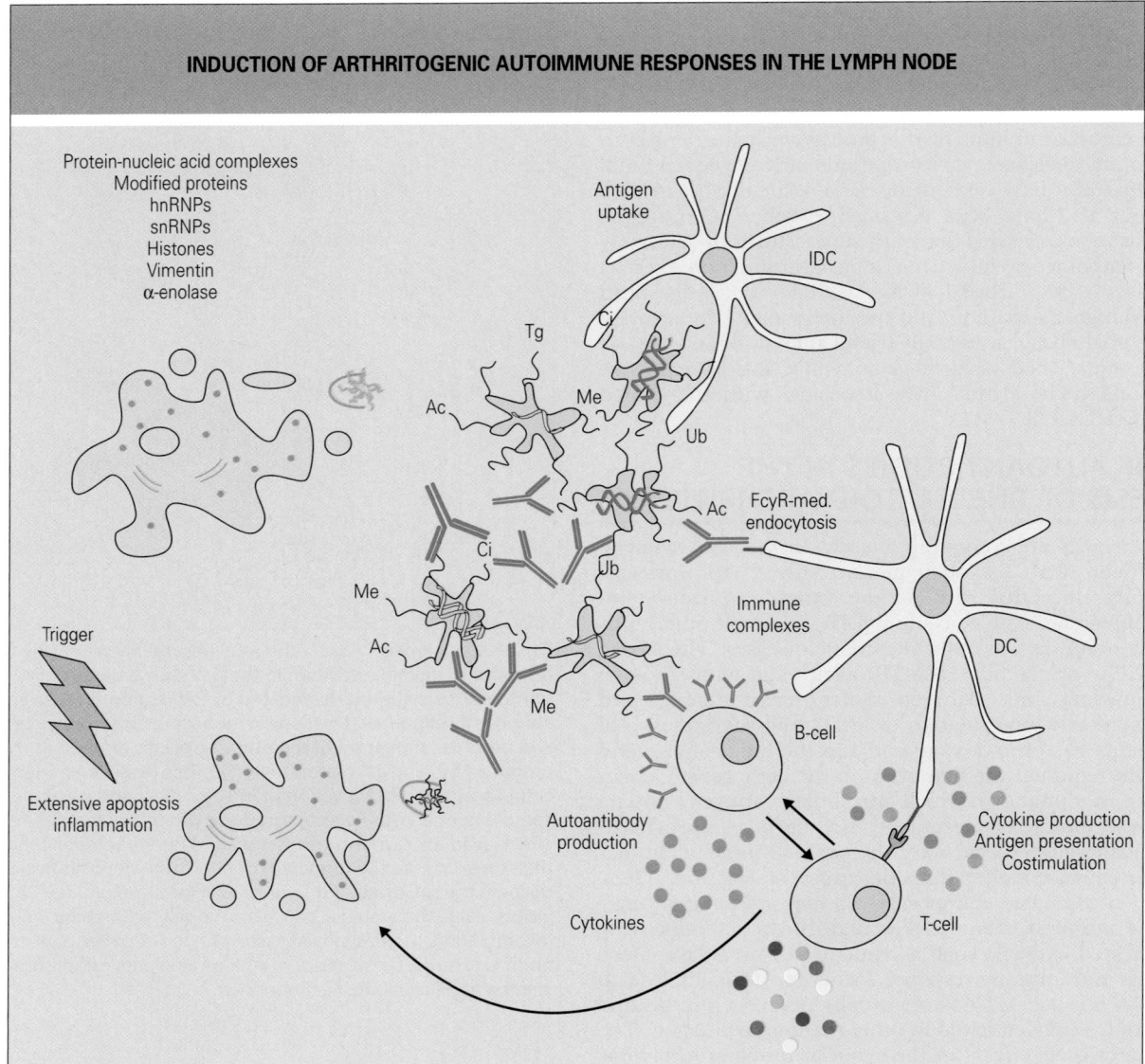

Fig. 88.10 Induction of arthritogenic autoimmune responses in the lymph node. An unknown trigger that may contain a danger signal provided by a pathogen or an intrinsic danger signal derived from exposed endogenous ligands initiates inflammation and subsequent apoptosis in secondary lymphoid organs. Insufficient removal of apoptotic cells leads to accumulation of apoptotic bodies containing nucleic acid–associated antigens and antigens modified during apoptosis such as histones, ribonucleoproteins, vimentin, or α-enolase, which are aberrantly engulfed by professional antigen-presenting cells such as immature dendritic cells (IDC). The nucleic acids (RNA in yellow, and DNA in red) associated with these antigens function as endogenous adjuvants that stimulate immune cells via Toll-like receptors (TLRs) and/or other endogenous receptors for RNA and DNA. The protein component is degraded in endosomes with subsequent membrane fusion to vesicles containing MHC class II molecules. Release of proinflammatory cytokines that upregulate expression of MHC class II and co-stimulatory molecules enhances the presentation of potentially pathogenic peptides to autoreactive T cells. These will subsequently activate autoreactive B cells leading finally to autoantibody production. Moreover, DNA- and RNA-associated autoantigens may directly activate autoreactive B cells via sequential engagement of the B-cell antigen receptor and TLR9 or TLR7, respectively. The formation of immune complexes further increases uptake of antigens via FcγR on dendritic cells. Autoreactive B and T cells emigrate from the lymph node to target organs where they recognize their respective autoantigens, setting off an inflammatory reaction that leads to further activation of autoreactive T and B cells in the affected organ where tertiary lymphoid organs may form. After enhanced tissue damage and increased production of apoptotic debris, a vicious circle is set in motion that may (dependent on the genetic background) result in the development of chronic autoimmune disease.

induced by the proinflammatory milieu within the joint. Thus, an increasing number of autoimmune reactions may be generated in the course of disease, all of which may contribute to the pathophysiology of RA.

Because of the exciting observations made in recent years, autoantibodies no longer can be regarded solely as useful diagnostic markers of otherwise little pathogenetic relevance. Identification of new auto-antigens and the characterization of the cellular and molecular processes underlying the pathologic autoimmune reactions against them has provided new insights into the pathogenesis of RA. A better understanding of the disease process will finally enable us to develop novel therapeutic concepts that may allow for treatment of RA in its initial stages in an antigen-specific manner and for a definitive cure for this debilitating disease.

KEY REFERENCES

1. Sutton B, Corper A, Bonagura V, Taussig M. The structure and origin of rheumatoid factors. Immunol Today 2000;21:177-183.
2. Westwood OM, Nelson PN, Hay FC. Rheumatoid factors: what's new? Rheumatology 2006;45:379-385.
3. Dorner T, Egerer K, Feist E, Burmester GR. Rheumatoid factor revisited. Curr Opin Rheum 2004;16:246-253.
4. Rantapaa-Dahlqvist S, de Jong BA, Berglin E, et al. Antibodies against cyclic citrullinated peptide and IgA rheumatoid factor predict the development of rheumatoid arthritis [see comment]. Arthritis Rheum 2003;48:2741-2749.
5. Nielen MMJ, van Schaardenburg D, Reesink HWR, et al. Specific autoantibodies precede the symptoms of rheumatoid arthritis: a study of serial measurements in blood donors. Arthritis Rheum 2004;50:380-386.
6. Jansen AL, van der Horst-Bruinsma I, van Schaardenburg D, et al. Rheumatoid factor and antibodies to cyclic citrullinated peptide differentiate rheumatoid arthritis from undifferentiated polyarthritis in patients with early arthritis. J Rheumatol 2002;29:2074-2076.
7. Nielen MM, van der Horst AR, van Schaardenburg D, et al. Antibodies to citrullinated human fibrinogen (ACF) have diagnostic and prognostic value in early arthritis. Ann Rheum Dis 2005;64:1199-1204.
8. Sinclair D, Hull RG. Why do general practitioners request rheumatoid factor? A study of symptoms, requesting patterns and patient outcome. Ann Clin Biochem 2003;40:131-137.
9. Nell V, Machold KP, Stamm TA, et al. Autoantibody profiling as early diagnostic and prognostic tool for rheumatoid arthritis. Ann Rheum Dis 2005;64:1731-1736.
10. Symmons DP. Classification criteria for rheumatoid arthritis—time to abandon rheumatoid factor? [see comment]. Rheumatology 2007;46:725-726.
11. Jonsson T, Steinsson K, Jonsson H, et al. Combined elevation of IgM and IgA rheumatoid factor has high diagnostic specificity for rheumatoid arthritis. Rheumatol Int 1998;18:119-122.
12. Bas S, Genevay S, Meyer O, Gabay C. Anti-cyclic citrullinated peptide antibodies, IgM and IgA rheumatoid factors in the diagnosis and prognosis of rheumatoid arthritis. Rheumatology 2003;42:677-680.
13. Greiner A, Plischke H, Kellner H, Gruber R. Association of anti-cyclic citrullinated peptide antibodies, anti-citrulline antibodies, and IgM and IgA rheumatoid factors with serological parameters of disease activity in rheumatoid arthritis. Ann N Y Acad Sci 2005;1050:295-303.
14. Scott DL. Prognostic factors in early rheumatoid arthritis. Rheumatology 2000;39(Suppl 1):124-129.
15. Lindqvist E, Eberhardt K, Bendtzen K, et al. Prognostic laboratory markers of joint damage in rheumatoid arthritis. Ann Rheum Dis 2005;64:196-201.
16. Turesson C, Jacobsson LT, Sturfelt G, et al. Rheumatoid factor and antibodies to cyclic citrullinated peptides are associated with severe extra-articular manifestations in rheumatoid arthritis. Ann Rheum Dis 2007;66:59-64.
17. Combe B, Landewe R, Lukas C, et al. EULAR recommendations for the management of early arthritis: report of a task force of the European Standing Committee for International Clinical Studies Including Therapeutics (ESCISIT) [see comment]. Ann Rheum Dis 2007;66:34-45.
18. Vossenaar ER, van Venrooij WJ. Citrullinated proteins: sparks that may ignite the fire in rheumatoid arthritis. Arthritis Res Ther 2004;6:107-111.
19. Vincent C, Nogueira L, Clavel C, et al. Autoantibodies to citrullinated proteins: ACPA. Autoimmunity 2005;38:17-24.
20. Raptopoulou A, Sidiropoulos P, Katsouraki M, Boumpas DT. Anti-citrulline antibodies in the diagnosis and prognosis of rheumatoid arthritis: evolving concepts. Crit Rev Clin Lab Sci 2007;44:339-363.
21. Youinou P, Serre G. The antiperinuclear factor and antikeratin antibody systems. Int Arch Allergy Immunol 1995;107:508-518.
22. Schellekens GA, de Jong BA, van den Hoogen FH, et al. Citrulline is an essential constituent of antigenic determinants recognized by rheumatoid arthritis-specific autoantibodies. J Clin Invest 1998;101:273-281.
23. Girbal Neuhauser E, Durieux JJ, Arnaud M, et al. The epitopes targeted by the rheumatoid arthritis–associated antifilaggrin autoantibodies are posttranslationally generated on various sites of (pro) filaggrin by deimination of arginine residues. J Immunol 1999;162:585-594.
24. Union A, Meheus L, Humbel RL, et al. Identification of citrullinated rheumatoid arthritis–specific epitopes in natural filaggrin relevant for antifilaggrin autoantibody detection by line immunoassay. Arthritis Rheum 2002;46:1185-1195.
25. Schellekens GA, Visser H, de Jong BA, et al. The diagnostic properties of rheumatoid arthritis antibodies recognizing a cyclic citrullinated peptide. Arthritis Rheum 2000;43:155-163.
26. Zendman AJ, van Venrooij WJ, Pruijn GJ. Use and significance of anti-CCP autoantibodies in rheumatoid arthritis. Rheumatology 2006;45:20-25.
27. Bizzaro N, Tonutti E, Tozzoli R, Villalta D. Analytical and diagnostic characteristics of 11 2nd- and 3rd-generation immunoenzymatic methods for the detection of antibodies to citrullinated proteins. Clin Chem 2007;53:1527-1533.
28. Masson-Bessiere C, Sebbag M, Girbal-Neuhauser E, et al. The major synovial targets of the rheumatoid arthritis–specific antifilaggrin autoantibodies are deiminated forms of the alpha- and beta-chains of fibrin. J Immunol 2001;166:4177-4184.
29. Vossenaar ER, Smeets TJ, Kraan MC, et al. The presence of citrullinated proteins is not specific for rheumatoid synovial tissue. Arthritis Rheum 2004;50:3485-3494.
30. Chapuy-Regaud S, Sebbag M, Baeten D, et al. Fibrin deimination in synovial tissue is not specific for rheumatoid arthritis but commonly occurs during synovitides. J Immunol 2005;174:5057-5064.
31. Vander Cruyssen B, Cantaert T, Nogueira L, et al. Diagnostic value of anti-human citrullinated fibrinogen ELISA and comparison with four other anti-citrullinated protein assays. Arthritis Res Ther 2006;8:R122.
32. Hill JA, Al-Bishri J, Gladman DD, et al. Serum autoantibodies that bind citrullinated fibrinogen are frequently found in patients with rheumatoid arthritis [see comment]. J Rheumatol 2006;33:2115-2119.
33. Vossenaar ER, Despres N, Lapointe E, et al. Rheumatoid arthritis specific anti-Sa antibodies target citrullinated vimentin. Arthritis Res Ther 2004;6:R142-R150.
34. Rodriguez-Mahou M, Lopez-Longo FJ, Sanchez-Ramon S, et al. Association of anti-cyclic citrullinated peptide and anti-Sa/citrullinated vimentin autoantibodies in rheumatoid arthritis. Arthritis Rheum 2006;55:657-661.
35. Bang H, Egerer K, Gauliard A, et al. Mutation and citrullination modifies vimentin to a novel autoantigen for rheumatoid arthritis. Arthritis Rheum 2007;56:2503-2511.
36. Tilleman K, Van Steendam K, Cantaert T, et al. Synovial detection and autoantibody reactivity of processed citrullinated isoforms of vimentin in inflammatory arthritides. Rheumatology 2008;47:597-604.
37. Kinloch A, Tatzer V, Wait R, et al. Identification of citrullinated alpha-enolase as a candidate autoantigen in rheumatoid arthritis. Arthritis Res Ther 2005;7:R1421-R1429.
38. Pratesi F, Tommasi C, Anzilotti C, et al. Deiminated Epstein-Barr virus nuclear antigen 1 is a target of anti-citrullinated protein antibodies in rheumatoid arthritis. Arthritis Rheum 2006;54:733-741.
39. Shi J, Sun X, Zhao Y, et al. Prevalence and significance of antibodies to citrullinated human papillomavirus-47 E2345-362 in rheumatoid arthritis. J Autoimmun 2008;31:131-135.
40. Burkhardt H, Sehnert B, Bockermann R, et al. Humoral immune response to citrullinated collagen type II determinants in early rheumatoid arthritis. Eur J Immunol 2005;35:1643-1652.
41. Suzuki A, Yamada R, Ohtake-Yamanaka M, et al. Anti-citrullinated collagen type I antibody is a target of autoimmunity in rheumatoid arthritis. Biochem Biophys Res Commun 2005;333:418-426.
42. Lundberg K, Kinloch A, Fisher BA, et al. Antibodies to citrullinated alpha-enolase peptide 1 are specific for rheumatoid arthritis and cross-react with bacterial enolase. Arthritis Rheum 2008;58:3009-3019.
43. Uysal H, Bockermann R, Nandakumar KS, et al. Structure and pathogenicity of antibodies specific for citrullinated collagen type II in experimental arthritis. J Exp Med 2009;206:449-462.
44. Masson Bessiere C, Sebbag M, Durieux JJ, et al. In the rheumatoid pannus, anti-filaggrin autoantibodies are produced by local plasma cells and constitute a higher proportion of IgG than in synovial fluid and serum. Clin Exp Immunol 2000;119:544-552.
45. Klareskog L, Padyukov L, Ronnelid J, Alfredsson L. Genes, environment and immunity in the development of rheumatoid arthritis. Curr Opin Immunol 2006;18:650-655.
46. van der Helm-van Mil AH, Verpoort KN, Breedveld FC, et al. The HLA-DRB1 shared epitope alleles are primarily a risk factor for anti-cyclic citrullinated peptide antibodies and are not an independent risk factor for development of rheumatoid arthritis. Arthritis Rheum 2006;54:1117-1121.
47. Gourraud PA, Dieude P, Boyer JF, et al. A new classification of HLA-DRB1 alleles differentiates predisposing and protective alleles for autoantibody production in rheumatoid arthritis. Arthritis Res Ther 2007;9:R27.
48. Verpoort KN, Cheung K, Ioan-Facsinay A, et al. Fine specificity of the anti-citrullinated protein antibody response is influenced by the shared epitope alleles. Arthritis Rheum 2007;56:3949-3952.
49. Fritsch R, Eselböck D, Skriner K, et al. Characterization of autoreactive T cells to the autoantigens RA33 (hnRNP A2) and filaggrin in patients with rheumatoid arthritis. J Immunol 2002;169:1068-1076.
50. Auger I, Sebbag M, Vincent C, et al. Influence of HLA-DR genes on the production of rheumatoid arthritis-specific autoantibodies to citrullinated fibrinogen. Arthritis Rheum 2005;52:3424-3432.

REFERENCES

Full references for this chapter can be found on www.expertconsult.com.

Cellular immunity in rheumatoid arthritis

J. S. Hill Gaston

89

- Components of the immune system, particularly T cells, are prominent within the rheumatoid synovial membrane.
- Susceptibility to autoantibody-positive disease correlates strongly with major histocompatibility complex antigens, the function of which is to control immune responses, particularly at the level of T-cell recognition.
- Therapies directed against several components of the immune system can alleviate symptoms and prevent disease progression.

INTRODUCTION

Although the immune system is centrally involved in rheumatoid arthritis (RA), the precise immune functions critical in its pathogenesis continue to be debated. What are the respective roles of the innate versus the acquired immune response, and which is dominant? Does RA require an antigen-specific immune response; and if so, what antigens are involved? Are they exogenous (e.g., from viruses or bacteria) or are they autoantigens? Alternatively, does RA result from activation of the immune system by stimuli that are not related to the joint or inherently arthritogenic? In this case the specificity of lymphocytes found at the site of disease would be irrelevant and chronic inflammation would be maintained by non-specific mechanisms, such as the antigen-independent interactions between activated T cells and synoviocytes, which can produce proinflammatory cytokines. In addition, given that immune responses to foreign or autoantigens do not usually give rise to a pathologic process, particularly chronic unresolved inflammation, is the defect in RA a failure to regulate or terminate immune responses that would normally be manageable? Such failures could reflect imbalances in cytokine production or a particular pattern of cytokine production that would favor chronic inflammation. On the other hand, they could represent a lack of an adequate response by regulatory T or B cells.

Each of these questions will be considered in this chapter. Often animal models of RA will be used to illustrate the kinds of processes that can give rise to joint inflammation and destruction, but it must be emphasized that "rodents don't get RA," that is, observations in animal models need validation in human disease.

POSSIBLE ANTIGENIC TARGETS OF THE IMMUNE RESPONSE IN RA

Autoantigens

RA has no "obvious" cause, such as a preceding specific infection. This, together with the observation of autoimmunity in the shape of rheumatoid factor (the first autoantibody to be described) led to the assumption the disease is autoimmune. However, unlike other autoimmune diseases, RA has lacked autoimmune responses that are obviously causal in the sense that tissue-specific autoantibodies and T-cell responses can be clearly seen to result in the tissue-specific destruction or stimulation so characteristic of other autoimmune diseases such as diabetes and thyroid disease. The generation of rheumatoid factors, antibodies to the Fc portion of IgG, cannot be straightforwardly linked

to synovitis or cartilage destruction. Indeed, rheumatoid factors commonly occur in chronic infections (e.g., endocarditis) without giving rise to arthritis. At first glance the same lack of tissue specificity applies to the more recently described anti-citrullinated peptide antibodies (ACPAs) (so named because they are measured using artificially constructed citrullinated cyclic peptides), which are a more specific marker of RA because proteins at many sites outside joints have post-translational modification of arginine residues to citrulline carried out by peptidyl arginine deiminases (PADs).

Nevertheless, in pursuit of the notion that RA is indeed autoimmune, several putative target antigens have been considered (Table 89.1).

Joint components

Type II collagen

Arthritis can readily be induced in rodents and primates by immunization with heterologous or homologous native type II collagen. Extensive studies of this model show that the arthritis requires both collagen-specific B and T cells. Susceptibility depends on major histocompatibility complex (MHC) antigens, and the disease can be modulated by interventions such as depletion of specific T cells, vaccination against T cells, and induction of tolerance by oral administration of type II collagen.[1] Despite the attractiveness of the model and the lessons learned from it, the importance of immune responses to type II collagen in RA remains unclear. Collagen-specific T and B cells can be isolated from RA patients[2] but only from a minority; these cells may be easier to find in synovial tissue but even here are not invariable. The possibility that they arise secondary to joint destruction, and exposure of otherwise cryptic epitopes in type II collagen to the immune system, has not been discounted, although a correlation between the degree of destruction and the presence of collagen-specific B cells in synovial fluid has not been found.[3] Finally, attempts to induce oral tolerance to type II collagen did not produce consistent effects on RA activity.[4,5] Together these findings do not greatly support the idea of type II collagen as the target autoantigen in RA. However, recent interest in immune responses to citrullinated peptides reopen this question, since type II collagen can be citrullinated. Antibodies to citrullinated type II collagen are more common in RA than antibodies to unmodified collagen, similar in frequency to ACPA and highly correlated with them.[6] In addition, experimentally citrullinated type II collagen induces more severe arthritis in rats than the native protein.[7]

Proteoglycans and chondrocyte proteins

Mice immunized with the human cartilage proteoglycan aggrecan develop erosive arthritis; but because they also have marked spondylitis, autoimmunity to proteoglycan may be a model of ankylosing spondylitis rather than of RA.[8] Indeed, proteoglycan-specific T cells have been identified in ankylosing spondylitis.[9] In addition to aggrecan, other cartilage proteoglycan molecules, such as biglycan and decorin, could, in principle, be targets of autoimmunity in RA but have yet to be investigated extensively. One additional chondrocyte protein has attracted attention: human cartilage glycoprotein 39 (HCgp39) is secreted in quantity by chondrocytes in arthritic joints but not those in normal joints. Again, immunizing mice with HCgp39 produces a mild arthritis, and certain HCgp39-derived peptides bind strongly to the RA-associated human leukocyte antigen (HLA) allele DRB1*0401 and can be recognized by T cells from some RA patients.[10] However, synovial HCgp39-specific T cells could not be identified in most DR4+ RA patients, using tetramers of specific HCgp39-derived peptide bound

TABLE 89.1 CANDIDATE ANTIGENS THAT COULD DRIVE THE IMMUNE RESPONSE IN RA

Autoantigens

Type II collagen
Proteoglycans
Human cartilage glycoprotein 39
Citrullinated proteins
Vimentin
Fibrinogen
α-Enolase
Type II collagen
Heat-shock proteins
Glucose-6-phosphate isomerase

Foreign antigens

Bacteria
Viruses
Superantigens

TABLE 89.2 SEQUENCE OF EVENTS IN THE DEVELOPMENT OF A MODEL OF EXPERIMENTAL ARTHRITIS CAUSED BY AUTOIMMUNE RECOGNITION OF A NORMAL CELLULAR ENZYME

1. A mouse T-cell receptor (termed KRN) was characterized that recognizes an experimental antigen (bovine ribonuclease) presented by the class II MHC antigen, I-A^k.
2. I-A^k mice transgenic for the KRN T-cell receptor were produced (i.e., all their T cells express the same receptor): mice were completely healthy.
3. KRN T-cell receptor transgenic mice expressing a different class II MHC antigen (I-A^{g7}) developed an aggressive RA-like inflammatory arthritis (the "K/BxN" mouse).
4. Arthritis was produced because the KRN T-cell receptor can recognize a peptide from an autoantigen, presented by I-A^{g7}—i.e., an "accidental" cross-reactivity of the T cell receptor.
5. The autoantigen was identified as a ubiquitous cellular enzyme: glucose-6-phosphate isomerase.
6. Both antibody and T-cell responses to the autoantigen are required to produce arthritis (no disease occurs in B-cell–deficient mice), and disease can be transferred with serum.

to DRB1*0401.[11] Thus, the status of HCgp39 as a target antigen is unclear.

Proteins not restricted to the joint

Given the relative lack of success in implicating a joint constituent as an autoantigen in RA, consideration has been given to antigens outside the joint that have been implicated in animal models of arthritis. This can also be justified by increasing evidence of a "pre-arthritis" phase of RA when autoantibodies such as rheumatoid factors and ACPAs are present without joint inflammation—often for years.[12,13]

Glucose-6-phosphate isomerase

An elegant murine model, the K/BxN mouse, has been influential as a convincing example of arthritis induced by an autoimmune response directed at a ubiquitous cellular antigen, a glycolytic enzyme, glucose-6-phosphate isomerase (G6PI).[14,15] The sequence of events leading to this fascinating discovery is detailed in Table 89.2. The arthritis has both T-cell–mediated and antibody-mediated components; mice that are B cell deficient fail to develop disease, and arthritis disease can be transferred with serum from arthritic mice. However, disease after passive transfer is transient as compared with that which develops in the T-cell receptor (TCR) transgenic mice (see Table 89.2). The model is highly artificial; in essence it stems from the accidental ability of a specific TCR, generated to recognize a non-self peptide, to recognize an autoantigenic peptide when presented by a different class II MHC allele, but it is still instructive in relation to our understanding of RA. The target of the autoimmune T-cell response, G6PI, is ubiquitous, and there is no evidence that it is overexpressed in the joint or on joint-derived antigen-presenting cells. Nevertheless, the inflammatory response is confined to the joint (and salivary glands). Furthermore, the initial defect, an autoreactive T cell, drives arthritis via the production of autoantibodies (again specific for G6PI), which, in turn, form immune complexes and activate both synoviocytes and mast cells in a complement-dependent fashion. Thus, RA need not require an immune response directed against a joint-specific antigen. Suggestions that the same antigen, G6PI, might be involved in RA have not been confirmed[16] and never seemed likely in view of the "accidental" event at the heart of the mouse model.

Citrullinated proteins

The discovery that autoantibodies that react with citrullinated proteins are a highly specific feature of RA is a major advance in our understanding of the pathogenesis of the disease.[17] Whereas most ACPA-positive patients are also rheumatoid factor positive, ACPAs have higher specificity for RA. They are also associated with erosive disease. Indeed, there is now compelling evidence to regard ACPA-positive and ACPA-negative "RA" as two quite separate diseases, with non-overlapping genetic and environmental factors in their pathogenesis and differing outcomes on treatment.[18,19] Although recognition of ACPAs came from work on autoantibodies to keratin (which has a large number of

deimidated arginine residues), the physiologic target of the "ACPA" response is still debated. Mention has already been made of immune responses to citrullinated type II collagen, but other joint-unrelated proteins have been examined. Antibodies to a range of citrullinated proteins are detected in RA, including vimentin, fibrinogen, heat shock proteins, and, intriguingly, α-enolase.[20] Data on α-enolase show that the immunodominant citrullinated peptide recognized is conserved in α-enolase from the bacterium *Porphyromonas gingivalis*, an etiologic agent of dental caries. Enolases are common targets of the immune response to bacteria.

Most work on immune response to citrullinated peptides has concerned autoantibodies, but because the antibodies are of high affinity and class switched, involvement of T cells in generating these responses can be assumed. T cells have been shown to recognize post-translationally modified peptides, specifically, citrullinated peptides,[21] and HLA-DR alleles containing the shared epitope bind citrullinated peptides more strongly than equivalent peptides containing unmodified arginine (Fig. 89.1).[22]

Heat-shock proteins

Heat-shock proteins (hsp), similar to G6PI and α-enolase, are ubiquitous cellular constituents; hsp control the correct folding, transport, and assembly of cellular proteins. Interest in immune responses to hsp as causes of arthritis stemmed from work on rat adjuvant arthritis, where mycobacterial hsp60 was shown to be an important T-cell target. Although adjuvant arthritis is acute and self-limiting, resembling reactive arthritis more than RA, the extensive sequence identity between bacterial and eukaryotic hsp60 led to the proposal that T cells, initially triggered to recognize bacterial hsp60 in the course of infection, could cross-react with the mammalian protein and thus initiate arthritis (the "molecular mimicry hypothesis" [see later]). Cross-reactive T cells of this kind have been described but are not confined to patients with arthritis. In adjuvant arthritis, the idea that the mycobacterial hsp60 epitope recognized by an arthritogenic T cell was conserved in rat hsp60, and therefore the target of an autoimmune response, has been shown to be incorrect. Indeed, more recent work suggests that autoimmune responses to hsp may ameliorate rather than initiate arthritis and initiate regulatory T-cell responses. Thus, rats previously immunized with mycobacterial hsp60 become resistant to induction of adjuvant arthritis, and the T cells conferring this resistance are the ones that cross-react with rat hsp60.[23,24] These findings for hsp60 may apply to other hsp; self-hsp70–specific T cells also protect in adjuvant arthritis. Together the findings on hsp as antigens point away from a simplistic idea of assuming that an autoimmune response inevitably gives rise to a pathologic process, whereas it is the nature of the response to an autoantigen that determines its influence on immunopathology. It is now evident that CD4+CD25+Foxp3+ regulatory cells[25] commonly recognize autoantigens, having been selected in the thymus on the

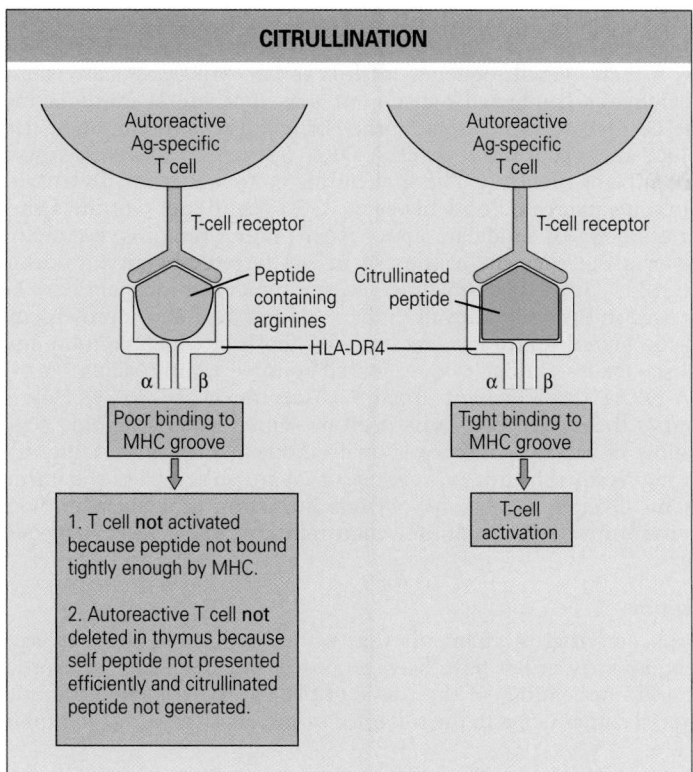

CITRULLINATION

Autoreactive
Ag-specific
T cell

Autoreactive
Ag-specific
T cell

T-cell receptor

T-cell receptor

Peptide
containing
arginines

Citrullinated
peptide

HLA-DR4

α | β

α | β

Poor binding to
MHC groove

Tight binding to
MHC groove

1. T cell **not** activated
because peptide not bound
tightly enough by MHC.

2. Autoreactive T cell **not**
deleted in thymus because
self peptide not presented
efficiently and citrullinated
peptide not generated.

T-cell
activation

Fig. 89.1 Citrullinated self peptides bind tightly to class II MHC alleles such as HLA-DR4 and can be presented to autoreactive T cells, whereas weakly binding unmodified peptides do not occupy HLA-DR4 molecules for long enough to stimulate autoreactive T cells. Likewise, the autoreactive T cells are not deleted in the thymus and are available in the periphery if only the weakly binding unmodified peptide is available for presentation and the citrullinated peptide is absent. Citrullination requires specific enzymes (peptidyl arginine deaminases [PADs]), which may not be available in the thymus.

basis of recognition of self peptides with an affinity low enough to avoid deletion but high enough to avoid death by neglect.

Unidentified self antigens

Another example of arthritis arising in the context of autoimmunity that is not joint specific is provided by the SKG mouse, which has a mutation in the ZAP-70 signaling molecule that interferes with efficient negative selection of T cells in the thymus.[26,27] Thus, a variety of high-affinity autoreactive T cells, which would normally have been efficiently eliminated in the thymus, escape to the periphery. The antigens recognized by these cells have not been characterized, but the mice develop a T-cell–mediated arthritis, in which high titers of rheumatoid factor and antibodies to type II collagen are both produced. However, unlike the K/BxN mouse, disease is not transferable by serum, and, indeed, in the absence of critical cytokines (e.g., IL-6), high titers of rheumatoid factors are observed in the absence of arthritis.

Summary

No autoantigen has been shown to be central to the pathogenesis of RA. If parallels with insulin-dependent diabetes mellitus and multiple sclerosis hold true, different joint antigens might be involved at various stages in the autoimmune process, perhaps through a process of "epitope spreading," in which autoimmune responses to one self epitope are followed later in disease by responses to separate epitopes in the same autoantigen or responses to other antigens in the same tissue. Some of the responses to autoantigens that have been documented in RA may arise as a consequence of joint destruction and subsequent display to the immune system of joint components not normally accessible to it (e.g., chondrocyte antigens). Moreover, a search for T-cell responses to autoantigens may be hampered by the chronic inflammatory process, because prolonged exposure to tumor necrosis factor (TNF)-α decreases T-cell responsiveness.[28] In addition, sites of inflammation recruit T cells non-specifically, so that a

disease-initiating, antigen-specific T-cell population in the joint will usually be swamped by large numbers of trafficking T cells of irrelevant specificity and hence be difficult to detect. Even in type II collagen-induced arthritis in mice, a disease that absolutely requires the presence of type II collagen-specific T cells, it is difficult to demonstrate these cells in the affected joints.

Exogenous antigens

An infective etiology for RA has often been postulated, but as yet no organism has been convincingly implicated.

Bacteria

Bacteria are attractive sources of putative RA-inducing antigens; myco-bacterial and streptococcal antigens are good inducers of experimental inflammatory arthritis, as are organisms derived from normal gut flora. Because RA does not show the epidemiologic features of a classic infectious disease, a candidate etiologic agent should be ubiquitous and well tolerated by the majority of those infected. Disease would then only occur in those with susceptibility genes, such as class II MHC alleles containing the shared epitope (e.g., *HLA-DR4*) and other susceptibility genes (e.g., *PTPN22*, *PADI4*), and/or additional environmental exposures. The relationship between peptic ulcer disease and *Helicobacter* infection is a useful illustration: even when there is a high incidence of infection by *Helicobacter* in the population, ulcer disease mainly occurs in association with risk factors such as smoking.

Reverse transcriptase polymerase chain reaction (RT-PCR) has been used to look for bacteria within RA synovium. By targeting bacterial rRNA the technique combines high sensitivity (because each organism has multiple copies of rRNA) and the ability to amplify unknown organisms. This is because all bacterial rRNA genes have stretches of highly conserved sequence, so that primers specific for these regions reliably amplify any bacterial rRNA present in the tissue. Sequencing the products identifies bacteria according to the unique regions within their rRNA sequences (by reference to the huge library of known bacterial rRNA genes) or can indicate the presence of a novel organism. This technique has shown that a plethora of bacterial rRNA sequences are present in RA synovium,[29] including occasionally mycobacterial sequences; the findings are unlikely to represent artifactual contamination. However, no unique "RA-associated" organism was identified. Instead, their presence correlated with inflammation rather than diagnosis and normal synovium did not contain bacterial rRNA. This suggests that inflamed synovium is colonized by bacteria (or bacterial nucleic acids), particularly from gut and skin commensals, which could be brought to the joint within phagocytic cells, since the synovium continuously recruits monocytes and dendritic cells. Although the organisms are probably viable for some time within synovium (bacterial rRNA has a short half-life), they do not replicate, and the joint remains sterile by conventional culture.

Although secondary "colonization" of inflamed synovium by bacteria and bacterial products may be common, it could still contribute to pathogenesis. Bacteria components are potent activators of the innate immune system and serve as adjuvants that allow adaptive T- and B-cell responses to be made. These components include lipopolysaccharide, peptidoglycan, and bacterial DNA, all of which act via Toll-like receptors (TLRs) to induce monokine secretion and upregulation of co-stimulatory molecules on antigen-presenting cells.[30] TLR9, which recognizes bacterial DNA, may be particularly important, because this mechanism has been shown to induce TNF-α–dependent arthritis in animal models.[31] Activation of antigen-presenting cells such as dendritic cells by bacterial DNA and other TLR ligands (i.e., an adjuvant function) might allow responses to self antigens to be generated in the joint. Lastly, given the interesting findings with respect to recognition of α-enolase, bacteria with α-enolases containing the same epitope as that found in *P. gingivalis* could contribute to joint inflammation on transport to the joint, particularly if tissue PAD enzymes are able to convert arginines in the bacterial α-enolase to citrullines, something that *P. gingivalis* can do without the need for exogenous PADs.[20]

Viruses

Several viruses cause joint inflammation in humans (e.g., rubella, parvovirus B19, arboviruses). As with bacteria, polymerase chain reaction has been used to detect viruses in RA synovium; generally this has produced either negative or inconsistent results. Herpesviruses, such as Epstein-Barr virus (EBV), cause ubiquitous lifelong infection, so an abnormal immune response to a persistent herpesvirus such as EBV has been an attractive idea to explore in RA. Abnormal immune responses to certain EBV antigens have previously been described in RA, particularly to Epstein-Barr nuclear antigen (EBNA)-1. This antigen contains a region of glycine-arginine repeats similar to those seen in several citrullinated autoantigens (e.g., keratin, fibrillarin). EBNA-1 can be citrullinated intracellularly when PAD is activated, and citrullinated EBNA is readily bound by ACPA from RA patients.[32] Although expansions of EBV-specific T cells, particularly CD8+ T cells, have been identified in RA synovium,[33] this is not surprising because the joint is enriched for memory T cells, and those recognizing persistent viruses such as EBV dominate the CD8+ T-cell repertoire. Thus, a role for EBV infection in RA pathogenesis remains unproven.

Molecular mimicry

Although bacterial or viral infection might be a direct cause of arthritis, it has often been postulated that disease could occur when foreign antigens "mimic" autoantigens present in the joint, because of similarity in their amino acid sequences. In this way immune responses correctly directed against components of a pathogen could cross-react with self proteins and lead to autoimmunity. When first formulated, the idea was thought of in terms of antibody cross-reactivity, which can be demonstrated by showing antibodies that bind to short linear peptides derived from a bacterial or viral protein and also to an autoantigen (Fig. 89.2). Mimicry is also possible in respect of shared conformational epitopes (those not determined by simple similarity between linear peptides).

However, when molecular mimicry at a T-cell level is considered, the situation is more complex. T cells recognize short linear peptides bound to MHC, but only a small number of amino acids within a peptide are actually necessary for T-cell recognition: those that allow binding to MHC and those that make contact with the TCR (see Fig. 89.2).[34] This means that two peptides with a very low level of overall sequence identity can both stimulate a given T cell, provided that these critical residues are conserved; indeed, any given TCR can recognize a large number of different peptides. For binding to MHC there is usually a set of preferred amino acids, so the main determinants of specificity are the small number of amino acids that influence interaction with the TCR, and these are not usually contiguous. Thus, whereas searching protein databases for bacterial or viral peptides that share a high degree of sequence identity with a self protein can reveal epitopes that are candidate mimics as far as antibody recognition is concerned, for

molecular mimicry at the T-cell level it is necessary to identify the critical residues and then look for peptides that have these features, even if their overall sequence identity is not striking. As an example, a search was conducted for self antigens that would mimic a major HLA-DR4–restricted epitope in the *Borrelia* ospA protein, and perhaps explain the occurrence of HLA-DR4–associated antibiotic-resistant chronic Lyme arthritis. The first mimic epitope identified was within a molecule expressed on leukocytes, CD18, but later work has shown a multiplicity of candidate epitopes in human proteins, but with no clear evidence that any of these is in fact targeted by an autoimmune process.[35,36] Several possible instances of molecular mimicry have been proposed in RA, including an *Escherichia coli* heat-shock protein, dnaJ, and the hemolysin of *Proteus mirabilis*, both of which contain amino acid sequences similar to the "shared epitope" (amino acids 70-74) in HLA-DRB1*0401, which confers susceptibility to RA.[37] However, whether the shared epitope is itself presented as an antigenic peptide to allow molecular mimicry is far from clear; it is much more likely that it governs the antigenic peptides that are presented to the immune system. Overall, despite its obvious attraction as an explanation of autoimmunity, the idea of molecular mimicry has lacked experimental support.[38]

Summary

Several potential mechanisms that would implicate infectious agents in the etiology of RA have been proposed, but none has been proven. The full implications of the traffic of phagocyte-associated bacteria or bacterial components to the inflamed synovium have yet to be explored.

ANTIGEN-INDEPENDENT EFFECTS OF T CELLS IN RHEUMATOID ARTHRITIS

The most abundant cytokines in the joint, and those that correlate with cartilage and joint destruction, are the monokines TNF-α and interleukin (IL)-1. Transgenic overexpression of TNF-α produces synovitis in mice,[39] as does the absence of the natural inhibitor of IL-1, IL-1 receptor antagonist.[40] In RA, unlike these experimental transgenic systems, monokine production is unlikely to be autonomous, at least in the early stages of synovitis, and is considered to be under T-cell control. However, mechanisms have been described whereby T cells give rise to monokine production other than after recognition of specific antigen. T cells that display the activation phenotype characteristic of synovial T cells (CD69+, HLA-DR+ [see later]) elicit monokine production from monocyte/macrophages[41] and can also interact with fibroblast-like synoviocytes to induce production of metalloproteinases. The mechanisms underlying these effects remain unclear, but cell-cell contact is required and T-cell membrane preparations are as effective as intact T cells. T cells may acquire this capacity as a result of the cytokine environment to which they are exposed within the joint. It has been shown that treatment with various "cocktails" of cytokines (e.g., IL-2, IL-6, and TNF-α)[42] can produce T cells capable of stimulating monokine production by monocytes or synoviocytes. Many of these cytokines are present in the RA joint and might therefore contribute to an antigen-independent activation of T cells. T cells eluted from RA synovial membrane have properties similar to those activated *in vitro* by cytokines in terms of their ability to induce TNF-α production by monocytes. Interestingly, the signaling pathways induced in monocytes by T cells activated via their TCR or via cytokines (IL-2, IL-6, and TNF-α) differ; NF-κB is critical to the latter but not the former, whereas PI3 kinase is required for the effects of TCR-stimulated T cells. Inhibiting PI3 kinase actually enhances the effects of cytokine-activated T cells. The same effects were observed with synovium-derived T cells. The introduction of PI3 kinase inhibitors that may be tested in RA might shed light on whether cytokine-activated, as distinct from antigen-activated, T cells are important in RA pathology.

PROPERTIES OF SYNOVIAL T CELLS IN RHEUMATOID ARTHRITIS

Leaving to one side the question of what activates T cells in RA, it might be possible to obtain clues on pathogenesis by examining

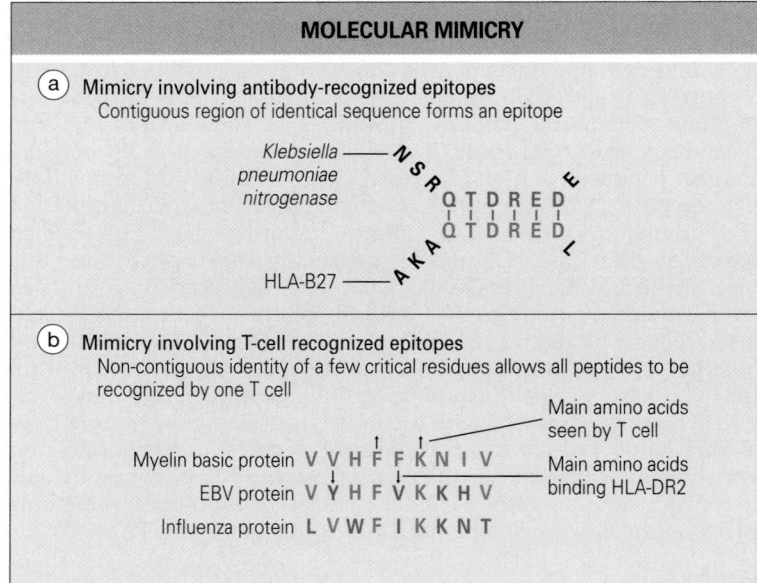

MOLECULAR MIMICRY

(a) Mimicry involving antibody-recognized epitopes
Contiguous region of identical sequence forms an epitope

Klebsiella pneumoniae nitrogenase — N S R Q T D R E D E
HLA-B27 — A K A Q T D R E D L

(b) Mimicry involving T-cell recognized epitopes
Non-contiguous identity of a few critical residues allows all peptides to be recognized by one T cell

Main amino acids seen by T cell
Main amino acids binding HLA-DR2

Myelin basic protein   V V H F F K N I V
EBV protein   V Y H F V K K H V
Influenza protein   L V W F I K K N T

Fig. 89.2 Molecular mimicry of self peptides by foreign peptides has different requirements for antibody and T-cell recognition.

different aspects of the phenotype of lymphocytes in RA, especially at sites of disease. The features examined include antigen-specific receptors, expression of activation and differentiation markers, and cytokine production.

TCR studies in RA

The use of TCR genes by peripheral blood or synovial T cells has been studied to determine whether RA patients possess a disease-specific population of T cells expressing identical or related receptors.[43] The TCR is made up of two chains, α and β (or γ and δ), and rearrangement of TCR genes (V, D, and/or J genes) is involved in each case to produce unique α and β chains and hence a unique αβ or γδ TCR. Random recruitment of T cells to the joint would produce a population expressing many different TCRs, whereas recruitment of T cells all recognizing a small number of peptide epitopes would result in over-representation of identical or related TCRs (i.e., an oligoclonal rather than a polyclonal T-cell population). In experimental autoimmune diseases, autoantigen-specific T cells often use a restricted number of TCR genes, and in early studies oligoclonality was also found in synovium, but these results likely reflected in-vitro expansion of particular clones rather than the in-vivo situation and have been discounted. Dominance of T cells using one TCRBV gene, but with differing CDR3 sequences would indicate the involvement of a superantigen in RA; these are often produced by bacteria. The CDR3 region is formed by the joining of V, D, and J genes, together with addition/deletion of further nucleotides and is the part of the TCR that contacts antigenic peptides. In contrast, superantigens stimulate T cells by binding specific TCRBV gene products, irrespective of their CDR3 sequence. However, no consistent expansions of particular TCR gene families have been documented and involvement of a superantigen seems unlikely.

Studies of surface phenotype of lymphocytes in RA

The RA joint contains both natural killer (NK) cells and T cells. The typical synovial NK cells are CD56[bright] and CD16−, an NK cell subset that secretes cytokines, especially interferon (IFN)-γ, rather than mediating cytotoxicity,[44] but the role of NK cells in RA has not yet been clarified.

Within the T-cell population, memory T cells predominate, which inevitably produces differences in functional tests between synovial fluid–derived T cells and those of peripheral blood, because the latter contains equal proportions of naive and memory cells. Because T cells differentiate from the naive to the memory subset after encounter with antigens, they alter their expression of different isoforms of the CD45 surface marker (termed RA, RB, RC, RO). Naive cells are CD45-RA+, RO−, RB[bright], whereas memory cells are CD45-RA−, RO+, RB[dull]. Judged by their expression of the CD45-RB isoform, synovial T cells are particularly highly differentiated, because they have very low levels, similar to those seen in vitro after several rounds of cell division (Fig. 89.3).[45] They have shorter telomeres, also reflecting increased numbers of divisions,[46] although a deficiency in telomerase (the enzyme that can maintain telomere length) has also been postulated. Normally, such "end-stage" cells are very likely to undergo apoptosis because they express high levels of the apoptosis-promoting molecule Fas and low levels of the apoptosis-protecting molecule bcl-2. Despite this phenotype, few synovial T cells can be shown to be undergoing apoptosis. They are protected from dying by factors within the synovial environment, including type I interferons and IL-15, a cytokine produced by synovial macrophages and fibroblasts.[47-49] Resistance to apoptosis has also been shown to be a feature of CD4+ T cells that have lost expression of CD28. This CD28− subset is enriched in synovium and has been proposed to be pathogenic. The cells are autoreactive, produce IFN-γ, and have cytolytic potential[50]; they also express several kinds of the HLA class I recognizing receptors (killer immunoglobulin-like receptors) common to T cells and NK cells, including the activatory receptor CD158b. This might allow their activation in an antigen-independent manner.

This preponderance of memory T cells in the joint reflects recruitment to the synovium because, by virtue of their expression of adhesion molecules, memory cells have preferential access to inflamed

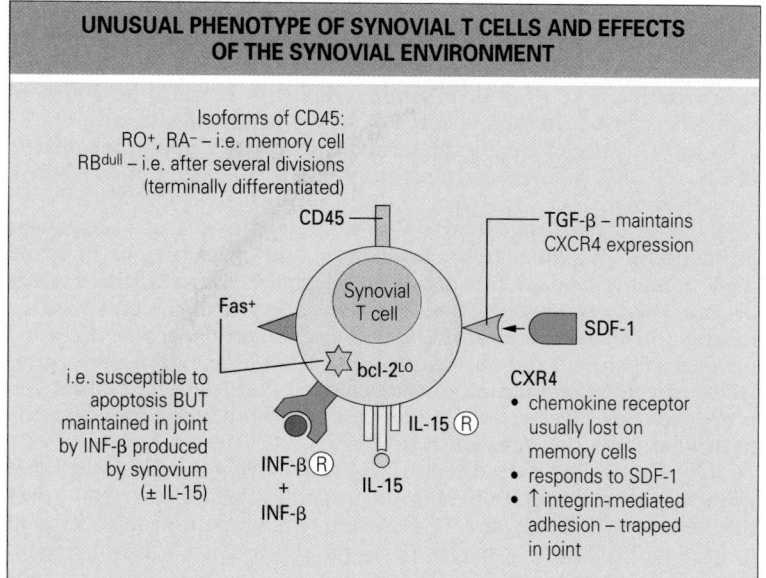

Fig. 89.3 Unusual phenotype of synovial T cells and effects of the synovial environment. CXCR4, CXC chemokine receptor 4; SDF-1, stromal-derived factor (CXCL12).

tissues. Synovial T cells are recruited and also retained in the joint through the actions of chemokines. The expression of some chemokines is aberrant in RA synovium and different from other inflammatory tissues. Unusually, memory T cells in synovium continue to express several chemokine receptors, particularly CXCR4, which are normally lost during differentiation from naive cells. Continued expression of CXCR4 may be stimulated by transforming growth factor (TGF)-β produced in the joint. Thus, T cells remain susceptible to the action of the CXCR4 ligand, CXCL12 (SDF-1), itself produced by synovial fibroblasts.[51] This results in their retention within the tissue, where they may exert the antigen-independent effects noted earlier, inducing synoviocytes to produce monokines and matrix metalloproteinases.

Cytokine production in RA

When it was proposed that joint inflammation in RA was driven by T-cell recognition of antigen, there was an expectation that synovial T cells would be actively dividing, secreting cytokines, and expressing surface activation markers such as the IL-2 receptor. In fact, only a small proportion of synovial T cells are actively dividing and, although they express some activation markers (CD69, HLA-DR), others, particularly the IL-2 receptor, are relatively infrequent. This phenotype is unusual, because in conventional in-vitro activation CD69 is expressed early and for a short period whereas HLA-DR occurs late after activation; this finding suggests an important influence of the microenvironment in maintaining this unusual "frustrated activation" phenotype. Such activated T cells may induce cytokine production in antigen-independent ways, and, as noted earlier, CD69 has been implicated in this process.

Initial studies of the cytokines made by synovial T cells were also surprising, particularly within the paradigm of two major T-cell subsets: T-helper type 1 (Th1) cells (proinflammatory, making IFN-γ, lymphotoxin, and IL-2) and T-helper type 2 (Th2) cells (allergy-related, making IL-4, IL-5, IL-10, and IL-13). RA was expected to be driven by Th1 cells, but IFN-γ concentrations in synovial fluid were scarcely detectable in comparison with the readily detected monokines IL-1 and TNF-α, and IFN-γ+ CD4+ T cells, detected by intracellular staining, were only present in small numbers. Interestingly, a similarly low proportion of IFN-γ–secreting T cells is seen in murine collagen-induced arthritis, a model known to be completely T cell dependent. IL-4+ cells were also absent from the synovial T-cell population in established RA, although investigation of very early arthritis has shown IL-4 and IL-13 (and IL-17) to be among those cytokines predictive of progression to established RA[52]; these cytokines were not present at later time points. These puzzling observations have been clarified by the discovery of an additional T-cell subset, Th17 cells, whose signature cytokine is IL-17.[53] IL-17, unlike IFN-γ, is essential for collagen-induced arthritis; in fact, absence of IFN-γ exacerbates disease. Th17 cells have also been clearly implicated in two other important models of RA: the SKG mouse[27] and gene-targeted mice deficient in IL-1 receptor antagonist.[54]

IL-17 is a particularly attractive candidate as a T-cell–dependent arthritogenic cytokine. It shares many of the properties of IL-1 and TNF-α, including induction of cartilage degradation, and shows synergy of action with these cytokines. It is also relevant to the erosive bone destruction of RA because it can induce expression of RANK ligand (osteoprotegerin ligand) by osteoblasts; RANK ligand is the critical factor in the differentiation of osteoclasts.[55] IL-17 levels in joints and proportions of Th17 cells in joints and peripheral blood have recently been reported to be elevated in RA.[56,57]

If Th17 cells are indeed central to RA pathogenesis, the factors that influence their generation become important. Although still under investigation, IL-6/IL-1 and TGF-β seem to be important in generation of human Th17 cells, whereas IL-23 influences their survival, expansion, and pathogenicity.[58] IL-23 is made particularly by dendritic cells and macrophages in response to TLR agonists,[59] cells that also secrete the Th1-driving cytokine IL-12. Thus, influences on dendritic cells that alter proportions of IL-12 and IL-23 that they make may in turn affect RA pathogenesis.

REGULATORY T CELLS IN RA

T cells within the joint have been assumed to be pathogenic since they are not present in normal synovium. However, in view of the evidence for regulatory T-cell subsets, particularly CD4+CD25+ cells, which protect from autoimmune disease and chronic inflammation, it is possible that some of the synovial CD4+ T-cell population could be beneficial, although they are obviously inadequate. Regulatory T cells (Treg) in peripheral blood have been thoroughly characterized[60]; they are CD4+ CD25[hi], express a transcription factor, Foxp3, that is critical to their regulatory function, and suppress both proliferation and cytokine production in a contact-dependent manner (Table 89.3). Mutations in FOXP3 genes are associated with severe spontaneous inflammatory and autoimmune disease in mice and humans. A relationship between generation of Th17 and Treg cells has been suggested, because both require TGF-β, but the presence of IL-6 favors Th17 generation over Treg.[61] Thus, an inflammatory cytokine environment containing IL-6 could enhance generation of Th17 cells and increase inflammation while at the same time decreasing the generation of the Treg subset that could otherwise downregulate the inflammatory response.

Like synovial T cells, Treg are resistant to in-vitro stimulation and commonly make IL-10, although this is not required for their regulatory function. Distinguishing Treg in synovial fluid is difficult, because activated human T cells are now known to express Foxp3, previously thought to be a specific marker of Treg. Thus, increased numbers of CD4+ CD25+ cells have been reported in synovial fluid and, in addition to the previously noted expression of CD69 and HLA-DR, were positive for other markers associated with Treg (CTLA-4 and GITR), although these also appear on activated T cells.[62] They showed regulatory function in in-vitro assays but may nevertheless be a form of induced Treg. Other studies suggested a defect in peripheral blood Treg function[63] and showed that treatment with anti–TNF-α (specifically infliximab) could reverse the functional defect, particularly the

TABLE 89.3 PROPERTIES OF EFFECTOR AND REGULATORY CD4+ T CELLS

	Regulatory CD4+ T cells	Effector CD4+ T cells
CD25 expression	Constitutive high level	Only on activation
CLTA-4 expression	High, constitutive	Late, post-activation
Responses to mitogens and anti-CD3	Poor	Vigorous
Foxp3 expression	Positive	Negative, except on activation
Typical cytokines	IL-10, TGF-β	IL-2, IFN-γ, IL-4, IL-17
Thymus dependent	Yes	Yes
Specificity	Self peptides on class II MHC	Non-self peptides on class II MHC
Affinity for self antigens	Moderate	Low

ability to inhibit TNF-α production. However, this proved to be due to the appearance of "induced" Treg cells, mediating suppression through IL-10 and TGF-β production, rather than by the contact-dependent mechanism used by "classic" Treg.[64,65] They also had an altered surface phenotype compared with classic Treg, with reduced expression of CCR7 and CD62L. Thus, within the joint, both pathogenic proinflammatory T cells and Treg populations (whether natural or induced) are likely to coexist. Their proportions may vary both in different phases of disease and in response to different treatments and, therefore, influence activity and progression of disease. Measures to manipulate Treg function and thereby influence disease activity are under investigation.

CONCLUSION

Cell-mediated immune responses, particularly those involving T cells, are strongly implicated in RA pathogenesis both by the association of disease with HLA-DR and the presence and properties of T cells in the synovium.

Whether the critical immune response in RA is directed against autoantigens or exogenous antigens is still not determined definitively. Experimental models of arthritis show that ubiquitous self-antigens, as well as those expressed preferentially in the joint, can be responsible for driving arthritis.

Synovial T cells are enriched for memory cells and are maintained in a highly differentiated state, reflecting recruitment to the joint and factors in the local environment that inhibit apoptosis. They are activated but make little IL-2 or IFN-γ. The proinflammatory cytokine IL-17 is produced, and this in conjunction with IL-1 or TNF-α can bring about cartilage and bone destruction.

Cytokines produced by macrophage-like synoviocytes, especially TNF-α, IL-1, and IL-6, dominate RA synovium. Their production could be brought about by either antigen-specific T cells or by T cells acting in an antigen-independent fashion, following activation by cytokines, or through other receptors (e.g., killer immunoglobulin-like receptors).

The synovial T-cell population also includes regulatory T cells, which can turn off proinflammatory T-cell–mediated responses; persistence of RA may relate to a failure in this regulatory mechanism.

KEY REFERENCES

1. Holmdahl R, Bockermann R, Backlund J, Yamada H. The molecular pathogenesis of collagen-induced arthritis in mice—a model for rheumatoid arthritis. Ageing Res Rev 2002;1:135-147.
6. Burkhardt H, Sehnert B, Bockermann R, et al. Humoral immune response to citrullinated collagen type II determinants in early rheumatoid arthritis. Eur J Immunol 2005;35:1643-1652.

7. Lundberg K, Nijenhuis S, Vossenaar ER, et al. Citrullinated proteins have increased immunogenicity and arthritogenicity and their presence in arthritic joints correlates with disease severity. Arthritis Res Ther 2005;7:R458-R467.
8. Glant T, Mikecz K, Arzoumanian A, Poole A. Proteoglycan induced arthritis in BALB/c mice: clinical features and histopathology. Arthritis Rheum 1987;30:201-212.

10. Cope AP, Patel SD, Hall F, et al. T cell responses to a human cartilage autoantigen in the context of rheumatoid arthritis-associated and nonassociated HLA-DR4 alleles. Arthritis Rheum 1999;42:1497-1507.
11. Kotzin BL, Falta MT, Crawford F, et al. Use of soluble peptide-DR4 tetramers to detect synovial T cells specific for cartilage antigens in patients with rheumatoid arthritis. Proc Nat Acad Sci U S A 2000;97:291-296.

12. Rantapää-Dahlqvist S, deJong BAW, Berglin E, et al. Antibodies against cyclic citrullinated peptide and IgA rheumatoid factor predict the development of rheumatoid arthritis. Arthritis Rheum 2003;48:2741-2749.

13. Nielen MMJ, van Schaardenburg D, Reesink HW, et al. Specific autoantibodies precede the symptoms of rheumatoid arthritis—a study of serial measurements in blood donors. Arthritis Rheum 2004;50:380-386.

14. Matsumoto I, Staub A, Benoist C, Mathis D. Arthritis provoked by linked T and B cell recognition of a glycolytic enzyme. Science 1999;286:1732-1735.

15. Matsumoto I, Maccioni M, Lee DM, et al. How antibodies to a ubiquitous cytoplasmic enzyme may provoke joint-specific autoimmune disease. Nat Immunol 2002;3:360-365.

17. Klareskog L, Ronnelid J, Lundberg K, et al. Immunity to citrullinated proteins in rheumatoid arthritis. Annu Rev Immunol 2008;26:651-675.

18. Klareskog L, Stolt P, Lundberg K, et al. A new model for an etiology of rheumatoid arthritis: smoking may trigger HLA-DR (shared epitope)-restricted immune reactions to autoantigens modified by citrullination. Arthritis Rheum 2006;54:38-46.

19. Kallberg H, Padyukov L, Plenge RM, et al. Gene-gene and gene-environment interactions involving HLA-DRB1, PTPN22, and smoking in two subsets of rheumatoid arthritis. Am J Hum Genet 2007;80:867-875.

20. Lundberg K, Kinloch A, Fisher BA, et al. Antibodies to citrullinated alpha-enolase peptide 1 are specific for rheumatoid arthritis and cross-react with bacterial enolase. Arthritis Rheum 2008;58:3009-3019.

21. Ireland J, Herzog J, Unanue ER. Cutting edge: unique T cells that recognize citrullinated peptides are a feature of protein immunization. J Immunol 2006;177:1421-1425.

22. Hill JA, Southwood S, Sette A, et al. Cutting edge: the conversion of arginine to citrulline allows for a high-affinity peptide interaction with the rheumatoid arthritis-associated HLA-DRB1*0401 MHC class II molecule. J Immunol 2003;171:538-541.

23. Anderton SM, van der Zee R, Prakken B, et al. Activation of T cells recognizing self 60-kD heat shock protein can protect against experimental arthritis. J Exp Med 1995;181:943-952.

24. Prakken BJ, Roord S, Ronaghy A, et al. Heat shock protein 60 and adjuvant arthritis: a model for T cell regulation in human arthritis. Springer Semin Immunopathol 2003;25:47-63.

25. Shevach EM, DiPaolo RA, Andersson J, et al. The lifestyle of naturally occurring CD4+ CD25+ Foxp3+ regulatory T cells. Immunol Rev 2006;212:60-73.

26. Hata H, Sakaguchi N, Yoshitomi H, et al. Distinct contribution of IL-6, TNF-alpha, IL-1, and IL-10 to T cell-mediated spontaneous autoimmune arthritis in mice. J Clin Invest 2004;114:582-588.

27. Hirota K, Hashimoto M, Yoshitomi H, et al. T cell self-reactivity forms a cytokine milieu for spontaneous development of IL-17+ Th cells that cause autoimmune arthritis. J Exp Med 2007;204:41-47.

28. Cope AP, Londei M, Chu NR, et al. Chronic exposure to tumor necrosis factor (TNF) in vitro impairs the activation of T cells through the T cell receptor CD3 complex: reversal in vivo by anti-TNF antibodies in patients with rheumatoid arthritis. J Clin Invest 1994;94:749-760.

29. Kempsell KE, Cox CJ, Hurle M, et al. Reverse transcriptase-PCR analysis of bacterial rRNA for detection and characterization of bacterial species in arthritis synovial tissue. Infect Immun 2000;68:6012-6026.

30. Medzhitov R, Janeway CA. Decoding the patterns of self and nonself by the innate immune system. Science 2002;296:298-300.

32. Pratesi F, Tommasi C, Anzilotti C, et al. Deiminated Epstein-Barr virus nuclear antigen 1 is a target of anti-citrullinated protein antibodies in rheumatoid arthritis. Arthritis Rheum 2006;54:733-741.

34. Rose NR. Infections, mimics, and autoimmune disease. J Clin Invest 2001;107:943-944.

36. Hemmer B, Gran B, Zhao YD, et al. Identification of candidate T-cell epitopes and molecular mimics in chronic Lyme disease. Nat Med 1999;5:1375-1382.

39. Kontoyiannis D, Pasparakis M, Pizarro TT, et al. Impaired on/off regulation of TNF biosynthesis in mice lacking TNF AU-rich elements: implications for joint and gut-associated immunopathologies. Immunity 1999;10:387-398.

40. Horai R, Saijo S, Tanioka M, et al. Development of chronic inflammatory arthropathy resembling rheumatoid arthritis in interleukin 1 receptor antagonist-deficient mice. J Exp Med 2000;191:313-320.

42. Brennan FM, Foey AD, Feldmann M. The importance of T cell interactions with macrophages in rheumatoid cytokine production. Curr Top Microbiol Immunol 2006;305:177-194.

43. Goronzy JJ, Zettl A, Weyand CM. T cell receptor repertoire in rheumatoid arthritis. Int Rev Immunol 1998;17:339-363.

46. Salmon M, Akbar AN. Telomere erosion: a new link between HLA DR4 and rheumatoid arthritis? Trends Immunol 2004;25:339-341.

49. Buckley CD, Filer A, Haworth O, et al. Defining a role for fibroblasts in the persistence of chronic inflammatory joint disease. Ann Rheum Dis 2004;63:ii92-ii95.

50. Warrington KJ, Takemura S, Goronzy JJ, Weyand CM. CD4+, CD28– T cells in rheumatoid arthritis patients combine features of the innate and adaptive immune systems. Arthritis Rheum 2001;44:13-20.

51. Burman A, Haworth O, Hardie DL, et al. A chemokine-dependent stromal induction mechanism for aberrant lymphocyte accumulation and compromised lymphatic return in rheumatoid arthritis. J Immunol 2005;174:1693-1700.

52. Raza K, Falciani F, Curnow SJ, et al. Early rheumatoid arthritis is characterized by a distinct and transient synovial fluid cytokine profile of T cell and stromal cell origin. Arthritis Res Ther 2005;7:R784-R795.

53. Gaston JS. Cytokines in arthritis—the "big numbers" move centre stage. Rheumatology (Oxford) 2008;47:8-12.

54. Cho ML, Kang JW, Moon YM, et al. STAT3 and NF-kappa B signal pathway is required for IL-23–mediated IL-17 production in spontaneous arthritis animal model IL-1 receptor antagonist–deficient mice. J Immunol 2006;176:5652-5661.

55. Kotake S, Udagawa N, Takahashi N, et al. IL-17 in synovial fluids from patients with rheumatoid arthritis is a potent stimulator of osteoclastogenesis. J Clin Invest 1999;103:1345-1352.

56. Shahrara S, Huang Q, Mandelin A, Pope RM. TH-17 cells in rheumatoid arthritis. Arthritis Res Ther 2008;10:R93.

57. Daoussis D, Solomou EE, Karampetsou M, et al. Th17 cells are increased in patients with active rheumatoid arthritis. Ann Rheum Dis 2008;67(Suppl II):152.

58. McGeachy MJ, Chen Y, Tato CM, et al. The interleukin 23 receptor is essential for the terminal differentiation of interleukin 17-producing effector T helper cells in vivo. Nat Immunol 2009;10:314-324.

59. Hunter CA. New IL-12-family members: IL-23 and IL-27, cytokines with divergent functions. Nat Rev Immunol 2005;5:521-531.

60. Schwartz RH. Natural regulatory T cells and self-tolerance. Nat Immunol 2005;6:327-330.

61. Bettelli E, Carrier Y, Gao W, et al. Reciprocal developmental pathways for the generation of pathogenic effector T(H)17 and regulatory T cells. Nature 2006;441:235-238.

62. van Amelsfort JM, Jacobs KM, Bijlsma JW, et al. CD4(+) CD25(+) regulatory T cells in rheumatoid arthritis: differences in the presence, phenotype, and function between peripheral blood and synovial fluid. Arthritis Rheum 2004;50:2775-2785.

63. Flores-Borja F, Jury EC, Mauri C, Ehrenstein MR. Defects in CTLA-4 are associated with abnormal regulatory T cell function in rheumatoid arthritis. Proc Natl Acad Sci U S A 2008;105:19396-19401.

64. Ehrenstein MR, Evans JG, Singh A, et al. Compromised function of regulatory T cells in rheumatoid arthritis and reversal by anti-TNFalpha therapy. J Exp Med 2004;200:277-285.

65. Nadkarni S, Mauri C, Ehrenstein MR. Anti-TNF-alpha therapy induces a distinct regulatory T cell population in patients with rheumatoid arthritis via TGF-beta. J Exp Med 2007;204:33-39.

REFERENCES

Full references for this chapter can be found on www.expertconsult.com.

Angiogenesis in rheumatoid arthritis

90

Zoltán Szekanecz and Alisa E. Koch

- Angiogenesis, the formation of new blood vessels, is important in the maintenance and perpetuation of leukocyte ingress into the synovium in rheumatoid arthritis.
- The outcome of neovascularization is highly dependent on the imbalance between angiogenic and angiostatic mediators including growth factors, cytokines, chemokines, cell adhesion molecules, and extracellular matrix components.
- Soluble and cell surface-bound factors involved in the pathogenesis of arthritis may regulate synovial angiogenesis, in part via by modulating the production of angiogenic mediators.
- Synovial inflammation and angiogenesis may be controlled by the blockade of angiogenic mediators or by the administration of angiogenesis inhibitors.

ABSTRACT

Angiogenesis is the formation of new capillaries from preexisting vessels. A number of soluble and cell-bound factors may stimulate neovascularization. The perpetuation of angiogenesis involving numerous soluble and cell surface-bound mediators has been associated with rheumatoid arthritis (RA). These angiogenic mediators, among others, include growth factors, primarily vascular endothelial growth factor (VEGF) and hypoxia-inducible factors (HIFs), as well as proinflammatory cytokines, various chemokines, matrix components, cell adhesion molecules, proteases, and others. Among the several potential angiogenesis inhibitors, targeting of VEGF, HIF-1, angiogenic chemokines, tumor necrosis factor-α, and the $\alpha_v\beta_3$ integrin may attenuate the action of angiogenic mediators and thus synovial angiogenesis. In addition, some naturally produced or synthetic compounds including angiostatin, endostatin, paclitaxel, fumagillin analogues, 2-methoxyestradiol, and thalidomide may be included in the management of RA.

INTRODUCTION

Endothelial cells lining blood vessels are involved in leukocyte ingress into inflammatory sites. Angiogenesis, involving endothelial proliferation and the formation of new vessels, is involved in organ development, tissue repair, and reproductive processes. In addition, the perpetuation of neovascularization is associated with inflammatory conditions and malignancies. Thus RA may also be considered as an "angiogenic disease": Increased neovascularization plays an important role in the pathogenesis of the disease, and, on the other hand, therapeutic control of angiogenesis may be beneficial for the outcome of RA (reviewed in references 1 to 5). In this chapter, we review current issues regarding the angiogenic process, its mediators and inhibitors, and the clinical relevance of angiogenesis in RA.

ANGIOGENESIS IN RHEUMATOID ARTHRITIS

Inflammatory leukocytes migrate through the fenestrated endothelia of vessels into the rheumatoid synovium. There is intensive neovascularization in the inflamed synovium indicated by the great number of newly formed vessels as opposed to osteoarthritic or normal synovial tissues. Soluble and cell surface-bound angiogenic factors enhance vessel formation and thus, indirectly, leukocyte extravasation and synovitis.[1-6] Synovial macrophages and angiogenic mediators produced by these cells are key players of this process.[7] These mediators of angiogenesis include most growth factors, some proinflammatory cytokines, chemokines, components of the extracellular matrix, matrix-degrading enzymes, and cellular adhesion molecules.[1-3,5,7] Most of these mediators have been detected in the RA synovium and have been implicated in the pathogenesis of RA, anyway.[1-3,5,7] On the other hand, some anti-inflammatory cytokines and chemokines, antirheumatic drugs, and other compounds inhibit synovial neovascularization and thus may suppress arthritis.[4,6] Therefore angiogenesis research has important clinical aspects. Angiogenesis and the expression of some angiogenic factors such as integrins have been correlated with the metastatic potential of some types of cancer. Similarly, the extent of neovascularization may reflect the degree of inflammation and may be a prognostic marker in RA.[1,2,5] Regarding therapy, small molecular agents and biologics that suppress synovial angiogenesis may be included in the management of RA and other types of arthritis.[2,4,6]

ANGIOGENIC PROCESS

Neovascularization is a complex process that includes several sequential steps. New capillaries develop from existing blood vessels.[1,5] First, angiogenic mediators described later in this chapter activate endothelial cells. This is associated with the production of matrix-degrading metalloproteinase (MMP) enzymes. These proteases degrade the basement membrane of the endothelium and the interstitium, thus enabling endothelial outgrowth. There are more than 20 known MMPs in addition to membrane-type MMPs (MT-MMP). Among these enzymes, collagenase (MMP-1) and gelatinases (MMP-2 and MMP-9) seem to be the most relevant for angiogenesis. In addition to MMPs, other enzymes termed *serine proteases* including tissue- and urokinase-type plasminogen activators (tPAs and uPAs) are also involved in neovascularization. The migration of loose endothelial cells results in the formation of capillary sprouts. Endothelial cells in the midsection of the sprout undergo mitosis, whereas others at the tip of the sprout only migrate but do not proliferate. This is followed by lumen formation within the sprout. Two sprouts then anastomose with each other, thus forming capillary loops. New basement membrane is then synthesized. The continuous emigration of endothelial cells results in the development of second and further generation of new vessels (Fig. 90.1).[1,5]

ANGIOGENIC MEDIATORS IN THE RHEUMATOID SYNOVIUM

Some relevant mediators implicated in RA-associated angiogenesis are included in Table 90.1. Some of the more important molecules are discussed as follows in more detail.

Growth factors

VEGF is probably the most well-known angiogenic factor associated with RA, other types of chronic inflammation, and malignancies.[8-10] VEGF directly induces angiogenesis. In addition, several other angiogenic mediators including interleukin-6 (IL-6), IL-17, IL-18, nitric oxide, hepatocyte growth factor (HGF), macrophage migration inhibitory factor (MIF), endothelin-1 (ET-1), and prostanoids act via VEGF-dependent mechanisms.[9,10] VEGF, HGF, basic fibroblast growth factor (bFGF), and acidic fibroblast growth factor (aFGF) are bound to heparin

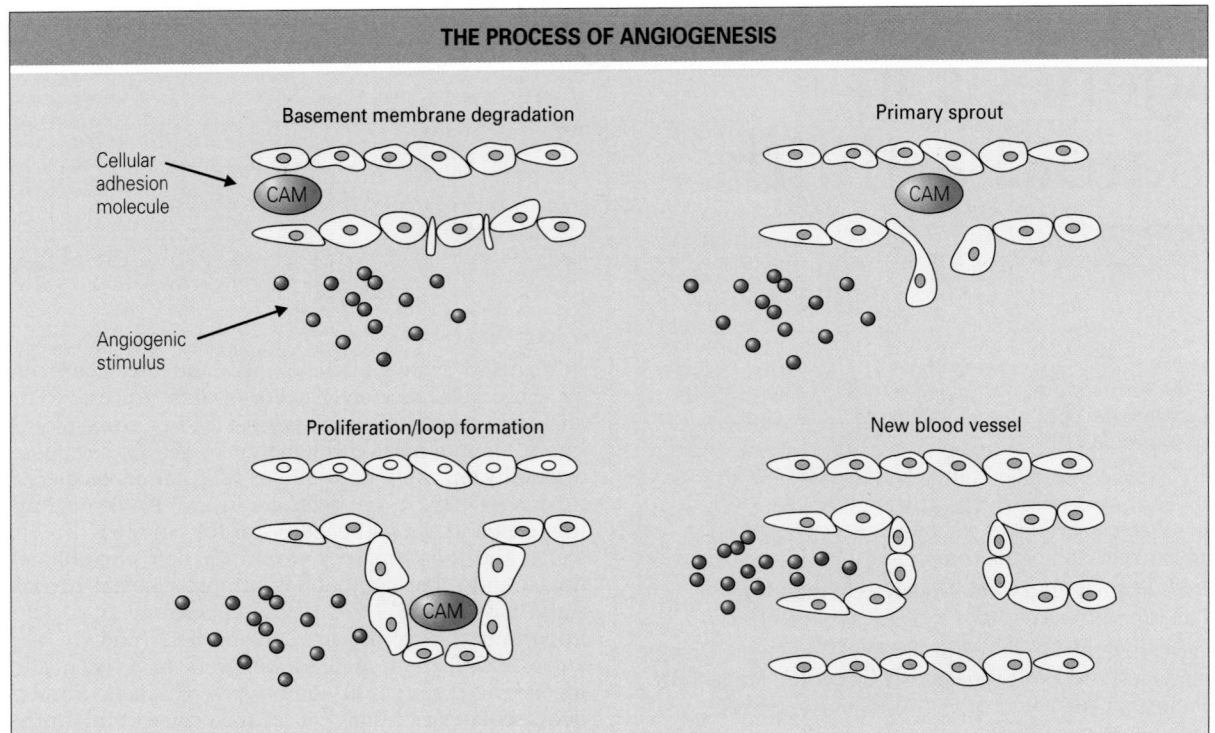

Fig. 90.1 The process of angiogenesis. Neovascularization consists of several distinct steps including basement membrane degradation, the emigration and proliferation of endothelial cells, sprouting, lumen formation, and basement membrane synthesis.

and heparan sulfate in the synovial interstitium. These growth factors are mobilized by heparinase and plasmin during neovascularization.[1,5,9,10] Hypoxia is a feature of the RA joint. Hypoxia itself stimulates the production of VEGF. In addition, HIF-1α and HIF-2α, which regulate VEGF gene transcription, have also been implicated in angiogenesis.[11] The angiopoietin-1 (Ang1)/Tie-2 complex interacts with VEGF during the stabilization of newly formed blood vessels, whereas in contrast, Ang2 inhibits vessel maturation.[2,5,9,10] Survivin, an apoptosis inhibitor, is also involved in VEGF-induced angiogenesis.[5,10]

Non-heparin–binding growth factors include platelet-derived (PDGF), platelet-derived endothelial cell (PD-ECGF), epidermal (EGF), insulin-like (IGF-I), keratinocyte (KGF), placenta (PIGF), and transforming (TGF)-β.[1,2,5] TGF-β may exert both stimulatory and inhibitory effects on angiogenesis, which is dose dependent.[12]

Cytokines

Among proinflammatory cytokines, tumor necrosis factor-α (TNF-α), IL-1, IL-6, IL-15, IL-17, IL-18, oncostatin M, MIF, granulocyte- (G-CSF), and granulocyte-macrophage colony-stimulating factors (GM-CSF) are involved in angiogenesis. These cytokines are abundantly produced in the sera and synovial fluid of RA patients.[1,2,5,12]

Chemokines and chemokine receptors

CXC chemokines containing the ELR (glutamyl-leucyl-arginyl-) amino acid motif stimulate synovial angiogenesis.[13] These chemokines include IL-8/CXCL8, epithelial neutrophil activating protein-78 (ENA-78/CXCL5), growth-related oncogene α (groα/CXCL1), and connective tissue activating protein-III (CTAP-III/CXCL6).[3,13] In contrast, other CXC chemokines lacking the ELR sequence suppress neovascularization.[3,13] Stromal cell–derived factor-1 (SDF-1/CXCL12) may be the only CXC chemokine that lacks the ELR motif but is still angiogenic.[3,14] SDF-1/CXCL12 is a key regulator of synovial lymphoid neogenesis.[14] Among CC chemokines, MCP-1/CCL2 promotes angiogenesis by supporting the activity of growth factors during angiogenesis.[3,5] Fractalkine/CX$_3$CL1 also promotes neovascularization.[3] These chemokines are also involved in leukocyte recruitment into the synovium in RA.[3,13]

Among chemokine receptors, CXCR2 may be the most important receptor for ELR$^+$ angiogenic CXC chemokines such as IL-8/CXCL68,

ENA-78/CXCL5 and groα/CXCL1 on endothelial cells.[3,5] CCR2-MCP-1/CCL2 interactions have also been implicated in RA-associated angiogenesis.[3,5]

Extracellular matrix components and cell adhesion molecules

Several matrix components including type I collagen, fibronectin, laminin, vitronectin, tenascin, thrombospondin, and proteoglycans play a role in endothelial cell adhesion and migration during neovascularization.[15] The role of matrix-degrading enzymes in angiogenesis is discussed earlier.

Cellular adhesion molecules are involved in leukocyte adhesion to endothelial cells and to matrix components. These molecules play a crucial role in leukocyte emigration into the RA synovium and synovial angiogenesis.[16,17] Among adhesion receptors expressed on endothelial cells, β_1 and β_3 integrins, E-selectin, the L-selectin ligand CD34, selectin-related glycoconjugates including Lewis^y/H and MUC18, vascular cell adhesion molecule-1 (VCAM-1), intercellular adhesion molecule-2 (ICAM-2), platelet-endothelial cell adhesion molecule-1 (PECAM-1; CD31), endoglin (CD105), and junctional cell adhesion molecules (JAM-A and JAM-C) mediate cellular adhesion during synovial angiogenesis.[16-19]

Other angiogenic mediators

The cyclooxygenase (COX)/prostaglandin system including prostaglandin E$_2$ itself is involved in VEGF-dependent neovascularization. Other angiogenic factors relevant for RA include angiogenin, angiotropin, ET-1, serum amyloid A (SAA), pleiotrophin, platelet-activating factor (PAF), histamine, substance P, erythropoietin, adenosine, prolactin, and thrombin.[1,2,5]

REGULATION OF SYNOVIAL ANGIOGENESIS

The outcome of angiogenesis and thus inflammatory leukocyte recruitment into the synovium through the newly formed vessels depends on the imbalance between angiogenic mediators and inhibitors of neovascularization (Fig. 90.2). A regulatory network consisting of numerous interactive mechanisms and feedback loops exists in the RA synovium.

TABLE 90.1 RELEVANT MEDIATORS AND INHIBITORS OF ANGIOGENESIS IN RHEUMATOID ARTHRITIS*

	Mediators	Inhibitors
1. **Growth factors**	VEGF, aFGF, bFGF, HGF, HIF-1, HIF-2, PDGF, EGF, KGF, IGF-I, TGF-β, PlGF	—
2. **Cytokines**	TNF-α, IL-1, IL-6, IL-8, IL-15, IL-17, IL-18, G-CSF, GM-CSF, oncostatin M, MIF	IFN-α, IFN-γ, IL-4, IL-12, LIF
3. **Chemokines/receptors**	IL-8/CXCL8, ENA-78/CXCL5, groα/CXCL1, CTAP-III/CXCL6, SDF-1/CXCL12, MCP-1/CCL2, fractalkine/CX3CL1, CXCR2, CXCR4, CCR2	PF4/CXCL4, MIG/CXCL9, IP-10/CXCL10, SLC/CCL21, CXCR3
4. **Matrix molecules**	Type 1 collagen, fibronectin, laminin, vitronectin, tenascin, proteoglycan	Thrombospondin-1, -2
5. **Cell adhesion molecules**	β1 and β3 integrins, E-selectin, VCAM-1, ICAM-2, CD34, Lewis^y/H, MUC18, PECAM-1, endoglin, JAM-A, JAM-C	—
6. **Proteolytic enzymes**	MMPs, plasminogen activators	TIMPs, PAIs
7. **Antirheumatic drugs**	—	Dexamethasone, rofecoxib, classical DMARDs, thalidomide, minocycline, anti-TNF biologics
8. **Antibiotic derivatives**	—	Minocycline, fumagillin analogues, deoxyspergualin, clarithromycin
9. **Environmental factors**	Hypoxia	—
10. **Others**	Angiopoietin 1/Tie-2, angiotropin, pleiotrophin, angiogenin, survivin, COX/prostaglandin E2, PAF, nitric oxide (NO), endothelin-1, serum amyloid A, histamine, substance P, adenosine, erythropoietin, prolactin, thrombin	Angiopoietin 2, angiostatin, endostatin, kallistatin, type 4 collagen derivatives, paclitaxel, 2-methoxyestradiol, osteonectin, opioids, troponin I, chondromodulin

See text for abbreviations. Abbreviations not mentioned in text: JAM, junctional adhesion molecule.

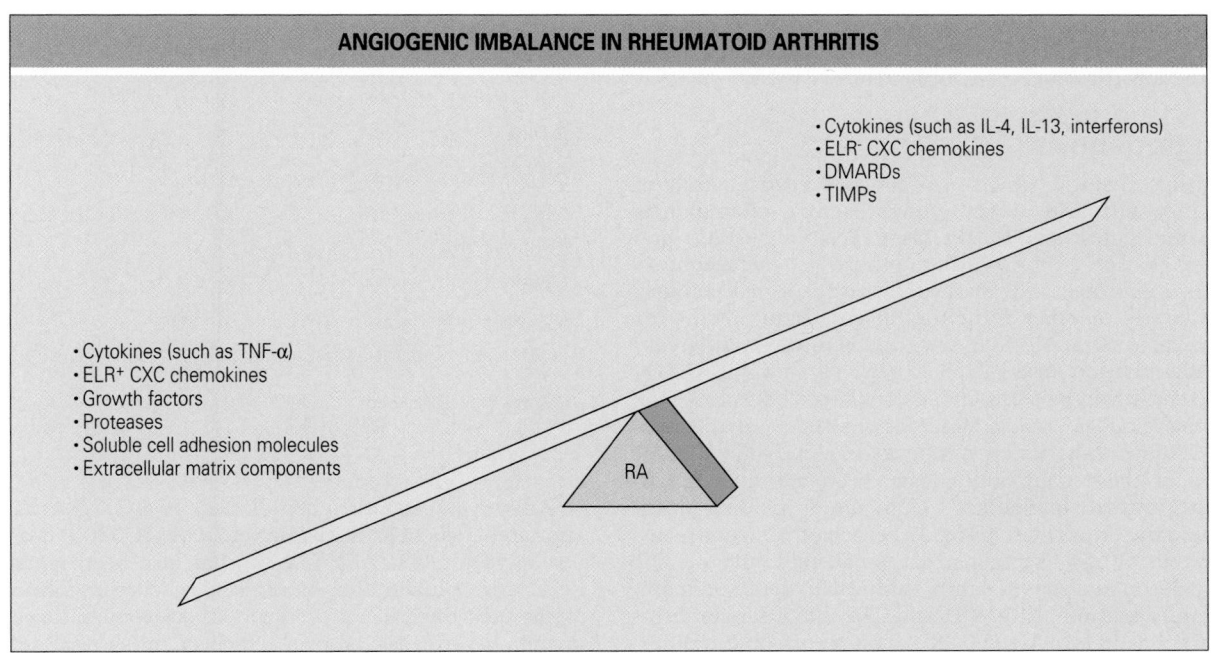

Fig. 90.2 Angiogenic imbalance in rheumatoid arthritis (RA). An imbalance in RA favors the abundance of angiogenic mediators over angiostatic factors. DMARDs, disease-modifying antirheumatic drug; RA, rheumatoid arthritis; TIMPs, tissue inhibitors of metalloproteinases; TNF, tumor necrosis factor.

For example, soluble and cell surface-bound angiogenic factors may interact with each other: VEGF, in part, acts via integrin-dependent pathways.[1,2,10] Other regulatory mechanisms include the balance between specific antagonistic pairs such as MMPs and tissue inhibitors of MMPs (TIMPs); the stimulation of angiostatic factors by angiogenic mediators (negative feedback); suppression of angiogenic mediator production by antagonists; and interactions between angiostatic molecules. The use of synthetic compounds in order to inhibit neovascularization is also a method of regulation, which is also relevant for antiangiogenic therapy.[2,4-6]

ANGIOGENESIS INHIBITION FOR THE TREATMENT OF RHEUMATOID ARTHRITIS

Angiogenesis inhibitors

Angiostatic factors that may be relevant for RA are listed in Table 90.1. Most inhibitors act by suppressing the action of angiogenic mediators, primarily VEGF, HIFs, and the α_vβ_3 integrin. Angiostatic cytokines include interferon-α (IFN-α), IFN-γ, IL-4, IL-12, and leukemia inhibitory factor (LIF).[1,5,12] As described earlier, ELR⁻ CXC chemokines such as platelet factor-4 (PF4/CXCL4), monokine induced by interferon-γ (MIG/CXCL9), and interferon-γ-inducible protein (IP-10/CXCL10) inhibit synovial neovascularization.[3,13] As IP-10/CXCL10 and MIG/CXCL9 bind to CXCR3, this receptor confers angiostasis.[3,13]

Protease inhibitors such as TIMPs and plasminogen activator inhibitors antagonize the effects of proteases. Heparin-binding factors such as thrombospondin-1 (TSP1), TSP2, and the PF4/CXCL4 chemokine block growth factor binding to heparin.[1,2,5]

A number of antirheumatic agents currently used for the treatment of RA have been shown to suppress endothelial cell migration and neovascularization. These compounds include dexamethasone, gold salts, chloroquine, sulfasalazine, methotrexate, azathioprine, cyclophosphamide, leflunomide, thalidomide, minocycline, anti-TNF agents, and possibly cyclosporine A.[1,4,6] Thalidomide is a potent TNF-α antagonist that inhibits angiogenesis.[4]

Some antibiotics and their derivatives may suppress angiogenesis via the inhibition of VEGF or MMP action. Apart from minocycline mentioned earlier, TNP-470 and PPI-2458—angiostatic analogues of fumagillin—decrease serum levels of VEGF and inhibit angiogenesis. Deoxyspergualin and clarithromycin also inhibit neovascularization.[1,4,6]

Angiostatin, a fragment of plasminogen; endostatin, a fragment of type XIII collagen; and their derivatives block $\alpha_V\beta_3$ integrin-dependent angiogenesis.[4-6] Endostatin also interferes with VEGF receptor 2 signaling.[6] Other derivatives such as protease-activated kringles 1-5 (K1-5), kallistatin, arresten, canstatin, and tumstatin also inhibit neovascularization.[4-6]

2-Methoxyestradiol (2-ME), a natural metabolite of estrogen with low affinity for estrogen receptors, inhibits angiogenesis by disrupting microtubules and by suppressing HIF-1α activity.[4-6] Paclitaxel (taxol) is a microtubule disrupting agent that diminishes HIF-1α expression and activity and thus indirectly inhibits angiogenesis.[4-6]

Other angiogenesis inhibitors include osteonectin, opioids, angiopoietin-2, retinoids, opioids, troponin I, and cartilage-derived natural inhibitors including chondromodulin-1.[4-6] Some of these agents gave promising results in cancer therapy trials and preclinical arthritis studies.[4-6]

Targeting angiogenesis

Future antiangiogenic therapy, which also controls synovial inflammation in RA, may primarily target growth factors, chemokines, cellular adhesion molecules, and MMPs, as well as angiostatin and endostatin (Table 90.2).[4,6,9,10,20-25] Either otherwise endogenously produced, natural inhibitors and their derivatives or exogenously administered antibodies or other inhibitors of angiogenic mediators could be used (see Table 90-2).[4-6] VEGF targeting is in the mainstream of cancer and inflammation research.[4,6,9,10] One can inhibit VEGF-mediated neovascularization by using monoclonal antibodies to VEGF or VEGF receptors (VEGFR), soluble VEGFR constructs, small molecule VEGF and VEGFR inhibitors, or inhibitors of VEGF and VEGFR signaling.[5,9] Some of these compounds have been administered to cancer and, recently, arthritis patients.[4-6,9] Compounds yielding promising results include the anti-VEGF antibody bevacizumab, some anti-VEGFR antibodies, the VEGF-Trap construct, small molecule VEGFR tyrosine kinase inhibitors such as vatalanib, sunitinib malate, sorafenib, vandetanib, cediranib, axatinib, KRN-951 and CEP-7055, semaphorin-3A, and soluble Fas ligand (sFasL, CD178).[9] The peroxisome-proliferator-activated receptor-γ (PPARγ) agonists rosiglitazone and pioglitazone, currently used to treat diabetes, inhibit VEGF- and bFGF-induced synovial angiogenesis.[20] There have been attempts to target HIF-1 signaling in inflammatory bowel disease.[6,11] Imatinib mesylate, a specific inhibitor of PDGF receptor activation, inhibits the development of murine arthritis and synovial angiogenesis (see Table 90.2).[4-6]

As discussed earlier, currently used antirheumatic agents including classic DMARDs and anti-TNF biologics, among other beneficial anti-inflammatory effects, also suppress synovial neovascularization.[4-6] For example, infliximab treatment reduced synovial VEGF expression and vascularity.[5] The anti-IL-6 receptor antibody tocilizumab, which has recently been approved for the treatment of RA, decreased serum levels of VEGF.[21] Thalidomide and its analogue, CC1069, effectively suppress synovial angiogenesis; however, thalidomide exerted moderate efficacy in RA and lupus trials (see Table 90.2).[4-6,22]

TABLE 90.2 POTENTIAL ANGIOGENESIS TARGETING STRATEGIES IN ARTHRITIS*

Compound	Reference(s)
Endogenous (natural) inhibitors	
Angiostatin	4, 5, 6
Endostatin	4, 5, 6
Protease-activated kringles 1-5 (K1-5) (angiostatin analogue)	4, 6
Kallistatin	4, 6
Thrombospondin-1, -2	4, 6
Interleukin-4, -13 gene	4, 5, 6
PF4/CXCL4 chemokine	3
2-methoxyestradiol (2-ME)	4, 6
Exogenous inhibitors	
Anti-VEGFR1 antibody	9
Vatalanib (VEGF-R tyrosine kinase inhibitor)	9
Imatinib mesylate (PDGF receptor signaling)	4, 6
Soluble Fas ligand	4, 6, 9
Bicyclam (AMD3100)	4, 14
Vitaxin (anti-$\alpha_V\beta_3$ integrin)	6, 13
Traditional DMARDs (methotrexate, sulfasalazine, etc.)	1, 4, 6
Rofecoxib	4, 5
Infliximab	5, 6
Tocilizumab	21
Thalidomide	4, 6, 22
CC1069 (thalidomide analogue)	4, 6
TNP-470 (fumagillin analogue)	4, 6
PPI2458 (fumagillin analogue)	4, 6
Statins	23
Endothelin-1 antagonists	25
Paclitaxel	4, 6
Minocycline	4, 6
Clarithromycin	4, 5
Deoxyspergualin	4, 5
PPARγ agonists (pioglitazone, rosiglitazone)	20

*See text for abbreviations.

Among angiostatic chemokines, PF4/CXCL4 has been tried in animal models of arthritis. Bicyclam (AMD3100) is a selective antagonist of SDF-1/CXCL12. CXCR2 has also been targeted in cancer.[3,4,6] Regarding cellular adhesion molecules, Vitaxin, a humanized antibody to the $\alpha_V\beta_3$ integrin suppressed leukocyte migration and neovascularization in arthritis models; however, it showed little efficacy in a human phase 1 RA trial.[4-6,18] Statins also modify endothelial function and adhesion receptor expression.[23] Numerous protease inhibitors including TIMPs and plasminogen activator inhibitors (PAIs) that antagonize the effects of proteases have been tried in angiogenesis models.[24] Angiostatin and endostatin also became primary targets. The administration of angiostatin and endostatin abrogated arthritis in various rodent models.[1,4-6] Endothelin (ET)-1 antagonists currently used in the treatment of scleroderma-associated pulmonary hypertension may also exert antiangiogenic effects (see Table 90.2).[25]

Among antibiotics, minocycline and clarithromycin showed some efficacy in human RA, and deoxyspergualin and the fumagillin analogues TNP-470 and PPI-2458 suppressed the development of arthritis in rodent models.[4-6] Theoretically, most angiostatic agents may have therapeutic relevance for arthritis- and tumor-associated angiogenesis (see Table 90.2).

REFERENCES

1. Koch AE. Angiogenesis: implications for rheumatoid arthritis. Arthritis Rheum 1998;41:951-962.
2. Szekanecz Z, Koch AE. Vascular involvement in rheumatic diseases: "vascular rheumatology". Arthritis Res Ther 2008;10:224.
3. Szekanecz Z, Koch AE. Chemokines and angiogenesis. Curr Opin Rheumatol 2001;13:202-208.
4. Lainer-Carr D, Brahn E. Angiogenesis inhibition as a therapeutic approach for inflammatory synovitis. Nat Clin Pract Rheumatol 2007;3:434-442.
5. Szekanecz Z, Koch AE. Mechanism of disease: angiogenesis in inflammatory diseases. Nat Clin Pract Rheumatol 2007;3:635-643.
6. Veale DJ, Fearon U. Inhibition of angiogenic pathways in rheumatoid arthritis: potential for therapeutic targeting. Best Pract Res Clin Rheumatol 2006;20:941-947.
7. Szekanecz Z, Koch AE. Macrophages and their products in rheumatoid arthritis. Curr Opin Rheumatol 2007;19:289-295.
8. Fava RA, Olsen NJ, Spencer-Green G, et al. Vascular permeability factor/endothelial growth factor (VPF/VEGF): accumulation and expression in human synovial fluids and rheumatoid synovial tissue. J Exp Med 1994;180:341-346.
9. Kiselyov A, Balakin KV, Tkachenko SE. VEGF/VEGFR signaling as a target for inhibiting angiogenesis. Expert Opin Investig Drugs 2007;16:83-107.
10. Shibuya M. Vascular endothelial growth factor-dependent and -independent regulation of angiogenesis. BMB Rep 2008;41:278-286.
11. Giatromanolaki A, Sivridis E, Maltezos E, et al. Upregulated hypoxia inducible factor-1α and -2α pathway in rheumatoid arthritis and osteoarthritis. Arthritis Res Ther 2003;5:R193-R198.
12. Brennan F, Beech J. Update on cytokines in rheumatoid arthritis. Curr Opin Rheumatol 2007;19:296-301.
13. Strieter RM, Polverini PJ, Kunkel SL, et al. The functional role of the ELR motif in CXC chemokine-mediated angiogenesis. J Biol Chem 1995;270:27348-27357.
14. Petit I, Jin D, Rafii S. The SDF-1-CXCR4 signaling pathway: a molecular hub modulating neo-angiogenesis. Trends Immunol 2007;28:299-307.
15. Jakobsson L, Claesson-Welsh L. Vascular basement membrane components in angiogenesis—an act of balance. Scientific World J 2008;8:1246-1249.
16. Agarwal SK, Brenner MB. Role of adhesion molecules in synovial inflammation. Curr Opin Rheumatol 2006;18:268-276.
17. Szekanecz Z, Szegedi G, Koch AE. Cellular adhesion molecules in rheumatoid arthritis. Regulation by cytokines and possible clinical importance. J Invest Med 1996;44:124-135.
18. Brooks PC, Clark RA, Cheresh DA. Requirement of vascular integrin alpha v beta 3 for angiogenesis. Science 1994;264:569-571.
19. Koch AE, Halloran MM, Haskell CJ, et al. Angiogenesis mediated by soluble forms of E-selectin and vascular cell adhesion molecule-1. Nature 1995;376:517-519.
20. Aljada A, O'Connor L, Fu YY, Mousa SA. PPARγ ligands, rosiglitazone and pioglitazone inhibit bFGF- and VEGF-mediated angiogenesis. Angiogenesis 2008;11:361-367.
21. Dessein PH, Joffe BI. Suppression of circulating interleukin-6 concentrations is associated with decreased endothelial activation in rheumatoid arthritis. Clin Exp Rheumatol 2006;24:161-167.
22. D'Amato RJ, Loughnan MS, Flynn E, Folkman J. Thalidomide is an inhibitor of angiogenesis. Proc Natl Acad Sci USA 1994;91:4082-4085.
23. McCarey DW, Sattar N, McInnes IB. Do the pleiotropic effects of statins in the vasculature predict a role in inflammatory diseases? Arthritis Res Ther 2005;7:55-61.
24. Skotnicki JS, Zask A, Nelson FC, et al. Design and synthetic considerations of matrix metalloproteinase inhibitors. Ann N Y Acad Sci 1999;878:61-72.
25. Koch AE, Distler O. Vasculopathy and disordered angiogenesis in selected rheumatic diseases: rheumatoid arthritis and systemic sclerosis. Arthritis Res Ther 2007;9(Suppl 2):S3.

REFERENCES

Full references for this chapter can be found on www.expertconsult.com.

The rheumatoid joint: synovitis and tissue destruction

91

Ellen M. Gravallese and Paul A. Monach

- Synovial tissues in rheumatoid arthritis (RA) are markedly expanded by the recruitment and retention of inflammatory cells, with the formation of villous projections and the generation of pannus tissue that invades and destroys cartilage and bone.

- Pathogenic events in RA probably occur in stages, and mechanisms leading to initiation of the disease appear to be distinct from those involved in the perpetuation of inflammation and the eventual destruction of joint tissues.

- Chronic synovitis is maintained by the interactions of cell types native to the joint and inflammatory cells recruited to the joint, with the subsequent establishment of cytokine "networks."

- Cartilage destruction results from the production of enzymes that destroy components of the cartilage extracellular matrix by cells within synovial tissues and by chondrocytes; osteoclasts contribute to destruction of articular bone.

INTRODUCTION

Inflammation of joints lined by synovium (synovitis) is the hallmark of rheumatoid arthritis (RA). Associated with synovitis is a propensity to destroy articular cartilage and bone, the structural components of the joint. Consequently, joint tissues from patients with RA have been the subject of extensive research, leading to tremendous advances in our understanding of the pathogenesis of synovitis and the subsequent rational development of effective new therapies. In this chapter, a review of the pathologic changes seen in RA synovium is followed by a detailed summary of the phenotypical and functional changes that occur in synovitis in RA, including the cell types and inflammatory mediators responsible for establishing and maintaining chronic inflammation. Mechanisms of joint destruction are reviewed. Finally, this information is synthesized with discussion of the current theories of RA pathogenesis, and a unifying hypothesis that integrates knowledge gained from the study of synovial tissues, animal models of arthritis, and insights from clinical trials is proposed.

NORMAL SYNOVIUM

In the normal joint, the synovium is a thin membrane that derives from cells of the embryonic mesenchyme and lines the fibrous joint capsule (Fig. 91.1). The synovium and joint capsule attach to skeletal tissues at the interface of cartilage and bone. Normal synovial tissues do not encroach on articular cartilage. The most superficial layer of the synovium, lying adjacent to the joint cavity, is known as the synovial intima or synovial lining cell layer. Electron microscopic (EM) images have demonstrated that the cells within this layer are loosely adherent to the synovial subintimal or sublining tissues and that these cells form a discontinuous layer lacking a true basement membrane.[1]

Cells within the synovial lining layer are 6 to 12 μm in diameter, excluding the numerous finger-like projections extending from the cell surface. Two distinct populations of cells have been identified by EM: the type A or macrophage-like synoviocyte and the type B or fibroblast-like synoviocyte (FLS). Type A synoviocytes contain filopodia, a prominent Golgi apparatus, lysosomes, and vacuoles.[1] These cells have a sparse endoplasmic reticulum, because these are primarily phagocytic cells that are presumably present in the joint to clear particulate matter

from the joint cavity. In addition, they express receptors for the Fc domains of IgG. In contrast, type B synoviocytes are fibroblast-like cells that contain abundant protein synthetic machinery and fewer filopodia and vacuoles and lack Fc receptors (Fig. 91.2).[1]

Type B synoviocytes produce hyaluronic acid and lubricin, which assist in normal joint motion. In addition, they synthesize proteins, including fibronectin and collagen. Type B synoviocytes can be identified using cytochemistry for uridine diphosphoglucose dehydrogenase activity (UDPGD) and by staining for CD55 (decay-accelerating factor [DAF]), whereas type A synoviocytes express monocyte-macrophage lineage cell surface markers (including CD14, CD11b, and CD68), as well as non-specific esterase activity (Fig. 91.3). Cells within the synovial lining layer lack tight junctions and desmosomes that would allow for stable cell-cell contact and maintenance of the structure of the lining layer. However, cadherin-11 has been shown to mediate homotypic interactions between type B synoviocytes and may contribute to adhesion between these cells.[2]

Cells within the synovial lining layer are loosely adherent to the sublining tissues, which are composed of connective tissue that becomes denser in areas closer to the joint capsule. This sublining tissue contains blood vessels (arterioles, capillaries, and postcapillary venules) as well as lymphatic vessels and nerves. It has been assumed that synovial tissues derived from healthy subjects are devoid of any significant number of inflammatory cells. However, a recent study of 12 healthy subjects undergoing needle biopsy of knee synovium demonstrated the presence of T cells in perivascular areas and/or diffusely in 9 of 10 cases. Macrophages were present in all cases, as were human leukocyte antigen (HLA)-DR–positive cells. Interestingly, B cells were not present in any case.[3] These results suggest that, in normal subjects, subclinical joint inflammation can occur, probably in response to stimuli within the joint, but it does not progress to overt arthritis.

SYNOVIUM IN RHEUMATOID ARTHRITIS

In RA, chronic, clinically significant synovial inflammation develops, leading to eventual destruction of cartilage and bone. At the gross level, inflamed synovial tissues in RA demonstrate a marked expansion, with the synovial surface thrown into innumerable hyperemic and edematous villous projections that extend into the joint cavity. The microscopic changes seen in the synovium of patients with RA are not unique to this disease and can be seen in other inflammatory arthritides. However, characteristic histologic findings can support the clinical diagnosis. These include hyperplasia of the synovial lining layer, a mixed inflammatory cell infiltrate in the subsynovium with follicle and germinal center formation in some cases, neovascularization, and, in clinically active disease, the deposition of fibrin (Fig. 91.4).

In RA the synovial lining layer may be up to 12 cells in thickness and individual cells may appear hypertrophic. Much of this increase is due to recruitment of cells of the monocyte-macrophage lineage from bone marrow. Evidence for recruitment of these cells into normal synovial tissues comes from studies of radiation chimeras of normal and beige mice. In beige mice, giant secondary lysosomes are present in cells of the monocyte-macrophage lineage. After bone marrow cells from beige mice were engrafted into normal irradiated histocompatible recipient mice, giant granules were identified in up to 7% of type A synovial lining cells.[4] Because macrophages are present in the sublining as tissue macrophages as well as in the lining as type A synoviocytes, it is not entirely clear whether the greatly increased numbers seen in rheumatoid synovial tissues arise from division of local precursors or

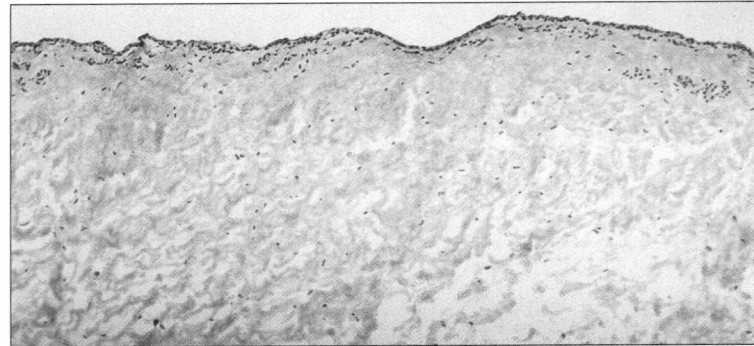

Fig. 91.1 Normal synovium. Low-power view of a normal synovial tissue. The intimal lining shown at the top of this section is only one or two cell layers deep, and sublining blood vessels and mononuclear cells are sparse.

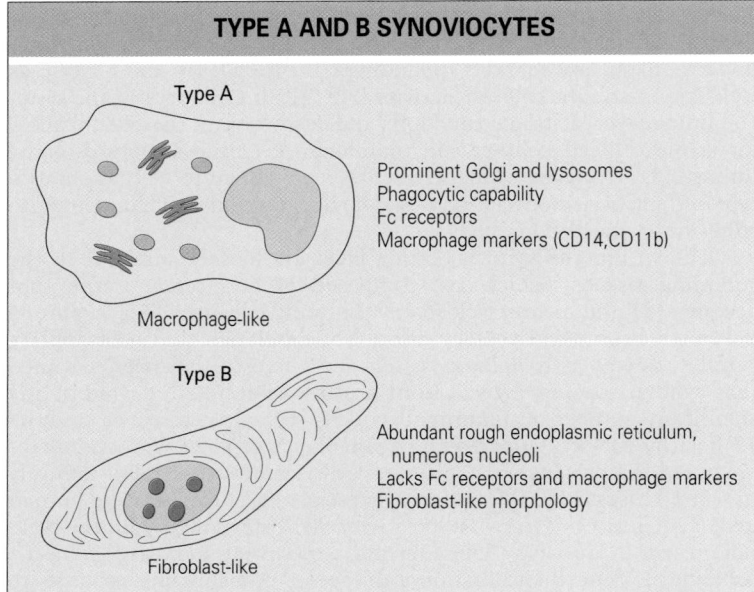

TYPE A AND B SYNOVIOCYTES

Type A

Prominent Golgi and lysosomes
Phagocytic capability
Fc receptors
Macrophage markers (CD14,CD11b)

Macrophage-like

Type B

Abundant rough endoplasmic reticulum, numerous nucleoli
Lacks Fc receptors and macrophage markers
Fibroblast-like morphology

Fibroblast-like

Fig. 91.2 Type A and B synoviocytes. Features of type A (macrophage-like) and type B (fibroblast-like) synoviocytes.

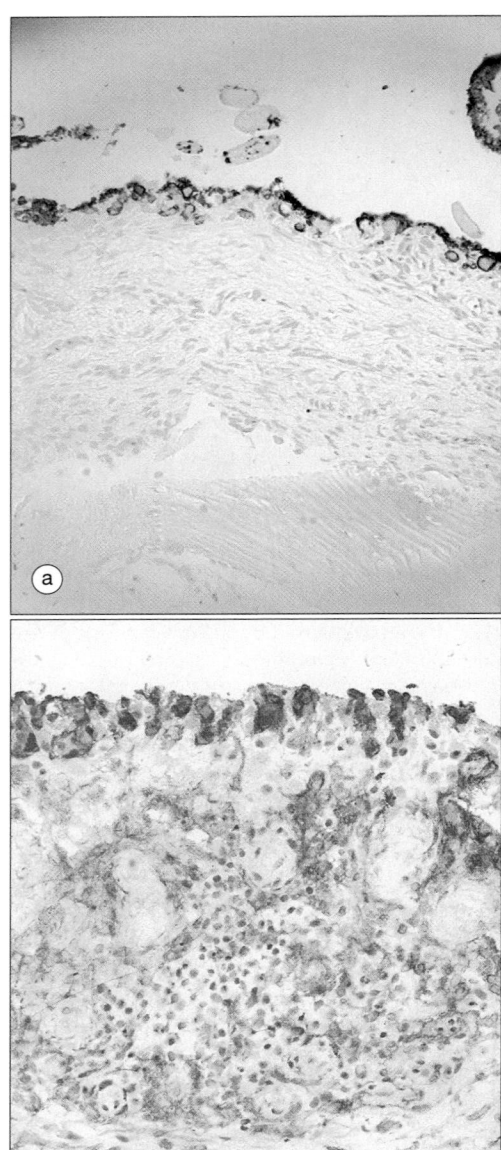

Fig. 91.3 Immunohistochemical staining in rheumatoid synovium. (a) Staining (brown) for CD55, demonstrating type B (fibroblast-like) synoviocytes in the lining layer. (b) Staining (red) for CD14, demonstrating type A (macrophage-like) synoviocytes in the lining layer as well as macrophages in the sublining tissue.

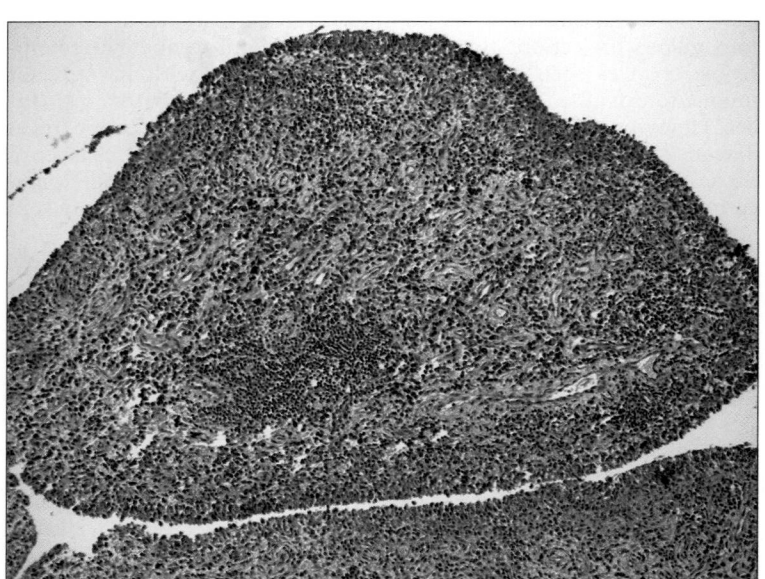

Fig. 91.4 Histology of synovium in chronic RA demonstrating hyperplasia of the synovial lining layer, infiltration of a heterogeneous admixture of mononuclear cells, including lymphocytes and plasma cells in the sublining tissue, and numerous blood vessels.

differentiate from newly recruited blood monocytes, but the latter mechanism is presumed to be the major source. The degree to which *in-situ* division of resident cells in synovial tissues occurs and contributes to lining layer hyperplasia is still a matter of debate, but markers of cell proliferation, including proliferating cell nuclear antigen (PCNA), have been identified in type B synoviocytes in the lining layer, demonstrating that some cell division does occur.[5] The increase in the numbers of synovial lining cells in RA is significant, because these cells are a source of a panoply of cytokines and other inflammatory mediators that contribute to chronic inflammation, as well as a source of matrix-degrading enzymes.

The inflammatory infiltrate within synovium in patients with established RA is heterogeneous and is composed of T and B cells, plasma cells, and macrophages, as well as lesser numbers of dendritic cells (DCs), mast cells, natural killer (NK) cells, and, occasionally, neutrophils. Neutrophils are more commonly seen in synovial fluid but can be present in significant numbers in synovial tissues during an acute flare of disease. Most studies demonstrate a predominance of CD4+ over CD8+ T cells, with CD4+ cells being present diffusely, in aggregates, and in perivascular areas. B cells are also present diffusely and in aggregates; and immunoglobulin-producing plasma cells, some of which produce rheumatoid factor (RF), are the predominant infiltrating cells in some cases. Macrophages are usually present in significant numbers between and sometimes within lymphoid aggregates. Although macrophages may act as antigen-presenting cells to resident T cells, DCs, which are more potent antigen-presenting cells, have also been shown to interdigitate among T-cell aggregates. In addition, resident B cells may also serve as antigen-presenting cells, particularly for antigens internalized via their surface Ig receptors.

There is a definite heterogeneity of histologic findings among patients with RA. However, there are distinct patterns of cellular infiltration that have only recently been categorized. Although cells within the synovium can move through the tissue in a dynamic fashion, synovial tissues from patients with RA typically have one of three histologic patterns of inflammatory cell infiltration, and these patterns appear to be preserved over time. Furthermore, these patterns of inflammation have been associated with typical and distinct cytokine profiles and may therefore have clinical relevance.[6]

The most common histologic pattern is that of a diffuse inflammatory infiltrate, in which infiltrating immune cells, predominantly lymphocytes and macrophages, are interspersed in a haphazard way among resident synovial fibroblasts and blood vessels. This form of synovitis is associated with low levels of messenger RNA (mRNA) for interferon-γ (IFN-γ) and interleukin-4 (IL-4), as well as low levels of tumor necrosis factor (TNF) and IL-1β mRNA. In addition, patients with this form of synovitis tend to have clinically milder disease. A second pattern is that of follicle formation, in which infiltrating T and B cells are arranged in distinct follicles or aggregates. In some cases, these follicles become highly organized into true, functionally competent germinal centers similar to those present in lymph nodes.[7] Finally, in the rarest form of synovitis, seen in only a few percent of cases, there is a granulomatous inflammatory infiltrate in which granulomas resembling rheumatoid nodules are present within synovial tissues. Both IFN-γ and IL-4 mRNA are charactersitically produced in this form of synovitis, as are high levels of TNF and IL-1β, suggesting that these tissues are associated with significant T-cell and macrophage stimulation. Patients with granulomas in synovial tissues also typically have rheumatoid nodules in the skin.[6]

MECHANISMS OF CHRONIC SYNOVITIS IN RHEUMATOID ARTHRITIS

Mechanisms for the recruitment and retention of inflammatory cells in chronic inflammatory diseases, including RA, have been the subject of intense investigation in recent years. The influx of inflammatory cells into synovial tissues occurs primarily through tethering of cells via selectins; upregulation of adhesion molecules including vascular cell adhesion molecule-1 (VCAM-1), intercellular adhesion molecules-1 and -2 (ICAM-1 and -2), and others on postcapillary venules; and chemokine-chemokine receptor interactions, which act as cellular "homing signals." Proinflammatory cytokines produced within RA

synovial tissues, including TNF and others, can induce the expression of several adhesion molecules on vascular endothelium.

Once inflammatory cells have served their purpose at a site of injury there is normally a clearance of these cells, via apoptosis or emigration of these cells from the site. In RA, however, chronic inflammation persists, reflecting an imbalance between cell recruitment, proliferation, and retention on the one hand and cell death and emigration from the tissue on the other hand. Exciting recent data suggest that cells migrating into a site of inflammation can transition from a "migratory" phenotype to a "stationary" phenotype based on changes in cellular receptor expression induced by interactions with stromal cells resident in the tissues they encounter. In the case of RA, interactions between T cells and stromal cells in synovial tissues favor inhibition of T-cell apoptosis[8] via the expression of IFN-β by resident synovial macrophages and fibroblasts. T-cell retention is also favored. One proposed mechanism for this retention is upregulation of the chemokine receptor CXCR4 on T cells, induced by locally expressed transforming growth factor (TGF)-β. The ligand for CXCR4 is stromal cell–derived factor-1 (SDF-1 or CXCL12), expressed on synovial cells and upregulated on RA synovial fibroblasts as compared with osteoarthritic (OA) synovial fibroblasts. SDF-1 is also a chemoattractant for other mononuclear cells expressing Mac-1 and CXCR4 and is a potent proangiogenic factor. The importance of SDF-1/CXCR4 interactions in RA was demonstrated in murine collagen-induced arthritis, where an antagonist of the interaction between SDF-1 and CXCR4 led to a decreased incidence of arthritis, a delay in onset of disease, and decreased clinical severity.[9]

Pannus

A characteristic histologic feature seen in patients with RA is the presence of a distinctive tissue located at the interface between synovium and cartilage/bone at sites of joint destruction. This tissue is known as *pannus*, which is Latin for "cloth" or "covering." Pannus tissue, not seen in this exact form in other inflammatory or non-inflammatory arthritides, was so named because of its location, draped over cartilaginous surfaces and adherent to these surfaces. It is derived from the synovial membrane and is thought to mediate the process of tissue destruction. EM studies of the cellular composition of pannus have demonstrated that fibroblast-like cells predominate in this tissue, especially on the surface, but that in deeper layers, and admixed with fibroblasts, are cells with the EM appearance of macrophages.[10] There are fewer lymphocytes and other inflammatory cells within pannus tissue compared with synovial tissues remote from bone, although these cells are often present (Fig. 91.5).

Fibroblasts in pannus tissue have an invasive nature owing at least in part to their ability to express proteinases that degrade the extracellular matrix components of cartilage. An additional cell termed a *pannocyte*, characterized by intense expression of VCAM-1 and a prolonged lifespan in culture,[11] has been isolated from pannus tissues. Whether the pannocyte represents a unique cell type or a phenotypical variant of the synovial fibroblast is not known. Finally, cells with the full phenotype of osteoclasts are present at the interface between pannus and bone and these cells are critical to the process of bone erosion.

Early rheumatoid arthritis

Histopathologic changes in synovium are seen within the first few weeks in the clinical course of RA. Attempts to obtain synovial tissues from patients with very early RA were initiated in the hope that unique pathologic changes would be identified that would provide clues to the events involved in disease initiation. Although initial studies suggested the presence of some unique histologic features such as vascular changes with evidence of endothelial cell damage, more recent studies have demonstrated that the pathologic changes in early RA are very similar to those in chronic disease (Fig. 91.6). Studies of synovium obtained from knee joints within 6 weeks of the onset of clinical disease in RA demonstrated an infiltration of T cells in all cases, with a predominance of CD4+ over CD8+ cells. B cells were seen in fewer numbers but were present in the majority of cases. Inflammatory infiltrates were perivascular and were localized to the superficial areas within the sublining, and no lymphocyte aggregates were present in

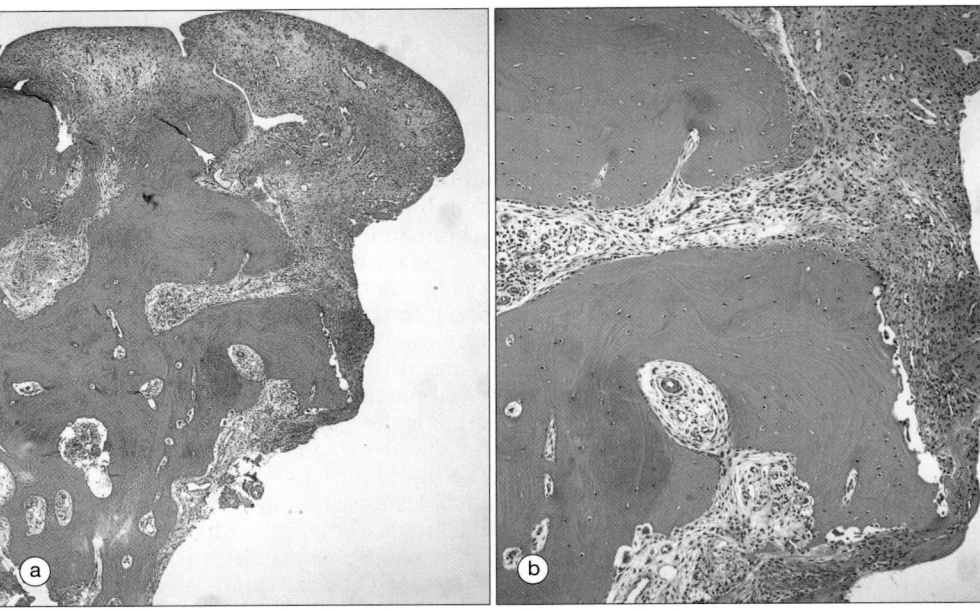

Fig. 91.5 Histology of the pannus/bone interface. (a) Low-power view demonstrating invasion of pannus tissue into cartilage and bone. (b) High-power detail demonstrating multinucleated osteoclast-like cells at the interface of pannus and bone.

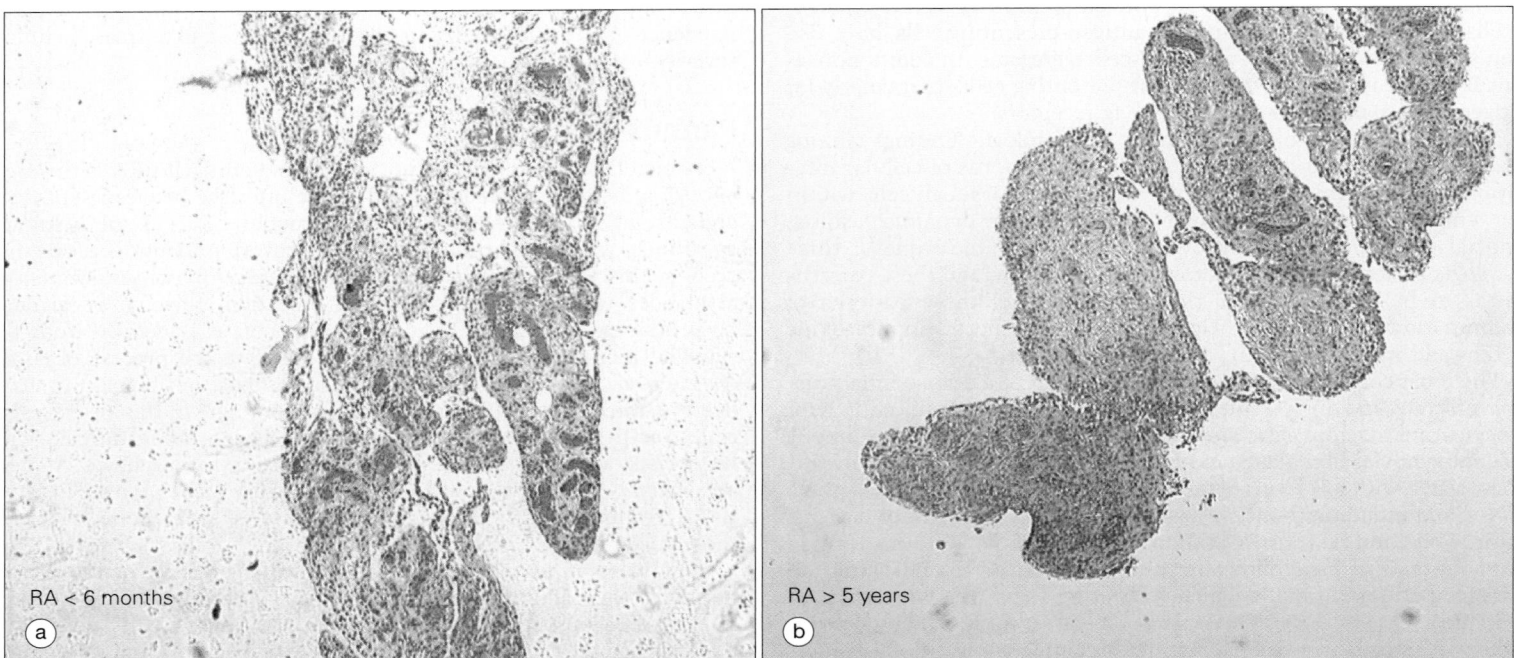

RA < 6 months

RA > 5 years

Fig. 91.6 RA synovium in early and late disease. Typical RA synovitis with synovial lining hyperplasia, increased numbers of blood vessels, and infiltration of the sublining with mononuclear cells. Early (a) and chronic (b) disease exhibit many of the same histologic features. *(Courtesy of Dr. P. P. Tak.)*

these early tissue samples.[12] In addition, inflammation has been shown to be present in synovial tissues in clinically uninvolved joints from patients with long-standing RA when biopsy samples are obtained and examined.[13] These data suggest that histologic inflammation of the synovium is an early and widespread event in RA and that the full clinical manifestation of arthritis requires additional pathologic events such as an increase in vascular permeability and activation of pain pathways.

COMPONENTS OF RHEUMATOID SYNOVIUM
Difficulties with analysis

Because synovitis is the characteristic feature of RA, it remains reasonable to hope that key insights into pathogenesis may be obtained by detailed analysis of inflamed synovial tissues. Unfortunately, however, no single analytical technique exists whereby the integrated function of diverse cell types can be evaluated comprehensively, with attention

to all possible genes, proteins, and other products. Thus, investigations have been conducted at several different levels and with different model systems, each with its own strengths and weaknesses. As shown in Figure 91.7, examination of intact or sectioned synovial tissue samples has the virtue of allowing the study of a biologic system with all of its components intact, but the proscription against manipulation inevitably brings uncertainty regarding the relationships between the structures seen and the functions proposed. Conversely, model systems produced by isolating cells and controlling experimental conditions allow for more detailed and scientifically rigorous dissection of mechanisms but suffer from potential artifacts from manipulation and oversimplification.

Not shown in Figure 91.7 is the role of animal models in clarifying disease mechanisms. Animal models offer the strengths of both *in-vivo* and *in-vitro* approaches and allow for detailed analyses of disease mechanisms, but their direct relevance to human RA remains uncertain. Despite these difficulties, it is important to note that it was through examination of data obtained by a combination of methods at

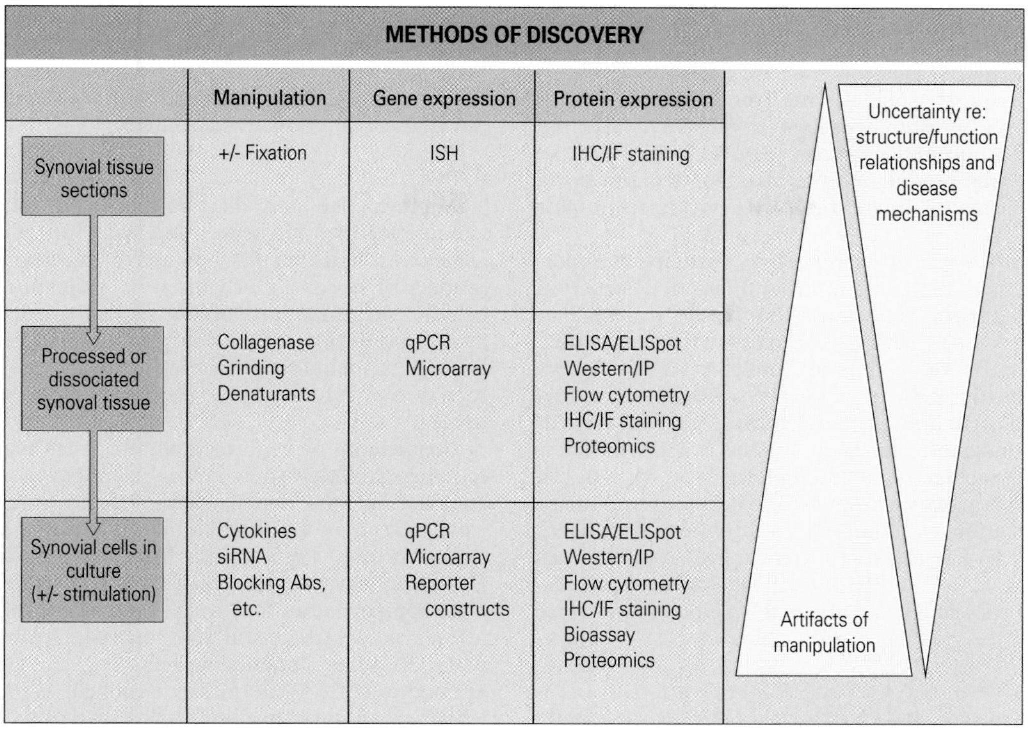

METHODS OF DISCOVERY				
	Manipulation	Gene expression	Protein expression	
Synovial tissue sections	+/- Fixation	ISH	IHC/IF staining	Uncertainty re: structure/function relationships and disease mechanisms
Processed or dissociated synovial tissue	Collagenase Grinding Denaturants	qPCR Microarray	ELISA/ELISpot Western/IP Flow cytometry IHC/IF staining Proteomics	
Synovial cells in culture (+/- stimulation)	Cytokines siRNA Blocking Abs, etc.	qPCR Microarray Reporter constructs	ELISA/ELISpot Western/IP Flow cytometry IHC/IF staining Bioassay Proteomics	Artifacts of manipulation

Fig. 91.7 Methods of evaluation of inflamed synovium or synovial fluid. Note that most gene-based techniques rely on hybridization of mRNA (or complementary DNA synthesized from it) to specific complementary nucleic acid sequences and that most protein-detecting techniques rely on binding by specific antibodies. siRNA, small interfering RNA—a short RNA sequence that binds to a specific mRNA transcript, leading to its degradation within cells. ISH, *in-situ hybridization*—a method for localizing and measuring specific mRNA transcripts using labeled specific DNA or RNA sequences. qPCR, quantitative polymerase chain reaction—a method for quantifying expression levels of specific mRNA transcripts by amplifying the region between two specific sequences and detecting amplified product. Microarray—a method for simultaneously quantifying thousands of mRNA transcripts by hybridization to a microscopic array of specific DNA sequences. Reporter constructs—attachment of regulatory sequences that normally control the transcription of a gene of interest to a gene encoding a product easily identified by color, fluorescence, or luminescence. IHC, immunohistochemistry—a method for localization and quantitation of protein and other structures using specific antibodies conjugated to enzymes that allow for detection via colored deposits. IF, immunofluorescence—analogous to IHC but using antibodies conjugated to molecules fluorescent in various colors. ELISA, enzyme-linked immunosorbent assay—quantifies a factor in solution by capture using a specific antibody, then detection using a second, enzyme-conjugated antibody that produces a soluble colored product. ELISpot—antibody-mediated capture of factors secreted by cells in culture, then detection using a precipitating enzyme product that allows for quantification of the number of cells making a factor. Western blot—detection, using enzyme-conjugated specific antibodies, of proteins previously separated by electrophoresis; correct identification of a protein is confirmed by its location after electrophoretic separation. IP, immunoprecipitation—capture of a factor from solution using specific antibodies, followed by capture of the complex on beads; it allows for quantification of relatively rare factors due to concentrating effect. Flow cytometry—quantification of cell surface and some intracellular proteins of individual cells in suspension, using fluorescently labeled specific antibodies; it allows for measurement of multiple proteins simultaneously via the use of different colored fluorophores. Bioassay—measurement of the response of living cells to added factors or cells used to follow complex interactions thought to be of biologic relevance. Proteomics—quantitative determination of total protein content or a large subset thereof that relies on separation of proteins and identification using mass spectrometry, multiple specific antibodies, and other techniques.

each of these levels of detail and manipulation that the central role of TNF in inflammatory arthritis was discovered, leading to an important advance in the treatment of RA.

Cells of rheumatoid synovium

Macrophages

Macrophages are abundant in rheumatoid synovium and are readily identified in tissue sections or after dispersion of tissue into cell suspensions, by their morphology and by surface markers such as CD14 and CD68. The number of macrophages on biopsy correlates with risk of radiographic joint destruction.[14] Although there is undoubtedly heterogeneity, cells of this lineage in rheumatoid synovium and synovial fluid show evidence of activation, such as surface markers characteris-

tic of mature phagocytic cells and high levels of major histocompatibility complex (MHC) class II molecules important for the presentation of peptide antigens to CD4+ T cells.

Macrophages within the lining layer appear to differ from those in the sublining in their expression of adhesion molecules and secreted mediators.[14] By analysis of tissue sections or freshly dispersed synovium, macrophages, especially those in the lining layer, appear to be a major source of numerous cytokines, including two known to be critically involved in the pathophysiology of RA, TNF, and IL-1,[15-18] as well as other cytokines that have well-described effects on immune and inflammatory responses, either stimulatory (IL-6, IL-12, IL-15, granulocyte-macrophage colony stimulating factor [GM-CSF]) or inhibitory (IL-1 receptor antagonist [IL-1ra], TGF-β).[15,16,19,20] Many cell surface receptors influence the activity of macrophages.[21] Notable examples expressed on synovial macrophages *in vivo* include the p55 and p75

TNF receptors, the low-affinity IgG receptors FcγRII and FcγRIII, and adhesion molecules CD31 and CD44. Investigation is ongoing into the expression by synovial macrophages of more recently described inflammatory mediators and receptors, such as the ligand-receptor pair of high mobility group box chromosomal protein-1 (HMGB-1) and the receptor for advanced glycation end products (RAGE),[22] the Toll-like receptors (TLRs) for microbial products, novel interleukins, and novel members of the TNF superfamily, including B-lymphocyte stimulator (BLyS).

Although macrophages have the machinery to participate importantly in the synthesis of lipid mediators of inflammation, destruction of cartilage and bone, and antigen presentation to T cells, it is unclear how their contribution to these activities compares with that of FLS (for the former two functions) or of DCs and B cells (for the latter). Macrophage cell lines derived from synovial tissue have been relatively difficult to obtain. Instead, macrophages derived from synovial fluid or from peripheral blood monocytes have been studied in vitro to determine the effects of various mediators on macrophage expression of cell surface molecules, proinflammatory cytokines, and effector functions.[23] At a level of great simplification, cytokines that stimulate macrophages include TNF, IL-1, IL-15, IL-17, and IL-18 and suppressive cytokines include IL-1ra, IL-4, IL-10, IL-11, and IL-13.[23-25] Macrophages are also stimulated by cell surface molecules on activated T cells, even if those T cells have been killed.[26]

Fibroblast-like synoviocytes

Like type A synoviocytes, type B synoviocytes or FLS are greatly expanded in number in rheumatoid synovium, although type A cells remain more abundant. Most of our knowledge of the function of FLS in RA has come from in-vitro studies because, unlike macrophages from synovial tissues, these cells can be readily passaged from culture of synovium. FLS in the normal synovial lining differ from fibroblasts in the sublining and other tissues, most notably by the expression of VCAM-1, cadherin-11, and the intracellular enzyme UDPGD.[2,27] The quintessential function of normal FLS is the production of proteoglycans for the synovial fluid and extracellular matrix, explaining the expression of the enzyme UDPGD, which catalyzes the rate-limiting step in the synthesis of a monosaccharide essential for the subsequent synthesis of hyaluronic acid. Rheumatoid FLS are notable for their ability to produce enzymes with the capacity to degrade cartilage (see later under Joint Destruction). Other pathologic functions that have been ascribed to FLS include differentiation into follicular dendritic cells (FDC), which organize germinal centers for B-cell maturation,[28] and an ability to present superantigens (bacterial proteins that bind MHC and the T-cell receptor [TCR] outside the usual interface), but not necessarily conventional peptide antigens, to T cells.[29]

FLS are strikingly active within the innate immune system, based on responsiveness to and secretion of various cytokines and other mediators. IL-1 and TNF appear to be the major stimulators of FLS and have been used in many in-vitro studies; receptors for these cytokines are also detectable on FLS in tissue sections.[18,30] Bacterial products such as lipopolysaccharide (LPS) and peptidoglycan are also stimulatory, presumably through specific receptors such as TLR-4 and TLR-2, respectively. Under such stimulation, FLS secrete IL-6,[31] the related cytokine IL-11,[32] and numerous chemotactic cytokines (chemokines) capable of acting on a variety of hematopoietic cell types.[33] Some of these products are also made at detectable levels without exogenous stimulation. There is evidence for FLS being the predominant source of other mediators, such as IL-16 and nitric oxide.

For many years, the concept of rheumatoid pannus as a benign tumor has been discussed, focusing on the FLS as a "partially transformed" cell. Rheumatoid FLS indeed share many features of transformed cells, such as anchorage-independent growth in vitro and expression of proto-oncogenes and telomerase. Genetic analysis of individual cells suggests division of FLS or precursor clones in erosive pannus.[34] However, these features are characteristic not only of premalignant cells but also of otherwise normal cells that have the potential to divide and are not terminally differentiated. Although there is evidence of genetic instability in FLS based on the loss or duplication of chromosomal markers, this is equally true of FLS derived from OA or RA patients.[35] Thus, although FLS from RA do have durable phenotypi-

cal changes, based on their growth properties in vitro as well as on their ability to degrade cartilage in vivo when co-transplanted with normal cartilage into severe combined immunodeficient (SCID) mice,[36] the use of the terms benign tumor and partially transformed suggests a potential that remains unsubstantiated.

B cells

The prevalence and distribution of B cells are two of the most variable features of rheumatoid synovium. Circulating autoantibodies are characteristic of RA but are of uncertain pathologic significance. Studies of B cells in rheumatoid synovium have therefore focused heavily on local production of autoantibodies and evidence for local maturation of antibody-producing cells. B cells have other functions, including presentation of antigens to CD4+ T cells and secretion of cytokines, but the importance of such functions in RA is unclear.

Sequencing of immunoglobulin genes expressed in RA synovium has suggested that there is local clonal expansion of B cells, but recent studies have questioned whether the lymphoid follicles and germinal centers seen in some rheumatoid synovia promote maturation and expansion of antigen-specific B cells as they do in lymphoid organs.[37-39] Determining what antigens might be recognized by synovial B cells has been approached in four ways. First, the levels of specific autoantibodies in synovial tissue and fluid have been compared with those in blood from the same patients. Levels of RF and anti-citrullinated peptide antibodies (ACPA) are locally enriched according to these studies,[40,41] which are quantitative but do not distinguish between local synthesis and local deposition. Second, synthesis of antibodies has been measured in tissue explants, with use of biosynthetic labeling or inhibition of protein synthesis to differentiate between local synthesis and deposition. Rheumatoid synovium synthesizes a large amount of IgG, IgM, and IgA, comparable to that produced by explanted lymphoid organs. Synovial B cells produce RF of all three of these isotypes and in higher relative concentrations than do peripheral blood B cells from RA patients.[42]

Third, the ability of individual synovial B cells to produce antibodies of particular specificities has been assessed by plaque-forming cell and enzyme-linked immunosorbent spot (ELISpot) assays. Large numbers of B cells secreting antibodies to type II collagen and C1q have been detected in the majority of synovia from both RF-seropositive and RF-seronegative patients.[43] Notably, none of these patients had detectable circulating antibodies to these autoantigens. Fourth and finally, hybridomas have been made from synovial B cells and the monoclonal antibodies produced by these cells have been evaluated for binding to antigens. Cells making antibodies to cartilage oligomeric matrix protein (COMP), the bacterial heat-shock protein hsp60, and several other proteins have been thus identified.[44] This apparent diversity of local autoantibodies makes it clear that evaluation of serum may greatly underestimate synovial levels of potentially pathogenic antibodies.

T cells

T cells are the dominant lymphocyte infiltrating the rheumatoid joint, and CD4+ cells predominate over CD8+ cells in most RA patients, as is true in lymph nodes and blood. A key role for CD4+ T cells in the pathogenesis of RA is suggested by the strong genetic linkage of disease susceptibility to HLA-DR alleles. However, various findings regarding synovial T cells have led to disagreement about their role in chronic disease, as discussed later in this chapter.

Many synovial T cells express surface markers suggesting prior activation, such as particular CD45 isoforms, CD44, and MHC class II molecules.[45,46] There is no clear evidence demonstrating that activation occurs locally, despite the various potential antigen-presenting cells in inflamed synovium. Previously activated T cells home nonspecifically to inflamed sites by virtue of their expression of particular adhesion molecules. Therefore, previously activated T cells are likely to be recruited into the synovium from peripheral blood independent of their antigen specificity.

Despite expression of activation markers, T cells from RA patients are paradoxically hyporesponsive to further stimulation through the TCR in vitro. First described in circulating cells, this observation has been extended to cells from synovial fluid and tissue.[47] Synovial T cells have decreased levels of the ζ chain of the TCR, a key element of antigen-driven signaling[48,49]; this abnormality has also been found in systemic lupus erythematosus (SLE) and other chronic inflammatory states, as well as in an animal model of chronic infection, suggesting that it is a generic response to chronic immune stimulation. Other defects in intracellular signaling[48,49] and cell surface phenotype characterize synovial T cells, but whether these changes are all part of a single differentiation program is unknown. Strikingly, at least some of these defects can be produced by chronic stimulation of normal T cells *in vitro* with TNF.[48]

Once immunologic studies had defined subsets of CD4+ T cells that secrete distinct panels of cytokines, often falling into the patterns of Th1 cells (expressing IL-2, IFN-γ, lymphotoxin-α [LT-α]) and Th2 cells (expressing IL-4, -5, -10 and -13), it became important to determine the expression of specific cytokines by T cells in rheumatoid synovium, because these cytokine panels have very different influences on immune responses. The salient finding of these studies is the dearth of T cell–derived cytokines (Table 91.1), whether measured by *in-situ* hybridization or immunostaining of tissue sections[50,51] or by Northern blot or polymerase chain reaction (PCR) of either whole synovium[19] or T cells isolated from synovium.[52] Low numbers of cells staining for IFN-γ are found in both early (<1 year) and late (>5 years) RA.[50] Nevertheless, cytokine-producing T cells are present in synovial tissues and were originally reported to demonstrate a Th1 pattern of cytokine expression, but with some deviation from that paradigm. Thus, IFN-γ and LT-α are expressed and IL-4 is not[51,52]; however, IL-2, a product

of Th1 cells, is not found whereas IL-10, a product of Th2 cells, is expressed.[52] Expression of the chemokine receptors CCR5 and CXCR3, associated with the Th1 phenotype, by the majority of synovial T cells also suggested Th1 dominance,[53] and discordant results were obtained regarding production of IL-6 by synovial T cells.

The paradigm of predominance of Th1 over Th2 cells in rheumatoid synovium has been challenged by the more recent discovery of a new CD4+ effector T-helper cell subset, the Th17 cell.[54] Th17 cells express IL-17A and IL-17F, along with IL-6, TNF, GM-CSF, and other cytokines. Much of the work in defining the Th17 cell has been performed in mice, where this subset is most clearly distinguished from Th1 and Th2 cells. Th17 cells have also been identified in humans, although the cytokine expression pattern of human Th17 cells is somewhat less distinct from that of other T-helper cell subsets. Differentiation factors for Th17 cells in mice (predominantly TGF-β, and IL-6) also differ from those in humans (IL-1β and IL-23).[55] Th17 cells have been implicated in the pathogenesis of several autoimmune disorders, including experimental allergic encephalitis and RA.[56] IL-17 has been identified in RA synovial fluid at higher levels than in OA fluid.[57] Further evidence for a role for IL-17 in the pathogenesis of RA includes *in-vivo* studies in mice, demonstrating that inflammation in collagen-induced arthritis is suppressed in IL-17–deficient mice,[58] and blockade of IL-17 during the early phase of arthritis suppresses arthritis onset.[59]

Regulatory T cells (Treg) are a recently defined subset of T cells that are important for prevention of autoimmune disease and control of inflammation, via secretion of IL-10, TGF-β, and also by mechanisms dependent on cell-cell contact.[60] The transcription factor Foxp3 is the

TABLE 91.1 CYTOKINES THAT HAVE BEEN INTENSIVELY STUDIED IN RHEUMATOID ARTHRITIS*

	Pro/anti-inflammatory	Increased in RA?	Clinical trial support	Cytokine cellular sources	Salient effects, stimulatory	Salient effects, inhibitory
TNF	Pro	+	+	**Mθ**, many others	COX, IL-1, TNF, IL-6, chemo, MMP	
IL-1	Pro	+	+	**Mθ**, many others	COX, TNF, IL-6, chemo, MMP, endo	Proteoglycans
IL-2	Pro	−		Th1	T-cell proliferation, NK	
IL-4	Anti	−		Th2	Abs	IL-1, TNF
IL-6	Pro/anti	+	+	**Mθ**, FLS, chond	Abs, acute phase, FLS prolif	IL-1, TNF, chemo
IL-10	Anti	+	−	**Mθ**, Th2, B	Abs	IL-1, TNF, chemo, COX, MMP
IL-11	Anti	±		**FLS**	Acute phase	IL-1, TNF
IL-13	Anti	±		Th2		IL-1, TNF, COX
IL-15	Pro	+		**Mθ**, FLS, endo	T cell prolif, TNF, chemo	
IL-17	Pro	+		**Th17**	COX, chemo, osteoclasts	
IL-18	Pro	+		Mθ, FLS, chond	TNF, Th1	
IFN-αβ	Pro/Anti	NR	−	DC		
IFN-γ	Pro/Anti	±	±	Th1, NK	TNF	IL-1, COX, MMP
GM-CSF	Pro	+		Mθ, many others	Nθ/Mθ Differentiation/ activation	
M-CSF		±		FLS, chond	Osteoclast precursors	
TGF-β	Anti	+		Mθ, many others	FLS prolif, ECM	IL-1, TNF, T cells
Chemokines	Pro	+		**Mθ, FLS**, endo, others	Leukocyte chemotaxis	
RANKL		+		T, FLS, osteoblasts	Osteoclasts	

*Antagonists such as IL-1ra and soluble (decoy) receptors are not shown.
Pro/anti-inflammatory: indicates predominant effect of cytokine.
Increased in RA?: increased (+) or not (−) vs. OA or normal synovium. ± indicates small differences or conflicting results; NR = not reported.
Clinical trial support: importance established (+) or (−) by clinical trials involving the cytokine itself (e.g., IL-10, IFN-αβ) or an agent that blocks its activity (e.g., TNF, IL-1, IL-6, IFN-γ). ± indicates uncertain result.
Cellular sources: major sources of factors clearly upregulated in RA synovium are indicated in bold. Mθ, macrophage; FLS, fibroblast-like synoviocyte; Th1, Th2, subsets of CD4+ T cells; B, B lymphocyte; chond, chondrocyte; DC, dendritic cell; endo, vascular endothelial cell; NK, natural killer cell.
Salient effects: stimulatory or inhibitory for the production of the factors or activity of the cells listed. COX, cyclo-oxygenase-2 enzyme; chemo, chemokines; Nθ, neutrophils; Abs, antibodies; ECM, extracellular matrix; MMP, matrix metalloproteinases.

most specific marker for Treg, but they also express high levels of CD25, which has been used more frequently due to greater ease of detection. Data obtained by quantifying or manipulating cells using CD25 carry the caveat that this marker is also expressed on activated T cells at a somewhat lower level. Reports differ as to whether Treg circulate at higher levels in patients with RA than healthy controls,[61-65] but increased numbers have been consistently found in synovial fluid compared with blood.[62-65] However, the in-vitro suppressive function of circulating Treg from RA patients is reduced by a mechanism dependent on TNF, because suppressive function is restored by anti-TNF therapy[66] and addition of TNF to Treg from healthy donors reduces suppressive activity.[67]

The interaction of human T cells with other cell types infiltrating inflamed tissues, most notably monocytes/macrophages, has been studied in vitro. Work on co-cultures of normal human T cells and monocytes has shown that previously activated T cells induce production of monocyte mediators such as IL-1, TNF, IL-10, and MMPs and that such induction involves both contact-dependent and contact-independent signals.[68] Effects on monocytes differ depending on whether the T cells are activated by stimulation through the TCR or by incubation with cytokines. Cytokine-activated T cells stimulate release, from monocytes/macrophages, of TNF but not IL-10, whereas TCR-activated T cells stimulate production of both cytokines.[68] Most interestingly, T cells freshly isolated from rheumatoid synovium behave like cytokine-stimulated and unlike TCR-stimulated T cells by this assay,[69] which has helped to bolster the provocative hypothesis that antigen-specific T-cell activation is of little relevance in established RA.

Indeed, evidence for local expansion of antigen-specific T cells within the synovium has been difficult to obtain. Synovial T cells have been described that react to peptides derived from the bacterial heat-shock protein dnaJ[70] and to peptides from the matrix protein gp39,[71] but, in general, the search for autoreactive T cells has not been as fruitful as that for autoantibodies. Indirect evidence of skewed recruitment or local expansion of T cells has been sought by comparison of TCR variable-region gene usage in synovial versus peripheral blood T cells in RA patients and controls, with the results summarized in a thorough review as "notable for their contradictory and confusing nature."[45]

Despite these results, it is important to note that even in known antigen-driven responses, the percentage of antigen-specific T cells within an inflammatory lesion is quite low, owing to the non-specific homing of previously activated cells to inflammatory sites, and the techniques used thus far may simply not be sensitive enough to detect an adaptive immune response, even one that is functionally important. Because previously activated T cells home non-specifically to inflamed sites, the discovery of reactivity to common pathogens within inflamed tissues such as RA synovium must also be interpreted cautiously.

Neutrophils

Neutrophils are the predominant cell type in rheumatoid synovial fluid but are present only sparsely in inflamed synovium and pannus, although they have been located by EM at the cartilage-pannus junction.[72] Neutrophils can, however, predominate in synovial tissues early in an acute flare of RA; and the histopathology of a synovial biopsy taken at this time may resemble that of a septic joint. Many synovial fluid neutrophils express surface markers indicative of activation by cytokines, such as the high-affinity IgG receptor FcγRI, the complement receptor CR3, and lactoferrin. In addition, synovial fluid contains antimicrobial peptides thought to be derived specifically from neutrophil granules.[73] There is little reason to propose that activation of neutrophils in rheumatoid joints differs from that in other inflamed but uninfected sites, but the recent description of different functional subsets of activated neutrophils in mice[74] may lead to more investigation of this issue. Likewise, interaction of circulating neutrophils with endothelial cells in the joint is thought to use the same set of adhesion molecules as in other sites. Initial tethering and rolling are mediated by selectins (L-selectin on neutrophils, E-selectin on endothelial cells) interacting with receptors containing sialyl-Lewis^x carbohydrate moieties. Tight adhesion is mediated by interaction of the β_2 integrins on neutrophils (LFA-1/CD11aCD18 and Mac-1/CD11bCD18) with ICAM-1 and ICAM-2 on endothelium.[75] Neutrophils do not express the integrin VLA-4, which may explain why they

do not remain in synovial tissue, where the expression of its counter-receptor VCAM-1 appears to be important in the retention of other kinds of leukocytes.

Details about the chemotaxis and activation of neutrophils have been gleaned from analyses of normal peripheral blood neutrophils cultured in vitro. IL-8/CXCL8, other ligands for the chemokine receptors CXCR1 and CXCR2, and TGF-β have been identified as important chemotactic factors for neutrophils.[75] Normal neutrophils can be induced to express cytokines, including IL-1β, IL-8, and oncostatin M (OSM), in vitro.[76,77] IL-1 and IL-8, in turn, induce neutrophil effector functions such as degranulation, phagocytosis, and the respiratory burst.[75] In the case of IL-8, these effects are likely to be direct but the priming of neutrophil functions by IL-1, more prominently seen in vivo than in vitro, is likely secondary to upregulation of the adhesion molecules E-selectin and ICAM-1 on endothelium,[75] rather than to a direct effect of IL-1 on neutrophils.

Dendritic cells

DCs, the cells most potent at presenting peptide antigens to T cells, are derived from precursors that migrate into joints and other tissues from peripheral blood. DCs make up 1% to 5% of the cells in rheumatoid synovial fluid[78] and can be isolated from synovial tissue as well. DCs can be distinguished from monocyte-derived cells by differences in surface markers, such as lower levels of CD14,[79] and absence of phagocytic capacity. Synovial DCs express the co-stimulatory molecule CD40 and high levels of MHC class I and II molecules,[79] although divergent results have been obtained for expression of the co-stimulatory molecule CD80/B7-1.[79,80] Thus, like other leukocytes in inflamed synovium, DCs appear to be activated. Considering the two predominant DC subtypes, the ratio of myeloid (mDC) to plasmacytoid DC (pDC) is higher in RA than non-RA synovium.[81] The role of DCs in initiating and perpetuating RA through the presentation of antigen to synovial T cells is a point of ongoing investigation and debate.[82]

Mast cells

Mast cells are found in small numbers in rheumatoid synovium but perhaps at an increased density compared with normal tissues.[83] Interest in a potential role for mast cells in RA has been aroused by their importance in a mouse model of IgG-mediated inflammatory arthritis[84] and by their ability to secrete tryptases and other proteases, preformed cytokines, and vasoactive and chemotactic factors. It is possible that mast cell phenotypes are more diverse and tissue specific than the classic delineation of connective tissue and mucosal subtypes. For example, mast cells in RA synovium differ from those in normal or OA synovium in expression of surface markers, such as the corticotropin-releasing hormone (CRH) receptor 1 and the chemokine receptor CXCR3.

Natural killer cells

NK cells are a lymphoid subpopulation characterized by their ability to mediate MHC-independent cytotoxicity, most notably by recognizing cells that have downregulated MHC class I molecules. These cells also have immunoregulatory functions that are being actively investigated, including the ability to suppress immunoglobulin production. NK cells and NK activity are not prominent in rheumatoid synovium. This finding suggests on its surface that NK cells do not play a significant role in synovitis but, alternatively, that their scarcity could represent a failure of regulation and contribute to chronic inflammation in the rheumatoid joint.

Chondrocytes

In addition to their complex structural role in cartilage, chondrocytes, the cellular elements of articular cartilage, have been found to be surprisingly interactive with inflammatory mediators. Most studies supporting this conclusion have been performed in vitro on cells cultured from OA or normal cartilage or on immortalized chondrocyte cell lines, but studies on intact OA cartilage have also demonstrated the production of cytokines including IL-1, TNF, and IL-6 by chondrocytes. It is therefore likely that chondrocytes in the rheumatoid joint are immunologically active. Chondrocyte production of IL-6 is stimulated in vitro by IL-1, TNF, IFN-γ, and TGF-β,[85] and production of IL-8 is induced by IL-1, TNF, TGF-β, and bacterial LPS.[86] Therefore, chondrocytes could participate in the cytokine networks proposed to be integral to RA (see later). IL-1 also inhibits synthesis of proteoglycans and type II collagen by cultured OA chondrocytes,[87] and IL-1 in synergy with TNF can upregulate the production of cartilage matrix-degrading enzymes by chondrocytes. These may be direct mechanisms by which cytokines contribute to cartilage destruction.

Endothelial cells

Vascular endothelial cells proliferate in rheumatoid synovium, as reviewed in Chapter 90, but whether they do so in proportion to the marked expansion of synovial tissue has been a subject of debate. Rheumatoid endothelial cells are activated to promote influx of inflammatory cells by expression of adhesion molecules (see earlier under Neutrophils and T cells),[88] and high endothelial venules, analogous to those important in the egress of lymphocytes from blood into lymphoid tissues, form in RA synovium.[89] Endothelial cells express a number of chemokines, degradative enzymes and cytokines, and receptors, including TNF, IL-1, and their receptors.[17,18,30,88] Anti-TNF treatment decreases expression of proinflammatory adhesion molecules, but it is not known whether this occurs by a direct effect or after a cascade of other anti-inflammatory actions.

SOLUBLE FACTORS IN THE RHEUMATOID SYNOVIUM

Interactions between the various cell types just described are critical for the development and maintenance of synovitis. Cellular communication is mediated by a large number of membrane-bound and secreted factors; the secreted factors have been easier to identify and manipulate and are therefore better understood. Protein mediators secreted by inflammatory cells are categorized as cytokines, chemokines, or growth factors based on the activity they most prominently display: modulation of immunologic activity, chemotaxis, or cell growth and division, respectively. However, the classification is artificial and many factors have characteristics of two or all three categories. Detailed knowledge of the function of individual cytokines and other factors in RA has generally come from the study of genetically manipulated animal models or from studies manipulating the activity of only one or two mediators in explanted synovial tissue or dispersed synovial cells, an environment that may or may not resemble that of unmanipulated tissue.

In this section, we will approach rheumatoid synovitis from the viewpoint of the role of soluble mediators in pathogenesis, with particular attention to those that have been investigated both *ex vivo* (in synovial extracts or sections) and *in vitro* (using explants and cell lines) and that have also been assessed in animal models of inflammatory arthritis. The key roles predicted for a few mediators have been convincingly confirmed using specific inhibitors in patients with RA, demonstrating the value of basic scientific investigation in the development of therapies. Table 91.1 provides a summary of cytokines that are relevant to RA pathogenesis, their cellular sources, and salient effects.

TNF

TNF is the prototype of a large family of cytokines. The simplified name TNF is now preferred over the former designation TNF-α, because the corresponding term TNF-β, an alternative name for LT, is now obsolete. TNF and other family members are active as trimers, some being secreted and some membrane bound. TNF itself is synthesized first as a membrane-bound protein and is subsequently cleaved to a soluble form, primarily by an enzyme known as TNF-α converting enzyme (TACE). Both forms of TNF are biologically active. There are two cell surface receptors for TNF: TNF-RI (p55) and TNF-RII (p75). Both receptors are ubiquitously expressed,[30] either constitutively (TNF-RI) or inducibly (TNF-RII). Both receptors can be cleaved from the cell surface to produce soluble proteins that can neutralize TNF and thus play a regulatory role. Soluble p55 and p75 TNF-Rs are found in both the blood and synovial fluid of RA patients, with concentrations greater in synovial fluid. TNF production is regulated to a remarkable degree at the posttranscriptional level by a network of positive and negative regulators that act on the 3' end of its mRNA.

TNF is produced by a wide variety of cell types but most prominently by cells of the monocyte-macrophage lineage. These cells appear to be the major producers of TNF in the rheumatoid joint,[17] in which this cytokine is readily detected by various methods.[17,19,90] TNF production by macrophages *in vitro* is induced by various pathogens and cytokines, including, but not limited to, IL-1, IFN-γ, and TNF itself. In turn, TNF has a wide range of effects on various cell types and induces the production of numerous cytokines by immune cells, with a net proinflammatory effect. In cultured rheumatoid synovial explants, addition of TNF induces expression of IL-6, IL-8, and IL-10 and blockade of TNF greatly reduces production of IL-1 and GM-CSF.[91] Salient effects of TNF on cultured FLS include induction of prostaglandin E$_2$, MMPs, and chemokines, including IL-8/CXCL8; TNF and IL-1 often act synergistically in these processes.[92]

TNF is a critical player in all animal models of inflammatory arthritis in which it has been evaluated, usually by using neutralizing antibodies or soluble receptors or using mice deficient in TNF.[93] The most dramatic demonstration of the ability of TNF to cause arthritis has come from a transgenic mouse aberrantly expressing human TNF due to deletion of the aforementioned negative regulatory sequences in its mRNA. This mouse expresses TNF at high levels in synovium and develops destructive inflammatory arthritis, even in the absence of lymphocytes.[94] IL-1, however, is still essential in this model.

Blockade of TNF using either monoclonal antibodies (infliximab, adalimumab) or a soluble p75-TNF-R (etanercept) has proved to be highly effective in treating patients with RA and several other inflammatory diseases. Several features of anti-TNF therapy will be notable as we consider the pathogenesis of RA later in this chapter: prompt improvement in symptoms in the majority of patients, marked improvement in synovial pathology with a significant decrease in the number of activated macrophages, and usually prompt return of disease when anti-TNF therapy is discontinued.

Other TNF superfamily members

Of the many secreted and cell surface members of the TNF superfamily, those that have received the most attention as potential contributors in the cytokine network of rheumatoid synovitis, have been LT, LIGHT, and BLyS/BAFF. LT exists in two similar isoforms, LT-α and LT-β, with the β isoform notable for being produced by Th1 CD4+ T cells. The LT isoforms were collectively known previously as TNF-β and have many overlapping functions with TNF, but a striking function specific for both LT isoforms in mice is an essential role in the formation of lymph nodes and ectopic lymphoid structures. LT proteins are not prominent in RA synovium,[16] but, interestingly, mRNA levels correlate with the presence of the ectopic germinal centers found in a substantial minority of RA patients.[7]

LIGHT (TNFSF14) is an LT-related mediator, best known as a product of activated T cells, that binds both the LT-β receptor and TNFSFR14, is important in T-cell activation, and when overexpressed in mice produces autoimmune disease.[95] LIGHT is also expressed by synovial macrophages and B cells from RA but not OA patients, and RA synovial macrophages or FLS stimulated *in vitro* by LIGHT secrete inflammatory cytokines and proteases.[96-98] A role for LIGHT and/or LT in murine collagen-induced arthritis was shown by reduction of disease in mice pretreated with a solubilized receptor fusion protein, LTβR-Ig, that binds both molecules. Treatment was only effective in the induction (i.e., immunization) phase of disease,[99] which differs from results obtained with TNF blockade.

BLyS, also known as BAFF (B cell–activating factor of the TNF family), is critical for mouse B-cell development and maintenance and elevated levels lead to humoral autoimmune disease in mice. BLyS/BAFF operates within a regulatory system that involves the similar molecule APRIL (a proliferation-inducing ligand) and multiple receptors, including BCMA (B-cell maturation antigen) and TACI (transmembrane activator and calcium modulator and cyclophilin ligand interactor). BLyS/BAFF and APRIL are both present at greater levels in inflammatory than in non-inflammatory synovial fluid and are locally produced within the joint. Macrophages appear to be the major source, but cleavage of membrane-bound BLyS/BAFF from neutrophils may be another mechanism of release.[100,101] Local production of these factors may enhance the survival and expansion of antibody-producing B cells, and/or B cells that promote T-cell activation, within arthritic joints. Neutralization of BLyS/BAFF and APRIL with the solubilized receptor TACI-Fc blocks disease in mouse collagen-induced arthritis, probably by inhibiting both B- and T-cell responses.[102]

IL-1

Like TNF, IL-1 is the prototype of a phylogenetically ancient family of cytokines, which includes IL-1α, IL-1β, IL-1ra, IL-18, and at least six others of little-known function.[92] IL-1α is primarily a cytosolic protein and is thought to act in an autocrine manner. It is only released from cells during cell death and therefore circulates in tiny amounts. IL-1β is also initially cytosolic but is then secreted by a novel and undefined mechanism after cleavage by a specific protease, the IL-1–converting enzyme (ICE). In addition to this posttranslational regulation, IL-1 production is also transcriptionally and post-transcriptionally regulated.

IL-1 is produced by many cell types relevant in rheumatoid synovitis, including FLS, endothelial cells, lymphocytes, and neutrophils, but monocytes and macrophages appear to be the major source. IL-1 is readily detected in the rheumatoid joint (Fig. 91.8), both in synovial fluid (IL-1β) and within cells (IL-1α > IL-1β[18]). Synthesis of IL-1 by monocytes *in vitro* is induced by activated T cells and by a variety of cytokines, including TNF and IL-1 itself. Numerous cell types express IL-1RI, and the effects of IL-1 are similar to those of TNF, that is, broadly proinflammatory. Of relevance in the rheumatoid joint, IL-1 stimulates prostaglandin, MMP, and chemokine (IL-8/CXCL8 and others) release from FLS; nitric oxide and prostaglandin production and adhesion molecule expression by endothelial cells; secretion of TNF (and further IL-1) by macrophages; and production of IL-6 and IL-8 but reduced synthesis of proteoglycans by chondrocytes.[103] In addition, IL-1 and TNF are synergistic in the induction of proteinases, prostaglandins, and cytokines by FLS. Although IL-1 and TNF upregulate their own and each other's expression, it has been argued that IL-1 is functionally downstream of TNF in the cytokine network of the rheumatoid synovium, because blockade of IL-1 does not reduce synthesis of either TNF or IL-1 in synovial explants,[104] whereas blockade of TNF markedly reduces production of IL-1.[91] Blockade of IL-1 in this system does reduce the synthesis of other factors, including IL-6 and IL-8.[105]

The activity of circulating IL-1 (primarily IL-1β) is regulated by a remarkable array of naturally occurring inhibitors. IL-1ra, a member of the IL-1 family, is secreted by the conventional endoplasmic reticulum-to-Golgi route; it binds to IL-1RI but does not activate signaling. A second cell surface receptor for IL-1, IL-1RII, appears to be devoid of signaling potential and thus is viewed as a decoy receptor for excess IL-1. Both IL-1RI and especially IL-1RII also circulate in soluble forms

and are thought to perform a similar decoy function.[103] Finally, antibodies that neutralize IL-1 are induced during immune responses at sufficient levels to have dampening effects.[105] The overall balance of IL-1 agonists and inhibitors is thought to be the critical factor in whether IL-1 contributes to an inflammatory state. Indeed, although IL-1ra is detectable in the rheumatoid joint, the ratio of IL-1 to IL-1ra favors IL-1 and inflammation.[15]

Animal models have indicated a central role for IL-1 in inflammatory arthritis. Expression of human IL-1β in rabbit knee joints causes synovial inflammation,[106] and local or systemic administration of IL-1 exacerbates arthritis in several mouse models. Mice deficient in IL-1ra develop inflammatory diseases that differ depending on genetic background and possibly also on environment; the BALB/c strain develops inflammatory polyarthritis.[107] Mice deficient in IL-1 or IL-1RI, or treated with IL-1ra or IL-1 blocking antibodies, are highly resistant to induction of experimental arthritis in a wide range of models.[93] Data from these studies suggest that, in mice, IL-1 and TNF both play important roles in inflammation but that IL-1 is more important in joint destruction.

IL-1ra (anakinra) has been shown to be modestly effective in patients with RA and interferes with both inflammation and joint destruction. Based on studies in animal models, it might have been predicted that IL-1 blockade would be as effective as TNF blockade in controlling inflammation, which has not been borne out in humans. This discrepancy may reflect either unfavorable pharmacokinetics and pharmacodynamics of current methods of IL-1 blockade or fundamental differences in pathogenic mechanisms between animal models and human RA.

IL-2

IL-2 is a T-cell product and is best known as an autocrine or paracrine growth factor for T cells. However, it also activates NK cells and modulates the function of other cell types that populate rheumatoid synovium, including B cells, macrophages, and FLS. In addition, the role of IL-2 in T-cell function is complex, because recent studies have shown that it is important in the development of regulatory T cells (Treg), which downregulate immune responses and are essential in mouse models for preventing autoimmune inflammatory diseases. To the extent that antigen-specific T cells are involved in the pathogenesis of RA, IL-2 is likely to be involved at some level as well, but IL-2 production is not prominent in patients with established disease. Circulating T cells from RA patients produce little IL-2 when stimulated. Reports differ on whether mRNA for IL-2 is found at all in rheumatoid synovium, and the amount of IL-2 protein is low or undetectable in synovial fluid and in supernatants of synovial explant cultures.[108] Analysis of cytokine production by individual T cells from rheumatoid synovium has not revealed any IL-2–producing cells.[52] Cyclosporine markedly decreases IL-2 production and has activity in RA, but this drug reduces synthesis of many other cytokines as well. Thus, the role of IL-2 in RA is likely to be limited to the onset of autoimmunity and/or the imbalance of effector and regulatory T cell subsets, because there is little evidence to support its role in the interplay between adaptive and innate immune cells and resident synovial cells.

IL-4, IL-5, and IL-13

Production of IL-4, IL-5, and IL-13 (along with IL-10, to be discussed separately) is characteristic of the subset of CD4+ T cells termed *Th2 cells*, which are specialized for generating antiparasitic, allergic, and anti-inflammatory responses in other immune cells. Th1 cells, in contrast, help propagate cell-mediated immune responses. Levels of IL-4 and IL-5 in rheumatoid synovium, synovial fluid, and synovial T cells are very low or undetectable.[52,109] Some, but not all,[110] investigators have detected IL-13 in synovial fluid and serum of RA patients at higher levels than in OA patients and healthy controls.[101] IL-4 and IL-13 both decrease the production of TNF, IL-1, and other inflammatory mediators by macrophages and FLS *in vitro*.[24] Administration of IL-4 or IL-13, by way of gene therapy or transduced cells, has attenuated disease in several rodent models of RA. However, in mouse arthritis induced by local induction of immune complexes, IL-13 exacerbated inflammation but reduced cartilage damage.[111]

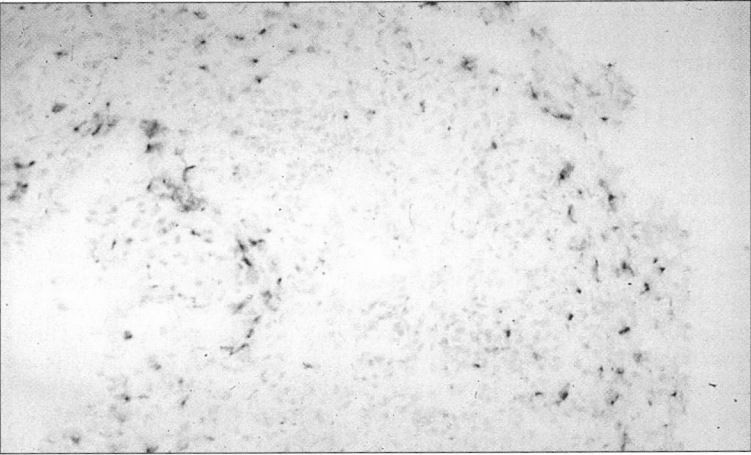

Fig. 91.8 IL-1 in RA synovial tissue. Distribution of IL-1 protein in RA synovial tissue using an immunoperoxidase technique on a section lacking counterstain. Prominent staining (brown) is seen in perivascular regions, with less staining in the intimal lining. *(Courtesy of Dr. M. Field.)*

IL-6

IL-6 is the prototype of a family of cytokines that share a common signal transduction pathway. Its receptor consists of two chains: a ligand-specific IL-6R that is found on most hematopoietic and some non-hematopoietic cells, and a signal-transducing chain, gp130, that is found on most cell types and is used by all the IL-6 superfamily members. A soluble form of the IL-6R (sIL-6R) exists and serves to promote signaling when bound by IL-6, rather than functioning as a blocking or decoy receptor as do the soluble receptors for TNF and IL-1. IL-6 has many effects, both pro- and anti-inflammatory, on hematopoietic and non-hematopoietic cells. It is perhaps best known for stimulating B cells to increase IgG production and differentiate into plasma cells. IL-6 is an endogenous pyrogen and a potent inducer of the acute-phase response in the liver.

In RA, IL-6 is produced by FLS[31] and by chondrocytes,[16] but the major local source is probably macrophages (Fig. 91.9).[16,112] Production is induced synergistically by TNF and IL-1. In turn, however, IL-6 decreases expression of TNF and IL-1, as well as the neutrophil-attracting chemokines CXCL8/IL-8 and CXCL1/MIP-2.[113] Levels of IL-6 are elevated in synovial fluid and serum of RA patients and serum levels correlate with levels of acute-phase reactants.[114]

Blockade of IL-6 activity reduces or prevents arthritis in several mouse models but only in those that include a phase of induction of autoimmunity after immunization. IL-6 has not been found to have a role in the effector phase of experimental arthritis after the production of autoantibodies.[93] Interestingly, a blocking antibody against the human IL-6R has been shown to be effective in improving both symptoms and inflammatory markers (especially C-reactive protein) in RA in several controlled clinical trials.[115]

IL-6 superfamily (OSM, IL-11, LIF, CNTF, CT-1)

Oncostatin M (OSM), IL-11, leukemia inhibitory factor (LIF), ciliary neurotrophic factor (CNTF), and cardiotropin-1 (CT-1) are all structurally related to IL-6 and there is substantial overlap with IL-6 in their effects, including induction of the acute-phase response and stimulation of myeloma cell proliferation. OSM, IL-11, and LIF are synthesized at high enough levels to be detected in the circulation and have been studied in RA.

OSM levels are increased in rheumatoid synovial fluid,[31,116] probably owing to production by both macrophages and neutrophils.[77,116] OSM is notable for its ability to synergize with IL-1 in promoting cartilage breakdown, both *in vitro*[116] and in mice. Blockade of OSM ameliorates arthritis in two mouse models, collagen- and pristine-induced arthritis,[117] but addition of OSM prevents arthritis induced by anti-collagen antibodies.[118]

In contrast to OSM, IL-11 is found at increased levels in both OA and RA synovial fluids.[31] FLS appear to be the major source, with secretion

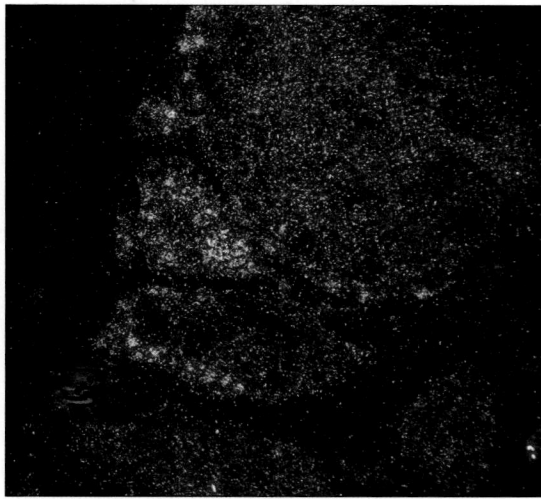

Fig. 91.9 Darkfield view of *in-situ* hybridization identifying IL-6 messenger RNA expression in RA synovium.

induced by TNF and IL-1.[32] Like IL-6, IL-11 decreases synthesis of IL-1 and TNF but there is stronger evidence for IL-11 having a net anti-inflammatory effect, at least in murine collagen-induced arthritis.[119]

LIF is detectable in synovial fluid, more in RA than OA,[30] and its expression is induced from both FLS and chondrocytes by TNF and IL-1.[31,85] Its role in mouse models of inflammatory arthritis has not been determined.

IL-10

More clearly than the IL-4 family members, IL-10 is a predominantly anti-inflammatory cytokine. Although initially described as a characteristic product of the Th2 subtype of CD4+ T cells, IL-10 is made in larger amounts by macrophages and is also produced by Treg and other cell types. Non–T cells, presumably macrophages, appear to be the major producers of IL-10 in rheumatoid synovium.[120] IL-10 levels are higher in RA than OA synovial fluid,[120] and increased IL-10 levels are inversely correlated with joint destruction.[121] In cultures of synovial fluid mononuclear cells, blockade of IL-10 increases, and addition of IL-10 decreases, production of IL-1, TNF, and other inflammatory mediators.[122] The actions of IL-10 are not universally immunosuppressive, however, because this cytokine can stimulate B cells to proliferate and to differentiate into plasma cells *in vitro*.

IL-10 has been extensively studied in animal models. IL-10–deficient mice spontaneously develop an inflammatory bowel disease that is dependent on TNF and IL-1. Collagen-induced arthritis is more severe in IL-10–deficient mice, but arthritis induced by anti-collagen antibodies is, surprisingly, less severe.[123] Addition of IL-10 by gene transfer in the active immunization model of collagen-induced arthritis decreases inflammation, but only if therapy is begun before clinical evidence of disease.[124] IL-10 gene therapy also decreases invasion of pannus into cartilage in a model in which human cartilage and synovium are co-transplanted into immunodeficient SCID mice.[125] Efforts to use recombinant IL-10 to treat established human RA have been disappointing.

IL-19, IL-20, and IL-22 are homologs of IL-10 but have proinflammatory activities. All of these cytokines are expressed in RA synovium,[126-128] but their roles, if any, in RA or in animal models are not yet known.

IL-12 and IL-23

IL-12 is primarily of macrophage origin and is considered a major driver of Th1 differentiation and of secretion of IFN-γ by both T cells and NK cells. IL-12 is a heterodimer composed of two subunits, p40 and p35. The p40 subunit is also used by the more recently described IL-23 and, indeed, mice lacking p40 or treated with antibodies that block p40 are deficient in IL-23 as well as IL-12. Nevertheless, this pair of cytokines is still clearly paramount in Th1 differentiation and promotion of cellular immunity.

IL-12 is expressed in rheumatoid synovium but whether at levels greater than those found in OA is unclear.[129] IL-23 has not been specifically examined, nor has IL-27, another member of this cytokine family. Divergent results have been reported with manipulation of IL-12 in the mouse model of collagen-induced arthritis, before the distinction between IL-12 and IL-23 was recognized. A recent study comparing mice lacking either IL-12 or IL-23, but not both, has helped to clarify this issue. IL-23–deficient mice were completely resistant to collagen-induced arthritis, whereas IL-12–deficient mice developed more severe disease,[130] suggesting that IL-23 is an essential mediator of arthritis, whereas IL-12 protects against it.

IL-15

IL-15 invites comparison with IL-2 by virtue of their shared signaling apparatus, but IL-15 and its receptor are much more widely expressed.[131] Based on the phenotype of IL-15–deficient mice, the salient function of IL-15 is as a survival factor for naive T cells, particularly CD8+ cells, but this cytokine has other, generally proinflammatory effects as well.

In rheumatoid synovium, IL-15 is prominently expressed by lining macrophages but is also found in FLS and endothelial cells,[20] and it is secreted in sufficient amounts to be detectable in synovial fluid in RA but not OA. Studies in patients with RA have demonstrated a significant relationship between levels of IL-15 and TNF in synovial fluid (Fig. 91.10). *In vitro*, IL-15 is important in the contact-dependent stimulation by T cells of TNF production from macrophages[132] and in the stimulation of T cells by FLS. In mice, recombinant IL-15 can replace adjuvant in the induction of collagen-induced arthritis, obviating the need for the immunostimulatory mycobacterial products present in complete Freund adjuvant. Conversely, blockade of IL-15 or IL-15R decreases the severity of collagen-induced arthritis.[133,134]

IL-17

IL-17[135,136] has proinflammatory effects on a variety of cell types, leading to the induction of prostaglandins, nitric oxide, cytokines, and chemokines. Six IL-17 family members have been identified (IL-17A-F), and IL-17A is a proinflammatory cytokine whose importance in the pathogenesis of RA has already been highlighted. IL-17A and F are produced by Th17 cells. IL-17 induces IL-1 and TNF production in synovial macrophages and fibroblasts[137,138] and can synergize with IL-1 in the upregulation of certain inflammatory mediators produced by FLS. Some unusual activities ascribed to IL-17 include induction of osteoclastogenesis, through upregulation of RANKL on osteoblasts and synovial fibroblasts,[139] and stimulation of synthesis of complement components by fibroblasts.

Synovial explants from the great majority of RA patients, but from few OA and non-arthritic patients, secrete IL-17.[140] Expression is high in T cell–rich areas, as expected.[140] In these explants, production of IL-17 is inhibited by addition of two of the cytokine products of Th2 cells, IL-4 or IL-13, and IL-17 appears to be important for the local production of IL-6.[140] The IL-17 receptor (IL-17R) uniquely binds IL-17 and is expressed on various synovial cell types in different arthritides, most notably in endothelial cells and chondrocytes.

Blockade of IL-17 reduces inflammation, joint damage, and systemic levels of IL-6 in the mouse model of collagen-induced arthritis. Importantly, this therapeutic effect occurs even if treatment is started after onset of clinical disease, indicating that the proinflammatory, rather than solely the immunomodulatory, effects of IL-17 are important in this model.[136]

IL-18

IL-18 is related in structure to IL-1 and also has broadly proinflammatory actions. In the rheumatoid joint, macrophages,[141] FLS,[142] and chondrocytes all can produce IL-18, although there is some disagreement as to whether macrophages are the predominant cell type producing this cytokine (Fig. 91.11).[141,142]

The IL-18 receptor is a heterodimer of α and β chains and its intracellular signaling is similar or identical to that of the IL-1R. Soluble splice variants of the IL-18Rα chain are secreted, can block the activity of the cytokine, and thus may play a role in regulation.[142] The IL-18R is expressed on many cell types potentially relevant to synovitis, including naive T cells, NK cells, macrophages, neutrophils, and chondrocytes. Notably, however, the β chain is not expressed on rheumatoid FLS.[143] Based on experiments in mice and *in vitro*, IL-18 promotes Th1 responses and IFN-γ secretion (particularly in combination with IL-12), RANKL expression, and osteoclastogenesis through actions on T cells and macrophage production of TNF and the innate immune receptors TLR2 and TLR4.

IL-18 mRNA and protein are found at higher levels in RA than in OA synovium,[25] and IL-18 levels correlate with other markers of disease activity.[144] In synovial explants, addition of TNF and IL-1 induces production of IL-18 and addition of IL-18 induces TNF, IFN-γ, GM-CSF, and nitric oxide.[25] Thus, IL-18, like IL-1, likely plays an important role in the cytokine network in rheumatoid synovitis. In mice, IL-18 can promote collagen-induced arthritis by substituting for adjuvant.[25] IL-18–deficient mice have a decreased incidence of collagen-induced arthritis, with defects in both the priming and effector phases of disease,[145] and anti-IL-18 antibodies inhibit arthritis induced by injection of streptococcal cell wall material.[146] In addition, IL-18 is a chemoattractant for T cells, derived from RA synovium, that express IL-18R.

Macrophage migration inhibitory factor

Among proinflammatory cytokines, macrophage migration inhibitory factor (MIF) is unique in that its synthesis is induced by modest doses of glucocorticoids.[147] In RA, MIF levels are elevated in synovial fluid.[148,149] Synovial production by macrophages, FLS, and T cells has been described,[148,149] but the major cellular source is uncertain, and other cell types such as DC may also produce MIF.[150] MIF induces multiple proinflammatory functions in macrophages, promotes both Th1 and Th2 T-cell responses, and promotes chemotaxis of a variety of leukocyte subtypes through induction of multiple chemokines.[147] In RA FLS, MIF induces proliferation[151] and synthesis of IL-8, VEGF, and multiple MMPs.[152-154] In mice, severity of collagen-induced arthritis is reduced by blockade or absence of MIF, owing to both reduced anti-collagen immunity and reduced inflammation induced by anti-collagen antibodies.[155,156] A similar role is seen in antigen-induced arthritis, and in that model exogenous MIF can reverse the anti-inflammatory effects of glucocorticoids.[157,158] A polymorphism has been identified in the MIF promoter that affects levels of expression.[159] Alleles associated with high expression have been reported as associated either with diagnosis of RA[160,161] or with severity or age at onset of RA[160,161] in different cohorts.

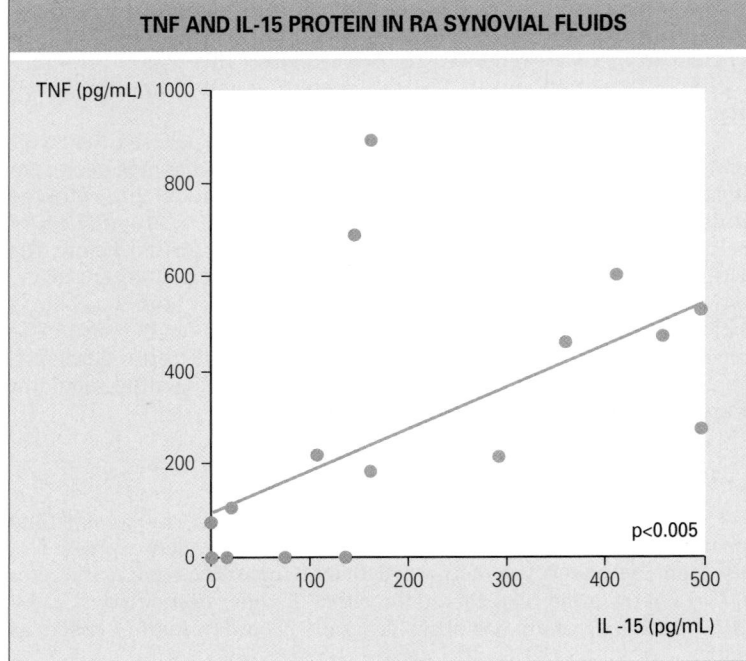

TNF AND IL-15 PROTEIN IN RA SYNOVIAL FLUIDS

TNF (pg/mL)

p<0.005

IL-15 (pg/mL)

Fig. 91.10 ELISA demonstrating the simultaneous detection of IL-15 and TNF in RA synovial fluids. *(Courtesy of Drs. B. P. Leung and I. B. McInnes.)*

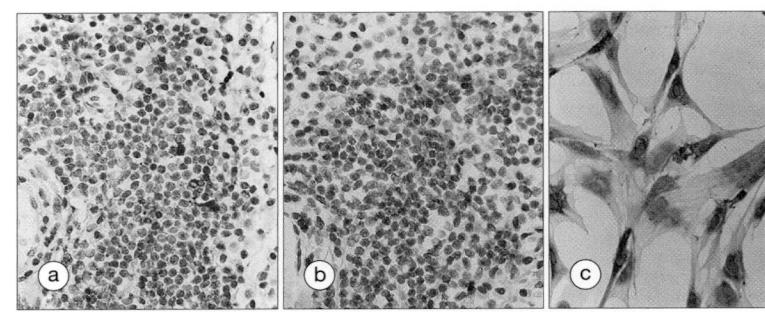

Fig. 91.11 Immunohistochemistry demonstrating IL-18 staining in RA synovium. (a) IL-18–expressing cells (brown) in lymphoid aggregate. (b) Neutralization of staining with recombinant IL-18. (c) IL-18 expression in cultured synovial fibroblasts. *(Courtesy of Drs. J. A. Gracie and I. B. McInnes.)*

Type I interferons

The type I interferons include many isoforms of IFN-α and one of IFN-β, all of which use the same receptor. IFN-α and IFN-β modulate immune responses in complex ways and it is difficult to characterize them as pro- or anti-inflammatory. In considering potential roles in RA, it is worth noting that SLE is characterized by evidence of high systemic type I IFN activity, that IFN-β is used to treat multiple sclerosis, and that treatment of chronic hepatitis C infection or malignancy with IFN-α has been associated with new-onset autoimmune disease, including inflammatory polyarthritis.[162]

Interest in using IFN-β to treat RA came from the observations that it inhibits monocyte synthesis of TNF, IL-1β, and IL-6[163] and increases production of IL-1ra and the soluble TNF-R. However, a sizeable clinical trial of IFN-β1a in RA patients showed no clinical benefit and no change in synovial inflammation.[164]

Interferon-γ

Interferon-γ is produced by Th1 T cells and NK cells and is the quintessential cytokine of cell-mediated immune responses by virtue of its ability to activate macrophages; in mice, it is important for eradication of intracellular bacteria and parasites but less important for protection against viruses.

On the basis of its macrophage-activating activity, IFN-γ was predicted to be a prominent player in RA but subsequent data in support of this hypothesis have been equivocal at best. IFN-γ was not detected by in-situ hybridization of rheumatoid synovium in an early study,[19] and levels in synovial fluid and tissue were subsequently found to be low. In further studies, IFN-γ transcripts have been detected but at minimally different levels in RA and OA synovium and IFN-γ has been detected in an only modest percentage of T cells purified from RA synovium.[52] However, stimulation of synovially derived cells in vitro with a T-cell mitogen induces production of IFN-γ, confirming that T cells capable of producing this cytokine are present in RA synovium. Surprisingly, assignment of IFN-γ as a proinflammatory cytokine has become as problematic as for type I interferons, because IFN-γ can either promote or inhibit arthritis in different animal models.[165]

The colony-stimulating factors: GM-CSF, G-CSF, M-CSF, IL-3

Granulocyte-macrophage colony stimulating factor (GM-CSF), granulocyte colony-stimulating factor (G-CSF), and macrophage colony stimulating factor (M-CSF) were initially described on the basis of their ability to promote the development of granulocytes and/or macrophages from progenitor cells.

Although GM-CSF is usually thought of as primarily a T-cell product, in RA synovium it localizes to macrophages, endothelial cells, and chondrocytes,[16] and FLS can produce it in vitro after stimulation with IL-1 or TNF. GM-CSF is present at higher levels in synovial fluid from RA than OA patients.[166,167] M-CSF is also found at higher levels in RA, but only modestly so. In vitro, M-CSF is produced by FLS, increasing after stimulation with other cytokines, and also by chondrocytes. M-CSF is notable for its ability to expand the osteoclast precursor pool, promoting the differentiation of osteoclasts in vitro. G-CSF has been detected in synovial fluids from various diseases,[166] but IL-3 has not been detected in RA synovial fluid.[108]

GM-CSF contributes to arthritis in murine collagen-induced arthritis, because antibodies to GM-CSF reduce the severity of disease even when started after arthritis is clinically detectable.[168] Analogous results have been obtained with G-CSF and M-CSF in murine collagen-induced arthritis, with addition of either cytokine exacerbating disease[169] and genetically deficient mice found to be resistant.[170] G-CSF appears to be important for neutrophil trafficking in this model.[170]

Some support for a role for G-CSF in promoting human RA has come from case reports describing exacerbation of disease in patients receiving G-CSF to treat neutropenia from various causes, but it is unclear whether the correction of neutropenia per se or other actions of the cytokine on neutrophils or other cells are responsible.

TGF-β

Transforming growth factor-β is the prototype of a large family of mediators that includes the bone morphogenic proteins (BMPs). It is broadly immunosuppressive and anti-inflammatory, but, as an example of its complex actions, it can both stimulate and inhibit angiogenesis under different conditions. TGF-β increases production and decreases breakdown of extracellular matrix and is thought to be a major factor in both physiologic wound healing and pathologic fibrosis.

TGF-β activity is readily detectable in rheumatoid synovial fluid,[109] and by immunohistochemistry TGF-β1 is present at increased levels in RA compared with OA synovial tissues,[171] apparently produced by macrophages, FLS, endothelial cells,[171] chondrocytes,[16] and DCs[172]; TGF-β2 and TGF-β3 appear to be made at lower levels.[172] TGF-β has many effects when added to FLS in vitro, including an increase in the synthesis of fibronectin-rich matrix, decrease in secretion of hyaluronic acid, and inhibition of induced apoptotic cell death. Reports of effects on production of inflammatory cytokines have been inconsistent. Beyond the well-known suppressive effects of TGF-β on proliferation of and cytokine production by T cells, it has been proposed that induction of the chemokine receptor CXCR4 by TGF-β contributes to accumulation of T cells in RA synovium.[173]

The importance of TGF-β isoforms in development has been shown using gene knockout mice. Disruption of TGF-β2, β3 or, in at least one strain background, β1 leads to fetal or perinatal demise. In a different strain background, TGF-β1 deficiency leads to widespread autoimmune inflammatory disease that is fatal before adulthood. Thus, suppressive effects of TGF-β on experimental arthritis have been shown using the purified cytokine or blocking antibodies. Mice engineered so that TGF-β signaling is defective only in T cells are more susceptible to collagen-induced arthritis.[174] Conversely, local injection of TGF-β into affected knee joints in murine arthritis induced by zymosan (a direct activator of complement) does not decrease inflammation but does restore the proteoglycan content of cartilage.[175] In addition, some investigators have found a genetic association between a polymorphism in the TGF-β1 gene and incidence or severity of human RA.

Other growth factors: PDGF, FGF, EGF

Several of the classic growth factors have been examined in rheumatoid synovium due to the prominence of fibroblast expansion and angiogenesis (see Chapter 90) arising in that tissue. Space limitations prevent us from discussing these mediators in detail, but it is worth noting that the distinction between cytokines and growth factors is somewhat arbitrary. Just as cytokines influence the growth and function of non-immune cells in the RA joint, so these growth factors also influence immune cells and the network of inflammatory mediators.

Chemokines

Chemokines, the name being an abbreviation of the term *chemotactic cytokines*, are protein mediators that cause the migration of various cell types, usually toward the source or highest concentration of the stimulus. Forty-eight human chemokine genes and 19 chemokine receptors have been described, with multiple ligands binding to a given receptor and, for additional complexity, multiple receptors often binding a given ligand. Both are grouped into four families—CC, CXC, C, and CX₃C—based on the positions of conserved cysteine residues.

What is known of the biology of chemokines is so complex as to make detailed discussion here impractical. In RA, chemokines likely promote chemotaxis of leukocyte subsets infiltrating the joint. In addition, chemokines can activate leukocytes and promote angiogenesis and have been implicated as playing roles in the formation of lymphoid follicles and in fibrosis. The potential roles for specific chemokines in RA have been reviewed in detail.[176] Numerous chemokines and receptors have been found at higher levels in synovial tissues in RA than in OA,[177] and several of these factors (CCL2/MCP-1, CCL5/RANTES, CXCL1/GROα, CXCL5/ENA-78, CXCL8/IL-8, CXCL10/IP-10, CXCL12/SDF-1, and CX₃CL1/Fractalkine) have also been shown to be important in the chemotactic activity of rheumatoid synovial fluid toward neutrophils, monocytes, or T cells (Table 91.2). Many chemo-

TABLE 91.2 CHEMOKINES ELEVATED IN SYNOVIAL TISSUES AND FLUIDS IN RHEUMATOID ARTHRITIS

Major target	CC ligands	CXC ligands	CX₃C ligands
Monocytes	CCL2, CCL3, CCL4, **CCL5**		**CX₃CL1**
Neutrophils		**CXCL1, CXCL5, CXCL8**	
T cells (esp. Th1)	**CCL2, CCL5**, CCL20	**CXCL10**, CXCL11, **CXCL12**	
B cells		CXCL13	
Endothelial cells		CXCL8, **CXCL12**	

Chemokines important for the chemotactic activity of synovial fluid for the listed cell type, based on experiments using blocking antibodies or other antagonists in vitro, are listed in bold. Note: older names include CCL4, MIP-1b; CCL20, LARC; CXCL11, ITAC; CXCL12, SDF-1a and b; CXCL13, BCA-1; CX₃CL1, Fractalkine; others are listed in the text.
Summary courtesy of Dr. A. Luster.

kine ligands are produced either constitutively or inducibly by macrophages and FLS; fewer have been noted to be produced by T cells, DCs, endothelial cells, and platelets, although this could merely indicate that these cell types have not been studied as closely. Chemokine receptors are expressed on various subpopulations of leukocytes, but FLS also express multiple chemokine receptors and migrate and proliferate in response to chemokines.[178-180] As a broad generalization, CXCLs are notable for being chemotactic for neutrophils but some can promote lymphocyte and monocyte migration as well and several appear to be important in either the promotion or inhibition of angiogenesis. CCLs are notable for monocyte chemotaxis but are often also active on lymphocytes.[176]

In light of the striking redundancy of the system, it is somewhat surprising that several individual chemokines and receptors have been shown to be important in various animal models of inflammatory arthritis. Blockade of CXCL8/IL-8, a product of macrophages and FLS and a powerful attractant for neutrophils, reduces the severity of various types of arthritis in rabbits. Although mice have no homolog of this chemokine, murine collagen-induced arthritis is inhibited by antagonism of CXCL1/GROα, CXCL12/SDF-1, CCL3/MIP-1α, or CCL5/RANTES, by combined blockade of CCR1 and CCR5, or by an agonist of the antiangiogenic mediator CXCL4/PF-4.[176] However, work with gene knockout mice has made this picture less rather than more clear. For example, mice lacking CCR5 are still susceptible to collagen-induced arthritis.[181] In addition, blockade of CCR1 and CCR5 or of their ligand CCL5/RANTES has no effect on adjuvant arthritis in rats.[182] Mice lacking CCR2 are unusually susceptible to collagen-induced arthritis,[181] and the effect of anti-CCR2 treatment depends on its timing.[183] Different chemokines are expressed at different times during the course of experimental arthritis, and further delineation of these events is an active area of research.

The application of chemokine blockade in human RA is in its early stages.[184] An antagonist of CCR1 reduced inflammation and produced some clinical improvement in a short phase I trial,[185] but an antagonist of CCR2 showed no benefit in a phase II trial.[186] Of interest, a polymorphism in CCR5 that leads to loss of function has been associated with a decreased incidence of RA, suggesting that CCR5 may be a viable target in the treatment of RA.

Arachidonic acid metabolites

Prostaglandins and leukotrienes are lipid mediators that are generally proinflammatory but have a complex biology. There are four known receptors for prostaglandin E_2 (PGE$_2$), an important prostaglandin in RA synovium, and individual receptors for the other prostaglandins. The COX-2 enzyme is expressed in rheumatoid but not normal synovium and is found in FLS, macrophages, endothelial cells, and other cell types.[187,188] Expression of COX-2 and, subsequently, PGE$_2$ is induced in FLS by proinflammatory mediators such as TNF and IL-1 and suppressed by anti-inflammatory cytokines such as IL-4, IL-10, and IL-13. Cyclooxygenase-2 (COX-2) and PGE$_2$ likely play as important a role in OA as in RA; COX-2 is found in OA cartilage,[188] and

PGE$_2$ is produced *in vitro* by OA FLS and is inducible *in vitro* from normal chondrocytes.

The described effects of PGE$_2$ that are potentially relevant to RA (and OA) are numerous and include increased cartilage degradation, chondrocyte apoptosis, angiogenesis, production of MMPs, and decreased collagen synthesis. PGE$_2$ also contributes to inflammation, and prostaglandins as a group are important in animal models of inflammatory arthritis; non-steroidal anti-inflammatory drugs (NSAIDs) or COX-2 selective inhibitors, which block the production of prostaglandins, prevent or treat disease in several models. COX-2 selective inhibitors have been as effective as non-selective inhibitors in several animal models of arthritis. However, in mouse arthritis induced by antibodies to glucose-6-phosphate isomerase (GPI), COX-1 but not COX-2 is required, challenging the paradigm that the COX-2 isoenzyme is the critical one in the synovium.[189] In any case, it is notable that although NSAIDs have a long track record in treating the symptoms of RA, they do not appear to be disease modifying, as might have been expected from animal models.

LTB$_4$, the most studied leukotriene, and other lipoxygenase metabolites are found at higher levels in rheumatoid than in non-inflamed synovial fluid and tissue.[190] Beyond the expected synthesis of LTB$_4$ by such proinflammatory cells as mast cells, FLS can synthesize it *in vitro*; reports differ, however, as to whether neutrophils in synovial fluid secrete more or less LTB$_4$ than do circulating neutrophils. LTB$_4$ acts through two receptors, the higher-affinity BLT1 and lower-affinity BLT2. BLT2, found on many cell types, appears to be more highly expressed than BLT1 in RA synovium, and BLT2 is not found in OA synovium. BLT1 remains the dominant receptor on synovial fluid cells.[191] Leukotrienes are best known for promoting vascular permeability and chemotaxis of inflammatory cells, but they likely have other effects in the rheumatoid joint. Antagonism of leukotriene synthesis or specific blockade of LTB$_4$ receptors reduces the severity of murine collagen-induced arthritis,[192] but some authors have found that dual blockade of both leukotriene and prostaglandin synthesis is more effective. LTB$_4$ and BLT1 are required in anti-GPI autoantibody-induced arthritis.[193,194] Reports of the use of leukotriene inhibitors and antagonists in RA have been few and preliminary.

Ligands for Toll-like receptors

TLRs are a family of membrane-associated receptors that are activated by a variety of unique microbial products and play an important role in "innate" immunity, that is, antimicrobial defense that does not require development of antigen-specific T- or B-cell responses. Activation of TLRs stimulates proinflammatory pathways[195] in leukocytes, endothelial cells, and parenchymal cells, and also promotes antigen-specific immune responses both directly in B cells[196] and indirectly via antigen presentation to and co-stimulation of T cells. In addition to microbial products, endogenous molecules (e.g., hyaluronic acid, HMGB1, heat-shock proteins, chromatin, and fibrinogen) have been shown to interact with and activate TLRs *in vitro*. Because these endogenous molecules are released in association with cell death and tissue damage, settings in which host defense needs to be activated, their binding to TLRs is likely relevant *in vivo* as well, and particularly in chronic inflammatory diseases.[197]

All of these putative endogenous TLR ligands are abundant in joints in established RA. In addition, bacterial products have been detected in a majority of inflamed joints of different etiologies.[198] TLRs are expressed on multiple cell types in RA synovium. For example, TLRs1 through 6 but not TLR7 to TLR10 are expressed by FLS,[199] and expression of TLRs2, 3, and 4 is higher in RA than control fibroblasts.[199,200] Stimulation of TLR2 induces secretion of several chemokines, VEGF, MMPs, and IL-15 by FLS.[201-204] Expression of TLR2 and TLR4 is also elevated on macrophages in inflamed synovium,[205,206] and ligation of these receptors leads to production of TNF and IL-8.[206] Not surprisingly, complexity in TLR-mediated responses in RA is emerging; for example, stimulation of TLR4 on DCs leads to increased production of MIF, whereas stimulation of TLR3 or TLR7 leads to decreased MIF production.[150]

TLRs play complex roles in mouse models of RA as well. Certain TLR ligands can produce inflammatory arthritis after intra-articular injection: hypomethylated CpG-containing DNA via TLR9[207] and streptococcal cell walls via TLR2.[208] Stimulation of TLR4 by bacterial LPS facilitates induction of arthritis by antibodies to type II collagen or GPI,[50,209] and blockade or absence of TLR4 reduces the severity of collagen-induced arthritis, chronic streptococcal cell wall–induced arthritis, and spontaneous arthritis arising in mice genetically lacking IL-1ra.[210-212] On the other hand, stimulation of TLR9 or TLR3 ameliorates different autoantibody-mediated arthritides via induction of type I interferons,[50,213] and absence of TLR2 is associated with more severe arthritis in mice lacking IL-1ra.[212]

A genetic polymorphism in TLR4 that is associated with hyporesponsiveness to stimulation *in vitro*[214] has been investigated for association with reduced risk of RA, but an association reported in one cohort[215] has not been confirmed in others.[216,217] Interference with signaling via the endosomally localized TLR3, TLR7, and TLR9 has been proposed as an important mechanism of action of antimalarial agents in autoimmune inflammatory diseases.[218]

Complement and immune complexes

Circulating complement is depleted in RA only in the setting of rheumatoid vasculitis. However, RA is apparently unique among the arthritides in the depletion of complement in the synovial fluid in comparison to blood.[219,220] In addition, complement degradation products are found in rheumatoid synovial fluid. Deposits containing both immunoglobulin and C3 are readily detected in articular cartilage of RA patients (Fig. 91.12). Similar deposits are found in articular cartilage in various mouse models; in the K/BxN mouse model, these deposits also contain the specific target antigen GPI.[221] Arthritis in several mouse models is dependent on the complement cascade and particularly on C5. Together, these findings suggest that immune complexes form and/or

are deposited in RA joints and locally activate complement, with the likely consequence of chemotaxis and activation of leukocytes by the cleavage products C3a and C5a. Which autoantibodies participate in the formation of these immune complexes is unknown; antibodies of several specificities, including RF, ACPA, and anti-type II collagen, are found at higher concentrations in synovial tissues than in the circulation, but whether this finding indicates local deposition in addition to local synthesis is unclear.

Arthritis in several mouse models is also dependent on the low-affinity stimulatory receptor for IgG, FcγRIII. The low-affinity inhibitory FcR, FcγRII, plays a protective role against arthritis in these models. The high-affinity receptor, FcγRI, is apparently not required. Because the low-affinity FcRs bind to aggregated but not monomeric IgG, their importance provides evidence for a key role in the handling of either immune complexes or surface-bound IgG in these models. Although roles for the FcRs have not been directly investigated in RA, polymorphisms in the genes for FcγRIIIA and FcγRIIA (both stimulatory, low-affinity FcRs) have been linked to susceptibility or severity of RA by several groups.

JOINT DESTRUCTION

Enzymatic destruction of components of the extracellular matrix (ECM) is the major mechanism proposed for cartilage, ligament, and tendon destruction in RA. In particular, cartilage destruction has been attributed to the combined actions of several distinct families of proteinases, each of which has a defined substrate specificity. Proteinases are produced by cells within the invasive pannus tissue, by cells in the synovium remote from bone, and by chondrocytes themselves under certain conditions of activation. These enzymes represent a potential therapeutic target for the protection from joint destruction in RA.

Matrix metalloproteinases

Perhaps the best studied family of enzymes implicated in joint destruction in RA is the MMP family, whose member interstitial collagenase (MMP-1) was the first to be identified in media from cultured RA synovial tissues.[222] Subsequently, studies utilizing *in-situ* hybridization of whole synovial tissues identified synoviocytes within the synovial lining layer as the exclusive sources of mRNA for MMP-1 and another MMP family member, stromelysin-1 (MMP-3), in RA synovium (Fig. 91.13).[223] In addition, MMP-1 and MMP-3 proteins have been demonstrated in synovium remote from bone as well as at sites of cartilage erosion.[224] Several additional MMP family members have now been identified as being expressed in RA synovial tissues and/or in synovially derived pannus tissues invading into cartilage. MMPs can act at neutral

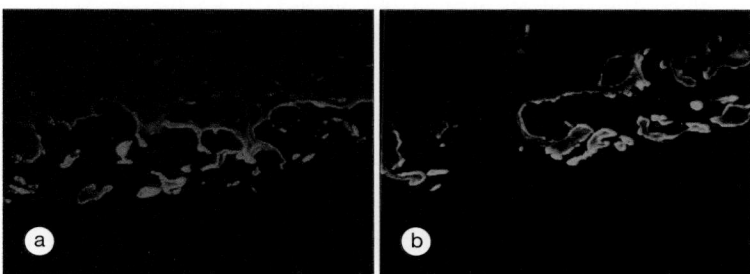

Fig. 91.12 Deposition of IgG (a, red) and C3 (b, green) on the cartilage surface of the knee, as shown by immunofluorescence staining. The patient was an 82-year-old woman with a 10-year history of RF-positive RA.

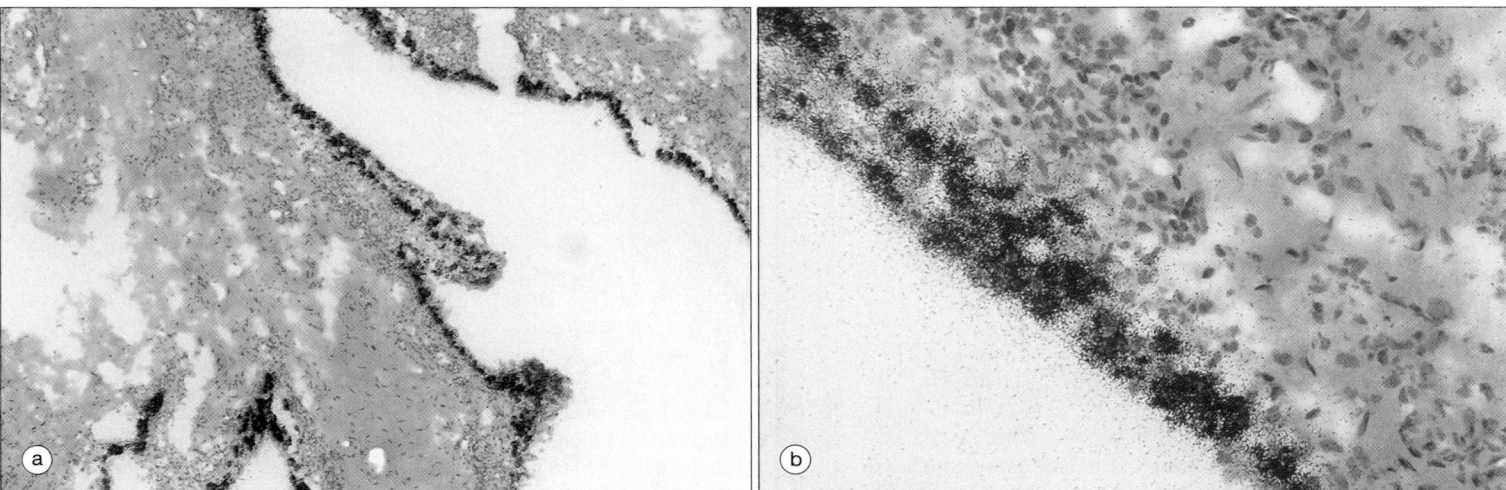

Fig. 91.13 Brightfield images of *in-situ* hybridization in RA synovial tissue. (a) Low-power view demonstrating abundant expression of mRNA (black dots) for MMP-3 (stromelysin-1). (b) High-power view demonstrating that MMP-3 mRNA expression is limited to cells within the synovial lining layer. *(From Gravallese EM, Darling JM, Ladd AL, et al. In situ hybridization studies of stromelysin and collagenase messenger RNA expression in rheumatoid synovium. Arthritis Rheum 1991;34:1076-1084. Reprinted with permission of Wiley-Liss, Inc., Wiley Publishing, Inc., a subsidiary of John Wiley & Sons, Inc.)*

pH and have the ability, in aggregate, to degrade the components of the ECM of cartilage.

The MMP family comprises 25 members. Classification of an enzyme as a member of this family depends on the presence of conserved "pro" and "catalytic" domains (Fig. 91.14). These enzymes are named "metallo" because of the presence of a zinc ion in the active site of the catalytic domain. Within the pro-domain there is a conserved cysteine residue that interacts with Zn^{2+} in the catalytic domain. When this interaction is disrupted by removal of the pro-peptide via proteolytic cleavage, the enzyme's active site becomes available and the enzyme is thus activated (see Fig. 91.14). Expression of the MMP enzymes is regulated at several steps, including at the levels of gene transcription, activation of the pro-enzyme to the active enzyme, focality of expression within tissues, and, finally, enzyme inactivation.[225]

Collagenases

Collagenases were the first of the MMP enzymes to be implicated in the process of cartilage destruction in RA. This group of enzymes cleaves the collagen triple helix at a defined site near its amino terminus. As such, the major substrates of the collagenases are native interstitial collagens types I and II, the latter being the predominant collagen component of cartilage.[225] Members of this group include fibroblast or interstitial collagenase (collagenase-1, MMP-1), neutrophil collagenase (collagenase-2, MMP-8), and collagenase-3 (MMP-13). Expression of MMP-1 has been demonstrated to be quantitatively greater in synovium from patients with RA as compared with those with OA.[223,226] Collagenase gene expression is regulated in part by the AP-1 family of transcription factors, which are also expressed in cells of the synovial lining layer (Fig. 91.15). In cultured FLS, TNF and IL-1 are potent synergistic inducers of MMP-1 gene transcription, with upregulation of MMP-1 mRNA occurring within hours of stimulation.

Neutrophil collagenase (MMP-8) and collagenase-3 (MMP-13) have also been implicated in joint destruction in RA. In particular, MMP-13 is expressed by cells within RA synovium as well as by chondrocytes in areas of cartilage damage. Because MMP-13 is efficient in cleaving native collagens as well as aggrecan and because gene expression for MMP-13 is also upregulated by TNF and IL-1, this enzyme has been implicated as a uniquely important therapeutic target for the protection of cartilage destruction in RA.

Stromelysins

The stromelysin group of MMPs has a broad substrate specificity for components of the ECM. This group of enzymes degrades non-collagen connective tissue components, including proteoglycans, fibronectin, and laminin, as well as some of the minor collagens. In addition, MMP-3 has the ability to cleave and activate pro-collagenase, thereby providing additional matrix-degrading capability. The rat homolog of stromelysin-1, transin, was originally cloned from transformed fibroblasts, and its expression in tumors has been shown to correlate with the invasive phenotype.[227]

The first observation of the potential importance of MMP-3 in inflammatory arthritis was the demonstration, in Lewis rats with streptococcal cell wall-induced arthritis, of transin protein in the synovial lining layer and in the underlying stroma.[228] In this model there is significant destruction of cartilage, implicating this MMP family member in joint destruction and suggesting, by correlation to the proposed role of transin in tumor invasion, that FLS expressing transin demonstrate a partially "transformed" phenotype. However, when collagen-induced arthritis was generated in MMP-3–deficient mice, severe inflammation and cartilage and bone destruction resulted, demonstrating that MMP-3 is not unique in its matrix-degrading capabilities.[229]

Of the three members of the stromelysin group (stromelysin-1 [MMP-3], stromelysin-2 [MMP-10], and stromelysin-3 [MMP-11]), MMP-3 is by far the most abundantly expressed in RA. *In-situ* hybridization studies demonstrate that, like MMP-1, gene expression for MMP-3 is greater in RA than in OA synovium.[223] Although very low levels of MMP-3 are expressed by unstimulated synoviocytes, TNF and IL-1 are potent stimulators of MMP-3 gene expression, as are fibronectin fragments through engagement and cross-linking of fibronectin receptors on synviocytes.

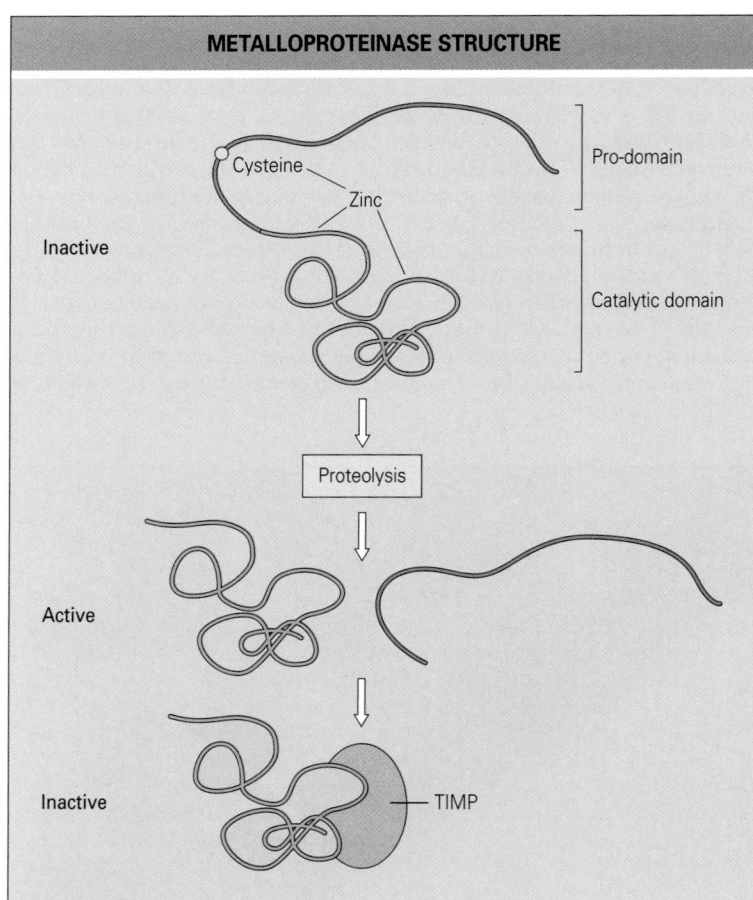

Fig. 91.14 Metalloproteinase structure. Schematic representation of metalloproteinase activation by limited proteolysis. After cleavage, the zinc cation is no longer complexed with the cysteine residue in the enzyme's pro domain and is available to catalyze the enzymatic reaction. Modification of the cysteine thiol group can also convert the enzyme to an active form. TIMPs can bind to the active enzyme and inhibit metalloproteinase activity.

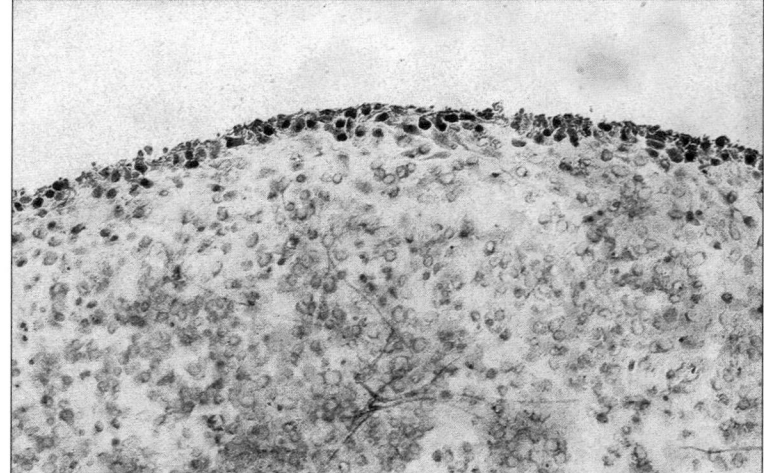

Fig. 91.15 Immunohistochemistry in RA synovium demonstrating intranuclear staining for the Fos family members (components of the AP-1 transcription factor complex) in cells within the synovial lining layer. *(From Handel ML, McMorrow LB, Gravallese EM. Nuclear factor-kappa B in rheumatoid synovium: localization of p50 and p65. Arthritis Rheum 1995;38:1762-1770. Reprinted with permission of Wiley-Liss, Inc., Wiley Publishing Inc., a subsidiary of John Wiley & Sons, Inc.)*

Other MMPs and related enzymes

Other MMP family members have been implicated in the process of cartilage destruction in RA, including the gelatinases: gelatinase A (72-kDa gelatinase, MMP-2) and gelatinase B (92-kDa gelatinase, MMP-9). These enzymes are expressed in RA synovium and can degrade partially cleaved collagens (gelatins). In an analysis of the expression of 16 MMP mRNAs in RA synovium versus synovium from patients with joint trauma, MMP-1, MMP-9, and MMP-14 (MT1-MMP) were expressed in all RA samples but in far fewer of the trauma samples. In addition, MMP-13 and the membrane-bound MT2-MMP were found exclusively in RA, implicating these enzymes specifically in joint destruction in RA.[230]

Aggrecan is a major proteoglycan component of articular cartilage. The cleavage of the aggrecan core protein in cartilage leads to destabilization of the protein, with subsequent loss of cartilage compressibility. Although several MMPs can cleave aggrecan, it has long been clear that another enzyme or enzymes must also be responsible for cleavage, because products were found in which cleavage took place between Glu373 and Ala374, a site that none of the known MMPs is able to cleave. A related but distinct family of enzymes was thus identified that may also play a role in cartilage destruction in RA. This is the ADAMTS (a disintegrin and metalloproteinase with thrombospondin motifs) family of proteinases. ADAMTS enzymes are involved in cell-cell interactions, ectodomain shedding, and other protein-processing events (including collagen processing), hemostasis, and inhibition of angiogenesis, as well as playing a role in developmental processes. Two members of this family implicated in cartilage destruction are aggrecanase-1 and aggrecanase-2, both of which are expressed in synoviocytes and synovial tissues in RA and OA.

Role of MMPs in inflammation

What is the exact role of the MMP family of enzymes in the pathogenesis of joint destruction in RA? This question has not been fully answered, in part because of the large number of MMPs and other proteases expressed by cells within RA synovium and cartilage. In addition, although MMPs have long been considered to be enzymes whose purpose is to remodel and degrade the components of the ECM, fascinating new data have demonstrated that these enzymes also play an important role in regulating the process of inflammation. It has become clear that many MMPs can also act on non-matrix proteins, including cytokines, chemokines, and their receptors and play a role in the innate immune system and in tissue repair.[225] The role of MMPs in the inflammatory process is evident from the results of experiments in which mice deficient in certain MMPs were challenged with inducers of arthritis. Surprisingly, MMP-2–deficient and MMP-3–deficient mice developed a more severe immune-mediated arthritis than did their control littermates,[229,231] suggesting that these enzymes may actually provide protection from inflammation, whereas MMP-9–deficient mice developed less severe arthritis.[231] Studies have further demonstrated that MMP-2 and MMP-3 can cleave certain chemokines, thus blocking their chemotactic activities and inhibiting the inflammatory process. Therefore, it will be critical to gain a better understanding of the role of the various MMPs in inflammation before targeting them for the prevention of joint destruction in arthritis.

Protease inhibitors

In addition to the regulatory mechanisms described earlier, the activity of MMP enzymes is also regulated by naturally occurring inhibitors. These include the tissue inhibitors of metalloproteinases (TIMPs), of which there are four family members (TIMP-1 to TIMP-4). Specific TIMPs have affinity for specific MMP family members and act by binding with high affinity to the catalytic domain of the enzyme in a 1:1 stoichiometry to render it inactive. Interestingly, in contrast to the marked upregulation of the production of certain MMPs in RA as compared with OA, TIMP-1 mRNA is expressed in similar amounts in synovial lining cells from patients with RA or OA.[226] Thus, in RA there is an apparent overexpression of MMPs that overwhelms the constitutive and induced inhibitors, including TIMPs. Two other known inhibitors of MMP activity are α_2-macroglobulin, which binds active MMP enzyme in the circulation, and RECK (reversion including cysteine-rich protein with kazal motifs), which inhibits the function of MMP-2, MMP-9, and MMP-14. The α_2-macroglobulin molecule forms a covalent link with the protease to render it inactive and is the main inhibitor of collagenase activity in serum. Neutrophil-derived elastases and serine proteinases can in turn inactivate α_2-macroglobulin.

Cysteine and serine proteases

Since the discovery of the MMP family of enzymes in RA synovium and pannus, several other classes of enzymes have also been described to be expressed by cells within RA synovial tissues and/or pannus tissues and have been implicated in cartilage destruction in arthritis. Included among these are the cysteine protease family of enzymes, especially cathepsins B, L, and K. Expression of two of the cathepsins, B and L, has been demonstrated by cells within the RA joint.[232] Cathepsin B is expressed by cells within pannus and attached to cartilage at sites of cartilage erosion. In synovial fluid there is greater expression of cathepsin B in RA than in OA or in normal control fluids. Cathepsin L is also expressed at the cartilage/pannus junction. As a class, the cathepsins have a wide range of substrate specificities, including native collagens, proteoglycans, fibronectin, fibrinogen, elastin, and laminin. Cathepsin K is another family member implicated in joint destruction. This enzyme is secreted in high amounts by osteoclasts and is largely responsible for the degradation of type I collagen in bone by these cells. Cathepsin K is also expressed by synovial fibroblasts in RA. The serine proteinases, including granzymes, neutrophil elastase, and mast cell chymases, have also been implicated in joint destruction in RA. In addition, several of these enzymes have the ability to activate pro-MMPs. Serine proteinase inhibitors (SERPINs) are present in plasma and synovial fluid and serve to block extracellular matrix degradation by this class of enzymes.

Bone destruction

Although the action of proteinases in degrading the various components of the ECM probably plays a major role in the destruction of cartilage, tendon, and ligament in RA, the destruction of bone requires removal of the mineralized bone matrix. In physiologic bone remodeling associated, for example, with microfracture or altered mechanical loading, removal of bone is accomplished by the osteoclast. Osteoclasts are specialized cells, differentiated from cells of the monocyte-macrophage lineage, that have the capacity to bind to the surface of bone, creating a tight "attachment zone" via interactions between integrins, including $\alpha_v\beta_3$, on the osteoclast membrane and matrix components in bone, including bone sialoprotein and osteopontin. The creation of this tight seal with bone allows the osteoclast to generate an acidic environment through the action of carbonic anhydrase II and a proton pump, leading to the removal of mineral from the bone. Osteoclasts also release lysosomal proteinases into this acidic environment, perhaps the most important of which is cathepsin K, as well as enzymes of the MMP group, including MMP-9, which lead to the degradation of the organic component of the bone matrix (Fig. 91.16).

A role for osteoclasts in focal bone erosion in RA was suspected initially on the basis of indirect evidence, including the identification of multinucleated cells at sites of erosion in subchondral bone and at the pannus/bone interface in tissue samples from patients with RA (Fig. 91.17).[233] Studies utilizing immunohistochemistry and in-situ hybridization have demonstrated that these multinucleated cells express characteristic markers of osteoclasts, including a marker unique to osteoclasts.[234] Similarly, osteoclasts have been identified at erosive surfaces in arthritic joints in numerous animal models of RA.

Our understanding of the pathogenesis of bone erosion and the role of osteoclasts in RA was greatly augmented by the discovery of a cytokine system now known to be the key regulatory system of osteoclast differentiation and activation. Receptor activator of nuclear factor-kappa B (NF-κB) ligand (RANKL, also known as osteoprotegerin ligand [OPGL], osteoclast differentiation factor [ODF], and TNF-related activation-induced cytokine [TRANCE]) is a cytokine initially identified as important in the regulation of interactions between DCs and T lymphocytes, as well as regulating lymph node organogenesis and lymphocyte development.[235,236] It was also recognized that RANKL is

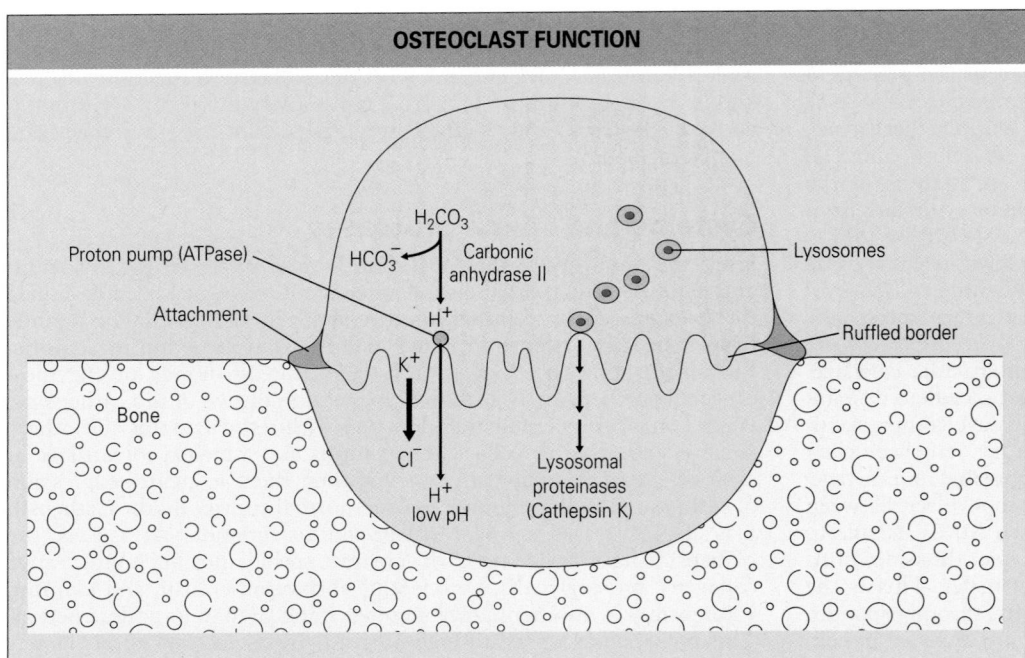

OSTEOCLAST FUNCTION

Fig. 91.16 The osteoclast. Protons generated by carbonic anhydrase II are pumped into the area adjacent to the bone surface to form an acidic environment that allows for the removal of bone mineral. Lysosomal enzymes and other proteinases contribute to the degradation of the bone matrix.

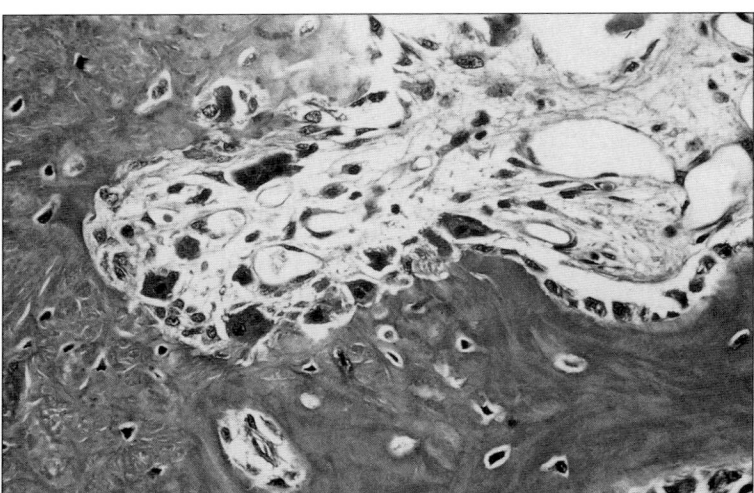

Fig. 91.17 Focal subchondral bone erosion in RA. Note that osteoclasts are present at a site of resorption. *(From Gravallese EM, Goldring SR. Cellular mechanisms and the role of cytokines in bone erosion in rheumatoid arthritis. Arthritis Rheum 2000;43:2143-2151. Reprinted with permission of Wiley-Liss, Inc., Wiley Publishing Inc., a subsidiary of John Wiley & Sons Inc.)*

essential for osteoclast differentiation and activation, providing a link between the immune system and bone. RANKL binds to its receptor, receptor activator of NF-κB (RANK), present on osteoclast precursor cells, to effect its biologic functions. Osteoprotegerin (OPG), a decoy receptor for RANKL, is the third member of this cytokine system. OPG can bind to RANKL with high affinity, thus preventing the binding of RANKL to RANK and blocking the biologic activity of RANKL (Fig. 91.18). The expression of RANKL protein relative to OPG protein at a given site is the critical determinant of the degree to which osteoclast-mediated bone resorption occurs at that site.

Several lines of experimental evidence have implicated the RANKL/RANK/OPG system in the pathogenesis of osteoclast-mediated bone erosion in RA. RANKL is expressed by two cell types within rheumatoid synovial tissue: FLS and T cells.[237] Cells isolated from cultured RA synovium also generate multinucleated cells that can resorb bone,[238] a definitive demonstration that these multinucleated cells are osteoclasts. Bone resorption is inhibited in these cultures by OPG, demonstrating that this is a RANKL-dependent process. In addi-

tion, the degree to which bone is resorbed strongly correlates with the ratios of RANKL/OPG mRNA levels in the RA synovial tissue samples studied.[238] Finally, RANKL is expressed at sites of bone resorption in tissues from patients with RA (Fig. 91.19). Taken together, these studies support a role for the RANKL/RANK/OPG system in bone erosion in RA.

The first definitive demonstration of the critical role of RANKL and osteoclasts in bone erosion in arthritis was reported in studies using the rat adjuvant-induced arthritis model, a model in which activated T cells have been shown to express RANKL protein. Treatment of arthritic rats with OPG was initiated at disease onset, and it was demonstrated that although levels of inflammation were similar in treated and untreated rats there was complete protection from bone erosion in arthritic rats treated with OPG.[239] Furthermore, studies in mice deficient in osteoclasts (due to deficiencies in different factors critical to osteoclastogenesis), including RANKL-deficient mice[240] and c-fos–deficient mice,[241] have demonstrated a dramatic protection from bone erosion in models of experimental arthritis driven by autoantibodies or by overexpression of TNF, respectively. These data provide further support for the importance of the RANKL/RANK/OPG system and of osteoclasts in the process of bone erosion in RA and suggest that therapeutic strategies that block osteoclast differentiation and/or function may be beneficial in protection from articular bone destruction in this disease.

In addition to the RANKL/RANK/OPG system, other cytokines and growth factors produced by synovial tissues and/or pannus tissues in RA can influence the differentiation and activation of osteoclasts. Factors that can play a direct role in osteoclast differentiation include TNF, which is a potent differentiation factor for osteoclast precursor cells in synergy with RANKL; M-CSF, which expands the pool of osteoclast precursor cells; and IL-1, which prevents apoptosis of osteoclasts and augments their bone-resorbing potential.[242,243] Therapeutic blockade of IL-1 or TNF in patients with RA can modulate both inflammation and bone erosion.[244,245] In addition, factors produced by RA synovial tissues, including IL-1, TNF and parathyroid hormone-related protein (PTHrP), may act indirectly on osteoclastogenesis and activity by increasing the RANKL/OPG expression ratio in the local bone microenvironment. T cells within the rheumatoid lesion may also contribute to osteoclast-mediated bone resorption, not only by expression of RANKL by activated T cells but also by production by a subset of T cells of IL-17, which is a potent stimulator of osteoclastogenesis by indirect mechanisms. The rheumatoid synovium is also a source of factors that can inhibit osteoclastogenesis, including IL-4, IL-10, and IFN-β and IFN-γ.

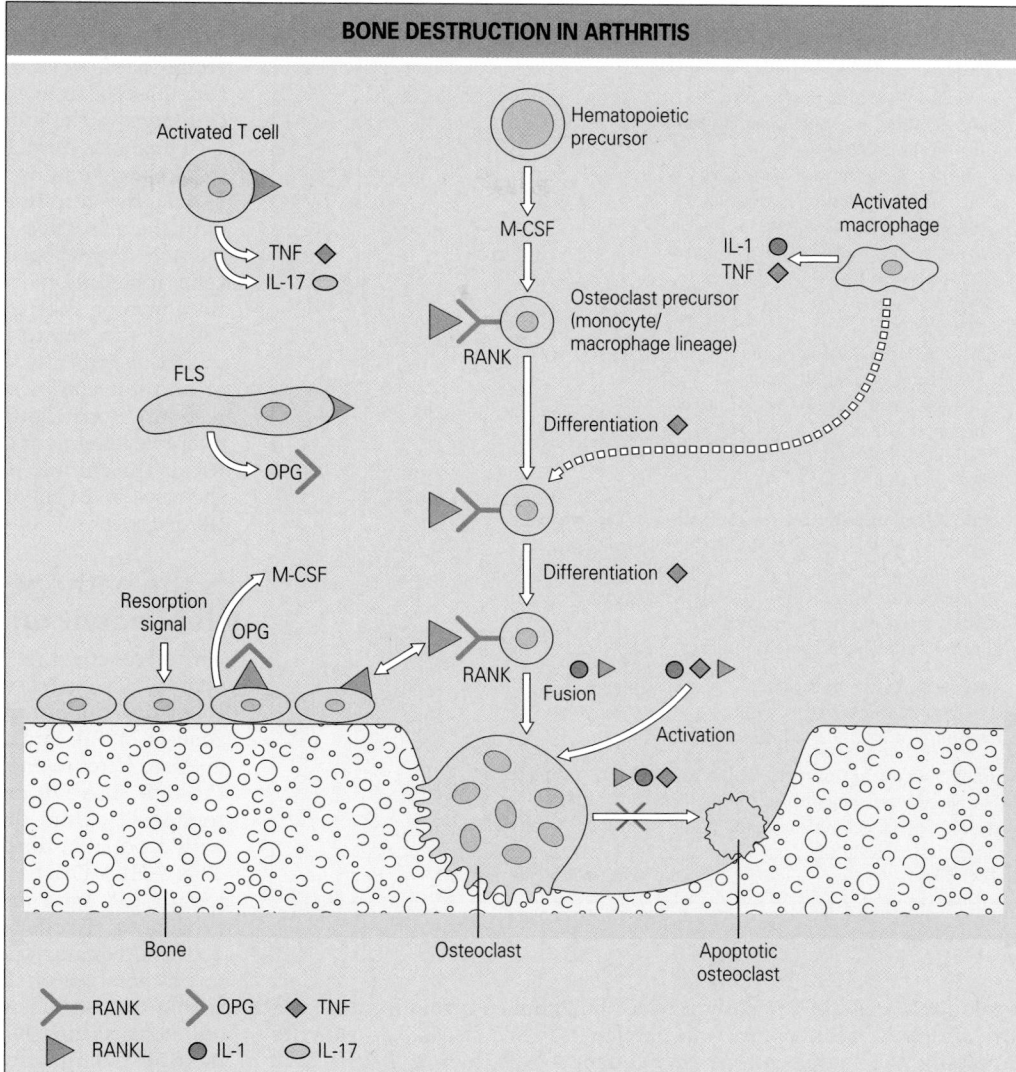

BONE DESTRUCTION IN ARTHRITIS

Fig. 91.18 Mechanisms of bone destruction in arthritis. Osteoclasts are derived from cells of the monocyte-macrophage lineage. Macrophage colony-stimulating factor (M-CSF) derived from bone lining (stromal) cells induces expansion of the osteoclast precursor pool and expression of RANK. Binding of RANKL to RANK leads to osteoclast differentiation, fusion, and activation. Tumor necrosis factor (TNF) can synergize with RANKL to induce osteoclast differentiation. Possible sources of RANKL in RA include bone lining cells, fibroblast-like synoviocytes (FLS), and activated T cells. Bone stromal cells and FLS are also sources of the RANKL decoy receptor OPG. Cells from RA synovium produce factors that could influence osteoclast differentiation, fusion, and activation at a number of steps. In addition, activated macrophages from synovial tissues can act as osteoclast precursor cells.

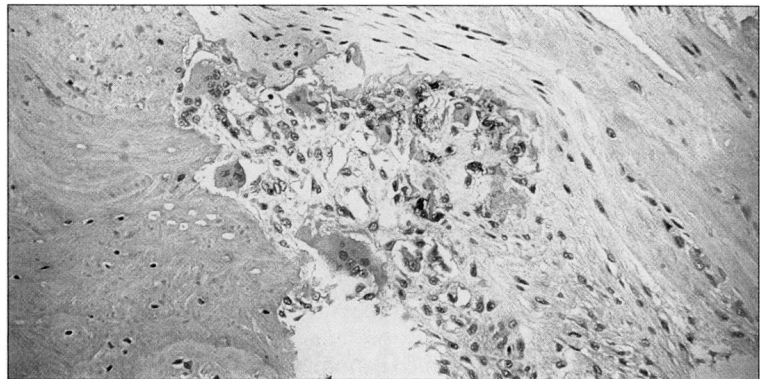

Fig. 91.19 Immunohistochemistry of pannus/bone interface in RA, demonstrating cells expressing RANKL (brown) in areas of osteoclast-mediated bone resorption.

PATHOGENESIS

Any theory of the pathogenesis of RA must extend beyond observations of synovial pathology and consider the epidemiology and clinical features of the disease as well. Although patients with RA often have extra-articular features, the dominant and defining clinical manifestation of this disease is chronic inflammation of joints lined by synovium. This fact undoubtedly holds a significant clue to the pathogenic mecha-

nisms underlying RA. One can propose a host of factors that could contribute to the joint-specific nature of RA, including unique structural features of the joint and the proximity of synovium to cartilage and bone, unique cell populations within the joint, and the organization of these cell types, tropism of pathogens to the joint, and joint-specific antigens (Box 91.1). Contributions from these factors are not mutually exclusive, and it is likely that some, or many, may play a role in the initiation and/or chronicity of this disease.

Twin studies have suggested that there is a genetic influence in RA, as well as the influence of non-genetic (environmental or "chance") factors. In addition, early *in-vitro* studies demonstrated that in allogeneic mixed lymphocyte cultures the lymphocytes from patients with RA proliferated normally when cultured with lymphocytes from normal donors but proliferation was significantly blunted when RA lymphocytes were cultured with cells from other RA patients. These studies suggested that there are genetic similarities among patients with RA.[246] The first real breakthrough in our understanding of RA pathogenesis came from studies demonstrating a genetic link of this disease to the HLA-DR genes, located in the MHC complex.[247]

The genetic influence in RA is more specifically associated with certain DRB1 alleles that share a common five amino acid sequence: QKRAA (or QRRAA), located at position 70-74 in the third hypervariable region of the peptide-binding cleft of the DR β chain. This sequence has been called the "shared epitope"[248] and has been associated with both disease susceptibility and severity. The shared epitope is found in several RA-associated DR genes, including DR1, DR4, and DR14. Because these genes produce proteins involved in antigen presentation to CD4+ T cells, the discovery of the shared epitope strongly suggested

---

BOX 91.1 FACTORS THAT COULD CONTRIBUTE TO THE JOINT-SPECIFIC NATURE OF RHEUMATOID ARTHRITIS

Structural features of the joint
Synovial fluid = unique plasma ultrafiltrate
Unique vasculature
    Trapping of immune complexes
    Response to immune complexes
    (Response to vasoactive mediators)
Proximity of tissue-specific cell types
    Chondrocytes
    Osteoclasts
    Osteoblasts
Cartilage = acellular surface
    Trapping of positively charged molecules
    (Dysregulated complement activation)
Chronic trauma
    (Proinflammatory byproducts)
Low oxygen tension

Unique cell populations/organization in synovium
Type A synoviocytes (and sublining macrophages)
Type B synoviocytes
Propensity to form ectopic germinal centers
(Tropism of lymphocyte subsets)
(Peripheral nervous system interactions)

Interaction with pathogens
Tropism of chronic pathogens: example = *Borrelia*
Trapping of bacterial products

Joint-specific antigens to which tolerance could be lost
Native antigens: examples = type II collagen, gp39
Neoantigens: example = citrullinated proteins

Those factors that are plausible but have little or no experimental support are in parentheses.

---

a role for T cells in RA pathogenesis and implied a role for one or a few antigenic peptides that initiate or "drive" disease in patients expressing the shared epitope. Subsequent to this finding, T cells have fallen in and out of favor as the cells responsible for orchestrating the disease process in RA and no specific "RA antigen" has been identified. In considering the roles of MHC alleles in the pathogenesis of diseases, it is sobering to note that no single peptide antigen has been identified to underlie the strong association of ankylosing spondylitis with HLA-B27. In fact, the HLA-B27 protein has been shown to have unusual biochemical features beyond the structure of its peptide-binding groove that may actually be more important in disease pathogenesis.

One additional clinical feature of RA that must be taken into account in any discussion of pathogenic mechanisms of disease is the presence of circulating autoantibodies including RF, ACPA, and others that are not in general clinical use. Strikingly, recent studies have shown that detectable serum RF and ACPA usually precede the clinical onset of RA, often by many years.[249] The best interpretation of these data is that humoral autoimmunity, with an early breakdown of T-cell tolerance, precedes chronic inflammation in RA and suggests that autoantibodies and possibly immune complexes play a role in disease pathogenesis. To gain further insight into the pathogenic mechanisms involved in RA, investigators have turned to animal models in an attempt to define both the events that may initiate the disease and those that can produce a state of chronic synovitis that leads eventually to the destruction of joint structures.

Lessons from animal models

All animal models of RA differ in important ways from the human disease, most notably in their rapidity of onset and progression, the details of the autoimmunity, and the requirement for either immunization or an overt genetic defect or manipulation (see Chapter 87). Starting from the perspective that models help define what could cause a human disease, rather than what does or does not, the first important lesson from study of the large and growing number of animal models

of RA is that there are many ways to cause a pathologic process that resembles the human disease. Second, these studies clearly demonstrate that TNF and IL-1 are critical players in all the models in which they have been evaluated,[93] and dysregulated overexpression of these cytokines in the joint is sufficient to cause chronic arthritis.[94,106]

Thus, any mechanism leading to excess TNF and IL-1 in the joint would likely produce RA-like disease. This task can be readily achieved by adaptive immunity to autoantigens or foreign antigens, beginning with the activation of T cells and leading in many models to the production of pathogenic autoantibodies. Activation of innate immune cells, including macrophages, mast cells, and neutrophils, may prime the joint for subsequent inflammation. Moreover, it is essential that cells of the innate immune system, to different degrees in different models, be recruited to the joint to mediate the proinflammatory effects of immune complexes and/or T cells. However, the adaptive immune response is critical for the production of TNF and IL-1 and the subsequent development of arthritis in most models.[93] How, then, in human RA, is the chronic production of TNF and IL-1 achieved and what are the roles of T cells, B cells, autoantibodies, and immune complexes in the pathogenesis of this disease?

Is the pathogenesis of rheumatoid arthritis dependent on T cells?

The discovery of the shared epitope, along with histopathologic studies demonstrating T cell–rich infiltrates in the synovium of patients with RA, led to the initial assumption that T cells are critical to the pathogenesis of RA and that antigen-specific T-cell responses are driving disease. Circumstantial evidence to support this hypothesis included the rich HLA-DR expression on synovial lining cells, DCs, and macrophages within the sublining of RA synovial tissues, consistent with a possible role for these cells in antigen presentation to T cells. These HLA-DR–bearing cells are often in close proximity to T cells within the synovium, which would facilitate cell-cell interactions. Products of T cells activated by antigen could then mediate the further activation of macrophages, fibroblasts, and synovial lining cells, leading to proliferation of these cells, activation and differentiation of B cells within the joint, as well as induction of adhesion molecule expression on endothelium. The latter event would allow for the further recruitment of inflammatory cells to the joint. This scenario could, in fact, explain many of the observed pathologic events in the chronic phase of RA.

Studies attempting to identify a specific arthritogenic peptide in RA, however, have not been fruitful; and clonal expansion of specific T-cell subsets, as might be expected in a disease driven by a unique antigen, has not been convincingly demonstrated. Advances in molecular and biochemical techniques have allowed for the identification of cytokines produced within RA synovial tissues. Cytokines derived from activated macrophages and fibroblasts, including not only TNF and IL-1 but also IL-6, IL-8, IL-15, and IL-18 and others, have been found to be abundantly expressed, whereas T-cell–derived cytokines, such as IFN-γ, IL-2, IL-4, and IL-5, have been detected in low amounts, if at all.[250]

Furthermore, the role of the shared epitope in RA may differ from that originally proposed. The shared epitope may be responsible for the targeting and activation of autoreactive T cells through molecular mimicry with proteins from pathogens, including Epstein-Barr virus–encoded proteins and heat-shock proteins. Recent evidence from the crystal structure of the DR molecule, however, demonstrates that the amino acid residues within the shared epitope are not located directly within the peptide-binding groove and therefore may not influence the exact peptides presented by these molecules. Possible alternative contributions of the shared epitope include the shaping of the T-cell repertoire to allow for the survival of autoreactive clones and the enhancement of T-cell reactivity due to unique contact points between DR molecules bearing the shared epitope and the T-cell receptor.[250] Finally, there remains the possibility that the shared epitope is not, in fact, a disease susceptibility/severity-associated gene but that genes closely linked to the MHC locus are actually playing a role in disease susceptibility/severity.

Taken as a whole, these data suggest that in the chronic phase of RA, specific activation of T cells by a unique "RA antigen," is not the primary mechanism of disease. However, T cells may participate in

RA pathogenesis in a number of alternative ways. T cells in chronic RA may be activated by antigens present locally within the joint, including either native proteins—such as type II collagen, heat-shock proteins, aggrecan, and proteoglycans—or neo-epitopes (self-antigens not normally seen by T cells during their development), such as citrullinated proteins generated by inflammation.[251] In addition, T cells may contribute to disease pathogenesis in ways that are independent of antigen.

Cell-cell and cytokine interactions in the perpetuation of inflammation in rheumatoid arthritis

Based on studies in animal models of RA, both the initiation and perpetuation of TNF and IL-1 production within inflamed synovial tissues as well as the maintenance of an activated phenotype of synovial lining cells and sublining fibroblasts and macrophages for the continued production of these and other critical proinflammatory cytokines are essential to the pathogenesis of RA. It has been hypothesized that the chronic inflammatory state in RA is maintained by complex interactions and positive feedback loops between cell types resident within and recruited to the synovium. Many of the cytokines and growth factors previously described in this chapter, most notably TNF, IL-1, IL-6, IL-17, prostaglandins, and chemokines, contribute to these feedback loops. T cells themselves also play a role in these complex interactions. An alternative mechanism by which T cells may contribute to the maintenance of chronic inflammation in RA through antigen-independent mechanisms is by direct cell-cell interaction of previously activated T cells with macrophages and/or fibroblasts, leading to the augmented production of effector molecules, including TNF and joint-damaging enzymes. For example, membranes from synovially derived T-cell clones have been shown to stimulate the production of MMP-1 and PGE$_2$, but not the inhibitor TIMP-1, in long-term culture.[252]

Recently, an important role has also been established for IL-15 in the perpetuation of chronic inflammation in RA, owing to the ability of this cytokine to regulate synovial TNF production. As previously discussed, IL-15 is produced predominantly by synovial lining layer macrophages, although FLS and endothelial cells also produce IL-15. In early studies it was demonstrated that cell-cell contact between mitogen-activated synovial T cells and macrophages led to the production of proinflammatory mediators by these cells.[253] Similarly, T cells freshly isolated from RA synovium induce synovially derived macrophages to produce TNF *in vitro* through cell-cell contact, an effect that is maintained by the addition of IL-15. Furthermore, IL-15, expressed on the membrane of RA FLS and upregulated by T cell/fibroblast contact, induces the production of the proinflammatory cytokines TNF,[132] IFN-γ, and IL-17 by T cells in culture through mechanisms dependent on cell-cell contact. These T-cell–derived cytokines can, in turn, activate FLS to produce increased levels of membrane-bound IL-15, as well as IL-6 and IL-8.

IL-18 induces the production of TNF, as well as GM-CSF and IFN-γ, by RA synovial macrophages, an effect that is enhanced by IL-15, as well as by IL-12. IL-18 has direct activating effects on both synovial macrophages and T cells and has a potent enhancing effect on TNF production induced by T cell/monocyte interactions. Interactions between T cells and synovial macrophages and fibroblasts are mediated through CD69, LFA-1/ICAM-1 (CD54), and other ligand-receptor interactions. Figure 91.20 demonstrates interactions between resident FLS and monocytes/macrophages that produce cytokines, chemokines, and other factors that activate cells in the local environment and maintain the chronic inflammatory state. Adhesion molecules on endothelial cells are upregulated by these products, leading to the further recruitment to the synovium of inflammatory cells expressing the proper chemokine receptors. These interactions could also augment T-cell activation and stimulate B cells to produce antibodies.

Autoantibodies and immune complexes

Since the discovery of RF by Rose and Waaler and the subsequent identification of RF as an autoantibody directed against the Fc portion of IgG, autoantibodies have been thought to play a role in the pathogenesis of RA. Early theories suggested that RF might initiate disease in RA via immune complex deposition in the joint, with the subsequent fixation of complement components, the generation of chemotactic factors including C5a, and the influx of inflammatory cells to the joint. This theory was slowly abandoned, however, because RF is

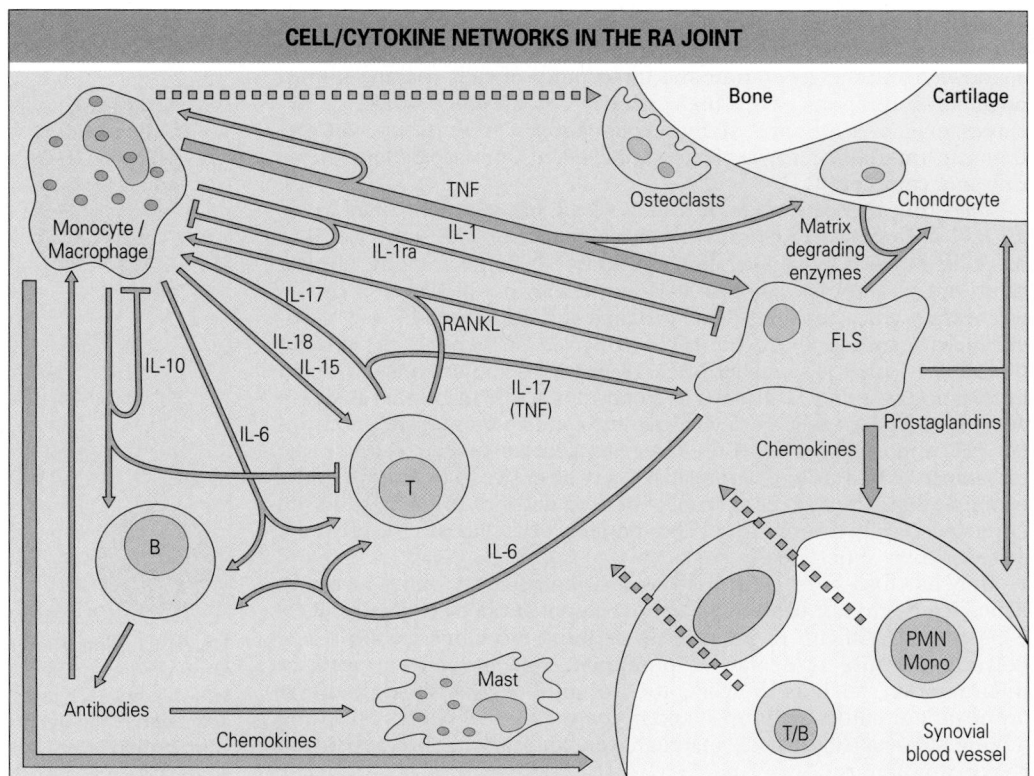

Fig. 91.20 Schematic showing some of the key cytokines and other soluble factors and the local cellular interactions that mediate rheumatoid synovitis and joint destruction. Cells are recruited into the synovium from the vasculature. Chronic inflammation in RA synovium leads to the activation of macrophages and fibroblast-like synoviocytes, resulting in joint destruction. Dashed lines depict either movement of cells (i.e., transmigration across the vascular endothelium) or differentiation of cells (i.e., differentiation of monocytes into osteoclasts). FLS, fibroblast-like synoviocyte; PMN, polymorphonuclear leukocyte (neutrophil); Mono, monocyte; Mast, mast cell.

not specific for RA. RF is present in some healthy individuals and in patients with other chronic inflammatory diseases that are not associated with synovitis, and it is absent in about 20% of patients with RA.

However, the notion that autoantibodies and immune complexes play an important role in disease pathogenesis remains plausible. Intracellular and extracellular deposits containing both immunoglobulin and C3 have been identified in synovium and on the cartilage surface in patients with RA, and there is evidence for local complement activation in RA synovial fluid. Such deposits could facilitate recruitment of inflammatory cells and activation of phagocytes. Finally, in several rodent models of RA, immune complexes or antibodies binding to endogenous components of cartilage initiate disease that is similar in many respects to human RA.[221,254]

Lessons from treatment of human RA

The importance of TNF in human RA has been demonstrated by the clinical efficacy of TNF-neutralizing agents. This finding does not, of course, illuminate the cause(s) behind excess production of TNF in the joint. Furthermore, blockade of TNF is also effective in other diseases, including ankylosing spondylitis, psoriatic arthritis, and Crohn disease, diseases that have pathogenic mechanisms that are both overlapping with and distinct from RA. However, treatment with TNF-neutralizing agents has allowed (admittedly imperfect) testing of the hypothesis that established networks of proinflammatory mediators in synovitis are self-perpetuating: in many patients with long-standing RA, synovitis improves or resolves with anti-TNF therapy, yet in most of these patients, discontinuation of effective anti-TNF treatment leads to relapse. Thus, the driving force behind the creation of the proinflammatory network remains intact and it is not adequate to simply "interrupt" the network.

The effectiveness of CTLA4-Ig (abatacept), which blocks co-stimulation of T cells by antigen-presenting cells, in established RA suggests that antigen presentation to T cells remains important in RA pathogenesis. However, because CTLA4-Ig interacts with other cells, such as macrophages, that are also clearly involved in networks of inflammation, it is possible that this agent is effective for reasons independent of co-stimulation of T cells. Similarly, the effectiveness of B-cell depletion in patients with long-standing RF-positive RA is the best evidence that autoantibodies are pathogenic but also has an alternative interpretation. B cells not only produce antibody but also present antigen to CD4+ T cells and likely participate in cytokine networks. Notably, however, B cells are only effective at presenting antigens internalized via the surface immunoglobulin receptor, so that it would be problematic to invoke the antigen-presenting function of B cells without acknowledging the generation and importance of cells making immunoglobulin receptors with high affinity for specific antigens. RF-expressing B cells are particularly adept at antigen presentation, because they can internalize any molecule attached to immunoglobulin in an immune complex.[255]

The clinical effectiveness of IL-1 blockade has also confirmed a role for IL-1 in human RA. Compared with blockade of TNF, however, IL-1 blockade in RA is not, in general, as effective in controlling the clinical signs and symptoms of disease. It is now clear that blockade of IL-1 is remarkably efficacious in several pediatric inflammatory diseases associated with mutations in the cryopyrin (*NALP3*) gene,[256] the protein product of which is involved in IL-1β processing. This has led many to question whether IL-1 plays as important a role in human RA as it does in rodent models. Nevertheless, it would be premature to diminish the importance of IL-1 in the pathogenesis of RA, because the imbalance of IL-1 and its antagonists may be easier to overcome in the pediatric diseases and the efficiency of drug delivery to the critical site (almost certainly the joint in RA but possibly other sites in the pediatric diseases) may differ greatly.

IL-6 has also been confirmed as an important cytokine in established RA by clinical trials using a monoclonal antibody to the IL-6R.[115] This effect is difficult to interpret in defining mechanisms of disease, however, because IL-6 plays a prominent role in many aspects of inflammation, such as the generation of antibody responses and systemic inflammatory responses, and in the cytokine networks operating among synovial fibroblasts, macrophages, and other cell types in the rheumatoid joint.

Unifying hypothesis

A unifying hypothesis for RA pathogenesis must attempt to incorporate information obtained from both human RA and from animal models of disease. What seems clear is that RA can best be conceptualized in stages that include disease initiation, establishment and maintenance of chronic inflammation, and joint tissue destruction (Fig. 91.21), the latter two of which certainly coexist temporally. The event or events that initiate RA are likely to be distinct from those responsible for the establishment and perpetuation of chronic inflammation in the synovium, and the destruction of joint structures proceeds by distinct mechanisms that are driven by chronic synovial inflammation.

Recent evidence from animal models suggests that a variety of autoimmune responses to joint-associated, but not necessarily joint-specific, antigens can initiate RA-like disease. The appearance of RF and ACPA significantly before clinical onset of disease in humans suggests that there is a breakdown of T-cell tolerance early in disease, providing help for autoantibody production. Several possible pathways could be invoked for the initiation of autoimmunity, including molecular mimicry (the cross-reaction of T cells initially activated by foreign peptides with self-peptides) or the generation of neo-epitopes within the joint through joint trauma or other mechanisms (Fig. 91.22). Certain individuals may be genetically susceptible to these events, either through the expression of specific MHC alleles or by other genetic factors predisposing to autoimmunity. Autoantibodies produced very early in disease could form immune complexes in synovium and/or on the surface of joint cartilage or deposit in the synovial vasculature, leading to activation and recruitment of cells of the innate immune system, including neutrophils, mast cells, and macrophages. Bacterial products including DNA containing CpG motifs and/or cell wall fragments containing peptidoglycans, which have been demonstrated to be present in RA synovial tissues, could engage TLRs on resident macrophages and DCs, leading to activation of these cells and the subsequent production of proinflammatory mediators and possibly antigen presentation to T cells. Stimulation through TLR2 could contribute to the early activation of FLS in RA. Mediators produced by cells of the innate immune system could augment vascular permeability and promote the generation of adaptive immune responses by T and B cells, setting up the potential for amplification of immune responses.

Once disease is initiated, the chronic inflammatory phase ensues. Deposition of autoantibodies in immune complexes, and/or local acti-

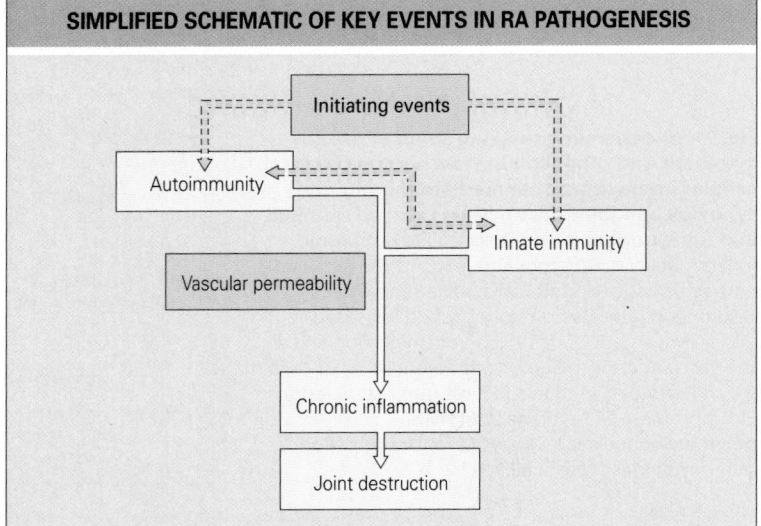

Fig. 91.21 Simplified schematic of key events in RA pathogenesis. Dotted arrows reflect pathways that are plausible but for which there is no detailed information, such as the origins of autoimmunity, the source of initial activation of innate immune cells in the synovium, and the possible contribution of activation of innate immune cells to the initiation or amplification of autoimmune responses.

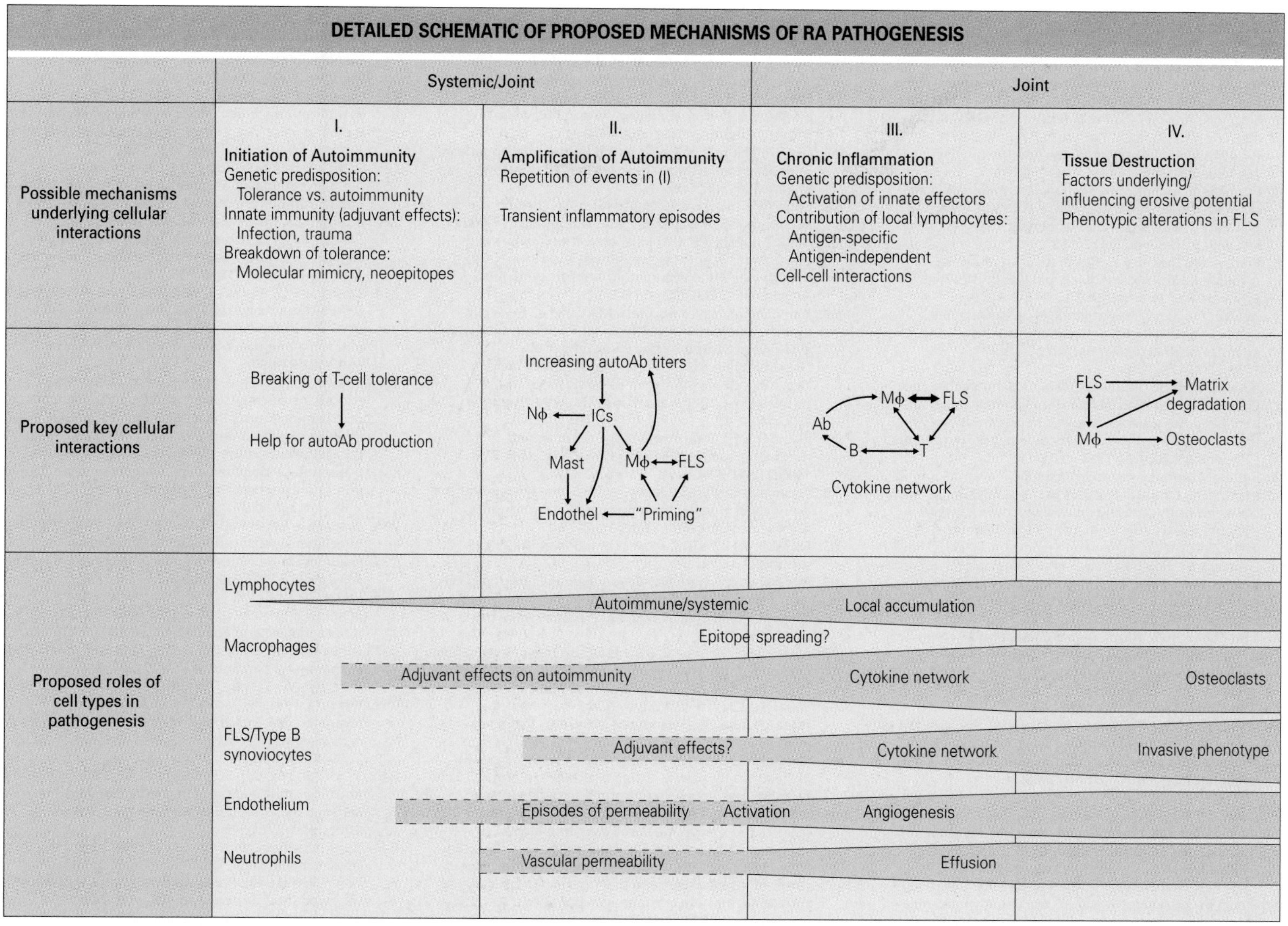

Fig. 91.22 **Detailed schematic of proposed mechanisms of RA pathogenesis.** The early phases of RA pathogenesis are speculative but probably involve initiation of autoimmunity and activation of the innate immune system (stage I) and amplification of autoimmunity (stage II). These events take place both systemically and within the joint. Pathogenic events in the joint-based chronic inflammatory phase (stage III) are better established. Contributions of immune complexes, antigen-reactive T cells, and antigen-independent T cells likely vary among patients. Tissue destruction (stage IV) coexists temporally with chronic inflammation (stage III). Changes in the numbers and activity of various cell types over time in the pathogenesis of RA are depicted in the bottom panel, with events depicted in stages I and II being speculative.

vation of antigen-specific T cells, could lead initially to the production of cytokines, with subsequent induction of neo-angiogenesis and the further influx of inflammatory cells to the synovium. Cell-cell interactions within synovial tissues result in the amplification of cytokine production and activation of synovial macrophages and fibroblasts. T cells could provide help to B cells for local antibody production, which would likely diversify to include additional autoantigens in a phenomenon known as "epitope spreading." However, T cells could also play a role in the chronic inflammatory phase of disease by mechanisms, described earlier, that are antigen independent. By a combination of such events that may differ among patients, cytokine networks are established, leading to the chronic production of critical mediators such as TNF and IL-1 (see Fig. 91.22). In the stage of tissue destruction, activated FLS adopt an invasive phenotype and elaborate degradative enzymes that destroy cartilage. In addition, production of RANKL, IL-17, TNF, IL-1, and other factors creates a pro-osteoclastogenic envi-

ronment, leading to the differentiation and activation of osteoclasts and the destruction of bone.

CONCLUSION

Tremendous progress has been made in understanding the pathogenic mechanisms involved in RA, particularly with regard to the mechanisms involved in the chronic phase of this disease. Out of this work have come new and effective targeted therapeutic interventions that have benefited RA patients, as well as new concepts for future therapies. However, there are still many unanswered questions, especially with regard to the initiating events in RA and the exact pathway involved in the establishment of chronic disease. The inroads that have now been made both in the clinical and basic science arenas certainly set the stage for further investigation and a clearer understanding of these mechanisms in the future.

KEY REFERENCES

1. Barland P, Novikoff AB, Hamerman D. Electron microscopy of the human synovial membrane. J Cell Biol 1962;14:207-220.

3. Singh JA, Arayssi T, Duray P, Schumacher HR. Immunohistochemistry of normal human knee synovium: a quantitative study. Ann Rheum Dis 2004;63:785-790.

4. Edwards JC, Willoughby DA. Demonstration of bone marrow–derived cells in synovial lining by means of giant intracellular granules as genetic markers. Ann Rheum Dis 1982;41(2):177-182.

6. Klimiuk PA, Goronzy JJ, Bjornsson J, et al. Tissue cytokine patterns distinguish variants of rheumatoid synovitis. Am J Pathol 1997;151:1311-1319.

11. Zvaifler NJ, Tsai V, Alsalameh S, et al. Pannocytes: distinctive cells found in rheumatoid arthritis articular cartilage erosions. Am J Pathol 1997;150:1125-1138.

12. Singh JA, Pando JA, Tomaszewski J, Schumacher HR. Quantitative analysis of immunohistological features of very early rheumatoid synovitis in disease modifying antirheumatic drug- and corticosteroid-naive patients. J Rheumatol 2004;31:1281-1285.

13. Soden M, Rooney M, Cullen A, et al. Immunohistological features in the synovium obtained from clinically uninvolved knee joints of patients with rheumatoid arthritis. Br J Rheumatol 1989;28:287-292.

15. Firestein GS, Boyle DL, Yu C, et al. Synovial interleukin-1 receptor antagonist and interleukin-1 balance in rheumatoid arthritis. Arthritis Rheum 1994;37:644-652.

16. Chu CQ, Field M, Allard S, et al. Detection of cytokines at the cartilage/pannus junction in patients with rheumatoid arthritis: implications for the role of cytokines in cartilage destruction and repair. Br J Rheumatol 1992;31:653-661.

17. Chu CQ, Field M, Feldmann M, Maini RN. Localization of tumor necrosis factor alpha in synovial tissues and at the cartilage-pannus junction in patients with rheumatoid arthritis. Arthritis Rheum 1991;34:1125-1132.

18. Deleuran BW, Chu CQ, Field M, et al. Localization of interleukin-1 alpha, type 1 interleukin-1 receptor and interleukin-1 receptor antagonist in the synovial membrane and cartilage/pannus junction in rheumatoid arthritis. Br J Rheumatol 1992;31:801-809.

19. Firestein GS, Alvaro-Gracia JM, Maki R, Alvaro-Garcia JM. Quantitative analysis of cytokine gene expression in rheumatoid arthritis. J Immunol 1990;144:3347-3353.

23. Kinne RW, Brauer R, Stuhlmuller B, et al. Macrophages in rheumatoid arthritis. Arthritis Res 2000;2:189-202.

26. Brennan F, Foey A. Cytokine regulation in RA synovial tissue: role of T cell/macrophage contact-dependent interactions. Arthritis Res 2002;4(Suppl 3):S177-S182.

30. Deleuran BW, Chu CQ, Field M, et al. Localization of tumor necrosis factor receptors in the synovial tissue and cartilage-pannus junction in patients with rheumatoid arthritis: implications for local actions of tumor necrosis factor alpha. Arthritis Rheum 1992;35:1170-1178.

31. Okamoto H, Yamamura M, Morita Y, et al. The synovial expression and serum levels of interleukin-6, interleukin-11, leukemia inhibitory factor and oncostatin M in rheumatoid arthritis. Arthritis Rheum 1997;40:1096-1105.

32. Mino T, Sugiyama E, Taki H, et al. Interleukin-1alpha and tumor necrosis factor alpha synergistically stimulate prostaglandin E2-dependent production of interleukin-11 in rheumatoid synovial fibroblasts. Arthritis Rheum 1998;41:2004-2013.

45. Fox DA. The role of T cells in the immunopathogenesis of rheumatoid arthritis: new perspectives. Arthritis Rheum 1997;40:598-609.

48. Cope AP. Studies of T-cell activation in chronic inflammation. Arthritis Res 2002;4(Suppl 3):S197-S211.

52. Nanki T, Lipsky PE. Cytokine, activation marker and chemokine receptor expression by individual CD4(+) memory T cells in rheumatoid arthritis synovium. Arthritis Res 2000;2(5):415-423.

69. Brennan FM, Hayes AL, Ciesielski CJ, et al. Evidence that rheumatoid arthritis synovial T cells are similar to cytokine-activated T cells: involvement of phosphatidylinositol 3-kinase and nuclear factor kappaB pathways in tumor necrosis factor alpha production in rheumatoid arthritis. Arthritis Rheum 2002;46:31-41.

75. Pillinger MH, Abramson SB. The neutrophil in rheumatoid arthritis. Rheum Dis Clin North Am 1995;21:691-714.

79. Thomas R, Davis LS, Lipsky PE. Rheumatoid synovium is enriched in mature antigen-presenting dendritic cells. J Immunol 1994;152:2613-2623.

83. Nigrovic PA, Lee DM. Mast cells in inflammatory arthritis. Arthritis Res Ther 2005;7:1-11.

88. Middleton J, Americh L, Gayon R, et al. Endothelial cell phenotypes in the rheumatoid synovium: activated, angiogenic, apoptotic and leaky. Arthritis Res Ther 2004;6:60-72.

93. Monach PA, Benoist C, Mathis D. The role of antibodies in mouse models of rheumatoid arthritis and relevance to human disease. Adv Immunol 2004;82:217-248.

103. Dinarello CA. The IL-1 family and inflammatory diseases. Clin Exp Rheumatol 2002;20(5 Suppl 27):S1-13.

108. Firestein GS, Xu WD, Townsend K, et al. Cytokines in chronic inflammatory arthritis: I. Failure to detect T cell lymphokines (interleukin 2 and interleukin 3) and presence of macrophage colony-stimulating factor (CSF-1) and a novel mast cell growth factor in rheumatoid synovitis. J Exp Med 1988;168:1573-1586.

109. Miossec P, Naviliat M, Dupuy d'Angeac A, et al. Low levels of interleukin-4 and high levels of transforming growth factor beta in rheumatoid synovitis. Arthritis Rheum 1990;33:1180-1187.

135. Toh ML, Miossec P. The role of T cells in rheumatoid arthritis: new subsets and new targets. Curr Opin Rheumatol 2007;19:284-288.

140. Chabaud M, Durand JM, Buchs N, et al. Human interleukin-17: a T cell–derived proinflammatory cytokine produced by the rheumatoid synovium. Arthritis Rheum 1999;42:963-970.

142. Liew FY, Wei XQ, McInnes IB. Role of interleukin 18 in rheumatoid arthritis. Ann Rheum Dis 2003;62(Suppl 2):ii48-ii50.

166. Bell AL, Magill MK, McKane WR, et al. Measurement of colony-stimulating factors in synovial fluid: potential clinical value. Rheumatol Int 1995;14:177-182.

176. Koch AE. Chemokines and their receptors in rheumatoid arthritis: future targets? Arthritis Rheum 2005;52:710-721.

221. Matsumoto I, Maccioni M, Lee DM, et al. How antibodies to a ubiquitous cytoplasmic enzyme may provoke joint-specific autoimmune disease. Nat Immunol 2002;3:360-365.

223. Gravallese EM, Darling JM, Ladd AL, et al. In situ hybridization studies of stromelysin and collagenase messenger RNA expression in rheumatoid synovium. Arthritis Rheum 1991;34:1076-1084.

225. Parks WC, Wilson CL, Lopez-Boado YS. Matrix metalloproteinases as modulators of inflammation and innate immunity. Nat Rev Immunol 2004;4:617-629.

229. Mudgett JS, Hutchinson NI, Chartrain NA, et al. Susceptibility of stromelysin 1-deficient mice to collagen-induced arthritis and cartilage destruction. Arthritis Rheum 1998;41:110-121.

230. Konttinen YT, Ainola M, Valleala H, et al. Analysis of 16 different matrix metalloproteinases (MMP-1 to MMP-20) in the synovial membrane: different profiles in trauma and rheumatoid arthritis. Ann Rheum Dis 1999;58:691-697.

232. Keyszer G, Redlich A, Haupl T, et al. Differential expression of cathepsins B and L compared with matrix metalloproteinases and their respective inhibitors in rheumatoid arthritis and osteoarthritis: a parallel investigation by semiquantitative reverse transcriptase-polymerase chain reaction and immunohistochemistry. Arthritis Rheum 1998;41:1378-1387.

234. Gravallese EM, Harada Y, Wang JT, et al. Identification of cell types responsible for bone resorption in rheumatoid arthritis and juvenile rheumatoid arthritis. Am J Pathol 1998;152:943-951.

235. Lacey DL, Timms E, Tan HL, et al. Osteoprotegerin ligand is a cytokine that regulates osteoclast differentiation and activation. Cell 1998;93:165-176.

237. Gravallese EM, Manning C, Tsay A, et al. Synovial tissue in rheumatoid arthritis is a source of osteoclast differentiation factor. Arthritis Rheum 2000;43:250-258.

239. Kong YY, Feige U, Sarosi I, et al. Activated T cells regulate bone loss and joint destruction in adjuvant arthritis through osteoprotegerin ligand. Nature 1999;402:304-309.

240. Pettit AR, Ji H, Von Stechow D, et al. TRANCE/RANKL knockout mice are protected from bone erosion in a serum transfer model of arthritis. Am J Pathol 2001;159:1689-1699.

244. Jiang Y, Genant HK, Watt I, et al. A multicenter, double-blind, dose-ranging, randomized, placebo-controlled study of recombinant human interleukin-1 receptor antagonist in patients with rheumatoid arthritis: radiologic progression and correlation of Genant and Larsen scores. Arthritis Rheum 2000;43:1001-1009.

245. Lipsky PE, Van Der Heijde DM, St Clair EW, et al. Infliximab and methotrexate in the treatment of rheumatoid arthritis. Anti-Tumor Necrosis Factor Trial in Rheumatoid Arthritis with Concomitant Therapy Study Group. N Engl J Med 2000;343:1594-1602.

248. Gregersen PK, Silver J, Winchester RJ. The shared epitope hypothesis: an approach to understanding the molecular genetics of susceptibility to rheumatoid arthritis. Arthritis Rheum 1987;30:1205-1213.

249. Rantapaa-Dahlqvist S, De Jong BA, Berglin E, et al. Antibodies against cyclic citrullinated peptide and IgA rheumatoid factor predict the development of rheumatoid arthritis. Arthritis Rheum 2003;48:2741-2749.

250. Firestein GS. Evolving concepts of rheumatoid arthritis. Nature 2003;423:356-361.

REFERENCES

Full references for this chapter can be found on www.expertconsult.com.

Evaluation and management of early inflammatory polyarthritis

Klaus P. Machold

92

- Early institution of DMARD therapy in rheumatoid arthritis (RA) can prevent joint damage and long-term disability.
- Recognition of RA early is important to interfere with persistence and especially damage by instituting DMARD therapy early.
- Differential diagnostic support comes from number of involved joints, duration of symptoms, and presence of serologic markers such as acute-phase reactants and autoantibodies.
- The ACR/EULAR classification criteria for RA will likely support early diagnosis.
- Early referral of patients with synovitis to the rheumatologist is a prerequisite for early diagnosis and therapy.

THE CONCEPT OF EARLY POLYARTHRITIS

Many inflammatory rheumatic diseases are characterized by a chronic course, spanning years or even decades. From this perspective, the "early" period of arthritis was (rather arbitrarily) assumed to be in the range of up to several years.[1-3]

Research in early arthritis patient cohorts over the past years, however, has demonstrated a remarkably short period of time during which an arthritis (in particular, rheumatoid arthritis [RA]) may be regarded as "early."[2,4,5] This period has also been named the "window of opportunity," implying that interventions such as treatment with disease-modifying antirheumatic drugs (DMARDs) would have a much greater effect compared with DMARDs initiated at a later time during the "disease career."

Among the (chronic) inflammatory arthritides, RA is considered the most problematic, owing to its characteristics of joint destruction, functional impairment, disability, and, finally, premature mortality.[6] In addition, several other arthritides with destructive potential, most notably psoriatic arthritis, may show similar courses and outcomes.[7] Retardation or prevention of progression of the destructive processes is possible both in early and later disease stages,[8,9] mainly by use of corticosteroids, "conventional" DMARDs, biologic agents, or combinations thereof.

Studies showing different cytokine patterns in the synovium of patients with early arthritis[10] support the hypothesis that the early months of (rheumatoid) arthritis are characterized by a different pathophysiology compared with later stages. This suggests that the pathogenetic events may change in the course of the disease. These observations are corroborated by clinical studies showing that, in RA, remission was more frequently induced in patients with disease duration of 4 months or less compared with longer duration.[11] Likewise, delayed radiologic progression was demonstrated if DMARD treatment was instituted early after symptom onset as compared with delayed therapy.[12] In contrast to these observations, other studies comparing early RA (defined as a symptom duration of <1 year) and established RA were unable to demonstrate any differences between early and long-standing disease by immunohistologic analysis of the synovium, including an assessment of the composition of cellular infiltrates as well as cytokine expression.[13,14]

Given the cumulative nature of (radiologic) damage that may occur in chronic destructive arthritis, it is also possible to define "early (poly-) arthritis" as a disease (stage) in which this damage, which is typical not only for RA but also for other entities such as psoriatic arthritis,

has not yet occurred. Thus, "early" is not defined by a certain time threshold, which, despite the mentioned advances in our knowledge, has to be somewhat arbitrary, but by the opportunity to preserve joint integrity by timely intervention. In clinical practice, a substantial majority of rheumatologists now adhere to a definition of "early RA," which limits its duration at 3 months.[15] It has been hypothesized, however, that the threshold for good clinical response may be even shorter, about 8 weeks.[16] In any case, even if destruction has already occurred, and thus the destructive nature of the disease been documented, immediate institution of an effective treatment strategy (see later) is mandatory to delay the pace of further damage.

This pace of damage occurring in RA varies widely. The majority of patients who developed erosive disease did so within the first year after symptom onset, and approximately 75% of RA patients had joint erosions at 2 years.[17,18] These findings underscore the necessity to consider effective treatment well before the first year of symptoms has elapsed. On the other hand, in a sizable minority of patients with overt synovitis, arthritis went on to run a relatively benign course with self-limiting disease and/or little, if any, damage.[18,19] Likewise, long-term patterns of progression in those patients who develop destructive/erosive disease are quite variable.[20] Sharp and associates[21] suggested that the pace of progression of radiologic damage slows down after longer duration. However, this slowing was only modest and did not appear before the third decade after disease onset. At this time a substantial proportion of the joints (approximately 20%) of these patients already were described to show "maximum erosion scores." This observation further supports the requirement of DMARD treatment as early as possible to prevent this catastrophic outcome.

CRITERIA FOR EARLY ARTHRITIS

At the time of first presentation to a physician, patients with arthritis have substantial variability in clinical signs and symptoms as well as in the presence or absence of laboratory or imaging abnormalities.[20,22] Well-validated criteria that would allow early differentiation of groups of patients with regard to their arthritis at this stage currently do not exist. Current classification criteria for "established" RA[23] (as well as other rheumatic diseases such as the vasculitides, systemic lupus erythematosus, psoriatic arthritis, osteoarthritis, and so on) have been developed with the clinical researcher in mind and are intended not primarily for diagnosis but rather should be used to separate groups of patients with a given disease from those with other diseases and to standardize the characteristics of these patients for clinical studies. Evaluation of an individual patient early in her or his disease has to account for many more features that characterize the clinical picture of an individual's arthritis and are useful primarily for the physician to guide further diagnostic evaluation and therapeutic decisions. In addition, given the inherent variability not only of RA but also of most other arthritides that may present clinically in a similar fashion to RA and other rheumatic diseases at onset, prognostication is an important aim for the clinician and the patient to select the appropriate therapy.[24] With this knowledge in mind, recent efforts have been directed primarily at identifying sets of risk factors that would help define "early RA," or, as has been done in the development of the newly proposed RA classification criteria by the American College of Rheumatology (ACR) and the European League Against Rheumatism (EULAR), patients who would have to be treated with DMARDs (e.g., methotrexate).

The Leiden group has analyzed a cohort suffering from undifferentiated arthritis (i.e., arthritis that could not be classified according to

TABLE 92.1 ACR/EULAR 2010 CLASSIFICATION CRITERIA FOR RHEUMATOID ARTHRITIS*

Joints (0-5)	
1 large joint	0
2-10 large joints	1
1-3 small joints (large joints not counted)	2
4-10 small joints (large joints not counted)	3
>10 joints (at least one small joint)	5
Serology (0-3)	
Negative RF *and* negative ACPAs	0
Low-positive RF *or* low-positive ACPAs	2
High-positive RF *or* high-positive ACPAs	3
Symptom duration (0-1)	
<6 weeks	0
≥6 weeks	1
Acute-phase reactants (0-1)	
Normal CRP *and* normal ESR	0
Abnormal CRP *or* abnormal ESR	1

*Cutpoint for RA: ≥6/10).
RF, rheumatoid factor; ACPAs, anticitrullinated peptide antibodies; CRP, C-reactive protein; ESR, erythrocyte sedimentation rate.

ACR criteria and lasting <1 year) and developed a scoring system to predict RA. This system was externally validated using a control group with identical characteristics (undifferentiated arthritis of up to 1 year's duration). The prediction score includes easily determinable clinical and laboratory characteristics (age, gender, distribution and symmetry of arthritis, morning stiffness, tender and swollen joint counts, C-reactive protein (CRP), rheumatoid factor (RF), and anticitrullinated peptide antibodies (ACPAs) and yielded positive and negative predictive values in the validation group in the vicinity of 90%.[25] This prediction system, although not fully and thoroughly validated in different settings, may guide treatment decisions and thus fulfill the requirement of both avoiding overtreatment and initiate (even very aggressive) treatment in patients who are highly likely to develop RA. The recently developed ACR/EULAR criteria for RA classification took a slightly different approach insofar as the criteria were developed using data from over 3000 patients who were determined to be (or not to be) in need of DMARD treatment by an expert panel from both North America and Europe. This set of criteria thus aims at identifying the necessity for DMARD treatment rather than "diagnosis" and encompasses the pattern of joint involvement (large vs. medium vs. small as well as number of joints), serology (RF and ACPA), duration of synovitis, and acute-phase reactants. These new criteria are shown in Table 92.1 and will need validation over the next years.[26]

CLINICAL DETECTION OF SYNOVITIS

Arthritis is usually painful; conversely, joint pain does not always correspond to synovial inflammation. The hallmark of synovial inflammation—swelling—is frequently subtle or hidden beneath other tissues such as muscle or bone (hip and shoulder) or subcutaneous fat (in obese patients). This clinical problem leads to considerable variability and uncertainty in clinical assessment of synovitis with high inter-observer variability.[27] In particular, ultrasonography has been consistently shown to be more sensitive than clinical examination in detecting synovial fluid accumulation.[28-30] However, because this technique is still not universally available, is time consuming, and is costly, in clinical practice one has to rely on clinical examination, which, at least for the purpose of evaluating joints longitudinally, should be done in a "standardized" way. EULAR has issued an illustrated guidebook of clinical assessment offering instructions on joint examination.[31] Because inflamed joints are usually painful and pain may be present even if joint swelling is subtle, a positive metatarsophalangeal (MTP)/

metacarpophalangeal (MCP) joint compression test (Gaenslen test) offers additional clinical evidence for involvement of MCP and MTP joints. In fact, a positive compression test provides a major contribution to diagnostic algorithms in early arthritis and is present in more than 60% of the patients who will be diagnosed as having RA. Stiffness after rest (frequently referred to as "morning stiffness") of long (more than several minutes) duration is another typical symptom of inflammatory joint disease. The 1982 classification criteria for established RA require a duration of at least 1 hour. Typically, in other disorders, such as osteoarthritis, stiffness is in general much shorter and only in the order of a few minutes. Therefore, morning stiffness of more than 30 minutes and definitely more than 45 minutes may be seen as characteristic for an inflammatory joint disease such as RA.[25]

Many patients who subsequently will be diagnosed as having RA have low numbers of swollen and/or tender joints ("joint counts") at disease onset or at first presentation to the physician. In one study on a cohort of very early arthritis patients, more than 25% of the individuals who became erosive within 1 year had 5 or fewer swollen joints at first presentation, employing a 28-joint count.[18] In another recent study, early arthritis patients who developed RA had a median of 4 swollen joints and more than 25% had only up to four tender joints using a 44-joint count. Recognizing the implications of these observations, recommendations of a task force of the EULAR suggested the consideration of early RA even with only one persistently swollen joint.[25,32] Nevertheless, the proposed algorithms for early detection of RA[25,33] as well as the ACR/EULAR classification criteria for RA[26] assigned more weight to polyarthritis as compared with arthritis in fewer joints.

EVALUATION AND DIFFERENTIAL DIAGNOSIS OF EARLY ARTHRITIS

Arthritis is a clinical manifestation of many diseases, such as metabolic, degenerative, infectious, and neoplastic disorders. In evaluating arthritis, special attention should be directed to the history of the patient, extra-articular signs of disease, the pattern of joint involvement, and serologic and imaging studies.

In the light of the lack of validated recommendations as to which studies need (or need not) to be performed in early arthritis, clinicians may adhere to either of two sets of recommendations concerning early arthritis. One of these calls for rapid referral to a rheumatologist in the event of clinical suspicion of RA.[34] According to these guidelines, clinical suspicion needs to be supported by the presence of three characteristics: greater than or equal to 3 swollen joints, positive compression (Gaenslen) test on MCPs or MTPs, and morning stiffness of more than 30 minutes. The other expert panel recommends referral of patients with one or more swollen joint within 6 weeks of symptom onset to a rheumatologist (to prevent a longer delay of referral of patients with potential RA). Careful history-taking and clinical and laboratory examinations to exclude other diseases are also suggested. It is emphasized that the probability of persistence increases with the number of swollen and tender joints, with the presence of acute-phase reactants, and with the autoantibody (RF, ACPA) levels; radiographs should be taken to reveal erosive disease.[32]

History and extra-articular clinical signs

Transient arthritis (with viral infections being the most frequent cause) is usually easily differentiated from RA owing to its self-limiting character. Therefore, in a patient whose arthritis has been present for only several days (up to a few weeks), it may be sufficient, in addition to the joint examination, to take a thorough history with special attention to exposure to infectious agents (such as contact with people such as children with a rash or a febrile illness), preceding infection or rash in the patient herself/himself, fever, weight loss, or previous arthritis episodes (such as may occur in crystal arthritis).

Once the duration of arthritis exceeds a few weeks (with the threshold most likely lying between 6 and 12 weeks), the differential diagnosis becomes much broader. Therefore, in this instance, seronegative spondyloarthropathies such as reactive arthritis, ankylosing spondylitis, arthritis associated with inflammatory bowel disease, and psoriatic arthritis have to be considered. In addition, sarcoidosis with arthritis (Löfgren syndrome), connective tissue diseases, rheumatic fever, gout, and pseudogout (the "crystal arthropathies"), as well as osteoarthritis (with inflammatory activity) need to be included in the differential diagnosis. Thus, the examination and history have to include signs of psoriasis (or patients may have a family member diagnosed with psoriasis), urogenital tract or gastrointestinal infection, which is frequently accompanied by abdominal symptoms, and "inflammatory" (low) back pain. Extra-articular involvement (e.g., of eyes, mucous membranes, skin) may be subtle and needs to be sought and inquired about. Erythema nodosum may be a characteristic sign of sarcoidosis or inflammatory bowel disease, and the arthritis frequently involves the ankle joints symmetrically. In addition, in sarcoidosis typical changes are present in the chest radiograph, and upper or lower gastrointestinal endoscopy frequently reveals typical changes for Crohn disease or ulcerative colitis. The rare connective tissue diseases generally show additional clinical manifestations such as myalgias, skin changes (e.g., an ultraviolet light–induced rash, alopecia, sclerosis, telangiectasia, Raynaud phenomenon), lymphadenopathy, and manifestations of internal organ involvement. A history of an untreated upper respiratory tract infection (e.g., tonsillitis) may be suggestive of rheumatic fever (or a reactive arthritis, if the lag time between the infection and the arthritis is less than 1 or 2 weeks). The characteristic history of crystal arthropathies (including acute onset of gout after heavy meals or alcohol intake, immobilization, chemotherapy, and preceding episodes of a similar arthritis) is usually diagnostic.

Patterns of joint involvement

Chronic arthritis may show a number of more or less distinct "joint patterns" (Fig. 92.1). This has also been recognized in the development of the new algorithms for risk stratification mentioned earlier. Monarthritis or oligoarthritis (i.e., involvement of two to four joints), although not included in the topic of this chapter and considered a sign of less aggressive disease course, may nevertheless represent the initial presentation of a chronic destructive arthritis. Involvement of small joints such as of the hands, in particular, is considered highly suggestive of a high probability of a destructive arthritis. Clinical manifestation of arthritis mostly in large joints, asymmetric involvement, and early spinal symptoms may be indicative of a seronegative spondyloarthropathy. In addition (inflammatory/active) osteoarthritis of the hands may present as an oligoarticular or polyarticular arthritis, albeit usually with clinically detectable preexisting changes indicative of bony appositions (Bouchard or Heberden nodes). Although these patterns are sometimes quite characteristic and may be diagnostic (e.g., if psoriatic lesions are present), exceptions and sometimes "overlap" manifestations (e.g., development of classic seropositive RA in an older individual with already preexisting Bouchard nodes) are frequent.

Laboratory and imaging studies

In a patient with early polyarthritis, careful history and clinical examination with special attention to synovitic swelling and its distribution may allow a preliminary classification and thus an appropriate estimate of risk for chronic or destructive/disabling disease. Laboratory and imaging studies, however, not only provide additional information with regard to this risk but may also occasionally show unexpected results, such as evidence for crystal deposits on radiographs or ultrasonography or high-titer antinuclear antibodies in a patient with symmetric polyarthritis of the hands. Therefore, all classification, stratification, and diagnostic criteria also include recommendations to perform a minimum set of laboratory investigations as well as imaging studies to exclude other disease entities than RA. In addition, if the clinical "index of suspicion" is high enough, extended laboratory investigations (e.g., screen for antinuclear antibodies, infections, metabolic disease, and genotyping, e.g., for HLA-B27 and other genetic traits) may be justified. Most criteria recommend performing tests for acute-phase reactants and for RF as well as, more recently, ACPAs.

RF, an antibody specific for IgG, has been known to be one of the characteristics of RA. It has been used to diagnose, classify, and characterize patients with this disease. Between 46% and 75% of patients with early RA test positive for RF.[18,35] However, RF is not

pathognomonic for RA and frequently occurs in other disorders, such as connective tissue diseases and chronic infections, and in healthy individuals, mostly in low titers.[36] High-titer RF (RF > 50 IU/mL), in contrast, has been shown to be highly discriminative between RA and non-RA in patients with early arthritis.[37] More recently, ACPAs have been described to occur relatively specifically in RA[38]; ACPA are found in the sera of about 50% of patients with early arthritis diagnosed subsequently as RA and may be present in patients even before symptom onset. Probably even more importantly, RF and/or ACPAs also give some prognostic information: the presence of these antibodies is highly predictive of erosive disease and associated with more rapid progression of joint destruction.[18,38] Moreover, RF is associated with persistence of arthritis.[39]

In addition to these (relatively specific) autoantibodies, an elevated acute-phase response is another, albeit non-specific, hallmark of early inflammatory arthritis. Laboratory testing usually reveals higher acute-phase parameters, such as CRP or ESR, in early arthritis patients destined to suffer from RA than in those who do not develop RA.[25] Characteristically, in the seronegative spondyloarthritides, the acute-phase reaction appears to be less pronounced. However, the variability between patients is considerable and makes the distinction difficult for individual patients owing to the broad overlap. Moreover, initially normal or negative tests for inflammatory markers do not rule out later evolution of erosive disease. On the other hand, joint damage in early RA increases with increasing acute-phase reactant levels.[18]

Because the genetic background of RA as well as reactive arthritis, ankylosing spondylitis, systemic lupus erythematosus, and other rarer rheumatic diseases is quite characteristic,[40,41] at least in white populations, it is tempting to use these tests for differential diagnosis. However, costs of accurate analyses as well as the complexities of the influences of the genetic background of a given individual currently preclude the use of genetic testing as a diagnostic or prognostic tool in most cases.

Currently, the only standard technique for visualizing the typical changes associated with RA and other destructive arthritides is conventional radiography. Unfortunately, this technique is notoriously insensitive to small and/or early changes.[28] Magnetic resonance imaging (MRI) and ultrasonography may allow detection of erosions earlier than traditional radiographic techniques.[42] However, these modalities have not yet been sufficiently validated and their diagnostic value is not undisputed.[43] Nevertheless, both MRI and ultrasonography are more sensitive than clinical examination to identify synovitis and joint effusions. Importantly, if the clinical presentation raises suspicion of a shoulder joint or spinal involvement (e.g., sacroiliitis in the context of psoriatic arthritis or ankylosing spondylitis), MRI is currently probably the most sensitive and accurate method for confirming such a diagnosis.

It is also important to recognize that the diagnosis of erosions by radiography also depends on the experience of the reader. Thus, only a specialist (radiologist, rheumatologist) experienced in assessing RA radiographs should perform the reading. The presence of erosions, which occur in a majority of RA patients, is very characteristic, albeit not to be expected in the very early stages of the disease. Occurrence of erosions early after onset of symptoms is indicative of RA[33]; however, at a mean of 8 weeks from symptom onset, these radiographic changes are found in only up to 10% of patients.[18] Therefore, this cannot be considered a characteristic of early RA. More importantly, the very aim of early diagnosis and treatment is the prevention of erosions and other signs of (possibly irreversible) joint destruction. Thus, the diagnosis needs to be made before the appearance of evidence for joint destruction.

PROGNOSTICATION IN EARLY ARTHRITIS

The major purpose of diagnosing a disease in a given patient is to guide treatment decisions on the basis of prognosis of the disease. This prognosis, in turn, determines the timing of treatment as well as its intensity. Furthermore, the necessary frequency of reassessment and follow-up will depend on these decisions. From the patients' view, this prognosis will also determine the risk that has to be taken through potentially toxic drugs or unpleasant or time-consuming treatments, such as wearing splints, undergoing physical therapy, or performing

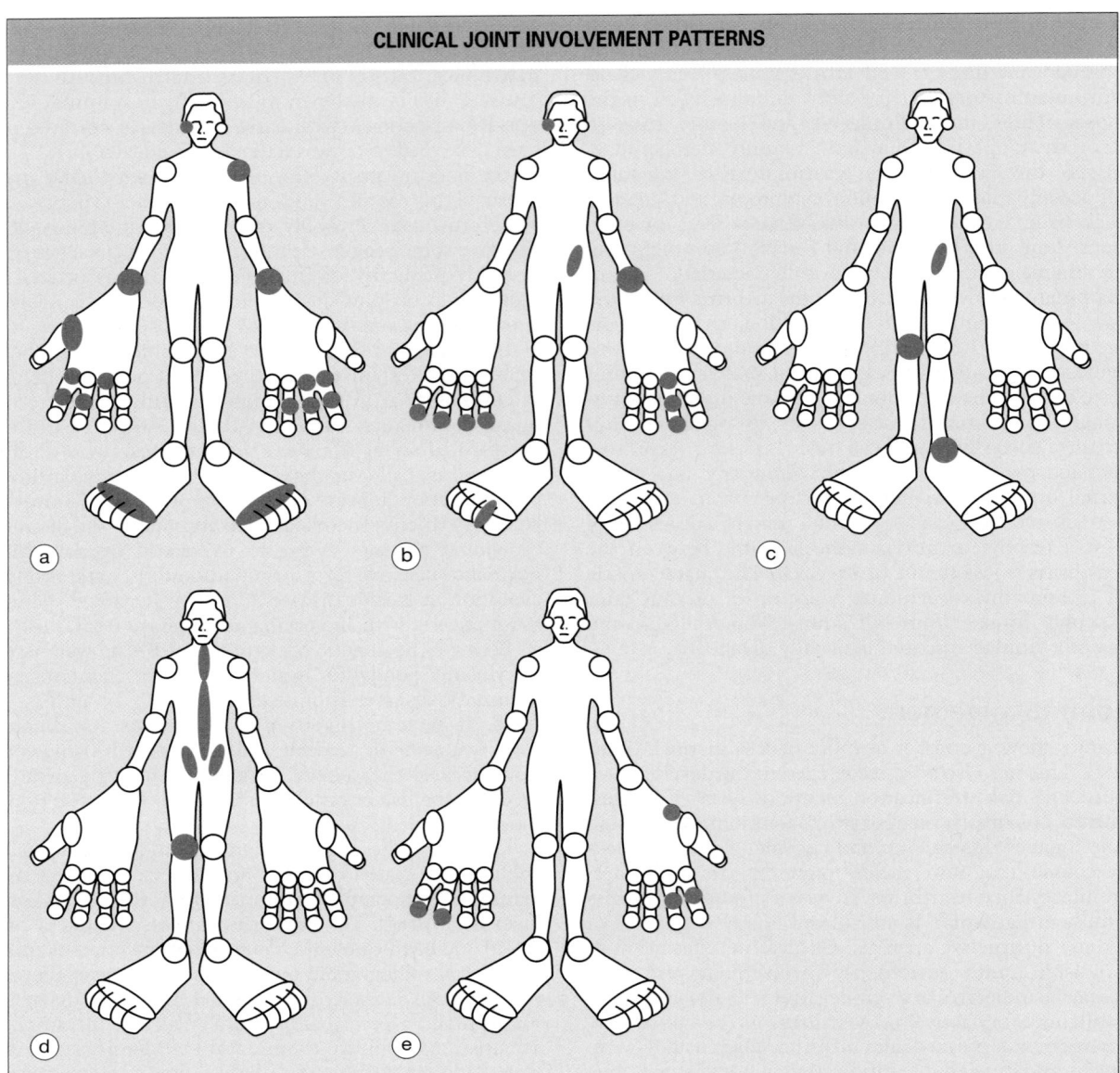

CLINICAL JOINT INVOLVEMENT PATTERNS

Fig. 92.1 Clinical joint involvement patterns. (a) "RA pattern": in rheumatoid arthritis, symmetric involvement of small joints (in particular, hand and feet joints) is considered characteristic. Involvement of larger joints and temporomandibular joints, however, may occur. "Symmetry" is not always absolute: in particular, involvement of "joint regions" such as "MCP joints" or "PIP joints" rather than individual joints is observed. Distal interphalangeal joints are usually spared. (b) "PsA pattern": psoriatic arthritis typically affects joints in a "longitudinal" ("ray", left side) or "transversal" (right side) pattern. DIP involvement, in contrast to the RA pattern, is found. In addition, involvement of axial joints (e.g., sacroiliac joints, frequently asymmetric) is common. Inflammation of periarticular soft tissues and enthesitis (inflammation of insertions of tendons or ligaments) together with skin changes and arthritis may lead to dactylitis, the so-called sausage digits (as on the right second toe of the panel). (c) "ReA pattern": reactive arthritis typically is a monarthritis or oligoarthritis, with predominance of large joints (mostly of the lower extremities) or sacroiliitis. (d) "AS pattern": inflammation of the joints of the axial skeleton and, in particular, symmetric sacroiliitis, is the hallmark of ankylosing spondylitis. In addition, enthesitis such as in PsA and large joint involvement may occur. (e) Osteoarthritis of the hands is characterized by bony enlargement (osteophytes) of affected joins, which are frequently the second and third DIP or PIP joints as well as the first carpometacarpal joint. In the affected joints, inflammatory activation with bony destruction may occur, making differentiation from RA or PsA difficult.

regular exercise. Early diagnosis with support of the new ACR/EULAR criteria (see Table 92.1) should allow identifying patients who may benefit most from appropriate therapeutic intervention and separate them from individuals who might sustain more harm than benefit from possibly toxic treatment.

TREATMENT OF EARLY ARTHRITIS

Non-steroidal anti-inflammatory drugs (NSAIDs) and non-medicinal therapies

As already mentioned, up to 60% of all patients presenting with early arthritis may have a self-limiting or benign course.[19,33] These patients only require temporary relief of their symptoms, which is usually accomplished by use of NSAIDs, which also may shorten the duration of the arthritis. NSAIDs do not alter the course of the arthritis and its outcome; their long-term use may be associated with considerable side effects.

In all types of arthritis, physical measures such as application of cold packs and (partial) immobilization using splints to prevent mechanical irritation have been advocated as temporary or long-term measures. Evidence for effectiveness of these measures, however, is still not sufficient or even negative.[44,45] Given the lack of side effects and possible individual benefits, however, most authors conclude to recommend the use of these treatments as palliative therapy or as an adjunct measure combined with exercises.

Glucocorticoids

Before an arthritis has reached the threshold for "persistence," that is, during the first few weeks or months, DMARDs may not be appropriate, because they are prescribed for longer periods of time and may have toxicities that outweigh the risk of a self-limiting condition. In clinical practice, glucocorticoids are often used, either as local intra-articular or as systemic intramuscular applications. Alternatively, short courses of oral glucocorticoids may be prescribed in these very early arthritis patients. In one of the few studies explicitly addressing the issue of treatment of very early (not necessarily rheumatoid) arthritis, Green and colleagues administered a single dose of a depot-glucocorticoid (120 mg methylprednisolone), either intra-articularly or intramuscularly. The results of this open study suggested that this approach was safe and resulted in a significant number of disease remissions.[5] Recently, two additional studies dealing with the value of glucocorticoids in the management of such very early arthritis patients have been published,[16,46] with slightly differing results: although the STIVEA study by Verstappen and colleagues demonstrated a small, although significant benefit of three weekly injections of depot glucocorticoids in a population of early (<12 weeks' duration) undifferentiated arthritis, the SAVE study, which used only a single injection in a very similar patient population, could not confirm these findings.

Unlike maintenance therapy with oral glucocorticoids, their short-term intermittent use is considered safe, although there is limited scientific evidence to underscore this.[47]

Disease-modifying anti-rheumatic drugs

Persistent early arthritis (i.e., once the clinically apparent arthritis has been continuously present for more than 6 weeks to 3 months) represents a situation in which DMARD therapy, either as a single measure or in combination with glucocorticoids (and NSAIDs, if needed), is deemed appropriate and necessary. Glucocorticoids have, in this situation, been advocated as both safe and efficacious in addition to DMARD therapy.[48,49] In this setting, effectiveness and superiority of early initiation of DMARDs compared with delayed treatment or treatment with NSAIDs alone has been conclusively demonstrated.[12] Because bone erosions or cartilage destruction, which are characteristic for RA as well as for psoriatic arthritis, rarely, if ever, heal[50,51] and thus damage accumulates over time, it is obvious that these agents will have better effects on outcome the earlier they are started.

As in established RA, methotrexate is regarded to be the drug of first choice,[24] considering its favorable risk-benefit ratio. Other DMARDs such as leflunomide, or sulfasalazine and sometimes (hydroxy-)chloroquine (in mild cases), may be considered in case of contraindications to methotrexate.[52] Other contraindications, such as the desire to become pregnant or significant co-morbidities such as liver or kidney disease, have to be accounted for appropriately. Likewise, at least in patients who at these stages were classified as having RA, a combination of glucocorticoids with DMARDs appears to offer additional benefits in terms of clinical response as well as radiologic outcomes,[48,53] although these findings have not been universally reproducible.[54]

More recently, "aggressive" treatment strategies have been proposed that used combinations of DMARDs and/or the addition of tumor necrosis factor (TNF) antagonists to "conventional" DMARDs in early "criteria positive" RA.[2,35,55,56] In these randomized trials, superior outcomes of combination therapies and/or the addition of "biologic" drugs compared with less aggressive "conventional" approaches were demonstrated. It is important to mention that some, but not all, combinations of (conventional) DMARDs may be superior to using the same DMARDs singly.[57] Furthermore, an important limitation of interpreting the results of these trials is the fact that none of them has included patients who did not fulfill the 1987 ACR RA criteria at the time of inclusion. Thus it remains unclear whether the possibly higher risk associated with more aggressive strategies is warranted at least in the subset of patients with less destructive diseases.

Biologic agents

Biologic drugs are currently only licensed for established RA and only after failure of at least one DMARD. The BeSt trial has revealed that the use of TNF blockade in early RA leads to good clinical results, although combination therapy with DMARDs plus intermediate-dose glucocorticoids led to similar clinical, functional, and radiographic results.[56] Currently, trials are in progress that employ TNF antagonists in early undifferentiated arthritis with substantial potential for destruction or persistence (e.g., RF or ACPA positivity or inflammatory arthritis for a minimum duration). The aim of these studies is to clarify whether such extremely early intense intervention might substantially and possibly permanently influence long-term outcomes or even prevent development of "full blown" RA (etanercept: EMPIRE and RIVERA trial, listed in the controlled-trials.com registry under ISRCTN 55428162 and ISRCTN 49682259, and infliximab: DINORA-trial, ISRCTN 21272423).

A recent analysis has revealed that the fate of any DMARD treatment (methotrexate or biologic agent) can be predicted within 3 to 6 months from start of therapy. Thus, starting patients with early RA with a more traditional therapeutic approach and then switching rapidly to another compound may be the most practical strategy.

CONCLUSION

Early inflammatory arthritis represents a substantial challenge to the clinician in everyday practice. The clinician has to discriminate as quickly as possible (usually within few weeks) between relatively benign disease and cases that call for urgent initiation of highly active treatment. Also, the intensity of treatment to avoid subjecting patients to the excessive risk associated with at least some of the therapies needs to be taken into consideration. Because in terms of the underlying pathogenetic (inflammatory) processes earlier intervention may be more effective before their mechanisms are "fully established" and have not reached an "autonomous" stage that is thought to prevail in later phases of RA, it seems advisable to start treatment as early as possible, ideally even before damage (defined as the visualized destruction of cartilage and/or bone) has occurred. The only, albeit still unresolved, obstacle to early therapy remains early diagnosis and/or prognostication. In recent years, however, both our knowledge and our appraisal of risk factors have been advanced and thus aided in refining the criteria on which to base therapeutic decisions. In particular, certain disease features appear to be indicative of an unfavorable prognosis: patients presenting with a higher number (more than 4 of 10) of swollen joints, positive MCP/MTP compression test, RF greater than or equal to 50 IU/mL or a positive ACPA test, and an elevated CRP value appear to be at a very high risk to develop persistent (and erosive) disease. In addition, the presence of erosions on initial radiographs would confirm the destructive nature of the arthritis. Persistence of arthritis (>12 weeks) and/or (initial) oligoarthritis accompanied by serologic evidence of inflammation or an RF greater than or equal to 50 IU/mL (or ACPA) are likewise regarded as indicators of a high risk for developing chronic and destructive joint disease. In all instances, other diseases associated with arthritis should have been excluded (see earlier). If these criteria are met, prompt institution of DMARD therapy is advisable to prevent further persistence, joint damage, and disability. Indeed, the ACR/EULAR classification criteria have accounted for most of these items using both an evidence- and a consensus-based approach.[26] In addition, expert consensus calls for rapid referral to a rheumatologist in the event of clinical suspicion of persistent arthritis and/or RA (within 6 weeks of symptom onset).

KEY REFERENCES

1. Ferraccioli GF, Della Casa-Alberighi O, Marubini E, et al. Is the control of disease progression within our grasp? Review of the GRISAR study (Gruppo Reumatologi Italiani Studio Artrite Reumatoide). Br J Rheumatol 1996;35(Suppl 2):8-13.

2. Korpela M, Laasonen L, Hannonen P, et al. Retardation of joint damage in patients with early rheumatoid arthritis by initial aggressive treatment with disease-modifying antirheumatic drugs—five-year experience from the FIN-RACo study. Arthritis Rheum 2004;50:2072-2081.

3. van der Horst-Bruinsma IE, Speyer I, Visser H, et al. Diagnosis and course of early-onset arthritis: results of a special early arthritis clinic compared to routine patient care. Br J Rheumatol 1998;37:1084-1088.

4. Van der Heide A, Jacobs JW, Bijlsma JW, et al. The effectiveness of early treatment with "second-line" antirheumatic drugs: a randomized, controlled trial. Ann Intern Med 1996;124:699-707.

5. Green M, Marzo-Ortega H, McGonagle D, et al. Persistence of mild, early inflammatory arthritis: the importance of disease duration, rheumatoid factor, and the shared epitope. Arthritis Rheum 1999;42:2184-2188.

6. Sokka T, Abelson B, Pincus T. Mortality in rheumatoid arthritis: 2008 update. Clin Exp Rheumatol 2008;26:S35-S61.

7. Gladman DD, Shuckett R, Russell ML, et al. Psoriatic arthritis (PSA)—an analysis of 220 patients. Q J Med 1987;62:127-141.

8. Pincus T, Ferraccioli G, Sokka T, et al. Evidence from clinical trials and long-term observational studies that disease-modifying anti-rheumatic drugs slow radiographic progression in rheumatoid arthritis: updating a 1983 review. Rheumatology 2002;41:1346-1356.

9. Bukhari MAS, Wiles NJ, Lunt M, et al. Influence of disease-modifying therapy on radiographic outcome in inflammatory polyarthritis at five years. Arthritis Rheum 2003;48:46-53.

10. Raza K, Falciani F, Curnow SJ, et al. Early rheumatoid arthritis is characterized by a distinct and transient synovial fluid cytokine profile of T cell and stromal cell origin. Arthritis Res Ther 2005;7:R784-R795. Epub 2005 Apr 7.

11. Mottonen T, Hannonen P, Korpela M, et al. Delay to institution of therapy and induction of remission using single-drug or combination-disease-modifying antirheumatic drug therapy in early rheumatoid arthritis. Arthritis Rheum 2002;46:894-898.

12. Finckh A, Liang MH, van Herckenrode CM, de Pablo P. Long-term impact of early treatment on radiographic progression in rheumatoid arthritis: a meta-analysis. Arthritis Rheum 2006;55:864-872.

14. Tak PP, Smeets TJM, Daha MR, et al. Analysis of the synovial cell infiltrate in early rheumatoid synovial tissue in relation to local disease activity. Arthritis Rheum 1997;40:217-225.

15. Aletaha D, Eberl G, Nell VPK, et al. Attitudes to early rheumatoid arthritis: changing patterns: results of a survey. Ann Rheum Dis 2004;63:1269-1275.

16. Machold KP, Landewé R, Smolen JS, et al. The Stop Arthritis Very Early (SAVE) trial, an international multi-center,randomized, double-blind, placebo controlled trial on glucocorticoids in very early arthritis. Ann Rheum Dis 2010;69:495-502.

17. Brook A, Corbett M: Radiographic changes in early rheumatoid disease. Ann Rheum Dis 1977;36:71-73.

18. Machold KP, Stamm TA, Nell VPK, et al. Very recent onset rheumatoid arthritis: clinical and serological patient characteristics associated with radiographic progression over the first years of disease. Rheumatology 2007;46:342-349.

19. Quinn MA, Green MJ, Marzo-Ortega H, et al. Prognostic factors in a large cohort of patients with early undifferentiated inflammatory arthritis after application of a structured management protocol. Arthritis Rheum 2003;48:3039-3045.

20. Plant MJ, Jones PW, Saklatvala J, et al. Patterns of radiological progression in early rheumatoid arthritis: results of an 8 year prospective study. J Rheumatol 1998;25:417-426.

21. Sharp JT, Wolfe F, Mitchell DM, Bloch DA. The progression of erosion and joint space narrowing scores in rheumatoid arthritis during the first twenty-five years of disease. Arthritis Rheum 1991;34:660-668.

22. Rantapaa-Dahlqvist S. Diagnostic and prognostic significance of autoantibodies in early rheumatoid arthritis. Scand J Rheumatol 2005;34:83-96.

23. Arnett FC, Edworthy SM, Bloch DA, et al. The American Rheumatism Association 1987 revised criteria for the classification of Rheumatoid Arthritis. Arthritis Rheum 1988;31:315-324.

24. Smolen JS, Sokka T, Pincus T, Breedveld FC. A proposed treatment algorithm for rheumatoid arthritis: aggressive therapy, methotrexate, and quantitative measures. Clin Exp Rheumatol 2003;21:S209-S210.

25. van der Helm-van Mil AHM, Detert J, le Cessie S, et al. Validation of a prediction rule for disease outcome in patients with recent-onset undifferentiated arthritis. Arthritis Rheum 2008;58:2241-2257.

26. Aletaha D, Neogi T, Silman A, Funovits J, Felson D, et al. The 2010 American College of Rheumatology/European League Against Rheumatism Classification Criteria for Rheumatoid Arthritis. Ann Rheum Dis 2010; in press.

27. Wood L, Peat G, Wilkie R, et al. A study of the noninstrumented physical examination of the knee found high observer variability. J Clin Epidemiol 2006;59:512-520.

28. Backhaus M, Kamradt T, Sndrock D, et al. Arthritis of the finger joints: a comprehensive approach comparing conventional radiography, scintigraphy, ultrasound, and contrast-enhanced magnetic resonance imaging. Arthritis Rheum 1999;42:1232-1245.

29. Kane D, Balint PV, Sturrock RD. Ultrasonography is superior to clinical examination in the detection and localization of knee joint effusion in rheumatoid arthritis. J Rheumatol 2003;30:966-971.

30. Luukkainen RK, Saltyshev M, Koski JM, Huhtala HS. Relationship between clinically detected joint swelling and effusion diagnosed by ultrasonography in metatarsophalangeal and talocrural joints in patients with rheumatoid arthritis. Clin Exp Rheumatol 2003;21:632-634.

31. The EULAR standing committee for international clinical studies including therapeutic trials—ESCISIT. In: van Riel PLCM, Scott DL, eds. EULAR handbook of clinical assessments in rheumatoid arthritis, 4th ed. Alphen aan den Rijn: Van Zuiden Communications B.V., 2004.

32. Combe B, Landewe R, Lukas C, et al. EULAR recommendations for the management of early arthritis: report of a task force of the European Standing Committee for International Clinical Studies Including Therapeutics (ESCISIT). Ann Rheum Dis 2007;66:34-45.

33. Visser H, le Cessie S, Vos K, et al. How to diagnose rheumatoid arthritis early: a prediction model for persistent (erosive) arthritis. Arthritis Rheum 2002;46:357-365.

34. Emery P, Breedveld FC, Dougados M, et al. Early referral recommendation for newly diagnosed rheumatoid arthritis: evidence based development of a clinical guide. Ann Rheum Dis 2002;61:290-297.

35. Boers M, Verhoeven AC, Markusse HM, et al. Randomised comparison of combined step-down prednisolone, methotrexate and sulphasalazine with sulphasalazine alone in early rheumatoid arthritis. Lancet 1997;350:309-318.

36. Steiner G, Smolen JS. Autoantibodies in rheumatoid arthritis, 2nd ed. In: Firestein GS, Panayi GS, Wollheim FA, eds. Rheumatoid arthritis. Oxford: Oxford University Press, 2006:193-198.

37. Nell VPK, Machold KP, Stamm TA, et al. Autoantibody profiling as early diagnostic and prognostic tool for rheumatoid arthritis. Ann Rheum Dis 2005;64:1731-1736.

38. van Venrooij WJ, Zendman AJ, Pruijn GJ: Autoantibodies to citrullinated antigens in (early) rheumatoid arthritis. Autoimmun Rev 2006;6:37-41.

39. Tunn EJ, Bacon PA: Differentiating persistent from self-limiting symmetrical synovitis in an early arthritis clinic. Br J Rheumatol 1993;32:97-103.

41. Plenge RM. Recent progress in rheumatoid arthritis genetics: one step towards improved patient care. Curr Opin Rheumatol 2009;21:262-271.

42. Ostergaard M, Ejbjerg B, Szkudlarek M. Imaging in early rheumatoid arthritis: roles of magnetic resonance imaging, ultrasonography, conventional radiography and computed tomography. Best Pract Res Clin Rheumatol 2005;19:91-116.

43. Boutry N, Hachulla E, Flipo RM, et al. MR imaging findings in hands in early rheumatoid arthritis: comparison with those in systemic lupus erythematosus and primary Sjögren syndrome. Radiology 2005;236:593-600.

46. Verstappen SM, McCoy MJ, Roberts C, et al. The beneficial effects of a 3 week course of intramuscular glucocorticoid injections in patients with very early inflammatory polyarthritis: results of the STIVEA trial. Ann Rheum Dis 2010;69:503-509.

48. Kirwan JR, and the Arthritis and Rheumatism Council low-dose glucocorticoid study group: the effects of glucocorticoids on joint destruction in rheumatoid arthritis. N Engl J Med 1995;333:142-146.

49. Wassenberg S, Rau R, Steinfeld P, Zeidler H. Very low-dose prednisolone in early rheumatoid arthritis retards radiographic progression over two years—a multicenter, double-blind, placebo-controlled trial. Arthritis Rheum 2005;52:3371-3380.

50. Sharp JT, van der Heijde D, Boers M, et al. Repair of erosions in rheumatoid arthritis does occur: Results from 2 studies by the OMERACT subcommittee on healing of erosions. J Rheumatol 2003;30:1102-1107.

REFERENCES

Full references for this chapter can be found on www.expertconsult.com.

Evaluation and outcomes of patients with rheumatoid arthritis

Daniel Aletaha and Josef S. Smolen

93

- Assessments in rheumatoid arthritis (RA) are aiming to evaluate or prognosticate the disease process or disease outcome.

- The 2010 classification criteria for RA have been developed jointly by the American College of Rheumatology (ACR) and the European League Against Rheumatism (EULAR) to allow treatment and assessment of patients with very early as well as established disease.

- Core sets of individual measures of the disease process have been defined and include joint swelling and tenderness, the acute-phase response, pain, patient global, and evaluator global.

- These individual measures can be effectively integrated into composite indices that allow determination of actual disease activity as well as disease activity states.

- In clinical practice, disease activity (process) is the immediate target of therapeutic interventions, whereas the goal of treatment is improvement of disease outcomes and health-related quality of life.

- In clinical trials, disease activity states and responses, as well as their time of onset and sustainment, should be reported.

- The typical proxy for disease outcome is radiographic damage, which is a surrogate for the accrued joint destruction and can be assessed by a variety of quantitative scores.

- Impairment of physical function (disability) is another important outcome and can be assessed by questionnaires, typically the Health Assessment Questionnaire (HAQ), or direct functional performance tests, such as grip strength.

- Physical function is influenced by both disease activity and joint damage; functional disability related to joint damage is currently considered to be irreversible.

INTRODUCTION

Over the past 2 to 3 decades the approach to treating patients with rheumatoid arthritis (RA) has undergone a spectacular evolution that still continues to advance and has led to unprecedented outcomes. It is a consequence of better insights into the natural history of the disease, better understanding of pathogenic pathways, a burst of novel therapies, innovative clinical trial design, recognition of the importance of treatment strategies over and above mere application of drugs, and the development of tools to assess RA and its progression reliably.[1] It is particularly the latter that has allowed one to comprehend many aspects of the natural as well as the therapeutically modified course of RA, to design elegant clinical trials, and to develop and modify strategic targets in RA therapy. Many of the instruments developed can be quite easily applied in clinical practice, signifying the translation of clinical trial results into the reality of daily patient care. In this chapter we discuss the various ways to assess patients with RA. However, before assessment of RA can be discussed, patients need to be adequately diagnosed or classified. In this regard, the 2010 American College of Rheumatology (ACR)/European League Against Rheumatism (EULAR) classification criteria for RA have been published.[2-4] In the first section of this chapter, we will provide a brief overview of these new criteria.

2010 ACR/EULAR CLASSIFICATION CRITERIA FOR RHEUMATOID ARTHRITIS

Until 2010, the classification criteria for RA in use were those by the American Rheumatism Association from 1987. These criteria have been increasingly debated in the recent past, because of their lack of sensitivity in early disease, given that they had been derived using mostly patients with long-standing, established RA. The best example is the inclusion of erosions in these criteria as a feature for diagnosis, which over the time contradicted the clinical practice of preventing erosions in RA by timely introduction of adequate therapy. In addition, nodules are rarely seen in early disease, and therefore even more weight is put on the remaining six variables, including erosions.

The joint Working Group of the ACR and the EULAR aimed to develop new classification criteria for RA that would replace the 1987 criteria. From July 2007 to June 2010 the Working Group engaged in a three-step approach that included a data analysis phase using early arthritis cohorts, a consensus science phase, and a refinement phase that led to three publications detailing the process and the final criteria.[2-4] Whereas the new criteria have been validated using early arthritis cohorts not utilized for their derivation, further prospective validation in many additional cohorts is awaited and expected.

As shown in Table 93.1, the 2010 criteria comprise four domains, including the number and type of the affected joints, rheumatoid factor (RF), and anticitrullinated peptide/protein antibodies (ACPAs), acute-phase reactants (C-reactive protein [CRP] and erythrocyte sedimentation rate [ESR]), and the duration of symptoms. For evaluation of a patient, the highest category within each domain is taken and the four respective numbers are added. The maximum possible score is 10, where any score of equal or greater than 6 indicates the presence of definitely classifiable RA. Another way to classify RA, based on the same rules, is by the tree algorithm depicted in Figure 93.1.

The 2010 criteria should be applied to any patient who presents with at least one clinically swollen joint, for which another disease is not the most likely cause. These classification criteria, although especially useful for groups of patients entering clinical trials, can just like other criteria be applied to facilitate diagnosis of RA and, in particular, an earlier diagnosis of RA, so that newly presenting patients would have the shortest possible delay in initiation of treatment. Once the diagnosis has been made and appropriate therapy considered or instituted, it is of utmost importance to observe patients regularly with respect to their disease activity and outcome. These aspects are discussed in the next sections of this chapter.

CONCEPTS

From pathogenesis to measurement

It is currently not possible to capture the cellular and molecular events leading to RA at the site of involvement, such as the joint or lymphatic organs. Even if we could routinely obtain snapshots of the expectedly manifold and heterogeneous interactions of pathogenic cells and molecules, their hierarchy or relative dominance would not yet be evident for us. As a consequence, measurements have to rely on phenomena that are further downstream to these pathogenetic events.

For example, the acute-phase reactant CRP is known to be induced by interleukin (IL)-6, which in turn can be activated by tumor necrosis factor (TNF), IL-1, and other pathways. Thus, CRP and other acute-phase reactants, which are easily measurable in peripheral blood,

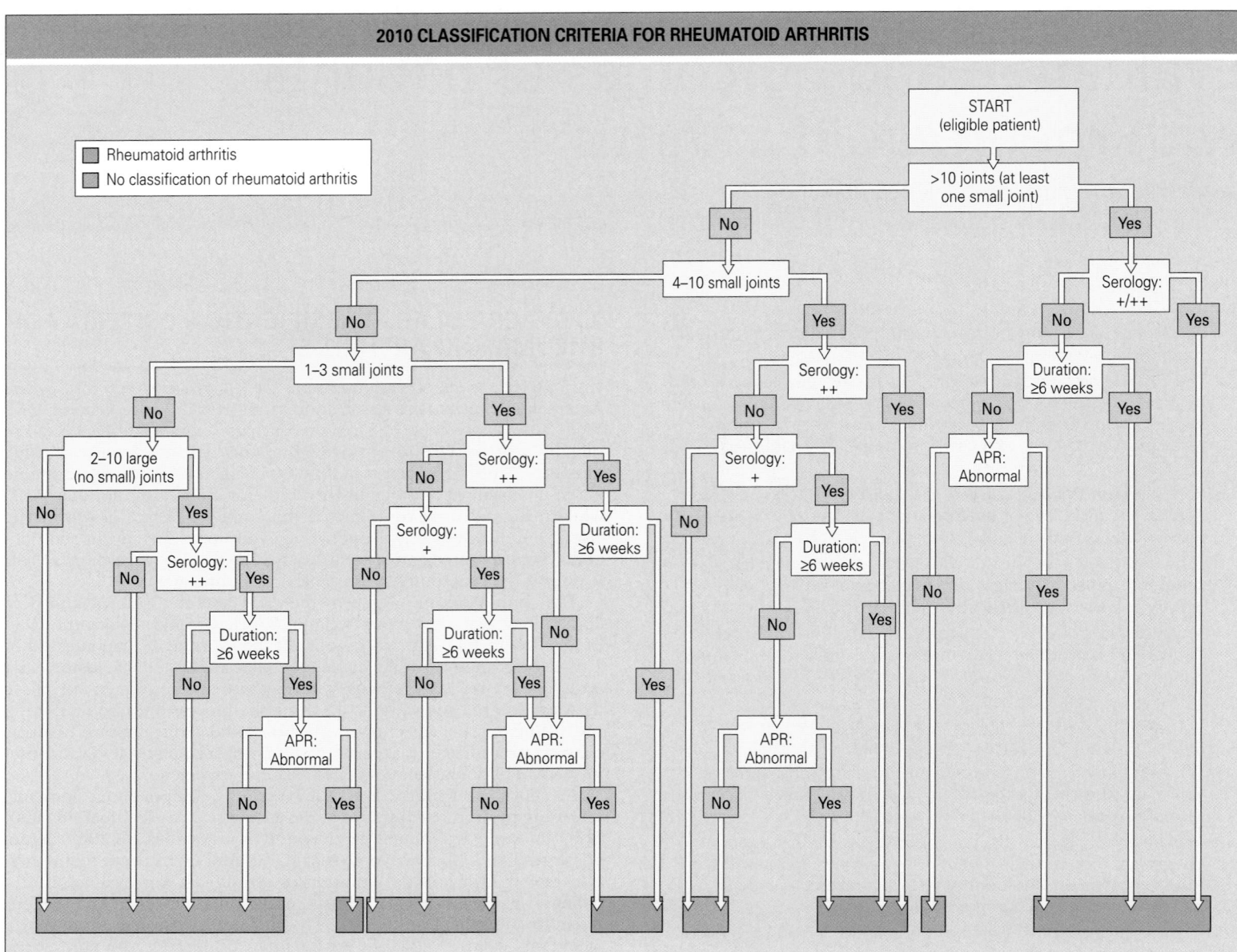

2010 CLASSIFICATION CRITERIA FOR RHEUMATOID ARTHRITIS

Fig. 93.1 Tree algorithm to classify definite rheumatoid arthritis (green boxes) or to exclude its current presence (red boxes) in patients who present with at least one swollen joint not otherwise explainable. Detailed definitions of domains and categories are provided in the footnotes to Table 93.1. *(From Aletaha D, Neogi T, Silman AJ, et al. The 2010 American College of Rheumatology/European League Against Rheumatism Classification Criteria for Rheumatoid Arthritis.)*

constitute downstream manifestations of cytokine activation. Likewise, joint swelling constitutes the downstream ("clinical") expression of synovial inflammation and, consequently, of the totality of the underlying inflammatory events, not just for a particular segment such as cytokine activation. Another example is joint destruction, which is elicited by osteoclasts on the one hand (bony damage) and chondrocytes and metalloproteases on the other hand (cartilage damage), both of which are induced during the active disease process. Currently, we are likewise unable to directly visualize this process as it occurs, but radiographic scores constitute the cumulative downstream markers of these events. Novel imaging techniques, such as methods of molecular and cellular imaging, may shift this upstream in the future and allow earlier detection and measurements.

The previous list could be broadly expanded but was just meant to exemplify the difficulty in depicting the basic pathogenetic pathways and the need to use their downstream expressions, ideally in some kind of combination, to best summarize the basic events, which are currently still enigmatic, at least from the perspective of accurate measurement.

Validity

Assessment is all about measurement and its employment to characterize attributes of a disease, including its outcome and prognosis. Any

measurement employed to evaluate aspects of a disease, be it laboratory tests or clinical measurement tools, must comply with a variety of requirements. It should reflect an important aspect of the disease (as judged by investigators and/or patients), be reliable, be sensitive to change, and thus fulfill the fundamental validity criteria (Table 93.2) and should be practical and easy to use (feasibility).

Disease process ("disease activity") and consequence ("disease outcome")

In the context of the assessment of patients with RA it is essential to bear in mind that RA, like many other disorders, has several facets that need to be captured. The cardinal elements are disease activity and joint damage, which are both reflections of the underlying pathobiology. At the same time, they are intimately associated with other important attributes, such as impairment of physical function, reduction in quality of life, extra-articular manifestations, systemic effects on patient well-being, co-morbidity, societal and economic aspects, and mortality (Fig. 93.2). It is legitimate to focus on some of these facets more than on others, because, first, there is a hierarchy within this diversity; second, they are all intertwined; and, third, some are relatively specific for RA, whereas others are common to many disorders. However, all of these components must be taken into account when evaluating RA and each of them has a discrete complexity.

TABLE 93.1 ACR/EULAR CLASSIFICATION CRITERIA FOR RHEUMATOID ARTHRITIS*

	Score
Joint involvement (0-5)[1]	
1 medium-large[2] joint	0
2-10 medium-large joints	1
1-3 small[3] joints (with or without involvement of large joints)	2
4-10 small joints (with or without involvement of large joints)	3
>10 joints[4] (at least one small joint)	5
Serology[5] (0-3)[†]	
Negative RF *and* negative ACPAs	0
Low-positive RF *or* low-positive ACPAs	2
High-positive RF *or* high-positive ACPAs	3
Acute-phase reactants[6] (0-1)[†]	
Normal CRP *and* normal ESR	0
Abnormal CRP *or* abnormal ESR	1
Duration of symptoms[7] (0-1)	
<6 weeks	0
≥6 weeks	1

**Score-based algorithm for classification in an eligible patient (cut-point for RA: ≥6/10).*
[†]*Individuals only should be scored by these criteria if at least one serologic test and at least one acute-phase reactant test result is available. When a value for a serologic test or acute-phase reactant is not available, that test should be considered as "negative/normal."*
[1]*Joint involvement refers to any swollen or tender joint on examination, or evidence of synovitis on magnetic resonance imaging or ultrasonography. Distal interphalangeal joints (DIPs), first carpometacarpal (CMC) joint, and first metatarsophalangeal (MTP) joint are excluded from assessment. Categories of joint distribution are classified according to the location and number of the involved joints, with placement into the highest category possible based on the pattern of joint involvement.*
[2]*Medium to large joints refer to shoulders, elbows, hips, knees, and ankles.*
[3]*Small joints refer to the metacarpophalangeal (MCP) joints, proximal interphalangeal (PIP) joints, metatarsophalangeal (MTP) joints 2 to 5, thumb interphalangeal (IP) joints, and wrists.*
[4]*In this category, at least one of the involved joints must be a small joint; the other joints can include any combination of large and additional small joints, as well as other joints not specifically listed elsewhere (e.g., temporomandibular, acromioclavicular, sternoclavicular).*
[5]*Negative refers to international unit (IU) values that are less than or equal to the upper limit of normal (ULN) for the laboratory and assay; low-positive refers to IU values that are greater than the ULN but less than or equal to three times the ULN for the laboratory and assay; high-positive refers to IU values that are more than three times the ULN for the laboratory and assay. When RF is only available as positive or negative, a positive result should be scored as "low-positive".*
[6]*Normal/abnormal is determined by local laboratory standards.*
[7]*Duration of symptoms refers to patient self-report of the duration of signs or symptoms of synovitis (e.g., pain, swelling, tenderness) of joints that are clinically involved at the time of assessment.*
RF, rheumatoid factor; ACPAs, anti-citrullinated protein/peptide antibodies; ULN, upper limit of normal; ESR, erythrocyte sedimentation rate; CRP, C-reactive protein.
From Aletaha D, Neogi T, Silman AJ, et al. The 2010 American College of Rheumatology/European League Against Rheumatism Classification Criteria for Rheumatoid Arthritis.

TABLE 93.2 CHARACTERIZATION OF MEASUREMENT: VALIDITY, RELIABILITY, AND FEASIBILITY

Characteristic	Definition	Examples/comments
Validity	The instrument measures what it is supposed to measure.	
Construct validity	The measure behaves in relation to other measures as one would expect if it was really measuring what it is supposed to measure; it changes in the same direction as the patient changes clinically.	
Content validity	The components of a composite measure capture all relevant aspects and should provide discrete, non-duplicated information.	Inclusion of measures of joint inflammation, acute phase, and pain in an activity index
Face validity	The measure appears sensible ("makes sense") (to both patients and physicians).	Assessment of joint swelling to evaluate disease activity of an arthritic condition
Criterion validity	The measure predicts a long-term outcome of importance (e.g., organ damage, functional impairment, death).	Acute-phase response has criterion validity given its association with joint damage progression over time.
Discriminant validity	The measure is responsive; it is sensitive to change (see definition below) when the true status changes and not if the true status remains stable; it therefore discriminates between effective and non-effective interventions.	The ACR20 response criteria well discriminate active drug and placebo in clinical trials of RA.
Reliability (reproducibility, precision)	Repeated testing in stable patients produces more or less the same results; the measure can be used by several individuals independently (inter-rater stability) and provide similar results when used by one individual repeatedly on the same subject (intra-rater stability).	Acute-phase response is relatively stable if measured by the same method repeatedly; radiographic scoring of two experienced readers have a low inter-rater variability.
Accuracy	A measurement is unbiased, i.e., free of a systematic error	Well-calibrated scales are usually accurate.
Responsiveness (sensitivity to change)	Clinically important changes can be detected even if these changes are small (overlap with the concept of discriminant validity).	Measures the ratio of the change produced by a treatment of known benefit to the within-subject variability in stable patients
Feasibility	The measure is easy to apply or calculate.	Can be applied reliably in clinical trials and daily practice without complexity in its calculation

Process variables reflect the actual pathophysiologic events and thus constitute mostly instant measures of disease activity, such as swollen joint counts or acute-phase reactant levels. Outcome variables measure the long-term consequences (or sum) of the disease process and include joint damage and physical disability.[5,6] However, many variables constitute mixtures of both, adding another layer of complexity (see Fig. 93.2). Thus, several process variables, when integrated over time, reflect outcome and several outcome measures reflect actual disease activity, at least in part. Impairment in physical function or quality of life, for example, will not only be a long-term product of the process but also result from actual manifestations, such as pain, joint swelling, and stiffness.

Measures of *disease activity* may therefore be better defined as those variables reflecting the underlying events that can fluctuate rapidly, spontaneously or upon treatment, and have the principal potential to normalize. In contrast, measures of *disease outcome*, even if they may additionally mirror the actual disease process at an individual point in time, reflect an abnormality that may become fixed in the course of the disease and then not any longer bears the potential to improve, let alone to normalize. In other words, *outcome* relates to (a varying degree of) irreversibility (with the ultimate, worst outcome being death) and *disease activity* relates to reversibility, amenability to interventions, and possible prevention of bad outcome. The disease process ("disease activity") and disease outcome are linked by a temporal relationship (see Fig. 93.2). The strength of this link might be predetermined in individual patients, and prognostic markers may help to define subgroups of patients (Fig. 93.3).

Effective treatment includes a reversal of symptoms caused by disease activity *and* the prevention of the natural course of RA leading to bad outcome, that is, structural, functional, and all other consequences of the disease. Sometimes, disease activity markers are used as surrogate markers of the disease outcome, because their presence reflects the future presence of bad outcome. Here, the concept of prognostication mixes into the mere evaluation process.

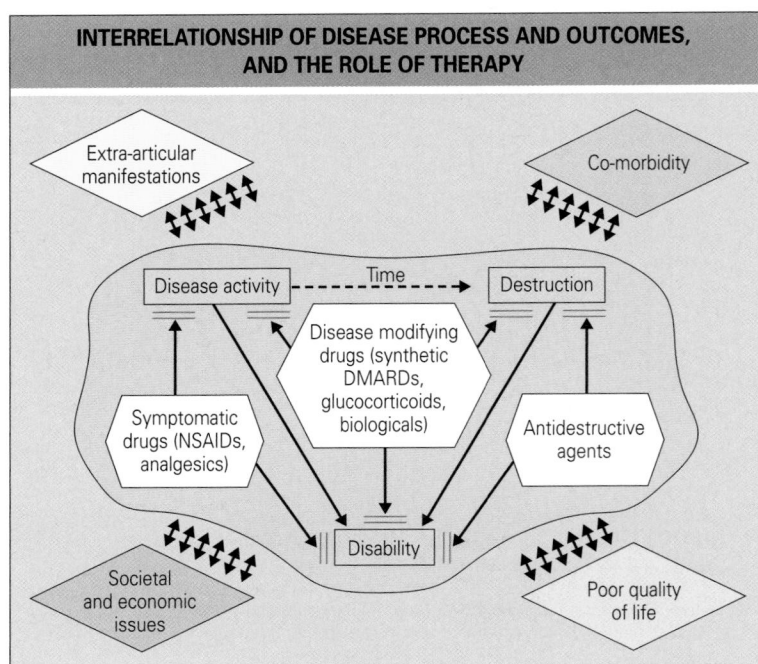

Fig. 93.2 Inter-relationship of disease process and outcomes and the role of therapy. Disease activity, destruction, and functional disability are the central determinants of outcomes assessment in rheumatoid arthritis and are interrelated (arrows). Different therapeutic modalities (white hexagons) affect these outcomes differently (blocking arrows). A number of contextual aspects contribute to this system.

Evaluation vs. prognostication

An important concept that needs to be derived from the mentioned link between process and outcome is the distinction between evaluation and prognostication. Although evaluation of disease activity at a given time is aiming at improving outcome, that is, at changing prognosis, this is practically different from the concept of prognostication

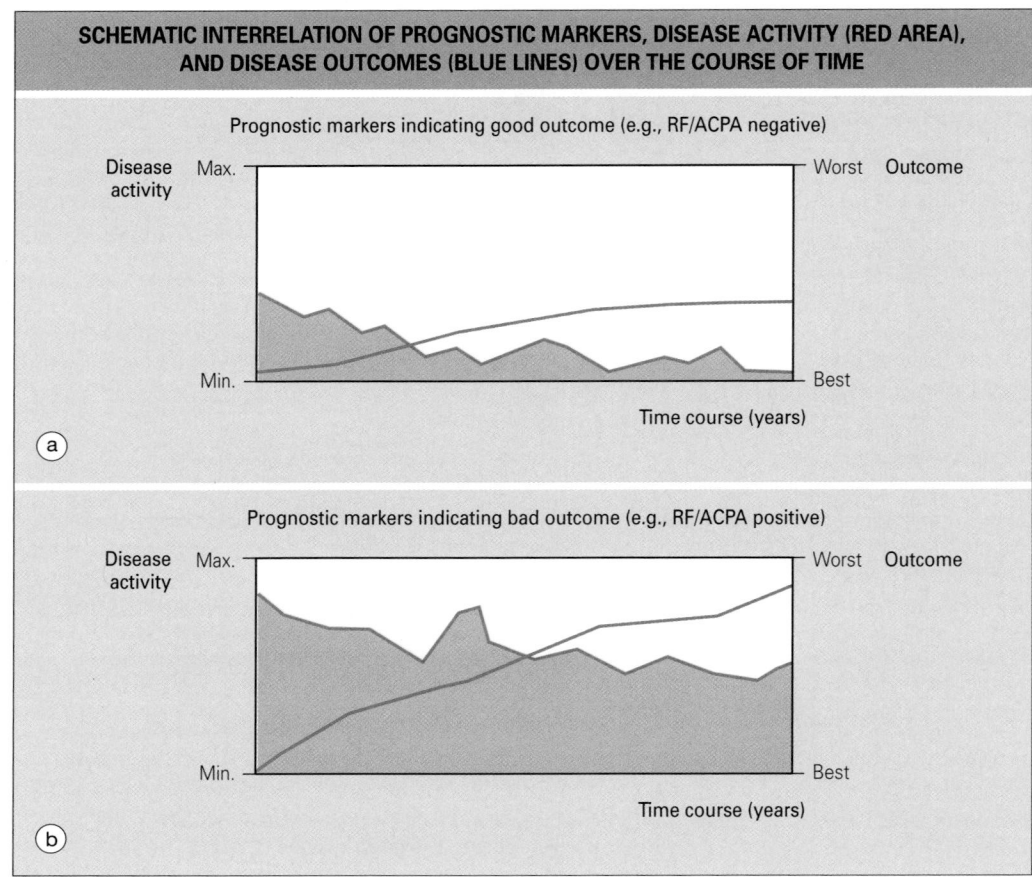

Fig. 93.3 Schematic interrelation of prognostic markers, disease activity (red area), and disease outcomes (blue lines) over the course of time.
(a) Example of a patient with good markers.
(b) Example of a patient with bad markers.

by measurement of specific markers: a prognostic marker is generally thought to be relatively constant ("fixed") and therefore relatively consistent if evaluated repeatedly or at different times, whereas an evaluative marker is supposed to vary, especially in the course of treatment, although again some markers may be valuable for both evaluation and prognostication. The evaluative markers are the main content of this chapter. Typical examples of "fixed" prognostic markers are genetic markers, but sometimes also autoantibodies can be regarded as such, given the information provided by their presence or absence at baseline or at the time of diagnosis, although they might still change over the course of the disease. For completeness, the aims and types of prognostic markers are discussed in the following section.

Two questions have historically been always important in this regard: "Will early undifferentiated arthritis evolve into persistent erosive disease?" and "Will patients with established rheumatoid arthritis develop severe disease?"

A number of prognostic factors for disease severity have been found. They comprise the presence and titer of autoantibodies, such as RF or ACPAs, (early) joint damage, and the HLA-DRB1 shared epitope alleles. The prognostic value of the last entity for severely destructive RA probably reflects an indirect relationship due to the association with autoantibody production rather than a stand-alone genetic risk factor.

Another group of prognostic factors relates to demographic variables. Women have worse radiographic and functional outcome than men, and this is further aggravated in the postmenopausal state. This may be partly due to the usually lower bone mineral density of women compared with men, particularly when postmenopausal, because lower bone mineral density is associated with more severe destruction in RA. A further, partly independent risk factor for joint damage is a low body mass index. Additional risk factors are smoking, no pregnancies, educational level, and psychological and social states.

Predicting the disease course in an individual patient is essential for the interaction between rheumatologist and patient and in the context of therapeutic decision-making. Prognostic indicators can be weighted and combined, and algorithms allowing one to recognize patients who will develop persistent destructive arthritis among those with early undifferentiated arthritis have been published but need further validation. However, many of the evaluative markers of the disease process, such as joint counts, acute-phase reactants, and others, collected in untreated patients at baseline also have prognostic value.[7]

Individual measures versus composite indices

Each individual measure of disease activity may only relate to a portion of it. Also, individual patients differ with regard to the presentation and course of their disease and even within an individual patient the disease expression may vary during its course. Moreover, each of the surrogates casts particular emphasis on one aspect of the disease and the evaluation of any one of these aspects over time will not allow reliable identification of a patient's disease activity and response to therapy. In clinical trials, the independent evaluation of each variable is afflicted with methodologic difficulties.[8] Composite indices of disease activity overcome these problems[9,10] by allowing more consistent follow-up of patients in clinical practice, which will improve outcomes of the disease (Fig. 93.4). In addition, also the patients' compliance will be improved by the enhanced understanding of the treatment targets, which can be expressed by a single number. In clinical trials, sample size requirements will be reduced by having more power provided by a pooled index.

The value of pooling is not limited to disease activity measures, as can be seen by the current ways to evaluate joint damage. Joint damage affects both cartilage and bone, and the mechanisms underlying destruction of these two compartments are largely different. Although cartilage and bone damage are scored separately, it is important to combine them into a total score[11] to reflect the overall structural consequences of the disease process (see later) and structural effects of an intervention. Likewise, impairment of physical function may affect the upper or the lower extremity and some activities may be more important to patients than others. Looking at these factors individually may be misleading in either direction. The combination of all

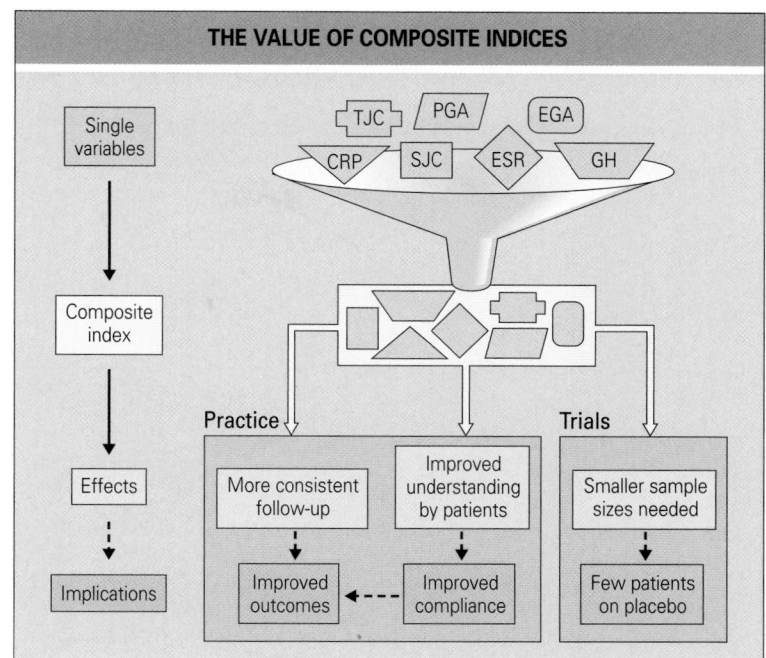

Fig. 93.4 The value of composite indices. Integration of individual variables into composite indices has beneficial effects in clinical practice and clinical trials.

important aspects into a single index warrants a most unbiased judgment (see later).[5]

Definition and evaluation of treatment targets in clinical practice

It has been recognized over the years that joint damage can occur already very early in the disease course and that the initiation of joint destruction is particularly prominent during the first 1 to 2 years, even if therapy has been instituted.[12] Therefore, it is of paramount importance to start effective treatment in the very early stages of disease,[13,14] thus preventing or at least delaying or mitigating the accrual of joint damage. Early referral strategies have been developed, as have recommendations for the management of early RA,[15] but classification criteria for early rheumatoid arthritis are currently still missing.

However, once therapy is instituted, a clear therapeutic target needs to be defined. It has become evident that adapting therapy to a predefined target value of a disease activity index (e.g., low disease activity) is by far superior to an unstructured change of treatment.[16,17] Likewise, the lower the disease activity state and the earlier this is achieved, the lesser joint damage will be.[18] Thus, employment of dynamic treatment strategies aiming to reach (individualized) predefined goals is one of the most recent innovative steps.

Another important strategic aspect of outcomes assessment is the notion that treatment should aim at reduction of disease activity to a certain level or state rather than for mere levels of change. Respective evidence comes from secondary analysis of clinical trial data, in which patients with ACR 50% or ACR 70% response rates (see later) had worse radiographic outcomes if they achieved only a moderate disease activity state when compared with those who achieved a low disease activity state or remission[19]; additional evidence comes from patient reported outcomes in observational studies, in which patients judged their disease to have undergone major improvement only if a low moderate disease activity state had been attained, irrespective of the baseline disease activity.[20]

Given that the long-term response to therapy can be predicted already after 3 to 6 months from its start,[21] therapy should be switched or adapted if the predefined goal is not achieved within this time frame (Fig. 93.5). Consequently, especially after the start of treatment or with active disease, follow-up examinations using the appropriate instruments for disease activity assessment need to be performed at least

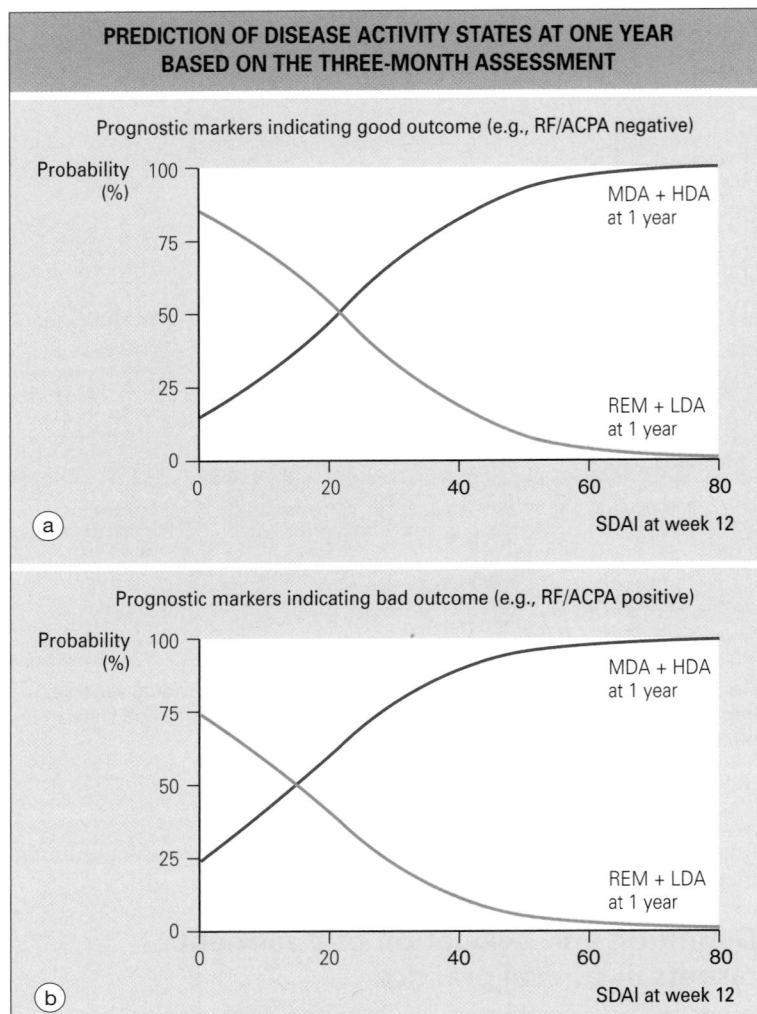

PREDICTION OF DISEASE ACTIVITY STATES AT ONE YEAR BASED ON THE THREE-MONTH ASSESSMENT

Prognostic markers indicating good outcome (e.g., RF/ACPA negative)

(a) Probability (%) — MDA + HDA at 1 year / REM + LDA at 1 year — SDAI at week 12

Prognostic markers indicating bad outcome (e.g., RF/ACPA positive)

(b) Probability (%) — MDA + HDA at 1 year / REM + LDA at 1 year — SDAI at week 12

Fig. 93.5 Prediction of disease activity states at 1 year based on the 3-month assessment. Using the 3 months SDAI levels (x-axis), one can estimate the probability of a patient to reach a good disease activity state at 1 year (i.e., remission and low disease activity, REM+LDA, green lines) or a bad disease activity state (moderate and high disease activity, MDA+HDA, red lines). The left panel shows the model for early arthritis; the right panel shows the results for established RA. For example, if a patient has an SDAI greater than or equal to 40 at 3 months, the probability of this patient to have moderate or high disease activity at 1 year is more than 80% (red curves); vice versa, the probability of this patient to achieve remission or low disease activity at 1 year is less than 20% (green curves).

every 3 months to decide on the continuation or adaptation of treatment. Outcome measures, such as joint radiographs, are less frequently needed, although functional evaluation may complement insights gained from disease activity assessment.

Assessment strategies in clinical trials

Whereas in clinical practice the ultimate goal is to measure each individual patient's disease activity most accurately, this focus shifts a little bit when it comes to measuring disease activity in clinical trials. The purpose of clinical trials is to show that interventions work on the *group* level when compared with another group treated differently. For clinical trial reporting, core set variables have been defined internationally[22-24] and criteria for improvement have been established.[25,26] More recently, the ACR and the EULAR have developed a minimal standard of core information to be provided when reporting on clinical trials, which include the presentation of baseline *and* endpoint data for core set variables *and* composite scores *as well as* response *and* state data including proportions of patients in low disease activity and remission (Table 93.3).[27,28] Inherent in these recommendations is the goal to

TABLE 93.3 EUROPEAN LEAGUE AGAINST RHEUMATISM (EULAR)/AMERICAN COLLEGE OF RHEUMATOLOGY (ACR) RECOMMENDATIONS ON REPORTING CLINICAL TRIAL RESULTS IN RHEUMATOID ARTHRITIS*

Preamble

There are several domains that are important in reporting clinical trials: disease activity, function and damage. For each of these domains response and state should be assessed and reported in clinical trials, where appropriate. However, the following recommendations will deal specifically with *disease activity*.

1. Each trial should report both the disease activity response and disease activity states.
   a. *Response:* ACR and EULAR response criteria.
   b. *States:* Continuous composite indices of disease activity with cut-points to define various disease activity states: they include DAS/DAS28, CDAI, and SDAI. Appropriate descriptive statistics of the baseline, the endpoint, and change of the composite indices should be reported.
2. Each trial should report the appropriate descriptive statistics of the baseline, the endpoint, and change of the single variables included in the core set.
3. Each trial should report the baseline disease activity levels, which could have relevance when interpreting the results.
4. Each trial should report the percentage of patients achieving a low disease activity state and remission.
   a. Definitions that should be used for *low disease activity* include cut-points for low disease activity for DAS/DAS28, CDAI, SDAI, and MDA.
   b. Definitions that could be used for *remission* include preliminary ARA remission criteria and respective cut-points for DAS/DAS28, CDAI, and SDAI.
5. Each trial should report the time to onset of the primary outcome (a particular response or a certain disease activity state).
6. Each trial should consider and report the sustainability of the primary outcome (as opposed to evaluating it at a single predefined time point during the trial).
7. Each trial should report on fatigue.

For the definition of the various instruments, please see the respective sections of the chapter. Adapted from Aletaha D, Landewe R, Karonitsch T, et al. Reporting disease activity in clinical trials of patients with rheumatoid arthritis: EULAR/ACR collaborative recommendations. Arthritis Rheum 2008;59:1371-1377; and Aletaha D, Landewe R, Karonitsch T, et al. Reporting disease activity in clinical trials of patients with rheumatoid arthritis: EULAR/ACR collaborative recommendations. Ann Rheum Dis 2008;67:1360-1364.

achieve trial reporting in RA that is consistent across clinical trials rather than varying depending on selected endpoints and also meaningful from the clinical rheumatologist's perspective, rather than merely by statistical properties of a specific measure.

INSTRUMENTS TO ASSESS DISEASE ACTIVITY

Joint swelling and tenderness, pain, as well as the global impression of disease activity by the patient and the person evaluating the patient, and laboratory measures of the acute-phase response are regarded as the major (core) variables for disease activity assessment. These measures have been defined in respective core sets of the various organizations (see later). In addition, there exist a variety of other variables, such as morning stiffness, squeeze pain, or fatigue, that deserve being addressed in this context.

The core sets of disease activity variables

In the early 1990s, efforts to select a minimal set of measures to be included for disease activity assessment in RA clinical trials arrived at similar results across various international organizations. The core sets comprise tender and swollen joint counts (TJC, SJC), patient assessment of pain (PP) and of global disease activity (PGA), evaluator's assessment of global disease activity (EGA), acute-phase reactants (CRP and/or ESR), physical function, and radiographic assessment of joint damage. The derivation of these measures was data driven, was supported by consensus, and showed validity in all respects (see Table 93.3). The ACR and WHO/ILAR core sets were identical, originally asking for 66 SJC and 68 TJC and for physical function as disease activity assessment, while radiographic changes were the sole outcome measurement. The EULAR core set did not comprise EGA and used 28 joint counts for SJC and TJC. Subsequently, the ACR also approved

TABLE 93.4 VARIOUS JOINT COUNTS IN RHEUMATOID ARTHRITIS

	Ritchie	Lansbury	ACR joint count	CSSRD	44 joint count	Reduced joint survey	32 joint count	28 joint count	18 joint count	16 joint count
Characteristics of the joint score										
Year of publication	1968	1956	1965	1983	1992	1985	NN	1989	2001	2001
Swollen (S)/tender (T)	T	S/T	S/T	S/T	S	S/T	S/T	S/T	S/T	S/T
Number of assessed joints	78	86	68/66	60	46/44	36	32	28	18	16
Joints effectively evaluated			68/66	60	54/52	36	40	28	42	40
Graded	0-3*	0-4	†	0-3						
Weighted		X						‡		
Included joint regions (number of counts on both sides)										
DIP (4 joints)		8	8							
PIP/IP1 (hands) (5 joints)	2	10	10	10	10	10	10	10	2	2
MCP (5 joints)	2	10	10	10	10	10	10	10	2	2
Carpometacarpal (5 joints)		2								
Carpus		2								
Wrist	2	2	2	2	2	2	2	2	2	2
Elbow	2	2	2	2	2	2	2	2	2	2
Shoulder	2	2	2	2	2		2	2	2	2
DIP (feet) (5 joints)		8								
PIP/IP1 (feet) (5 joints)		10	10	10	2 (IP1)					
MTP (5 joints)	2	10	10	10	2	10	2		2	
Tarsometatarsal (5 joints)	2	2								
Tarsus	2	6	2	2	4					
Ankle	2	2	2	2	2		2		2	2
Knee	2	2	2	2	2	2	2	2	2	2
Hip	2	2	2	2					2	2
Acromioclavicular	1	2	2	2	2					
Sternoclavicular	1	2	2	2	2					
Temporomandibular	1	2	2	2	2					
Cervical spine	1									

*Modified by Hart et al. to exclude grading of severity.
†The 66/68 joint counts were initially graded for the degree of tenderness and swelling.
‡A weighting of the 28 joint count has been proposed but has never been established in practice.
Adapted from Aletaha D, Smolen JS. The definition and measurement of disease modification in inflammatory rheumatic diseases. Rheum Dis Clin North Am 2006;32:9-44.

the application of reduced joint counts. Moreover, EULAR regarded functional assessment as an outcome measure, in addition to joint damage, rather than an activity measurement. In the context of this chapter we will separately discuss the activity measures, damage, and physical function, because we believe in the conceptually distinct, though intertwined, nature of activity (process), damage (structural changes), and function, with the latter constituting a hybrid measure comprising the two former and more (see Fig. 93.2).

Swollen and tender joint counts

Joint involvement is the fundamental hallmark of RA. Joints are the "organ involved" for the patient and the "organ of interest" for the rheumatologist. It is therefore virtually obligatory to assess the organ joint at every patient visit. The inflammation of the joint leads to soft tissue swelling (synovitis, effusion), tenderness, pain on motion, and reduced range of motion and, in the longer term, deformity. Several joint counts and indices have been developed over the decades, differing by the number of joints assessed or by the way joints are aggregated into joint regions.

The 66/68 joint count assesses, among many other joints, the distal interphalangeal (DIP) joints of the hands, which are usually not involved in RA but frequently affected in osteoarthritis and psoriatic arthritis. The 28 joint count spares these joints as well as the joints of the ankles and feet, which are often painful and tender due to other reasons than RA; also, these regions are often swollen due to co-morbid conditions, entailing the possibility of misjudgment. Moreover, the 28 joint count captures frequently involved joints and reflects the complete joint count very well. Importantly, however, using the 28 joint count for disease activity assessment does not negate the importance of other joints, particularly those of the feet, which clearly need to be evaluated in the course of thorough follow-up. A variety of other joint counts have been published in the literature, some of which are presented in Table 93.4, which is adapted from a recent review.[29] However, the 28 joint count seems to be the most established reduced joint counts, at present. Indeed, the 28 joint count is simple and fast to assess and has all validity attributes.

Joint counts differ not only by the number of joints assessed but also by the fact that some (older) scales weight joints by surface area (usually referred to as "weighted" joint counts), whereas other indices weight joints by severity of swelling and tenderness (usually referred to as "graded" joint counts) (see Table 93.4). The first joint index, the *Lansbury Index*, graded swelling and tenderness in 86 joints (minimal, slight, moderate, or maximal) and also weighted for joint surface area. Another early index, the *Ritchie Articular Index*, assesses graded tenderness in 26 joint areas and was later simplified by Hart to exclude the grading by severity, which is a major cause of inter-rater disagreement. The comprehensive *66/68 Joint Count*, as suggested by the American Rheumatism Association (ARA; now American College of Rheumatology [ACR]) in 1965, and the Cooperative Systemic Studies of Rheumatic Diseases (CSSRD) joint count are both time consuming and therefore limited in their use in clinical practice. Importantly, neither do expanded joint counts convey more information than reduced ones nor does weighting or grading provide added value. Rather than that, inter-observer error increases with the use of more complex means to evaluate joint involvement, which is indeed one of the major problems afflicted with joint counts. However, within a single observer, joint counts are reliable. This is also the case with self-assessed joint counts, but the differences to assessor-derived joint counts are tremendous; therefore, patient assessment of joint counts is not recommended.[30]

TJCs and SJCs may run common as well as disparate courses. Although TJCs and SJCs correlate with each other, TJCs correlate with pain and are more sensitive to change. TJCs also correlate with disability. In contrast, SJCs correlate much better than TJCs with progression of joint damage, suggesting that they reflect the pathogenetic events typical of RA more accurately. Likewise, SJCs correlate well with acute-phase reactants.

Pain

Pain is a prominent symptom in RA. It is mostly assessed on 100-mm horizontal visual analog scales (VAS), typically evaluating the period of the last week. Numerical or verbal rating scales are also used, frequently as 5-point scales. Horizontal and vertical VAS scales are well correlated, but vertical scales tend to produce systematically higher values, although there is considerable heterogeneity in the patients' ability to complete a VAS. In this respect, 11-point numerical rating scales of pain seem to be similarly reliable and responsive but are easier to use for patients. The ACR recommends the use of a 10-cm horizontal VAS with "no pain" at one end and "worst possible pain" at the other, without intermediate categories, or the Likert scale (1 = asymptomatic, 2 = mild, 3 = moderate, 4 = severe, 5 = very severe) to assess current pain in clinical trials.

Patient and evaluator assessment of global disease activity

Global disease activity rated by a patient or the physician (or practically any other third person evaluating the patient, i.e., the "evaluator") is also typically assessed on a 10-cm VAS. In addition to the PGA, sometimes the global health scale is evaluated, which essentially includes also all possible domains of health outcomes that are not directly related to "disease activity." The subjective PGA and the integrative and more objective EGA are usually assessed in combination. Patients tend to rate their disease activity to be higher than their evaluators, a systematic difference, which is a good argument for evaluating both in common ("averaging" effect). One reason for this difference might be that patients relate their disease state to the experience with their disease while evaluators relate an individual patient's disease status to their experience with all their patients. The responsiveness of measures of global disease activity is good, and they discriminate well between different levels of response and treatment groups.

Acute-phase reactants

The most frequently used and most reliable biomarkers in RA are the acute-phase reactants CRP and the ESR. Although many other biomarkers, especially proinflammatory cytokines, also reflect the events ongoing in active RA and may even more directly mirror the disease process and response to treatment, they have not been shown to provide superior information to the acute-phase reactants. Indeed, also biomarkers reflecting joint damage or synovial inflammation have not been shown to provide superior information to that conveyed by CRP. The acute-phase reactants, however, correlate well with SJCs, and the time-integrated acute-phase reactants also correlate well with radiographic progression. However, within composite indices, acute-phase reactants, especially CRP, add only little information (unless they are heavily weighted such as in the DAS28 [see later]), although they increase the content validity of a score by encompassing an "objective" laboratory measure. However, acute-phase reactant levels are also prone to elevations due to other reasons, such as infection, while they are normal in many patients with RA at their first presentation.

Composite indices of core set measures

The composite measures of disease activity are able to capture the spectrum of the disease despite its variations. This is relevant because RA has a very heterogeneous presentation across individuals and even within individuals when they are assessed longitudinally. Many features of disease activity are providing overlapping information, but they are still complementary in some respects. Thus, the evaluation of any single measure does not allow sufficiently accurate determination of the present level of a patient's disease activity or response to therapy. In addition, it is difficult to decide which single measure should be used as a disease activity marker in clinical trials, whereas the independent evaluation of all variables has methodologic problems.[31] Composite indices are a solution to this problem, because they provide a single result but are based on a combination of several measures. The indices differ in terms of what they measure (i.e., current disease activity or change) and their scales (e.g., continuous or ordinal). Continuous measures usually allow one to determine an "absolute" value of disease activity at any point in time, or—by virtue of established cut-points—the current disease activity state, such as remission.

The composition of various composite scores is shown in Table 93.5. Older scores, such as the ones by Steinbrocker and Lansbury, included additional features related to disease activity, such as anemia. The Mallya index includes tender joints, morning stiffness, ESR, hemoglobin, pain, and grip strength. The Stoke index comprises acute-phase reactants, morning stiffness, synovitis score, and tender joint score and showed good correlation with evaluator's and patient's global assessment of disease activity. The Mallya and the Stoke indices are measured on ordinal scales.

The *Disease Activity Score* (DAS) has been statistically derived based on physicians' decision to start or stop disease-modifying antirheumatic drugs (DMARDs). This was related to states of high and low disease activity, respectively.[32] The DAS therefore employs a complex formula, using transformations and weighting of variables (see Table 93.5). Whereas the original DAS employed the graded Ritchie Articular Index to evaluate joint tenderness and a 44 swollen joint count (see Table 93.4), its modification, the DAS28, includes condensed 28 joint counts.[33] The DAS and the DAS28 have also been modified to include CRP instead of ESR (DAS-CRP and DAS28-CRP) or to exclude assessment of global health (DAS-3 and DAS28-3) and cut-points for disease activity states have been derived (Table 93.6). For the DAS28, cut-points between high disease activity, moderate disease activity, low disease activity, and remission are 5.1, 3.2, and 2.6, respectively. Although in high ranges of composite indices the likelihood is high that all or most components contribute fairly equally to the result, this is different in the lower ranges of the DAS/DAS28. There, a single component, such as an acute-phase reactant or a patient assessment of disease activity, may dominate the score and might misinform on the overall disease activity. In fact, in DAS28 remission many patients may have significant residual disease activity, especially a high number of swollen joints, because of the low weight of swollen joints in the formula.[33] Moreover, because the ESR is also strongly weighted, small changes in ESR, even within the normal range, may bring patients into remission even in the presence of many swollen joints. Therefore, in states of low disease activity, a separate look at the contributing components may be worthwhile before drawing therapeutic conclusions. Given the complex formula of the DAS and the DAS28 and the computational need to calculate it, simpler indices were sought.

The variables of the *Simplified Disease Activity Index* (SDAI)[34] (see Table 93.6) were selected based on the core set of the ACR and the EULAR.[35,36] It was the first index for RA to employ a linear sum of variables that were untransformed and unweighted, a concept based on previous studies on reactive arthritis. The SDAI has been widely

TABLE 93.5 INDICES FOR EVALUATION OF RHEUMATOID ARTHRITIS ACTIVITY

	Steinbrocker therapeutic scorecard	Lansbury systemic manifestations	Mallya–Mace*	Paulus criteria	DAS/DAS 28 (4 items)	RADAR	ACR response criteria	RADAI	SDAI	CDAI
Year published	1946	1956	1981	1990	1990-1995	1992	1995	1995	2003	2003-2005
Number of swollen joints	X			X	X	X†	X	X†	X	X
Number of tender joints	X		X	X	X	X†,‡	X	X†,‡	X	X
Joint motion/Pain on motion	X	X								
Morning stiffness		X	X	X				X		
ESR/CRP	ESR	ESR	ESR	ESR	ESR/CRP§		Either		CRP	
Hemoglobin (Hb)/Anemia (An)	Hb	An	Hb							
Weight	X									
Fever		X								
Pain	X	X	X			X	X	X		
Global health	X				X‖					
Patient global disease activity				X		X¶	X	X¶	X	X
Evaluator global disease activity				X			X		X	X
Function	X					X	X			
Grip strength			X							
Muscle weakness		X								
Fatigue		X								

ESR, erythrocyte sedimentation rate; CRP, C-reactive protein.
*The index was later modified by van Riel and colleagues to include only the number of tender joints, morning stiffness, Hb, and ESR.
†Overall swelling and tenderness in joints is graded by patient.
‡List of joint regions, graded for tenderness from 0-3.
§The DAS/DAS28 were originally calculated using ESR and subsequently modified to also allow for CRP instead of ESR.
‖Global health excluded in the three-variable DAS/DAS28.
¶Global disease activity over the past 6 months
Adapted from Aletaha D, Smolen JS. The definition and measurement of disease modification in inflammatory rheumatic diseases. Rheum Dis Clin North Am 2006;32:9-44.

TABLE 93.6 CALCULATION, CUT-POINTS, AND RANGES OF COMPOSITE INDICES

DAS*	4	ESR†	$= 0.54 \times \sqrt{(Ritchie)} + 0.065 \times SJC44 + 0.33 \times \log_{nat}(ESR) + 0.0072 \times GH$	REM < 1.6 LDA < 2.4 MDA < 3.7 HDA ≥ 3.7	0.23-9.87
	4	CRP†	$= 0.54 \times \sqrt{(Ritchie)} + 0.065 \times SJC44 + 0.17 \times \log_{nat}(CRP+1) + 0.0072 \times GH + 0.45$		0.57-9.58
	3	ESR	$= 0.54 \times \sqrt{(Ritchie)} + 0.065 \times SJC44 + 0.33 \times \log_{nat}(ESR) + 0.22$		0.45-9.37
	3	CRP	$= 0.54 \times \sqrt{(Ritchie)} + 0.065 \times SJC44 + 0.17 \times \log_{nat}(CRP+1) + 0.65$		0.77-9.06
DAS28*	4	ESR	$= 0.56 \times \sqrt{(TJC28)} + 0.28 \times \sqrt{(SJC28)} + 0.70 \times \log_{nat}(ESR) + 0.014 \times GH$	REM < 2.6 LDA < 3.2 MDA < 5.1 HDA ≥ 5.1	0.49-9.07
	4	CRP	$= 0.56 \times \sqrt{(TJC28)} + 0.28 \times \sqrt{(SJC28)} + 0.36 \times \log_{nat}(CRP+1) + 0.014 \times GH + 0.96$		1.21-8.47
	3	ESR	$= [0.56 \times \sqrt{(TJC28)} + 0.28 \times \sqrt{(SJC28)} + 0.70* \times \log_{nat}(ESR)] \times 1.08 + 0.16$		0.68-8.44
	3	CRP	$= [0.56 \times \sqrt{(TJC28)} + 0.28*\sqrt{(SJC28)} + 0.36* \log_{nat}(CRP+1)] \times 1.10 + 1.15$		1.42-7.87
SDAI	5	CRP	SJC28 + TJC28 + PGA + EGA + CRP	REM ≤ 3.3 LDA ≤ 11 MDA ≤ 26 HDA > 26	0-100
CDAI	4	—	SJC28 + TJC28 + PGA + EGA	REM ≤ 2.8 LDA ≤ 10 MDA ≤ 22 HDA > 22	0-76

*Formulae for the DAS and the DAS28 variations obtained from the website: http://www.das-score.nl/www.das-score.nl/index.html, accessed August 2009.
†Range of ESR assumed as 2-100 mm/hr, and range of CRP assumed as 0-24 mg/dL.
DAS, Disease Activity Score; DAS28, DAS based on 28 joint counts; Ritchie, Ritchie Articular Index; SJC28, SJC44, swollen joint counts based on the evaluation of 28 or 44 joints, respectively; TJC28, tender joint count based on 28 joints; ESR, erythrocyte sedimentation rate; CRP, C-reactive protein; GH, global health; PGA, EGA, patient and evaluator global; REM, remission; LDA, low disease activity; MDA, moderate disease activity; HDA, high disease activity.
Adapted from Aletaha D, Smolen JS. The definition and measurement of disease modification in inflammatory rheumatic diseases. Rheum Dis Clin North Am 2006;32:9-44.

validated, and definitions of states of remission and of low, moderate, and high disease activity have been elaborated.[37] The SDAI, DAS, and DAS28 require the availability of an acute-phase reactant (CRP or ESR), which frequently precludes the immediate assessment owing to unavailable laboratory results. However, even in the absence of CRP values, the resulting score comprising the residual SDAI components was shown to have correlational and construct validity as well as sensitivity to change.[34] The statistical rationale and validity of such a clinical index, then named the *Clinical Disease Activity Index* (CDAI), was subsequently shown (see Table 93.6).[38] The value of the CDAI lies particularly in allowing the treating physician to make prompt treatment decisions based on the actual levels of disease activity. Similar to the DAS28, cut-points between the states of high disease activity, moderate disease activity, low disease activity, and remission have been defined as 26, 11, and 3.3, respectively, for the SDAI, and as 22, 10, and 2.8, respectively, for the CDAI (see Table 93.6). The SDAI and CDAI are both stringent measures of remission, allowing only a maximum sum of two swollen or tender joints (2+0, 1+1, or 0+2, respectively).

A variety of patient-reported questionnaires for disease activity evaluation in RA have been published. The *Rapid Assessment of Disease Activity in Rheumatology* (RADAR)[39] is a brief, two-page, patient self-assessed questionnaire including six items (see Table 93.5). The RADAR requires expert interpretation of its individual items, or use of other studies as references, but does not provide a single "total" result. Another instrument developed for clinical practice is the *Rheumatoid Arthritis Disease Activity Index* (RADAI),[40] a five-item questionnaire (see Table 93.5). The RADAI requires the use of a calculator, and its agreement with scores encompassing physician assessment is low. Both the RADAR and the RADAI are rarely used in clinical practice and clinical trials; rather, patient self-assessment of physical function is frequently employed. Another series of summary measures based primarily on patient report, called the Routine Assessment of Patient Index Data (RAPID) scores, have been published recently and include three to five of such measures.[41] RAPID-3 includes three patient reported measures: physical function, pain, and global estimate; RAPID-4 adds a self-report joint count from the RADAI (see earlier); RAPID-5 adds a physician estimate of global status. Thus, RAPID does not include a formal evaluator-assessed joint count and comprises physical function, which may be partly irreversible and therefore limited in its sensitivity to change (see later).

Improvement criteria

Assessing improvement to treatment is important in clinical trials but also in clinical practice. The term *improvement* incorporates a time component and implies that disease activity is assessed and compared with the baseline activity. In clinical trials, the baseline usually is the trial baseline, whereas in clinical practice this is often less clearly defined. Often it will be the start of a therapeutic segment, which can be the presentation of a patient to a specific clinic or (more often) the start of DMARD treatment.

Improvement can be assessed by looking at absolute or relative changes from the baseline. However, improvement can also be evaluated by looking at whether a patient has achieved a good clinical state. This evaluation principally does not any more depend on the comparison to the baseline and, therefore, is more feasible in clinical practice. Finally, there is also the option to assess improvement by combining a change with achievement of a particular disease activity state.

The *Paulus* criteria define improvement if four of six of the following conditions are fulfilled: improvement of greater than or equal to 20% for morning stiffness, ESR, joint pain/tenderness score, and joint swelling score and more than two grades on a five-grade scale (or moving from grade 2 to grade 1) for PGA and EGA.[42] The Paulus criteria do not account for the level of disease activity at baseline.

The *ACR improvement criteria*[25] are a modification of the Paulus criteria and have been widely used in clinical trials of the past decade. They require 20% improvement ("ACR20") in SJCs and TJCs and three of the five remaining core set variables (patient and evaluator global assessments, pain assessment, physical function, and acute-phase reactant level). These criteria were developed to best discriminate the effects of active drug from placebo in clinical trials. The minimal

improvement is a 20% response (ACR20), but the criteria have also been applied to study more profound responses, such as ACR50 and ACR70 response rates, although the latter do not discriminate better between placebo and active medication and may even have less statistical power. Similar to the Paulus criteria, the ACR criteria do not consider a patient's disease activity starting point and provide only a dichotomous "yes/no" result. The numerical ACR response, the *ACR-N*, has been developed to create a continuous scale ranging from 0% to 100% using the original structure of the ACR response criteria. The readout is the smallest relative improvement of three measures: SJC, TJC, and the median of the five remaining core set variables.[43] One point of criticism regarding the ACR type of response criteria is the issue of neglecting worsening (0% is the minimum). In addition, the ACR-N response cannot be assessed over time (area under the curve), because the results may be inflated owing to calculation of response in comparison to the baseline at every time point. It should be emphasized that an area under the curve analysis of continuous composite indices (cumulative disease activity over time) can be useful to determine differences between treatment groups when rapidity of response is an issue.

Recently, the ACR response criteria have been modified and the ACR has adopted the so-called Hybrid-ACR criteria as their new official response measure.[44] The *Hybrid-ACR* is a pseudo-continuous index that is based on the traditional ACR response assessment. To obtain the Hybrid-ACR, first the average percentage improvement in core set measure needs to be determined, while in the case of worsening, the percentage is censored by 100%, even if the respective measure deteriorated by much more. Thereafter, two outcomes are determined: first, the average of the percent changes across all core set measures and, second, the level of traditional ACR response (i.e., ACR non-response, ACR20, ACR50, or ACR70 response). The Hybrid-ACR then is the first of these two (the mean percent change across the core set variables), except if it does not fall within the respective range of the traditional ACR response. In that case the response is categorized to values of 19.99, 49.99, and 69.99 if mean core sets are lying above the traditional ACR categories achieved or they are set to 20, 50, or 70, if the mean core sets are lying below the respective ACR categories. The Hybrid-ACR is therefore a rather complex index with an unusual distribution with natural peaks at the mentioned values. Its statistical properties will need to be determined in future studies. However, it has been adopted because it discriminated active drug from comparator in RA clinical trials at the highest level of statistical significance.

The *EULAR response criteria* require not only a certain degree of improvement but also attainment of a good (or moderate) disease activity state (Fig. 93.6).[26] The EULAR criteria are based on DAS or DAS28 measurements. They classify improvement into no, moderate, or good response. In clinical trials, good plus moderate response tends to be somewhat higher than the ACR20 response, and a good EULAR response is usually more frequent than ACR50 response.

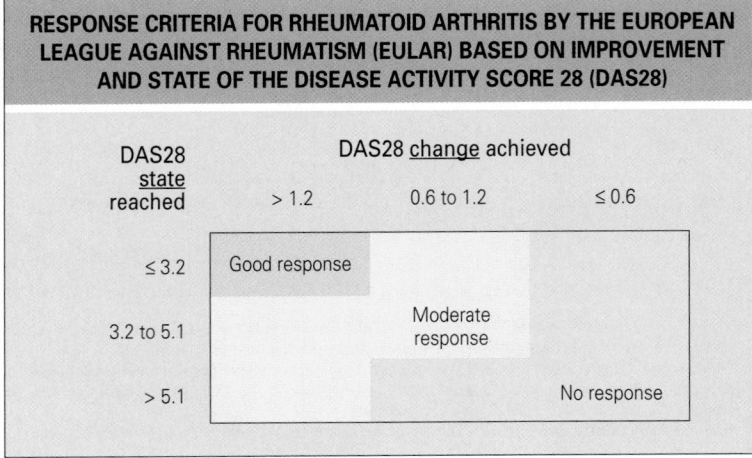

Fig. 93.6 Response criteria for rheumatoid arthritis by the European League Against Rheumatism (EULAR) based on improvement and state of the Disease Activity Score 28 (DAS28).

Finally, Scott has proposed a *simple index* compiling a predefined maximal value in certain domains (morning stiffness ≤ 15 minutes, ≤ 3 tender joints, ≤ 3 swollen joints, ESR ≤ 30 mm) plus greater than or equal to 50% reduction of pain and greater than or equal to 40% improvement of functional impairment.[45] Each of these six criteria is given 1 point, and the sum can be 0 to 6.

In summary, indices differ by the scale of measurement that they are using: many use a continuous scale (e.g., the Lansbury systemic index, the DAS/DAS28, SDAI, CDAI, or the pooled index); others use ordinal scales (e.g., the Mallya-Mace index, Stoke index, the Paulus criteria, the ACR criteria, Simple index, EULAR response criteria). They may also differ in their structure as being measures of disease activity (Lansbury, DAS/DAS28, SDAI, CDAI, Mallya/Mace, Stoke) and disease activity states (DAS/DAS28, SDAI, CDAI) or measures of response (Pooled index, Paulus criteria, ACR response criteria) or both (Simple index, EULAR response criteria).

INSTRUMENTS TO ASSESS PHYSICAL FUNCTION

Physical function is a central aspect of life of patients with rheumatoid arthritis and thus a major focus of RA patient care. Physical function can be regarded as one domain within the wider concept of health status and a key driver of a patient's quality of life (QoL). Improving functional outcomes is therefore a central goal of RA therapy. Assessment of physical function can most directly be done by subjecting individuals to performance tests. These are often too complex to implement in a broader group of patients or assess function only of specific body parts, such as hand function. Therefore, function most commonly is evaluated using questionnaires.

Questionnaires

There exist a large number of questionnaires that can be used to assess physical disability or quality of life in patients with RA. For a comprehensive view of these, the reader is referred to relevant review articles.[46] We will briefly touch on the most commonly used ones. The Medical Outcomes Study Short Form-36 (SF-36)[47] is the most commonly used generic (i.e., non-disease specific) measure that includes physical function as one of its eight scales (domains). From its 36 items, eight subscales can be calculated based on 2 to 10 items of the questionnaire), which include physical functioning, physical role, pain, and general health, as well as vitality, emotional role, social functioning, and mental health. Two summary measures, the physical component score (PCS) and the mental component score (MCS), can be calculated for the first and the latter four, respectively, whereas one item on reported health transition stands alone. Each scale is expressed with values from 0 to 100, and a lower score indicates poorer health. PCS and MCS scores are expressed using norm transformed domain scores that yield normative values of 50, with a standard deviation of 10, allowing comparison across populations, although this normalization may reduce the degree of potential change. The minimal clinically important difference (MCID) for the PCS is 5 to 10 points in individual domains and 2.5 to 5 points for the MCS domains. As a generic tool, the SF-36 is useful because it allows the comparison of patients with different diseases and with the normal population. It is a valid and reliable tool with good psychometric properties.

The Health Assessment Questionnaire (HAQ)[48] is a more disease-specific functional instrument. The "full" HAQ includes the assessment of discomfort, drug side effects, costs, mortality, and the Disability Index (HAQ-DI). Only the latter is in widespread use. The HAQ-DI evaluates the ability to perform activities of daily living. It comprises 20 questions on activities involving the upper and/or lower extremity, which are organized in eight categories (dressing, rising, eating, walking, hygiene, reach, grip, and usual activities). For each question there is a four-level difficulty scale ranging from 0 to 3, representing no difficulty ("0"), some difficulty ("1"), much difficulty ("2"), and inability to do ("3"). The final HAQ score is the mean of the highest scores across the eight categories and ranges from 0 to 3, with higher levels indicating more disability. Since its introduction, many modifications of the original HAQ have been published; Pincus and colleagues developed the modified HAQ (MHAQ), simplifying the scoring for daily clinical care, although the original HAQ remains the most widely used

instrument. In the MHAQ the questions from the original HAQ were reduced to one or two per category, also deriving its total score by taking the average of the eight categories. In 1999, Pincus introduced the multi-dimensional HAQ (MDHAQ), amending the 8-item MHAQ to 14 items. These additional items improved the floor effect that had been noticed with the use of the MHAQ. Because the intervals between scores at different points of the HAQ scale did not translate into similar changes in functional impairment, Wolfe and colleagues recently developed the HAQ-II, in which this psychometric problem has been addressed.

The MCID of the HAQ has been suggested to be 0.22. However, recent studies showed that the potential for change of HAQ scores may differ depending on the average duration of RA. The amount of underlying damage may reduce the reversibility of HAQ scores in individual patients. Likewise, in highly active RA, HAQ scores vary little with respect to differences in underlying damage owing to the great impact of activity on the HAQ, with an average HAQ score of about 1.3 (and up to a mean of 1.9 in trials), whereas in remission HAQ scores differ considerably but were mostly less than 0.6. Thus, it is important to bear in mind that the HAQ as a measure of functional limitation is determined by both activity (reversible component) and accrued damage (irreversible component). In early stages of RA the HAQ score is usually fully reversible, although this may not at all be the case in very late stages. It has been well established that the HAQ-DI increases with duration of RA, reflecting the accumulated joint damage, and even more directly by the fact that over the longer term the correlation between HAQ-DI and radiographic damage increases.

The Arthritis Impact Measurement Scale (AIMS)[49] includes nine domains, each of which is comprised of 4 to 7 questions, totaling to 49 questions. Different versions of the original AIMS have been published, including the longer AIMS2 (12 domains and 78 questions) and the shorter AIMS2-short form (5 domains and 26 questions). In one study, the AIMS2-SF has shown to reduce the completion time while maintaining the properties of the longer AIMS2. Wolfe and colleagues developed the clinical HAQ (CLINHAQ), which, in addition to the eight categories of the original HAQ, borrowed the depression and anxiety scales from the AIMS and included five additional visual analog scales and a pain diagram. The Euro-QoL 5-D (EQ-5D) is a simple standardized self-report questionnaire for use as a measure of health outcome ("health states").[50]

Functional tests

In contrast to questionnaires, measures that assess the strength, precision, or swiftness of various aspects of locomotor function constitute a more direct way of assessing functioning.[51] Grip strength is usually assessed using a vigorimeter or a dynamometer, and a measurement on the pressure attained by squeezing a compressible rubber bulb is taken. The Moberg picking-up test is a standardized timed assessment of the ability to pick up small items randomly placed in three lines on the table and to put them into a box. In the button test, patients are timed while undoing and re-buttoning five buttons on a board with one hand. The walking time is a timed measurement of the patient's ability to walk a particular distance. It has been shown that, using standardized protocols, all these instruments have good reliability and predict long-term morbidity and mortality in patients with RA.

INSTRUMENTS TO ASSESS STRUCTURAL PROGRESSION

Scoring of radiographs

Radiographic damage is the hallmark of rheumatoid arthritis, and it usually progresses over time. Most scoring methods of radiographs are based on assessment of hands and feet, joint areas that are thought to be representative of overall radiographic damage. Because measurement error is an issue in radiographic scoring, it is recommended to train readers and calculate the mean of two independent readers. If the purpose is assessing structural damage, annual radiographs of the hands and feet are generally satisfactory, but for particular research questions or in early RA, smaller intervals and/or the inclusion of more joints might be appropriate. It is still a matter of debate whether

TABLE 93.7 RADIOGRAPHIC SCORING METHODS FOR RHEUMATOID ARTHRITIS							
	Level of assessment	Scale/joint	Joints/regions assessed	Total score	Hands	Feet	Year
Steinbrocker	Patient	—	—	0-4	X		1949
Kellgren	Patient	—	—	0-5	X		1963
Sievers	Patient	—	—	0-8	X		1965
Berens	Patient	—	—	0-5	X		1969
Scores based on the method developed by Sharp							
Sharp	Features	0-5 ERO; 0-4 JSN	54 ERO; 54 JSN	0-486	X		1971
Sharp (modified Sharp)	Features	0-5 ERO; 0-4 JSN	46 ERO, 48 JSN [42 JSN]	0-422 [-398]	X	X	2000
Genant (modified Sharp)	Features	0-3.5 (steps of 0.5) ERO; 0-4 JSN	28 ERO; 13 JSN	0-150	X	X	1983
Bluhm (modified Sharp)	Features	0-5 ERO; 0-4 JSN	34 ERO; 36 JSN	0-314	X		1983
Nance/Kaye (modified Sharp)	Features	0,2-4 ERO; 0,2-5 JSN; 0,2-4 MLG	22 ERO; 28 JSN; 30 MLG	0-348	X		1986
van der Heijde (modified Sharp)	Features	0-5(10)* ERO; 0-4 JSN	32 ERO; 30 JSN	0-448	X	X	1989
Simple Erosion Narrowing Score (SENS)	Features	0-1 ERO; 0-1 JSN	22 ERO; 21 JSN	0-86	X	X	1999
Scores based on the method developed by Larsen							
Larsen	Joint	0-5	22 (-28)	0-110 (-140)	X	X	1974
Gofton (modified Larsen)	Joint	0-4 ERO	48 ERO	0-192	X		1982
Scott (modified Larsen)	Joint	0-5	22 (-28)	0-110 (-140)	X	X	1995
Rau (modified Larsen)	Features	0-5 ERO	38 ERO	0-190	X		1995
Kaarela/Kautiainen (modified Larsen)	Joint	0-5	20	0-100	X	X	1997

*Erosions of the feet are scored on the proximal and distal aspect of the joint, resulting on a possible score per joint of 10. ERO, erosions; JSN, joint space narrowing.
Adapted from Aletaha D, Smolen JS. The definition and measurement of disease modification in inflammatory rheumatic diseases. Rheum Dis Clin North Am 2006;32:9-44.

radiographs should be read in random or chronologic order, because reading radiographs in random order reduces expectation bias (improving signal-to-noise ratio) but decreases the ability to determine small changes. There are a large number of instruments in use for radiographic scoring that can be categorized into three groups (Table 93.7): (1) instruments assigning a single radiographic grade to a patient (no longer in use); (2) those that provide an overall score for a given joint and sum the scores of multiple joints; and (3) those that separately score two or more features of each joint and then sum multiple joints into the radiographic score (by feature or as a total sum of scores on different features).

The first index, published by Steinbrocker, assigned radiographic damage to four stages based on the joint with the greatest abnormality, translating the degree of damage of a single, worst affected joint into a crude summary for a patient. Subsequent scoring methods refining the grading of radiographic abnormalities had similar limitations with respect to sensitivity to change and are essentially no longer in use. Later, wider scales employed summary ratings of individual joints instead of global ratings of patients. Scores with wider ranges had the advantage of increased sensitivity to change but were less reliable, because raters were more prone to be inconsistent in their scoring.

The most prominent scoring method that combines all features of a particular joint globally is the Larsen method (soft tissue swelling or osteoporosis = 1; erosions of increasing extent = 2-5). Standard atlas radiographs are provided for all joints as a comparative means. The method was later modified by Larsen to remove soft tissue swelling and osteoporosis.[52] In the new method, a score of 1 already required erosions or joint space narrowing to be present. Since its development, the Larsen score was modified manifold (see Table 93.7).

The Sharp score[53] was the first instrument to include a separate scoring for erosions and joint space narrowing (see Table 93.7) as a reflection of bone and cartilage damage, respectively, which may provide independent information. It initially evaluated only joints of the hands and wrists but was further modified by Sharp to enable the evaluation of the feet as well (see Table 93.7). A further modification of the Sharp score by van der Heijde[54] also introduced the 10 metatarsophalangeal joints and the interproximal joints of the big toes, whereas some areas of the wrist were excluded because of the difficulty of their

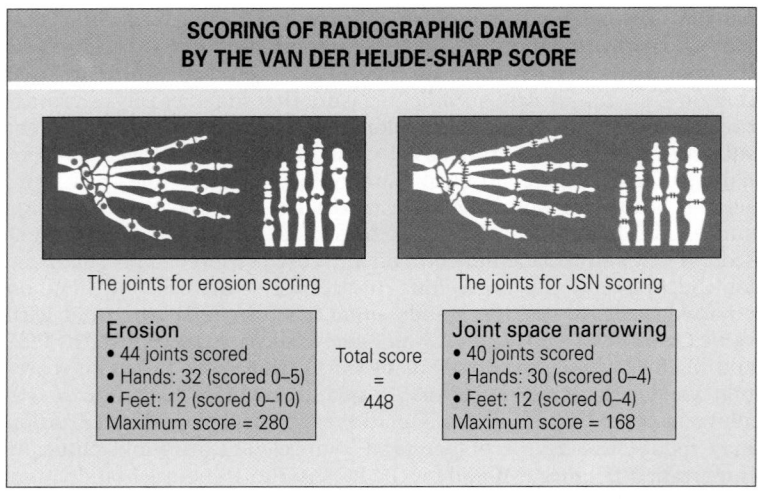

SCORING OF RADIOGRAPHIC DAMAGE BY THE VAN DER HEIJDE-SHARP SCORE

The joints for erosion scoring   The joints for JSN scoring

Erosion	Total score = 448	Joint space narrowing
• 44 joints scored • Hands: 32 (scored 0–5) • Feet: 12 (scored 0–10) Maximum score = 280		• 40 joints scored • Hands: 30 (scored 0–4) • Feet: 12 (scored 0–4) Maximum score = 168

Fig. 93.7 Scoring of radiographic damage by the van der Heijde–Sharp score. Separate evaluation of erosions (0-5) and joint space narrowing (0-4) in the joints of the hands and the feet. *(Adapted from van der Heijde DM, Van't Hof MA, van Riel PL, et al. Validity of single variables and composite indices for measuring disease activity in rheumatoid arthritis. Ann Rheum Dis 1992;51:177-181.)*

assessment. The Sharp–van der Heijde (SvdH) score is widely used now (Fig. 93.7). In this score, erosions of the feet are scored 0 to 10 (see Table 93.7). Another score that has been used in recent clinical trials is the Genant modified Sharp score, which assesses fewer joint regions than the Sharp and SvdH scores, uses a scale of 0 to 3.5 for erosions and 0 to 4 for joint space narrowing and spans from 0 to 150 rather than ranging beyond 400 (see Table 93.7). A Simple Erosion and Narrowing Score (SENS) counts the number of eroded joints and the number of joints exhibiting narrowing and sums them. Several other modifications use different joint regions or other features, such as malalignment, in addition to erosion and joint space narrowing (see Table 93.7). In general, the Sharp and the Larsen methods provide similar estimates of radiographic severity but the Sharp score and its modifications are more sensitive to change.

A single radiograph in conjunction with the knowledge of a patient's duration of RA allows estimation of a patient's annual progression rate. This rate integrates an individual patient's history (RA severity and treatment) as a benchmark to assess structural effects of subsequent therapeutic regimens.

Other imaging modalities

Radiographic scoring appears to be a crude way to determine joint damage, and more sophisticated modalities are therefore of significant interest. Magnetic resonance imaging (MRI) and ultrasonography are two of these. By using contrast media (MRI) and power Doppler imaging, the vascularity of a lesion, such as synovial membrane, can be easily determined. Ultrasonography also allows one to assess cartilage thickness and to depict some erosions. MRI enables seeing erosions relatively early. However, none of these methods has been sufficiently validated as being meaningful to outcome. Also, both have a number of limitations. Although ultrasonography is cost effective, it is very time consuming if one wanted to depict all joints that are evaluated by hand and foot radiographs. Also, the handling of the transducer is investigator-dependent and the angle may differ even within an individual patient with differing states of joint swelling or stiffness. Also, some areas may escape visibility by ultrasonography. With MRI, on the other hand, aside from its costs, it is still difficult to depict cartilage changes. Furthermore, the currently employed MRI scoring system, the RA-MRI score (RAMRIS) and its recent modification,[55] looks at wrist and metacarpophalangeal joints and thus does not account for proximal interphalangeal joints, which are frequently involved in RA and included in the radiographic scores. Interestingly, in a recent trial, radiographic scores were as sensitive to change as the RAMRIS.[56] Moreover, on a group level, radiographic changes can be depicted within 3 months of start of treatment,[57] suggesting that radiographic assessment in RA is currently not inferior to other imaging modalities in its sensitivity to change or time to detectability of change, whereas other modalities are still more expensive, more time consuming, or both. Most importantly, although radiographic changes have been associated with time-integrated disease activity on the one hand and disability on the other hand, these data still need to be provided and validated for ultrasonography and MRI.

OTHER INSTRUMENTS: FATIGUE, WORK PRODUCTIVITY, AND CO-MORBIDITY

We have already mentioned that one of the many features of RA is fatigue. Although the mechanisms underlying fatigue are not clear but might comprise direct or indirect consequences of cytokine release on the central nervous system, or may be related to pain, depression, anemia or other aspects of the disease, it is a fact that clinical improvement generally leads to improvement in fatigue. Various scales have been employed, among them simple VAS or the more complex FACIT fatigue scale,[58] which ranges from 0 to 52, with higher scores meaning less fatigue and an MCID of 4.

Another important outcome relates to work productivity. A variety of instruments have been developed and validated and are increasingly used in clinical trials, addressing the impact of the disease and consequences of therapeutic interventions on the ability to work. The data provide one of the bases for health economic analyses. Providing information on these instruments would go beyond the scope of this chapter, and the reader is referred to recent review articles.[59]

Likewise, co-morbidities not only influence disease outcome but also frequently limit the applicability of certain therapies. Several instruments are available.[60] Although their value in RA has not yet been sufficiently validated, the assessment of co-morbidity may provide additional important insights in our understanding of RA and response to therapy. Finally, a very important aspect of caring for patients with chronic disease is prevention of drug toxicity. Clinical trials usually report on the more frequent adverse events within the short-term horizon of the respective studies, but observational studies and registries have been set up to identify rarer events and long-term consequences of therapy. There is currently no uniform method of toxicity assessment, especially when feasibility is an issue, such as in clinical practice.

CONCLUSION

Rheumatoid arthritis is a complex systemic disease. Outcomes assessment in RA therefore is also more complex than in other chronic diseases. The three main areas of outcomes are disease activity, joint damage, and functional impairment. Each of these areas is represented by various domains, each of which again can be assessed using various instruments. This makes the field not easily transparent at first sight. Consistently, however, in the past until now, disease activity has been found to be reflected best by using the core set of measures, that include joint counts, global scales, pain scores, and acute-phase response. Ideally, however, in clinical trials and clinical practice, these measures need to be combined into single summary measures (scores, indices), so that clear targets for treatment can be defined. The benefit of treatment strategies targeted at specific outcomes has only been elucidated in the past few years and cannot be overemphasized. At the same time, the level of functional capacity and radiographic damage need to be considered when outcomes are assessed or treatment decisions are made. All three areas—activity, function, and damage—are linked with one influencing the other, and all three are determinants of the most important outcome, which is a patient's quality of life.

KEY REFERENCES

1. Smolen JS, Aletaha D, Koeller M, et al. New therapies for treatment of rheumatoid arthritis. Lancet 2007;370:1861-1874.
2. Aletaha D, Neogi T, Silman AJ, et al. The 2010 American College of Rheumatology/European League Against Rheumatism Classification Criteria for Rheumatoid Arthritis.
3. Neogi T, Aletaha D, Silman AJ, et al. The American College of Rheumatology/European League Against Rheumatism Classification Criteria for Rheumatoid Arthritis—Methodological Report Phase 2. Arthritis Rheum
4. Funovits J, Aletaha D, Bykerk V, et al. The American College of Rheumatology/European League Against Rheumatism Classification Criteria for Rheumatoid Arthritis: Methodological Report Part I. Ann Rheum Dis.
5. Fries JF, Spitz P, Kraines RG, Holman HR. Measurement of patient outcome in arthritis. Arthritis Rheum 1980;23:137-145.
6. van Riel PL, Fransen J. Established rheumatoid arthritis: clinical assessments. Best Pract Res Clin Rheumatol 2007;21:807-825.
7. van der Helm-van Mil AH, Detert J, Le Cessie S, et al. Validation of a prediction rule for disease outcome in

patients with recent-onset undifferentiated arthritis: moving toward individualized treatment decision-making. Arthritis Rheum 2008;58:2241-2247.
8. Tugwell P, Bombardier C. A methodologic framework for developing and selecting endpoints in clinical trials. J Rheumatol 1982;9:758-762.
9. van der Heijde DM, Van't Hof MA, van Riel PL, et al. Validity of single variables and composite indices for measuring disease activity in rheumatoid arthritis. Ann Rheum Dis 1992;51:177-181.
10. Goldsmith CH, Smythe HA, Helewa A. Interpretation and power of a pooled index. J Rheumatol 1993;20:575-578.
11. Sharp JT, Lidsky MD, Collins LC, Moreland J. Methods of scoring the progression of radiologic changes in rheumatoid arthritis: correlation of radiologic, clinical and laboratory abnormalities. Arthritis Rheum 1971;14:706-720.
12. van der Heijde DM. Joint erosions and patients with early rheumatoid arthritis. Br J Rheumatol 1995;34(Suppl 2):74-78.
13. van der Heide A, Jacobs JW, Bijlsma JW, et al. The effectiveness of early treatment with "second-line" antirheumatic drugs: a randomized, controlled trial. Ann Intern Med 1996;124:699-707.

14. Nell V, Machold KP, Eberl G, et al. Benefit of very early referral and very early therapy with disease-modifying anti-rheumatic drugs in patients with early rheumatoid arthritis. Rheumatology (Oxford) 2004;43:906-914.
15. Combe B, Landewe R, Lukas C, et al. EULAR recommendations for the management of early arthritis: report of a task force of the European Standing Committee for International Clinical Studies Including Therapeutics (ESCISIT). Ann Rheum Dis 2006; Jan 5 [Epub ahead of print].
16. Grigor C, Capell H, Stirling A, et al. Effect of a treatment strategy of tight control for rheumatoid arthritis (the TICORA study): a single-blind randomised controlled trial. Lancet 2004;364:263-269.
17. Verstappen SM, Jacobs JW, van der Veen, MJ, et al. Intensive treatment with methotrexate in early rheumatoid arthritis: aiming for remission. Computer Assisted Management in Early Rheumatoid Arthritis (CAMERA, an open-label strategy trial). Ann Rheum Dis 2007;66:1443-1449.
18. Smolen JS, Han C, Van der Heijde DM, et al. Radiographic changes in rheumatoid arthritis patients attaining different disease activity states with methotrexate monotherapy and infliximab plus

methotrexate: the impacts of remission and TNF-blockade. Ann Rheum Dis 2008; Jul 7 [Epub ahead of print].

19. Aletaha D, Funovits J, Smolen JS. The importance of reporting disease activity states in clinical trials of rheumatoid arthritis. Arthritis Rheum 2008;58:2622-2631.

20. Aletaha D, Funovits J, Ward MM, et al. Perception of improvement in patients with rheumatoid arthritis varies with disease activity levels at baseline. Arthritis Rheum 2009 Mar 15;61(3):313-320

21. Aletaha D, Funovits J, Keystone EC, Smolen JS. Disease activity early in the course of treatment predicts response to therapy after one year in rheumatoid arthritis patients. Arthritis Rheum 2007;56:3226-3235.

22. Felson DT, Anderson JJ, Boers M, et al. The American College of Rheumatology preliminary core set of disease activity measures for rheumatoid arthritis. The Committee on Outcome Measures in Rheumatoid Arthritis Clinical Trials. Arthritis Rheum 1993;36:729-740.

23. Smolen JS. Report of the EULAR Standing Committee on International Clinical Studies Including Therapeutic Trials. Rheumatol Eur 1994;23:37-39.

24. Boers M, Tugwell P, Felson DT, et al. World Health Organization and International League of Associations for Rheumatology core endpoints for symptom modifying antirheumatic drugs in rheumatoid arthritis clinical trials. J Rheumatol Suppl 1994;41:86-89.

25. Felson DT, Anderson JJ, Boers M, et al. American College of Rheumatology preliminary definition of improvement in rheumatoid arthritis. Arthritis Rheum 1995;38:727-735.

26. van Gestel AM, Prevoo MLL, van't Hof MA, et al. Development and validation of the European League Against Rheumatism response criteria for rheumatoid arthritis: comparison with the preliminary American College of Rheumatology and the World Health Organization/International League Against Rheumatism Criteria. Arthritis Rheum 1996;39:34-40.

27. Aletaha D, Landewe R, Karonitsch T, et al. Reporting disease activity in clinical trials of patients with rheumatoid arthritis: EULAR/ACR collaborative recommendations. Arthritis Rheum 2008;59:1371-1377.

28. Aletaha D, Landewe R, Karonitsch T, et al. Reporting disease activity in clinical trials of patients with rheumatoid arthritis: EULAR/ACR collaborative recommendations. Ann Rheum Dis 2008;67:1360-1364.

29. Aletaha D, Smolen JS. The definition and measurement of disease modification in inflammatory rheumatic diseases. Rheum Dis Clin North Am 2006;32:9-44.

30. Prevoo ML, Kuper IH, van't Hof MA, et al. Validity and reproducibility of self-administered joint counts: a prospective longitudinal followup study in patients with rheumatoid arthritis. J Rheumatol 1996;23:841-845.

31. Tugwell P, Bombardier C. A methodologic framework for developing and selecting endpoints in clinical trials. J Rheumatol 1982;9:758-762.

32. van der Heijde DM, van't Hof MA, van Riel PL, et al. Judging disease activity in clinical practice in rheumatoid arthritis: first step in the development of a disease activity score. Ann Rheum Dis 1990;49:916-920.

33. Prevoo ML, van't Hof MA, Kuper HH, et al. Modified disease activity scores that include twenty-eight-joint counts: development and validation in a prospective longitudinal study of patients with rheumatoid arthritis. Arthritis Rheum 1995;38:44-48.

34. Smolen JS, Breedveld FC, Schiff MH, et al. A simplified disease activity index for rheumatoid arthritis for use in clinical practice. Rheumatology 2003;42:244-257.

35. Smolen JS. The work of the EULAR Standing Committee on International Clinical Studies Including Therapeutic Trials (ESCISIT). Br J Rheumatol 1992;31:219-220.

36. Felson DT, Anderson JJ, Boers M, et al. The American College of Rheumatology preliminary core set of disease activity measures for rheumatoid arthritis clinical trials. The Committee on Outcome Measures in Rheumatoid Arthritis Clinical Trials. Arthritis Rheum 1993;36:729-740.

37. Aletaha D, Ward MM, Machold KP, et al. Remission and active disease in rheumatoid arthritis: defining criteria for disease activity states. Arthritis Rheum 2005;52:2625-2636.

38. Aletaha D, Nell VK, Stamm T, et al. Acute phase reactants add little to composite disease activity indices for rheumatoid arthritis: validation of a clinical activity score. Arthritis Res Ther 2005;7:R796-R806.

39. Mason JH, Anderson JJ, Meenan RF, et al. The rapid assessment of disease activity in rheumatology (RADAR) questionnaire: validity and sensitivity to change of a patient self-report measure of joint count and clinical status. Arthritis Rheum 1992;35:156-162.

40. Stucki G, Liang MH, Stucki S, et al. A self-administered rheumatoid arthritis disease activity index (RADAI) for epidemiologic research: psychometric properties and correlation with parameters of disease activity. Arthritis Rheum 1995;38:795-798.

41. Pincus T, Yazici Y, Bergman M, et al. A proposed approach to recognise "near-remission" quantitatively without formal joint counts or laboratory tests: a patient self-report questionnaire routine assessment of patient index data (RAPID) score as a guide to a "continuous quality improvement" s. Clin Exp Rheumatol 2006;24(6 Suppl 43):S60-S65.

42. Paulus HE, Egger MJ, Ward JR, Williams HJ. Analysis of improvement in individual rheumatoid arthritis patients treated with disease-modifying antirheumatic drugs, based on the findings in patients treated with placebo. The Cooperative Systematic Studies of Rheumatic Diseases Group. Arthritis Rheum 1990;33:477-484.

43. Siegel JN, Zhen B-G. Use of the American College of Rheumatology N (ACR-N) index of improvement in rheumatoid arthritis: argument in favor. Arthritis Rheum 2005;52:1637-1641.

44. A proposed revision to the ACR20: the hybrid measure of American College of Rheumatology response. Arthritis Rheum 2007;57:193-202.

45. Scott DL. A simple index to assess disease activity in rheumatoid arthritis. J Rheumatol 1993;20:582-584.

46. Scott DL, Garrood T. Quality of life measures: use and abuse. Baillieres Best Pract Res Clin Rheumatol 2000;14:663-687.

47. Ware JE Jr, Sherbourne CD. The MOS 36-item short-form health survey (SF-36): I. Conceptual framework and item selection. Med Care 1992;30:473-483.

48. Fries JF, Spitz P, Kraines RG, Holman HR. Measurement of patient outcome in arthritis. Arthritis Rheum 1980;23:137-145.

49. Meenan RF, Gertman PM, Mason JH. Measuring health status in arthritis: the arthritis impact measurement scales. Arthritis Rheum 1980;23:146-152.

50. Kind P. The EuroQoL instrument: an index of health-related quality of life. In: Spilker B, ed. Quality of life and pharmacoeconomics in clinical trials, 2nd ed. Philadelphia: Lippincott-Raven, 1996:191-201.

REFERENCES

Full references for this chapter can be found on www.expertconsult.com.

Management of rheumatoid arthritis: synovitis

94

Jon T. Giles and Joan M. Bathon

- Complete remission of rheumatoid arthritis (RA) disease activity should be the ultimate goal for treatment in all RA patients.
- Early, aggressive treatment of synovitis is desirable in order to have the greatest impact in preventing damage and disability.
- Patients with risk factors for poor prognosis warrant the most aggressive suppression of synovitis.
- Step-up combination approaches, beginning with rapidly titrated methotrexate, are the best studied and most commonly used strategies in clinical practice.
- With further study, first-line combinations of biologic and non-biologic disease-modifying antirheumatic drugs may be warranted in patients with the poorest prognosis.
- Emerging targeted therapies hold great therapeutic promise and may alter current treatment paradigms in the future.
- The use of bridging and/or low-dose corticosteroids, non-steroidal anti-inflammatory drugs and simple analgesics is often required to maximally manage symptoms.

Rheumatoid arthritis (RA) is a systemic disease with both articular and extra-articular features. The primary pathology is inflammation and hypertrophy of the synovial lining of diarthrodial joints. The inflamed rheumatoid synovium directly invades and destroys articular and periarticular structures (described in detail in Chapter 17), a process manifested clinically by joint swelling, pain, and tenderness, collectively referred to as *synovitis*. Chronic synovitis, if left untreated or inadequately suppressed, will result in joint destruction and dysfunction.

Synovitis is thus a cardinal feature of RA. Demonstration of synovitis is essential for the diagnosis of RA,[1] and reduction in the burden of synovitis constitutes a critical component of the response and remission criteria that are widely used in clinical trials of RA to evaluate the efficacy of new therapies.[2,3] In general, treatment strategies that successfully suppress synovitis are associated with improvements in articular pain, stiffness, and physical functioning, as well as reduction of joint deformity, disability, and, possibly, mortality.[4,5] In contrast, treatment strategies with little capacity to reduce synovitis (i.e., non-steroidal anti-inflammatory drugs [NSAIDs] and narcotic analgesics) have limited ability to modify the outcomes listed earlier.

The currently available therapeutic agents that are used for the treatment of RA have been discussed in detail in previous chapters (Chapters 44 to 67). The goal of this chapter is to outline management strategies for RA that take into account not only characteristics of these individual therapies or classes of therapies but also features of the disease and of the patient that will influence outcomes and response to treatment. The important roles of physical and occupational therapy (Chapter 46), pain control (Chapter 48), joint surgery (Chapter 66), patient education (Chapter 44), complementary therapies (Chapter 47), and a multidisciplinary approach to rheumatoid arthritis (Chapter 95) are reviewed in detail in other sections of this book.

HISTORIC BACKGROUND

Finding safe and effective strategies to suppress synovitis, in order to reduce or prevent disability and pain, has always been the primary aim of the pharmacologic management of RA. However, it has only been in the past several decades, with the evolution of molecular biology and a concomitant explosion in large-scale randomized clinical trials, that therapies with favorable benefit-to-risk profiles have been identified or confirmed (Fig. 94.1).

The use of high doses of salicylates and glucocorticoids in the first half of the 20th century, although revolutionary, was accompanied by unacceptable degrees of toxicity. From the mid-20th century until the mid-1980s, a slow, cautious approach to the treatment of RA, known as the *pyramid approach*, was most widely practiced. This consisted of a prolonged period of treatment with NSAIDs, with or without glucocorticoids, before adding a disease-modifying antirheumatic drug (DMARD). The prescription of one of a limited array of DMARDs available at the time (e.g., gold salts, penicillamine) was often delayed because of their limited efficacy, risk of major toxicities, and potential to lose their effectiveness over time.[6] If the DMARD of choice was ineffective in controlling synovitis, it was discontinued in favor of an alternative DMARD. Not surprisingly, the pyramid approach inevitably resulted in some degree of joint destruction and disability in nearly all RA patients.

By the 1980s, the introduction and gradual acceptance of low-dose weekly methotrexate as a highly effective treatment for RA with relatively low toxicity prompted the abandonment of the pyramid approach in favor of much earlier DMARD use in RA patients. The use of DMARDs in combination and the recent introduction of biologic DMARDs have moved the notion of early, aggressive treatment of RA forward such that complete remission of RA disease activity should be the ultimate goal for treatment in all RA patients.

PATIENT CHARACTERISTICS THAT AFFECT TREATMENT DECISIONS

Because inflammation is a relatively constant feature of RA throughout the course of the disease, joint damage will continue to accrue over time if treatment is not adequate. More than half of patients will develop erosions on plain radiographs within just 2 years of disease onset, and some data suggest that the rate of radiographic damage may be higher in the first years of disease.[7] Thus early treatment is desirable in order to have the greatest impact in preventing damage and disability,[8] yet treatment initiated or ramped up at any phase of the disease will still be capable of decreasing inflammation and preventing additional damage.[9,10] For these reasons, the most recent ACR guidelines for the use of biologic and non-biologic DMARDs in RA include treatment algorithms for patients with early disease (<6 months' duration).[11]

WHAT IS AGGRESSIVE THERAPY?

The importance of "aggressive" management of RA is now generally accepted.[12] A reasonable definition of aggressive management is a treatment strategy that rapidly and maximally suppresses synovitis without inducing an unacceptable burden of adverse side effects. The evidence-based ACR 2008 recommendations for DMARD use in RA organize treatment algorithms for initiating or resuming DMARDs on the basis of the duration of disease, level of disease activity, and features of poor prognosis (described later).[11] Under these guidelines, in a patient presenting with modest disease activity and few risk factors for poor prognosis (see later), early initiation and rapid dose escalation of a single DMARD may be sufficient to effectively control disease activity.

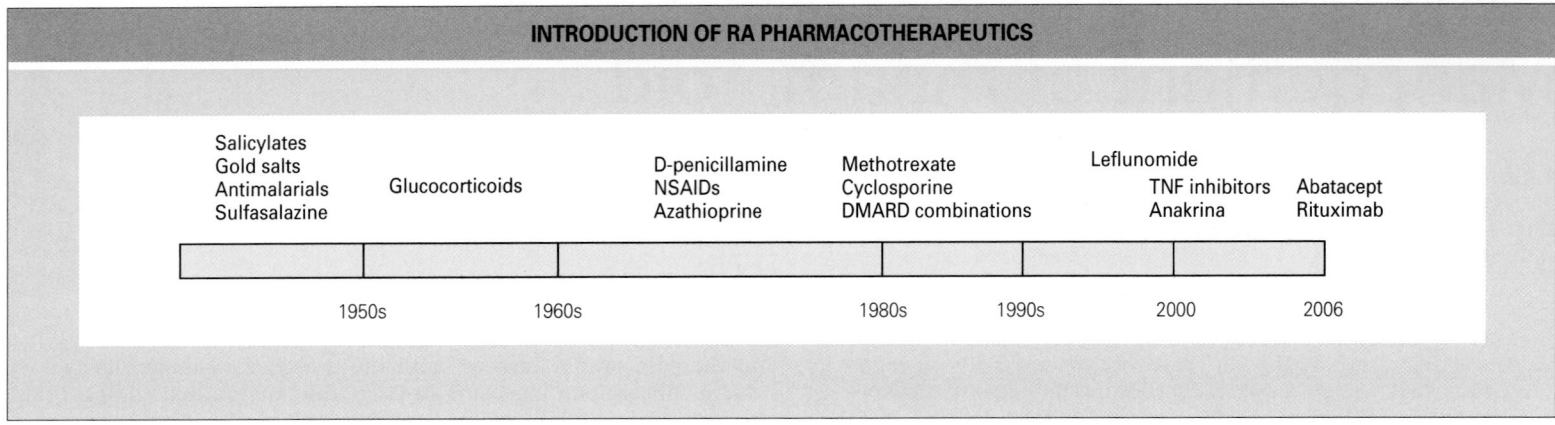

Fig. 94.1 Timeline: introduction of rheumatoid arthritis pharmacotherapeutics.

In contrast, in a patient presenting with high disease activity and many risk factors for an unfavorable outcome, early initiation of a combination of DMARDs is recommended. In this instance, concomitant corticosteroids may also be necessary. Thus the notion of aggressive management is somewhat relative, referring to the choice of agent(s), the number of agents, and the rapidity of dose escalation of each of the agents, and these are dictated, in turn, by the profile of the patient being treated.

For each individual, the choice of treatment depends on an analysis of the benefit the patient is expected to gain from that treatment versus the potential risks that the treatment, or combination of treatments, poses. The ability early in disease to differentiate patients with a poor prognosis from those with a good prognosis will allow for individual tailoring of therapeutic regimens that have the highest benefit-to-risk ratio for each patient.

PREDICTORS OF POOR OUTCOME

There is no single clinical, laboratory, or imaging parameter that is sufficiently sensitive to clearly identify patients who are at the highest risk for a poor outcome (e.g., disability). However, prediction models based on combinations of factors have been developed.[13,14] In most longitudinal studies on which prediction models have been based, radiographic progression of erosive disease serves as the surrogate for poor outcome because periarticular erosions are relatively specific for RA, can be inexpensively assessed over a relatively short period of time (6 to 12 months), accumulate in proportion to burden of disease, and predict long-term disability.[15,16]

Several patient characteristics assessed early in disease (usually within the first 2 to 3 years of symptoms) have been associated consistently with the likelihood of developing erosive damage. The factors with the strongest predictive value include presence and titer of autoantibodies (e.g., rheumatoid factor [RF] and anticyclic citrullinated peptides [anti-CCP]); genetic factors (the presence of HLA-DRB1 "shared epitope" alleles, especially HLA-DRB1*0401 and HLA-DRB1*0404); radiographic factors (the presence of erosive disease on plain radiographs at presentation); elevated inflammatory markers (e.g., C-reactive protein [CRP] and erythrocyte sedimentation rate [ESR]); and degree of functional disability (measured using the Health Assessment Questionnaire [HAQ]).[17-19] All these variables are easily and inexpensively assessed in the routine clinical setting. However, because the shared epitope status correlates closely with the other clinical risk factors (e.g., RF) and thus adds minimal additional predictive value, it is not routinely assessed in clinical practice.[14] Numerous additional factors,[20-22] including enzymes (e.g., granzyme B); other autoantibodies (e.g., anti-type II collagen, anti-BiP, PAD4); breakdown products of bone and cartilage (e.g., CTX-I and -II); and genetic polymorphisms of proteins involved in immune function (e.g., tumor necrosis factor-α [TNF-α]),[23] have been linked to an increased risk for erosive disease; however, their utility in clinical practice is limited by expense, lack of commercial availability, and failure to provide additional predictive power over and above routine clinical testing. Other baseline clinical parameters, such as early age of onset, low body mass

index (BMI),[24] and the number of swollen and tender joints, have been associated, albeit less potently or consistently, with the potential for radiographic progression of erosive disease.

Although the presence of these factors increases the risk of erosive disease, their absence does not guarantee a benign course. For example, seroconversion of RF may occur after disease presentation.[25] Thus if seropositivity is weighted heavily in an algorithm of risk factors for treatment, some seronegative patients will likely be undertreated.

Imaging modalities with greater sensitivity for detecting erosions may help to stratify patients at risk for progressive articular destruction earlier than can be determined using plain radiography. The role of magnetic resonance imaging (MRI) and ultrasound in detecting early erosive disease has been explored in this regard[26] and is discussed in detail in Chapter 39. However, given the expense of MRI and operator variability in ultrasound acquisitions, these imaging techniques are currently used primarily for research purposes.

TREATMENT STRATEGIES

Rationale

As with clinical outcomes, no single clinical, laboratory, or radiographic parameter has been identified to date that will reliably predict a favorable response to a particular DMARD.[27] Furthermore, the paucity of head-to-head comparisons of different DMARDs does not allow for the rank ordering, as yet, of individual DMARDs, or combinations of DMARDs, for safety and efficacy. Nonetheless, a number of highly effective treatment strategies have been identified through clinical trials in RA that allow the clinician to organize the selection, order, and dosing of DMARDs for an individual patient.

There are three general strategies for DMARD treatment of RA:

1. sequential monotherapy
2. step-up combination therapy
3. initial combination (induction) therapy

The last two approaches use combinations of DMARDs consisting of non-biologics only, biologics only, or a combination of both. All three approaches can be applied early or late in disease, although most commonly these strategies are discussed in reference to patients with early (DMARD-naive) disease.

Criteria for assessing response to therapy have been developed for use in clinical trials and are discussed in detail in Chapter 93. Among these, the disease activity score (DAS), measured as a continuous variable, is the most useful in the clinical practice setting.[28] The European League Against Rheumatism (EULAR) cut-offs for a "good" response (DAS < 2.4 and a decrease from baseline DAS by > 1.2) and for "remission" (DAS < 1.6) may be helpful in guiding treatment decisions. In clinical practice, using the DAS and EULAR cutoffs for disease activity and response can be cumbersome. Recently, efforts have been made to validate simpler methods of assessing RA disease activity, including composite measures consisting entirely of patient-reported domains, with a primary aim at streamlining and promoting the use of quantitative outcomes in clinical care.[29]

Sequential monotherapy, as discussed previously, consists of discontinuation of an ineffective DMARD (e.g., gold) and replacement with an alternative DMARD (e.g., penicillamine), a process that can be repeated until all available DMARDs are exhausted. This approach has largely been abandoned in light of extensive data showing the superiority of step-up and induction approaches. The step-up approach is currently the most widely practiced strategy in clinical practice for the management of RA[30] and is the strategy used in the majority of clinical trials in RA to date. In this approach, a second DMARD (e.g., sulfasalazine or a TNF inhibitor) is added to the first DMARD (e.g., methotrexate) if a response to the first DMARD is inadequate. In most published step-up combination approaches, methotrexate serves as the "anchor" DMARD. The advantage of the step-up strategy is that it permits graded escalation of therapy up to the desired level of control of synovitis without exposing the patient to more DMARDs than are necessary. The disadvantage is that a lag time, depending on how many "steps" are required, must elapse before disease control is attained. During this time, irreversible articular damage may occur. As such, the "model" step-up strategy outlined in the 2008 ACR Guidelines for the Management of RA[11] advocates frequent evaluation and rapid escalation of therapy in the face of incomplete response.

In contrast, in induction therapy (modeled after cancer chemotherapy strategies) the patient is started immediately on a combination of DMARDs. Once maximal or acceptable control of synovitis is achieved, the combination may be continued indefinitely or "stepped down" to a single DMARD for maintenance. The theoretical advantage of induction therapy is more rapid control of synovitis and thus less accumulation of joint damage compared with the monotherapy and step-up approaches. The disadvantages of the induction approach are potential overtreatment and exposure to unnecessary toxicities in patients in whom disease may have been adequately controlled by a single DMARD; in addition, there can be difficulty in attribution of an adverse event to a specific drug.

A landmark induction with step-down study was the Dutch Combinatietherapie Bij Rheumatoide Artritis (COBRA) trial.[31] In this trial, patients with early RA were randomized to initial treatment with sulfasalazine alone or to a combination of sulfasalazine + methotrexate + high-dose prednisolone with taper of high-dose to low-dose prednisolone by week 6 and taper to sulfasalazine monotherapy by 6 months. Radiographic outcomes in the induction/step-down group were superior to the monotherapy group at the end of 6 months. Furthermore, the rate of new radiographic damage continued to be lower in the induction/step-down group through 5 years of follow-up compared with the monotherapy group, even though the randomized treatment phase had long since ended. Similar clinical and radiologic results were reported in the Finnish Rheumatoid Arthritis Combination Therapy Study (FIN-RACo)[32,33] in which treatment with combination DMARDs with step-down was compared with DMARD monotherapy over 5 years of follow-up.

The results from these studies and others[8,9] have led to the speculation that a "window of opportunity" exists early in the disease, during which aggressive treatment may serve to permanently slow, or even "turn off," disease activity.[34] Although this concept is difficult to prove, subsequent clinical trials in patients with early RA have at least corroborated the superiority of combination induction regimens to stable monotherapy, although most of these trials have not included a step-down phase. A summary of these trials, including those with anti-TNF therapy, is provided later in the section "Stepping up therapy."

A head-to-head comparison of induction versus step-up versus sequential monotherapy strategies was evaluated in the Behandel-Strategieën in Reumatoïde Artritis (Treatment Strategies in Rheumatoid Arthritis: BeST) trial.[35] Data from this study indicate that two different induction regimens (1. the COBRA induction/step-down regimen of non-biologic DMARDs; and 2. combination of infliximab + methotrexate) were superior to sequential monotherapy or step-up combinations in slowing radiographic progression over 12 months. However, all of the treatment strategies studied resulted in comparable percentages of patients in a low-disease activity state at 12 months. In particular, because many of the patients in the initial combination with infliximab group were able to discontinue their TNF inhibitor within the first years of the study and maintain a low-disease activity state,

the initial investment of combination therapy may actually be cost saving in the long term without sacrificing efficacy.

Finally, "individualized targeted tight control" is a variant on each of these approaches in which the rapid attainment of a numerically low disease activity score and/or a percent improvement in baseline disease activity is set as the goal of therapy. A treatment algorithm is established that mandates an increase in dose or number of DMARDs at specified intervals of time until this numeric goal has been achieved. The prototype of this approach is the Tight Control for Rheumatoid Arthritis (TICORA) trial[36] in which treatment in an "aggressively managed" group was escalated at each study visit if the DAS score was greater than 2.4. In contrast, in the "routine care" group, the DAS score was not a part of the clinical decision making and these patients received therapy at the discretion of the treating rheumatologist. At the end of 18 months of treatment, patients treated intensively had superior clinical responses and fewer radiographic erosions than those in the routine care group.

In summary, the evidence to date suggests that "aggressive" treatment to rapidly achieve a low level of disease activity, which often necessitates a combination of agents, has superior efficacy to conservative approaches that involve sequential, low-dose monotherapy. Given the expense of combination therapy, especially with the biologic DMARDs and the current environment of cost containment, the step-up combination approach remains the most common in clinical practice.[30] However, the ACR 2008 treatment guidelines[11] do include the use of initial combination regimens of non-biologic DMARDs with or without a TNF inhibitor for patients with high disease activity and features of poor prognosis. The recommendations do not, however, provide guidance on how and when to step up or step down from initial therapeutic decisions nor on drug switching within a class of agents. In contrast, EULAR recommendations for the management of early RA recommend the initial use of methotrexate in all patients at risk for disease persistence, unless contraindicated.[37] The remainder of the chapter focuses on specific DMARDs (Table 94.1) and DMARD combinations with the step-up approach in mind.

CHOICE OF THE INITIAL DISEASE-MODIFYING ANTIRHEUMATIC DRUG

In most cases, except where there are specific contraindications or there is very high disease activity, a non-biologic DMARD is recommended as the initial therapy in a DMARD-naïve patient with early disease.[11] Although biologic DMARDs are also effective in early disease, their significantly higher cost generally limits their use as first-line agents. Of the non-biologic DMARDs, methotrexate, sulfasalazine, leflunomide, hydroxychloroquine, and minocycline are the most commonly used. The first three of these agents were shown in placebo-controlled randomized clinical trials[38,39] to be relatively comparable in their abilities to reduce articular signs and symptoms of RA, improve physical function, and retard radiographic progression (see Chapters 52 to 54). Minocycline and hydroxychloroquine (see Chapters 52 and 56) also improve joint pain, swelling, and physical functioning, but their effects are considerably less potent than those of the other three oral DMARDs.[8,40] For this reason, the ACR 2008 treatment recommendations advise that minocycline or hydroxychloroquine as monotherapy should be limited to patients with the mildest disease.[11]

Monotherapy: methotrexate as the "standard" first-line DMARD

The last several decades have seen the gradual acceptance of methotrexate as the first-line DMARD of choice, even in Europe where sulfasalazine was previously preferred. This is due to its marked efficacy, safety, tolerability, and sustainable effect (discussed in Chapter 53). Consequently, most clinical trials have tested the safety and efficacy of new drugs in combination with methotrexate.

Aggressive dose escalation of methotrexate (MTX) has gained relatively widespread acceptance in recent years, particularly in the United States and Western Europe, on the basis of its favorable safety profile. A paradigm for rapid escalation was provided by the Early RA (ERA) study[41] in which methotrexate treatment was initiated at a dose of 10

TABLE 94.1 DISEASE-MODIFYING ANTIRHEUMATIC DRUGS

DMARD	Mechanism of action	Annual retail cost, brand (generic) USD*
Conventional DMARDs		
Methotrexate	Inhibition of purine biosynthesis/cytokine expression. Induction of monocyte apoptosis	790-2632 (166-555)
Sulfasalazine	Inhibition of cytokine expression/neutrophil migration	421-1264 (139-416)
Leflunomide	Inhibition of pyrimidine biosynthesis/cytokine expression/neutrophil migration	6645-6935 (487-799)
Hydroxychloroquine	Unknown	2112 (438)
Azathioprine	Active metabolite, 6-mercaptopurine, interferes with adenine and guanidine biosynthesis	1235-6174 (341-1703)
Cyclosporine	Inhibition of T-cell response via calcineurin inhibition	1947-5840 (1825-5475)
Cyclophosphamide	Lymphocyte cytotoxicity	1534-4599 (1341-4022)
D-penicillamine	Unknown	845-3380
Injectable gold salts	Unknown	
Auranofin	Unknown	3398
Minocycline	Inhibition of metalloproteinases—exact mechanism unknown	7415 (560)
Biologic DMARDs		
Etanercept	Soluble 75kDa TNF receptor: inhibits biologic effects of TNF-α	19,838
Infliximab	Chimeric anti-TNF-α antibody: inhibits biologic effects of TNF-α. Cell lysis of TNF-α expressing cells	Variable
Adalimumab	Human anti-TNF-α antibody: inhibits biologic effects of TNF-α	21,627-43,254
Anakinra	Recombinant IL-1 receptor agonist: inhibits biologic effects of IL-1	18,562
Rituximab	Anti-CD20 monoclonal antibody: depletes B cells	Variable
Abatacept (CTLA4Ig)	Inhibits T-cell co-stimulation	Variable

*www.drugstore.com.
DMARD, disease-modifying antirheumatic drug; TNF, tumor necrosis factor; USD, U.S. dollars.

mg per week and escalated by 5 mg every 4 weeks until a weekly dose of 20 to 25 mg was achieved, provided that side effects did not necessitate stopping at a lower dose. In practice, many patients tolerate an initial dose of 15 mg per week. In this study and others in patients with either early[41-43] or advanced[44] RA, aggressively titrated methotrexate monotherapy was comparable with anti-TNF monotherapy in reducing clinical signs and symptoms of RA, although cumulative radiographic joint damage over several years was somewhat higher in the methotrexate group at 1 to 2 years of follow-up.

Because of the slow onset of action of MTX, an interval of 4 to 6 weeks is generally required to determine whether a patient has responded to a dose increase. Thus using the dosing strategy described earlier, an interval of approximately 2 to 3 months is recommended to evaluate the initial response to methotrexate monotherapy. If the response at 2 to 4 months is minimal, the addition of a second DMARD is recommended at this point. If, on the other hand, the response is robust, methotrexate may be continued as monotherapy, perhaps with additional dose adjustment, recognizing that the maximal effect of the drug may not be fully realized for an additional month or two.

For patients who have had an inadequate response to 20 to 25 mg per week of oral methotrexate, substitution of an equivalent dose of subcutaneous (SC) or intramuscular (IM) methotrexate may be more efficacious,[45] although this conclusion has been called into question.[46] Given the availability of an array of other DMARDs on the market, the addition of a second DMARD is the preferred next step in most patients failing oral methotrexate.

Although the majority of patients will tolerate rapid escalation of methotrexate, dose-limiting side effects related to drug-induced folate deficiency, such as hepatic transaminitis, stomatitis, nausea, cytopenias, and hair loss (discussed in detail in Chapter 53), may present barriers to continuing or escalating the drug. Methotrexate-induced folate deficiency has also been implicated as a contributor to the enhanced risk for cardiovascular disease in RA patients.[4] Consequently, supplementation with folate (in the form of folic or folinic acid) is recommended in all methotrexate-treated patients because this appears

to reduce side effects with minimal compromise of overall efficacy.[47] Although methotrexate is generally appropriate for most patients, absolute contraindications to it include active liver disease (including chronic hepatitis B and C infection), alcohol abuse, pregnancy, and breastfeeding. Alternative DMARD choices for these patients are discussed next.

First-line monotherapy with non-biologic DMARDs: alternatives to methotrexate

Leflunomide, a pyrimidine synthesis inhibitor (discussed in detail in Chapter 54), has been shown in head-to-head trials in established RA to have equivalent efficacy to methotrexate or sulfasalazine in suppressing synovitis and inhibiting radiographic progression,[38,39] although it could be argued that both methotrexate and sulfasalazine were underdosed in these trials. The usual dose of leflunomide is 20 mg a day but can be reduced to 10 mg per day in cases of toxicity. Its contraindications for use (alcoholism, pregnancy, active liver disease, and renal impairment) and adverse effect profile (requiring routine monitoring of transaminases) are similar to methotrexate. A generic formulation of leflunomide is now available in the United States, substantially reducing its cost differential compared with the other non-biologic DMARDs.

The efficacy of sulfasalazine (discussed in detail in Chapter 52) in the treatment of RA was first recognized in the 1940s, although its mechanism of action in RA has never been clearly elucidated. In Europe it was the preferred first-line DMARD until recently, having been displaced by methotrexate. Head-to-head studies have shown relative equivalence in efficacy compared with methotrexate and leflunomide,[48,49] although (as noted earlier) methotrexate was relatively underdosed in these studies relative to current clinical practice. The usual dose of sulfasalazine for the treatment of RA is 1 to 3 g per day in divided doses. Sulfasalazine is contraindicated in patients with sulfa allergy or G6PD deficiency. Potential advantages of sulfasalazine over methotrexate include its reduced cost, relative safety during pregnancy, and low incidence of hepatotoxicity and bone marrow toxicity.

Sulfasalazine is an important option for RA patients with chronic hepatitis C infection or other liver conditions. Comparative disadvantages include a higher rate of early discontinuation due to intolerance (usually gastrointestinal [GI]) and the potential for lower patient compliance because of the need for twice-daily dosing.

Neither leflunomide nor sulfasalazine has been studied in combination with other non-biologic and biologic DMARDs as rigorously as methotrexate. For these and the other reasons cited earlier, methotrexate remains the most commonly used first-line DMARD for RA, although both leflunomide and sulfasalazine are excellent alternatives.

Hydroxychloroquine (see Chapter 52) has a long track record of use in the treatment of RA. Its low toxicity profile, ease of administration (oral QD or BID), low cost (comparable with methotrexate and sulfasalazine), and apparent safety in pregnancy make it an attractive agent for use in RA. However, head-to-head studies versus the other conventional DMARDs discussed earlier[8,40] confirm that hydroxychloroquine is a comparatively less potent DMARD, especially in its ability to slow radiographic progression. Thus its use as monotherapy is generally restricted to patients with very mild disease with few or no risk factors for poor prognosis, a setting in which it can be surprisingly effective.[50] Given these limitations, hydroxychloroquine is most commonly used as adjunctive therapy rather than monotherapy for RA. The usual dose is 200 to 400 mg per day with yearly monitoring for retinal toxicity. Dose loading of up to 1200 mg per day for the first 6 weeks of therapy has been shown to safely hasten the onset of action[51]; however, this strategy has not undergone long-term evaluation and is not widely practiced. Additional benefits of hydroxychloroquine on metabolic and cardiovascular risk profiles have been reported.[52,53]

First-line monotherapy: biologic DMARDs

Three TNF inhibitors (etanercept, infliximab, and adalimumab) and one interleukin-1 (IL-1) inhibitor (anakinra) are U.S. Food and Drug Administration (FDA) approved for the treatment of RA (see Chapter 61). Each has been demonstrated to be efficacious as monotherapy for the treatment of RA, although anakinra is a relatively weak agent compared with the TNF inhibitors and infliximab is recommended only in conjunction with methotrexate (in order to suppress antichimeric antibodies). Compared with aggressively dosed methotrexate, neither etanercept monotherapy nor adalimumab monotherapy shows superiority in reducing clinical signs and symptoms of disease, although each does exhibit modest superiority in reducing radiographic progression.[41,43,44] Nonetheless, this modest advantage is offset by the high costs of these agents such that methotrexate remains the preferred first-line DMARD. There are patients, however, in whom first-line monotherapy with etanercept or adalimumab is preferred, such as those with multiple contraindications to non-biologic DMARDs. Evolving clinical experience suggests that TNF inhibitors may be relatively safe during conception and pregnancy,[54] although more study is required before their use under these circumstances can be recommended. Insofar as the most common use of TNF inhibitors is in combination with MTX,[12] these drugs are addressed in greater detail later in the discussion on "step-up" therapy.

First-line monotherapy with anakinra or either of the newer approved biologic DMARDs, abatacept and rituximab, has not been studied. First-line therapy with abatacept in combination with methotrexate has been recently evaluated (see later).

First-line monotherapy: other non-biologic DMARDs

Several additional non-biologic DMARDs remain available on the market for the treatment of RA. These include oral and injected gold (see Chapter 52), D-penicillamine, minocycline (see Chapter 56), cyclosporine, tacrolimus, cyclophosphamide, azathioprine (see Chapter 55). In view of the greater convenience, lower toxicity profiles, and quicker onset of action of methotrexate, leflunomide, and sulfasalazine, coupled with the emergence in 1998 of the TNF inhibitors, these older non-biologic DMARDs have been virtually abandoned in developed countries for the treatment of RA, at least as monotherapies. However, some combination therapies (e.g., cyclosporine +

methotrexate) may be practical in some circumstances (see later) and these drugs remain viable affordable alternatives in less developed countries.

Stepping up therapy: inadequate response to DMARD monotherapy

Approximately 50% of patients will have an inadequate response to monotherapy with an aggressively dosed non-biologic DMARD.[38,39,41,42,49] In these patients, adding a DMARD (or DMARDs) (step-up combination) is preferable to sequential monotherapy. As always, the addition of any new DMARD poses additional risks that must be weighed against the potential benefit of additional treatment. It is often productive, at the initial visit, to introduce the concept that a combination of DMARDs may be necessary, that this need can be ascertained within the first 2 to 4 months of monotherapy, and that therapies with various routes of administration are available. This allows adequate time for the treating rheumatologist and patient to discuss expected benefits, side effects, and preferences for route of administration.

Biologic DMARDs: TNF inhibitors

For patients with an inadequate response to several months of aggressively dosed methotrexate, the addition of a TNF inhibitor is a highly effective and generally safe strategy for further reducing synovitis. That the combination of a TNF inhibitor plus methotrexate is superior to monotherapy with methotrexate in reducing signs, symptoms, and radiographic progression of disease in patients with early and/or advanced RA has been demonstrated for etanercept in the TEMPO trial,[44] for infliximab in the ASPIRE and ATTRACT trials,[55,56] and for adalimumab in the PREMIER and ARMADA trials.[43,57] Their ability to effect robust, rapid, and sustainable clinical responses in many patients has overshadowed, but not eclipsed, concerns about short- and long-term toxicities. These toxicities include enhanced risk of serious and opportunistic infections, induction of autoantibodies, and risk of inducing or exacerbating symptoms of congestive heart failure and of demyelinating diseases (discussed in detail in Chapter 61). Fortunately, the incidence of these potential side effects is uncommon. The superior efficacy of adding a TNF inhibitor (infliximab) to methotrexate over the addition of sulfasalazine/hydroxychloroquine in early RA patients was recently confirmed in the SWEFOT trial.[58] The increasing prescription of TNF inhibitors over the years since FDA approval has proven that self-injection and intravenous infusion are acceptable routes of administration for treatment of patients with RA. In patients at high risk for joint damage, the high cost of anti-TNF therapy is expected to be balanced or offset in the long term by a reduction in joint surgeries, disability, and unemployment. Thus their position as the ideal choice for second-line therapy for patients with moderate to severe residual disease activity on background MTX is now relatively commonplace.

No evidence suggests that one TNF inhibitor is superior to another. Furthermore, potential adverse effects are generally comparable among the three, although infliximab treatment has been associated with a higher incidence of opportunistic infection.[59] Therefore the selection of TNF inhibitor is often based on patient preference. Etanercept and adalimumab are self-administered via subcutaneous injection (50 mg once per week or 25 mg twice per week for etanercept; 40 mg every 1 to 2 weeks for adalimumab). Higher doses of etanercept were not shown to increase response.[60] Infliximab is administered as an intravenous infusion every 8 weeks (after an initial loading regimen). The standard dose of infliximab, 3 mg per kilogram body weight, can be titrated up to 10 mg per kilogram if needed and/or the dosing interval can be decreased (to every 6 or every 4 weeks). It is recommended that infliximab be administered concurrently with methotrexate (at least 7.5 mg per week) to prevent the development of neutralizing antibodies, although other mechanisms might be relevant with respect to the enhanced efficacy of infliximab in combinations with MTX because the efficacy of other TNF inhibitors is also increased by combination with MTX, and infliximab is effective as monotherapy in psoriatic arthritis and ankylosing spondylitis. Limited data suggest that the combination of a TNF inhibitor with non-biologic DMARDs other than methotrexate (e.g., leflunomide and/or sulfasalazine) is safe and perhaps efficacious as well.[61,62] Formal drug interaction studies, however, have not been done with these drugs and the anti-TNF therapies. However, combining TNF inhibitors or combinations of TNF inhibitors with other biologic DMARDs is not recommended[11] because of the risk of enhanced infection and other toxicities.

In general, the onset of action of TNF inhibitors is more rapid than non-biologic DMARDs, with many patients achieving a clinical response after only 8 to 12 weeks of therapy. However, some patients may be slower to respond and, similar to methotrexate, approximately 50% of patients fail to have a robust response to anti-TNF therapy at all.[41,42,56,57] The factors responsible for this variability are not known, although pharmacogenetic studies are under way to investigate the issue.

Biologic DMARDs: T-cell costimulatory modulators

The T-cell costimulatory modulator abatacept (see Chapter 58) has been shown to have clinical efficacy as monotherapy in moderate to severe RA patients with an inadequate response to methotrexate,[63] and in combination with methotrexate in patients who have failed methotrexate monotherapy,[64] other non-biologic DMARDs,[65] and/or TNF inhibitors.[66] Reduction in radiographic progression compared with placebo has also been observed uniformly across these studies. A recent study showed that early, very active, DMARD-naïve RA patients treated with the combination of abatacept + methotrexate were significantly more likely to achieve clinical remission at 1 year compared with those treated with methotrexate alone.[67] However, an abatacept monotherapy arm was not included in this study. In the only head-to-head trial assessing efficacy of abatacept against a TNF inhibitor, clinical response outcomes were similar over 1 year for active RA patients randomized to receive abatacept versus infliximab,[68] although infliximab was only allowed at the minimum (3 mg/kg) dose.

Overall, the safety profile of abatacept from clinical trial data is modestly superior to TNF inhibitors. Infusion reactions were lower in abatacept-treated patients compared with infliximab-treated patients[68] and no cases of tuberculosis or other opportunistic infections have been associated with abatacept. However, compared with the TNF inhibitors, long-term and safety registry data on the incidence of serious infections and malignancies with abatacept are limited. In particular, a potential signal for lung cancer and pulmonary exacerbations in patients with COPD noted in a large safety trial (ASSURE)[65] has not been replicated in subsequent studies but warrants additional confirmation and investigation into mechanism.

Abatacept is administered according to weight and a loading regimen is recommended. Thereafter, infusions are administered every 4 weeks. Because the onset of clinical effect can be delayed, a recent consensus statement recommends continuing abatacept for at least 16 weeks before evaluating efficacy.[69]

Optimal placement of abatacept in the sequence of RA therapeutics has not been firmly established. Although clinical trials data indicate efficacy at most stages of disease, the lack of long-term efficacy and safety data generally relegate abatacept to a position behind the TNF inhibitors as second-line agents. However, it is an appealing option in patients who have failed TNF inhibitors or those with contraindication to TNF inhibitors. Abatacept should not be combined with TNF inhibitors because the combination was associated with higher infection rates without improved efficacy.[70]

Biologic DMARDs: B-cell depletion

Rituximab, a chimeric monoclonal antibody directed against CD20 (see Chapter 59), has been shown to be efficacious in combination with methotrexate in reducing the signs and symptoms of active RA and in slowing radiographic progression of disease in patients with inadequate responses to methotrexate and/or TNF inhibitors.[71-73] Rituximab is currently FDA approved in the United States only for use in RA patients who have had an inadequate response to TNF inhibitors. It has not been specifically studied in early RA, in combination with other biologic DMARDs, or with other non-biologic DMARDs except methotrexate and cyclophosphamide. The best evidence for its efficacy is in populations selected on RF seropositivity[71,72]; however, it has been applied with success in seronegative patients,[73] suggesting that the

mechanism of action of the drug is not dependent on reduction in autoantibodies.

The safety profile for the first treatment course (paired infusions 2 weeks apart) of rituximab is generally favorable, with few serious infections and no opportunistic infections noted in clinical trials. Infusion reactions are more frequent with rituximab than the other infused biologic DMARDs, necessitating the recommendation for pretreatment corticosteroids. Infusion reactions tend to diminish with repeated infusions. Reductions in immunoglobulin levels have been noted over two to three courses of treatment; however, these decreases have not been associated with an increased risk for infection to date. Open label studies will provide information as to whether longer-term treatment will result in progressive and clinically important depletion of immunoglobulins that might limit length of treatment. Sporadic cases of progressive multifocal leukoencephalopathy (PML) have been reported in patients receiving rituximab for non-Hodgkin lymphoma, systemic lupus erythematosus, and RA,[74] although additional concomitant immunosuppressing agents have generally been present in these cases.

Rituximab administered as two doses of 1000 mg separated by 2 weeks is the current FDA licensed dosage, although one study showed nearly equivalent efficacy with two 500-mg doses.[72] The duration of effect is variable but is typically greater than 6 months.[75] Durable responses of 18 and greater months have been reported.[76] In some cases, subsequent infusions result in longer duration of response. Although peripheral B cells are rapidly diminished after treatment in most cases, reemergence of B cells does not predict loss of response and continued depletion does not guarantee maintenance of response. Importantly, patients who do not achieve a response with the first treatment course do not benefit from repeated treatments.[77]

Related to its licensing in the United States, rituximab is usually reserved as third-line therapy in patients who have failed other biologics, although it may be a good option for patients with specific contraindications to other therapies. Some concern has been raised about the safety of initiating therapy with other biologics in patients with depleted B cells but an inadequate clinical response to rituximab. However, preliminary evidence suggests that starting a TNF inhibitor in this scenario may be safe.[78]

Biologic DMARDs: IL-1 inhibitors

There is only one FDA-approved inhibitor of IL-1 (anakinra) on the market for the treatment of RA. Anakinra (see Chapter 60) is administered as a once-daily subcutaneous injection. It has been shown, both as monotherapy and in combination with methotrexate, to be superior to placebo in reducing signs, symptoms, and radiographic progression in patients with advanced RA. Although generally safe when used in combination with non-biologic DMARDs other than methotrexate in patients with comorbid illnesses, there was a modest increase in incidence of serious infections in anakinra-treated, compared with placebo-treated, patients in a large clinical trial.[79] The combination of anakinra with etanercept (or presumably other TNF inhibitors) is not recommended, however, because it was associated with a significantly higher rate of serious infections (compared with etanercept monotherapy) without enhancing efficacy.[80] Although anakinra has not been compared directly with any of the TNF inhibitors, its efficacy in clinical trials is consistently and substantially lower than that of the TNF inhibitors. This, coupled with the inconvenient dosing schedule, has placed anakinra as a distant choice for step-up therapy in clinical practice. However, it is a reasonable alternative in patients with inadequate responses to the available biologic DMARDs or in patients with contraindications to TNF inhibitors such as moderate to severe congestive heart failure or multiple sclerosis.

Non-biologic DMARD combinations

As noted previously, combinations of non-biologic DMARDs using the "induction" approach have substantial superiority over monotherapy for the treatment of RA. This is also demonstrated in clinical trials for the "step-up" approach. For example, the combination of sulfasalazine + hydroxychloroquine + methotrexate was superior to methotrexate alone, to sulfasalazine alone, and to the dual combinations[81] for reducing signs and symptoms of disease, although radiographic assessments were not performed in these studies. This strategy, termed "triple therapy," is generally well tolerated and is relatively low in cost. Disadvantages include a dosing schema that may present barriers to adherence in some patients and the potential for a negative effect of sulfasalazine + methotrexate due to sulfasalazine's inhibition of cellular uptake of methotrexate by the reduced folate carrier.[82]

The addition of leflunomide to methotrexate in patients with an inadequate response to methotrexate was also associated with enhanced clinical improvement compared with methotrexate alone, but no radiographic endpoints were assessed.[83] Drug-related toxicities associated with the combination are relatively low; however, careful monitoring of hepatic function is advocated in patients receiving this combination. Suggested ways to minimize toxicity are the elimination of the loading dose of leflunomide, initiation of leflunomide at the lower (10 mg per day) dose, and reduction of the dose of methotrexate. As with triple therapy, head-to-head comparisons of methotrexate + leflunomide against regimens containing a TNF inhibitor have not been performed. For these reasons, these combinations are often selected in patients with contraindications to TNF inhibitors (e.g., patients with recurrent serious infections) or those with an aversion to self-injection or infusion.

Other step-up combination regimens that have demonstrated favorable clinical efficacy in randomized, blinded, placebo-controlled trials include methotrexate + IM gold[84] and methotrexate + cyclosporine.[85] Although of some clinical merit, the potential toxicity profiles of both these combination regimens limit their application in the current environment, where safer and possibly more effective treatment strategies are available.

Third-line therapy: when initial biologics fail

Although the 2008 ACR treatment recommendations do not indicate a preference between TNF inhibitors, abatacept, or rituximab for RA patients with active disease of more than 6 months' duration with poor prognostic features who have failed initial therapy with non-biologics,[11] typically a TNF inhibitor will be used first. Thereafter, there is little evidence to guide treatment decisions if an adequate response is not achieved because no head-to-head studies have been conducted of the available biologic choices in patients who have failed a prior biologic. Although a switch to a biologic with a different mechanism of action would seem appropriate, observational data suggest that overall drug survival rates for a second TNF inhibitor are similar to those for the first when the first was discontinued due to inefficacy.[86] Thus switching to an alternate TNF inhibitor is advocated in a recent multinational consensus statement.[69]

Glucocorticoids

Glucocorticoids (see Chapter 51) are potent anti-inflammatory drugs that constitute important adjunctive therapy for RA but should never suffice as monotherapy for any prolonged period of time. In general, the prescription of glucocorticoids should be at as low a dose and for as short a time as possible. They can be administered orally or by intra-articular injection, intravenous infusion, or intramuscular injection. Glucocorticoids are particularly useful at the onset of disease because they produce a rapid and substantial reduction in synovitis,[31] thus reducing patient discomfort while the slower acting DMARD(s) takes effect. This "bridging" strategy, in which glucocorticoids are tapered and discontinued as the DMARD takes full effect, can also be applied during disease flares.[87] Frequent flares requiring repeated short bursts of glucocorticoid therapy, however, should alert the clinician that the disease is inadequately controlled and, in these situations, the dose or number of DMARDs should be increased or other DMARD strategies employed.

Some RA patients have severe disease that is not well controlled despite aggressive management with multiple DMARDs and NSAIDs. In these patients, chronic low-dose prednisone (<10 mg daily) is frequently necessary to enhance comfort. Low-dose prednisone also slows joint damage (assessed radiographically),[88] although its effect is considerably more modest than that of the DMARDs and appears to diminish with prolonged use. Intra-articular injection of a glucocorticoid is indicated for the patient in whom the disease is well controlled except for

a single joint or two, after first establishing that the joint is not infected (see Chapter 51). In view of the adverse effects associated with chronic glucocorticoid administration, some of which have been underappreciated (e.g., accelerated atherosclerosis, osteoporosis), the treating rheumatologist must always take into account the benefit versus risk of toxicity associated even with low doses of chronic glucocorticoid.

Non-steroidal anti-inflammatory drugs

The rapid onset of the anti-inflammatory and analgesic effects of NSAIDs makes them the preferred first line of anti-inflammatory treatment in RA. However, NSAIDs are not disease modifying, so their use as monotherapy for any prolonged period of time should be avoided. Continued prescription of an NSAID throughout the course of RA, in conjunction with DMARDs, is common.[89] Many NSAIDs are commercially available and are discussed in detail in Chapter 50. Along with well-recognized GI side effects, recent concerns for an increased risk of cardiovascular events associated with the COX-2 selective NSAIDs (and even non-selective NSAIDs) have drawn into question the widespread use of this class of drugs.[90] In RA patients with well-controlled synovitis, lowering the dose and/or frequency or even complete discontinuation of NSAID may be advantageous.

Maintenance of the treatment response

RA is a chronic disease that rarely remits spontaneously. Consequently, DMARD treatment must be continued indefinitely because its discontinuation will generally lead to reemergence of signs and symptoms of disease within weeks to months. Patients who have been treated according to an "induction" regimen may tolerate a simplification of their treatment regimen to a single DMARD. Many patients will experience a flare in disease activity over the course of their illness, necessitating an adjustment in treatment, usually in the form of increased dose or number of DMARDs.

Future

A subset of RA patients with very destructive disease will not respond adequately to aggressive management with multiple DMARDs, low-dose steroids, and NSAIDs. Data from clinical trials have shown that 30% to 50% of patients do not achieve clinically meaningful response, for example, to the combination of a TNF inhibitor and methotrexate. Fortunately, a number of new drugs have novel mechanisms of action (see Chapters 61 to 63) that hopefully will provide alternatives for these patients. Additional TNF inhibitors, second-generation B-cell depleting therapies, and novel biologic inhibitors of IL-6, BLyS, TACI, and small molecule inhibitors of enzymes in inflammatory pathways (e.g., kinases) are all in various phases of clinical investigation. In the coming years, clinical research will establish where these agents fit in the evolving treatment algorithms for RA.

OTHER CONSIDERATIONS

Swelling with or without fever in a single joint in an RA patient in whom disease has been previously well controlled should raise the possibility of a septic joint. Aspiration and culture of the fluid are critical before a decision to readjust the DMARD regimen or to perform a corticosteroid injection is made. Similarly, the sudden emergence of generalized musculoskeletal pain should prompt consideration of a systemic infection, particularly in patients receiving biologics or broad immunosuppressants. Some patients will continue to complain of intractable pain even in the face of well-controlled synovitis. In these cases, non-inflammatory pain syndromes such as fibromyalgia or regional pain syndromes such as tendonitis should be considered as possible etiologies for the pain and treated appropriately. Escalation of DMARDs is not appropriate in these patients.

BARRIERS TO AGGRESSIVE MANAGEMENT

The ability to escalate therapy to the desired level in an individual RA patient may be limited by one or more comorbid illnesses and/or patient behaviors. Comorbidities such as recurrent infections, chronic liver disease, and moderate-to-severe congestive heart failure are relative contraindications to the use of some biologic or non-biologic DMARDs as discussed earlier and in other chapters. In some patients, non-adherence to medications and/or laboratory monitoring may necessitate the choice of a treatment regimen with simpler dosing schemes or lower risk of toxicity. Educating the patient about RA and their medications and an attempt to understand the patient's barriers to adherence (e.g., fear of medications, lack of understanding of the potential destructiveness of the disease) may help to overcome these limitations. Finally, the high cost of biologic DMARDs limits their use in a significant subset of patients.

CONCLUSION

The treatment of RA has changed dramatically in the past 10 years. The initiation of treatment very early in disease, the use of combinations of DMARDs, and the emergence of the biologic inhibitors of TNF-α have made it possible to achieve control of synovitis and improvement in the quality of life in the majority of RA patients. Complete remission of disease (on therapy) should be the goal of treatment, even if not always achievable, in all RA patients. Indeed, emerging clinical and epidemiologic data suggest that excellent long-term control of synovitis will result in significant reductions in rates of unemployment, joint surgeries, disability, and mortality in RA patients.

KEY REFERENCES

1. Arnett FC, Edworthy SM, Bloch DA, et al. The American Rheumatism Association 1987 revised criteria for the classification of rheumatoid arthritis. Arthritis Rheum 1988;31:315-324.
2. Felson DT, Anderson JJ, Boers M, et al. American-College-Of-Rheumatology Preliminary Definition of Improvement in Rheumatoid-Arthritis. Arthritis Rheum 1995;38:727-735.
3. van der Heijde DMFM, Vanthof MA, Vanriel PLCM, et al. Judging Disease-Activity in Clinical-Practice in Rheumatoid-Arthritis—1st Step in the Development of a Disease-Activity Score. Ann Rheum Dis 1990;49:916-920.
4. Choi HK, Hernan MA, Seeger JD, et al. Methotrexate and mortality in patients with rheumatoid arthritis: a prospective study. Lancet 2002;359:1173-1177.
5. Pincus T, Ferraccioli G, Sokka T, et al. Evidence from clinical trials and long-term observational studies that disease-modifying anti-rheumatic drugs slow radiographic progression in rheumatoid arthritis: updating a 1983 review. Rheumatology 2002;41:1346-1356.
6. Aletaha D, Smolen JS. Effectiveness profiles and dose dependent retention of traditional disease modifying antirheumatic drugs for rheumatoid arthritis. An observational study. J Rheumatol 2002;29:1631-1638.
7. Fuchs HA, Kaye JJ, Callahan LF, et al. Evidence of significant radiographic damage in rheumatoid arthritis within the first 2 years of disease. J Rheumatol 1989;16:585-591.
8. Lard LR, Visser H, Speyer I, et al. Early versus delayed treatment in patients with recent-onset rheumatoid arthritis: comparison of two cohorts who received different treatment strategies. Am J Med 2001;111:446-451.
9. Verstappen SM, Jacobs JW, Bijlsma JW, et al. Five-year followup of rheumatoid arthritis patients after early treatment with disease-modifying antirheumatic drugs versus treatment according to the pyramid approach in the first year. Arthritis Rheum 2003;48:1797-1807.
10. van Aken J, Lard LR, le Cessie S, et al. Radiological outcome after four years of early versus delayed treatment strategy in patients with recent onset rheumatoid arthritis. Ann Rheum Dis 2004;63:274-279.
11. Saag KG, Teng GG, Patkar NM, et al. American College of Rheumatology 2008 recommendations for the use of nonbiologic and biologic disease-modifying antirheumatic drugs in rheumatoid arthritis. Arthritis Rheum 2008;59:762-784.
12. Aletaha D, Eberl G, Nell VPK, et al. Attitudes to early rheumatoid arthritis: changing patterns. Results of a survey. Ann Rheum Dis 2004;63:1269-1275.
13. Visser H, le Cessie S, Vos K, et al. How to diagnose rheumatoid arthritis early—a prediction model for persistent (erosive) arthritis. Arthritis Rheum 2002;46:357-365.
14. Drossaers-Bakker KW, Zwinderman AH, Vlieland TP, et al. Long-term outcome in rheumatoid arthritis: a simple algorithm of baseline parameters can predict radiographic damage, disability, and disease course at 12-year followup. Arthritis Rheum 2002;47:383-390.
15. Clarke AE, St Pierre Y, Joseph L, et al. Radiographic damage in rheumatoid arthritis correlates with functional disability but not direct medical costs. J Rheumatol 2001;28:2416-2424.
16. Hulsmans HM, Jacobs JW, van der Heijde DM, et al. The course of radiologic damage during the first six years of rheumatoid arthritis. Arthritis Rheum 2000;43:1927-1940.

17. Goronzy JJ, Matteson EL, Fulbright JW, et al. Prognostic markers of radiographic progression in early rheumatoid arthritis. Arthritis Rheum 2004;50:43-54.
18. Jansen LMA, Horst-Bruinsma IE, van Schaardenburg D, et al. Predictors of radiographic joint damage in patients with early rheumatoid arthritis. Ann Rheum Dis 2001;60:924-927.
19. van Gaalen FA, Linn-Rasker SP, van Venrooij WJ, et al. Autoantibodies to cyclic citrullinated peptides predict progression to rheumatoid arthritis in patients with undifferentiated arthritis: a prospective cohort study. Arthritis Rheum 2004;50:709-715.
20. Garnero P, Landewe R, Boers M, et al. Association of baseline levels of markers of bone and cartilage degradation with long-term progression of joint damage in patients with early rheumatoid arthritis: the COBRA study. Arthritis Rheum 2002;46:2847-2856.
21. Goldbach-Mansky R, Suson S, Wesley R, et al. Raised granzyme B levels are associated with erosions in patients with early rheumatoid factor positive rheumatoid arthritis. Ann Rheum Dis 2005;64:715-721.
22. Harris ML, Darrah E, Lam GK, et al. Association of autoimmunity to peptidyl arginine deiminase type 4 with genotype and disease severity in rheumatoid arthritis. Arthritis Rheum 2008;58:1958-1967.
23. Khanna D, Wu H, Park G, et al. Association of tumor necrosis factor alpha polymorphism, but not the shared epitope, with increased radiographic progression in a seropositive rheumatoid arthritis inception cohort. Arthritis Rheum 2006;54:1105-1116.
24. Westhoff G, Rau R, Zink A. Radiographic joint damage in early rheumatoid arthritis is highly dependent on body mass index. Arthritis Rheum 2007;56:3575-3582.
25. Nielen MM, van Schaardenburg D, Reesink HW, et al. Specific autoantibodies precede the symptoms of rheumatoid arthritis: a study of serial measurements in blood donors. Arthritis Rheum 2004;50:380-386.
26. McQueen FM, Benton N, Crabbe J, et al. What is the fate of erosions in early rheumatoid arthritis? Tracking individual lesions using x rays and magnetic resonance imaging over the first two years of disease. Ann Rheum Dis 2001;60:859-868.
27. Hider SL, Buckley C, Silman AJ, et al. Factors influencing response to disease modifying antirheumatic drugs in patients with rheumatoid arthritis. J Rheumatol 2005;32:11-16.
28. Vanderheijde DMFM, Vanthof MA, Vanriel PLCM, et al. Judging Disease-Activity in Clinical-Practice in Rheumatoid-Arthritis—1st Step in the Development of A Disease-Activity Score 1. Ann Rheum Dis 1990;49:916-920.
29. Pincus T, Swearingen CJ, Bergman M, Yazici Y. RAPID3 (Routine Assessment of Patient Index Data 3), a rheumatoid arthritis index without formal joint counts for routine care: proposed severity categories compared to disease activity score and clinical disease activity index categories. J Rheumatol 2008;35:2136-2147.
30. Wolfe F, Rehman Q, Lane NE, Kremer J. Starting a disease modifying antirheumatic drug or a biologic agent in rheumatoid arthritis: standards of practice for RA treatment. J Rheumatol 2001;28:1704-1711.
31. Boers M, Verhoeven AC, Markusse HM, et al. Randomised comparison of combined step-down prednisolone, methotrexate and sulphasalazine with sulphasalazine alone in early rheumatoid arthritis. Lancet 1997;350:309-318.
32. Mottonen T, Hannonen P, Leirisalo-Repo M, et al. Comparison of combination therapy with single-drug therapy in early rheumatoid arthritis: a randomised trial. FIN-RACo trial group. Lancet 1999;353:1568-1573.

33. Korpela M, Laasonen L, Hannonen P, et al. Retardation of joint damage in patients with early rheumatoid arthritis by initial aggressive treatment with disease-modifying antirheumatic drugs: five-year experience from the FIN-RACo study. Arthritis Rheum 2004;50:2072-2081.
34. Boers M. Understanding the window of opportunity concept in early rheumatoid arthritis. Arthritis Rheum 2003;48:1771-1774.
35. De Vries-Bouwstra JK, Goekoop-Ruiterman YPM, Van Zeben D, et al. A comparison of clinical and radiological outcomes of four treatment strategies for early arthritis: results of the BeST trial. Ann Rheum Dis 2004;63:58.
36. Grigor C, Capell H, Stirling A, et al. Effect of a treatment strategy of tight control for rheumatoid arthritis (the TICORA study): a single-blind randomised controlled trial. Lancet 2004;364:263-269.
37. Combe B, Landewe R, Lukas C, et al. EULAR recommendations for the management of early arthritis: report of a task force of the European Standing Committee for International Clinical Studies Including Therapeutics (ESCISIT). Ann Rheum Dis 2007;66:34-45.
38. Smolen JS, Kalden JR, Scott DL, et al. Efficacy and safety of leflunomide compared with placebo and sulphasalazine in active rheumatoid arthritis: a double-blind, randomised, multicentre trial. European Leflunomide Study Group. Lancet 1999;353:259-266.
39. Strand V, Cohen S, Schiff M, et al. Treatment of active rheumatoid arthritis with leflunomide compared with placebo and methotrexate. Arch Intern Med 1999;159:2542-2550.
40. Tsakonas E, Fitzgerald AA, Fitzcharles MA, et al. Consequences of delayed therapy with second-line agents in rheumatoid arthritis: a 3 year followup on the hydroxychloroquine in early rheumatoid arthritis (HERA) study. J Rheumatol 2000;27:623-629.
41. Bathon JM, Martin RW, Fleischmann RM, et al. A comparison of etanercept and methotrexate in patients with early rheumatoid arthritis. N Engl J Med 2000;343:1586-1593.
42. St Clair EW, van der Heijde DM, Smolen JS, et al. Combination of infliximab and methotrexate therapy for early rheumatoid arthritis: a randomized, controlled trial. Arthritis Rheum 2004;50:3432-3443.
43. Breedveld FC, Weisman MH, Kavanaugh AF, et al. The PREMIER study: a multicenter, randomized, double-blind clinical trial of combination therapy with adalimumab plus methotrexate versus methotrexate alone or adalimumab alone in patients with early, aggressive rheumatoid arthritis who had not had previous methotrexate treatment. Arthritis Rheum 2006;54(1):26-37.
44. Klareskog L, van der HD, de Jager JP, et al. Therapeutic effect of the combination of etanercept and methotrexate compared with each treatment alone in patients with rheumatoid arthritis: double-blind randomised controlled trial. Lancet 2004;363:675-681.
45. Braun J, Kastner P, Flaxenberg P, et al. Comparison of the clinical efficacy and safety of subcutaneous versus oral administration of methotrexate in patients with active rheumatoid arthritis: results of a six-month, multicenter, randomized, double-blind, controlled, phase IV trial. Arthritis Rheum 2008;58:73-81.
46. Lambert CM, Sandhu S, Lochhead A, et al. Dose escalation of parenteral methotrexate in active rheumatoid arthritis that has been unresponsive to conventional doses of methotrexate: a randomized, controlled trial. Arthritis Rheum 2004;50:364-371.
47. Hornung N, Ellingsen T, Stengaard-Pedersen K, Poulsen JH. Folate, homocysteine, and cobalamin status in

patients with rheumatoid arthritis treated with methotrexate, and the effect of low dose folic acid supplement. J Rheumatol 2004;31: 2374-2381.

48. Haagsma CJ, van Riel PL, de Jong AJ, van de Putte LB. Combination of sulphasalazine and methotrexate versus the single components in early rheumatoid arthritis: a randomized, controlled, double-blind, 52 week clinical trial. Rheumatology 1997;36:1082-1088.

49. Dougados M, Combe B, Cantagrel A, et al. Combination therapy in early rheumatoid arthritis: a randomised, controlled, double blind 52 week clinical trial of sulphasalazine and methotrexate compared with the single components. Ann Rheum Dis 1999;58:220-225.

50. Matteson EL, Weyand CM, Fulbright JW, et al. How aggressive should initial therapy for rheumatoid arthritis be? Factors associated with response to "non-aggressive" DMARD treatment and perspective from a 2-yr open label trial. Rheumatology 2004;43:619-625.

REFERENCES

Full references for this chapter can be found on www.expertconsult.com.

Multidisciplinary approach to rheumatoid arthritis

95

Ingvild Kjeken, Hanne Dagfinrud, Turid Heiberg, and Tore K. Kvien

- Patient education may improve pain, functional ability, depression, coping, and self efficacy and should be a cornerstone in the multidisciplinary care of persons with rheumatoid arthritis (RA).

- Nursing care provides continuity and the opportunity for shared decision making and focuses on the patient's coping strategies.

- Persons with RA have increased risk of cardiovascular diseases and osteoporosis. Health professionals should therefore promote physical activity and guide patients in achieving and maintaining a healthy lifestyle.

- Dynamic exercises are safe and beneficial for patients with RA, but patients with extensive joint damage or joint prostheses should be careful with high-intensity weight-bearing exercises.

- Physical modalities are a possible adjunctive method with uncertain positive but no harmful effects.

- Orthopedic shoes, insoles, wrist orthoses and splints correcting for foot or hand deformities, and assistive devices may decrease pain and improve function.

- Persons with RA should follow a healthy diet, avoid certain foods if they have allergies or intolerance, and consult a nutritionist if they want to try any special diet.

- Persons at risk of being work disabled should have rapid access to vocational rehabilitation because prevention of work disability is probably more effective than correction of work disability after work loss.

- Team care such as comprehensive inpatient and day patient programs is more effective than regular outpatient care to control disease activity and improve functional ability.

- Transdisciplinary models, in which clinicians take on extended roles, may in many occasions be at least as effective as and more cost effective than extensive team care.

INTRODUCTION

Over the past decades, new medical and surgical treatments have improved prognosis and quality of life in people with RA. Still, most patients will experience periods with pain, fatigue, and loss of function and benefit from therapeutic interventions from a variety of health professionals. The expectations for level of functioning and participation in society have also been raised with the new opportunities for improvement.

A consumer-centered approach is now widely applied in the disease management. Individual goals and treatment plans are jointly set by the patient and the rest of the team. The roles and areas of expertise of the potential team members[1] are described in Table 95.1. Even if each profession has different areas of expertise, a common goal will always be to reduce and control disease activity, to maintain or improve function and work ability, and to enhance coping strategies and the quality of life of the patient and his or her family. How a team of health professionals work together will, to a large degree, depend on the problems of the patient, the treatment setting, and the treatment goals. Traditionally, two models of care have been distinguished: a multidisciplinary approach, in which different team members cooperate on a regular basis while staying within their professional boundaries, and

an interdisciplinary team model, in which the members analyze, synthesize, and harmonize links between disciplines to establish a shared basis of knowledge and common goals in the treatment or rehabilitation of the patient.[2] Although patients with an aggressive disease, multiple problems, and/or a complex life situation may profit from the latter model, the multidisciplinary team model may be appropriate for patients with a stable disease and life situation. Also, some patients may prefer to relate to one or a few health professionals rather than an extensive team, and the involvement of fewer persons is likely to assist communication and partnership with the patient.[1]

Lately, a third so-called *transdisciplinary model* has emerged. In this approach, members transcend their traditional boundaries and take on extended roles to be able to meet a patient's need for more rapid access to care, to provide more time and continuity in care, or to provide a more optimal treatment when funding or human resources are limited. Examples of such models are clinical nurse specialists who conduct examinations and monitor treatment usually performed by a rheumatologist, and the primary therapist model, in which specially trained physical or occupational therapists function as multiskilled health professionals working in consultation with or with referral to peers or other services when necessary.[2]

Published recommendations for disease management often divide the recommendations into pharmacologic and non-pharmacologic interventions, even if the recent American College of Rheumatology recommendations only focused on drug therapy in RA.[3] Health professionals primarily work with non-pharmacologic interventions. This chapter reports the evidence for such interventions and discusses different care models.

Non-pharmacologic interventions

Successful multidisciplinary care depends on the availability of skilled health professionals, as well as timely and coordinated delivery of the relevant interventions.

Patient education

The primary target of patient education is the disease consequences: symptoms and disability. Independence, feeling in control, and confidence are also major targets. The implication is that cognitive-behavioral skills must be addressed in addition to disability and symptoms.

Patients want and are entitled to get the information that they need, both in written and oral form. However, self-management and shared decision making are important means to cope with the disease consequences.[4] Interactive computerized patient education may be a valuable supplement today, also to improve cognitive-behavioral outcomes. Lorig[5] developed and implemented patient education programs in arthritis on the basis of the concept of self-efficacy (grade A).[‡] Lorig's arthritis self-management programs (ASMPs) have been disseminated internationally, and evidence supports that increased self-efficacy

---

[‡]Grade A* Systematic review and meta-analysis of randomized trials. Grade A: If there is not a systematic review and/or meta-analysis "on point", then the authors should cite data from individual randomized controlled trials to support the recommendations. Recommendations based on results from observation studies (Grade B) and/or case series (Grade C) should be used only when the data from randomized controlled trials are not available.

TABLE 95.1 ROLES AND AREAS OF EXPERTISE OF THE POTENTIAL MEMBERS OF A MULTIDISCIPLINARY TEAM*

Profession	Roles and area of expertise
Clinical pharmacist	The clinical pharmacist identifies, solves, and prevents drug-related problems such as unnecessary drug use, non-optimal drug or dosage, need for additional drug, interaction between drugs, adverse drug reactions, and need for more information or therapy discussion.
Nurse	The nurse assists the patient in the performance of health-promoting activities to meet needs when altered ways of self-care are required due to disease or treatment. Nurses focus on activities that the patient would perform unaided given the skill, will or knowledge, and thus the mobilization, strengthening, or compensation of these resources. Optimal levels of physical, mental, and social coping and symptom relief are important targets.
Nutritionist/dietician	The nutritionist/dietician assesses, diagnoses, and treats nutrition-related problems and gives practical guidance regarding diets to individuals and to the public health. He or she is qualified to treat a range of medical conditions with dietary therapy on the basis of current literature, scientific evidence, best practices, and the individual needs of the person.
Occupational therapist	The occupational therapist evaluates the impact of rheumatic diseases on function and performance of daily tasks and valued life roles, using interviews, observation, and standardized assessments. Personal goals, interests, and resources are screened to develop an individualized program aimed at assisting adjustment to new or modified life roles, and the home/school/work environment is assessed to determine if adjustments are necessary to enhance the person's abilities. The most important interventions in occupational therapy are patient education concerning ergonomic principles and energy conservation, therapeutic exercise, and activity programs, provision of orthoses and assistive technology, and environmental and task modifications.
Orthopedic surgeon	An orthopedic surgeon trained in the treatment of people with RA will be responsible for performance of surgical procedures and, together with the patient, rheumatologist, and relevant team members, will establish a plan for surgical procedures that should be coordinated with the timing of other interventions.
Podiatrist/orthopedic shoemaker/orthotist	The orthopedic shoemaker evaluates the foot and ankle in order to define deformities, instabilities, and painful areas. Custom-made insoles, prefabricated orthopedic shoes, and custom-made shoes are common interventions in pain relief and stabilization of an unstable and/or painful rheumatoid foot and ankle. The orthotist can apply prefabricated or custom-made orthoses for all body parts in order to prevent or correct deformities, reduce pain, or increase function. Lightweight and soft materials with an easy closure system are preferred. Because rheumatoid arthritis usually affects multiple joints, it is important to have an overall and integrated view when planning the orthotic treatment.
Psychologist	The role of the clinical psychologist is to assist the patient and family in managing emotional and psychological stress and to assist living and coping with a chronic disease. On the basis of an evaluation, the psychologist tailors a treatment plan to meet the needs of the patient. The clinical psychologist provides a wide range of interventions designed to enhance coping, including cognitive therapy, pain, sleep, and stress management; sexual and relationship counseling; and psychotherapy. The psychologist may also have a consultation role with the interdisciplinary team.
Physical therapist	The physical therapist assists patients in achieving optimal function, pain relief, and physical recovery. On the basis of an evaluation of physical and functional status, the physical therapist uses therapeutic exercises and manual techniques to improve patients' muscle strength, joint mobility, and cardiovascular function. Physical modalities such as heat, cold, electrical therapy, and hydrotherapy may also be used to achieve temporary pain relief and reduce muscle spasm, thus preparing the patient for exercise and activity.
Rheumatologist	The rheumatologist is primarily responsible for diagnosis and the total management. His or her main responsibility is usually pharmacologic interventions and disease monitoring. The rheumatologist will work with the patient and members of the multidisciplinary team to identify needs for non-pharmacologic interventions.
Social worker	Social workers play a role in preventing and solving personal problems and problems regarding networks of interpersonal relation in the family and outside the family. They also address economic problems and limitations regarding education, work, and/or a professional career.

Based on descriptions found on the Web sites of the specific professions and the Association of Rheumatology Health Professions (www.rheumatology.org).

TABLE 95.2 EFFECT OF PATIENT EDUCATION INTERVENTIONS ON VARIOUS OUTCOMES AT FIRST AND LAST FOLLOW-UP VISITS*

Outcome measure	First follow-up		Last follow-up	
	Exp/control	SMD (95% CI)	Exp/control	SMD (95% CI)
Pain	1119/1000	−0.08 (−0.16, 0.00)	530/543	−0.07 (−0.019, 0.05)
Functional disability	1153/1122	−0.17 (−0.25, −0.09)	651/657	−0.09 (−0.20, 0.02)
Joint count	585/573	−0.13 (−0.24, −0.01)	484/490	−0.08 (−0.22, 0.07)
Patient Global Assessment	181/177	−0.28 (−0.49, −0.07)	302/316	−0.06 (−0.22, 0.10)
Psychological status	561/577	−0.16 (−0.28, −0.04)	392/402	0.04 (−0.10, 0.19)
Anxiety	671/657	−0.04 (−0.15, 0.07)	481/509	0.01 (−0.12, 0.13)
Depression	899/871	−0.14 (−0.23, −0.05)	564/579	−0.09 (−0.21, 0.02)
Disease activity	326/321	−0.03 (−0.19, 0.12)	359/359	−0.05 (−0.20, 0.10)

Modified from Riemsma RP, Taal E, Kirwan JR, Rasker JJ. Systematic review of rheumatoid arthritis patient education. Arthritis Rheum 2004;51:1045-1059.
CI, confidence interval; SMD, standardized mean difference.

TABLE 95.3 RECOMMENDATIONS FOR DIFFERENT TYPES OF PHYSICAL ACTIVITY FOR PATIENTS WITH RHEUMATOID ARTHRITIS[16]

Goal	Frequency, days per week	Duration, minutes	Intensity, % of APM*	Intensity, according to Borg's RPE scale†	Weight, % of 1 RM‡
Maintenance, secondary prophylactic	4-7	30	50-70	10-14	—
Improved aerobic capacity	3	30-60	60-80	11-15	—
Improved strength	2-3				50-80
Improved endurance	2-3				30-40

*Age predicted maximal heart rate.
†Rating of perceived exertion, Borg scale 6-20 (maximal exertion).
‡Repetition maximum (the maximum amount of weight one can lift in a single repetition for a given exercise).
APM, Age-predicted maximal heart rate; RPE, rating of perceived exertion, Borg scale 6-20 (maximal exertion); RM, repetition maximum (the maximum amount of weight one can lift in a single repetition for a given exercise).

mediates improvement in perception of control, health behaviors, and health status (grade A).[6]

A systematic review has shown that patient education is more effective on symptoms and health status than on disease activity and anxiety, and that the efficacy was mostly seen only at the first follow-up visit (grade A) (Table 95.2).[7] Another systematic review highlighted that educational programs improved knowledge and compliance, without improvement in health status, whereas psychoeducational programs improved coping behavior. Further, short-term effects in program targets were generally observed, whereas long-term changes in health status were not convincingly demonstrated (grade A).[8]

Almost all persons with RA use medications, and in a Norwegian study, up to 60% of patients with RA or polyarthritis reported using five or more drugs when admitted to a hospital.[9] Not surprisingly, issues concerning medication and side effects are frequently raised in studies exploring unmet health care needs in this patient population. Clinical pharmacists are educated to identify and prevent drug-related problems.[9] Counseling with pharmacists should thus be available on an individual basis, as well as in group-based patient education programs.

Joint protection is a self-management program that aims to maintain functional ability by teaching participants to use altered movement patterns, alternative working methods, assistive devices, and activity pacing.[10] Studies of such programs using standard methods of information and training have shown little or no effect. However, improvement in several outcomes was observed in individuals with early RA exposed to a joint protection program based on educational-behavioral teaching methods, compared with those who received a program based on traditional practice (grade A).[10] This suggests that joint protection programs can help slow the progression of the effects of RA over and above the effects of drug therapy alone.

In conclusion, patient education should be an integrated part of the total management of RA. Elements that focus on aspects like self-efficacy and coping behavior seem to increase the likelihood of an effect on symptoms and health status.

Nursing care

Nursing care for patients with RA includes emotional support for adaptation to the new diagnosis, knowledge about the disease, consequences, and treatment, as well as discussions on the self-management in general and on symptoms. This type of care was previously performed only in the setting of hospitalization, but the principles are increasingly transferred into day care or outpatient clinics. It is not known whether nurse-led clinics can prevent or reduce the impact of the disease, but significant increases in patient satisfaction have been recorded (grade A).[11]

Assessments in nursing care should address needs on the basis of what is most important to the patients. Pain, physical functioning, and fatigue are the most frequently reported prioritized symptoms and areas of disease impact. The assessment of patients' own resources is equally important. Knowledge and confidence in the ability to influence health and daily activities have been measured with a patient knowledge questionnaire and RA-specific self-efficacy scales or RA attitude index, respectively. Nursing care aims to mobilize, strengthen, or compensate deficiencies in dimensions of self-care.

Physical activity

Physical activity, exercises, and physiotherapy are important components to optimize non-pharmacologic care. These three terms describe different concepts. *Physical activity* is defined as any bodily movement produced by skeletal muscles that results in energy expenditure, whereas *exercises* are a subset of physical activity that is planned, structured, and repetitive, with the objective of improvement or maintenance of physical fitness (grade B).[12] In addition, *physiotherapy* includes treatment options addressing disease symptoms like pain and joint mobility such as massage, mobilization, manipulative techniques, and different physical modalities.

Due to fear of aggravating disease activity and symptoms, people with RA were earlier advised to limit their amount of physical activity and protect their joints when exercising physically. However, current strong evidence supports that people with RA should be encouraged to be physically active in order to maintain or improve physical and mental health and reduce the risk of co-morbidities. In general, physical activity is associated with better physical and mental health, prevention of disease, and reduced risk of all-cause mortality. Deconditioning and low muscle strength predict earlier mortality in both diseased and normal populations at levels of significance similar to or greater than biomedical predictors (grade B).[13,14] Patients with RA are shown to have reduced muscle strength, endurance, and aerobic capacity compared with age-matched controls.[15]

On the basis of consistent findings in the literature, physical activity is both safe and beneficial and should be considered an important part of the management of RA. Recommendations for physical activity summarized in Table 95.3 are based on a systematic review of randomized controlled trials (RCTs) addressing the effect of training in people with RA.[16] The recommendations are similar to those for the general population except from some special considerations that may be necessary for people with RA:

- Careful progression of intensity and individual adjustments of program may be necessary due to disease fluctuations and/or disease activity.
- Cautions should be made for increased risk of fractures due to osteoporosis or treatment with glucocorticoids.
- Patients with joint replacements should be careful with heavy loads.
- In phases with high disease activity, flexibility and range of motion exercises together with strength training of large muscles are preferred.

Exercise therapy

Exercising is one of the most important behavioral interventions that can have major beneficial health effects. In a systematic review including six RCTs examining the effects of dynamic exercise programs, the overall conclusion was that dynamic exercise is effective with respect to improvement of aerobic capacity and muscle strength in patients with RA. More research is necessary to evaluate the long-term effects of dynamic exercise therapy on radiologic progression and functional ability, but it is important to notice that no detrimental effects on disease activity and pain were reported in this review (grade A*).[17]

The positive effects of dynamic exercise on aerobic capacity and muscle strength were confirmed in a review of literature published up to 2005. Nine RCTs provided a high level of evidence regarding the effects of dynamic exercise therapy in RA patients older than 18 years of age (grade A).[18] The authors also concluded that the clinical and laboratory safety profiles were good, but conclusions concerning functional ability, physical capacity, quality of life, and structural damages could not be drawn. Therefore a randomized, controlled trial was conducted, comparing a 4-week dynamic exercise program with a conventional joint rehabilitation group. Fifty patients with RA were included, and the results after 1 month indicated that dynamic exercises were more effective than conventional joint rehabilitation in improving functional status (HAQ), quality of life, and aerobic fitness, but the statistically significant differences between the groups were not maintained at the 6-month follow-up (grade A).[19]

The evidence of beneficial effects of exercises were supported in a review of 15 clinical trials evaluating aerobic and strengthening exercises (grade A).[16] The reviewers concluded that aerobic capacity and strength improved without negative effects on pain and disease activity, but specific effects of exercises on activities of daily living, health-related quality of life, and disease progression remain unclear. On the basis of their findings, the authors provide the following recommendations for aerobic exercises: the intensity level should be moderate to hard (i.e., 60% to 85% of maximum heart rate), and exercises should be performed three times weekly for a duration of 30 to 60 minutes.[16] The benefit of high-intensity exercises was further supported in a large multicenter study in the Netherlands, including 300 patients with RA. The effectiveness and safety of a high-intensity program were compared with usual care, and the experimental program was found to be most effective in improving functional ability of RA patients (grade A).[20] Further, it is important to notice that the progression of radiographic joint damage of the small joints of hands and feet did not increase by the long-term, high-intensity, weight-bearing exercises.

Most of the studies on effects of exercise interventions comprise patients with established, stable RA, but a randomized controlled study conducted in Finland included patients with early RA (grade A).[21] In this study, a strength training program was compared with a program of range-of-motion exercises, and during the 2-year training period, muscle strength and functional capacity improved statistically more in the strength training group.

The results of this study indicate that, also in patients with early RA, dynamic strength training should be preferred before stretching and range-of-motion exercises. However, in order to maintain adequate joint flexibility, range-of-motion exercises should be part of exercise programs for patients with RA, even if high-quality studies evaluating the effect of such exercises are lacking.

Many of the activity limitations seen in persons with RA are explained by impaired hand function, with grip force as the most important determinant.[22] Thus hand exercises have been a recommended strategy to improve hand function. In 2004 a systematic review concluded that there is some, but limited, evidence that long-term hand exercise may increase grip strength in patients with RA (grade A).[23] Recent studies have further confirmed that intensive hand exercise programs are well tolerated and more effective in improving hand function in terms of decreased pain and increased grip strength, compared with a traditional conservative program (grade B).[24] Also, in a randomized controlled study of hot paraffin bath and hand exercises, the authors concluded that wax baths followed by hand exercises were more effective to improve joint mobility and grip function than hand exercises alone, whereas a wax bath alone had no significant effect on hand function (grade A).[25] However, more research is necessary to determinate the optimal combinations of different kinds of exercises, variations in resistance, repetitions, and daily or weekly frequency for patients with early or established RA.

Recently, several studies have focused on cardiovascular risk factors in RA patients, underlining that this represents an excess burden of morbidity and mortality. In a recent cross-sectional study, the authors reported that physically inactive RA patients have a significantly worse cardiovascular disease (CVD) risk profile compared with physically active patients (grade B).[26] A review of studies investigating exercise interventions in relation to cardiovascular disease in RA provided strong evidence that exercise from low to high intensity of various modes is effective in improving disease-related characteristics and functional ability in RA patients, but future studies are required to investigate the effects of exercise in improving the cardiovascular status of this patient population (grade A).[27]

In summary, dynamic exercises are safe and beneficial for patients with both early and established RA. For most patients, no harmful effects on radiologic damage of the joints were reported, but patients with extensive joint damage should be careful with high-intensity weight-bearing exercises. Due to the increased risk of co-morbidities such as cardiovascular diseases and osteoporosis, it is of importance that health professionals promote physical activity and guide patients in achieving and maintaining a healthy lifestyle (grade B).[28]

Physical modalities

Physical modalities such as thermotherapy, hydrotherapy, electrotherapy, and laser are frequently used in physiotherapy practice for patients with RA to enhance pain relief and increase joint flexibility.

Thermotherapy includes a variety of local or whole-body applications of cold or heat. Since Hippocratic times, heat treatments have been appreciated as treatment for musculoskeletal and rheumatic disorders. Superficial moist heat and cryotherapy can be used as palliative therapy. Paraffin wax baths combined with exercises can be recommended for beneficial short-term effects for arthritic hands, but the conclusions are limited by methodologic considerations such as the poor quality of trials (grade A).[29]

Overall there is insufficient evidence that *balneotherapy* is more effective than no treatment, that one type of bath is more effective than another, or that one type of bath is more effective than mudpacks, exercises, or relaxation therapy. Many studies suffer from poor methodology and "positive findings" should therefore be considered with caution (grade A).[30]

Electrotherapy is based on therapeutic use of different forms of electric current, most often applied by surface electrodes. Transcutaneous electrical nerve stimulation (TENS) is used for pain control or muscle stimulation. Electric stimulation (ES) has been shown to have a clinically beneficial effect on grip strength for RA patients with muscle atrophy of the hand, but more well-designed studies are needed to provide further evidence of the efficacy of ES in RA (grade A).[31]

Low-level *laser therapy* is a light source that generates extremely pure light of a single wavelength and was introduced in the treatment of RA about 20 years ago. Low-level laser therapy has been shown to reduce pain and improve health status in chronic joint disorders, but the heterogeneity in patient samples, treatment procedures, and trial design calls for cautious interpretation of the results (grade A).[32]

Ultrasound in combination with some other treatment modalities (exercises, faradic current, and wax baths) was not found to be effective in a Cochrane review. However, some studies, mostly of poor quality, indicated that ultrasound alone on the hand may have beneficial effect on grip strength, wrist motion, morning stiffness, and joint counts. No harmful effects have been reported (grade A).[33]

The Ottawa Panel has recommended the use of low-level laser therapy, therapeutic ultrasound, thermotherapy, electrical stimulation, and transcutaneous electrical nerve stimulation for the management of rheumatoid arthritis (grade A).[34] However, in summary, the role of electrotherapy is limited to a possible adjunctive therapeutic approach, and more well-conducted and adequately powered clinical trials are needed.

Hand orthoses

The wrists and finger joints are the most frequently involved joints in persons with RA. Thus hand splints or orthoses are often prescribed to reduce pain and/or swelling, prevent contractures and deformities, and increase joint stability. Working wrist orthoses, resting splints for the wrist and hand, and splints to correct for specific deformities are three commonly used hand orthoses in RA (Fig. 95.1). A systematic review of splints and orthoses for treatment of RA concluded that working wrist splints have no positive short- or long-term effect on pain, grip strength, or range of motion (grade A).[35] Still, the authors recommended that patients try inexpensive, ready-made wrist orthoses because studies indicate that they may provide pain relief for some

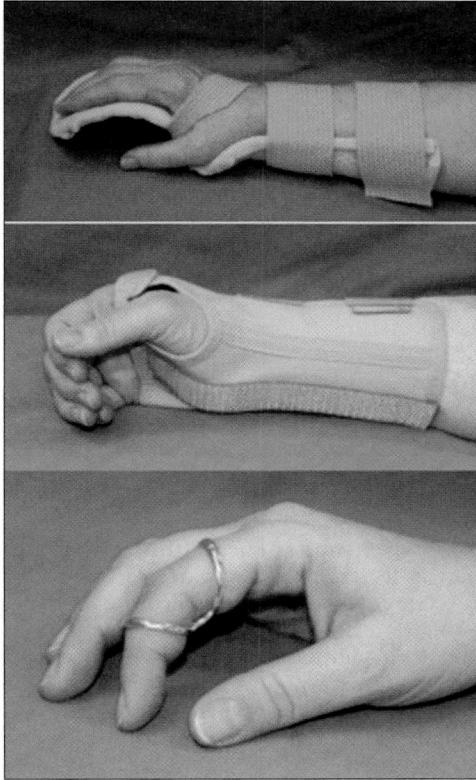

Fig. 95.1 Hand orthoses may decrease pain and correct for deformities. From top to bottom: a resting splint that restricts motion and maintains a functional position, a functional wrist splint that supports the wrist during hand activities, and a silver ring splint that corrects and/or prevents deformities.

patients in some activities. This recommendation was later supported by a randomized controlled study in which pain scores decreased by 32% after 4 weeks in the splinting group and increased by 17% in the control group (grade A).[36]

The authors of a systematic review of orthoses concluded that recommendations regarding the use of resting hand splints to reduce pain and swelling could not be given on the basis of current evidence, even if patients in one of the two studies preferred wearing the splints to not wearing them (grade A).[35] Unfortunately, two randomized controlled studies published in 2008 do not add evidence in either direction.

Small custom-made splints have been shown to correct deformities and improve pain, while specially designed silver ring splints may improve dexterity in patients with swan neck or boutonnière deformities.

Foot orthoses, insoles, and orthopedic shoes

More than 85% of people with established RA have involvement of the joints in the foot, which can lead to pain, joint instability and deformities, walking difficulties, and limitations in performance of daily activities.[41] In addition, joint abnormalities in the foot may alter walking patterns and thereby the biomechanics of the entire lower extremity. Persons with RA therefore often use foot orthoses, insoles, or orthopedic shoes to relieve foot pain and normalize gait. A variety of prefabricated and custom-made orthoses and shoes are available. Soft insoles made of viscoelastic materials may attenuate shock during walking, semirigid orthoses are made to enhance a more uniform pressure distribution in the foot, and rigid foot orthoses are designed to reduce unwanted motion and maintain desired structural alignment. Orthopedic shoes are made with extra depth in the shoe box, greater foot stability, and/or padded heel collars for improved fit. Often, a combination of orthopaedic shoes, orthoses, and soles is used to give an optimal effect (Fig. 95.2).

In general, current research supports use of these interventions. The results of a systematic review of interventions for foot disease in RA indicates that extra-depth shoes have beneficial effects on pain and function and that the benefit is greater if combined with orthoses (grade

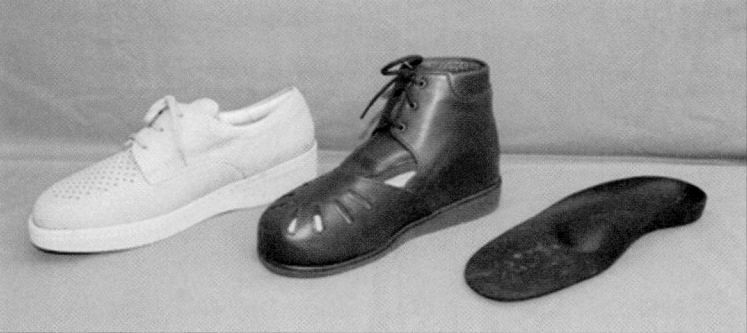

Fig. 95.2 Foot orthoses and orthopedic shoes may reduce pain and improve functional ability. From left to right, a prefabricated orthopedic shoe, a custom-made orthopedic shoe, and a custom-made insole.

A).[37] Strong evidence supports that orthoses in the rheumatoid foot contribute to pain reduction and improved functional ability. Some evidence supports that orthoses may slow down the progression of hallux valgus deformities (grade A).[38] Treatment effect was reached during the first 6 weeks and maintained as long as patients used their orthoses, but studies have not clearly shown which type of foot orthoses is most effective.

Assistive technology

Assistive technology is prescribed and used as a means to reduce pain and compensate for impairment and environmental demands, and it is one of the most frequent self-help strategies reported by persons with RA.[39] It includes a wide range of products, from low-tech devices to technologically complex equipment, some of which is designed for the general population, whereas others are developed to meet the needs of people with functional limitations or disabilities (Fig. 95.3). Studies indicate that two thirds of all persons with arthritis use assistive devices on a daily basis and that use of such technology is associated with a more severe disease, a longer disease duration, and loss of grip strength and functional ability. However, even if provision of assistive devices is a widely used multidisciplinary intervention, there is a general lack of studies evaluating the effect of such devices. Only one small study assessing the effect of an eye drop delivery device met the inclusion criteria of a review of assistive technology in RA (grade A).[39] One reason for the small number of studies and low level of formal evidence may be that the effect of some assistive devices seems rather obvious, such as the benefit of using raised seats, grab bars, or canes or crutches to ease safe transfer or mobility.

Psychological interventions

Living with a persistent and chronic disease like RA may lead to psychological distress and reduced quality of life. Psychological interventions are therefore often used to improve pain, anxiety, and/or depression. These interventions may consist of one or a combination of modalities such as relaxation strategies (e.g., progressive muscle relaxation), biofeedback therapy for reduction of muscle tension, cognitive-behavioral strategies (e.g., cognitive reconstruction, pain coping), and patient education. Research indicates that these approaches may be effective adjuncts to conventional medical management. In a review based on data from 25 randomized controlled studies, there were statistically significant improvement in pain, functional ability, depression, coping, and self-efficacy immediately following psychological treatment, but the effect sizes were small (grade A),[40] and these significant effects were not maintained to the follow-up examinations after an average of 8.5 months. Subgroup analyses revealed that psychological interventions may be more effective in patients with shorter disease duration.

Nutrition

People with RA may try to replace their traditional food with special diets.[41] The most common diets are vegetarian (usually eliminating meat and fish), vegan (eliminating meat, fish, eggs, and milk),

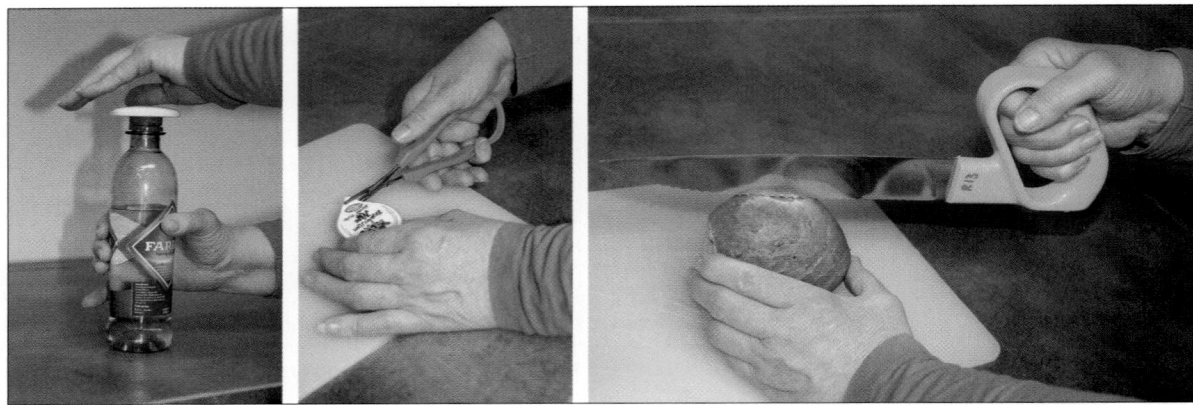

Fig. 95.3 Use of assistive devices is one of the most frequent self-help strategies reported by persons with rheumatoid arthritis. From left to right: an enlarged grip for opening bottles, a self-opening scissor tong, and a bread knife with an ergonomic handle.

Mediterranean (including small amounts of meat and more fish, fruits, vegetables, and olive oil), and elemental or elimination diets. Elemental diets are usually liquid diets that contain nutrients that are broken down to make digestion easier, whereas elimination diets are used to exclude foods that might worsen the disease. A systematic review of dietary interventions in RA concluded that effects of diet on pain, stiffness, and physical function were uncertain (grade A).[41] However, the results from the included single trial in this review indicated that both fasting followed by a vegetarian diet and a Cretan Mediterranean diet may improve pain when compared with an ordinary diet (grade A), whereas elemental diets have no significant positive effect (grade A), and the effects of vegan and elimination diets are uncertain (grade A).

Many dietary interventions are in line with what may be considered a healthy diet, with a focus on fiber, fruits, vegetables, antioxidants, fish, moderate amounts of lean meat, and reduction of saturated fat and sugar. In general, persons with RA should therefore be given the same advice as the general population, which is to follow a healthy diet, avoid certain foods that may cause allergies or intolerance, and consult a nutritionist if they want to try any special diet.

Vocational rehabilitation

Functional limitations may cause productivity loss in terms of work disability, work loss (synonymous with absenteeism or short-term sick leave), or work limitation (reduction in productivity while still present at work). A systematic review concerning productivity loss due to RA showed that RA-related work disability rates were similar in the United States and European countries, and that a median of 66% of employed RA subjects had experienced work loss due to RA for a medium duration of 39 days in the previous year (grade A).[42] However, the times from RA diagnosis until a 50% probability of being work disabled varied from 4.5 to 22 years. The results also showed that the prevalence of RA-related work disability has decreased over time, which may be due to advances in drug treatment of RA, a general decrease in the proportion of people engaged in manual or physically demanding work, or changes in social policies, level of education, age, and disease duration (grade A).

To enable persons with RA to maintain or return to work, multidisciplinary vocational rehabilitation programs have been developed. These programs may involve many professionals including physiotherapists, occupational therapists, psychologists, social workers, vocational trainers, job counselors, case managers, and job placement agencies. The formal evidence of the efficacy of such programs is limited.[43] Even if five of the six studies in this systematic review demonstrated some positive effect on vocational status, the authors concluded that the proof of the effect was limited because all included studies were uncontrolled trials and five had a retrospective design (grade B).

Prevention of work disability is probably more effective than correction of work disability after work loss. One program included self-management group sessions combined with individual professional assessments and interventions, with a follow-up by telephone 1 month after completion of the program. As a consequence, participants were more able to adapt their work to their arthritis, and improved fatigue, self-efficacy, and at-work productivity over 12 months were shown (grade B).[44] Another randomized controlled study compared job loss between individuals with early RA who were randomized to adalimumab combined with methotrexate versus methotrexate alone. The proportion with job loss after 56 weeks was significantly lower in the group receiving combination therapy (grade A).[45] This current evidence indicates that more attention should be directed to rapid identification and treatment of persons at risk of being work disabled.

Multiple disciplinary team care

Access to a multidisciplinary team is in many countries considered a part of the standard care for patients with RA. However, access to services from health professionals differs and may be influenced not only by socioeconomic factors but also by factors such as awareness of doctors about treatment opportunities, availability of health professionals, waiting lists, living in rural areas, and insufficient funding for effective services.[46]

A randomized Swedish study published in the late 1980s suggested that outpatient multidisciplinary team care was effective in RA (grade A).[47] Further, a review of effects of comprehensive rehabilitation concluded that inpatient and day patient programs were equally effective with regard to disease activity and functional ability (grade A).[48]

In many countries, a clinical nurse practitioner care model exists. Nurse practitioners have extended their roles to incorporate some of the services that usually have been offered by the rheumatologist or other health professionals, and nurse-led clinics intend to assist the access to services and the clinical communication for patients with rheumatic diseases. The number of studies evaluating clinical nurse practitioner models are few, but in a recent randomized controlled trial, the clinical effectiveness of three different care models was compared (i.e., care delivered by a clinical nurse specialist, inpatient team care, and day patient team care) (grade A).[49] Care provided in nurse-led clinics showed similar clinical outcomes regarding disease activity, functional ability, and quality of life when compared with inpatient and day patient team care, but at a significantly lower cost. Although all patients reported to be highly satisfied with multidisciplinary care, patients who attended a nurse-led clinic were slightly less satisfied than those who received inpatient or day patient team care. The authors concluded that the choice of management strategy should depend on the availability of facilities and health care providers, the preferences of patients, and economic considerations. In a 2-year follow-up of this study, no significant differences in medical treatment, use of services of other health professionals, introduction of adaptive equipment, or number of hospitalizations were observed and long-term clinical outcomes were similar. Thus nurse-led clinics appear to be an effective innovation in the care for patients with RA.[49]

The primary therapist model is another transdisciplinary model, in which trained health professionals assume the roles of case managers and health care providers rather than generic therapists.[50] If considered safe, they will consult their colleagues, rather than transferring a patient to the other discipline for completion of a rehabilitation regimen. In this way, they transcend their professional boundaries and take on extended roles and responsibilities. The model has been tested in a randomized controlled study with 111 participants. The effect of 6 weeks of services from a primary therapist (primary therapist model [PTM]) was compared with traditional care from physical therapists and/or occupational therapists.[50] After 6 months, a significantly greater proportion of patients in the PTM group were clinical responders and the PTM group also had larger improvement in quality-adjusted life years (QALYs) but with higher costs. The authors concluded that the PTM has the potential to be an alternative to traditional physical/occupational therapy, and further research should focus on strategies to reduce costs of the model and assess the long-term economic consequences in managing RA.

In summary, team care, defined as care provided by a group of health professionals with different professional backgrounds, seems to be beneficial for patients with RA (i.e., comprehensive inpatient and day patient programs seem to be more effective than regular outpatient care regarding disease activity and functional ability). Further, it appears that similar effects, but at lower costs, may be achieved by transdisciplinary models, in which clinicians take on extended roles coordinating multidisciplinary care in an outpatient setting. Flexible models of care should be provided for patients with RA, meeting the varying needs and preferences of people with different age, gender, and life and disease stages. Future research should address the effect of the content and constitution of the team care on relevant outcomes and identify patients and contextual factors that enhance or limit the efficacy of team care interventions.

KEY REFERENCES

1. Vliet Vlieland TP, Li LC, MacKay C, et al. Does everybody need a team? J Rheumatol 2006 Sep;33:1897-1899.
2. Choi BC, Pak AW. Multidisciplinarity, interdisciplinarity, and transdisciplinarity in health research, services, education and policy: 2. Promotors, barriers, and strategies of enhancement. Clin Invest Med 2007;30:E224-E232.
3. Saag KG, Teng GG, Patkar NM, et al. American College of Rheumatology 2008 recommendations for the use of nonbiologic and biologic disease-modifying antirheumatic drugs in rheumatoid arthritis. Arthritis Rheum 2008;59:762-784.
4. Lorig KR, Sobel DS, Stewart AL, et al. Evidence suggesting that a chronic disease self-management program can improve health status while reducing hospitalization: a randomized trial. Med Care 1999;37:5-14.
5. Lorig K, Chastain RL, Ung E, et al. Development and evaluation of a scale to measure perceived self-efficacy in people with arthritis. Arthritis Rheum 1989;32:37-44.
6. Barlow JH, Turner AP, Wright CC. A randomized controlled study of the Arthritis Self-Management Programme in the UK. Health Educ Res 2000;15:665-680.
7. Riemsma RP, Taal E, Kirwan JR, Rasker JJ. Systematic review of rheumatoid arthritis patient education. Arthritis Rheum 2004;51:1045-1059.
8. Niedermann K, Fransen J, Knols R, Uebelhart D. Gap between short- and long-term effects of patient education in rheumatoid arthritis patients: a systematic review. Arthritis Rheum 2004;51:388-398.
9. Viktil KK, Enstad M, Kutschera J, et al. Polypharmacy among patients admitted to hospital with rheumatic diseases. Pharm World Sci 2001;23:153-158.
10. Hammond A, Freeman K. The long-term outcomes from a randomized controlled trial of an educational-behavioural joint protection programme for people with rheumatoid arthritis. Clin Rehabil 2004;18:520-528.
11. Hill J. Patient satisfaction in a nurse-led rheumatology clinic. J Adv Nurs 1997;25:347-354.
12. Caspersen CJ, Powell KE, Christenson GM. Physical activity, exercise, and physical fitness: definitions and distinctions for health-related research. Public Health Rep 1985;100:126-131.
13. Sokka T, Hakkinen A, Kautiainen H, et al. Physical inactivity in patients with rheumatoid arthritis: data from twenty-one countries in a cross-sectional, international study. Arthritis Rheum 2008;59:42-50.
14. Andersen LB, Schnohr P, Schroll M, et al. All-cause mortality associated with physical activity during leisure time, work, sports, and cycling to work. Arch Intern Med 2000;160:1621-1628.
15. Sokka T, Hakkinen A. Poor physical fitness and performance as predictors of mortality in normal populations and patients with rheumatic and other diseases. Clin Exp Rheumatol 2008;26(Suppl 51):S14-S20.

16. Stenstrom CH, Minor MA. Evidence for the benefit of aerobic and strengthening exercise in rheumatoid arthritis. Arthritis Rheum 2003;49:428-434.
17. van den Ende CH, Vliet Vlieland TP, Munneke M, et al. Dynamic exercise therapy in rheumatoid arthritis: a systematic review. Br J Rheumatol 1998;37:677-687.
18. Gaudin P, Leguen-Guegan S, Allenet B, et al. Is dynamic exercise beneficial in patients with rheumatoid arthritis? Joint Bone Spine 2008;75:11-17.
19. Baillet A, Payraud E, Niderprim VA, et al. A dynamic exercise programme to improve patients' disability in rheumatoid arthritis: a prospective randomized controlled trial. Rheumatology (Oxford) Epub 2009 Feb 11.
20. de Jong Z, Munneke M, Zwinderman AH, et al. Long term high intensity exercise and damage of small joints in rheumatoid arthritis. Ann Rheum Dis 2004;63:1399-1405.
21. Hakkinen A, Sokka T, Hannonen P. A home-based two-year strength training period in early rheumatoid arthritis led to good long-term compliance: a five-year followup. Arthritis Rheum 2004;51:56-62.
22. Thyberg I, Hass UA, Nordenskiold U, et al. Activity limitation in rheumatoid arthritis correlates with reduced grip force regardless of sex: the Swedish TIRA Project. Arthritis Rheum 2005;53:886-896.
23. Wessel J. The effectiveness of hand exercises for persons with rheumatoid arthritis: a systematic review. J Hand Ther 2004;17:174-180.
24. Rønningen A, Kjeken I. Effect of an intensive hand exercise programme in patients with rheumatoid arthritis. Scand J Occup Ther 2008;15:173-183.
25. Dellhag B, Wollersjo I, Bjelle A. Effect of active hand exercise and wax bath treatment in rheumatoid arthritis patients. Arthritis Care Res 1992;5:87-92.
26. Metsios GS, Stavropoulos-Kalinoglou A, et al. Association of physical inactivity with increased cardiovascular risk in patients with rheumatoid arthritis. Eur J Cardiovasc Prev Rehabil 2009;16:188-194.
27. Metsios GS, Stavropoulos-Kalinoglou A, et al. Rheumatoid arthritis, cardiovascular disease and physical exercise: a systematic review. Rheumatology (Oxford) 2008;47:239-248.
28. van den Berg MH, de Boer I, le Cessie S, et al. Are patients with rheumatoid arthritis less physically active than the general population? J Clin Rheumatol 2007;13:181-186.
29. Robinson V, Brosseau L, Casimiro L, et al. Thermotherapy for treating rheumatoid arthritis. Cochrane Database Syst Rev 2002;(2):CD002826.
30. Verhagen AP, Bierma-Zeinstra SM, Cardoso JR, et al. Balneotherapy for rheumatoid arthritis. Cochrane Database Syst Rev 2003;(4):CD000518.
31. Brosseau LU, Pelland LU, Casimiro LY, et al. Electrical stimulation for the treatment of rheumatoid arthritis. Cochrane Database Syst Rev 2002;(2):CD003687.

32. Bjordal JM, Couppe C, Chow RT, et al. A systematic review of low level laser therapy with location-specific doses for pain from chronic joint disorders. Aust J Physiother 2003;49:107-116.
33. Casimiro L, Brosseau L, Robinson V, et al. Therapeutic ultrasound for the treatment of rheumatoid arthritis. Cochrane Database Syst Rev 2002;(3):CD003787.
34. Ottawa Panel Evidence-Based Clinical Practice Guidelines for Electrotherapy and Thermotherapy Interventions in the Management of Rheumatoid Arthritis in Adults. Phys Ther 2004;84:1016-1043.
35. Egan M, Brosseau L, Farmer M, et al. Splints and orthoses in the treatment of rheumatoid arthritis. Cochrane Database Syst Rev 2003;(1):CD004018.
36. Veehof MM, Taal E, Heijnsdijk-Rouwenhorst LM, et al. Efficacy of wrist working splints in patients with rheumatoid arthritis: a randomized controlled study. Arthritis Rheum 2008;59:1698-1704.
37. Farrow SJ, Kingsley GH, Scott DL. Interventions for foot disease in rheumatoid arthritis: a systematic review. Arthritis Rheum 2005;53:593-602.
38. Clark H, Rome K, Plant M, et al. A critical review of foot orthoses in the rheumatoid arthritic foot. Rheumatology (Oxford) 2006;45:139-145.
39. Tuntland H, Kjeken I, Nordheim L, et al. Assistive technology for rheumatoid arthritis. Cochrane Database of Systematic Reviews 2009; Accepted for publication.
40. Astin JA, Beckner W, Soeken K, et al. Psychological interventions for rheumatoid arthritis: a meta-analysis of randomized controlled trials. Arthritis Rheum 2002;47:291-302.
41. Hagen KB, Byfuglien MG, Falzon L, et al. Dietary interventions for rheumatoid arthritis. Cochrane Database Syst Rev 2009;(1):CD006400.
42. Burton W, Morrison A, Maclean R, et al. Systematic review of studies of productivity loss due to rheumatoid arthritis. Occup Med (Lond) 2006;56(1):18-27.
43. de Buck PD, Schoones JW, Allaire SH, et al. Vocational rehabilitation in patients with chronic rheumatic diseases: a systematic literature review. Semin Arthritis Rheum 2002;32:196-203.
44. Lacaille D, White MA, Rogers PA, et al. A proof-of-concept study of the "Employment and Arthritis: Making It Work" program. Arthritis Rheum 2008;59:1647-1655.
45. Bejarano V, Quinn M, Conaghan PG, et al. Effect of the early use of the anti-tumor necrosis factor adalimumab on the prevention of job loss in patients with early rheumatoid arthritis. Arthritis Rheum 2008;59:1467-1474.
46. Jacobi CE, Mol GD, Boshuizen HC, et al. Impact of socioeconomic status on the course of rheumatoid arthritis and on related use of health care services. Arthritis Rheum 2003;49:567-573.

REFERENCES

Full references for this chapter can be found on www.expertconsult.com.

7

PEDIATRIC RHEUMATOLOGY

Evaluation of musculoskeletal complaints in children

96

Nora G. Singer and Angelo Ravelli

■ This chapter highlights the approach to assessing the following:
- Symptoms of musculoskeletal and rheumatic diseases in childhood
- The use of physical examination to distinguish between inflammatory rheumatic and mechanical musculoskeletal diseases of children
- Distinguishing Legg-Calvé-Perthes disease and slipped capital femoral epiphysis as distinct causes of hip pain
- Specific clinical maneuvers that can be used to identify the range of disorders of the knee that may cause pain but that are not manifestations of systemic disease

INTRODUCTION

The diagnosis of musculoskeletal complaints that begin during childhood or adolescence requires clinical skill, recognizing when the findings of the physical examination are abnormal and then distinguishing features that differentiate mechanical from inflammatory diseases. The aims of this chapter are to (1) outline questions during the history taking that should alert the clinician that a diagnosis of musculoskeletal disease is possible; (2) list some key physical abnormalities that may be found in common non-inflammatory musculoskeletal disorders of the hip and knee; (3) suggest radiologic investigations that may help in diagnosing common disorders of the hip and knee; and (4) delineate the spectrum of musculoskeletal conditions that can occur in children and adolescents, emphasizing the clinical reasoning leading to a diagnosis.

When considering a diagnosis of musculoskeletal or rheumatic disease in a child, the history is of principal importance in distinguishing whether the complaints or physical findings are more likely related to congenital or acquired abnormalities of the developing musculoskeletal system or due to autoinflammatory or autoimmune disorders with tissue-specific manifestations. Overdiagnosis of mechanical musculoskeletal "disorders" in children, such as the variations of normal alignment in the growing skeleton, can be avoided through recognition of normal findings during an examination. In contrast, prompt recognition of abnormalities is key, because delay in diagnosis of rheumatic disease may have adverse consequences and incorrect diagnoses of mechanical disorders may delay directed therapy and/or result in treatments more specific for autoimmune disease.

In children, in general, and adolescents, in particular, transient musculoskeletal complaints are common, as are sports-related complaints or non-inflammatory conditions of the musculoskeletal system compared with inflammatory rheumatic disease. Almost every musculoskeletal symptom that children complain of, or parents report, can indicate a rheumatic disease. Systemic symptoms such as fever, rash, headache, listlessness or lethargy, limping, weakness, anorexia, or pain, all of which are usually associated with both transient and chronic inflammatory disease, should lead the examiner away from mechanical and non-inflammatory disorders as the primary cause of the complaints. Knowledge of broad differential diagnostic categories (Table 96.1) will also help to focus the diagnostic strategy. Additionally, it is important to be aware of the spectrum of pediatric diseases primarily involving other body systems that are associated with musculoskeletal or rheumatic complaints (Table 96.2). The astute clinician should understand the role of symptom combinations in clinical reasoning leading to a correct diagnosis, rather than isolated symptoms or laboratory examinations; disease features such as peripheral joint swelling increase the likelihood of a rheumatic diagnosis, whereas demonstration of joint instability, pain with maneuvers to isolate specific structures, and absence of local inflammation and/or systemic symptoms is more suggestive of non-inflammatory rheumatic disease (Table 96.3).

HISTORY

Children of all ages should be spoken to directly, honestly, and at an age-appropriate level. In this manner, reassurance can be given, both verbally and non-verbally, by an explanation of what the visit will entail. For very young children fear may be assuaged by talking first to their parents while they are held in their parents lap. Major sources of anxiety for many children are fear of the unknown and fear of pain, such as might occur during physical examination or laboratory testing, and telling the child what is required of him or her establishes trust in the long term even though it may be stressful at the initial encounter. The role of the parent in providing historical details is clearly dependent on the age of the patient; adolescents should be encouraged to provide their own history, perhaps with the parent not even being present in the examination room; for younger children the sense of time and pain localization may be difficult to elicit directly from the patients themselves. Disparity in the historical narrative between the patient and parent should be noted and may lead to future clues as to the underlying problems. Discrepancies may be due to genuine mistakes, inaccurate recall, errors of interpretation, or manifestations of a serious underlying problem, such as abuse. Child abuse at any level (physical, psychological, or sexual) may present as rheumatic complaints, particularly musculoskeletal pain.

Constitutional features

Most chronic inflammatory diseases are accompanied by a constellation of relatively non-specific but potentially important constitutional features, such as lethargy and/or fatigue, mood change, irritability, reduced appetite, and weakness. Fever is a prominent indication of inflammation. Examples include the evening fevers of systemic arthritis, the low-grade fever that may occur in other forms of juvenile idiopathic arthritis (JIA), systemic lupus erythematosus (SLE), and, occasionally, in juvenile dermatomyositis (JDM), and the episodic nature of fevers seen in the periodic fever syndromes such as familial Mediterranean fever (FMF), TNF-receptor associated periodic syndrome (TRAPS), and others. Complaints of muscle weakness are common in inflammatory disease, whereas complaints of muscle pain may accompany infectious and postinfectious inflammatory myopathy (e.g., pyomyositis, influenza associated) or in the absence of weakness may point toward complex regional or generalized pain disorders. Specific muscle strength testing may reveal localizing features such as proximal myopathy, which have important diagnostic implications.

Joint pain

Joint pain is a key clinical feature of musculoskeletal and inflammatory rheumatic diseases. Its description should include whether it interferes with function (e.g., walking, running, or writing), aggravating and relieving factors, diurnal variation, and progression. It is important to be aware that most children have difficulty in describing pain, although pain reporting can be improved through use of an age-appropriate visual analog scale such as one with happy and sad faces. The presence of pain may also be deduced by observing a child's pain avoidance behavior, rather than a direct and accurate description of the pain itself. Enlisting the parent's assistance in choosing the right terms for the child is often helpful. Beware that many children with the most dramatic complaints of musculoskeletal pain may have an important psychological component to their pain. The pain associated with inflammation tends to be mild to moderate in intensity, whereas the pain of infection is, in general, severe (see Table 96.1).

Joint swelling

Joint swelling may be reported during the history but may not be present at the time of examination. Sites of reported swelling should be assessed and confirmed during the physical examination (see later).

Joint stiffness

Joint stiffness is the reporting of reduced, uncomfortable range of joint movement. In chronic inflammatory disease, it often seems to be at its worst on awakening in the mornings ("early morning stiffness") and improves throughout the day, although "gelling" may occur after prolonged inactivity, such as sitting in a car or at a desk. The duration of early morning stiffness may be less reproducible in children compared with adults but may still correlate with levels of systemic inflammation.

PHYSICAL EXAMINATION

Examination of all children and adolescents should take place in an appropriately decorated, secure, sensitive, and confidential environment,

TABLE 96.1 THE RELATIVE CONTRIBUTION OF MUSCULOSKELETAL CLINICAL FEATURES IN DIFFERENTIAL DIAGNOSIS IN CHILDREN

	Inflammatory disease	Mechanical disorder	Amplified pain disorders
Pain*	+/–	+	+++
Joint stiffness	++	–	+
Joint swelling	+++	+/–	+/–
Joint instability	+/–	++	+/–
Sleep disturbance	+/–	–	++
Physical signs†	++	+	+/–

*May depend both on the age of the child and the age appropriateness of the tool used to measure pain.
†Changes in temperature may be found in inflammatory disease and in amplified pain disorders but are more frequently accompanied by complaints of dysesthesia in the latter.
From: Southwood TR. Evaluating musculoskeletal and rheumatic disorders in children. In: Hochberg M, Silman AJ, Smolen JS, et al, eds. Rheumatology, Philadelphia: Mosby-Elsevier, 2007:961-973.

TABLE 96.2 SOME MAJOR PEDIATRIC DISEASES THAT MAY HAVE MUSCULOSKELETAL MANIFESTATIONS

Disease	Musculoskeletal manifestation
Cystic fibrosis	Large and small joint arthropathy
Down syndrome	Carpal osteolysis
Diabetes	Cheiroarthropathy
Hypo/hyperthyroidism	Musculoskeletal pain
Hemophilia	Intra-articular and muscle hemorrhage
Hemoglobinopathies	Avascular necrosis, septic arthritis
Pancreatitis	Osteolytic lesions
Inflammatory bowel disease	Erythema nodosum, large joint arthritis, spondyloarthritis
Cyanotic congenital heart disease	Hypertrophic osteoarthropathy
Malignancies	Metastases, hypertrophic osteoarthropathy

From: Southwood TR. Evaluating musculoskeletal and rheumatic disorders in children. In: Hochberg M, Silman AJ, Smolen JS, et al, eds. Rheumatology, Philadelphia: Mosby-Elsevier, 2007:961-973.

TABLE 96.3 MANEUVERS THAT MAY BE USED TO DIAGNOSE MECHANICAL DISORDERS OF THE KNEE

Maneuver name	Structure(s) tested	Description
Patellar apprehension	Patella (laxity)	Performed by placing the knee in relaxed flexion (30°) and subluxing the patella laterally using gentle pressure (not so much pressure as could displace patella)
Lachman	Anterior cruciate ligament integrity (ACL)	Knee is flexed to 20°; the examiner holds the distal thigh above the knee pressing down with that hand while simultaneously grasping the tibia with the other hand and pulling it forward. Excess motion or no sharp stop compared with the other side indicates possible injury to the ACL.
Anterior drawer	ACL	Knee is flexed to 90° with foot stabilizing the knee. The proximal tibia is held with both hands, thumbs in front reaching circumferentially; the tibia is displaced anteriorly. Excess laxity compared with the other side is considered a positive test, although asymmetric pain and any abnormal movement should be noted.
McMurray	Menisci	With a thumb and fingers placed over the medial and lateral joint line, the knee is moved through range of motion by holding the foot with the other hand and applying medial or lateral rotational pressure. The knee is extended passively and the procedure repeated to detect pain at the joint line. Pain, sometimes accompanied by a "thunk," suggests the presence of meniscal abnormality.
Valgus stress	Medial collateral ligament (MCL)	With an extended knee, the upper hand is placed above the knee laterally and the lower hand over the gastrocnemius on the medial aspect. Pressure is applied outward on the calf, and laxity and pain are noted if MCL is not functioning normally.
Varus stress	Lateral CL (LCL)	With an extended knee, the upper hand is placed above the knee medially, the lower hand over the gastrocnemius laterally. Pressure is applied inward on the calf, and laxity and pain are noted if LCL is not functioning normally.
Posterior drawer	Posterior CL (PCL)	Performed in the same manner as the anterior drawer test except the tibia is forced posteriorly.
Ober test	IT bands	Performed by placing the patient on the non-painful side. The affected hip is placed in a slightly extended position with the hip flexed and pain or limitation are observed when the affected leg is no longer held in the air by the examiner but instead returns to the surface.
Thomas test	Quadriceps flexibility	Performed by placing a hand under the lumbar lordosis and asking the patient to flex one knee to the chest; if the other hip flexes this suggests tightness of the quadriceps.

TABLE 96.4 THE FUNCTIONAL MUSCULOSKELETAL EXAMINATION

Position	Musculoskeletal features examined
Sitting cross-legged	Hip abduction, external rotation and flexion, knee flexion
Rising to stand straight	Leg extension, back extension, lower limb muscle power
Bending forward	Anterior spinal curvature, scoliosis
Removing shoes/socks	Hip/knee flexion, hand and wrist function
Removing top	Shoulder and elbow range of movement
Walking normally	Gait phases: stance, toe off, swing, heel strike
Tiptoe walking	Toe extension, ankle plantarflexion, muscle power
Heel walking	Ankle dorsiflexion, knee extension, pain at enthesis
Hands pronated, arms extended	Elbow extension, shoulder power
Making a fist	Finger flexion
The "hands praying" position	Wrist extension, elbow flexion, finger extension
Arms up above the head, reaching	Shoulder flexion
Looking over each shoulder	Cervical spine rotation

From: Southwood TR. Evaluating musculoskeletal and rheumatic disorders in children. In: Hochberg M, Silman AJ, Smolen JS, et al, eds. Rheumatology, Philadelphia: Mosby-Elsevier, 2007:961-973.

in the presence of an independent chaperone if necessary. The child should be changed into non-restrictive clothing for examination to maximize observation but in such a manner as not to embarrass the child or parent. A single encounter may not be sufficient for a thorough examination of all joints depending on the child's level of cooperativeness; engaging the child in play is often helpful. Much functional musculoskeletal evaluation can be achieved through observation of the child at play (Table 96.4).

NORMAL VARIATIONS IN SKELETAL DEVELOPMENT AND ANATOMY OF SELECTED STRUCTURES

Growth velocity in childhood is not strictly linear and minor degrees of asymmetry may be detected on examination, most commonly in the size of the feet and length of the legs, which often goes unnoticed unless there is a specific complaint.

The hip socket (acetabulum) consists of parts of the ischium, ilium, and pubis surrounding the femoral head to create a ball-and-socket type joint. The growth of the proximal femur and acetabulum are interdependent. The concave shape of the acetabulum develops in response to the presence of a spherical femoral head as a stimulus.[1] Acetabular development is determined by about 8 years of age. In the infant, the proximal femur is composed entirely of cartilage, with three main growth areas: the physeal plate, the growth plate of the greater trochanter, and the plate on the femoral neck isthmus.[2,3] The developmental growth of the structure is affected by muscle pull, weight bearing, joint nutrition, circulation, and muscle tone.[1] Approximately 30% of growth of the overall length of the femur is from the proximal femoral physeal plate. The depth of the acetabulum increases at puberty, with development of three secondary centers of ossification in the hyaline cartilage surrounding the acetabular cartilage.[4,5]

Knee deformities

Substantial changes in skeletal alignment such as knock knees (genu valgum) and bow legs (genu varum) frequently bring children to the attention of musculoskeletal clinicians. Infants are normally born with

a varus knee angle that gradually straightens to achieve neutral alignment between 18 months and 2 years of age. Further normal growth usually results in a progressive change in knee alignment to a valgus position that is maximal between 5 and 7 years (up to 15 degrees), resulting in an intermalleolar distance at the ankles of up to 5 cm. Children with JIA may develop increasing knee valgus due to differential overgrowth of the medial femoral condyle as a consequence of the inflammatory process. If the intermalleolar distance progresses beyond 10 cm, surgical correction may be necessary.

Foot and ankle anatomy

There is variation in the normal posture of the foot. At birth, most infants do not have a discrete medial longitudinal foot arch or a stable hindfoot position. Thus, ankle valgus and a "flat foot" (pes planus) are frequently noticed once the infant begins walking. The adult foot posture slowly develops throughout childhood. If a child of approximately 10 years or over continues to have pes planus and ankle valgus (overpronation) in association with lower limb, back, or generalized musculoskeletal pain, a diagnosis of benign joint hypermobility syndrome may be considered. In general, children are more flexible than adults and the range of normal joint movement in children is greater. However, the combination of skeletal malalignment and increased muscle tension to maintain posture may result in joint or muscle pain in some children.

Examination of the musculoskeletal system

The general appearance of the child, including recording of growth and percentiles, skin color and condition, overall nutritional status, muscle bulk, vital signs (temperature, blood pressure), and joint movement when playing can help to form an overall assessment of whether the child is well or sick. Musculoskeletal and rheumatic symptoms may be the initial manifestations of a wide range of pediatric diseases heightening the importance of a careful general physical examination. Careful assessment of the eyes and peripheral pulses should also be included as part of the routine physical examination of these children (see Table 96.4).

Joint assessment

For each joint, a standardized approach will minimize the risk of omission (always remembering to compare side to side). Many clinicians perform head to toe joint examination so as not to forget to examine any joints, except in a very young child when starting with examination of the extremities may be less threatening to the child.

Suggested steps in the joint examination include:

1. *Looking:* inspect the position of the joint at rest, its surface anatomy, contours, color, scar, size and muscle bulk, and limb length.
2. *Feeling:* palpating for skin warmth, joint swelling, and tenderness. Swelling includes any increase in joint size that alters the normal surface markings of the joint. The key sites for observing swelling are dependent on the particular joint and the nature of the swelling itself. Swelling may be due to intra-articular effusion, periarticular collection of fluid, soft tissue changes (generalized edema, thickening of the joint capsule, and inflammation of muscle, ligament, and subcutaneous or cutaneous tissues), or bony changes. Also note joint margin tenderness and other tender spots, including the presence of enthesitis (tenderness and inflammation at the site of insertion into bone of ligament, fascia, or joint capsule).
3. *Moving:* by the examiner (passive range of motion [ROM]) and by the patient (active ROM), noting any pain or irritability on motion (POM) especially at the end range of joint motion.
4. Next, assess joint stability, particularly for the stability ligaments of the knee (cruciate and collateral ligaments), and pain referable to other joint structures such as the menisci and associated structures such as the iliotibial bands and bursa.

Young children, in particular, may find that a musculoskeletal examination that begins with the toes and feet is the least upsetting. Examining the most painful areas at the end of the examination often facilitates a complete examination.

Feet and ankles

With the child supine, observe the leg lengths carefully for any discrepancy. Ask the patient to curl the toes to observe the flexion and extension range of metatarsal and interphalangeal joint movement. Carefully squeeze the metatarsophalangeal joints in such a manner as not to cause alarm; and if tenderness is noted, assess each joint for synovitis by gently palpating the joint margins while moving the joint through its range of movement. Examine the midtarsal joints by stabilizing the calcaneus while inverting and everting the forefoot. Assess the subtalar joints by inverting and everting the calcaneus (hindfoot) and the ankle joints (tibiotalar) by dorsiflexion and plantarflexion at the ankle. Synovitis of subtalar and ankle joints may be poorly localized and occasionally only visible from the posterior aspect; observation from the posterior view also allows assessment as to whether the Achilles tendon(s) is thickened. Palpate for tenderness at the insertion of the plantar fascia to metatarsal heads, fifth metatarsal base, calcaneus, and Achilles tendon insertion into the posterior aspect of the calcaneus to detect enthesitis.

Knees

Observe for any loss of vastus medialis muscle bulk and/or bulk in the gastrocnemius suggesting muscle atrophy due to reduced use in association with a painful joint. Also inspect for subtle loss of knee extension using "relaxed passive extension" of both knees by lifting the patient's feet gently up off the bed (Fig. 96.1). Mild swelling frequently obscures the medial and lateral contours of the patella and can be confirmed by palpating and inspecting for a synovial fluid wave or bulge sign (medial compression followed by lateral "re-expression" of the swelling) and by balloting the patella. Joint margin tenderness is often maximal just medial to the lower patellar border. Key points for palpation of entheses are at the tibial tuberosity and 2-, 6-, and 10-o'clock positions around the patella. Assessment of knee stability is important, particularly if the patient is complaining of "mechanical" symptoms of knee locking or giving way. The most useful examination techniques for medial and lateral collateral ligament integrity are the application of gentle valgus and varus pressure, respectively, on the knee (while held in 5 degrees of flexion), which may result in abnormal abduction or adduction. The anterior cruciate ligament is also vulnerable to sports injuries in children and young people; that, and the posterior cruciate, can be assessed using anterior and posterior drawer tests. These and other tests to elicit derangement or tightness of structures in and around the knee are listed in Table 96.3.

Hips

Detection of intra-articular effusion requires ultrasonography or magnetic resonance imaging (MRI). Screening for hip disease on physical examination is detected by passive internal and external rotation with the hip and knee flexed at 90 degrees. Greater than 45 degrees of internal rotation can usually be elicited in the normal hip. Extension range, which is normally 30 degrees beyond neutral when the patient is lying prone, also tends to be lost early in hip arthritis. Loss of flexion

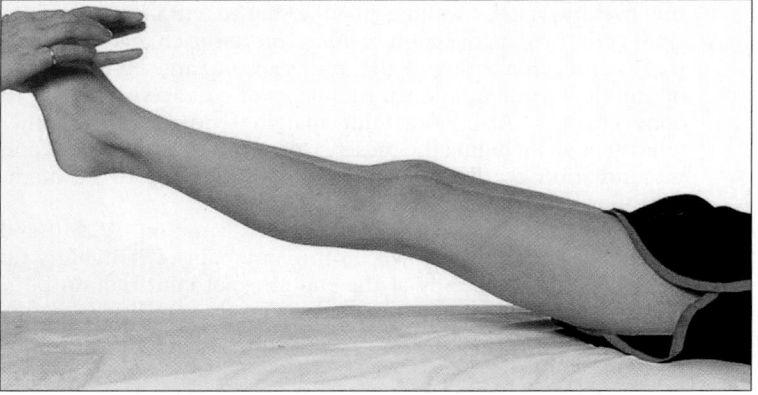

Fig. 96.1 Relaxed passive extension of the knees. The right knee has subtle loss of relaxed passive extension indicating loss of joint range secondary to JIA. *(From: Southwood TR. Evaluating musculoskeletal and rheumatic disorders in children. In: Hochberg M, Silman AJ, Smolen JS, et al, eds. Rheumatology, Philadelphia: Mosby-Elsevier, 2007:961-973.)*

in the hip generally indicates more advanced disease. Enthesitic points that should be examined include the greater trochanter and anterior superior iliac spines.

Hands and wrists

Examination of the hands and wrists is undertaken with the child sitting up with hands held out in front of the body. Observation begins with inspection of the dorsal aspect of the hands and fingers (including looking for the nail pitting seen in some children with psoriasis) and active finger flexion to "make fists" and "bury the fingernails." Joint swelling can be palpated with the hands in a prone position, noting also joint margin tenderness and passive range of joint movement. Rotation of the wrists at the distal radioulnar joint allows inspection of the palmar surface of the hands and fingers. Active finger flexion at the interphalangeal joints should normally result in the fingertips making contact with the palms overlying the metacarpal joints. Using the "prayer" position with palms placed together, finger flexion or wrist extension deformities can be detected, which has the advantage of highlighting asymmetry at the wrists and small joints of the hand.

Elbows and shoulders

The elbows are extended fully with hands reaching toward the ceiling (sometimes called "reaching for the sky" will also demonstrate shoulder flexion) and then lowered in an extended position to allow palpation of the olecranon bursa itself (which is rarely swollen in children except in injury or infection) and either side of the olecranon process. Functional elbow flexion can be demonstrated by placing the hands to the mouth. Pronation/supination of hands with the elbows at 90 degrees of flexion may reveal disruption of the proximal radioulnar joint. Assessment of the glenohumeral joint itself may proceed by palpating the joint margin with the humerus abducted to 90 degrees and rotated internally and externally (using the forearm as a lever down and up, respectively). The sternoclavicular joints should be palpated for tenderness and/or swelling.

Cervical spine and temporomandibular joints

Detection of limitation in motion in these joints may raise the possibility of systemic arthritis even if the child does not have complaints specifically referable to these joints (e.g., a teenager with ankylosing spondylitis as a cause of hip joint space narrowing may complain of hip pain but also have restricted neck motion). The movements of lateral rotation and extension are most likely to be lost early if the cervical spine is affected by arthritis. Rotation can be evaluated by asking the patient to place the chin on each shoulder. The normal extension range on tipping the head back is greater than 20 degrees. Having the child place the ear on the shoulder will allow assessment of lateral flexion. The face should be inspected carefully for asymmetry or mandibular hypoplasia. The temporomandibular joints can be palpated just anterior to the tragus of the ear, where tenderness may be demonstrated and asymmetric movement detected, particularly on asking the patient to open the mouth widely.

Spine and gait

The spine is best examined with the patient standing on bare feet and viewed from behind. Observe the position of the feet for loss of medial longitudinal arch contour (pes planus) and hindfoot for overpronation, suggesting hypermobility (Fig. 96.2). Check that the pelvis is horizontal; leg-length discrepancy is best assessed clinically when the patient is standing. Assess for scoliosis by noting the symmetry of the spine in standing and gentle forward flexion. Palpation over the sacroiliac joints may reveal tenderness, although this is a rather insensitive test for inflammation. The lateral profile of the spine should also be observed while the patient remains in the flexed position, checking particularly for abnormal flattening of the lumbar spine, which might suggest spondylitis. The presence of such an abnormality can be supported by the finding of pain on hyperextension of the spine, which puts the only synovial joints (the apophyseal joints) in the spine on the stretch. The gait is best assessed when the patient is wearing shorts and walks with bare feet. Note is made of each of the gait phases (heel strike, stance, toe off, and swing phases), looking for antalgia, Trendelenburg abnormality (a waddling gait due to weakness of hip stability muscles), and any other asymmetry.

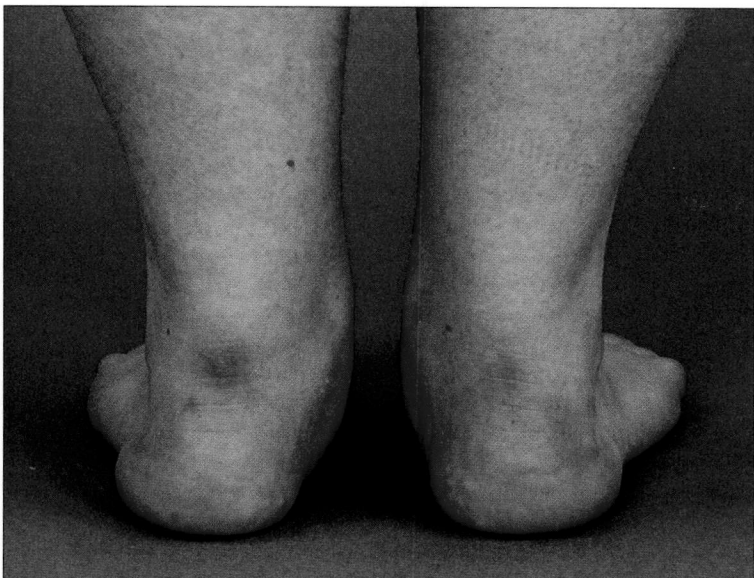

Fig. 96.2 Overpronation of both ankles associated with hypermobility. *(From: Southwood TR. Evaluating musculoskeletal and rheumatic disorders in children. In: Hochberg M, Silman AJ, Smolen JS, et al, eds. Rheumatology, Philadelphia: Mosby-Elsevier, 2007:961-973.)*

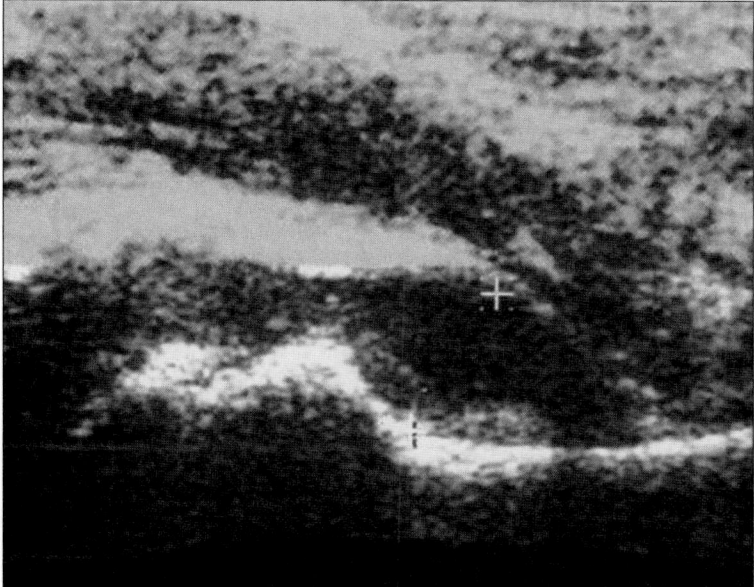

Fig. 96.3 Ultrasound image of the hip showing effusion distorting the joint capsule away from the neck of the femur. *(From: Southwood TR. Evaluating musculoskeletal and rheumatic disorders in children. In: Hochberg M, Silman AJ, Smolen JS, et al, eds. Rheumatology, Philadelphia: Mosby-Elsevier, 2007:961-973.)*

Laboratory and imaging studies

Imaging

Imaging studies are extremely useful when normal. Plain radiographs of any affected joints (and occasionally contralateral joints for comparison) may help to rule out fracture, avascular necrosis, periostitis, osteomyelitis, benign bone cysts, bone neoplasia, and bone dysplasia. Ultrasound evaluation of the hip joints is useful to confirm effusion (Fig. 96.3), and abdominal ultrasonography may help to exclude neuroblastoma. A technetium-99m bone scintiscan may highlight unsuspected skeletal trauma or a hot spot suggestive of osteoid osteoma (especially in the child with pain predominantly at night) and may be useful in the evaluation of Legg-Calvé-Perthes disease (see later). Increasing availability of MRI has illustrated the value of determining the anatomic detail of abnormalities in the musculoskeletal system.

Laboratory investigations

Laboratory studies will be determined by the possible differential diagnoses. Any suggestion that the child has a septic arthritis must be

investigated with aspiration of the affected joint to obtain synovial fluid for microscopy and culture and sensitivity studies, whereas in non-inflammatory causes of effusion the white blood cell count would be expected to be very low. Blood cultures may be drawn if hematogenous spread of infection is postulated to have resulted in joint inflammation. In the absence of an obvious orthopedic disorder, other blood tests for initial assessment might include a complete blood cell count, immunoglobulins to ascertain IgA deficiency, anti-streptolysin O titer for rheumatic fever, a search for serologic evidence of infection in cases of suspected reactive arthritis (e.g., Lyme disease), and, on occasion, a bone marrow aspiration to exclude leukemia. Coagulation studies can detect clotting disorders, particularly hemophilia, and an antinuclear antibody panel will be helpful if a connective tissue disease is suspected or to give expectant guidance regarding the frequency of slit-lamp examinations in JIA patients at risk for uveitis. Relevant biochemical tests for muscle abnormalities, endocrinopathies, and inborn errors of metabolism may be indicated depending on the clinical picture. Evaluation of urinary catecholamines should be considered to exclude neuroblastoma for children in an appropriate age group presenting with features suggestive of systemic arthritis. Tests for acute-phase reactants (erythrocyte sedimentation rate [ESR] and C-reactive protein [CRP]) may be normal in children with inflammatory arthritis. In contrast, many normal children, especially those with intercurrent viral infections, will have elevated ESR and CRP values even if they do not have inflammatory rheumatic disease (low specificity for rheumatic disease).

SELECTED MUSCULOSKELETAL DISORDERS DURING CHILDHOOD AND ADOLESCENCE

Childhood musculoskeletal diseases may in part be discerned by the age at onset of the symptoms. Understanding the spectrum of disorders that present in different age groups is helpful in focusing the clinician to a working diagnosis. Because the differential diagnosis of musculoskeletal complaints is wide, it is important to remember all the possibilities. The acronym ARTHRITIS, proposed by Taunton Southwood, is a helpful mnemonic (Box 96.1). In the review that follows the most important disorders of non-inflammatory etiology are described in the typical age group of presentation (Table 96.5).

Disorders presenting at birth or in the neonatal period

Talipes equinovarus (clubfoot) refers to a condition in which the foot is inverted and supinated and the forefoot is adducted. It is frequently bilateral, and the affected foot is shorter with less calf muscle bulk than normal. During plantarflexion the heel rotates inward. It occurs approximately twice as frequently in male infants as female infants, and its incidence approaches 1 in 1000 live births. Oligohydramnios may precede this condition as may spina bifida and other congenital disorders. Physiotherapy, positional splinting, and surgical correction may be required. Talipes equinovarus should be differentiated from talipes calcaneovalgus in which the foot is dorsiflexed and everted. The

TABLE 96.5 NON-INFLAMMATORY MUSCULOSKELETAL DISORDERS: SYMPTOM COMBINATIONS AND PIVOTAL CLINICAL FEATURES

"Typical" symptom combinations	Pivotal clinical features	Possible diagnoses
"Clunk" on hip movement screening, limping in an older infant	Asymmetric upper leg skin folds, limited hip abduction	Developmental dysplasia of hip
Nocturnal awakening with leg pain in young child	Normal child	"Growing pains" Osteoid osteoma
Sudden limping in an otherwise well young child	Unilateral restricted hip movement	Toxic synovitis
Joint effusion with or without pain	Effusion with hemorrhagic fluid on aspiration	Hemarthrosis after trauma or if recurrent Pigmented villonodular synovitis (PVNS)
Hip pain in a preadolescent boy > girl	Loss of joint range, pain on motion, may be bilateral	Legg-Calvé-Perthes disease
Hip pain in an obese preadolescent boy	Unilateral hip restriction	Slipped Upper femoral epiphysis
Hip pain and limp in adolescent girl	Unilateral pain and stiffness	Idiopathic chondrolysis
"Snapping" hip	Sensation of internal or external hip	Internal movement of the iliopsoas muscle over iliopectineal eminence, lesser trochanter, or anterior superior iliac spine. External movement of the iliotibial band over the greater trochanter hip
Localized pain	Point tenderness ± localized swelling	Stress fracture
Anterior knee pain	Pain with stairs (ascending or descending), stiffness	Patellofemoral syndromes
	Tenderness over the tibial tuberosity	Osgood-Schlatter disease (apophysitis of the tibial tuberosity)
	Tenderness over inferior pole patella	Sinding-Larsen-Johansson syndrome Apophysitis of the inferior pole of the patella
	Pain over patellar tendon or quadriceps tendon	Extensor tendinitis
Lateral knee pain	Pain where iliotibial band courses over lateral femoral epicondyle; also may radiate proximally into iliotibial band	Iliotibial band syndrome
	Pain over lateral joint line, may have positive McMurray test	Lateral meniscal injury
Medial knee pain	Intermittent pain-effusion ± locking, usually ↑ w/ activity	Osteochondritis dissecans
	Popping or snapping medially when extending from flexion	Medial plica syndrome
	Pain inferior to medial joint line/tibia	Pes anserine bursitis

latter usually self-corrects, but passive foot exercises are sometimes advised. Positional talipes from intrauterine compression is common. If the deformity is mild and the foot of normal size, it can be corrected to the neutral position with passive manipulation/exercises.

Skeletal dysplasias and inherited disorders of connective tissue are covered in Section 17.

Disorders beginning during childhood

As indicated earlier, the diagnosis of juvenile idiopathic arthritis is based on the exclusion of other causes of the child's symptoms. In the review that follows there is a brief summary of the most important disorders, with the exception of JIA and related disorders, which are covered in other chapters.

Arthritic disorders
Septic arthritis
Septic or infectious arthritis is a serious infection of the joint space that can rapidly lead to joint destruction, occasionally within 24 hours of onset if appropriate treatment is not initiated. Monarticular disease is much more common than polyarticular disease with most organisms, the most notable exception being gonococcal arthritis in teenagers. The hip joint is most commonly affected in young children, and this is more common in boys. *Staphylococcus aureus* is the most common bacteria causing septic arthritis since the routine use of *Haemophilus influenzae* vaccine has drastically reduced the incidence of *H. influenzae*–related invasive disease. Underlying and predisposing illnesses should increase the suspicion of septic arthritis, such as immunodeficiency and sickle cell disease. Children with infected joints

generally look unwell and sometimes "toxic" in appearance, with high fever and often inability to bend the affected joint due to severe pain. Aspiration of the joint space is the definitive test. Septic arthritis usually results from hematogenous spread but may also occur after a puncture wound or infected skin lesions (e.g., chickenpox). In young children, it may result from spread from adjacent osteomyelitis into joints where the capsule inserts below the epiphyseal growth plate. It is preferable that intravenous antibiotics begin after blood cultures and joint aspirations have been performed unless to do so would delay therapy unacceptably. Coexistent osteomyelitis is common and occurs in up to 15% of affected children.

Reactive or postinfectious arthritis
Reactive arthritis is the most common form of arthritis in childhood. It is defined as time-limited joint swelling (usually <6 weeks) following (or rarely accompanying) evidence of extra-articular infection. The enteric bacteria (*Salmonella*, *Shigella*, *Campylobacter*, and *Yersinia*) are implicated in most pediatric cases of reactive arthritis. Other etiologic agents include prior infection with (or vaccination against) rubella, parvovirus B19, influenza, herpesviruses and coxsackieviruses, *Mycoplasma*, and *Borrelia* (controversy remains regarding the relative contribution of persistence of infection versus immune response to prior infection in chronic Lyme arthritis).[6,7] Acute rheumatic fever and post-streptococcal reactive arthritis may be classified within the broader category of reactive arthritis. If *Streptococcus*-associated joint symptoms occur in the setting where streptococcal infection was not recognized or treated, then antibiotic therapy is used to eradicate the organism and symptomatic treatment with non-steroidal anti-inflammatory drugs (NSAIDs) or, more rarely, salicylates is used.

Regional syndromes

Benign limb pain (growing pains)

Benign limb pains, also known as "growing pains," occur in about 10% of children between the ages of 4 and 14 years. The relationship with growth is uncertain because this period is not when maximum linear growth occurs. Children typically awaken at night with deep thigh or calf pain that responds to analgesics, massage, and heat and there may be a family history of similar problems in one of the parents. The information that the child resumes full normal activities immediately after the episode and normal findings on physical examination are helpful in distinguishing benign limb pain from a more serious cause of night pain (e.g., osteoid osteoma or malignancy-associated limb pain). No further workup is needed if there is a typical history and absence of any physical abnormalities. Atypical presentations may require further workup with laboratory tests and/or radiologic imaging to exclude more serious problems.[8] "Growing pains" frequently remit, although intermittent night pain may continue over many years.[8]

Hypermobility

Joint pain secondary to hypermobility (see Chapter 206) is the most common non-inflammatory diagnosis in patients newly referred to a pediatric rheumatology clinical service. The diagnosis of hypermobility, however, should only be made in the knowledge of the normal range of joint flexibility in childhood, which varies with age, gender, and ethnic background. In general, it is normal for younger children to be more flexible than adolescents and girls to be more flexible than boys. There are also major ethnic differences. A hypermobility index called the Beighton score has been validated in Dutch children, although the cut-point differs for children depending on whether they are 10 years of age or older.[9] Hypermobility should be considered in older child or adolescent with musculoskeletal pain principally confined to the lower limbs and back who lack objective evidence of joint swelling. Common lower limb findings of hypermobility are pes planus, out-toeing gait, overpronated feet (secondary to ankle hypermobility), and genu recurvatum, all of which may be improved through using ready-made or custom orthotics that support the longitudinal foot arch and stabilize the ankle. Mechanical causes of joint pain tend to be worse after exercise and as the day goes on, but early morning stiffness 1 or 2 days after exercise may be a feature. Diffuse idiopathic musculoskeletal pain syndromes, such as fibromyalgia, have also been associated with hypermobility in schoolchildren. Important differential diagnoses include the inherited collagen disorders such as Marfan and Ehlers-Danlos syndromes.[9]

Hip disorders

Developmental dysplasia of the hip

This is a spectrum of disorders with a number of predisposing factors: positive family history for developmental dysplasia of the hip (DDH), female gender, first-born children, breech presentation, and oligohydramnios. Early detection, institution of corrective treatment, and the prevention of long-term disability are the aims of screening programs at birth and the routine 6-week postnatal checkup, but when the levels of evidence were examined to justify screening and intervention, the evidence level was fair to poor, confounded by the knowledge that a substantial proportion of hips initially labeled as DDH will resolve spontaneously without intervention.[10] The techniques of examination vary but usually involve examining one hip at a time while steadying the contralateral pelvis with the other hand. The upper portion of the femur is carefully rocked back and forth to check if the hip can be dislocated posteriorly out of the acetabulum (Barlow maneuver) or relocated back into the acetabulum on abduction (Ortolani maneuver). It is important not to exert excessive forces during these maneuvers. Presentation in later childhood may be detected by observing asymmetry of skinfolds around the hip, limited abduction of the hip, shortening of the affected leg, or a limp or abnormal gait (Fig. 96.4). Ultrasound screening on all neonates, which is highly specific for detecting the condition, is expensive and has a high rate of false-positive findings. If DDH is suggested, an orthopedic consultation is indicated. The affected infant may be placed in a positioning device that puts the hips in abduction for several months. Progress is then monitored by ultrasonography or radiography. If the hip has not stabilized or the condition is diagnosed late, hip abduction using traction and a further period of splinting (in a plaster hip spica) may be tried. Weight bearing on a dislocated hip should be avoided

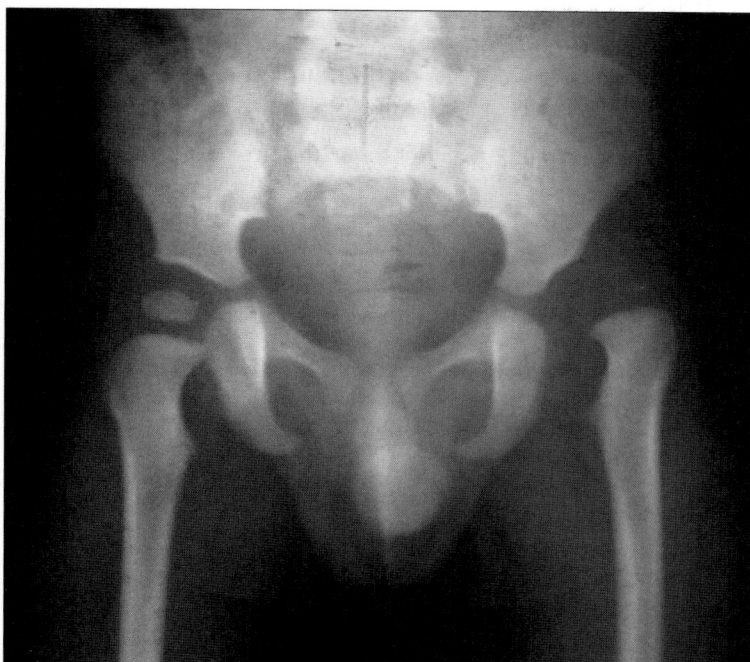

Fig. 96.4 Developmental dysplasia of the left hip with failure of acetabular formation and "telescoping" of the left femur. *(From: Southwood TR. Evaluating musculoskeletal and rheumatic disorders in children. In: Hochberg M, Silman AJ, Smolen JS, et al, eds. Rheumatology, Philadelphia: Mosby-Elsevier, 2007:961-973.)*

because it causes damage to the femoral head and acetabulum. Open reduction and derotation femoral osteotomy will be required if conservative measures fail. The risk of both closed and surgical procedures is that of aseptic necrosis of the femoral head.

Transient (toxic) synovitis (irritable hip)

This is the most common cause of acute hip pain in children, occurring in those aged 2 to 12 years. It often follows or is accompanied by a viral infection. Presentation is with sudden onset of pain in the hip or a limp. There is no pain at rest, but there is decreased range of movement; like septic arthritis, the hip may be held in the position of greatest comfort, in external rotation. The pain may be referred to the knee. The child has a mild fever or is afebrile and does not appear ill. The neutrophil count and acute-phase reactants are normal or slightly raised. Blood cultures are negative, and the radiograph of the joint is normal but there may be a small joint effusion on ultrasound evaluation (Fig. 96.5). The most important differential diagnosis is septic arthritis, but this is usually distinguished from transient synovitis by the presence of high fever, severe illness, pain at rest, minimal or no movement of the hip, and marked elevation of the neutrophil count and acute-phase reactants.[11] If there is any suspicion of septic arthritis, the joint should be aspirated under ultrasound guidance. Frequently, aspiration of the hip joint may temporarily relieve most or all of the symptoms. In a small proportion of children, transient synovitis is assumed to underlie the presentation of Legg-Calvé-Perthes disease or slipped capital femoral epiphysis. Management of transient synovitis is with bed rest if tolerated. It usually improves within a few days.

Legg-Calvé-Perthes disease

Legg-Calvé-Perthes (LCP) disease was described independently by Legg, Calvé, Perthes, and Waldenstrom.[12] It is generally considered a non-inflammatory disease of the hip of unknown etiology that is more common in boys than girls. The peak incidence is between 4 and 10 years of age. Presentation is insidious with onset of a limp or persistent hip or knee pain. Approximately 13% of children have bilateral involvement, often with the second hip being asymptomatic.[13] The bilateral involvement is usually synchronous but may occur up to 8 to 10 years later.[14] However, even with synchronous involvement, the hips are usually in different stages of disease with ischemia of the femoral epiphysis, resulting in avascular necrosis, followed by revascularization, and reossification over 18 to 36 months. Recent evidence from a two families suggests that mutation in the *COL2A1* gene (encodes precursor of type II collagen α1 chain) was associated with LCP as was premature osteoarthritis of the hip and avascular necrosis of the hip.[15,16] Why the phenotypic expression of the mutation differs within a single family is not yet understood.[16] There appears to be no significant gender difference regarding severity of involvement and long-term risk, even though girls constitute fewer than 20% of the patients.[17] Children are generally afebrile. Routine laboratory tests such as a complete blood cell count and ESR are normal.

Imaging

Although the *initial* radiographs may be normal, radiographs usually show increased density in the femoral head, which subsequently becomes fragmented (Fig. 96.6) during revascularization and irregular, resulting in superior and lateral subluxation. By 3 to 6 months after symptom onset, the size of the proximal femoral epiphysis is decreased: it is smaller and denser and the joint space wider than in the normal hip (Fig. 96.7). As demonstrated by plain radiographs there are four stages of the pathologic process: initial, fragmentation, healing, and reossification. The apparent widening of the medial joint space may be the result of continued cartilage growth in the absence of bone growth. Healing is manifested by new bone formation and reossification, with or without residual deformity. Changes in the acetabulum are important in the long term, and the radius of the acetabulum may be the most sensitive measurement representing the pathologic

changes.[18] A classification system divides LCP into four groups on the basis of the extent of femoral head involvement: group I, less than 25%; group II, 25% to 50%; group III, 50% to 75%; and group IV, greater than 75%.[19] Although widely adopted, studies eventually showed that the results were difficult to reproduce and led to a lateral pillar classification based on the height of the lateral epiphysis on anteroposterior radiographs: in group A 100% of the pillar height was maintained; in group B, more than 50%; and in group C, less than 50%. Further use required the addition of a fourth or B/C group for hips with exactly 50% maintenance of lateral pillar height. With this addition, good reproducibility has been reported.[20]

Even if the initial radiograph is normal, a repeat radiograph may be required if clinical symptoms persist. Because the extent of femoral head involvement and the degree of lateral subluxation are such important prognostic factors, assessment often requires MRI. Bone scintigraphy and arthrography were used in the past but have largely been replaced by MRI in practice. In one comparative study, MRI was superior to conventional radiography and bone scintigraphy in determining the extent of involvement in the femoral head, the location of the head involvement, and the degree of lateral subluxation. Arthrography was as good as or better than MRI in defining the shape of the articular surfaces and the presence of lateral subluxation.[18]

Before MRI, technetium-based bone scintigraphy had long been considered the gold standard for this disease. There is reduced uptake

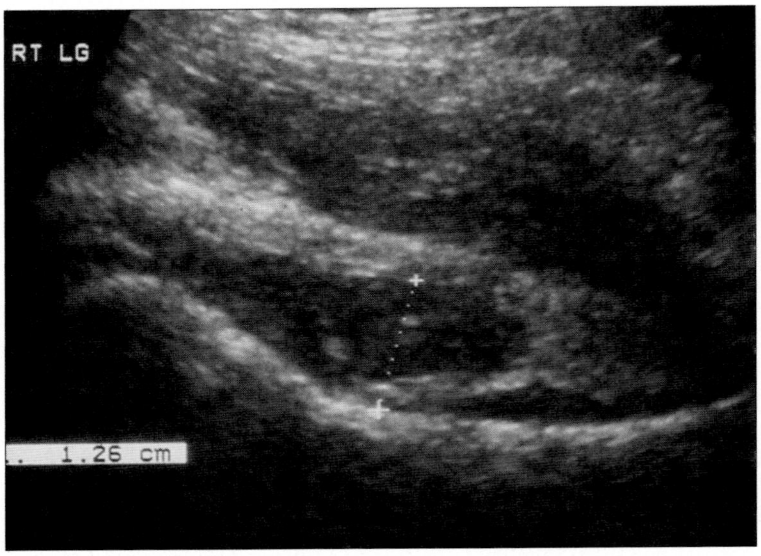

Fig. 96.5 Ultrasound image in irritable hip (transient synovitis of the hip) demonstrating effusion. *(From: Southwood TR. Evaluating musculoskeletal and rheumatic disorders in children. In: Hochberg M, Silman AJ, Smolen JS, et al, eds. Rheumatology, Philadelphia: Mosby-Elsevier, 2007:961-973.)*

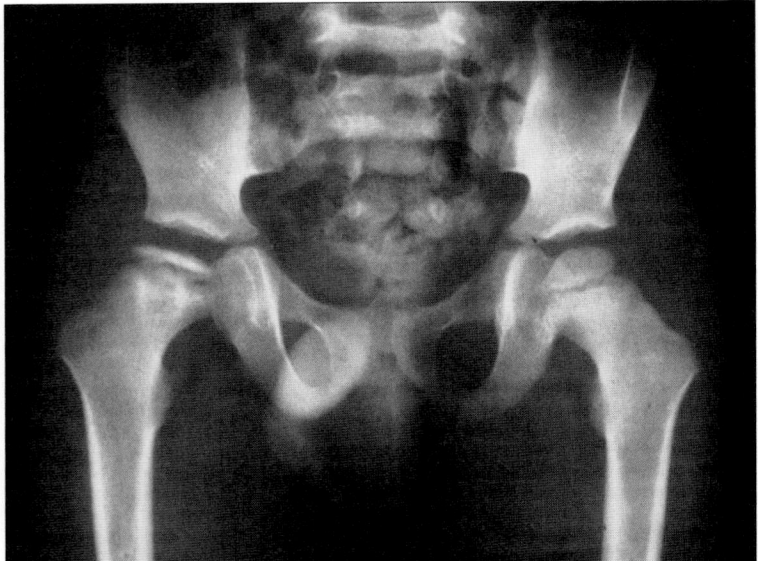

Fig. 96.6 Avascular necrosis of the right hip. *(From: Southwood TR. Evaluating musculoskeletal and rheumatic disorders in children. In: Hochberg M, Silman AJ, Smolen JS, et al, eds. Rheumatology, Philadelphia: Mosby-Elsevier, 2007:961-973.)*

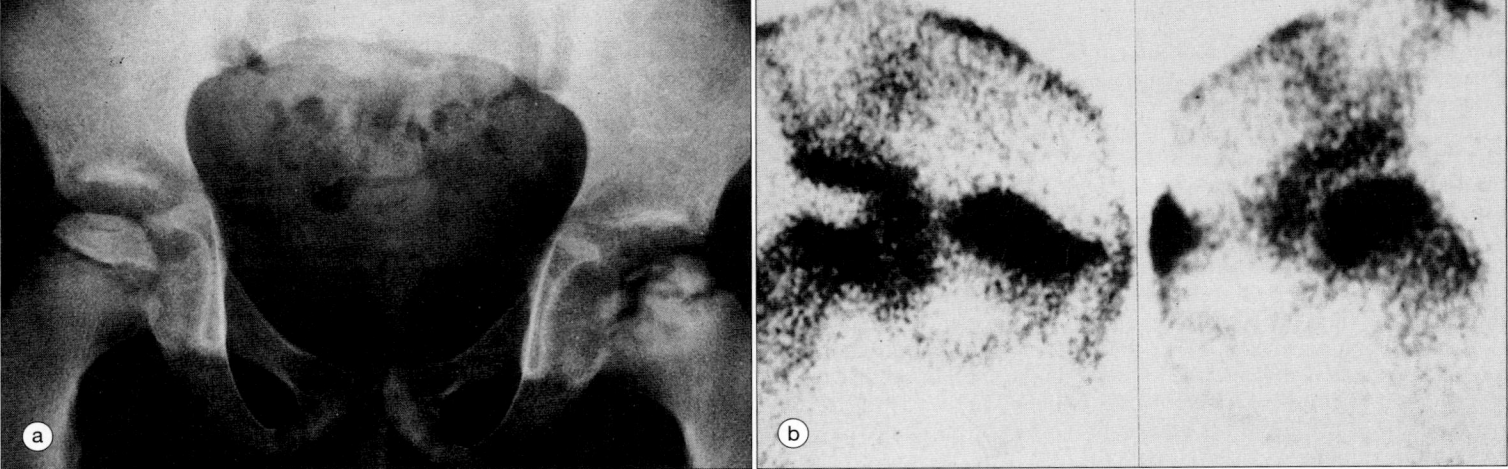

Fig. 96.7 Pelvic radiograph and technetium bone scintiscan in an 8-year-old with Legg-Calvé-Perthes disease. (a) The child has early involvement of the right hip, with relatively subtle changes on the radiograph. (b) However, the bone scintiscan shows complete blood loss in the right femoral head, consistent with osteonecrosis. The left hip shows classic, more advanced stages of Legg-Calvé-Perthes disease (in the revascularization phase), with return of normal blood flow visible on the scintiscan. *(From: Southwood TR. Evaluating musculoskeletal and rheumatic disorders in children. In: Hochberg M, Silman AJ, Smolen JS, et al, eds. Rheumatology, Philadelphia: Mosby-Elsevier, 2007:961-973.)*

initially but increased accumulation in part of the femoral head as revascularization occurs. It is an early and sensitive indicator of femoral head involvement, preceding plain radiographic changes by approximately 3 months and allowing earlier diagnosis and treatment.[21] However, in practice, bone scintigraphy is often deferred and MRI ordered for the evaluation of LCP.

MRI adds additional anatomic visualization. In early disease there is low signal intensity at the superior and lateral aspect of the femoral head on the T1-weighted (T1W) images and an area with a secondary double line of low and high signal intensity on T2-weighted (T2W) images. Widening of the medial joint space may be due to either overgrown cartilage in the initial stage or both overgrown cartilage and widened true medial joint space at the fragmentation stage and widened true medial joint space in the healing stage. Subchondral fracture line on MRI has been suggested to be a better predictor of eventual necrosis than the extent of necrosis in the early stage.[22] Gadolinium-enhanced subtraction MRI can improve sensitivity in early diagnosis. MRI has also been found to be of value in monitoring changes in the femoral epiphysis over time and led to the development of a new classification system using MRI abnormalities.[23] When subluxation is being evaluated, MRI is more sensitive than plain radiographs. MRI studies showed evidence of synovitis in all 72 patients with a correlation between the severity of the synovitis and the severity of the necrosis.[23] Synovitis was evident for 6 to 60 months after diagnosis.[23-25] Cartilaginous physeal and metaphyseal abnormalities are common and frequently associated with growth arrest.

Pathophysiology

Metaphyseal histology by core biopsy performed in conjunction with surgery in 22 patients in one study showed fat necrosis, vascular proliferation, and focal fibrosis indicative of earlier episodes of ischemia.[26] Ischemic necrosis precedes collapse of the head and subsequent repair of the femoral capital epiphysis. The initial event is silent clinically, and with collapse and repair of the bone, pain and limitation of motion, particularly abduction and internal rotation, develop to varying degrees.[17,27] The extent of subsequent growth disturbance of the proximal femur where the epiphyseal and physeal cartilage are located depends on the extent of the avascular event. The pathogenesis involves a disruption or interruption of the blood supply to the femoral head (Fig. 96.8). A leading current theory is that there is thrombophilia (enhanced ability to form clots), hypofibrinolysis (decreased clot breakdown), or both. LCP with thrombophilia secondary to protein C and S deficiency as well as Leiden V mutation has been reported.[28-30] The recent reports of LCP in a family with premature hip osteoarthritis and avascular necrosis of the hip with *COL2A1* mutations has not been reproduced in single patient cohorts.[15,16,30]

Treatment

Many children with LCP have mild disease and do not require treatment. They can be observed and managed symptomatically with activity restriction and physical therapy. This low-risk group includes children who maintain good hip motion (at least 30 degrees of abduction) or who are younger than 6 years of age. However, about 60% will require mechanical treatment, which is based on the principle of containment of the femoral head within the acetabulum so that, during healing, the head is molded by the acetabulum. Containment is sought by bracing, or by surgical intervention using an innominate osteotomy (Salter), femoral osteotomy, or a combination of the two.

Prognosis

In most children, the prognosis is good, particularly in those younger than 6 years of age with less than half the epiphysis involved. When over half the epiphysis is affected and the child is older than 6 years old, deformity of the femoral head and metaphyseal damage are more likely, resulting in secondary osteoarthritis in adult life. When the condition is identified early and less than half the femoral head is affected, only bed rest and traction may be required. In more severe disease, the femoral head needs to be covered by the acetabulum to act as a mold for the reossifying of the epiphysis. This is achieved by maintaining the hip in abduction with plaster or calipers or by performing femoral or pelvic osteotomy. Age determinations show chronologic age to exceed the pelvis bone age and the hand-wrist bone age in both sexes with LCP.[31] The Stulberg classification of I to V uses several radiographic parameters of the hip at maturity as predictors but is based primarily on femoral head sphericity, or lack of it, and is used to predict propensity to develop degenerative changes.[32,33]

Long-term follow-up

A review of 20- to 40-year follow-up studies found that 70% to 90% of patients are active and pain free, regardless of treatment.[1] Radiographs are not usually normal, but patients have good range of motion. Chronic pain and loss of motion and function occur primarily in patients with irregular, flattened femoral heads at the time of primary healing and in patients with premature closure of the epiphysis, neck shortening, head deformity, and trochanteric overgrowth. Growth studies in children followed longitudinally show that affected children are slightly shorter at birth and that they remain shorter over the entire growth period. The difference is significant: 4.4 cm in boys and 2.5 cm in girls.[34] The femoral head and neck deformity can lead to a "functional retroversion," causing an externally rotated gait.[35]

Slipped capital femoral epiphyses

Slipped capital femoral epiphyses (SCFE) occurs typically in preteen and early teenage boys with an incidence of 0.7 to 3.4 pre 100,000.[36,37] Boys are affected at least two to five times the rate of that in girls.[37] Peak age incidence is 11.5 years in girls and 13 years for boys.[38] Acute SCFE occurs up to 10% to 15% of the time.[39,40] The slip occurs at the weakest part of the physeal plate and results in the head being displaced from the metaphysis. Risk factors for SCFE include obesity, hypothyroidism, and hypoparathyroidism and perhaps therapy with growth hormone.

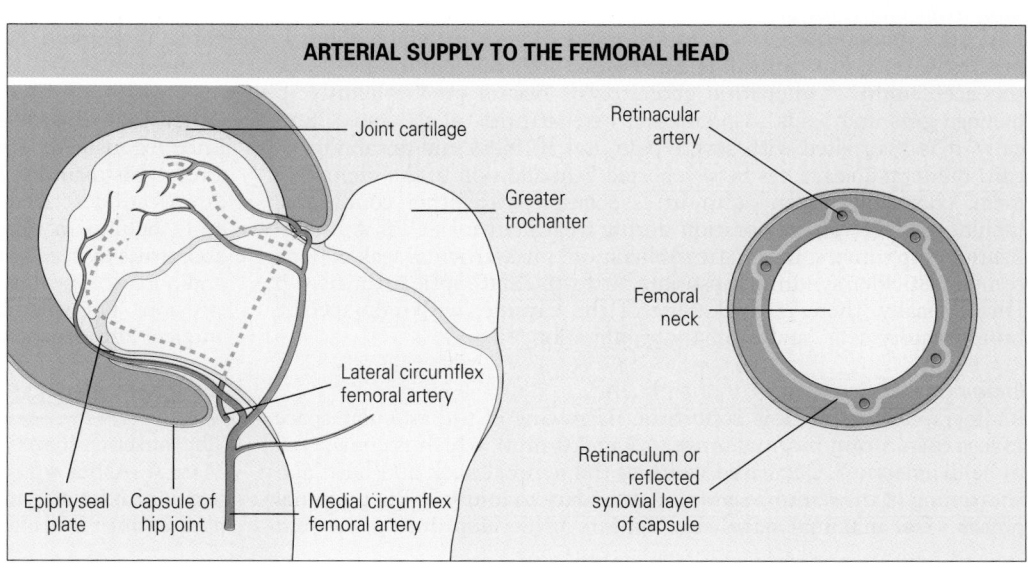

Fig. 96.8 Arterial supply to the femoral head in a 4-year-old child. A blockage of this blood supply, as yet not fully understood, leads to Legg-Calvé-Perthes disease. *(From: Southwood TR. Evaluating musculoskeletal and rheumatic disorders in children. In: Hochberg M, Silman AJ, Smolen JS, et al, eds. Rheumatology, Philadelphia: Mosby-Elsevier, 2007:961-973.)*

ARTERIAL SUPPLY TO THE FEMORAL HEAD

Joint cartilage

Retinacular artery

Greater trochanter

Femoral neck

Lateral circumflex femoral artery

Retinaculum or reflected synovial layer of capsule

Epiphyseal plate

Capsule of hip joint

Medial circumflex femoral artery

Clinical findings

Patients may present without pain; patients with pain may have 1 to 3 months of subclinical symptoms. The slip itself usually occurs during the preadolescent growth spurt and is more common in obese children. Up to 25% to 40% of children have bilateral slips, and up to half of children with bilateral slips may be asymptomatic for the slip in the side without pain. SCFE should be in the differential diagnosis for hip, thigh, or knee pain in children ages 10 to 15. An acute or unstable SCFE is defined as an SCFE resulting in a child who cannot walk or cannot walk without crutches and usually presents as severe pain of acute onset comparable to that of a displaced femoral neck fracture.[39] A history of mild trauma is frequently present.[39] The prognosis is guarded in an unstable slip because a proportion of children with unstable SCFE go on to develop avascular necrosis of the femoral head.

Imaging

In acute SCFE an anteroposterior pelvis may be the only radiograph the child tolerates initially and confirms the finding of an abrupt displacement of the epiphysis on the metaphysis. If the acute slip is additive to a chronic clinically unnoticed slip, then there will be metaphyseal remodeling along the superior and anterior femoral neck.[39] A cross-table lateral view of the hip but not a frog-legged lateral (which could exacerbate the slip) may help assess the presence of anterior physeal separation, a risk factor for avascular necrosis; a cross-table frog-legged view of the contralateral hip should also be obtained.[39] Bone scans may be helpful in predicting prognosis because "cold spots" on technetium bone scan in acute SCFE may represent ischemia and therefore are thought to be related to the risk of avascular necrosis. Because avascular necrosis is not usually seen in stable SCFE, bone scans are not usually performed.

Treatment

Operative treatment of acute SCFE is controversial with regard to the operative timing, method (internal fixation with one or two screws), bone graft epiphysiodesis, reduction of the hip, decompression of the hip joint, and the role of femoral osteotomy.[39] In addition, controversy also exists about whether there exists a role for prophylactic pinning of the contralateral hip. A recent open-label observational trial suggested a potential role for intravenous therapy with bisphosphonates as adjunctive therapy for acute SCFE that had been operatively fixed.[40] Only patients with "cold spots" on technetium bone scintigraphy, which have a high correlation with avascular necrosis, were offered entry into the trial because "hot spots" on bone scintiscans are not correlated with decrease in vascular supply and thus avascular necrosis.[41] The rationale for use of bisphosphonates as adjunctive therapy was that it may slow resorption of necrotic bone and allow for revascularization with new bone formation.[41] Currently there is no effective therapy for traumatic femoral head necrosis in adolescents.[41] Side effects were typical of what has been seen with intravenous use of bisphosphonates; flu-like symptoms were seen, but no cases of osteonecrosis of the jaw were observed.[41]

Idiopathic chondrolysis

Idiopathic chondrolysis is an uncommon disease in which there is progressive necrosis of hyaline cartilage of both the femoral head and the acetabulum.[42] Idiopathic chondrolysis occurs predominantly in teenage girls and leads to premature osteoarthritis of the hip. Clinically, it is associated with severe pain and stiffness and an abnormal gait. Bilateral disease has been reported.[43] In addition to the idiopathic form, chondrolysis can occur in association with other conditions, including SCFE, pin perforation during treatment for SCFE, immobilization, hip tumors, traumatic subluxation, intra-articular leak of bone cement, Stickler syndrome, psoriatic arthritis, and septic arthritis.[44,45] Histologically, there is thickening of the capsule, with non-specific inflammatory cells, and capillary proliferation.[46]

Imaging

Radiographically, there is concentric narrowing of the articular space to less than 3 mm (normal range, 3.5 to 7.0 mm), which is considered to be diagnostic.[47] Decreased width of the femoral neck and head and shortening of the femur may occur secondary to injury to the proximal physis. The maximal narrowing appears to develop during the first

year, with some increase in joint space and motion over the first few years followed by progressive osteoporosis, osteophyte formation, and sometimes protrusio acetabuli. Both the size of the head and the width of the neck are diminished; technetium bone scan shows marked periarticular uptake and premature fusion of the epiphysis of the greater trochanter and may precede the abnormalities seen on MRI and plain radiographs.

Treatment and prognosis

The prognosis is generally poor and many patients eventually require hip replacement. A single case has been reported in which the patient was treated with etanercept and improved rapidly despite having not responded to NSAIDs or methotrexate.[48]

Knee disorders

The physical examination of the knee is described in detail in Chapter 74. A summary table (see Table 96.3) is provided in this chapter for convenience of use when examining children and adolescents with complaints referable to the knee.

Patellofemoral dysfunction

Also known as patellofemoral pain syndrome, this syndrome is extensively described in Chapter 80 and is a common cause of pain in adolescents and in some children.

Chondromalacia patellae

This condition results from softening of the articular cartilage of the patella. It commonly affects adolescent females, and pain can be reproduced when the patella is tightly apposed to the femoral condyles, as in standing up from sitting or on walking up stairs. Treatment is conservative with rest and physical therapy for quadriceps muscle strengthening.

Malignant tumors, including osteogenic sarcoma and Ewing tumor, may present as pain or swelling or with pathologic fracture and are fortunately rare. Osteoid osteoma is a benign tumor affecting adolescents, especially boys, usually involving the femur or tibia. The pain is thought to be due to local release of prostaglandins, is more severe at night, and often improves with NSAID therapy. The radiograph is usually diagnostic, the radiologic appearance being that of a sharply demarcated radiolucent focus of osteoid tissue surrounded by sclerotic bone. If the radiograph is normal, CT or MRI is required. Treatment is by surgical removal/curettage. Tumors of bone are described in more detail in Chapter 208.

Osgood-Schlatter disease

Osgood-Schlatter disease is a traction apophysitis seen primarily in boys from ages 11 to 17. Physical examination frequently shows tenderness and/or protuberance of the tibial tuberosity. The bone at the ages described is thought to be more susceptible to repetitive injury than the patellar tendon, resulting in fragmentation of the bone. Disease may be unilateral or bilateral. Treatment is with icing after activity. NSAIDs to control pain are used as needed but not at such doses as to ease the way for further overuse. Physical therapy to increase flexibility of the thigh muscles accompanied by core strengthening is helpful. Rarely, casting or surgical excision of ossicles is required.

Other knee disorders

Knee extensor tendinitis (jumper's knee) may be seen in young athletes. This disorder, pes anserine bursitis, and the iliotibial band syndrome are described in Chapter 80. Performing the Ober test can be quite helpful in diagnosing iliotibial band syndrome. Finally, osteochondritis dissecans is another common cause of knee pain in children and adolescents that typically presents as intermittent knee pain and effusion. The subchondral bone is involved. Treatment is frequently surgical and depends on the size of the lesion.

ACKNOWLEDGMENTS

The authors thank Taunton R. Southwood, Carol B. Lindsley, and Marc A. Asher who authored chapters in the previous editions of this text for materials published in the fourth edition that have been incorporated into this chapter.

REFERENCES

1. Weinstein SL. Natural history and treatment outcomes of childhood hip disorders. Clin Orthop Relat Res 1997;344:227-242.
2. Siffert RS. Patterns of deformity of the developing hip. Clin Orthop 1981;160:14-29.
3. Watanabe RS. Embryology of the human hip. Clin Orthop Relat Res 1974;98:8-26.
4. Harrison TJ. The growth of the pelvis in the rat: a mensural and morphological study. J Anatomy 1958;92:236-260.
5. Southwood TR. Evaluating musculoskeletal and rheumatic disorders in children. In Hochberg MC, Silman AL, Smolen SJ, et al, eds. Rheumatology, 4th ed. Edinburgh Philadelphia, Mosby-Elsevier, 2007.
6. Hartwig NG. How to treat acute musculoskeletal infections in children. Adv Exp Med Biol 2006;582:191-200.
7. Nau R, Christen HJ, Eiffert HE. Lyme disease—current state of knowledge. Dtsch Arztebl Int 2009;106:72-81; quiz 82.
8. Lowe RM, Hashkes PJ. Growing pains: a non-inflammatory pain syndrome of early childhood. Nat Clin Pract Rheumatol 2008;4:542-549.
9. van der Giessen LJ, Liekens D, Rutgers KJM, et al. Validation of Beighton score and prevalence of connective tissue signs in 773 Dutch children. J Rheumatol 2001;28:12.
10. Shipman SA, Helfand M, Moyer VA, et al. Screening for developmental dysplasia of the hip: a systematic literature review for the U.S. Preventative Services Task Force. Pediatrics 2006;117:e557-e576.
11. Kocher MS, Zurakowski D, Kasser JR. Differentiating between septic arthritis and transient synovitis of the hip in children: an evidence-based clinical prediction algorithm. J Bone Joint Surg Am 1999;81:1662-1670.
12. Catterall A. The natural history of Perthes' disease. J Bone Joint Surg 1987;53B:37-53.
13. Guille JT, Lipton GE, Szoke G, et al. Legg-Calvé-Perthes disease in girls: a comparison with those seen in boys. J Bone Joint Surg Am 1998;80:1256-1263.
14. Canale ST, D'Anca AF, Cotler SM, et al. Innominate osteotomy in Legg-Calvé-Perthes. J Bone Joint Surg Am 1972;54:25-40.
15. Miyamoto Y, Matsuda T, Kitoh H, et al. A recurrent mutation in type II collagen gene causes Legg-Calvé-Perthes disease in a Japanese family. Hum Genet 2007;121:625-629.
16. Su P, Li R, Liu S, et al. Age at onset-dependent presentations of premature hip osteoarthritis, avascular necrosis of the femoral head, or Legg-Calvé-Perthes disease in a single family, consequent upon a p.Gly1170Ser mutation of COL2A1. Arthritis Rheum 2008;58:1701-1706.
17. Myers MT, Thompson GH. Imaging the child with a limp. Pediatr Clin North Am 1997;44:637-658.
18. Grasemann H, Nicolai RD, Patsalis T, et al. The treatment of Legg-Calvé-Perthes disease: to contain or not to contain. Arch Orthop Trauma Surg 1997;116:50-54.
19. Christensen F, Soballe K, Ejsted R, et al. The Catteral classification of Perthes disease: an assessment of reliability. 1986;68:614-615.
20. Herring JA, Kim HT, Browne R, et al. Legg-Calvé-Perthes disease: I. Classification of radiographs with use of the modified lateral pillar and Stulberg classifications. J Bone Joint Surg Am 2004;86:2103-2120.
21. Eggl H, Drekonja T, Kaiser B, et al. Ultrasonography in the diagnosis of transient synovitis of the hip and Legg-Calvé-Perthes disease. J Pediatr Orthop B 1999;8:177-180.
22. Song HR, Lee SH, Na JB, et al. Comparison of MRI with subchondral fracture in evaluation of the extent of epiphyseal necrosis in the early stage of Legg-Calvé-Perthes disease. J Pediatr Orthop 1999:19: 70-75.
23. Hochbergs P, Eckerwall G, Egund N, et al. Synovitis in Legg-Calve-Perthes disease. Evaluation with MR imaging in 84 hips. Acta Radiol 1988;39(5):532-537.
24. Wingstand H. Significance of synovitis in Legg-Calvé-Perthes disease. J Pediatr Orthop B 1999;8:156-160.
25. Ozonoff MB. Pediatric orthopaedic radiology, 2nd ed. Philadelphia: WB Saunders, 1992.
26. Kay RM, Morrissy RT, Kehl DK. Late metachronous involvement of the contralateral hip in Legg-Calvé-Perthes disease. J Pediatr Orthop 1997;18:807-810.
27. Thompson GH, Slater RB. Legg-Calvé-Perthes disease: current concepts and controversies. Orthop Clin North Am 1987;18:617-635.
28. Glueck CJ, Tracy T, Wang P. Legg-Calvé-Perthes disease, venous and arterial thrombi, and the factor V Leiden mutation in a four-generation kindred. J Pediatr Orthop 2007;27:834-837.
29. Gallistl S, Reitinger T, Linhart W, et al. The role of inherited thrombotic disorders in the etiology of Legg-Calvé-Perthes disease. J Pediatr Orthop 1999;19:82-83.
30. Kenet G, Ezra E, Wientroub S, et al. Perthes' disease and the search for genetic associations: collagen mutations, Gaucher's disease and thrombophilia. J Bone Joint Surg Br 2008;90:1507-1511.
31. Matsumato T, Enomoto H, Takahashi K, et al. Decreased levels of IGF binding protein-3 in serum from children with Perthes disease. Acta Orthop Scand 1998;69:125-128.
32. Stulberg SD, Cooperman DR, Wallenstein R. The natural history of Legg-Calvé-Perthes disease. J Bone Joint Surg Am 1981;63:1095-1108.
33. Herrin JA, Williams JJ, Neustadt JS, et al. Evolution of femoral head deformity during the healing phase of Legg-Calvé-Perthes. J Pediatr Orthop 1993;13:41-45.
34. Eckerwall G, Wingstrand H, Hägglund, et al. Growth in 110 children with Legg-Calvé-Perthes disease: a longitudinal infancy childhood puberty growth\model study. J Pediatr Orthop B 1996;5:181-184.
35. Kim HT, Wenger DR. "Functional retroversion" and "functional coxa vara" in late Legg-Calvé-Perthes disease and epiphyseal dysplasia; correction of deformity defined by new imaging modalities. J Pediatr Orthop 1997;17:247-254.
36. Stanitski CL. Acute slipped capital femoral epiphysis. J Am Acad Othop Surg 1994;2:96-106.
37. Busch MT, Morissy RT. Slipped capital femoral epiphysis. Orthop Clin North Am 1987;18:637-647.
38. Carney BT, Weinstein SL, Noble JN. Long-term follow-up of slipped capital femoral epiphysis. J Bone Joint Surg Am 1991;73:1109-1113.
39. Loder RT. Controversies in slipped capital femoral epiphysis. Orthop Clin North Am 2006;37:211-221.
40. Boyer DW, Mickelson MR, Ponsetu IV. Slipped capital femoral epiphysis: long-term follow-up and study of one hundred and twenty one patients. J Bone Joint Surg Am 1982;63:1109-1113.
41. Ramachandran M, Ward K, Brown RR, et al. Intravenous bisphosphonate therapy for traumatic osteonecrosis of the femoral head in adolescents. J Bone Joint Surg Am 2007;89:1727-1734.
42. Jones BS. Adolescent chondrolysis of the hip. S Afr Med J 1971;45:196-202.
43. Rachinsky I, Boguslavsky L, Cohen E, et al. Bilateral idiopathic chondrolysis of the hip: a case report. Clin Nucl Med 2000;25:1007-1009.
44. Donnan L, Einoder B. Idiopathic chondrolysis of the hip. Aust NZ J Surg 1996;66:569-571.
45. Rowe LJ, Ho EK. Idiopathic chondrolysis of the hip. Skeletal Radiol 1996;25:178-182.
46. Bleck EE. Idiopathic chondrolysis of the hip. J Bone Joint Surg Am 1983;65:1266-1275.
47. Del Couz, Garla A, Fernández PL, et al. Idiopathic chondrolysis of the hip: long-term evolution. J Pediatr Orthop 1999;19:449-454.
48. Appleyard DV, Schiller JR, Eberson CP, et al. Idiopathic chondrolysis treated with etanercept. Orthopedics 2009;32:214.

Classification and epidemiology of juvenile idiopathic arthritis

Kirsten Minden

- Chronic arthritides of childhood represent a clinically heterogeneous group of disorders.
- Childhood arthritis has undergone multiple classifications.
- Because of the lack of a single diagnostic gold standard test, all classifications have relied on clinical and laboratory features for disease definition and subtype classification.

HISTORICAL DEVELOPMENT OF CHILDHOOD ARTHRITIS CLASSIFICATION

The study of childhood arthritic diseases has a relatively short history, although references to the occurrence of swollen, dysfunctional joints can be found in both portraiture and literature over the past 500 years. By the end of the 19th century at least 38 case reports of arthritis in children had been published and reviewed by Diamant-Berger. He recognized differing subtypes of disease and attempted to classify at least three different patterns (i.e., acute, slow, and partial forms) of childhood arthritis. In 1897, the pinnacle of description of childhood arthritis occurred, when George Frederic Still reported on 22 children with chronic arthritis and commented that childhood arthritis was more than one disease and mostly different from chronic arthritis as described in adults. Since these first publications, different names have been used for the description of childhood arthritic diseases and different classification systems have been developed (Table 97.1).

Two major classification systems have been accepted worldwide: in North America, the classification of the American College of Rheumatology (ACR; in former times, the American Rheumatism Association [ARA]) gave the term *juvenile rheumatoid arthritis* (JRA),[1] whereas the European League Against Rheumatism (EULAR) classification gave the term *juvenile chronic arthritis* (JCA).[2] Both were based on the concept of classification by mode of onset and distinguished the same subgroups: systemic arthritis, oligoarthritis, and polyarthritis. However, the two classifications did not include identical spectra of disease (Table 97.2), impeding the comparison of epidemiologic, clinical, serologic, and genetic data.

THE ILAR CLASSIFICATION OF CHILDHOOD ARTHRITIS

In an effort to overcome the limitations of the preexisting, somewhat discordant classification systems and to replace them with one unified, internationally accepted classification, in 1995 the International League of Associations for Rheumatology (ILAR) Task Force on the Classification of Childhood Arthritis proposed a new classification using the term *juvenile idiopathic arthritis* (JIA) for all chronic childhood arthritides of unknown cause.[3-5] JIA was defined as definite arthritis of unknown origin that begins before the age of 16 years and persists for at least 6 weeks.

Accordingly, arthritides for which there is a known cause do not fall into the ILAR classification scheme. This applies to the reactive arthritides, for example, after enteric infection with *Salmonella*, *Yersinia* species, *Shigella*, or *Campylobacter* or after genitourinary tract infection with *Chlamydia trachomatis*. Acute rheumatic fever after

pharyngeal infection with group A *Streptococcus* and Lyme disease that results from infection with *Borrelia burgdorferi* are also both considered separately. Similarly, arthritis accompanying disorders of connective tissues, metabolic, and other genetic diseases is not regarded as JIA.

According to the ILAR classification, JIA can be diagnosed as early as 6 weeks after the onset of symptoms, whereas the allocation to a specific JIA category requires the duration of the disease to be up to 6 months. The ILAR criteria were not developed for clinical decision-making, and, therefore, their use for clinical diagnosis is inappropriate. The ILAR criteria are based on inclusion and exclusion criteria and seek to define groups of patients with a high degree of internal homogeneity without overlap among the six specific categories. The JIA categories (Table 97.3) are distinguished on the basis of clinical features over the first 6 months of disease, especially the number of affected joints, but also the presence of extra-articular manifestations and rheumatoid factor (RF). The number "4" as the criterion for the assignment to oligoarthritis or polyarthritis is an arbitrary value; however, in the evaluation study of the ACR criteria, Cassidy and colleagues showed by cluster analyses that the involvement of more than four joints is the most important variable associated with outcome in polyarthritis.[6]

A number of "descriptors" have also been proposed to gather further information about the pattern of these diseases (e.g., age at onset, antinuclear antibody [ANA] positivity, chronic or acute uveitis), but they are not part of the JIA classification.

Many papers have acknowledged that the ILAR classification defines immunogenetically distinct groups of patients, with different clinical presentations, different treatment responses, and different disease courses and outcomes.[7-9] In particular, systemic arthritis has some distinctive markers that set it apart from the other JIA categories. It is characterized by prominent systemic features; and data about its pathogenesis highlight the relevance of an uncontrolled innate immune system as an important mechanism for this disease. This indicates that systemic arthritis is primarily an autoinflammatory rather than autoimmune disease, which might change its classification in the future.[10]

Even though the ILAR classification yielded greater clarity and homogeneity than previous classifications, different disease categories of JIA, such as oligoarthritis, RF-negative polyarthritis, or psoriatic arthritis, still include heterogeneous patient collectives.[11,12]

The family of juvenile spondylarthritides, which includes juvenile ankylosing spondylitis, reactive arthritis, psoriatic arthritis, enteropathic arthritis, and undifferentiated juvenile spondylarthritis, is not completely encompassed under the term JIA. Diseases included in the juvenile spondylarthritides group share common features, such as asymmetric involvement of large joints of the lower extremities, enthesopathy, HLA-B27 positivity, and a family history of this group of diseases. Most children presenting with such features, especially those with isolated forms of arthritis and the seronegative enthesopathy and arthropathy (SEA) syndrome and those with juvenile ankylosing spondylitis, are classified as having enthesitis-related arthritis in the ILAR approach to classification. Patients with juvenile psoriatic arthritis are considered as having a distinct entity, and those with reactive arthritis are excluded according to the ILAR. This is in contrast to the European Spondylarthropathy Study Group (ESSG) classification,[13] which covers the whole spectrum of juvenile spondylarthritides and represents an alternative approach to classify this patient group. Enthesitis-related arthritis and ESSG criteria perform differently because they refer to different concepts. Even though both sets may properly classify

TABLE 97.1 MILESTONES IN THE CLASSIFICATION OF CHILDHOOD ARTHRITIS

1864	First detailed description of juvenile arthritis by Cornil
1891	First classification of childhood arthritis into three forms by Diamant-Berger
1897	Description of childhood arthritis as being more than a single disease by Still
1959	Description of different disease-onset patterns by Ansell and Bywaters
1968	Criteria for the diagnosis of Still's disease (Taplow criteria)
1972	American Rheumatism Association (ARA) criteria for the classification of juvenile rheumatoid arthritis (JRA)
1977	Revision of ARA criteria for JRA[1]
1978	European League Against Rheumatism (EULAR) criteria for juvenile chronic arthritis (JCA)[2]
1995	International League of Associations for Rheumatology (ILAR) criteria for juvenile idiopathic arthritis (JIA), Santiago, 1994[3]
1998	Vancouver criteria for juvenile psoriatic arthritis
1998	First revision of the ILAR criteria, Durban, 1997[4]
2004	Second revision of the ILAR criteria, Edmonton, 2001[5]

TABLE 97.2 CLASSIFICATIONS OF CHILDHOOD ARTHRITIS

Classification according to:	ACR	EULAR	ILAR
Term	Juvenile rheumatoid arthritis (JRA)	Juvenile chronic arthritis (JCA)	Juvenile idiopathic arthritis (JIA)
Age at arthritis onset	<16 yr	<16 yr	<16 yr
Duration of arthritis	>6 wk	>3 mo	>6 wk
Onset types	3	3	7
Exclusion	Juvenile ankylosing spondylitis, juvenile psoriatic arthritis, arthritis of inflammatory bowel disease	Seropositive polyarthritis	Reactive arthritis

TABLE 97.3 CURRENT ILAR CLASSIFICATION OF JUVENILE IDIOPATHIC ARTHRITIS

Category	Definition	Exclusions*
1. Systemic arthritis	Arthritis with or preceded by daily fever of at least 2 weeks' duration that is documented to be quotidian for at least 3 days and accompanied by one or more of: 1) Evanescent, non-fixed erythematous rash 2) Generalized lymph node enlargement 3) Hepatomegaly and/or splenomegaly 4) Serositis	a, b, c, d
2. Oligoarthritis	Arthritis affecting one to four joints during the first 6 months of disease	a, b, c, d, e
Persistent	Arthritis affecting no more than four joints throughout the disease course	
Extended	Arthritis affecting a total of more than four joints after the first 6 months of disease	
3. Polyarthritis (RF-negative)	Arthritis affecting more than four joints during the first 6 months of disease; tests for RF are negative	a, b, c, d, e
4. Polyarthritis (RF-positive)	Arthritis affecting more than four joints during the first 6 months of disease; tests for RF are positive (on at least two occasions more than 3 months apart)	a, b, c, e
5. Psoriatic arthritis	Arthritis and psoriasis, or arthritis and at least two of: 1) Dactylitis 2) Nail abnormalities (pitting or onycholysis) 3) Psoriasis in a first-degree relative	b, c, d, e
6. Enthesitis-related arthritis	Arthritis and enthesitis, or arthritis or enthesitis with at least two of: 1) Presence or a history of sacroiliac joint tenderness and/or inflammatory lumbosacral pain 2) Presence of HLA-B27 3) Onset of arthritis in a male older than 6 years of age 4) Acute (symptomatic) anterior uveitis 5) History of ankylosing spondylitis, enthesitis-related arthritis, sacroiliitis with inflammatory bowel disease, Reiter's syndrome, or acute anterior uveitis in a first-degree relative	a, d, e
7. Other arthritis	Arthritis that fulfills criteria in no category or in two or more of the above categories	

*Exclusions:
a) Psoriasis or a history of psoriasis in the patient or a first-degree relative
b) Arthritis in an HLA-B27–positive male beginning after the sixth birthday
c) Ankylosing spondylitis, enthesitis-related arthritis, sacroiliitis with inflammatory bowel disease, Reiter's syndrome, or acute anterior uveitis or a history of one of these disorders in a first-degree relative
d) Presence of IgM RF on at least two occasions at least 3 months apart
e) Presence of systemic juvenile idiopathic arthritis
Data from Petty RE, Southwood TR, Manners P, et al. International League of Associations for Rheumatology classification of juvenile idiopathic arthritis: second revision, Edmonton, 2001. J Rheumatol 2004;31:390-392.

children with spondylarthritides, enthesitis-related arthritis criteria correspond better to the clinical picture of juvenile-onset spondylarthritides because the relevance of enthesopathy in the whole group is much greater than that of inflammatory back pain. The latter is the major diagnostic criterion, besides synovitis, according to ESSG, but is an infrequent event in children with recent-onset disease.

Validity of the ILAR criteria

The proposed ILAR classification has been evaluated in more than 15 studies, of which the majority compared the Durban criteria[4] with other published classification sets. In these studies, comprising almost 3500 children, the performance of the ILAR classification has not been adequately analyzed, however. The reliability and precision of the criteria have not been tested, and their feasibility has been rated as relatively low. Berntson and colleagues reported on the difficulties of fulfilling the specified exclusion criteria in clinical work.[14] The face validity of the ILAR classification was, however, affirmed, despite some concern being expressed regarding the high number of patients

(2% to 23%) who were unclassifiable. This issue was addressed by the second revision of the ILAR classification (Edmonton criteria)[5] through a refinement of the exclusion criteria. The ILAR classification is, like its predecessors, based on published literature and expert opinions. The criteria have not been tested against non-rheumatic disease control groups and rheumatic disease control groups; thus its sensitivity and specificity are unknown.

Nevertheless, the ILAR classification constitutes the current international diagnostic standard for chronic childhood arthritides of unknown etiology. The proposed classification has restrictions intrinsic to any classification founded on clinical criteria, but it will probably be modified as progress is made in the understanding of the pathophysiology and phenotypic expression of childhood arthritides.

TABLE 97.4 PREDOMINANTLY POPULATION-BASED STUDIES ON THE PREVALENCE AND/OR INCIDENCE OF CHILDHOOD CHRONIC ARTHRITIS IN MAINLY WHITE POPULATIONS, PUBLISHED AFTER 1990

Case ascertainment	Study	Classification system	Incidence (per 100,000 under risk and year)	Prevalence (per 100,000 under risk)
Population-survey and specialist examination	Mielants et al, Belgium, 1993[16]	EULAR	—	167/100*
	Manners et al, Australia, 1996[16]	EULAR	—	400
Practitioner (or register)-based	Andersson Gäre et al, Sweden, 1992[16]	EULAR	11	86/64*
	Peterson et al, U.S., 1996[18]	ACR	12	86-94
	Von Koskull et al, Germany, 2001[19]	EULAR	7	15
	Huemer et al, Austria, 2001[20]	ACR	4	—
	Kaipiainen-Seppänen et al, Finland, 2001[21]	ACR	20	—
	Savolainen et al, Finland, 2003[22]	ILAR	23	—
	Berntson et al, Norway, Finland, Sweden, Denmark, Iceland, 2003[17]	ILAR	15	—
	Hanova et al, Czech Republic, 2006[23]	ILAR	13	140
	Danner et al, France, 2006[24]	ILAR	3	20
	Pruunsild et al, Estonia, 2007[25,26]	ILAR	22	84
	Riise et al, Norway, 2008[27]	ILAR	14	—
Clinic-based	Oen et al, Canada, 1995[28]	ACR	5	97
	Symmons et al, U.K., 1996[16]	EULAR	10	—
	Malleson et al., Canada, 1996[16]	ACR	3	—
	Kiessling et al, Germany, 1998[16]	EULAR	4	20
	Moe et al, Norway, 1998[16]	EULAR	23	148

*Active cases.

EPIDEMIOLOGY

The epidemiologic attributes of JIA have been subject to considerable study. However, available data on the occurrence of chronic childhood arthritis, disease characteristics, risk factors, and the natural course of the disease are difficult to compare and interpret because of the heterogeneity of the disease, differences in the classification criteria used for definition and inclusion, and differences in source populations and case ascertainment. Here, the terms JIA, JCA, or JRA will be used corresponding to the criteria that were used to define the respective study group.

Incidence and prevalence

JIA is the most common chronic inflammatory rheumatic disease experienced in childhood. It occurs worldwide, but studies on the incidence and prevalence of chronic childhood arthritis conducted in different parts of the world show substantial variation. The published incidence rates vary between 0.8 to 23 per 100,000, and the prevalence rates range from 7 to 400 per 100,000 children younger than the age of 16 years of age. Differences in case ascertainment contribute, among others, to these variances, whereas differences in the classification criteria applied contributed only marginally to the variation.[15-17] Population surveys yielded the highest prevalence values (Table 97.4), pointing to a significant number of undiagnosed children in a community.

It is assumed, however, that true differences in JIA occurrence exist. On the one hand, JIA seems to occur more frequently in children of European descent than in children of African, Asian, or East Indian origin.[29] In fact, the prevalence rate of 0.83/100,000 children in Japan is among the lowest documented.[30] On the other hand, a north-south gradient in the incidence of juvenile arthritis in Europe is demonstrated.[17]

Trends in the incidence of JIA have been reported. An increasing incidence of JIA, as might be expected due to the increasing knowledge, awareness, and availability of diagnostic and treatment resources, was observed in some areas of Estonia and Finland.[21,25] However, several other studies could not confirm this.[16] The Rochester Epidemiology database even suggested a decreasing incidence of chronic arthritis in children between the 1960s and the 1980s.[18] Hence, a clear time trend in JIA incidence has not been unequivocally documented.

Disease characteristics

The picture of JIA differs around the world, suggesting true differences in disease manifestations pertaining to immunogenetic or environmental factors, or a combination of both.

In white populations from Europe and North America, oligoarthritis constitutes at least half of all incident JIA cases; approximately 20% have polyarticular disease and less than 10% a systemic onset of disease (Table 97.5). Progression to a polyarticular disease course, labeled as extended oligoarthritis, has been described in 20% to 50% of patients with oligoarthritis.[33,34]

Overall, more girls than boys are affected by JIA, but the sex distribution varies with disease subtype, with a striking female predominance in oligoarticular and polyarticular onset (girl-to-boy-ratio of approximately 3:1), an even distribution of sexes in systemic onset disease, and male predominance (male-to-female ratio of 2-3:1) in enthesitis-related arthritis.

The different JIA subtypes have characteristic distributions of age at onset. Oligoarthritis is typically a disease of young children, although onset before 6 months of age is highly unusual. The peak age at onset in oligoarthritis is at 2 to 3 years of age, whereas enthesitis-related arthritis and RF-positive polyarthritis occur predominantly in children over the age of 8 years. In juvenile psoriatic arthritis, however, the age at onset is biphasic, with peaks occurring at approximately 2 years of age and again in later childhood.[12] In general, there have been two major peaks in JIA onset observed at 2 to 3 years and between the ages of 11 and 12 years.

Antinuclear antibodies (for the most part of unknown specificity) are the most frequently detected autoantibodies in JIA (in ~50% of cases). They are most frequently seen in patients with oligoarthritis. IgM rheumatoid factors are rarely found in JIA (<5%) and, by

TABLE 97.5 AVERAGE RELATIVE FREQUENCIES OF JIA SUBGROUPS IN INCEPTION COHORTS OF PREDOMINANTLY WHITE ORIGIN,* AND SUBGROUP CHARACTERISTICS, BASED ON LARGE JIA COHORTS OF MORE THAN 500 CASES, RESPECTIVELY†

JIA subgroup	%	Age at onset, years (median)	Girls (%)	ANA positive (%)	HLA-B27 positive (%)
Systemic arthritis	4-7	4-7	48-70	12-19	4-11
Oligoarthritis	46-54	4-5	66-78	67-73	11-17
RF-negative polyarthritis	13-21	4-7	76-80	43-50	10-11
RF-positive polyarthritis	1-4	11-12	83-92	56-57	8-18
Psoriatic arthritis	3-7	8-10	57-69	50-51	8-21
Enthesitis-related arthritis	4-14	10-12	9-38	23-31	67-76
Total	100	6-7	65-66	52-56	17-21

*See references 17, 25, 29, and 31.
†See references 8, 29, 31, and 32.

definition, are only found in those with RF-positive polyarthritis or other arthritis.

Extra-articular features differ among the various JIA subtypes. As the name implies, systemic manifestations characterize the systemic-onset JIA form and enthesitis is a distinguishing feature of enthesitis-related arthritis. Dactylitis is most frequently seen in juvenile psoriatic arthritis.[12] Uveitis can be observed most frequently in patients with the extended oligoarthritis course type (cumulative incidence 25%-30%), followed by persistent oligoarthritis (16%-18%), and seronegative polyarthritis (4%-14%) or psoriatic arthritis (10%-12%).[35,36] Several studies have shown that positivity for antinuclear antibody (ANA), age younger than 6 years at onset of JIA, and subtype of JIA are independent risk factors of uveitis. Uveitis develops in about 90% of cases within the first 4 years of JIA and presents mainly as anterior uveitis but is mainly asymptomatic in the most affected JIA subgroups.

The picture of JIA is very different for different populations. In Asia, oligoarthritis is reported to be relatively uncommon. In an analysis of 570 patients with JRA in Japan, Fujikawa and Okuni found that 54% of the cases had systemic-onset disease, 25% had polyarticular disease, and only 21% had oligoarticular-onset disease.[37] Saurenmann and colleagues confirmed significant differences in JIA subtype distribution among different ethnic groups in their multiethnic cohort study from Toronto, comprising over 800 children and adolescents. They found that patients of Asian origin, but also of North American origin and African origin, were less likely to have oligoarticular JIA than patients in other ethnic groups.[29] On the other hand, the authors observed an overrepresentation of polyarticular JIA among children of African, native North American, or Latin American origin. In particular, an increased prevalence of seropositive polyarthritis (16%-20%) was found in comparison with children of European descent (2%). This is consistent with the findings of other studies, suggesting that predisposing genetic factors exist.

Risk factors

Evidence suggests that JIA develops as untoward consequence of interactions between genetic susceptibility and environmental risk factors, in a manner hitherto incompletely understood.

Genetic factors

Compelling evidence for the genetic component in childhood arthropathies results from twin, family, and association studies. Studies of affected sibling pairs have shown a concordance rate of 25% in monozygotic twins for a disease with a population prevalence of 0.1%, implying a relative risk of 250 for a monozygotic twin.[38] The sibling recurrence risk (λs) was estimated to be 15, a value similar to those for other autoimmune diseases. Affected sibling pairs are genetically concordant for clinical phenotype, age at onset, as well as human leukocyte antigen (HLA) haplotypes, which strengthens the evidence that genetic factors play an important role, not only in determining susceptibility to but also in the expression of JIA.[39]

The most well-established susceptibility locus for JIA is the HLA region. Several associations between JIA and variants of HLA class I and class II genes have been unequivocally established, although both the strength of the associations and the associated alleles vary between subtypes (Table 97.6). Generally, JIA appears to be influenced by genetic factors within and outside the HLA region. It is presumed that a combination of several susceptibility genes culminates in the loss of tolerance to self and a resulting autoimmune or autoinflammatory pathology with specific JIA phenotypes.

The most consistent associations have been found for oligoarthritis and include at least three different regions of the HLA system: one class I HLA (A2), a second from DR/DQ (DRB1*08, *11, *13), and a third from DP (DPB1*0201). The RF-negative polyarthritis is associated with DRB1*08, DRB1*11, and DPB1*03, while the RF-positive polyarticular JIA is associated with DRB1*04. DRB1*04 is strongly associated with adult RA, and its association with RF-positive polyarthritis supports that this subtype is the juvenile equivalent of adult RA. Although DRB1*04 is a risk factor for RF-positive polyarthritis, it is associated with decreased odds ratios in many other subtypes of JIA. Although some associations appear to be secondary to linkage disequilibrium, most associations are not explained by linkage disequilibrium, suggesting that several HLA loci independently contribute to susceptibility to JIA or its subtypes. There appears to be a window of susceptibility during which children with predisposing HLA alleles or combination of alleles are maximally susceptible to the development of JIA.[40] For example, susceptibility from HLA-B27, which is known to increase the risk for enthesitis-related arthritis, appears to start by 6 to 7 years of age in boys and not before 15 years of age in girls.

Association studies have estimated that 17% of the genetic risk comes from the HLA-DR region. Genetic variants outside the HLA region also influence susceptibility to JIA. Although there are numerous reports of associations between non-HLA genes and JIA overall or its subtypes, independent confirmations have been found for only a few of candidate genes that play roles in immune regulations and functions. Among them are the genes encoding the protein tyrosine phosphatase 22 (*PTPN22*), interleukin-2 receptor antagonist (IL2RA)/CD25, the macrophage migration inhibitory factor (MIF), the cytokines interleukin-6 and tumor necrosis factor-α, and *SLC11A1* (formerly *NRAMP1*). Most of these gene polymorphisms have only modest odds ratios of about 1.5 and are not unique to JIA but have also been associated with various other autoimmune disorders.[41] It is therefore not surprising that autoimmune diseases cluster in JIA patients, as well as in families. An increased prevalence of other autoimmune disorders, such as autoimmune thyroid disease, diabetes mellitus, or celiac disease, has been found in patients with JIA, as a history of autoimmunity has been demonstrated in 12.6% of first- and second-degree relatives of JIA patients, compared with 4% of the control population.[42] Prahalad and colleagues reported a higher prevalence of autoimmunity in maternal versus paternal relatives of children with JIA. They additionally found a significantly increased prevalence of autoimmune

TABLE 97.6 ASSOCIATIONS BETWEEN JIA SUBTYPES AND DIFFERENT HLA ALLELES

JIA subgroup	Alleles conferring susceptibility	Protective alleles
Systemic arthritis	DRB1*04, DRB1*11, DQA1*05	—
Oligoarthritis, persistent	DRB1*08, DRB1*11, DRB1*13, DPB1*0201, DQA1*0103, DQA1*04, DQA1*05, DQB1*04	DRB1*04, DRB1*07, DQA1*02, DQA1*03
Oligoarthritis, extended	A2, DRB1*01, DRB1*08, DRB1*11, DPB1*0201, DQA1*04, DQB1*04	DRB1*04, DQA1*0102, DQA1*03
RF-negative polyarthritis	A2, DRB1*08, DPB1*03, DQA1*04	—
RF-positive polyarthritis	DRB1*04, DQA1*03, DQB1*03	DRB1*07, DQA1*02
Psoriatic arthritis	DRB1*01, DQA1*0101, DQB1*05	DRB1*04, DQA1*03
Enthesitis-related arthritis	B27, DRB1*01, DQA1*0101, DQB1*05	DPB1*0201

Data from Thomson W, Barrett JH, Donn R, et al. British Paediatric Rheumatology Study Group. Juvenile idiopathic arthritis classified by the ILAR criteria: HLA associations in UK patients. Rheumatology (Oxford) 2002;41:1183-1189; and Prahalad S, Glass DN. A comprehensive review of the genetics of juvenile idiopathic arthritis. Pediatr Rheumatol Online J 2008;6:11.

diseases in maternal relatives of JIA cases compared with relatives of controls, which suggests a maternal parent-of-origin effect in JIA.

Environmental factors

Some epidemiologic studies support the concept of environmental triggers. Seasonal variation in the incidence of systemic JIA and changes in incidence of JIA in general over time have been observed.[16,18,21,28] Oen and coworkers correlated yearly incidence trends in Manitoba, Canada, with the occurrence of infections to *Mycoplasma pneumoniae*.[28] Other support for the role of infectious agents includes the detection of rubella virus and parvovirus B19 in children with JRA or JIA. Moreover, a few studies point to a link between exposure to infections in early life (in utero or during infancy) and later disease risk. For example, Pritchard and colleagues noted an association between intrauterine or neonatal exposure to influenza A and the much later development of polyarticular JCA.[43] A Swedish nationwide register-based case-control study demonstrated an increased risk of later-onset JIA in children being hospitalized for any infection during the first year of life (odds ratio 1.9).[44]

Other environmental factors investigated included nutrition, substance use, and socioeconomic parameters. One study of infant feeding patterns concluded that children who were breast fed had a lower incidence of JRA than those who were fed cow's milk, but this could not be confirmed in another study. In a Finnish birth cohort study, an association between fetal exposure to tobacco smoke products and a higher risk of JRA in general was found. The risk of JRA was twofold higher for all children and even threefold higher for girls whose mothers

had smoked more than 10 cigarettes per day in pregnancy, compared with children of non-smoking mothers.[45] A national Danish cohort study of incident JCA cases found an effect of socioeconomic variables on the risk of JCA, with an eight times higher risk of arthritis in an only child, living in an apartment, with high income parents compared with a child with siblings, living on a farm, with low income parents.[46] The influence of sibship size on JIA occurrence could not be confirmed by others, nor could any association of birth order, maternal age, birth weight, preterm delivery, multiple births, season of birth, and civil status with the risk of JIA.

Altogether, conflicting data exist regarding each environmental factor that has been investigated and no final conclusions on environmental risk factors for JIA can be drawn so far. The scarce data available support the hypothesis that environmental exposures early in life, which might induce changes in functional development, are important in the etiology of JIA.

Course and prognosis

JIA is associated with increased mortality, significant morbidity, chronic disability, and restricted participation in society.

Two population-based studies reported a roughly fourfold increase in overall mortality in patients with JIA compared with the general population. Thomas and colleagues estimated that the standardized mortality ratio (SMR) in women and men with JIA was 5 and 3, respectively, and therewith even twice as high as those calculated for men and women with RA.[47]

Epidemiologic studies in the 21st century that evaluated the outcomes of juvenile arthritis patients from North America and Europe showed that inactive arthritis or clinical remission is present in 40% to 60% of patients after a disease duration of 10 to 28 years. There are substantial differences regarding the persistence of active disease among the various subgroups. Using life-table analyses, patients with oligoarthritis were found to have the highest projected remission rates at 10 years (approximately 50%), whereas remission rates were about 40% in patients with systemic-onset JIA and 15% in patients with polyarticular JIA.[48] After 15 years of disease duration, more than one third of young people with JIA have experienced significant articular and/or extra-articular damage, such as radiographic joint changes, growth disturbances, osteopenia, osteoporosis, and visual loss.

Despite the long-term persistence of disease activity in most patients, a pronounced improvement in functional outcome has been documented. In the 1970s, the percentage of patients with serious functional disability (ARA functional classes III and IV) ranged from 17% to 22%, whereas a lower percentage of patients with serious functional disability of 2% to 10% have been observed since the 1990s. According to the results from a more sensitive measure of function, the Health Assessment Questionnaire (HAQ), approximately 40% of young adults with JIA are somewhat limited in their functional capacity (HAQ > 0) and 10% are in need of assistance and/or aids to manage their daily routines.[49] There is also a negative effect on general health status and quality of life, and despite better than average educational achievements there are lower employment rates for patients with JIA.

Several indicators of poor JIA outcome have been identified, including greater severity or extension of arthritis at onset, symmetric disease, early wrist or hip involvement, the presence of rheumatoid factor, and persistent active disease. However, the prediction of long-term prognosis remains imperfect.[50]

REFERENCES

1. Brewer EJ, Bass J, Baum J, et al, and the JRA Criteria Subcommittee of the Diagnostic and Therapeutic Criteria Committee of the American Rheumatism Association Section of the Arthritis Foundation. Current proposed revision of JRA criteria. Arthritis Rheum 1977;20(Suppl):195-199.
2. Wood PHN. Special meeting on nomenclature and classification of arthritis in children. In: Munthe E, ed. The care of rheumatic children: summarised reports of papers, discussions, and recommendations of the EULAR/WHO workshop on the care of rheumatic children, March 21-24, 1977, Oslo. Basel: EULAR Publishers, 1978:47-50.
3. Fink CW, and the Task Force for Classification Criteria: Proposal for the development of classification criteria for idiopathic arthritides of childhood. J Rheumatol 1995;22:1566-1569.
4. Petty RE, Southwood TR, Baum J, et al. Revision of the proposed classification criteria for juvenile idiopathic arthritis, Durban, 1997. J Rheumatol 1998;25:1991-1994.
5. Petty RE, Southwood TR, Manners P, et al. International League of Associations for Rheumatology classification of juvenile idiopathic arthritis: second revision, Edmonton, 2001. J Rheumatol 2004;31:390-392.
6. Cassidy JT, Levinson JE, Bass JC, et al. A study of classification criteria for a diagnosis of juvenile rheumatoid arthritis. Arthritis Rheum 1986;29: 274-281.
7. Thomas E, Barrett JH, Donn RP, et al. Subtyping of juvenile idiopathic arthritis using latent class analysis. British Paediatric Rheumatology Group. Arthritis Rheum 2000;43:1496-1503.
8. Thomson W, Barrett JH, Donn R, et al. British Paediatric Rheumatology Study Group. Juvenile idiopathic arthritis classified by the ILAR criteria: HLA associations in UK patients. Rheumatology (Oxford) 2002;41: 1183-1189.
9. Ravelli A, Martini A. Juvenile idiopathic arthritis. Lancet 2007;369:767-778.

10. Frosch M, Roth J. New insights in systemic juvenile idiopathic arthritis—from pathophysiology to treatment. Rheumatology (Oxford) 2008;47:121-125.

11. Ravelli A, Felici E, Magni-Manzoni S, et al. Patients with antinuclear antibody-positive juvenile idiopathic arthritis constitute a homogeneous subgroup irrespective of the course of joint disease. Arthritis Rheum 2005;52:826-832.

12. Stoll ML, Lio P, Sundel RP, Nigrovic PA. Comparison of Vancouver and International League of Associations for rheumatology classification criteria for juvenile psoriatic arthritis. Arthritis Rheum 2008;59:51-58.

13. Dougados M, van der Linden S, Juhlin R, et al. The European Spondylarthropathy Study Group preliminary criteria for the classification of spondyloarthropathy. Arthritis Rheum 1991;34:1218-1227.

14. Berntson L, Fasth A, Andersson Gäre B, et al, Nordic Study Group. Construct validity of ILAR and EULAR criteria in juvenile idiopathic arthritis: a population-based incidence study from the Nordic countries. International League of Associations for Rheumatology. European League Against Rheumatism. J Rheumatol 2001;28:2737-2743.

15. Oen KG, Chang M. Epidemiology of chronic arthritis in childhood. Semin Arthritis Rheum 1996;26:575-591.

16. Manners PJ, Bower C. Worldwide prevalence of juvenile arthritis: why does it vary so much? J Rheumatol 2002;29:1520-1530.

17. Berntson L, Andersson Gäre B, Fasth A, et al, Nordic Study Group. Incidence of juvenile idiopathic arthritis in the Nordic countries: a population-based study with special reference to the validity of the ILAR and EULAR criteria. J Rheumatol 2003;30:2275-2282.

18. Peterson LS, Mason T, Nelson AM, et al. Juvenile rheumatoid arthritis in Rochester, Minnesota, 1960-1993. Is the epidemiology changing? Arthritis Rheum 1996;39:1385-1390.

19. Von Koskull S, Truckenbrodt H, Holle R, Hörmann A. Incidence and prevalence of juvenile arthritis in an urban population of southern Germany: a prospective study. Ann Rheum Dis 2001;60:940-945.

20. Huemer C, Huemer M, Dorner T, et al. Incidence of pediatric rheumatic diseases in a regional population in Austria. J Rheumatol 2001;28:2116-2119.

21. Kaipiainen-Seppänen O, Savolainen A. Changes in the incidence of juvenile rheumatoid arthritis in Finland. Rheumatology (Oxford) 2001;40:928-932.

22. Savolainen E, Kaipiainen-Seppänen O, Kröger L, Luosujärvi R. Total incidence and distribution of inflammatory joint diseases in a defined population: results from the Kuopio 2000 arthritis survey. J Rheumatol 2003;30:2460-2468.

23. Hanova P, Pavelka K, Dostal C, et al. Epidemiology of rheumatoid arthritis, juvenile idiopathic arthritis and gout in two regions of the Czech Republic in a descriptive population-based survey in 2002-2003. Clin Exp Rheumatol 2006;24:499-507.

24. Danner S, Sordet C, Terzic J, et al. Epidemiology of juvenile idiopathic arthritis in Alsace, France. J Rheumatol 2006;33:1377-1381.

25. Pruunsild C, Uibo K, Liivamägi H, et al. Incidence of juvenile idiopathic arthritis in children in Estonia: a prospective population-based study. Scand J Rheumatol 2007;36:7-13.

26. Pruunsild C, Uibo K, Liivamägi H, et al. Prevalence and short-term outcome of juvenile idiopathic arthritis: a population-based study in Estonia. Clin Exp Rheumatol 2007;25:649-653.

27. Riise ØR, Handeland KS, Cvancarova M, et al. Incidence and characteristics of arthritis in Norwegian children: a population-based study. Pediatrics 2008;121:e299-e306.

28. Oen K, Fast M, Postl B. Epidemiology of juvenile rheumatoid arthritis in Manitoba, Canada, 1975-92: cycles in incidence. J Rheumatol 1995;22:745-750.

29. Saurenmann RK, Rose JB, Tyrrell P, et al. Epidemiology of juvenile idiopathic arthritis in a multiethnic cohort: ethnicity as a risk factor. Arthritis Rheum 2007;56:1974-1984.

30. Fujikawa S, Okuni M. A nationwide surveillance study of rheumatic diseases among Japanese children. Acta Paediatr Jpn 1997;39:242-244.

31. Adib N, Hyrich K, Thornton J, et al. Association between duration of symptoms and severity of disease at first presentation to paediatric rheumatology: results from the Childhood Arthritis Prospective Study. Rheumatology (Oxford) 2008;47:991-995.

32. Minden K, Niewerth M. Juvenile idiopathic arthritis— clinical subgroups and classification. Z Rheumatol 2008;67:100-110.

33. Oen K, Malleson PN, Cabral DA, et al. Disease course and outcome of juvenile rheumatoid arthritis in a multicenter cohort. J Rheumatol 2002;29:1989-1999.

34. Guillaume S, Prieur AM, Coste J, Job-Deslandre C. Long-term outcome and prognosis in oligoarticular-onset juvenile idiopathic arthritis. Arthritis Rheum 2000;43:1858-1865.

35. Heiligenhaus A, Niewerth M, Ganser G, et al. Prevalence and complications of uveitis in juvenile idiopathic arthritis in a population-based nation-wide study in Germany: suggested modification of the current screening guidelines. Rheumatology (Oxford) 2007;46:1015-1019.

36. Saurenmann RK, Levin AV, Feldman BM, et al. Prevalence, risk factors, and outcome of uveitis in juvenile idiopathic arthritis: a long-term followup study. Arthritis Rheum 2007;56:647-657.

37. Fujikawa S, Okuni M. Clinical analysis of 570 cases with juvenile rheumatoid arthritis: results of a nationwide retrospective survey in Japan. Acta Paediatr Jpn 1997;39:245-249.

38. Savolainen A, Saila H, Kotaniemi K, et al. Magnitude of the genetic component in juvenile idiopathic arthritis. Ann Rheum Dis 2000;59:1001.

39. Prahalad S, Glass DN. A comprehensive review of the genetics of juvenile idiopathic arthritis. Pediatr Rheumatol Online J 2008;6:11.

40. Murray KJ, Moroldo MB, Donnelly P, et al. Age-specific effects of juvenile rheumatoid arthritis-associated HLA-alleles. Arthritis Rheum 1999;42:1843-1853.

41. Phelan JD, Thompson SD. Genomic progress in pediatric arthritis: recent work and future goals. Curr Opin Rheumatol 2006;18:482-489.

42. Prahalad S, Shear ES, Thompson SD, et al. Increased prevalence of familial autoimmunity in simplex and multiplex families with juvenile rheumatoid arthritis. Arthritis Rheum 2002;46:1851-1856.

43. Pritchard MH, Matthews N, Munro J. Antibodies to influenza A in a cluster of children with juvenile chronic arthritis. Br J Rheumatol 1988;27:176-180.

44. Carlens C, Jacobsson LT, Brandt L, et al. Perinatal characteristics, early life infections, and later risk of rheumatoid arthritis and juvenile idiopathic arthritis. Ann Rheum Dis 2008; Oct 28. [Epub ahead of print].

45. Jaakkola JJ, Gissler M. Maternal smoking in pregnancy as a determinant of rheumatoid arthritis and other inflammatory polyarthropathies during the first 7 years of life. Int J Epidemiol 2005;34:664-671.

46. Nielsen HE, Dorup J, Herlin T, et al. Epidemiology of juvenile chronic arthritis: risk dependent on sibship, parental income, and housing. J Rheumatol 1999;26:1600-1605.

47. Thomas E, Symmons DP, Brewster DH, et al. National study of cause-specific mortality in rheumatoid arthritis, juvenile chronic arthritis, and other rheumatic conditions: a 20 year followup study. J Rheumatol 2003;30:958-965.

48. Oen K. Long-term outcomes and predictors of outcomes for patients with juvenile idiopathic arthritis. Best Pract Res Clin Rheumatol 2002;16:347-360.

49. Flato B, Lien G, Smerdel A, et al. Prognostic factors in juvenile rheumatoid arthritis: a case-control study revealing early predictors and outcome after 14.9 years. J Rheumatol 2003;30:386-393.

50. Adib N, Silman A, Thomson W. Outcome following onset of juvenile idiopathic inflammatory arthritis: II. predictors of outcome in juvenile arthritis. Rheumatology (Oxford) 2005;44:1002-1007.

Presentations, clinical features, and special problems in children

98

Boel Andersson Gäre and Anders Fasth

DEFINITION

- Juvenile idiopathic arthritis (JIA) is defined as arthritis of unknown etiology that begins before the 16th birthday and persists for at least 6 weeks, provided other known conditions are excluded.
- JIA is the most commonly diagnosed rheumatic disease in children and an important cause of disability and blindness.

CLINICAL FEATURES

- The clinical features of JIA are heterogeneous. Using the ILAR criteria for classification, six major clinical subtypes can be identified. Different clinical pictures at onset and during the course of the disease can provide guidance for treatment and prediction of outcome.

INTRODUCTION

Juvenile idiopathic arthritis (JIA), previously referred to as juvenile rheumatoid arthritis (JRA) in the United States and juvenile chronic arthritis (JCA) in Europe, is the most commonly diagnosed rheumatic disease in children and can be an important cause of disability, impaired vision, and even blindness. The classification of juvenile arthritis has been a challenge because of the heterogeneity of the disease. The International League of Associations for Rheumatology (ILAR) developed and revised a classification system that was published in 2004.[1] This new classification aims at defining biologically more homogeneous groups than the formerly used American College of Rheumatology (ACR)[2] and European League against Rheumatism (EULAR)[3] criteria, in order to enhance scientific and clinical communication globally. However, the ILAR criteria represent a change not only in terminology but also in definition of the subtypes (Table 98.1). Because most studies published to date have used the ACR or EULAR criteria, it is still important to be aware of these differences in definitions.[4-6]

The ILAR classification is outlined according to the second revision in Box 98.1, definitions of terms for clinical signs and symptoms are presented in Box 98.2, and clinical characteristics of the different JIA subtypes are listed in Table 98.2. The classification and the descriptive epidemiology of JIA are reviewed in Chapter 97.

The occurrence of JIA is common compared with other pediatric-onset chronic illnesses. It is thus 4 times more common than sickle cell disease and cystic fibrosis and 10 times more common than muscular dystrophy, hemophilia, or lymphoblastic leukemia.[7]

PRESENTATION AT ONSET

Symptoms and signs

In the diagnosis of JIA a careful history and physical examination are the key elements.

The main clinical feature in JIA, arthritis, is defined as "swelling within a joint or limitation in range of joint movement with joint pain or tenderness, which persists for at least 6 weeks, is observed by a physician and which is not due to primary mechanical disorders or to other identifiable causes."[1]

Children with chronic arthritis most commonly present with complaints of joint swelling and/or gait disturbance. Although musculoskeletal pain is the most common reason for referral to pediatric rheumatology clinics, isolated musculoskeletal pain is seldom a presenting complaint in children with chronic forms of arthritis.[8] Pain is, on the other hand, an important component in the management of JIA (see later). A more detailed discussion of differential diagnosis follows in a later section, and the clinical features of each subgroup of JIA are presented separately.

Laboratory investigations

Laboratory investigations have only a supportive role in diagnosing JIA, mainly allowing the exclusion of other diseases such as acute lymphatic leukemia or septic arthritis. Neither antinuclear antibodies (ANAs) nor rheumatoid factor (RF) have any discriminatory ability to identify children with JIA, that is, they are mainly useful in the further classification of children with diagnosed chronic arthritis. Erythrocyte sedimentation rate (ESR) and C-reactive protein (CRP) are useful tests in delineating children with JIA from children with non-inflammatory disorders. However, a normal ESR and/or CRP should not be used to rule out JIA when convincing clinical signs are present, because almost half of the children have normal levels at onset of the disease in a population-based setting.[9]

In children diagnosed with JIA, laboratory abnormalities mainly reflect the extent of the inflammatory response. In the systemic- and polyarticular-onset subgroups the ESR and CRP can be very high and thrombocytosis may be present. Anemia can occur in all forms of JIA but is also more pronounced in the systemic- and polyarticular-onset groups. Usually the anemia is secondary to the chronic disease, as reflected by low serum iron, low iron-binding capacity, and normal hemosiderin stores. Serum ferritin may be elevated and mirrors inflammatory activity and not iron stores. Specifically, in systemic-onset JIA very high ferritin levels can be found and could signal complications with macrophage activation syndrome (or secondary hemophagocytosis).[10]

Treatment with corticosteroids and non-steroidal anti-inflammatory drugs (NSAIDs) may cause intestinal blood loss; usually the anemia will respond to iron supplements. Anemia quickly resolves if the disease remits.

Leukocytosis up to 15,000 to 25,000/mm^3 with a neutrophil predominance is seen in 80% of the children with systemic-onset JIA and is also common in polyarticular-onset JIA. Thrombocytopenia is not part of JIA, but if it is found, a workup for systemic lupus erythematosus (SLE) or malignancy, especially acute lymphatic leukemia, should be done. Serum immunoglobulins can be elevated, as can the antistreptolysin O (ASO) titer, even though there is no evidence for a recent streptococcal infection. Occasionally, selective IgA deficiency is seen in association with JIA.

IgM RF is almost exclusively present in teenagers presenting with polyarticular JIA only and not in other subgroups. ANAs occur in 40% to 85% of early-onset oligoarticular JIA, and this is associated with chronic uveitis. ANA positivity in teenagers with arthritis should lead to investigation for SLE. The presence of anti-citrullinated protein antibodies (ACPAs) has a limited role in JIA. ACPAs are found in teenagers with late-onset polyarticular JIA and parallel the results of IgM RF testing.[11]

Synovial fluid shows white blood cell counts ranging from 41,000 to 100,000 cells/mm.^{3} The fluid may also show decreased glucose and glycosaminoglycan levels and hyaluronic acid and chondroitin sulfate levels similar to those found in adult patients with RA.

TABLE 98.1 CLASSIFICATION OF JIA AND SUBTYPE DISTRIBUTION IN INCIDENCE CASES

Characteristic	JIA (ILAR)*	%	JRA (ACR)*	%	JCA (EULAR)*	%
Age at onset	<16 yr		<16 yr		<16 yr	
Minimum duration of arthritis	6 wk		6 wk		3 mo	
Subtypes	Systemic arthritis	4-15	Systemic onset	7	Systemic onset	4
	Oligoarthritis	35-43	Pauciarticular	68	Pauciarticular	66
	Persistent	17-38				
	Extended	5-17				
	Polyarthritis (RF−)	7-15	Polyarticular (RF does not alter classification)	25	Polyarticular	23
	Polyarthritis (RF+)	2				
	Enthesitis-related arthritis	4-7	Excluded		Juvenile ankylosing spondylitis	2
					Arthritis with inflammatory bowel disease	3
	Psoriatic arthritis	3-4	Excluded		Juvenile psoriatic arthritis	2
	Other	20				

Classifications according to: juvenile idiopathic arthritis (JIA)—International League of Associations for Rheumatology classification of juvenile idiopathic arthritis (ILAR)[1]; juvenile rheumatic arthritis (JRA)—American College of Rheumatology (ACR)[2]; and juvenile chronic arthritis (JCA)—European League against Rheumatism (EULAR).[3] Subgroup distribution for JIA,[4-5] JRA,[6] JCA,[4] studies that include mainly white populations in Europe and the United States.

BOX 98.1 ILAR CLASSIFICATION OF JUVENILE IDIOPATHIC ARTHRITIS: SECOND REVISION, EDMONTON, 2001

Systemic arthritis
Definition: Arthritis in one or more joints with or preceded by fever of at least 2 weeks' duration that is documented to be daily ("quotidian") for at least 3 days and accompanied by one or more of the following:
1. Evanescent (non-fixed) erythematous rash
2. Generalized lymph node enlargement
3. Hepatomegaly and/or splenomegaly
4. Serositis
Exclusions: a, b, c, d

Oligoarthritis
Definition: Arthritis affecting one to four joints during the first 6 months of disease. Two subcategories are recognized:
1. Persistent oligoarthritis: affecting not more than four joints throughout the disease course
2. Extended oligoarthritis: affecting a total of more than four joints after first 6 months of disease
Exclusions: a, b, c, d, e

Polyarthritis (rheumatoid factor negative)
Definition: Arthritis affecting five or more joints during the first 6 months of disease; a test for RF is negative.
Exclusions: a, b, c, d

Polyarthritis (rheumatoid factor positive)
Definition: Arthritis affecting five or more joints during the first 6 months of disease; two or more tests for RF at least 3 months apart during the first 6 months of disease are positive.
Exclusions: a, b, c, e

Psoriatic arthritis
Definition: Arthritis and psoriasis or arthritis and at least two of the following:
1. Dactylitis
2. Nail pitting or onycholysis
3. Psoriasis in a first-degree relative
Exclusions: b, c, d, e

Enthesitis-related arthritis
Definition: Arthritis and enthesitis or arthritis or enthesitis with at least two of the following:

1. The presence of or a history of sacroiliac joint tenderness and/or inflammatory lumbosacral pain
2. The presence of HLA-B27 antigen
3. Onset of arthritis in a male older than 6 years of age
4. Acute (symptomatic) anterior uveitis
5. History of ankylosing spondylitis, enthesitis-related arthritis, sacroiliitis with inflammatory bowel disease, Reiter's syndrome, or acute anterior uveitis in a first-degree relative
Exclusions: a, d, e

Undifferentiated arthritis
Definition: Arthritis that fulfills criteria in no category or in two or more of the above categories

---

Descriptors
A number of "descriptors" have been proposed to gather further information on the patterns of the clinical picture. These include age at onset, further description of the arthritis (large joints, small joints, symmetry, upper or lower limb predominance, and individual joint involvement), disease course (number of joints), presence of antinuclear antibodies, chronic or acute anterior uveitis, and the HLA allelic associations. The potential value of antinuclear antibodies as a diagnostic criterion has received a great deal of attention, but there is insufficient evidence to support its inclusion at this time. The descriptors are not part of the classification of JIA, but new data about them may allow reclassification in the future.
Exclusions
The principle of this classification is that all categories of JIA are mutually exclusive. This principle is reflected in the list of possible exclusions for each category:
a. Psoriasis or a history of psoriasis in the patient or first-degree relative
b. Arthritis in a HLA-B27–positive male beginning after the sixth birthday
c. Ankylosing spondylitis, enthesitis-related arthritis, sacroiliitis with inflammatory bowel disease, Reiter's syndrome, or acute anterior uveitis or a history of one of these disorders in a first-degree relative
d. The presence of IgM rheumatoid factor on at least two occasions at least 3 months apart
e. The presence of systemic JIA in the patient
The application of exclusions is indicated under each category and may change as new data become available.

From Petty RE, Southwood TR, Manners P, et al. International League of Associations for Rheumatology classification of juvenile idiopathic arthritis: second revision, Edmonton, 2001. J Rheumatol 2004;31:390-392.

TABLE 98.2 CHARACTERISTICS OF JIA SUBTYPES

Subtype	Age at onset	Joints affected	Systemic features	Major complication(s)
Oligoarticular, persistent	Early childhood	Large joints, asymmetric (knee, ankle, wrist, elbow, temporomandibular joint, cervical spine)	No	Chronic uveitis Local growth disturbances
Oligoarticular, extended	Early childhood	Same as above, but > 4 joints affected at 6 months after onset	No	Local growth disturbances
Polyarticular, RF-negative	Throughout childhood	Any, often symmetric	Malaise, subfebrile	
Polyarticular, RF-positive	Teenage	Any, typically symmetric and involving small joints	Malaise, subfebrile	
Systemic	Throughout childhood	Any or none	High fever, rash, polyserositis, marked acute-phase response	Acute: macrophage activating syndrome Chronic: amyloidosis, general growth disturbance
Psoriatic	Late childhood	Spine, lower extremities, distal interphalangeal joints		Psoriasis
Enthesitis related	Late childhood	Spine, sacroiliac, lower extremities, thoracic cage joints	Inflammatory bowel disease	Acute painful uveitis Inflammatory bowel disease

BOX 98.2 DEFINITION OF TERMS IN THE ILAR CLASSIFICATION

Arthritis: Swelling within a joint or limitation in the range of joint movement with joint pain or tenderness that persists for at least 6 weeks, is observed by a physician, and is not due to primarily mechanical disorders or to other identifiable causes

Dactylitis: Swelling of one or more digits, usually in an asymmetric distribution that extends beyond the joint margin

Enthesitis: Tenderness at the insertion of a tendon, ligament, joint capsule or fascia to bone

Inflammatory lumbosacral pain: Lumbosacral spinal pain at rest with morning stiffness that improves on movement

Nail pitting: A minimum of two pits on one or more nails at any time

Number of affected joints: Joints that can be individually evaluated clinically are counted as separate joints.

Positive test for rheumatoid factor (RF): At least two positive results (as routinely defined in an accredited laboratory), at least 3 months apart, during the first 6 months of disease

Psoriasis: As diagnosed by a physician (but not necessarily a dermatologist).

Quotidian fever: Fever that rises to ≥39°C once a day and returns to ≤37°C between fever peaks

Serositis: Pericarditis and/or pleuritis and/or peritonitis

Sacroiliac joint arthritis: Presence of tenderness on direct compression over the sacroiliac joints

Spondyloarthropathy: Inflammation of entheses and joints of the lumbosacral spine

Uveitis: Chronic anterior uveitis as diagnosed by an ophthalmologist

From Petty RE, Southwood TR, Manners P, et al. International League of Associations for Rheumatology classification of juvenile idiopathic arthritis: second revision, Edmonton, 2001. J Rheumatol 2004;31:390-392.

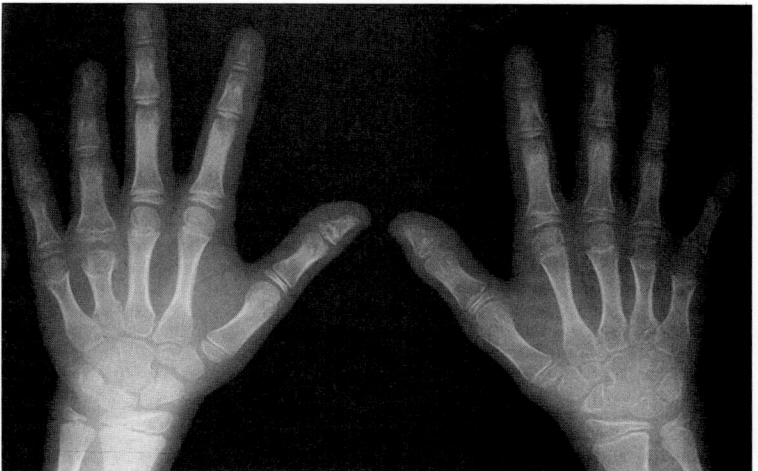

Fig. 98.1 Oligoarticular-onset JIA in an 8-year old. Epiphyseal destruction and undergrowth of the third metacarpophalangeal joint of the left hand are seen, as well as overgrowth of the carpal bones of the right wrist compared with the left wrist. Also note the widened appearance of the third phalanges caused by periosteal new bone formation.

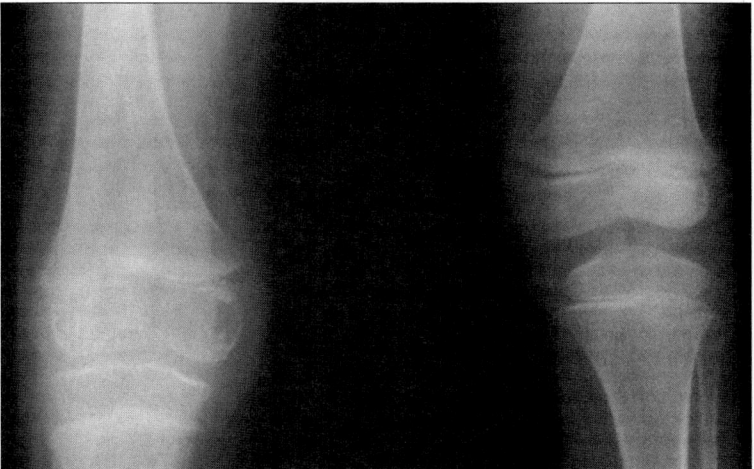

Fig. 98.2 Oligoarticular-onset JIA involving the left knee with overgrowth of the leg and widening of the epiphysis.

Imaging in differential diagnosis and follow-up

Radiographic changes during the course of JIA are common. Early changes include soft tissue swelling around affected joints and juxtaarticular osteopenia and periosteal new bone formation (Fig. 98.1), resulting in a widened midportion of the phalanges. Ballooning of the epiphysis also occurs (Fig. 98.2). In contrast to adult RA, erosions are a late finding because much of the cartilage in growing joints is not calcified; the visualization of erosions is possible only after the cartilage has calcified. Joint space narrowing is an early sign that cartilage has been eroded. Erosions or joint space narrowing can be found as early as a couple of years from the onset of active arthritis in a child with systemic- or polyarticular-onset JIA.

Cartilage that has been destroyed during the course of severe JIA can be replaced with fibrocartilage if the disease becomes quiescent (Fig. 98.3). Growth arrest lines may result from temporary loss of

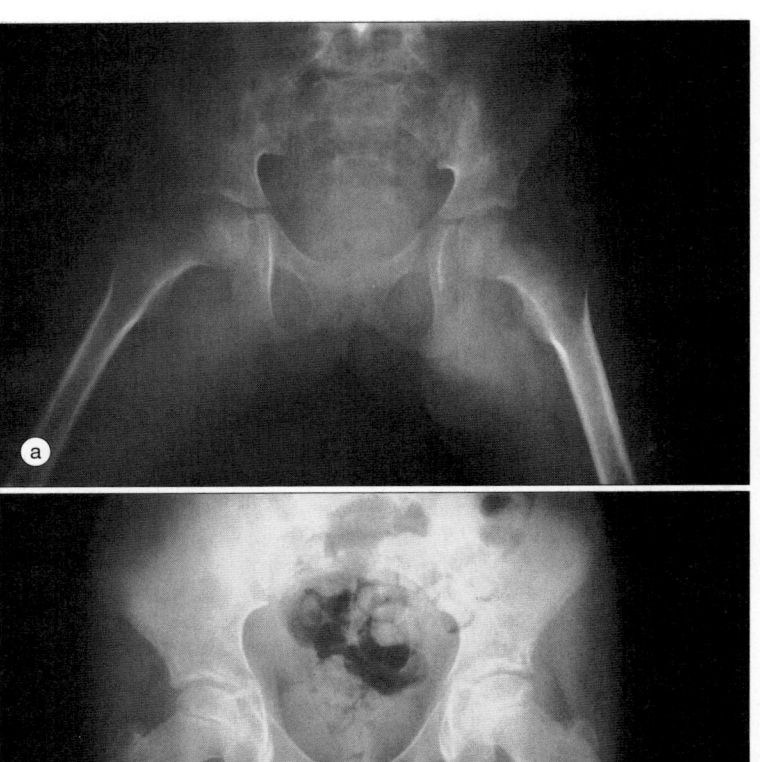

Fig. 98.3 Systemic-onset JIA with polyarticular course. (a) There is hip joint space narrowing bilaterally. (b) There was recovery of joint space 2 years later (standing view).

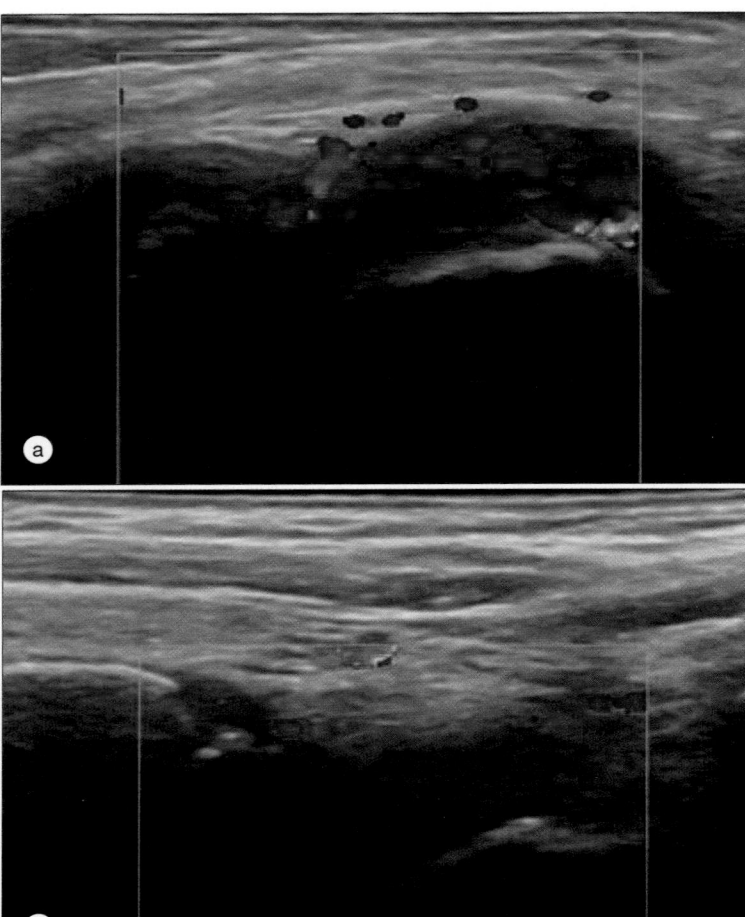

Fig. 98.5 Ultrasound images of the tibiotalar joint, longitudinal view. (a) Before intra-articular injection of corticosteroids note synovial hypertrophy and marked hyperemia revealed by color Doppler imaging. (b) Four weeks later there was no hyperemia and less hypertrophy. *(Courtesy of L. Laurell.)*

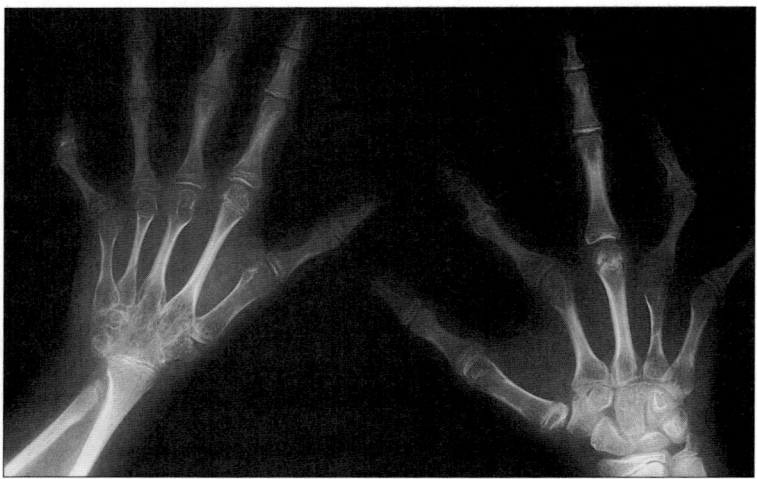

Fig. 98.4 RF-negative polyarticular-onset JIA in a 12-year-old who was diagnosed at age 4. Note the asymmetry and obvious fusion and growth abnormalities of the left wrist compared with the right wrist.

growth velocity and are frequently seen around the knee. Bony anky-losis, more common in children with arthritis than adults, is seen most frequently in the carpal and tarsal bones (Fig. 98.4). Radiographic changes in the sacroiliac joints in children are difficult to interpret because of the open epiphysis at the sacroiliac joints.

Radiographs usually show no abnormalities early in the course of JIA. In such circumstances magnetic resonance imaging (MRI) can be

an excellent adjunct for demonstrating the articular cartilage, fluid, and soft tissue structures in the joint. Post–gadolinium-diethylenetriamine pentaacetic acid (Gd-DTPA) sequences are valuable because they can demonstrate synovitis before conventional radiographic abnormalities appear.[12] MRI is, however, expensive and time consuming, and general anesthesia is often necessary in young children, thus, it should be reserved for the difficult-to-diagnose cases.

Dynamic MRI can be used to demonstrate sacroiliitis in children with clinical characteristics consistent with spondyloarthropathy. In one report, dynamic MRI demonstrated sacroiliitis in 16 children who had normal conventional radiographs of the sacroiliac joints.[13]

Ultrasonography, which can be done at the bedside,[14] is helpful in visualizing joint effusions, synovitis, and other soft tissue inflamma-tions, including enthesitis, and has the advantage of being easier to do and with no need for general anesthesia. It can be used to guide the needle for intra-articular injections, avoiding unnecessary radiation, and if equipped with power Doppler function it is possible to follow synovial inflammation during the disease course and interventions (Fig. 98.5). Musculoskeletal ultrasonography in children is still a rela-tively unexplored field but should have the same possibilities as for adults with rheumatic disorders.

DIFFERENTIAL DIAGNOSIS

JIA is a diagnosis of exclusion[15] and must be considered among the many causes of arthritis/arthralgia in children (Table 98.3). Making the diagnosis of arthritis in a child can be difficult because children frequently cannot describe their problems and, as stated earlier, rarely complain of pain.

TABLE 98.3 CONDITIONS WITH ARTHRALGIA/ARTHRITIS THAT MIGHT BE CONFUSED WITH JIA

Type of condition	Examples
Infections	Viral and mycoplasmal
	Bacterial
	Aseptic arthritis associated with bacterial infections (osteomyelitis)
	Borrelia infection (Lyme disease)
	Tuberculosis
Post infectious	Rheumatic fever
	Post-streptococcal
	Post-dysenteric arthritis (*Salmonella, Campylobacter*)
Non-inflammatory	Hypermobility
	Ehlers-Danlos disease
	Trauma/overuse
	Foreign body synovitis
	Patellar femoral syndrome
	Osteochondrosis
	Slipped capital femoral epiphysis
	Camptodactyly/arthropathy/coxa vara/pericarditis syndrome (CACP)
	Other congenital and genetic disorders of supportive tissue
Hematologic disorders	Sickle cell anemia
	Hemophilia
	Von Willebrand disease
Systemic inflammatory disorders	Systemic lupus erythematosus
	Juvenile dermatomyositis
	Mixed connective tissue disease
	Scleroderma
	Vasculitis (e.g., Henoch-Schönlein purpura, Kawasaki disease, Behçet's syndrome)
	Chronic multifocal osteomyelitis
Autoinflammatory disorders	CINCA/NOMID
	Blau syndrome
	Familial Mediterranean fever and others
Malignancy	Leukemia, acute lymphatic
	Neuroblastoma
	Localized bone tumors
Pain	Complex regional pain syndrome (CRPS)
	Fibromyalgia
	Musculoskeletal pain of non-somatic etiology (e.g., depression, severe family situation, bullying, incest)
Miscellaneous	Primary immunodeficiency
	Sarcoidosis

TABLE 98.4 COMMON MUSCULOSKELETAL CAUSES OF LIMP IN CHILDREN

Cause	Age		
	1-4 yr	5-10 yr	11-15 yr
Vascular		Legg-Calvé-Perthes disease, Köhler's disease and similar diseases	Freiberg's disease Osteochondritis dissecans
Infection	Septic arthritis	*Borrelia* arthritis (any age)	Septic arthritis (gonococcal)
	Osteomyelitis		
	Discitis		
Trauma	Fracture		Osgood-Schlatter disease
	Child abuse		
Tumor	Leukemia		Osteosarcoma
			Osteoid osteoma
Anomaly	Hip dysplasia	Discoid meniscus	Tarsal coalition
Metabolic	Rickets		Osteoporosis
	Renal disease		
Inflammatory	Oligoarticular JIA	Polyarticular JIA	Polyarticular JIA
	Polyarticular JIA	Oligoarticular JIA	Enthesitis-associated JIA
			Psoriasis JIA
Neuromuscular	Cerebral palsy		
	Muscular dystrophy		

such as septic arthritis, osteomyelitis, Legg-Calvé-Perthes disease, slipped capital femoral epiphysis, neoplasia, osteoid osteoma, and, less commonly, sickle cell disease and hemophilia.

The initial diagnostic steps include a history and physical examination, complete blood cell count, differential leukocyte count, CRP or ESR, urinalysis, a throat swab for *Streptococcus pyogenes*, and serology for *Borrelia burgdorferi*.

Toxic synovitis of the hip

This disorder may present as low-grade fever, a slightly increased leukocyte count, and a moderately increased ESR/CRP. Effusions and synovitis of the hip can be shown by ultrasonography (Fig. 98.6). In the presence of persistent fever, hip joint aspiration should be performed to rule out septic arthritis, especially if clinical signs worsen or if a high spiking fever is associated with severe hip pain and limitation at the initial presentation.

Legg-Calvé-Perthes disease

This disease predominantly affects boys aged 3 to 12 years and is bilateral in 10% of cases. On the initial radiographs, one should look for early signs, which include subchondral translucency of the femoral epiphysis and a smaller epiphysis on the affected side.

Slipped capital femoral epiphysis

A slipped capital femoral epiphysis should be suspected in the obese or the tall, slim young patient. The clinical course is prolonged if not treated, and initial radiographs show widening of the epiphyseal line and irregular demineralization of the adjacent area.

Osteoid osteomas

Osteoid osteomas occur mainly in the proximal half of the femur and may simulate synovitis when near the hip joints. On radiographs, a central nidus circumscribed by a thin translucent peripheral rim, which in turn is surrounded by a zone of dense bone sclerosis, is typical of osteoid osteoma.

The child presenting with a limp

Because limping is one of the most common presentations for childhood musculoskeletal problems, understanding the differential diagnosis of the child with a limp is essential (Table 98.4). Limping associated with painful limitation of motion in the hip is also common in children. JIA rarely presents as hip monarthritis and therefore remains a diagnosis of exclusion. The most common cause of hip pain is toxic synovitis of the hip (simplex coxitis), but other conditions can occur,

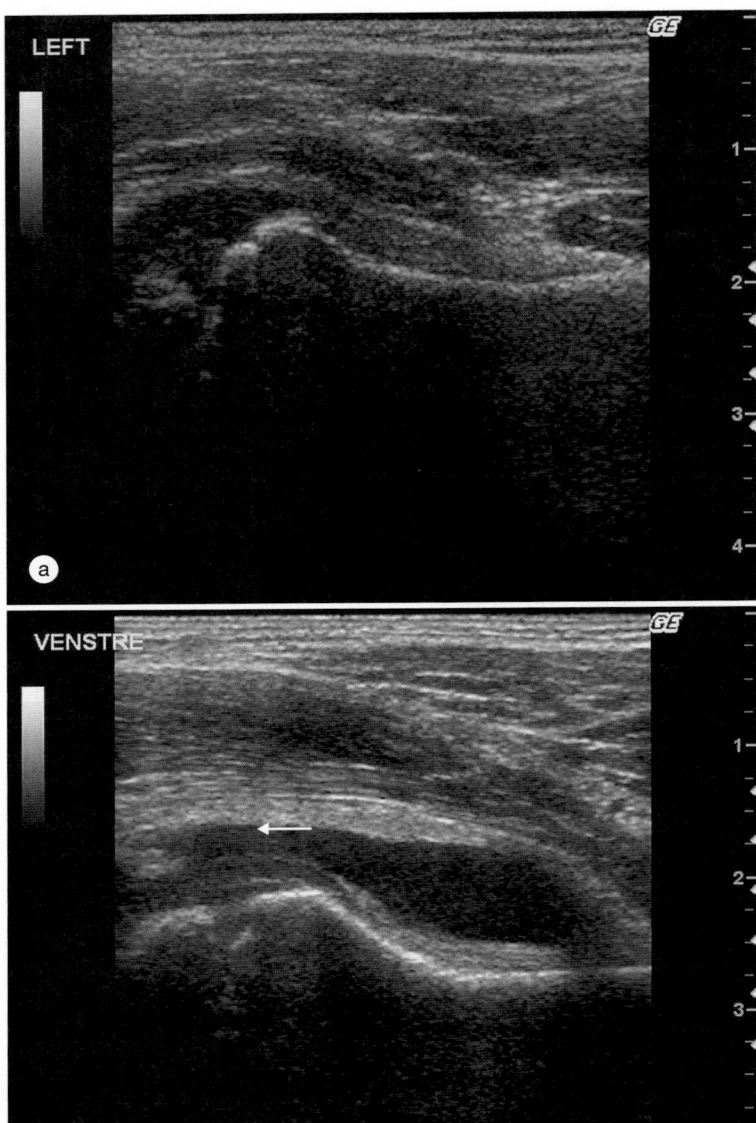

Fig. 98.6 Ultrasound images of the hip. (a) Normal. (b) With effusion.

Other causes of joint symptoms in children

The pattern of arthritis such as monarticular versus polyarticular or migratory versus non-migratory and the presence or absence of fever will help differentiate the causes of the arthritis. A child with JIA is likely to have a warm, swollen joint that is non-tender and generally does not look systemically ill, although an important exception is the systemic-onset subtype.

Infection

Most children with infectious arthritis appear systemically ill with fever and usually have a monarthritis. There are notable exceptions, such as gonorrhea, which has an early migratory phase before settling in one joint. Infection with *Borrelia burgdorferi* acquired by a tick bite can masquerade as JIA, particularly because it tends to be migratory over several months to years, and a combination of clinical judgment and careful interpretation of serologic test results is needed to make the correct diagnosis.

Back syndromes

Children rarely complain of low back pain without a mechanical cause,[16] so processes such as spondylolysis, Scheuermann's disease, discitis, and disc herniation must be excluded. Avulsion fractures can masquerade as enthesopathies associated with spondyloarthropathy.

Non-specific joint pains

The common non-rheumatic condition of "growing pains of childhood" should be considered in a child with bilateral lower extremity pain that is worse in the evening but leaves the child active during the day. Laboratory investigations are normal. Musculoskeletal pain syndromes including fibromyalgia do occur in children and are a common cause for referral in older children and teenagers. They should be considered in the evaluation of the achy child[17] and, importantly, can in children, as in adults, be secondary to rheumatic disease.

Malignancy

Malignancy can masquerade as JIA for several months.[18] In a child with painful joints and fever, acute lymphoblastic leukemia and neuroblastoma are the most common malignancies seen. Clues to the diagnosis include thrombocytopenia rather than the expected thrombocytosis, anemia more severe than expected, and (rarely) neutropenia. Blast cells on the peripheral blood smear are frequently absent. Radiographs may be normal or show pathologic fractures, lytic lesions, or a periosteal reaction. Bone scintigraphy may be useful to demonstrate metastases.

Other inflammatory syndromes

One disease that can be difficult to differentiate from systemic-onset JIA is rheumatic fever. Usually, the patient with rheumatic fever has a sustained fever, the migratory arthritis is exquisitely painful in contrast to systemic JIA, and the rash migrates.

Henoch-Schönlein purpura, Kawasaki disease, and SLE are other systemic inflammatory diseases commonly diagnosed in pediatric rheumatology clinics. Confirmation of SLE may take several years: a child can present with polyarthritis and a negative ANA test but develop other signs of SLE months to years later and convert negative serology to positive for ANAs and anti-DNA antibodies.[19] Dermatomyositis and scleroderma can also present as arthritis, but the associated features of the disease result in a correct diagnosis. When a child has delayed growth and anemia, the diagnosis of inflammatory bowel disease should be considered even in the absence of diarrhea. Autoimmune syndromes, such as familial Mediterranean fever, chronic infantile neurologic cutaneous and articular (CINCA) syndrome, and Blau syndrome, can also mimic systemic-onset JIA.

CLINICAL FEATURES OF DIFFERENT SUBGROUPS

Systemic arthritis

The designation of systemic-onset subtype is recognized in the ILAR as well as the ACR and EULAR criteria. This is the subtype most often associated with serious short- and long-term morbidity as well as increased mortality. It typically comprises 5% of the total unselected JIA population and is defined by its extra-articular features of fever and rash. Girls and boys are equally affected, and onset can occur throughout childhood. The extra-articular manifestations may precede the articular signs by weeks or months, or even years. The fevers typically rise to greater than 39°C daily and return to less than 37°C between fever peaks for at least 2 weeks before this diagnosis is considered. Fever usually occurs daily or twice daily and often appears late in the afternoon or evening, returning to normal or below normal in the morning (Fig. 98.7).

Classically, the child appears toxic with the fever and can have accompanying shaking chills, but not rigors, and then the temperature returns to normal or subnormal each day. In 90% of cases a characteristic evanescent salmon-colored macular or maculopapular rash (Fig. 98.8) occurs on the trunk and thighs, that is, under the clothing, most commonly when the fever is present. The rash can be brought out by scratching the skin (Köbner phenomenon) or a hot bath and is occasionally pruritic. Fifty to 75 percent of patients will have generalized lymphadenopathy and hepatosplenomegaly. The lymph nodes are usually firm, movable, and non-tender and on biopsy show follicular hyperplasia and, rarely, necrotizing lymphadenitis. The child may complain of abdominal pain secondary to hepatomegaly. There can be mild associated transaminitis, although fulminant hepatic failure is rare.[20] Polyserositis is common, with about one third of patients having

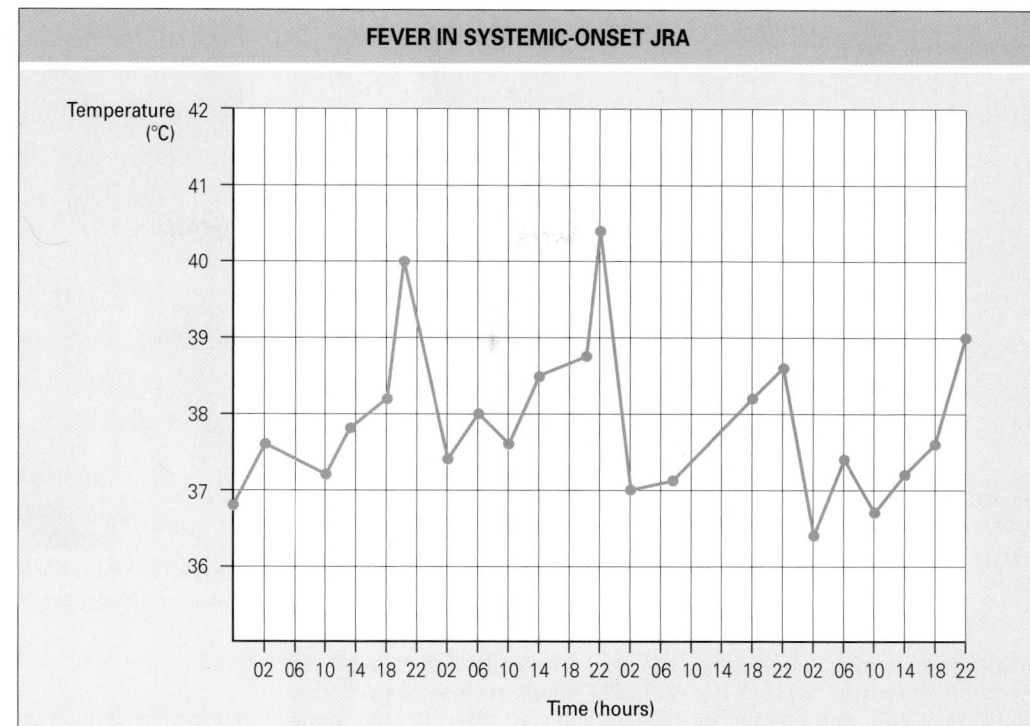

FEVER IN SYSTEMIC-ONSET JRA

Fig. 98.7 Fever in systemic-onset JIA. An example of the typical fever curve seen in systemic-onset disease.

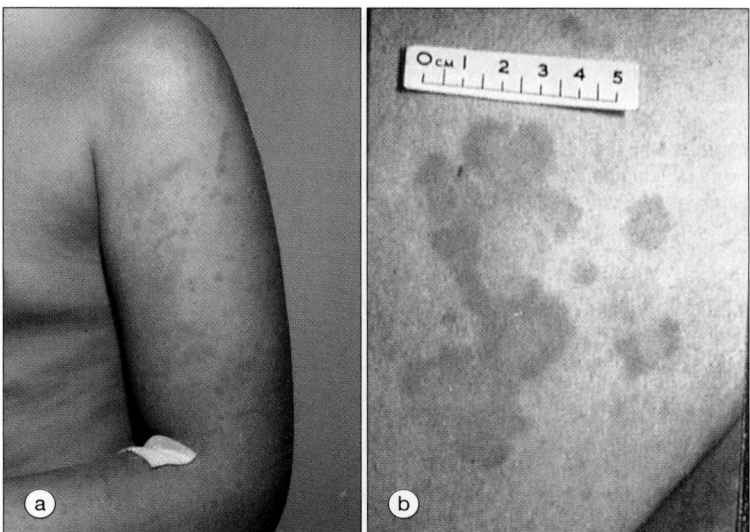

Fig. 98.8 The rash of systemic-onset JIA. (a) Larger lesions are becoming confluent. This must be differentiated from erythema marginatum (b), which is characteristic of the rash seen in rheumatic fever.

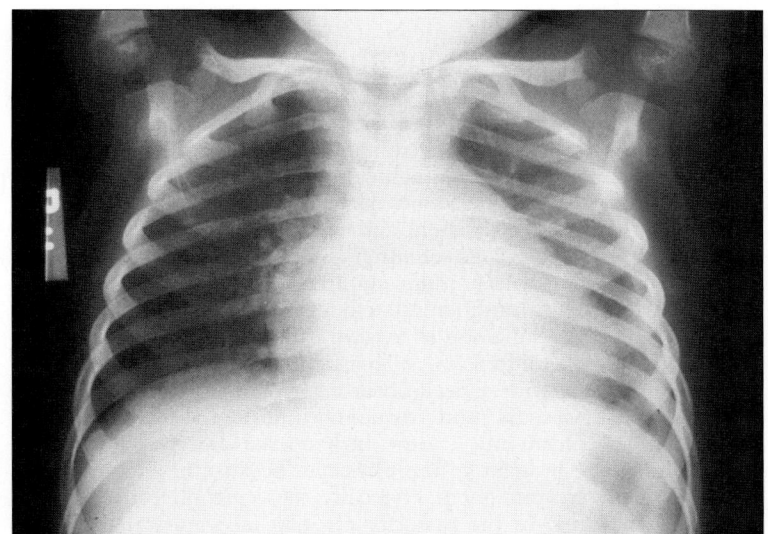

Fig. 98.9 Radiograph of a 3-year old with systemic-onset JIA who presented with pericardial effusion.

documented pericarditis (Fig. 98.9).[21] Most pericardial involvement is subclinical. Tamponade and myocarditis[22] can occur but are rare. Pulmonary disease is equally unusual and can manifest as pneumonitis, pleural effusion, or pulmonary fibrosis.[23] Central nervous system involvement with coma and meningitis has been described, but it is very unusual.[24]

Approximately 50% of children with systemic-onset JIA develop polyarthritis within 3 to 12 months of the onset of the fever. The wrists, knees, and ankles are most commonly involved, with the cervical spine, hips, temporomandibular joints, and hands also being affected. Cricoarytenoid arthritis resulting in hoarseness and laryngeal stricture has been reported.[25]

Recurring periodic fevers without chronic arthritis but often arthralgias, stomatitis, or peritonitis are more consistent with a group of autoimmune syndromes such as familial Mediterranean fever, mevalonate kinase deficiency (hyper-IgD syndrome), and cyclic neutropenia, for some of which the genetics have been elucidated.

A mild consumption coagulopathy has been described in systemic-onset JIA without sequelae.[26] In contrast, a serious but rare complication that occurs in the setting of systemic-onset JIA is macrophage activation syndrome or reactive hemophagocytic lymphohistiocytosis. Macrophage activation syndrome is also seen in infections, such as mononucleosis, and in malignancy. It is characterized by the rapid development of fever, rash, and encephalopathy; rapid rise of liver transaminase levels; disseminated intravascular coagulopathy; neutropenia; thrombocytopenia; increased triglycerides; low albumin; and a low ESR associated with hypofibrinogenemia. A coagulopathy is present with an increase in fibrin degradation products and prolonged prothrombin time and partial thromboplastin time. Macrophage activation syndrome in JIA has been reported without and with

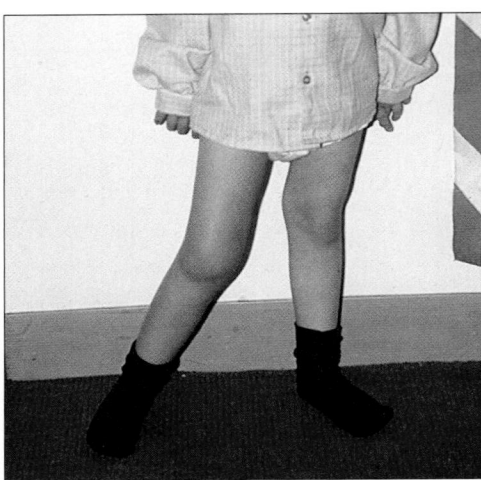

Fig. 98.10 Oligoarticular-onset JIA in a 2-year-old girl that was affecting her right knee.

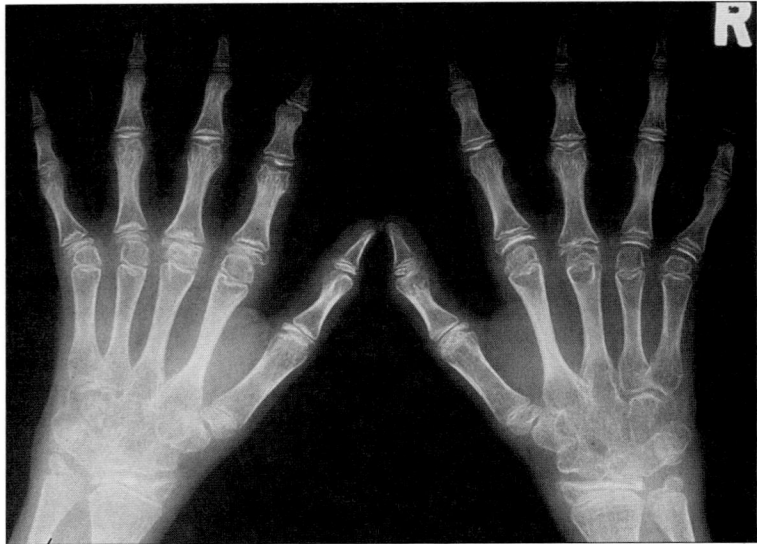

Fig. 98.11 An 11-year old with IgM RF JIA has erosions at several metacarpophalangeal joints and carpal bone fusion in the wrist.

medication changes. The diagnosis is made clinically and is supported by very high ferritin levels (>10,000 mg/L), soluble transferrin receptor (sCD25),[27] and demonstration of hemophagocytosis in the bone marrow, liver, and/or spleen. Because the mortality has been as high as 50% in some series, prompt treatment with corticosteroids and, if poor response, also with etoposide[27] or anti-thymocyte globulin and cyclosporine is necessary.[10]

Oligoarthritis: persistent and extended

This is the most common subtype of JIA and is defined as arthritis that presents as involvement of fewer than five joints (see Table 98.2). Several different approaches to subtyping of oligoarticular-onset JIA have been identified. These include those presenting with lower-extremity arthritis usually before the age of 5 years, which can be further subdivided into persistent and extended oligoarticular JIA, and those presenting in older children with or without sacroiliitis (enthesitis-related arthritis). Many children with oligoarthritis are also found in the group "undifferentiated arthritis" because they fulfill criteria for no other subgroup or for two or more subgroups.[4]

The majority of children with oligoarticular-onset JIA present before the age of 5 years, with a peak onset between 1 and 3 years of age. Oligoarticular JIA occurs more frequently in girls, the ratio being 2:1 for the persistent form and 5:1 for the extended subtype. Commonly, such children are brought to the physician because of a limp[9]; complaints of pain are infrequent. Typically there are no constitutional signs or symptoms. In the majority of cases laboratory findings are normal, with no increase of CRP and ESR and no leukocytosis, except for ANA positivity. If the joint is painful and red, the child has a fever, or there is a marked inflammatory response, a more likely diagnosis is septic arthritis. The knee (Fig. 98.10) is the most commonly affected joint (47%), followed by the ankle and then either the small joints of the hand or the elbow. Involvement of the temporomandibular joint and cervical spine is also common, while involvement of other joints occurs less frequently. Arthritis limited to the hip is extremely rare in this subgroup, and if it is present the diagnosis should be questioned.

ANAs are present in 40% to 85% of children with oligoarticular-onset JIA, both persistent and extended, and are largely associated with chronic anterior uveitis. The association with chronic anterior uveitis is particularly strong for the young child (<5 years) with ANA-positive oligoarticular arthritis, regardless of sex. The child with uveitis is asymptomatic, thus making routine eye examination essential.

Polyarthritis

Approximately 25% of children with JIA have polyarticular onset, with five or more joints involved in the first 6 months of disease. This subtype is divided into those who have persistent serum IgM rheumatoid factor (RF) and those who do not.

RF-negative polyarticular-onset JIA

This type may involve low-grade fevers and mild hepatosplenomegaly and occurs throughout childhood. The joints tend to be symmetrically involved, with the knees, wrists, and ankles being most commonly affected. In the hands the metacarpophalangeal and proximal interphalangeal joints are involved and there is flexor tenosynovitis. The cervical spine is often involved and occasionally patients will present with torticollis. Hip and shoulder involvement occurs usually after at least 1 year of polyarthritis in those who present young and have persistently active disease.

RF-positive polyarticular-onset JIA

This presentation is very similar to that of seropositive adult-onset RA. Most patients are female and present between the ages of 12 and 16 years. Symmetric small joint involvement is most typical, including the metacarpophalangeal (Fig. 98.11), proximal interphalangeal, and metatarsophalangeal joints as well as sometimes the distal interphalangeal joints. Large joints tend to be involved only in association with small joint involvement. Flexor tenosynovitis is common and often results in trigger fingers. Children with early involvement of the small joints, unremitting inflammatory activity, nodules similar to those seen in adult RA, and early development of erosions on radiographs are more likely to have IgM RF and ACPAs,[11] persistence of disease, and poor outcome. Systemic features are rare.

The complications of this form of arthritis include growth retardation and delay in sexual maturation, protein-calorie malnutrition, osteopenia, carpal tunnel syndrome, Sjögren's syndrome, and, mainly after childhood, aortic regurgitation, pulmonary fibrosis, vasculitis, sometimes associated with digital calcification, atlantoaxial subluxation with neurologic impairment, and Felty's syndrome.

Psoriatic arthritis

When the ACR and EULAR classifications were originally proposed, juvenile psoriatic arthritis and spondylarthritis were considered to be very rare disorders and presented no problem to the classification. Only later was the complex relationship between psoriasis and arthritis also revealed in children. About 30% of patients with psoriasis will have onset of the skin disease before the age of 15; and because psoriasis is more common than JIA among older children, it is difficult to distinguish the "random" co-occurrence of psoriasis and JIA from "true" psoriatic JIA. Furthermore, as with enthesitis-related arthritis, the full picture of the arthritis might only develop in adulthood. Dactylitis, nail

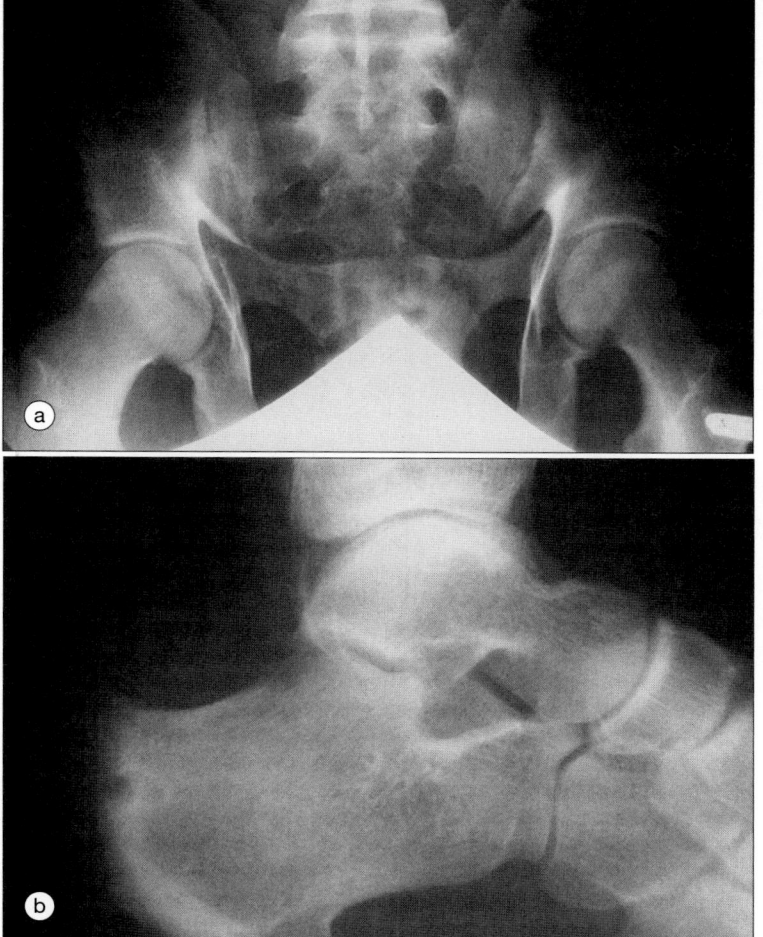

Fig. 98.12 A 19-year old presented with bilateral heel pain since the age of 9 years. (a) Sacroiliitis is evident in the left sacroiliac joint. The patient was still without back symptoms. (b) Erosion in the right heel was noted 10 years after onset of heel pain.

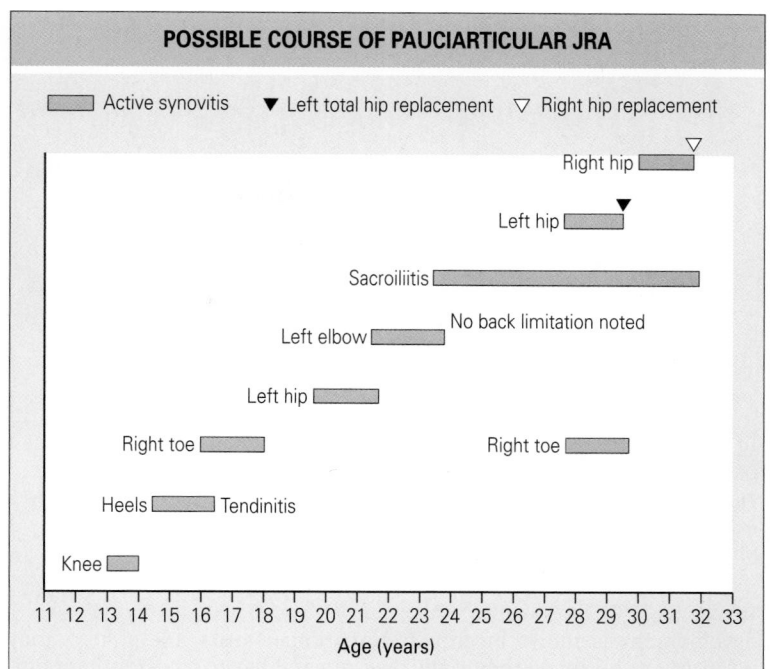

Fig. 98.13 Pauciarticular-onset JRA with evolution into juvenile spondyloarthropathy.

pitting, distal interphalangeal arthritis, and asymmetric RF-negative peripheral arthritis are typical findings, as in adult psoriatic arthritis. A significant proportion of children have inflammatory back disease, including spondylarthritis and sacroiliitis. ANA positivity was found in one third of children fulfilling the ILAR criteria for psoriatic arthritis in one epidemiologic study from Scandinavia.[4] In a long-term follow-up of JIA patients the following early predictors of juvenile psoriatic arthritis were identified: psoriasis in a first-degree relative or in the patient, dactylitis, and toe and/or ankle involvement within the first 6 months. After 23 years the juvenile psoriatic arthritis patients had poorer physical health than those with either oligoarthritis or polyarthritis.[28]

Enthesitis-related arthritis

This subtype of JIA affects boys more than girls and presents most commonly after the age of 9 years. In a recent Scandinavian report the boy-to-girl ratio was 4 : 1, and the median age at onset was 11 years.[4] The lower extremity tends to be involved (especially the knee and ankle) but, in contrast to the younger-onset oligoarticular group, the hip can also be affected.[29] Enthesitis, defined by ILAR as "tenderness at the insertion of the tendon, ligament, joint capsule or fascia to bone,"[1] occurs frequently and is commonly seen as plantar fasciitis, Achilles tendinitis, Osgood-Schlatter patellar tendon enthesis, or back pain. Enthesitis can be difficult to differentiate from arthritis, especially in the child with back pain. Many of these children develop sacroiliitis several years later (Fig. 98.12), and some will evolve into ankylosing spondylitis or other spondyloarthropathies (Fig. 98.13).

The enthesitis-related arthritis group of disorders in children with JIA incorporates those conditions traditionally viewed as spondyloarthropathies in adults, including juvenile ankylosing spondylitis, the syndrome of seronegative enthesopathy and arthropathy (SEA syndrome),[29] and arthritis associated with inflammatory bowel disease.[30]

Enthesitis-related arthritis is very difficult to diagnose correctly during childhood because the features defining the subgroup typically develop over many years of disease. The full picture might not be seen until the child has moved on to adult rheumatology. Also, this is a subgroup in which pain in the form of diffuse back pain might be the initial symptom bringing the teenager to seek medical advice. Many years may elapse before the definitive diagnosis of inflammatory back disease is made, causing much frustration for the family and doctor. The association with HLA-B27 is strong; and those with HLA-B27, a family history of spondyloarthropathy, and definite arthritis are more likely to develop a definite spondyloarthropathy at follow-up.[30] Iritis, usually acute and symptomatic, occurs in 15% to 25% of this group. Another major complication can be severe hip disease, requiring early total hip replacement. In this subgroup, inflammatory bowel disease must be considered once septic arthritis has been excluded, especially if there is a persistent fever associated with the arthritis.

Undifferentiated arthritis

This rather unsatisfactory subgroup is a result of the goal of the present ILAR classification to form homogeneous subgroups. Patients are excluded from the other subgroups either because they fulfill criteria for two or more subgroups or because an exclusion criterion did not allow them to be put into any subgroup. In the previously mentioned Scandinavian epidemiologic study using an earlier problematic version of the ILAR criteria, about a fifth of the children with JIA could not be classified into subgroups.[4] Almost all of them had oligoarthritis, extended or persistent, or enthesitis-related arthritis, and the main reason for exclusion was for a family history of psoriasis. The present revision of the ILAR criteria, in which psoriasis among second-degree relatives is no longer an exclusion criterion, should substantially diminish the proportion allocated to this subgroup.

SPECIAL PROBLEMS OF ARTHRITIS IN THE CHILD

Children and adolescents with rheumatic diseases have specific problems that do not pertain to adults. For example, delayed physical

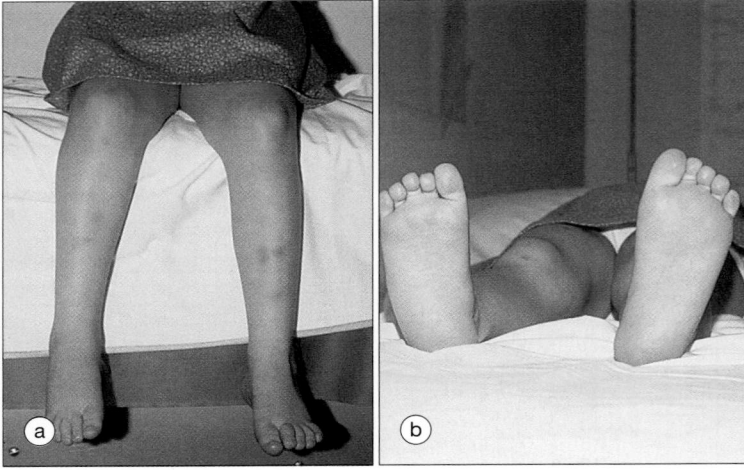

Fig. 98.14 Oligoarticular-onset JIA in the right ankle. (a) A shorter leg length from the knee to the ankle is seen. (b) The right foot is smaller, with underdevelopment of the right forefoot due to disuse.

development as shown by growth, nutritional status, and puberty may occur in all childhood rheumatic diseases and has to be carefully monitored. Growth disturbances can be local or general. Osteopenia in the growing individual can result in later osteoporosis. The chronic uveitis that may occur in children with arthritis is specific for young age at onset. Quality of life for the growing individual may be affected by pain and sleep disturbances, which can interfere with psychosocial adjustment. One should be aware that the problems are mainly linked to ongoing inflammation and can to a large extent be ameliorated by the active treatment and management that are possible today.[31] However, the inflammatory activity of the disease in some patients may not respond to the treatment available (see later).

Local growth disturbances

Local factors that influence bone growth include cytokines produced as the result of the joint inflammation. The cytokines stimulate osteoblasts to epiphyseal growth but also, if of long standing, to maturation and closure of the epiphysis. Also, muscle spasm, capsular and ligamentous contracture or rupture, destructive synovitis eroding articular surfaces, and subluxed articular surfaces can influence local growth.

The knee

The most frequent site for overgrowth is the inflamed knee. This results in leg-length inequality, with the longer leg on the side of the involved knee, particularly if the disease begins before the age of 3 years (see also Figs. 98.2 and Fig. 98.10).[32,33] A leg-length inequality greater than 0.5 cm is clinically significant and, to prevent functional scoliosis, shoe lifts should be prescribed to equalize the difference in the leg lengths.

If the inflammation in the joint is controlled, the leg lengths will equalize as the child grows. The local growth disturbance can result in early epiphyseal closure, causing a permanently shorter leg on the side of the involved knee. Another cause for undergrowth or delayed bone and soft tissue maturity is disuse (Fig. 98.14).

Wrist and hand

The next most common joint to experience growth abnormalities is the wrist. In contrast to the knee, many growth defects seen radiographically in the wrist are not observed clinically. The wrist can show increased bone age with early disease onset (see Fig. 98.1) and carpal bone fusion with long-standing involvement. Growth defects are also seen in the ulna and the fourth and fifth metacarpal bones. The ulna, because of epiphyseal undergrowth, can be shorter than the radius, resulting in ulnar migration of the carpal bones, subluxation, and severe deformity. Brachydactyly can occur in the fingers or toes as a result of early epiphyseal closure (see Fig. 98.1). In polyarticular disease, especially if RF positive, radiologic abnormalities of the wrist and hand

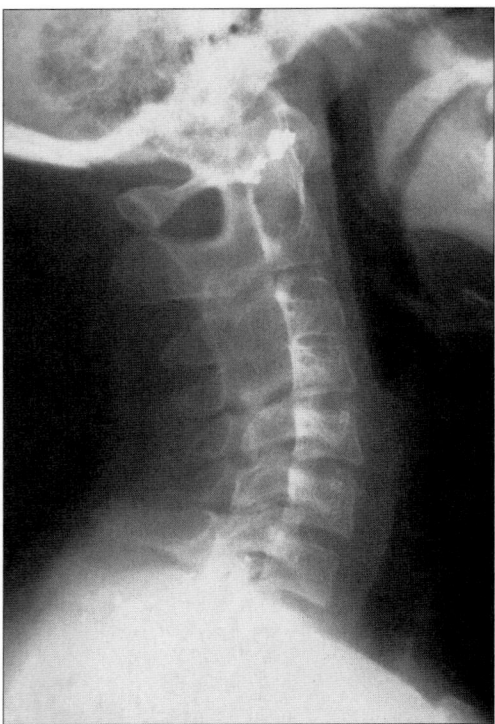

Fig. 98.15 Systemic-onset JIA in a child who had a polyarticular course. Her neck shows apophyseal fusion of C2-C4 and undergrowth of adjacent vertebrae.

can be seen at onset of disease, which highlights the need for timely diagnosis and early treatment in JIA.[34]

The hip

The hip demonstrates some growth abnormalities in a third of children with JIA. There may be lack of growth of the iliac bone and a coxa valga deformity, with either widening of the femoral neck and/or premature fusion leading to stunting of the femoral neck.

The cervical spine

The cervical spine can develop growth abnormalities that result in apophyseal joint space narrowing and bony ankylosis (especially C2-C3) with a secondary decrease in the vertical and anteroposterior size of the adjacent vertebral bodies (Fig. 98.15). Similar findings are not seen in the dorsal lumbar spine, but compression fractures of the thoracic spine do occur, particularly in those children taking corticosteroids.

Temporomandibular joint (TMJ)

TMJ involvement is often overlooked because small children have difficulties in describing subjective symptoms from the area. Thus, clinical signs of mandibular dysfunction such as reduced opening of the mouth, TMJ crepitations, and restricted horizontal movements are important to identify at an early stage. In a population-based study of JCA, more than 50% of the patients 7 years or older reported symptoms of mandibular dysfunction. Moreover, 30% of all the children had clinical signs of TMJ involvement when evaluated by a dentist and 40% had radiographic changes elucidated by a tomographic method.[35] Unilateral TMJ disease can result in deviation to the affected side of the jaw on opening the mouth. In the just-described population, 20% had either frontal facial asymmetry or a small chin or both. Mandibular hypoplasia may be due to inflammation/destruction in the TMJ, reduced mandibular growth, and adjacent disease of the spine (Figs. 98.16 and 98.17).

TMJ involvement occurs in all subgroups: systemic, 67%; oligoarticular persistent, 39%; oligoarticular extended, 75%; polyarticular RF-positive, 33%; RF-negative, 59%; enthesitis-related, 13%; and psoriatic arthritis, 33%. Regular evaluation by a pedodontist or orthodontist of all children with JIA is thus recommended to enable early detection and intervention.[36]

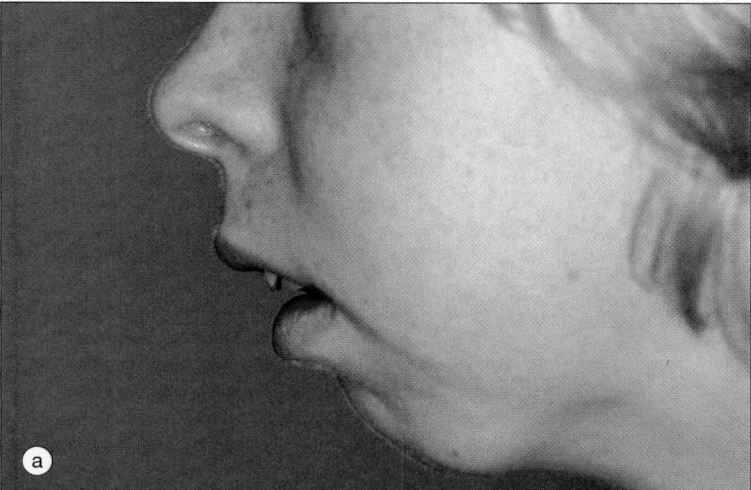

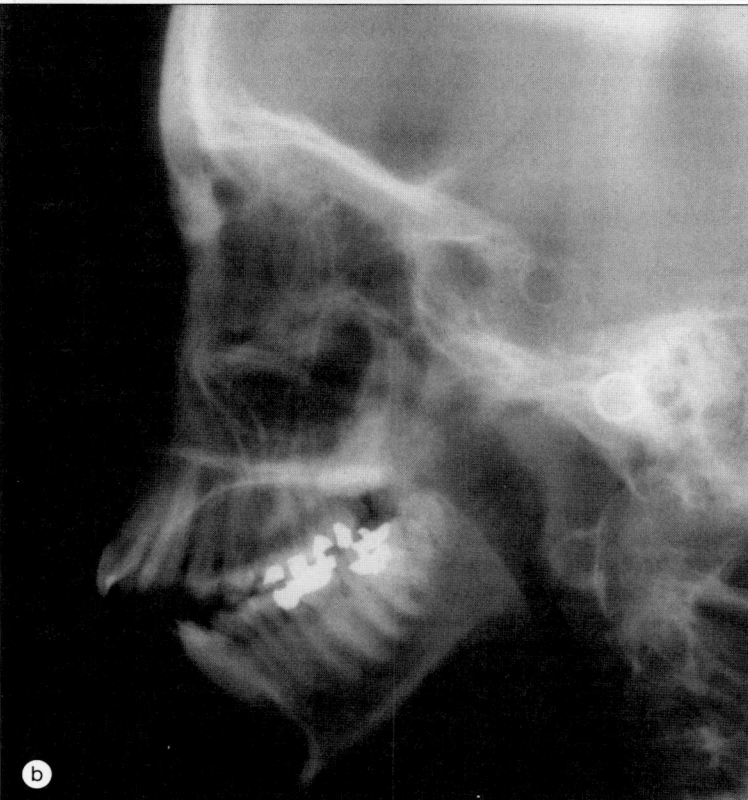

Fig. 98.16 TMJ involvement. Note growth failure of lower jaw (a) and malocclusion on the radiograph (b).

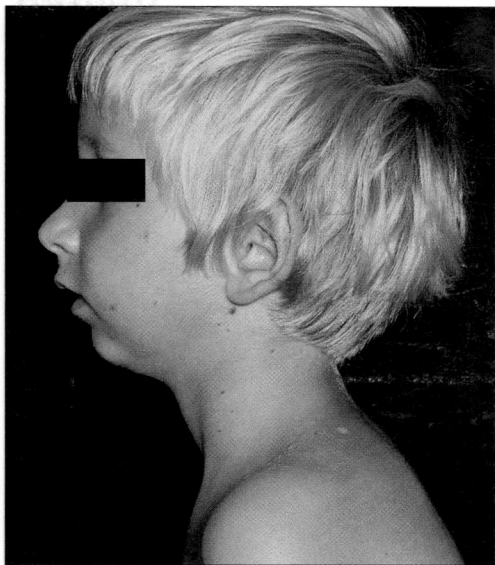

Fig. 98.17 Failure of development of the lower jaw some 5 years after systemic onset of disease. The neck is short and slightly flexed.

General growth disturbance

Generalized growth disturbance has been observed in children with active disease and is related to active disease intensity and duration. During quiescent periods of the disease, height can return to normal in 2 or 3 years if premature closure of the epiphysis has not occurred.

The etiology of delayed growth and low weight is unclear, but it is tightly linked to the level of general inflammation. Studies suggest that severe weight loss or lack of weight gain may also contribute to the lack of growth in height. Nutritional studies have suggested that decreased caloric intake, increased metabolic needs beyond recommended daily requirements, or lack of essential vitamins could result in decreased weight and height.[37] In older studies a substantial proportion of the patients showed growth retardation, whereas in more recent studies fewer, 5% to 10%, are afflicted, probably owing to better control of general disease activity/inflammation with active treatment.[38-40] Mainly patients with systemic and unremitting extended oligoarticular or polyarticular course diseases develop growth retardation.

Corticosteroid therapy also inhibits growth in height but usually not skeletal maturation (Fig. 98.18). Growth retardation is likely to occur with corticosteroid doses greater than 5 mg/m²/day for 6 months or more.[41]

Levels of growth hormone and insulin-like growth factor (IGF)-1 and IGF-2 are usually normal but occasionally are reduced.[42] Levels of IGF-1 have been found to be inversely correlated with interleukin-6 levels in systemic disease.[43] Growth hormone (GH) has been given to children with normal GH levels and JIA at doses of 1.4 IU/kg/wk, resulting in a mean height velocity increase of 3.5 cm/yr and an accompanying 12% increase in lean body mass. In that study, at the end of 1 year the height velocity returned to the pretest levels. Other studies have shown that there was no correlation between GH levels and response to GH.[42] Response to GH is best when the disease is inactive and no or very low doses of corticosteroids are used.[44]

It is equally important to monitor the overall nutrition of the child. Growth retardation and decreased bone mineralization occur during active disease and are exacerbated by anorexia and inanition. Nutritional and vitamin supplementation are often needed. Assessment of nutritional status should be a part of every patient's evaluation.[45]

Osteopenia

Osteopenia, or low bone mass for age, is now recognized as a major complication of JIA. An important determinant of future fracture risk is the attainment of a high peak bone mass, which is completed in adolescence. Peak bone mass is determined by genetics as well as nutrition, exercise and hormones, especially estrogen. In children with JIA, active disease, poor nutrition such as low calcium and vitamin D intake, drugs such as corticosteroids, lack of exercise, and delayed menarche can all affect the peak bone mass.[46] Bone mineral density has been found to be low at all sites in children with JIA, but the cortical bone is frequently affected the most. Recently, treatment with bisphosphonates has been shown to increase bone density by dual-energy x-ray absorptiometry bone measurement, but the long-term effects on growing bone are unknown.

Uveitis

According to population-based series of JIA, uveitis occurs in 3% to 16% of patients, with predominance among those with oligoarticular arthritis.[4,47-50] In the majority of cases the uveitis is "silent" and asymptomatic. More girls than boys are affected, and 50% to 80% are ANA positive. Interestingly, some geographic areas (e.g., Costa Rica, India, and South Africa) report very few or no patients with ANA-positive oligoarthritis associated with uveitis,[49] suggesting true differences in

GROWTH CHART OF A GIRL WITH SYSTEMIC JIA

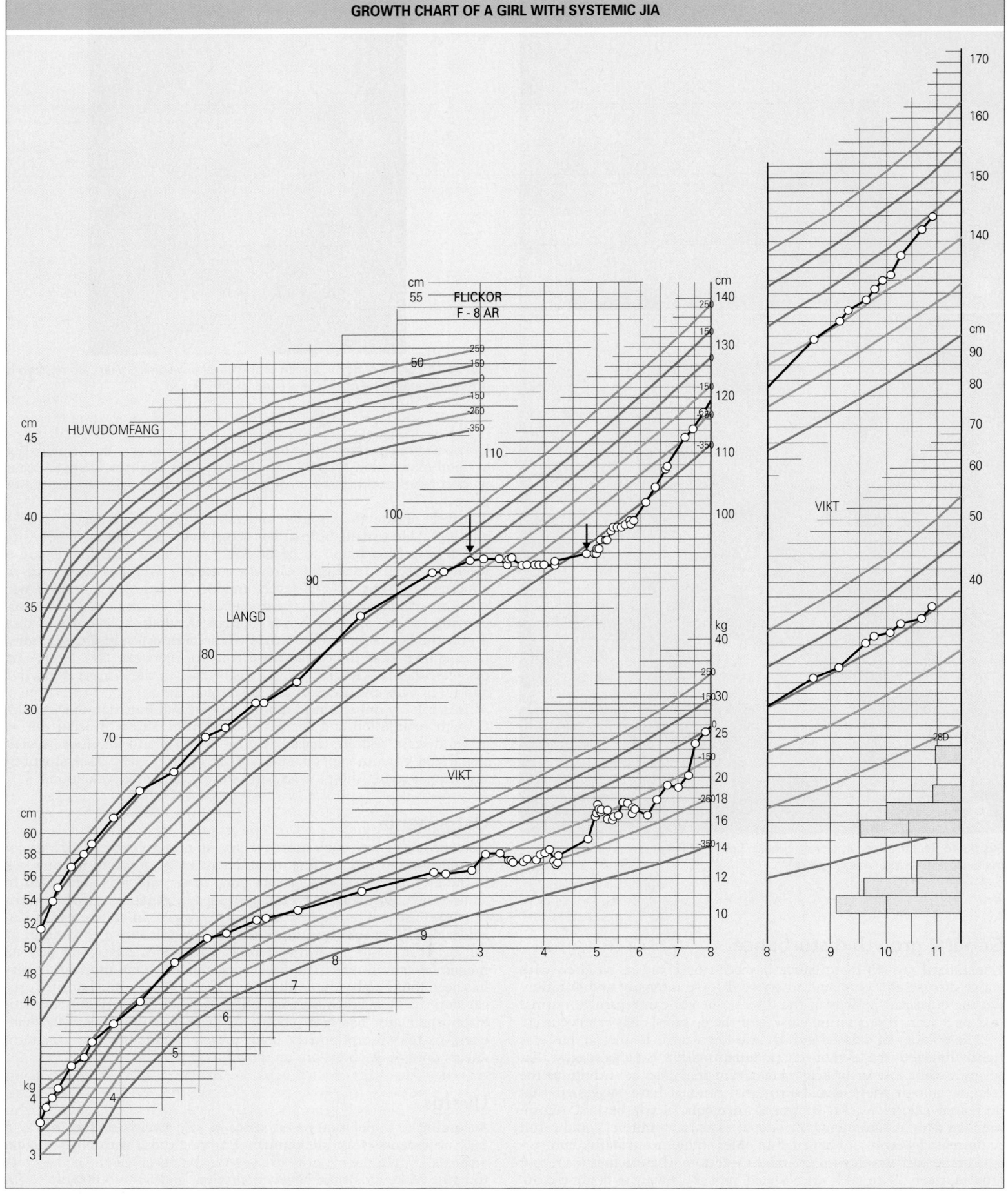

Fig. 98.18 A growth chart of a girl with systemic JIA. First arrow indicates start of corticosteroid treatment. Second arrow indicates time for autologous stem cell transplantation.

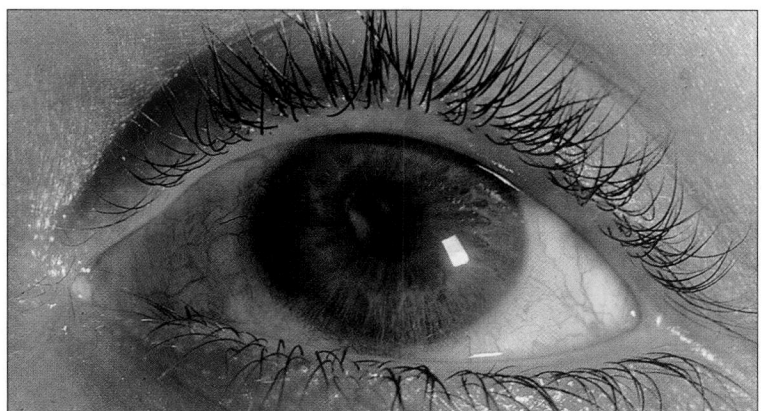

Fig. 98.19 Iritis demonstrating cataract and irregular pupil secondary to posterior synechiae. *(Courtesy of J. J. Kanski.)*

<table>

BOX 98.3 **AMERICAN ACADEMY OF PEDIATRICS GUIDELINES FOR SCREENING EYE EXAMINATIONS IN JRA FROM 1993**

JRA onset subtype	Age at onset	
	<7 years	>7 years
Systemic	Annual	Annual
Polyarticular		
ANA-positive	Every 3-4 months for 4 years, then every 6 months for 3 years, then annually	Every 6 months for 4 years, then annually
ANA-negative	Every 6 months for 4 years, then annually	
Pauciarticular		
ANA-positive	Every 3-4 months for 4 years, then every 6 months for 3 years, then annually	Every 6 months for 4 years, then annually
ANA-negative	Every 6 months for 4 years, then annually	

ANA, antinuclear antibodies.
From American Academy of Pediatrics. Section on Rheumatology. Guidelines for ophthalmologic examinations in children with juvenile rheumatoid arthritis. Pediatrics 1993;92:295-296.

disease manifestations pertaining to immunogenetics or environmental factors or a combination of both. Symptomatic cases occur more often among boys, are more often HLA-B27 positive, and are associated with enthesitis-related arthritis.[48]

According to population-based data, the median age at onset of JIA associated with uveitis is 5 years (range, 1-16 years). At least half of the patients have onset of uveitis close to arthritis onset, but late cases may occur. In most children, however, the eye disease occurs within 7 years of the onset of arthritis. The uveitis is bilateral in 50% to 60% of the cases.

A slit-lamp examination is necessary for early detection of eye involvement. In late disease the iris may also demonstrate irregularity due to posterior synechiae when a bright light is shone into the pupil (Fig. 98.19). The outcome is worse in patients in whom uveitis occurs before or at the onset of JIA, who have severe disease at onset that is continually active.[50] Complications to ongoing active inflammation and prolonged local corticosteroid treatment are synechiae, band keratopathy, cataracts, and glaucoma.

Early detection and intensive treatment seem to have improved considerably the prognosis for vision. Older studies, from ophthalmology clinics where probably mainly severe cases were seen, reported 30% to 40% blindness in JRA-related uveitis. In contrast, in recent population-based studies from Finland and the United States (Minnesota), the prognosis is less gloomy. In the Finnish study, with a median follow-up of 7 years, one third of patients still had active uveitis but only 3% had severe visual loss. In the study from Olmsted County, Minnesota, 3% developed uveitis, none of whom had visual impairment after 8 to 24 years' follow-up. The course of the eye disease is unrelated to the course of the arthritis and may persist after the arthritis has remitted.[51]

In conclusion, the importance of screening for uveitis, intensive treatment of inflammation when found, and the active treatment of complications from uveitis must be stressed. However, a few patients who do not respond even to the intensive treatments available today, will still develop severely impaired vision.

The American Academy of Pediatrics sections on rheumatology and ophthalmology have recommended a schedule for regular eye examinations (Box 98.3).[52]

Amyloidosis

In the assessment of JIA, any patient with persistent activity of the disease who develops proteinuria and a rising ESR with a falling hemoglobin and serum albumin level should be considered for serum amyloid P protein scan,[53] which currently is the most sensitive method for demonstrating deposition of amyloid. The incidence of amyloidosis, however, is declining according to recent studies, probably owing to the more aggressive anti-inflammatory therapy given today. In early studies mortality ranged from 4% to 7% in JIA, whereas in more recent reports it is usually close to 0% except for in systemic JIA. [9,41,54,55] In a large series of patients with systemic disease, two deaths among 122 patients were reported.[54]

Pain

Pain is a frequent complaint in all children. Headache, abdominal pain, and musculoskeletal pain are the most frequent. Girls and older children experience pain more often than boys and younger children. Many factors influence the experience of pain in the child such as experience, development, disease severity, daily mood, beliefs, and family function. In one investigation, schoolchildren had musculoskeletal pain at least once a week.[56] Girls generally report higher anxiety about pain, and boys may underestimate pain to appear brave. Biologic differences might also underlie gender differences because lower pain threshold has been found in girls compared with boys.

In research by Sällfors and coworkers[57,58] on pain experienced by children with JCA, a strong influence on daily life was obvious. Pain created an uncertainty because the older children never could predict if it would be a "good" day with little pain or a "terrible" day with severe pain. Also, the fact that pain is not able to be seen made the understanding from peers difficult. The uncertainty came from the many social consequences, such as not being able to predict if the teenager would be able to go to school that particular day, if it would be possible to take part in physical education, and the increased dependence on parents at an age when increasing independence is the norm.

Good pain control is thus not only highly desirable but very important for the normal social function of the child with JIA. If antirheumatic drugs do not give enough pain control, it is as important to add analgesics, when needed, as it is to investigate coping strategies, mood changes, and family attitudes to pain and chronic disease.

Sleep disturbance and fatigue

Sleep is of primary importance for physical and intellectual growth, and sleep disturbances that begin in childhood may persist into adulthood. Studies of sleep patterns in children with JIA have shown differences in multiple sleep domains when compared with children without disease. The background to the disturbances is multifactorial but leads to a common endpoint of sleep fragmentation and/or deprivation. Factors that may contribute include anxiety, pain, breathing problems owing to micrognathia and cervical spine compromise, and autonomic nervous system imbalance. Children's self-reports reveal that sleep disturbance correlates well with pain, whereas parents' reports do not. This puts emphasis on both the importance of listening to the child's own experience and the need for good pain management programs. The effect of sleep disturbance experienced by children with JIA is also multifactorial. It leads to daytime fatigue and irritability, which in turn have effects on social life and school performance. It may also interfere with growth hormone secretion and thus affect growth.[59,60]

Assessment of fatigue in adult rheumatology has received empirical attention, whereas in pediatric rheumatology it has so far not been deeply explored. However, Varni and associates studied the PedsQL Multidimensional Fatigue Scale in pediatric patients with rheumatic diseases and confirmed that the instrument has good validity and reliability. It distinguished between healthy children and children with rheumatic disease, was associated with greater disease severity, and could thus be helpful in further studies of the impact of fatigue in JIA and in the evaluation of therapeutic interventions.[61] The first clinical follow-up study that used this instrument showed that children with active polyarticular JIA had lower scores on all the domains of the PedsQL Multidimensional Fatigue Scale compared with children with inactive disease.[62]

OUTCOME

Outcome in chronic disease such as JIA is a complex phenomenon that needs to be viewed from many perspectives. Most studies have focused on traditional disease-centered outcomes, including clinical remission, physical disability, and structural damage. Lately, broader perspectives on outcome, for example, psychosocial well-being or "quality of life" and socioeconomic attainments, have been given attention.[61] A common misconception has been that most childhood arthritis would disappear in adulthood. However, when reviewing data from the past 4 decades there is no indication that JIA is a benign disease.[31] In follow-up studies published after 1994, the percentage of patients with inactive or disease in remission varies from 45% to 60%, indicating that roughly half of the patients have ongoing active disease when entering adulthood. On the other hand, the functional outcome seems to have improved considerably over the past decades. In studies published before 1980 the proportion of patients classified in Steinbrocker class III or IV was 30% to 55%, whereas the proportion in studies published after 1990 was 5% to 15%.[31] A recent study of a tertiary center cohort of JIA patients showed an even lower fraction, 3.6%. This decline in the frequency of patients with severe functional disability is likely to be due to more active treatment with disease-modifying antirheumatic drugs such as methotrexate and, lately, biologic medications, intra-articular corticosteroids, and team-based comprehensive care. However, changes in natural history of the disease or better general health status in children are possible contributing factors.[55]

The outcome of JIA is variable depending on the subtype and course of disease. The remission rate is highest in persistent oligoarticular arthritis, at 50% to 80%,[9,39,63] whereas it is lower in polyarticular disease, at 20% to 30%, especially among RF-positive patients. Remission rates in studies on systemic disease are more variable, 0% to 50%, probably owing to the heterogeneity of this subtype. The long-term remission rates in enthesitis-related arthritis as well as in juvenile psoriatic arthritis seem to be low at 0% to 30% and 30% to 40%, respectively.[9,28,39,63-66]

Functional outcomes in individual subtypes are fairly distinct when evaluated by the Child Health Assessment Questionnaire (CHAQ), one of the six components used in the core set of outcome for JIA.[67] Overall, 80% of those with persistent oligoarticular-onset JIA

are without difficulty at 15-year follow-up.[39] However, of those with an oligoarticular onset who develop extended arthritis, roughly 50%, the majority have some functional disability at 15-year follow-up. A major cause of morbidity in oligoarticular-onset JIA is uveitis (see earlier). Patients with enthesitis-related arthritis may develop acute uveitis, some with a chronic course.

In patients with polyarticular onset, more than half will develop some functional disability, and it is mainly in this subgroup that we find those with severe functional limitations: 18% among RF-positive patients and 8% among those who are RF negative.[64] Attainment of inactive disease at least once in the first 5 years has been found to be associated with less long-term joint damage and a trend toward less functional impairment.[68] Poor functional outcome can also be seen in patients with systemic onset who develop polyarticular disease. At higher risk for having a poor functional outcome in systemic disease are those with disease onset before age 5 years, with persistent disease activity for the first 5 years, accelerated radiologic changes, pericarditis, and thrombocytosis.[65]

Among risk factors for continued disease activity in JIA, the most consistent are polyarticular onset and disease course, especially in females, elevated inflammatory markers at onset, and positive RF. Predictors for disability and joint damage are similar (i.e., continuous disease activity, polyarticular disease course, female sex, articular severity score, and RF positivity).[66,68]

To better categorize outcome, the pediatric medical community has developed a core set of outcome variables.[67] These have provided a way to objectively define and monitor disease activity, disease improvement, and disease flare.[69] Patient, parent, and physician global assessment, the CHAQ,[70] the number of active joints, and the ESR make up the core outcome variables. The Juvenile Arthritis Damage Index (JADI), another tool with the aim of scoring all forms of long-term articular and extra-articular morbidity in patients with JIA, has also been developed and found valuable.[29,68,71] Early treatment with drugs demonstrated to decrease joint destruction as well as new methods to monitor disease activity and improvement are likely to improve the long-term outcome of JIA.

Even with aggressive treatment, 10% to 20% of children with JIA continue to have poor health, psychosocial, and educational outcomes. A 25-year population-based follow-up study of JRA patients compared with sex- and age-matched non-disabled peers showed that those with JRA had greater disability, more pain, increased fatigue, poorer health perception and decreased physical functioning, lower rates of employment, and less involvement with exercise.[72] Similarly, raised levels of depression,[73] anxiety, isolation,[74] and lack of serious relationships with young people of the opposite sex have been reported in a significant proportion of selected JRA populations.[75,76]

Because of these findings and the fact that many young people have continued active disease into adulthood, this group needs continuity of care in the transition period from child-centered to adult-oriented systems. They need health care providers who can help the young person and the family to move through the appropriate developmental milestones and navigate the difficult transitions from school to tertiary education and work, home to independence, and pediatric to adult health care. Transition is not an event but a process. Careful planning is essential so that these patients become successful members of adult society. Several reviews are available that outline the process and the particular issues faced by adolescents as they make the transition to adult systems.[77]

KEY REFERENCES

1. Petty RE, Southwood TR, Manners P, et al. International League of Associations for Rheumatology classification of juvenile idiopathic arthritis: second revision, Edmonton, 2001. J Rheumatol 2004;31:390-392.
4. Berntson L, Andersson Gäre B, Fasth A, et al. Incidence of juvenile idiopathic arthritis in the Nordic countries: a population-based study with special reference to the validity of the ILAR and EULAR criteria. J Rheumatol 2003;30:2275-2282.
6. Towner SR, Michet CJ, O'Fallon, et al. The epidemiology of juvenile arthritis in Rochester, Minnesota 1960-1979. Arthritis Rheum 1983;26:1208-1213.

8. McGhee JL, Burks FN, Sheckels JL, Jarvis JN. Identifying children with chronic arthritis based on chief complaints: absence of predictive value for musculoskeletal pain as an indicator of rheumatic disease in children. Pediatrics 2002;110:354-359.
9. Andersson Gäre B, Fasth A. The natural history of juvenile chronic arthritis: a population-based cohort study: I. Onset and disease process. J Rheumatol 1995;22:295-307.
10. Ravelli A. Macrophage activation syndrome. Curr Opin Rheumatol 2002;14:548-552.

12. Lamer S, Sebag GH. Magnetic resonance imaging and ultrasound in children with juvenile idiopathic arthritis. Eur J Radiol 2000;33:85-93.
17. Sherry DD. An overview of amplified musculoskeletal pain syndromes. J Rheumatol 2000;58:44-48.
25. Lomater C, Gereloni V, Gattinara M, et al. Systemic onset juvenile idiopathic arthritis: a retrospective study of 80 consecutive patients followed for 10 years. J Rheumatol 2000;27:491-496.
28. Flatø B, Lien G, Smerdel-Ramoya A, Vinje O. Juvenile psoriatic arthritis: long-term outcome and differentiation from other subtypes of juvenile

idiopathic arthritis. J Rheumatol 2009;36: 642-650.

29. Cabral DA, Oen KG, Petty RE. SEA syndrome revisited: a long-term follow up of children with a syndrome of seronegative enthesopathy and arthropathy. J Rheumatol 1992;19:1282.

30. Petty RE. HLA-B27 and rheumatic diseases of childhood. Perspect Pediatr Rheum 1990;17(Suppl 26):7-10.

31. Ravelli A. Toward an understanding of the long-term outcome of juvenile idiopathic arthritis. Clin Exp Rheumatol 2004;22:271-275.

32. Moskowitz A. Scoliosis and JRA. Spine 1990;15:46-49.

36. Twilt M, Mobers SMLM, Arends LR, et al. Temporomandibular involvement in juvenile idiopathic arthritis. J Rheumatol 2004;31:1418-1422.

39. Flatö B, Aasland A, Vinje O, Förre Ö. Outcome and predictive factors in juvenile rheumatoid arthritis and juvenile spondylarthropathy. J Rheumatol 1998;25:366-375.

40. Minden K, Nieworth M, Listing J, et al. Long-term outcome in patients with juvenile idiopathic arthritis. Arthritis Rheum 2002;46:2392-2401.

44. Simon D. Management of growth retardation in juvenile idiopathic arthritis. Horm Res 2007;68(Suppl 5):122-125.

46. Cassidy JT. Osteopenia and osteoporosis in children. Clin Exp Rheumatol 1999;17:245-250.

47. Carvounis PE, Herman DC, Cha SS, Burke JP. Ocular manifestations of juvenile rheumatoid arthritis in Olmsted County, Minnesota: a population-based study. Graefes Arch Clin Exp Ophtalmol 2005;243:217-221.

48. Kotaniemi K, Kaipianien-Seppänen O, Savolainen A, Karma A. A populations-based study on uveitis in juvenile rheumatoid arthritis. Clin Exp Rheumatol 1999;17:119-122.

50. Edelsten C, Lee V, Bently CR, et al. An evaluation of baseline factors predicting severity in juvenile idiopathic arthritis–associated uveitis and other chronic anterior uveitis in early childhood. Br J Ophthalmol 2002;86:51-56.

51. Skarin A, Elborgh R, Edlund E, Bengtsson-Stigmar E. Long-term follow-up of patients with uveitis associated with juvenile idiopathic arthritis: a cohort study. Ocul Immunol Inflamm 2009;17:104-108.

54. Spiegel LR, Schneider R, Lang BA, et al. Early predictors of poor functional outcome in systemic-onset juvenile rheumatoid arthritis: a multicenter cohort study. Arthritis Rheum 2000;43:2402-2409.

55. Solari N, Viola S, Pistorio A, et al. Assessing current outcomes of juvenile idiopathic arthritis: a cross-sectional study in a tertiary center sample. Arthritis Rheum 2008;59:1571-1579.

58. Sällfors C, Hallberg LR-M, Fasth A. Coping with chronic pain: in-depth interviews with children suffering from juvenile chronic arthritis. Scand J Dis Res 2001;3:3-20.

60. Bloom BJ, Owens JA, McGuinn M, et al. Sleep and its relation to pain, dysfunction and disease activity in juvenile rheumatoid arthritis. J Rheumatol 2002;29:169-173.

61. Varni JW, Burwinkle TM, Szer IS. The PedsQL multidimensional fatigue scale in pediatric rheumatology: reliability and validity. J Rheumatol 2004;31:2494-2500.

62. Ringold S, Wallace CA, Rivara FP. Health-related quality of life, physical function, fatigue, and disease activity in children with established polyarticular juvenile idiopathic arthritis. J Rheumatol 2009;36:1330-1336.

63. Minden K, Kiessling U, Listing J, et al. Prognosis of patients with juvenile chronic arthritis and juvenile spondylarthropathy. J Rheumatol 2000;27: 2256-2263.

64. Oen K, Malleson PN, Cabral DA, et al. Disease course and outcome of juvenile chronic arthritis in a multicenter cohort. J Rheumatol 2002;29:1989-1999.

65. Schneider R, Lang BA, Reilly BJ, et al. Prognostic indicators of chronic destructive arthritis in systemic onset JRA. Arthritis Rheum 1989;32:S83.

66. Andersson Gäre BA, Fasth A. The outcome of juvenile idiopathic arthritis. Curr Paediatrics 2003;13:327-334.

68. Magnani A, Pistorio A, Magni-Manzoni S, et al. Achievement of a state of inactive disease at least once in the first 5 years predicts better outcome of patients with polyarticular juvenile idiopathic arthritis. J Rheumatol 2009;36:628-634.

69. Lovell DJ, Giannini EH, Reiff A, et al. Etanercept in children with polyarticular juvenile rheumatoid arthritis. Pediatric Rheumatology Collaborative Study. N Engl J Med 2000;342:763-769.

71. Sarma PK, Misra R, Aggarwal A. Physical disability, articular, and extra-articular damage in patients with juvenile idiopathic arthritis. Clin Rheumatol 2008;27:1261-1265.

73. David J, Cooper C, Hickey L, et al. The functional and psychological outcomes of juvenile chronic arthritis in young adulthood. Br J Rheumatol 2004;33:876-881.

76. Ostensen M, Almberg K, Koksvik H. Sex, reproduction and gynecological disease in young adults with a history of juvenile rheumatoid arthritis. J Rheumatol 2000;27:1783.

77. White PH. Transition to adulthood. Curr Opin Rheumatol 1999;11:408-411.

REFERENCE

Full references for this chapter can be found on www.expertconsult.com.

Etiology and pathogenesis of juvenile idiopathic arthritis

99

Rachelle Donn

- Juvenile idiopathic arthritis (JIA) represents several subgroups that have distinct clinical, immunologic, and genetic differences.
- JIA subgroups are each complex traits with contributions from both genetic and environmental parameters.
- Synovium and cartilage are both affected. Triggers for the initiation and progression of the pathology that manifests as JIA have not been identified.
- Association and linkage to HLA loci have been confirmed for certain JIA subgroups.
- Only a limited number of non-HLA loci have been shown to be significant in conferring susceptibility to JIA.

INTRODUCTION

Juvenile idiopathic arthritis (JIA) is the most common rheumatic disease of childhood. It encompasses a heterogeneous group of chronic arthropathies, all of which share persistent idiopathic inflammation of one or more synovial joints. The subtypes of JIA differ in their clinical manifestations, prognosis, and specific autoimmune characteristics.

The classification of chronic arthritis of childhood onset remains problematic. Different classifications exist in the literature be that of the International League of Associations for Rheumatology (i.e., JIA), European League Against Rheumatism (i.e., juvenile chronic arthritis [JCA]), or American College of Rheumatology (i.e., juvenile rheumatoid arthritis [JRA]) naming conventions (see Chapter 97). This makes comparisons of the research literature difficult. This chapter essentially focuses on JIA (as defined by the ILAR)[1] but refers to the naming as cited in the original articles throughout.

PATHOLOGY

JIA is an inflammatory disorder that primarily affects synovial joints. The clinical characteristics of joint involvement vary across the different JIA subgroups but generally present as swelling, stiffness, pain, and/or loss of function of the affected joint. The disease process of JIA includes synovial hyperplasia causing soft tissue swelling, joint effusion, and cartilage destruction that result in bone erosions. Lymphocytes, plasma cells, macrophages, and dendritic cells are all present in increased numbers within the inflamed JIA joint.[2] A schematic representation of the pathology of the JIA joint is shown in Figure 99.1.

The immunopathogenic mechanisms underlying JIA have been the subject of intensive study but have not yet been elucidated. The detection of T cells and chronic synovial inflammation has indicated cellular mediation, whereas the finding of immune complexes and complement has suggested a possible B-cell–mediated response.

Synovial fluid

The volume of synovial fluid in affected joints is increased in JIA, with viscosity being decreased mainly because of reduced concentrations of hyaluronic acid. Synovial fluid contains various inflammatory cells, including neutrophils, plasma cells, dendritic cells, and a high proportion of T cells expressing markers of activation.[3] These cells are most likely extravasated from the inflamed synovial lining. Mediators of inflammation such as cytokines and cleavage products of the complement system are also abundant.

Synovial tissue

One of the hallmarks of the pathology of JIA, and in particular for the rheumatoid factor (RF)-positive polyarticular JIA presentation, is the tumor-like expansion of inflamed synovial tissue, or pannus, which causes much of the joint damage in this disease.[4] With the progression of the disease, pannus spreads over the synovial space and adheres to intra-articular cartilage. It is in the areas of pannus/cartilage junction that the cartilage eventually degrades (Fig. 99.2). Such expansion results from the invasion of the synovial tissue by inflammatory cells recruited from the peripheral circulation and the proliferation of synoviocytes.

Cartilage

Cartilage is a primary target organ that is affected as part of the pathogenic process of JIA.[5-7] Superficial cartilage thinning is a feature of early and untreated JIA. Complete cartilage destruction and cartilage erosions leading to bone erosions can occur with long-standing disease.[8,9] Magnetic resonance imaging (MRI) enhanced with gadolinium-tetraazacyclododecanetetraacetic acid (Gd-DOTA) increases the sensitivity for the detection of inflammatory changes in JIA (Fig. 99.3).[10]

T cells and JIA

CD4+ T lymphocytes are the predominant cell population in the JRA synovium and exhibit phenotypic and functional characteristics of cells that have undergone prior activation *in vivo*.[4] These characteristics include expression of interleukin (IL)-2 receptors (CD25), early activation antigen CD69, CD45RO (memory phenotype), very late activation antigen type 1 (VLA-1), and HLA class II antigens.[3] It has been suggested that such activation might be induced by an autoantigen located in the inflamed joints.

Analysis of several experimental antigen-driven models has shown that antigen-specific T cells often make up only a very small proportion of all T cells present at the site of the immune response, suggesting that most of the other cells are recruited in a non-specific manner. The extrapolation of these data to JRA pathogenesis suggests that the numbers of T cells critical to the autoimmune response in inflamed joints may be very small.

Regulatory T cells, Th17 cells, and JIA

CD4+ T helper (Th) cells help to regulate the immune response. Effector Th cell subsets, characterized by their differential cytokine production, have resulted in the Th1-Th2 paradigm. Th1 cells produce interferon-γ and regulate antigen presentation and immunity against intracellular pathogens. Th2 cells produce IL-4, IL-5, and IL-13 and mediate some humoral responses and immunity against parasites. However, observations by several different groups described the proinflammatory cytokines IL-17 and IL-17F to be expressed by distinct Th cells, which did not express either interferon-γ or IL-4. This has resulted in the discovery of Th17 cells as a Th lineage independent of Th1 or Th2 cells.

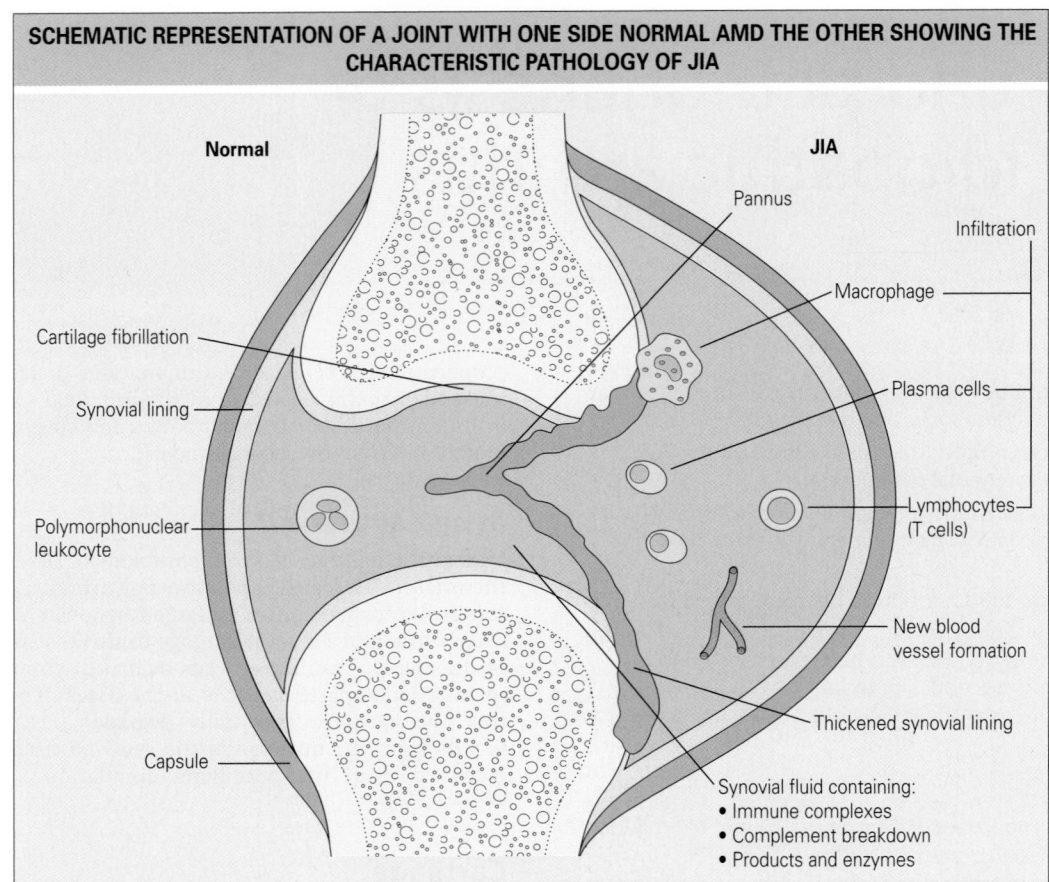

SCHEMATIC REPRESENTATION OF A JOINT WITH ONE SIDE NORMAL AMD THE OTHER SHOWING THE CHARACTERISTIC PATHOLOGY OF JIA

Normal

JIA

Pannus

Infiltration

Macrophage

Cartilage fibrillation

Plasma cells

Synovial lining

Lymphocytes (T cells)

Polymorphonuclear leukocyte

New blood vessel formation

Thickened synovial lining

Capsule

Synovial fluid containing:
• Immune complexes
• Complement breakdown
• Products and enzymes

Fig. 99.1 Schematic representation of a joint with one side normal and the other showing the characteristic pathology of JIA. *(Modified from Chapel H, Haeney M, Misbah S, et al. Essentials of clinical immunology. Oxford: Blackwell Science, 1999.)*

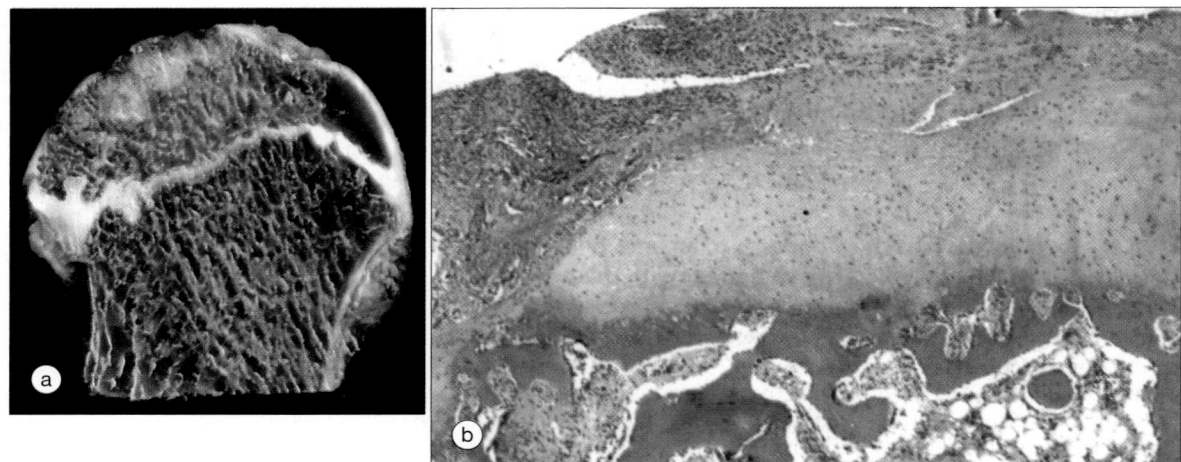

Fig. 99.2 Destructive inflammatory pannus in JRA. (a) Photograph of a frontal section taken through the femoral head of a child with JRA. Extensive destruction of the articular cartilage has occurred, with associated erosion of the subchondral bone. (b) Photomicrograph of a section taken at the articular margin of the specimen demonstrated in (a), showing a destructive inflammatory pannus extending onto the articular surface. *(With permission from Bullough PG. Orthopaedic pathology, 3rd ed. London: Mosby-Wolfe, 1997.)*

Regulatory T cells (Treg) have the phenotype CD4+CD25+. These spontaneously occurring T cells can actively and dominantly prevent the activation and effector function of autoreactive T cells that escape other mechanisms of tolerance. A role for CD4+CD25+ Treg cells in JIA pathogenesis has been considered by a number of groups.[11-14] More recently, a role for IL-17–producing T cells has been shown. IL-17–positive T cells are enriched within the joints of JIA patients, and the number of such cells was found to be higher in patients with extended oligoarthritis as compared with patients with the milder persistent oligoarthritis. An inverse relationship between IL-17+ T cells and Fox3P+ Treg cells was found.[15] This suggests that the Th17 cells are contributing to the joint pathology of JIA and that the balance between IL-17+ T cells and Treg cells may influence disease outcome.

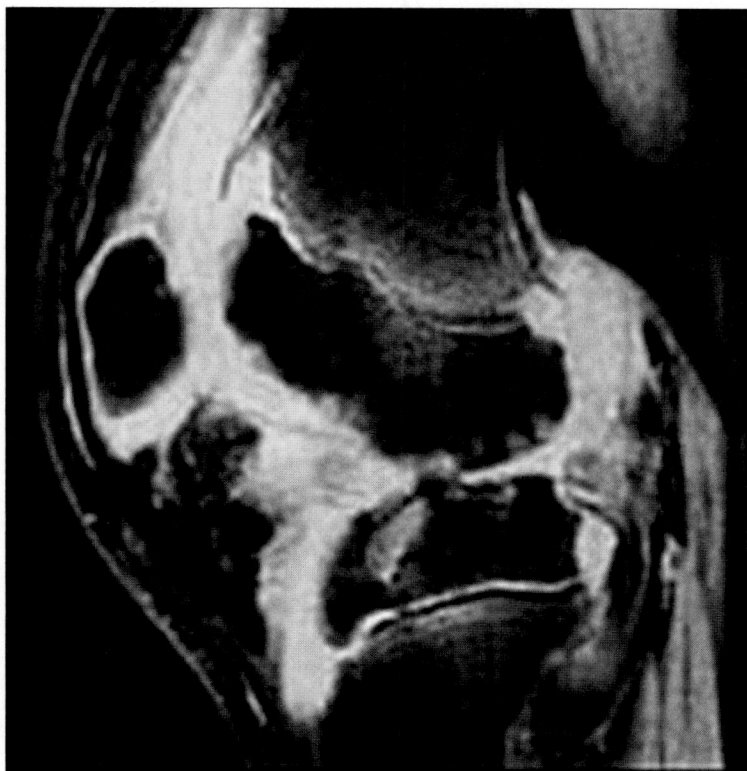

Fig. 99.3 A T2-weighted fat-suppressed MR image in a 10-year-old child shows high signal intensity from both the synovium and synovial fluid, which are difficult to distinguish. Numerous erosions, cartilage loss, and fat pad irregularity are seen on this image. *(Reproduced, with permission, from Gardner-Medwin J, Southwood T. Current developments in juvenile arthritis. Topical Reviews No. 5, Reports on Rheumatic Diseases, Series 4, 2001, published by the Arthritis Research Campaign [www.arc.org.uk].)*

Macrophage and fibroblast contribution to JIA pathogenesis

Increased numbers of macrophages, dendritic cells, and proliferation of fibroblast-like and macrophage-like synoviocytes are typical features of JRA synovium.[4] The abundance of cytokines secreted by these cells provides further evidence for the major role of these cells in the perpetuation of the synovial inflammation. Martini and coworkers, in 1986, noted high spontaneous production of IL-1 by mononuclear cells derived from peripheral blood of patients with juvenile arthritis.[16] More recently, an abundance of IL-1–producing macrophages has also been demonstrated in inflamed JRA synovial tissues.[17]

Analysis of tumor necrosis factor (TNF) expression and the distribution of the TNF receptors in JRA synovial tissues provided strong evidence for the role of both TNF-α and TNF-β in the amplification of the synovial inflammation in JRA.[18] Numerous cells staining for TNF-α were found in the majority of synovial tissue samples, and the pattern of distribution of TNF-α⁺ cells was similar in nature to the distribution of macrophages. The level of expression of TNF-α correlated closely with the degree of inflammatory infiltration of the synovial membrane.

IL-6, another macrophage-derived product, has been consistently found in the synovial fluids of patients with JIA. More importantly, in systemic-onset JIA, IL-6 concentrations are increased not only in the synovial compartment but also in serum, and the serum concentrations of IL-6 protein correlate with the extent of joint involvement and peripheral thrombocytosis. High levels of expression of IL-6 in synovial tissue samples have been shown to distinguish patients with systemic JRA, even at later stages of the disease.[19,20] An important role for IL-6 in the pathogenesis of systemic-onset disease is supported by genetic findings (see later).

B-cell contribution to the disease pathogenesis of JIA

B-cell activity

Although macrophages and T cells are usually more numerous in inflamed synovial tissue, B-cell activity appears also to be enhanced in both the peripheral blood and synovial compartment. Lindblad and colleagues[21] described synovial tissue specimens from patients with juvenile arthritis in which there were significantly increased numbers of focally aggregated immunoglobulin-synthesizing cells. As a consequence of increased B-cell activity, hyperglobulinemia and circulating immune complexes, antinuclear antibodies (ANAs), and RFs are common findings in many patients with JIA.

Rheumatoid factor

Rheumatoid factor, an autoantibody directed against the Fc region of human IgG, is found in the serum and synovial fluid of the majority of patients with RA. RF can only rarely be detected in patients with JIA by the classic Rose-Waaler reaction or latex fixation method, although the probability of finding it increases with the age and the duration of the disease. Allen and Kunkel[22] demonstrated a so-called hidden RF defined as IgM 19S antiglobulin. This antiglobulin is "hidden" because of its occupied binding sites. Gel filtration at acid pH dissociates IgM from IgG and allows IgM RF to fix complement in hemolytic assay. This technique makes it possible to detect the presence of RF in a much larger proportion of JIA patients, specifically the polyarticular subgroup.

Antinuclear antibodies (ANAs)

The reported incidence of ANAs in patients with juvenile arthritis varies from 4% to 88%, depending on the clinical subtype and the laboratory technique used.[23] ANAs are uncommon in systemic-onset disease, whereas more than 50% of children with oligoarticular JCA have ANAs in their serum. Children who are ANA positive carry an especially high risk of developing chronic anterior uveitis.

The full specificity of these antibodies remains to be determined. Some studies indicated that ANAs in most patients are directed to a ribonucleoprotein that requires both RNA and protein components for antigenic integrity. Szer and associates[24] concluded that ANA specificity profiles were highly individual and did not appear to correlate with disease subtype or activity. Several studies revealed that antibodies to many antigens typical for other rheumatic diseases—for example, the extractable nuclear protein, centromere proteins, scleroderma Scl-70, Ro, La, and double-stranded DNA—are generally absent in JIA. More recently, the antibodies to the 45-kDa DEK nuclear antigen, a putative oncoprotein, have been associated with the oligoarticular type of JCA, particularly in patients with a history of iridocyclitis. However, the presence of these antibodies does not appear to be limited to or specific for JIA.

Anti-citrullinated peptide antibodies

Citrulline is a translational modification of the amino acid arginine by peptidyl arginine deiminase (PAD). Citrulline becomes part of a protein after post-translational modification by PAD enzymes. Antibodies to citrullinated proteins have been shown to aid in the determination of disease prognosis in adult RA patients. The autoantibody system involved includes antiperinuclear factor, antikeratin antibodies, antifilaggrin antibodies, anticitrullinated fibrin antibodies, and anti-Sa (citrullinated vimentin) antibodies. A number of studies have now evaluated anti-citrullinated peptide antibody (ACPA) levels in JIA patients. These studies show that ACPA positivity is only significantly raised in the RF-positive polyarticular JIA cases. Specifically, Ferucci and coworkers found ACPA formation in HLA-DR4–positive cases and the ACPA antibodies were associated with polyarticular onset and erosive disease.[25]

ENVIRONMENTAL FACTORS

In an attempt to identify the causative agent(s) implicated in the etiopathogenesis of juvenile arthritis, associations with a number of potential viral and bacterial pathogens have been sought. A self-limiting polyarthritis can follow a wide variety of viral infections, including those caused by coxsackievirus B, Epstein-Barr virus, parvovirus, and rubella virus.[26,27] Studies reporting positive findings of viral antigens in JCA patients, however, are limited. Rubella virus has been implicated for some time,[28] and a small proportion of individuals who received rubella immunizations develop arthritis very similar to that of pauciarticular JCA. Chantler and colleagues isolated rubella particles from the synovial fluid and/or blood mononuclear cells from 1 of 5 children with systemic-onset JCA, 2 of 2 with polyarticular JCA, 2 of 6 with pauciarticular JCA, and 2 of 6 with spondyloarthropathy. The virus was identified two or more times in 4 of the 7 originally positive patients. All 16 controls, 8 of whom had other connective tissue disorders or mechanical joint effusions and 8 normal subjects included in the study, were negative for rubella.[29]

Pritchard and associates noted birth-date clustering among polyarticular JCA patients who developed progressive disease after the appearance of influenza A H3N2 in 1977.[30] These patients had all been born in 1963, a year in which an epidemic of influenza A H3N2 had occurred. Raised levels of antibody to H3N2, the strain of influenza A prevalent at the time at which they were born, were recorded in this cohort. This led to the suggestion that these individuals developed their arthritis in 1977 because they had been pre-sensitized to influenza A by contact with the earlier strain when *in utero*. In a follow-up study on a similar cohort, influenza-specific cytotoxic T-cell clones were identified in the blood and synovial fluid but no evidence of sequestration to the joints of such clones was found.[31]

Clinical features of systemic-onset JIA are particularly suggestive of a viral origin, and rising antibody titers to coxsackievirus B4 were found during the acute stages of illness.[32] Feldman and colleagues addressed the seasonal difference in the onset of systemic-onset JRA by examining data collected from all patients with systemic-onset disease from 1980 to 1992 who presented to pediatric rheumatology clinics across Canada. The onset pattern of systemic-onset JRA was then compared with the incidence data on viral infection.[33] Across Canada the onset of systemic-onset JRA was found to be constant across the seasons. Whereas in the prairie region there was a significant seasonal pattern, with peaks occurring in the autumn and early spring, there was no evidence that viral infection correlated with disease incidence. Furthermore, a large multicenter European study failed to show a seasonal pattern to the onset of systemic or any other form of JCA.[34]

Clustering of pauciarticular arthritis in Connecticut, in the United States, led to the description of Lyme arthritis, later called Lyme disease.[35] The pathogenic agent is the spirochete *Borrelia burgdorferi*, transferred to humans by infected ticks. A number of studies have similarly tried to identify a microorganism, bacterium, or mycoplasma associated with JIA. Oen and associates noted a correlation between the number of *Mycoplasma pneumoniae* infections recorded and the incidence of JRA between 1985 and 1990 in the province of Manitoba, Canada.[36]

HLA-B27–associated forms of JCA may be triggered by bacterial infections. A bacteria-specific synovial cellular immune response was found in spondyloarthritis patients to *Chlamydia trachomatis* and *Yersinia enterocolitica*, organisms known to be important in reactive arthritis.[37] Also, an immunodominant epitope, Gro EL of *Escherichia coli* heat-shock proteins, is one target of immune responsiveness in HLA-B27–positive JCA.[38]

Cellular immune responses to dnaJ, an *E. coli* heat-shock protein, were found to be related to disease activity in a study of 25 JRA patients.[39] No immunologically cross-reactive human homologue to this bacterial dnaJ has yet been identified.

Specific humoral reactivity against two proteins from Epstein-Barr virus, Bolf1 and Balf2, have been described in oligoarticular JIA cases. These viral proteins share sequence homologies with HLA antigens known to be associated with this patient subgroup.[40]

GENETIC FACTORS

Evidence for a genetic component to a disease can come from a variety of sources, such as twin, family, or case-control association studies. The degree of disease concordance in monozygotic (MZ) twins gives an indication of the level of involvement of genetic factors within a given disease. An alternative estimate of the genetic component of a disease can be obtained from family studies using the sibling recurrence risk (λs). This is calculated as the prevalence of the disease in siblings of affected individuals divided by the prevalence of the disease in the general population.

The largest study of both affected sibling pairs (ASPs) and of twins with JRA comes from the National Institute of Arthritis, Musculoskeletal and Skin Diseases' (NIAMS)–sponsored Research Registry for JRA. Of 118 ASPs on the register in 2000, there were 14 pairs of twins in which both twins have arthritis.[41] One pair comprised a girl with polyarticular JRA and a boy with pauciarticular JRA. The other 13 pairs (11 monozygotic [MZ] and 2 of unknown zygosity) were concordant for gender (9 female, 4 male), disease onset (10 pauciarticular, 3 polyarticular), and disease course (8 pauciarticular, 5 polyarticular).

In a recent Finnish study of JIA multicase families, eight sets of twins were identified, two of which were concordant for arthritis. A concordance rate of 25% for a disease with a population prevalence of 1 per 1000 implies a relative risk of JIA of a staggering 250 for an MZ twin.[42] By comparison, for adult RA the risk to an MZ twin has been reported to be 12 to 62.[43]

As noted earlier, the largest series of ASPs have been collected as part of NIAMS' JRA registry. In 1997 the registry contained a series of 71 ASPs; 63% were concordant for gender and 76% for onset type, which was higher than expected based on comparisons with non-ASP populations. This study gave an estimate of the λs for JRA of approximately 15, a value similar to that seen in insulin-dependent diabetes mellitus and multiple sclerosis. It also provided evidence that this value is likely to differ between subtypes, with the strongest genetic component being attributable to the pauciarticular JRA subtype.[44,45] The most recent report from the registry includes 183 ASPs from 164 families, 19 of which are twin pairs.[46] There is a relatively high degree of disease-onset type concordance between the ASPs, 53% concordant for pauciarticular onset and 19% for polyarticular onset. The concordance is, however, markedly less for systemic-onset disease. The clinical manifestations seen within the ASPs is very similar to those of a comparative simplex JRA study population, with the exception of the number of affected joints at JRA onset among the polyarticular-onset disease group.[46] Among the ASPs, age at JRA onset (sibling 1 vs. sibling 2) was not significantly different. However, the ASPs do not develop their disease at the same point in real time (mean real-time difference of 5.1 years). Familial aggregation was marked for tenosynovitis (λs 29.5), leukocytosis (λs 25), and RF (λs 11). Such familial aggregation of clinical features among the ASPs adds strongly to the evidence of a genetic background to the disease.

Similarly, from Finland, 49 ASPs from 37 families were identified from a population of approximately 2000 JIA cases. Within the ASPs there was little difference found for either onset type (57% concordance in ASPs) or disease course (61% concordance in ASPs) when compared with a population-based JIA series. Given a population prevalence of JIA in Finland of approximately 1 per 1000, this study suggests that the λs for JIA is around 25, again supporting the idea of a substantial genetic component in the etiology of JIA.[47]

HLA associations

Much of the genetic work in the past 3 decades has centered round HLA genes. A complete description of the HLA system can be found in Chapter 14. The fact that HLA molecules play a central role in the immune system has led to HLA genes being considered as candidates in association studies in many diseases, particularly those thought to have an immune basis such as JIA.

The majority of the HLA studies in juvenile arthritis have been in children classified according to either the EULAR or ACR criteria and have been reviewed by Donn and Ollier.[48] A large cohort of U.K. patients classified using the ILAR system has also been reported.[49] A summary of HLA class I and class II associations with different subgroups of juvenile arthritis is listed in Table 99.1.

HLA linkage and JIA

A number of recent studies have been able to confirm the HLA associations by establishing linkage. Moroldo and associates showed linkage to both HLA class I and class II using the transmission disequilibrium

TABLE 99.1 HLA CLASS I AND CLASS II ASSOCIATIONS

HLA association	Patient subgroup
Class I	
HLA-B27	Male late-onset pauciarticular Enthesitis-related arthritis (ERA)
HLA-A2	Pauciarticular and young age at disease onset
Class II	
HLA-DRB1*11 (a subtype of HLA-DR5) and HLA-DRB1*08	Early-onset pauciarticular/oligoarthritis
†HLA-DRB1*04 and HLA-DRB1*07	Early-onset pauciarticular/oligoarthritis
HLA-DPB1*0201	Early-onset pauciarticular Persistent and extended oligoarthritis
HLA-DR8/HLA-DRB1*08	RF-negative polyarthritis
HLA-DQ4 (DQA1*0401/DQB1*0402)	RF-negative polyarthritis
HLA-DP3/DPB1*0301	RF-negative polyarthritis
HLA-DR4	RF-positive polyarthritis
HLA-DR5 and HLA-DR8 HLA-DRB1*11	Systemic onset Systemic onset
HLA-DR4	Systemic onset

All the HLA associations listed confer increased risk of susceptibility except for (†) decreased risk of susceptibility.

test (TDT) in pauciarticular-onset JRA patients.[50] HLA-A2, HLA-B27 and B35, and HLA-DR5 and DR8 all showed excess transmission, whereas HLA-DR4 was undertransmitted. A second study confirmed linkage using the TDT in a U.K. cohort of oligoarticular JIA.[51] Here, HLA-A2, HLA-DRB1*08, and DRB1*11 were overtransmitted and HLA-A3 and HLA-DRB1*04 and 07 undertransmitted. This study demonstrated that the effects at these two loci were independent. Finally, linkage analysis utilizing the ASPs within the NIAMS-sponsored registry for JRA has confirmed linkage of pauciarticular JRA and HLA-DR and established linkage also for polyarticular JRA and HLA-DR.[52] Prahalad and colleagues estimated that the proportion of the sibling recurrence risk attributable to HLA (λs_{HLA}) is 2.5, indicating that HLA accounts for 17% of the total genetic component of pauciarticular JIA. Hence, other non-HLA genes must play a role in susceptibility.[52]

Non-HLA genes and JIA

Multiple different non-HLA genetic loci have been investigated in children with arthritis.[53] Arguably, any association reported is only of value in helping to decipher the etiopathogenesis of JIA if the genetic findings are replicated, providing robust evidence of a true effect. Taking this approach substantially curtails the non-HLA genetic loci currently of potential relevance to JIA susceptibility. To date, replication has been achieved for only a handful of genes. Two of these are cytokine genes—IL-6 and macrophage migration inhibitory factor (MIF)—and two are not related to cytokine production—SLC11A2 (formally NRAMP1), important in macrophage-mediated natural resistance to a variety of intracellular pathogens, and WISP3 (wnt1-inducible signaling pathway protein 3), important for cell growth and differentiation.

Interleukin-6

A single nucleotide polymorphism (SNP) at position −174 in the regulatory region of the IL-6 gene, which determines transcriptional response of the IL-6 gene to IL-1 and LPS, was identified by Fishman and associates.[54] The wild-type GG genotype was shown to have significantly higher serum IL-6 levels than the mutant CC genotype. Furthermore, there was a significant lack of the protective genotype

(CC: low producer of IL-6 on stimulation by IL-1/LPS) in children who develop systemic-onset JCA.[54] A multicenter TDT study confirmed IL-6 G allele as a susceptibility factor for systemic arthritis.[55] These findings have recently been extended by Fife and coworkers, who showed a four-marker haplotype across the IL-6 promoter to be significantly overtransmitted to patients with systemic arthritis.[56]

Macrophage migration inhibitory factor

Macrophage MIF is a unique molecule that has proinflammatory, hormonal, and enzymatic properties.[57] A novel polymorphism in the 5′ flanking region (−173) of the macrophage migration inhibitory factor gene (MIF) was reported to be associated initially with systemic-onset JIA[58] and subsequently with susceptibility to all JIA subgroups.[59] Donn and colleagues replicated their initial association study of MIF and JIA using the TDT test. This work revealed that a particular promoter haplotype of the MIF gene (CATT₇-MIF-173*C) is both linked and associated with an increased risk of JIA susceptibility.[60]

The mutant allele, that is, MIF-173*C, results in higher endogenous MIF production in the serum of healthy individuals and in higher MIF production in both the serum and synovial fluids of JIA patients. Furthermore, this same promoter polymorphism of MIF (MIF-173*C) has also been shown to be predictive of disease outcome in patients with systemic-onset JIA.[61] More specifically, De Benedetti and coworkers found that carriage of the MIF-173*C polymorphism was correlated with raised serum and synovial fluid levels of MIF protein and predictive of the duration of response to intra-articular injection of triamcinolone hexacetonide (TXA). Those individuals with a mutant allele at −173 (MIF-173*C) experienced relapse more quickly than individuals with the MIF-173 GG wild-type genotype.[61] This effect has now been demonstrated also for the response to intra-articular TXA injection in patients with an oligoarticular phenotype, the most common presentation of JIA. Again, the duration of clinical response to the corticosteroid treatment (months with no clinical evidence of synovitis) was significantly shorter in patients carrying an MIF-173*C allele (median, 6 months; range, 1-39 months) than in the MIF-173*GG homozygotes (median, 9 months; range, 2-62 months).[62]

SLC11A1 (NRAMP1)

A study of persistent oligoarticular and RF-negative polyarticular JIA patients and controls from Latvia and a more limited number of Russian patients and controls found an association with the microsatellite marker D2S1471 (~80 kb downstream of the SLC11A1 locus) and a functional polymorphism in the natural resistance associated macrophage protein gene.[63] Runstadler and associates, in a large study of Finnish JIA nuclear families and controls, studied the same D2S1471 marker, additional intergenic SNPs, and an insertion deletion. This study again found evidence of association of the D2S1471 microsatellite marker with these subgroups of JIA and additionally found haplotypical associations spanning the SLC11A1 locus as a risk factor independent of the known HLA associations that occur in these JIA subgroups.[64]

Wnt1-inducible signaling pathway protein 3 (WISP3)

Mutations of the WISP3 gene are known to cause progressive pseudorheumatoid dysplasia, a rare syndrome that can clinically mimic polyarticular JIA.[65] Lamb and associates investigated SNPs of WISP3 in two independent polyarticular-course JIA patient cohorts and controls. Replication of association with a SNP within the first intron of the WISP3 gene (WISP3*G84A) was found.[66]

The era of whole genome association studies

The results of the first whole genome linkage scan, based on 247 JRA cases from 121 families, were published.[67] In addition to the HLA region, this study identified five putative regions (1p36, 1q31, 15q21, 19p13, and 20q13) important in JRA as a whole. Four of these regions overlap peaks of linkage described in other autoimmune diseases. This is particularly interesting in light of the findings of Prahalad and colleagues, who showed an increased prevalence of familial auto-immunity, and in particular Hashimoto thyroiditis, in simplex and multiplex families with JRA.[68] The genomic regions identified represent putative leads that will need fine mapping to potentially identify any genes involved in JIA susceptibility.

Whole-genome association studies (WGAS) examine hundreds of thousands of single nucleotide (SNP) variants in a large number of unrelated cases and controls. In 2007, the Wellcome Trust Case Control Consortium published its seminal manuscript detailing a genome-wide association study of 14,000 cases of seven common diseases and 3000 shared controls.[69] This represented a turning point in complex disease genetics, with most now agreeing that, for any given disease, the most informative way forward is by a WGAS approach. Several groups are currently undertaking such studies for JIA. To date, however, only one genome-wide association analysis in JIA has been published. Hinks and colleagues performed a genome-wide association study using Affymetrix GeneChip 100K arrays in 279 cases and 184 controls. By current standards this is a low-density SNP array and the sample numbers used are small. However, the authors were able to replicate an association with SNPs in the *VTCN1* gene.[70] This is a potentially interesting locus for involvement in JIA susceptibility because *VTCN1* is expressed on activated T cells, B cells, and monocytes and may be involved in the attenuation of the inflammatory response.[71]

There is also a current trend, post WGAS, to look at associated loci in different diseases, where there is some clinical or pathologic evidence of disease overlap. Taking this approach, Hinks and colleagues have looked at the *IL2RA/CD25* gene that encodes for the IL-2 receptor α chain. Association of SNPs within this gene have already been shown with type I diabetes mellitus, Graves' disease, rheumatoid arthritis, and multiple sclerosis, suggesting it as a pan-autoimmune locus. A large U.K. sample set of 654 JIA cases compared with 3849 controls was studied. Evidence of association of the rs2104286 SNP was seen. With the use of an independent cohort of samples from North America (747 JIA cases and 1161 controls), weak evidence of replication was found. This SNP appears to confer protection from JIA susceptibility with an odds ratio of around 0.8.[72]

CONCLUSION

JIA is an intriguing collection of phenotypes. Many diverse features occur along with a limited number of unifying ones (onset before 16 years of age, chronic synovitis of joints). Much research still needs to be done to elucidate the etiopathogenesis of JIA. Utilization of homogeneous patient groups, international collaborations to enhance patient numbers, and the application of emerging technologies, in particular the use of high-density SNP arrays and proteomic screening for biomarkers of JIA outcomes, is the way forward. Also, analysis of gene/gene as well as potential gene/environment interactions needs to be studied. Such approaches should accelerate productive research findings for these important groups of arthritides.

KEY REFERENCES

10. Johnson K, Wittkop B, Haigh F, et al. The early magnetic resonance imaging features of the knee in juvenile idiopathic arthritis. Clin Radiol 2002;57:466-471.
15. Nistala K, Moncrieffe H, Newton KR, et al. Interleukin-17-producing T cells are enriched in the joints of children with arthritis, but have a reciprocal relationship to regulatory T cell numbers. Arthritis Rheum 2008;58:875-887.
16. Martini A, Ravelli A, Notarangelo LD, et al. Enhanced interleukin 1 and depressed interleukin 2 production in juvenile arthritis. J Rheumatol 1986;13:598-603.
17. Harjacek M, Diaz-Cano S, Alman BA, et al. Prominent expression of mRNA for proinflammatory cytokines in synovium in patients with juvenile rheumatoid arthritis or chronic Lyme arthritis. J Rheumatol 2000;27:497-503.
18. Grom AA, Thompson SD, Luyrink L, et al. Dominant T-cell-receptor beta chain variable region V beta 14+ clones in juvenile rheumatoid arthritis. Proc Natl Acad Sci U S A 1993;90:11104-11108.
21. Lindblad S, Klareskog L, Hedfors E, et al. Phenotypic characterization of synovial tissue cells in situ in different types of synovitis. Arthritis Rheum 1983;26:1321-1332.
22. Allen JC, Kunkel HG. Hidden rheumatoid factors with specificity for native gamma globulins. Arthritis Rheum 1966;9:758-768.
24. Szer W, Sierakowska H, Szer IS. Antinuclear antibody profile in juvenile rheumatoid arthritis. J Rheumatol 1991;18:401-408.
25. Ferucci ED, Majka DS, Parrish LA, et al. Antibodies against cyclic citrullinated peptide are associated with HLA-DR4 in simplex and multiplex polyarticular-onset juvenile rheumatoid arthritis. Arthritis Rheum 2005;52:239-246.
29. Chantler JK, Tingle AJ, Petty RE. Persistent rubella virus infection associated with chronic arthritis in children. N Engl J Med 1985; 313:1117-1123.
30. Pritchard MH, Matthews N, Munro J. Antibodies to influenza A in a cluster of children with juvenile chronic arthritis. Br J Rheumatol 1988;27:176-180.
32. Heaton DC, Moller PW. Still's disease associated with Coxsackie infection and haemophagocytic syndrome. Ann Rheum Dis 1985;44:341-344.
33. Feldman BM, Birdi N, Boone JE, et al. Seasonal onset of systemic-onset juvenile rheumatoid arthritis. J Pediatr 1996;129:513-518.
34. Prieur A, Listrat V, Dougados M. Evaluation of the possible seasonal onset in juvenile arthritis from 2954 cases obtained from a multicentre European survey. Clin Exp Rheumatol 1994;12:S124.
35. Steere AC, Malawista SE, Snydman DR, et al. Lyme arthritis: an epidemic of oligoarticular arthritis in

children and adults in three Connecticut communities. Arthritis Rheum 1977;20:7-17.
36. Oen K, Fast M, Postl B. Epidemiology of juvenile rheumatoid arthritis in Manitoba, Canada, 1975-92: cycles in incidence. J Rheumatol 1995;22:745-750.
38. Life P, Hassell A, Williams K, et al. Responses to gram negative enteric bacterial antigens by synovial T cells from patients with juvenile chronic arthritis: recognition of heat shock protein HSP60. J Rheumatol 1993;20:1388-1396.
39. Albani S, Ravelli A, Massa M, et al. Immune responses to the *Escherichia coli* dnaJ heat shock protein in juvenile rheumatoid arthritis and their correlation with disease activity. J Pediatr 1994;124:561-565.
40. Massa M, Mazzoli F, Pignatti P, et al. Proinflammatory responses to self HLA epitopes are triggered by molecular mimicry to Epstein-Barr virus proteins in oligoarticular juvenile idiopathic arthritis. Arthritis Rheum 2002;46:2721-2729.
41. Prahalad S, Ryan MH, Shear ES, et al. Twins concordant for juvenile rheumatoid arthritis. Arthritis Rheum 2000;43:2611-2612.
42. Savolainen A, Saila H, Kotaniemi K, et al. Magnitude of the genetic component in juvenile idiopathic arthritis. Ann Rheum Dis 2000;59:1001.
43. Seldin MF, Amos CI, Ward R, Gregersen PK. The genetics revolution and the assault on rheumatoid arthritis. Arthritis Rheum 1999;42:1071-1079.
44. Moroldo MB, Tague BL, Shear ES, et al. Juvenile rheumatoid arthritis in affected sibpairs. Arthritis Rheum 1997;40:1962-1966.
45. Glass DN, Giannini EH. Juvenile rheumatoid arthritis as a complex genetic trait. Arthritis Rheum 1999;42:2261-2268.
46. Moroldo MB, Chaudhari M, Shear E, et al. Juvenile rheumatoid arthritis affected sibpairs: extent of clinical phenotype concordance. Arthritis Rheum 2004;50:1928-1934.
47. Saila HM, Savolainen HA, Kotaniemi KM, et al. Juvenile idiopathic arthritis in multicase families. Clin Exp Rheumatol 2001;19:218-220.
48. Donn RP, Ollier WE. Juvenile chronic arthritis—a time for change? Eur J Immunogenet 1996;23:245-260.
49. Thomson W, Barrett JH, Donn R, et al. Juvenile idiopathic arthritis classified by the ILAR criteria: HLA associations in UK patients. Rheumatology (Oxford) 2002;41:1183-1189.
50. Moroldo MB, Donnelly P, Saunders J, et al. Transmission disequilibrium as a test of linkage and association between HLA alleles and pauciarticular-onset juvenile rheumatoid arthritis. Arthritis Rheum 1998;41:1620-1624.

51. Zeggini E, Donn RP, Ollier WER, The BPRG Study Group, Thomson W. Genetic dissection of the major histocompatibility complex in juvenile oliogoarthritis. Arthritis Rheum 2002;46:S272.
52. Prahalad S, Ryan MH, Shear ES, et al. Juvenile rheumatoid arthritis: linkage to HLA demonstrated by allele sharing in affected sibpairs. Arthritis Rheum 2000;43:2335-2338.
53. Rosen P, Thompson S, Glass D. Non-HLA gene polymorphisms in juvenile rheumatoid arthritis. Clin Exp Rheumatol 2003;21:650-656.
54. Fishman D, Faulds G, Jeffery R, et al. The effect of novel polymorphisms in the interleukin-6 (IL-6) gene on IL-6 transcription and plasma IL-6 levels, and an association with systemic-onset juvenile chronic arthritis. J Clin Invest 1998;102:1369-1376.
55. Ogilvie EM, Fife MS, Thompson SD, et al. The −174G allele of the interleukin-6 gene confers susceptibility to systemic arthritis in children: a multicenter study using simplex and multiplex juvenile idiopathic arthritis families. Arthritis Rheum 2003;48:3202-3206.
56. Fife MS, Ogilvie EM, Kelberman D, et al. Novel IL-6 haplotypes and disease association. Genes Immun 2005;6:367-370.
57. Donn RP, Ray DW. Macrophage migration inhibitory factor: molecular, cellular and genetic aspects of a key neuroendocrine molecule. J Endocrinol 2004;182:1-9.
58. Donn RP, Shelley E, Ollier WE, Thomson W. A novel 5′-flanking region polymorphism of macrophage migration inhibitory factor is associated with systemic-onset juvenile idiopathic arthritis. Arthritis Rheum 2001;44:1782-1785.
59. Donn R, Alourfi Z, De Benedetti F, et al. Mutation screening of the macrophage migration inhibitory factor gene: positive association of a functional polymorphism of macrophage migration inhibitory factor with juvenile idiopathic arthritis. Arthritis Rheum 2002;46:2402-2409.
60. Donn R, Alourfi Z, Zeggini E, et al. A functional promoter haplotype of macrophage migration inhibitory factor is linked and associated with juvenile idiopathic arthritis. Arthritis Rheum 2004;50:1604-1610.
61. De Benedetti F, Meazza C, Vivarelli M, et al. Functional and prognostic relevance of the −173 polymorphism of the macrophage migration inhibitory factor gene in systemic-onset juvenile idiopathic arthritis. Arthritis Rheum 2003;48:1398-1407.
62. De Benedetti F, Vivarelli M, Lamb R, et al. Association of the −173 SNP of the macrophage migration inhibitory factor (MIF) gene with response to intraarticular glucocorticoids in oligoarticular JIA. Arthritis Rheum 2003;48:S254.

63. Sanjeevi CB, Miller EN, Dabadghao P, et al. Polymorphism at NRAMP1 and D2S1471 loci associated with juvenile rheumatoid arthritis. Arthritis Rheum 2000;43:1397-1404.
64. Runstadler JA, Saila H, Savolainen A, et al. Association of SLC11A1 (NRAMP1) with persistent oligoarticular and polyarticular rheumatoid factor-negative juvenile idiopathic arthritis in Finnish patients: haplotype analysis in Finnish families. Arthritis Rheum 2005;52:247-256.
65. Lamb R, Thomson W, Ogilvie E, Donn R. Wnt-1-inducible signaling pathway protein 3 and susceptibility to juvenile idiopathic arthritis. Arthritis Rheum 2005;52:3548-3553.
66. Thompson SD, Moroldo MB, Guyer L, et al. A genome-wide scan for juvenile rheumatoid arthritis in affected sibpair families provides evidence of linkage. Arthritis Rheum 2004;50:2920-2930.
67. Prahalad S, Shear ES, Thompson SD, et al. Increased prevalence of familial autoimmunity in simplex and multiplex families with juvenile rheumatoid arthritis. Arthritis Rheum 2002;46:1851-1856.
68. Wellcome Trust Case Control Consortium. Genome-wide association study of 14,000 cases of seven common diseases and 3,000 shared controls. Nature 2007;447:661-678.
69. Hinks A, Barton A, Shephard N, et al. Identification of a novel susceptibility locus for juvenile idiopathic arthritis by genome-wide association analysis. Arthritis Rheum 2009;60:258-263.
70. Sica GL, Choi IH, Zhu G, et al. B7-H4, a molecule of the B7 family, negatively regulates T cell immunity. Immunity 2003;18:849-861.
71. Hinks A, Ke X, Barton A, et al. Association of the IL2RA/CD25 gene with juvenile idiopathic arthritis. Arthritis Rheum 2009;60:251-257.

REFERENCES

Full references for this chapter can be found on www.expertconsult.com.

Management of juvenile idiopathic arthritis

100

Philip J. Hashkes and Ronald M. Laxer

MEDICAL MANAGEMENT

- The treatment approach to JIA has changed in recent years from the pyramidal approach to early aggressive therapy.
- The treatment is individualized according to subtype of JIA and the presence of uveitis.
- Many new medications are available in children, especially biologic modifiers, with effects on varying immunologic pathways.

SURGICAL MANAGEMENT

- The need for surgical therapy may be decreasing as a result of improved medical management.
- The role of synovectomy in the treatment of JIA, particularly oligoarthritis, is still not clear.
- There are several issues specific to children in arthroplasty surgery.

OTHER ISSUES OF MANAGEMENT

- Greater attention needs to be given to the treatment of pain.
- Issues of bone health and growth need to be addressed.
- Physical and occupational therapy as well as assistive devices, splints, and orthotics are an important part of therapy (addressed in detail in Chapter 103).

INTRODUCTION

The treatment of juvenile idiopathic arthritis (JIA) has changed dramatically in the past 20 years. Until the late 1980s, aspirin and other non-steroidal anti-inflammatory drugs (NSAIDs) were the predominant medications used to treat children with JIA, with additional use of systemic corticosteroids, gold, hydroxychloroquine, and D-penicillamine. The first change occurred in the late 1980s with the increasing use of intra-articular corticosteroid injections in children with oligoarthritis and of methotrexate (MTX) in those with polyarthritis. The second major change occurred in the late 1990s with the development of biologic modifiers, first anti–tumor necrosis factor (TNF) medications and later biologic modifiers targeting other cytokines involved in the inflammatory process or lymphocyte receptors.

The discovery of new effective medications was facilitated by the development of research networks. The Pediatric Rheumatology Collaborative Study Group (PRCSG) in North America and the Pediatric Rheumatology International Trials Organization (PRINTO) in Europe and elsewhere have conducted high-quality, multicenter, multinational controlled trials. Another important development was the validation of efficacy outcome measures (Table 100.1). The American College of Rheumatology (ACR) Pediatric 30 (Pediatric ACR30) defines patients as responders or non-responders (Table 100.2).[1] This outcome measure has been modified for systemic arthritis studies (includes the absence of fever and characteristic rash) and to define a flare outcome in drug withdrawal studies, used mainly in studies of rapid-acting biologic modifiers. Because of the advent of powerful biologic-modifying medications, patients and physicians expect to achieve much better responses than those of the Pediatric ACR30. Thus, most new studies also report the Pediatric ACR50/70/90 and even ACR100 response criteria. Recently, preliminary definitions of remission have been reported with three levels: inactive disease, clinical remission on medication, and clinical remission off medication (Table 100.3).[2] New tools to assess disease activity as a composite numeric score based on modified joint counts, parental and physical global assessment, and inflammatory markers are being developed. Long-term outcome tools including specific radiographic composite scores and clinical damage index tools are in the process of validation.[3] Several functional tools and quality of life tools have been validated and adapted for JIA.

The treatment philosophy of JIA has also undergone a transformation. In the past, treatment was based on the "pyramid" approach, initially using various types of NSAIDs and corticosteroids and gradually advancing to other medications.[4] Studies in the late 1980s indicated that earlier assumptions on the course and outcome of JIA were incorrect. Radiologic joint damage, previously thought to occur late in the disease course, occurs in most patients with systemic arthritis and polyarthritis within 2 years and in oligoarthritis within 5 years of disease onset[5] and perhaps earlier as shown by magnetic resonance imaging (MRI).

The assumption that JIA will usually resolve by adulthood is also incorrect. Studies have shown that between 50% and 70% of patients with polyarthritis or systemic arthritis and 40% to 50% of patients with oligoarthritis will continue to have active disease in adulthood.[5,6] Only a minority of patients will even attain clinical remission off medications for at least 2 years, and only 4% attained a remission for at least 5 years.[6] Between 30% and 40% of patients have significant long-term disabilities, including unemployment, and between 25% and 50% need major surgery, including joint replacement.[7] Patients with oligoarthritis frequently develop leg-length inequality and muscle atrophy near affected joints.[8] Patients with systemic arthritis have an increased mortality rate, mainly from amyloidosis (almost exclusively in Europe) and the macrophage activation syndrome. Thus, the burden of disease to the patient, family, and, ultimately, society, is large; and it is crucial to recognize the disease and treat it early and aggressively, before soft tissue deformities and joint damage become irreversible.

Several predictors of a poor outcome can help determine patients requiring early aggressive therapy. Patients with polyarthritis and positive rheumatoid factor (RF), anti-citrullinated peptide antibodies (ACPAs), the presence of HLA-DR4, nodules, and early-onset symmetric small joint involvement have a worse prognosis. Patients with systemic arthritis who are corticosteroid dependent for control of systemic symptoms and have a platelet count greater than 600,000/mm^3 after 6 months of disease have a worse outcome.[9]

The treatment of JIA depends to a large extent on the disease subtype and combines anti-inflammatory and immunomodulatory medications with physical and occupational therapy, an occasional need for surgery, nutritional support, and psychosocial and educational partnership with patients and parents. The treatment plan should try to be as simple as possible based on studies showing relatively low adherence to recommendations, both to medications and, to a larger extent, physical therapy and exercise.[10] Fortunately, many of the modern JIA medications are given once weekly or less (many by injection), making it easier to adhere to the treatment plan. The increased efficacy has decreased the rate of many complications and deformities, thus somewhat diminishing the roles of rehabilitation therapy and surgery as compared with the past. In this chapter we will present guidelines for the medical treatment (Table 100.4) and other therapies for JIA (including uveitis) and offer a rational approach for the treatment of the various subtypes of disease.

NON-STEROIDAL ANTI-INFLAMMATORY DRUGS

The actual efficacy of NSAIDs (Table 100.5) is unknown because none of the studies was placebo controlled. In a summary of studies, only

TABLE 100.1 ASSESSMENT AND OUTCOME MEASURE TOOLS FOR JIA

Domain	Assessment tools
Disease activity	Active joint count, acute-phase reactants
Global assessment	Physician, patient visual analog scale
Functional assessment	Childhood Health Assessment Questionnaire (CHAQ), Juvenile Arthritis Functional Assessment Report (JAFAR), Juvenile Arthritis Functional Status Index (JASI)
Quality of life assessment	Childhood Health Questionnaire (CHQ), Peds-Quality of Life (QOL)—Rheumatology subset, pain visual analog scale
Radiologic damage	Poznanski, Dijkstra scores
Disease-related irreversible damage	Juvenile Arthritis Damage Index (JADI)
Clinical trial outcome measures	American College of Rheumatology Pediatric 30 (Pediatric ACR30) (modified for systemic arthritis and flare), criteria for inactive disease or clinical remission

TABLE 100.2 THE PEDIATRIC ACR30 FOR JIA TRIALS

1. Active joint count (joints with swelling or tender/pain on motion)
2. Joints with limited range of motion
3. Parent/patient global assessment (measured on 0-10 visual analog scale)
4. Physician global assessment (measured on 0-10 visual analog scale)
5. Laboratory measure of inflammation (erythrocyte sedimentation rate, C-reactive protein)
6. Functional assessment (Childhood Health Assessment Questionnaire)

NOTE: A patient's disease is considered to have responded if there has been an improvement in at least three variables by at least 30% and worsening in not more than one variable by more than 30%.
From Giannini EH, Ruperto N, Ravelli A, et al. Preliminary definition of improvement in juvenile arthritis. Arthritis Rheum 1997;40:1202-1209.

TABLE 100.3 CRITERIA AND TYPES OF REMISSION IN JIA

1. No active arthritis
2. No fever, rash, serositis, splenomegaly, or generalized lymphadenopathy attributable to JIA
3. No active uveitis
4. Normal erythrocyte sedimentation rate or C-reactive protein
5. Physician's global assessment of disease activity at the best score possible for the instrument used

Clinical remission on medication: 6 continuous months of inactive disease on medication
Clinical remission off medication: 12 months of inactive disease off all anti-arthritis (and anti-uveitis) medications.
From Wallace CA, Ruperto N, Giannini E, et al. Preliminary criteria for clinical remission for select categories of juvenile idiopathic arthritis. J Rheumatol 2004;31:2290-2294.

TABLE 100.4 MAJOR MEDICATIONS AND INDICATIONS FOR TREATMENT OF JIA

Medication	Arthritis subtype	Indication
NSAIDs	All types	Symptomatic: pain, stiffness, anti-inflammatory in mild cases
Intra-articular corticosteroids	All types, mainly oligoarthritis	Injection of few active joints
Systemic corticosteroids	Systemic, polyarthritis	Fever, serositis, bridging medication, macrophage activation syndrome
Methotrexate	All types, less effective in systemic and enthesitis-related axial disease	Disease-modifying
Leflunomide	Polyarthritis	Disease-modifying
Sulfasalazine	Oligoarthritis, polyarthritis, enthesitis-related peripheral disease	Disease-modifying
Cyclosporine	Systemic	Macrophage activation syndrome
Thalidomide	Systemic	Biologic modifier
Anti-TNF (etanercept infliximab, adalimumab)	Polyarthritis, enthesitis-related Uveitis (infliximab, adalimumab), less effective in systemic	Biologic modifier
Abatacept	Polyarthritis, including anti-TNF failure	Biologic modifier
Anti-IL-1 (anakinra, rilonacept, canakinumab)	Systemic	Biologic modifier
Anti-IL-6 (tocilizumab)	Systemic	Biologic modifier
IVIg	Systemic	Steroid-sparing

NSAIDs, non-steroidal anti-inflammatory drugs; TNF, tumor necrosis factor; IL, interleukin; IVIg, intravenous immunoglobulin.

treatment of JIA. It is important to consider the dosing schedule and form of giving NSAIDs, with a preference to once- or twice-daily dosing because recent studies showed a low compliance of patients taking NSAIDs, with as many as half of the patients adherent less than 80% of the time.[10] Suspension preparations are available for naproxen, ibuprofen, meloxicam, and indomethacin; and celecoxib is available as sprinkable capsules.

NSAIDs approved by the U.S. Food and Drug Administration (FDA) for use in JIA include tolmetin, naproxen, ibuprofen, meloxicam, and celecoxib (Table 100.5). Other NSAIDs that underwent controlled studies include diclofenac, ketoprofen, indomethacin, fenoprofen, sulindac, and rofecoxib.[11,12] Comparative efficacy of nabumetone was reported in an open study.[13] Rofecoxib was approved by the FDA for JIA but was removed from the market because of cardiovascular adverse events in adults.

Serious gastrointestinal adverse effects of NSAIDs are rare, although as many as 28% of children develop gastrointestinal symptoms. Of these, 34% to 75% were found to have gastritis and/or duodenitis.[4] There was not a significant reduction in the incidence of gastrointestinal adverse effect with the cyclooxygenase-2 selective celecoxib compared with naproxen.[12] These adverse effects can often be prevented by taking NSAIDs with food, but, if not, switching to another NSAID or using proton pump inhibitors or misoprostol may improve symptoms. Another important adverse effect is the development of pseudoporphyria, which is most often associated with the use of naproxen (prevalence up to 11.4%)[14] in fair-haired white patients when used for oligoarthritis and usually occurs within 2 years of use. The scarring

25% to 33% of the patients, mainly those with oligoarthritis, showed a significant response to NSAIDs.[4] A 4-week trial of an individual NSAID is necessary to assess its efficacy. Because NSAIDs were not shown to alter the disease course or prevent joint damage, they are used more to treat pain, stiffness, and the fever associated with systemic arthritis. No individual NSAID has been shown to have a clear advantage over others in treating arthritis, although there are suggestions that indomethacin may be more beneficial for treatment of the fever and pericarditis of systemic arthritis and enthesitis-related arthritis. The need to administer aspirin four times per day and to monitor serum levels, the association of Reye syndrome with salicylates, and other aspirin-related side effects (mainly liver enzyme abnormalities) have largely resulted in other NSAIDs replacing aspirin in the

TABLE 100.5 DOSAGE AND SPECIAL CHARACTERISTICS OF NSAIDS COMMONLY USED TO TREAT JIA

NSAID	Dose			How supplied	Special characteristics
	In mg/kg	Max.	Times per day		
Acetylsalicylic acid	80-100	4000	3-4	Tablet	Need to measure levels, liver enzyme abnormalities, risk for Reye syndrome
Naproxen*	15-20	1000	2	Tablet, suspension	Pseudoporphyria
Ibuprofen*	30-50	2400	3-4	Tablet, suspension	
Indomethacin	1.5-3.0	200	1-2	Capsule, suspension	More gastrointestinal and neurologic adverse events, perhaps more beneficial for fever, pericarditis in systemic and enthesitis-related arthritis
Tolmetin*	20-30	1800	3	Tablet	
Sulindac	4-6	400	2	Tablet	Fewer renal adverse events
Diclofenac	2-3	200	2	Tablet	
Piroxicam	0.2-0.3	20	1	Tablet	More gastrointestinal adverse effects
Etodolac	10-20	1000	2	Tablet, capsule	
Meloxicam*	0.25-0.375	15	1	Tablet, suspension	
Nabumetone	30	2000	1	Tablet	
Celecoxib*	3-6	200	2	Capsule	Use for bleeding disorders, cross-reacts with sulfa allergies

NSAID, Non-steroidal anti-inflammatory drug.
*Approved by the U. S. Food and Drug Administration for the treatment of JIA.

resulting from pseudoporphyria may not resolve for years. Central nervous system adverse effects may occur, including headaches and disorientation, especially from indomethacin. Renal adverse effects, particularly papillary necrosis or tubular function abnormalities, are uncommon in children but are more frequent during concurrent use of more than one NSAID. The issue of cardiovascular adverse effects was not addressed, but there are no reports of these events in children with JIA; however, only two NSAID studies (naproxen, meloxicam) prospectively followed JIA patients for at least 6 months.[11]

CORTICOSTEROIDS

Because of many deleterious effects, especially the effect on bone and growth, pediatric rheumatologists try to minimize the use of systemic corticosteroids for JIA. There is no evidence that systemic corticosteroids are disease modifying. The main indications for the use of systemic corticosteroids are severe fever, serositis, and the macrophage activation syndrome in patients with systemic arthritis. They are also frequently used as a bridging medication until other disease-modifying medications take effect. In some patients periodic intravenous pulses of corticosteroids (30 mg/kg/dose, maximal 1 g, usually given for 1-3 consecutive days) are used instead of high-dose daily oral corticosteroids, although there are no controlled studies showing fewer adverse effects of this modality in children and the effect is short lived. High-dose alternate-day corticosteroids may be an alternative to daily corticosteroids in systemic arthritis, with one series showing equal efficacy and fewer adverse events.[15] One controlled study showed that the use of intravenous "mini-pulses" of corticosteroids in the first week of using corticosteroids to treat systemic arthritis resulted in lower daily and cumulative doses at 6 months when compared with traditional initial oral doses of corticosteroids.[16]

There is better evidence for the efficacy of intra-articular injections of corticosteroids, mainly in patients with oligoarthritis. A Markov decision-analysis model comparing various modalities of treatment for knee monoarthritis found that an initial intra-articular corticosteroid injection was associated with the best patient outcome in terms of efficacy, duration of active arthritis, and adverse effects.[17] As many as 70% of patients with oligoarthritis do not have reactivation of disease in the injected joint for at least 1 year, and in 40% to 60% of patients this can be for more than 2 years.[18] Radiographic and MRI studies have shown a marked decrease in synovial volume after injection without deleterious effects on the cartilage. There were significantly fewer patients with leg-length discrepancies in a practice advocating repeated

early intra-articular corticosteroid injections when compared with a practice rarely employing intra-articular injections.[8] The efficacy is less in patients with systemic arthritis. Two studies found that systemic and oligoarthritis patients with the 173-C macrophage migration inhibitory factor gene polymorphism responded less well to intra-articular corticosteroids. Several controlled studies, including a study of simultaneous injections of bilateral inflamed joints in individual patients, have found that long-acting triamcinolone hexacetonide was more effective and had a longer effect than other forms of injectable corticosteroids.[19] Other reported factors associated with a longer remission after intra-articular injections include injection of the knee (as opposed to other joints), concomitant use of MTX, and the use of general anesthesia for the procedure. Intra-articular corticosteroid injections are also useful in the treatment of temporomandibular joint (TMJ) arthritis. For some joints it may be preferable to inject using radiologic guidance, particularly joints with difficult access, such as the hip, subtalar or temporomandibular joints, or complex multiple joints like the wrist.[20] Studies in adults have shown a lack of equal distribution of corticosteroid throughout the wrist joints when injection is performed without radiologic guidance.

There are few adverse effects associated with these injections, most often the development of periarticular subcutaneous atrophy and/or asymptomatic intra-articular calcifications (Fig. 100.1). In some joints, especially the subtalar joint, this may occur in as many as 53% of injections. This may be prevented by injecting small amounts of saline into the joint after the injection and by applying pressure to the injection site. Repeated injections to an individual joint (generally not more than every 3 months) were not found to be associated with joint or cartilage damage. Patients must be warned about the risks of infection, although this is extremely rare when done in aseptic conditions. Occasional cases of aseptic necrosis more likely result from severe underlying disease than the joint injection.

Younger children, or children needing multiple joint injections, usually require sedation during the procedure. Various types of sedation have been employed, including nitrous oxide, various methods of conscious sedation, and general anesthesia. The use of lidocaine-based cream before the procedure was found in a controlled study not to be beneficial in pain reduction.[21]

METHOTREXATE

The use of MTX is the cornerstone of the treatment plan for most patients with polyarthritis (Table 100.6).[22-24] A large, open, randomized

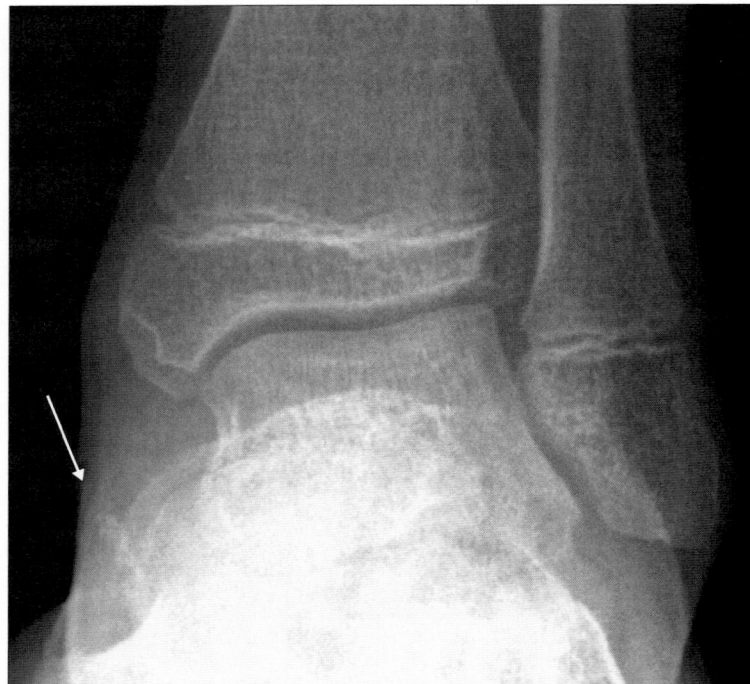

Fig. 100.1 Radiograph of ankle joint demonstrating calcifications secondary to corticosteroid injection.

TABLE 100.6 DOSAGES AND MAJOR ADVERSE REACTIONS OF OTHER MAJOR MEDICATIONS USED TO TREAT JIA

Medication	Dose	Main adverse reactions
Methotrexate	10-15 mg/m²/wk (parenteral if >12.5 mg/m²), max. 30 mg	Gastrointestinal symptoms, mouth sores, liver enzymes, cytopenia
Sulfasalazine	30-50 mg/kg/day, max. 3000 mg, divided in 2 doses	Gastrointestinal symptoms, rashes (Stevens-Johnson syndrome), cytopenia
Leflunomide	<20 kg: 10 mg every other day	Gastrointestinal symptoms, increased liver enzymes
	20-40 kg: 10 mg/day	
	>40 kg: 20 mg/day	
Etanercept	0.8 mg/kg, max. 50 mg, SC injection once weekly or 0.4 mg/kg twice weekly	Injection site reaction, upper respiratory symptoms, infections
Adalimumab	<30 kg: 20 mg SC injection every other week ≥30 kg: 40 mg SC injection every other week	Injection site reaction, upper respiratory symptoms, infections
Infliximab	6 mg/kg, intravenously at weeks 0, 2, 6 then every 6-8 weeks (may need to administer every 4 weeks)	Infusion reactions (allergic), infections
Anakinra	1-2 mg/kg/day SC injection, max. 100 mg	Injection site reaction, upper respiratory symptoms, infections
Abatacept	10 mg/kg, intravenous at week 0, 2, 4 then every 4 weeks, max. 1000 mg	Infections
Tocilizumab	<20 kg: 12 mg/kg, intravenous every 2 weeks ≥20 kg: 8 mg/kg, intravenous every 2 weeks	Infections, liver enzymes, hypercholesterolemia
Triamcinolone hexacetonide	For large joints: 1 mg/kg IA injection, max. 40 mg	Potential for infection, subcutaneous atrophy, intra-articular calcifications

study showed that increasing the dose of MTX to 15 mg/m²/wk and giving it by subcutaneous injection was effective for most patients not responsive to 10 mg/m²/wk given orally. There was no additional advantage in giving higher doses up to 30 mg/m²/wk.[25]

The efficacy of MTX differs by the subtype of JIA, with the greatest efficacy seen in patients with extended oligoarthritis and much lower effects in patients with systemic arthritis.[23] The presence of the 1298C allele in the methylenetetrahydrofolate reductase (*MTHFR*) gene was associated with increased efficacy compared with the A allele.[26] MTX may exhibit a disease-modifying effect because the radiologic damage progression rate was decreased in two small uncontrolled series. MTX treatment was also found to improve growth parameters at 1 and 3 years, both for height and weight, among prepubertal children who responded to MTX.[27] The early response to MTX may be predictive of the long-term outcome. Patients with a Pediatric ACR70 response to MTX by 6 months had significantly less active joints and joints with limitation of motion than patients with a lesser or no response years later. MTX also improves the health-related quality of life.

It is not clear when MTX should be discontinued in patients who have responded. Patients with JIA may experience a flare in up to 60% of cases after discontinuing MTX, usually by 18 months. One retrospective survey found that continuing MTX for more than 1 year after inactive disease was associated with a lower rate of flare, but another study did not find differences between patients who discontinued MTX 3 months after disease inactivity and at 1 year. The level of myeloid-basic protein 14 was a better measure to predict which patients would experience a flare when MTX was discontinued.[28] Nearly 90% of the patients responded when MTX was restarted. There is no good evidence about the preferred method of tapering MTX before discontinuation.

Because food decreases the bioavailability of MTX it is advised to give MTX on an empty stomach. At doses of 10 mg/m²/wk there is no difference in the efficacy of MTX whether administered orally or parenterally, although parenteral MTX may be better tolerated. MTX at greater doses is usually given by subcutaneous or intramuscular injection, because oral MTX is not absorbed well at doses greater than or equal to 12 mg/m².

MTX should be administered with folic acid, 1 mg/day, or folinic acid, 25% to 50% of the MTX dose, given once weekly the day after MTX. A controlled study of folic acid and a retrospective study of folinic acid found decreased adverse effects of nausea, oral ulcerations, and perhaps liver enzyme abnormalities without decreasing the efficacy of MTX.[29]

Nausea and other gastrointestinal symptoms are frequent. Strategies to decrease the severity of these phenomena include taking MTX before bed, switching the mode of administration (oral to parenteral), and using antiemetics. Many children, especially adolescents, develop a psychological aversion to MTX, which may include anticipatory nausea or behavioral distress before the administration of MTX. This adverse effect may be alleviated by behavioral therapy, including teaching relaxation or self-hypnosis techniques. Although mild elevations of liver enzymes occur frequently through the course of treatment, no cases of severe, irreversible liver fibrosis have been reported in JIA.[30] Routine liver biopsies are not recommended. Persistent liver enzyme abnormalities and obesity are associated with more significant liver histology changes, including mild fibrosis, and liver biopsies should be considered in those patients. The presence of the 677T allele in the *MTHFR* gene was associated with more adverse effects (nausea, liver enzyme abnormalities, and hair loss) than the C allele in one study.[26]

Tests to monitor for MTX toxicity, complete blood cell counts, liver enzymes, and renal function are recommended, although the optimal frequency of testing is unclear. Although most pediatric rheumatologists follow adult ACR guidelines in testing every 4 to 8 weeks, one study reported that tests at 3-month intervals at doses up to 15 mg/m²/wk detected significant hematologic and liver enzyme abnormalities as often as testing at monthly intervals. Pulmonary toxicity is very rare in children. Nodulosis has rarely been reported. Very few severe infections have been reported in children. Recent studies showing efficacy of mumps, measles, and rubella vaccine without causing disease flare have resulted in many pediatric rheumatologists modifying previous recommendations that children avoid live vaccinations while using MTX.[31] Non-live vaccinations are safe to be given, and seasonal influenza vaccine is recommended. The issue of varicella vaccine has not been studied. If possible, children should receive varicella vaccine before starting MTX, although it is not clear how long after it is necessary to wait before starting MTX. Rare cases of Hodgkin's and non-Hodgkin's lymphoma have been reported in children treated with MTX, in one case associated with Epstein-Barr virus infection. Although no formal studies were done, current data do not suggest that the rate of malignancies is greater than in the general child population. There does not seem to be any long-term impact on fertility.

OTHER DISEASE-MODIFYING ANTI-RHEUMATIC DRUGS (DMARDS) AND IMMUNOSUPPRESSIVE MEDICATIONS (Tables 100.6 and 100.7)

Most controlled studies in children did not find hydroxychloroquine, oral gold, or D-penicillamine to be significantly effective in the treatment of JIA, although one study using less rigorous outcome measures found that D-penicillamine was more effective than placebo in the treatment of oligoarthritis and polyarthritis.[4,11] A subsequent study could not find differences between responders and non-responders to those drugs.[4] One study did not find parenteral gold to be more effective than D-penicillamine or hydroxychloroquine.[11]

Most studies of sulfasalazine were not controlled. One controlled study showed that sulfasalazine is effective in the treatment of oligoarthritis and polyarthritis,[32] and an earlier introduction of treatment may result in better long-term outcomes. A follow-up of 61 of 68 patients in that study for a median of 9 years reported that the effectiveness of those who received sulfasalazine persisted, with 77% of the sulfasalazine group still considered at follow-up to be responders by the

TABLE 100.7 EFFICACY OF COMMON MEDICATIONS USED TO TREAT JIA

Medication	Efficacy		
	Persistent Oligoarthritis	Polyarticular-onset JIA	Systemic-onset arthritis
NSAID	Mild-moderate	Mild	Mild
Intra-articular corticosteroids	Significant	Moderate	Mild-moderate
Methotrexate	Significant	Significant	Mild
Leflunomide	Unknown	Significant	Unknown
Sulfasalazine	Unclear	Moderate	Contraindicated[†]
Etanercept	Unknown	Significant	Moderate
Infliximab	Unknown	Significant*	Moderate
Adalimumab	Unknown	Significant	Unknown
Abatacept	Unknown	Significant	Unknown
Anakinra	Unknown	Moderate*	Moderate-significant
Rilonacept	Unknown	Unknown	Moderate-significant
Tocilizumab	Unknown	Unknown	Significant

Mild: effective in up to 25% of patients; Moderate: effective in 25%-50% of patients; Significant: effective in more than 50% of patients. For intra-articular corticosteroids, efficacy was measured as benefit for more than 6 months.
NSAID, non-steroidal anti-inflammatory drug.
NOTE: Non-effective medications (i.e., hydroxychloroquine, penicillamine, oral gold, azathioprine) or medications not commonly used (cyclophosphamide, intravenous immunoglobulin, thalidomide, collagen) or not studied in children (rituximab, minocycline) were not included in this table. Evidence is lacking on the utility of medications in the other types of JIA.
*Was not significantly more effective than placebo in controlled study.
†Sulfasalazine is associated with development of macrophage activation syndrome in patients with systemic disease.

Pediatric ACR30 versus none of the original placebo group, even though 83% of the placebo group received sulfasalazine when the randomized phase was completed. The sulfasalazine group also reported improved well-being and had more patients in remission off medication after 9 years than the placebo group.[33] Sulfasalazine may also have disease-modifying effects on radiologic progression.[3]

In a small placebo-controlled study of juvenile spondyloarthropathy comparing sulfasalazine with chloroquine in oligoarthritis and polyarthritis, no significant differences were found.[11] In many of the open studies sulfasalazine was most effective in older males with oligoarthritis, representing, perhaps, children with enthesitis-related arthritis. Adverse reactions were frequently reported, especially rashes, gastrointestinal symptoms, and leukopenia, and sulfasalazine was discontinued in nearly one third of the patients. The dose of sulfasalazine is usually gradually increased to prevent some of these adverse events. Adverse effects may be especially severe in patients with systemic arthritis, with the potential for the development of macrophage activation syndrome. Sulfasalazine is contraindicated in patients with porphyria and glucose-6-phosphate dehydrogenase deficiency.

In a controlled study comparing leflunomide to MTX for patients with polyarthritis, significantly more responders were found in the MTX group, although high response rates were also found with leflunomide.[34] Many of the leflunomide non-responders were in the younger group receiving 10 mg every other day. Indeed, pharmacokinetic studies showed a lower steady-state concentration of the active metabolite of leflunomide in children weighing less than 40 kg, suggesting that some of the smaller children may have responded to a higher dose.[35] Most of the patients responsive to leflunomide maintained their response in a 2-year open label extension study. No significant differences in adverse effects were found. A controlled study of azathioprine in JIA did not find a significantly greater efficacy than placebo.[11] There are no studies of minocycline use in JIA.

There are no controlled studies of cyclosporine in JIA. Small series have shown cyclosporine to be efficacious in some patients refractory to MTX. However, in a large international phase 4 post-marketing study of the use of cyclosporine in 329 patients, remission was reported in only 9% of patients, whereas 61% continued to have moderate to severe arthritis and discontinued the medication due to lack of efficacy.[36] Cyclosporine may be more beneficial for fever control and corticosteroid dose reduction than for the treatment of patients with systemic arthritis and may be especially effective in patients with the macrophage activation syndrome.[37] There were many adverse effects, especially renal, associated with cyclosporine.[36]

One large, open series showed chlorambucil to be beneficial in patients with refractory JIA, especially those with amyloidosis, but the high mortality rate (6%), including the development of leukemia, precludes using the drug other than as a last resort.[38]

Two multicenter series found that thalidomide was effective for 26 of 32 patients with refractory systemic arthritis, both for systemic features and arthritis, with most patients able to significantly reduce their corticosteroid use and obtaining at least a Pediatric ACR30 response.[39] However, 5 patients developed peripheral neuropathy (2 clinically and 3 by electromyography monitoring). Therefore, besides the teratogenic effect, careful observation for the development of peripheral neuropathy is necessary. Drowsiness may be significant and may require dose reduction or discontinuation.

There are no controlled studies of combination DMARD therapy with or without MTX in JIA. In a series of 17 patients with polyarthritis refractory to MTX, treated with MTX and cyclosporine, 8 (47%) met the Pediatric ACR30 criteria for improvement. In a study of 18 patients with systemic arthritis an excellent response rate was found in all patients treated with a combination of intravenous pulse corticosteroids and cyclophosphamide, 400 mg/m^2, given every 3 months with MTX, 10 mg/m^2/wk, when treated early in the disease course for 1 year. However no long-term results have been reported.[11]

BIOLOGIC-MODIFYING MEDICATIONS

Anti-TNF medications

Three anti-TNF medications are currently used in JIA: (1) etanercept, a genetically engineered p75-soluble TNF receptor fused to the Fc domain fragment of human IgG1; (2) adalimumab, a humanized TNF antibody; and (3) infliximab, a murine-based TNF antibody.

Etanercept and adalimumab both have been approved by the FDA for use in polyarticular-onset JIA after they were found to be effective in two-phase withdrawal studies.[40,41] One study found that patients with the 308GG polymorphism in the TNF promoter gene responded significantly more frequently to etanercept than those with 308GA or AA.[42] Several uncontrolled studies and surveys have suggested that etanercept and infliximab are less effective in patients with systemic arthritis and that the initial response is often not sustained in these patients.[43] An excellent response to anti-TNF medications has been reported in uncontrolled studies of patients with juvenile spondyloarthropathies.[44] These agents usually have a rapid onset of action, but the maximal effect may take several months.

The dose of etanercept is either 0.4 mg/kg (max: 25 mg) given subcutaneously twice weekly or 0.8 mg/kg (max: 50 mg) once weekly and is approved from the age of 2 years. Adalimumab is given subcutaneously at a dose of 20 mg every other week in children weighing less than 30 kg and 40 mg every other week in children larger than 30 kg and is approved from the age of 4 years. In the controlled study, infliximab did not attain statistical significance compared with placebo for the primary outcome, mainly owing to study design and conduct issues, but it still was effective in the majority of patients.[45] Infliximab is given intravenously, initially at a dose of 6 mg/kg at weeks 0, 2, and 6 and then every 8 weeks. This dose is associated with fewer adverse effects than 3 mg/kg, especially infusion reactions and the development of human anti-chimeric antibodies to infliximab.[45]

Open-label extension studies of the original pivotal study etanercept cohort for up to 8 years as well as other registries have shown continued efficacy in the majority of patients, although MTX was added to many of the patients and prednisone to some.[46] More than 50% of patients on anti-TNF medications have a response greater than the Pediatric ACR70 level. These and other studies have shown a survival of the first anti-TNF medications of 50% to 60% after 4 years, with the major cause of discontinuation being lack of efficacy in 20% to 30% of patients and adverse events in 22% of infliximab-treated patients and 7% of those treated with etanercept. Nearly a similar survival rate was found in about the one third of patients switched to another anti-TNF medication.[47]

No controlled studies were published on the combination of etanercept with MTX versus etanercept or MTX alone, although in the German registry data there was a higher Pediatric ACR30/50/70 response in patients receiving the MTX-etanercept combination as opposed to etanercept monotherapy.[48] However, there may be greater adverse effects in the combination group with more infections and non-infectious serious adverse effects reported in the combination group, including three malignancies, as compared with the monotherapy group. Similar efficacy results were found in the pivotal adalimumab study with a tendency for greater response when combined with MTX, although the study was not powered for this outcome.[41] A controlled study comparing the use of etanercept-MTX combination therapy (with low-dose prednisone in the first 4 months) versus MTX monotherapy for early polyarthritis is in advanced stages of enrollment.

Initial signs of a disease-modifying effect of anti-TNF medications have been found, including slower radiologic progression measured by the Poznanski score among 40 patients compared with a historic MTX cohort of 67 patients.[49] Other improved outcome measures related to anti-TNF therapy include significant increase in bone strength measured by ultrasound among etanercept responders after a year of treatment, improved growth velocity independent of corticosteroid dose and pubertal stage, and improved functional status and quality of life.

Adverse effects of anti-TNF medications, although potentially severe, are generally mild, mainly injection site reactions, upper respiratory infections, and headaches.[40,41,45,46] However, in a series of 61 patients with polyarthritis and systemic arthritis, 12 (20%) discontinued etanercept due to adverse effects, including neurologic symptoms, psychiatric problems, severe infections, cutaneous vasculitis, and pancytopenia. One case of aseptic meningitis complicating varicella and other bacterial infections needing hospitalization has been reported. One patient developed group A β-hemolytic streptococcal sepsis that resulted in amputation of a foot.[40] Rare cases of tuberculosis and histoplasmosis were reported in the use of anti-TNF medications for JIA. Rare cases of malignancy, mainly lymphoma, have been reported in children and young adults treated with anti-TNF for JIA and Crohn's disease, but it is not clear whether the rate is greater than that expected in population or disease-cohort studies.[48] The FDA has issued an updated boxed warning highlighting the increased risk of cancer, including lymphoma, leukemia, and melanoma, in children and adolescents who receive anti-TNF agents. Autoimmune phenomena have been reported in several children or young adults with JIA, including the development of diabetes mellitus after 2 months of etanercept therapy, drug-induced lupus, cutaneous vasculitis, and central nervous system demyelination. Administering infliximab at a dose of 6 mg/kg as well as premedication with acetaminophen, diphenhydramine, and, occasionally, hydrocortisone may prevent or minimize infusion reactions that may rarely result in anaphylaxis. Overall, the rate of serious adverse effects from anti-TNF medications is estimated at 0.03 to 0.12 events per patient-year of treatment.[46] Several cases of a uveitis flare or the new development of uveitis were reported during use of etanercept. Adult screening guidelines for tuberculosis, at a minimum using purified protein derivative (PPD) skin testing before anti-TNF therapy are generally adopted in pediatric practice. Although one small study suggested it may be safe, current recommendations are to avoid live vaccines with anti-TNF therapy. Attention should be paid to a family history of demyelinating disease, and consultation with a neurologist should be obtained if symptoms and signs consistent with demyelination develop.

Abatacept

Abatacept, a selective T-cell co-stimulator inhibitor (CTLA-4Ig), was found to be effective in polyarticular-onset JIA in a controlled two-phase withdrawal study among 190 patients treated with 10 mg/kg (max: 1000 mg) intravenously at week 0, 2, 4 and then every 4 weeks.[50] Although abatacept was more effective in anti-TNF–naive patients, nearly 40% of patients who were anti-TNF failures were considered Pediatric ACR30 responders. Adverse effects were generally mild with rare infectious serious adverse events reported. Abatacept has been approved by the FDA for use in polyarticular-onset JIA from age 4 years.

Anti-Interleukin (IL)-1 medications

There are three anti-IL-1 medications on the market or in development: anakinra, an IL-1 receptor antagonist; rilonacept, an IL-1 trap (soluble receptor); and canakinumab, an IL-1 antibody. Most trials and clinical experience have been with anakinra.

In a controlled withdrawal study of anakinra given at 1 mg/kg/day (max: 100 mg) subcutaneously to 86 patients with polyarticular-onset JIA there was no evidence of a significantly decreased flare rate among the anakinra group compared with the placebo group, although the study was underpowered.[51] Adverse events were mild and were mainly pain at the injection site and reactions. No differences were seen in children treated with or without concurrent MTX.

However, anakinra may have an important role in systemic-onset JIA. Several studies have shown benefit for both the systemic and articular components, including patients not responsive to anti-TNF medications. Indeed, in the study of polyarthritis, patients with systemic-onset disease showed a more favorable response than those with polyarthritis or oligoarthritis onset: 79% vs. 67% vs. 52%, respectively.[51] Pascual and coworkers reported complete remission in 7 of 9 patients refractory to other medications, including anti-TNF in 4 patients and a partial response in another 2 patients. Sera from 4 of these patients were shown to stimulate IL-1 gene expression and production in mononuclear blood cells from healthy individuals, whereas IL-6 gene stimulation was demonstrated in only 1 of these patients.[52] However, it seems that not all patients with systemic-onset JIA respond to anakinra. In studies from Europe it appears that there are two subsets of patients in regard to response to anakinra, with about 50% exhibiting a dramatic response while others have a small or lack of response.[53,54] It was not possible to predict who would respond based on initial clinical presentation and IL-1 secretion levels before therapy.[53] A recent study was able to distinguish the gene expression profile of patients with systemic arthritis from those with other febrile diseases as well as to show the difference before and after anti-IL-1 therapy.[55] This study found 88 systemic arthritis specific genes with 12 accurately predicting those with systemic features of fever and rash. It appears that IL-1 plays an important role in systemic arthritis and many patients respond dramatically to therapy.

A small pilot phase 1 study of rilonacept for systemic arthritis showed that it was safe at a dose of 2.2 mg/kg/day administered subcutaneously (max: 160 mg), but only about 50% were responders. In the controlled phase of this trial (not designed primarily for efficacy) there were no significant differences with the placebo group.[56] Further increase of the dose to 4.4 mg/kg/day did not result in improved efficacy. Further studies of rilonacept and canakinumab are underway as well as gene expression studies to attempt to predict anti-IL-1 therapy responders.

Anti-IL-6

IL-6 is an important cytokine in the pathogenesis of systemic arthritis, especially for systemic symptoms, thrombocytosis, osteoporosis, and growth retardation. A controlled two-phase withdrawal study of tocilizumab, an antibody to the IL-6 receptor, for systemic arthritis, given intravenously at a dose of 8 mg/kg every 2 weeks, with a 48-week open extension, showed a Pediatric ACR30 response rate of 91% and a Pediatric ACR70 rate of 68%.[57] Flares were significantly increased in the placebo withdrawal group. Serious adverse events have included anaphylaxis, gastrointestinal perforation, and non-opportunistic infections. Hyperlipidemia may also occur. There is another ongoing controlled study in systemic arthritis that has just completed enrollment.

Intravenous immunoglobulin

Two controlled studies did not find intravenous immunglobulin (IVIg) to be effective in the treatment of the arthritis component of systemic- and polyarthritis JIA.[11] However, both studies were small and had insufficient power to detect significant differences. There may be more benefit for IVIg in the first year of the disease and for the treatment of the systemic features of systemic-onset arthritis, but this has not been examined in a controlled study. IVIg is often used in the treatment of macrophage activation syndrome at a dose of 2 g/kg.

Rituximab

There are only rare case reports of the use of rituximab (anti-CD20 mature B-cell antibodies) for JIA.

Autologous stem cell transplantation (ASCT)

There is substantial evidence that abnormal autoreactive T-cell clones have an important role in the pathogenesis of JIA. Wulffraat and associates first reported in 1999 on 4 Dutch children with long-standing and unresponsive systemic and polyarthritis JIA who underwent ASCT with non-autoreactive T-cell precursors. The same group has reported on 34 patients (most with systemic arthritis), with a mean follow-up of 29 months (range: 12-60 months).[58] Complete drug-free remission was reported in 18 (53%) patients, partial response according to the Pediatric ACR30 in 6 (18%) patients, and no improvement in 7 (21%). There were 5 (15%) deaths after ASCT, 3 from early post-ASCT infection-associated macrophage activation syndrome (triggered by Epstein-Barr virus, cytomegalovirus, and *Toxoplasma*) and 2 non-responsive patients, 13 and 16 months post ASCT. In responsive patients there were marked changes in the synovial cellular and cytokine profile, restoration of perforin and natural killer cell function, and decrease in the secretion of myeloid-related proteins. However, 5 responders of 20 patients followed for a median of 80 months experienced a relapse of their disease, 2 of whom died of infections after renewal of immunosuppressive medications.

There are still many unknown issues regarding patient selection, conditioning protocol, graft preparation, and post-transplant care. Therefore, ASCT must still be regarded as an experimental procedure for selected patients with severe and unremitting disease.

THERAPY FOR UVEITIS

Topical therapy for uveitis with corticosteroid drops and mydriatics to prevent posterior synechiae is the treatment of choice. Other local therapies include subtenon corticosteroid injections or long-acting corticosteroid implants. However, it is often hard to wean patients with JIA-related uveitis from topical therapy, and many patients develop treatment-related complications of cataract and glaucoma. Unfortunately, despite the known complications of JIA-related uveitis and topical corticosteroid treatment, until recently the majority of patients with uveitis were not treated with corticosteroid-sparing medications. One study showed only 9 of 44 (20%) patients were treated with MTX or other immunosuppressive medications. The utility of disease-modifying therapy, especially MTX, was reported in several uncontrolled studies.[59] Most patients respond to therapy and more than 50% attain remission while on MTX. In a 20-year series, early immunosuppressive therapy (mostly with MTX) was associated with an improved visual acuity outcome compared with a late initiation of therapy ($P < .005$) with near normalization of visual acuity in patients entering remission within 3 years of starting therapy.[60] However, not all patients respond to MTX, and some even develop uveitis during MTX therapy.

Etanercept, unfortunately, does not appear to be effective in the treatment of JIA-related uveitis. A small, controlled, double-blind study of 12 patients as well as uncontrolled studies did not find etanercept to be effective.[61] For patients non-responsive to MTX or other immunosuppressive medications, several series have found infliximab and adalimumab to be effective in inducing remission, including discontinuation of topical corticosteroids for most patients.[62-64] In a retrospective, comparative study from Toronto of 25 children with uveitis, including 15 with JIA, patients treated with infliximab were more likely to have a better clinical response and fewer eye complications, including cataract or glaucoma, than those treated with etanercept.[62] However, a recent adult study showed that for many patients the effect of infliximab wore off with time. In one study, 35% of patients previously treated with infliximab responded to adalimumab.[64] In some patients it is necessary to give weekly adalimumab. For very severe cases chlorambucil has been used. A recent paper found little value for cyclosporine for JIA uveitis, with only one fourth of the patients treated with cyclosporine monotherapy developing inactive uveitis. There are little data on the effect of mycophenolate mofetil or azathioprine in JIA-related uveitis. However, in a small series it appears that mycophenolate was not as effective in JIA-related uveitis as for other types of uveitis.[65]

MANAGEMENT OF PAIN

Pain, the most common symptom in children with JIA, is an important determinant of physical function and quality of life. Even modest reduction in pain can result in an improvement in the quality of life of children with JIA.[66]

Control of inflammation is critical to the management of pain. Because there are multiple factors leading to pain, specific treatment above and beyond anti-inflammatory treatment, including pharmacologic and psychosocial approaches, should be pursued. Cognitive behavioral therapy approaches with an experienced psychologist/pain management team may often assist with strategies and pain coping.[67] Several interventions in children with JIA[68,69] can improve fitness and may reduce disease activity and pain. Because poor sleep may be a contributing factor to pain, sleep hygiene should be monitored.[70]

Pharmacologic approaches to pain control have traditionally used a "step-up" approach, beginning with acetaminophen, progressing to non-steroidal anti-inflammatory drugs and opioids. Most pediatric rheumatologists are reluctant to prescribe opioids for fear of their side effects and potential for addiction despite evidence that addiction is not a problem when these medications are used appropriately and prescribed by experienced practitioners in a well-controlled and monitored environment.[71] The development of localized and diffuse pain syndromes such as fibromyalgia in patients with JIA must also be addressed. While pharmacologic approaches with tricyclic antidepressants may offer short-term relief, drug therapy alone is generally ineffective. Amitriptyline, 25 mg before bedtime, was not found to be effective in treatment of pain for active polyarticular-onset JIA.[72] Care must be taken if prescribing selective serotonin reuptake inhibitors and serotonin-norepinephrine reuptake inhibitors owing to their potential risk of suicide ideation. Pregabalin (Lyrica) has recently been approved for adult fibromyalgia, but reports of use in children are limited.

REHABILITATION

The principles of rehabilitation in children with JIA are discussed in detail in Chapter 103. Physical and occupational therapists are integral members of the team and play critical roles in working with the child and family to preserve and improve range of motion and muscle strength. Because of the chronicity of disease, slow improvements, and pain induced by exercise, adherence with an exercise regimen is often a challenge and techniques to improve adherence must be used.[73] An experienced occupational therapist can be of great benefit in working with the child to find ways to improve function and provide assistive devices, such as ring splints for inflamed fingers and orthotics for inflamed and deformed feet and to enhance the activities of daily living. Customized semirigid foot orthotics were found to be superior to both prefabricated "off-the-shelf" shoe inserts and supportive athletic shoes in pain reduction, speed of ambulation, and level of disability for patients with JIA and foot pain.[74]

Multiple reports demonstrate the safety of increased exercise intensity for most children with JIA, with improved range of motion, increased muscle strength, and some improvements in aerobic fitness. However, high-intensity exercise does not seem to confer added benefits to function or fitness relative to less strenuous exercise.[75] Hydrotherapy may not offer sufficient benefit to support its use.[76]

A Cochrane review reported that although exercise therapy is safe and does not exacerbate JIA, it did not result in significant effects on functional ability, health-related quality of life, aerobic capacity, or pain over the short term. However, the long-term benefits are unknown.[77] An algorithm that outlines an approach to physical activity and participation in sports in children with JIA has been published.[75]

CALCIUM SUPPLEMENTATION

Several studies have shown that patients with JIA have low bone mineral density, even when not treated with corticosteroids. A controlled study performed to investigate the effect of calcium supplementation in JIA patients not treated with corticosteroids found only a marginal increase in bone density.[78] Calcium and vitamin D supplementation should be given to all JIA patients treated with corticosteroids for more than very brief courses. There are only small studies on the use of bisphosphonates in JIA; a review of these studies reported that the increase in bone mineral density ranges from 4.5% to 19.1%, with only minor safety issues.[79]

GROWTH RETARDATION

There are a significant number of patients with JIA who develop growth failure, particularly those with systemic arthritis who are treated with corticosteroids. Nutrition assessment and support is necessary to increase calorie intake in those patients with lack of weight gain. Some of those patients may benefit from night-time tube feeding. Nutrition consultation is also needed for those on corticosteroids on issues of calorie restriction, adequate calcium and vitamin D, and low sodium intake.

Several studies, including controlled studies, have been published showing the benefit of growth hormone in increasing height growth velocity, even in patients treated with corticosteroids.[80] One study showed a beneficial long-term effect on the final height attained by JIA patients, although the final height was still below the population mean.[81] In most studies no significant flares were found, although we and other physicians have noticed flares in some patients with disease that is not completely controlled.

SURGICAL INTERVENTIONS

Synovectomy

The removal of inflamed synovial tissue might theoretically be beneficial in children with only one or a few persistently active joints despite appropriate therapy. In general, however, the effect of synovectomy is transient. In one study only about one third of patients remained in remission after a mean follow-up of 65 months. Factors predicting a more sustained response were persistent, unique, isolated monarticular disease; shorter disease duration; and normal acute-phase reactants. No side effects were observed.[82] A high recurrence rate post synovectomy was also seen in a group of patients who did not receive intra-articular corticosteroids after the procedure.[83] Elbow synovectomy in 19 patients with juvenile rheumatoid arthritis (JRA) resulted in excellent or good subjective outcome in 72% of patients but no significant improvement in functional ability or range of motion, and complete pain relief was achieved in only 44% of patients.[84] Open hip joint synovectomies performed in 67 hips of 56 patients with both early and late disease provided significant improvements in pain, mobility, walking ability, and function. A 94% hip survival rate at a mean of 4 years post synovectomy was reported.[85] Although there may not be long-term efficacy, the benefit of arthroscopic synovectomy, at least in the hip, may be to temporize while systemic medications such as methotrexate or biologic agents are taking effect.

Epiphysiodesis

With the early institution of more "aggressive" medical management, including intra-articular corticosteroids, the development of leg-length discrepancy and progressive valgus deformity of the knee is less common than in the past. Appropriately timed epiphysiodesis with temporary stapling of the femoral, with or without tibial epiphyses, has resulted in excellent short- and long-term outcomes in correcting leg-length discrepancy with few complications.[86] Patients must be followed closely to avoid overcorrection. This procedure is preferable to surgical epiphysiodesis, which is not reversible. Epiphysiodesis with stapling may also be considered in patients with valgus deformity of the knee, a common knee deformity in JIA. This can be considered when the intermalleolar distance exceeds 10 cm and the physeal growth plates are still open. Although the possible benefit in postponing the need for total-knee arthroplasty appears to be limited, it may ultimately make the procedure easier by reducing the soft tissue and bony imbalance. Both short- and long-term outcomes of this procedure are generally good.[87,88]

Complications from stapling may arise if the staples are inserted incorrectly and they may damage the growth plate, leading to progressive deformity. Deep infection is another possible, although unusual, complication.

Arthroplasty

Although current approaches to treatment have led to marked improvements in outcomes, a small number of children still develop significant joint damage, debilitating pain, and loss of function. It is for these indications that joint replacement surgery may be contemplated. When this is considered, a number of specific issues relevant to the pediatric patient must be considered. Because of the extensive rehabilitation required and the necessity of adhering to a rehabilitation regimen, the emotional and psychosocial state of the child and family must be assessed to ensure that compliance with the program will be maintained. Special attention must be paid to joint contractures and soft tissue management at the time of surgery, requiring release of soft tissues and correction of bony changes. The effect of the disease on growth may result in small bones and difficulty getting a standard prosthesis, and therefore custom-made prostheses are often required. Finally, bone quality is often poor owing to the underlying disease activity, poor nutrition, immobility, and sometimes corticosteroid therapy. This may result in difficulties using the generally preferred uncemented prosthesis. In general, attempts should be made to delay surgery until the child has stopped growing. However, this must be balanced with the degree of disability and pain. It is important to keep all these principles in mind when considering total joint replacement in patients with JIA.

Results of total hip and knee arthroplasty are generally quite good. Improvements in pain, function, and range of motion are expected after hip arthroplasty.[89,90] Revisions may be necessary owing to aseptic loosening with functional impairment. Even in experienced hands, revision surgery is difficult.[91]

With total-knee arthroplasty, improvement in functional score and decrease in pain is observed, although improvement in range of motion is not as significant.[92,93] A number of postoperative complications related to poor range of motion of the knee and continuing anterior knee pain may be seen.[93]

When the disease is bilateral, simultaneous procedures should be done if possible. Hip replacement should precede knee replacement to improve the chances of successful rehabilitation. Bilateral combined hip and knee arthroplasty in young patients with JRA has been reported with good success.[94] Despite apparent poor outcome on some of the functional scales, adults with JIA report that total-knee arthroplasty had a major positive impact on their quality of life.[95]

Results with shoulder arthroplasty are limited. Pain relief is the major goal of shoulder arthroplasty and can be achieved.[96] A small improvement in range of motion may have a significant impact on function. The results of total elbow arthroplasty are not as satisfactory as with other joints and are associated with significant early and late complications.[97]

Surgical treatment of temporomandibular joint deformities

Surgical treatment of TMJ deformities involves a team consisting of dentist, orthodontist, and craniofacial surgeon in addition to the rheumatologist. Most case series have reported both improved occlusion and facial aesthetics postoperatively. Some patients may still be left with TMJ pain, and numbness of the lip, chin, teeth, and gums may develop. A number of different procedures have all been reported to have good outcomes.[98-100]

SUMMARY OF TREATMENT EVIDENCE FOR THE SUBTYPES OF JIA

Oligoarthritis

One fourth to one third of patients with mild disease will respond to NSAIDs. In patients not responsive to NSAIDs after 4 to 6 weeks, or in patients presenting with local complications including flexion contractures and leg-length discrepancies, intra-articular corticosteroid injections, especially with triamcinolone hexacetonide, are effective for the majority of patients (Fig. 100.2). Patients not responsive to corticosteroid injections or patients with extended oligoarthritis or with small joint involvement should be treated as patients with polyarthritis.

Polyarthritis, RF-negative

NSAIDs are not effective as disease-modifying medications and should not be used as a sole medication (Fig. 100.3). The use of NSAIDs is more for symptom control. MTX should be started early initially at 10 mg/m²/wk and, if not effective, increased to 15 mg/m²/wk, with the route of administration changed from oral to parenteral. Other DMARD options include the use of sulfasalazine, particularly in older boys, and leflunomide. If these agents are not effective, then anti-TNF medications or abatacept should be used, although there is still no evidence whether a combination of MTX and anti-TNF medications or abatacept is more effective than only anti-TNF medications alone. Currently, etanercept, adalimumab, and abatacept are approved by the FDA. In patients who fail one anti-TNF, changing to either another anti-TNF medication or to abatacept is an option.

Intra-articular corticosteroid injections can be used as an adjunct for one or few very painful or swollen joints. Occasionally, systemic corticosteroids may be necessary as a bridging medication or during flares, although there is no evidence that systemic corticosteroids are disease modifying.

Polyarthritis, RF-positive

These patients have a poor outcome and should be treated aggressively per algorithms for rheumatoid arthritis in adults, including the early

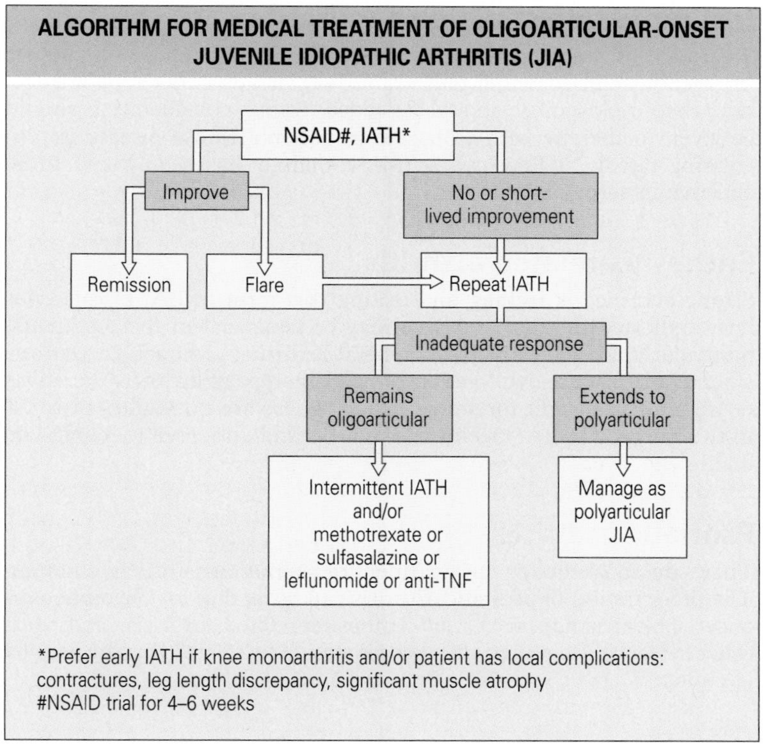

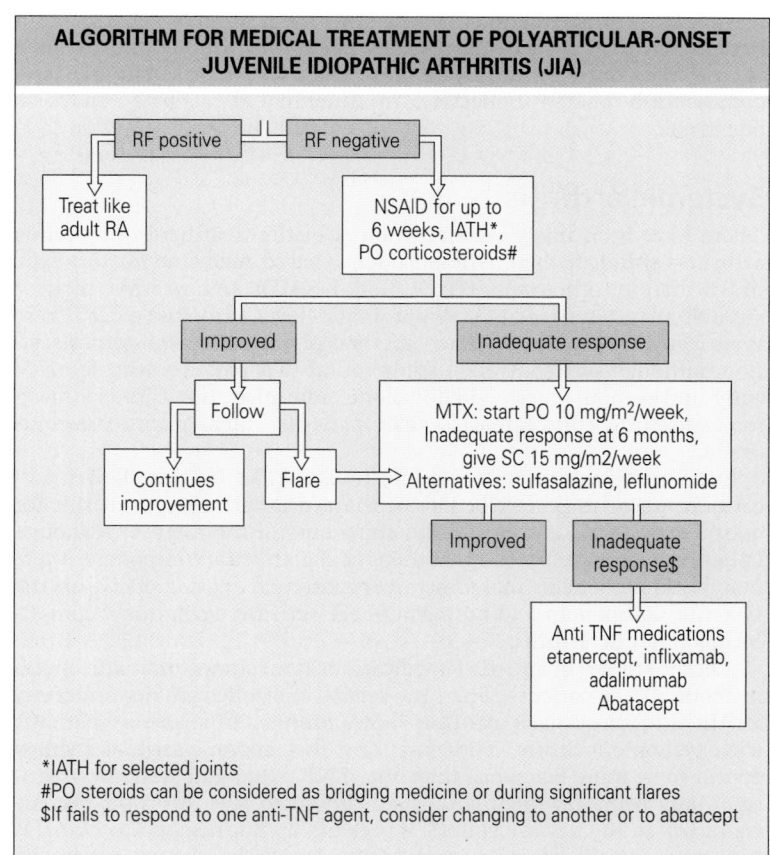

Fig. 100.3 Algorithm for medical treatment of polyarticular-onset JIA. NSAID, non-steroidal anti-inflammatory drug; IATH, intra-articular triamcinolone hexacetonide; MTX, methotrexate; TNF, tumor necrosis factor; PO, oral; SC, subcutaneous.

Fig. 100.2 Algorithm for medical treatment of oligoarticular-onset JIA. NSAID, non-steroidal anti-inflammatory drug; IATH, intra-articular triamcinolone hexacetonide; TNF, tumor necrosis factor.

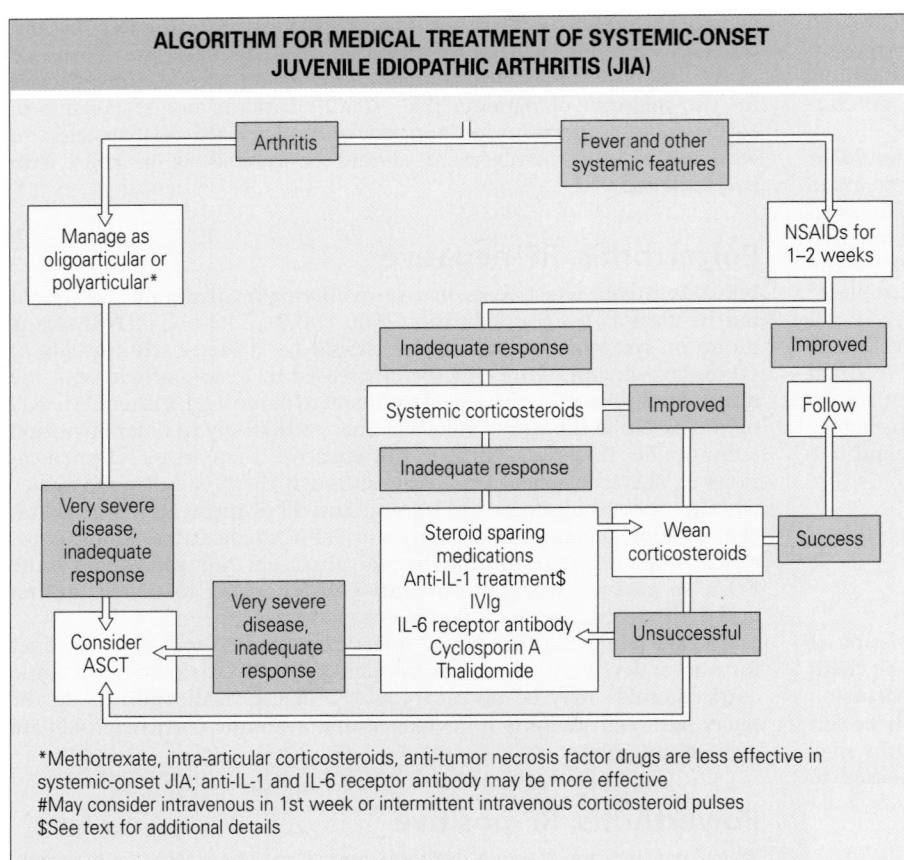

ALGORITHM FOR MEDICAL TREATMENT OF SYSTEMIC-ONSET JUVENILE IDIOPATHIC ARTHRITIS (JIA)

Fig. 100.4 Algorithm for medical treatment of systemic-onset JIA. NSAID, non-steroidal anti-inflammatory drug; IVIg, intravenous immunoglobulin; ASCT, autologous stem cell transplantation; IL, interleukin; TNF, tumor necrosis factor.

use of MTX and addition of anti-TNF medication or abatacept in patients with an inadequate response to MTX. Although not studied in children, other medications (e.g., rituximab or tocilizumab) and combination therapy effective in rheumatoid arthritis may be beneficial.

Systemic arthritis

There have been many recent advances in the treatment of systemic arthritis, although there is less evidence-based medicine for this type of JIA than for other types (Fig. 100.4). NSAIDs and systemic corticosteroids are often needed for symptomatic (fever, serositis) relief. There is no evidence on the preferred method of corticosteroid administration, although one controlled study found that patients who received early intravenous methylprednisolone administration needed fewer total systemic corticosteroids than patients starting corticosteroids orally.

Intra-articular corticosteroid injections, MTX, and anti-TNF medications appear to be less beneficial than in other subtypes of JIA, for both the systemic and arthritis components of the disease. Although IVIg is not effective for the treatment of the arthritis component, there may be some benefit, including a corticosteroid-sparing effect, on the systemic component and on macrophage activation syndrome complicating systemic arthritis.

Recent studies of anti-IL-1 medications have shown dramatic effects in about 50% of patients. There are several controlled studies underway for these medications. Anti-IL-6 shows promise in refractory patients with systemic arthritis. Therefore, anti-IL-1 and/or anti-IL-6 therapy appear to be more beneficial than anti-TNF therapy in systemic arthritis. Many pediatric rheumatologists choose to give anti-IL-1 therapy very early in the disease course, if patients do not respond to NSAIDs or become steroid dependent even before use of other disease-modifying or anti-TNF medications. Thalidomide or early treatment with a combination of cyclophosphamide, MTX, and intravenous pulse corticosteroids may be an alternative in unresponsive patients; but with the increased and early use of anti-IL-1 and anti-IL-6 therapy the use of

these medications should not be needed. For patients with severe, unresponsive systemic and polyarthritis JIA, ASCT may be used as a last resort, although there is a high proportion of mortality associated with this therapy.

Macrophage activation syndrome

Treatment of macrophage activation syndrome includes high-dose intravenous corticosteroid pulses and IVIg; if this is not rapidly effective, then cyclosporine should be added. Strong consideration should be given to therapy with etoposide in patients whose disease is progressing rapidly.[101] Recently, anti-IL-1 therapy has been found to be effective in some patients.

Enthesitis-related arthritis

Strong evidence is lacking for treating this form of JIA. Open series have indicated that sulfasalazine may be beneficial in these patients, particularly older boys with peripheral arthritis, although in the one small controlled study of patients with this type of arthritis there was no significant benefit for sulfasalazine. There are no studies of MTX in this subtype of JIA. Open series have found anti-TNF therapy to be highly effective.

Psoriatic arthritis

There are no studies of the treatment of psoriatic arthritis in children. The presentation of psoriatic arthritis can be as that for oligoarticular-onset, polyarticular-onset, and enthesitis-related arthritis, and until other evidence is reported this disease should be treated like the parallel JIA subset.

Uveitis

The early use of MTX in topical corticosteroid-dependent disease appears to be warranted. For patients not responsive to MTX, infliximab and adalimumab appear to be effective, but not etanercept. Cyclosporine does not appear to be very effective. Mycophenolate mofetil has not been adequately studied in JIA-related uveitis.

CONCLUSION

The development of new therapies has already markedly increased our ability to effectively treat children with JIA, and the future appears promising, especially for difficult patients with systemic-onset and polyarticular arthritis. However, there is still a lack of evidence-based medicine in the treatment of JIA, especially for enthesitis-related and psoriatic arthritis and systemic-onset arthritis to a lesser degree. Recent sobering studies have shown our inability to induce long-term medication-free remission in most patients, even with modern therapy. The study of the effect of early aggressive therapy on the disease course, including the potential use of combination "induction" therapy, has just begun. The long-term disease-modifying effects of methotrexate and of the new "biologic" medications on remission rates, radiologic changes, bone strength, growth, functional capabilities, quality of life, and prevention of surgery are still mostly unknown, although there are initial signals of benefits in many of these outcomes. It is necessary to study the long-term adverse effects of these medications, especially if used as combination therapy. Future multicenter controlled studies and post-marketing surveillance with large registries are necessary to address these issues.

KEY REFERENCES

1. Giannini EH, Ruperto N, Ravelli A, et al. Preliminary definition of improvement in juvenile arthritis. Arthritis Rheum 1997;40:1202-1209.
2. Wallace CA, Ruperto N, Giannini E, et al. Preliminary criteria for clinical remission for select categories of juvenile idiopathic arthritis. J Rheumatol 2004;31:2290-2294.
4. Giannini EH, Cawkwell GD. Drug treatment in children with juvenile rheumatoid arthritis. Pediatr Clin North Am 1995;42:1099-1125.
5. Wallace CA, Levinson JE. Juvenile rheumatoid arthritis: outcome and treatment for the 1990s. Rheum Dis Clin North Am 1991;17:891-905.
8. Sherry DD, Stein LD, Reed AM, et al. Prevention of leg-length discrepancy in young children with pauciarticular juvenile rheumatoid arthritis by treatment with intra-articular steroids. Arthritis Rheum 1999;42:2330-2334.
11. Hashkes PJ, Laxer RM. Medical treatment of juvenile idiopathic arthritis. JAMA 2005;294:1671-1684.
12. Foeldvari I, Szer IS, Zemel LS, et al. A prospective study comparing celecoxib with naproxen in children with juvenile rheumatoid arthritis. J Rheumatol 2009;36:174-182.
14. Schad SG, Kraus A, Haubitz I, et al. Early onset pauciarticular arthritis is the major risk factor for naproxen-induced pseudoporphyria in juvenile idiopathic arthritis. Arthritis Res Ther 2007;9:R10.
17. Beukelman T, Guevara JP, Albert DA: Optimal treatment of knee monarthritis in juvenile idiopathic arthritis: a decision analysis. Arthritis Rheum 2008;59:1580-1588.
18. Padeh S, Passwell JH: Intraarticular corticosteroid injections in the management of children with chronic arthritis. Arthritis Rheum 1998;41:1210-1214.
19. Zulian F, Martini G, Gobber D, et al. Triamcinolone acetonide and hexacetonide intra-articular treatment of symmetrical joints in juvenile idiopathic arthritis: a double-blind trial. Rheumatology 2004;43:1288-1291.
20. Beukelman T, Arabshahi B, Cahill AM, et al. Benefit of intra-articular corticosteroid injection under fluoroscopic guidance for subtalar arthritis in juvenile idiopathic arthritis. J Rheumatol 2006;33:2330-2336.
22. Giannini EA, Brewer EJ, Kuzmina N, et al. Methotrexate in resistant juvenile rheumatoid arthritis: results of the U.S.A.-U.S.S.R. double-blind, placebo-controlled trial. N Engl J Med 1992;326:1043-1049.
23. Woo P, Southwood TR, Prieur AM, et al. Randomized, placebo-controlled, crossover trial of low-dose oral methotrexate in children with extended oligoarticular or systemic arthritis. Arthritis Rheum 2000;43:1849-1857.
24. Takken T, Van Der Net J, Helders PJ: Methotrexate for treating juvenile idiopathic arthritis. Cochrane Database Syst Rev 2001;3:CD003129.
25. Ruperto N, Murray KJ, Gerloni V, et al. A randomized trial of parenteral methotrexate comparing an intermediate dose with a higher dose in children with juvenile idiopathic arthritis who failed to respond to standard doses of methotrexate. Arthritis Rheum 2004;50:2191-2201.
26. Schmeling H, Biber D, Heins S, et al. Influence of methylenetetrahydrofolate reductase polymorphisms on efficacy and toxicity of methotrexate in patients with juvenile idiopathic arthritis. J Rheumatol 2005;32:1832-1836.

30. Hashkes PJ, Balistreri WF, Bove KE, et al. The long-term effect of methotrexate therapy on the liver in patients with juvenile rheumatoid arthritis. Arthritis Rheum 1997;40:2226-2234.
31. Heijstek MW, Pileggi GC, Zonneveld-Huijssoon E, et al. Safety of measles, mumps and rubella vaccination in juvenile idiopathic arthritis. Ann Rheum Dis 2007;66:1384-1387.
32. Van Rossum MAJ, Fiselier TJW, Franssen MJAM, et al. Sulfasalazine in the treatment of juvenile chronic arthritis: a randomized double-blind placebo-controlled, multicenter study. Arthritis Rheum 1998;41:808-816.
33. van Rossum MA, van Soesbergen RM, Boers M, et al. Long-term outcome of juvenile idiopathic arthritis following a placebo-controlled trial: sustained benefits of early sulfasalazine treatment. Ann Rheum Dis 2007;66:1518-1524.
34. Silverman E, Mouy R, Spiegel L, et al. Leflunomide or methotrexate for juvenile rheumatoid arthritis. N Engl J Med 2005;352:1655-1666.
36. Ruperto N, Ravelli A, Castell E, et al. Cyclosporine A in juvenile idiopathic arthritis: results of the PRCSG/PRINTO phase IV post marketing surveillance study. Clin Exp Rheumatol 2006;24:599-605.
37. Mouy R, Stephan JL, Pillet P, et al. Efficacy of cyclosporine A in the treatment of macrophage activation syndrome in juvenile arthritis: report of five cases. J Pediatr 1996;129:750-754.
40. Lovell DJ, Giannini EH, Reiff A, et al. Etanercept in children with polyarticular juvenile rheumatoid arthritis. N Engl J Med 2000;342:763-769.
41. Lovell DJ, Ruperto N, Goodman S, et al. Adalimumab with or without methotrexate in juvenile rheumatoid arthritis N Engl J Med 2008;359:810-820.
43. Quartier P, Taupin P, Bourdeaut F, et al. Efficacy of etanercept for the treatment of juvenile idiopathic arthritis according to the onset type. Arthritis Rheum 2003;48:1093-1101.
44. Tse SM, Burgos-Vargas R, Laxer RM. Anti–tumor necrosis factor alpha blockade in the treatment of juvenile spondyloarthropathy. Arthritis Rheum 2005;52:2103-2108.
45. Ruperto N, Lovell DJ, Cuttica R, et al. A randomized, placebo-controlled trial of infliximab plus methotrexate for the treatment of polyarticular-course juvenile rheumatoid arthritis. Arthritis Rheum 2007;56:3096-3106.
46. Lovell DJ, Reiff A, Ilowite NT, et al. Safety and efficacy of up to eight years of continuous etanercept therapy in patients with juvenile rheumatoid arthritis. Arthritis Rheum 2008;58:1496-1504.
47. Tynjälä P, Vähäsalo P, Honkanen V, et al. Drug survival of the first and second course of anti-tumour necrosis factor agents in juvenile idiopathic arthritis. Ann Rheum Dis 2009;68:552-557.
48. Horneff G, De Bock F, Foeldvari I, et al. Safety and efficacy of combination of etanercept and methotrexate compared to treatment with etanercept only in patients with juvenile idiopathic arthritis (JIA): preliminary data from the German JIA Registry. Ann Rheum Dis 2009;68:519-525.
49. Nielsen S, Ruperto N, Gerloni V, et al. Preliminary evidence that etanercept may reduce radiographic progression in juvenile idiopathic arthritis. Clin Exp Rheumatol 2008;26:688-692.

50. Ruperto N, Lovell DJ, Quartier P, et al. Abatacept in children with juvenile idiopathic arthritis: a randomized, double-blind, placebo-controlled withdrawal trial. Lancet 2008;372:383-391.
51. Ilowite N, Porras O, Reiff A, et al. Anakinra in the treatment of polyarticular-course juvenile rheumatoid arthritis: safety and preliminary efficacy results of a randomized multicenter study. Clin Rheumatol 2008;28:129-137.
52. Pascual V, Allantaz F, Arce E, et al. Role of interleukin-1 (IL-1) in the pathogenesis of systemic onset juvenile idiopathic arthritis and clinical response to IL-1 blockade. J Exp Med 2005;201:1479-1486.
53. Gattorno M, Piccini A, Lasigliè D, et al. The pattern of response to anti-interleukin-1 treatment distinguishes two subsets of patients with systemic-onset juvenile idiopathic arthritis. Arthritis Rheum 2008;58:1505-1515.
54. Lequerré T, Quartier P, Rosellini D, et al. Interleukin-1 receptor antagonist (anakinra) treatment in patients with systemic-onset juvenile idiopathic arthritis or adult-onset Still disease: preliminary experience in France. Ann Rheum Dis 2008;67:302-308.
57. Yokata S, Imagawa T, Mori M, et al. Efficacy and safety of tocilizumab in patients with systemic-onset juvenile idiopathic arthritis: a randomized, double-blind, placebo-controlled, withdrawal phase III trial. Lancet 2008;371:998-1006.
58. Brinkman DM, de Kleer IM, ten Cate R, et al. Autologous stem cell transplantation in children with severe progressive systemic or polyarticular juvenile idiopathic arthritis: long-term follow-up of a prospective clinical trial. Arthritis Rheum 2007;56:2410-2421.
59. Foeldvari I, Wierk A. Methotrexate is an effective treatment for chronic uveitis associated with juvenile idiopathic arthritis. J Rheumatol 2005;32:362-365.
61. Smith JA, Thompson DJ, Whitcup SM, et al. A randomized, placebo-controlled double-masked clinical trial of etanercept for the treatment of uveitis associated with juvenile idiopathic arthritis. Arthritis Rheum 2005;53:18-23.
62. Saurenmann RK, Levin AV, Rose JB, et al. Tumour necrosis factor alpha inhibitors in the treatment of childhood uveitis. Rheumatology 2006;45:982-989.
63. Tynjälä P, Kotaniemi K, Lindahl P, et al. Adalimumab in juvenile idiopathic arthritis-associated chronic anterior uveitis. Rheumatology (Oxford) 2008;47:339-344.
71. Kimura Y, Walco GA. Treatment of chronic pain in pediatric rheumatic disease. Nat Clin Pract Rheumatol 2007;3:210-218.
75. Klepper SE. Exercise in pediatric rheumatic diseases. Curr Opin Rheumatol 2008;20:619-624.
77. Takken T, van Brussel M, Engelbert RH, et al. Exercise therapy in juvenile idiopathic arthritis. Cochrane Database Syst Rev 2008;16:CD005954.
80. Simon D, Prieur AM, Quartier P, et al. Early recombinant human growth hormone treatment in glucocorticoid-treated children with juvenile idiopathic arthritis: a 3-year randomized study. J Clin Endocrinol Metab 2007;92:2567-2573.
82. Toledo MM, Martini G, Gigante C, et al. Is there a role for arthroscopic synovectomy in oligoarticular juvenile idiopathic arthritis? J Rheumatol 2006;33:1868-1872.
90. Kitsoulis PB, Stafilas KS, Siamopoulou A, et al. Total hip arthroplasty in children with juvenile chronic arthritis: long-term results. J Pediatr Orthop 2006;26:8-12.

REFERENCES

Full references for this chapter can be found on www.expertconsult.com.

INDEX

Note: Page numbers followed by *b* indicate boxes; *f*, figures; *t*, tables.